Foye's

PRINCIPLES OF MEDICINAL CHEMISTRY

8TH EDITION

Foye's

PRINCIPLES OF MEDICINAL CHEMISTRY

8TH EDITION

VICTORIA F. ROCHE, PHD
Professor of Pharmacy Sciences
School of Pharmacy and Health Professions
Creighton University
Omaha, Nebraska

S. WILLIAM ZITO, PHD
Professor Pharmaceutical Sciences
College of Pharmacy and Health Sciences
St. John's University
Jamaica, New York

THOMAS L. LEMKE, PHD
Professor Emeritus
College of Pharmacy
University of Houston
Houston, Texas

DAVID A. WILLIAMS, PHD
Professor Emeritus of Chemistry
School of Pharmacy
MCPHS University
Boston, Massachusetts

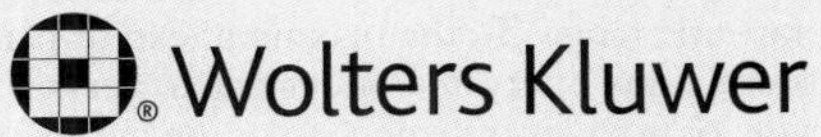

Philadelphia • Baltimore • New York • London
Buenos Aires • Hong Kong • Sydney • Tokyo

Acquisitions Editor: Matt Hauber
Senior Development Editor: Amy Millholen
Editorial Coordinator: Kerry McShane
Production Project Manager: Bridgett Dougherty
Marketing Manager: Jason Oberacker
Design Coordinator: Joan Wendt
Art Director: Jennifer Clements
Prepress Vendor: TNQ Technologies

Eighth Edition

9 8 7 6 5 4 3 2 1

Printed in China

Library of Congress Cataloging-in-Publication Data

ISBN-13:978-1-4963-8502-4

Cataloging in Publication data available on request from publisher.

This work is provided "as is," and the publisher disclaims any and all warranties, express or implied, including any warranties as to accuracy, comprehensiveness, or currency of the content of this work.

This work is no substitute for individual patient assessment based upon healthcare professionals' examination of each patient and consideration of, among other things, age, weight, gender, current or prior medical conditions, medication history, laboratory data and other factors unique to the patient. The publisher does not provide medical advice or guidance and this work is merely a reference tool. Healthcare professionals, and not the publisher, are solely responsible for the use of this work including all medical judgments and for any resulting diagnosis and treatments.

Given continuous, rapid advances in medical science and health information, independent professional verification of medical diagnoses, indications, appropriate pharmaceutical selections and dosages, and treatment options should be made and healthcare professionals should consult a variety of sources. When prescribing medication, healthcare professionals are advised to consult the product information sheet (the manufacturer's package insert) accompanying each drug to verify, among other things, conditions of use, warnings and side effects and identify any changes in dosage schedule or contraindications, particularly if the medication to be administered is new, infrequently used or has a narrow therapeutic range. To the maximum extent permitted under applicable law, no responsibility is assumed by the publisher for any injury and/or damage to persons or property, as a matter of products liability, negligence law or otherwise, or from any reference to or use by any person of this work.

shop.lww.com

CCS0719

This textbook is dedicated to students of all ages who have been blessed with a love of learning and an appreciation for the elegant beauty of the chemical sciences. It was written for those with the drive to understand how and why drugs behave as they do, and who have a calling to serve others through drug design/discovery or the practice of the profession of pharmacy. It is offered with gratitude to academic colleagues who contributed to its development and/or will use it in the education of the next generation of pharmacists and pharmaceutical scientists.

Victoria F. Roche

S. William Zito

Thomas L. Lemke

David A. Williams

Dedication to William O. Foye

William O. Foye, Sawyer Professor of Medicinal Chemistry at the MCPHS University (formerly Massachusetts College of Pharmacy), Boston, MA, was born in 1923 in western Massachusetts. He received his BA (1944) in chemistry from Dartmouth College and PhD in Organic Chemistry (M. Carmack) from Indiana University in 1948. He served in the U.S. Navy during World War II as a chemical warfare instructor. He joined DuPont (Delaware) as a research scientist, then in 1950 joined the School of Pharmacy at the University of Wisconsin as assistant professor of pharmaceutical chemistry. In 1955, he moved to MCPHS University, Boston, as Professor of Chemistry, where he brought a new vision of pharmaceutical chemistry (medicinal chemistry) to the pharmacy curriculum. As department chair, he advocated for organic medicinal chemistry in the pharmacy curriculum.

The impetus for a new text in medicinal chemistry, grounded on Alfred Burger's two-volume *Medicinal Chemistry*, came from Dr. Norman Doorenbos, College of Pharmacy University of Maryland (Baltimore), who had made arrangements with Lea & Febiger (forerunner of Wolters Kluwer) for publishing a companion text to Wilson & Gisvold's *Textbook of Organic Medicinal and Pharmaceutical Chemistry*. Because Dr. Doorenbos was moving to chair the new Pharmacognosy Department at the School of Pharmacy, University of Mississippi, he relinquished the job of editing this text to Dr. Foye. During this time, a number of teachers and researchers in medicinal chemistry felt that a text on drugs that included biochemical mechanisms of action, aimed primarily at professional students, should be written. Although other pharmaceutical and medicinal chemistry books had been written during this time (*The Chemistry of Organic Medicinal Products*, Jenkins and Hartung, and *Textbook of Organic Medicinal and Pharmaceutical Chemistry*, Wilson and Gisvold), these authors organized their books according to the accepted scheme of chemical classification of the more important organic medicinal compounds, their methods of synthesis, properties and descriptions, and their uses and modes of administration. Therefore, this "Principles" text provided a contemporary basis for the biochemical understanding of drug action that included the principles of structure-function relationships and drug metabolism. Dr. Foye assembled authors who were experts in their respective fields and published the first edition of *Principles of Medicinal Chemistry* in 1972.

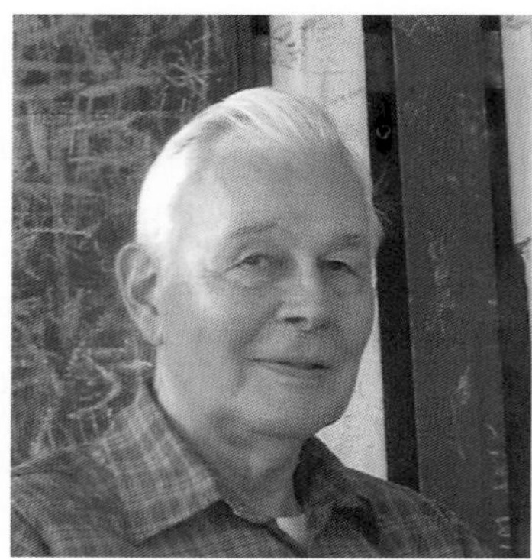

The authors of the eighth edition of *Foye's Principles of Medicinal Chemistry* have embraced Dr. Foye's original concept of a textbook of significant value to pharmacy students. Today, even more than when the original text appeared in 1972, the complex nature of disease states and their biochemical/physiological origins needs to be explored and understood at the molecular level for healthcare professionals to ensure maximal benefits for patients. All editions of this text have had a primary goal to both meet students' short-term need for a contemporary medicinal chemistry education and stimulate a lifelong desire to know more about how the chemicals we call drugs work.

Dr. Foye had a long and creative career in medicinal chemistry with more than 150 refereed scientific publications, book chapters, and editor of Cancer Chemotherapeutic Agents ACS Monograph Series. His research focused on numerous areas especially the SAR of antiradiation organosulfur compounds, anticancer agents, and chelation as mechanism of drug action. He was elected Fellow of the AAPS and Fellow of APhA, received the APhA Foundation Research Achievement Award in Medicinal Chemistry, and was an emeritus member of AAAS, ACS, APhA, and AAPS. He was one of the founding members of the Medicinal Chemistry Group of the Northeast Section of the American Chemical Society (1968). He retired in 1995. In addition to being Chair of the Department of Chemistry, he was also the Dean of Faculties and Dean of Graduate Studies at the MCPHS University. Dr. Foye traveled widely and was an invited participant at numerous meetings.

Not only was Dr. Foye a distinguished scientist, he was an avid fly-fisherman, outdoorsman, and environmentalist. He published several books about the western Massachusetts wilderness, *Trout Waters: Reminiscence with Description of the Upper Quabbin Valley* (1992) and *North Quabbin Wilds: A Populous Solitude* (2005). He was a dedicated supporter of the arts in Boston. He married Lila Siddons in 1974 and has a son Owen and stepson Kenneth. Dr. Foye died in 2014.

David A. Williams, PhD

Preface

Welcome to the Eighth Edition of Foye's Principles of Medicinal Chemistry

It has been a true labor of love by the editorial team and the multitude of authors and contributors to bring this Eighth Edition of *Foye's Principles of Medicinal Chemistry* to inquiring minds everywhere. While it has been specifically designed to be of value to those actively engaged in the science and practice of Pharmacy (including those studying to be officially admitted into this respected profession), it is our hope that its impact will be felt beyond that highly important, yet also limited, realm. In truth, this book is for anyone interested in knowing how the chemicals we call drugs really work; how medicinal chemists discern, define, and refine the intimate relationship between structure and biologic activity (termed Structure-Activity Relationships, or SAR); and how pharmacists can harness their understanding of the chemical basis of drug action and translate it into improved patient care. For, as we are fond of reminding our pharmacy students, the study of medicinal chemistry is a "logical" component of their professional preparation. Playing off the familiar "If A is B, and B is C, then A is C" (an example of deductive reasoning), if drugs are chemicals, and pharmacists are the drug experts, then pharmacists are the chemical experts of the healthcare team. Since no student ever argues with the first two clauses, it becomes impossible to argue against the truly unique and highly valuable role pharmacists play in patient care. This realization can be the epiphany that forever changes the way students look at the practice of the profession and their responsibility to be scientifically grounded in the science of drug chemistry for as long as they practice.

So, to all who have been blessed with the gift of intellectual curiosity and have picked up Foye's Eighth Edition for medicinal chemistry enlightenment, welcome to our world; we're glad you're here.

A Brief History of the Discipline

The first chapter of this text introduces readers to the medicinal chemistry discipline and provides an overarching summary of its evolution to the patient care–relevant reputation it enjoys in schools and colleges of pharmacy today. While the emphasis on what pharmacists can do (indeed, are expected to do) with a firm grounding in this science may be relatively contemporary, much of the traditional emphasis on what the science entails remains critical. In other words, the "new" has not replaced the "old" but, rather, has enriched it and provided clinical meaning to students seeking to care for people as their life's work.

As effectively summarized by Drs. Lemke and Williams in the Preface to the Seventh Edition, medicinal chemistry education in pharmacy programs was historically rooted in the long-standing recognition of the impact of drug functional groups and stereochemistry on observed drug action. SAR, first conceptualized in the mid-1800s, was studied in isolation, often because the chemical nature of the target receptor was not known and the importance of integrating this knowledge with what was learned in Pharmacology, Pharmacokinetics, and Pharmacotherapeutics courses was not yet universally appreciated. In the early days, students focused on the memorization of structure, SAR rules, and lists of activities for specific drugs, rather than making critical connections between SAR and biologically linked realities. However, as the 20th century progressed, so did the approach to teaching and learning medicinal chemistry. Seminal discoveries relating to the SAR of corticosteroids, prostaglandins, and sex steroids allowed for the development of potent and selective anti-inflammatory agents and contraceptives. Explorations into the chemistry of histamine receptors led to the rational design of the first H_2 antagonist used to treat peptic ulcers (cimetidine), a drug that was optimized based on SAR to generate analogues that were not only more effective, but also chemically constructed to have fewer problematic drug-drug interactions. The elucidation of multiple opioid receptor subtypes led to the design of morphine analogues that targeted the strongly analgesic, but less addictive, kappa receptor. Proton pump inhibitors were elegantly designed to take full advantage of (1) pK_a differences of key amines and (2) the vulnerability of sulfenic acid intermediates to nucleophilic attack by H^+, K^+-ATPase cysteine sulfhydryl groups to essentially halt gastric acid secretion, making them useful in the treatment of gastro/duodenal ulcers and gastroesophageal reflux disease (GERD). Among the more recent of medicinal chemistry's critical contributions to mechanism-driven drug design are cancer chemotherapies that target the complex entanglement of aberrant biochemical pathways at work in neoplastic cells. By teasing out the genetic underpinnings of these pathways and identifying the disease-promoting genes and proteins for targeted chemotherapy, patients and their loved ones have been given the gifts of an enhanced quality of life and legitimate hope. These are only a few of myriad examples of the explosion of medicinal chemistry–led drug design, discovery, and development efforts that have advanced our collective understanding of disease and scientifically grounded approaches to treating them.

High-throughput screening techniques that became widely available as the 21st century dawned allowed for the rapid evaluation of millions of compounds against a particular therapeutic target or a pharmacologic or genetic process, allowing chemists to quickly home in on promising compounds (known as "hits") to further develop into leads that could be optimized, evaluated through clinical trials, and brought to market. Today, the "omic" sciences, including genomics, proteomics, and metabolomics, contribute to drug discovery initiatives by allowing medicinal chemists to mine information relative to the comprehensive makeup of (1) the human genome, (2) the proteins that are produced by those genes, and (3) the specific proteins that serve as metabolizing enzymes within the human organism in order to achieve therapeutic benefits for patients.

Natural products chemistry (once fondly known as "weeds and seeds") was pivotal to the education of pharmacists in the first half of the 20th century, then briefly fell out of favor when computer-facilitated drug design strategies emerged on the scene. However, medicinal chemists did not abandon the treasure trove of drug structure templates found in the world's plants, animals, and soils, and continue to tap this rich source of compounds for rational development based on an ever-expanding understanding of the biochemical mechanisms of disease and the three-dimensional structure of target proteins and nucleic acids. Natural medicines and nutraceuticals are of keen interest to many patients seeking holistic care for themselves or loved ones, and many of these products have meaningful culturally-rooted histories that can heal spirits as well as bodies. Appropriately, this content has found its way back into contemporary curricula, both in required courses and through focused elective offerings. Given the fragile state of the planet and the ease with which medicinal species can be lost forever, it is essential that this important body of knowledge continue to be respected, expanded, and preserved.

THE ESSENTIAL SCIENCE

The role of the pharmacist as an integral member of the healthcare team was driven home with force in the early 1990s when the mandate to provide pharmaceutical care was *the* topic of conversation at gatherings of practitioners and educators. While the terms used to describe the professional expectation to take proactive responsibility for patient care outcomes and quality of life have changed, the goal has not. Indeed, this goal has been unilaterally embraced and championed across the profession. The emphasis on the pharmacist as an educator, communicator, interprofessional collaborator, patient advocate, and decision-maker demanded new skills and the opportunity to hone them prior to licensure. In response, academic institutions began to reform curricula to accommodate expanded pharmacotherapeutics coursework and experiential education requirements, most commonly within a traditional 6-year comprehensive educational timeframe. Biomedical and pharmaceutical sciences coursework was scrutinized for clinical relevance and courses that could be taken at the undergraduate level often moved to preprofessional programs of study.

As the curricular pendulum swung, some feared that medicinal chemistry might fall victim to professional education restructuring if faculties failed to recognize how strongly this science fosters the critical thinking and analytical reasoning skills demanded by contemporary practice. However, to academic pharmacy's credit, medicinal chemistry remains a mandated component of a pharmacist's education, and for good reason. In addition to allowing students to discern both significant and subtle differences in pharmacologic action based on critical changes in the structure of existing drugs, this science provides a foundational framework to evaluate the therapeutic potential and liability of drugs developed long after the completion of formal medicinal chemistry coursework. Medicinal Chemistry is the science that asks *why* drugs behave as they do, and then provides the molecular evidence needed to answer that all-important question. As such, it is the heart and soul of a pharmacy student's professional preparation. Simply put, understanding drug action at this deepest mechanistic level is a nonnegotiable expectation for anyone claiming terminal credentials in the discipline: Technicians of pharmacy know what, Doctors of Pharmacy know why.

The profession recognizes that understanding drugs for the biologically active chemicals they are, and using this understanding to predict therapeutic and adverse activities that inform sound patient care decisions, is more important now than ever before. Our discipline is standing strong because we are now purposefully integrating our component of the comprehensive drug action/therapeutic use story with other disciplines so that our students see one interconnected picture related to how drugs work to treat disease and/or promote wellness. Collaboration with other disciplines builds content bridges and promotes mutual respect for what each area of pharmaceutical and clinical science study brings to patient care, and that elevates the profession and those who practice it beyond measure.

ORGANIZATIONAL PHILOSOPHY

Foye's Eighth Edition is organized into four major sections: Principles, Receptor Targets, Pharmacodynamic Agents, and Disease State Management.

The **Principles** chapters set the learning stage with descriptive discussions on the evolution of the discipline, foundational medicinal chemistry principles and functional groups, drug metabolism, drug transporters, and biotechnology-derived proteins and nucleotides. The **Receptor Targets** chapters that follow provide an in-depth discussion of the chemistry, topography, and function of pharmacologically relevant binding sites, using selected representative ligands to exemplify the binding and activity of agonists, inverse agonists, and antagonists. The discussions are robust, and readers should refer back to these chapters as appropriate when reading Pharmacodynamic Agents chapters (and, indeed, are often directed to do so by those authors).

In keeping with the ever-increasing integration of medicinal chemistry into "Drugs and Disease" types of courses that also include pharmacology, pathophysiology, and pharmacotherapeutics content, **Pharmacodynamic Agents** chapters are organized around disease states rather than being strictly focused on drugs within given pharmacologic and/or chemical classes. Authors were asked to include detailed discussions of the chemistry of the most commonly used drugs to treat the disease state(s) addressed in the chapter, along with less detailed and/or tabularized descriptions of therapeutic agents not used as commonly in patient care. Drugs no longer in widespread clinical use are mentioned if they have historical importance or have served as templates for contemporary drug development.

While authors were given the freedom to organize their chapters in a way that best tells the chemical stories of the drugs under discussion, readers will find consistency in content coverage within this section. Chapters will provide a pharmacologic and therapeutic overview to their agents, followed by in-depth discussions of chemical mechanisms of action, physicochemical and pharmacokinetic properties, receptor binding, SAR, metabolism, and clinically important interactions and adverse effects (particularly those driven by the drug's chemistry).

The **Disease State Management** chapters review key SAR and other chemically relevant aspects of drugs most commonly used in the treatment of the disease state in question. These chapters were written to showcase how rigorous, in-depth medicinal chemistry content can be effectively incorporated into integrated Disease State Module–based courses where chemistry content must be coordinated with content from other disciplines. The three disease states selected to be exemplified by a Disease State Management chapter include coronary artery disease, rheumatoid arthritis, and obesity.

As in the Seventh Edition, all chapters begin with a roster of drugs discussed within the chapter and a listing of the abbreviations used. The use of red coloration to draw attention to structural elements of importance in figures, schemes, and other graphics has also been retained.

SPECIAL FEATURES

The **Clinical Significance** sections introduced in the Seventh Edition have been retained in the Eighth Edition. These important preambles to each chapter provide a clinical expert's view of the importance of a working knowledge of medicinal chemistry to the therapeutic use of the drugs covered within the chapter. The Clinical Significance boxes have been refreshed from the Seventh Edition either through an updated discussion by a previous clinical contributor or by sharing the thoughts and opinions of new pharmacy practice colleagues.

Every **Pharmacodynamic Agents** and **Disease State Management** chapter now concludes with a learning assessment exercise that allows readers to test themselves on retention of key concepts. The **clinical scenarios** and **medicinal chemistry case studies** that were included in all Seventh Edition chapters focused on drug therapy are now two options for authors to use to strategically showcase how readers can use their understanding of drug chemistry to address therapeutic problems and advance patient well-being. A third learning assessment exercise option is the **Structure Challenge**, in which readers are presented with the structures of several drugs covered in the chapter and asked five or more therapeutically focused multiple choice/multiple answer questions that can be answered through an analysis of drug chemistry. The answers to these learning assessment exercises are provided after the Reference section.

Acknowledgments

The editorial team gratefully acknowledges the dedicated collaboration of our publication partners at Wolters Kluwer, in particular Kerry McShane (Editorial Coordinator), Amy Millholen (Senior Development Editor), and Matt Hauber (Acquisitions Editor). Their unfailing support and assistance throughout this major undertaking has been truly noteworthy and did much to assure the quality of the final product. In addition, the support of colleagues and administrators at the Pharmacy programs at Creighton and St. John's Universities (where two of the editors were employed during at least part of the book's development) is recognized with sincere appreciation. Of course, this book would not exist without the commitment of our chapter authors to craft contemporary narratives that are scholarly yet readable, comprehensive yet focused, as well as effectively organized and engagingly illustrated. Our clinical contributors who wrote the Clinical Significance sections and/or collaborated on Clinical Scenario learning assessment exercises are also acknowledged for their important contribution to the goal of making this text explicitly relevant to patient care.

Finally, the editors acknowledge with love and gratitude the spouses whose patience and support was unwavering throughout what was effectively an intense 2.5-year commitment: Edward (Ted) Roche, Julie Zito, Patricia Lemke, and Gail Williams.

Victoria F. Roche, PhD
S. William Zito, PhD
Thomas L. Lemke, PhD
David A. Williams, PhD

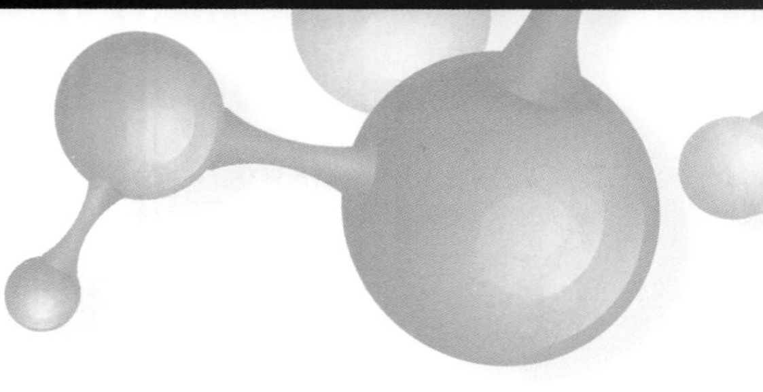

Contributors

Ali R. Banijamali, PhD
Atlantiks Pharma Consulting
Boston, Massachusetts

Kimberly Beck, PhD
College of Pharmacy and Health Sciences
Butler University
Indianapolis, Indiana

Swati Betharia, PhD
School of Pharmacy
MCPHS University
Boston, Massachusetts

Raymond G. Booth, PhD
School of Pharmacy
Northeastern University
Boston, Massachusetts

Kristopher E. Boyle, PhD
School of Pharmacy
Loma Linda University
Loma Linda, California

Clinton E. Canal, PhD
College of Pharmacy
Mercer University
Atlanta, Georgia

Andrew Coop, PhD
School of Pharmacy
University of Maryland, Baltimore
Baltimore, Maryland

Christopher W. Cunningham, PhD
School of Pharmacy
Concordia University
Mequon, Wisconsin

Gregory D. Cuny, PhD
College of Pharmacy
University of Houston
Houston, Texas

James T. Dalton, PhD
College of Pharmacy
University of Michigan
Ann Arbor, Michigan

E. Kim Fifer, PhD
College of Pharmacy
University of Arkansas for Medical Sciences
Little Rock, Arkansas

Elmer J. Gentry, PhD
College of Pharmacy
Chicago State University
Chicago, Illinois

Helmut B. Gottlieb, PhD
Feik School of Pharmacy
University of the Incarnate Word
San Antonio, Texas

Robert K. Griffith, PhD
School of Pharmacy
West Virginia University
Morgantown, West Virginia

Marc W. Harrold, PhD
School of Pharmacy
Duquesne University
Pittsburgh, Pennsylvania

Peter J. Harvison, PhD
Philadelphia College of Pharmacy
University of the Sciences
Philadelphia, Pennsylvania

David A. Johnson, PhD
School of Pharmacy
Duquesne University
Pittsburgh, Pennsylvania

Stephen G. Kerr, PhD
School of Pharmacy
MCPHS University
Boston, Massachusetts

Dan Kiel, PhD
School of Pharmacy
MCPHS University
Boston, Massachusetts

James J. Knittel, PhD
College of Pharmacy and Health Sciences
Western New England University
Springfield, Massachusetts

Srikanth Kolluru, PhD
School of Pharmacy and Health Sciences
Keck Graduate Institute
Claremont, California

Vijaya L. Korlipara, PhD
College of Pharmacy and Health Sciences
St. John's University
Queens, New York

Thomas L. Lemke, PhD
College of Pharmacy
University of Houston
Houston, Texas

Timothy J. Maher, PhD
School of Pharmacy
MCPHS University
Boston, Massachusetts

Michael L. Mohler, PharmD, PhD
GTx, Inc.
Memphis, Tennessee

Nader H. Moniri, PhD
College of Pharmacy
Mercer University
Atlanta, Georgia

Marilyn E. Morris, PhD
School of Pharmacy and Pharmaceutical Sciences
The State University of New York at Buffalo
Buffalo, New York

Bridget L. Morse, PharmD, PhD
Eli Lilly and Company
Indianapolis, Indiana

Ramesh Narayanan, PhD
College of Pharmacy
University of Tennessee Health Science Center
Memphis, Tennessee

E. Jeffrey North, PhD
School of Pharmacy and Health Professions
Creighton University
Omaha, Nebraska

Edward B. Roche, PhD
College of Pharmacy
University of Nebraska
Omaha, Nebraska

Victoria F. Roche, PhD
School of Pharmacy and Health Professions
Creighton University
Omaha, Nebraska

Anand Sridhar, PhD
Wegmans School of Pharmacy
St. John Fisher College
Rochester, New York

Tanaji T. Talele, PhD
College of Pharmacy and Health Sciences
St. John's University
Queens, New York

David Wallace, PharmD
College of Pharmacy
University of Houston
Houston, Texas

Abby J. Weldon, PhD
School of Pharmacy
William Carey University
Biloxi, Mississippi

David J. Weldon, PhD
School of Pharmacy
William Carey University
Biloxi, Mississippi

Jennifer L. Whetstone, PhD
College of Pharmacy
The Ohio State University
Columbus, Ohio

David A. Williams, PhD
School of Pharmacy
MCPHS University
Boston, Massachusetts

Patrick M. Woster, PhD
College of Pharmacy
Medical University of South Carolina
Charleston, South Carolina

Raghunandan Yendapally, PhD
Feik School of Pharmacy
University of the Incarnate Word
San Antonio, Texas

Sabesan Yoganathan, PhD
College of Pharmacy and Health Sciences
St. John's University
Queens, New York

Robin M. Zavod, PhD, FAPhA
Chicago College of Pharmacy
Midwestern University
Downers Grove, Illinois

S. William Zito, PhD
College of Pharmacy and Health Sciences
St. John's University
Jamaica, New York

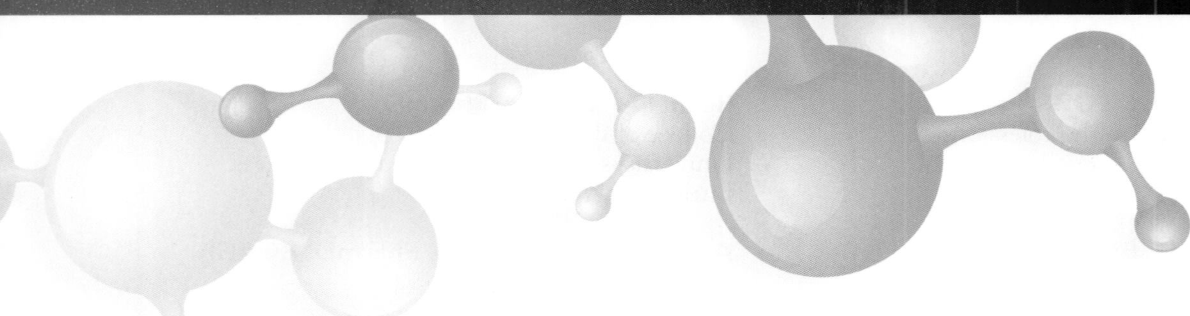

Clinical Contributors

Emily M. Ambizas, PharmD, MPH
College of Pharmacy and Health Sciences
St. John's University
Queens, New York

Alexander J. Ansara, PharmD, BCPS-AQ Cardiology
College of Pharmacy and Health Sciences
Butler University
Indianapolis, Indiana

Sean N. Avedissian, PharmD
Chicago College of Pharmacy
Midwestern University
Downers Grove, Illinois

Kathryn A. Connor, PharmD, BCPS, BCNSP
Wegmans School of Pharmacy
St. John Fisher College
Rochester, New York

Christopher J. Destache, PharmD, FCCP
School of Pharmacy and Health Professions
Creighton University
Omaha, Nebraska

Joseph V. Etzel, PharmD
College of Pharmacy and Health Sciences
St. John's University
Queens, New York

Michelle M. Hughes, PharmD, BCPS, BCACP
Neighborhood Healthcare
Escondido, California

Bethany A. Kalich, PharmD, BCPS–AQ Cardiology
Feik School of Pharmacy
University of the Incarnate Word
San Antonio, Texas

Tina J. Kanmaz, PharmD, AAHIVE, BCMAS
College of Pharmacy and Health Sciences
St. John's University
Queens, New York

Justin Kinney, PharmD
School of Pharmacy
Loma Linda University
Loma Linda, California

Sum Lam, PharmD, BCPS, BCGP
College of Pharmacy and Health Sciences
St. John's University
Queens, New York

Susan W. Miller, PharmD, BCGP, FASCP
College of Pharmacy
Mercer University
Atlanta, Georgia

Kathryn Neill, PharmD
College of Pharmacy
University of Arkansas for Medical Sciences
Little Rock, Arkansas

Kelly K. Nystrom, PharmD, BCOP
School of Pharmacy and Health Professions
Creighton University
Omaha, Nebraska

Kathleen A. Packard, PharmD, BCPS
School of Pharmacy and Health Professions
Creighton University
Omaha, Nebraska

Michael W. Perry, PharmD, BCPS, BCCCP
School of Pharmacy
Duquesne University
Pittsburgh, Pennsylvania

Amy M. Pick, PharmD, BCOP
School of Pharmacy and Health Professions
Creighton University
Omaha, Nebraska

Paul L. Price, PharmD, BCPP
School of Pharmacy and Health Professions
Creighton University
Omaha, Nebraska

Gigi Shafai, PharmD
Boston, Massachusetts

Jeffrey T. Sherer, PharmD, MPH, BCPS, BCGP
College of Pharmacy
University of Houston
Houston, Texas

Douglas Slain, PharmD, BCPS, FCCP, FASHP
School of Pharmacy
West Virginia University
Morgantown, West Virginia

Tracy Sprunger, PharmD, BCPS
College of Pharmacy and Health Sciences
Butler University
Indianapolis, Indiana

Rachel A. Stafford, PharmD
College of Pharmacy
University of Arkansas for Medical Sciences
Little Rock, Arkansas

Autumn Stewart-Lynch, PharmD, BCACP
School of Pharmacy
Duquesne University
Pittsburgh, Pennsylvania

Ernest S. Stremski, MD, MBA
School of Pharmacy
Concordia University
Mequon, Wisconsin

Sheila Wang, PharmD, BCPS-AQID
Chicago College of Pharmacy
Midwestern University
Downers Grove, Illinois

Trisha D. Wells, PharmD
College of Pharmacy
University of Michigan
Ann Arbor, Michigan

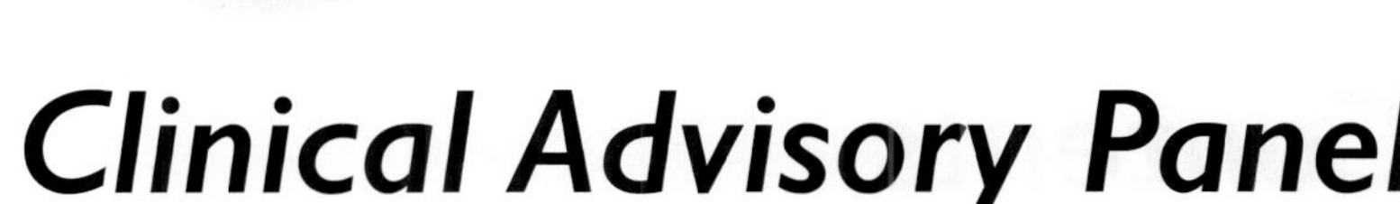

Clinical Advisory Panel

Michael Angelini, PharmD, BCPP
School of Pharmacy
MCPHS University
Boston, Massachusetts

Judy Cheng, PharmD, FCCP, BCPS
School of Pharmacy
MCPHS University
Boston, Massachusetts

Joseph V. Etzel, PharmD
College of Pharmacy and Health Sciences
St. John's University
Queens, New York

Michael P. Kane, PharmD, FCCP, BCPS, BCACP
Albany College of Pharmacy and Health Sciences
Albany, New York

Kamala Nola, PharmD
College of Pharmacy
Lipscomb University
Nashville, Tennessee

Kelly K. Nystrom, PharmD, BCOP
School of Pharmacy and Health Professions
Creighton University
Omaha, Nebraska

Contents

PART I

PRINCIPLES

CHAPTER 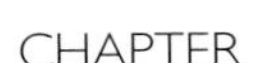

Introduction to Medicinal Chemistry

Andrew Coop

Abbreviations

P-gp P-glycoprotein
GCPRs G protein–coupled receptors
SAR structure-activity relationships
CNS central nervous system

INTRODUCTION

Medicinal chemistry has as many definitions as those doing the defining, and is complicated by the concurrent use of terms such as pharmaceutical chemistry, drug chemistry, bioorganic chemistry, chemical biology, and the list goes on. The question of "What is medicinal chemistry?" has been thoroughly discussed,[1,2] and this author views medicinal chemistry as "the application of chemistry to the continuous improvement of health." With such a general definition, it is clear that medicinal chemistry forms a critical component of the world's health care systems, but it is an area that many practitioners do not have a deep understanding of and one that can be initially overwhelming for learners. This short chapter explains the key components of medicinal chemistry and the skills required to fully comprehend the topic and is designed to remove the apprehension often observed by those new to medicinal chemistry.

Medicinal Chemistry is not Just Synthesis and Pushing Electrons

Traditional undergraduate teaching of chemistry is often overwhelming for students; it is a seemingly endless list of named reactions, along with "pushing electrons," filling an alphabet soup of electron shells, and mathematical equations describing statistical analysis of where electrons are while admitting we have no idea where they are![3] It is therefore of no surprise to this author that some students fear any topic that includes the name chemistry. As an introduction to medicinal chemistry, it needs to be remembered that the whole area originates from the use of natural products to treat conditions, where traditional remedies were handed down through the generations. As scientific understanding of the specific active components increased, the area evolved to one where the active ingredient was extracted, followed by making chemical modifications resulting in new drugs. It is therefore not unexpected that medicinal chemistry education in pharmacy schools was focused on extraction and chemical synthesis, areas close to undergraduate chemistry. However, medicinal chemistry has continued to evolve, and the health care professional needs to bring a new range of chemical skills to the table.

The Components of Medicinal Chemistry

A medicinal chemist can seem a magician to one not trained in the area. Simply by looking at patterns of hexagons and pentagons, with a few letters (e.g., C, N, O, S), along with charges (+ and −), the medicinal chemist can predict

- the effects of that drug on the human body, including magnitude of effect and duration
- the potential for interactions with other drugs
- possible adverse effects of the drug
- optimal methods of administration of the drug
- how to change the drug to eliminate or attenuate unwanted effects
- how to store the drug to ensure prolonged effectiveness
- how a drug may be misused (abused)

Obviously to be able to predict all such actions, the medicinal chemist must be skilled in many avenues of science, including organic chemistry, inorganic chemistry, physical chemistry, computational chemistry, pharmacology, metabolism, biology, biochemistry, mathematics, and, yes, psychology. That a medicinal chemist is required to apply and integrate all these differing scientific disciplines in order to make drug design decisions is what causes the apprehension for learners, but also what places it as a central discipline in health care. For that reason alone, the discipline of medicinal chemistry should excite learners relative to how they might bring a professionally unique and critically needed skill set to the interprofessional care team and the patient care environment.

So, Where to Start?

If we consider the first bullet above, the effects of the drug depend on the chemical constituents of the molecule, including how they interact with proteins, nucleic acids, or other macromolecules in the human body, what specific macromolecules they interact with, how they are degraded by enzymes in the body, how they facilitate transport of the drug across membranes, and how they facilitate solubility in aqueous media, among others. It is important to remember that all atoms in all molecules follow simple predictable rules and that all drugs are molecules and will behave as their chemistry dictates they must. Many molecules are small (e.g., aspirin [Chapter 15]); several are large (paclitaxel) (Chapter 33) (Fig. 1.1); and biologics are simply very large molecules or mixtures of large molecules. However, they are all molecules that follow the same rules.

Solubility

Let us consider aqueous (water-based) solubility as an area to apply this metric. Solubility under aqueous conditions is a critical component of the action of a drug, as the human body is mostly water and all life occur in aqueous systems. Whether we consider aspirin or paclitaxel in terms of solubility, we are considering the same principles: do the polar groups overcome the lipophilic groups to allow solubility in the polar solvent of water? If, like aspirin and paclitaxel, the answer is no, the second question is "Are there acidic and/or basic groups that could be utilized to yield an ionized species?" as the introduction of ionization increases polarity. In the case of aspirin, the answer is "yes," but in the case of paclitaxel, it is "no," making aspirin the more water soluble of the two drugs. The theory and application of acid/base principles is involved, but the fundamental concept remains the same for all drugs—is it polar enough to be water soluble?

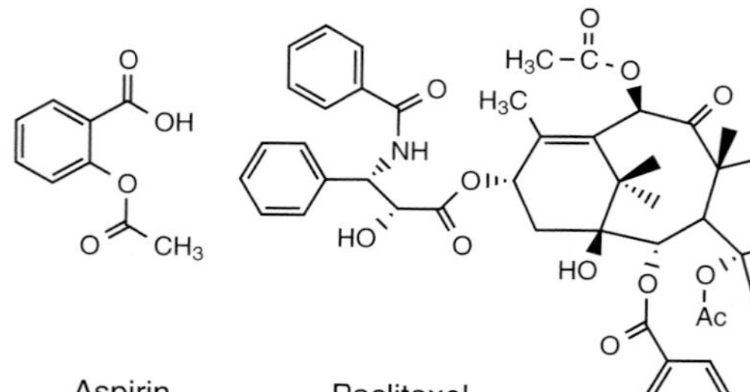

Figure 1.1 Example of a small and large drug molecule.

Crossing Membranes

Biological membranes exist at the surface of cells but also form barriers that drugs are required to cross to reach their target biological system (see below). Membranes are lipids, and this lipophilic character is in contrast to the aqueous environment outside the membrane. One confounding factor that many learners confront is the fact that if a drug is soluble in the aqueous environment, how can it enter the membrane to cross passively? One must remember that there are extremes, such as the opioid antagonist methylnaltrexone that is always fully ionized and designed not to cross the blood-brain barrier to limit actions centrally (Chapter 14) and others that are extreme in terms of lipophilicity, such as short-acting barbiturates (Chapter 12), fentanyl analogues (Chapter 14), or the triglyceride-lowering drug fenofibrate (Chapter 19). However, most drugs are designed at a "happy medium" with a sufficient balance of aqueous and lipid solubility that allows them to traverse the disparate barriers they will encounter in distributing from the site of administration to the site of action and ultimately to the site of elimination.

Interaction With Biological Systems

The majority of drugs exert their effects through direct action on biological systems. These interactions are again consistent for all drugs and all biological systems—a simple effect of thermodynamics. How energetically favorable are the dipole-dipole interactions between biological system (the target receptor or enzyme) and drug compared to the same interaction between drug and the aqueous environment, which includes considering the entropy of both drug-target and drug-water complexes? Again, the science behind the multiple effects is involved, but the fundamental principle is constant. Indeed, it is also the same principle that determines whether the drug interacts with (or binds to) other unwanted biological targets, which leads to adverse effects that can limit therapeutic utility.

The interactions can be modeled using computational chemistry, or a pattern of chemical substituents that lead to stronger interactions can be determined through the analysis of a large set of differing drug analogues. The development of an activity pattern from a large set of drugs is what is called structure-activity relationships (SAR). SAR is a powerful tool, allowing the prediction of the activity of a new drug, but this author's experience is that learners often fall into the trap of thinking that SAR is a hard and fast "law" and are frustrated by compounds that are active but do not satisfy SAR rules. This, again, is where a grasp of the principles behind the terms is required. SAR is a pattern that chemists have developed to help explain the action of drugs and is therefore a model based on known knowledge. All models have limitations, and anything based on current knowledge is one new data point away from no longer being accurate. Thus, this author considers SAR as more of an art than a science, a useful guide that helps predict activity, but not a "set in stone" law. Indeed, even the author has proposed SAR for a class of compounds that was shown not to be accurate for all compounds in that class!

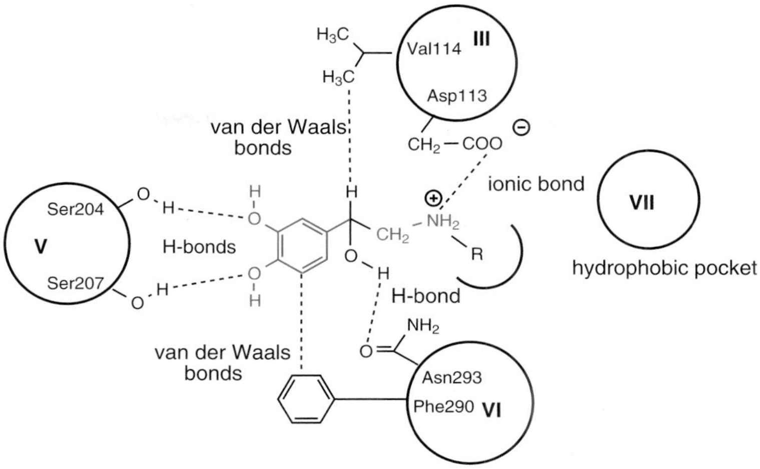

Figure 1.2 Norepinephrine binding to key residues in the adrenergic receptor.

Functional Activity at Receptors

The interaction with biological systems mentioned above is simply recognition or binding between drug and macromolecular receptors (Fig. 1.2). This correlates very well with enzyme inhibitory function, but medicinal chemists also need to understand how receptors function. G protein–coupled receptors (GPCRs) are one main type of receptor which spans cell membranes and functions to translate the message from the drug to the inside of the cell (readers are directed to Chapters 6-9 of this text for more in-depth information on drug receptors). The pharmacology of such receptors and intracellular pathways are complicated, but again, the learner should not lose sight that a drug can bind and activate the receptor (an agonist) or bind and not activate the receptor (an antagonist). Within the pages of this text, you will encounter a range of other activities associated with drugs (ligands), such as inverse agonists, partial agonists, and allosteric binders, but all interact and either activate a receptor macromolecule in some way or inactivate it.

Metabolism

One key component of the action of a drug is length of duration. As with the topics above, duration is complicated, but many of the factors that limit duration are due to metabolism. Metabolism is the natural enzymatic modification of molecules by the body, with the goal of increasing polarity for excretion through, for instance, the urine (see Chapter 3). Understanding that metabolism is aimed at increasing polarity and having a grasp of the functional groups that are both prone and resistant to metabolism allow one to predict the rate of metabolism of each group and to design a new molecule that is not prone to metabolism but still satisfies the SAR. The metabolic pathways by all the metabolic enzymes are numerous but can be broken down into Phase 1 (hydrolysis, oxidation, and reduction), Phase 2 (conjugation), and efflux (see below), which is sometimes referred to as Phase 3. Thus, a grasp of the chemistry of the functional groups in a molecule allows an analysis of the rate of metabolism and methods to prevent the actions of the metabolizing enzyme or, in the case of prodrugs that require metabolic activation, to harness them. There are many approaches you will encounter in this textbook; however, many are simply the replacement of a "hydrogen" that is prone to oxidation through hydroxylation with a metabolism-resistant substituent. A common metabolically vulnerable hydrogen is the *p*-hydrogen on an aromatic ring (Fig. 1.3). Thus, when looking through structures of therapeutics, please take note of the large number that contains *p*-halogens (such as haloperidol [Chapter 11] shown below, with *p*-halogens in red). It may well not be noted that the halogens eliminate such metabolism, but that is a major reason why such halogens are a common feature in drugs.

Active Transporters

The passive crossing of membranes was discussed above in terms of lipophilicity, but active transporters also exist–biological molecules that span membranes and actively transport the drug both into (influx) and out of (efflux) the cell. Amino acid transporters are a well-described class of transporters that facilitate influx of chemical species that would not passively cross membranes. P-glycoprotein (P-gp) is a well-described example of an efflux transporter (Chapter 4). P-gp is again a complicated protein, and how it truly functions remains open to debate, but the fundamental principle is that it removes exogenous chemical

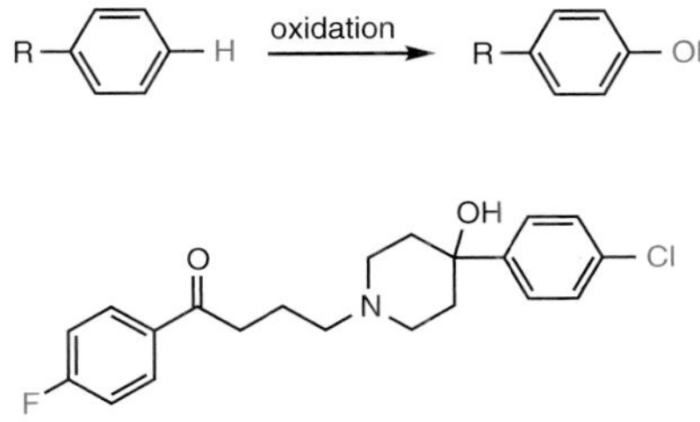

Figure 1.3 Example of hydrogen replacement with halogens to block oxidative metabolism to extend drug duration of action.

species from the body. This was obviously beneficial to remove toxins from eating poisonous berries during human evolution but works against us with drugs. P-gp recognizes a broad range of molecular species (its SAR contains many different functional groups that lead to transport) and is actually upregulated in many cancer cells. Thus, low activity as a substrate for P-gp is critical for many central nervous system (CNS) agents and anticancer drugs. By way of example, cancer cells initially responsive to the antimitotic agents paclitaxel and docetaxel can develop resistance to these drugs by upregulating (generating more molecules of) P-gp. However, the newest taxane antimitotic, cabazitaxel, has a lower affinity for this efflux protein and retains efficacy in malignant cells that no longer respond to other taxanes (Chapter 33). On the downside, because cabazitaxel is not rapidly ejected from cells by P-gp, it can accumulate in enterocytes, causing significant diarrhea (an adverse effect of therapy).

Abuse Liability

What is generally true in life can also be true in medicinal chemistry: a problem is often an opportunity. Drugs of abuse tend to function by acting on targets in the CNS. Thus, the fact that high P-gp substrate activity limits access to the CNS is one reason why the antidiarrheal loperamide has the actions of an opioid (such as morphine) when tested in cells but has very limited central opioid activity (and thus addiction potential with accompanying abuse liability) when taken by patients at recommended doses (Chapter 14). Figure 1.4 shows the relationship between morphine and loperamide; at first, they appear to be very different structures. However, as highlighted in red, they both share a phenylpropyl pattern of atoms; such a common feature between molecules with the same biological actions is termed a pharmacophore, essentially a special form of SAR. This does not mean that all molecules that

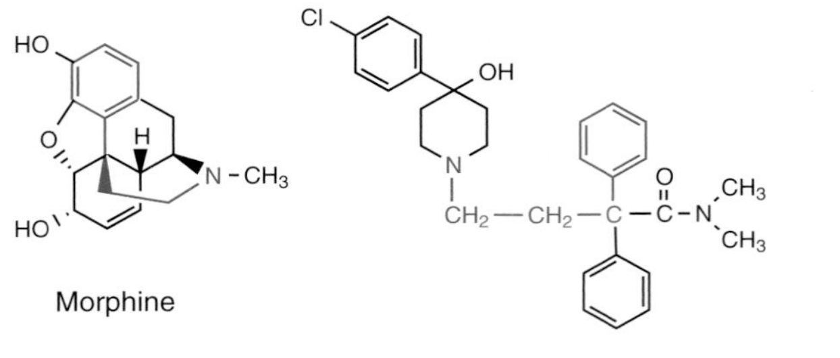

Figure 1.4 Comparison of morphine and loperamide showing the common phenylpropyl moiety.

contain a phenylpropyl are opioids (remember SAR is not a "law"), but common pharmacophores are a useful guide when determining the biological activity of a molecule.

SUMMARY

The short paragraphs above are an introduction to the various aspects of medicinal chemistry, and all will be discussed in greater detail in the various chapters within this text. The goal of this introductory chapter is to bring clarity to many of the concepts and terms and is intended as a starting point from which to progress. Enjoy the journey!

REFERENCES

1. Faruk Khan MO, Deimling MJ, Philip A. Medicinal chemistry and the pharmacy curriculum. *Am J Pharm Educ*. 2011;75(8):161.
2. Erhardt PW. Medicinal chemistry in the new millennium. A glance into the future. *Pure Appl Chem*. 2002;74:703-785.
3. Griffiths DJ, Schroeter DF. *Introduction to Quantum Mechanics*. 3rd ed. Cambridge: Cambridge University Press; 2018.

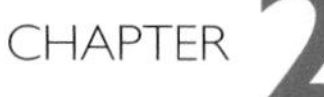

CHAPTER 2

Foundational Principles and Functional Group Impact on Activity

James J. Knittel and Robin M. Zavod

Abbreviations

BCRP breast cancer resistance protein
HCl hydrochloric acid
HPT-1 human peptide transporter 1
IV intravenous
MRP2, MRP3 multiresistance associated proteins 2 & 3
MW molecular weight
NaOH sodium hydroxide
OAT organic anion transporter
OCT organic cation transporter
PABA *p*-aminobenzoic acid
PepT1 peptide transporter 1
PHTs polyhistidine triad
P-gp P-glycoprotein
QSAR quantitative structure-activity relationship
SAR structure-activity relationship
USP U.S. Pharmacopeia

Medicinal chemistry is an interdisciplinary science at the intersection of organic chemistry, biochemistry (bio-organic chemistry), computational chemistry, pharmacology, pharmacognosy, molecular biology, and physical chemistry. This branch of chemistry is involved with the identification, design, synthesis, and development of new drugs that are safe and suitable for therapeutic use in humans and pets. It includes the study of marketed drugs, their biologic properties, and their quantitative structure-activity relationships (QSARs).

Medicinal chemists study how chemical structure influences biologic activity. As such, it is necessary to understand not only the mechanism by which a drug exerts its effect but also how the molecular and physicochemical properties of the molecule influence the drug's pharmacokinetics (absorption, distribution, metabolism, toxicity, and elimination) and pharmacodynamics (what the drug does to the body). The term "physicochemical properties" refers to how the functional groups present within a molecule influence its acid-base properties, water solubility, partition coefficient, crystal structure, stereochemistry, and ability to interact with biologic systems, such as enzyme active sites and receptor binding sites. To design better medicinal agents, the relative contribution that each functional group (i.e., pharmacophore) makes to the overall physicochemical properties of the molecule must be evaluated. Studies of this type involve modification of the molecule in a systematic fashion followed by a determination of how these changes affect biologic activity. Such studies are referred to as structure-activity relationships (SARs)—that is, the relationship of how structural features of the molecule contribute to, or take away from, the desired biologic activity. Because of the foundational nature of the content of this chapter, there are numerous case studies presented throughout the chapter (as boxes).

INTRODUCTION

Chemical compounds, usually derived from plants and other natural sources, have been used by humans for thousands of years to alleviate pain, diarrhea, infection, and various other maladies. Until the 19th century, these "remedies" were primarily crude preparations of plant material of unknown constitution. The revolution in synthetic organic chemistry during the 19th century produced a concerted effort toward identification of the structures of the active constituents of these naturally derived medicinals and synthesis of what were hoped to be more efficacious agents. By determining the molecular structures of the active components of these complex mixtures, it was thought that a better understanding of how these components worked could be elucidated.

RELATIONSHIP BETWEEN MOLECULAR STRUCTURE AND BIOLOGIC ACTIVITY

Early studies of the relationship between chemical structure and biologic activity were conducted by Crum-Brown and Fraser[1] in 1869. They demonstrated that many compounds containing tertiary amine groups exhibited activity as muscle relaxants when converted to quaternary ammonium compounds. Molecules with widely differing pharmacologic properties, such as strychnine (a convulsant), morphine (an analgesic), nicotine (a deterrent, insecticide), and atropine (an anticholinergic), could be converted to muscle relaxants with properties similar to those of tubocurarine when methylated (Fig. 2.1). Crum-Brown and Fraser therefore concluded that muscle relaxant activity required the presence of a quaternary ammonium group within the structure. This initial hypothesis was later

Tubocurarine
(muscle relaxant)

Morphine
(analgesic)

N-Methylmorphine
(muscle relaxant)

Nicotine
(insecticide)

N-Methylnicotine
(muscle relaxant)

Atropine
(mydriatic)

N-Methylatropine
(muscle relaxant)

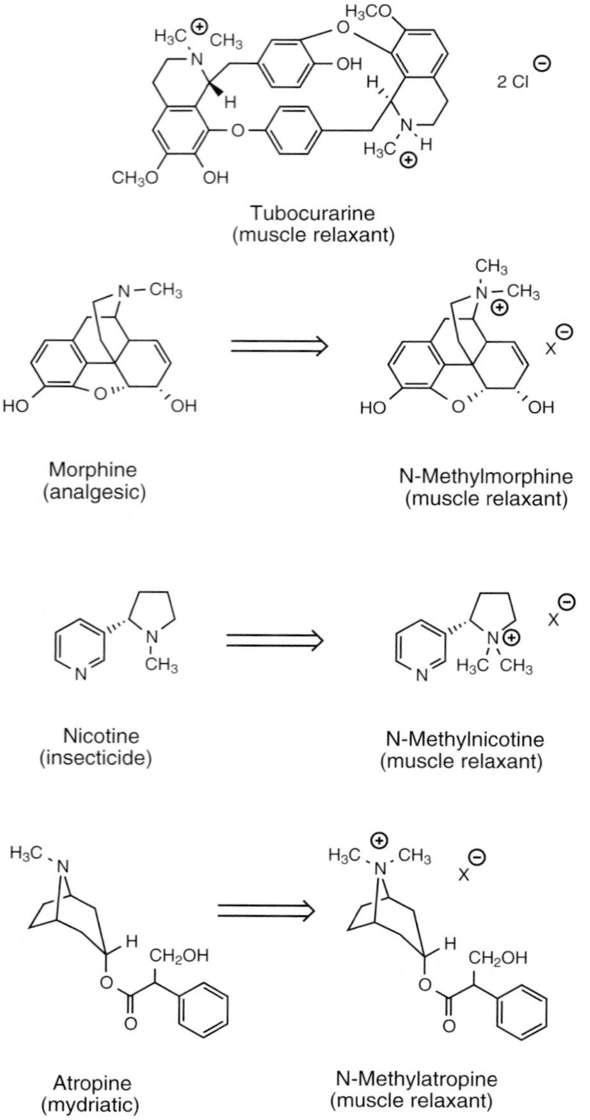

Figure 2.1 Effects of methylation on biologic activity.

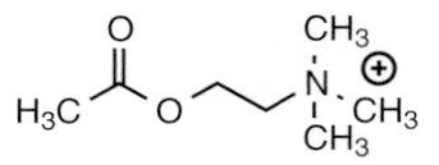

Figure 2.2 Acetylcholine, a neurotransmitter and muscle relaxant.

disproven by the discovery of the natural neurotransmitter and activator of muscle contraction, acetylcholine (Fig. 2.2). Even though Crum-Brown and Fraser's initial hypothesis that related chemical structure with action as a muscle relaxant was incorrect, it demonstrated the concept that molecular structure influences the biologic activity of chemical entities and that alterations in structure produce changes in biologic action.

With the discovery by Crum-Brown and Fraser that quaternary ammonium groups could produce molecules with muscle relaxant properties, scientists began to look for other functional groups that produce specific biologic responses. At the time, it was thought that specific chemical groups, or nuclei (rings), were responsible for specific biologic effects. This led to the postulate, which took some time to disprove, that "one chemical group gives one biological action."[2] Even after the discovery of acetylcholine by Loewi and Navrati,[3] which effectively dispensed with Crum-Brown and Fraser's concept of all quaternary ammonium compounds being muscle relaxants, this was still considered to be dogma and took a long time to refute.

SELECTIVITY OF DRUG ACTION AND DRUG RECEPTORS

Although the structures of many drugs or xenobiotics, or at least their functional group composition, were known at the start of the 20th century, how these compounds exerted their effects was still a mystery. Using his observations with regard to the staining behavior of microorganisms, Ehrlich[4] developed the concept of drug receptors. He postulated that certain "side chains" on the surfaces of cells were "complementary" to the dyes (or drug) and suggested that the two could therefore interact with one another. In the case of antimicrobial compounds, interaction of the chemical with the cell surface "side chains" produced a toxic effect. This concept was the first description of what later became known as the receptor hypothesis for explaining the biologic action of chemical entities. Ehrlich also discussed selectivity of drug action via the concept of a "magic bullet." He suggested that this selectivity permitted eradication of disease states without significant harm coming to the organism being treated (i.e., the patient). This was later modified by Albert[5] and today is referred to as "selective toxicity." An example of poor selectivity was demonstrated when Ehrlich developed organic arsenicals that were toxic to trypanosomes as a result of their irreversible reaction with thiol groups (-SH) on vital proteins. The formation of As-S bonds resulted in death of the target organism. Unfortunately, these compounds were toxic not only to the target organism but also to the host once certain blood levels of arsenic were achieved.

The "paradox" that resulted after the discovery of acetylcholine, how one chemical group can produce two different biologic effects (i.e., muscle relaxation and muscle contraction), was explained by Ing[6] using the actions of acetylcholine and tubocurarine as his examples. Ing hypothesized that both acetylcholine and tubocurarine act at the same receptor, but that one molecule fits the receptor in a more complementary manner and "activates" it, causing muscle contraction. (Ing did not elaborate just how this activation occurred.) The blocking effect of the larger molecule, tubocurarine, could be explained by its occupation of part of the receptor, thereby preventing acetylcholine, the smaller molecule, from interacting with the receptor. With both molecules, the quaternary ammonium functional group is a common structural feature and interacts with the same region of the receptor. If one closely examines the structures of other molecules with opposing effects on the same pharmacologic system, this appears to be a common theme: Molecules that block the effects of natural neurotransmitters, such as norepinephrine, histamine, dopamine, or serotonin, for example, are called antagonists and are usually larger in size than the native compound, which is not the case for antagonists of peptide neurotransmitters and hormones such as cholecystokinin, melanocortin, or substance P. Antagonists to these peptide molecules are usually smaller in size. However, regardless of the type of neurotransmitter (biogenic amine or peptide), both agonists and antagonists share common structural features with the neurotransmitter that they influence. This provides support to the concept that the structure of a molecule, its composition and arrangement of functional groups, determines the type of pharmacologic effect that it possesses (i.e., SAR). For example, compounds that are muscle relaxants acting via the cholinergic nervous system possess a quaternary ammonium or protonated tertiary ammonium group and are larger than acetylcholine (compare acetylcholine in Fig. 2.2 with tubocurarine in Fig. 2.1).

SARs are the underlying principle of medicinal chemistry. Similar molecules exert similar biologic actions in a qualitative sense. A corollary to this is that structural elements (functional groups) within a molecule most often contribute in an additive manner to the physicochemical properties of a molecule and, therefore, to its biologic action. One need only peruse the structures of drug molecules in a particular pharmacologic class to become convinced (e.g., histamine H_1 antagonists, histamine H_2 antagonists, β-adrenergic antagonists). In the quest for better medicinal agents (drugs), it must be determined which functional groups within a specific structure are important for its pharmacologic activity and how these groups can be modified to produce more potent, more selective, and safer compounds.

An example of how different functional groups can yield chemical entities with similar physicochemical properties is demonstrated by the sulfanilamide antibiotics. In Figure 2.3, the structures of sulfanilamide and *p*-aminobenzoic acid (PABA) are shown. In 1940, Woods[7] demonstrated that PABA reverses the antibacterial action of sulfanilamide (and other sulfonamide-based antibacterials) and both PABA and sulfanilamide have similar steric and electronic properties. Both molecules contain acidic functional groups, with PABA containing an aromatic carboxylic acid (Ar-COOH) and sulfanilamide an aromatic sulfonamide (Ar-SO_2NH_2). When ionized at physiologic pH, both compounds have a similar electronic configuration, and the distance between the ionized acid and the weakly basic amino group is also very similar. It should be no surprise that sulfanilamide acts as an antagonist to PABA metabolism in bacteria.

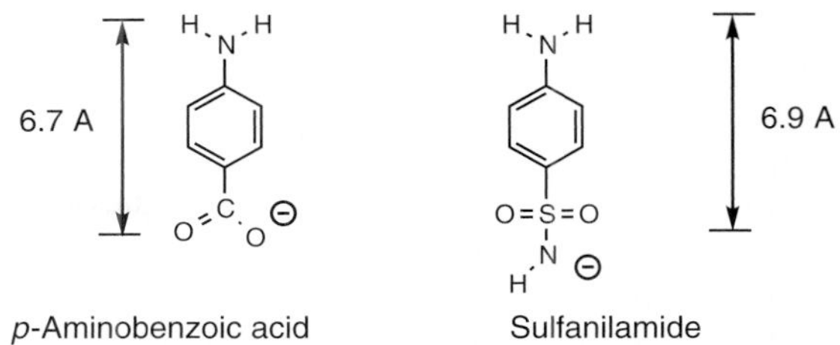

Figure 2.3 Ionized forms of *p*-aminobenzoic acid (PABA) and sulfanilamide, with comparison of the distance between amine and ionized acids of each compound. Note how closely sulfanilamide resembles PABA.

Biologic Targets for Drug Action

In order for drug molecules to exhibit their pharmacologic activity, they must interact with a biologic target, typically a receptor, enzyme, nucleic acid, excitable membrane or other biopolymer. These interactions occur between the functional groups found in the drug molecule and those found within each biologic target. The relative fit of each drug molecule with its target is a function of a number of physicochemical properties including acid-base chemistry and related ionization, functional group shape and size, and three-dimensional spatial orientation. The quality of this "fit" has a direct impact on the biologic response produced. In this chapter, functional group characteristics are discussed as a means to better understand overall drug molecule absorption, distribution, metabolism, and excretion, as well as potential interaction with a biologic target.

PHYSICOCHEMICAL PROPERTIES OF DRUGS

Acid-Base Properties

The human body is 70%-75% water, which amounts to approximately 51-55 L of water for a 160-lb (73-kg) individual. For an average drug molecule with a molecular weight of 200 g/mol and a dose of 20 mg, this leads to a solution concentration of approximately 2×10^{-6} M (2 μM). When considering the solution behavior of a drug within the body, we are dealing with a dilute solution, for which the Brönsted-Lowry[8] acid-base theory is most appropriate to explain and predict acid-base behavior. This is a very important concept in medicinal chemistry, because the acid-base properties of drug molecules determine the ionization state of the molecule at a given pH therefore directly affecting absorption, excretion, and compatibility with other drugs in solution. According to the Brönsted-Lowry theory, an "acid" is any substance capable of yielding a proton (H^+), and a "base" is any substance capable of accepting a proton. When an acid gives up a proton to a base, it is converted to its "conjugate base." Similarly, when a base accepts a proton, it is converted to its "conjugate acid" (Equations (2.1) and (2.2)):

Eq. 2.1

$$CH_3COOH + H_2O \rightleftharpoons CH_3COO^{\ominus} + H_3O^{\oplus}$$

Acid (acetic acid) · Base (water) · Conjugate Base (acetate) · Conjugate Acid (hydronium ion)

Eq. 2.2

$$CH_3NH_2 + H_2O \rightleftharpoons CH_3NH_3^{\oplus} + {}^{\ominus}OH$$

Base (methylamine) · Acid (water) · Conjugate Acid (methyl ammionium ion) · Conjugate Base (hydroxide ion)

Note that when an acidic functional group loses its proton (often referred to as having undergone "dissociation"), it is left with an extra electron and becomes negatively charged. This is the "ionized" form of the acid. The ability of the ionized functional group to participate in an ion-dipole interaction with water (see the Water Solubility of Drugs section) enhances its water solubility. Many functional groups behave as acids (Table 2.1). The ability to recognize these functional groups and their relative acid strengths helps to predict absorption, distribution, excretion, and potential incompatibilities between drugs.

When a basic functional group is converted to the corresponding conjugate acid, it too becomes ionized. In this instance, however, the functional group becomes positively charged due to the extra proton. Most drugs that contain basic functional groups contain primary, secondary, and tertiary amines or imino amines, such as guanidines and amidines. Other functional groups that are basic are shown in Table 2.2. As with the acidic groups, it is important to become familiar with these functional groups and their relative strengths.

Table 2.1 Common Acidic Organic Functional Groups and Their Ionized (Conjugate Base) Forms

Acids (pK_a)	Acid	Conjugate base form	Conjugate Base
Phenol (9-11)	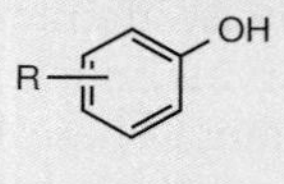 R–C₆H₄–OH	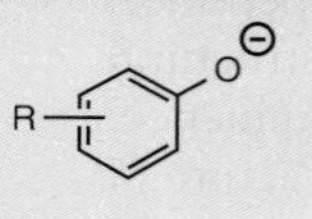 R–C₆H₄–O⊖	Phenolate
Sulfonamide (9-10)	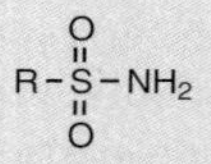 R-SO₂-NH₂	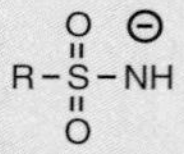 R-SO₂-NH⊖	Sulfonamidate
Imide (9-10)	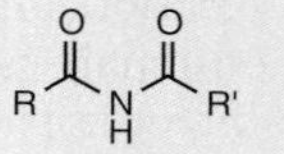 RC(O)NHC(O)R'	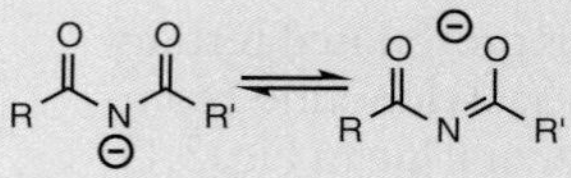 RC(O)N⊖C(O)R' ⇌ RC(O⊖)=NC(O)R'	Imidate
Alkylthiol (10-11)	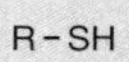 R-SH	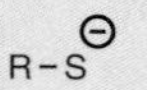 R-S⊖	Thiolate
Thiophenol (9-10)	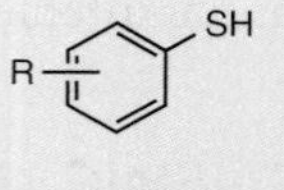 R–C₆H₄–SH	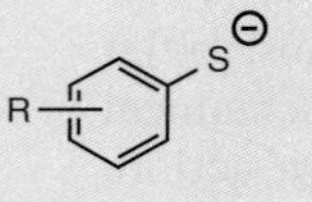 R–C₆H₄–S⊖	Thiophenolate
N-Arylsulfonamide (6-7)	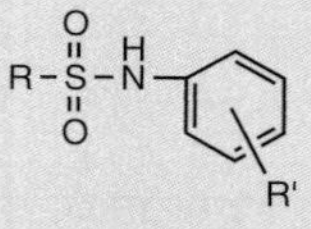 R-SO₂-NH-C₆H₄-R'	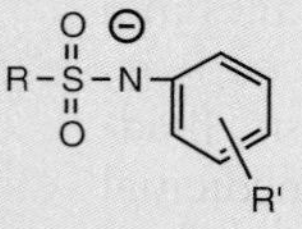 R-SO₂-N⊖-C₆H₄-R'	N-Arylsulfonamidate
Sulfonimide (5-6)	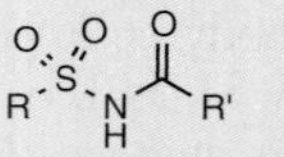 RSO₂NHC(O)R'	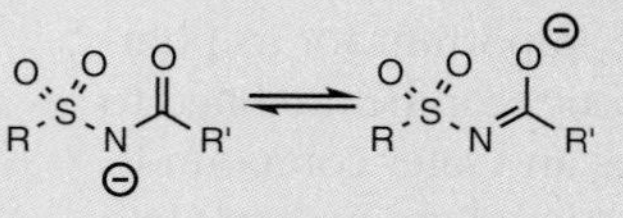 RSO₂N⊖C(O)R' ⇌ RSO₂N=C(O⊖)R'	Sulfonimidate
Alkylcarboxylic acid (5-6)	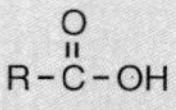 R-C(O)-OH	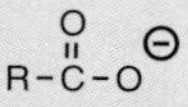 R-C(O)-O⊖	Alkylcarboxylate
Arylcarboxylic acid (4-5)	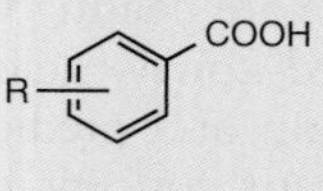 R–C₆H₄–COOH	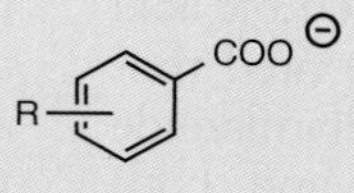 R–C₆H₄–COO⊖	Arylcarboxylate
Sulfonic acid (0-1)	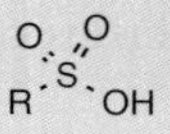 RSO₂OH	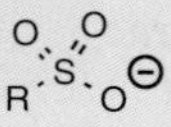 RSO₂O⊖	Sulfonate

Acid strength increases as one moves down the table.

Table 2.2 Common Basic Organic Functional Groups and Their Ionized (Conjugate Acid) Forms

Base			Conjugate Acid (pK_aHB^+)
Arylamine	R–C₆H₄–NH₂	R–C₆H₄–$NH_3^{\oplus}$	Arylammonium (9-11)
Aromatic amine	R–pyridine (N)	R–pyridinium (NH⊕)	Aromatic ammonium (5-6)
Imine	R-CH=NH	R-CH=$NH_2^{\oplus}$	Iminium (3-4)
Alkylamines	piperidine (NH); R-NH_2	piperidinium ($NH_2^{\oplus}$); R-$NH_3^{\oplus}$	Alkylammonium (2°—10-11) (1°—9-10)
Amidine	R-C(=NH)-NH_2	R-C(=$NH_2^{\oplus}$)-NH_2	Amidinium (10-11)
Guanidine	R-NH-C(=NH)-NH_2	R-NH-C(=$NH_2^{\oplus}$)-NH_2	Guanidinium (12-13)

Functional groups that cannot give up or accept a proton are considered to be "neutral" (or "nonelectrolytes") with respect to their acid-base properties. Common neutral functional groups are shown in Table 2.3. Quaternary ammonium compounds are neither acidic nor basic and are not electrically neutral. Additional information about the acid-base properties of the functional groups listed in Tables 2.1-2.3 can be found in Lemke.[9]

A molecule can contain multiple functional groups with acid-base properties and, therefore, can possess both acidic and basic character. For example, ciprofloxacin (Fig. 2.4), a fluoroquinolone antibacterial agent, contains a secondary alkylamine, two tertiary arylamines (aniline-like amines), and a carboxylic acid. The two arylamines are weakly basic and, therefore, do not contribute significantly to the acid-base properties of ciprofloxacin under physiologic conditions. Depending on the pH of the physiologic environment, this molecule will either accept a proton (secondary alkylamine), donate a proton (carboxylic acid), or both. Thus, it is described as amphoteric (both acidic and basic) in nature. Figure 2.5 shows the acid-base behavior of ciprofloxacin in two different environments. Note that at a given pH (e.g., pH 1.0-3.5), only one of

Table 2.3 Common Organic Functional Groups That are Considered Neutral Under Physiologic Conditions

R-CH_2-OH **Alkyl Alcohol**	R-O-R' **Ether**	R-C(=O)-O-R' **Ester**	R-S(O_2)-O-R' **Sulfonic Acid Ester**
R-C(=O)-NH_2 Amide	R-C₆H₄-NH-C₆H₄-R' Diarylamine	R-C≡N Nitrile	R-$N^{\oplus}$(R')(R'')-R''' Quaternary ammonium
R-N(R')(R'')→O Amine oxide	R-C(=O)-R' Ketone and Aldehyde	R-S-R' Thioether	R-S(=O)-R' R-S(O_2)-R' Sulfoxide sulfone

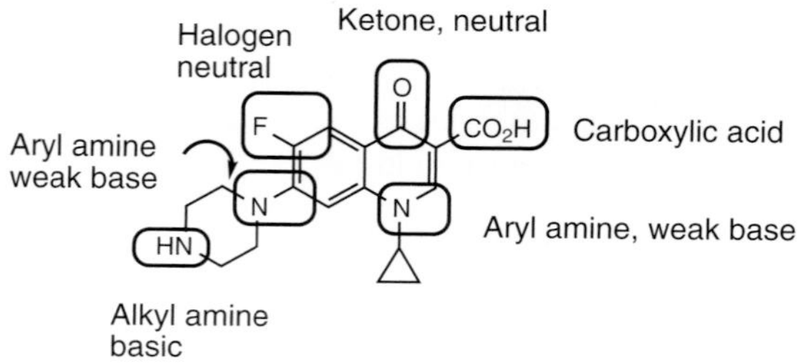

Figure 2.4 Chemical structure of ciprofloxacin showing the various organic functional groups.

the functional groups (the alkylamine) is significantly ionized. To be able to make this prediction, an appreciation for the relative acid-base strength of both the acidic and basic functional groups is required. Thus, one needs to know which acidic or basic functional group within a molecule containing multiple functional groups is the strongest and which acidic or basic functional group is the weakest. The concept of pK_a not only describes relative acid-base strength of functional groups but also allows one to calculate, for a given pH, the relative percentages of the ionized and un-ionized forms of the drug. As stated earlier, this helps to predict relative water solubility, absorption, and excretion for a given compound.

Relative Acid Strength (pK_a)

Strong acids and bases completely donate (dissociate) or accept a proton in aqueous solution to produce their respective conjugate bases and acids. For example, mineral acids, such as hydrochloric acid (HCl), or bases, such as sodium hydroxide (NaOH), undergo 100% dissociation in water, with the equilibrium between the ionized and un-ionized forms shifted completely to the right (ionized), as shown in Equations (2.3) and (2.4):

Eq. 2.3 $$HCl + H_2O \rightleftharpoons Cl^{\ominus} + H_3O^{\oplus}$$

Eq. 2.4 $$NaOH + H_2O \rightleftharpoons Na^{\oplus} + OH^{\ominus} + H_2O$$

Acids and bases of intermediate or weak strength, however, incompletely donate (dissociate) or accept a proton, and the equilibrium between the ionized and un-ionized forms lies somewhere in the middle, such that all possible species can exist at any given time. Note that in Equations (2.3) and (2.4), water acts as a base in one instance and as an acid in the other. Water is therefore *amphoteric*—that is, it can act as an acid or a base, depending on the prevailing pH of the solution. From a physiologic perspective, drug molecules are always present as a dilute aqueous solution. The strongest base that is present is OH^-, and the strongest acid is H_3O^+. This is known as the "leveling effect" of water. Thus, some functional groups that have acidic or basic character do not behave as such under physiologic conditions in aqueous solution. For example, alkyl alcohols, such as ethyl alcohol, are not sufficiently acidic to become significantly ionized in an aqueous solution at a physiological pH. Water is not sufficiently basic to remove the proton from ethyl alcohol to form the ethoxide ion (Equation (2.5)). Therefore, under physiologic conditions, alcohols are neutral with respect to acid-base properties:

Eq. 2.5 $$CH_3CH_2OH + H_2O \not\rightleftharpoons CH_3CH_2O^- + H_3O^{\oplus}$$

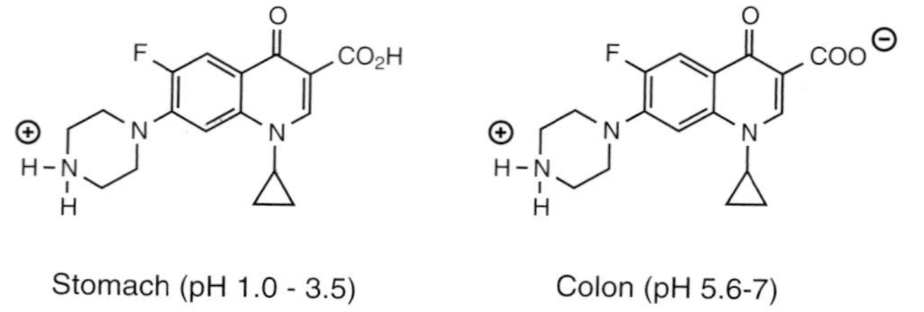

Stomach (pH 1.0 - 3.5)   Colon (pH 5.6-7)

Figure 2.5 Predominate forms of ciprofloxacin at two different locations within the gastrointestinal tract.

Predicting the Degree of Ionization of a Molecule

By knowing if there are acidic and/or basic functional groups present in a molecule, one can predict whether a molecule is going to be predominantly ionized or un-ionized at a given pH. To be able to quantitatively predict the degree of ionization of a molecule, the pK_a values of each of the acidic and basic functional groups present and the pH of the environment in which the molecule will be located must be known. The magnitude of the pK_a value is a measure of relative acid or base strength, and the Henderson-Hasselbalch equation (Equation (2.6)) can be used to calculate the percent ionization of a compound at a given pH (this equation was used to calculate the major forms of ciprofloxacin in Fig. 2.5):

Eq. 2.6 $$pK_a = pH + \log \frac{[\text{acid form}]}{[\text{base form}]}$$

The key to understanding the use of the Henderson-Hasselbalch equation for calculating percent ionization is to realize that this equation relates a constant, pK_a, to the ratio of the acidic form of a functional group to its conjugate base form (and conversely, the conjugate acid form to its base). Because pK_a is a constant for any given functional group, the ratio of acid to conjugate base (or conjugate acid to base) will determine the pH of the solution. A sample calculation is shown in Figure 2.6 for the sedative hypnotic amobarbital.

When dealing with a basic functional group, one must recognize the conjugate acid represents the ionized form

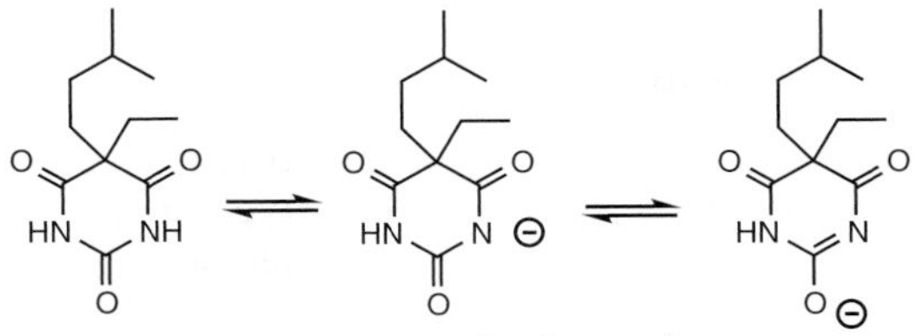

Question: At a pH of 7.4, what is the percent ionization of amobarbital?

Answer: $8.0 = 7.4 + \log\frac{[\text{acid}]}{[\text{base}]}$

$0.6 = \log\frac{[\text{acid}]}{[\text{base}]}$

$10^{0.6} = \frac{[\text{acid}]}{[\text{base}]} = \frac{3.98}{1}$

$\%\ \text{acid form} = \frac{3.98 \times 100}{4.98} = 79.9\%$

Figure 2.6 Calculation of percent ionization of amobarbital. Calculation indicates that 80% of the molecules are in the acid (or protonated) form, leaving 20% in the conjugate base (ionized) form.

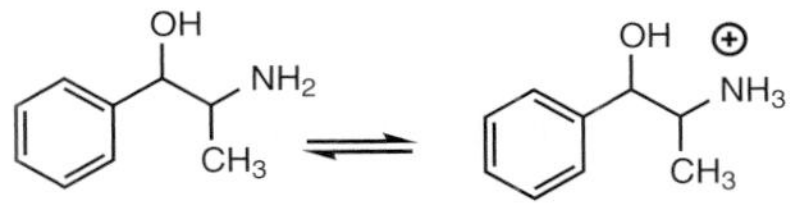

Question: What is the % ionization (acid form) of phenylpropanolamine at pH 7.4?

Answer: $7.4 = 9.4 + \log\frac{[\text{acid}]}{[\text{base}]}$

$2.0 = \log\frac{[\text{acid}]}{[\text{base}]}$

$10^{2} = \frac{[\text{acid}]}{[\text{base}]} = \frac{100}{1}$

$\%\ \text{ionization} = \frac{100 \times 100}{101} = 99\%$

Figure 2.7 Calculation of percent ionization of phenylpropanolamine. Calculation indicates that 99% of the molecules are in the conjugate acid form, which is the same as the percent ionization.

of the functional group. Figure 2.7 shows the calculated percent ionization for the decongestant phenylpropanolamine. It is very important to understand that for a base, the pK_a refers to the conjugate acid or ionized form of the compound. To thoroughly comprehend this relationship, calculate the percent ionization of an acidic functional group and a basic functional group at different pH values and carefully observe the trend.

Water Solubility of Drugs

The solubility of a drug molecule in water greatly affects the routes of administration that are available, as well as its absorption, distribution, and elimination. Two key concepts to keep in mind when considering the water (or fat) solubility of a molecule are the potential for hydrogen bond formation and ionization of one or more functional groups within the molecule.

Hydrogen Bonds

Each functional group capable of donating or accepting a hydrogen bond contributes to the overall water solubility of the compound and increases the hydrophilic (water-loving) nature of the molecule. Conversely, functional groups that cannot form hydrogen bonds do not enhance hydrophilicity and will contribute to the hydrophobic (water-fearing) nature of the molecule. Hydrogen bonds are a special case of what are usually referred to as dipole-dipole interactions. A permanent dipole occurs as a result of an unequal sharing of electrons between two atoms within a covalent bond. This unequal sharing of electrons only occurs when these two atoms have significantly different electronegativities. When a permanent dipole is present, a partial charge is associated with each of these atoms along a single bond (one atom has a partial negative charge, and one atom has a partial positive charge). The atom with a partial negative charge has higher electron density than the other atom. When two functional groups containing one or more permanent dipoles approach one another, they align such that the negative end of one dipole is electrostatically attracted to the positive end of the other. When the positive end of the dipole is a hydrogen atom, this interaction is referred to as a "hydrogen bond" (or H-bond). Thus, for a hydrogen bonding interaction to occur, at least one functional group must contain a dipole with an electropositive hydrogen. The hydrogen atom must be covalently bound to an electronegative atom, such as oxygen (O), nitrogen (N), sulfur (S), or selenium (Se). Of these four elements, only oxygen and nitrogen atoms contribute significantly to the dipole, and we will therefore concern ourselves only with the hydrogen-bonding capability (specifically as hydrogen bond donors) of functional groups that contain a bond between oxygen and hydrogen atoms (e.g., alcohols) and functional groups that contain a bond between nitrogen and hydrogen atoms (e.g., primary and secondary amines and amides) (e.g., NH and CONH groups).

Case Study

ABSORPTION/ACID-BASE CASE

A long-distance truck driver comes into the pharmacy complaining of seasonal allergies. He asks you to recommend an agent that will act as an antihistamine but will not cause drowsiness. He regularly takes TUMS for indigestion due to the bad food he eats while on the road.

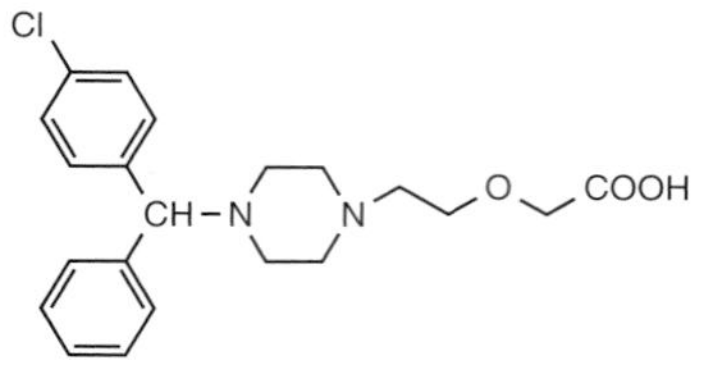

Cetirizine (Zyrtec)

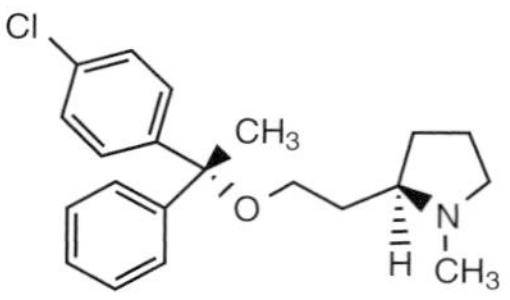

Clemastine (Tavist)

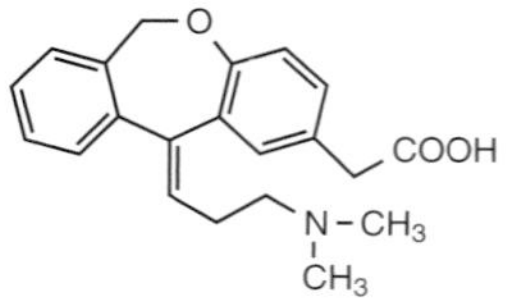

Olopatadine (Patanol)

1. Identify the functional groups present in Zyrtec and Tavist, and evaluate the effect of each functional group on the ability of the drug to cross lipophilic membranes (e.g., blood-brain barrier). Based on your assessment of each agent's ability to cross the blood-brain barrier (and, therefore, potentially cause drowsiness), provide a rationale for whether the truck driver should be taking Zyrtec or Tavist.
2. Patanol is sold as an aqueous solution of the hydrochloride salt. Modify the structure present in the box to show the appropriate salt form of this agent. This agent is applied to the eye to relieve itching associated with allergies. Describe why this agent is soluble in water and what properties make it able to be absorbed into membranes that surround the eye.
3. Consider the structural features of Zyrtec and Tavist. In which compartment (stomach [pH 1] or intestine [pH 6-7]) will each of these two drugs be best absorbed?
4. TUMS neutralizes stomach acid to pH 3.5. Based on your answer to question 3, determine whether the truck driver will get the full antihistaminergic effect if he takes his antihistamine at the same time he takes his TUMS. Provide a rationale for your answer.

Case Solution found immediately after References.

Case Study

ACID-BASE CHEMISTRY/COMPATIBILITY CASE

The intravenous (IV) technician in the hospital pharmacy gets an order for a patient that includes the two drugs drawn below. She is unsure if she can mix the two drugs together in the same IV bag and is not certain how water soluble the agents are.

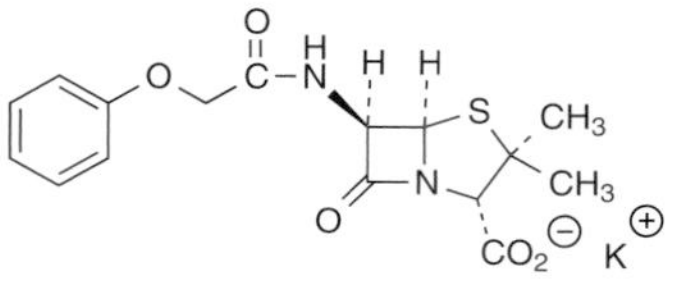

Penicillin V potassium

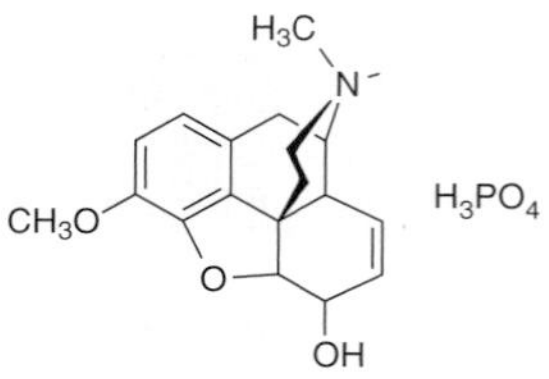

Codeine

1. Penicillin V potassium is drawn in its salt form, whereas codeine phosphate is not. Modify the given structure above to show the salt form of codeine phosphate. Determine the acid-base character of the functional groups in the two molecules drawn above as well as the salt form of codeine phosphate.
2. As originally drawn above, which of these two agents is more water soluble? Provide a rationale for your selection that includes appropriate structural properties. Is the salt form of codeine phosphate more or less water soluble than the free base form of the drug? Provide a rationale for your answer based on the structural properties of the salt form of codeine phosphate.
3. What is the chemical consequence of mixing aqueous solutions of each drug in the same IV bag? Provide a rationale that includes an acid-base assessment.

Case Solution found immediately after References.

Even though the energy associated with each hydrogen bond is small (1-10 kcal/mol/bond), it is the additive nature of multiple hydrogen bonds that contributes to the overall water solubility of a given drug molecule. This type of interaction is also important in the interaction between a drug and its biologic target (e.g., receptor). Figure 2.8 shows several types of hydrogen bonding interactions that can occur with a couple of functional groups and water. As a general rule, the more hydrogen bonds that are possible between a drug molecule and water, the greater the water solubility of the molecule. Table 2.4 lists several common functional groups and the number of hydrogen bonds in which they can potentially participate. Note that this table does not

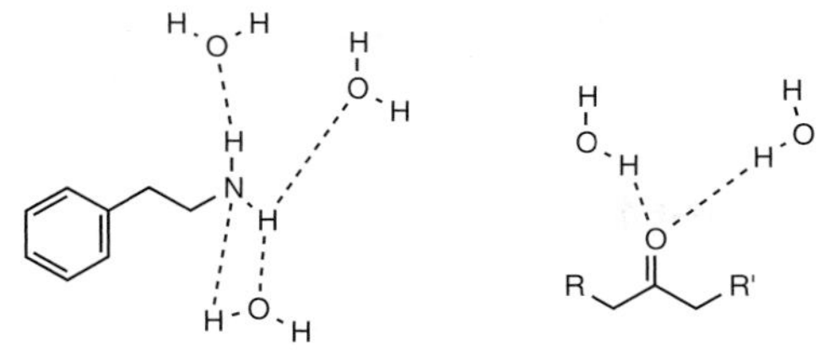

Figure 2.8 Examples of hydrogen bonding between water and hypothetical drug molecules.

Table 2.4 Common Organic Functional Groups and Their Hydrogen-Bonding Potential

Functional Groups	Number of Potential H-Bonds
R-OH	3
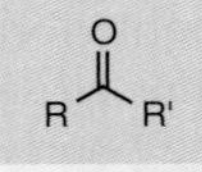 R-C(=O)-R'	2
$R-NH_2$	3
R-NH-R'	2
R-N(R')-R"	1
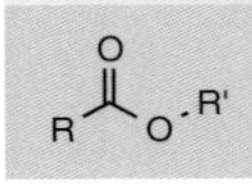 R-C(=O)-O-R'	2

Case Study

ABSORPTION/BINDING INTERACTIONS CASE

A 24-year-old man comes into the pharmacy and asks you to recommend a treatment for the itching and burning he has recently noticed on both feet. He indicates that he would prefer a cream rather than a spray or a powder. Your recommendation to this patient is to use Lamisil (terbinafine), a very effective topical antifungal agent that is sold over the counter.

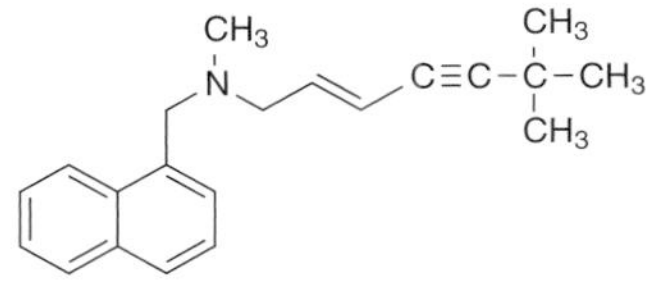

Terbinafine (Lamisil)

1. Identify the structural characteristics and the corresponding properties that make terbinafine an agent that can be used topically.
2. The biologic target of drug action for terbinafine is squalene epoxidase. Consider each of the structural features of this antifungal agent and describe the type of interactions that the drug will have with the target for drug action. Which amino acids are likely to be present in the active site of this enzyme?

Case Solution found immediately after References.

take into account the possibility of intramolecular hydrogen bond formation. Each intramolecular hydrogen bond decreases water solubility (and increases lipid solubility) because there is one less interaction possible with water.

Ionization

In addition to the hydrogen-bonding capacity of a molecule, another type of interaction plays an important role in determining water solubility: the ion-dipole interaction. This type of interaction can occur with organic salts. Ion-dipole interactions occur between either a cation and the partially negatively charged atom found in a permanent dipole (e.g., the oxygen atom in water) or an anion and the partially positively charged atom found in a permanent dipole (e.g., the hydrogen atoms in water) (Fig. 2.9).

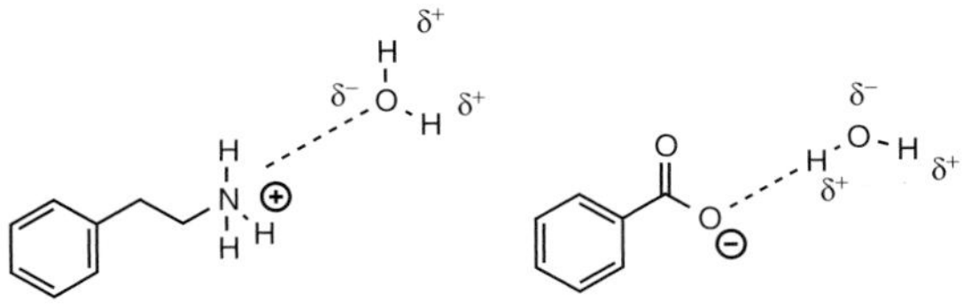

Figure 2.9 Examples of ion-dipole interactions.

Organic salts are composed of a drug molecule in its ionized form and an oppositely charged counterion. For example, the salt of a carboxylic acid is composed of the carboxylate anion (ionized form of the functional group) and a positively charged ion (e.g., Na^+), and the salt of a secondary amine is composed of the ammonium cation (ionized form of the functional group and a negatively charged ion; e.g., Cl^-). Not all organic salts are very water soluble. To associate with enough water molecules to become soluble, the salt must be highly dissociable; in other words, the cation and anion must be able to separate and interact independently with water molecules. Highly dissociable salts are those formed from strong acids with strong bases (e.g., sodium chloride), weak acids with strong bases (e.g., sodium phenobarbital), or strong acids with weak bases (e.g., atropine sulfate). Examples of strong acids (strong acids are 100% ionized in water [i.e., no ionization constants or pK_a- values >1]) include the hydrohalic (hydrochloric, hydrobromic, and hydrofluoric), sulfuric, nitric, and perchloric acids. All other acids (e.g., phosphoric, tartaric, acetic, and other organic acids and phenols) are partially ionized with pK_a values from 1 to 14 and are, therefore, considered to be moderate or weak acids. Hydroxides of sodium, potassium, and calcium are strong bases because they are 100% ionized, whereas other bases, such as amines, are of moderate or weak strength. The salt formed by a carboxylic acid with an alkylamine is the salt of a weak acid and weak base, respectively. This salt does not dissociate appreciably and cannot significantly contribute to the overall water solubility of a given drug molecule. In general, low-molecular-weight salts are water soluble, and high-molecular-weight salts are water insoluble. Examples of common organic salts used in pharmaceutical preparations are provided in Figure 2.10.

The extent to which ionized molecules are soluble in water is also dependent on the presence of intramolecular ionic interactions. Molecules with ionizable functional groups of opposite charge have the potential to interact with each other rather than with water molecules. When this occurs, these molecules often become water insoluble. A classic example is the amino acid tyrosine (Fig. 2.11). Tyrosine contains three very polar functional groups, two of which are ionizable (the alkylamine and carboxylic acid) depending on the pH of the environment.

The phenolic hydroxyl group is also ionizable (pK_a 9-10); however, it does not contribute significantly to the ionization of tyrosine under pharmaceutically or physiologically relevant conditions (<1% ionized at pH 7). Because of the presence of three very polar functional groups (two of them being ionizable), one would expect tyrosine to be very soluble in water, yet its solubility is only 0.45 g/1000 mL. The basic alkylamine (pK_a (HB^+) 9.1 for the conjugate acid) and the carboxylic acid (pK_a 2.2) are both ionized at physiologic pH, and a zwitterionic molecule results. These two charged groups are sufficiently close that a strong ion-ion interaction occurs, thereby keeping each group from participating in ion-dipole interactions with surrounding water molecules. This lack of interaction between the ions and the dipoles found in water results in a molecule that is very water insoluble (Fig. 2.12). Not all zwitterions or multiply charged molecules demonstrate this behavior; only those that contain ionized functional groups close enough for an ionic interaction to occur will be poorly

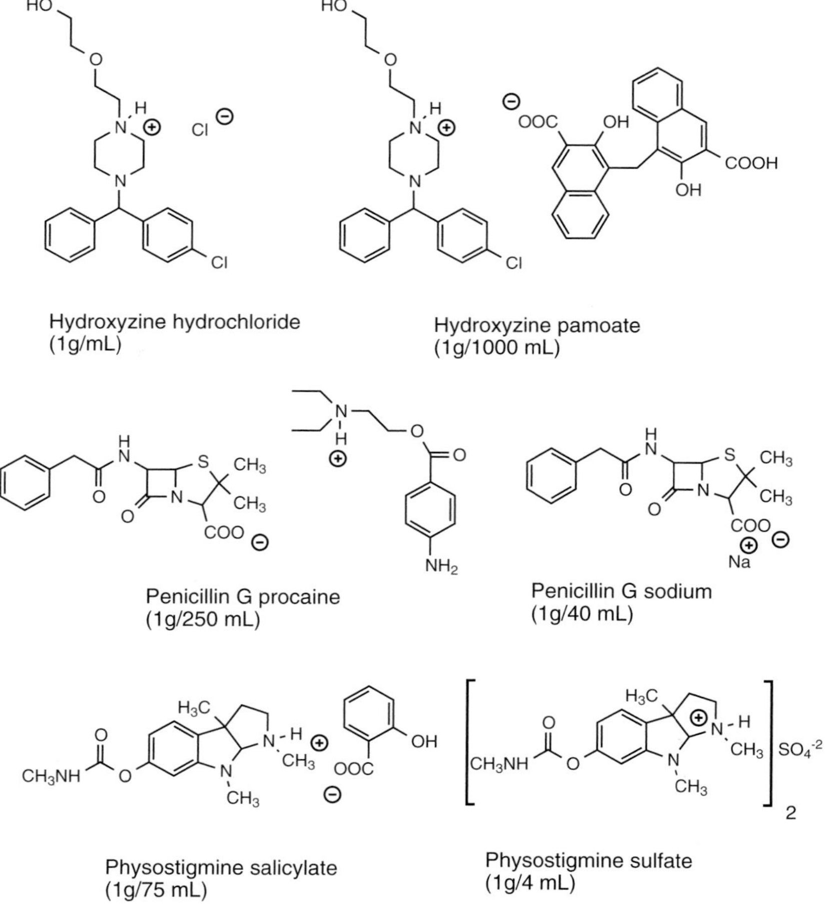

Figure 2.10 Water solubilities of different salt forms of selective drugs.

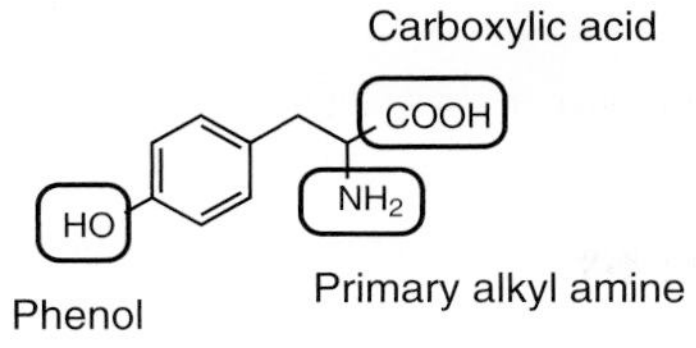

Figure 2.11 Functional groups present in tyrosine (see text for pK_a values).

soluble. Generally, the greater the separation between charges, the more highly water soluble one anticipates the molecule will be. This is only true, however, up to a certain number of carbon atoms. This will be discussed in more detail later.

Predicting Water Solubility: The Empirical Approach

Lemke[9] developed an empiric approach to predicting the water solubility of molecules based on the carbon-solubilizing potential of several functional groups. In his approach, if the solubilizing potential of the functional groups exceeds the total number of carbon atoms present, then the molecule is considered to be water soluble. Otherwise, it is considered to be water insoluble. Participation in intramolecular hydrogen bonding or ionic interactions decreases the solubilizing potential of a given functional group. It is difficult to quantitate how much such interactions will decrease a molecule's overall water solubility.

Table 2.5 shows the water-solubilizing potential for several functional groups common to many drugs. Because most drug molecules contain more than one functional group (i.e., are polyfunctional), the second column in the table will be of more utility. To demonstrate Lemke's method, consider the structure of anileridine. Anileridine (Fig. 2.13) is an opioid analgesic containing three functional groups that contribute to water solubility: an aromatic amine (very weak base), a tertiary alkylamine (weak base), and an ester (neutral). There are a total of 22 carbon atoms in the molecule and a solubilizing potential from the three functional groups of 9 carbon atoms. Since the solubilizing potential of the functional groups is less than the total number of carbons present, it is predicted that anileridine is insoluble in water. This is, indeed, the case: The solubility of anileridine is reported in the U.S. Pharmacopeia (USP) as 1 g/10,000 mL, or 0.01%. Now consider the

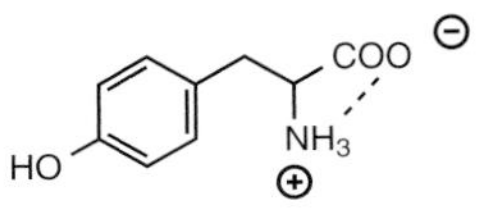

Figure 2.12 Zwitterionic form of tyrosine showing ion-ion bond.

Table 2.5 Water-Solubilizing Potential of Organic Functional Groups in a Mono- or Polyfunctional Molecule

Functional Group	Monofunction Molecule	Polyfunctional Molecule
Alcohol	5-6 carbons	3-4 carbons
Phenol	6-7 carbons	3-4 carbons
Ether	4-5 carbons	2 carbons
Aldehyde	4-5 carbons	2 carbons
Ketone	5-6 carbons	2 carbons
Amine	6-7 carbons	3 carbons
Carboxylic acid	5-6 carbons	3 carbons
Ester	6 carbons	3 carbons
Amide	6 carbons	2-3 carbons
Urea, carbonate, carbamate		2 carbons

Water solubility is defined as greater than 1% solubility.[9]

hydrochloride salt of anileridine. Not only do the three functional groups contribute a solubilizing potential of 9 carbon atoms, the positive charge of the alkylammonium also contributes to its water solubility. Lemke[9] estimates that each ionized functional group (cationic or anionic) found within a drug molecule contributes a solubilizing potential of 20-30 carbon atoms. Thus, the solubilizing potential for all of the functional groups in anileridine hydrochloride is 29-39 carbon atoms, which is more than the total number of carbon atoms in the molecule. This salt should therefore be soluble in water, and it is to the extent of 0.2 g/mL, or 20%. Solubility data for drug molecules can be found in the USP. In most instances, discrepancies between approximate and actual water solubilities can be rationalized by careful inspection of the chemical structure.

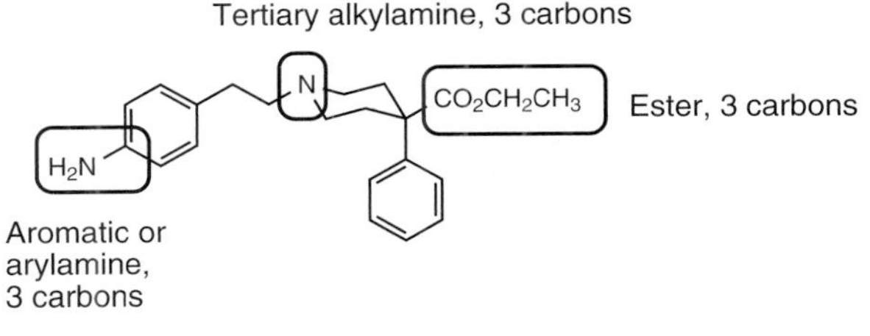

Figure 2.13 Identification of functional groups in anileridine.

Case Study

BINDING INTERACTIONS CASE

Each of these drug molecules interacts with a different biologic target and elicits a unique pharmacologic response. For each of the three molecules, list the types of interactions that are possible with a biologic target. For each type of interaction, provide one example of an amino acid that could participate in that interaction.

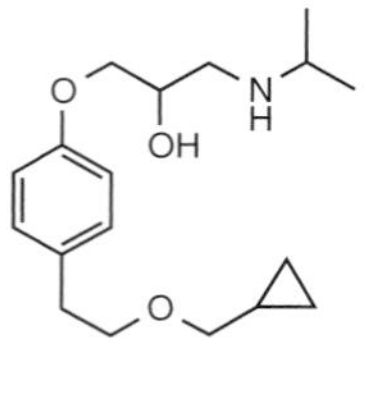

Betaxolol (Betoptic)

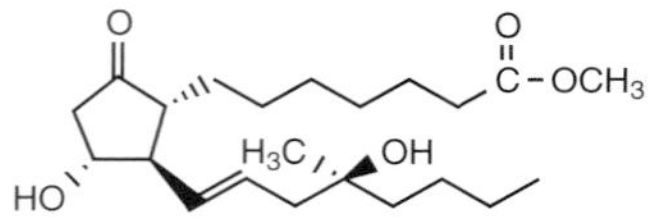

Misoprostol (Cytotec)

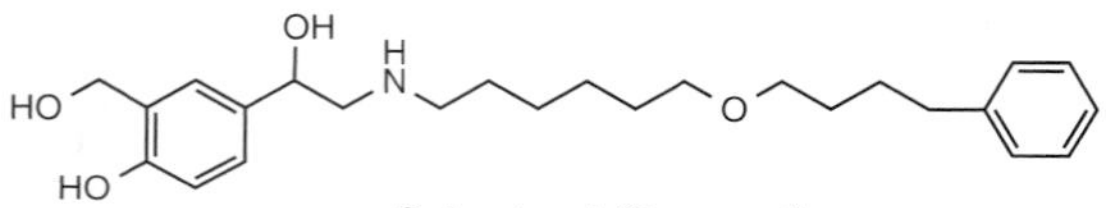

Salmeterol (Serevent)

Example: Binding interaction: Van der Waals
Amino acid: leucine

Case Solution found immediately after References.

Case Study

WATER/LIPID SOLUBILITY CASE

When you look at any drug molecule, there are a number of functional groups present that contribute to the properties of that drug molecule. Identify the types of functional groups in each molecule and to which physical properties (water/lipid solubility) each contributes.

1. Structural feature — Physical property

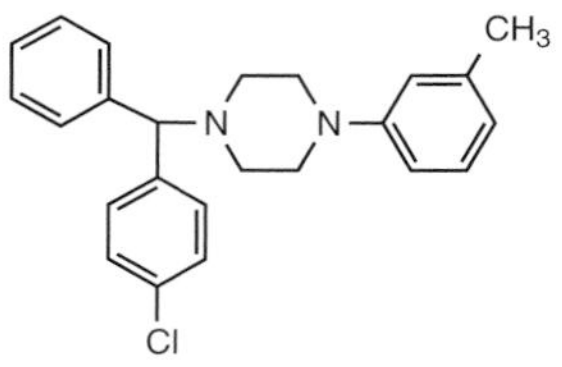

Meclizine (Antivert)

2. Structural feature — Physical property

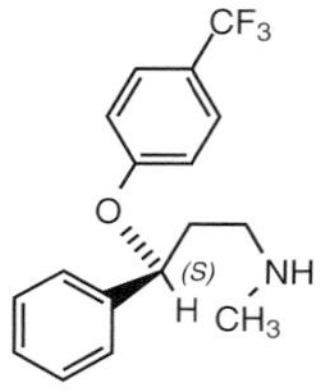

Fluoxetine (Prozac)

3. Structural feature — Physical property

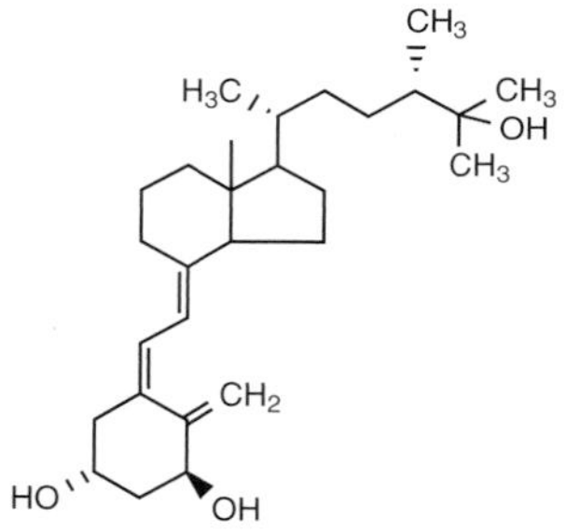

1,25-Dihydroxy Vit D_2

Case Solution found immediately after References.

Predicting Water Solubility: Analytical/ Quantitative Approach

Another method for predicting water solubility involves calculation of an approximate log P, or log of the partition coefficient for a molecule. This approach is based on an approximation method developed by Cates[10] and discussed in Lemke.[9] In this approach, one sums the hydrophobic or hydrophilic properties of each functional group present in the molecule. Before we can calculate log P values, a brief explanation of the concept of partition coefficient is necessary.

In its simplest form, the partition coefficient, P, refers to the ratio of drug concentration in octanol (C_{oct}) to that in water (C_{water}) (Equation (2.7)). Octanol is used to mimic the amphiphilic nature of lipid, because it has a polar head group (primary alcohol) and a long hydrocarbon chain, or tail, similar to the fatty acid tail that makes up part of a lipid membrane. Because P is logarithmically related to free energy,[11] P is generally expressed as log P and is, therefore, the sum of the hydrophobic and hydrophilic characteristics of the functional groups that make up the structure of a molecule. Thus, log P is a measure of the lipid/water solubility characteristics of the entire molecule. Because each functional group contained within the molecule contributes to its overall hydrophilic/hydrophobic character, a hydrophilic/hydrophobic value (the hydrophobic substituent constant, π) can be assigned to each functional group. Equation (2.8) defines this relationship:

Case Study

INTERACTIONS/SOLUBILITY CASE STUDY

J.K. presents a prescription for her 6-month-old daughter for Donatussin Drops. She wants to know if this medication will have an effect on her daughter's alertness.

Components of Donatussin:

1. Identify the structural features/functional groups of phenylephrine and guaifenesin that contribute to improved water solubility (medication given as drops). List the type(s) of interactions that these groups have with water, and draw an example of these interactions (with appropriate labels).
2. Evaluate each of the three molecules, and determine if each molecule contains any functional groups that will allow the drug to cross the blood-brain barrier and have an effect on this child's alertness (create a list of relevant functional groups for each molecule). Based on your evaluation, which agent is likely to have the most significant effect? Identify what property is necessary for these agents to cross this biologic membrane.
3. Identify the binding interactions that chlorpheniramine and guaifenesin could have with their respective targets for drug action. Be sure to identify which functional groups will participate in each of these binding interactions.

Case Solution found immediately after References.

Eq. 2.7 $$P = C_{oct} / C_{water}$$

Eq. 2.8 $$\text{LogP} = \sum \pi \text{ (fragments)}$$

When calculating log P from hydrophobic substituent constants, the sum is usually referred to as log P_{calc} or Clog P (for software sources to calculate Clog P, see Ref. 15) to distinguish it from an experimentally determined value (Mlog P or log P_{meas}). Over the years, extensive tables of π values have been compiled for organic functional groups and molecular fragments[11-14] Table 2.6 is a highly abbreviated summary of π values from Lemke,[9] based largely on the manuscript by Cates.[10] Using the values in this table, a fairly reasonable estimate for the water solubility of many organic compounds (shown as log P) can be determined.

Again, we will consider the structure of the opioid analgesic anileridine to demonstrate the calculation of log P (Fig. 2.14). This compound has a total of 22 carbon atoms, some aliphatic and some aromatic. We need to distinguish between the aliphatic and aromatic carbon atoms because the delocalized π orbitals for the sp^2-hybridized aromatic carbon atoms make them more polar than aliphatic carbons. The compound also contains one tertiary alkylamine, one aromatic or arylamine, and one ester. Evaluation of esters and amides requires that the oxygen, nitrogen, and ester/amide carbon atoms are counted in this π value. The remaining aliphatic carbons are then counted. Figure 2.14 summarizes the log P calculation for anileridine. The calculation gives a Clog P value for anileridine of +7.00. Water solubility as defined by the USP is solubility greater than 3.3%, which equates to an approximate log P of +0.5. Log P values less than +0.5 are therefore considered to be water soluble, and those greater than +0.5 are considered to be water insoluble. According to our calculation, anileridine would be predicted to be insoluble in water. This calculation agrees with the empiric procedure discussed earlier.

Other sample calculations are shown in Figure 2.15. In Figure 2.15, Mlog P values (when available) and Clog P values[15] are included for comparison purposes (see Appendix A for additional Clog P values). Even though the π values from Table 2.6 are not as extensive as those in the computer program, there is good general agreement with most of these compounds with respect to their solubility (or insolubility) in water. In addition, other programs besides Clog P are available to predict log P values; some of these programs are available on the Internet. One must keep in mind that due to the assumptions made in these programs, they cannot produce results that are in total agreement with measured values or other prediction programs. Clog P values calculated from ACDLog P[15] are generally considered to be more accurate. Other programs for calculating log P values, such as Molinspiration,[16] use different methods and assumptions and, and therefore, do not always agree with Clog P predictions or experimentally determined values. This is not to say that other programs do not give accurate results. Often, one or all of the available programs will have reasonable agreement with measured values, but greater disagreement tends to occur as the number of functional groups in the molecule that participate as hydrogen-bond acceptor and/or hydrogen-bond donor groups increases. This increases the likelihood that intramolecular interactions will occur—something that is not always taken into account with these programs.

Table 2.6 Hydrophilic-Lipophilic Values (πV) for Organic Fragments

Functional Group	π Value (Aliphatic)	π Value (Aromatic)
H		0.00
Alkane	0.50	0.56 (CH_3); 1.02 (CH_2CH_3)
Alkene		0.82
C_6H_5 (phenyl)	2.15	1.96
Br, Cl, F, I	0.60; 0.39; −0.17; 1.00	0.86; 0.71; 0.14; 1.12
NO_2	−0.85	−0.28
NH_2 (primary amine)	−1.19	−1.23
NHR (secondary amine)	−0.67	0.47
NR_2 (tertiary amine)	−0.30	0.18
–NHC = OR (amide)	−0.97	
SC_6H_5	2.32	
OH	−1.12	−0.67
OCH_3		−0.02
–OC = OR (ester)	−0.27	−0.64
CHO (aldehyde)		−0.65
C = OCH_3 (ketone)		−0.55
CO_2H		−0.32
SO_2 NH_2 (sulfonamide)		−1.82

Based on Cates LA. Calculation of drug solubilities by pharmacy students. *Am J Pharm Ed.* 1981;45:11-13.

Fragments	≠
1 primary arylamine	-1.23
1 tertiary alkylamine	-0.30
9 aliphatic carbons	+4.5
2 phenyl rings	+4.30
1 ester	-0.27
logP	+7.0

Figure 2.14 Calculation of log P for anileridine.

The ability to predict the percent ionization or water solubility of a molecule should not be viewed as an exercise in arithmetic, but rather as a way to understand the solution behavior of molecules, especially as it relates to admixtures and the pharmacokinetic differences among molecules. The ionization state of a molecule not only influences its water solubility but also its ability to traverse membranes and, therefore, its ability to be absorbed. The distribution of the drug and its ability to bind to proteins other than its target are also greatly influenced by the ionization state and the hydrophilic/hydrophobic nature of the molecule.

DRUG ABSORPTION

A variety of routes for administration of drugs exist varying from intravenous (IV), subcutaneous (SC), and intramuscular (IM) injection. Nasal, buccal, inhalation, and rectal administration have also been used. By far the most common, and desirable from a compliance point of view, is that of oral administration: swallowing a tablet, capsule, liquid, or syrup. Each of these approaches to delivery of medications has its advantages and disadvantages, but from a patient perspective the oral route is preferred. As a result, the physical chemical properties of the medication greatly influence the absorption properties of the compound as well as its stability as it traverses the gastrointestinal tract. The type of formulation is also influenced by the physical chemical properties of the compound and will enhance absorption, protect from degradation, or affect the rate of absorption. Because the oral route of drug administration is so important and desirable for drug delivery, a discussion of gastrointestinal physiology is necessary in order to understand the complexities of the conditions encountered by the medication as it passes through this region.

Gastrointestinal Physiology

When administered orally, a drug molecule encounters many physical and chemical barriers to its absorption into the systemic circulation. Figure 2.16 is a diagram of these barriers to absorption and the complexities involved. The stomach is divided into two major anatomical regions: the body of the stomach and the pylorus. The former region secrets pepsin and hydrochloric acid (HCl) and is also muscular, and contractions of these muscles allow for mechanical breakdown of ingested food. By breaking food particles into smaller pieces a larger surface area is obtained allowing for additional digestion to occur with pepsin and HCl. The pyloric region is the mucus-secreting area. This mucus serves as a protective layer preventing damage to the stomach lining by pepsin and HCl. That is, it helps prevent the stomach from digesting itself. It also lubricates the gastrointestinal tract allowing freer movement of solid material. Within the stomach the dosage form begins to disaggregate and some dissolution of the drug may begin to occur, except in the case of enteric-coated formulations which do not breakdown under acidic conditions and pass through the stomach. These types of formulations will be discussed in later chapters with specific compounds. Depending upon

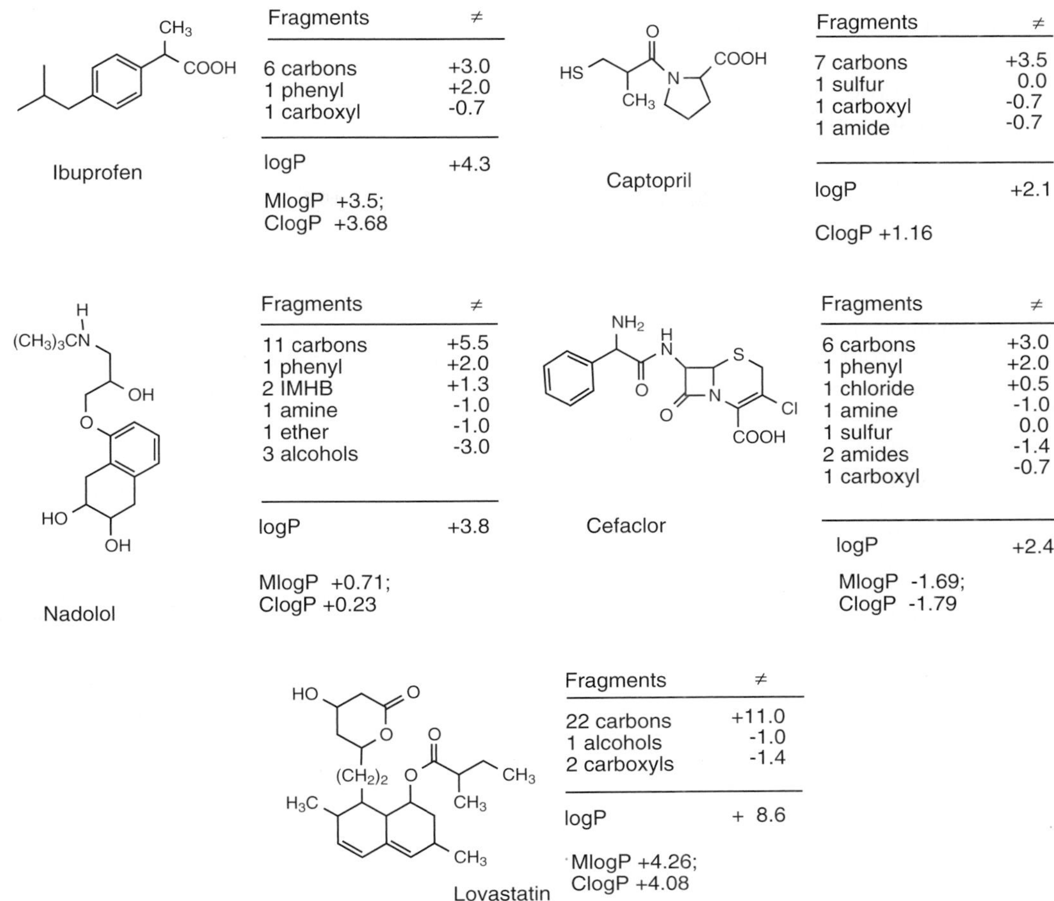

Figure 2.15 Clog P calculations for selected compounds.

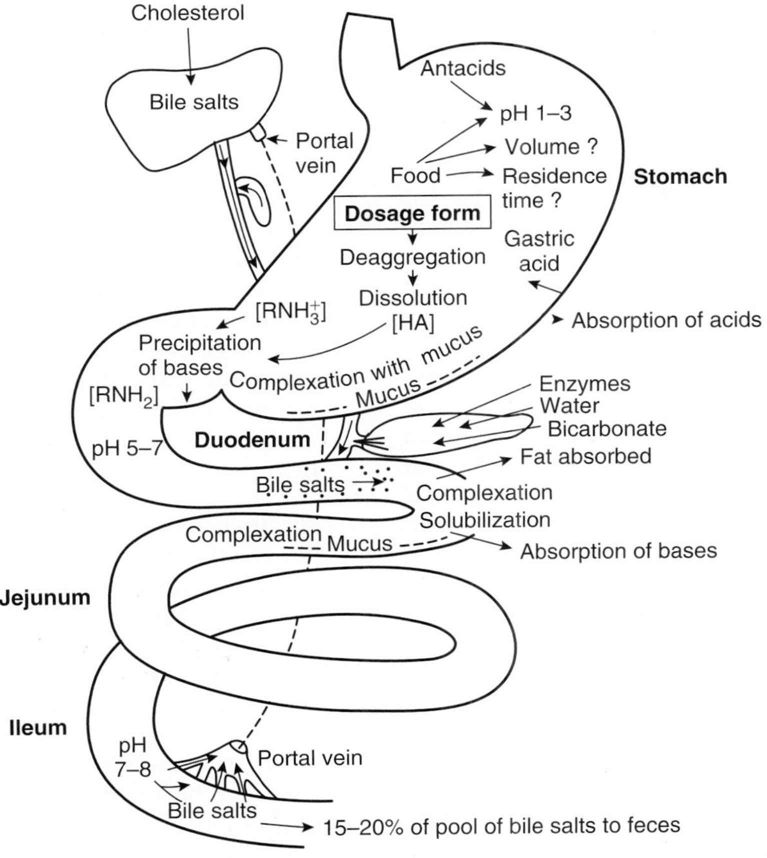

Figure 2.16 **Processes occurring along with drug absorption when drug molecules travel down the gastrointestinal tract and the factors that affect drug absorption.** Reprinted with permission from Florence AT, Attwood D. *Physiochemical Principles of Pharmacy*. 5th ed. New York: Chapman & Hall; 2011.

the physical chemical properties of the compound, some dissolution may occur within the stomach. Significant absorption generally does not occur within the stomach due to the low surface area, acidity, and possible association with other contents of the stomach such as fiber, metal ions, etc.

Passage into the small intestine is accompanied by a significant change in pH and in the anatomical structure of the region. The small intestine comprises three distinct regions: duodenum, jejunum, and ileum. Within this region the pH changes from approximately 5 (duodenum) to 7-8 (ileum) and significantly affects the solubility of drugs. Acidic molecules now become ionized and more water soluble, while basic molecules become less ionized and may even begin to precipitate. Because the epithelium of the small intestine is highly convoluted, the nutrients (and drugs) here are efficiently absorbed due to the large surface area that results. Because bases are less ionized within this region, they are more lipophilic and therefore able to cross the cell membranes more efficiently. Basic molecules therefore undergo more rapid absorption in the small intestine. All is not perfect, however. The presence of bile acids, mucus, and food particles can prevent absorption by forming complexes or adsorbing the drug. Such an action results in some drugs passing through the gastrointestinal tract and being excreted in the feces.

In order to get to the systemic circulation, the drug must traverse biomembranes of the epithelial cells lining the lumen of the intestine, pass through the cells and through another membrane to reach the blood. This requires the drug to be hydrophilic enough to be soluble in water (the major constituent within the gastrointestinal tract) to be able to come into contact with the membrane and hydrophobic enough to be able to cross the membrane. Thus there is a delicate balance between being too hydrophilic or too hydrophobic to be able to be absorbed into the systemic circulation. To complicate matters even more, the presence on the drug of functional groups that are acidic, basic, or both will influence solubility and therefore absorption. Obviously, these barriers can be overcome; otherwise we would not have orally administered medications in our formularies.

The processes of disaggregation and dissolution of drug formulations are beyond the scope of this chapter, and the reader will become acquainted with this area of physical pharmacy in other parts of the curriculum. For now we will concentrate on what occurs once the drug is in solution within the gastrointestinal tract and how even ionized molecules are able to cross biological membranes. We will mainly concentrate on the process of passive diffusion of drugs across membranes. Other processes will also be mentioned, but will be discussed in more detail in other chapters within this text.

PASSIVE DIFFUSION

Nonionized Drugs

The simplest case to consider is that of a drug that is neither basic nor acidic with sufficient water solubility to have contact with the membranes of epithelial cells lining the intestine. With this process the molecule is simply undergoing diffusion across the membrane from a region of high drug concentration to that of low concentration. Such diffusion may occur through the membrane lipid layer (Fig. 2.17A) or via a channel protein (Fig. 2.17B). In either case no energy expenditure is involved and this is referred to as passive diffusion (Fig. 2.17).

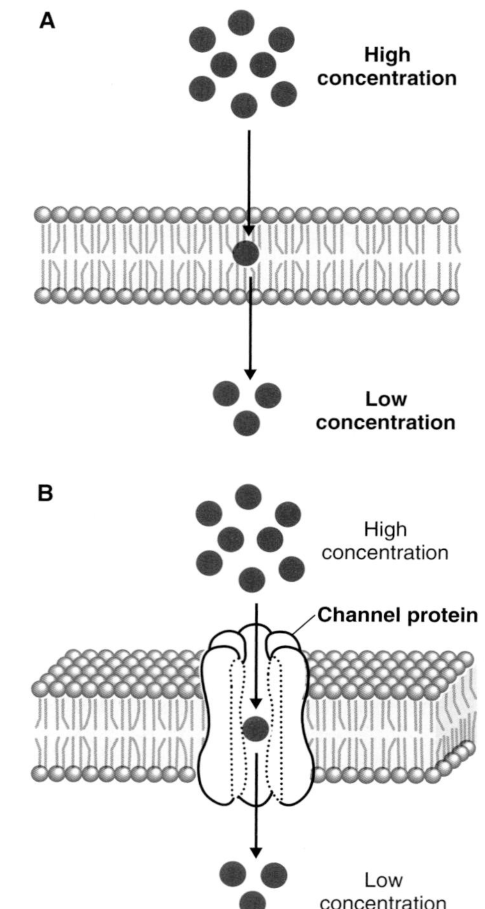

Figure 2.17 A, Simple diffusion. B, Membrane channels. Adapted with permission from Smith C, Marks A, Lieberman M, eds. *Basic Medical Biochemistry*. 2nd ed. Baltimore: Lippincott Williams & Wilkins; 2004.

Acidic Drugs

Acidic drugs encounter an increasingly basic environment as they pass through the gastrointestinal tract that results in an increase in the percentage of ionized drug. Absorption of the acidic drug occurs within the stomach primarily due to the protonated un-ionized species predominating there. However, the greatest absorption occurs just below the stomach, in the duodenum, due to the greater surface area of the microvilli of the brush border. Efficient absorption can still occur even though a significant amount of drug may be ionized due to the equilibria shown in Figure 2.18, with HA representing the protonated, un-ionized, drug and A^- the deprontonated ionized species.

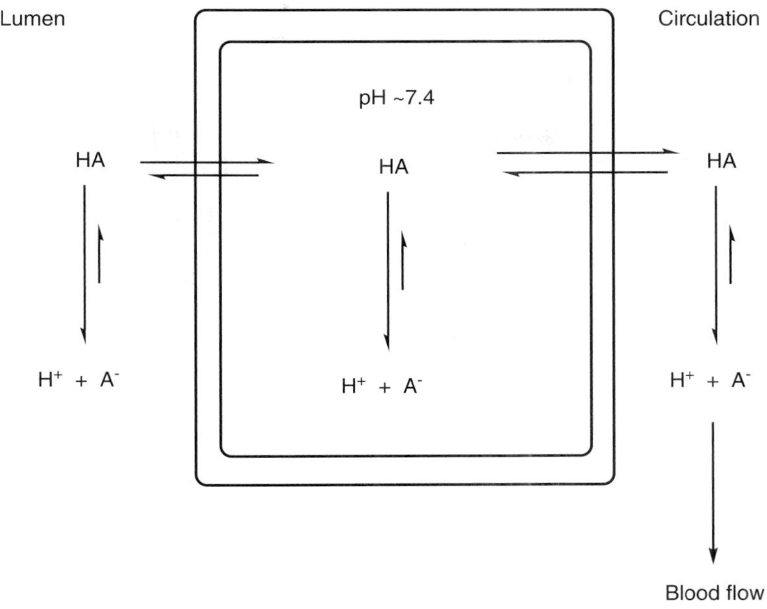

Figure 2.18 Equilibria involved in absorption of an acidic drug from the gastrointestinal tract.

In the duodenum the compound is ionized with the equilibrium shifted toward A^-. However, there is always some HA present which can partition through the membrane into the epithelial cell of the brush border. Once through the membrane, another equilibrium is established within the cytoplasm of the cell due to the pH (~7.4). As HA partitions through the membrane and into the cell, the equilibrium in the intestinal lumen must shift to form more HA. This is an example of Le Chatelier's principle from your first year chemistry course. The equilibrium within the lumen of the duodenum must be maintained. More HA forms which can now cross the membrane into the cytoplasm of the epithelial cell. But something else must be occurring to keep HA partitioning across the membrane. For this we now need to consider what is happening within the epithelial cell of the brush border.

Within the cell the pH causes deprotonation of the drug resulting in a second equilibrium which is shifted toward A^-. This decreases the amount of HA within the cell causing a shift in the equilibrium across the cell membrane. The HA within the cytoplasm can pass through the membrane of the epithelial cell into the circulation where two things occur. First, due to the pH of the blood, a fourth equilibrium occurs between HA and A^- and is shifted toward A^-. Second, the circulation carries both HA and A^- away which causes the equilibrium across the membrane to shift allowing more HA to cross into the circulation. In summary, Le Chatelier's principle is at play here. As the equilibria shift in response to changes in pH and relative concentrations of un-ionized and ionized drug, absorption of the drug into the systemic circulation occurs.

Basic Drugs

With the increasing basicity in the jejunum and ileum, absorption of basic drugs becomes more efficient. As shown in Figure 2.19, as the pH increases the equilibrium between the conjugate acid (BH+) and free base (B) form shifts to favor the latter. Following the same line of reasoning as above with acidic drugs, the free base form crosses the membranes and reestablishes equilibria with the conjugate acid form within the cytoplasm and subsequently within the circulation. As the equilibria shift to form more B, and as HB^+ and B are removed by the circulation, diffusion of the drug from high to low concentration occurs.

Active Transport (Influx and Efflux Transporters)

As discussed above, passive diffusion is the passage of a drug from a region of high concentration to that of low concentration and is an energy neutral process. Active transport requires energy and is generally a process of transporting the drug against a concentration gradient. Because active transport requires the drug to be "recognized" by a transport protein that normally mediates movement of a molecule of similar structure across the membrane, it is also a saturable process. That is, at high drug concentrations the ability to transport the drug plateaus due to the limited number of transport proteins available. Another difference is that the structural specificity required to be recognized and transported can result in competition with other compounds of similar structure. These could be natural substances that normally are transported by these proteins, or other drugs.[19] These will be discussed in more detail below (Fig. 2.20).

Some membrane transporters enhance the passage of drugs across membranes (influx), while others reverse absorption (efflux transporters). All transporters (influx and efflux) are membrane associated proteins that have multiple transmembrane regions and require energy for the process. Some transporters recognized a broad range of structures, while others are very specific.

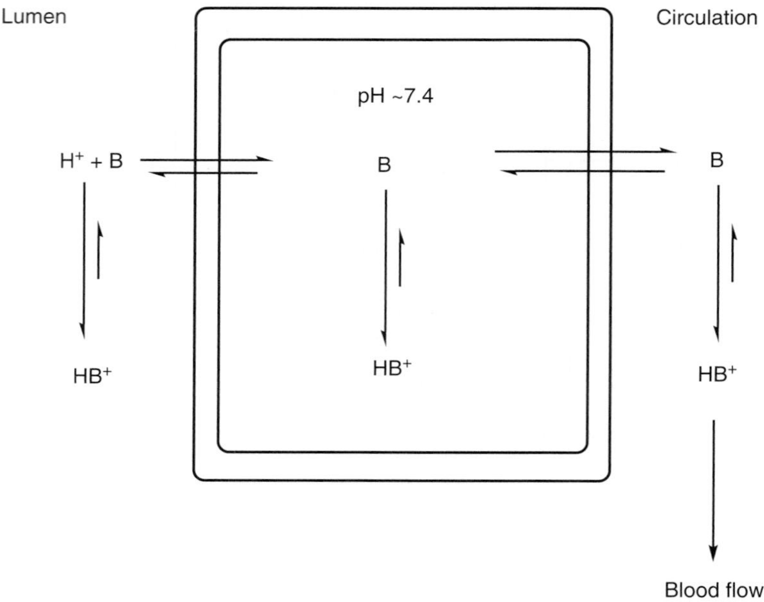

Figure 2.19 Equilibria involved in absorption of a basic drug from the gastrointestinal tract.

Influx Transporters

Several types of influx transporters with differing substrate selectivity exist within the luminal surface of the intestinal mucosa and can influence the rate of oral absorption (see Chapter 4 for more discussion). Peptide transporters such as the peptide transporter 1 (PepT-1) and human peptide transporter 1 (HPT-1) are responsible for the transport of many diverse peptide and peptide mimetic substrates such as β-lactam antibiotics, ACE inhibitors, and amino acid conjugated drugs (e.g., valacyclovir). Other transporters within the intestinal tract include the bile acid, nucleoside, organic cation/anion (OCTP and OATP, respectively) and fatty acid transporters. Just as with PepT-1 and HPT-1, drugs that structurally resemble the natural substrates for these may have enhanced absorption in addition to passive diffusion. Throughout this text, the influence of influx transporters on intestinal absorption of specific drugs will be discussed when relevant.

Efflux Transporters

Drug efflux into the intestinal lumen is influenced by P-glycoprotein (P-gp), multiresistance associated proteins 1 and 2 (MRP1 and MRP2), and breast cancer resistance protein (BCRP) (see Chapter 4). These transporters prevent the influx and accumulation of many drugs into the general circulation as well as specific organs: e.g., transport into bile, preventing blood-brain barrier (BBB) penetration, and tumor tissue. P-gp appears to be the most ubiquitous of these efflux proteins returning a portion of drug entering the intestinal mucosa back to the lumen in a concentration-dependent manner. Two types of P-gp have been shown to exist in mammals: drug-transporting and phospholipid transporting P-gp. Localization of P-gp in the intestine, kidney, and liver suggest that it is a leading player in excreting xenobiotics into the intestinal lumen, urine, and bile. The number of drugs shown to be substrates increases each year and includes HIV protease inhibitors and verapamil. The latter also acts as an inhibitor of P-gp increasing intestinal permeabilities.

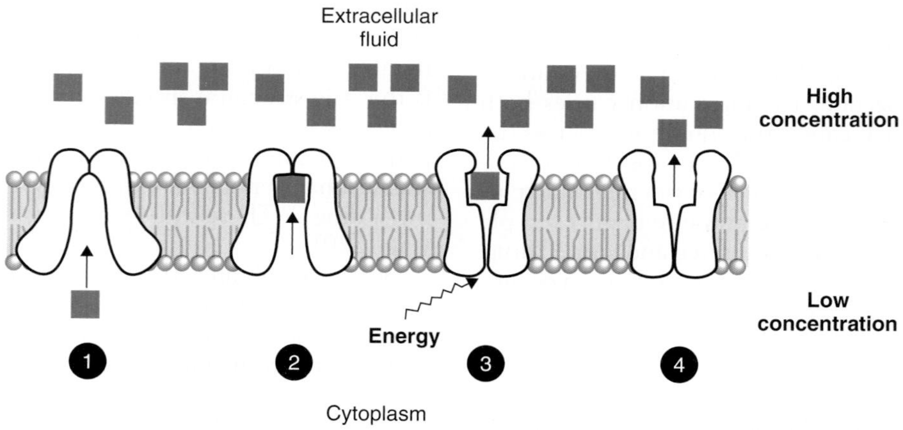

Figure 2.20 **Active transport.** Adapted with permission from Smith C, Marks A, Lieberman M, eds. *Basic Medical Biochemistry*. 2nd ed. Baltimore: Lippincott Williams & Wilkins; 2004.

PRODRUGS

By definition prodrugs are compounds that undergo metabolic or chemical conversion to produce a biologically active substance. That is, the ingested compound is not pharmacologically active and must first be converted via action of an enzyme or chemical degradation to produce the active species. Some prodrugs have been developed because the pharmacologically active form has poor oral bioavailability, usually due to poor absorption in the gastrointestinal tract. Other prodrugs are highly water-soluble derivatives of compounds that are too hydrophobic to be dissolved in aqueous to be given intravenously. Examples of well-known prodrugs include omeprazole, simvastatin, levastatin, enalapril, clopidogel, valacyclovir, acyclovir, and oseltamivir (Fig. 2.21).

Other reasons for developing prodrugs may be chemical instability, unacceptable odor or taste, gastric irritation, inadequate BBB permeability, presystemic metabolism, or toxicity. The most common approach to prodrug design is to use an ester linkage to the drug (e.g., lovastatin, simvastatin, oseltamivir, clopidogrel, valcyclovir and enalapril in Fig. 2.21). As you will learn in Chapter 3, esters are readily hydrolyzed by ubiquitous esterases within the systemic circulation. The rates at which these esters are hydrolyzed can be influenced via steric or electronic effects of substituents on either side of the ester bond following basic organic chemical principles. The ester may be hydrophobic (i.e., alkyl esters) to improve diffusion across membranes; ionizable (e.g., succinates or amino acids) to improve aqueous solubility; or sterically hindered to slow hydrolysis providing an acceptable rate for "release" of the active drug.

STEREOCHEMISTRY AND DRUG ACTION

Stereoisomers are molecules that contain the same number and kinds of atoms, the same arrangement of bonds, but different three-dimensional structures; in other words, they only differ in the three-dimensional arrangement of atoms in space. There are two types of stereoisomers: enantiomers and diastereoisomers. Enantiomers are pairs of molecules for which the three-dimensional arrangement of atoms represents nonsuperimposable mirror images. Diastereoisomers represent all of the other stereoisomeric compounds that are not enantiomers. Thus, the term "diastereoisomer" includes compounds that contain double bonds (geometric isomers) and ring systems. Unlike enantiomers, diastereoisomers exhibit different physicochemical properties, including, but not limited to, melting point, boiling point, solubility, and chromatographic behavior. These differences in physicochemical properties allow the separation of individual diastereoisomers from mixtures with the use of standard chemical separation techniques, such as column chromatography or crystallization. Enantiomers cannot be separated using

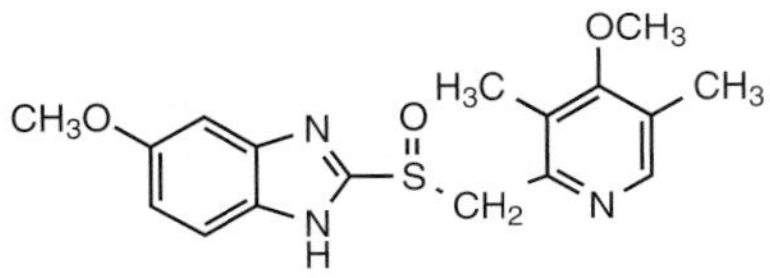

Omeprazole (Prilosec)

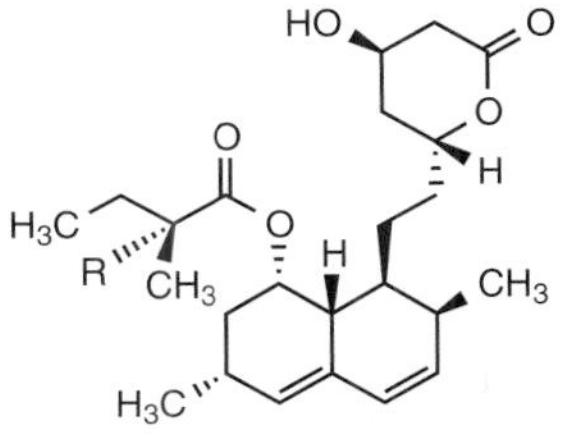

Lovastatin (Mevacor, R = H)
Simvastatin (Zecor, R = CH_3)

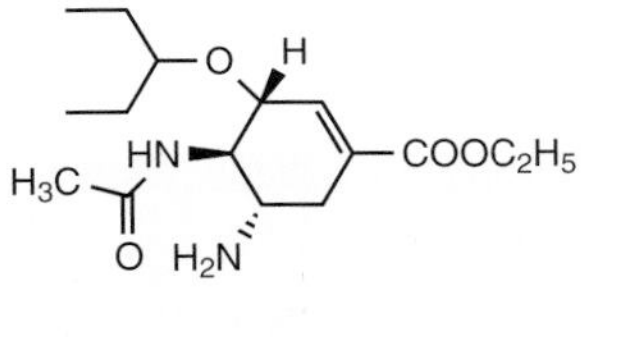

Oseltamivir (Tamiflu)

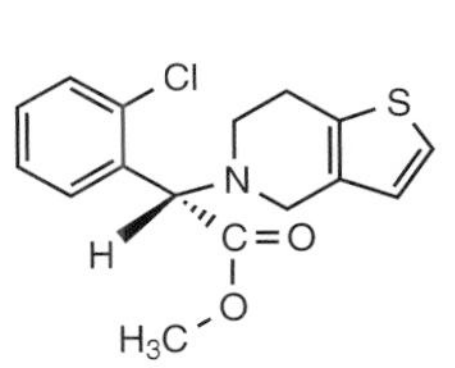

Clopidogrel (Plavix)

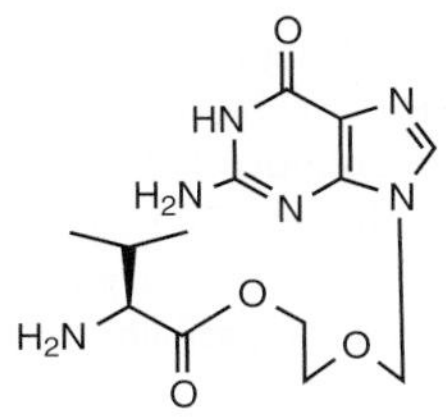

Valacyclovir (Valtrex)

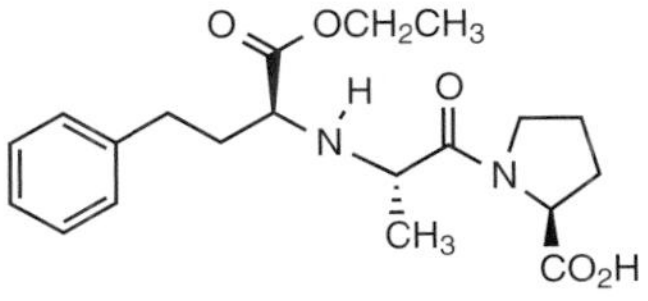

Enalapril (Vasotec)

Figure 2.21 Commercially available blockbuster prodrugs and their structures.

such techniques unless a chiral environment is provided or if they are first converted to diastereoisomers (e.g., salt formation with another enantiomer). Examples of enantiomers and diastereoisomers are provided in Figure 2.22.

The physicochemical properties of a drug molecule are dependent not only on what functional groups are present in the molecule but also on the spatial arrangement of these groups. This becomes an especially important factor when the environment that a molecule is in is asymmetric, such as the human body. Proteins and other biologic targets are asymmetric in nature. How a particular drug molecule interacts with these macromolecules is determined by the three-dimensional orientation of the functional groups present. If critical functional groups in the drug molecule do not occupy the proper spatial region, then productive interactions with the biologic target will not be possible. As a result, it is possible that the desired pharmacologic activity will not be achieved. If, however, the functional groups within a drug molecule are located in the proper three-dimensional orientation, then the drug can participate in multiple key interactions with its biologic target. It is important to understand not only which functional groups contribute to the pharmacologic activity of a drug, but also the importance of the three-dimensional nature of these functional groups in predicting drug potency and potential side effects.

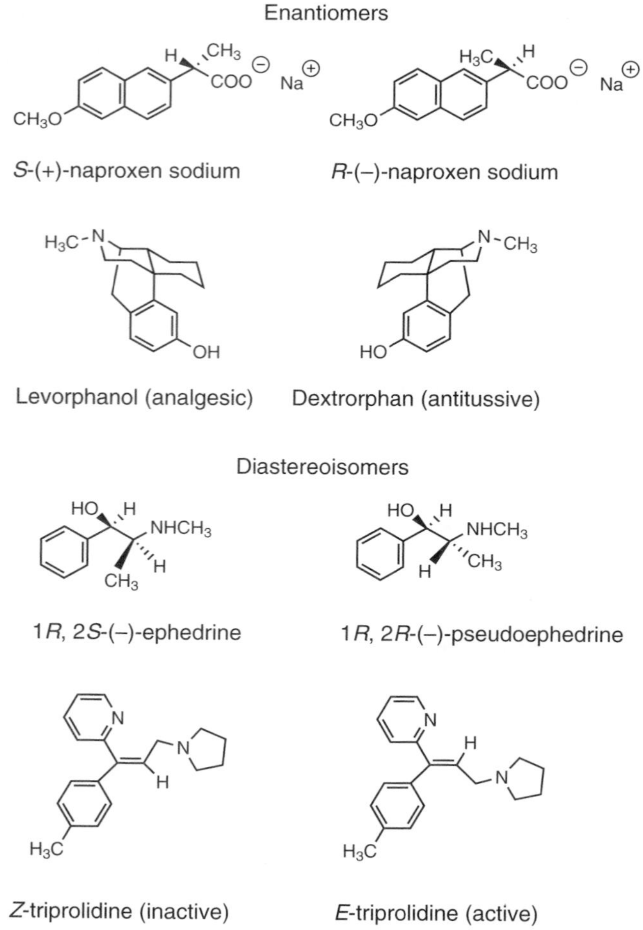

Enantiomers

S-(+)-naproxen sodium

R-(−)-naproxen sodium

Levorphanol (analgesic)

Dextrorphan (antitussive)

Diastereoisomers

1*R*, 2*S*-(−)-ephedrine

1*R*, 2*R*-(−)-pseudoephedrine

Z-triprolidine (inactive)

E-triprolidine (active)

Figure 2.22 Examples of stereoisomers.

Approximately one in every four drugs currently on the market is some type of isomeric mixture. For many of these drugs, the biologic activity may reside in one isomer (or at least predominate in one isomer). The majority of these isomeric mixtures are termed "racemic mixtures" (or "racemates"). A racemic mixture is comprised of equal amounts of both possible drug enantiomers. As mentioned earlier in this chapter, when enantiomers are introduced into an asymmetric, or chiral, environment, such as the human body, they display different physicochemical properties. This can lead to significant differences in their pharmacokinetic and pharmacodynamic behavior, resulting in adverse side effects or toxicity. For example, individual isomers in a racemic mixture can exhibit significant differences in absorption (especially active transport), serum protein binding, and metabolism. As it relates to drug metabolism, it is certainly possible that only one of the isomers can be converted into a toxic substance or can influence the metabolism of another drug (Chapter 3). Since stereochemistry can have a profound effect on both the pharmacokinetic and pharmacodynamic properties of a drug, it is important to review the foundational concepts.

STEREOCHEMICAL DEFINITIONS

Designation of Absolute Configuration

At first, enantiomers were distinguished by their ability to rotate the plane of polarized light. Isomers that rotate the plane of polarized light to the right, or in a clockwise direction, were designated as dextrorotatory, indicated by a (+)-sign before the chemical name (e.g., (+)-amphetamine or dextroamphetamine). The opposite designation, levorotatory or (−)-, was assigned to molecules that rotate the plane of polarized light to the left, or in a counterclockwise direction. The letters d- and l- are also used to indicate (+)- and (−)-, respectively. A racemate (racemic mixture)—that is, a 1:1 mixture of enantiomers—is indicated by placement of a (±)- before the compound name. This nomenclature is based on a physical property of the molecule and does not describe the absolute configuration or three-dimensional arrangement of atoms around the chiral center.

QUESTIONS WE CAN NOW ANSWER ABOUT ANY DRUG MOLECULE

Based on your knowledge of acid-base chemistry, from where will this drug primarily be absorbed?

What is the solubility of the drug in the stomach, plasma, or an aqueous IV?

What are the possible interactions that the drug could have with its respective target for drug action?

What is the compatibility of the drug if mixed with other drugs?

How should this drug be delivered? Is it stable in stomach acid?

D-(+)-Glyceraldehyde L-(−)-Glyceraldehyde

D-(+)-Serine L-(−)-Serine

Figure 2.23 Relationship of optical isomers of serine to D- and L-glyceraldehyde.

In the late 19th century, Fisher and Rosanoff developed a system of nomenclature based on the structure of glyceraldehyde (Fig. 2.23). Since there were no methods at that time to determine the absolute three-dimensional arrangement of atoms in space, the two isomers of glyceraldehyde were arbitrarily assigned the designation of D-(+)- and L-(−). It was not until the 1950s that the absolute configurations of these molecules were determined (Fisher had fortuitously guessed correctly). The configurations of other molecules were then assigned based on their relationship to D- or L-glyceraldehyde via synthetic methods or chemical degradation. Thus, via chemical degradation, it was possible to determine that (+)-glucose, (−)-2–deoxyribose, and (−)-fructose had the same terminal configuration as D-(+)-glyceraldehyde and, therefore, were assigned the D-absolute configuration. Amino acid configurations were assigned based on their relationship to D-(+)- and L-(−)-serine (Fig. 2.23). Unfortunately, this system becomes very cumbersome with molecules that contain more than one chiral center.

LEARNING THE LINGO: DRUG MOLECULE EVALUATION

Analysis of individual functional groups:
- Name of functional group
- Shape of functional group
- Hydrophobic vs. hydrophilic character
- Polar vs. nonpolar character
- Acidic vs. basic (pK_a) character
- Binding interactions
- Chemical/enzymatic stability

Analysis of the whole drug molecule:
- Looking for functional group balance: water solubility and absorption
- Ionization issues: effect on solubility and absorption
- Drug combinations: acid-base interactions
- Drug interactions with biologic target: good fit or not?
- Stability and bioavailability: route of administration

In 1956, a new system of stereochemical nomenclature was introduced by Cahn, Ingold, and Prelog[20] and is known as the Sequence Rule or CIP system. With this system, atoms attached to a chiral center are ranked based on their atomic number. Highest priority is given to the atom with the highest atomic number, and subsequent atoms are ranked accordingly, from highest to lowest. When a decision cannot be made in the assignment of priority—for example, two atoms with the same atomic number attached to the chiral center—this evaluation extends to the next atom until a priority can be established. When the molecule is then viewed from the side opposite to the lowest-priority atom, the priority sequence from highest to lowest can then be determined. If the priority sequence proceeds to the right, or in a clockwise direction, the chiral center is designated with an *R*-absolute configuration. The designation is *S* when the priority sequence proceeds to the left, or in a counterclockwise direction. An example of this is seen in the neurotransmitter norepinephrine.

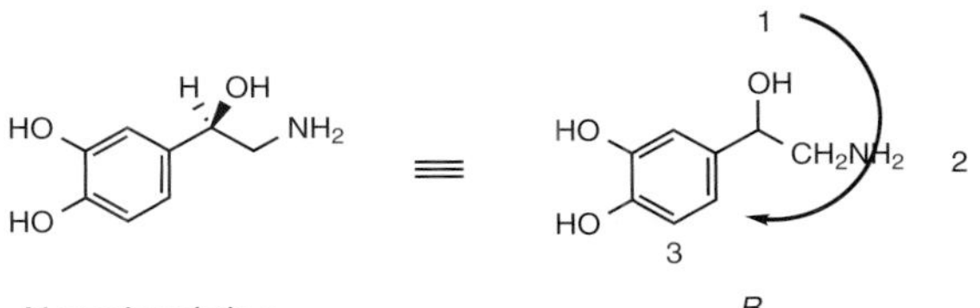

Norepinephrine *R*

Degradation studies demonstrate that (−)-norepinephrine is related to D-(−)-mandelic acid; therefore, it was given the D-designation using the Fisher system. With the CIP system, norepinephrine is assigned the *R*-absolute configuration.

It should be noted that the CIP nomenclature system uses a set of arbitrary rules and, therefore, should be viewed as a system that tracks absolute configuration only. In many instances, two molecules can have different absolute configurations as designated by the CIP system, but the same relative orientation of the functional groups relevant for biologic activity. An example of this is demonstrated when the absolute configuration of the nonselective β-adrenergic antagonist propranolol is compared to norepinephrine. Because of the presence of the ether oxygen atom, the priority sequence of the functional groups about the chiral center results in the assignment of the *S*-absolute configuration for the more active enantiomer of propranolol. Close inspection of both *R*-norepinephrine and *S*-propranolol, however, shows that the hydroxy group, basic amine, and aromatic rings of both compounds occupy the same regions in three-dimensional space.

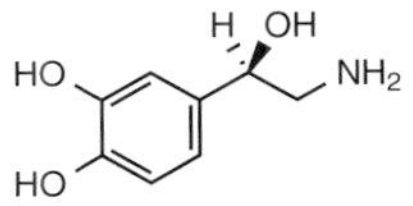

(*R*)-Norepinephrine 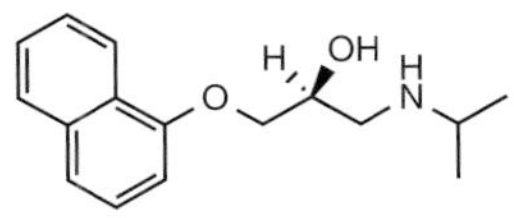 (*S*)-Propranolol

Stereochemistry and Biologic Activity

Easson-Stedman Hypothesis

In 1886, Piutti[21] reported different physiologic actions for the enantiomers of asparagine, with (+)-asparagine having a sweet taste and (−)-asparagine a bland one. This was one of the earliest observations that enantiomers can

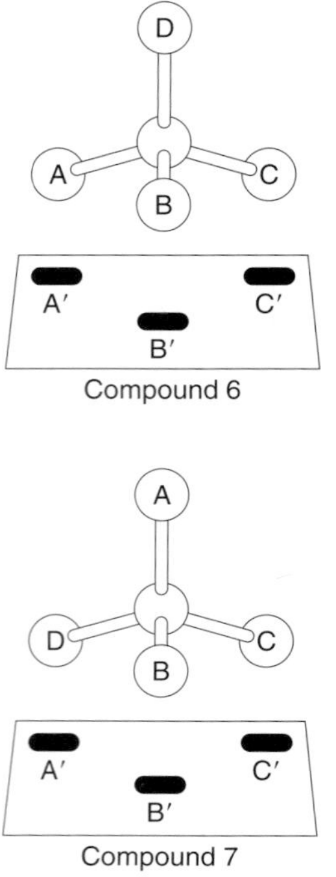

Figure 2.24 Optical isomers. Only in compound 6 do the functional groups A, B, and C align with the corresponding sites of binding on the asymmetric surface.

exhibit differences in biologic action. In 1933, Easson and Stedman[22] reasoned that differences in biologic activity between enantiomers resulted from selective reactivity of one enantiomer with its receptor. They postulated that such interactions require a minimum of a three-point fit to the receptor. This is demonstrated in Figure 2.24 for two hypothetical enantiomers. In Figure 2.24, the letters A, B, and C represent hypothetical functional groups that can interact with complementary sites on the hypothetical receptor surface, represented by A′, B′, and C′. Only one enantiomer is capable of attaining the correct special orientation to enable all three functional groups to interact with their respective sites on the receptor surface. The inability of the other enantiomer to achieve the same number of interactions with the hypothetical receptor surface explains its reduced biologic activity. The Easson-Stedman hypothesis states that the more potent enantiomer must be involved in a minimum of three intermolecular interactions with the surface of the biologic target and that the less potent enantiomer only interacts with two sites. This can be illustrated by looking at the differences in vasopressor activity of *R*-(−)-epinephrine, *S*-(+)-epinephrine, and the achiral N-methyldopamine (Fig. 2.25). With *R*-(−)-epinephrine, the three points of interaction with the receptor site are the substituted aromatic ring, β-hydroxyl group, and the protonated secondary ammonium group. All three functional groups interact with their complementary sites on the receptor surface, resulting in receptor stimulation (in this case). With *S*-(+)-epinephrine, only two interactions are possible (the protonated secondary ammonium and the substituted aromatic ring). The β-hydroxyl group is located in the wrong place in space and, therefore, cannot interact properly with the receptor. N-methyldopamine can achieve the same interactions with the receptor as *S*-(+)-epinephrine; therefore, it is not surprising that its vasopressor response is the same as that of *S*-(+)-epinephrine and less than that of *R*-(−)-epinephrine.

Not all stereoselectivity seen with enantiomers can be attributed to differences in the ability of the drug molecule to interact with its biologic target. Differences in biologic activity can also result from differences in the ability of each enantiomer to reach the biologic target. Because the biologic system encountered by the drug is asymmetric, each enantiomer can experience selective penetration into membranes, metabolism, absorption at sites of loss (e.g., adipose tissue), and/or excretion. Figure 2.26 shows various phases that enantiomers can encounter before reaching the biologic target. An enantiomer may not encounter stereoselective environments at each of these points; however, enantioselectivity at any point can provide enough of an influence to cause one enantiomer to produce a significantly better pharmacologic effect than the other. Conversely, such processes can also contribute to untoward effects of a particular enantiomer. Differences in pharmacologic action among stereoisomers provide an

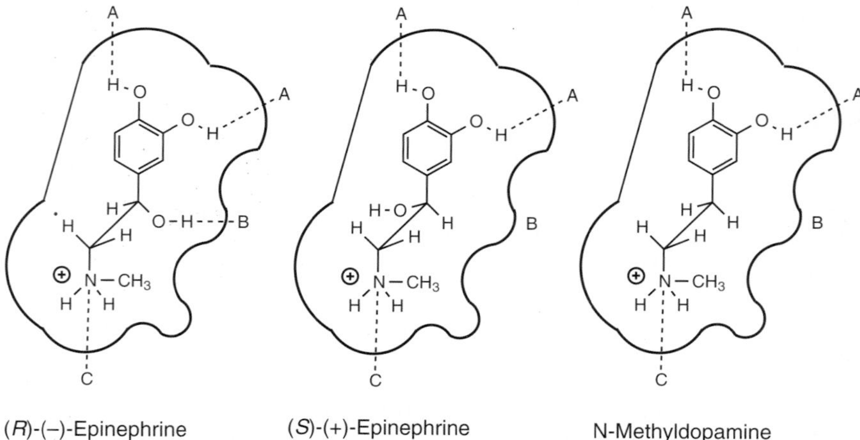

Figure 2.25 Drug receptor interaction of *R*-(−)-epinephrine, *S*-(+)-epinephrine, and N-methyldopamine.

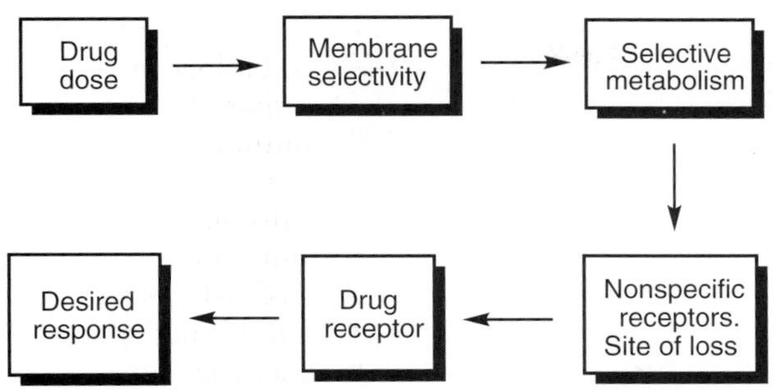

Figure 2.26 Selective phases to which optical isomers can be subjected before biologic response.

excellent example of how not all pharmacologic effects of a drug are necessarily beneficial to the patient. Although there is no regulatory prohibition on the development of racemic agents, it is reasonable that single enantiomer drugs will become the overwhelming therapeutic choice in the future.

Diastereomers

As mentioned earlier, diastereoisomers are molecules that are nonsuperimposable, nonmirror images. This type of isomer can result from the presence of more than one chiral center in the molecule, double bonds, or ring systems. These isomers have different physicochemical properties, and as a result, it is possible that they can have differences in biologic activity.

Molecules that contain more than one chiral center probably are the most common type of drug-based diastereoisomers. Classic examples are the diastereoisomers ephedrine and pseudoephedrine (Fig. 2.27). When a molecule contains two chiral centers, there can be as many as four possible stereoisomers consisting of two sets of enantiomeric pairs. When considering an enantiomeric pair of molecules, there is inversion of all chiral centers. In diastereomers, there is inversion of one or more, but not all chiral centers. Figure 2.28 shows several examples that contain two or more chiral centers and, therefore, are diastereoisomeric.

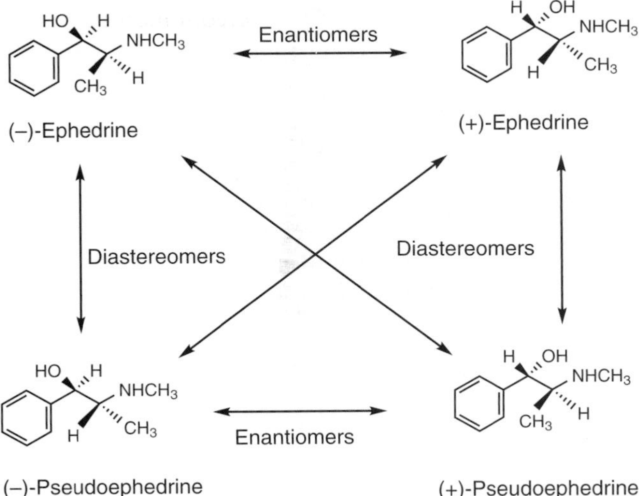

Figure 2.27 Relationship between the diastereomers of ephedrine and pseudoephedrine.

Restricted bond rotation caused by carbon-carbon double bonds (alkenes or olefins) and similar systems, such as imines (C = N), can produce stereoisomers. These are also referred to as geometric isomers, although they more properly are classified as diastereoisomers. In this situation, substituents can be oriented on the same side or on opposite sides of the double bond. The alkene 2-butene is a simple example.

H H
H_3C CH_3

cis or *Z* isomer

H_3C H
H CH_3

trans or *E* isomer

With 2-butene, it is readily apparent that the methyl groups can be on the same or on opposite sides of the double bond. When they are on the same side, the molecule is defined as the *cis*- or *Z*-isomer (from the German *zusammen*, meaning "together"); when they are on opposite sides, the designation is *trans*- or *E*- (from the German *entgegen*, meaning "opposite"). With simple compounds, such as 2-butene, it is easy to determine which groups in the molecule are *cis* or *trans* to one another. This becomes more difficult to determine, however, with more complex structures, where it is less obvious which substituents should be referred to when naming the compound. In 1968, Blackwood et al.[23] proposed a system for the assignment of "absolute" configuration with respect to double bonds. Using the CIP sequence rules, each of the two substituents attached to the carbon atoms comprising the double bond is assigned a priority of 1 or 2, depending on the atomic number of the atom attached to the double bond. When two substituents of higher priority are on the same side of the double bond, this isomer is given the designation of *cis* or *Z*. When the substituents are on opposite sides, the designation is *trans* or *E*. The histamine H_1-receptor antagonist triprolidine (Fig. 2.29) is a good example for demonstrating how this nomenclature system works. The *E*-isomer of triprolidine is more active both in vitro and in vivo, indicating that the distance between the pyridine and pyrrolidine rings is critical for binding to the receptor.

Diastereoisomers (as well as enantiomers) can also be found in cyclic molecules. For example, the cyclic alkane 1,2-dimethylcyclohexane can exist as *cis*/*trans*-diastereoisomers, and the *trans* isomer can also exist as an enantiomeric pair. In Figure 2.30, each of the *trans*-enantiomorphs is depicted in the two possible chair conformations for the cyclohexane ring. Since cyclohexane rings can exhibit significant conformational freedom, this allows for the possibility of conformational isomers. Isomers of this type will be discussed in the next section. When two or more rings share a common bond (e.g., decalin), rotation around the bonds is even more restricted. This prevents ring "flipping" from occurring, and as a result, diastereoisomers and enantiomers are generated.

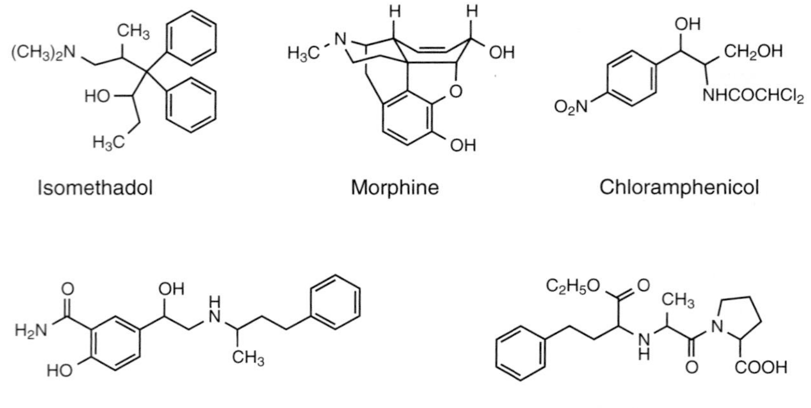

Figure 2.28 Examples of chiral drugs with two or more asymmetric centers.

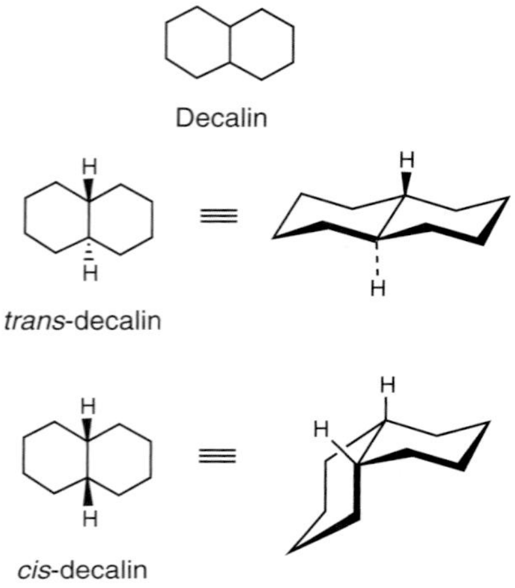

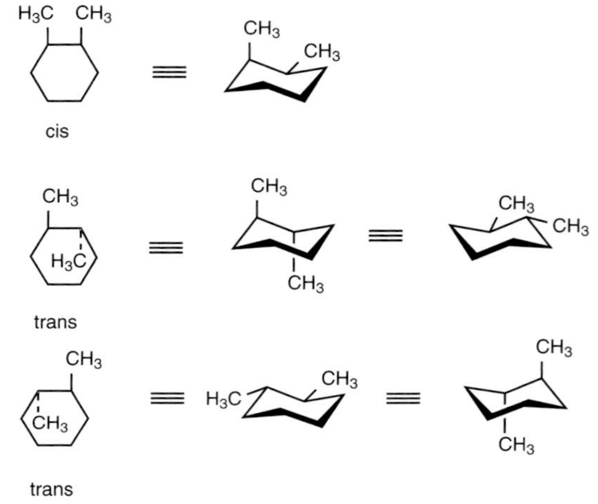

Figure 2.30 Diastereomers of 1,2-dimethylcyclohexane.

In the case of decalin, a two-ring system, the rings are fused together via a common bond in either the *trans* or *cis* configuration as shown. Steroids, a class of medicinally important compounds that consist of four fused rings (three cyclohexanes and one cyclopentane) exhibit significantly different biologic activity when the first two cyclohexane rings are fused into different configurations, referred to as the 5α- or 5β-isomers (Fig. 2.31). The α-designation indicates that the hydrogen atom in the 5-position is below the "plane" of the ring system; the β-designation refers to the hydrogen atom being above this plane. What appears to be a very minor change in orientation for the substituent results in a very drastic change in the three-dimensional shape of the molecule and in its biologic activity. Figure 2.31 shows the diastereoisomers 5α-cholestane and 5β-cholestane as examples. The chemistry and pharmacology of steroids will be discussed in more detail in later chapters.

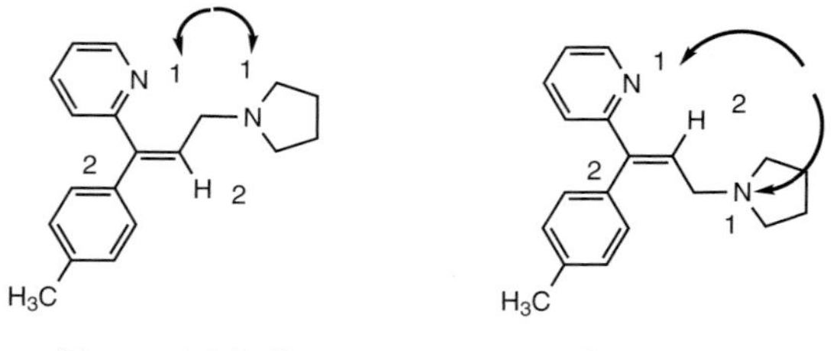

Figure 2.29 Geometric isomers of triprolidine.

Conformational Isomerism

Conformational isomerism takes place via rotation about one or more single bonds. Such bond rotation results in nonidentical spatial arrangement of atoms in a molecule. This type of isomerism does not require much energy because no bonds are broken. In the conversion of one enantiomer into another (or diastereoisomer), bonds are broken, which requires significantly more energy. The neurotransmitter acetylcholine can be used to demonstrate the concept of conformational isomers.

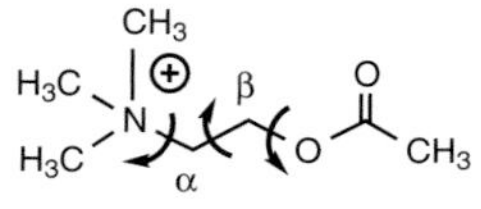

Acetylcholine

Each single bond within the acetylcholine molecule is capable of undergoing rotation, and at room

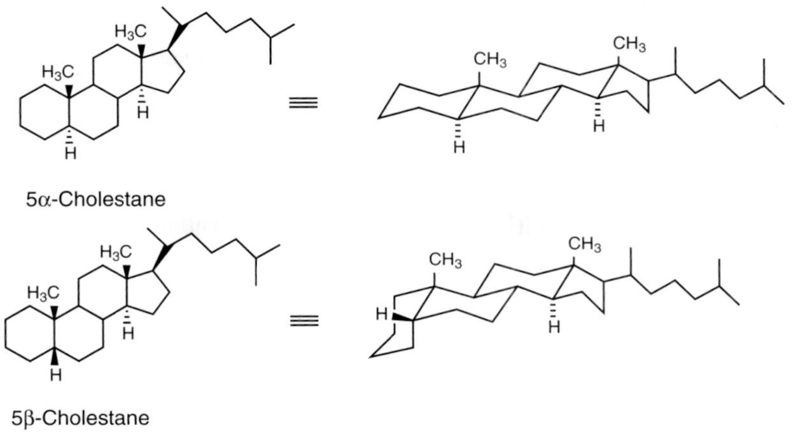

Figure 2.31 The 5α and 5β conformations of the steroid nucleus cholestane.

temperature, such rotations readily occur. Rotation around single bonds Cα-Cβ bond of acetylcholine was shown by Kemp and Pitzer[24] in 1936 not to be free but, rather, to have an energy barrier, which is sufficiently low that at room temperature acetylcholine exists in many interconvertible conformations. Rotation around the central Cα-Cβ bond produces the greatest spatial rearrangement of atoms compared to rotation around any other bond. Since the atoms at the end of some of the bonds within acetylcholine are identical, rotation about several of these bonds produces redundant structures when viewed along the Cα-Cβ bond and can be depicted in the sawhorse or Newman projections, as shown in Figure 2.32. When the ester and trimethylammonium groups are 180° apart, the molecule is said to be in the anti-, or staggered, conformation (or conformer or rotamer). This conformation allows maximum separation of the functional groups and is the most stable conformation energetically. It is possible that other conformations are more stable if factors other than steric interactions are considered (e.g., intramolecular hydrogen bonds). Rotation of one end of the Cα-Cβ bond by 120° or 240° results in the two gauche, or skew, conformations shown in Figure 2.32. These are less stable than the anticonformer, although some studies suggest that an electrostatic attraction between the electron-poor trimethylammonium and electron-rich ester oxygen atom stabilizes this conformation. Rotation by 60°, 180°, and 240° produces the least stable conformations in which all of the atoms overlap, what are referred to as eclipsed conformations.

Drug Design: Discovery and Structural Modification of Lead Compounds

Process of Drug Discovery

The process of drug discovery begins with the identification of new, previously undiscovered, biologically active compounds, often called "hits," which are typically found by screening many compounds for the desired biologic properties. We will next explore the various approaches used to identify "hits" and how these are converted into "lead" compounds and, subsequently, into drug candidates suitable for clinical trials. Sources of "hits" can originate from natural sources, such as plants, animals, or fungi; from synthetic chemical libraries, such as those created through combinatorial chemistry or historic chemical compound collections; from chemical and biologic intuition from years of chemical-biologic training; from targeted/rational drug design; or from computational modeling of a target site such as an enzyme. Chemical or functional group modifications are then performed in order to improve the pharmacologic, toxicologic, physiochemical, and pharmacokinetic properties of a "hit" compound to ultimately obtain a "lead" compound. The lead compound to be optimized should be of a known chemical structure and possess a known mechanism of action, including knowledge of its functional groups (pharmacophoric groups) that are recognized by the receptor/active site and are responsible for that molecule's affinity at the targeted receptor site. "Lead optimization" is the process whereby modifications of the

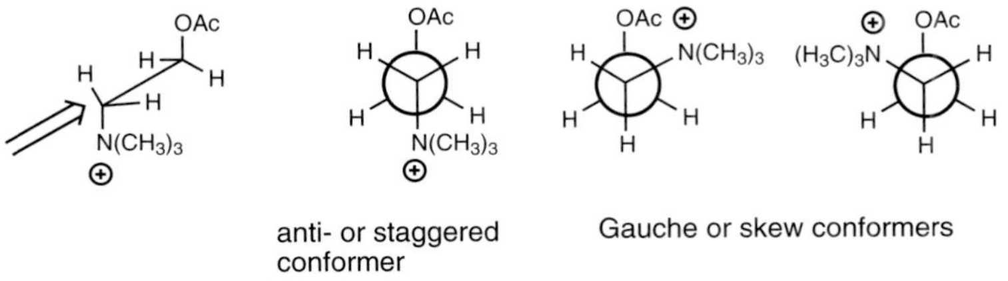

Figure 2.32 Anti- and gauche conformations of acetylcholine.

functional groups of the lead compound are carried out in order to improve its recognition, affinity, and binding geometries of the pharmacophoric groups for the targeted site (a receptor or enzyme); its pharmacokinetics; or its reactivity and stability toward metabolic degradation. The final step of the drug discovery process involves rendering the lead compound into a drug candidate that is safe and suitable for use in human clinical trials, including the preparation of a suitable drug formulation.

Natural Product Screening

Perhaps the most difficult aspect of drug discovery is that of lead discovery. Until the late 19th century, the development of new chemical entities for medicinal purposes was achieved primarily through the use of natural products, generally derived from plant sources. As the colonial powers of Europe discovered new lands in the Western Hemisphere and colonized Asia, the Europeans learned from the indigenous peoples of the newly discovered lands of remedies for many ailments derived from plants and animals. Salicylic acid was isolated from the bark of willow trees after learning that Native Americans brewed the bark to treat inflammatory ailments. Structural optimization of this lead compound (salicylic acid) by the Bayer Corporation of Germany resulted in acetylsalicylic acid, or aspirin, the first nonsteroidal anti-inflammatory agent. South American natives used a tea obtained by brewing Cinchona bark to treat chills and fever. Further study in Europe led to the isolation of quinine and quinidine, which subsequently were used to treat malaria and cardiac arrhythmias, respectively. Following "leads" from folklore medicine, chemists of the late 19th and early 20th centuries began to seek new medicinals from plant sources and to assay them for many types of pharmacologic actions. This approach to drug discovery is often referred to as "natural product screening." Before the mid-1970s, this was one of the major approaches to obtaining new chemical entities as "leads" for new drugs. Unfortunately, this approach fell out of favor and was replaced with the rational approaches to drug design developed during that period (see the next section). Heightened awareness of the fragility of ecosystems, especially the rainforests, has fueled a resurgence of screening products from plants before they become extinct. A new field of pharmacology, called "ethnopharmacology," which is the discipline of identifying potential natural product sources with medicinal properties based on native lore, has emerged as a result.

Compounds isolated from natural sources are usually tested in one or more bioassays for the ailment(s) that the plant material has been purported to treat. Interestingly, the treatment of different ailments can require different methods of preparation (e.g., brewing, chewing, or direct application to wounds) or different parts of the same plant (e.g., roots, stem, leaves, flowers, or sap). As it turns out, each method of administration or part of the plant used can produce one or more different chemical compounds that are necessary to generate the desired outcome.

Drug Discovery via Random Screening of Synthetic Organic Compounds

The random screening of synthetic organic compounds approach to the discovery of new chemical entities for a particular biologic action began in the 1930s, after the discovery of the sulfonamide class of antibacterials. All compounds available to the investigator (natural products, synthetic molecules), regardless of structure, were tested in the pharmacologic assays available at the time. This random screening approach was also applied in the 1960s and 1970s in an effort to find agents that were effective against cancer. Some groups did not limit their assays to identify a particular type of biologic activity but, rather, tested compounds in a wide variety of assays. This large-scale screening approach of drug "leads" is referred to as high-throughput screening, which involves the simultaneous bioassay of thousands of compounds in hundreds to thousands of bioassays. These types of bioassays became possible with the advent of computer-controlled robotic systems for the assays and combinatorial chemistry techniques for the synthesis of large numbers of compounds in small (milligram) quantities. This type of random screening eventually gave way to targeted dedicated screening and rational design techniques.

Drug Discovery From Targeted Dedicated Screening and Rational Drug Design

Rational drug design is a more focused approach that uses greater knowledge (structural information) about the drug receptor (targets) or one of its natural ligands as a basis to design, identify, or create drug "leads." Testing is usually done with one or two models (e.g., specific receptor systems or enzymes) based on the therapeutic target. The drug design component often involves molecular modeling and the use of quantitative structure-activity relationships (QSARs) to better define the physicochemical properties and the pharmacophoric groups that are essential for biologic activity. The development of QSARs relies on the ability to examine multiple relationships between physical properties and biologic activities. In classic QSAR (e.g., Hansch-type analysis), an equation defines biologic activity as a linear free-energy relationship between physicochemical and/or structural properties. It permits evaluation of the nature of interaction forces between a drug and its biological target, as well as the ability to predict activity in molecules. These approaches are better for the development of a lead compound into a drug candidate than for the discovery of a lead compound.

Drug Discovery via Drug Metabolism Studies

New drug entities have been "discovered" as drug leads through investigation of the metabolism of drug molecules that already are clinical candidates or, in some instances, are already on the market. In this method, metabolites of known drug entities are isolated and assayed for biologic

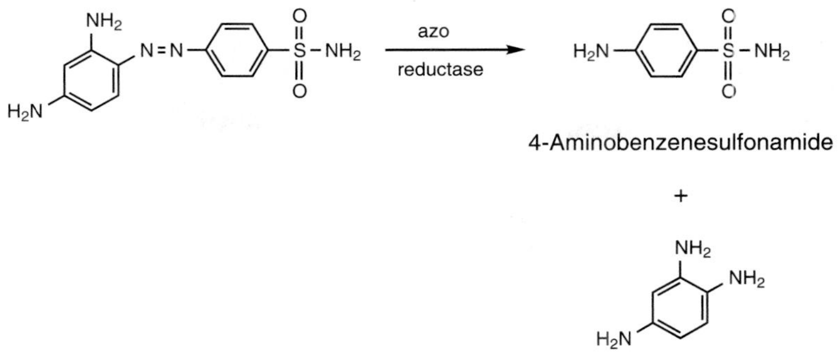

Figure 2.33 Metabolic conversion of prontosil to 4-aminobenzenesulfonamide.

activity using either the same target system or broader screen target systems. The broader screening systems are more useful if the metabolite under evaluation is a chemical structure that was radically altered from the parent molecule through some unusual metabolic rearrangement reaction. In most cases, the metabolite is not radically different from the parent molecule and, therefore, would be expected to exhibit similar pharmacologic effects. One advantage of evaluating this type of drug candidate is that a metabolite can possess better pharmacokinetic properties, such as a longer duration of action, better oral absorption, or less toxicity with fewer side effects (e.g., terfenadine and its antihistaminic hydroxylated metabolite, fexofenadine). As it turns out, the sulfonamide antibacterial agents were discovered in this way. The azo dye prontosil was found to have only antibacterial action in vivo. It was soon discovered that this compound required metabolic activation via reduction of the diazo group to produce the active metabolite 4-aminobenzenesulfonamide (Fig. 2.33). The sulfonamide mimics the physicochemical properties of PABA, a crucial component in microbial metabolism. It is no surprise that the sulfonamide acts as a competitive inhibitor of the enzyme for which PABA is a substrate.

Drug Discovery From the Observation of Side Effects

An astute clinician or pharmacologist can detect a side effect in a patient or animal model that could lead, on further development, to a new therapeutic use for a particular chemical entity. Discovery of new lead compounds via exploitation of side-effect profiles of existing agents is discussed below.

One of the more interesting drug development scenarios is that of the phenothiazine antipsychotics (see Chapter 11). Molecules with this type of biologic activity can be traced back to the first histamine H_1-receptor antagonists developed in the 1930s. In 1937, Bovet and Staub[25] were the first to recognize that it should be possible to antagonize the effects of histamine and, thereby, treat allergic reactions. They tested compounds that were known to act on the autonomic nervous system and, eventually, discovered that benzodioxanes (Fig. 2.34) significantly antagonized the effects of histamine. During an attempt to improve the antihistaminergic action of the benzodioxanes, it was discovered that phenyl substituted ethanolamines

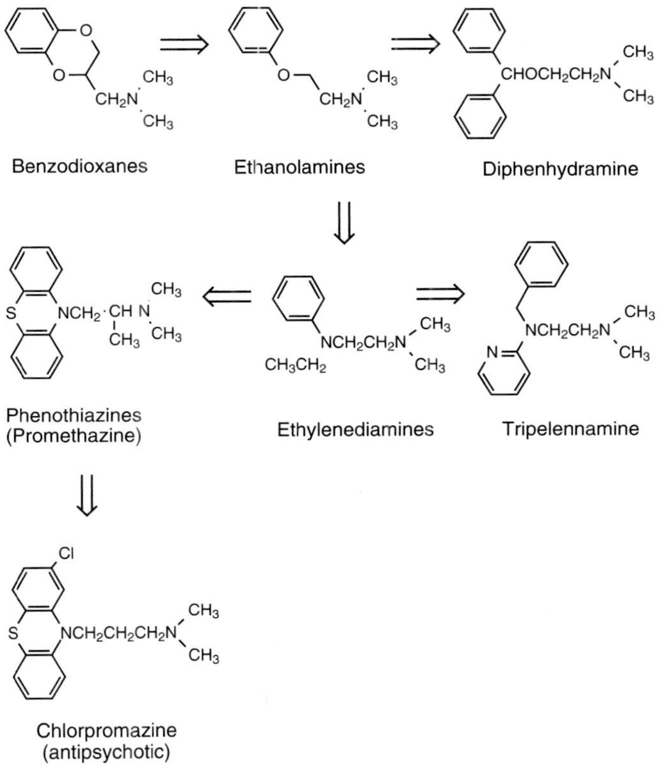

Figure 2.34 Development of phenothiazine-type antipsychotic drugs.

also demonstrated significant antihistaminergic activity. Further development of this class generated two different classes of antihistamines: the diphenhydramine class of antihistamines represented by diphenhydramine and the ethylenediamine class, represented by tripelennamine (Fig. 2.34) (see also Chapter 25).

Incorporation of the aromatic rings of the ethylenediamines into the rigid and planar tricyclic phenothiazine structure produced molecules (e.g., promethazine) with good antihistaminergic action and relatively strong sedative properties (see also Chapters 11 and 12). At first, these compounds were found to be useful as antihistamines, but their very strong sedative properties led to their use as potentiating agents for anesthesia.[26] Further development to increase the sedative properties of the phenothiazines resulted in the development of chlorpromazine in 1950.[27]

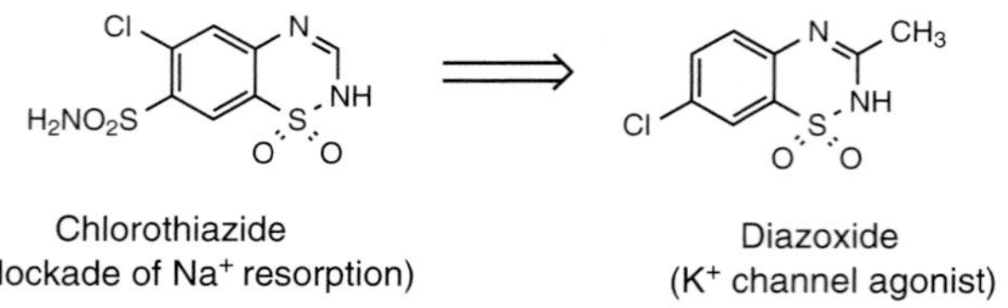

Figure 2.35 Structural similarity of chlorothiazide (a diuretic) and diazoxide (an antihypertensive that acts via opening of K^+ channels).

Chlorpromazine was found to produce a tendency for sleep, but unlike the antihistamine phenothiazines, it also produced a disinterest in patients with regard to their surroundings (i.e., tranquilizing effects). In patients with psychiatric disorders, an ameliorative effect on the psychosis and a relief of anxiety and agitation were noted. These observations suggested that chlorpromazine had potential for the treatment of psychiatric disorders. Thus, what started out as an attempt to improve antihistaminergic activity ultimately resulted in an entirely new class of chemical entities useful in the treatment of an unrelated disorder.[28]

Another example of how new chemical entities can be derived from biologically unrelated molecules is illustrated by the development of the potassium channel agonist diazoxide (Fig. 2.35). This molecule was developed as a result of the observation that the thiazide diuretics, such as chlorothiazide, not only exhibited diuretic activity, due to inhibition of sodium absorption in the distal convoluted tubule, but also demonstrated a direct effect on the renal vasculature. Structural modification to enhance this direct effect led to the development of diazoxide and related potassium channel agonists for the treatment of hypertension (see Chapter 17).

Refinement of the Lead Structure

Determination of the Pharmacophore

Once a "hit" compound has been discovered for a particular therapeutic use, the next step is to identify the pharmacophoric groups. The pharmacophore of a drug molecule is that portion of the molecule that contains the essential functional group(s) that directly bind with the active site of the biologic target to produce the desired biologic activity. Because drug-target interactions can be very specific (think of a lock [receptor] and key [drug] relationship), the pharmacophore can constitute a small portion of the molecule. In many cases, a very structurally complex molecule can be "stripped down" to a simpler structure with retention of the pharmacophoric groups while maintaining the desired biologic action. An example of this is the opioid analgesic morphine, a tetracyclic compound with five chiral centers. Not only would structure simplification possibly provide molecules with fewer side effects, but a reduction in the number of chiral centers would greatly simplify the synthesis of morphine derivatives. Figure 2.36 shows how the morphine structure has been simplified in the search for molecules with fewer deleterious side effects, such as respiratory depression and addiction potential. Within each class are analogues that are less potent, equipotent, and many times more potent than

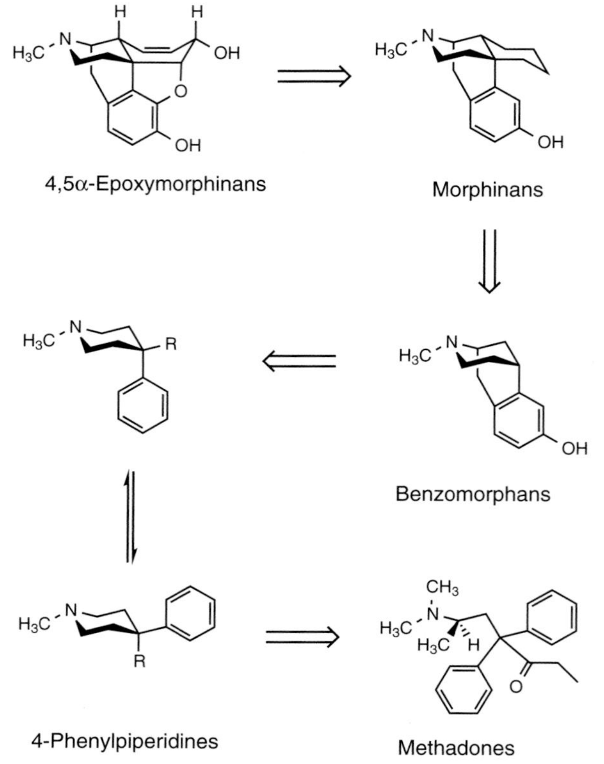

Figure 2.36 Morphine pharmacophore and its relationship to analgesic derivatives.

morphine. As shown in the figure, the pharmacophore of morphine consists of a tertiary alkylamine that is at least four atoms away from an aromatic ring. A more detailed discussion of the chemistry and pharmacology of morphine can be found in Chapter 14.

Alterations in Alkyl Chains: Chain Length, Branching, and Rings

An increase or decrease in the length of an alkyl chain (homologation), branching, and alteration of ring size can have a profound effect on the potency and pharmacologic activity of the molecule. A change in the length of an alkyl chain by one CH_2 unit or branch alters the lipophilic character of the molecule and, therefore, its properties of absorption, distribution, and excretion. If the alkyl chain is directly involved in an interaction with the biologic target, then this type of alteration can influence the quality of those interactions. Molecules that are conformationally flexible can become less flexible if branching is introduced at a key position of an alkyl chain or the alkyl chain is incorporated into a ring equivalent. Changes in conformation can alter the spatial relationship between the pharmacophoric (functional) groups in the molecule and thereby influence interactions with the biologic target. Small structural changes are important to consider in the design of structural analogues.

An example that demonstrates how an increase in hydrocarbon chain length has significant effects not only on potency but also on drug action (agonist

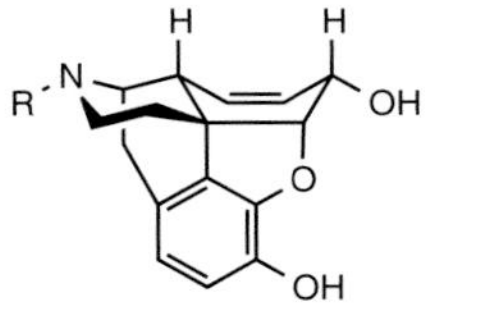

R	Pharmacological activity
$-CH_3$	Analgesic (morphine)
$-CH_2CH_3$	Opioid agonist activity decreased
$-CH_2CH_2CH_3$	Opioid antagonist activity increased
$-CH_2CH_2CH_2CH_3$	Inactive as opioid agonist or antagonist
$-CH_2CH_2CH_2CH_2CH_3$	Opioid antagonist activity increased
$-CH_2CH_2CH_2CH_2CH_2CH_3$	Opioid antagonist activity increased
$-CH_2CH_2-C_6H_5$ 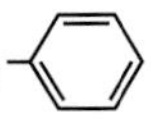	14X potency of morphine

Figure 2.37 Effect of alkyl chain length on bioactivity of morphine.

vs. antagonist) is provided by a series of N-alkyl morphine analogues (Fig. 2.37). In this series, homologation of R = CH_3 (morphine) to R = $CH_2CH_2CH_3$ (N-propylnormorphine) produces a pronounced decrease in agonist activity and an increase in antagonist activity. When further homologated by one methylene unit R = $CH_2CH_2CH_2CH_3$ (N-butylnormorphine), the resulting analogue is totally devoid of agonist or antagonist activity (i.e., the compound is inactive). Additional increases in chain length (R = $CH_2CH_2CH_2CH_2CH_3$ and R = $CH_2CH_2CH_2CH_2CH_2CH_3$) produce compounds with increasing potency as agonists. When R is β-phenylethyl, the compound is a full agonist, with a potency approximately 14-fold that of morphine.[29,30]

Branching of alkyl chains can also produce drastic changes in potency and pharmacologic activity. If the mechanism of action is closely related to the lipophilicity of the molecule, then hydrocarbon chain branching will result in a less lipophilic compound and a significant alteration in biologic effect. This decrease in lipophilicity is a result of the alkyl chain becoming more compact and causes less disruption of the hydrogen-bonding network of water. If the hydrocarbon chain is directly involved in interactions with its biologic target, then branching can produce major changes in pharmacologic activity. For example, consider the phenothiazines promethazine and promazine.

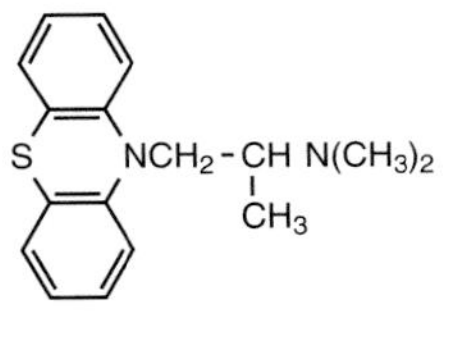

Promethazine: $NCH_2-CH(CH_3)N(CH_3)_2$

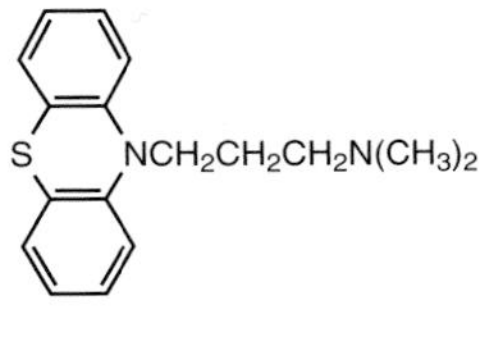

Promazine: $NCH_2CH_2CH_2N(CH_3)_2$

The primary pharmacologic activity of promethazine is that of an antihistamine, whereas promazine is an antipsychotic. The only difference between the two molecules is the alkylamine side chain. In the case of promethazine, there is an isopropylamine side chain, whereas promazine contains an *n*-propylamine. In this case, simple modification of one carbon atom from a branched to a linear hydrocarbon radically alters the pharmacologic activity.

Positional isomers of aromatic ring substituents can also possess different pharmacologic properties. Substituents on aromatic rings can alter the electron distribution throughout the ring, which, in turn, can influence how the ring interacts with the biologic target. Aromatic ring substituents can also influence the conformation of the flexible portion of a molecule, especially if the substituents are located ortho to the same carbon attached to the flexible side chain. Ring substituents influence the conformations of adjacent substituents via steric interactions and can significantly alter interactions with the biologic target.

Functional Group Modification: Bioisosterism

Bioisosterism

When a lead compound is first discovered, it often lacks the required potency and pharmacokinetic properties suitable for making it a viable clinical candidate. These can include undesirable side effects, physicochemical properties, other factors that affect oral bioavailability, and adverse metabolic or excretion properties. These undesirable properties are often the result of the presence of specific pharmacophoric (functional) groups in the molecule. Successful modification of the compound to reduce or eliminate these undesirable features without losing the desired biologic activity is the goal. Replacement or modification of specific pharmacophoric (functional) groups with other groups having similar properties is known as "isosteric replacement" or "bioisosteric replacement."

In 1919, Langmuir[31,32] first developed the concept of chemical isosterism to describe the similarities in physical properties among atoms, functional groups, radicals, and molecules. The similarities among atoms described by Langmuir resulted primarily from the fact that these atoms contained the same number of valence electrons and came from the same columns within the periodic table. This concept of isosterism was limited to elements in adjacent rows and columns, inorganic molecules, ions, and small organic molecules, such as diazomethane and ketene. Table 2.7 shows a comparison of the physical properties of N_2O and CO_2 to illustrate Langmuir's concept.

To account for similarities between functional groups with the same number of valence electrons but different numbers of atoms, Grimm[33] developed his hydride displacement law. This is not a "law" in the strict sense but, rather, more an illustration of similar physical properties among closely related functional groups. Table 2.8 presents an example of Grimm's hydride displacement. Descending diagonally from left to right in the table, hydrogen atoms are progressively added to maintain the same number of

Table 2.7 Comparison of Physical Properties of N_2O and CO_2

Property	N_2O	CO_2
Viscosity at 20°C	148×10^6	148×10^6
Density of liquid at 10°C	0.856	0.858
Refractive index of liquid, D line 16°C	1.193	1.190
Dielectric constant of liquid at 0°C	1.593	1.582
Solubility in alcohol at 15°C	3.250	3.130

valence electrons for each group of atoms within a column (thus the term "hydride"). Within each column, the groups are considered to be "pseudoatoms" with respect to each another. Thus, NH_2 is considered to be isosteric to OH, and so on. This early view of isosterism did not consider the actual location, motion, and resonance of electrons within the orbitals of these functional group replacements. Careful observation of this table reveals that some groups do share similar physicochemical properties, but others have very different properties, despite having the same number of valence electrons. For example, OH and NH_2 share similar hydrogen-bonding properties and, therefore, should be interchangeable if that is the only important criterion. The NH_2 group is basic, whereas the OH is neutral. Hence, at physiologic pH, the NH_2 group exists in its protonated or conjugate acid form and the molecule becomes positively charged. If OH is being replaced by NH_2, the additional positive charge could have a significant effect on the overall physicochemical properties of the molecule in which it is being introduced. The difference in physicochemical properties of the CH_3 group relative to the OH and NH_2 groups is even greater. In addition to acid-base character, this "law" fails to take into account other important physicochemical parameters, such as electronegativity, polarizability, bond angles, size, shape of molecular orbitals, electron density, and partition coefficients, all of which contribute significantly to the overall physicochemical properties of a molecule.

Instead of considering only partial structures, Hinsberg[34] applied the concept of isosterism to entire molecules. He developed the concept of "ring equivalents"—that is, functional groups that can be exchanged for one another in aromatic ring systems without drastic changes in

Table 2.8 Grimm's Hydride Displacement "Law"

C	N	O	F	Ne
	CH	NH	OH	FH
		CH_2	NH_2	OH_2
			CH_3	NH_3

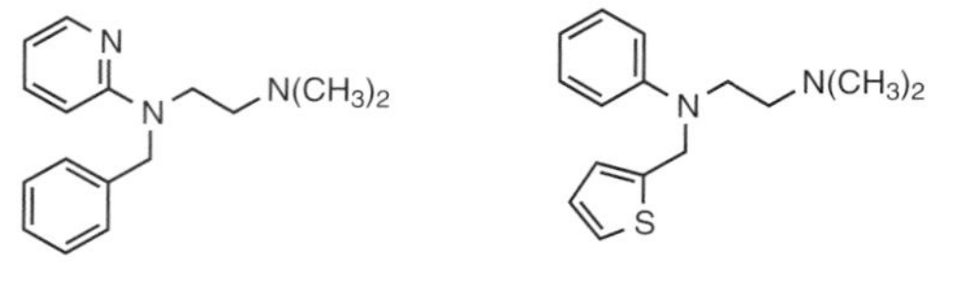

Tripelennamine Methaphenilene

Figure 2.38 Isosteric substitution of thiophene for benzene and benzene for pyridine.

physicochemical properties relative to the parent structure. Benzene, thiophene, and pyridine illustrate this concept (Fig. 2.38). A –CH = CH– group in benzene is replaced by the divalent sulfur, -S-, in thiophene, and a –CH = is replaced by the trivalent –N = to give pyridine. The physical properties of benzene and thiophene are very similar. For example, the boiling point of benzene is 81.1°C, and that of thiophene is 84.4°C (at 760 mm Hg). Pyridine, however, deviates, with a boiling point of 115-116°C. Hinsberg therefore concluded that divalent sulfur (-S- or thioether) must resemble –C = C– in shape, and these groups were considered to be isosteric. Note that hydrogen atoms are ignored in this comparison. Today, this isosteric relationship is seen in many drugs e.g., H_1-receptor antagonists (Fig. 2.38).

It is difficult to relate biologic properties to physicochemical properties of individual atoms, functional groups, or entire molecules, because many physicochemical parameters are involved simultaneously and, therefore, are difficult to quantitate. Simple relationships as described earlier often do not hold up across the many types of biologic systems seen with medicinal agents. That is, what can work as an isosteric replacement in one biologic system cannot work in another. Because of this, it was necessary to introduce the term "bioisosterism" to describe functional groups related in structure that have similar biologic effects. Friedman[35] introduced the term bioisosterism and defined it as follows: "Bioisosteres are (functional) groups or molecules that have chemical and physical similarities producing broadly similar biological properties." Burger[36] expanded this definition to take into account biochemical views of biological activity: "Bioisosteres are compounds or groups that possess near equal molecular shapes and volumes, approximately the same distribution of electrons, and which exhibit similar physical properties such as hydrophobicity. Bioisosteric compounds affect the same biochemically associated systems as agonist or antagonists and thereby produce biological properties that are related to each other."

Classical and Nonclassical Bioisosteres

Bioisosteric groups can be subdivided into two categories: classical and nonclassical bioisosteres. Functional groups that satisfy the original conditions of Langmuir and Grimm are referred to as classical bioisosteres. Nonclassical bioisosteres do not obey steric and electronic definitions of classical bioisosteres and do not necessarily have the same number of atoms as the functional group that they replace. A wider set of compounds and functional groups are encompassed by nonclassical bioisosteres that produce, at the molecular level, qualitatively similar agonist or antagonist action. In animals, many hormones and neurotransmitters with very similar structures and biologic actions can be classified as bioisosteres. An example is the insulins isolated from various mammalian species. Even though these insulins can differ by several amino acid residues, they still produce the same biologic effects. (If this did not occur, the use of insulin to treat diabetes would have had to wait another 60 years for recombinant DNA technology to allow production of human insulin.)

What can be a successful bioisosteric replacement for a given molecule that interacts with a particular biologic target quite has often no effect or abolishes biologic activity in another. Thus, the use of bioisosteric replacement (classical or nonclassical) in the design of new chemical entities (drug discovery) is highly dependent on the biologic system under investigation. No hard-and-fast rules exist to determine which bioisosteric replacement is going to work with a given molecule, although as the following tables and examples demonstrate, some generalizations are possible. Each category of bioisostere can be further subdivided as shown below, and examples are provided in Tables 2.9 and 2.10:

1. Classical bioisosteres
   a. Monovalent atoms and groups
   b. Divalent atoms and groups
   c. Trivalent atoms and groups
   d. Tetrasubstituted atoms
   e. Ring equivalents
2. Nonclassical bioisosteres
   a. Exchangeable groups
   b. Rings versus noncyclic structure

Table 2.9 Classical Bioisosteres (Groups Within the Row Can Replace Each Other)

Monovalent Bioisosteres
F, H
OH, NH
F, OH, NH, or CH_3 for H
SH, OH
Cl, Br, CF_3

Divalent bioisosteres
—C=S, —C=O, —C=NH, —C=C—

Trivalent atoms or groups:
—CH=, —N=
—P=, —As=

Tetrasubstituted atoms:
$—N^{+}—$, —C—, $—P^{+}—$, $—As^{+}—$

Ring equivalents:
(benzene, thiophene, pyridine, furan)

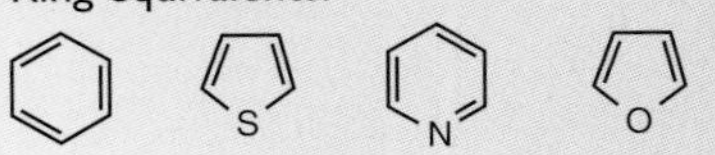

Table 2.10 Nonclassical Bioisosteric Replacements

Compounds	Bioisosteric Replacement	References
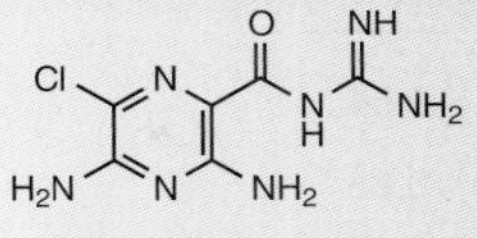 (amiloride-type pyrazine acylguanidine)	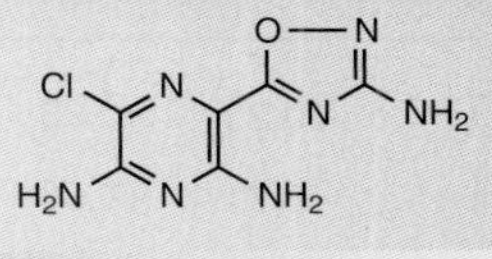 (1,2,4-oxadiazole analog)	40
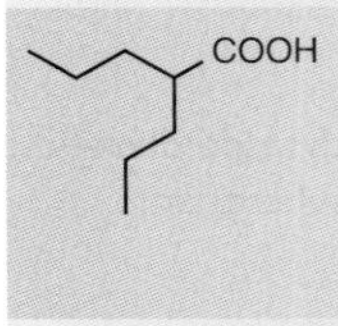 (2-propylpentanoic acid, COOH)	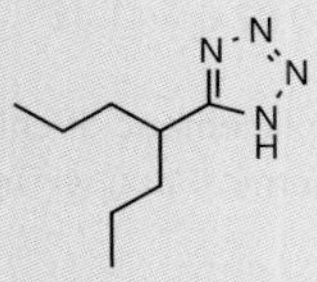 (tetrazole analog)	41
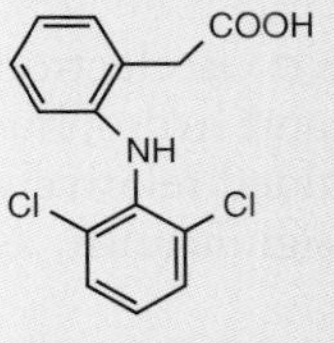 (diclofenac, COOH)	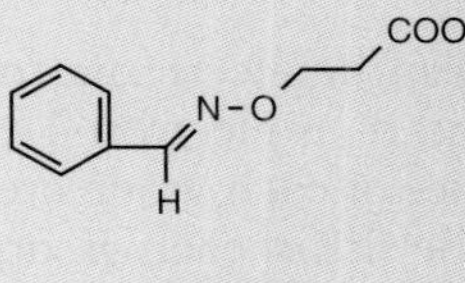 (oxime ether, N-O, COOH)	42
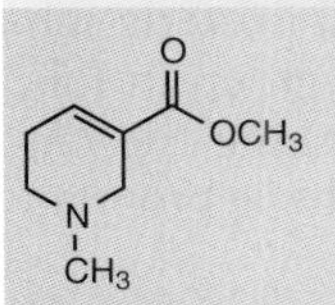 (arecoline, OCH_3, N-CH_3)	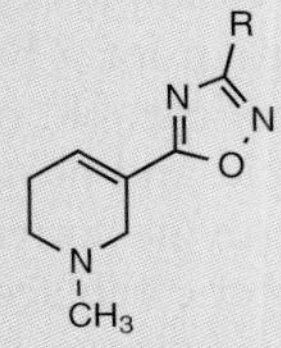 (1,2,4-oxadiazole, R, N-CH_3)	43
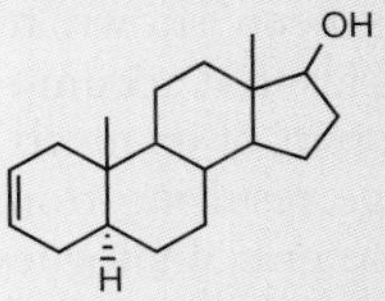 (steroid, OH)	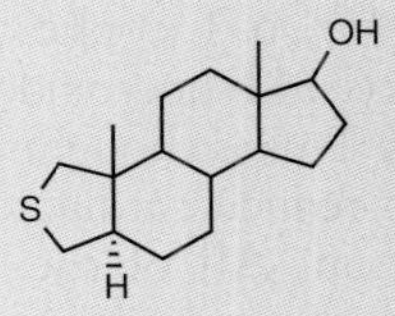 (thia-steroid, S, OH)	44
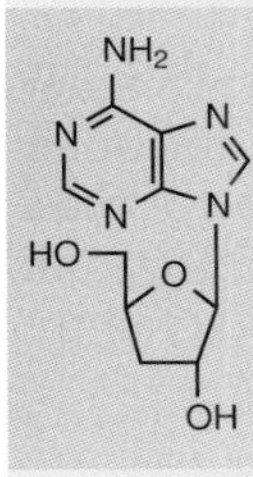 (adenosine, NH_2, HO, OH)	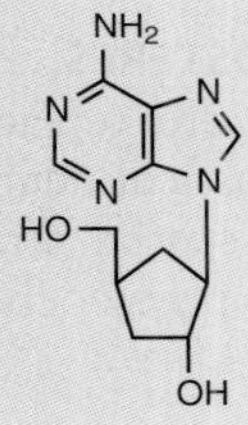 (carbocyclic adenosine analog, NH_2, HO, OH)	45
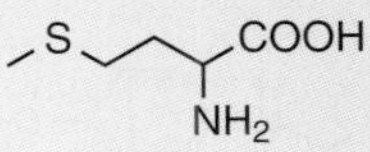 (methionine: S, COOH, NH_2)	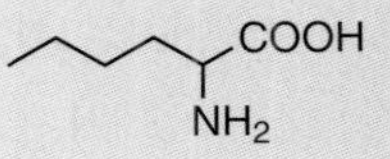 (norleucine: COOH, NH_2)	46

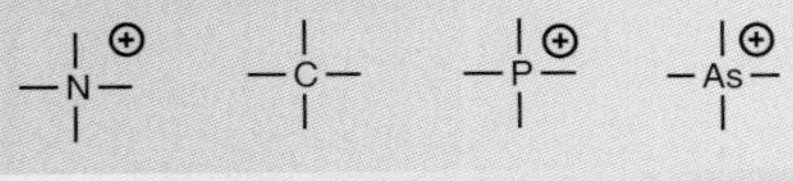

CLASSICAL BIOISOSTERES. Substitution of hydrogen with fluorine is a common monovalent isosteric replacement. Sterically, hydrogen and fluorine are quite similar, with their van der Waals radii measuring 1.2 and 1.35 Å, respectively. Because fluorine is the most electronegative element in the periodic table, any differences in biologic activity resulting from replacement of hydrogen with fluorine can be attributed to this property.

A classic example of hydrogen replacement by fluorine is development of the antineoplastic agent 5-fluorouracil from uracil. Another example is shown in Figure 2.39, in which the chlorine of chlorothiazide has been replaced with bromine or a trifluoromethyl group. For each of

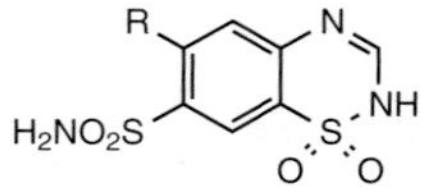

R =	Cl	Br	CF_3
σ	+0.23	+0.23	+0.54
π	+0.71	+0.86	+0.88
E_s	-0.97	-1.16	-2.40

Figure 2.39 Isosteric replacement of chlorine in thiazide diuretics. Comparison of physicochemical properties of the substituents.

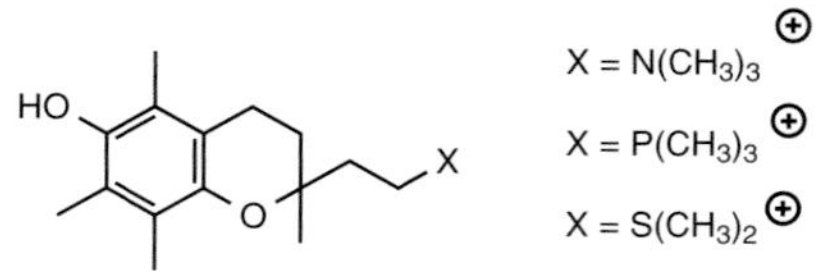

the substitutions, the electronic (σ, where σ^+ is electron withdrawing and σ^- is electron donating) and hydrophobic (π) properties of each group are maintained relatively constant, but the size of each group varies significantly, as indicated by the Taft steric parameter (E_s).

Figure 2.40 shows an example of classical isosteric substitution of an amino group for a hydroxyl group in folic acid. The amino group is capable of mimicking the tautomeric forms of folic acid and providing the appropriate hydrogen bonds to the enzyme active site.

A tetravalent bioisosteric replacement study was conducted by Grisar et al.[37] with a series of α-tocopherol analogues (Fig. 2.41). α-Tocopherol has been shown to scavenge lipoperoxyl and superoxide radicals that accumulate in heart tissue. This is thought to be part of its mechanism of action to reduce cardiac damage resulting from myocardial infarction. All of the bioisosteric analogues were found to produce similar biologic activity.

Nonclassical Bioisosteres. As mentioned earlier, nonclassical bioisosteres are replacements of functional groups not defined by classical definitions. Some of these groups, however, mimic spatial arrangements, electronic properties, or some other physicochemical property of the

X = $N(CH_3)_3^{\oplus}$
X = $P(CH_3)_3^{\oplus}$
X = $S(CH_3)_2^{\oplus}$

α-Tocopherol X = $C_{14}H_{29}$

Figure 2.41 Tetravalent bioisosteres of α-tocopherol.

molecule or functional group critical for biologic activity. One example is the use of a double bond to position essential functional groups into a particular spatial configuration critical for activity. This is shown in Figure 2.42 with the naturally occurring hormone estradiol and the synthetic analogue diethylstilbestrol. The *trans* isomer of diethylstilbestrol has approximately the same potency as estradiol, whereas the *cis* isomer is only one-fourteenth as active. In the *trans* configuration, the phenolic hydroxy groups mimic the correct orientation of the phenol and alcohol in estradiol.[38,39] This is not possible with the *cis* isomer, and more flexible analogues (Fig. 2.42) have little or no activity.[40,41]

Another example of a nonclassical replacement is that of a sulfonamide group for a phenol in catecholamines (Fig. 2.43). With this example, steric factors appear to have less influence on receptor binding than acidity and hydrogen-bonding potential of the functional group on the aromatic ring. Both the phenolic hydroxyl of isoproterenol and the acidic proton of the arylsulfonamide have nearly the same pK_a (~10).[42] Both groups are weakly acidic and capable of losing a proton and interacting with the biologic target as anions (Fig. 2.43). Because the replacement is not susceptible to metabolism by catechol O-methyltransferase, it has also the added advantage of increasing the duration of action and making the compound orally active. Other examples of successful bioisosteric replacements are shown in Table 2.10, and a more detailed description of the role of bioisosterism can be found in the review by Patani and LaVoie.[43]

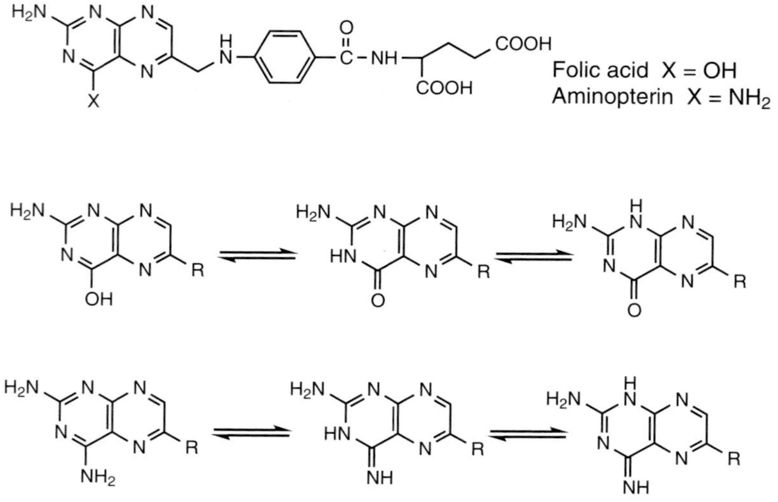

Folic acid X = OH
Aminopterin X = NH_2

Figure 2.40 Isosteric replacement of OH by NH_2 in folic acid and possible tautomers of folic acid and aminopterin.

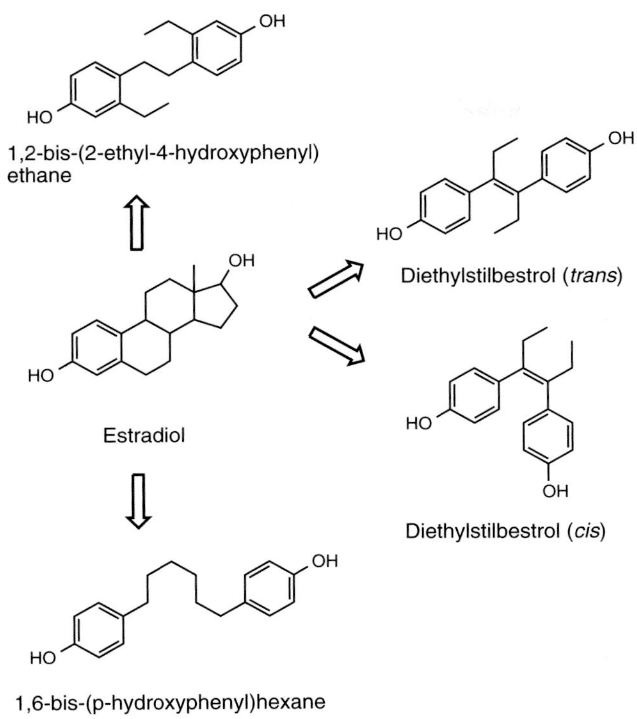

Figure 2.42 Noncyclic analogues of estradiol.

PEPTIDE AND PROTEIN DRUGS

Not all drugs are small molecules as described thus far. Some very important therapeutic agents are peptidic in nature (e.g., insulin, calcitonin) and, due to their physical chemical properties, generally cannot be delivered orally and must be administered parenterally. Peptides and proteins are very similar in that they are made up of units, or residues, of amino acids that are linked by amide bonds, also referred to as peptide bonds. There is no definitive number of amino acid residues that delineates a peptide from a protein. However, the term peptide refers generally to molecules that contain 15-50 amino acids. Molecules composed of more than 50 residues are generally referred to as proteins.

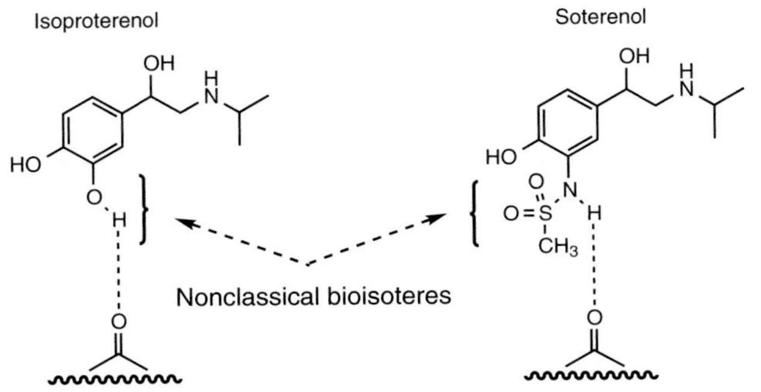

Figure 2.43 Bioisosteric replacement of *m*-OH of isoproterenol with a sulfonamido group and similar hydrogen-bonding capacity to a possible drug receptor.

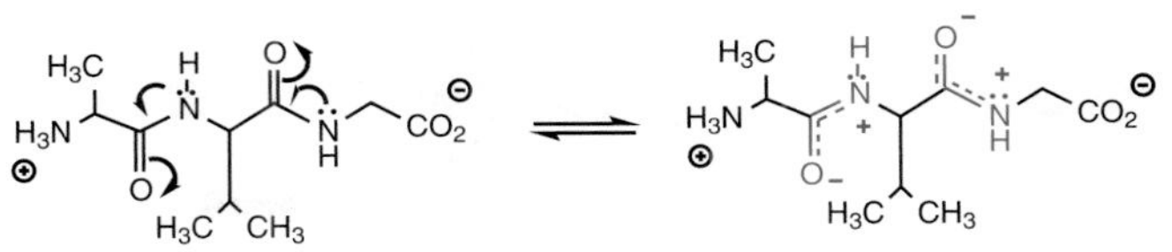

Figure 2.44 A tripeptide, Ala-Val-Gly, indicating the planarity of the peptide bonds caused by the restricted rotation around the amide bond.

There are 20 naturally occurring amino acids that serve as the building blocks for both peptide and protein drugs (Table 2.11). Each amino acid contains a common functional group "backbone" that includes a basic amine attached to the α-carbon of an acidic carboxylic acid. The α-carbon for each amino acid is substituted with a unique side chain. The amino acid side chains contribute significantly to the physical chemical properties of the peptide that is formed from a unique sequence of amino acids.

As previously mentioned, the amino acid residues are linked by amide bonds, as shown in Figure 2.44. Each carboxylic acid forms an amide bond with the amine group of the next amino acid in the sequence. As with other amide bonds, conjugation between the lone pair of electrons on the nitrogen atom and the adjacent carbonyl group results in the amide bond having partial double-bond character due to a resonance structure as shown in Figure 2.44. This property has two major consequences: (1) the amide bond is therefore co-planar; and (2) there is restricted rotation around the C-N bond (Fig. 2.44). Because of this restricted rotation, there are two conformations possible, *cis* and *trans* (Fig 2.45). The *trans*-conformation is lower in energy due to fewer steric interactions (similar to that found with a carbon-carbon double bond) and is favored. When proline is one of the amino acid residues, the *cis*-conformation can be favored as a result of the amine group being part of a pyrrolidine ring. For this reason, the presence of proline in peptides and proteins is associated with a "kink" or bend in the overall conformation of the peptide chain.

Physical Chemical Properties of Peptides

Since the α-amine and α-carboxylic acid of each amino acid are involved in the peptide backbone (except at each terminus of the chain), the basic and acidic nature of these functional groups does not contribute to the overall physical chemical properties of the molecule. The functional groups found within the amino acid side chains are what are integral to the physicochemical properties of the peptide or protein and represent important

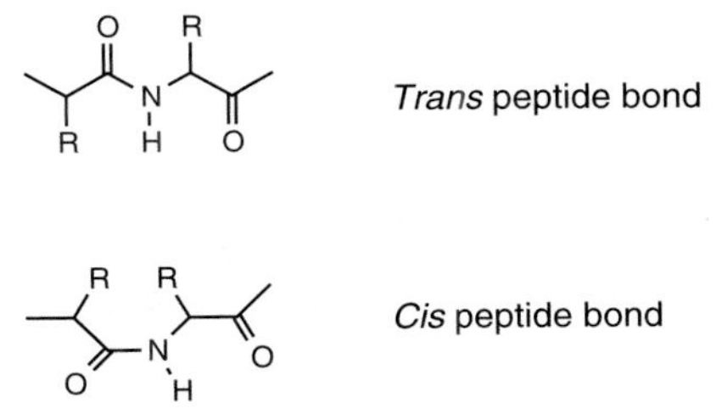

Figure 2.45 *Cis/trans* peptide bond configuration.

Table 2.11 The Twenty Natural Occurring Amino Acids

General Structure: $H_2N-CH(R)-CO_2H$

Name	Three-Letter Code	Single-Letter Code	Structure R =	pK_a of Side Chain
Glycine	Gly	G	-H	None
Alanine	Ala	A	$-CH_3$	None
Valine	Val	V	$-CH(CH_3)_2$	None
Isoleucine	Ile	I	$-CH(CH_3)CH_2CH_3$	None
Leucine	Leu	L	$-CH_2CH(CH_3)_2$	None
Proline	Pro	P	(pyrrolidine ring: N–H, CO_2H)	(Acidic) ~4
Phenylalanine	Phe	F	$-CH_2-C_6H_5$	None
Tryptophan	Trp	W	$-CH_2$–(indole, N–H)	None
Methionine	Met	M	$-CH_2CH_2SCH_3$	None
Cysteine	Cys	C	$-CH_2SH$	(Acidic) ~8
Serine	Ser	S	$-CH_2OH$	None
Threonine	Thr	T	$-CH(CH_3)OH$	None
Tyrosine	Tyr	Y	$-CH_2-C_6H_4-OH$	(Acidic) ~10
Arginine	Arg	R	$-CH_2CH_2CH_2-NH-C(=NH)-NH_2$	(Basic) ~12.5
Lysine	Lys	K	$-CH_2CH_2CH_2NH_2$	(Basic) ~10.5
Histidine	His	H	$-CH_2$–(imidazole, N, NH)	(Basic) ~6
Asparagine	Asn	N	$-CH_2CONH_2$	None
Glutamine	Gln	Q	$-CH_2CH_2CONH_2$	None
Aspartic acid	Asp	D	$-CH_2COOH$	(Acidic) ~3.8
Glutamic acid	Glu	E	$-CH_2CH_2COOH$	(Acidic) ~4

points of interaction with the corresponding biologic target. Examination of Table 2.11 shows that the functional groups found within the amino acid side chains can be basic (e.g., amine, guanidine, imidazole), acidic (e.g., carboxylic acid, phenol, thiol), neutral (e.g., thioether, amide), or hydrocarbon (e.g., alkyl, aromatic rings) in nature. All of the functional groups found in amino acid side chains were discussed previously as components of small-molecule drugs. The primary differences in physical chemical properties between peptides and small molecules are due to their large size (molecular weight [MW]) and, as a result, the sheer number of different side chains (i.e., functional groups) present in a given structure. As might be expected, the types and number of functional groups present in the side chains dictate how much more or less polar the peptide is compared to a small-molecule drug. It is certainly plausible that peptide-based drugs will not have optimal log P values for passive absorption across membranes and, given their large MW, will not readily cross membranes.

Metabolism/Degradation of Peptide and Protein Drugs

Peptides and proteins are metabolized extensively by enzymes in the gastrointestinal tract, blood, interstitial fluid, vascular bed, and cell membranes, which results in very poor oral absorption and a short half-life for these molecules. The primary route of metabolism of peptides and proteins involves hydrolysis of the peptide bonds that link the amino acids by enzymes called peptidases. Some of these peptidases exhibit specificity for certain amino acid sequences or have specificity for either the amino or carboxyl terminus of the peptide (exopeptidase). For example, carboxypeptidases cleave off one C-terminal residue, dipeptidyl carboxypeptidases cleave dipeptides from the C terminus, aminopeptidases cleave off one N-terminal residue, and amidases (endopeptidases) cleave internal peptide bonds. There are also peptidase subclasses that exhibit specificity for certain amino acid sequences within the peptide or at either of the termini. Some peptidases (e.g., dipeptidyl peptidase IV) have been found to catalyze the degradation of naturally occurring peptides (e.g., GLP-1) (Fig. 2.46) (see also Chapters 5 and 20).

SUMMARY

Medicinal chemistry involves the discovery of new chemical entities and the systematic study of the SARs of these compounds for disease state management. Such studies provide the basis for development of better and therapeutically safer medicinal agents from lead compounds found from natural sources, random screening, systematic screening, and focused rational design. Drug design goals include increasing the potency and duration of action of newly discovered compounds and decreasing adverse side effects.

For the pharmacist, it is also important to understand how the physicochemical properties influence the pharmacokinetic properties of the medicinal agents being dispensed. Such knowledge will help the pharmacist not only to better understand the clinical properties of these compounds but also to anticipate the properties of newly marketed agents. An understanding of the chemical properties of the molecule will allow the pharmacist to anticipate formulation problems (especially IV admixtures), as well as potential adverse interactions with other drugs as the result of serum protein binding and metabolism.

Subject to proteolytic degradation catalyzed by dipeptidyl peptidase

↓

His-Ala-Glu-Gly-Thr-Phe-Thr-Ser-Asp-Val-Ser-Ser-Tyr-Leu-Glu—

Gly-Gln-Ala-Ala-Lys-Glu-Phe-Ile-Ala-Trp-Leu-Val-Lys-Gly-Arg

GLP-1

Figure 2.46 GLP-1 degradation by dipeptidyl peptidase IV.

REFERENCES

1. Crum-Brown A, Fraser TR. On the connection between chemical constitution and physiological action. Part 1: on the physiological action of the ammonium bases derived from Strychia, Brucia, Thebia, Codeia, Morphia, and Nicotia. *Trans R Soc Edinburgh.* 1869;25:257-274.
2. Ariëns EJ. A general introduction to the field of drug discovery. In: Ariëns EJ, ed. *Drug Design.* New York: Academic Press; 1971:689-696.
3. Loewi O, Navrati E. Über humorale übertragbarkeit der herznervenwirkung XI mitteilung. über den mechanismus der vaguswirkung von physostigmin und ergotamine. *Plugers Arch Ges Physiol Menshen Tiere.* 1926;214:689-696.
4. Ehrlich P. On immunity with special reference to cell life. In: Himmelweit F, ed. *Collected Papers of Paul Ehrlich.* London: Pergamon; 1957:178-195.
5. Albert A. The long search for valid structure–action relationships in drugs. *J Med Chem.* 1982;25:1-5.
6. Ing HR. The curariform action of onium salts. *Physiol Rev.* 1936;16:527-544.
7. Woods DD. The relation of p-aminobenzoic acid to the mechanism of the action of sulfanilamide. *Br J Exp Pathol.* 1940;21:74-90.
8. Kauffman GB. The Brönsted-Lowry acid-base concept. *J Chem Ed.* 1988;85:28-31.
9. Lemke TL. *Review of Organic Functional Groups: Introduction to Medicinal Organic Chemistry.* 5th ed. Philadelphia, PA: Lippincott Williams & Wilkins; 2012.
10. Cates LA. Calculation of drug solubilities by pharmacy students. *Am J Pharm Ed.* 1981;45:11-13.
11. Fujita T. The extrathermodynamic approach to drug design. In: Hansch C, ed. *Comprehensive Medicinal Chemistry.* Vol. 4. New York: Pergamon Press; 1990:497-560.
12. Tute MS. Principles and practice of Hansch analysis: a guide to structure–activity correlation for the medicinal chemist. In: Harper NJ, Simons AB, eds. *Advances in Drug Research.* London: Academic Press; 1971:1-77.
13. Hansch C, Leo A. *Substituent Constants for Correlation Analysis in Chemistry and Biology.* New York: John Wiley; 1979.
14. Hansch C, Leo A. *Exploring QSAR: Hydrophobic, Electronic, and Steric Constants.* Washington, DC: American Chemical Society; 1995.
15. ClogP. BioByte Corp. Claremont, CA; ACDLogP®, Advanced Chemistry Development Toronto Canada; KOWWIN®, Chemaxon, Budapest, Hungary; CSLogP, ChemSilico, Tewksbury, MA.
16. Molinspiration Chemoinformatics. http://www.molinspiration.com. Accessed 6 February 2018.
17. Florence AT, Attwood D. *Physiochemical Principles of Pharmacy.* 5th ed. New York: Chapman & Hall; 2011.
18. Smith C, Marks A, Lieberman M, eds. *Basic Medical Biochemistry.* 2nd ed. Baltimore: Lippincott Williams & Wilkins; 2004.
19. Kunta JR, Sinko PJ. Intestinal drug transporters: in vivo function and clinical importance. *Curr Drug Metabo.* 2004; 5:109-124.
20. Cahn RS, Ingold CK, Prelog V. The specification of asymmetric configuration in organic chemistry. *Experientia.* 1956;12:81-94.
21. Piutti A. Su rune nouvelle espec d'asparagine. *Compt Red.* 1886;103:134-138.
22. Easson LH, Stedman E. Studies on the relationship between chemical constitution and physiological action. V. Molecular dissymmetry and physiological activity. *Biochem J.* 1933;27:1257-1266.
23. Blackwood JE, Gladys CL, Loening KL, et al. Unambiguous specification of stereoisomerism about a double bond. *J Am Chem Soc.* 1968;90:509-510.
24. Kemp JD, Pitzer KS. Hindered rotation of the methyl groups in ethane. *J Chem Phys.* 1936;4:749.
25. Bovet D, Staub A. Action protectice des ethers phenoliques au cours de l'intoxication histaminique. *C R Soc Biol (Paris).* 1937;124:547-549.

26. Laborit H, Huguenard P, Alluaume R. Un nouveau stabilisateur vegetatif, le 4560 RP. *Presse Med.* 1952;60:206-208.
27. Charpentier P, Gaillot P, Jacob R, et al. Recherches sur les dimethylaminopropyl N-phenothiazines. *C R Acad Sci (Paris)*. 1952;325:59-60.
28. Delay J, Deniker P, Hurl JM. Utilisation en thirapeutique psychiatrique d'une phenothiazine d'action centrale elective. *Ann Med Psychol (Paris)*. 1952;110:112-117.
29. McCawley EL, Hart ER, Marsh DF. The preparation of N-allylnormorphine. *J Am Chem Soc.* 1941;63:314.
30. Clark RL, Pessolano AA, Weijlard J, et al. N-substituted epoxymorphinans. *J Am Chem Soc.* 1953;75:4964-4967.
31. Langmuir I. The arrangement of electrons in atoms and molecules. *J Am Chem Soc.* 1919;41:868-934.
32. Langmuir I. Isomorphism, isosterism, and covalence. *J Am Chem Soc.* 1919;41:1543-1559.
33. Grimm HG. Über ban und grösse der nichtmetallhydride. *Z Elekrochemie.* 1925;31:474-480.
34. Hinsberg O. The sulfur atom. *J Prakt Chem.* 1916;93:302-311.
35. Friedman HL. *Influence of isosteric replacements upon biological activity*. In: *Symposium on Chemical–Biological Correlation. Publication 206*. Vol. 206. Washington, DC: National Academy of Science; 1951:295-358.
36. Burger A. Isosterism and bioisosterism in drug design. *Prog Drug Res.* 1991;37:288-371.
37. Grisar JM, Marciniak G, Bolkenius FN, et al. Cardioselective ammonium, phosphonium, and sulfonium analogues of α-tocopherol and ascorbic acid that inhibit in vitro and ex vivo lipid peroxidation and scavenge superoxide radicals. *J Med Chem.* 1995;38:2880-2886.
38. Dodds EC, Goldberg L, Lawson W, et al. Estrogenic activity of certain synthetic compounds. *Nature.* 1938;141:247-248.
39. Walton E, Brownlee G. Isomers of stilbestrol and its esters. *Nature.* 1943;151:305-306.
40. Blanchard EW, Stuart AH, Tallman RC. Studies on a new series of synthetic estrogenic substances. *Endocrinology.* 1943;32:307-309.
41. Baker BR. Some analogues of hexestrol. *J Am Chem Soc.* 1943;65:1572-1579.
42. Larsen AA, Gould WA, Roth HR, et al. Sulfonanilides. II. Analogues of catecholamines. *J Med Chem.* 1967;10:462-472.
43. Patani GA, LaVoie EJ. Bioisosterism: a rational approach in drug design. *Chem Rev.* 1996;96:3147-3176.

Case Study

ABSORPTION/ACID-BASE CASE SOLUTION

I.

Name of Functional Group	Drug in Which Functional Group Is Present	Character: Hydrophilic or Hydrophobic	Function: ↑ Aqueous Solubility or Drug Absorption	Character: Acidic, Basic or Neutral	Function: Contributes to Ability of Drug to Cross BBB?
Aromatic hydrocarbon	Zyrtec, Tavist, Patanol	Hydrophobic	↑ Absorption	Neutral	Yes
Halogenated aromatic hydrocarbon	Zyrtec	Hydrophobic	↑ Absorption	Neutral	Yes
Alkene	Patanol	Hydrophobic	↑ Absorption	Neutral	Yes
Tertiary amine	Zyrtec, Tavist, Patanol	Hydrophobic (R) Hydrophilic (N)	↑ Absorption ↑ Solubility	Basic (pK_a = 9-11)	Yes (in un-ionized form to a limited extent via R groups)
Ether	Zyrtec, Patanol	Hydrophobic (R) Hydrophilic (O)	↑ Absorption ↑ Solubility (limited)	Neutral	Yes (via R groups)
Carboxylic Acid	Zyrtec, Patanol	Hydrophilic	↑ Solubility	Acidic (pK_a = 2-5)	No

Cetirizine is a second-generation H_1 antagonist and is purported to be nonsedating. Clemastine is a first-generation H_1 antagonist and is considered to be a sedating antihistamine. Based on the structure evaluation process, both cetirizine and clemastine contain several hydrophobic functional groups that would facilitate their passive diffusion across the blood-brain barrier. Both molecules contain an ionizable amine that will be predominantly ionized in the plasma (pH = 7.4). A key structural difference between these drug molecules is the presence of a carboxylic acid in cetirizine. This functional group is very hydrophilic and will also be predominantly ionized in the plasma (pH = 7.4) and therefore may limit the extent of absorption across the blood-brain barrier. Though both of these drugs will be predominantly ionized at pH = 7.4, it is important to remember that ionizable functional groups exist in equilibrium with their unionized forms. In the case of clemastine, it is possible that for a small fraction of time there will be some unionized drug available to cross the blood-brain barrier. In the case of cetirizine, with multiple ionizable functional groups, it is highly unlikely that the drug will exist in its un-ionized form. In order to limit the degree of drowsiness, it would be appropriate to recommend cetirizine (Zyrtec®) for this patient.

Case Study—Continued

2.

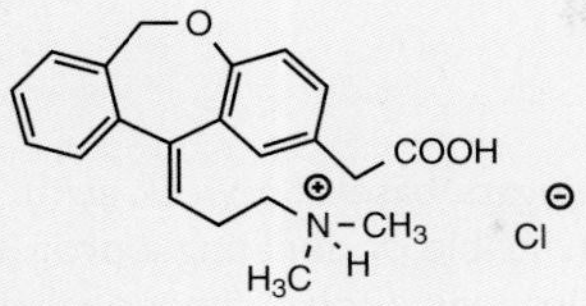

Olopatadine contains functional groups (e.g., aromatic hydrocarbons, alkene, R groups of ethers and amines) with hydrophobic character. Since hydrophobic character contributes to the ability of a drug to cross lipophilic membranes (e.g., the membranes that surround the eye) passively, then it is no surprise based on our evaluation thus far that there is the potential for this agent to be absorbed.

The next set of functional groups to evaluate are those that exist predominantly in their ionized form at physiological pH. Olopatadine contains both an ionizable amine (pK_a = 9-11) and an ionizable carboxylic acid (pK_a = 3-5) that will be predominantly ionized in the ocular fluid. These ionizable functional groups contribute to the drug's ability to be soluble in an aqueous environment, including in the aqueous eye drop formulation. These same functional groups limit the ability of the drug to be absorbed passively into the membranes of the eye.

3.

Assumptions:	pK_a (tertiary amine) = 9.5	
	pK_a (carboxylic acid) = 3.0	
	pH = 1 (stomach)	pH = 10 (intestine)
Tertiary amine (basic)	Predominantly ionized	Close to 50/50% ionized/unionized
Carboxylic acid (acidic)	Unionized	Predominantly ionized

Zyrtec: In both compartments there will be at least one ionized functional group. In the intestine roughly 50% of the time there will be two functional groups ionized that will limit the extent of absorption from this compartment. Zyrtec is probably absorbed from both sites but is probably absorbed from the stomach to a greater extent.

Tavist: Absorbed best in the intestine where it exists in its un-ionized form ~50% of the time.

4. If the truck driver takes Zyrtec at the same time that he takes his TUMs, then the pH of the stomach will be elevated to 3.5 from pH = 1. At this pH the carboxylic acid will become ionized and the extent of absorption from the stomach may be decreased to a limited extent. The truck driver may not receive the full antihistaminergic effect if he takes these two medications at the same time.

Assumptions:	pK_a (tertiary amine) = 9.5	
	pK_a (carboxylic acid) = 3.0	
	pH = 3.5 (stomach + TUMS)	pH = 10 (intestine)
Tertiary amine (basic)	Predominantly ionized	Close to 50/50% ionized/unionized
Carboxylic acid (acidic)	Close to 50/50% ionized/unionized	Predominantly ionized

Case Study

ACID-BASE CHEMISTRY/COMPATIBILITY CASE SOLUTION

1. *Acid/base evaluation of codeine phosphate:*
   Ethers—neutral
   Secondary alcohol—neutral
   Aromatic hydrocarbon—neutral
   Cycloalkenes—neutral
   Tertiary amine (in salt form)—acidic (conjugate acid of a weak base)
   Tertiary amine (as parent drug)—basic (capable of accepting a proton)
2. *Acid/base evaluation of penicillin V potassium:*
   Aromatic hydrocarbon—neutral

Case Study—Continued

Thioether—neutral
Amide/lactam—neutral
Ether—neutral
Alkane—neutral
Carboxylic acid (in salt form)—basic (conjugate base of a weak acid)
Carboxylic acid (as parent drug)—acidic (capable of donating a proton)

3. Penicillin V potassium contains several hydrophilic (polar) functional groups (amide, lactam, potassium salt of carboxylic acid) and only a moderate amount of hydrophobic character (aromatic hydrocarbon, thioether, alkane). Codeine phosphate (as parent drug) contains a tertiary amine and an alcohol that are hydrophilic in character. It contains a couple of functional groups that have mixed hydrophobic/hydrophilic character (ethers) and a fair amount of hydrophobic character (aromatic hydrocarbon, cycloalkane, alkene). In order for a drug to be water soluble it must be able to interact with water *via* hydrogen bonding or an ion/dipole interaction. Hydrophilic functional groups can typically participate in these types of interactions. Considering the structural features of both agents, Penicillin V potassium will be more water soluble due to the presence of several hydrophilic functional groups, including an ionized functional group. The ionized form of codeine is more water soluble than the free base/parent form since the ionized tertiary amine can participate in ion/dipole interactions with water (a strong interaction).
4. If these two salts are mixed in the same IV bag, then it is anticipated that the salts will dissociate in the aqueous environment. In their dissociated forms, the free forms of the drugs (Penicillin V potassium is an acid in its free form and codeine phosphate is a base in its free form) may not be as water soluble as their salt forms. Reduced aqueous solubility could result in one or both of these agents forming a precipitate. Since they are in the same IV bag, it is certainly possible that these drugs (acid + base) could form a complex (ionic). This complex is not likely to be particularly water soluble and may very well form a precipitate in the IV bag.

Case Study

ABSORPTION/BINDING INTERACTIONS CASE SOLUTION

Name of Functional Group	Character: Hydrophilic and/Or Hydrophobic	Function: ↑ Aqueous Solubility or Drug Absorption	Function: Contributes to Ability of Drug to Penetrate Skin	Binding Interactions Possible with Enzyme	Amino Acids that Could Interact with Group
Aromatic hydrocarbon	Hydrophobic	↑ Absorption	Yes	Hydrophobic Stacking interactions	Phenylalanine Tyrosine
Alkene	Hydrophobic	↑ Absorption	Yes	Hydrophobic	Isoleucine Leucine Valine Alanine Methionine
Alkane	Hydrophobic	↑ Absorption	Yes	Hydrophobic (too bulky for Van der Waals)	Isoleucine Leucine Valine Alanine Methionine
Alkyne	Hydrophobic	↑ Absorption	Yes	Hydrophobic	Isoleucine Leucine Valine Alanine Methionine

Case Study—Continued

Name of Functional Group	Character: Hydrophilic and/Or Hydrophobic	Function: ↑ Aqueous Solubility or Drug Absorption	Function: Contributes to Ability of Drug to Penetrate Skin	Binding Interactions Possible with Enzyme	Amino Acids that Could Interact with Group
Tertiary amine	Hydrophobic (R) Hydrophilic (N)	↑ Absorption (R) ↑ Solubility (N)	Yes (to a limited extent via the R groups)	H-bonding Dipole/dipole Ion/dipole Ionic	Serine Threonine Cysteine Tyrosine Glutamic acid, etc.

1. Those functional groups that are hydrophobic in character will facilitate the absorption of this medication into the skin.
2. Selection of the amino acids is based on the types of interactions that are possible with the particular functional group. With the tertiary amine it is essential to consider the ionization of this functional group prior to pairing with an amino acid. For the ion/dipole interaction it is important to determine whether the drug is participating as the ion or the dipole when coupling potential amino acids to this type of functional group.

Case Study

BINDING INTERACTIONS CASE SOLUTION

Name of Functional Group	Drugs in Which Functional Group Is Present	Binding Interactions Possible with Enzyme	Amino Acids that Could Interact with Group
Aromatic hydrocarbon	Betaxolol Salmeterol	a. Hydrophobic b. Stacking interactions	a. Phenylalanine b. Tyrosine
Alkane	Betaxolol Misoprostol Salmeterol	Hydrophobic (too bulky for Van der Waals)	Leucine
Ether	Betaxolol Salmeterol	a. H-bonding b. Dipole/dipole c. Hydrophobic	a. Serine b. Threonine c. Valine
Ketone	Misoprostol	a. H-bonding b. Dipole/dipole c. Ion/dipole	a. Cysteine b. Lysine c. Glutamic acid (in ionized form)
Secondary amine	Betaxolol Salmeterol	a. H-bonding b. Dipole/dipole c. Ion/dipole d. Ionic	a. Histidine b. Glutamine c. Cysteine d. Aspartic acid
Ester	Misoprostol	a. H-bonding b. Dipole/dipole c. Ion/dipole	a. Serine b. Threonine c. Arginine
Phenol	Salmeterol	a. H-bonding b. Dipole/dipole c. Ion/dipole d. Ionic	a. Tyrosine b. Threonine c. Cysteine d. Lysine

Case Study—Continued

Name of Functional Group	Drugs in Which Functional Group Is Present	Binding Interactions Possible with Enzyme	Amino Acids that Could Interact with Group
Primary alcohol	Salmeterol	a. H-bonding b. Dipole/dipole c. Ion/dipole	a. Glutamic acid b. Glutamine c. Arginine
Secondary alcohol	Betaxolol Salmeterol Misoprostol	a. H-bonding b. Dipole/dipole c. Ion/dipole	a. Aspartic acid b. Glutamine c. Lysine
Tertiary alcohol	Misoprostol	a. H-bonding b. Dipole/dipole c. Ion/dipole	a. Glutamic acid b. Asparagine c. Arginine

Case Study

WATER/LIPID SOLUBILITY CASE SOLUTION

Name of Functional Group	Drugs in Which Functional Group Is Present	Character: Hydrophilic and/Or Hydrophobic	Function: ↑ Aqueous Solubility or Drug Absorption
Aromatic hydrocarbon	Meclizine Fluoxetine	Hydrophobic	↑ Absorption
Cycloalkane	1,25 di (OH) Vit D_2	Hydrophobic	↑ Absorption
Halogenated aromatic hydrocarbon	Meclizine	Hydrophobic	↑ Absorption
Halogen (F)	Fluoxetine	Hydrophilic	↑ Solubility
Ether	Fluoxetine	Hydrophobic (R) Hydrophilic (O)	↑ Absorption (R) ↑ Solubility (O)
Alkene	1,25-di(OH) vit D_2	Hydrophobic	↑ Solubility
Secondary or tertiary amine	Meclizine Fluoxetine	Hydrophobic (R) Hydrophilic (N)	↑ Absorption (R) ↑ Solubility (N)
Alcohol	1,25-di(OH) vit D_2	Hydrophobic (R) Hydrophilic (OH)	↑ Absorption (R) ↑ Solubility (OH)

Case Study

INTERACTIONS/SOLUBILITY CASE SOLUTION

1.

Name of Functional Group	Drugs in Which Functional Group Is Present	Character: Hydrophilic and/Or Hydrophobic	Function: ↑ Aqueous Solubility and/Or ↑ Absorption Across BBB	Binding Interactions Possible with Target of Drug Action
Aromatic hydrocarbon	Phenylephrine Chlorpheniramine Guaifenesin	Hydrophobic	↑ Absorption	Hydrophobic stacking interactions
Halogenated aromatic hydrocarbon (Cl)	Chlorpheniramine	Hydrophobic	↑ Absorption	Hydrophobic stacking interactions Dipole-dipole
Ether	Guaifenesin	Hydrophobic (R) Hydrophilic (O)	↑ Absorption (R) ↑ Solubility (O)	H-bonding Dipole-dipole Ion-dipole
Secondary or tertiary amine	Phenylephrine Chlorpheniramine	Hydrophobic (R) Hydrophilic (N)	↑ Absorption (R) ↑ Solubility (N)	H-bonding Dipole-dipole Ion-dipole Ionic
Primary or secondary alcohol	Phenylephrine Guaifenesin	Hydrophobic (R) Hydrophilic (OH)	↑ Absorption (R) ↑ Solubility (OH)	H-bonding Dipole-dipole Ion-dipole
Phenol	Phenylephrine	Hydrophobic Hydrophilic (OH)	↑ Absorption (R) ↑ Solubility (OH)	H-bonding Dipole-dipole Ion-dipole Ionic

Functional groups that contribute to aqueous solubility are hydrophilic in character and are able to interact with water *via* hydrogen bonding or dipole-dipole interactions. If the functional group is ionizable (e.g., carboxylic acids), then the group can participate in an ion-dipole interaction with water.

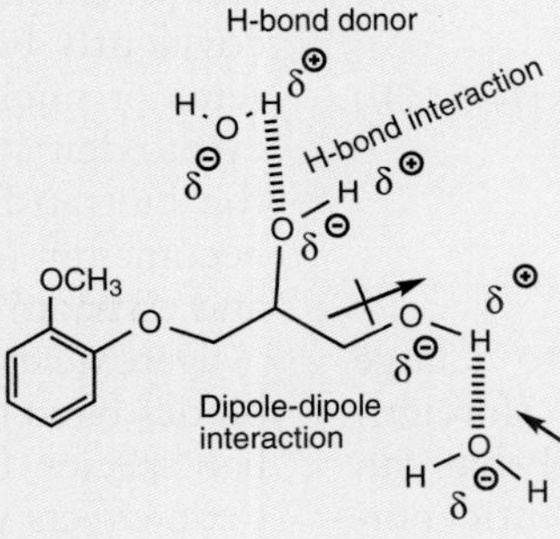

2. The agent that has the most hydrophobic character is the one that is most likely to cross the lipophilic blood-brain barrier and have an effect on the child's alertness. Of these agents, chlorpheniramine has the most hydrophobic character (see list of structural features above).

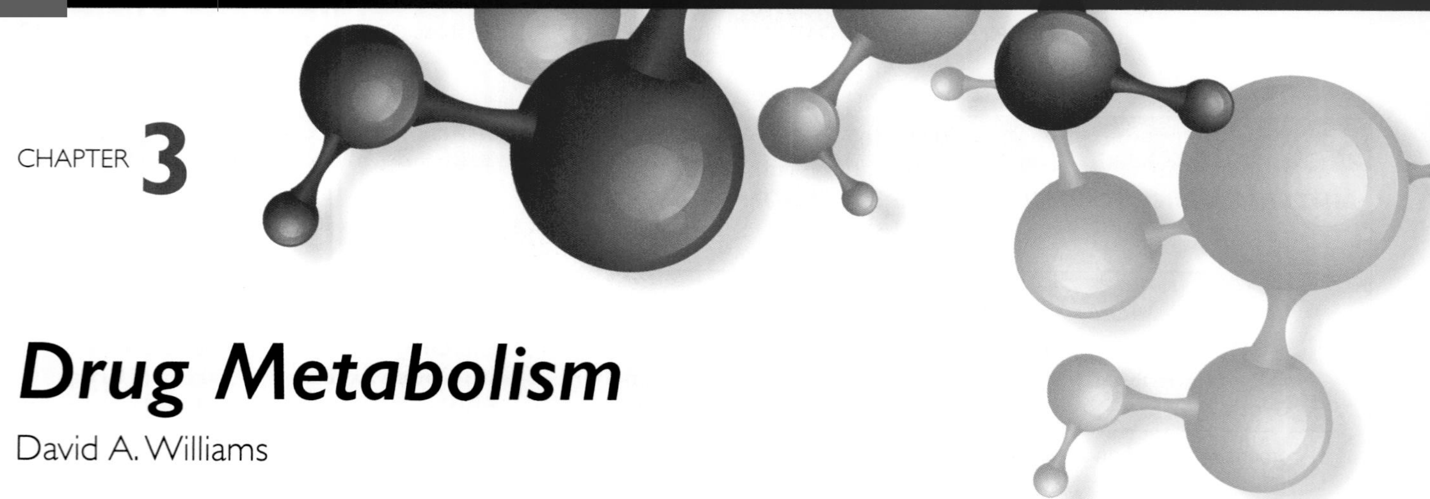

CHAPTER 3

Drug Metabolism

David A. Williams

Abbreviations

ADH alcohol dehydrogenases
AhR aromatic hormone receptor
ALHD aldehyde dehydrogenases
ATP adenosine triphosphate
CAR constitutive androstane receptor
CNS central nervous system
BBB blood-brain barrier
EHC extrahepatic cycling
EM fast or extensive metabolizer
ER endoplasmic reticulum
FAD flavin dinucleotide
$FADH_2$ reduced form of flavin dinucleotide
FDA U.S. Food and Drug Administration
FMN flavin mononucleotide
$FMNH_2$ reduced form of flavin mononucleotide
FMO flavin-containing monooxygenase
GIT gastrointestinal tract
GST glutathione S-transferases
IDR idiosyncratic drug reaction
IM intermediate metabolizer
MAO monoamine oxidase
NAT N-acetyltransferase
NAD+ nicotinamide adenine dincucleotide
NADH the reduced form of nicotinamide adenine dinucleotide
NADP+ nicotinamide adenine dinucleotide phosphate
NADPH the reduced form of nicotinamide adenine dinucleotide phosphate
P450 cytochrome P450 monooxygenase (P450 genes are in italics)
PAH polycyclic aromatic hydrocarbon
PAPS 3′-phosphoadenosine-5′-phosphosulfate
P-gp P-glycoprotein
PM poor metabolizer
ROS reactive oxygen species
SULT sulfotransferase
UGT UDP-glucuronosyl transferase
UM ultrafast metabolizer

What is a poison?
All substances are poisons;
There is none that is not a poison.
The right dose differentiates a poison from a drug.

Paracelsus (1493-1541)

INTRODUCTION

Humans are exposed throughout their lives to a large variety of drugs and nonessential exogenous (foreign) compounds (collectively termed "xenobiotics") that can pose health hazards. Drugs taken for therapeutic purposes, as well as exposures to vapors of volatile chemicals or solvents, pose possible health risks; smoking and drinking lead to the absorption of large amounts of xenobiotics with potentially adverse health effects. Furthermore, ingestion of natural toxins in vegetables and fruits, pesticide residues in food, and carcinogenic pyrolysis products from fats and protein formed during the charbroiling of meat poses additional health risks. Most of these exogenous substances undergo enzymatic biotransformations by xenobiotic-metabolizing enzymes in the liver and extrahepatic tissues and are eliminated by excretion as hydrophilic metabolites. In some cases, especially during oxidative metabolism, numerous chemical procarcinogens form reactive metabolites capable of covalently binding to critical biopolymers, such as proteins or nucleic acids, which can lead to mutagenicity, cytotoxicity, and carcinogenicity. Therefore, insight into the biotransformation and bioactivation of xenobiotics becomes an indisputable prerequisite to assess drug safety and estimate risks associated with chemicals and drugs.

Detoxication and toxic effects of drugs and other xenobiotics have been studied extensively in various mammalian species. Frequently, differences in sensitivity to these toxic effects were observed and can now be attributed to genetic differences between species in the isoenzyme/isoforms of cytochrome P450 monooxygenases (P450). The level of expression of the P450 enzymes is regulated by genetics and by a variety of endogenous factors such as hormones, gender, age, and disease, as well as the presence of environmental factors, such as inducing agents. Drugs were developed and prescribed under the old paradigm that "one dose fits all," which ignored largely the fact that humans (both adults and children) are genetically and metabolically different, resulting in variable responses to drugs and risks of drug-drug interactions.

Drugs can no longer be regarded as chemically stable entities that elicit the desired pharmacological responses and then are excreted from the body. Drugs undergo a variety of chemical changes in humans brought about by enzymes of the liver, intestine, kidney, lung, and other tissues, with subsequent alterations of their pharmacological activities, durations of activity, and toxicities. Thus, the pharmacological and toxicological activities of a drug (or xenobiotic) are, in many ways, consequences of its metabolism.

The practice of simultaneous prescriptions of several drugs has become common. Thus, an awareness of possible drug-drug interactions is essential to avoid catastrophic synergistic effects and chemical, enzymic, and pharmacokinetic interactions that can produce toxic adverse effects.

The study of xenobiotic metabolism has developed rapidly during the past few decades.[1-10] These studies have been fundamental in the assessment of drug efficacy and safety and in the design of dosage regimens; in the development of food additives and the assessment of potential hazards of contaminants; in the evaluation of toxic chemicals; and in the safety development of pesticides and herbicides and the assessment of their metabolic fates in insects, other animals, and plants. The metabolism of drugs and other xenobiotics is fundamental to many toxic processes, such as carcinogenesis, teratogenesis, and tissue necrosis. Often the same enzymes involved in drug metabolism also carry out the regulation and metabolism of endogenous substances such as steroids, vitamin D, prostaglandins, and lipids. Consequently, the inhibition and induction of these enzymes by drugs and xenobiotics can have a profound effect on the normal processes of intermediary metabolism, such as tissue growth and development, hematopoiesis, calcification, and lipid metabolism.

Familiarity with the mechanisms of drug metabolism can often aid the prediction of the consequences of drug-drug interactions, drug-food interactions, and herbal drug-drug interactions and help to explain patients' adverse responses to drug regimens. Incorporating pharmacogenomics into the selection of drug regimens will change the way in which drugs are prescribed. Selection based on a patient's individual genetic makeup could eliminate previously unpredictable responses to drug treatment caused by genetic polymorphisms that affect metabolism, clearance, and tolerance. Pharmacogenomic testing to determine a patient's phenotype (i.e., poor metabolizer) and thus, his or her ability to metabolize drugs, will become common in the future. Such knowledge will assure improved selection of proper drug regimens and doses before therapy begins.

The increased knowledge of drug metabolism, fed by the need for better safety evaluations of drugs and chemicals, has resulted in a proliferation of publications (e.g., *Drug Metabolism Reviews*, *Drug Metabolism and Disposition*, and *Xenobiotica*) and a series of monographs that present the current state of knowledge of foreign compound metabolism from biochemical and pharmacological viewpoints.[3-10]

PATHWAYS OF METABOLISM

The goals of drug metabolism are to change/terminate the physical and pharmacological properties of a drug/xenobiotic through metabolic biotransformations (and therefore its action and effectiveness), and to effectively remove these apparently chemically stable drugs from the body. The metabolite thus becomes less lipophilic, more water-soluble (hydrophilic), and possibly more easily eliminated (increased body clearance) by multiple routes (e.g., urine, feces).

To accomplish these goals, drug metabolism changes the molecular structure and shape of the drug/xenobiotic by the addition or exposure of a "handle" so that the substance no longer binds to its receptors/enzymes. The "handle" often increases molecular hydrophilicity to ensure increased water solubility by oxidation and conjugation and ensures elimination from the body by one or more routes. Common handles include alcoholic or phenolic hydroxyl groups, ionic carboxyl groups, ionic glucuronides, ionic sulfate esters, and ionic mercapturates.

The term "detoxication" describes the result of these metabolic biotransformations. Although, as a rule, drug metabolism leads to detoxication, the processes of oxidation, reduction, glucuronidation, sulfonation (sulfo-conjugation), and other enzyme-catalyzed reactions can lead to the formation of metabolites having therapeutic or toxic effects from inactive parent drugs. This process is often referred to as "bioactivation." One of the earliest discoveries of bioactivation to an active metabolite was the reduction of prontosil to the antibacterial agent sulfanilamide. Further examples of drug bioactivation to active metabolites include the hydroxylation of the peripheral analgesic acetanilide to acetaminophen, the N-demethylation of the antidepressant imipramine to form desipramine, and conversion of the anxiolytic diazepam to desmethyldiazepam. The insecticide parathion is desulfurized by both insects and mammals to form the toxic metabolite paraoxon.

Most drugs and other xenobiotics are metabolized by enzymes normally associated with the metabolism of endogenous constituents (e.g., steroids and biogenic amines). The liver is the primary site of drug metabolism, although other xenobiotic-metabolizing enzymes are found in nervous tissue, kidney, lung, plasma, and the gastrointestinal tract (GIT; digestive secretions, bacterial flora, and the intestinal wall).

Although hepatic metabolism continues to be the most important route of metabolism for xenobiotics and drugs, other biotransformation pathways play a significant role in the metabolism of these substances. Among the more active extrahepatic tissues capable of metabolizing drugs are the intestinal mucosa, kidney, and lung (see section Extrahepatic Metabolism). The ability of the liver and extrahepatic tissues to metabolize substances to either pharmacologically inactive or bioactive metabolites before they achieve systemic blood levels is termed "first-pass metabolism" or the "presystemic first-pass effect." Other metabolite reactions occurring in the GIT are associated with bacteria and other microflora in the tract. The bacterial flora can affect metabolism through: (1) production of toxic metabolites, (2) formation of carcinogens from inactive precursors, (3) detoxication, (4) exhibition of species differences in drug metabolism, (5) exhibition of individual differences in drug metabolism, (6) production of pharmacologically active metabolites from inactive precursors, and (7) production of metabolites not formed by animal tissues.

Phase I Reactions

The pathways of xenobiotic metabolism are divided into three major categories. Phase 1 reactions (biotransformations) include oxidation, hydroxylation, reduction, and hydrolysis. In each of these enzymatic reactions, a new functional group is introduced into the substrate molecule, an existing functional group is modified, or a functional group or acceptor site for Phase 2 transfer reactions is exposed, thus making the xenobiotic more polar and, therefore, more readily excreted.

Phase 2 Reactions

Phase 2 reactions (conjugation) are enzymatic syntheses whereby a functional group, such as an alcohol, a phenol, an amine, or a carboxylic acid, is masked by the addition of a new group, such as acetyl, sulfate, glucuronic acid, or certain amino acids, which usually increases the polarity of the drug or xenobiotic. Most substances undergo both Phase 1 and Phase 2 reactions sequentially.

Those xenobiotics that are resistant to metabolizing enzymes or are already hydrophilic are excreted largely unchanged. This basic pattern of xenobiotic metabolism is common to all animal species, including humans, but species can differ in details of the reaction and enzyme control.

Phase 3 Transporters

Once xenobiotics have been converted into low-toxicity and water-soluble metabolites by the combination of Phase 1 and Phase 2 reactions, these metabolites must be transported against a concentration gradient out of the cell into the interstitial space between cells, and then into the bloodstream for filtration by the kidneys. The biggest hurdle is the transport of these hydrophilic metabolites out of the cell. Charged Phase 2 metabolites will be effectively "ion-trapped" in the cell, as the cell membrane is highly lipophilic and is an effective barrier to the exit, as well as entry, of most hydrophilic molecules. In addition, failure to remove the hydrophilic products of conjugation reactions can lead to toxicity.

Consequently, an array of multipurpose membrane-bound transport carrier systems has evolved which can actively remove hydrophilic metabolites and many other low-molecular-weight drugs and toxins from cells (see Chapter 4). Thus, the term of Phase 3 metabolism has been applied to the study of this essential arm of the detoxification process. Efflux transporters transport hydrophilic substrates out of cells into interstitial fluid, blood, kidneys, and the GIT. Influx transporters transport hydrophilic substrates into cells from the bloodstream.

FACTORS AFFECTING METABOLISM

Drug therapy is becoming oriented more toward controlling metabolic, genetic, and environmental illnesses rather than short-term therapy associated with infectious diseases. In most cases, drug therapy lasts for months or even years, and the problems of drug-drug interactions and chronic toxicity from long-term drug therapy have become more serious. Therefore, a greater knowledge of drug metabolism is essential. Several factors influencing xenobiotic metabolism include:

- *Genetic polymorphism*. Genetic polymorphisms of drug-metabolizing enzymes give rise to distinct subgroups in the population that differ in their ability to perform certain drug biotransformation reactions. Polymorphisms are generated by mutations in the genes for these enzymes, which cause decreased, increased, or absent enzyme expression or activity by multiple molecular mechanisms. Individual differences in drug effectiveness (drug sensitivity or drug resistance), drug-drug interactions, and drug toxicity can depend on racial and ethnic characteristics impacting the population frequencies of the many polymorphic genes and the expression of the metabolizing enzymes. Pharmacogenetics focuses primarily on genetic polymorphisms (mutations) responsible for interindividual differences in drug metabolism and disposition. Genotype-phenotype correlation studies have validated that inherited mutations result in two or more distinct phenotypes causing very different responses following drug administration. The genes encoding for CYP2A6, CYP2C9, CYP2C19, and CYP2D6 are functionally polymorphic; therefore, at least 30% of P450-dependent metabolism is performed by polymorphic enzymes. For example, mutations in the *CYP2D6* gene result in poor (PM), intermediate (IM), or ultrarapid (UM) metabolizers of more than 30 cardiovascular and central nervous system (CNS) drugs. Thus, each of these phenotypic subgroups experiences different responses to drugs extensively metabolized by the CYP2D6 pathway ranging from severe toxicity to complete lack of efficacy (see section Genetic Polymorphism).
- *Physiologic factors*. Age is a factor, as both very young and old have impaired metabolism. Hormones (including those induced by stress), sex differences, pregnancy, changes in intestinal microflora, diseases (especially those involving the liver), and nutritional status can also influence drug and xenobiotic metabolism.

Because the liver is the principal site for xenobiotic and drug metabolism, liver disease can modify the pharmacokinetics of drugs hepatically metabolized. Liver disease affects the elimination half-life of some drugs but not of others, even if they all undergo hepatic biotransformation. Some studies have shown that the capacity for drug metabolism is impaired in chronic liver disease, which could lead to unintentional drug overdosage. Because of the unpredictability of drug effects in the presence of liver disorders, drug therapy in these circumstances is complex, and more than usual caution is needed.

Protein deficiency leads to reduced hepatic microsomal protein and lipid metabolism, and oxidative metabolism is decreased due to an alteration in endoplasmic reticulum (ER) membrane permeability affecting electron transfer. Protein deficiency would increase the toxicity of drugs and xenobiotics by reducing their oxidative P450 metabolism and clearance from the body.

- *Pharmacodynamic factors*. Dose, frequency, and route of administration, plus tissue distribution and protein binding of a drug, affect its metabolism.
- *Environmental factors*. Competition of ingested environmental substances for metabolizing enzymes and poisoning of enzymes by toxic chemicals such as carbon monoxide can alter drug and other xenobiotic metabolism. Induction of enzyme expression (in which the number of enzyme molecules is increased, while the activity is constant) by other drugs and xenobiotics is another consideration. Environmental factors can change not only the kinetics of an enzyme reaction but also the whole pattern of metabolism, thereby altering bioavailability, pharmacokinetics, pharmacological activity, and/or toxicity of a xenobiotic. Species differences in response to xenobiotics must be considered in the extrapolation of pharmacological and toxicological data from animal experiments to predict effects in humans.

DRUG BIOTRANSFORMATION PATHWAY (PHASE 1)

Human Hepatic Cytochrome P450 Enzyme System

Introduction

Oxidation, the most common reaction in xenobiotic metabolism, is catalyzed by a group of membrane-bound monooxygenases found in the smooth ER of the liver and other extrahepatic tissues, termed the "cytochrome P450 monooxygenase enzyme system" (hereafter, abbreviated as P450). P450 has also been called a mixed-function oxidase or microsomal hydroxylase. The tissue homogenate fraction containing the smooth ER is called the microsomal fraction. P450 functions as a multicomponent electron-transport system, responsible for the oxidative metabolism of a variety of endogenous substrates (e.g., steroids, fatty acids, prostaglandins, and bile acids) and xenobiotics including drugs, carcinogens, insecticides, plant toxins, environmental pollutants, and other foreign chemicals. Central to the functioning of this unique superfamily of heme proteins is an iron protoporphyrin. The iron protoporphyrin is coordinated to the sulfur of cysteine and can form a complex with carbon monoxide, resulting in a complex which has its primary absorption maximum at 450 nm (thus the title of these metabolizing P450 enzymes). P450 has an absolute requirement for NADPH (the reduced form of nicotinamide adenine dinucleotide phosphate) and molecular oxygen (dioxygen). The rate at which various compounds are metabolized by this system depends on the animal species, strain, nutritional status, type of tissue, age, and pretreatment of animals. P450 has the ability to catalyze the C–H oxidation of a wide range of structurally dissimilar functional groups. All of these reactions have a common characteristic: H atom abstraction mechanism from C–H, with the resultant formation of a hydroxyl group via oxygen rebound.[11] The same active enzyme site binds to structurally dissimilar substrates, resulting in indiscriminate substrate binding. The variety of reactions catalyzed by P450 (Table 3.1) include the oxidation of alkanes and aromatic compounds; the epoxidation of alkenes, polycyclic hydrocarbons, and halogenated benzenes; the dealkylation of secondary and tertiary amines and ethers; the deamination of amines; the conversion of amines to N-oxides, hydroxylamine, and nitroso derivatives; and the dehalogenation of halogenated hydrocarbons. It also catalyzes the oxidative cleavage of organic thiophosphate esters, the sulfoxidation of some thioethers, and the reduction of azo and nitro compounds to primary aromatic amines. A nonheme, microsomal flavoprotein monooxygenase is responsible for the oxidation of certain nitrogen- and sulfur-containing organic compounds. Substrate and inhibitor promiscuity have an impact on drug-drug interactions.

While all P450 enzymes share a common tertiary protein structure, the flexibility and functional amino acids around the active site account for the ability of P450 enzymes to accommodate a vast number of structurally dissimilar substrates and support a wide range of selective oxidations. The P450 superfamily has a remarkable adaptability (plasticity) for substrate recognition and regio- and stereoselectivity in the catalytic chemistry. This is possibly due to secondary protein structural features surrounding the P450 active site. Not only do these features differ between enzymes, but they change even between different states of individual enzymes.

The most important function of P450 is to "activate" molecular oxygen (dioxygen) to a ferric iron-oxene intermediate, permitting the incorporation of one atom of oxygen into an organic substrate molecule concomitant with the reduction of the other atom of oxygen to water. The introduction of a hydroxyl group into the hydrophobic substrate provides a site for subsequent conjugation with hydrophilic compounds (Phase 2), thereby increasing the aqueous solubility of the product for transport and excretion from the body. The P450 enzyme system not only catalyzes xenobiotic transformations in ways that lead typically to detoxication but, in some cases, in ways that lead to products having greater cytotoxic, mutagenic, or carcinogenic properties.

Components of P450

P450 consists of at least two protein components: a heme protein called P450 and a flavoprotein called NADPH-P450 reductase, containing both flavin mononucleotide (FMN) and flavin dinucleotide (FAD). P450 is the substrate- and oxygen-binding site of the enzyme system, whereas the reductase serves as an electron carrier, shuttling electrons from NADPH to P450. A third component essential for electron transport from NADPH to P450 is a phospholipid, phosphatidylcholine, which facilitates the transfer of electrons from NADPH-P450 reductase to P450.[6] Although the phospholipid does not function in the system as an electron carrier, it has a great influence on the P450 monooxygenase system. The phospholipid constitutes approximately one-third of the hepatic ER and contributes to a negatively charged environment at physiological pH.

Table 3.1 Hydroxylation Mechanisms Catalyzed by Cytochrome P450

Aromatic hydroxylation	$CH_3CO{-}NH{-}C_6H_5 \xrightarrow{[OH]} CH_3CO{-}NH{-}C_6H_4{-}OH$
Aliphatic hydroxylation	$R{-}CH_3 \xrightarrow{[OH]} R{-}CH_2{-}OH$
Deamination	$R{-}CH(NH_2){-}CH_3 \xrightarrow{[OH]} (R{-}C(OH)(NH_2){-}CH_3) \longrightarrow R{-}COCH_3 + NH_3$
O-Dealkylation	$R{-}O{-}CH_3 \xrightarrow{[OH]} (R{-}O{-}CH_2{-}OH) \longrightarrow R{-}OH + CH_2O$
N-Dealkylation	$R{-}N(CH_3)_2 \xrightarrow{[OH]} (R{-}N(CH_2OH)(CH_3)) \longrightarrow R{-}NH{-}CH_3 + CH_2O$
	$R{-}NH{-}CH_3 \xrightarrow{[OH]} (R{-}NH{-}CH_2OH) \longrightarrow R{-}NH_2 + CH_2O$
N-Oxidation	$(CH_3)_3{-}N \xrightarrow{[OH]} ((CH_3)_3{-}NOH) \longrightarrow (CH_3)_3{-}NO + H^{\oplus}$
Sulfoxidation	$R{-}S{-}R' \xrightarrow{[OH]} (R{-}\overset{+}{S}(O^-){-}R') \longrightarrow R{-}S(=O){-}R' + H^{\oplus}$

Of the three components involved in microsomal oxidative xenobiotic metabolism, P450 is important due to its vital role in oxygen activation and substrate binding. P450 is an integral protein embedded in the membrane matrix. The electron components of P450 are located on the cytoplasmic side of the ER membrane, and the hydrophobic active site is oriented toward the lumen of the ER.[6] The active site of P450 consists of a hydrophobic substrate-binding domain in which is embedded an iron protoporphyrin (heme) prosthetic group. This group is exactly like that of hemoglobin, peroxidase, and the *b*-type cytochromes. The iron in the iron protoporphyrin is coordinated with four nitrogens via a tetradentate link to the porphyrin ring. X-ray studies reveal that in the ferric state, the two nonporphyrin ligands are water and cysteine (Fig. 3.1). The cysteine thiolate ligand (proximal) is absolutely essential for the formation of the reactive ferric oxenoid intermediate. The sixth (distal) coordination position is occupied by an easily exchangeable ligand, most likely water, which is labile and readily displaced by stronger drug or xenobiotic ligands. The ferrous form loses the water ligand completely, leaving the sixth position open for binding ligands such as oxygen and carbon monoxide.

The vast array of xenobiotics presents a unique challenge to the human body to metabolize these many lipophilic foreign compounds. This makes it impractical to have one enzyme to metabolize each compound or each class of compounds. Therefore, whereas most cellular functions are normally very specific, oxidation of xenobiotics necessitates P450s with diverse substrate specificities and regioselectivities (i.e., multiple sites of oxidation). Several types of P450 enzymes can be found in a single animal species. Humans have 57 genes and more than 59 pseudogenes divided among 18 families and 43 subfamilies of P450 genes, each coding for a different version of the enzyme (isoform) so that, together, the P450s can metabolize almost any lipophilic compound to which the individual is exposed.

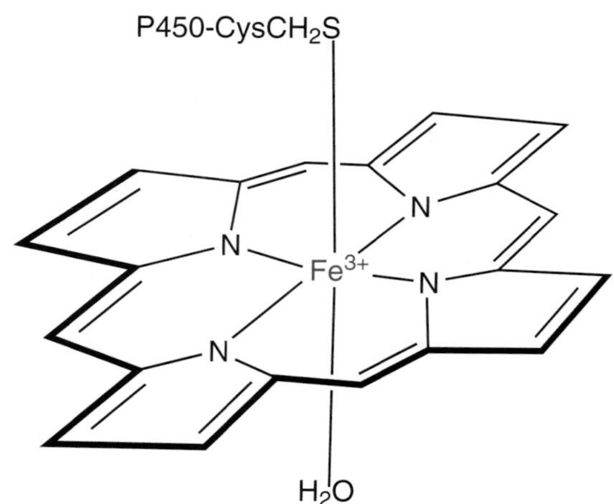

Figure 3.1 Ferric heme thiolate catalytic center of CYP450. The porphyrin side chains are deleted for clarity.

Classification of the P450 Multigene Family

Nebert et al.[12,13] classified the P450 supergene family on the basis of structural (evolutionary) relationships. P450 monooxygenases resulting from this supergene family have been subdivided into families, which possess greater than 40% amino acid homology, with subfamilies possessing greater than 55% homology.[12,13] The P450s are named with the root symbol CYP followed by an Arabic numeral designating the family (e.g., CYP1, CYP2, or CYP3), a letter denoting the subfamily (e.g., CYP1A, CYP2C, CYP2D, or CYP2E), and another Arabic numeral representing the individual gene (e.g., CYP3A4). Names of genes are written in italics. The nomenclature system is based solely on sequence similarity among the P450s and does not indicate the properties or functions of individual P450s. Of the more than 17 P450 isoforms that have been identified so far, the primary isoforms responsible for drug metabolism in the liver are presented in Figure 3.2. It is evident that the CYP3A and CYP2C families are the isoforms most involved in the metabolism of clinically relevant drugs, while the CYP1A2 isoform is predominantly involved in the bioactivation of environmental substances.

P450s initially evolved for the regulation of endogenous substances, such as the metabolism of cholesterol necessary to maintain membrane integrity, and for steroid biosynthesis and metabolism, rather than for metabolizing toxic xenobiotics. P450s are either located in the inner mitochondrial membrane and involved in highly specific steroid hydroxylations or bound to the ER of the cell and have broad substrate specificity. In evolutionary terms, P450s evolved from a common ancestor, and only more recently (during the last 100 million years) have P450 genes taken on the role of producing enzymes to metabolize a vast array of lipophilic foreign compounds. The xenobiotic P450 genes probably emerged from the steroidogenic P450s to enhance animal survival by synthesizing new P450s to metabolize plant toxins concentrated in the food chain. It is not surprising that animals and humans possess a vast array of P450 enzymes capable of handling a multitude of xenobiotics. Interindividual variation in the expression of xenobiotic P450 genes (genetic polymorphism) or in their inducibility can be associated with differences such as individual susceptibilities to cigarette smoke–induced carcinogenesis. Certain P450 isoforms that clearly exhibit genetic polymorphisms are known to metabolize (and as a rule inactivate) therapeutic agents. The extent of P450 polymorphism in humans is being investigated to determine the potential for protection against cancers. Food mutagens are typically carcinogens in tissues, but they are activated by CYP1A2 and CYP3A in the liver. Specific forms of P450 in hepatic microsomes are regulated by hormones (e.g., the CYP3A subfamily) and are induced or inhibited by drugs, food toxins, or other environmental xenobiotics (see section Induction and Inhibition of Cytochrome P450 Isoforms). Identification of a specific P450 isoform as the primary form responsible for the metabolism of a specific drug in humans permits reconciliation of the drug's toxicity and/or other pharmacological effects.

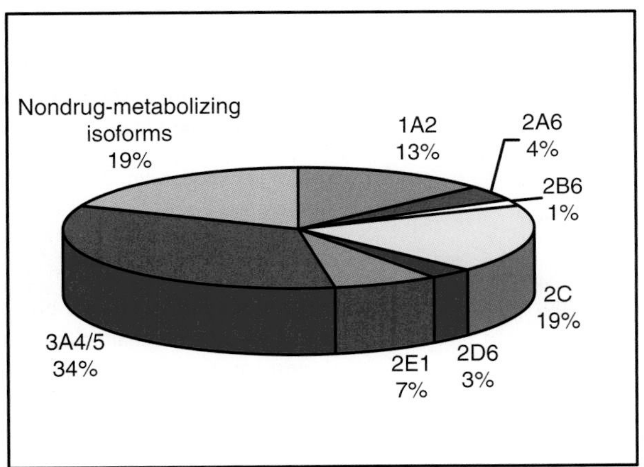

Figure 3.2 Total human CYP450 isoforms expressed in the liver that metabolize drugs.

Substrate Specificity

The substrate specificities, affinities, regioselectivities, and rates of hydrogen abstraction are probably consequences of the conformational changes resulting from ligand binding at the site of hydroxylation. Protein-protein interactions and amino acid side chains play a key role in substrate cooperativity, as well as flexible and dynamic arrangements that change depending upon the presence of substrate, cofactor, and oxidation state.[14,15] Because a primary function of these enzymes is the metabolism of hydrophobic substrates, it is likely that hydrophobic forces are important in the binding of many substrates to the apoproteins. Nonspecific binding is consistent with the multiple substrate orientations at the active site necessary for the broad regioselectivities observed. A specific binding requirement would decrease the diversity of substrates. Some P450 isoforms have constrained binding sites, thus they metabolize only small organic molecules (e.g., CYP2E1). CYP1A1/2 isoforms have planar binding sites and metabolize only aromatic planar compounds (i.e., polycyclic aromatic hydrocarbons [PAHs]). CYP2D6 exhibits high affinity for specific apoprotein interactions (hydrogen bonds, ion-pair formation) with specific substrates such as lipophilic amines. CYP3A4 has a broader affinity for a variety of lipophilic substrates with molecular weights of 200-1200 daltons. If P450 isoforms are tightly membrane bound, substrate access to the active sites is limited to compounds that can diffuse through the membranes. P450 isoforms that are less tightly bound will metabolize hydrophilic compounds.

The site of hydroxylation is determined by accessibility to, and topography of, the active site of the protein, the degree of steric hindrance encountered by substrate to the heme ferric-oxenoid species at the site of reaction, the ease of H atom abstraction or electron transfer from the compound (metabolic soft spot), and the stability of the carbon center radical, which follows the carbocation (C+) stability; tertiary > secondary > primary > CH_3.[15,16] Alkyl groups are electron donating so they neutralize the positive charge on the C+. The more alkyl substituents attached to the C+, the greater the surface area over which to spread the positive charge. The lower charge density translates to greater stability. Since the tertiary carbons are electron donating, this will stabilize a partial negative charge on an electronegative atom.

The P450s were often referred to as having broad and overlapping specificities, but it became apparent that the broad substrate specificity could be attributed to multiple isoenzymic forms of P450. The phenotype of an individual with respect to the forms and amounts of individual P450s expressed in the liver can determine the rate and pathway of the metabolic clearance of a compound (see section Genetic Polymorphism). Significant differences exist between humans and other animal species with respect to the catalytic activities and regulation of expression of hepatic drug-metabolizing P450s. These differences often make it difficult to extrapolate results of P450-mediated metabolism studies performed experimentally in animal species to humans. Caution is warranted in the extrapolation of rodent data to humans, as some isoforms are similar between species (e.g., CYP1A and CYP3A subfamilies) whereas others are different (e.g., CYP2A, CYP2B, CYP2C, and CYP2D subfamilies). The unique and diverse characteristics of the P450 ensure that predicting the metabolism of xenobiotics will be difficult.

Other P450 Isoforms

Other P450 isoforms catalyzing the oxidation of steroids, bile acids, fat-soluble vitamins, and other endogenous substances are shown in Table 3.2.

Cytochrome P450 Isoforms Metabolizing Drugs/Xenobiotics

Figure 3.3 shows the % participation of the hepatic P450 isoforms in the metabolism of drugs and xenobiotics. P450s are the most important enzymes responsible for phase 1 drug metabolism.[17] The polymorphic nature of the P450s influences individual drug responses and drug-drug interactions and induces adverse drug reactions. The crystal structures of eight mammalian P450s (CYP2C5, CYP2C8, CYP2C9, CYP3A4, CYP2D6, CYP2B4, CYP2A6, and CYP1A2) have been published. Approximately one-third of all drugs are metabolized by one isoform, CYP3A4, increasing the potential for drug-drug interactions.[17] When two drugs are metabolized by the same isoform, only one drug can serve as a substrate at a time at an individual enzyme active site, increasing the likelihood of a drug-drug interaction, especially if one drug has a low therapeutic threshold.

Family 1

CYP 1 consists of three isoforms, CYP1A1, CYP1A2, and CYP1B1, three genes, and one pseudogene. The human CYP1A subfamily has an integral role in the metabolism of estrogens and two important classes of environmental carcinogens, PAHs and arylamines (Tables 3.3 and 3.4). The PAHs are commonly present in the environment through industrial combustion processes and tobacco products. Several potent carcinogenic arylamines result from the pyrolysis of amino acids in cooked meats and cause colon cancer in rats. Environmental and genetic factors can alter the expression of this subfamily of enzymes.

Table 3.2 Other Cytochromes With Indicated Specificities and Actions

CYP450s	Activity	Location	Actions
CYP4	ω-hydroxylases		ω-Hydroxylation of fatty acids, leukotrienes, eicosanic acids
CYP5	Thromboxane A2 synthase		Arachidonic acid to thromboxane A_2 effecting platelet aggregation
CYP7A	7α-Hydroxylase		Cholesterol to bile acids formation
CYP7B	7α-Hydroxylase	Brain	Neurosteroids formation: 7α-hydroxydehydroepiandrosterone and 7α-hydroxypregnenolone
CYP8A	Prostacyclin synthase		Synthesis of prostaglandin I2 regulating hemostasis
CYP8B	12α-Hydroxylase		Catalyzes bile acid biosynthesis
CYP11A1	Steroid 20α-/22-hydroxylase	Adrenal mitochondria	Catalyzes mitochondrial steroid biosynthesis via 17-side chain cleavage of cholesterol to pregnenolone—lack of leads to feminization and hypertension
CYP11B1	11β- Hydroxylase	Adrenal cortex	Catalyzes 11-deoxycortisol to hydrocortisone or 11-deoxycorticosterone to corticosterone

Table 3.2 Other Cytochromes With Indicated Specificities and Actions (Continued)

CYP450s	Activity	Location	Actions
CYP11B2	18-Hydrolyase	Adrenal zona glomerulosa	Hydroxylates corticosterone at the 18-position leading to aldosterone
CYP17A1	17α-Hydroxylase and 17,20-lyase	ER of adrenal cortex	Production of testosterone and estrogen—lack of affects sexual development
CYP19A	Aromatase	ER of gonads, brain, adipose tissue	Aromatization of ring A of testosterone leading to estrogen—lack of causes estrogen deficiency
CYP21A1	C21 steroid hydroxylase	Adrenal cortex	17-hydroxyprogesterone to cortisol
CYP24	24-Hydroxylase	Mitochrondria	Catalyzes the degradation/inactivation of vitamin D metabolites
CYP26A1	*Trans*-retinoic acid hydroxylase		Terminates retinoic acid signal
CYP26B1	Retinoic acid hydroxylase		Catalyzes the hydroxylation of *cis*-retinoic acids
CYP26C	Retinoic acid hydroxylase		Unknown
CYP27A1	27-hydroxylase		Catalyzes the oxidation of the cholesterol in bile acid biosynthesis
CYP27B1	Vitamin D_3 1-α-hydroxylase	Mitochrondria	Activates vitamin D3
CYP27C1			Unknown
CYP39			Catalyzes the 7-hydroxylation of 24-hydroxy cholesterol
CYP46	Cholesterol 24-hydroxylase		Unknown
CYP51	Lanosterol 14α-demethylase		Converts lanosterol into cholesterol

CYP1A1. The CYP1A1 isoform (also called aromatic hydrocarbon hydroxylase) is expressed primarily in extrahepatic tissues, the small intestine, placenta, skin, and lung as well as in the liver in response to the presence of CYP1A1 inducers such as PAHs (i.e., in cigarette smoke and the carcinogen 3-methylcholanthrene), α-naphthoflavone (a noncarcinogenic inducer related to dietary flavones), and indole-3-carbinol (found in Brussels sprouts and related vegetables). CYP1A1 metabolizes a range of PAHs, including a large number of procarcinogens and promutagens (Table 3.4). Interindividual variations in the inducible expression of CYP1A1 might be related to genetic differences in aromatic hydrocarbon receptor (AhR) expression, which could explain differences in individual susceptibilities to cigarette smoke–induced lung cancer. Therefore, genetic factors appear to be important in the expression of the *CYP1A1* gene in humans and its involvement in human carcinogenesis. Women who smoke are at greater risk than men to develop lung cancer (adenocarcinoma) and chronic obstructive pulmonary disease.

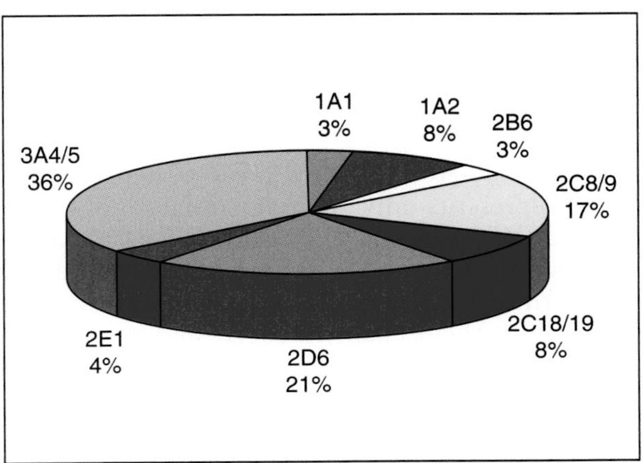

Figure 3.3 Percentage of clinically important drugs metabolized by human CYP450 isoforms.

The mechanism for induction of the *CYP1A1* gene begins with binding of the inducing agents to a cytosolic receptor protein, the AhR, which is then translocated to the nucleus where it binds to the DNA of the *CYP1A1* gene, thus enhancing the rate of transcription. The presence of the Ah receptor in hepatic and intestinal tissues can have implications beyond xenobiotic metabolism and can have a role in the induction of other genes for the control of cellular growth and differentiation. On

Table 3.3 Some Substrates and Reaction Type for Human Subfamily CYP1A2[a]
Acetaminophen (Iminoquinone)
Amitriptyline (N-demethylation)
Caffeine (N1- and N3-demethylation)
Chlordiazepoxide
Clomipramine (N-demethylation)
Clopidogrel
Clozapine
Cyclobenzaprine
Desipramine (N-demethylation)
Diazepam
Duloxetine
Erlotinib
Estradiol (2- and 4-hydroxylation)
Flutamide
Fluoroquinolones (3′-hydroxylation of piperazine ring)
Fluvoxamine
Haloperidol
Imipramine (N-demethylation)
Levobupivacaine
Mexiletine
Mirtazapine
Naproxen
Nortriptyline
Olanzapine
Ondansetron
Propafenone
Propranolol
Ramelteon
Riluzole
Ropinirole
Ropivacaine
Tacrine
Theophylline
Tizanidine
Verapamil
R-Warfarin
Zileuton
Zolmitriptan

[a]Drugs in bold italic have been reported to cause drug-drug interactions.

the other hand, CYP1A1 can metabolize procarcinogens to hydroxylated inactive compounds that are not mutagenic.

CYP1A2. The CYP1A2 isoform (also known as phenacetin O-deethylase, caffeine demethylase, or antipyrine N-demethylase) is one of the major P450s in human liver metabolizing approximately 8% of the clinically important drugs (Fig. 3.3) and catalyzes the oxidation (and in some cases the bioactivation) of arylamines, nitrosamines and aromatic hydrocarbons, the bioactivation of promutagens and procarcinogens, estrogens and other substances (Table 3.4). CYP1A2 is expressed in the liver (13%) (Fig. 3.2), intestine, and stomach and is induced by smoking and polyaromatic hydrocarbons. CYP1A2 is primarily responsible for the activation of the carcinogen aflatoxin B1 found in contaminated peanuts. CYP1A2 is subject to reversible and/or irreversible inhibition by a number of drugs, natural substances, and other compounds. The CYP1A2 gene expresses a 515-residue protein with a molecular mass of 58.3 KDa.

The CYP1A2 structure exhibits a relatively compact and planar active site cavity that is highly adapted for the size and shape of its substrates. A large interindividual variability in the expression and activity of CYP1A2 has been observed, which is largely caused by genetic, epigenetic, and environmental factors (e.g., smoking). CYP1A2 is primarily regulated by the AhR. Induction or inhibition of CYP1A2 may provide a partial explanation for some clinical drug interactions. More than 15 variant alleles of the CYP1A2 gene have been identified and some of them have been associated with altered drug clearance and response and disease susceptibility. Evidence for polymorphism of this isoform has been reported, and it is likely that low CYP1A2 activity will be associated with altered susceptibility to the bioactivation of procarcinogens, promutagens, and other xenobiotic substrates. The expression of the *CYP1A2* gene in the stomach becomes an important issue for gastric carcinogenesis, which is induced by smoking and by the metabolic activation of the procarcinogenic arylamines to mutagens.[18]

Family 2

The human CYP2 family comprises 16 isoforms, CYP2A6, CYP2A7, CYP2A13, CYP2B6, CYP2C8, CYP2C9, CYP2C18, CYP2C19, CYP2D6, CYP2E1, CYP2F1, CYP2J2, CYP2R1, CYP2S1, CYP2U1, CYP2W1, 16 genes, and 16 pseudogenes. CYP2A7 is nonfunctional.

CYP2A6. CYP2A6 has a low level of hepatic expression and represents only approximately 4% of the total of hepatic P450 isoforms (Fig. 3.3). It is also expressed at low level in lung and nasal epithelium and exhibits high interindividual variability (polymorphism). Lung CYP2A6 bioactivates many tobacco-smoke-specific carcinogens, procarcinogens, and nitrosoamines. Mutant alleles of this isoenzyme have been associated with an elevated risk for small cell lung cancer. Hepatically, CYP2A6 is the major enzyme catalyzing the 7-hydroxylation of coumarin (coumarin 7-hydroxylase) and the C5 oxidation of nicotine to cotinine (nicotine

Table 3.4 Some Procarcinogens and Other Toxins Activated by Human Cytochrome P450s

CYP1A1	CYP1A2	CYP2E1	CYP3A4
Benzo[a]pyrene and other polycyclic aromatic hydrocarbons	4-Aminobiphenyl	Benzene	Aflatoxin B1
	2-Naphthylamine	Styrene	Aflatoxin G1
	2-Aminofluorene	Acrylonitrile	Estradiol
	2-Acetylaminofluorene	Vinyl bromide	6-Aminochrysene
	2-Aminoanthracene	Trichloroethylene	Polycyclic hydrocarbons
	Heteropolycyclic amines (2-aminoquinolines)	Carbon tetrachloride	Dihydrodiols
		Chloroform	
	Aflatoxin B1	Methylene chloride	
	Ipomeanol	1,2-Dichloropropane	
		Ethyl carbamate	

C-oxidase) (Table 3.5). Other substrates include aflatoxin B1, naproxen, tacrine, clozapine, mexiletine, and cyclobenzaprineas.

In vitro studies with human microsomes and expressed human CYP2A6 have shown that selegiline and its desmethyl metabolite are mechanism-based CYP2A6 inhibitors of nicotine metabolism, and inhibition of nicotine metabolism by selegiline could increase plasma nicotine in vivo. There is overlapping substrate specificity with CYP2A13. CYP2A6 exhibits polymorphism with an incidence of 2% in the Caucasian population, a population characterized as PMs. Smokers with a defective *CYP2A6* gene smoke fewer cigarettes, implicating a genetic factor in nicotine dependence.

CYP2A13. CYP2A13 is expressed highest in nasal epithelium, followed by lung and trachea with high interindividual variability. CYP2A13 activates tobacco-smoke-specific carcinogens, procarcinogens, and nitrosoamines into DNA-altering compounds that cause lung cancer. Individuals with a high level of CYP2A13 expression could likely have an increased risk of developing tobacco-smoking-related lung cancers. Although CYP2A13 and CYP2A6 are 93.5% identical in amino acid sequence, CYP2A13 exhibits higher affinity for metabolizing tobacco smoke carcinogens than does CYP2A6. A comparison of the crystal structures of CYP2A13 and CYP2A6 has shown them to be very similar and, like CYP2A6, the CYP2A13 active site cavity is small and highly hydrophobic with a cluster of phenylalanine residues. Amino acid differences between CYP2A6 and CYP2A13 at key positions could be the cause of the significant variations observed in ligand binding and catalysis.

Table 3.5 Some Substrates for CYP2A6

Acetaminophen	Nicotine
Cisapride	Omeprazole
Clomethiazole	Pilocarpine
Cyclophosphamide	Promazine
Disulfiram	Propofol
Efavirenz	Tamoxifen
Etodolac	Tretinoin
Ifosfamide	Zidovudine
Methoxsalen	

Adapted from Di YM, Chow VD, Yang LP, et al. Structure, function, regulation and polymorphism of human cytochrome CYP2A6. *Curr Drug Metab.* 2009;10:754-780.

CYP2B6. The CYP2B6 subfamily has not been as fully characterized at the molecular level as other members of the human P450 family. This family represents less than 1% of the total of hepatic P450 isoforms (Fig. 3.2), and its level of expression in the liver is low. This enzyme exhibits polymorphic and ethnic differences in expression and therefore could be important in drug-drug interactions. CYP2B6 metabolizes approximately 3% of the clinically used drugs (Fig. 3.3) (Table 3.6). CYP2B6 also metabolizes arachidonic acid, lauric acid, 17β-estradiol, estrone, ethinyl estradiol, and testosterone and can also bioactivate several procarcinogens and toxicants. CYP2B6 is closely regulated by the androstane receptor which can activate CYP2B6 expression upon ligand binding. Pregnane X receptor and glucocorticoid receptor also have a role in the regulation of CYP2B6.

Induction of CYP2B6 may partially explain some clinically relevant drug-drug interactions observed. For example, coadministered carbamazepine decreases the blood levels of bupropion. There is a wide interindividual variability in the expression and activity of CYP2B6. Such a large variability is the result of genetic polymorphisms and exposure to drugs that are inducers or inhibitors of CYP2B6. CYP2B6 substrates are by and large small nonplanar molecules, unionized or weakly basic, highly lipophilic with one or two hydrogen-bond acceptors, and frequently active in the CNS. Phenobarbital appears to induce its formation.

CYP2C. The CYP2C subfamily is the most complex subfamily, consisting of three isoforms, CYP2C8, CYP2C9, and CYP2C19, metabolizing approximately 25% of the clinically important drugs (Fig. 3.3) (Table 3.7). The CYP2C subfamily represents approximately 20% of the total of P450 isoforms in the liver (Fig. 3.2). CYP2C8 is expressed primarily in extrahepatic tissues (kidney, adrenal, brain, uterus, breast, ovary, and intestine) and metabolizes the tricyclic antidepressants, diazepam and verapamil. Its level of expression is less than that of the other CYP2C9 and CYP2C19 isoforms.

CYP2C9 metabolizes approximately 15% of clinically relevant drugs (Table 3.7). CYP2C9, a highly polymorphic isoform, also metabolizes endogenous compounds such as

Table 3.6 Some Substrates for Human Subfamily CYP2B6

Amitriptyline	Diclofenac	Methadone	Sevoflurane
Artemisinin	Diphenhydramine	Methoxyflurane	S-mephenytoin
Bupropion	Disulfiram	Mianserin	S-mephobarbital
Carbamazepine	Efavirenz	Nevirapine	Tamoxifen
Carbaryl	Fluoxetine	Nicotine	Temazepam
Clomethiazole	Haloperidol	Prasugrel	Thiotepa
Clopidogrel	Ifosfamide	Promazine	Tramadol
Cyclophosphamide	Imipramine	Propofol	Tretinoin
Desmethylselegiline	Ketamine	Selegiline	Valproic acid
Diazepam	Meperidine	Sertraline	Verapamil

Adapted from Mo SL, Liu YH, Duan W, et al. Substrate specificity, regulation, and polymorphism of human cytochrome CYP2B6. *Curr Drug Metab.* 2009;10:730-753.

steroids, melatonin, retinoids, and arachidonic acid. Many CYP2C9 substrates are weak acids, but CYP2C9 has also the capacity to metabolize un-ionized, highly lipophilic compounds. Ligand-based and homology models of CYP2C9 have been reported which have provided insights into how its substrates are bound to the active site of CYP2C9. The resolved crystal structure of CYP2C9 has confirmed the importance of substrate specificity and ligand orientation. CYP2C9 is subject to induction by rifampin, phenobarbital, and dexamethasone, indicating the involvement of pregnane X receptor, the androstane receptor and the glucocorticoid receptor in the regulation of CYP2C9.

A number of compounds inhibit CYP2C9, which could provide an explanation for some clinically important drug-drug interactions. Tienilic acid, suprofen, and silybin are mechanism-based inhibitors of CYP2C9. Given the importance of CYP2C9 in drug metabolism and the presence of polymorphisms, it is important to identify drugs as potential substrates, inducers, or inhibitors of CYP2C9.

CYP2C19 is found primarily in the liver and intestine. The expression of CYP2C19 in the liver is less than that of CYP2C9 and also exhibits polymorphism. Differences in the DNA sequence for the *CYP2C* gene changes the enzyme's ability to metabolize substrates (i.e., PM phenotype). Because of this genetic difference in expressing CYP2C isoforms, it is important to be aware of a person's race when prescribing and/or dispensing drugs that are commonly metabolized differently by different racial populations (see section Genetic Polymorphism). This allows pharmacists to be proactive in evaluating the potential risk to patients who may be of the PM phenotype by assessing their reaction to previously prescribed CYP2C substrates and encouraging communication if the patient experiences adverse reactions. CYP2C19 (S-mephenytoin hydroxylase) is the isoform associated with the 4′-hydroxylation of S-mephenytoin. The CYP2C subfamily is apparently not inducible in humans.

CYP2D6. CYP2D6 polymorphism is the most studied P450. This enzyme is responsible for at least 30 different drug oxidations, representing approximately 21% of clinically important drugs (Fig. 3.3). CYP2D6 is only 3% expressed in the liver and minimally expressed in the intestine, and it does not appear to be inducible. Because there might not be any other way to clear drugs metabolized by CYP2D6 from the system, PMs of CYP2D6 substrates can be at severe risk for adverse drug reactions or drug overdoses. This isoform metabolizes a wide variety of lipophilic amines (Table 3.8) and is probably the only P450 for which a charged or ion-pair interaction is important for substrate binding. It appears also to preferentially catalyze the hydroxylation of a single enantiomer (stereoselectivity) in the presence of enantiomeric mixtures.

Quinidine is an inhibitor of CYP2D6 and its concurrent administration with CYP2D6 substrates results in increased blood levels and toxicities for these substrates. If the pharmacological action of the CYP2D6 substrate depends on the formation of active metabolites, 2D6 inhibition results in a lack of a therapeutic response. The competition of two substrates for CYP2D6 can prompt a number of clinical responses. For example, when substrates have unequal affinities for CYP2D6, the first-pass hepatic metabolism of a substrate (drug) with high affinity for CYP2D6 will inhibit binding of a second substrate which has a lower affinity for this enzyme. The result will be a rapid absorption of the second nonmetabolized substrate leading to a higher plasma concentration and to the increased potential for an adverse reaction or toxicity.

CYP2E1. Few drugs are metabolized by CYP2E1; however, this isoform has a major role in the metabolism of numerous halogenated hydrocarbons (including volatile general anesthetics) and of a range of low-molecular-weight organic compounds including dimethyformamide, acetonitrile, acetone, ethanol, and benzene, as well as in the activation of acetaminophen to its reactive metabolite, N-acetyl-p-benzoquinoneimine[19] (Table 3.9). CYP2E1 is of high interest because of the oxidation of ethanol into its reactive products, acetaldehyde and 1-hydroxyethyl radicals, and its ability to activate low-molecular-weight products into electrophilic reactive metabolites which result in

Table 3.7 Some Substrates and Reaction Type for Human Subfamily CYP2C[a]

CYP2C8	CYP2C9	CYP2C9 (cont.)	CYP2C19
Amiodarone	Amitriptyline	Losartan (hydroxymethyl to carboxylic acid)	Amitriptyline
Amodiaquine	Bosentan	Mefenamic acid	Carisoprodol
Benzphetamine	Buprenorphine	Meloxicam	Cilostazol
Carbamzepine	Carvedilol	*R*-Mephenytoin	Citalopram
Docetaxel	Celecoxib	Mestranol	Clomipramine
Fluvastatin	Chlorpheniramine	Montelukast	***Clopidogrel***
Isotretinoin	Chloramphenicol	Naproxen	Cyclophosphamide
Paclitaxel	Clomipramine	Nateglinide	Desipramine
Phenytoin	Chlorpropamide	Omeprazole	***Diazepam*** (N-demethylation)
Pioglitazone	Clopidogrel	Phenobarbital	Escitalopram
Repaglinide	Dapsone	***Phenytoin*** (4′-hydroxylation)	Esomeprazole
Retinol	Desogestrel	Phenylbutazone (4-hydroxylation)	Formoterol
Rosiglitazone	Diclofenac (4′-hydroxylation)	Piroxicam	Hexobarbital
Tolbutamide	***Diazepam***	Prasugrel	Imipramine (N-demethylation)
Torsemide	Diphenhydramine	***Ramelteon***	Indomethacin
Verapamil	Donepezil	Rosiglitazone	Lansoprazole
Zopiclone	Dorzolamide	Rosuvastatin	Loratadine (N-descarbethoxyation)
	Dronabinol	Sildenafil	*S*-Mephenytoin (4′-hydroxylation)
	Eletriptan	Sulfamethoxazole	*R*-Mephenytoin (N-demethylation)
	Etodolac	Sulfinpyrazone (aromatic hydroxylation)	*R*-Mephobarbital
	Fluoxetine	Suprofen	Moclobemide
	Flurbiprofen (4′-hydroxylation)	Tamoxifen	Nelfinavir
	Fluvastatin	Tenoxicam	Nilutamide
	Formoterol	Terbinafine	Omeprazole (hydroxylation)
	Glibenclamide	Tienilic acid (thiophene ring hydroxylation)	Pantoprazole
	Gliclazide	Tolbutamide (p-methyl-hydroxylation)	Pentamidine
	Glimepiride	Tolterodine	Phenobarbital
	Glipizide	Torsemide	***Phenytoin*** (ring hydroxylation)
	Glyburide	Δ^1-THC (7-hydroxylation)	Progesterone
	Halothane	Testosterone (16α-hydroxylation)	Proguanil (cyclization)
	Hexobarbital (3′-hydroxylation)	Trimethadione	Propranolol (side chain hydroxylation)
	Ibuprofen (i-butylmethyl-hydroxylation)	Valdecoxib	Rabeprazole
	Imipramine	Vardenafil	Teniposide
	Indomethacin	Valproic acid	***Thioridazine***
	Irbesartan	Valsartan	Tolbutamide
	Irinotecan	Voriconazole	***Voriconazole***
	Ketamine	*S*-warfarin (7′-hydroxylation)	*R*-Warfarin
	Lornoxicam	Zafirlukast	
		Zileuton	
		Zopiclone	

[a] Drugs in bold italic have been reported to cause drug-drug interactions.

toxicity and carcinogenicity. This enzyme then oxidizes acetaldehyde produced from ethanol to acetic acid. This isoform is only 7% expressed in the liver (Fig. 3.2) and expressed also in the kidney, intestine, and lung.

CYP2E1 is inducible under diverse pathophysiological conditions including diabetes, obesity, fasting, cancer, alcoholic liver disease, and nonalcoholic liver disease and by the chemical substances ethanol, isoniazid, and 4-methylpyrazole, among others (Table 3.9). Mitochrondrial CYP2E1 induces the formation of reactive oxygen species (ROS) which is associated with oxidative stress, lipid peroxidation, and it augments ethanol-induced hepatocellular injury. CYP2E1 is also known as the microsomal ethanol-oxidizing system, benzene hydroxylase, or aniline hydroxylase. CYP2E1 is induced in alcoholics and there is a polymorphism associated with this isoform which is most common in Chinese people. This isoform appears also to be involved

Table 3.8 Some Substrates and Reaction Type for Human CYP2D6 Isoform[a]

Alprenolol (4-Hydroxylation)	Dexfenfluramine	Lidocaine (3-hydroxylation)	Pindolol
Amitriptyline (10-hydroxylation)	***Dextromethorphan*** (O-demethylation)	Maprotiline	Promethazine (ring hydroxylation, S-oxidation, N-demethylation)
Amphetamine	Diphenhydramine (N-demethylation, ring hydroxylation, cleavege ether bond)	***Meperidine***	***Propafenone*** (4-hydroxylation)
Aripiprazole	Dolasetron (hydroxylation of indole ring)	***Methadone***	***Propoxyphene***
Atomoxetine	***Donepezil***	Methamphetamine	Propranolol (4′-hydroxylation)
Bufuralol (1′-hydroxylation)	***Doxepin***	Methoxyamphetamine (4-hydroxylation, N-demethylation)	Quetiapine
Bisoprolol	***Duloxetine***	Metoclopramide	Quinidine (hydroxylation)
Captopril	Encainide (N-demethylation, O-demethylation)	Metoprolol (O-demethylation)	Ranolazine
Carvedilol	Fenfluramine	***Mexiletine*** (4-hydroxylation and methyl hydroxylation)	Risperidone
Cevimeline	Fluphenazine	Minaprine	Ritonavir
Chlorpheniramine (N-demethylation, ring hydroxylation, deamination)	***Fentanyl***	Mirtazapine	Sertraline
Chlorpromazine	***Flecainide*** (O-dealkylation)	Morphine	S-metoprolol
Chlorpropamide	Fluoxetine(N-dealkylation)	Nebivolol	Sparteine (N-oxidation)
Clemastine	Fluvoxamine	***Nortriptyline*** (10-hydroxylation)	Tamoxifen
Clomipramine (hydroxylation)	Formoterol	Olanzapine	**Thioridazine** (aromatic hydroxylation)
Clozapine (aromatic hydroxylation)	Galantamine	Ondansetron (hydroxylation of indole ring)	Timolol (O-dealkylation)
Codeine (O-demethylation)	Guanoxan (6- and 7-hydroxylation)	***Oxycodone*** (O-demethylation)	Tolterodine (2-hydroxylation)
Cyclobenzaprine	***Haloperidol***	Paroxetine	***Tramadol*** (O-demethylation)
Darifenacin	***Hydrocodone***	Perhexiline (4′-hydroxylation)	***Trazodone***
Debrisoquine (4-hydroxylation)	Hydroxyzine (ring hydroxylation)	Perphenazine (aromatic hydroxylation)	Tripelennamine
Desipramine	***Imipramine*** (2-hydroxylation)		Tropisetron (hydroxylation of indole ring)
	Indoramin (6-hydroxylation)		Venlafaxine

[a]Drugs in bold italic have been reported to cause drug-drug interactions.

Table 3.9 Some Substrates and Reaction Type for Human CYP2E1 Isoform[a]

Acetaminophen (p-benzoquinoneimine)
Styrene (epoxidation)
Theophylline (8-oxidation)
Disulfiram
Halogenated hydrocarbons
Dehalogenation of chloroform, methylene chloride
Volatile anesthetics (fluorinated hydrocarbons)
Enflurane, halothane, methoxyflurane, sevoflurane, desflurane
Miscellaneous organic solvents
Ethanol (to acetaldehyde)
Glycerin
Dimethylformamide (N-demethylation)
Acetone
Diethylether
Benzene (hydroxylation)
Aniline (hydroxylation)
Acetonitrile (hydroxylation to cyanohydrin)
Pyridine (hydroxylation)

[a]Drugs in bold italics have been reported to cause drug-drug interactions.

in smoking-induced cancer (c.f., CYP1A2). Most of the compounds that induce CYP2E1 are also substrates for this enzyme.

The induction of this enzyme in humans can cause enhanced susceptibility to the toxicity and carcinogenicity of CYP2E1 substrates. Some evidence shows interindividual variation in the in vitro liver expression of this isoform. The mechanism of induction appears to be a combination of an increase in CYP2E1 transcription, mRNA translation efficiency, and stabilization of CYP2E1 against proteolytic degradation. The induction of CYP2E1 resulting from ketosis (i.e., due to starvation, a high-fat diet, uncontrolled diabetes or obesity) or from exposure to alcoholic beverages or other xenobiotics can be detrimental to individuals simultaneously exposed to halogenated hydrocarbons (increased hepatotoxicity because of exposure to halothane or chloroform).[20] Chronic alcohol intake is known to enhance the hepatotoxicity of halogenated hydrocarbons. Testosterone appears to regulate CYP2E1 levels in the kidney, and pituitary growth hormone regulates hepatic levels of CYP2E1.

Family 3

The human CYP3 family comprises one subfamily, four isoforms, CYP3A4, CYP3A5, CYP3A7, CYP3A43, four genes, and two pseudogenes.

CYP3A4. The CYP3A subfamily includes the most abundantly expressed P450s in the human liver and intestine (extrahepatic metabolism) (Fig. 3.2). Although CYP3A4 is responsible for approximately two-thirds of CYP3A-mediated drug metabolism, the other minor isoforms also (CYP3A5, CYP3A7, and CYP3A43) contribute.

Approximately one-third of the total CYP450 in the liver and two-thirds in the intestine are CYP3A4. This isoform is responsible for the metabolism of testosterone and more than one-third of clinically important drugs (Table 3.10) and is inhibited by a number of xenobiotics (Table 3.11). CYP3A4 appears also to activate aflatoxin B1 and, possibly, to metabolize benzo[a]pyrene. The interindividual differenes reported for metabolism of nifedipine, cyclosporine, triazolam, and midazolam are probably related to changes in induction and not to polymorphism. CYP3A4 is expressed in the intestine, lung, placenta, kidney, uterus, and brain and is glucocorticoid-inducible.

Binding to CYP3A4 is predominantly lipophilic. Drugs known to be substrates for CYP3A4 have low and variable oral bioavailabilities that might be explained by prehepatic metabolism by a combination of intestinal CYP3A4 and P-glycoprotein (P-gp) in the enterocytes of the intestinal wall (see section Presystemic First-Pass Metabolism). Therefore, it is the expression and function of CYP3A4 that governs the rate and extent of metabolism of the substrates for the CYP3A subfamily. The induction of the CYP3A subfamily by phenobarbital in humans could ultimately be responsible for many of the well-documented interactions between barbiturates and other drugs.[14,15]

CYP3A5 is the best studied of the minor CYP3A isoforms, with 85% sequence identity with CYP3A4. Approximately 20% of human livers express this isoform. The expression of CYP3A5 shows ethnic differences, with the wild-type *CYP3A5*1* allele more common in Africans than in Caucasians or Asians. In individuals who express CYP3A5, 17%-50% of the total hepatic CYP3A is this isoform. Additionally, CYP3A5 is also expressed in a range of extrahepatic tissues (kidney, small intestine, lung, adrenal glands) and is inducible via the pregnane X receptor. Both CYP3A4 and CYP3A5 exhibit significant overlap in substrate specificity but can differ in catalytic activity and regioselectivity. Results from a comparison of CYP3A4 and CYP3A5 enzyme kinetics indicate that CYP3A5 has different enzymatic characteristics than CYP3A4 in some CYP3A-catalyzed reactions. The enzyme kinetics of CYP3A5 suggests faster substrate turnover than that observed with CYP3A4.[6,7]

CYP3A7 is predominantly expressed in fetal liver (approximately 50% of total fetal CYP450 enzymes) but is also found in some adult livers and extrahepatically. CYP3A7 has a specific role in the hydroxylation of retinoic acid, 16α-hydroxylation of steroids, and hydroxylation of allylic and benzylic carbons, and, therefore, it is relevant in both normal development and in carcinogenesis.

Family 4

The human CYP450 4 family consists of 6 subfamilies and 13 CYP450 4 proteins, of which the CYP4A, 4B and 4F subfamilies have been most studied. The CYP4A subfamily (fatty acid hydroxylases) catalyzes the hydroxylation of

Table 3.10 Substrates and Reaction Type for Human CYP3A4 Isoform[a]

Alfentanyl	Clomipramine	Dronabinol	Isradipine	***Odansetron***	***Solifenacin***	Δ^1-THC
Alfuzosin	Clonazepam	Dutasteride	(aromatization)	***Omeprazole***	Sorafenib	(6β-hydroxylation)
Almotriptan	***Clopidogrel***	Efavirenz	***Itraconazole***	***Oral contraceptives/***	Steroids	Theophylline (8-oxidation)
Alprazolam	Clozapine	***Eplerenone***	***Ketoconazole***	***progestins***	Testosterone	***Tiagabine***
Amitriptyline	Cocaine	***Ergotamine***	Lansoprazole	Oxybutynin	(6β-hydroxylation)	Tinidazole
Amiodarone	Codeine	***Erlotinib***	Letrozole	***Paclitaxel***	Progesterone	***Tipranavir***
(N-deethylation)	(N-demethylation)	***Erythromycin***	***Lidocaine***	Pantoprazole	(6β-hydroxylation)	***Tolterodine***
Amlodipine	***Colchicine***	(N-demethylation)	(N-deethylation)	Pioglitazone	***Estradiol*** (2- and	(N-demethylation)
Amprenavir	Cyclophosphamide	Esomeprazole	Lopinavir	Prasugrel	4-hydroxylation)	Toremifene
Aprepitant	***Cyclosporine***	***Eszopiclone***	Loratadine	Propranolol	***17α-ethinyl estradiol***	Tramadol
Aripiprazole	(N-demethylation	***Ethinyl estradiol***	***Lovastatin***	***Quetiapine***	(2- and	***Trazodone***
Astemizole	and methyl	***Ethosuximide***	(6-hydroxylation)	***Quinidine***	4-hydroxylation)	***Triazolam***
Atazanavir	oxidation)	Etonogestrel	***Methadone***	(3-hydroxylation)	***Norethisterone***	Trimetrexate
Atorvastatin	Dapsone (N-oxide)	***Etoposide***	***Midazolam***	Quinine	(2-hydroxylation)	Valdecoxib
"Azole" antifungals	***Darifenacin***	Exemestane	(methyl	Rabeprazole	Hydrocortisone	Valproic acid
Bepridil	Delavirdine	***Felodipine***	hydroxylation)	***Ramelteon***	(6-hydroxylation)	(hydroxylation and
Bromocriptine	Desogestrel	***Fentanyl***	***Mifepristone***	***Ranolazine***	Methylprednisolone	dehydrogenation)
Budesonide	Dextromethorphan	Fexofenadine	***Mirtazapine***	Repaglinide	***Prednisone***	***Vardenafil***
Buprenorphine	(N-demethylation)	Finasteride	***Modafinil***	Rifampin, ***rifabutin***	(6β-hydroxylation)	***Verapamil***
Buspirone	Diazepam (C7	Flutamide	***Mometasone***	and related	***Prednisolone***	(N-demethylation)
Cafergot	hydroxylation)	***Fluticasone***	***Montelukast***	compounds	(6β-hydroxylation)	***Vinblastine***
Caffeine	***Dihydroergotamine***	Galantamine	Nateglinide	***Ritonavir***	Dexamethasone	***Vincristine***
Cannabinoids	***Disopyramide***	Gleevec	***Nelfinavir***	Salmeterol	***Sunitinib***	***Voriconazole***
Carbamazepine	***Diltiazem***	Haloperidol	Nevirapine	***Saquinavir***	***Tacrolimus***	***R-Warfarin***
(epoxidation)	(N-deethylation)	Hydrocodone	***Nicardipine***	***Sertraline***	***Tadalafil***	Zaleplon
Cevimeline	Docetaxel	Imatinib	(aromatization)	Sibutramine	***Tamoxifen***	***Zileuton***
Chlorpheniramine	Dofetilide	Imipramine	***Nifedipine***	***Sildenafil***	(N-demethylation)	***Ziprasidone***
Cilostazol	Dolasetron (N-oxide)	(N-demethylation)	***Nisoldipine***	***Simvastatin***	***Telithromycin***	Zolpidem
Citopram	Domperidone	***Indinavir***	Nitrendipine	***Sirolimus***	Temazepam	***Zonisamide***
Clarithromycin	Donepezil	Irinotecan	Norethindrone			
Clindamycin	Doxorubicin					

[a]Drugs in bold italic have been reported to cause drug-drug interactions.

Table 3.11 Cytochrome P450 Inhibitors[a]

CYP1A2	CYP2B6	CYP2C8	CYP2C19	CYP2C9	CYP2D6	CYP2E1	CYP3A4/5/7
Amiodarone	Amiodarone	Anastrozole	Cimetidine	***Amiodarone***	***Amiodarone***	Diethyl dithiocarbamate	***Amiodarone***
Atazanavir	Amlodipine	***Gemfibrozil***	Citalopram	Atazanavir	Bupropion	Disulfiram	***Amprenavir***
Cimetidine	Azelastine	Glitazones	Delavirdine	***Cimetidine***	Celecoxib		***Aprepitant***
Ciprofloxacin	Citalopram	Montelukast	Efavirenz	Clopidogrel	Chloroquine		***Atazanavir***
Citalopram	Clotrimazole	Nicardipine	Felbamate	Cotrimoxazole	Chlorpheniramine		***Cimetidine***
Clarithromycin	Desipramine	Sulfinpyrazone	Fluconazole	Delavirdine	Chlorpromazine		Ciprofloxacin
Diltiazem	Disulfiram	Trimethoprim	***Fluoxetine***	Disulfiram	***Cimetidine***		***Clarithromycin***
Enoxacin	Doxorubicin		Fluvastatin	Efavirenz	***Cinacalcet***		***Cyclosporine***
Erythromycin	Ethinyl estradiol		***Fluvoxamine***	Fenofibrate	Citalopram		Danazol
Ethinyl Estradiol	Fluoxetine		Indomethacin	***Fluconazole***	Clemastine		***Delavirdine***
Fluoroquinolones	Fluvoxamine		Isoniazid	Fluorouracil	Clomipramine		Diethyl dithiocarbamate
Fluvoxamine	Isoflurane		Ketoconazole	***Fluoxetine***	Cocaine		***Diltiazem***
Interferon	Ketoconazole		Lansoprazole	Fluvastatin	***Darifenacin***		***Efavirenz***
Isoniazid	Mestranol		Modafinil	***Fluvoxamine***	Desipramine		***Erythromycin***
Ketoconazole	Methimazole		Omeprazole	Gemfibrozil	Diphenhydramine		Ethinyl estradiol
Methoxsalen	Miconazole		Oxcarbazepine	Imatinib	Doxepin		***Fluconazole***
Mibefradil	Nelfinavir		Probenecid		Doxorubicin		Fluoxetine
	Orphenadrine		Ticlopidine	Itraconazole	***Duloxetine***		***Fluvoxamine***
	Paroxetine		Topiramate	Ketoconazole	Escitalopram		Gestodene
	Sertraline			Leflunomide	***Fluoxetine***		Imatinib
	Sorafenib			Lovastatin	Fluphenazine		***Indinavir***
	Tamoxifen			Methoxsalen	Halofantrine		***Isoniazid***
	Ticlopidine			***Metronidazole***	Haloperidol		***Itraconazole***
	Thiotepa			Mexiletine	Hydroxychloroquine		***Ketoconazole***
	Venlafaxine			Modafinil	Hydroxyzine		Methylprednisolne

(continued)

Table 3.11 Cytochrome P450 Inhibitors[a] (Continued)

Nalidixic acid	Imatinib	***Metronidazole***
Norethindrone	Levomepromazine	Mibefradil
Norfloxacin	Methadone	***Miconazole***
Omeprazole	Metoclopramide	Mifepristone
Oral contraceptives	Mibefradil	***Nelfinavir***
Paroxetine	Midodrine	Nicardipine
Phenylbutazone	Moclobemide	***Nifedipine***
Probenecid	Norfluoxetine	Norethindrone
Sertraline	***Paroxetine***	***Norfloxacin***
Sulfamethoxazole	Perphenazine	Norfluoxetine
Sulfaphenazole	Propafenone	Oxiconazole
Sulfonamides	Propoxyphene	Prednisone
Tacrine	***Propranolol***	***Quinine***
Teniposide	Quinacrine	***Ranolazine***
Ticlopidine	***Quinidine***	***Ritonavir***
Tipranavir	Ranitidine	***Roxithromycin***
Troleandomycin	Ranolazine	***Saquinavir***
Voriconazole	***Ritonavir***	***Sertraline***
Zafirlukast	***Sertraline***	***Telithromycin***
Zileuton	Terbinafine	***Troleandomycin***
	Thioridazine	***Verapamil***
	Ticlopidine	***Voriconazole***
	Tipranavir	***Zafirlukast***
	Tripelennamine	***Zileuton***
		Zolpidem

Data from *Stockley's Drug Interactions: A Source Book of Interactions, Their Mechanisms, Clinical Importance and Management*. 11th ed. London and Chicago: Pharmaceutical Press; 2016.

[a]P450 isoform inhibitors presented in bold italics have been associated with drug-drug interactions of clinical relevance or with drug-drug interaction warnings that can require dosage adjustment.

the terminal ω-carbon and, to a lesser extent, the ω-1 position of saturated and unsaturated fatty acids, as well as the ω-hydroxylation of various prostaglandins. The *CYP4A1*, *A2*, and *A3* genes are expressed mostly in the liver and kidney and their expression is induced by a class of chemicals known as peroxisome proliferators. Induction of CYP4A expression by fibrate antihyperlipidemic agents is due to transcriptional activation, mediated possibly via a peroxisome proliferator-activated receptor (PPAR). CYP4A gene expression is hormonally regulated. There is a close association between microsomal CYP4A1 induction, peroxisome proliferation, and induction of the peroxisomal fatty acid metabolizing system.

The CYP4A subfamily is involved in the metabolism of eicosanoic acids (e.g., arachidonic acid) leading to the formation of physiologically important metabolites involved in processes such as blood flow in the kidney, cornea, and brain. CYP4B1 is a major bioactivating factor catalyzing the formation of reactive metabolites, such as the pneumotoxin and 4-ipomeanol. The CYP4F subfamily consists of seven proteins, ω-hydroxylases which function as eicosanoid regulators. This family is responsible for inactivating the vascular effects of leukotrienes, omega-3 fatty acids, and tocopherols (vitamin E analogues).

Clearly, no one animal model or combination of animal models represents the metabolic capabilities of humans. By having a complete understanding of the factors (e.g., inducers, inhibitors, and effects of disease states) that alter the expression and activity of an enzyme responsible for the metabolism of a particular compound, and by a determination of responsible isoforms and patient phenotyping, it might be possible to predict drug-drug interactions and metabolic clearance.

An alphabetical listing of the clinically important drugs and the CYP450 isoforms catalyzing their oxidative metabolism is presented in Table 3.12.

Oxygen Activation

Elemental oxygen (dioxygen) is a relatively unreactive form of oxygen that exists as an unpaired diradical in the triplet form. Dioxygen activation by P450s requires the sequential addition of two single electrons to the P450 from NAD(P)H through the redox partners.

$$R\text{–}H + O_2 + 2\,NAD(P)H + 2\,H^{\oplus} \rightarrow R\text{–}OH + H_2O + 2\,NADP^{\oplus}$$

Table 3.12 Some Substrates for the P450 Isoforms Catalyzing Their Metabolism

Acetaminophen	1A2, 2E1, 3A4, 2C9	Caffeine	1A2
Albendazole	3A4, 1A2	Cannabinoids	3A4
Alfentanil	3A4	Carbamazepine	2C8, 3A4, 2B6
Alprazolam	3A4	Carisoprodol	2C19
Amiodarone	3A4, 2C9	Carvedilol	2C9, 2D6
Amitriptyline	1A2, 2C9, 2D6, 3A4, 2C19	Celecoxib	2C9
Amlodipine	3A4	Cevimeline	2D6
Amphetamine	2D6	Chlordiazepoxide	1A2
Aripiprazole	2D6, 3A4	Chloroquine	3A4
Anastrozole	3A4	Chlorpromazine	2D6, 3A4
Astemizole	3A4	Chlorzoxazone	2E1
Atomoxetine	2D6	Cimetidine	3A4
Atorvastatin	3A4	Cisapride	3A4
Bepridil	3A4	Citalopram	2C19, 3A4
Bisoprolol	2D6	Clarithromycin	3A4
Bosentan	2C9	Clindamycin	3A4
Bupropion	2C9, 2B6, 2A6, 1A2	Clomipramine	1A2, 2C9, 2C19, 2D6, 3A4
Busulfan	3A4	Clopidogrel	2C19, 2C9, 1A2, 3A4/5

(continued)

Table 3.12 Some Substrates for the P450 Isoforms Catalyzing Their Metabolism (Continued)

Clonazepam	3A4	Estrogens, oral	3A4
Clozapine	1A2, 2D6, 2C19, 3A4	Ethanol	2E1
Cocaine	3A4	Ethinyl estradiol	3A4
Codeine	2D6, 3A4	Etodolac	2C9
Cyclobenzaprine	1A2, 2A6, 2D6, 3A4	Etoposide	3A4
Cyclophosphamide	2B6, 2C19, 3A4	Felodipine	3A4
Cyclosporine	3A4	Fenfluramine	2D6
Dapsone	2C9, 3A4	Fentanyl	2D6, 3A4
Delavirdine	3A4	Fexofenadine	3A4
Desipramine	1A2, 2C19, 2D6	Finasteride	3A4
Desogestrel	2C9	Flecainide	2D6
Dexamethasone	3A4	Fluconazole	3A4
Dexfenfluramine	2D6	Flurbiprofen	2C9
Dextromethorphan	2D6, 3A4	Fluoxetine	2C9, 2D6, 2B6
Diazepam	1A2, 2C19, 2C9, 3A4	Fluvastatin	2C8, 2C9
Diclofenac	2C8, 2C9	Fluphenazine	2D6
Diltiazem	3A4	Flutamide	1A2, 3A4
Diphenhydramine	2C9	Fluvoxamine	1A2, 2D6
Disopyramide	3A4	Formoterol	2C9, 2C19, 2D6
Divalproex sodium	2C19	Galantamine	2D6
Docetaxel	2C8, 3A4	Glimepiride	2C9
Dolasetron	2D6, 3A4	Glipizide	2C9
Donepezil	2D6, 3A4, 2C9	Glyburide	2C9, 3A4
Dorazolamide	2C9	Granisetron	3A4
Doxepin	2D6	Halofantrine	3A4
Doxorubicin	3A4	Haloperidol	1A2, 2D6
Dronabinol	2C9	Halothane	2E1, 2C9
Efavirenz	2B6	Hydrocodone	2D6, 3A4
Eletriptan	2C9	Hydrocortisone	2D6, 3A4
Enalapril	3A4	Ibuprofen	2C9
Encainide	2D6	Ifosfamide	2B6, 3A4
Enflurane	2E1	Imipramine	1A2, 2C19, 2C9, 2D6, 3A4
Ergot alkaloids	3A4	Indinavir	2D6, 3A4
Erythromycin	3A4	Indomethacin	2C9, 2C19
Esomeprazole	2C19	Irbesartan	2C9
Estradiol	1A2	Isoflurane	2E1,.2B6

Table 3.12 Some Substrates for the P450 Isoforms Catalyzing Their Metabolism (Continued)

Isotretinoin (retinoids)	1A2, 2C8, 3A4	Nelfinavir	2B6, 3A4
Isradipine	3A4	Nevirapine	3A4
Itraconazole	3A4	Nicardipine	3A4
Ketamine	2B6, 2C9	Nicotine	2A6, 2B6, 2A13
Ketoconazole	3A4	Nifedipine	3A4/5
Labetalol	2D6	Nilutamide	2C19
Lansoprazole	2C19, 3A4	Nimodipine	3A4
Lidocaine	2D6, 3A4	Nisoldipine	3A4
Leflunomide	1A2, 2C9. 2C19	Nitrendipine	3A4
Losartan	2C9, 3A4	Nortriptyline	1A2, 2D6
Lovastatin	3A4	Olanzapine	1A2, 2D6, 3A4
Maprotiline	2D6	Omeprazole	2C19, 2C9, 3A4
Moclobemide	2C19	Ondansetron	1A2, 2D6, 2E1, 3A4
Mefenamic acid	2C9	Oral contraceptives	3A4
Mefloquine	3A4	Oxycodone	2D6
Meloxicam	2C9	Paclitaxel	2C8, 3A4
Meperidine	2D6, 2B6	Pantoprazole	2C19
Mephenytoin	2C19	Paroxetine	2D6
Mephobarbital	2C9, 2B6	Perphenazine	2D6
Mestranol	2C9	Phenol	2E1
Methadone	1A2, 2D6, 2B6	Phenobarbital	2B6, 2C9
Methamphetamine	2D6	Phenytoin	2C19, 2C8, 2C9
Metoprolol	2D6	Pimozide	3A4
Mexiletine	1A6, 2D6, 2A6	Pindolol	2D6, 3A4
Mibefradil	3A4	Pioglitazone	2C8, 3A4
Miconazole	3A4	Piroxicam	2C18, 2C9
Midazolam	3A4	Prasugrel	3A4, 2B6, 2C9
Mirtazapine	1A2, 2D6, 3A4	Pravastatin	3A4
Modafinil	3A4	Praziquantel	2B6, 3A4
Montelukast	2C9	Prednisone	3A4
Morphine	2D6	Progesterone	3A4, 2C19
Naproxen	1A2, 2C18, 2C9, 2A6	Proguanil	2C18, 2C19
Nateglinide	2C9	Propafenone	1A2, 2D6, 3A4
Navelbine	3A4	Propofol	2B6, 2C9
Nefazodone	3A4	Propoxyphene	2D6

(continued)

Table 3.12 Some Substrates for the P450 Isoforms Catalyzing Their Metabolism (Continued)

Propranolol	1A2, 2C18, 2C19, 2D6	Terfenadine	3A4
Quetiapine	3A4	Testosterone	3A4
Quinidine	3A4	Δ^9-THC	2C9
Quinine	3A4	Thiabendazole	1A2
Rabeprazole	2C19	Timolol	2D6
Rapaglinide	2C8	Tolbutamide	2C8, 2C9, 2C19
Retinoic acid	2C8	Tolterodine	2D6, 2C9
Rifabutin	3A4	Torsemide	2C9
Rifampin	3A4	Tramadol	2D6
Riluzole	1A2	Trazodone	2D6
Risperidone	2D6, 3A4	Tretinoin	2C8, 3A4
Ritonavir	2A6, 2C19, 2C9, 2D6, 2E1, 3A4	Triazolam	3A4
Ropinirole	1A2	Troleandomycin	3A4
Ropivacaine	1A2, 2D6	Tropisetron	2D6
Rosiglitazone	2C8, 2C9	Valsartan	2C9
Rosuvastatin	2C9	Valproic acid	2C9, 2A6, 2B6
Salmeterol	3A4	Valdecoxib	2C9
Saquinavir	3A4	Vardenafil	3A4
Selegiline	2D6, 2B6, 2A6	Venlafaxine	2D6
Sertindole	2D6	Verapamil	1A2, 3A4, 2C8
Sertraline	2D6, 2C19, 3A4, 2B6	Vinblastine	3A4
Sevoflurane	2E1	Vincristine	3A4
Sildenafil	2C9, 3A4	Voriconazole	2C9
Simvastatin	3A4	Warfarin	2C18, 2C9
Sufentanil	3A4	R-warfarin	1A2
Suprofen	2C9	S-warfarin	2C9, 2C18
Sulfamethoxazole	2C9	Yohimbine	2D6
Tacrine	1A2, 2A6	Zafirlukast	2C9
Tacrolimus	3A4	Zaleplon	3A4
Tamoxifen	1A2, 2A6, 2B6, 2D6, 2E1, 3A4	Zileuton	1A2, 2C9, 3A4
Temazepam	3A4	Zolpidem	3A4
Teniposide	3A4, 2C19	Zopiclone	2C8, 2C9, 3A4
Terbinafine	2C9		

The function of CYP450 monooxygenases is mostly hydroxylation of a substrate. A reactive radical-like iron oxenoid intermediate is generated that is reactive enough to split aliphatic C–H bonds, add to C–H bonds α to heteroatoms, or remove single electrons from heteroatoms to produce radical-cations. The reactive oxygen intermediate has been spectroscopically observed.[20,21]

Catalytic Cycle of Cytochrome P450: Steps of the Catalytic Cycle

Many variant CYP450 isoforms that have been isolated show a remarkable uniformity for the catalytic mechanism. The net C–H hydroxylation reaction is an insertion of oxygen with a ferric-oxenoid complex into a

C–H bond to produce an alcohol or phenol. The ease with which P450 enzymes perform hydroxylation in unreactive substrates such as hydrocarbons indicates a highly reactive enzyme intermediate capable of mediating such chemistry. A major determinant in the regioselectivity of hydroxylation is the hydrogen atom abstraction and the stability of the radical intermediate being formed.[10,20,21]

The current view illustrating the cyclic ("wheel") mechanism for reduction and oxygenation of P450 with stepwise interactions with substrate molecules, electron donors, and oxygen is shown in Figure 3.4 and can be summarized as follows.[21,22]

The catalytic P450 cycle

Step 1. The resting [Fe^{3+}-P450] complex binds reversibly with a molecule of the substrate (RH) displacing the distal water resulting in a complex resembling enzyme-substrate complex [Fe^{3+}-P450*RH]. The binding of the substrate triggers/facilitates the first one-electron reduction step from NADPH.

Step 2. The substrate complex of [Fe^{3+}-P450*RH] undergoes reduction to a [Fe^{2+}-P450*RH] substrate complex by an electron originating from its redox partner by the flavoprotein [NADPH-P450 reductase $FNMH_2$/FADH complex].

Step 3. The reduced [Fe^{2+}-P450*RH] substrate complex readily binds dioxygen as the sixth ligand of Fe^{2+} to form a [dioxy-Fe^{2+}-P450*RH] substrate complex.

Step 4. The [dioxy-Fe^{2+}-P450*RH] complex rearranges by resonance because of the strong electronegativity of O_2 to form the [Fe^{3+}-P450*RH-superoxide anion $^{\bullet}O_2^{-1}$] complex.

Step 5. The [Fe^{3+}-P450*RH-superoxide] complex undergoes further reduction by accepting a second electron from NADPH-P450 reductase to form the equivalent of a two-electron reduced [peroxy-Fe^{3+}-P450*RH] (hydroperoxide anion) complex (the step where O_2 is split into an oxygen atom). If the electron is not delivered rapidly, this complex dissociates and is aborted (uncoupled) from subsequent substrate

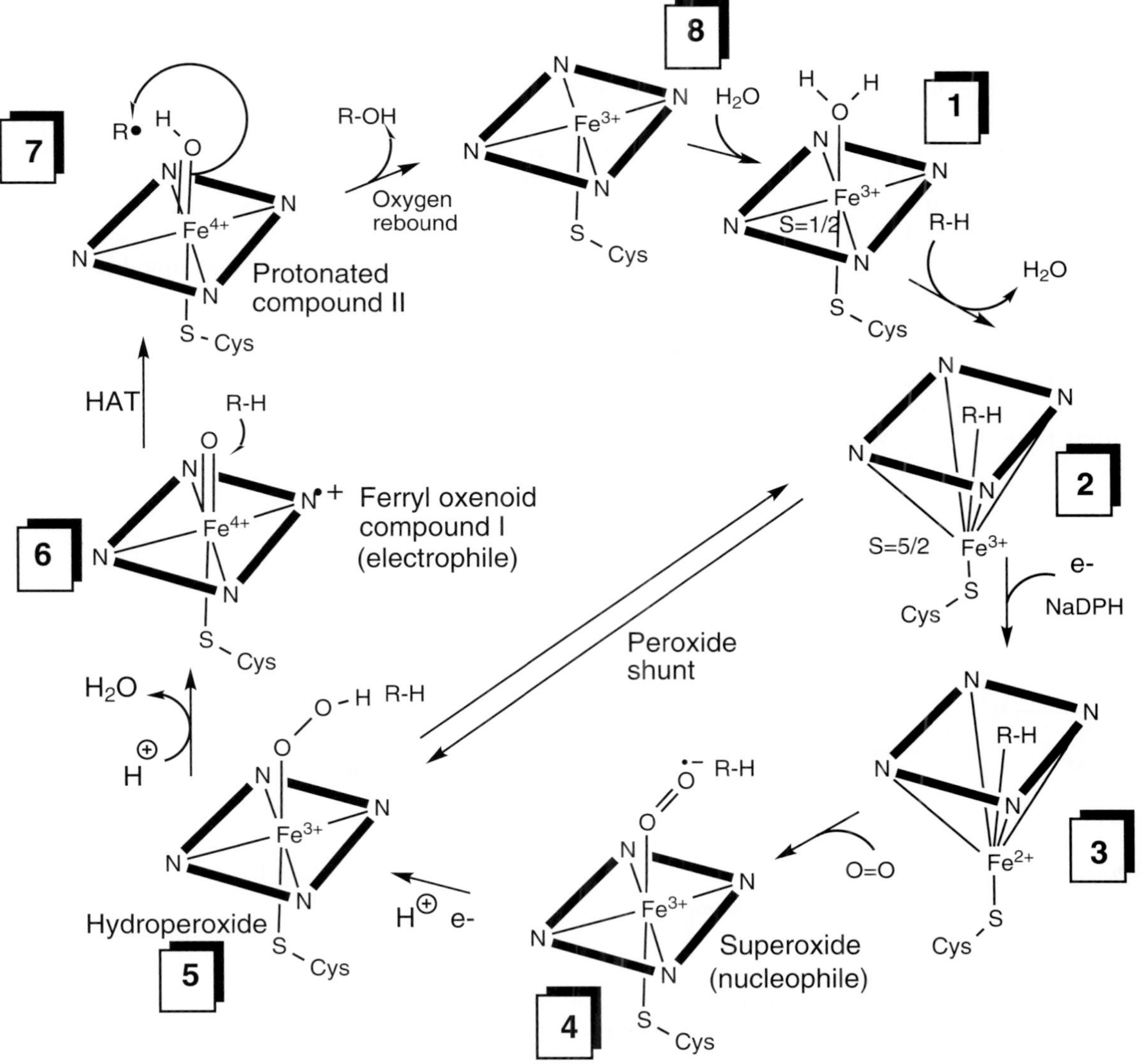

Figure 3.4 Generalized cyclic mechanism for CYP450.

hydroxylation at this step by xenobiotics which can cause release of superoxide, which decomposes to hydrogen peroxide and dioxygen with regeneration of the starting point of the cycle, the Fe^{3+}-P450 complex.

Step 6. The unstable [Fe^{3+}-peroxy-P450*RH) complex undergoes heterolytic cleavage of peroxide anion upon protonation to form water and a highly electrophilic porphyrin-radical cation intermediate (ferryl oxenoid species, Fe^{4+}=O) (Compound I, the more favorable oxygen-cysteine-porphyrin radical cation resonance-stabilized complex). The Fe^{4+}=O species represents the catalytically active oxygenation species. One role of the cysteine sulfur ligand is thought to be electron donation (push) that weakens the peroxide O–O bond, causing peroxide bond scission to produce a highly reactive and strong oxidizing intermediate (Compound I).

Step 7. Abstraction of a hydrogen atom (HAT) from the substrate (RH) by the electrophilic [Fe^{4+}=O*RH] species to produce either a carbon-centered radical, radical addition to a π-bond, or single electron transfer (SET) from a heteroatom to form a heteroatom-centered radical-cation ferryl intermediate. Subsequent radical recombination with the ferric-bound hydroxyl radical [Fe^{4+} *OH] (step 7/8, oxygen rebound) or single electron-transfer (SET, deprotonation) yields the carbon oxidized hydroxylated product (Compound II) and the regeneration of the initial Fe^{3+}-P450 enzyme complex (Fig. 3.5).[23,24]

Until the final step, the oxidizable substrate has been an inactive spectator in the chemical events of oxygen activation. None of the peroxide or superoxide intermediates in the cycle are sufficiently reactive to abstract hydrogen from the substrate. The ferryl oxenoid complex (Step 7) is a good hydrogen abstractor, even for relatively inert terminal methyl groups on hydrocarbon chains. The ferric-oxenoid complex exhibits regioselectivity in its choice of hydrogen atoms, balancing stability of the resulting carbon radical with stereochemical constraints. The reactivity of C–H abstraction depends on carbon radical stability. Some of the factors that stabilize carbon radicals include neighboring carbon atoms, neighboring carbon–carbon multiple bonds, and neighboring heteroatoms with lone pairs of electrons, e.g., oxygen, nitrogen. Carbon radicals are electron deficient and are seeking electrons and therefore are stabilized by nearby electron-donating groups. Because the inert aliphatic region of the substrate has been converted to a highly reactive radical, the process is described as substrate activation.[25]

Oxidations Catalyzed by Cytochrome P450 Isoforms

Aliphatic and Alicyclic Hydroxylations

The accepted mechanism of hydroxylation of alkane C–H bonds is shown in Figure 3.6 and has been reviewed in detail elsewhere.[25-27] The principal metabolic pathway of the methyl group is oxidation to the hydroxymethyl derivative followed by microsomal oxidation to the carboxylic acid (e.g., tolbutamide) (Fig. 3.7). On the other hand, some methyl groups are oxidized only to the hydroxymethyl derivative, without further oxidation to the acid. Where there are several equivalent methyl groups, as a rule only one methyl group is oxidized. In the case of aromatic methyl groups, the para-methyl is the most vulnerable because it is less sterically hindered.

Alkyl side chains exhibit regioselectivity and are often hydroxylated on the terminal or penultimate (secondary) carbon atoms (e.g., pentobarbital) (Fig. 3.7). The isopropyl group is an interesting side chain which is hydroxylated at the tertiary carbon and at either of the equivalent

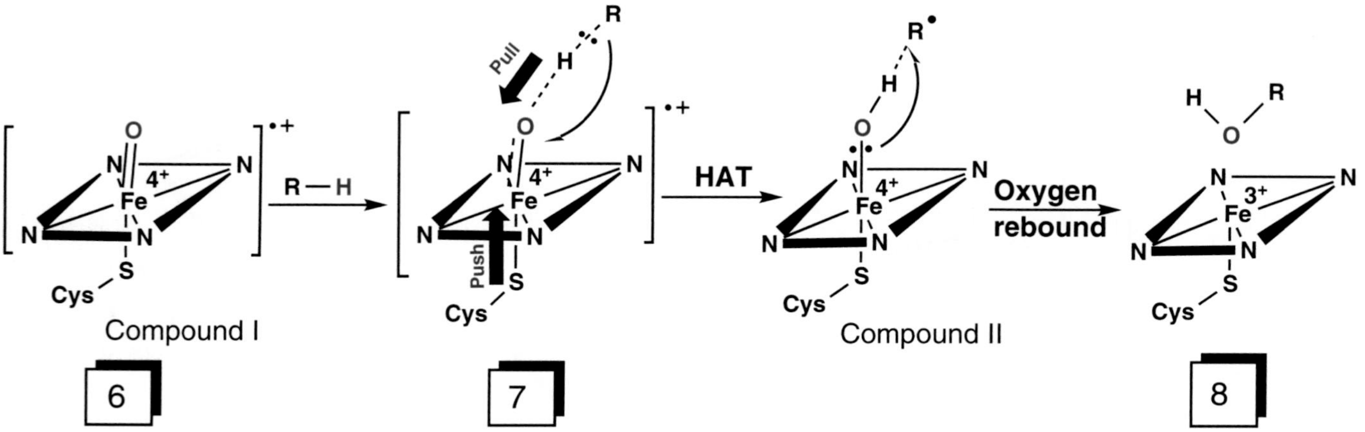

Figure 3.5 Oxygen rebound: a two step mechanism: the electrophilic ferryl oxenoid species [Fe^{4+}=O] abstracts a hydrogen (step 7) from the substrate (R–H) to give a carbon radical intermediate (R•) that recombines with the ferric-bound hydroxyl radical [Fe^{4+}·OH] (step 7/8) to give the final hydroxyl product.

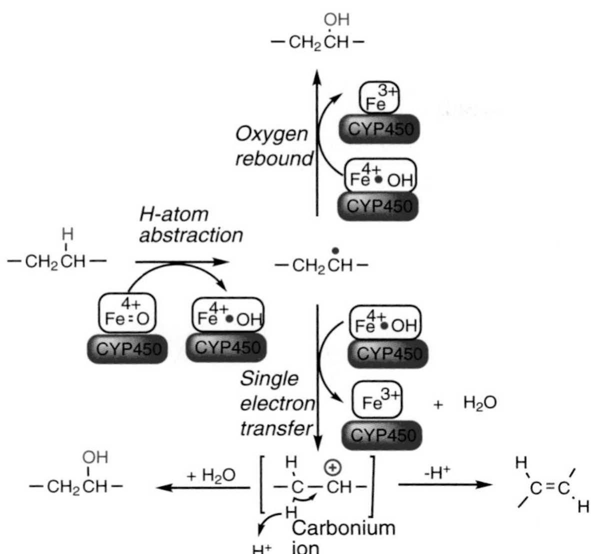

Figure 3.6 Proposed mechanisms for the hydroxylation and dehydrogenation of alkanes.

methyl groups (e.g., ibuprofen) (Fig. 3.7). Hydroxylation of alkyl side chains attached to an aromatic ring does not follow the general rules for alkyl side chains, because the aromatic ring activates the α-position of hydroxylation (Fig. 3.7). Oxidation occurs preferentially on the benzylic methylene group and, to a lesser extent, at other positions on the side chain.

The methylene groups of an alicycle are readily hydroxylated, usually at the least hindered position, or at an activated position; for example, α to a carbonyl (cyclohexanone), α to a double bond (cyclohexene), or α to a phenyl ring (tetralin). The products of hydroxylation often show regioselectivity and stereoisomerism. Nonaromatic heterocycles normally undergo oxidation at the α-carbon adjacent to the heteroatom (e.g., phenmetrazine) (Fig. 3.7).[27]

In addition to hydroxylation reactions, P450s can catalyze the dehydrogenation of an alkane to an alkene (olefin). The reaction is thought to involve formation of a carbon radical and electron transfer to the ferryl complex of CYP450, which produces a carbocation that is deprotonated to a dehydrogenated product alkene (Fig. 3.7).[27-29] An example of the ability of CYP450 to function as both a dehydrogenase and a monooxygenase has been demonstrated with the antiseizure drug valproic acid. Whereas the major metabolic products in humans are formed by β-oxidation and Phase 2 acyl glucuronidation, several alkenes are also formed, including (*E*)2-ene isomer (Fig. 3.7).[26] Presumably, the CYP3A subfamily catalyzes these reactions. The factors which determine whether CYP450 catalyzes hydroxylation (oxygen rebound/recombination) or dehydrogenation (electron transfer) remain unknown, but hydroxylation is usually favored. In some instances, the product of dehydrogenation can be the primary product (e.g., 6,7-dehydrogenation of testosterone).

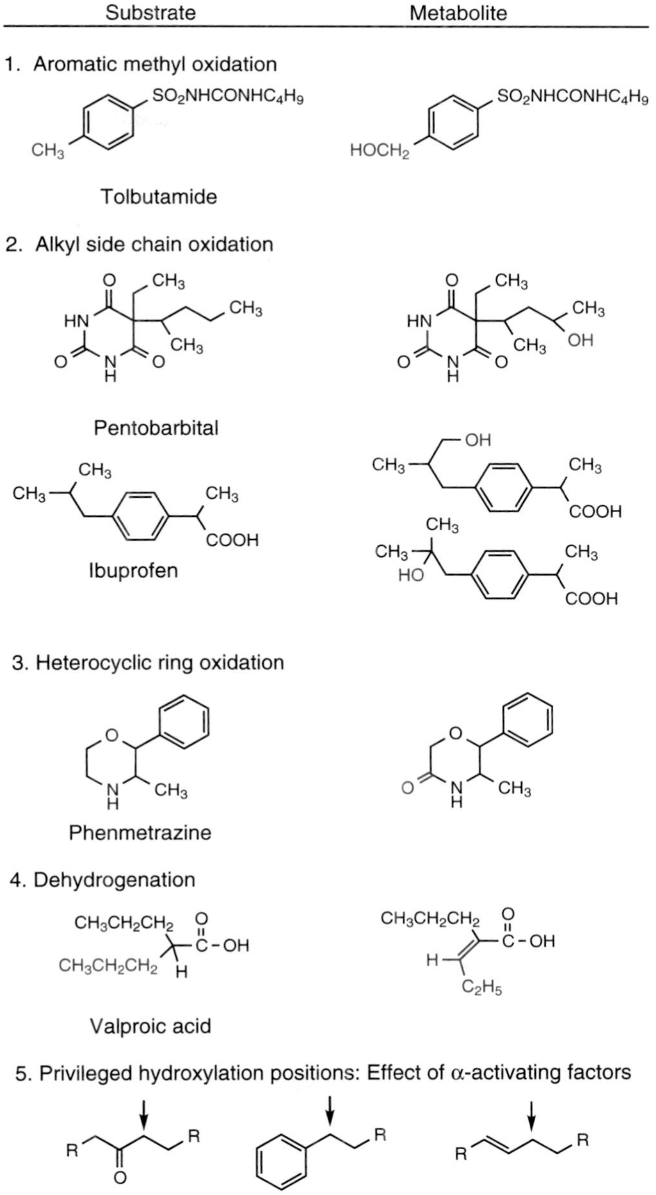

Substrate — Metabolite

1. Aromatic methyl oxidation

Tolbutamide (CH_3–C_6H_4–$SO_2NHCONHC_4H_9$ → $HOCH_2$–C_6H_4–$SO_2NHCONHC_4H_9$)

2. Alkyl side chain oxidation

Pentobarbital

Ibuprofen

3. Heterocyclic ring oxidation

Phenmetrazine

4. Dehydrogenation

Valproic acid

5. Privileged hydroxylation positions: Effect of α-activating factors

Figure 3.7 Examples of oxidative metabolism of aliphatic and alicyclic hydrocarbons catalyzed by CYP450.

Alkene and Alkyne Hydroxylation

The proposed mechanism for the oxidation of π-bonds in alkenes is a stepwise sequence of one-electron transfers between the radical complex and the ferryl oxenoid intermediate [Fe^{+4}=O], leading to alkene oxidation (Fig. 3.8).[27] Following the initial formation of an unsaturated CYP450 π-complex, the one-electron transfer either (1) yields a radical σ-complex which can collapse either to an arene or to an alkene epoxide (step a or d, Fig. 3.8), (2) undergoes a 1,2-group migration to form a carbonyl product (steps a and b, Fig. 3.8), or (3) produces a vinyl hydroxylated product (step c, Fig. 3.8) or a σ-complex which can break down to a phenol (step e, Fig. 3.8). The presence of a hydroxyl radical in the porphyrin ring allows some substrate radicals to covalently bond by

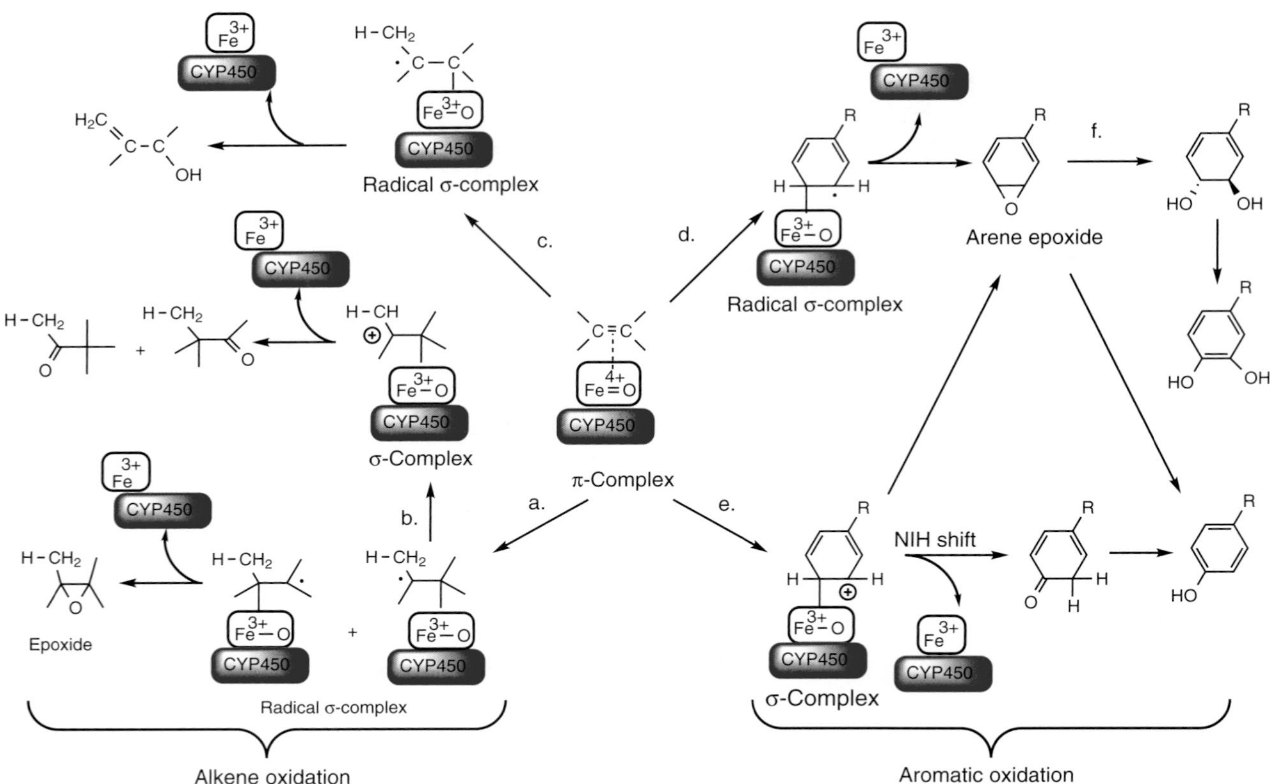

Figure 3.8 Proposed mechanisms for the oxidation of alkene and aromatic compounds.

N-alkylation of a pyrrole nitrogen rather than recombination with $(Fe–OH)^{+3}$ radical. This deviation from the normal course of reaction explains the suicide inhibition exhibited by some xenobiotics, such as the oral contraceptives, erythromycin, and paroxetine.[26,27]

The oxidation of alkenes yields primarily epoxides and a series of products derived from 1,2-migration (Fig. 3.8). The stereochemical configuration of the alkene is retained during epoxidation. The epoxides can differ in reactivity. Those that are highly reactive undergo either pH-catalyzed hydrolysis to excretable vicinal dihydrodiols or covalent reactions (alkylation) with macromolecules such as proteins or nucleic acids, which lead to tissue necrosis or carcinogenicity. Moreover, the ubiquitous epoxide hydrolase can catalyze the rapid hydrolysis of epoxides to nontoxic vicinal dihydrodiols. Several drugs (carbamazepine, cyproheptadine, and protriptyline), however, were found to form stable epoxides at the 10,11-position during biotransformation (Fig. 3.9). The fact that these epoxides could be detected in the urine indicates that these oxides are not particularly reactive and should not readily react covalently with macromolecules.

The epoxidation of terminal alkenes is accompanied by the mechanism-based ("suicide") N-alkylation of the heme-porphyrin ring. If the π-complex attaches to the alkene at the internal carbon, the terminal carbon of the double bond can irreversibly N-alkylate the pyrrole nitrogen of the porphyrin ring.[29] The heme adduct formation is observed mostly with monosubstituted, unconjugated alkenes (i.e., 17α-ethylenic steroids and 4-ene metabolite of valproic acid) (Fig. 3.9).

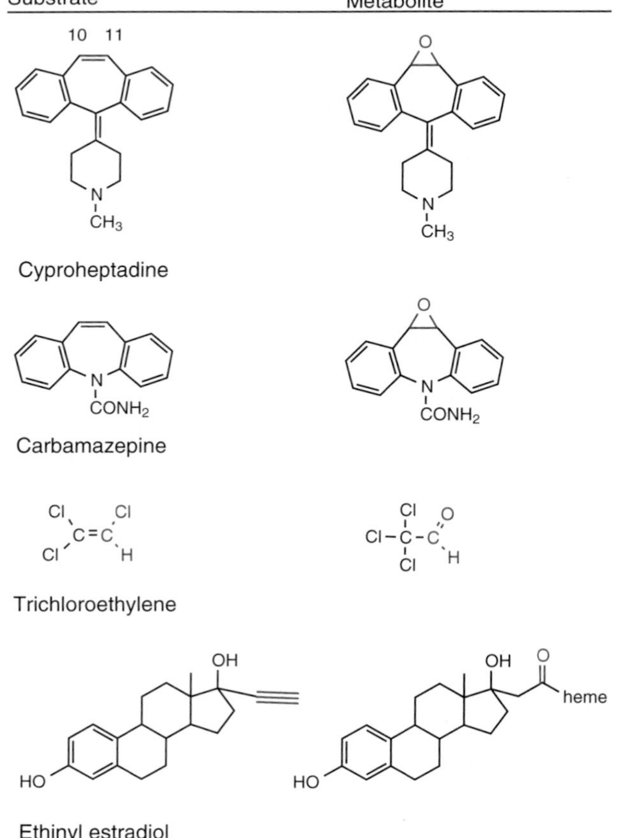

Figure 3.9 Examples of oxidative metabolism of alkenes and alkynes catalyzed by CYP450.

In addition to the formation of epoxides, heme adducts, and hydroxylated products, carbonyl products are also created. These latter products result from the migration of atoms to adjacent carbons (i.e., 1,2-group migration). For example, during the P450-catalyzed oxidation of trichloroethylene, a 1,2-shift of chloride occurs to yield chloral (Fig. 3.9).

Like the alkenes, alkynes (acetylenes) are readily oxidized, but usually faster.[29] Depending on which of the two alkyne carbons are attacked, different products are obtained. If attachment of P450 occurs on the terminal alkyne carbon, a R2 group migrates, forming a ketene intermediate that readily hydrolyzes with water to form an acid or that alkylates nucleophilic protein side chains (i.e., lysinyl or cysteinyl) to form a protein adduct (Fig. 3.10). The effect of attaching the ferryl oxygen at the internal alkenyl carbon is N-alkylation of a pyrrole nitrogen in the porphyrin ring by the terminal acetylene carbon, with the formation of a keto heme adduct (Fig. 3.11). This mechanism has been proposed for the irreversible inactivation of CYP3A4 with 17α-alkenyl steroids (i.e., 17α-ethinyl estradiol).

Aromatic Hydroxylation

In the case of aromatic oxidations (Fig. 3.8),[6,25,26] following the initial formation of an arene CYP450 π-complex, one-electron transfer yields either a π-complex or a radical σ-complex. The radical σ-complex can collapse to the arene epoxide (Fig. 3.8, step d) or the π-complex can proceed to a σ-complex followed by a NIH shift (1,2-group migration) to a phenolic product (Fig. 3.8, step e). Arene oxides are highly unstable entities and rearrange (NIH shift) nonenzymatically to phenols or hydrolyze enzymatically with epoxide hydrolase to 1,2-dihydrodiols (*trans* configuration) (Fig. 3.8, step f), which subsequently are dehydrogenated to 1,2-diphenols (catechols). The oxidation of aromatic compounds can be highly specific to individual CYP450 isoforms, suggesting that substrate binding and orientation at the active site can dominate the mechanism of oxidative catalysis.

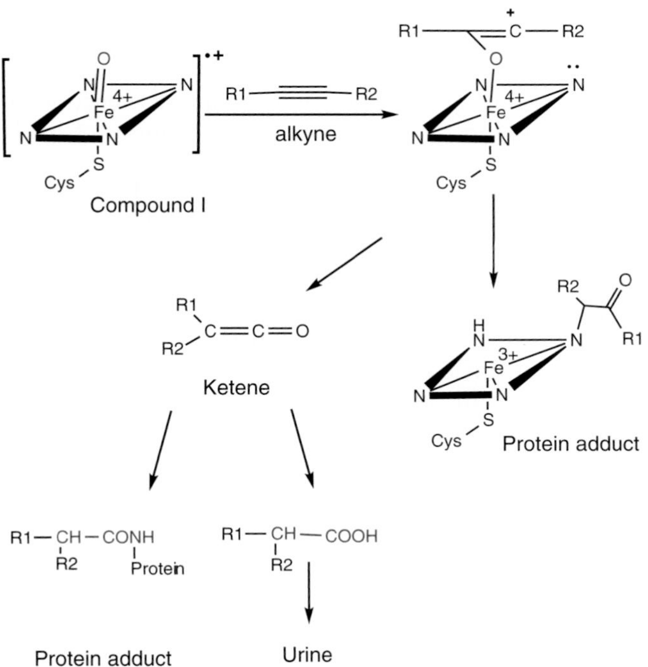

Figure 3.10 Alkyne oxidation catalyzed by CYP450.

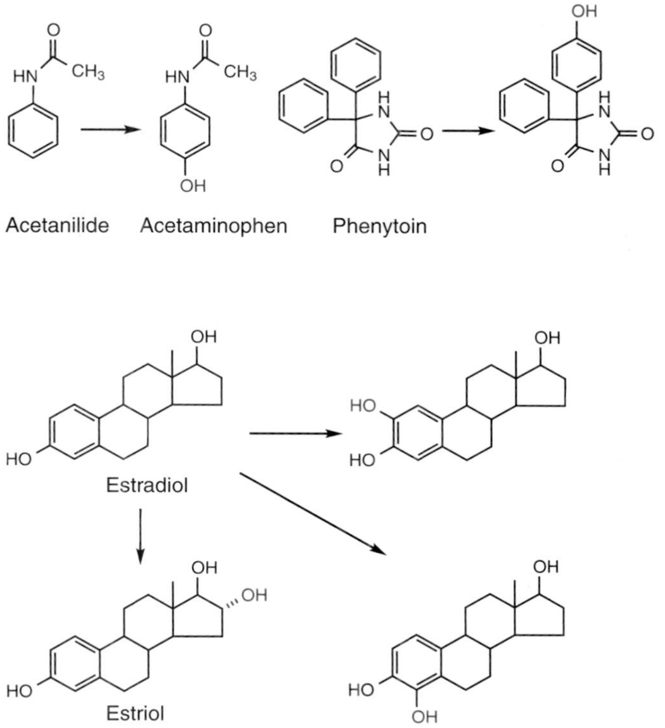

Acetanilide Acetaminophen Phenytoin

Estradiol

Estriol

Figure 3.11 Examples of oxidative metabolism of aryl compounds catalyzed by CYP450.

The metabolic oxidation of aromatic carbon atoms by P450 depends on both the isoform catalyzing the oxidation and the oxidation potential of the aromatic compound. The products are typically phenolic and the position of hydroxylation can be activated/deactivated by the type of substituents on the ring, according to the theories of aromatic electrophilic substitution (Fig. 3.8). For example, electron-donating substituents enhance *o*- and *p*-hydroxylation, whereas electron-withdrawing substituents reduce or prevent *o*- or *p*-hydroxylation. Moreover, steric factors must also be considered, since oxidation occurs mostly at the least hindered position. For monosubstituted benzene compounds, *p*-hydroxylation frequently predominates, with some ortho product also formed (Fig. 3.11). When more than one phenyl ring is present, only one ring is typically hydroxylated (e.g., phenytoin).

Traditionally, hydroxylation of aromatic compounds by P450 has been thought to be mediated by an arene oxide (epoxide) intermediate, followed by the NIH shift as discussed previously[6,26] (Fig. 3.8). The formation of phenols and the isolation of urinary dihydrodiols, catechols, and Phase 2 glutathione conjugates (mercapturic acid derivatives), implicate arene oxides as intermediates in the metabolism of both benzene and substituted benzenes. Arene oxides are also prone to conjugate with glutathione to form premercapturic acids (see section Glutathione Conjugation and Mercapturic Acid Synthesis).

The CYP1A and CYP3A subfamilies are important contributors to 2- and 4-hydroxylation of estradiol, and CYP3A4 is an important contributor to 2-hydroxylation of the synthetic estrogens (e.g., 17α-ethinyl estradiol). The principal metabolite (as much as 50%) for estradiol is 2-hydroxyestradiol, with 4-hydroxy and 16α-hydroxyestradiol as minor metabolites (Fig. 3.11). The 2-hydroxy metabolite of both estradiol and ethinyl estradiol have limited or no estrogenic activity, whereas the C4 and C16 α-hydroxy metabolites have a potency similar to that of estradiol. In humans, 16α-hydroxyestradiol (estriol) is the primary estrogen metabolite both in pregnancy and in breast cancer. The metabolites 16α-hydroxyestrone and 4-hydroxyestrone can be carcinogenic in specific cells since they are capable of damaging cellular proteins and DNA after activation to quinone intermediates.

Xenobiotic-metabolizing enzymes not only detoxify xenobiotics but also cause the formation of active intermediates (bioactivation), which in certain circumstances can elicit a multitude of toxicities, including mutagenesis, carcinogenesis, and hepatic necrosis.[29,30] In addition to glutathione, some nucleophiles such as other sulfhydryl compounds (most effective), alcohols, and phosphates can react with arene oxides. Many of these nucleophiles are found in proteins and nucleic acids. The covalent binding of these bioactive epoxides to intracellular macromolecules provides a molecular basis of these toxic effects (see the discussion of toxicity due to oxidative metabolism).

N-*Dealkylation, Oxidative Deamination, and* N-*Oxidation*

The accepted mechanism of oxidative N-, O-, and S-dealkylations involves two competing mechanisms: single electron transfer (SET) or hydrogen atom abstraction (HAT) (Fig. 3.12).[6,25,26] Heteroatom-containing substrates most commonly undergo hydroxylation adjacent (α) to the heteroatom, as compared to other positions. Reactions of this type include N-, O-, and S-dealkylations as well as dehydrohalogenations and oxidative deamination reactions. The SET pathway involves abstraction of an electron from the heteroatom to produce a radical cation, while the HAT pathway involves hydrogen abstraction. Both pathways are followed by the loss of the α-proton from the more labile α carbon to generate a carbon radical which can recombine with the ferric hydroxyl radical intermediate (oxygen rebound) to generate an unstable geminal hydroxy heteroatom-substituted intermediate (e.g., carbinolamine, halohydrin, hemiacetal, hemiketal, or hemithioketal) that breaks down, releasing the dealkylated heteroatom and forming a carbonyl compound. The resultant carbon radical is stabilized by the heteroatom. However, if the recombination reaction with the ferric hydroxyl radical intermediate (oxygen rebound) is faster than the deprotonation of the α-proton from the adjacent α-carbon, the oxidation will simply result in oxidation of the heteroatom, as in the formation of N-oxides or oxidation of sulfides to sulfoxides and/or sulfones. Therefore, whether N-dealkylation metabolism occurs by HAT or SET depends on the substrate.

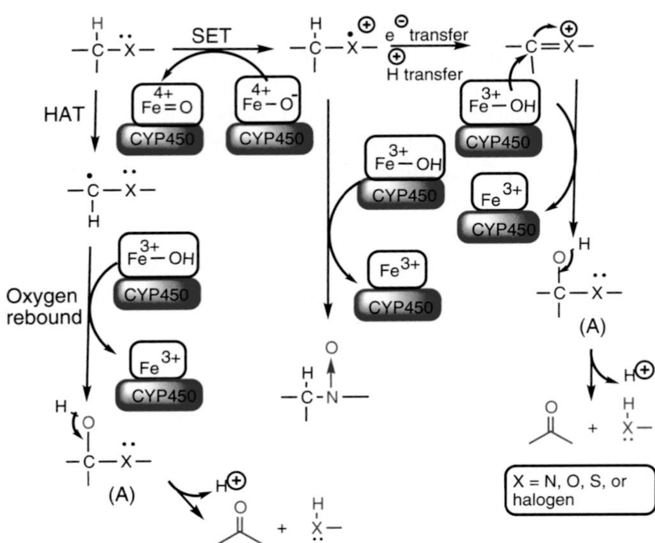

Figure 3.12 Proposed mechanism for heteroatom-compound oxidation, dealkylation, and dehalogenation.

Xenobiotics containing heteroatoms (N and S) can also be metabolized by heteroatom oxidation to their corresponding heteroatom oxides (tertiary amines to N-oxides, sulfides to sulfoxides and/or sulfones). Heteroatom oxidation can also be attributed to a microsomal flavin-containing monooxygenase (FMO). As is the case with heteroatom α-hydroxylation, one-electron oxidation of the heteroatom occurs as the first step to form the heteroatom ferric-hydroxide radical intermediate. This reaction is favored by the absence of α-hydrogens and by the stability of the heteroatom radical-cation, which cannot lose a proton, and collapses to generate the heteroatom oxide.

N-DEALKYLATION.

Dealkylation of secondary and tertiary amines to yield primary and secondary amines, respectively, is one of the most important and frequently encountered reactions in drug metabolism.[25,26] The proposed mechanism of oxidative N-dealkylation involves α-hydrogen abstraction or an electron abstraction from the nitrogen by the ferryl oxenoid and has been previously discussed (Fig. 3.12).

Typical N-substituents removed by oxidative dealkylation are methyl, ethyl, *n*-propyl, isopropyl, *n*-butyl, allyl, and benzyl. Dealkylation occurs most readily with a smaller alkyl group. Substituents that are more resistant to dealkylation include *t*-butyl (no α-hydrogen) and cyclopropylmethyl. In general, tertiary amines are dealkylated to secondary amines faster than secondary amines are dealkylated to primary amines. This rate difference has been correlated with lipid solubility. Appreciable amounts of secondary and primary amines accumulate as metabolites which are more polar than the parent amine, thus slowing the rate at which the amines diffuse across membranes and reducing their accessibility to receptors. Frequently, these amine metabolites contribute to the pharmacological activity of the parent substance (e.g., imipramine) (Fig. 3.13), or they produce unwanted side effects, such as hypertension that results from the N-dealkylation of N-isopropylmethoxamine to methoxamine. The design of an analogous drug without these unwanted metabolites can be achieved by proper choice of replacement substituents, such as substitution of the N-isopropyl group in N-isopropylmethoxamine with a tert-butyl (N-tert-butylmethoxamine or butoxamine).

N-dealkylation of substituted amides and aromatic amines occurs in a similar manner to aliphatic amines. N-substituted nonaromatic nitrogen heterocycles undergo oxidation on the α-carbon to a lactam (e.g., nicotine to cotinine) as well as N-dealkylation (e.g., nicotine to nornicotine, cotinine, and norcotinine) (Fig. 3.13).

OXIDATIVE DEAMINATION. The mechanism of oxidative deamination follows a pathway similar to that of N-dealkylation. Initially, oxidation to the imminium ion occurs, followed by decomposition to the carbonyl metabolite and ammonia. Oxidative deamination can occur with α-substituted amines, exemplified by amphetamine (Fig. 3.13). Disubstitution of the α-carbon inhibits deamination

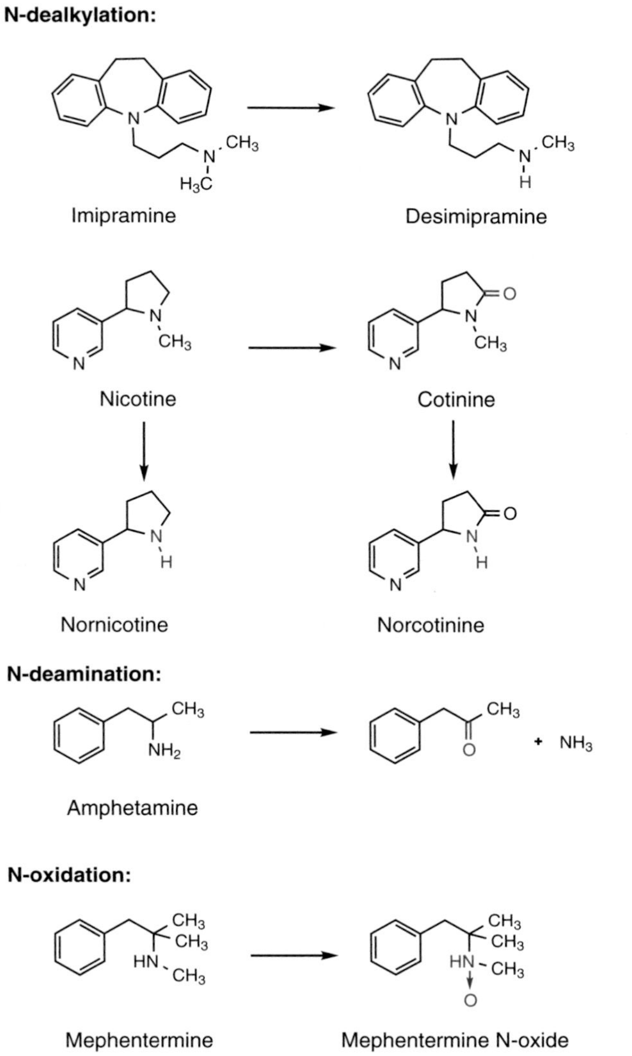

N-dealkylation:

Imipramine → Desimipramine

Nicotine → Cotinine

Nornicotine, Norcotinine

N-deamination:

Amphetamine → + NH_3

N-oxidation:

Mephentermine → Mephentermine N-oxide

Figure 3.13 Examples of N-dealkylation, oxidative deamination, and N-oxidation reactions catalyzed by CYP450.

(e.g., phentermine). Some secondary and tertiary amines, as well as amines substituted with bulky groups, can undergo deamination directly without N-dealkylation (e.g., fenfluramine). Apparently, this behavior is associated with increased lipid solubility.

N-OXIDATION.

In general, N-oxygenation of amines forms stable N-oxides with tertiary amines and amides and hydroxylamines with primary and secondary amines. This reaction predominates when no α-protons are available (e.g., mephentermine and arylamines) (Fig. 3.13). Tertiary amines having one or more hydrogens on the adjacent carbon dealkylate via the N-oxide. Rearrangement of the N-oxide forms a carbinolamine, which subsequently collapses to produce the secondary amine. Amine metabolites can be N-conjugated, increasing their rate of excretion.

O- AND S-DEALKYLATION.

Oxidative O-dealkylation of ethers is a common metabolic reaction with a mechanism analogous to N-dealkylation; oxidation of the α-carbon and subsequent decomposition of the unstable hemiacetal to an alcohol (or phenol) and a carbonyl product. S-dealkylation of thioethers to hemithioacetals is a minor pathway in comparison to the major direct CYP450 oxidation of sulfur to sulfoxides and/or sulfones.

The majority of ether groups in drug molecules are aromatic ethers (e.g., codeine, prazocin, and verapamil). For example, codeine is O-demethylated to morphine (Fig. 3.14). The rate of O-dealkylation is a function of chain length (i.e., increasing chain length or branching reduces the rate of dealkylation). Steric factors and aromatic ring substituents influence the rate of dealkylation but are complicated by electronic effects. Some drug molecules contain more than one ether group, in which case, only one ether is dealkylated. The methylenedioxy group undergoes variable rates of dealkylation to the 1,2-diphenolic metabolite. Metabolism of such a group is also being capable of forming a stable complex with (and inhibiting) CYP450.

By analogy to O- and N-dealkylations, esters and amides can also be oxidized by CYP450. In these reactions, the carbon next to the ether oxygen of an ester or the nitrogen of an amide (termed the α-carbon) is attacked by the enzyme. This reaction is minor due to the significantly more common hydrolysis of esters and amides.

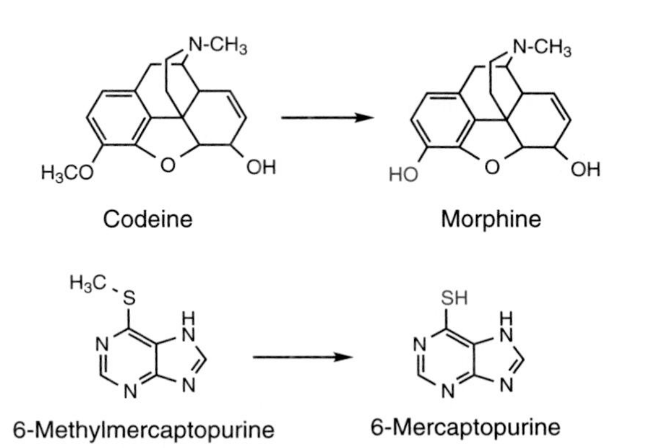

Codeine → Morphine

6-Methylmercaptopurine → 6-Mercaptopurine

Figure 3.14 Examples of O- and S-dealkylations catalyzed by CYP450.

Aliphatic and aromatic methyl thioethers undergo S-dealkylation to thiols and carbonyl compounds. For example, 6-methylthiopurine is demethylated to give the active anticancer drug 6-mercaptopurine (Fig. 3.14). Other thioethers are oxidized to sulfoxides or sulfones (see N- and S-oxidations).

Oxidative Dehalogenation

Many halogenated hydrocarbons, such as insecticides, pesticides, general anesthetics, plasticizers, flame retardants, and commercial solvents, undergo a variety of different dehalogenation biotransformations.[31,32] Because of our potential exposure to these halogenated compounds as drugs and environmental pollutants in air, soil, water, or food, it is important to understand the interactions between metabolism and toxicity.

When the carbon bearing the halogen also contains a hydrogen, carbon-centered hydroxylation (C–OH) occurs. The hydroxylated products are unstable and react with loss of the halogen to give an aldehyde or a ketone. Halogenated hydrocarbons differ in their chemical reactivity because of the electron-withdrawing properties of the halogens on adjacent carbon atoms, resulting in the α-carbon developing electrophilic character that promotes carbon-centered oxidation (C–OH). The halogen atoms also have the ability to stabilize α-carbon cations, free radicals, carbanions, and carbenes. If other halogens are also present in the molecule, then acyl halides result (Fig. 3.12). Acyl halides can react with macromolecules (protein) and cause hepatotoxicity or immunogenicity. These acyl halides have been implicated in the toxicity of chloroform and halothane. Some halogenated hydrocarbons form glutathione or mercapturic acid conjugates, whereas others undergo oxidative dehydrohalogenation (elimination of hydrogen halide) and reductive dehalogenation catalyzed by CYP2E1. In many cases, reactive intermediates, including radicals, anions, and cations, are produced that can react with a variety of molecules in tissues, resulting in hepatotoxicity or immunogenicity.

Oxidative dehydrohalogenation is a common metabolic pathway of many halogenated hydrocarbons. P450-catalyzed oxidative dehydrohalogenation generates the transient *gem*-halohydrin (analogous to alkane hydroxylation) that can eliminate the hydrohalic acid to form carbonyl derivatives (aldehydes, ketones, acyl halides, and carbonyl halides) (Fig. 3.15). This reaction requires the presence of at least one halogen and one α-hydrogen. *gem*-Trihalogenated hydrocarbons are more readily oxidized than are the *gem*-dihalogenated and monohalogenated compounds. The acyl and carbonyl halides formed are reactive metabolites that can react either with water to form carboxylic acids or nonenzymatically with tissue molecules (with a potential for eliciting increased toxicity).

Oxidative dehydrohalogenation leading to significant hepatotoxicity and nephrotoxicity is seen with the fluorinated inhalation anesthetics halothane, enflurane, isoflurane, desflurane, and methoxyflurane, but not sevoflurane[31,32] (Fig. 3.15). The fluranes are metabolized by CYP2E1 to reactive intermediates that produce trifluoroacetylated immunogenic protein adducts. The severity of hepatotoxicity is associated with the degree of hepatic metabolism. The hepatotoxicity of halothane and the other fluranes is related to their metabolism to either an acid chloride (or fluoride) or a trifluoroacetate intermediate.[31,32] The hydroxylated intermediate decomposes spontaneously to reactive intermediates, an acid chloride (or

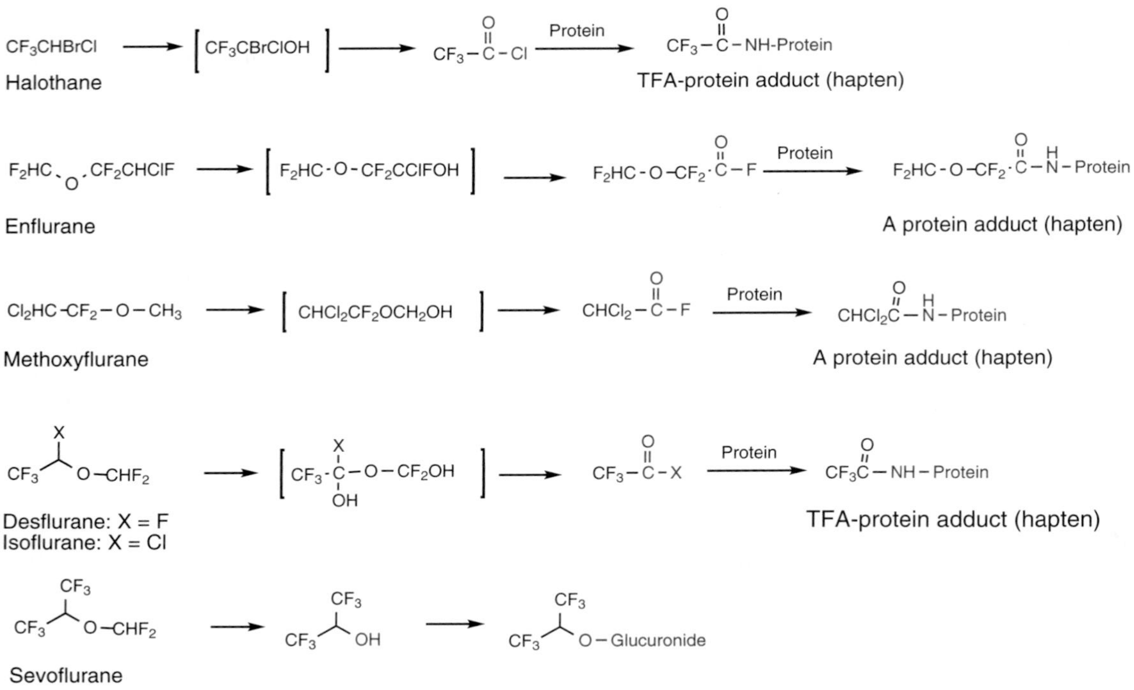

Figure 3.15 CYP2E1-catalyzed metabolism of fluorinated volatile anesthetics to antigenic proteins.

fluoride) or trifluoroacetate, that can either react with water to form halide anions and a fluorinated carboxylic acid or bind covalently to tissue proteins to produce an acylated protein. The acylated protein becomes a "hapten," stimulating an immune response and a hypersensitivity reaction.

Halothane has received the most attention because of its ability to cause "halothane-associated" hepatitis. This immunologic reaction occurs after repeated exposure in surgical patients to trifluoroacetylate protein. After subsequent exposure to a fluorinated anesthetic, the antigenic trifluoroacetylate protein stimulates an immunogenic response, producing halothane-like hepatitis. For this reason, halothane is no longer used in general anesthesia in humans.

Because of the common metabolic pathway involving CYP2E1 for enflurane, isoflurane, desflurane, and methoxyflurane, halothane-exposed patients who have halothane hepatitis can show cross-sensitization to one of the other fluranes, triggering an idiosyncratic hepatotoxicity. The formation of antigenic protein is related to the amount of CYP2E1-catalyzed metabolism of each agent: halothane (20%-40%) > enflurane (2%-8%) > isoflurane (0.2%-1.0%) > desflurane (<0.1%).[31,32] Enough fluoride ion is generated from oxidative dehalogenation during flurane anesthesia to produce subclinical nephrotoxicity. For patients with preexisting liver dysfunction, isoflurane, desflurane, or sevoflurane may be better choices of general anesthetic.

Unlike halothane and the other halogenated anesthetics, sevoflurane is not significantly metabolized to hepatotoxic trifluoroacetylated proteins but, rather, is metabolized by O-dealkylation to hexafluoroisopropanol and readily eliminated as the glucuronide. Approximately 90% of administered sevoflurane is eliminated intact in the patient's expired air. The glucuronide is mostly excreted in urine within 12 hours after anesthesia, whereas trifluoroacetic acid is detectable in urine for up to 12 days after anesthesia.

In today's environment, most humans have been exposed to many CYP2E1-inducing agents (including recreational, industrial, and agricultural chemicals and alcohol). This exposure has an unknown effect on hepatic toxicity from administered volatile anesthetics. Enhanced activity of CYP2E1 has been observed in obesity, isoniazid therapy, ketogenic diets, and alcoholism.

Azo and Nitro Reduction

In addition to the oxidative systems, liver microsomes also contain enzyme systems that catalyze the reduction of azo and nitro compounds to primary amines. A number of azo compounds, such as prontosil and sulfasalazine (Fig. 3.16) are converted to aromatic primary amines by azoreductase, an NADPH-dependent enzyme system in the liver microsomes. Evidence exists for the participation of CYP450 in some reductions. Nitro compounds (e.g., chloramphenicol and nitrobenzene) are reduced to aromatic primary amines by a nitroreductase, presumably through nitrosamine and hydroxylamine intermediates. These reductases are not solely responsible of reduction of azo and nitro compounds; reduction by the bacterial flora in the anaerobic environment of the intestine can also occur.

In summary, all known oxidative reactions catalyzed by CYP450 monooxygenases can be described in the context of a mechanistic scheme which involves the ability of a high-valent ferric iron oxenoid species to bring about the stepwise one-electron oxidation through the abstraction of hydrogen atoms, abstraction of electrons from heteroatoms, or addition to π-bonds. A series of radical recombination reactions completes the oxidation process.

Induction and Inhibition of Cytochrome P450 Isoforms

Induction

Many of the enzymes involved in drug metabolism can be upregulated by exposure to drugs and environmental chemicals or by other coingested/inhaled compounds. This leads to increased rates of drug metabolism, thereby altering pharmacological and toxicological effects.[33-35] Prolonged administration of some drugs or xenobiotics can enhance their own metabolism, along with a wide variety of other compounds. This phenomenon is known as enzyme induction, a dose-dependent phenomenon.

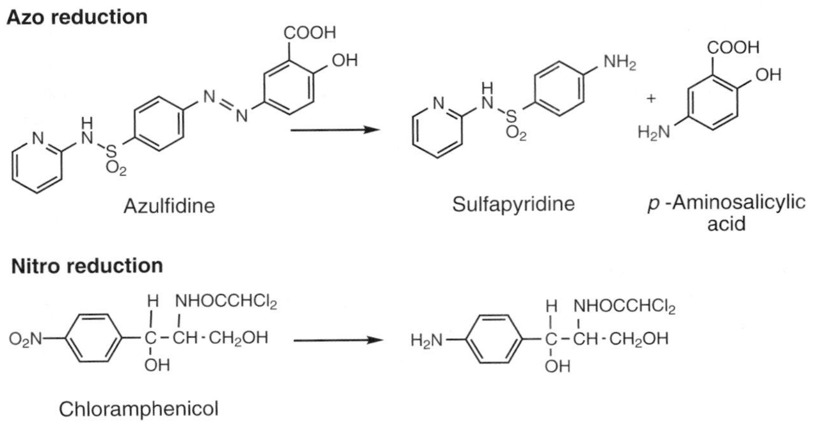

Azo reduction

Azulfidine → Sulfapyridine + *p*-Aminosalicylic acid

Nitro reduction

Chloramphenicol

Figure 3.16 CYP450-catalyzed reduction of azo and nitro compounds.

Drugs and xenobiotics exert this effect by inducing transcription of CYP450 mRNA and synthesis of xenobiotic-metabolizing enzymes in the smooth ER of the liver and other extrahepatic tissues.[33-35] Enzyme induction is an adaptive response associated with increases in liver weight, induction of gene expression, and morphological changes in hepatocytes. Induction is the process whereby the rate of enzyme synthesis is increased relative to the rate of enzyme synthesis in the uninduced organism. In many older studies of mammalian systems, the term "induction" was inferred from an increase in enzyme activity, but the amount of enzyme protein had not been determined.

Enzyme induction is important to interpret the results of chronic toxicities, mutagenicities, or carcinogenesis and to explain certain unexpected drug-drug interactions in patients. Enzyme inducers trigger pathways involving the constitutive androstane receptor (CAR), the peroxisome proliferator-activated receptor (PPAR), the aryl hydrocarbon receptor (AhR), and the pregnane-X-receptor (PXR).[35] CAR is a member of the nuclear receptor superfamily and, along with PXR, upregulates the expression of P450 proteins responsible for the metabolism and excretion of these xenobiotics, and thus it is a key regulator of xenobiotic CYP450 metabolism.

Many drugs and xenobiotics induce/stimulate the upregulation of CYP450 isoforms, as shown in Table 3.13. These inducers have nothing in common so far as their pharmacological activities or chemical structures are concerned, but they are all metabolized by one or more of the CYP450 isoforms. Most are lipid soluble at physiological pH. Polycyclic aromatic hydrocarbons in cigarette smoke, xanthines and flavones in foods, halogenated hydrocarbons in insecticides, polychlorinated biphenyls, and food additives are but a few of the environmental chemicals that alter the activities of CYP450 enzymes.[34]

Enzyme induction, which can last as long as 1-3 weeks to allow for drug blood levels to decrease, can alter the pharmacokinetics and pharmacodynamics of a drug, with clinical implications for the therapeutic actions of the drug as well as increased potential for drug-drug interactions. Because of induction, a drug can be metabolized more rapidly to metabolites that are more potent, more toxic, or less active than the parent drug. Induction can also enhance the activation of procarcinogens or promutagens.

Not all inducing agents enhance their own metabolism; for example, phenytoin induces CYP3A4 but is hydroxylated by CYP2C9. Some of the more common enzyme inducers of CYP450 subfamilies, which can also be substrates for the same P450 isoforms, include phenobarbital (CYP2B6, CYP2C, and CYP3A4), rifampicin (CYP3A4), and cigarette smoke (CYP1A1/2) (Table 3.13). The broad range of drugs metabolized by these CYP450 subfamilies (Table 3.12) that are also affected by these enzyme inducers raise the issue of clinically significant drug-drug interactions and their clinical implications. Examples of a clinically significant CYP450 drug-drug interaction and an herbal drug-drug interaction are rifampin and oral contraceptives, and St. John's wort and oral contraceptives, respectively. Both rifmapin and St. John's wort induce the expression of CYP3A4. This reduces the serum levels of the oral contraceptive due to increased oxidative metabolism of the oral contraceptives by CYP3A4 to less active metabolites, thereby increasing the risk for pregnancy. Drugs poorly metabolized by CYP450 enzymes are less affected by enzyme induction.

Inducers of CYP450 isoforms also stimulate oxidative metabolism and the synthesis of endogenous substances: for example, the hydroxylation of androgens,

Table 3.13 Drugs That Induce the Expression of P450 Isoforms[a]

Drug	Isoforms	Drug	Isoforms
Amprenavir	3A4	4-Methylpyrazole	2E1
Aprepitant	2C9	Modafinil	1A2, 2B6, 3A4
Barbiturates	3A4, 2C9, 2C19, 2B6	Nevirapine	3A4, 2B6
		Norethindrone	2C19
Carbamazepine	1A2, 3A4, 2C8, 2C9, 2D6, 2B6	Omeprazole	1A1/2, 3A4
		Oxcarbazepine	3A4
Charbroiled meats	1A1/2,	***Phenobarbital***	3A4, 2C, 2B6, 2D6, 1A2
Cigarette smoke	1A1/2	***Phenytoin***	3A4, 1A2, 2B6, 2C8, 2C19, 2D6
Clotrimazole	1A1/2, 3A4	Primidone	3A4, 2C9, 1A2, 2B6, 2D6
Ethanol	2D6, 2E1	Psoralen	1A1/2
Efavirenz	3A4	***Ethosuximide***	3A4
Erythromycin	3A4	Polycyclic aromatic hydrocarbons	1A1/2
Glucocorticoids (Dexamethasone, prednisone)	3A4, 2A6, 2C19	Rifampin	2C8, 2C9, 2C19, 2D6, 3A4, 2B6
		Rifampicin	2C8
		Rifabutin	2C8, 3A4
		Rifapentine	3A4
Griseofulvin	3A4	Ritonavir	2D6, 3A4
		St. Johns wort	1A2, 2C9, 3A4
Lansoprazole	1A1/2, 3A4		
Mephenytoin	2B6	Topiramate	3A4

[a]Drugs in bold italic have been reported to cause drug-drug interaction.

estrogens, progestational steroids (synthetic oral contraceptives), and glucocorticoids, which decreases their biological activity. These enzyme inducers might also be implicated in deficiencies associated with these steroids. For example, the induction of C2 hydroxylation of estradiol and synthetic estrogens by phenobarbital, dexamethasone, or cigarette smoking in women results in the increased formation of the principal and less active metabolite of these estrogenic substances, reducing their effectiveness. Thus, cigarette smoking in premenopausal women could result in an estrogen deficiency, increasing the risks of osteoporosis and early menopause. Postmenopausal women who smoke and take estrogen replacement therapy risk decreasing the effectiveness of the estrogen.

In addition to enhancing the metabolism of other drugs, many compounds, when chronically administered, stimulate their own metabolism, thereby decreasing their therapeutic activity and producing a state of apparent tolerance. This self-induction can explain some of the changes in drug toxicity observed during prolonged treatments. The duration of the sedative action of phenobarbital, for example, becomes shorter with repeated doses, and this can be explained, in part, on the basis of increased metabolism via enzyme induction.

The time course of induction varies with different inducing agents and with different P450 isoforms. CYP1A induction always involves the AhR. Increased transcription of CYP450 mRNA has been detected as early as 1 hour after administration of phenobarbital, with maximum induction occurring after 48-72 hours. After administration of PAH such as 3-methylcholanthrene and benzo[a]pyrene, maximum induction of the CYP1A subfamily is reached within 24 hours. Less potent inducers of hepatic drug metabolism can take as long as 6-10 days to produce maximum induction.[33]

Exposure to a variety of different xenobiotics can increase the hepatic content of specific isoforms of CYP450.[33-35] Therefore, the process of enzyme induction involves the adaptive increase in the content of specific enzymes in response to the enzyme-inducing agent. Other inducible Phase 2 metabolizing enzymes include uridine diphosphate (UDP)-glucuronosyl transferase and glutathione transferase.

Specific Inducers

PHENOBARBITAL AND RIFAMPIN.
Phenobarbital and rifampin are enzyme inducers which have been most extensively studied. These drugs alter the pharmacokinetics and pharmacodynamics of many concurrently administered drugs listed in Tables 3.7 (CYP2C) and 3.10 (CYP3A4), which raises the issue of clinically significant drug-drug interactions.

CIGARETTE SMOKE. Cigarette smoke has been shown to increase the hydrocarbon-inducible isoforms CYP1A1 and CYP1A2 in the lungs, liver, small intestine, and placentas. A stimulation of the CYP1A1/2 metabolism of several drugs, and a decrease in their pharmacological action, is the end result. Cigarette smoking has been reported to lower blood levels of drugs metabolized by CYP1A1/2, including theophylline, imipramine, estradiol, pentazocine, and propoxyphene. Smoking also decreases urinary excretion of nicotine and the drowsiness caused by chlorpromazine, diazepam, and chlordiazepoxide.

ALCOHOL. Alcoholics show an increase in CYP2E1 enzyme activity, leading to more rapid clearance of drugs and xenobiotics that are substrates for this isoform. As discussed previously, hepatic CYP2E1 oxidizes ethanol, and chronic ethanol intake increases the activity of CYP2E1 through enzyme induction.[19] The changes in drug metabolism in alcoholics can also be attributed to other factors, such as malnutrition, coadministered drugs, and the trace chemicals that are sources of flavors and odors of particular alcoholic beverages. Heavy drinkers metabolize phenobarbital, tolbutamide, and phenytoin more rapidly than nonalcoholics, which can be clinically important when adjusting drug therapies for alcoholics.

Inhibition

Another method to alter in vivo effects of xenobiotics metabolized by P450s is the use of inhibitors (Table 3.11). The CYP450 inhibitors can be divided into three categories according to their mechanisms of action: reversible inhibition, metabolite intermediate complexation of P450, or mechanism-based inactivation of CYP450.[35,36] The polysubstrate nature of CYP450 is responsible for the large number of documented interactions associated with the inhibition of drug oxidation and drug biotransformation.

Reversible Inhibition

Reversible inhibition of CYP450 is the result of reversible interactions at the heme-iron active center of P450, the lipophilic sites on the apoprotein, or both. The interaction occurs before the oxidation steps of the catalytic cycle and the effects dissipate quickly when the inhibitor is discontinued. The most effective reversible inhibitors are those that interact strongly with both the apoprotein and the heme iron. It is widely accepted that inhibition has an important impact on the oxidative metabolism and pharmacokinetics of drugs which have a metabolism that cosegregates with that of an inhibitor (Tables 3.3 and 3.7-3.10).[35,36] Some drugs that interact reversibly with CYP450 are shown in Table 3.11. The imidazole-based azole antifungals are potent inhibitors of CYP3A4 and of the CYP450-mediated biosynthesis of endogenous steroid hormones. The azole antifungals noted in this Table exert their fungiostatic effects through inhibition of fungal P450, inhibiting the oxidative biosynthesis of lanosterol to ergosterol, thereby affecting the integrity and permeability of the fungal membranes.

CYP450 COMPLEXATION INHIBITION. Some alkylamine drugs have the ability to undergo P450-mediated oxidation to nitrosoalkane metabolites, which have high affinities for the P450 heme iron active center and form stable complexes with the reduced (ferrous) heme-P450 intermediates of the CYP2B, CYP2C, and CYP3A subfamilies. This process is termed "metabolite intermediate complexation."[6,8] Thus the CYP450 isoform is unavailable for further oxidation, and synthesis of the new enzyme is required to restore CYP450 activity. The process relies on at least one iteration of the CYP450 catalytic cycle to generate the required heme intermediate.

The macrolide antibiotics troleandomycin, erythromycin, and clarithromycin, as well as their analogues, are selective inhibitors of CYP3A4 and are capable of inducing expression of hepatic and extrahepatic CYP3A4 mRNA and of inducing their own biotransformation into nitrosoalkane metabolites. The clinical significance of this inhibition with CYP3A4 is the long-lived impairment of metabolism of a large number of coadministered substrates of this isoform, and the potential for drug-drug interactions and time-dependent nonlinearities in their pharmacokinetics upon long-term administration (Tables 3.11 and 3.12). For macrolides to be so metabolized, they must possess an unhindered dimethylamino sugar and the compound itself must be lipophilic. A second example is methylenedioxyphenyl compounds (i.e., the antidepressant paroxetine, the insecticide synergist piperonyl butoxide, and the flavoring agent isosafrole), which generate metabolite intermediates which form stable complexes with both the ferric and ferrous state of P450.

Mechanism-Based Inhibition. Certain drugs that are not inhibitors of CYP450 contain functional groups that, when oxidized by P450, generate metabolites that irreversibly bind to the enzyme.[34,37] This process is termed "mechanism-based inhibition" ("suicide inhibition") and requires at least one catalytic CYP450 cycle either during or subsequent to the oxygen-transfer step, when the drug is activated to the inhibitory species. Alkenes and alkynes were the first functionalities found to inactivate P450 by generation of a radical intermediate that alkylates the heme structure (see section Alkene and Alkyne Hydroxylation). Iron is lost from the heme and abnormal N-alkylated porphyrins are produced. Drugs that are mechanism-based inhibitors of CYP450 include (1) the 17α-acetylenic estrogen 17α-ethinyl estradiol,[37] the 17α-acetylenic progestin norethindrone (norethisterone), and their radical intermediates that N-alkylate the heme of CYP3A4; (2) cyclophosphamide and its generated acrolein and phosphoramide mustard that alkylates CYP2B6 apoprotein; (3) spironolactone and its 7-thio metabolite that alkylates heme; (4) 8-methoxypsoralen (a furocoumarin) and its epoxide metabolite that alkylates the CYP450 apoprotein of CYP2A6; (5) nicotine (CYP1A6 and 1A13 isoforms); (6) isoniazide that alkylates CYP1A2, 2A6, 2C19, and 3A4 isoforms; (7) 21-halosteroids; (8) halocarbons; and (9) secobarbital. The selectivity of CYP450 isoform destruction by several of these inhibitors indicates involvement of specific isoforms in the bioactivation of such drugs.[38,39]

Oxidations Catalyzed by Flavin Monooxygenase

Flavin-containing monooxygenase (FMO) oxidizes drugs, xenobiotics, and environmental chemicals containing a soft-nucleophile, usually nitrogen or sulfur. A soft-nucleophile is a group that is less electronegative, is more polarizable, and has a weak tendency to donate or share their electrons. FMO is a monooxygenase but, unlike P450, utilizes the two electron reducing equivalents of NADPH (as hydride anion) in one step to reduce one atom of molecular oxygen to water, while the other oxygen atom is used to oxidize the substrate. Because oxygen activation occurs in two steps before substrate addition, any compound binding to 4α-hydroperoxyflavin, the enzyme-bound monooxygenating FMO intermediate, is a potential substrate. The products formed from FMO-catalyzed oxidation are consistent with a two-electron oxidation of the heteroatom. Unlike P450, FMO does not catalyze epoxidation reactions or hydroxylation reactions at unactivated carbon atoms of xenobiotics. FMO and P450 also exhibit similar tissue and cellular location, molecular weight, and substrate specificity and exist as multiple enzymes.

Humans express five different flavin monooxygenases (FMO1, FMO2, FMO3, FMO4, and FMO5) in a tissue-specific manner, with different substrate specificities. Unlike P450, the human FMO functional gene family consists of five families each expressing a single protein. Three of the five expressed human FMO genes, *FMO1*, *FMO2*, and *FMO3*, exhibit genetic polymorphisms. FMO3 is the prominent form in adult human liver that is likely to be associated with the bulk of FMO-mediated metabolism and contributes to the disease known as trimethylaminuria. FMO2 is largely found in the lung. Because of their low expression, little is known about the substrate specificity for FMO3 and FMO4. Thus, these enzymes do not contribute significantly (<10%) to human drug metabolism.

The catalytic cycle of FMO and P450 is very different. For example, FMO does not require a reductase to transfer electrons from NADPH. Another distinction is the lack of induction of FMOs by xenobiotics. In general, P450 is the major contributor to oxidative xenobiotic metabolism. However, FMO activity may be of significance in a number of reactions involving N or S (see below) and should not be overlooked. FMO and P450 have overlapping substrate specificities but often yield different metabolites with potentially diverse toxicological/pharmacological consequences.

The physiological function(s) of FMO are poorly understood.[40] Unlike P450 which exhibits interindividual variation in expression to both genetic and environmental factors, FMO is not regulated by environmental factors and interindividual variability in FMO enzyme expression would be predominately genetic in origin.

N- and S-Oxidations

FMO constitutes an alternative biotransformation pathway for converting N- and S-containing lipophilic drugs and xenobiotics to more polar metabolites that are more efficiently excreted in the urine. Typically, FMO catalyzes oxygenation of the N- and S-heteroatoms (soft nucleophiles) (Fig. 3.17), excluding heteroatom dealkylation reactions. FMO is not normally inducible by phenobarbital, nor is it affected by P450 inhibitors. With few exceptions, however, xenobiotic substrates of FMO are also substrates of the P450 isoforms, producing similar oxidation products. Which monooxygenase is responsible for the oxidation can be readily determined, because FMO is thermally labile in the absence of NADPH, whereas P450 is stable.

Of the many nitrogen functional groups in xenobiotics, only secondary and tertiary acyclic, cyclic and arylamines, as well as hydroxylamines and hydrazines, are oxidized by FMO and excreted in urine (Fig. 3.17). The tertiary amines form stable amine oxides (N-oxides) which are highly polar, hydrophilic, and less basic compounds, and which can be reduced back to the parent tertiary amine in the GIT. On the other hand, secondary amines are sequentially oxidized to hydroxylamines, nitrones, and a complex mixture of products. Secondary N-alkylarylamines can be N-oxygenated to reactive N-hydroxylated metabolites, which are responsible for the toxic, mutagenic, and carcinogenic activity of these compounds. For example, the chemically unstable hydroxylamine intermediates of aromatic amines degrade into bladder carcinogens (see discussion of this type of toxic mechanism in section Glucuronic

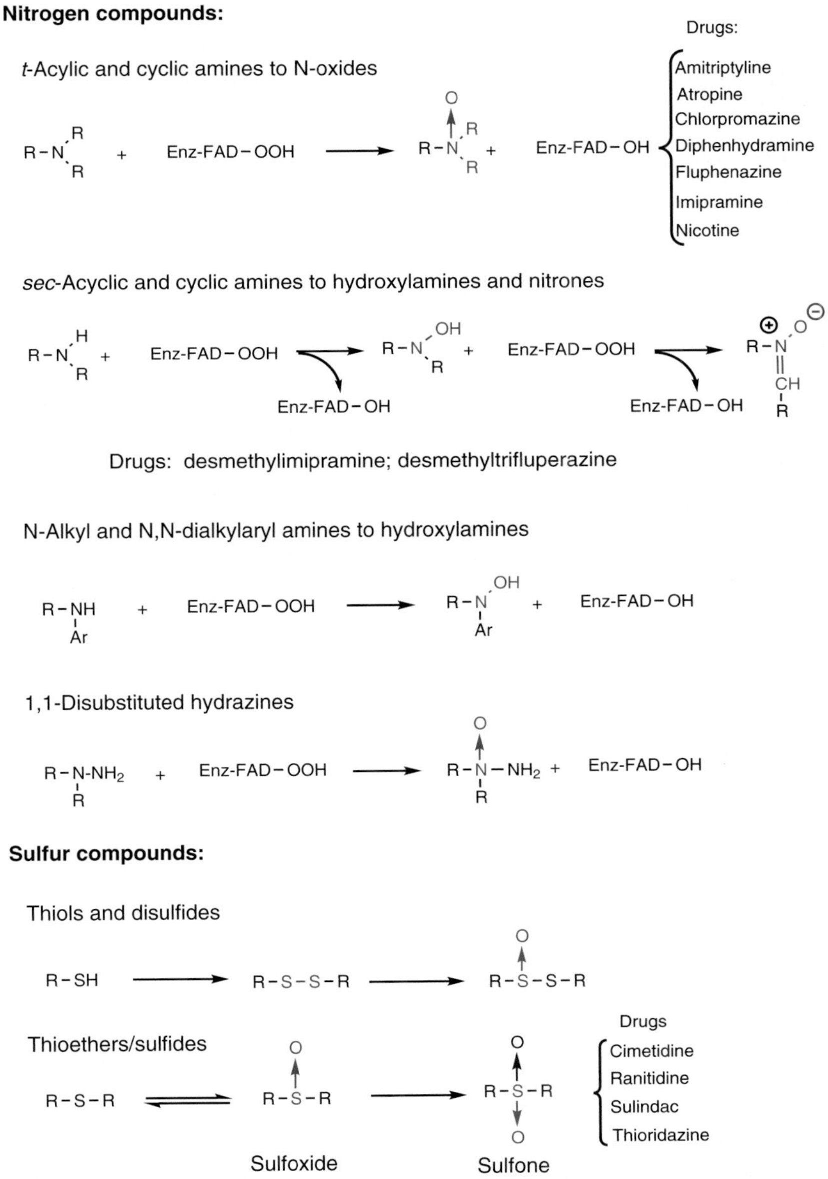

Nitrogen compounds:

t-Acylic and cyclic amines to N-oxides

$R-NR_2$ + Enz-FAD−OOH ⟶ $R-N(\rightarrow O)R_2$ + Enz-FAD−OH

Drugs: Amitriptyline, Atropine, Chlorpromazine, Diphenhydramine, Fluphenazine, Imipramine, Nicotine

sec-Acyclic and cyclic amines to hydroxylamines and nitrones

$R-NH-R$ + Enz-FAD−OOH ⟶ (Enz-FAD−OH) $R-N(OH)-R$ + Enz-FAD−OOH ⟶ (Enz-FAD−OH) $R-N^{+}(O^{-})=CH-R$

Drugs: desmethylimipramine; desmethyltrifluperazine

N-Alkyl and N,N-dialkylaryl amines to hydroxylamines

$R-NH-Ar$ + Enz-FAD−OOH ⟶ $R-N(OH)-Ar$ + Enz-FAD−OH

1,1-Disubstituted hydrazines

$R-N(R)-NH_2$ + Enz-FAD−OOH ⟶ $R-N(\rightarrow O)(R)-NH_2$ + Enz-FAD−OH

Sulfur compounds:

Thiols and disulfides

R−SH ⟶ R−S−S−R ⟶ $R-S(\rightarrow O)-S-R$

Thioethers/sulfides

R−S−R ⇌ $R-S(\rightarrow O)-R$ (Sulfoxide) ⟶ $R-S(\rightarrow O)_2-R$ (Sulfone)

Drugs: Cimetidine, Ranitidine, Sulindac, Thioridazine

Figure 3.17 Examples of flavin monooxygenase (FMO) oxidations.

Acid Conjugation), and the hydroxamic acid intermediates of N-arylacetamides are bioactivated into liver carcinogens. Hepatic FMO, however, will not catalyze the oxidation of primary alkyl- or arylamines, except for the carcinogenic N-hydroxylated derivatives of 2-aminofluorene, 2-aminoanthracene, and other amino PAHs.

S-oxidation occurs almost exclusively by FMO (Fig. 3.17). Sulfides are oxidized to sulfoxides and sulfones; thiols to disulfides and thiocarbamates; mercaptopyrimidines and mercaptoimidazoles (i.e., the antithyroid drug methimazole) via sulfenates (RSOH) to sulfinates (R-SO-OH), all of which are eliminated in urine. FMO S-oxygenates a number of sulfur-containing substrates. The hepatotoxicity of thioureas (e.g., the antimycobacterial drug ethionamide) is the result of metabolic bioactivation through FMO3-dependent S-oxidation to produce toxic sulfinic acid metabolites. Metabolic bioactivation of ethionamide by bacterial FMOs may be its antimycobacteral mechanism of action.

Primary aromatic amines and amides, aromatic heterocyclic amines and imines, and the aliphatic primary amine phentermine are N-oxidized by P450 to hydroxylamines.

Catalytic Cycle for Flavin Monooxygenase

The major steps in the catalytic cycle for FMO are shown in Figure 3.18.[40-42] Like most of the other monooxygenases, FMO requires NADPH and oxygen as cofactors to catalyze the oxidation of the xenobiotic substrate. Unlike P450, however, the xenobiotic being oxidized does not need to be bound to the 4α-hydroperoxyflavin intermediate (FAD-OOH) for oxygen activation to occur. FMO is present within the cell in its enzyme-bound activated hydroperoxide (Enz-FAD-OOH) state, ready to oxidize any suitable lipophilic substrate that binds to it. The FMO uses a nonradical, nucleophilic displacement type of mechanism binding dioxygen with a reduced flavin. The reactive oxygen intermediate is a reactive derivative of hydrogen peroxide, flavin-4α-hydroperoxide (Fig. 3.18, insert), which is reactive enough to successfully attack a lone electron pair on a heteroatom, such as nitrogen or sulfur, but not reactive enough to abstract a hydrogen atom from a typical C–H bond. Studies suggest the xenobiotic substrate interacts with the 4α-hydroperoxyflavin form of FMO and is oxidized by oxygen transfer from Enz-FAD-OOH to form the oxidized product. Steps 2-5 in Figure 3.18 simply regenerate the oxygenating agent Enz-FAD-OOH from Enz-FAD-OH, NADPH, oxygen, and a proton. Any compound readily crossing cell membranes and penetrating to the FMO-bound hydroperoxyflavin intermediate is a potential substrate, thus explaining the broad substrate specificity exhibited by FMO. The fact that the xenobiotic substrate is not required for activation of the FMO-hydroperoxyflavin state distinguishes FMO from P450 monooxygenases, in which substrate binding initiates the P450 catalytic cycle and activation of oxygen to the ferryl oxenoid intermediate. It is not unusual for FMO oxidation products to undergo reduction to the parent xenobiotic, which can enter into repeated redox reactions (termed "metabolic cycling").

Results of substrate specificity studies suggest that the number of ionic groups on endogenous substrate is an important factor in enabling FMO to distinguish between xenobiotic and endogenous substrates, thus preventing the indiscriminate oxidation of physiologically important amine and sulfur compounds.[43] Without exception, FMO readily catalyzes the oxidation of uncharged amines or sulfur compounds (in equilibrium with its respective monocation or monoanion; for sulfur compounds, the charge is on sulfur atom). The FMO will not catalyze the oxidation of dianions (e.g., thiamine pyrophosphate), dications (e.g., polyamines), dipolar ions (e.g., amino acids and peptides), or other polyionic compounds with one or more anionic groups (e.g., COO^-) distal to the heteroatom (e.g., coenzyme A).

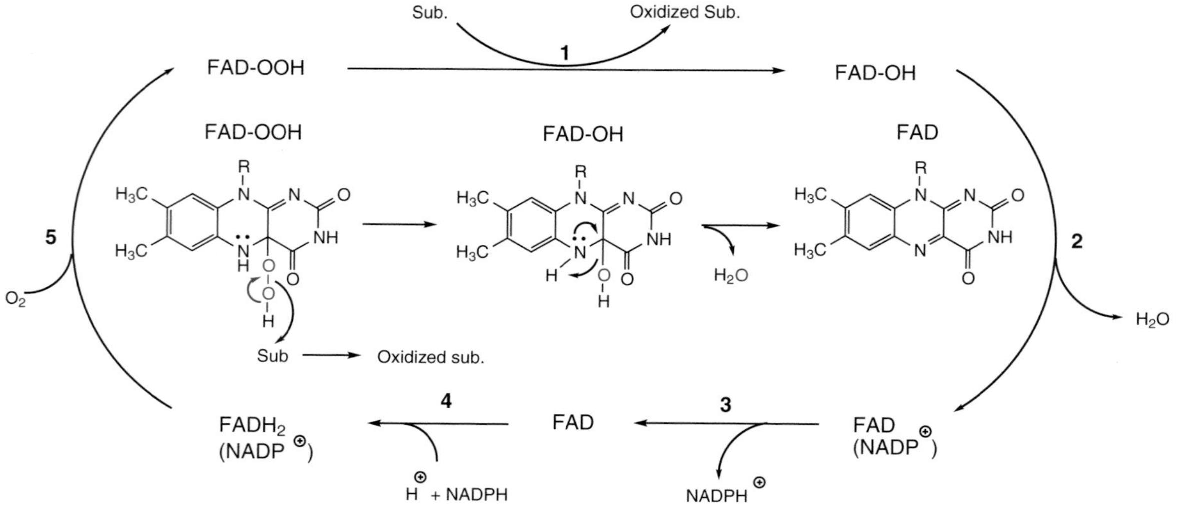

Figure 3.18 Flavin monooxygenase (FMO) catalytic cycle. Oxygenated substrate is formed by nucleophilic attack of a substrate (Sub.) by the terminal oxygen of the enzyme-bound hydroperoxyflavin (FAD-OOH), followed by heterolytic cleavage of the peroxide (1). The release of H_2O (2) or of $NADP^+$ (3) is rate-limiting for reactions catalyzed by liver FMO. Reduction of flavin by NADPH (4) and addition of oxygen (5) complete the cycle by regeneration of the oxygenated FAD-OOH.

Unlike the P450 system, only three isoforms of hepatic FMO have been characterized in the adult human liver (FMO1, FMO2, FMO3).[42,43] FMO1 is the major form in fetal liver. The availability of different forms of FMO can be of clinical importance in the pharmacological and toxicological properties of FMO-dependent drug oxidations.

The substrate specificity for FMO3 is distinct from that of FMO1. FMO3 N-oxygenates primary, secondary, and tertiary amines, whereas FMO1 is only efficient at N-oxygenating tertiary amines. FMO3 is sensitive to steric features of the substrate, and aliphatic amines with linkages of at least five carbons between the nitrogen atom and a large aromatic group (e.g., phenothiazines) are N-oxygenated significantly more efficiently than substrates with a two or three carbon spacer. Amines with smaller aromatic substituents (e.g., phenethylamines) are often efficiently N-oxygenated by FMO3. Interindividual variation in FMO3-dependent metabolism of drugs, xenobiotics, and environmental chemicals is therefore more likely because of genetic differences, rather than environmental effects.

Certain mutations of the FMO3 gene have been associated with deficient N-oxygenation of trimethylamine, which results in an inherited genetic condition called trimethylaminuria. Allelic variations of FMO3 might cause abnormal metabolism of drugs, which has clinical implications for human drug metabolism. For example, (*S*)-Nicotine N1′-oxide formation is a highly stereoselective product of FMO3 for adult humans who smoke cigarettes. Thus, FMO3 genetic polymorphism and poor metabolism phenotype in certain human populations could contribute to adverse drug reactions or exaggerated clinical response to certain medications. *FMO3* may be another example of an environmental gene that participates in a protective mechanism to help shield humans from potentially toxic exposure to chemicals.

Peroxidases and Other Monooxygenases

Peroxidases are hemoproteins that are closely related enzymes to P450 monooxygenase.[44,45] The differences between peroxidase and P450 include the replacement of the cysteine axial ligand of P450 with a histidine residue and the inclusion of polar amino acids within proximity of the heme-active site. These polar amino acid differences in the peroxidase heme-active site allow the peroxidase to rapidly catalyze the reduction of hydroperoxides to alcohol (water in the case of hydrogen peroxide) and the simultaneous reoxidation of peroxidase. The normal course of peroxide (ROOH)-catalyzed oxidation involves the formation of the ferryl-oxo-intermediate, analogous to the ferryl oxenoid complex in P450. Thus, the catalytic cycle of peroxidases is simpler than that of P450. Unlike P450 which is capable of abstracting a hydrogen atom from almost any type of substrate, peroxidase-catalyzed oxidation of drugs and xenobiotics is limited to electron-rich substrates that are easily oxidized (e.g., heteroatom oxygenation, aromatization [oxidation] of 1,4-dihydropyridines [calcium channel blockers] and arylamines).

ROOH + [dihydropyridine: Cl, Cl, C_2H_5OOC, $COOCH_3$, H_3C, N–H, CH_3] —([FeO]$^{3+}$ → Fe^{3+}; H_2O)→ ROH + [pyridine: Cl, Cl, C_2H_5OOC, $COOCH_3$, H_3C, N, CH_3]

Cyclooxygenase (COX, also known as prostaglandin synthase or prostaglandin endoperoxide synthetase) is a widely-distributed heme-peroxidase enzyme responsible for the formation of important biological mediators, called prostanoids, from arachidonic acid. These essential prostanoids include prostaglandins, prostacyclin, and thromboxane. COX catalyzes the heme-peroxidation of arachidonic acid by means of hydrogen atom abstraction by a tyrosine radical generated by a ferryl-oxo-heme-intermediate to hydroperoxy endoperoxide prostaglandin G_2 (PGG_2), which is then reduced to prostaglandin H_2, regenerating the COX. Two oxygen molecules then react with the arachidonic acid radical to produce PGG_2. During the reduction of prostaglandin G_2 (PGG_2) to prostaglandin H_2, drug substrates can be oxidized. Three COX isoenzymes are known: COX-1, COX-2, and COX-3. Inhibitors of COX are the nonsteroidal anti-inflammatory drugs (NSAIDs).

Myeloperoxidase (MPO) is a heme-peroxidase enzyme most abundantly present in neutrophil granulocytes (a subtype of white blood cells). MPO differs from P450 and other peroxidases in that the substrates are hydrogen peroxide and chloride anion. The chloride anion is oxidized to hypochlorous acid (HOCl) in the granulocyte, which is cytotoxic and very effective in killing bacteria, viruses, and other pathogens: the natural function of neutrophils. HOCl is also used to disinfect drinking water. HOCl can oxidize drugs to reactive intermediates (e.g., nitrenium ions) which can be responsible for causing agranulocytosis. Examples of HOCl-generated reactive intermediates associated with agranulocytosis are the atypical antipsychotic clozapine, the antimalarial amodiaquine, and the phosphodiesterase cardiotonic vesnarinone.

Other peroxidases include horseradish peroxidase (found in plants), lactoperoxidase found in breast milk, and thyroid peroxidase found in the thyroid gland to produce thyroid hormones from iodide.

Other monooxygenases catalyzing oxidation reactions similar to P450 include dopamine β-monooxygenase, a mammalian copper-containing enzyme catalyzing carbon hydroxylation, epoxidation, S-oxygenation, and N-dealkylation reactions, and nonheme iron–containing enzymes from bacteria and plants.

Nonmicrosomal Oxidations

In addition to the microsomal monooxygenases, other oxidases and dehydrogenases that catalyze oxidation reactions are present in the mitochondrial and soluble fractions of tissue homogenates.

Oxidation of Alcohols

Alcohol dehydrogenases (ADH) are a family of NAD-specific dehydrogenase enzymes that occur in many organisms and are responsible for catalyzing the oxidation of primary and secondary alcohols to aldehydes and ketones, respectively, with concurrent reduction of NAD+ to NADH. ADHs can also catalyze the reverse reaction, oxidizing NADH to NAD+. In humans and many other animals, genetic evidence suggests that early on in evolution, ADHs were effective for metabolizing endogenous and exogenous formaldehyde and metabolizing naturally occurring toxic alcohols contained in foods or produced by bacteria in the digestive tract.

In humans, ADH exists as a dimer with a mass of 80 kDa and is encoded by at least seven different genes. There are five classes (1-5) of alcohol dehydrogenases, but the hepatic form that is primarily present in humans is class 1. Class 1 consists of A, B, and C subunits that are encoded by the genes *ADH1A*, *ADH1B*, and *ADH1C*. The human genes that encode class 2, 3, 4, and 5 ADHs are *ADH4*, *ADH5*, *ADH7*, and *ADH6*, respectively. The large number of ADH classes gives the body the capability to metabolize/detoxify a variety of primary and secondary alcohols.

Human ADH is present at high levels in the liver and the lining of the stomach and exhibits a broad specificity for alcohols. Most primary alcohols are readily oxidized to their corresponding aldehydes. Some secondary alcohols are oxidized to ketones, whereas other secondary and tertiary alcohols are excreted either unchanged or as their glucuronide conjugate metabolite. Some secondary alcohols show also mixed activity due to steric factors and a lack of substrate affinity for the enzyme. The mechanism of dehydrogenation involves abstraction and transfer of a hydride anion from the alcohol to NAD+, reducing NAD+ to NADH, with the subsequent formation of an aldehyde. ADH contains a two Zn^{+2} ions in each subunit (Fig. 3.19). One of those Zn ions is located at the catalytic site and binds the hydroxyl group of the alcohol in place for dehydrogenation to occur. Alcohol dehydrogenase is located in the soluble fraction of tissue homogenates.

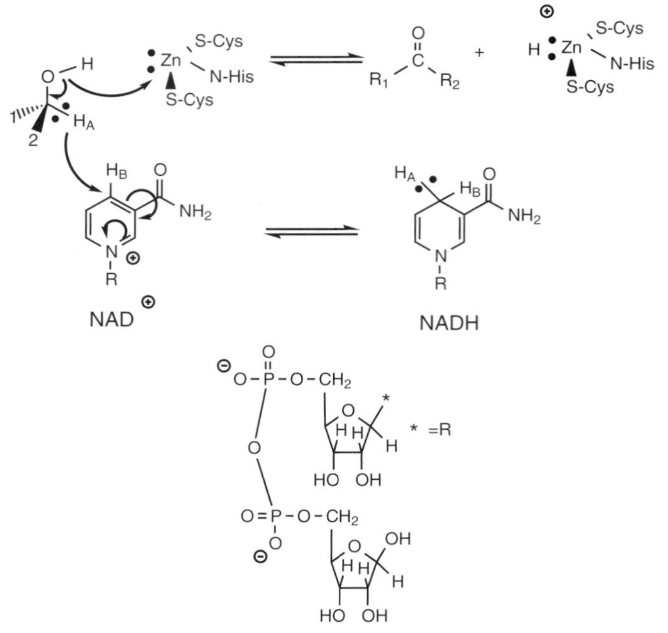

Figure 3.19 Alcohol dehydrogenase oxidation mechanism.

Oxidation by ADH is the principal pathway for ethanol metabolism, but the microsomal isoform CYP2E1 has also a significant role in ethanol metabolism and tolerance. Two-thirds of ingested ethanol is oxidized by ADH and the remainder by CYP2E1 (Fig. 3.20). During intoxication, however, ethanol induces the expression of CYP2E1. The induction of CYP2E1 contributes to the activation of other drugs and xenobiotics, increasing the vulnerability of heavy drinkers to anesthetic drugs, over-the-counter analgesics, prescription drugs, and chemical carcinogens. In turn, the excessive amounts of acetaldehyde generated cause hepatotoxicity, lipid peroxidation of membranes, formation of protein adducts, and other hepatocellular changes.

The toxicity of methanol and ethylene glycol in humans has long been recognized, but frequent reports of such toxicity are not surprising given the number of consumer products containing these alcohols (e.g., automotive antifreeze). Methanol (wood alcohol or methyl alcohol) is commonly used as a solvent in organic synthetic procedures and is available to consumers in a variety of products, ranging from solid fuels (Sterno), paint removers, motor fuels, antifreeze to alcoholic beverages (an adulterant in wines or an unintentional ingredient). Oral methanol toxicity in humans is characterized by its rapid absorption from the gut, followed by a latent period of many hours before metabolic acidosis (lowered blood pH and bicarbonate levels) and ocular toxicity are evident. The metabolic acidosis and blindness result from the excessive accumulation of formic acid and the inability of the hepatic tetrahydrofolate pathway to oxidize formate to carbon dioxide. The rate of elimination of methanol from the blood is relatively slow compared to the rapid rate for

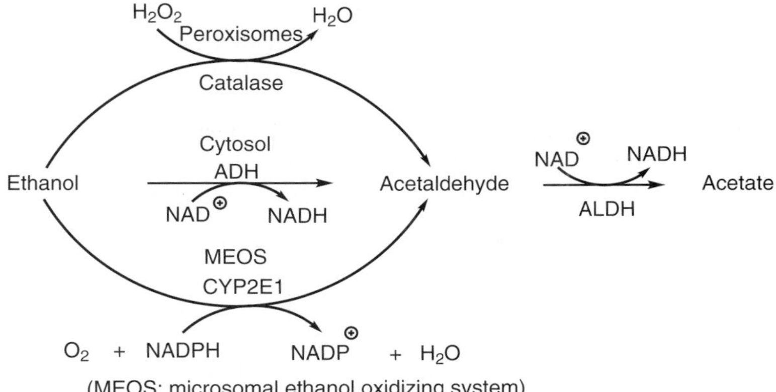

Figure 3.20 Ethanol metabolism in humans.

ethanol, accounting for its long latency period. Its half-life ranges from 2 to 3 hours at low blood concentration to 27 hours at high blood concentration. Research supports the singular role of liver ADH in the metabolism of methanol to formaldehyde, although it is oxidized slowly by ADH (approximately one-sixth the rate of ethanol).

The demonstration that methanol is a substrate for ADH provides a rational basis for the use of ethanol in the treatment of methanol toxicity. Ethanol depresses the rate of methanol oxidation by acting as a competitive substrate for ADH, reducing the formation of formaldehyde. On the other hand, formaldehyde is not customarily detected in the blood because of its rapid metabolism by ADH to formate. Although human exposure to methanol vapor is less prevalent, methanol is rapidly absorbed through the skin or by inhalation, and depending on the severity of exposure, this can result in methanol poisoning.

Ethylene glycol is oxidized to hydroxyacealdehyde and glyoxal and, subsequently, to oxalate by ADH. When eliminated into the urine, oxalate forms calcium oxalate crystals that can block the renal tubules. 4-Methylpyrazole (Fomepizole) is an alcohol dehydrogenase inhibitor that is used as an antidote for the treatment of methanol or ethylene glycol poisoning. 1,4-Butanediol is a solvent that has become known to the public as a date-rape drug and drug-of-abuse due to its metabolism to γ-hydroxybutyrate. The oxidized metabolite binds to the γ-hydroxybutyrate receptor, which in turn produces CNS sedation with amnesia.

Alcohol dehydrogenase functions also as a reductase when it catalyzes the reduction of an aldehyde or ketone to an alcohol. In addition, other NADP- or NAD-dependent dehydrogenases in the cytosol are capable of reducing a variety of ketones. Ketones are stable to further oxidation and, consequently, yield reduction products as major metabolites. Examples of reduction include the sedative-hypnotic chloral hydrate to trichloroethanol, the opioid antagonist naltrexone to 6B-β-hydroxynaltrexol, the opioid analgesic methadone to α-methadol, the antipsychotic haloperidol to hydroxyhaloperidol, and the antiemetic dolasetron to dihydrodolasetron. These alcohol metabolites are all pharmacologically active.

Aldehyde Dehydrogenase

Aldehyde dehydrogenases (ALHD) (not to be confused with aldehyde oxidase) are a family of polymorphic NAD+-specific enzymes that catalyze the NAD+-dependent oxidation (dehydrogenation) of aldehydes to carboxylic acids, which are subsequently metabolized by the body's muscle and heart. There are three mammalian classes of these enzymes: class 1 (low K_m, cytosolic ALDH1), class 2 (low K_m, mitochondrial ALDH2), and class 3 (high K_m, such as those expressed in tumors, stomach, and cornea). In all the three classes, constitutive (an enzyme whose activity is constant and active) and inducible forms exist. ALDH1 and ALDH2 are the most important enzymes for aldehyde oxidation and both are tetrameric enzymes composed of 54 kDA subunits. These enzymes are found in many tissues of the body but are at the highest concentration in the liver.

ALDH1, along with ADH, is responsible for the metabolism of retinol to retinoic acid. ALDH2 catalyzes the bioactivation of nitroglycerin (glyceryl trinitrate) in blood vessels, resulting in vasodilation by nitric oxide (NO). ALDH2 has a major role in the hepatic detoxication of acetaldehyde and other aldehydes produced from oxidation of ethanol and other primary alcohols, and the oxidation of endogenous aldehydes, such as those produced by the oxidation of biogenic amines (norepinephrine, serotonin, dopamine). These aldehydes can be toxic and health problems arise when the aldehyde cannot be cleared. The accumulation of unmetabolized acetaldehyde in the blood has been shown to be a carcinogen in lab animals.

For example, when high levels of acetaldehyde occur in the blood, symptoms of facial flushing, light-headedness, palpitations, nausea, and general "hangover" symptoms occur. These symptoms are indicative of a disease known as "Asian flush" or "Oriental flushing syndrome," which is due to a mutant form of ALDH2 termed *ALDH2*2*. In the protein expressed by this mutant, a lysine residue replaces a glutamate in the active site, yielding an enzyme with about 8% of the activity of the wild-type (normal) *ALDH*2* allele. The mutant allele shows a higher km for NAD+ than the wild-type allele. This mutation is common in Japan, where 41% of a nonalcoholic control group were *ALDH2* (wild-type) deficient, and where only 2%-5% of an alcoholic group were ALDH2 deficient. In Taiwan, the numbers are similar, with 30% of the nonalcoholic control group showing the wild-type deficiency and 6% of alcoholics displaying the deficiency. The ALDH2 wild-type deficiency is manifested by slow acetaldehyde removal and low alcohol tolerance, which may lead to a lower frequency of alcoholism. These acetaldehyde toxicity symptoms are similar to those observed in people who drink ethanol while being treated with the drug disulfiram (Antabuse), which is why it is used to treat alcoholism in patients seeking recovery. These patients show higher blood levels of acetaldehyde and become violently ill upon consumption of even small amounts of alcohol. Several other drugs (e.g., metronidazole) cause a similar reaction known as "disulfiram-like reaction."

Disulfiram → Diethyldithiocarbamic acid

CH_3-S(O)-CH_3 → CH_3-S-CH_3

Dimethylsulfoxide → Dimethylsulfide

Molybdenum Hydroxylases

Molybdenum hydroxylases are non-P450 enzymes capable of catalyzing the oxidation of drugs. The molybdenum hydroxylases, which include aldehyde oxidase, xanthine oxidase, and xanthine dehydrogenase, are more commonly found in the cytosol of mammalian liver and carry out the oxidation and detoxification of structurally different azaheterocycles[46-48] (Fig. 3.21). The efficient oxidation of endogenous purine nucleosides suggests that their metabolism and detoxification might be an important physiological role of the molybdenum hydroxylases. Among the azaheterocycles metabolized are derivatives of pyridine, quinoline, pyrimidine, purine, quinazoline, and pteridines.

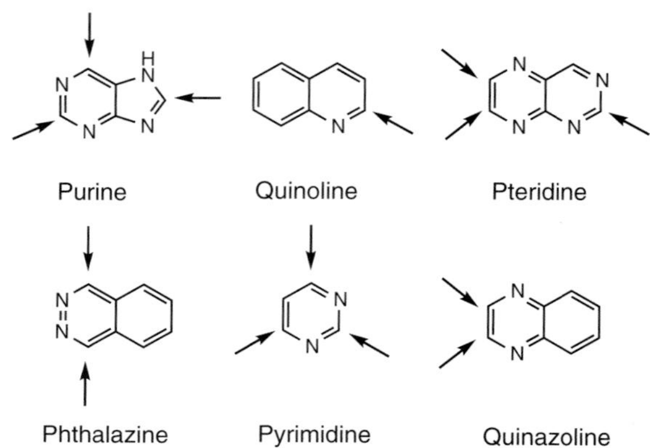

Figure 3.21 Heterocycle substrates for aldehyde oxidase.

These hydroxylases as a rule oxidize the α-carbon to the nitrogen of the azaheterocycle to oxo metabolites (also known as lactams).

The molybdenum hydroxylases are cytosolic with a common electron-transfer system in each enzyme subunit: a molybdopterin (a pyranopteridine ligand) cofactor that binds the single molybdenum (Mo) ion, two iron-sulfur centers, and an FAD molecule. The Mo is an essential component of the enzyme and, along with FAD, is required for enzyme catalysis. The enzyme is biologically inactive until it becomes complexed by the pterin to form the tetracyclic pteridine complex termed "MoCo." The pterin moiety positions the catalytic Mo correctly within the active site of the enzyme to participate in electron transfer to and from the Mo atom. The molybdenum hydroxylases catalyze their reactions differently than P450 and other hydroxylase enzymes, requiring water rather than molecular oxygen as the source of the oxygen atom incorporated into the metabolite, and with the concomitant reduction of molecular oxygen to superoxide.[47] The active sites possess a catalytically labile Mo^{V}-OH group that is transferred to the substrate during the hydroxylation reaction.

ALDEHYDE OXIDASE. Aldehyde oxidase (AO) is an enzyme located in the cytosol of cells and is similar to the xanthine oxidase (XO) family of molybdoenzymes that requires a molybdenum cofactor (MoCo) for the catalytic activity. The physiological role of AO remains unclear, but in humans, it plays an important role in the clearance of drug compounds containing aldehydes and N-containing heterocyclic aromatic compounds. It generates carboxylic acids from aldehydes in the presence of oxygen. Although aldehydes are not often present in drug compounds, they can be a product of biotransformation reactions by P450s and MAO, which can be subsequently oxidized to a carboxylic acid by AO. In addition to metabolizing some aldehydes, aldehyde oxidase also oxidizes a variety of azaheterocycles but excludes thia- or oxaheterocycles. Of the various purine nucleosides metabolized by aldehyde oxidase, the 2-hydroxy- and 2-amino derivatives are more efficiently metabolized. The typical order of N9 substituent preference of the acyclic nucleosides is as follows: 9-[(hydroxy-alkyloxy)methyl]-purines > 2′-arabinofuranosyl > H. The kinetic rate constants for purine analogues reveal that the pyrimidine portion of the purine ring system is more important for substrate affinity than the imidazole portion. Aldehyde oxidase is inhibited by potassium cyanide and menadione (synthetic vitamin K).

Aldehyde oxidase metabolizes an assortment of azaheterocycles, including the short-acting sedative-hypnotic drug zaleplon (a pyrazolo[1,5α] pyrimidine derivative) to its 5-oxo metabolite; the anticancer drug thioguanine to 8-oxothioguanine; the α_2-adrenergic agonist brimonidine (a pyrimidine derivative) to its 2-oxo-, 3-oxo-, and 2,3-dioxo- metabolites; quinine and quinidine to their 2-quinolone metabolites; the pro-antiviral drug famiclovir (a purine derivative) to its active 6-oxo metabolite (penciclovir); O6-benzylguanine to its 8-oxo metabolite (also formed primarily from CYP3A4); and the antiseizure drug zonisamide (a 1,2-benzisoxazole derivative), primarily by reductive cleavage of the 1,2-benzisoxazole ring to 2-sulfamoylacetylphenol. Although the azaheterocycles thiazole and oxazole are not metabolized by aldehyde oxidase, their carbocyclic analogues, benzothiazole, benzoxazole, and 1,2-benzisoxazole, are. On the other hand, the heterocycles, benzothiophene and benzofuran, which do not contain a nitrogen atom, are not metabolized by, nor do they inhibit, aldehyde oxidase. Both aldehyde oxidase and xanthine oxidase contribute to the first-pass hepatic metabolism of orally administered methotrexate (a 2,4-diaminopteridine) to its 7-hydroxymethotrexate metabolite.

Potent inhibitors of aldehyde oxidase include the selective estrogen receptor modulator raloxifene, tamoxifen, estradiol, and ethinyl estradiol. Other classes of drugs that demonstrate inhibition of aldehyde oxidase included phenothiazines, tricyclic antidepressants, tricyclic atypical antipsychotic agents, dihydropyridine calcium channel blockers, loratadine, ondansetron, propafenone, domperidone, quinacrine, verapamil, and salmeterol. Thus, the possibility of clinical drug interactions mediated by inhibition of this aldhyde oxidase could be observed between these drugs, and drugs for which aldehyde oxidase is the primary route of metabolism.

XANTHINE OXIDASE AND XANTHINE DEHYDROGENASE. The properties of AO and XO are closely related. Both enzymes are present in the cytosol. The primary difference between the two enzymes is that XO can exist in two interconvertible forms, xanthine oxidase (XO) and xanthine dehydrogenase, while AO exists only in the oxidase form. AO utilizes only molecular oxygen as an electron acceptor in contrast to XO, which can transfer electrons to both oxygen and NAD^+. The key physiological function of XO has been recognized as the oxidative metabolism of purines into the terminal metabolite uric acid (Fig. 3.22).

XO and xanthine dehydrogenase represent different forms of the same gene product. Xanthine dehydrogenase can be interconverted to XO by reversible sulfhydryl oxidation. These two enzyme forms and their reactions often are referred to as xanthine oxidoreductase. XO is the rate-limiting enzyme in human purine catabolism of hypoxanthine to uric acid and can also generate reactive oxygen species. XO is a cytosolic 370 kDa molybdoflavoenzyme that requires a molydopterin cofactor, two iron-sulfur centers, and FAD.

Both XO and xanthine dehydrogenase have important roles in the metabolism of purine anticancer drugs to their active and inactive metabolites. Although XO is strongly inhibited by the antigout drug allopurinol, AO also oxidizes allopurinol to oxypurinol. Only xanthine dehydrogenase requires NAD^+ as an electron acceptor for the oxidation of azaheterocycles. 6-Mercaptopurine is metabolized by XO to 6-mercapturic acid. In humans, XO is normally found in the liver and not free in the blood. Xanthinuria is a rare genetic disorder where the lack of XO leads to high concentration of xanthine in blood and can cause health problems such as renal failure. There is no specific treatment for this disorder except to avoid foods high in purine and to maintain a high fluid intake.

Oxidative Deamination of Amines

Monoamine oxidase (MAO) catalyzes the oxidative deamination of amines to aldehydes in the presence of oxygen. The aldehyde products can be metabolized further to the corresponding acid or alcohol by aldehyde oxidase or dehydrogenase.

Monoamine Oxidase

MAO is a mitochondrial membrane flavin-containing enzyme that catalyzes the oxidative deamination of monoamines, where oxygen is used to remove an amine group from a monoamine substrate resulting in the formation of the corresponding aldehyde and ammonia[48] (Fig. 3.23).

Substrates for this enzyme include primary amines and secondary and tertiary amines in which the amine substrates are methyl groups. The amine must be attached to an unsubstituted methylene group. Compounds having a single substitution at the α-carbon atom are poor substrates

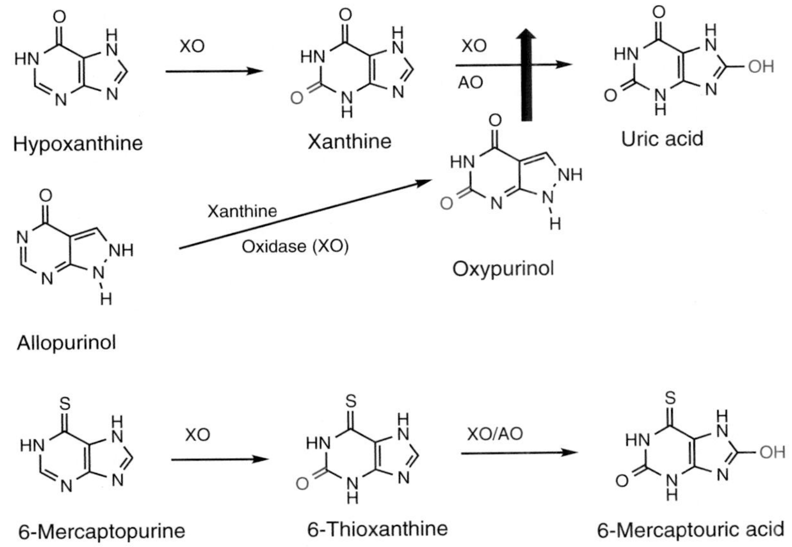

Figure 3.22 Xanthine oxidase reactions.

$$RCH_2NH_2 \underset{}{\overset{\text{E-FAD} \rightarrow \text{E-FADH}}{\rightleftharpoons}} RCH_2\overset{\bullet+}{N}H_2 \xrightarrow{\text{E-FADH} \rightarrow \text{E-FADH}_2,\ H^{\oplus}} RCH{=}\overset{\oplus}{N}H_2 \xrightarrow{H_2O} NH_4^{\oplus} + RCH{=}O$$

Regeneration of E-FAD:

$$\text{E-FADH}_2 + O_2 \longrightarrow \text{E-FAD} + H_2O_2$$

Figure 3.23 MAO oxidation of monoamines.

for MAO (e.g., aniline, amphetamine, and ephedrine) but can be oxidized by the microsomal P450 enzymes. For secondary and tertiary amines, alkyl groups larger than a methyl and branched alkyl groups (i.e., isopropyl, *t*-butyl, or β-phenylisopropyl) inhibit MAO oxidation, but such substrates can function as reversible inhibitors of this enzyme. Nonselective irreversible inhibitors of MAO include hydrazides (phenelzine) and tranylcypromine and the MAO-B selective inhibitors pargyline and selegiline. Monoamine oxidase is important in regulating the metabolic degradation of catecholamines and serotonin in neural tissues. Hepatic MAO has a crucial defensive role in inactivating circulating monoamines, or those originating in the GIT and absorbed into the systemic circulation (e.g., tyramine).

There are two types of MAO: MAO-A and MAO-B. They show dissimilar substrate preferences and different sensitivities to inhibitors. MAO-A, found mainly in peripheral adrenergic nerve terminals but also in the liver, GIT, and placenta, shows substrate preference for 5-hydroxytryptamine, norepinephrine, and epinephrine. MAO-B is found principally in platelets and shows selectivity for nonphenolic, lipophilic β-phenethylamines. Common substrates to both MAO-A and MAO-B are dopamine, tyramine, and other monophenolic phenylethylamines.

A contaminant in the synthesis of reversed esters of meperidine, 1-methyl-4-phenyl-1,2,3,6-tetrahydropyridine (MPTP), was discovered to be a highly selective neurotoxin for dopaminergic cells, producing parkinsonism.[49] The neurotoxicity of MPTP is associated with cellular destruction in the substantia nigra along with severe reductions in the concentration of dopamine, norepinephrine, and serotonin. The remarkable neurotoxic action for MPTP involves a sequence of events beginning with the metabolic activation of MPTP to the toxic metabolite MPP^+ (1-methyl-4-phenylpyridinium ion) by MAO-B, specific uptake and accumulation of MPP^+ in the nigrostriatal dopaminergic neurons, and ending with the inhibition of oxidative phosphorylation. This inhibition results in mitochondrial injury depriving the sensitive nigrostriatal cells of oxidative phosphorylation with their eventual cell death (neurotoxic actions of MPP^+). The MAO-B inhibitors (e.g., deprenyl) blocked this biotransformation.

MPTP MPP^+

Because of the vital role that MAOs have in the inactivation of neurotransmitters, MAO dysfunction (too much or too little MAO activity) is thought to be responsible for a number of neurological disorders. For example, unusually high or low levels of MAOs in the body have been associated with depression, schizophrenia, substance abuse, attention deficit disorder, and migraines. Monoamine oxidase inhibitors (MAOIs) are one of the major classes of drugs prescribed for the treatment of depression, although they are last-line treatment due to risk of the drug's interaction with dietary constituents (e.g., tyramine) or other drugs. Excessive levels of catecholamines (epinephrine, norepinephrine, and dopamine) may lead to a hypertensive crisis, and excessive levels of serotonin may lead to serotonin syndrome, both of which are potentially fatal.

Miscellaneous Reductions

Various studies on the biotransformation of xenobiotic ketones have established that ketone reduction is an important metabolic pathway in mammalian tissue.[50] Because carbonyl compounds are lipophilic and can be retained in tissues, their reduction to the hydrophilic alcohols and subsequent conjugation are critical to their elimination. Although ketone reductases (carbonyl reductases) can be closely related to the alcohol dehydrogenases, they have distinctly different properties and use NADPH as the cofactor. Carbonyl reductase participates in arachidonic acid metabolism. The metabolism of xenobiotic ketones to free alcohols or conjugated alcohols has been demonstrated for aromatic, aliphatic, alicyclic, and unsaturated ketones (e.g., naltrexone, naloxone, hydromorphone, and daunorubicin). The carbonyl reductases are distinguished by the stereospecificity of their alcohol metabolites.

Hydrolysis

In general, esters and amides are hydrolyzed by enzymes in the blood, liver microsomes, intestine, kidneys, and other tissues. Esters and certain amides are rapidly hydrolyzed by a group of enzymes termed "carboxylesterases." The more lipophilic the amide, the more favorable it is as a substrate for this enzyme. In most cases, the hydrolysis of an ester or amide bond in a toxic substance results in bioinactivation to hydrophilic metabolites that are readily excreted. Some of these metabolites can yield conjugated metabolites (i.e., glucuronides). Amides are very common in food as proteins and peptides we eat. Not surprisingly, there are a large number of proteolytic enzymes in the GIT called amino endopeptidases and amino exopeptidases that hydrolyze ingested proteins into amino acids.

Carboxylesterases include cholinesterase (pseudocholinesterase), arylcarboxyesterases, liver microsomal carboxylesterases, and other unclassified liver carboxylesterases. Cholinesterase hydrolyzes choline-like esters (e.g., actylcholine, succinylcholine) and procaine as well as acetylsalicylic acid. Genetic variant forms of cholinesterase have been identified in human serum (e.g., succinylcholine toxicity results when administered as a ganglionic blocker for muscle relaxation to patients with the variant form of cholinesterase). Meperidine is hydrolyzed only by liver microsomal carboxylesterases (Fig. 3.24). Diphenoxylate is hydrolyzed to its active metabolite diphenoxylic acid within 1 hour (Fig. 3.24). Presumably, the lack of a central pharmacological action of diphenoxylate is attributed to the formation of a zwitterionic diphenoxylic acid, which is readily eliminated in the urine.

Sterically hindered esters are hydrolyzed more slowly and can appear unchanged in the urine. For example, approximately 50% of a dose of atropine appears unchanged in the urine of humans, and the remainder consists of unhydrolyzed biotransformed products.

As a rule, amides are more stable to hydrolysis than are esters and it is not surprising to find amides of drugs excreted largely unchanged. This fact has been exploited in developing the antiarrhythmic drug procainamide. Procaine is not useful as an antiarrhythmic because of its rapid esterase-catalyzed hydrolysis, but 60% of a dose of procainamide was recovered unchanged from the urine of humans, with the remainder being mostly N-acetylprocainamide. On the other hand, the deacylated metabolite of indomethacin (a tertiary amide) is one of the major metabolites detected in human urine. Amide hydrolysis of phthalylsulfathiazole and succinylsulfathiazole by bacterial enzymes in the colon releases the antibacterial agent sulfathiazole.

SUMMARY

In summary, Phase 1 metabolic transformations introduce new and polar functional groups into the molecule, which can produce one or more of the following changes:

1. Decreased pharmacological activity (deactivation)
2. Increased pharmacological activity (activation)
3. Increased toxicity (carcinogenesis, mutagenesis, cytotoxicity)
4. Altered pharmacological activity

Drugs exhibiting increased activity or activity different from the parent drug usually undergo further metabolism and conjugation resulting in deactivation and excretion of the inactive conjugates.

DRUG CONJUGATION PATHWAYS (PHASE 2)

Conjugation reactions (Fig. 3.25) represent probably the most important xenobiotic biotransformation. Xenobiotics are as a rule lipophilic, well absorbed into tissues from the blood, but excreted slowly in the urine.[5] Only after conjugation (Phase 2) reactions have added an ionic hydrophilic moiety, such as glucuronic acid, sulfate ester, or glycine to the xenobiotic, is water solubility significantly increased and lipid solubility decreased enough to make urinary elimination possible. The major proportion of the administered drug dose is excreted as conjugates into the urine and bile. Conjugation reactions can be preceded by Phase 1 reactions. For xenobiotics with a functional group available for Phase 2 metabolism, conjugation can be its fate.

Common Features of Phase 2 Pathways

Phase 2 conjugation commonly creates anionic metabolites (e.g., glucuronides, sulfate esters, glycine conjugates, glutathione conjugates) that are then actively excreted into the bile via biliary transporters, or into the renal proximal tubules by renal transporters.[5,7,51] Conjugated metabolites often have higher elimination clearance than the parent drug, due in part to active excretion/transport into urine and/or bile, and are expected to have a half-life shorter than that of the parent drug. Cofactor depletion can occur at high drug doses. Biliary excretion of glucuronide and sulfate ester conjugates with higher molecular weight (e.g., >325) is increased.

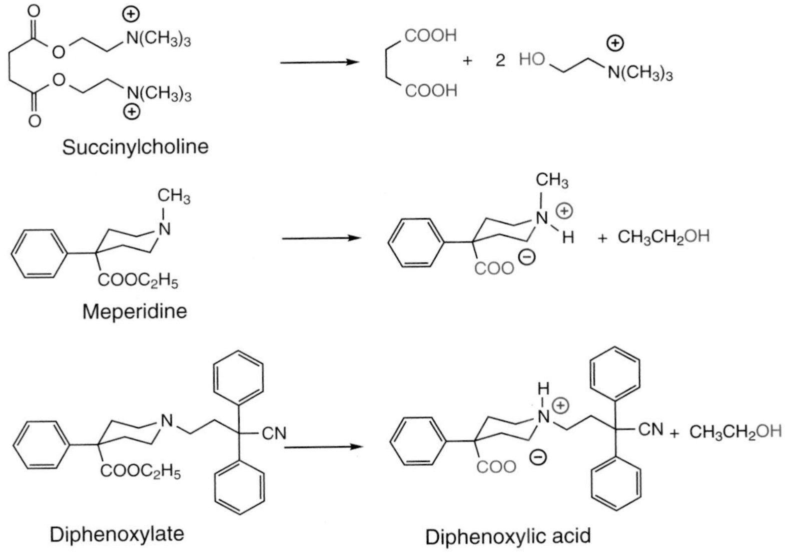

Figure 3.24 Examples of hydrolysis reactions.

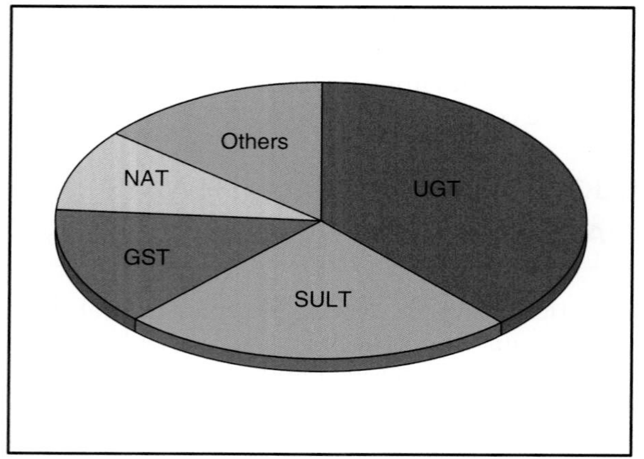

Figure 3.25 Phase 2 pathways contributing to drug metabolism (new).

The major conjugation reactions (glucuronidation and sulfonation) were traditionally thought to terminate pharmacological activity by transforming the parent drug or Phase 1 metabolites into readily excreted ionic polar products. Moreover, these terminal metabolites were assumed to have no significant pharmacological activity due to poor cellular diffusion and poor affinity for the active drug's receptor. This long-established view has changed with the discoveries that morphine 6-glucuronide has more analgesic activity than morphine in humans, and that minoxidil sulfate is the active metabolite for the antihypertensive minoxidil. For most xenobiotics, however, conjugation is an inactivating and detoxification mechanism. However, some compounds could form reactive intermediates that have been implicated in carcinogenesis, allergic reactions, and tissue damage.

Sequential conjugation of the same drug substance produces multiple conjugated products, for example, *p*-aminosalicylic acid in Figure 3.26. Thus, the drug or xenobiotic can be a substrate for more than one metabolizing enzyme. Different conjugation pathways could compete for the same functional group with the outcome being an array of metabolites excreted in the urine or feces. Factors determining the outcome of this interplay include availability of cofactors, enzyme kinetics (V_{max}), affinity of the drug/xenobiotic (K_m) for the metabolizing enzyme, and type of tissues (e.g., hepatic, kidney, lung). When a cofactor is low or depleted, the competing conjugation reactions can take control. The reactivity of the functional group is determined also by all subsequent conjugation reactions. For example, major competing conjugation reactions are sulfonation, ether glucuronidation, and methylation for the phenolic hydroxyl groups; acetylation, sulfonation, and

Acetylation / N-glucuronidation (H_2N)
O-glucuronidation / O-sulfation (OH)
Acyl glucuronidation / Glycine conjugation (COOH)

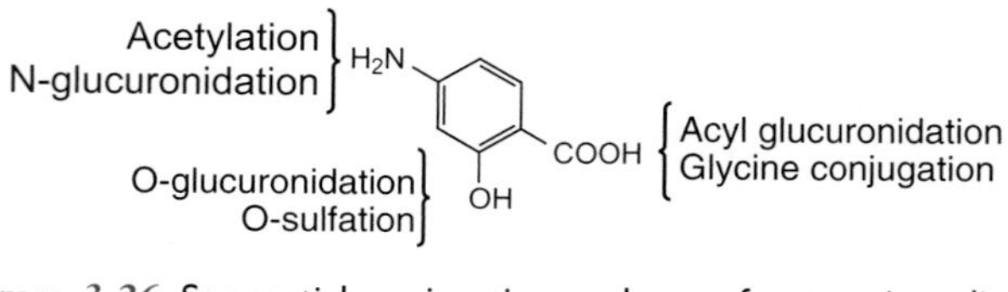

Figure 3.26 Sequential conjugation pathways for *p*-aminosalicylic acid.

glucuronidation for amine groups; and amino acid conjugation, CoA conjugation, and ester glucuronidation for carboxyl groups.

Conjugation enzymes can show stereospecificity toward enantiomers when a racemic drug is administered. The metabolite pattern of a drug when administered orally can be different when the same drug is administered intravenously because of the avoidance of presystemic intestinal conjugation via the latter route.

Glucuronic Acid Conjugation

Glucuronide formation is the most common route for Phase 2 metabolism to water-soluble metabolites, accounting for approximately 35% of drug conjugation and the major share of the conjugated metabolites found in the urine and bile.[51] The significance of glucuronidation lies in the available supply of glucuronic acid (oxidized glucose) in the liver and in the many functional groups capable of forming glucuronide conjugates (e.g., phenols, alcohols, carboxylic acids, and amines).

Mechanism of Glucuronide Conjugation

Glucuronide conjugation involves the direct condensation of the xenobiotic (or its Phase 1 metabolite) with the activated form of glucuronic acid, UDP-glucuronic acid (UDPGA). The overall scheme of the glucuronide conjugation reaction is shown in Figure 3.27. The SN_2 reaction between UDPGA requires a nucleophile or "handle" on the drug or xenobiotic acceptor compound and is catalyzed by a family of UDP-glucuronosyltransferases (UGT), a multigene family of isozymes located along the ER of the liver, epithelial cells of the intestine, and other extrahepatic tissues.[5] Its unique location in the ER, along with the P450 isoforms, has important physiologic effects in the conjugation of reactive metabolites generated by the P450 isoforms and in controlling the levels of reactive metabolites present in these tissues. Transporters carry the UDPGA and xenobiotics from the cytosol into the ER lumen and then transport the glucuronide metabolite from the ER lumen into the cytosol. The presence of the active site for UGT toward the ER lumen catalyzes the reaction between the substrate and UDPGA.[51]

Glucuronidation is a low-affinity (a higher concentration of the xenobiotic is required for full enzyme activity) and high-capacity (high rate of xenobiotic turnover) Phase 2 reaction. The resultant glucuronide has the β-configuration about carbon 1 of glucuronic acid. With the attachment of the hydrophilic carbohydrate moiety containing an easily ionizable carboxyl group (pK_a = 3-4), a lipid-soluble substance is converted into a conjugate that is reabsorbed poorly by the renal system.

Endogenous substances that readily conjugate with glucuronic acid include catecholamines, steroids, bilirubin, and thyroxine. Not all glucuronides are excreted by the kidneys. Some are excreted into the intestinal tract with bile (enterohepatic cycling), where β-glucuronidase in the intestinal flora hydrolyzes the C^1-O-glucuronide

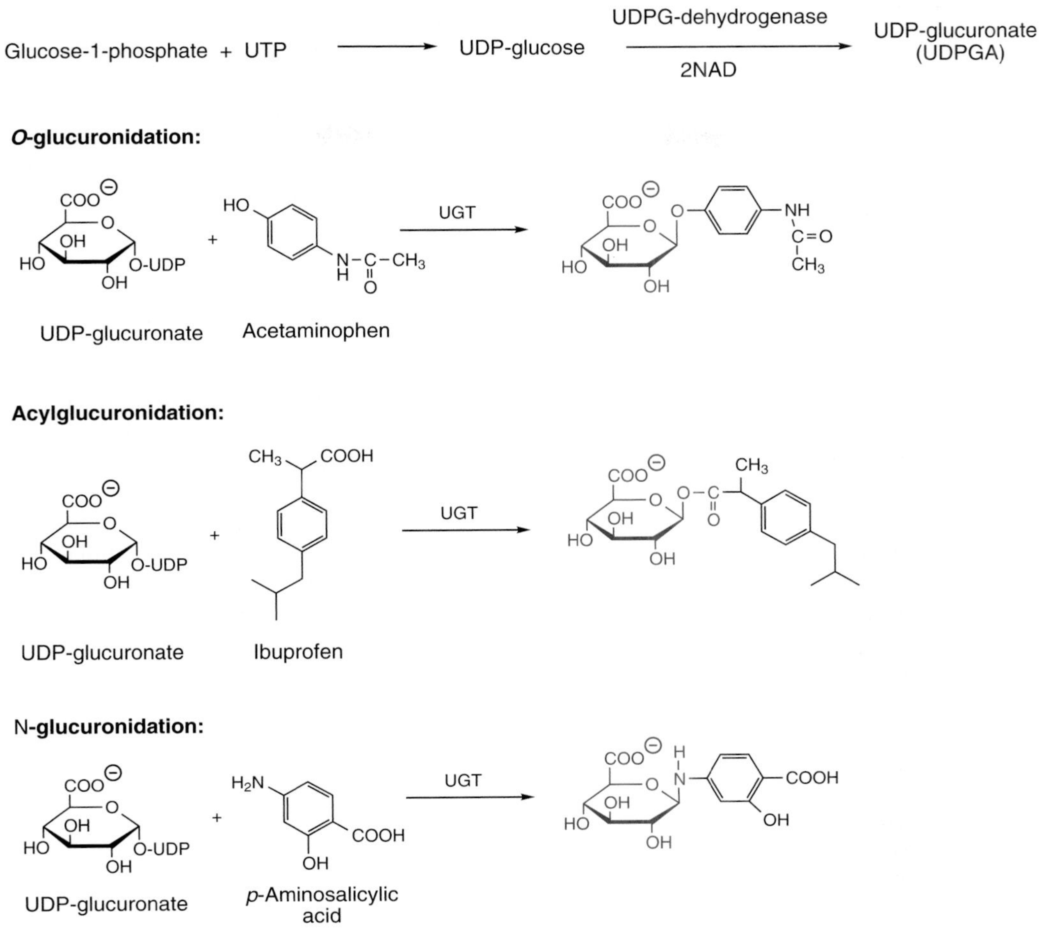

Glucose-1-phosphate + UTP ⟶ UDP-glucose ⟶ (UDPG-dehydrogenase, 2NAD) UDP-glucuronate (UDPGA)

***O*-glucuronidation:**

UDP-glucuronate + Acetaminophen ⟶(UGT)

Acylglucuronidation:

UDP-glucuronate + Ibuprofen ⟶(UGT)

N-glucuronidation:

UDP-glucuronate + *p*-Aminosalicylic acid ⟶(UGT)

Figure 3.27 Glucuronidation pathways catalyzed by UDP-glucuronosyltransferases (UGTs).

to the aglycone (xenobiotic or their metabolites) for reabsorption into the portal circulation (see section Enterohepatic Cycling of Drugs). A summary of drug functional groups commonly glucuronidated is provided in Figure 3.28.

UGT Families

UGTs have been classified into families according to similarities in amino acid sequences, analogous to the P450 family.[51] The human UGT family is divided into two subfamilies, UGT1 (UGT1A1, 1A2, 1A3, 1A4, 1A5, 1A6, 1A7, 1A8, 1A9, and 1A10) and UGT2 (UGT2B4, 2B7, 2B10, 2B11, 2B15, 2B17, and 2B28).[5,7,51] Considerable overlap in substrate specificities exists between the two families. The UGT1A1 isoform is primarily responsible for the glucuronidation of bilirubin, estradiol, and other estrogenic steroids; UGT1A3 and UGT1A4 catalyze the glucuronidation of drugs with tertiary amines to form quaternary glucuronides and hydroxylated xenobiotics; UGT1A6 exhibits limited substrate specificity for planar phenolic substances; UGT1A9 has a wide range of substrate specificity and can glucuronidate nonplanar phenols, plant substances (e.g., anthraquinones and flavones), steroids, other phenolic drugs, and C-glucuronidate phenylbutazoine; and UGT1A10 glucuronidates mycophenolic acid, an inhibitor of inosine monophosphate dehydrogenase. Human family 2 isoform UGT2B4 is homologous to UGT2B7 and catalyzes the glucuronidation of the 6α-hydroxyl group of bile acids; UGT2B7 glucuronidates the largest number of substrates including the 3- and 6-glucuronidation of morphine and 6-glucuronidation of codeine; UGT2B11 glucuronidates a wide range of planar phenols, bulky alcohols, and polyhydroxylated estradiol metabolites; and UGT2B15 catalyzes the glucuronidation of the 17α-hydroxyl group of dihydrotestosterone and other steroidal compounds. UGT1A isoforms are inducible with 3-methylcholanthrene and cigarette smoking, and the UGT2B family is inducible by barbiturates. Approximately 40% of the glucuronides are produced by UGT2B7, 20% by UGT1A4, and 15% by UGT1A1.

UGT Distribution

The human liver is the most important tissue for all routes of Phase 1 and Phase 2 metabolism. The UGTs expressed in the intestine include UGT1A1 (bilirubin-glucuronidating isoform), UGT1A3, UGT1A4, UGT1A6, UGT1A8, UGT1A9, and UGT1A3. Substrate specificities of intestinal UGT isoforms are comparable to those in the liver. The UGT isoforms in the intestine can glucuronidate orally administered drugs, such as morphine, acetaminophen,

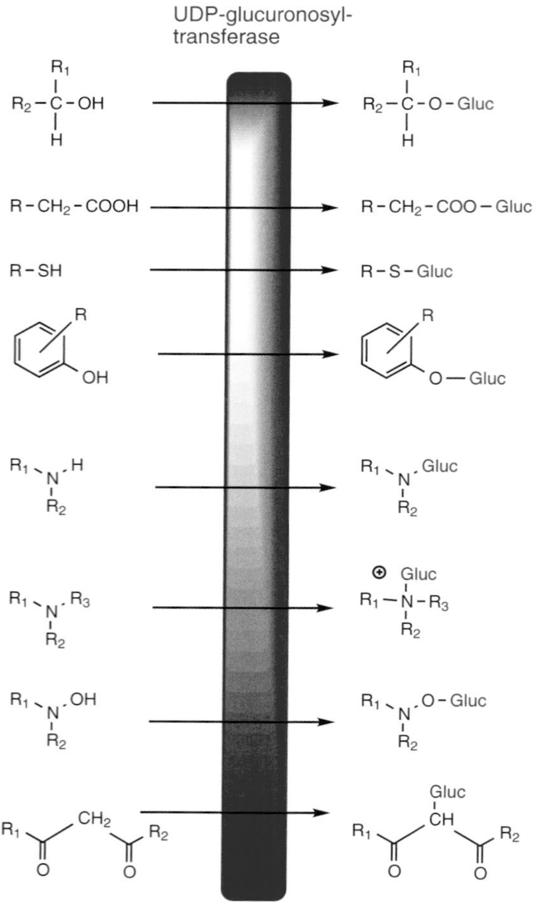

Figure 3.28 Phase 2 glucuronidation pathways contributing to drug metabolism (new).

α- and β-adrenergic agonists, and other phenolic phenethanolamines, as well as other dietary xenobiotics, reducing their oral bioavailability (first-pass metabolism). Although UGT isoforms are found in the kidney, brain, nasal epithelia, and lung, they are not uniformly distributed, with UGT1A6 being the isoform that is ubiquitous in extrahepatic tissue.

O-, N-, and S-Glucuronides

The xenobiotics that contain an electron-rich nucleophilic (heteroatom) O, N, or S or some extremely electophillic carbons form glucuronides. In humans, almost 40%-70% of clinically used drugs are subjected to O-glucuronidation, with alcohols and phenols producing ether O-glucuronides. O-phenolic glucuronides predominate over alcohol hydroxy O-glucuronidation because of the greater nucleophilicity of phenols (pK_a 7-10), efficiencies, and turnover rates. Aromatic and some aliphatic carboxylic acids form ester (acyl) glucuronides. Aromatic amines form N-glucuronides and sulfhydryl compounds form S-glucuronides, both of which are more labile to acid as compared with the O-glucuronides (Fig. 3.27). Some tertiary amines (e.g., tripelennamine) have been reported to form quaternary ammonium N-glucuronides. Substances containing a 1,3-dicarbonyl structure (e.g., phenylbutazone) can undergo formation of C-glucuronides by direct conjugation without previous metabolism. The acidity of the methylene carbon of the 1,3-dicarbonyl group determines the degree of C-glucuronide formation.

Acyl Glucuronides

Drug-acyl glucuronides are reactive conjugates of carboxylic acids at physiologic pH.[52] The acyl group of the C1-acyl glucuronide can migrate via transesterification from the original C1 position of the glucuronic acid to the C2, C3, or C4 positions (Fig. 3.27). The resulting positional isomers are not hydrolyzed by β-glucuronidase, giving the appearance of a new unknown conjugate. However, under physiologic or weakly alkaline conditions, the C1-acyl glucuronide can hydrolyze in the urine to produce the parent substance (aglycone) or undergo acyl migration to an acceptor macromolecule, forming an immunoreactive hapten. The pH-catalyzed migration of the acyl group from the drug C1-O-acyl glucuronide to a protein or other cellular constituent occurs with the formation of a covalent bond to the protein. The acylated protein becomes a "hapten" and could stimulate an immune response against the drug, resulting in the expression of a hypersensitivity reaction or other forms of immunotoxicity. A high incidence of idiosyncratic/immunotoxic reactions has been reported for several NSAIDs; for example, benoxaprofen, zomepirac, indoprofen, alclofenac, ticrynafen, and ibufenac, all of which have been removed from the market. All of these NSAIDs are metabolized by humans to acyl glucuronides. Similar reactions have been reported for other NSAIDs, including tolmetin, sulindac, ibuprofen, ketoprofen, and acetylsalicylic acid. The frequency of the immunotoxic response can be related to the stability of the acyl glucuronide, the chemical rate kinetics for the migration of the acyl group, and the concentration and stability/half-life of the antigenic protein.

When the acyl glucuronide is the primary metabolite in patients with decreased renal function (i.e., elderly individuals) or when probenecid is coadministered, renal cycling of the unconjugated (aglycone) parent drug or metabolite is likely to occur, resulting in the plasma accumulation of the aglycone. The reduced elimination of the acyl glucuronide increases its hydrolysis to either the aglycone or the migration of the C1-O-acyl group to an acceptor macromolecule, as previously described.

Bioactivation and Toxic Glucuronides

As a rule, glucuronides are biologically and chemically less reactive than their parent molecules and are readily eliminated without interaction with intracellular substances. However, some glucuronide conjugates are more pharmacologically active than the parent drug.[53] Morphine, for example, forms the 3-O- and 6-O-glucuronides in the intestine and in the liver. The 3-O-glucuronide is the primary glucuronide metabolite of morphine with a blood concentration 20-fold that of morphine. Pharmacologically, it is an opioid antagonist. On the other hand, 6-O-glucuronide is a more potent μ-receptor agonist than morphine and, whether administered orally or parentally, is 650-fold more analgesic than morphine in humans. Thus, the analgesic effects of morphine are the result of a complex interaction of the drug and its two glucuronide metabolites with the opioid receptor. The 6-O-glucuronide is transported into the brain via an anion-transport system.

Glucuronidation is also capable of causing hepatotoxicity and carcinogenesis by facilitating the formation of reactive electrophilic (electron-deficient) intermediates and their transport into target tissues.[54] As previously described, the major metabolic biotransformations for carboxylic acids include conjugation with glucuronic acid, which are bioactivated via UGT-catalyzed conjugation with glucuronic acid to acyl glucuronides. The reactive acyl glucuronides are electrophilic and, therefore, can contribute to the acylation of target proteins (see section Reactive Metabolites Resulting from Bioactivation), resulting in idiosyncratic reactions.

The induction of bladder carcinogenesis by aromatic amines can result from the O-glucuronidation of the N-hydroxylarylamine[54] (Fig. 3.29). These O-glucuronides become concentrated in the urine, where they are either hydrolyzed by the acid pH of the urine to produce N-hydroxylarylamines or eliminate water from the N-hydroxylarylamine under these acidic conditions to form an electrophilic arylnitrenium species (see Fig. 3.29, metabolite 4). This reactive species binds covalently with endogenous cellular constituents (e.g., nucleic acids and proteins), initiating carcinogenesis.

Sulfonation and glucuronidation occur side by side, often competing for the same substrate (most commonly phenols, i.e., acetaminophen). The balance between sulfonation and glucuronidation is influenced by factors such as animal species, dose, availability of cofactors, and inhibition and induction of the respective transferases.

Sulfonation (Sulfoconjugation)

Sulfonation (sulfoconjugation) is an important conjugation reaction in the biotransformation of steroid hormones, catecholamine neurotransmitters, thyroxine, bile acids, phenolic drugs, and other xenobiotics.[7,55,56] The major physiologic consequence of sulfonation of a drug or xenobiotic is its increased aqueous solubility and excretion. Because the pK_a of the sulfate group is approximately 1, sulfate esters are completely ionized in physiologic solution and possess a smaller volume of distribution than unconjugated steroids and drugs. Thus a lipid-soluble substance is converted into a conjugate that is reabsorbed poorly by the renal system. For some drugs, sulfonation can result in their bioactivation to reactive electrophiles (molecules that accept an electron pair to make a covalent bond) or therapeutically active conjugates (e.g., minoxidil sulfate). Cytosolic sulfotransferases are, in general, associated with the sulfonation of phenolic steroids, neurotransmitters, and xenobiotics. Membrane-bound sulfotransferases are localized in the Golgi apparatus of most cells and are responsible for the sulfonation of glycosaminoglycans, glycoproteins, and the tyrosinyl group of peptides and protein but are usually not associated with xenobiotic metabolism.

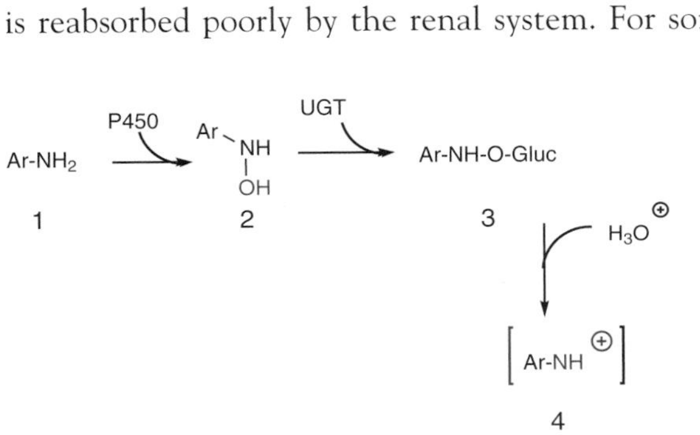

Ar-NH2 —P450→ Ar-NH-OH —UGT→ Ar-NH-O-Gluc —$H_3O^{\oplus}$→ [Ar-NH$^{\oplus}$]

1 2 3 4

Figure 3.29 Bioactivation of arylamines.

Mechanism of Sulfonation

Xenobiotics are sulfonated by the transfer of a sulfonic group ($-SO_3^-$) from 3′-phosphoadenosine-5′-phosphosulfate (PAPS) to the acceptor molecule, a cytosolic reaction catalyzed by a family of multigene sulfotransferases (Fig. 3.30); PAPS is formed enzymatically from adenosine triphosphate (ATP) and inorganic sulfate. Sulfonation is a reaction principally of phenols and to a lesser extent, of alcohols to form highly ionic and hydrophilic sulfate esters ($R\text{-}O\text{-}SO_2H$). The availability of PAPS and its precursor inorganic sulfate determines the sulfonation reaction rate.

The total pool of sulfate is frequently limited and can be readily exhausted due to the large number of substrates. Sulfonation is a high-affinity and low-capacity Phase 2 reaction which works in conjunction with glucuronidation on overlapping substrates. Thus, sulfonation predominates at low substrate concentrations and glucuronidation at high substrate concentrations.[55] When sulfonation becomes saturated from increasing doses of a drug, sulfonation becomes a less predominant pathway and the rate of glucuronidation increases until it reaches saturation. At that point, either the drug is excreted unchanged or other metabolism pathways become activated. For example, at high doses of acetaminophen, glucuronidation predominates over sulfonation, which prevails at low doses. When PAPS, inorganic sulfate, or the sulfur amino acids are low or depleted, or when a substrate for sulfonation is given in high doses, competing reactions with glucuronidation can take control. Additionally, O-methylation is a competing reaction for a catechol.

Sulfotransferase Family

In humans, sulfotransferases are divided into two families, SULT1 and SULT2.[55] SULT1A1, SULT1A2, and SULT1A3 catalyze the sulfonation of many phenolic drugs, catecholamine, hormones, aromatic amines, and other xenobiotics. SULT1A3 displays stereoselectivity in the sulfonation of chiral phenolic phenethanolamines. This isoform can be responsible, in part, for the enantiomer-specific metabolism observed for the β-adrenergic agonists. For example, the (+)-enantiomers of terbutaline and isoproterenol and the (−)-enantiomer of albuterol are selectively sulfonated.

SULT1A1/2 (formerly known as phenol sulfotransferase thermally stable) preferentially sulfonates small planar phenols in the micromolar concentration range,

SO_4^{2-} + ATP —(1. ATP-sulfurylase; 2. APS-phosphokinase)→ 3-Phosphoadenosine-5'-phosphosulfate (PAPS) + ADP + PPi

PAPS + Acetaminophen —(Sulfotransferase)→ + PAP

Figure 3.30 Sulfonation pathways.

estradiol and synthetic estrogens, phytoestrogens, acetaminophen, N-hydroxyaromatic and heterocylic amines. The crystal structure for SULT1A1 has provided insights into this enzyme's substrate specificity and catalytic function, including its role in the sulfonation of endogenous substrates such as estrogens. SULT1A3 (formerly known as phenol sulfotransferase thermally labile) selectively sulfonates the catecholamines dopamine, norepinephrine, and epinephrine, as well as the N-oxide of minoxidil, thyroid hormones, but not estrogenic steroids and other hydroxy steroids. SULT1B1 catalyzes the sulfonation of the thyroid hormones, while SULT1C1 is involved with the bioactivation of procarcinogens via sulfonation. SULT1E1 (formerly known as estrogen sulfotransferase) preferentially sulfonates estradiol in the nanomolar range. SULT2A1 (formerly known as dehydroepiandrosterone [DHEA] sulfotransferase) conjugates DHEA, estradiol (micromolar range), the synthetic estrogens, and other estrogen metabolites. Finally, SULT2B1 (formerly known as hydroxysteroid sulfotransferase) sulfonates DHEA and pregnenolone. A summary of drug functional groups commonly sulfonated is provided in Figure 3.31.

Sulfonation is an important reaction in the transport and metabolism of steroids. Sulfonation decreases the biological activity of the steroid because the steroid sulfate esters are not capable of binding to their receptors. It provides for the transport of an inactive form of the steroid to its target tissue, where the active steroid is regenerated by sulfatases at the target tissue.

Sulfotransferase Distribution

The SULT1A families are abundantly expressed in the liver, small intestine, brain, kidneys, and platelets.[55] For example, phenol is sulfonated by a sulfotransferase in the liver, kidneys, and intestines, whereas steroids are sulfonated only in the liver. The broad diversity of compounds sulfonated in human tissues results, in part, from the multi-isoforms of the cytosolic sulfotransferases and their overlapping substrate specificities. Sulfate esters are almost totally ionized and, therefore, are excreted mostly in the urine, via transporters but biliary elimination is common for steroids. When biliary sulfate esters are hydrolyzed in the intestine by sulfatases, the parent drug (or xenobiotic) or its metabolites can be reabsorbed into the portal circulation to be resulfonated for eventual elimination in the urine as a sulfate ester (enterohepatic cycling). The rate of sulfonation appears to be age dependent, decreasing with age.

An important site of sulfonation, especially after oral administration, is the intestine. The result is a presystemic first-pass effect, decreasing drug bioavailability of several drugs for which the primary route of conjugation is sulfonation. Drugs such as isoproterenol, albuterol, steroid hormones, α-methyldopa, acetaminophen, and fenoldopam are sulfonated in the gut. Competition for intestinal sulfonation between coadministered substrates can influence their bioavailability with either an enhancement of or a decrease in therapeutic effects. An example would be the coadministration of a 500-mg dose of acetaminophen and 0.03-mg dose of the oral contraceptive ethinyl estradiol. This interaction could result in increased toxicity of ethinyl estradiol because of less sulfonation in the gut.

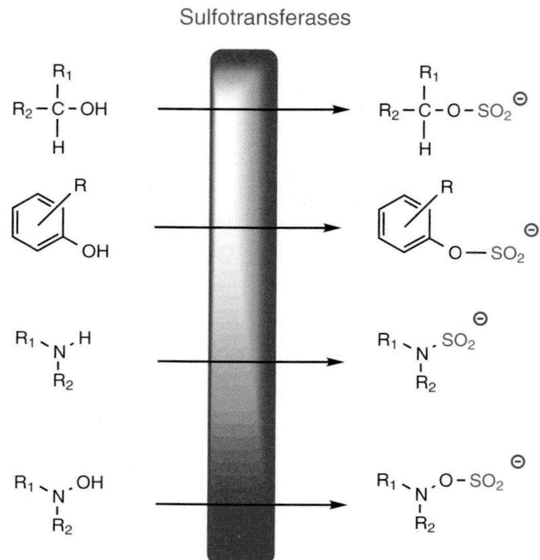

Figure 3.31 Phase 2 sulfonation pathways contributing to drug metabolism (new).

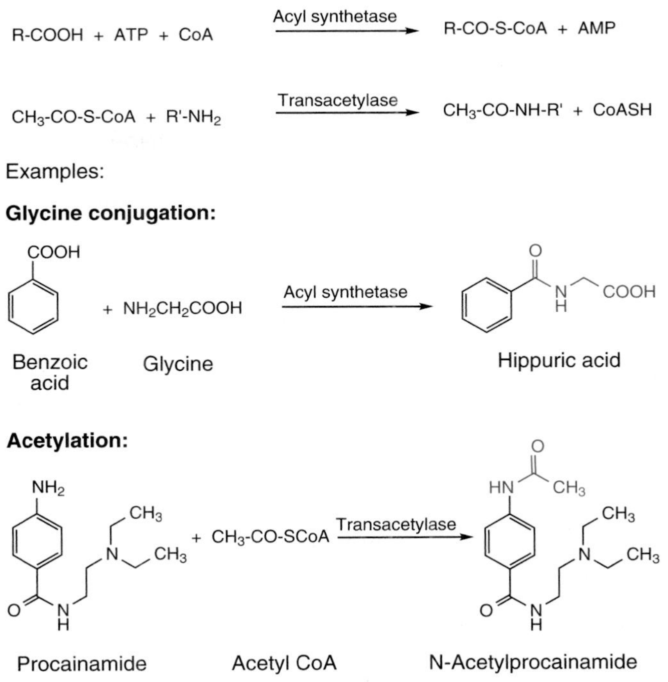

Bioactivation and Toxicity

Sulfonation is a common final step in the biotransformation of xenobiotics and is traditionally associated with inactivation, although sulfate esters have been reported to be pharmacologically active (e.g., minoxidil sulfate, dehydroepiandrosterone sulfate, and morphine 6-sulfate). However, the sulfate ester group is electron-withdrawing and may be cleaved off in some molecules, leading to an electrophilic cation forming reactive intermediates implicated in carcinogenesis and tissue damage.[56] Sulfotransferase-mediated toxicity has been demonstrated for numerous benzylic alcohols derived from polycyclic aromatic hydrocarbons and various aromatic hydroxylamines. For example, 1′-hydroxysafrole (an allylic/benzylic alcohol) is bioactivated to reactive metabolites by sulfotransferases. SULT1A1 can also sulfonate procarcinogens such as hydroxymethyl polycyclic aromatic hydrocarbons, producing reactive intermediates capable of forming DNA adducts, potentially resulting in mutagenesis. Sulfonation of an alcohol generates a good leaving group and can be an activation process for alcohols to produce a reactive electrophilic species.[55] However, like the N-glucuronides, N-sulfates are capable of promoting cytotoxicity by facilitating the formation of reactive electrophilic intermediates. Sulfonation of N-oxygenated aromatic amines is an activation process for some arylamines which can eliminate sulfate to produce an electrophilic species capable of reacting with proteins or DNA (e.g., 2-acetylaminofluorene). N-sulfonation of arylamines to arylsulfamic acids ($R\text{-}NHSO_3H$) is a minor pathway.

Conjugation with Amino Acids

Conjugation with amino acids is an important metabolic route in the metabolism of drug or xenobiotic carboxylic acids before elimination involving CoA thioesters.[5,7] Glycine, the most common amino acid, forms water-soluble ionic conjugates with aromatic, arylaliphatic, and heterocyclic carboxylic acids. These glycine conjugates are usually less toxic than their precursor acids and are readily excreted into the urine and bile. These reactions involve the formation of an amide or peptide bond between the xenobiotic carboxylic acid and the amino group of glycine. The xenobiotic is first activated to its CoA thioester before reacting with the amino group (Fig. 3.32). The formation of the xenobiotic acyl CoA thioester is of critical importance in intermediary metabolism of lipids, as well as intermediate- and long-chain fatty acids.

The major metabolic biotransformations for xenobiotic carboxylic acids include conjugation with either glucuronic acid or glycine. Carboxylic acids can be bioactivated via two distinct pathways: UGT-catalyzed conjugation with glucuronic acid to acyl glucuronides, or acyl CoA synthetase–catalyzed formation of acyl CoA thioesters.[52,57] The reactive acyl glucuronides and CoA thioester intermediates of carboxylic acids are electrophilic and, therefore, can contribute to the acylation of target proteins (see section Reactive Metabolites Resulting from Bioactivation). Acyl CoA thioester serves as an obligatory

$$\text{R-COOH} + \text{ATP} + \text{CoA} \xrightarrow{\text{Acyl synthetase}} \text{R-CO-S-CoA} + \text{AMP}$$

$$CH_3\text{-CO-S-CoA} + \text{R'-}NH_2 \xrightarrow{\text{Transacetylase}} CH_3\text{-CO-NH-R'} + \text{CoASH}$$

Examples:

Glycine conjugation:

Benzoic acid + NH_2CH_2COOH (Glycine) —Acyl synthetase→ Hippuric acid

Acetylation:

Procainamide + $CH_3\text{-CO-SCoA}$ (Acetyl CoA) —Transacetylase→ N-Acetylprocainamide

Figure 3.32 Amino acid conjugation pathway of carboxylic acids with glycine and acetylation pathway catalyzed by acetyltranferases.

intermediate in the formation of glycine conjugates and carnitine esters, which are involved in mitochondrial acyl transfer or elimination of acyl groups into urine. Therefore, their appearance in metabolism studies and urine is of significance because they serve as biomarkers for the formation acyl CoA thioesters, which can provide the link between protein-reactive acyl CoA thioesters and the rare and unpredictable idiosyncratic drug reactions in humans. Unlike CYP and UGT, which are localized in the SER, the enzymes of amino acid conjugation reside in mitochondria of the liver and kidney.

Glycine conjugation has generally been assumed to be a detoxification mechanism, increasing the water solubility of organic acids in order to facilitate their urinary excretion as compared to glucuronidation. However, glycine conjugation does not significantly increase the water solubility of aromatic acids. The role of glycine conjugation is to dispose of the end products of benzoic acid metabolism into hippuric acid products.[57]

The metabolic fate of these carboxylic acids depends on the size and type of substituents adjacent to the carboxyl group. Most unbranched aliphatic acids are completely oxidized by β-oxidation to acetic acids and do not typically form conjugates. Branched aliphatic and arylaliphatic acids are resistant to β-oxidation and form glycine or acyl glucuronide conjugates: substitution of the α-carbon favors glucuronidation over glycine conjugation. Benzoic and heterocyclic aromatic acids are mostly conjugated with glycine. Glycine conjugation is preferred for xenobiotic carboxylic acids at low doses, and glucuronidation is preferred at high doses with broad substrate selectivity. In humans, glutamine can also form a conjugate with phenylacetic acids and related arylacetic acids.

Bile acids form conjugates with glycine and taurine by the action of enzymes in the microsomal fraction rather than in the mitochondria.

In contrast to the enhanced reactivity and toxicity of the various glucuronides, sulfate ester, acetyl and glutathione conjugates, amino acid conjugates have not proven to be toxic. However, organic acids can be toxic if they are not a substrate for glycine conjugation with CoASH.[57] Carboxylic acids have been associated with adverse reactions linked to the metabolic activation of the carboxylic acid moiety of the compounds. It has been proposed that amino acid conjugation is a detoxication pathway for reactive acyl CoA thioesters.

Several carboxylic acid–containing drugs (e.g., zomiperac and benzoxaprofen) have been implicated in rare but serious adverse reactions. These carboxylic acids were withdrawn in the late 1980s from the market as a result of unpredictable idiosyncratic reactions that could have been caused by carboxylic acid-protein adducts formed by reaction of their reactive acyl glucuronide or acyl CoA thioesters with endogenous proteins.

Acetylation

Acetylation is principally a reaction of amino groups involving the transfer of acetyl CoA to primary aliphatic and aromatic amines, amino acids, hydrazines, or sulfonamide groups. The liver is the primary site of acetylation, although extrahepatic sites have been identified. Antimicrobial sulfonamides (e.g., sulfisoxazole), being difunctional, can form either N1 or N4 acetyl derivatives. Secondary amines are not acetylated. Acetylation can produce conjugates that retain the pharmacological activity of the parent drug (e.g., N-acetylprocainamide) (Fig. 3.32).

Acetylation, a nonmicrosomal form of metabolism, also exhibits polymorphisms and was first demonstrated in the acetylation of isoniazid. Several forms of N-acetyltransferase (NAT1 and NAT2) occur in humans. NAT1 (arylamine N-acetyltransferase) is widely distributed and catalyzes the N-acetylation of acidic arylamines, such as *p*-aminobenzoic acid and *p*-aminosalicylic acid; therefore its expression levels in the body have toxicological importance with regard to drug toxicitry and cancer risk (e.g., bladder cancer and colorectal cancer).

NAT2 is found predominatly in the liver. Clinically used drugs undergoing NAT2-catalyzed N-acetylation include isoniazid, procainamide, hydralazine, phenelzine, dapsone, caffeine, and the carcinogenic secondary N-alkylarylamines (2-aminofluorene, benzidine, and 4-aminobiphenyl). Substituents ortho to the amino group sterically block acetylation. Polymorphisms in the NAT2 gene in human populations can be segregated into fast, intermediate, and slow acetylator phenotypes. Polymorphisms in NAT2 are also associated with higher incidences of cancer and drug toxicity. Intestinal N-acetyltransferase appears not to be polymorphic (i.e., 5-aminosalicylic acid). The proportion of the fast acetylation phenotype is approximately 30%-45% in Caucausians, 89%-90% in the Oriental population, and 100% in Canadian Eskimos. Drug-induced systemic lupus erythematosus from chronic procainamide therapy is more likely to appear with slow acetylators.

Acetylation polymorphism has been associated with differences in human drug toxicity between slow and fast acetylator phenotypes. Slow acetylators are more prone to drug-induced toxicities and accumulate higher blood concentrations of the unacetylated drug than do fast acetylators. Examples of toxicities that can result include hydralazine- and procainamide-induced lupus erythematosus, isoniazid-induced peripheral nerve damage, and sulfasalazine-induced hematologic disorders. Fast acetylators eliminate the drug more rapidly by conversion to its relatively nontoxic N-acetyl metabolite. However, for some drug substances, fast acetylators can pose a greater risk of liver toxicity than slow acetylators because fast acetylators produce toxic metabolites more rapidly. The possibility arises that genetic differences in acetylating capacity can confer differences in susceptibility to chemical carcinogenicity from arylamines.

The tumorigenic activity of arylamines (1 in Fig. 3.33) can be the result of a complex series of sequential metabolic reactions commencing with N-acetylation (2 in Fig. 3.33), subsequent oxidation to arylhydroxamic acids (3 in Fig. 3.33), and metabolic transformation to acetoxyarylamines by N,O-acyltransferase (4 in Fig. 3.33).[54] The acetoxyarylamine can eliminate the acetoxy group to form the reactive arylnitrenium ion (5 in Fig. 3.33), which is capable of covalently binding to nucleic acids and proteins, thus increasing the risk for development of bladder and liver tumors.[54] The rapid acetylator phenotype is expected to form the acetoxyarylamine metabolite at a greater rate than the slow acetylator and thereby, to present a greater risk for development of tumors compared with the slow acetylator.

Glutathione Conjugation and Mercapturic Acid Synthesis

Mercapturic acids are S-derivatives of N-acetylcysteine synthesized from glutathione (GSH).[5,58,59] The mercapturic acid pathway appears to have evolved as a protective (scavenger) mechanism against xenobiotic-induced hepatotoxicity or carcinogenicity, serving to detoxify a large number of noxious substances that we inhale or ingest or that are produced daily in the human body. Most xenobiotics that are metabolized to mercapturic acids first undergo

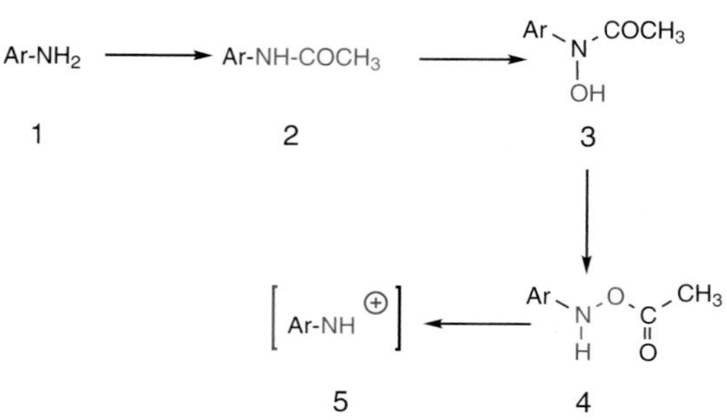

Figure 3.33 Bioactivation of acetylated arylamines.

conjugation with GSH catalyzed by the enzyme glutathione S-transferase (GST), a multigene isoenzyme family that is abundant in the soluble supernatant liver fractions. In humans, the GST family consists of cytosolic dimeric isoenzymes of 45-55 kDa size that have been assigned to at least seven classes: alpha (five members), kappa (one member), mu (six members), omega (two members), pi (one member), theta (two members), zeta (one member), and microsomal (three members). The principal drug substrates for the mu family are the nitrosourea and mustard-type anticancer drugs. The theta isoform metabolizes small organic molecules, such as solvents, halocarbons, and electrophilic compounds (e.g., α,β-unsaturated carbonyl compounds). The GSH conjugation reaction to mercapturic acid metabolites is depicted in Figure 3.34.

GST increases the ionization of the thiol group of GSH, increasing its nucleophilicity toward electrophiles (a group or ion that accepts an electron pair to make a covalent bond such as a carbocation or acyl ion) and thereby increasing the rate of conjugation with these potentially harmful electrophiles. In this way, GSH conjugation protects other vital nucleophilic centers in the cell, such as nucleic acids and proteins, from these electrophiles. Glutathione is also capable of reacting nonenzymatically with nucleophilic sites on neighboring macromolecules (Fig. 3.34) (see also section Metabolic Activation). Once conjugated with GSH, the electrophiles are excreted in the bile and urine.

A range of functional groups yields thioether conjugates of GSH, as well as products other than thioethers (Fig. 3.34). The nucleophilic attack by GSH occurs on electrophilic carbons with leaving groups (e.g., halogen [alkyl, alkenyl, aryl, or aralkyl halides], sulfonates [alkylmethanesulfonates] and nitro [alkyl nitrates] groups), ring opening of small ring ethers (epoxides and β-lactones, e.g., β-propiolactone), and the Michael-type addition to the activated β-carbon of an α,β-unsaturated carbonyl compound (e.g., acrolein) (see section Reactive Metabolites Resulting from Bioactivation). The lack of substrate specificity gives argument to the fact that glutathione transferase has undergone adaptive changes to accommodate the variety of xenobiotics to which it is exposed. The conjugation of an electrophilic compound with GSH is usually a reaction of detoxication, but in some cases carcinogens have been activated through conjugation with GSH.[58,59]

The enzymatic conjugation of GSH with epoxides provides a mechanism for protecting the liver from injury caused by certain bioactivated intermediates (see section Reactive Metabolites Resulting from Bioactivation). Not all epoxides are substrates for this enzyme, but the more chemically reactive epoxides appear to be better substrates. Important among the epoxides that are substrates for this enzyme are those produced from halobenzenes and polycyclic aromatic hydrocarbons through the action of a P450 monooxygenase. Epoxide formation represents bioactivation because the epoxides are reactive and potentially toxic, whereas their GSH conjugates are inactive. Conjugation of GSH with the epoxides of aryl hydrocarbons eventually results in the formation of hydroxymercapturic acids (premercapturic acids) which undergo acid-catalyzed dehydration to the mercapturic acids. The halobenzenes are typically conjugated in the *p*-position.

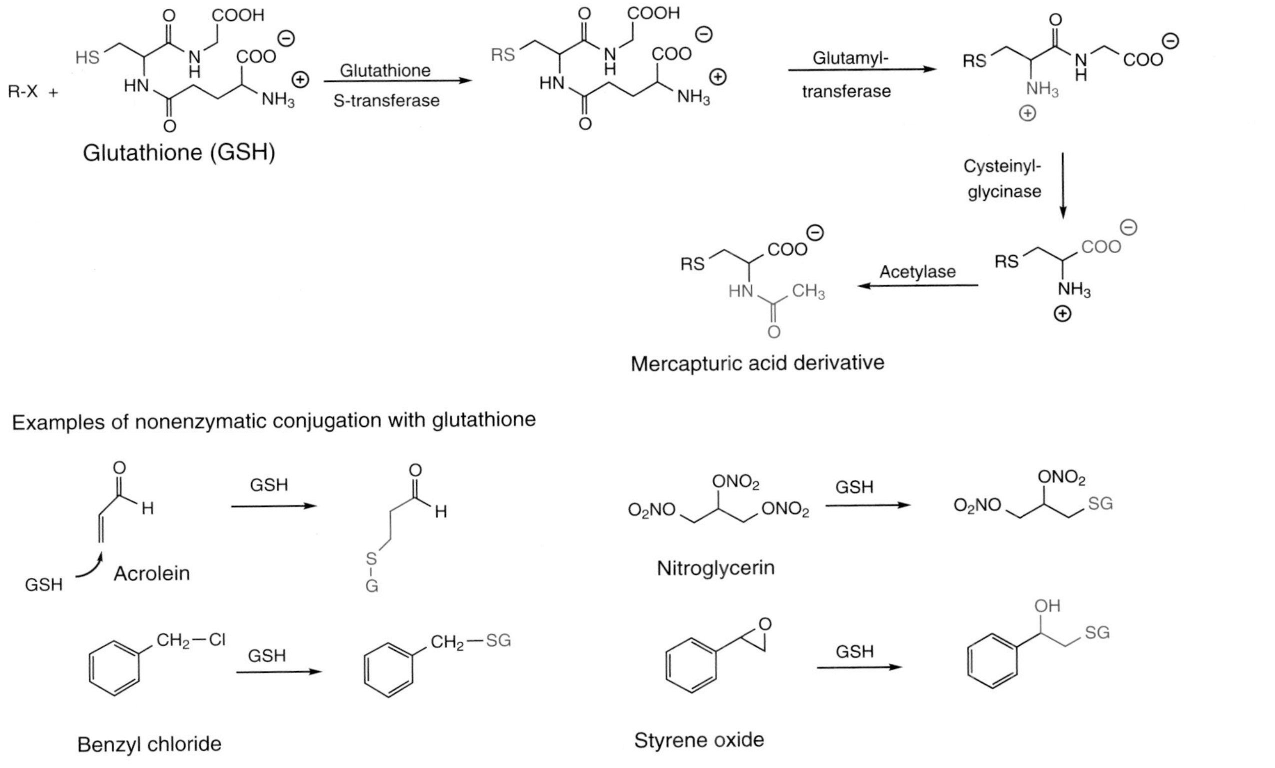

Figure 3.34 Glutathione and mercapturic acid conjugation pathways.

Monohalogenated, *gem*-dihalogenated, and vicinal dihalogenated alkanes undergo glutathione transferase–catalyzed conjugation reactions to produce S-substituted glutathione derivatives that are metabolically transformed into the more stable and less toxic mercapturic acids. This common route of metabolism occurs through nucleophilic displacement of a halide ion by the thiolate anion of glutathione. The mutagenicity of the 1,2-dihaloethanes (e.g., the pesticide and fumigant ethylene dibromide) has been attributed to GSH displacing bromide with the formation of the S-(2-haloethyl) glutathione, which subsequently rearranges to a reactive episulfonium ion electrophile that, in turn, alkylates DNA. Many of the halogenated hydrocarbons exhibiting nephrotoxicity undergo the formation of similar S-substituted cysteine derivatives.

A correlation exists between the hepatotoxicity of acetaminophen and levels of GSH in the liver. The probable mechanism of toxicity that has emerged from animal studies is that acetaminophen is oxidized by CYP1A2 and CYP2E1 to the N-acetyl-p-benzoquinonimine intermediate, which conjugates with and depletes hepatic GSH levels (Fig. 3.35). This action allows the benzoquinonimine to bind covalently to tissue macromolecules. The mercapturic acid derivative of acetaminophen represents approximately 2% of the administered dose of acetaminophen. Thus, the possibility exists that those toxic metabolites that are mostly detoxified by conjugating with GSH exhibit their hepatotoxicity (or, perhaps, carcinogenicity) because the liver has been depleted of GSH and is incapable of inactivating them. Pretreatment of animals with phenobarbital often hastens the depletion of GSH by increasing the formation of epoxides or other reactive intermediates.

Methylation

Methylation is a common biochemical reaction but appears to be of greater significance in the metabolism of endogenous compounds than for drugs and other xenobiotics. Methylation differs from other conjugation processes in that the O-methyl metabolites formed can, in some cases, have as great or greater pharmacological activity and lipophilicity than the parent molecule (e.g., the conversion of norepinephrine to epinephrine). Methionine is involved in the methylation of endogenous and exogenous substrates, because it transfers its methyl group via the activated intermediate S-adenosylmethionine to the substrate under the influence of methyltransferases (Fig. 3.36). Methylation results principally in the formation of O-methylated, N-methylated, and S-methylated products.

O-Methylation

O-methylation is catalyzed by the magnesium-dependent enzyme catechol-O-methyltransferase (COMT), which transfers a methyl group primarily to the *m*- or 3-hydroxy group of the catechol moiety (3,4-dihydroxylphenyl moiety) of norepinephrine, epinephrine, or dopamine, resulting in inactivation. Less frequently, the *p*- or 4-hydroxy group of these catecholamines is methylated (regioselectivity), along with their deaminated metabolites. COMT does not methylate monophenols or other dihydroxy non-catechol phenols. The *m:p* product ratio depends greatly on the type of substituent attached to the catechol ring. Substrates specific for COMT include the aforementioned catecholamines norepinephrine, epinephrine, and dopamine; the catechol amino acids L-DOPA and α-methyl-DOPA; and 2- and 4-hydroxyestradiol (catechol-like) metabolites of estradiol. It is found in liver, kidneys, nervous tissue, and other tissues.

Hydroxyindole-O-methyltransferase, which O-methylates N-acetylserotonin, serotonin, and other hydroxyindoles, is found in the pineal gland and is involved in the formation of melatonin, a hormone associated with the dark-light diurnal cycle in humans. This enzyme differs from COMT in that it does not methylate catecholamines and has no requirement for magnesium ion.

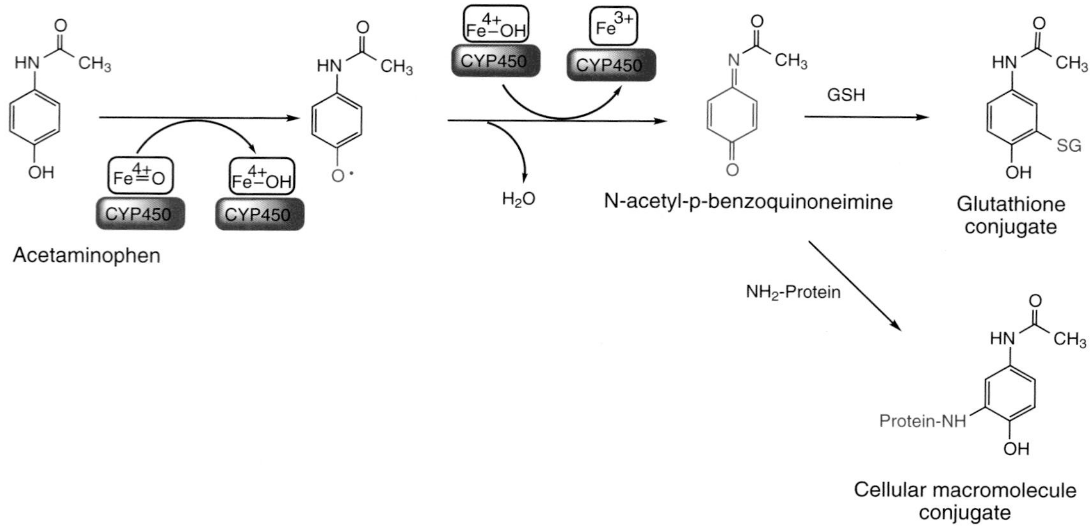

Figure 3.35 Proposed mechanism for the CYP450-catalyzed oxidation of acetaminophen to its N-acetyl-p-benzoquinoneimine intermediate, which can further react with either glutathione (GSH) or cellular macromolecules (NH_2-protein).

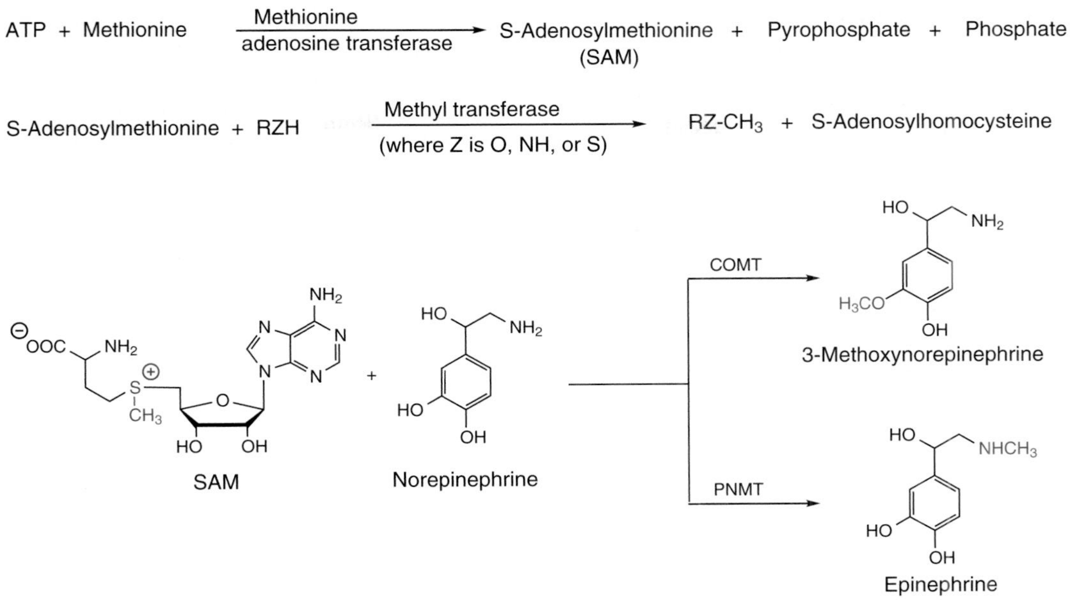

ATP + Methionine —(Methionine adenosine transferase)→ S-Adenosylmethionine (SAM) + Pyrophosphate + Phosphate

S-Adenosylmethionine + RZH —(Methyl transferase; where Z is O, NH, or S)→ $RZ\text{-}CH_3$ + S-Adenosylhomocysteine

SAM + Norepinephrine —COMT→ 3-Methoxynorepinephrine

SAM + Norepinephrine —PNMT→ Epinephrine

Figure 3.36 Methylation pathways.

N-*Methylation*

N-Methylation is among several conjugation pathways for metabolizing amines. Specific N-methyltransferases catalyze the transfer of active methyl groups from S-adenosylmethionine to the acceptor substance. Phenylethanolamine-N-methyltransferase methylates a number of endogenous and exogenous phenylethanolamines (e.g., normetanephrine, norepinephrine, and norephedrine) but does not methylate phenylethylamines. Histamine-N-methyl transferase methylates specificially histamine, producing the inactive metabolite N1-methylhistamine. Amine-N-methyltransferase will N-methylate a variety of primary and secondary amines from a number of sources, including endogenous biogenic amines (serotonin, tryptamine, tyramine, and dopamine) and drugs (desmethylimipramine, amphetamine, and normorphine). Amine-N-methyltransferases seem to have a role in recycling N-demethylated drugs.

S-*Methylation*

As a rule, thiols are toxic, and the role of thiol S-methyltransferases is a nonoxidative detoxification pathway of these compounds. S-methylation of sulfhydryl compounds also involves a microsomal enzyme requiring S-adenosylmethionine. Although a wide range of exogenous sulfhydryl compounds are S-methylated by this microsomal enzyme, none of the endogenous sulfhydryl compounds (e.g., cysteine and GSH) can function as substrates. S-methylation represents a detoxication step for thiols. Dialkyldithiocarbamates (e.g., disulfiram) and the antithyroid drugs (e.g., 6-propyl-2-thiouracil), mercaptans, and hydrogen sulfide (from thioglycosides as natural constituents of foods, mineral sulfides in water, fermented beverages, and bacterial digestion) are S-methylated. Other drugs undergoing S-methylation include captopril, thiopurine, azaprine, penicillamine, and 6-mercaptopurine.

Thiopurine methyltransferase or thiopurine S-methyltransferase (TPMT) catalyzes the S-methylation of thiopurine drugs, such as azathioprine, 6-mercaptopurine, and 6-thioguanine. Interindividual variations in sensitivity and toxicity to thiopurine are correlated with TPMT genetic polymorphisms. Defects in the TPMT gene result in decreased methylation and decreased inactivation of the thiopurine drugs, leading to enhanced bone marrow toxicity. The clinical result may be myelosuppression, anemia, bleeding tendency, leukopenia, and infection. Approximately, 5% of all thiopurine therapies will fail due to toxicity related to TPMT polymorphism.

ELIMINATION PATHWAYS

Most xenobiotics are lipid-soluble and are altered chemically by the metabolizing enzymes, usually into less toxic and more water-soluble substances, before being excreted into the urine or, in some cases, bile. The formation of conjugates with sulfonate, amino acids, and glucuronic acid is particularly effective in increasing the hydrophilicity of drug molecules. The principal route of excretion of drugs and their metabolites is via the urine. If drugs and other compounds foreign to the body are not metabolized in this manner, substances with a high lipid-water partition coefficient could be reabsorbed readily from the urine through the renal tubular membranes and into the plasma. Therefore, such substances would continue to be recirculated and their pharmacological or toxic effects would be prolonged. Very polar or highly ionized drug molecules often are excreted in the urine unchanged. Urine is not the only route for excreting drugs and their metabolites from the body. Other routes include bile, saliva, lungs, sweat, and milk. The bile and biliary efflux transporters have been recognized as major routes of excretion for many endogenous and exogenous compounds.

Enterohepatic Cycling of Drugs

The liver is the principal organ for the metabolism and eventual elimination of xenobiotics from the human body in either the urine or the bile. When eliminated in the bile, steroid hormones, bile acids, drugs, and their respective conjugated metabolites are available for reabsorption from the duodenal-intestinal tract into the portal circulation, undergoing the process of enterohepatic cycling (EHC) (Fig. 3.37).[60] Nearly all drugs are excreted in the bile, but only a few are concentrated in the bile. For example, the bile salts are efficiently concentrated in the bile and reabsorbed from the GIT, such that the entire body pool of bile acids/salts are recycled multiple times per day. Therefore, EHC is responsible for the conservation of bile acids, steroid hormones, thyroid hormones, and other endogenous substances. In humans, compounds excreted into the bile typically have a molecular weight greater than 500 Da. In humans, metabolites with a molecular weight between 300 and 500 Da are excreted in both urine and bile. Compounds excreted into bile are, as a rule, hydrophilic substances that can be either charged (anionic) or uncharged (e.g., cardiac glycosides and steroid hormones). Biotransformation of these compounds by means of Phase 1 and Phase 2 reactions would produce a conjugated metabolite, which is anionic and hydrophilic with a molecular weight greater than that of the parent compound. The conjugated metabolites are most often glucuronides, because glucuronidation adds 176 Da to the molecular weight of the parent compound. Unchanged drug in the bile is either excreted with the feces, metabolized by the bacterial flora in the intestinal tract, or reabsorbed into the portal circulation via EHC.

The bacterial intestinal flora is directly involved in EHC and the recycling of drugs through the portal circulation.[61] A conjugated drug and metabolites excreted via the bile can be hydrolyzed by enzymes of the bacterial flora, releasing the parent drug or its Phase 1 metabolite for reabsorption into the portal circulation. Among the numerous compounds metabolized in the enterohepatic circulation are the estrogenic and progestational steroids, digitoxin, indomethacin, diazepam, pentaerythritol tetranitrate, mercurials, arsenicals, and morphine. The oral ingestion of xenobiotics inhibiting the gut flora (i.e., nonabsorbable antibiotics) can affect the pharmacokinetics of drugs.

The impact of EHC on the pharmacokinetics and pharmacodynamics of a drug depends on the importance of biliary excretion relative to renal clearance and on the efficiency of gastrointestinal absorption. The EHC becomes dominant when biliary excretion is the major clearance mechanism for the drug. Because the majority of the bile is stored in the gallbladder and released on the ingestion of food, intermittent spikes in the plasma drug concentration is observed following reentry of the drug from the bile via EHC. From a pharmacodynamic point of view, the net effect of EHC is to increase the duration of a drug in the body and to prolong its pharmacological action.

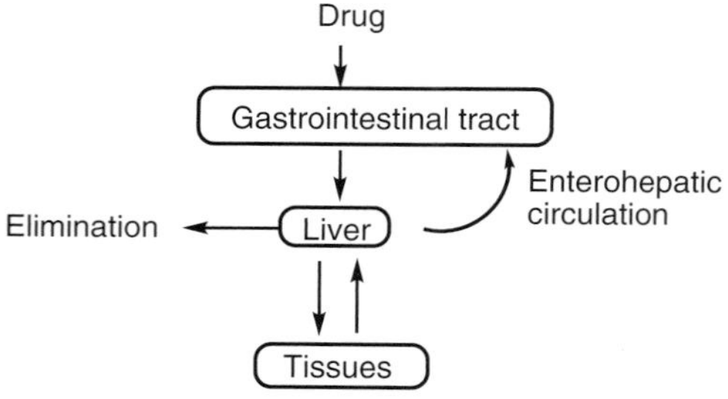

Figure 3.37 Enterohepatic cycling.

DRUG METABOLISM AND AGE

Metabolism in the Elderly

The widespread use of medications in the elderly increases the potential for an increased incidence of drug-related interactions, which can be related to changes in drug metabolism and clearance from the body (Table 3.14).[62,63] The interpretation of the age-related alteration in drug response must consider the contributions of absorption, distribution, metabolism, and excretion. Drug therapy in

Table 3.14 Effect of Age on the Clearance of Some Drugs

No Change	Decrease
Acetaminophen[a]	Alprazolam
Aspirin	Amitriptyline
Diclofenac	Chlordiazepoxide
Diphenhydramine	Chlormethiazole
Ethanol	Diazepam
Flunitrazepam	Labetalol
Midazolam	Lidocaine
Nitrazepam	Lorazepam
Oxazepam	Morphine
Phenytoin[a]	Meperidine
Prazosin	Nifedipine and other dihydropyridines
Propylthiouracil	Norepinephrine
Temazepam	Nortriptyline
Thiopental[a]	Phenytoin
Tolbutamide[a]	Piroxicam
Warfarin	Propranolol
	Quinidine
	Quinine
	Theophylline
	Verapamil

[a]Drugs for which clearance is disputable but can be increased

the elderly is expected to become one of the more significant problems for clinical medicine. It has been well documented that the metabolism of many drugs and their elimination is impaired in the elderly.

The decline in drug metabolism due to advancing age is associated with physiological changes that have pharmacokinetic implications affecting the steady-state plasma concentrations and renal clearance for the parent drug and its metabolites. Those changes relevant to the bioavailability of drugs in the elderly are decreases in hepatic blood flow, glomerular filtration rate, hepatic P450 activity, plasma protein binding, and body mass. Because the rate of a drug's elimination from the blood through hepatic metabolism is determined by hepatic blood flow, protein binding, and intrinsic clearance, a reduction in hepatic blood flow can lead to an increase in drug bioavailability and decreased clearance, with the symptoms of drug overdose and toxicity as the outcome (e.g., warfarin in patients with congestive heart failure[63,64]). Those orally administered drugs exhibiting a reduction in first-pass metabolism in the elderly include antihypertensives, diuretics, and antidepressants.

Age-related changes in drug metabolism are a complicated interplay between the age-related physiological changes, genetics, environmental influences (diet and nutritional status, smoking, and enzyme induction), concomitant diseases states, and drug intake. In most studies, the elderly appear to be just as responsive to drug-metabolizing enzyme activity (Phase 1 and Phase 2) as young individuals. Given the number of factors that determine the rate of drug metabolism, it is not surprising that the effects of aging on drug elimination by metabolism have yielded variable results, even for the same drug. The fact that drug elimination can be altered in old age suggests that doses of metabolized drugs should be initially reduced in older patients and then adjusted according to the clinical response. A decrease in hepatic drug metabolism coupled with age-related alterations in clearance, volume of distribution, and receptor sensitivity can lead to prolonged plasma half-life and increased drug toxicity.

Those P450 substrates reported to cause drug-drug interactions are shown in Tables 3.3-3.10 in bold italics.

Drug Metabolism in the Fetus and During Pregnancy

Over two-thirds of women receive prescription drugs while pregnant, with treatment and dosing strategies based on data from healthy male volunteers and nonpregnant women, and with little adjustment for the complex physiology of pregnancy and its unique disease states. Pregnancy influences hepatic metabolism of drugs in a CYP-dependent manner. Hormone levels in the plasma which rise during pregnancy are capable of regulating expression of hepatic drug metabolism enzymes. These hormones include estrogens, progesterone, cortisol, and prolactin. Studies are needed to examine the role of pregnancy hormones in altered drug metabolism during pregnancy.

The activities of CYP3A4, CYP2A6, CYP2D6, and CYP2C9 are all increased during pregnancy. Changes in CYP3A4 activity lead to increased metabolism of drugs (Table 3.10). By contrast, CYP1A2 and CYP2C19 appear to undergo a gradual decrease in activity with advancing gestation,[63,64] though with uncertain effects on drug therapy. The activity of Phase 2 enzymes, including uridine 5′-diphosphate glucuronosyltransferases (UGTs), is also altered during pregnancy, with a 200% increase in UGT1A4 activity during the first and second trimesters and a 300% increase during the third trimester.[63,64] This change leads to lower concentrations of UGT1A4 substrates such as lamotrigine, leading directly to poorer seizure control with advancing gestation in the absence of appropriate dose titration.

Knowledge of drug transporter function during pregnancy is necessary for a complete understanding of drug absorption, distribution, elimination, and effect.[63] In addition, fetal development is dependent upon the transport of nutrients by the placenta toward the fetal side, and that of products of fetal metabolism transported away from the fetus for elimination by the mother.[65] The placenta produces and secretes hormones that affect the maternal physiology and endocrine state. Compounds transported between the mother and the fetus are carried by the maternal circulation within the uterine vasculature.

The ability of the human fetus and placenta to metabolize xenobiotics is well established. Drug-metabolizing enzymes expressed in the placenta include CYP1A1, 2E1, 3A4/5, 3A7, 4B1, epoxide hydrolase, alcohol dehydrogenase, glutathione transferase, UGTs, sulfotransferases, and N-acetyltransferase. The majority of the drugs used in pregnancy readily cross the placenta, thus exposing the fetus to a large number of xenobiotic agents. The human fetus is at special risk from these substances due to the presence of the P450 system which is capable of metabolizing xenobiotics during the first part of gestation. Placentas of tobacco smokers have shown a significant increase in the rate of placental CYP1A activity. Concern for this CYP1A activity is increasing because this enzyme system is known to catalyze the formation of reactive metabolites capable of covalently binding to macromolecules, producing permanent effects (e.g., teratogenicity, hepatotoxicity, or carcinogenicity) in the fetus and newborn. A more disturbing fact is that the conjugation enzymes (i.e., glucuronosyltransferases, glutathione transferase, and sulfotransferase), which are important for the formation of Phase 2 conjugates of these reactive metabolites, are found in low to negligible levels in the fetus and newborn, increasing the exposure of these infants to these potentially toxic metabolites.

The placenta is not a barrier protecting the fetus from xenobiotics; almost every drug present in the maternal circulation will cross the placenta and reach the fetus. For some drugs, however, the placental efflux transport protein P-gp functions as a maternofetal barrier, pumping drugs and Pgp substrates out of the fetal circulation back into the maternal circulation[65] and protecting the fetus from exposure to potentially harmful teratogenic xenobiotics/drugs and endogenous substances that have been absorbed through the placenta. The P-gp inhibitors should be carefully evaluated for their potential to increase fetal susceptibility to drug/chemical-induced teratogenesis. On the other hand, selective inhibition of P-gp could be used clinically to improve pharmacotherapy of the unborn child. Because metabolites are usually more water soluble than the parent substance, drug metabolites formed in the fetus can be trapped and accumulate on the fetal side of the placenta. Such accumulation can result in drug-induced toxicities or developmental defects. The activity of CYP3A isoenzymes in the human fetal liver is similar to that seen in adult liver microsomes. The fetal activity for CYP3A7 is unusual, as most other fetal isoenzymes of P450 exhibit activity 5%-40% of the adult isoenzymes. Fetal and neonatal drug-metabolizing enzyme activities can differ from those in the adult.

Most xenobiotics cross the placental barrier by simple diffusion. Protein binding, degree of ionization, lipid solubility, and molecular weight can affect placental transport. In fact, small, lipid-soluble, ionized, and poorly protein-bound molecules cross the placenta easily. For other substrates, the placenta facilitates maternal to fetal transport through the polarized expression of various transporters.[65] Transporters enable transport of specific endogenous substrates (such as cytokines, nucleoside analogues, and steroid hormones); however, exogenous compounds with similar structures may also interact with them.

From the day of birth, the neonate is exposed to drugs and other foreign compounds persisting from pregnancy, as well as those transferred via breast milk. Fortunately, many of the drug-metabolizing enzymes operative in the neonate developed during the fetal period. The routine use of therapeutic agents during labor and delivery, as well as during pregnancy, is widespread, and consideration must be given to the fact that potentially harmful metabolites can be generated by the fetus and newborn. Consequently, the use of drugs capable of forming reactive metabolic intermediates should be avoided during pregnancy, delivery, and the neonatal period. The activity of Phase 1 and Phase 2 drug-metabolizing enzymes is high at birth but decreases to normal levels with increasing age. Evidence suggests increased activity of drug-metabolizing enzymes in liver microsomes of neonates resulting from treatment of the mother during the pregnancy with enzyme inducers (e.g., phenobarbital).

GENETIC POLYMORPHISM

The reality of drug therapy is that many drugs do not work in all patients.[66] By current estimates, the percentage of patients who will react favorably to a specific drug ranges from 20% to 80%. Drugs have been developed and dosage regimens prescribed under the old paradigm that "one dose fits all," which largely ignores the fact that humans are genetically different, resulting in interindividual differences in drug metabolism and disposition.[66] It is widely accepted that genetic factors have an important impact on the oxidative metabolism and pharmacokinetics of drugs. Genotype-phenotype correlation studies (pharmacogenetics) have shown that inherited mutations in P450 genes (alleles) result in distinct phenotypic subgroups. For example, mutations in the *CYP2D6* gene result in poor (PM), intermediate (IM), extensive (EM), and ultrarapid (UM) metabolizers of CYP2D6 substrates[67] (Table 3.8). Each of these phenotypic subgroups experiences different responses to drugs extensively metabolized by the CYP2D6 pathway, ranging from severe toxicity to complete lack of efficacy. Genetic studies confirm that "one dose does not fit all," leaving the question of why we would continue to develop and prescribe drugs under the old paradigm. The regulatory agencies have recognized that identifying genetic polymorphisms might allow the safe dosing, marketing, and approval of drugs that would otherwise not be approved and advised pharmaceutical companies to incorporate the knowledge of genetic polymorphisms into drug development. Importantly, pharmacogenomic testing (the study of heritable traits affecting patient response to drug treatment) can significantly increase the likelihood of developing drug regimens that benefit most patients without severe adverse events. Pharmacists play a vital role in the development of patient-specific dosing regimens based on metabolizing phenotype.

Polymorphisms are expressed for a number of metabolizing enzymes, but the polymorphic P450 isoforms that are most important for drug metabolism include CYP2A6, CYP2A13, CYP2B6, CYP2C9, CYP2C19, and CYP2D6.[68-71] These isoforms have been studied extensively and, despite their low abundance in the liver, they have been found to catalyze the metabolism of many drugs. Most gene variants are expressed into inactive, truncated proteins or they fail to express any protein. There is no clear information about CYP1A1 and CYP3A4/5 polymorphism. These polymorphic isoforms give rise to phenotypic subgroups in the population differing in their ability to perform clinically significant biotransformation reactions with obvious clinical ramifications.[66] Metabolic polymorphism can have several consequences; for example, when enzymes that metabolize drugs used either therapeutically or socially are deficient, adverse or toxic drug reactions can occur in these individuals.

The discovery of genetic polymorphism resulted from the observation of increased frequency of adverse effects or no drug effects after normal doses of drugs to some patients (e.g., hyper-CNS response from the administration of the antihistamine doxylamine or no analgesic response with codeine). Polymorphism is a difference in DNA sequence found at 1% or greater in a population and expressed as an amino acid substitution in the protein sequence of an enzyme resulting in changes in its rate of activity (V_{max}) or affinity (K_m). Thus, mutant DNA sequences can lead to interindividual differences in drug metabolism. Furthermore, the polymorphisms do not occur with equivalent frequency in all racial or ethnic groups. Because of these differences, it is important to be aware of a person's race and ethnicity when giving drugs that are metabolized differently by different populations, although practitioners must guard against stereotyping.[66] Because no other way may exist to adequately clear these drugs from the body, PMs can be at greater risk for adverse drug reactions or toxic overdoses. The signs and symptoms of these overdoses are primarily extensions of the drug's common adverse effects or pharmacological effects (Table 3.15).[66] The level of adverse reactions or overdosage depends very much on the overall contribution of the mutant isoform to the drug's metabolism. Perhaps the most interesting explanation for the various mutant isoforms is that they evolved as protective mechanisms against

Table 3.15 Impact of Human P450 Polymorphisms on Drug Treatment in Poor Metabolizers

Polymorphic Enzyme	Decreased Clearance	Adverse Effects (Overdosage)	Reduced Activation of Coadministered Prodrug
CYP2C9	*S*-warfarin	Bleeding	Losartan
	Phenytoin	Ataxia	
	Losartan		
	Tolbutamide	Hypoglycemia	
	NSAIDs	GI bleeding	
CYP2C19	Omeprazole		Proguanil
	Diazepam	Sedation	
CYP2D6	Tricyclic antidepressants	Cardiotoxicity	Tramadol
	SSRIs	Serotonin syndrome	Codeine
	Anti-arrythmic drugs	Arrythmias	Ethylmorphine
	Perhexiline	Neuropathy	
	Haloperidol	Parkinsonism	
	Perphenazine		
	Zuclopenthixol		
	S-Mianserin		
	Tolterodine		
CYP2A6	Nicotine		

alkaloids and other common substances in the food chain for the different ethnicities. Although much effort has gone into finding polymorphisms of *CYP3A4* and *CYP1A2* genes, none has yet to be discovered.

Occasionally, one derives benefit from an unusual P450 phenotype. For example, cure rates for peptic ulcer treated with omeprazole are substantially greater in individuals with defective CYP2C19 due to the sustained high plasma levels achieved.

CYP2A6

CYP2A6 is of particular importance because it activates a number of procarcinogens to carcinogens and is the major isoform metabolizing the anticoagulant warfarin and nicotine.[69] Approximately 15% of Asians express the *CYP2A6*4del* allele and 2% of Caucasians express the other *CYP2AD6*2* allele. Both these alleles express either no enzyme or a nonfunctional enzyme, and individuals carrying these alleles are referred to as having the PM phenotype. A benefit from being a PM of CYP2A6 substrates might be the protection against some carcinogens, including cigarette smoke due to the high plasma levels of nicotine achieved with fewer cigarettes.

CYP2B6

CYP2B6 is of special interest due to its wide interindividual variability in expression and activity.[70] Such a large variability for an enzyme that is not highly expressed is probably because of genetic polymorphisms and exposure to drugs that are inducers or inhibitors of CYP2B6. Variant alleles resulting from splicing defects or gene deletions have been identified in PM individuals with altered metabolic activity or impaired enzyme function. At least 28 allelic variants and some subvariants of *CYP2B6* have been shown to have an effect on drug clearance and drug response. For example, HIV-infected African-American individuals with a defective variant of *CYP2B6* are PMs of efavirenz and have plasma levels approximately 3-fold higher than individuals with the normal *CYP2B6* gene. A different variant of *CYP2B6* is associated with approximately 2-fold greater plasma levels of nevirapine in HIV-infected patients. A benefit from being a PM of CYP2B6 antiviral drugs might be enhanced HIV protection because of the higher plasma levels of the antiviral drugs achieved with lower dosages. Smokers with another variant of *CYP2B6* may be more vulnerable to abstinence symptoms and relapse following treatment with bupropion (a CYP2B6 substrate) as a smoking cessation agent.

CYP2C9 and CYP2C19

CYP2C9 and CYP2C19 metabolize approximately 15% of clinically used drugs, such as phenytoin, *S*-warfarin, tolbutamide, losartan, and many NSAIDs.[71] Although CYP2C19 metabolizes fewer drugs than CYP2D6, the drugs that

CYP2C19 does metabolize are clinically important (Table 3.7). The deficit of CYP2C19 found in the PM phenotype is only seen in 8%-13% of Caucasians, 20%-30% of the Asian population (11%-23% of Japanese and 5%-37% of Chinese), up to 20% of the black African-American population, 14%-15% of Saudi Arabians and Ethiopians, and up to 70% of Pacific Islanders.[71] The more common mutant allele in these individuals is *CYP2C19*2*, which expresses an inactive enzyme. The large interindividual variability observed in the therapeutic response to the antiseizure drug mephenytoin is attributed to CYP2C19 polymorphism, which catalyzes the *p*-hydroxylation of the *S*-stereoisomer.[71] The *R*-enantiomer is N-demethylated by CYP2C8 with no difference in its metabolism between PMs and EMs.

CYP2C9 is highly polymorphic with at least 33 variants identified. *CYP2C9*2* is frequent among Caucasians with ~1% of the population being homozygous carriers and 22% heterozygous. The corresponding homozygous/heterozygous figures for the *CYP2C9*3* allele are 0.4% and 15%, respectively. Clinical studies have addressed the importance of the *CYP2C9*2* and **3* alleles as a determining factor for drug clearance and drug response. P450 2C9 polymorphisms are relevant for the efficacy and adverse effects of numerous NSAIDs, sulfonylurea antidiabetic drugs, and, most critically, oral anticoagulants belonging to the class of vitamin K epoxide reductase inhibitors (e.g., warfarin).[71] A deficiency of this isoform is seen in 8%-13% of Caucasians, 2%-3% of African-Americans, and 1% of Asians. Individuals with the PM phenotype who possess this deficient isoform variant are ineffective in clearing S-warfarin (so much so that they can be fully anticoagulated on just 0.5 mg of warfarin per day) and in the clearance of phenytoin, which has a potentially very toxic narrow therapeutic range. On the other hand, the prodrug losartan will be poorly activated and ineffective.

CYP2D6

CYP2D6 is of specific importance because it metabolizes a wide range of commonly prescribed drugs, including antidepressants, antipsychotics, β-adrenergic blockers, and antiarrhythmics (Table 3.8).[67,68] CYP2D6 deficiency is a clinically important genetic variation of drug metabolism characterized by three phenotypes: UM, EM, and PM. About 10% of Caucasians have gene variants that result in a functionally deficient CYP2D6 enzyme, and these PMs often respond inadequately to drugs, such as codeine, that are activated by CYP2D6. The PM phenotype is inherited as an autosomal recessive trait, with 5 of 30 of the known *CYP2D6* gene mutations leading to either zero expression or the expression of a nonfunctional enzyme.[68] Approximately 12%-20% of Caucasians express the *CYP2D6*4* allele and 5% express the other *CYP2D6* alleles. Up to 34% of African-Americans express the *CYP2D6*17* allele and 5% express the other *CYP2D6* alleles. Up to 50% of Chinese express the *CYP2D6*10* allele and 5% express the other *CYP2D6* alleles (these individuals are all referred to as PM).[67,68] Conversely, the 20%-30% of Saudi Arabians and Ethiopians who express the *CYP2D6*2XN* allele are known as UMs of CYP2D6 substrates, because they express excess enzyme because of having multicopies of the gene.[72] Inasmuch as CYP2D6 is not inducible, many individuals of Ethiopian and Saudi Arabian descent have developed a genetically different strategy to cope with the (presumed) high load of alkaloids and other substances in their diet, thus the high expression of CYP2D6 using multiple copies of the gene.

Those individuals who are deficient in CYP2D6 will be predisposed to adverse effects or drug toxicity from antidepressants or neuroleptics caused by inadequate metabolism, leading to long half-lives, but the metabolism of CYP2D6-dependent prodrugs in these patients will be ineffective due to lack of activation (e.g., codeine, which must be metabolized by O-demethylation to morphine). In contrast, individuals with the UM phenotype will require a dose of drugs inactivated by CYP2D6 that is much higher than normal to attain therapeutic drug plasma concentrations (e.g., one patient required a daily dose of approximately 300 mg of nortryptyline to achieve therapeutic plasma levels; the usual dose is 25 mg) or a lower dose for prodrugs that require metabolic activation. Individuals with the PM phenotype are also characterized by loss of CYP2D6 stereoselectivity in hydroxylation reactions. It can be anticipated that large differences in steady-state concentration for CYP2D6 substrates will occur between individuals with the different phenotypes when they receive the same dose. Depending on the drug and reaction type, a 10- to 30-fold difference in blood concentrations can be observed in the PM-phenotype polymorphism.[68]

Other Polymorphic Metabolizing Enzymes

CYP2E1 polymorphism is expressed more frequently in individuals of Chinese ancestry than in Caucasians. Those with the CYP2E1 PM phenotype exhibit tolerance to alcohol and less toxicity from halohydrocarbon solvents.

Polymorphism has been associated with serum cholinesterases, alcohol dehydrogenases, aldehyde dehydrogenases, epoxide hydrolase and xanthine oxidase. Approximately 50% of the Oriental population lack aldehyde dehydrogenase, resulting in high levels of acetaldehyde following ethanol ingestion and causing nausea and flushing. People with genetic variants of cholinesterase respond abnormally to succinylcholine, procaine, and other related choline esters. The clinical consequence of reduced enzymatic activity of cholinesterase is that succinylcholine and procaine are not hydrolyzed in the blood, resulting in prolongation of their respective pharmacological activities (e.g., skeletal muscle paralysis in the case of succinylcholine).

Increasing knowledge of genetic polymorphism has contributed a great deal to our understanding about interindividual variation in the metabolism of drugs, including how to change dose regimens accordingly to minimize drug toxicity and improve therapeutic efficacy.

Presystemic First-Pass Metabolism

Although hepatic metabolism continues to be the most important route for xenobiotics, the ability of the liver and intestine to metabolize substances to either pharmacologically inactive or bioactive metabolites before reaching the systemic circulation is called presystemic first-pass metabolism. This metabolic process results in low systemic availability for orally susceptible drugs. Sulfonation and glucuronidation are major pathways of presystemic intestinal first-pass metabolism in humans. For example, oral acetaminophen, phenylephrine, terbutaline, albuterol, fenoterol, or isoproterenol exhibits approximately 5% bioavailability because of sulfonation and glucuronidation.

The discovery that CYP3A4 is found in the mucosal enterocytes of the intestinal villi signifies its role as a key determinant in the oral bioavailability of its numerous drug substrates (Table 3.10). Drugs known to be substrates for CYP3A often have a low and/or variable oral bioavailability that can be explained by presystemic first-pass metabolism by the small intestine P450 isoforms.[68] The concentration of functional intestinal CYP3A is influenced by genetic disposition, induction, and inhibition, which to a great extent determines drug blood levels and therapeutic response. Xenobiotics when ingested orally can modify the activity of intestinal CYP3A enzymes by induction and inhibition. By modulation of the isoform pattern in the intestine, a xenobiotic could alter its own metabolism and that of others in a time- and dose-dependent manner.

The concentration of CYP3A in the intestine is comparable to that of the liver. The oral administration of dexamethasone induces the formation of CYP3A and erythromycin inhibits it. The glucocorticoid inducibility of CYP3A4 can also be a factor in differences of metabolism between males and females. Studies have suggested that intestinal CYP3A4 C2 hydroxylation of estradiol contributed to the oxidative metabolism of endogenous estrogens circulating with the enterohepatic recycling pool.[72] Norethisterone has a low oral bioavailability of 42% due to oxidative CYP3A first-pass metabolism, but levonorgestrel is completely available in women, having no conjugated metabolites.

Several clinically relevant drug-drug interactions between orally coadministered drugs and CYP3A4 can be explained by a modification of drug metabolism at the P450 level. If a drug has high presystemic elimination (low bioavailability) and is metabolized primarily by CYP3A4, then coadministration with a CYP3A4 inhibitor can be expected to alter the drug's pharmacokinetics by reducing its metabolism, thus increasing its plasma concentration. Drugs and some foods (e.g., grapefruit juice) that are known inhibitors, inducers, or substrates for intestinal CYP3A4 can potentially interact with the metabolism of a coadministered drug, affecting its area under the curve and rate of clearance (Tables 3.10-3.12). Inducers can reduce absorption and oral bioavailability, whereas these same factors are increased by inhibitors. For example, erythromycin can enhance the oral absorption of another drug by inhibiting its metabolism in the small intestine by CYP3A4. Because they are competitive substrates for CYP3A4, prednisone, prednisolone, and methylprednisolone (but not dexamethasone) are competitive inhibitors of synthetic glucocorticoid metabolism. This is because a major metabolic pathway for synthetic glucocorticoids involves CYP3A4. In addition to coadministered drugs, metabolic interactions with exogenous CYP3A4 substrates secreted in the bile are possible. The poor oral bioavailability for cyclosporine is attributed to a combination of intestinal metabolism by CYP3A4 and efflux by P-gp.[73]

Because the intestinal mucosa is enriched with glucuronosyltransferases, sulfotransferases, and glutathione transferases, presystemic first-pass metabolism for orally administered drugs susceptible to these conjugation reactions results in their low oral bioavailability. Presystemic metabolism often exceeds liver metabolism for some drugs. For example, more than 80% of intravenously administered albuterol is excreted unchanged in urine, with the balance presenting as glucuronide conjugates, whereas when albuterol is administered orally, less than 5% is systemically absorbed because of intestinal sulfonation and glucuronidation. Presystemic metabolism is a major pathway in humans for most β-adrenergic agonists, such as glucuronides or sulfate esters of terbutaline, fenoterol, albuterol and isoproterenol, morphine (3-O-glucuronide), acetaminophen (O-sulfate and O-glucuronide), and estradiol (3-O-sulfate). The bioavailability of orally administered estradiol or ethinyl estradiol in females is approximately 50% because of conjugation. Mestranol (3-methoxyethinyl estradiol) has greater oral bioavailability because, as a nonphenol, it is not significantly conjugated. Levodopa has a low oral bioavailability because of its metabolism by intestinal L-aromatic amino acid decarboxylase. Drugs subject to first-pass metabolism are included in Table 3.16.

The extensive presystemic first-pass sulfonation of phenolic drugs, for example, can lead to increased bioavailability of other drugs by competing for the available sulfate pool, resulting in the possibility of drug toxicity. Concurrent oral administration of acetaminophen with phenolic drugs could result in an increase in drug blood levels. Ascorbic acid, which is sulfonated, also increases the bioavailability of concurrently administered phenolic drugs. Sulfonation and glucuronidation occur side by side, often competing for the same substrate, and the balance between sulfonation and glucuronidation is influenced by several factors, such as species, doses, availability of cosubstrates, inhibition, and induction of the respective transferases.

EXTRAHEPATIC METABOLISM

Because the liver is the primary tissue for xenobiotic metabolism, it is not surprising that our understanding of mammalian P450 monooxygenase is based chiefly on hepatic studies. Although the tissue content of P450s is highest in the liver, P450 enzymes are found in the lung, nasal epithelium, intestinal tract, kidney, adrenal tissues, and brain. It is possible that the expression of the polymorphic genes and induction of the isoforms in the extrahepatic tissues can affect the activity of the P450 isoforms in the metabolism of endogenous steroids, drugs, and other xenobiotics. Therefore, characterization of P450, UGT, SULT, and other polymorphic drug-metabolizing enzymes

Table 3.16 Examples of Drugs Exhibiting Presystemic Metabolism

Acetaminophen	Isoproterenol	Oxprenolol
Albuterol	Lidocaine	Pentazocine
Alprenolol	Meperidine	Propoxyphene
Aspirin	Methyltestosterone	Propranolol
Cyclosporin	Metoprolol	Salicylamide
Desmethylimipramine	Dihydropyridines (nifedipine)	Terbutaline
Fluorouracil	Nortriptyline	Verapamil
Hydrocortisone	Organic nitrates	
Imipramine		

in extrahepatic tissues is important to our overall understanding about the biological importance of these isoform families to improved drug therapy, design of new drugs and dosages forms, toxicity, and carcinogenicity.

The mucosal surfaces of the GIT, the nasal passages, and the lungs are major portals of entry for xenobiotics into the body and, as such, are continuously exposed to a variety of orally ingested or inhaled airborne xenobiotics, including drugs, plant toxins, environmental pollutants, and other chemical substances. As a consequence of this exposure, these tissues represent a major target for tumorigenesis and other chemically induced toxicities. Many of these toxins and chemical carcinogens are relatively inert substances that must be bioactivated to exert cytotoxicity and tumorigenicity. The epithelial cells of these tissues are capable of metabolizing a wide variety of exogenous and endogenous substances, and these cells provide the principal and initial source of biotransformation for these xenobiotics during the absorptive phase. The consequences of such presystemic biotransformation is either (1) a decrease in the amount of xenobiotics available for systemic absorption by facilitating the elimination of polar metabolites or (2) toxification by activation to carcinogens, which can be one determinant of tissue susceptibility for the development of intestinal cancer. The risk of colon cancer can depend on dietary constituents that contain either procarcinogens or compounds modulating the response to carcinogens.

Intestinal Metabolism

As noted earlier, many of the clinically relevant aspects of P450 can, in fact, occur at the level of the intestinal mucosa and can account for differences among patients in dosing requirements. The intestinal mucosa is enriched especially with the CYP3A4 isoform, glucuronosyltransferases, sulfotransferases, and GSTs, making it particularly important for orally administered drugs susceptible to oxidation and/or Phase 2 glucuronidation, sulfonation, or glutathione conjugation pathways. The highest concentrations of P450s occur in the duodenum, with gradual tapering into the ileum. In the human intestine, CYP2E, CYP3A, CYP2C8, CYP2C9, CYP2C19, and CYP2D6 have been identified. Therefore, intestinal P450 isoforms provide potential presystemic first-pass metabolism of ingested xenobiotics affecting their oral bioavailability (e.g., hydroxylation of naloxone) or bioactivation of carcinogens or mutagens. It is not surprising that dietary factors can affect the intestinal P450 isoforms. For example, a 2-day dietary exposure to cooked Brussels sprouts significantly decreased the 2α-hydroxylation of testosterone, yet induced CYP1A2 activity for PAH metabolism. An 8-oz. glass of grapefruit juice inhibited the sulfoxidation metabolism of omeprazole (CYP3A4) but not its hydroxylation (CYP2C19), thus increasing its systemic blood concentrations. These types of interactions between a drug and a dietary inhibitor could result in a clinically significant drug interaction.

Intestinal UGT isoforms can glucuronidate orally administered drugs, such as morphine, acetaminophen, α- and β-adrenergic agonists, and other phenolic phenethanolamines and dietary xenobiotics, resulting in a reduction of their oral bioavailability (increasing first-pass metabolism), thus altering their pharmacokinetics and pharmacodynamics. The UGTs expressed in the intestine include UGT1A1 (bilirubin-glucuronidating isoform), UGT1A3, UGT1A4, UGT1A6, UGT1A8, UGT1A9, and UGT1A3. Substrate specificities of intestinal UGT isoforms are comparable to those in the liver. Glucuronidase hydrolysis of biliary glucuronide conjugates in the intestine can contribute to EHC of the parent drug.

Likewise, the sulfotransferases in the small intestine can metabolize orally administered drugs and xenobiotics for which the primary route of conjugation is sulfonation (e.g., isoproterenol, albuterol, steroid hormones, α-methyldopa, acetaminophen, and fenoldopam), decreasing their oral bioavailability and, thus, altering their pharmacokinetics and pharmacodynamics. Competition for intestinal sulfonation between coadministered substrates can influence their bioavailability with either an enhancement or a decrease of therapeutic effects. Sulfatase hydrolysis of biliary sulfate esters in the intestine can contribute to EHC of the parent drug.

Plants contain a variety of protoxins, promutagens, and procarcinogens, and the occurrence of intestinal P450 enzymes and bacterial enzymes in the microflora allows the metabolic conversion of relatively stable environmental pollutants and food-derived xenobiotics into mutagens and carcinogens. For example, cruciferous vegetables (Brussels sprouts, cabbage, broccoli, cauliflower, and spinach) are all rich in indole compounds (e.g., indole 3-carbinol) which, with regular and chronic ingestion, are capable of inducing some intestinal P450s (CYP1A subfamily) and inhibiting others (CYP3A subfamily). It is likely that these vegetables would also alter the metabolism of food-derived mutagens and carcinogens. For example, heterocyclic amines produced during the charbroiling of meat are P450 N-hydroxylated and become carcinogenic in a manner similar to arylamines.

Intestinal Microflora

When drugs are orally ingested, or there is considerable biliary excretion of a drug or its metabolites into the GIT, such as with a parentally administered drug (EHC or recirculation), the intestinal bacterial microflora can have a significant metabolic role. The microflora has an important role in the enterohepatic recirculation of xenobiotics via their conjugated metabolites (e.g., digoxin, the oral contraceptives norethisterone and ethinyl estradiol and chloramphenicol) and endogenous substances (steroid hormones, bile acids, folic acid, and cholesterol), which reenter the gut via the bile. Compounds eliminated in the bile are conjugated with glucuronic acid, glycine, sulfate, and glutathione and, once secreted into the small intestine, the bacterial β-glucuronidase, sulfatase, nitroreductases, and various glycosidases catalyze the hydrolysis of the conjugates. The activity of orally administered conjugated estrogens (e.g., Premarin) involves the hydrolysis of the sulfate esters by sulfatases, releasing estrogens to be reabsorbed from the intestine into the portal circulation. The clinical use of oral antibiotics (e.g., erythromycin, penicillin, clindamycin, and aminoglycosides) has a profound effect on the gut microflora and the enzymes responsible for the hydrolysis of drug conjugates undergoing EHC. Bacterial reduction includes nitro reduction of nitroimidazole, azo reduction of azides (sulfasalazine to 5-aminosalicylic acid and sulfapyridine), and reduction of the sulfoxide to its sulfide. The sulfoxide of sulindac is reduced by both gut microflora and hepatic P450s. Other ways in which bacterial flora can affect metabolism include the following: (1) production of toxic metabolites, (2) formation of carcinogens from inactive precursors, (3) detoxication, (4) exhibition of species differences in drug metabolism, (5) exhibition of individual differences in drug metabolism, (6) production of pharmacologically active metabolites from inactive precursors, and (7) production of metabolites not formed by animal tissues. In contrast to the predominantly hepatic oxidative and conjugative metabolism of the liver, gut microflora is largely degradative, hydrolytic, and reductive, with a potential for both metabolic activation and detoxication of xenobiotics.

Lung Metabolism

Some of the hepatic xenobiotic biotransformation pathways are also operative in the lung. Because of the differences in organ size, the total content of the pulmonary xenobiotic-metabolizing enzyme systems is usually lower than in the liver, creating the impression of a minor role for the lung in xenobiotic elimination. CYP2E1 is expressed in the lung to the greatest extent. The expression of other P450s, FMO, epoxide hydrolase, and the Phase 2 conjugation pathways are comparable to those in the liver. Thus, the lungs can have a significant role in the metabolic elimination or activation of low-molecular-weight inhaled xenobiotics.

When drugs are injected intravenously, intramuscularly, or subcutaneously, or after skin absorption, the drug initially enters the pulmonary circulation, after which the lung becomes the organ of first-pass metabolism for the drug. The blood levels and therapeutic response of the drug are influenced by genetic disposition, induction, and inhibition of the pulmonary metabolizing enzymes. By modulation of the P450 isoform pattern in the lung, a xenobiotic could alter its own metabolism and that of others in a time- and dose-dependent manner. Because of its position in the circulation, the lung provides a second-pass metabolism for xenobiotics and their metabolites exiting from the liver, but it is also susceptible to the cytotoxicity or carcinogenicity of hepatic activated metabolites. Antihistamines, β-blockers, opioids, and tricyclic antidepressants are among the basic amines known to accumulate in the lungs because of their binding to surfactant phospholipids in lung tissue. The significance of this relationship to potential pneumotoxicity remains to be seen.

Nasal Metabolism

The nasal olfactory mucosa is recognized as a first line of defense for the lung against airborne environmental xenobiotics because the mucosa is constantly exposed to the airborne external environment.[74] Drug metabolism in the olfactory nasal epithelium represents a major metabolic pathway for protecting the CNS and brain against the entry of drugs, inhaled environmental pollutants, or other volatile chemicals. In some instances, these enzymes can biotransform a given drug or environmental or airborne xenobiotic into more reactive and potentially toxic metabolites, increasing the risk of carcinogenesis in the nasopharynx and lung (e.g., procarcinogens and nitrosamines in cigarette smoke). P450 activity is high in olfactory tissue and olfactory-specific isoforms have been identified, which include CYP1A2, CYP2A6, CYP2A13, CYP2E1, CYP3A4, and the olfactory-specific CYP2G1 isoform, as well as several isoforms of the flavin-dependent monooxygenases. Phase 2 enzymes found in the olfactory mucosa include UGTs, glutathione-S-transferases, carboxylesterases, aldehyde oxidases, and epoxide hydrolases. The most striking feature of the nasal epithelium is that the P450 catalytic activity per gram of tissue is higher than in any other extrahepatic tissue or in the liver. Nasal decongestants, essences, anesthetics, alcohols, nicotine, and cocaine have been shown to be metabolized in vitro by P450 enzymes from the nasal epithelium. Because the P450s in the nasal mucosa are active, first-pass metabolism should be considered when delivering susceptible drugs intranasally.

The nasal mucosa is also exposed to a wide range of odorants. Odorants, which are mostly small lipophilic molecules, enter the mucosa and reach the odorant receptors on sensory neurons by a transient process requiring signal termination, which could be provided by biotransformation of the odorant in the epithelial supporting cells. Thus metabolism of odorants could be involved in both the termination and initiation of olfactory stimuli.

Brain Metabolism

The metabolism of endogenous neurochemicals and neurotransmitters by brain CYPs may help explain variations in mood, aggression, personality disorders, and other psychiatric conditions.[75-77] The role of brain CYP metabolism in neurotoxicity may also contribute to our understanding of the underlying mechanisms of diseases such as Parkinson's disease. Knowledge of CYP isoforms and transporter function in the blood-brain barrier (BBB) may increase our ability to deliver active forms of drugs specifically to the brain.

The isoforms of P450s and their regulation in the brain are of interest in defining the possible involvement of P450s in CNS toxicity and carcinogenicity. The expression level of P450 in the brain is approximately 0.5%-2% of that in liver, too low to significantly influence the overall pharmacokinetics of drugs and hormones in the periphery.[75,77] Brain CYPs can impact acute and chronic drug response and susceptibility to damage by neurotoxins and are associated with altered personality, behavior, and risk of neurological disease. The functional role for brain CYP enzyme activity can impact CNS drug activation, protection against neurotoxicity, regulate neurotransmitter metabolism, chronic (e.g., nicotine dependence) response to drugs, and are associated with altered personality and behavior, and risk of neurological disease. Expression on a g/tissue basis can be as high as levels in hepatocytes. However, while hepatic CYPs are expressed primarily in the endoplasmic reticulum, brain expression is found in the mitochondrial and plasma membrane fraction and other cell membrane compartments. CYP1A1, CYP2B6, CYP2D6, CYP2E1, and CYP3A, are predominantly found in neurons and glial cells. CYP3A4 and CYP2C19 are expressed in human prefrontal cortex, hippocampus, and amygdala, areas that may mediate the behavioral effects of testosterone. Human CYP1B1 is found at the blood-brain interface, where it may act in conjunction with transporters, such as ATP-binding cassette transporters, to regulate passage of xenobiotics in and/or out of the brain. The interaction of a variety of transporters, in addition to local CYP-mediated metabolism, may play an important role in regulating the levels of centrally acting drugs in the brain and, thereby, their therapeutic effects.

The expression of brain CYPs levels vary among different brain regions. For example, in the human brain, CYP2B6 protein expression varies significantly among brain regions with a 2.5-fold range.[75] Brain CYP2D6 can metabolize endogenous neurochemicals, such as tyramine to dopamine and 5-methoxytryptamine to serotonin, while the metabolism of the endogenous cannabinoid anandamide, the neurosteroid progesterone, and testosterone (to 16α-hydroxytestosterone) is catalyzed by CYP2B6.[75] Thus these enzymes may play a functional role in the brain. CYP2C19 can metabolize the sex hormones testosterone, progesterone, and estradiol that are known to affect brain function and personality traits, such as aggression and anxiety. CYP2E1 can metabolize the fatty acid neural signaling molecule arachidonic acid, which is abundant in the brain and is required for neurologic health, and CYP19 aromatase can metabolize testosterone to estradiol, both of which can influence personality traits, including aggression, impulsivity, and anxiety. The differences in expression of specific brain CYPs can cause shifts in the neurochemical homeostasis in the brain.

Individuals with a CYP2D6 PM genotype are at greater risk for parkinsonism, and this risk is even greater with exposure to neurotoxic pesticides.[75] CYP2D6 metabolizes and inactivates a number of compounds that can cause parkinsonian symptoms, including MPTP, a Parkinson-causing compound, and its neurotoxic metabolite MPP+. CYP2D6 is expressed in human brain regions affected by Parkinson's disease, such as the substantia nigra. The impaired ability of CYP2D6 PMs to inactivate these neurotoxic metabolites may contribute to their increased risk for Parkinson's disease. In contrast to CYP2D6 PMs, smokers are at lower risk for Parkinson's disease since nicotine is neuroprotective. In humans, CYP2D6 expression levels are higher in the brains of smokers than in those of nonsmokers, while induction of brain CYP2D6 by nicotine or smoking may reduce an individual's relative risk for the disease. These data support a contributing role for lower brain CYP2D6 in the increased risk for Parkinson's disease, likely through modulation of local neurotoxin metabolism.[75]

Nicotine is the main component of cigarette smoke that causes tobacco dependence, and genetic variation in brain CYP2B6, CYP2D6, and CYP2E1 can affect smoking behaviors.[75,76] CYP2B6 slow metabolizers (IMs) progress to tobacco dependence more quickly and have more difficulty quitting than normal (EM) metabolizers. Brain CYP2B6 metabolizes nicotine and other endogenous substrates, such as serotonin and neurosteroids. Nicotine and smoking induces the brain expression of CYP2B6, CYP2D6, and CYP2E1, all of which affect smoking behaviors. Smokers have higher levels of brain CYP2D6, but unchanged levels of hepatic CYP2D6. Individuals exposed to nicotine through smoking or through nicotine replacement therapy are likely to have increased CYP2D6-mediated brain metabolism of centrally acting drugs, neurotoxins, and endogenous neurochemicals, increasing risk of drug interactions and neurotoxicity. Brain levels of CYP2D6 enzymes and activity may be contributing factors to the clinical observations of personality differences with chronic nicotine administration between CYP2D6 EM and PM phenotypes. Preliminary data suggest that reducing brain CYP2B and CYP2D6 activity increases the rewarding properties of nicotine by altering brain levels of nicotine and its metabolites.

Metabolism in Other Tissues

P450s in the kidney and adrenal tissues include isoforms primarily involved in the hydroxylation of steroids, arachidonic acid, and 25-hydroxycholcalciferol.

STEREOCHEMICAL ASPECTS OF DRUG METABOLISM

In addition to the physicochemical factors that affect xenobiotic metabolism, stereochemical factors have an important role in the biotransformation of drugs. This involvement is not unexpected, because the xenobiotic-metabolizing enzymes are also the same enzymes that metabolize certain endogenous substrates which, for the most part, are chiral molecules. Most of these CYP isoforms show stereoselectivity but not stereospecificity; in other words, one stereoisomer enters into biotransformation pathways preferentially but not exclusively. Metabolic stereochemical reactions can be categorized as follows: substrate stereoselectivity, in which two enantiomers of a chiral substrate are metabolized by CYP isoforms at different rates; product stereoselectivity, in which a new chiral center is created in a symmetric molecule and one enantiomer is metabolized preferentially; and substrate-product stereoelectivity, in which a new chiral center of a chiral molecule is metabolized preferentially to one of two possible diastereomers.

An example of substrate stereoselectivity is the preferred decarboxylation of (*S*)-α-methyldopa to (*S*)-α-methyldopamine, with almost no reaction for (*R*)-α-methyldopa. Another example is the (*S*)-ketamine enantiomer, which is preferentially N-demethylated by CYP2B6 to (*S*)-norketamine, whereas the (*R*) enantiomer is N-demethylated by CYP3A4. The reduction of ketones to stereoisomeric alcohols and the hydroxylation of enantiotropic protons or phenyl rings by P450 are examples of product stereoselectivity. For example, phenytoin undergoes aromatic *p*-hydroxylation of only one of its two phenyl rings to create a chiral center at C5 of the hydantoin ring; methadone is reduced preferentially to its α-diastereometric alcohol and naltrexone is reduced to its 6-β-alcohol. Two examples of substrate-product stereoselectivity are the reduction of the enantiomers of warfarin, and the β-hydroxylation of (*S*)-α-methyldopamine to (1*R*,2*S*)-α-methylnorepinephrine ((*R*)-α-methyldopamine is hydroxylated only to a negligible extent). In vivo studies of this type often can be confused by the further biotransformation of one stereoisomer, giving the false impression that only one stereoisomer was formed preferentially. Moreover, some compounds show stereoselective absorption, distribution, and excretion, which proves the importance of performing in vitro studies.

Although studies regarding the stereoselective biotransformation of drug molecules are not yet extensive, those that have been done indicate that stereochemical factors have an important role in drug metabolism. In some cases, stereoselective biotransformation could account for the differences in pharmacological activity and duration of action between enantiomers.

METABOLIC BIOACTIVATION: ROLE IN HEPATOTOXICITY, IDIOSYNCRATIC REACTIONS, AND CHEMICAL CARCINOGENESIS

Drug-Induced Hepatotoxicity

Drug-induced hepatotoxicity is the leading cause of hepatic injury, accounting for approximately half of all cases of acute liver failure in the U.S. Recent studies have shown that drug-induced hepatotoxicity represents a larger percentage of adverse drug reactions than reported previously, and that the incidence and severity of drug-induced liver injury is underestimated among the general population.

Acetaminophen overdose is the leading cause for calls to poison control centers (>100,000 calls/year) and accounts for more than 56,000 emergency room visits, 2600 hospitalizations, and an estimated 458 deaths from acute liver failure each year. Among the listed drugs in Table 3.17, acetaminophen is the most frequently implicated hepatotoxic agent and can cause extensive hepatic necrosis with as little as 10-12 g (30-40 tablets). Chronic alcohol intake enhances acetaminophen hepatotoxicity more than five times as compared to acute alcohol intake, yet acetaminophen is heavily marketed for its safety as compared to nonsteroidal analgesics (NSAIDs). U.S. drug manufacturers continue to market and promote extra-strength acetaminophen products (500-750 mg/tablet) and a variety of Extra-strength acetaminophen-drug combination products. Self-poisoning with acetaminophen (paracetamol) is also a common cause of hepatotoxicity in the Western world. To reduce the number of acetaminophen poisonings in the UK, over-the-counter (nonprescription) sales of acetaminophen are limited to 16 tablets per packet.

Drug-induced hepatotoxicity is also the most frequent reason that new therapeutic agents are not approved by the FDA (e.g., ximelagatran in 2004) and the most common adverse drug reaction leading to withdrawal of a drug from the market (Table 3.17). Hepatotoxicity almost always involves metabolism with Phase 1 P450 enzymes rather than Phase 2 enzymes. More than 600 drugs, chemicals, and herbal remedies can cause hepatotoxicity, of which more than 30 drugs have either been withdrawn from the U.S. market because of hepatotoxicity or have carried a black box warning for hepatotoxicity since 1990. Table 3.17 includes some of the more common drugs that have exhibited drug-induced hepatotoxicity ranging from severe, requiring the drug's regulatory withdrawal from the market (bold in Table 3.17); moderate to severe, requiring black box warning restrictions (italics in Table 3.17); or mild to moderate, requiring frequent liver function monitoring.

Table 3.17 Some Drugs Causing Hepatic Injury[a]

Acarbose	*Felbamate*	Methotrexate	Ritonavir
Acetaminophen	Fenofibrate	Methsuximide	Rosiglitazone
Allopurinol	*Fluconazole*	Methyldopa	Rosuvastatin
Amiodarone	*Flutamide*	Nabumetone	*Saquinavir*
Amprenavir	Fluvastatin	Naproxen	Simvastatin
Anagrelide	Gemfibrozil	**Nefazodone (2005)**	Sulindac
Atomoxetine	Gemtuzumab	*Nevirapine*	*Tacrine*
Atorvastatin	Griseofulvin	Niacin (SR)	Tamoxifen
Azathioprine	*Halothane*	Nitrofurantoin	**Tasosartan (1998)**
Bicalutamide	Imatinib	Olanzapine	*Terbinafine*
Bosentan	Indinavir	Oxaprozin	Testosterone
Bromfenac (1998)	*Infliximab*	**Pemoline (2005)**	Thioguanine
Carbamazepine	Isoflurane	Pentamidine	Tizanidine
Celecoxib	Isotretinoin	Pioglitazone	*Tolcapone*
Dapsone	Itraconazole	Piroxicam	**Troglitazone (2000)**
Diclofenac	*Ketoconazole*	Pravastatin	*Trovafloxacin*
Disulfiram	*Ketorolac*	*Pyrazinamide*	*Valproic acid*
Duloxetine	Lamivudine	Ribavirin	Voriconazole
Efavirenz	*Leflunomide*	Rifabutin	**Ximelagatran (2004)**
Ethotoin	Lovastatin	*Rifampin*	*Zileuton*
Ethosuximide	Meloxicam	Riluzole	*Zafirlukast*

[a]Drugs in **bold** have exhibited severe drug-induced hepatotoxicity and were withdrawn either voluntarily or by a regulatory agency (year given). Drugs in *italics* have exhibited moderate-severe drug-induced hepatotoxicity requiring a black box warning restricting their use. The other drugs have exhibited mild to moderate drug-induced hepatotoxicity that can need frequent liver transaminase testing for those at risk (see Table 3.18).

However, Watkins[78] reported that one-third of 106 patients taking a maximum daily acetaminophen dose of 4 g for 8 days, either alone or in combination with hydrocodone, exhibited a 3-fold increase in liver enzymes associated with acetaminophen-induced liver injury. This 3-fold increase in transminase levels is a signal for potential liver safety concerns in those individuals who are at risk of acetaminophen-induced liver toxicity. Drugs reported to cause hepatocellular necrosis include acetaminophen, methyldopa, valproic acid, trazodone, nefazodone, venlafaxine, and lovastatin. Drug-induced liver damage occurs after a prolonged period of drug administration.

The most commonly used indicators of hepatotoxicity (i.e., liver injury) are increased levels of the liver transaminases, aspartate aminotransferase (AST), and alanine aminotransferase (ALT).[79] Drug-induced hepatotoxicity can develop rapidly, often before abnormal laboratory tests are noticed, which are characterized by rapid elevations in ALT and AST of 8-500 times the upper normal limit, with variable elevations in bilirubin. Drugs causing acute liver injury (hepatocellular necrosis) exhibit elevations in hepatic transaminases ranging from 50 to 100 times higher than the normal level. On the other hand, the elevations of ALT and AST in alcoholic liver disease are two to three times higher than normal. Some hepatotoxins, however, do not elevate transaminases, whereas nonhepatic toxins can elevate ALT.

Most drug-induced hepatotoxicity is of an idiosyncratic nature, occurring in a small percentage of patients (1 in 5000) who ingest the drug.[80-82] These reactions tend to be of two distinct types: (1) hypersensitivity reactions that are immune mediated, occurring within the first 4-6 weeks and are associated with fever, rash, eosinophilia, and a hepatitis-like picture (e.g., phenytoin, sulindac, and allopurinol); and (2) metabolic idiosyncratic reactions that tend to occur at almost any time during the first year of treatment (e.g., troglitazone). The incidence of overt idiosyncratic liver diseases varies with the drug, ranging from approximately 1 in 1000 with phenytoin, to 1 in 10,000 or more with sulindac and troglitazone and 1 in 100,000 with diclofenac. To detect a single case of drug-induced hepatotoxicity with 95% confidence requires the number of patients studied to be 3-fold the incidence of the reaction (i.e., for one adverse drug reaction in 10,000 patients, at least 30,000 patients need to be evaluated). Thus, many drugs are approved before liver toxicity is observed. It is the responsibility of postmarketing surveillance and monitoring of liver transaminases to identify potential cases of liver-adverse drug reactions.

Risk factors (Table 3.18) for drug-induced liver injury, such as age, gender, genetic predisposition, multiple drugs, or dietary supplements and degree of alcohol consumption, appear to increase the susceptibility to drug-induced hepatotoxicity.[80,81] However, the drugs in Table 3.17 should be used with caution in these high-risk patients, because such patients can have altered metabolism of these drugs and, therefore, can be at increased risk for liver injury. The coadministration of drugs in Table 3.17 with enzyme inducers, such as phenobarbital, phenytoin, ethanol, and/or cigarette smoke, can induce hepatic enzymes, resulting in the enhancement of hepatotoxicity.

Most hepatic adverse effects associated with drugs occur in adults rather than children. Drug-induced liver injury occurs at a higher rate in patients older than 50 years and drug-associated jaundice occurs also more frequently in the geriatric population.[80,81] This age-risk can be the result of increased frequency of drug exposure, multidrug therapy, and age-related changes in drug metabolism.

For reasons that are unclear, drug-induced liver injury affects females more than males. Females accounted for approximately 79% of all reactions to acetaminophen and 73% of all idiosyncratic drug-induced reactions. Females exhibit increased risk of hepatic injury from drugs such as atorvastatin, nitrofurantoin, methyldopa, and diclofenac.[81]

Genetic factors because of enzyme polymorphism in affected individuals can decrease the ability to metabolize or eliminate drugs, thus increasing their duration of action and drug exposure and/or decreasing the ability to modulate the immune response to drugs or metabolites. Chronic ingestion of alcohol can also predispose many patients to increased hepatotoxicity from drugs by lowering the store of glutathione (a detoxifying mechanism), which prevents trapping of the toxic metabolites as mercapturate conjugates that are excreted in the urine.

Drug-induced hepatotoxicity can be categorized as intrinsic (predictable) or idiosyncratic (unpredictable) reactions.[82] Most drugs involved in hepatotoxicity belong to the idiosyncratic group. Intrinsic hepatotoxins produce liver injury in a dose-related manner when a toxic

Table 3.18 Risk Factors for Drug-Induced Liver Injury

Race	Some drugs exhibit different toxicities based on race because of individual P450 polymorphism. For example, blacks and Hispanics can be more susceptible to isoniazid (INH) toxicity.
Age	Elderly persons are at increased risk of hepatic injury due to decreased clearance, drug-drug interactions, reduced hepatic blood flow, variation in drug binding, and lower hepatic volume. In addition, poor diet, infections, and multiple hospitalizations are important reasons for drug-induced hepatotoxicity. Hepatic drug reactions are rare in children (e.g., acetaminophen, halogenated general anesthetics).
Gender	Although the reasons are unknown, hepatic drug reactions are more common in females. Females are more susceptible to hepatotoxicity from acetaminophen, halothane, nitrofurantoin, diclofenac, and sulindac.
Alcohol	Alcoholics are susceptible to drug toxicity because alcohol induces liver injury and cirrhotic changes that alter drug metabolism. Alcohol causes depletion of glutathione (hepatoprotective) stores, making the person more susceptible to toxicity by drugs (e.g., acetaminophen, statins).
Liver disease	Patients with chronic liver disease are not uniformly at increased risk of hepatic injury. Although the total P450 level is reduced, some patients can be affected more than others. The modification of doses in persons with liver disease should be based on knowledge of the specific P450 isoform involved in the metabolism. Patients with HIV infection who are coinfected with hepatitis B or C virus are at increased risk for hepatotoxic effects. Similarly, patients with cirrhosis are at increased risk to hepatotoxic drugs (e.g., methotrexate, methyldopa, valproic acid).
Genetic factors	Genetic (polymorphic) differences in the formation of P450 isoforms (2C family and 2D6) can result in abnormal reactions to drugs, including idiosyncratic reactions
Other comorbidities	Patients with AIDS, renal disease, diabetes mellitus, persons who are malnourished, and persons who are fasting can be susceptible to drug reactions because of low glutathione stores.
Pharmacokinetics	Long-acting drugs can cause more injury than shorter-acting drugs, as well as sustained-release drug product formulation.
Drug adulterants	Contaminants are often found in noncertified herbal supplements (e.g., hepatitis C).

amount of drug is ingested without bioactivation, such as the toxins found in the *Amanita* mushroom. Idiosyncratic hepatotoxicity is the result of the toxic effects of a drug's metabolites.

The common trigger for both mild and severe forms of hepatotoxicity is bioactivation of relatively inert functional groups to reactive electrophilic intermediates, which is considered to be an obligatory event in the etiology of many drug-induced idiosyncratic hepatotoxicity.[83,84] Research now shows that reactive metabolites are formed from drugs known to cause idiosyncratic hepatotoxicity, but how these toxic species initiate and propagate tissue damage remains poorly understood. However, the relationship between bioactivation and the occurrence of hepatic injury is not simple. For example, many drugs at therapeutic doses undergo bioactivation in the liver but are not hepatotoxic. The tight coupling of bioactivation with bioinactivation pathways can be one reason for the lack of hepatotoxicity with these drugs. Examples of bioinactivation (detoxification) pathways include glutathione conjugation of quinones by glutathione S-transferases (GSTs) and hydration of arene oxides to dihydrodiols by epoxide hydrolases. When reactive metabolites are poor substrates for such detoxifying enzymes, they can escape bioinactivation and, thereby, damage proteins and nucleic acids, prompting hepatotoxicity.

Most drugs, however, are not directly chemically reactive but, through the normal process of drug metabolism, can form electrophilic, chemically reactive metabolites. Formation of chemically reactive metabolites is mainly catalyzed by P450 enzymes (Phase 1), but products of Phase 2 metabolism (e.g., acylglucuronides, acyl CoA thioesters, or N-sulfates) can also lead to toxicity. However, if Phase 1 drug bioactivation is closely coupled with Phase 2 bioinactivation (e.g., glutathione conjugation to mercapturates), then the net chemical process is one of detoxification if the final product is rapidly cleared.

Toxicity can accrue when accumulation of a chemically reactive metabolite, if not detoxified, leads to covalent modification of biological macromolecules. The identity of the target macromolecule and the functional consequence of its modification will dictate the resulting toxicological response. P450 enzymes are present in many organs, mainly the liver but also the kidney and lung, and thus can bioactivate chemicals to cause organ-specific toxicity. Evidence for the formation of reactive metabolites was found for 5 of the 6 drugs that have been withdrawn from the market since 1995 and for 8 of the 15 drugs that have black box warnings (Table 3.17). Evidence for reactive metabolite formation has been found for acetaminophen, bromfenac, diclofenac, clozapine and troglitazone. Acetaminophen is the most studied hepatotoxin.

The current hypotheses of how reactive metabolites lead to liver injury suggest that hepatic (target) proteins can be modified by reactive metabolites. Much more clinically important is the identification of the target proteins modified by these toxic metabolites and how these reactions alter the function of those proteins. Additionally, it is important to note that the toxicity of reactive metabolites can also be mediated by noncovalent binding mechanisms, which can have profound effects on normal liver physiology. Such information should dramatically improve our understanding of drug-induced hepatotoxic reactions. Moreover, covalent binding per se does not necessarily lead to drug hepatotoxicity. The regioisomer of acetaminophen, 3-hydroxyacetanilide, becomes covalently bound to hepatic proteins in rodents without inducing hepatotoxicity.[85]

It therefore is necessary to identify targets for these reactive metabolites (i.e., covalently modified macromolecules) that are critical to the toxicological process. Unfortunately, no simple rules predict the target macromolecules for a particular chemically reactive metabolite or the biological consequences of a particular modification. Furthermore, noncovalent interactions also have a role, because covalent binding of hepatotoxins is not indiscriminate with respect to proteins. Even within a single protein, there can be selective modification of an amino acid side chain found repeatedly in the primary structure. Thus, the microenvironment (e.g., pK_a and hydrophobicity) of the amino acid in the tertiary structure appears to be the crucial determinant of selective binding and, therefore, the impact of covalent binding on protein function. In turn, the extent of binding and the biochemical role of the protein will determine the toxicological insult of drug bioactivation. The resulting pathological consequences will be a balance between the rates of protein damage and the rates of protein replacement and cellular repair.

Drug-Induced Idiosyncratic Reactions

Idiosyncratic drug reactions (IDR; type B adverse drug reactions) occur in from 1 in 1000 to 1 in 50,000 patients, are not predictable from the known pharmacology or toxicology of the drug, are not produced experimentally in vitro and in vivo, and are dose independent. The occurrence of IDRs during late clinical trials or after a drug has been released can lead to severe restriction of its use and even its withdrawal. IDRs do not as a rule result from the drug itself because most people can tolerate the drug, but rather from a unique set of patient characteristics, including gender, age, genetic predisposition, and a lack of drug-metabolizing enzymes that can increase the risk of these adverse drug reactions. Most IDRs are caused by hypersensitivity reactions and can result in hepatocellular injury. The hepatic injury occurs within 1 week to 12 months after initiation of drug therapy and is often accompanied by systemic characteristics of allergic drug reactions, such as rash and fever. Signs of hepatic injury reappear with subsequent administration of the same drug with only one or two doses. Hypersensitivity reactions can be severe and associated with fatal reactions as a multiorgan clinical syndrome characterized by the following: (1) fever; (2) rash; (3) gastrointestinal symptoms (e.g., nausea, vomiting, diarrhea, or abdominal pain); (4) generalized malaise, fatigue, or achiness; and (5) respiratory symptoms (e.g., dyspnea, cough, or pharyngitis). Examples of drugs causing IDRs through a hypersensitivity mechanism include penicillin, methyldopa, chlorpromazine, erythromycin, azathioprine toxicity in thiopurine methyltransferase–deficient individuals, sulfonamide and acetaminophen hepatotoxicity in alcoholics and in UGT1A6-deficient cats, ivermectin neurotoxicity in Collie dogs deficient in P-gp, perhexilene hepatotoxicity in CYP2D6-deficient individuals, phenytoin toxicity in CYP2C9-deficient individuals, and valproic acid hepatotoxicity.

The clinical features of some cases of drug-induced idiosyncratic hepatotoxicity strongly suggest an involvement of the immune system.[83,84] These clinical characteristics include the following: (1) concurrence of rash, fever, and eosinophilia; (2) delay of the initial reaction (1-8 weeks) or requirement of repeated exposure to the culprit drug; (3) rapid recurrence of toxicity on reexposure to the drug; and (4) presence of antibodies specific for native or drug-modified hepatic proteins. Our current understanding of drug-induced adaptive immune responses is largely based on the hapten hypothesis.

Idiosyncratic drug reactions that are connected with hepatotoxicity involve the formation of reactive metabolites.[83,84] Such reactions are not predictable, but current bioanalytical technology have enabled the in vivo identification of the formation of reactive metabolites, as evidenced by the detection of biomarkers (i.e., mercapturate or cysteine adducts) in urine, drug-specific antibodies, or antibodies to P450 isoforms.[84] As a result, some drugs known to cause hepatic injury continue to be used because the drug's benefit outweighs its risk and no alternative efficacious drug exists. Additionally, NSAIDs, including cyclooxygenase-2 inhibitors (e.g., celecoxib), commonly are associated with idiosyncratic liver injury. Most of the idiosyncratic toxins listed in Table 3.19 that have been studied to date produce reactive metabolites.

Current hypotheses regarding IDRs suggest that metabolic activation of a drug to a reactive metabolite is a necessary step in the generation of an idiosyncratic reaction.[83] Evidence for this hypothesis comes from drugs that are associated with hepatotoxicity (Table 3.19) and the detection of drug-metabolite specific antibodies in affected patients.

For the other drugs that have been associated with idiosyncratic hepatotoxicity but that do not have black box warnings, either evidence for hepatotoxicity was not available or suitable studies had not been carried out. High doses increase the risk for an IDR (e.g., cloazapine at 300 mg/d vs. olanzapine 20 mg/d).

The hapten hypothesis proposes that the reactive metabolites of hepatotoxic drugs act as haptens and bind covalently to endogenous proteins to form immunogenic drug-protein adducts triggering either antibody or cytotoxic T-cell responses.[84] The hapten hypothesis is supported by the detection of antibodies that recognize drug-modified hepatic proteins in the sera of drug-induced liver injury patients. For example, antibodies that recognize trifluoroacetate-altered hepatic proteins have been detected in the sera of patients with halothane-induced hepatitis. Such drug-specific antibodies that recognize native liver proteins have also been found in patients with liver injury caused by other drugs, such as diclofenac. Most drugs are small molecules and are unlikely to form haptens. Electrophilic acylators can react with the lysine ω-amino residues of the target protein or guanosine residues of DNA. Halothane is the most studied molecule for supporting this hypothesis regarding IDRs.[84] Therefore, it is not surprising that irreversible chemical modification of a protein, which has a profound effect on function, is a mechanism of idiosyncratic hepatotoxicity. However, it is important to note that a number of drugs (e.g., penicillins, aspirin, and omeprazole) rely on covalent binding to proteins for their efficacy; thus, prevention of their covalent binding through chemical modification of the compound can also, inadvertently, lead to loss of efficacy.

Table 3.19 Some Examples of Idiosyncratic Toxins

Abacavir	Hypersensitivity
Acetaminophen	Hepatotoxicity
Amiodarone	Hepatotoxicity
Aromatic anticonvulsants	Hypersensitivity
Cefaclor	Hepatotoxicity
Clozapine	Agranulocytosis
Diclofenac	Hepatotoxicity
Felbamate	Aplastic anemia
Fibrates	Hepatotoxicity
Halothane	Hepatotoxicity
Indomethacin	Hepatotoxicity
Isoniazid	Hepatotoxicity
Levamisole	Hepatotoxicity
Nefazodone	Hepatotoxicity
Nevirapine	agranulocytosis
Oral contraceptives	Hepatotoxicity
Paroxetine	Hepatotoxicity
Penicillinamine[a]	Hypersensitivity
Phenytoin	Hepatotoxicity
Statins	Hepatotoxicity
Sulfonamides	Stevens-Johnson syndrome
Tamoxifen	Hepatotoxicity
Tacrine	Hepatotoxicity
Tienilic acid	Hypersensitivity
Ticlopidine	Agranulocytosis
Troglitazone	Hepatotoxicity
Valproic acid	Hepatotoxicity
Vesnarinone	Agranulocytosis

[a]Does not produce reactive metabolites.

Reactive Metabolites Resulting From Bioactivation

Electrophiles

The concept that small organic molecules can undergo bioactivation to electrophiles (an electron-deficient group or ion that accepts an electron pair to make a covalent bond, such as carbocations and acyl ions) and free radicals, and can elicit toxicity by chemical modification of cellular macromolecules, has its basis in chemical carcinogenicity and the pioneering work of the Millers[86] and Gillette et al.[87] Electrophiles are reactive because they possess electron-deficient centers (polarization-activated double bonds or positive-charge acylators) (Fig. 3.38) and can form covalent bonds with electron-rich biological nucleophiles such as the thiol groups in either glutathione or cysteine residues within proteins. A number of different types of reactive metabolites exist; however, they can be broadly classified as either electrophiles (Fig. 3.38) or free radicals (Fig. 3.39).[88] These reactive metabolites are short-lived, with half-lives of usually less than 1 minute, and they are not normally detectable in plasma or urine except as Phase 2 conjugates or other biomarkers.

Activated double bonds are electrophilic intermediates. Examples of activated double bond electrophiles include α,β-unsaturated carbonyl compounds, quinones, quinoneimines, quinonemethides, and diiminoquinones as shown in Figure 3.40. These electrophilic intermediates are highly polarized and can react with nucleophiles in a 1,4-Michael-type addition at the more electrophilic β-carbon of the activated double bond intermediate to generate the addition product (Fig. 3.40A). Specific examples of activated double bond electrophiles that have been proposed for the anticancer drug leflunomide, acetaminophen, the antiandrogen flutamide, the anticonvulsant felbamate, and the cytotoxic cyclophosphamide are shown in Figure 3.40C. The bioinactivation pathways for these electrophilic intermediate can involve direct addition, with or without GSH or epoxide transferases, depending upon the degree of polarization and reactivity of the electrophilic intermediate.[89]

Other commonly found electrophilic intermediate for drug molecules in Figure 3.38 include ketenes from the bioactivation of acetylenic groups (e.g., ethinyl estradiol) (2 in Fig. 3.38); isocyanates from thiazolidinediones (e.g., the "glitazones") (4 in Fig. 3.38)[88]; acylonium ions from halogenated hydrocarbons (e.g., halothane) (3 in Fig. 3.38)[88] and carboxylic acids; β-dicarbonyl from furans (e.g., furosemide) (5 in Fig. 3.38)[88]; activated thiophene-S-oxide from thiophenes, such as ticlopidine and tenoxicam which cause an IDR, agranulocytosis (6 in Fig. 3.38)[88]; and epoxides and arene oxides from olefins and aromatic compounds (7 in Fig. 3.38).[88]

Drugs possessing structural features prone to metabolic epoxidations are abundant. Therefore the incidence of epoxide metabolites in mediating adverse biologic effects has aroused concern about clinically used drugs known to be metabolized to epoxides. Metabolically produced epoxides have been reported for allobarbital, secobarbital, protriptyline, carbamazepine, and cyproheptadine and are implicated with 8-methoxypsoralen and other furanocoumarins (6,7-dihydroxybergamottin in grapefruit juice), phenytoin, phensuximide, phenobarbital, mephobarbital, lorazepam, and imipramine.[89,90] The alarming biologic effects of some epoxides, however, do not imply that all epoxides have similar effects. Epoxides vary greatly in molecular geometry, stability, electrophilic reactivity, and relative activity as substrates for epoxide-transforming enzymes (e.g., epoxide hydrolase, glutathione S-transferase, and others).

Some carboxylic acid–containing drugs have been implicated in rare IDRs, which was the basis for the market withdrawal of the NSAIDs zomiperac and benzoxaprofen.[57,91] These drugs (e.g., NSAIDs, fibrates, "statins," and valproic acid) can be bioactivated to acyl glucuronides or acyl CoA thioesters[57] (1 and 5 in Fig. 3.41). These products are electrophilic acylators that can acylate target proteins if they escape inactivation by S-glutathione-thioester formation.[92] A crucial factor is the concentration of acyl glucuronides in hepatocytes due to their transport by conjugate export pumps, where acylglucuronides can selectively acylate hepatic membrane proteins. Acyl CoA esters can be either rapidly hydrolyzed or further metabolized in hepatocytes. Evidence is accumulating that acyl glucuronides can alter cellular function by haptenation of peptides, target protein acylation or glycation, or direct stimulation of neutrophils and macrophages. The role of acyl CoA reactive metabolites is less clear. It should be noted that some noncarboxylic acid drugs can be biotransformed by oxidative metabolism in the liver to the respective carboxylic acids.[93]

Free Radicals

P450 activates molecular dioxygen to generate reactive oxygen species (ROS), such as singlet oxygen ($^1O_2$) or superoxide. Reactive metabolites that possess an odd unpaired electron are free radicals that can react with molecular oxygen (ground state triplet) to generate intracellular oxidative stress damage.[94] Free radicals abstract a hydrogen atom from other molecules rather than becoming covalently bound. Free radical reactions can be self-propagating by abstracting a hydrogen atom from the double bond of a lipid that initiates a chain reaction leading to lipid peroxidation, oxidative stress, or other types of modification of biological molecules.

Some examples of free radicals generated by the bioactivation of drug molecules are shown in Figure 3.39. Isoniazid is acetylated to its major metabolite acetylisoniazid, which is hydrolyzed to acetylhydrazine and isonicotinic acid (1 in Fig. 3.39). Acetylhydrazine is further metabolized by the CYP2E1 to an N-hydroxy intermediate that hydrates into an acetyl radical, which can then initiate the process that leads to hepatic necrosis. Other carbon-centered radicals are formed from hydrazines such as the antihypertensive hydralazine and thio-radicals from the ACE inhibitor captopril (3 in Fig. 3.39).

Bioinactivation Mechanisms

Several enzyme systems exist as cellular defense (detoxification) pathways against the chemically reactive metabolites

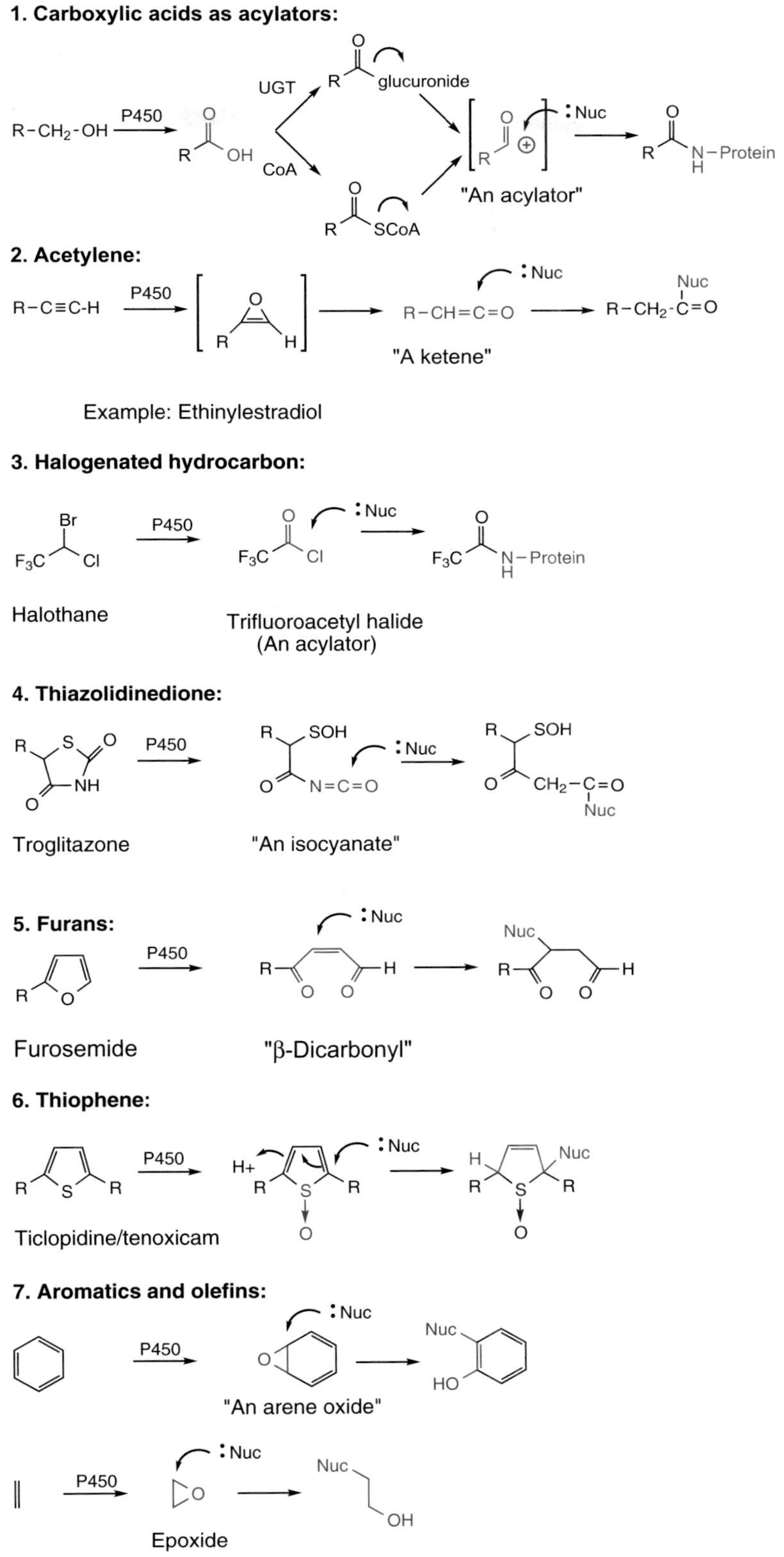

Figure 3.38 Some examples of electrophilic intermediates resulting from bioactivation. *NUC*, nucleophiles.

generated by P450 metabolism. These include GST, epoxide hydrolase, and quinone reductase, as well as catalase, glutathione peroxidase, and superoxide dismutase, which detoxify the peroxide and superoxide by-products of metabolism. The efficiency of the bioinactivation process is dependent on the inherent chemical reactivity of the electrophilic intermediate, its affinity and selectivity of the reactive metabolite for the bioinactivation enzymes, the tissue expression of these enzymes, and the rapid upregulation of these enzymes, and cofactors mediated by the cellular

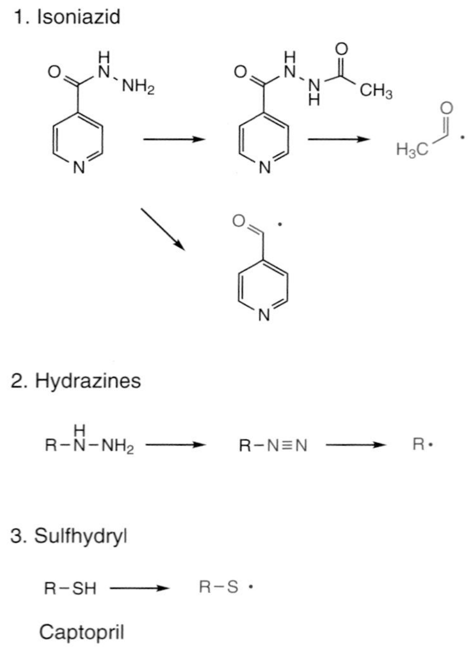

1. Isoniazid

2. Hydrazines

$R{-}NH{-}NH_2 \longrightarrow R{-}N{\equiv}N \longrightarrow R\cdot$

3. Sulfhydryl

$R{-}SH \longrightarrow R{-}S\cdot$

Captopril

Figure 3.39 Drug bioactivation to free radicals.

A. 1,4-Addition of a nucleophile in a Michael-type reaction:

(X = O, N C - activated)

B. Examples of activated double bonds:

Quinone Quinonemethide Iminoquinones 3-Alkylindole

C. Reactive intermediates from drugs that form activated double bonds:

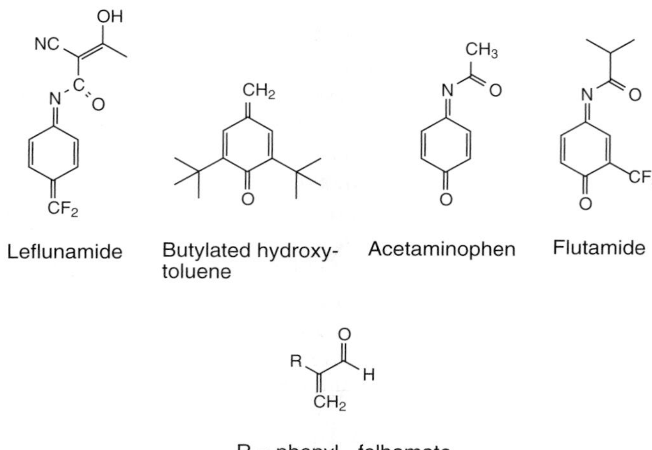

R = phenyl - felbamate
R = H - acrolein from cyclophosphamide

Figure 3.40 Examples of activated double bonds to electrophilic reactive intermediates.

sensors of chemical stress. The reactive metabolites that can evade these defense systems can damage target proteins and nucleic acids by either oxidation or covalent modification.

The most abundant agents of cellular defense are thiols. Glutathione will only react noncatalytically with electrophiles, such as activated double bonds (Fig. 3.40). Glutathione conjugation to mercapturates is one of the most important defenses against hepatocellular injury.[58,59] Glutathione protects cellular enzymes and membranes from toxic metabolites, and its inadequate stores can compromise efficient detoxification of the reactive metabolites. The subsequent inability to detoxify the reactive metabolites can result in hepatocellular injury. The rate-limiting factor for glutathione synthesis is the intracellular concentration of cysteine. N-acetylcysteine is often used as an alternative to glutathione to trap the iminoquinone intermediate in the treatment of acute acetaminophen toxicity and in preventing nephrotoxicity from ifosfamide-generated chloroacetaldehyde. Glutathione has a protective role in the hepatic tissue injury produced by acetaminophen, but not by furosemide.

The relationship between bioactivation, bioinactivation, and DNA adduct formation has been well established for a number of hepatocarcinogens.[94] Glutathione conjugation of carcinogens becomes more efficient when catalyzed by GSTs, an important example being the detoxification of the hepatocarcinogen aflatoxin. Aflatoxin, a hepatocarcinogen and a hepatotoxin found in mold growing on peanuts, is converted into aflatoxin B1 epoxide in rodents, which is more readily detoxified by GST enzymes than by epoxide hydrolase. The balance between these transferase reactions explains the greater DNA damage in humans compared with rodents, because human forms of GST are less able to catalyze the conjugation of aflatoxin epoxide compared with the rodent forms. Transgenic knockout mice have been used to establish the role of bioactivation by P450 and bioinactivation by GSTs for a number of carcinogenic polyaromatic hydrocarbons.

Substances that detoxify free radicals include the antioxidants vitamin C, vitamin E, and carotene, which scavenge free radicals, including reactive metabolites and reactive oxygen species generated as a consequence of chemical stress.

Specific Examples

Some examples of bioactivation to hepatotoxic or IDR electrophilic intermediates are shown in Figure 3.41. Bioactivation can occur by both oxidation and conjugation reactions, such as those with diclofenac, which undergoes the formation of an acyl glucuronide to produce iminoquinones via formation of a phenol intermediator (1 in Fig. 3.41).[92] The anticonvulsant carbamazepine is 2-hydroxylated and the elimination of the amide group yields the

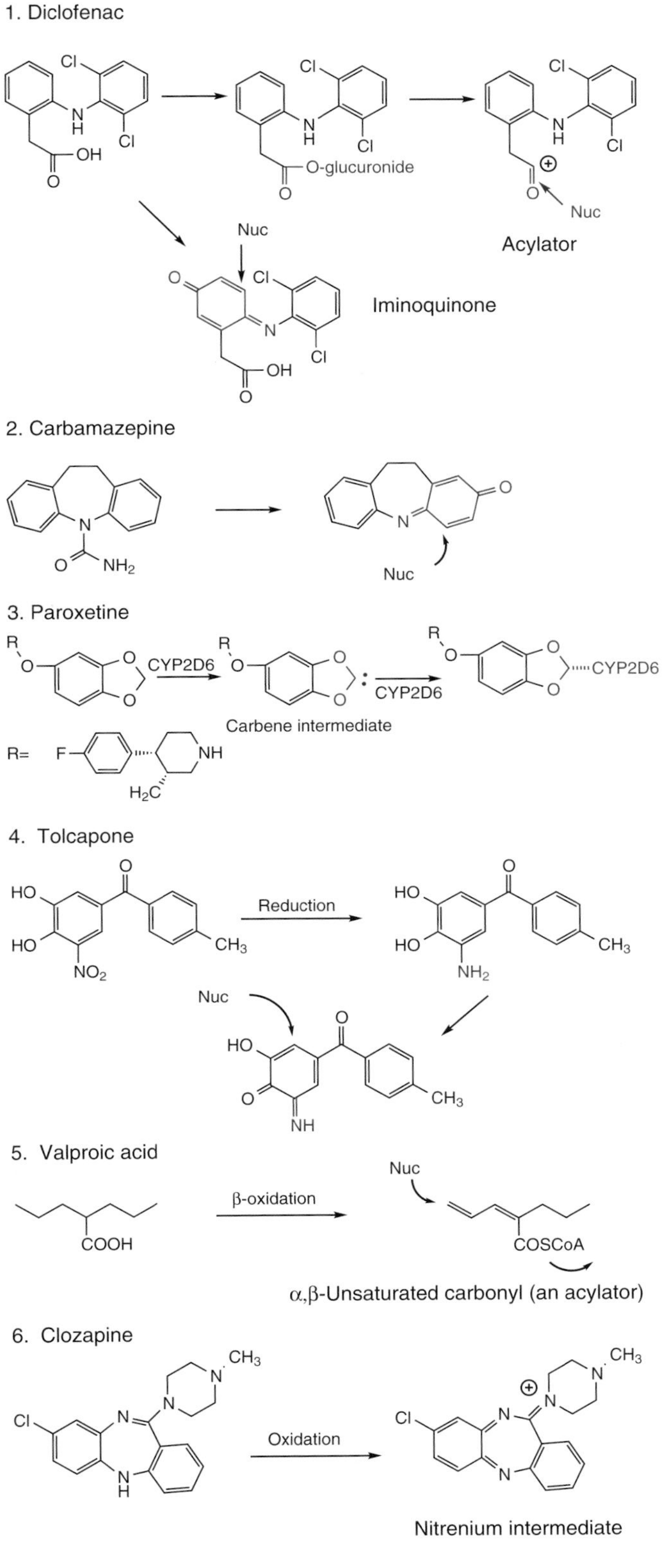

Figure 3.41 Examples of drug bioactivation to hepatotoxic intermediates.

reactive quinoneimine intermediate (2 in Fig. 3.41). The antidepressant paroxetine and other xenobiotics with the common methylenedioxyphenyl nucleus undergo methylene oxidation to a p-quinoid intermediate (3 in Fig. 3.41). The nitro group of the COMT inhibitor tolcapone, used in the treatment of parkinsonism, is first reduced to an amine, then oxidized to an *o*-quinoneimine (4 in Fig. 3.41). The mitochondrial/hepatotoxicity of the anticonvulsant valproic acid results from the formation of an activated α,β-unsaturated CoA thioester via mitochrondrial β-oxidation, most commonly associated with the oxidation of fatty acids (5 in Fig. 3.41). The agranulocytosis resulting from the ingestion of the antipsychotic clozapine is bioinitiated by oxidation by hypochlorous acid in neutrophils to a nitrenium intermediate (6 in Fig. 3.41).[93]

The effect of structure modification for troglitazone that reduced its hepatotoxicity is shown in Figure 3.42. The p-dihydroxy groups of the chroman ring nucleus (outlined in red in Fig. 3.42) of troglitazone is bioactivated to an activated double bond (*p*-quinone) was replaced with a pyridine ring that is not bioactivated, although the thiazolidone ring can be bioactivated to an isocyanate (Fig. 3.42).[91]

The oxidation of acetaminophen to the chemically reactive N-acetyl-p-benzoquinoneimine (Fig. 3.36) is catalyzed by the isoforms CYP1A2 and CYP2E1. The reactive quinoneimine can react covalently either with glutathione to form an inactive product or with cellular macromolecules, initiating the processes leading to hepatic necrosis (Fig. 3.36).[93] The usual route for acetaminophen metabolism is glucuronidation. If insufficient UDP-glucuronic acid is present, then bioactivation will dominate.

Furosemide, a frequently used diuretic drug, is reportedly a human hepatocarcinogen. The hepatic toxicity apparently results from metabolic activation of the furan ring to a β-dicarbonyl intermediate (5 in Fig. 3.38).[93] Ticlopidine and tenoxicam, reported to cause agranulocytosis, do so via metabolic activation of the thiophene ring to an S-oxide (6 in Fig. 3.38).[92] The agranulocytosis resulting from the ingestion of clozapine is via its bioactivation to a nitrenium ion intermediate (6 in Fig. 3.41).[93,94]

Drug-Induced Chemical Carcinogenesis

The mechanism whereby xenobiotics are transformed into chemical carcinogens is usually accepted as bioactivation to reactive metabolites, which are responsible for initiating carcinogenicity.[86,87] Many carcinogens elicit their cytotoxicity through a covalent linkage to DNA. This process can lead to mutations and, potentially, to cancer. Most chemical carcinogens of concern are chemically inert but require activation by the xenobiotic-metabolizing enzymes before they can undergo reaction with DNA or proteins (cytotoxicity). There are many ways to bioactivate procarcinogens, promutagens, plant toxins, drugs, and other xenobiotics (Fig. 3.43).

Oxidative bioactivation reactions are by far the most studied and common. Conjugation reactions (Phase 2), however, are also capable of activating these xenobiotics to produce electrophiles, in which the conjugating derivative acts as a leaving group. These reactive metabolites are mostly electrophiles, such as epoxides, quinones, or free radicals formed by the P450 enzymes or FMO. The reactive metabolites tend to be oxygenated

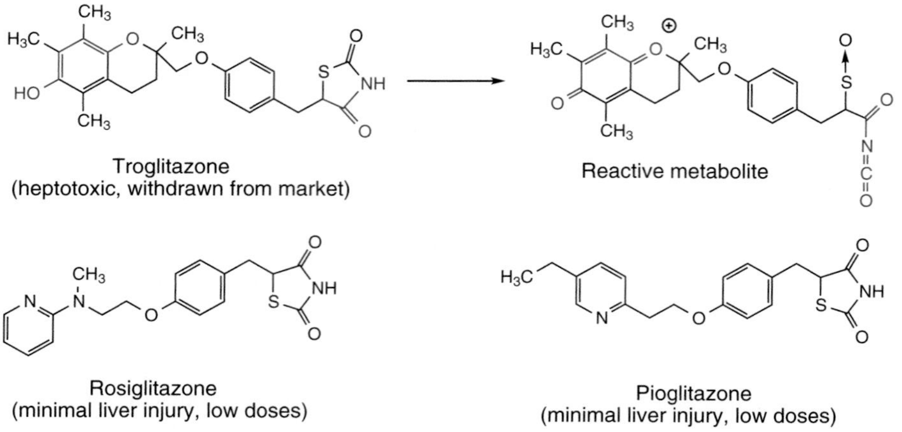

Troglitazone
(heptotoxic, withdrawn from market)

Reactive metabolite

Rosiglitazone
(minimal liver injury, low doses)

Pioglitazone
(minimal liver injury, low doses)

Figure 3.42 The effect of structure modification on drug-induced hepatotoxicity of troglitazone.

in sterically hindered positions, making them poor substrates for subsequent bioinactivation enzymes, such as epoxide hydrolase and GST. Therefore, their principal fate is formation of covalent linkage to intracellular macromolecules, including enzyme proteins and DNA.[91,92] Experimental studies indicate that the CYP1A subfamily can oxygenate aromatic hydrocarbons (e.g., PAHs) in sterically hindered positions to arene oxides. Activation by N-hydroxylation of polycyclic aromatic amines (e.g., aryl N-acetamides) appears to depend on either FMO or P450 isoforms. The formation of chemically reactive metabolites is important, because they frequently cause a number of different toxicities, including tumorigenesis, mutagenesis, tissue necrosis, and hypersensitivity reactions.

Our understanding of these reactions was advanced by the studies of the Millers[86] and Gillette et al.[87] They proposed that the proportion of the dose that binds covalently to critical macromolecules could depend on the quantity of the reactive metabolite is formed.

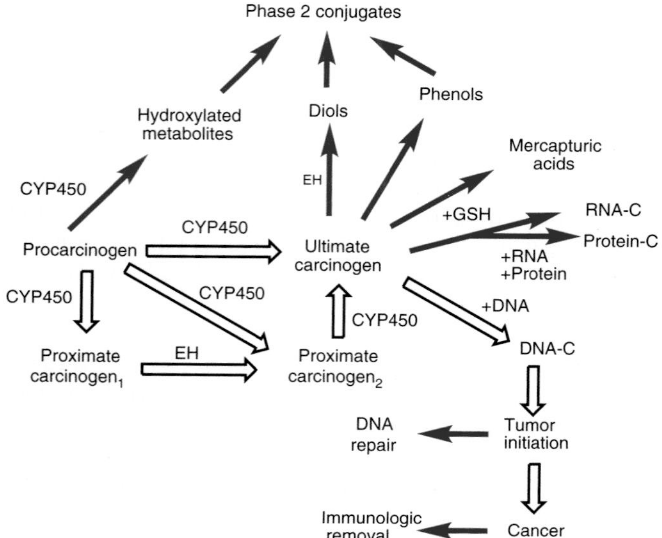

Figure 3.43 The bioactivation of procarcinogens and a proposed mechanism of chemical carcinogenesis.

A scheme illustrating the complexities of drug-induced chemical carcinogenesis is shown in Figure 3.43. Reactions that proceed via the open arrows eventually lead to neoplasia. Some carcinogens can form the "ultimate carcinogen" directly through P450 isoform bioactivation; others, like the PAHs (e.g., benzo[a]pyrene), appear to involve a multistep reaction sequence forming an epoxide, reduction to a diol by epoxide hydrolase, and perhaps the formation of a second epoxide group on another part of the molecule. Other procarcinogens form the N-hydroxy intermediate that requires transferase-catalyzed conjugation (e.g., O-glucuronide and O-sulfate) to form the "ultimate carcinogen." The quantity of "ultimate carcinogen" formed should relate directly to the proportion of the dose that binds or alkylates DNA.

The solid-arrow reaction sequences in Figure 3.43 are intended to show detoxification mechanisms, which involve several steps. First, the original chemical can form less active products (phenols, diols, mercapturic acids, and other conjugates). Second, the "ultimate carcinogen" can rearrange to be prevented from its reaction with DNA (or whatever the critical macromolecule is). Third, the covalently bound DNA can be repaired. Fourth, immunologic removal of the tumor cells can occur. Several mechanisms within this scheme could regulate the quantity of covalently bound carcinogen: (1) The activity of the rate-limiting enzyme, such as epoxide hydrolase, P450 isoform, or one of the transferases, could be involved; (2) the availability of cofactors, such as glutathione, UDP-glucuronic acid, or PAPS, can be rate-limiting; (3) relative P450 activities for detoxification and activation must be considered; (4) availability of alternate reaction sites for the ultimate carcinogen (e.g., RNA and protein can be involved); (5) and possible specific transport mechanisms that deliver either the procarcinogen or its ultimate carcinogen to selected molecular or subcellular sites.

It is well established that numerous organic compounds that are essentially nontoxic as long as their structure is preserved can be converted into cytotoxic, teratogenic, mutagenic, or carcinogenic compounds by normal biotransformation pathways in both animals and humans.

The reactive electrophilic intermediate involves reaction with cellular DNA constituents forming either detoxified products or covalent bonding with essential macromolecules, initiating processes that eventually lead to the toxic effect. A better understanding of the mechanisms underlying these reactions can lead to more rational approaches to the development of nontoxic therapeutic drugs. Special attention to risk factors is required for drugs that will be used for long periods in the same patient.

DRUG-DRUG INTERACTIONS

Drug-drug interactions represent a common clinical problem, which has been compounded by the introduction of many new drugs and the expanded use of herbal medicines. Such interactions do significant harm, prompting anywhere from 1.9 to 5 million patient visits to hospital emergency departments per year according to data from the Medication Safety Program at the Centers for Disease Control and Prevention. Approximately 50% of these serious drug-drug interactions involved P450 inhibition. The problem is likely to grow in the future as the population ages and more people take multiple medications.

Drug-drug interactions occur when the efficacy or toxicity of a medication is changed by coadministration of another substance, drug, food (i.e., grapefruit), or herbal product.[95,96] Pharmacokinetic interactions often occur because of a change in drug metabolism. For example, CYP3A4 oxidizes more than 30% of the clinically used drugs with a broad spectrum of structural features, and its location in the small intestine and liver permits an effect on both presystemic and systemic drug disposition. Some drug-drug interactions with CYP3A4 substrates/inhibitors can also involve inhibition of P-gp. Other clinically important sequelae due to drug-drug interactions resulting from coadministration of CYP3A4 substrates or inhibitors include rhabdomyolysis with the coadministration of some 3-hydroxy-3-methylglutaryl-CoA reductase inhibitors ("statins"), symptomatic hypotension with some dihydropyridine calcium antagonists, excessive sedation from benzodiazepine or nonbenzodiazepine hypnosedatives, ataxia with carbamazepine, and ergotism with ergot alkaloids.

The clinical importance of any drug-drug interaction depends on factors that are drug-, patient-, and administration-related. Drugs with low oral bioavailability or high first-pass metabolism are particularly susceptible to drug-drug interactions when inhibitors that alter absorption, distribution, and elimination are coadministered. In general, a doubling or more of the plasma drug concentration has the potential for enhanced adverse or beneficial drug response. Less pronounced pharmacokinetic drug interactions can still be clinically important for drugs with a steep concentration-response relationship or narrow therapeutic index. In most cases, the extent of drug interaction varies markedly among individuals; this is likely to be dependent on interindividual differences in P450 content (polymorphism), preexisting medical conditions, and possibly age. Drug-drug interactions can occur under single-dose conditions or only at steady state. The pharmacodynamic consequences may or may not closely follow pharmacokinetic changes. Drug-drug interactions can be most apparent when patients are stabilized on the affected drug and the P450 substrates or inhibitors are then added to the regimen. One reason for the increased incidence of drug-drug interactions is the practice of simultaneously prescribing several potent drugs, as well as concurrently ingesting nonprescription products and herbal products that compete for, inhibit, or induce metabolizing enzymes.

Although drug-drug interactions constitute only a small proportion of adverse drug reactions, they have become an important issue in health care. Many of the drug-drug interactions can be explained by alterations in the metabolic enzymes in the liver and other extrahepatic tissues, and many of the major pharmacokinetic interactions between drugs are caused by hepatic P450 isoenzymes being affected by coadministration of other drugs. Some drugs act as potent enzyme inducers, whereas others are inhibitors. Drug-drug interactions involving enzyme inhibition, however, are much more common. Understanding these mechanisms of enzyme inhibition or induction is extremely important to appropriately administer multidrug therapies. Individuals at greatest risk for drug-drug interactions and adverse events need to be identified and treated based upon their specific pharmacogenomic-related needs.

P450s have a dominant role in the metabolism and elimination of drugs from the body, and their substrates are shown in Tables 3.3 and 3.7-3.10. Drugs in bold italics have been associated with clinically relevant drug-drug interactions. Inhibitors of P450 are shown in Table 3.11. Pharmacokinetic interactions can arise when the biotransformation and elimination of a drug are impaired by coadministered drugs. Thus, drugs can compete for biotransformation by a common P450. Adverse drug reactions, including toxicity, can occur if elimination is dependent on a P450 that exhibits defective gene variants. Thus, the genetic makeup of the individual (see section Genetic Polymorphism) has a major influence on the duration of drug action, as well as on drug efficacy and safety.

P450 pharmacogenetics affects the tendency for certain drug-drug interactions to occur. Thus, the future safe use of drug combinations in patients can require genotyping and phenotyping of individuals before the commencement of therapy. Identification of subjects who metabolize drugs in a different fashion from the general population should minimize the impact of pharmacogenetic variation on drug pharmacokinetics.

Metabolism-Based Enzyme Inhibition

Many drug-drug interactions are the result of inhibition or induction of P450 enzymes. Metabolism-based enzyme inhibition involves mostly reversible competition between two drugs for the enzyme-active site. Metabolic drug-drug interactions occur when drug A (or its metabolite) alters the pharmacokinetics of a coadministered drug B by inhibiting, activating, or inducing the activity of the enzymes that metabolize drug B. Inhibitory drug-drug interactions could result in serious adverse effects, including fatalities in patients receiving multiple medications. This process is competitive and begins with the first dose of the inhibitor, with the extent of inhibition correlating with their relative affinities for the enzymes and the metabolic half-lives of the drugs involved. On the other hand, mechanism-based (irreversible) inhibition results from a metabolite that binds irreversibly to the enzyme through a covalent bond, rendering the enzyme inactive.[36]

Enzyme-specific P450 inhibitors, including metabolism- and mechanism-based inhibitors, or drugs that are metabolized by specific P450 isoforms, are by and large excluded from further consideration for new drug development. Not only is CYP3A4 the most abundant isoform in human liver, it also metabolizes more than 30% of the drugs in clinical use, which renders CYP3A4 highly susceptible to both metabolism- (reversible) and mechanism-based inhibition. The CYP3A subfamily is involved in many clinically significant drug-drug interactions and therefore metabolism-based inhibition of CYP3A can cause clinically significant drug-drug interactions, such as those involving nonsedating antihistamines and the GI motility stimulant cisapride that can result in cardiac dysrhythmias. An excellent example of a metabolism-based inhibition drug-drug interaction that resulted in a life-threatening ventricular arrhythmia associated with QT prolongation (torsades de pointes) occurred when CYP3A4 substrates or inhibitors were coadministered with terfenadine, astemizole, cisapride, or pimozide. This potentially lethal drug interaction led to the withdrawal of terfenadine and cisapride from clinical use and to the approved marketing of fexofenadine, the active metabolite of terfenadine, which does not have this interaction.

Inhibitors of CYP3A4 can increase the risk of toxicity from many drugs, including carbamazepine, cyclosporine, ergot alkaloids, lovastatin, protease inhibitors, rifabutin, simvastatin, tacrolimus, and vinca alkaloids. Furthermore, inhibitors of CYP1A2 can increase the risk of toxicity from clozapine or theophylline. Inhibitors of CYP2C9 can increase the risk of toxicity from phenytoin, tolbutamide, and oral anticoagulants (e.g., warfarin). Inhibitors of CYP2D6 can increase risk of toxicity of many antidepressants, opioid analgesics, and psychotherapeutic agents. Examples of enzyme inducers include barbiturates, carbamazepine, glutethimide, griseofulvin, phenytoin, primidone, rifabutin, and rifampin. Some drugs, such as ritonavir, can act as either an enzyme inhibitor or an enzyme inducer, depending on the situation. Drugs metabolized by CYP3A4 or CYP2C9 are particularly susceptible to enzyme induction.

Mechanism-Based Enzyme Inhibition

Mechanism-based inhibition differs from metabolism-based (reversible) inhibition in that the inhibitors require enzymatic activation by the target enzyme prior to exerting their inhibitory effect.[36] This initial activation step leads to the formation of an active inhibitor, often referred to as the metabolite-intermediate complex (MIC). The MIC can then exert its inhibitory effect by either forming a direct covalent link with the enzyme or forming a noncovalent tight binding complex. Mechanism-based inhibition is characterized by NADPH-, time-, and concentration-dependent enzyme inactivation, occurring when some drugs are converted by P450s to reactive metabolites.[36] Mechanism-based inactivation of CYP3A4 by drugs can be the result of chemical modification of the heme, the apoprotein, or both, because of covalent binding of the modified heme to the protein. The clinical pharmacokinetic effect of a mechanism-based CYP3A4 inhibitor is a function of its enzyme kinetics (i.e., K_m and V_{max}) and the rate of synthesis of new or replacement enzyme. Predicting drug-drug interactions involving CYP3A4 inactivation is possible when pharmacokinetic principles are followed. Such prediction can become difficult, however, because the clinical outcomes of CYP3A4 inactivation depend on many factors associated with the enzyme, the drugs, and the patients.

Some of the clinically important drugs that have been identified to be mechanism-based CYP3A4 inhibitors include antibacterials (e.g., clarithromycin, erythromycin, isoniazid), anticancer drugs (e.g., irinotecan, tamoxifen, raloxifene), antidepressants (e.g., fluoxetine and paroxetine), anti-HIV agents (e.g., ritonavir and delavirdine), antihypertensives (e.g., dihydralazine and verapamil), steroids and their receptor modulators (e.g., ethinyl estradiol, gestodene, and raloxifene), dihydrotestosterone reductase inhibitors (e.g., finasteride), and some herbal constituents (e.g., bergamottin and glabridin). Drugs inactivating CYP3A4 often possess several common moieties such as a tertiary amine, furan ring, or an acetylene group. The chemical properties of a drug critical to CYP3A4 inactivation include formation of reactive metabolites by P450 isoenzymes, P450 inducers, P-gp substrates, or inhibitors and the occurrence of clinically significant pharmacokinetic interactions with coadministered drugs.

Compared to the more common metabolism-based (reversible) inhibition, mechanism-based inhibitors of CYP3A4 more frequently cause pharmacokinetic-pharmacodynamic drug-drug interactions and are often the cause for unfavorable drug-drug interactions because the inactivated CYP3A4 must be replaced by newly synthesized CYP3A4 protein.[95,96] The resultant drug interactions may lead to adverse drug effects, including some fatal events. For example, raloxifene, a drug approved for the treatment of osteoporosis and chemoprevention of breast cancer in postmenopausal women at high risk for invasive breast cancer, has demonstrated the ability to act as a mechanism-based inhibitor of CYP3A4 by forming adducts with the apoprotein. It has been established that 3′-hydroxyraloxifene is produced exclusively via CYP3A4-mediated oxygenation to produce a reactive diquinone methide, excluding the alternative arene oxide pathway.

However, predicting drug-drug interactions involving CYP3A4 inactivation is difficult, since the clinical outcomes depend on a number of factors that are associated with drugs and patients. The apparent pharmacokinetic effect of a mechanism-based inhibitor of CYP3A4 would be a function of its enzyme kinetics and the synthesis rate of new or replacement enzyme. Most CYP3A4 inhibitors are also P-gp substrates/inhibitors, confounding the in vitro to in vivo extrapolation. The clinical significance of CYP3A inhibition for drug safety and efficacy warrants an in-depth understanding of the mechanisms for each inhibitor. Furthermore, such inactivation may be exploited for therapeutic gain in certain circumstances. Clinicians should have good knowledge about these CYP3A4 inhibitors and avoid their combination.

Although CYP2D6 constitutes a relatively minor fraction of the total hepatic P450 content (Fig. 3.2), the contribution of this isoform is significant because of its role in the metabolism and clearance of many therapeutic agents that target the cardiovascular and CNS (Fig. 3.3) (Table 3.8). In addition, clinically significant polymorphisms in the CYP2D6 gene have been identified in a variety of populations with altered metabolic activity as PMs or individuals with impaired enzyme function resulting from splicing defects or gene deletions. On the other hand, EMs (individuals with normal enzyme function) are heterozygous or homozygous for the wild-type allele. In vivo clearance of CYP2D6 substrates in PMs is usually much lower than in EMs, leading to higher plasma concentrations and the potential for clinical toxicities with therapeutic doses. For example, paroxetine is a selective serotonin reuptake inhibitor that is both a substrate for and an inhibitor of CYP2D6. Paroxetine is metabolized by CYP2D6 via the formation of a carbene intermediate of the methylenedioxy group yielding an irreversible complex with CYP2D6 (Fig. 3.41).[97] Also, an in vitro study with 3,4-methylenedioxy-methamphetamine (MDMA, ecstasy) suggested that a typical recreational MDMA dose could inactivate most hepatic CYP2D6 within an hour, and the return to a basal level of CYP2D6 could take at least 10 days, impacting its pharmacokinetics.

Because of the pivotal role of P450 isoenzymes in drug metabolism, significant inactivation of these isoforms, and particularly the major human hepatic and intestinal CYP3A4 and hepatic CYP2D6, could result in drug-drug interactions and adverse drug reactions. Compared with the reversible inhibition of CYP3A4 and CYP2D6, mechanism-based inhibitors of these isoenzymes more frequently cause pharmacokinetic/pharmacodynamic drug-drug interactions, as the inactivated isoenzyme has to be replaced by newly synthesized P450 protein. Pharmacokinetic interactions often occur because of a change in drug metabolism. For example, the macrolide antibiotics increase the plasma concentrations of therapeutic agents that are substrates of CYP3A4 (Table 3.10). Diltiazem has been shown to inhibit the metabolism of a variety of coadministered drugs including carbamazepine, quinidine, midazolam, and lovastatin (Table 3.10). Inhibition of CYP3A by ritonavir explains, in part, the remarkable elevation of blood concentrations and area under the plasma concentration-time curve (AUC) of other concomitantly administered drugs that are extensively metabolized by CYP3A4 and have significant first-pass metabolism. These drugs include rifabutin (400%), clarithromycin (77%), ketoconazole, saquinavir (5000%), amprenavir (210%), nelfinavir (152%), lopinavir (7700%), and indinavir (380%).[96] Furthermore, such inactivation can be exploited for therapeutic gain in certain circumstances, e.g., extended duration of action of the protease inhibitors ritinovir/indinavir used in the treatment of AIDS.

Beneficial Drug-Drug Interactions

By understanding the unique functions and characteristics of these isoenzymes, health care practitioners can better anticipate and manage drug-drug interactions. They can also predict or explain an individual's response to a particular therapeutic regimen. A beneficial drug interaction, for example, is the coadministration of a CYP3A4 inhibitor with cyclosporine. By inhibiting CYP3A4, the plasma concentrations of cyclosporine (a CYP3A4 substrate) are increased which allows a reduction of the cyclosporine dosage thereby improving clinical efficacy and reducing its cost. Similarly, certain HIV protease inhibitors, such as saquinavir, have a low oral bioavailability due to intestinal CYP3A4 metabolism. The oral bioavailability of saquinavir can be profoundly increased by the addition of a low dose of the mechanism-based CYP3A4 inhibitor, ritonavir. This concept of altering drug pharmacokinetics by adding a low, subtherapeutic dose of a mechanism-based CYP3A4 inhibitor (ritonavir) to increase the oral bioavailability of another protease inhibitor, lopinavir (CYP3A4 substrate), led to the marketing of Kaletra, a new drug combination of lopinavir and ritonavir.

Another beneficial mechanism-based inhibition is of the P2Y12 receptor (a protein found on the surface of blood platelet cells and an important regulator in blood clotting) by the antiaggregating platelet prodrugs, clopidogrel and prasugrel. Clopidogrel is bioactivated to its reactive metabolite by CYP2C19, CYP1A2, and CYP3A4, whereas prasugrel is bioactivated by CYP3A4 and CYP2B6. The bioactivated metabolites can then react with the P2Y12 receptor protein.

Grapefruit Juice-Drug Interactions

Historical Significance of Grapefruit Juice

The discovery that grapefruit juice can markedly increase the oral bioavailability of CYP3A4 drugs was based on an unexpected observation from an interaction study between the dihydropyridine calcium channel antagonist felodipine and ethanol in which grapefruit juice was used to mask the taste of the ethanol. Subsequent investigations confirmed that grapefruit juice significantly increased the oral bioavailability of felodipine by reducing presystemic felodipine metabolism through selective inhibition of CYP3A4 expression in the intestinal wall.[98]

Grapefruit juice is a beverage often consumed at breakfast for its health benefits and to mask the taste of drugs or foods. Unlike other citrus fruit juices, however, grapefruit juice can significantly increase the oral bioavailability of drugs that are metabolized primarily by intestinal CYP3A4, causing an elevation in their serum concentrations (Table 3.20). Those drugs with high oral bioavailabilities (>60%), however, are all likely safe to be taken with grapefruit juice because their high oral bioavailability leaves little room for elevation by grapefruit juice. The importance of the interaction appears to be influenced by individual patient susceptibility, type and amount of grapefruit juice, and administration-related factors.

Grapefruit juice can alter oral drug pharmacokinetics by different mechanisms. Irreversible inactivation of intestinal CYP3A4, which can persist up to 24 hours, is produced by grapefruit juice given as a single, normal, 200- to 300-mL drink or by whole fresh fruit segments (Table 3.20). As a result, presystemic metabolism is reduced and oral drug bioavailability increased. Enhanced oral drug bioavailability can occur up to 24 hours after juice consumption, so taking CYP3A4 vulnerable drugs with water or other liquids within 24 hours of consuming grapefruit juice can still result in an interaction. Inhibition of P-gp is a possible mechanism by which grapefruit juice, and perhaps grapefruit oil, increases oral drug bioavailability by reducing intestinal and/or hepatic efflux transport. Inhibition of organic anion–transporting polypeptides by grapefruit juice and apple juice has been observed; intestinal uptake transport appeared to be decreased as oral drug bioavailability was reduced.

Numerous medications used in the prevention or treatment of coronary artery disease and its complications have been observed or predicted to interact with grapefruit juice. Such drug-drug interactions can increase the risk of rhabdomyolysis when dyslipidemia is treated with the HMG-CoA reductase inhibitors ("statins"). Such drug-drug interactions could also cause excessive vasodilatation when hypertension is managed with the dihydropyridines felodipine, nicardipine, nifedipine, nisoldipine, or nitrendipine. An alternative agent could be amlodipine. The therapeutic effect of the angiotensin II type I receptor antagonist losartan can be reduced by grapefruit juice. Grapefruit juice interacting with the antidiabetic agent repaglinide can cause hypoglycemia, and interaction with the appetite suppressant sibutramine can cause elevated blood pressure and heart rate. In angina pectoris, administration of grapefruit juice could result in atrioventricular conduction disorders with verapamil or attenuated antiplatelet activity with clopidogrel. Grapefruit juice can enhance the drug toxicity for antiarrhythmic agents, such as amiodarone, quinidine, disopyramide, or propafenone and for the congestive heart failure drug carvedilol. Some drugs used for the treatment of peripheral or central vascular disease also have the potential to interact with grapefruit juice. Interaction with sildenafil, tadalafil, or vardenafil for erectile dysfunction can cause serious systemic vasodilatation, especially when

Table 3.20 Some CYP3A4 Substrates and Interactions With Grapefruit Juice

Drug	Interaction[a]	Drug	Interaction[a]	Drug	Interaction[a]
Calcium channel blockers		**HIV protease inhibitors**		**CNS drugs**	
Amlodipine	Y	Indinavir	N?	Buspirone	Y
Felodipine	Y	Nelfinavir	N?	Carbamazepine	Y
Nifedipine	Y	Ritonavir	N?	Diazepam	Y
Nimodipine	Y	Saquinavir	Y	Midazolam	Y
Nisoldipine	Y	**Macrolides**		Triazolam	Y
Nitrendipine	Y	Clarithromycin	N	**Immunosuppressants**	
Pranidipine	Y	**HMG-CoA reductase inhibitors**		Cyclosporine	Y
Antiarrhythmics		Atorvastatin	Y	Tacrolimus	Y?
Diltiazem	N	Fluvastatin	N?	**Other**	
Verapamil	N	Lovastatin	Y	Methadone	Y
Quinidine	N	Pravastatin	N?	Sildenafil	Y
Antihistamines		Simvastatin	Y		
Ebastine	Y?				
Loratadine	Y?				

[a] Y (yes) and N (no) indicate published evidence of the presence or absence of an interaction with grapefruit juice. Y? and N? indicate expected findings based on available data. Those drugs with Y or Y? should not be consumed with grapefruit juice in an unsupervised manner.

combined with a nitrate. In stroke, interaction with nimodipine can cause systemic hypotension.

If a drug has low inherent oral bioavailability from presystemic metabolism by CYP3A4 or efflux transport by P-gp and the potential to produce serious overdose toxicity, avoidance of grapefruit juice entirely during pharmacotherapy appears mandatory. Although altered drug response is variable among individuals, the outcome is difficult to predict and avoiding the combination will guarantee that toxicity is prevented.

The mechanism by which grapefruit juice produces its effect is through inhibition of the enzymatic activity and a decrease in the intestinal expression of CYP3A4. The P-gp efflux pump also transports many CYP3A4 substrates; thus, the presence of inhibitors of P-gp in grapefruit juice (e.g., 6′,7′-dihydroxybergamottin and other furanocoumarins) could be a related factor for drug-grapefruit juice interactions.[99] Numerous studies have shown that grapefruit juice consumed in normal (single glass) quantities acts on intestinal CYP3A4, not at the hepatic level.

Does the quantity of juice matter? The majority of the presystemic CYP3A4 inhibition is obtained following ingestion of one glass of grapefruit juice; however, 24 hours after ingestion of a glass of grapefruit juice, 30% of its effect is still present.[99] The reduction in intestinal CYP3A4 concentration is rapid: a 47% decrease occurred in a healthy volunteer within 4 hours after consuming grapefruit juice. Daily ingestion of grapefruit juice results in a loss of CYP3A4 from the small intestinal epithelium. Consumption of very large quantities of grapefruit juice (six to eight glasses/day) can lead to inhibition of hepatic CYP3A4.

The active constituents found in grapefruit juice responsible for its effects on CYP3A4 include flavonoids (e.g., naringenin and naringin) and furanocoumarins (e.g., bergamottin and 6′,7′-dihydroxybergamottin).[90]

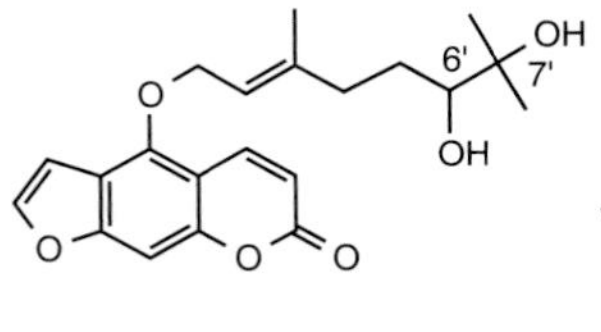

6′,7′-Dihydroxybergamottin

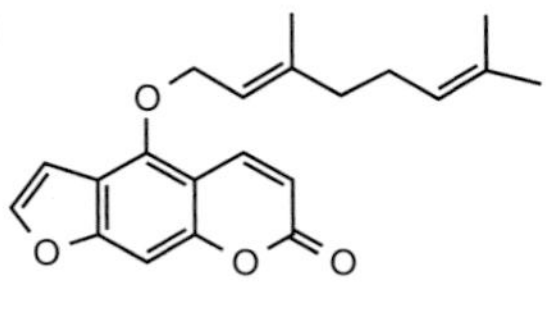

Bergamottin

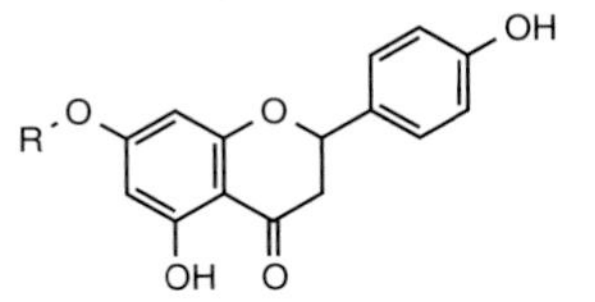

Naringin R: rhamnose-glucoside-
Naringinin R: H-

The majority of studies to date have used either freshly squeezed grapefruit juice, reconstituted frozen juice, commercial grapefruit juice, grapefruit segments, or grapefruit extract; all are capable of causing drug-drug interactions with CYP3A4 substrates (blended grapefruit juices have not yet been investigated). The active constituents in grapefruit juice are present not just in the juice but also in the pulp, peel, and core of the fruit and are responsible for its flavor. Bergamottin and 6′,7′-dihydroxybergamottin are potent mechanism-based inhibitors of CYP3A4 and naringenin isomers are competitive inhibitors of CYP3A4. Higher concentrations of 6′,7′-dihydroxybergamottin are present in grapefruit segments. Thus, any therapeutic concern for a drug interaction with grapefruit juice should now be extended to include whole fruit and other products derived from the grapefruit peel. The difference in the in vitro CYP3A4 inhibition between grapefruit juice and orange juice is that orange juice contained no measurable amounts of 6′,7′-dihydroxybergamottin. The nutraceutical grapefruit oil contains minor amounts of bergamottin, therefore grapefruit oil has the potential to cause drug ineractions with CYP3A4 substrates.

If a patient has been taking medication with grapefruit juice for some time without ill effects, is it safe to continue to do so? Much of this unpredictability results from the inconsistency of the juice concentrations and the sporadic manner in which grapefruit juice is consumed, suggesting that this approach cannot be entirely safe. Given the unpredictability of the effect of grapefruit juice on the oral bioavailability of the drugs in Table 3.20, patients should be advised to avoid this combination, thus preventing the onset of potential adverse effects. Each patient's situation should be considered, and advice should be based on consumption history and the specific medications involved. The benefits of increased and controlled drug bioavailability by grapefruit juice can, in the future, be achieved through either standardizing the constituents or coadministration of the isolated active ingredients. This would then lead to a safe, effective, and cost-saving means to enhance the absorption of many therapeutic agents.

P-Glycoprotein-Drug Interactions

P-gp–mediated transport has an important role in pharmacokinetic-mediated drug-drug interactions. The effect of P-gp inhibition is to increase the oral bioavailability of CYP3A4 substrates so that the later actions of CYP3A4 inhibition will be increased. One of the best examples is the interaction between digoxin and quinidine. Quinidine blocks P-gp in the intestinal mucosa and in the proximal renal tubule; thus, digoxin elimination into the intestine and urine is inhibited, increasing the plasma digoxin concentration to toxic levels. Another example is loperamide, which is an opioid antidiarrheal normally kept out of the brain by the P-gp pump. Inhibition of P-gp allows accumulation of loperamide in the brain, leading to respiratory depression as a result of central μ opioid receptor agonism.

The components of grapefruit juice reportedly inhibit P-gp, and this can be one of the mechanisms for the increase in bioavailability of drugs that are substrates for P-gp.

Drug-Dietary Supplement Interactions

The increasing use of dietary supplements presents a special challenge in health care; thus, there is an increasing need to predict and avoid these potential adverse drug-dietary supplement interactions.[99] The present interest and widespread use of herbal remedies has created the possibility of interaction between them and over-the-counter or prescription drugs if they are used simultaneously. As herbal medicines become more popular, herbal hepatotoxicity is being increasingly recognized. Females appear to be predisposed to hepatotoxicity, and coadministered agents that induce P450 enzymes (e.g., St. Johns wort) can also increase individual susceptibility to some dietary supplements. Nearly one in five adults taking prescription medicines is also taking at least one dietary supplement. The mechanisms for drug-dietary supplement interactions are similar to those for drug-drug interactions affecting the pharmacokinetics of the respective drug. Little is known regarding the pharmacokinetic properties of many of the substances in dietary supplements. Therefore, the potential for drug-dietary supplement interactions has greatly increased.

A commonly reported drug-dietary supplement interaction is between St. John's wort and HIV protease inhibitors, leading to drug resistance and treatment failure. St. John's wort is a popular dietary supplement often used for depression. Of the two substances found in St. John's wort, hypericin and hyperforin, hyperforin appears to be the main constituent, with in vitro selective serotonin reuptake inhibitor (SSRI) activity. Hyperforin appears also to be the more potent inducer of CYP3A enzymes based on in vitro and in vivo studies.

Other Dietary Supplements Exhibiting Drug-Induced Heptatotoxicity

DHEA and androstenedione are dietary testosterone precursors that have been associated with hepatic toxicity and should not be taken by those with hepatic disease. Co-ingestion with other potentially hepatotoxic products or enzyme inducers that might increase the risk of liver damage should also be avoided.

Black cohosh, commonly used by women for menopausal symptoms, including hot flashes and sleep disorders, forms quinone metabolites in vitro, but no mercapturate conjugates were detected in urine samples from women who consumed multiple oral doses of up to 256 mg of a standardized black cohosh extract. At moderate doses of black cohosh, the risk of liver injury is minimal.

Silybum marianum (milk thistle) is used in the treatment of chronic or acute liver disease, as well as in protecting the liver against toxicity. Silybum is cited as one of the oldest known herbal medicines. The active constituents of milk thistle are flavonolignans, which are known collectively as silymarin.

Miscellaneous Drug-Drug Interactions

The ability of drugs and other foreign substances to induce metabolism of other drugs has already been discussed. Phenobarbital, for example, stimulates metabolism of a variety of drugs (e.g., phenytoin and coumarin anticoagulants). Stimulation of bishydroxycoumarin metabolism can create a problem in patients undergoing anticoagulant therapy. If phenobarbital administration is stopped, the rate of metabolism of the anticoagulant decreases, resulting in greater plasma concentrations of bishydroxycoumarin and enhanced anticoagulant activity, increasing the possibility of hemorrhage. Serious side effects have resulted from this type of interaction. These observations indicate that combined therapy of a potent drug (e.g., bishydroxycoumarin) and an inducer of drug metabolism (e.g., phenobarbital) can create a hazardous situation if the enzyme inducer is withdrawn and therapy with the potent drug is continued without an appropriate decrease in dose.

Serious reactions have been reported in patients treated with an MAO inhibitor such as tranylcypromine because they are, as a rule, sensitive to a subsequent dose of a sympathomimetic amine (e.g., amphetamine) or a tricyclic antidepressant (e.g., amitriptyline), which is metabolized by MAO.

Allopurinol, a xanthine oxidase inhibitor used for the treatment of gout, inhibits metabolism of 6-mercaptopurine and other drugs metabolized by this enzyme. A serious drug interaction results from the concurrent use of allopurinol for gout and 6-mercaptopurine to block the immune response from a tissue transplant or as antimetabolite in neoplastic diseases.

Gender Differences in Drug Metabolism

Although numerous gender differences have been described in humans, so far most clinical research has been carried out with the questionable view that the male can fulfill the function of the true representative of the human species. However, in spite of the increasing evidence pointing out physiological and pathological differences between the sexes, beyond those related to reproduction, women differ from men in gene expression and regulation, in the susceptibility to and risk for many medical conditions, and in the response to numerous drugs.[100,101] Gender difference in drug response may explain, at least in part, the interindividual variations occurring in therapeutic response and toxicity, especially considering that female sex has been shown to be a risk factor for the development of adverse drug reactions (ADRs). Nonetheless, current studies indicate that gender differences in pharmacological response are more widespread than originally believed and involve pharmacodynamics and pharmacokinetics, with pharmacokinetic being the most investigated.

The role of pharmacokinetics versus pharmacodynamics is not yet completely appreciated, and only a few contributions have evaluated the impact of genetics, hormonal variations, and their relative interactions.[100] The role of gender as a contributor to variability in xenobiotic metabolism and IDRs, which are more common in women than in men, is not clear, but increasing numbers of reports show differences in metabolism between men and women, raising the intriguing possibility that endogenous sex hormones, hydrocortisone, or their synthetic equivalents can influence the activity of inducible

CYP3A. N-demethylation of erythromycin was significantly higher in females than males, which was persistent throughout adulthood. In contrast, males exhibited unchanged N-demethylation values.

Gender-dependent differences of metabolic rates have been detected for some drugs. Side-chain oxidation of propranolol was 50% faster in males than in females, but no differences between genders were noted in aromatic ring hydroxylation. N-demethylation of meperidine was depressed during pregnancy and for women taking oral contraceptives. CYP1A2 shows a higher activity in men, and therefore, clearance of antidepressant, antipsychotic drugs, and theophylline is faster in men than in women. CYP1A2 activity is decreased during pregnancy. Other examples of drugs cleared by CYP3A4 more rapidly in men than in women include chlordiazepoxide and lidocaine. Diazepam, prednisolone, caffeine, and acetaminophen are metabolized slightly faster by women than by men. No gender differences have been observed in the clearance of phenytoin, nitrazepam, and trazodone, which interestingly are not substrates for the CYP3A subfamily. CYP3A4 activity is higher in women than in men. Drugs such as cyclosporine, erythromycin, nimodipine, and cortisol are substrates of CYP3A4, showing faster clearance among women. Although CYP3A4 is also responsible for about 60% of CYP-mediated metabolism of zolpidem, its overall clearance is actually slower in women than in men, requiring a FDA-recommended 50% dose reduction. Gender differences in the rate of glucuronidation have been noted. Men show a faster clearance of drugs that are primarily eliminated by glucuronidation. Thus, oxazepam, metabolized mainly by UGT2B15, has a longer half-life in women than in men. Gender differences are also found in other pharmacokinetic parameters such as drug absorption, drug distribution, and excretion.

Historically, women were less enrolled in clinical trials because both the pharmacokinetics and pharmacodynamics of a drug can be influenced by menstrual cycle phases, hormonal fluctuations, use of oral contraceptives, and hormonal therapy. There was also concern about life events such as pregnancy and lactation, including the potential negative impact of investigational drugs on the fetus or nursing neonate.[100] The number of trials enrolling women has increased after an FDA request to include a fair representation of both genders as participants, but overall, women are still underrepresented. Women are generally treated with doses that essentially reflect the results obtained by trials carried out mainly in men.

Despite the differences in drug pharmacokinetics between men and women, sex-specific recommendations in dosage do not exist for most drugs.[101] Pharmacists need to recognize the underrepresentation of women in clinical trials and take the responsibility to inform consumers and emphasize to clinicians that women can differ significantly from men with respect to metabolism, absorption, distribution, and excretion of drugs. Pharmacists also need to be aware that pregnancy, oral contraceptive use, and hormonal replacement therapy can significantly change drug metabolism and drug clearance. If a woman consistently experiences more adverse drug events or less therapeutic effect from a particular drug, it may be necessary to discuss with her physician the possibility of changing the dosing regimen or switching to a different medication. Even in postmenopausal women, CYP3A function can be altered and influenced by the lack of estrogen or the presence of androgens.

Compared to men, there are more women in the population, more women with chronic diseases, and more women visiting physicians. It is, therefore, obvious that there needs to be more interest in knowing how women react to drugs. Ultimately, a better understanding of sex-related influences on drug responses will help to improve drug safety and efficacy and will also permit to practitioners to "tailor" pharmacological treatments both in men and women.

MAJOR PATHWAYS OF METABOLISM

Table 3.21 contains an extensive list of commonly used drugs and the P450 isoforms that catalyze their metabolism. In addition, Phase 1 and Phase 2 metabolic pathways for some common drugs are listed in Table 3.21.

Table 3.21 Metabolic Pathways of Common Drugs

Drug	Pathway	Drug	Pathway
Amphetamines [structure: CH_3, α, NHR, β, phenyl]	Deamination (followed by oxidation and reduction of the ketone formed) N-oxidation N-dealkylation Hydroxylation of the aromatic ring Hydroxylation of the β-carbon atom Conjugation with glucuronic acid of the acid and alcohol products from the ketone formed by deamination	Barbiturates [structure: R_5, R_5', O, 6, 5, 4, O, R_1N, 2, NR_3, 1, 3, O]	Oxidation and complete removal of substituents at carbon 5 N-dealkylation at N1 and N3 Desulfuration at carbon 2 (thiobarbiturates) Scission of the barbiturate ring at the 1:6 bond to give substituted malonylureas

(continued)

Table 3.21 Metabolic Pathways of Common Drugs (Continued)

Drug	Pathway	Drug	Pathway
Phenothiazines 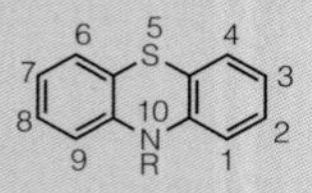	N-dealkylation in the N10 side chain N-oxidation in the N10 side chain Oxidation of the heterocyclic S atom to sulfoxide or sulfone Hydroxylation of one or both aromatic rings Conjugation of phenolic metabolites with glucuronic acid or sulfate Scission of the N10 side chain	Sulfonamides 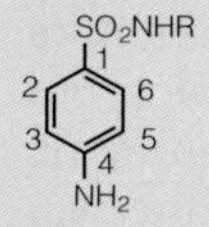	Acetylation at the N4 amino group Conjugation with glucuronic acid or sulfate at the N4 amino group Acetylation or conjugation with glucuronic acid at the N1 amino group Hydroxylation and conjugation in the heterocyclic ring, R
Phenytoin 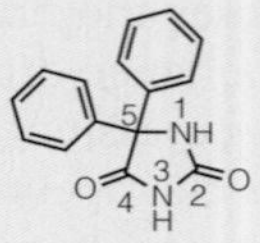	Hydroxylation of one aromatic ring Conjugation of phenolic products with glucuronic acid or sulfate Hydrolytic scission of the hydantoin ring at the bond between carbons 3 and 4 to give 5,5-diphenylhydantoic acid	Meperidine 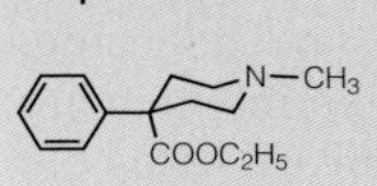	Hydrolysis of ester to acid N-dealkylation Hydroxylation of aromatic ring N-oxidation Both N-dealkylation and hydrolysis Conjugation of phenolic products
Pentazocine 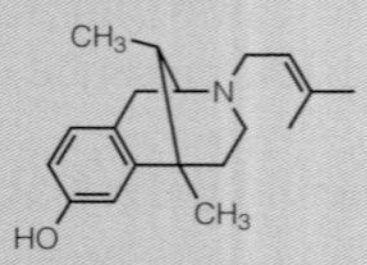	Hydroxylation of terminal methyl groups of the alkenyl side chain to give *cis* and *trans* (major) alcohols Oxidation of hydroxymethyl product of the alkenyl side chain to carboxylic acids Reduction of alkenyl side chain and oxidation of terminal methyl group	Cocaine 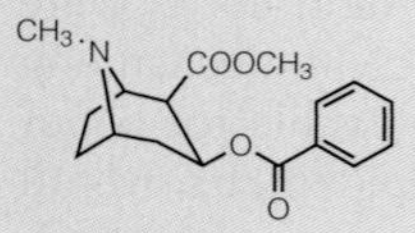	Hydrolysis of methyl ester Hydrolysis of benzoate ester N-dealkylation Both hydrolysis and N-dealkylation
Phenmetrazine 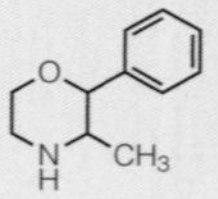	Oxidation to lactam Aromatic hydroxylation N-oxidation Conjugation of phenolic products	Ephedrine 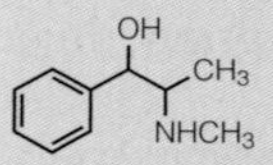	N-dealkylation Oxidative deamination Oxidation of deaminated product to benzoic acid Reduction of deaminated product to 1,2-diol
Propranolol 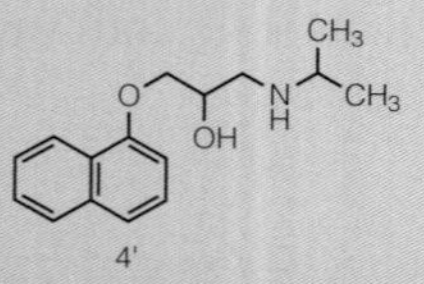	Aromatic hydroxylation at C4′ N-dealkylation Oxidative deamination Oxidation of deaminated product to naphthoxylactic acid Conjugation with glucuronic acid O-dealkylation	Indomethacin 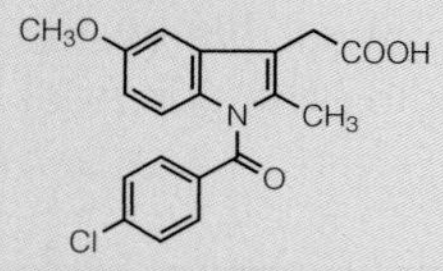	O-demethylation N-deacylation of p-chlorobenzoyl group Both O-dealkylation and N-deacylation Conjugation of phenolic products with glucuronic acid Other conjugation products
Diphenoxylate 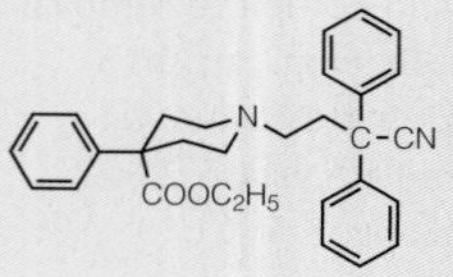	Hydrolysis of ester to acid Hydroxylation of one aromatic ring attached to the N-alkyl side chain	Diazepam 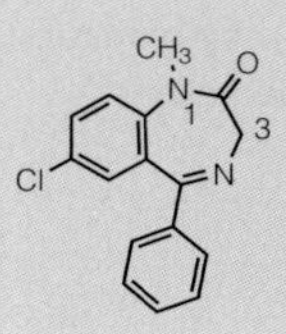	N-dealkylation at N1 Hydroxylation at carbon 3 Conjugation with glucuronic acid Both N-dealkylation of N1 and hydroxylation at carbon 3

Table 3.21 Metabolic Pathways of Common Drugs (Continued)

Drug	Pathway	Drug	Pathway
Prostaglandins 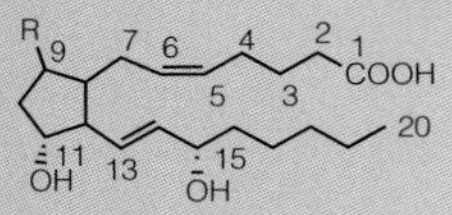	Reduction of double bonds at carbons 5 and 6 and 13 and 14 Oxidation of 15-hydroxyl to ketone β-Oxidation of carbons 3, 5 and 7 ω-Oxidation of carbon 20 to acid	Cyproheptadine 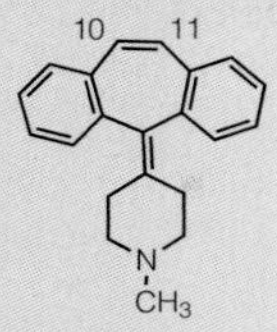	N-dealkylation 10,11-Epoxide formation Both N-dealkylation and 10,11-epoxidation
Hydralazine 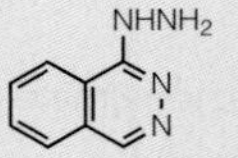	N-acetylation with cyclization to a methyl-S-triazolophthalazine N-formylation with cyclization to an S-triazolo- phthalazine Aromatic hydroxylation of benzene ring Oxidative loss of hydrazinyl group to 1-hydroxy Hydroxylation of methyl of methyl-S-triazolophthalazine Conjugation with glucuronic acid	Methadone 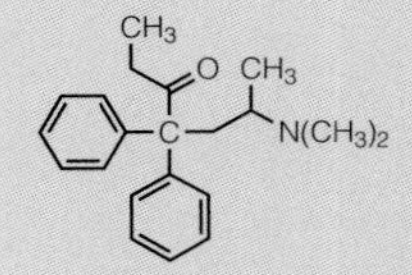	Reduction of ketone to hydroxyl Aromatic hydroxylation of one aromatic ring N-dealkylation of alcohol product N-dealkylation with cyclization to pyrrolidine
Lidocaine 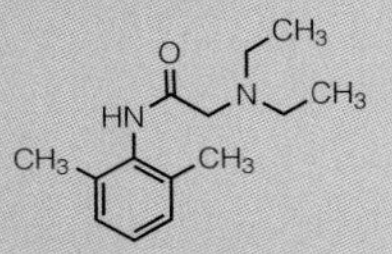	N-dealkylation Oxidative cyclization to a 4-imidazolidone N-oxidation of amide N Aromatic hydroxylation ortho to methyl Hydrolysis of amide	Imipramine 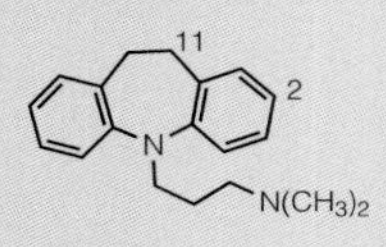	N-dealkylation Hydroxylation at C11 Aromatic hydroxylation (C2) N-oxidation Both N-dealkylation and hydroxylation
Cimetidine 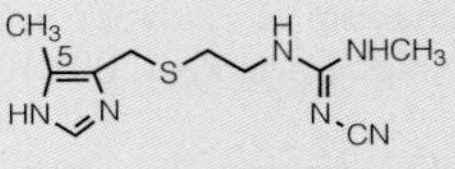 2	S-oxidation Hydroxylation of 5-methyl	Valproic acid 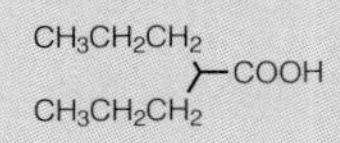	CoA thioester Dehydrogenation to (E) 2-ene Dehydrogenation to (E) 2,4-diene Dehydrogenation to 4-ene 3-Hydroxylation
Piroxicam 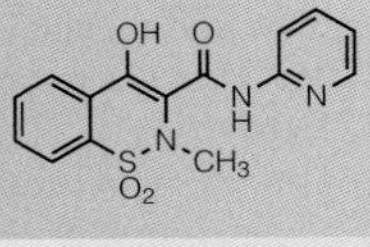 4	Pyridine 3′-hydroxylation Hydrolysis of amide Decarboxylation	Caffeine 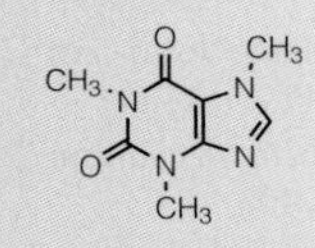	N3-demethylation N1-demethylation N7-demethylation to theophylline C8 oxidation to uric acids Imidazole ring opened
Theophylline 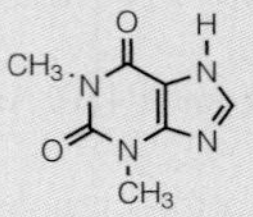	N3-demethylation N1-demethylation C8 oxidation to uric acids Imidazole ring opened 1-Me xanthine to 1-Me uric acid—xanthine oxidase	Nicotine 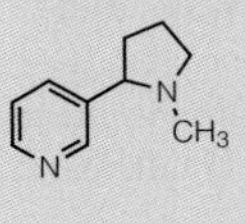	Pyrrolidine 5′-hydroxylation to cotinine Pyrrolidine N-oxidation (FMO) N-demethylation (nornicotine and norcotinine) Pyridine N-methylation 3′-Hydroxylation of cotinine
Ibuprofen 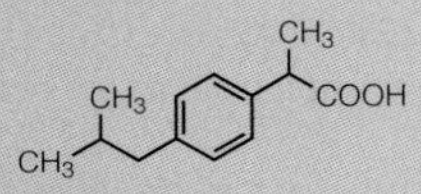 8	CoA thioester and epimerization of R- to S+ enantiomer Methyl hydroxylation to CH_2OH CH_2OH to COOH Acylglucuronide	Tamoxifen 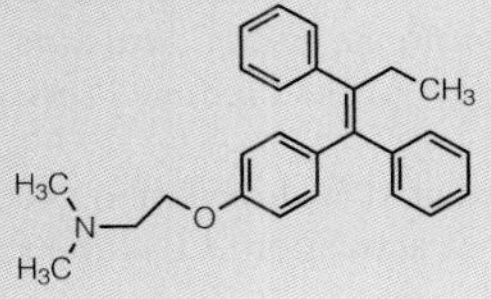	N-demethylation 4′-Hydroxylation N-oxidation (FMO) 4′-O-sulfate 4′-O-glucuronide

(continued)

Table 3.21 Metabolic Pathways of Common Drugs (Continued)

Drug	Pathway	Drug	Pathway
Lovastatin 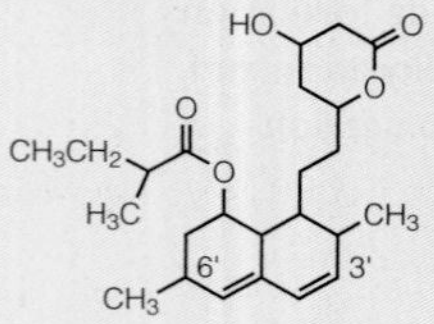	6′-Hydroxylation 3′-Side chain hydroxylation 3′-Hydroxylation β-oxidation of lactone O-glucuronides	Ciprofloxacin 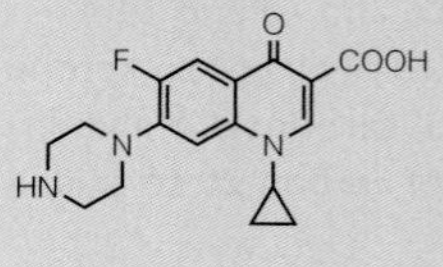	Piperazine 3′-hydroxylation N-sulfonation
Labetalol 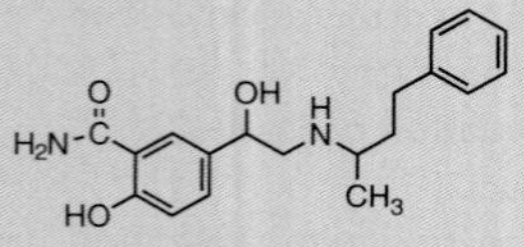	O-sulfate (major) O-glucuronide	Acetaminophen 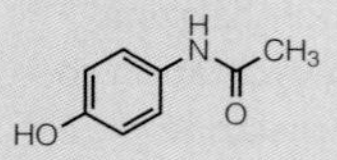	O-glucuronide O-sulfate Oxidation to N-acetyl-p-benzoquinoneimine Conjugation of N-acetyl-*p*-benzoquinoneimine with glutathione
Tripelennamine 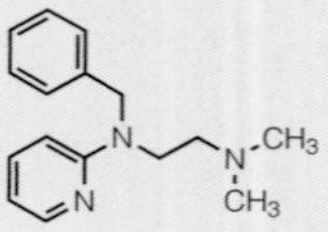	*p*-Hydroxylation Benzylic C-hydroxylation N-depyridinylation N-debenzylation	Felodipine 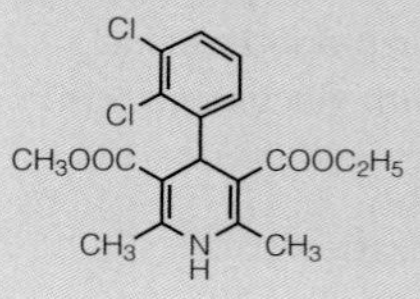	Aromatization Ester hydrolysis Methyl hydroxylation

REFERENCES

1. Williams RT. *Detoxication Mechanisms*. 2nd ed. New York: John Wiley and Sons; 1959.
2. Anders M, ed. *Bioactivation of Foreign Compounds*. New York: Academic Press; 1983.
3. Jakoby W, ed. *Enzymatic Basis of Detoxication*. Vols. I and II. New York: Academic Press; 1980.
4. Jakoby W, Bend JR, Caldwell J, eds. *Metabolic Basis of Detoxication—Metabolism of Functional Groups*. New York: Academic Press; 1982.
5. Mulder GJ, ed. *Conjugation Reactions in Drug Metabolism: An Integrated Approach*. London: Taylor and Francis; 1990.
6. Ortiz de Montellano PR, ed. *Cytochrome P450: Structure Mechanism and Biochemistry*. 2nd ed. New York: Plenum Press; 1993.
7. Testa B, Krämer SD. *The Biochemistry of Drug Metabolism Volume 1: Principles, Redox Reactions, Hydrolyses and Volume 2: Conjugations, Consequences of Metabolism, Influencing Factors*. New York: Wiley-VCH; 2003.
8. Rodrigues A. *Drug-drug interactions. Drugs and the Pharmaceutical Sciences*. Vol. 179, 2nd ed. New York: Informa Healthcare; 2008.
9. Pearson PG, Wienkers LC. *Handbook of drug metabolism. Drugs and the Pharmaceutical Sciences*. Vol. 186, 2nd ed. New York: Informa Healthcare; 2008.
10. Groves JT. Models and mechanisms of cytochrome P450. In: Ortiz de Montellano PR, ed. *Cytochrome P450: Structure Mechanism and Biochemistry*. 3rd ed. New York: Plenum Press; 2005:1-44.
11. Huang X, Groves JT. Beyond ferryl-mediated hydroxylation: 40 years of the rebound mechanism and C-H activation. *J Biol Inorg Chem*. 2017;22:185-207.
12. Nebert DW, Nelson DR, Coon MJ, et al. The P450 superfamily: update on new sequences, gene mapping and recommended nomenclature. *DNA Cell Biol*. 1991;10:1-14.
13. Gonzalez FJ, Gelboin HV. Human cytochromes P450: evolution and cDNA-directed expression. *Environ Health Perspect*. 1992;98:810-883.
14. Rendic S, DiCarlo FJ. Human cytochrome P450 enzymes: a status report summarizing their reactions substrates inducers and inhibitors. *Drug Metab*. 1997;29:413-580.
15. Guengerich FP. Enzymatic oxidation of xenobiotic chemicals. *Crit Rev Biochem Mol Biol*. 1990;25:97-153.
16. Meunier B, de Visser SP, Shaik S. Mechanism of oxidation reactions catalyzed by cytochrome P450 enzymes. *Chem Rev*. 2004;104:3947-3980.
17. Guengerich FP. Human cytochrome P450 enzymes. In: Ortiz de Montellano PR, ed. *Cytochrome P450: Structure Mechanism and Biochemistry*. 3rd ed. New York: Plenum Press; 2005:377-530.
18. Traber PG, McDonnell WM, Wang R. Expression and regulation of cytochrome P450I genes (CYP1A1 and CYP1A2) in the rat alimentary tract. *Biochim Biophys Acta*. 1992;1171:167-173.
19. Koop DR. Oxidative and reductive metabolism of cytochrome P4502E1. *FASEB J*. 1992;6:724-730.
20. Raucy JL, Kraner JC, Lasker JM. Bioactivation of halogenated hydrocarbons by cytochrome P4502E1. *Crit Rev Toxicol*. 1993;23:1-20.
21. White RE, Coon MJ. Oxygen activation by cytochrome P450. *Ann Rev Biochem*. 1980;49:315-356.
22. Makris TM, Denisov L, Schlichting L, et al. Activation of molecular oxygen by cytochrome P450 enzymes. In: Ortiz de Montellano PR, ed. *Cytochrome P450: Structure Mechanism and Biochemistry*. 3rd ed. New York: Plenum Press; 2005:149-182.
23. Groves JT. Key elements of the chemistry of cytochrome P450. The oxygen rebound mechanism. *J Chem Educ*. 1985;62:928-931.
24. Groves JT. Enzymatic C-H bond activation: using push to get pull. *Nat Chem*. 2014;6(2):89-91.
25. Ortiz de Montellano PR, DeVoss JJ. Substrate oxidation by cytochrome P450 enzymes. In: Ortiz de Montellano PR, ed. *Cytochrome P450: Structure Mechanism and Biochemistry*. 3rd ed. New York: Plenum Press; 2005:193-198.
26. Guengerich FP, MacDonald TL. Mechanisms of cytochrome P450 catalysis. *FASEB J*. 1990;4:2453-2459.
27. Ortiz de Montellano PR. Cytochrome P-450 catalysis: radical intermediates and dehydrogenation reactions. *Trends Pharmacol Sci*. 1989;10:354-359.

28. Ballie TA. Metabolism of valproate to hepatotoxic intermediates. *Pharm Weekbl [Sci]*. 1992;14:122-123.
29. Ortiz de Montellano PR. Alkenes and alkynes. In: Anders M, ed. *Bioactivation of Foreign Compounds*. New York: Academic Press; 1985, 121-153.
30. Guengerich FP. Metabolic activation of carcinogens. *Pharmacol Ther*. 1992;54:17-61.
31. Thummel KE, Kharasch ED, Podoll, et al. Human liver microsomal enflurane defluorination catalyzed by cytochrome P-450 2E1. *Drug Metab Dispos*. 1993;21:350-356.
32. Kharasch ED, Hankins DC, Thummel KE. Human kidney methoxyflurane and sevoflurane metabolism. Intrarenal fluoride production as a possible mechanism of methoxyflurane nephrotoxicity. *Anesthesiology*. 1995;82:689-699.
33. Williams SN, Dunkan E, Bradfield CA. Induction of cytochrome P450 enzymes. In: Ortiz de Montellano PR, ed. *Cytochrome P450: Structure Mechanism and Biochemistry*. 3rd ed. New York: Plenum Press; 2005:323-346.
34. Okey AB. Enzyme induction in the cytochrome P450 system. *Pharmacol Ther*. 1990;45:241-298.
35. Barry M, Feely J. Enzyme induction and inhibition. *Pharmacol Ther*. 1992;48:71-94.
36. Correia MA, Ortiz de Montellano PR. Inhibition of cytochrome P450 enzymes. In: Ortiz de Montellano PR, ed. *Cytochrome P450: Structure Mechanism and Biochemistry*. 3rd ed. New York: Plenum Press; 2005:247-322.
37. Martucci CP, Fishman J. P450 enzymes of estrogen metabolism. *Pharmacol Ther*. 1993;57:237-257.
38. Murray M, Reidy GF. Selectivity in the inhibition of mammalian cytochromes P-450 by chemical agents. *Pharmacol Rev*. 1990;42:85-101.
39. Murray M. P450 enzymes. *Clin Pharmacokinet*. 1992;23:132-146.
40. Zeigler DM. Flavin-containing monooxygenases. *Drug Metab Rev*. 1988;19:1-32.
41. Zeigler DM. Flavin-containing monooxygenases: enzymes adapted for multisubstrate specificity. *Trends Pharmacol Sci*. 1990;11:321-324.
42. Krueger SK, Williams DE. Mammalian flavin-containing monooxygenases: structure/function, genetic polymorphisms and role in drug metabolism. *Pharmacol Thera*. 2005;106:357-387.
43. Cashman JR, Wang Z, Yang L, et al. Stereo- and regioselective N- and S-oxidation of tertiary amines and sulfides in the presence of adult liver microsomes. *Drug Metab Dispos*. 1993;21:492-501.
44. Hollenberg PF. Mechanism of cytochrome P450 and peroxide-catalyzed xenobiotic metabolism. *FASEB J*. 1992;6:686-694.
45. Marnett LJ, Kenned TY. Comparison of the peroxidase activity of hemeproteins and Cytochrome P450. In: Ortiz de Montellano PR, ed. *Cytochrome P450: Structure Mechanism and Biochemistry*. 3rd ed. New York: Plenum Press; 2005:49-80.
46. Hille R. Molybdenum enzymes. *Essays Biochem*. 1999;34:125-137.
47. Kitamura S, Sugihara K, Ohta S. Drug-metabolizing ability of molybdenum hydroxylases. *Drug Metab Pharmacokinetics*. 2006;21:83-98.
48. Lang D, Kalgutkar AS. Non-P450 mediated oxidative metabolism of xenobiotics. In: Lee JS, Obach RS, Fisher MB, eds. *Drug Metabolizing Enzymes: Cytochrome P450 and Other Enzymes in Drug Discovery and Development*. New York: FontisMedia-Marcel Dekker; 2003:483-539.
49. Singer TP, Ramsay RR. Mechanism of neurotoxicity of MPTP. *FEBS Lett*. 1990;274:1-8.
50. Malatkova P, Wsol V. Carbonyl reduction pathways in drug metabolism. *Drug Metab Rev*. 2014;46:96-123.
51. Burchell B, Mcgurk K, Brierly CH, et al. UDP-glucuronosyltransferases. In: Guengerich FP, ed. *Comprehensive Toxicology*. Vol. 3. New York: Pergamon–Elsevier Science; 1997:449-473.
52. Spahn-Langguth H, Benet LZ. Acylglucuronides revisited: is the glucuronidation process a toxification as well as a detoxication mechanism. *Drug Metab Rev*. 1992;24:5-48.
53. Mulder GJ. Pharmacological effects of drug conjugates: is morphine 6-glucuronide an exception. *Trends Pharmacol Sci*. 1992;13:302-304.
54. Nelson SD. Arylamines and arylamide: oxidation mechanisms. In: Anders M, ed. *Bioactivation of Foreign Compounds*. New York: Academic Press; 1985:349-373.
55. Falani CN. Enzymology of human cytosolic sulfotransferases. *FASEB J*. 1997;11:206-216.
56. Lindsay J, Wang LL, Li Y, Zhou SF. Structure, function and polymorphism of human cytosolic sulfotransferases. *Curr Drug Metab*. 2008;9:99-103.
57. Skonberg C, Olsen J, Madsen KG, Hansen SH, Grillo MP. Metabolic activation of carboxylic acids. *Expert Opin Drug Metab Toxicol*. 2008;4:425-438.
58. Mannervik B, Danielson UH, Ketterer B. Glutathione transferases—structure and catalytic activity. *Crit Rev Biochem*. 1988;23:283-337.
59. Liu Y, Hyde AS, Simpson MH, Barycki JJ. Emerging regulatory paradigms in glutathione metabolism. *Adv Cancer Res*. 2014;122:69-101.
60. Dobrinska MR. Enterohepatic circulation of drugs. *J Clin Pharmacol*. 1989;29:577-580.
61. Ilett KF, Tee LBG, Reeves PT, et al. Metabolism of drugs and other xenobiotics in the gut lumen and wall. *Pharmacol Ther*. 1990;46:67-93.
62. Schmucker DL. Aging and drug disposition: an update. *Pharmacol Rev*. 1985;37:133-143.
63. Durnas C, Loi CM, Cusack BJ. Hepatic drug metabolism and aging. *Clin Pharmacokinet*. 1990;19:359-389.
64. Woodhouse K, Wynne HA. Age-related changes in hepatic function: implications for drug therapy. *Drugs Aging*. 1992;2:243-246.
65. Smit JW, Huisman MT, van Tellingen O, et al. Absence or pharmacological blocking of placental P-glycoprotein profoundly increases fetal drug exposure. *J Clin Invest*. 1999;104:1441-1447.
66. Ingelmann-Sundberg M, Oscarson M, McLellan RA. Polymorphic human cytochrome P450 enzymes: an opportunity for individualized drug treatment. *Trends Pharmacol Sci*. 1999;20:342-349.
67. Zhou SF. Polymorphism of human cytochrome P450 2D6 and its clinical significance: Part I. *Clin Pharmacokinet*. 2009;48:689-723.
68. Ingelman-Sundberg M. Genetic polymorphisms of cytochrome P450 2D6 (CYP2D6): clinical consequences, evolutionary aspects and functional diversity. *Pharmacogenomics J*. 2005;5:6-13.
69. Di YM, Chow VD, Yang LP, Zhou SF. Structure, function, regulation and polymorphism of human cytochrome CYP2A6. *Curr Drug Metab*. 2009;10:754-780.
70. Mo SL, Liu YH, Duan W, et al. Substrate specificity, regulation, and polymorphism of human cytochrome CYP2B6. *Curr Drug Metab*. 2009;10:730-753.
71. Zhou SF, Zhou ZW, Huang M. Polymorphisms of human cytochrome CYP2C9 and the functional relevance. *Toxicology*. 2010;278:165-188.
72. Kaminsky LS, Fasco MJ. Small intestinal cytochromes P450. *Crit Rev Toxicol*. 1991;21:407-422.
73. Kane GC, Lipsky JJ. Drug–grapefruit juice interactions. *Mayo Clin Proc*. 2000;75:933-942.
74. Sarkar MA. Drug metabolism in the nasal mucosa. *Pharmacol Res*. 1992;9:1-8.
75. Miksys S, Tyndale RF. Cytochrome P450–mediated drug metabolism in the brain. *J Psychiatry Neurosci*. 2013;38:152-163.
76. McMillan DM, Tyndale RF. CYP-mediated drug metabolism in the brain impacts drug response. *Pharmacol Ther*. 2018;184:189-200.
77. Toselli F, Dodd PR, Gillam E. Emerging roles for brain drug-metabolizing cytochrome P450 enzymes in neuropsychiatric conditions and responses to drugs. *Drug Metabol Rev*. 2013;48(3):379-404.
78. Watkins PB. Role of cytochrome P450 in drug metabolism and hepatotoxicity. *Semin Liver Dis*. 1990;10:235-250.

79. Watkins PB, Kaplowitz N, Slattery JT, et al. Aminotransferase elevations in healthy adults receiving 4 grams of acetaminophen daily. *JAMA*. 2006;296:87-93.
80. Park BK, Kitteringham NR, Maggs JL, et al. The role of metabolic activation in drug-induced hepatotoxicity. *Annu Rev Pharmacol Toxicol*. 2005;45:177-202.
81. Williams DP, Kitteringham NR, Naisbitt DJ, et al. Are chemically reactive metabolites responsible for adverse reactions to drugs? *Curr Drug Metab*. 2002;3:351-366.
82. Navarro VJ, Senior JR. Drug-related hepatotoxicity. *N Engl J Med*. 2006;354:731-739.
83. Ju C, Uetrecht JP. Mechanism of idiosyncratic drug reactions: reactive metabolite formation, protein binding and the regulation of the immune system. *Curr Drug Metab*. 2002;3:367-377.
84. Hussaini SH, Farrington EA. Idiosyncratic drug-induced liver injury: an overview. *Expert Opin Rug Saf*. 2007;6:673-684.
85. Myers TG, Dietz EC, Anderson N, et al. A comparative study of mouse liver proteins arylated by reactive metabolites of acetaminophen and its nonhepatotoxic regioisomer, 3'-hydroxyacetanilide. *Chem Res Toxicol*. 1995;8:403-413.
86. Miller EC, Miller JA. Mechanisms of chemical carcinogenesis. *Cancer*. 1981;47:1055-1064.
87. Gillette JR. The problem of chemically reactive metabolites. *Drug Metab Rev*. 1982;13:941-961.
88. Kalgutkar AS, Gardner I, Obach RS, et al. A comprehensive listing of bioactivation pathways of organic functional groups. *Curr Drug Metab*. 2005;6:161-223.
89. Oesch F. Metabolic transformation of clinically used drugs to epoxides: new perspectives in drug–drug interactions. *Biochem Pharmacol*. 1976;25:1935-1937.
90. Reed DJ. Cellular defense mechanisms against reactive metabolites. In: Anders M, ed. *Bioactivation of Foreign Compounds*. New York: Academic Press; 1985:71-108.
91. Nelson SD, et al. Role of metabolic activation in chemical-induced tissue injury. In: Jerina DM, ed. *Drug Metabolism Concepts. ACS Symposium Series 44*. Washington, DC: American Chemical Society; 1977:155-183.
92. Uetrecht J. Bioactivation. In: Lee JS, Obach RS, Fisher M, eds. *Drug-metabolizing Enzymes: Cytochrome P450 and Other Enzymes in Drug Discovery and Development*. Weimar, TX: Culinary and Hospitality Industry Publications Services; 2003:87-143.
93. Boelsterli UA. Xenobiotic acyl glucuronides and acyl CoA thioesters as protein-reactive metabolites with the potential to cause idiosyncratic drug reactions. *Curr Drug Metab*. 2002;3:439-450.
94. Zhou S, Yung Chan S, Cher Goh B, et al. Mechanism-based inhibition of cytochrome CYP3A4 by therapeutic drugs. *Clin Pharmacokinet*. 2005;44:279-304.
95. Dressor GK, Spence JD, Bailey DG. Pharmacokinetic–pharmacodynamic consequences and clinical relevance of cytochrome CYP3A4 inhibition. *Clin Pharmacokinet*. 2000;38:41-57.
96. Murray M. Mechanisms of inhibitory and regulatory effects of methylenedioxyphenyl compounds on cytochrome P450-dependent drug oxidation. *Curr Drug Metab*. 2000;1:67-84.
97. Bailey DG, Dresser GK, Kreeft JH, et al. Grapefruit–felodipine interaction: effect of unprocessed fruit and probable active ingredients. *Clin Pharmacol Ther*. 2000;68:468-477.
98. Evans AM. Influence of dietary components on the gastrointestinal metabolism and transport of drugs. *Ther Drug Monit*. 2000;22:131-136.
99. Franconi F, Brunelleschi S, Steardo L, Cuomo V. Gender differences in drug responses. *Pharmacol Res*. 2007;55:81-95.
100. Chu T. Gender differences in pharmacokinetics. *US Pharm*. 2014;39:40-43.
101. Soldin OP, Mattison DR. Sex differences in pharmacokinetics and pharmacodynamics. *Clin Pharmacokinet*. 2009;48:143-157.

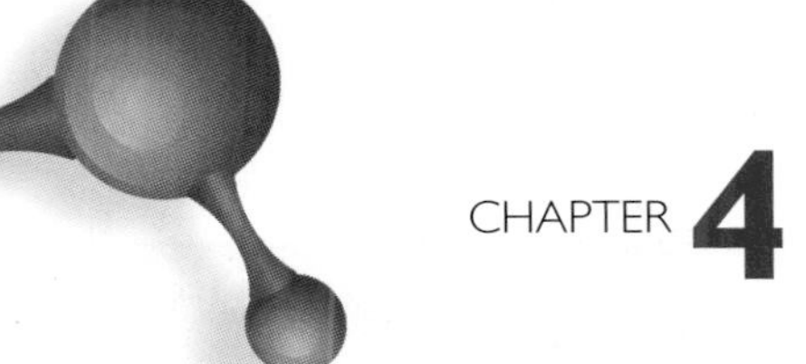

CHAPTER **4**

Membrane Drug Transporters

Marilyn E. Morris and Bridget L. Morse

Drugs covered in this chapter:

- Acyclovir
- Adefovir
- Atorvastatin
- Cerivastatin
- Cidofovir
- Cisplatin
- Cyclosporine
- Dabigatran
- Digoxin
- Dofetilide
- Doxorubicin
- Erythromycin
- Fexofenadine
- Furosemide
- Gabapentin
- Gabapentin enacarbil
- Gemfibrozil
- Lamivudine
- Metformin
- Methotrexate
- Morphine
- Mycophenolate mofetil
- Nitrofurantoin
- Olmesartan
- Oxaliplatin
- Paclitaxel
- Penicillin
- Pravastatin
- Probenecid
- Repaglinide
- Rifampin
- Rosuvastatin
- Simvastatin
- Sumatriptan
- Tenofovir
- Topotecan
- Valacyclovir
- Valsartan
- Verapamil

Abbreviations

ABC ATP-binding cassette
ACE angiotensin-converting enzyme
ATP adenosine triphosphate
AUC area under the curve
BBB blood-brain barrier
BCRP breast cancer resistance protein
BSEP bile salt export pump
CNT concentrative nucleoside transporter
ENT equilibrative nucleoside transporter
FXR farnesoid X receptor
GI gastrointestinal
GHB γ-hydroxybutyrate
HMG-CoA 3-hydroxy-3-methyl-glutaryl-coenzyme A
LAT l-type amino acid transporter
MATE multidrug and toxin extrusion protein
MCT monocarboxylate transporter
MDR multidrug resistance
MRP multidrug resistance–associated protein
OAT organic anion transporter
OATP organic anion transporting polypeptide
OCT organic cation transporter
OCTN organic cation/carnitine transporter
P-gp P-glycoprotein
PEPT peptide transporter
PHT peptide/histidine transporter
PXR pregnane X receptor
SLC solute carrier
SMCT sodium-coupled monocarboxylate transporter
SNP single nucleotide polymorphism

INTRODUCTION

THE OBJECTIVES OF THE CHAPTER ARE:

- Emphasize the significance of transport in pharmacokinetics and pharmacodynamics
- Provide an overview of transport mechanisms and classification of drug transporters
- Summarize transporters relevant to drug disposition and their drug substrates
- Provide evidence and mechanisms for transport interactions clinically relevant in therapeutics
- Provide an understanding of mechanisms underlying interindividual variability in the pharmacokinetics of drug transporter substrates

Transporters have fundamental roles in cell homeostasis and physiologic function by facilitating the movement of molecules across biological membranes. Transporters are responsible for maintaining ionic and osmotic gradients necessary for normal cell activity. Transporters facilitate the oxygen binding and release in red blood cells, and they are necessary for the transport of nutrients to vital organs. The primary function of transporters is to transport endogenous substances, such as hormones, glucose, and amino acids; however, many of these transporters also transport xenobiotics. It is these drug transporters that are of importance when considering drug disposition and drug response.

Drug transporters are localized to barrier membranes of the body responsible for xenobiotic entry and exit. They are expressed in organs of absorption, such as the intestine, and clearance organs including the liver and kidney. Transporters are also expressed on membranes that separate particularly susceptible organs from the rest of the body, including the blood-brain and blood-placenta barriers, where they facilitate the influx of nutrients and efflux of potentially harmful xenobiotics. Because of their location on barrier membranes, transporters have an important role in drug pharmacokinetics and pharmacodynamics. Transporters can have a role in drug absorption and can facilitate or prevent drug entry into the body. Transporters also have a role in drug distribution, as they facilitate the movement of drugs between the blood and peripheral tissues. The role of transporters in drug distribution can also affect drug response by allowing or preventing drug access to the site of action. One of the most interesting roles of drug transporters is their indirect effects on drug metabolism. Transporters can restrict or allow a drug's distribution into organs that contain drug-metabolizing enzymes, particularly the liver and the intestine. In this regard, there can be extensive transport-metabolism interplay, and transport or metabolism can be the rate-limiting process controlling drug elimination. Transporters are also responsible for transport and removal of drug metabolites. Finally, transporters have a significant role in drug excretion, as they are present in the kidney and on the canalicular membrane of the liver where they can facilitate drug elimination into the urine or bile, respectively.

Because transporters can have a significant effect on drug absorption, distribution, and clearance, changes in the function of these transporters can significantly alter drug pharmacokinetics and pharmacodynamics. Factors leading to changes in transporter function include interactions with other drugs, disease states, and genetic variability in expression. Understanding transporter effects and the effects of changes in transporter function is important for effective therapeutic use of drugs that interact with transporters.

MECHANISMS OF MEMBRANE TRANSPORT

Membrane transport is essential for almost every drug to be therapeutically effective. This can be achieved by different mechanisms of transport (Fig. 4.1). Passive diffusion is the simplest way for a drug to pass through a membrane and depends only on the existence of a concentration gradient for a molecule across the membrane. Because of the lipophilicity of biologic membranes, diffusion is energetically unfavorable for drugs that are relatively hydrophilic, particularly for drugs that are predominantly ionized at physiologic pH, and these molecules require facilitated transport. Facilitated transport refers to any transport aided by a facilitating protein. Similar to diffusion, passive facilitated transport depends only on the existence of a concentration gradient and involves movement of molecules down this gradient. Active transport uses a separate energy source to move molecules against their concentration gradient. Drug transporters can use either passive or active transport mechanisms. Paracellular transport (transfer of substances between cells of an epithelial cell layer) and transcytosis (vesicular transfer of substances across the interior of a cell) are less commonly used mechanisms of membrane transport. Mannitol can pass through membranes via paracellular transport and can be used as a probe for this type of transport. Transcytosis is often receptor mediated and is a mechanism of transport for endogenous substances such as insulin and transferrin.

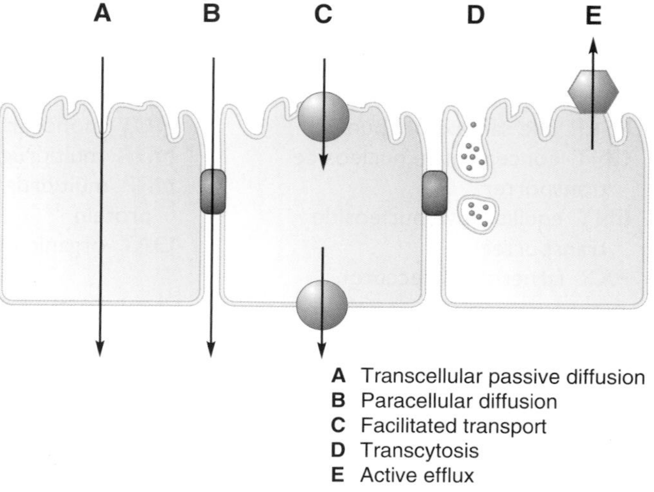

Figure 4.1 Mechanisms of membrane transport. Transport mechanisms most commonly affecting therapeutic agents include passive diffusion, facilitated transport and active efflux.

Molecules can use one or more of these mechanisms to cross biological membranes. Transporter processes are saturable and substrates are often lipophilic and capable of passive diffusion; therefore, drug transport can often be described with the following equation:

$$J = \frac{V_{max} \times C}{K_m + C} + P \times C$$

where J is the rate of total drug transport, V_{max} is the maximum rate of the saturable transporter system, K_m reflects the affinity of a drug substrate for the transporter system, P is the rate of nonsaturable transport or passive diffusion, and C is the drug concentration. The importance of a transporter depends on to what extent transporter-mediated transport (V_{max}/K_m) is responsible for membrane passage of a drug compared to other mechanisms like passive diffusion (P). Transporter-mediated transport becomes particularly important when the need is present to move a molecule against its concentration gradient, as this type of transport can only be achieved by active transporters.

When considering drug transport, it is important to consider the polarization of biological membranes, in that different membranes can have different properties relating to their function as a barrier, including the expression of different transporters. The membrane facing the systemic circulation is referred to as the basolateral membrane, or the sinusoidal membrane in the liver. The membrane facing the exterior, such as the gut lumen, is referred to as the apical membrane. The apical membrane is also called the brush border membrane in the kidney or intestine and the canalicular membrane in the liver. Transport across membranes is actually a two-step process in which molecules must be transported across the apical then basolateral membrane or vice versa. Drug transport is a concerted action between transporters expressed on both membranes.

CLASSIFICATION OF TRANSPORTERS

Facilitative Versus Active Transporters

Although all transporters are facilitating proteins, the terms facilitative and active transporters refer to transporters that transport substrates down their concentration gradients and against their concentration gradients, respectively. Transporters that are classified as facilitative transporters only move molecules down their concentration gradient, without the use of a separate energy source. The transporters of this type should not be confused with channels. Channels also facilitate the movement of ions and hydrophilic molecules across membranes and down their concentration gradient; however, channels control transport or flow of substrates by gating mechanisms, whereas transporters bind to their substrates and undergo a conformational change to transport the substrate across a membrane.

Primary Versus Secondary Active Transporters

Most drug transporters are active transporters that use an energy source other than the drug's concentration gradient to transport substrates across membranes from a region of lower concentration to a region of higher concentration (i.e., against its concentration gradient). Active transporters are further classified as primary or secondary active transporters. Primary active transporters most commonly use adenosine triphosphate (ATP) as an energy source for substrate transport. Secondary active transporters use the concentration gradient of another substance, such as protons or sodium ions, but also other ionic endogenous substances as energy sources to drive transport. The concentration gradients that drive secondary active transport are generally created by primary active transporters; an example of interplay between the two types of transporters is depicted in Figure 4.2. As shown, primary active transport by the Na^+/K^+ ATPase results in a concentration gradient of Na^+ ions. This concentration gradient drives secondary active transport by the Na^+/H^+ exchanger, and the resulting proton gradient drives transport of the drug substrate against its concentration gradient. The Na^+/K^+ ATPase and Na^+/H^+ exchanger do not transport drug substrate but are involved in drug transport by producing the sodium and proton gradients used as driving forces. Molecules used to drive secondary active transport are also substrates for the secondary active transporter and are simultaneously transported across the membrane. This simultaneous transport may be in the same direction, referred to as *symport*, or in opposite directions, referred to as *antiport*.

Influx Versus Efflux Transporters

Influx transporters transport substrates from extracellular spaces into cells. Efflux transporters transport substrates out of cells. Transporters are usually responsible for either drug influx or drug efflux, but in some cases facilitate both types of transport.

Secretory Versus Absorptive Transporters

Secretory transporters facilitate drug clearance and are responsible for transport of drugs from the blood, such as excretion into the urine. Absorptive transporters allow a drug access into the blood, such as those facilitating absorption in the gut or reabsorption in the kidney. A transporter can be both secretory and absorptive depending on its physiologic locations. The same transporter is often expressed at both the site responsible for drug absorption and that responsible for drug clearance; hence, the transporter would serve both secretory and absorptive functions. When considering transport across membranes of the brain and placenta, the terms secretion and absorption are applied differently. With respect to these sites, absorptive transporters allow access into the sites and out of the circulation, and secretory transporters efflux drugs out of these sites and back into the blood circulation.

ABC Versus SLC Transporters

Drug transporters have been classified into two families, namely the ABC (ATP-binding cassette) and SLC (solute carrier) families. Members of the ABC family are primary active transporters that use ATP as an energy source. Most SLC transporters are secondary active transporters, using the concentration gradients of several different molecules

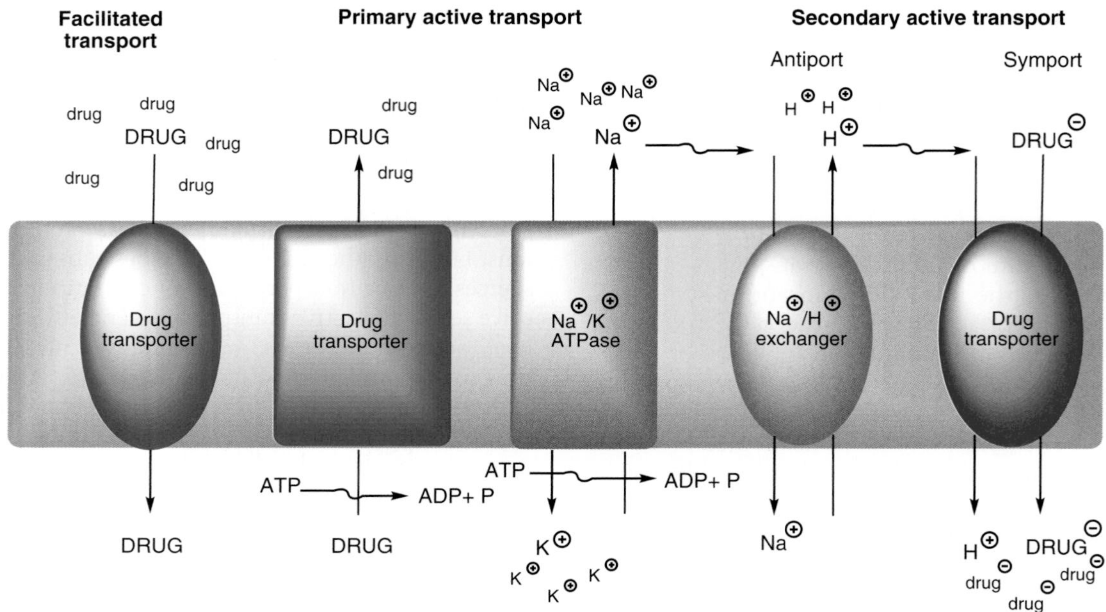

Figure 4.2 Types of drug transporters. Primary active transporters use ATP and have the ability to transport substrates against their concentration gradient. Secondary active transporters use gradients created by primary active transport to transport drug substrates. Facilitated transporters only transport substrates down their concentration gradient. Transporters that transport drug substrates are shown in *red*, whereas those shown in *gray* provide driving forces for drug transport.

as a driving force for transport. The SLC family also includes a handful of facilitative transporters. Many members of each family have a role in drug disposition, and these transporters are summarized in Table 4.1.

ABC Transporters

ABC transporters are efflux transporters, many of which are located on the apical side of biological membranes, facilitating drug secretion. ABC transporters are primary active transporters and use ATP as an energy source. The widespread physiologic expression of ABC transporters and their extensive range of substrates make it inevitable for these transporters to have effects on drug pharmacokinetics and elicit clinically significant drug interactions. Substrates and inhibitors for ABC transporters are given in Table 4.2.

MULTIDRUG RESISTANCE PROTEINS (ABCB)

MDR1 (*ABCB1*). MDR1, more commonly known as P-glycoprotein (P-gp), is the most extensively characterized of all drug transporters. The structure of P-gp consists of two homologous halves each with six transmembrane-spanning domains and one ATP binding site (Fig. 4.3). Transport by P-gp is notably complicated, with at least two binding sites and three different proposed mechanisms by which it transports substrates.[1,2]

P-gp is expressed in most tissues and is involved in drug transport in the intestine, liver, kidney, brain, and placenta, as well as in tumor cells. This is one reason P-gp has been, and remains, a transporter of clinical interest. The ability of P-gp to transport a wide range of substrates is another remarkable feature. These substrates span many therapeutic areas and drug classes, making it difficult to determine the structure-activity relationship for P-gp–mediated transport, though much progress has been made in this area in recent years.[3] Digoxin serves as a probe for P-gp in both in vitro and in vivo studies.[4] Other substrates include many chemotherapeutic drugs, other cardiovascular agents, and HIV protease inhibitors. One common feature of P-gp substrates is that they are generally lipophilic (Fig. 4.4). The relative lipophilicity of these molecules implies that most P-gp substrates may also have high rates of passive diffusion. This means that P-gp transport must be efficient to have an effect on the passage of its substrates across membranes, and P-gp transport does not always result in clinically relevant effects. P-gp substrates are rarely specific and are also often substrates of other transporters and drug-metabolizing enzymes, particularly CYP3A4, making it difficult to attribute in vivo pharmacokinetic effects or interactions to P-gp alone. Mouse models of P-gp knockout indicate intestinal efflux by P-gp contributes to the low bioavailability of many compounds.[5] Accordingly, significant drug-drug interactions have also been demonstrated involving P-gp in humans at the intestine, as well as in the kidneys.[6,7] P-gp is also likely important in pregnancy in that it protects the fetus from xenobiotics by effluxing them back into the maternal blood circulation.[8] In addition, as the original name "multidrug resistance protein" (MDR) implies, P-gp is also recognized as a potential factor for chemotherapeutic drug resistance due to its overexpression in tumor cells. While clinical studies evaluating P-gp inhibition to overcome resistance have had varying results, this continues to be considered as potential concurrent treatment with chemotherapy.[9] Similarly while single nucleotide polymorphisms (SNPs) in the *MDR1* gene have been identified, the impact of these on drug disposition remains controversial.[10]

Table 4.1 Drug Transporters

Transporter Family	Family Member	Gene Name	Location	Role in Drug Disposition
MDR	MDR1	*ABCB1*	Intestine, liver, kidneys, brain, heart, placenta	• Role in oral absorption, biliary clearance, renal secretion, and drug penetration of blood-brain barrier • Drug-drug interactions • Known polymorphisms • Role in multidrug resistance
MRP	MRP1	*ABCC1*	Intestine, brain	• Role in multidrug resistance • Facilitates basolateral drug efflux
	MRP2	*ABCC2*	Intestine, liver, kidney	• Role in oral absorption, biliary clearance, and renal secretion of drugs and drug conjugates • Known polymorphisms that affect drug disposition
	MRP3	*ABCC3*	Liver, intestine, brain	• Facilitates sinusoidal efflux of bile acids, drugs and drug conjugates
	MRP4	*ABCC4*	Kidney, liver, brain	• Facilitates renal secretion and sinusoidal efflux of bile acids, drugs and drug conjugates
BCRP	BCRP1	*ABCG2*	Intestine, liver, kidney, brain, heart, placenta	• Role in oral absorption, biliary secretion, and drug penetration of blood-brain barrier • Drug-drug interactions • Known polymorphisms that affect drug disposition • Role in multidrug resistance
OCT	OCT1	*SLC22A1*	Liver	• Facilitates sinusoidal uptake • Drug-drug interactions • Known polymorphisms that affect drug disposition
	OCT2	*SLC22A2*	Kidney	• Facilitates renal secretion • Drug-drug interactions • Known polymorphisms that affect drug disposition
OCTN	OCTN1	*SLC22A4*	Kidney, intestine	• Role in oral absorption and renal reabsorption
	OCTN2	*SLC22A5*	Kidney, intestine, liver, brain, muscle, lung	• Role in oral absorption and renal reabsorption • Known polymorphisms
OAT	OAT1	*SLC22A6*	Kidney	• Facilitates renal secretion • Drug-drug interactions
	OAT2	*SLC22A7*	Liver	• Facilitates sinusoidal uptake and renal secretion
	OAT3	*SLC22A8*	Kidney	• Facilitates renal secretion • Drug-drug interactions
	OAT4	*SLC22A11*	Kidney	• Facilitates renal reabsorption

(continued)

Table 4.1 Drug Transporters (Continued)

Transporter Family	Family Member	Gene Name	Location	Role in Drug Disposition
OATP	OATP1A2	*SLCO1A2*	Brain	• Role in brain uptake
	OATP1B1	*SLCO1B1*	Liver	• Facilitates sinusoidal uptake • Drug-drug interactions • Known polymorphisms that affect in vivo drug disposition
	OATP1B3	*SLCO1B3*	Liver	• Facilitates sinusoidal uptake • Known polymorphisms
	OATP2B1	*SLCO2B1*	Intestine, liver	• Role in oral absorption and sinusoidal uptake
	OATP4C1	*SLCO4C1*	Kidney	• Facilitates renal secretion
MATE	MATE1	*SLC47A1*	Kidney, liver	• Role in renal and biliary secretion • Drug-drug interactions • Known polymorphisms that affect in vivo drug disposition
	MATE2-K	*SLC47A2*	Kidney	• Facilitates renal secretion
MCT	MCT1	*SLC16A7*	Ubiquitous	• Role in oral absorption and renal reabsorption • Overexpression in tumor cells
PEPT	PEPT1	*SLC15A1*	Intestine, kidney	• Facilitates oral absorption • Drug-drug interactions
	PEPT2	*SLC15A2*	Kidney	• Facilitates renal reabsorption
CNT	CNT1	*SLC28A1*	Intestine, kidney, liver	• Role in absorption and disposition of nucleoside analogues
	CNT2	*SLC28A2*	Intestine, kidney, liver	• Role in absorption and disposition of nucleoside analogues
	CNT3	*SLC28A3*	Kidney, brain, placenta	• Role in distribution and renal reabsorption of nucleoside analogues
ENT	ENT1	*SLC29A1*	Ubiquitous	• Role in absorption and disposition of nucleoside analogues
	ENT2	*SLC29A2*	Ubiquitous	• Role in absorption and disposition of nucleoside analogues
Bile acid	BSEP	*ABCB11*	Liver	• Role in biliary secretion of bile acids • Known polymorphisms
	NTCP	*SLC10A1*	Liver	• Sinusoidal uptake of bile acids
	OSTαβ	*OSTA/B*	Liver	• Compensatory efflux of bile acids on sinusoidal membrane during cholestasis
	ASBT	*SLC10A2*	Intestine	• Role in absorption of bile acids

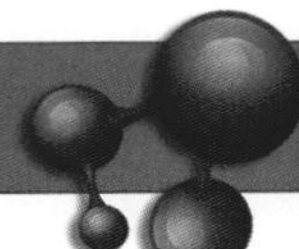

CLINICAL SIGNIFICANCE

P-GP AND DIGOXIN

Digoxin undergoes little metabolism in humans, and transport by P-gp is the primary determinant of digoxin pharmacokinetics. One of the first drug interactions noted with digoxin was that with cyclosporine, leading to decreased digoxin clearance and digoxin-associated arrhythmias.[11] It was later discovered that cyclosporine and other therapeutic agents decrease digoxin clearance due to inhibition of P-gp–mediated renal secretion.[12] Nonrenal clearance of digoxin is minimal; however, P-gp inhibitors have similarly been demonstrated to decrease digoxin biliary excretion.[13] P-gp function also affects digoxin absorption, and concomitant oral administration of clarithromycin was demonstrated to increase digoxin bioavailability along with decreasing digoxin renal clearance.[6] Because in vivo P-gp inhibition can affect both absorption and clearance, there exists substantial risk of elevated digoxin plasma concentrations and digoxin-associated toxicity with concomitant inhibitor administration.

P-gp induction can also affect digoxin pharmacokinetics. In a study of human volunteers, chronic rifampin administration resulted in a 3.5-fold increase in duodenal P-gp expression leading to a decrease in digoxin bioavailability.[14] P-gp expression correlated well with digoxin area under the curve (AUC) in this study, emphasizing the significance of intestinal P-gp on digoxin exposure.

Table 4.2 Relevant Drug Substrates and Inhibitors of ABC Transporters

Transporter	Substrates	Inhibitors
MDR1	Atorvastatin, cyclosporine, dabigatran, daunorubicin, dexamethasone, digoxin, diltiazem, docetaxel, doxorubicin, erythromycin, etoposide, fexofenadine, ketoconazole, loperamide, methadone, mitoxantrone, morphine, paclitaxel, phenytoin, rifampin, ritonavir, saquinavir, simvastatin, tacrolimus, talinolol, verapamil, vinblastine, vincristine	Clarithromycin, cyclosporine, elacridar, quinidine, verapamil
MRP2	Ampicillin, ceftriaxone, cisplatin, daunomycin, doxorubicin, etoposide, fluorouracil, glucuronide conjugates, glutathione conjugates, irinotecan, methotrexate, mitoxantrone, olmesartan, pravastatin, ritonavir, rosuvastatin, saquinavir, SN-38-glucuronide, valsartan, vinblastine, vincristine	Cyclosporine, probenecid, efavirenz, emtricitabine
MRP3	Bile acids, fexofenadine, glucuronide conjugates, methotrexate	Efavirenz, emtricitabine
MRP4	Adefovir, furosemide, methotrexate, rosuvastatin, tenofovir, topotecan	Diclofenac
BCRP	Atorvastatin, ciprofloxacin, imatinib, irinotecan, methotrexate, mitoxantrone, nitrofurantoin, rosuvastatin, sorafenib, topotecan	Elacridar

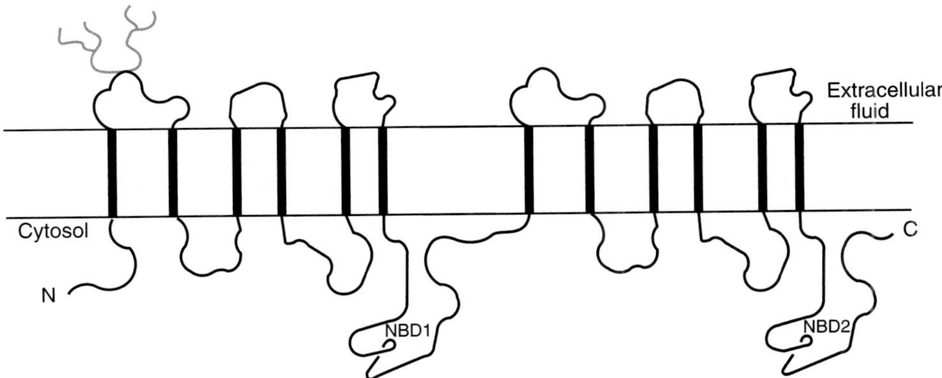

Figure 4.3 Structure of P-glycoprotein including 12 transmembrane-spanning domains and two nucleotide-binding domains (NBDs).

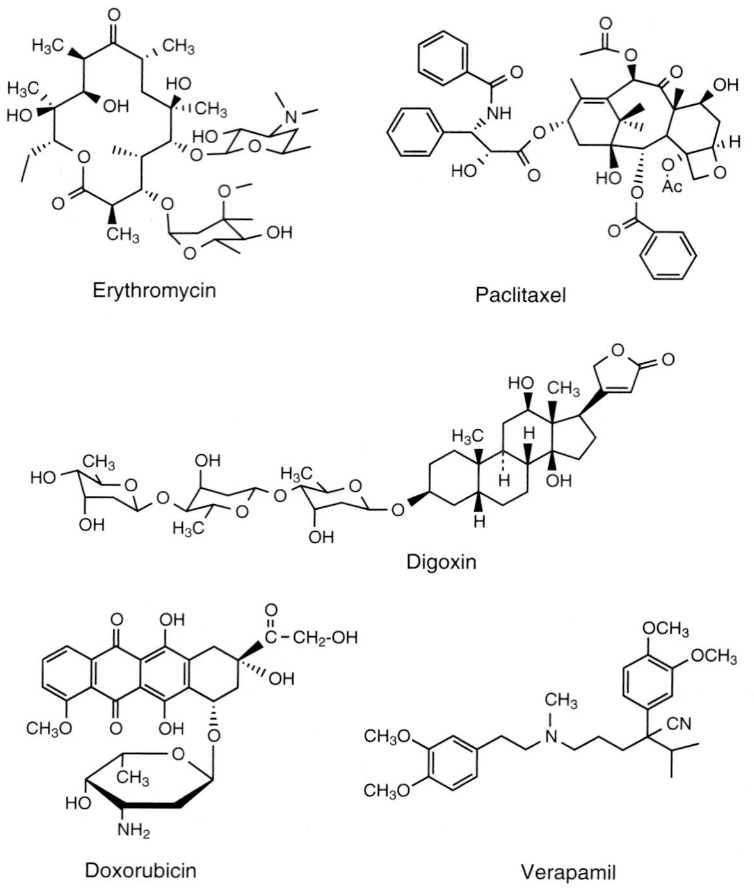

Erythromycin

Paclitaxel

Digoxin

Doxorubicin

Verapamil

Figure 4.4 Examples of P-gp substrates/inhibitors.

MULTIDRUG RESISTANCE–ASSOCIATED PROTEINS (ABCC)

MRP2 (*ABCC2*). Multidrug resistance–associated protein 2 (MRP2) is primarily localized to three apical membrane barriers, the liver canalicular membrane, the brush border membrane in the kidney, and the apical membrane of the gut, where it serves to excrete substrates into the bile, urine, and back into the gut lumen, respectively. The major substrates of MRP2 are conjugates, including glucuronide, glutathione, and sulfate conjugates, and the primary endogenous function of MRP2 is the secretion of bilirubin and bile acid conjugates across the canalicular membrane into the bile. In addition to phase 2 drug metabolites, MRP2 substrates also include many unconjugated therapeutic drugs including vinca alkaloids. Glutathione symport is often required for transport of unconjugated substances.[15] MRP2 can contribute to the renal secretion of some drug substrates; however, the main role of MRP2 in drug disposition appears to be hepatobiliary transport.[1,16] Due to transport of drug conjugates, MRP2 has an important role in enterohepatic cycling. MRP2 transports conjugates into the bile, which empties into the gut lumen. Bacteria in the gut metabolize the conjugate back to the parent drug, which can then be reabsorbed back into the systemic blood circulation. In this way, MRP2 can be responsible for maintaining plasma concentrations of drugs that are not substrates, due to transport of their conjugated metabolites. P-gp is also expressed on the canalicular membrane, although it does not appear to have a role in biliary secretion of drug conjugates. Because of overlapping specificity of MRP2 substrates and inhibitors with P-gp, it can sometimes be difficult to attribute in vivo pharmacokinetic effects to MRP2 alone. SNPs in MRP2 have been identified, resulting in a condition called Dubin-Johnson syndrome. While not leading to severe pathology, subjects with this condition display increased plasma levels of endogenous MRP2 substrates such as conjugated bilirubin.[17]

Other MRPs. In contrast to the apical expression of MRP2, MRPs 1, 3, 4, 5, and 6 are basolateral efflux transporters. MRP1 is another ABC transporter that can be overexpressed in cancer cells, resulting in resistance to chemotherapy.[15] MRP3 has an important role in the transport of conjugated drug metabolites in the liver, particularly glucuronide conjugates. Located on the sinusoidal membrane, MRP3 serves to efflux metabolites out of hepatocytes into the plasma, resulting in conjugate excretion into the urine. Although the bile acid transporters discussed below play a primary adaptive role in response to cholestasis, MRP3 also transports conjugated bile acids and can be induced in cholestatic conditions.[18] MRP3 protein has also been detected in the intestine.[19] MRP4 is expressed on the brush border membrane of the kidney and has a role in anionic drug secretion into the urine.[16] Similar to

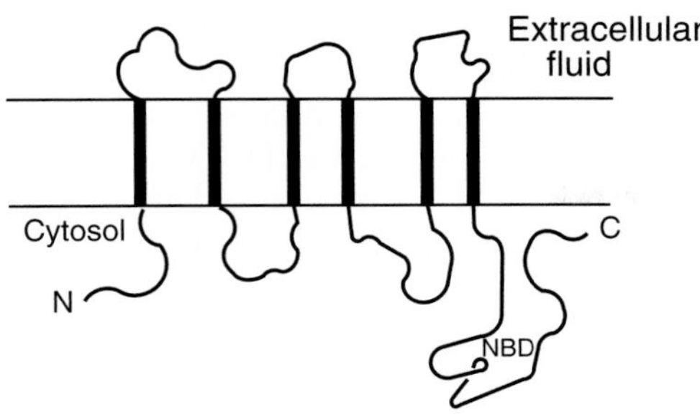

Figure 4.5 Structure of BCRP. BCRP is regarded as a half transporter due to its structure including only six transmembrane-spanning domains and one nucleotide-binding domain (NBD).

MRP3, it has a postulated compensatory role in effluxing substrates from the liver during cholestasis or other forms of liver injury.[20] MRP4 and MRP5 also transport cGMP and cAMP and therefore play a role in maintaining the intracellular concentrations of these molecules.[21]

Breast Cancer Resistance Protein

BCRP (*ABCG2*). Breast cancer resistance protein (BCRP) is actually a "half" transporter, in that it consists of only six transmembrane-spanning domains and one ATP binding site (Fig. 4.5). Like P-gp, BCRP expression is widespread. Its highest expression is in the placenta, and it is present in the intestine, liver, kidney, brain, heart, testes, and ovaries.[22] Also similar to P-gp, multiple binding sites have been proposed for BCRP. As its name implies, BCRP has been attributed with causing chemotherapeutic drug resistance due to overexpression in tumor cells, and among its substrates are several chemotherapeutic agents. BCRP shares many substrates with P-gp and is commonly localized with P-gp, making it difficult to attribute drug transport or inhibition to BCRP. However, the use of BCRP inhibitors, Bcrp knockout animals, and identification of SNPs in the *ABCG2* gene have demonstrated the importance of BCRP in drug disposition. Significant effects of BCRP transport have been demonstrated on drug absorption, biliary clearance, and interestingly on drug transport in the mammary gland, mediating the transport of some drugs into breast milk.[23-25] BCRP has a similar role as P-gp in pregnancy, as it is highly expressed at the blood-placenta barrier, where it also serves a protective function to efflux potentially harmful xenobiotics.[8] Likewise, given their co-localization and shared substrate specificity, synergism between P-gp and BCRP has been demonstrated at other particularly vulnerable physiologic barriers, such as those in the brain and testes in P-gp/Bcrp knockout animal models.[26]

SLC Transporters

Members of the SLC transporter family are secondary active transporters and, as such, use the concentration gradients of many other substances to transport drug substrates. The concentration gradients of these other substances generally facilitate drug influx, although in some physiologic locations they can facilitate efflux, and some transporters can be capable of transport in both directions. Like the ABC transporters, SLC transporters are physiologically expressed throughout the body. They transport many different xenobiotics along with many endogenous substances, leading to effects on drug disposition and drug interactions. Substrates and inhibitors of SLC transporters are given in Table 4.3.

Organic Anion Transporting Polypeptides (SLCO)

OATP1B1 (SLCO1B1). This transporter is one of the most clinically relevant in that its substrates include drugs such as the 3-hydroxy-3-methyl-glutaryl-coenzyme A (HMG-CoA) reductase inhibitors, or statins, which are widely prescribed. This transporter is localized specifically on the sinusoidal membrane of the liver, where it serves to influx substrates into hepatocytes, where they can be metabolized or transported into bile. The driving force of organic anion transporter polypeptide (OATP) 1B1 and other OATPs is unclear, but it is proposed that they are antiporters, potentially using the high intracellular concentration of glutathione as a driving force. Although the name implies anion transport, OATPs are also capable of transporting cationic and unionized compounds, with OATP1B1 displaying the broadest substrate specificity overall. OATP1B1 transports many endogenous substrates including conjugates of bilirubin and estrogen. Common drug substrates of OATP1B1 and other OATPs are given in Figure 4.6. Inhibitors of this transporter are also commonly used in the clinic for similar or concomitant disease states. Rifampin and cyclosporine potently inhibit OATP1B1 in vivo and are used in the clinic for assessment of interactions with potential OATP substrates. Interactions with these inhibitors can result in very large increases in substrate exposure. Recent findings may help explain the large magnitude of these interactions in that long-lasting inhibition has been demonstrated in vitro and in vivo, at least in rats, particularly for cyclosporine.[27,28] This transporter has also gained attention due to the recognition that it is highly polymorphic, with a large number of SNPs having been identified in the *SLCO1B1* gene. Many of these SNPs translate into decreased hepatic uptake in vivo, resulting in decreased clearance of OATP1B1 substrates.[29]

TRANSPORTER POLYMORPHISMS: ROLE IN STATIN DISPOSITION

The effect of OATP1B1 polymorphisms on statin pharmacokinetics and response further emphasizes the significance of OATP-mediated uptake for the hepatic clearance of these compounds. Studies of subjects with the common SLCO1B1 c.521CC genotype have reported increases in plasma AUC from 65% with rosuvastatin to 221% with simvastatin, compared to subjects carrying the wild-type allele.[29] Likely the most prominent finding with regard to statin myopathy was the genome-wide association study which found this polymorphism to be the strongest predictor of the toxicity of simvastatin.[30] A recent study also found the SLCO2B1 c.1475CT polymorphism had an effect on rosuvastatin lipid-lowering effect, although this has yet to be replicated.[31] Given that many statins are also substrates for BCRP and there are known polymorphisms in ABCG2, studies have also evaluated the effect of the

ABCG2 c.388GA polymorphism on statin exposure. The greatest effect has been demonstrated for rosuvastatin; the increased plasma exposure associated with this SNP may involve increased bioavailability and/or decreased biliary secretion by BCRP.[32] Increased effect of rosuvastatin was also demonstrated in this particular study. Alterations in the function of both OATPs and BCRP can significantly affect the safe and effective use of statins. Algorithms for statin dosing incorporating SLCO1B1 and ABCG2 genotyping are currently proposed for individualizing statin therapy.[33]

Other OATPs. Like OATP1B1, OATP1B3 is expressed exclusively on the sinusoidal membrane of the liver. The substrates for OATP1B3 are generally shared by OATP1B1, although there are compounds, such as telmisartan, to which OATP1B3 transport is attributed to be predominant.[34] Therefore, OATP1B3 may act as a compensatory transport mechanism when transport by OATP1B1 is deficient due to inhibition or genetic polymorphisms. The other OATPs with identified drug substrates and effects on drug disposition include OATP1A2, 2B1, and 4C1. OATP1A2 is expressed in the brain and may be responsible for blood-brain barrier transport of drugs and endogenous substances. OATP2B1 is also expressed on the sinusoidal membrane of the liver with OATP1B1 and 1B3; however, unlike these transporters, it is also expressed in other tissues including the intestine.[19] OATP4C1 is expressed on the basolateral membrane of the kidney. Among its substrates are digoxin and the antidiabetic drug sitagliptin; however, the role of this transporter in the in vivo disposition or drug interactions of these drugs is as of yet unclear.[35]

Organic Anion Transporters (*SLC22A*)

The organic anion transporters (OATs) are highly expressed in the kidney where they have a significant role in the renal clearance of many anionic drugs. The driving

Table 4.3 Relevant Drug Substrates and Inhibitors of SLC Transporters

Transporter	Substrates	Inhibitors
OATP1B1	Atorvastatin, bosentan, caspofungin, cerivastatin, enalapril, erythromycin, fexofenadine, fluvastatin, methotrexate, olmesartan, pravastatin, repaglinide, rifampin, rosuvastatin, simvastatin, SN-38, valsartan	Cyclosporine, erythromycin, gemfibrozil, rifampin, ritonavir, saquinavir, tacrolimus
OATP1B3	Digoxin, docetaxel, fexofenadine, olmesartan, paclitaxel, rifampin, telmisartan	Cyclosporine, erythromycin, rifampin, ritonavir
OATP1A2	Digoxin, erythromycin, fexofenadine, imatinib, levofloxacin, methotrexate, pitavastatin, rocuronium, rosuvastatin, saquinavir, sumatriptan	Grapefruit juice, rifampin, ritonavir, saquinavir, verapamil
OATP2B1	Atorvastatin, bosentan, fexofenadine, pravastatin, rosuvastatin	Grapefruit juice, cyclosporine, gemfibrozil, rifampin
OAT1	Acyclovir, adefovir, cidofovir, ciprofloxacin, lamivudine, methotrexate, penicillins, tenofovir, zidovudine	Probenecid, NSAIDs
OAT2	Ketoprofen, theophilline	
OAT3	Bumetanide, cefaclor, ceftizoxime, furosemide, methotrexate, NSAIDs, penicillins	Probenecid, NSAIDs
OCT1	Metformin, morphine, ondansetron, oxaliplatin, sumatriptan	Erlotinib, propranolol, quinidine, verapamil
OCT2	Cisplatin, lamivudine, metformin, oxaliplatin, procainamide	Cimetidine, pyrimethamine, vandetanib, dolutegravir
MATE1	Cisplatin, metformin, oxaliplatin	Cimetidine, cobicistat, famotidine, quinidine, pyrimethamine, trimethoprim, vandetanib
MCT1	Atorvastatin, salicylic acid, valproic acid, γ-hydroxybutyric acid	Dietary flavonoids
PEPT1	Captopril, cefadroxil, cephalexin, enalapril, valacyclovir	Glycyl-proline, zinc
PEPT2	Captopril, cefadroxil, cephalexin, enalapril, valacyclovir	Fosinopril
CNT/ENT	Clofarabine, ribavirin, other nucleoside analogues	Dipyridamole
NTCP	Atorvastatin, pravastatin, rosuvastatin	Bosentan, cyclosporine, gemfibrozil

NSAIDs, nonsteroidal anti-inflammatory drugs.

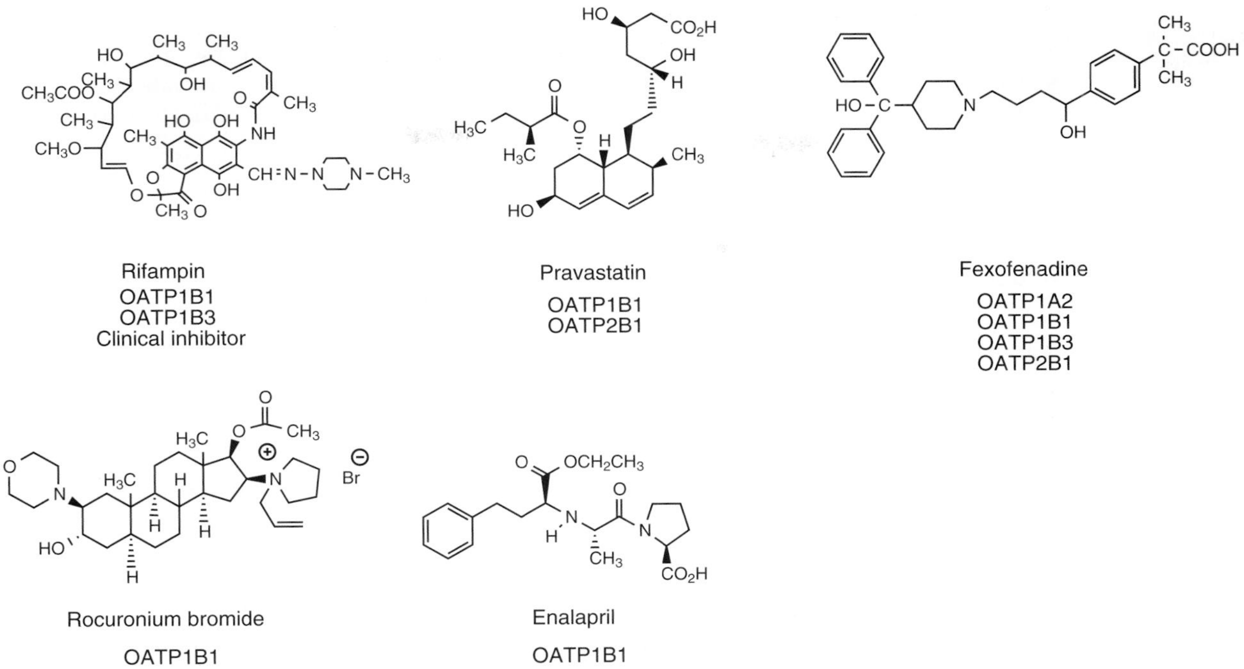

Rifampin
OATP1B1
OATP1B3
Clinical inhibitor

Pravastatin
OATP1B1
OATP2B1

Fexofenadine
OATP1A2
OATP1B1
OATP1B3
OATP2B1

Rocuronium bromide
OATP1B1

Enalapril
OATP1B1

Figure 4.6 Common OATP substrates/inhibitors.

forces and polarized renal expression of OATs support renal secretion of drug substrates from the blood circulation into the urine. OAT1 is expressed primarily in the kidney, on the basolateral membrane of renal tubule cells, along with OAT3. These transporters facilitate anion transport into renal tubule cells through antiport with intracellular dicarboxylates like α-ketoglutarate. Located on the apical membrane, OAT4 can transport drugs from the tubule cells into the urine, but it is likely primarily responsible for renal reabsorption.[36] OATs transport an expansive range of drugs, and the importance of OAT expression in the kidney has been demonstrated with numerous clinically relevant drug interactions. Coadministration of OAT inhibitors can lead to decreased renal secretion of OAT substrates including penicillin antibiotics and diuretic agents (Tables 4.3 and 4.4).[16] Along with renal transport, OATs can also mediate hepatic anion transport. The primary location of OAT2 is on the liver sinusoidal membrane, where it facilitates anion uptake into hepatocytes. OAT2 expression has also recently been demonstrated in the kidney and has been implicated to play a role in the renal excretion of creatinine.[37] OATs are also present on the choroid plexus (a structure in the brain where cerebrospinal fluid [CSF] is produced), where they can have a role in transfer of drugs between the blood and CSF.[38]

Organic Cation/Carnitine Transporters (*SLC22A*)

Organic cation transporters (OCTs) are electrogenic uniporters, which use only the negative membrane potential as a driving force and require no co-substrate. OCT1 is expressed primarily in the liver and OCT2 in the kidney, both on the basolateral membrane. Although they are named cation transporters, these transporters are also capable of transporting some anionic and unionized compounds. SNPs in OCT1 have demonstrated effects on the plasma exposure of multiple OCT1 substrates.[39] Drug interactions and drug toxicity have been attributed to OCT2-mediated transport, due to a substrate range that includes commonly prescribed therapeutic agents, such as metformin (Table 4.3). Coadministration of OCT2 inhibitors and genetic variation in OCT2 has been demonstrated to increase plasma concentrations of metformin due to its decreased renal secretion (Table 4.4).[40-42] Renal transport of cisplatin by OCT2 has also been identified as a significant factor in cisplatin-induced nephrotoxicity.[43] OCT3 transports monoamines and is located in the brain and placenta, where its primary role can be to eliminate catecholamines from the fetal blood circulation.[44] Decreased OCT3 transport has also been suggested to be related to cases of preeclampsia.[45]

Organic cation/carnitine transporter (OCTN) 1 and OCTN2 are proton antiporters expressed in the kidney, where they are localized on the apical membrane. Expression of human OCTN1/2 mRNA has also been detected in the intestine.[46] OCTN2 is responsible for carnitine transport into tissues and is widely expressed, including in the skeletal muscle, liver, brain, and lung.[47] These transporters share substrates with OCTs, and their apical expression may allow for the concerted movement of these substrates across membranes in which they are co-expressed. These transporters are of particular importance in the placenta, as they are responsible for transporting carnitine to the fetus.[44] Some antiepileptics, like valproate, inhibit OCTNs, and it has been suggested that inhibition of carnitine transport can be partly responsible for teratogenicity and other adverse effects associated

Table 4.4 Select Clinically Relevant Drug Interactions Involving Transporters

Transporter	Substrate	Inhibitor(s)	Effect on Substrate Pharmacokinetics
MDR1	Digoxin	Clarithromycin, cyclosporine, ritonavir, verapamil	↑ plasma AUC (↓ Cl_r, ↓ Cl_{bile}, and/or ↑ F)
		Rifampin, St. John's wort	↓ plasma AUC, ↓ F (induction)
	Fexofenadine	Erythromycin, itraconazole, lopinavir/ritonavir	↑ F
	Dabigatran	Clarithromycin, verapamil	↑ plasma AUC, ↑ F
BCRP	Topotecan	Elacridar	↑ plasma AUC, ↑ F
	Rosuvastatin	Atazanavir/ritonavir, cyclosporine	↑ plasma AUC, ↑ F and/or ↓ Cl_{bile}
MRP2	Mycophenolic acid (glucuronide conjugates)	Cyclosporine	↓ Cl_{bile} of conjugates leading to ↓ enterohepatic circulation
OATP1B1/1B3	Statins	Cyclosporine, gemfibrozil, lopinavir/ritonavir, rifampin	↑ plasma AUC, ↓ Cl
	Bosentan	Cyclosporine, lopinavir/ritonavir, rifampin	↑ plasma AUC, ↓ Cl
	Repaglinide	Cyclosporine, gemfibrozil	↑ plasma AUC, ↓ Cl
OATP2B1	Rosuvastatin	Ronacaleret	↓ plasma AUC, ↓ F
OAT1/3	Acyclovir, cephalosporins, cidofovir, ciprofloxacin, furosemide, methotrexate, penicillins	Probenecid	↑ plasma AUC, ↓ Cl_r
OCT2/MATE1	Dofetilide, metformin	Cimetidine, dolutegravir, pyrimethamine, vandetanib	↑ plasma AUC, ↓ Cl_r

AUC, area under the curve; Cl, clearance; Cl_{bile}, biliary clearance; Cl_r, renal clearance; F, bioavailability.

with valproate use.[48] Mutations in OCTN2 lead to systemic carnitine deficiency syndrome, causing early-onset cardiomyopathy, including congestive heart failure.[49] The anticholinergic drugs ipratropium and tiotropium are transported primarily by OCTN2 and, to a lesser extent, by OCTN1, by bronchial epithelial cells.[50] These findings are consistent with the pharmacologic activity of the drugs after administration via inhalation.

Multidrug and Toxin Extrusion Transporters (*SLC47A*)

Multidrug and toxin extrusion transporter (MATE) 1 and MATE2-K are cation transporters that use proton antiport as a driving force. MATE1 is located primarily on the apical membrane of the kidney and canalicular membrane of the liver. MATE2-K is kidney specific, and recently it was found that expression even in human proximal tubule cells of kidney is low, leading to ambiguity of its in vivo relevance given that substrates are often shared with MATE1.[51] The significance of MATE1 transport in metformin pharmacokinetics was characterized in Mate1 knockout mice, in which the renal clearance of metformin was decreased to less than 20% that of controls, indicating the importance of this transporter for metformin renal secretion.[52] Drug interactions with metformin and other substrates in humans involve MATE inhibition in kidney (Table 4.4).[53] Inhibition of Mate1 in mice increased the liver accumulation of metformin, and SNPs with decreased function in the *SLC47A* gene have been associated with increased metformin response.[54,55] MATE1 has a role in the renal secretion and nephrotoxicity of platinum agents, where MATE1 secretion appears protective due to the prevention of renal cell accumulation.[56,57] Many drug substrates and inhibitors of these transporters have been identified and can be cationic, unionized, or anionic at physiologic pH.[53] MATE substrates and inhibitors are often shared with those of OCT2, and sometimes OAT1 or OAT3, which can lead to drug-drug interactions involving both uptake and efflux into proximal tubule cells, discussed in further detail below.[58]

Monocarboxylate Transporters (*SLC16A* and *SLC5A*)

The first discovered monocarboxylate transporters (MCTs) were proton coupled, transporting monocarboxylates via symport. Because the transport of substrates by

MCTs is driven by the proton gradient, these transporters can influx or efflux substrates depending on this gradient. The MCTs are ubiquitously expressed, and their role in the transport of endogenous substances, including lactate and pyruvate, has been extensively characterized.[59] Many therapeutic agents have also been identified as substrates; however, the clinical relevance of MCT transport of these agents is unclear (Table 4.3). A relevant therapeutic aspect of MCT1 is its high expression in the intestine, making this transporter a target as a means for facilitating oral drug absorption.[60] MCT1 has also been identified to be overexpressed in tumor cells, and inhibition of this transporter represents a possible therapeutic strategy for some cancers.[61] The drug of abuse γ-hydroxybutyrate (GHB) has been identified as a MCT substrate, and the relevance of MCT transport of this drug has been established. Inhibition of the MCT-mediated renal reabsorption of GHB has been demonstrated to increase its renal and total clearance, making MCT inhibition a possible strategy for the treatment of GHB overdose.[62,63] Other MCTs have been less well studied, but both MCT8 and MCT10 have demonstrated affinity for thyroid hormones.[64]

MCT1 AND ORAL DRUG DELIVERY

The antiepileptic agent, gabapentin, has unfavorable oral pharmacokinetics, with low, dose-dependent bioavailability and poor rates of clinical response. In an effort to improve the oral delivery of gabapentin, a prodrug, gabapentin enacarbil, was designed to target absorption by MCT1. In a pilot study comparing the pharmacokinetics of gabapentin to the prodrug, gabapentin displayed dose-dependent bioavailability ranging from 27%-65%, whereas gabapentin enacarbil displayed bioavailability above 68% for all doses and dose-proportional oral exposure.[65] Gabapentin enacarbil resulted in higher plasma concentrations of gabapentin at similar doses compared to gabapentin itself. This case emphasizes the utility of high-capacity transporters like MCT1 for facilitating oral drug delivery and achieving clinically desirable drug pharmacokinetics.

Another subset of MCTs has been identified that use sodium for monocarboxylate symport and are referred to as sodium-coupled MCTs (SMCTs). Expression of SMCTs is also widely distributed, including the apical membranes of the intestine and kidney, where they likely act in conjunction with proton-coupled MCTs to transport monocarboxylates across membranes.

Peptide Transporters (*SLC15A*)

Peptide transporters (PEPTs) mediate the transport of di- and tripeptides via proton symport. PEPT1 has very high expression on the apical membrane of the intestine and, as such, is used for drug delivery.[19] Transport mediated by PEPT1 facilitates sufficient oral absorption to allow oral administration for many therapeutic drugs and prodrugs structurally designed to target this transporter (Fig. 4.7 and Table 4.3).[60] PEPT1 is also present at lower levels on the brush border membrane of the kidney; however, PEPT2 is the major peptide transporter at this site. PEPT2 is also localized to the apical membrane where it serves mainly to reabsorb peptides from the urine in renal tubule cells. It also facilitates transport of drug substrates similar to PEPT1, including β-lactam antibiotics and angiotensin-converting enzyme (ACE) inhibitors (Table 4.3).[66] Two peptide/histidine transporters (PHTs) were recently identified, PHT1 and PHT2. Expression of these transporters has been demonstrated in the intestine, and they likely have a role in peptide absorption, along with PEPT1. Expression of mRNA for these transporters has also been identified in several other human tissues.[67] The role of the PHTs in drug disposition has yet to be elucidated.

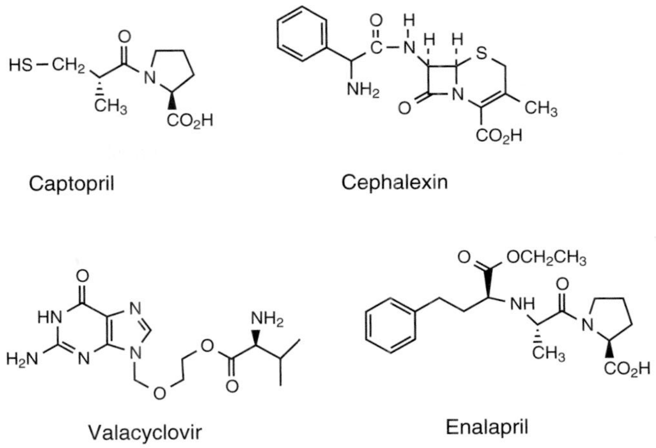

Figure 4.7 Drug substrates of peptide transporters.

Nucleoside Transporters (*SLC28* and *SLC29*)

Two nucleoside transporter groups exist, the concentrative nucleoside transporters (CNTs) and the equilibrative nucleoside transporters (ENTs). CNTs are present on the apical membrane of cells and are sodium dependent, whereas ENTs are facilitative and located primarily on basolateral membranes.[68] These two groups of transporters work together to achieve vectorial transport of purines and pyrimidines. The expression of both groups of transporters is widespread, and although their primary function is to facilitate cellular uptake of nucleosides, they also transport many nucleoside analogues (Fig. 4.8), and these transporters are associated with toxicity and therapeutic response to these drugs (Table 4.3).[68,69]

Bile Acid Transporters (*ABCB11*, *SLC10A*, and *OSTA/B*)

The human in vivo bile acid pool is highly conserved due to enterohepatic recirculation; therefore, the bile acid transporters involved in this process have been well characterized.[70] It has been recently demonstrated, however, that these transporters can also transport xenobiotics. NTCP (sodium-taurocholate cotransporting polypeptide) is

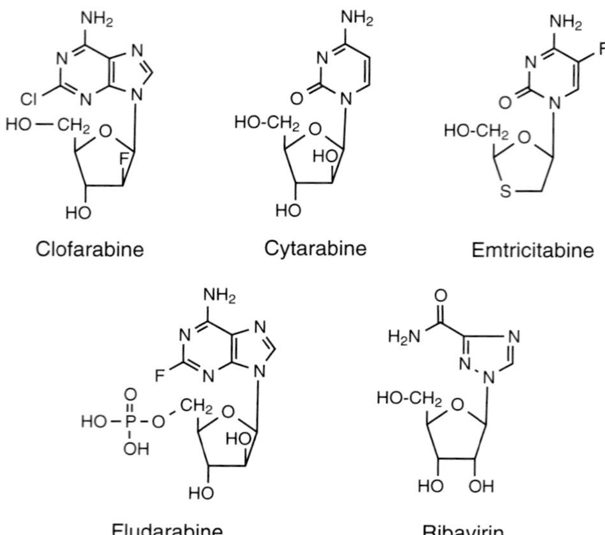

Figure 4.8 Drug substrates of nucleoside transporters.

primarily responsible for the hepatic uptake of bile acids, and this transporter has been demonstrated to transport some of the statins. Many drugs are also known to inhibit NTCP.[71] The bile salt export pump (BSEP) is likely the most notable bile acid transporter that interacts with drugs, as it has been shown that inhibitors of this transporter often lead to hepatotoxicity.[72] Recently, other transporters in the liver have also been recognized to be involved in bile acid–induced hepatotoxicity such as MRP3/4 and Ostα/Ostβ. These transporters are expressed on the basolateral membrane of the liver and their role is compensatory to BSEP inhibition in that bile acid accumulation/liver injury leads to their upregulation.[18,73] Many inhibitors of BSEP also inhibit these compensatory transporters, which further explains the resulting hepatotoxicity observed with these compounds.[74] There are also bile acid transporters in the intestine which are responsible for reabsorption of bile acids in the gut following their export by BSEP into the bile, and drugs can also interact with these transporters, both as substrates and inhibitors. Inhibition of the apical sodium-dependent bile acid transporter (ASBT) in the gut in particular has been postulated as potential therapy for hypercholesterolemia and diabetes by preventing the conservation of bile acids.[75]

EVALUATING TRANSPORTER EFFECTS IN VIVO

Many transporters share substrates with other transporters and with drug-metabolizing enzymes, making it difficult to attribute in vivo effects to a specific transporter. The use of probe substrates and specific inhibitors makes this identification easier, but these are not available for most transporters or may not be suitable for in vivo use. Knockout animals can be used to assess the effects of a specific transporter in vivo, whereas transfected cell lines or oocytes and specific silencing of a transporter using small interfering double-stranded RNA can be useful to assess effects in vitro. Assessment of the effects of transporter polymorphisms can be useful to allow some determination of a transporter's role in the disposition of a drug in humans. When evaluating the effects of drug transport on bioavailability, it can be difficult to attribute effects to transport in the intestine alone, as changes in both bioavailability and clearance can affect plasma concentrations after oral administration. It is necessary to assess administration of substrates and inhibitors both orally and intravenously to determine if transport primarily affects substrate bioavailability or systemic clearance. Often both parameters are affected by changes in transport because the same transporters are responsible for both processes. Significant effects on absorption cannot always be demonstrated with efflux transporter substrates in vivo. This can be due to the very high luminal concentrations of substrate causing transporter saturation and to the passive membrane permeability of these compounds. A lack of effect can also be due to shared transporter substrates, allowing compensatory transport by one transporter when another is inhibited.

EFFECT OF TRANSPORT ON DRUG PHARMACOKINETICS AND DRUG-DRUG INTERACTIONS

Intestinal Transport

The importance of transporter-mediated influx or efflux in the intestine depends primarily on two factors. The first is the contribution of transporter-mediated transport compared to the other mechanisms of drug passage across the gut wall. The second is drug concentration. Drug concentrations are generally much higher in the gut lumen compared to the systemic blood circulation due to a lower volume of distribution. This causes the concentration gradient driving diffusion to be very large but, more importantly, can lead to transporter saturation. This can result in low bioavailability due to saturation of influx transporters and nonlinearity in drug absorption. Transporter saturation can also aid in drug absorption in that high drug concentrations in the enterocyte can saturate efflux transporters. High drug concentrations in the gut also increase the risk of drug interactions affecting oral absorption of other drugs. The U.S. Food and Drug Administration–recommended Biopharmaceutics Classification System names solubility and permeability as determining factors of oral absorption,[76] factors which can be translated into effects on drug concentration (C) and nonsaturable transport (P) in the intestine. Considering these factors, the predicted effects of drug transporters on oral absorption are given in Figure 4.9.[77]

The polarized expression of relevant drug transporters in the intestine is illustrated in Figure 4.10. Clinical relevance of drug transport is determined not only by the presence of transporters on a biologic membrane but also by their relative expression. The transporters with highest intestinal expression include BCRP, PEPT1, P-gp, and

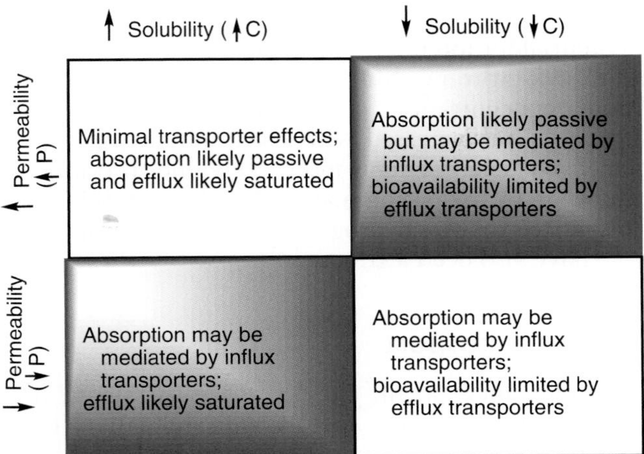

Figure 4.9 Role of transporters in drug absorption. High aqueous drug solubility will result in high luminal drug concentrations, allowing for possible transporter saturation. High permeability results in high passive diffusion, allowing these drugs to be orally absorbed without dependence on transporters. Adapted from Shugarts S, Benet LZ. The role of transporters in the pharmacokinetics of orally administered drugs. *Pharm Res.* 2009;26:2039-2054.

MCT1.[19,78] High expression of influx transporters, such as PEPT1 and MCT1, allows the use of these high-capacity transporters as a drug delivery mechanism. High expression of efflux transporters makes these transporters important in limiting drug bioavailability.

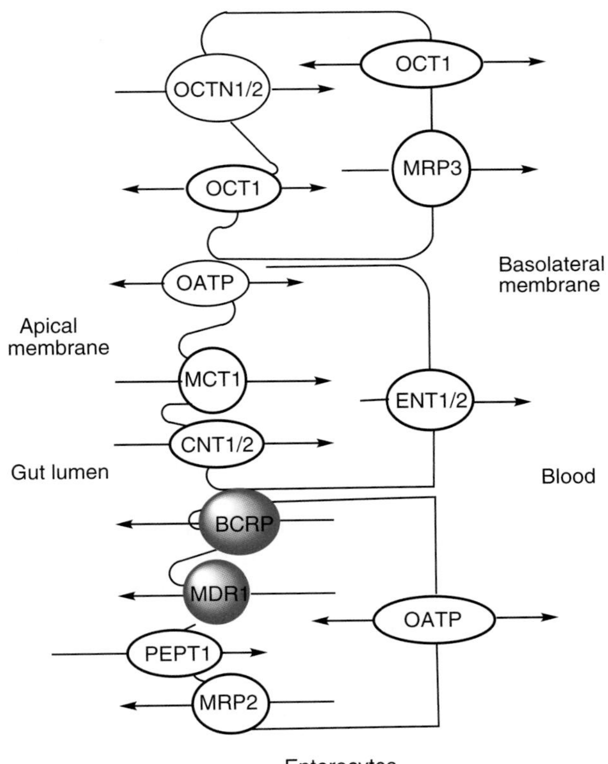

Figure 4.10 Polarized expression of drug transporters in the intestine. Transporters most relevant to drug disposition are shown in *red*.

Along with drug transporters, drug-metabolizing enzymes, including phase 1 and phase 2 enzymes, are present in the enterocytes forming the gut wall. First-pass metabolism in the gut can be a reason for low oral bioavailability. Transporters often share substrates with drug-metabolizing enzymes, and the intestine is one site in which substantial transport-metabolism interplay has been recognized. In particular, it has been noted that P-gp shares many substrates with the enzyme CYP3A4, and it is proposed that P-gp can prevent oral absorption through drug efflux and by facilitating drug metabolism by CYP3A4.[79] Effects on metabolism likely occur by multiple mechanisms, including decreasing intracellular substrate concentrations preventing saturation of metabolism, and by the cycling of substrates through the gut lumen and enterocytes, allowing enzymes such as CYP3A4 multiple opportunities to metabolize their substrates.[80] This interplay is depicted in Figure 4.11.

Efflux Transporters and Drug Bioavailability

Studies using specific P-gp inhibitors and Mdr1 knockout animals have demonstrated the importance of P-gp in the oral bioavailability of drugs, including HIV protease inhibitors, β-receptor antagonists, morphine, and many other therapeutic agents.[81] Many of the drug interactions in the intestine with P-gp or other efflux transporters involve inhibition of transport, resulting in increased bioavailability of the transporter substrate. Efflux transporters, specifically P-gp, may also be induced, resulting in decreased bioavailability (Table 4.5). Administration of P-gp inhibitors and inducers has demonstrated clinically significant effects on the bioavailability of P-gp substrates, including digoxin, paclitaxel, and dabigatran.[12,14]

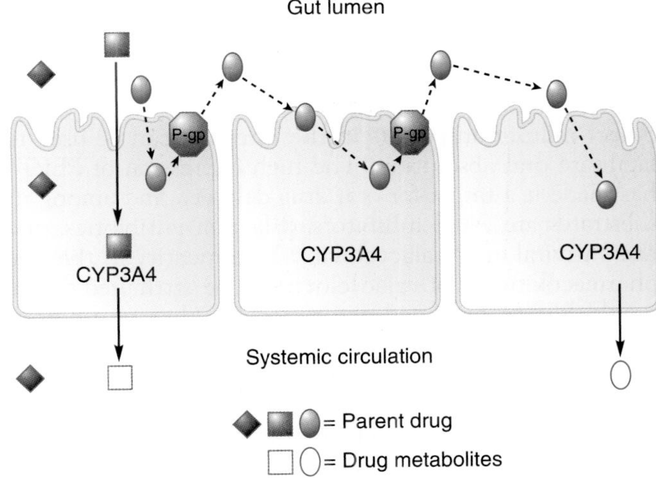

Figure 4.11 Transport-metabolism interplay in the intestine. Drugs may be orally absorbed without undergoing metabolic conversion. Drugs may undergo metabolism in the gut, and this may occur upon initial entry into the enterocyte or after cycling between the gut lumen and the enterocyte. P-gp facilitates CYP3A4 metabolism by decreasing intracellular substrate concentrations preventing enzyme saturation and by allowing the enzyme multiple opportunities for drug metabolism, as demonstrated by the molecule shown in red. Adapted from Benet LZ. The drug transporter-metabolism alliance: uncovering and defining the interplay. *Mol Pharm.* 2009;6:1631-1643.

Table 4.5 Nuclear Receptors Involved in Transporter Regulation

Nuclear Receptor or Transcription Factor	Agents That Act on Receptor	Transporters Affected
Pregnane X receptor (PXR)	Rifampin, cytokines	MDR1, MRP2, MRP3, OATP1B1
Constitutive androstane receptor (CAR)	Phenobarbital	MDR1, MRP2, MRP3, MRP4
Farnesoid X receptor (FXR)	Bile acids	MRP2, MRP1, OATP1B1, OATP1B3, NTCP, Ost$\alpha\beta$

Drug bioavailability can also be limited by BCRP. Administration of the P-gp/BCRP inhibitor elacridar increased the bioavailability of topotecan sixfold in Mdr1 knockout mice, and oral coadministration with elacridar has been shown to increase the bioavailability of topotecan in humans to almost 100%.[23,24] Similarly, oral coadministration of the statin rosuvastatin, a BCRP substrate, and the antivirals atazanavir/ritonavir, known to inhibit BCRP, significantly increased rosuvastatin exposure in humans, most likely due to inhibition of BCRP-mediated intestinal efflux and biliary secretion.[82] Polymorphisms in the *ABCG2* gene can also affect the plasma exposure of rosuvastatin and other BCRP substrates.

Influx Transporters and Drug Bioavailability

Select influx transporters in the intestine can be used to facilitate oral absorption. The high expression of PEPT1 has made it a target for oral drug delivery, and among its substrates are ACE inhibitors, β-lactam antibiotics, and the antiviral drug valacyclovir.[66] Nonlinearity in the oral pharmacokinetics of valacyclovir can be attributed to saturable PEPT1-mediated absorption.[83] Other transporters involved in oral drug delivery include OATPs and MCT1.[60]

Influx transporters can also be responsible for drug interactions in the intestine, although fewer drug interactions have been noted compared with efflux transporters. Specifically interactions have been attributed to OATP transport in the intestine. Originally, it was thought that OATP1A2 was the primary OATP expressed in the intestine; however, recent data indicate measurable expression of OATP2B1 with concurrent negligible OATP1A2 expression.[19] Decreased oral exposure of rosuvastatin was recently attributed to inhibition of OATP2B1 in the intestine by ronacaleret.[84] While this interaction was supported by inhibition of OATP2B1 by ronacaleret in vitro, recent data in CaCo-2 cells, a human colon carcinoma epithelial cell line, indicate OATP2B1 expression on the basolateral rather than apical membrane, leaving a potential for interaction with another transporter prior to rosuvastatin reaching the basolateral membrane.[85] Plasma concentrations of fexofenadine, another OATP substrate, are decreased with concomitant ingestion of grapefruit juice.[86] This is most likely due to transporter inhibition by the naringin and other flavonoids in grapefruit juice, to which drug interactions with intestinal P-gp have also been attributed.[87]

Hepatic Transport

As a clearance organ, the liver can eliminate drugs through two pathways, metabolism and biliary excretion. Uptake into the liver is necessary for both of these processes, and for hydrophilic drugs that are primarily ionized at blood pH, this is often a transporter-mediated process. Active transport is also necessary for biliary excretion, as diffusion of drugs into the bile is unlikely due to the low volume of the bile canaliculus resulting in high drug concentrations on the biliary side of the canalicular membrane. As with the intestine, there exists transporter-metabolism interplay in the liver because transporters regulate the distribution of drug substrates into the liver and therefore their access to drug-metabolizing enzymes. Just as the significance of a transporter on a drug's membrane permeability is determined by the contribution of that process to overall transport, uptake by transporters or by limited diffusion needs to be rate-limiting for uptake to be a significant factor in drug elimination. The intrinsic clearance of drugs in the liver has traditionally been thought of as simply the rate of metabolism, therefore:

$$Cl_{int} = Cl_{met}$$

i.e., the hepatic intrinsic clearance (Cl_{int}) can be defined as solely the intrinsic ability of the liver to metabolize a drug (metabolic clearance, Cl_{met}). It is now recognized that for drugs which undergo active uptake by drug transporters, multiple processes need to be incorporated to define its intrinsic clearance, namely those in the "extended clearance" equation:

$$Cl_{int} = Cl_{met/bile} \bullet \frac{Cl_{active} + Cl_{passive}}{Cl_{passive} + Cl_{met/bile}}$$

where $Cl_{met/bile}$ is the combined metabolic and biliary clearances and Cl_{active} and $Cl_{passive}$ represent the active transporter-mediated and passive diffusion clearances in the liver, respectively.[88] Cl_{int} can then be incorporated into a hepatic clearance model incorporating other physiologic parameters to derive the in vivo hepatic clearance from Cl_{int}.[89] The transporters facilitating both drug uptake and biliary excretion in the liver are depicted in Figure 4.12. As shown in the figure, while it is known that efflux transporters are present not only on the canalicular membrane but also on the sinusoidal membrane of hepatocytes, there is as of yet limited knowledge of the role or clinical relevance of these transporters in drug disposition or drug-drug interactions.

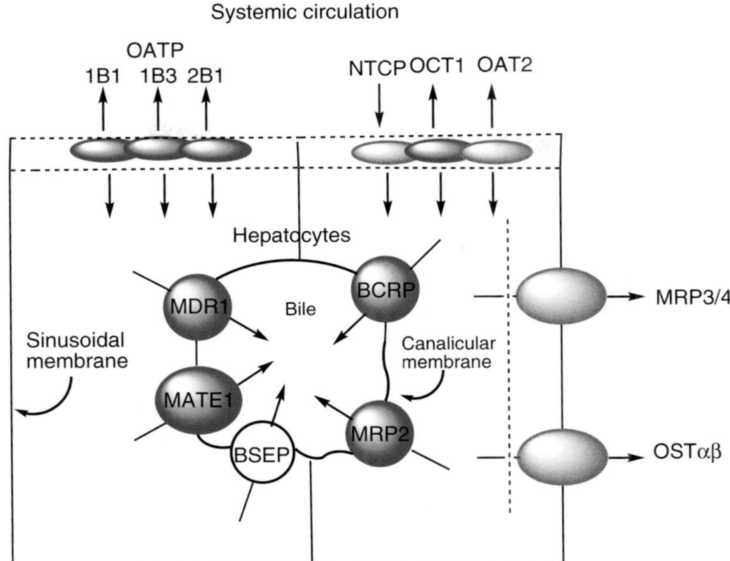

Figure 4.12 Drug transporter expression in hepatocytes. Transporters most relevant to drug disposition are shown in *red*.

Role of Transporters in Hepatic Clearance and Drug Interactions at the Sinusoidal Membrane

Of the transporters present on the sinusoidal membrane, the greatest number of drug-drug interactions has been demonstrated with the OATPs. One of the first interactions noted was the severalfold increase in cerivastatin plasma concentrations following gemfibrozil administration, resulting in severe cases of rhabdomyolysis.[90,91] This drug interaction was determined to be due to inhibition of OATP1B1 and CYP2C8 by gemfibrozil and its glucuronide metabolite and eventually contributed to cerivastatin being withdrawn from market.[91] Gemfibrozil increases the plasma AUC of other statins which undergo little metabolism (e.g., rosuvastatin), indicating the significance of OATP-mediated transport.[29,92] Similar effects on statin pharmacokinetics have been demonstrated with other OATP1B1 inhibitors, including cyclosporine and rifampin.[93-95] OATP-mediated hepatic uptake may not only relate to the pharmacokinetics of drugs, it can impact pharmacodynamics as well, given they allow the statins access to their site of action, the liver. Drug interactions resulting in OATP1B1 inhibition, and numerous polymorphisms in the *SLCO1B1* gene, demonstrate decreased clearance of statins as well as other OATP substrates, including repaglinide, methotrexate, and the active metabolite of irinotecan, SN-38.[29,96] While OATP-mediated transport put the concept of uptake rate-limited hepatic clearance on the map, more recently clinical relevance of other hepatic transporters has surfaced, specifically that of OCT1. Polymorphisms have been identified in the *SLC22A1* gene that have reduced uptake of OCT1 substrates.[39] Clinical studies have shown homozygous carriers of OCT1 variants with reduced function to affect the plasma exposure of sumatriptan, morphine, and 5HT-3 antagonists.[97-99] While metformin is not eliminated by metabolism or biliary clearance and therefore is cleared completely by the kidneys, OCT1-mediated uptake of metformin is another example of hepatic transporters having a role in pharmacodynamics. Carriers of reduced function *SLC22A1* variants have reduced response to metformin; a similar reduction has been observed with inhibition of OCT1 by verapamil.[100,101]

Role of Transporters in Biliary Drug Excretion and the Effect of Drugs on Canalicular Membrane Transport

It can be difficult to attribute clearance to biliary excretion in vivo, given that sampling bile is very technically challenging and, in the absence of this, drug excreted into bile ends up in the feces and is therefore indistinguishable from unabsorbed drug following oral absorption. Fecal drug amounts following IV administration can be evaluated and other methods for sampling drug in the duodenum and/or via noninvasive imaging methods are becoming useful. Accordingly, bile duct-cannulated mice, including transporter knockout mice, are often relied upon to identify this route and mechanism of elimination for drugs. Some of the first drug interactions discovered to affect biliary clearance of drugs in humans involved the ABC transporter P-gp. It was demonstrated that quinidine and verapamil, known P-gp inhibitors, significantly decreased the biliary clearance of digoxin, resulting in increased digoxin plasma concentrations.[13,102] P-gp efflux also has a role in the biliary excretion of doxorubicin, as demonstrated by an 80%-90% decrease in doxorubicin biliary clearance in Mdr1 knockout mice.[103] Fecal excretion is also a significant elimination pathway for doxorubicin in humans suggesting biliary clearance. MRP2 also mediates biliary excretion of doxorubicin and other therapeutic agents, including pravastatin and valsartan (Table 4.3).[104-106] MRP2 has a significant role in the biliary excretion of drug conjugates, resulting in their enterohepatic cycling. There is a clear in vivo drug-drug interaction between cyclosporine and mycophenolic acid, which has been attributed to inhibition of MRP2-mediated biliary secretion of the glucuronide conjugate leading to decreased hydrolysis of the conjugate in the intestinal tract and reabsorption of mycophenolic acid itself.[107] BCRP has a more significant role in the excretion of sulfate conjugates, along with its role in secreting unconjugated drugs. Decreased biliary excretion of acetaminophen sulfate and other sulfate conjugates has been reported in mice lacking Bcrp but not in those lacking Mdr2.[108,109] BCRP knockout or inhibition results in decreased biliary clearance of therapeutic agents in mice, including topotecan, nitrofurantoin, and ciprofloxacin.[24,25,110] In addition, polymorphisms in the *ABCG2* gene have been shown to correlate with increased response to rosuvastatin, which may be explained by increased concentrations in the liver, the site of action, due to decreased biliary excretion by BCRP, along with increased absorption.[32] As mentioned above efflux transporters MRP2 and BSEP are also primarily responsible for the biliary secretion of endogenous substances, and drug interactions may also interfere with these processes through inhibition of these transporters (Table 4.3).

Renal Transport

Renal clearance is mediated by three primary pathways: glomerular filtration, tubular secretion, and renal reabsorption. Small molecules that are not protein bound will be filtered at the glomerulus. Drugs that undergo glomerular filtration can have negligible renal clearance if they are sufficiently lipophilic to be passively reabsorbed from the tubular lumen back into systemic circulation. Drugs that undergo filtration and are hydrophilic or ionized will be excreted into the urine unless they are actively reabsorbed by transporters. Drugs can have extensive renal clearance (Cl_r), sometimes much greater than the glomerular filtration rate, if they undergo renal secretion. The following equation can be used to determine renal clearance considering the possibility of all three processes:

$$Cl_r = (GFR^* f_{up} + Cl_{rs})(1 - FR)$$

where GFR is the glomerular filtration rate; f_{up} is the fraction unbound in the plasma; Cl_{rs} is the clearance by renal secretion; and FR is the fraction of unchanged drug that is filtered and secreted in the urine, which is reabsorbed. Given that urine is a biological sample easily collected, renal clearance and the net contribution of active secretion or reabsorption are readily calculable; transporters are involved whenever active secretion or active reabsorption occur. Secretion and reabsorption require transport of drug across both apical and basolateral membranes, and the polarized expression of organic anion and organic cation transporters on both membranes allows directional transport of ionized substrates. The transporters responsible for active secretion and active reabsorption and their polarized expression in the kidney are illustrated in Figure 4.13.

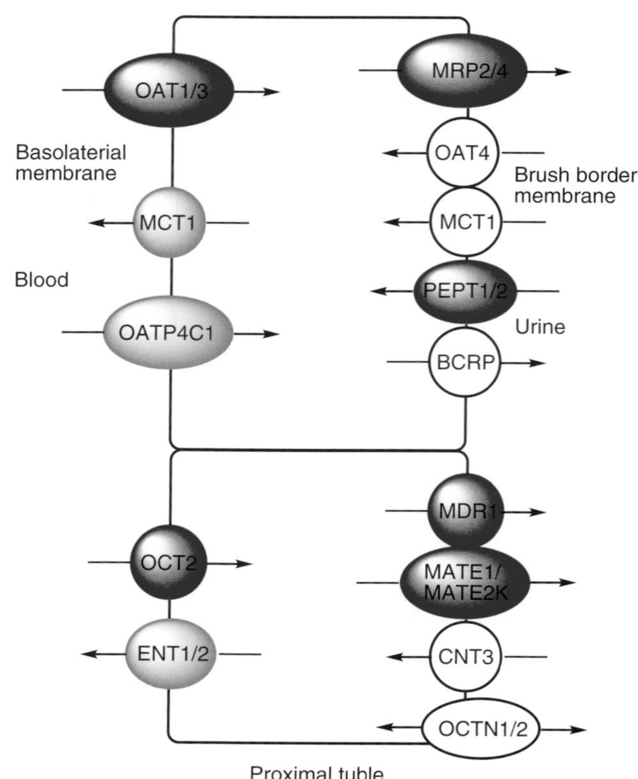

Figure 4.13 Drug transporter expression in the renal proximal tubule. Transporters most relevant to drug disposition are shown in *red*.

Renal Clearance of Anions

Tubular secretion of anions across the basolateral membrane is mediated primarily by OAT1 and OAT3. Substrates of these transporters include β-lactam antibiotics, nonsteroidal anti-inflammatory drugs, and many other anionic therapeutic agents (Table 4.3). Probenecid is a known inhibitor of OATs, and coadministration with OAT substrates leads to decreased renal clearance of these substrates. One of the most highly recognized transporter interactions is that between probenecid and penicillin derivatives, and coadministration of probenecid has been demonstrated to decrease the renal clearance of numerous drugs of this class, including piperacillin, nafcillin, ticarcillin, and others.[16] Inhibition of OAT transport by probenecid also causes decreased renal clearance of diuretics like furosemide and results in diminished diuretic effect due to decreased tubular drug concentrations.[111,112] OAT-mediated drug interactions affect renal secretion of many other OAT substrates including methotrexate, acyclovir, and zidovudine.[16] Secretion of anions across the renal brush border membrane is primarily mediated by MRP2 and MRP4. Probenecid is also an MRP2 inhibitor, and some of its effects on renal clearance can be due to combined inhibition of OATs and MRP2. MRP4 is present at similar levels to MRP2 in human kidney, and Mrp4 knockout mice display significant renal cell accumulation of the nucleotide phosphonates adefovir and tenofovir.[51,113] Additionally, case reports exist in which administration of MRP4 inhibitors have been associated with nephrotoxicity of tenofovir.[114] Interestingly, cidofovir does not appear to be transported by MRP4, and this may be a reason for the significant nephrotoxicity associated with this drug. These drugs are also OAT substrates, and OAT inhibition may have therapeutic potential for preventing renal accumulation and toxicity with these agents.[113]

RENAL CLEARANCE BY OCT2/MATE: CISPLATIN TOXICITY

The platinum agents are used clinically for treatment of a variety of cancers. Treatment with cisplatin has been limited by its adverse effects, including nephrotoxicity, ototoxicity, and neurotoxicity.[115] Transport by OCT2 has been attributed with facilitating cisplatin toxicity in the kidney, demonstrated by decreased nephrotoxicity with coadministration of OCT2 inhibitors and in Oct2 knockout animals.[116] Genetic polymorphism in OCT2 has also been correlated with decreased serum creatinine concentrations in patients undergoing cisplatin treatment, suggesting decreased nephrotoxicity.[43] Oxaliplatin, another OCT2 substrate, is not associated with severe nephrotoxicity. Oxaliplatin is efficiently transported by MATE1 and MATE2-K, allowing for secretion of this drug from tubule cells into the urine.[57] Cisplatin, a poor MATE substrate, has been demonstrated to accumulate in renal tubule cells.[117] Carboplatin, another platinum-based agent, is a substrate for neither OCT2 nor MATE transporters and, similarly to oxaliplatin, does not display nephrotoxicity.[57] It is apparent that the effects of cisplatin in the kidney can be attributed to OCT2-mediated influx followed by inefficient apical efflux, resulting in renal cell accumulation and toxicity. Recently, OCT2 was also found to be present in the cochlea, and Oct2 knockout prevented cisplatin-induced ototoxicity, along with reducing nephrotoxicity.[118] OCT2 inhibition represents a potentially clinically relevant therapy for the prevention of both toxicities during cisplatin therapy; however, selective inhibition of OCT2 over MATE1 is essential.

Renal Clearance of Cations

While not always true, renal secretion of cations generally involves transport across the basolateral membrane by OCT2 followed by transport across the brush border membrane by MATE1 or possibly P-gp. Cations can be substrates of OATs as well, and MATE1 can also be involved in the secretion of anions.[53] Metformin is a substrate of both OCT2 and MATE1, and drug interactions involving either or both of these transporters result in significant decreases in metformin renal clearance (Table 4.4).[40,119] As mentioned previously, inhibitor specificity is often, but not always, shared between OCT2 and MATEs. Genetic variants of both OCT2 and MATE1 have also been correlated with decreased metformin clearance and/or increased glucose-lowering effects with metformin treatment.[42,55,120] Platinum-based chemotherapeutic agents also use the OCT2/MATE transport system, and this transport is a factor in toxicity of these agents. A topic of great recent interest in drug development is the inhibition of OCT2 or MATEs by compounds leading to increased serum creatinine, due to its decreased active secretion.

RENAL TRANSPORTERS AND CREATININE CLEARANCE

Monitoring of endogenous creatinine clearance has traditionally been used as a surrogate for measurement of glomerular filtration rate (GFR) and kidney injury, given the negligible protein binding of creatinine and its complete excretion unchanged into urine. In recent years, however, it has been recognized that changes in serum creatinine and creatinine clearance can occur without changes in other biomarkers of renal injury or without change in other markers of GFR, such as iohexol or cystatin C. Creatinine has been shown to be taken up by cationic renal transporters OCT2, MATE1, and MATE-2K, and there are multiple clinical examples in which the administration of drugs that inhibit these transporters result in an elevation of serum creatinine or decrease in creatinine clearance.[121] Although it has been well documented that creatinine renal clearance is indeed higher than GFR, indicating that creatinine undergoes renal secretion, there is still controversy over which transporters are truly most important for this process in vivo. Recently creatinine has been determined a substrate of OAT2, with some reports indicating affinity for this transporter to be much greater than the cationic transporters; however, further clinical evidence is required to determine if inhibitors of OAT2 solely decrease creatinine renal secretion.[37,122]

Blood-Brain Barrier and Blood-Cerebrospinal Fluid Barrier Transport

The blood-brain barrier (BBB) serves an important protective function for the CNS and presents both structural and metabolic barriers for xenobiotic penetration into the brain. The endothelial cells of the BBB form tight junctions with minimal fenestrations, limiting BBB penetration to drug molecules that are capable of transcellular diffusion. For entry of polar or charged essential nutrients such as amino acids and glucose, transport processes are necessary. Transporters present on the BBB for this function have been exploited to facilitate brain penetration of agents like levodopa, one of the most commonly used agents in Parkinson's disease, which is transported into the brain by the L-type amino acid transporter (LAT) 1.[123] MCT1 is also expressed at the BBB, and along with its role in the renal reabsorption of GHB, it is responsible for distribution of GHB into the brain, where it elicits its euphoric effects.[124] Other influx transporters expressed at the BBB include ENTs and OCTs, which have known drug substrates and may therefore be involved in brain distribution of these drugs.[38] It should be noted that drug concentrations in the brain are not easily measured, and changes in brain concentrations do not generally result in any changes in plasma concentrations of the drug, making it difficult to assess the in vivo importance of transporters at the BBB. However, preclinical knockout models are particularly useful in this case, although extrapolation to humans is uncertain as knockout models represent an extreme scenario. These models have aided in assigning a clear limitation of brain penetration to transport by efflux transporters expressed at the BBB, including P-gp, BCRP, and MRPs. Mdr1 knockout mice display substantially higher brain/plasma concentration ratios for many P-gp substrates, with over 10-fold increases exhibited for digoxin, paclitaxel, and protease inhibitors compared to wild-type animals.[125,126] Inhibition of P-gp has been used as a strategy to increase BBB penetration and has been demonstrated to be effective in animal models.[126,127] The use of P-gp inhibitors in studies with human subjects shows similar, but much more modest, effects on brain penetration. This decreased effect is due in part to the lower inhibitor concentrations reached at doses used in human subjects.[128] Bcrp knockout animals have demonstrated the ability of this efflux transporter to limit brain penetration of drugs such as sorafenib.[129] Many anticancer drugs are co-substrates for P-gp and BCRP, and knockout of both transporters has demonstrated synergistic effects on brain accumulation of these drugs.[26,129,130] The use of co-inhibitors represents a potential strategy for improving treatment of brain tumors with these agents.[127] There are various influx and efflux transporters present on the blood-cerebrospinal fluid barrier (BCSFB) as well, including P-gp and MCT1, as well as others not present at the BBB, such as PEPT2.[38] Given that the CSF is occasionally sampled in clinical studies as a surrogate for the rest of the CNS, it is important to recognize there are differences in transporter expression at the BBB and the BCSFB, and even those transporters expressed on both barriers may be present to different extents and may serve different functions. For example, for P-gp substrates, it has been shown that P-gp serves to keep drug out of the brain at the BBB; however, it also pumps drug into the CSF, resulting in a disparity in the CSF-to-plasma and brain-to-plasma ratios for P-gp substrates.[38,131,132]

Regulation of Transporters and Interindividual Variability

While inherent polymorphisms in transporter genes can be one factor in the interindividual variability of transporter substrate pharmacokinetics, other factors such as transcriptional regulation of transporters, effects mediated by nuclear receptors, can also contribute. While there is little evidence of in vivo induction with most transporters, there are nuclear receptors implicated to affect transporter expression in vitro or in human tissue samples (Table 4.5).[133,134] One exception among these is P-gp, for which there are multiple examples of in vivo drug-drug interactions as a result of induction. Rifampin, a strong agonist of the nuclear receptor pregnane X (PXR), induces the expression of several enzymes and transporters including CYP3A4 and MDR1. During rifampin treatment, decreased drug exposure is observed with CYP3A4/MDR1 co-substrates such as cyclosporine, calcium channel blockers, and chemotherapeutic agents, leading to a complete loss of response for some of these substrates.[135,136] Rifampin and other PXR agonists also result in interactions with P-gp substrates that are not metabolized by CYP3A4, such as digoxin, dabigatran, talinolol, and fexofenadine, demonstrating the in vivo relevance of P-gp induction.[14,137-139] There also exists some in vitro and in vivo evidence for induction of OATPs by rifampin.[140-142] (Note that inhibitor vs. inductive effects of rifampin can be determined with single- and multiple-dose rifampin administration, respectively.) Rifampin also increased the effect of metformin on blood glucose, suggesting induction of OCT1 in the liver as well.[143] While there is no in vitro evidence to support rifampin effects on renal transporters, renal secretion of metformin also increased in this study, suggesting induction of OCT2 or MATE1. While effects at nuclear receptors may be mediated by concomitant drugs, interesting effects on transporter and enzyme regulation also occur in the presence of disease states. As mentioned above, during cholestasis hepatic transporter expression changes facilitate bile acid secretion into the plasma by MRPs and Ostαβ and decrease secretion into the bile by MRP2 and BSEP. This change in transporter function has been attributed to the effect of bile acids on the farnesoid X receptor (FXR), as well as PXR, causing upregulation of sinusoidal efflux transporters and downregulation of those at the canalicular membrane.[144] Changes in enzyme and transporter expression have also been demonstrated in other disease states, including cancer, chronic renal failure, inflammation, and epilepsy, which display considerable interindividual variability.[145-147] Current literature supports the involvement of select nuclear receptors in the regulation of affected proteins in some of these conditions.[145] Along with changes in gene expression or structure, transporter function can also be affected by posttranslational modifications, such as glycosylation or phosphorylation, which can lead to rapid changes in transporter activity.[70] Understanding the role of these posttranscriptional modifications in interindividual variability is ongoing, along with regulatory effects with the aforementioned diseases, and the mechanisms by which transporter functions are altered will aid in the accurate dosing of drugs in patient populations.

Conclusions

Transporters have important roles in the pharmacokinetics of many therapeutic agents. Transport can result in drug-drug interactions, nonlinear pharmacokinetics, and interindividual variability. Changes in transporter function can translate into drug toxicity, although transporter interactions also have the potential to be beneficial for drug therapy by increasing bioavailability or decreasing clearance. Application of transport principles and understanding the effects of transport on drug substrate concentrations promote the safe and effective use of therapeutic agents. Further investigation of transporter effects in vivo and mechanisms in vitro is expected to reveal additional significant effects of drug transporters on drug disposition.

Acknowledgment

Supported in part by National Institutes of Health Grant DA 023223 for MEM.

REFERENCES

1. Hoffmann U, Kroemer HK. The ABC transporters MDR1 and MRP2: multiple functions in disposition of xenobiotics and drug resistance. *Drug Metab Rev*. 2004;36:669-701.
2. Zhou SF. Structure, function and regulation of P-glycoprotein and its clinical relevance in drug disposition. *Xenobiotica*. 2008;38:802-832.
3. Liu H, Ma Z, Wu B. Structure-activity relationships and in silico models of P-glycoprotein (ABCB1) inhibitors. *Xenobiotica*. 2013;43:1018-1026.
4. Giacomini KM, Huang SM, Tweedie DJ, et al. Membrane transporters in drug development. *Nat Rev Drug Discov*. 2010;9:215-236.
5. Chan LM, Lowes S, Hirst BH. The ABCs of drug transport in intestine and liver: efflux proteins limiting drug absorption and bioavailability. *Eur J Pharm Sci*. 2004;21:25-51.
6. Rengelshausen J, Goggelmann C, Burhenne J, et al. Contribution of increased oral bioavailability and reduced nonglomerular renal clearance of digoxin to the digoxin-clarithromycin interaction. *Br J Clin Pharmacol*. 2003;56:32-38.
7. Ding R, Tayrouz Y, Riedel KD, et al. Substantial pharmacokinetic interaction between digoxin and ritonavir in healthy volunteers. *Clin Pharmacol Ther*. 2004;76:73-84.
8. Hutson JR, Koren G, Matthews SG. Placental P-glycoprotein and breast cancer resistance protein: influence of polymorphisms on fetal drug exposure and physiology. *Placenta*. 2010;31:351-357.
9. Joshi P, Vishwakarma RA, Bharate SB. Natural alkaloids as P-gp inhibitors for multidrug resistance reversal in cancer. *Eur J Med Chem*. 2017;138:273-292.
10. Wolking S, Schaeffeler E, Lerche H, et al. Impact of genetic p-olymorphisms of ABCB1 (MDR1, P-glycoprotein) on drug disposition and potential clinical implications: update of the literature. *Clin Pharmacokinet*. 2015;54:709-735.
11. Dorian P, Strauss M, Cardella C, et al. Digoxin-cyclosporine interaction: severe digitalis toxicity after cyclosporine treatment. *Clin Invest Med*. 1988;11:108-112.
12. Koren G, Woodland C, Ito S. Toxic digoxin-drug interactions: the major role of renal P-glycoprotein. *Vet Hum Toxicol*. 1998;40:45-46.
13. Hedman A, Angelin B, Arvidsson A, et al. Digoxin-verapamil interaction: reduction of biliary but not renal digoxin clearance in humans. *Clin Pharmacol Ther*. 1991;49:256-262.
14. Greiner B, Eichelbaum M, Fritz P, et al. The role of intestinal P-glycoprotein in the interaction of digoxin and rifampin. *J Clin Invest*. 1999;104:147-153.
15. Schinkel AH, Jonker JW. Mammalian drug efflux transporters of the ATP binding cassette (ABC) family: an overview. *Adv Drug Deliv Rev*. 2003;55:3-29.
16. Masereeuw R, Russel FG. Therapeutic implications of renal anionic drug transporters. *Pharmacol Ther*. 2010;126:200-216.
17. Keppler D. The roles of MRP2, MRP3, OATP1B1, and OATP1B3 in conjugated hyperbilirubinemia. *Drug Metab Dispos*. 2014;42:561-565.
18. Scheffer GL, Kool M, de Haas M, et al. Tissue distribution and induction of human multidrug resistant protein 3. *Lab Invest*. 2002;82:193-201.
19. Drozdzik M, Groer C, Penski J, et al. Protein abundance of clinically relevant multidrug transporters along the entire length of the human intestine. *Mol Pharm*. 2014;11:3547-3555.
20. Kock K, Ferslew BC, Netterberg I, et al. Risk factors for development of cholestatic drug-induced liver injury: inhibition of hepatic basolateral bile acid transporters multidrug resistance-associated proteins 3 and 4. *Drug Metab Dispos*. 2014;42:665-674.
21. Keppler D. Multidrug resistance proteins (MRPs, ABCCs): importance for pathophysiology and drug therapy. *Handb Exp Pharmacol*. 2011:299-323.
22. Mao Q, Unadkat JD. Role of the breast cancer resistance protein (BCRP/ABCG2) in drug transport–an update. *AAPS J*. 2015;17:65-82.
23. Kruijtzer CM, Beijnen JH, Rosing H, et al. Increased oral bioavailability of topotecan in combination with the breast cancer resistance protein and P-glycoprotein inhibitor GF120918. *J Clin Oncol*. 2002;20:2943-2950.
24. Jonker JW, Smit JW, Brinkhuis RF, et al. Role of breast cancer resistance protein in the bioavailability and fetal penetration of topotecan. *J Natl Cancer Inst*. 2000;92:1651-1656.
25. Merino G, Jonker JW, Wagenaar E, et al. The breast cancer resistance protein (BCRP/ABCG2) affects pharmacokinetics, hepatobiliary excretion, and milk secretion of the antibiotic nitrofurantoin. *Mol Pharmacol*. 2005;67:1758-1764.
26. Kodaira H, Kusuhara H, Ushiki J, et al. Kinetic analysis of the cooperation of P-glycoprotein (P-gp/Abcb1) and breast cancer resistance protein (Bcrp/Abcg2) in limiting the brain and testis penetration of erlotinib, flavopiridol, and mitoxantrone. *J Pharmacol Exp Ther*. 2010;333:788-796.
27. Taguchi T, Masuo Y, Kogi T, et al. Characterization of long-lasting oatp inhibition by typical inhibitor cyclosporine A and in vitro-in vivo discrepancy in its drug interaction potential in rats. *J Pharm Sci*. 2016;105:2231-2239.
28. Shitara Y, Sugiyama Y. Preincubation-dependent and long-lasting inhibition of organic anion transporting polypeptide (OATP) and its impact on drug-drug interactions. *Pharmacol Ther*. 2017;177:67-80.
29. Kalliokoski A, Niemi M. Impact of OATP transporters on pharmacokinetics. *Br J Pharmacol*. 2009;158:693-705.
30. Group SC, Link E, Parish S, et al. SLCO1B1 variants and statin-induced myopathy–a genomewide study. *N Engl J Med*. 2008;359:789-799.
31. Kim TE, Shin D, Gu N, et al. The effect of genetic polymorphisms in SLCO2B1 on the lipid-lowering efficacy of rosuvastatin in healthy adults with elevated low-density lipoprotein. *Basic Clin Pharmacol Toxicol*. 2017;121:195-201.
32. Lee HK, Hu M, Lui S, et al. Effects of polymorphisms in ABCG2, SLCO1B1, SLC10A1 and CYP2C9/19 on plasma concentrations of rosuvastatin and lipid response in Chinese patients. *Pharmacogenomics*. 2013;14:1283-1294.
33. DeGorter MK, Tirona RG, Schwarz UI, et al. Clinical and pharmacogenetic predictors of circulating atorvastatin and rosuvastatin concentrations in routine clinical care. *Circ Cardiovasc Genet*. 2013;6:400-408.
34. Ishiguro N, Maeda K, Kishimoto W, et al. Predominant contribution of OATP1B3 to the hepatic uptake of telmisartan, an angiotensin II receptor antagonist, in humans. *Drug Metab Dispos*. 2006;34:1109-1115.
35. Chu XY, Bleasby K, Yabut J, et al. Transport of the dipeptidyl peptidase-4 inhibitor sitagliptin by human organic anion transporter 3, organic anion transporting polypeptide 4C1, and multidrug resistance P-glycoprotein. *J Pharmacol Exp Ther*. 2007;321:673-683.
36. Ekaratanawong S, Anzai N, Jutabha P, et al. Human organic anion transporter 4 is a renal apical organic anion/dicarboxylate exchanger in the proximal tubules. *J Pharmacol Sci*. 2004;94:297-304.
37. Shen H, Liu T, Morse BL, et al. Characterization of organic anion transporter 2 (SLC22A7): a highly efficient transporter for creatinine and species-dependent renal tubular expression. *Drug Metab Dispos*. 2015;43:984-993.
38. Morris ME, Rodriguez-Cruz V, Felmlee MA. SLC and ABC transporters: expression, localization, and species differences at the blood-brain and the blood-cerebrospinal fluid barriers. *AAPS J*. 2017;19:1317-1331.
39. Lozano E, Herraez E, Briz O, et al. Role of the plasma membrane transporter of organic cations OCT1 and its genetic variants in modern liver pharmacology. *Biomed Res Int*. 2013;2013:692071.
40. Somogyi A, Stockley C, Keal J, et al. Reduction of metformin renal tubular secretion by cimetidine in man. *Br J Clin Pharmacol*. 1987;23:545-551.
41. Song IS, Shin HJ, Shim EJ, et al. Genetic variants of the organic cation transporter 2 influence the disposition of metformin. *Clin Pharmacol Ther*. 2008;84:559-562.

42. Hou W, Zhang D, Lu W, et al. Polymorphism of organic cation transporter 2 improves glucose-lowering effect of metformin via influencing its pharmacokinetics in Chinese type 2 diabetic patients. *Mol Diagn Ther*. 2015;19:25-33.
43. Filipski KK, Mathijssen RH, Mikkelsen TS, et al. Contribution of organic cation transporter 2 (OCT2) to cisplatin-induced nephrotoxicity. *Clin Pharmacol Ther*. 2009;86:396-402.
44. Ganapathy V, Prasad PD. Role of transporters in placental transfer of drugs. *Toxicol Appl Pharmacol*. 2005;207:381-387.
45. Ciarimboli G. Organic cation transporters. *Xenobiotica*. 2008;38:936-971.
46. Koepsell H, Lips K, Volk C. Polyspecific organic cation transporters: structure, function, physiological roles, and biopharmaceutical implications. *Pharm Res*. 2007;24:1227-1251.
47. Tamai I. Pharmacological and pathophysiological roles of carnitine/organic cation transporters (OCTNs: SLC22A4, SLC22A5 and Slc22a21). *Biopharm Drug Dispos*. 2013;34:29-44.
48. Wu SP, Shyu MK, Liou HH, et al. Interaction between anticonvulsants and human placental carnitine transporter. *Epilepsia*. 2004;45:204-210.
49. Tein I. Carnitine transport: pathophysiology and metabolism of known molecular defects. *J Inherit Metab Dis*. 2003;26:147-169.
50. Nakanishi T, Hasegawa Y, Haruta T, et al. In vivo evidence of organic cation transporter-mediated tracheal accumulation of the anticholinergic agent ipratropium in mice. *J Pharm Sci*. 2013;102:3373-3381.
51. Prasad B, Johnson K, Billington S, et al. Abundance of drug transporters in the human kidney cortex as quantified by quantitative targeted proteomics. *Drug Metab Dispos*. 2016;44:1920-1924.
52. Tsuda M, Terada T, Mizuno T, et al. Targeted disruption of the multidrug and toxin extrusion 1 (mate1) gene in mice reduces renal secretion of metformin. *Mol Pharmacol*. 2009;75:1280-1286.
53. Nies AT, Damme K, Kruck S, et al. Structure and function of multidrug and toxin extrusion proteins (MATEs) and their relevance to drug therapy and personalized medicine. *Arch Toxicol*. 2016;90:1555-1584.
54. Hume WE, Shingaki T, Takashima T, et al. The synthesis and biodistribution of [(11)C]metformin as a PET probe to study hepatobiliary transport mediated by the multi-drug and toxin extrusion transporter 1 (MATE1) in vivo. *Bioorg Med Chem*. 2013;21:7584-7590.
55. Stocker SL, Morrissey KM, Yee SW, et al. The effect of novel promoter variants in MATE1 and MATE2 on the pharmacokinetics and pharmacodynamics of metformin. *Clin Pharmacol Ther*. 2013;93:186-194.
56. Nies AT, Koepsell H, Damme K, et al. Organic cation transporters (OCTs, MATEs), in vitro and in vivo evidence for the importance in drug therapy. *Handb Exp Pharmacol*. 2011:105-167.
57. Yonezawa A, Inui K. Organic cation transporter OCT/SLC22A and H(+)/organic cation antiporter MATE/SLC47A are key molecules for nephrotoxicity of platinum agents. *Biochem Pharmacol*. 2011;81:563-568.
58. Tanihara Y, Masuda S, Sato T, et al. Substrate specificity of MATE1 and MATE2-K, human multidrug and toxin extrusions/H(+)-organic cation antiporters. *Biochem Pharmacol*. 2007;74:359-371.
59. Merezhinskaya N, Fishbein WN. Monocarboxylate transporters: past, present, and future. *Histol Histopathol*. 2009;24:243-264.
60. Varma MV, Ambler CM, Ullah M, et al. Targeting intestinal transporters for optimizing oral drug absorption. *Curr Drug Metab*. 2010;11:730-742.
61. Kennedy KM, Dewhirst MW. Tumor metabolism of lactate: the influence and therapeutic potential for MCT and CD147 regulation. *Future Oncol*. 2010;6:127-148.
62. Morris ME, Hu K, Wang Q. Renal clearance of gamma-hydroxybutyric acid in rats: increasing renal elimination as a detoxification strategy. *J Pharmacol Exp Ther*. 2005;313:1194-1202.
63. Morris ME, Morse BL, Baciewicz GJ, et al. Monocarboxylate transporter inhibition with osmotic diuresis increases gamma-hydroxybutyrate renal elimination in humans: a proof-of-concept study. *J Clin Toxicol*. 2011;1:1000105.
64. Jones RS, Morris ME. Monocarboxylate transporters: therapeutic targets and prognostic factors in disease. *Clin Pharmacol Ther*. 2016;100:454-463.
65. Cundy KC, Sastry S, Luo W, et al. Clinical pharmacokinetics of XP13512, a novel transported prodrug of gabapentin. *J Clin Pharmacol*. 2008;48:1378-1388.
66. Rubio-Aliaga I, Daniel H. Peptide transporters and their roles in physiological processes and drug disposition. *Xenobiotica*. 2008;38:1022-1042.
67. Herrera-Ruiz D, Wang Q, Gudmundsson OS, et al. Spatial expression patterns of peptide transporters in the human and rat gastrointestinal tracts, Caco-2 in vitro cell culture model, and multiple human tissues. *AAPS PharmSci*. 2001;3:E9.
68. Huber-Ruano I, Pastor-Anglada M. Transport of nucleoside analogs across the plasma membrane: a clue to understanding drug-induced cytotoxicity. *Curr Drug Metab*. 2009;10:347-358.
69. Endres CJ, Moss AM, Govindarajan R, et al. The role of nucleoside transporters in the erythrocyte disposition and oral absorption of ribavirin in the wild-type and equilibrative nucleoside transporter 1−/− mice. *J Pharmacol Exp Ther*. 2009;331:287-296.
70. Stieger B. The role of the sodium-taurocholate cotransporting polypeptide (NTCP) and of the bile salt export pump (BSEP) in physiology and pathophysiology of bile formation. *Handb Exp Pharmacol*. 2011:205-259.
71. Dong Z, Ekins S, Polli JE. Structure-activity relationship for FDA approved drugs as inhibitors of the human sodium taurocholate cotransporting polypeptide (NTCP). *Mol Pharm*. 2013;10:1008-1019.
72. Dawson S, Stahl S, Paul N, et al. In vitro inhibition of the bile salt export pump correlates with risk of cholestatic drug-induced liver injury in humans. *Drug Metab Dispos*. 2012;40:130-138.
73. Schaffner CA, Mwinyi J, Gai Z, et al. The organic solute transporters alpha and beta are induced by hypoxia in human hepatocytes. *Liver Int*. 2015;35:1152-1161.
74. Morgan RE, van Staden CJ, Chen Y, et al. A multifactorial approach to hepatobiliary transporter assessment enables improved therapeutic compound development. *Toxicol Sci*. 2013;136:216-241.
75. Chen L, Yao X, Young A, et al. Inhibition of apical sodium-dependent bile acid transporter as a novel treatment for diabetes. *Am J Physiol Endocrinol Metab*. 2012;302:E68-E76.
76. Amidon GL, Lennernas H, Shah VP, et al. A theoretical basis for a biopharmaceutic drug classification: the correlation of in vitro drug product dissolution and in vivo bioavailability. *Pharm Res*. 1995;12:413-420.
77. Shugarts S, Benet LZ. The role of transporters in the pharmacokinetics of orally administered drugs. *Pharm Res*. 2009;26:2039-2054.
78. Englund G, Rorsman F, Ronnblom A, et al. Regional levels of drug transporters along the human intestinal tract: co-expression of ABC and SLC transporters and comparison with Caco-2 cells. *Eur J Pharm Sci*. 2006;29:269-277.
79. Benet LZ. The drug transporter-metabolism alliance: uncovering and defining the interplay. *Mol Pharm*. 2009;6:1631-1643.
80. Shi S, Li Y. Interplay of drug-metabolizing enzymes and transporters in drug absorption and disposition. *Curr Drug Metab*. 2014;15:915-941.
81. Mealey KL. Therapeutic implications of the MDR-1 gene. *J Vet Pharmacol Ther*. 2004;27:257-264.
82. Busti AJ, Bain AM, Hall RG II, et al. Effects of atazanavir/ritonavir or fosamprenavir/ritonavir on the pharmacokinetics of rosuvastatin. *J Cardiovasc Pharmacol*. 2008;51:605-610.
83. Bolger MB, Lukacova V, Woltosz WS. Simulations of the nonlinear dose dependence for substrates of influx and efflux transporters in the human intestine. *AAPS J*. 2009;11:353-363.

84. Johnson M, Patel D, Matheny C, et al. Inhibition of intestinal OATP2B1 by the calcium receptor antagonist ronacaleret results in a significant drug-drug interaction by causing a 2-fold decrease in exposure of rosuvastatin. *Drug Metab Dispos*. 2017;45:27-34.
85. Keiser M, Kaltheuner L, Wildberg C, et al. The organic anion-transporting peptide 2B1 is localized in the basolateral membrane of the human jejunum and Caco-2 monolayers. *J Pharm Sci*. 2017;106:2657-2663.
86. Dresser GK, Kim RB, Bailey DG. Effect of grapefruit juice volume on the reduction of fexofenadine bioavailability: possible role of organic anion transporting polypeptides. *Clin Pharmacol Ther*. 2005;77:170-177.
87. Shirasaka Y, Suzuki K, Nakanishi T, et al. Differential effect of grapefruit juice on intestinal absorption of statins due to inhibition of organic anion transporting polypeptide and/or P-glycoprotein. *J Pharm Sci*. 2011;100:3843-3853.
88. Varma MV, Steyn SJ, Allerton C, et al. Predicting clearance mechanism in drug discovery: extended clearance classification system (ECCS). *Pharm Res*. 2015;32:3785-3802.
89. Zuegge J, Schneider G, Coassolo P, et al. Prediction of hepatic metabolic clearance: comparison and assessment of prediction models. *Clin Pharmacokinet*. 2001;40:553-563.
90. Backman JT, Kyrklund C, Neuvonen M, et al. Gemfibrozil greatly increases plasma concentrations of cerivastatin. *Clin Pharmacol Ther*. 2002;72:685-691.
91. Shitara Y, Hirano M, Sato H, et al. Gemfibrozil and its glucuronide inhibit the organic anion transporting polypeptide 2 (OATP2/OATP1B1:SLC21A6)-mediated hepatic uptake and CYP2C8-mediated metabolism of cerivastatin: analysis of the mechanism of the clinically relevant drug-drug interaction between cerivastatin and gemfibrozil. *J Pharmacol Exp Ther*. 2004;311:228-236.
92. Schneck DW, Birmingham BK, Zalikowski JA, et al. The effect of gemfibrozil on the pharmacokinetics of rosuvastatin. *Clin Pharmacol Ther*. 2004;75:455-463.
93. Kostapanos MS, Milionis HJ, Elisaf MS. Rosuvastatin-associated adverse effects and drug-drug interactions in the clinical setting of dyslipidemia. *Am J Cardiovasc Drugs*. 2010;10:11-28.
94. Neuvonen PJ, Niemi M, Backman JT. Drug interactions with lipid-lowering drugs: mechanisms and clinical relevance. *Clin Pharmacol Ther*. 2006;80:565-581.
95. Lau YY, Huang Y, Frassetto L, et al. Effect of OATP1B transporter inhibition on the pharmacokinetics of atorvastatin in healthy volunteers. *Clin Pharmacol Ther*. 2007;81:194-204.
96. Fahrmayr C, Fromm MF, Konig J. Hepatic OATP and OCT uptake transporters: their role for drug-drug interactions and pharmacogenetic aspects. *Drug Metab Rev*. 2010;42:380-401.
97. Matthaei J, Kuron D, Faltraco F, et al. OCT1 mediates hepatic uptake of sumatriptan and loss-of-function OCT1 polymorphisms affect sumatriptan pharmacokinetics. *Clin Pharmacol Ther*. 2016;99:633-641.
98. Tzvetkov MV, Saadatmand AR, Bokelmann K, et al. Effects of OCT1 polymorphisms on the cellular uptake, plasma concentrations and efficacy of the 5-HT(3) antagonists tropisetron and ondansetron. *Pharmacogenomics J*. 2012;12:22-29.
99. Tzvetkov MV, dos Santos Pereira JN, Meineke I, et al. Morphine is a substrate of the organic cation transporter OCT1 and polymorphisms in OCT1 gene affect morphine pharmacokinetics after codeine administration. *Biochem Pharmacol*. 2013;86:666-678.
100. Shu Y, Sheardown SA, Brown C, et al. Effect of genetic variation in the organic cation transporter 1 (OCT1) on metformin action. *J Clin Invest*. 2007;117:1422-1431.
101. Cho SK, Kim CO, Park ES, et al. Verapamil decreases the glucose-lowering effect of metformin in healthy volunteers. *Br J Clin Pharmacol*. 2014;78:1426-1432.
102. Angelin B, Arvidsson A, Dahlqvist R, et al. Quinidine reduces biliary clearance of digoxin in man. *Eur J Clin Invest*. 1987;17:262-265.
103. van Asperen J, van Tellingen O, Beijnen JH. The role of mdr1a P-glycoprotein in the biliary and intestinal secretion of doxorubicin and vinblastine in mice. *Drug Metab Dispos*. 2000;28:264-267.
104. Vlaming ML, Mohrmann K, Wagenaar E, et al. Carcinogen and anticancer drug transport by Mrp2 in vivo: studies using Mrp2 (Abcc2) knockout mice. *J Pharmacol Exp Ther*. 2006;318:319-327.
105. Yamazaki M, Akiyama S, Ni'inuma K, et al. Biliary excretion of pravastatin in rats: contribution of the excretion pathway mediated by canalicular multispecific organic anion transporter. *Drug Metab Dispos*. 1997;25:1123-1129.
106. Yamashiro W, Maeda K, Hirouchi M, et al. Involvement of transporters in the hepatic uptake and biliary excretion of valsartan, a selective antagonist of the angiotensin II AT1-receptor, in humans. *Drug Metab Dispos*. 2006;34:1247-1254.
107. Kuypers DR, Ekberg H, Grinyo J, et al. Mycophenolic acid exposure after administration of mycophenolate mofetil in the presence and absence of cyclosporin in renal transplant recipients. *Clin Pharmacokinet*. 2009;48:329-341.
108. Zamek-Gliszczynski MJ, Nezasa K, Tian X, et al. The important role of Bcrp (Abcg2) in the biliary excretion of sulfate and glucuronide metabolites of acetaminophen, 4-methylumbelliferone, and harmol in mice. *Mol Pharmacol*. 2006;70:2127-2133.
109. Chen C, Hennig GE, Manautou JE. Hepatobiliary excretion of acetaminophen glutathione conjugate and its derivatives in transport-deficient (TR-) hyperbilirubinemic rats. *Drug Metab Dispos*. 2003;31:798-804.
110. Ando T, Kusuhara H, Merino G, et al. Involvement of breast cancer resistance protein (ABCG2) in the biliary excretion mechanism of fluoroquinolones. *Drug Metab Dispos*. 2007;35:1873-1879.
111. Walshaw PE, McCauley FA, Wilson TW. Diuretic and non-diuretic actions of furosemide: effects of probenecid. *Clin Invest Med*. 1992;15:82-87.
112. Honari J, Blair AD, Cutler RE. Effects of probenecid on furosemide kinetics and natriuresis in man. *Clin Pharmacol Ther*. 1977;22:395-401.
113. Imaoka T, Kusuhara H, Adachi M, et al. Functional involvement of multidrug resistance-associated protein 4 (MRP4/ABCC4) in the renal elimination of the antiviral drugs adefovir and tenofovir. *Mol Pharmacol*. 2007;71:619-627.
114. Morelle J, Labriola L, Lambert M, et al. Tenofovir-related acute kidney injury and proximal tubule dysfunction precipitated by diclofenac: a case of drug-drug interaction. *Clin Nephrol*. 2009;71:567-570.
115. de Jongh FE, van Veen RN, Veltman SJ, et al. Weekly high-dose cisplatin is a feasible treatment option: analysis on prognostic factors for toxicity in 400 patients. *Br J Cancer*. 2003;88:1199-1206.
116. Katsuda H, Yamashita M, Katsura H, et al. Protecting cisplatin-induced nephrotoxicity with cimetidine does not affect antitumor activity. *Biol Pharm Bull*. 2010;33:1867-1871.
117. Yokoo S, Yonezawa A, Masuda S, et al. Differential contribution of organic cation transporters, OCT2 and MATE1, in platinum agent-induced nephrotoxicity. *Biochem Pharmacol*. 2007;74:477-487.
118. Ciarimboli G, Deuster D, Knief A, et al. Organic cation transporter 2 mediates cisplatin-induced oto- and nephrotoxicity and is a target for protective interventions. *Am J Pathol*. 2010;176:1169-1180.
119. Elsby R, Chidlaw S, Outteridge S, et al. Mechanistic in vitro studies confirm that inhibition of the renal apical efflux transporter multidrug and toxin extrusion (MATE) 1, and not altered absorption, underlies the increased metformin exposure observed in clinical interactions with cimetidine, trimethoprim or pyrimethamine. *Pharmacol Res Perspect*. 2017;5:e00357.
120. Chen Y, Li S, Brown C, et al. Effect of genetic variation in the organic cation transporter 2 on the renal elimination of metformin. *Pharmacogenet Genomics*. 2009;19:497-504.

121. Chu X, Bleasby K, Chan GH, et al. The complexities of interpreting reversible elevated serum creatinine levels in drug development: does a correlation with inhibition of renal transporters exist? *Drug Metab Dispos*. 2016;44:1498-1509.
122. Lepist EI, Zhang X, Hao J, et al. Contribution of the organic anion transporter OAT2 to the renal active tubular secretion of creatinine and mechanism for serum creatinine elevations caused by cobicistat. *Kidney Int*. 2014;86:350-357.
123. Pinho MJ, Serrao MP, Gomes P, et al. Over-expression of renal LAT1 and LAT2 and enhanced L-DOPA uptake in SHR immortalized renal proximal tubular cells. *Kidney Int*. 2004;66:216-226.
124. Roiko SA, Felmlee MA, Morris ME. Brain uptake of the drug of abuse gamma-hydroxybutyric acid in rats. *Drug Metab Dispos*. 2012;40:212-218.
125. Schinkel AH, Wagenaar E, van Deemter L, et al. Absence of the mdr1a P-glycoprotein in mice affects tissue distribution and pharmacokinetics of dexamethasone, digoxin, and cyclosporin A. *J Clin Invest*. 1995;96:1698-1705.
126. Kemper EM, van Zandbergen AE, Cleypool C, et al. Increased penetration of paclitaxel into the brain by inhibition of P-glycoprotein. *Clin Cancer Res*. 2003;9:2849-2855.
127. Breedveld P, Beijnen JH, Schellens JH. Use of P-glycoprotein and BCRP inhibitors to improve oral bioavailability and CNS penetration of anticancer drugs. *Trends Pharmacol Sci*. 2006;27:17-24.
128. Eyal S, Ke B, Muzi M, et al. Regional P-glycoprotein activity and inhibition at the human blood-brain barrier as imaged by positron emission tomography. *Clin Pharmacol Ther*. 2010;87:579-585.
129. Agarwal S, Sane R, Ohlfest JR, et al. The role of the breast cancer resistance protein (ABCG2) in the distribution of sorafenib to the brain. *J Pharmacol Exp Ther*. 2011;336:223-233.
130. Zhou L, Schmidt K, Nelson FR, et al. The effect of breast cancer resistance protein and P-glycoprotein on the brain penetration of flavopiridol, imatinib mesylate (Gleevec), prazosin, and 2-methoxy-3-(4-(2-(5-methyl-2-phenyloxazol-4-yl)ethoxy) phenyl)propanoic acid (PF-407288) in mice. *Drug Metab Dispos*. 2009;37:946-955.
131. Shen J, Carcaboso AM, Hubbard KE, et al. Compartment-specific roles of ATP-binding cassette transporters define differential topotecan distribution in brain parenchyma and cerebrospinal fluid. *Cancer Res*. 2009;69:5885-5892.
132. Venkatakrishnan K, Tseng E, Nelson FR, et al. Central nervous system pharmacokinetics of the Mdr1 P-glycoprotein substrate CP-615,003: intersite differences and implications for human receptor occupancy projections from cerebrospinal fluid exposures. *Drug Metab Dispos*. 2007;35:1341-1349.
133. Tirona RG. Molecular mechanisms of drug transporter regulation. *Handb Exp Pharmacol*. 2011:373-402.
134. Klaassen CD, Aleksunes LM. Xenobiotic, bile acid, and cholesterol transporters: function and regulation. *Pharmacol Rev*. 2010;62:1-96.
135. Harmsen S, Meijerman I, Beijnen JH, et al. The role of nuclear receptors in pharmacokinetic drug-drug interactions in oncology. *Cancer Treat Rev*. 2007;33:369-380.
136. Niemi M, Backman JT, Fromm MF, et al. Pharmacokinetic interactions with rifampicin: clinical relevance. *Clin Pharmacokinet*. 2003;42:819-850.
137. Hartter S, Koenen-Bergmann M, Sharma A, et al. Decrease in the oral bioavailability of dabigatran etexilate after co-medication with rifampicin. *Br J Clin Pharmacol*. 2012;74:490-500.
138. Westphal K, Weinbrenner A, Zschiesche M, et al. Induction of P-glycoprotein by rifampin increases intestinal secretion of talinolol in human beings: a new type of drug/drug interaction. *Clin Pharmacol Ther*. 2000;68:345-355.
139. Bosilkovska M, Samer CF, Deglon J, et al. Geneva cocktail for cytochrome p450 and P-glycoprotein activity assessment using dried blood spots. *Clin Pharmacol Ther*. 2014;96:349-359.
140. Markert C, Ngui P, Hellwig R, et al. Influence of St. John's wort on the steady-state pharmacokinetics and metabolism of bosentan. *Int J Clin Pharmacol Ther*. 2014;52:328-336.
141. Varma MV, Lin J, Bi YA, et al. Quantitative prediction of repaglinide-rifampicin complex drug interactions using dynamic and static mechanistic models: delineating differential CYP3A4 induction and OATP1B1 inhibition potential of rifampicin. *Drug Metab Dispos*. 2013;41:966-974.
142. Williamson B, Dooley KE, Zhang Y, et al. Induction of influx and efflux transporters and cytochrome P450 3A4 in primary human hepatocytes by rifampin, rifabutin, and rifapentine. *Antimicrob Agents Chemother*. 2013;57:6366-6369.
143. Cho SK, Yoon JS, Lee MG, et al. Rifampin enhances the glucose-lowering effect of metformin and increases OCT1 mRNA levels in healthy participants. *Clin Pharmacol Ther*. 2011;89:416-421.
144. Jonker JW, Liddle C, Downes M. FXR and PXR: potential therapeutic targets in cholestasis. *J Steroid Biochem Mol Biol*. 2012;130:147-158.
145. Morgan ET, Goralski KB, Piquette-Miller M, et al. Regulation of drug-metabolizing enzymes and transporters in infection, inflammation, and cancer. *Drug Metab Dispos*. 2008;36:205-216.
146. Dreisbach AW. The influence of chronic renal failure on drug metabolism and transport. *Clin Pharmacol Ther*. 2009;86:553-556.
147. Potschka H. Modulating P-glycoprotein regulation: future perspectives for pharmacoresistant epilepsies? *Epilepsia*. 2010;51:1333-1347.

CHAPTER **5**

Principles of Biotechnology-Derived Drugs

Tanaji T. Talele and Vijaya L. Korlipara

Drugs covered in this chapter:

- Abciximab
- Ado-trastuzumab emtansine
- Alemtuzumab
- Ave9633
- Axicabtagene
- Bevacizumab
- Brentuximab vedotin
- Capromab pendetite
- Catumaxomab
- Cetuximab
- Clopidogrel
- Codeine
- Eculizumab
- 5-Fluorouracil
- Gemtuzumab ozogamicin
- Imgn901
- Imiciromab pentetate
- Infliximab
- Inotuzumab ozogamicin
- Irinotecan
- Isoniazid
- 6-Mercaptopurine
- Niraparib
- Nofetumomab
- Olaparib
- Pegloticase
- Rucaparib
- SAR3419
- Satumomab
- Tamoxifen
- Technetium-99m-arcitumomab
- Tisagenlecleucel
- Tolterodine
- Trastuzumab
- Trastuzumab-MCC-DM1
- Vemurafenib
- Voretigene neparvovec-rzyl
- Warfarin

Abbreviations

AAV adeno-associated virus
ABC ATP-binding cassette
ADC antibody-drug conjugate
BRCA breast cancer–associated gene
Cas9 CRISPR-associated protein9
CDR complementarity-determining region
CRISPR clustered regularly inter-spaced short palindromic repeats
DAR drug-to-antibody ratio
DPD dihydropyrimidine dehydrogenase
DSB double strand break
G6PD glucose-6-phosphate dehydrogenase
HAMA human anti-mouse antibody
HDR homology-directed repair
HGP human genome project
MAb monoclonal antibody
NAT N-acetyl transferase
PARP poly (ADP-ribose) polymerase
PCR polymerase chain reaction
PEG polyethylene glycol
SNP single nucleotide polymorphism
TALEN transcription activator–like effector nuclease
TPMT thiopurine methyl transferase
UDP uridine diphosphate
UGT UDP glucuronyl transferase
URE upstream regulatory elements
ZFN zinc finger nuclease

INTRODUCTION

Pharmaceutical biotechnology generates basic scientific knowledge, useful therapeutic and diagnostic products, and promising methodologies for future research and clinical applications. The techniques of biotechnology lead to the development of novel therapeutics, improved methods of manufacturing pharmaceuticals, and significant contributions to our understanding of disease etiology, pathophysiology, and biochemistry. Genomics, transcriptomics, proteomics, pharmacogenomics, and metabolomics, the core approaches to pharmaceutical biotechnology, are making major contributions in three areas:

1. Identification of new genes
2. Identification of drug targets
3. Development of "personalized medicine"

Although many of the first biotechnology-derived therapeutics were initially used in acutely ill, hospitalized patients, the products of today's pharmaceutical biotechnology have an impact on patient populations with chronic diseases such as rheumatoid arthritis, gout, and cancer.

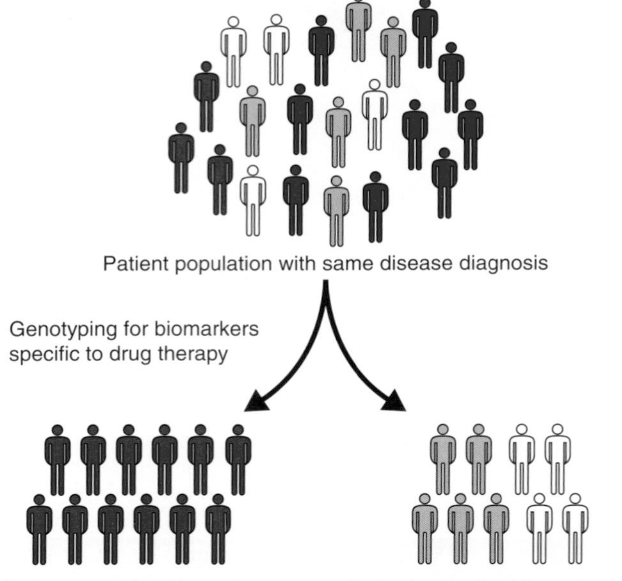

Figure 5.1 Manipulating therapeutic outcomes. Manipulating therapeutic outcomes through pharmacogenetic analysis of a population with the same disease diagnosis to eliminate patients with genetic biomarkers indicating an adverse response to a particular drug therapy.

PHARMACOGENETICS

The Human Genome Project (HGP), funded by the DOE (Department of Energy) and NIH (the National Institutes of Health), began in the early 1990s and was completed in the early 2000s.[1] The application of genetic information gained from the HGP to disease diagnosis and drug therapy is a major development that is bringing about a wealth of change including the potential to develop drugs for hundreds of rare, inherited Mendelian disorders. A major benefit of pharmacogenetic screening is a reduction in the health care costs resulting from more effective treatments with fewer side effects and higher cure rates achieved from the patients' treatment targeted to the molecular etiology of their disease. Mutations are the result of heritable, permanent changes in DNA base sequence. These usually come about by one of the following three mechanisms: substitution, addition, or deletion. The number of base pair changes involved in a single gene mutation can vary from a single base pair change or single nucleotide polymorphism (SNP) to a large number of gross changes in the gene structure involving insertion, deletion, or rearrangements of a very large number of base pairs.

Mutations result in a variety of changes to the gene product. If the base change occurs within the reading frame of the gene product, it may alter the amino acid sequence of the gene product (protein). SNPs have been defined as single base mutations that occur in 1% or more of the population.[2,3] Many of these SNPs may be responsible for the production of a malfunctioning gene product that, in turn, is responsible for a serious disease. The well-used example is the A → T mutation in the β-globin gene, in which the GAG glutamic acid codon is changed to the GTG valine codon, resulting in abnormal aggregation of the hemoglobin molecules and causing sickle cell anemia. Another example is one form of β-thalassemia that results from a mutation of a CAG glutamine codon to the TAG stop codon early in the DNA sequence, resulting in premature termination of the translation process and total loss of the β-subunit of the adult hemoglobin molecule.

In principle, one is able to manipulate the therapeutic outcome of a patient population by separating patients who will not respond normally to a particular drug therapy from those who will, based on an analysis of established genetic biomarkers related to the drug's metabolic profile (Fig. 5.1). Patients who are homozygous for the genetic biomarkers indicating poor metabolism of the recommended therapeutic agent may, depending on the therapeutic window of the drug, exhibit a response resembling an overdose to the normal drug dose and require a reduced dose to achieve therapeutic levels, whereas patients carrying the biomarkers indicating extensive metabolism may exhibit a lack of efficacy at normal doses and require an increased dose of the drug to achieve therapeutic activity. The patients who are homozygous or heterozygous for the normal (wild-type) genetic biomarker may require no alteration of the "normal" dose of the drug for adequate therapeutic outcome.

The action of a drug on the body is a complex interaction involving the metabolism of drugs, the transport of drugs throughout the body, and the interaction of the drug with its target. The application of genetic variation to drug therapy centered on the variations seen in a number of drug metabolism enzymes, and much of the pharmacogenetic research has developed with the phase I (oxidative) and phase II (conjugative) metabolic enzymes. Currently, considerable data relate SNPs in the coding and regulatory regions of these genes to poor metabolism of particular drugs that have the potential to result in drug overdoses in patients carrying the genetic variations and given the "normal" dose of drug. Transport proteins, such as the ATP-binding cassette (ABC) transporters, that move drugs through membrane barriers are critical in the absorption, distribution, and excretion of drugs and drug metabolites. Drug targets as well as the biochemical pathways following the drug-receptor interaction influence the drug response. Thus, the candidate genes for the therapeutic drug pathway include the genes for drug metabolism, drug transport, and drug response (Table 5.1).

Table 5.1 Specific Examples of the Application of Allelic Variation in Drug Therapy

Protein	Action	Drug	Therapy	Efficacy/toxicity
CYP450 2D6	Drug metabolism	Codeine	Pain	Efficacy
CYP450 2C9	Drug metabolism	Warfarin	Coagulation	Toxicity (hemorrhage)
Thiopurine S-methyltransferase	Drug metabolism	Mercaptopurine	Acute lymphoblastic leukemia	Toxicity (myelotoxic)
HER2/neu	Drug target	Herceptin	Breast cancer	Efficacy
BCR/ABL	Drug target	Gleevec	Chronic myelogenous leukemia	Efficacy
EGFR	Drug target	Erbitux	Colon cancer	Efficacy
Apolipoprotein E4	Marker	Tacrine	Alzheimer disease	Efficacy
Cholesteryl ester transferase	Marker	Statins	Atherosclerosis	Efficacy
ATP-binding cassette B1	Drug transport	Saquinavir	HIV	Efficacy
		Indinavir	Leukemia	
		Ritonavir		
		Daunorubicin		
		Etoposide		
UDP-glucuronosyltransferase 1A1	Drug metabolism	Irinotecan	Cancer	Toxicity (myelotoxic)
N-Acetyltransferase 2	Drug metabolism	Isoniazid	Tuberculosis	Toxicity (hepatotoxic)
Pseudocholinesterase	Drug metabolism	Suxamethonium	Muscle relaxation during surgery	Toxicity (prolonged apnea)
CYP3A4/CYP2D6	Drug metabolism	Tamoxifen	Cancer	Efficacy
CYP2C19	Drug metabolism	Clopidogrel	Antithrombotic	Cardiovascular toxicity
CYP3A4/CYP2D6	Drug metabolism	Tolterodine	Antimuscarinic	Efficacy
Dihydropyrimidine dehydrogenase	Drug metabolism	5-Fluorouracil	Cancer	Toxicity
BRAF V600E	Drug target	Vemurafenib	Metastatic melanoma	Efficacy
BRCA-deficiency	Synthetic lethality	Olaparib, niraparib, rucaparib	BRCA-mutated cancers	Efficacy

ATP, adenosine triphosphate; BRCA, breast cancer–associated gene; EGFR, epidermal growth factor receptor; HER2, human epidermal growth factor receptor 2; HIV, human immunodeficiency virus.

Genomics

Genomics is the study of the full complement of genetic information, both coding and noncoding, in an organism's genome. The main genomics technique is the use of SNPs as biomarkers to inform clinicians about subtypes of disease that require differential treatments and provide pharmacists with information for selection of the best therapeutic methodology to effectively manage the disease as well as provide an indication of the patients at risk of experiencing adverse reactions or those who will not respond to a given drug dose. The general genotyping procedure for detecting known SNPs consists of polymerase chain reaction (PCR) amplification of the region of interest in the genome, discrimination of the alleles in that region, and detection of the discrimination products.

Transcriptomics

Transcriptomics is the technology behind the study of the full complement of messenger RNA (mRNA) transcripts in the cell's transcriptome and also is known as expression profiling. Methods of expression profiling are either "open" or "closed." Open systems do not require any advance knowledge of the sequence of the genome being examined; closed systems require some advance knowledge and usually involve the use of

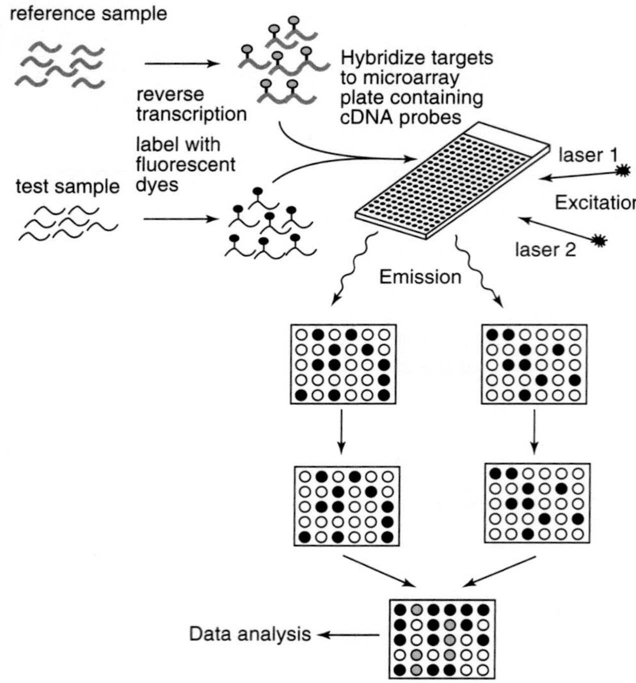

Figure 5.2 cDNA chip. Schematic representation of a cDNA microarray chip. Probes of interest are obtained from DNA clones and printed on coated glass microscope slides. Analysis of mRNA expression is carried out by taking total messenger RNA (mRNA) from both a test and control sample, fluorescently labeling the samples with either Cy3- or Cy5-dUTP during a single round of reverse transcription, pooling the fluorescent targets, and hybridizing to the immobilized probes on the array under very stringent conditions. Laser excitation of the incorporated targets yields an emission with a characteristic spectrum, which is measured using a scanning confocal laser microscope and analyzed using a computer program. From Duggan DJ, Bittner M, Chen Y, et al. Expression profiling using cDNA microarrays. *Nat Genet.* 1999;21(suppl 1):10-14.

oligonucleotide or complementary DNA (cDNA) array hybridization technologies (the gene chip) and quantitative PCR (Fig. 5.2).

The cDNA arrays are prepared by spotting gene-specific PCR products, including full-length cDNAs, collections of partially sequenced cDNAs, or randomly chosen cDNAs from any library of interest onto a glass, silicon, gel, or bead matrix or a nylon or nitrocellulose membrane. The matrix (most often glass) is coated with polylysine, amino silanes, or amino-reactive silanes to assist in the attachment of the cDNA probes. The PCR products of the clones are purified and spotted onto the matrix by robots through contact printing or noncontact piezo or ink-jet devices. After cross-linking the probe to the matrix by ultraviolet irradiation, the probe is made single stranded by heat or alkali treatment. The mRNA target is prepared from both a test and reference sample by reverse transcription to produce cDNA, which is then labeled with fluorescent probes (one for the test and another for the reference). The fluorescent targets are pooled and hybridized to the probe array under very stringent conditions. Laser excitation of the hybridized samples on the matrix and comparison of the fluorescence intensity of the reference sample with the fluorescence intensity of the test sample using computer algorithms yield an emission characteristic of the increase or decrease of mRNA expression under test conditions.

CRISPR Technologies and Therapeutic Applications

Clustered regularly interspaced short palindromic repeats (CRISPR)-CRISPR-associated protein (Cas9) complex, a genome editing tool that holds promise for human gene therapy, was named as the "Breakthrough of the Year" by *Science* magazine in 2015.[4] CRISPR technology is comprised of three components: (1) a guide RNA that targets a specific locus in the gene; (2) a Cas9 nuclease, which creates a DNA break at the locus; and (3) a DNA repair template to enable gene replacements and insertions.[5] The use of this technology offers the ability to genetically manipulate the patient-derived stem cells to generate various disease models, including cystic fibrosis, Parkinson's disease, cardiomyopathy, and ischemic heart disease. CRISPRs, together with Cas9 RNA–guided endonuclease proteins, can be easily targeted to virtually any genomic location of choice by a short RNA guide. The guide sequence within these CRISPR RNAs typically corresponds to phage sequences, which constitute the natural mechanism by which CRISPR produces antiviral defense; however, it can be easily replaced by a sequence of interest to retarget the Cas9 nuclease. The principle behind CRISPR is illustrated in Figure 5.3.[6]

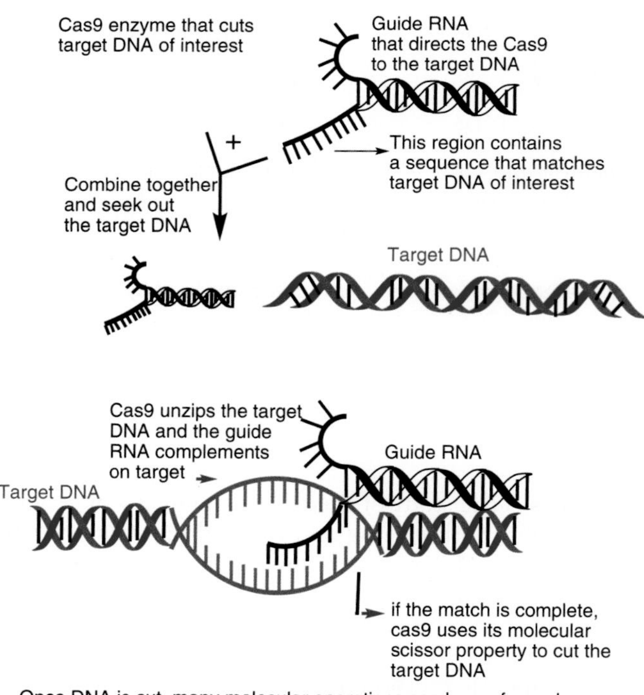

Figure 5.3 CRISPR (clustered regularly interspaced short palindromic repeats) technology.

Some applications of CRISPR technologies include homology-directed repair (HDR), gene silencing, pooled genome-scale knockout screening, transient activation of endogenous genes (CRISPRa or CRISPRon), transient gene silencing or transcriptional repression (CRISPRi), DNA-free CRISPR-cas9 gene editing, and embryonic stem cells and transgenic animals.[6]

CRISPR technology–based modified bacteriophages can be developed as a delivery vehicle for a CRISPR-cas9 gene editing system that targets and inactivates either virulence genes or the resistance genes themselves, leaving the rest of the microbiome intact. In another application, CRISPR can be used to target known bacterial resistance genes to deactivate them *in situ* and resensitize virulent bacteria, thus making existing antibiotics effective again.[7]

Although promising, CRISPR-based therapeutic development has a number of challenges that remain to be addressed. These include (1) a potential for the induction of off-target mutations at sites other than the intended target, (2) considerable safety concerns for CRISPR use in humans, (3) ethical concerns, (4) the fact that most diseases are not caused by single mutations, and (5) availability of safe carrier systems for CRISPR-cas9 delivery to human cells *in vivo*.

Proteomics

The array of proteins found within the cell, their interactions, and modifications hold the key to understanding biologic systems. The proteome is defined as a protein population of a cell characterized in terms of localization, posttranslational modification, interactions, and turnover, at any given time. The complexity of the proteome surpasses that of the genome. Proteomics is the technology behind the study of the total protein complement of a genome or the complete set of proteins expressed by a cell, tissue, or organism. The presence of an open reading frame in a DNA sequence indicates the presence of a gene, but it does not indicate gene transcription, RNA editing, translation, or posttranslational modification and the presence of isoforms. Analysis of the transcriptome does not indicate alteration of protein levels by proteolysis, recycling, and sequestration. Therefore, it is important to determine protein levels, protein expression, and protein-protein interactions directly.

Proteomics is divided into three main areas[8]:

1. Microcharacterization for large-scale identification of proteins and posttranslational modifications.[8]
2. Differential gel electrophoresis for comparison of protein levels.[9]
3. Protein-protein interaction studies using protein chips,[10] mass spectrometry isotope-coded affinity tag technology,[11] and the yeast two-hybrid system.[12]

Metabolomics

Metabolomics is the technology behind the measurement of metabolite concentrations, fluxes, and secretions in cells and tissues (metabolome). Metabolomics is at the cross-roads of genotype/phenotype interactions, where the interrelationship of metabolic pathways is considered to be the fundamental component of an organism's phenotype. Metabolomics is distinguished by the fact that metabolites are not directly linked to the genetic code but actually are products of a concerted action of many enzyme networks and other regulatory proteins.[13,14] Metabolites also are more complex than nucleic acids, which are composed of four nucleotides, or proteins, which in turn are composed of 20 different amino acids. As a result, metabolites cannot be sequenced like genes and proteins, and so their characterization requires that the structure of each metabolite be determined individually through description of elemental composition and stereochemical orientation of functional groups.

Metabolites are more than just products of enzyme-catalyzed reactions. They also are sensors and regulators of complex molecular interactions in the organism, and as a result, the composition of the metabolome can be altered by changes in the individual's environment. Therefore, a study of the metabolome is complicated not only by the uniqueness of the individual's genome but also by the uniqueness of the individual's environment. On the other side of the coin, however, one could consider the metabolome to be a very sensitive indicator of the individual's phenotype.[15,16]

Metabolomics can be approached by using several different but related strategies:

1. Target analysis investigates the primary metabolic effect of a genetic variation, in which the analysis usually is limited to the substrate and/or product of the protein expressed by the altered gene.
2. Metabolic profiling limits the investigation to a number of predefined metabolites, usually in a specific metabolic pathway.
3. Metabolomics is a comprehensive analysis (both identification and quantification) of metabolites in a biologic system, which investigates the effect of multiple genetic variations on many different biochemical pathways.
4. Metabolic fingerprinting is a strategy to screen a large number of metabolites for biologic relevance in diagnostic or other analytical procedures in which it is important to rapidly distinguish between individuals in a population. Metabolic fingerprinting is the ultimate characterization of an individual's phenotype for disease diagnosis and drug therapy. Once the technologic problems of high-throughput metabolic analysis are developed, it will be a major competitor of SNP analysis in pharmacogenomics.

The analytical technologies used in metabolomic investigations are nuclear magnetic resonance and mass spectrometry alone or in combination with liquid or gas chromatographic separation of metabolites. Other techniques include thin-layer chromatography, Fourier transform infrared spectrometry, metabolite arrays, and Raman spectroscopy.

Pharmaceutical Biotechnology Methods

Pharmaceutical biotechnology is defined, at its most basic level, as the manipulation of nucleic acids in the production of therapeutic and diagnostic agents. In order to understand both DNA and RNA, the fundamental genetic material, it is important to understand the basic process that moves information from DNA to RNA. This process starts with transcription.

Transcription

The genetic information in DNA is transcribed to the intermediate RNA molecule that moves to the cytoplasm, where it directs the synthesis of the gene product it encodes using ribosomes. RNA differs chemically from DNA in that the deoxyribose sugar molecule in DNA is replaced by ribose and the thymine in DNA is replaced by uracil in RNA. Structurally, RNA contains both single-stranded runs and short, double helical regions.

There are several types of RNA molecules in the cell, three of which are highlighted here. Messenger RNA (mRNA) is transcribed from a particular DNA sequence. Transfer RNAs (tRNAs) are covalently linked to specific amino acids and carry the anticodon triplet that recognizes a complementary trinucleotide sequence of the mRNA that is specific for the amino acid that it carries. The ribosome contains both ribosomal RNA (rRNA) and proteins.

Several differences exist in the mechanism of transcription between prokaryotes and eukaryotes. These differences are important when evaluating if recombinant expression of a protein should be carried out in a eukaryotic or prokaryotic system. For our purposes, we describe transcription in a eukaryotic system.

Transcription is carried out by RNA polymerases, of which there are three types in eukaryotes. RNA pol I catalyzes the synthesis of rRNAs, RNA pol II is responsible for the synthesis of mRNA, and RNA pol III synthesizes tRNA. All three polymerases are large enzymes containing 12 or more subunits.

Each eukaryotic RNA polymerase copies DNA from the 3′ end, thus catalyzing mRNA formation in the 5′ → 3′ direction and synthesizing RNA complementary to the antisense DNA template strand. The reaction requires the precursor nucleotides adenosine triphosphate (ATP), guanosine triphosphate (GTP), cytidine triphosphate (CTP), and uridine triphosphate (UTP) and does not require a primer for initiation of transcription. The five stages of eukaryotic transcription include initiation, elongation and termination, capping, polyadenylation, and splicing.

Initiation

Eukaryotes have different RNA polymerase–binding promoter sequences than prokaryotes. The TATA consensus sequence of the eukaryotic promoter region is located 25-35 base pairs upstream from the transcription start site (Fig. 5.4). The low activity of basal promoters is greatly increased by the presence of upstream regulatory elements (UREs) located 40-200 base pairs upstream of the promoter sequence and includes the SP1 box, the CCAAT box, and the hormone response elements. Transcription from many eukaryotic promoters can be stimulated by control elements, called enhancers, located many thousands of base pairs away from the transcription start site.

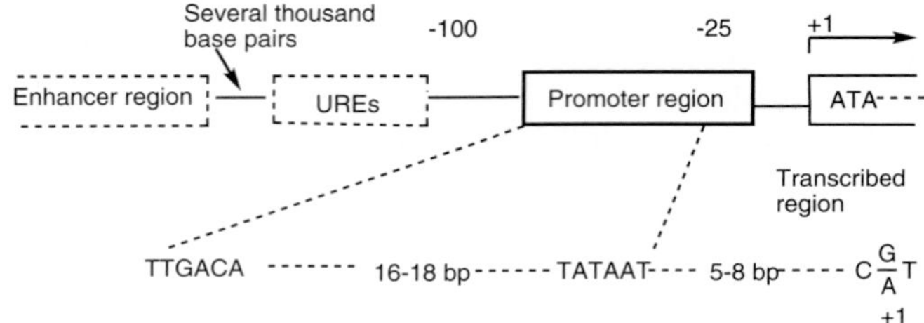

Figure 5.4 **Schematic representation of the eukaryotic transcription unit showing the relationship between the promoter, upstream regulatory elements (UREs), and enhancer region. Note that transcription usually starts with a purine base in the 1 position.** Adapted from Turner PC, McLennan AG, Bates AD, White MRH. *Instant Notes in Molecular Biology*. New York: BIOS Scientific Publishers Ltd, Springer-Verlag; 1997; with permission.

Elongation and Termination

RNA polymerase moves along the DNA template until a terminator sequence is reached. The RNA molecule made from a protein-coding gene by RNA pol II in eukaryotes is called pre-mRNA. The pre-mRNA from a eukaryotic protein-coding gene is extensively processed within the nucleus before export to the cytoplasm.

Capping

At the end of polymerization, the 5′ end of the pre-mRNA molecule is modified by addition of an N7-methyl guanine molecule (Fig. 5.5).

Polyadenylation

The 3′ end of the pre-mRNA is generated by nuclease catalyzed cleavage followed by the addition of a run, or tail, of 100-200 adenosine nucleotides, resulting in what is called the poly (A) tail. Cleavage and polyadenylation require

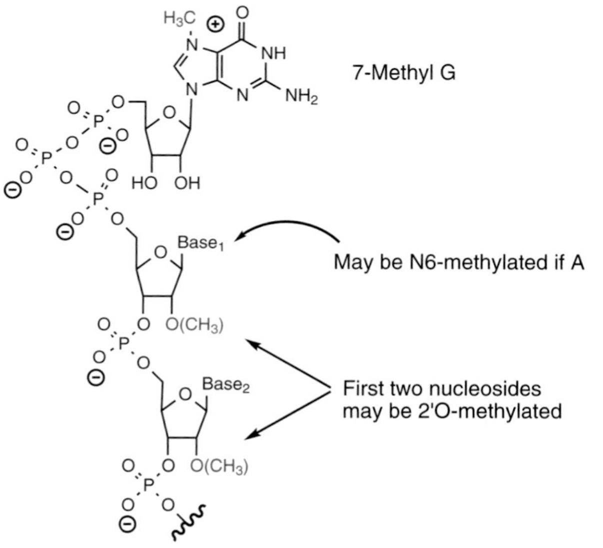

Figure 5.5 **Chemical structure of the 5′-cap of mRNA (messenger RNA). Cap 0 consists of the 7-methylguanosine triphosphate attached to the 5′ end of the mRNA. Cap 1 consists of the 7-methylguanosine and 2′O-methylation of the 5′ base. Cap 2 consists of the 7-methylguanosine and the 2′O-methylation of the first two bases in the sequence.**

specific sequences in the DNA and its pre-mRNA transcript that are part of the transcription termination signal. The poly (A) tail helps stabilize the mRNA molecule, reducing its sensitivity to 3′-nuclease activity.

RNA Splicing

Splicing is the precise excision of the intron sequences and joining of exons to produce a functional mRNA molecule.

Translation

Once the fully processed mRNA has been transported from the nucleus to the cytoplasm, protein synthesis occurs. The triplet genetic code carried on the mRNA is translated into a protein sequence by the ribosome. Amino acids are delivered to the ribosome by tRNAs that carry specific amino acids attached to their 3′-terminus based on the tRNA anticodon sequence. The anticodon complements the triplet codon sequence in mRNA, and 61 triplet sequences code for the 20 amino acids (Table 5.2). Three codons are nonsense or stop codons that terminate translation. The code is degenerate with 18 of the 20 common amino acids coded for by more than one codon. Two amino acids, Met (AUG) and Trp (UGG), have one unique codon each. From a fixed start point on the mRNA (start codon, AUG), which establishes the open reading

Table 5.2 The Genetic Code

First Position	Second Position				Third Position
	U	C	A	G	
U	**Phe** UUU	**Ser** UCU	**Tyr** UAU	**Cys** UGU	U
	Phe UUC	**Ser** UCC	**Tyr** UAC	**Cys** UGC	C
	Leu UUA	**Ser** UCA	**Stop** UAA	**Stop** UGA	A
	Leu UUG	**Ser** UCG	**Stop** UAG	**Trp** UGG	G
C	**Leu** CUU	**Pro** CCU	**His** CAU	**Arg** CGU	U
	Leu CUC	**Pro** CCC	**His** CAC	**Arg** CGC	C
	Leu CUA	**Pro** CCA	**Gln** CAA	**Arg** CGA	A
	Leu CUG	**Pro** CCG	**Gln** CAG	**Arg** CGG	G
A	**Ile** AUU	**Thr** ACU	**Asn** AAU	**Ser** AGU	U
	Ile AUC	**Thr** ACC	**Asn** AAC	**Ser** AGC	C
	Ile AUA	**Thr** ACA	**Lys** AAA	**Arg** AGA	A
	Met AUG	**Thr** ACG	**Lys** AAG	**Arg** AGG	G
G	**Val** GUU	**Ala** GCU	**Asp** GAU	**Gly** GGU	U
	Val GUC	**Ala** GCC	**Asp** GAC	**Gly** GGC	C
	Val GUA	**Ala** GCA	**Glu** GAA	**Gly** GGA	A
	Val GUG	**Ala** GCG	**Glu** GAG	**Gly** GGG	G

frame, each group of three bases in the coding region of the mRNA represents a codon that is recognized by a complementary triplet on the tRNA molecule.

There are four stages in the protein synthesis in both prokaryotes and eukaryotes:

1. *Initiation*—assembly of the ribosome on an mRNA molecule.
2. *Elongation*—repeated cycles of amino acid addition.
3. *Termination*—recognition of the stop codon, release of the new protein chain, and breakdown of the synthetic complex.
4. *Posttranslational modification*—usually includes protein cleavage by carboxy or aminopeptidases and chemical modification such as acetylation, sulfonylation, phosphorylation, hydroxylation, lipidation, and/or addition of polysaccharides.

Genes

A gene is the segment of genomic DNA (gDNA) involved in producing a polypeptide chain. The mRNA assembled from the gene includes regions preceding (the leader or 5′-untranslated region) and following (the trailer or 3′-untranslated region) the coding region as well as intervening sequences such as introns that are removed in the processing of the pre-mRNA. With the discovery of other processes that contribute to the penultimate sequence of the mature mRNA, the definition of a gene is evolving.[17]

Cloning and the Preparation of DNA Libraries

Two discoveries in the early 1970s provided breakthroughs in nucleic acid chemistry: the discovery of bacterial enzymes capable of cleaving nucleic acids at specific, palindromic (symmetrical) base sequences (Figs. 5.6 and 5.7) and the discovery of bacterial plasmids as vehicles (vectors) to amplify and carry the gene fragments produced by those restriction enzymes. Plasmids are small, circular, extrachromosomal nucleic acid molecules in bacteria that replicate independently within the bacterial cell. Restriction enzymes (and now PCR) are used to produce relatively small DNA fragments that are inserted into bacterial plasmid vectors, forming recombinant DNA (rDNA) molecules. The rDNA vectors are inserted into bacterial hosts, where the plasmid replicates with the bacteria, producing a large number of identical rDNA molecules known as clones, thus completing the process known as DNA cloning.

SEQUENCING DNA FRAGMENTS. The two previous methods of nucleic acid sequencing, the Maxam and Gilbert method (chemical method)[18] and Sanger's dideoxy method,[19] have been superseded by the far faster massive parallel sequencing methods. In short, high-throughput sequencing involves breaking up gDNA into fragments and placing the individual fragments onto specially designed microbeads where the many copies of each fragment have been amplified. The amplified fragments are then loaded into the small wells of a substrate. As the wells are loaded with sample, reagents are pumped across the plate. The addition of the reagents results in an enzymatic reaction between complimentary bases in the DNA fragments, and a fluorescent signal is released and read by a computational sequence analyzer.[20]

SYNTHESIZING OLIGONUCLEOTIDES. The need for short oligonucleotides of known sequence has grown tremendously with the need for radiolabeled and fluorescently labeled probes to isolate and characterize nucleic acids. The phosphite triester and the phosphotriester methods are convenient solid-phase automated techniques for the synthesis of oligonucleotides (Fig. 5.8).[21]

POLYMERASE CHAIN REACTION (PCR). Working with small quantities of nucleic acids isolated from cell and tissue sources is difficult, and there is often a need to amplify these sequences. PCR is used to amplify fragments of DNA

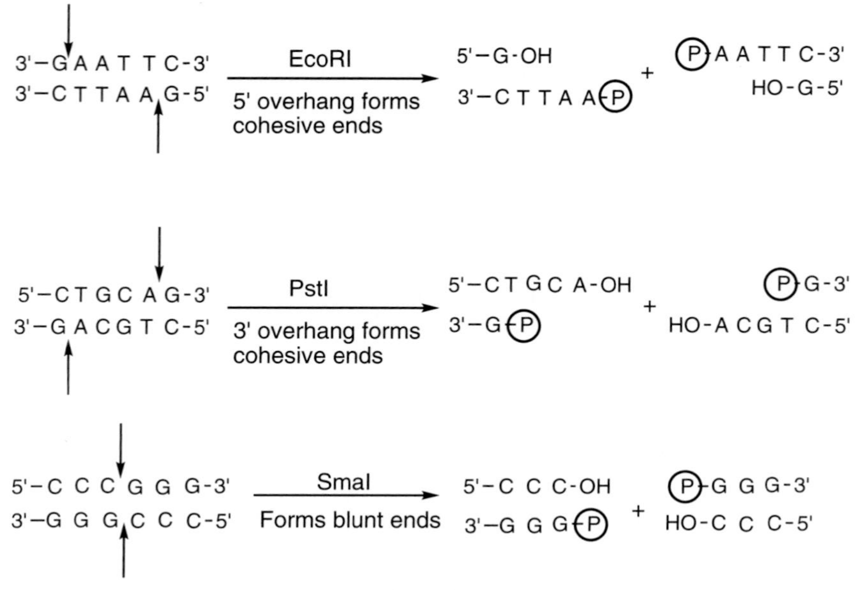

3'–GAATTC-3' / 3'–CTTAAG-5' → EcoRI (5' overhang forms cohesive ends) → 5'–G-OH / 3'–CTTAA(P) + (P)AATTC-3' / HO-G-5'

5'–CTGCAG-3' / 3'–GACGTC-5' → PstI (3' overhang forms cohesive ends) → 5'–CTGCA-OH / 3'–G(P) + (P)G-3' / HO-ACGTC-5'

5'–CCCGGG-3' / 3'–GGGCCC-5' → SmaI (Forms blunt ends) → 5'–CCC-OH / 3'–GGG(P) + (P)GGG-3' / HO-CCC-5'

Figure 5.6 Actions of restriction endonucleases EcoRI, PstI, and SmaI at their recognition sequences. Note that EcoRI and PstI enzymes produce "sticky ends" with overlapping sequences, whereas SmaI produces "blunt ends" or nonoverlapping sequences.

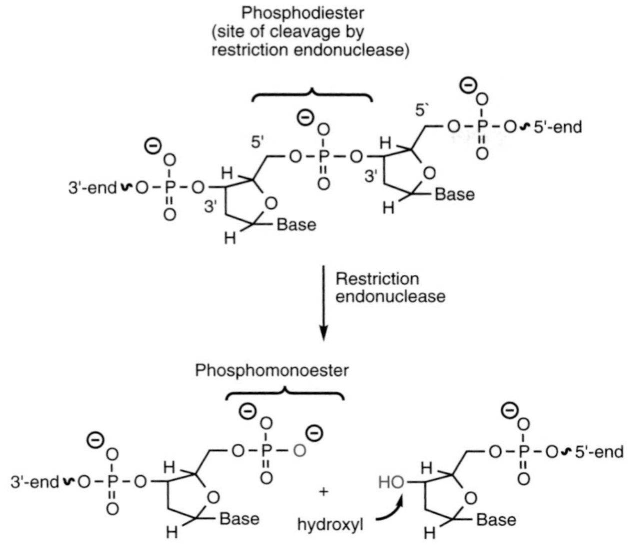

Figure 5.7 Cleavage by restriction endonuclease.

without the need for cloning. The process can amplify samples that contain as little as a single nucleotide fragment used as template. There is a requirement for the sequences flanking the boundaries of the fragment to be amplified so that oligonucleotide primers can be prepared.[22]

PROTEIN SYNTHESIS THROUGH RECOMBINANT DNA. Once the gene coding for the desired protein has been identified and isolated (Fig. 5.9), the genetic material is introduced into cells on a vector capable of DNA replication and initiation of transcription. A cloning vector is a carrier molecule, the vehicle that is used to insert foreign DNA into a host cell. Typically, vectors are genetic elements that can be replicated in a host cell separately from that cell's chromosomes. Bacterial plasmids are circular DNA of only a few thousand base pairs that replicate freely within the cells and are ideal for carrying the gene into the host organism. DNA fragments coding for the desired protein can be cloned from gDNA or cDNA and inserted into the vector that carries the code to synthesize the protein in the host.

The vector containing the code for the target protein is then inserted into the host. Host cells are typically bacteria (e.g., *Escherichia coli*), eukaryotic yeast (e.g., *Saccharomyces cerevisiae* [baker's yeast]), or mammalian cell lines. The choice of host system is influenced primarily by the type of protein to be expressed and by the key differences among the various host cells. Overall protein yields generally are much lower in mammalian cells, but in some cases, this may be the only system that produces the specific protein of interest. It should be noted that recombinant proteins produced in gram-negative bacteria may contain endotoxins.

The host cells containing the vector are grown under selection to identify a clone that contains the desired gene and is able to produce the best protein. The selected cloned cells are used as inoculum first for a small-scale cell culture/fermentation, which is then followed by larger fermentations in bioreactors. The medium is carefully controlled to enhance cell reproduction and protein synthesis. The host produces its natural proteins along with the desired

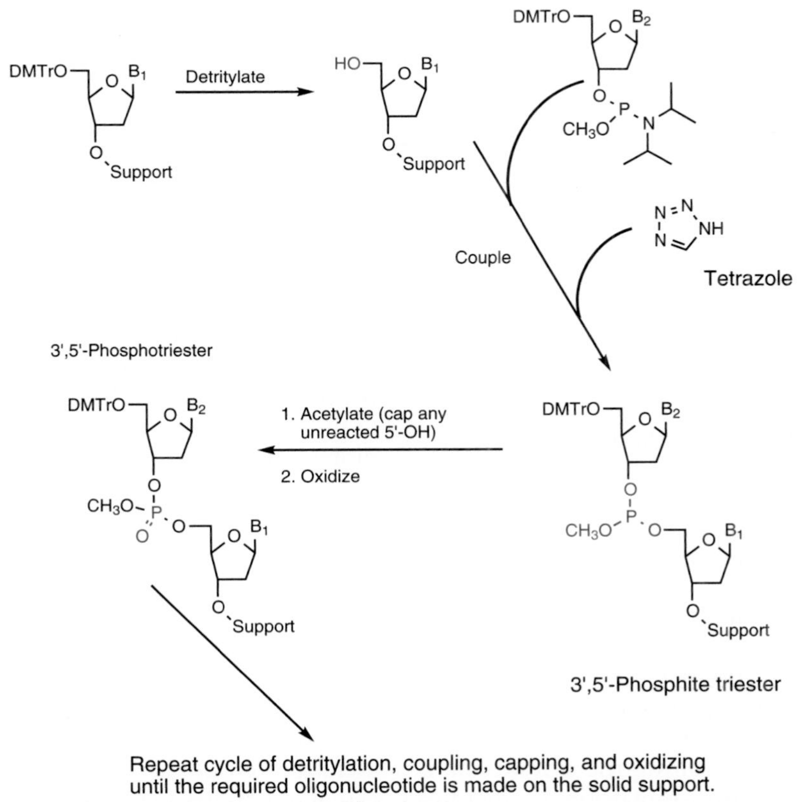

Figure 5.8 Solid-phase phosphate and phosphite triester method of oligodeoxyribonucleotide synthesis. DMTr, 4,4-dimethoxytrityl

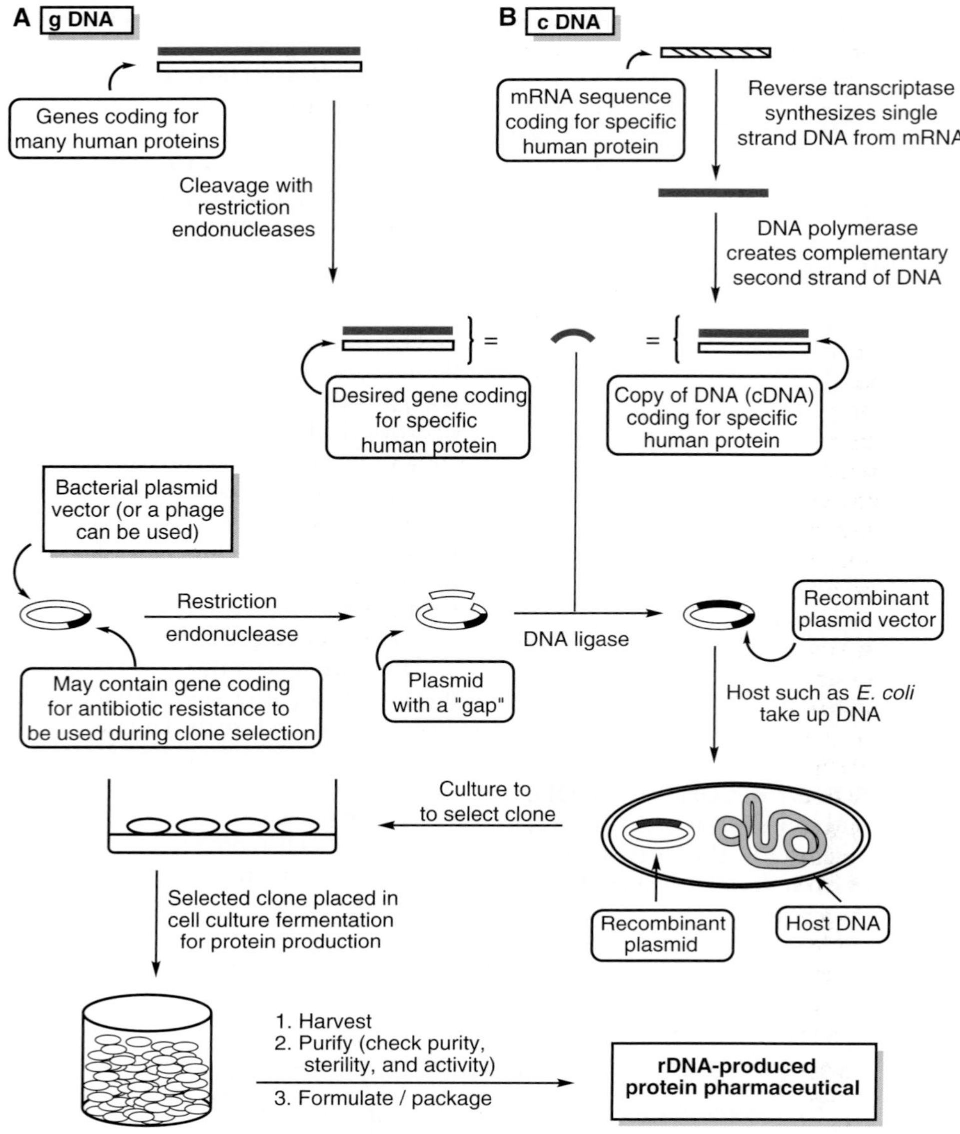

Figure 5.9 Summary of typical rDNA production of a protein from either (A) genomic DNA or (B) cDNA.

protein, which may be secreted into the growth medium. The protein of interest can then be isolated from the fermentation, purified, and formulated to give a potential rDNA-produced pharmaceutical.

PROTEIN ISOLATION AND PURIFICATION. The isolation and purification of the final protein product from the complex mixture of cells, cellular debris, medium nutrients, and other host metabolites is a challenging task. The structure, purity, potency, and stability of the recombinant protein must be considered. Often, sophisticated filtrations, phase separations, precipitation, and complex multiple-column chromatographic procedures are required to obtain the desired protein. Although isolation of the recombinant protein, produced in culture in relatively large amounts, generally is easier than isolating the native protein, ensuring the stability and retention of the bioactive three-dimensional structure (correct protein folding) of any biopharmaceutical is a more arduous task. In addition, recombinant proteins from bacterial hosts require removal of endotoxins, whereas viral particles may need to be removed from mammalian cell culture products. A discussion of these techniques is beyond the scope of this chapter; however, useful reviews on the analysis and chromatography[23] of biotechnology products are available as a resource for further information.

GENERAL PROPERTIES OF BIOTECHNOLOGY-PRODUCED MEDICINAL AGENTS

rDNA and hybridoma technologies have made it possible to produce large quantities of highly pure, therapeutically useful proteins. The rDNA-derived proteins and monoclonal antibodies (MAbs) are not dissimilar to the other protein pharmaceuticals or biopharmaceuticals that pharmacists have dispensed in the past. As polymers of amino acids joined by peptide bonds, the properties of these proteins differ generally from those of small organic molecule pharmaceuticals.

Stability of Biotech Pharmaceuticals

The instability of proteins, including protein pharmaceuticals, can be separated into three distinct classes. Chemical instability results from bond formation or cleavage yielding a modification of the protein and a new chemical entity. Photoinstability of protein drugs upon exposure to light results in chemical and physical instability. Physical instability involves a change to the secondary or higher order structure of the protein rather than a covalent bond–breaking modification.[24-26]

Chemical Instability

A variety of reactions give rise to the chemical instability of proteins, including hydrolysis, oxidation, racemization, β-elimination, and disulfide exchange (Fig. 5.10). Each of these changes may cause a loss of biologic activity. Proteolytic hydrolysis of peptide bonds results in fragmentation of the protein chain. It is well established that in dilute acids, aspartic acid residues in proteins are hydrolyzed at a rate at least 100-fold faster than that of other peptide bonds because of the mechanism of the reaction.

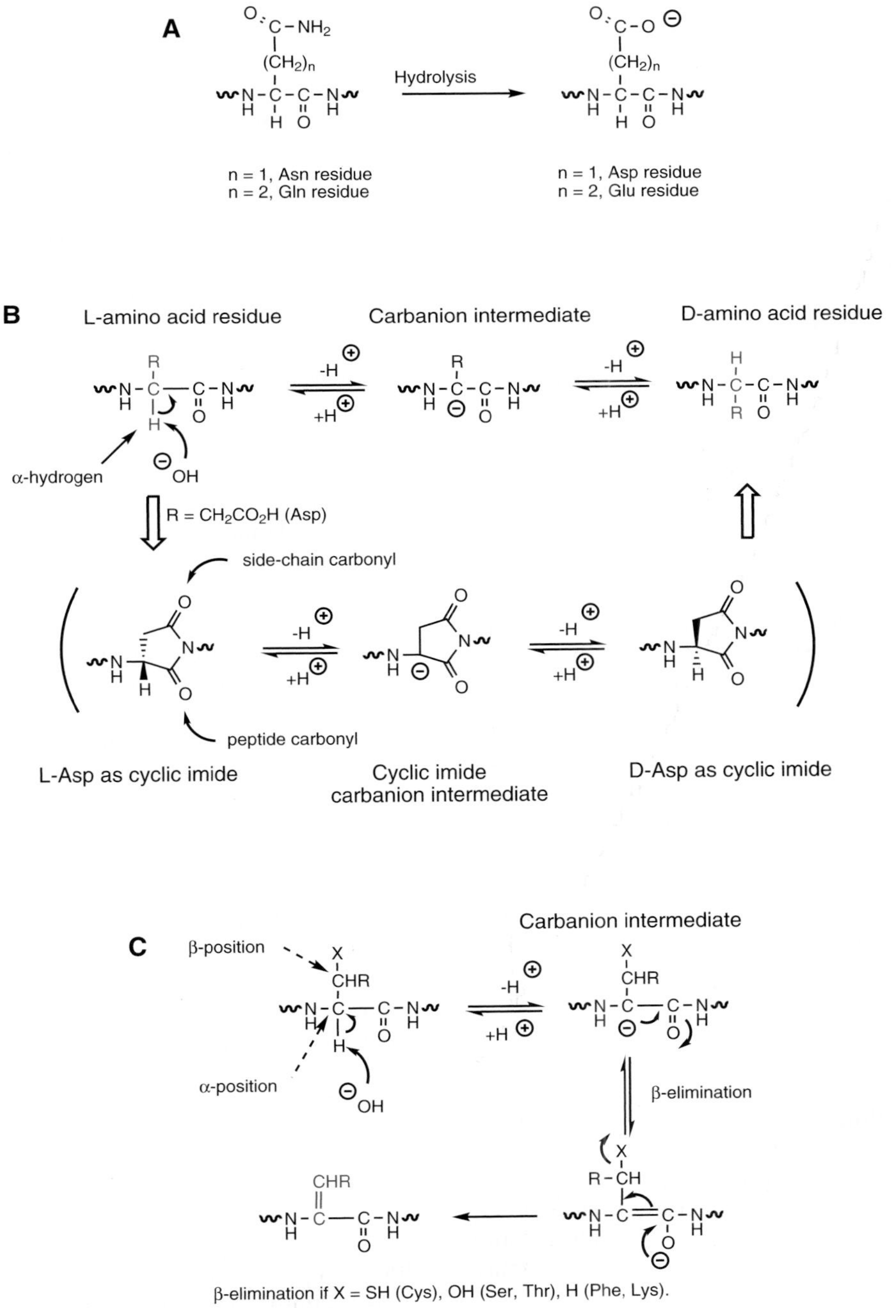

Figure 5.10 Chemical instability of protein biopharmaceuticals. (A) Hydrolysis, (B) base-catalyzed racemization, and (C) β-elimination.

An additional hydrolysis reaction is the deamidation of the neutral residue of asparagine and glutamine side chain linkages, forming the ionizable carboxylic acid residues aspartic acid and glutamic acid (Fig. 5.10A). This conversion may be considered primary sequence isomerization.[26]

Oxidative degradative reactions can occur to the side chains of sulfur-containing methionine and cysteine residues and the aromatic amino acid residues histidine, tryptophan, and tyrosine in proteins during their isolation and storage. The weakly nucleophilic thioether group of methionine ($R\text{-}S\text{-}CH_3$) can be oxidized at low pH by hydrogen peroxide as well as by oxygen in the air to the sulfoxide ($R\text{-}SO\text{-}CH_3$) and the sulfone ($R\text{-}SO_2\text{-}CH_3$). The thiol (sulfhydryl, R-SH) group of cysteine can be successively oxidized to the corresponding sulfenic acid (R-SOH), disulfide (R-SS-R), sulfinic acid ($R\text{-}SO_2H$), and, finally, sulfonic acid ($R\text{-}SO_3H$). A number of factors, including pH, influence the rate of this oxidation. Oxidation of histidine, tryptophan, and tyrosine residues is believed to occur with a variety of oxidizing agents, resulting in the cleavage of the aromatic rings.

Base-catalyzed racemization reactions may occur in any of the amino acids except achiral glycine to yield residues in proteins with mixtures of L- and D-configurations. The α-methine hydrogen is removed to form a carbanion intermediate (Fig. 5.10B). The degree of stabilization of this intermediate controls the rate of this reaction. Racemization generally alters the proteins' physicochemical properties and biologic activity. Also, racemization generates nonmetabolizable D-configuration forms of the amino acids. Aspartate residues in proteins racemize at a 10^5-fold faster rate than when free, in contrast to the 2- to 4-fold increase for the other residues. The facilitated rate of racemization for aspartic acid residues is believed to result from the formation of a stabilized cyclic imide.

Proteins containing cysteine, serine, threonine, phenylalanine, and lysine are prone to β-elimination reactions under alkaline conditions (Fig. 5.10C). The reaction proceeds through the same carbanion intermediate as racemization. The reaction is influenced by a number of additional factors, including temperature and the presence of metal ions.

The interrelationships of disulfide bonds and free sulfhydryl groups in proteins are important factors influencing the chemical and biologic properties of protein pharmaceuticals. Disulfide exchange can result in incorrect pairings and major changes in the higher order structure (secondary and above) of proteins. The exchange may occur in neutral, acidic, and alkaline media.

Photoinstability

The exposure of proteins to light and the ensuing chemical and physical degradation have been studied extensively for many years.[26] The peptide backbone, tryptophan, tyrosine, phenylalanine, and cysteine are the primary targets of photodegradation in proteins. Primary or type I photodegradation begins with absorption of light, resulting in excitation of an electron to higher energy singlet states. Absorption occurs through either the peptide backbone or by the amino acid side chains of tryptophan, tyrosine, phenylalanine, and cysteine. In aqueous solution, the absorption wavelengths are 180-230 nm for the peptide backbone, 280-305 nm for tryptophan, 260-290 nm for tyrosine, 240-270 nm for phenylalanine, and 250-300 nm for cysteine. Although tryptophan is present in relatively low abundance in proteins, it has the highest molar absorption coefficients and is therefore a major player in the photodegradation of protein drugs.

The major photolytic pathways of tryptophan in proteins are shown in Figure 5.11. Following absorption of light, the excited state tryptophan will relax to the lowest energy singlet state followed by fluorescence, undergo intersystem crossing to the triplet state (^{3}tryptophan), or eject an electron with formation of a tryptophan radical cation that will rapidly deprotonate to form the neutral tryptophan radical. The tryptophan radical may extract a hydrogen from a nearby tyrosine, repairing the tryptophan and forming a tyrosine phenoxy radical; react with oxygen, if present, forming a peroxy radical on the Trp; or react with nearby amino acids.

The ejected electron can become solvated forming an e^-_{aq} or migrate along the peptide backbone and react with cystine residues, forming a disulfide radical anion as discussed below. Under anaerobic conditions, the tryptophan triplet state generally either relaxes back to the ground state with formation of light at 420-500 nm or electron transfers to a nearby cystine with subsequent reactions as discussed earlier. In the presence of oxygen, formation of the tryptophan-based peroxy radical can undergo further reaction to produce N-formylkyneurenine and kyneurenine. Interestingly, the N-formylkyneurenine and kyneurenine absorb light at longer wavelengths than Trp, thereby acting as photosensitizers to visible light, causing additional damage to the protein. Likewise, photodegradation of tyrosine, phenylalanine, cysteine, and histidine residues in proteins can occur.

Changes in the primary structure of the protein can result in changes in the secondary and tertiary structures, impacting long-term stability, bioactivity, and immunogenicity of the peptide and protein drugs. Complete protection of the proteins from light is the only method to prevent photodegradation. This is achieved with primary and secondary packaging containers such as cardboard boxes that block incoming light to the protein. Addition of excipients such as methionine is also used to further reduce the protein aggregation as in the case of darbepoetin alfa formulation. Methionine is known to react with peroxide to form methionine sulfoxide and likely reduces protein aggregation through its effect as a peroxide scavenger. Because photodegradation reactions occur through generation of singlet oxygen species, which are generated during the photolytic process by reaction of molecular dioxygen, some biopharmaceutical products, both liquid and lyophilized, are packaged in inert atmospheres.

Physical Instability

Generally not encountered in most small organic molecules, physical instability is a consequence of the polymeric nature of proteins. Proteins adopt secondary, tertiary, and quaternary structures, which influence

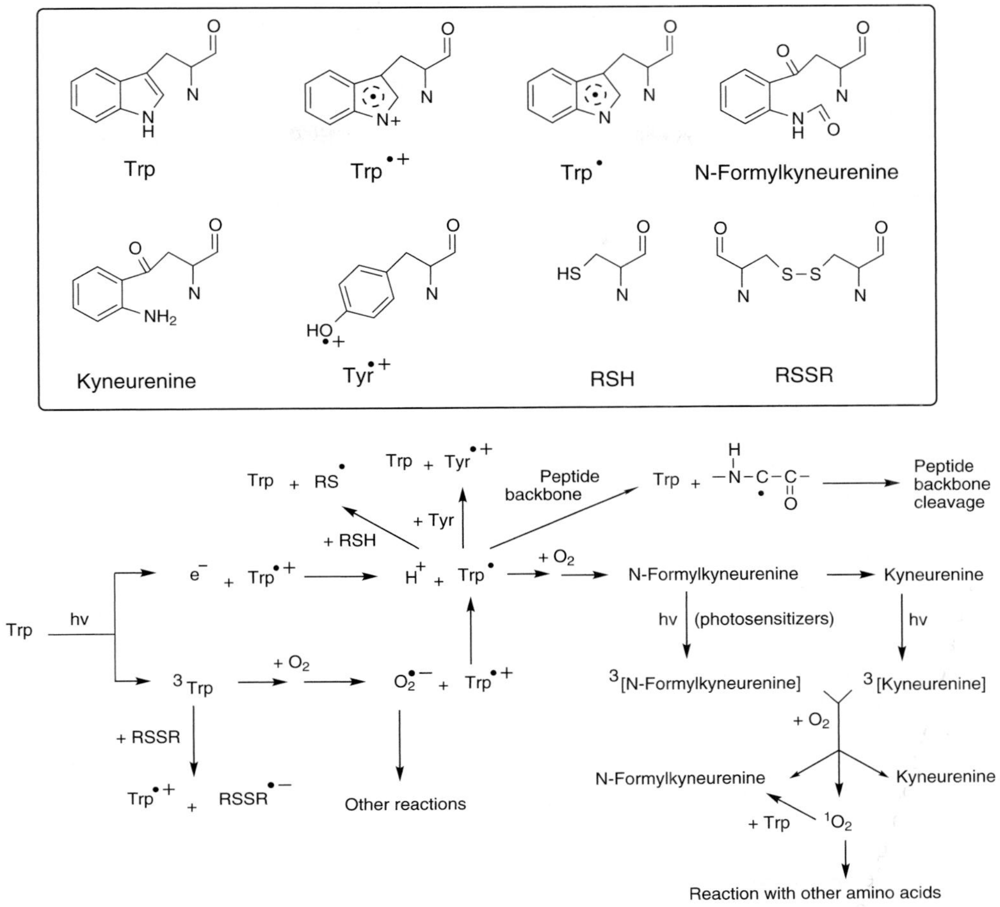

Figure 5.11 Structure of tryptophan (Trp), tyrosine (Tyr), and common photolytic pathways.

their three-dimensional shape and, therefore, their biologic activity. Any change to the higher order structure of a protein may alter both. Physical instability includes denaturation, adsorption to surfaces, and noncovalent self-aggregation (soluble and precipitation). The most widely studied aspect of protein instability is denaturation. Noncovalent aggregation, however, is one of the primary mechanisms of protein degradation.[27]

A protein, in principle, can be folded into a virtually infinite number of conformations. Denaturation occurs by disrupting the weaker noncovalent interactions that hold a protein together in its secondary and tertiary structures. Temperature, pH, and the addition of organic solvents and solutes may cause denaturation. The process can be reversible or irreversible. In general, denaturation affects the protein by decreasing aqueous solubility, altering the three-dimensional molecular shape, increasing susceptibility to enzymatic hydrolysis, and causing the loss of the native protein's biologic activity.

Handling and Storage of Biotechnology-Produced Products

The preparation and administration of protein drugs of synthetic, recombinant, or hybridoma origin are dissimilar to the nonprotein pharmaceuticals. Proteins generally have more limited shelf stability. The average shelf life for a biotechnology product is 12-18 months, compared with more than 36 months for a low-molecular-weight drug. Although each individual biotechnology drug may be different, several generalizations can be made.

Proper storage of the lyophilized and the reconstituted drug is essential. Most of these drugs are expensive, so special care must be taken not to inactivate the therapeutic protein during storage and handling. The human proteins have limited chemical and physical stability, which is shortened on reconstitution. Expiration dating ranges from 2 hours to 30 days. The self-association of either native state or misfolded protein subunits may readily occur under certain conditions. This can lead to aggregation and precipitation and results in a loss of biologic activity. Self-association mechanisms depend on the conditions of formulation and may occur as a result of hydrophobic interactions.

Many of the biotechnology-produced drugs are stored refrigerated, but not frozen (2-8°C). In general, temperature extremes must be avoided. One example is the rDNA-produced, blood clot–dissolving drug alteplase. A recombinant version of a naturally occurring human tissue-type plasminogen activator, lyophilized alteplase is stable at room temperature for several years if protected from light. Freezing or exposure to excessive heat decreases the physical stability of the protein. Anything that causes denaturation or self-aggregation, even though labile peptide bonds are not broken, may inactivate the protein. Some pharmacy facilities may need to increase cold storage capacity to accommodate biotech storage needs. If the patient must travel any distance home after receiving the medication, the pharmacist should help package the biotechnology product according to the manufacturer's directions. This may mean supplying a reusable cooler for the patient's use. Because the protein drug should not be frozen, the cooler should contain an ice pack rather than dry ice.

Some rDNA-derived pharmaceuticals, particularly the cytokines (e.g., the interferons, interleukin-2, and colony-stimulating factors), require human serum albumin in their formulation to prevent adhesion of the protein drug to the glass surface of the vial, which results in loss of protein. The amount of human serum albumin added varies with the biotech product. The vials should not be shaken to prevent foaming of the albumin, which causes protein loss or inactivation of the biotechnology-derived proteins. Care must be exercised in reconstituting protein pharmaceuticals. The diluent used for reconstitution of biotechnology drugs varies with the product and is specified by the manufacturer. Diluents can include normal saline, bacteriostatic water, and 5% dextrose. Several reviews of biotechnology drugs written for pharmacists contain additional information on the subjects of handling and storage.

Pharmacokinetic Considerations of Biotechnology-Produced Proteins

The processes of absorption into, distribution within, metabolism by, and excretion from the body (i.e., ADME) of biotechnology-produced pharmaceuticals are important factors affecting the time course of their pharmacologic effect. To deliver quality pharmaceutical care with biotech products, a pharmacist must be able to apply pharmacokinetic principles to establish and maintain a nontoxic, therapeutic effect. The pharmacokinetics of protein and peptide drugs differs in some pharmacokinetic aspects from those of the small molecule organic agents with which we are most familiar. Although a lengthy discussion of this topic is beyond the scope of this chapter, a brief overview of metabolism follows. Useful reviews are also available for further information.[28,29]

The plasma half-life of most administered proteins and peptides is relatively short because they are susceptible to a wide variety of metabolic reactions. The enzymes involved in peptide bond hydrolysis and, thus, the degradation of peptides and proteins are known as peptidases and can be found in the blood, in the vascular bed, in the interstitial fluid, on cell membranes, and within cells. These enzymes include carboxypeptidases (cleaves C-terminal residues), dipeptidyl carboxypeptidases (cleaves dipeptides from the C-terminus), aminopeptidases (cleaves N-terminal residues), and amidases (cleaves internal peptide bonds). For the most part, these enzymes are all specific for the natural amino acids of the L-configuration. Overall, the metabolic products of most proteins and peptides are not considered to be a safety issue. They generally are broken down into amino acids and reincorporated into new, endogenously biosynthesized proteins.

Metabolic oxidation reactions may occur to the side chains of sulfur-containing residues, similar to that observed for in vitro chemical instability. Methionine can be oxidized to the sulfoxide, whereas metabolic oxidation of cysteine residues forms a disulfide. Metabolic reductive cleavage of disulfide bridges in proteins may occur, yielding free sulfhydryl groups.

Biotechnology Drug Delivery

Protein-based pharmaceuticals, whether produced by biotechnology or isolated from traditional sources, present challenges to drug delivery because of the unique demands imposed by their physicochemical and biologic properties. Although a detailed discussion of this topic is beyond the scope of this chapter, a brief overview follows. Useful reviews also are available for further information.[30-32]

Delivery of high-molecular-weight, biotechnology-produced drugs into the body is difficult because of the poor absorption of these drugs, the acid lability of peptide bonds, and the rapid enzymatic degradation of these drugs in the body. In addition, protein pharmaceuticals are susceptible to physical instability, complex feedback control mechanisms, and peculiar dose-response relationships.

Given the limitations of today's technology, the strongly acidic environment of the stomach, the peptidases in the gastrointestinal tract, and the barrier to absorption presented by gastrointestinal mucosal cells preclude successful oral administration of most protein and peptide drugs. Therefore, administration of all the biotechnology-produced protein drugs and some natural or synthetic peptides currently is parenteral (by intravenous, subcutaneous, or intramuscular injections) to provide a better therapeutic profile. Manufacturers supply most of these drugs as sterile solutions without a preservative. In such cases, it is recommended that only one dose be prepared from each vial to prevent bacterial contamination.

Novel solutions to overcome delivery problems associated with biotechnology protein products and natural or synthetic peptide drugs are being explored. Oral drug delivery approaches in development for proteins and peptide drugs include conjugated systems (e.g., PEGylation with polyethylene glycol), amino acid substitution, liposomes, microspheres, erythrocytes as carriers, and viruses as drug carriers.

PEGylation is frequently used to improve the pharmacokinetic properties of biotechnology-produced drugs.[33] This method involves the attachment of a flexible strand or strands of polyethylene glycol (PEG) to a protein. PEG is a simple, water-soluble, nontoxic polymer that is nonimmunogenic, is readily cleared from the body, and has been approved for human administration by mouth, injection, and topical application. The most common process used for PEGylation of protein is to activate the PEG with functional groups suitable for reaction with lysine and N-terminal amino groups. PEGylated proteins are less rapidly broken down by the body's enzymes than are the unmodified proteins. PEG can extend the duration of action of proteins and peptides in the body from minutes, to hours, to days, depending on the PEG molecule used. By increasing the biologic half-life and improving the efficacy of proteins in the body, these modifications can reduce the frequency of injections a patient requires. They also reduce the rapidity and intensity of the body's immune reaction against molecules such as interferon. Several PEGylated protein products (e.g., pegvisomant, certolizumab pegol, peginterferon α2a) are currently marketed, and many are under development.

When metabolism studies indicate a predominant cleavage site, attempts can be made to replace that residue with another that retains the receptor-binding activity of the protein/peptide drug while yielding enhanced resistance to peptidase activity. Often, this can be accomplished by replacing the offending L-residue with its enantiomer, the D-amino acid, or another D-residue. Many peptidases are unable to cleave peptide bonds consisting of a "fraudulent" D-amino acid, and peptides containing such changes are designed as a means to increase their half-life. Also, the replacement of an L-amino acid with L-proline or N-methylation of the amide nitrogen offers the possibility of generating a peptide that is more resistant to enzymatic hydrolysis. The introduction of pseudopeptide bonds[34] and the design of retro-inverso peptides[35] are two examples of strategies that can afford peptidase resistance to peptide drugs.

Adverse Effects

An important consideration in the pharmaceutical care of a patient being administered a biotechnology-produced medicinal agent is the potential for adverse reactions. Many of the protein drugs are biotechnology-derived versions of endogenous human proteins normally present, on stimulus, in minute quantities near their specific site of action. Therefore, the same protein administered in much larger quantities may cause adverse effects not commonly observed at normal physiologic concentrations. Careful monitoring of patients administered biotechnology-produced drugs is critical for the health care team.

Immunogenicity

The immune system may respond to an antigen, such as a protein pharmaceutical, by triggering the production of antibodies. Biotechnology-derived proteins may possess a different set of antigenic determinants (i.e., regions of a protein recognized by an antibody) because of structural differences between the recombinant protein and the natural human protein.[36] Factors that can contribute to this immunogenicity include lack of or incorrect glycosylation, amino acid modifications, and amino acid additions and deletions. A number of recombinant proteins produced with bacterial vectors contain an N-terminal methionine in addition to the natural human amino acid sequence. Bacterial vector-derived recombinant protein preparations also may contain small amounts of immunoreactive bacterial polypeptides as possible contaminants. Additionally, immunogenicity may result from proteins that are misfolded, denatured, or aggregated.

Production of Peptide and Protein Drugs

The production of many of important peptides and proteins, via synthetic procedures as well as through biotechnology, involves the pharmaceutical industry. Of necessity, peptides of low to moderate molecular weight, chemically modified peptides, and those containing pseudopeptide bonds or fraudulent amino acids will continue to be made by synthetic procedures rather than through biotechnology. Many of these peptides and proteins are available as chemical analogs, and these also are discussed, particularly the chemical changes made and the implications of these changes to the resulting biologic action (see Chapter 34).

MONOCLONAL ANTIBODIES

Introduction to Antibodies

The cell-mediated branch of the immune system includes the antibody-secreting B cells or plasma cells.[37] Antibodies or immunoglobulins are soluble proteins that are produced in response to an antigenic stimulus. As part of the normal immune system, each B cell produces as many as 100 million antibody proteins (polyclonal antibodies) directed against bacteria, viruses, and other foreign invaders. Antibodies act by binding to a particular antigen, thereby "tagging" it for removal or destruction by other immune system components.

The production of antigen-"neutralizing" antibodies or immunoglobulins and the detection of a sufficient antibody titer are important concepts for an understanding of vaccinations and exposure to antigens. The humoral response to an antigen involves the creation of memory B cells and the transformation of B lymphocyte into plasma cells that serve as factories for the production of secreted antibodies. Approximately 4 days after initial contact with an antigen (immunization), immunoglobulin M (IgM) antibodies (one of five types of immunoglobulin structure) appear and then peak approximately 4 hours later. Approximately 7 days after exposure, IgG, the major class of circulating immunoglobulin, appears. The antibodies bind to the antigen and affect additional immune system–mediated events, "neutralizing" the antigen and leading to its elimination. The concentration of an immunoglobulin specific for a given antigen at a given time is referred to as the antibody titer and may be a measure of the effectiveness of the initial antigen exposure/vaccination to elicit immunologic memory.

MAbs are monovalent antibodies that bind to the same epitope and are produced from a single B-lymphocyte clone. Some of the improvements that can be done on Abs include minimizing immunogenicity and enhancing antigen-binding affinity, effector function, and pharmacokinetic profile.[38] One can reduce immunogenicity by minimizing nonhuman sequences by creating chimeric, humanized, or human versions of Abs. Antigen-binding affinity can be enhanced by using phage display libraries to isolate MAbs with strong affinities to the antigen.

Antibody Structure

Antibodies are glycoproteins. The simplest structure of an immunoglobulin molecule consists of two identical long peptide chains (the heavy chains) and two identical short polypeptide chains (the light chains) interconnected by several disulfide bonds. The selectivity of any immunoglobulin for a particular antigen is determined by its structure and, specifically, by the variable or antigen-binding regions (Fig. 5.12). Enzymatic digestion of the antibody with papain yields the functional human antibody (Fab) fragment, which contains the antigen-binding sites, and the Fc fragment, which specifies the other biologic activities of the molecule.

Hybridoma Technology

MAbs are ultrasensitive, hybrid immune system–derived proteins designed to recognize specific antigens. Nobel Laureates Kohler and Milstein first reported MAbs in 1975.[39] MAbs have been used in laboratory diagnostics, site-directed drugs, and home test kits. The B lymphocyte produces a wide range of structurally diverse antibody proteins with varying degrees of specificity in response to a single antigen stimulus. Because of their structural diversity, these antibodies would be called polyclonal antibodies. MAbs are homogeneous hybrid proteins produced by a selected, single clone of an engineered B lymphocyte. They are designed to recognize specific sites or epitopes on antigens.

Hybridoma technology (the technology used to produce MAbs) consists of combining or fusing two different cell lines: a myeloma cell (generally from a mouse) and a plasma spleen cell (B lymphocyte) capable of producing an antibody that recognizes a specific antigen (Fig. 5.13). The resulting fused cell, or hybridoma, possesses some of the characteristics of both original cells: the myeloma cell's ability to survive and reproduce in culture (immortality) and the plasma spleen cell's ability to produce antibodies to a specific antigen.

Monoclonal antibodies are more attractive than polyclonal antibodies for diagnostic and therapeutic applications because of their increased specificity of antigen recognition. Thus, they can serve as target-directed "homing devices" to find and attach to the targeted antigen. Developments in hybridoma technology have led to highly specific diagnostic agents for home use in pregnancy testing and ovulation prediction kits; laboratory use in detection of colorectal cancer, ovarian cancer, and others; and design of site-directed therapeutic agents, such as trastuzumab to combat metastatic breast cancer and abciximab as an adjunct for the prevention of cardiac ischemic complications.

Monoclonal Antibody Immunogenicity

Nearly 25 years after the pioneering work of Kohler and Milstein, MAbs began to realize their therapeutic potential.[40] Until recently, most MAbs were murine proteins based on their production. Initial clinical trials of murine MAbs showed that these mouse proteins were highly immunogenic in patients after just a single dose. Human patients formed antibodies to combat the foreign MAb that was administered. The human anti-mouse antibody response is known as HAMA. So, far from being the "magic bullets" that were proposed, immunogenic murine MAbs were useless in chronic therapy. Thus, a different approach was needed to eliminate the unwanted immune response (HAMA) in patients.

The variable regions of an immunoglobulin must be of a specific chemical structure with the ability to bind to the antigen they "recognize." The part within the variable region that forms the intermolecular interactions with the antigen is the complementarity-determining region (CDR). The variable domains of antibody light and heavy chains contain three CDRs each.

It was determined that immune responses against the mouse-produced MAbs were directed against both the variable and the constant regions of the antibody. Human and murine antibodies are very homologous in

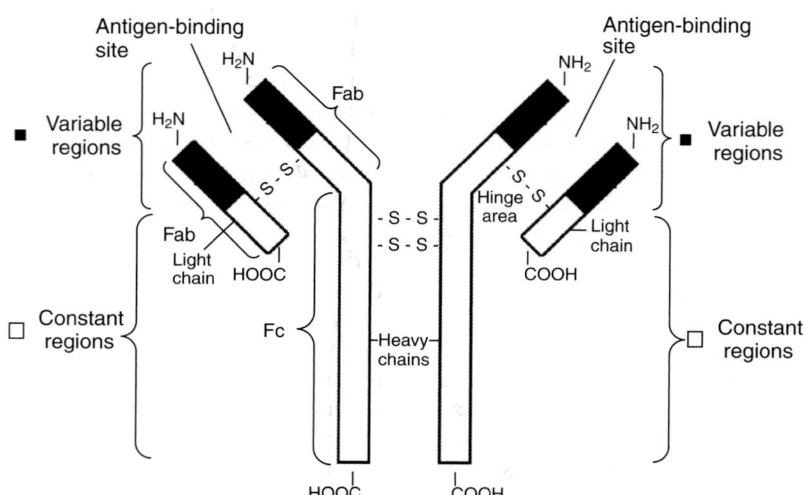

Figure 5.12 Schematic model of an antibody molecule.

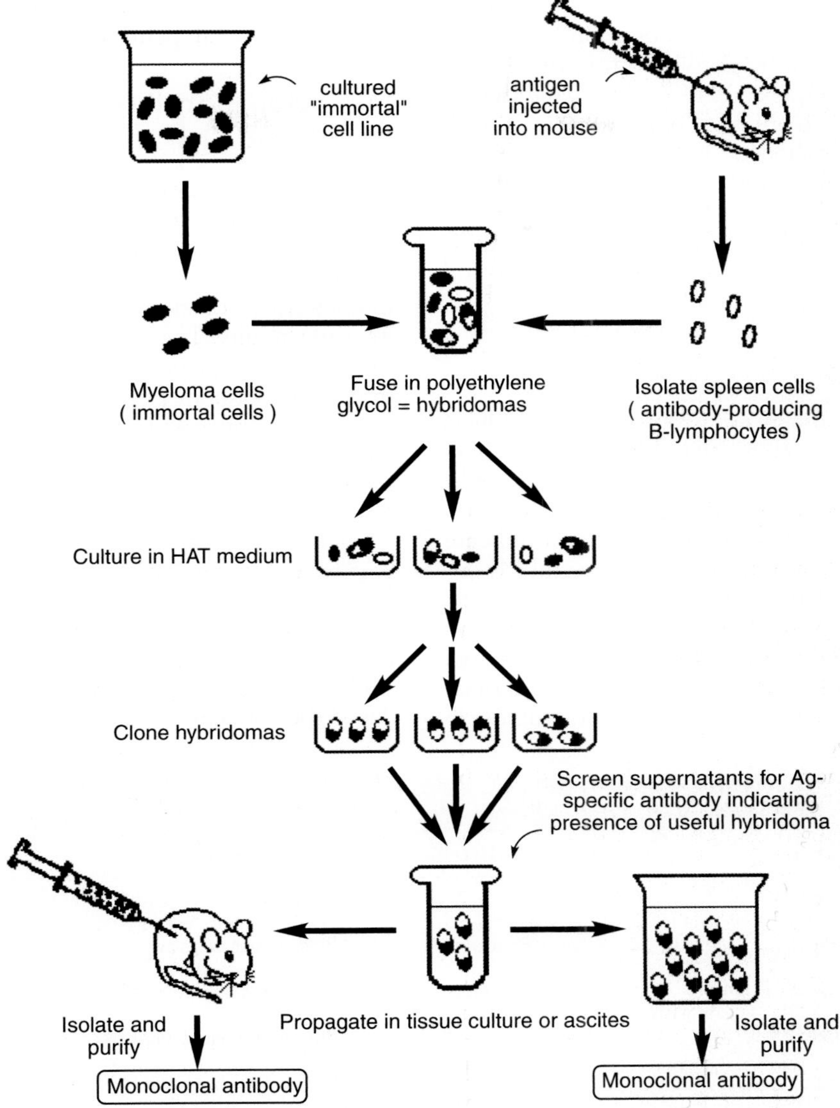

Figure 5.13 Outline of hybridoma creation and monoclonal antibody (MAb) production.

chemical structure. Thus, a MAb with decreased immunogenicity can be engineered by replacing the mouse constant regions of an IgG with human constant regions, making the antibody less mouselike. In practice, what generally occurs is that the variable heavy chain and variable light chain domains (CDRs) of human immunoglobulins are replaced with those of a murine antibody, which possesses the requisite antigen specificity. This "chimeric" MAb will retain its ability to recognize the antigen (a property of the murine MAb) and retain the many effector functions of an immunoglobulin (both murine and human) but will be much less immunogenic (a property of a human immunoglobulin). A chimeric MAb, containing approximately 70% human sequence, will have a longer half-life than its murine counterpart in a human patient. Therapeutic MAbs that are chimeric include catumaxomab (for malignant ascites), cetuximab (for colorectal cancer), and infliximab (for Crohn's disease).

The discovery of the conserved structure of antibodies, particularly IgGs, across many species suggested the possibility of chimeric antibodies, and the realization that the homology extended to the antigen-binding site facilitated the engineering of humanized immunoglobulins. Advances in phage display technology and the production of transgenic animals has led to the production of humanized or fully human MAbs.[39] Functional human antibody fragments (e.g., Fab fragments) can be displayed on the surface of bacteriophages. A bacteriophage, also called a phage, is a virus that infects bacteria. The expression of these human antibody fragments on the phage surface has facilitated efficient screening of large numbers of phage clones (phage display) for antigen-binding specificity.[41] Once a fragment with the requisite antigen specificity is selected, it can be isolated and engineered into a humanized MAb (replacing up to 95% of the murine protein sequence) or a fully human MAb (100% human sequence). Transgenic strains of mice have been genetically engineered to possess most or all of the essential human antibody genes. Thus, on immunization with a foreign antigen, the transgenic mice will develop humanized or fully human antibodies in response. Both of these techniques, although very complex and expensive, have yielded FDA-approved, humanized antibody pharmaceuticals, such as alemtuzumab (for lymphocytic leukemia), bevacizumab (for metastatic colorectal cancer), eculizumab (for paroxysmal nocturnal hemoglobinemia), and trastuzumab (for refractory breast cancer). The half-life of humanized antibodies is dramatically enhanced (from hours to weeks), and immunogenicity is drastically reduced.

Monoclonal Antibody Diagnostic Agents

Several ultrasensitive diagnostic MAb-based products have enjoyed great success; these include a variety of imaging agents for the detection of blood clots and cancer cells. A monoclonal Fab fragment, technetium-99m-arcitumomab (CEA-Scan), can detect the presence and indicate the location of recurrent and metastatic colorectal cancer. Colorectal cancer and ovarian cancer can be detected with satumomab pendetide (OncoScint CR/OV). Capromab pendetide (ProstaScint) is used for detection, staging, and follow-up of patients with prostate adenocarcinoma. Small-cell lung cancer can be detected with nofetumomab (Verluma). The first imaging MAb for myocardial infarction is imiciromab pentetate (MyoScint).

Monoclonal Antibody–Based, In-Home Diagnostic Kits

The strong trend toward self-care, coupled with a heightened awareness by the public of available technology and an emphasis on preventive medicine, has increased the use of in-home diagnostics. MAb specifically minimizes the possibilities of interference from other substances that might yield false-positive test results. The antigen being selectively detected by MAb-based pregnancy test kits is human chorionic gonadotropin, the hormone produced if fertilization occurs and that continues to increase in concentration during the pregnancy. Table 5.3 lists some examples of MAb-containing in-home pregnancy test kits as well as some examples of MAb-based, in-home ovulation prediction kits.

ANTIBODY-DRUG CONJUGATES

Paul Ehrlich, in late 1800s and early 1900s, pioneered the studies in immunology as well as chemotherapy and introduced the concept of "magic bullets." It is now known that

Table 5.3 Some MAb-Based In-Home Test Kits

Manufacturer	Product Distributor	Positive End Point
Pregnancy		
Answer Plus	Carter Products	Plus in test window = +
Answer Quick & Simple	Carter Products	Plus in test window = +
Clear Blue Easy	Unipath	Blue line in large window = +
Clear Blue Easy One Min.	Unipath	Blue line in large window = +
Conceive	Quidel	Pink to purple test line = +
I Step E.P.T.	Warner Lambert	Pink color in test and control = +
Ovulation		
Answer Quick & Simple	Carter Products	Purple stick line darker than reference = +
Conceive I Step	Quidel	Pink to purple test line darker than reference = +
First Response I Step	Carter Products	Purple test line darker than reference = +
Clear Plan Easy	Unipath	Blue test line in large window similar or darker than line in small window = +
Ovukit Self Test	Quidel	White to shades of blue compared to LH surge guide = +
OvuQuick	Quidel	Test spot appears darker than reference = +
Q Test	Quidel	Purple test line darker than reference = +

Data from Pray W. *Nonprescription Product Therapeutics*. 2nd ed. Philadelphia: Lippincott Williams & Wilkins; 2006:778-780; Quattrocchi E, Hove I. Ovulation & pregnancy home testing products. *U.S. Pharmacist*. 1998;23:54-63; and Rosenthal WM, Briggs GC. Home testing and monitoring devices. In: Allen LV Jr, Berardi RR, DeSimone EM II, et al., eds. *Handbook of Nonprescription Drugs*. Washington, D.C.: American Pharmaceutical Association; 2000:917-942.
LH, luteinizing hormone; MAb, monoclonal antibody.

cancer cells differ from normal cells as a consequence of genomic mutations in oncogenes and/or tumor suppressor genes.[42] Consequently, certain antigens are specifically expressed on the surface of human tumor cells, which can be targeted by MAbs. Binding of MAbs to such tumor cells surface antigens is highly specific and triggers cell death by many mechanisms, including abrogation of tumor cell signaling and apoptosis, complement-dependent cytotoxicity, and inhibition of tumor vasculature. Despite many cell-killing mechanisms, MAbs often have limited antitumor activity as single agents, particularly against solid tumors.[43] Conventional chemotherapeutic agents on the other hand suffer from systemic toxicity and a lack of tumor specificity. This has paved the way for the development of antibody-drug conjugates (ADCs).[44] ADCs are tripartite drugs containing a tumor-specific MAb conjugated to a potent cytotoxic agent via a stable linker. Advantage of an ADC is that it selectively delivers a cytotoxic agent to the cancer cells while sparing the normal cells offering a better balance between safety and efficacy.

There has been an explosion in ADC research over the last 10 years.[45] Early attempts to develop ADCs were plagued with limited success due to low drug potency, high antigen expression on normal cells, and unstable nature of the linker used for attaching the drug to the MAb.[46] Currently two ADCs are approved by the US FDA for the treatment of cancer: ado-trastuzumab emtansine (Kadcyla) and brentuximab vedotin (Adcetris), and more than 30 are in clinical development.

Various Aspects of Designing ADCs

The selected MAb should target a well-defined antigen that is highly expressed at the tumor site but minimally expressed in the normal tissue to ensure efficient killing of tumor cells by ADCs while limiting general toxicity. Bifunctional linkers carrying attachment sites for both the MAb and cytotoxic drug are used to join the two components. Existing linker attachment strategies typically depend on the modification of solvent-accessible cysteine or lysine residues on the MAb, which leads to heterogeneous ADC populations with variable drug:MAb ratios. While low drug loading reduces potency, high drug loading can negatively impact pharmacokinetics (PK). The drug:MAb ratios can also significantly influence the efficacy of ADCs. Moreover, the linker must remain stable in systemic circulation to minimize adverse effects yet rapidly cleave once ADC binds to its intended target antigen. Once antigen is recognized and ADC binds to it, ensuing ADC-antigen complex is internalized via a receptor-mediated endocytosis.[47] Once inside the cell, the drug is released by one of several mechanisms, including nonenzymatic hydrolysis or enzymatic cleavage of the linker or via degradation of the antibody.

Linker technology and stability:

The two major classes of linkers being widely used in ADC drug development include cleavable and noncleavable linkers that utilize different mechanisms for release of the drug payload from the MAb (Fig. 5.14). The cleavable linkers are of three types: (1) lysosomal protease–sensitive linkers, (2) acid-sensitive linkers, and (3) glutathione-sensitive linkers.

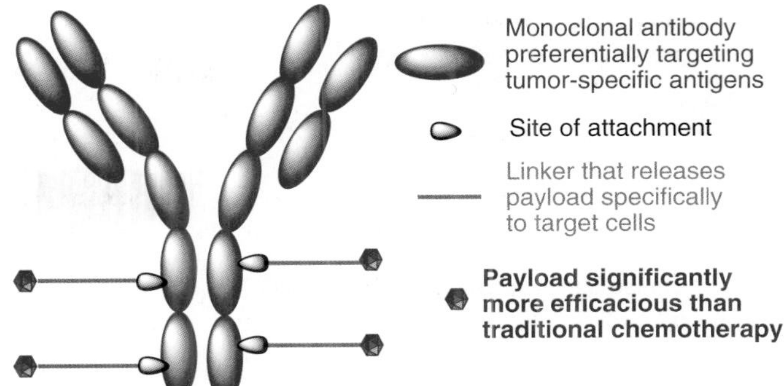

Figure 5.14 Schematic representation of key components of an antibody-drug conjugate (ADC).

1. Lysosomal protease–sensitive linkers. Lysosomal proteases such as cathepsin B particularly recognize and cleave a dipeptide bond as in a valine-citrulline linker (Fig. 5.15) to release the free drug from the ADC.[48] Several ADCs evaluated in the clinic including FDA-approved brentuximab vedotin (for Hodgkin lymphoma) contain such a linker because it provided optimal balance between plasma stability and subsequent cleavage by intracellular protease.[49]
2. Acid-sensitive linkers (Fig. 5.15). These types of linkers exploit the low pH (~5) in the lysosomal compartment to initiate hydrolysis of an acid-labile hydrazone group of the linker and subsequent release of the drug payload from the ADC. Hydrazone linkers have been used in the discovery and development of Mylotarg (anti-CD33 calicheamicin conjugate) and in inotuzumab ozogamicin (anti-CD22 calicheamicin conjugate)[50,51]; however, both of these ADCs were withdrawn from the market due to toxicities related to the unstable nature of the hydrazone linker.[52]
3. Glutathione-sensitive linkers (Fig. 5.15). These linkers take advantage of the higher concentration of glutathione inside the cell relative to that in the plasma. Therefore, a disulfide bond in these linkers is relatively stable in the bloodstream; however, it is capable of undergoing reduction by intracellular glutathione, which ultimately leads to release of the free drug from ADCs. The increased plasma stability of a disulfide bond in the circulation is a result of insertion of a sterically crowded *gem*-dimethyl group adjacent to the disulfide bond to prevent premature cleavage in the plasma.[53,54] Similar to other linkers described above, glutathione-sensitive linkers are also used in several clinical ADC candidates, including SAR3419 (anti-CD19 maytansine conjugate), IMGN901 (anti-CD56 maytansine conjugate), and AVE9633 (anti-CD33 maytansine conjugate).[51]

The noncleavable linker strategy depends on complete degradation of the MAb upon internalization of the ADC, which results in release of free drug molecules that

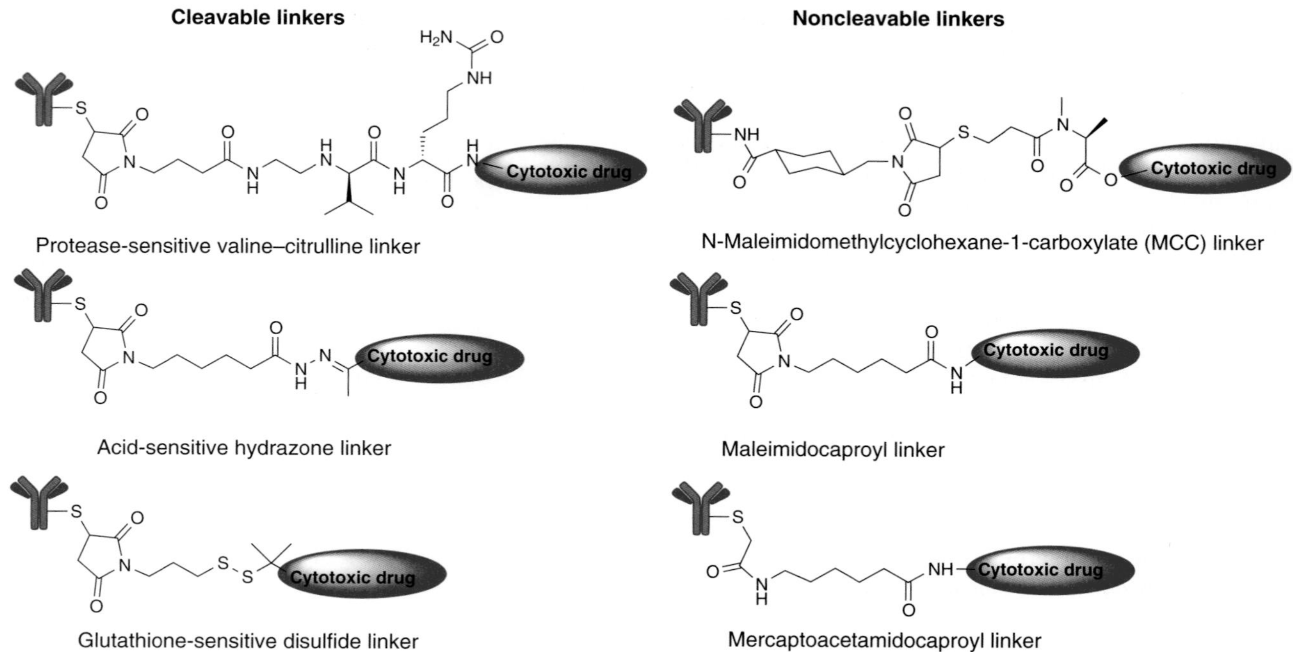

Figure 5.15 A snapshot of cleavable and noncleavable linkers used in antibody-drug conjugate (ADC) development.

still carry a linker moiety and amino acid residue from the MAb (Fig. 5.15). Noncleavable linker strategies are useful to those payloads that exert their antitumor effect despite being chemically modified. Noncleavable linker strategy has been effectively used in the development of Kadcyla (trastuzumab-MCC-DM1, for metastatic breast cancer), wherein the released modified payload (lysine-MCC-DM1) demonstrated comparable potency to DM1 alone.[55] Noncleavable linkers have greater stability in the plasma as compared to cleavable linkers.

Conjugation Strategies: Chemical Conjugation

This strategy involves covalent bonding of a reactive moiety pendant to the drug-linker to the target antibody via an amino acid residue side chain, usually the ε-amine of lysine. This strategy has been successfully used for the development of gemtuzumab ozogamicin (Mylotarg; for acute myeloid leukemia).[56] Another approach involves a two-step process wherein surface lysine residues on the target antibody are first modified to insert a reactive functional group such as a maleimide, and subsequent conjugation to the drug-linker moiety containing a suitable reactive handle such as thiol group.[57] This strategy was used for the development of trastuzumab-MCC-DM1 (Kadcyla; for metastatic breast cancer). Yet another approach involves controlled reduction of existing disulfide bonds in the target antibody to liberate free cysteine residues, which are further reacted with a maleimide attached to the drug-linker. This approach was successfully used in development of brentuximab vedotin (Adcetris; for Hodgkin lymphoma).[58] The abovementioned approaches are random and as a result produce heterogeneous mixtures of conjugated antibodies with highly variable drug-to-antibody ratios (DARs). Therefore, techniques that allow production of site-specific conjugation with robust DARs are highly desirable.

Site-specific Conjugation

This strategy allows production of homogeneous ADCs. Three major strategies for site-specific conjugation are (1) insertion of cysteine residues in the target antibody sequence by site-directed mutagenesis, (2) insertion of an unnatural amino acid residue with a bio-orthogonal reactive handle, and (3) enzymatic conjugation. As compared to conventional conjugation-derived ADCs, ADCs generated through drug-linker conjugation with the surface cysteine residues showed minimal heterogeneity, defined DAR, and improved pharmacokinetic and pharmacodynamic parameters.

Bystander Killing by ADCs

A bystander killing mechanism operates when cytotoxic species comes out of the tumor cell and diffuse and kill nearby cancer cells.[59]

Vaccines

There are two types of immunization: active immunization and passive immunization. Active immunization is the induction of an immune response either through exposure to an infectious agent or by deliberate immunization with a vaccine (vaccination) made from the microorganism or its products to develop protective immunity. Passive immunization involves the transfer of products produced by an immune animal or human (preformed antibody or sensitized lymphoid cells) to a previously nonimmune recipient host, usually by injection. Sufficient active immunity may take days, several weeks, or even months to induce (possibly including booster vaccinations), but it generally is long-lasting (even lifelong) through the clonal selection of genetically specific immunologic memory B and T lymphocytes. Passive immunity, although often providing effective protection against some infection, is relatively brief, lasting only until the injected immunoglobulin or lymphoid cells have disappeared (a few weeks or months). Thus, vaccines enable the body to resist diseases caused by infectious agents. In response to an injection of vaccine, the immune system makes antibodies, which recognize surface antigens found in the vaccine. If the subject is later exposed to a virulent form of the virus, the immune system is primed and ready to eliminate it. Many viral vaccines are produced from the antigens isolated from pooled human plasma of virus carriers. Vaccinations are among the most cost-effective and widely used public health interventions. Although generally safe, the minimal risk of vaccine-produced infections can be eliminated by administration of highly purified vaccine antigens of recombinant origin. The different types of vaccines are described below, and the vaccines currently available in the Unites States are listed in Table 5.4.

Live, Attenuated Vaccines

To make a live, attenuated vaccine, the disease-causing organism is grown under special laboratory conditions that cause it to lose its virulence or disease-causing properties.

Inactivated Vaccines

Inactivated vaccines are produced by killing the disease-causing microorganism with chemicals or heat.

Subunit Vaccines

Sometimes vaccines developed from antigenic fragments are able to evoke an immune response, often with fewer side effects than might be caused by a vaccine made from the whole organism.

Toxoid or Inactivated Toxins

A toxoid is an inactivated toxin, the harmful substance produced by a microbe. Many of the microbes that infect people are not themselves harmful. It is the powerful toxins they produce that can cause illness. To inactivate such powerful toxins, vaccine manufacturers treat them by chemical means (formalin solution) and irradiation to completely cripple any disease-causing ability.

Conjugate Vaccines

The bacteria that cause some diseases, such as pneumococcal pneumonia and certain types of meningitis, have special outer coats. These coats disguise antigens so that the immature immune systems of infants and younger children are unable to recognize these harmful bacteria. In a conjugate vaccine, proteins or toxins from a second type of organism, one that an immature immune system can recognize, are linked to the outer coats of the disease-causing bacteria. This enables a young immune system to respond and defend against the disease agent.

DNA Vaccines or Naked Vaccine

Genes encoding antigens of an infectious organism are expressed by the host's own cells. Genes are inserted into a bacterial plasmid under the control of a mammalian promoter. The chimeric plasmid is either directly injected into muscle or the DNA is conjugated to a solid matrix such as gold particles.

Recombinant Vector Vaccines

A vaccine vector, or carrier, is a weakened virus or bacterium into which harmless genetic material from another disease-causing organism can be inserted.

PHARMACOGENOMICS AND PERSONALIZED MEDICINE

Personalized medicine is defined as the utilization of molecular biomarkers from an individual's genome, transcriptome, proteome, and metabolome under the influence of the individual's envirome in the assessment of predisposition to disease, screening and early diagnosis of disease, assessment of prognosis, pharmacogenomic prediction of therapeutic drug efficacy and risk of toxicity, and monitoring of illness until the final therapeutic outcome is determined. Biomarkers serve as critical tools for disease detection and subsequent monitoring. For example, gene mutations, alterations in gene transcription and translation, and alterations in their protein products can all serve as specific biomarkers for disease.[60] Furthermore, mass spectrometry–driven proteomic analysis plays an important role in rapid detection of disease-specific biomarkers and proteomic patterns of various tissues and body fluids.[61]

The concept of personalized medicine was anticipated by Sir William Osler (1849-1919), a well-known Canadian physician during his time. He recognized that "variability is the law of life, and as no two faces are the same, so no two bodies are alike, and no two individuals react alike and behave alike under the abnormal conditions we know as disease." Personalized medicine has rapidly advanced the prediction of disease incidence as well as the prevention of prescribing the incorrect drug based on a person's clinical, genetic, and environmental information. The goal of personalized medicine is optimizing the medical care and outcomes for each patient.[62]

Pharmacogenomics uses genomic tools to understand the genotype effects of relevant genes on the behavior of a drug, as well as the effects of a drug on gene expression. The best examples of successful pharmacogenomic applications are presented below.

Drug efficacy is not solely influenced by variations in drug-metabolizing genes but also by polymorphisms in genes that encode drug receptors and transporters. Polymorphisms and alleles in major phase I drug-metabolizing enzymes (CYP450s) and phase II drug

Table 5.4 Some FDA-Approved Vaccines

Generic Name	Trade Name	Vaccine Type	Protection Against
Anthrax	BioThrax	Inactivated	Anthrax
Chicken pox	Varivax	Live attenuated	Chicken pox
Diphtheria	Pediarix	Toxoid	Diphtheria
Haemophilus influenza type b (Hib)	ActHib, PedvaxHib	Conjugate	*H. influenza*
Hepatitis A	Havrix, Vaqta	Inactivated	Hepatitis A
Hepatitis B	Engerix-B, Recombivax	Recombinant subunit	Hepatitis B
HepA-HepB	Twinrix	Inactivated recombinant	Hepatitis A and B
Herpes zoster	Zostavax	Live attenuated	Herpes zoster
Human papilloma virus	Gardasil, Cervarix	Recombinant	Cervical cancer
Influenza	Fluarix, Fluvirin, Fluzone, Flulaval, Afluria, Agriflu, FluMist	Inactivated live attenuated	Influenza
Japanese encephalitis	Ixiaro, JE-Vax	Inactivated	Japanese encephalitis
Measles	Attenuvax	Live attenuated	Measles
Meningococcal conjugate	Menactra, Menomune, Menveo	Inactivated	Meningococcal
Mumps	Mumpsvax	Live attenuated	Mumps
Pertussis	Boostrix	Subunit	Pertussis
Pneumococcal	Prevnar, PCV13, Pneumovax23	Conjugate	Pneumococcal
Polio	Ipol	Inactivated	Polio
Sipuleucel-T	Provenge	Autologous	Prostate cancer
Rabies	Imovax, Rabavert	Inactivated	Rabies
Rotavirus	Rotarix, RotaTeq	Live attenuated	Rotavirus
Rubella	Meruvax	Live attenuated	Measles
Tetanus toxoid (TT)		Toxoid	Tetanus
Typhoid	Typherix, Vivotif Berna, Typhim Vi	Inactivated	Typhoid
Varicella	Varivax	Live attenuated	Varicella
Vaccinia (smallpox)	ACAM2000	Live attenuated	Smallpox
Yellow fever	YF-Vax	Live attenuated	Yellow fever

metabolizing-enzymes (UDP-glucuronyl transferases, thiopurine S-methyltransferases [TPMT]) can be genotyped to aid physicians in individualizing treatment doses for patients on therapeutics metabolized through the products of these genes.

The oral anticoagulant warfarin is prescribed for the long-term treatment and prevention of thromboembolic events. An investigation of the pharmacokinetic and pharmacodynamic drug properties of warfarin indicated the additive involvement of two genes when determining the dosage. One of these genes encodes for CYP2C9, which is responsible for the metabolic clearance (~80%) of the pharmacologically potent S-enantiomer of warfarin (Fig. 5.16). There are three allele types, wild-type CYP2C9*1 and nonsynonymous polymorphisms *2 and *3, and both CYP2C9*2 and *3 code for CYP2C9 enzymes with reduced enzymatic activity leading to increased warfarin half-life and subsequent significant clinical influence on warfarin sensitivity and severe bleeding events.[63] A 10-fold difference in warfarin clearance was observed between groups of individuals having the genotype of the highest metabolizer (CYP2C9*1 homozygote) and lowest metabolizer (CYP2C9*3 homozygote).[64]

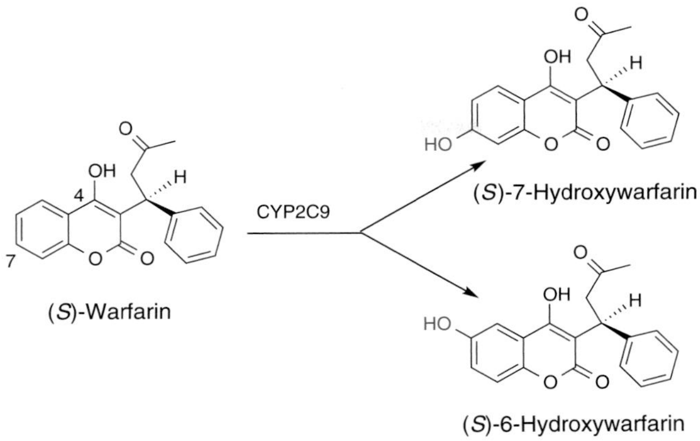

Figure 5.16 Warfarin metabolic inactivation.

Tamoxifen is a prodrug that is metabolized by members of the CYP450 family into two active metabolites: 4-hydroxy tamoxifen (4OH-TAM) and 4-hydroxyl-*N*-desmethyltamoxifen (endoxifen) (Fig. 5.17). CYP3A4/5 is responsible for the conversion of tamoxifen into N-desmethyltamoxifen, which is then converted into its active metabolite, endoxifen, by CYP2D6. CYP2D6 is also responsible for the conversion of tamoxifen into 4OH-TAM. In a recent study of steady-state levels of tamoxifen and active tamoxifen metabolites, there was interpatient variability for all three metabolites. A recent study investigating the *CYP2D6*4* allele (inactive enzyme), a poor metabolizer that is common in Caucasians, in patients being treated with tamoxifen found that individuals who were homozygous for *CYP2D6*4* had significantly lower endoxifen levels than patients who had the wild-type gene. This study clearly indicates that genotyping of patients with impaired CYP2D6 function may be beneficial in a clinical setting to determine which patients will derive the most benefit from tamoxifen therapy.[65]

Tolterodine [(*R*)-N,N-diisopropyl-3-(2-hydroxy-5-methylphenyl)-phenylpropanamine] is an antimuscarinic drug for the treatment of urinary urge incontinence and other symptoms associated with an overactive bladder. Two different oxidative metabolic pathways, hydroxylation and N-dealkylation, have been identified in humans (Fig. 5.18). Hydroxylation to the pharmacologically active 5-hydroxymethyl metabolite (5-HM) is catalyzed by CYP2D6, whereas the N-dealkylation pathway is catalyzed by CYP3A4. Further oxidation of 5-HM catalyzed by alcohol and aldehyde dehydrogenases yields the carboxylic acid of tolterodine and its N-dealkylated form, along with N-dealkylated 5-HM. As described previously, CYP2D6 is subject to genetic polymorphism, with important implications for drugs that are metabolized by this enzyme such as tolterodine. Clinical studies have demonstrated that individuals with reduced CYP2D6-mediated metabolism represent a high-risk group in the population, with a propensity to develop adverse drug effects. In fast metabolizers, the mean systemic clearance of tolterodine was found to be 44 L/h, yielding a half-life of 2-3 hours. In contrast, poor metabolizers have a fivefold lower clearance and a mean half-life of 9 hours, which results in a sevenfold higher maximum serum concentration of tolterodine at steady state.[66]

Codeine is a prodrug whose analgesic property is primarily due to its metabolic conversion to the central analgesic morphine (Fig. 5.19). This metabolic conversion

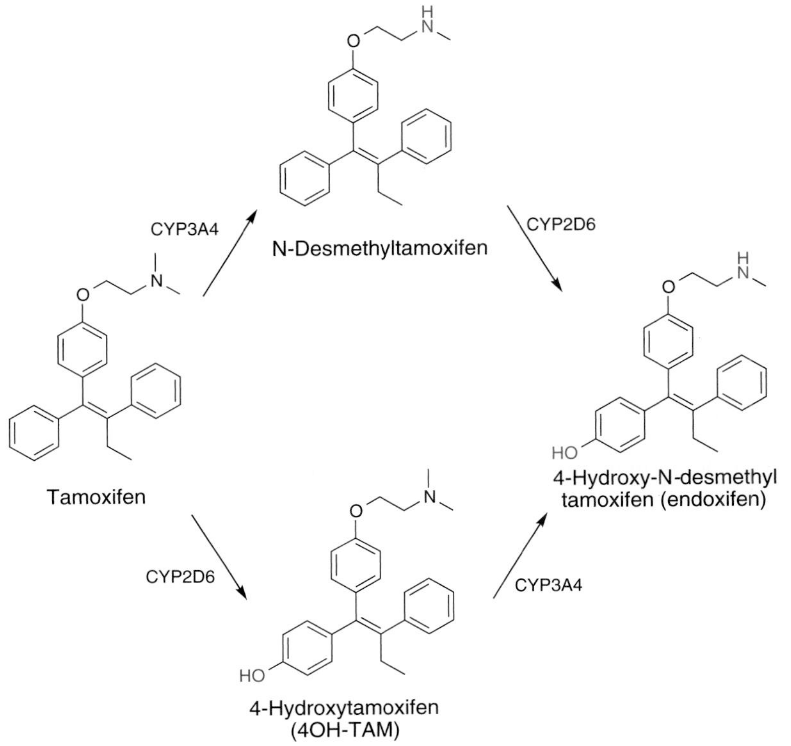

Figure 5.17 Tamoxifen metabolic pathway.

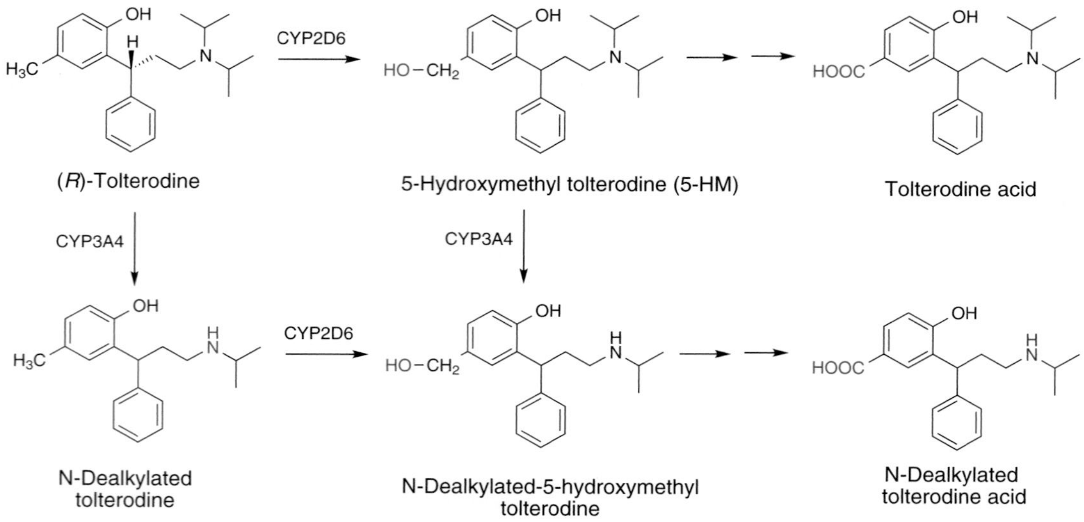

Figure 5.18 Tolterodine metabolic pathway.

is catalyzed by CYP2D6 enzyme. Loss-of-function variations in CYP2D6 can lead to a poor analgesic response, and patients carrying such a variation are considered poor metabolizers and receive little therapeutic benefit from codeine. About 5%-10% of Caucasians are CYP2D6 poor metabolizers; the percentage is approximately 2%-3% in other racial and ethnic groups.[67] On the other hand, variations that result in increased metabolic activity of CYP2D6 will lead to enhanced conversion of codeine to morphine with concomitant increased analgesic response. Patients who carry such variations are at risk for opioid toxicity, which includes moderate to severe central nervous system depression. Therefore, drugs containing codeine such as CYP2D6 ultrarapid metabolizers carry a product label that include warnings such as "may experience overdose symptoms such as extreme sleepiness, confusion or shallow breathing, even at labeled dosage regimens," and encourages physicians to "choose the lowest effective dose for the shortest period of time and inform their patients about the risks and the signs of morphine overdose".

Clopidogrel, a thienopyridine derivative, is used for the prevention of recurrent thrombosis in patients with myocardial infarction and percutaneous coronary intervention with stent implantation. Clopidogrel response has been shown to vary widely, both interindividually and interethnically. CYP2C19 metabolizes clopidogrel to its pharmacologically active metabolite (Fig. 5.20). Therefore, patients who carry the loss-of-function *CYP2C19*2* alleles are particularly at higher risk for producing major cardiovascular events such as bleeding as compared to noncarriers.[68]

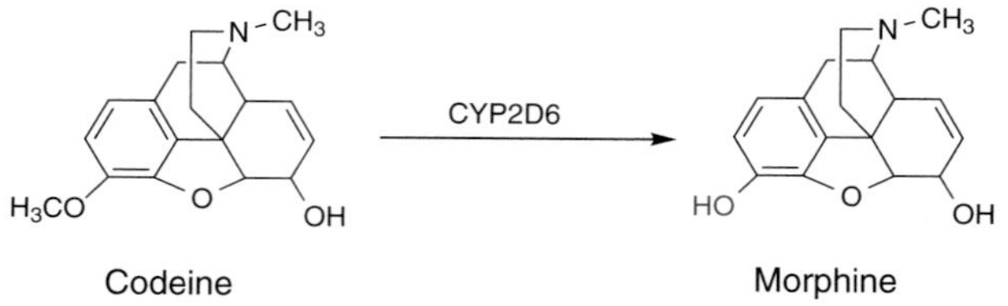

Figure 5.19 Codeine metabolism to morphine.

Irinotecan (also known as CPT-11 or Camptosar) is an approved topoisomerase I inhibitor used to treat patients with metastatic colon cancer. Acute and delayed diarrhea and neutropenia often occur after treatment with irinotecan. Diarrhea following treatment with irinotecan occurs due to the excretion of an active metabolite (SN-38:10-hydroxy-7-ethyl-camptothecin) initially into the bile and subsequently the colon (Fig. 5.21; for more details, see Chapter 33: Drugs Used to Treat Neoplastic Diseases). Irinotecan treatment is associated with an increased frequency of severe and potentially life-threatening toxicity among patients with genetic polymorphisms that markedly reduce glucuronidation of SN-38. Patients with decreased capacity to glucuronidate SN-38 (e.g., patients homozygous for specific UDP-glucuronosyl transferase 1A1 [UGT1A1] genotypes such as *UGT1A1*28* [TA7]) are at increased risk for severe neutropenia after treatment with irinotecan or SN-38 than patients with the wild-type sequence.[69]

TPMT is a key enzyme involved in the metabolism of azathioprine (AZA) and 6-mercaptopurine (6-MP), two widely used drugs to treat leukemia, rhematic diseases,

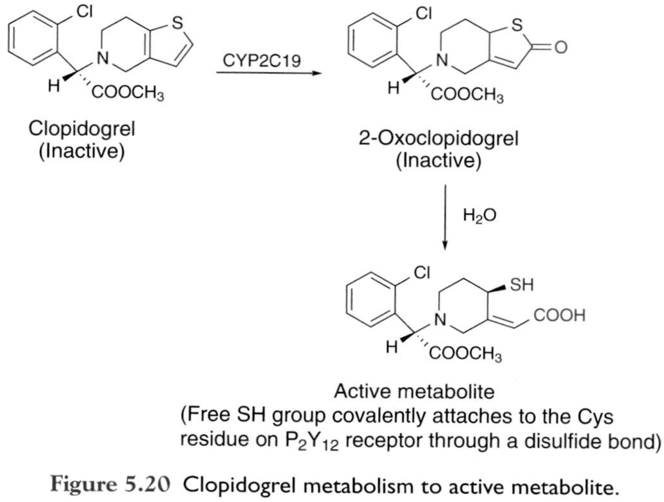

Figure 5.20 Clopidogrel metabolism to active metabolite.

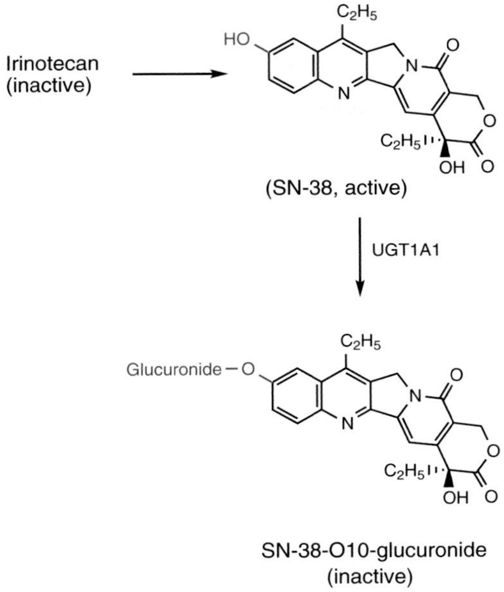

Figure 5.21 Metabolic activation of irinotecan.

inflammatory bowel disease, and solid organ transplantation.[70] AZA is metabolized to 6-MP, the active metabolite of AZA. 6-MP can be inactivated by either xanthine oxidase (XO) or TPMT to nontoxic metabolites (Fig. 5.22). TPMT-deficient patients carrying the nonfunctional TPMT∗2, TPMT∗3A, and TPMT∗3C alleles are at higher risk for producing severe hematologic toxicity, and consequently TPMT-deficient patients require substantial reduction in dose.[71]

Dihydropyrimidine dehydrogenase (DPD) is the rate-limiting enzyme that metabolizes 5-fluorouracil (5-FU), a widely used anticancer drug (Fig. 5.23). A genetic deficiency of the DPD enzyme can lead to toxicity to 5-FU due to reduced clearance, and thus, this drug should not be used in patients with DPD deficiency.[72,73]

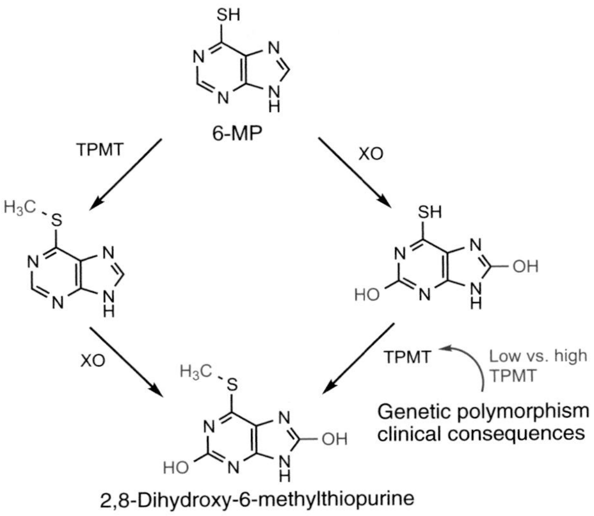

Figure 5.22 Metabolism of 6-mercaptopurine (6-MP) by thiopurine methyl transferase (TPMT) and xanthine oxidase (XO).

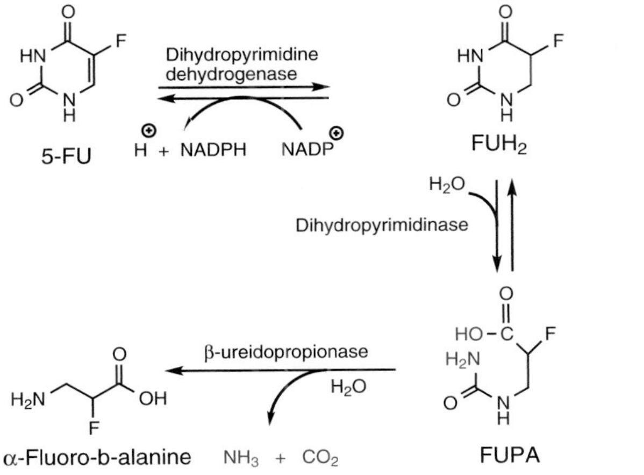

Figure 5.23 5-Fluorouracil (5-FU) inactivation by dihydropyrimidine dehydrogenase (DPD).

The human N-acetyl transferases (NATs) are responsible for the catalytic transfer of an acetyl group from acetyl coenzyme A to arylhydrazines as in isoniazid (Fig. 5.24).[74] Functional polymorphisms have been observed in two human NAT genes, *NAT1* and *NAT2*, leading to altered enzyme activity. Based on NAT activity, patients can be classified into two phenotypes: fast acetylators (wild-type NAT acetylation activity) and slow acetylators (reduced NAT enzyme activity). Polymorphisms in the *NAT1* (i.e., *NAT1*14*, **15*, **17*, **19*, and **22*) and *NAT2* (e.g., *NAT2*5*, **6*, **7*, **10*, **14*, and **17*) result in slow acetylation phenotype.[75] Since NAT2 plays an important role in deactivation of isoniazid, its response is dependent on the presence/absence of a particular NAT2 genotype. Slow acetylators are presented with increased risk of isoniazid-induced hepatitis.[76]

Trastuzumab is a MAb that specifically targets breast cancers overexpressing the *HER2/neu* gene and thus is marketed solely for the subset of breast cancer patients overexpressing the *HER2/neu* gene (~10%). Because trastuzumab was developed for marker-positive individuals who comprise a rather low proportion of breast cancer patients, trastuzumab therapy may be one of the best examples of a genomic technology paving the way for personalized medical treatment.[77]

Vemurafenib is specifically indicated for the treatment of metastatic melanoma with *BRAF* V600E mutation.[78] It is not indicated for patients with wild-type *BRAF* melanoma. A newly developed diagnostic kit, Cobas® 4800 BRAF V600 mutation test, was approved by the US FDA to identify patients who will respond to vemurafenib treatment.

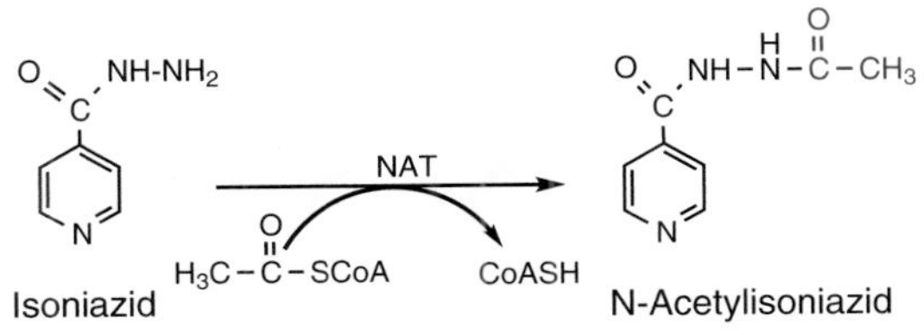

Figure 5.24 Metabolism of isoniazid by N-acetyltransferase (NAT).

Compounds that pharmacologically inhibit the nuclear poly (ADP-ribose) polymerase (PARP) family of enzymes are a novel class of anticancer drugs targeting the DNA repair activity of PARP-1, the principal member of the PARP family. PARP inhibitors (PARPi) as single agents are efficacious in treating tumors deficient in homologous recombination (HR) components, including breast cancer–associated genes (*BRCA*)1/2. *BRCA1/2* and other tumor suppressor genes are crucial for accurate HR-mediated DNA double strand break (DSB) repair mechanism (Fig. 5.25). Restoration of BRCA function leads to resistance to PARPi. The US FDA–approved PARPi such as olaparib/Lynparza, niraparib/Zejula, and rucaparib/Rubraca (Fig. 5.26) are primarily used as a single drug to treat *BRCA*-deficient tumors based on the synthetic lethality concept. (**Synthetic lethality:** cancer cells that have lost key *BRCA* gene functions depend on backup DNA repair pathways such as PARP, and by inhibiting PARP, such dependence is exploited to preferentially kill the cancer cells while sparing normal cells.)[79]

Pegloticase (Krystexxa), a pegylated uricase enzyme approved for the treatment of chronic gout, metabolizes uric acid to allantoin, a highly water soluble product that is easily excreted by the kidney (Fig. 5.27). With each molecule of uric acid degradation there is a simultaneous production of one molecule of hydrogen peroxide, which leads to overwhelming oxidative stress and subsequent hemolytic anemia and methemoglobinemia. Normally, oxidative stress is counteracted by the presence of glucose-6-phosphate dehydrogenase (G6PD) through production of cellular reducing equivalents such as NADH and glutathione. Pegloticase treatment of patients with G6PD deficiency is thus precluded.[80]

GENE THERAPY

Translation of gene therapy concepts to patient care began nearly three decades ago.[81] In principle, gene therapy can produce a lasting and potentially curative clinical benefit. After numerous setbacks due to therapy-related toxicities, the studies are bearing fruit with approvals of gene therapy products by the US FDA beginning in 2017.[82] A major problem encountered in gene therapy was similar to the problem encountered in all forms of drug therapy—the assurance of drug efficacy through efficient delivery of the therapeutic agent to its biologic target in a fully functional form. Gene therapy is unique in the sense that it is the product of gene expression, the protein, and not the gene itself that is the therapeutic agent. Hence, we must not only deliver the gene to its proper target but also assure that when the gene reaches its target, it will arrive in a form that will produce the therapeutic agent in such a form that it, too, will be assured of reaching its specified target.[83-85]

Gene therapy studies have traditionally focused on direct *in vivo* administration of viral vectors such as replication-defective retroviruses and adeno-associated virus (AAV). The steps (administration, delivery, and expression) involved in the delivery of the therapeutic gene are shown in Figure 5.28.[86] The field is further fueled by the availability of robust gene editing technologies such as CRISPR, zinc finger nuclease (ZFN), and transcription activator–like effector nuclease (TALEN) and *ex vivo* approaches using genetically engineered T cells[87] and hematopoietic stem cells. Three gene therapy products have been approved by the US FDA

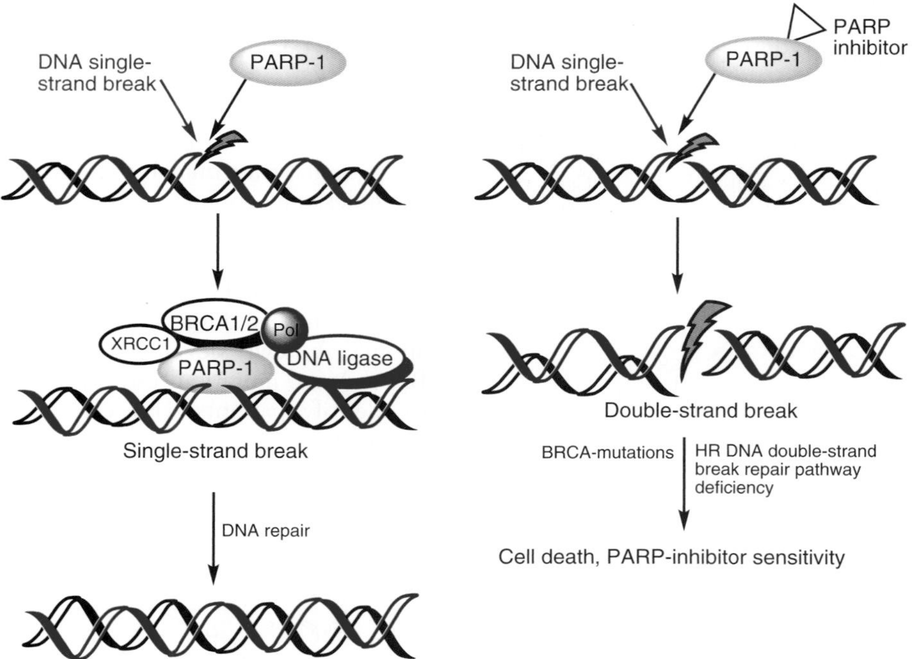

Figure 5.25 Role of poly (ADP-ribose) polymerase-1 (PARP-1) in DNA single-strand break repair and PARP-inhibitor sensitivity in patients with breast cancer–associated gene (BRCA) mutations (homologous recombination [HR] deficiency).

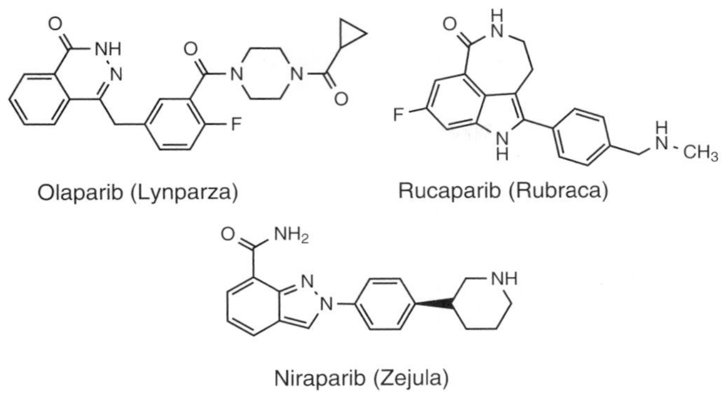

Olaparib (Lynparza)

Rucaparib (Rubraca)

Niraparib (Zejula)

Figure 5.26 Structures of FDA-approved PARP-1 (poly [ADP-ribose] polymerase-1) inhibitors.

since August 2017, ushering in a new approach to the treatment of serious and life-threatening diseases. Tisagenlecleucel (Kymriah) and axicabtagene ciloleucel (Yescarta) are chimeric antigen receptor T-cell immunotherapies, in which patient's immune cells are removed, injected with DNA outside the body, and returned to the bloodstream for the treatment of B-cell malignancies. Voretigene neparvovec-rzyl (Luxturna), the latest gene therapy product to be approved, is an AAV vector for *in vivo* treatment of congenital blindness. In addition, a number of gene therapy products are under various phases of clinical investigation for different disease conditions including severe combined immunodeficiency disease due to adenosine deaminase deficiency ($CD34^+$ cells transduced with adenosine deaminase gene), glioblastoma (Toca511, a retroviral replicating vector), age-related macular degeneration (AAV2-sFLT01), Parkinson's disease (CERE-120: AAV delivery of neurturin), advanced osteocarcinoma (Her2 chimeric antigen receptor expressing T cells), chronic lymphocytic leukemia (CLL) (autologous T lymphocytes engrafted with a chimeric antigen receptor targeting the kappa light chain), Alzheimer disease (CERE-110: AAV delivery of nerve growth factor), acute lymphoblastic leukemia (ALL) (LV CD19 4-1BB CAR-T), multiple myeloma (gamma-RV BCMA CD28 CAR-T), HIV (ZFN CCR5 electroporation), beta-thalassemia (LV antisickling beta-hemoglobin), and hemophilia B (AAV8-Factor IX).[82,88]

SUMMARY

Completion of the HGP in 2003 resulted in the elucidation of the entire sequence of the 3 billion base pairs in the human genome, estimated to contain some 25,000

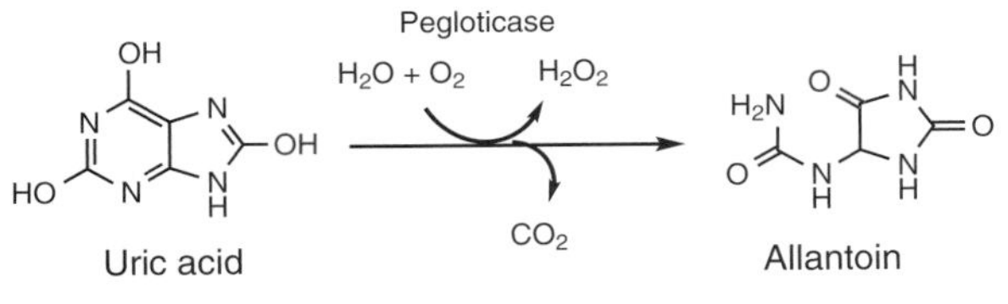

Pegloticase

$H_2O + O_2$ → H_2O_2, CO_2

Uric acid → Allantoin

Figure 5.27 Degradation of uric acid by pegloticase.

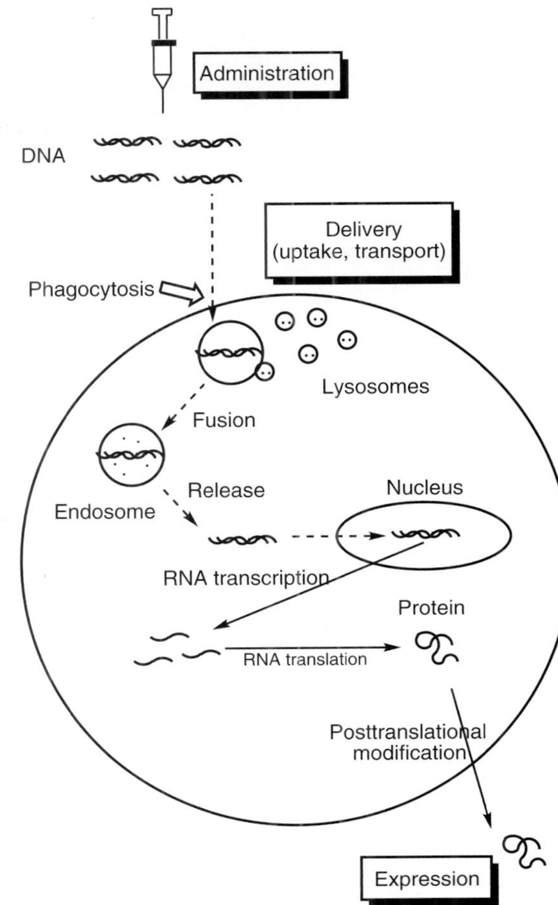

Figure 5.28 Steps in gene therapy. Gene therapy involves the steps of administration, delivery, and expression. (Note: dashed arrows represent uptake and transport.)

genes. The full impact that this scientific advance will have on our lives has yet to be determined, but the social, legal, ethical, and economic issues are certain to be extensive and complex. The manipulation and analysis of the genomic information obtained from the HGP is paving the path for transformative biomedical developments. DNA-based tests are among the first commercial medical applications. Gene tests can be used to diagnose and confirm disease, provide prognostic information about the course of disease, and predict the risk of future disease in healthy individuals.

Knowledge of genes involved in diseases, disease pathways, and drug response sites will result in the discovery of novel therapeutic targets beyond the 500 or so that were known prior to the completion of the HGP, providing a tremendous opportunity for the discovery of drugs that work through previously unexplored mechanisms.

Discovery of genomic biomarkers can help determine the type of drug therapy. For example, one of the most commonly used predictive biomarkers in cancer is immunohistochemical staining for the presence of the estrogen receptor in breast cancer. Only estrogen receptor–positive breast tumors are likely to respond to antihormonal therapy.

Table 5.5 FDA-Approved Biosimilars

Drug Name	Approval Date	Indication
Zarxio (filgrastim)	March 2015	Increases white blood cells to reduce the risk of infection
Inflectra (infliximab)	April 2016	As a tumor necrosis factor blocker to treat inflammatory diseases
Erelzi (etanercept)	August 2016	As a tumor necrosis factor blocker to treat inflammatory diseases
Amjevita (adalimumab)	September 2016	As a tumor necrosis factor blocker to treat inflammatory diseases
Renflexis (infliximab)	May 2017	As a tumor necrosis factor blocker to treat inflammatory diseases
Cyltezo (adalimumab)	August 2017	As a tumor necrosis factor blocker to treat inflammatory diseases
Mvasi (bevacizumab)	September 2017	Vascular endothelial growth factor–specific angiogenesis inhibitor to treat wide range cancers
Ogivri (trastuzumab)	December 2017	HER2/neu receptor antagonist for treating breast and gastric cancers
Ixifi (infliximab)	December 2017	As a tumor necrosis factor blocker to treat inflammatory diseases

Data from https://www.fda.gov/Drugs/DevelopmentApprovalProcess/HowDrugsareDevelopedandApproved/ApprovalApplications/TherapeuticBiologicApplications/Biosimilars/ucm580432.htm.

Identification of biomarkers for various diseases can help in the selection of patients most likely to benefit from a potential drug, which in turn will speed the design of clinical trials that are more efficient and have the potential to reduce drug approval time and associated costs. Predicting toxicity is another important outcome of the availability of the genomic information. For example, patients who have mutations in the TPMT gene will metabolize the chemotherapeutic mercaptopurine drugs at a reduced rate and can be overdosed on their treatment. Similarly, an SNP in the coding region of genes expressing drug-metabolizing CYP450 enzymes results in either poor (overdose) or fast (subtherapeutic dose) metabolism of drugs.

The future will see an altered form of health care using a genetic information infrastructure to contain costs and predict outcomes, create advanced personalized therapies, and develop a predict-and-manage paradigm of health care. Recent years have witnessed the introduction of a steady stream of biotechnology-derived drugs. The trend is expected to continue for the foreseeable future. The expiration of patents on biotechnology-derived drugs will introduce an era of more affordable biosimilars or follow-on biologics.[89] A biosimilar is defined by the World Health Organization as a biotherapeutic agent, which is similar in terms of quality, safety, and efficacy to an already licensed biotherapeutic (innovator) product. Unlike small molecules, biologics are much more complex and produced in living cells through rDNA technologies rendering their exact replication impossible. Consequently, the approval process of a biosimilar is highly regulated and requires a comparability exercise between biosimilar and innovator product in terms of physicochemical and biological comparability (quality studies), preclinical comparability (*in vitro* and *in vivo* studies), and clinical comparability.[90,91] The first biosimilar product, Zarxio (filgrastim), was FDA approved in 2015. Eight additional biosimilars were approved by the end of 2017 as shown in Table 5.5.

ACKNOWLEDGMENT

The authors wish to acknowledge the work of Drs. Ronald E. Reid and Robert D. Sindelar, who authored the content used within this chapter in a previous edition of this text.

REFERENCES

1. Hefti MM, Beck AH. The human genome project and personalized medicine. *Pathobiology of Human Disease: A Dynamic Encyclopedia of Disease Mechanisms*. 2014:3418-3422.
2. Wang DG, Fan JB, Siao CJ, et al. Large-scale identification, mapping, and genotyping of single-nucleotide polymorphisms in the human genome. *Science (New York, NY)*. 1998;280:1077-1082.
3. https://www.cancer.org/content/dam/cancer-org/research/cancer-facts-and-statistics/annual-cancer-facts-and-figures/2017/cancer-facts-and-figures-2017.pdf.
4. Travis J. Genetic engineering. Germline editing dominates DNA summit. *Science (New York, NY)*. 2015;350:1299-1300.
5. Scott A. How CRISPR is transforming drug discovery. *Nature*. 2018;8:555.
6. Hsu PD, Lander ES, Zhang F. Development and applications of crispr-cas9 for genome engineering. *Cell*. 2014;157:1262-1278.
7. Greene AC. Crispr-based antibacterials: transforming bacterial defense into offense. *Trends Biotechnol*. 2018;36:127-130.
8. Pandey A, Mann M. Proteomics to study genes and genomes. *Nature*. 2000;405:837-846.
9. Tonge R, Shaw J, Middleton B, et al. Validation and development of fluorescence two-dimensional differential gel electrophoresis proteomics technology. *Proteomics*. 2001;1:377-396.
10. Zhu H, Snyder M. Protein arrays and microarrays. *Curr Opin Chem Biol*. 2001;5:40-45.
11. Smolka MB, Zhou H, Purkayastha S, Aebersold R. Optimization of the isotope-coded affinity tag-labeling procedure for quantitative proteome analysis. *Anal Biochem*. 2001;297:25-31.

12. Uetz P, Giot L, Cagney G, et al. A comprehensive analysis of protein-protein interactions in saccharomyces cerevisiae. *Nature*. 2000;403:623-627.
13. Saghatelian A, Cravatt BF. Global strategies to integrate the proteome and metabolome. *Curr Opin Chem Biol*. 2005;9:62-68.
14. Clish CB. Metabolomics: an emerging but powerful tool for precision medicine. *Cold Spring Harbor Mol Case Studies*. 2015;1:a000588.
15. Bino RJ, Hall RD, Fiehn O, et al. Potential of metabolomics as a functional genomics tool. *Trends Plant Sci*. 2004;9:418-425.
16. Fiehn O. Metabolomics–the link between genotypes and phenotypes. *Plant Mol Biol*. 2002;48:155-171.
17. Gerstein MB, Bruce C, Rozowsky JS, et al. What is a gene, post-encode? History and updated definition. *Genome Res*. 2007;17:669-681.
18. Maxam AM, Gilbert W. A new method for sequencing DNA. *Proc Natl Acad Sci USA*. 1977;74:560-564.
19. Sanger F, Nicklen S, Coulson AR. DNA sequencing with chain-terminating inhibitors. *Proc Natl Acad Sci USA*. 1977;74:5463-5467.
20. Tucker T, Marra M, Friedman JM. Massively parallel sequencing: The next big thing in genetic medicine. *Am J Hum Genet*. 2009;85:142-154.
21. Lonnberg H. Solid-phase synthesis of oligonucleotide conjugates useful for delivery and targeting of potential nucleic acid therapeutics. *Bioconjug Chem*. 2009;20:1065-1094.
22. Arnheim N, Erlich H. Polymerase chain reaction strategy. *Annu Rev Biochem*. 1992;61:131-156.
23. Briggs J, Panfili PR. Quantitation of DNA and protein impurities in biopharmaceuticals. *Anal Chem*. 1991;63:850-859.
24. Li S, Schoneich C, Borchardt RT. Chemical instability of protein pharmaceuticals: Mechanisms of oxidation and strategies for stabilization. *Biotechnol Bioeng*. 1995;48:490-500.
25. Frokjaer S, Otzen DE. Protein drug stability: a formulation challenge. *Nat Rev Drug Discovery*. 2005;4:298-306.
26. Kerwin BA, Remmele RL Jr. Protect from light: photodegradation and protein biologics. *J Pharm Sci*. 2007;96:1468-1479.
27. Rathore N, Rajan RS. Current perspectives on stability of protein drug products during formulation, fill and finish operations. *Biotechnol Prog*. 2008;24:504-514.
28. Buckley ST, Hubalek F, Rahbek UL. Chemically modified peptides and proteins – critical considerations for oral delivery. *Tissue Barriers*. 2016;4:e1156805.
29. Pisal DS, Kosloski MP, Balu-Iyer SV. Delivery of therapeutic proteins. *J Pharm Sci*. 2010;99:2557-2575.
30. Goldberg M, Gomez-Orellana I. Challenges for the oral delivery of macromolecules. *Nat Rev Drug Discovery*. 2003;2:289-295.
31. Bayley H. Protein therapy-delivery guaranteed. *Nat Biotechnol*. 1999;17:1066-1067.
32. Orive G, Hernandez RM, Rodriguez Gascon A, Dominguez-Gil A, Pedraz JL. Drug delivery in biotechnology: Present and future. *Curr Opin Biotechnol*. 2003;14:659-664.
33. Dozier JK, Distefano MD. Site-specific pegylation of therapeutic proteins. *Int J Mol Sci*. 2015;16:25831-25864.
34. Gentilucci L, De Marco R, Cerisoli L. Chemical modifications designed to improve peptide stability: Incorporation of non-natural amino acids, pseudo-peptide bonds, and cyclization. *Curr Pharm Des*. 2010;16:3185-3203.
35. Chorev M, Goodman M. A dozen years of retro-inverso peptidomimetics. *Acc Chem Res*. 1993;26:266-273.
36. Dingermann T. Recombinant therapeutic proteins: production platforms and challenges. *Biotechnol J*. 2008;3:90-97.
37. Kwakkenbos MJ, van Helden PM, Beaumont T, Spits H. Stable long-term cultures of self-renewing b cells and their applications. *Immunol Rev*. 2016;270:65-77.
38. Dostalek M, Gardner I, Gurbaxani BM, Rose RH, Chetty M. Pharmacokinetics, pharmacodynamics and physiologically-based pharmacokinetic modelling of monoclonal antibodies. *Clin Pharmacokinet*. 2013;52:83-124.
39. Hoogenboom HR. Selecting and screening recombinant antibody libraries. *Nat Biotechnol*. 2005;23:1105-1116.
40. Bakhtiar R. Therapeutic recombinant monoclonal antibodies. *J Chem Edu*. 2012;89:1537-1542.
41. Gai SA, Wittrup KD. Yeast surface display for protein engineering and characterization. *Curr Opin Struct Biol*. 2007;17:467-473.
42. Chow AY. Cell cycle control by oncogenes and tumor suppressors: driving the transformation of normal cells into cancerous cells. *Nature Educ*. 2010;3:7.
43. Reichert JM. Monoclonal antibodies in the clinic. *Nat Biotechnol*. 2001;19:819-822.
44. Lambert JM. Drug-conjugated antibodies for the treatment of cancer. *Br J Clin Pharmacol*. 2013;76:248-262.
45. Nathan LT. Thinking small and dreaming big: medicinal chemistry strategies for designing optimal antibody-drug conjugates (adcs). *Med Chem Rev*. 2016;52:363-381.
46. Petersen BH, DeHerdt SV, Schneck DW, Bumol TF. The human immune response to ks1/4-desacetylvinblastine (ly256787) and ks1/4-desacetylvinblastine hydrazide (ly203728) in single and multiple dose clinical studies. *Cancer Res*. 1991;51:2286-2290.
47. Ritchie M, Tchistiakova L, Scott N. Implications of receptor-mediated endocytosis and intracellular trafficking dynamics in the development of antibody drug conjugates. *mAbs*. 2013;5:13-21.
48. Dubowchik GM, Firestone RA. Cathepsin b-sensitive dipeptide prodrugs. 1. A model study of structural requirements for efficient release of doxorubicin. *Bioorg Med Chem Lett*. 1998;8:3341-3346.
49. Dubowchik GM, Firestone RA, Padilla L, et al. Cathepsin b-labile dipeptide linkers for lysosomal release of doxorubicin from internalizing immunoconjugates: Model studies of enzymatic drug release and antigen-specific in vitro anticancer activity. *Bioconjug Chem*. 2002;13:855-869.
50. Hamann PR, Hinman LM, Hollander I, et al. Gemtuzumab ozogamicin, a potent and selective anti-cd33 antibody-calicheamicin conjugate for treatment of acute myeloid leukemia. *Bioconjug Chem*. 2002;13:47-58.
51. Sapra P, Hooper AT, O'Donnell CJ, Gerber HP. Investigational antibody drug conjugates for solid tumors. *Expert Opin Investig Drugs*. 2011;20:1131-1149.
52. Ducry L, Stump B. Antibody-drug conjugates: Linking cytotoxic payloads to monoclonal antibodies. *Bioconjug Chem*. 2010;21:5-13.
53. Saito G, Swanson JA, Lee KD. Drug delivery strategy utilizing conjugation via reversible disulfide linkages: role and site of cellular reducing activities. *Adv Drug Deliv Rev*. 2003;55:199-215.
54. Talele TT. Natural-products-inspired use of the gem-dimethyl group in medicinal chemistry. *J Med Chem*. 2018;61:2166-2210.
55. Erickson HK, Widdison WC, Mayo MF, et al. Tumor delivery and in vivo processing of disulfide-linked and thioether-linked antibody-maytansinoid conjugates. *Bioconjug Chem*. 2010;21:84-92.
56. Bross PF, Beitz J, Chen G, et al. Approval summary: Gemtuzumab ozogamicin in relapsed acute myeloid leukemia. *Clin Cancer Res*. 2001;7:1490-1496.
57. Junutula JR, Raab H, Clark S, et al. Site-specific conjugation of a cytotoxic drug to an antibody improves the therapeutic index. *Nat Biotechnol*. 2008;26:925-932.
58. Senter PD. Potent antibody drug conjugates for cancer therapy. *Curr Opin Chem Biol*. 2009;13:235-244.
59. Staudacher AH, Brown MP. Antibody drug conjugates and bystander killing: Is antigen-dependent internalisation required? *Brit J Cancer*. 2017;117:1736.
60. Srinivas PR, Kramer BS, Srivastava S. Trends in biomarker research for cancer detection. *Lancet Oncol*. 2001;2:698-704.
61. Wulfkuhle JD, Liotta LA, Petricoin EF. Proteomic applications for the early detection of cancer. *Nat Rev Cancer*. 2003;3:267-275.
62. Hong KW, Oh B. Overview of personalized medicine in the disease genomic era. *BMB Rep*. 2010;43:643-648.
63. Klein TE, Altman RB, Eriksson N, et al. Estimation of the warfarin dose with clinical and pharmacogenetic data. *N Engl J Med*. 2009;360:753-764.
64. Voora D, McLeod HL, Eby C, Gage BF. The pharmacogenetics of coumarin therapy. *Pharmacogenomics*. 2005;6:503-513.

65. Rofaiel S, Muo EN, Mousa SA. Pharmacogenetics in breast cancer: steps toward personalized medicine in breast cancer management. *Pharmgenomics Pers Med*. 2010;3:129-143.
66. Postlind H, Danielson A, Lindgren A, Andersson SH. Tolterodine, a new muscarinic receptor antagonist, is metabolized by cytochromes p450 2d6 and 3a in human liver microsomes. *Drug Metab Dispos*. 1998;26:289-293.
67. Rollason V, Samer C, Piguet V, Dayer P, Desmeules J. Pharmacogenetics of analgesics: Toward the individualization of prescription. *Pharmacogenomics*. 2008;9:905-933.
68. Mega JL, Simon T, Collet JP, et al. Reduced-function cyp2c19 genotype and risk of adverse clinical outcomes among patients treated with clopidogrel predominantly for pci: A meta-analysis. *JAMA*. 2010;304:1821-1830.
69. Gagne JF, Montminy V, Belanger P, Journault K, Gaucher G, Guillemette C. Common human ugt1a polymorphisms and the altered metabolism of irinotecan active metabolite 7-ethyl-10-hydroxycamptothecin (SN-38). *Mol Pharmacol*. 2002;62:608-617.
70. Eichelbaum M, Ingelman-Sundberg M, Evans WE. Pharmacogenomics and individualized drug therapy. *Annu Rev Med*. 2006;57:119-137.
71. Whirl-Carrillo M, McDonagh EM, Hebert JM, et al. Pharmacogenomics knowledge for personalized medicine. *Clin Pharmacol Ther*. 2012;92:414-417.
72. Gonzalez FJ, Fernandez-Salguero P. Diagnostic analysis, clinical importance and molecular basis of dihydropyrimidine dehydrogenase deficiency. *Trends Pharmacol Sci*. 1995;16:325-327.
73. van Kuilenburg AB. Screening for dihydropyrimidine dehydrogenase deficiency: To do or not to do, that's the question. *Cancer Invest*. 2006;24:215-217.
74. Blum M, Grant DM, McBride W, Heim M, Meyer UA. Human arylamine N-acetyltransferase genes: Isolation, chromosomal localization, and functional expression. *DNA Cell Biol*. 1990;9:193-203.
75. Sim E, Lack N, Wang CJ, et al. Arylamine N-acetyltransferases: Structural and functional implications of polymorphisms. *Toxicology*. 2008;254:170-183.
76. Huang YS, Chern HD, Su WJ, et al. Polymorphism of the N-acetyltransferase 2 gene as a susceptibility risk factor for antituberculosis drug-induced hepatitis. *Hepatology (Baltimore, MD)*. 2002;35:883-889.
77. Ross JS, Schenkein DP, Pietrusko R, et al. Targeted therapies for cancer 2004. *Am J Clin Pathol*. 2004;122:598-609.
78. Chapman PB, Robert C, Larkin J, et al. Vemurafenib in patients with brafv600 mutation-positive metastatic melanoma: final overall survival results of the randomized brim-3 study. *Ann Oncol*. 2017;28:2581-2587.
79. Lord CJ, Ashworth A. Parp inhibitors: synthetic lethality in the clinic. *Science (New York, NY)*. 2017;355:1152-1158.
80. Owens RE, Swanson H, Twilla JD. Hemolytic anemia induced by pegloticase infusion in a patient with g6pd deficiency. *J Clin Rheumatol*. 2016;22:97-98.
81. Keeler AM, ElMallah MK, Flotte TR. Gene therapy 2017: progress and future directions. *Clin Transl Sci*. 2017;10:242-248.
82. Dunbar CE, High KA, Joung JK, Kohn DB, Ozawa K, Sadelain M. Gene therapy comes of age. *Science (New York, NY)*. 2018;359.
83. Terazaki Y, Yano S, Yuge K, et al. An optimal therapeutic expression level is crucial for suicide gene therapy for hepatic metastatic cancer in mice. *Hepatology (Baltimore, MD)*. 2003;37:155-163.
84. Goverdhana S, Puntel M, Xiong W, et al. Regulatable gene expression systems for gene therapy applications: progress and future challenges. *Mol Ther*. 2005;12:189-211.
85. Chen P, Tian J, Kovesdi I, Bruder JT. Promoters influence the kinetics of transgene expression following adenovector gene delivery. *J Gene Med*. 2008;10:123-131.
86. Ledley FD. Nonviral gene therapy: the promise of genes as pharmaceutical products. *Hum Gene Ther*. 1995;6:1129-1144.
87. Sadelain M, Riviere I, Riddell S. Therapeutic t cell engineering. *Nature*. 2017;545:423-431.
88. Naldini L. Gene therapy returns to centre stage. *Nature*. 2015;526:351-360.
89. Dahodwala H, Sharfstein ST. Biosimilars: imitation games. *ACS Med Chem Lett*. 2017;8:690-693.
90. Agarwal AB, McBride A. Understanding the biosimilar approval and extrapolation process-a case study of an epoetin biosimilar. *Crit Rev Oncol Hematol*. 2016;104:98-107.
91. Blandizzi C, Meroni PL, Lapadula G. Comparing originator biologics and biosimilars: a review of the relevant issues. *Clin Ther*. 2017;39:1026-1039.

PART II

Receptor Targets

CHAPTER 6

G Protein–Coupled Receptors

Timothy J. Maher and Dan Kiel

Drugs covered/mentioned in this chapter:

- Acetylcholine
- Atropine
- Butorphanol
- Cimetidine
- Dihydromorphinone
- Diphenhydramine
- Dopamine
- Doxepin
- Epinephrine
- Fexofenadine
- Isoproterenol
- Mechlorethamine
- Morphine
- Muscarine
- Nalbuphine
- Naloxone
- Naltrexone
- Norepinephrine
- Pentazocine
- Pilocarpine
- Pirenzepine
- Propranolol
- Ranitidine
- Risperidone
- Sufentanil
- Tiprolisant

Abbreviations

ATP adenosine triphosphate
cAMP cyclic adenosine monophosphate
cGMP cyclic guanosine monophosphate
BBB blood-brain barrier
DAG diacylglycerol
DAT dopamine transporter
ERK extracellular signal-regulated kinase
GABA γ-aminobutyric acid
GI gastrointestinal
GDP guanosine diphosphate
GPCRs G protein–coupled receptors
Grb2 growth factor receptor-bound protein 2
GSK-3 glycogen synthase kinase 3
GTP guanosine triphosphate
HTS high-throughput screening
IP_3 inositol 1,4,5-triphosphate
JAK Janus kinase
LGIC ligand-gated ion channel
MAPK mitogen-activated protein kinase
MEK MAPK kinase
PKC protein kinase C
PLC phospholipase C
STAT signal transducer and activator of transcription

INTRODUCTION

Historical Perspectives

For years it had been known that some drugs were capable of producing their effects by acting at specific sites within the body. Claude Bernard was the first to demonstrate this in the mid-1800s, with his classical experiments involving curare.[1] He demonstrated that this neuromuscular blocking agent, which was used as an arrow poison by the South American natives, was capable of preventing skeletal muscle contraction following nerve stimulation but was without effect when the muscle was stimulated directly. This work demonstrated for the first time a localized site of action for a drug and, most importantly, suggested that a gap, now termed a synapse, existed between the nerve and the muscle. From these findings, he postulated that some chemical substance normally communicated the information between the nerve and the target tissue—in this case, the muscle. These findings established the foundations for what is known today as "chemical neurotransmission," a process frequently disrupted by diseases and, likewise, the target of many therapeutic agents.

Investigations by J.N. Langley[2] in the early 1900s established the initial foundations for the interaction of drugs with specific cellular components, later to be identified and termed "receptors." Before this time, many leading experts believed that most drugs acted nonselectively on virtually all the cells in the body to produce their biologic responses, with a response resulting from their general physical characteristics (e.g., molecular size, lipid solubility) and not related to specific three-dimensional structural features of the compound. Langley noted that the natural product pilocarpine, which acts to mimic the parasympathetic division of the autonomic nervous system and which utilizes acetylcholine as the endogenous neurotransmitter, was very selective and also extremely potent. Additionally, the natural product atropine was capable of blocking, in a rather selective fashion, the effects of pilocarpine and parasympathetic nervous system stimulation. Importantly, he concluded that these two compounds interacted with the same component of the cell.

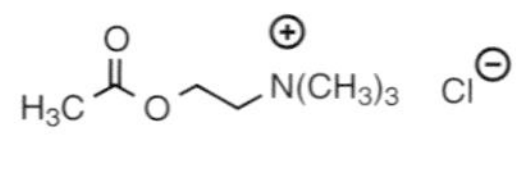

Acetycholine chloride

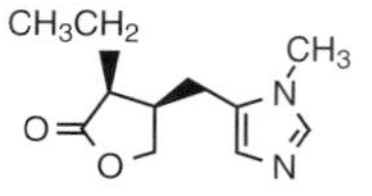

Pilocarpine

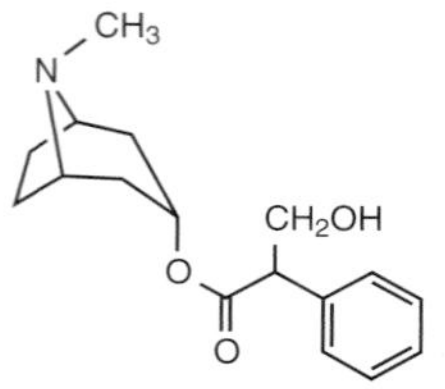

Atropine

Paul Ehrlich,[3] a noted microbiologist during the late 19th and early 20th centuries, is credited with coining the term "receptive substance," or "receptor." His observations that various organic compounds appeared to produce their antimicrobial effects with a high degree of selectivity led him to speculate that drugs produced their effects by binding to such a receptive substance. The interaction or binding of the drug with the receptor was analogous to a "lock" (the receptor) and a "key" (the drug), which gave rise to the "lock and key" fit theory for drug receptors. Thus, certain organic compounds would properly fit into the receptor and activate it, leading to a high degree of specificity. Although such a situation might be considered ideal for drug therapy, few drugs actually interact only with their intended receptors. The frequency of side effects is not always associated with a simple extension of their desired pharmacologic actions; instead, drug molecules can also bind with other receptors or nonreceptor entities on or within cells to produce a host of other—and often undesirable—effects.

A small number of drugs produce their desired therapeutic effects without interacting with a specific receptor. For example, osmotic diuretics produce their pharmacologic effects simply by creating an osmotic gradient in the renal tubules promoting the elimination of water in the urine, and antacids produce their beneficial effects by chemically neutralizing the hydrochloric acid found in the stomach. More sophisticated mechanisms can also be involved in the non–receptor-mediated actions of older antineoplastic agents (e.g., the nitrogen mustard mechlorethamine), which act to alkylate a number of nucleophilic sites on DNA.

There are four major categories or superfamilies of receptors identified to date: (1) G protein–coupled receptors (GPCRs), (2) transmembrane catalytic receptors (Chapter 9), (3) ion-channel receptors (Chapter 8), and (4) intracellular cytoplasmic/nuclear receptors (Chapter 7). This chapter will discuss the GPCRs.

TRANSMEMBRANE G PROTEIN–COUPLED RECEPTORS

The GPCRs are a family of large membrane-bound proteins that share a well-conserved structure and transduce their signal via the activation of an intracellular guanine nucleotide–binding protein (G protein). This family of proteins has seven hydrophobic (heptahelical) transmembrane domains (TMD) that span the plasma membrane, and its shape has a serpentine structure (Fig. 6.1). The extracellular region of the protein is composed of the amino terminus and several loops (EC1 through EC3) which comprise the ligand-binding site. The seven transmembrane domains are composed primarily of lipophilic amino acids arranged in α-helices connected by regions of hydrophilic amino acids. The hydrophilic regions form loops on the intracellular and extracellular faces of the membrane. Smaller sized ligands tend to bind deep within the transmembrane regions, close to the plasma membrane, whereas larger sized molecules have binding sites that are more superficial.

The carboxy end of the receptor is located in the area of the protein that protrudes into the cytoplasm. The intracellular side of the receptor also includes the binding site for the G protein, which usually binds to the protein on the third loop between TMD 6 and 7. Close to the carboxy terminus are Ser and Thr residues, which are targets for adenosine triphosphate (ATP)–dependent phosphorylation.

More than 100 different GPCRs bind to a variety of ligands encompassing biogenic amines, such as norepinephrine, dopamine, serotonin, histamine, and acetylcholine; amino acid neurotransmitters, such as glutamate and γ-aminobutyric acid (GABA); peptide neurotransmitters, neuromodulators, and hormones, such as endogenous opioids, angiotensin II, and somatostatin; and other neurotransmitters such as the endocannabinoids. There are oftentimes multiple GPCR types for a single ligand; in some cases as many as 12! The result is the possibility that a single ligand can activate a variety of transduction pathways and produce a multiplicity of cellular responses. Thus, a receptor is defined not only by which ligand binds to it but also by how the signal is transduced and the nature of the resultant physiologic response.

As an example, at least nine different adrenergic receptor (adrenoceptor) subtypes exist. Norepinephrine can bind to the β_1 adrenoceptor, which is coupled to a G protein (designated G_s). Following receptor stimulation of G_s, there is activation of the enzyme adenylyl cyclase, leading

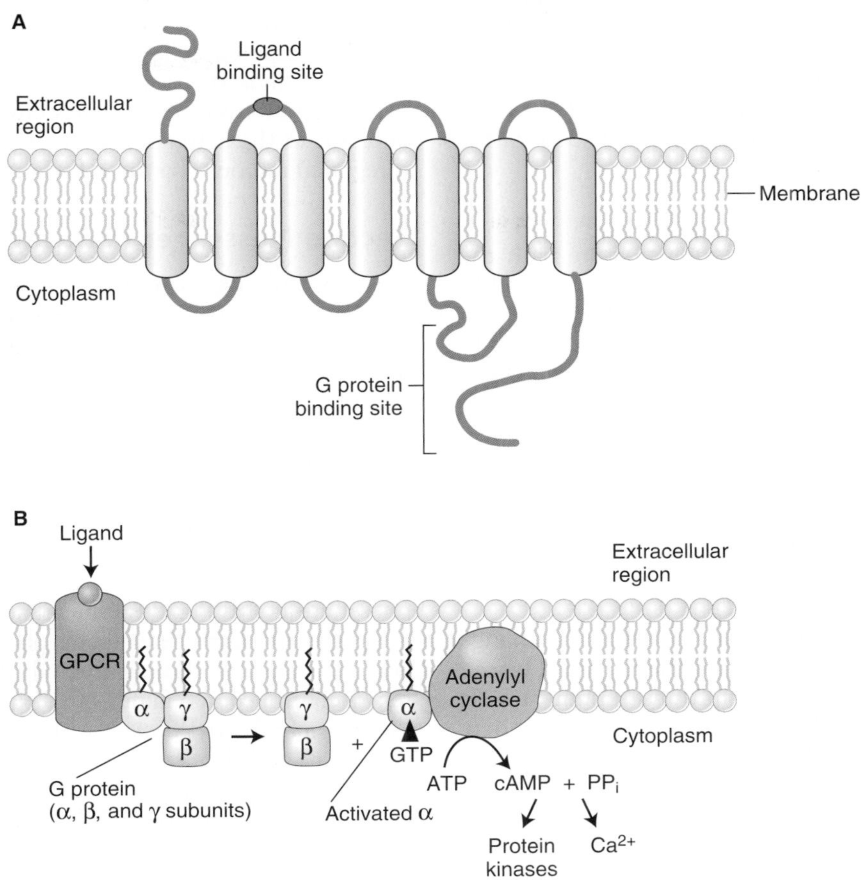

Figure 6.1 General GPCR structure and activation by agonist. A, Diagram of a GPCR showing the extracellular N-terminus, three extracellular loops (one of which binds ligands) and the seven transmembrane regions. Three intracellular loops and the C-terminus are also depicted with the interface between intracellular loop 3 and the C-terminus representing the site of G protein recognition. B, Activation of a Gs linked GPCR leads to dissociation of the three G protein subunits and the subsequent stimulation of adenylyl cyclase by the GTP-bound α-subunit. Adenylyl cyclase converts ATP into cAMP which activates protein kinase A. From Pandit N, Soltis R. *Introduction to the Pharmaceutical Sciences.* 2nd ed. Baltimore: Lippincott Williams & Wilkins; 2011, with permission.

ultimately to an increase in heart rate and force of contraction. Norepinephrine binding to α_1-adrenoceptors, on the other hand, results in the binding to a different G protein (G_q), which activates the production of the second messengers inositol 1,4,5-triphosphate (IP_3) and diacylglycerol (DAG), which then can initiate a cascade of intracellular events leading to smooth muscle contraction. Therefore, a single ligand can induce a wide range of responses as a consequence of coupling receptors to different G proteins. Which G protein is activated depends on factors such as the presence and availability of individual G proteins within a particular cell type, kinetic issues (e.g., the binding affinity of the G protein for the receptor protein), and, finally, the affinity of the activated G protein subunits for signal transduction enzymes.

A number of experimental findings over the last 20 years have demonstrated that the "lock and key" model for GPCR activation is inadequate. The demonstration that systems overexpressing GPCRs have low but measurable basal activity, and that certain ligands termed "inverse agonists" reduce this activity, cannot be explained by the "lock and key" model. Thus the "two-state" receptor model has replaced it. This postulates that a population of any GPCR exists in at least two conformations, an active and an inactive form.[4] The active form spontaneously couples to G proteins while the inactive form does not. With no ligand present, the vast majority of the receptors are in the inactive form but a small percentage is in the active form, thus generating the basal activity. Agonists are defined as ligands that selectively bind to the active receptor; the more the number of agonists added to cells, the greater the population of receptors that shifts to the active conformation. Inverse agonists are those ligands that have affinity for the inactive conformation, and as concentrations of inverse agonists are increased, the basal activity decreases as those few active receptors shift into the inactive conformation. Partial agonists are defined as having preferential affinity for the active receptor but still having some affinity for inactive receptors. Thus, as the concentration of partial agonist is increased, the cell becomes activated because the net effect is that more receptors shift into the active conformation than the inactive. But as the ligand also binds the inactive conformation, all the receptors cannot convert to the active conformation no matter how much partial agonist is added. This results in a partial agonist activating a system but with a lower maximal effect compared to a full agonist. Some ligands bind with equal affinity for the active and inactive conformations of the receptor and are termed neutral antagonists. These ligands will not change the basal activity of the biological system but will block the binding and actions of both agonists and inverse agonists.

G Proteins

The G proteins are heterotrimeric in structure with the subunits (in decreasing size) designated as α, β, and γ. Many types of these G proteins have been identified, with as many as 17 varieties of the α-subunits, five of the β-subunits, and 11 of the γ-subunits. The characteristics of the α-subunit are what largely determine the designation of the G protein and are thus the most widely studied.[5] Some of the more common α-subunits characterized are termed G_s, G_i, G_o, and $G_{q/11}$. Individual G proteins transduce the receptor activation signal via one of a number of second messenger systems discussed below. The best understood second messenger systems associated with each G protein family are summarized in Table 6.1.

Receptor activation leads to a conformational change in the associated G protein, triggering the release of bound guanosine diphosphate (GDP) from the α-subunit, which is then replaced by a molecule of guanosine triphosphate (GTP). With the binding of GTP, the α-subunit GTP complex dissociates from the βγ subunits and binds to a particular target enzyme, resulting in its activation or inhibition. Within a short period of time, the α-subunit catalyzes the dephosphorylation of the associated GTP molecule to GDP, resulting in the reassociation of the α subunit with the βγ subunits and, thus, the return of the G protein to the inactivated state. Variations on this scheme include the activation of proteins such as G protein–gated ion channels by dissociated βγ subunits and the ability of receptor proteins to activate more than a single G protein. The simultaneous activation of more than one type of GPCR results in the initiation of multiple signals, which can then interact with one another (a phenomenon commonly referred to as cross-talk). This interaction can be of several types: If both receptors use a common signal transduction pathway, the activation can result in an additive response by the cell. Conversely, if simultaneous receptor activation triggers opposing signal transduction pathways, the outcome will be an attenuated cellular response. Other types of interactions include the desensitization or activation of other receptor proteins or second messenger pathways. The final outcome of the activation of multiple signals is an overall integrated response by the cell (Fig. 6.2).

Table 6.1 G Protein Transducers and Second Messengers

G Protein Transducer Family	Second Messenger System
G_s	Stimulates adenylyl cyclase activity and Ca^{2+} channels
$G_{i/o}$	Inhibits adenylyl cyclase activity and activates K^+ channels
G_q	Stimulates phospholipase C activity
G_{12}	Modulates sodium/hydrogen ion exchanger

Second Messenger Pathways

As previously discussed, in response to receptor activation, G proteins activate plasma membrane–bound enzymes, which then trigger a metabolic cascade that results in a cellular response.[5] The products of these enzymatic actions are termed "second messengers" because they mobilize other enzymatic and structural proteins, which then ultimately produce the cellular response. The enzymes catalyzing the synthesis of second messengers fall generally into two categories: those that convert the purine triphosphates ATP and GTP into their respective cyclic monophosphates (e.g., cyclic adenosine monophosphate [cAMP], cyclic guanosine monophosphate [cGMP]) and enzymes that synthesize second messengers from plasma membrane phospholipids (e.g., DAG and IP_3). The most thoroughly studied second messenger system is controlled by a family of 10 plasma membrane–bound isozymes of adenylyl cyclase which catalyze the conversion of ATP to cAMP (Fig. 6.1B). Adenylyl cyclase is activated by the G_s family of G proteins and inhibited by the G_i family. Following synthesis, cAMP activates cAMP-dependent protein kinases by triggering the dissociation of regulatory subunits from catalytic subunits. The catalytic subunits then activate other target proteins via phosphorylation, which then trigger the cellular response (Fig. 6.3). The magnitude of the cellular response is proportional to the concentration of cAMP. Degradation of cAMP occurs via phosphodiesterases or by reducing cAMP concentration via active transport out of the cell. The result is termination of the signal.

A similar, although less ubiquitous, second messenger pathway is associated with guanylyl cyclase. Guanylyl cyclase is activated in response to some other non-GPCR catalytic receptors selective for ligands including atrial natriuretic factor and nitric oxide. When stimulated, guanylyl cyclase catalyzes the synthesis of cGMP from GTP. The formed cGMP subsequently activates cGMP-dependent protein kinases, which then activate other proteins. The actions of cGMP are terminated by enzymatic degradation of the second messenger by the same phosphodiesterases mentioned above or the dephosphorylation of substrates. One effect of this second messenger pathway is relaxation of smooth muscle via the dephosphorylation of myosin light chain kinases.

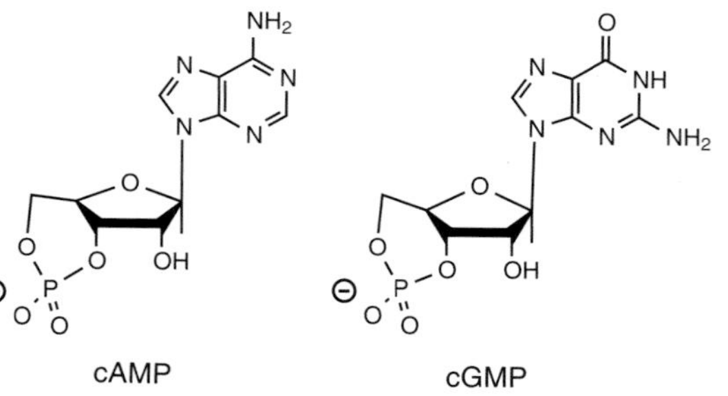

cAMP cGMP

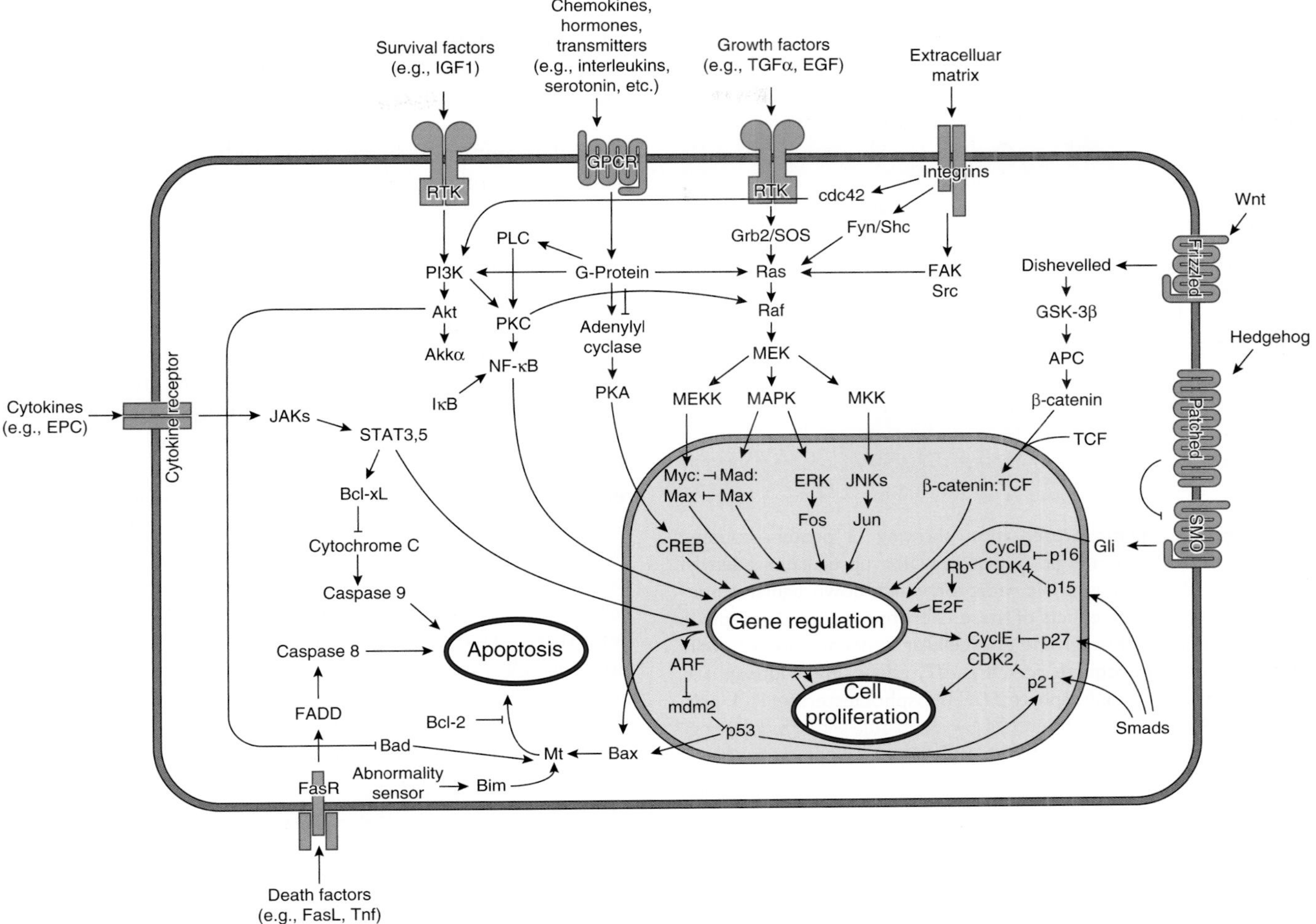

Figure 6.2 **Signal transduction cascades that regulate gene expression and apoptosis.** From Wikipedia. *Mitogen-Activated Protein Kinase. Available at http://en.wikipedia.org/wiki/Mitogen-activated_protein_kinase.*

The generation of second messengers from plasma membrane phospholipids is mediated primarily by G protein activation of phospholipase C (PLC).[6] There are three families of PLC, designated PLC-β, PLC-γ, and PLC-δ. PLC-β can be activated by the α subunit of the G_q family of G proteins or the βγ subunits of other G proteins. PLC-γ is activated via tyrosine kinase receptors, but the mechanism for PLC-δ is not yet well understood.

On activation, PLC hydrolyzes phosphatidyl inositol-4,5-bisphosphate to DAG and IP_3. The water-soluble IP_3 diffuses into the cytoplasm, where it triggers the release of calcium (Ca^{2+}) from intracellular stores. Intracellular calcium then binds to the protein calmodulin (CaM) and also to protein kinase C (PKC), both of which then stimulate, via protein phosphorylation, a broad range of enzymes and other proteins, including specific kinases. The other product of PLC, DAG, is lipid soluble and remains in the plasma membrane, where it facilitates the activation of PKC by calcium (Fig. 6.4). The signal is terminated via inactivation of IP_3 by dephosphorylation, whereas DAG is inactivated by phosphorylation to phosphatidic acid or deacetylation to fatty acids. The concentration of intracellular calcium is reduced by sequestration within cytoplasmic organelles or transport out of the cell.

Activation of phospholipase D hydrolyzes phosphatidylcholine to phosphatidic acid, which can then be metabolized to DAG via phosphatidate phosphohydrolase. This pathway prolongs the duration of elevated levels of DAG. Phospholipase A_2 is activated by increased concentrations of intracellular calcium and metabolizes phosphatidylcholine to arachidonic acid. Arachidonic acid then functions as a substrate for the synthesis of autocoids, including prostaglandins, thromboxane A_2, and leukotrienes.

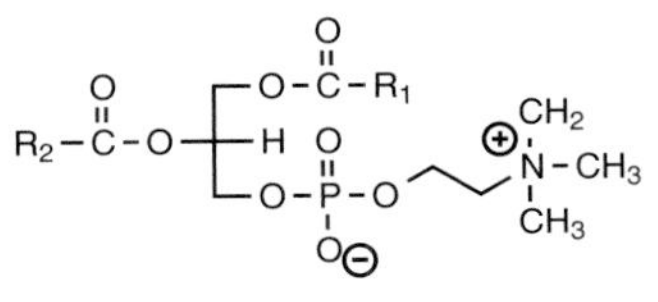

Phosphatidyl choline

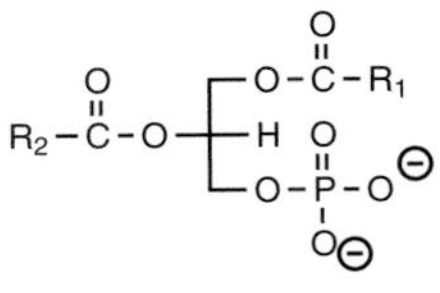

Phosphatidic acid

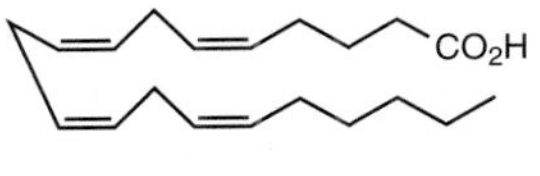

Arachidonic acid

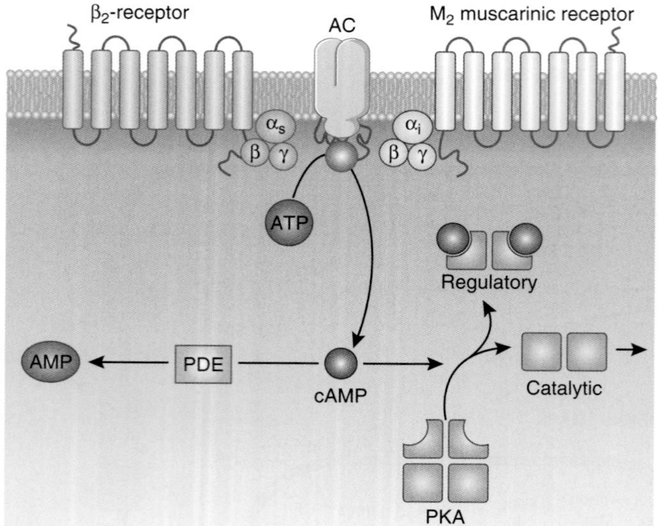

Figure 6.3 Schematic presentation showing G protein–coupled receptors; the β_2 adrenergic receptor, which upregulates adenylyl cyclase; and the M_2 muscarinic receptor, which downregulates adenylyl cyclase (AC). The effects of these G protein–coupled receptors are then mediated through the intercellular concentration of cyclic adenosine monophosphate (cAMP). *ATP*, adenosine triphosphate; *AMP*, adenosine monophosphate; *PDE*, phosphodiesterase; *PKA*, protein kinase A. From Flood P, Rathmell J, Shafer S. *Stoelting's Pharmacology & Physiology in Anesthetic Practice*. 5th ed. Baltimore: Lippincott Williams & Wilkins; 2014, with permission.

Abundantly expressed in the brain, G_o is related to G_i and regulates various ion channels. Receptors that couple to G_i often couple to G_o as well and include somatostatin receptors and the therapeutically important opioid receptors. Activation of G_o leads to inhibition of voltage-dependent calcium channels and the opening of potassium channels. These effects result in reduced release of neurotransmitter and hyperpolarization of neurons leading to reduced cellular activity. The effect of G_o on adenylyl cyclase may not be as clear-cut as G_i, but in vitro studies suggest that some species of G_o may inhibit adenylyl cyclase.

Frizzled is another family of GPCR proteins that regulate functions such as embryonic development, the formation of neural synapses, and cell polarity via a signal transduction cascade composed of protein kinases such as glycogen synthase kinase 3 (GSK-3), phosphatases, and proteolytic enzymes. A target molecule for this cascade is β-catenin, which promotes specific gene expression.

With the development of screening assays of cDNA libraries, a number of GPCRs have been identified for which there is no known endogenous ligand. These receptors are termed "orphan receptors." When the endogenous ligand is identified, the receptor is said to be "adopted." Strategies for identifying the ligand of orphan receptors include (1) expression of the GPCR in a recombinant assay system, (2) screening candidate ligands against the receptor, (3) detecting active ligands by activation of signal transduction cascades, and (4) further testing of the ligand against other GPCRs to determine selectivity (Fig. 6.5). An example of an adopted orphan GPCR is Axor 35, which was ultimately characterized as the histamine H_4 receptor.[7]

Dynamic Nature of GPCRs

The GPCRs, as is characteristic of most individual components of living systems, are not static but, rather, are constantly in a state of dynamic adaptation. One could

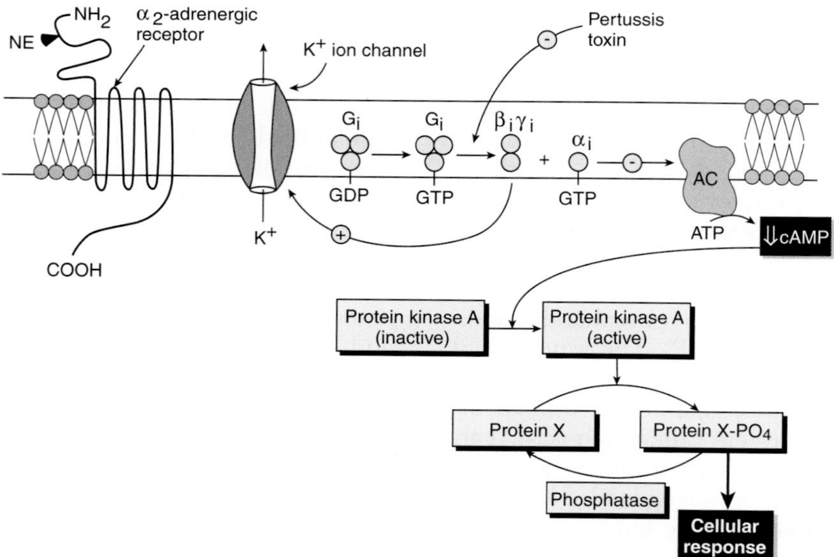

Figure 6.4 Activation of the α_2-adrenergic receptor. Stimulation of a G_i-linked receptor results in the dissociation of the G protein into the α- and βγ-subunits. The βγ-subunits bind to potassium channels increasing their open state leading to potassium efflux and hyperpolarization of the cell. The α-subunit bound to GTP inhibits adenylyl cyclase, thus decreasing intracellular cAMP and reducing activation of protein kinase A. Pertussis toxin is used as a tool to modify subunits of Gi preventing them from inhibiting adenylyl cyclase. *AC*, adenylate cyclase; *ACh*, acetylcholine; *CaM*, Ca^{2+}/calmodulin-dependent protein kinase; *DAG*, diacylglycerol; *IP_3*, inositol triphosphate; *NE*, norepinephrine; *PIP2*, phosphatidylinositol biphosphate; *PLC*, phospholipase C; *SER*, smooth endoplasmic reticulum. From Dudek R. *High-Yield Histopathology*. 2nd ed. Baltimore: Lippincott Williams & Wilkins; 2010, with permission.

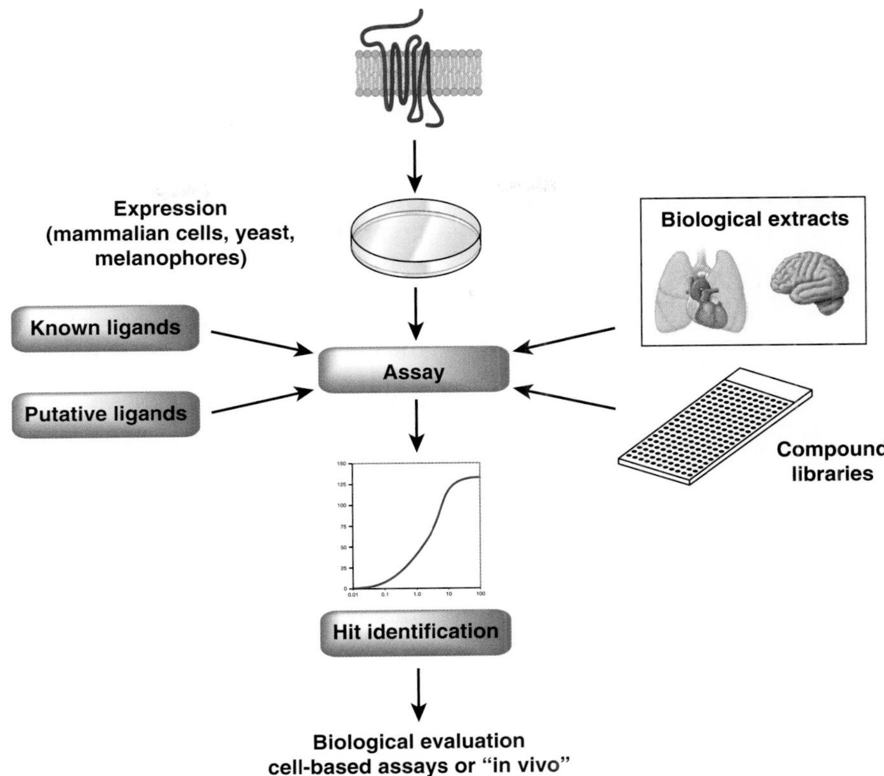

Figure 6.5 Strategy for the identification of ligands for orphan G protein–coupled receptors (GPCRs). Orphan GPCRs are expressed in a recombinant expression system, such as mammalian cells, yeast, or *Xenopus* melanophores. Following expression, it is usual to generate an assay amenable to the screening of candidate ligands in microtiter plate formats. The identification of an activating ligand is detected according to the activation of an intracellular signaling cascade. An activating ligand is identified according to its ability to cause a concentration-dependent increase in the activity of a signaling cascade. Once identified, the ligand can be further characterized against other GPCRs to determine its activity and selectivity profile prior to being used in cell-based, tissue, and, in some cases, whole-animal experiments in order to study the physiologic role of the newly liganded receptor.

envision these protein molecules floating within the fluid mosaic of the biologic membrane, awaiting interaction with normal physiologic signals. The function of such receptors, once stimulated, involves attempts to respond to perturbations of the normal physiology of the cell or organism. The role in maintaining homeostasis within the organism requires constant adaptation of receptor number and/or sensitivity in response to the changing environment in the vicinity of the receptor.

One approach to controlling receptor activation is by regulating the concentration of neurotransmitter at the receptor binding site. This is oftentimes accomplished by the modulation of neurotransmitter release via activation of presynaptic receptors; this modulation can be either an increase or a decrease. Altering the rate of synthesis, degradation, or efficiency of the enzymes that create or degrade neurotransmitter molecules is also used to regulate neurotransmitter concentrations at the receptor. An example of this is seen when, in response to product feedback inhibition, the activity of the enzyme tyrosine hydroxylase (which catalyzes the rate-limiting step of catecholamine synthesis) is modulated via phosphorylation by protein kinases or dephosphorylation by phosphatases. This and other control mechanisms allow for a strict minute-to-minute regulation of catecholamine synthesis and, thus, neurotransmission.[8]

A second mechanism for modulating the cellular response to receptor activation is to alter postsynaptic receptor number and/or sensitivity. The process is best understood for GPCRs but has also been characterized for other receptor types, such as the ion channel nicotinic receptor. The alteration in the availability or functional capacity of a given receptor constitutes an adaptive mechanism whereby the cell or organism is protected from agonist overload. For example, the chronic administration of a β-adrenoceptor agonist, such as isoproterenol, is known to produce a desensitization of the β-adrenoceptors in the heart.[9] During the period of overstimulation, the receptor becomes desensitized to further activation via phosphorylation by protein kinase A or G protein–coupled kinases, such as β-adrenoceptor kinase (βARK), at Ser and Thr residues on the C-terminal domain that interferes with G_s binding (Fig. 6.6). Desensitization can also occur at other receptors with analogous phosphorylation sites (heterologous desensitization).

A more prolonged or powerful overstimulation typically results in a decrease in receptor number and is termed "downregulation." In these GPCRs, downregulation initiated by phosphorylation of amino acids near the intracellular C-terminal domain results in binding to β-arrestins that facilitate their internalization via a clathrin-dependent pathway. Following internalization, the receptor can either

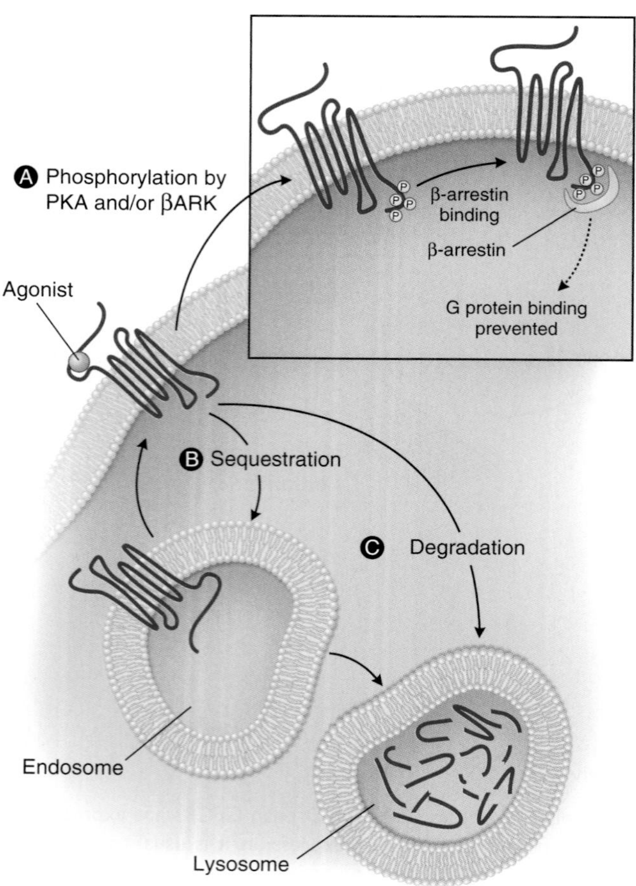

Figure 6.6 Adrenergic receptor regulation. Agonist-bound adrenergic receptors activate G proteins, which then stimulate adenylyl cyclase activity (not shown). A, Repeated or persistent stimulation of the receptor by agonist results in phosphorylation of amino acids at the C-terminus of the receptor by protein kinase A (PKA) and/or adrenergic receptor kinase (ARK). Arrestin then binds to the phosphorylated domain of the receptor and blocks Gs binding, thereby decreasing adenylyl cyclase (effector) activity. B, Binding of arrestin also leads to receptor sequestration into endosomal compartments via clathrin-mediated endocytosis (not shown), effectively neutralizing adrenergic receptor signaling activity. The receptor can then be recycled and reinserted into the plasma membrane. C, Prolonged receptor occupation by an agonist can lead to receptor downregulation and eventual receptor degradation. Cells can also reduce the number of receptors by inhibiting the transcription or translation of the gene coding for the receptor (not shown). From Golan D. *Principles of Pharmacology*. 4th ed. Baltimore: Lippincott Williams & Wilkins; 2012, with permission.

be recycled back into the plasma membrane via endosomes or degraded by lysosomes (Fig. 6.6). Reduced receptor numbers can also be accomplished via changes in the transcription and/or translation of genes that code for the receptor. Changes in receptor number or efficiency of receptors that lead to diminished responses and, thus, diminished efficacy of a drug with repeated or long-term use are examples of pharmacodynamic tolerance. As a general principle, the body will always attempt to maintain homeostasis, whether perturbed by environmental challenges, disease processes, or even the administration of drugs. Actually, the body interprets the administration of drugs as a perturbation of homeostasis and may attempt to counter the effects of the drug by invoking receptor adaptations. Often, however, with appropriate dosing schedules, drugs can be used with little observed receptor adaptation such that the desired pharmacologic effect continues to be observed.

In a similar fashion to the example described above, chronic administration of the β-adrenoceptor antagonist propranolol leads to a state of receptor supersensitivity or upregulation. The cells within the tissue, such as the heart, sense an alteration in the normal rate of basal β-adrenoceptor stimulation and, thus, respond by either increasing the number or the affinity of the receptors for their endogenous agonists, norepinephrine and epinephrine. An enhanced efficiency of the interaction between the receptor and its transducing systems can also account for a portion of the observed supersensitivity. The knowledge that such a receptor adaptation occurs has paramount practical therapeutic implications, as abrupt withdrawal of this class of agents can precipitate acute myocardial infarction due to activation of a very high number of β-receptors, and thus, this practice should be scrupulously avoided.

Some pathophysiologic states are characterized by perturbations in receptor dynamics. Prinzmetal angina is thought to be characterized by an imbalance between vasodilatory β_2-adrenoceptor function and vasoconstrictor α_1-adrenoceptor function. In this disease state, the excessive α vasoconstriction of coronary arteries leads to myocardial ischemia and pain. The inadvertent use of a β-adrenoceptor antagonist, which can be safely employed in typical angina pectoris to prevent β-adrenoceptor vasodilation, can leave unopposed α-adrenoceptor–mediated vasoconstrictor inputs and actually precipitate anginal pain. Thus, an understanding of the role that receptors have in physiology, pathophysiology, and pharmacology is essential for optimal therapeutic interventions.

Major classes of therapeutic agents interact with GPCRs to produce their desired effects. Some of these are now discussed in greater detail.

ADRENOCEPTORS

Adrenoceptors were initially subclassified by Ahlquist[10] in 1948 into α- and β-adrenoreceptor classes according to their responses to different adrenergic receptor agonists, principally norepinephrine, epinephrine, and isoproterenol. These catecholamines are able to stimulate α-adrenoceptors in the following descending order of potency: epinephrine > norepinephrine > isoproterenol. In contrast, β-adrenoceptors are stimulated in the following descending order of potency: isoproterenol > epinephrine > norepinephrine.

HO, HO, OH, NHR

Norepinephrine, R = H
Epinephrine, R = CH_3
Isoproterenol, R = $CH(CH_3)_2$

Since this original classification, additional small-molecule agonists and antagonists have been used to allow further subclassification of α- and β-receptors into the α_1 and α_2 subtypes of α-adrenoceptors and the β_1, β_2, and β_3 subtypes of β-adrenoceptors. The human β_2-adrenoceptor was one of the first to be cloned and extensively studied[11] (Fig. 6.7).

The powerful tools of molecular biology have been used to clone, sequence, and identify even more subtypes of α-adrenoceptors for a total of six. Currently, three types of α_1-adrenoceptors, termed α_{1A}, α_{1B}, and α_{1D}, are known. (There is no α_{1C} because identification of a supposed α_{1C} was found to be incorrect.) Currently, three subtypes of α_2, known as α_{2A}, α_{2B}, and α_{2C}, are also known. An example of the α_2-adrenoceptor from human kidney is depicted in Figure 6.8. This time, the α_1-, α_2-, β_1-, β_2- and β_3-adrenoceptor subtypes are sufficiently well differentiated by their small-molecule binding characteristics to be clinically significant in pharmacotherapeutics.

Salient features of the extensively studied β_2-adrenoreceptor are indicated in Figure 6.7. Binding studies with selectively mutated β_2-adrenoceptors have provided strong evidence for binding interactions between agonist functional groups and specific residues in the transmembrane domains of adrenoceptors. Such studies indicate that Asp113 in TMD3 of the β_2-adrenoceptor is the acidic residue that forms a bond, presumably ionic or a salt bridge, with the positively charged amino group of catecholamine agonists. An Asp residue is also found in a comparable position in all the other adrenoceptors, as well as other known GPCRs that bind substrates having positively charged nitrogen atoms in their structures. Elegant studies with mutated receptors and analogues of isoproterenol demonstrated that Ser204 and Ser207 of TMD5 are the residues that form hydrogen bonds with the catechol hydroxyls of β_2-agonists.[12] Furthermore, the evidence indicates that Ser204 interacts with the *m*-hydroxyl group of the ligand, whereas Ser207 interacts specifically with the *p*-hydroxyl group. Serine residues are found in corresponding positions in TMD5 of the other known adrenoceptors. Evidence indicates that Phe on TMD6 is also involved in ligand-receptor bonding with the catechol ring. Studies such as these and others that indicated the presence of specific disulfide bridges between Cys residues of the β_2-adrenoceptor lead to receptor binding.

Structural differences exist among the various adrenoceptors with regard to their primary structure, including the actual peptide sequence and length. Each of the adrenoceptors is encoded on a distinct gene, and this information was crucial to the proof that each adrenoceptor is, indeed, distinct (although related). The amino acids that make up the seven transmembrane regions are highly conserved among the various adrenoceptors, but the hydrophilic portions are quite variable. The largest differences occur in the third intracellular loop connecting TMD5 and TMD6, which is the site of linkage between the receptor and its associated G protein. Compare the diagram of the β_2-receptor in Figure 6.7 with that of the α_2-receptor in Figure 6.8.

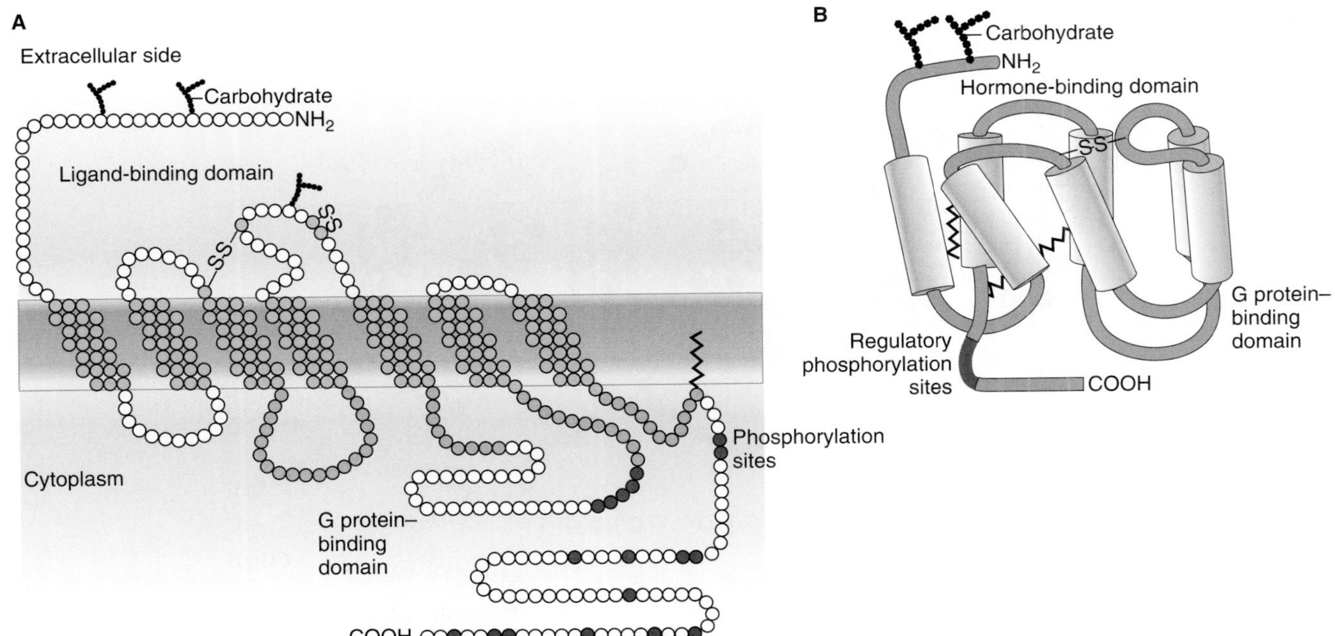

Figure 6.7 β_2-adrenergic receptor. The receptor has seven α-helical domains that span the membrane and is therefore a member of the heptahelical class of receptors. A, The transmembrane domains are drawn in an extended form. The amino terminus (residues 1 through 34) extends out of the membrane and has branched high-mannose oligosaccharides linked through N-glycosidic bonds to the amide of asparagine. Part of the receptor is anchored in the lipid plasma membrane by a palmitoyl group that forms a thioester with the -SH residue of a cysteine. The -COOH terminus, which extends into the cytoplasm, has several serine and threonine phosphorylation sites. B, The seven transmembrane helices (shown as tubes) form a cylindrical structure. Loops connecting helices form the hormone binding site on the external side of the plasma membrane, and a binding site for a G protein is on the intracellular side. From Lieberman M. *Marks' Essentials of Medical Biochemistry*. 5th ed. Philadelphia: Wolters Kluwer; 2017, with permission.

Each adrenoceptor is coupled through a G protein to an effector mechanism; all the α_1 adrenoceptors are linked to $G_{q/11}$, all the α_2 adrenoceptors to $G_{i/o}$, and all the β_1 and β_2-adrenoceptors to G_s, while the β_3-adrenoreceptor is linked to either G_s (adipocytes and bladder smooth muscle) or G_i (myocardial atrial cells).

Receptor Localization

The generalization made in the past about synaptic locations of adrenoceptor subtypes was that all α_1-, β_1-, β_2-, and β_3-adrenoceptors are postsynaptic receptors linked to stimulation of biochemical processes in the postsynaptic cell. Presynaptic β-adrenoceptors, however, are known to occur, although their function is unclear. Traditionally, the α_2-adrenoceptor has been viewed as a presynaptic receptor that resides on the outer membrane of the nerve terminus or presynaptic cell and interacts with released neurotransmitter. The α_2-adrenoceptor serves as a sensor or "autoreceptor" and modulator of the quantity of neurotransmitter present in the synapse at any given moment, and thus, during periods of rapid nerve firing and neurotransmitter release, the α_2-adrenoceptor is stimulated and causes an inhibition of further release of neurotransmitter. This is a well-characterized mechanism for modulation of neurotransmission. However, not all α_2-adrenoceptors are presynaptic, but the physiologic significance of postsynaptic α_2-receptors is less well understood.[13]

SEROTONIN RECEPTORS

Initially, serotonin (5-hydroxy-tryptamine; 5-HT) was thought to interact with what were termed 5-HT receptors. Today, seven distinct families or populations of serotonergic receptors have been identified, 5-HT_1 through 5-HT_7, and several are divided into subpopulations (Table 6.2). With the exception of the 5-HT_3 receptor (Chapter 8), which is an ion channel–type receptor, all of the 5-HT receptors are members of the GPCR superfamily. The discovery of the individual populations and subpopulations of 5-HT receptors follows the approximate order of their numbering and, as a consequence, more is known about 5-HT_1 and 5-HT_2 receptors than about 5-HT_6 and 5-HT_7 receptors. A factor contributing to our current lack of understanding about the function of certain 5-HT receptor populations (e.g., 5-HT_{1E} or 5-HT_5 receptors) is the absence of agonists and/or antagonists with selectivity for these receptors.

NH_2

HO

N H

Serotonin (5-HT)

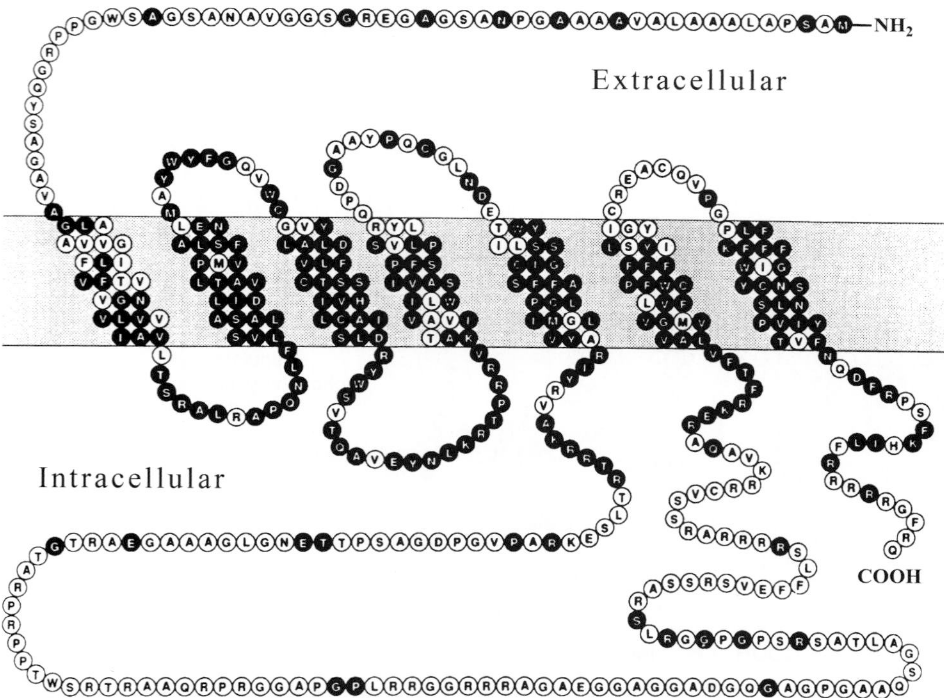

Figure 6.8 Human kidney α_2-adrenergic receptor: amino acid sequence of the human kidney α_2 receptor showing the seven transmembrane domains and the connecting intracellular and extracellular loops. Note particularly the large third intracellular loop, which is the G protein–binding site. The arrows point to the sites of glycosylation. Amino acids in black circles are those identical to the amino acids in the human platelet α_2 receptor. From Regan JW, Kobilka TS, Yang-Feng TL, et al. Cloning and expression of a human kidney cDNA for an α_2 -adrenergic receptor subtype. *Proc Natl Acad Sci USA*. 1988;85:6301-6305, with permission.

Table 6.2 Classification and Nomenclature for the Various Populations of 5-HT Receptors

Populations and Subpopulations	Second Messenger System[a]	Currently Accepted Name[b]	Comments
5-HT_1			
5-HT_{1A}	AC(−)	5-HT_{1A}	Cloned and pharmacologic 5-HT_{1A} receptors
5-HT_{1B}	AC(−)	5-HT_{1B}	Rodent homolog of 5-HT_{1B} receptors
$5\text{-HT}_{1B\beta}$			A mouse homolog of $h5\text{-HT}_{1B}$ receptors
5-HT_{1D}			Sites identified in binding studies using human and calf brain homogenates
$5\text{-HT}_{1D\alpha}$	AC(−)	$h5\text{-HT}_{1D}$	A cloned human 5-HT_{1D} subpopulation
$5\text{-HT}_{1D\beta}$	AC(−)	$h5\text{-HT}_{1B}$	A second cloned human 5-HT_{1D} subpopulation; human counterpart of rat 5-HT_{1B}
5-HT_{1E}	AC(−)	5-HT_{1E}	Sites identified in binding studies using brain homogenates and cloned receptors
$5\text{-HT}_{1E\alpha}$			An alternate name that has been used for cloned human 5-HT_{1E} receptors
$5\text{-HT}_{1E\beta}$	AC(−)	5-ht_{1F}	A cloned mouse homolog of 5-HT_{1F} receptors
5-HT_{1F}			A cloned human 5-HT_1 receptor population
5-HT_2			
5-HT_2	PI	5-HT_{2A}	Original "5-HT_2" (sometimes called $5\text{-HT}_{2\alpha}$) receptors
5-HT_{2F}	PI	5-HT_{2B}	5-HT_2–like receptors originally found in rat fundus
5-HT_{1C}	PI	5-HT_{2C}	Originally described as 5-HT_{1C} ($5\text{-HT}_{2\beta}$) receptors
5-HT_3			
5-HT_3	Ion channel	5-HT_3	An ion channel receptor
5-HT_4	AC(+)	5-HT_4	5-HT_4 population originally described in functional studies
5-HT_{4S}			Short form of cloned 5-HT_4 receptors
5-HT_{4L}			Long form of cloned 5-HT_4 receptors
$5\text{-HT}_{4(b)–4(d)}$			Recently identified human 5-HT_4 receptor isoforms
5-HT_5			
5-HT_{5A}	?	5-HT_{5A}	Cloned mouse, rat, and human 5-HT_5 receptors
5-HT_{5B}	?	5-HT_{5A}	Cloned mouse and rat 5-HT_{5A}–like receptor
5-HT_6			
5-HT_6	AC(+)	5-HT_6	Cloned rat and human 5-HT receptor
5-HT_7			
5-HT_7	AC(+)	5-HT_7	Cloned rat, mouse, guinea pig, and human 5-HT receptors

[a]*AC*, adenylyl cyclase; (–), negatively coupled; (+), positively coupled; *PI*, phospholipase coupled.
[b]Currently accepted names are taken from Hoyer et al.[9]

Table 6.2 lists the receptor classification and nomenclatures that have been employed for serotonergic receptors. Care should be used when reading the older primary literature because 5-HT receptor nomenclature has changed so dramatically and, often, can be confusing and very frustrating to comprehend.

All of the six 5-HT GPCR populations (and subpopulations) have been cloned and, together with the cloning of other neurotransmitter receptors, has led to generalizations regarding amino acid sequence homology.[14] Any two receptors with amino acid sequences that are approximately 70%-80% identical in their transmembrane-spanning segments are called the *intermediate-homology group*. This group of receptors could be members of the same subfamily and have highly similar to nearly indistinguishable pharmacologic profiles or second messenger systems. A *low-homology group* (~35%-55% transmembrane homology) consists of distantly related receptor subtypes from the same neurotransmitter family, and a *high-homology group* (~95%-99% transmembrane homology) consists of species homologs from the same gene in different species.[14] Species homologs of the same gene reveal high sequence conservation in regions outside the transmembrane domains, whereas intraspecies receptor subtypes usually are quite different.[14] Current 5-HT receptor classification and nomenclature require that several criteria be met before a receptor population can be adequately characterized. Receptor populations must be identified on the basis of drug binding characteristics (*operational* or *recognitory criteria*), receptor-effector coupling (*transductional criteria*), and gene and receptor structure sequences for the nucleotide and amino acid components, respectively (*structural criteria*).[14-16]

The 5-HT receptors are linked to G proteins as follows: 5-HT_{1A}, 5-HT_{1B}, 5-HT_{1D}, 5-HT_{1E}, 5-HT_{1F}, and 5-HT_5 are linked to $G_{i/o}$; 5-HT_{2A}, 5-HT_{2B}, and 5-HT_{2C} are linked to $G_{q/11}$; and 5-HT_4, 5-HT_6, and 5-HT_7 are linked to G_s.

CHOLINERGIC MUSCARINIC RECEPTORS

The endogenous neurotransmitter acetylcholine can interact with two major cholinergic receptor classes: nicotinic (Chapter 8) and muscarinic. The cholinergic receptors at the parasympathetic neuroeffector site are termed muscarinic receptors (mAChRs) because muscarine, a natural alkaloid, demonstrated activity at these sites while having none at the nicotinic sites (neuromuscular junction and autonomic ganglia) where nicotine had activity.

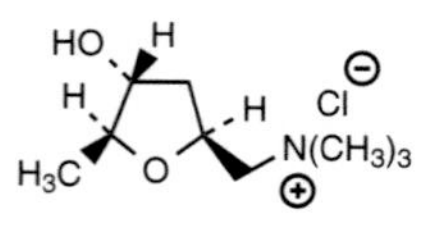

L(+)-Muscarine chloride

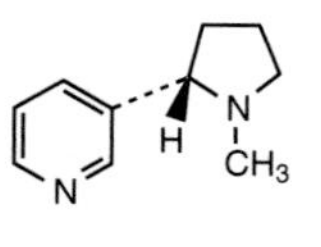

S(−)-Nicotine

Prior to the discovery that mAChR were members of the GCPR family, early SAR studies regarding affinity and efficacy of cholinergic agonists provided the basis for models (as depicted in Fig. 6.9) indicating the importance of the binding of an ester functional group and a quaternary ammonium group separated by two carbons. This model depicts ionic bonding between the positively charged quaternary nitrogen of acetylcholine and a negative charge at the anionic site of the mAChR. The negative charge was suggested to result from a carboxylate ion from the free carboxyl group of a dicarboxylic amino acid (e.g., aspartate or glutamate) at the binding site on the receptor protein. This model also involved a hydrogen bond between the ester oxygen of acetylcholine and a hydroxyl group contributed by the esteratic site of the receptor.

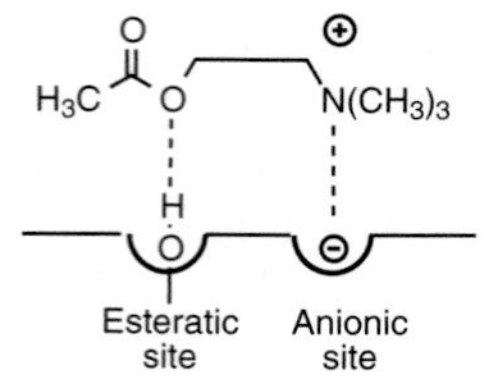

Esteratic site

Anionic site

Figure 6.9 Original representation of the muscarinic acetylcholine receptor (mAChR).

Although this early mAChR model accounted for two important SAR requirements for muscarinic agonists, it failed to explain the following: (1) at least two of the alkyl groups bonded to the quaternary nitrogen must be methyl groups; (2) the known stereochemical requirements for agonist binding to the receptor; and (3) the fact that all potent cholinergic agonists have only five atoms between the quaternary nitrogen and the terminal hydrogen atom. This last point is known as Ing's "Rule of Five."[17]

Heterogeneity in the mAChR population was first suggested in the late 1970s during pharmacologic studies using the muscarinic antagonist pirenzepine. At the time, pirenzepine was the only muscarinic antagonist to block gastric acid secretion at concentrations that did not block the effects of muscarinic agonists. This observation initiated research that ultimately led to discovery of mAChR subtypes, designated as M_1, M_2, and M_3 based on their pharmacologic responses to various ligands. Rapid advances in molecular biology led to cloning of cDNAs that encoded for five mAChRs, designated as m_1 through m_5; m_1, m_2, and m_3 correspond to the respective M_1 through M_3 receptors identified by their pharmacologic specificity. The International Union of Pharmacology Committee on Receptor Nomenclature and Drug Classification has recommended that the uppercase nomenclature M_1 through M_5 be used to designate both pharmacologic and molecular subtypes.[18]

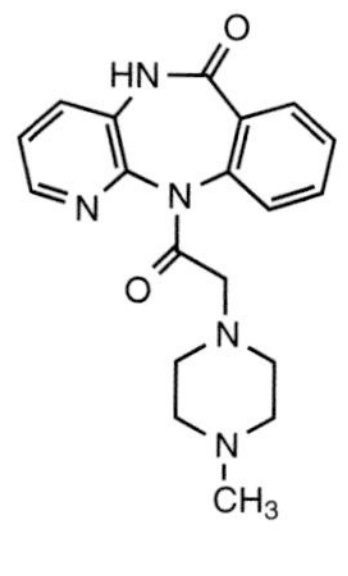

Pirenzepine

All mAChR subtypes (M_1 to M_5) are found in the CNS, and other tissues can contain more than one. These receptors are summarized in Table 6.3. As more mAChR subtypes have been discovered, it has become apparent that there is a lack of known antagonists and agonists exhibiting very high subtype selectivity. Thus, proof for involvement of any one receptor subtype in a given system currently requires use of more than one antagonist. Additionally, if the selectivity of a novel muscarinic antagonist or putative agonist is to be assessed, it should be through use of recombinant mAChRs expressed in cell lines, rather than with native receptors.

Computer-assisted molecular modeling has made it possible to obtain three-dimensional representations of the mAChR[19]; a proposed top-view model of the M_1 mAChR is shown in Figure 6.10.[20] This model suggests that the quaternary nitrogen of acetylcholine participates in an ionic bond with the free carboxylate group of an aspartate residue (Asp105 in TMD 3)—one of the receptor functional groups that was originally hypothesized to be involved in receptor binding of acetylcholine.

Signal transduction at the stimulatory "odd-numbered" mAChRs (i.e., M_1, M_3, and M_5) is via coupling with a $G_{q/11}$ protein that is involved with mobilization of intracellular calcium. The M_1, M_3, and M_5 receptors also stimulate phospholipase A_2 and phospholipase D. Activation of phospholipase A_2 results in release of arachidonic acid, with subsequent synthesis of eicosanoids (C_{20} fatty acids).

The "even-numbered" mAChR subtypes (i.e., M_2 and M_4) are coupled to G_i/G_o proteins, whose activation inhibits adenylyl cyclase. This results in a decrease in cAMP, inhibition of voltage-gated calcium channels, and

Table 6.3 Muscarinic Acetylcholine Receptor Subtypes

Receptor	G Protein	Tissue Location	Cellular Response	Function
M_1	$G_{q/11}$	CNS, gastric and salivary glands, autonomic ganglia, enteric nerves	PLC activation (↑IP_3 and ↑DAG → ↑Ca^{2+} and PKC); depolarization and excitation (↑sEPSP); PLA_2 and PLD_2 activation; ↑AA	↑ Cognitive function ↑ Seizure activity ↑ Secretions ↑ Autonomic ganglia depolarization ↓ DA release and locomotion
M_2	G_i/G_o	Autonomic nerve terminals; CNS; heart; smooth muscle	Inhibition of adenylyl cyclase (↓cAMP) & voltage-gated Ca^{2+} channels; activation of inwardly rectifying K^+ channels	↓ Heart rate ↑ Smooth muscle contraction Neural inhibition in periphery via autoreceptors and heteroreceptor ↓ Ganglionic transmission Neural inhibition in CNS ↑ Tremors, hypothermi,a & analgesia
M_3	$G_{q/11}$	CNS (less than other mAChRs), smooth muscle, glands, heart	Same as M_1	↑ Smooth muscle contraction (e.g., bladder) ↑ Salivary gland secretion ↑ Food intake, body fat deposits Inhibits dopamine release Synthesis of nitric oxide
M_4	G_i/G_o	CNS	Same as M_2	Inhibition of autoreceptor-and heteroreceptor-mediated transmitter release in CNS Analgesia Cataleptic activity Facilitates dopamine release
M_5	$G_{q/11}$	Low levels in CNS and periphery; predominate mAChRs in dopaminergic neurons of substantia nigra and ventral tegmentum area	Same as M_1	Mediates dilation of cerebral arteries Facilitates dopamine release Augments drug-seeking behavior and reward

Adapted from Westfall TC, Westfall DP. Neurotransmission: the autonomic and somatic motor nervous systems. In: Brunton LL, Lazo JS, Parker KL, eds. *Goodman and Gilman's the Pharmacological Basis of Therapeutics*. 11th ed. New York: McGraw-Hill; 2006:137-181; with permission.

AA, arachidonic acid; cAMP, cyclic adenosine monophosphate; CNS, central nervous system; DAG, diacylglycerol; IP_3, inositol-1, 4, 5- triphosphate; mAChRs, muscarinic acetylcholine receptor subtypes; PKC, protein kinase C; PLA, phospholipase A; PLC, Phospholipase C; PLD_2 phospholipase D; sEPSP, slow excitatory postsynaptic potential; VTA, ventral tegmentum area.

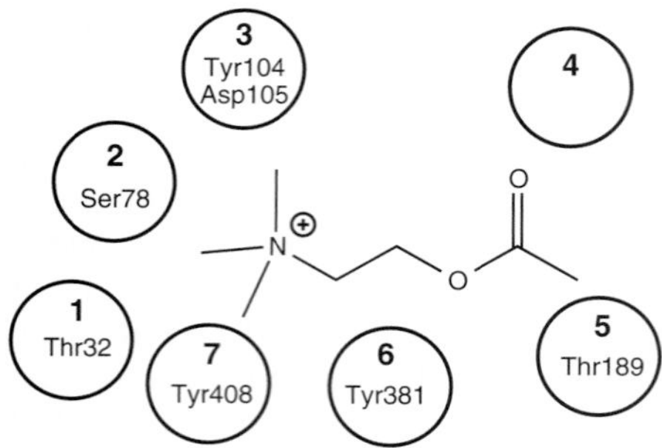

Figure 6.10 Model of acetylcholine interaction with muscarinic M_1 receptor. Circles represent seven transmembrane domains.

activation of inwardly rectifying potassium channels. The result is hyperpolarization and inhibition of these excitable membranes.

The M_1 receptors are sometimes described as "neural" due to their abundance in the cerebral cortex, hippocampus, and striatum. M_1 receptors have been implicated in Alzheimer disease and are thought to be involved with memory and learning. Early studies suggested that the agonist McN-A-343 was selective for the M_1 receptor, but more recent evidence indicates otherwise. It can show moderate selectivity for M_4 receptors. Additionally, M_1 receptors are found at autonomic ganglia, enteric nerves, and salivary and gastric glands. Agonists at M_1 receptors show the greatest promise for treatment of the cholinergic deficit associated with Alzheimer disease.

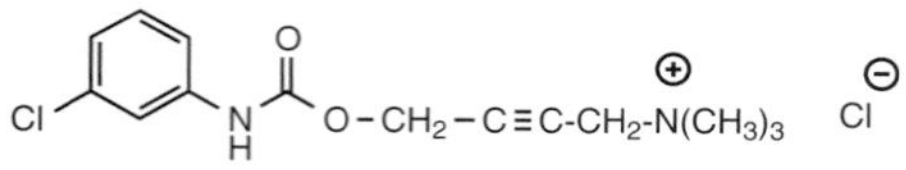

Cl–C6H4–NH–C(=O)–O-CH2-C≡C-CH2-$N^{+}(CH_3)_3$ Cl^{-}

McN-A-343

M_2 receptors are found in abundance in the heart, where activation exerts both negative chronotropic and inotropic actions, and stimulates contraction of smooth muscle. Activation of M_2 autoreceptors located on nerve terminals affords neural inhibition by decreasing acetylcholine release.

M_3 receptors are found in abundance in smooth muscle and glands, where their stimulation leads to contraction and secretion, respectively. Knowledge of this effect on smooth muscle of the bladder has led to development and subsequent approval of several M_3 receptor antagonists for treatment of overactive bladder. Although widely distributed in the CNS, their concentration in the CNS is lower than those of other mAChRs. M_3 mAChRs function to decrease neurotransmitter release.

M_4 receptors are found in the striatum and basal forebrain, where they decrease transmitter release in both the CNS and periphery. Their activation in smooth muscle and secretary glands leads to inhibition of potassium and calcium channels.

M_5 receptors are the least characterized of the mAChRs, and there is evidence for their existence in the CNS and periphery, where they can regulate dopamine release in the CNS.

Opioid Receptors

While scientists had postulated for some time based on the rigid structural and stereochemical requirements essential for the analgesic actions of morphine and related opioids that binding to specific receptors was required, the endogenous ligands for such receptors were unknown until the discovery by Hughes et al.[21] of the two pentapeptides, Tyr-Gly-Gly-Phe-Met (Met-enkephalin) and Tyr-Gly-Gly-Phe-Leu (Leu-enkephalin), that caused the opioid activity (Fig. 6.11). Because these endogenous compounds were isolated from brain tissue they were named enkephalins after the Greek word *Kaphale*, which translates as "from the head." Shortly after this discovery additional endogenous opioids were identified including other endogenous opioid peptides β-endorphin,[22] the dynorphins,[23] and the endomorphins.[24] All of the endogenous opioid peptides are synthesized as part of the structures of large precursor proteins.[25]

Identification of multiple opioid receptors has depended on the discovery of selective agonists and antagonists, the identification of sensitive assay techniques,[26] and, ultimately, the cloning of the receptor proteins.[27] The techniques that have been especially useful are the radioligand binding assays on brain tissues and the electrically stimulated peripheral muscle preparations. Rodent brain tissue contains all three opioid receptor types, and special evaluation procedures (computer-assisted line fitting) or selective blocking (with reversible or irreversible binding agents) of some of the receptor types must be used to sort out the receptor selectivity of test compounds. The myenteric plexus–containing longitudinal strips of guinea pig ileum contain μ- and κ-opioid receptors. The contraction of these muscle strips is initiated by electrical stimulation and is inhibited by opioids. The vas deferens from mouse contains μ, δ, and κ receptors and reacts similarly to the guinea pig ileum to electrical stimulation and to opioids. Homogenous populations of opioid receptors are found in rat (μ), hamster (δ), and rabbit (κ) vas deferentia, and all interact with receptors that belong to the GPCR superfamily.

Met-enkephalin = Tyr-Gly-Gly-Phe-Met
Leu-Enkephalin = Tyr-Gly-Gly-Phe-Leu
β-Endorphin = Tyr-Gly-Gly-Phe-Met-Thr-Ser-Glu-Lys-Ser10-Gln-Thr-Pro-Leu-Val-Thr-Leu-Phe-Lys- Asn20-Ala-Ile-Ile-Lys-Asn-Ala-Tyr-Lys-Lys-Gly-GluOH31
Dynorphin(dyn$^{1-17}$) = Tyr-Gly-Gly-Phe-Leu-Arg-Arg-Ile-Arg-Pro-Lys-Leu-Lys-Trp-Asp-Asn-Gln
Dynorphin(dyn$^{1-8}$) = Tyr-Gly-Gly-Phe-Leu-Arg-Arg-Ile
Dynorphin(dyn$^{1-13}$) = Tyr-Gly-Gly-Phe-Leu-Arg-Arg-Ile-Arg-Pro-Lys-Leu-Lys
α-Neoenodorphin = Tyr-Gly-Gly-Phe-Leu-Arg-Lys-Tyr-Pro-Lys
β-Neoendorphin = Tyr-Gly-Gly-Phe-Leu-Arg-Lys-Tyr-Pro
Nociceptin = Phe-Gly-Gly-Phe-Thr-Gly-Ala-Arg-Lys-Ser-Ala-Arg-Lys-Leu-Ala-Asn-Gln

Figure 6.11 Precursor proteins to the endogenous opioid peptides.

All three of the receptor types have been well characterized and cloned.[27] The signal transduction mechanism for these three opioid receptor subtypes is through $G_{i/o}$ proteins resulting in inhibition of adenylyl cyclase activity, leading to decreased cAMP production, efflux of potassium ions, and closure of voltage-gated Ca^{2+} channels. The net result is cellular hyperpolarization and cell firing inhibition.[28]

As with many other receptors during the initial stages of discovery and characterization, the nomenclature usually evolves as more research is conducted. A system for consistent nomenclature adopted by the International Union of Pharmacology (IUPHAR) in 2000, named the receptors as MOP-μ, DOP-δ, and KOP-κ. In current literature, however, the opioid receptors often are referred to as DOR (δ), KOR (κ), and MOR (μ). There is evidence for subtypes of each of these receptors; however, the failure of researchers to find genomic evidence for additional receptors indicates that the receptor subtypes are posttranslational modifications (splice variants) of known receptor types.[29] Receptor subtypes may also be known receptor types that are coupled to different signal transduction systems.

Table 6.4 lists the opioid receptor types, their known physiologic functions, and selective agonists and antagonists for each of the receptors. All three of the major opioid receptor types are located in human brain or spinal cord tissues, and each has a role in the mediation of pain. See Chapter 14 for a summary of key binding interactions of μ and κ receptor agonists and antagonists.

As with other GPCRs, opioid receptors can undergo dimerization to form homo- and heterodimers (e.g., DOR-MOR, DOR-KOR) with a resultant lower affinity for very selective agonists. Additionally, these heterodimers tend to display an altered cellular signaling in response to agonists. Interestingly, antagonism of DOR receptors or DOR knock-out animals, where no DOR dimers can exist, results in reduced tolerance that develops on chronic administration of the MOR agonist morphine, suggesting a possible link between tolerance and opioid receptor dimerization.[30]

Mu (μ)-Opioid Receptors

Endomorphin-1 (Tyr1-Pro-Trp-Phe4-NH_2) and endomorphin-2 (Tyr1-Pro-Phe-Phe4-NH_2) are endogenous opioid peptides with a high degree of selectivity for μ (MOP) receptors. A number of therapeutically useful compounds have been found that are selective for μ-opioid receptors (Fig. 6.12). All of the opioid alkaloids and most of their synthetic derivatives are μ-selective agonists (see Chapter 14). Morphine, normorphine, and dihydromorphinone have 10- to 20-fold μ-receptor selectivity and were particularly important in early studies to differentiate the opioid receptors. Sufentanil and the peptides DAMGO and dermorphin,[31] all with 100-fold selectivity for μ over other opioid receptors, are frequently used in laboratory studies to demonstrate μ-receptor selectivity in cross-tolerance, receptor binding, and isolated smooth muscle assays. Studies with μ-receptor knockout mice have confirmed that all the major pharmacologic actions observed on injection of morphine (e.g., analgesia, respiratory depression, tolerance, withdrawal symptoms, decreased gastric motility, and emesis) occur by interactions with μ receptors.[32]

There is evidence that μ_1 receptors are high-affinity binding sites that mediate pain neurotransmission, whereas μ_2 receptors control respiratory depression. Naloxonazine is a selective inhibitor of μ_1-opioid receptors.[33] Naloxone and naltrexone are antagonists that have weak (5- to 10-fold) selectivity for μ receptors.

Using μ-opioid receptor ligands, investigators have demonstrated that opioid binding is generally rather superficially located and exposed to that portion of the receptor that is on the extracellular surface. This superficial binding location may help to partially account for the rather rapid dissociation half-lives of many of the potent opioids as compared with other ligands that bind to other nonopioid receptors (e.g., some muscarinic and β-adrenoceptors).[34] Both agonists and antagonists bind to the μ-opioid receptor such that the OH and N^+ groups of the tyramine moiety found in alkaloid ligands interact within the binding pocket with Asp7 in TMIII and His20 in TMVI. With cyclic peptide opioids a similar interaction with the receptor occurs, but this involves H-bonding via the Tyr found in the opioid peptides.[35]

Ethylketazocine and bremazocine are 6,7- benzazocine derivatives with κ-opioid receptor selectivity (Fig. 6.13). These two compounds were used in early studies to investigate κ (KOP) receptors, and the "k" in ethyl**k**etocyclazocine gave the κ receptor its name. They are not highly selective, however, and their use in research has diminished. A number of arylacetamide derivatives having a high selectivity for κ over μ or δ receptors have been discovered. The first of these compounds, (±)-U50488, has a 50-fold selectivity for κ over μ receptors and has been extremely important in the characterization of κ-opioid activity.[36] Other important agents in this class are (±) PD-117302[37] and (−) CI-977.[38] Each of these agents has 1,000-fold selectivity for κ over μ or δ receptors. Evidence suggests that the arylacetamides bind to a subtype of κ receptors.

In animals, including humans, κ agonists produce analgesia. Other prominent effects are diuresis, sedation, and dysphoria. Compared to μ agonists, κ agonists were initially thought to have less respiratory depressant, constipating and addictive (euphoria and physical dependence) properties. It was hoped that κ agonists would become useful strong analgesics that lacked addictive properties; however, clinical trials with several highly selective and potent κ agonists were aborted because of the occurrence of unacceptable sedative and dysphoric side effects. Pentazocine, butorphanol, and nalbuphine are κ agonists that provide only mild analgesia (see Chapter 14). κ-Selective opioids with only a peripheral action have been shown to be effective in relieving inflammation and the pain associated with it.[39] Scientific evidence suggests there are κ_1, κ_2, and κ_3 subtypes of κ receptors; however, the physiologic effects initiated by the κ receptor subtypes are not well defined.[40]

The peptides related to dynorphin are the natural agonists for κ receptors, but their selectivity for κ over μ receptors is not very high. Synthetic peptide analogues have been reported that are more potent and more selective

Table 6.4 Opioid Receptors

Receptor Subtype	δ (delta, DOP)	Κ (kappa, KOP)	μ (mu, MOP)	NOP (N/OFQ peptide)
Transduction Mechanism	Inhibition of adenylyl cyclase, activation of inwardly rectifying K^+ channels, inhibition of Ca^{2+} channels, phospholipase C stimulation			
G protein	$G_{i/o}$	$G_{i/o}$	$G_{i/o}$	$G_{i/o}$
Localization	Olfactory bulb Nucleus accumbens Caudate putamen neocortex	Cerebral cortex Nucleus accumbens hypothalamus	CNS (neocortex, thalamus, nucleus accumbens, hippocampus, amygdala Vas deferens Myenteric gut neurons	Cortex, olfactory nucleus, hypothalamus, hippocampus, substantia nigra, locus coerulus, spinal cord, amygdala,
Endogenous ligand	Enkephalins β-Endorphin	Dynorphins β-Endorphin	Endomorphin 1 Endomorphin 2 β-Endorphin	N/OFQ peptide
Likely physiological roles	Analgesia GI motility Olfaction Immune stimulation Respiratory depression (rate) Cognitive function Motor integration	Regulation of nociception Analgesia Sedation Miosis Diuresis Dysphoria Neuroendocrine secretions	Analgesia (morphine-like) Euphoria Increased gastrointestinal transit time thermo regulation Immune suppression Respiratory depression (volume) Emetic effects Tolerance Physical dependence	Motor and balance control Reinforcement and reward Nociception Stress response Sexual behavior Aggression Autonomic control of physiological processes
Key selective agonists	DADLE (D-Ala2-D-Leu5-enkephalin) DSLET (Tyr-D-Ser-Gly-Phe-Leu-Thr) DPDPE (D-Pen2-D-Pen5-DADLE (δ_2) D-Ala2-deltorphin II (δ_2)	Ethylketocyclazocine (EKC) Bremazocine Mr2034 Dyn (1-17) Trifluadom U-50,488 (κ_1) Spiradoline (U-62,066) (κ_1) U-69,593 (κ_1) PD 117302 (κ_1) Dyn (1−17) (κ_1) NalBzOH (κ_1)	Morphine Sufentanil DAMGO (Tyr-D-Ala-MePhe-NH-$(CH_2)_2$ OH PLO17 (Tyr-Pro-MePhe-D-Pro-NH_2 BIT (affinity label) Meptazinol (μ_1 high affinity) Etonitazene	N/OFQ peptide Nociceptin (1-13)
Key Selective Antagonists	ICI 174864 FIT (affinity label) SUPERFIT (affinity label) Naltrindole (NTI) BNTX Naltriben (NTB) Naltrindol isothiocyanate (NTII)	TENA nor-BNI UPHIT	Naloxone Naltrexone CTOP Cyprodime β-FNA (affinity label) Naloxonazine	(N-phe1)-Nociceptin (1−13) J-113397 UFP-101

CNS, central nervous system; GI, gastrointestinal; nor-BNI, norbinaltorphimine.

than dynorphin for κ receptors. The major antagonist with good selectivity for κ receptors is norbinaltorphimine (Fig. 6.13).[41] This compound has approximately 100-fold selectivity for κ over δ receptors and an even greater selectivity for κ over μ receptors when tested during competitive binding studies in monkey brain homogenate. No medical use for a κ antagonist has been found.

Delta (δ)-Opioid Receptors

Enkephalins, the natural ligands at δ (DOP) receptors, are only slightly selective for δ over μ receptors. Changes in the amino acid composition of the enkephalins can give compounds with high potency and selectivity for δ receptors. The peptides most often used as selective δ receptor ligands are (D-Ala2, D-Leu5) enkephalin (DADLE),[42]

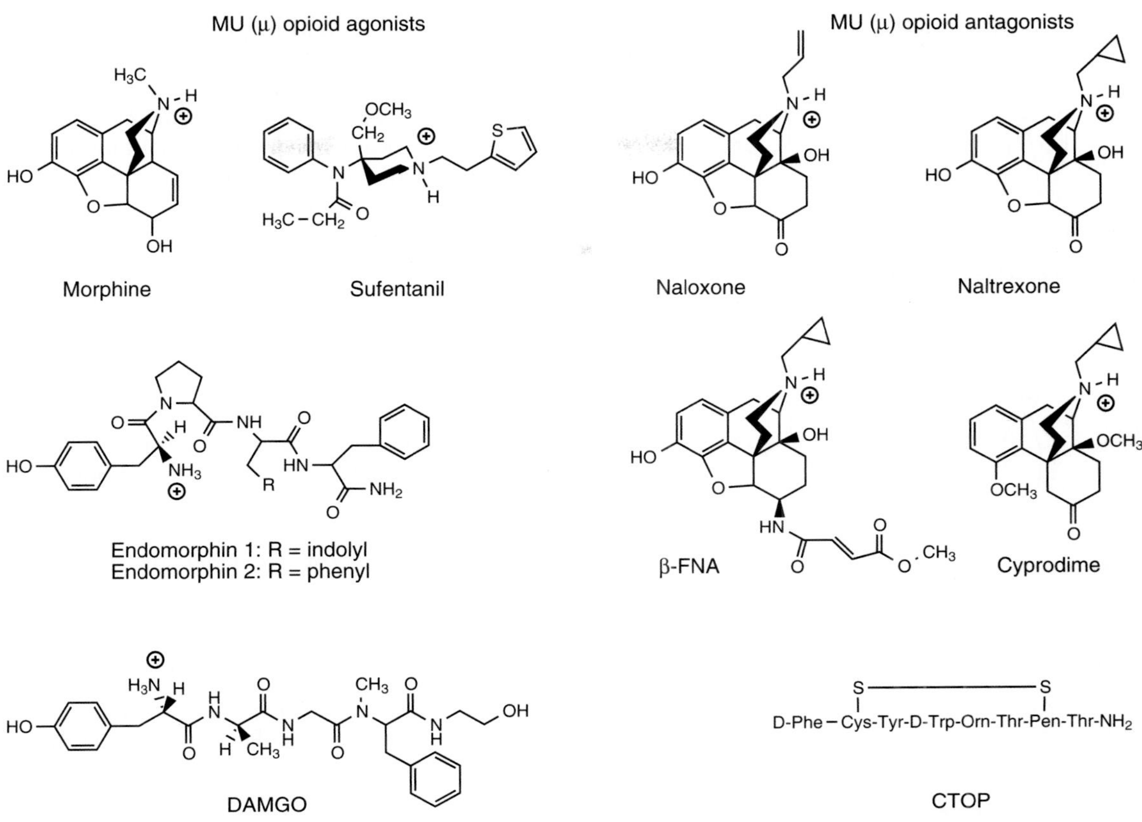

Figure 6.12 Structures of compounds selective for μ (OP3) opioid receptors.

(D-Ser2, Leu5) enkephalin-Thr (DSLET),[43] and the cyclic peptide (D-Pen2, D-Pen5) enkephalin (DPDPE)[44] (Fig. 6.14) These and other δ-receptor selective peptides have been useful for in vitro studies, but their metabolic instability and poor distribution properties (penetration of the blood-brain barrier [BBB] is limited by their hydrophilicity) have limited their usefulness for in vivo studies.

Nonpeptide agonists that are selective for δ receptors have been reported. Derivatives of morphindoles (e.g., nor-OMI, Fig. 6.14) were the first nonpeptide molecules to show δ selectivity in in vitro assays.[45] SNC-80 (Fig. 6.14) is a newer and more selective δ-opioid receptor agonist.[46] This compound produces analgesia after oral dose in several rodent models, and side effects appear minimal. Clinical trials with SNC-80 and other nonpeptide δ receptor agonists were attempted and aborted, primarily because of the convulsant action of δ receptor agonists.

Naltrindole[47] and naltriben[48] (Fig. 6.14) are highly selective nonpeptide antagonists for δ receptors. Naltrindole penetrates the CNS and displays antagonist activity that is selective for δ receptors in in vitro and in vivo systems. The δ-opioid receptor antagonists have shown clinical potential as immunosuppressants and in treatment of cocaine abuse.

NOP Receptor

A fourth opioid receptor named after its endogenous ligand N/OFQ peptide (NOP; OP_4) has been identified and cloned based on homology with the cDNA sequence of the known (μ, δ, and κ) opioid receptors.[49,50] Despite the homology in cDNA sequence with known opioid receptors, NOP did not bind the classical opioid peptide or nonpeptide agonists or antagonists with high affinity. Thus, the receptor was initially called the orphan opioid receptor or opioid-like receptor (OPLR-1). In subsequent studies, two research groups found a heptadecapeptide (Phe-Gly-Gly-Phe-Thr-Gly-Ala-Arg-Lys-Ser-Ala-Arg-Lys-Leu-Ala-Asn-Gln) to be the endogenous peptide for this receptor and named it nociceptin because it caused hyperalgesia (nociception) after intracerebral ventricular injection in mice.[51] Another research group[52] named the heptapeptide orphanin FQ, after its affinity for the "orphan opioid receptor" and after the first and last amino acids in the peptide's sequence (i.e., F = Phe and Q = Gln). Thus, the OPRL-1 receptor was renamed the NOP or N/OFQ peptide receptor, and the current name for the endogenous ligand is N/OFQ peptide. Human N/OFQ peptide is derived from a precursor protein, preproN/OFQ (ppN/OFQ), which consists of 176 amino acids and resembles dynorphin-A in structure, with the most notable difference being the replacement of the N-terminus Tyr1 for dynorphin A with Phe1.[52]

Conflicting results have been published regarding the ability of N/OFQ peptide to produce hyperalgesia versus analgesia in rodent pain assay models. One study has established this compound to be a potent initiator of pain signals in the periphery, where it acts by releasing substance P from nerve terminals.[53] N/OFQ peptide is thought to be an endogenous antagonist of dopamine transport that may act either directly on dopamine or by inhibiting GABA to affect

Kappa (κ) opioid agonists

(±) Ethylketazocine

(±) PD 117302

(±) Bremazocine

(±) U 50488

Kappa (κ) opioid antagonists

(±) Norbinaltorphimine

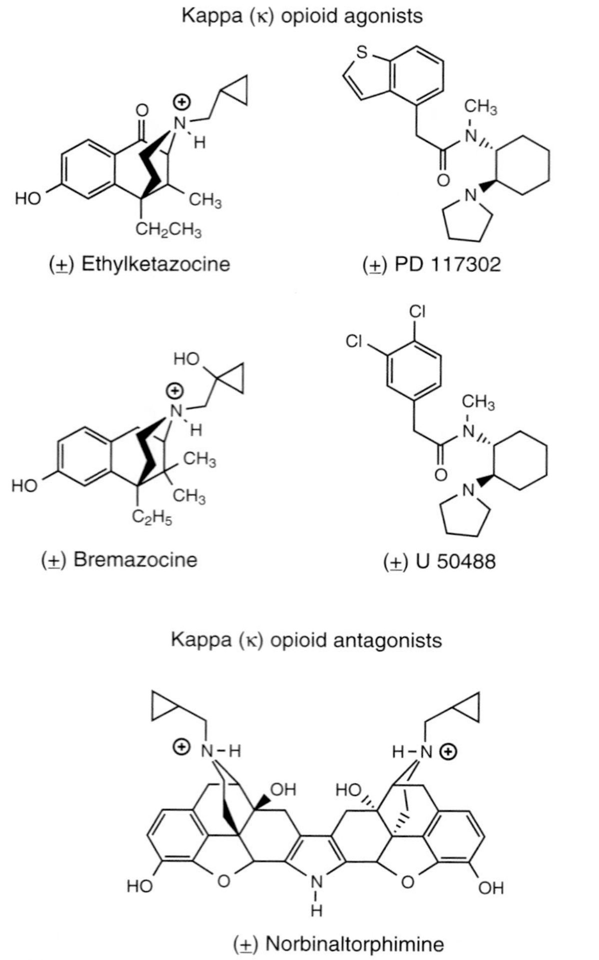

Figure 6.13 Structures of compounds selective for κ (OP2) opioid receptors. (−)-Stereoisomers are the most active compounds.

dopamine levels.[54] Within the CNS, the actions of N/OFQ can be either similar or opposite to those of opioids depending on the location. It controls a wide range of biologic functions ranging from nociception to food intake, from memory processes to cardiovascular and renal functions, from spontaneous locomotor activity to gastrointestinal (GI) motility, and from anxiety to the control of neurotransmitter release at peripheral and central sites.[51] Several commonly used opioid drugs, including etorphine and buprenorphine, have been demonstrated to bind to nociceptin receptors, but this binding is relatively insignificant compared to their binding at other opioid receptors. More recently, a range of selective ligands for NOP have been developed that show little or no affinity to other opioid receptors, which allows NOP-mediated responses to be studied in isolation.[55] Injection of an N/OFQ peptide antagonist into the brains of laboratory animals results in an analgesic effect, raising hope for the use of these agents in the management of pain.[51]

The NOP receptors are widely distributed in the brain, and it is not surprising that many central actions of N/OFQ peptide have been suggested from animal studies, including supraspinal hyperalgesia, spinal analgesia, hyperphagia, depression, and inhibitions of anxiety, epilepsy, cough, motor activity, and learning and memory, as well as the regulation of cardiovascular, urogenital, GI, and immune systems. Many efforts have been expended in the development of agonists or antagonists of this novel member of the opioid receptor family. Table 6.4 identifies the major NOP receptor agonists and antagonists developed thus far.

HISTAMINE RECEPTORS

Histamine is an endogenous amine involved in a variety of functions in the human body. It functions peripherally as an autacoid and centrally as a neurotransmitter. Histamine

Delta (δ) opioid agonists

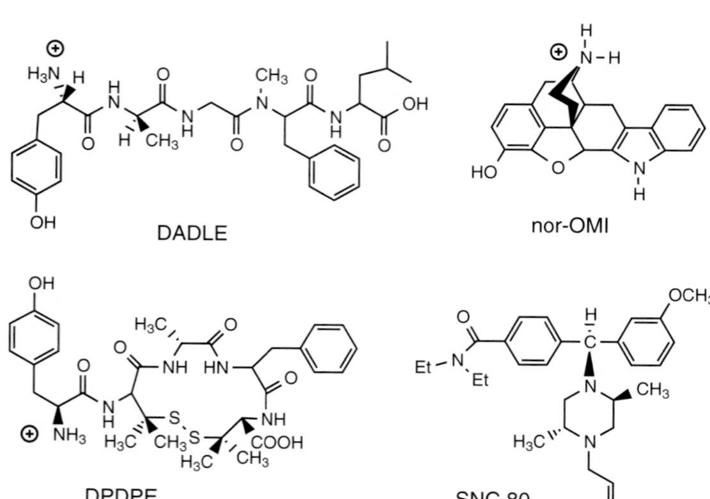

nor-OMI

Delta (δ) opioid antagonists

Naltrindol (X = NH)
Naltriben (X = O)

TIPP-g

Figure 6.14 Structures of compounds selective for δ (OP1) opioid receptors.

produces these effects through activation of at least four different GPCRs named H_1, H_2, H_3, and H_4 receptors. The potency of histamine for activating its receptors is highest for the H_3 and H_4 receptors, followed by the H_2 receptor and lastly the H_1 receptor. The development of receptor ligands displaying selectivity for each of these receptor subtypes has helped elucidate the functions of these various receptors.

H_1 Receptors

H_1 receptors mediate the classical effects of histamine associated with allergic symptoms and are the targets of "antihistamines" which have been commercially available for over 60 years, even though the H_1 receptor was not cloned until the early 1990s. Activation by histamine results in constriction of smooth muscle, including the airway smooth muscle during anaphylaxis. Vasodilation leading to shock is the result of H_1-mediated nitric oxide production from vascular endothelial cells. H_1 receptors are widespread throughout the brain, and receptor knockout studies in mice link these receptors to the cortical activation during waking. Thus, H_1 receptor antagonists that cross the BBB produce pronounced sedation by blocking histamine signaling in the brain.

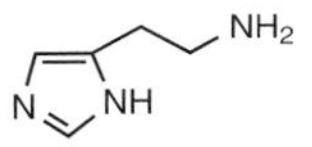

NH_2 N NH

Histamine

As befitting a monoamine receptor, the H_1 receptor shares certain structural and binding features with other biogenic amine receptors, most notably the β-adrenergic receptors, including ligand binding within a pore formed by TM3, TM5, and TM6 as determined by site-directed mutagenesis studies and X-ray crystallography.[56] Coupled primarily to $G_{q/11}$ and $G_{i/o}$ in a few systems, increased intracellular calcium is the main response to H_1 receptor stimulation.

Antihistamines, or H_1 receptor inverse agonists, are classified into the older "first-generation" antihistamines and the newer "second-generation" drugs. First-generation antihistamines, characterized by diphenhydramine (Benadryl), are more lipophilic and less selective (considerable antagonism of muscarinic receptors) compared to the newer peripherally selective ("nonsedative") drugs such as fexofenadine (Allegra).

The molecular determinants of antihistamine binding to the H_1 receptor have been identified through the crystal structure of the H_1 receptor bound to the first-generation antihistamine doxepin.[57] As predicted, doxepin binds within the pore created by TM3, TM5, and TM6, which is a well-conserved binding pocket among adrenergic receptors and also the site of histamine binding. Doxepin directly interacts with Trp428, a highly conserved residue. Affinity for these binding determinants, common in many monoamine receptors, is thought to be the basis for the poor selectivity of the first-generation antihistamines. Modeling of second-generation antihistamines with the H_1 receptor shows that fexofenadine can form a salt bridge with Lys191 which is found in TM5 near the extracellular surface and is not conserved among monoaminergic receptors. This may be the basis for the greater selectivity of the second-generation antihistamines.

CH_3 H C-O N CH_3 — H N CH_3 CH_3 — H H_3C N CH_3

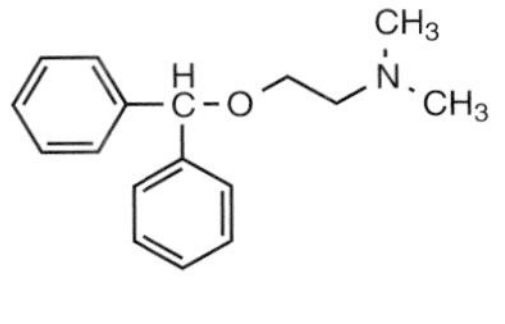

Diphenhydramine

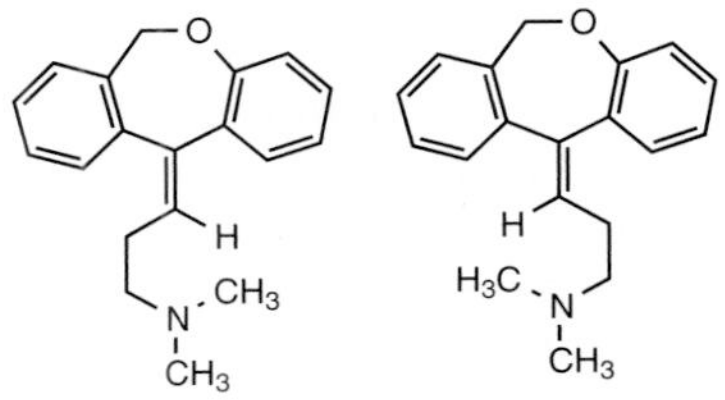

E-isomer Z-isomer

Doxepin (*E/Z* = 85/15%)

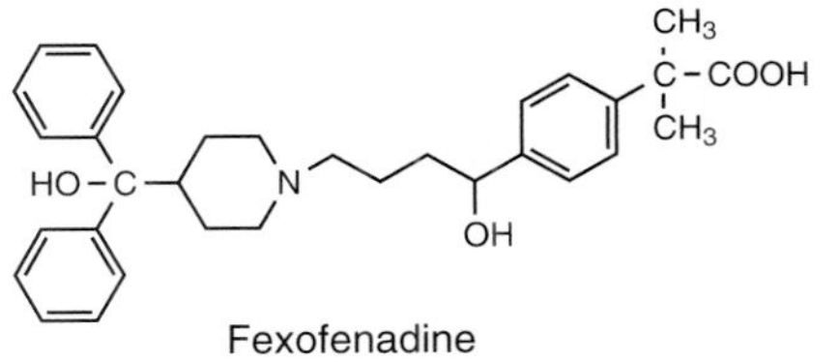

CH_3 C-COOH CH_3 HO-C N OH

Fexofenadine

H_2 Receptors

The inability of classical antihistamines to reduce histamine-induced gastric acid secretion led to the identification of H_2 histamine receptors in the 1970s. Linked mainly to G_s, activation of H_2 receptors leads to increased cAMP. Expression is highest in stomach and brain. H_2 antagonists such as cimetidine and ranitidine have been demonstrated to be inverse agonists as they reduce constitutive activity. Although they have been largely replaced by proton pump inhibitors recently, the development and commercialization of H_2 antagonists reduced the need for surgical intervention in the management of gastric ulcers.

The search for H_2 receptor antagonists began by modifying the structure of histamine and testing compounds in bioassays. This approach ultimately yielded cimetidine, which shares the imidazole ring of histamine but with a longer side chain. Mutagenesis data with the H_2 receptor supports a model where Asp186 in TM5 of the H_2 receptor is essential for cimetidine binding, probably through an interaction between the negatively charged amino acid and the imidazole ring.[58] This residue is not necessary for binding of histamine, but a nearby Thr190 is required for the agonist binding and activity.

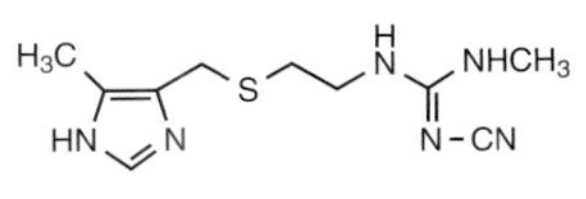

H_3C S H N $NHCH_3$ HN N N-CN

Cimetidine

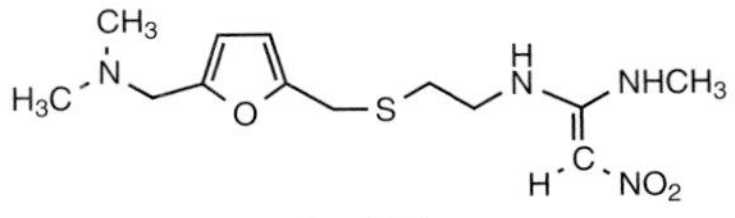

CH_3 H_3C N O S H N $NHCH_3$ H C NO_2

Ranitidine

H_3 Receptors

The H_3 receptors differ from the H_1 and H_2 receptors in a number of ways. There is low overall homology between the H_3 and either the H_1 or H_2 receptors; no blockbuster drugs target this receptor; and it is one of the few GPCRs that display considerable in vivo constitutive signaling. High constitutive signaling is indicative of a receptor population where a greater than usual proportion of receptors are in the active conformation in the absence of ligands. The ability of pertussis-toxin to inhibit H_3-mediated effects suggested linkage to $G_{i/o}$, and activation of H_3 receptors is coupled to a reduction in intracellular cAMP.

The H_3 receptor primarily functions as a presynaptic autoreceptor-regulating histamine synthesis and release in various areas of the brain. Evidence also suggests that H_3 receptors may function as heteroreceptors regulating release of neurotransmitter from adrenergic, serotonergic, cholinergic and dopaminergic neurons. Consequently, a number of inverse agonists at the H_3 receptor have been developed and clinically tested in a variety of neurological disorders including sleep disorders, ADHD, and Alzheimer's disease. The inverse agonist tiprolisant is the first H_3 ligand and is awaiting FDA approval. It promotes wakefulness and is indicated for treating narcolepsy, presumably by increasing the release of histamine in the brain.

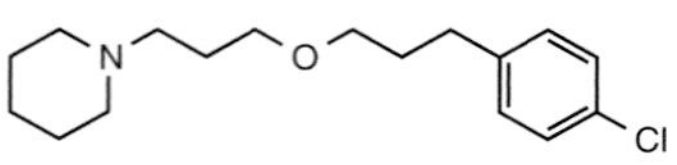

N O Cl

Tiprolisant

H_4 Receptors

The most recently discovered histamine receptor is the H_4 receptor. It is most similar to the H_3 receptor in terms of secondary structure, histamine binding and G protein selectivity ($G_{i/o}$). Receptor expression seems highest in the bone marrow and hematopoietic cells. H_4 receptor antagonists have demonstrated clinical efficacy in pruritic conditions including psoriasis and atopic dermatitis.

Dopamine Receptors

Dopamine mediates a variety of central and peripheral effects including vessel tone, voluntary movement, sensory gating, and reward behavior via activation of D_1, D_2, D_3, D_4, or D_5 receptors, which are found in a wide variety of central and peripheral locations. There is considerable homology between the D_1 and the D_5 receptors, and also between the D_2, D_3, and D_4 receptors. The D_1 class (D_1 and D_5 receptors) activates G_s and is primarily postsynaptic while the D_2 class (D_2 through D_4 receptors) activates G_i and include both presynaptic and postsynaptic locations. Ligands of varying selectivity have been developed for most of the receptors with the exception of the D_5 receptor.

Agonists at the D_2 receptors have been developed to treat Parkinson's disease while antagonists at this receptor are the traditional antipsychotics (e.g., haloperidol) or the atypical antipsychotics (e.g., risperidone) which also bind the $5HT_{2A}$ receptor. The crystal structure of the D_2 receptor complexed with risperidone revealed that risperidone binds in a deep binding pocket between TM3, TM5, and TM6 and interacts with a number of amino acids in these regions.[59] Ligands that bind to the D_3 or D_4 receptors do not bind as deeply into those receptors. Importantly, many of the residues required for risperidone binding to the D_2 receptor are also present in the $5HT_{2A}$ receptor.

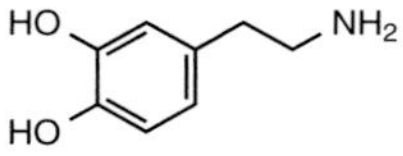

HO HO NH_2

Dopamine

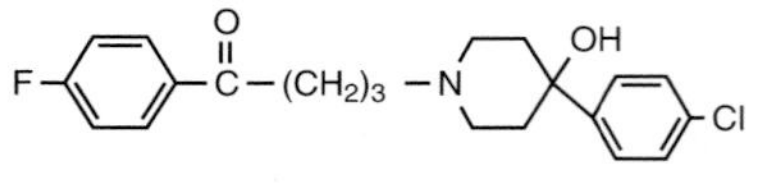

F O C $-(CH_2)_3-$ N OH Cl

Haloperidol

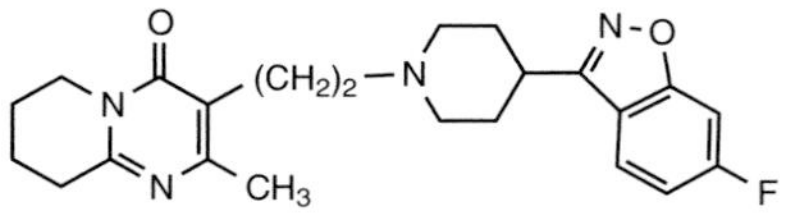

O N N $(CH_2)_2-$ N CH_3 N-O F

Risperidone (Risperdal)

Dopamine receptors represent one of a handful of GPCRs for which "biased ligands" have been developed. This concept holds that a GPCR activated by one ligand may cause activation of the associated G protein, but the same GPCR is activated by a different ligand and may cause the receptor to activate other signaling pathways. One such pathway involves signaling through β-arrestin, a protein involved in the homologous desensitization of receptors. A number of studies have demonstrated that D_2 receptor-induced β-arrestin activation leads to stimulation of Akt/GSK3 signaling.

Compounds such as UNC9975 and UNC9994, analogues of the antipsychotic aripiprazole, have been demonstrated to act as β-arrestin–biased D_2 receptor ligands.[60] These compounds promote signaling via the β-arrestin pathways while inhibiting signaling via the canonical G_i pathway. UNC9975 reportedly demonstrated antipsychotic properties in mice without the extrapyramidal adverse effects characteristic of most D_2 receptor antagonists. Thus, the development of biased ligands may improve the benefit-to-risk ratio of antipsychotics.

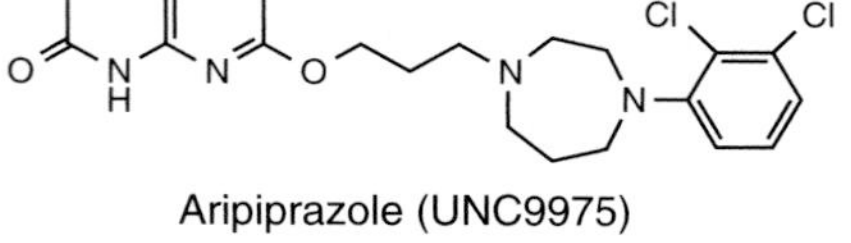

O N H N O N N Cl Cl

Aripiprazole (UNC9975)

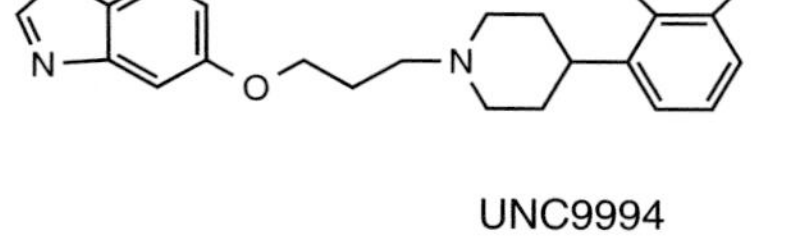

S N O N Cl Cl

UNC9994

ACKNOWLEDGMENTS

The authors wish to acknowledge the works of Malgorzata Dukat, PhD, Richard A. Glennon, PhD, Robert K. Griffith, PhD., Wendel L. Nelson, PhD, Edward B. Roche, PhD, Victoria F. Roche, PhD, and David A. Williams, PhD who authored content used within this chapter in a previous edition of this text.

REFERENCES

1. Leake CD. *A Historical Account of Pharmacology in the 20th Century*. Springfield, IL: Charles C. Thomas; 1975.
2. Langley JN. On the reaction of cells and nerve endings to certain poisons. *J Physiol*. 1905;33:374-413.
3. Ehrlich P. In: Himmelweit F, ed. *Collected Papers of Paul Ehrlich*, Vol. III. London: Pergamon; 1957.
4. Gether U, Kobilka BK. G protein-coupled receptors II mechanism of agonist activation. *J Biol Chem*. 1998;273:17979-17982.
5. Gilman AG. G proteins: transducers of receptor-generated signals. *Annu Rev Biochem*. 1987;56:615-649.
6. Berridge MJ. Inositol triphosphate and diacylglycerol: two interacting second messengers. *Ann Rev Biochem*. 1987;56:159-193.
7. Wise A, Jupe SC, Rees S. The identification of ligands at orphan G-protein coupled receptors. *Annu Rev Pharmacol Toxicol*. 2004;44:43-66.
8. Tekin I, Roskoski R Jr, Carkaci-Salli N, et al. Complex molecular regulation of tyrosine hydroxylase. *J Neural Transm*. 2014;121:1451-1481.
9. Tattersfield AD. Tolerance to β-agonists. *Bull Eur Physiopathol Respir*. 1985;21:1S-5S.
10. Ahlquist RP. A study of the adrenotropic receptors. *Am J Physiol*. 1948;153:586-600.
11. Kobilka BK, Dixon RA, Frielle T, et al. cDNA for the human β2-adrenergic receptor: a protein with multiple membrane-spanning domains and encoded by a gene whose chromosomal location is shared with that of the receptor for platelet-derived growth factor. *Proc Natl Acad Sci USA*. 1987;84:46-50.
12. Strader CD, Candelore MR, Hill WE, et al. Identification of two serine residues involved in agonist activation and the β-adrenergic receptor. *J Biol Chem*. 1989;264:13572-13578.
13. Starke K. Presynaptic α-autoreceptors. *Rev Physiol Biochem Pharmacol*. 1987;107:73-146.
14. Hartig PR, Branchek TA, Weinshank RI. A subfamily of 5-HT1D receptor genes. *Trends Pharmacol Sci*. 1992;3:152-159.
15. Hoyer D, Hannon JP, Martin GR. Molecular, pharmacological, and functional diversity of 5-HT receptors. *Pharmacol Biochem Behav*. 2002;71:533-534.
16. Hoyer D, Clarke DE, Fozard JR, et al. International union of pharmacology nomenclature and classification of receptors for 5-hydroxytryptamine (serotonin). *Pharmacol Rev*. 1994;46:157-203.
17. Ing HR. The structure–action relationships of the choline group. *Science*. 1949;109:264-266.
18. Caulfield JP, Birdsall NJM. International Union of Pharmacology. XVII. Classification of muscarinic acetylcholine receptors. *Pharmacol Rev*. 1998;50:279-290.
19. Nordvall G, Hacksell U. Binding-site modeling of the muscarinic m1 receptor: a combination of homology-based and indirect approaches. *J Med Chem*. 1993;36:967-976.
20. Humblet C, Mirzadegan T. Three-dimensional models of G protein-coupled receptors. *Annu Rep Med Chem*. 1992;27: 291-300.
21. Hughes J, Smith TW, Kosterlitz HW, et al. Identification of two related pentapeptides from the brain with potent opiate agonist activity. *Nature*. 1975;258:577-579.
22. Li CH, Lemaire S, Yamashiro D, et al. The synthesis and opiate activity of β-endorphin. *Biochem Biophys Res Commun*. 1976; 71:19-25.
23. Goldstein A, Tachibana S, Lowney LI, et al. Procaine pituitary dynorphin: complete amino acid sequence of the biologically active heptadecapeptide. *Proc Natl Acad Sci USA*. 1979;76:6666-6670.
24. Zadina JE, Hackler L, Ge LJ, et al. A potent and selective endogenous agonist for the μ-opiate receptor. *Nature*. 1997;386:499-502.
25. Akil H, Watson SJ, Young E, et al. Endogenous opioids: biology and function. *Annu Rev Neurosci*. 1984;7:233-255.
26. Leslie FM. Methods used for the study of opioid receptors. *Pharmacol Rev*. 1987;39:197-249.
27. Satoh M, Minami M. Molecular pharmacology of the opioid receptors. *Pharmacol Ther*. 1995;68:343-364.
28. Connor M, Christie MD. Opioid receptor signaling mechanisms. *Clin Exp Pharmacol Physiol*. 1999;26:493-499.
29. Pan L, Xu J, Yu R, et al. Identification and characterization of six new alternatively spliced variants of the human mu opioid receptor gene, *Oprm*. *Neuroscience*. 2005;133;209-220.
30. Zhu Y, King MA, Schuller AG, et al. Retention of supraspinal delta-like analgesia and loss of morphine tolerance in delta opioid receptor knockout mice. *Neuron*. 1999;24:243-252.
31. Negri L, Erspamer GF, Severini C, et al. Dermorphin-related peptides from the skin of *Phyllomedusa bicolor* and their amidated analogues activate two μ opioid receptor subtypes that modulate antinociception and catalepsy in the rat. *Proc Natl Acad Sci USA*. 1992;89:7203-7207.
32. Keiffer BL. Opioids: first lessons from knockout mice. *Trends Pharmacol Sci*. 1999;20:19-25.
33. Paul D, Pasternak GW. Differential blockade by naloxonazine of two mu opiate actions: analgesia and inhibition of gastrointestinal transit. *Eur J Pharmacol*. 1988;149:403-404.
34. Manglik A, Kruse AC, Kobilka TS, et al. Crystal structure of the μ-opioid receptor bound to a morphine antagonist. *Nature*. 2012;485:321-326.
35. Pogozheva ID, Lomize AL, Mosberg HI. Opioid receptor three-dimensional structures from distance geometry calculations with hydrogen bonding constraints. *Biophys J*. 1998;75:612-634.
36. Szmuszkovicz J, Von Voigtlander PF. Benzenecetamide amines: structurally novel non-μ opioids. *J Med Chem*. 1982;25:1125-1126.
37. Clark CR, Halfpenny PR, Hill RG, et al. Highly selective κ opioid analgesics. Synthesis and structure-activity releationships of novel *N*-[(2-aminocyclohexyl)aryl]acetamide and *N*-[(2-aminocyclohexyl) aryloxy]acetamide derivatives. *J Med Chem*. 1988;31:831-836.
38. Hunter JC, Leighton GE, Meecham KG, et al. CI-977, a anovel and selective agonist for the κ-opioid receptor. *Br J Pharmacol*. 1990;101:183-189.
39. Barber A, Bartoszyk GD, Bender HM, et al. A pharmacological profile of the novel, peripherally-selective κ-opioid receptor agonist, EMD 61753. *Br J Pharmacol*. 1994;113:843-851.
40. Rothman RB, Bykov V, de Costa BR, et al. Evidence for four opioid κ binding sites in Guinea pig brain. *Prog Clin Bio Res*. 1990;328:9-12.
41. Portoghese PS, Lipkowski AW, Takemori AE. Bimorphinans as highly selective, potent κ opioid receptor antagonists. *J Med Chem*. 1987;30:238-239.
42. James IF, Goldstein A. Site-directed alkylation of multiple opioid receptors. I. Binding selectivity. *Mol Pharmacol*. 1984;25:337-342.
43. Gacel C, Fournie-Zaluski M-C, Roques BP. D-Tyr-Ser-Gly-Phe-Leu-Thr, a highly preferential ligand for δ-opiate receptors. *FEBS Lett*. 1980;118:245-247.
44. Mosberg HI, Hurst R, Hruby VJ, et al. Bis-penicillamine enkephalins possess highly improved specificity toward δ opioid receptors. *Proc Natl Acad Sci USA*. 1983;80:5871-5874.
45. Portoghese PS, Larson DL, Sultana M, et al. Opioid agonist and antagonist activities of morphindoles related to naltrindole. *J Med Chem*. 1992;35:4325-4329.
46. Bilsky EJ, Calderon SN, Wang T, et al. SNC 80, a selective, nonpeptidic, and systemically active opioid δ agonist. *J Pharmacol Exp Ther*. 1995;273:359-366.
47. Portoghese PS, Sultana M, Takemori AE. Naltrindole, a highly selective and potent nonpeptide δ opioid receptor antagonist. *Eur J Pharmacol*. 1988;146:185-186.

48. Takemori AE, Sultana M, Nagase H, et al. Agonist and antagonist activities of ligands derived from naltrexone and oxymorphone. *Life Sci*. 1992;149:1-5.
49. Henderson G, McKnight AT. The orphan opioid receptor and its endogenous ligand—nociceptin/orphanin FQ. *Trends Pharmacol Sci*. 1997;18:293-300.
50. Meunier JC, Mollereau C, Toll L, et al. Isolation and structure of the endogenous agonist of opioid receptor-like OR1 receptor. *Nature*. 1995;377:532-535.
51. Zeilhofer HU, Calo G. Nociceptin/orphanin FQ and its receptor – potential targets for pain therapy. *J Pharmacol Exp Ther*. 2003;306:423-429.
52. Chiou LC, Liao YY, Fan PC, et al. Nociceptin/orphanin FQ peptide receptors: pharmacology and clinical implications. *Curr Drug Targets*. 2007;8:117-135.
53. Portoghese PS, Larson DL, Sayre LM, et al. A novel opioid receptor site directed alkylating agent with irreversible narcotic antagonistic and reversible agonistic activities. *J Med Chem*. 1980;23:233-234.
54. Calo G, Guerrini R, Rizzi A, et al. Pharmacology of nociceptin and its receptor: a novel therapeutic target. *Br J Pharmacol*. 2000;129:1261-1283.
55. Lambert DG. The nociceptin/orphanin FQ receptor: a target with broad therapeutic potential. *Nat Rev Drug Discov*. 2008;7:694-710.
56. Cordova-Sintjago TC, Fang L, Bruysters M, et al. Molecular determinants of ligand binding at the human histamine H1 receptor: site-directed mutagenesis results analyzed with ligand docking and molecular dynamics studies at H1 homology and crystal structure models. *J Chem Pharm Res*. 2012;4(6):2937-2951.
57. Shimamura T, Shiroishi M, Weyand S, et al. Structure of the human histamine H1 receptor complex with doxepin. *Nature*. 2011;475:65-70.
58. Gantz I, DelValle J, Wang LD, et al. Molecular basis for the interaction of histamine with the histamine H_2 receptor. *J Biol Chem* 1992;267:20840-20843.
59. Wang S, Che T, Levit A, et al. Structure of the D_2 dopamine receptor bound to the atypical antipsychotic drug risperidone. *Nature*. 2018;555:269-273.
60. Allen JA, Yost JM, Setola V, et al. Discovery of β-arrestin-biased dopamine D_2 ligands for probing signal transduction pathways essential for antipsychotic efficacy. *Proc Natl Acad Sci USA*. 2011;108(45):18488-18493.

CHAPTER 7

Nuclear Receptors

David A. Johnson

Abbreviations

9CRA 9-*cis*-retinoic acid
AF1 hormone-independent transactivation function 1
AF2 ligand-dependent activation function 2
APL acute promyelocytic leukemia
AR androgen receptor
ARE androgen response element
ATRA *all-trans*-retinoic acid
DBD DNA-binding domain
DHT dihydrotestosterone
DNA deoxyribonucleic acid
DR direct repeat
ER estrogen receptor
ERE estrogen response element
GLU glutamic acid
GRE glucocorticoid response element
LBD ligand-binding domain
MR mineralocorticoid receptors
mRNA messenger RNA
NCOA1 nuclear receptor coactivator 1
NRs nuclear receptors
NTD N-terminal domain
PPAR peroxisome proliferator–activated receptors
RAR retinoic acid receptors
RARE retinoic acid response element
RNA ribonucleic acid
T testosterone
TR thyroid receptors
TRE thyroid response element
T3 triiodothyronine
T4 thyroxine
VDR vitamin D receptor
VDRE vitamin D response element
WHI Women's Health Initiative

INTRODUCTION

Definitions

Nuclear receptors (NRs) are ligand-activated transcription factors located in the cytoplasm and nuclei of the cells of animals that regulate a wide range of physiological functions including cell mitosis and differentiation, embryonic development, cellular and organ system metabolism, and homeostasis. When agonists activate NRs, the receptor initiates gene expression by binding to specific DNA response elements. Following binding of activated NRs to a response element, other proteins are recruited to the site to initiate gene transcription.

Classification

There are over 300 protein molecules included in the superfamily of nuclear receptors; however, only 49 are found in humans. Nuclear receptors are divided into 6 subfamilies that include receptors for steroidal hormones, thyroid hormone, bile acids, and vitamins A and D. In addition, NRs include receptors discovered by screening DNA libraries called "orphan receptors" that have no known ligand.[1]

Structure and Functions

Nuclear receptor proteins are composed of a single peptide chain comprising five domains (Fig. 7.1).

N-*Terminal Domain and AF-1*

The N-terminal domain (NTD), Domain A/B (see Fig. 7.1), is a highly variable amino terminal region that contains a hormone-independent transactivation function (AF-1). AF-1 can bind coactivator or corepressor proteins that modulate receptor activation without ligand. In addition, the NTD contains phosphorylation sites that can facilitate or inhibit gene transcription by modulating NR dimerization and the recruitment of coactivators or corepressors and other regulators of gene expression.

DNA-Binding Domain

Domain C, the DNA-binding domain (DBD) is composed of a 66-amino-acid core including two loops coordinated by "zinc fingers" that play a key role in DNA binding[2] and a "D-box" involved in receptor dimerization and a "P-box" that binds the NR to specific half-element DNA sequences.[3] NRs usually bind to DNA as homodimers for steroid NRs or heterodimers for nonsteroid NRs. The DBD binds to DNA response elements. Selectivity for

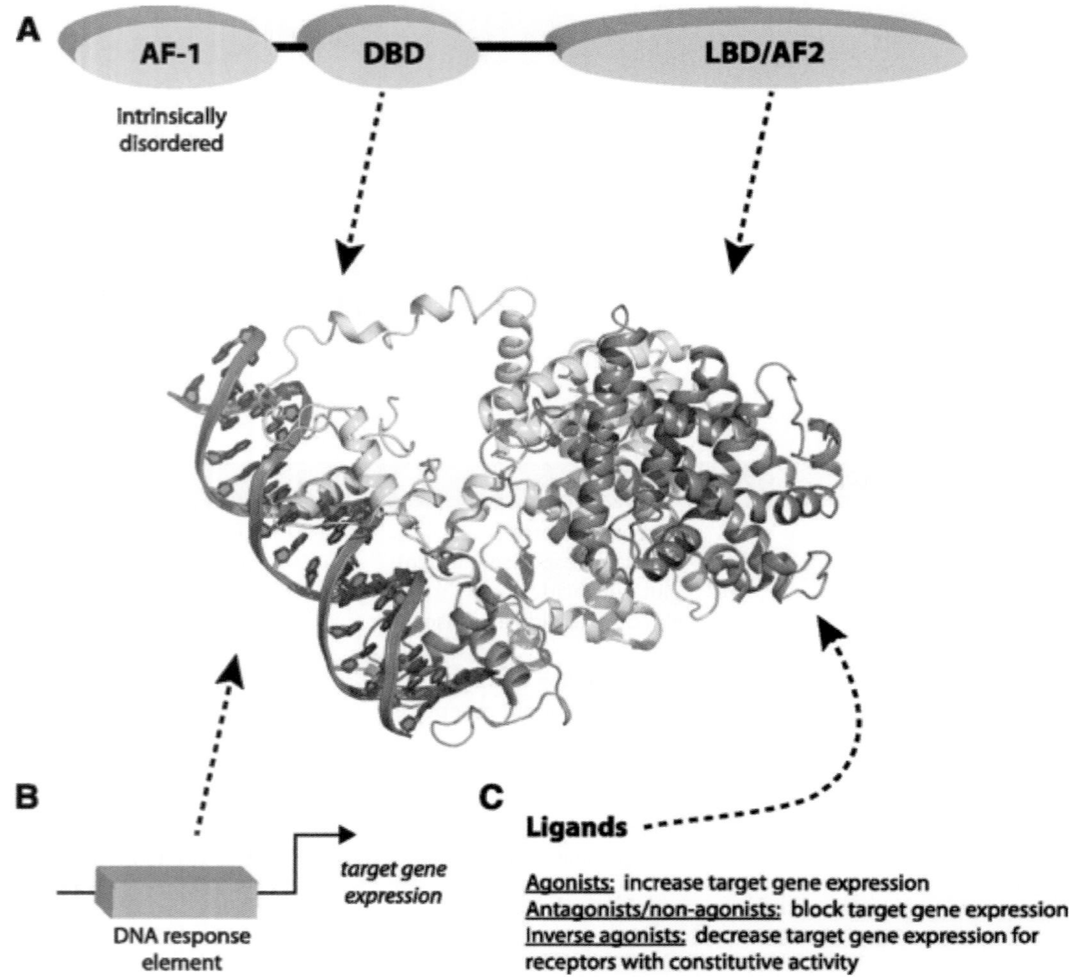

Figure 7.1 Nuclear receptor structure. Nuclear receptors are single peptide chains comprising five domains: (1) Domain A/B, the N-terminal domain (NTD), that functions in the allosteric binding of coactivator and corepressor proteins that participate in receptor activation; (2) Domain C, the DNA-binding domain (DBD), that selectively docks the NR to specific DNA response elements to initiate the process of gene transcription; (3) Domain D, the hinge domain that links the DBD to the ligand-binding domain; (4) Domain E, the ligand-binding domain (LBD) that contains the primary hormone binding site and allosteric sites for binding coactivators and repressors; (5) Domain F, function is not well understood. A, The order and relative size of domains within the nuclear receptor protein. B, Nuclear receptors bind to particular response elements of DNA to trigger gene translation and expression. C, Ligands bind to the LBD domain to regulate receptor activation and gene expression.

DNA response element binding is achieved through variations in the arrangement of nucleotides in the response element and the degree of separation between "half-sites." The response element for nonsteroid receptor dimers is composed of six nucleotide sequences arranged as direct repeats separated by a variable number of "spacer" nucleotides (DR1-DR5). For steroid NRs the half-site nucleotide sequence is typically arranged as inverted repeats and always separated by three spacer nucleotides (DR3).

Domain D: The Hinge Domain, Domain E: The Ligand-Binding Domain, and Domain F

Domain D is a variable "hinge domain" that links the DBD to Domain E, the ligand-binding domain (LBD). The LBD includes the ligand-dependent activation function 2 (AF-2), containing the ligand binding site of the NR. AF-2 comprises a sandwich of 12 alpha-helices (H1-H12), arranged in an antiparallel three-layer sandwich fold that forms a hydrophobic binding pocket comprising helices H3, H4/5, H7, and H11.[4] The binding of an agonist shifts the orientation of H12 and stabilizes the LBD in a conformation that is favorable for binding coactivators to AF-2. Antagonists do not stabilize AF-2 or stabilize the domain in a conformation that recruits corepressors to suppress activation. Partial agonists can recruit either coactivators or corepressors. The variability of NR response to activation in different tissues is a consequence of the differential expression of coactivators and corepressors in different cell types. Domain F is not found in every NR, and the function of this domain is not well understood.

NR Activation

Unbound steroid receptors are located in the cytoplasm. Following ligand binding, they dimerize and are transported

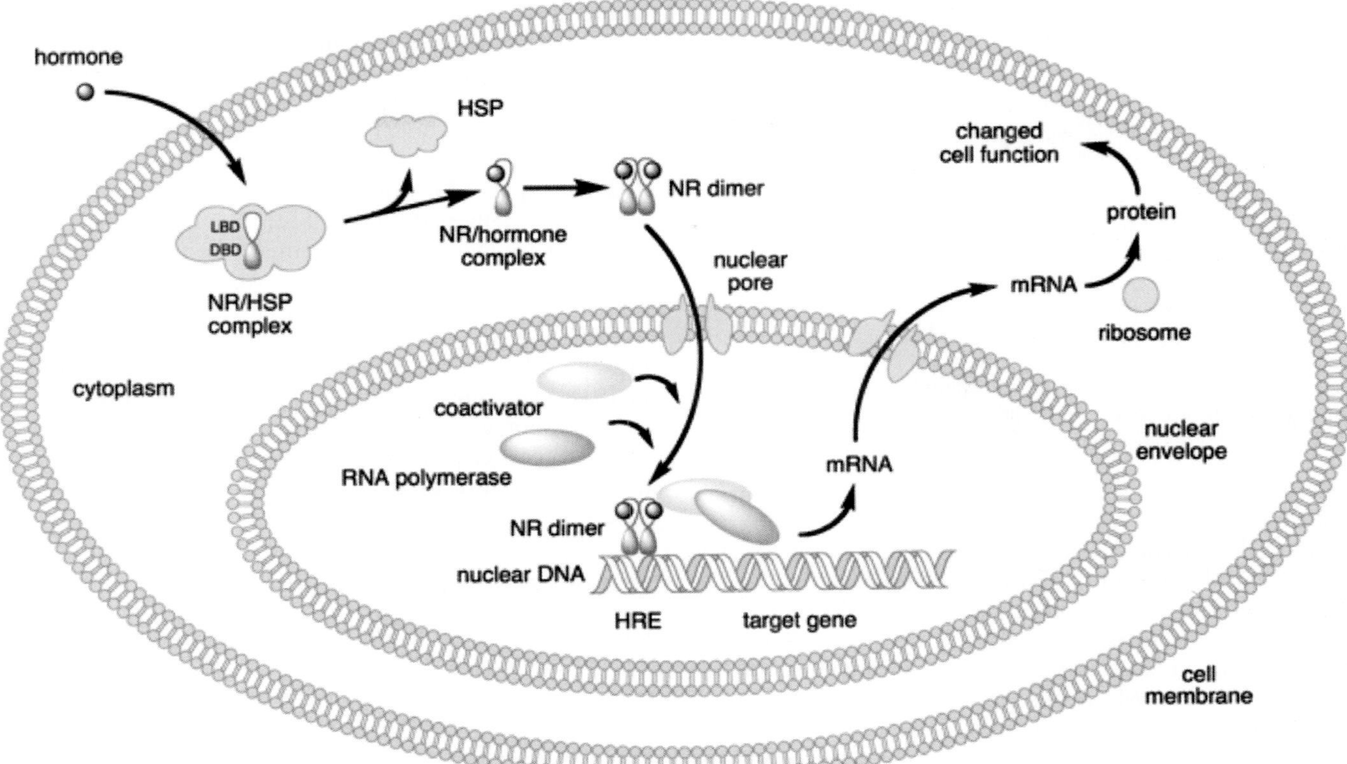

Figure 7.2 **Nuclear receptor ligand binding: translocation and DNA docking.** The steps in NR activation, translocation to the nucleus, and DNA docking: (1) the steroid hormone diffuses or is transported into the cytoplasm where it binds to the NR bound to chaperone heat shock proteins (SHP); (2) the HSP chaperones dissociate from the NR-hormone complex; (3) the NR-hormone complex is translocated to the cell nucleus where it binds to coactivator and/or corepressor proteins; (4) the complex docks with the DNA response element and recruits additional proteins including RNA polymerase to initiate gene transcription.

to the nucleus via molecular chaperones. Once in the nucleus, steroid NR homodimers selectively bind to DNA response elements and recruit coactivators and other proteins involved in regulating gene transcription (Fig. 7.2). Inactive nonsteroid NRs are located in the nucleus as hetero- or homodimers bound to a response element and corepressors that inhibit gene transcription. When an agonist binds to the dimer, the corepressors are exchanged for coactivators, and gene transcription is initiated.

Transactivation and Transrepression

The binding of an NR to a DNA response element can also facilitate the transcription of adjacent genes by enhancing the binding of coactivators or the binding of NRs to DNA response elements. Nuclear receptors can also inhibit adjacent gene expression by decreasing the availability of coactivators and transcription factors. In addition, NRs can inhibit gene expression by functioning as corepressor proteins or by slowing the degradation of corepressors.

ESTROGEN RECEPTORS

Estrogens are principle hormones in women involved in the regulation of the estrous cycle, pregnancy, breast development, and secondary sex characteristics. Estrogens also affect cognition and mood, bone density, fat distribution, and other functions. There are two isoforms of the estrogen receptor (ER), ERα and ERβ. The two receptors have a relatively close amino acid sequence homology in the LBD and DBD; however, the amino acid sequence in the NTD has only 24% homology.[5] The relative distribution of ERα and ERβ can vary both within and between tissues. Moreover, the variability of tissue responsiveness to estrogens may, in part, be due to the presence of differing numbers and abundance of ER subtypes and splice variants, which can alter the binding affinity of proteins resulting in increased or decreased responsiveness to estrogen.

Ligand Binding

Activation of ERs following the binding of an agonist involves a shift in the orientation of the H12 loop in AF-2 to facilitate the binding of coactivators, while the binding of antagonists repositions H12 to sterically hinder coactivator binding and/or facilitate the binding of corepressors. For binding to the ER, estrogens are unique in having a 3-hydroxyl group on the A-ring of the steroid core. This structural distinction provides selectivity for ligand binding to the ER. Estrogens bind to the receptor utilizing hydrogen bonds with the 3-hydroxyl group to glutamate-353

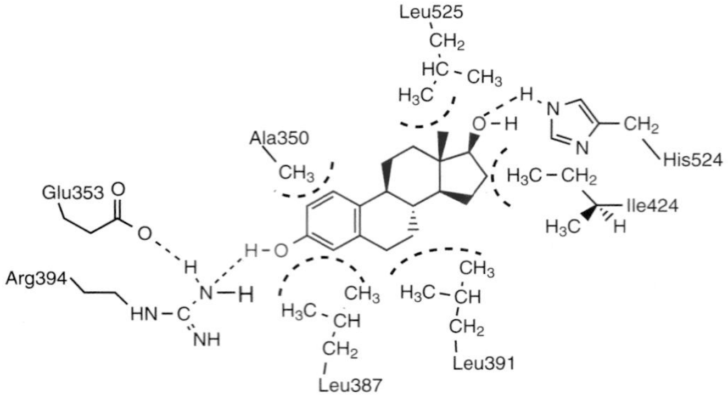

Figure 7.3 Crystal structure of the ligand-binding domain of the estrogen receptor bound to estradiol.

and arginine-394. In addition, amino acids with neutral side chains provide van der Waals interactions with rings A, B, and C of the steroid core. An additional hydrogen bond occurs between the 17-hydroxyl group of the D-ring and the δ nitrogen of histidine-524[6] (Fig. 7.3).

Estrogen receptors, especially ERα, can also be activated by coactivators binding to AF-1 independent of estrogen binding. Moreover, phosphorylation of sites in the amino-terminal region enables "cross talk" interactions between ERs and other signal transduction pathways.

Estrogen Receptor Binding to the DNA Estrogen Response Element

Once the ER dimer has translocated to the nucleus, it binds to the estrogen response element (ERE). Binding of the receptor to the ERE triggers the binding of nuclear coactivators which then recruit enzymes that modify the chromatin to allow greater accessibility to DNA for transcription by RNA-polymerase. Estrogen receptor dimers can also modulate the transcription of other genes via cooperativity with other NRs such as progesterone receptors (PRs) and the recruitment of enzymes to facilitate gene transcription. Moreover, ERs can repress gene activation by binding to particular transcription factors and repress activation of other genes by inhibiting DNA interactions or the activity of other factors.[7]

Progesterone Receptors

Progesterone is a hormone released by the ovaries, testis, adrenal cortex, and to a lesser extent in brain and adipose tissue and is a metabolic precursor for other steroids including aldosterone, testosterone, and estrogens. Physiologically, progesterone is important for female reproductive organs, such as the uterus and breast, and PR antagonists are effective for treating endometriosis and benign uterine tumors. Aside from female reproductive organs, progesterone modulates neurotransmission in the brain and plays a role in smooth muscle and skin.[8] There are two progesterone receptor (PR) subtypes, PRA and PRB, that share high amino acid sequence homology in the DBD and LBD domains. PRA and PRB are nearly identical except in the A/B domain where PRB has an additional 165 amino acids that comprise an upstream segment, AF3.[9] PRA and PRB target distinct genomic sites and bind different coregulators. In normal tissues, PRA and PRB are expressed in equimolar amounts; however, knockout models demonstrate that PRA plays a significant role in mammary gland development, while PRB is predominantly involved in ovarian and uterine functions.[10] In cancer cells there can be a differential level of expression of the PR isotypes. As an example, in breast cancers, either PRA or PRB can dominate; however, tumors in which PRB is overexpressed tend to be relatively unresponsive to treatment with the progesterone antagonist mifepristone.[11] Breast cancers that have a high PRA to PRB ratio have increased resistance to ER selective modulators and therefore increased mortality.[12]

Progesterone Receptor Binding

Unlike ERs, the PR forms a hydrogen bond via glutamine-725 with the 3-keto group of the A-ring of progesterone. Analogous to the ER binding pocket, Arginine-766 serves to properly orient Gln-725 via water-mediated hydrogen bonds and Phe-778 interacts with the A-ring of progesterone via van der Waals contacts. There is no well-defined binding of the 17-methyl-keto moiety on the D-ring of progesterone[13] (Fig. 7.4).

PR-ER Interactions

There is significant cross-talk between PRs and ERs. It is well established that PRs bound to either progestin agonists or antagonists can suppress ER-mediated gene expression, and PRA activation or inhibition of PR can shift ER signaling. The use of progestin agonists and antagonists in the treatment of breast cancer is controversial. The Women's Health Initiative (WHI) found that postmenopausal women receiving hormone replacement therapy containing estrogens and progestin had a higher incidence of breast cancer.[14] Other studies found that progesterone antagonists, by suppressing ER signaling, could slow the growth of ER positive tumors.[15]

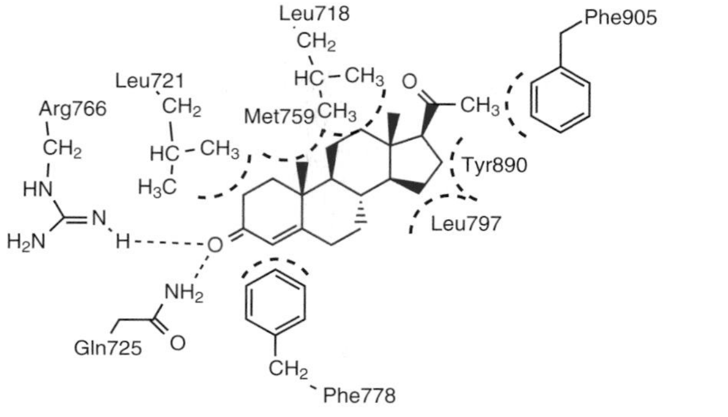

Figure 7.4 Crystal structure of the ligand-binding domain of the progesterone receptor bound to progesterone.

Table 7.1 Nuclear Receptor Superfamily: Receptors and Ligands

Subfamily	Receptor (Including Subtypes)	Ligand
1	Thyroid receptor α, β Retinoic acid receptor α, β, γ Peroxisome proliferator–activated receptor α, β/δ, γ Vitamin D receptor	Thyroid hormone Retinoic acid Fatty acids, eicosanoids Calcitriol
2	Retinoid X receptor α, β, γ	9-*cis*-retinoic acid unsaturated fatty acids
3	Estrogen receptor α, β Progesterone receptor A, B Androgen receptor Glucocorticoid receptor α, β Mineralocorticoid receptor	Estrogens Progesterone Testosterone, DHT Cortisol, aldosterone Aldosterone, cortisol
4	Neuron-derived orphan	Orphan
5	Steroidogenic factor–like	Orphan
6	Germ cell nuclear factor	Orphan

ANDROGEN RECEPTORS

The androgens, testosterone (T) and dihydrotestosterone (DHT) are steroid hormones that promote the development of primary and secondary sex characteristics of male anatomy and physiology. Testosterone is synthesized primarily in the testicles under regulation by the hypothalamic-pituitary-gonadal axis and circulates in the blood bound to carrier proteins such as sex hormone binding hormone and albumin. Upon reaching target tissues, unbound T passively diffuses into cells where it is converted by the enzyme 5α reductase to the more active metabolite, DHT. Androgen effects are mediated by the androgen receptor (AR), a member of subfamily 3, of the NR superfamily (Table 7.1). The gene for AR is widely expressed across organ systems. Aside from male reproductive organs and sexual functions, androgens affect the skin, bone development and density, muscle and fat distribution, and cardiovascular, neuro, and immune function.[16]

Androgen Receptor Structure

The AR, like other NRs, has a modular structure made up of NTD, DBD, hinge, and LBD domains. The NTD is relatively long and has a variable amino acid sequence that contains AF1.[17] In addition, the NTD has polymeric glutamine repeats that can affect cellular sensitivity to androgens. The nucleotide half-site sequence for AR comprises two 6-base-pair asymmetrical elements separated by a 3-BP spacer.[18] A C-terminal extension functions to selectively bind the androgen response element (ARE). The LDB of the AR is similar to other NRs being composed of 12 α-helices. The binding of ligand changes the conformation of helix 12 to allow for binding of coactivators.

Androgen Receptor Binding

Androgens bind to the AR with affinity in the nanomolar range with DHT having an approximately 2-fold higher affinity than T and a dissociation rate that is 5-fold slower. The binding of T to the AR is similar to progesterone binding to the PR receptor except that the 3-keto group on the A-ring has hydrogen binding interactions with arginine-752. In addition, the hydroxyl group on the D-ring binds to asparagine-705 and threonine-877. Aside from hydrogen binding there are a number of van der Walls interactions between the steroid ring core structure and neutral amino acids including methionine, tryptophan, leucine, and phenylalanine[19] (Fig. 7.5).

AR Signal Transduction

The AR without ligand is located in the cytosol bound to chaperone proteins. When androgens bind to the receptor, there is a conformational change and the receptor dissociates from chaperone proteins and translocates into the nucleus where it binds to the ARE on the promoter region of target genes. Once bound, coregulator proteins promote transcription by remodeling histones and attracting general transcription factors to initiate gene transcription.

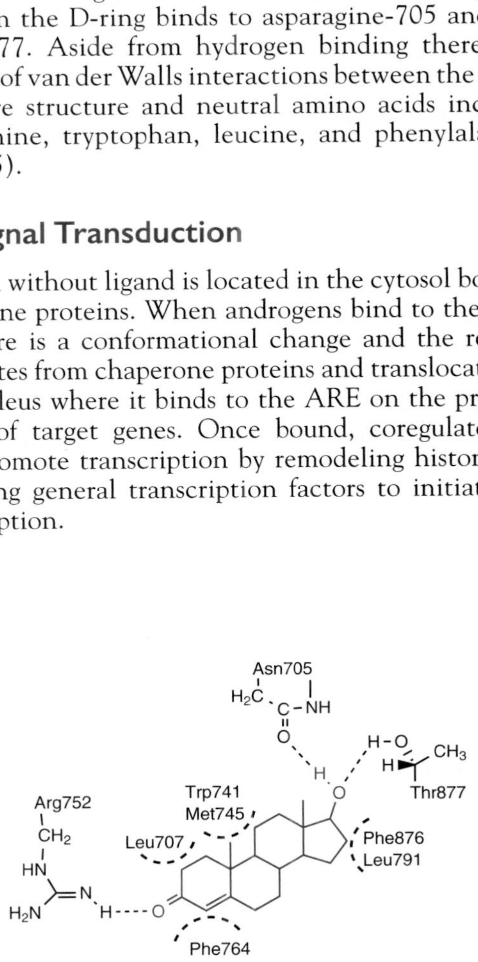

Figure 7.5 Crystal structure of the ligand-binding domain of the androgen receptor bound to testosterone.

Clinical Applications

AR receptor antagonists are utilized clinically to treat prostate cancer. However, in later stages of the disease, tumor cells can become resistant to antiandrogen therapy. Mechanisms for resistance include upregulation of AR receptor number or sensitivity, and in approximately 10% of cancers, the expression of ARs with point mutations provides a growth advantage to the tumor by decreasing selectivity of ligand binding or conferring intrinsic agonist activity to the antagonists.[20]

GLUCOCORTICOID RECEPTORS

Cortisol is a primary human stress hormone released from the adrenal cortex. Glucocorticoids are involved in maintaining organ system and cellular homeostasis during normal function and in response to stressful physiological challenges. Cortisol produces its effects through regulation of metabolism, and immune, reproductive, and neuronal systems. Glucocorticoid receptors (GR) are found in almost all cell types consistent with the wide-ranging role that glucocorticoids play in regulating physiological functions.[21] Drugs that interact with the GR are among the most commonly prescribed drugs in the world. Glucocorticoids are effective in treating inflammatory and autoimmune diseases, preventing organ transplant rejection, and the treatment of certain cancers.[22] While the GR is derived from a single gene, there are many isoforms resulting from alternative gene splicing as well as variations in mRNA translation. The variety of GR isoforms provides a range of responses to glucocorticoids within particular tissues and different organs.

GR Structure

The glucocorticoid receptor structure, like other steroid NRs, comprises ATD, DBD, hinge region, and LBD. In addition, GRs have two nuclear localization signals, NL1 and NL2, to selectively bind the receptor to the GRE and an LBD that facilitates the shuttling of the GR from the cytosol to the nucleus.[23] Alternative splicing results in two isoforms, GRα and GRβ. The GRα isoform mediates the actions of glucocorticoids, while the GRβ isoform contains an additional 15 amino acids, which does not bind agonists but resides constitutively in the cell nucleus. By competing for transcriptional coregulators, a GRα-GRβ heterodimer is inhibitory when bound to the GR response element (GRE)[24] and as a consequence, the heterodimer may play a role in glucocorticoid resistance and hypersensitivity to proinflammatory factors.[25] GRβ can also decrease the response to glucocorticoids via recruitment of histone deacetylases that repress gene expression.[26] There are eight translational isoforms of GRα that provide selectivity for gene expression within a particular cell line. Moreover, posttranslational phosphorylation of AF-1 can increase or decrease gene transcription depending on the particular phosphorylation site.

GR Binding

The cellular response and tissue sensitivity to corticosteroids is dependent on the intracellular concentration of the hormone. Following diffusion into the cytosol, cortisol concentration is regulated by enzymes that maintain an equilibrium between cortisol and the inactive metabolite cortisone. For cortisol binding to the GR, in addition to hydrophobic interactions, cortisol has four hydrogen bonds formed between the hydrophilic groups of the steroid and the polar amino acids of the binding pocket[27] (Fig. 7.6).

Signal Transduction

The binding of cortisol to GR results in dissociation of chaperone proteins and translocation to the nucleus where it binds to the GRE. The GRE is palindromic and comprises 6-base pair half-sites separated by a spacer of three nucleotides. As with other NRs, once GR is bound to GRE, coregulators are recruited to facilitate gene transcription. The result is the transcription of genes regulated by GRE and the potential suppression of other genes. The range of gene expression under the control of GREs varies from tissue to tissue, and hence responses to glucocorticoids are also variable. As an example, activation of GRE can enhance the expression of β arrestin 1 but inhibit β arrestin 2. Decreasing the expression of β arrestin 2 slows the downregulation of β-adrenergic receptors.[28] This is thought to be a mechanism for synergism between glucocorticoids and β-adrenergic agonists in treating respiratory diseases such as COPD. The GR can also influence the transcription of genes regulated by other NRs. As an example, GR binds to proinflammatory transcription factors AP1 and NF-κB to inhibit transfection of inflammatory cytokines and ultimately suppress inflammation.

MINERALOCORTICOID RECEPTORS

Mineralocorticoid receptors (MR) were first identified in 1974.[22] Activation of MRs promotes renal sodium reabsorption and potassium excretion.[29] However, activation of MRs is also associated with a number of pathological conditions including promotion of inflammation and

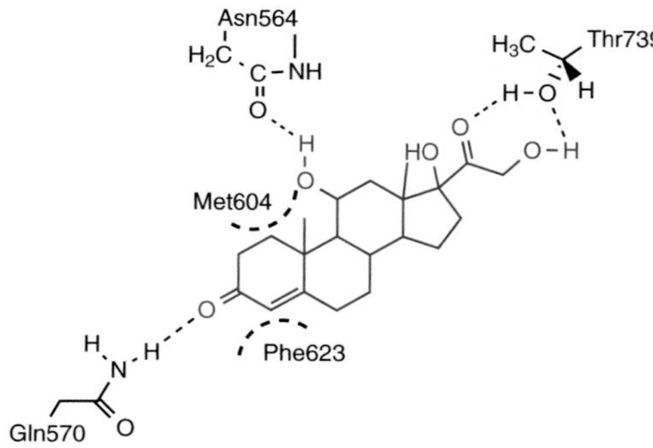

Figure 7.6 Crystal structure of the ligand-binding domain of the glucocorticoid receptor bound to cortisol.

fibrosis in the aortic endothelium,[30] proliferation of smooth muscle cells,[31] cardiac remodeling,[32] and thermogenesis.[33] The single gene for the MR produces several transcription isoforms and variants that provide for diverse responses to receptor activation in different tissues. Aldosterone, the primary endogenous MR ligand, is released from the adrenal cortex in response to activation of angiotensin II and ACTH receptors and serum potassium concentrations. Glucocorticoids can also activate MRs; however, activation is limited by enzymes that metabolize glucocorticoid hormones to structures that lack significant binding affinity for the MR. The MR antagonist spironolactone has been employed clinically for decades as an adjunct for patients with hypertension treated with potassium-depleting diuretic agents such as furosemide and hydrochlorothiazide. More recently, spironolactone has also been prescribed for patients with heart failure to inhibit the myocardial remodeling associated with that disorder.

MR Structure

MR has a longer N terminal domain than other steroid receptors and contains two AF1 domains and a domain that can inhibit transactivation by AF-1.[33] There is a high degree of homology between the MR DBD domain and those of GR, PR, and AR. The DBD "D-box" facilitates homodimerization or heterodimerization with other steroid receptors especially GR and AR.[34] The MR response element is composed of an inverted repeat separated by three nucleotides. The LBD of the MR is structurally similar to other steroid receptors and contains a ligand dependent AF-2 domain, which can interact with coactivator proteins. Posttranslational modifications to the MR include phosphorylation that facilitates cytoplasmic to nuclear transport and MR degradation.

MR Receptor Binding

Aldosterone binding to MR is stronger than cortisol binding to CR. While the K_D values are in the same order of magnitude, aldosterone dissociates more slowly. Moreover, the ED_{50} for MR activation is approximately 100-fold lower than for cortisol.[35] Hydrogen bond interactions between aldosterone and MR include the 3-keto group and Gln776 and Arg817, the 20-keto group and Cys942, and 21-hydroxyl group with Asn770[36] (Fig. 7.7).

THYROID RECEPTORS

Thyroid hormones are regulated by the hypothalamus through the release of thyrotropin-releasing hormone (TRH), which triggers the release of thyroid-stimulating hormone (TSH) from the anterior pituitary gland. TSH stimulates the thyroid gland to synthesize and release thyroid hormones triiodothyronine (T3) and thyroxine (T4) from iodinated tyrosine residues of the protein thyroglobulin. Following release from the thyroid gland, T3 circulates in the blood bound to transport proteins, enters the nucleus of cells, and binds to the thyroid nuclear receptor

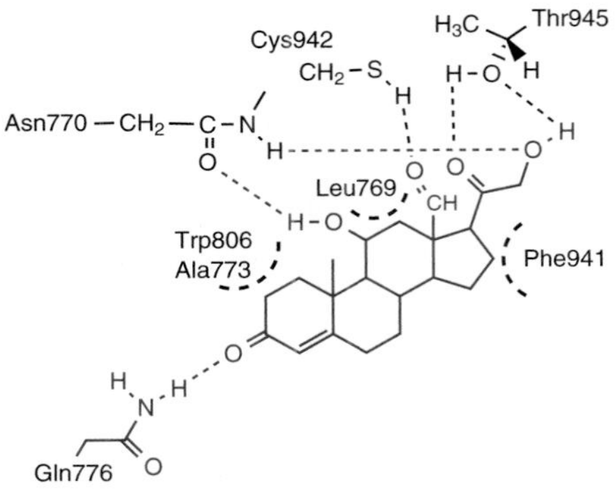

Figure 7.7 Crystal structure of the ligand-binding domain of the mineralocorticoid receptor bound to aldosterone.

(TR). Binding of T3 to TR alters the conformation of the receptor and triggers the thyroid DNA response element (TRE) to initiate target gene transcription. Physiologic responses to receptor activation include regulation of brain development, thermogenesis, increased cardiac function, and increased cellular metabolism.

Thyroid Receptor Structure

The structure of TR is consistent with the modular domains of other NRs. TR subtypes designated TRα and TRβ are the product of two distinct genes. Each TR transcript is subject to alternative spicing that results in three isoforms of TRα and two of TRβ.[37] The amino-terminal domain is the least conserved among NRs and as a result of gene splicing is markedly different between isoforms. As with other NRs, the binding of corepressors and activators to the AF1 region plays an important role in ligand dependent and independent activation. Variations in the amino-terminal domain of TR isoforms provide selectivity in receptor dimerization and hence in gene transcription in different tissues based on expression of the particular TR isoform and the relative availability of coactivator or corepressor proteins.

TR Ligand Binding

As with other NRs the ligand binding pockets of TRα and TRβ are largely composed of amino acids with neutral side chains. However, two polar regions of the binding pocket provide hydrogen bonding opportunities at the opposite ends of ligands. Histidine-435 forms a hydrogen bond with the phenolic hydroxyl of T3, while arginine-282 provides hydrogen binding to the carboxylate group at the other end of the molecule[38] (Fig. 7.8).

TR Signal Transduction

Thyroid receptors generally form homodimers or heterodimers with different TR isoforms or the retinoid X receptor (RXR), employing dimerization surfaces in the LBD and DBD. Particular dimers will bind selectively to TREs of target genes. Characteristics of TRE include 4 spacer base pairs between half-sites arranged as direct repeats.[39]

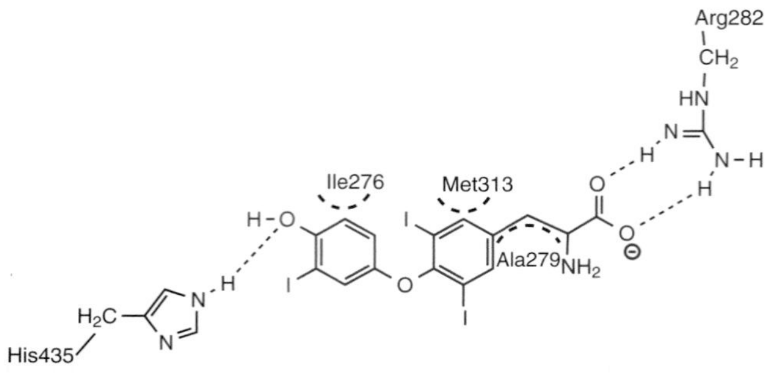

Figure 7.8 Crystal structure of the ligand-binding domain of the thyroid hormone receptor bound to triiodothyronine (T3).

The two zinc finger modules of the DBD mediate selective DNA sequence recognition and spacing between half-sites of the TRE. The hinge regions of the two receptors provide flexibility for the dimer to bind to TREs with different half-site orientations. When not bound to ligand, TR dimers repress gene transcription by binding to the TRE while complexed with corepressors. The conformational change that results from ligand binding facilitates the release of corepressors and the binding of coactivators resulting in reorientation of the chromatin by coactivators and upregulation of transcription of the target gene. Mutations to TRβ isoforms can result in the loss of sensitivity of T3 in select tissues via inhibition of the recruitment of coactivators that can produce genetic diseases characterized by resistance to T3, elevated blood levels of T3 and TSH, and goiter. Mutations to TRα are associated with growth retardation and constipation.

PEROXISOME PROLIFERATOR–ACTIVATED RECEPTORS

Peroxisome proliferator–activated receptors (PPAR), belong to subfamily 1 of NRs. The name of the receptor comes from first being identified in *Xenopus* frogs having the ability to increase cellular peroxisome numbers.[40] There are three receptor isotypes designated, PPARα, PPARβ/δ, and PPARγ, each derived from a separate gene. The α isotype is abundant in brown adipose tissue, liver, heart, kidney, and intestine—organs that are involved in lipid catabolism.[41] The γ isotype has two isoforms γ1 and γ2; γ2 is found in high concentrations in adipose tissues, while γ1 and PPARβ/δ are broadly distributed.[42]

PPAR Function

PPARs are involved in a wide array of functions including carbohydrate metabolism and storage, insulin sensitivity, cell proliferation and differentiation, tissue repair and inflammation. The primary function of PPARα is regulation of lipid metabolism, including hepatic fatty acid catabolism and gluconeogenesis.[43] In the liver, PPARα increases fatty acid oxidation, lipolysis, and high-density lipoprotein synthesis, leading to enhanced reverse cholesterol transport. It also attenuates inflammation by inhibiting leukocyte recruitment and adhesion to endothelial cells. Increased fatty acid oxidation mediated by PPARα lowers plasma triglycerides, liver and muscle steatosis, reduces adiposity, and enhances insulin sensitivity. Fibrate drugs such as fenofibrate and gemfibrozil activate PPARα to lower plasma triglycerides and decrease the progression of atherosclerosis. PPARα also decreases the synthesis of very-low-density lipoproteins resulting in decreased plasma triglycerides and low-density lipids. In addition, activation of PPARα enhances the release of the vasodilator nitric oxide.[44] Overall, the effects of PPARα activation is vasoprotection from atherosclerosis.[45] In coronary heart disease, fibrates were effective in lowering cardiovascular disease risk in patients with type 2 diabetes. Overall, the activation of PPARα promotes vasoprotection from atherosclerosis.

PPARβ/δ receptors are involved in cell proliferation, differentiation, and tissue repair.[46] Inflammation increases the expression of PPARβ/δ and the ligands that activate the receptor. Increased receptor activity decreases apoptosis following injury and facilitates the rate of wound healing. PPARγ is expressed primarily in adipose tissue and is associated with adipocyte differentiation leading to increased numbers of adipocytes and increased cell size. Receptor activation is also associated with fluid retention and edema.

Drugs that activate PPARγ have clinical utility in treating type 2 diabetes.[47] The thiazolidinediones, pioglitazone and rosiglitazone are PPARγ agonists and effective for enhancing insulin sensitivity and increasing plasma glucose uptake into skeletal muscle and adipose tissues. Also, via actions at adipocytes, there is increased fatty acid clearance and reduced lipolysis. Thiazolidinediones also have hepatic effects including enhanced hepatic glucose uptake and decreased gluconeogenesis. Adverse effects associated with PPARγ activation include weight gain and edema; therefore thiazolidinediones are contraindicated in patients with heart failure.

PPAR Receptor Structure

PPARs have the same general structural features common to NRs including a highly conserved DBD and an LBD containing the binding pocket and surfaces for coactivator and corepressor binding. Interestingly, the binding cavity for PPARα and PPARγ are larger than for PPAR β/δ, which allows for binding of a wider array of ligands. PPARs also form heterodimers with the RXR receptor independent of ligand binding.

PPAR Signal Transduction

When activated, the receptor binds to a PPAR response element (PPARE) located in the promoter region of the target gene. The response element is direct repeat half-sites separated by a single nucleotide spacer. Selectivity for the particular PPAR isotype is mediated by the 5′-flanking region of the PPRARE. Activation of the dimer requires the binding of coactivators. Seventeen coactivators have currently been identified for PPARγ.

RETINOIC ACID RECEPTORS

Vitamin A, retinol, is metabolized via alcohol dehydrogenase to retinaldehyde, which is then oxidized to *all-trans*-retinoic acid (ATRA) by retinaldehyde dehydrogenase. The *all-trans*-retinoic acid metabolite is the most potent natural ligand acting at retinoic acid receptors (RARs). ATRA and metabolites regulate a number of functions during embryonic development including organogenesis, cellular differentiation, and apoptosis.[48] The effects are mediated through one of three RAR subtypes designated RARα, RARβ, and RARγ. The LBD of each subtype has a single amino acid substitution that provides selectivity for subtype-specific binding[49] (see Fig. 7.9 for receptor binding to ATRA[50]).

RARs form heterodimers with one of three subtypes of the retinoid X receptor (RXR). The dimer binds to retinoic receptor response elements (RARE), located in the promoter region of target genes. The RARE is composed of direct repeat binding half-sites and separated by 1, 2, or 5 nucleotide spacers (DR1, 2, 5). In the absence of agonist, the RXR-RAR heterodimer binds corepressors that inhibit gene transcription. When an agonist binds to the dimer, a conformational change occurs, and the corepressors are released and replaced by coactivators that facilitate gene transcription.[51] Interestingly, while the dimer will initiate gene transcription following the binding of an RAR agonist, the binding of an RXR agonist will not result in transcription without the binding of an RAR agonist that will initiate dissociation of corepressors from the RXR receptor.[52] The RAR-RXR dimer is also subject to "cross talk" from other signal transduction pathways via phosphorylation at AF-1 and AF-2 domains.

Abnormal signaling involving genes for RARα and genes for promyelocyte leukemia proteins results in a fusion protein with high binding affinity for corepressors. The result leads to acute promyelocytic leukemia (APL). Fortunately, APL is responsive to treatment with ATRA, which dissociates the corepressors from RAR and facilitates gene transcription and differentiation of immature leukemic promyelocytes, ultimately triggering spontaneous apoptosis. ATRA has also shown effectiveness for patients diagnosed with cutaneous T-cell malignancies and juvenile chronic myelogenous leukemia.[53] Aside from cancer, retinoids including ATRA, 9-*cis*-retinoic acid, and the synthetic compounds isotretinoin and etretinate are effective in treating dermatologic diseases such as acne and psoriasis.

RXR RECEPTORS

Retinoid X receptors selectively bind 9-*cis*-retinoic acid (9CRA) with high affinity (Fig. 7.10).[54]

There are three subtypes (RXRα, RXRβ, and RXRγ) derived from different genes. The expression of RXR subtypes is dependent on cell type and the degree of cell differentiation.[55] Natural ligands for RXRα include unsaturated fatty acids including arachidonic and oleic acids.[56] 9CRA binds with high affinity to both RAR and RXR; however, the conformations of the ligand binding pockets between the two receptors are substantially different, which provide selectivity for ligand binding. Drugs that target RXR heterodimers are utilized in the treatment of a number of diseases including cancer, endocrine disorders, dermatologic diseases, and metabolic syndrome.[57] RXRα is expressed in the epidermis, intestine, liver, and kidney, while RXRγ is found primarily in the brain and muscle cells. RXRβ is broadly expressed across cell types. RXR receptors can form heterodimers with a number of NRs and can also form homodimers, but the role of RXR-RXR homodimers in gene expression is not well understood. RXR facilitates the binding of heterodimer partners to response elements found in the promoter regions of target genes and is necessary for the dimer to initiate gene expression following ligand binding.[58,59] The specificity of the RXR heterodimer for a particular response element is dependent on the number of spacer base pairs between response element half-sites. As examples, the RXR-RAR heterodimer requires 5-base pair spacing (DR-5), while the RXR-PPAR heterodimer requires a DR1 spacing. Flanking nucleotides adjacent to the response element can also enhance the selectivity of dimer binding. The activation of RXR heterodimers can be "permissive" or "nonpermissive," meaning that for certain heterodimer partners such as PPARs, activation of the dimer will occur with ligand binding to either the PPAR receptor or the RXR receptor or both. However, for other nonpermissive heterodimers such as RAR and TR, ligand binding to the RXR receptor will not result in activation unless the partner is bound to an agonist as well. This phenomenon is referred to as subordination.

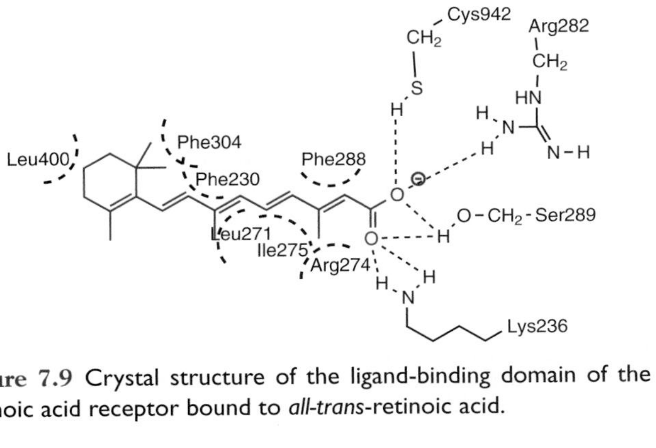

Figure 7.9 Crystal structure of the ligand-binding domain of the retinoic acid receptor bound to *all-trans*-retinoic acid.

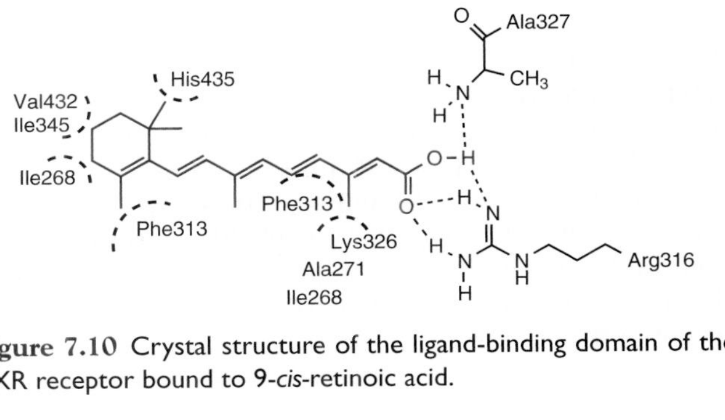

Figure 7.10 Crystal structure of the ligand-binding domain of the RXR receptor bound to 9-*cis*-retinoic acid.

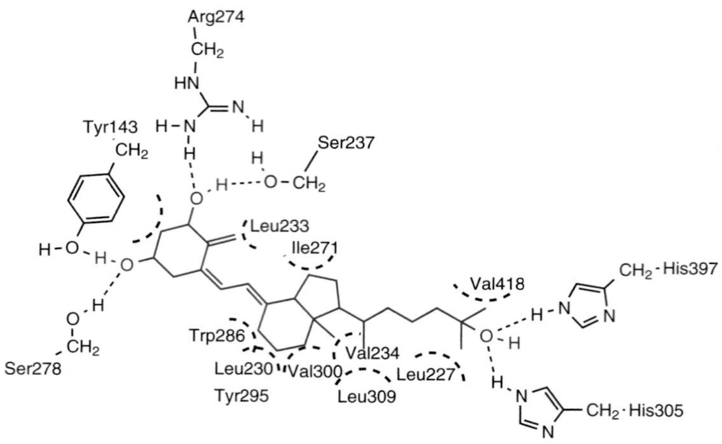

Figure 7.11 Crystal structure of the ligand-binding domain of the vitamin D receptor bound to vitamin D.

VITAMIN D RECEPTORS

D-vitamins include D_2, ergocalciferol, and D_3, cholescalciferol. Vitamin D is a fat-soluble vitamin with a steroidlike structure that, in addition to magnesium and phosphate, regulates blood calcium levels via facilitation of calcium absorption from the gastrointestinal tract and resorption of calcium from the bone. In addition to calcium transport, calcitriol (1,25-dihydroxycholecalciferol) is associated with a number of physiologic functions including inhibition of the synthesis of parathyroid hormone,[60] regulation of keratinocyte differentiation,[61] hair follicle cycling,[62] immune function,[63] cardiac function,[64] skeletal muscle,[65] breast development,[66] and lung development.[67]

Although D vitamins are constituents of the diet, a major source of the vitamin is via synthesis from 7-dehydrocholesterol in the skin following exposure to UV-radiation. Vitamin D_3 is transported to the liver and metabolized to calcifediol and subsequently transported to the kidneys where it is metabolized to the most metabolically active form, calcitriol. Calcitriol binds to the vitamin D receptor (VDR), triggering the transcription of target genes[68] (Fig. 7.11).

There are two isoforms of the receptor resulting from different transcription start sites. Individuals with the shorter isoform tend to have lower bone density than those with the longer isoform. As with other NRs the DBD of VDR is highly conserved with two zinc fingers: the N-terminal finger providing selectivity for binding to the VDR response element (VDRE), and the C-terminal finger facilitating heterodimerization with RXR and other NR receptors. Although there are variations in conformation, the VDRE generally comprises two direct repeat half-sites separated by three nucleotides. RXR binds to the upstream half- site and VDR binds to the downstream site. The LBD, aside from providing surfaces for dimerization, contains AF-2, the ligand binding site for calcitriol and coactivators and corepressors.[69]

REFERENCES

1. Aranda A, Pascual A. Nuclear hormone receptors and gene expression. *Physiol Rev*. 2001;81:1269-1204.
2. Rastinejad F. Structure and function of the steroid and nuclear receptor DNA binding domain. In: Freedman L, ed. *Molecular Biology of Steroid and Nuclear Hormone Receptors*. Boston: Birkhauser; 1998:105-131.
3. Freedman LP. Anatomy of the steroid receptor zinc finger region. *Endocr Rev*. 1992;13(2):129-145.
4. Wurtz JM, Bourguet W, Renaud JP, et al. A canonical structure for the ligand-binding domain of nuclear receptors. *Nat Struct Biol*. 1996;3:87-94.
5. Nagy L, Schwabe JW. Mechanism of the nuclear receptor molecular switch. *Trends Biochem Sci*. 2004;29:317-324.
6. Brozowski AM, Pike AC, Dauter Z, et al. Molecular basis of agonism and antagonism in the oestrogen receptor. *Nature*. 1997;389:753-758.
7. Harrington R, Sheng S, Barnett DH. Activities of estrogen receptor alpha- and beta-selective ligands at diverse estrogen responsive gene sites mediating transactivation or transrepression. *Mol Cell Endocrinol*. 2013;1-2:13-22.
8. Graham JD, Clarke CL. Physiological action of progesterone in target tissues. *Endocr Rev*. 1997;18:502-519.
9. Sartorius CA, Melville MY, Hovland AR, et al. A third transactivation function (AF3) of human progesterone receptors located in the unique N-terminal segment of the B-isoform. *Mol Endocrinol*. 1994;8:1347-1360.
10. Conneely OM, Mulac-Jericevic B, DeMayo F, et al. Reproductive functions of progesterone receptors. *Recent Prog Horm Res*. 2002;57:339-355.
11. Mote PA, Gompel A, Howe C, et al. Progesterone receptor A predominance is a discriminator of benefit from endocrine therapy in the ATAC trial. *Breast Cancer Res Treat*. 2015;151(2):309-318.
12. Singhal H, Greene ME, Zarnke AL, et al. Progesterone receptor isoforms, agonists, and antagonists differentially reprogram estrogen signaling. *Oncotarget*. 2018;9(4):4282-4300.
13. Williams SP, Sigler PB. Atomic structure of progesterone complexed with its receptor. *Nature*. 1998;393:392-396.
14. Chlebowski RT, Anderson GL, Gass M, et al. Estrogen plus progestin and breast cancer incidence and mortality in postmenopausal women. *JAMA*. 2010;304:1684-1692.
15. Mohammed H, Russell IA, Stark R, et al. Progesterone receptor modulates ERα action in breast cancer. *Nature*. 2015;523:313-317.
16. MacLean HE, Chu S, Warne GL, Zajac JD. Related individuals with different androgen receptor gene deletions. *J Clin Invest*. 1993;91:1123-1128.

17. Lavery DN, McEwan IJ. The human androgen receptor AF1 transactivation domain: interactions with transcription factor IIF and molten-globule-like structural characteristics. *Biochem Soc Trans.* 2006;34:1054-1057.
18. Roche PJ, Hoarse SA, Parker MG. A consensus DNA-binding site for the androgen receptor. *Mol Endocrinol.* 1992;6(12):2229-2235.
19. Askew EB, Gampe RT, Stanley TB, et al. Modulation of androgen receptor activation function 2 by testosterone and dihydrotestosterone. *J Biol Chem.* 2007:25801-26816.
20. Joseph JD, Lu N, Qian J, et al. A clinically relevant androgen receptor mutation confers resistance to second-generation antiandrogens enzalutamide and ARN-509. *Cancer Discov.* 2013;3(9):1020-1029.
21. Rhen T, Cidlowski JA. Antiinflammatory action of glucocorticoids–new mechanisms for old drugs. *N Engl J Med.* 2005;353(16):1711-1723.
22. Marver D, Stewart J, Funder JW, et al. Renal aldosterone receptors: studies with (3H)aldosterone and the anti-mineralocorticoid (3H)spirolactone (SC-26304). *Proc Natl Acad Sci USA.* 1974;71:1431-1435.
23. Grad I, Picard D. The glucocorticoid responses are shaped by molecular chaperones. *Mol Cell Endocrinol.* 2007;275(1-2):2-12.
24. Uhlenhaut NH, Barish GD, Yu RT, et al. Insights into negative regulation by the glucocorticoid receptor from genome-wide profiling of inflammatory cistromes. *Mol Cell.* 2013;49(1):158-171.
25. Reddy TE, Gertz J, Crawford GE, et al. The hypersensitive glucocorticoid response specifically regulates period 1 and expression of circadian genes. *Mol Cell Biol.* 2012;32(18):3756-3767.
26. Kelly A, Bowen H, Jee YK, et al. The glucocorticoid receptor beta isoform can mediate transcriptional repression by recruiting histone deacetylases. *J Allergy Clin Immunol.* 2008;121(1):203-208.
27. He Y, Yi W, Suino-Powell KM, et al. Crystal structure of cortisol-bound glucocorticoid receptor ligand binding domain. *Cell Res.* 2014;24:713-726.
28. Surjit M, Ganti KP, Mukherji A, et al. Widespread negative response elements mediate direct repression by agonist-liganded glucocorticoid receptor. *Cell.* 2011;145(2):224-241.
29. Penton D, Czogalla J, Loffing J. Dietary potassium and the renal control of salt balance and blood pressure. *Pflugers Arch.* 2015;467:513-530.
30. Nakamura Y, Suzuki S, Suzuki T, et al. MDM2: a novel mineralocorticoid-responsive gene involved in aldosterone-induced human vascular structural remodeling. *Am J Pathol.* 2006;169:362-371.
31. Fejes-Toth G, Naray-Fejes-Toth A. Early aldosterone-regulated genes in cardiomyocytes: clues to cardiac remodeling? *Endocrinology.* 2007;148:1502-1510.
32. Viengchareun S, Penfornis P, Zennaro MC, Lombes M. Mineralocorticoid and glucocorticoid receptors inhibit UCP expression and function in brown adipocytes. *Am J Physiol Endocrinol Metab.* 2001;280:E640-E649.
33. Pascual-Le Tallec L, Kirsh LMC, Lecomte MC, et al. Protein inhibitor of activated signal transducer and activator of transcription 1 interacts with the N-terminal domain of mineralocorticoid receptor and represses its transcriptional activity: implication of small ubiquitin-related modifier 1 modification. *Mol Endocrinol.* 2003;17:2529-2542.
34. Liu W, Wang J, Sauter NK. et al. Steroid receptor heterodimerization demonstrated *in vitro* and in vivo. *Proc Natl Acad Sci USA.* 1995;92:12480-12484.
35. Rupprecht R, Arriza JL, Spengler D, et al. Transactivation and synergistic properties of the mineralocorticoid receptor relationship to the glucocorticoid receptor. *Mol Endocrinol.* 1993;7:597-603.
36. Bledsoe RK, Madauss KP, Holt JA, et al. Mineralocorticoid receptor with bound aldosterone. *J Biol Chem.* 2005;280:31283-31293.
37. Lazar MA. Thyroid hormone receptors: multiple forms, multiple possibilities. *Endocr Rev.* 1993;14:184-193.
38. Nascimento AS, Dias SMG, Nunes FM, et al. Structural rearrangements in the thyroid hormone receptor hinge domain and their putative role in receptor function. *J Mol Biol.* 2006;360:586-598.
39. Brent GA, Williams GR, Harney JW, et al. Capacity for cooperative binding of thyroid hormone (T3) receptor dimers defines wild type T3 response elements. *Mol Endocrinol.* 1992;6(4):502-514.
40. Dreyer C, Krey G, Keller H, et al. Control of the peroxisomal beta-oxidation pathway by a novel family of nuclear hormone receptors. *Cell.* 1992;68(5):879-887.
41. Mandard S, Muller M, Kersten S. Peroxisome proliferator-activated receptor alpha target genes. *Cell Mol Life Sci.* 2004;61:393-416.
42. Chawla A, Schwarz EJ, Dimaculangan DD, et al. Peroxisome proliferator- activated receptor (PPAR) gamma: adipose-predominant expression and induction early in adipocyte differentiation. *Endocrinology.* 1994;135:798-800.
43. Reddy JK, Hashimoto T. Peroxisomal beta-oxidation and peroxisome proliferator-activated receptor alpha: an adaptive metabolic system. *Annu Rev Nutr.* 2001;21:193-230.
44. Goya K, Sumitani S, Xu X, et al. Peroxisome proliferatoractivated receptor agonists increase nitric oxide synthase expression in vascular endothelial cells. *Arterioscler Thromb Vasc Biol.* 2004;24:658-663.
45. Marx N, Duez H, Fruchart JC, et al. Peroxisome proliferator-activated receptors and atherogenesis: regulators of gene expression in vascular cells. *Circ Res.* 2004;94:1168-1178.
46. Tan NS, Michalik L, Desvergne B, et al. Peroxisome proliferator activated receptor-beta as a target for wound healing drugs. *Expert Opin Ther Targets.* 2004;8:39.
47. Staels B, Fruchart JC. Therapeutic roles of peroxisome proliferatoractivated receptor agonists. *Diabetes.* 2005;54:2460-2470.
48. Petkovich M, Brand NJ, Krust A, Chambon P. A human retinoic acid receptor which belongs to the family of nuclear receptors. *Nature.* 1987;330:444-450.
49. Kastner P, Mark M, Chambon P. Nonsteroid nuclear receptors: what are genetic studies yelling us about their role in real life? *Cell.* 1995;83:859-869.
50. Renaud JP, Rochel N, Ruff M. Crystal structure of the RAR-gamma ligand-binding domain bound to all-trans retinoic acid. *Nature.* 1995;378:681-689.
51. Bastien J, Rochette-Egly C. Nuclear retinoid receptors and the transcription of retinoid-target genes. *Gene.* 2004;328:1-16.
52. Smith MA, Parkinson DR, Cheson BD, et al. Retinoids in cancer therapy. *J Clin Oncol.* 1992;10(5):839-864.
53. Heller EH, Siffman NJ. Synthetic retinods in dermatology. *Can Med Assoc J.* 1985;132(10):1129-1136.
54. Egea PF, Mitschler A, Rochel N. Crystal structure of the human RXR alpha ligand binding domain bound to 9-*cis*-retinoic acid. *EMBO J.* 2000;19:2592-2601.
55. Mangelsdorf DJ, Borgmeyer U, Heyman RA, et al. Characterization of three RXR genes that mediate the action of 9-cis retinoic acid. *Genes Dev.* 1992;6:329-344.
56. Fan Y-Y, Spencer TE, Wang N, et al. Chemopreventive n-3 fatty acids activate RXRα in colonocytes. *Carcinogenesis.* 2003;24:1541-1548.
57. Dawson MI. Synthetic retinoids and their nuclear receptors. *Curr Med Chem Anticancer Agents.* 2004;4:199-230.
58. Shulman AI, Mangelsdorf DJ. Retinoid X receptor heterodimers in the metabolic syndrome. *N Engl J Med.* 2005;353:604-615.
59. Westin S, Kurokawa R, Nolte RT, et al. Interactions controlling the assembly of nuclear-receptor heterodimers and co-activators. *Nature.* 1998;395:199-202.
60. Germain P, Iyer J, Zechel C, et al. Coregulator recruitment and the mechanism of retinoic acid receptor synergy. *Nature.* 2002;415:187-192.
61. van Etten E, Mathieu C. Immunoregulation by 1,25-dihydroxyvitamin D3: basic concepts. *J Steroid Biochem Mol Biol.* 2005;97:93-101.
62. Cantley LK, Russell J, Lettieri D, et al. 1,25-Dihydroxyvitamin D3 suppresses parathyroid hormone secretion from bovine parathyroid cells in tissue culture. *Endocrinology.* 1985;117:2114-2119.
63. Hsieh JC, Sisk JM, Jurutka PW, et al. Physical and functional interaction between the vitamin D receptor and hairless corepressor, two proteins required for hair cycling. *J Biol Chem.* 2003;278:38665-38674.

64. Weishaar RE, Kim SN, Saunders DE, et al. Involvement of vitamin D3 with cardiovascular function. III. Effects on physical and morphological properties. *Am J Physiol.* 1990;258:E134-E142.
65. Girgis CM, Clifton-Bligh RJ, Hamrick MW, et al. The roles of vitamin D in skeletal muscle: form, function, and metabolism. *Endocr Rev.* 2013;34:33-83.
66. Lopes N, Paredes J, Costa JL, et al. Vitamin D and the mammary gland: a review on its role in normal development and breast cancer. *Breast Cancer Res.* 2012;14:211.
67. Nguyen TM, Guillozo H, Marin L, et al. 1,25-dihydroxyvitamin D3 receptors in rat lung during the perinatal period: regulation and immunohistochemical localization. *Endocrinology.* 1990;127(4):1755-1762.
68. Rochel N, Wurtz JM, Mitschler A, et al. The crystal structure of the nuclear receptor for vitamin D bound to its natural ligand. *Mol Cell.* 2000;5(1):173-179.
69. Prufer K, Racz A, Lin GC, Barsony J. Dimerization with retinoid X receptors promotes nuclear localization and subnuclear targeting of vitamin D receptors. *J Biol Chem.* 2000;275:41114-41123.

CHAPTER **8**

Ion Channel Receptors

Swati Betharia and Timothy J. Maher

Drugs covered/mentioned in this chapter:

- Acetylcholine
- Amantadine
- D-(-)-2-Amino-5-phosphonopentanoic acid (D-AP5)
- Anandamide
- 2-Arachidonylglycerol
- Aspartate
- Atracurium
- Bicuculline
- Carbachol
- Chloroquine
- Clozapine
- Curare
- Cyclothiazide
- Cytisine
- Dextromethorphan
- Dextorphan
- Diltiazem
- Dizocilpine
- Domoic Acid
- 1,1-Dimethyl-4-phenylpiperazinium iodide (DMPP)
- Ivermectin
- Felbamate
- Flumazenil
- Gamma-aminobutyric acid (GABA)
- Gaboxadol
- Glutamate
- Glycine
- Granisetron
- Hexamethonium
- Homoquinolinic acid
- Indiplon
- Irinotecan
- Isoguvacine
- Ivermectin
- Ketamine
- Lidocaine
- Mecamylamine
- Memantine
- Methacholine
- MK-801
- Muscimol
- Nicotine
- N-Methyl-D-aspartate (NMDA)
- Ondansetron
- Pancuronium
- Phaclofen
- Phencyclidine
- Picrotoxin
- Piracetam
- Pregnenolone sulfate
- Quinine
- Ramosetron
- (*R*)-HA-966 (*R*-(+)-3-Amino-1-hydroxypyrrolidin-2-one)
- Ro19-4603
- D-Serine
- Serotonin
- Spermine
- Spermidine
- Strychnine
- Succinylcholine
- Δ9-Tetrahydrocannabinol (THC)
- Tetramethylammonium (TMA)
- TPMPA (1,2,5,6-Tetrahydropyridin-4-yl)-methylphosphinic acid)
- Trimethaphan
- Tubocurarine
- Varenicline
- Vecuronium
- Zaleplon
- Zolpiclone
- Zolpidem

Abbreviations

5-HT 5-Hydroxytryptamine
5-HT$_3$R 5-HT receptor subtype 3
AMPA α-Amino-3-hydroxy-5-methyl-4-isoxazole propionic acid
ATP Adenosine triphosphate
cAMP Cyclic adenosine monophosphate
CNS Central nervous system
EAA Excitatory amino acid
GABA Gamma-aminobutyric acid
GLU Glutamate
GluR Glutamate receptor
GLY Glycine
GPCR G protein–coupled receptors
HVA High-voltage activated
IAA Inhibitory amino acid
IP$_3$ Inositol-1,4,5-triphosphate
LGIC Ligand-gated ion channel
LTD Long-term depression
LTP Long-term potentiation
LVA Low-voltage activated
mAChR Muscarinic acetylcholine receptor
mRNA Messenger ribonucleic acid
nAChR Nicotinic acetylcholine receptor
NMDA N-Methyl-D-aspartate
PLC Phospholipase C
TM Transmembrane
ZAC Zinc-activated channel

INTRODUCTION

Signal transduction can occur through various receptor types present on the cellular transmembrane surface. These include ligand-gated ion channels (LGICs), G protein–coupled receptors (GPCRs), and catalytic receptors or enzyme-coupled receptors (Fig. 8.1). Voltage-gated ion channels, while also found on the transmembrane surface, are not categorized as receptors in the classical sense, as they do not require ligand binding for activation. A fourth receptor type, known as nuclear receptors, is located intracellularly and is not found on the transmembrane surface (Fig. 8.1).

LIGAND-GATED ION CHANNELS

The most rapid cellular responses to receptor activation are mediated via LGICs. The majority of LGICs are categorized into the Cys-loop family of pentameric receptors. These plasma membrane–spanning proteins are composed of five peptide subunits with a central ion-conducting pore. Each subunit is comprised of an extracellular ligand-binding N-terminus, four transmembrane loops (TM1 to TM4), a large cytoplasmic domain, and an extracellular C-terminus. A characteristic Cys-loop is formed in the N-terminus when the two Cys terminal ends of an approximately 13 amino acid chain form an internal disulfide bond.[1] The nicotinic acetylcholine receptor (nAChR), serotonin (5-hydroxytryptamine, 5-HT) receptor 5-HT_3R, γ-aminobutyric acid (GABA) receptor, glycine receptor (GLY), and the zinc-activated channel (ZAC) all belong to the Cys-loop family of receptors. They share a similar structural conformation and function, except for the specificity of the ligand-binding site and selectivity of the channel for particular ions. Exceptions in the LGICs are the GluR family and the adenosine triphosphate (ATP)–gated purinergic receptors (P2X), which do not belong to the Cys-loop pentameric receptor family and are tetrameric and trimeric proteins, respectively.

The binding of a ligand (neurotransmitters, exogenous molecules, or allosteric modulators) results in a conformational change in the receptor protein structure, allowing for the central pore to conduct specific ions down their electrochemical gradient. The primary reason for the rapidity (milliseconds) of the cellular response with LGICs is that the transduction of the signal requires the activation of a single molecule. Therefore, this transduction mechanism is especially suited for physiologic processes needing an immediate response, such as the stimulation of nerves and muscle fibers. A survey of ligand-gated ion channels is provided in Table 8.1, and the structures of their endogenous ligands are shown in Figure 8.2.

Nicotinic Acetylcholine Receptors

Structure and Function

The nAChRs are perhaps the best characterized LGICs. These receptors are found at the skeletal neuromuscular junction, adrenal medulla, and autonomic ganglia. They are composed of five distinct subunits, two α and, depending on the receptor subtype, various combinations of additional α, β, γ, and δ subunits. A total of 17 subunit types have been identified to date (α1-α10, β1-β4, γ, δ, and ε). The five subunits of each nAChR protein are arranged around a central pore that serves as the ion channel.[2] Based on molecular modeling of the deduced primary structure of the individual subunits, it has been proposed that each subunit (α, β, γ [or ε], and δ) possesses a hydrophilic extracellular N-terminus, a hydrophilic extracellular C-terminus, and four α helical hydrophobic transmembrane domains (TM1 to TM4) (Fig. 8.3). A pentameric arrangement of these five amphipathic subunits makes up the walls of the ion channel.[3] Two binding sites for the endogenous ligand acetylcholine exist on the extracellular domain of the nAChR molecule. In Figure 8.3, one binding site is located on each α subunit at the αγ and αδ interfaces. The binding sites show a positive cooperativity, meaning that ligand binding to one site facilitates binding to the other. The ability of the sites to communicate exists even though the binding sites

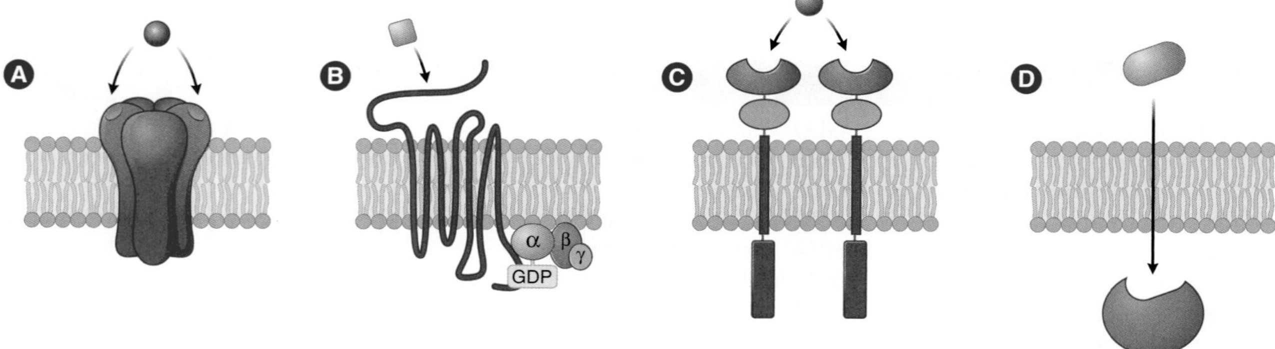

Figure 8.1 Major classes of drug receptors. A, Transmembrane ligand-gated ion channel receptor. B, Transmembrane G protein–coupled receptor (GPCR). C, Transmembrane catalytic receptor or enzyme-coupled receptors. D, Intracellular cytoplasmic/nuclear receptor. From Golan DE, Armstrong EJ, Armstrong AW, eds. Chapter 1: Drug–receptor interactions. In: *Principles of Pharmacology:* The Pathophysiologic Basis of Drug Therapy. Baltimore: Lippincott Williams & Wilkins; 2012:1-3, with permission.

Table 8.1 Survey of Ligand-Gated Receptor Subtypes

Receptor Class	Subtype	Selective Agonist	Antagonist	Effector
Excitatory amino acid receptors	NMDA	NMDA	D-AP5	↓Na^+/Ca^{2+}
	AMPA	AMPA	CNQX	↑Na^+
	Kainate	Kainate	CNQX	↑Na^+/K^+
GABA receptors	$GABA_A$	Muscimol	Bicuculline	↑Cl^-
	$GABA_c$	*cis*-4-Aminocrotonic acid	TPMPA	↑Cl^-
Glycine (GLY) receptors		Glycine	Strychnine	↑Cl^-
Nicotinic receptors	N_{muscle}	?	Decamethonium	↑Na^+/Ca^{2+}
	$N_{neuronal}$	?	Hexamethonium	↑Na^+/Ca^{2+}
P2X receptors	$P2X_1$-$P2X_7$	ATP	TNP-ATP triethylammonium salt	↑$Na^+/K^+/Ca^{2+}$
Serotonin receptors (5-HT)	$5\text{-}HT_3$	m-Chlorophenylbiguanide hydrochloride	Ondansetron	↑$Na^+/K^+/Ca^{2+}$
Zinc activated channel (ZAC)		Copper ions	Tubocurarine	↑$Na^+/K^+/Cs^+$

?, no known selective compounds available; cloned, receptor subtype has been cloned and the amino acid structure is known. Chemical abbreviations used: AMPA, D, L-α-amino-3-hydroxy-5-methyl-4-isoxalone propionic acid; ATP, adenosine triphosphate; CNQX, 6-cyano-7-nitroquinoxaline-2, 3-dione; D-AP5, D-amino-5-phosphonopentanoate; GABA, γ-aminobutyric acid; 5-HT, 5-hydroxytryptamine, serotonin; IP_3, inositol 1,4,5-triphosphate; NMDA, N-methyl-D-aspartate; and TPMPA, 1,2,5,6-tetrahydropyridin-4-yl.

are not adjacent to each other in the pentameric receptor.[4] Ligand binding induces a conformational change in the receptor, opening the ion channel and allowing the passage of sodium (Na^+) and potassium (K^+) ions through the center of the protein. The result is depolarization of the surrounding plasma membrane.

The multiplicity of nAChRs is based on different structural requirements for agonists and antagonists acting at the autonomic ganglia and the skeletal neuromuscular junction and is supported by research in molecular biology.[5] The two types of nAChRs, namely ganglionic neuronal (N_N) and neuromuscular (somatic muscle) (N_M), are both classified as LGICs. Central and peripheral nAChR subtypes with different subunit compositions are summarized in Table 8.2.[6] The nAChR of skeletal (somatic) muscle tissue is a transmembrane glycoprotein consisting of four types of subunits; α, β, γ (or ε), and δ. Only the α_1 subtype of the subunit is

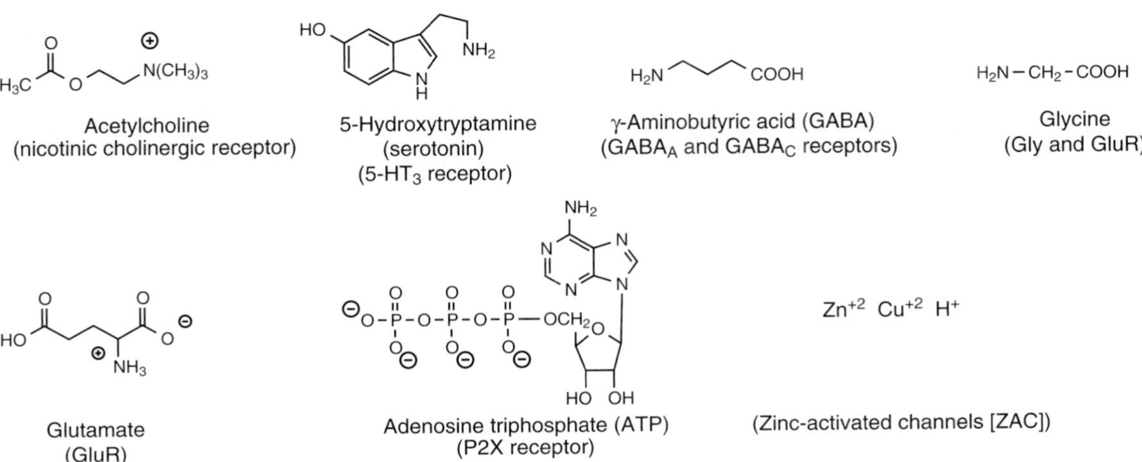

Figure 8.2 Natural ligands of ion channel receptors. Acetylcholine for nicotinic cholinergic receptors, 5-hydroxytryptamine (serotonin) for $5\text{-}HT_3$ receptors, gamma-amino butyric acid (GABA) for $GABA_A$ and $GABA_C$ receptors, GLY for glycine and GluR, GLU for GluR, and ATP for P2X receptors. Zn^{2+}, Cu^{2+}, and H^+ serve as natural ligands for the zinc-activated channels.

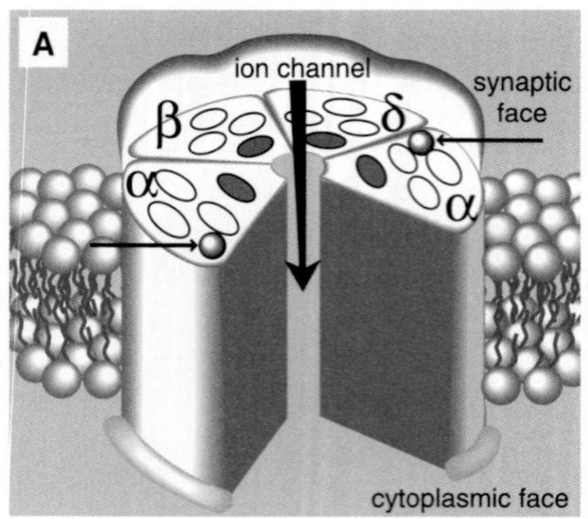

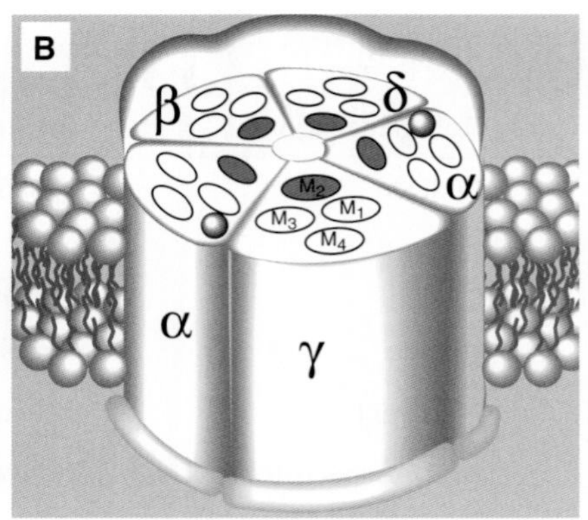

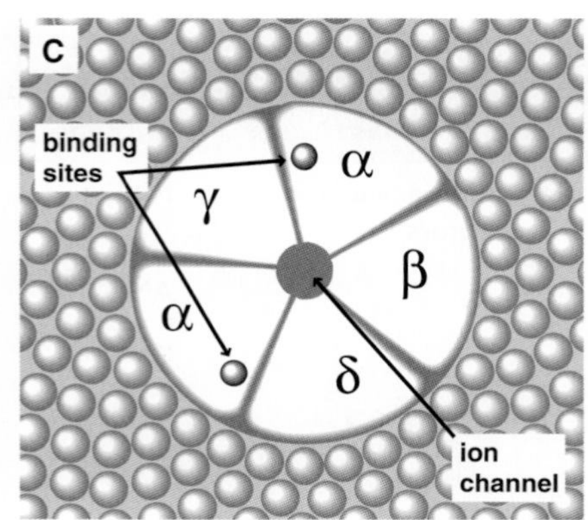

Figure 8.3 nAChR (nicotinic acetylcholine receptor): A, Longitudinal view (γ subunit removed) showing the internal ion channel. Acetylcholine binding sites on the α subunits are indicated by the arrows. These are located at the αγ and αγ interfaces. B, Each of the five transmembrane subunits (α, α, β, δ, and γ) are composed of four hydrophobic membrane-spanning segments (M_1 to M_4). C, Top view of the nAChR showing the subunits surrounding the ion channel.

present in muscle. In a mature muscle end plate, the γ subunit is replaced by an ε subunit. This change in gene expression encoding the γ and ε subunits affects ligand selectivity, along with receptor turnover and/or tissue location. One class of neuronal nAChRs exists as a heteromeric pentamer composed of α (α_2 to α_6) and β (β_2 to β_4) subunits—for example, $\alpha_4\beta_3$ with a stoichiometry of two α_4 and three β_3 subunits. Another class of functional homomeric nAChRs is composed of α_7 through α_{10} subunits. The diversity of the subunits and the pentameric structure suggest that a large number of nAChR subtypes can exist.[3]

Nicotinic Receptor Agonists

The nAChRs have been the focus of intensive research, even though the majority of clinically effective cholinergic medicinal agents are either muscarinic agonists or antagonists. The best known nicotinic agonist is nicotine, which is an alkaloid obtained from the *Nicotiana tabacum* plant with minimal effects on the cholinergic muscarinic receptors. Other nAChR agonists such as acetylcholine, carbachol, and methacholine are nonselective and also activate the muscarinic receptors. Full (nicotine) and partial (varenicline and cytisine) agonists for the nAChRs have been used in the treatment of tobacco addiction.[7]

Table 8.2 Nicotinic Acetylcholine Receptor Subtypes

Receptor	Location	Membrane Response	Molecular Mechanism	Agonists	Antagonists
Neuromuscular (N_M) $(\alpha_1)_2\beta_1\varepsilon\delta$ $(\alpha_1)_2\beta_1\gamma\delta$	Skeletal (somatic) neuromuscular junction (postjunctional)	Excitatory; end plate depolarization; contraction (skeletal muscle)	Increased Na^+ and K^+ permeability	ACh; nicotine; succinylcholine	Atracurium; Vecuronium; *d*-tubocurarine; pancuronium; α-conotoxin; α-bungarotoxin
Ganglionic neuronal (N_N) $(\alpha_3)_2(\beta_4)_3$	Autonomic ganglia; adrenal medulla	Excitatory; depolarization firing of postganglionic neuron; depolarization and secretion of catecholamines	Increased Na^+ and K^+ permeability	ACh; nicotine; epibatidine; dimethylphenyl-piperazinium	Trimethaphan; mecamylamine; dihydro-β erythrodine; erysodine lophotoxin
Central neuronal $(\alpha_4)_2(\beta_4)_3$ (α-bungarotoxin insensitive)	CNS; pre- and postjunctional	Pre- and postsynaptic excitation; prejunctional control of transmitter release	Increased Na^+ and K^+ permeability	Cytisine; epibatidine; Anatoxin A	
$(\alpha_7)_5$ (α-bungarotoxin sensitive)	CNS; pre- and postsynaptic	Same as central neuronal	Increased Ca^{2+} permeability	Anatoxin A	Methyllycaconitine α-conotoxin; α-bungarotoxin

Reprinted with permission from Westfall TC, Westfall DP. Neurotransmission: the autonomic and somatic motor nervous systems. In: Brunton LL, Hilal-Dandan R, Knollmann BC, eds. *Goodman and Gilman's The Pharmacological Basis of Therapeutics*. 13th ed. New York: McGraw-Hill; 2018:191.

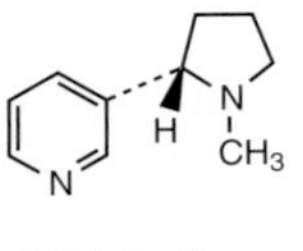

S(-)-Nicotine 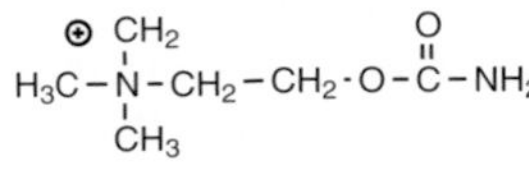 Carbachol 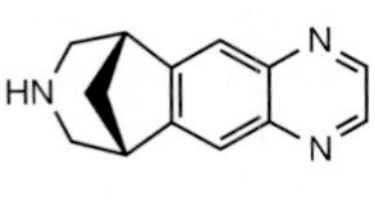 Varenicline

Nicotinic Receptor Antagonists

Nicotinic antagonists are chemical compounds that bind to nAChRs but have no intrinsic activity. All therapeutically useful nicotinic antagonists are competitive antagonists; in other words, their effects are reversible with acetylcholine. There are two subclasses of nicotinic antagonists—skeletal neuromuscular blocking agents and ganglionic blocking agents—classified according to the two populations of nAChRs, N_M and N_N, respectively.

NEUROMUSCULAR NICOTINIC RECEPTOR BLOCKING AGENTS. In terms of the historical perspective, tubocurarine, the first known neuromuscular blocking drug, was as important to the understanding of nicotinic antagonists as atropine was to that of muscarinic antagonists. The neuromuscular blocking effects of extracts of curare were first reported as early as 1510, when explorers of the Amazon River region of South America found natives using these plant extracts as arrow poisons. Early research with these crude plant extracts indicated that the active components caused muscle paralysis by effects on either the nerve or the muscle (remember that the concept of neurochemical transmission was not introduced until the late 19th century). In 1856, however, Bernard described the results of his experiments, which demonstrated unequivocally that curare extracts prevented skeletal muscle contractions by an effect at the neuromuscular junction, rather than the nerve innervating the muscle or the muscle itself.[8]

Much of the early literature concerning the effects of curare is confusing and difficult to interpret. This is not at all surprising considering that this research was performed using crude extracts, many of which came from different plants. It was not until the late 1800s that scientists recognized that curare extracts contained quaternary ammonium salts. This knowledge prompted the use of other quaternary ammonium compounds to explore the neuromuscular junction. In the meantime, curare extracts continued to be used to block the effects of nicotine and acetylcholine at skeletal neuromuscular junctions and to explore the nAChRs.

In 1935, King isolated a pure alkaloid, which he named *d*-tubocurarine, from a tube curare of unknown botanical origin.[9] The word "tube" refers to the container in which the South American natives transported their plant extract. It was almost 10 years later that the botanical source for *d*-tubocurarine was clearly identified as *Chondrodendron tomentosum*. The structure that King assigned to tubocurarine possessed two nitrogen atoms, both of which were quaternary ammonium salts (i.e., a bis-quaternary ammonium compound). It was not until 1970 that the correct structure was reported by Everett et al.[10] The correct structure has only one quaternary ammonium nitrogen; the other nitrogen is a tertiary amine salt. Nevertheless, the incorrect structure of tubocurarine served as the model for the synthesis of all the neuromuscular blocking agents in use today. These compounds have been of immense therapeutic value for surgical and orthopedic procedures and have been essential to research that led to the isolation and purification of nAChRs.

By the 1980's, important developments in the characterization of the nAChR resulted from research on two unlikely animal sources. The finding that the electric eel, *Torpedo californica*, contained a rich source of nAChR that could be isolated allowed for the purification of large quantities of the receptor for study.[11] Additionally, it was found that the venom from a snake, the Southeast Asian banded krait, *Bungarus multicinctus*, contained the 74-amino acid peptide, α-bungarotoxin which binds competitively and almost irreversibly with very high affinity to the two $\alpha 7$ subunits of the nAChR to prevent channel opening. When exposed to α–bungarotoxin, the nAChRs in the skeletal muscles responsible for normal respiration are antagonized, leading to respiratory paralysis and, if not treated, death.[12] These two findings were essential to our understanding of the structure and binding requirements of the nAChR.

The potential therapeutic benefits of the neuromuscular blocking effects of tubocurarine, as well as the difficulty in obtaining pure samples of the alkaloid, encouraged medicinal chemists to design structurally related compounds possessing nicotinic antagonist activity. Using the incorrectly assigned bis-quaternary ammonium structure of tubocurarine as reported by King[9] as a guide, a large number of compounds were synthesized and evaluated. It became apparent that a bis-quaternary ammonium compound having two quaternary ammonium salts separated by 10-12 carbon atoms (similar to the distance between the nitrogen atoms in tubocurarine) was a requirement for neuromuscular blocking activity. The rationale for this structural requirement was that, in contrast to muscarinic acetylcholine receptor (mAChRs), nAChRs possessed two anionic-binding sites, both of which had to be occupied for a neuromuscular blocking effect. It is important to observe that the current transmembrane model for the nAChR protein has two anionic sites in the extracellular domain.

Some of the new bis-quaternary ammonium agents, such as the dicholine ester succinylcholine produced depolarization of the postjunctional membrane at the neuromuscular junction before causing blockade; other compounds, such as tubocurarine, did not produce this initial depolarization. Thus, the structural features of the remainder of the molecule determined whether the nicotinic antagonist was a depolarizing or a nondepolarizing neuromuscular blocker.

Neuromuscular blocking agents are used primarily as an adjunct to general anesthesia. They produce skeletal muscle relaxation that facilitates operative procedures such as abdominal surgery. Furthermore, they reduce the depth requirement for general anesthetics; this decreases the overall risk of a surgical procedure and shortens the postanesthetic recovery time. Muscles producing rapid movements are the first to be affected by neuromuscular blocking agents. These include muscles of the face, eyes, and neck. Muscles of the limbs, chest, and abdomen are affected next, with the diaphragm (respiration) being affected last. Recovery generally is in the reverse order. Neuromuscular blocking agents have also been used in the correction of dislocations and the realignment of fractures. Short-acting neuromuscular blocking agents, such as the depolarizing blocker succinylcholine, are routinely used to assist in tracheal intubation. Other neuromuscular agents that act by a nondepolarizing mechanism (similar to tubocurarine) include pancuronium and vecuronium, which structurally are aminosteroids, and atracurium, a benzylisoquinoline.[13]

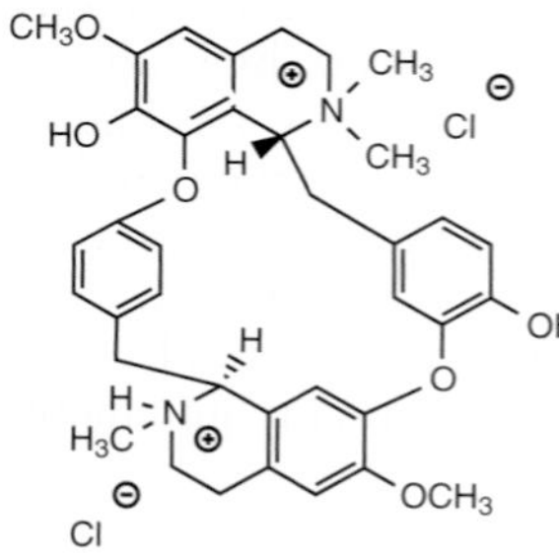

d-Tubocurarine chloride

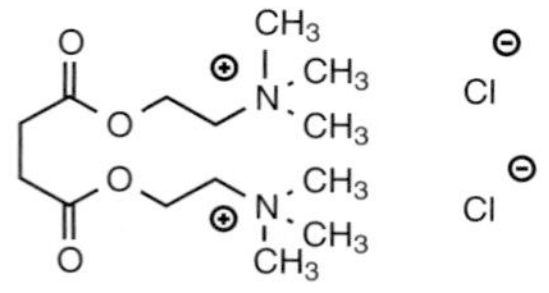

Succinylcholine chloride

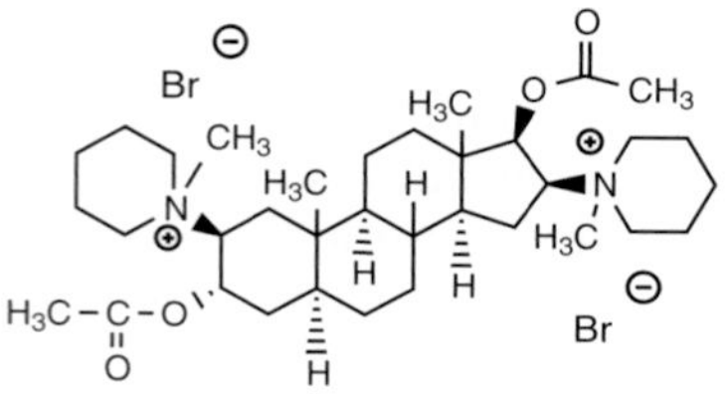

Pancuronium bromide

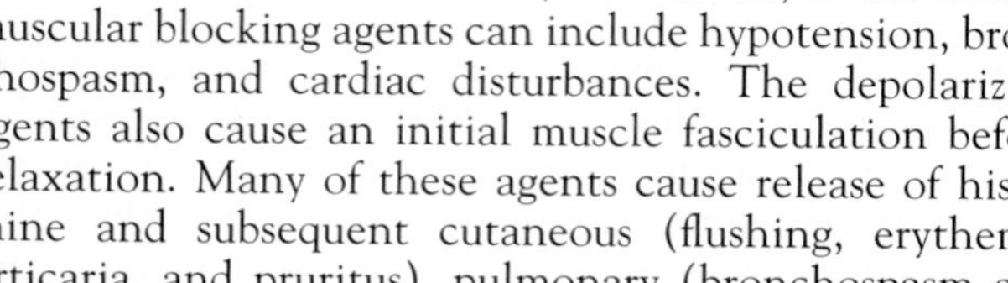

Atracurium besylate

Adverse reactions to most, but not all, of the neuromuscular blocking agents can include hypotension, bronchospasm, and cardiac disturbances. The depolarizing agents also cause an initial muscle fasciculation before relaxation. Many of these agents cause release of histamine and subsequent cutaneous (flushing, erythema, urticaria, and pruritus), pulmonary (bronchospasm and wheezing), and cardiovascular (hypotension) effects. For more information on neuromuscular blockers, refer to Chapters 10 and 12.

NEURONAL (GANGLIONIC) NICOTINIC RECEPTOR AGONISTS AND ANTAGONISTS. While the blockade of the neuromuscular nAChRs was observed to require a separation of nitrogen atoms by 10-12 carbons, the blockade of the neuronal nAChRs in the ganglia can be observed with a separation of six carbon atoms, indicating the differences in antagonist binding requirements. Thus, hexamethonium is rather selective for the neuronal nAChR with little activity at the neuromuscular nAChRs or the mAChRs. Other so-called ganglionic antagonists include trimethaphan and mecamylamine.

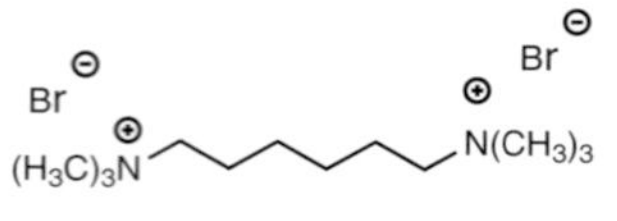

Hexamethonium bromide

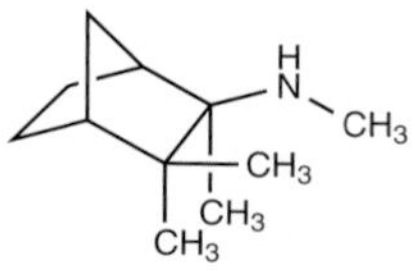

Mecamylamine

While nicotine initially acts as an agonist and stimulates the ganglionic nAChRs, which is followed by blockade, there are agonists at this site that do not also block the receptor. These include tetramethylammonium (TMA) and 1,1-dimethyl-4-phenylpiperazinium iodide (DMPP).

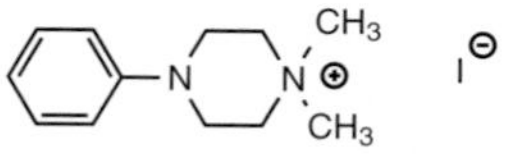

1,1-Dimethyl-4-phenylpiperazinium iodide (DMPP)

Serotonergic Receptors

Seven classes of 5-HT receptors (5-HTRs) have been identified, of which only the 5-HT_3R is an excitatory, cationic LGIC belonging to the Cys-loop receptor family. Five subunit types, namely 5-HT_3A through 5-HT_3E, have been cloned in humans. However, the functional 5-HTRs are only found as homopentamers of subunit A, depicted as (5-HT_3A)5, or as heteropentamers of subunits A and B, depicted as 5-HT_3AB, implying that subunit A is required to constitute functional receptors.[14] Each subunit is comprised of extracellular, transcellular, and intracellular domains. Binding of the natural ligand 5-HT at the orthosteric binding site (extracellular domain) results in the opening of the ion pore permeable to Na^+, K^+, and calcium (Ca^{2+}) ions. This cationic movement results in net membrane depolarization, and in the case of presynaptic 5-HT_3R present on GABAergic or glutamatergic neurons, the synaptic release of corresponding neurotransmitters.[15]

5-HT_3Rs are located centrally in regions of the brain stem, forebrain, olfactory tract, and prefrontal cortex.[16] Activation of these receptors located in the vomiting center leads to emesis. Varenicline, a partial agonist at nAChRs noted earlier, is also a partial agonist at the 5-HT_3R, which could explain the nausea associated with its use as a smoking cessation therapy.[14] Competitive antagonists which also bind to the extracellular receptor domain have therefore been used as antiemetic agents in chemotherapy- and pregnancy-associated vomiting.[17] Examples include ondansetron, granisetron, and ramosetron ("setron" family). Some additional compounds that have also been found to have a competitive antagonistic effect at the 5-HT_3R include chloroquine (antimalarial), clozapine (antipsychotic), irinotecan (anticancer), and tubocurarine (neuromuscular blocker).

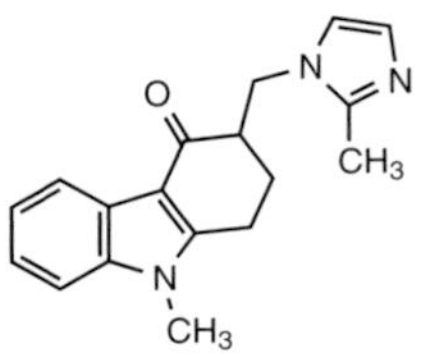

Ondansetron

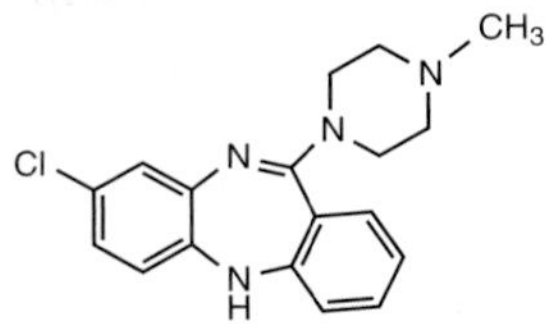

Clozapine

Noncompetitive antagonists which bind to the TM domain as opposed to the 5-HT binding extracellular domain of the receptor have also been identified. These vary in their selectivity for the homopentamer and heteropentamer 5-HT_3Rs based on the differences in the transmembrane amino acid residues in these two receptor subtypes. Examples of noncompetitive antagonists include picrotoxin ($GABA_A$ receptor antagonist), diltiazem (calcium channel blocker), quinine (antimalarial), and Δ9-tetrahydrocannabinol (cannabinoid). 5-HT_3 receptor antagonists have been explored for their use in the treatment of irritable bowel syndrome, schizophrenia, anxiety, substance abuse, pain, and inflammation. Additionally, general anesthetics (e.g., ethanol, chloroform) can bind to distinct binding sites on the extracellular or TM domains and serve as positive allosteric modulators.[14]

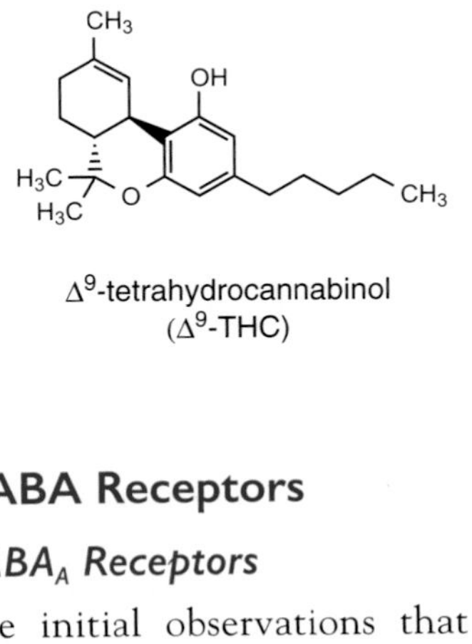

Δ^9-tetrahydrocannabinol (Δ^9-THC)

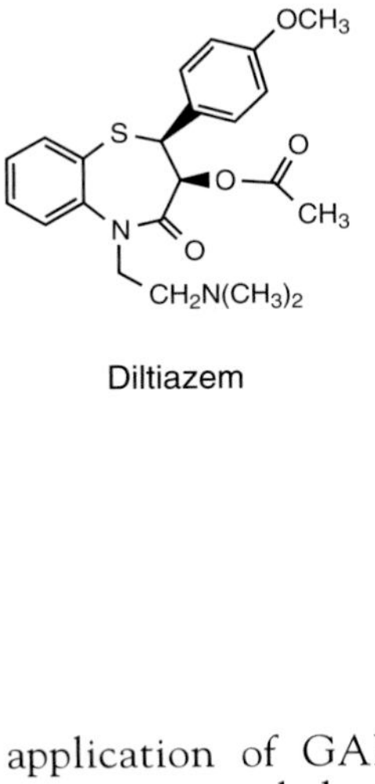

Diltiazem

GABA Receptors

$GABA_A$ Receptors

The initial observations that application of GABA was capable of hyperpolarizing neurons, coupled with the lack of activity of structurally related amino acids and other compounds, suggested that a specific receptor likely mediated this response. There have been at least three different families of GABA receptors identified to date. These are referred to as $GABA_A$, $GABA_B$, and $GABA_C$. While $GABA_A$ and $GABA_C$ are LGICs, $GABA_B$ belongs to the GPCR family of receptors.

The $GABA_A$ receptor was the first identified and found to be an LGIC that, when activated, allows for the entry of chloride ion (Cl^-) into the cell, thereby hyperpolarizing the neuron and making cell firing more difficult. The $GABA_A$ receptor is also a member of the Cys-loop family of receptors and is a heteropentamer containing various combinations of subunits termed α, β, γ, δ, ε, π, ρ, and θ. Various subunit isoforms have been identified with 6 αs, 3 βs, 3 γs, and 3 ρs (some have suggested that the ρ subunits are found only in the $GABA_C$ receptor). Each subunit is a four transmembrane-spanning protein that, when arranged pseudosymmetrically, form the ion channel with a diameter of about 8 nm. One of the most common $GABA_A$ receptor conformations in the mammalian central nervous system (CNS) consists of a pair of α1 subunits, a pair of β subunits, and a single γ2 subunit. Other identified conformations contain α1, α2, α3, α5, forms of the β subunit, and typically the γ2 subunit, and are always in a 2:2:1 stoichiometry.[18] The binding of two molecules of GABA, probably to the individual β subunits near the α-β interface, is believed to be required for normal receptor activation.

A major class of compounds that modulate $GABA_A$ receptor function is the benzodiazepines. The binding site for benzodiazepines (e.g., diazepam) is likely the α subunits in proximity to the β subunit. The form of the γ subunit appears to help determine the affinity of the individual benzodiazepine for the receptor. The benzodiazepines bind better to receptors containing γ2 than to the γ1 subunit. Similarly, very low affinity binding is observed if a receptor contains the α6 subunit. In fact, the α6 subunit seems to confer binding preference to inverse agonists such as Ro19-4603. The benzodiazepines do not bind to the GABA recognition site on the receptor and can only produce effects if presynaptic GABA has been released and is present at the receptors. Via an allosteric modulation of the $GABA_A$ receptor, the benzodiazepines appear to increase the frequency of the Cl^- channel opening when GABA is bound, which potentiates the response of exogenously released GABA.

Clinically, the benzodiazepines are very safe when used alone in the absence of CNS depressants, as they are not active on GABA receptors alone. This is in contrast to the barbiturates, which can directly activate the $GABA_A$ receptor when present in much a higher concentration than therapeutic concentrations and thus have a much lower therapeutic index. However, a benzodiazepine receptor antagonist flumazenil is available, which is used for the treatment of severe benzodiazepine overdose. Flumazenil competitively antagonizes the binding and allosteric effects of benzodiazepine agonists as well as benzodiazepine inverse agonists, such as the β-carboline DMCM (methyl 4-ethyl-6,7-dimethoxy-9*H*-pyrido[5,4-b] indole-3-carboxylate).

Using molecular biological techniques, point mutations of the α subunits have revealed that the sedative effects of the benzodiazepines are due to an interaction with the α1 subunit, while the anxiolytic effects are due to an interaction at the α2 subunit.[19,20] Nonbenzodiazepine receptor agonists such as indiplon, zaleplon, zolpiclone, and zolpidem are α1 subunit–preferring ligands that are used as sedative-hypnotics.[21]

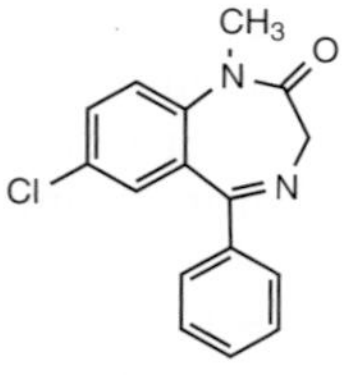

Diazepam

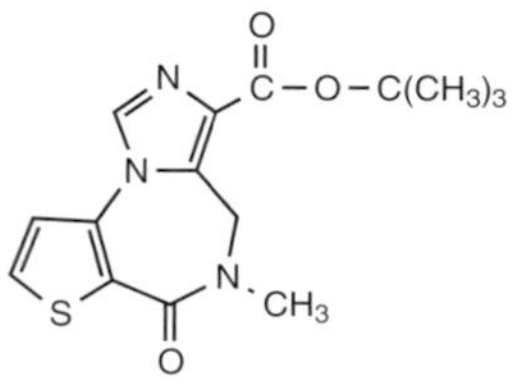

Ro19-4603

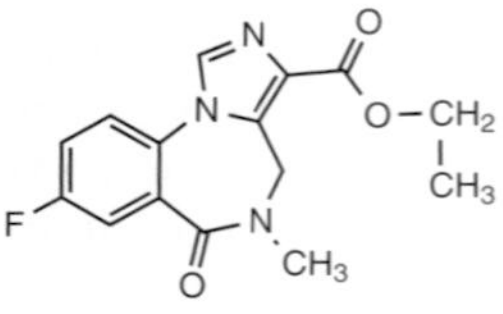

Flumazenil

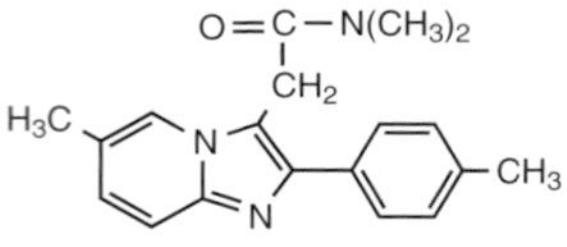

Zolpidem

An agent that acts on the $GABA_A$ receptor that does not interact with the benzodiazepine binding site is gaboxadol (previously called THIP; 4,5,6,7-tetrahydroisoxazolo[4,5-c]pyridine-3-ol). This sedative-hypnotic binds with high affinity to the extrasynaptic $\alpha4\beta\delta GABA_A$ receptor and does not alter sleep onset or REM sleep as the benzodiazepines do. On the other hand, gaboxadol increases slow wave sleep.[22]

The barbiturates bind to a different portion of the $GABA_A$ receptor and, similar to the benzodiazepines, enhance the activity of GABA. However, this leads to an increase in the duration of Cl^- channel opening, rather than frequency as seen with the benzodiazepines. Higher concentrations of the barbiturates can directly activate the $GABA_A$ receptor and open the Cl^- channel, explaining why overdoses of barbiturates can lead to life-threatening CNS-mediated respiratory and cardiovascular depression.

A number of compounds are known to directly activate the $GABA_A$ receptor. Of these compounds, muscimol and isoguvacine are the most well-known. Unlike GABA which does not cross the blood-brain barrier, these agents do enter the CNS and display GABA-mimetic activity following peripheral administration. Additionally, a number of compounds can bind to the $GABA_A$ receptor and antagonize the actions of GABA. Bicuculline, by binding to the GABA recognition site and preventing GABA from binding, produces convulsions in experimental animals. Picrotoxin, via its active metabolite picrotoxinin binds in the Cl^- channel to prevent ion flow when the receptor is activated by GABA. Picrotoxin does not alter GABA binding, but instead prevents ions from flowing and is a potent convulsant.

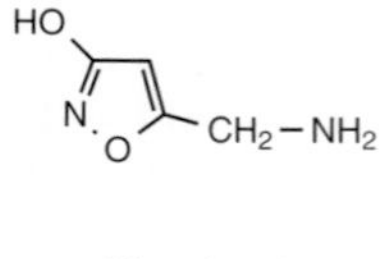

Muscimol

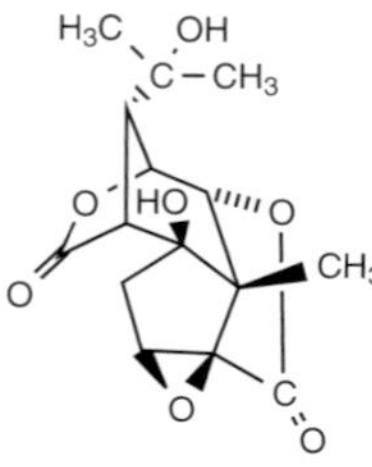

Picrotoxin

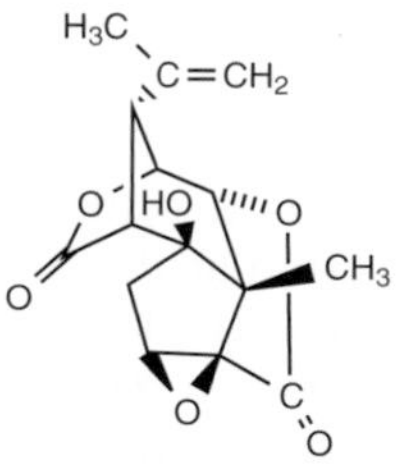

Picrotoxinin

With the many possible assembly sequences of $GABA_A$ receptors, advances in medicinal chemistry may someday be able to design compounds that target specific pentameric subunit assemblies to preferentially produce specific effects.[23] For instance, located on the base of the dendritic spines of hippocampal pyramidal cells are $GABA_A$ receptors with an $\alpha5$ subunit composition. These receptors are thought to counteract the excitatory input due to glutamatergic N-methyl-D-aspartate (NMDA) receptor activation involved in learning and memory. Activation of $GABA_A$ receptors in this area disrupts learning and memory, while NMDA receptor activation improves these critical skills. Administration of an inverse agonist of the $GABA_A$ receptor with selectivity for the $\alpha5$ subunit improves memory performance in experimental animals.[24] Additionally, $\alpha3$ selective agonists may be useful in treating schizophrenia, as this subtype of $GABA_A$ receptor appears to play a role in decreasing the release of dopamine from overactive neurons in the mesolimbic system.[25]

General anesthetics also appear to have interactions with the $GABA_A$ receptor in producing their various anesthetic effects, including immobilization, respiratory depression, and hypnosis via binding to hydrophobic pockets within the receptor. Using point-mutated knock-in mice, agents such as enflurane, etomidate, and propofol have been found to interact with the $\beta3$ subunit of the $GABA_A$ receptor to produce immobilization and hypnosis.[26] However, the heart-rate– and body temperature–depressant effects of etomidate and propofol do not appear to be mediated by the $\beta3$ subunit. Studies are underway to improve our understanding of the molecular mechanisms of this chemically varied group of agents used as general anesthetics.

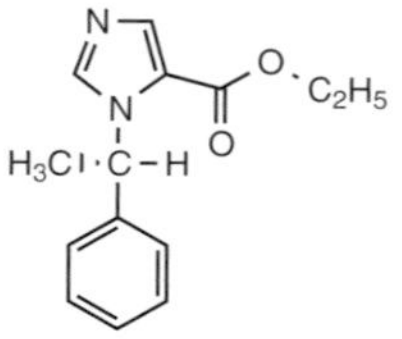

Etomidate

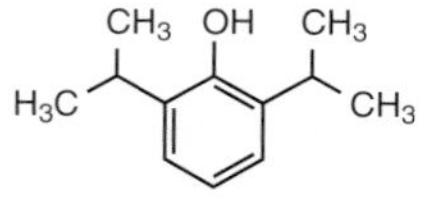

Propofol

Neurosteroids are also capable of modulating the activity of GABA at the $GABA_A$ receptor by binding to a site distinct from that utilized by GABA, benzodiazepines, and barbiturates. These steroids, including the progesterone metabolites pregnanolone (3α-hydroxy-5β-pregnan-20-one), allopregnanolone (3α-hydroxy-5α-pregnan-20-one), and allotetrahydrodeoxycorticosterone (3α,21-dihydroxy-5α-pregnan-20-one), enhance GABA-mediated inhibitory activity. The presence of the δ subunit in the pentameric $GABA_A$ receptor greatly increases the affinity of steroid binding and efficacy. High concentrations of these steroids can also result in direct activation of the receptor. Thus, it may be possible in the future to selectively target the various modulatory sites on the $GABA_A$ receptor to produce preferential pharmacological effects; for instance, benzodiazepines that are anxiolytic without sedative effects, antischizophrenic agents that lack sedation and extrapyramidal side effects, and general anesthetics that do not alter respiratory and/or heart rates.

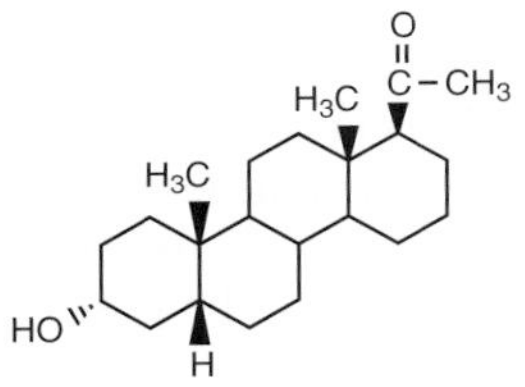

Pregnanolone

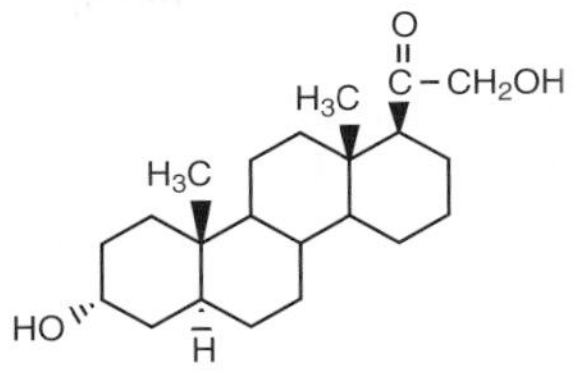

Allotetrahydrodeoxycorticosterone

$GABA_C$ Receptors

Another receptor that binds GABA, but is not antagonized by bicuculline (a $GABA_A$ antagonist) or phaclofen (a $GABA_B$ antagonist) and is not influenced by either the benzodiazepines or barbiturates, is termed the $GABA_C$ receptor. The endogenous neurotransmitter GABA is an order of magnitude more potent on the $GABA_C$ receptor as compared with the $GABA_A$ receptor, and the responses to activation of the $GABA_C$ receptor are much slower and sustained as compared with the rapid and brief responses following $GABA_A$ receptor activation. The $GABA_C$ receptor is most abundant in the retina, with significant levels in the spinal cord and pituitary gland. A pentamer of subunits form the Cl^- ion channel. As noted earlier, the ρ subunit may be unique to the $GABA_C$ receptor.[27] On the extracellular domain there appears to be binding sites for zinc, which is a potent modulator of receptor activity.

The most well-described $GABA_C$ receptor antagonist is TPMPA ([1,2,5,6-tetrahydropyridin-4-yl]-methylphosphinic acid). Interestingly, isoguvacine, an agonist at the $GABA_A$ receptors, acts as an antagonist at the $GABA_C$ receptor. Much information regarding the location, function, and pharmacology of the $GABA_C$ receptor is needed to begin to take advantage of this receptor for therapeutic purposes.

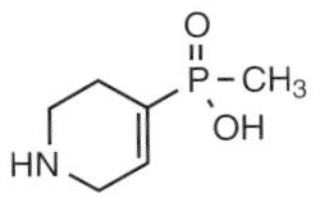

TPMPA

Glycine Receptors

The receptor mediating the actions of the inhibitory amino acid (IAA) GLY is similar to the $GABA_A$ receptor and other members of the Cys-loop family in being a pentameric ion-channel that allows for the conduction of Cl^-.[28] However, unlike the GABA receptors, the inhibitory GLY receptor can be a homopentamer of α subunits or a heteropentamer comprised of 3 α subunits and 2 β subunits. There have been four isoforms of the α subunit identified, while only one β subunit is known. The inhibitory neurotransmitter GLY, in addition to taurine, D-alanine, L-alanine, β-alanine, hypotaurine, L-serine, and β-aminobutyric acid, can activate the receptor by binding to any of the three α subunits. Positive modulators of the inhibitory GLY receptor include zinc, neurosteroids, propofol, ethanol, and volatile anesthetics such as isoflurane.[29]

The best described antagonist of the inhibitory GLY receptor is the convulsant **strychnine**. Strychnine binds to a different site from that which recognizes GLY. Sometimes the inhibitory GLY receptor is referred to as the "strychnine-sensitive" GLY receptor to distinguish it from the GLY modulatory site on the glutaminergic NMDA receptor. The $GABA_A$ receptor antagonist picrotoxin can also inhibit the GLY receptor. More recently the endocannabinoids such as anandamide and 2-arachidonylglycerol have been shown to antagonize the activity of GLY at this receptor. Agents that act as agonists at the IAA GLY receptor may find utility as anticonvulsants, muscle relaxants, sedatives, and general anesthetics.

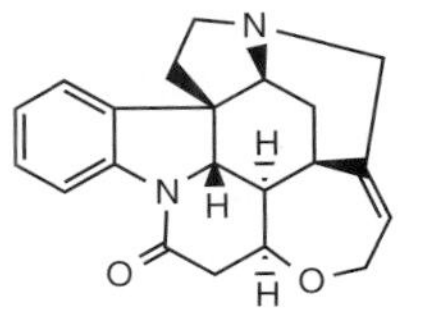

Strychnine

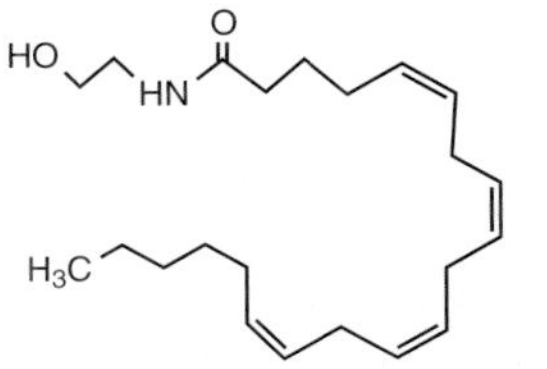

Anandamide

Zinc-Activated Channel

As another member of the Cys-loop family of receptors, the ZAC is yet to be fully characterized. It exists as a homopentamer with four transmembrane loops and is activated by divalent zinc (Zn^{2+}) and copper (Cu^{2+}) ions and by proton (H^+). Contrary to its name, Cu^{2+} and H^+ have been found to be more potent at activating this channel compared to Zn^{2+}. When open, the central pore of the ZAC is permeable to monovalent cations such as Na^+, K^+, and cesium (Cs^+) but is impermeable and inactivated by high concentrations of extracellular Ca^{2+} and magnesium (Mg^{2+}).[30] In the adult human brain, ZAC messenger RNA (mRNA) has been located in hippocampus, striatum, thalamus, and amygdala. In the periphery, ZAC mRNA is expressed in the lungs, trachea, thyroid, and prostate.[31] These channels show constitutive activity which can be blocked by tubocurarine, but their physiological roles are still under investigation.[32]

Excitatory Amino Acid Receptors

The receptors for GLU and the other excitatory amino acids (EAAs) are categorized into two major groups: ionotropic and metabotropic. The three ionotropic receptor types are classified based on their originally preferred synthetic agonist: NMDA, α-amino-3-hydroxy-5-methyl-4-isoxazole propionic acid (AMPA), and kainate. Distinct from the pentameric Cys-loop receptor family, these LGIC receptors are composed of homo- or heterotetramers of individual subunits that confer cation selectivity. Each subunit has an extracellular N-terminus with three TM domains, an intramembrane reentrant "p-loop" between the first and third TM domains, and an intracellular C-terminus.[33] The metabotropic GluRs belong to the larger family of GPCRs (see Chapter 6). When activated, these receptors can alter the activity of effector proteins such as adenylyl cyclase and phospholipase C (PLC). To date, there appears to be at least eight distinct EAA metabotropic receptor subtypes. The EAA receptors, in balance with the receptors for the IAAs, are likely crucial for the regulation of neuronal plasticity, including long-term potentiation (LTP) and long-term depression (LTD).

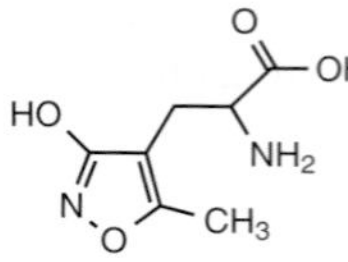

AMPA 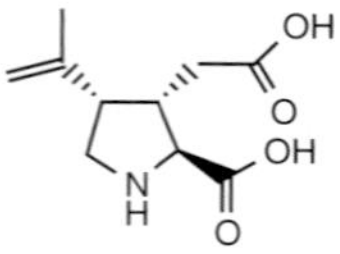 Kainic acid 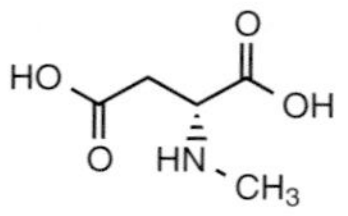 N-Methyl-D-aspartic acid (NMDA)

NMDA Receptor

The NMDA receptor is a heterotetramer comprised of a number of subunit forms termed GLUN1, GLUN2A, GLUN2B, GLUN2C, GLUN2D, GLUN3A, and GLUN3B that can confer unique pharmacology to individual receptors. Additionally, splice variants can lead to a number of isoforms of the above subunits with the potential of changing the binding characteristics and functions of the receptor. Activation of the NMDA receptor requires the binding of two agonists: GLU to the GLUN2 subunit and GLY to a binding site on the GLUN1 subunit.[34] Glycine GLY appears to act as an important coagonist-positive modulator at a unique recognition site, and unlike the actions of GLY as an IAA neurotransmitter, this recognition site is not sensitive to blockade by strychnine (see above). Thus, this GLY binding site is often referred to as the strychnine-insensitive receptor site.

Agonists at the GLU binding site include NMDA, L-glutamate, L-aspartate, and homoquinolinic acid. The best characterized antagonist at this site is D-(-)-2-Amino-5-phosphonopentanoic acid (D-AP5). In addition to GLY, D-serine is a well-known agonist at the GLY site. D-Serine, which is normally only found in glia and astrocytes, is synthesized from L-serine via serine racemase, and is thought to be one of the important modulators of NMDA receptor activity.

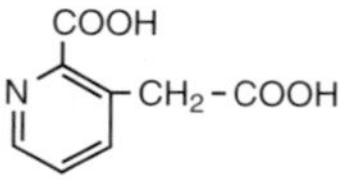

Homoquinolinic acid 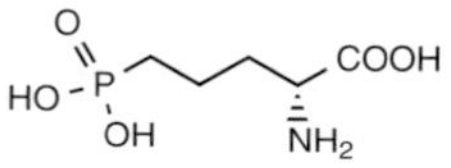 D-AP5

The NMDA receptor also has many sites for channel modulation by pharmacological agents. Endogenous inhibitory channel modulators include Mg^{2+}, Zn^{2+}, and H^{+}. Neurosteroids can either inhibit or potentiate NMDA receptor channel function depending upon the subunit forms comprising the tetrameric structure. For instance, pregnenolone sulfate inhibits NMDA receptors assembled as GLUN1/GLUN2C but potentiates those assembled as GLUN1/GLUN2A and GLUN1/GLUN2B.[35] Polyamines such as spermine and spermidine are known to be positive channel modulators.

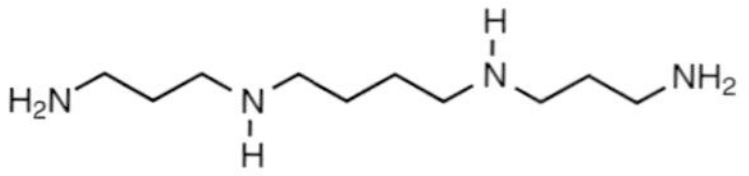

Spermine 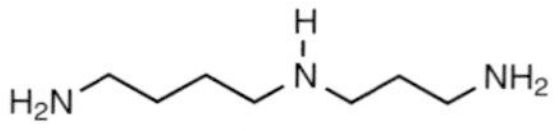 Spermidine

A number of important NMDA channel antagonists also exist and include amantadine (an antiviral agent that also releases dopamine and is used in Parkinson's disease), ketamine (a dissociative anesthetic agent that acts via the NMDA receptor), phencyclidine (a psychoactive drug of abuse also known as "PCP"), and memantine (recently approved for the treatment of Alzheimer's disease). While the antitussive agent dextromethorphan, via its metabolite dextrorphan, is known to block the NMDA channel, its cough-suppressant activity is likely not due to its action at this site. However, the psychotomimetic effects observed with the abuse of this compound could likely be NMDA receptor mediated. An endogenous antagonist of the NMDA receptor is the Mg^{2+} ion, which normally prevents the flow of Ca^{2+} through the channel. However, when both glutamate (or another suitable agonist) and glycine bind, the inhibition normally maintained by Mg^{2+} is relieved, Ca^{2+} can flow, and the cell can depolarize. Some studies in experimental animals have demonstrated the NMDA receptor–mediated neuroprotective effects of Mg^{2+} in models of stroke and other CNS insults.

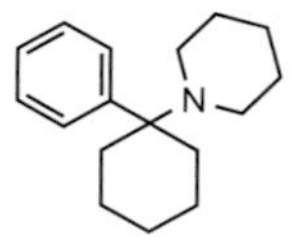

Phencyclidine (PCP) 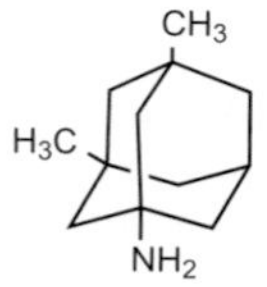 Memantine 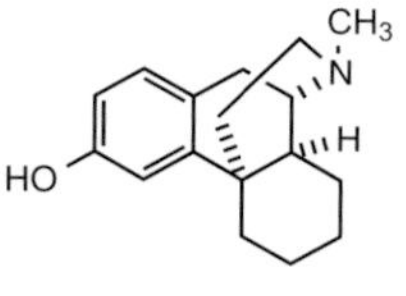 Dextrorphan

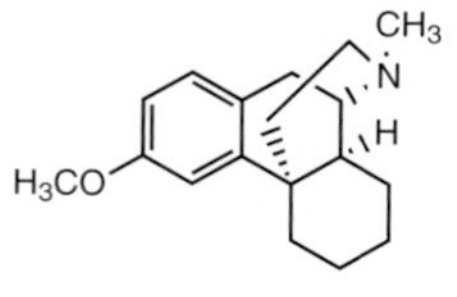

Dextromethorphan

One of the first NMDA receptor antagonists to be identified was dizocilpine, commonly known as MK-801. Much excitement was initially generated with the discovery of MK-801, as the ability to block the excessive intracellular cation flow (Ca^{2+}, Na^+) that follows neuronal hypoxic insults following cerebral vascular accidents (stroke) or head trauma might lead to effective treatments for such pathologic conditions. While MK-801 was very effective in decreasing infarct size in various rodent models of stroke, poor efficacy was noted in humans. Additionally, the generation of severe psychotic behaviors was deemed unacceptable.[36]

The strychnine-insensitive binding site on the NMDA receptor has also been a target for researchers, since an agent that would antagonize this binding site might be useful in preventing the neuronal damage that occurs following hypoxic insults leading to excessive GLU release or in controlling electrical neuronal dysfunction associated with epilepsy. One agent, (R)-HA-966 (*R*-(+)-3-amino-1-hydroxypyrrolidin-2-one), is a GLY receptor antagonist that, unfortunately, has not been used therapeutically due to its NMDA receptor–unrelated hepatotoxic properties. While the anticonvulsant felbamate (2-phenyl-1,3-propanedioldicarbamate) produces part of its activity by allosterically altering the binding of GLY at the NMDA GLY binding site, it also has interactions at the AMPA and kainate receptors which contribute to its anticonvulsant activity.[37]

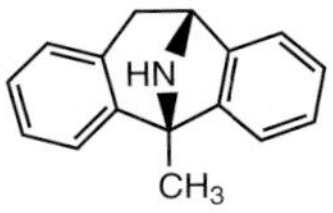

Dizocilpine

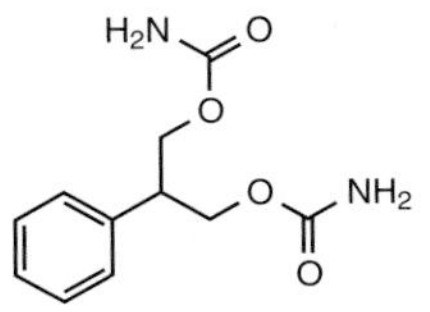

Felbamate

AMPA Receptors

Another ionotropic EAA receptor is preferentially activated by AMPA. While at one time this receptor was referred to as the quisqualate receptor, the AMPA receptor (as it is now known) mediates fast synaptic activity via the influx of Na^+ and, in some neurons, K^+ efflux. The AMPA receptor, in high abundance in the cerebral cortex and hippocampus, is comprised of subunits GluR1, GluR2, GluR3, and GluR4. One of these subunits, GluR2, when present prevents the formation of an ionophore that can efficiently conduct Ca^{2+}. However, when the AMPA receptor does not contain a GluR2 subunit, Ca^{2+} can be conducted through the ion channel. On the extracellular loop between TM3 and TM4, there exists a region termed the "flip-flop" that is sensitive to splice variants of the gene coding for each subunit. Such splice variants can lead to significant differences in the desensitization kinetics of the receptor.[38] Additionally, intracellular sites on the C-terminus, where modulatory proteins such as NSF (N-ethylmaleimide-sensitive fusion protein) and PICK (protein interacting with C kinase) can bind, allow for another important site where regulation of receptor trafficking can be influenced.

The discovery that some of the 2,3-benzodiazepines (e.g., GYK1 53655) can selectively bind the AMPA receptor has aided in studies to understand its location and functions, especially where mixed populations of EAA receptors are present.[39] Agents known to potentiate AMPA receptor activity include piracetam (2-oxo-1-pyrrolidine acetamide), a cyclic derivative of GABA, and the benzothiazide cyclothiazide (6-chloro-3,4-dihydro-3[2-norbornen-5-yl]-2H-1,2,4-benzothiadiazine-7-sulfonamide). Additionally, some evidence suggests that certain barbiturates and volatile anesthetics have binding sites on the AMPA receptor. Agents that positively modulate the AMPA receptor have been termed "ampakines" and have been suggested in various studies to improve memory, enhance the activity of certain antipsychotic agents, improve attention-deficit hyperactivity disorder, improve Parkinson's disease symptoms, and provide neuroprotection following CNS ischemic insults.[40]

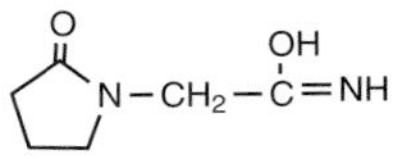

Piracetam

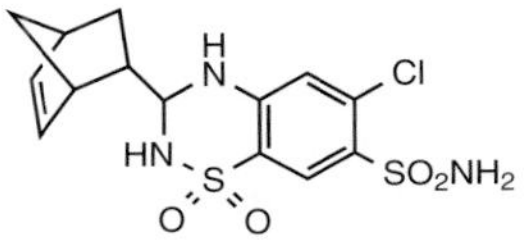

Cyclothiazide

Kainate Receptors

The ionotropic kainate receptor is a heterotetramer comprised of subunits GluR5, GluR6, GluR7, KA1, and KA2. While GluR5-7 can form functional homo- and heteromeric receptors, the KA1 and KA2 subunits require the presence of the Glu5-7 subunits to assemble into functional receptors. Similarities exist between the binding characteristics of AMPA receptors and kainite receptors, such that few pharmacological agents are available that effectively differentiate between the two.[41] Kainate receptors tend to be more sensitive to the kainic acid analog domoic acid than AMPA receptors.

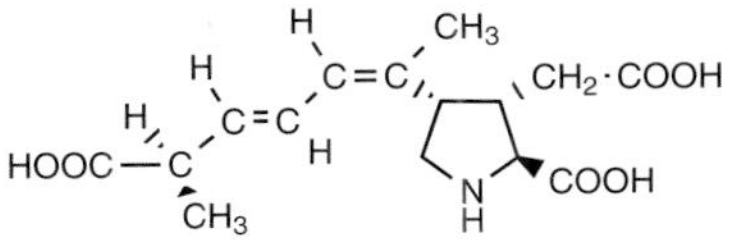

Domoic acid

While kainate receptors are located postsynaptically and mediate neuronal excitation (as do NMDA and AMPA receptors), kainate receptors have also been found presynaptically. Such presynaptic receptors appear to act to regulate the release of GABA in the hippocampus and GLU in other brain regions. Additionally, some kainate receptors have been shown to be linked to a pertussis toxin–sensitive G protein which, via interaction with PLC, in turn, may act to influence nearby voltage-dependent Ca^{2+} channels.[42] This dual signaling capability of kainate receptors appears unique for an EAA ionotropic receptor and may facilitate the role of this receptor subtype in influencing both short- and long-term synaptic plasticity in the CNS.

P2X Receptors

Purinergic P2X receptors occur as trimeric proteins with agonist-binding extracellular domains, the pore-forming transmembrane (TM1-TM2) domains, and intracellular domains. Seven functional isoforms (P2X1-P2X7) have been identified to date in mammals, varying from homotrimers to heterotrimers.[43] These receptors are gated by adenosine-5′-triphosphate (ATP), at least three molecules of which are needed to open this channel, and nucleotide analogs of ATP have been found to have agonistic effects. Pore opening allows for the flow of Na^+, K^+, and Ca^{2+} ions. Prolonged ATP binding leads to receptor desensitization to varying degrees between the seven receptor subtypes. A number of allosteric modulators (e.g., zinc, copper) have been found to have varying effects on receptor activation based on the modulator concentration and receptor subtype.[44] Ivermectin (an antihelminthic agent used to treat river blindness in humans and commonly used in veterinary medicine for heart worms; also known to bind to GABA and GLY receptors) interacts with P2X4 as a positive modulator potentiating ATP-gated currents.[45] Because these receptors are involved in the release of inflammatory molecules, selective antagonists for the P2X7 and P2X3 have been explored for their use in inflammatory pain with mixed results.

R =
$B_{1\alpha}$ = C_2H_5
$B_{1\beta}$ = CH_3

Ivermectin

Voltage-Gated and Second Messenger–Gated Channels

Although not considered receptors since they are not ligand dependent, there are other ion channels that are controlled by either voltage changes or second messenger molecules. An example of a voltage-gated channel includes the Na^+ channels responsible for impulse conduction in sensory nerve fibers that transmit information about pain and temperature. Following administration, the local anesthetic lidocaine enters the nerve cell via diffusion in its free base form. Once inside the nerve cell, lidocaine is protonated and, in this charged form, is capable of blocking the sodium (Na^+) channel from the intracellular side. Some second messenger molecules (e.g., cAMP and IP_3) generated following the activation of GPCRs can influence the degree of channel opening or closing. The most common channels influenced by these second messengers include those for Ca^{2+} and K^+.

Mechanisms of Calcium Movement and Storage

The regulation of cytosolic Ca^{2+} levels occurs via specific influx, efflux, and sequestering mechanisms (Fig. 8.4). The influx of Ca^{2+} can occur through receptor-operated channels (site 1), the Na^+/Ca^{2+} exchange process (site 2), "leak" pathways (site 3), and potential-dependent channels (site 4). Influx via either receptor-operated or voltage-dependent channels has been proposed to be the major entry pathway for Ca^{2+}. Receptor-operated channels have been defined as those associated with cellular membrane receptors and activated by specific agonist-receptor interactions. In contrast, potential-dependent channels, also known as voltage-dependent or voltage-gated calcium channels, have been defined as those activated by membrane depolarization. The Na^+/Ca^{2+} exchange process can promote either influx or efflux because the direction of Ca^{2+} movement depends on the relative intracellular and extracellular ratios of Na^+ and Ca^{2+}. The "leak" pathways, which include unstimulated Ca^{2+} entry as well as entry during the fast-inward Na^+ phase of an action potential, play only a minor role in Ca^{2+} influx.

Efflux can occur through either an ATP-driven membrane pump (site 5) or via the Na^+/Ca^{2+} exchange process previously mentioned (site 2). In addition to these influx and efflux mechanisms, the sarcoplasmic reticulum (site 6) and the mitochondria (site 7) function as internal storage/release

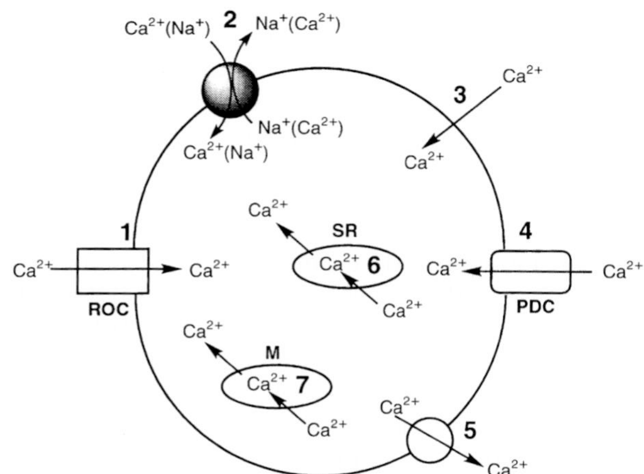

Figure 8.4 Cellular mechanisms for the influx, efflux, and sequestering of Ca^{2+}. M, mitochondria; PDC, potential-dependent Ca^{2+} channels; ROC, receptor-operated Ca^{2+} channels; and SR, sarcoplasmic reticulum.

sites. These storage sites work in concert with the influx and efflux processes to assure that cytosolic Ca^{2+} levels are appropriate for cellular needs. Although influx and release processes are essential for excitation-contraction coupling, efflux and sequestering processes are equally important for terminating the contractile process and for protecting the cell from the deleterious effects of Ca^{2+} overload.[46,47]

Potential-Dependent Calcium Channels

The pharmacologic class of agents known as calcium channel blockers produces their effects through interaction with potential-dependent channels. To date, six functional subclasses, or types, of potential-dependent Ca^{2+} channels have been identified: T, L, N, P, Q, and R. These types differ in location and function and can be divided into two major groups: low-voltage–activated (LVA) channels and high-voltage–activated (HVA) channels. Of the six types, only the T (transient, tiny) channel can be rapidly activated and inactivated with small changes in the cell membrane potential. It is thus designated as an LVA channel. All of the other types of channels require a larger depolarization and are thus designated as HVA channels.

The L (long-lasting, large) channel is the site of action for currently available calcium channel blockers and, therefore, has been extensively studied. It is located in skeletal, cardiac, and smooth muscle and, thus, is highly involved in organ and vessel contraction within the cardiovascular system. The N channel is found in neuronal tissue and exhibits kinetics and inhibitory sensitivity distinct from both L and T channels. The functions, sensitivities, and properties of the other three types of channels are not as well known. The P channel has been named for its presence in the Purkinje cells, whereas the Q and R channels have been characterized by their abilities to bind to certain polypeptide toxins.[48,49]

The L channel is a pentameric complex consisting of α_1, α_2, β, γ, and δ polypeptides (Fig. 8.5). The α_1 subunit is a transmembrane-spanning protein that consists of four domains and functions as the pore-forming subunit. The α_1 subunit also contains binding sites for all the currently available calcium channel blockers. The other four subunits surround the α_1 portion of the channel and contribute to the overall hydrophobicity of the pentamer. This hydrophobicity is important in that it allows the channel to be embedded in the cell membrane. Additionally, the α_2, δ, and β subunits modulate the α_1 subunit.

Other types of potential-dependent channels are similar to the L channel. They all have a central α_1 subunit; however, molecular cloning studies have revealed that there are at least six α_1 genes: α_{1S}, α_{1A}, α_{1B}, α_{1C}, α_{1D}, and α_{1E}. Three of these genes, α_{1S}, α_{1C}, and α_{1D}, have been associated with L channels. The L channels found in skeletal muscle result from the α_{1S} gene; those in the heart, aorta, lung, and fibroblast result from the α_{1C} gene; and those in endocrine tissue result from the α_{1D} gene. Both α_{1C} and α_{1D} are used for L channels in the brain. Thus, there are some differences among the L channels located in different organs and tissues. Additionally, differences in α_1 genes and differences among the other subunits are responsible for the variations seen among the other five types of potential-dependent channels. As an example, the N channel lacks the γ subunit and contains an α_1 subunit derived from the α_{1B} gene.[48] A number of calcium channel blockers are currently available for use in cardiovascular disorders (see Chapter 15).

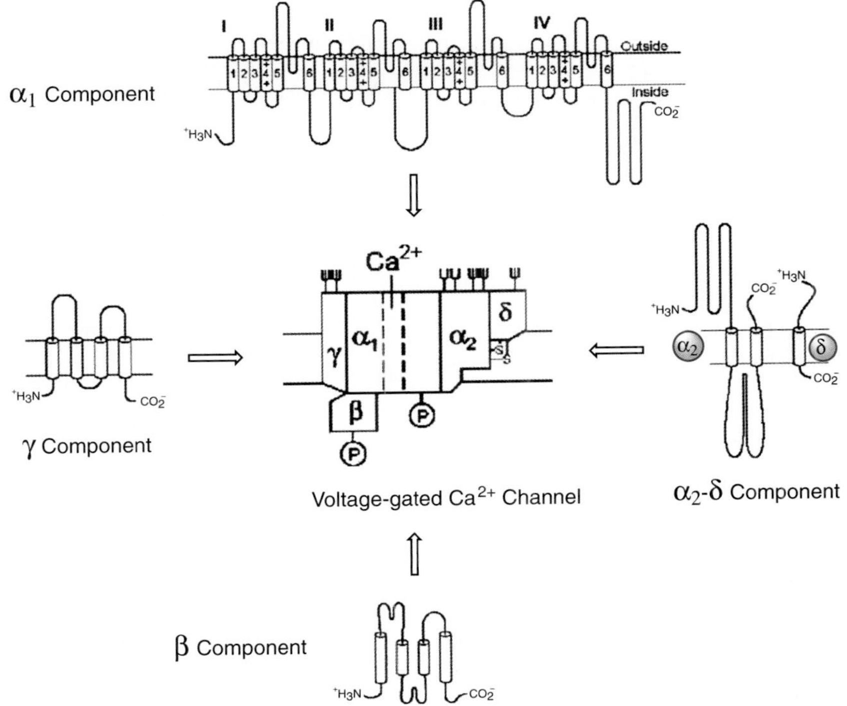

Figure 8.5 Representation of the structure of the voltage-gated Ca^{2+} channel (L channel) composed of several subunits—α_1, $\alpha_2\delta$, β, γ—organized as depicted in the central area.

ACKNOWLEDGMENTS

The authors wish to acknowledge the work of E. Kim Fifer, PhD, and Mark Harrold, PhD, who authored the content used within this chapter in a previous edition of this text.

REFERENCES

1. Sparling BA, DiMauro EF. Progress in the discovery of small molecule modulators of the Cys-loop superfamily receptors. *Bioorg Med Chem Lett*. 2017;27(15):3207-3218.
2. Albuquerque EX, Pereira EF, Alkondon M, et al. Mammalian nicotinic acetylcholine receptors: from structure to function. *Physiol Rev*. 2009;89:73-120.
3. Papke RL. Merging old and new perspectives on nicotinic acetylcholine receptors. *Biochem Pharmacol*. 2014;89:1-11.
4. Taylor P, Brown JH. Nicotinic receptors. In: Siegel GJ, Agranoff BW, Albers RW, et al, eds. *Basic Neurochemistry: Molecular, Cellular and Medical Aspects*. 6th ed. Philadelphia: Lippincott-Raven; 1999.
5. Lindstrom J, Anand R, Peng X, et al. Neuronal nicotinic receptor subtypes. *Ann NY Acad Sci*. 1995;757:100-116.
6. Westfall TC, Macarthur H, Westfall DP. Neurotransmission: the autonomic and somatic motor nervous systems. In: Brunton LL, Lazo JS. Parker KL, eds. *Goodman and Gilman's the Pharmacological Basis of Therapeutics*. 13th ed. New York: McGraw-Hill; 2018:115-148.
7. Crooks PA, Bardo MT, Dwoskin LP. Nicotinic receptor antagonists as treatments for nicotine abuse. *Adv Pharmacol*. 2014;69:513-551.
8. McIntyre AR. History of curare. In: Cheymol J, ed. *International Encyclopedia of Pharmacology and Therapeutics, Section 14*. Vol. 1. Oxford: Pergamon Press; 1972:187-203.
9. King H. Curarie alkaloids. I. Tubocurarine. *J Chem Soc*. 1935:1381-1389.
10. Everett AJ, Lowe AJ, Wilkinson S. Revision of the structures of (+)-tubocurarine chloride and (+)-chondrocurine. *J Chem Soc*. 1970;16:1020-1021.
11. Kistler J, Stroud RM. Crystalline arrays of membrane-bound acetylcholine receptor. *Proc Natl Acad Sci USA*. 1981;78:3678-3682.
12. Barnard EA, Coates V, Dolly JO, et al. Binding of α-bungarotoxin and cholinergic ligands to acetylcholine receptors in the membrane of skeletal muscle. *Cell Biol Int Rep*. 1977;1:99-106.
13. Raghavendra T. Neuromuscular blocking drugs: discovery and development. *J R Soc Med*. 2002;95(7):363-367.
14. Thompson AJ. Recent developments in 5-HT3 receptor pharmacology. *Trends Pharmacol Sci*. 2013;34:100-109.
15. Gupta D, Prabhakar V, Radhakrishnan M. 5HT3 receptors: target for new antidepressant drugs. *Neurosci Biobehav Rev*. 2016;64:311-325.
16. Parker RM, Barnes JM, Ge J, et al. Autoradiographic distribution of [3H]-(S)zacopride-labelled 5 HT-3 receptors in human brain. *J Neurol Sci*. 1996;144:119-127.
17. Walstab J, Rappold G, Niesler B. 5-HT3 receptors: role in disease and target of drugs. *Pharmacol Ther*. 2010;128:146-169.
18. Rudolph U, Mohler H. GABA-based therapeutic approaches: GABAA receptor subtype functions. *Curr Opin Pharmacol*. 2006;6:18-23.
19. Rudolph U, Crestani F, Benke D, et al. Benzodiazepine actions mediated by specific gamma-aminobutyric acid(A) receptor subtypes. *Nature*. 1999;401:796-800.
20. Löw K, Crestani F, Keist R, et al. Molecular and neuronal substrates for the selective attenuation of anxiety. *Science*. 2000;290:131-134.
21. Foster AC, Pelleymounter MA, Cullen MJ, et al. In vivo pharmacological characterization of indipion, a novel pyrazolopyrimidine sedative-hypnotic. *J Pharmacol Exp Ther*. 2004;311:547-559.
22. Lancel M, Langebartels A. Gamma-aminobutyric acid(A) agonist 4,5,6,7-tetrahydroisoxazolo[4,5-c] pyridine-3-ol persistently increases sleep maintenance and intensity during chronic administration to rats. *J Pharmacol Exp Ther*. 2000;293:1084-1090.
23. Whiting PJ. GABA-A receptors: a viable target for novel anxiolytics? *Curr Opin Pharmacol*. 2006;6:24-29.
24. Sternfeld F, Carling RW, Jelley RA, et al. Selective, orally active gamma-aminobutyric acidA alpha5 receptor inverse agonists as cognition enhancers. *J Med Chem*. 2004;47:2176-2179.
25. Yee BK, Keist R, von Boehmer L, et al. A schizophrenia-related sensorimotor deficit links α3-containing GABAA receptors to a dopamine hyperfunction. *Proc Natl Acad Sci USA*. 2005;102:17154-17159.
26. Jurd R, Arras M, Lambert S, et al. General anesthetic actions in vivo strongly attenuated by point mutation in the GABA(A) receptor beta3 subunit. *FASEB J*. 2003;17:250-252.
27. Seighart W, Sperk G. Subunit composition, distribution and function of GABA(A) receptor subtypes. *Curr Top Med Chem*. 2002;2:795-816.
28. Breitinger HG, Becker CM. The inhibitory glycine receptor-simple views of a complicated channel. *Chembiochem*. 2003;3:1042-1052.
29. Lobo IA, Harris RA. Sites of alcohol and volatile anesthetic action on glycine receptors. *Int Rev Neurobiol*. 2005;65:53-87.
30. Trattnig SM, Gasiorek A, Deeb TZ, et al. Copper and protons directly activate the zinc-activated channel. *Biochem Pharmacol*. 2016;103:109-117.
31. Houtani T, Munemoto Y, Kase M, et al. Cloning and expression of ligand-gated ion-channel receptor L2 in central nervous system. *Biochem Biophys Res Commun*. 2005;335:277-285.
32. Davies PA, Wang W, Hales TG, et al. A novel class of ligand-gated ion channel is activated by Zn^{2+}. *J Biol Chem*. 2003;278:712-717.
33. Dingdledine R, Borges K, Bowie D, et al. The glutamate receptor ion channels. *Pharmacol Rev*. 1999;51:7-61.
34. Erreger K, Chen PE, Wyllie DJ, et al. Glutamate receptor gating. *Crit Rev Neurobiol*. 2004;16:187-224.
35. Maleyev A, Gibbs TT, Farb DH. Inhibition of the NMDA response by pregnenolone sulphate revels subtype selective modulation of NMDA receptors by sulphated steroids. *Br J Pharmacol*. 2002;135:901-909.
36. Huettner JE, Bean BP. Block of N-methyl-D-aspartate-activated current by the anticonvulsant MK-801: selective binding to open channels. *Proc Natl Acad Sci USA*. 1988;85:1307-1311.
37. Subramaniam S, Rho JM, Penix L, et al. Felbamate block of the N-methyl-D-aspartate receptor. *J Pharmacol Exp Ther*. 1995;273:878-886.
38. Brorson JR, Li D, Suzuki T. Selective expression of heteromeric AMPA receptors driven by flip-flop differences. *J Neurosci*. 2004;24:3461-3470.
39. Paternain AV, Morales M, Lerma J. Selective antagonism of AMPA receptors unmasks kainate receptor-mediated responses in hippocampal neurons. *Neuron*. 1995;14:185-189.
40. Lynch G. Glutamate-based therapeutic approaches: ampakines. *Curr Opin Pharmacol*. 2006;6:82-88.
41. Lerma J, Paternain AV, Rodriguez-Moreno A, et al. Molecular physiology of kainate receptors. *Physiol Rev*. 2001;81:971-998.
42. Lerna J. Kainate receptor physiology. *Curr Opin Pharmacol*. 2006;6:89-97.
43. North RA. Molecular physiology of P2 receptors. *Physiol Rev*. 2002;82:1013-1067.
44. Stojilkovic SS, Leiva-Salcedo E, Rokic MB, et al. Regulation of ATP-gated P2X channels: from redox signaling to interactions with other proteins. *Antioxid Redox Signal*. 2014;21:953-970.
45. Pasqualetto G, Brancale A, Young MT. The molecular determinants of small-molecule ligand binding at P2X receptors. *Front Pharmacol*. 2018;9:58.
46. Janis RA, Triggle DJ. New developments in Ca^{2+} channel antagonists. *J Med Chem*. 1983;26:775-785.
47. Swamy VC, Triggle DJ. Calcium channel blockers. In: Craig CR, Stitzel RE, eds. *Modern Pharmacology With Clinical Applications*. 6th ed. Lippincott Williams & Wilkins; 2004:218-224.
48. Varadi G, Mori Y, Mikala G, et al. Molecular determinants of Ca^{2+} channel function and drug action. *Trends Pharmacol Sci*. 1995;16:43-49.
49. Gilmore J, Dell C, Bowman D, et al. Neuronal calcium channels. *Annu Rep Med Chem*. 1995;30:51-60.

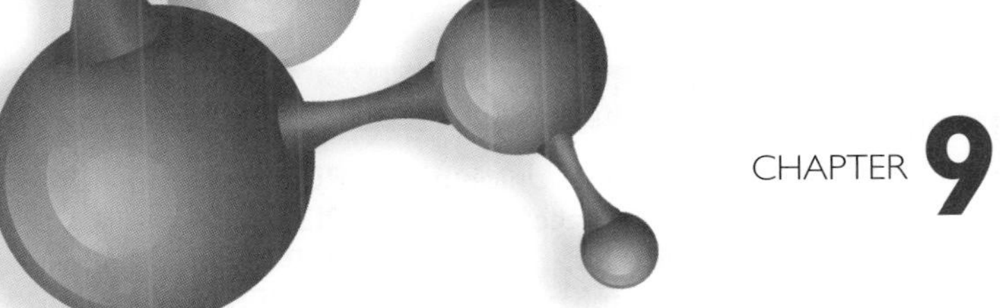

CHAPTER **9**

Enzyme/Catalytic Receptors

Stephen G. Kerr

Drugs covered in this chapter:

- Acetylcholine
- Alisertib
- Amoxicillin
- Ara C
- Azidothymidine
- Barasertib
- Bosutinib
- Captopril
- Cilomilast
- Cilostazol
- Clavulanic acid
- Coformycin
- Dabrafenib
- Danusertib
- Dasatinib
- Deoxycoformycin
- Dideoxycytidine
- Dipyridamole
- Enalaprilat
- Enalapril
- Everolimus
- Finasteride
- Fluorodeoxyuridine monophosphate
- Fluorouracil
- Gabaculin
- Gefitinib
- Ibrutinib
- Imatinib
- Inamrinone
- Methotrexate
- Milrinone
- Nevirapine
- Penicillin
- Physostigmine
- Prontosil
- Rapamycin
- Roflumilast
- Sildenafil
- Sirolimus
- Sulfanilamide
- Sunitinib
- Taladafil
- Temsirolimus
- Thiacytidine
- Thymidine
- Trametinib
- Vardenafil
- Vemurafenib
- Zaprinast

Abbreviations

ACE angiotensin-converting enzyme
AChE acetylcholinesterase
Akt protein kinase B
AMP adenosine monophosphate
ANP atrial natriuretic peptide
Ara-C cytosine arabinoside
ATP adenosine triphosphate
AZT azidothymidine
cAMP cyclic adenosine monophosphate
cGMP cyclic guanosine monophosphate
CML chronic myelogenous leukemia
dC deoxycytidine
ddC 2′,3′-dideoxycytidine
DFG aspartate-phenyl-glycine
DHFR dihydrofolate reductase
dNTP deoxynucleotide triphosphate
E enzyme
EC Enzyme Commission
EGFR epidermal growth factor receptor
E.I. enzyme-inhibitor complex
E.S. enzyme-substrate complex
FDA US Food and Drug Administration
FdUMP 5-fluorodeoxyuridine monophosphate
5-FU 5-fluorouracil
GABA-T γ-aminobutyric acid transaminase
GTP guanosine triphosphate
HGNC Human Genome Nominating Committee
k_{cat} catalytic or first-order rate constant
K_d enzyme-substrate dissociation constant
K_i inhibition constant
k_{inact} inactivation rate constant
K_p partition ratio
k_{diff} diffusion rate constant
KLIFS kinase-ligand interaction fingerprints and structures
K_m Michaelis-Menten constant or apparent substrate-enzyme dissociation constant
M moles/L
mTOR mammalian target of rapamycin

Abbreviations—Continued

NC-IUPHAR International Union of Basic and Clinical Pharmacology
NDA new drug application
NTP nucleoside triphosphate
cNMP cyclic nucleoside monophosphate
P product
Pi inorganic phosphate
PAP 2-phenylaminopyrimidine
PDE phosphodiesterase
PI3K phosphoinositide-3-kinase
PLP pyridoxal phosphate
PDGFR platelet-derived growth factor receptor
PTP protein tyrosine phosphatases
RT reverse transcriptase
RTK receptor tyrosine kinases
S substrate
SAR structure-activity relationship
3-TC 3-thiacytidine
TKI tyrosine kinase inhibitor
TLCK tosyl-lysyl-chloromethyl-ketone
TPCK tosyl-phenylalanyl-chloromethyl-ketone
v velocity or rate of enzyme reaction
V_{max} maximum velocity or rate of enzyme reaction

INTRODUCTION

Overview of Catalytic Receptors and Enzymes: A Perspective

The sequencing of the human genome has resulted in an explosive growth into the research and understanding of receptors. Furthermore, it has also spawned the adoption of select nomenclature to categorize receptors.[1] The NC-IUPHAR (International Union of Basic and Clinical Pharmacology) works closely with the Human Genome Nominating Committee (HGNC) to standardize the receptor nomenclature. In elementary terms, a receptor may be defined as a biomacromolecule (protein, nucleic acid, polysaccharide, or lipid aggregate) that on binding a ligand results in some biological effect. Receptors may be present on the cell surface, be cytoplasmic or in extracellular fluid. Those present on the cell surface, on binding a ligand, transmit a signal resulting in some cellular action. Catalytic receptors are specifically those cell surface receptors whose binding to a ligand causes conformational changes, such as dimeric action or oligomerization, which results in a chemical reaction (usually phosphorylation) leading to activation of downstream signaling events. The NC-IUPHAR has described three major catalytic receptors which include many subtypes. The major catalytic receptors are the cytokine receptors, pattern receptors, receptor kinases inclusive of the tyrosine kinase and serine/threonine kinases or tyrosine-like kinases.[1] Catalytic receptors have been subdivided based on their specific catalytic reaction, and there are five major transmembrane receptors with catalytic activity. These are the receptor tyrosine kinases (RTK)—the largest group which on being activated by a ligand, dimerize and phosphorylate tyrosine residues on the cytosolic side of the receptor; the tyrosine phosphatases which can dephosphorylate (or hydrolyze) phosphorylated tyrosine residues; tyrosine-associated receptor kinases (nonreceptor tyrosine kinases) that phosphorylate cytosolic proteins; the receptor serine/threonine kinases which can phosphorylate serine/threonine residues on cytosolic proteins; and the receptor guanylyl cyclases that catalyze the formation of cGMP from GTP on the cytosolic side to induce signaling. See Figure 9.1 for a brief depiction of the various catalytic receptors.[2] More general types of receptors, however, are the biological catalysts, which are more commonly known as enzymes, since they bind substrates (ligands) and in essence transmit a "biological signal" through product formation of the chemical reaction being catalyzed which results in some specific action. It is often the dysregulation of these receptors either through genetic mutation or through over/under-expression that results in various disease states (e.g., cancer, autoimmune disease, diabetes) as homeostasis gets disrupted and signaling mechanisms are compromised. During infections of the host, it is the expression or presence of foreign substances—proteins, lipids, nucleic acids, and other factors, that result in the pathogenesis. For either of the above scenarios, in order to ameliorate the disease state, the design of molecules (drugs) to counterbalance the dysregulation or neutralize the pathogen has long been a continuous developmental strategy.

The concept of using small molecules that specifically target one or more enzymatic systems in the body is not new. Historically, compounds that were extracted from natural products have been used as medicinal agents. Subsequently, they have been shown to have their therapeutic effect by targeting certain systemic enzymes.[3] A classic example is the bark of the willow tree, known since ancient days to have antipyretic and analgesic effects. Its active ingredient, salicin, a glycoside, is metabolized in vivo to salicylic acid, which is a known inhibitor of cyclooxygenase, a key enzyme in the formation of prostaglandins, which are mediators of pain and fever. Similarly, physostigmine, isolated from the West African Calabar bean, was used as a treatment for glaucoma in the mid-1800s.

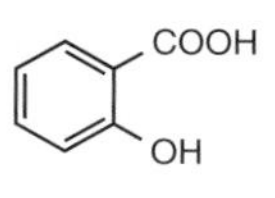

Salicylic acid 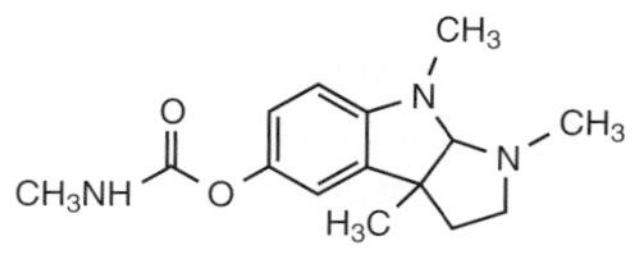 Physostigmine

Physostigmine's mechanism of action was only later determined to be inhibition of acetylcholinesterase.[3] Inhibition of acetylcholinesterase in the eye leads to

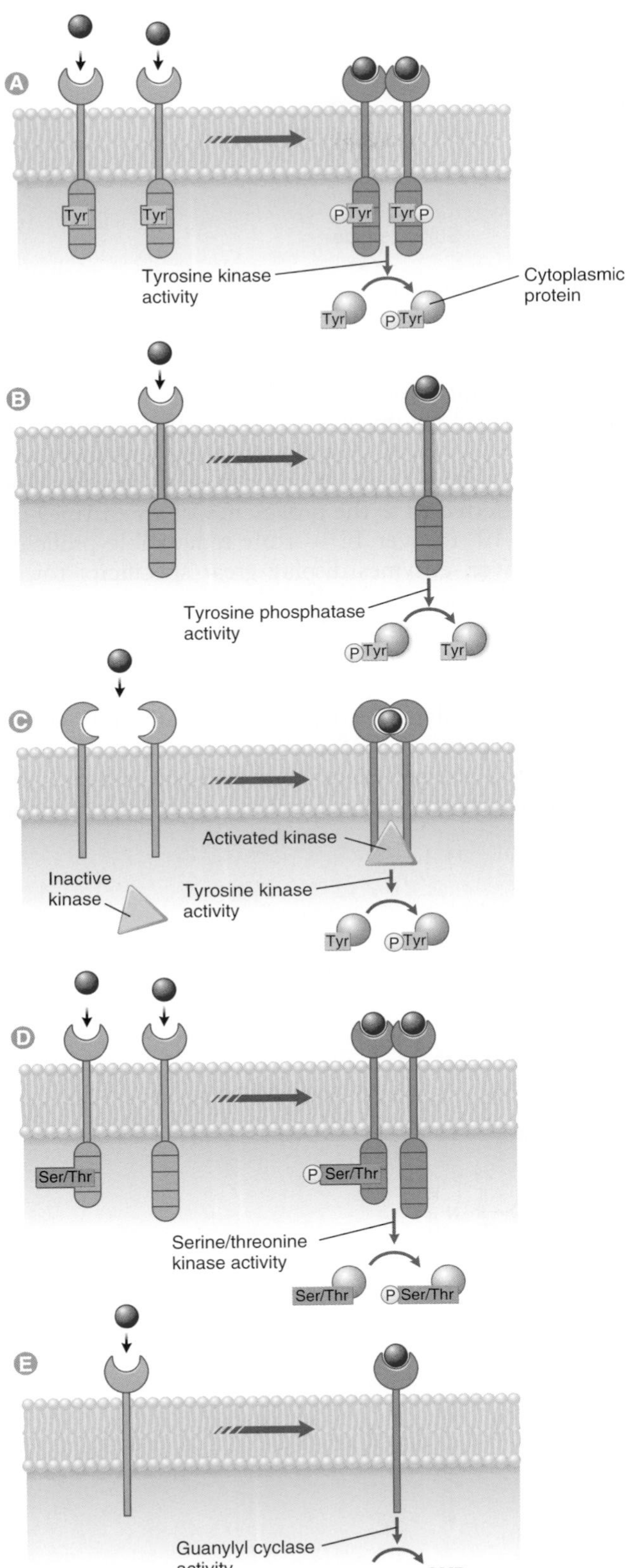

Figure 9.1 Major types of transmembrane receptors with linked enzymatic domains. A, The receptor tyrosine kinases. B, Tyrosine phosphatases. C, Tyrosine kinase-associated receptors. D, Receptor serine/threonine kinases. E, Receptor guanylyl cyclases. Reprinted with permission from Golan DE, Armstrong EJ, Armstrong AW, eds. *Principles of Pharmacology: The Pathophysiologic Basis of Drug Therapy.* 4th ed. Wolters Kluwer; 2017:12: chap 1.

improved drainage and, thus, a decrease in the intraocular pressure giving relief to glaucoma patients. It was only in the 20th century, with the concept of the "magic bullet" having selective toxicity, introduced by Ehrlich as a rational approach to chemotherapy,[4] that the concept of rational design and discovery of enzyme inhibitors followed. The discovery of the antibacterial activity of the azo dye prontosil in 1935 by Domagk,[4] and the subsequent explanation[5] of its metabolic reduction to sulfanilamide, an antimetabolite of *p*-aminobenzoic acid, in 1940 by Woods, finally paved the way for the rational design of enzyme inhibitors (Fig. 9.2). *p*-Aminobenzoic acid is an essential metabolite used in the bacterial synthesis of folic acid. Sulfanilamide, by its structural resemblance to *p*-aminobenzoic acid, competes for and selectively inhibits the bacterial enzyme dihydropteroate synthase (Fig. 9.3). In the absence of dihydropteroic acid, the bacteria are unable to synthesize tetrahydrofolic acid, an essential cofactor in one-carbon transfers that is involved in the de novo synthesis of purines and in the synthesis of thymidylate.

This concept of designing drugs as antimetabolites, or structural analogues of essential metabolites, became the hallmark for the development of enzyme inhibitors. This was especially important in cancer therapy during the early days of rational drug design.[6] As mechanisms of enzymes became better understood, the inhibitor design strategy grew more sophisticated, resulting in more potent and selective inhibitors being developed. The present-day focus on drug design through enzyme inhibition makes use of the antimetabolite theory as well as detailed kinetic and mechanistic information about the enzymatic pathways. These strategies use sophisticated assays, enzyme crystal structures and active site environments, site-directed mutagenesis experiments of catalytic residues of enzymes, and molecular docking experiments employing computers. It must be mentioned, however, that in the drug design process, designing a potent inhibitor of an enzyme is only the first step in the long and difficult process of drug development. Other factors, including pharmacokinetic profile of the inhibitor, toxicities and side effects, and animal and preclinical studies, must all be satisfactorily completed or addressed before the inhibitor can even enter clinical studies as a new drug candidate. Thus, even though an enormous amount of data exist regarding enzyme inhibitors, only a selected few turn out to be marketable drugs (Table 9.1).

In the succeeding paragraphs, an overview of enzymes as catalytic receptors and general concepts of enzyme inhibitors and their rational design into drugs will be discussed with selected examples. Enzymes catalyze chemical reactions involved in the biosynthesis and degradation of many cellular products. Moreover, all catalytic receptors have enzymatic activity and are involved in group transfer reactions with amino acid side chains on polypeptides resulting in products that propagate a cellular signal. Historically, enzymes derive their name from Greek, where "enzyme" means "in yeast" and the term was used to distinguish the "whole" microorganism, such as yeast ("organized ferments"), from the "extracts" of the whole microorganisms ("unorganized ferments"). Although the vast majority of enzymes are proteins, certain nucleic acids

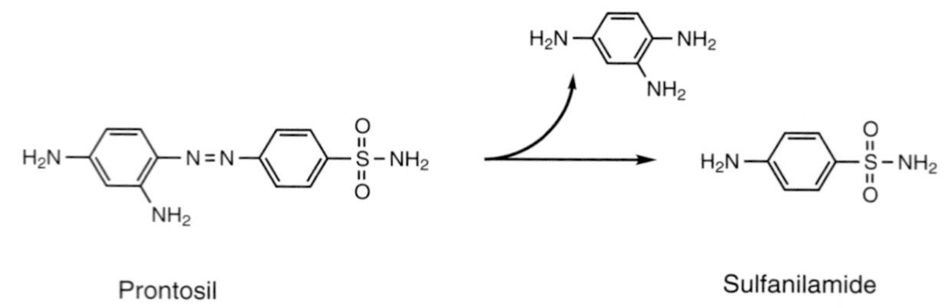

Figure 9.2 Metabolic reduction of prontosil to sulfanilamide.

(RNAs) also possess enzymatic activity (i.e., ribozymes). Enzymes are the most efficient catalysts known in nature because they have the ability to enhance reaction rates by enormous factors.[7] Like all catalysts, enzymes have the ability to lower the activation energy of reactions, and the tremendous catalytic power they posses results from their inherent ability to provide stabilization to the reacting molecules at their activated complex states. From a preliminary enquiry, enzymatic rates for reactions in physiological solutions are limited by the diffusion rate constant of water. This implies that the second-order rate constant of an enzyme (k_{cat}/K_m) is approximately 10^9 M^{-1} s^{-1} (diffusion rate constant of water),[8] a value that infers that every collision of a reactant molecule (substrate) with the enzyme leads to product formation. Because for many enzymes K_m (the Michaelis or apparent substrate-enzyme dissociation constant) values are in the micro- or sub-micromolar range (10^{-4} M), one can compute the k_{cat} (the catalytic or first-order rate constant) value to be approximately 10^5/s. Estimates[9] for uncatalyzed reactions in water have ranged from 10^{-1} to 10^{-20}/s; thus, the rate enhancements for enzyme-catalyzed reactions over the noncatalyzed reaction (also referred to as the proficiency of an enzyme) can range from 10^6 to over 10^{25}—truly remarkable proficiencies. Moreover, enzymes display great specificity toward particular chemical bonds (bond specificity; e.g., peptidases for peptide bonds) or functional groups (group specificity; e.g., esterases for esters), or they display absolute specificity toward a single molecule (e.g., carbonic anhydrase, which catalyzes the hydration of carbon dioxide or decomposition of carbonic acid). Furthermore, this specificity and catalytic proficiency is carried out, in most cases, at ambient temperatures and normal pressures in aqueous solutions.

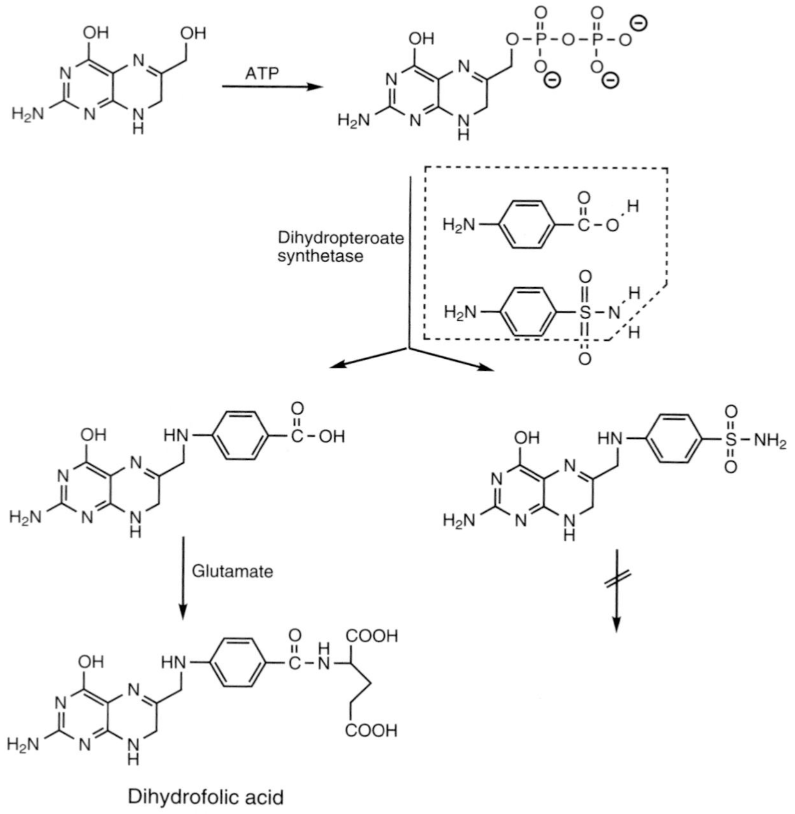

Figure 9.3 Metabolic pathway leading to dihydrofolic acid and its inhibition by sulfanilamide. This figure shows the structural resemblance to *p*-aminobenzoic acid.

Table 9.1 A Partial Listing of Enzyme Inhibitor Presently Used as Drugs

Inhibitor (Drug)	Enzyme Inhibited	Use	Organism
Caspofungin	1,3-β-Glucan synthase	Antifungal	Fungal
Trilostane	3-(or 17)β-Hydroxysteroid dehydrogenase	Breast cancer	Human
Sildenafil	3′,5′-Cyclic GMP phosphodiesterase	Erectile dysfunction	Human
Theophylline	3′,5′-Cyclic nucleotide phosphodiesterase	Asthma	Human
Nitisinone	4-Hydroxyphenylpyruvate dioxygenase	Tyrosinemia	Human
Finasteride	Steroid 5α-reductase	Benign prostatic hyperplasia	Human
Pyridostigmine	Acetylcholinesterase	Myasthenia gravis	Human
Pentostatin	Adenosine deaminase	Cancer	Human
Cycloserine	Alanine racemase	Tuberculosis	Bacterial
Fomepizole	Alcohol dehydrogenase	Alcoholism	Human
Disulfiram	Aldehyde dehydrogenase	Alcoholism	Human
Acarbose	α-Amylase	Diabetes	Human
Miglitol	α-Glucosidase	Diabetes	Human
Ethambutol	Arabinosyltransferase	Tuberculosis	Bacterial
Zileuton	Arachidonate 5-lipoxygenase	Inflammation	Human
Carbidopa	Aromatic L-amino acid decarboxylase	Parkinson disease	Human
Clavulanic acid	β-Lactamase	In combination with penicillins	Bacterial
Acetazolamide	Carbonate dehydratase (carbonic anhydrase)	Glaucoma	Human
Entacapone	Catechol O-methyltransferase	Parkinson disease	Human
Miglustat	Ceramide glucosyltransferase	Gaucher disease	Human
Methotrexate	Dihydrofolate reductase	Cancer	Human
Trimethoprim	Dihydrofolate reductase	Antibacterial	Bacterial
Sulfamethoxazole	Dihydropteroate synthase	Antibacterial	Bacterial
Topotecan	DNA topoisomerase	Cancer	Human
Ciprofloxacin	DNA gyrase	Antibacterial	Bacterial
Acyclovir	DNA-directed DNA polymerase	Antiviral (anti-HSV)	Viral
Rifampin	DNA-directed RNA polymerase	Antibacterial	Bacterial
Bacitracin	Dolichyl phosphatase	Antibacterial	Bacterial
Isoniazid	Fatty acid enoyl reductase	Tuberculosis	Bacterial
Oseltamivir	Viral neuraminidase	Anti-influenza	Viral
Fondaparinux	Factor Xa	Thrombosis	Human

(continued)

Table 9.1 A Partial Listing of Enzyme Inhibitor Presently Used as Drugs (Continued)

Inhibitor (Drug)	Enzyme Inhibited	Use	Organism
Alendronate	Farnesyl-diphosphate farnesyltransferase	Osteoporosis	Human
Pyrazinamide	Mycobacterial fatty acid synthase	Tuberculosis	Bacterial
Valproic acid	Histone acetyltransferase	Seizures	Human
Nelfinavir	HIV protease	AIDS (anti-HIV)	Viral
Esomeprazole	H^+/K^+-ATPase	Gastroesophageal reflux disease	Human
Atorvastatin	HMG-CoA reductase	Hyperlipidemia	Human
Mycophenolate	IMP dehydrogenase	Immune suppression	Human
Propylthiouracil	Iodide peroxidase	Hyperthyroid	Human
Cilastatin	Renal dehydropeptidase	In combination with imipenem	Human
Eflornithine	Ornithine decarboxylase	Trypanosomes	Parasitic
Allopurinol	Xanthine oxidase	Gout	Human
Captopril	Peptidyl-dipeptidase A (angiotensin-converting enzyme)	Hypertension	Human
Pemetrexed	Phosphoribosylglycinamide formyltransferase	Cancer	Human
Aprotinin	Plasma kallikrein	Thrombosis	Human
Aminocaproic acid	Plasmin	Thrombosis	Human
Etodolac	Prostaglandin-endoperoxide synthase (cyclooxygenase)	Inflammation	Human
Bortezomib	Proteasome endopeptidase complex	Myeloma	Human
Imatinib	Protein-tyrosine kinase	Cancer	Human
Gemcitabine	Ribonuleoside-diphosphate reductase	Cancer	Human
Ribavirin	IMP dehydrogenase	Anti-viral (broad spectrum)	Viral
Azidothymidine	HIV reverse transcriptase	AIDS (anti-HIV)	Viral
Lamivudine	Reverse transcriptase	AIDS, hepatitis B	Viral
Penicillin	Serine-type D-Ala—Ala carboxypeptidase	Antibiotic	Bacterial
Digitoxin	Na^+/K^+-ATPase	Congestive heart failure	Human
Terbinafine	Squalene monooxygenase	Antifungal	Fungal
Itraconazole	Sterol 14 α-demethylase	Antifungal	Fungal
Lepirudin	Thrombin	Thrombosis	Human
Floxuridine	Thymidylate synthase	Cancer	Human
Orlistat	Triacylglycerol lipase	Obesity	Human
Metyrosine	Tyrosine 3-monooxygenase	Pheochromocytoma	Human

Table 9.1 A Partial Listing of Enzyme Inhibitor Presently Used as Drugs (Continued)

Inhibitor (Drug)	Enzyme Inhibited	Use	Organism
Fosfomycin	UDP-N-acetylglucosamine 1-carboxyvinyltransferase	Antibacterial	Bacterial
Aminoglutethimide	Monooxygenase	Breast cancer	Human
Acetohydroxamic acid	Urease	Gastritis	Bacterial
Dicumarol	Vitamin K epoxide reductase	Thrombosis	Human

Adapted from Robertson J. Mechanistic basis of enzyme-targeted drugs. *Biochemistry.* 2005;44:5561-5771, with permission.

Enzymes have been classified on the type of reaction catalyzed, and six major classes (families) of enzymes, numbered from 1 to 6, have been assigned by the Enzyme Commission (EC) of the International Union of Biochemistry and Molecular Biology.[9] These classes are (1) oxidoreductases (e.g., dehydrogenases); (2) transferases (group transfer enzymes; e.g., kinases); (3) hydrolases (hydrolytic reactions; e.g., esterases); (4) lyases (formation or removal of double bonds; e.g., hydratase—addition of water across a double bond); (5) isomerases (e.g., mutarotation of glucose by mutases); and (6) ligases (joining of two substrates at the expense of energy, also referred to as synthetases). All presently discovered enzymes are identified by the prefix EC followed by an Arabic numeral based on the major class of reaction catalyzed, as indicated above. Furthermore, this is followed by a series of three more Arabic numerals, which indicate the subclass (functionality), sub-subclass (specific bond type), and serial number of the enzyme in that class, respectively. For example, the enzyme, acetylcholinesterase has been given the following assignment, EC 3.1.1.7. As can been seen in this example, the numeral 3 indicates that this enzyme belongs to the family of hydrolases, the first 1 indicates that the nature of the bond being hydrolyzed is an ester, the second 1 indicates that specific ester bond is a carboxylic acid ester, and the last number is the serial number of this enzyme in this sub-subclass.

Many enzymes make use of cofactors, which enable them to carry out the catalysis. These small molecules (including ions) are intimately bound to the enzyme and are essential to the functioning of the enzyme. As macromolecular receptors, enzymes have the inherent ability to bind ligands (substrates). In effecting the transformation of these substrates to products (catalyzing the chemical reaction), enzymes use all the necessary tools in the chemical bonding arsenal to hold these substrates extremely tightly as the transformation occurs. Because all chemical reactions require bond breakage and formation, the substrate must go through a transition state, or an "activated complex," which is a destabilizing event, because bonds are being polarized and there is partial charge development. It is the inherent ability of the enzyme to greatly stabilize such activated complexes that give them their role in nature and allows their phenomenal catalytic power.

Pauling first proposed the stabilization theory of the activated complex by enzymes.[10] He concluded that the active site of the enzyme is complementary to the structure of the activated complex so that the binding of the enzyme to the activated complex is extremely tight. The ability to stabilize such complexes and correspondingly reduce the activation energy of the reaction and, thus, enhance the reaction rate is caused by many factors, both noncovalent and covalent.[11] Noncovalent influences include entropic effects, such as proximity and orientation; restricted motion, where enzymes, by their evolvement, have the inherent ability to bring reacting molecules closer together and in the correct orientation for bonds to form; desolvation effects, to strip solvent (water) molecules from the reactants; transition state electrostatic stabilization, to stabilize the partial charges being developed in the activated complex; induced-fit effects, in which the flexibility of the enzyme can accommodate the substrate, intermediate, and/or product; strain and distortion effects, to increase the reactivity of compounds; and many other such ancillary effects. Moreover, covalent influences (effects) also play a vital role in the enzyme's catalytic role. "Covalent effects" imply a covalent bond being made by the enzyme (or its cofactor) to the substrate being transformed. These covalent effects would include general acid-base catalysis, in which amino acid residues partake in the overall reaction through proton donation (general acid) or proton abstraction (general base), as well as nucleophilic and electrophilic catalysis, in which there is bond formation with an amino acid side-chain residue (or cofactor) to the substrate.

It should be mentioned here that "covalent catalysis" has traditionally implied a group transfer reaction between one substrate and another being facilitated through an enzyme-residue intermediate (e.g., the enzyme sucrose phosphorylase transfers a glucose residue from sucrose to phosphate giving the products glucose-1-phosphate and fructose through an enzyme-glucosyl intermediate). Many amino acid side-chain residues (i.e., acidic and basic amino acids, e.g., Asp, Glu, His, Lys, Arg, Tyr, and Cys) as well as nucleophilic amino acid residues allow such covalent effects. Recent analysis of enzyme rate enhancements has postulated that noncovalent effects allow an increase of as many as 11 orders of magnitude over the noncatalyzed reaction, whereas for those enzymes with rate enhancements exceeding 11 orders of magnitude (over noncatalyzed reactions), it is covalent catalysis in the transition state that accounts for this exceptional increase in rate enhancement.[12]

Noncovalent effects like proximity and orientation may be explained on the basis that enzymes have the inherent ability to affect the order of reactions by the "effective concentration" principle—for example, to change a second-order reaction to a first-order one by bringing the reacting molecules closer to each other so that there is a lower amount of entropic loss for the reacting substrates. In the example shown in Figure 9.4, which is taken from physical-organic chemical studies,[13,14] one can consider the hydrolysis of a nitrophenyl ester by an amine in two scenarios: reaction (i), with two individual molecules reacting (i.e., amine and ester), versus reaction (ii), with a single molecule having an "in-built" amine on the ester molecule. If the reaction rate constants are compared (one needs to keep in mind that we are comparing a first-order rate constant for (ii), with a second-order rate constant for (i), which may not be a true comparison, because mechanisms are likely to be different), however, one finds that the first-order rate reaction (reaction (ii)) has a rate enhancement over the reaction (i) by a factor of ~5,000 M attributed to the fact that reaction (i) needs to give up more degrees of freedom (as compared to reaction (ii)) to react (i.e., form productive collision complexes, leading to product formation). This proximity effect indicates that by using such a system (bringing the reacting centers closer to each other), one can effectively increase the concentration of the reactants by this factor, resulting in a faster reaction. This enhancement factor of 5,000 M (i.e., effectively changing a second-order reaction to that of a first-order one) has been termed the "effective concentration" because this is an unrealistic increase in the concentration of the reactants, which gives rise to the higher rate constant (i.e., it is impossible to make a solution of 5,000 M of the reactants—consider the concentration of water is only 55 M).

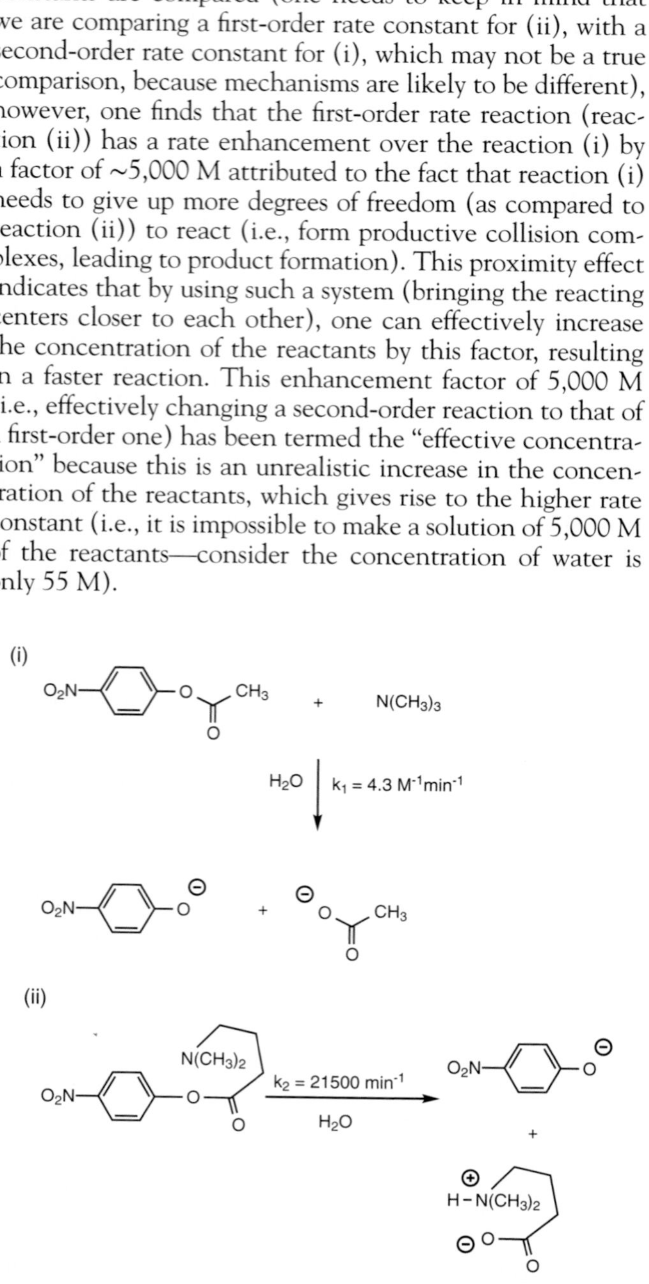

Effective concentration = k_2/k_1 = 5000 M (approx.)

Figure 9.4 Concept of proximity and effective concentration.

The next example, which is shown in Figure 9.5, illustrates that besides the proximity factor, one also can use "orientation" effects to bring about an increase in the reaction rate constant.[14] For example, as shown in Figure 9.5, one may use alkyl groups to sterically hinder rotation about single bonds, effectively freezing the molecule in a particular conformation to provide maximum orbital overlap for bonding. Thus, using a "dimethyl lock" system in molecule II, which restricts rotation, ensures that lactonization for molecule II is faster by a factor of 4×10^4 than molecule I. Both of these effects, proximity and orientation, are thought to be part of an enzyme's arsenal of tools in allowing enzymes to lower the activation energy for reactions.

Other noncovalent effects, such as desolvation of the reactant molecules, also can be effectively achieved by enzymes. Enzymes have the capacity, by lining their exterior and/or interior surfaces with appropriately situated hydrophobic amino acids, to effectively strip away water molecules from substrates as they enter into the active site of the enzyme through such channels. Thus, no further expense of energy is required to desolvate the substrate before the reaction.

As mentioned previously, enzymes also use covalent chemistry as a means to effect catalysis. Indeed, it has been recently postulated that covalent chemistry plays a far greater role in enzyme catalysis than previously thought.[12] Nucleophilic catalysis by hydrolytic enzymes, such as the serine proteases or esterases, is a classic example of covalent effects in enzyme catalysis. In such systems, for example, as in the case of the serine protease chymotrypsin, which hydrolyzes peptide bonds containing aromatic amino acids (e.g., phenylalanine and tyrosine), the covalent effects occur at the level of general acid, general base, and nucleophilic covalent catalysis. Figure 9.6 illustrates an accepted mechanism for such enzymes. It should be noted that all serine proteases contain a "catalytic triad" of the amino acids, designated as Ser195, His57, and Asp102 (numerals represent the amino acid position in the protein primary structure), which are present in the active sites of these proteases. The catalysis is effected by making the hydroxyl functionality of the serine residue

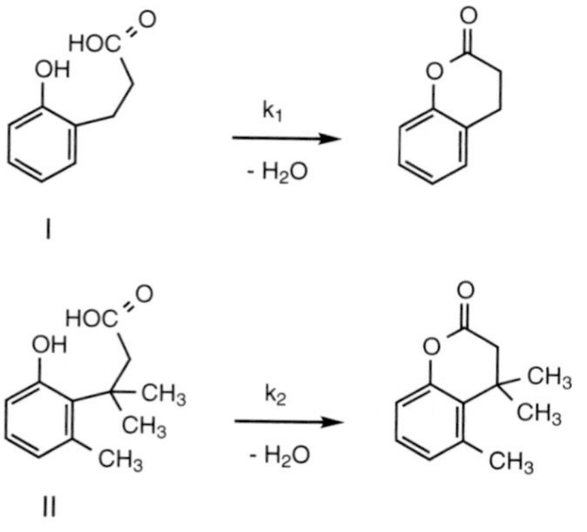

Relative rate, $k_2/k_1 = 4 \times 10^4$

Figure 9.5 Concept of orientation.

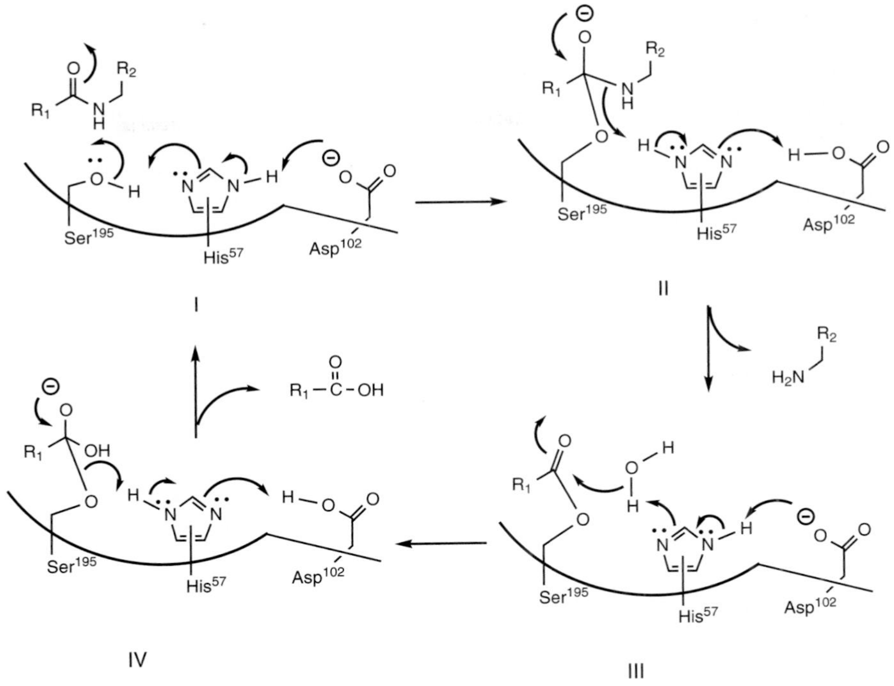

Figure 9.6 Acid, base, and nucleophilic covalent catalysis by chymotrypsin.

more nucleophilic for attack at the carbonyl center of the peptide bond. One should recall that in general, hydroxyl groups have pK_a values in the range of greater than 14 and, as such, are not acidic and unable to ionize at physiological pH. Because of catalytic triad, however, the proton from the serine hydroxyl group is transferred to the aspartate residue through the histidine residue in a "charge relay system" such that the serine hydroxyl group can be made into the highly nucleophilic alkoxide ion. This is achieved by the aspartate residue acting as a general base to pick up the proton from histidine, which also can abstract a proton from the serine-hydroxyl group (see I in Fig. 9.6). Thus, histidine behaves as a tautomeric catalyst in this enzyme (i.e., acts as both a general acid and a general base) and, in essence, relays the proton from serine to aspartate. The serine (as its alkoxide) is now a much more powerful nucleophile and can attack the peptidyl carbonyl group to generate a "tetrahedral oxy-anion intermediate" (see II in Fig. 9.6), which collapses to liberate a new amino terminus of the peptide and the acylated serine enzyme (see III in Fig. 9.6). The next part of the reaction involves a water molecule (which also is made more nucleophilic by a similar mechanism; see III in Fig. 9.6) that goes on to hydrolyze, through a tetrahedral intermediate (see IV in Fig. 9.6), the serine-acyl bond to liberate the new carboxyl terminus of the peptide (R_1COOH) and the free enzyme, which can be recycled for another round of catalysis.

Knowledge of the mechanisms and interactions, both noncovalent and covalent, that allow enzymes to function as such efficient catalysts provides the medicinal chemist with insights to design molecules that achieve selective inhibition of the enzyme. Such knowledge also paves the way to the design and discovery of drugs.

General Concepts of Enzyme Inhibition

The body is composed of thousands of different enzymes, many of them acting in concert to maintain homeostasis. Although disease states may arise from the malfunctioning of a particular enzyme, or the introduction of a foreign enzyme through infection by microorganisms, inhibiting a specific enzyme to alleviate a disease state is a challenging process. Most bodily functions occur through a cascade of enzymatic systems, and it becomes extremely difficult to design a drug molecule that can selectively inhibit an enzyme and result in a therapeutic benefit. To address the problem, however, the basic mechanism of enzyme action needs to be understood. Once knowledge of a particular enzymatic pathway is determined and the mechanism and kinetics are worked out, the challenge is then to design a suitable inhibitor that is selectively used by the enzyme causing its inhibition.

As outlined above, enzymes (E) represent the best-known chemical catalysts because they are uniquely designed to carry out specific chemical reactions in a highly efficient manner.[8,11] They initially act by binding a substrate (S) to form an enzyme-substrate complex [E·S], which undergoes specific chemistry (catalysis) to give the enzyme-product complex [E·P], followed by dissociation of product (P) and free enzyme (E). Equation (9.1) represents a simplified version of this scenario:

Eq. 9.1 $$E + S \underset{}{\overset{K_d \text{ (or } K_m)}{\rightleftharpoons}} [E{\cdot}S] \overset{k_{cat}}{\rightleftharpoons} [E{\cdot}P] \rightleftharpoons E + P$$

where K_d is the enzyme-substrate dissociation constant and k_{cat} represents the rate constant for the catalytic step (chemical modification step or slowest step in the overall pathway). If the binding step of E + S to form [E·S] is relatively fast as compared to the catalytic step and one assumes steady-state conditions, then K_m, the Michaelis constant, (the substrate concentration at half-maximum velocity $[V_{max}/2]$), may be equated to the K_d, as shown in Equation (9.2)):

Eq. 9.2

$$\text{Michaelis-Menten equation: } v = \frac{V_{max}[S]}{K_m + [S]}$$

$$\text{Lineweaver-Burk equation: } \frac{1}{v} = \frac{K_m}{V_{max}} \times \frac{1}{[S]} + \frac{1}{V_{max}}$$

where v is the velocity of the reaction.

The rate of the reaction can then be derived in terms of K_m and V_{max} (or $k_{cat} = V_{max}/[E]$). From the knowledge of the dissociation constant ($K_{m(d)}$) and the rate constant for catalysis (k_{cat}), it is then possible to compare inhibitors and the dissociation constant for the inhibitors, K_i, in relation to the natural substrates and the effect on the catalytic rates. These kinetic parameters, k_{cat} and $K_{m(d)}$ (or K_i), can then give an indication as to the affinity (K_i vs. $K_{m(d)}$) and specificity (k_{cat}/K_i or $k_{cat}/K_{m(d)}$) of the inhibitor for a particular enzyme. Equation (9.3a and b) represents the general scheme of reversible inhibition, competitive and non-competitive, respectively, and Figure 9.7 illustrates graphically and mathematically the relationship of the velocity of the enzyme reaction to the substrate [S] and inhibitor [I] concentration as well as the kinetic parameters K_m, K_i, and V_{max} (or $k_{cat} = V_{max}/[E]$):

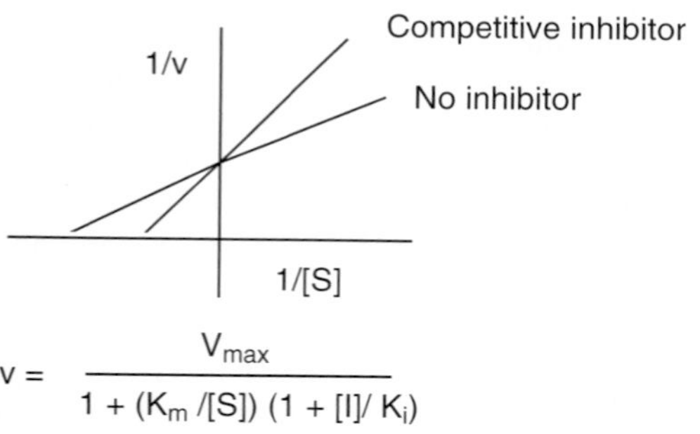

$$v = \frac{V_{max}}{1 + (K_m/[S])(1 + [I]/K_i)}$$

(K_m increases, V_{max} unchanged)

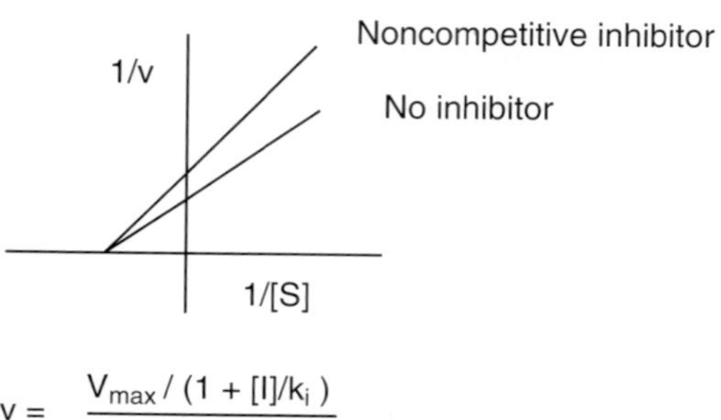

$$v = \frac{V_{max}/(1 + [I]/K_i)}{1 + (K_m/[S])}$$

(K_m unchanged, V_{max} decreases)

Figure 9.7 Graphic representation of competitive and noncompetitive enzyme inhibition.

Eq. 9.3a Competitive Inhibition:

$$E + S \underset{}{\overset{K_m}{\rightleftharpoons}} [E{\cdot}S] \overset{k_{cat}}{\rightleftharpoons} E + P$$

$$E + I \overset{K_i}{\rightleftharpoons} [E{\cdot}I] \not\rightarrow P$$

Eq. 9.3b Non-competitive Inhibition:

$$E + S \overset{K_m}{\rightleftharpoons} [E{\cdot}S] \overset{I}{\rightleftharpoons} [ESI]$$

$$E + I \overset{K_i}{\rightleftharpoons} [E{\cdot}I] \overset{S}{\rightleftharpoons} [ESI]$$

Inhibition of enzymes may be broadly classified under two categories—reversible and irreversible inhibitors—as shown in Equation (9.4):

Eq. 9.4

$$E + I \overset{K_i}{\rightleftharpoons} [E{\cdot}I] \quad \text{(Reversible inhibition)}$$

$$E + I \overset{K_i}{\longrightarrow} E\text{–}I \quad \text{(Irreversible inhibition)}$$

In the presence of inhibitor, the enzyme-substrate complex, [E·S], is replaced by the enzyme-inhibitor complex, [E·I], which may block or retard the formation of product. In the presence of a reversible inhibitor, the enzyme is tied up and the reaction, retarded or stopped; however, the enzyme can be subsequently regenerated from the enzyme-inhibitor complex, [E·I], to react again with substrate and produce product (see Equation (9.3)). On the other hand, irreversible inhibition implies that the enzyme cannot be regenerated, and the only way for catalysis to proceed would be if new molecules of the enzyme are generated from gene transcription and translation. Irreversible inhibition is commonly associated with covalent bond formation between inhibitor and enzyme [E—I], which *cannot* be easily broken and often is defined as a time-dependent loss of enzyme activity. Reversible inhibition, on the other hand, does not necessarily imply noncovalent bond formation. In many instances, reversible inhibition can occur through covalent bond formation, but these bonds can be hydrolyzed to regenerate free enzyme and inhibitor. Thus, for a reversible enzyme inhibitor, there is no time-dependent loss of activity, and enzyme activity can always be recovered. There are instances when reversible inhibition tends to look kinetically like irreversible inhibition. This scenario results whenever there is a tight binding of a reversible inhibitor to the enzyme; consequently, the dissociation of the enzyme from this enzyme-inhibitor complex is extremely slow. Kinetically, it is extremely difficult to distinguish this type of inhibition from an irreversible inhibitor, because over time, the enzyme does tend to look like it loses its activity and, for all practical purposes, the enzyme behaves as if it were irreversibly tied up. To differentiate between tight-binding reversible and irreversible inhibitors, one can dialyze the enzyme-inhibitor complex. In case of the reversible inhibitor, on dialysis, the inhibitor will be removed from the enzyme, resulting in recovery of the enzyme activity; however, this is not so with the irreversible one.

Reversible Enzyme Inhibition

Reversible enzyme inhibition may be classified under two main headings, competitive and noncompetitive, with both following Michaelis-Menten kinetics. Competitive inhibition, by definition, requires that the inhibitor competes with the substrate for binding to the enzyme at the active site, and this binding is mutually exclusive. That is, if the inhibitor binds to the enzyme, the substrate will not be able to bind, and vice versa. Competitive inhibition also, however, suggests that the inhibition can be reversed in the presence of saturating amounts of substrate, because in this case, all enzyme active sites will be occupied by substrate-displacing inhibitor. In contrast, noncompetitive inhibition implies independent binding (i.e., both inhibitor and substrate may bind to the enzyme at different sites). Because binding of the inhibitor to the enzyme is at a site other than the active site, noncompetitive inhibition cannot be reversed by increasing the concentration of substrate. Graphing the kinetics of inhibition (Fig. 9.7), the Lineweaver-Burk plot of $1/V$ versus $1/[S]$ shows distinguishing characteristics between the two types of inhibition. In competitive inhibition, there is no change in the maximum velocity of the reaction (V_{max}; the intercept on the *y*-axis remains constant in the presence of inhibitor). However, the slope of the curve (K_m/V_{max}) is different with the inhibitor present, and K_m changes because of the presence of the competitive inhibitor (Fig. 9.7, competitive inhibition). In the case of noncompetitive inhibition, only the V_{max} of the reaction decreases, while the K_m remains unchanged (intercept on the *x*-axis unchanged with inhibitor, Fig. 9.7, noncompetitive inhibition).

Most of the rationally designed and clinically useful reversible inhibitors are competitive inhibitors. Table 9.1 gives a listing of several currently approved drugs that act as enzyme inhibitors. The majority of enzyme inhibitors generally bear some structural resemblance to the natural substrate of the enzyme. The design of such inhibitors would thus seem to be a logical and rational task which is uniquely suited to the medicinal chemist who can use the principles of bioisosteric modification of natural enzyme substrates and metabolites, or modification of "lead" structures and structure activity relationships, to create selective and potent inhibitors. There are pitfalls in this endeavor, however, because even the most rationally designed drug must still overcome transport and other cellular barriers before exerting its effects. In the case of the noncompetitive inhibitors, the design is not as straightforward. These inhibitors can have widely differing structures, which in many instances bear no resemblance to the natural substrate. In general, inhibitors of the noncompetitive type have been obtained primarily through random screening of chemically novel molecules followed by further synthetic manipulation of the pharmacophore to optimize their inhibitory effects.

Examples of Reversible Inhibitors

The design of enzyme inhibitors has included random screening of synthetic chemical agents, natural products, and combinatorial libraries followed by molecular optimization or structure-activity relationships of so-called lead structures as well as bio-isosteric analogues of the enzyme substrates themselves. Drugs (e.g., finasteride) also have been developed for one indication but, based on observed side effects, have led to other uses.

The rational approach in the design of enzyme inhibitors is greatly aided if the enzymatic reaction is characterized in terms of its kinetic mechanism. Such a characterization would include the knowledge of the kinetic parameters (rate constants and dissociation constants) of individual steps in the overall reaction pathway as well as the characterization of (any) intermediates involved in these individual steps. Examples of such "rational" inhibitors include both reversible and irreversible inhibitors of enzymes.

USES OF FINASTERIDE

Finasteride (Proscar) an inhibitor of steroid 5α-reductase, an enzyme involved in the catalytic reduction of testosterone to dihydrotestosterone, was originally developed as an agent to treat prostate hyperplasia. In addition to this original use, finasteride also currently is indicated as an agent (Propecia) to stimulate hair growth for treatment of male pattern baldness. This benefit was recognized as a useful side effect during clinical trials of finasteride as an antiprostate agent.

ANTIMETABOLITES. Antimetabolites are agents that interfere with the functioning of an essential metabolite and that most often are designed as structural analogues of the natural metabolite. As described earlier, the mechanism of action of sulfanilamide is that of a competitive inhibitor of *p*-aminobenzoic acid. In the case of sulfanilamide, however, the mechanism was only determined after the bacterial inhibitory action was noted. This often is the case when a drug is discovered to have a certain therapeutic effect and, later, this effect is "rationalized" as being caused by an enzyme-inhibitory action. Other classic examples of a competitive inhibitor acting as an antimetabolite include a number of nucleoside analogues used as antiviral and anticancer agents. These agents again bear structural resemblance to natural nucleosides, which in their triphosphate form are substrates for nucleic acid polymerases involved in the synthesis of nucleic acids. Nucleic acid polymerases catalyze the condensation of the free 3′-hydroxy end of a nucleic acid with an incoming 5′-triphosphate derivative of a nucleoside (dNTP), resulting in a 3′,5′-phosphodiester linkage. Hence, nucleoside analogues, to compete with the natural substrate in the synthesis of nucleic acid, must be converted intracellularly to their mono-, di-, and finally, triphosphate derivative before exerting their inhibitory effects on nucleic acid synthesis. Certain drug design strategies incorporate a "masked" phosphate group on the nucleoside such that once absorbed, they enter into the systemic circulation as the monophosphate.[15] The majority of these analogues are designed such that they lack the 3′-hydroxy group and are dideoxy derivatives of the natural substrate. These analogues thus ensure that once they are incorporated into nucleic acid, further extension of the nucleic acid is prevented because of the lack of a 3′-hydroxy group.

INHIBITION OF HIV-REVERSE TRANSCRIPTASE ***Azidothymidine (AZT)***. The advent of AIDS stimulated a great interest in designing inhibitors against the essential viral polymerase—HIV-reverse transcriptase (HIV-RT). AZT is a potent inhibitor of HIV-RT,[16] the retroviral polymerase that catalyzes the formation of proviral DNA from viral RNA. Structurally, AZT is similar to the natural nucleoside thymidine but has an azide group (–N_3) rather than a hydroxy group (–OH) at the 3′-position of the sugar deoxyribose (Fig. 9.8).

AZT is activated intracellularly to its triphosphate and competes with thymidine triphosphate for uptake by HIV-RT into DNA.[17] Once incorporated, further chain extension of the DNA is prevented, because there is no 3′-hydroxyl group to continue the DNA synthesis. In this fashion, AZT is an effective chain terminator of viral DNA synthesis.

Dideoxycytidine (ddC [Zalcitabine]) and 3-thiacytidine (3-TC [Lamivudine]). 2′,3′-Dideoxycytidine is another antiretroviral agent used against HIV-RT. In this case, ddC resembles the natural metabolite, deoxycytidine (dC), and as in the case of AZT, it is a 3′-deoxy analogue of dC, where the 3′-OH group of dC is replaced by a hydrogen atom. Similarly, 3-TC is another anti-HIV agent that resembles dC. In this example, however, rather than replacing the 3′-hydroxyl functionality as in ddC, the 3′-carbon position of the sugar has been substituted by a sulfur atom.

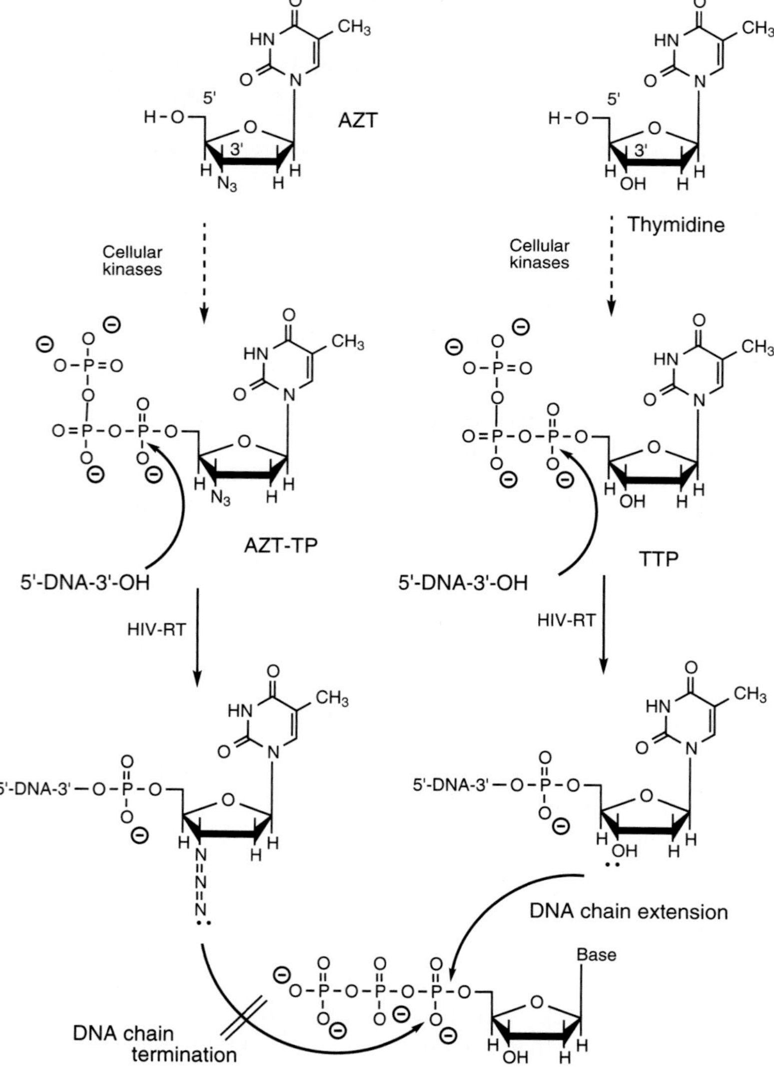

Figure 9.8 Activation, incorporation, and chain-terminating action of azidothymidine (AZT), a thymidine analogue, as a reversible inhibitor of human immunodeficiency virus-reverse transcriptase (HIV-RT).

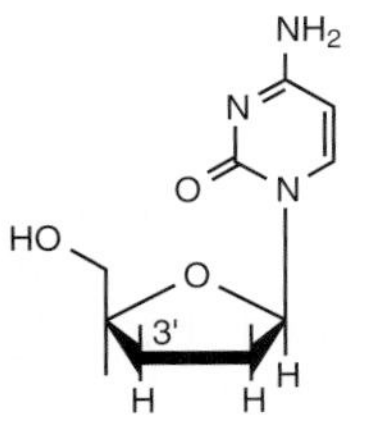

HISTORICAL DEVELOPMENT OF AZT

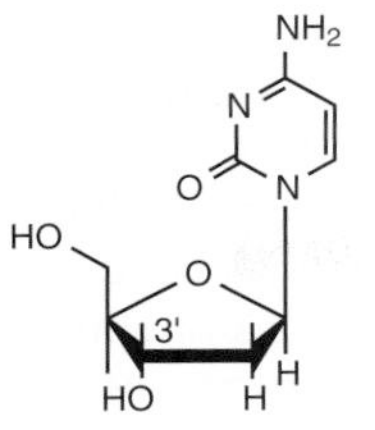

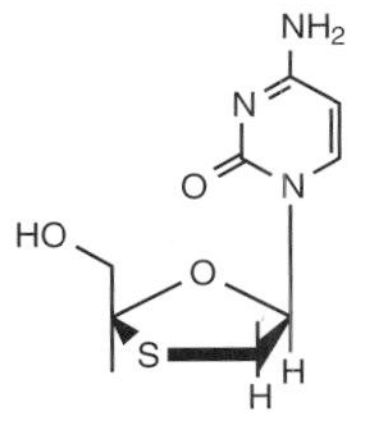

Interestingly, AZT was originally synthesized as an anticancer agent to inhibit cellular DNA synthesis, but it was found to be too toxic. Subsequently, in the mid-1980s, during a random screening of nucleoside agents for potential inhibitory effects against HIV-RT, AZT was found to have selectivity for HIV-RT.[16] As such, its effects on host cell polymerases result in its dose-limiting bone marrow toxicity.

Nevirapine. An example of a potent noncompetitive inhibitor of HIV-RT is the drug nevirapine, a benzodiazepine analogue,[18] which is extremely tight-binding to the enzyme, having a K_i in the nanomolar range. As can be seen in the structure of nevirapine, the drug bears no resemblance to any of the natural nucleotide substrates and was discovered through a random screening program. X-ray crystallographic studies of HIV-RT complexed with nevirapine have shown it binding in a hydrophobic pocket at a site adjacent to and slightly overlapping the nucleotide-binding site of HIV-RT.[19] Kinetic studies with the enzyme have revealed an extremely slow binding rate for the drug; however, once bound, the polymerization rate for the reaction is effectively reduced.[20]

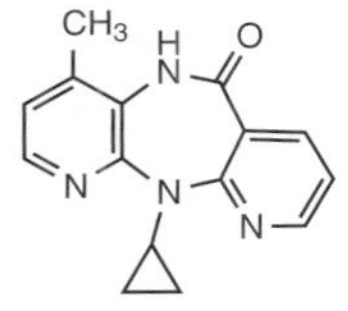

A drawback for nevirapine, however, is that the virus can develop resistance very rapidly, through mutation of the amino acid residues in the binding pocket.[20,21] Thus, its usefulness is limited to combination therapy with other antiretroviral agents rather than single-drug therapy.

Reversible Inhibitors Used in Cancer Therapy

The design of several anticancer agents has been based on the antimetabolite theory. Because cancer results in overproliferation and uncontrolled cell growth, drugs designed against cancer have been based on inhibiting DNA synthesis in the cell. Thus, these drugs have been targeted against those enzymes, including nucleic acid polymerases, thymidylate synthase, and dihydrofolate reductase (DHFR), that play a role in DNA synthesis. Examples of drugs that have been designed against nucleic acid polymerases include cytosine arabinoside (Ara-C) and 5-fluorouracil (5-FU) (Fig. 9.9). Cytosine arabinoside is first converted to its triphosphate, and as such, it functions as an antimetabolite of deoxycytidine triphosphate (deoxy CTP) to inhibit DNA polymerase. As can be seen from its structure, Ara-C is the arabino isomer of cytidine. That is, the 2′-hydroxyl functionality in Ara-C is in the arabino configuration rather than the ribo configuration of cytidine. Because of this stereochemical change in the placement of the 2′-hydroxyl function, Ara-C tends to resemble deoxycytidine rather than cytidine. In this way, Ara-C inhibits DNA polymerases by competing with deoxycytidine. 5-FU is an analogue of the pyrimidine base uracil, where the hydrogen at the 5-position in uracil has been substituted by an isosteric fluorine (F)

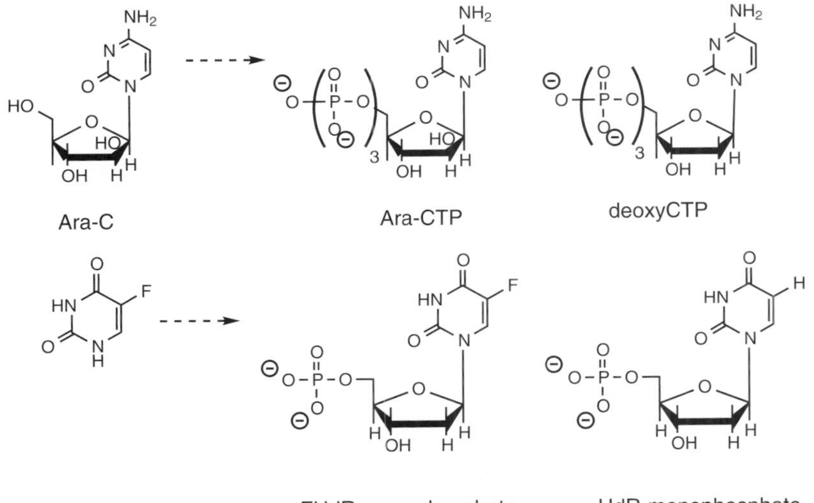

Figure 9.9 Structures of pyrimidine antimetabolites used in cancer chemotherapy.

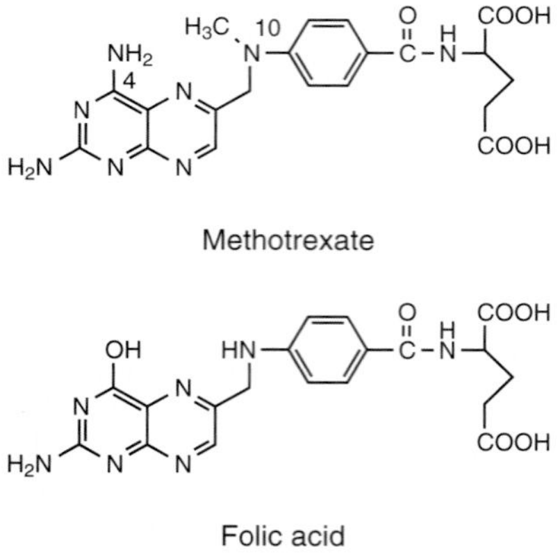

Figure 9.10 Methotrexate, the antimetabolite of folic acid.

atom. This makes 5-FU look very similar to uracil. 5-FU, after conversion to 5-fluorodeoxyuridine monophosphate (FdUMP), is an inhibitor of thymidylate synthase, the enzyme involved in the de novo synthesis of thymidylate. In this case, FdUMP is an antimetabolite of deoxyuridine monophosphate.

Methotrexate is a potent inhibitor of DHFR, the enzyme responsible for the reduction of folic acid to dihydro- and tetrahydrofolic acid, precursors to one-carbon donation in purine and pyrimidine de novo synthesis. Methotrexate is an analogue of folic acid where the 4-hydroxyl group (–OH) on the pteridine ring of folic acid has been replaced by an amino (–NH_2) functionality and the nitrogen atom at the 10-position is methylated (Fig. 9.10). These substitutions led to methotrexate having an affinity for DHFR orders of magnitude greater than that for the natural metabolite, folic acid, and allows it to be an extremely potent inhibitor.

Inhibition of Acetylcholinesterase

Acetylcholinesterase (AChE) is the enzyme that catalyzes the catabolism of the neurotransmitter acetylcholine to acetate and choline. Thus, inhibition of AChE would lead to increased concentrations of acetylcholine and a prolonged action of the neurotransmitter. Inhibitors of AChE have found use in cases of myasthenia gravis, glaucoma, and Alzheimer's disease. To appreciate the design of these inhibitors, it is useful to first understand the mechanism of action of AChE. AChE has an anionic site that can bind the positively charged quaternary ammonium group of the choline functionality and an active esteratic site that contains a nucleophilic serine residue involved in the hydrolysis of the ester bond (Fig. 9.11). The mechanism involves the attack of the nucleophilic serine hydroxy group on the carbonyl group of acetylcholine to form a tetrahedral intermediate that breaks down, resulting in the release of choline and an intermediate, acetylated serine that subsequently hydrolyzes to release AChE.

Physostigmine has been used in the treatment of glaucoma. It is an alkaloid with a carbamate moiety that resembles the ester linkage of acetylcholine. Being an alkaloid, it is protonated at physiological pH and, thus, can bind to the anionic site of AChE. Following the mechanism of AChE, the serine residue of the enzyme can attack the carbonyl group of physostigmine, and in the process, the serine is carbamylated (Fig. 9.12). This carbamyl serine intermediate is more stable to enzymatic hydrolysis than is acetylated SER and subsequent hydrolysis by water occurs extremely slowly. The carbamylated enzyme is only slowly regenerated, with a half-life of 38 minutes—more than seven orders of magnitude slower than that for the natural substrate, acetylcholine. This is an example of a reversible inhibitor involved in covalent bond formation with the enzyme that ultimately gets hydrolyzed.

Inhibitors of Angiotensin-Converting Enzyme

Angiotensin-converting enzyme (ACE) is a carboxypeptidase having a zinc ion as a cofactor and is involved in the renin-angiotensin cascade of blood pressure control.[22] The design of the antihypertensive drug captopril, a clinically important and potent reversible inhibitor of ACE, is an example of one of the early endeavors and successes of a rationally designed enzyme inhibitor (see Chapter 17). The design of captopril was based on several factors. These included the knowledge that ACE was similar in its enzymatic mechanism to carboxypeptidase A, except that ACE cleaved off a dipeptide, whereas carboxypeptidase A cleaved single amino acid residues from the carboxyl end of the protein; the discovery of L-benzylsuccinic acid

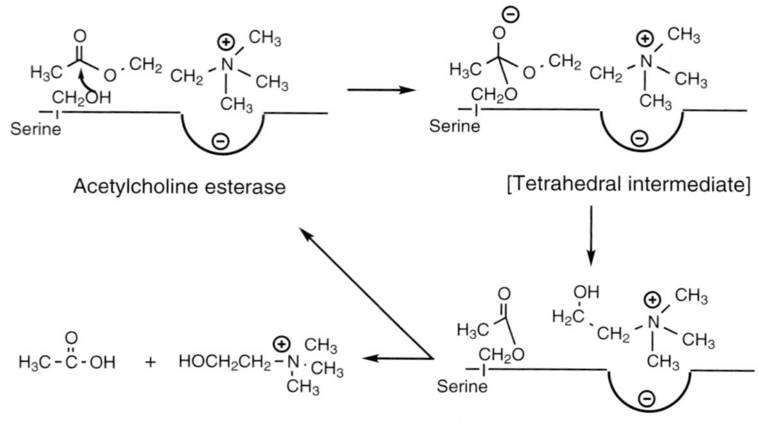

Figure 9.11 Mechanism of hydrolysis of acetylcholine by acetylcholine esterase.

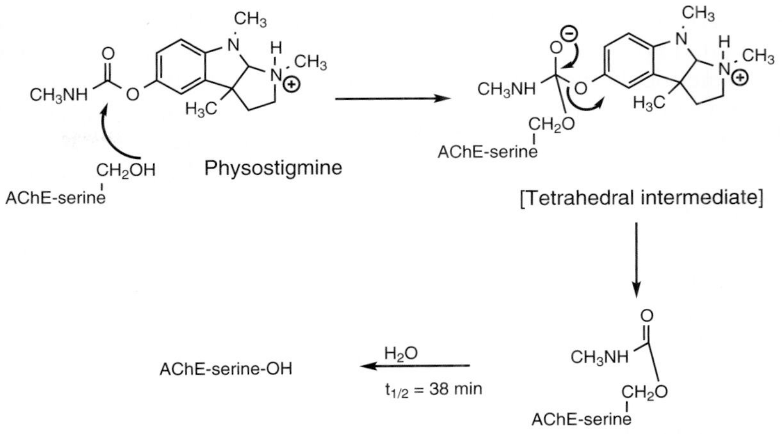

Figure 9.12 Mechanism of inhibition of acetylcholine esterase by physostigmine.

as a potent inhibitor of carboxypeptidase A; and, studies of a potent pentapeptide inhibitor of ACE, $BPP_{5\alpha}$ (Glu-Lys-Trp-Ala-Pro), from the venom of the Brazilian viper (*Bothrops jararaca*), which showed that the N-terminal peptide fragments, including tetra-, tri-, and dipeptide fragments (Ala-Pro) of $BPP_{5\alpha}$, retained some inhibitory activity. Benzylsuccinic acid has been described as a by-product inhibitor of carboxypeptidase A, wherein its design was based on the combination of the products of the peptidase reaction (i.e., the two peptide fragments, one with a free carboxyl end that coordinates the zinc ion of the protease and the other with a free amino terminus; Fig. 9.13).[23,24] In the case of benzylsuccinic acid, the amino ($-NH_2$) functionality is replaced by the isosteric methylene ($-CH_2-$) group. Using the above concepts, it was rationalized that succinyl amino acids could similarly behave as by-product inhibitors of ACE. Starting with a succinyl-proline moiety, the structural activity developmental effort finally resulted in captopril with the substitution of the stronger zinc coordinating mercapto functionality in place of the carboxylic residue (of succinic acid) and a stereospecific R methyl group on the succinyl function to represent the

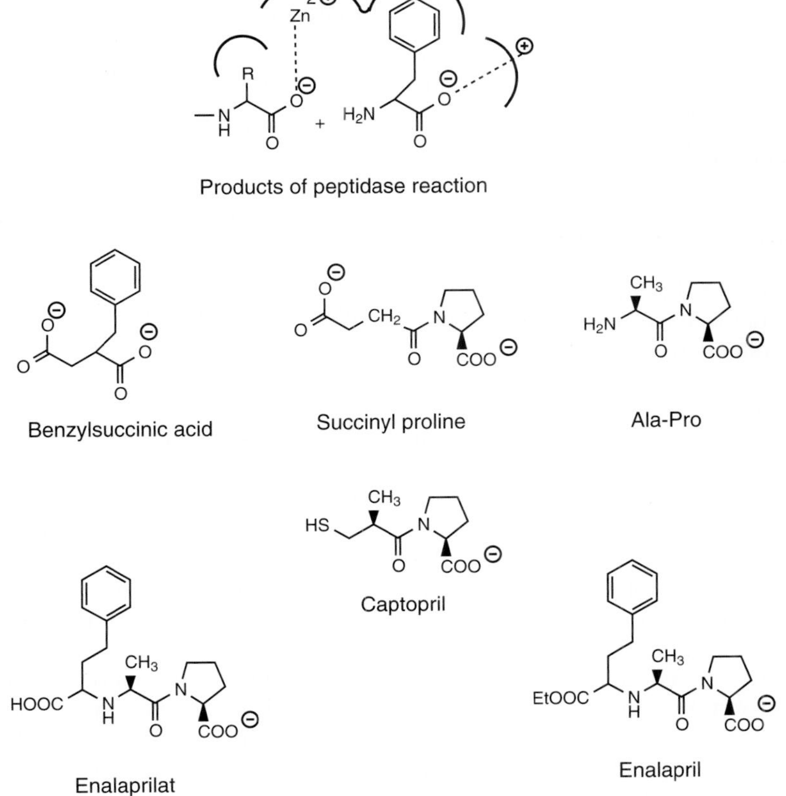

Figure 9.13 Angiotensin-converting enzyme (ACE) inhibitors and efforts that led to their development.

methyl group on the natural L-Ala residue in Ala-Pro (the dipeptide fragment that had previously shown inhibitory activity). Captopril soon became highly successful in the clinic as an antihypertensive agent and, in combination with diuretics, has proved to be the treatment of choice in controlling hypertension.

Following on the heels of captopril was another by-product ACE inhibitor, enalaprilat. Enalaprilat incorporated a phenylethyl moiety with the *S*-configuration and made use of a hydrophobic binding pocket in ACE that was overlooked during the design of captopril.[25] Recalling that the tripeptide fragment of $BPP_{5\alpha}$ (Trp-Ala-Pro) contained the aromatic tryptophan residue and showed weak inhibitory properties suggested the benefit of an aromatic binding site. Substituting the tryptophan residue with a phenyl group allowed the design of enalaprilat, which retained the carboxylic group as the coordinating ligand for zinc and resulted in a 20-fold increase in potency over captopril. However, enalaprilat, a diacid, was poorly absorbed from the gastrointestinal tract; thus, a pro-drug ethyl ester of enalaprilat, called enalapril, was developed. Enalapril had superior pharmacokinetics to enalaprilat and was rapidly metabolized to the active drug.

Transition-State Analogues

Transition-state analogues are compounds that resemble the substrate portion of the hypothetical transition state of an enzymatic reaction. All chemical reactions progressing from substrate to product must cross an energy barrier and proceed through a transition state or activated high-energy complex. This energy barrier is described as the activation energy. In the case of enzyme-catalyzed reactions, it is accepted that the enzyme reduces this energy barrier as compared to the nonenzyme-catalyzed reaction. Factors contributing to this reduced energy barrier are several and include stabilization of the transition state and intermediate forms of the reaction during the course of transition from substrate to product as well as conformational effects of distortion of the substrate while traversing toward the product. In 1948, Pauling initially suggested that compounds resembling the transition state of an enzyme-catalyzed reaction would be effective inhibitors of the enzyme, because the substrate transition state should have the greatest affinity for the enzyme.[10] Later, Wolfenden proposed that thermodynamically, it is possible to relate the hypothetical equilibrium dissociation constants between substrate and its transition state of an enzyme-catalyzed reaction with that of the nonenzyme-catalyzed one.[26] Using such an analysis, he showed that the ratio of the hypothetical transition state dissociation constants of nonenzyme-catalyzed reaction to that of the enzyme-catalyzed one is equal to the ratio of the first-order rate constants of formation of transition state for enzyme-catalyzed reaction to noncatalyzed reaction. Because the ratio of the enzyme-catalyzed rate constant to that of the noncatalyzed one ranges from 10^7 to 10^{10}, it follows that the substrate transition state would bind the enzyme 10^7- to 10^{10}-fold more tightly than the substrate itself.[27] Hence, transition-state analogues that resemble the substrate would be extremely tight-binding compounds. To design a transition-state inhibitor, knowledge of the enzyme chemistry and its mechanism is a basic requirement. It must be understood, however, that these substrate transition states are, by nature, unstable transient species existing for no longer than a few picoseconds. Nevertheless, experimental evidence has shown that even crudely designed transition-state inhibitors resembling the substrate are extremely potent inhibitors.[27]

TRANSITION-STATE INHIBITOR OF ADENOSINE DEAMINASE. Adenosine deaminase is the enzyme that hydrolyzes adenosine (or deoxyadenosine) to inosine (or deoxyinosine) and is important for purine metabolism. High levels of adenosine are toxic to B cells of the immune system and can result in an immunocompromised state. Also, people who lack the gene for adenosine deaminase have the genetic condition of severe combined immunodeficiency and are extremely susceptible to opportunistic infections. Many cancer and antiviral agents also are degraded by this enzyme; hence, there is a role for the development of inhibitors of this enzyme.[28] The mechanism proposed for adenosine deaminase is a nucleophilic attack of water at the 6-position of the purine base to form a tetrahedral intermediate (Fig. 9.14). The transition state presumably resembles this intermediate.

During the course of the deaminase reaction, the hybridization of the G-carbon changes from an sp^2-hybridized state to an sp^3 state. Subsequently, there is a loss of ammonia to give the product inosine. To develop a transition-state inhibitor for this enzyme, one would have to factor in this change in the hybridization of the substrate molecule; thus, molecules having an sp^3-hybridized carbon at this position and resembling the substrate would potentially be candidates for transition-state inhibitors. The compound 1,6-dihydro-6-hydroxymethylpurine has such geometry, and its potent inhibitory properties of adenosine deaminase ($K_i < 1$ μM, as compared to a K_m for adenosine of 31 M) has been rationalized as being a transition-state inhibitor.[29] Two compounds that nature has provided, coformycin and its deoxyribose analogue, deoxycoformycin (Fig. 9.14), are extremely potent inhibitors of adenosine deaminase (K_i = 0.002 nM). Both of these compounds contain a seven-member ring structure, which through its flexibility is presumed to resemble the hypothesized distorted sp^2–sp^3 transition state that forms during the addition of water to adenosine.[30]

Irreversible Enzyme Inhibition

As previously described, irreversible enzyme inhibition is defined as "time-dependent inactivation of the enzyme," which implies that the enzyme has, in some way or form, been permanently modified, because it can no longer carry out its function. This modification is the result of a covalent bond being formed with the inhibitor and some amino acid residue in the protein. Furthermore, this bond is extremely stable and, for all practical purposes, is not hydrolyzed to give back the enzyme in its original state or structure. In most examples of irreversible inhibition, a new enzyme must be generated through gene transcription and translation for the enzyme to continue its normal catalytic action. Basically, there are two types of irreversible enzyme inhibitors, the

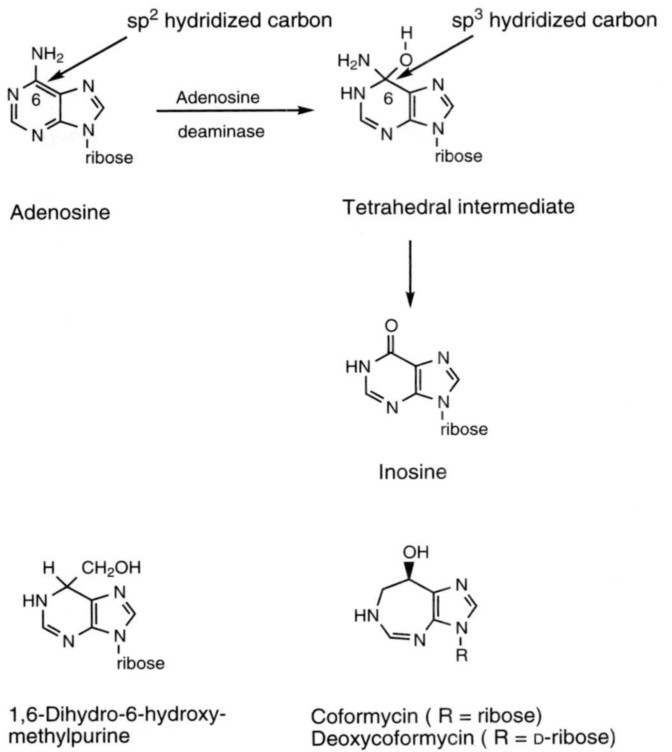

Figure 9.14 Mechanism and transition-state inhibitors of adenosine deaminase.

affinity labels or active site–directed irreversible inhibitors, and the mechanism-based irreversible enzyme inactivators.

AFFINITY LABELS AND ACTIVE SITE–DIRECTED IRREVERSIBLE INHIBITORS. The affinity labels are those chemical entities that are inherently reactive and can target any nucleophilic residue in the enzyme, especially those residing in and around the catalytic center of the protein. These agents generally resemble the substrate so that they may bind in the active site of the enzyme. In most examples, these agents also contain an electrophilic functional group, which includes groups such as halo-methyl ketones (X-CH_2C=O, where X = halide), sulfonyl fluorides (SO_2F), nitrogen mustards (($ClCH_2CH_2)_2NH$), diazoketones ($COCHN_2$), alpha beta unsaturated carbonyls (e.g., Michael Acceptors), and other such reactive groups, that can "label," or alkylate, a nucleophilic amino acid residue in the enzyme. They generally tend to be indiscriminate in their action and have little therapeutic value, because they are nonselective and, thus, inherently toxic. They have been used mainly as biochemical tools to probe active sites of enzyme to discern the types of amino acid residues both in and around the catalytic center of an enzyme. The classic example of an affinity label is TPCK (tosyl-phenylalanyl-chloromethyl-ketone), an irreversible inhibitor of the serine protease chymotrypsin.[31] Because TPCK resembles the amino acid phenylalanine, it can bind to the active site of the chymotrypsin, the selectivity of which is for such hydrophobic amino acid residues (Phe and Tyr). During the course of normal peptide hydrolysis, the reactive chloromethyl-ketone labels the nucleophilic histidine residue present as part of the catalytic triad (Ser-His-Asp) in the active site of the protease (Fig. 9.15). Another similarly designed affinity label is TLCK (tosyl-lysyl-chloromethyl-ketone), the specificity of which is for the protease trypsin. Trypsin cleaves peptide bonds adjacent to the basic amino acids, lysine and arginine. It was found that TLCK was a specific inhibitor of trypsin but had no activity for chymotrypsin. On the other hand, TPCK, although extremely specific for chymotrypsin, showed no activity for trypsin. However, there are some examples of such molecules (e.g., Michael acceptors) being developed as useful drugs—see discussion on Tyrosine Kinase Inhibitors (see Chapter 33).

TosHN TosHN H2N Cl Cl O O

TPCK TLCK

Because of the inherent reactivity and nonselectivity of many affinity labels and their limited utility in drug therapy, B.R. Baker extended this concept to design inhibitors that would have greater selectivity and specificity and, thus, be potential drug candidates.[32] He designed several analogues, termed active site–directed irreversible inhibitors, targeted toward thymidylate synthase, a key enzyme involved in the de novo metabolism of thymidylate. These analogues contained a substrate-binding region linked to a reactive group, such as a halomethyl ketone, by a tether whose chain length could be manipulated. The substrate portion of the analogue ensures both affinity and rapid binding to

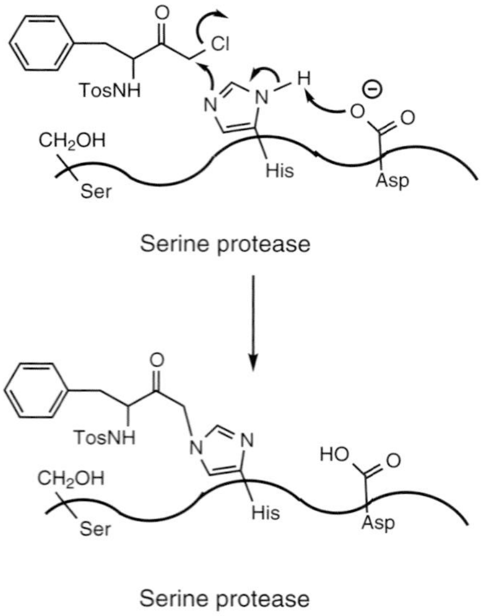

Figure 9.15 Mechanism of affinity label of serine protease with TPCK (tosyl-phenylalanyl-chloromethyl-ketone).

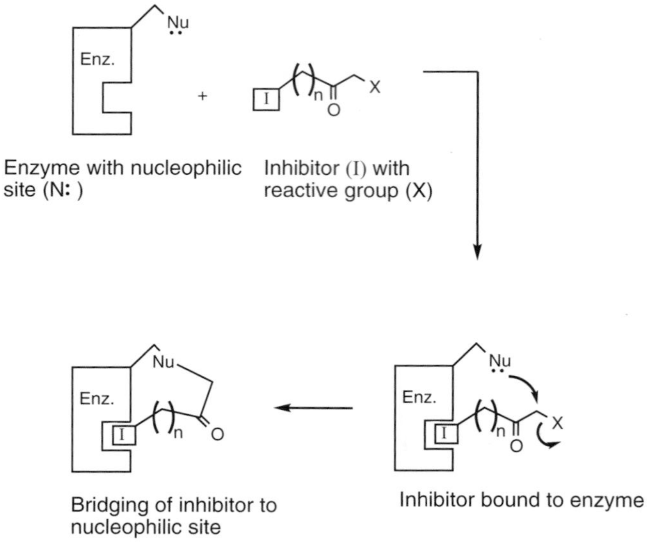

Figure 9.16 Model showing Baker's[32] active site–directed irreversible inhibitors.

the enzyme active site. Once bound, areas in and around the binding site and on the surface of the enzyme could be probed for nucleophilic amino acid residues. By manipulating the length of the tether, ideal inhibitors could then be designed such that any suitably located, sufficiently nucleophilic amino acid residue on the surface of the enzyme could potentially be alkylated by the halomethyl ketone (Fig. 9.16). Once alkylated, the tether "bridges" the active site with the labeled amino acid residue, thus "tying up" and preventing further catalysis by the enzyme.

Mechanism-Based Irreversible Enzyme Inactivators

Overview. The mechanism-based irreversible inhibitors also have been termed as "suicide substrates," "k_{cat} inhibitors," "Trojan horse inhibitors," or "latent alkylating agents." These inhibitors are inherently unreactive but, on normal catalytic processing by the enzyme, are activated into highly reactive moieties.[33–35] These reactive functionalities can then irreversibly alkylate a nucleophilic amino acid residue or cofactor in the enzyme and, in essence, cause the enzyme's death ("suicide"). Basically, these inhibitors have a latent reactive functionality that only becomes apparent after binding and acted on by the normal catalytic machinery of the enzyme. This type of inhibitor design differs from the preceding one in that these inhibitors have one more level of built-in selectivity. The kinetic scheme for such inhibition is shown in Equation (9.5), in which enzyme, E, binds with inhibitor, S, to give an [E–S] complex with dissociation constant of K_m (or K_i):

$$\mathrm{E + S} \underset{}{\overset{K_m}{\rightleftharpoons}} [\mathrm{E{\cdot}S}] \overset{k_{cat}}{\rightleftharpoons} [\mathrm{E{\cdot}S^*}] \xrightarrow{k_{inact}} \mathrm{E\text{-}S^*} \text{ (Enzyme inactivated)}$$

$$[\mathrm{E{\cdot}S^*}] \xrightarrow{k_{diff}} \mathrm{E + S^*} \xrightarrow{+\ddot{\mathrm{N}}\mathrm{u}} \mathrm{Nu\text{-}S^*} \text{ (Nonselective inactivation)} \qquad \text{Eq. 9.5}$$

$$K_p \text{ (partition ratio)} = k_{diff}/k_{inact}$$

Next, the [E·S] complex is converted into a highly activated complex [E·S*] by the catalytic machinery (k_{cat}) of the enzyme, which can then go on to alkylate the enzyme, [E-S*]. Note that it is possible for the reactive species [S*] to diffuse (dissociate) from the enzyme and react with some other (off) target nucleophilic species (Nu), that is, the system is "leaky." If this happens, however, the inhibitor cannot be classified as a true suicide substrate, because specificity is lost.

Several requirements need to be met by these inhibitors for them to be classified as suicide substrates. These include the following: (1) inactivation should be time dependent (reaction should be irreversible), (2) kinetics should be first order, (3) the enzyme should show saturation phenomenon, (4) the substrate should be able to protect the enzyme, and (5) stoichiometry of the reaction should be 1:1 (one active site to one inhibitor), and if stoichiometry is not 1:1, then the partition

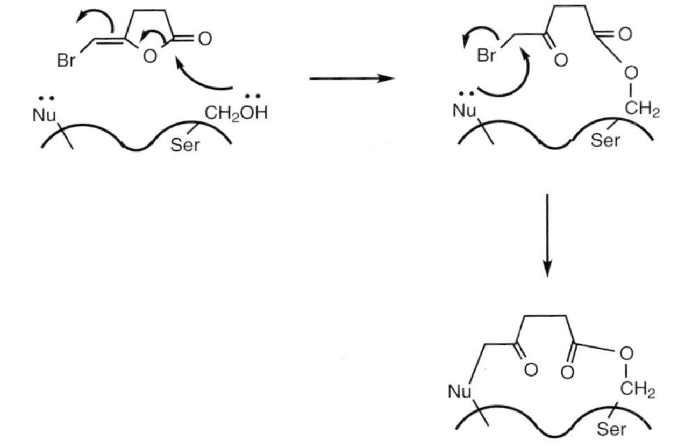

Figure 9.17 Mechanism-based inhibition of serine proteases by Katzenellenbogen's halo enol lactone.

ratio, ratio of the inactivation step to the diffusion step ($K_p = k_{diff}/k_{inact}$), should not change with increasing inhibitor concentrations.

EXAMPLES OF SUICIDE SUBSTRATES. During the past three decades, besides the rational design of hundreds of molecules that have been synthesized and tested as suicide substrates, it also has come to light that nature itself has known about this mechanistic mode of enzyme inhibition and provided us with several extremely potent mechanism-based suicide inactivators. Below are a few selected examples to demonstrate the mode of action of these inhibitors.

Halo enol lactones. Halo enol lactones are an example of suicide inhibitors for serine proteases. These analogues were developed by Katzenellenbogen and coworkers at the University of Illinois.[35] On normal catalytic processing by the serine hydroxyl functionality, they give rise to a reactive halo-methyl ketone, which subsequently alkylates a nearby nucleophilic residue on the enzyme (Fig. 9.17). Other suicide inactivators for the serine proteases have been designed by various researchers.[34]

Clauvulinic acid. Clavulanic acid, a natural product synthesized by certain *Streptomyces* bacteria is a potent inhibitor of bacterial β-lactamase.[36] This enzyme is a serine protease and can hydrolyze β-lactams, such as the penicillin antibiotics. It is the principal enzyme responsible for penicillin-resistant bacteria. Clavulanic acid itself is a β-lactam and, if given in combination with penicillin, is preferentially taken up by β-lactamase and hydrolyzed. During the process of hydrolysis, however, the molecule undergoes a cleavage, leading to the formation of a "Michael acceptor," which subsequently alkylates a nucleophilic residue on β-lactamase, causing irreversible inhibition (Fig. 9.18). Such combinations of a β-lactamase inhibitor and a penicillin have resulted in clinically useful agents (clavulanic acid plus amoxicillin [Augmentin]).

Gabaculin. Gabaculin, a naturally occurring neurotoxin, is a potent mechanism-based inhibitor of the enzyme γ-aminobutyric acid transaminase (GABA-T) with an interesting mechanism of action.[37] GABA-T is a pyridoxal phosphate (PLP)–dependent enzyme involved in the catabolism (transamination) of the excitatory neurotransmitter, GABA, to succinate semialdehyde and pyridoxamine. As part of the normal catalytic mechanism of PLP-dependent enzymes, the amino group of gabaculin first forms a Schiff base with the aldehyde of PLP (Fig. 9.19). Next, this adduct undergoes an aromatization reaction, resulting in an extremely stable covalent bond with the cofactor, PLP. Hence, in this case, rather than an enzymatic nucleophilic residue being alkylated, the cofactor is "tied up," resulting in the inhibition.

Finasteride. Finasteride is a clinically useful agent in the treatment of prostate hyperplasia and male pattern baldness. It is a potent inhibitor of human steroid-5α-reductase, the enzyme responsible for the reduction of testosterone to dihydrotestosterone (Fig. 9.20). The inhibitory action of finasteride has been attributed both to its similarity in structure to testosterone, which allows it to bind to the enzyme and be reduced to dihydrofinasteride in place of testosterone, as well as to its ability to act as a mechanism-based inhibitor, during which it can tie up the cofactor, NADPH, by forming a covalent NADP-dihydrofinasteride adduct (Fig. 9.20) (see Chapter 24). This adduct very slowly releases dihydrofinasteride with a half-life of 1 month.[38]

Inhibitors of Clinically Important Enzymes

Cyclic Nucleotide Phophodiesterase Inhibitors

Phosphodiesterases belong to a large family of enzymes which hydrolyze phosphate-ester bonds (viz. ester bonds

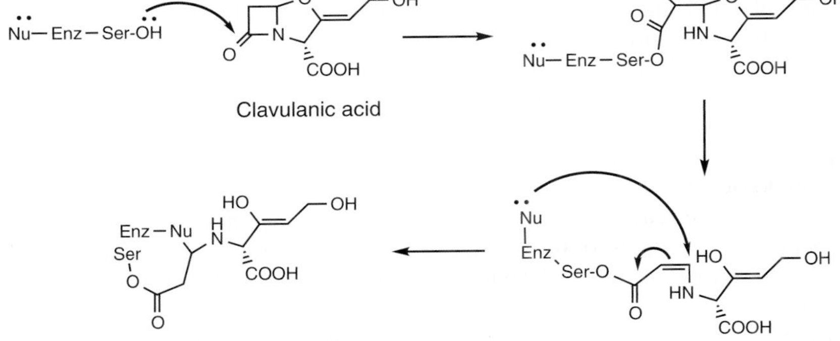

Clavulanic acid

Figure 9.18 Mechanism-based inhibition of β-lactamases by clavulanic acid.

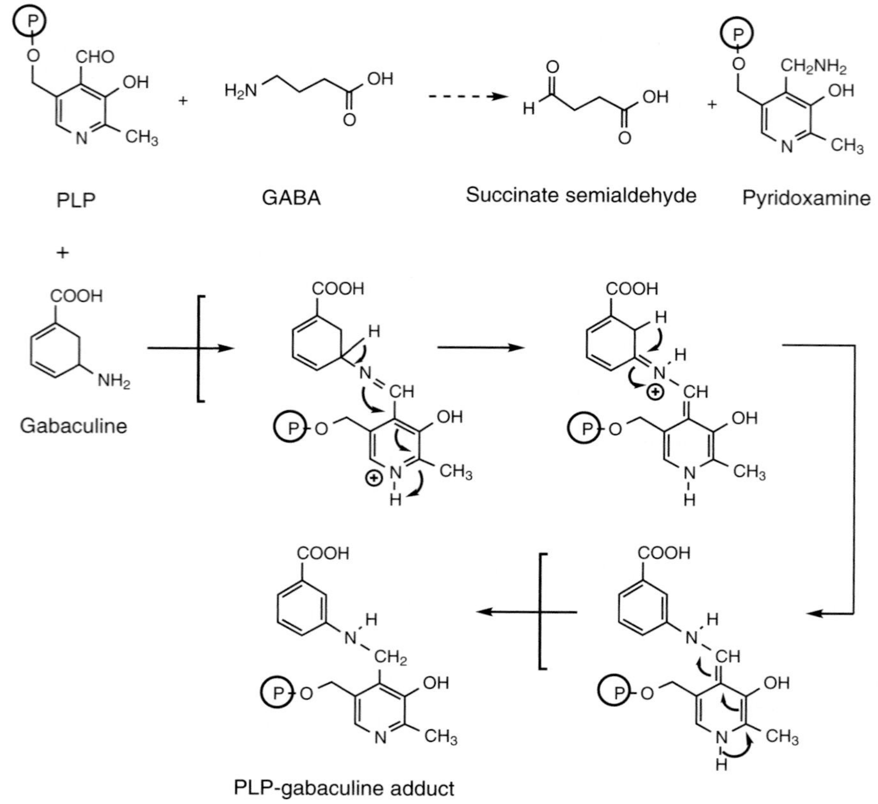

Figure 9.19 Pyridoxal phosphate–dependent γ-aminobutyric acid transaminase (GABA-T) reaction and the mechanism of suicide inhibition by gabaculin.

between two hydroxyl functionalities with phosphoric acid). In nature there are numerous biomolecules containing such phosphodiester bonds including glycerol-phosphates (phosphor-lipids), sugar phosphates, inositol phosphates, nucleic acids, and nucleotides including the cyclic nucleotides. While all of these molecules are essentially hydrolyzed by a phosphodiesterase, however, the specific name of phosphodiesterase (PDE) has been reserved for enzymes that hydrolyze the cyclic nucleotide monophosphate (cNMP), viz. cyclic adenosine monophosphate (cAMP) and cyclic guanosine monophosphate (cGMP), both molecules involved in signal transduction and second messenger cell signaling (Fig. 9.21). Enzymes that hydrolyze the phosphodiester bonds other than the cyclic nucleotides are known by other names, e.g., nucleases (DNAses or RNAses, for nucleic acids) and phopholipases for glycerol phosphates.

The cyclic nucleotide phosphodiesterases (PDEs) hydrolyze the 3′-5′ phosphodiester bond of cAMP and cGMP leading to the formation of AMP (5′-adenosine monophosphate) and GMP (5′-guanosine monophosphate). The PDEs can bind either cyclic nucleotide with selectivity depending on the particular isozyme. These cyclic nucleotide (cAMP and cGMP), substrates for PDEs, are formed from their precursor nucleotide triphosphates, NTP (ATP and GTP, respectively) by nucleotide cyclases (Fig. 9.21). There are many different isoforms of the PDEs present in cells which allow for great diversity in substrate specificity and cell regulation.

This diversity further governs specific roles for each of these PDEs in various cellular locales, physiological and pathological conditions. Currently the PDEs have been classified into eleven different families based upon gene products (amino acid homology) and are estimated to comprise over 100 different mRNAs from 21 different genes due to alternative splicing and transcription start sites.[39–41] The nomenclature of these PDE families are based upon the species of origin, the gene and the variant discovered. For example, HsPDE2A3 signifies that the origin is from *Homo sapiens* (Hs), PDE denotes that it is a cyclic nucleotide phosphodiesterase, the 2A indicates that it is from the PDE gene 2 family A, and 3 indicates that it is the third variant that was reported in the gene database.

The different PDEs have been shown to regulate various cellular activities, and hence because of this diverse functional ability, one could develop drugs to control these PDEs in a selective manner (Table 9.2).[42,43] Structural studies of several of these PDEs have shown that they all contain a "catalytic domain" with a consensus sequence denoting a metal ion binding site (a phosphorylase sequence, containing a signature recognition sequence for all PDEs) of two histidines and two aspartates that bind Zn^{2+}/Mg^{2+}; a "glutamine switch" which accounts for the substrate specificity (cAMP or cGMP) where an invariant glutamine amino acid residue can rotate to either H-bond with cAMP or cGMP (utilizing either cNMP as substrate) or is constrained from binding to one of the cNMPs thus favoring binding to the other nucleotide; and a "regulatory

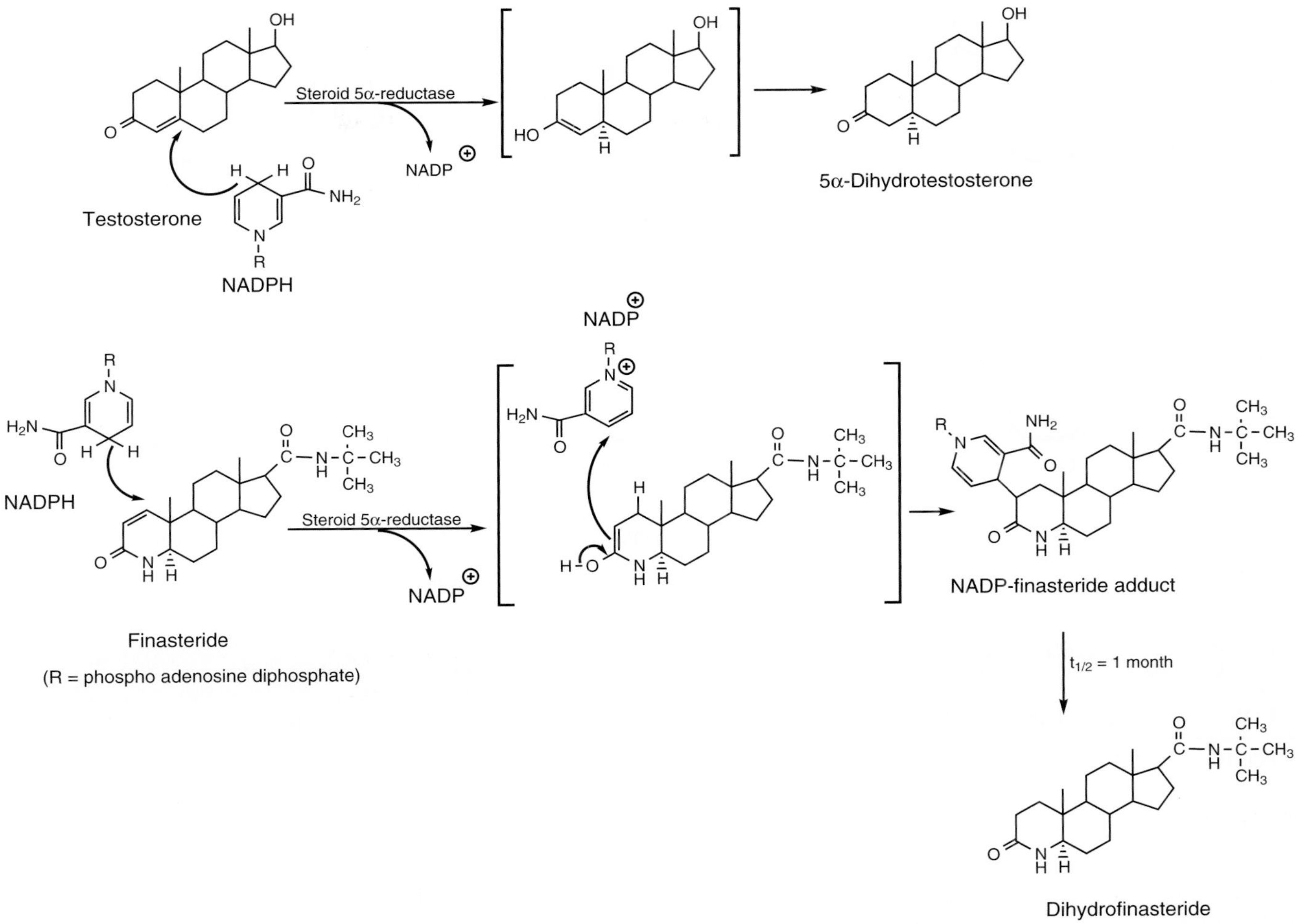

Figure 9.20 Mechanism of steroid reductase reduction on finasteride and testosterone and the structure of hypothesized NADPH-dihydrofinasteride adduct.[38]

domain" based upon the specific PDE family (e.g., Ca^{2+}—calmodulin binding site for PDE1) as well as an allosteric binding sites for cGMP.[40,41]

X-ray crystallographic studies with inhibitors bound with the protein have indicated that there are several binding modes for inhibition and the active site architecture is often unique for different PDEs. Inhibitors can bind to the protein through H-bonds with amino acid residues that make up the active site for cNMP binding, with residues that line the channel leading to the active site as well as by H-bonding with water to residues that bind to the active site metal ions. Moreover, because of the order of magnitude differences in cellular concentrations of the cyclic nucleotides (as compared to its precursor, NTP molecule, <1-10 μM for cAMP/cGMP vs. mM concentrations for ATP/GTP), these PDEs become attractive targets to design drugs[40] (since competitive inhibition for a natural substrate whose cellular concentration is 1 μM is achieved much more easily than if the substrate concentration was 1 mM!). Structural knowledge of the different binding modes for inhibitors with the PDEs has given rise to the rapid development of selective PDE inhibitors to allow for specific interactions along regulatory pathways involving such PDEs. While inhibitors of PDEs have been known for quite some time, e.g., caffeine and theophylline have been in use as therapeutic agents for many decades (as nonselective inhibitors of PDE), the development of drugs to selectively inhibit a particular PDE is a more recent phenomenon. Moreover, selective inhibitors would also have a better safety profile as one would expect a decreased amount of side/toxic effects. For example, theophylline, a nonselective PDE inhibitor, is known to have a narrow therapeutic index because of its interaction with multiple PDEs.

PDE5 SELECTIVE INHIBITORS. The impetus for the development of PDE inhibitors arose from the knowledge that vasodilation (for treatment of high blood pressure) could be achieved through the stimulation of atrial natriuretic peptide (ANP), an endogenous peptide which allows for renal excretion of sodium/water. Furthermore, it was also known that ANP stimulated the synthesis of cGMP through its activation of guanylyl cylcase. Hence inhibition of cGMP hydrolysis (i.e., PDE activity) was a rational target for the development of these vasodilators. Since ANP worked in the kidney, the idea was to target the specific PDE in the kidney. The lead compound for the development of

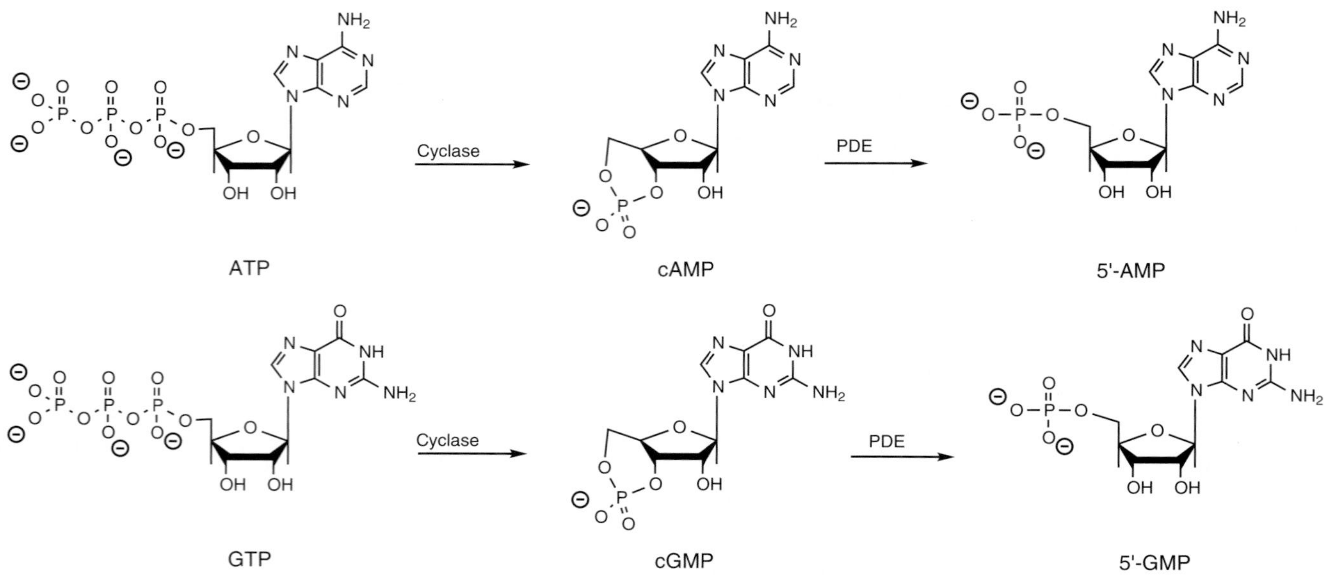

Figure 9.21 Enzymatic interconversions of cyclic and linear nucleotides.

Table 9.2 Specificity and Potency of PDE Inhibitors

PDE	Specificity	Inhibitor	IC_{50}[a] (nM)	PDE	Specificity	Inhibitor	IC_{50}[a] (nM)
PDE1B	Duel	Rolipram	>200,000	PDE6	cGMP	Sildenafil	50[b]
		Cilomilast	87,000			Vardenafil	11[c]
		Roflumilast	>200,000			Tadalafil	2,000[b]
		Sildenafil	1,500	PDE7B	cAMP	Rolipram	>2,000,000
		Vardenafil	300			Cilomilast	44,000
		Tadalafil	50,000			Roflumilast	>200,000
PDE2A	Duel	Rolipram	>200,000			Sildenafil	78,000
		Cilomilast	160,000			Vardenafil	1,900
		Roflumilast	>200,000			Tadalafil	74,000
		Sildenafil	35,000	PDE8A	cAMP	Rolipram	>200,000
		Vardenafil	3,100			Cilomilast	7,000
		Tadalafil	130,000			Roflumilast	>200,000
PDE3B	cAMP > cGMP	Rolipram	>200,000			Sildenafil	>200,000
		Cilomilast	87,000			Vardenafil	57,000
		Roflumilast	>200,000			Tadalafil	>200,000
		Sildenafil	15,000	PDE9A	cGMP	Rolipram	>200,000
		Vardenafil	580			Cilomilast	>200,000
		Tadalafil	280,000			Roflumilast	>200,000
PDE4B	cAMP	Rolipram	570			Sildenafil	5,600
		Cilomilast	25			Vardenafil	680
		Roflumilast	0.84			Tadalafil	150,000
		Sildenafil	20,000	PDE10A	cAMP<cGMP	Rolipram	140,000

Table 9.2 Specificity and Potency of PDE Inhibitors (Continued)

PDE	Specificity	Inhibitor	IC_{50}[a] (nM)	PDE	Specificity	Inhibitor	IC_{50}[a] (nM)
		Vardenafil	3,800			Cilomilast	73,000
		Tadalafil	9,200			Roflumilast	>200,000
PDE4D	cAMP	Rolipram	1,100			Sildenafil	6,800
		Cilomilast	11			Vardenafil	880
		Roflumilast	0.68			Tadalafil	19,000
		Sildenafil	14,000	PDE11A	Duel	Rolipram	>200,000
		Vardenafil	3,900			Cilomilast	21,000
		Tadalafil	19,000			Roflumilast	25,000
PDE5A	cGMP	Rolipram	>200,000			Sildenafil	6,100
		Cilomilast	53,000			Vardenafil	240
		Roflumilast	17,000			Tadalafil	10
		Sildenafil	2.2				
		Vardenafil	1.0				
		Tadalafil	1.2				

[a]Data are from Sutherland and Rall[40] unless stated otherwise. The numbers shown in the table are the 50% inhibition concentration (IC50). The cAMP and cGMP; concentrations used were far below the K_m of all the PDEs assayed except for PDE9A, in which case it was close to the K_m. The IC50s obtained are good approximations of the inhibition constant K_i. Selectivities of an inhibitor may be determined by taking ratios of the numbers given in the table.
[b]K_i values are from Card et al.[42]
[c]Value from Hatzelmann and Schudt.[43]

these PDE inhibitors was a xanthine derivative, zaprinast (Fig. 9.22), previously shown to demonstrate weak PDE inhibition.[44] Analysis of the heterocyclic ring of zaprinast and comparison with the purine heterocycle of cGMP led to the development of a number of derivatives displaying PDE5 inhibitory activity, including the design of one containing a pyrazolopyrimidinone which ultimately resulted in the development of the potent PDE5 inhibitor, Sildenafil.[45] During clinical trials of Sildenafil as an antihypertensive and vasodilatory agent, it was found to have a (beneficial) side effect in erectile dysfunction. This pharmacological effect was recognized, appreciated, and commercialized into a new line of therapeutic agents to treat the condition, erectile dysfunction. Inhibition of cGMP hydrolysis (PDE5) in the corpus cavernosum results in elevated levels of cGMP leading to increased smooth muscle relaxation and improved blood flow and maintenance of an erection. Presently, PDE5 selective inhibitors include the drugs sildenafil (Viagra), vardenafil (Levitra), and tadalafil (Cialis). They have been one of the most widely marketed and commercially successful drugs in recent years to treat erectile dysfunction in males and also more recently have been approved to treat pulmonary hypertension. These drugs have high selectivity to inhibit PDE5 over the other PDE classes. PDE5 is a phosphodiesterase that specifically hydrolyzes cGMP to GMP at low substrate levels and also has a high affinity binding site for cGMP on its regulatory domain.

The enzyme, originally isolated from platelets, was later found to be a regulator in vascular smooth muscle contraction present in the lungs and brains. The drugs are all reversible inhibitors of PDE5 where they bind in the active site of PDE5, the heterocyclic nucleus of the inhibitors binding in the space reserved for the purine ring (of cGMP). Side effects include hypotension, and also, since the active site structures of PDE5 and PDE6 are similar in architecture, some cross inhibition to PDE6 enzymes has been observed. PDE6 enzymes regulate the phototransduction cascade where PDE6 rapidly reduces the steady-state concentration of cGMP in response to light stimuli. Thus side effects of these PDE5 inhibitors include decreased vision in some patient populations. The drug, tadalafil, however, is about 1000-fold more selective for PDE5 versus PDE6. Several other selective competitive PDE inhibitors are approved for use, and these include the PDE4 inhibitors, cilomilast and roflumilast for treatment of COPD (Fig. 9.23) as well as the PDE3 inhibitors, dipyridamole and cilostazol, as antiplatelet drugs (Fig. 9.24), and inamrinone and milrinone as positive inotropic agents (Fig. 9.25).

Protein Kinase Inhibitors

Protein kinases belong to the family of group transfer phosphorylating enzymes that transfer a phosphate group from ATP onto amino acid residues of proteins. It is estimated that there are over 500 of these kinases encoded by the

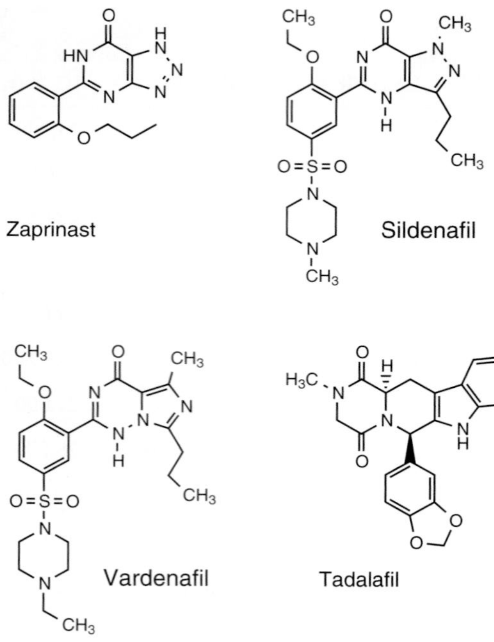

Zaprinast Sildenafil Vardenafil Tadalafil

Figure 9.22 Inhibitors of PDE5.

Dipyridamole Cilostazol

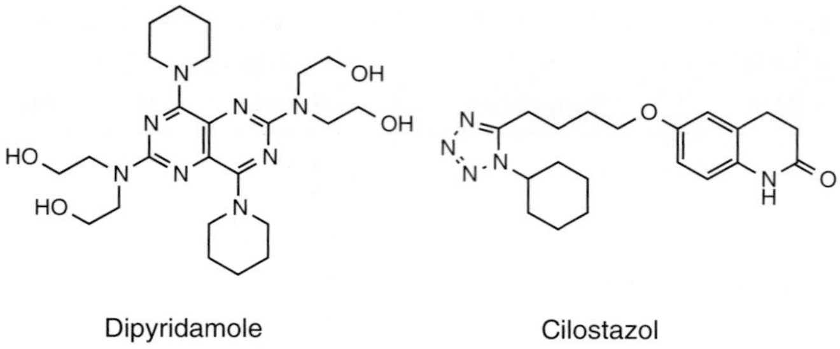

Figure 9.24 Antiplatelet inhibitors of PDE3.

human genome (the kinome), and this kinase reaction when coupled with a phosphatase (dephosphorylation) reaction, i.e., reversible phosphorylation of proteins, offers cells a precise regulatory mechanism to control its differentiation, maturation, proliferation, apoptosis, and other cellular functions.[46] The substrate amino acid residues on proteins that are phosphorylated belong largely to the hydroxyl bearing amino acids such as serine, threonine, and tyrosine. Hence, these kinases are referred to as either serine/threonine kinases or tyrosine kinases. Similarly, the phosphatases are referred to as serine/threonine or tyrosine phosphatases of which the tyrosine phosphatases predominate. Since these proteins are involved in regulatory functions of the cell, it becomes intuitive that mutations or aberrations of expression of these proteins can lead to dysregulation of cellular functions giving rise to tumors and cancers and other diseases. Indeed, research has shown that of the 518 kinase genes present in the human genome, 244 map to disease loci and cancer.[46] Moreover, targeting these enzymes with inhibitors would be a way to selectively target cancers without the noxious side effects seen with conventional anticancer drugs such as the alkylating agents or antitumor antibiotics. Research over the last decade has provided this as a rationale to develop selective (targeted) anticancer therapy where such kinases which manifest themselves in certain cancers have been specifically targeted for inhibition resulting in dramatic declines of cancer cells and greater survival times for the patient.[47] Examples of such targeted anticancer drugs have involved primarily the development of the tyrosine kinase inhibitors (TKIs) several of which are FDA approved (see Chapter 33); however, more recently, inhibitors of serine/threonine kinases have entered the clinical market while inhibitors of the tyrosine phosphatases are in development.

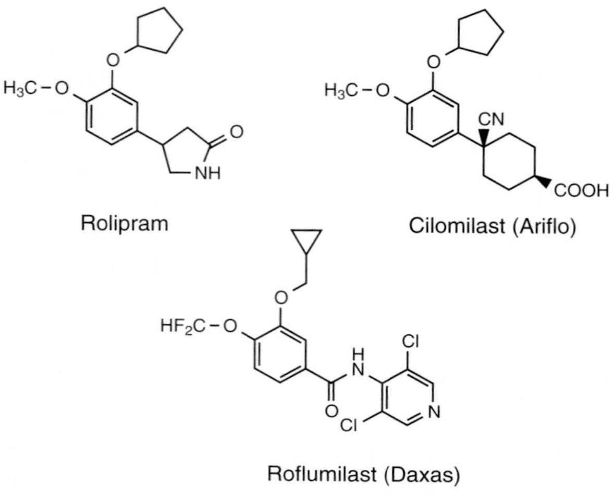

TYROSINE KINASE INHIBITORS. The tyrosine kinases are a group of enzymes responsible for signal transduction and intracellular signaling functions many of which are involved in cell differentiation and proliferation. They can be divided into two major types depending upon where they act in the cell, viz. receptor tyrosine kinases (RTK), a membrane spanning protein having an extracellular ligand binding domain and an intracellular catalytic (kinase) domain involved in the transduction of extracellular signals from the membrane to the cytoplasm, and the nonreceptor tyrosine kinases involved in cytosolic signaling events.[47,48] Inhibitors for these have been developed for both types and have shown excellent and selective activity in cancers manifested by aberrant expression of these proteins. The design for selective inhibitors has been based on determining important binding regions to the protein. The kinase domain has a C-terminal domain linked via a "hinge region" to the N-terminal domain, and structural studies have indicated that ATP is known to bind to the backbone of this hinge region (ATP binding pocket). These kinases all have an "activation loop" which contains a tyrosine

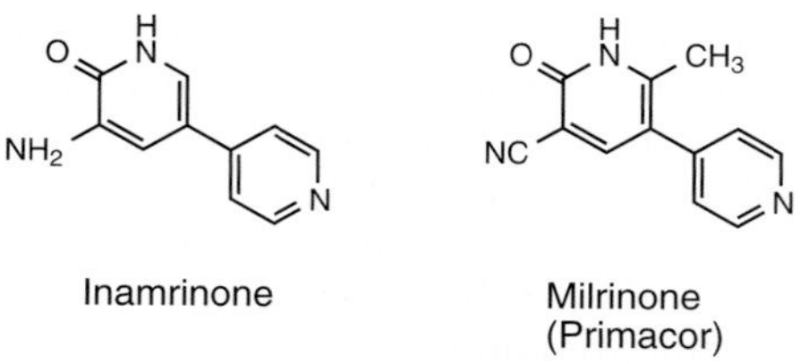

Rolipram Cilomilast (Ariflo) Roflumilast (Daxas)

Figure 9.23 Competitive inhibitors of PDE4.

Inamrinone Milrinone (Primacor)

Figure 9.25 PDE3 inhibitors with cardiac and pulmonary effects.

residue (Tyr393), the major phosphorylated residue that allows switching the kinase from inactive to active forms and allowing for ATP binding. The large majority of the TKIs bind to this region via H-bonding. Areas of the protein that have been identified as important for the function of kinases include a glycine-rich loop (G-loop), ATP binding pocket, a gate-keeper residue (an amino acid preceding the hinge region), and the DFG activation motif. Most of the inhibitors that have been developed tend to bind to the ATP binding pocket and have been classified based on their binding motif. The Type I inhibitors bind the "DFG-in" motif of the activation loop (the active form of the kinase, where the kinase is poised for the phosphoryl transfer) and is a more conserved region, while the Type II inhibitors bind the inactive (DFG-out) motif which is a region of less conserved residues but would allow for greater specificity. Type III and Type IV inhibitors bind to regions outside of the ATP binding pocket (distal sites) and are classified as allosteric inhibitors. The kinase-ligand interaction fingerprints and structures (KLIFS) is a useful database that identifies the binding pocket for Type I to Type IV inhibitors which includes the gatekeeper residues for various kinases and is often used to aid medicinal chemists in designing new kinase inhibitors.

The development of a tyrosine kinase inhibitor (TKI) to selectively treat a cancer, chronic myelogenous leukemia, CML, was the impetus leading to the large number of presently available TKIs. CML in the majority of patients is due to a reciprocal translocation of chromosomes 9 and 22 resulting in a fusion of the *abl* (Abelson leukemia virus) gene of chromosome 9 to the *bcr* (breakpoint cluster) gene of chromosome 22 leading to the *bcr-abl* fusion gene (the Philadelphia chromosome). While the *abl* gene normally produces a nonreceptor tyrosine kinase whose activity is highly regulated, the *bcr-abl* fusion gene produces a tyrosine kinase that is constitutively active and whose activity is required for the transformation of cells to become malignant.[49] The knowledge of this direct correlation between expression of the abnormal fusion protein and CML allowed for the development of specific inhibitors for this protein and other such dysregulated kinases that are overexpressed in many cancers. Using a high-throughput screening program to develop inhibitors for receptor tyrosine kinases as a possible treatment for such cancers, 2-phenylaminopyrimidine (PAP) became a lead compound. Further structure activity optimization and refinement of this lead led to Imatinib (Fig. 9.26), the first targeted drug for treatment of CML.[49–51] Note, the structure optimization to imatinib included addition of a pyridine, a methyl as well as a benzamide to enhance the potency of the basic PAP nucleus. The piperazinyl functionality helped to increase water solubility allowing for better "drug-like" properties. Imatinib also proved to be inhibitory in many other cancers with overexpressed kinases, such as gastrointestinal stromal tumors (GIST) (which overexpress *c-kit*), myelodysplastic diseases associated with platelet-derived growth factor receptor (PDGFR) as well as in Philadelphia chromosome-positive adult lymphoblastic leukemia.[50] X-ray crystallographic studies with imatinib co-cyrstallized with the TK expressed from *abl* showed that imatinib binds to the

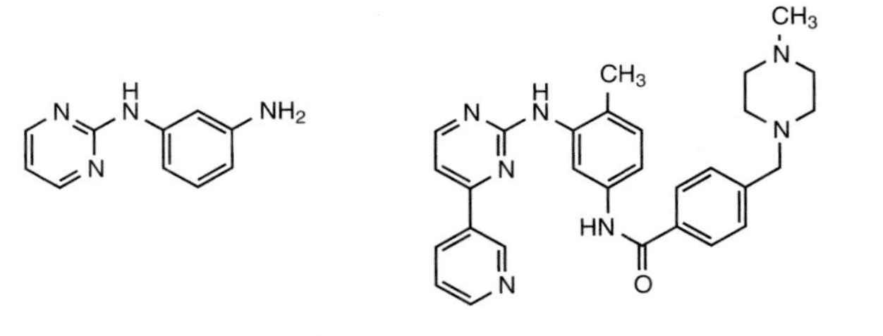

2-Phenylaminopyrimidine Imatinib

Figure 9.26 Structures of 2-phenylaminopyrimidine and imatinib.

ATP binding site of the protein in its inactive conformation (DFG-out form—Type II), and this binding prevented the kinase from achieving its productive binding conformation with ATP.[49] Studies showed that with the protein-bound imatinib, Tyr393 was not phosphorylated and the conformation of this activation loop in the nonphosphorylated protein changed to that resembling substrate (ATP) being bound to the kinase. In this way, the altered geometry brought about by imatinib binding to the protein prevented the protein from binding its true substrate, ATP.

Resistance develops to imatinib due to mutations (in the hydrophobic pocket, gate keeper residue being mutated to a larger residue) that prevent access of imatinib to the protein in the off state, thus allowing for the kinase to bind ATP and cancer to progress. TKIs dasatinib and bosutinib have also been developed to bind the kinase in its "on" (active conformation, Type-I) where the drugs can access hydrophobic regions in the ATP binding pocket as well as drugs that can bind both "on" and "off" forms—dual mode inhibitors which are more potent than imatinib.[52–54] It has been more than 15 years since the introduction of imatinib, and today many other TKI drugs have been developed for related tyrosine kinases such as epidermal growth factor receptor (EGFR), platelet-derived growth factor receptor (PDGFR), and vascular endothelial growth factor receptor (VEGFR). The inhibitors make use of differences in the variable region of the protein surrounding the ATP binding pocket which allows for specific binding interactions with the various functionalities present on the individual inhibitors. Resistance to these inhibitors manifest themselves due to mutations to these variable regions on the protein as well as to cellular efflux pumps being activated. While the vast majority of these clinically used drugs are reversible inhibitors of the Type I and II, more recently Type III inhibitors have been introduced in the clinic. Furthermore, irreversible inhibitors of Type I which employ the "Michael acceptor" functionality to irreversibly alkylate an active site cysteine residue have also been introduced. Examples of these inhibitors such as dasatinib (Type I for imatinib resistance), sunitinib (Type I, inhibitor of VEGFR), gefitinib (Type I, inhibitor of EGFR), trematinib (Type III, inhibitor of MEK), and the irreversible Type I inhibitor, Ibrutinib with the α,β unsaturated system (Michael acceptor) are shown in Figure 9.27.

SERINE/THREONINE KINASE INHIBITORS. The serine/threonine kinases are a family of enzymes that phosphorylate the hydroxyl groups of serine and threonine present

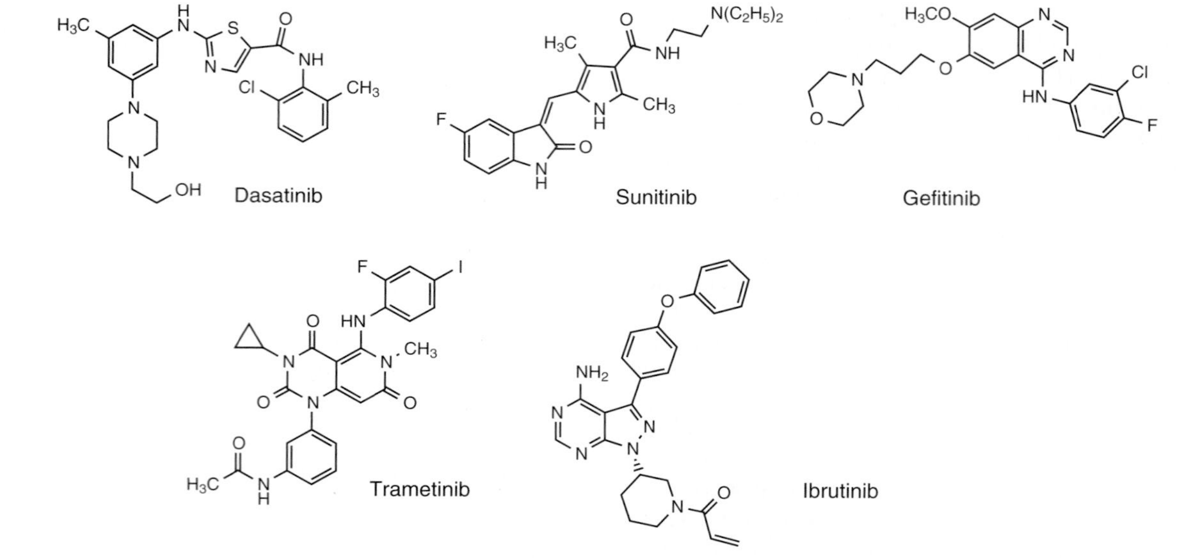

Figure 9.27 Structures of the tyrosine kinase inhibitors, dasatinib, sunitinib, gefitinib, and ibritutinib.

on proteins. There are a number of such serine/threonine kinases that are important regulators of cell proliferation and survival and whose dysregulation often lead to cancer and tumorigenesis. Protein kinase C is perhaps the most well-studied system, whose activation results in the formation of diacylglycerol (DAG), phosphatidylinositol-3,4,5-triphosphate (PIP3), and concomitant increase in intracellular calcium, leading to various signal transduction events in the cell through activation of the mitogen-activated protein kinase (MAPK) family.[55] Furthermore, other serine/threonine kinase proteins such as PI3K (phosphoinositide-3-kinase), Akt (protein kinase B), and mTOR (mammalian target of Rapamycin) are part of an intracellular signaling pathway that is important for regulation of cell proliferation, migration, and survival. Initial events leading to cell proliferation via the PI3K-Akt-mTOR have been shown to begin with growth factor or hormonal activation of a receptor tyrosine kinase which leads to activation of PI3K. This activation results in the release of PIP3 which in turn leads to phosphorylation and further activation of Akt and mTOR. Inhibitors of mTOR include rapamycin (sirolimus) and its derivatives, everolimus and temsirolimus. Rapamycin is a macrolide originally isolated from a microbe on Easter Island and primarily used as an immunosuppressant drug while its derivatives, everolimus and temsirolimus, have been used to treat renal cell carcinoma.

Additional development of molecules to specifically inhibit the PI3K-Akt pathway include copanlisib, which was recently introduced to treat follicular lymphoma, and duvelisib, a first-in-class inhibitor of PI3K that has recently received FDA new drug application (NDA) status to treat chronic lymphocytic leukemia (Fig. 9.28). Additional serine/threonine kinase function is also observed during mitosis, which is a highly regulated process with multiple checkpoints encountered during the chromosomal segregation stage of cell division. The phosphorylation of specific serine/threonine residues by these mitotic kinases (also known as Aurora A and Aurora B kinases) serves as important checkpoints during mitosis. These Aurora kinases interact with many proteins, including tumor suppressors and activators from the mitotic entry stage all the

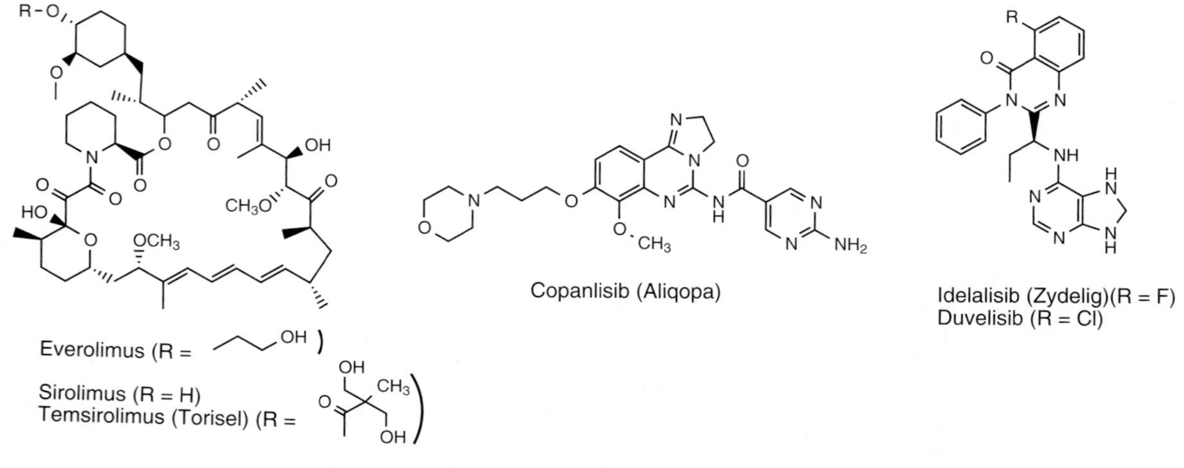

Figure 9.28 Structures of mTOR and PI3K-Akt serine/threonine kinase inhibitors.

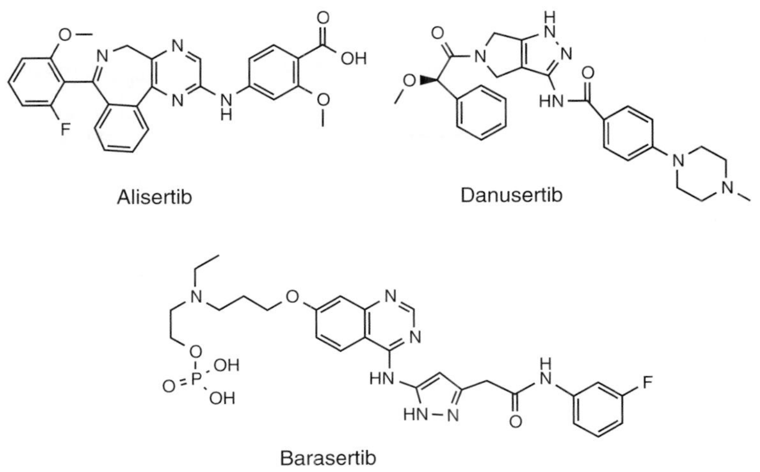

Alisertib

Danusertib

Barasertib

Figure 9.29 Structures of Aurura kinase inhibitors.

way to cytokinesis. It is not surprising then that they are overexpressed in many tumors (breast, colon, gastric, ovarian, and pancreatic) and thus have become an attractive target for anticancer drug development.[56,57] Examples of some of these inhibitors include alisertib, danusertib, and a phosphate-based prodrug currently under development, barasertib (Fig. 9.29).

Other serine/threonine kinases include the RAF proteins which are involved in the MAPK activation cascade during cell growth. B-RAF is one member of the RAF family where mutations (specifically the V600E) have resulted in dysregulation of the cascade leading to many cancers. Specific clinically used inhibitors of the V600E B-RAF mutated protein include vemurafenib and dabrafenib (Fig. 9.30) used to treat metastatic melanoma.[58]

PROTEIN TYROSINE PHOSPHATASES. The PTP is another family of proteins that is important for maintaining homeostasis where levels and extent of protein phosphorylation/dephosphorylation bring about changes in cellular activity. Recent estimates from proteonomic data suggest that the bulk of cellular proteins get phosphorylated at serine/threonine and/or tyrosine residues at some time or another during their tenure. This implies that dephosphorylation (phosphatase activity) must also occur in order to control the overall level of protein phosphorylation.[59] The extent and variation of phosphorylation would result in changes at the cellular level to protein-protein interactions, protein localization, migration, protein stability, gene transcription, apoptosis, protein signaling, and other types of cellular interactions. Thus phosphatases, in conjunction with the kinases, provide a mechanism for precise control of cellular activities. It is evident then that any dysregulation in kinase and/or phosphatse activity would likely lead to various disease states including cancer, diabetes, and autoimmune diseases. The mechanism of action of PTPs involve nucleophilic covalent catalysis by an active site cysteine residue on the phosphorous atom of the phosphorylated tyrosine to form a thiophosporyl intermediate, which is subsequently hydrolyzed by general base catalysis to release the free cysteine.[59] Moreover, the active sites of the PTPS are remarkably conserved, and so it becomes a challenge to design inhibitors directed to the active site to achieve specificity. However, studies have also shown that the activity of PTPS may be regulated by several mechanisms including·gene transcription, protein localization, and oligomerization (dimerization), as well as the oxidation state of the thiol group of the active site cysteine. Dimerization of the PTPs results in preventing the substrate from binding to the PTP active site.[59] Additionally, the catalytic activity of the active site cysteine thiol group is regulated by intracellular hydrogen peroxide. The –SH (thiol) group of the active site cysteine is easily oxidized by H_2O_2 to the nonnucleophilic, sulfenate (–SOH), thus inhibiting the phosphorylase activity. Figure 9.31 A and B depicts the mechanism of the phosphatase activity as well as the redox regulation of the free cysteine. It should be remembered that the sulfenate can be easily reduced

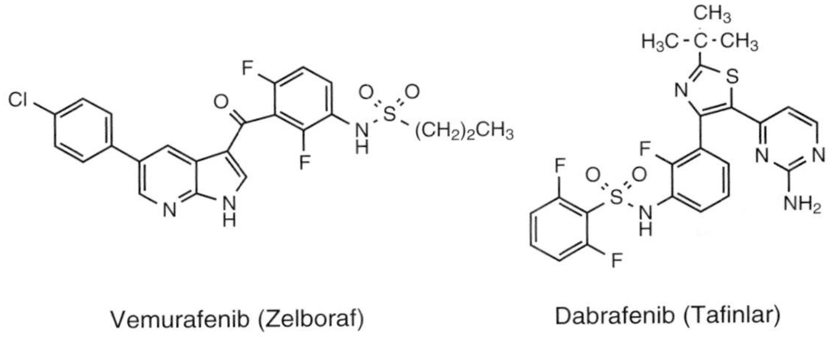

Vemurafenib (Zelboraf)

Dabrafenib (Tafinlar)

Figure 9.30 Structures of B-RAF inhibitors.

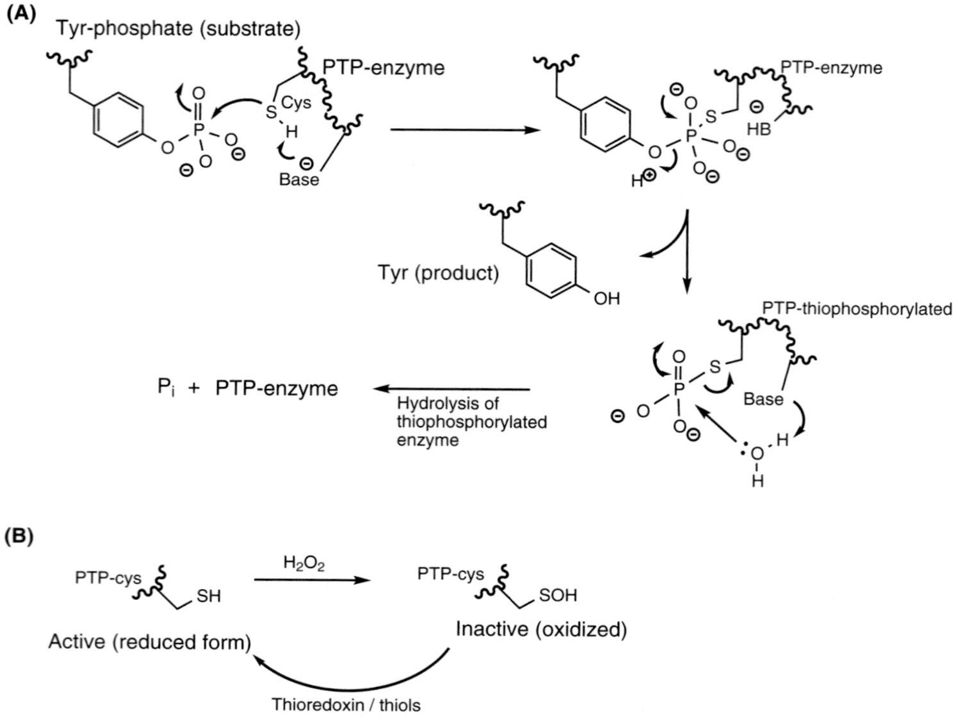

Figure 9.31 A, Mechanism of PTP phosphatase action. B, Oxidation of free thiol of cysteine by hydrogen peroxide.

back to the active thiol by cytosolic thioredoxin or other small-molecule thiols.

This redox mechanism controlling the activity of the PTPs may then be exploited in order to design specific inhibitors. Efforts aimed to design inhibitors of the PTPs include molecules that interfere with the dimerization of the PTPs (compound 211 and SHP099) as well as those that can capture the sulfenate forms of active site cysteines (1,3-diketones and dimedone; see Fig. 9.32).[60]

CONCLUSION

This chapter has attempted to give the reader an overview of catalytic receptors and enzyme catalysis. Based on the properties and mechanisms of enzyme action, the essentials of the drug design process and discovery through enzyme inhibition with a few examples have been outlined. The reader is referred to suggested reading material for some of the historical efforts as well as more detailed explanations and insights regarding the rationale and design strategies of enzyme inhibitors. In conclusion, catalytic receptors and enzymes continue to be an area that is exploited to develop therapies for human diseases. There will always be the need to elucidate receptor and enzyme mechanisms and based on this discovery, to design more selective and potent inhibitors in an effort to increase the therapeutic benefit to patients. It is hoped that this chapter has given the reader an insightful perspective into this fascinating area of medicinal chemistry.

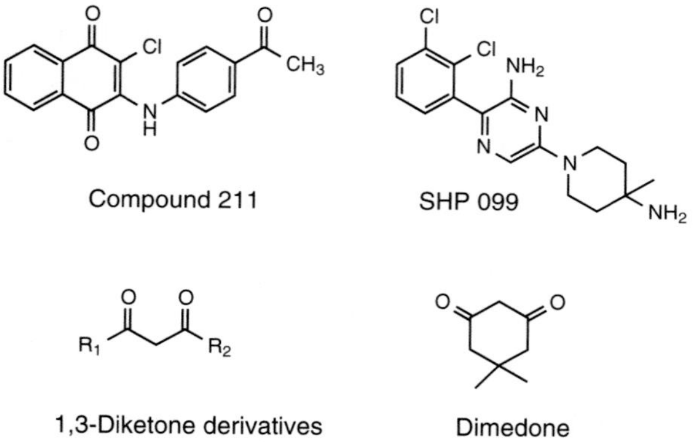

Figure 9.32 Structures of PTP inhibitors.

REFERENCES

1. Catalytic Receptors. IUPHAR/BPS Guide to Pharmacology. http://www.guidetopharmacology.org/GRAC/FamilyDisplayForward?familyId=862. Accessed 12 April 2018.
2. Golan DE, Armstrong EJ, Armstrong AW, eds. *Principles of Pharmacology: The Pathophysiologic Basis of Drug Therapy*. 4th ed. Wolters Kluwer; 2017:12: chap 1.
3. Albert A. *Selective Toxicity—The Physicochemical Basis of Therapy*. 7th ed. New York: Chapman & Hall; 1985.
4. Domagk G. Ein beitrag zur chemotherapie der bakteriellen infektionen. *Dtsch Med Wochenschr*. 1935;61:250-253.
5. Woods DD. Relation of *p*-aminobenzoic acid to mechanism of action of sulfanilamide. *Br J Exp Pathol*. 1940;21:74-90.
6. Albert A. Chapter 9. In: *Selective Toxicity—The Physicochemical Basis of Therapy*. 7th ed. New York: Chapman & Hall; 1985.
7. Fersht A. *Structure and Mechanism in Protein Science: A Guide to Enzyme Catalysis and Protein Folding*. 3rd ed. New York: W.H. Freeman; 2000.
8. Lad C, Williams H, Wolfenden R. The rate of hydrolysis of phosphomonoester dianions and the exceptional catalytic proficiencies of protein and inositol phosphatases. *Proc Natl Acad Sci USA*. 2003;100:5607-5610.

9. Available at http://www.sbcs.qmul.ac.uk/iubmb/enzyme/. Accessed 4 April 2018.
10. Pauling L. The nature of forces between large molecules of biological interest. *Nature*. 1948;161:707-709.
11. Garcia-Viloca M, Gao J, Karplus M, et al. How enzymes work: analysis by modern rate theory and computer simulations. *Science*. 2004;303:186-195.
12. Zhang X, Houk KN. Why enzymes are proficient catalysts: beyond the Pauling paradigm. *Acc Chem Res*. 2005;38:379-385.
13. Bruice TC, Benkovic SJ. A comparison of the bimolecular and intramolecular nucleophilic catalysis of the hydrolysis of substituted phenyl acylates by the dimethylamino group. *J Am Chem Soc*. 1963;85:1-8.
14. Michael C, Gaston S. Formation and hydrolysis of lactones of phenolic acids. *J Am Chem Soc*. 1980;102:4815-4821.
15. Sastry JK, Nehete PN, Khan S, et al. Membrane-permeable dideoxyuridine 5′-monophosphate analogue inhibits human immunodeficiency virus infection. *Mol Pharmacol*. 1992;41:441-445.
16. Mitsuya H, Weinhold KJ, Furman PA, et al. 3′-Azido-3′-deoxythymidine (BW A509U): an antiviral agent that inhibits the infectivity and cytopathic effect of human T-lymphotropic virus type III/lymphadenopathy-associated virus in vitro. *Proc Natl Acad Sci USA*. 1985;82:7096-7100.
17. Furman PA, Fyfe JA, St. Clair MH, et al. Phosphorylation of 3″-azido-3′-deoxythymidine and selective interaction of the 5′-triphosphate with human immunodeficiency virus reverse transcriptase. *Proc Natl Acad Sci USA*. 1986;83:8333-8337.
18. Grob PM, Wu JC, Cohen KA, et al. Nonnucleoside inhibitors of HIV-1 reverse transcriptase: nevirapine as a prototype drug. *AIDS Res Hum Retrovir*. 1992;8:145-152.
19. Kohlstaedt LA, Wang J, Friedman JM, et al. Crystal structure at 3.5 A resolution of HIV-1 reverse transcriptase complexed with an inhibitor. *Science*. 1992;256:1783-1790.
20. Spence RA, Kati WM, Anderson KS, et al. Mechanism of inhibition of HIV-1 reverse transcriptase by nonnucleoside inhibitors. *Science*. 1995;267:988-993.
21. Mellors JW, Dutschman GE, Im GJ, et al. In vitro selection and molecular characterization of human immunodeficiency virus-1 resistant to nonnucleoside inhibitors of reverse transcriptase. *Mol Pharmacol*. 1992;41:446-451.
22. Harvison P, Harrold M. Chapter 16. In: Roche V, Zito S, Lemke T, Williams DA, eds. *Foye's Principles of Medicinal Chemistry*. 8th ed. Kluwers Wolters; 2019.
23. Cushman DW, Cheung HS, Sabo EF, et al. Design of potent competitive inhibitors of angiotensin-converting enzyme. Carboxyalkanoyl and mercaptoalkanoyl amino acids. *Biochemistry*. 1977;16:5484-5491.
24. Byers LD, Wolfenden R. Binding of the by-product analogue benzylsuccinic acid by carboxypeptidase A. *Biochemistry*. 1973;12:2070-2078.
25. Patchett AA, Harris E, Tristram EW, et al. A new class of angiotensin-converting enzyme inhibitors. *Nature*. 1980;288:280-283.
26. Wolfenden R. Transition-state analogues for enzyme catalysis. *Nature*. 1969;223:704-705.
27. Wolfenden R. Transition-state analogues as potential affinity labeling agents. *Methods Enzymol*. 1977;46:15-28.
28. Shannon WM, Schabel FM. Antiviral agents as adjuncts in cancer chemotherapy. *Pharmacol Ther*. 1980;11:263-390.
29. Evans BE, Wolfenden RJ. A potential transition-state analogue for adenosine deaminase. *J Am Chem Soc*. 1970;92:4751-4752.
30. Nakamura H, Koyama G, Iitaka Y, et al. Structure of Coformycin, an unusual nucleoside of microbial origin. *J Am Chem Soc*. 1974;96:4327-4328.
31. Walpole CSJ, Wrigglesworth R. Enzyme inhibitors in medicine. *Nat Prod Rep*. 1989;63:311-346.
32. Baker BR. *Design of Active Site Directed Irreversible Enzyme Inhibitors*. New York: Wiley; 1967.
33. Walsh C. Recent developments in suicide substrates and other active site–directed inactivating agents of specific target enzymes. *Horiz Biochem Biophys*. 1977;3:36-81.
34. Abeless RH. Suicide enzyme inactivators. *Chem Eng News*. 1983;61(38):48-55.
35. Kraft GA, Katzenellenbogen JA. Synthesis of halo enol lactones. Mechanism-based inactivators of serine proteases. *J Am Chem Soc*. 1981;103:5459-5466.
36. Charnas RL, Knowles JR. Inactivation of RTEM β-lactamase from *Escherichia coli* by clavulanic acid and 9-deoxyclavulanic acid. *Biochemistry*. 1981;20:3214-3219.
37. Rando RR. Mechanisms of naturally occurring irreversible enzyme inhibitors. *Acc Chem Res*. 1975;8:281-288.
38. Bull HG, Garcia-Calvo M, Andersson S, et al. Mechanism-based inhibition of human steroid 5α-reductase by finasteride: enzyme-catalyzed formation of NADP-dihydrofinasteride, a potent bisubstrate analogue inhibitor. *J Am Chem Soc*. 1996;118:2359-2365.
39. Bender AT, Beavo JA. Cyclic nucleotide phosphodiesterases: molecular regulation to clinical use. *Pharmacol Rev*. 2006;58:488-520.
40. Lugnier C. Cyclic nucleotide phosphodiesterase (PDE) superfamily: a new target for the development of specific therapeutic agents. *Pharmacol Ther*. 2006;109:366-398.
41. Sutherland EW, Rall TW. Fractionation and characterization of a cyclic adenine ribonucleotide formed by tissue particles. *J Biol Chem*. 1958;232:1077-1091.
42. Card GI, England BP, Suzuki Y, et al. Structural basis for the activity of drugs that inhibit phosphodiesterases. *Structure (Camb)*. 2004;12:2233-2247.
43. Hatzelmann A, Schudt C. Anti-inflammatory and immunomodulatory potential of the novel PDE4 inhibitor roflumilast in vitro. *J Pharmacol Exp Ther*. 2001;297:267-279.
44. Emmons PR, Harrison MJG, Honour AJ, et al. Effect of dipyridamole on human platelet behavior. *Lancet*. 1965;2:603-606.
45. Terrett NK, Bell AS, Brown P, et al. Sildenafil (Viagara®), a potent and selective inhibitor of type 5 cGMP phosphodiesterase with utility for the treatment of male erectile dysfunction. *Bioorg Med Chem Lett*. 1996;6:1819-1824.
46. Manning G, Whyte DB, Martinez R, et al. The protein complement of the human genome. *Science*. 2002;298:1912-1934.
47. Noble MEM, Endicott JA, Johnson LN. Protein kinase inhibitors: insights into drug design from structure. *Science*. 2004;303:1800-1805.
48. Sawyers C. Chronic myeloid leukemia. *N Eng J Med*. 1999;340:1330-1340.
49. Schindler T, Bornmann W, Pellicena P et al. Structural mechanism for STI-571 inhibition of Abelson tyrosine kinase. *Science*. 2000;289:1938-1942.
50. Druker BJ, Tamura J, Buchdunger E et al. Effects of a selective inhibitor of the ABL tyrosine kinase on the growth of the Bcr-Abl positive cells. *Nat Med*. 1996;2:561-566.
51. Aurora A, Scholar EM. Role of tyrosine kinase inhibitors in cancer therapy. *J Pharmacol Exp Ther*. 2005;315:971-979.
52. Nagar B, Bornmann WG, Pellicena P et al. Crystal structures of the kinases domain of c-Abl in comples with the small molecule inhibitors PD173955 and imatinib (STI-571). *Can Res*. 2002;62:4236-4243.
53. Wu P, Neilson TE, Cluasen MH. FDA appoved small molecule kinase inhibitors. *Trends Pharm Sci*. 2015. 36(7). 422-439.
54. Kooistra AJ, Kanev GK, van Linden OPJ. et al. KLIFS: a structural kinase-ligand interaction database. *Nucleic Acids Res*. 2016;44(Database issue):D365-D371.
55. Spitaler M, Cantrell DA. Protein kinase C and beyond. *Nat Immunol*. 2004;5:785-790.
56. Vader G, Lens SMA. The Aurora family in cell division and cancer. *Biochem Biophys Acta*. 2008;1786:60-72.
57. Katayama H, Sen S. Aurora kinase inhibitors as anticancer molecules. *Biochem Biophys Acta*. 2010;1799:829-839.
58. Hertzman Johansson C, Egyhazi Brage S. BRAF inhibitors in cancer therapy. *Pharmacol Ther*. 2014;142:176-182.
59. Sharma K, D'Souza RCJ, Tyanova S, et al. Ultradeep human phosphoproteome reveals a distinct regulatory nature of Tyr and Ser/Thr-based signaling. *Cell Rep*. 2014;8:1583-1594.
60. Yu ZH, Zhang ZY. Regulatory mechanisms and novel therapeutic targeting strategies for protein tyrosine phosphatases. *Chem. Rev*. 2018;118:1069-1091.

SUGGESTED READINGS

Abeless RH. Suicide enzyme inactivators. *Chem Eng News*. 1983;61(38):48-55.

Albert A. *Selective Toxicity—The Physicochemical Basis of Therapy*. 7th ed. New York: Chapman & Hall; 1985.

Baker BR. *Design of Active Site Directed Irreversible Enzyme Inhibitors*. New York: Wiley; 1967.

Kalman TI, ed. *Drug Action & Design—Mechanism-Based Enzyme Inhibitors*. New York: Elsevier Science; 1979.

Seiler N, Jung MJ, Kock-Weser J, eds. *Enzyme-Activated Irreversible Inhibitors*. New York: Elsevier North Holland; 1978.

Silverman RB, Holladay MW. *The Organic Chemistry of Drug Design and Drug Action*. 3rd ed. New York: Elsevier–Academic Press; 2014.

Silverman RB. *The Organic Chemistry of Enzyme Catalyzed Reactions*. Revised ed. London: Academic Press; 2002.

Smith JS, ed. *Smith and Williams' Introduction to the Principles of Drug Design and Action*. 3rd ed. Amsterdam: Harwood Academic Press; 1998.

Sneader W. *Drug Discovery – A History*. John Wiley & Sons; 2005.

Walpole CSJ, Wrigglesworth R. Enzyme inhibitors in medicine. *Nat Prod Rep*. 1989;63:311-346.

Wolfenden R. Transition-state analogues as potential affinity labeling agents. *Methods Enzymol*. 1977;46:15-28.

PART III

PHARMACODYNAMIC AGENTS

SECTION I

Drugs Impacting the Central Nervous System

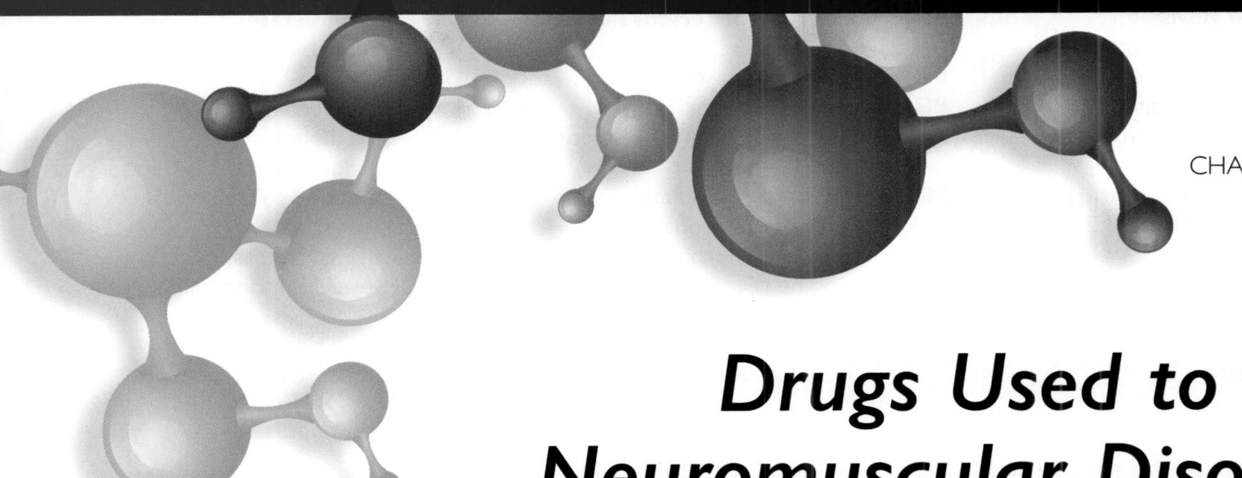

CHAPTER 10

Drugs Used to Treat Neuromuscular Disorders

Gregory D. Cuny

Drugs covered in this chapter:

- Alemtuzumab
- Amantadine
- Apomorphine
- Baclofen
- Botulinum toxin type A
- Bromocriptine
- Cabergoline
- Carbidopa
- Carisoprodol
- Cyclobenzaprine
- Dalfampridine
- Dantrolene
- Deflazacort
- Diazepam
- Dimethyl fumarate
- Edaravone
- Entacapone
- Eteplirsen
- Fingolimod
- Glatiramer
- Interferon beta-1a
- Interferon beta-1b
- L-Dopa
- Metaxalone
- Methocarbamol
- Natalizumab
- Neostigmine
- Nusinersen
- Ocrelizumab
- Peginterferon beta-1a
- Pramipexole
- Pyridostigmine
- Rasagiline
- Riluzole
- Ropinirole
- Rotigotine
- Safinamide
- Selegiline
- Sugammadex
- Teriflunomide
- Tetrabenazine
- Tizanidine
- Tolcapone
- Valbenazine

Abbreviations

AAAD aromatic L-amino acid decarboxylase
AD aldehyde dehydrogenase
ALS amyotrophic lateral sclerosis
AUC area under the plasma concentration curve
BCRP breast cancer resistant protein
BBB blood-brain barrier
COMT catechol-O-methyltransferase
C_{max} concentration maximum
CNS central nervous system
CP cerebral palsy
CYP450 cytochrome P450
DβH dopamine β-hydroxylate
DOPAC 3,4-dihydroxyphenylacetic acid
DOPAL 3,4-dihydroxyphenylacetaldehyde
DMD Duchenne muscular dystrophy
FAD flavin adenine dinucleotide
GABA gamma-aminobutyric acid
HVA homovanillic acid
IgG immunoglobulin G
JAK/STAT Janus kinase/signal transducers and activators of transcription
KEAP-1 Kelch-like erythroid cell–derived associated protein-1
LRRK2 leucine-rich repeat kinase 2
MAO monoamine oxidase

Abbreviations—Continued

MBP myelin basic protein
MG myasthenia gravis
MHC major histocompatibility complex
MND motor neuron disease
MPDP 1-methyl-4-phenyl-2,3-dihydropyridinium
MPP⁺ 1-methyl-4-phenylpyridinium
MPTP 1-methyl-4-phenyl-1,2,3,6-tetrahydropyridine
MS multiple sclerosis
MTA 3-methoxytyramine
NADP nicotinamide adenine dinucleotide phosphate
NMDA N-methyl-*D*-aspartate
Nrf2 nuclear factor (erythroid derived 2)-like 2
PD Parkinson's disease
PDB Protein Data Bank
PENT phenylethanolamine-N-methyltransferase
PINK1 PTEN-induced putative kinase 1
PLP pyridoxal-5′-phosphate
RLS restless leg syndrome
RYR ryanodine receptor
SAM *S*-adenosyl methionine
SMA spinal muscular atrophy
SMN spinal muscular neuron
SOD superoxide dismutase
SULT sulfotransferase
TDP-43 TAR-DNA binding protein 43
TH tyrosine hydroxylase
T_{max} time maximum
UGT UDP-glucuronosyltransferase
VCAM-1 vascular cell adhesion molecule 1
VMA vanillylmandelic acid
VMAT-2 vesicular monoamine transporter 2
VPS35 vacuolar protein sorting-associated protein 35

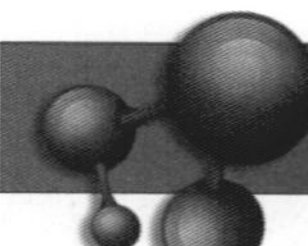

CLINICAL SIGNIFICANCE

Jeffrey T. Sherer, PharmD, MPH, BCPS, BCGP

Drugs to treat Parkinson's disease (PD) are a diverse group with vastly differing mechanisms of action. The introduction of new drugs and dosage forms has dramatically increased the number of therapeutic options for patients suffering from this often difficult movement disorder, but it has also created new controversies regarding the appropriate management of PD. Because the pharmacotherapy of PD must be individualized based on patient and disease factors, pharmacists should be aware of the chemistry of the various drug classes and specific agents within each class in order to maximize the likelihood that patients will receive therapy that is likely to help and unlikely to result in adverse effects.

The dopamine precursor L-Dopa, combined with the peripheral decarboxylase inhibitor (*S*)-carbidopa, remains the most effective treatment available for motor symptoms of PD. Most clinicians use this combination as first-line therapy when the motor symptoms significantly affect quality of life. While earlier concerns about oxidative stress and accelerated disease progression in patients receiving L-Dopa have been largely disproven, most patients will experience complications such as a shorter duration of action ("wearing-off effect") and motor fluctuations ("on-off effect") within 8 years of starting therapy. Therefore, other agents such as the direct dopamine agonists, catechol-O-methyltransferase inhibitors, and monoamine oxidase-B (MAO-B) inhibitors are commonly used as well.

The MAO-B inhibitors are particularly interesting from a chemistry standpoint, and understanding differences within this class is critically important. The first-generation agent selegiline, which has been approved in the United States since 1989, has been studied and found to improve motor symptoms in patients with PD but does not appear to slow the progression of the disease. Some literature suggests rasagiline, a second-generation MAO-B inhibitor first approved in 2006, may both treat motor symptoms and affect disease progression, while other literature has shown that the drug only improves symptoms. Since PD is a progressive disease and no currently approved agents have been definitively proven to arrest or slow this progression, recognizing the differences between these two agents—as well as the newly (2017) approved safinamide—may provide insights about how future drugs may help achieve this vitally important outcome.

Muscle relaxants and other agents to treat pain and spasticity are commonly prescribed and often not well tolerated due to their prominent anticholinergic effects and general central nervous system depression. Recognizing how the available agents differ structurally and how these differences may affect their adverse-effect profiles is important for choosing the most appropriate agent for an individual patient. It may also provide insight into developing more effective and safer medications to treat pain associated with spasticity, particularly in the current climate where the risks of long-term opioid use are becoming more apparent.

Other neuromuscular conditions including multiple sclerosis, Duchenne muscular dystrophy, myasthenia gravis, and amyotropic lateral sclerosis are less common but can have devastating effects on sufferers. Progress has been made in the area of pharmacotherapy for these diseases, but much work remains. As new treatments are researched and introduced, understanding the chemistry of these agents and the rationale for their use is vitally important, as many have novel mechanisms of action.

Overview of Neuromuscular Disorders

Neuromuscular disorders are a broad classification of conditions for which chemotherapeutic agents are available for only a subset of maladies. This chapter will cover the neurodegenerative movement disorder Parkinson's disease (PD) and the autoimmune disease multiple sclerosis (MS). In addition, several neuromuscular disorders for which drug treatments have only more recently become available will also be described, including amyotrophic lateral sclerosis (ALS) and Duchenne muscular dystrophy (DMD). However, pharmacotherapy for these aliments remains far from ideal. Although advances are being made in understanding the cause and pathogenesis of these diseases, prophylactic or curative therapies are not currently available.

The second group of conditions examined includes muscle spasticity disorders, which broadly cover maladies characterized by tonic stretch reflexes, flexor muscle spasms, and muscle weakness. Spasticity may accompany a number of disorders but is often associated with cerebral palsy, multiple sclerosis, spinal cord injury, and stroke. A number of chemotherapeutics are available to treat these ailments. But their mechanism of action, and in some cases their efficacy, is less clear. Recently approved chemotherapeutic agents for reversing anesthetic drug–induced nondepolarizing neuromuscular blockage that have also been used for treating myasthenia gravis (MG) will be described. Finally, drugs to treat chorea associated with Huntington's disease and tardive dyskinesia, which can occur in patients on long-term neuroleptic medication treatment, will be presented.

Parkinson's Disease

Therapeutic Context Overview

PD is a chronic and progressive movement disorder that presents with symptoms of (1) resting tremor of the hands, arms, legs, jaw, and/or face; (2) bradykinesia or slow initiation and paucity of voluntary movements; (3) rigidity of the limbs and trunk; and (4) postural instability, including impaired balance and coordination. Many PD patients also suffer from dementia and psychiatric conditions, including hallucinations and depression.[1]

PD is a neurodegenerative disease most prominently afflicting the extrapyramidal dopaminergic neurons that have cell bodies in the *substantia nigra pars compacta* located in the midbrain with nerve terminals extending into the corpus striatum (Fig. 10.1). These regions of the brain play significant roles in motor control. PD results from progressive dysfunction and cell death of these neurons causing a deficiency of dopamine in the nerve terminals in the corpus striatum.[1]

Like many other neurodegenerative diseases, PD is characterized by diagnostic histopathological features. One of the most prominent facets is Lewy bodies, which are intracellular protein aggregates that form spherical deposits within neurons. However, Lewy bodies are not confined to the *substantia nigra pars compacta* or corpus striatum, but can also be found in other areas of the brain. Furthermore, these aggregates are present in other neurological conditions,[2] such as dementia with Lewy bodies and multiple system atrophy. The primary component of the aggregates is alpha-synuclein, an abundant protein found mainly in the brain and in lesser amounts in other tissues. The functions of alpha-synuclein are not well understood. However, it may play a role in regulating dopamine homeostasis, including modulation of dopamine synthesis (e.g., interacting with tyrosine hydroxylase), release, and reuptake at nerve terminals.[3,4] However, its neurotoxicity may stem from synaptic dysfunction, mitochondrial impairment, defective endoplasmic reticulum function and autophagy-lysosomal pathways, and nuclear dysfunction.[5] In addition, oligomeric forms of the protein are also thought to be involved in neurotoxicity mechanisms.[6]

The etiology of PD is unknown. However, in some cases genetics appears to play a critical role. Epidemiologic studies have found age is the most prominent risk factor

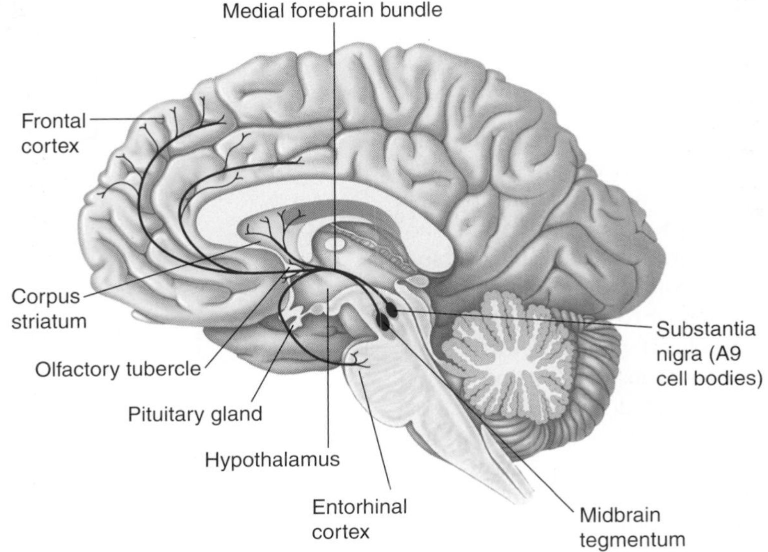

Figure 10.1 Depiction of brain regions and dopaminergic pathways involved in PD.

for developing PD followed by a family history of the disease.[7,8] Genetic forms of PD have been found in a small portion of cases (<10%), most involving early disease onset. For example, autosomal dominant mutations in the alpha-synuclein gene (e.g., *SNCA*) have been described in several families.[9,10] Mutations in other genes have also been found to be associated with PD, including those that encode leucine-rich repeat kinase 2 (LRRK-2), VPS35, parkin, PINK1, and DJ-1.[11]

Mutations in the *PARK8* gene, which encodes for LRRK2, have been linked to early onset PD. Individuals who inherit the G2019S mutation in LRRK2 from either parent have a significant increased risk for developing PD with increasing age. In addition, up to 40% of people of North African Arab ancestry and 25% of Ashkenazi Jewish people with PD have this particular mutation.[12] LRRK2 is a complex protein containing domains with GTPase, kinase, and scaffolding functions. LRRK2 (wild-type and mutants) has been implicated in a host of neurotoxic mechanisms, such as apoptosis induction, autophagy and mitochondrial dysfunction, which could contribute to PD.

A mutation (D620N) in the vacuolar protein sorting-associated protein 35 (VPS35) subunit of the retromer complex, which is involved in retrograde transport of proteins from endosomes to the Golgi, was identified as a rare cause of autosomal dominant familial PD.[13,14] The VPS35 D620N mutation exhibits both gain and loss of functions that could contribute to PD.[15]

Loss-of-function mutations in the *PARK2* gene, which encodes the protein parkin, cause autosomal recessive juvenile PD. Loss of the protein may lead to synaptic damage and dysfunction resulting in dopaminergic neuron loss.[16] Parkin appears to also be recruited to impaired mitochondria where it can promote autophagy, which is an intracellular degradation system that delivers cytoplasmic constituents to the lysosome for catabolism.[17,18]

Autosomal recessive mutations have been found in the *PARK6* gene, which encodes the PTEN-induced putative kinase 1 (e.g., PINK1), a mitochondrial serine/threonine protein kinase. This protein appears to function in mitochondrial quality control since mutations in this gene have been shown to compromise mitochondrial integrity.[19,20]

Finally, autosomal recessive mutations have been reported in the *PARK7* gene (also known as the *DJ-1* gene), which encodes the protein DJ-1. In the context of PD, this protein is thought to function as a redox-dependent molecular chaperone of alpha-synuclein.[21,22] While its functions in cells are not fully understood, it appears to provide neurons protection against oxidative stress.[23] Although an array of protein mutations have been associated with PD, most cases are considered to be sporadic.[24]

Environmental factors also appear to play an important role in the etiology of PD. It has been well recognized that exposure to certain chemicals can cause PD symptoms or significantly increase the risk of developing the disease. One of the most direct connections of chemical exposure and PD involves the compound MPTP (1-methyl-4-phenyl-1,2,3,6-tetrahydropyridine). This material induces a PD-like condition in humans and primates that is similar in neuropathology and motor abnormalities seen in the idiopathic form of the disease,[25] which came to light through tragic cases of illicit designer drug use involving a derivative of meperidine where the ester was reversed.[26,27] In this case it is not the parent compound that is the culprit for the neurotoxicity, but a reactive metabolite (Fig. 10.2). Since MPTP has low molecular weight and contains a lipophilic tertiary amine, it readily crosses the blood-brain barrier (BBB), where it undergoes oxidative metabolism to the unstable intermediate $MPDP^+$, which is further oxidized to MPP^+,[28,29] a pyridinium cation that is a reactive electrophile. The metabolism is monoamine oxidase B (MAOB) mediated, as inhibitors of this enzyme have been shown to block the reaction pathway.[30] Furthermore, MPP^+ is taken up by dopamine transporters present in catecholamine neurons, including those in the *substantia nigra*, and elicits neurotoxicity by inhibition of mitochondrial complex I.[31] Other chemicals have similarly been linked to PD, including the herbicide paraquat (which is structurally similar to MPP^+),[32] the natural product rotenone,[33,34] and manganese.[35]

Interestingly, some environmental factors appear to reduce the risk of developing PD. For example, cigarette smokers have a lower incidence of PD than nonsmokers.[36,37] It has been proposed that tobacco smoke may contain MAO inhibitors[38,39] or that nicotine might play a role.[40] Coffee consumption is also correlated with a lower risk of developing PD[41] possibly due to caffeine's antagonism of adenosine receptors.[42]

PD typically presents after age 55 and affects approximately 1%-2% of the population over age 65. However, after age 84 the incidence of PD increases to 3%-5% per year.[43] Very little prevalence differences are seen in the incidence of PD between men and women, as well as geographical location.[44]

As the second most common neurodegenerative disease, PD accounts for significant national economic burdens. In the United States, the cost associated with PD exceeded

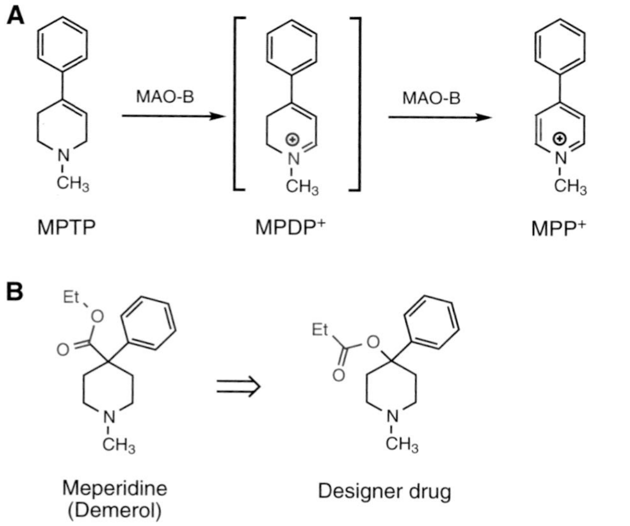

A

MAO-B → MAO-B

CH_3 MPTP — [$MPDP^+$] — MPP^+

B

Meperidine (Demerol) ⇒ Designer drug

Figure 10.2 (A) Metabolism of MPTP to MPP+, a neurotoxin that causes a PD-like condition. (B) Structures of meperidine and a designer drug where the ester of meperidine is reversed.

US$14.4 billion in 2010 (approximately US$22,800 per patient). This burden is projected to grow substantially over the next few decades as the size of the elderly population increases.[45] Similar trends are likely throughout the world where the size of the elderly population is increasing. According to the Parkinson's Foundation, the estimated per patient medication cost for treating PD is US$2500 per year.[46]

Pharmacology Overview

Since the most consequential tissue affected by PD is extrapyramidal dopaminergic neurons in the *substantia nigra pars compacta* and corpus striatum, it is perhaps not surprising that most current pharmacological therapies for the treatment of PD have a connection to the neurotransmitter dopamine. However, direct administration of dopamine to PD patients is not an effective treatment mainly due to the inability of peripheral dopamine to penetrate the BBB. Although dopamine has low molecular weight, it is a relatively polar molecule and is not subjected to active transport into the brain.

In order to understand the rationale for the development of dopamine-based PD drugs, it is first important to review the biosynthesis and catabolism of this neurotransmitter (Fig. 10.3). The essential amino acid L-tyrosine is converted to L-Dopa by tyrosine hydroxylase (TH), which is found peripherally and in the central nervous system (CNS).[47] The primary route of metabolism of L-Dopa is decarboxylation to dopamine by an aromatic L-amino acid decarboxylase (AAAD, e.g., L-Dopa decarboxylase), again in both the periphery and CNS, although a minor pathway generating 3-methoxy-4-hydroxyphenyllactic acid also occurs. Dopamine is further metabolized via two primary pathways. The first route involves MAO-mediated oxidation to DOPAL (3,4-dihydroxyphenylacetaldehyde) that is further oxidized by aldehyde dehydrogenase (AD) to DOPAC (3,4-dihydroxyphenylacetic acid), which is

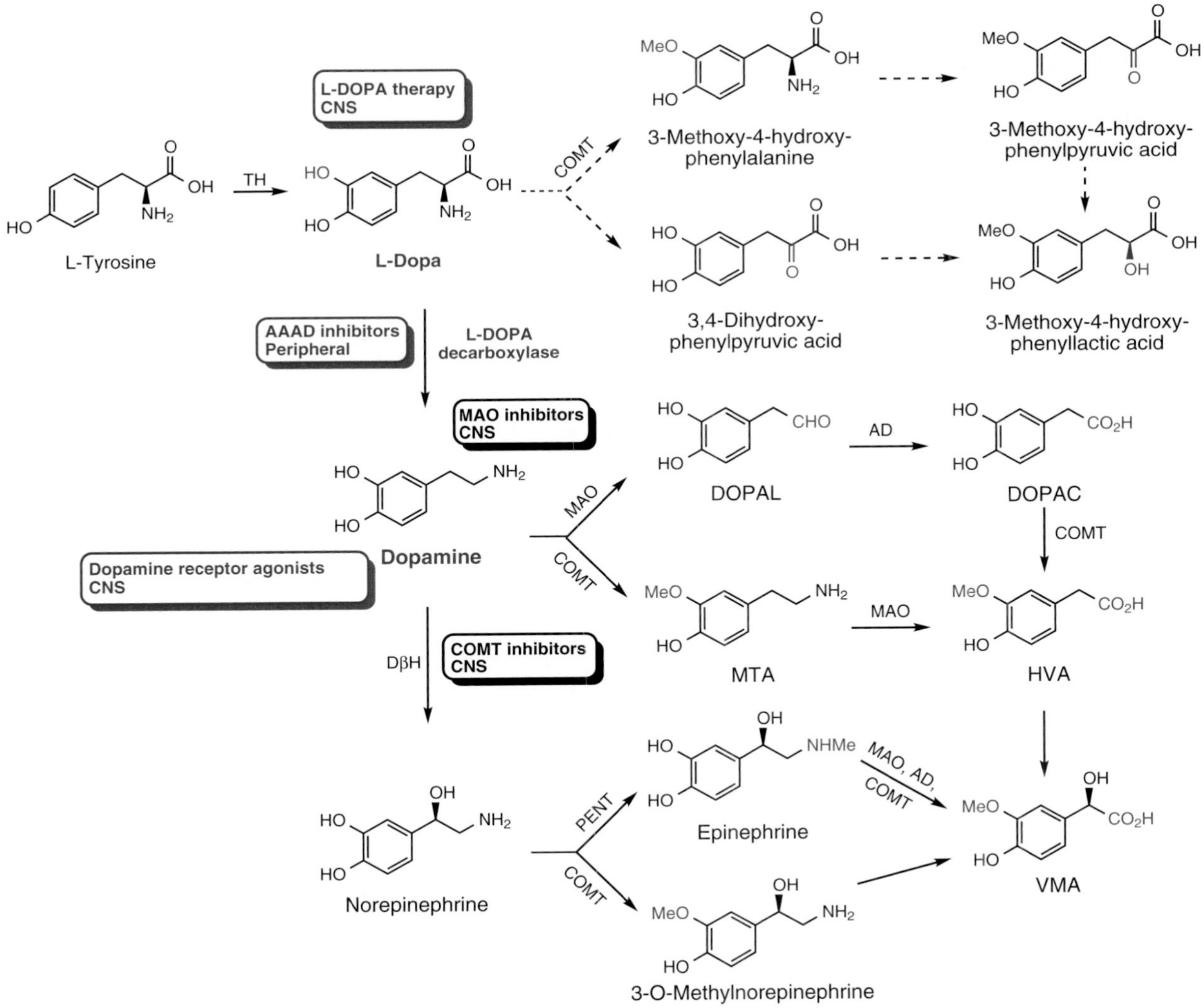

Figure 10.3 Biosynthesis and catabolism of dopamine. Intervention points to increase brain dopamine concentration and/or neurotransmitter function are highlighted. Dash arrows indicate minor routes. *AAAD*, aromatic L-amino acid decarboxylase; *AD*, aldehyde dehydrogenase; *CNS*, central nervous system; *COMT*, catechol-O-methyltransferase; *DH*, dopamine β-hydroxylase; *DOPAC*, 3,4-dihydroxyphenylacetic acid; *DOPAL*, 3,4-dihydroxyphenylacetaldehyde; *HVA*, homovanillic acid; *MAO*, monoamine oxidase; *MTA*, 3-methoxytyramine, *PENT*, phenylethanolamine-N-methyltransferase; *VMA*, vanillylmandelic acid.

methylated on the 3-hydroxy by catechol-O-methyltransferase (COMT) to generate HVA (homovanillic acid). Alternatively, dopamine is converted to MTA via COMT and then oxidized by MAO to generate HVA. The second pathway involves dopamine β-hydroxylate (DβH) oxidation of dopamine to norepinephrine, which is converted to vanillylmandelic acid (VMA) via a series of enzyme-mediated reactions.

The nature of the oxidative metabolism of dopamine is also believed to play a contributing role in the neurotoxicity observed in PD via several different mechanisms. For example, in the synthesis of dopamine, L-tyrosine is converted to L-Dopa via hydroxylation of the 3-position of the phenol. This reaction may proceed directly via C-H bond insertion, circumventing highly electrophilic and reactive intermediates (Fig. 10.4A). Alternatively, the process can generate an epoxide intermediate, as is seen in the metabolic conversion of benzene to phenol.[48] This intermediate can rearrange to a hydroxyl ketone intermediate that can tautomerize to L-Dopa. However, this same intermediate can potentially be oxidized to an *ortho*-quinone intermediate. Both the epoxide and *ortho*-quinone intermediates are electrophilic and highly reactive toward nucleophilic functional groups, such as those present in proteins, RNA, DNA, or other biomolecules, which can lead to neurotoxicity.[49] In addition, dopamine can auto-oxidize to the hydroxyl ketone and *ortho*-quinone intermediates.[50,51] Finally, during MAO catalysis of dopamine (and other monoamine neurotransmitters, like norepinephrine and serotonin) hydrogen peroxide is generated (Fig. 10.4B) that can undergo a redox reaction (e.g., Haber-Weiss reaction) with superoxide to form the cytotoxic hydroxy radical (e.g., $OH^\bullet$).

It was recognized several decades ago that dopamine concentrations in the corpus striatum of PD patient's brains were only 20% of normal levels.[52] Thus, the biosynthesis and catabolism of dopamine presented several intervention points to increase dopamine concentration and/or the function of the neurotransmitter in affected brain areas. One of the most direct strategies to do this was to administer L-Dopa. Birkmayer and Hornykiewicz found that high oral doses of racemic Dopa to PD patients were effective.[53] Subsequent clinical trials with racemic and enantiomeric pure L-Dopa demonstrated the benefits of this therapeutic strategy.[54-56] Although L-Dopa is more polar than dopamine and, based on its physiochemical properties, would not be expected to cross the BBB, it is actively transported into the brain primarily by L-type amino acid transporters and then decarboxylated to dopamine in situ.[57]

Although L-Dopa can be efficacious as a single agent, only about 1% of an orally administered dose reaches the brain.[58] The remainder undergoes rapid decarboxylation in peripheral tissues to generate dopamine, which does not cross the BBB. However, the peripheral decarboxylation

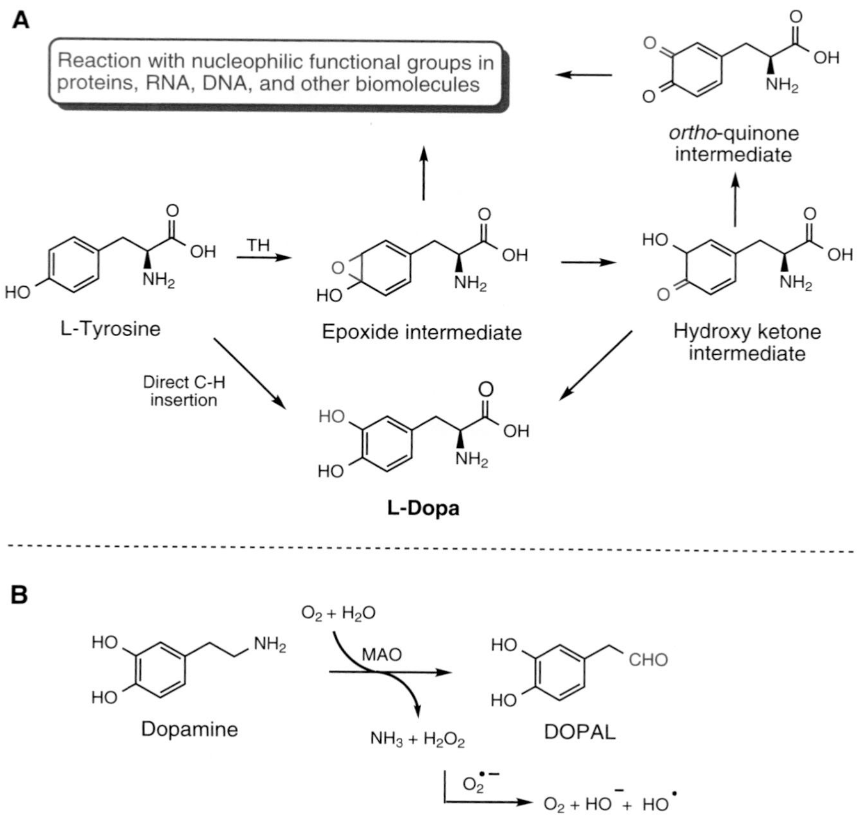

Figure 10.4 (A) Potential mechanism for the conversion of L-tyrosine to L-Dopa and reactive intermediates that could contribute to neurotoxicity in PD. (B) Potential mechanisms for the generation of cytotoxic hydroxy radical (e.g., OH) during MAO mediated oxidation of dopamine to DOPAL.

of L-Dopa can be competitively inhibited by coadministration of a DOPA decarboxylase inhibitor.[59] Furthermore, the DOPA decarboxylase inhibitors were designed to restrict permeability across the BBB. Thus, these compounds prevent decarboxylation of L-Dopa selectively in the periphery, but not in the CNS. Overall, this combination therapy markedly increases (by 2.5- to 30-fold) the amount of L-Dopa that reaches the brain where it is converted to dopamine.[60]

Two other therapeutic strategies for the treatment of PD involve inhibition of dopamine-metabolizing enzymes. As previously mentioned, once dopamine is generated in the brain it is subjected to three routes of metabolism. One of these pathways is the conversion of dopamine to norepinephrine via benzylic oxidation by DβH. However, this is not a process for which inhibitors have been developed for the treatment of PD. But blocking the conversion of dopamine to DOPAL via MAO and to MTA via COMT have become effective means of increasing brain levels of dopamine that provides symptomatic relief for PD patients.

The final dopamine-related therapeutic approach is the use of dopamine agonists to mimic the actions of the depleted endogenous neurotransmitter. Although these drugs do not increase brain levels of dopamine, they bind to various dopamine receptors and act as functional agonists, stimulating signaling pathways normally activated by dopamine. Although these drugs can provide symptomatic relief for PD patients, they do not impact the underlying disease progression.

The last common pharmacotherapy approach currently available for the treatment of PD is the use of non-dopamine-related drugs. These agents have a variety of functions that may offer neuroprotective effects that can provide benefit for PD and/or the associated dyskinesias induced by L-Dopa therapy. Although a number of genetic links have been made to PD as discussed above, to date these targets and associated pathways have yet to be translated into effective pharmacotherapy. Research activities into these various molecular targets continue with the hope that new and potentially disease modifying agents will emerge for clinical testing.

Many PD pharmacotherapies are associated with common adverse effects. For example, patients receiving drugs that increase dopamine levels or function report falling asleep while engaged in activities of daily living, including driving or operating machinery. Although many of these patients reported somnolence, some perceived that they had no warning signs. Other common adverse effects of anti-PD drugs include hyperpyrexia and confusion, impulse control and compulsive behaviors, hallucinations/psychotic-like behavior, dyskinesia, and depression. Interestingly, studies have shown that PD patients have a higher risk (2- to 6-fold) of developing melanoma, a malignant skin cancer. It is unclear if this increased risk is due to the neurodegenerative disease or drug treatment. Also, since many drugs used to treat PD increase dopamine levels or agonize dopamine receptors, they can modulate the function of dopamine antagonists, such as antipsychotics.

In addition, some PD pharmacotherapies are associated with drug-drug interactions. For example, concomitant use of nonselective or selective MAO inhibitors with antidepressants, including selective serotonin reuptake inhibitors, serotonin-norepinephrine reuptake inhibitors, and tricyclics, as well as opioid analgesics such as meperidine, tramadol, methadone, and propoxyphene, can cause serotonin syndrome. This condition can range in severity from mild to life-threatening, typically consisting of signs broadly characterized as altered mental status, abnormal neuromuscular tone, and autonomic hyperactivity.[61] These symptoms can include high body temperature (>40 °C), agitation, increased reflexes, tremor, sweating, dilated pupils, and diarrhea, potentially resulting in seizure. Another example of drug-drug interactions is the modulation of MAO and COMT that are involved in the biosynthesis and catabolism of catecholamines, as well as the metabolism of xenobiotics (see Chapter 3). Inhibitors of these enzymes can have an impact on catecholamine levels and the metabolism of concomitant drug treatment. Therefore, drugs known to be metabolized by MAO or COMT should be administered with caution in patients receiving MAO or COMT inhibitors.

Dopamine and Dopamine Receptor–Related Therapy

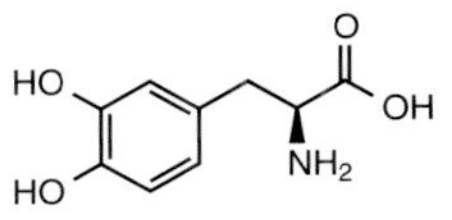

L-Dopa
(Levodopa)

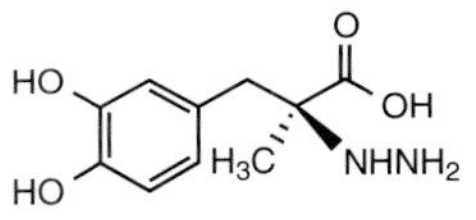

Carbidopa
(Lodosyn)

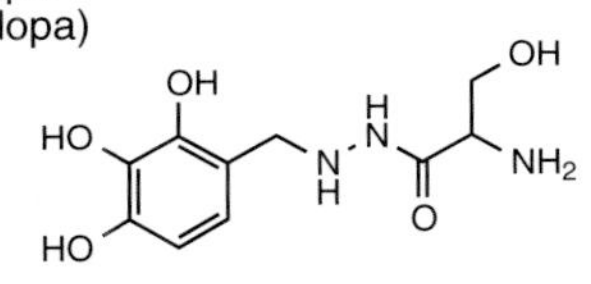

Benserazide

L-Dopa decarboxylase inhibitors.

L-Dopa

L-Dopa is an amino acid ((S)-3,4-dihydroxyphenylalanine) that has been used as dopamine replacement therapy since it is capable of crossing the BBB and undergoing decarboxylation to generate dopamine in the brain. However, L-Dopa is currently coadministered/coformulated with a DOPA decarboxylase inhibitor (e.g., carbidopa or benserazide). In patients with an average age of 71, L-Dopa has an oral bioavailability of 63%, a plasma clearance of 14.2 mL/min/kg, and a volume of distribution of 1.01 L/kg (Table 10.1). In the presence of carbidopa, the area under the plasma concentration curve (AUC) after oral administration of L-Dopa significantly increases (2926 ng hr/mL to 4530 ng hr/mL) due to lower systemic clearance.[62] In addition, the plasma elimination half-life of L-Dopa increases from 50 minutes to 1.5 hours. L-Dopa undergoes extensive peripheral metabolism with <1% of an oral dose being eliminated as the parent drug in the urine.[63]

Table 10.1 Pharmacokinetic Parameters of Drugs Used to Treat PD

Drug Class	Drug	Plasma Elimination Half-life	Clearance	Volume of Distribution	Oral Bioavailability	Plasma Protein Binding
Dopamine and dopamine receptor–related therapy	L-Dopa	50 min-1.5 hr	14.2 mL/min/kg	1.01 L/kg	63%	10%-30%
	Carbidopa	2 hr			60%	36%
Monoamine oxidase inhibitors	Rasagiline	3 hr		87 L	36%	88%-94%
	Selegiline	1.5 hr	59 L/min	1854 L	10%	
	Safinamide	20-26 hr	4.6 L/hr	165 L	95%	88%-90%
Catechol-O-methyl transferase inhibitors	Entacapone	2.4 hr			35%	98%
	Tolcapone		7 L/hr		65%	>99.9%
Dopamine receptor agonists	Apomorphine	40 min	223 L/hr	218 L	–	
	Bromocriptine	4.9 hr				>90%
	Carbergoline	63-109 hr				40%
	Pramipexole	8-12 hr	400 mL/min	500 L	>90%	15%
	Ropinirole	6 hr	47 L/hr	7.5 L/kg	45%-55%	40%
	Rotigotine	5-7 hr		84 L/kg		90%
Nondopamine related therapy	Amantadine	12-17 hr	0.28 L/hr/kg	3-8 L/kg		

Carbidopa

Carbidopa is used in combination with L-Dopa for the treatment of PD. Although carbidopa is structurally similar to L-Dopa, it has two notable differences. First, the amine in L-Dopa has been replaced with a hydrazine moiety, while the absolute stereochemistry (e.g., S) has been retained. Second, the carbon that the hydrazine is attached to is further substituted with a methyl group. Both of these changes provide a hydrazine that can readily react with a cofactor in the active site of L-Dopa decarboxylase (see below). Carbidopa is formulated as a monohydrate that is a white crystalline solid and slightly soluble in water. Benserazide, although not approved for use in the United States, is another L-Dopa decarboxylase inhibitor used in other countries for the same purpose. Structurally it is quite different from carbidopa. It is comprised of the racemic form of the amino acid serine linked through an acyl hydrazine, which is further substituted with pyrogallol attached through a methylene. Benserazide is readily hydrolyzed in plasma to trihydroxybenzylhydrazine that readily reacts with a cofactor in the active site of L-Dopa decarboxylase (see below).[64]

Carbidopa itself has not been demonstrated to have any additional pharmacodynamic activity in the treatment of PD. Since it does not cross the BBB, it does not affect the metabolism of L-Dopa within the CNS. However, carbidopa reduces the amount of L-Dopa required for therapeutic response by about 75% by increasing both the plasma level and half-life of L-Dopa, and decreasing plasma and urinary dopamine and homovanillic acid levels.

A cocrystal structure of a carbidopa derivative containing a hydrazone linkage to its cofactor pyridoxal-5′-phosphate (PLP) bound to L-Dopa decarboxylase has been reported (Fig. 10.5).[65] The structure reveals key engagements including a hydrogen bond and an ionic-dipole interaction between the catechol and the alcohol side-chain of Thr82 (e.g., threonine residue 82) and the phosphate of PLP, respectively, and interactions between the carboxylate of carbidopa and the imidazole side-chain of His192. A cocrystal structure of benserazide with DOPA decarboxylase has not been reported.

Both carbidopa and L-Dopa have relatively low plasma protein binding of 36% and 10%-30%, respectively (Table 10.1). Carbidopa has an oral bioavailability of 60% and a terminal phase plasma elimination half-life of 2 hours. A similar terminal phase elimination half-life of L-Dopa, in the presence of carbidopa, is also observed. About 30% of a carbidopa dose is eliminated unchanged in urine. Carbidopa is metabolized to generate α-methyl-3,4-dihydroxyphenylpropionic acid (Fig. 10.6) via reduction of the hydrazine.[66,67] This metabolite is then converted to α-methyl-3-methoxy-4-hydroxyphenylpropionic acid, presumably by COMT. The catechol metabolite also undergoes a rather unusual transformation of being reduced to α-methyl-3-hydroxyphenylpropionic acid. All three of these metabolites

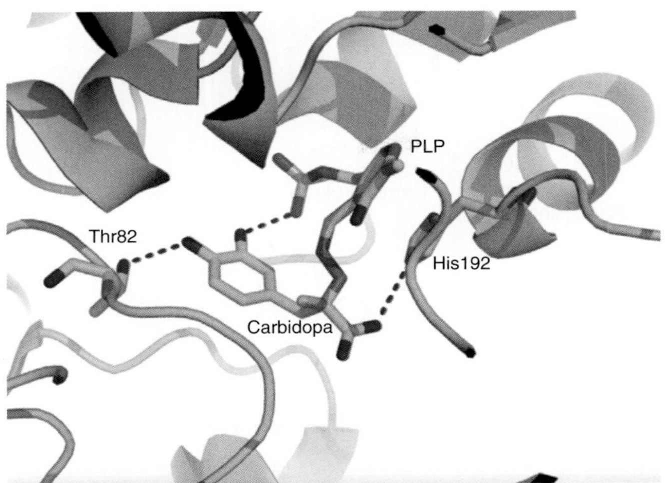

Figure 10.5 Cocrystal structure of carbidopa-pyridoxal-5′-phosphate (PLP) hydrazone with L-Dopa decarboxylase (PDB: 1JS3). Hydrogen bonding interactions shown with red dashes.

participate in conjugation with glucuronic acid with subsequent elimination in urine, although the structures of the gucuronides have not been reported. Finally, 3,4-dihydroxyphenylacetone has also been isolated from urine after administration of carbidopa. This compound may arise via oxidative decarboxylation of α-methyl-3-methoxy-4 hydroxyphenylpropionic acid. However, it may also form directly by auto-oxidation of the parent drug.[68]

Several drug-drug interactions can occur with carbidopa. For example, iron salts (including in multivitamins) can chelate carbidopa reducing its bioavailability.[69] Also carbiodopa can have a drug-drug interaction with isoniazid since both inhibit tryptophan oxygenase and kynureninase.[70] Carbidopa concomitantly administered with L-Dopa is contraindicated with nonselective MAO inhibitors. When carbidopa is administered concomitantly with L-Dopa, the most common adverse reactions in early PD patients are nausea, dizziness, headache, insomnia, abnormal dreams, dry mouth, dyskinesia, anxiety, constipation, vomiting, and orthostatic hypotension. In advanced PD patients the most common adverse events include nausea and headache.

Monoamine Oxidase Inhibitors

In addition to dopamine replacement therapy, another widely used strategy for the treatment of PD is to block the conversion of dopamine to DOPAL via inhibition of the enzyme MAO. Three drugs, rasagiline, selegiline, and safinamide, operate through this mechanism of action.

Rasagiline (Azilect)

Selegiline (Eldepryl)

Safinamide (Xadago)

Monoamine oxidase inhibitors.

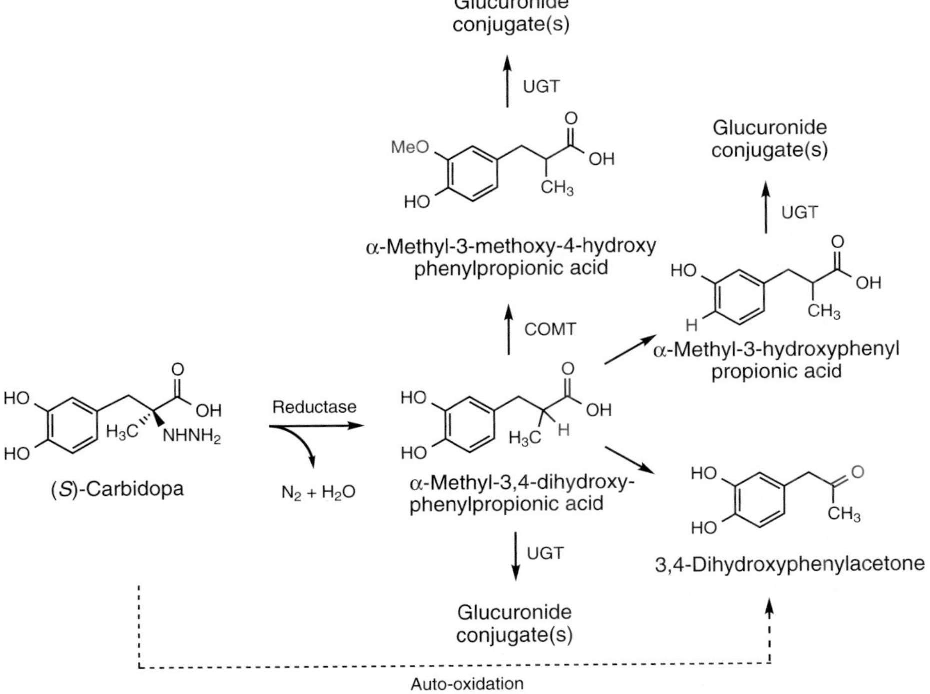

Figure 10.6 Metabolism of carbidopa.

Rasagiline

Rasagiline is indicated as a monotherapy or as adjunct therapy in PD patients taking L-Dopa. Rasagiline is a secondary amine that is substituted with two hydrophobic groups, a propargyl (e.g., type of alkyne) and an indane. It also contains one chiral center with an (*R*)-configuration. Rasagiline is formulated as a mesylate salt and is a white powder that is freely soluble in water or ethanol, but sparingly soluble in isopropanol.

Rasagiline acts as a selective inhibitor of MAO-B. However, it does not block the enzyme activity by reversibly binding to the active site. Instead, rasagiline is initially a substrate for MAO-B and is converted to a reactive intermediate that then forms a covalent irreversible adduct with the enzyme co-factor FAD. The chemistry is shown in Figure 10.7A.[71] MAO-B oxidation activates the propargyl amine to undergo nucleophilic attack by one of the nitrogen atoms of FAD. The resulting adduct of this reaction can be seen in a reported rasagiline·MAO-B·FAD cocrystal structure (Fig. 10.7B).[72]

Rasagiline is readily soluble and permeable resulting in rapid absorption (T_{max} of 1 hr) following oral administration.[73] The drug is subjected to first pass metabolism. As a result it has an oral bioavailability of only 36% (Table 10.1). The drug's steady-state plasma elimination half-life is 3 hours. However, there is no correlation of its pharmacokinetics with its pharmacological outcome due to its irreversible inhibition of MAO-B. Food does not affect the time to maximum plasma concentration (e.g., T_{max}), but the maximum plasma concentration (C_{max}) and exposure (AUC) are decreased by approximately 60% and 20%, respectively, when the drug is taken with a high-fat meal. Rasagiline demonstrates plasma protein binding of 88%-94% and a moderate volume of distribution of 87 L.

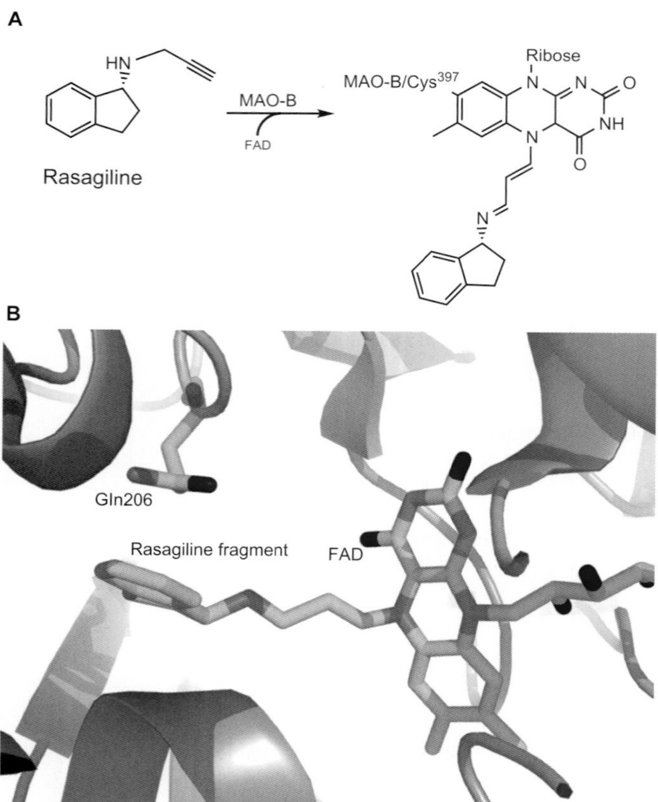

Figure 10.7 (A) Covalent interaction between rasagiline, MAO-B, and FAD. (B) Cocrystal structure of rasagiline covalently bonded to FAD and complexed with MAO-B (PDB: 1S2Q).

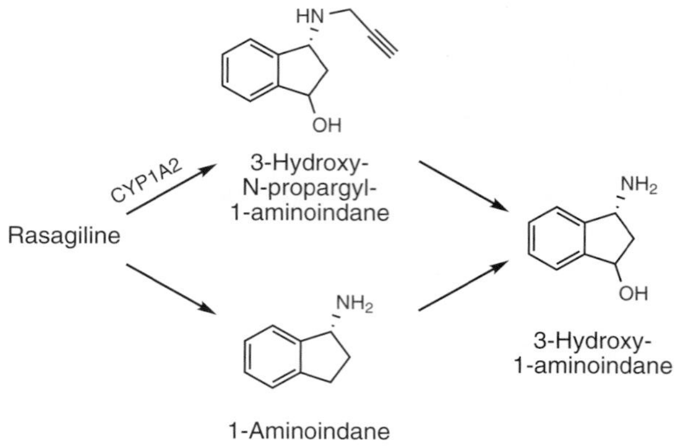

HN
OH
CYP1A2
3-Hydroxy-
N-propargyl-
1-aminoindane
Rasagiline
NH_2
1-Aminoindane
NH_2
OH
3-Hydroxy-
1-aminoindane

Figure 10.8 Phase I metabolism of rasagiline.

Rasagiline is highly metabolized and undergoes almost complete biotransformation in the liver prior to excretion. The parent drug is N-dealkylated to yield 1-aminoindane (Fig. 10.8). It also undergoes benzylic oxidation to form 3-hydroxy-N-propargyl-1-aminoindane. Both of these metabolites can be further oxidized to 3-hydroxy-1-aminoindane. All of these metabolic reactions are CYP450 mediated, with CYP1A2 being the major isoenzyme involved. These phase 1 metabolites also undergo glucuronidation before subsequent urinary excretion.

Given the extensive CYP450-mediated metabolism of rasagiline, especially via the CYP1A2 isozyme, patients taking concomitant ciprofloxacin or other CYP1A2 inhibitors are advised not to exceed a dose of 0.5 mg once daily. In addition, patients with mild hepatic impairment should also not exceed this dose. Rasagiline can also exacerbate hypertension. The most common adverse effects of rasagiline are somnolence, hypotension, dyskinesia, psychotic-like behavior, compulsive behaviors, withdrawal-emergent hyperpyrexia, and confusion.

Selegiline

Selegiline (also known as L-deprenyl) is approved as an adjunct therapy in the management of parkinsonian patients being treated with L-Dopa/carbidopa who exhibit deterioration in the quality of their response to dopamine replacement therapy. Selegiline has not demonstrated beneficial effect in the absence of concurrent L-Dopa/carbidopa therapy. It is also formulated for transdermal delivery and is used for the treatment of depression. Selegiline is structurally related to rasagiline, except that it contains a tertiary amine and a 2-phenpropyl in place of the indane. The drug is formulated as a hydrochloride salt, which is a white crystalline solid that is readily soluble in water. Similar to rasagiline, selegiline is a substrate for MAO-B oxidation and subsequent reactivity with FAD to form a covalent adduct. Hence, it is a selective irreversible inhibitor of MAO-B.

Selegiline is readily soluble and permeable resulting in rapid absorption (T_{max} < 1 hr) following oral administration.[74] It is subjected to extensive first pass metabolism. As a result, it has an oral bioavailability of only 10% (Table 10.1). The pharmacokinetics of selegiline is highly variable. An oral 10 mg dose results in a maximum plasma concentration of 2 μg/L and plasma elimination half-life of 1.5 hours. The drug has a large volume of distribution of 1854 L and a clearance of 59 L/min, which is higher than liver blood flow and indicative of extrahepatic elimination.[75] Following multiple administration, accumulation of both the parent drug and its metabolites have been reported.[76]

Selegiline undergoes extensive metabolism to (*R*)-methamphetamine, via oxidative dealkylation of the propargyl, as the major plasma metabolite (Fig. 10.9). A minor metabolite is N-desmethylselegiline, which is also an irreversible MAO-B inhibitor that is not surprising given its structural similarity to both selegiline and rasagiline.[77] N-Desmethylselegiline is further metabolized to (*R*)-amphetamine again via oxidative dealkylation of the propargyl. Both (*R*)-methamphetamine and (*R*)-amphetamine undergo aromatic hydroxylation to (*R*)-4-hydroxymethamphetamine and (*R*)-4-hydroxyamphetamine, respectively, which are found as their corresponding glucuronide phase II metabolites in urine.[78]

Selegiline is contraindicated for use with meperidine and other opioids due to increased risk of serotonin syndrome. CNS toxicity can occur with the combination of tricyclic antidepressants and selegiline. CNS toxicity can also be observed with the combination of selegiline and selective serotonin reuptake inhibitors. The most common adverse effects of selegiline include nausea, hallucinations, confusion, depression, loss of balance, insomnia, orthostatic hypotension, increased akinetic involuntary movements, agitation, arrhythmia, bradykinesia, chorea, delusions, hypertension, new or increased angina pectoris, and syncope.

Safinamide

Safinamide is the latest MAO-B inhibitor to be introduced for the treatment of PD.[79] It is approved as an adjunct therapy to L-Dopa/carbidopa and has resulted in improved motor function without involuntary movements. The drug has not been shown to be effective as a monotherapy for PD. It is structurally different from both selegiline and rasagiline. Its composition is based on the amino acid alanine. It has a primary amide, a benzyl amine and ether, and one chiral center with an (*S*)-configuration. Safinamide is formulated as the mesylate salt, which is a white crystalline solid that is highly soluble in water. Safinamide's aqueous solubility is pH dependent, showing greatest solubility at pH 1.2-4.5, but with low solubility (<0.4 mg/mL) at pH ≥ 6.8.

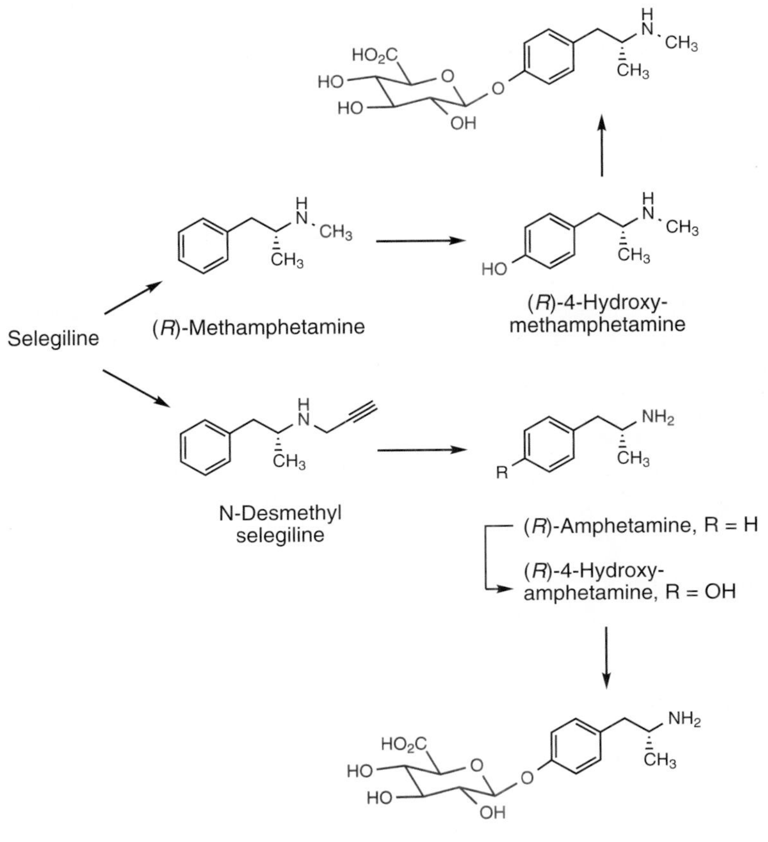

Selegiline
(*R*)-Methamphetamine
(*R*)-4-Hydroxy-methamphetamine
N-Desmethyl selegiline
(*R*)-Amphetamine, R = H
(*R*)-4-Hydroxy-amphetamine, R = OH

Figure 10.9 Metabolism of selegiline.

The mechanism of action of safinamide for inhibition of MAO-B is also different than that of selegiline and rasagiline. It is a reversible MAO-B inhibitor and consequently does not form a covalent bond with the enzyme or the FAD cofactor. But this mode of inhibition still results in increased levels of dopamine. It has 5000-fold selectivity over inhibition of MAO-A. Several molecular interactions contribute to the binding of safinamide to MAO-B, which occur close to the bound FAD. These engagements include van der Waal interaction of the 3-fluorobenzyloxy moiety and hydrogen bonding of the amide and secondary amine of safinamide with Gln206 and an ordered water molecule (Fig. 10.10).[80] Safinamide also inhibits glutamate release and dopamine reuptake, as well as blocks sodium and calcium channels. However, these latter two properties probably do not contribute to the drug's pharmacodynamic effects in the treatment of PD.

Safinamide is readily absorbed following oral administration and is not subjected to extensive first pass metabolism resulting in a bioavailability of 95% (Table 10.1).[81] It reaches maximum plasma concentration about 2-3 hours after administration. The drug has plasma protein binding of 88%-90%, a long terminal plasma elimination half-life of 20-26 hours, a moderate volume of distribution of 165 L, and total clearance of 4.6 L/hr. A slight delay in maximum plasma concentration is observed in the fed verses fasted state, but this has no effect on exposure ($AUC_{0-\infty}$) or maximum plasma concentration (C_{max}). Although safinamide avoids first pass metabolism, it does eventually undergo extensive metabolism with only about 8.5% of the parent drug being excreted unchanged in urine and feces. Safinamide undergoes amidase-mediated hydrolysis of the primary amide to the corresponding carboxylic acid, which is N-dealkylated to a primary amine (Fig. 10.11). Alternatively, the parent drug is directly N-dealkylated to generate the same primary amine. This metabolite is deaminated via MAO-A oxidation to the corresponding aldehyde, which is oxidized via AD to the carboxylic acid, which is the primary metabolite found in plasma. In addition, this metabolite undergoes phase 2 UGT-mediated glucuronidation. The metabolites of safinamide are primarily excreted via the kidney. Furthermore, none of these metabolites appear to exhibit biological activity responsible for the pharmacodynamic effects of the parent drug in the treatment of PD.

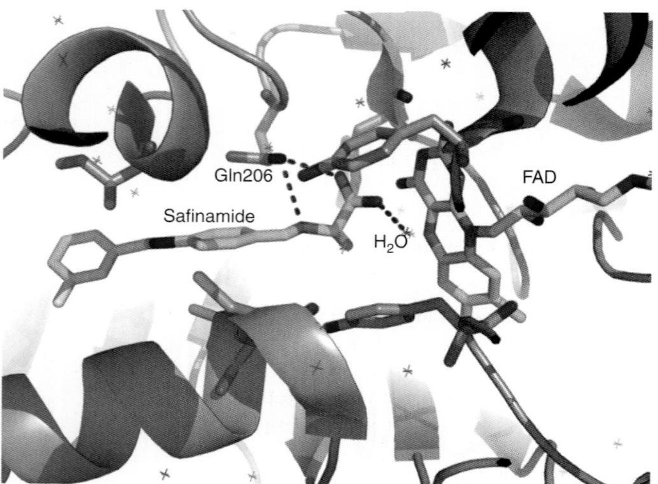

Figure 10.10 Cocrystal structure of safinamide with MAO-B and FAD (PDB: 2V5Z). Hydrogen bonding interactions are depicted with red dashes.

Animal and human studies have not revealed an increased risk of drug-drug interaction with safinamide. Although safinamide does undergo CYP450 metabolism, the prototypic CYP3A4 inhibitor ketoconazole did not alter the formation and clearance of safinamide metabolites to a clinically relevant extent.[82] However, individuals with severe liver problems as well as those using dextromethorphan, other MAO inhibitors, opioids, St. John's wort, antidepressants, or cyclobenzaprine should not use safinamide. The most common adverse effects of safinamide include uncontrolled involuntary movements, nausea, insomnia, and falls.

Catechol-O-Methyltransferase Inhibitors

An alternative strategy used for the treatment of PD is to block the conversion of dopamine to MTA by inhibition of the enzyme COMT. Two drugs, entacapone and tolcapone, operate through this mechanism of action.

Entacapone (Comtan)

Tolcapone (Tasmar)

Entacapone

Entacapone is approved for the treatment of PD as an adjunct therapy to L-Dopa/carbidopa. The structure of entacapone has an (*E*)-alkene substituted with a tertiary amide, nitrile, and nitro-containing catechol. The drug is a crystalline solid that is only sparingly soluble in water. Its mechanism of action is selective and reversible inhibition of COMT.

Entacapone's pharmacokinetic properties are independent of coadministered L-Dopa/carbidopa. The drug is readily absorbed following oral administration reaching maximum plasma concentrations within 1 hour.[83] However, first pass metabolism limits oral bioavailability to 35% (Table 10.1). Food does not affect the pharmacokinetics of entacapone. The elimination of entacapone is biphasic, with a plasma elimination half-life of 0.4-0.7 hours based on the β-phase and 2.4 hours based on the γ-phase. After a single 200 mg oral dose of entacapone, the maximum plasma concentration is 1.2 µg/mL. The drug's volume of distribution is low, limiting tissue concentrations due to high plasma protein binding (e.g., 98%).

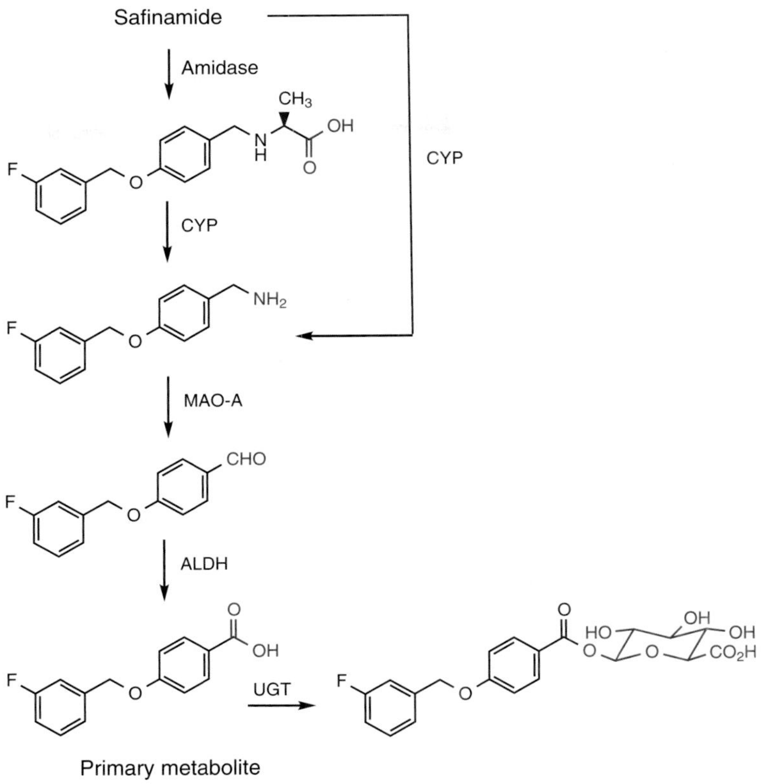

Safinamide
Amidase
CYP
CYP
MAO-A
ALDH
UGT
Primary metabolite

Figure 10.11 Metabolism of safinamide.

Entacapone is significantly metabolized prior to excretion, with only 0.2% of the parent drug found unchanged in urine and 10% in feces. Entacapone undergoes alkene isomerization to the inactive Z-isomer. Interestingly, (Z)-entacapone is the only phase 1 metabolite found in human plasma. The parent drug is also metabolized via glucuronidation predominately by UGT1A9 to generate two regioisomeric metabolites.[84] The isomerized phase 1 metabolite also undergoes glucuronidation. The resulting glucuronides from the parent and the alkene isomer represent about 70% and 25%, respectively, of the urinary metabolites (Fig. 10.12).[85] Curiously, the nitro group appears to block COMT-mediated methylation of the catechol.

One precautionary note about entacapone is that the exposure (AUC) and maximum plasma concentration (C_{max}) can significantly increase in patients with hepatic impairment. The most common adverse effects of entacapone are urine discoloration, nausea, hyperkinesia, abdominal pain, vomiting, and dry mouth.

Tolcapone

Similar to entacapone, tolcapone is indicated for the treatment of PD as an adjunct therapy to L-Dopa/carbidopa. The two compounds also have a structural resemblance since they both contain a nitro-substituted catechol. However, tolcapone has another benzene ring linked through a ketone as opposed to an alkene. Tolcapone is a yellow crystalline solid that is poorly soluble in water.

Tolcapone is a selective and reversible inhibitor of COMT. As can be seen in the tolcapone·SAM·COMT·Mg^{+2} cocrystal structure,[86] the catechol of tolcapone forms an interaction with the Mg^{+2} ion as well as a hydrogen bond to Asn170 and an ionic-dipole interaction with Glu199 (Fig. 10.13). Furthermore, the SAM methyl group that normally is transferable to the substrate is positioned close to the para-hydroxyl group of tolcapone. However, transfer does not occur likely due to the strong electron-withdrawing effect of the nitro group, although some methylation of the other hydroxyl group is observed as a minor metabolite (see below).

Tolcapone's pharmacokinetic properties are linear and independent of L-Dopa/(S)-carbidopa coadministration. The drug is readily absorbed after oral administration and demonstrates moderate bioavailability of 65% reaching maximum plasma concentration in 2 hours (Table 10.1).[87] Food delays and decreases the absorption of tolcapone by about 10%-20%. After oral doses of 100 or 200 mg, maximum plasma concentrations of 3 and 6 µg/mL, respectively, are obtained. Tolcapone has high plasma protein binding (>99.9%). Consequently, it has moderate systemic clearance (7 L/hr) and does not distribute widely into tissues.

Tolcapone is extensively metabolized prior to excretion, with only 0.5% of the dose found unchanged in urine and 60% and 40% of the metabolites excreted in urine and feces, respectively. The primary metabolite of tolcapone is the glucuronide of the more sterically accessible phenol (Fig. 10.14). Several minor metabolites are also formed, including oxidation of the benzylic position (via CYP3A4 and 2A6) to an alcohol that is subsequently oxidized to the corresponding carboxylic acid, reduction of the nitro to an aniline that is subsequently acetylated, and COMT-mediated methylation to 3-O-methyl-tolcapone, as mentioned above.

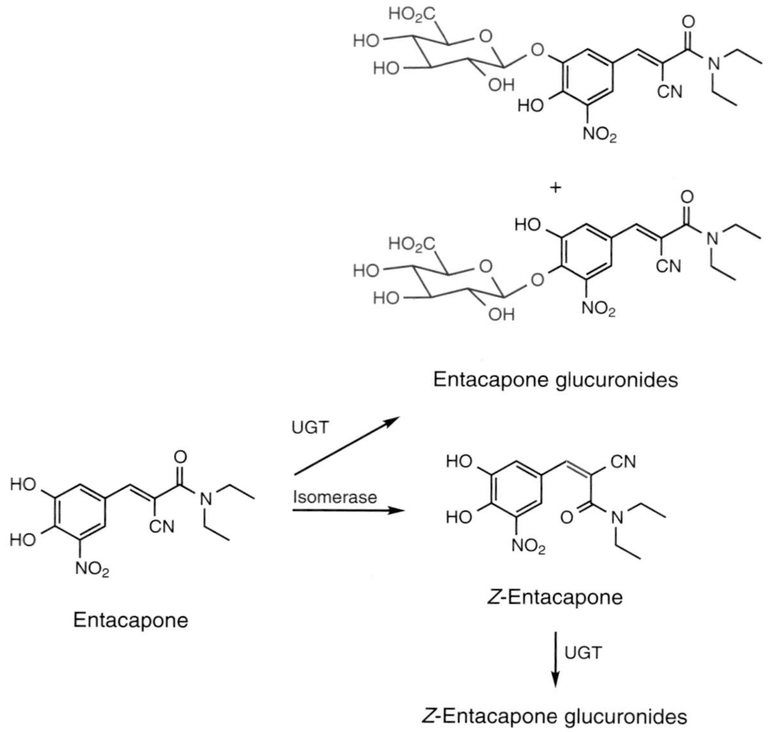

Entacapone glucuronides

UGT

Isomerase

Entacapone

Z-Entacapone

UGT

Z-Entacapone glucuronides

Figure 10.12 Metabolism of entacapone.

Tolcapone is contraindicated in patients with liver disease or in patients who were withdrawn from tolcapone treatment because of drug-induced hepatocellular injury. Hepatic failures have been observed leading to its market withdrawal in some countries, as well as restriction in the United States to only those patients not responsive to other therapies and who can be appropriately monitored for hepatic toxicity. It is also contraindicated in patients with a history of nontraumatic rhabdomyolysis or hyperpyrexia and/or confusion possibly related to medication. The most common adverse effects of tolcapone are nausea, anorexia, sleep disorder, vomiting, urine discoloration, dystonia, and sweating.

Dopamine Receptor Agonists

Another strategy for the treatment of PD is through agonism of dopamine receptors, particularly postsynaptic D_2-types. Six drugs, apomorphine, bromocriptine, carbergoline, pramipexole, ropinirole, and rotigotine, work via this mode, providing symptomatic relief to PD patients.

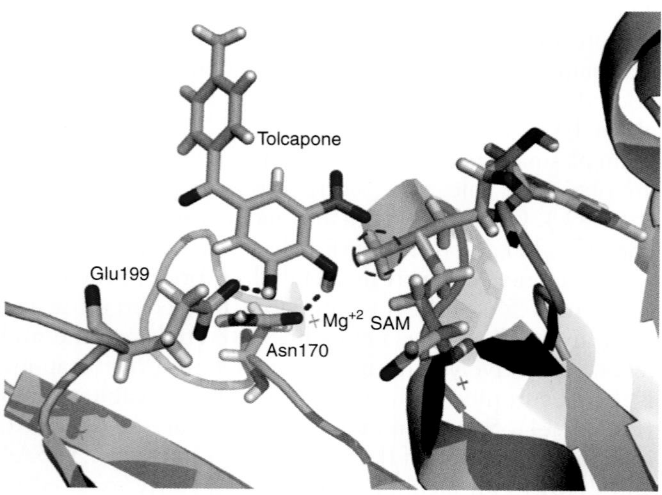

Figure 10.13 Tolcapone·SAM·COMT·Mg^{+2} cocrystal structure (PDB: 3S68). Hydrogen bonding interactions are shown with red dashes. The transferable methyl on SAM is highlighted with a red dashed circle. Residues 3-12 and 21-56 have been deleted for clarity.

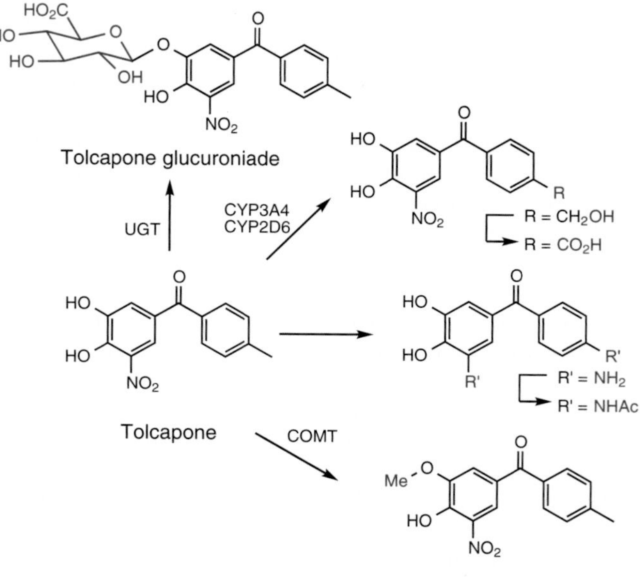

Figure 10.14 Metabolism of tolcapone.

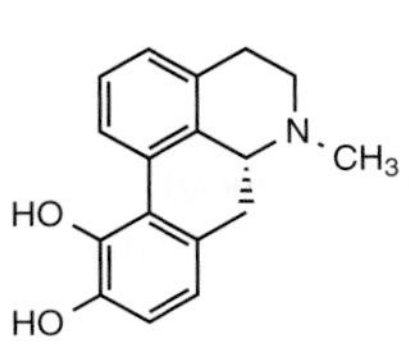

Apomorphine (Apokyn)　Bromocriptine (Parlodel)　Cabergoline (Dostinex)

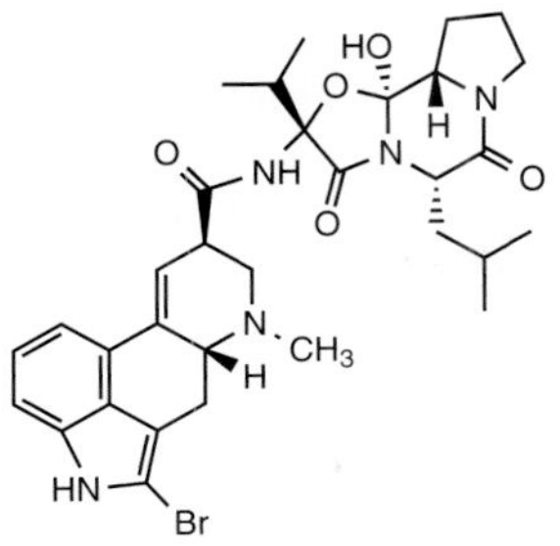

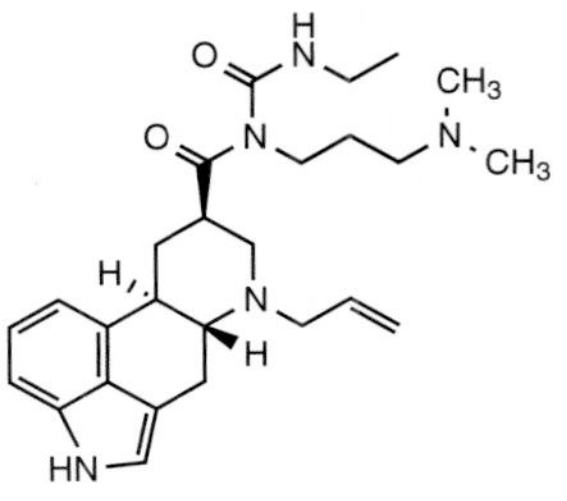

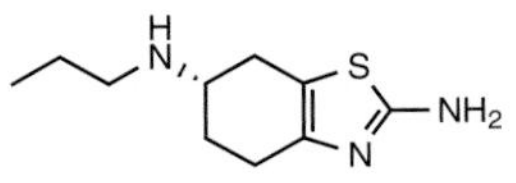

Pramipexole (Mirapex)　Ropinirole (Requip)　Rotigotine (Neupro)

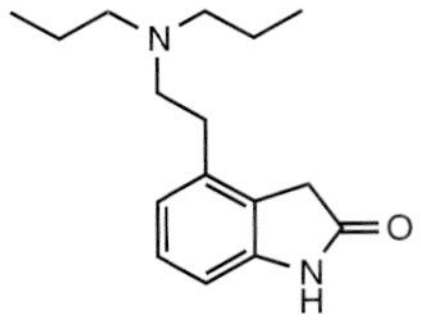

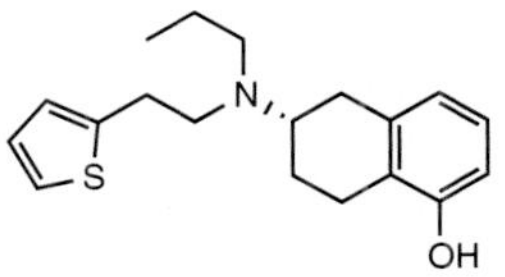

Dopamine receptor agonists.

Apomorphine

Apomorphine is indicated for the acute, intermittent treatment of hypomobility, or "off" episodes (e.g., times when other PD medications, such as L-dopa/carbidopa, are not working well) in patients with advanced PD. It is a synthetic compound related to a class of alkaloids called aporphines that are found in a wide variety of plants. Apomorphine contains a tertiary amine and has a catechol that makes up part of the aporphine tetracyclic scaffold and one chiral center with an (*R*)-configuration. The drug is formulated as a hydrochloride salt that forms white crystals or is a white powder. It is administered by subcutaneous injection.

Apomorphine's mechanism of action in the treatment of PD is postulated to occur via stimulation of postsynaptic dopamine D_2-type receptors within the caudate-putamen region of the brain. Apomorphine has high in vitro binding affinity for the D_4 receptor and moderate affinity for D_2, D_3, and D_5, and adrenergic α_{1D}, α_{2B}, α_{2C} receptors.[88] The rigid tetracyclic structure and hydroxyl groups at C10 and C11 of (*R*)-apomorphine mimic the *trans*-α-conformational isomer of dopamine (Fig. 10.15) likely representing the binding conformation.[89] In contrast, (*R*)-isoapomorphine that displays the structure of dopamine in the *trans*-β-conformational isomer has less activity. Finally, (*R*)-1,2-dihydroxyaporphine that displays the structure of dopamine in the *cis*-α-conformational isomer is inactive as a dopamine receptor agonist.[90]

Apomorphine hydrochloride is rapidly absorbed following subcutaneous administration into the abdominal wall and reaches a maximum plasma concentration in 10-60 minutes.[91] The drug exhibits linear pharmacokinetics over a dose range of 2-8 mg following a single subcutaneous injection. It also demonstrates an apparent volume of distribution of 218 L, apparent clearance of 223 L/hr, and a relatively short mean terminal plasma elimination half-life of 40 minutes (Table 10.1). The major excreted metabolites are apomorphine sulfate and apomorphine glucuronide.[92]

Apomorphine is contraindicated in patients using concomitant 5-HT_3 antagonists, including antiemetics (e.g., ondansetron, granisetron, dolasetron, palonosetron) and

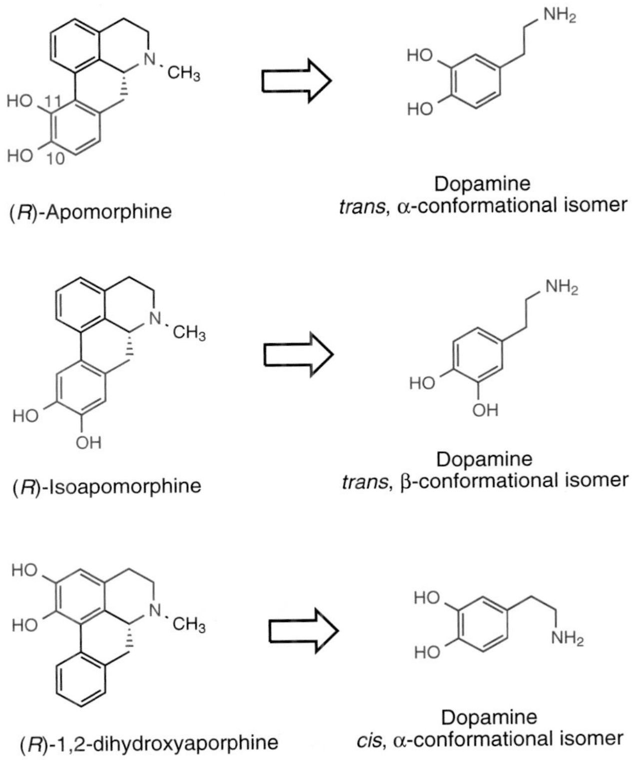

(*R*)-Apomorphine　Dopamine *trans*, α-conformational isomer

(*R*)-Isoapomorphine　Dopamine *trans*, β-conformational isomer

(*R*)-1,2-dihydroxyaporphine　Dopamine *cis*, α-conformational isomer

Figure 10.15 Comparison of conformational restricted dopamine analogues (*R*)-apomorphine, (*R*)-isoapomorphine, and (*R*)-1,2-dihydroxyaporphine with the *trans*-α-, *trans*-β-, and *cis*-α-conformational isomers of dopamine.

alosetron used to treat severe diarrhea-predominant irritable bowel syndrome, due to increased risk of hypotension that can result in loss of consciousness. The drug dose should also be reduced in patients with mild or moderate renal impairment, as well as mild or moderate hepatic impairment. In both cases apomorphine exposure can increase in these patients. The most common adverse effects of apomorphine are nausea and vomiting, coronary events, QT prolongation, proarrhythmia, and priapism.

Bromocriptine

Bromocriptine is indicated for the treatment of idiopathic or postencephalitic PD, as well as hyperprolactinemia-associated dysfunctions and acromegaly. It is a structurally complex synthetic compound related to naturally occurring ergot alkaloids. Bromocriptine contains a tertiary amine that allows the free base to be formulated as a mesylate salt. Although salt formation increases aqueous solubility, it still remains low (<1 mg/mL).

Bromocriptine is a partial agonist at D_2 and D_3 receptors[93] with selective over D_1, D_4, and D_5 receptors.[88] It also has potent to moderate binding affinity for α_{1A}, α_{1B}, α_{1D}, α_{2A}, α_{2B}, α_{2C}, 5-HT_{1A}, and 5-HT_{1D} receptors.[88] The drug was the first direct dopamine agonist indicated for the treatment of PD, after its development for use at lower doses as a prolactin inhibitor.[94]

The enteral absorption of bromocriptine is incomplete (~30%-40% in rats and monkeys) possibly due to its high molecular weight, poor aqueous solubility, and/or permeability. Following an oral dose (2 × 2.5 mg) of bromocriptine mesylate, a maximum plasma concentration of 465 pg/mL is achieved in 2.5 hours. Bromocriptine is highly protein bound (>90%) and has a plasma elimination half-life of 4.9 hours (Table 10.1).[95]

The drug undergoes extensive first pass metabolism with the main route of elimination in bile (80%-93% of the absorbed dose) with little parent drug excreted in urine and feces. It appears that two primary pathways are responsible for metabolism of bromocriptine[96,97]: hydrolysis and epimerization generating 2-bromolysergic acid and the epimer 2-bromoisolysergic acid via the intermediate amides (Fig. 10.16). The second metabolism route involves oxidation of C8 in the proline fragment. Further oxidation of the C9 position, as well as formation of the 8-O- and 9-O-glucuronides, occurs. These metabolites are likely also susceptible to hydrolysis and epimerization. Interestingly, the lysergic acid portion of bromocriptine and its metabolites seems quite stable to metabolism.

Caution should be used when coadministering bromocriptine with drugs that inhibit CYP3A4. The concomitant use of macrolide antibiotics, such as erythromycin, can increase the plasma levels of bromocriptine.[98] In addition, bromocriptine should not be used during the postpartum period in women with a history of coronary artery disease and other severe cardiovascular conditions due to an increased risk of vasospastic reactions. The most common adverse effects of bromocriptine with concomitant reduction in the dose of L-dopa/carbidopa are nausea, abnormal involuntary movements, hallucinations, confusion, "on-off" phenomenon, dizziness, drowsiness, faintness/fainting, vomiting, asthenia, abdominal discomfort, visual disturbance, ataxia, insomnia, depression, hypotension, shortness of breath, constipation, and vertigo.

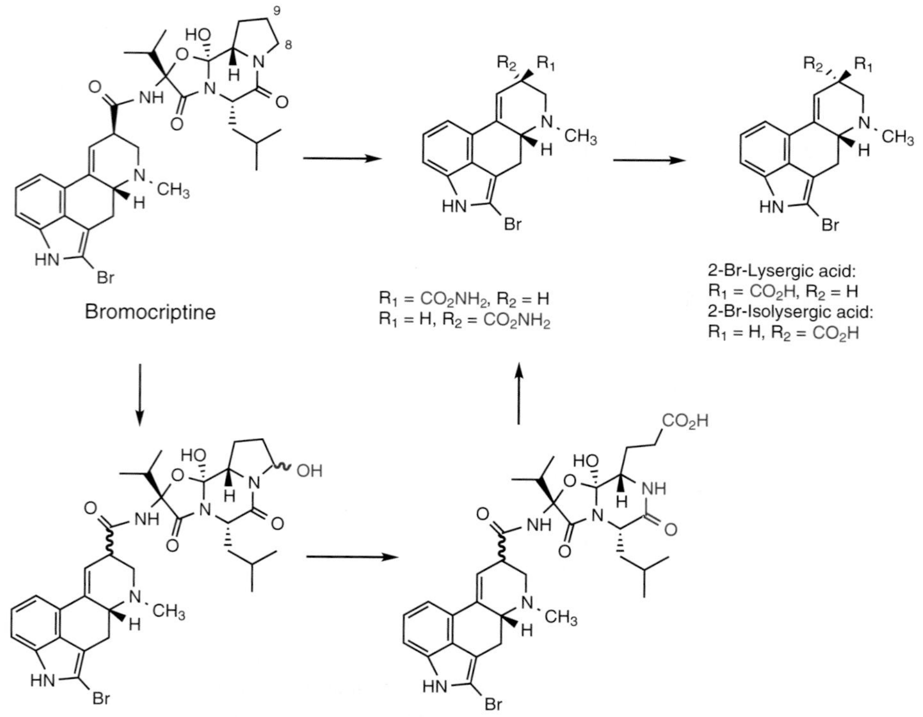

Bromocriptine

$R_1 = CO_2NH_2$, $R_2 = H$
$R_1 = H$, $R_2 = CO_2NH_2$

2-Br-Lysergic acid:
$R_1 = CO_2H$, $R_2 = H$
2-Br-Isolysergic acid:
$R_1 = H$, $R_2 = CO_2H$

Figure 10.16 Metabolism of bromocriptine.

Cabergoline

Carbergoline is indicated for the treatment of early phase PD, as well as a number of other conditions including hyperprolactinemic disorders (e.g., idiopathic or due to pituitary adenomas). It is structurally related to bromocriptine. However, the secondary amide in carbergoline has been significantly simplified, the N-alkyl group has been changed, the alkene has been saturated, and the bromine on the indole has been removed. Cabergoline is a white powder slightly soluble in 0.1 N hydrochloric acid but insoluble in water. Its mechanism of action is also similar to bromocriptine, demonstrating full agonism at D_2 receptors and partial agonism at D_3 and D_4 receptors, without appreciable activity at D_1 receptors.[88,93] It also has potent binding affinity for α_{2D}, and 5-HT_{1D}, 5-HT_{2A}, and 5-HT_{2B} receptors.[88]

Following oral administration, cabergoline reaches maximum plasma levels in 2-3 hours and has a long elimination plasma half-life of 63-109 hours (Table 10.1).[99] Cabergoline is moderately bound to human plasma proteins (~40%). The drug is extensively metabolized by the liver, with fecal excretion of metabolites as the main route of elimination over a prolonged period of time. Two hydrolysis routes of the acylurea account for the predominate metabolism of cabergoline (Fig. 10.17). In the first, the urea moiety is hydrolyzed to generate a secondary amide. Alternatively, the acylurea bond is broken to produce the carboxylic acid. But, similar to bromocriptine, the tetracyclic scaffold is quite resistant to metabolism.

Cabergoline is contraindicated in patients with a history of cardiac valvular disorders, as well as pulmonary, pericardial, or retroperitoneal fibrotic disorders. The drug's most common adverse effects are headache, nausea, and vomiting.

Pramipexole

Pramipexole is indicated for the treatment of PD. It is structurally distinct from bromocriptine and cabergoline in that it is unrelated to ergot alkaloids. Its structure consists of a 2-aminothiazole fused to cyclohexyl hydrocarbon that is further substituted with a secondary amine as the (S)-enantiomer. It is formulated as the dihydrochloride monohydrate salt that is a white powder with more than 20% by weight solubility in water. Mechanistically, it is a D_2 receptor agonist with affinity for the D_3 and D_4 receptor subtypes, but low affinity for the D_1 receptor. However, it demonstrates lower in vitro binding affinity versus adrenergic and serotonin receptors compared to apomorphine, bromocriptine, and cabergoline.[88]

Pramipexole's low molecular weight and good aqueous solubility, coupled with permeability and resistance to first pass metabolism, result in excellent oral bioavailability of >90% (Table 10.1).[100] It reaches maximum plasma concentration in 2 hours after oral administration, although this can increase to 3 hours if taken with food. Pramipexole is only about 15% bound to plasma proteins contributing to its extensive tissue distribution (e.g., volume of distribution of 500 L). Pramipexole is not extensively metabolized, contributing to a long terminal plasma elimination half-life of 8-12 hours, with 90% excreted in urine unchanged with clearance of 400 mL/min.

Pramipexole does not significantly inhibit CYP450 enzymes and does not appear to participate in drug-drug interactions. However, given its dependence on renal clearance, elimination can be significantly lower in patients with moderate to severe kidney impairment. Finally, the most common adverse effects of pramipexole are nausea, dizziness, somnolence, insomnia, constipation, asthenia, and hallucinations.

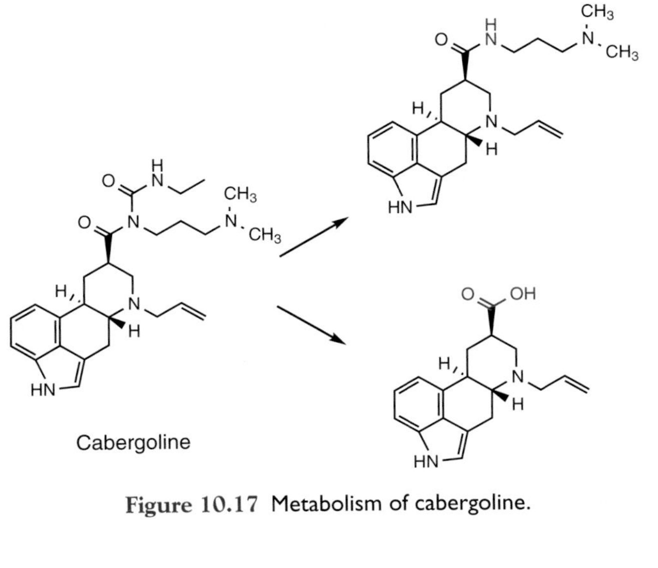

Cabergoline

Figure 10.17 Metabolism of cabergoline.

Ropinirole

Ropinirole, which is structurally similar to pramipexole, is also indicated for the treatment of PD. It contains an oxindole tethered via an ethylene linker at the 4-position to a tertiary amine. This later functional group is used to formulate ropinirole as a hydrochloride salt, which is a white to yellow solid with excellent water solubility of 133 mg/mL. Ropinirole is a D_2 agonist with weaker binding affinities to D_3, D_4, 5-HT_2, and α_2 receptors.[101]

Ropinirole, with a low molecular weight and good aqueous solubility, is rapidly absorbed after oral administration reaching maximum plasma concentrations in 1-2 hours, which can increase to 4 hours (along with concomitant decrease in maximum plasma concentration of 25%) when taken with food.[102] However, ropinirole is more susceptible to first pass metabolism compared to pramipexole, likely contributing to a lower absolute bioavailability of 45%-55% (Table 10.1). Ropinirole is modestly bound to plasma proteins (e.g., 40%) with a high apparent volume of distribution of 7.5 L/kg, clearance of 47 L/hr, and plasma elimination half-life of 6 hours. The primary route of elimination is in urine with <10% of the administered dose of ropinirole excreted unchanged.

Ropinirole is extensively metabolized by the liver. The predominant route of metabolism is via N-depropylation.[103] This metabolite is further transformed by hydroxylation at C-7 followed by glucuronidation (Fig. 10.18). In addition, N-depropylropinirole is converted to a carboxylic acid metabolite and an N-carbamylglucuronide, a rather uncommon type of metabolite.

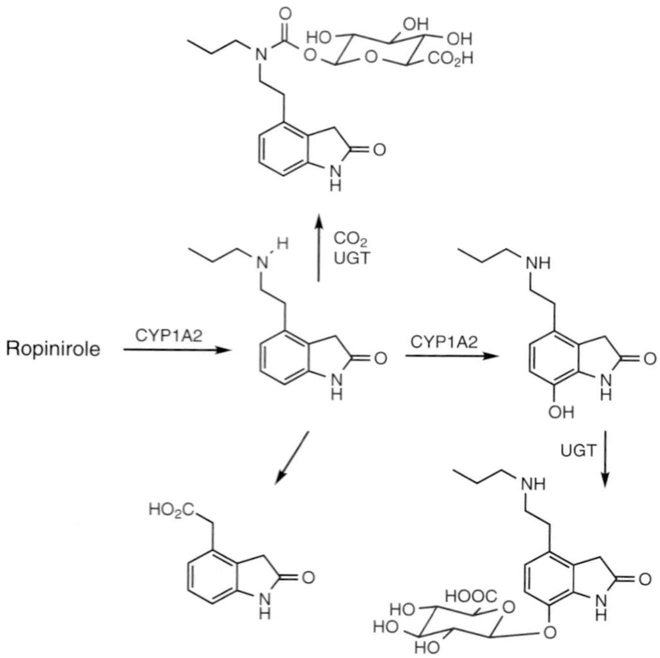

Figure 10.18 Metabolism of ropinirole.

The primary CYP450 isozyme responsible for the phase 1 metabolism of ropinirole is CYP1A2.[104] Consequently, coadministration with CYP1A2 inhibitors, such as ciprofloxacin, can increase exposure (e.g., AUC) and maximum plasma concentration (e.g., C_{max}) of ropinirole. On the other hand, cigarette smoking is expected to decrease exposure to ropinirole since CYP1A2 is known to be induced by smoking, which may require drug dose adjustment. The most common adverse effects of ropinirole are nausea, somnolence, dizziness, syncope, asthenic condition (i.e., asthenia, fatigue, and/or malaise), viral infection, leg edema, vomiting, and dyspepsia.

Rotigotine

Rotigotine is indicated for the treatment of both early and advanced PD. It is administered by transdermal patch.[105] Like ropinirole and pramipexole, rotigotine does not resemble ergot alkaloids and contains a phenol fused to a cyclohexyl, which is tethered via an ethylene linker to a tertiary amine, again as the (*S*)-enantiomer. The amine is also connected to a thiophene. Rotigotine's mechanism of action is similar to ropinirole and pramipexole, specifically, D_1, D_2, and D_3 receptor agonism.[106]

Rotigotine is relatively highly bound to human plasma proteins (e.g., ~90%). The drug has a high apparent volume of distribution of 84 L/kg (Table 10.1). After removal of the patch, drug levels decrease with a terminal plasma elimination half-life of 5-7 hours. Rotigotine is primarily excreted in urine (~71%) and feces (~23%).[107] It is metabolized by multiple CYP450 isozymes to N-desproply and N-desthienylethyl phase 1 metabolites, which undergo sulfonation of the phenol. The parent drug is also a substrate for SULT and UGT, generating metabolites resulting from sulfonation and glucuronidation of the phenol (Fig. 10.19).[108]

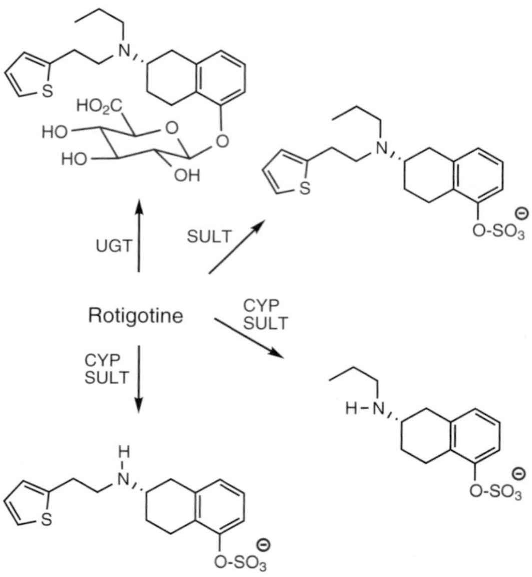

Figure 10.19 Metabolism of rotigotine.

Since rotigotine is metabolized by multiple CYP450, SULT, and UGT isoforms, it has low risk of interacting with other drugs. The most common adverse effects of rotigotine are nausea, vomiting, somnolence, application site reactions, dizziness, anorexia, hyperhidrosis, insomnia peripheral edema, and dyskinesia.

The three dopamine agonists pramipexole, ropinirole and rotigotine are also indicated for the treatment of restless leg syndrome (RLS), also known as Willis-Ekbom disease, which is a neuromuscular condition associated with abnormal sensations in the legs particularly during sleep. Although the cause is not known, RLS appears to involve brain iron deficiency. Surprisingly, overall brain dopamine is actually increased in RLS patients. However, dopamine has a circadian activity pattern decreasing in the evening/night and increasing in the morning. Therefore, overcompensation of postsynaptic adjustment to increased dopamine stimulation during the daytime may cause deficient dopamine response at night.[109] Thus, dopamine agonists may help dampen the effects of lower nocturnal dopamine responsiveness. In addition to dopamine agonists, calcium channel alpha-2-delta antagonists (e.g., gabapentin, gabapentin enacarbil, and pregabalin) are also used as first-line treatments and in some cases are preferred.[110]

Nondopamine-Related Therapy

The mainstay of current PD chemotherapy is focused on dopamine, through replacement, agumentation of its catabolism, or functional agonism of postsynaptic dopamine receptors. However, nondopamine-based therapies have also been assessed as alternative strategies. One drug that has been approved for the treatment of PD that does not elicit its effects via dopamine-related mechansims is amantadine.

Amantadine

Amantadine (Symmetrel) Memantine (Namenda)

Amantadine is indicated in the treatment of PD and drug-induced extrapyramidal reactions. Interestingly, it was originally developed and indicated for the prophylaxis and treatment of influenza A virus infections. The drug contains a primary amine attached to the bulky and hydrophobic cyclic hydrocarbon adamantane. It is formulated as the hydrochloride salt, which is a white crystalline solid that is readily soluble in water.

Amantadine is an NMDA glutamate receptor antagonist that might provide neuroprotective effects in PD. The drug has been shown to cause dopamine and norepinephrine release from intraneuronal storage sites and to block dopamine reuptake.[111] It may provide moderate benefit early in PD by enhancing the effects of L-Dopa and limiting the severity of dyskinesias induced by L-Dopa therapy.[112] Although the drug was originally developed as an antiviral agent, PD patients appeared to have improvements of symptoms.[113] However, others have cast doubt on the efficacy of amantadine in the treatment of PD, concluding that randomized controlled clinical trials did not provide sufficient evidence of efficacy and safety in the treatment of idiopathic PD.[114] Memantine is a close structural derivative that demonstrates similar pharmacology but is indicated for the treatment of moderate to severe dementia of the Alzheimer's type.

Amantadine is well absorbed following oral administration, reaching maximum plasma concentrations in about 3 hours.[115] The drug has a clearance of 0.28 L/hr/kg with a large volume of distribution of 3-8 L/kg and a long plasma elimination half-life of 12-17 hours (Table 10.1). It is primarily excreted unchanged (65%-85% of the dose) in urine. However, a number of metabolites are observed following therapeutic dosing (Fig. 10.20). The major metabolite of amantadine is the N-acetylated derivative (5%-15% of the dose). However, several other minor metabolites have been identified.[116]

Amantadine can accumulate in patients with renal dysfunction. However, it does not appear to interact with other drugs.[117] The most common adverse effects of amantadine are nausea, dizziness, and insomnia.

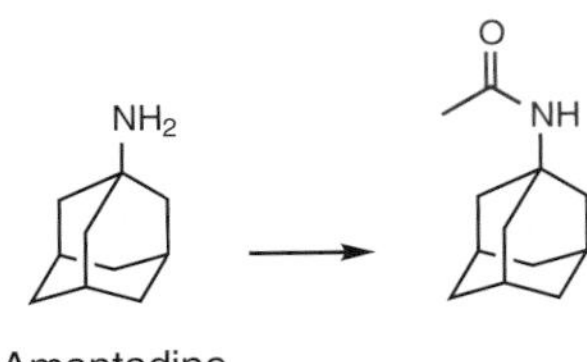

Figure 10.20 Metabolism of amantadine.

MULTIPLE SCLEROSIS

Therapeutic Context Overview

Multiple sclerosis (MS) is a chronic disease that involves demyelination of nerve cells (e.g., oligodendrocytes) in the brain and spinal cord. The condition leads to a variety of symptoms including vision difficulties, fatigue, coordination problems, spasticity, as well as cognitive and behavioral changes. The disease takes two forms: progressive and relapsing-remitting. This latter form of MS is most common (80%-90% of cases), with about half of the patients eventually entering a degenerative progressive phase.

Although the cause of MS is not known, there are two general hypotheses that have influenced current MS chemotherapeutic development.[118] The most widely accepted premise is the autoimmune hypothesis. According to this hypothesis, myelin basic protein (MBP) antigen-specific CD4-positive T cells are first primed by dendritic cells in peripheral CNS-draining lymph nodes. This leads to differentiation into Th17 cells by interleukin-23. Th17 cells enter the cerebral spinal fluid, where they are reactivated by MHC class II-expressing macrophages or dendritic cells, followed by entry into the CNS. Here these autoreactive leukocytes initiate disease leading to neuroinflammation that results in oligodendrocyte demyelination. The other premise is the oligodendrogliopathy hypothesis, where the disease starts with oligodendroglial apoptosis initiated from undetermined causes resulting in demyelination. The associated neuroinflammation is a secondary event in response to the oligodendroglial apoptosis.[119]

MS typically presents in adults 20-50 years of age and is the most common cause of nontraumatic disability in young adults. The disease afflicts approximately 2-2.5 million people worldwide, with the highest prevalence (100-200 cases per 100,000) in populations of Northern European origin.[120] Furthermore, the prevalence ratio of MS in women to men has increased markedly during the last decades (2.3-3.5:1).[121] In the United States, the annual costs per patient of disease-modifying therapies have dramatically increased and are currently >$70,000 a year.[122]

Pharmacology Overview

Given the complex pathological processes involving different cell types in both the periphery and CNS that result in MS, it is not surprising that diverse therapeutic strategies have emerged. However, the assortment of available chemotherapeutics also extends to the chemical matter that comprises MS drugs, from low-molecular-weight organic molecules, to a polymeric composition to monoclonal antibodies.

The pharmacology of MS drugs falls into several categories. The first group comprises agents that either (1) replace or mimic the action of endogenous interferon beta resulting in upregulation of immunomodulatory genes, or (2) enhance the production of the anti-inflammatory cytokines interleukin 4 and 5, as well as induce an antioxidative stress response. The second set of agents can broadly be defined as those altering the modulation (e.g., reduced activation or proliferation, or induced lysis) of T and/or B cells through a number of different mechanisms. The third category of drugs either results in sequestration of lymphocytes in lymph nodes or prevents their migration from the periphery into the CNS. The fourth class of drugs does not directly target the underlying neuropathology of MS per se. Instead it blocks potassium channels restoring axonal conduction that improved mobility of MS patients.

Interferon Beta-1a, Interferon Beta-1b, and Peginterferon Beta-1a

Interferon beta-1a (Avonex), interferon beta-1b (Betaseron), and peginterferon beta-1a (Plegridy) are indicated for the treatment of patients with relapsing forms of MS. Interferon beta-1a is administered via intramuscular injection, while interferon beta-1b and peginterferon beta-1a are given by subcutaneous injection. The structure of interferon beta-1a consists of a 166-amino-acid glycosylated protein (molecular weight ~22.5 kDa) that is identical to human interferon beta. Interferon beta-1b is similar, but with several modifications, including serine in place of the cysteine residue at position 17, one less amino acid, and no carbohydrate side chains, resulting in a lower molecular weight (~18 kDa). Peginterferon beta-1a is a derivative of interferon beta-1a in which a single linear 20 kDa methoxy poly(ethyleneglycol)-O-2-methylpropionaldehyde is covalently attached near the N-terminus of the protein, which reduces clearance. These drugs are manufactured using recombinant DNA technology genetically engineered into either Chinese hamster ovary cells or *Escherichia coli*. For peginterferon beta-1a, a subsequent step is needed to attach the polymer chain.

Interferon beta is an endogenous cytokine that is produced in response to biological and chemical stimuli. It binds to type I interferon receptors that signal through the Janus kinase/signal transducers and activators of transcription (JAK/STAT) pathway, resulting in the modulation of gene expression for a host of biological molecules culminating in immunomodulatory, antiviral, and antitumor effects.[123] With regard to the mechanism of action for interferon beta-1a, interferon beta-1b, and peginterferon beta-1a in the treatment of MS, it is the immunomodulatory role that is likely critical. These molecules reduce peripheral myeloid dendritic cells, T-cell responses, and antigen presentation by microglia and monocytes.

Interferon beta-1a reaches maximum plasma concentrations 3-15 hours after administration with a plasma elimination half-life of 10 hours. For interferon beta-1b, plasma concentrations are not detectable following subcutaneous administration of low dose (e.g., ≤0.25 mg). At higher dose (e.g., 0.5 mg) maximum plasma concentrations were reached within 1-8 hours. Peginterferon beta-1a reaches maximum plasma concentration within 1-1.5 days and has a volume of distribution of 481 L, a plasma elimination half-live of 78 hours, and a clearance of 4.1 L/hr. The drugs are catabolized and excreted by the kidneys.

These drugs are contraindicated in patients sensitive to stabilizers used in the formuations, such as albumin and mannitol. Some of the most common adverse effects of these agents are flu-like symptoms including injection site reaction, myalgia, asthenia, lymphopenia, leukopenia, neutropenia, increased liver enzymes, insomnia, abdominal pain, asthenia, pyrexia, and arthralgia.

Glatiramer

Glatiramer (Copaxone) is indicated for reduction of the frequency of relapses in patients with relapsing-remitting MS. Structurally this drug is quite unique. It consists of a synthetic polymer of L-glutamic acid, L-alanine, L-lysine, and L-tyrosine in an average molar fraction of 0.141, 0.427, 0.095, and 0.338, respectively. The material is formulated as an acetate salt (e.g., $(Glu, Ala, Lys, Tyr)_x{\cdot}xCH_3COOH$). The polymeric drug has an average molecular weight of 5-9 kDa.

The polymeric drug is believed to elicit its effects in MS by mimicking MBP. In this way the drug competes with MBP, reducing the number of antigen-specific CD4-positive T cells, which interrupts the autoimmune cascade.[124] Glatiramer may also modulate the activity of MHC antigen-presenting cells.[125] These mechanisms are distinct from those elicited by interferon beta-1a, interferon beta-1b, and peginterferon beta-1a.[126]

A significant portion of the subcutaneously administered dose is partially hydrolyzed near the injection site. A portion of the injected material, either intact or partially hydrolyzed, likely enters the lymphatic circulation with some entering the systemic circulation. The most common adverse effects of glatirmer are injection site reactions, vasodilatation, rash, dyspnea, and chest pain.

Ocrelizumab, Alemtuzumab, and Natalizumab

Three human monoclonal antibodies have also been developed for the treatment of MS. Ocrelizumab (Ocrevus) is indicated for the treatment of patients with relapsing form of MS. It is also the first drug approved for the treatment of the primary progressive form of MS. Ocrelizumab is a humanized anti-CD20 IGg1 glycosylated monoclonal antibody with a molecular weight of 145 kDa that is administered via intravenous infusion. The antibody binds to CD20 on the cell surface of B-lymphocytes, causing antibody-dependent cellular cytolysis and complement-mediated cell lysis. The efficacy of ocrelizumab in the treatment of MS highlights the important role of B lymphocytes as precursors of antibody-secreting plasma cells and as antigen-presenting cells for the activation of T cells.[127] The residence time of ocrelizumab is long, requiring maintenance doses of 600 mg every 6 months for relapsing-remitting MS patients or two 300 mg infusions separated by 14 days every 6 months for primary progressive MS patients.[128] The drug has a volume of distribution of 2.78 L, a clearance of 0.17 L/d, and terminal plasma elimination half-life of 26 days with metabolism via catabolism. Ocrelizumab is contraindicated for use in patients with active hepatitis B virus infection. The most common adverse effects of ocrelizumab are respiratory tract and skin infections, as well as infusion reactions.

Alemtuzumab (Lemtrada) is indicated for the treatment of patients with relapsing forms of MS. It is a recombinant humanized anti-CD52 IGg1κ monoclonal antibody with a molecular weight of 150 kDa that is administered via intravenous infusion. The drug binds to CD52, a cell surface antigen present on T and B lymphocytes, natural killer cells, monocytes, and macrophages. Binding results in antibody-dependent cellular cytolysis and complement-mediated lysis. The drug is primary distributed to the blood and interstitial space with a volume of distribution of 14.1 L.[129] It has a plasma elimination half-life of 2 weeks and is undetectable after 30 days. Alemtuzumab is contraindicated in human immunodeficiency virus patients. It has several associated warnings including causing serious autoimmune conditions, life-threatening infusion reactions, and increased risk of malignancies, such as thyroid cancer and melanoma. In addition, the drug has an array of common adverse effects, such as rash, headache, pyrexia, nasopharyngitis, nausea, urinary tract infection, fatigue, insomnia, upper respiratory tract infection, herpes viral infection, urticaria, pruritus, thyroid gland disorders, fungal infection, arthralgia, pain in extremity, back pain, diarrhea, sinusitis, oropharyngeal pain, paresthesia, dizziness, abdominal pain, flushing, and vomiting.

Natalizumab (Tysabri) is indicated for the treatment of patients with relapsing forms of MS, as well as those with moderate to severe active Crohn's disease. It is a recombinant humanized anti-α4 integrin IGg1κ monoclonal antibody with a molecular weight of 149 kDa that is administered via intravenous infusion. The drug binds the α4-subunit of α4β1 and α4β7 integrins expressed on all leukocytes except neutrophils. This binding prevents the leukocytes from associating with vascular cell adhesion molecule 1 (VCAM-1) on the surface of vascular brain and spinal cord endothelial cells, blocking entry of leukocytes into the CNS.[130,131] Natalizumab has a mean plasma elimination half-life of 11 days, volume of distribution of 5.7 L, and clearance of 16 mL/hr.[132] The drug should not be used concomitant with chronic immunosuppressant or immunomodulatory therapies. It is also contraindicated in patients who have or have had progressive multifocal leukoencephalopathy. Several warnings are associated with natalizumab, including hypersensitivity reactions, increased the risk for certain infections, and hepatotoxicity. The most common adverse effects of natalizumab in MS patients are headache, fatigue, arthralgia, urinary tract infections, lower respiratory tract infections, gastroenteritis, vaginitis, depression, pain in extremities, abdominal discomfort, diarrhea, and rash.

Dimethyl Fumarate

MeO₂C–CH=CH–CO₂Me — Dimethyl fumarate (Tecfidera)

MeO₂C–CH=CH–CO₂H — Monomethyl fumarate

Dimethyl fumarate is indicated for the treatment of patients with relapsing forms of MS. The drug is structurally simple with a low molecular weight and consists of two methyl esters attached to an alkene in an E-orientation. It is a white powder that is highly soluble in water.

Dimethyl fumarate appears to act as a prodrug, with its hydrolysis metabolite monomethyl fumarate being the active component. Monomethyl fumarate modulates a number of immune-related properties that could contribute to its efficacy in the treatment of the relapsing forms of MS.[133] For example, it is able to enhance anti-inflammatory interleukin 4 and 5 production in stimulated peripheral mononuclear blood cells.[134] The drug also appears able to induce an antioxidative stress response that may contribute to its efficacy. It binds Kelch-like erythroid cell-derived associated protein-1 (KEAP-1), dissociating it from nuclear factor (erythroid-derived 2)-like 2 (Nrf2). This transcription factor translocates to the nucleus resulting in transcription of antioxidative genes, including hemoxygenase-1, nicotinamide adenine dinucleotide phosphate (NADP), and quinoline oxidoreductase-1.[135]

After oral administration, dimethyl fumarate undergoes rapid presystemic hydrolysis to its active metabolite monomethyl fumarate, which reaches maximum plasma concentration in 2-2.5 hours.[136] Taking the drug with a high-fat meal decreases maximum plasma concentrations by 40% and delays the time to reach maximum plasma concentration to 5.5 hours. Monomethyl fumarate has relatively low plasma protein binding of 27%-45% and a volume of distribution of 53-73 L. The drug does not undergo CYP450 metabolism. Instead it enters the tricarboxylic acid cycle and is metabolized to fumaric acid, citric acid, and glucose with exhalation of CO_2 as the primary route of elimination. The plasma elimination half-life of monomethyl fumarate is 1 hour.

Neither dimethyl fumarate nor its active metabolite monomethyl fumarate appears to participate in drug-drug interactions. The most common adverse effects of dimethyl fumarate are flushing, abdominal pain, diarrhea, and nausea.

Fingolimod

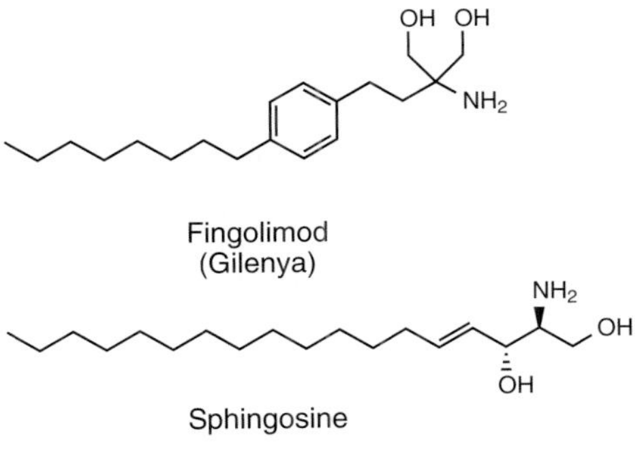

OH OH NH₂

Fingolimod (Gilenya)

NH₂ OH OH

Sphingosine

Fingolimod is indicated for the treatment the relapsing forms of MS. Structurally the drug is related to sphingosine and consists of a hydrophobic *n*-octyl substituted phenyl that is connected to a hydrophilic fragment made up of a primary amine and two alcohols. Fingolimod is formulated as a hydrochloride salt that is a white powder and readily soluble in water.

Fingolimod acts as a prodrug that is rapidly converted to fingolimod phosphate, which binds to the sphingosine-1-phosphate receptor 1 as a receptor modulator. This results in the internalization of the receptor causing sequestration of lymphocytes in lymph nodes, which prevents them from infiltrating the CNS. However, additional effects of sphingosine-1-phosphate receptor modulation may also contribute to efficacy.[137]

Fingolimod is readily absorbed after oral administration with a bioavailability of >90% and is unaffected by dietary intake.[138] The drug reaches maximum plasma concentrations in 12-16 hours. Fingolimod and its active metabolite fingolimod phosphate are highly protein bound (>99%). In addition, the parent drug is highly distributed in red blood cells resulting in a large volume of distribution of about 1200 L.[139] Fingolimod and its active metabolite are cleared very slowly with a terminal plasma half-life of 5-6 days.[140] Fingolimod is converted to fingolimod phosphate via sphingosine kinase type 2 (Fig. 10.21). One of the metabolic pathways of fingolimod phosphate is dephosphorylation by lipid phosphate phosphohydrolases and sphingosine 1-phosphate phosphatase.[141] A second metabolic pathway is alkyl oxidation (CYP4F mediated) to produce a primary alcohol metabolite, as well as six other alkyl hydroxyl metabolites, and oxidation to a butanoic acid metabolite, which is the major metabolite found in urine.[142] Finally, fingolimod undergoes biotransformation by (dihydro)ceramide synthase to produce ceramides.

Fingolimod is contraindicated in patients with a variety of cardiovascular and related conditions, including recent myocardial infarction, unstable angina, stroke, transient ischemic attack, heart failure, history of atrioventricular block, sick sinus syndrome, or QT prolongation since it is known to induce a transient decrease in heart rate during intial dosing possibly by enhancing cardiac parasympathetic activity.[143] The most common adverse effects of fingolimod are headache, liver transaminase elevation, diarrhea, cough, influenza, sinusitis, back pain, abdominal pain, and pain in extremities.

Teriflunomide

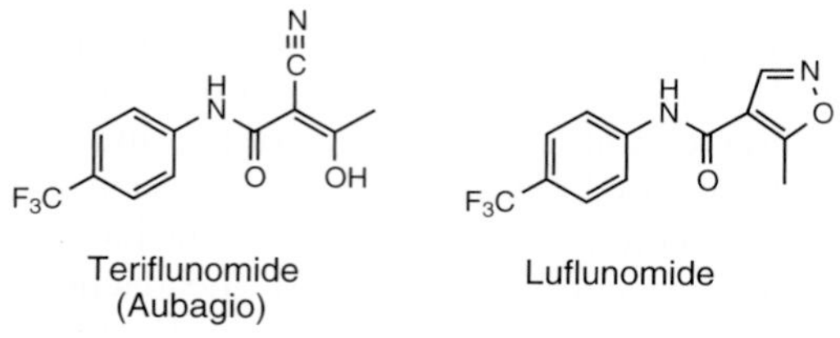

Teriflunomide (Aubagio)

Luflunomide

Teriflunomide is indicated for the treatment of patients with relapsing forms of MS. The structure of the drug consists of a para-trifluoromethyl-substituted anilide that also contains a nitrile Z-substituted enol. It is the active metabolite of leflunomide, which is used in the treatment of rheumatoid and psoriatic arthritis. Teriflunomide is a white powder that is practically insoluble in water. Teriflunomide is a selective and reversible inhibitor of dihydroorotate dehydrogenase, a key mitochondrial enzyme in the de novo pyrimidine synthesis pathway. Inhibition of this enzyme leads to reduced proliferation of activated T and B lymphocytes.[144]

Teriflunomide reaches maximum plasma concentration in about 5 hours after oral administration.[145] The drug is extensively bound to plasma protein (>99%), which limits its distribution primarily to plasma with a very long plasma elimination half-life.[146] The parent drug is primary eliminated unchanged in feces. Although the drug is not extensively metabolized, 2-oxo-2-[[4-(trifluoromethyl) phenyl]amino]acetic acid is a minor metabolite found in

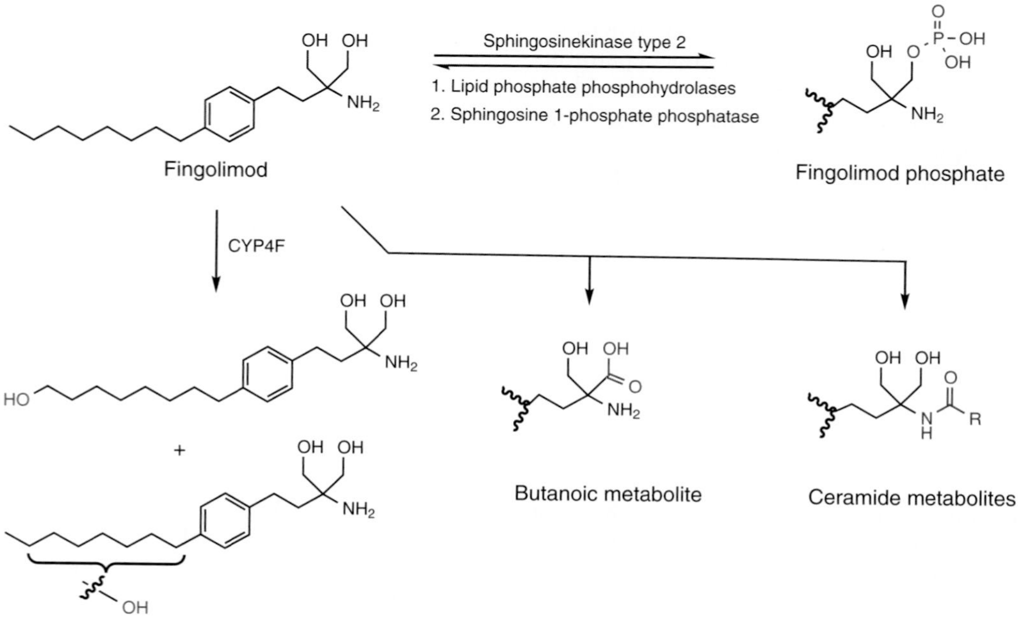

Sphingosinekinase type 2

1. Lipid phosphate phosphohydrolases
2. Sphingosine 1-phosphate phosphatase

Fingolimod

Fingolimod phosphate

CYP4F

Butanoic metabolite

Ceramide metabolites

Figure 10.21 Metabolism of fingolimod.

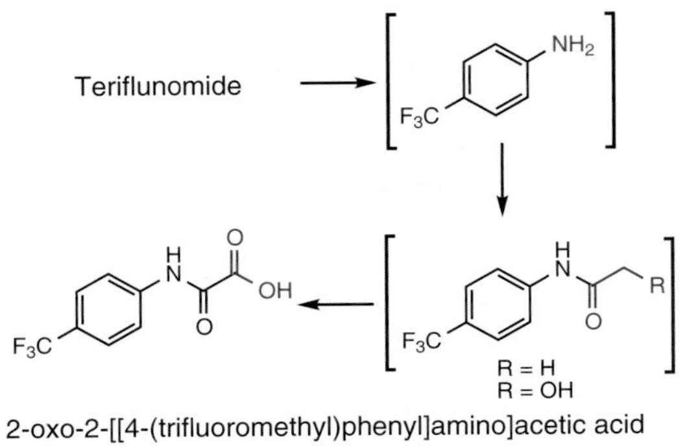

Figure 10.22 Metabolism of teriflunomide.

plasma with renal excretion.[147] This metabolite may be formed by hydrolysis to the corresponding aniline (Fig. 10.22), which is known to be acylated and oxidized to 2-oxo-2-[[4-(trifluoromethyl)phenyl]amino]acetic acid in rodents.[148]

Teriflunomide participates in a number of potential drug-drug interactions. For example, it is a substrate of the efflux transporter breast cancer resistant protein (BCRP) and thus BCRP inhibitors may increase exposure of teriflunomide. It also can interact with drugs metabolized by CYP 2C8 and 1A2. The drug is contraindicated for use in patients with severe hepatic impairment and also has a significant risk to cause hepatotoxicity. Teriflunomide presents a risk of teratogenicity and should not be used during pregnancy.

Dalfampridine

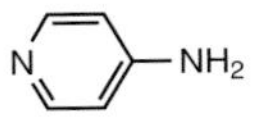

Dalfampridine is indicated to improve walking in adult patients with MS. Structurally it is a 4-aminopyridine, which is a white powder. Dalfampridine's mechanism of action is proposed to be its ability to block potassium channels that become exposed during axonal demyelination. This blockage restores axonal conduction resulting in improved walking speed and MS patient–reported perceptions of walking.[149]

Dalfampridine is rapidly absorbed after oral administration with a bioavailability of 96% and reaches maximum plasma concentration in 3-4 hours.[150] The drug has very low plasma protein binding (≤3%), a volume of distribution of 2.6 L/kg, a plasma elimination half-life of 5-6 hours, and a majority of the dose is excreted in urine as parent drug. Dalfampridine does undergo CYP2E1-mediated oxidation to 3-hydroxy-4-aminopyridine, which is conjugated by SULT to 3-hydroxy-4-aminopyridine sulfate (Fig. 10.23).

Dalfampridine is contraindicated in patients taking oct2 transporter inhibitors, such as cimetidine. The most common adverse effects of dalfampridine are urinary tract infection, insomnia, dizziness, headache, nausea, asthenia, back pain, balance disorder, multiple sclerosis relapse, paresthesia, nasopharyngitis, constipation, dyspepsia, and pharyngolaryngeal pain.

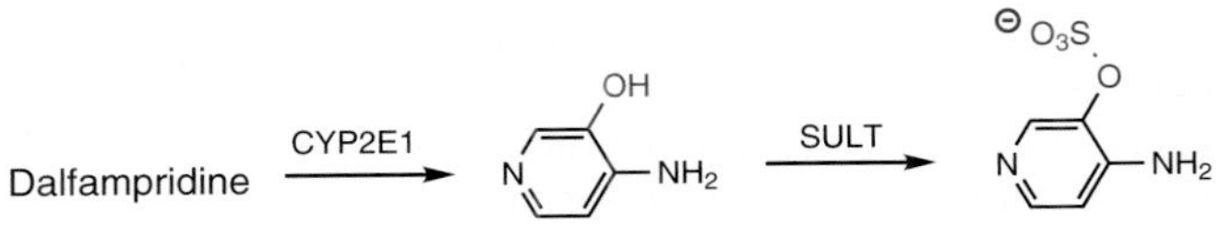

Figure 10.23 Metabolism of dalfampridine.

AMYOTROPHIC LATERAL SCLEROSIS

Therapeutic Context Overview

Amyotrophic lateral sclerosis (ALS), also called Lou Gehrig's disease in the United States and motor neuron disease (MND) in the United Kingdom, is a neurodegenerative condition that results in the death of corticospinal neurons with cell bodies in the motor cortex region of the brain and descending axons in the brainstem and lateral spinal cord, as well as cell death of spinal motor neurons that innervate voluntary skeletal muscles. The disease initially presents with subtle cramping or weakness in limbs, which then progresses to paralysis of most skeletal muscles, ultimately resulting in death usually within 3-5 years after onset, most commonly from respiratory failure.

The prevalence of ALS in the United States is around 4-5 cases per 100,000. Overall, ALS is more common among Caucasians, males, and persons aged 60-69 years.[151] Although the disease can strike most age groups, the mean age of onset is 55 years. Similar to other neurodegenerative diseases, most cases of ALS appear to be idiopathic. However, about 10% of ALS patients have a clear genetic link. In 1993, the first gene connected to ALS, superoxide dismutase-1 (SOD1), was reported.[152] SOD1 is a homodimeric Cu/Zn-containing enzyme that catalyzes the disproportionation of highly reactive superoxide to hydrogen peroxide and dioxygen (e.g., $2O_2^{\cdot-} + 2H^+ \rightarrow H_2O_2 + O_2$). SOD1 appears to play a prominent role in cellular response to oxidative stress. Consequently, loss of function for this enzyme (e.g., by mutations) could hinder a cell's ability to cope with oxidative stress, resulting in dysfunction or death. Over 170 ALS-causing SOD1 mutations have now been identified. However, no correlation between reduced superoxide dismutase enzyme activity and age of disease onset or disease progression has been found, suggesting that the toxic properties of SOD1 are due to other factors.[153]

Since the discovery of SOD1 mutations, other potential ALS genes have been proposed, including those involved in protein quality control, RNA stability, function and metabolism, as well as cytoskeletal dynamics.[154] Even in sporadic cases of ALS, 1%-3% of patients have missense SOD1 mutations.[155] Furthermore, genetic alterations may also contribute to disease susceptibility and progression. Like other neurodegenerative diseases, aggregated protein deposits appear as inclusions in affected cells in ALS patients. In this case the spinal motor neurons accumulate deposits of ubiquitinated TAR DNA-binding protein 43 (TDP-43).[156] However, the clinical significance of TDP-43 neuropathology on duration of disease or rate of progression is not obvious.[157]

The economic encumbrance of ALS is significant. A recent study in 2015 found that the annual total cost per ALS patient in the United States was US$69,475, with the national economic burden estimated at US$279-472 million. These per patient costs were greater than for most other neurological diseases.[158] Medication costs per year vary from US$14,400 (estimated nonsubsidized 2011 cost) for the older drug riluzole approved in the United States in 1995 compared to $145,000 (estimated nonsubsidized 2017 cost) for the newly introduced drug edaravone.[159,160]

Pharmacology Overview

The pharmacology of current therapies for the treatment of ALS is not particularly clear. It is possible that the drugs elicit their effects through a complex set of interactions and functions that are difficult to reduce to a few molecular targets. This is similarly reflected in the emerging array of genes and mutations associated with a subset of familial ALS patients. The net result has been great difficulty assigning mechanism of actions for currently available drugs and for crafting therapeutic strategies necessary for the development of new chemotherapeutic approaches for treating this devastating neuromuscular degenerative disease.

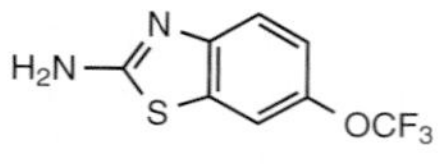

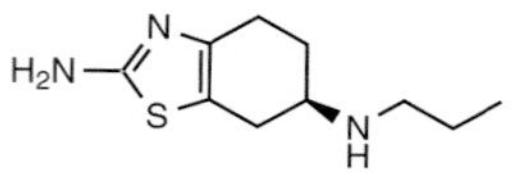

Riluzole

Riluzole is indicated for the treatment of patients with ALS. Although riluzole extends survival and/or time to tracheostomy, measures of muscle strength and neurological function do not show a benefit. Riluzole contains a 2-aminobenzothiazole substituted with a trifluoromethyl ether. It is a white to faintly yellow powder that is slightly soluble in water.

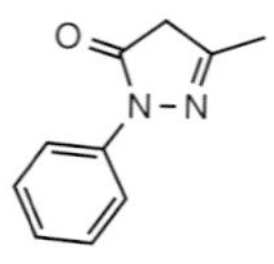

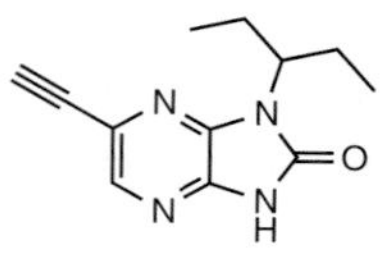

The mechanism of action of riluzole is unclear and may be multifactorial. It may be related to inhibitory effects on neurotransmitter (e.g., glutamate) release, including interference with intracellular events that follow transmitter binding at excitatory amino acid receptors, inactivation of voltage-dependent sodium channels (e.g., Na^+ current and repetitive firing), and/or potentiation of calcium-dependent K^+ current.[161] Interestingly in 2013, a structurally related compound called dexpramipexole (the enantiomer of the PD drug (*S*)-pramipexole), failed in a phase 3 clinical trial for ALS due to insufficient efficacy, highlighting the continued lack of understanding for this class of therapeutic agents.

Riluzole is quite hydrophobic, which contributes to it being well absorbed (~90%) with an oral bioavailability of 60%.[162] However, intersubject variation in plasma concentrations of the drug can be large (e.g., 30%-100%), likely resulting from variable first pass metabolism. After oral administration, riluzole reaches maximum plasma concentrations within 1-1.5 hours and has a mean plasma elimination half-life of 12 hours. A high-fat meal decreases absorption with reduced exposure (e.g., AUC and C_{max} decrease 20% and 45%, respectively).

Riluzole undergoes only limited first pass metabolism and is excreted predominantly unchanged in urine.[163] The phase 1 reactions that do occur appear to be mediated by CYP1A2 and extrahepatic CYP1A1 isozymes. These reactions include N-hydroxylation, oxidation of the benzene portion of the heterocyclic system in the 4-, 5-, and 7-positions generating phenols, as well as dealkylation of the trifluoromethyl ether (Fig. 10.24). These phase 1 metabolites are subjected to phase 2 glucuronidation with the resulting glucuronides accounted for >85% of the metabolites in urine.

Riluzole should be used with caution in patients with concomitant liver insufficiency. The most common adverse effects associated with this drug are asthenia, nausea, dizziness, decreased lung function, diarrhea, abdominal pain, pneumonia, vomiting, vertigo, circumoral paresthesia, anorexia, and somnolence.

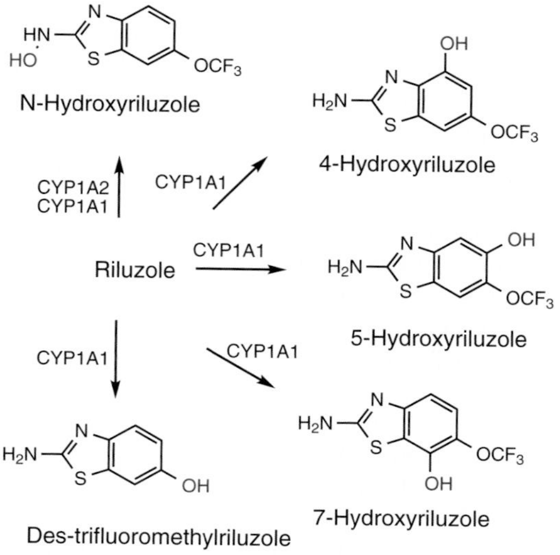

Figure 10.24 Phase I metabolism of riluzole.

Edaravone

Edaravone is indicated for the treatment of ALS as an intravenous infusion, receiving approval in the United States in May 2017. The drug consists of a 5-pyrazolone connected to a phenyl. It is a white crystalline powder that is only slightly soluble in water.

Although the precise mechanism of action for edaravone is not known, one potential pathway might be the ability of the compound to reduce oxidative stress. In vitro and in vivo data suggest that edaravone may possess broad free radical scavenging activity, which protects neurons, glia, and vascular endothelial cells.[164]

Edaravone has high human protein binding of 92% and a terminal plasma elimination half-life of 4.5-6 hours. The drug mainly undergoes phase 2 metabolism with glucuronidation and sulfonation on the oxygen atom to form the corresponding pyrazole metabolites (Fig. 10.25). The sulfonate conjugate is the primary metabolite detected in plasma. However, in the urine the drug is excreted as its glucuronide conjugate (70%-90% of the dose) and sulfonate conjugate (5%-10% of the dose) with only 1% of the parent drug remaining unchanged.[165]

Edaravone is not expected to participate in drug-drug interactions since it has not demonstrated significant affects on CYP450 isozymes, UGT enzymes, or major transporters. The most common adverse effects reported for this drug are contusion, gait disturbance, and headache.

Tirasemtiv

Tirasemtiv (also known as CK-2017357) is an experimental compound that has progressed into phase 2 clinical trials for the treatment of ALS. Its structure contains a central imidazo[4,5-*b*]pyrazin-2-one substituted with an alkyne and a hydrophobic 3-pentyl group. The compound's mechanism of action appears to involve activation of the fast skeletal muscle troponin complex, increasing its sensitivity to calcium resulting in increased skeletal muscle force and power while delaying the time to muscle fatigue.[166] The compound has demonstrated positive results for muscle function and performance in ALS mouse models.[167] In clinical trials the most common adverse effects of tirasemtiv have been dizziness and general fatigue.[168]

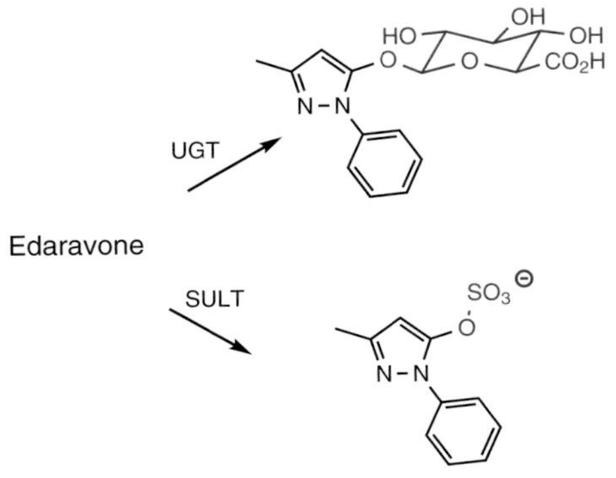

Edaravone

UGT

HO OH OH O O CO_2H N-N

SULT

$SO_3^{\ominus}$ O N-N

Figure 10.25 Metabolism of edaravone.

DUCHENNE MUSCULAR DYSTROPHY

Therapeutic Context Overview

Duchenne muscular dystrophy (DMD) is a progressive neuromuscular disorder involving the gene that encodes for the protein dystrophin.[169,170] This condition severely affects males (but is mild or asymptomatic in females) and is characterized by progressive muscle degeneration and weakness. About two-thirds of cases are inherited from the mother as an X-linked mutation (e.g., an exon deletion/frame-shift mutation—most common, a point mutation, or a duplication), while the remainder arises from noninherited mutations of the dystrophin gene. Symptoms usually begin to appear around age 3-4 years as muscle weakness of the hips, pelvis, thighs, and shoulders. As the disease progresses, voluntary skeletal muscles in the arms, legs, and trunk begin to be impacted followed by heart and respiratory muscles. Death usually occurs in the second to fourth decade of life, with the most common cause being heart failure from cardiomyopathy.

Dystrophin is a large (e.g., 427 kDa) cytoplasmic protein that is part of a complex that connects the cytoskeleton of muscle fibers to the surrounding extracellular matrix. Dystrophin links actin filaments to another support protein that resides on the inside surface of the muscle fiber's plasma membrane. Functionally, dystrophin supports muscle fiber strength. Therefore, mutations in this protein can compromise functional properties of the muscle leading to progressive muscle weakness and other pathological conditions, including severe myocardial fibrosis and cardiac hypertrophy.

DMD is the most common muscular dystrophy, with an incidence in boys of about 200 per million births.[171] DMD presents a significant public health burden with average annual patient health care costs of US$23,005. These costs significantly increase for patients aged 14-29 years to US$40,132.[172] Although drugs for the treatment of DMD have only very recently been approved in the United States, per patient costs are significant, ranging from US$35,000 to US$300,000 per year, which will certainly increase the future average annual patient health care costs.

Pharmacology Overview

Few chemotherapeutic options are available for the treatment of DMD. One approach is the use of glucocorticoids. These compounds bind to the glucocorticoid nuclear receptor and have been shown to increase muscle strength in DMD patients.[173] However, this action is in contrast to their direct effect on myofibers resulting in decreased protein synthesis and increased protein catabolism, causing muscle weakness and atrophy.[174] The purported explanation for these opposing mechanisms for glucocorticoids is that the clinical outcome of increased muscle strength, although mitigated to some extent by adverse effects on myofibers, provides an overall benefit to DMD patients.[175]

The second pharmacological approach for the treatment of DMD is very recently developed and is applicable to only a subset of patients with a specific exon deletions/

frame-shift mutation. The drug causes excision of an exon during pre-mRNA splicing that partially corrects the reading frame of the dystrophin mRNA, resulting in production of partially functional dystrophin protein.

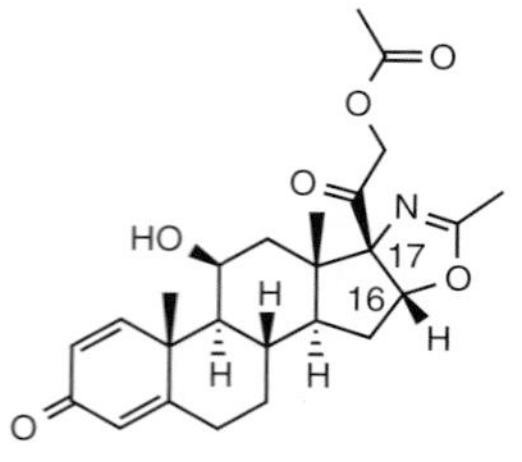

Deflazacort
(Emflaza)

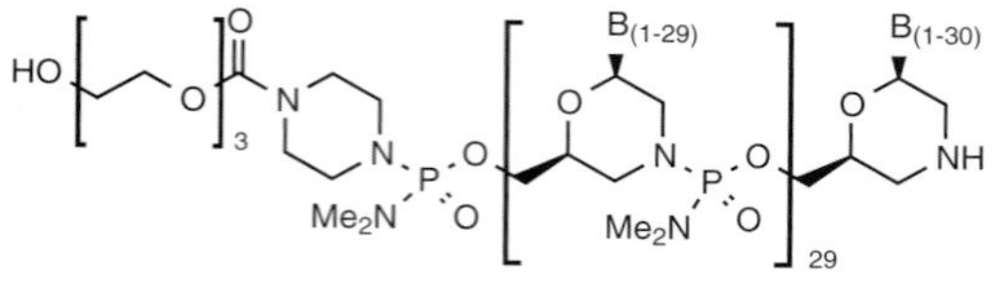

B(1-30): C-T-C-C-A-A-C-A-T-C-A-A-G-G-A
-A-G-A-T-G-G-C-A-T-T-T-C-T-A-G

(where A: adenine, C: cytosine, G: guanine, T: thymine)

Eteplirsen
(Exondys 51)

Deflazacort

Deflazacort is indicated for the treatment of DMD in patients who are ≥5 years of age. It consists of a glucocorticoid structure with a dihydrooxazole fused to carbons 16 and 17 and an ester protected alpha-hydroxy ketone on carbon 17. Deflazacort is a white powder with poor water solubility (<1 mg/mL). However, the pharmacologically active metabolite 21-desDFZ is more soluble in water (1.4 mg/mL) due to the exposed primary alcohol.

Deflazacort is a prodrug that is rapidly converted by esterases to 21-desDFZ (Fig. 10.26). This metabolite likely elicits it pharmacology through the glucocorticoid receptor to exert anti-inflammatory and immunosuppressive effects, although the precise mechanism by which it exerts therapeutic properties in DMD is not entirely clear.

After oral administration, deflazacort is readily absorbed, reaching maximum plasma concentration within 1 hour.[176] Following a 0.65 mg/kg dose of deflazacort, the maximum plasma concentration of 21-desDFZ is 0.28 μg/mL and is reached in 2 hours. The plasma elimination half-life of this metabolite is 1.94 hours, its volume of distribution is 1.5 L, and its clearance is 0.53 L/hr. The active metabolite 21-desDFZ is about 40% plasma protein bound and urinary excretion is the predominant route of elimination. 21-desDFZ is metabolized by CYP3A4 to several inactive metabolites, including oxidation to 6β-hydroxy 21-desDFZ.[177] Another interesting metabolite found in plasma and urine forms from ketone reduction and stereoselective alkene epoxidation.[178]

Deflazacort should be used with caution in patient's coadministered moderate to potent CYP3A4 inhibitors and avoided in patients coadministered moderate or potent CYP3A4 inducers. The most common adverse effects of deflazacort are typical for glucocorticoids, including Cushingoid appearance, weight gain, increased appetite, upper respiratory tract infection, cough, pollakiuria, hirsutism, central obesity, and nasopharyngitis.

Eteplirsen

Eteplirsen is indicated for the treatment of DMD in patients with a confirmed mutation of the DMD gene that is amenable to exon 51 skipping (~13% of DMD patients). The drug

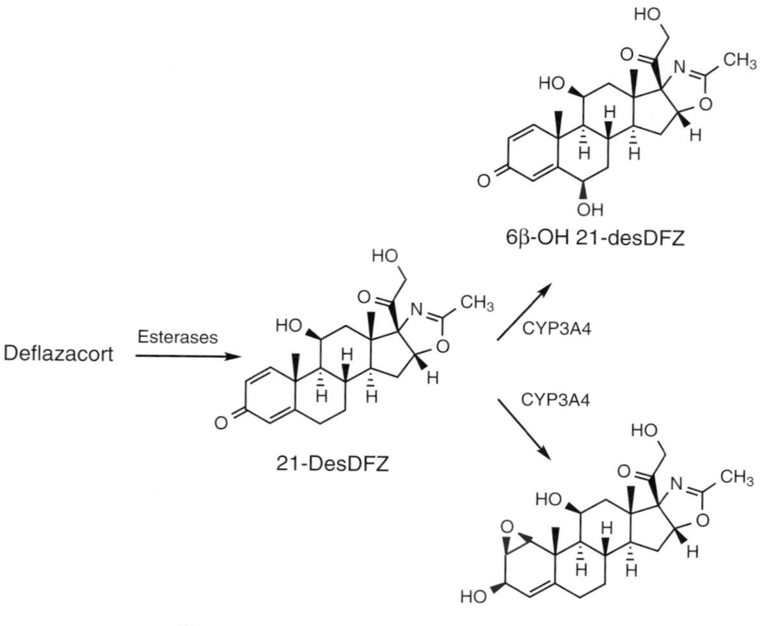

Deflazacort → Esterases → 21-DesDFZ → CYP3A4 → 6β-OH 21-desDFZ; 21-DesDFZ → CYP3A4 → (epoxide metabolite)

Figure 10.26 Metabolism of deflazacort.

is administered by intravenous infusion. Eteplirsen is a synthetic molecule that has a complex chemical structure consisting of 30 subunits of morpholino phosphorodiamidate, each linked to an oligonucleotide, terminating in a carbamate capped piperazine. The morpholino phosphorodiamidates replace the five-membered ribofuranosyls found in DNA and RNA. Eteplirsen binds to the splice-donor region of exon 51 of dystrophin pre-mRNA inducing skipping of exon 51 that yields an in-frame, truncated, and partially functional dystrophin protein, which causes a less severe form of the disease.[179]

The maximum plasma concentrations of eteplirsen occurred near the end of infusion. The drug has low plasma protein binding (e.g., 6%-17%) with a volume of distribution of 600 mL/kg.[180] Eteplirsen is almost completely eliminated within 24 hours of administration with no accumulation observed. The clearance of eteplirsen is 339 mL/hr/kg following 12 weeks of therapy with 30 mg/kg/wk and a plasma elimination half-life of 3-4 hours. The primary route of elimination is renal clearance. Due to eteplirsen's low plasma protein binding, lack of CYP450 metabolism, and lack of interaction with drug transporters, it is expected to have a low potential for drug-drug interactions. The most common adverse effects of the drug were balance disorder and vomiting.

Spinal Muscular Atrophy

Therapeutic Context Overview

Spinal muscular atrophy (SMA) is a rare genetic neuromuscular disorder with an incidence of 1 in 6-10,000 live births.[181] The disease involves loss of motor neurons in the spinal cord with progressive muscle wasting. The age of symptom onset correlates with disease severity.[182] For example, children who display symptoms at birth or during infancy (referred to as type 1) usually have the most severe outcome oftentimes not surviving beyond age 5 with death most likely caused by respiratory failure, making SMA the most common genetic cause of infant death. Conversely, SMA onset in teens or adults (referred to as type 4) commonly correlates with higher levels of motor function and normal life expectancy.

The survival motor neuron 1 (SMN1) gene encodes for the SMN protein, which plays a key role in the subsistence of motor neurons.[183] A related gene, SMN2, undergoes alternative splicing with only 10%-20% of SMN2 transcripts coding fully functional SMN protein, whereas the remaining transcripts result in a truncated protein (SMNΔ7) that is rapidly degraded. SMA is caused by homozygous mutations of the SMN1 gene, generally showing the absence of exon 7. This results in SMN protein deficiency causing death of motor neurons in the anterior horn of the spinal cord and brain. Consequently, decreased impulse transmissions to muscles via the motor neurons leads to decreased muscle contractility and progressive muscle atrophy.

Pharmacology Overview

The principle strategy pursued for chemotherapeutic treatment of SMA has been to identify mechanisms for circumventing the alternative splicing of the SMN2 transcript in order to enhance the production of fully functional SMN protein.[184] This approach has been clinically successful using an antisense oligonucleotide, while additional mechanisms for achieving a similar outcome are activity being investigated. A number of other approaches are also currently being pursued at the preclinical stage and in clinical trials, including activation of the SMN2 gene, SMN1 gene replacement, and SMN protein stabilization. Finally, the identification of potential disease-modifying factors underlying motor neuron vulnerability and subsequent muscle weakness may offer additional therapeutic modalities.[185]

Nusinersen

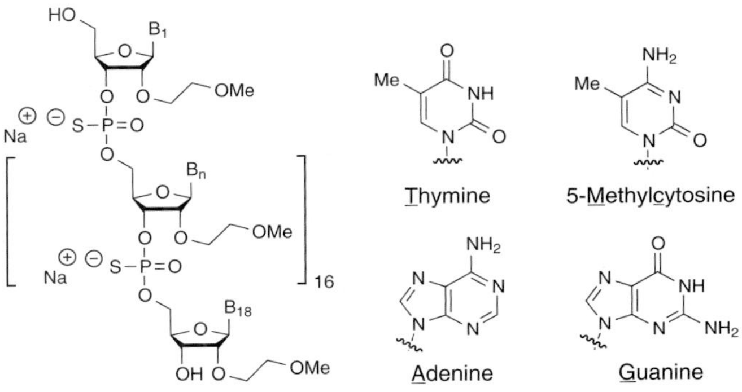

HO, B_1, OMe, Na, S–P=O, B_n, OMe, Na, S–P=O, 16, B_{18}, OH, OMe

Me, O, NH, N, O — Thymine

Me, NH_2, N, N, O — 5-Methylcytosine

NH_2, N, N, N, N — Adenine

O, N, NH, N, N, NH_2 — Guanine

$B_{1\text{-}18}$: T-MC-A-MC-T-T-T-MC-A-T-A-A-T-G-MC-T-G-G

Nusinersen
(Spinraza)

Nusinersen is indicated for the treatment of SMA in pediatric and adult patients. The structure of nusinersen is an antisense oligonucleotide derivative consisting of 18 subunits in which the ribofuranosyl 2′-hydroxys and phosphates found in oligonucleotides are replaced with 2′-O-2-methoxyethyls and phosphorothioates, respectively. The drug is supplied as a solution for intrathecal administration. Nusinersen increases exon 7 inclusions in SMN2 messenger ribonucleic acid transcripts resulting in enhanced production of full-length SMN protein.

Upon intrathecal administration, nusinersen distributes to both CNS and peripheral tissues with maximum plasma concentrations reached within 1.7-6.0 hours.[186] The plasma terminal elimination half-life is 63-87 days, while the terminal elimination half-life in cerebral spinal fluid is 135-177 days. Nusinersen is metabolized via exonuclease (3′-and 5′)-mediated hydrolysis with elimination of the parent drug and chain-shortened metabolites via urinary excretion. Nusinersen is not an inhibitor or inducer of CYP450 enzymes.

Nusinersen increases the risk of coagulation abnormalities and thrombocytopenia, as well as renal toxicity, including fatal glomerulonephritis. The most common adverse effects of the drug are lower and upper respiratory infections, as well as constipation.

SPASTICITY DISORDERS

Therapeutic Context Overview

Spasticity is characterized by skeletal muscle spasms and an increase in tonic stretch reflexes that causes muscle stiffness. This can interfere with normal movement and gait, as well as speech. Other common symptoms can include muscle stiffness, muscle and joint deformities, muscle fatigue, and longitudinal muscle growth deficits. The origin of the spasticity is usually injury to the portion of the brain or spinal cord that controls voluntary movement.[187] This impairment can lead to changes in signaling between the nervous system and muscles often involving damage to descending pathways in the spinal cord that results in hyperexcitability of motor neurons.[188] However, the detailed pathophysiology of spasticity is not well understood. In addition, assessing the effectiveness of antispasmodic drugs is difficult.[189,190] Since spasticity is frequently associated with pain, antispasmodic drugs may elicit efficacy via skeletal muscle relaxation as well as through analgesia.[191,192]

Spasticity disorders afflict more than 12 million people worldwide, thus representing a significant public health burden. It is also commonly occurs in patients with cerebral palsy (CP) and multiple sclerosis (MS). For example, about 80% of CP and MS patients have spasticity. In addition, many other maladies have associated spasticity disorders, including traumatic brain and spinal cord injuries and stroke, which contributes to its overall prevalence.

Several other conditions related to spasticity will also be covered in this chapter. This includes chemotherapeutics that reverse anesthetic drug-induced nondepolarizing neuromuscular blockage that have also been used to treat myasthenia gravis (MG). Finally, new agents used to treat the neuromuscular conditions of chorea associated with Huntington's disease and tardive dyskinesia, which can result in some patients after long-term use of neuroleptic medications, will be presented.

Pharmacology Overview

Several classes of drugs are used to treat spasticity disorders and can generally be categorized as those indicated for the relief of discomfort associated with musculoskeletal conditions and those indicated for the treatment of spasticity. The oldest class of skeletal muscle relaxants indicated for the relief of discomfort associated with musculoskeletal conditions are those based on 3-phenoxy-1,2-propanediol. These molecules appear to elicit muscle relaxant properties similar to that of sedative-hypnotics. However, the 3-phenoxy-1,2-propanediol class of drugs have greater selectivity for modulating effects mediated by the spinal cord, thus producing less sedation than general sedative-hypnotics. Nonetheless, this class of drugs has common side effects related to CNS depression, including sedation and dizziness, as well as muscle weakness.

Another class of skeletal muscle relaxants used in the relief of discomfort associated with musculoskeletal conditions are alkanediols and derivatives. These molecules may modulate $GABA_A$ receptors in addition to producing benzodiazepine-like sedative and anxiolytic effects. Consequently, drugs of this class can have abuse and dependency liabilities.[190]

Several other drugs have been marketed for relief of discomfort associated with musculoskeletal conditions. For example, chlorzoxazone appears to provide skeletal muscle relaxation via central nervous system depression. However, it is associated with idiosyncratic hepatotoxicity and several sensitivity reactions (e.g., urticaria, erythema, and pruritus) that limits it use.[190] Orphenadrine is a drug that has been used as a muscle relaxant that likely elicits its therapeutic effects through blocking acetylcholine in the central and peripheral nervous systems.

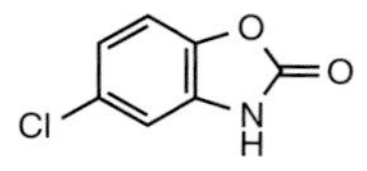

Chlorzoxazone (Paraflex)

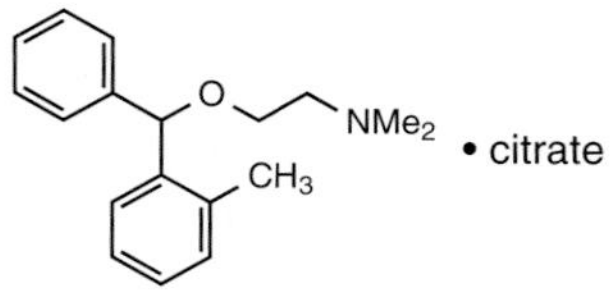

Orphenadrine citrate (Norflex)

A number of small molecule drugs, as well as a protein therapeutic, are indicated (or used off-label) for the treatment of spasticity. These drugs elicit their pharmacology through an array of mechanisms, including adrenergic receptor agonism, serotonin receptor antagonism, modulation of $GABA_B$ receptor, interfering with the release of Ca^{+2} from the sarcoplasmic reticulum (possibly due to antagonizing ryanodine receptor channels), or blocking acetylcholine release at neuromuscular junctions. In many cases the precise mechanism of drug action is unknown or debatable.

Finally, a drug has recently been approved to reverse the effects of neuromuscular blockade induced by the aminosteroid anesthetics rocuronium bromide and vecuronium bromide. The drug sequesters these two agents through noncovalent interactions preventing them from binding their intended target. Peripherally acting acetylcholinesterase inhibitors have been used for the same indication, as well as for the treatment of the neuromuscular condition myasthenia gravis. Other drugs recently introduced for the treatment of chorea associated with Huntington's disease and tardive dyskinesia elicit therapeutic effects via inhibition of the vesicular monoamine transporter 2.

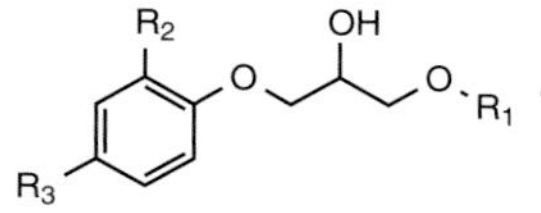

Antodyne ($R_1 = R_2 = R_3 = H$)
Mephenesin ($R_2 = CH_3$, $R_1 = R_3 = H$)
Chlorphenesin carbamate (Maolate) ($R_1 = C(=O)NH_2$, $R_2 = H$, $R_3 = Cl$)
Methocarbamol (Robaxin) ($R_1 = C(=O)NH_2$, $R_2 = OCH_3$, $R_3 = H$)

Methocarbamol

Methocarbamol is indicated for the relief of discomfort associated with acute, painful musculoskeletal conditions. Structurally it consists of a glycerol unit substituted on one terminus with a 2-methoxyphenyl ether and with a carbamate on the other. It belongs to the broader class of drugs based on 3-phenoxy-1,2-propanediol pharmacophore. The first drug recognized to exhibit spasmolytic activity from this class was antodyne. However, it had too short of plasma half-life for clinical use. The close structurally related derivative mephenesin was a widely prescribed skeletal muscle relaxant, but it is no longer used.[193] The primary alcohol is not required for antispasmolytic activity. It could be replaced with a carbamate resulting in chlorphenesin carbamate and methocarbamol, although the former is no longer prescribed. Methocarbamol is chiral with the *R*-enantiomer demonstrating greater muscle relaxant activity in mice.[194] However, the drug is currently only available in racemic form. Methocarbamol is a white powder with low aqueous solubility.

The mechanism of action of methocarbamol as a skeletal muscle relaxant is not known, but appears to be indirect. It seems to be a CNS depressant with sedative properties that result in musculoskeletal relaxation. Interestingly, it has no direct action on the contractile mechanism of striated muscle, the motor end plate, or nerve fibers.

Methocarbamol is readily absorbed following oral administration and reaches maximum plasma concentrations in 1.4 hours. The drug has plasma protein binding of 50%, a moderate volume of distribution of 0.48 L/kg, plasma clearance of 0.20-0.80 L/hr/kg, and a fairly rapid plasma elimination half-life of 1.2 hours (Table 10.2).[195] A small amount of the parent drug is excreted in the urine, while its metabolites are also eliminated by renal clearance. Methocarbamol is metabolized via demethylation of the ether and hydroxylation of the *para*-position on the benzene ring (Fig. 10.27). Extensive conjugation (e.g., glucoronidation and sulfonation) of methocarbamol and its phase 1 metabolites also occurs.[196] Several of the glucuronides have been identified and characterized in rodents.[197]

The clearance of methocarbamol can be reduced in renal or hepatic impaired patients. Since methocarbamol possesses CNS depressant effects, it may cause drowsiness and therefore should be used with caution in combination with alcohol and other CNS depressants and in situations where patients are performing activities requiring mental alertness. Other adverse effects include dizziness, ataxia, nausea, flushing, blurred vision, and fever.

Metaxalone

Metaxalone
(Skelaxin)

Metaxalone is indicated as an adjunct to rest, physical therapy, and other measures for relief of discomforts associated with acute, painful musculoskeletal conditions. Structurally it is closely related to methocarbamol, except that the phenyl is substituted differently and it contains a cyclic carbamate (2-oxazolidinone), demonstrating that the secondary alcohol present in the 3-phenoxy-1,2-propanediol structure is not required. Although it does contain a chiral center, the drug is only available in racemic form. Metaxalone is a white crystalline solid with low aqueous solubility. The mechanism of action of methocarbamol again appears to be indirectly acting as CNS depressant with sedative properties that result in musculoskeletal relaxation.

After oral administration, metaxalone reaches peak plasma concentration in 3 hours.[198] The drug's very large volume of distribution of approximately 800 L is indicative of extensive tissue distribution, and its plasma elimination half-life is 5 hours (Table 10.2). If taken with a high-fat meal, the maximum plasma concentration can increase

Table 10.2 Pharmacokinetic Parameters of Several Drugs Used to Treat Spasticity Disorders

Drug	Plasma Elimination Half-life	Clearance	Volume of Distribution	Oral Bioavailability
Methocarbamol	1.2 hr	0.20-0.80 L/hr/kg	0.48 L/kg	
Metaxalone	5 hr		800 L	
Carisoprodol	1.7-2.0 hr		0.93-1.3 L/kg	92%
Cyclobenzaprine	18 hr	0.7 L/min		33%-55%
Baclofen	3-4 hr		0.7 L/kg	70%-80%
Dantrolene	12 hr			70%
Tizanidine	2.5 hr		2.4 L/kg	40%
Diazepam	1-3 hr; $t_{1/2}\beta$ 1-2 d		0.8-1.0 L/kg	

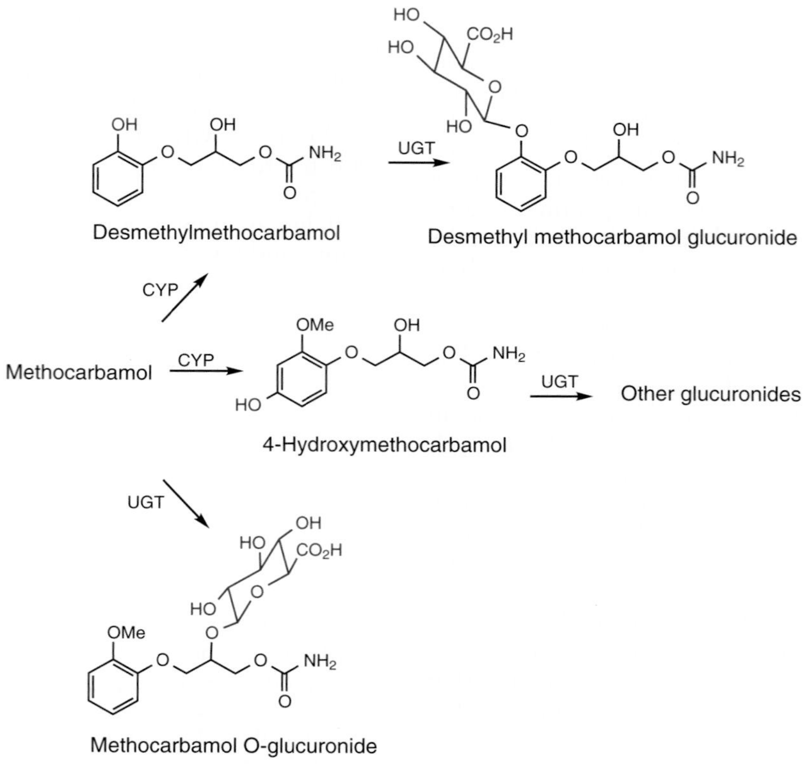

Figure 10.27 Metabolism of methocarbamol.

23% and the time to maximum plasma concentration can be 8 hours. The major route of metaxalone metabolism is benzylic oxidation to give the corresponding carboxylic acid (Fig. 10.28). In this phase 1 metabolism CYP1A2, CYP2D6, CYP2E1, and CYP3A4 are the primary isozymes involved. The carboxylic acid undergoes phase 2 conjugation to the glucuronide. A minor route of metaxalone metabolism is cleavage of the ether, which again is CYP450 mediated.[199]

Metaxalone does not significantly inhibit or induce major CYP450 enzymes. Consequently, it may not be prone to drug-drug interactions. However, the drug should be administered with caution to patients with mild to moderate hepatic and renal impairment. Metaxalone is contraindicated in patients with known tendency to drug-induced, hemolytic, or other anemias. Again, since metaxalone possesses CNS-depressant effect, it should be used with caution in combination with other CNS depressants. Other adverse effects include drowsiness, dizziness, headache, nervousness, nausea, vomiting, and gastrointestinal upset.

Carisoprodol

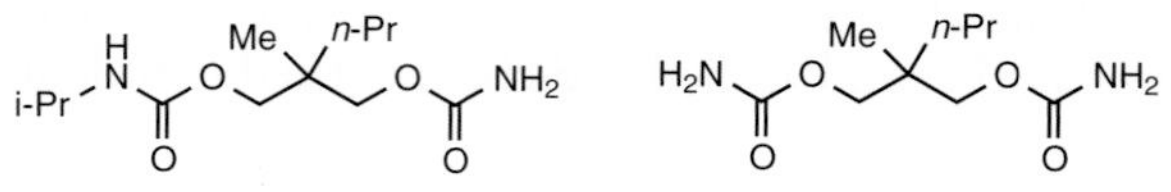

Carisoprodol (Rela, Soma)

Meprobamate (Equanil, Miltown)

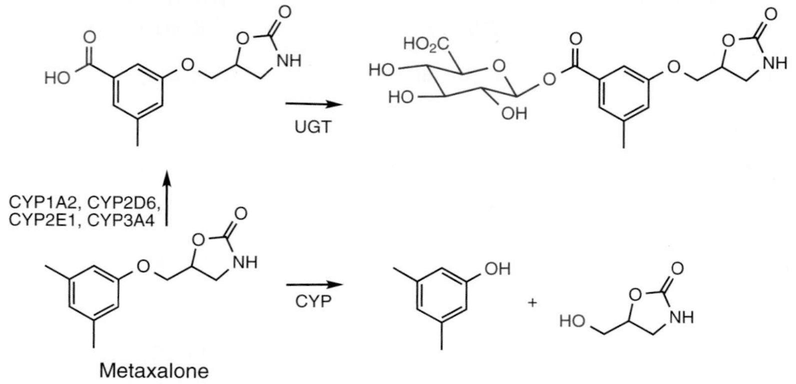

Figure 10.28 Metabolism of metaxalone.

Carisoprodol is indicated for the relief of discomforts associated with acute, painful musculoskeletal conditions. It is a bis-carbamate of a substituted 1,3-propanediol that is a prodrug of meprobamate. Carisoprodol is a white crystalline solid that is slightly soluble in water.

Although the mechanism of action of carisoprodol is not fully understood, its ability to modulate $GABA_A$ receptors likely plays a role in muscle relaxation.[200] In addition, the primary metabolite, meprobamate, has comparable properties producing sedative and anxiolytic effects similar to benzodiazepines.[201,202]

Carisoprodol is well absorbed and quickly reaches maximum plasma levels within 1.5-1.7 hours after oral administration. It is not subjected to extensive first metabolism, thus providing excellent oral bioavailability of 92% (Table 10.2). Although its terminal plasma elimination half-life is only 1.7-2.0 hours, terminal plasma elimination half-life for its metabolite meprobamate is 3.6-4.5 hours, which reaches maximum plasma levels in 9.7 hours.[203] Pharmacokinetic modeling of carisoprodol and meprobamate disposition estimates a moderate volume of distribution for the parent prodrug to be 0.93-1.3 L/kg and meprobamate to be 1.4-1.6 L/kg.[204]

Carisoprodol is metabolized via dealkylation of the isopropyl attached to the carbamate (Fig. 10.29) in the liver by CYP2C19 to meprobamate.[205] In addition, meprobamate has been shown to undergo additional metabolism in rats and rabbits, including oxidation of the *n*-propyl group to a carboxylic acid and secondary alcohol. This secondary alcohol can undergo further oxidation to the corresponding ketone and conjugation to the corresponding glucuronide. Finally, meprobamate also undergoes glucuronidation on the nitrogen atom of the carbamate.[206]

Carisoprodol can participate in drug-drug interactions. Coadministration of CYP2C19 inhibitors (e.g., omeprazole or fluvoxamine) with carisoprodol can result in increased exposure of carisoprodol and decreased exposure of meprobamate. Coadministration of CYP2C19 inducers (e.g., rifampin, St. John's wort, or aspirin) with carisoprodol can result in decreased exposure of carisoprodol and increased exposure of meprobamate. The drug is also contraindicated in patients with a history of acute intermittent porphyria. Given the modulation of carisoprodol and its principle metabolite on $GABA_A$ receptor and their benzodiazepine-like effects, carisoprodol has liabilities for dependence, withdrawal, and abuse with prolonged use.[190] The most common adverse effects of carisoprodol are drowsiness, dizziness, and headache.

Cyclobenzaprine

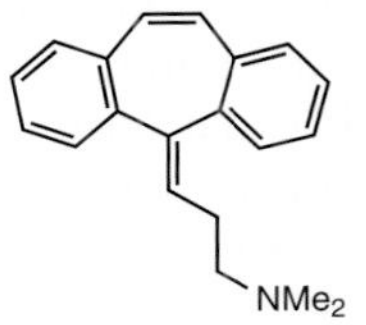

NMe2

Cyclobenzaprine
(Flexaril)

Cyclobenzaprine is indicated for relief of muscle spasm associated with acute, painful musculoskeletal conditions. Structurally, it contains a dibenzo[*a*,*d*][7] annulene core, which is attached to a tertiary amine through an alkene-linked propyl group. Due to the basic amine, it is formulated as the hydrochloride salt that is a white crystalline solid with very good water solubility (e.g., >200 mg/mL).

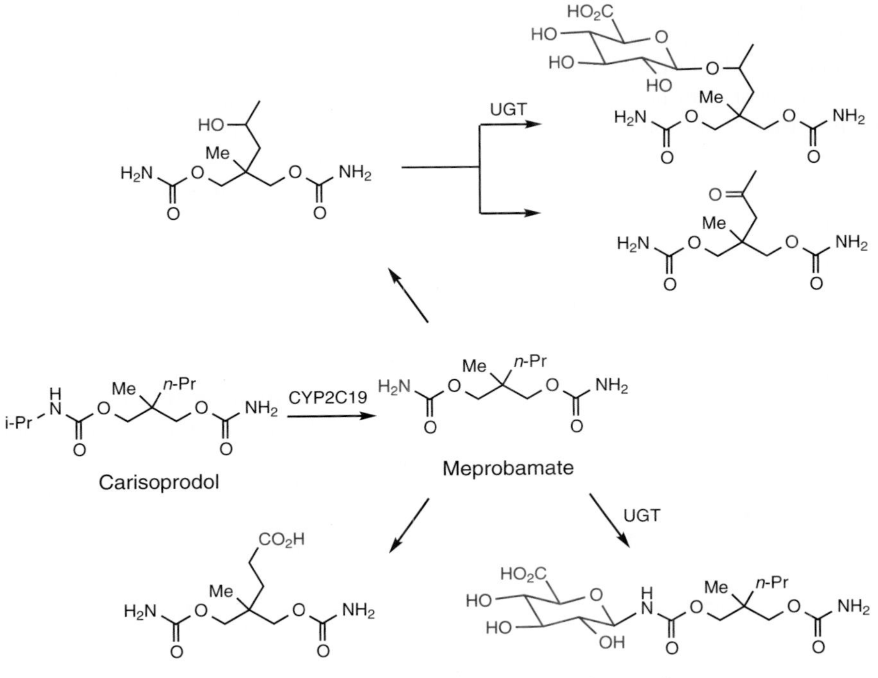

UGT
CYP2C19
Carisoprodol
Meprobamate
UGT

Figure 10.29 Metabolism of carisoprodol and meprobamate.

Cyclobenzaprine is able to provide relief from skeletal muscle spasm of local origin without interfering with muscle function. It is not effective in treating muscle spasm due to central nervous system disease, although the efficacy for skeletal muscle spasm is likely centrally mediated. Although the mechanism of action of cyclobenzaprine is unclear, it has been postulated to act via α_2 agonism. However, other mechanisms have been proposed, including via 5-HT_2 antagonism.[207] Pharmacological studies in animals show a similarity between the effects of cyclobenzaprine and structurally related tricyclic antidepressants.

Cyclobenzaprine is well absorbed after oral administration but is subject to first pass metabolism that reduces it oral bioavailability to 33%-55% (Table 10.2).[208] The drug also participates in enterohepatic circulation, is highly bound to plasma proteins, and accumulates reaching steady state within 3-4 days upon multiple dosing. Cyclobenzaprine is eliminated slowly, with a plasma half-life of 18 hours and a plasma clearance of 0.7 L/min. The drug is metabolized by CYP450-mediated oxidation (e.g., 3A4, 1A2, and, to a lesser extent, 2D6) of the alkene present in the dibenzo[*a*,*d*][7]annulene, likely to an intermediate epoxide that undergoes hydrolysis to the cis-10,11-dihydroxyl metabolite (Fig. 10.30).[209] Although the trans-diol metabolite has not been reported for cyclobenzaprine, it has been observed in the metabolism of amitriptyline, a structurally related compound.[210] Cyclobenzaprine also undergoes glucuronidation of the tertiary amine. These metabolites are excreted primarily via the kidneys.

Cyclobenzaprine should be used with caution in the elderly, where increased exposure has been observed likely due to diminished metabolic activity, and patients with hepatic impairment. The drug is contraindicated with concomitant use of MAO inhibitors or within 14 days after MAO inhibitor discontinuation due to increased risk of hyperpyretic crisis seizures. Cyclobenzaprine has also been associated with the development of serotonin syndrome. Given its structural similarity to tricyclic antidepressants, it also may enhance the effects of alcohol, barbiturates, and other CNS depressants. The most common adverse effects of cyclobenzaprine are drowsiness, dry mouth, and dizziness.

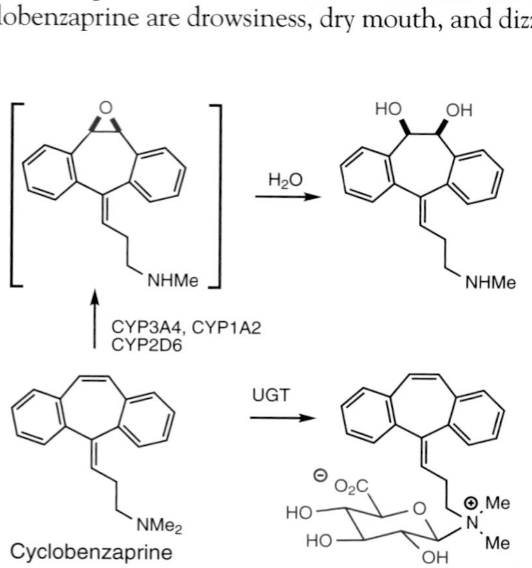

Figure 10.30 Metabolism of cyclobenzaprine.

Baclofen

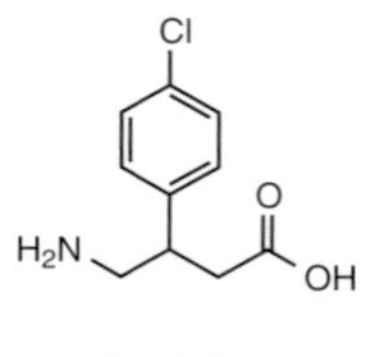

Baclofen
(Lioresal)

Baclofen is indicated for suppression of voluntary muscle spasm in multiple sclerosis and spinal lesions caused by trauma, infections, degeneration, neoplasm, and unknown origins that cause skeletal hypertonus, as well as spastic and dyssynergic bladder dysfunction. However, it is not recommended in PD or spasticity arising from stroke, cerebral palsy, or rheumatoid disorders. Structurally, baclofen is related to the inhibitory neurotransmitter GABA (gamma-aminobutyric acid), except it contains a 4-chlorophenyl substituent on the beta-carbon. It also contains one chiral center. Although the (*R*)-enantiomer is the more active isomer, only the racemate is approved for clinical use. Baclofen is a white crystalline solid that is slightly soluble in water.

Baclofen's antispastic activity is believed to result from receptor binding in the spinal cord, effectively reducing muscle hypertonia. In contract, its adverse effects (e.g., depressant properties) are likely centrally mediated. Hence, intrathecal administration using an indwelling pump can provide direct delivery to the site of action within the spinal cord, while limiting systemic exposure potentially reducing adverse effects.[211] Baclofen depresses monosynaptic and polysynaptic reflex transmission via agonism of $GABA_B$ receptors.[212] This stimulation in turn inhibits the release of excitatory amino acids, such as glutamate and aspartate. Baclofen also displays antinociceptive activity,[213] although the clinical significance of this is not clear. In neurological diseases associated with skeletal muscle spasm, baclofen can cause muscle relaxation and pain relief.

Despite having two ionizable functional groups, baclofen is rapidly and completely absorbed following oral administration, reaching maximum plasma concentration in 2-4 hours.[214] It is subjected to some first pass metabolism resulting in an oral bioavailability of 70%-80% (Table 10.2). Baclofen has plasma protein binding of 30%, a moderate volume of distribution of 0.7 L/kg, and a plasma elimination half-life of 3-4 hours.[215] The charged state of baclofen at physiologic pH does limit its ability to cross into the CNS and spinal cord. As a result, cerebrospinal fluid concentrations are 8.5 times lower than in plasma. Approximately 70% of baclofen is eliminated in the urine unchanged, whereas 15% of the dose is metabolized in the liver and excreted in the urine and feces. The primary metabolism pathway for baclofen is deamination to β-4-chlorophenyl-γ-hydroxybutyric acid (Fig. 10.31).[216] More recently, it has been shown that this metabolic process is more extensive for the (*S*)-enantiomer.[217]

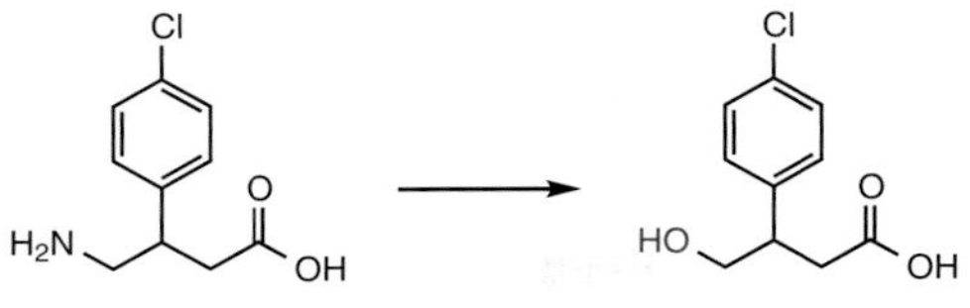

Figure 10.31 Metabolism of baclofen.

Baclofen should be used cautiously in patients with psychiatric and nervous system disorders. In addition, caution is advised in patients with epilepsy or other convulsive conditions, cortical or subcortical brain damage, or significant electroencephalography abnormalities, since the drug can lower the convulsion threshold. In addition, baclofen should be used with caution in patients with impaired renal function. The most common adverse effects for baclofen are sedation, somnolence, and nausea.

Dantrolene

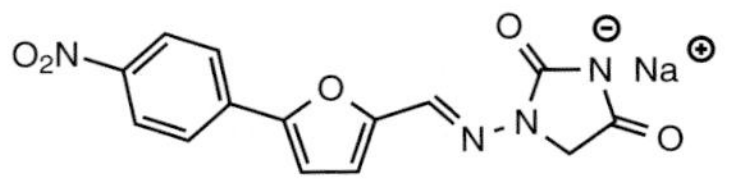

Dantrolene sodium
(Dantrium)

Dantrolene is indicated for the treatment of spasticity resulting from upper motor neuron disorders, such as spinal cord injury, stroke, cerebral palsy, or multiple sclerosis. It is also indicated for preoperative prevention or attenuation of malignant hyperthermia. Structurally, the drug contains a *p*-nitrophenyl substituted furan that is linked via an imine to 1-aminohydantoin. This latter component contains an imide with a pK_a of 7.5. This functional group can be deprotonated under basic conditions. Thus, dantrolene is formulated as a sodium salt, which is a hydrate (~15% water) and is an orange powder. Although it is a salt, the drug is poorly soluble in water, presenting difficulties for rapid preparation of intravenous solutions in emergency situations. In addition, intravenous formulations require a pH of 9.5 to ensure solubility, which can be highly irritating to peripheral veins, thus requiring injection into a large vein or use of a fast running infusion.[218] Although dantrolene contains a hydantoin, it does not have local anesthetic or anticonvulsant activities.[219]

Dantrolene appears to produce skeletal muscle relaxation by affecting the contractile response beyond the myoneural junction. It dissociates the excitation-contraction coupling, probably by interfering with the release of Ca^{+2} from the sarcoplasmic reticulum, and is more pronounced in fast muscle fibers. More recently, dantrolene has been shown to block ryanodine receptor (RYR) channels inhibiting Ca^{+2} release from sarcoplasmic reticulum. The drug displays selectivity for RYR1 (skeletal muscle) and RYR3 (brain) isoforms over RYR2 (myocardium).[220]

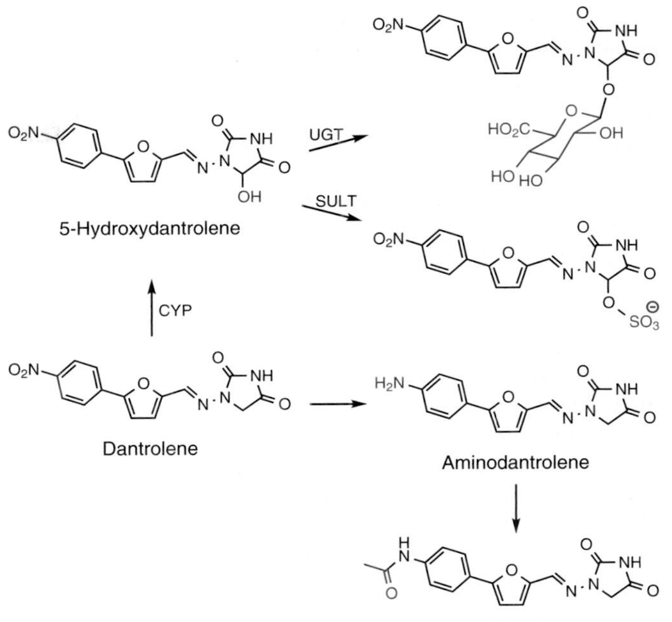

Figure 10.32 Metabolism of dantrolene.

Dantrolene is well absorbed following oral administration, with a bioavailability of 70% and maximum plasma concentration reached in 6 hours. The plasma elimination half-life of the drug is 12 hours (Table 10.2). Dantrolene undergoes oxidation to 5-hydroxydantrolene (Fig. 10.32), a potent skeletal muscle relaxant, which undergoes conjugation to the corresponding glucuronide and sulfate.[221] In addition, dantrolene is metabolized by nitroreductases to aminodantrolene, which is acetylated. The reduction process appears to form electrophilic intermediates that generate mercapturic acid metabolites.[222] Such intermediates could increase risk for hepatotoxicity that has resulted in a blackbox warning. Dantrolene and its metabolites are excreted mainly in urine and bile.

Dantrolene is contraindicated in patients with hepatic disease, such as hepatitis and cirrhosis. It can cause idiosyncratic or hypersensitive liver disorders. The drug is also contraindicated in patients where spasticity is utilized to sustain upright posture and balance in locomotion. The most common adverse effects of dantrolene are drowsiness, dizziness, weakness, general malaise, fatigue, and diarrhea.

Tizanidine

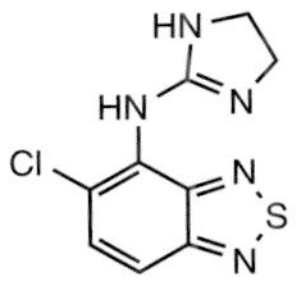

Tizanidine
(Zanaflex)

Tizanidine is indicated for the management of spasticity. This short-acting drug is comparable to baclofen or diazepam, with global tolerability data favoring tizanidine.[223] Structurally it contains a benzo[c][1,2,5]thiadiazole that is substituted with a chlorine atom and a guanidine (e.g., the aminoimidazoline), a basic functional group. The drug is formulated as the hydrochloride salt that is a white crystalline solid with slight water soluble. Tizanidine readily crosses the BBB where it functions as a α_2-adrenergic agonist reducing spasticity by increasing presynaptic inhibition of motor neurons.

Tizanidine is well absorbed following oral administration. However, its absolute oral bioavailability is only 40% due to first pass hepatic metabolism (Table 10.2).[224] It reaches maximum plasma concentration in 1.0 hour, but the parent drug has a relatively short plasma elimination half-life of 2.5 hours. Tizanidine also has relatively low plasma protein binding (30%) and a large volume of distribution (2.4 L/kg) indicative of extensive tissue exposure.

Approximately 95% of an orally administered dose of tizanidine is metabolized primarily by CYP1A2. Very little parent drug is excreted unchanged (0.4% in urine). Tizanidine is oxidized to the sulfuric diamide TZD-1(Fig. 10.33).[225] The parent compound also undergoes oxidation of the imidazoline to generate TZD-2, which is hydrolyzed to intermediate TZD-3 that is dealkylated to TZD-4. Furthermore, the parent drug is oxidized to intermediate TZD-5, which leads to intermediate TZD-6 that is conjugated to glucuronide TZD-7 and sulfate TZD-8. Finally, the epoxide intermediate also undergoes reaction with glutathione and further enzyme-mediated processing to metabolite TZD-9. The metabolites are slowly eliminated, with plasma elimination half-lives of 20-40 hours, via the urine (70%) and feces (30%).

Tizanidine is contraindicated with concomitant use of CYP1A2 inhibitors, such as fluvoxamine or ciprofloxacin. Cigarette smoking is expected to decrease exposure to tizanidine, which may require drug dose adjustment. The drug should also be used with caution in patients with renal insufficiency or hepatic impairment. Since tizanidine is a α_2-adrenergic agonist, it can result in hypotension and syncope. The most frequent adverse events with tizanidine are dry mouth, somnolence/sedation, asthenia (e.g., weakness, fatigue, and/or tiredness), and dizziness.

Diazepam

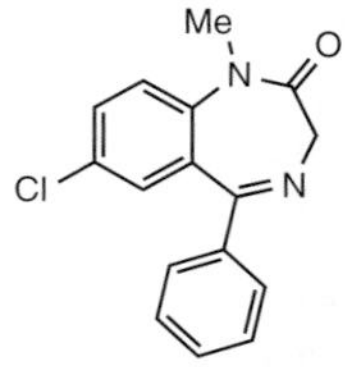

Diazepam
(Valium)

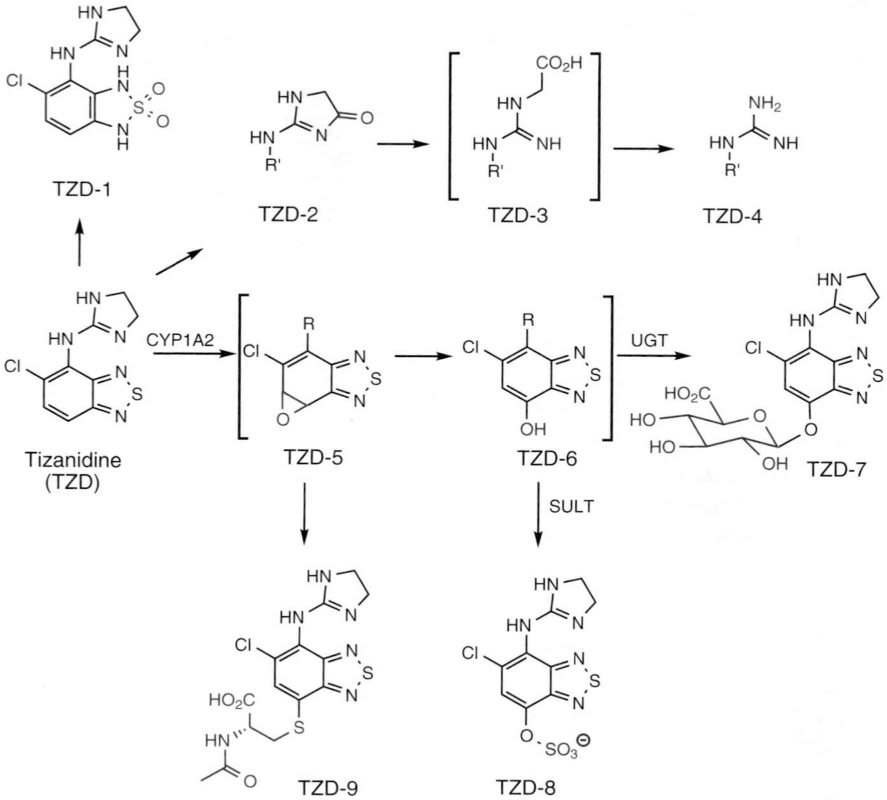

Figure 10.33 Metabolism of tizanidine.

Diazepam is indicated for the management of anxiety disorders. However, it is a useful adjunct therapy for the relief of skeletal muscle spasm due to reflex spasm to local pathology (e.g., inflammation of muscles) and spasticity caused by upper motor neuron disorders. In addition, it is useful for treating acute alcohol withdrawal and adjunctively in convulsive disorders. Structurally diazepam is a benzodiazepine derivative that contains a tertiary amide and substituted with a chlorine atom and phenyl, which contribute to its hydrophobicity. It is a colorless to light yellow crystalline compound that is insoluble in water. Diazepam, being a benzodiazepine, is a positive allosteric modulator of the $GABA_A$ receptor, with high affinity likely for the α2 and α3 subunits.[226,227] Consequently, binding of diazepam and GABA increases chloride ion influx that hyperpolarizes the neuron's membrane potential increasing the difference between resting and threshold potentials. For the treatment of spasticity disorders, this likely results in decreased neuronal firing in the spinal cord.[228] However, diazepam does not appear to be more efficacious than carisoprodol, cyclobenzaprine, or tizanidine.[189,190]

Diazepam is well absorbed (>90%) after oral administration and reaches a maximum plasma concentration in 1-1.5 hours.[229] Taking the drug with food delays absorption and the time to reach maximum plasma concentration, while decreasing maximum plasma concentration (e.g., 20% reduction in C_{max}) and exposure (e.g., AUC decreased 27%). Diazepam is highly plasma protein bound (98%) and has a moderate volume of distribution 0.8-1.0 L/kg and biphasic elimination with the first phase being 1-3 hours (Table 10.2). However, the terminal plasma elimination half-life (e.g., $t_{1/2\beta}$) can be 1-2 days.[230]

The major diazepam metabolite found in plasma is N-desmethyldiazepam (Fig. 10.34) via CYP450-mediated N-demethylation.[231] In addition, the parent drug also undergoes CYP450 alkyl oxidation on the carbon between the amide and imine functional groups to yield temazepam. Both of these metabolites can be further oxidized to oxazepam. The N-demethylation reactions appear to be catalyzed by 2C19 and 3A4 isozymes, whereas the hydroxylation is mediated by 3A4.[232] All three of these phase 1 metabolites are active as positive allosteric modulators of the $GABA_A$ receptor. In addition, temazepam and oxazepam are conjugated with glucuronic acid before renal excretion.

Diazepam has the potential to participate in drug-drug interactions with drug modulating CYP 3A and 2C19. The drug is contraindicated in patients with myasthenia gravis, severe respiratory insufficiency, severe hepatic insufficiency, and sleep apnea. It is also not recommended in the treatment of psychotic patients and should not be used concomitant with alcohol or CNS depressants.

Botulinum Toxin Type A

Botulinum toxin type A is indicated for the treatment of upper limb spasticity in adult patients, as well as prophylaxis of headaches in adult patients with chronic migraine, cervical dystonia in adult patients, severe

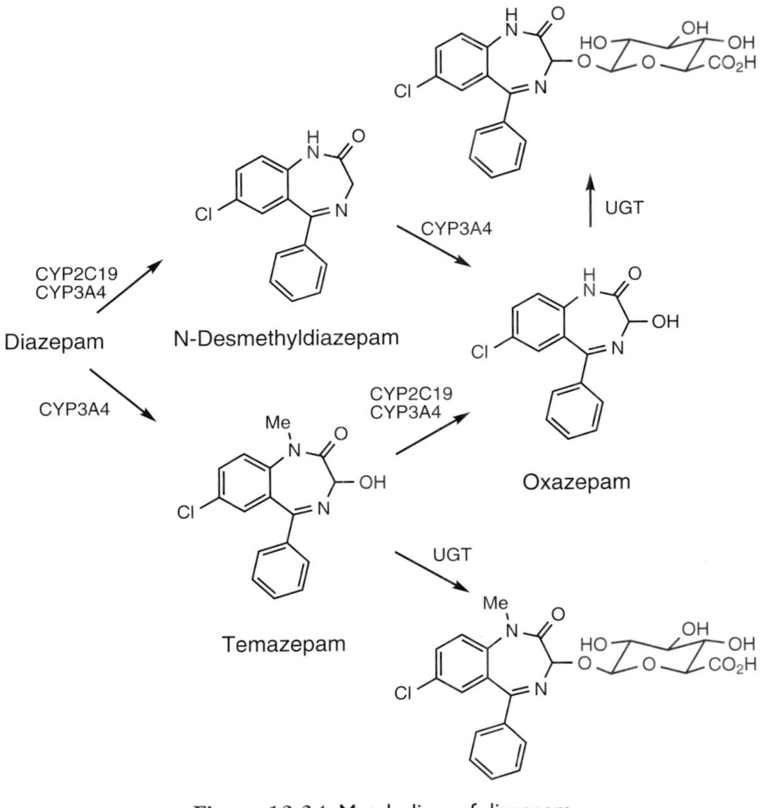

Figure 10.34 Metabolism of diazepam.

axillary hyperhidrosis, blepharospasm associated with dystonia, and strabismus. Botulinum toxin type A is one of seven immunologically distinct forms of botulinum neurotoxin. All forms consisting of a 100-kDa heavy chain and a 50-kDa light chain.[233] The C-terminal region binds to synaptic vesicle protein 2 receptors expressed on presynaptic acetylcholine motor nerve endings before being endocytosed.[234] Once in the cytoplasm, the light chain, a zinc-containing protease, targets synaptobrevin proteins that mediate fusion of acetylcholine-containing synaptic vesicles.[235,236] This process results in inhibition of acetylcholine release at the neuromuscular junction, blocking motor end-plate potential[237] and causing temporary muscle denervation and relaxation, which can be used to treat involuntary muscle spasticity. Botulinum toxin type A is injected into target muscles, but generally does not diffuse beyond 2 cm,[236] although distant spreading of the toxin is a risk. Patients with compromised respiratory status being treated for upper limb spasticity should be closely monitored. The clinical effect is observed about 4 days after injection and lasts 3-4 months.[238] Coadministration of botulinum toxin type A and drugs that interfere with neuromuscular transmission (e.g., aminoglycosides) should be done with caution, as the effect of the toxin may be potentiated. Anticholinergic drugs may also potentiate systemic anticholinergic effects of botulinum toxin type A.

Sugammadex

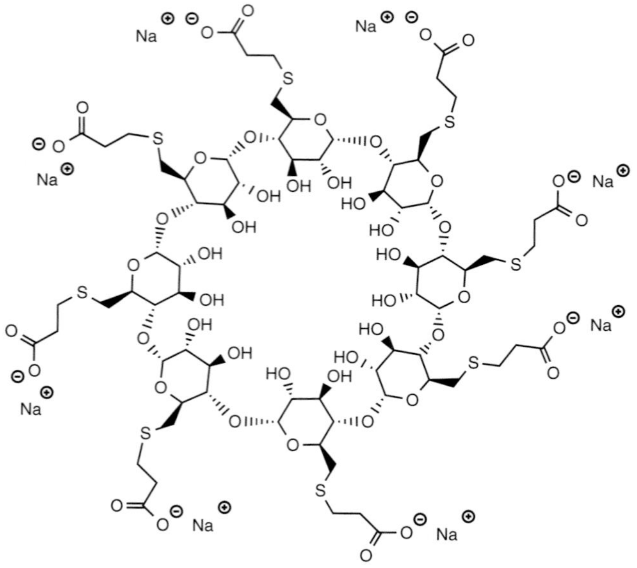

Sugammadex
(Bridion)

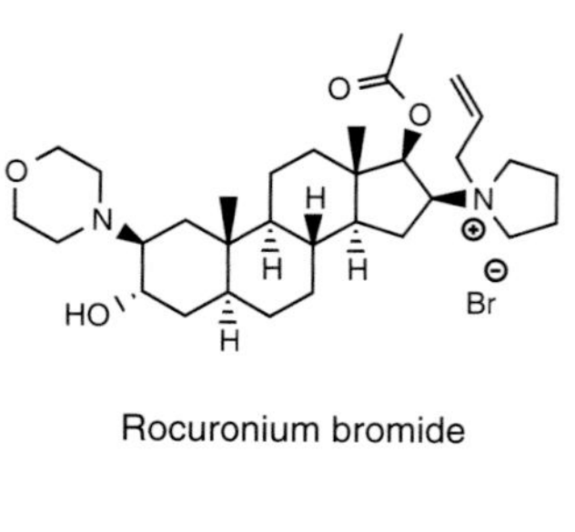

Rocuronium bromide

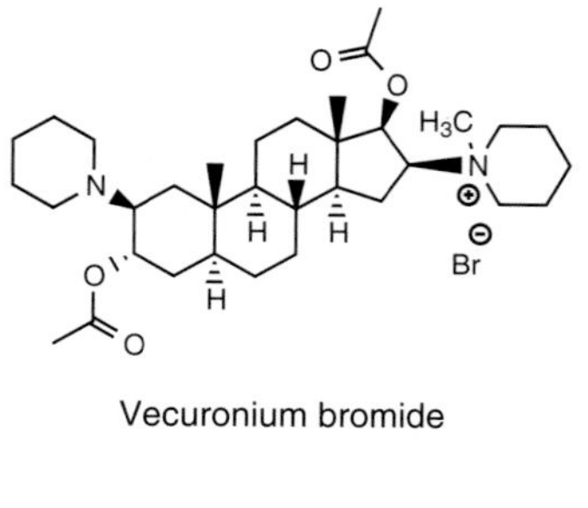

Vecuronium bromide

Sugammadex is indicated for intravenous use for the reversal of neuromuscular blockade by the nicotinic acetylcholine receptor antagonists rocuronium bromide and vecuronium bromide in adults undergoing surgery. The structure of this drug consists of a γ-cyclodextrin, which is made up of eight dextrose residues connected into a macrocycle that provides a lipophilic core and a hydrophilic periphery, with each sugar subunit attached to a propionate linked through thioethers. The hydroxyl and propionate groups on the outer surface of the cyclodextrin core impart excellent water solubility. Sugammadex is associated with the aminosteroids through van der Waal and ionic interactions to form stable complexes.[239] Overall, this results in a reduction of free aminosteroid concentration, which in turn allows acetylcholine binding to nicotinic acetylcholine receptors at neuromuscular junctions.[240]

Sugammadex does not have appreciable binding to plasma proteins and has a volume of distribution of 18 L.[241] In adult anesthetized patients with normal renal function, the plasma elimination half-life is 2 hours. In vivo the drug is quite stable, does not undergo metabolism, and is primarily excreted in urine unchanged.[242] Drug-drug interactions are possible with the selective estrogen receptor modulator toremifene and hormonal contraceptives, which have relatively high binding affinities for sugammadex. Most common adverse effects of the drug are vomiting, pain, nausea, hypotension, and headache.

Neostigmine and Pyridostigmine

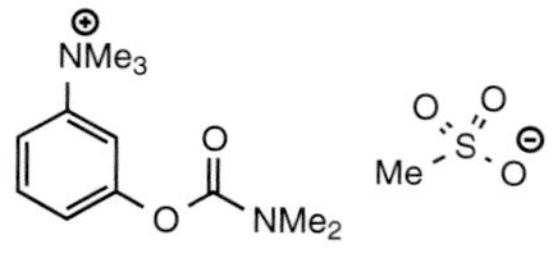

Neostigmine methylsulfate
(Bloxiverz)

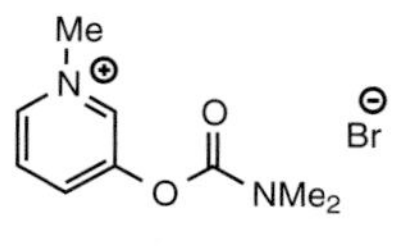

Pyridostigmine bromide
(Mestinon)

Neostigmine is indicated for the reversal of the effects of nondepolarizing neuromuscular blocking agents after surgery and for the treatment of myasthenia gravis (MG), both via parenteral administration. This latter condition is an autoimmune disease in which IgG1-dominant antibodies disrupt nicotinic acetylcholine receptors at neuromuscular junctions (as well as muscle-specific kinase or lipoprotein-related protein 4), resulting in muscle weakness that affects the eyes, face, head, and neck, causing difficulties swallowing, speaking, and eating. In addition, limb and respiratory muscles can also be affected. MG is association with thymomas (e.g., benign or malignant tumors arising in epithelial cells of the thymus) in 20% of patients, as well as other autoimmune diseases such as hyperthyroidism and Hashimoto's disease.[243] The estimated prevalence of MG is 25-142 per million.[244] Neostigmine is a competitive cholinesterase inhibitor that increases acetylcholine in the neuromuscular junctions, which enhances nerve impulse transmission. As a quaternary amine, the drug does not have CNS effects due to its inability to cross the BBB.

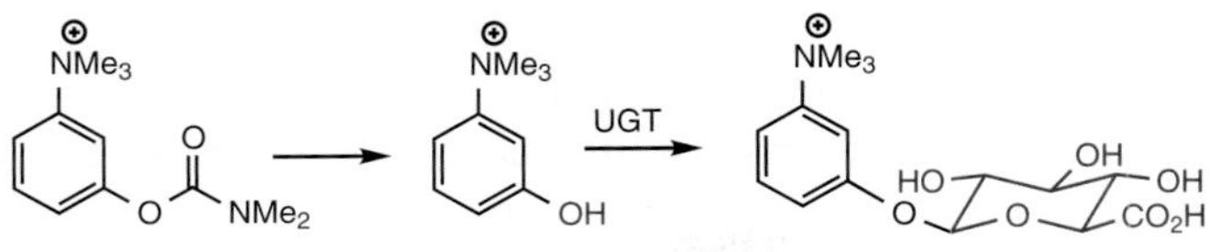

Neostigmine

UGT

Figure 10.35 Metabolism of neostigmine.

Structurally neostigmine consists of benzene substituted with a quaternary amine and a carbamate. It is formulated as a methylsulfate salt that is a highly water-soluble white crystalline solid.

Neostigmine has relatively low plasma protein binding (15%-25%). Following intravenous injection, the drug has a rapid distribution half-life of <1 minutes,[245] plasma elimination half-life of 24-113 minutes, clearance of 1.14-16.7 mL/min/kg, and volume of distribution of 0.12-1.4 L/kg. The drug is metabolized to the corresponding phenol, which is subjected to glucuronidation (Fig. 10.35).[246] Neostigmine is contraindicated in patients with peritonitis or mechanical obstruction of the intestinal or urinary tract. The most common adverse effects of the drug are bradycardia, nausea, and vomiting.

Pyridostigmine is a structurally related drug with a similar mechanism of action that is also indicated for the treatment of MG. It contains an N-methylpyridinium substituted with a carbamate and formulated as the bromide salt that is orally or intravenously administered. The drug's oral bioavailability is 12%-20%. Its plasma elimination half-life is 200 minutes, which is twice as long as the terminal plasma elimination half-life (97 min) after intravenous infusion. This suggests that absorption may proceed at a slower rate than elimination.[247] Pyridostigmine, like neostigmine, is primarily metabolized by hydrolysis of the carbamate to the corresponding phenol followed by glucuronidation.[248] This drug has the same contraindication as neostigmine, and the most common adverse effects are nausea, vomiting, upset stomach, diarrhea, abdominal cramps, increased saliva/mucus, decreased pupil size, and increased urination.

In addition to neostigmine and pyridostigmine, another chemotherapeutic treatment of MG is the use of immunomodulators. For example, both azathioprine[249] and cyclosporine[250] have been shown to be efficacious and safe in the treatment of MG. Azathioprine is an orally bioavailable prodrug converted by reductive cleavage of the thioether to 6-mercaptopurine, which has immunosuppressive properties. Azathioprine is indicated as an adjunct for the prevention of rejection in renal homotransplantations and for the management of active rheumatoid arthritis.[251] Cyclosporine is an orally bioavailable macrocylic peptide that has potent immunosuppressive properties. It is indicated for kidney, liver, and heart transplantation; rheumatoid arthritis; and psoriasis.[252] Finally, the immunomodulator mycophenolate mofetil is used in the treatment of MG. However, its efficacy for this indication is not clear.[253] Mycophenolate mofetil is a prodrug that is readily hydrolyzed to mycophenolic acid, which is a potent inhibitor of inosine monophosphate dehydrogenase, an enzyme involved in guanine nucleotide synthesis. It is indicated for kidney, liver, and heart transplantation.[254]

Tetrabenazine

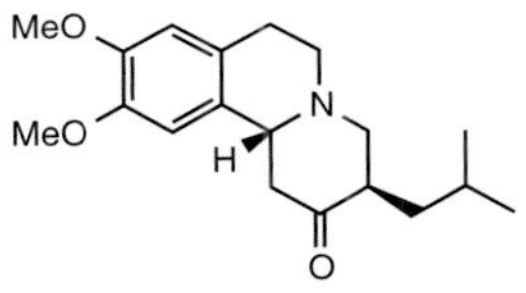

Tetrabenazine
(Xenazine)

Tetrabenazine is indicated for the treatment of chorea, an abnormal involuntary movement disorder, associated with Huntington's disease. Structurally, the drug consists of a benzoquinolizine with two dimethoxyethers on the benzo-portion and a ketone on the piperidine fragment, as well as two chiral centers. The drug is currently marketed

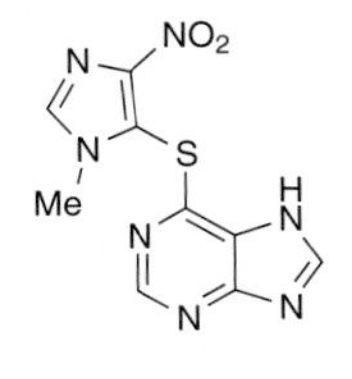

Azathioprine
(Imuran)

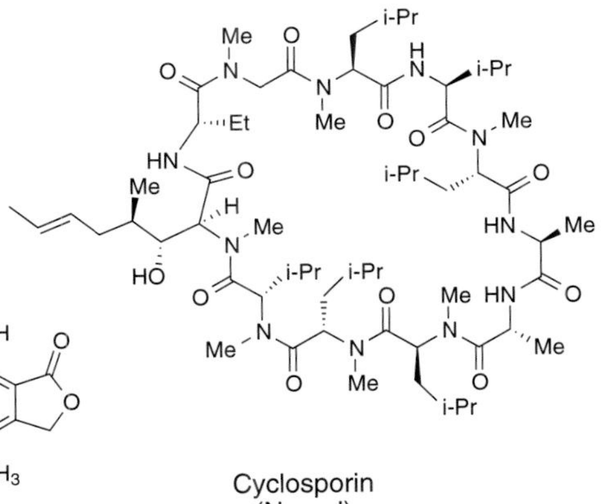

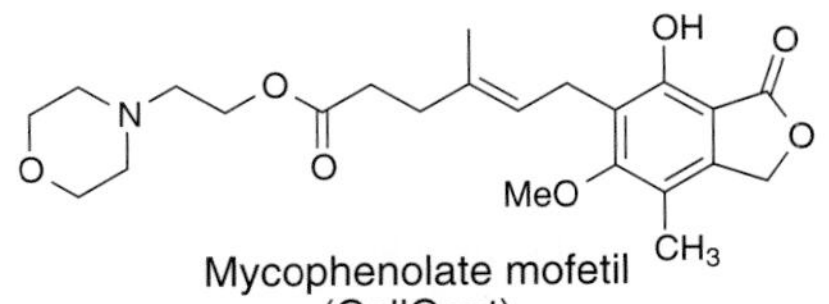

Mycophenolate mofetil
(CellCept)

Cyclosporin
(Neoral)

as a racemate. Although it contains a basic tertiary amine, it is formulated as the free-base that is a white to slightly yellow crystalline solid with low water solubility.

The mechanism of action of tetrabenazine and its active metabolites (e.g., α- and β-dihydrotetrabenazine resulting from ketone reduction) is via reversible and selective inhibition of vesicular monoamine transporter 2 (VMAT2). This transporter participates in the regulation of monoamine (particularly dopamine) uptake from the cytoplasm to the synaptic vesicle for storage and release.[255] Thus, the drug's efficacy for the treatment of chorea associated with Huntington's disease presumably stems from blocking dopamine release via inhibition of VMAT2. The tetrabenazine eutomer has high binding affinity for VMAT2 (K_i = 4.5 nM), while the distomer demonstrates significantly less affinity (K_i = 36,400 nM). The active metabolites α- and β-dihydrotetrabenazines also bind with high affinity to VMAT2 (K_i = 4.0 and 13.4 nM, respectively).[256]

Tetrabenazine has moderate absorption (75%) after oral administration but undergoes rapid and extensive hepatic metabolism by carbonyl reductase to α- and β-dihydrotetrabenazines (Fig. 10.36), which reach maximum plasma concentrations in 1 hour. Very little of the parent drug makes it into systemic circulation and it is not detectable in urine.[257] Tetrabenazine and α- and β-dihydrotetrabenazines have moderate plasma protein binding (59%-85%). The plasma elimination half-lives of the parent drug and the two metabolites are 2.1, 7.6, and 5.9 hours, respectively.[258] Both α- and β-dihydrotetrabenazines are further metabolized by CYP2D6 via dealkylation to the corresponding 9-O-desmethyl metabolites, with 9-O-desmethyl-β-dihydrotetrabenazine having a plasma elimination half-life of 12 hours. All four of the oxoreductase metabolites are conjugated to give an array of glucuronide and sulfonate phase 2 metabolites. The primary route of elimination of all of the metabolites appears to be renal.

Tetrabenazine is contraindicated in patients with hepatic impairment and those taking MAO inhibitors or reserpine. It is also not recommended in combination with other drugs that prolong the QT interval and should be used with caution with other drugs that induce CYP2D6. The drug can increase risk for depression and suicidal thoughts, as well as lead to parkinsonism, dysphagia, and neuroleptic malignant syndrome. The most common adverse effects of tetrabenazine are sedation, somnolence, fatigue, insomnia, depression, akathisia, anxiety, and nausea.

Valbenazine

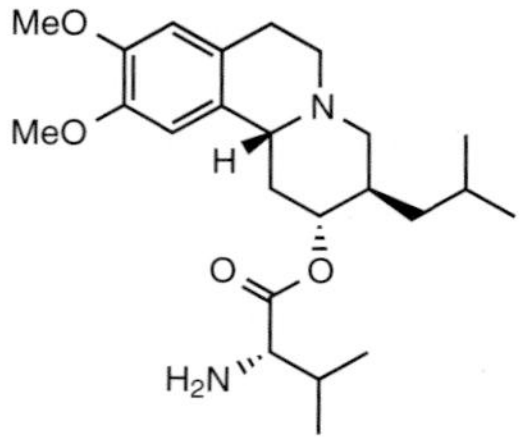

MeO MeO H N O O H_2N

Valbenazine
(Ingrezza)

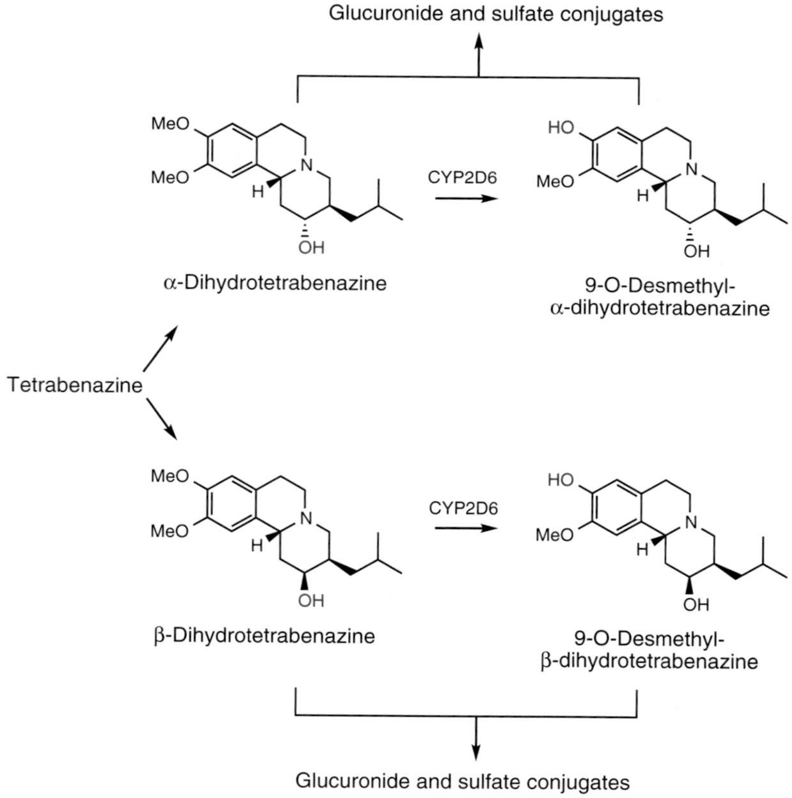

Glucuronide and sulfate conjugates

MeO MeO H N OH — CYP2D6 → HO MeO H N OH

α-Dihydrotetrabenazine

9-O-Desmethyl-
α-dihydrotetrabenazine

Tetrabenazine

MeO MeO H N OH — CYP2D6 → HO MeO H N OH

β-Dihydrotetrabenazine

9-O-Desmethyl-
β-dihydrotetrabenazine

Glucuronide and sulfate conjugates

Figure 10.36 Metabolism of tetrabenazine.

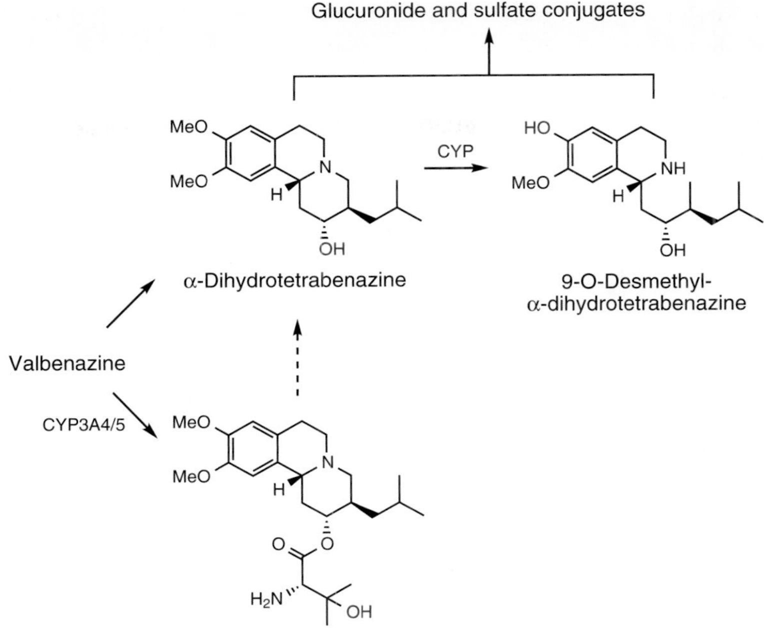

Figure 10.37 Metabolism of valbenazine. Dashed arrow indicates a presumed reaction.

Valbenazine is indicated for the treatment of adults with tardive dyskinesia, which is believed to arise from neuroleptic-induced dopamine hypersensitivity. The drug is also being evaluated as a treatment for Tourette's syndrome. Structurally, valbenazine is similar to tetrabenazine, except that the ketone is replaced with a secondary alcohol (resulting in one additional chiral center) that is formed into a valine ester prodrug. Given that the drug has two basic amines, it is formulated as a ditosylate salt that is slightly soluble in water. Similar to tetrabenazine, both valbenazine and its active metabolite (e.g., α-dihydrotetrabenazine) are reversible and selective inhibitors of VMAT2. However, the parent drug demonstrates lower binding affinity (K_i = 150 nM).[259]

Valbenazine reaches maximum plasma concentration in 0.5-1.0 hours after oral administration with a bioavailability of 49%. The active metabolite α-dihydrotetrabenazine, formed by ester hydrolysis (Fig. 10.37), reaches maximum plasma concentration 4-8 hours after administration. Taking the drug with a high-fat meal decreases maximum plasma concentration (C_{max}) and exposure (AUC) of the parent drug by 47% and 13%, respectively. The parent drug is highly plasma protein bound (99%), while the active metabolite is less strongly bound (64%). Both the parent drug and active metabolite are slowly eliminated, resulting in long plasma elimination half-lives (15-22 hr). In addition to being hydrolyzed to the active metabolite, valbenazine is also subjected to CYP3A4/5-mediated oxidation on the valine ester portion of the molecule.[260]

Valbenazine may cause an increase in the QT interval and should not be used in patients with congenital long QT syndrome or with arrhythmias associated with a prolonged QT interval. The most common adverse effect of valbenazine is somnolence.

ACKNOWLEDGMENT

The author wishes to acknowledge the work of Raymond G. Booth, PhD, who authored content used within this chapter in a previous edition of this text.

Structure Challenge

The following are structures of eight drugs described in this chapter. For each patient described indicate (a) two drugs that would be appropriate to use based on the indication, (b) from among these two drugs, the drug of choice, and (c) your rationale for selecting the drug of choice.

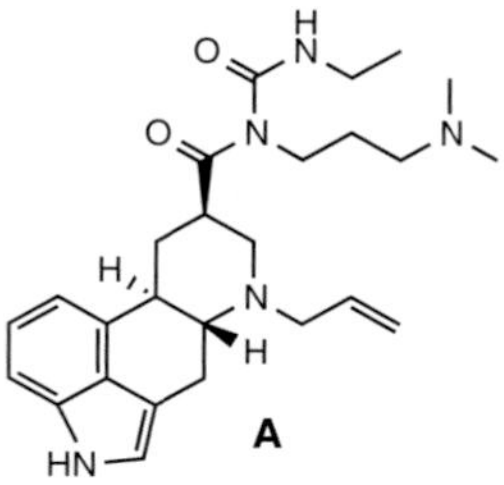

A B C D E F G H

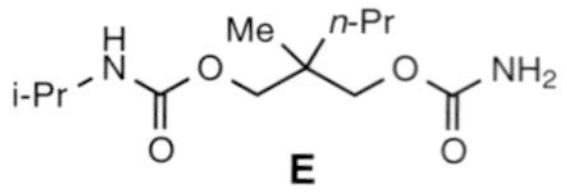

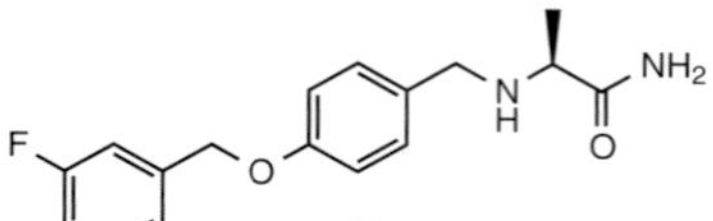

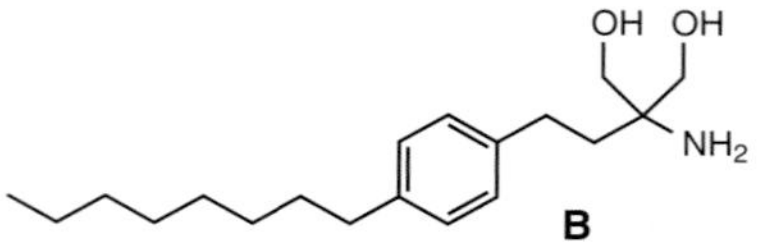

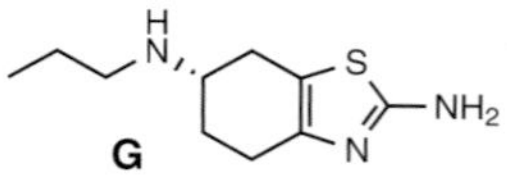

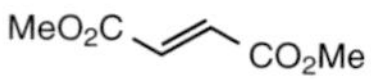

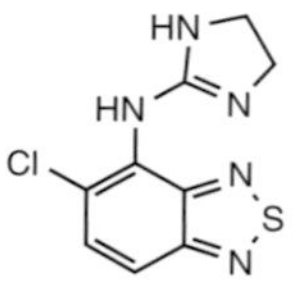

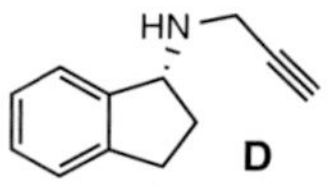

1. A patient with Parkinson's disease who would benefit from adjuvant MAO-B inhibitor treatment who is also currently taking cimetidine.
2. A patient who would benefit from treatment for relapsing multiple sclerosis who has a history of cardiovascular problems, including a prior heart attack.
3. A patient with Parkinson's disease, whose occupation is a long-haul truck driving, would benefit from adjuvant dopamine agonist treatment.
4. A patient, who has a history of drug dependence, has muscle spasms.

Chemical Structure answers found immediately after References.

REFERENCES

1. Olanow CW, Stern MB, Sethi K. The scientific and clinical basis for the treatment of Parkinson disease. *Neurology*. 2009;72(21 suppl 4):S1-S136.
2. Galasko D. Lewy body disorders. *Neurol Clin*. 2017;35(2):325-338.
3. Norris EH, Giasson BI, Lee VM. α-Synuclein: normal function and role in neurodegenerative diseases. *Curr Top Dev Biol*. 2004;60:17-54.
4. Ozansoy M, Başak AN. The central theme of Parkinson's disease: α-synuclein. *Mol Neurobiol*. 2013;47(2):460-465.
5. Wong YC, Krainc D. α-Synuclein toxicity in neurodegeneration: mechanism and therapeutic strategies. *Nat. Med*. 2017;23; 1-13.
6. Bengoa-Vergniory N, Roberts RF, Wade-Martins R, et al. Alpha-synuclein oligomers: a new hope. *Acta Neuropathol*. 2017;134(6):819-838.
7. Semchuk KM, Love EJ, Lee RG. PD: a test of the multifactorial etiologic hypothesis. *Neurology*. 1993;43:1173-1180.
8. Gwinn-Hardy K. Genetics of parkinsonism. *Mov Disord*. 2002;17:645-656.
9. Polymeropoulos MH, Lavedan C, Leroy E, et al. Mutation in the α-synuclein gene identified in families with PD. *Science*. 1997;276:2045-2047.
10. Kruger R, Kuhn W, Muller T, et al. Ala30Pro mutation in the gene encoding α-synuclein in PD. *Nat Genet*. 1998;18:106-108.
11. Lill CM. Genetics of Parkinson's disease. *Mol Cell Probes*. 2016;30(6):386-396.
12. Ozelius LJ, Senthil G, Saunders-Pullman R, et al. LRRK2 G2019S as a cause of Parkinson's disease in Ashkenazi Jews. *N Engl J Med*. 2006;354:424-425.
13. Vilariño-Güell C, Wider C, Ross OA, et al. VPS35 mutations in Parkinson disease. *Am J Hum Genet*. 2011;89(1):162-167.
14. Zimprich A, Benet-Pagès A, Struhal W, et al. A mutation in VPS35, encoding a subunit of the retromer complex, causes late-onset Parkinson disease. *Am J Hum Genet*. 2011;89(1):168-175.

15. Mohan M, Mellick GD. Role of the VPS35 D620N mutation in Parkinson's disease. *Parkinsonism Relat Disord*. 2017;36:10-18.
16. Sassone J, Serratto G, Valtorta F, et al. The synaptic function of Parkin. *Brain*. 2017;140(9):2265-2272.
17. Narendra D, Tanaka A, Suen DF, et al. Parkin is recruited selectively to impaired mitochondria and promotes their autophagy. *J Cell Biol*. 2008;183:795-803.
18. Mizushima N. Autophagy: process and function. *Genes Dev*. 2007;21:2861-2873.
19. Clark IE, Dodson MW, Jiang C, et al. Drosophila pink1 is required for mitochondrial function and interacts genetically with Parkin. *Nature*. 2006;441:1162-1166.
20. Park J, Lee SB, Lee S, et al. Mitochondrial dysfunction in Drosophila PINK1 mutants is complemented by Parkin. *Nature*. 2006;441:1157-1161.
21. Shendelman S, Jonason A, Martinat C, et al. DJ-1 is a redox-dependent molecular chaperone that inhibits alpha-synuclein aggregate formation. *PLoS Biol*. 2004;2(11):e362.
22. Zhou W, Zhu M, Wilson MA, et al. The oxidation state of DJ-1 regulates its chaperone activity toward alpha-synuclein. *J Mol Biol*. 2006;356:1036-1048.
23. Biosa A, Sandrelli F, Beltramini M, et al. Recent findings on the physiological function of DJ-1: beyond Parkinson's disease. *Neurobiol Dis*. 2017;108:65-72.
24. Gasser T. Genetics of PD. *Curr Opin Neurol*. 2005;18:363-369.
25. Burns RS, Chiueh CC, Markey SP, et al. A primate model of parkinsonism: selective destruction of dopaminergic neurons in the pars compacta of the substantia nigra by N-methyl-4-phenyl-1,2,3,6-tetrahydropyridine. *Proc Natl Acad Sci USA*. 1983;80:4546-4550.
26. Davis GC, Williams AC, Markey SP, et al. Chronic parkinsonism secondary to intravenous injection of meperidine analogues. *Psychiatr Res*. 1979;1:249-254.
27. Langston JW, Ballard P, Tetrud JW, et al. Chronic parkinsonism in humans due to a product of meperidine-analog synthesis. *Science*. 1983;219:979-980.
28. Chiba K, Trevor A, Castagnoli N. Metabolism of the neurotoxic tertiary amine, MPTP, by brain monoamine oxidase. *Biochem Biophys Res Commun*. 1984;120:574-578.
29. Salach JI, Singer TP, Castagnoli N, et al. Oxidation of the neurotoxic amine 1-methyl-4-phenyl-1,2,3,6-tetrahydropyridine (MPTP) by monoamine oxidases A and B and suicide inactivation of the enzymes by MPTP. *Biochem Biophys Res Commun*. 1984;125:831-835.
30. Langston JW, Irwin I, Langston EB, et al. Pargyline prevents MPTP-induced parkinsonism in primates. *Science*. 1984;225:1480-1482.
31. Storch A, Ludolph AC, Schwarz J. Dopamine transporter: involvement in selective dopaminergic neurotoxicity and degeneration. *J Neural Transm (Vienna)*. 2004;111(10-11):1267-1286.
32. Brooks AI, Chadwick CA, Gelbard HA, et al. Paraquat elicited neurobehavioral syndrome caused by dopaminergic neuron loss. *Brain Res*. 1999;823:1-10.
33. Miller GW. Paraquat: the red herring of Parkinson's disease research. *Toxicol Sci*. 2007;100:1-2.
34. Hatcher JM, Pennell KD, Miller GW. Parkinson's disease and pesticides: a toxicological perspective. *Trends Pharmacol Sci*. 2008;29:322-329.
35. Graham DG. Catecholamine toxicity: a proposal for the molecular pathogenesis of manganese neurotoxicity and Parkinson's disease. *Neurotoxicology*. 1984;5:83-95.
36. Kessler II, Diamond EL. Epidemiologic studies of PD. I. Smoking and PD: a survey and explanatory hypothesis. *Am J Epidemiol*. 1971;94:16-25.
37. Tanner CM, Goldman SM, Aston DA, et al. Smoking and PD in twins. *Neurology*. 2002;58:581-588.
38. Yu PH, Boulton AA. Irreversible inhibition of monoamine oxidase by some components of cigarette smoke. *Life Sci*. 1987;41:675-682.
39. Khalil AA, Davies B, Castagnoli N. Isolation and characterisation of a monoamine oxidase B selective inhibitor from tobacco smoke. *Bioorg Med Chem*. 2006;14:3392-3398.
40. Chapman MA. Does smoking reduce the risk of PD through stimulation of the ubiquitin-proteasome system? *Med Hypotheses*. 2009;73:887-891.
41. Hernan MA, Takkouche B, Caamano-Isorna F, et al. A meta-analysis of coffee drinking, cigarette smoking, and the risk of Parkinson's disease. *Ann Neurol*. 2002;52:276-284.
42. Trevitt J, Kawa K, Jalali A, et al. Differential effects of adenosine antagonists in two models of parkinsonian tremor. *Pharmacol Biochem Behav*. 2009;94:24-29.
43. Alves G, Forsaa EB, Pedersen KF, et al. Epidemiology of PD. *J Neurol*. 2008;255(suppl 5):18-32.
44. Pringsheim T, Jette N, Frolkis A, et al. The prevalence of Parkinson's disease: a systematic review and meta-analysis. *Mov Disord*. 2014;29(13):1583-1590.
45. Kowal SL, Dall TM, Chakrabarti R, et al. The current and projected economic burden of Parkinson's disease in the United States. *Mov Disord*. 2013;28(3):311-318.
46. http://parkinson.org/Understanding-Parkinsons/Causes-and-Statistics/Statistics. Last accessed 4 January 2018.
47. Nagatsu T. Tyrosine hydroxylase: human isoforms, structure and regulation in physiology and pathology. *Essays Biochem*. 1995;30:15-35.
48. Soloway AH. Potential endogenous epoxides of tyrosine: causative agents in initiating idiopathic Parkinson's disease? *Med Hypotheses Res*. 2009;5:19-26.
49. Soloway AH. Potential endogenous epoxides of steroid hormones: initiators of breast and other malignancies? *Med Hypoth*. 2007;69:1225-1229.
50. Graham DG, Tiffany SM, Bell WR, et al. Autoxidation versus covalent binding of quinones as the mechanism of toxicity of dopamine, 6-hydroxydopamine, and related compounds toward C1300 neuroblastoma cells in vitro. *Mol Pharmacol*. 1978;14:644-653.
51. Jenner P. Oxidative stress in PD. *Ann Neurol*. 2003;53(suppl 3):S26-S36.
52. Ehringer H, Hornykiewicz O. Distribution of noradrenaline and dopamine(3-hydroxytyramine) in the human brain and their behavior in diseases of the extrapyramidal system. *Wien Klin Wochenschr*. 1960;38:1236-1239.
53. Birkmayer W, Hornykiewicz O. The L-3,4-dioxyphenylalanine (DOPA)-effect in Parkinson-akinesia. *Wien Klin Wochenschr*. 1961;73:787-788.
54. Barbeau A. Biochemistry of Parkinson's disease. *Proc Seventh Int Congr Neurol*. 1961;2:925.
55. Barbeau A. L-DOPA therapy in Parkinson's disease: a critical review of nine years' experience. *Can Med Assoc J*. 1969;101:59-68.
56. Cotzias GC, Papavasiliou PS, Gellene R. Modification of Parkinsonism—chronic treatment with L-DOPA. *N Engl J Med*. 1969;280:337-345.
57. Sampaio-Maia B, Serrão MP, Soares-da-Silva P. Regulatory pathways and uptake of L-DOPA by capillary cerebral endothelial cells, astrocytes, and neuronal cells. *Am J Physiol Cell Physiol*. 2001;280(2):C333-C342.
58. Vogel WH. Determination and physiological disposition of p-methoxyphenylethylamine in the rat. *Biochem Pharmacol*. 1970;19:2663-2665.
59. Burkard WP, Gey KF, Pletscher A. Inhibition of decarboxylase of aromatic amino acids by 2,3,4-trihydroxybenzylhydrazine and its seryl derivative. *Arch Biochem Biophys*. 1964;107:187-196.
60. Standaert DG, Young AB. Treatment of central nervous system degenerative disorders. In: Brunton LL, Lazo JS, Parker KL, eds. *Goodman and Gilman's the Pharmacological Basis of Therapeutics*. New York: McGraw-Hill; 2006:527-546.
61. Iqbal MM, Basil MJ, Kaplan J, et al. Overview of serotonin syndrome. *Ann Clin Psychiatry*. 2012;24(4):310-318.
62. Robertson DR, Wood ND, Everest H, et al. The effect of age on the pharmacokinetics of levodopa administered alone and in the presence of carbidopa. *Br J Clin Pharmacol*. 1989;28(1):61-69.
63. Abrams WR, Coutino CB, Leon AS, et al. Absorption and metabolism of levodopa. *J Am Med Assoc*. 1971;218:1912-1914.

64. Schwartz DE, Brandt R. Pharmacokinetic and metabolic studies of the decarboxylase inhibitor benserazide in animals and man. *Arzneimittelforschung*. 1978;28:302-307.
65. Burkhard P, Dominici P, Borri-Voltattorni C, et al. Structural insight into Parkinson's disease treatment from drug-inhibited DOPA decarboxylase. *Nat Struct Biol*. 2001;8:963-967.
66. Vickers S, Stuart EK, Bianchine JR, et al. Metabolism of carbidopa (1-(-)-alpha-hydrazino-3,4-dihydroxy-alpha-methylhydrocinnamic acid monohydrate), an aromatic amino acid decarboxylase inhibitor, in the rat, rhesus monkey, and man. *Drug Metab Dispos*. 1974;2(1):9-22.
67. Vickers S, Stuart EK, Hucker HB. Further studies on the metabolism of carbidopa, (minus)-L-alpha-hydrazino-3,4-dihydroxy-alpha-methylbenzenepropanoic acid monohydrate, in the human, Rhesus monkey, dog, and rat. *J Med Chem*. 1975;18(2):134-138.
68. Chase TN, Watanabe AM. Methyldopahydrazine as an adjunct to L-dopa therapy in parkinsonism. *Neurology*. 1972;22(4):384-392.
69. Campbell NR, Hasinoff BB. Iron supplements: a common cause of drug interactions. *Br J Clin Pharmacol*. 1991;31(3):251-255.
70. Bender DA. Inhibition in vitro of the enzymes of the oxidative pathway of tryptophan metabolism and of nicotinamide nucleotide synthesis by benserazide, carbidopa and isoniazid. *Biochem Pharmacol*. 1980;29(5):707-712.
71. Hubálek F, Binda C, Li M, et al. Inactivation of purified human recombinant monoamine oxidases A and B by rasagiline and its analogues. *J Med Chem*. 2004;47(7):1760-1766.
72. Binda C, Hubálek F, Li M, et al. Crystal structures of monoamine oxidase B in complex with four inhibitors of the N-propargylaminoindan class. *J Med Chem*. 2004;47(7):1767-1774.
73. https://www.accessdata.fda.gov/drugsatfda_docs/label/2014/021641s016s017lbl.pdf. Last accessed 3 January 2018.
74. https://www.accessdata.fda.gov/drugsatfda_docs/label/2008/020647s006s007lbl.pdf. Last accessed 3 January 2018.
75. Mahmood I. Clinical pharmacokinetics and pharmacodynamics of selegiline. An update. *Clin Pharmacokinet*. 1997;33:91-102.
76. Barrett JS, Rohatagi S, DeWitt KE, et al. The effect of dosing Regimen and food on the bioavailability of the extensively metabolized, highly variable drug Eldepryl(®) (selegiline hydrochloride). *Am J Ther*. 1996;3(4):298-313.
77. Heinonen EH, Anttila MI, Karnani HL, et al. Desmethylselegiline, a metabolite of selegiline, is an irreversible inhibitor of monoamine oxidase type B in humans. *J Clin Pharmacol*. 1997;37:602-609.
78. Shin HS. Metabolism of selegiline in humans. Identification, excretion, and stereochemistry of urine metabolites. *Drug Metab Dispos*. 1997;25:657-662.
79. Caccia C, Maj R, Calabresi M, et al. Safinamide: from molecular targets to a new anti-Parkinson drug. *Neurology* 2006;67(7 suppl 2):S18-S23.
80. Binda C, Wang J, Pisani L, et al. Structures of human monoamine oxidase B complexes with selective noncovalent inhibitors: safinamide and coumarin analogs. *J Med Chem*. 2007;50:5848-5852.
81. https://www.accessdata.fda.gov/drugsatfda_docs/label/2017/207145lbl.pdf. Last accessed 3 January 2018.
82. Krösser S, Marquet A, Gallemann D, et al. Effects of ketoconazole treatment on the pharmacokinetics of safinamide and its plasma metabolites in healthy adult subjects. *Biopharm Drug Disp*. 2012;33(9):550-559.
83. https://www.pharma.us.novartis.com/sites/www.pharma.us.novartis.com/files/comtan.pdf. Last accessed 3 January 2018.
84. Lautala P, Ethell BT, Taskinen J, et al. The specificity of glucuronidation of entacapone and tolcapone by recombinant human UDP-glucuronosyltransferases. *Drug Metab Dispos*. 2000;28(11):1385-1389.
85. Wikberg T, Vuorela A, Ottoila P, et al. Identification of major metabolites of the catechol-O-methyltransferase inhibitor entacapone in rats and humans. *Drug Metab Dispos*. 1993;21:81-92.
86. Ellermann M, Lerner C, Burgy G, et al. Catechol-O-methyltransferase in complex with substituted 3'-deoxyribose bisubstrate inhibitors. *Acta Crystallogr D Biol Crystallogr*. 2012;68(Pt 3):253-260.
87. https://www.accessdata.fda.gov/drugsatfda_docs/label/2013/020697s004lbl.pdf. Last accessed 3 January 2018.
88. Millan MJ, Maiofiss L, Cussac D, et al. Differential actions of antiparkinson agents at multiple classes of monoaminergic receptor. I. A multivariate analysis of the binding profiles of 14 drugs at 21 native and cloned human receptor subtypes. *J Pharmacol Exp Ther*. 2002;303(2):791-804.
89. Giesecke J. The absolute configuration of apomorphine. *Acta Cryst*. 1977;B33:302-303.
90. Neumeyer JL, McCarthy M, Battista S, et al. Aporphines. 9. The synthesis and pharmacological evaluations of (±)-9,10-dihyroxyaporphine, ([±]-isoapomorphine), (±)-, (−)-, and (+)-1,2-dihydroxyaporphine, and (+)-1,2,9,10 tetrahydroxyaprophine. *J Med Chem*. 1973;16:1228-1233.
91. https://www.accessdata.fda.gov/drugsatfda_docs/label/2014/021264s010lbl.pdf. Last accessed 3 January 2018.
92. van der Geest R, van Laar T, Kruger PP, et al. Pharmacokinetics, enantiomer interconversion, and metabolism of R-apomorphine in patients with idiopathic Parkinson's disease. *Clin Neuropharmacol*. 1998;21(3):159-168.
93. Newman-Tancredi A, Cussac D, Audinot V, et al. Differential actions of antiparkinson agents at multiple classes of monoaminergic receptor. II. Agonist and antagonist properties at subtypes of dopamine D(2)-like receptor and alpha(1)/alpha(2)-adrenoceptor. *J Pharmacol Exp Ther*. 2002;303:805-814.
94. Blanchet PJ. Rationale for use of dopamine agonists in Parkinson's disease: review of ergot derivatives. *Can J Neurol Sci*. 1999;26(suppl 2):S21-S26.
95. Schran HF, Bhuta SI, Schwartz HJ, et al. The pharmacokinetics of bromocriptine in man. *Adv Biochem Psychopharmacol*. 1980;23:125-139.
96. Maurer G, Schreier E, Delaborde S, et al. Fate and disposition of bromocriptine in animals and man. I: structure elucidation of the metabolites. *Eur J Drug Metab Pharmacokinet*. 1982;7(4):281-292.
97. Maurer G, Schreier E, Delaborde S, et al. Fate and disposition of bromocriptine in animals and man. II: absorption, elimination and metabolism. *Eur J Drug Metab Pharmacokinet*. 1983;8(1):51-62.
98. Nelson MV, Berchou RC, Kareti D, et al. Pharmacokinetic evaluation of erythromycin and caffeine administered with bromocriptine. *Clin Pharmacol Ther*. 1990;47(6):694-697.
99. Del Dotto P, Bonuccelli U. Clinical pharmacokinetics of cabergoline. *Clin Pharmacokinet*. 2003;42(7):633-645.
100. http://docs.boehringer-ingelheim.com/Prescribing%20Information/PIs/Mirapex%20ER/MirapexER.pdf. Last accessed 3 January 2018.
101. Eden RJ, Costall B, Domeney AM, et al. Preclinical pharmacology of ropinirole (SK&F 101468-A) a novel dopamine D2 agonist. *Pharmacol Biochem Behav*. 1991;38(1):147-154.
102. https://www.gsksource.com/pharma/content/dam/GlaxoSmithKline/US/en/Prescribing_Information/Requip/pdf/REQUIP-PI-PIL.PDF. Last accessed 3 January 2018.
103. Ramji JV, Keogh JP, Blake TJ, et al. Disposition of ropinirole in animals and man. *Xenobiotica*. 1999;29(3):311-325.
104. Bloomer JC, Clarke SE, Chenery RJ. In vitro identification of the P450 enzymes responsible for the metabolism of ropinirole. *Drug Metab Dispos*. 1997;25(7):840-844.
105. Hutton JT, Metman LV, Chase TN, et al. Transdermal dopaminergic D(2) receptor agonist therapy in Parkinson's disease with N-0923 TDS: a doubleblind, placebo-controlled study. *Mov Disord*. 2001;16:459-463.
106. Morgan JC, Sethi KD. Rotigotine for the treatment of Parkinson's disease. *Expert Rev Neurother*. 2006;6:1275-1282.
107. https://www.accessdata.fda.gov/drugsatfda_docs/label/2012/021829s001lbl.pdf. Last accessed 3 January 2018.
108. Cawello W, Braun M, Boekens H. Absorption, disposition, metabolic fate, and elimination of the dopamine agonist rotigotine in man: administration by intravenous infusion or transdermal delivery. *Drug Metab Dispos*. 2009;37(10):2055-2060.

109. Allen RP. Restless leg syndrome/Willis-Ekbom disease pathophysiology. *Sleep Med Clin*. 2015;10(3):207-214.
110. Wijemanne S, Ondo W. Restless legs syndrome: clinical features, diagnosis and a practical approach to management. *Pract Neurol*. 2017;17(6):444-452.
111. Le DA, Lipton SA. Potential and current use of N-methyl-D-aspartate (NMDA) receptor antagonists in diseases of aging. *Drugs Aging*. 2001;18:717-724.
112. Paci C, Thomas A, Onofrj M. Amantadine for dyskinesia in patients affected by severe Parkinson's disease. *Neurol Sci*. 2001;22:75-76.
113. Schwab RS, Poskanzer DC, England AC, et al. Amantadine in the treatment of Parkinson's disease. Review of more than two years' experience. *JAMA*. 1972;222:792-795.
114. Crosby N, Deane KH, Clarke CE. Amantadine in Parkinson's disease. *Cochrane Database Syst Rev*. 2003;(1):CD003468.
115. https://www.accessdata.fda.gov/drugsatfda_docs/label/2009/016023s041, 018101s016lbl.pdf. Last accessed 3 January 2018.
116. Köppel C, Tenczer J. A revision of the metabolic disposition of amantadine. *Biomed Mass Spectrom*. 1985;12(9):499-501.
117. Aoki FY, Sitar DS. Clinical pharmacokinetics of amantadine hydrochloride. *Clin Pharmacokinet*. 1988;14(1):35-51.
118. Nakahara J, Maeda M, Aiso S, et al. Current concepts in multiple sclerosis: autoimmunity versus oligodendrogliopathy. *Clin Rev Allergy Immunol*. 2012;42(1):26-34.
119. Nakahara J, Aiso S, Suzuki N. Autoimmune versus oligodendrogliopathy: the pathogenesis of multiple sclerosis. *Arch Immunol Ther Exp (Warsz)*. 2010;58(5):325-333.
120. Milo R, Kahana E. Multiple sclerosis: geoepidemiology, genetics and the environment. *Autoimmun Rev*. 2010;9(5):A387-A394.
121. Harbo HF, Gold R, Tintoré M. Sex and gender issues in multiple sclerosis. *Ther Adv Neurol Disord*. 2013;6(4):237-248.
122. Hartung DM. Economics and cost-effectiveness of multiple sclerosis therapies in the USA. *Neurotherapeutics*. 2017;14(4):1018-1026.
123. Haji Abdolvahab M, Mofrad MR, Schellekens H. Interferon beta: from molecular level to therapeutic effects. *Int Rev Cell Mol Biol*. 2016;326:343-372.
124. Fridkis-Hareli M, Teitelbaum D, Gurevich E, et al. Direct binding of myelin basic protein and synthetic copolymer 1 to class II major histocompatibility complex molecules on living antigen-presenting cells – specificity and promiscuity. *Proc Natl Acad Sci USA*. 1994;91(11):4872-4876.
125. Weber MS, Hohlfeld R, Zamvil SS. Mechanism of action of glatiramer acetate in treatment of multiple sclerosis. *Neurotherapeutics*. 2007;4(4):647-653.
126. Yong VW. Differential mechanisms of action of interferon-beta and glatiramer aetate in MS. *Neurology*. 2002;59(6):802-808.
127. Lehmann-Horn K, Kronsbein HC, Weber MS. Targeting B cells in the treatment of multiple sclerosis: recent advances and remaining challenges. *Ther Adv Neurol Disord*. 2013;6(3):161-173.
128. https://www.accessdata.fda.gov/drugsatfda_docs/label/2017/761053lbl.pdf. Last accessed 3 January 2018.
129. https://www.accessdata.fda.gov/drugsatfda_docs/label/2007/103948s5070lbl.pdf. Last accessed 3 January 2018.
130. Yednock TA, Cannon C, Fritz LC, et al. Prevention of experimental autoimmune encephalomyelitis by antibodies against alpha 4 beta 1 integrin. *Nature*. 1992;356(6364):63-66.
131. Léger OJ, Yednock TA, Tanner L, et al. Humanization of a mouse antibody against human alpha-4 integrin: a potential therapeutic for the treatment of multiple sclerosis. *Hum Antibodies*. 1997;8(1):3-16.
132. https://www.accessdata.fda.gov/drugsatfda_docs/label/2012/125104s0576lbl.pdf. Last accessed 3 January 2018.
133. Bomprezzi R. Dimethyl fumarate in the treatment of relapsing-remitting multiple sclerosis: an overview. *Ther Adv Neurol Disord*. 2015;8(1):20-30.
134. de Jong R, Bezemer AC, Zomerdijk TP, et al. Selective stimulation of T helper 2 cytokine responses by the anti-psoriasis agent monomethylfumarate. *Eur J Immunol*. 1996;26(9):2067-2074.
135. Chen H, Assmann JC, Krenz A, et al. Hydroxycarboxylic acid receptor 2 mediates dimethyl fumarate's protective effect in EAE. *J Clin Invest*. 2014;124(5):2188-2192.
136. https://www.accessdata.fda.gov/drugsatfda_docs/label/2013/204063lbl.pdf. Last accessed 3 January 2018.
137. Groves A, Kihara Y, Chun J. Fingolimod: direct CNS effects of sphingosine 1-phosphate (S1P) receptor modulation and implications in multiple sclerosis therapy. *J Neurol Sci*. 2013;328(1-2):9-18.
138. https://www.pharma.us.novartis.com/sites/www.pharma.us.novartis.com/files/gilenya.pdf. Last accessed 3 January 2018.
139. David OJ, Kovarik JM, Schmouder RL. Clinical pharmacokinetics of fingolimod. *Clin Pharmacokinet*. 2012;51(1):15-28.
140. Kovarik JM, Hartmann S, Bartlett M, et al. Oral-intravenous crossover study of fingolimod pharmacokinetics, lymphocyte responses and cardiac effects. *Biopharm Drug Dispos*. 2007;28(2):97-104.
141. Zollinger M, Gschwind HP, Jin Y, et al. Absorption and disposition of the sphingosine 1-phosphate receptor modulator fingolimod (FTY720) in healthy volunteers: a case of xenobiotic biotransformation following endogenous metabolic pathways. *Drug Metab Dispos*. 2011;39(2):199-207.
142. Jin Y, Zollinger M, Borell H, et al. CYP4F enzymes are responsible for the elimination of fingolimod (FTY720), a novel treatment of relapsing multiple sclerosis. *Drug Metab Dispos*. 2011;39(2):191-198.
143. Li K, Konofalska U, Akgün K, et al. Modulation of cardiac autonomic function by fingolimod initiation and predictors for fingolimod induced bradycardia in patients with multiple sclerosis. *Front Neurosci*. 2017;11:540.
144. Bar-Or A, Pachner A, Menguy-Vacheron F, et al. Teriflunomide and its mechanism of action in multiple sclerosis. *Drugs*. 2014;74(6):659-674.
145. https://www.accessdata.fda.gov/drugsatfda_docs/label/2012/202992s000lbl.pdf. Last accessed 3 January 2018.
146. Parekh JM, Vaghela RN, Sutariya DK, et al. Chromatographic separation and sensitive determination of teriflunomide, an active metabolite of leflunomide in human plasma by liquid chromatography-tandem mass spectrometry. *J Chromatogr B Analyt Technol Biomed Life Sci*. 2010;878(24):2217-2225.
147. Wiese MD, Rowland A, Polasek TM, et al. Pharmacokinetic evaluation of teriflunomide for the treatment of multiple sclerosis. *Expert Opin Drug Metab Toxicol*. 2013;9(8):1025-1035.
148. Wilson ID, Macdonald CM, Fromson JM, et al. Species differences in the metabolism of 14C-p-trifluoromethylaniline: production of an oxanilic acid as the major metabolite by the rat. *Biochem Pharmacol*. 1985;34(11):2025-2028.
149. Blight AR, Henney HR, Cohen R. Development of dalfampridine, a novel pharmacologic approach for treating walking impairment in multiple sclerosis. *Ann NY Acad Sci*. 2014;1329:33-44.
150. https://www.accessdata.fda.gov/drugsatfda_docs/label/2013/022250s006lbl.pdf. Last accessed 3 January 2018.
151. Mehta P, Kaye W, Bryan L, et al. Prevalence of amyotrophic lateral sclerosis – United States, 2012-2013. *MMWR Surveill Summ*. 2016;65(8):1-12.
152. Rosen DR, Siddique T, Patterson D, et al. Mutations in Cu/Zn superoxide dismutase gene are associated with familial amyotrophic lateral sclerosis. *Nature*. 1993;362:59-62.
153. Cleveland DW, Laing N, Hurse PV, et al. Toxic mutants in Charcot's sclerosis. *Nature*. 1995;378:342-343.
154. Taylor JP, Brown RH, Cleveland DW. Decoding ALS: from genes to mechanism. *Nature*. 2016;539(7628):197-206.
155. Gamez J, Corbera-Bellalta M, Nogales G, et al. Mutational analysis of the Cu/Zn superoxide dismutase gene in a Catalan ALS population: should all sporadic ALS cases also be screened for SOD1? *J Neurol Sci*. 2006;247:21-28.
156. Neumann M, Sampathu DM, Kwong LK, et al. Ubiquitinated TDP-43 in frontotemporal lobar degeneration and amyotrophic lateral sclerosis. *Science*. 2006;314:130-133.
157. Cykowski MD, Powell SZ, Peterson LE, et al. Clinical significance of TDP-43 neuropathology in amyotrophic lateral sclerosis. *J Neuropathol Exp Neurol*. 2017;76(5):402-413.

158. Gladman M, Zinman L. The economic impact of amyotrophic lateral sclerosis: a systematic review. *Expert Rev Pharmacoecon Outcomes Res*. 2015;15(3):439-450.
159. http://web.alsa.org/site/PageServer?pagename=ALSA_Ask_Dec2011. Last accessed 3 January 2018.
160. https://www.forbes.com/sites/matthewherper/2017/05/05/fda-approves-first-new-drug-to-treat-als-in-22-years/#305578337fb3. Last accessed 3 January 2018.
161. Bellingham MC. A review of the neural mechanisms of action and clinical efficiency of riluzole in treating amyotrophic lateral sclerosis: what have we learned in the last decade? *CNS Neurosci Ther*. 2011;17(1):4-31.
162. Le Liboux A, Lefebvre P, Le Roux Y, et al. Single- and multiple-dose pharmacokinetics of riluzole in white subjects. *J Clin Pharmacol*. 1997;37(9):820-827.
163. Sanderink GJ, Bournique B, Stevens J, et al. Involvement of human CYP1A isoenzymes in the metabolism and drug interactions of riluzole in vitro. *J Pharmacol Exp Ther*. 1997;282(3):1465-1472.
164. Takei K, Watanabe K, Yuki S, et al. Edaravone and its clinical development for amyotrophic lateral sclerosis. *Amyotroph Lateral Scler Frontotemporal Degener*. 2017;18(sup1):5-10.
165. Komatsu T, Nakai H, Takamatsu Y, et al. Pharmacokinetic studies of 3-methyl-1-phenyl-2-pyrazolin-5-one (MCI-186): metabolism in rats, dogs and human. *Drug Metab Pharmacokinet*. 1996;11:451-462.
166. Russell AJ, Hartman JJ, Hinken AC, et al. Activation of fast skeletal muscle troponin as a potential therapeutic approach for treating neuromuscular diseases. *Nat Med*. 2012;18(3):452-455.
167. Hwee DT, Kennedy A, Ryans J, et al. Fast skeletal muscle troponin activator tirasemtiv increases muscle function and performance in the B6SJL-SOD1G93A ALS mouse model. *PLoS One*. 2014;9(5):e96921.
168. Shefner J, Cedarbaum JM, Cudkowicz ME, et al. Safety, tolerability and pharmacodynamics of a skeletal muscle activator in amyotrophic lateral sclerosis. *Amyotroph Lateral Scler*. 2012;13(5):430-438.
169. Monaco AP, Neve RL, Colletti-Feener C, et al. Isolation of candidate cDNAs for portions of the Duchenne muscular dystrophy gene. *Nature*. 1986;323(6089):646-650.
170. Hoffman EP, Brown RH, Kunkel LM. Dystrophin: the protein product of the Duchenne muscular dystrophy locus. *Cell*. 1987;51(6):919-928.
171. Stark AE. Determinants of the incidence of Duchenne muscular dystrophy. *Ann Transl Med*. 2015;3(19):287.
172. Thayer S, Bell C, McDonald CM. The direct cost of managing a rare disease: assessing medical and pharmacy costs associated with Duchenne muscular dystrophy in the United States. *J Manag Care Spec Pharm*. 2017;23(6):633-641.
173. Biggar WD, Politano L, Harris VA, et al. Deflazacort in Duchenne muscular dystrophy: a comparison of two different protocols. *Neuromuscul Disord*. 2004;14(8-9):476-482.
174. Hoffman EP, Nader GA. Balancing muscle hypertrophy and atrophy. *Nat Med*. 2004;10(6):584-585.
175. Hoffman EP, Reeves E, Damsker J, et al. Novel approaches to corticosteroid treatment in Duchenne muscular dystrophy. *Phys Med Rehabil Clin N Am*. 2012;23(4):821-828.
176. https://www.accessdata.fda.gov/drugsatfda_docs/label/2017/208684s000, 208685s000lbl.pdf. Last accessed 3 January 2018.
177. Assandri A, Buniva G, Martinelli E, et al. Pharmacokinetics and metabolism of deflazacort in the rat, dog, monkey and man. *Adv Exp Med Biol*. 1984;171:9-23.
178. Huber EW, Barbuch RJ. Spectral analysis and structural identification of a major deflazacort metabolite in man. *Xenobiotica*. 1995;25(2):175-183.
179. Mendell JR, Rodino-Klapac LR, Sahenk Z, et al. Eteplirsen for the treatment of Duchenne muscular dystrophy. *Ann Neurol*. 2013;74(5):637-647.
180. https://www.accessdata.fda.gov/drugsatfda_docs/label/2016/206488lbl.pdf. Last accessed 3 January 2018.
181. D'Amico A, Mercuri E, Tiziano FD, et al. Spinal muscular atrophy. *Orphanet J Rare Dis*. 2011;6:71.
182. Kolb SJ, Kissel JT. Spinal muscular atrophy. *Neurol Clin*. 2015;33(4):831-846.
183. Ahmad S, Bhatia K, Kannan A, et al. Molecular mechanisms of neurodegeneration in spinal muscular atrophy. *J Exp Neurosci*. 2016;23;10:39-49.
184. Parente V, Corti S. Advances in spinal muscular atrophy therapeutics. *Ther Adv Neurol Disord*. 2018. doi: 10.1177/1756285618754501.
185. Tu WY, Simpson JE, Highley JR, et al. Spinal muscular atrophy: factors that modulate motor neurone vulnerability. *Neurobiol Dis*. 2017;102:11-20.
186. https://www.accessdata.fda.gov/drugsatfda_docs/label/2016/209531lbl.pdf. Last accessed 25 February 2018.
187. http://www.aans.org/Patients/Neurosurgical-Conditions-and-Treatments/Spasticity. Last accessed 4 January 2018.
188. Elbasiouny SM, Moroz D, Bakr MM, et al. Management of spasticity after spinal cord injury: current techniques and future directions. *Neurorehabil Neural Repair*. 2010;24:23-33.
189. Montane E, Vallano A, Laporte JR. Oral antispastic drugs in nonprogressive neurologic diseases: a systematic review. *Neurology*. 2004;63:1357-1363.
190. Beebe FA, Barkin RL, Barkin S. A clinical and pharmacologic review of skeletal muscle relaxants for musculoskeletal conditions. *Am J Ther* 2005;12:151-171.
191. Delgado MR, Hirtz D, Aisen M, et al. Practice parameter: pharmacologic treatment of spasticity in children and adolescents with cerebral palsy (an evidence-based review): report of the quality Standards Subcommittee of the American Academy of Neurology and the Practice Committee of the Child Neurology Society. Quality Standards Subcommittee of the American Academy of Neurology and the Practice Committee of the Child Neurology Society. *Neurology* 2010;74:336-343.
192. Chou R. Pharmacological management of low back pain. *Drugs*. 2010;70:387-402.
193. Berger FM, Bradley W. The pharmacological properties of an alpha, betadihydroxy-gama-(2-methylphenoxy)-propane (Myanesisn). *Br J Pharmacol Chemother*. 1946;1:265-272.
194. Souri E, Sharifzadeh M, Farsam H, et al. Muscle relaxant activity of methocarbamol enantiomers in mice. *J Pharm Pharmacol*. 1999;51:853-855.
195. Forist AA, Judy RW. Comparative pharmacokinetics of chlorphenesin carbamate and methocarbamol in man. *J Pharm Sci*. 1971;60(11):1686-1688.
196. Bruce RB, Turnbull LB, Newman JH. Metabolism of methocarbamol in the rat, dog, and human. *J Pharm Sci*. 1971;60(1):104-106.
197. Thompson RM, Gerber N, Seibert RA. Metabolism of methocarbamol (robaxin) in the isolated perfused rat liver and identification of glucuronides. *Xenobiotica*. 1975;5(3):145-153.
198. https://www.accessdata.fda.gov/drugsatfda_docs/label/2015/022503s000lbl.pdf. Last accessed 3 January 2018.
199. Bruce RB, Turnbull L, Newman J, et al. Metabolism of metaxalone. *J Med Chem*. 1966;9(3):286-288.
200. Gonzalez LA, Gatch MB, Taylor CM, et al. Carisoprodol-mediated modulation of GABAA receptors: in vitro and in vivo studies. *J Pharmacol Exp Ther*. 2009;329(2):827-837.
201. Rho JM, Donevan SD, Rogawski MA. Barbiturate-like actions of the propanediol dicarbamates felbamate and meprobamate. *J Pharmacol Exp Ther*. 1997;280(3):1383-1391.
202. Kumar M, Dillon GH. Assessment of direct gating and allosteric modulatory effects of meprobamate in recombinant GABAA receptors. *Eur J Pharmacol*. 2016;775:149-158.
203. Simon S, D'Andrea C, Wheeler WJ, et al. Bioavailability of oral carisoprodol 250 and 350 mg and metabolism to meprobamate: a single-dose crossover study. *Curr Ther Res Clin Exp*. 2010;71(1):50-59.

204. Lewandowski TA. Pharmacokinetic modeling of carisoprodol and meprobamate disposition in adults. *Hum Exp Toxicol.* 2017;36(8): 846-853.
205. Dalén P, Alvan G, Wakelkamp M, et al. Formation of meprobamate from carisoprodol is catalysed by CYP2C19. *Pharmacogenetics.* 1996;6(5):387-394.
206. Yamamoto A, Yoshimura H, Tsukamoto H. Metabolism of drugs. 28. Metabolic fate of meprobamate. (1). Isolation and characterization of metabolites. *Chem Pharm Bull.* 1962;10:522-528.
207. Kobayashi H, Hasegawa Y, Ono H. Cyclobenzaprine, a centrally acting muscle relaxant, acts on descending serotonergic systems. *Eur J Pharmacol.* 1996;311(1):29-35.
208. https://www.accessdata.fda.gov/drugsatfda_docs/label/2013/017821s051lbl.pdf. Last accessed 3 January 2018.
209. Hucker HB, Stauffer SC, Balletto AJ, et al. Physiological disposition and metabolism of cyclobenzaprine in the rat, dog, rhesus monkey, and man. *Drug Metab Dispos.* 1978;6(6):659-672.
210. Prox A, Breyer-Pfaff U. Amitriptyline metabolites in human urine. Identification of phenols, dihydrodiols, glycols, and ketones. *Drug Metab Dispos.* 1987;15(6):890-896.
211. Penn RD, Savoy SM, Corcos D, et al. Intrathecal baclofen for severe spinal spasticity. *N Engl J Med.* 1989;320:1517-1521.
212. Bowery NG. GABAB receptor: a site of therapeutic benefit. *Curr Opin Pharmacol.* 2006;6(1):37-43.
213. Wilson PR, Yaksh A. Baclofen is antinociceptive in the spinal intrathecal space of animals. *Eur J Pharmacol.* 1978;51:323-330.
214. https://www.google.com/search?ei=SDZNWs7BK8nJjwTMi-76wAg&q=baclofen+package+insert&oq=baclofen+package+insert&gs_l=psy-ab.3..0j0i7i30k1l2j0j0i7i30k1j0i5i30k1j0i7i5i30k1.4600.6545.0.6841.8.8.0.0.0.0.95.546.7.7.0....0...1c.1.64.psy-ab..1.7.543....0.WOfMi6TpuFU. Last accessed 3 January 2018.
215. Wuis EW, Dirks MJ, Termond EF, et al. Plasma and urinary excretion kinetics of oral baclofen in healthy subjects. *Eur J Clin Pharmacol.* 1989;37:181-184.
216. Faigle JW, Keberle H. The chemistry and kinetics of lioresal. *Postgrad Med J.* 1972;48(suppl 5):9-13.
217. Sanchez-Ponce R, Wang LQ, Lu W, et al. Metabolic and pharmacokinetic differentiation of STX209 and racemic baclofen in humans. *Metabolites.* 2012;2(3):596-613.
218. Krause T, Gerbershagen MU, Fiege M, et al. Dantrolene–a review of its pharmacology, therapeutic use and new developments. *Anaesthesia.* 2004;59(4):364-373.
219. Ward A, Chaffman MO, Sorkin EM. Dantrolene. A review of its pharmacodynamic and pharmacokinetic properties and therapeutic use in malignant hyperthermia, the neuroleptic malignant syndrome and an update of its use in muscle spasticity. *Drugs.* 1986;32:130-168.
220. Zhao F, Li P, Chen SR, et al. Dantrolene inhibition of ryanodine receptor Ca^{2+} release channels. *J Biol Chem.* 2001;276:13810-13816.
221. Ellis KO, Wessels FL. Muscle relaxant properties of the identified metabolites of dantrolene. *Naunyn Schmiedebergs Arch Pharmacol.* 1978;301(3):237-240.
222. Arnold TH, Epps JM, Cook HR, et al. Dantrolene sodium: urinary metabolites and hepatotoxicity. *Res Commun Chem Pathol Pharmacol.* 1983;39(3):381-398.
223. Kamen L, Henney HR, Runyan JD. A practical overview of tizanidine use for spasticity secondary to multiple sclerosis, stroke, and spinal cord injury. *Curr Med Res Opin.* 2008;24(2):425-439.
224. https://www.accessdata.fda.gov/drugsatfda_docs/label/2013/021447s011_020397s026lbl.pdf. Last accessed 3 January 2018.
225. Koch P, Hirst DR, von Wartburg BR. Biological fate of sirdalud in animals and man. *Xenobiotica.* 1989;19(11):1255-1265.
226. Crestani F, Low K, Keist R, et al. Molecular targets for the myelorelaxant action of diazepam. *Mol Pharmacol.* 2001;59:442-445.
227. Basile AS, Lippa AS, Skolnick P. Anxioselective anxiolytics: can less be more? *Eur J Pharmacol.* 2004;500:441-451.
228. Date SK, Hemavathi KG, Gulati OD. Investigation of the muscle relaxant activity of nitrazepam. *Arch Int Pharmacodyn Ther.* 1984;272(1):129-139.
229. https://www.accessdata.fda.gov/drugsatfda_docs/label/2008/013263s083lbl.pdf. Last accessed 3 January 2018.
230. Klotz U. Klinische Pharmakokinetik von Diazepam und seinen biologisch aktiven Metaboliten. *Klin Wochenschr.* 1978;56(18): 895-904.
231. Jack ML, Colburn WA. Pharmacokinetic model for diazepam and its major metabolite desmethyldiazepam following diazepam administration. *J Pharmaceut Sci.* 1983;72:1318-1323.
232. Jung F, Richardson TH, Raucy JL, et al. Diazepam metabolism by cDNA-expressed human 2C P450s: identification of P4502C18 and P4502C19 as low K(M) diazepam N-demethylases. *Drug Metab Dispos.* 1997;25(2):133-139.
233. Dolly JO, Aoki KR. The structure and mode of action of different botulinum toxins. *Eur J Neurol.* 2006;13(suppl 4):1-9.
234. Dolly JO, Black J, Williams RS, et al. Acceptors for botulinum neurotoxin reside on motor nerve terminals and mediate its internalization. *Nature.* 1984;307:457-460.
235. Schiavo G, Benfenati F, Poulain B, et al. Tetanus and botulinum-B neurotoxins block neurotransmitter release by proteolytic cleavage of synaptobrevin. *Nature.* 1992;359:832-835.
236. Koussoulakos S. Botulinum neurotoxin: the ugly duckling. *Eur Neurol.* 2009;61:331-342.
237. Dolly JO, Lande S, Wray DW. The effects of in vitro application of purified botulinum neurotoxin at mouse motor nerve terminals. *J Physiol.* 1987;386:475-484.
238. Ward AB. Spasticity treatment with botulinum toxins. *J Neural Transm.* 2008;115:607-616.
239. Bom A, Bradley M, Cameron K, et al. A novel concept of reversing neuromuscular block: chemical encapsulation of rocuronium bromide by a cyclodextrin-based synthetic host. *Angew Chem Int Ed Engl.* 2002;41:266-270.
240. Tarver GJ, Grove SJ, Buchanan K, et al. 2-O-substituted cyclodextrins as reversal agents for the neuromuscular blocker rocuronium bromide. *Bioorg Med Chem.* 2002;10:1819-1827.
241. Nag K, Singh DR, Shetti AN, et al. Sugammadex: a revolutionary drug in neuromuscular pharmacology. *Anesth Essays Res.* 2013;7(3):302-306.
242. Hemmerling TM, Zaouter C, Geldner G, et al. Sugammadex: a short review and clinical recommendations for the cardiac anesthesiologist. *Ann Card Anaesth.* 2010;13:206-216.
243. Berrih-Aknin S, Frenkian-Cuvelier M, Eymard B. Diagnostic and clinical classification of autoimmune myasthenia gravis. *J Autoimmun.* 2014;48-49:143-148.
244. Silvestri NJ, Wolfe GI. Myasthenia gravis. *Semin Neurol.* 2012;32(3):215-226.
245. Calvey TN, Wareing M, Williams NE, et al. Pharmacokinetics and pharmacological effects of neostigmine in man. *Br J Clin Pharmacol.* 1979;7(2):149-155.
246. Somani SM, Chan K, Dehghan A, et al. Kinetics and metabolism of intramuscular neostigmine in myasthenia gravis. *Clin Pharmacol Ther.* 1980;28(1):64-68.
247. Breyer-Pfaff U, Maier U, Brinkmann AM, et al. Pyridostigmine kinetics in healthy subjects and patients with myasthenia gravis. *Clin Pharmacol Ther.* 1985;37(5):495-501.
248. Zhao B, Moochhala SM, Lu J, et al. Determination of pyridostigmine bromide and its metabolites in biological samples. *J Pharm Pharm Sci.* 2006;9(1):71-81.
249. Gupta A, Goyal V, Srivastava AK, et al. Remission and relapse of myasthenia gravis on long-term azathioprine: an ambispective study. *Muscle Nerve* 2016;54(3):405-412.
250. Lavrnic D, Vujic A, Rakocevic-Stojanovic V, et al. Cyclosporine in the treatment of myasthenia gravis. *Acta Neurol Scand.* 2005;111(4):247-252.
251. https://www.accessdata.fda.gov/drugsatfda_docs/label/2011/016324s034s035lbl.pdf. Last accessed 19 February 2018.
252. https://www.accessdata.fda.gov/drugsatfda_docs/label/2009/050715s027, 050716s028lbl.pdf. Last accessed 19 February 2018.

253. Heatwole C, Ciafaloni E. Mycophenolate mofetil for myasthenia gravis: a clear and present controversy. *Neuropsychiatr Dis Treat.* 2008;4(6):1203-1209.
254. https://www.accessdata.fda.gov/drugsatfda_docs/label/2009/050722s021, 050723s019, 050758s019, 050759s024lbl.pdf. Last accessed 19 February 2018.
255. German CL, Baladi MG, McFadden LM, et al. Regulation of the dopamine and vesicular monoamine transporters: pharmacological targets and implications for disease. *Pharmacol Rev.* 2015;67(4):1005-1024.
256. Yao Z, Wei X, Wu X, et al. Preparation and evaluation of tetrabenazine enantiomers and all eight stereoisomers of dihydrotetrabenazine as VMAT2 inhibitors. *Eur J Med Chem.* 2011;46(5):1841-1848.
257. Mehvar R, Jamali F, Watson MW, et al. Pharmacokinetics of tetrabenazine and its major metabolite in man and rat. Bioavailability and dose dependency studies. *Drug Metab Dispos.* 1987;15(2):250-255.
258. Derangula VR, Pilli NR, Nadavala SK, et al. Liquid chromatography-tandem mass spectrometric assay for the determination of tetrabenazine and its active metabolites in human plasma: a pharmacokinetic study. *Biomed Chromatogr.* 2013;27(6):792-801.
259. https://www.accessdata.fda.gov/drugsatfda_docs/label/2017/209241lbl.pdf. Last accessed 3 January 2018.
260. Grigoriadis DE, Smith E, Hoare SRJ, et al. Pharmacologic characterization of valbenazine (NBI-98854) and its metabolites. *J Pharmacol Exp Ther.* 2017;361(3):454-461.

Structure Challenge Answers

1a. D and F, 1b. F, 1c. Safinamide (F) is less likely to have drug-drug interactions, whereas the metabolism of rasagiline (D) may be altered by Cimetidine, a known CYP1A2 inhibitor.

2a. B and C, 2b. C, 2c. Dimethyl fumarate (C) is not contraindicated in patients with cardiovascular conditions, whereas fingolimod (B) is.

3a. A and G, 3b. A, 3c. Dopamine agonists are known to cause somnolence. However, given the high molecular weight and the number of polar functional groups cabergoline (A) is less likely to cross the BBB compared to pramipexole (G).

4a. E and H, 4b. H. 4c. Tizanidine (H) is not known to cause drug dependence, whereas carisoprodol (E) and its metabolite Meprobate interact with $GABA_A$ receptor and have benzodiazepine-like effects potentially leading to dependence, withdraw, and abuse.

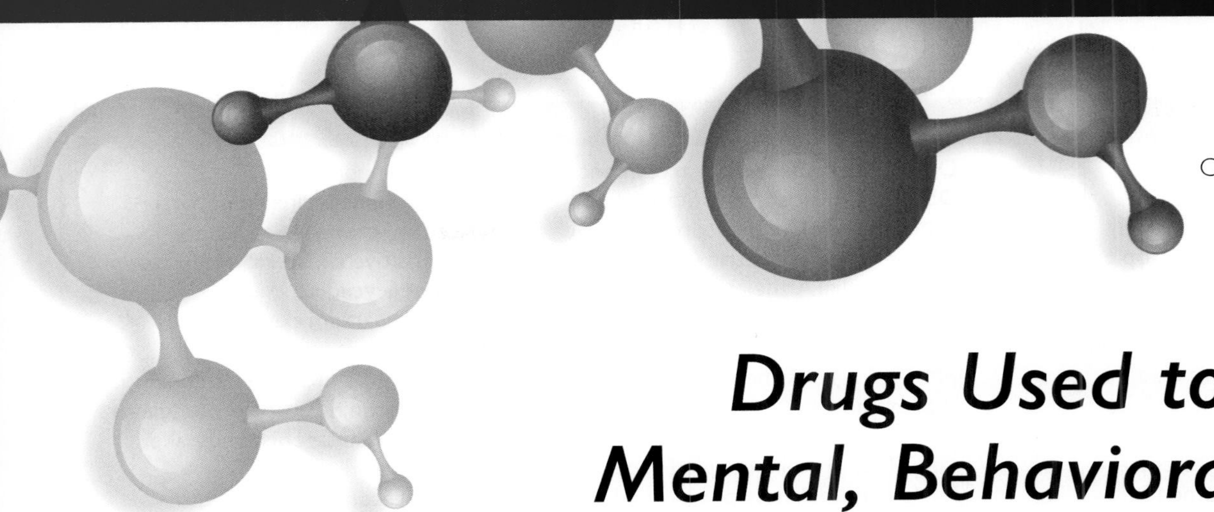

CHAPTER 11

Drugs Used to Treat Mental, Behavioral, and Cognitive Disorders

Clinton E. Canal, Raymond G. Booth, and David A. Williams

Drugs covered in this chapter:

ANTIPSYCHOTIC DRUGS

PHENOTHIAZINE/THIOXANTHENES
- Chlorpromazine
- Perphenazine
- Thiothixene
- Butyrophenone
- Droperidol
- Haloperidol
- Pimozide

DIARYLAZEPINES
- Asenapine
- Clozapine
- Loxapine
- Olanzapine
- Quetiapine

BENZISOXAZOLE/BENZISOTHIAZOLES
- Iloperidone
- Lurasidone
- Paliperidone
- Risperidone
- Ziprasidone

BENZAMIDE
- Amisulpride

PHENYLPIPERAZINES
- Aripiprazole
- Brexpiprazole
- Cariprazine

MISCELLANEOUS DRUGS
- Tetrabenazines for tardive dyskinesia
- Pimavanserin for Parkinson's disease psychosis

ANXIOLYTIC DRUGS ACTING AT GABA RECEPTORS

BENZODIAZEPINES
- Chlordiazepoxide
- Diazepam
- Flurazepam
- Oxazepam

NONBENZODIAZEPINE
- Eszopiclone
- Zaleplon
- Zolpidem

MISCELLANEOUS DRUGS
- Baclofen

ANTIDEPRESSANT DRUGS

TRICYCLIC TERTIARY AMINES
- Amitriptyline
- Doxepin
- Clomipramine
- Imipramine
- (+)-Trimipramine

TRICYCLIC SECONDARY AMINES
- Amoxapine
- Desipramine
- Maprotiline
- Nortriptyline
- Protriptyline

SELECTIVE SEROTONIN REUPTAKE INHIBITORS (SSRIS)
- (±)-Citalopram
- (+)-Escitalopram (S-citalopram)
- (±)-Fluoxetine
- Fluvoxamine
- (−)-Paroxetine
- (+)-Sertraline

ATYPICAL DRUGS
- (−)-Atomoxetine
- Bupropion
- Desvenlafaxine
- (−)-Duloxetine
- (−)-Levomirtazapine
- Trazodone
- Venlafaxine
- Vilazodone
- Vortioxetine
- Ketamine

NEUROACTIVE STEROID
- Brexanolone (allopregnanolone)

MONOAMINE OXIDASE INHIBITORS (MAOIS)
- Phenelzine
- Tranylcypromine

MOOD STABILIZERS
- Lithium carbonate

ALZHEIMER'S DISEASE DRUGS

CHOLINESTERASE INHIBITORS
- Donepezil
- Galantamine
- Rivastigmine

NMDA RECEPTOR ANTAGONISTS
- Memantine

ATTENTION-DEFICIT HYPERACTIVITY DISORDER (ADHD) DRUGS

NONSTIMULANT DRUGS FOR ADHD
- Atomoxetine
- Bupropion
- Clonidine
- Guanfacine
- Imipramine

STIMULANT DRUGS FOR ADHD
- Methylphenidate
- Dexmethylphenidate
- Dextroamphetamine
- Lisdexamphetamine

Abbreviations

5-HT serotonin
α, A alpha adrenergic
ACh acetylcholine
ACTH adrenocorticotropic hormone
ADHD attention-deficit hyperactivity disorder
AMPA α-amino-3-hydroxy-5-methyl-4-isoxazolepropionic acid
AUC area under the curve
Aβ amyloid-beta peptide
AChE acetylcholinesterase
AD Alzheimer's dementia
ADL activities of daily living
APP amyloid precursor protein
BuChE butyrylcholinesterase
CES1A1 carboxylesterase 1A1
CNS central nervous system
CRF corticotrophin-releasing factor
CYP cytochrome P450
D, DA dopamine
DAT dopamine transporter
DDI drug-drug interaction
DMT disease-modifying treatment
DSM-5 Diagnostic and Statistical Manual of Mental Disorders of the American Psychiatric Association
FAD familial Alzheimer's dementia
FDA U.S. Food and Drug Administration
FMRP fragile X mental retardation protein
GABA γ-aminobutyric acid
GPCR G protein–coupled receptor
HPA hypothalamus-pituitary-adrenal axis
LVM levomilnacipran
M muscarinic acetylcholine receptor
MAO monoamine oxidase
MAOI monoamine oxidase inhibitor
MDD major depressive disorder
nAChR nicotinic acetylcholine receptor
NaSSA noradrenergic and specific serotonergic antidepressant
NE norepinephrine
NET norepinephrine transporter
NMDA N-methyl-D-aspartate
PAM positive allosteric modulator
PCP phencyclidine
PDD postpartum depression
PMS premenstrual syndrome
SAD sporadic Alzheimer's dementia
SARI serotonin receptor modulators (serotonin antagonist/reuptake inhibitors)
SERT serotonin transporter
SMS serotonin modulators and stimulants
SNRI serotonin and norepinephrine reuptake inhibitor
SSRI selective serotonin reuptake inhibitor
TCA tricyclic amine antidepressant
VMAT vesicular monoamine transporter

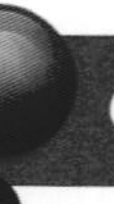

CLINICAL SIGNIFICANCE

Paul L. Price, PharmD, BCPP

In the evaluation and application of the principles of pharmacotherapeutics to psychiatric disease states, a clinician must have a thorough understanding of all the variables that contribute to the selection and application of drug therapies to this patient population. The practice of psychiatry does not have the luxury of predetermining what will be the best choice of drug for an individual patient. The clinician can only make selections based on the patient's or the patient's family members' history of psychotropic medication use, if available. Otherwise, the selection is determined by the evidence-based effectiveness in a disease state, adverse effect profiles of said entities, preexisting disease states present in the specific patient, other medications in the treatment of these disease states, and the potential for drug-drug and/or drug-disease state interactions that could limit treatment. The lack, to date, of head-to-head clinical trials of antidepressants, for example, can lead to the practitioner's assumption that, from an effectiveness perspective, all antidepressants are equal. This assumption necessitates the practitioner taking into consideration each drug's variant properties and clinically relevant aspects within therapeutic groups. Many other examples exist including the varying types of medications used to treat ADHD or cognitive disorders like Alzheimer's dementia.

The pharmacology/pharmacodynamics, pharmacokinetics, and adverse effects of psychotropic drugs are widely variant and dependent on each drug's chemical structure, receptor affinities, and actions. Understanding a drug's medicinal chemistry is critical to understanding effectiveness and the potential for adverse effects. For example, adverse effects with the atypical antipsychotic agents are linked to the chemical nature and variances of each medication. When comparing the side effect profiles of quetiapine (dibenzothiazepine) versus lurasidone (benzoisothiazole piperazine), quetiapine's side effect profile is less likely to cause extrapyramidal adverse effects compared with lurasidone. Antihistamine effects (sedation and weight gain) are much more common with quetiapine when compared with lurasidone. However, quetiapine is more likely to cause QTc prolongation when compared with lurasidone. Thus, the clinician can use structural clues to use-limiting adverse effects to select the atypical antipsychotic that the patient will best tolerate, fully aware of the potential toxicity risks. Another aspect to consider is the long-acting injectable prodrug of the atypical antipsychotic aripiprazole lauroxil. Once administered intramuscularly, aripiprazole lauroxil, via enzyme mediated hydrolysis, is converted to N-hydroxymethyl aripiprazole, which hydrolyzes to aripiprazole. This results in an extend release of the prodrug and a prolonged duration of action compared with free aripiprazole.

The principles of medicinal chemistry are critical in the application of the principles of pharmacotherapeutics. They are complementary sciences that, taken together, promote an in-depth scientific understanding of drug action that can inform rational decision-making in the care of patients with mental, behavioral, and cognitive disorders.

Overview of Drugs Used to Treat Mental, Behavioral, and Cognitive Disorders

Psychotherapeutic agents differ in their ability to treat unique psychiatric symptoms. Thus, an appropriate clinical diagnosis—currently founded on the presence of distinct symptoms—is critical to selecting an efficacious drug. The definitive diagnostic criteria for psychiatric disorders in the United States are described in the *Diagnostic and Statistical Manual of Mental Disorders of the American Psychiatric Association* (DSM-5).[1] This chapter focuses on the medicinal chemistry of drugs that treat psychotic disorders, anxiety disorders, depressive disorders, and attention-deficit hyperactivity disorder (ADHD). It also covers the medicinal chemistry of drugs that treat Alzheimer's dementia.

Psychoses and Anxiety Disorders

Psychotic disorders are arguably the most severe mental illnesses and are characterized foremost by hallucinations and/or delusions, wherein consensus reality is distorted or has disintegrated. Defined psychotic disorders include schizophrenia, schizoaffective disorder, schizophreniform disorder, delusional disorder, postpartum psychosis, psychosis associated with bipolar disorder or depression, psychosis caused by a general medical disorder (e.g., Parkinson's disease psychosis), and substance-induced psychosis. Lifetime prevalence of psychotic disorders is about 0.75%,[2] and recent studies reveal that about 6% of otherwise healthy people report isolated psychotic experiences—reports of hallucinations are much more common than delusions.[3] Schizophrenia, the most common psychotic disorder, has a prevalence of about 0.64%.[2] Schizophrenia's economic burden is estimated to be as high as 1.65% of gross domestic product.[4]

In anxiety disorders, the ability to comprehend reality is retained, but cognition and mood problems can be disabling. Anxiety can be defined as a sense of apprehensive expectation. In reasonable amounts and at appropriate times, anxiety is helpful (e.g., anxiety before an examination may motivate a student to initiate an appropriate study plan). Too much anxiety, however, can be deleterious. Anxiety can be considered pathological when it is either completely inappropriate to the situation or is in excess of what the situation normally should call for. An example of the former is nocturnal panic attacks—episodes of extreme anxiety that arise out of one of the most physiologically quiet times of the day, stage III/IV sleep. An example of the latter is an irrational fear of public spaces (agoraphobia). The estimates for lifetime morbid risk/12-month prevalence are 18%/12% for specific phobia, 13%/7% for social phobia, 9%/2% for generalized anxiety disorder, 7%/2% for panic disorder, and 4%/2% for agoraphobia.[5]

Schizophrenia

A thorough description of schizophrenia was reported 100 years ago by the German psychiatrist Emil Kraepelin. Patients presented with a severe, progressive and chronic type of mental enfeeblement, which was not caused by known infections or brain injury. Kraepelin carefully annotated symptoms that included hallucinations (e.g., hearing voices), delusions (e.g., being persecuted), incoherence of thought and thought disturbances (e.g., thoughts are "pushed" into mind or do not belong to the patient), stereotyped thinking (persistence of single ideas) and behaviors (e.g., echocholia), bizarre movements (e.g., "waxy flexibility"), inattention, inappropriate emotions, intellectual and behavioral negativism (e.g., knowingly responding incorrectly to questions or acting contrarily), blunted affect, avolition (e.g., catatonia) and loss of will power, susceptibility to influence, social withdrawal (autistic-like), and language or speech problems (e.g., paraphasia).[6] Kraepelin also described bodily symptoms, including sleep and appetite disturbances. Meanwhile, the Swiss psychiatrist Eugen Bleuler had coined this disorder "schizophrenia" as there was a perceived "schism" or splitting in mental functioning.[7]

The modern definition of schizophrenia as defined by the DSM-5[8] takes into account three major root characteristics: (1) chronicity and poor outcomes, as described by Kraepelin[6]; (2) dissociative and negative symptoms (diminished emotional expression or avolition), as described by Bleuler[7]; and (3) reality distortion or positive symptoms, as described by Schneider.[9] The diagnostic criterion for characteristic symptoms of schizophrenia, "Criterion A", requires two or more of the following to be present for a significant proportion of time during a 1-month period: (1) delusions, (2) hallucinations, (3) disorganized speech, (4) grossly disorganized or catatonic behavior, (5) negative symptoms. At least one of the characteristic symptoms must be delusions, hallucinations, or disorganized speech. In addition to Criterion A, there are two other criteria, "Criterion B" and "Criterion C." The former notes that "for a significant portion of the time since the onset of the disturbance, one or more major areas of functioning, such as work, interpersonal relations, or self-care, are markedly below the level achieved prior to the onset (or when the onset is in childhood or adolescence, failure to achieve expected level of interpersonal, academic, or occupational achievement)."[8] "Criterion C" states that continuous symptoms must persist for 6 months. Finally, before a diagnosis of schizophrenia is made, schizoaffective and mood disorders as well as psychotic symptoms caused by substances (e.g., medications or illicit drugs) or other medical conditions must be ruled out. The DSM-5 also introduced psychopathological dimensions—presence/absence of specific psychiatric symptoms and numerically categorized symptom severity—to improve the ability to describe the heterogeneity of schizophrenia in a valid and clinically useful manner.[10] DSM-5 criteria for schizophrenia do not take into account cognitive symptoms observed in schizophrenia, even though they are prominent and impair quality of life. These include deficits in working memory, attention, and verbal learning and memory.

Etiology of Schizophrenia

Schizophrenia is a neurodevelopmental disorder that often manifests during late adolescence. Although environmental factors influence the development of schizophrenia, heritability is about 80%.[11] Its genetic etiology involves numerous common alleles with small to moderate effect, and rare to ultrarare, but highly penetrant copy number variations.[12] A large (~150,000 subjects) genome-wide association study reported 108 schizophrenia-associated loci.[13] Genes within associated loci included *DRD2* (dopamine D_2 receptor), *CHRNA3*, *CHRNA5*, and *CHRNB4* (nicotinic acetylcholine receptors), as well as genes involved in glutamate (e.g., *GRM3*, glutamate mGluR3 receptor) and GABA (e.g., *IGSF9B*) neurotransmission, synaptic development and plasticity, and several others which encode mRNAs that interact with FMRP, the protein lost in fragile X syndrome (the most common monogenetic cause of intellectual disability and autism).[12-14]

Many of the genes implicated in schizophrenia map to glutamatergic pyramidal cells and GABAergic interneurons in the cortex and to dopamine D_1- and D_2-containing medium spiny neurons in the striatum,[15] inferring alterations in excitatory-inhibitory homeostasis as well as dysregulation of dopamine neurotransmission. These observations support the predominant theories of schizophrenia etiology (described below). Most of the genetic polymorphisms observed across studies, however, do not change exonic sequences; In other words, schizophrenia-associated genes likely alter splicing, transcription, and noncoding RNAs.

A revealing development from several massive, genome-wide association studies is that alterations in common loci observed in schizophrenia are also observed in other psychiatric disorders, including bipolar disorder, clinical depression, autism spectrum disorder, ADHD, and posttraumatic stress disorder, pointing to common underlying and/or interconnected pathologies.[16-18] Also revealing, the personality trait "neuroticism" associates with almost every psychiatric disorder, including schizophrenia.[19] Despite clarifications regarding the genetics of schizophrenia, recent findings have not yet converged on any new, well-defined targets for medicinal chemistry drug discovery.

Investigations of environmental influences have focused on prenatal and perinatal risk factors for abnormal brain development. For example, retrospective analyses show that schizophrenia is associated with influenza or other virus exposure and Rh factor incompatibility during prenatal development, and with obstetrical complications, such as asphyxia during childbirth. These environmental insults activate inflammatory processes including cytokines and brain microglia that likely contribute to gray matter loss in schizophrenia.[20] Genetic and environmental interactions—involving several common polymorphisms and a perturbed womb environment—may converge with precipitating factors such as psychosocial stress and synaptic pruning in the cortex during adolescence to cause schizophrenia.

Neuroanatomical changes associated with psychoses include loss of dendritic arbors and synaptic spines in cortical pyramidal neurons, thinning of cortical layers, decreased hippocampal CA1 volume, and enlargement of the brain's ventricular system. Also, neurochemical abnormalities, including changes in the central dopamine system, are well-documented in psychoses. Neuropathology in schizophrenia (e.g., overt loss of nerve cells), however, is not as striking as neurodegenerative diseases such as Parkinson's or Alzheimer's disease.

Models of Schizophrenia Etiology

There are three interrelated models for studying schizophrenia etiology: (1) the neurodevelopmental model, (2) the excitation-inhibition imbalance model, and (3) the "dopamine hypothesis"[21] (now well-tested and verified to be a model). Alterations of dopaminergic neurotransmission in psychoses have been studied for more than 50 years; thus there is substantially more knowledge surrounding the dopamine model (discussed in detail in the next section). The neurodevelopmental and the excitation-inhibition imbalance models have evolved more recently. Collectively, the models posit that schizophrenia is caused by disruptions in GABAergic and glutamatergic networks and perturbations in dopamine signaling in subcortical and cortical brain regions during critical periods of synaptic formation and rearrangement. The excitation-inhibition model of schizophrenia asserts that cortical pyramidal neurons are in a hyperexcited, disorganized state, creating neural noise that interferes with normal reality judgment. Cortical hyperexcitability results from a loss of inhibition from GABAergic interneurons. This model emerged in part from observations that glutamate N-methyl-D-aspartate (NMDA) receptor antagonists (e.g., phencyclidine, PCP or "angel dust") can cause a psychotomimetic state that includes positive and negative symptoms. Blockade of glutamate NMDA receptors expressed on GABAergic interneurons inhibits GABA neurotransmission, subsequently enhancing glutamate neurotransmission.[22] Neuroimaging studies in patients with schizophrenia support this model,[23] but thus far, no compounds that directly modify glutamate neurotransmission have succeeded in clinical trials for schizophrenia.

The Dopamine Model

According to the dopamine model of schizophrenia, psychosis symptoms result from aberrant dopamine neurotransmission—specifically, increased dopamine neurotransmission in the mesolimbic pathway (including the ventral striatum) and decreased dopamine neurotransmission in the mesocortical pathway (including the prefrontal cortex). The model arose initially from observations that the first effective antipsychotic drugs, the phenothiazines, e.g., chlorpromazine, affected brain dopamine metabolism.[24] Further support emanated from observations of elevated psychostimulant-induced dopamine release in the striatum, but reduced release in the prefrontal cortex in persons with schizophrenia. Also, acutely psychotic patients, as well as patients prodromal for schizophrenia, display increased presynaptic striatal dopamine synthesis.[25] Increases in expression of dopamine D_2 receptors, as well as genetic polymorphisms at a locus that includes the D_2 gene, *DRD2*, have also been observed.[13]

Many antipsychotic medications bind to D_2 receptors with high affinity (K_i < 10 nM) (see Table 11.1), and their affinities for D_2 strongly correlate with their average therapeutic doses.[26] Binding to dopamine D_2 receptors in vivo also correlates with clinical efficacy[27]; neuroimaging studies suggest about 65% occupancy of dopamine D_2 receptors is required for efficacy of typical antipsychotics. Although most antipsychotics block D_2 receptors, functional interactions are complex, involving competitive antagonism, inverse agonism, and partial agonism. Moreover, it is now realized that G protein–coupled receptors (GPCRs), including D_2, can couple to multiple, distinct, intracellular signaling pathways, and drugs can possess a bias for activating or inactivating certain pathways.[28] In other words, based on the unique chemical interactions they have with the receptor, ligands can stabilize unique receptor conformations, resulting in unique cellular effects.[29-31] Thus, the biochemical effects, and by extension, clinical and side effects of antipsychotics are likely not due to simple blockade of endogenous agonist (dopamine) access to the D_2 receptor. More likely, they reduce dopamine neuron activity via unique actions at D_2 receptors. Antipsychotic drug discovery programs are exploring D_2-biased agonists which might maximize efficacy while minimizing side effects.[32]

Dopamine Receptors in Schizophrenia

There are five genetically encoded dopamine receptors (D_1, D_2 [with short and long splice variants], D_3, D_4, and D_5) and each is a GPCR. Historically, there were few medicinal chemical probes specific enough to distinguish between the five subtypes; thus dopamine receptors often are classified as the D_1-type (includes D_5) that stimulates adenylyl cyclase, and the D_2-type (includes D_3 and D_4) that inhibits adenylyl cyclase. Several chemical probes are available that can distinguish between the general D_1-type and D_2-type receptor families (Fig. 11.1). The *R*-(+)-isomer of the benzazepine derivative, SKF 38393, is used for research as a selective D_1-type partial agonist. Meanwhile, the structurally related benzazepine derivative, *R*-(+)-SCH 23390, is used as a selective D_1-type receptor antagonist. Although not very selective for D_1-type over D_2-type receptors, the rigid benzophenanthridine derivative (+)-dihydrexidine is a useful research tool because it is a D_1-type full-efficacy agonist.[33] Although binding to dopamine D_1 receptors does not correlate with antipsychotic potencies, some studies suggest altered levels of cortical D_1 receptors in drug naïve patients with psychosis.[34] Since D_1 activation can improve cognitive function, such as working memory, which is impaired in schizophrenia, researchers are developing D_1-selective agonists to treat cognitive dysfunction in schizophrenia.[35] D_1 activation, however, is associated with nausea and vomiting.

D_2-type full agonists, such as the pyrazole derivative (−)-quinpirole, and D_2-type antagonists, such as (−)-sulpiride and raclopride, also are available to researchers, but these compounds do not distinguish D_2 and D_3 receptors well. The dopamine D_3 receptor has been of interest to neuropharmacologists and medicinal chemists since the early 1990s because of its preferential distribution in certain limbic regions of mammalian brain—notably in the nucleus accumbens (part of the ventral striatum) where it modulates glutamate and dopamine neurotransmission.[36] It was proposed that D_3-selective drugs might be developed as antipsychotic agents with preferential limbic

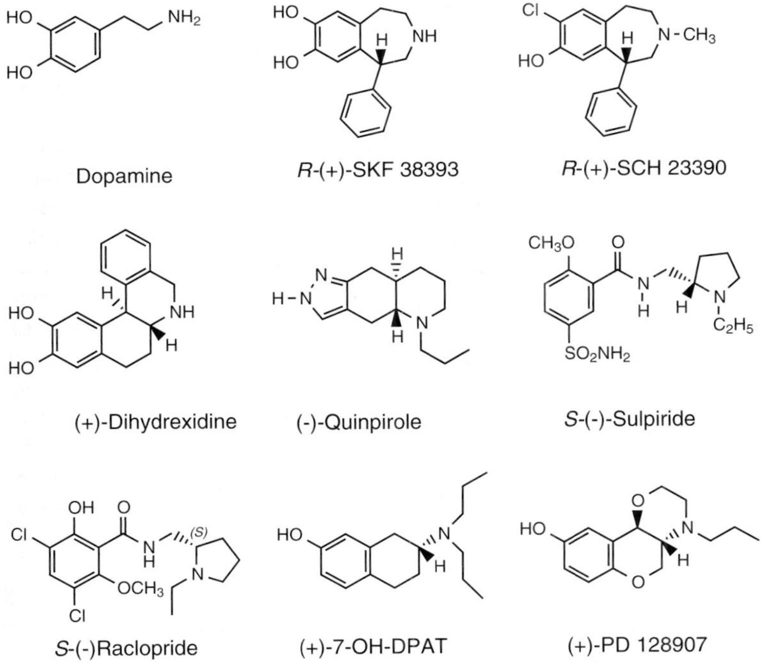

Figure 11.1 Structures of compounds useful for characterizing dopamine receptors.

antidopaminergic actions while sparing the extrapyramidal basal ganglia. Theoretically, this tactic would treat psychotic symptoms but prevent the neurological movement disorder side effects associated with antipsychotic drug therapy.

The D_3-preferring tetrahydronaphthalene, (+)-7-hydroxy-N,N-di-n-propyl-2-aminotetralin (7-OH-DPAT) helped to elucidate the distribution of D_3 receptors in the brain ex vivo, though in vivo, under conditions of high extracellular NaCl conditions, 7-OH-DPAT does not adequately discriminate D_3 from D_2.[36] (+)-PD 128907, a congener of 7-OH-DPAT, remains one of the most selective D_3 agonists for experimental purposes. Confirmatory results for targeting D_3 for schizophrenia were not observed until 2017, when F17464, a preferential D_3 antagonist, was shown to be efficacious in a placebo-controlled phase 2 study of patients with an acute exacerbation of schizophrenia.[37] The antipsychotics cariprazine, asenapine, and perphenazine bind D_3 with very high affinity ($K_i < 1$ nM) (Table 11.1), and there is some evidence that targeting D_3 may improve negative symptoms of schizophrenia, which are more difficult to treat than positive symptoms.

Enthusiasm for D_4 was sparked when it was found that the prototypical and highly effective second-generation antipsychotic, clozapine, had higher affinity at D_4 relative to all other dopamine receptors. D_4 ligands, however, failed in clinical trials for schizophrenia. Nevertheless, there remains a groundswell of interest in developing selective D_4 ligands as pharmacotherapies for Parkinson's disease, addiction, and other disorders.[38] A small number of human genetic studies have reported associations between the D_5 gene (*DRD5*) and schizophrenia, but there has been only limited interest from the medicinal chemistry community. An extremely high affinity ($K_i < 0.1$ nM), D_5 antagonist has been reported,[39] but there are no others.

The dopamine D_1-type and D_2-type receptor families are differentially distributed in mammalian forebrain dopaminergic pathways. The extrapyramidal nigrostriatal pathway, which plays a key role in locomotor coordination, consists of neurons with cell bodies in the A9 pars compacta of the substantia nigra in the midbrain. These neurons project to the basal ganglia structures caudate nucleus and putamen (collectively referred to as the dorsal striatum) in the forebrain (Fig. 11.2). Degeneration of neurons in the nigrostriatal pathway is the hallmark pathological feature of Parkinson's disease, clinically manifested as bradykinesia, muscular rigidity, resting tremor, and impairment of postural balance.

The mesolimbic and mesocortical pathway, involved in integrating emotions and perceptions, motivated behaviors, and executive functions, consist of neurons with cell bodies in the A8 and A10 ventral tegmentum area. These neurons project to limbic forebrain structures, including the nucleus accumbens (ventral striatum) and the amygdala, and to higher levels of cerebral function, such as the frontal cortex (Fig. 11.2). Reiterating, according to the dopamine model, increased dopaminergic neurotransmission in limbic pathways contributes to positive symptoms (e.g., hallucinations and delusions), but negative symptoms (e.g., catatonia) may be mediated by hypoactivity of dopaminergic signaling in the prefrontal cortex.

All antipsychotics, except pimavanserin, act in both extrapyramidal and limbic brain regions at D_2-type dopamine receptors that can be located postsynaptically (on cell bodies, dendrites, and nerve terminals of other neurons) as well as presynaptically on dopamine neurons. Dopamine receptors located presynaptically on dopamine cell bodies and nerve terminals are called autoreceptors and act to decrease dopamine synthesis and release and to decrease neuronal firing probability (Fig. 11.3). Low concentrations of certain dopamine agonists can stereospecifically activate dopamine D_2-type autoreceptors to decrease dopamine synthesis and release,[40,41] thus reducing dopaminergic neurotransmission. Consistent with the dopamine model of schizophrenia, selective dopamine autoreceptor agonists

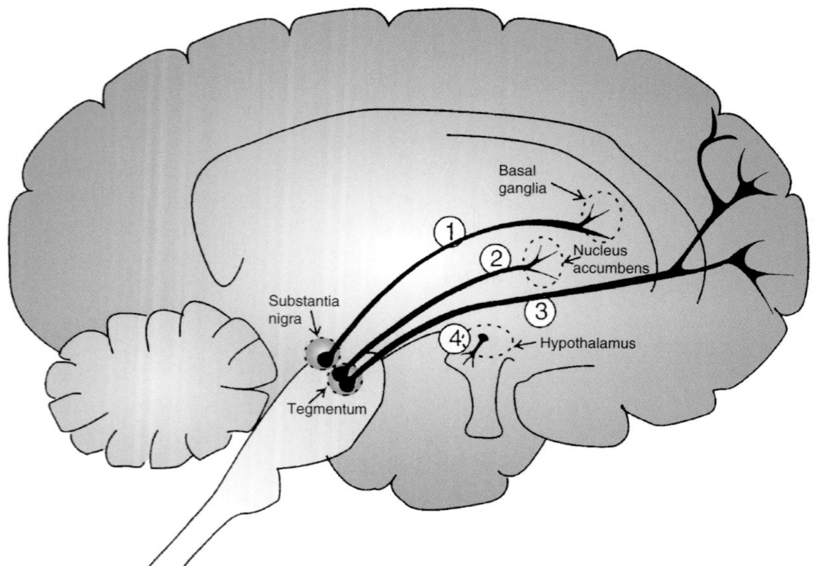

① **Nigrostriatal pathway:** projects from the substantia nigra to the basal ganglia

② **Mesolimbic pathway:** projects from the ventral tegmental area to the nucleus accumbens

③ **Mesocortical pathway**: projects from the ventral tegmental area to the prefrontal cortex

④ **Tuberoinfundibular pathway:** projects from the hypothalamus to the anterior pituitary gland

Figure 11.2 Dopamine pathways in human brain.

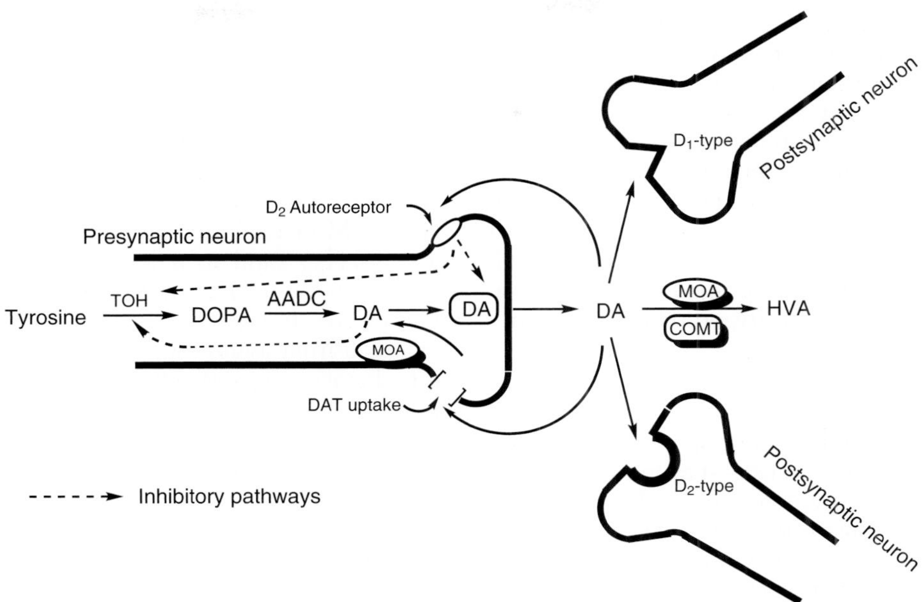

Figure 11.3 Tyrosine is hydroxylated in a rate-limiting step by tyrosine hydroxylase (TOH) to form dihydroxylphenylalanine (DOPA), which is decarboxylated by L-aromatic amino acid decarboxylase (AADC) to form dopamine (DA). Newly synthesized DA is stored in vesicles, from which release occurs into the synaptic cleft by depolarization of the presynaptic neuron in the presence of Ca^{2+}. The DA released into the synaptic cleft stimulates postsynaptic D_1- and D_2-type receptors enabling neurotransmission. Released DA also stimulates presynaptic D_2-type autoreceptors that modulate DA synthesis and release through negative feedback. The action of synaptic DA is inactivated largely via uptake into the presynaptic neuron by the DA transporter (DAT) located on the nerve terminal membrane. Cytoplasmic pools of DA may undergo metabolic deamination by monoamine oxidase (MAO), an enzyme bound to the outer membrane of mitochondria, to form dihydroxyphenylacetaldehyde, which oxides to didydroxyphenylacetate (DOPAC). The DA or DOPAC may undergo methylation by catechol-O-methyltransferase (COMT), ultimately forming homovanillic acid (HVA), a metabolite excreted in urine.

could, theoretically, be pharmacotherapeutic agents in schizophrenia and related mental illnesses, and indeed newer antipsychotics, including aripiprazole, brexpiprazole, and cariprazine, possess D_2 autoreceptor agonist activity.

Pharmacotherapy of Schizophrenia and Related Psychoses

Antipsychotic drugs were historically called neuroleptics. This term suggested they "take hold" (*lepsis*) of the central nervous system (CNS) to suppress movement in addition to psychotic symptoms. While treating psychosis, classic neuroleptics, such as haloperidol, also cause debilitating extrapyramidal movement side effects. Indeed, the term "neuroleptic" is so synonymous with neurologic side effects that later developed antipsychotic drugs, with reduced risk of extrapyramidal effects, such as clozapine, were coined atypical neuroleptic drugs or second-generation antipsychotics. All new antipsychotics since clozapine are now simply called atypical antipsychotics. Though, likely forthcoming is an updated nomenclature based on a therapeutic continuum that takes into account: (1) efficacy to treat distinct psychiatric and cognitive symptoms and (2) specific side effects and side effect severity.

Chemical classes of typical antipsychotics include the phenothiazines, thioxanthenes, and butyrophenones. Atypical antipsychotic drug classes include the dibenzodiazepines, benzisoxazoles, benzamides, and phenylpiperazines. In general, pharmacotherapy with either typical/first-generation or atypical/second-generation antipsychotics effectively treats positive symptoms of schizophrenia, whereas negative symptoms—which greatly impair quality of life—are not as appreciably affected despite concerted drug discovery efforts. There is some evidence that certain atypical antipsychotics, including clozapine, amisulpride, olanzapine, risperidone, and cariprazine, have better efficacy than the typical antipsychotic, haloperidol, in the treatment of negative symptoms. However, pivotal double-blind, randomized, clinical trials comparing a first-generation/typical antipsychotic (perphenazine) versus second-generation/atypical antipsychotics (olanzapine, quetiapine, risperidone, ziprasidone) revealed no substantial differences in overall efficacy. All medications were associated with high discontinuation rates due to intolerable side effects or inefficacy. Moreover, extrapyramidal side effects, unexpectedly, were not less frequent in patients treated with the atypical drugs. Clozapine was the most effective drug for individuals with a poor symptom response to previous antipsychotics.[42] Despite these findings, atypical antipsychotic prescriptions for new patients far exceed typical antipsychotic prescriptions.

A more recent and thorough meta-analysis showed superior efficacy of clozapine, amisulpride, olanzapine, and risperidone compared to several other antipsychotics, regardless of typical versus atypical designation. For example, clozapine and amisulpride (both atypicals) were more efficacious than lurasidone and iloperidone (both atypicals).[43] Differences between antipsychotic drugs are particularly evident in their side-effect profiles,[43,44] but again, they are not clearly parsed by typical versus atypical categorization. We urge students, therefore, to pay close attention to chemical structures and unique receptor pharmacology profiles to gain a clearer understanding of mechanisms and side effects of specific antipsychotics until further recategorization of antipsychotics occurs. Indeed, each antipsychotic, by nature of its structure, and hence engagement with targets (its affinity, on/off kinetics, functional biases), is unique.

Mechanism of Action of Antipsychotics

Given that the pathogenesis of schizophrenia and other psychotic disorders remains unclear—beyond burgeoning views involving neurocytoarchitecture development, synapse formation and pruning, coordination of excitation and inhibition processes, neuroinflammation, and alterations in dopamine function—it is perhaps naïve to describe how drugs act at the molecular level to relieve the symptoms of these disorders. Nevertheless, it generally is agreed that the mechanism of action of nearly all antipsychotics includes modulation of dopamine neurotransmission in the mesolimbic-mesocortical pathways via direct interaction with D_2 receptors. Though, all antipsychotics also have an affinity for 5-HT_{2A} receptors[45] (Table 11.1), which likely contributes to antipsychotic efficacy. Indeed, activation of 5-HT_{2A} receptors potentiates dopamine release and can disturb perception and cognition[46-48]—antipsychotics are 5-HT_{2A} inverse agonists[49,50] which block these effects. Most convincingly, pimavanserin selectively targets 5-HT_{2A} (and to a lesser extent 5-HT_{2C}) receptors as an inverse agonist and effectively treats psychosis in Parkinson's disease.[51]

Aside from affinity for D_2 and 5-HT_{2A}, receptor binding characteristics of different antipsychotics are unique (Table 11.1). For example, certain antipsychotics target other (non-D_2-type) dopamine receptors, serotonin 5-HT_{1A} and/or 5-HT_{2C}, acetylcholine muscarinic, and/or histamine H_1 receptors, all of which are known to modulate dopamine synthesis and/or release in striatal and cortical systems, potentially contributing to efficacy.[52-55]

Furthermore, activation of 5-HT_{2C} receptors (converse to activation of 5-HT_{2A} receptors) produces antipsychotic-like effects in various rodent models of schizophrenia,[48,54,56] and aripiprazole possesses 5-HT_{2C} partial agonist activity. The most recent antipsychotics approved for schizophrenia

Table 11.1 Representative FDA-approved Antipsychotics: Affinities at Receptor Targets Implicated in Therapeutic and Side Effects, Oral Doses and Half-lives

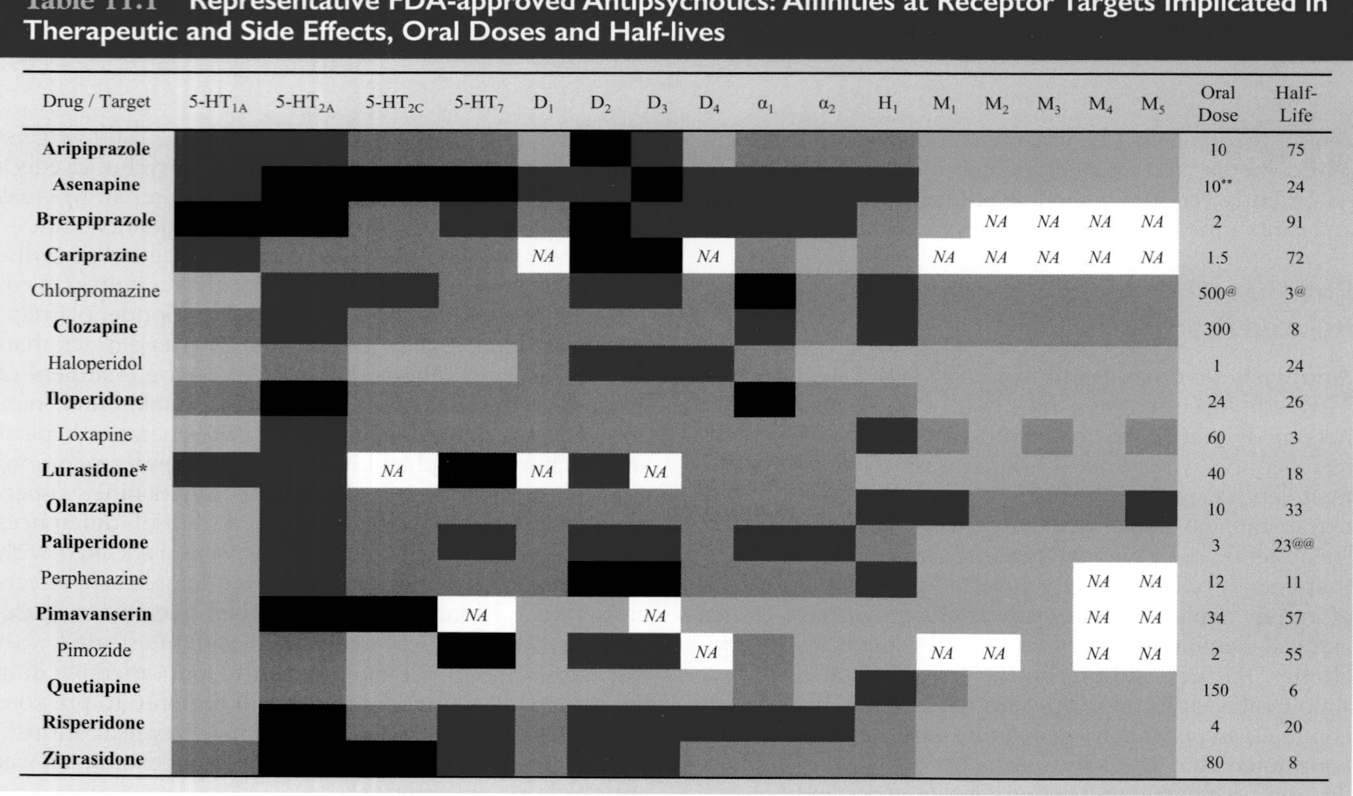

Drug / Target	5-HT_{1A}	5-HT_{2A}	5-HT_{2C}	5-HT_7	D_1	D_2	D_3	D_4	α_1	α_2	H_1	M_1	M_2	M_3	M_4	M_5	Oral Dose	Half-Life
Aripiprazole																	10	75
Asenapine																	10**	24
Brexpiprazole													*NA*	*NA*	*NA*	*NA*	2	91
Cariprazine					*NA*			*NA*				*NA*	*NA*	*NA*	*NA*	*NA*	1.5	72
Chlorpromazine																	500@	3@
Clozapine																	300	8
Haloperidol																	1	24
Iloperidone																	24	26
Loxapine																	60	3
Lurasidone*			*NA*		*NA*		*NA*										40	18
Olanzapine																	10	33
Paliperidone																	3	23@@
Perphenazine															*NA*	*NA*	12	11
Pimavanserin				*NA*			*NA*								*NA*	*NA*	34	57
Pimozide								*NA*				*NA*	*NA*		*NA*	*NA*	2	55
Quetiapine																	150	6
Risperidone																	4	20
Ziprasidone																	80	8

Black represents very high affinity (K_i < 1 nM). **Red** represents high affinity (K_i < 10 nM). **Gray** represents moderate affinity (K_i < 300 nM). **Light red** represents low affinity (K_i > 300 nM). *NA* denotes that data have not been reported. Values were culled from the PDSP website (Roth et al., 2000) in July 2018 or from the initial reported characterization of the drug and represent affinities at human cloned or human brain receptors, with the exception of * where some data are from rat or guinea pig brain tissue, as human data have not been reported. "Atypical" antipsychotics are emboldened. Half-life refers to approximate elimination half-life in hours, and oral dose is the lowest recommended target dose in mg/24 hr for adults with schizophrenia, provided in prescribing information. **Sublingual formulation. @ Not firmly established. @@ Extended-release formulation.

(cariprazine and brexpiprazole—see below) include 5-HT_{1A} partial agonist activity, similar to several other atypical antipsychotics. 5-HT_{1A} receptors are expressed at much higher densities in the cortex, relative to the striatum, and activation of 5-HT_{1A} receptors increases dopamine release in the cortex, potentially contributing to antipsychotic efficacy, especially regarding negative and cognitive symptoms.[57]

Structure-Activity Relationships

GPCR targets of antipsychotics share a three-dimensional structure consisting of a bundle of seven transmembrane alpha helices, connected by alternating intracellular and extracellular loops, with the N-terminus in the extracellular domain and C-terminus in the intracellular domain. Antipsychotics bind to the orthosteric (endogenous ligand) pocket inside of GPCRs. This pocket is characterized by many hydrophobic side chains from residues in transmembranes two, three, five, six, and seven. There is a fair to high degree of amino acid sequence overlap within the transmembrane helices between different GPCRs, and even more overlap in the sequences that form the binding sites of endogenous ligands. This contributes to the polypharmacology of antipsychotics, i.e., their high affinity for multiple GPCRs.

All extant antipsychotics possess a basic amine (a protonatable nitrogen atom) that forms a salt bridge with the side chain carboxylate of an aspartate residue in the third transmembrane, Asp3.32, present in all aminergic GPCRs. This interaction is crucial for binding.[58] Also, antipsychotics have hydrogen bond acceptors and donors, hydrophobic groups, and aromatic rings that form distinct interactions with GPCR residues. These interactions determine affinities and the functional activities of antipsychotics at GPCRs. The detailed molecular structure of the human dopamine D_3 receptor, in complex with eticlopride, a potent D_2/D_3 receptor antagonist, is resolved and illustrates: (1) how an antagonist binds to the receptor and (2) the shape of an inactive GPCR highly targeted by antipsychotics.[59] Canonical interactions include a disulfide bond bridging a cysteine in the second extracellular loop and a cysteine in transmembrane three (Cys3.25). Another interaction believed to be critical in stabilizing an inactive GPCR conformation is the ionic lock—a salt bridge between the charged Arg3.50 in the conserved "D[E]RY" (aspartic acid, [glutamic acid], arginine, tyrosine) motif and Asp6.30 (or Glu6.30) at the cytoplasmic side of transmembrane three and six.

Side Effects

Up to two-thirds of patients with psychoses are noncompliant or cease taking their antipsychotic medications, often because of obvious and serious side effects that include extrapyramidal symptoms, weight gain, sedation, lethargy, and emotional dampening that interfere with daily life functions and cause psychological distress. Though it is more apparent with some antipsychotics than others, sedation is a side effect of every antipsychotic agent. Since sedation can exacerbate negative symptoms of schizophrenia, such as avolition, it exemplifies a major challenge in treating both positive and negative symptoms.

Extrapyramidal side effects occur in up to 50% of patients taking antipsychotics. They tend to present within 8 weeks of initiating treatment, and despite the development of numerous atypical antipsychotics, they continue to be the greatest side-effect burden. Extrapyramidal side effects include akathisia, tardive dyskinesia, dystonia, such as facial grimacing, torticollis, and oculogyric crisis, and parkinsonian-type symptoms, such as bradykinesia, cogwheel rigidity, tremor, masked face, and shuffling gait. Akathisia, a feeling of inner restlessness or an urge to move, occurs in about 20% of patients on antipsychotics. Incidence in patients treated with haloperidol, aripiprazole, or quetiapine is about 60%, 18%, and 4%, respectively.[60] Tardive dyskinesia occurs in 20%-30% of patients on antipsychotics and is characterized by stereotyped, involuntary, repetitive, choreiform movements of the face, eyelids, mouth (grimaces), tongue, extremities, and trunk. A new medicine was recently developed to treat tardive dyskinesia—valbenazine, a highly selective vesicular monoamine transporter 2 inhibitor that modulates the packaging and release of dopamine[61] (covered in Specific Drugs).

Extrapyramidal side effects are caused by prolonged blockade of dopamine binding to D_2 receptors in the nigrostriatal pathway. Similarly, hyperprolactinemia (elevation of blood levels of the lactation hormone, prolactin) is caused by D_2 blockade in the tuberoinfundibular (connecting the hypothalamus to the pituitary gland) pathway and is a common side effect of various antipsychotics. Closely titrating antipsychotic dose or switching to a different antipsychotic is necessary to reduce the likelihood or severity of these side effects. Certain antipsychotics (e.g., clozapine, quetiapine) have a low incidence of extrapyramidal and hyperprolactinemia side effects; likely contributing factors include reduced affinity at D_2, and similarly, unique binding kinetics at D_2 receptors—namely unique association and dissociation rates.[62] An optimal kinetic profile for antipsychotics would permit endogenous dopamine to continue acting at the D_2 receptor, while also permitting the drug to sufficiently modulate the receptor's function. Insurmountable binding to D_2, for example, would completely block dopamine's ability to function, but slower on and faster off rates would allow time for dopamine to bind and function. This is notable, as in general, antipsychotics that are more potent on a dose basis produce more side effects, suggesting tighter binding to D_2.

Additional side effects of antipsychotics such as sedation, hypotension, tachycardia, and other autonomic effects reflect blockade of histamine H_1 and adrenergic α_1/α_2 receptors. Antimuscarinic (M_1-$_5$) actions of certain antipsychotics account for cardiac, ophthalmic, xerostomia, gastrointestinal, and genitourinary side effects. On the other hand, it has been proposed that modulation of muscarinic cholinergic activity might be beneficial in controlling negative symptoms in patients with schizophrenia. Also, the severity of extrapyramidal side effects increases with the ratio of antidopaminergic to anticholinergic potency, and anticholinergic medications can reverse some extrapyramidal side effects. For example, antimuscarinic alkaloids found in belladonna can be used in Parkinson's disease therapy.[63] Thus, antimuscarinic effects may also be favorable for preventing extrapyramidal symptoms.

Weight gain and general metabolic dysregulation that lead to type II diabetes and cardiovascular disease are problematic for many typical and atypical antipsychotic drugs. The mechanism for antipsychotic-induced weight gain and metabolic syndrome is not known for certain but might involve serotonin 5-HT_{2C} and histamine H_1 GPCR antagonism or inverse agonism.[64-66] It is notable that haloperidol and aripiprazole treatment is associated with relatively low incidence of weight gain[43]; haloperidol has no activity at 5-HT_{2C} receptors, whereas aripiprazole is a 5-HT_{2C} partial agonist. Meta-analyses consistently show that clozapine and olanzapine cause more weight gain and metabolic side effects,[43,67] and both are potent 5-HT_{2C} inverse agonists. Conversely, selective activation of 5-HT_{2C} receptors reduces food intake, and may improve metabolic function, as evidenced by the 5-HT_{2C} selective agonist, lorcaserin, approved for obesity.

Relatively common dermatologic reactions (e.g., urticaria and photosensitivity) are observed especially with the phenothiazines. Antipsychotics also can prolong QTc intervals which potentiates the risk of serious ventricular arrhythmias. Antipsychotics are associated with increased risk of seizures, especially at high doses, and they carry a black box warning of increased risk of mortality in elderly patients with dementia-related psychosis. Deaths are typically attributed to cardiovascular events or infection. Antipsychotics also cause a threefold increase in the risk of stroke in the elderly.

Development of the First Antipsychotic Drugs: Phenothiazines

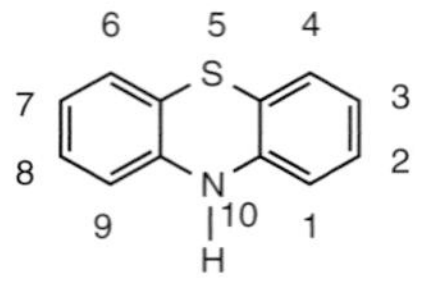

Phenothiazine

The phenothiazine nucleus was synthesized in 1883. It was used as an anthelmintic (antiparasitic) for many years, but it has no antipsychotic activity. The basic structure from which the phenothiazine antipsychotic drugs trace their origins is benzodioxane, and type I benzodioxanes are antihistamines (Fig. 11.4). In 1937, Bovet hypothesized that specific substances antagonizing histamine should exist, tried various compounds known to act on the autonomic nervous system, and was the first to recognize antihistamine activity with the discovery of piperoxan.[68] Starting with the benzodioxanes (Fig. 11.4 I), many molecular modifications were carried out in various laboratories in search of other types of antihistamines.

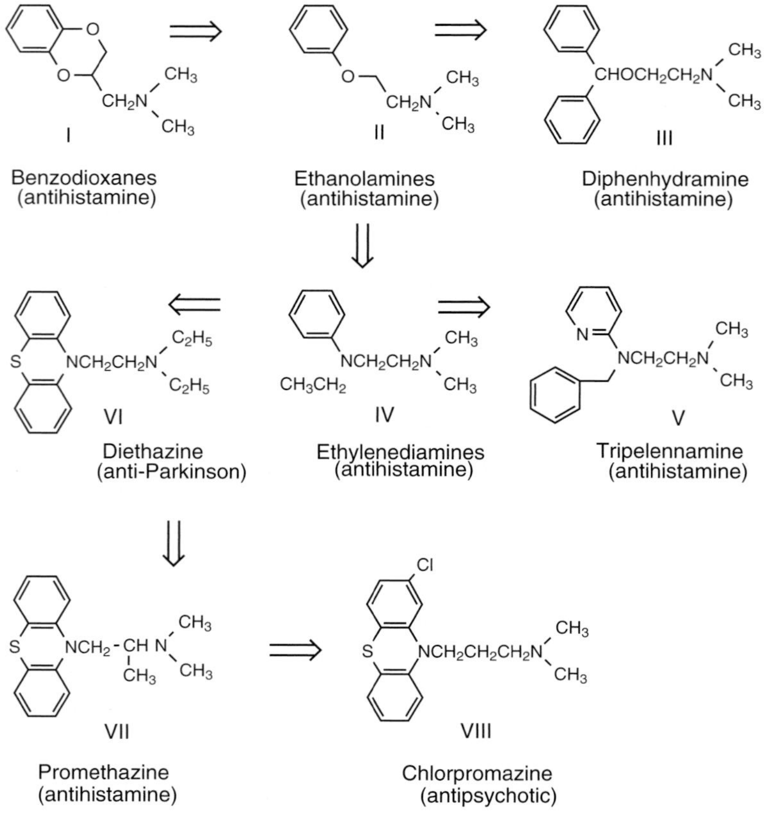

Figure 11.4 Development of phenothiazine-type antipsychotic drugs.

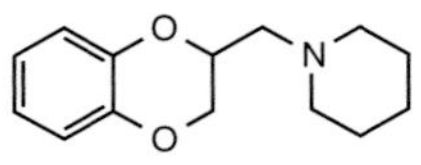

Piperoxan

The benzodioxanes led to ethers of ethanolamine (Fig. 11.4 II) which, after further modifications, led to the benzhydryl ethers that are characterized by the clinically useful antihistamine diphenhydramine (Fig. 11.4 III) or to ethylenediamine (Fig. 11.4 IV) which led to antihistamine drugs, such as tripelennamine (Fig. 11.4 V). Further modification of the ethylenediamine type of antihistamine resulted in the incorporation of one of the nitrogen atoms into a phenothiazine ring system which produced phenothiazine, a compound that was found to have antihistamine properties and, similar to many other antihistamines, a strong sedative effect. Diethazine (Fig. 11.4 VI) is more useful in the treatment of Parkinson's disease (because of its potent antimuscarinic action) than in allergies, whereas promethazine (Fig. 11.4 VII) is clinically used as an antihistamine. After it was discovered that promethazine prolongs barbiturate-induced sleep in rodents, the drug was introduced into clinical anesthesia as a potentiating agent.

To enhance the sedative effects of such phenothiazines, Charpentier and Courvoisier synthesized and evaluated many modifications of promethazine. This research effort eventually led to the synthesis of chlorpromazine (Fig. 11.4 VIII) in 1950 at the Rhône-Poulenc Laboratories. Soon thereafter, the French surgeon Laborit and his coworkers described the ability of this compound to potentiate anesthetics and produce artificial hibernation.[69] They noted that chlorpromazine, by itself, did not cause a loss of consciousness but did produce a tendency to sleep and a marked disinterest in the surroundings. The first attempts to treat mental illness with chlorpromazine were made in Paris in 1951 and early 1952 by Paraire and Sigwald.

In 1952, Delay and Deniker began their important work with chlorpromazine.[70] They were convinced that chlorpromazine achieved more than symptomatic relief of agitation or anxiety, and that this drug had an ameliorative effect on psychosis. Thus, what initially involved minor molecular modifications of an antihistamine that produced sedative side effects resulted in the development of a major class of drugs that initiated a new era in drug therapy for the mentally ill—chlorpromazine spawned the "psychopharmacological revolution."[71] More than anything else in the history of psychiatry, the phenothiazines and related drugs have positively influenced the lives of schizophrenic patients, enabling them to assume a greatly improved role in society.

More than 24 phenothiazine and the related thioxanthene derivatives are used in medicine, most of them for psychiatric conditions. The structures, generic and trade names, dose, and effects of phenothiazine-type and thioxanthene-type antipsychotics currently in use are listed in Table 11.2.

It is presumed that phenothiazine and thioxanthene antipsychotic drugs mediate their effects mainly through interactions at D_2-type dopamine receptors. Examination of the x-ray structures of dopamine (in the preferred *trans* α-rotamer conformation) and chlorpromazine shows that these two structures can be partly superimposed (Fig. 11.5).[72] In the preferred conformation of chlorpromazine, its side chain tilts away from the midline toward the chlorine-substituted ring.

The electronegative chlorine atom on ring "a" is responsible for imparting asymmetry to this molecule, and the attraction of the amine side chain (protonated at physiologic pH) toward the ring containing the chlorine atom indicates an important structural feature of such molecules. Phenothiazine and related compounds lacking a chlorine atom in this position are, in most cases, inactive as antipsychotic drugs. In addition to the ring "a" substituent, another major requirement for therapeutic efficacy of phenothiazines is that the side-chain amine contains three carbons separating the two nitrogen atoms (Fig. 11.5). Phenothiazines with two carbon atoms separating the two nitrogen atoms lack antipsychotic efficacy. Compounds such as promethazine (Fig. 11.4 VII) are primarily antihistamines and are less likely to assume the preferred conformation.

When thioxanthene derivatives that contain an olefinic double bond between the tricyclic ring and the side chain are examined, it can be seen that such structures can exist in either the *cis* or *trans* isomeric configuration. For example, the *cis* isomer of the antipsychotic thiothixene is several-fold more active than both the *trans* isomer and the compound obtained from saturation of the double bond. Structure D in Figure 11.5 shows that the active structure of dopamine does not superimpose with a *trans*-like conformer of chlorpromazine that would be predicted to be inactive.

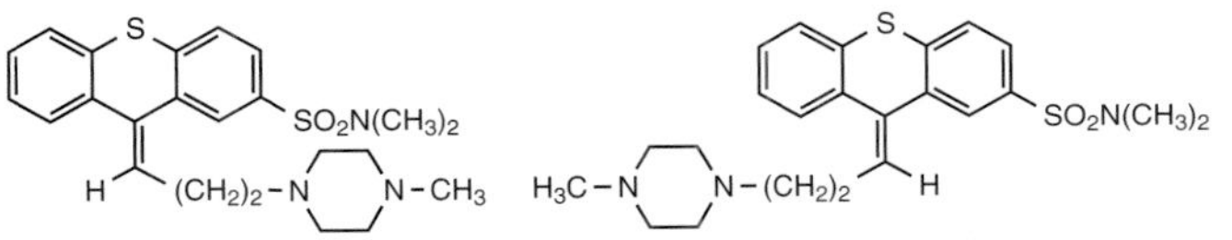

Cis isomer   *Trans* isomer

Thiothixene

Some metabolic pathways for chlorpromazine are shown in Figure 11.6. It should be kept in mind that during metabolism, several processes can and do occur for the same molecule. For example, chlorpromazine can be demethylated, sulfoxidized, hydroxylated, and glucuronidated to yield 7-O-glu-nor-chlorpromazine-sulfoxide. The combination of such processes leads to >100 identified metabolites. Evidence indicates that the 7-hydroxylated derivatives and possibly other hydroxylated derivatives as well as the mono- and di-desmethylated products (nor_1-chlorpromazine, nor_2-chlorpromazine) are active in vivo and at dopamine D_2 receptors, whereas the sulfoxide (chlorpromazine-sulfoxide) is inactive. Although the thioxanthenes are closely related to the phenothiazines in their pharmacological effects, there seems to be at least one major difference in metabolism—most of the thioxanthenes do not form ring-hydroxylated derivatives. Metabolic pathways for phenothiazines and thioxanthenes are significantly altered, both quantitatively and qualitatively, by a number of factors, including age, gender, interaction with other drugs, and route of administration.

Table 11.2 Phenothiazine- and Thioxanthene-type Antipsychotic Drugs

Generic Name	Trade Name	R_{10} (phenothiazine nucleus: S, N–R_{10}, R_2)	R_2	Adult Antipsychotic Oral Dose Range (mg/d)	Side Effects[a]: Sedative Effects	Side Effects[a]: Extrapyramidal Effects	Side Effects[a]: Hypotensive Effects	Other Effects
Phenothiazines Type								
Chlorpromazine hydrochloride	Generic	$(CH_2)_3N(CH_3)_2.HCl$	Cl	300-800	+++	++	Oral ++ IM +++	Antiemetic dose 10-25 mg every 4-6 hr
Thioridazine hydrochloride	Generic	$(CH_2)_2$– (piperidine) N ·HCl, N–CH_3	SCH_3	200-600	+++	+	++	
Perphenazine	Generic	$(CH_2)_3-N$ (piperazine) $N-CH_2CH_2OH$	Cl	8-32	++	+++	+	
Prochlorperazine edisylate maleate	Compro	$(CH_2)_3-N$ (piperazine) $N-CH_3$	Cl	75-100	++	+++	+	Antiemetic dose 5-10 mg every 4-6 hr
Fluphenazine hydrochoride	Generic	$(CH_2)_3-N$ (piperazine) $N-CH_2CH_2OH$ ·2HCl	CF_3	1-20	+	+++	+	
Trifluoperazine hydrochoride	Generic	$(CH_2)_3-N$ (piperazine) $N-CH_3$ ·2HCl	CF_3	6-20	+	+++	+	
Thioxanthene Type								
Thiothixene hydrochoride	Generic (presently unavailable)	(thioxanthene, S) $SO_2N(CH_3)_2$; H, $(CH_2)_2\cdot N$ (piperazine) $N-CH_3$ ·HCl		6-30	++	++	++	

[a] +++, high; ++, medium; +, low.

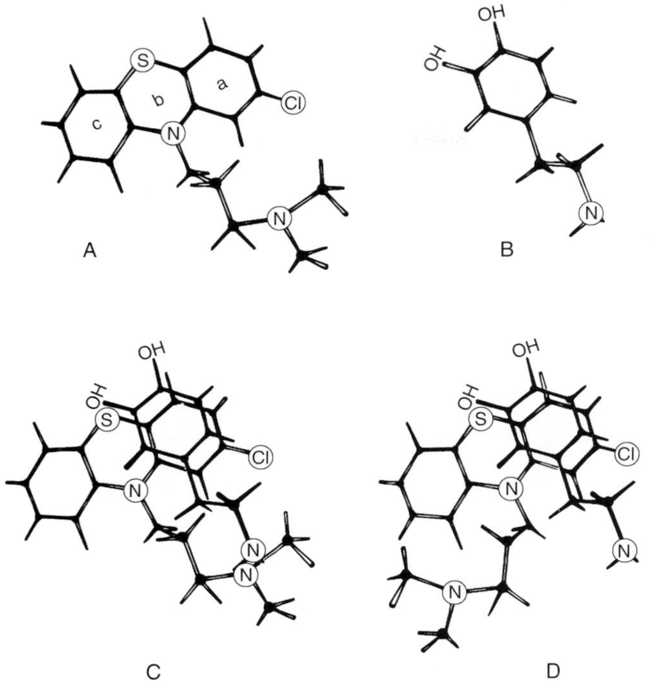

A B

C D

Figure 11.5 Conformations of chlorpromazine (A), dopamine (B), and their superposition (C) as determined by x-ray crystallographic analysis. The a, b, and c in (A) designate rings. Also shown (D) is another conformation in which the alkyl side chain of chlorpromazine is in the *trans* conformation (ring a and amino side chain), which is not superimposable onto dopamine. Adapted from Horn AS, Snyder SH. Chlorpromazine and dopamine: conformational similarities that correlate with the antischizophrenic activity of phenothiazine drugs. *Proc Natl Acad Sci USA*. 1971;68:2325-2328, with permission.

Development of Butyrophenone Antipsychotics

In the late 1950s, Janssen and coworkers synthesized the propiophenone and butyrophenone analogues of meperidine in an effort to increase its analgesic potency.[73] Both had greater analgesic potency than meperidine, but the butyrophenone analogue also displayed activity resembling that of chlorpromazine. The structure-activity results of Janssen and coworkers showed that it was possible to eliminate the analgesic activity and, simultaneously, enhance the chlorpromazine-like antipsychotic activity in the butyrophenone series.

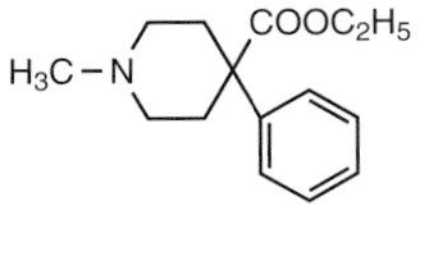

Meperidine 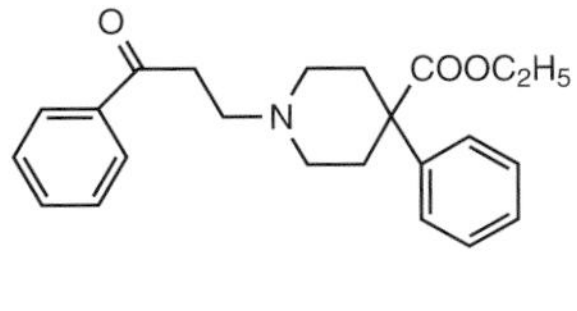 Propiophenone analogue

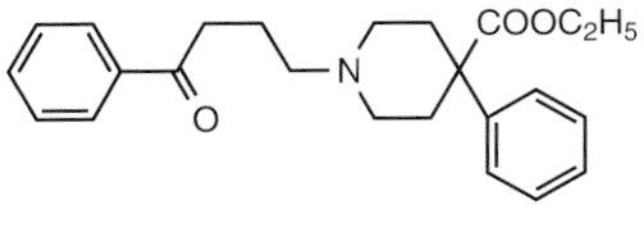

Butyrophenone analogue

All butyrophenone derivatives displaying high antipsychotic potency, including haloperidol, droperidol, and pimozide have the following general structure:

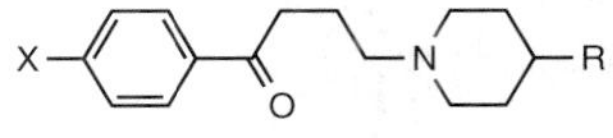

X = F or OCH_3

Butyrophenone scaffold

The attachment of a tertiary amino group to the fourth carbon of the butyrophenone skeleton is essential for antipsychotic activity; lengthening, shortening, or branching of the three-carbon propyl chain decreases antipsychotic potency. Replacement of the keto moiety (e.g., with the thioketone group as in the butyrothienones, with olefinic or phenoxy groups, or reduction of the carbonyl group) decreases antipsychotic potency. In addition, most potent butyrophenone compounds have a fluorine substituent in the para position of the benzene ring. Variations are possible in the tertiary amino group without loss of antipsychotic potency; for example, the basic nitrogen usually is incorporated into a six-membered ring (piperidine, tetrahydropyridine, or piperazine) that is substituted in the para position.

In most respects, the pharmacological effects of butyrophenones differ in degree, but not in kind, from those of the piperazine phenothiazines. Consistent with its higher affinity for dopamine D_2 receptors, haloperidol—the prototypical butyrophenone antipsychotic—is more potent and produces a higher incidence of extrapyramidal reactions than chlorpromazine, but sedative effects in moderate doses are less than that observed with phenothiazines. Butyrophenones have less prominent autonomic effects than the phenothiazine-type antipsychotic drugs, and only mild hypotension occurs. Also, haloperidol has less propensity to induce weight gain than chlorpromazine and most of the second-generation antipsychotic drugs.

Haloperidol was introduced for the treatment of psychoses in Europe in 1958 and in the United States in 1967. It is an effective alternative to phenothiazine antipsychotics and also is used for the manic phase of bipolar disorder. Haloperidol decanoate has been introduced as depot maintenance therapy. When injected every 4-6 weeks, the drug appears to be as effective as daily orally administered haloperidol. Other currently available (mostly in Europe) butyrophenones include the very potent spiperone (spiroperidol) as well as trifluperidol and droperidol (Fig. 11.7). Droperidol, a short-acting butyrophenone, is used in anesthesia for its sedating and antiemetic effects and sometimes in psychiatric emergencies as a sedative antipsychotic. Droperidol often is administered in combination with the potent narcotic analgesic fentanyl for pre-anesthetic sedation and anesthesia.

Modification of the haloperidol butyrophenone side chain by replacement of the keto functional group with a di-4-flourophenylmethane moiety results in diphenylbutyl piperidine antipsychotics, such as pimozide, penfluridol, and fluspirilene, which have a longer duration of action than the butyrophenone analogues. Pimozide also is used as a treatment for

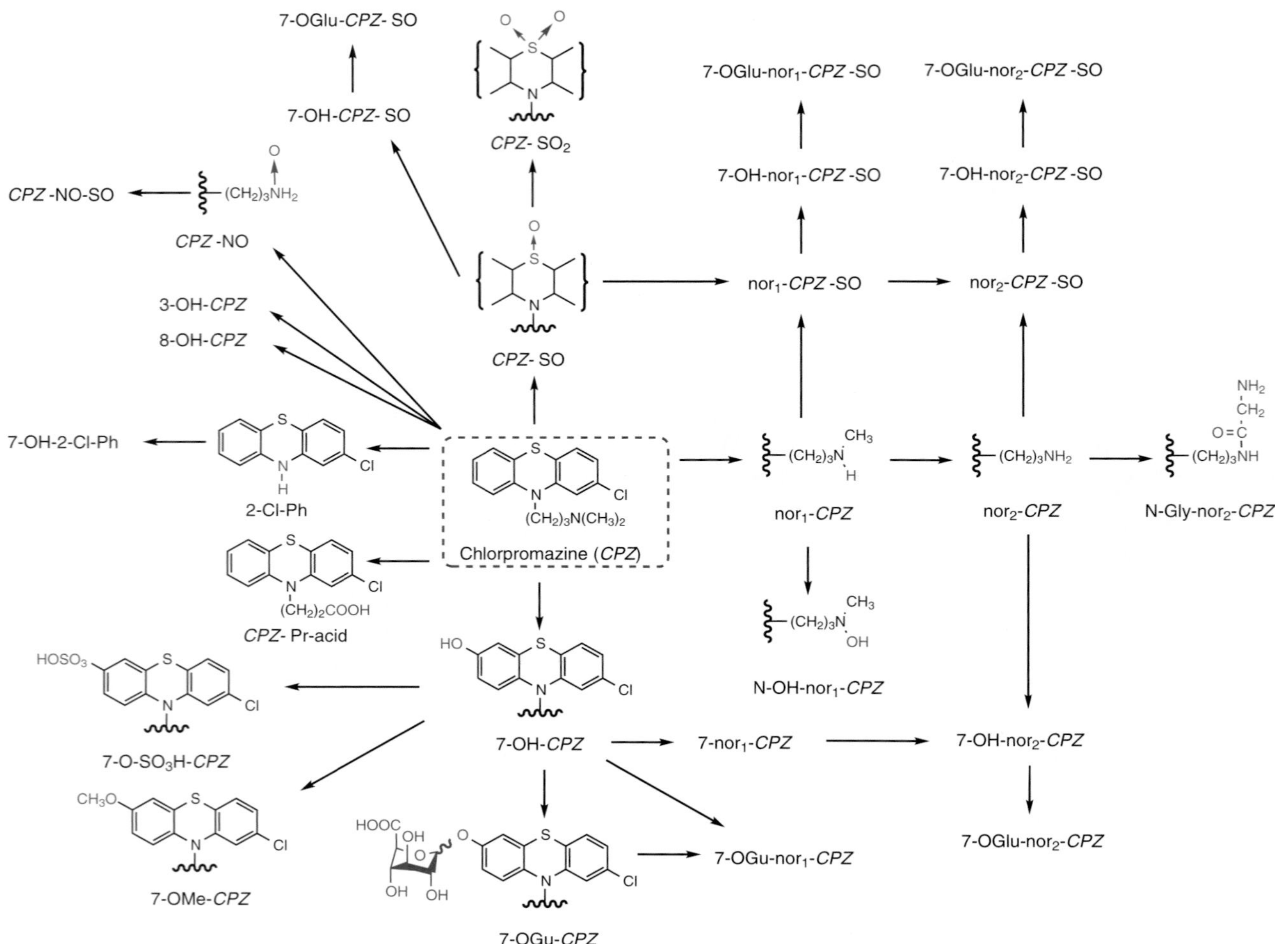

Figure 11.6 Metabolism of chlorpromazine. CPZ, chlorpromazine; NO, N-oxide; O-Glu, O-glucuronide; O-SO_3H, sulfate; Ph, phenothiazine; Pr-acid, propionic acid; SO, sulfoxide; SO_2, sulfone.

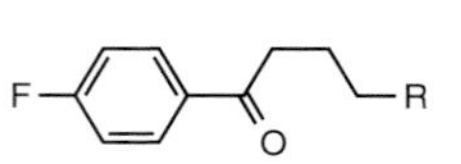

Generic names	Trade names	R
Haloperidol	Haldol	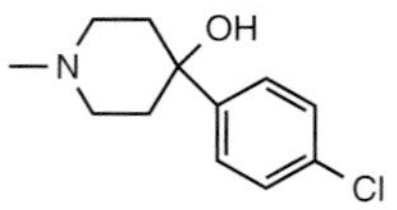
Haloperidol decanoate		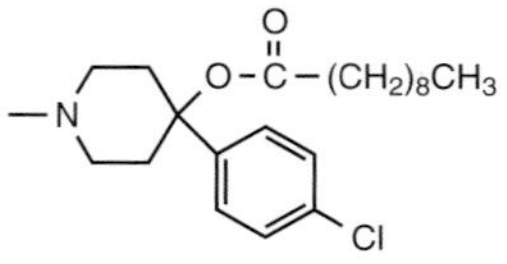
Droperidol	Inapsine	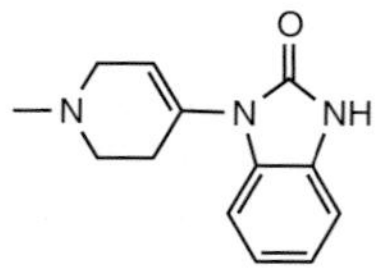
Pimozide	Orap	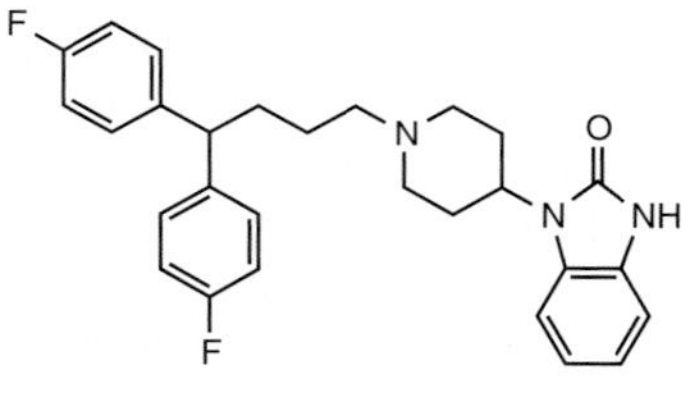

Figure 11.7 Haloperidol and its analogues.

Tourette's syndrome, a movement disorder that is characterized by facial tics, grimaces, emitting of strange and uncontrollable sounds, and sometimes, involuntary shouting of obscenities. This disorder can be misdiagnosed by clinicians as schizophrenia. Typically, the onset of Tourette's syndrome occurs at age 10, and standard treatment for Tourette's syndrome has been antipsychotics. Chronic treatment of Tourette's syndrome with pimozide and other typical antipsychotics carries the risk of producing tardive dyskinesia.

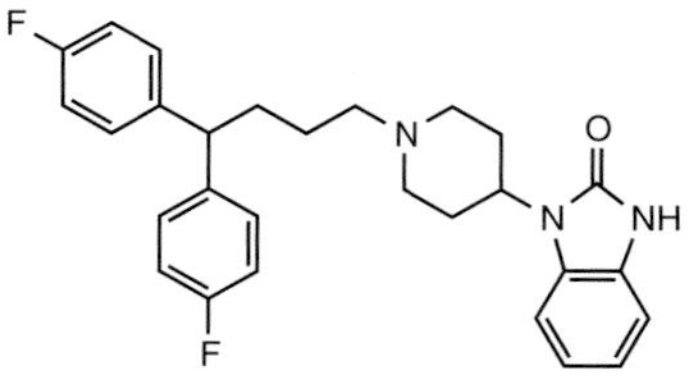

Pimozide

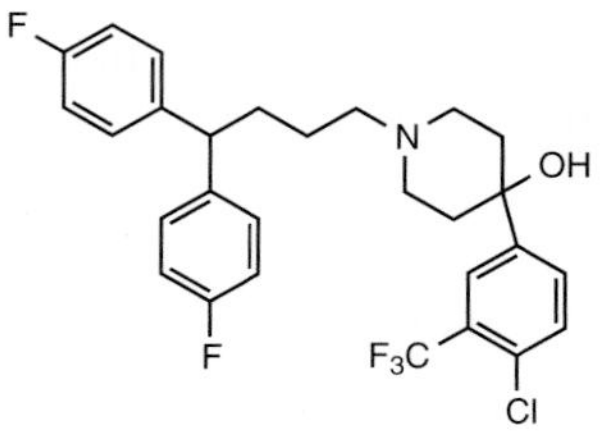

Penfluridol

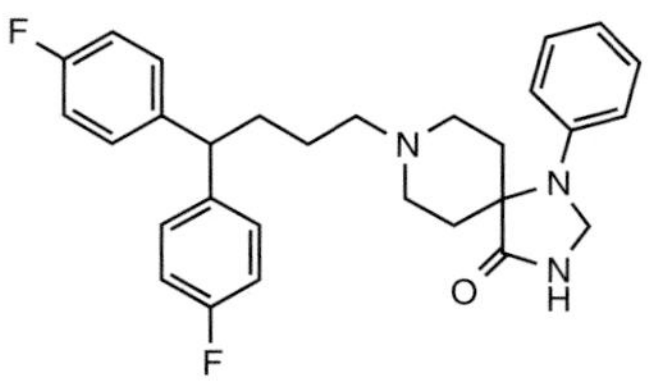

Fluspirilene

Haloperidol is readily absorbed from the gastrointestinal tract. The drug is concentrated in the liver and CNS and is mostly bound to plasma proteins.[74] Peak plasma levels occur 2-6 hours after ingestion. Approximately 15% of a given dose is excreted in the bile, and approximately 40% is eliminated through the kidney. Figure 11.8 shows the typical oxidative metabolic pathway of butyrophenones as exemplified by haloperidol.

NEUROTOXICOLOGY OF HALOPERIDOL

As discussed in the section on Side Effects of antipsychotics, untoward extrapyramidal effects occur in up to 50% of patients receiving standard doses of typical antipsychotics. The severe and sometimes irreversible dyskinesias associated with haloperidol pharmacotherapy are hypothesized to result from neurotoxicity involving dopaminergic systems. In fact, the central and peripheral biochemical and resulting pathophysiological features of haloperidol-induced movement disorders are similar to the potent dopaminergic neurotoxicant and parkinsonian-producing agent, 1-methyl-4-phenyl-1,2,3,6-tetrahydropyridine (MPTP).

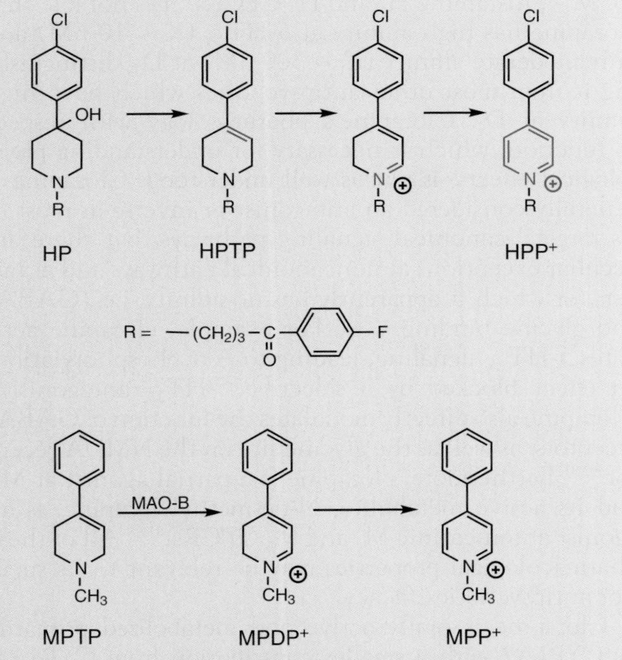

HP HPTP HPP+

R = —$(CH_2)_3$—C(=O)—C₆H₄—F

MPTP —MAO-B→ MPDP+ → MPP+

Proposed neurotoxicological mechanisms for haloperidol-induced dyskinesias similar to that of dopaminergic toxicant MPTP.

Microsomal-catalyzed dehydration of haloperidol (HP) yields the corresponding haloperidol 1,2,3,6-tetrahydropyridine derivative (HPTP) that is a close analogue of the parkinsonian-inducing neurotoxicant MPTP. Long-term (58-week) administration of HPTP to nonhuman primates alters both presynaptic and postsynaptic dopaminergic neuronal function, which may contribute to the parkinsonian-type side effects and tardive dyskinesia that are relatively common with haloperidol pharmacotherapy.[75] In baboons treated chronically with HPTP, animals developed orofacial dyskinesia, and histopathological studies revealed volume loss in the basal forebrain and hypothalamus, along with other neuronal cell loss that may be relevant to the pathophysiology of tardive dyskinesia.[76] In humans and baboons, HPTP is oxidized in vivo to the corresponding haloperidol pyridinium species (HPP^+) similar to the oxidation of MPTP to its ultimate neurotoxic species MPP^+. HPP^+ is neurotoxic to dopaminergic and, especially, serotonergic neurons in vivo in rats,[77] and HPP^+ has been identified in the urine of humans treated with haloperidol.[78] Furthermore, in a study involving psychiatric patients who were treated chronically with haloperidol, the severity of tardive dyskinesia and parkinsonism was associated with an increased serum concentration ratio of HPP^+ to haloperidol,[79] providing compelling clinical evidence for the neurotoxicity of HPP^+. Investigations continue to determine if antipsychotic-induced pathology of the extrapyramidal motor system, such as that associated with tardive dyskinesia, may be related to production of MPP^+/HPP^+-type species in humans.

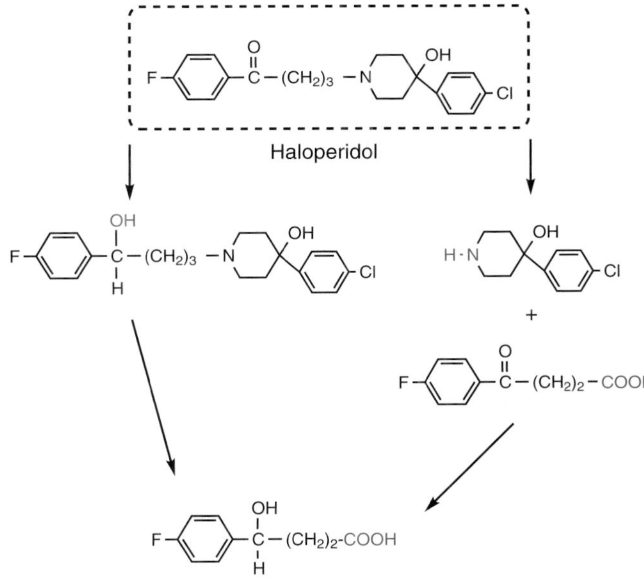

Haloperidol

Figure 11.8 Metabolism of haloperidol.

Second-Generation (Atypical) Antipsychotic Drugs

Atypical antipsychotic drugs emerged with the introduction of the diarylazepine derivative, clozapine. This was followed by approval of the first benzisoxazole and benzisothiazole derivatives such as risperidone (1994) and ziprasidone (2001). The arylpiperazine quinolinone derivative, aripiprazole (introduced in 2002), occasionally is referred to as a "third-generation" antipsychotic drug because its mechanism of action involves unique partial agonist and biased agonist (or functionally selective) activity at D_2 autoreceptors; however, no formal redesignation has been concluded. It is reiterated that the second-generation/atypical antipsychotic classification grew from observations that clozapine did not produce extrapyramidal movement disorder side effects like haloperidol. Many other atypical antipsychotics including risperidone and lurasidone, however, have a propensity to produce motor side effects, and akathisia is a common side effect of new antipsychotics, including the most recently approved medications, brexpiprazole, cariprazine, asenapine, and lurasidone. Other side effects, also, do not reliably define boundaries of classic, first-generation versus second-generation antipsychotics. Numerous investigators, therefore, suggest reclassification of antipsychotics.[80,81]

Diarylazepine and Related Analogues

The structures of the diarylazepine derivatives, clozapine, olanzapine, quetiapine, loxapine, amoxapine (an active metabolite of loxapine, indicated for symptoms of depression in patients with neurotic depressive disorders as well as psychotic depressions), and the related dibenzo-oxepine asenapine are shown in Figure 11.9.

CLOZAPINE. Clozapine is the quintessential, atypical antipsychotic drug. It carries minimal extrapyramidal side effects and does not produce tardive dyskinesia with long-term use. It is believed this is due to its selective targeting of limbic rather than striatal dopamine receptors, its receptor binding kinetics, and/or its activity at muscarinic receptors. Clozapine maintains superiority to nearly all other antipsychotics, effectively alleviating both positive and negative symptoms of schizophrenia.[82] Serious drawbacks to the use of clozapine, however, are metabolic effects (weight gain, hyperglycemia, diabetes, dyslipidemia), and with rarer incidence, potentially fatal agranulocytosis (decreased white blood cell count). Agranulocytosis is reported to occur in ~0.7% of patients and may be related to a rare mutation, which also affects agranulocytosis susceptibility related to other medications.[83] Because of this risk, clozapine is reserved only for (1) use in the treatment of severely ill patients with schizophrenia who fail to respond adequately to other antipsychotics or (2) for reducing recurrent suicidal behavior in patients with schizophrenia or schizoaffective disorder. All patients treated with clozapine must have a baseline white blood cell count and absolute neutrophil count before, and regularly during, treatment, and for at least four weeks after discontinuation.

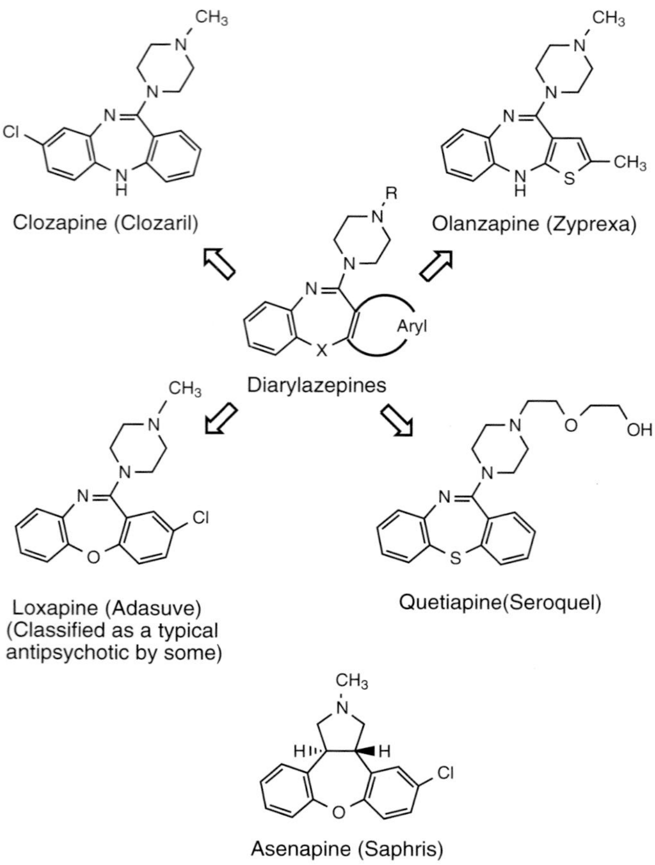

The GPCR profile for clozapine is well characterized with respect to binding. In addition to D_2 and 5-HT_{2A}, clozapine has high to moderate affinity at dopamine D_1, D_3, D_4, D_5, serotonin 5-HT_{1A}, 5-HT_{2B}, 5-HT_{2C}, 5-HT_3, 5-HT_6, 5-HT_7, adrenergic α_{1A}, α_{1B}, α_{2A}, α_{2B}, α_{2C}, cholinergic M_1-$_5$, histamine H_1 and H_2 GPCRs. It is notable that clozapine has high affinity at 5-HT_{2A} (K_i < 10 nM) and only moderate affinity ($K_i \sim 300$ nM) at D_2, distinguishing it from most other antipsychotics which have high affinity at D_2. Clozapine's pharmacology with respect to function, which is necessary for understanding physiological effects, is not as well understood. Clozapine is generally considered an antagonist or inverse at most of its targets' canonical signaling pathways, but there are peculiar exceptions at noncanonical pathways and at targets for which it apparently has no affinity, i.e., $GABA_B$ and glycine binding sites. For example, clozapine activates 5-HT_{2A} signaling, leading to Akt phosphorylation, an effect blocked by a selective 5-HT_{2A} antagonist.[84] Clozapine also directly modulates the function of $GABA_B$ receptors, as well as the glycine site on the NMDA receptor.[80,81] Furthermore, clozapine is a partial agonist at M_4, and its active metabolite, N-desmethylclozapine, is an agonist at muscarinic M_1 and M_4 GPCRs.[82,83] All of these pharmacological properties may be relevant to its superior antipsychotic efficacy.

Clozapine is orally active and metabolized primarily by CYP1A2 with a smaller contribution from CYP3A4, although there is a high degree of between-subject and within-subject variability [84] (Fig. 11.10). It has a half-life of about 8 hours. The main products of metabolism are inactive hydroxyl and N-oxide derivatives. N-desmethylclozapine has a receptor binding profile similar to clozapine, although with higher affinity at 5-HT_{1A}. It is noted that caffeine is metabolized primarily by CYP1A2, and it has been observed that some patients who consume caffeine-containing beverages while taking clozapine show signs of increased arousal and extrapyramidal symptoms; removal of caffeine results in resolution of these problems,[85]

Clozapine (Clozaril)
Olanzapine (Zyprexa)
Diarylazepines
Loxapine (Adasuve) (Classified as a typical antipsychotic by some)
Quetiapine(Seroquel)
Asenapine (Saphris)

Figure 11.9 Diarylazepine derivatives.

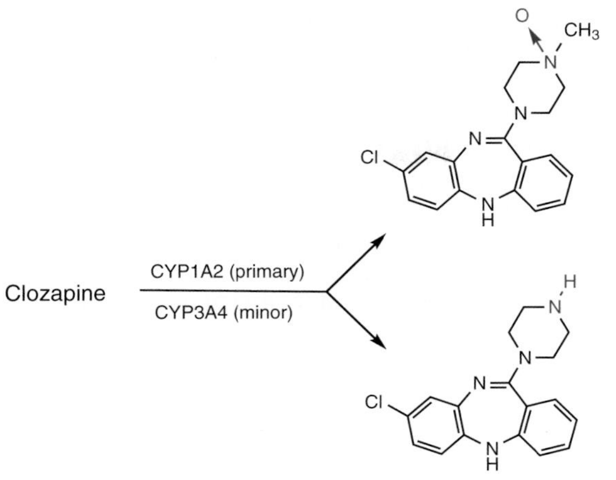

Figure 11.10 Metabolism of clozapine.

suggesting a clinically-relevant drug interaction. Also, cigarette smoking induces activity of CYP1A2, and patients who smoke while taking clozapine can have significantly lower serum levels of clozapine. [86,87]

OLANZAPINE. The thienobenzodiazepine olanzapine shares close structural resemblance to clozapine and has a similar receptor binding profile, except it has higher affinity at dopamine D_2 and serotonin 5-HT_{2A} receptors but lower affinity at 5-HT_{1A} and α-adrenergic receptors. Olanzapine is effective at treating positive and negative symptoms. Its side-effect profile is similar to that of clozapine, with the exception of agranulocytosis that is not usually seen with olanzapine use. Also, olanzapine causes serious weight gain. For example, prolonged use of olanzapine can cause some patients to gain 30 lbs. or more. Olanzapine is well absorbed after oral administration and is metabolized mainly by CYP1A2 to inactive metabolites similar to those seen with clozapine (N-oxide and N-demethylation) along with methyl oxidation and phase 2 glucuronidation[88,89] (Fig. 11.11). The drug has a variable half-life of approximately 20-50 hours. There is available a long-acting injectable formulation, olanzapine pamoate (Zyprexa Relprevv).

QUETIAPINE. Quetiapine is a dibenzothiazepine that binds with high affinity at histamine H_1 GPCRs, but with low to moderate affinity at most other targets. Quetiapine is 100% bioavailable, but first-pass metabolism yields at least 20 metabolites, with the major metabolites shown in Figure 11.12. The major products are the sulfoxide (catalyzed by CYP3A4) and the carboxylic acid.[90] N-desalkylquetiapine has high affinity at several GPCRs, is a 5-HT_{1A} agonist, and potently inhibits the norepinephrine transporter which may contribute to antidepressant activity.[91] It does not appear that CYP2D6 or CYP1A2 is involved in quetiapine metabolism, and cigarette smoking does not affect the pharmacokinetics of this drug. Relative to many other antipsychotics, but similar to clozapine, quetiapine has a short half-life, approximately 6 hours (Table 11.1). Also akin to clozapine, quetiapine carries a low incidence of extrapyramidal side effects, likely owing to its relatively low affinity at dopamine D_2 receptors.

LOXAPINE. The dibenzoxazepine loxapine has high affinity for dopamine D_2-type, serotonin 5-HT_2-type, and histamine H_1 GPCRs. It also has moderate affinity for 5-HT_6, 5-HT_7, α-adrenergic, M_1 and M_3 receptors. Loxapine has a short half-life of about 3 hours, undergoing phase I aromatic hydroxylation to yield several phenolic metabolites that have higher affinity for D_2-type receptors than the parent drug. Loxapine also undergoes N-desmethylation to form amoxapine. Similarly, aromatic hydroxylation of amoxapine produces metabolites that have D_2 antagonist activity similar to haloperidol. Unlike loxapine, amoxapine has moderate affinity for serotonin, norepinephrine, and dopamine neurotransporters and blocks reuptake of these neurotransmitters; it is used clinically as an antidepressant.

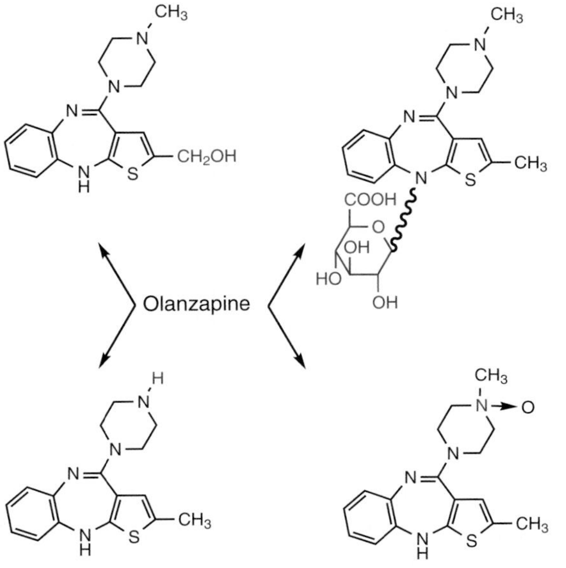

Figure 11.11 Metabolism of olanzapine.

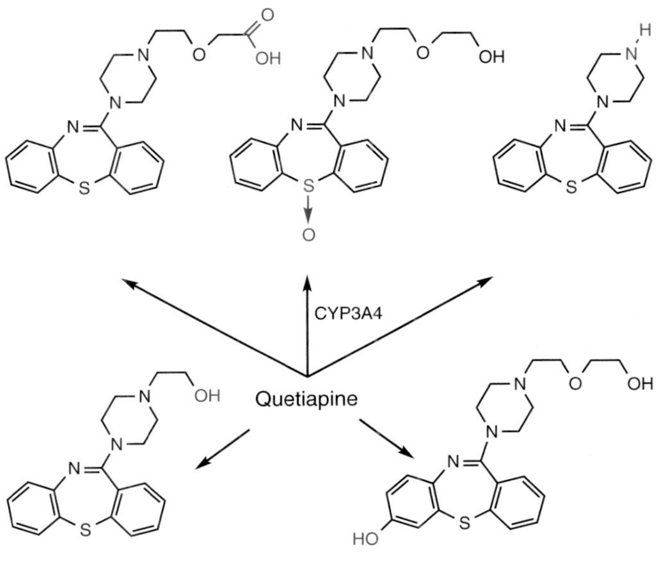

Figure 11.12 Major metabolic products of quetiapine.

ASENAPINE (SAPHRIS). Asenapine is a dibenzo-oxepino pyrrole that is unique in that it has very high to high affinity at several targets. These include 5-HT_{1A}, 5-HT_{1B}, 5-HT_{2A}, 5-HT_{2B}, 5-HT_{2C}, 5-HT_5, 5-HT_6, 5-HT_7, D_1, D_2, D_3, D_4, α_{1A}, α_{2A}, α_{2B}, α_{2C}, H_1, and H_2. It is reported that asenapine antagonizes all of its targets.[92] Also in contrast to other diarylazepines asenapine has essentially no affinity (K_i > 10 μM) for cholinergic muscarinic (M_1-M_5) GPCRs. Despite its unique polypharmacology, there does not appear to be any efficacy advantages for asenapine over other antipsychotic drugs (typical or atypical) for treating schizophrenia or bipolar disorder.[43] Moreover, its side-effect profile is similar to other antipsychotics, except it produces a lower incidence of extrapyramidal effects and prolactin secretion compared to haloperidol, and weight gain is less than with olanzapine. The most common adverse reactions are akathisia, oral hypoesthesia, and somnolence.

When given as a sublingual tablet, bioavailability is about 35% (<2%, orally) with a half-life of 24 hours. The drug is extensively metabolized to compounds with little or no contributing activity. Elimination is primarily by direct glucuronidation by UGT1A4, yielding asenapine-N-glucuronide, and by N-demethylation and aromatic oxidation (primarily by CYP1A2) followed by conjugation (Fig. 11.13). Approximately 50% of the administered dose is lost via the kidney and 40% via the fecal route.

BENZISOXAZOLE AND BENZISOTHIAZOLE DERIVATIVES. Because certain diarylazepine type antipsychotic agents with high affinity for 5-HT_{2A} receptors produce low extrapyramidal and prolactinemia side effects (i.e., clozapine), investigators predicted that combined, selective D_2 and 5-HT_{2A} receptor blockade would effectively treat schizophrenia without causing such adverse events. Linking the chemical features present in potent benzamide D_2 antagonists (e.g., remoxipride, discussed below) with those of the benzothiazolyl piperazine 5-HT_{2A} antagonists (e.g., tiospirone, Fig. 11.14) led to the development of the 3-(4-piperidinyl)-1,2-benzisoxazole nucleus present, for example, in risperidone and ziprasidone (Fig. 11.14). Postmarketing analyses of these medications have not supported the D_2 plus 5-HT_{2A} antagonist hypothesis for reduced extrapyramidal and prolactinemia side-effect risks.

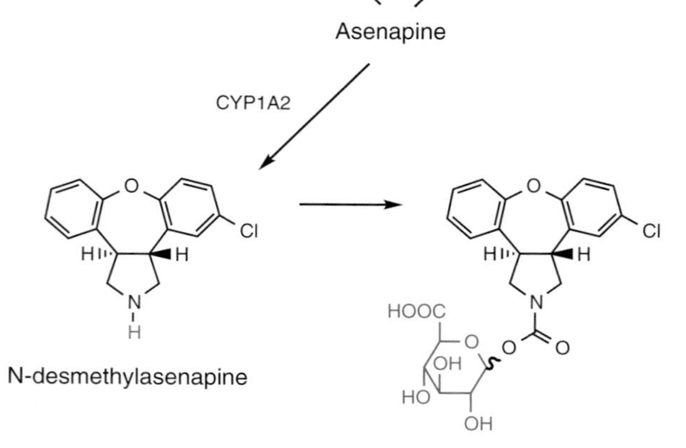

Figure 11.13 Major metabolic plasma products for asenapine.

RISPERIDONE AND PALIPERIDONE. Risperidone is a benzisoxazole piperidine that has very high affinity at serotonin 5-HT_{2A} and high affinity at dopamine D_2 GPCRs, where it has been shown to act as an antagonist or inverse agonist. Despite this pharmacology, risperidone and its active 9-OH metabolite, marketed as paliperidone (Fig. 11.14), demonstrate higher incidence of extrapyramidal side effects compared to clozapine and others, and no difference compared to amisulpride,[43] a benzamide discussed below that is a selective D_2-type antagonist with no activity at 5-HT_{2A}. Compared to haloperidol, extrapyramidal incidents are lower, but hyperprolactinemia incidents are higher with risperidone and paliperidone. Both produce significant weight gain on par with most other antipsychotics, excluding haloperidol, ziprasidone, and lurasidone which produce minimal weight gain. Other aspects of risperidone's and paliperidone's GPCR binding profile include high affinity at α_1- and α_2-type, and 5-HT_7 receptors, with moderate affinity at H_1, H_2, D_1, 5-HT_{2B}, and 5-HT_{2C} receptors.

Risperidone is well absorbed orally and undergoes hepatic CYP2D6- and CYP3A4-catalyzed N-dealkylation and 9-hydroxylation—paliperidone is the racemic version of the 9-hydroxy metabolite (Fig. 11.14). Paliperidone is not extensively metabolized by the liver and is excreted largely unchanged through the kidney. The half-lives of risperidone and paliperidone are approximately 23 hours. Patients differ regarding proportions of the (+)- and (−)-enantiomers of paliperidone produced in vivo, with the (+)-enantiomer arising from hydroxylation of risperidone by CYP2D6 and the (−)-enantiomer being formed mainly by action of CYP3A4.[93] There are no remarkable differences between risperidone and paliperidone regarding therapeutic activity, but reduced QTc prolongation with paliperidone compared to risperidone is a notable difference. Most clinical trials for both drugs were conducted versus placebo, but meta-analyses do not show superiority of these agents to other atypical antipsychotics.[43] Both drugs are available as long-acting injectable forms: risperidone in a physical complex with carbohydrate microspheres and paliperidone as the palmitate fatty acid ester.

Iloperidone. Like paliperidone, this benzisoxazole is very similar to risperidone regarding both its chemical structure and its GPCR binding profile—with the exception that iloperidone has additional moderate affinity for 5-HT_{1A} receptors. Iloperidone functions as an antagonist at all tested GPCRs. The affinities of the active metabolites P88 and P95 (Fig. 11.14) are similar to that of the parent compound.[94] In the few studies where iloperidone was compared to other antipsychotic drugs (haloperidol, risperidone, ziprasidone), there was no difference in antipsychotic efficacy. Iloperidone produces significant weight

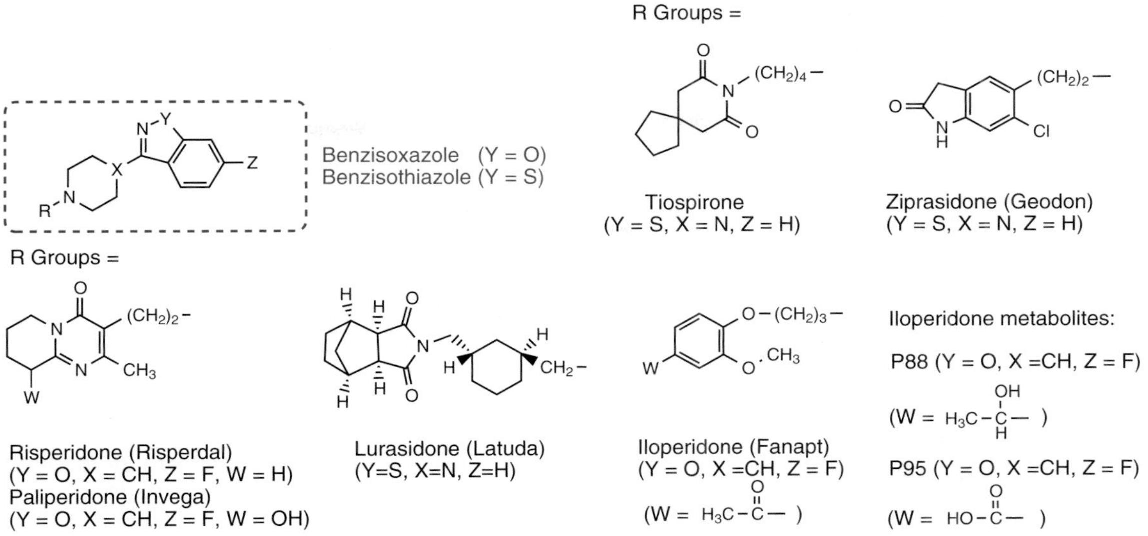

Figure 11.14 Benzisoxazole and benzisothiazole antipsychotic agents.

gain, more than risperidone (2.1 vs. 1.8 kg). Interestingly, iloperidone and risperidone have about the same affinity for serotonin 5-HT_{2C} and histamine H_1 receptors, which are thought to be responsible for antipsychotic-induced weight gain. Unlike risperidone and paliperidone, iloperidone is not associated with an increase in prolactin release. As is the case for risperidone, iloperidone is well absorbed orally and undergoes hepatic CYP2D6- and CYP3A4-catalyzed N-dealkylation. A majority of iloperidone is recovered unchanged in feces, indicating biliary excretion. Prescribing information reports that elimination half-lives for iloperidone, P88, and P95 in CYP2D6 extensive metabolizers are 18, 26, and 23 hours, respectively, whereas in poor metabolizers, half-lives are 33, 37, and 31 hours, respectively.

Ziprasidone. Ziprasidone is chemically similar to risperidone, but with a substitution of piperzinyl and benzisothiazole for piperidinyl and benzisoxazole and with minor aromatic modifications (Fig. 11.14) that impact its pharmacology and side effects. Like risperidone, ziprasidone has very high-affinity at 5-HT_{2A}, but also at 5-HT_{2C}, receptors. It has high affinity at 5-HT_{1B}, 5-HT_{1D}, 5-HT_7, α_{1B}, D_2, D_3, and moderate affinity at 5-HT_{1A}, 5-HT_{2B}, 5-HT_5, 5-HT_6, α_{1A}, α_{2A}, α_{2B}, α_{2C}, D_1, D_4, and H_1 GPCRs. Ziprasidone also has moderate affinity at the serotonin transporter and the norepinephrine transporter. Moreover, ziprasidone can activate 5-HT_{1A} receptors that regulate dopaminergic neurotransmission in brain regions involved in critical cognitive functions.[95] Ziprasidone can cause hyperprolactinemia and extrapyramidal side effects, but incidents of hyperprolactinemia are low, relative to risperidone and paliperidone. Akathisia incidents are very low. Ziprasidone has a relatively low propensity for inducing weight gain despite its significant affinity at histamine H_1 and serotonin 5-HT_{2C} receptors. Ziprasidone oral bioavailability is approximately 60%, which can be enhanced in the presence of fatty foods. It is extensively metabolized (<5% excreted unchanged) by aldehyde oxidase, which results in reductive cleavage of the S–N bond, and then by S-methylation. Ziprasidone also can undergo CYP3A4-catalyzed N-dealkylation and S-oxidation.[96] It has a half-life of about 8 hours.

Lurasidone (Latuda). Lurasidone is a benzoisothiazole piperazine structurally similar to ziprasidone. It has very high affinity at serotonin 5-HT_7 receptors; high affinity at 5-HT_{2A}, 5-HT_{1A}, and dopamine D_2; and moderate affinity at D_4, α_1- and α_2-type GPCRs. Lurasidone is an antagonist at these receptors, with the exception of 5-HT_{1A} where it behaves as a partial agonist.[97] Lurasidone has a low incidence of weight gain but can cause significant extrapyramidal side effects and prolactin increases. Lurasidone, like paliperidone (and aripiprazole, discussed below), is unique among many antipsychotics because it carries a low risk of QTc prolongation. Metabolism is reported as oxidative N-dealkylation, hydroxylation of the norbornane ring, and S-oxidation, mainly by CYP3A4. It has a half-life of 18 hours and is suitable for once-daily dosing.

Benzamide Derivatives

Analogues of the benzamide antiemetic and gastroparesis medication, metaclopramide, in which the side chain is incorporated into a pyrrolidine ring include S-(−)-sulpiride, S-(−)-remoxipride, and racemic amisulpride. Each is a potent D_2 receptor antagonist that displays antipsychotic properties.

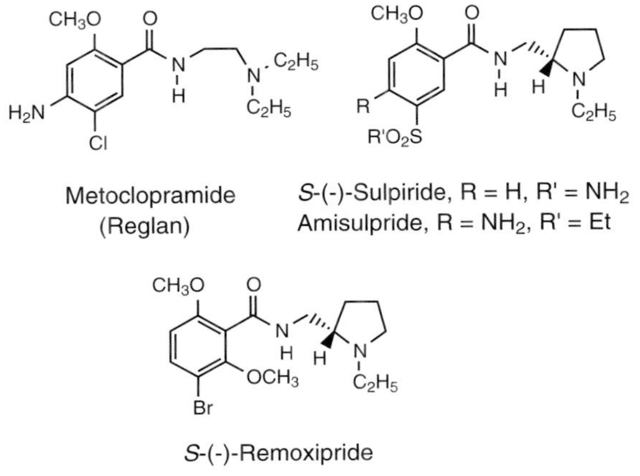

Benzamide derivatives

The hydrophilic properties of sulpiride might account for its poor oral absorption, limited penetration into the CNS and resulting low potency. Remoxipride was a promising antipsychotic that is comparable to haloperidol in potency and efficacy and has less incidence of extrapyramidal and autonomic side effects. Life-threatening aplastic anemia, however, was reported with remoxipride use, which prompted its withdrawal from the market.

AMISULPRIDE. The racemic para-amino congener of sulpiride, amisulpride, is used as an antipsychotic agent outside of the United States. It is distinguished from other antipsychotics, because it is has high affinity for dopamine D_2 and D_3 receptors, as well as 5-HT_{2B} and 5-HT_7 receptors (K_i < 15 nM); it has very low affinity (K_i = 1,000-10,000 nM) for all other common GPCR targets of antipsychotics, including 5-HT_{2A}.[98] A meta-analysis shows amisulpride to be the next most effective antipsychotic behind clozapine, and it can treat patients with predominant negative symptoms of schizophrenia.[43,99] Extrapyramidal effects, weight gain, sedation, and overall discontinuation rates are relatively low with amisulpride, especially at low doses that treat negative symptoms. Low extrapyramidal risk may be due to preferential blockade of mesolimbic compared to nigrostriatal D_2 and D_3 receptors, as shown in animal studies. QTc prolongation incidents with amisulpride treatment are high compared to most other antipsychotics. There are contraindications with citalopram and (*S*)-citalopram (escitalopram), because of increased risk of ventricular arrhythmia, particularly torsades de pointes. Amisulpride, like sulpiride, can also cause hyperprolactinemia.

Amisulpride bioavailability is 48%. It is poorly metabolized; two inactive metabolites account for only about 4% of the total amount of drug eliminated. Amisulpride is eliminated unchanged in the urine. Amisulpride does not accumulate, and its pharmacokinetics remain the same after repeated administration. The elimination half-life is approximately 12 hours after an oral dose.

Phenylpiperazines

ARIPIPRAZOLE. Aripiprazole (Fig. 11.15) is an arylpiperazine quinolinone derivative that has received a lot of attention in the clinical and basic science literature.

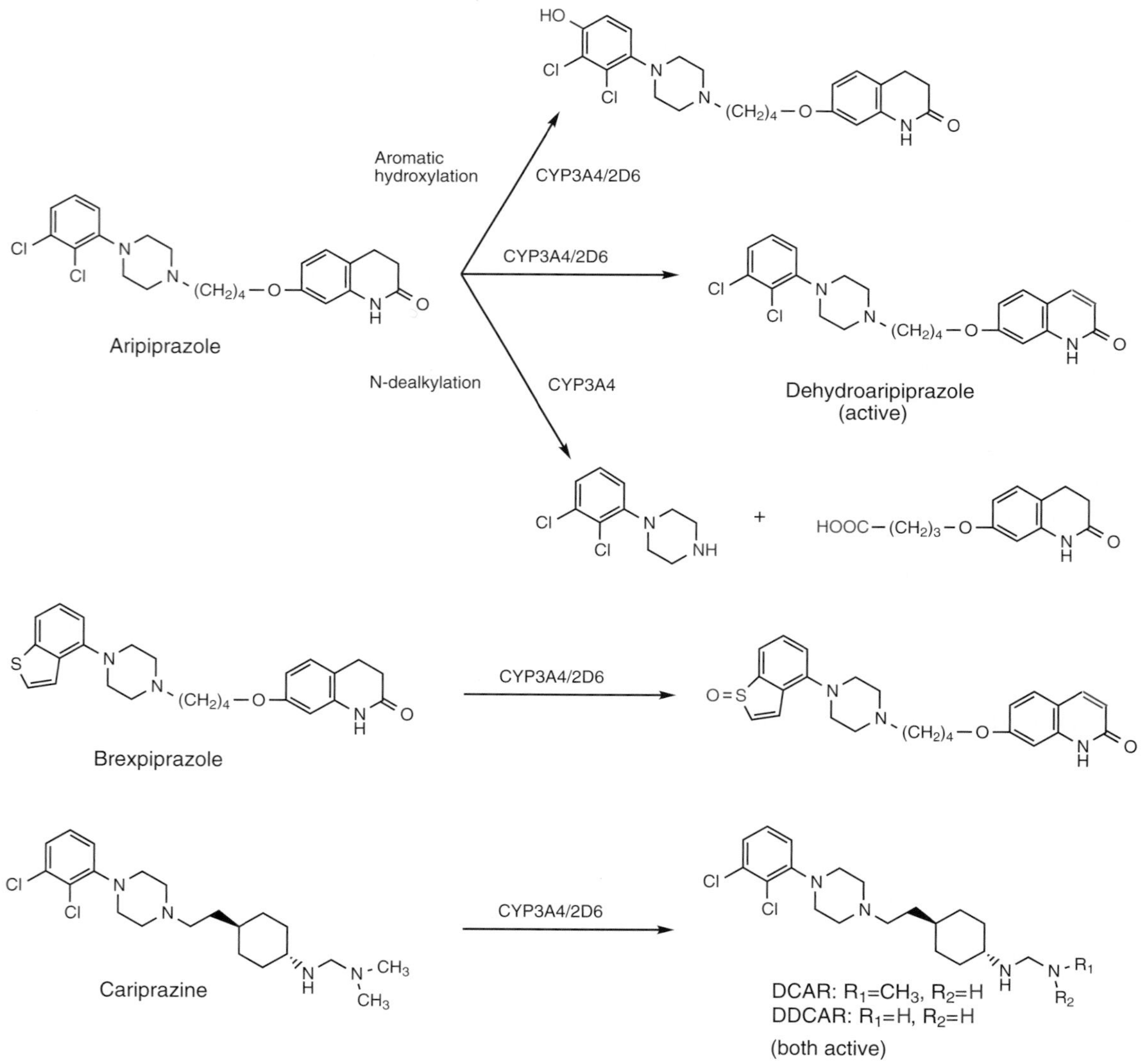

Figure 11.15 Structures and metabolism of aripiprazole, brexpiprazole, and cariprazine.

Aripiprazole has high affinity at 5-HT_{1A}, 5-HT_{2A}, and D_3 and very high affinity at D_2 receptors. Although its efficacy is not superior to other antipsychotic drugs, it has an improved side effect profile compared to many others. Aripiprazole does not prolong the QTc and causes relatively minimal weight gain.[43] Also, despite its very high affinity at dopamine D_2, aripiprazole has a relatively low propensity to cause extrapyramidal symptoms, with the exception of akathisia (affecting ~10% of patients), and does not increase prolactin.[43,100] Partly, this may be explained by its GPCR functional profile.

Aripiprazole is a partial agonist at dopamine D_2, D_3, serotonin 5-HT_{1A} and 5-HT_{2C} receptors—with efficacies depending on the cellular milieu—and is an antagonist at 5-HT_{2A} receptors.[57] Recall that prolonged D_2 blockade produces extrapyramidal and hyperprolactinemia side effects. As a D_2 receptor partial agonist with moderate intrinsic activity, aripiprazole may partially block D_2 receptor signaling in neural systems with high dopaminergic tone, that is, the striatal dopamine system of schizophrenic patients. Conversely, it may partially activate D_2 receptors in neural systems with low dopaminergic tone, that is, the mesocortical system in schizophrenic patients. This may account for its efficacy to treat psychoses.[80,101] Other proposed pharmacological mechanisms focus on aripiprazole's full agonism at presynaptic D_2 autoreceptors in vivo in animal models.[57,80,101-103] D_2 autoreceptors modulate dopamine neurotransmission via a negative feedback mechanism. For example, at relatively high dopamine concentrations (or during phasic dopamine release), presynaptic D_2 autoreceptors are activated to decrease dopamine synthesis and release, and somatodendritic D_2 autoreceptors decrease neuronal firing rate. Striatal dopamine neurons express high levels of D_2 autoreceptors, whereas they are scantly expressed in the mesocortical dopamine pathway. Thus, aripiprazole, by acting as a D_2 autoreceptor agonist, may decrease dopaminergic tone selectively in the striatum. Combined with antagonist activity at postsynaptic D_2 receptors in vivo, this pharmacology may contribute to its unique clinical effects. Finally, aripiprazole's functional effects at the D_2 receptor vary depending on signaling pathway, cell type, and cellular context, providing evidence that it may be a biased agonist at the D_2 receptor in vivo. Aripiprazole's partial agonist activity at 5-HT_{1A} and 5-HT_{2C} receptors might also contribute to its efficacy for treating negative symptoms, and to its low propensity to induce weight gain, respectively.

Aripiprazole has high oral bioavailability (90%) with a half-life of approximately 75 hours. It undergoes hepatic CYP3A4- and CYP2D6-catalyzed N-dealkylation and hydroxylation as well as dehydrogenation to dehydroaripiprazole (Fig. 11.17), which is an active metabolite with a half-life of about 90 hours. Recent preclinical data show that aripiprazole, as well as cariprazine (discussed below), and a common metabolite of each, 2,3-(dichlorophenyl) piperazine, inhibit cholesterol biosynthesis at the conversion of 7-dehydrocholesterol (7-DHC) to cholesterol.[104] The inhibition of this enzymatic step by mutations in the *DHCR7* gene leads to Smith-Lemli-Opitz syndrome, a severe developmental disorder that affects many parts of the body and causes intellectual and behavioral problems. Thus, risks associated with aripiprazole usage during pregnancy should be strongly considered.

BREXPIPRAZOLE (REXULTI). Brexpiprazole is a close analogue of aripiprazole and similarly, has been shown to be effective at treating positive and negative symptoms of schizophrenia. In addition to schizophrenia, brexpiprazole is also approved as an adjunctive treatment of major depressive disorder. Brexpiprazole has high affinity at many serotonin, α-adrenergic, and dopamine receptors. Brexpiprazole, compared to its predecessor aripiprazole, has ≥10-fold higher affinity at D_4, 5-HT_{1A}, 5-HT_{2A}, α_{1A}, α_{1B}, and α_{2C} and similar affinity at all other GPCRs tested.[105] Brexpiprazole exhibits D_2, D_3, 5-HT_{1A}, and 5-HT_{2C} partial agonism, similar to aripiprazole. However, brexpiprazole exhibits lower intrinsic activity at dopamine D_2 receptors relative to aripiprazole. Its functional activities at D_3 and 5-HT_{2C}, also, are very weak. It behaves as an antagonist at 5-HT_{2A}, 5-HT_{2B}, and α1- and α_2-type receptors. It also has inhibitory activity at the serotonin (IC_{50} = 29 nM) and norepinephrine (IC_{50} = 139 nM) transporters that is similar to fluoxetine.[105] This likely contributes to its antidepressant activity. Like aripiprazole, akathisia is a common adverse effect of brexpiprazole, but incidence is reportedly lower than aripiprazole—which might be due lower D_2 intrinsic activity. Other adverse events are comparable to placebo.

Brexpiprazole has high absolute bioavailability (95%), is highly bound to plasma protein (>99%), and undergoes CYP3A4 and CYP2D6 metabolic oxidation to the major inactive metabolite DM-3411, which apparently does not contribute to clinical effects. Various other oxidative metabolites have been reported. The terminal elimination half-lives of brexpiprazole and its major metabolite, DM-3411, are 91 hours and 86 hours, respectively.

CARIPRAZINE (VRAYLAR). Cariprazine is effective at treating both positive and negative symptoms of schizophrenia. A recent clinical trial reported superiority at treating negative symptoms compared to risperidone.[106] In addition to schizophrenia, cariprazine is also approved to treat manic or mixed episodes associated with bipolar I disorder in adults. Like its structurally similar counterparts, aripiprazole and brexpiprazole, cariprazine is a 5-HT_{1A}, dopamine D_2 and D_3 receptor partial agonist—with efficacies depending on cellular milieu. Cariprazine has very high affinity for both the D_2 and D_3 receptors but is unique among antipsychotics for possessing higher selectivity for the dopamine D_3 receptor (D_3 K_i < 0.1 nM; D_2 K_i < 1 nM). This was corroborated in a clinical trial that showed preferential binding to D_3 in patients with schizophrenia when administered at low doses.[107] At doses ≥1.5 mg/d, D_2 and D_3 receptor occupancy is ≥75%. In addition to the usual targets, cariprazine also shows moderate affinity for sigma σ1 receptors. Long-term administration of cariprazine changes the expression of dopamine, serotonin, and glutamate receptor subtypes in multiple brain regions.[108,109]

Cariprazine is metabolized by CYP3A4 and to a lesser extent by CYP2D6 to two clinically active metabolites, desmethyl-cariprazine and didesmethyl-cariprazine, which are excreted in the urine with only a small amount of the unchanged parent drug. Cariprazine has a half-life of 2-4 days, and didesmethyl-cariprazine has a terminal half-life of 2-3 weeks. At high doses (>6 mg/d), there is increased incidence of extrapyramidal effects (akathisia and Parkinson's disease symptoms) and hypertension.[110] Akathisia and other extrapyramidal symptoms were particularly high in patients treated with cariprazine—in some cases, 14% and 20% of patients reported these respective side effects (compared to 4% and 8% with placebo). Cariprazine (6 mg/d or less) showed no clinically relevant effects on QTc prolongation or prolactin elevation.

Long-Acting Antipsychotics

The duration of action of many of the antipsychotics with a free hydroxyl moiety (e.g., perphenazine and fluphenazine Table 11.2) can be considerably prolonged by the preparation of a long-chain fatty acid ester analogue (Table 11.3). Fluphenazine decanoate and fluphenazine enanthate were the first of such esters to appear in clinical use and are longer acting, with fewer side effects than the unesterified parent drug. The ability to treat patients with a single intramuscular injection every 1-2 weeks with the enanthate or every 2-3 weeks with the decanoate ester means that problems associated with patient compliance to the drug regimens and with drug malabsorption can be reduced. Table 11.3 lists long-acting forms of phenothiazine-type and thioxanthene-type antipsychotics that are derivatives available in the United States and other countries.

Aripiprazole also is available in a long-acting form, aripiprazole lauroxil (Aristada). It is an intramuscular injectable formulation administered monthly, every 6 weeks, or every 2 months, depending on dose. Aripiprazole lauroxil undergoes esterase-catalyzed hydrolysis to N-hydroxymethyl aripiprazole which is then hydrolyzed to aripiprazole[111] (Fig. 11.16).

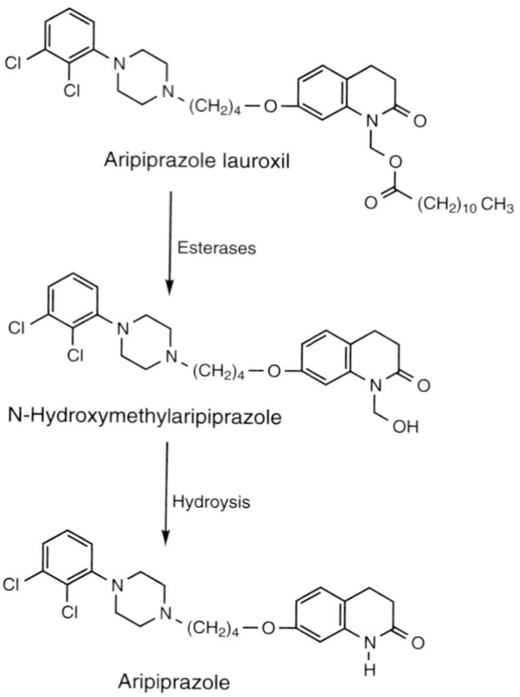

Aripiprazole lauroxil

Esterases

N-Hydroxymethylaripiprazole

Hydroysis

Aripiprazole

Figure 11.16 Hydrolysis of apripiprazole lauroxil to aripiprazole.

Miscellaneous Medications

VALBENAZINE (INGREZZA) FOR TARDIVE DYSKINESIA. Tetrabenazine and its pro-drug forms, deutetrabenazine and valbenazine (Fig. 11.17), are vesicular monoamine transporter 2 (VMAT2) inhibitors approved to treat tardive dyskinesia, a common extrapyramidal side effect of high-dose antipsychotics. Both tetrabenazine and deutetrabenazine also have been approved for treatment of chorea associated with Huntington's disease. The keto moiety of tetrabenazine (an enantiomeric mixture)

Table 11.3 Long-acting Phenothiazines and Thioxanthenes for Intramuscular Depot Injection

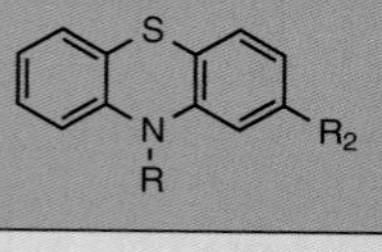

Generic Name	R	R_2	Dosage Range	Duration of Action
Phenothiazines				
Fluphenazine decanoate	$(CH_2)_3$-N(piperazine)N-CH_2CH_2O-C(=O)-$(CH_2)_8CH_3$	CF_3	25-200 mg	2-3 wk
Fluphenazine enanthate	$(CH_2)_3$-N(piperazine)N-CH_2CH_2O-C(=O)-$(CH_2)_5CH_3$	CF_3	Discontinued	
Perphenazine enanthate	$(CH_2)_3$-N(piperazine)N-CH_2CH_2O-C(=O)-$(CH_2)_5CH_3$	Cl	Discontinued	
Thioxanthene				
Flupentixol decanoate	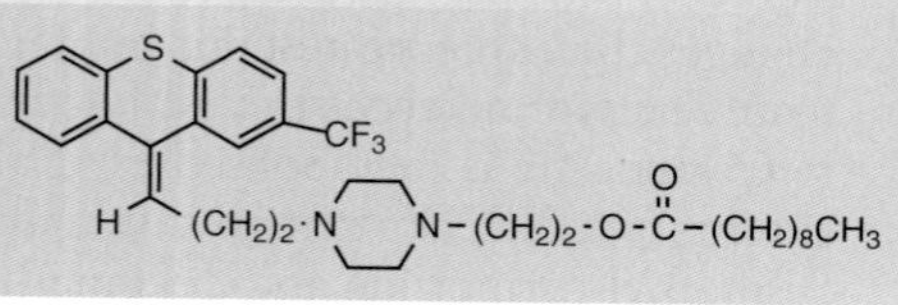 (thioxanthene, CF_3) =CH-$(CH_2)_2$-N(piperazine)N-$(CH_2)_2$-O-C(=O)-$(CH_2)_8CH_3$		Discontinued	

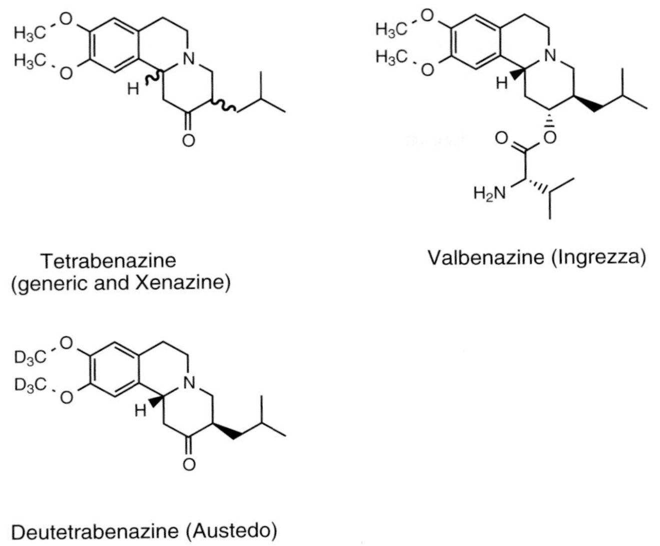

Tetrabenazine
(generic and Xenazine)

Valbenazine (Ingrezza)

Deutetrabenazine (Austedo)

Figure 11.17 Structures of tetrabenazine and its prodrug forms valbenazine and deutetrabenazine.

undergoes rapid and extensive hepatic metabolism by carbonyl reductase to an enantiomeric mixture of dihydrotetrabenazines (Fig. 11.18). Plasma concentrations of tetrabenazine are not detected after oral administration due to rapid metabolism to dihydrotetrabenazines. These then undergo oxidative demethylation by CYP2D6 to inactive metabolites that subsequently undergo phase-II metabolism to sulfates and glucuronidates (Fig. 11.18). The half-life for tetrabenazine is 10 hours, whereas the half-life of the active drug metabolite, (*R*,*R*,*R*)-α-dihydrotetrabenazine, is 2-8 hours.

(*R*,*R*,*R*)-α-dihydrotetrabenazine is active to inhibit VMAT2, an antiporter protein found within the membrane of dopamine vesicles. These vesicles regulate dopamine (and to a lesser extent serotonin and norepinephrine) uptake from the cytoplasm into synaptic vesicles, which

Tetrabenazine

Carbonyl reductase

α-Dihydrotetrabenazine
(reduction products are an enantiomeric mixture; the active enantiomer is shown)

CYP2D6

Sulfates + glucuronides

Inactive

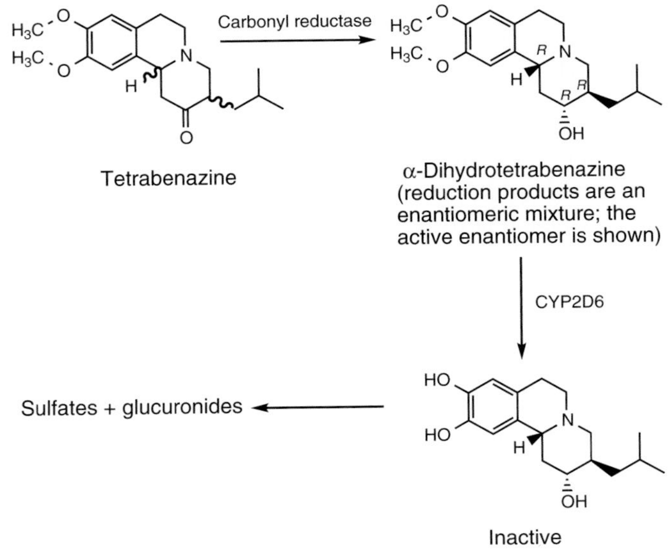

Figure 11.18 Metabolism of tetrabenazine.

stores neurotransmitters prior to their subsequent release into extracellular zones. Reversible binding of tetrabenazine to VMAT2 reduces storage and synaptic concentrations of dopamine. The reduction in synaptic dopamine levels is hypothesized to address the pathophysiology of tardive dyskinesia. Specifically, it is believed that prolonged antipsychotic drug blockade of dopamine receptors results in receptor hypersensitivity that leads to tardive dyskinesia. Reducing synaptic dopamine levels by VMAT2 inhibition decreases activity of dopamine receptors to alleviate tardive dyskinesia.

Valbenazine (Fig. 11.17) is a single enantiomer pro-drug form of tetrabenazine containing an L-valine ester moiety that is hydrolyzed in vivo to the single active enantiomer (*R*,*R*,*R*)-α-dihydrotetrabenazine.[112] The hydrolysis step occurs slowly; thus, valbenazine has a half-life of 15 hours. Deutetrabenazine[113] (Fig. 11.17) is the first deuterated drug approved by the Food and Drug Administration (2017). Analogously to tetrabenazine, deutetrabenazine undergoes reduction to an enantiomeric mixture of deutdihydrotetrabenazines, with the active drug being the (*R*,*R*,*R*) enantiomer of α-deutdihydrotetrabenazine. The substitution of carbon-hydrogen with carbon-deuterium on the methoxy moiety of (*R*,*R*,*R*)-α-deutdihydrotetrabenazine is presumed to slow CYP2D6-catalyzed oxidative demethylation, resulting in a half-life of 9 hours for the active drug and a reduced dosing frequency for prodrug deutetrabenazine.

Sedation is the most common adverse effect of tetrabenazine and its analogues. The incidence of extrapyramidal symptoms is low and includes mainly dyskinesia, not akathisia. Tetrabenazine and its analogues carry a black box warning of the potential for depression and suicidality. Additionally, deutetrabenazine is contraindicated in patients with hepatic impairment, in patients taking monoamine oxidase inhibitors and in patients taking reserpine.

PIMAVANSERIN (NUPLAZID) FOR PARKINSON'S DISEASE PSYCHOSIS[50]. Up to 60% of Parkinson's disease patients develop psychosis, which may be caused by dopamine agonist medications or may be related to pathology. Management often includes a reduction in dopaminergic medications or the introduction of an atypical antipsychotic medication, such as clozapine. The serious side effects associated with clozapine, such as metabolic syndrome, however, created an opportunity for new drug development that avoided direct targeting of dopamine receptors. Pimavanserin is a selective serotonin 5-HT_{2A} (and to a lesser extent 5-HT_{2C}) receptor inverse agonist approved for Parkinson's disease psychosis in 2016. In a randomized, double-blind, placebo-controlled study, pimavanserin improved psychotic symptoms in patients with Parkinson's disease, while also leading to improved sleep and decreased caregiver burden.[51] Pimavanserin is predominantly metabolized by CYP3A4 and CYP3A5; CYP3A4 is the major enzyme responsible for the formation of its major active metabolite. The half-life of pimavanserin is very long (54 hr), and it is recommended to reduce the dose by one-half if patients are also taking strong inhibitors of CYP3A4, such as ketoconazole.

Confusional state (6%), peripheral edema (7%), and hallucinations (7%, paradoxically) were reported side effects occurring in ≥5% of patients receiving pimavanserin that did not also occur at or above this frequency with placebo. There are no data on long-term efficacy and safety in Parkinson's disease patients, but it may prolong the QTc interval. Postmarketing side effects of pimavanserin reported include rash, urticaria, potential angioedema, and somnolence. Pimavanserin, like other antipsychotics, carries a black box warning of increased mortality in elderly patients with dementia-related psychosis. Pimavanserin is not currently approved for psychosis unrelated to Parkinson's disease; however, in a phase 2, randomized, placebo-controlled, double-blind study, it was effective for Alzheimer's disease psychosis after 6 weeks of treatment; effects did not endure to 12 weeks.[114]

Pimavanserin tartrate (Nuplazid)

Anxiety Disorders

In DSM-5, anxiety disorders include generalized anxiety disorder, separation anxiety disorder, social anxiety disorder (social phobia), specific phobia, panic disorder, agoraphobia, and selective mutism (a disorder in which a person normally capable of speech does not speak in specific situations or to certain people). Notably, anxiety disorders are considered separate from obsessive-compulsive disorders and trauma and stressor-related disorders (include post-traumatic stress disorder), albeit several of the drugs discussed in this chapter that target GABA receptors to treat anxiety disorders also are approved to treat obsessive-compulsive disorder. To meet general DSM-5 reference criteria, anxiety symptoms cannot be caused by an exogenous factor (e.g., caffeine) or a medical condition (e.g., hyperthyroidism), and at least three (one in children) of the following symptoms must occur more days than not for at least 6 months: restlessness, irritability, muscle tension, difficulty to concentrate, sleep disturbance, fatigue. Moreover, a diagnosis of anxiety disorder requires that the mental and/or physical symptoms impair social, occupational, and/or other important areas of functioning.

Etiology of Anxiety Disorders

Studies of patients with anxiety disorders have not revealed a general gross neuroanatomical lesion. In vivo functional imaging studies, however, show altered blood oxygen levels (as a manifestation of blood flow) or glucose utilization in specific brain areas in patients with anxiety conditions,[115,116] including panic disorder[117,118] and specific phobia,[119,120] mostly implicating the prefrontal cortex and limbic areas as being involved in pathologic anxiety. Although there is some evidence linking acid-sensitive channels and catechol-O-methyltransferase to panic disorder, genetic mechanisms underlying general symptoms of anxiety remain unclear. It is also important to note that there is significant comorbidity for anxiety and major depressive disorder in both children and adults,[121,122] suggesting mechanistic overlap between the disorders.

A variety of neurotransmitters, neuromodulators (e.g., adenosine), and neuropeptides (e.g., cholecystokinin, corticotropin-releasing factor, and neuropeptide Y) are suggested to be involved in the pathophysiology of anxiety. Abundant evidence exists to document the involvement of the neurotransmitters GABA, glutamate, norepinephrine, serotonin, and dopamine in anxiety. Notably, most drugs effective for anxiety disorders affect one or several of these neurotransmitters. Anxiety disorders, however, are not simply a deficiency or excess of one neurotransmitter or another—research increasingly is revealing that these neurotransmitter systems have complex anatomical and functional interrelationships. Such complexity helps to explain the unpredictable and sometimes paradoxical responses to medications.

GABA Receptors

The major inhibitory neurotransmitter in the mammalian CNS, GABA is widespread, with approximately one-third of all synapses in the CNS utilizing this neurochemical for intercellular communication. The two major classes of GABA receptors[123] are inotropic $GABA_A$ and metabotropic $GABA_B$ receptors. The so-called $\rho GABA_A$ receptor is the preferred term to describe a gene product that was identified, pre-cloning, as a GABA receptor-like protein with pharmacology distinct from $GABA_A$ and $GABA_B$ receptors.[124] Based on primary sequence and function, $\rho GABA_A$ appears closely related to $GABA_A$ receptors, and it is currently recommended by the International Union of Pharmacology to not use the term "$GABA_C$" receptor to describe $\rho GABA_A$ receptors.

$GABA_A$ Receptor

The $GABA_A$ receptor is a member of the gene superfamily of ligand-gated ion channels that is known as the "cys-loop" family because of the presence of a cysteine loop in their N-terminal domain.[123] These receptors exist as heteropentameric subunits arranged around a central ion channel (Fig. 11.19A). Each of the five polypeptide subunits is composed of an extracellular region, four membrane-spanning α-helical cylinders, and a large intracellular cytoplasmic loop.

The second of the four membrane-spanning α-helical cylinders, from each of the five subunits, forms the $GABA_A$ ion channel, which conducts chloride to hyperpolarize the cell, e.g., decreases the firing probability of a neuron. The first $GABA_A$ subunit was sequenced in 1987.[125] In humans, so far, 16 different genetically distinct subunits for the $GABA_A$ receptor have been isolated. These polypeptides are denoted as α_{1-6}, β_{1-3}, γ_{1-3}, δ, ε, π, and θ. The subunits can combine in varied proportions and alternatively spliced variants are common. Thus, many possible receptor subtypes may exist.

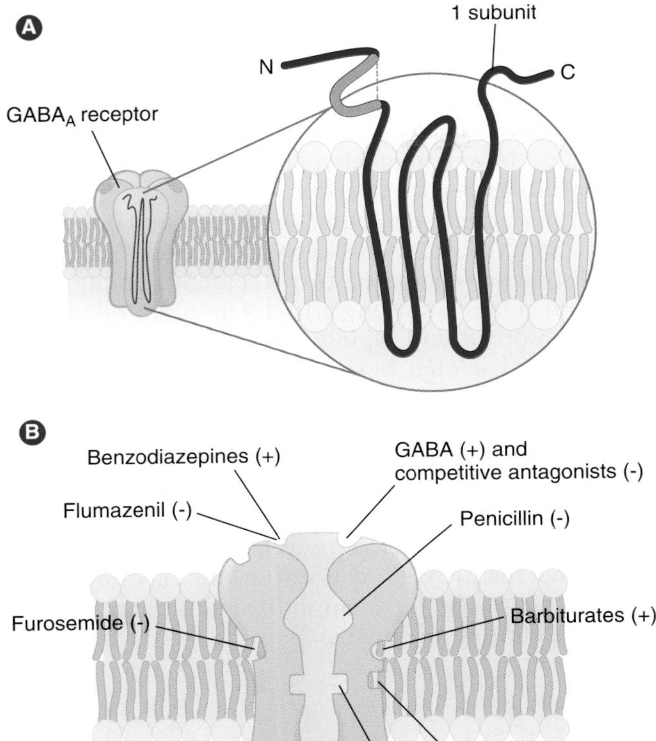

Figure 11.19 Schematic representation of the γ-aminobutyric acid$_A$ (GABA$_A$) receptor. A, GABA$_A$ receptors have a pentameric structure composed predominantly of α, β, and γ subunits arranged, in various proportions, around a central ion channel that conducts chloride. (refer to text) Each subunit has four membrane-spanning regions and a cysteine loop in the extracellular N-terminal domain (dashed line). B, There are several unique ligand binding sites on the GABA$_A$ receptor, where drugs can bind to impact GABA$_A$ receptor function. (From Chou J. Strichartz GR, Lo EA. Pharmacology of Excitatory and Inhibitory Neurotransmission. In: Golan DE, ed. *Principles of Pharmacology*. Philadelphia: Lippincott Williams & Wilkins; 2005:142; with permission.)

The major (60%) GABA$_A$ receptor isoform in human adult brain consists of two α_1 subunits, two β_2 subunits, and one γ_2 subunit.[126] Recently, cryo-electron microscopy structures with overall resolution of 3.9 Å of the human $\alpha_1\beta_2\gamma_2$ GABA$_A$ receptor, bound to GABA and flumazenil (an antagonist of the site on the GABA$_A$ receptor where benzodiazepines bind, see below), were reported.[127] In contrast to GABA$_A$ receptors, ρ subunits alone can form functional homo- and heteropentameric ρGABA$_A$ receptors. So far, three different human rho subunits ($\rho_{1\text{-}3}$) have been identified as structural components of the ρGABA$_A$ receptor.

The GABA$_A$ receptor contains many distinct binding sites (Fig. 11.19B), including a site for GABA (orthosteric site) as well as sites where neuroactive drugs, e.g., benzodiazepines, barbiturates, picrotoxin, ethanol, and neurosteroids (allosteric sites), bind—the recently resolved GABA$_A$ crystal structure also revealed several additional binding sites that will likely aid in the design of novel GABA$_A$ targeting medication candidates. The orthosteric, GABA binding site is at the interface between α and β subunits, whereas the allosteric binding site for benzodiazepines, commonly prescribed as anxiolytic and sedative agents, is defined by the α and γ subunits.[123] The distinct composition of α and γ subunits determines the affinity and efficacy of unique benzodiazepines.[128,129]

GABA$_B$ Receptors

The GABA$_B$ receptor is a class-C GPCR that can modulate (via $G\alpha_{i/o}$) activity of the effector proteins adenylyl cyclase, G protein–activated inwardly rectifying K^+ channels (GIRK) channels, and G protein–dependent neuronal Ca^{2+} channels.[130] Like GABA$_A$, neurophysiological effects of GABA$_B$ signaling include hyperpolarization of neurons and inhibition of neurotransmitter release. The GABA$_B$ GPCR exists as two major subtypes, GABA$_{B(1)}$ and GABA$_{B(2)}$. The GABA$_{B(1)}$ subtype can be expressed as GABA$_{B(1a)}$ and GABA$_{B(1b)}$ isoforms that differ in their extracellular NH_2-terminal domains but are derived from the same gene.[131] Interestingly, it was discovered early on that compared to native GABA$_B$ receptors, recombinant GABA$_{B(1a)}$ and GABA$_{B(1b)}$ receptors expressed in heterologous cells display 100- to 150-fold lower affinity for agonist ligands. Likewise, recombinant GABA$_{B(1a)}$ and GABA$_{B(1b)}$ receptors were shown to couple inefficiently to their effector systems. These surprising pharmacological findings were explained by the discovery that recombinant GABA$_{B(1a)}$ and GABA$_{B(1b)}$ receptors expressed in heterologous cells are retained in the endoplasmic reticulum. In fact, it turned out that GABA$_{B(1)}$ receptors do not traffic to the cell membrane surface in the absence of GABA$_{B(2)}$ receptors. This remarkable discovery that the GABA$_{B(2)}$ receptor co-expresses on the cell surface with the GABA$_{B(1a)}$ or GABA$_{B(1b)}$ receptor to form a functional heterodimeric GPCR was reported simultaneously by three research groups from the pharmaceutical industry in 1998.[132-134] GABA$_B$ receptors were the first GPCR shown to function not as a single protein but rather, as two distinct subunits, neither of which is functional by itself (Fig. 11.20). Recently, it was determined that the GABA$_B$ receptor also is expressed on

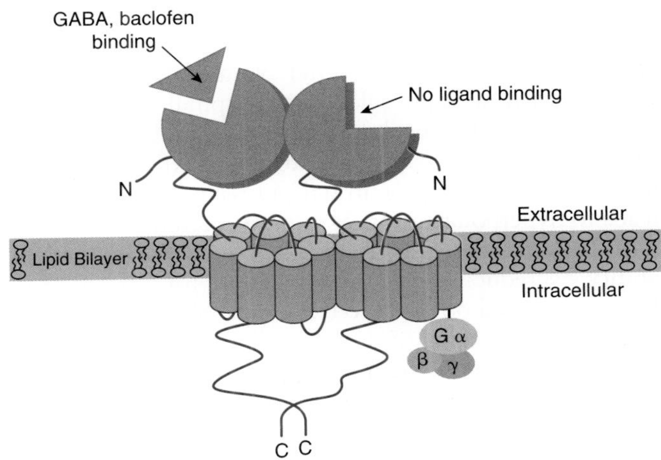

Figure 11.20 Schematic representation of the γ-aminobutyric acid$_B$ (GABA$_B$) receptor.

the cell surface as a large oligomeric complex.[135] Homo- and/or heterodimerization, as well as oligomerization, has been documented for many GPCRs and may account for the diverse signaling functionality for this protein family.

The solved structure[136] of the extracellular orthosteric ligand-binding region of the heterodimeric $GABA_{B(1b)}$/$GABA_{B(2)}$ GPCR is very different and considerably more complex in comparison to other aminergic GPCRs that are able to function as monomers.[130] In accordance with the Venus flytrap model for class-C GPCRs,[137] the extracellular domains of the $GABA_{B(1b)}$ and $GABA_{B(2)}$ subunits each are a pair of globular lobes, with a hinge region separating each lobe within the pair. Only the $GABA_{B(1b)}$ subunit binds orthosteric ligands, while the $GABA_{B(2)}$ unit couples with G protein. The $GABA_{B(2)}$ subunit also interacts with potassium channel tetramerization-domain proteins that modulate kinetic parameters of G protein signaling. Upon binding of an orthosteric agonist (e.g., GABA or the clinical drug baclofen) to the $GABA_{B(1b)}$ subunit, the flytrap closes and the $GABA_B$ receptor is activated. Binding of an antagonist ligand (usually containing a bulky chemical moiety) to the $GABA_{B(1b)}$ subunit sterically hinders flytrap closure and stabilizes an inactive conformation of receptor. The $GABA_{B(1a)}$ subunit is proposed to possess the same ligand-binding function within the heteromer as the $GABA_{B(1b)}$ subunit.

$GABA_B$ receptors are reported to play a role in the pathophysiology and perhaps pharmacotherapy of a variety of CNS diseases and disorders, including, Alzheimer's disease, addiction (especially ethanol), anxiety, autism spectrum disorder (including, fragile X syndrome),[138,139] depression, epilepsy, Huntington's disease, pain, Parkinson's disease, schizophrenia, and stroke, as well as muscle spasticity disorders and gastroesophageal reflux disease.[140-142] The only drug currently in clinical use that selectively interacts with the $GABA_B$ receptor is baclofen (β-*p*-chlorophenyl-GABA). Baclofen was first synthesized in 1962 and was shown to have potent muscle relaxant and analgesic activity. In 1972, the R/S racemate was marketed (Lioresal) to treat spasticity disorders. In 1980, the *R*-(−)-enantiomer of baclofen was shown to stereoselectively interact (as an agonist) with what is now known as the $GABA_B$ receptor. Currently, baclofen is indicated only for the relief of muscle spasticity in patients with multiple sclerosis and spinal cord injuries. It is proposed that baclofen inhibits spinal cord monosynaptic and polysynaptic reflexes via $GABA_B$ receptor–mediated opening of neuronal potassium channels that leads to hyperpolarization of primary afferent fiber terminals. In spinal motor neurons, baclofen suppresses excitability by reducing calcium persistent inward currents. Baclofen is used off-label to treat some of the many other conditions thought to involve $GABA_B$ receptors (as listed above), including anxiety, albeit there currently is not compelling evidence $GABA_B$ receptors play a major role in the pathophysiology or pharmacotherapy of anxiety disorders. Although baclofen is rapidly absorbed after oral administration, absorption is mainly limited to the upper small intestine, and therapeutic concentrations in brain are difficult to achieve because it is transported out of the brain via the organic acid transporter.[141] Baclofen also has a short duration of action (half-life 3-4 hr) and is rapidly cleared from circulation, largely eliminated unchanged, via renal excretion.

The investigational compound, arbaclofen placarbil, is a prodrug of (*R*)-baclofen developed to enhance oral absorption compared to the parent compound.[143] Afer oral administration, arbaclofen placarbil is efficiently absorbed and rapidly converted to *R*-baclofen. Although arbaclofen has been studied to treat symptoms of autism and fragile X syndrome ,[138,139] convincing efficacy has not been established and the prodrug has not been approved. Adverse effects with oral baclofen include muscle weakness, nausea, somnolence, and paraesthesia. Rapid tolerance to its therapeutic effects occurs. Intrathecal baclofen can bypass the difficulty to obtain therapeutic CNS concentrations via oral administration, allowing for a minimized dose and perhaps minimized untoward effects.[140]

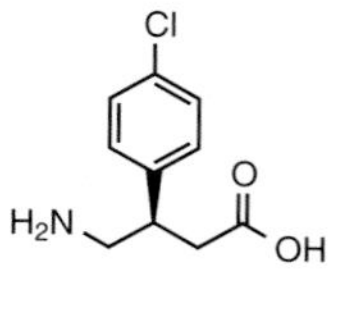

Cl H2N O OH

R(-)-Baclofen

Cl H N O O O O O OH

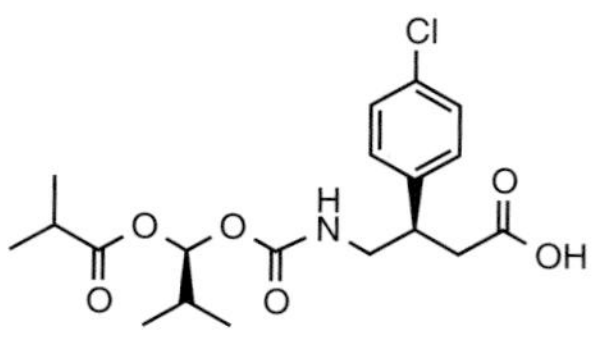

Arbaclofen placarbil

Drugs Targeting $GABA_A$ Receptors for the Treatment of Anxiety

Benzodiazepines

The benzodiazepines are efficacious drugs for treating anxiety disorders. Chlordiazepoxide was the first benzodiazepine to be marketed for clinical use in 1960. Its effectiveness and wide margin of safety were major advances over compounds, such as barbiturates, used previously. A variety of new benzodiazepines followed, each with minor differences, highlighted in marketing campaigns. The major factors to be considered when selecting an agent include rate and extent of absorption, presence or absence of active metabolites, and degree of lipophilicity. These factors help to determine how a benzodiazepine is marketed and used; for example, an agent that is rapidly absorbed and fast-acting, such as alprazolam, may be used to treat panic attacks, which are overwhelming bouts of fear that occur unexpectedly.

Development of Benzodiazepine Anxiolytics. In the 1950s, the medicinal chemist Sternbach noted that "basic groups frequently impart biological activity," and in accordance with this observation, he synthesized,

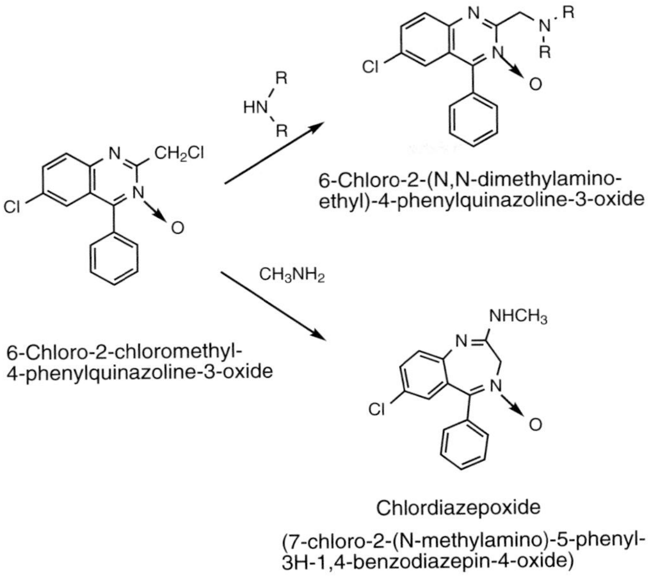

6-Chloro-2-chloromethyl-4-phenylquinazoline-3-oxide

6-Chloro-2-(N,N-dimethylamino-ethyl)-4-phenylquinazoline-3-oxide

Chlordiazepoxide (7-chloro-2-(N-methylamino)-5-phenyl-3H-1,4-benzodiazepin-4-oxide)

Figure 11.21 Synthesis of chlordiazepoxide.

at the New Jersey laboratories of Hoffman LaRoche, a series of compounds by treating various chloromethylquinazoline N-oxides with amines to produce what he hoped would be products with "tranquilizer" activity.[144,145] Sternbach's studies included the reaction of 6-chloro-2-chloromethyl-4-phenylquinazoline-3-oxide with methylamine, which yielded the unexpected rearrangement product 7-chloro-2-(N-methylamino)-5-phenyl-3H-1, 4,-benzodiazepin-4-oxide (Fig. 11.21). This product was given the code name RO 50690 and screened for pharmacological activity in 1957. Subsequently, Randall et al.[146,147] reported that RO 50690 was hypnotic and sedative and had antistrychnine properties similar to the propanediol meprobamate, a sedative that has tranquilizer (anxiolytic) properties only at intoxicating doses. Renamed chlordiazepoxide, RO 50690 was marketed in 1960 as Librium, a safe and effective anxiolytic agent.

Chlordiazepoxide turned out to have rather remarkable pharmacological properties and tremendous potential as a pharmacotherapeutic agent, but it possessed a number of unacceptable physical chemical properties. In an effort to enhance its "pharmaceutical elegance," structural modifications of chlordiazepoxide were undertaken that eventually led to the synthesis of diazepam in 1959. In contrast to the maxim that basic groups impart biological activity, diazepam contains no basic nitrogen moiety. Diazepam, however, was found to be 3- to 10-fold more potent than chlordiazepoxide and was marketed in 1963 as the anxiolytic drug Valium. Subsequently, thousands of benzodiazepine derivatives were synthesized, and more than two dozen benzodiazepines are in clinical use in the United States (Fig. 11.22).

BENZODIAZEPINE BINDING SITE LIGANDS

An endogenous ligand with affinity for the CNS benzodiazepine binding site of the $GABA_A$ receptor complex has not been identified conclusively. Several compounds of endogenous origin, however, that inhibit the binding of radiolabeled benzodiazepines to the benzodiazepine binding site have been reported. In 1980, Braestrup et al.[148] reported the presence of β-carboline-3-carboxylic acid ethyl ester (βCCE) in normal human urine, which has very high affinity for the benzodiazepine binding site complex. It was subsequently shown, however, that βCCE formed as an artifact from Braestrup's extraction procedure, during which the urine extract was heated with ethanol at pH 1, a condition favoring formation of the ethyl ester from β-carboline-3-carboxylic acid, a tryptophan metabolite.

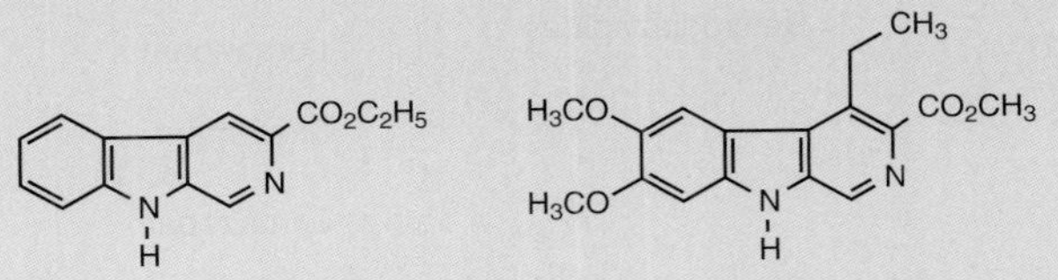

βCCE

DMCM

Betacarboline

Although βCCE actually was shown not to be of endogenous origin, its discovery as a high-affinity benzodiazepine binding site ligand stimulated research that led to the synthesis of a series of β-carboline derivatives with a variety of intrinsic activities, presumably mediated through the benzodiazepine binding site on the $GABA_A$ receptor. For example, although βCCE is considered to be a partial inverse agonist at this site, 6,7-dimethoxy-4-ethyl-β-carboline-3-carboxylic acid methyl ester (DMCM) appears to be a full inverse agonist.[149] In fact, βCCE blocks the convulsions produced by the very potent convulsant DMCM.[150] These effects are even more complex and interesting in light of the approximately 10-fold higher affinity that βCCE shows for the benzodiazepine binding site labeled by [^{3}H]diazepam when compared to DMCM.[151] The β-carbolines currently are important research tools to probe the agonist, competitive antagonist, inverse agonist, and partial agonist/inverse agonist pharmacophores of the benzodiazepine binding site/on the $GABA_A$ receptor.

A major advance in the benzodiazepine field was made in 1981 with the first report that the imidazobenzodiazepinone derivative, flumazenil, binds with high affinity to the benzodiazepine binding site and blocks the pharmacological effects of the classical benzodiazepines in vitro and in vivo.[152] Binding of [^{3}H]flumazenil to the benzodiazepine binding site is not affected

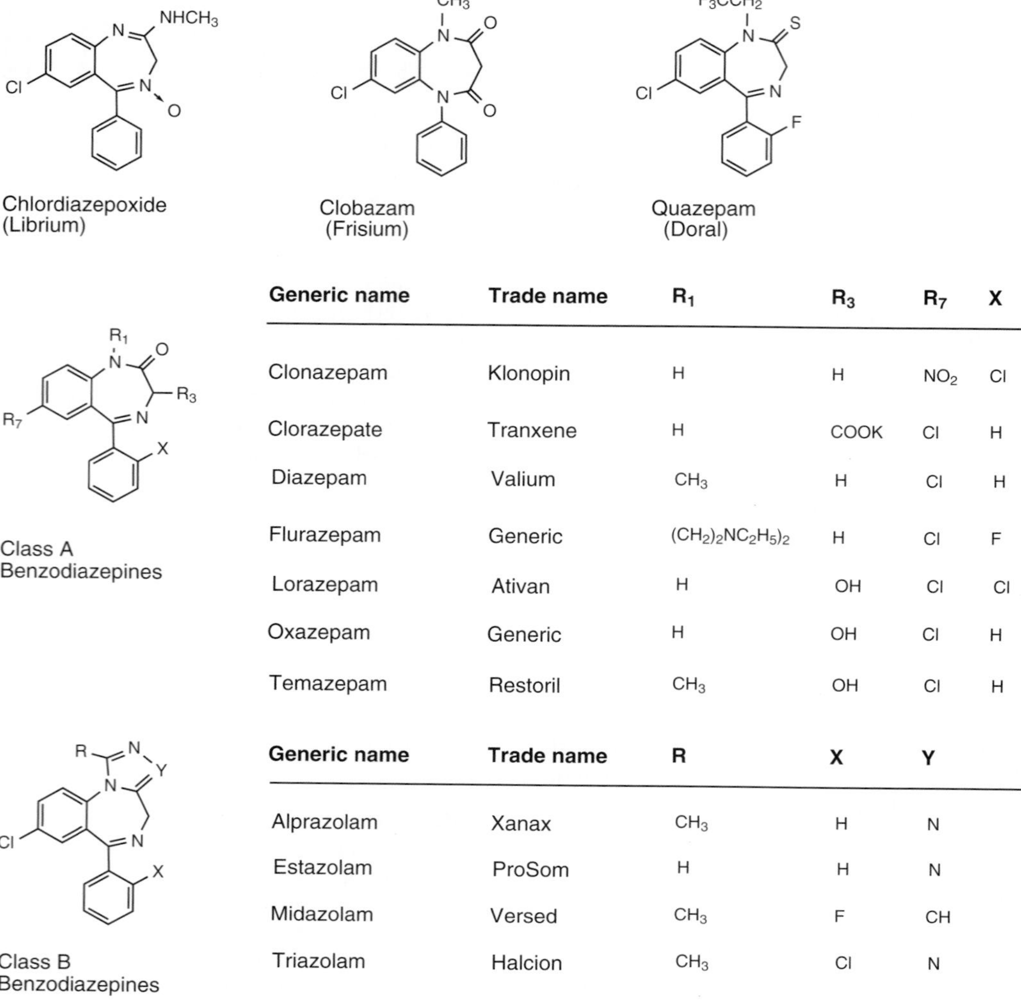

Generic name	Trade name	R_1	R_3	R_7	X
Clonazepam	Klonopin	H	H	NO_2	Cl
Clorazepate	Tranxene	H	COOK	Cl	H
Diazepam	Valium	CH_3	H	Cl	H
Flurazepam	Generic	$(CH_2)_2NC_2H_5)_2$	H	Cl	F
Lorazepam	Ativan	H	OH	Cl	Cl
Oxazepam	Generic	H	OH	Cl	H
Temazepam	Restoril	CH_3	OH	Cl	H

Generic name	Trade name	R	X	Y
Alprazolam	Xanax	CH_3	H	N
Estazolam	ProSom	H	H	N
Midazolam	Versed	CH_3	F	CH
Triazolam	Halcion	CH_3	Cl	N

Figure 11.22 Structures of some commercially available anxiolytic benzodiazepines.

by GABA and has no intrinsic activity of its own.[153] It is therefore a neutral antagonist. Flumazenil is used clinically to reverse benzodiazepine-induced sedation in overdose.

Flumazenil RO 15-4513

Mechanism of Action of Anxiolytic Benzodiazepines. A representation of the relationship between ligand interaction with the benzodiazepine binding site and intrinsic activity to modulate GABAA receptor function is shown in Figure 11.23. Anxiolytic benzodiazepines do not *directly* alter transmembrane chloride conduction to produce their anxiolytic effects. Rather, they are positive allosteric modulators (PAMs) of GABA binding to $GABA_A$. When an anxiolytic benzodiazepine binds to the benzodiazepine site, it greatly increases the affinity of GABA at $GABA_A$, which leads to a strong potentiation of chloride conductance through the channel and an increase in cell hyperpolarization (e.g., decreases activity of a neuron). Neutral antagonists benzodiazepines, such as flumazenil, bind to the benzodiazepine site, but have no effect on the intrinsic activity of the $GABA_A$ receptor. That is, they do not affect chloride conductance. Neutral antagonists, however, block access of other drugs (e.g., PAMs and negative allosteric modulators) to the site, e.g., RO 15-4513. Negative allosteric modulators (or inverse agonists), such as RO 15-4513, bind to the benzodiazepine site and decrease GABA binding, which decreases chloride conductance through the channel, leading to cell depolarization (e.g., increases activity of a neuron).

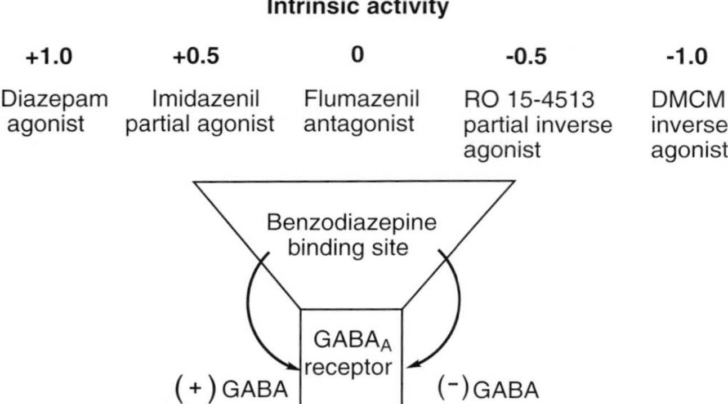

Figure 11.23 Ligand interaction with the γ-aminobutyric acid A ($GABA_A$)benzodiazepine binding site. Drugs with a range of different chemical structures, which produce different pharmacological activity, bind at the $GABA_A$ benzodiazepine binding site to modulate GABA binding at the $GABA_A$ receptor. Certain drugs (e.g., flumazenil) can block the binding of other drugs to the benzodiazepine binding site.

The benzodiazepine site can be rendered benzodiazepine-insensitive by a point mutation in the α subunit, replacing a critical histidine residue for arginine.[154] The affinity, intrinsic activity, and efficacy of benzodiazepines are determined by the nature of both the α and γ subunits. Different α and γ subunit compositions give rise to subtypes of the $GABA_A$ receptor that are pharmacologically distinct with regard to ligand affinity and intrinsic activity, providing a mechanistic basis for development of ligands that are anxioselective (i.e., anxiolysis in the absence of sedation, muscle relaxation, amnesia, and ataxia). Thus, current drug discovery approaches target specific α and γ molecular subunits of the $GABA_A$ receptor in the quest for benzodiazepine and nonbenzodiazepine (see below) drugs that demonstrate anxioselectivity. In studies using nonhuman primates, it was suggested several decades ago that $GABA_A$ α_2, α_3, and α_5 subunits mediate anxiolytic and muscle relaxant effects of benzodiazepines, whereas α_1 receptors mediate the sedative effects.[155] Currently used benzodiazepines, however, are not selective for particular α subtypes. Several putative anxioselective benzodiazepines have reached the clinic; however, they have not exhibited the degree of anxioselectivity predicted from preclinical testing and, usually, have lower efficacy than standard benzodiazepines.

STRUCTURE-ACTIVITY RELATIONSHIPS

Benzodiazepine structure

Thousands of benzodiazepine derivatives with a variety of substituents have been synthesized that interact with the benzodiazepine site, and structure-activity relationships for classical 5-phenyl-1,4-benzodiazepine-2-one anxiolytic agents are well-known. Most pharmacophore models that describe ligand functional activity are based on binding activity at a single benzodiazepine site, and this approach is used here to summarize the structure-activity relationship for benzodiazepine derivatives.

Ring A. In general, the minimum requirement for binding of 5-phenyl-1,4-benzodiazepin-2-one derivatives to the benzodiazepine site includes an aromatic or heteroaromatic ring (ring A), which is believed to participate in π-π stacking with aromatic amino acid residues of the receptor. Substituents on ring A have varied effects on binding of benzodiazepines to the benzodiazepine site, but such effects are not predictable on the basis of electronic or (within reasonable limits) steric properties. It is generally true, however, that an electronegative group (e.g., halogen or nitro) substituted at the 7-position markedly increases functional anxiolytic activity, albeit effects on binding affinity in vitro are not as dramatic. On the other hand, substituents at positions 6, 8, or 9 generally decrease anxiolytic activity. Other 1,4-diazepine derivatives in which ring A is replaced by a heterocycle generally show weak binding affinity in vitro and even less pharmacological activity in vivo when compared to phenyl-substituted analogues.

Ring B. A proton-accepting group is believed to be a structural requirement of both benzodiazepine and nonbenzodiazepine ligand binding to the $GABA_A$ receptor, putatively for interactions with a histidine residue that serves as a proton source in the $GABA_A$ α_1 subunit. For the benzodiazepines, optimal affinity occurs when the proton-accepting group in the 2-position of ring B (i.e., the carbonyl moiety) is in a coplanar spatial orientation with the aromatic ring A. Substitution of sulfur for oxygen at the 2-position may affect selectivity for binding to GABA receptors, but anxiolytic activity is maintained. Substitution of the methylene 3-position or the imine nitrogen is sterically unfavorable for antagonist activity but has no effect on PAM (i.e., anxiolytic) activity. Derivatives substituted with a 3-hydroxy moiety have comparable potency to nonhydroxylated analogues and are excreted faster. Esterification of a 3-hydroxy moiety also is possible without loss of potency. Neither the 1-position amide nitrogen nor its substituent is required for in vitro binding to the benzodiazepine site, and many clinically used analogues are not N-alkylated (Fig. 11.22). Although even relatively long N-alkyl side chains do not dramatically decrease affinity, sterically large substituents like tert-butyl drastically reduce receptor affinity and in vivo activity. Neither the 4,5-double bond nor the 4-position nitrogen (the 4,5-[methyleneimino] group) in ring B is required for in vivo anxiolytic activity, albeit in vitro affinity is decreased if the C=N bond is reduced to C–N. It is proposed that in vivo activity of such derivatives results from oxidation back to C=N. It follows that the 4-oxide moiety of chlordiazepoxide can be removed without loss of anxiolytic activity.

Ring C. Ring C (5-phenyl) is not required for binding to the benzodiazepine site in vitro. This accessory aromatic ring may contribute favorable hydrophobic or steric interactions to receptor binding, however, and its relationship to ring A planarity may be important. Substitution at the 4′-(para)-position of an appended 5-phenyl ring is unfavorable for PAM activity, but 2′-(ortho)-substituents are not detrimental, suggesting that limitations at the para position are steric, rather than electronic, in nature.

1,2-Annelation

s-Triazolo[4,3a][1,4]benzodiazepine Imidazo[1,5a][1,4]benzodiazepine

Annelation

Annelating the 1,2-bond of ring B with an additional "electron-rich" (i.e., proton acceptor) ring, such as *S*-triazole or imidazole, also results in pharmacologically active benzodiazepine derivatives with high affinity for the benzodiazepine site. For example, the *S*-triazolo-benzodiazepines triazolam, alprazolam, and estazolam and the imidazo-benzodiazepine midazolam are clinically effective anxiolytic agents (Fig. 11.22).

Stereochemistry

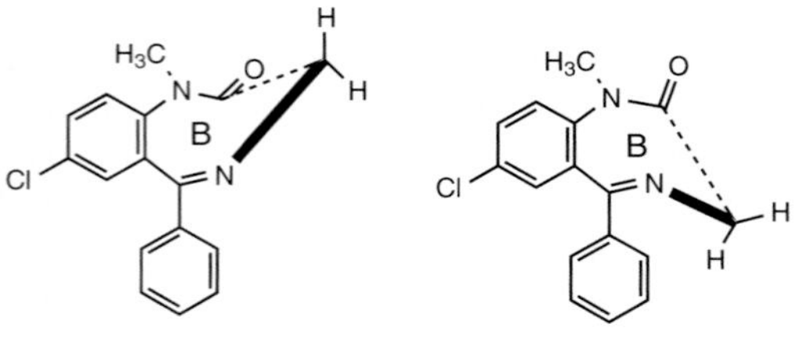

A B

Stereochemistry

Most clinically useful benzodiazepines do not have a chiral center; however, the seven-membered ring B may adopt one of two possible boat conformations, *a* and *b*, that are "enantiomeric" (mirror images) to each other. Nuclear magnetic resonance studies indicate that the two conformations can easily interconvert at room temperature, making it impossible to predict which conformation is active at the benzodiazepine site, a priori. Evidence for stereospecificity for binding to the benzodiazepine site was provided by introducing a 3-substituent into the benzodiazepine nucleus to provide a chiral center and enantiomeric pairs of derivatives.[151] In vitro binding affinity and in vivo anxiolytic activity of several 3-methylated enantiomers were found to reside in the *S*-isomer. Moreover, the *S*-enantiomer of 3-methyldiazepam was shown to stabilize conformation *a* for ring B, whereas the *R*-enantiomer stabilizes conformation *b*. Also, the 3-S configuration and *a* conformation for ring B is present in both the crystalline state[156] and in solution[157] for 3-methyldiazepam. In spite of the enantioselectivity demonstrated for benzodiazepines, the commonly used 3-hydroxylated derivatives (e.g., lorazepam and oxazepam) are commercially available only as racemic mixtures.

Physiochemical and Pharmacokinetics. The physiochemical and pharmacokinetic properties of the various benzodiazepines vary widely, and these properties have clinical implications. For example, depending on the nature of substituents, particularly with regard to electronegative substituents, the lipophilicity of the benzodiazepines may vary by more than three orders of magnitude, which affects absorption, distribution, and metabolism. In general, most benzodiazepines have relatively high lipid:water partition coefficients (Log P values) and are completely absorbed after oral administration and rapidly distributed to the brain and other highly perfused organs. A notable exception is clorazepate (Fig. 11.23), which is rapidly decarboxylated at the 3-position to N-desmethyldiazepam and, subsequently, quickly absorbed. Overall, chlorazepate clinical and pharmacokinetic properties are similar to chlordiazepoxide and diazepam (see below).

Most benzodiazepines and their metabolites bind to plasma proteins. The degree of protein binding is dependent on lipophilicity of the compound and varies from approximately 70% for more polar benzodiazepines, such as alprazolam, to 99% for very lipophilic derivatives, such as diazepam. As shown in Figure 11.24, hepatic microsomal oxidation, including N-dealkylation and aliphatic hydroxylation by a wide variety of CYP enzymes, accounts for the major metabolic disposition of most benzodiazepines. Subsequent conjugation of microsomal metabolites by glucuronyl transferases yields polar glucuronides that are excreted in urine. In general, the rate and product of benzodiazepine metabolism varies, depending on route of administration and the individual drug.

Specific Drugs

Chlordiazepoxide. Chlordiazepoxide is well absorbed after oral administration, and peak blood concentration usually is reached in approximately 4 hours. Intramuscular absorption of chlordiazepoxide, however, is slower and erratic. The half-life of chlordiazepoxide is variable but usually quite long (6-30 hr). Hepatic metabolism is mainly by CYP3A4 to give the initial N-desmethylation product, N-desmethylchloridiazepoxide. This metabolite undergoes deamination to form the demoxepam (Fig. 11.24), which is extensively metabolized, with less than 1% of a dose of chlordiazepoxide excreted as demoxepam. Demoxepam can undergo four different metabolic fates. Removal of the N-oxide moiety yields the active metabolite, N-desmethyldiazepam (desoxydemoxepam). This product is a metabolite of both chlordiazepoxide and diazepam and can be hydroxylated to yield oxazepam, another active metabolite that is rapidly glucuronidated

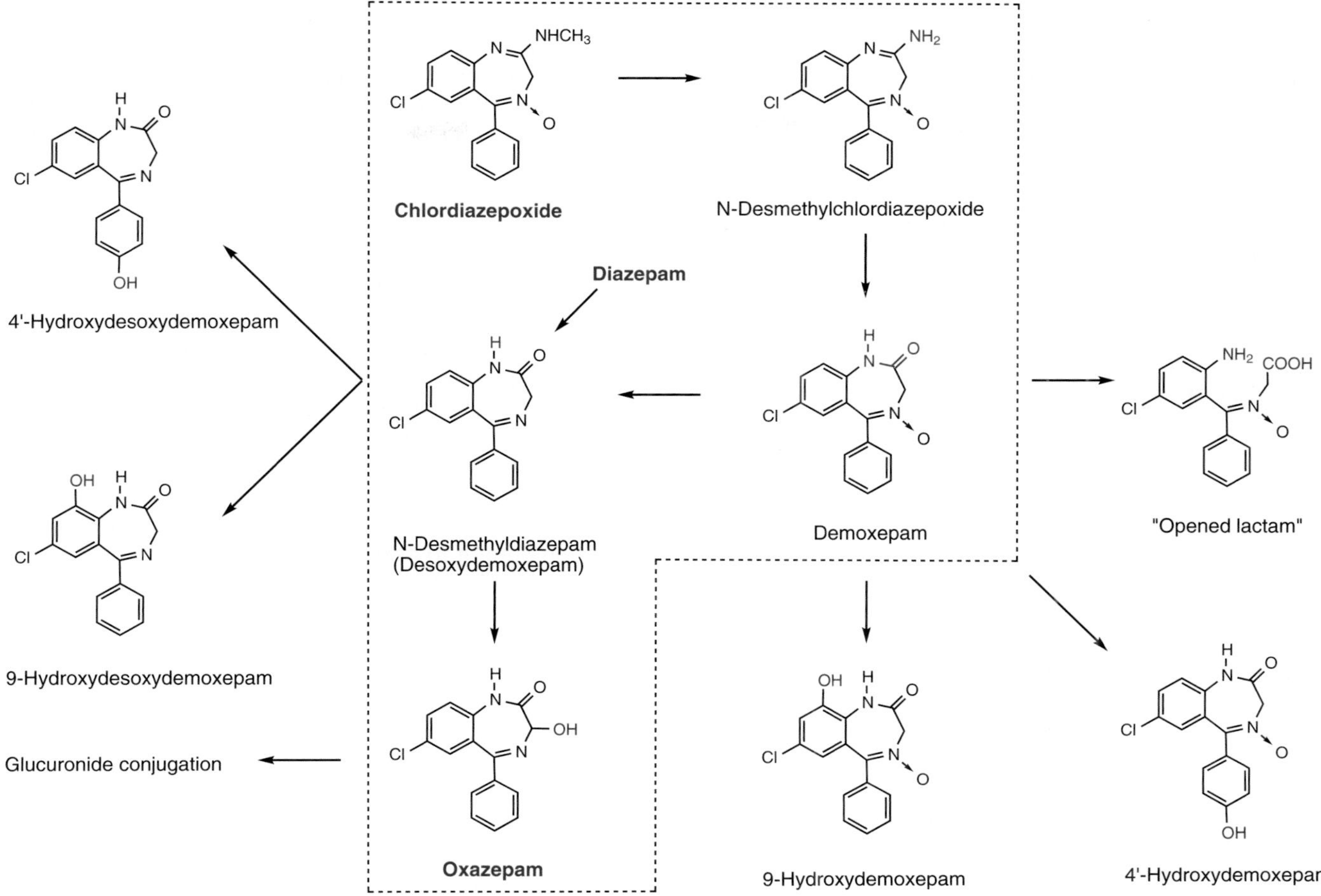

Figure 11.24 Metabolism of chlordiazepoxide and related benzodiazepines.

and excreted in the urine. Another possibility for metabolism of demoxepam is hydrolysis to the "opened lactam," which is inactive (Fig. 11.24). The two other metabolites of demoxepam are the products of ring A hydroxylation (9-hydroxydemoxepam) or ring C hydroxylation (4′-hydroxydemoxepam), both of which are inactive. The majority of a dose of chlordiazepoxide is excreted as glucuronide conjugates of oxazepam and other phenolic (9- or 4′-hydroxylated) metabolites. As with diazepam (see below), repeated administration of chlordiazepoxide can result in accumulation of parent drug and its active metabolites, which may have important clinical implications, including excessive sedation.

Diazepam. Diazepam is rapidly and completely absorbed after oral administration. Maximum peak blood concentration occurs in 2 hours, and elimination is slow, with a half-life of approximately 20-50 hours. As with chlordiazepoxide, the major metabolic product of diazepam (by CYP3A4) is N-desmethyldiazepam, which is pharmacologically active and undergoes even slower metabolism than its parent compound. Repeated administration of diazepam or chlordiazepoxide leads to accumulation of N-desmethyldiazepam, which can be detected in the blood for more than 1 week after discontinuation of the drug. Hydroxylation of N-desmethyldiazepam at the 3-position gives the active metabolite oxazepam (Fig. 11.24).

Oxazepam. Oxazepam is an active metabolite of both chlordiazepoxide and diazepam and is marketed separately, as a short-acting anxiolytic agent. Oxazepam is rapidly inactivated to glucuronidated metabolites that are excreted in the urine (Fig. 11.24). The half-life of oxazepam is approximately 4-8 hours, and cumulative effects with chronic therapy are much less than with long-acting benzodiazepines, such as chlordiazepoxide and diazepam. **Lorazepam** is the 2′-chloro derivative of oxazepam and has a similarly short half-life (2-6 hr) and pharmacological activity.

Flurazepam. Flurazepam (Fig. 11.22) is administered orally as the dihydrochloride salt. It is rapidly N-dealkylated (primarily by CYP3A4) to give the 2′-fluoro derivative of N-desmethyldiazepam, and it subsequently follows the same metabolic pathways as chlordiazepoxide and diazepam (Fig. 11.24). The half-life of flurazepam is fairly long (~7 hr). Consequently, it has the same potential as chlordiazepoxide and diazepam to produce cumulative clinical effects and side effects (e.g., excessive sedation) and residual pharmacological activity, even after discontinuation.

Midazolam. Midazolam has a pK_a of 6.2, making it one of the few benzodiazapines that is highly water soluble (pH <4), as well as, highly lipid soluble (pH >4). It is the most commonly used benzodiazepine as a premedication for anesthesia, with a quick onset (1-2 min) and recovery (20 min) after a bolus injection.[158] The time to full altertness after midazolam premedication, however, is about 40 minutes, which is much longer than for nonbenzodiazepine agents such as propofol (10 min). The intravenously administered preparation is a dihydrochloride salt preparation that is buffered to pH 3—at this pH, acid-catalyzed diazepine ring opening at the 4,5-double bond occurs that assists water solubility but renders the compound inactive. The dihydrochloride salt preparation consists of about 80%-85% of the ring-opened structure II and 15%-20% of the ring-closed form Ia.[159] The diazepine ring completely reforms to the active midazolam compound (I) upon intravenous injection, i.e., at pH 7.4.[158] Midazolam undergoes hepatic metabolism mainly by CYP3A4 and CYP3A5 to yield primarily hydroxylated derivatives that likely do not contribute to pharmacological activity at usual doses; these are subsequently excreted as glucuronide conjugates.[158]

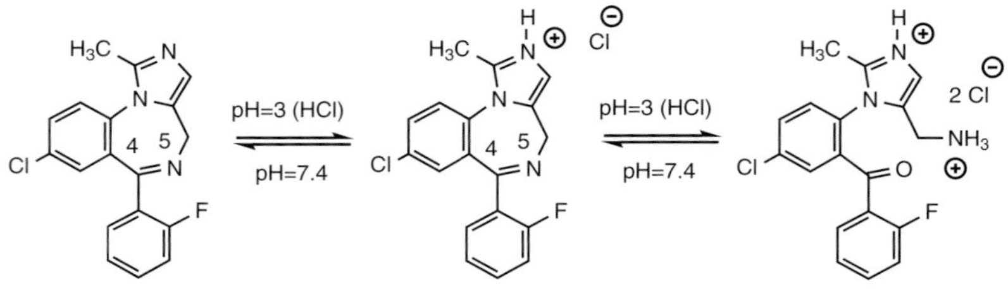

therapeutic and toxic effects may persist several days after discontinuation of chronically administered, long-acting benzodiazepines, such as chlordiazepoxide and diazepam. Thus, short-acting benzodiazepines, such as oxazepam, that are rapidly metabolized to inactive products should be considered in elderly or hepato-compromised patients.

Nonbenzodiazepine Agonists at the Benzodiazepine Site of the $GABA_A$ Receptor

Relatively few structural classes of nonbenzodiazepine compounds have clinically relevant affinity for the benzodiazepine site and show desired anxiolytic or other pharmacological activity in vivo. Representative drugs of these classes in current clinical use include the cyclopyrrolone eszopiclone, the pyrazolopyrimidine zaleplon, and the imidazopyridazine zolpidem (also see Chapter 12). These ligands show greater selectivity for $GABA_A$ receptors containing the α_1 subunit; however, it should be noted that the α_2, α_3, α_5, and γ subunits may be important in mediating anxiolytic effects.

I ⇌ Ia ⇌ II (pH=3 (HCl) / pH=7.4)

Midazolam

PHARMACOKINETICS OF BENZODIAZEPINES. Detailed pharmacokinetic analysis for most benzodiazepines is complex. Two-compartment models may be adequate to describe the disposition of most derivatives, but three-compartment models are necessary for highly lipophilic agents, such as diazepam. The distribution of such lipophilic drugs is further complicated by enterohepatic circulation. Thus, the usually stated elimination half-life of benzodiazepines may not adequately account for the pharmacodynamics of the distributive phase of the drug, which can be clinically important. For example, the distributive (α) half-life of diazepam is approximately 1 hour, whereas the elimination (β) half-life is approximately 1.5 days, acutely, and even longer after chronic dosing that results in accumulation of the drug. Furthermore, plasma concentration and clinical effectiveness of benzodiazepines is difficult to correlate, and only a twofold increase in clinically effective levels produces sedative side effects. Consequently, despite the long half-life of many benzodiazepines, they are not safe or effective when given in once-daily dose and usually are divided into two to four doses per day for treatment of daytime anxiety. Both

CYCLOPYRROLONES

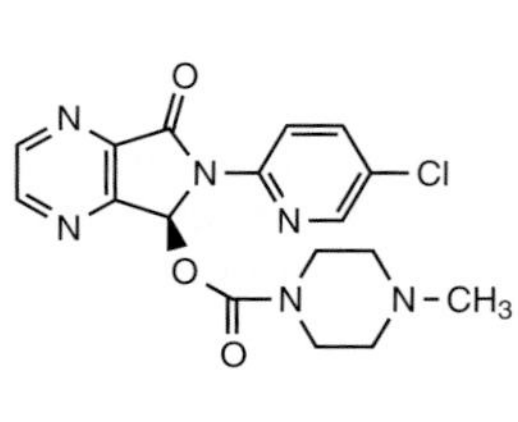

Eszopiclone

The cyclopyrrole zopiclone is described as a "superagonist" of the benzodiazepine site with the subunit composition $\alpha_1\ \beta_2\ \gamma_2$ and $\alpha_1\ \beta_2\ \gamma_3$ because it potentiates the GABA-gated current more than the benzodiazepine (flunitrazepam) reference agonist.[160] Racemic zopiclone has been available in Europe since 1992 and the higher-affinity *S*-enantiomer (eszopiclone) was marketed in the United States in 2005. It is used primarily to treat insomnia, because of its rapid onset and moderate duration (half-life, ~6 hr) of hypnotic-sedative effect.[161] Less than 10% of orally administered eszopiclone is excreted unchanged because it undergoes extensive CYP3A4- and CYP2E1-catalyzed oxidation and demethylation to metabolites excreted primarily in urine (see Chapter 12).

PYRAZOLOPYRIMIDINES

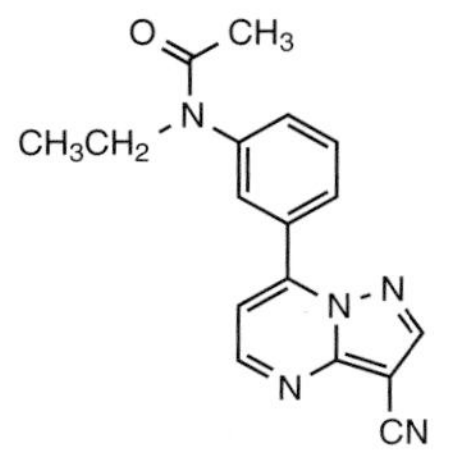

Zaleplon (Sonata)

The pyrazolopyrimidine zaleplon has selective high affinity for α_1-containing benzodiazepine sites but also produces effects at other $GABA_A$ binding sites. In patients with insomnia, zaleplon is effective to decrease sleep latency and does not appear to induce withdrawal symptoms or rebound insomnia on discontinuation. Zaleplon is absorbed rapidly and reaches peak plasma concentrations in approximately 1 hour, with a half-life approximately 1 hour as well. Less than 1% of a dose of zaleplon is excreted unchanged because most is oxidized by aldehyde dehydrogenase and CYP3A4 to inactive metabolites, which are converted to glucuronides and eliminated in urine (see Chapter 12).

IMIDAZOPYRIDINES

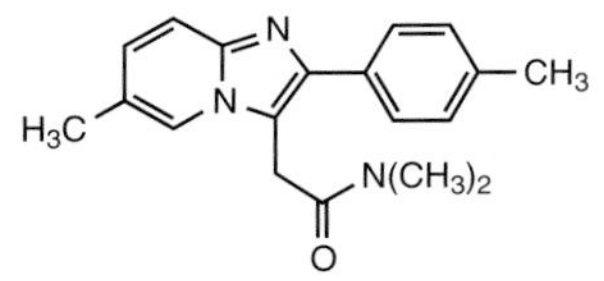

Zolpidem (Ambien)

The imidazopyridines, zolpidem and alpidem, represent another example of α_1 subunit-selective ligands of the benzodiazepine that have clinical profiles different from those of typical benzodiazepines. For example, although the activating effects of zolpidem on $GABA_A$ receptors qualitatively resemble those of benzodiazepines, clinically it shows a weaker anticonvulsant effect and a stronger sedative effect. Zolpidem was marketed as a sedative-hypnotic in the United States in 1993 and is effective in shortening sleep latency and prolonging total sleep time, without affecting sleep stages, in patients with insomnia.[162] Zolpidem is readily absorbed from the gastrointestinal tract and is extensively metabolized by the liver to inactive oxidized products, with a half-life of approximately 2 hours (see Chapter 12).

$GABA_A$ Partial Positive Allosteric Modulators

Partial agonists (partial PAMs) of the benzodiazepine site offer some theoretical and practical advantages over full agonists, including less side effects (sedation and ataxia) and abuse potential. For example, imidazenil is an imidazobenzodiazepine carboxamide that has higher affinity than diazepam but is only about half as efficacious at potentiating GABA effects on chloride currents. Consistent with the general pharmacological principle that partial agonists may show antagonist functional effects in competition with a more efficacious agonist, imidazenil blocks the sedative and ataxic effects of diazepam.[163] Interestingly, however, imidazenil does not block the anticonvulsant effects of diazepam; accordingly, it has been proposed as a better alternative to flumazenil in the alleviation of benzodiazepine-induced withdrawal symptoms.[163] In addition to imidazenil, several other structural classes of $GABA_A$ partial agonists have been evaluated; however, no $GABA_A$ partial agonist has reached the marketplace because data from clinical trials did not support promising preclinical results.[164]

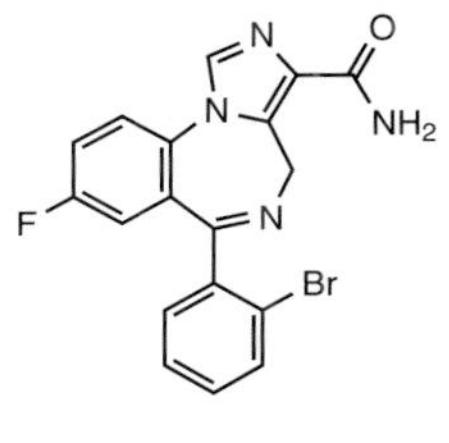

Imidazenil

DRUGS USED TO TREAT DEPRESSION

Canst thou not minister to a mind diseas'd
Pluck from the memory a rooted sorrow
Raze out the written troubles of the brain
And with some sweet oblivious antidote
Cleanse the stuff'd bosom of that perilous stuff
Which weighs upon the heart?

William Shakespeare

Depression is a common anxiety-mood disorder representing a social problem in the United States and worldwide, that is predicted to become the second largest cause of disability in 2020 by the World Health Organization (WHO).[165,166] Depression can be triggered by traumatic life events, hormone imbalance, lack of exercise, medications, drug and alcohol use, and several other factors. Whereas, a healthy lifestyle, including consuming a nutritious diet and exercising regularly is an effective preventive and/or treatment strategy for depression. However, engaging in a healthy lifestyle may not be effective enough, and medication therapy can help. The discovery of the first-generation antidepressants, i.e., monoamine oxidase inhibitors (MAOIs), tricyclic amine antidepressants (TCAs), followed by selective serotonin reuptake inhibitors (SSRIs), mixed-acting serotonin/norepinephrine reuptake inhibitors (SNRIs), atypical antidepressants, and a few others, improved significantly the treatment and the prognosis of depression in addition to promoting the investigation of biological mechanisms.[165,166] However, a long latency to therapeutic effect, the presence of side effects, and treatment resistance are still major problems with most antidepressant medications. For these reasons, the pharmacological treatment of depression is still far from being satisfactory. Other mechanisms are being explored in the attempt to discover novel and effective antidepressants (e.g. see discussion regarding ketamine).

Depression is an ancient and prevalent mental condition that has been referenced throughout history in song, poetry, and literature.[165,166] Clinical depression immobilizes a person, afflicting both men and women, rich and poor, and young and old alike. Depression symptoms include exhaustion, feelings of worthlessness, helpless ness, and hopelessness, and involves thoughts that often lead to suicidal ideation. Depression affects appetite and sleep, interfering with normal day-to-day functioning. Clinical depression is not the same as a passing blue mood. Without suitable treatment, depressive symptoms can last for weeks, months, or years. Appropriate treatment, however, can help most people who suffer from depression. Negative thinking fades as treatment begins to take effect. Unfortunately, many people do not recognize that *depression is a treatable illness*. Much of this suffering is unnecessary, because depression is one of the most treatable mental illnesses.

> *Depression is the flaw in love. The meaninglessness of every enterprise and every emotion, the meaninglessness of life itself, becomes self-evident. The only feeling left in this loveless state is insignificance.*
>
> *My depression had grown on me as that vine had conquered the oak; it had been a sucking thing that had wrapped itself around me, ugly and more alive than I. It had a life of its own that bit by bit asphyxiated all of my life out of me. My moods belonged to the depression as surely as the leaves on that oak tree's high branches belonged to the vine.*
>
> *Drug therapy hacks through the vine. You can feel it happening, how the medication seems to be poisoning the parasite so that bit by bit it withers away. You feel the weight going, feel the way that the branches can recover much of their natural bent. But even with the vine gone, you may still have a few leaves and shallow roots and the rebuilding of your self cannot be achieved with any drugs that now exist. Rebuilding of the self in and after depression requires love, insight and most of all, time.*
>
> **Andrew Solomon, The Noonday Demon: An Atlas of Depression**

One in four women and one in 10 men can expect to develop depression during their lifetime. In the United States alone, approximately 19 million adults are afflicted yearly with some type of depression, and at least 50% of those with major depression will suffer one or more repeated episodes during their adult lifetime.[165,166] Depression affects at least one in 50 children under the age of 12 years and one in 20 teenagers, mostly girls. The increased rate of depression among adolescent girls is related more to physical changes that occur during puberty, suggestive of hormonal changes. Further evidence of hormonal involvement is depression associated with premenstrual syndrome (PMS) and postpartum depression. About half of all cases of depression go unrecognized, and the annual suicide rate in the United States is over 13 in 100,000.

Depression in the elderly (17%-35%) often is dismissed as a normal part of aging and may go undiagnosed and untreated, causing needless suffering for the family and for the individual who could otherwise live a fruitful life. Often, the symptoms described usually are physical and the older person often is reluctant to discuss feelings of hopelessness, sadness, loss of interest in normally pleasurable activities, or extremely prolonged grief after a loss. Some symptoms may be the result of adverse (side) effects of medications that the elderly person is taking for other physical problems, or they may be caused by a concurrent illness. Improved recognition and treatment of depression will make life more enjoyable and fulfilling for the depressed elderly person, the family, and the caretakers.

The economic cost for depressive illnesses in the United States is estimated to be $210 billion per year, according to the newest data available from CDC 2014, but the cost in human suffering cannot be estimated. Approximately 6%-7% of full-time U.S. workers experienced clinical depression in 2016. In 2016, antidepressant drugs including TCAs, SNRIs, SSRIs, and atypical antidepressants ranked in the Top 50 drugs dispensed, third in total prescriptions written, and third in total dollar prescription sales, at approximately $12.5 billion (~5% of total prescription drug sales).

TYPES OF DEPRESSIVE DISORDERS

Major Depressive Disorder

Major depressive disorder (MDD; also called clinical depression) is manifested by depressed mood, thoughts, and physiological symptoms that impair the ability to work, study, sleep, eat, and enjoy once-pleasurable activities. It is heritable and often reoccurs multiple times during a lifetime.[165,166] The treatments for MDD are medication, psychotherapy, and in extreme cases, electroconvulsive therapy (ECT).

Dysthymia

This is a mild, chronic depression that lasts for 2 years (1 yr for children and adolescents) or longer and is characterized by chronic symptoms that do not disable but that keep one from functioning well or from feeling good about themselves.[165] Many of those with dysthymia also experience major depressive episodes at some point in their lives. Most people may not realize that they are depressed and continue to function at work or school, but often with the feeling that they are "just going through the motions." Antidepressants or psychotherapy can help.

Bipolar Disorder (Manic-Depressive Illness)

Bipolar disorders can be divided into bipolar I (episodes of severe mood swings from mania to depression), bipolar II (milder episodes of hypomania that alternate with depression), cyclothymia (milder episodes of bipolar II; low grade bipolar II), or rapid-cycling bipolar disorder (more than four episodes within a year affecting women more than men).[167] Clinical studies over the years have provided evidence that monoamine signaling and hypothalamic-pituitary-adrenal axis disruption are integral to the pathophysiology of bipolar disorder.[166,167] Bipolar disorders also appear to run in families and affects men and women equally. Not nearly as prevalent as the other forms of depressive disorders, bipolar disorders are characterized by cyclical periods of depression (lows) with periods of abnormal behavior (highs) known as either hypomania or mania. Sometimes, the mood switches are dramatic and rapid, but most often, they are gradual. When in the depressed cycle, an individual can exhibit the symptoms of a depressive disorder. When in the hypomanic/manic cycle, the individual may be overactive, be overtalkative, and have a great deal of energy. The hypomanic/manic cycle often affects thinking, judgment, and social behavior in ways that cause serious problems and embarrassment. For example, the individual in the hypomanic/manic cycle may feel elated, full of grand schemes that might range from unwise business decisions to romantic sprees. Lithium, carbamazepine, topiramide, and valproic acid are effective mood-stabilizing treatments for bipolar disorders.[167]

Other Types of Depressive Disorders

Other, less common types of depression include seasonal affective disorder. This disorder involves symptoms of depression that occur during the fall and winter seasons, when the days are shorter and there is less exposure to natural sunlight. When the spring and summer seasons begin and there is greater exposure to longer hours of daylight, the symptoms of depression disappear. Adjustment disorder with depressed mood is a type of depression that may result when a person experiences a life trauma (e.g., job loss or death of a partner). It generally fades as time passes and the person gets over whatever it was that happened.[165] Additional factors involved in its onset include stresses at home, work, or school and symptoms may persist for as long as 6 months.

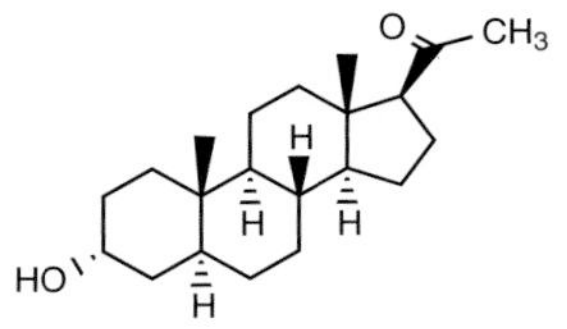

Allopregnanolone

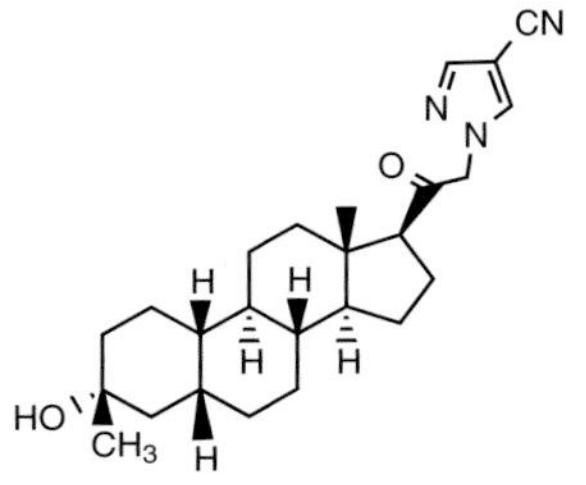

SAGE 217

Postpartum depression (PPD) is a common debilitating illness. It affects 15%-20% of women who experience significant depressive symptoms after the birth of a child.[168] Of these, 5%-10% experience severe depressive symptoms.[168,169] Low plasma levels of allopregnanolone have been implicated in the pathophysiology of mood disorders, such as PMS and PPD.

Because PPD is associated with morbidity, improved pharmacological treatment options are needed. The FDA recently approved brexanolone (Zulresso) (an IV infusion formulation of allopregnanolone) for the treatment of moderate to severe postpartum depression in women.[170,171] It is ideally suited for parenteral administration due to its low oral bioavailability. A 60-hour infusion of brexanolone returns levels of allopregnanolone (which drop precipitously after childbirth) to predelivery levels. The results at the end of the 60-hour infusion are dramatic. In a clinical trial, women treated with the active drug showed a marked response—full remission of symptoms—in comparison to one of 10 women who were treated with placebo. Importantly, the benefits of the drug were still apparent 30 days after the beginning of the infusion. The treatment was also well tolerated, and all achieved remission of depressive symptoms.[172]

Allopregnanolone (3α-hydroxy-5α-pregnan-20-one) is a neurosteroid metabolite of progesterone and functions as a PAM of $GABA_A$ receptors. As previously noted (Anxiety Disorders), $GABA_A$ receptor PAMs, e.g., benzodiazepines, have sedative and anxiolytic effects. Allopregnanolone also has strong sedative and anxiolytic properties, and low endogenous levels have been associated with depressed mood.[173] SAGE-217 is an investigational medication under development by SAGE Therapeutics for the treatment of major depressive disorder, postpartum depression, the tremor of Parkinson's disease, insomnia, and seizures. It is a synthetic, orally active, inhibitory pregnane neurosteroid, and like brexanolone acts as a PAM of the $GABA_A$ receptor. The candidate drug is being developed as an improvement over brexanolone with high oral bioavailability and a biological half-life suitable for once-daily administration.[173]

Allopregnanolone is synthesized in the CNS from progesterone, but the main sources of serum allopregnanolone in nonpregnant women are the corpus luteum and the adrenal cortex. Low oral bioavailability and oxidation of the 3α-hydroxyl to 3-ketone limit the oral therapeutic use of allopregnanolone. During the menstrual cycle, serum allopregnanolone concentrations vary between around 0.5 and 4-5 nmol/L. During pregnancy, fetoplacental synthesis causes the maternal serum concentrations of allopregnanolone to rise to reach more than 10 times the maximum menstrual cycle levels.[174] After baby delivery, the allopregnanolone level rapidly drops to 2 nmol/L within a few days. When intravenously administered to nonpregnant women, pregnancy-like allopregnanolone serum concentrations are sedative and this suggests that a tolerance to allopregnanolone develops during pregnancy.

Lower allopregnanolone plasma levels have been observed in women with depression compared to women with no history of depression, and additional studies have linked low levels of allopregnanolone to anxiety, anorexia, obesity, and posttraumatic stress disorder in women.[173] However, increased serum allopregnanolone has also been observed after unsuccessful treatment with antidepressants. Nevertheless, alterations in the metabolism of allopregnanolone from progesterone could serve as an "affective switch" in susceptible women.[174]

Biological Basis of Depression

Existing treatments for depression usually take weeks to months to achieve their effects, and about >30% of patients never show adequate improvement. In addition, increased risk of suicide attempts is a major public health concern during the first month of standard antidepressant therapy, especially among the youth. Thus, new antidepressant treatment strategies presenting a rapid improvement of depressive symptoms—within hours or even a few days—and whose effects are sustained would have an enormous impact on public health.

Monoamine Hypothesis

Although the underlying pathophysiology of depression has not been clearly defined, preclinical and clinical evidence indicate that neurotransmission disturbances in the monoamines, serotonin (5-HT), norepinephrine (NE), and dopamine (DA) in the CNS may be involved. Most available antidepressants act by one or more of the following mechanisms: inhibition of reuptake of 5-HT or NE and/or DA, or inhibition of monoamine oxidase.[175,176] All of these mechanisms serve to increase monoamine levels. NE plays a role in regulating cognition, motivation, and intellect, which are fundamental in social relationships.[177] Norepinephrine-deficit depressions are associated with decreased concentration, low motivation, poor energy, inattention, poor self-care, and cognitive difficulties, whereas serotonin-deficit depressions are associated with anxiety, suicidality, and appetite disturbances (Fig. 11.25). DA deficiencies are associated primarily with lack of motivation and listlessness.

Schildkraut et al.[178] postulated early on that depression arises as a consequence of a deficiency of NE and that the effects caused by catecholamine depletion can be reversed by the TCAs or the atypical SNRIs. Depression in animals following inhibition of the enzyme, tyrosine hydroxylase, with α-methyl-*p*-tyrosine,[175] can be reversed by TCAs or atypical SNRIs. These results suggested that the antidepressant effects were caused by an increase of NE. Studies in depressed patients in remission and no longer taking medication produced similar results as rat studies where α-methyl-*p*-tyrosine treatment resulted in rapid appearance of depressive symptoms. Also, functional deletion

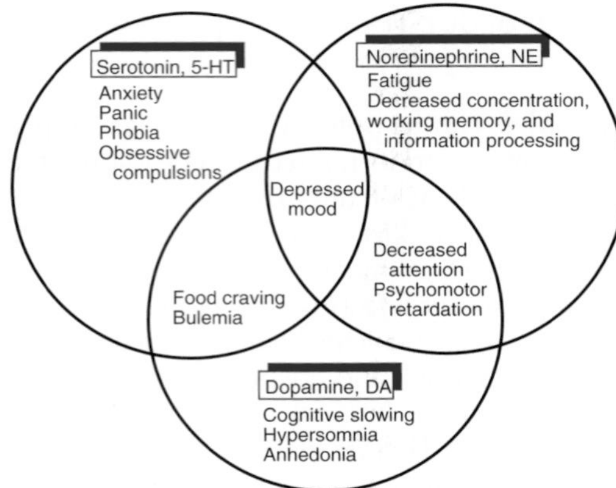

Figure 11.25 Neurotransmitter deficiency syndromes and their interactions.

(knockout) of the NE transporter in mice resulted in increased extracellular levels of NE,[176,179] and this model functionally mimics the therapeutic effects of selective NE antidepressants.

During the late 1960s, Kielholz, a Swiss psychiatrist, noted that different antidepressants had unique effects and argued that it was important to carefully select the right antidepressant for the right patient. He differentiated the TCAs based on whether they possessed the ability to sedate, e.g., trimipramine; to stimulate, e.g., desipramine or nortriptyline; or to improve mood, e.g., clomipramine. By the end of the decade, the broad consensus was that secondary amine TCAs such as desipramine or nortriptyline inhibited the reuptake of NE into noradrenergic neurons and that blocking 5-HT reuptake by tertiary amine TCAs such as clomipramine explained the mood elevation of some antidepressants.[179] The catecholamine hypothesis (which focused on NE) was then modified to include 5-HT in the etiology of depression.[180,181] Subsequent studies with inhibitors of monoamine biosynthesis supported Kielholz's and Schildkraut's ideas that clinical depression is the result of a deficiency in both 5-HT and NE (Fig. 11.25).

Inhibition of 5-HT biosynthesis reverses the therapeutic effects of treatment with antidepressants that have predominantly 5-HT reuptake inhibitory activity (e.g., fluoxetine) but less so with those that have predominantly NE reuptake inhibitory activity (e.g., desipramine).[177] Also, inhibition of 5-HT biosynthesis produced a relapse in depressed patients whose depression was successfully treated with imipramine or tranylcypromine, whereas inhibitors of DA or NE synthesis had no effect on these depressed patients.[176] A depletion of catecholamines reverses the therapeutic effects of desipramine more than that of fluoxetine or sertraline.[175,178] These studies appear to confirm the proposed mechanism that antidepressants work by regulating monoamine activity. Kielholz further reasoned that because NE reuptake inhibitors (activating antidepressants) were likely to trigger suicide and because 5-HT reuptake inhibitors would be less likely to lead to suicide, it would be worth developing drugs that selectively inhibited the reuptake of 5-HT for treatment of depression.[179]

Changes in NE and 5-HT levels do not affect mood in everyone. Some evidence also suggests that for a subset of patients, DA plays a role in depression.[182,183] Dopaminergic substances have been used as antidepressants when other measures have failed. The DA hypothesis of schizophrenia and the emphasis on other neurotransmitters, most notably NE and 5-HT, in the pathogenesis of depression have focused attention away from DA and its role in affective disorders. Recent clinical evidence shows involvement of DA in several subtypes of depression, psychomotor retardation and diminished motivation, and seasonal mood disorder.[183] The biochemical evidence in patients with depression indicates diminished DA turnover. In addition, a considerable amount of pharmacological evidence exists regarding the efficacy of antidepressants with dopaminergic effects in the treatment of depression. However, the role of DA in depression must be understood in the context of existing theories involving other neurotransmitters that may act independently and interact with DA and other neurochemicals to contribute to depression.[183]

In conclusion, although 5-HT has been the most studied neurotransmitter in depression, converging lines of evidence suggest that NE is of major importance in the pathophysiology and treatment of depressive disorder.[175] The limbic system is implicated in the NE regulation of emotions and cognition. Substantial functional biochemical differences exist in the NE system in postmortem brains from depressed patients and healthy controls. Chemical manipulation that depletes the brain of NE increases the susceptibility of recovered depressed patients to a depressive relapse. Therapeutic agents which specifically increase NE activity are effective antidepressants, and there is evidence that those acting simultaneously on 5-HT and NE neurotransmission (SNRIs) may have an antidepressant action superior to SSRIs.[182]

Limitations of the Monoamine Hypothesis

While the monoamine deficiency hypothesis of depression has been commonly used to explain the mechanism of actions of the antidepressant drugs, a growing body of evidence has been accumulating over the past two decades supporting alternative non-monoamine mechanisms of action including pertubations of the cholinergic[184] and glutamatergic systems and of neurohormones.[168]

Cholinergic Hypothesis of Depression

More than 40 years ago, the cholinergic theory of depression and mania hypothesized a balance between cholinergic and adrenergic systems,[179] suggesting that hyperactivity of the cholinergic system over the adrenergic system would lead to symptoms of depression, mediated through excessive neuronal nicotinic receptor (nAChR) activation.[184] Thus, the therapeutic actions of some antidepressants may be, in part, mediated through inhibition of nAChRs.[184] On the other hand, hypocholinergic activity would lead to the symptoms of mania. Consistent with this hypothesis, physostigmine a cholinesterase inhibitor (increases synaptic ACh levels), when administered to normal subjects, produces symptoms of depression, anxiety, irritability, aggressiveness, and hostility.[184] When physostigmine was administered to patients with MDD, these symptoms were more pronounced and longer lasting.[169] Physostigmine also induces depression in patients with acute mania. The hypercholinergic effects of physostigmine are mediated primarily through acetylcholine activation of neuronal nAChRs, not muscarinic receptors. Over the past 20 years, various groups have reported on the nAChR inhibitory actions of classic TCAs including imipramine, nortriptyline, amitriptyline, and desipramine; and the serotonin reuptake inhibitors including fluoxetine, sertraline, paroxetine, and citalopram.[184] nAChRs modulate not only the release of monoamines, but also GABA, glutamate, and various neuropeptides. Perhaps one of the most interesting antidepressants to have nAChR inhibitory activity is the atypical antidepressant, bupropion. Bupropion is unique because it is metabolized to hydroxybupropion which is an SNRI and a reuptake inhibitor of DA.

In addition, transdermal nicotine administration (patch) has been shown to substantially improve the depressive symptoms of patients with MDD, an effect believed to be due to nicotine's effects on nAChRs. These effects have been attributed primarily to nicotine-induced desensitization of nAChRs, leading to decreased function or inhibition, specifically, of a high-affinity nAChR subtype in the brain, the $\alpha_4\beta_2$ subunit, which is the predominant mammalian brain nAChR subtype. Thus, cigarette smoking may exert antidepressant effects in patients with MDD who were refractory to SSRI treatment,[184] supporting the view that depressed smokers self-medicate by smoking.

Evidence for hypercholinergic mechanisms in depression and hypocholinergic mechanisms in mania has been building over the last several decades, especially the clinical relationships between tobacco use and depression, which suggests important effects of nicotine in MDD. About 120 years ago, Willoughby (Lancet, 1889) first reported the use of pilocarpine (a cholinomimetic) to treat acute mania. During the 1970s, Janowski[184] and others hypothesized that a cholinergic imbalance (i.e., hypercholinergic tone) was a primary factor in depressive illnesses. Since that time, a number of key findings from both animal and human studies have supported this hypothesis, with focus specifically on central nACh rather than muscarinic pathways. Most clinically prescribed antidepressants target NE and 5-HT neurotransmitter systems; however, some of the drugs that target these systems also act as potent noncompetitive antagonists of nACHRs at clinically effective doses for treatment of clinical depression.[177] The rapid monoamine effects of the antidepressants but delayed therapeutic onset of action have led to reconsideration of alternative hypotheses regarding the mechanism of action of antidepressants.

There is a well-established connection between smoking and depression.[184] Depressed individuals are overrepresented among smokers, and ex-smokers often experience increased depressive symptoms immediately after stopping smoking. The effects of nicotine on depression-like behaviors support the idea that dysregulation of the cholinergic system might contribute to the etiology of major depressive disorder.[184] Thus, pharmacological agents that limit acetylcholine signaling through neuronal nAChRs might be promising for the development of novel antidepressant medications.

Hormonal Hypothesis

The hormonal hypothesis suggests that stress-induced changes in the hypothalamus-pituitary-adrenal axis (HPA) contribute to thought and mood disorders.[185] Environmental or psychological stress stimulates the hypothalamus to produce a hormone in the brain called corticotrophin-releasing factor (CRF), which in turn stimulates the pituitary gland to secrete adrenocorticotropic hormone (ACTH) into the blood, where it stimulates the adrenal glands to release hydrocortisone (cortisol), a glucocorticoid which prepares the body for dealing with stress. Stress also directly stimulates the adrenal gland to secrete epinephrine and NE. Prolonged, high levels of glucocorticoids can damage brain cells in the hippocampus and alter functional connectivity in the amygdala, which likely contribute to depression and anxiety. Approximately 50% of those with MDD have elevated hydrocortisone levels as a result of hyper-CRF activity. Moreover, one of the most replicated findings in biological psychiatry is that large numbers of unmedicated depressed patients exhibit HPA hyperactivity. Some evidence suggests that nAChRs play important roles in mediating stress-related and possibly depression-inducing neuroendocrine effects. Hypercholinergic activity, increased ACh in response to stress, can stimulate the HPA through activation of nAChRs. Thus, antidepressants may reduce symptoms of depression, in part, through blockade of nAChRs involved with stress-induced activation of the HPA.[184]

Living organisms are constantly adapting to environmental perturbations, and much of this work is performed by the autonomic and endocrine systems that have evolved to modulate rates of biochemical pathways to maintain homeostasis. One of the hallmarks of these regulatory systems is the short-lived nature of the nerve signals produced. The half-life of neurotransmitters is measured in seconds, whereas those of the circulating hormones may be minutes or hours. A rationale for the short-lived nature of the neurotransmitters is to permit these signaling pathways to quickly reset themselves to meet the next challenge. Readjustments (i.e., plasticity) in these systems include receptor desensitization or sensitization, degradation or increased expression of receptors, and up- and downregulation of signaling molecules that affect the primary signaling pathway. The hypotheses described in this section are not mutually exclusive but rather, form a general theory wherein disruptions in the orchestration of cellular communication of these regulatory systems likely contribute to psychiatric manifestations.

The Discovery of Antidepressant Medications

Before 1950, there were no antidepressants—at least not as we know them today. The two treatments for depressive illness were either amphetamine stimulants, which often were ineffective and had the general effect of increasing energy and activity, or ECT, which was effective but had the disadvantage of terrifying and often endangering the patient. Not until the late 1950s were the first generation of antidepressants discovered (the TCAs and MAOIs), not by design but by chance. While searching for "chlorpromazine-like" compounds to treat schizophrenia, imipramine was recognized by Kuhn[185] for its antidepressant properties, thus becoming the forerunner for the tricyclic class of monoamine reuptake inhibitor antidepressants (i.e., the TCAs). The second compound to be discovered was the antitubercular drug isoniazid,[186] which proved to have powerful mood-enhancing properties, becoming the forerunner of the MAOIs. With the introduction of imipramine and isoniazid, the theory and treatment of depression changed. These early studies still summarize much of our current knowledge regarding the therapeutic effects of antidepressant treatments.

Between 1960 and 1980, TCAs were the major pharmacological treatment for depression.[187] Certain TCAs, however, have many other actions in addition to blocking monoamine reuptake, including anticholinergic, antihistaminergic, and cardiotoxic side effects that are related to their affinity for muscarinic, H_1, and α_1-adrenergic receptors. Some TCAs also have off-target activity at sodium channels in cardiac tissue and in the CNS (Table 11.4). The improved safety, tolerability, and reuptake selectivity of the SSRIs, SNRIs, and serotonin modulators and stimulants (SMSs) have resulted in displacement of the TCAs as the first choice for the treatment of MDD. The TCAs, however, still occupy an important role in pharmacotherapy for MDD.

The early MAOIs irreversibly inhibited the oxidative deamination of the neurotransmitter monoamines. The biggest liability for these MAOIs was their potential to cause life-threatening hypertensive reactions, resulting from the irreversible inhibition of both MAO-A and MAO-B isoenzymes which decreases the intestinal and hepatic degradation of dietary sources of tyramine. The inhibition of MAO allows excessive amounts of dietary tyramine, a weak sympathomimetic vasoconstrictor, to be absorbed from food, resulting in increased blood pressure (refer to the section of MAOIs in this chapter for more details). Inhibition of MAOs also can alter

Table 11.4 FDA Approved Antidepressant Classes of Drugs: Generic Name, Trade Name, and Common Side Effects[a]

Generic Name	Trade Name	Amine Effects	Seizures	Sedation	Hypotension	Anticholinergic Effects	GI Effects	Sexual Effects	Cardiac Effects
Tricyclic Teriary Amines									
Amitriptyline	Elavil and generic	NE, 5-HT	2+	3+	3+	3+	+	2+	3+
Clomipramine	Anafranil	NE, 5-HT	3+	2+	2+	+	2+	3+	
Doxepine	Adapin, Sinequan	NE, 5-HT	2+	3+	2+	+	2+	3+	
Imipramine	Tofranil and generic	NE, 5-HT	2+	2+	2+	2+	+	2+	3+
(+)-Trimipramine	Surmontil	NE, 5-HT	2+	3+	2+	3+	+	2+	3+
Tricyclic Secondary Amines									
Amoxapine	Ascendin	NE, DA	2+	+	2+	+	+	+	2+
Desipramine	Norpramin	NE	+	+	+	+	+	2+	2+
Maprotiline	Ludiomil	NE	3+	2	2	0	+	2+	2
Nortryptyline	Pamelor	NE	+	+	+	0	+	2+	2+
Protriptyline	Vivactil	NE	2+	0	+	0	+	2+	2+
Selective Serotonin Reuptake Inhibitors (SSRIs)									
(±)-Citalopram	Celexa	5-HT	0	0/+	0	0	3+	3+	0
(+)-Escitalopram	Lexapro	5-HT	0	0/+	0	0	3+	3+	0
(±)-Fluoxetine	Prozac	5-HT	+	0/+	0	0	3+	3+	0
Fluvoxamine	Luvox	5-HT	0	0/+	0	0	3+	3+	0
(−)-Paroxetine	Paxil	5-HT	0	0/+	0	0	3+	3+	0
(+)-Sertraline	Zoloft	5-HT	0	0/+	0	0	3+	3+	0

(continued)

Table 11.4 FDA Approved Antidepressant Classes of Drugs: Generic Name, Trade Name, and Common Side Effects[a]—Cont'd

Generic Name	Trade Name	Amine Effects	Seizures	Sedation	Hypotension	Anticholinergic Effects	GI Effects	Sexual Effects	Cardiac Effects
Serotonin and Norepinephrine Reuptake Inhibitors (SNRIs)									
(−)-Atomoxetine	Strattera	NE	0	0	0	0	0	0	0
(+)-Duloxetine	Cymbalta	NE, 5-HT	0/+	0/+	0/+	0	0/+	0/+	0/+
Levomirtazapine	Fetzima	5-HT, NE	0	4+	0	0	0	0	0
(±)-Mirtazapine	Remeron	5-HT, NE	0	4+	0	0	0	0	0
(±)-Venlafaxine	Effexor	5-HT	0	+	0	0	3+	3+	0
Desvenlafaxine	Pristiq	5-HT	0	+	0	0	3+	3+	0
Serotonin Modulators and Stimulants (SMS and SARIs)									
Vilazodone	Viibryd	5-HT	0/+	+	0	0	3+	2+	1+
Vortioxetine	Brintellix	5-HT	0	0	0	2+	3+	3+	0
Trazodone	Desyrel	5-HT	0	0	3+	0	2+		
Norepinephrine and Dopamine Reuptake Inhibitors (NDRIs)									
Bupropion	Wellbutrin, Zyban, etc	NE, DA	3+	0	0	0/+	2+	0/+	0/+
Monoamine Oxidase Inhibitors (MAOIs)									
Phenelzine	Nardil	NE, 5-HT, DA	+	+	0	+	3+	0	
Tranylcypromine	Parnate	NE, 5-HT, DA	0	+	0	+	2+	0	

[a] 0, no effect; +, little effect; 2+, significant effect; 3+, major effect..

the pharmacokinetics of monoamine over-the-counter and prescription drugs, allowing them to accumulate in the blood and, thus, increasing their potential for causing adverse drug effects and drug-drug interactions. Minimizing drug and food interactions of these early MAOIs inspired the development of a new generation of MAOIs that are both reversible and selective for MAO-A. The demise of the early MAOIs allowed the TCAs to become the gold standard for the treatment of depressive disorders.

Discovery of SSRI Antidepressants

The discovery that certain antihistaminic agents without the condensed aromatic ring systems are selective inhibitors of 5-HT reuptake with little affinity for the other neuroreceptors and almost devoid of cardiotoxicity questioned the need for the 10,11-ethylene bridge for the TCAs. Thus, the search for inhibitors that selectively blocked 5-HT reuptake without the seven-membered central ring of the TCAs resulted in the synthesis of the diarylpropylamine analogues of the TCAs (Fig. 11.26). During the late 1960s and early 1970s, antihistamine molecules were structurally manipulated in the search for compounds that selectively inhibited 5-HT reuptake with greater potency. The initial breakthrough came with the synthesis of Z-zimeldine (the *cis*-isomer) (a.k.a., zimelidine, patented in 1971), the first SSRI that selectively inhibited the presynaptic reuptake of 5-HT without the adverse events associated with the multireceptor activities of the TCAs.[188,189] The design of zimeldine was based on manipulating the antihistamine pheniramine into a diaryl allylamine, the *cis*-isomer (rigid analogue) of the propylamine group (Fig. 11.26).[188]

Other structural changes that enhanced its potency and selectivity for blocking 5-HT reuptake were moving the regional position of the 2-pyridyl ring of pheniramine to the 3-pyridyl position and substitution of a halogen into the 4-position of the phenyl ring (2-substitutions selectively block NE reuptake). The secondary amine and primary metabolite, norzimeldine, is 15 times more potent than zimeldine for blocking 5-HT reuptake. On the other hand, (*E*)-zimeldine (the *trans*-isomer) is an inhibitor of both 5-HT and NE reuptake, whereas its corresponding secondary amine is a potent and selective inhibitor of NE reuptake. It is not unusual for geometric isomers to differ markedly from each other with regard to their receptor or transporter selectivity, affinity, and pharmacodynamic properties. Thus, zimeldine became the first SSRI to be marketed as an antidepressant, but unfortunately, several cases of Guillain-Barre syndrome (an autoimmune disorder attacking the peripheral nervous system) were associated with the use of this drug and led to its withdrawal from the market in 1983. During postmarketing clinical studies, zimeldine showed an increase in the number of suicide attempts than had been expected—this adverse event was to become a major issue with the SSRIs 20 years later.

The success of zimeldine as an SSRI led to the discovery and marketing of several nontricyclic SSRIs from multiple pharmaceutical companies worldwide.[190] Another manipulation of the antihistamines produced indalpine (patented in 1977 by Rhône Poulenc) (Fig. 11.26). It produced responses in patients who had not responded to the TCAs or MAOIs but then ran into trouble because clinical trials suggested that it might cause agranulocytopenia (a lowering of the white blood cell count). For the most part, this is not a serious problem, but in rare cases, if undetected, it can be fatal. It was removed from the European market in 1985 and was never marketed in the United States. Other SSRIs developed during this period that have become household words include paroxetine

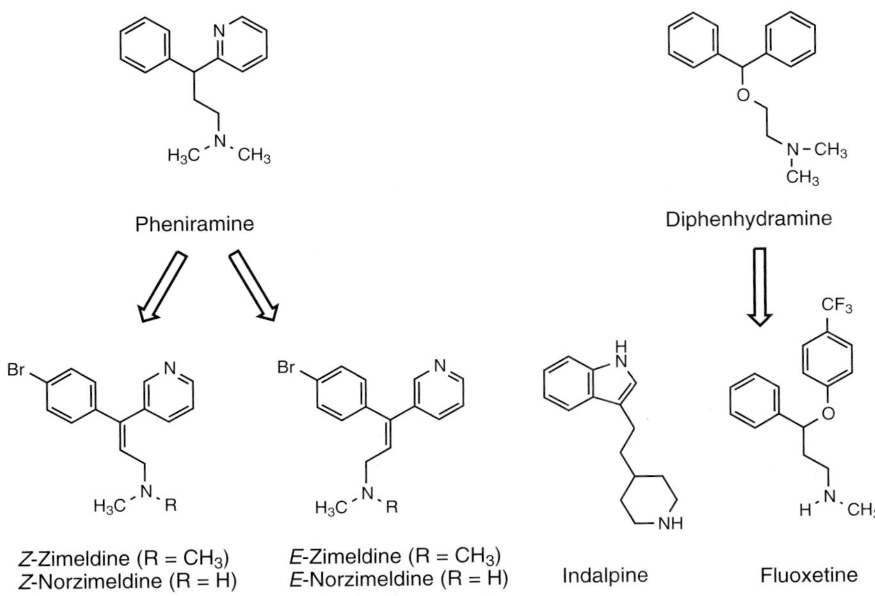

Pheniramine

Diphenhydramine

Z-Zimeldine (R = CH_3)
Z-Norzimeldine (R = H)

E-Zimeldine (R = CH_3)
E-Norzimeldine (R = H)

Indalpine

Fluoxetine

Figure 11.26 Development of and Structural relationship between antihistamines and antidepressants that block the reuptake of 5-HT.

(patented in 1975 by Ferrosan to SmithKlineBeecham then to GlaxoKline), citalopram (patented in 1979 by Lindberg, licensed to Forest Labs), fluoxetine (patented in 1982 by Lilly), and sertraline (patented in 1985 by Pfizer).

Scientists at Lilly Research Laboratories synthesized more than 50 phenoxypropylamines derived from the antihistamine diphenhydramine (Benadryl) before discovering fluoxetine[190-192] (Fig. 11.26). The first of these compounds was nisoxetine, a potent SNRI (see Fig. 11.26) that was clinically developed but never marketed. Other derivatives that have since been marketed by Lilly include atomoxetine and duloxetine, both atypical SNRIs.

Fluoxetine (Prozac) was heralded as the prototype for the next generation of SSRI antidepressants possessing fewer adverse effects and with a greater margin of safety when overdoses are consumed compared with the TCAs; it also lacked the food-interaction toxicity of MAOIs. Fluoxetine was marketed in 1987 and within a few years, it boasted worldwide sales of nearly $1.2 billion a year. During the past 20 years, nontricyclic selective NE or 5-HT reuptake inhibitors and TCA reuptake inhibitors of both NE and 5-HT as well as reversible selective MAOIs have been approved for use in depression. These newer additions allow exploration of the roles of NE versus 5-HT using treatments that are devoid of confounding receptor activities.

Conscious targeting of more than one neurotransmitter activity while retaining specificity is the target for the development of the next generation of antidepressants. The majority of tricyclic antidepressants in current use selectively inhibit the reuptake of 5-HT and NE. Based on the previously neglected role proposed for DA in depression, it has been hypothesized that a "broad-spectrum" antidepressants will produce a more rapid onset and/or higher efficacy than agents inhibiting the selective reuptake of 5-HT and/or NE.[29] Broad-spectrum antidepressants are compounds that inhibit the reuptake of NE, 5-HT, and DA, the three biogenic amines most closely linked to depression. However, cocaine and several cathinone psychostimulant drugs of abuse possess this pharmacology, so potential addictive effects must be carefully examined.

Traditionally, antidepressants have been classified according to their structure (i.e., secondary or tertiary amine TCAs) or their principal mechanism of action. With the appearance of increasing numbers of second- and third-generation antidepressants, however, a better way of classifying and describing the antidepressants was necessary. For the purposes of this chapter, the antidepressants are organized into seven classes (Table 11.4) and discussed according to their distinct and different mechanisms of action (Fig. 11.27). Considerable overlap exists in their mechanism of actions and uses, but these different classes of antidepressants work by distinct mechanisms, have different side-effect profiles, and may be favored for different types of depressive illnesses.

A key step that determines the intensity and duration of monoamine signaling at synapses is the reuptake of the released neurotransmitter into nerve terminals through high-affinity plasma membrane transporters.[193] Reuptake is the process of rapidly removing the monoamine neurotransmitters from the synaptic cleft and allowing most of the released neurotransmitter to be recycled for further use. The advantage of reuptake is that it is faster than passive diffusion through the membrane. Any monoamine neurotransmitter remaining in the synaptic cleft is then absorbed and metabolized into inactive metabolites. The monoamine reuptake transporter protein binds the released neurotransmitter in the extracellular fluid and transports the monoamine across the presynaptic plasma membrane back into the intracellular fluid of the presynaptic neuron (Fig. 11.28). Monoamine transporters (Fig. 11.29 and sidebar for more detail) are embedded in the plasma membrane of the nerve terminals (perisynaptically) of dopaminergic, noradrenergic, and serotonergic neurons rather than intrasynaptically (along the portion of the nerve terminal forming the synapse). They are members of a larger sodium-dependent transporter family and represent a major mechanism terminating the action of released monoamine neurotransmitters in the synaptic cleft. These transporters are important targets for many antidepressive drugs and substances of abuse (i.e., cocaine). Transporter proteins are specific to their respective neurotransmitter: serotonin reuptake transporter (SERT), NE reuptake transporter (NET), and dopamine reuptake transporter (DAT). None of the reuptake antidepressants exhibit significant affinity for DA transporters, which may be related to their ineffectiveness in types of depression that are resistant to the SNRIs and SSRIs. The TCAs and nontricyclic SNRIs block the reuptake transporters for both NE and 5-HT, and the SSRIs selectively block SERT. The antidepressant reuptake inhibitors also may contribute to relief of depression by decreasing the expression of their respective transporter proteins.

Figure 11.30 graphically illustrates the selectivity of the reuptake inhibitors for their respective transporters.[194,195] For example, a value of approximately 1 for amitriptyline means that amitriptyline will inhibit both NET and SERT at the same concentration (i.e., no selectivity with regard to their mechanism of antidepressant activity). The value of −30 for desipramine means that desipramine is 30 times more potent at inhibiting NET than SERT. The SSRIs with selectivity ratio values of greater than 100 are more than 100 times more potent at inhibiting SERT than NET. Furthermore, because the selectivity ratio for most SSRIs is more than 100, a plasma concentration of any SSRI that will produce inhibition of SERT will likely produce no physiologically meaningful inhibition of NET. The converse will be true regarding selectivity for NET. Clinically, such selectivity ratios of greater than 100 translate into being able to produce all the physiological effects mediated by inhibiting one transporter without causing any effects that will be produced by inhibiting the other uptake transporter. When the selectivity ratio is less than 30, such as with fluoxetine, the difference is small enough

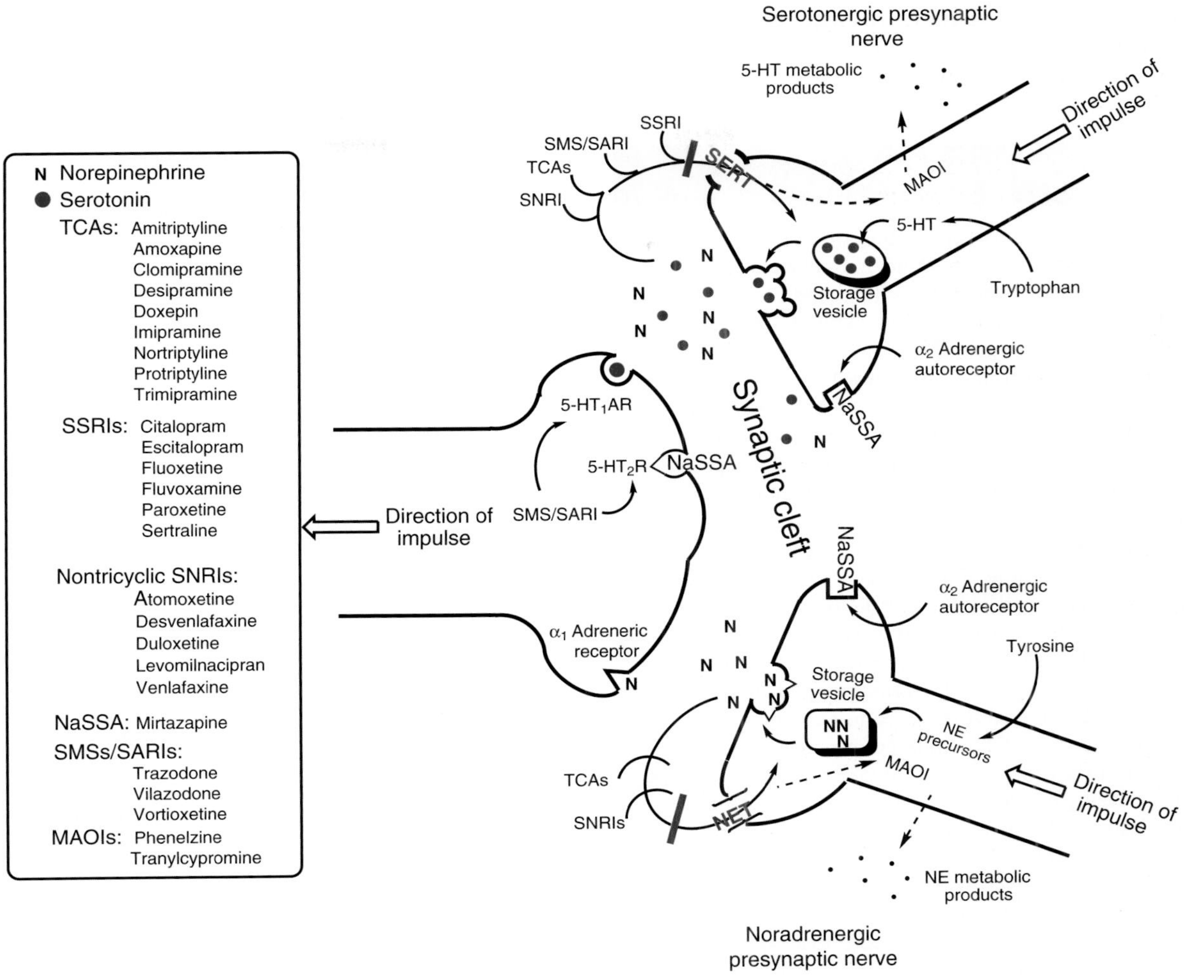

N Norepinephrine
● Serotonin
TCAs: Amitriptyline
Amoxapine
Clomipramine
Desipramine
Doxepin
Imipramine
Nortriptyline
Protriptyline
Trimipramine
SSRIs: Citalopram
Escitalopram
Fluoxetine
Fluvoxamine
Paroxetine
Sertraline
Nontricyclic SNRIs:
Atomoxetine
Desvenlafaxine
Duloxetine
Levomilnacipran
Venlafaxine
NaSSA: Mirtazapine
SMSs/SARIs:
Trazodone
Vilazodone
Vortioxetine
MAOIs: Phenelzine
Tranylcypromine

Serotonergic presynaptic nerve
5-HT metabolic products
SSRI
SMS/SARI
TCAs
SNRI
SERT
MAOI
Direction of impulse
5-HT
Storage vesicle
Tryptophan
α_2 Adrenergic autoreceptor
NaSSA
5-HT_1AR
5-HT_2R
SMS/SARI
Direction of impulse
Synaptic cleft
α_1 Adreneric receptor
Tyrosine
NE precursors
TCAs
SNRIs
NET
NE metabolic products
Noradrenergic presynaptic nerve

Figure 11.27 Sites of action of the antidepressants.

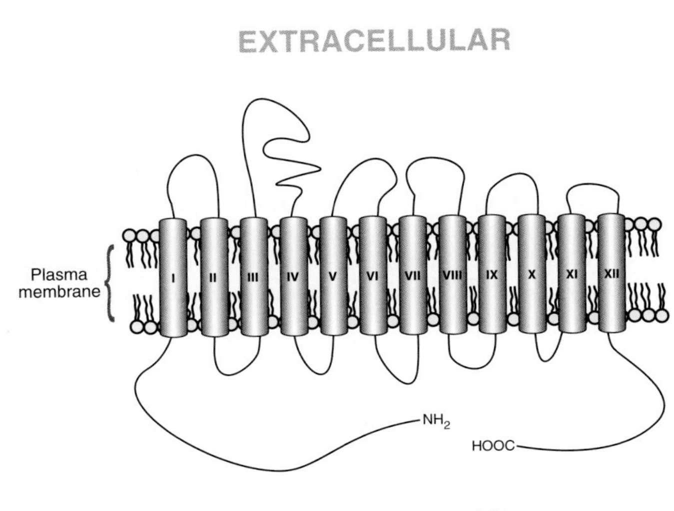

Figure 11.28 Monoamine reuptake transporter.

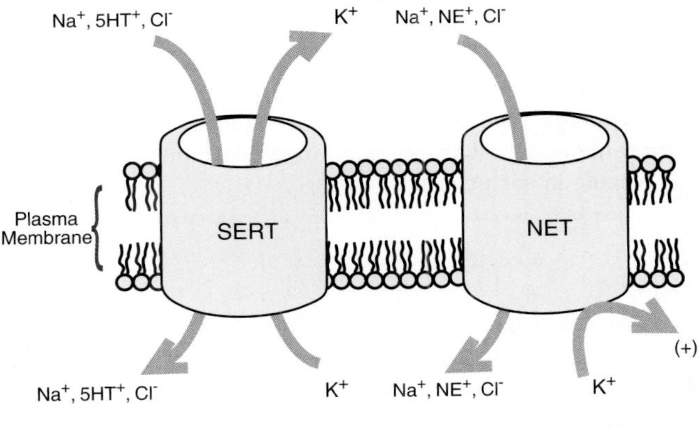

Figure 11.29 Model of the NET and SERT and the ion-coupled NE and 5-HT reuptake. Reuptake of 5-HT is dependent on the cotransport of Na^+ and Cl^- and countertransport of K^+. Reuptake of NE is dependent on the cotransport of Na^+ and Cl^- with intracellular K^+ stimulation but without K^+ efflux.

that inhibition of both reuptake transporters may occur under therapeutic doses, and might contribute to the antidepressant activity of the drug.

TRANSPORTER PROTEINS

The monoamine transporter protein (molecular weights, 60-80 kDa) is a string of amino acids that weaves in and out of the presynaptic membrane 12 times (Fig. 11.28)—that is, 12 transmembrane domains (TMs) with a large extracellular loop between TM3 and TM4. Both the N- and C-termini of the transporters are located within the cytoplasm. There are six potential sites of phosphorylation by protein kinase A and protein kinase C, which regulate the transporters. The large extracellular loop and the cytoplasmic parts of the N- and C-termini do not appear to be the target sites for the transporter inhibitors (i.e., antidepressants). Rather, the areas important for selective monoamine affinity appear to be localized within TM1 to TM3 and TM8 to TM12 that project into the synapse, and these areas of the transporters have a common binding site for the monoamine and many of its inhibitors (Fig. 11.28). To transport protonated 5-HT ($5\text{-}HT^+$), SERT cotransports one sodium ion (Na^+) and one chloride ion (Cl^-) while countertransporting a potassium ion (K^+) (Fig. 11.29). The SERT then flips inside the cell, releasing the $5\text{-}HT^+$ and the Na^+ and Cl^- into the cytoplasm of the neuron. On releasing the $5\text{-}HT^+$ and the Na^+ and Cl^-, SERT flips back out, with the unoccupied binding site exposed to the synaptic cleft, ready to receive and transport another $5\text{-}HT^+$ molecule. To transport protonated NE (NE^+), NET also cotransports Na^+ and Cl^- with intracellular K^+ stimulation and no K^+ efflux. The initial complex of the monoamine, Na^+ and Cl^- with the transporter protein creates a conformational change in the transporter protein. The driving force (electrical potential) for the energetically unfavorable transport of the monoamine is the Na^+ concentration gradient. The Na^+, K^+ transporter (Na^+, K^+-ATPase) maintains the extracellular Na^+ concentration as well as the intracellular K^+ concentration. The Na^+, K^+-ATPase transports three Na^+ ions for each two K^+ ions pumped into the cell. Unlike channels that stay open or closed, transporters undergo conformational changes (changes in their three-dimensional shape) and move one monoamine molecule in each cycle.

Most scientists agree that TCAs, MAOIs, SSRIs, and the atypical SNRIs improve depression by boosting the levels of NE and/or 5-HT in the brain, but what is not established is how increased concentrations of NE and 5-HT translate into reducing depression.[175] One problem with the original monoamine model was that whereas plasma concentrations of the antidepressant and binding to the monoamine transporter occur almost immediately, chronic administration of antidepressants is needed before clinical efficacy is attained.[187] The therapeutic effect of an

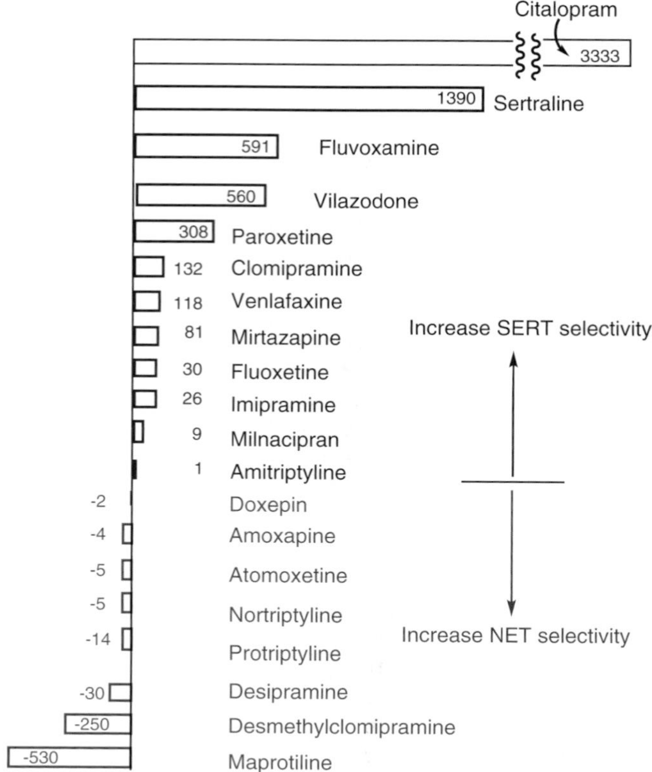

Figure 11.30 In vitro selectivity ratios for reuptake inhibitors.

antidepressant is almost always observed after a period of 3-6 weeks of treatment. This suggests that certain adaptive changes are occurring with chronic administration of these drugs that are important for their antidepressant action. Over the years, mechanisms such as alterations in the expression of NMDA receptors, desensitization of presynaptic α_2-adrenoceptors, downregulation of $5\text{-}HT_2$ receptors, desensitization of presynaptic $5\text{-}HT_{1A}$ receptors, and increased neurogenesis (e.g., birth of new neurons in the hippocampus) following antidepressant therapy have been cited either as the final common pathway or as one of many possible final common pathways.

It should be remembered that the neurotransmitter and downregulation hypotheses are incomplete explanations for how antidepressants work. Antidepressants most likely set off an intricate chain of reactions that occur between the time the patient first takes them and the following few weeks, when they finally produce their effect.[196] What the neurotransmitter and downregulation hypotheses do provide are useful—if simplistic—models for comprehending at least some of the basic biochemical processes triggered by antidepressants.

EFFICACY OF ANTIDEPRESSANT

Antidepressants are widely prescribed in primary and secondary care, along with psychological interventions such as cognitive behavioral therapy. The most effective antidepressants for adults, revealed in a major review of 522 antidepressant trials by Cipriani,[196] found that all of the 21 antidepressant drugs studied performed better than placebo in short-term trials measuring response to treatment. However, effectiveness varied widely and the researchers ranked drugs by effectiveness and acceptability after 8 weeks of treatment. Five antidepressants appear more effective and better tolerated than others and include escitalopram, paroxetine, sertraline, agomelatine (not available in the US), and mirtazapine. The most effective antidepressant compared to placebo was the tricyclic antidepressant amitriptyline, which increased the chances of treatment response more than twofold. The least effective was roboxetine (available in the UK), which is a selective NE inhibitor. People were 30% more likely to stop taking the tricyclic clomipramine than placebo or the SSRI fluoxetine. There has been uncertainty in recent years about the effectiveness of antidepressants. Their mode of action is poorly understood, and improvement in mood tends to be modest. A 2008 metaanalysis suggested that antidepressants gave little benefit over placebo for mild to moderate depression. However, it did not assess antidepressants compared to other treatments such as cognitive behavioral therapy, or treatments in combination. There is conflicting evidence to guide which antidepressants should be prescribed first-line, although SSRIs are generally first-line choices.

The introduction of the second-generation classes of antidepressants in the 1980s and 1990s (SSRIs, atypical SNRIs and serotonin receptor modulators [serotonin antagonist/reuptake inhibitors (SARIs) and noradrenergic and specific serotonergic antidepressants (NaSSA; mirtazapine)]) (Table 11.4, Fig. 11.27) has been regarded as the major pharmacological advance in the treatment of depression since the appearance of the TCAs and MAOIs. The SSRIs and atypical SNRIs have proven to be effective for a broad range of depressive illnesses, dysthymia, several anxiety disorders, and bulimia. In addition to being the usual first-line treatments for major depression, the SSRIs also are first-line treatments for panic disorder, obsessive-compulsive disorder, social phobia, posttraumatic stress disorder, and bulimia. They also may be the best medications for treatment of dysthymia and generalized anxiety disorder.

Differences in tolerability of the different classes of antidepressants and in their side-effect profiles are well known. Generally, compared with the TCAs, the SSRIs cause significantly more nausea, diarrhea, agitation, sexual dysfunction, anorexia, insomnia, nervousness, and anxiety, whereas the TCAs cause more cardiotoxicity, dry mouth, constipation, dizziness, sweating, and blurred vision.[187] Although the SSRIs and SNRIs possess improved safety margins and lesser cardiovascular adverse effects than tertiary TCAs, and utility for treating other nondepressive disorders, they offer no real gain in efficacy than the first-generation TCAs. Despite pharmacological differences in their mechanisms of actions, the general view has been that all antidepressants are of equal efficacy. Only within the last 10 years has this general assumption come under serious challenge from comparisons of antidepressants with dual mechanisms of action which can be acting in a complementary and perhaps synergistic manner to improve depression versus those with a single mechanism of action.[177] Often, a variety of antidepressants will be prescribed and the dosage adjusted before the most effective antidepressant or combination of antidepressants is found. Patient compliance can become an issue, because patients often stop medication too soon as a result of feeling better. Additionally, they may have problems with the adverse effects or they may think the medication is not helping at all. It is important for the patient to keep taking the antidepressant until it has a chance to work, although side effects often appear before antidepressant activity does. Once the individual is feeling better, it is important to continue the medication for at least 4-9 months (or longer) to prevent a recurrence of the depression. Antidepressants alter brain chemistry; therefore, they must be stopped gradually to give the brain time to readjust. For some individuals with bipolar disorder or chronic major depression, antidepressant therapy may need to be maintained indefinitely.[197] All patients who are prescribed antidepressants should be informed that discontinuation/withdrawal symptoms may occur on stopping, on missing doses, or occasionally, on reducing the dose of the drug. These symptoms usually are mild and self-limiting, but occasionally, they can be severe, particularly if the drug is stopped abruptly. Symptoms of antidepressant withdrawal include nausea, vomiting, anorexia, headache, restlessness, agitation, "chills," "brain zaps," insomnia, and sometimes, hypomania, panic and anxiety, and extreme motor restlessness, especially if an antidepressant (particularly an MAOI) is stopped suddenly after regular administration for 8 weeks or more.

In addition to the wide use of antidepressants to treat depression, chronic neuropathic pain disorders which include fibromyalgia, diabetic and other peripheral neuropathic syndromes, have responded at least partly to treatment with tertiary TCAs and the SNRIs duloxetine, milnacipran and venlafaxine. The SNRIs appear to be superior to the SSRIs. [196,198]

Effect of Physicochemical Properties and Stereochemistry on Antidepressant Efficacy

Small substituent changes in molecular structure can affect the pharmacokinetic and pharmacodynamic (clinical) properties of antidepressant drug molecules, resulting in profound differences between their transporter selectivity and their antidepressant effect. For example, a difference of a 2-chloro group between the structurally related antidepressants imipramine and clomipramine results in a >10-fold change in SERT affinity (affinity of clomipramine > imipramine), and the *o*- versus

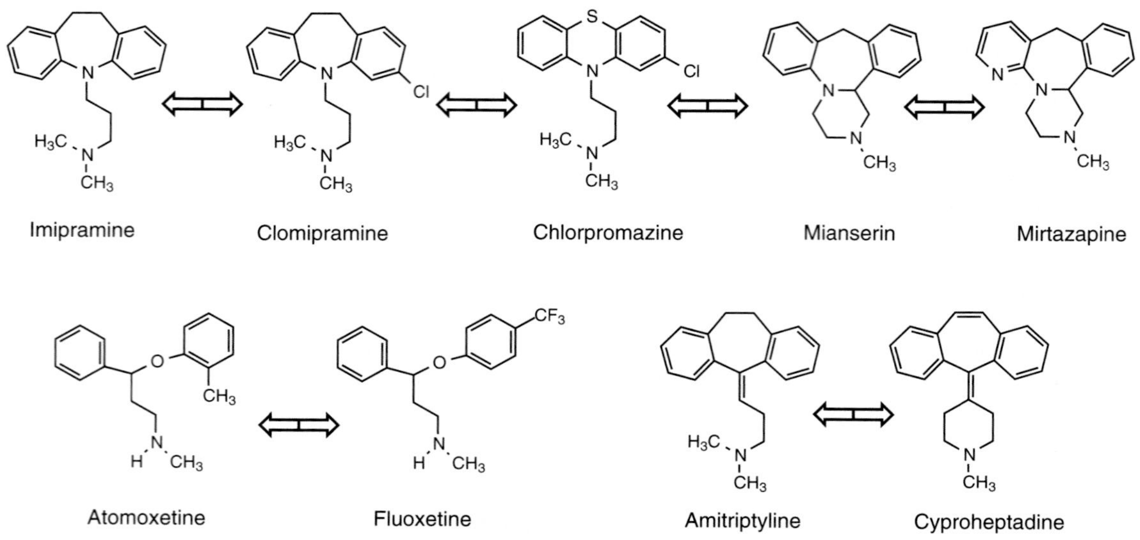

Imipramine Clomipramine Chlorpromazine Mianserin Mirtazapine

Atomoxetine Fluoxetine Amitriptyline Cyproheptadine

Figure 11.31 Structural relationship between selected molecular structures.

p-substituents between duloxetine (SNRI) and atomoxetine (SNRI) results in a >100-fold change in SERT affinity (affinity of duloxetine > atomoxetine) (Fig. 11.31). Furthermore, a seemingly simple isosteric replacement of a sulfur atom in the central ring of chlorpromazine with an ethylene group to give a seven-membered azepine ring (clomipramine) or the replacement of the methylpiperidylidene at the 5-position for the antihistamine/5-HT antagonist cyproheptadine with a dimethylaminopropylidene for the antidepressant reuptake inhibitor amitriptyline has profound effects on the physicochemical properties, pharmacokinetics, mechanisms of action, and therapeutic activities (Fig. 11.31). Other examples include mianserin and mirtazapine (Fig. 11.31).[199] The isosteric replacement of a benzene ring (mianserin) with a pyridine (mirtazapine) results in significant changes in their dipole moments, lipophilicity (Log P), pK_a values, and electronegativity, resulting in different mechanisms of action and regioselectivity in formation of hydroxylated metabolites.

Many antidepressants are stereoisomers and contain either a chiral center or a center of unsaturation by which chiral metabolites could result.[200,201] Often, such chiral drugs are marketed as a mixture of the resultant enantiomers (racemates) or of geometric isomers (e.g., levomilnacipran, *1S,2R*, and *1R,2S*). These enantiomers or geometric isomers may differ markedly from each other with regard to their pharmacodynamic and/or pharmacokinetic properties. Increased knowledge about the molecular structure of specific drug targets and an awareness of several possible advantages to using single enantiomers rather than racemic mixtures of drugs have led to an increased emphasis on understanding the role of chirality in drug development of antidepressant drugs. Several notable SSRI antidepressants currently are available in which the individual enantiomers or geometric isomers differ considerably with regard to binding to SERT and NET, interactions with receptors and metabolizing enzymes, and clearance rates from the body. Examples of the effects of chiral centers or geometric centers on such properties include racemic mixtures (e.g., (±)-fluoxetine, (±)-citalopram, (±)-bupropion, and (±)-trimipramine), single enantiomers (e.g., (+)-sertraline, (−)-paroxetine, (−)-escitalopram, and (−)-atomoxetine), or geometric isomers (e.g., 1*S*,2*R*-*cis*-levomilnapran, *Z*-zimeldine, *Z*-doxepin, and *E*-fluvoxamine). Recent developments in analytical and preparative resolution of racemic and geometric drug mixtures as well as increased interest in developing new drugs that interact with specific targets, which have been described in detail at the molecular level, have resulted in increased emphasis on stereochemistry in antidepressant drug development.

Structure-Activity Relationship of the TCAs

The tricyclic ring structure can be found in a variety of different drugs and, for the most part, represents a method for medicinal chemists to restrict the conformational mobility of two phenyl rings attached to a common carbon or hetero atom. The tricyclic ring structure is formed by joining the two phenyl rings into 6-6-6 or 6-7-6 ring systems, in which the central ring is either a six-membered or seven-membered carbocyclic or heterocyclic ring, respectively. Small molecular changes, such as ring flexibility, substituents, or heteroatoms in the tricyclic ring structure, can bring about significant changes in physicochemical, electronegativity (dipole moments), and pharmacodynamic properties (e.g., anticholinergics [antimuscarinic], cholinesterase inhibitors, antihistamine, antipsychotics, and antidepressants). This suggests that the tricyclic structure is not associated with affinity for any particular receptor but, rather, contributes to a range of multiple CNS pharmacodynamic (adverse) effects because of increased lipophilicity. The most

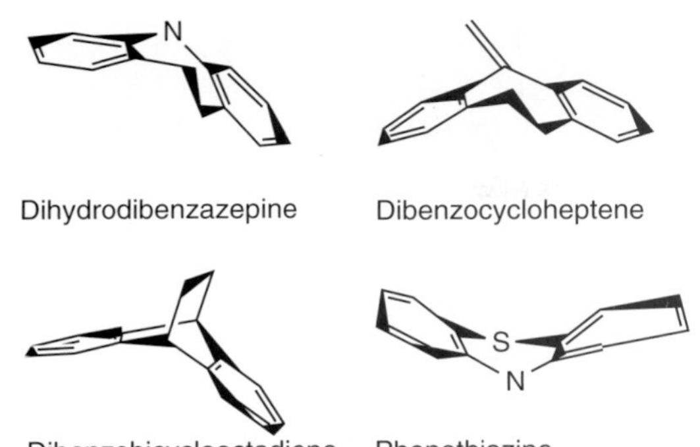

Figure 11.32 Three-dimensional models of the tricyclic and tetracyclic ring systems.

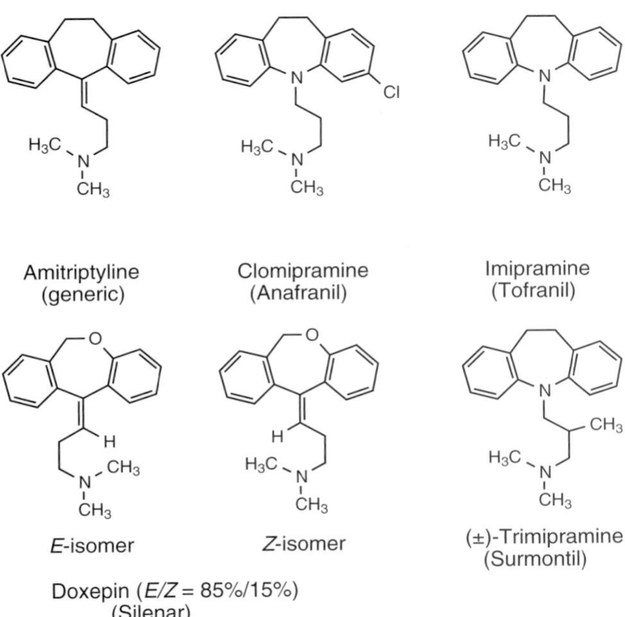

Figure 11.33 Tertiary amine tricyclic antidepressants.

common tricyclic ring found in drugs is the near-planar phenothiazine ring common to most of the antipsychotic drugs (Fig. 11.32). The TCAs are classified as such because they contain a 6-7-6 ring arrangement in which the central seven-membered ring is either carbocyclic or heterocyclic, saturated or unsaturated, which is fused to two phenyl rings (Figs. 11.33 and 11.35 for secondary amine TCAs). The side chain may be attached to any one of the atoms in the central seven-membered ring, but it must be three carbon atoms, either saturated (propyl) or unsaturated (propylidine) and have a terminal amine group (secondary or tertiary). The TCAs differ structurally from the antipsychotic phenothiazines in that the two phenyl (aromatic) rings are connected by a 2-carbon link to form a central seven-membered ring instead of a sulfur bridge.

The TCAs are subdivided into a dihydrodibenzazepine ring (a.k.a. iminodibenzyl, from which the name imipramine is derived), a dibenzocycloheptene ring whereby the ring nitrogen of imipramine is replaced by an exocyclic olefinic group (e.g., amitriptyline), a dibenzoxepin ring as a bioisosteric modification of imipramine (e.g., doxepin), a dibenzocycloheptriene ring which replaces the dihydroethylene group of imipramine with an olefinic ethylene group (e.g., protriptyline), or a tetracyclic (bicyclic ring, e.g., maprotiline) derivatives. The tricyclic ring system has little significance regarding selectivity for inhibiting the NET or SERT, but it appears to be important for DA transporter inhibition.

The secondary and tertiary amine TCAs differ markedly with regard to their selectivity ratios (Fig. 11.30) and their pharmacodynamic and/or pharmacokinetic properties (Tables 11.5 and 11.6). Substituting a halogen (i.e., chlorine; clomipramine) or cyano group into the 3-position of the dihydrodibenzazepine ring enhances preferential affinity for SERT. 3-Cyanoimipramine was investigated as a potent SSRI but was never marketed as an antidepressant agent. It is used as a research probe for studying 5-HT transporters. Branching the propyl side chain with a 2-methyl group (as in trimipramine) significantly reduces the affinity (~100 times) of imipramine for both the SERT and NET. The Z (*cis*) geometry for the propylidine group in chiral TCAs appears to be important for transporter selectivity and affinity (e.g., doxepin).

Studies correlating the binding of the TCAs with the SSRIs found that the TCAs and SSRIs bind to different sites on the transporter and that the TCAs may act as a modulator of monoamine reuptake by producing conformational changes in the transporter, affecting affinity for the monoamine neurotransmitter.[202]

Although similar in a two-dimensional plane to the antipsychotic phenothiazines, the ethylene bridge linking the two phenyl rings of the TCAs causes the two phenyl rings to be twisted out of the plane, leading to a less rigid and more conformationally mobile molecular structure than the phenothiazines (Fig. 11.32). The conformational mobility for the TCAs, including ring inversion of the tricyclic ring system, flexing of the CH_2-X bridge (X=CH_2, O, N, or S) in the central seven-membered ring, and flexibility of the alkyl side chain, can result in substantial changes in the overall shape of the molecules. This in turn can affect transporter affinity and selectivity, diverse neuroreceptor affinity, and the drug's physicochemical properties. The rate of ring flexibility seems to be correlated with their differences in clinical potency. A dibenzazepine ring system exhibits a greater degree of conformational ring flexing, whereas the dibenzocycloheptene ring system and inserting heteroatoms into the benzylic position reduce the rate of ring flexing in TCAs and their potency.[203] Thus, the differences in the pharmacological activity between these TCAs allow selective binding to their respective transporter proteins. The angle between the two aromatic rings ranges from 106 to 110° for the TCAs, and the large lipophilic ring enhances the affinity of TCA to block the CNS muscarinic, H_1-, and α_1-adrenergic receptors and to block sodium channels, contributing to its multiple pharmacodynamic effects.

Table 11.5 Pharmacokinetics of the Tricyclic Tertiary Amine Antidepressants

Parameters	Amitriptyline	Clomipramine	Doxepin	Imipramine	Trimipramine
Oral bioavailability (%)	31-61	~50	13-45	29-77	44
Lipophilicity (Log $D_{7.4}$)	2.96	3.31	2.50	2.68	3.04
Protein binding (%)	95	96-98	ND	89-95	95
Volume of distribution (L/kg)	12-18	17 (9-25)	12-28	23 (15-31)	~31
Elimination half-life (hr)	10-26	32 (19-37)	11-16	11-25	9-11
Cytochrome P450 major isoform	2D6	2D6	2D6 and 2C19	2D6 and 2C19	2D6 and 2C19
Major active metabolites	Nortriptyline	Desclomipramine (54-77 hr)	Nordoxepin (~30 hr)	Desipramine	Desmethyltrimipramine (30 hr)
Peak plasma concentration (hr)	2-12	2-6 (4.7)	<2	1-2	<2
Excretion (%)	Urine 25-50	Urine 51-60 (14 d)	Renal ~50	Urine ~40 (24 hr)	Urine <5
	Feces minor	Feces 24-32	Feces minor	Feces minor	Feces 80-90
Plasma half-life (hr)	21 (10-46)	34 (22-84)	8-24	18 (9-24)	9
Time to steady-state concentration	–	1-2 wk	ND	ND	ND

ND, not determined.

Table 11.6 Pharmacokinetics of the Tricyclic Secondary Amine Antidepressants

Parameters	Desipramine	Nortriptyline	Amoxapine	Protriptyline	Maprotiline
Oral bioavailability (%)	60-70	32-79	ND	77-93	66-75
Lipophilicity (Log $D_{7.4}$)	1.58	2.28	1.70	1.85	2.10
Protein binding (%)	91	92	92	92	88
Volume of distribution (L/kg)	17-42	14-22	ND	22	15-28
Elimination half-life (hr)	30 (12-30)	30 (18-44)	8 (8-30)	67-89	43 (27-58)
Major active metabolites	None	10-E-hydroxy-	8-OH (30 hr) 7-OH (6.5 hr)	None	(60-90 hr)
Peak plasma concentration (hr)	4-6	7-9	90 min	24-30	8-24
Excretion (%)	Urine	Urine 40	Urine 60 (6 d)	Urine 50 (16 d)	Urine 65 (21 d)
	Feces	Feces minor	Feces 7-18	Feces minor	Feces 30
Plasma half-life (hr)	14-62	18-93	8	54-198	21-52
Time to steady-state concentration	ND	ND	ND		7 d

ND, not determined.

Drug Metabolism and Drug-Drug Interactions

The incidence of adverse drug events associated with antidepressant treatment increases with patient age (e.g., in the elderly), with polypharmacotherapy (e.g., via drug-drug interactions), and with individual variability in drug metabolism (e.g., genetic factors, concurrent disease, diet, and eating habits). Pharmacokinetic drug-drug interactions occur when one medication (the precipitant drug) significantly affects the plasma concentration, half-life, or both of another medication (the object drug) by altering its absorption, distribution, metabolism, or elimination. For object drugs with narrow therapeutic indices, even small elevations in plasma drug concentration can cause potentially serious adverse reactions. Pharmacodynamic drug-drug interactions occur when the precipitant drug affects the ability of the object drug to bind with its therapeutic target (e.g., transporter protein or receptor). Some compounds compete directly for binding to a receptor; others indirectly affect the ability of an object drug to interact with its site of action. Many medications can bind to multiple receptor types (e.g., first-generation TCAs), causing diverse adverse reactions. Thus, before adding a new drug to an existing antidepressant regimen, it is wise to determine whether any medications can be eliminated. Reduction of total drug burden, adjustment of dose levels, and careful selection of an appropriate agent are important steps toward avoiding adverse drug interactions. In addition, the documented and potential drug interactions of the various classes of antidepressants—and of the specific drugs within each class—should be considered. Each patient should be treated individually and monitored carefully during the initiation and maintenance of antidepressant therapy.

The infamous, potentially lethal, drug-drug interactions between the antihypertensive, calcium channel blocker mibefradil (Propulsid) and antihistamine terfenadine (Seldane) and other drugs metabolized by CYP3A4 resulted in these drugs being withdrawn from the market, which placed a spotlight on hepatic drug metabolism as a significant participant in drug-drug interactions. Nearly all the antidepressants are metabolized by at least one CYP isoform, and these drugs and their metabolites may be substrates or inhibitors for the CYPs (Table 11.7).

When an antidepressant is metabolized by more than one CYP isoform in parallel, the antidepressant is unlikely to be affected by drug interactions or genetic polymorphisms and to cause clinically significant drug interactions via CYP isoform inhibition.[204] However, if the drug is metabolized (depending upon enzyme kinetics) primarily by CYP3A4 or the polymorphic CYP2C18 or CYP2D6 isoforms, the potential for drug-drug interactions increases. Therefore, knowledge regarding the metabolic pathways of antidepressants as well as knowledge about substrates and inhibitors of the CYP isoforms can assist in the selection of a proper drug and its dose, thus minimizing the risks of drug-drug interactions.[204]

Drug Safety

Clinical trials have concluded that two to four of every 100 children and teenagers treated with antidepressants might be at higher risk of suicidal behavior. Most of the risk is associated with SSRIs; however, data regarding suicidal behavior vary among the antidepressants, which leads to the conclusion that no antidepressant is free from risk at this time. Approximately 7% of antidepressant prescriptions are written for children. Thus, the FDA in 2007 approved that a "boxed warning" (sometimes called a black box warning) be included on antidepressant product packaging, alerting physicians of possible risks of suicidal behavior and to watch for signs of worsening depression or suicidal thoughts and behavior in children and young adults (up to age 24) who are taking any antidepressant. In 2018, the FDA directed manufacturers of all antidepressant drugs to revise the labeling for their products to include a "boxed warning" and expanded warning statements that alert health care providers to an increased risk of suicidality (suicidal thinking and behavior) in children and adolescents being treated with these antidepressants, and to include additional information about the results of pediatric studies. The FDA also informed these manufacturers that it has determined that it is appropriate for patients on antidepressants medications be given a medication guide which advises them (and their caregivers) of the risks and precautions involved in taking these medications. Medication guides are intended to be distributed by the pharmacist with each prescription or refill of a medication.

The risk of suicidality associated with antidepressant drugs was identified in a combined analysis of short-term (up to 4 mo) placebo-controlled trials of nine antidepressant drugs, including the SSRIs, SNRIs, and others, in children and adolescents with MDD, obsessive compulsive disorder, or other affective disorders. The analysis showed a greater risk of suicidality during the first few months of treatment in those receiving antidepressants. The average risk of such events was 4%, twice the placebo risk of 2%. Among the antidepressants, only Prozac (fluoxetine) is approved for use in treating MDD in pediatric patients. Fluoxetine, sertraline, fluvoxamine, and clomipramine are approved for obsessive compulsive disorder in pediatric patients. Pediatric patients being treated with antidepressants for any indication should be closely observed for clinical worsening, as well as agitation, irritability, suicidality, and unusual changes in behavior, especially during the initial few months of a course of drug therapy, or at times of dose changes, either increases or decreases.

Table 11.7 Cytochrome P450 (CYP) Metabolism[a]

Antidepressant	Major CYP	Minor CYP	Metabolism Pathway	CYP Inhibitor
Amitriptyline	2D6	3A4, 2C19, 2C9, 1A2, and 2B6	2D6, 3A4, 2C19, and 1A2 N-demethylation 2D6 and 2B6 *E*-10-hydroxylation	2D6, 2C19, 1A2, and 2C9[b]
Clomipramine	2D6	3A4, 2C19, 1A2, and 2C9	2D6, 3A4, 2C19, 2C9, and 1A2 N-demethylation 2D6 2- and 8-hydroxylation	2D6
Desipramine	2D6	1A2 and 2C19	1A2 and 2C19 N-demethylation 2D6 and 2C19 2-hydroxylation	2D6 and 2C19[b]
E-Doxepine	2D6 and 2C9	3A4, 1A2, and 2C19	2D6 and 2C9 hydroxylation 3A4 and 1A2 N-demethylation	
Z-Doxepine	2C19	2C9, 3A4, and 1A2	2C19 and 2C9 N-demethylation 3A4 and 1A2 N-demethylation	
Imipramine	2D6	3A4, 2C19, 1A2, 2B6, and 2C9	1A2 and 2C19 N-demethylation 2D6, 1A2, 3A4, and 2C19 2- and 10-hydroxylation	1A2, 2D6 and 2C19
Maprotiline	2D6	1A2	2D6 and 1A2 N-demethylation	
Nortriptyline	2D6	3A4, 2C19, and 1A2	2D6, 3A4, 2C19, and 1A2 N-demethylation 2D6 *E*-10-hydroxylation	2D6 and 2C19[b]
Trimipramine	2D6	2C9 and 2C19	2-hydroxyl, 10-hydroxyl, and N-demethylation	2D6
(±)-Citalopram	2C19	3A4, 2D6	2C19, 3A4 N-demethylation 2D6 N-oxidation	1A2[b] and 2D6[b]
Escitalopram	2D6	1A2 and 2C19	2D6, 2C19, and 3A4 N-demethylation 2D6 N-oxidation	
(±)-Fluoxetine	2D6	3A4, 2C9, 2C19, and 1A2	2D6 and 2C19 N-dealkylation 1A2 and 2C9 O-dealkylation	2D6 (*S*-fluoxetine) 1A2,[b] 2C19,[b] 3A4,[b] 2C9,[b] and 2D6[b]

Table 11.7 Cytochrome P450 (CYP) Metabolism[a] (Continued)

Antidepressant	Major CYP	Minor CYP	Metabolism Pathway	CYP Inhibitor
Sertraline	3A4	2D6 and 2C19	3A4, 2C19, 2D6, and 2C9 N-demethylation	2C19,[b] 3A4,[b] and 2D6[b]
Fluvoxamine	1A2	3A4, 2C19, and 2D6	2D6 and 1A2 O-dealkylation	2C19, 1A2,[b] and 3A4[b]
Paroxetine	2D6	3A4, 1A2, and 2C9	2D6 cleavage methylenedioxy	2D6,[c] 2C19,[b] and 3A4[b]
Venlafaxine	2D6	3A4, 2C19, and 2C9	2D6, 2C19, and 2C9 O-demethylation 2C19, 2C9, and 3A4 N-demethylation	2D6[b]
Atomoxetine	2D6	3A4, 2C19, and 1A2	2D6, 1A2, 2B6, and 2C19 4-hydroxylation 2C19, 3A4, and 2B6 N-demethylation	
Duloxetine	2D6	1A2	4- and 6-hydroxylation	2D6
Mirtazapine	2D6	3A4 and 1A2	2D6 and 1A2 8-hydroxylation 3A4 N-demethylation 3A4 and 1A2 N-oxidation	3A4[b] and 2D6[b]
Vilazodone	3A4/5	2C19, 2D6	6-Aromatic hydroxylation of indole ring	
Vortioxetine	2D6	2C9, 2C19, 3A4	2D6 and 2C19 methyl hydroxylation 2D6 and 2C9 aromatic hydroxylation 3A4 N- and *S*-oxidation	2D6
Bupropion	2B6	2E1, 3A4, and 2D6	Hydroxylation t-butyl group	2D6[b]
Trazodone	3A4	2D6	N-dealkylation to chlorophenylpiperazine Aromatic ring hydroxylation	
Tranylcypromine		3A4, 2A6, 2D6, 2C19, and 2C9	Aromatic ring hydroxylation	2A6[c]
Levomilnacipran	3A4		N-deethylation and *p*-hydroxylation	

[a]Rendic S. *Human P450 Metabolism Database*. Available at http://www.gentest.com/human_p450_database. Accessed July 11, 2003.
[b]Weak CYP inhibitor.
[c]Mechanism-based inhibition.

SSRIs are safer than the TCAs for older people because they do not disturb heart rhythms and rarely cause dizziness that may result in falls. But liver function is less efficient in older people, so there is a greater risk of drug interactions involving the CYP system (Table 11.7). For that reason, older people do best with rapidly metabolized SSRIs like sertraline.

SPECIFIC DRUGS

Tricyclic Tertiary Amine Antidepressants

Despite the current popularity of the SSRIs for the treatment of depression, the noradrenergic neurons should not be overlooked.[175] Deficits in noradrenergic neurotransmission appear to be associated with decreased concentration, energy, attention, self-care, and cognition, whereas deficits in serotonergic neurotransmission are associated with changes in mood, anxiety, suicidality, and appetite disturbances (Fig.11.25). Thus, the different symptoms of depression may benefit from drugs acting mainly on one or other of the neurotransmitter systems.[187] The secondary amine TCAs (Fig. 11.35), which act at NET and SERT, seem to be at least as effective as the SSRIs in the treatment of depressive illness[196]. Thus, the SSRIs and secondary amine TCAs influence depression by parallel, independent pathways. The secondary amine TCAs have a role in the treatment of depression, either alone or as adjunct therapy. The secondary amine TCAs are well tolerated but possess different adverse event profiles.

The selectivity ratios (Fig. 11.30) show that the TCAs, as a group, are potent inhibitors of the SERT and NET and that the secondary amine TCAs are substantially more potent with regard to their inhibition of NE reuptake in comparison to the SSRIs. Their in vitro affinity for inhibiting the NET essentially mirrors more or less their clinical efficacy as antidepressants[175,197]: desipramine > protriptyline > amitriptyline = nortriptyline > maprotiline > amoxapine > imipramine.

The tricyclic tertiary amines (Fig. 11.33) have a relatively low bioavailability suggesting first-pass metabolism (N-demethylation) to their secondary amine active metabolites (nor or desmethyl metabolites) and aromatic ring hydroxylation (Table 11.5). Despite the fact that steady-state serum plasma levels are reached within 1-2 days, their onset of antidepressant action typically is at least 2-3 weeks or longer. Their volume of distribution is very high, suggesting distribution into the CNS and protein binding (Table 11.5). Excretion is primarily as metabolites via renal elimination. Renal and liver function can affect the elimination and metabolism of the parent TCA and its metabolites, leading to increased potential for adverse effects, especially in those patients (e.g., elderly) with renal disease (Table 11.5). Meaningful differences between the TCA tertiary amines is largely related to their pharmacokinetics, metabolism to active metabolites, inhibition of CYP isoforms, potential for drug-drug interactions, and half-lives.

Mechanisms of Action Common to the TCA Tertiary Amines

The exact mechanism of action for the tertiary amine TCAs is unclear, but it is known that the parent tertiary amine TCA exhibits mixed inhibition of NET and SERT. The result is an increase in both NE and 5-HT concentrations in the synaptic cleft. The in vivo antidepressant activity for these TCAs is more complex, however, because of the formation of secondary amine TCA metabolites, which in many cases annuls the 5-HT affinity of the parent TCA, leading to NET selectivity. The plasma concentrations for the secondary amine metabolites usually are higher than that of their parent tertiary amine TCA because of rapid N-demethylation metabolism. Note that none of the tertiary amine TCAs have any significant affinity for the DA transporter. During chronic therapy with the tertiary amine TCAs, downregulation of the noradrenergic and serotonergic receptors occurs, which is caused by the continued high concentrations of NE and 5-HT at the receptors. Although they have inhibitory activity at SERT, the TCA tertiary amines are less potent inhibitors than the SSRIs.

Therapeutic Uses Common to Tricyclic Tertiary Amine Antidepressants

For the most part, the therapeutic uses for the tertiary amine TCAs are very similar as a group, but they may be used in different cases of depression based on their relative activities at NET and SERT and their adverse effects. The tertiary TCAs may offer an option in the treatment of MDD for patients who have failed treatment with or who do not tolerate SNRIs or SSRIs.

Adverse Effects Common to Tricyclic Tertiary Amine TCAs

Because of their potent and multiple pharmacodynamic effects at off-targets including H_1, muscarinic, and α_1-adrenergic receptors, the tertiary amine TCAs exhibit greater anticholinergic, antihistaminic, and hypotensive adverse effects than the secondary amine TCAs (Table 11.6). Increased cardiotoxicity or frequency of seizures is higher for the tertiary amine TCAs than for the secondary amine TCAs, because they are potent inhibitors of sodium channels, leading to changes in nerve conduction. Cardiotoxicity can occur at plasma concentrations approximately 5-10 times higher than therapeutic blood levels. These concentrations can occur in individuals who take an overdose of the tertiary amine TCA or who are slow metabolizers and develop higher plasma concentrations on what usually are therapeutic doses.

Drug-Drug Interactions Common to Tricyclic Tertiary Amine TCAs

For the most part, drug-drug interactions for the tertiary amine TCAs are very similar to those for the secondary amine TCAs. The concurrent use of tertiary amine TCAs with SSRIs and other serotonergic drugs may result in 5-HT syndrome (see the discussion of drug interactions of SSRIs). Coadministration of a tertiary amine TCA with an MAOI is potentially hazardous and may result in severe adverse effects associated with 5-HT syndrome.

Because protein binding of the tertiary amine TCAs is high, displacement interactions with other highly protein-bound drugs and drugs with narrow therapeutic indices, although not fully evaluated, may be important. That is, TCAs might displace other drugs bound to proteins, increasing their blood concentrations and bioavailability, potentially leading to toxic effects. Concurrent use of tertiary amine TCAs with anticholinergic drugs requires close supervision and careful adjustment of the dosage because of potential additive anticholinergic effects (i.e., spastic colon). An additional disadvantage of the tertiary amine TCAs is their toxicity from overdosage, especially in those who are being treated for depression having suicidal thoughts.

The plasma concentrations of tertiary amine TCAs usually are lower and plasma concentrations of their secondary amine metabolites higher, as a result of CYP1A induction.

Patient Information Common to the Tertiary Amine TCAs

Common patient information and recommendations are similar to those given to patients who are prescribed secondary amine TCAs (Table 11.8).

Unique Properties of Specific Tricyclic Tertiary TCAs

AMITRIPTYLINE. Amitriptyline is a tricyclic tertiary amine dibenzocycloheptadiene TCA with a propylidene side chain extending from the central carbocyclic ring (Fig. 11.33). The dimethylaminopropylidene moiety for amitriptyline makes it sensitive to photo-oxidation; therefore, its hydrochloride solutions should be protected from light to avoid ketone formation and precipitation.

Pharmacokinetics. Amitriptyline is rapidly absorbed from the gastrointestinal tract and from parenteral sites. Its pharmacokinetics is shown in Table 11.5. Amitriptyline and its active metabolite, nortriptyline, are distributed into breast milk. Amitriptyline is primarily (65%) metabolized via N-demethylation by CYP2D6 to nortriptyline and hydroxylation to its *E*-10-hydroxy metabolite. Nortriptyline is pharmacologically active as a secondary amine TCA. Amitriptyline shows modestly higher affinity for SERT compared to NET.

IMIPRAMINE. Imipramine is a 10,11-dihydrodibenzazepine tricyclic tertiary amine TCA (Fig. 11.33) that is marketed as hydrochloride and pamoate salts, both of which are administered orally. Although the hydrochloride salt may be administered in divided daily doses, imipramine's long duration of action suggests that the entire oral daily dose could be administered at one time. In line with this, imipramine pamoate usually is administered as a single daily oral dose. Imipramine preferentially inhibits 5-HT reuptake over NE; however, the formation of its N-desmethyl metabolite removes whatever 5-HT activity imipramine had, with the net result of enhanced noradrenergic activity from inhibition of NE reuptake at the presynaptic neuronal membrane. Imipramine shares the pharmacological and adverse-effect profile of the other tertiary TCAs.

The pharmacokinetics of imipramine is shown in Table 11.5. Imipramine is completely absorbed from the gastrointestinal tract. Imipramine is primarily metabolized by CYP2D6 to its 2- and 10-hydroxylated metabolites and N-demethylated via CYP2C11 and CYP1A2 to desipramine, its N-monodemethylated metabolite.

Therapeutic Uses. Besides being used in the clinical treatment of depression, imipramine also has been used for the treatment of functional enuresis in children who are at least 6 years of age (25 mg daily administered 1 hr before bedtime, not to exceed 2.5 mg/kg daily).

DOXEPIN. Doxepin is a tricyclic tertiary amine dibenzoxepine derivative with an oxygen replacing one of the

Table 11.8 Patient Information and Recommendations for Tricyclic Secondary Amines Antidepressants

Patient Information	Recommendations
Potential drug-drug and drug-health interactions	Share medical conditions, other medicines (including over-the-counter and herbal medicines), allergies to TCAs, fertility status, or breast-feeding with pharmacist
Seizures, breathing difficulties, fever and sweating, loss of bladder control, muscle stiffness, unusual weakness or tiredness	Discontinue therapy and consult physician (TCAs may increase risk of seizures)
Course of therapy	Complete full course of therapy
Discontinuance of therapy	Consult physician; abrupt discontinuance not recommended because it may cause nausea, headache, and malaise
Alcohol use	Avoid alcohol
Central nervous system depressants	May exacerbate TCAs
Drowsiness, dizziness, blurred vision	Avoid driving or performing tasks requiring alertness and coordination
Sun/sunlamp exposure	Avoid prolonged exposure because of photosensitivity

ethylene carbons in the bridge. The oxygen introduces asymmetry into the tricyclic ring system, resulting in the formation of two geometric isomers: *E* (*trans*) and *Z* (*cis*) (Fig. 11.33). No commercial attempt was made to separate the isomers; thus, doxepin is administered as an 85:15 mixture of *E*- and *Z*-stereoisomers, with the *Z*-isomer being the more active stereoisomer for inhibiting the reuptake of 5-HT.[205] The *E*-isomer inhibits the reuptake of NE.[206] Unless otherwise specified, the reported in vitro and in vivo studies with dioxepin were done with the 85:15 geometric mixture.

Mechanism of Action. Because doxepin is administered as an 85:15 mixture of geometric isomers, its mechanism of action and antidepressant properties reflect this ratio. Therefore, doxepin's selectivity for inhibiting presynaptic NE reuptake is most likely caused by the 85% presence of the *E*-isomer in the geometric mixture. Its antidepressant activity is similar to amitriptyline. Data suggest NE reuptake inhibitory potency comparable to imipramine and clomipramine; the fact that doxepin is an 85:15 mixture of *E*- and *Z*-geometric isomers clouds its true efficacy for SERT or NET. The formation of N-desmethyldoxepin results in inhibition of NET with enhanced activity. As a result of these mixed effects on the 5-HT and NE transporters (and off-target activity at histaminergic, serotonergic, muscarinic, and α_1-adrenergic GPCRs), doxepin shares the pharmacological and adverse-effect profile of other TCAs.

The pharmacokinetics of oral doxepin is described in Table 11.5. After oral dosing, no significant difference was found between the bioavailability of the *E*- and *Z*-isomers. The plasma concentrations of the doxepin isomers remained roughly those of the administered drug, whereas the ratio for the metabolites, *E*-N-desmethyldoxepin and *Z*-N-desmethyldoxepin, were approximately 1:1.[205,206] This similarity in ratios of metabolites is attributed to *E*-doxepine being primarily metabolized in parallel by CYP2D6 and CYP2C19, whereas *Z*-doxepine is primarily metabolized only by CYP2C19 and not at all by CYP2D6 (Table 11.5). Its *Z*-N-demethylated metabolite is pharmacologically more active than its *E*-metabolite as an inhibitor of SERT and NET.[204] Both isomers of doxepin showed large volumes of distribution and relatively short half-lives in plasma, suggestive of extensive distribution and/or tissue binding. Renal clearances did not differ for the isomers.[205]

CLOMIPRAMINE. This tricyclic tertiary dihydrodibenzazepine TCA, with actions on both NET and SERT and at several off-target GPCRs, was the last of the major TCAs to come to market. Initially, the FDA regarded it as another "me too" drug and accordingly, they did not license it. Subsequently, however, it was licensed for the treatment of obsessive compulsive disorder. Clomipramine differs from imipramine only by the addition of a 3-chloro group (Fig. 11.33).

Mechanism of Action. Clomipramine exhibits preferential selectivity for inhibiting SERT at the presynaptic neuronal membrane. Its antidepressant mechanism of action as a SERT inhibitor is reduced in vivo, however, because of the formation of its active metabolite, N-desmethylclomipramine, which inhibits the reuptake of NE. As a result of its common structure with the other TCAs, clomipramine shares the pharmacological and adverse-effect profile of other TCAs.

The efficacy of clomipramine relative to the other TCAs in the treatment of obsessive compulsive disorder may be related to its potency in blocking SERT at the presynaptic neuronal membrane. Clomipramine appears to decrease the turnover of 5-HT in the CNS, probably because of a decrease in the release and/or synthesis of 5-HT. Although in vitro studies suggest that clomipramine is approximately four times more potent than fluoxetine as a SERT inhibitor, in vivo studies suggest the opposite. This difference has been attributed to the relatively long elimination half-life for fluoxetine and its principal serotonergic metabolite norfluoxetine. In addition, metabolism of clomipramine to its N-desmethyl secondary amine metabolite decreases the potency and selectivity of 5-HT reuptake inhibition.

Pharmacokinetics. Clomipramine appears to be well absorbed from the gastrointestinal tract following oral administration, with an oral bioavailability of approximately 50%, suggesting some first-pass metabolism (Table 11.5). Food does not appear to substantially affect its bioavailability. Clomipramine and its active metabolite, N-desmethylclomipramine, exhibit nonlinear pharmacokinetics at 25-150 mg daily. At dosages exceeding 150 mg daily, their elimination half-lives may be considerably prolonged, allowing plasma concentrations of both to accumulate, which may increase the incidence of plasma concentration–dependent adverse effects, particularly seizures. Because of the relatively long elimination half-lives of clomipramine and N-desmethylclomipramine, their steady-state plasma concentrations generally are achieved within approximately 1-2 weeks. Plasma concentration of N-desmethylclomipramine generally is greater than that for chlomipramine at steady-state conditions. Clomipramine crosses the placenta and is distributed into breast milk.

Clomipramine is primarily metabolized by CYP2D6 N-dealkylation to its pharmacologically active metabolite (N-desmethylclomipramine), the 2- and 8-hydroxylated metabolites and their glucuronides and clomipramine N-oxide (Fig. 11.34). N-dealkylation also involves CYP3A4, CYP2C19, CYP2C9, and CYP1A2. Like all the other secondary amine TCAs, N-desmethylclomipramine is significantly more potent as an inhibitor of NE reuptake than clomipramine. Although N-desmethylclomipramine is pharmacologically active, its efficacy in obsessive compulsive disorder is not known. 8-Hydroxyclomipramine and 8-hydroxydesmethylclomipramine also are pharmacologically active, but their clinical importance remains unknown. The hydroxylation and N-demethylation of clomipramine highlight CYP2D6 polymorphism in healthy adults who were phenotyped as either extensive metabolizers or poor metabolizers of clomipramine.

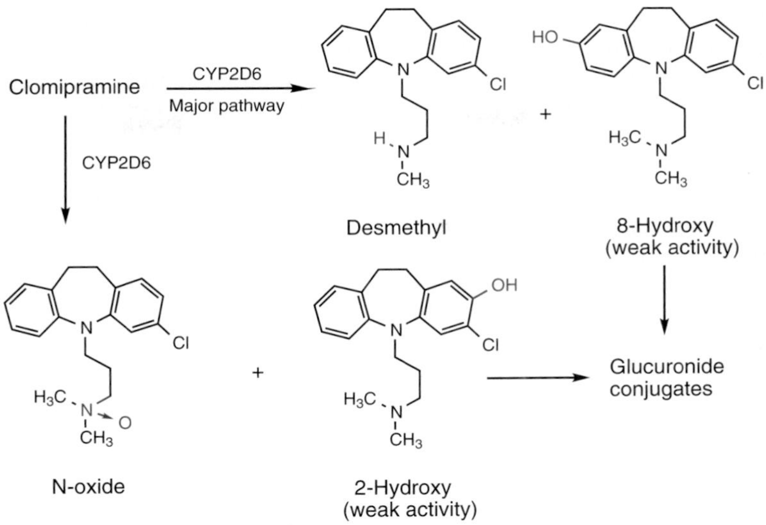

Figure 11.34 Metabolism of chlorimipramine.

Interindividual variation in plasma concentrations may be caused by genetic differences in the metabolism of the drug. In addition, CYP1A2 ring hydroxylates clomipramine. Less than 1% of an oral dose of clomipramine was excreted unmetabolized into the urine, with 8-hydroxyclomipramine glucuronide as the principal metabolite found in the urine. The effects of renal clearance suggest that clomipramine and desmethylclomipramine should be decreased in patients with renal impairment.

Pharmacogenetic differences in the metabolism of clomipramine after a single oral dose are apparent as increased plasma clomipramine concentrations in Indian and Pakistani patients compared with Caucasians. In Japanese patients, substantial interindividual variation in demethylation and hydroxylation of clomipramine was observed, although the prevalence of poor demethylators and poor hydroxylators of clomipramine has been estimated to be less than 1%.

If inhibition of SERT is critical to the desired clinical effect for clomipramine, then a patient may fail to respond, because of higher levels of N-desmethylclomipramine as opposed to the parent drug. On the other hand, if a patient who had responded well and was stabilized to a dose of clomipramine, the drug might lose efficacy if exposed to an environmental agent that is capable of inducing CYP1A or CYP3A4.

Adverse Effects. Patients taking clomipramine should be informed of sexual dysfunction as a side effect associated with antidepressants having significant serotonergic activity. Sexual dysfunction in men appears as ejaculatory incompetence, ejaculatory retardation, decreased libido, or inability to obtain or maintain an erection. Sexual dysfunction in women is similar to men, and includes decreased libido and orgasmic disturbances. Sexual dysfunction is dose-related and can be treated by simply lowering the drug dose.

TRIMIPRAMINE. Trimipramine is also a tertiary amine dihydrodibenzazepine TCA that differs structurally from imipramine in that the 5-propyl side chain is branched by a methyl group creating a chiral center (Fig.11.33). Trimipramine is marketed as a racemic mixture. No data are available regarding the activity of the enantiomers. Apparently, branching the propyl side chain reduces affinity by 100 times for both SERT and NET, but the selectivity ratio favors the 5-HT transporter. In fact, affinity for NET is rather low, compared to most other TCAs. Although trimipramine has the weakest binding affinity for the monoamine transporters, it shares the pharmacological and toxicity actions of the other TCAs and is used primarily in the treatment of depression. Its efficacy might be due to its potency at α_1-adrenergic GPCRs.

The pharmacokinetics for trimipramine is shown in Table 11.5. Trimipramine is rapidly absorbed. Trimipramine demonstrates stereoselectivity in its metabolism to its three major metabolites. (−)-Trimipramine is primarily metabolized via CYP2D6 hydroxylation to 2-hydroxytrimipramine, whereas (+)-trimipramine is preferentially metabolized by CYP2C19 N-demethylation to desmethyltrimipramine. Desmethyltrimipramine is further hydroxylated to 2-hydroxydesmethyltrimipramine. (−)-Trimipramine is metabolized by CYP3A4/5 to an unknown metabolite.[207,208] Most of the oral dose is excreted in urine in 72 hours, primarily as N-demethylated or hydroxylated and conjugated metabolites. The pharmacokinetics of trimipramine in geriatric individuals (≥65 yr of age) does not differ substantially from that in younger adults.

Trimipramine is one of the TCA antidepressants with the most pronounced differences in pharmacokinetics caused by the CYP2D6 genetic polymorphism.[205,207] Its bioavailability and systemic clearance depend significantly on the CYP2D6 isoform with a linear dose relationship. Its mean bioavailability was 44% in individuals without CYP2D6 (poor metabolizers) but 16 and 12% in those individuals with two and three active genes of CYP2D6 (fast and ultrafast metabolizers), respectively. Consequently, the mean total clearances of the oral dose were 27, 151, and 253 L/hr in poor, extensive, and ultrarapid metabolizers, respectively. The 44% bioavailability combined with low systemic clearance of trimipramine in poor metabolizers of CYP2D6 substrates results in a very high exposure to trimipramine with the risk of adverse drug reactions. On the other hand, the presystemic elimination may result in subtherapeutic drug concentrations in carriers of CYP2D6 gene duplications with a high risk of poor therapeutic response.[205,207]

Tricyclic Secondary Amine Antidepressants

Pharmacokinetics Common to Secondary Amine TCAs

The secondary amine TCAs are rapidly and well absorbed following oral administration. Although the pharmacokinetics is approximately similar within the tertiary and secondary amine groups, it is different between the two groups (Tables 11.5 and 11.6). The secondary amine TCAs have relatively high bioavailability. Their primary routes of hepatic metabolism are N-demethylation to inactive primary amine metabolites and aromatic ring hydroxylation (Table 11.6). Despite the fact that serum plasma levels are reached within 1-2 days, their onset of antidepressant action typically is at least 2-3 weeks or longer. Their volume of distribution is very high, suggesting distribution into the CNS and protein binding. Elimination is primarily as metabolites and their conjugates via renal elimination. Renal and liver function can affect the elimination and metabolism of the parent secondary amine TCA and its metabolites, leading to increased potential for adverse effects, especially in those patients (e.g., the elderly) with renal disease.

Mechanisms of Action Common to Secondary Amine TCAs

The exact mechanism of action for the secondary TCAs is unclear, but the secondary amine TCAs exhibit substantially more affinity than the SSRIs and the tertiary TCAs for inhibiting the NET. None of the secondary TCAs has significant affinity for DAT. Blocking the reuptake of NE increases its concentration in the synaptic cleft and its ability to interact with synaptic NE receptors. When drugs are selective for a transporter, differences in potency become clinically irrelevant because the plasma concentration can be dose-adjusted to achieve inhibition of the desired transporter without affecting the other transporters. During chronic therapy with the TCAs, adaptive changes at noradrenergic receptors occur, i.e., downregulation, as a result of prolonged, relatively high concentrations of NE in and around synaptic zones. Therapeutic effects are associated with changes of expression and function of α_1-adrenergic receptors. The antidepressant action of the NE-selective secondary amine tricyclic antidepressants such as desipramine and nortriptyline suggests a major involvement of NE neurotransmission in depression, although these compounds or their metabolites also have some action at SERT and certain GPCRs. The selective NET inhibitor, reboxetine, has demonstrated equivalent efficacy to the TCA (tricyclic antidepressants) in some studies.

Drug-Drug Interactions Common to the Secondary Amine TCAs

The secondary amine TCAs were once first-line therapy for depression because of their efficacy in a broad range of depressive disorders. Today, however, these agents generally are reserved for second-line treatment because of their narrow therapeutic-to-toxicity ratios and troublesome adverse-effect profiles. Even the better-tolerated nortriptyline is fatal in overdose and may have significant adverse effects at therapeutic dose levels. Most TCAs are metabolized by multiple CYP enzymes and, thus, are likely to be object drugs for many common medications. Because these TCAs have narrow therapeutic indices, any interference with their metabolism can lead to serious adverse reactions resulting from increased plasma concentrations (e.g., arrhythmias, seizures, and confusion). Such reactions are both more common and more likely to be life-threatening in elderly patients because of age-related pharmacokinetic alterations. Therefore, although specific secondary amine TCAs are useful for some conditions (e.g., major depression), coadministration with other drugs should be done cautiously.

Concurrent administration of TCAs and MAOIs is contraindicated and at least two weeks should elapse between discontinuance of TCA therapy and initiation of MAOI therapy and vice versa, to allow washout. Coadministration of SNRIs, TCAs, and MAOIs is potentially hazardous and may result in severe adverse effects associated with hypertension.

Because protein binding of secondary amine TCAs is high, displacement interactions with other highly protein-bound drugs with narrow therapeutic indices, although not yet fully evaluated, may be important. Concurrent use of the secondary amine TCAs with anticholinergics requires close supervision and careful adjustment of the dosage because of potential additive anticholinergic effects (i.e., spastic colon) and increased blood pressure and heart rate. An additional disadvantage of these TCAs is their toxicity from overdosage, especially in those being treated for depression who may have suicidal thoughts.

In addition, the secondary amine TCAs are inhibitors of sodium channels and, thus, can slow ventricular conduction at therapeutic doses. If the patient overdoses or drug interactions result in increased plasma concentration of the TCA, severe conduction block contributing to cardiotoxicity may result in ventricular arrhythmias. Also, changes in CNS conduction can result in seizures. Patients who are sensitive to one TCA may be sensitive to other TCAs.

The effect of smoking on the activity of CYP1A2 does not appear to have an effect on the plasma concentrations of the secondary TCAs. This is because CYP1A2 is not involved with the N-dealkylation to their primary amine metabolites.

For common patient information and recommendations, see Table 11.8.

Unique Properties for the Specific Secondary Amine TCAs

DESIPRAMINE. Desipramine is a dihydrodibenzazepine secondary amine TCA that is also the active metabolite of imipramine (Fig. 11.35). Desipramine appears to have a bioavailability comparable to the other secondary TCAs (Table 11.6). Desipramine is distributed into milk in concentrations similar to those present at steady state in maternal plasma. This drug is metabolized primarily by CYP2D6 to its 2-hydroxy metabolite and by CYP1A2 and CYP2C19 to its N-demethylated (primary amine) metabolite (Table 11.7).

Desipramine exhibits a greater potency and selectivity for NET than the other secondary TCAs do (Fig. 11.30). Its antidepressant effect results from increases in the level of NE in CNS synapses, and long-term administration causes a downregulation of α_1-adrenoceptors and desensitization of presynaptic α_2-receptors, equilibrating the noradrenergic system and, thus, correcting the dysregulated output of depressed patients. The SSRIs do not produce this effect. Desipramine also downregulates NET, but not SERT. Substantial loss of NET binding sites takes 15 days to occur and is accompanied by a marked reduction of NET function in vivo. Relative to NET, desipramine has weak effects on SERT.

NORTRIPTYLINE. Nortriptyline is a secondary amine dibenzocycloheptene TCA (Fig. 11.35) as well as the major metabolite of amitriptyline. Similar to desipramine, nortriptyline appears in mother's milk and is metabolized by CYP2D6 to the primary amine and by ring hydroxylation to its *E*-10-hydroxy metabolite (Table 11.6). Approximately one-third of a dose of nortriptyline is excreted in urine as metabolites within 24 hours and small amounts are excreted in feces via biliary elimination.

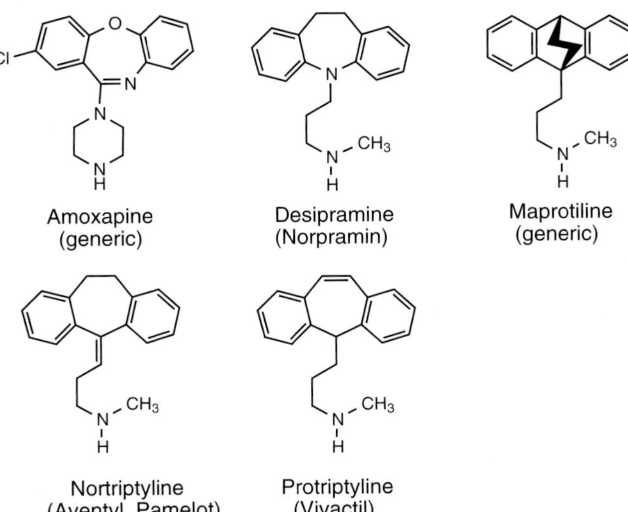

Figure 11.35 Secondary amine tricyclic antidepressants.

AMOXAPINE. Amoxapine is a dibenzoxazepine TCA (Fig. 11.35) with antidepressant and antipsychotic effects that has shown therapeutic effectiveness in patients with delusional depression. Additionally, it is the N-desmethyl metabolite of the antipsychotic loxapine. Amoxapine differs structurally from the other secondary TCAs in that it has both a nitrogen and an oxygen atom in its seven-membered central ring and a piperazinyl ring rather than a propylamino side chain attached to the central ring.

Amoxapine shares the toxic potentials of the TCAs, and the usual precautions of TCA administration should be observed. In addition to its activity at NET, amoxapine resembles antipsychotic drugs in that it potently antagonizes D_2 and 5-HT_2 receptors. Amoxapine is rapidly and almost completely absorbed from the GI tract. Its pharmacokinetics is shown in Table 11.6. Amoxapine and its 8-hydroxyamoxapine metabolite have been detected in human milk at concentrations below steady-state therapeutic concentrations. Amoxapine has the shortest elimination time (~8 hr) of the secondary TCAs. It is metabolized in the liver principally to 8-hydroxyamoxapine and to 7-hydroxyamoxapine. Both of these metabolites are pharmacologically active and have half-lives of 30 and 6.5 hours, respectively. The hydroxylation of amoxapine is inhibited by ketoconazole, suggesting the involvement of CYP3A4.

PROTRIPTYLINE. Protriptyline is a dibenzocycloheptriene TCA that differs from the other tricyclics by having an unsaturated ethylene bridge joining the two aromatic rings and a secondary aminopropyl side chain (Fig. 11.35). Protriptyline is completely absorbed from the GI tract and slowly eliminated. Its pharmacokinetic data are shown in Table 11.6. Metabolism data are limited for protriptyline, but it is most likely metabolized via the same pathways as the other TCAs are (Table 11.7). Very little drug is excreted in the feces via the bile. Protriptyline exhibits high selectivity for NET, but with less potency than desipramine (Fig. 11.35). Its mechanism of action is similar to that of desipramine.

MAPROTILINE. Maprotiline is a tetracyclic secondary amine dibenzobicyclooctadiene that differs structurally from certain other TCAs by having an ethylene bridge in its central ring, resulting in a rigid bicyclo-molecular skeleton (Fig. 11.32 and 11.35). The tetracyclics have diverse pharmacology and differ from TCAs in a number of ways. They are highly selective for NET (low nM K_is) over SERT (μM K_is). They block 5-HT_2 receptors, similar to TCAs, and they also block the α_1-adrenergic receptor. The tetracyclics also potently block the histamine H_1 receptor, with hardly any activity at other histamine receptors (H_2, H_3, H_4), and they tend to be stronger antihistamines than other TCAs. On the other hand, in contrast to almost all TCAs, they have only low affinity for the neuronal muscarinic receptors and, for this reason, are associated with few or no anticholinergic side effects.

Maprotiline exhibits the highest affinity and selectivity for NET (Fig. 11.30). Its antidepressant mechanism of action is similar to that of desipramine, with an onset of action of up to 2-3 weeks. Maprotiline is slowly but completely absorbed from the gastrointestinal tract and like the other TCAs, it is metabolized by CYP2D6 and CYP2C19 isoforms in the liver, primarily to pharmacologically active N-desmethylmaprotiline and to maprotiline-N-oxide. Its pharmacokinetics is shown in Table 11.6. Maprotiline is distributed into breast milk at concentrations similar to those found at steady state in maternal blood. The elimination half-life of maprotiline averages 43 hours (60-90 hours for its N-desmethyl metabolite).

Maprotiline shares the toxic potentials of the secondary TCAs, and the usual precautions of TCA administration should be observed. Although most of the TCAs have been reported to induce seizures, it is generally recognized that maprotiline may be associated with a higher incidence of dose-dependent seizures compared with the other secondary TCAs. Maprotiline has been reported to produce sedation in depressed patients and to reduce aggressive behavior in animals. At high concentrations, maprotiline also shares the anticholinergic and cardiovascular effects of the secondary TCAs and may cause electrocardiographic changes, tachycardia, and postural hypotension.

Therapeutic Uses Common to All TCAs

The efficacy of the secondary and tertiary amine TCAs in the clinical treatment of depressive illness is recommended for various conditions, including major depressive episodes, dysthymia, panic disorder, social phobia, bulimia, narcolepsy, attention-deficit disorder with or without hyperactivity, migraine headache and various other chronic pain syndromes, enuresis in children, and obsessive compulsive disorder (clomipramine). The TCAs possibly are useful as well for a broader range of depressive conditions described as dysthymia or depressive neurosis and even for prolonged or pathological mourning, agoraphobia without panic attacks, and some of the symptoms (e.g., nightmares) in post-traumatic stress disorder.

Adverse Effects Common to All TCAs

The family of TCAs has many undesirable side effects, owing to off-target activities. Depending on dose, they not only block the reuptake of NE and 5-HT (on-targets) but also can block muscarinic receptors (anticholinergic), α_1-adrenergic receptors (hypotension), H_1-receptors (antihistamine), certain serotonergic receptors, and sodium channels. The common adverse effects and appropriate responses are given in Table 11.9.

Table 11.9 Common Adverse Effects With Tricyclic Secondary Amine Antidepressants and Recommendations

Side Effects	Treatment Recommendations
Dry mouth	Drink sips of water; chew sugarless gum; clean teeth daily
Constipation	Diet rich in bran cereals, prunes, fruit and vegetables
Bladder complaints (weak urine stream, emptying difficulty, painful urination)	Consult physician
Sexual problems	Consult physician
Blurred vision	Should pass with time
Dizziness	Rise slowly from the bed or chair
Daytime drowsiness	Do not drive; take medication at bedtime; commonly will pass with time

Selective 5-HT Reuptake Inhibitors (SSRIs)

Serotonin Hypothesis of Depression

5-HT is a major player in depressive illness, and serotonergic pathways are closely related to mood disorders, especially depression (Fig. 11.25).[209-211] Thus, drugs affecting 5-HT levels in the neural synapse and serotonergic pathways may lead to effective antidepressant therapy.

5-HT is synthesized from tryptophan, packaged into vesicles and released into the synaptic cleft following an action potential. Once in the synaptic cleft, 5-HT interacts with both the pre- and postsynaptic serotonergic receptors. Evidence implicating multiple abnormalities in serotonergic pathways as a cause of depression include:

1. Low urinary concentrations of 5-HT's major metabolite, 5-hydroxyindoleacetic acid.
2. A low density of brain and platelet 5-HT transporters in depressed individuals.
3. A high density of brain and platelet 5-HT binding sites.
4. A low synaptic concentration of tryptophan, which is used in 5-HT synthesis. Of these, the low level of midbrain SERT in depressed patients has received the most attention in the development and synthesis of the SSRIs. The precise antidepressant mechanism of action for the SSRIs eludes neuroscientists, but most likely involves adaptive recalibration of several 5-HT receptors, including 5-HT_{1A}, 5-HT_{2A}, and 5-HT_{2C}. The SSRIs have been shown to alleviate depression and are the most commonly used drugs in the therapy for depression. Claims of

decreased adverse effects (adverse drug reactions) and less toxicity in overdose than both the MAOIs and the TCAs, together with increased safety, have led to their extensive use and several are ranked in the top 50 prescription drugs dispensed in the United States during the year 2016.

The SSRIs are proven treatments for depression, obsessive compulsive disorder, and panic disorder and are helpful in a variety of other conditions as well. The most substantial benefit to the SSRIs compared with the TCAs is their reduced adverse-effect profile and the fact that they are better tolerated. Although the SSRIs have become the most commonly prescribed drugs for depression, there are clinical situations in which TCAs may be more appropriate (e.g., melancholic depression, depression related to pain, and poor response to SSRIs). Meaningful differences between the individual SSRIs are largely related to their pharmacokinetics, metabolism to active metabolites, inhibition of CYP isoforms, effect of drug-drug interactions, and the half-life of the individual SSRI

Noncompliance with SSRIs (and most other psychotropic medications), because patients "feel better" and think medication is no longer needed, is an issue to be aware of. Persuading the patient to take his or her medication as prescribed is extremely important, because of the fact that depression can return. SSRIs also carry sexual side effects. Because of this, it is exceedingly important that patients receive the lowest effective dose of any drug they are prescribed to minimize side effects and maximize outcomes.

The Discovery of SSRIs

The early antidepressants indicated that 5-HT might play a significant role in depression. Therefore, medicinal chemists set out in search of the ideal SSRI with the goal of developing drugs with:

- High affinity and selectivity for the 5-HT uptake transporter.
- Ability to slow or inhibit the transporter when bound to it.
- Low affinity for the multiple neuroreceptors known to be responsible for many of the adverse effects of the TCAs (e.g., muscarinic, histaminergic and adrenergic receptors).
- No inhibition of the fast sodium channels which cause the cardiotoxicity problems associated with TCAs.

Initial success occurred with the synthesis of zimeldine, in which the central ring of amitriptyline was opened to form a diphenylpropylidine analogue. Z-zimeldine displayed selective inhibition of 5-HT reuptake, with minimal inhibition of NE reuptake. Most importantly, zimeldine was without the adverse-event profile exhibited by the TCAs. Thus, zimeldine became the template for the second-generation SSRIs shown in Figures 11.26, 11.36, and 11.37.

Mechanisms of Action Common to the SSRIs

The SSRIs preferentially act to inhibit SERT (the reuptake transporter for 5-HT) with minimal or no affinity for NE and DA transporters[177] (Fig. 11.30). These drugs block 5-HT from binding to SERT and being transported into presynaptic cells (Fig. 11.27). The excess 5-HT in the synaptic cleft means increased activation of serotonergic receptors. Over an extended period of time, this causes downregulation of pre- and postsynaptic receptors, a reduction in the amount of 5-HT produced in the CNS and a reduction in the number of SERTs expressed.

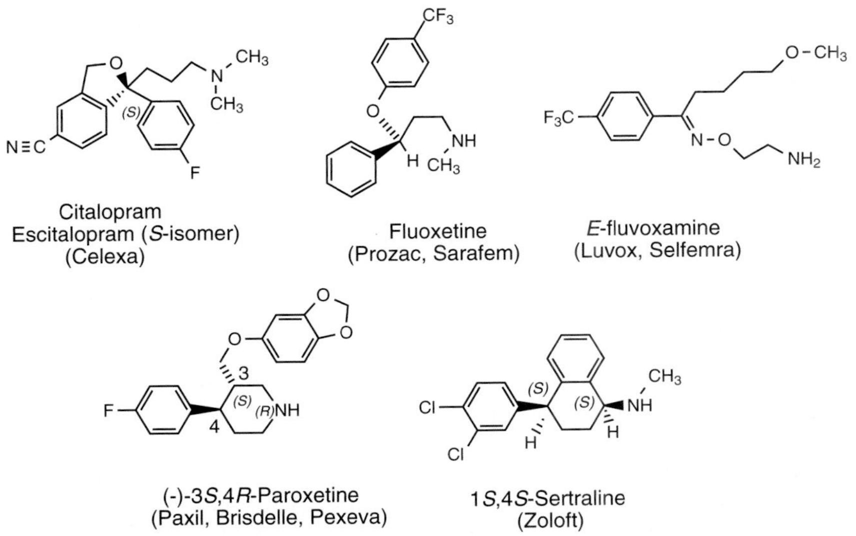

Citalopram
Escitalopram (S-isomer)
(Celexa)

Fluoxetine
(Prozac, Sarafem)

E-fluvoxamine
(Luvox, Selfemra)

(-)-3S,4R-Paroxetine
(Paxil, Brisdelle, Pexeva)

1S,4S-Sertraline
(Zoloft)

Figure 11.36 Selective serotonin reuptake inhibitors (SSRIs).

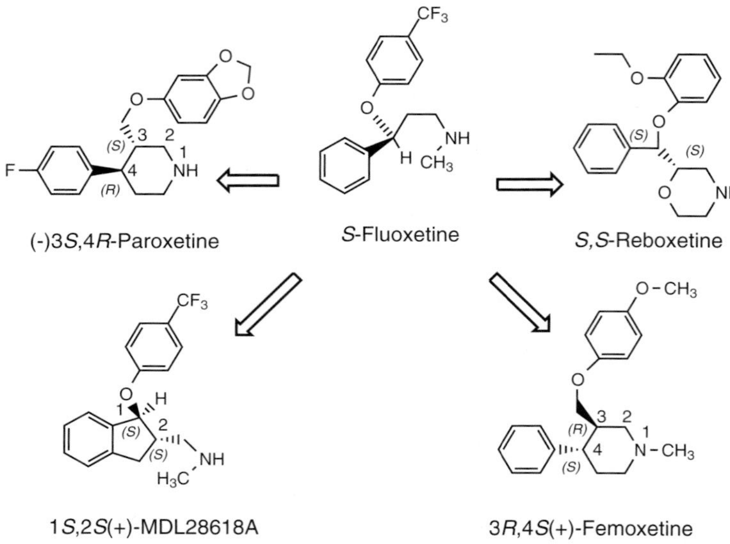

Figure 11.37 Development of and structural relationships for the phenoxyphenylalkylamines.

Long-term administration of SSRIs causes downregulation of SERT, but not NET. Substantial loss of SERT binding sites takes 15 days to occur and is accompanied by a marked reduction of SERT function in vivo. These compensatory responses at receptors and transporters are thought to produce the antidepressant effects of SSRIs. This onset delay may, in part, explain the delayed onset of action of SSRIs in the treatment of depression.[212,213] Similar to the binding of 5-HT, SSRIs likely bind to SERT at the same site as 5-HT, although it has not been determined conclusively. Although not as selective as the SSRIs, drugs of abuse, such as cocaine, are inhibitors of SERT. Other drugs, including the appetite suppressant fenfluramine and the entactogen 3,4-methylenedioxymethamphetamine ("Ecstasy") are SERT substrate–type serotonin releasers.

The affinity data for the SSRIs show that the SSRIs, as a group, are very potent and selective inhibitors for SERT compared with their affinity for NET and DAT (Fig. 11.30) and are more potent inhibitors of 5-HT reuptake than are the tertiary amine TCAs. None of the SSRIs has substantial effect on NET or DAT. Of the SSRIs, sertraline exhibits the most potent inhibition of DAT, although it is still 100 times less potent in terms of inhibiting DAT versus SERT. Therefore, the plasma concentration of sertraline would have to be increased by as much as 100 times to inhibit DAT. When drugs are this selective for the reuptake transporters, differences in potency become clinically irrelevant because the plasma concentration can be dose-adjusted to achieve inhibition of the desired transporter without affecting the other transporters. Clomipramine displays less affinity for SERT than citalopram, fluvoxamine, paroxetine, or sertraline does and is more potent than fluoxetine. In terms of the ability to inhibit NET, the SSRIs are two to three times less potent than the SNRI TCA, desipramine.The SSRIs have little or no affinity for α_1, α_2, H_1, and muscarinic receptors, which may explain the adverse-effect profile differences between TCAs and SSRIs.

Table 11.10 shows the therapeutic doses that produce approximately 60%-80% inhibition of SERT.[212-214] The inhibition of SERT is relevant to the antidepressant efficacy of the SSRIs and suggests that approximately 70%-80% inhibition of this transporter usually is necessary to produce an antidepressant effect. Higher doses of these drugs do not produce a greater antidepressant response on average (i.e., a flat dose-response curve for antidepressant efficacy) but do increase the incidence and severity of adverse effects mediated by excessive 5-HT reuptake inhibition, e.g., sexual side effects, fatigue, or tiredness. Obviously, the results shown in Table 11.10 pertain to the average patient. A patient who has a rapid clearance of the SSRI may need a higher-than-average dose to achieve an effective concentration, whereas a patient who has a slow clearance may do better in terms of the ratio of efficacy to adverse effects on a minimum dose.

The β-adrenergic blocker pindolol blocks presynapatic 5-HT_{1A} receptors, thereby increasing 5-HT neuronal transmission, and Bordet et al.[215] demonstrated an accelerated antidepressant response of pindolol with paroxetine. The theory is that downregulation of 5-HT_{1A} receptors after prolonged exposure (several weeks) to 5-HT, i.e., with SSRI treatment, contributes to antidepressant effects. So, to facilitate effects, combining SSRI treatment with a direct, 5-HT_{1A} inhibitor (mimicking functionally 5-HT_{1A} downregulation) may augment and accelerate antidepressant effects.

Pharmacokinetics Common to the SSRIs

The SSRIs share a number of pharmacokinetic characteristics[212-214] (Table 11.11). They are well absorbed orally, although the presence of food in the stomach may alter the

Table 11.10 Relationship Between Dose, Plasma Level, Potency, and Serotonin Uptake

SSRI	Dose (mg/d)	Plasma Level	In Vitro Potency (IC_{50})	Inhibition of SERT (%)
Citalopram	40	85 ng/mL (260 nM)	1.8	60
Fluoxetine	20	200 ng/mL (300 nM)[a]	3.8	70
Fluvoxamine	150	100 ng/mL (300 nM)	3.8	70
Paroxetine	20	40 ng/mL (130 nM)	0.29	80
Sertraline	50	25 ng/mL (65 nM)	0.19	80

[a]Plasma level for fluoxetine represents the total of fluoxetine plus norfluoxetine given comparable effects on SERT; parent SSRI alone shown for all others. Also, plasma levels are a total of both enantiomers for citalopram and fluoxetine. Values for the parent drug and for the respective major metabolite are in parentheses.

absorption of some SSRIs. Food, however, does not affect the area under the curve (AUC) and does not appear to affect clinical efficacy. The SSRIs are highly lipophilic and are highly plasma protein bound.

Current SSRIs tend to be characterized by high volumes of distribution, which results in relatively long plasma concentrations (typically 4-8 hr). The SSRIs display a range of elimination half-life values for the parent drugs, from half-life values of approximately 20 hours for paroxetine and fluvoxamine to 2 days for fluoxetine. Only sertraline and citalopram exhibit linear pharmacokinetics, whereas fluvoxamine, fluoxetine, and paroxetine exhibit nonlinear pharmacokinetics (i.e., changes in plasma concentration are not proportional to dose) as a result of their longer plasma half-lives within the usual therapeutic ranges (Table 11.11). Fluoxetine

Table 11.11 Pharmacokinetics of the Selective Serotonin Reuptake Inhibitors

Parameters	(±)-Fluoxetine	(−)-Sertraline	(−)-Paroxetine	E-Fluvoxamine	(±)-Citalopram [(+)-Escitalopram]
Oral bioavailability (%)	70	20-36	50	>50	80 (51-93)
Lipophilicity (Log $D_{7.4}$)	1.75	3.14	1.46	1.08	1.27
Protein binding (%)	95	96-98	95	77	~56 (70-80)
Volume of distribution (L/kg)	12-18	17 (9-25)	25 (12-28)	15-31	12-16
Elimination half-life (hr)	50	24 (19-37)	22	15-20	36 (27-32) Elderly ~48
Cytochrome P450 major isoform	2D6	3A4	2D6	2D6	2C19, 2D6, and 3A4
Major active metabolites	O-desmethyl-fluoxetine (240 hr) Norfluoxetine (96-364 hr)	N-desmethyl (62-104 hr)	None	None	Desmethylcitalopram (30 hr)
Peak plasma concentration (hr)	6-8	4-8	2-8	3-8	4 (1-6)
Excretion (%)	Urine 25-50 Feces minor	Urine 51-60 Feces 24-32	Renal ~50% Feces minor	Urine ~40% (24 hr) Feces minor	Urine <5% Feces 80%-90%
Plasma half-life (hr)	1-4 d (norfluoxetine 7-15 d)	22-35	24	7-63	36 (23-75)
Time to steady-state concentration (d)	~4 wk	7-10 d Elderly 2-3 wk	7-14 d	10 d	7 d

and fluvoxamine are least likely to penetrate into breast milk. Thus, the SSRI antidepressants best suited for pharmacokinetic optimization of therapy are the following: sertraline, fluvoxamine, and citalopram. All the SSRIs are extensively metabolized by CYP isoforms to pharmacologically active N-demethylated metabolites, which are then excreted in urine and feces. Except for sertraline, the drugs fluoxetine, paroxetine, and fluvoxamine are metabolized by polymorphic CYP isoforms, a matter of concern for poor and extensive metabolizers who may need dose adjustments. Citalopram, the most selective SERT inhibitor, is metabolized almost equally by CYP2C19, CYP2D6, and CYP3A4 (Table 11.11). Peak plasma levels usually are reached in approximately 6-8 hours and steady-state plasma levels in approximately 7-10 days except for fluoxetine (~4 wk). The half-lives are variable depending on the specific SSRI and the presence and plasma concentration of an active metabolite, but the half-lives tend to be prolonged. No evidence indicates that serum drug monitoring of SSRIs is a useful strategy to predict response. The SSRIs in general exhibit a flat, dose-independent antidepressant response curve (i.e., the antidepressant activity does not improve with increasing dose, only side effects increase).[214]

Some of the key differences among the SSRIs are the result of differences in their pharmacokinetic properties and metabolism to active metabolites (Table 11.11). Fluoxetine is unique because of its long half-life and the long half-life of its active metabolite norfluoxetine.[216] Although sertraline also has an active metabolite, it is 10 times less potent than sertraline and probably is not clinically relevant.[216] Fluvoxamine and paroxetine have no active metabolites. Because of the differences in half-lives and activities of metabolites, a much longer washout period is necessary when switching from fluoxetine (a long-acting SSRI) to another SSRI. These differences can cause considerable therapeutic delays in the treatment of refractory patients.

Adverse Effects Common to the SSRIs

The SSRIs are reported to have fewer side effects than the TCAs, which have strong anticholinergic and cardiotoxic properties.[212,213] Among the SSRIs, there are few differences in adverse effects. The adverse effects observed for the SSRIs include dry mouth, nausea, headaches, nervousness, restlessness, trouble sleeping, excessive sleepiness, sexual dysfunction, and anxiety. Fewer patients have discontinued SSRIs than TCAs (amitriptyline and imipramine and not nortriptyline, desipramine, doxepin, and clomipramine).

Sexual dysfunction is reported in both men and women, such as decreased libido, anorgasmia, ejaculatory incompetence, ejaculatory retardation, or inability to obtain or maintain an erection. The basic pharmacological similarities among the SSRIs suggest that the effects on sexual function should be comparable for each drug, but orgasm difficulties and impotence occur more frequently with paroxetine as compared with sertraline and fluoxetine. Evidence suggests that SSRI-induced sexual dysfunction may be dose-related and may be treated by simply lowering its dose. In patients who cannot have their SSRI dosage reduced, another option is simply to wait and reassess sexual function after several months. The addition of amantadine, cyproheptadine, yohimbine, or sildenafil has been reported to be effective in some patients with SSRI-induced sexual dysfunction. If the above measures are ineffective in managing SSRI-induced sexual dysfunction, the next step is to consider an alternative antidepressant without serotonergic activity (e.g., bupropion).

Drug Interactions Common to the SSRIs

The most serious drug-drug interaction for the SSRIs is their potential to produce the "serotonin syndrome" (i.e., hyperserotonergic effect), which typically develops within hours or days following the addition of another serotonergic agent to a drug regimen that already includes serotonergic-enhancing drugs. Symptoms of the 5-HT syndrome include agitation, diaphoresis, diarrhea, fever, hyperreflexia, incoordination, confusion, myoclonus, shivering, or tremor.

The 5-HT syndrome interaction between MAOIs and SSRIs is the most important drug interaction for the SSRIs, necessitating a washout ranging from 2 to 5 weeks depending on the plasma half-life of the SSRI. These differences in washout times for the SSRIs when switching to an MAOI are key differences between SSRIs and should be remembered if an MAOI is planned as a possible subsequent treatment in the event of SSRI failure. The differences among SSRIs are not important when a patient is switched from an MAOI to an SSRI. However, in this case, a 10- to 14-day washout for the MAOI is necessary, regardless of which SSRI is used, to allow regeneration of monoamine oxidase. The drug interaction between TCAs and SSRIs is of particular importance because of the potential for the development of toxic TCA concentrations, 5-HT syndrome, and subsequent adverse effects.[212,213]

Clinically, the potency of the SSRIs to inhibit CYP2D6 decreases from paroxetine to fluoxetine to norfluoxetine and then to fluvoxamine, with sertraline and citalopram being metabolized by CYP3A4 and CYP2C19, respectively, explaining the extent of differences in pharmacokinetic interactions between the SSRIs and other CYP2D6 substrates. Fluvoxamine is associated with drug interactions from its inhibition of CYP1A2, CYP2C9, CYP2C19, and CYP3A4. Because all the SSRIs are extensively metabolized in the liver, it is possible that other drugs that inhibit or induce hepatic CYP microsomal enzyme systems may alter SSRI plasma concentrations (AUCs) (Table 11.11). The SSRIs may inhibit or interfere with the metabolism of other frequently prescribed drugs that are CYP hepatically metabolized, increasing the potential for drug-drug interactions (Table 11.7). Although similar drug interactions are possible with other SSRIs, there is considerable variability among the drugs in the extent to which they inhibit CYP2D6. Fluoxetine and paroxetine appear to be more potent in this regard than sertraline. The extent to which this potential interaction may become clinically important depends on the extent of inhibition of CYP2D6 by the SSRI and the therapeutic index of the concurrently administered drug. The drugs for which this potential interaction is of greatest concern are those that are metabolized principally by CYP2D6 and have a narrow therapeutic index. Caution should be exercised whenever concurrent therapy with fluoxetine and other drugs metabolized by CYP2D6 is considered. The clinical significance of these possible interactions with the CYP isoforms is questionable, however, because there is no known correlation between plasma concentration and therapeutic response for any of the SSRIs.[213] If an interaction is suspected, the patient's SSRI dosage can be easily adjusted.

The SSRIs are highly protein bound and may affect the pharmacodynamic effect of other protein-bound drugs with narrow therapeutic indices (e.g., warfarin). The changes appear to be clinically significant, however, only for fluoxetine, fluvoxamine, and paroxetine. Close monitoring of prothrombin time and international normalized ratio is necessary if these drugs are used together.

The SSRIs have a high toxic to therapeutic ratio and, therefore, are safer than the TCAs or MAOIs in acute overdose. The SSRI overdoses can result in drowsiness, tremor, nausea, and vomiting, including seizures, electrocardiographic changes, and coma. Fatalities are uncommon with pure SSRI overdoses.

Therapeutic Uses Common to the SSRIs

The primary uses for the SSRIs include MDD, anxiety disorders, and obsessive compulsive disorder. Sertraline and paroxetine are approved for panic disorder. Sertraline is also approved for premenstrual dysphoric disorder. Fluoxetine is approved for bulimia nervosa and pediatric depression, and when combined with the antipsychotic, olanzapine, is also approved for depressive episodes associated with bipolar I disorder. Other indications treated with SSRIs, including off-label indications, include dysthymia, dysphoria, postpartum depression, post-traumatic stress disorder, obesity, borderline personality disorder, alcoholism, rheumatic pain, and migraine headache. Among the SSRIs, there are more similarities than differences; however, the differences between the SSRIs could be clinically significant.

Although the neurobiological mechanisms that contribute to antidepressant efficacy are still uncertain, they have effects on neuroplasticity and can increase neurogenesis in certain brain regions, including the hippocampus—these effects, succinctly, restructuring of circuits in the brain that regulate emotion and memory, may be important mediators, which are supported by several preclinical studies.

Phenoxyphenylalkylamine SSRIs

(±)-FLUOXETINE

Structure-activity Relationship. Fluoxetine is a 3-phenoxy-3-phenylpropylamine that exhibits selectivity and high affinity for human SERT and low affinity for NET (Fig. 11.36).[191] It is marketed as a racemic mixture of *R*- and *S*-fluoxetine. Its selectivity for SERT inhibition depends on the position of the substituent in the phenoxy ring (Table 11.12). Mono-substitution in the 4-(*para*) position of the phenoxy group (with an electron-withdrawing group, e.g., trifluoromethyl group, as in fluoxetine) results in selective inhibition of 5-HT reuptake. Disubstitution (2,4- or 3,4-disubstitution) results in loss of SERT selectivity. Constraining fluoxetine into semirigid analogues, such as MDL28618A or a phenylpiperidine (i.e., femoxetine), maintains selectivity for SERT, but both have approximately 10% of the affinity of fluoxetine for SERT[216] (Fig. 11.37). The *trans*-(1S,2S)-MDL28618A stereoisomer is approximately 10 times more potent than the *cis*-(−)-enantiomer.[216,217] The *trans*-(3*R*,4*S*)-(+)-enantiomer of femoxetine has approximately 10% the affinity of fluoxetine for SERT.[217] N-demethylation of femoxetine to its secondary amine enhances affinity for SERT by 10 times (comparable to fluoxetine). Femoxetine is not only an analogue of fluoxetine and paroxetine but also the (3*R*,4*S*)-diastereomer of a paroxetine analogue.

Table 11.12 Structure Activity Relationships for Atypical Phenoxyphenyl-Propylamines

R (phenyl)–O–CH(phenyl)–CH₂CH₂–NHCH₃

R (drug)	Inhibition of Reuptake (K_i nM) (28)	
	5-HT	NE
H	102	200
2-OCH_3 (nisoxetine)	1,371	2.4
2-SCH_3 (thionisoxetine)	130	0.2
2-CH_3 (atomoxetine)	390	3.4
2-F	898	5.3
2-I	25	0.4
2-CF_3	1,489	4,467
3-CF_3	16	1,328
4-CF_3 (fluoxetine)	17	2,703
4-CF_3 (norfluoxetine, NH_2)	17	2,176
4-CH_3	95	570
4-OCH_3	71	1,207
4-Cl	142	568
4-F	638	1,276

Mechanism of Action. Fluoxetine is a potent and selective inhibitor of 5-HT reuptake, but not of NE or DA uptake in the CNS. Its mechanism of action is common to the SSRIs. With the exception of moderate affinity for 5-HT_{2C} and 5-HT_{2A} receptors, fluoxetine does not interact directly with postsynaptic 5-HT receptors and has weak affinity for the other neuroreceptors. Both enantiomers of fluoxetine display similar affinities for human SERT. The NE/5-HT selectivity ratio, however, indicates that the *S*-enantiomer is approximately 100 times more selective for SERT inhibition than the *R*-enantiomer. The *R*-(+)-stereoisomer is approximately eight times more potent an inhibitor of SERT together with a longer duration of action than the *S*-(−)-isomer. However, the *S*-(−)-norfluoxetine metabolite is seven times more potent as an inhibitor of the 5-HT transporter than the *R*-(+)-metabolite, with a selectivity ratio approximately equivalent to that of *S*-fluoxetine.[216,217]

Pharmacokinetics. The pharmacokinetics of fluoxetine fits the general characteristics of the SSRIs (Table 11.11). Of particular importance is its long half-life contributing to its nonlinear pharmacokinetics. In vitro studies show that fluoxetine and norfluoxetine are potent inhibitors of CYP2D6 and CYP3A4 and less potent inhibitors of CYP2C9, CYP2C19, and CYP1A2. Fluoxetine is metabolized primarily by CYP2D6 N-demethylation to its active metabolite norfluoxetine and, to a lesser extent, O-dealkylation to form the inactive metabolite *p*-trifluoromethylphenol. Following oral administration, fluoxetine and its metabolites are excreted principally in urine, with approximately 73% as unidentified metabolites, 10% as norfluoxetine, 10% as norfluoxetine glucuronide, 5% as fluoxetine N-glucuronide, and 2% as unmetabolized drug.

Both *R*- and *S*-norfluoxetine were less potent than the corresponding enantiomers of fluoxetine as inhibitors of NE uptake. Inhibition of 5-HT uptake in cerebral cortex persisted for more than 24 hours after administration of *S*-norfluoxetine similar to fluoxetine. Thus, *S*-norfluoxetine is the active N-demethylated metabolite responsible for the persistently potent and selective inhibition of 5-HT uptake in vivo.[217]

The pharmacokinetics of fluoxetine in healthy geriatric individuals do not differ substantially from those in younger adults. Because of its relatively long half-life and nonlinear pharmacokinetics, the possibility of altered pharmacokinetics in geriatric individuals could exist, particularly those with systemic disease and/or in those receiving multiple medications concurrently. The elimination half-lives of fluoxetine and norfluoxetine do not appear to be altered substantially in patients with renal or hepatic impairment.

Drug Interactions. Fluoxetine and its norfluoxetine metabolite, like many other drugs metabolized by CYP2D6, inhibit the activity of CYP2D6 and, potentially, may increase plasma concentrations of concurrently administered drugs that also are metabolized by this enzyme. Fluoxetine may make normal CYP2D6 metabolizers resemble poor metabolizers. Fluoxetine can inhibit its own CYP2D6 metabolism, resulting in higher-than-expected plasma concentrations during upward dose adjustments. Therefore, switching from fluoxetine to another SSRI or other serotonergic antidepressant requires a washout period of at least 5 weeks or a lower-than-recommended initial dose with monitoring for adverse events.

Fluoxetine is highly protein bound and may affect the free plasma concentration and, thus, the pharmacological effect of other highly protein-bound drugs (e.g., warfarin sodium).

(-)-PAROXETINE

Structure-activity Relationship. Paroxetine is a constrained analogue of fluoxetine in which the linear phenylpropylamine group has been folded into a piperidine ring (Fig. 11.38). Paroxetine contains two chiral centers, with the possibility of four stereoisomers. One of these stereoisomers, the (3*S*,4*R*)-(−)-enantiomer is marketed as paroxetine. Paroxetine is a potent and selective inhibitor of SERT and displays high affinity for human SERT and moderate affinity for NET and DAT. Converting the secondary amine of the piperidine ring into a tertiary amine with a methyl group reduces affinity for SERT by 100 times (Fig. 11.38). Substituting the 4-fluoro with either a hydrogen or methyl reduces affinity for human SERT by approximately 10 times; replacing the 3,4-methylenedioxy group with a 4-methoxy group in the phenoxy ring also reduces affinity by a factor of 10. Stereochemical factors affect affinity of the paroxetine molecule for SERT. Therefore, substitution into the 2-(*ortho*) position of either aromatic ring decreases affinity for rat SERT by as much as 10- to 100 times, with the greatest loss occurring in the phenoxy ring. In vitro binding studies suggest that paroxetine is a more selective and potent inhibitor of 5-HT reuptake than fluoxetine. Paroxetine has very limited off-target liability, having only moderate to low affinity at certain muscarinic receptors—it maintains greater than 2000-fold selectivity for SERT, compared to muscarinic receptors, given its very high affinity for SERT (K_i ~0.1 nM). Therefore, activity

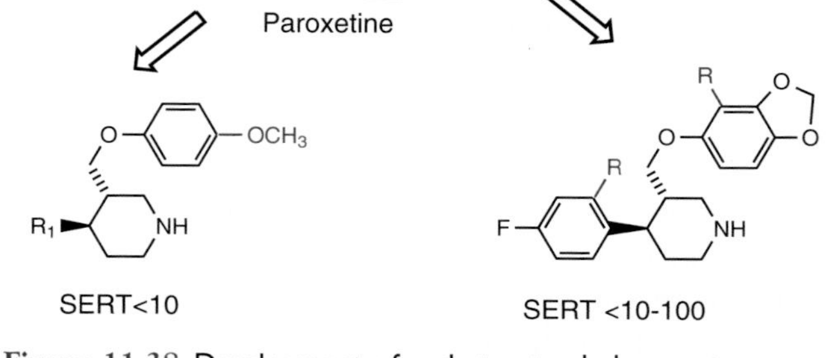

Figure 11.38 Development of and structural changes to paroxetine and effects on SERT affinity.

at muscarinic receptors is likely irrelevant at therapeutic concentrations. Its onset of action is 1-4 weeks.

Pharmacokinetics. Paroxetine appears to be slowly but well absorbed from the GI tract following oral administration with an oral bioavailability of approximately 50%, suggesting first-pass metabolism (Table 11.11), reaching peak plasma concentrations in 2-8 hours. Food does not substantially affect the absorption of paroxetine. Paroxetine is distributed into breast milk. Approximately 80% of an oral dose of paroxetine is oxidized by CYP2D6 to a catechol intermediate, which is then either O-methylated or O-glucuronidated. These conjugates are then eliminated in the urine.

Paroxetine exhibits a preincubation-dependent increase in inhibitory potency of CYP2D6 consistent with a mechanism-based inhibition of CYP2D6.[218] The inactivation of CYP2D6 occurs via the formation of an *o*-quinonoid reactive metabolite.

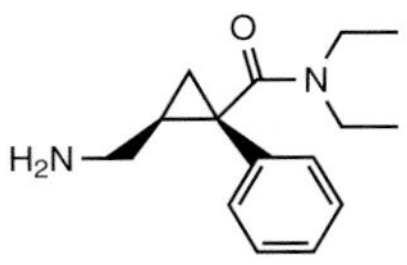

cis-Milnacipran (Fetzma, Savella)

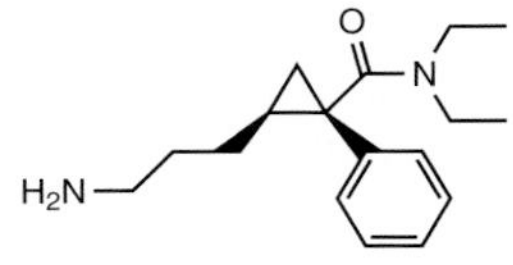

cis-1-Phenyl-2-[1-aminopropyl]-N,N-diethylcyclopropanecarboxamide

The methylenedioxy moiety has been associated with mechanism-based inactivation of other CYP isoforms.[219,220] [In contrast, fluoxetine, a potent inhibitor of CYP2D6 activity, did not exhibit a mechanism-based inhibition of CYP2D6.] As a result of mechanism-based inhibition, saturation of CYP2D6 at clinical doses appears to account for its nonlinear pharmacokinetics observed with increasing dose and duration of paroxetine treatment, which results in increased plasma concentrations of paroxetine at low doses. The elderly may be more susceptible to changes in doses and, therefore, should be started off at lower doses. Following oral administration, paroxetine and its metabolites are excreted in both urine and feces.

Oral administration of a single dose resulted in unmetabolized paroxetine accounting for 2% and metabolites accounting for 62% of the excretion products. The effect of age on the elimination of paroxetine suggests that hepatic clearance of paroxetine can be reduced, leading to an increase in elimination half-life (e.g., to ~36 hr) and increased plasma concentrations. The metabolites of paroxetine have been shown to possess no more than 2% of the potency of the parent compound as inhibitors of 5-HT reuptake; therefore, they are essentially inactive (Fig. 11.38).

Because paroxetine is a potent mechanism-based inhibitor of CYP2D6, this type of inhibition yields nonlinear and long-term effects on drug pharmacokinetics because the inactivated or complexed CYP2D6 must be replaced by newly synthesized CYP2D6 protein. Thus, coadministration of paroxetine with CYP2D6-metabolized medications should be closely monitored or, in certain cases, avoided, as should upward dose adjustment of paroxetine itself.

(±)-CITALOPRAM. In trying to create a new antidepressant to inhibit NE reuptake, Lundbeck chemists serendipitously synthesized two new compounds (talopram and tasulopram) having the phenylspiro-isobenzofuran nucleus (Fig. 11.39). These compounds were potent SNRIs, but considering that a number of suicide attempts were reported during clinical studies with these compounds, Lundbeck discontinued the studies. Undeterred, the chemists subsequently modified talopram by addition of a 5-cyano to the isobenzofuran ring and a 4-fluoro to the benzene ring in the formation of citalopram. Therapeutic activity for (±)-citalopram resides in the S-(+)-isomer. Citalopram was marketed in the United States in 1996 as the most selective SSRI and, therefore, is the least likely to cause the adverse effects associated with off-target activity, observed with most of the other antidepressants (Fig. 11.30).

Mechanism of Action. Citalopram, primarily through its *S*-enantiomer, selectively blocks 5-HT reuptake, leading to potentiation of serotonergic activity in the CNS. Citalopram exhibits the greatest in vitro selectivity for

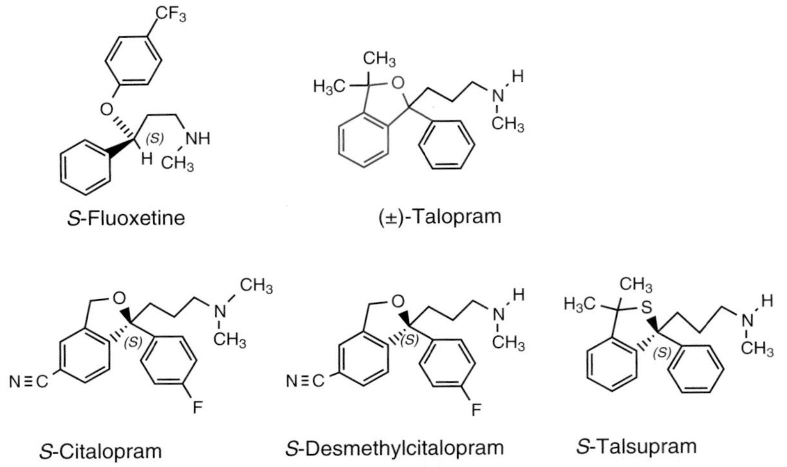

S-Fluoxetine

(±)-Talopram

S-Citalopram

S-Desmethylcitalopram

S-Talsupram

Figure 11.39 Discovery of and structural relationships for citalopram SSRIs.

5-HT reuptake inhibition compared with the other SSRIs (Fig. 11.30). The drug essentially has no effect on NE or DA reuptake, nor does it show affinity for other neuroreceptors.

Pharmacokinetics. The pharmacokinetics of citalopram is shown in Table 11.11. Unlike several of the other SSRIs, citalopram does not undergo first-pass metabolism; it has an oral bioavailability of approximately 80%. Food does not affect absorption. Citalopram is highly lipophilic and widely distributed throughout the body, including the blood-brain barrier. However, its metabolite, demethylcitalopram does not cross the blood-brain barrier well. The drug is metabolized via hepatic N-demethylation to its major metabolite, N-desmethylcitalopram, almost equally by CYP2C19, CYP2D6, and CYP3A4 (Table 11.7). The major metabolite exhibits approximately 50% of the potency of citalopram as an inhibitor of 5-HT reuptake. Because the metabolite concentration in the plasma is lower than that of citalopram, it should not add significantly to citalopram's antidepressant effects. Citalopram exhibits dose-proportional linear pharmacokinetics in a dosage range of 10-60 mg/d; plasma levels increase proportionately with each increasing dose. Approximately 12%-23% of an oral dose was recovered in the urine as unmetabolized drug and 10% in feces. The clearance of orally administered citalopram was reduced by 37 and 17% in patients with hepatic and renal function impairment, respectively.

Citalopram and its desmethyl metabolite are weak inhibitors of the CYP isoforms, suggesting a low potential for drug interactions. Although no relevant in vivo interactions between citalopram and CYP2D6-metabolized medications have been reported, caution is advised when coadministering citalopram with potential object drugs, especially those having narrow therapeutic indices, in elderly patients. Because citalopram is metabolized in parallel by CYP2C19, CYP2D6, and CYP3A4, it would have little inhibitory effect on the metabolism of other drugs metabolized by these isoenzymes. Citalopram is less highly protein bound than the other SSRIs, reducing the potential for drug interactions with protein-bound drugs having narrow therapeutic indices.

ESCITALOPRAM. Escitalopram is the *S*-enantiomer of citalopram that binds with high affinity and selectivity to the human SERT equivalent to (±)-citalopram. It has been reported that nearly all the activity resides in the *S*-enantiomer and that *R*-citalopram actually counteracts the action of the *S*-enantiomer.[58,59] Studies show that escitalopram exhibits twice the activity of citalopram and is at least 27 times more potent than the *R*-enantiomer. The *R*-enantiomer inhibits the *S*-enantiomer at the transporter.[221,222] Escitalopram's mechanism of action is common to the SSRIs.

The pharmacokinetics for escitalopram does not exhibit stereoisomer selectivity and, therefore, is similar to that for citalopram (Table 11.11). Likewise, it exhibits linear pharmacokinetics so that plasma levels increase proportionately and predictably with increased doses and its half-life of 27-32 hours is consistent with once-daily dosing. It also has been found that *R*-citalopram is cleared more slowly than the *S*-enantiomer. Therefore, when the drug is used as a racemic mixture (citalopram), the inactive isomer predominates at steady state. This is an added incentive for use of the enantiomerically pure escitalopram. Escitalopram has negligible effects on CYP isoforms, suggesting a low potential for drug-drug interactions.

Escitalopram is metabolized to *S*-desmethylcitalopram by CYP2C19 (37%), CYP2D6 (28%), and CYP3A4 (35%) and to *S*-didesmethylcitalopram (only by CYP2D6) in human liver microsomes and in expressed cytochromes. Escitalopram and its desmethyl metabolite were negligible inhibitors of CYP1A2, CYP2C9, CYP2C19, CYP2E1, and CYP3A and were weakly inhibited by CYP2D6. *R*-citalopram and its metabolites had properties very similar to those of the corresponding *S*-enantiomers. Because escitalopram is biotransformed by three CYP isoforms in parallel, escitalopram is unlikely to be affected by drug interactions or genetic polymorphisms and is unlikely to cause clinically important drug interactions via CYP inhibition.

Phenylalkylamine SSRIs

SERTRALINE. Sertraline is a phenylaminotetralin, in which the diphenylbutylamine nucleus is constrained into a rigid bicyclic ring system (Fig. 11.40). In the early work with the discovery of SSRIs at Pfizer, tametraline was initially synthesized in 1978. Animal studies showed it to be a stimulant and to block NE and DA uptake, a use that Pfizer was not interested in pursuing. Subsequently, one or two chlorine atoms were introduced into tametraline to produce new molecules that were potent inhibitors of 5-HT reuptake in the CNS. One of the dichloro compounds was to become known as sertraline.

Sertraline contains two chiral centers and only the *S,S*-(+)-diastereomer is marketed. The *R,R*-, *R,S*-, and *S,R*-diastereomers are significantly weaker as inhibitors of 5-HT reuptake. Sertraline was marketed in the United States in 1992, emphasizing its pharmacokinetic differences from the other SSRIs.

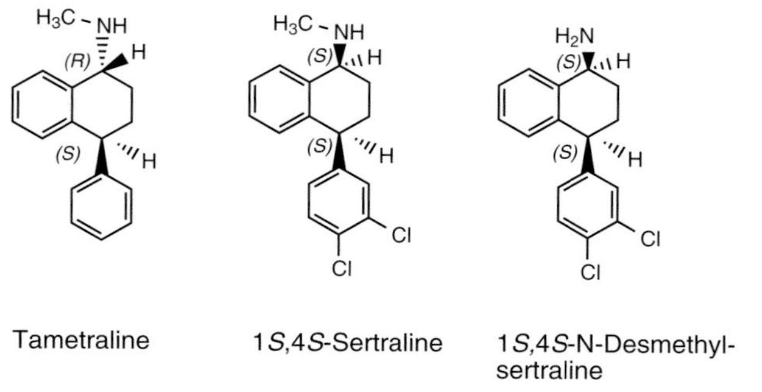

Tametraline | 1*S*,4*S*-Sertraline | 1*S*,4*S*-N-Desmethyl-sertraline

Figure 11.40 Structural relationships for the phenylalkylamine SSRIs.

Mechanism of Action. Sertraline is a potent and selective inhibitor of the neuronal reuptake 5-HT transporter. In vitro binding studies suggest that sertraline has a substantially higher selectivity for inhibiting 5-HT reuptake than tertiary TCAs, including clomipramine (Fig. 11.30). It has only weak effects on neuronal uptake of NE and DA. Its mechanism of action is common to the SSRIs. Sertraline is selective, lacking affinity for other neuroreceptors at therapeutic concentrations. At high doses, however, sertraline may interact with α1 receptors (K_i ~200 nM).

Pharmacokinetics. Sertraline appears to be well absorbed from the GI tract following oral administration with an oral bioavailability in humans from 20% to 36% (Table 11.11), suggesting extensive first-pass metabolism to its N-desmethylated metabolite. Food enhances its oral absorption, decreasing the time to achieve peak plasma concentrations from approximately 8 to 6 hours. Following multiple dosing, steady-state plasma sertraline concentrations are proportional and linearly related to dose (half-life: single dose, 24 hr; multiple dose, 24 hr). N-desmethylsertraline, sertraline's principal metabolite, exhibits dose-dependent pharmacokinetics. Sertraline and N-desmethylsertraline are distributed into breast milk. Protein binding is approximately 98%. Although in elderly patients the elimination half-life is increased to approximately 36 hours. This effect does not appear to be clinically important and does not warrant dosing alterations. Sertraline is primarily metabolized to N-desmethylsertraline through the action of CYP2B6[223] and to a minor extent by CYP2C9, CYP2C19, CYP2D6, and CYP3A4 (Fig. 11.41). N-desmethylsertraline is approximately 5-10 times less potent as an inhibitor of 5-HT reuptake than sertraline. The formation of sertraline ketone can occur through the action of either CYP or MAO, but studies have not been reported to indicate the role of either or both. The formation of sertraline N-carbamoyl glucuronide is a unique product which was shown to form in vitro through the action primarily by UGT2B7. The involvement of multiple enzymes in the metabolism of sertraline suggests that no single drug could significantly alter sertraline pharmacokinetics and produce any drug-drug interactions. Sertraline and N-desmethylsertraline undergo further metabolism via oxidative deamination and ring hydroxylation and glucuronide conjugation. N-desmethylsertraline has an elimination half-life approximately 2.5 times that of sertraline. Following oral administration, sertraline and its conjugated metabolites are excreted in both urine and feces and unmetabolized sertraline accounts for less than 5% of the oral dose. Plasma clearance of sertraline was approximately 40% lower in geriatric patients. The elimination half-life of sertraline in patients with hepatic disease was prolonged to a mean of 52 hours, compared with 22 hours in individuals without hepatic disease.

Drug Interactions. Sertraline is not a potent inhibitor of CYP3A4 and because CYP2D6 metabolism is a minor pathway for sertraline, drug-drug interactions with these isoforms is unlikely to be of clinical importance. Sertraline is metabolized by more than one CYP isoform in parallel; therefore, drug interactions or genetic polymorphisms are unlikely to cause clinically significant drug interaction via CYP isoform inhibition. Caution is advised, however, when coadministering sertraline with potential object drugs, especially those with narrow therapeutic indices in elderly patients. For example, sertraline has been shown to reduce the clearance of desipramine and imipramine as a result of CYP2D6 inhibition.

Because sertraline is highly protein bound, patients receiving it concurrently with any highly protein-bound drug should be observed for potential adverse effects associated with combined therapy.

Aralkylketone SSRI

FLUVOXAMINE. Fluvoxamine is a SERT inhibitor that is structurally unique among the SSRIs by being the (*E*)-isomer of a 2-aminoethyl oxime ether of an aralkylketone (Fig. 11.42). The C=N double bond is isosteric with the propylidene group in amitriptyline and, thus, imparts geometric *E* or *Z* stereoisomerism to fluvoxamine. The oxime ether is found in a previously marketed analogue of amitriptyline called noxiptilin (in 1966 by Bayer AG

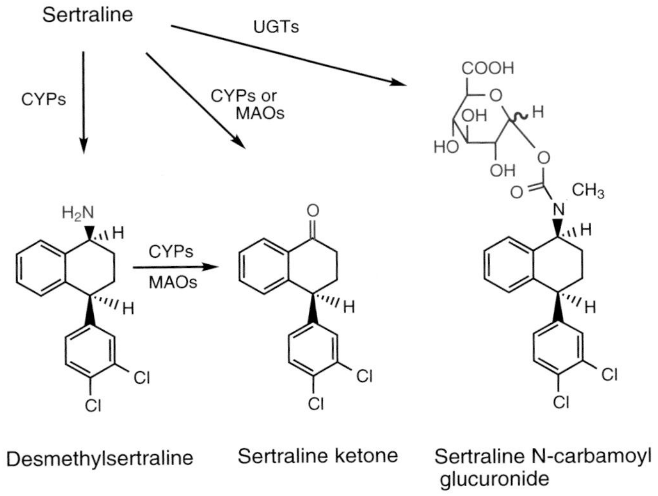

Figure 11.41 Metabolic products formed from sertraline metabolism.

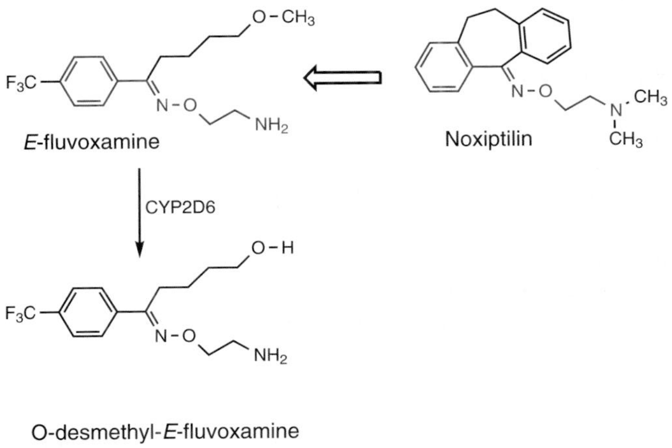

Figure 11.42 Structural relationships for fluvoxamine and its metabolism.

[Germany]). Thus, fluvoxamine may be considered to be an open-chain analogue of the tricyclic noxipitilin. The 4-trifluoromethyl group or other electronegative group is essential for SERT affinity and selectivity. The C=N double bond also enhances the susceptibility of fluvoxamine to photoisomerization by ultraviolet UV-B light (290-320 nm). When fluvoxamine solutions were exposed to UV-B light, photoisomerization to the pharmacologically inactive Z-isomer occurred. Thus, fluvoxamine solutions should be protected from sunlight to prevent loss of antidepressant efficacy. No studies have been reported regarding its solid-state stability to UV-B light.

Mechanism of Action. Fluvoxamine is a highly selective inhibitor of 5-HT reuptake at the presynaptic membrane. Potency data from in vitro affinity studies suggest that fluvoxamine is less potent than other SSRIs (e.g., paroxetine, sertraline, and citalopram). Its mechanism of action is similar to that of the other SSRIs. Fluvoxamine appears to have little or no effect on the reuptake of NE or DA. In vitro studies have demonstrated that fluvoxamine possesses virtually no affinity for other neuroreceptors. Its onset of action is similar to the other SSRIs (2-4 wk).

Pharmacokinetics. Fluvoxamine is well absorbed, with a bioavailability of approximately 50%, because of first-pass metabolism (Table 11.11). At steady-state doses, fluvoxamine demonstrates nonlinear pharmacokinetics over a dosage range of 100-300 mg/d, which results in higher plasma concentrations at higher doses than would be predicted by lower-dose kinetics (single dose, 15 hr; multiple dosing, 22 hr). Food does not significantly affect oral bioavailability. The mean apparent volume of distribution for fluvoxamine reflects its lipophilic nature, extensive tissue distribution, and protein binding. Fluvoxamine is distributed into breast milk. Fluvoxamine is preferentially metabolized by CYP2D6 by O-demethylation to its alcohol metabolite, which is subsequently oxidized to a carboxylic acid and on to a O-glucuronide. Oxidative deamination and nine other metabolites have been identified, none of which shows significant pharmacological activity.

Adverse Effects. The adverse effects for fluvoxamine include symptoms of drowsiness, nausea or vomiting, abdominal pain, tremors, sinus bradycardia, and mild anticholinergic symptoms. Toxic doses could produce seizures and severe bradycardia.

Drug Interactions. In vitro studies have shown fluvoxamine to be a potent inhibitor of CYP1A2, to inhibit CYP3A4 and CYP2C19 and to weakly inhibit CYP2D6. The bioavailability of fluvoxamine is significantly decreased in smokers compared with nonsmokers, possibly because of induction of CYP1A2 metabolism of fluvoxamine. Therefore, interactions with drugs that inhibit CYP1A2 also should be considered (e.g., theophylline and caffeine).

Therapeutic Uses. Fluvoxamine is approved for treatment of obsessive compulsive disorder.

Atypical Antidepressants

The atypical antidepressants are distinct from other classes of antidepressants that include SSRIs, TCAs, and MAOIs.[198] Atypical antidepressants are frequently used in patients with MDD who have inadequate responses or intolerable side effects during first-line treatment with SSRIs. However, atypical antidepressants are often first-line treatment if the drug has a desirable characteristic (e.g., sexual side effects occur less often with bupropion than SSRIs). Examples of atypical antidepressants include mirtazapine, bupropion, trazodone, vilazodone, and vortioxetine. Atypical antidepressants are unlike the SSRIs, TCAs, and MAOIs and act mainly as SNRIs, SMSs, and SARIs.[198]

Nontricyclic Serotonin and Norepinephrine Reuptake Inhibitors

Clinical studies suggest that compounds which increase the synaptic availability of both NE and 5-HT have greater efficacy than single-acting drugs such as SSRIs in the treatment of MDD.[224] Thus efforts began to design a drug that combined the properties of SSRIs and TCAs that only blocked SERT and NET without the unwanted adverse effects of TCAs,[224] i.e., effects related to off-target activities at certain GPCRs and sodium channels. Currently, the nontricyclic mixed inhibitors of 5-HT and NE uptake, i.e., SNRIs, are venlafaxine, desvenlafaxine, levomilnacipran, atomoxetine, and duloxetine (Fig. 11.44). Based on preclinical studies, venlafaxine, desvenflaxine, levomilnacipran, milnacipran, atomoxetine, and duloxetine inhibit the reuptake of 5-HT and NE both in vitro and in vivo in the following order of decreasing potency: duloxetine > levomilnacipran > venlafaxine > desvenlafaxine. All the mixed reuptake inhibitors exhibit low affinity at neuronal receptors of the other neurotransmitters, suggesting a low side-effect potential. Desvenlafaxine, levomilnacipran, atomoxetine, and duloxetine have been shown to be as efficacious as TCAs in treating MDD.[196] These nontricyclic antidepressants are reported to produce a faster and greater antidepressant response than an SSRI alone, suggesting that these mixed mechanisms of action can be synergistic in terms of mediating antidepressant efficacy. Meaningful differences between the nontricyclic

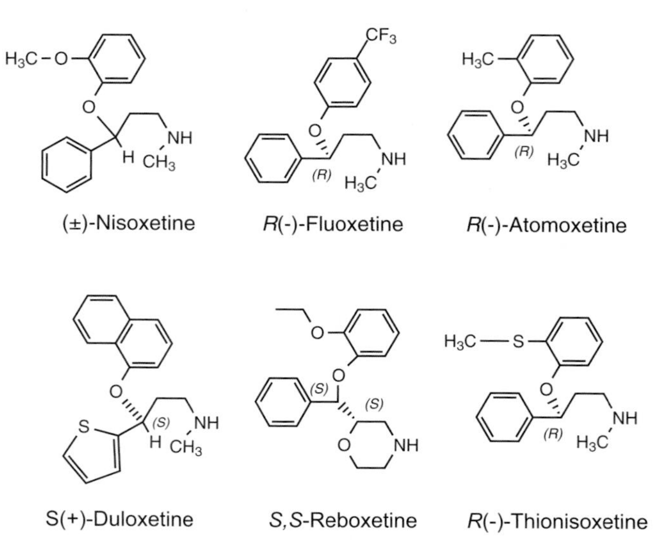

(±)-Nisoxetine R(-)-Fluoxetine R(-)-Atomoxetine

S(+)-Duloxetine S,S-Reboxetine R(-)-Thionisoxetine

Figure 11.43 Structural relationships for the nontricyclic SNRIs.

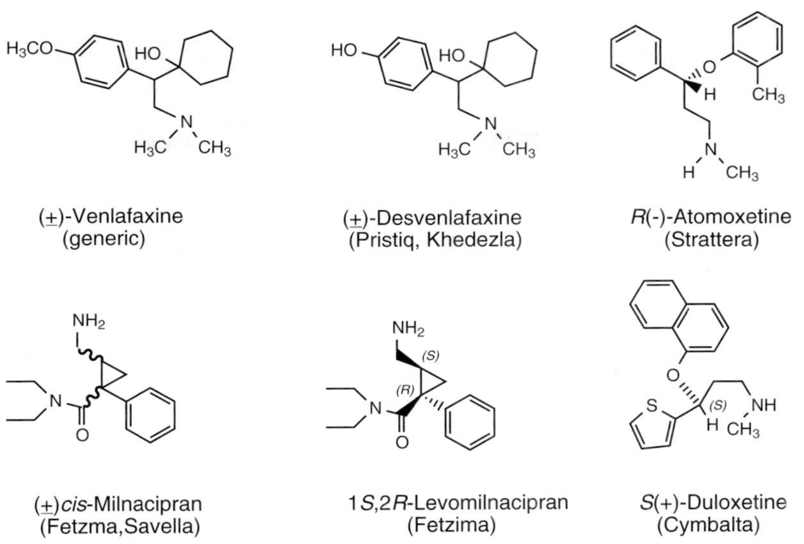

(±)-Venlafaxine (generic)

(±)-Desvenlafaxine (Pristiq, Khedezla)

R(-)-Atomoxetine (Strattera)

(±)cis-Milnacipran (Fetzma, Savella)

1S,2R-Levomilnacipran (Fetzima)

S(+)-Duloxetine (Cymbalta)

Figure 11.44 Nontricyclic SNRIs.

SNRIs are largely related to their pharmacokinetics, metabolism to active metabolites, inhibition of CYP isoforms, drug-drug interactions, and half-lives.[196]

VENLAFAXINE. Venlafaxine is a methoxyphenylethylamine antidepressant that resembles an open TCA with one of the aromatic rings replaced by a cyclohexanol ring and a dimethylaminomethyl group rather than a dimethylaminopropyl chain (Fig. 11.45).

Venlafaxine and its active metabolite, O-desmethylvenlafaxine (ODV), have mixed mechanisms of action, with preferential affinity for 5-HT reuptake and weak inhibition of NE and DA reuptake. Venlafaxine is approximately 30 times more potent as an inhibitor of SERT than of NET.[225] Because of the 30 times difference in transporter affinities, increasing the dose of venlafaxine from 75 to 375 mg/d can sequentially inhibit both SERT and NET. Thus, venlafaxine displays an ascending dose-dependent antidepressant response in contrast to the flat dose-antidepressant response curve observed with the SSRIs. This sequential action for venlafaxine also is consistent with its dose-dependent adverse-effect profile. Its mechanism of action is similar to imipramine.

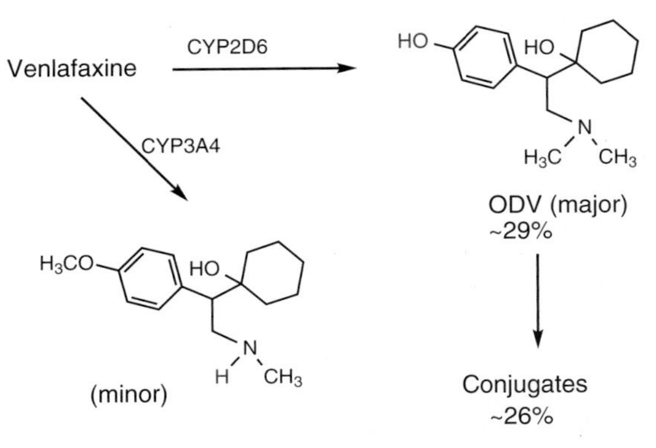

Venlafaxine → CYP2D6 → ODV (major) ~29% → Conjugates ~26%

Venlafaxine → CYP3A4 → (minor)

Figure 11.45 Metabolism of venlafaxine.

Venlafaxine is rapidly and well absorbed, but with a bioavailability of 45%, which has been attributed to first-pass metabolism (Table 11.13). Food delays its absorption but does not impair the extent of absorption. Venlafaxine is distributed into breast milk. Venlafaxine is primarily metabolized in the liver by CYP2D6 to its primary metabolite, ODV, which is approximately equivalent in pharmacological activity and potency to venlafaxine. In vitro studies indicate that CYP3A4 also is involved in the metabolism of venlafaxine to its minor and less active metabolite, N-desmethylvenlafaxine (Fig. 11.45). Protein binding for venlafaxine and ODV is low and is not a problem for drug interactions. In patients with hepatic impairment, elimination half-lives were increased by approximately 30% for venlafaxine and approximately 60% for ODV (Table 11.13). In patients with renal function impairment, elimination half-lives were increased by approximately 40%-50% for venlafaxine and for ODV. At steady-state doses, venlafaxine and ODV exhibit dose-proportional linear pharmacokinetics over the dose range of 75-450 mg/d. Steady-state concentrations of venlafaxine and ODV are attained within 3 days with regular oral dosing. Venlafaxine and its metabolites are excreted primarily in the urine (87%).

The potential for cardiotoxicity with venlafaxine during normal use and for various toxicities in overdose situations are key concerns. Venlafaxine displays minimal in vitro affinity for the other neural neurotransmitter receptors and, thus, a low probability for adverse effects. To minimize gastrointestinal upset (e.g., nausea), venlafaxine can be taken with food without affecting its GI absorption. Venlafaxine should be administered as a single daily dose with food at approximately the same time each day. The extended-release capsules should be swallowed whole with fluid and should not be divided, crushed, chewed, or placed in water.

Whenever venlafaxine is being discontinued after more than 1 week of therapy, it generally is recommended that

Table 11.13 Pharmacokinetics of the Nontricyclic SNRIs

Parameters	Venlafaxine	desvenlafaxine	Levomilnacipran	duloxe-tine	Atomoxetine
Oral bioavailability (%)	45	45	92	>90	70
Lipophilicity (cLog $D_{pH7.4}$)	1.93	1.93	-1.09	ND	1.06
Protein binding	27	30	22	>90	>97
Volume of distribution (L/kg)	7.5 ± 3.7	5.7 ± 1.8	387-473	1,640	93-328(250)
Elimination half-life (hr)	5	11	12	12	4 (3-6) (EM) 17-21 (PM)
Major active metabolites	Desvenlafaxine (ODV)	None	None	none	none
Peak plasma concentration (hr)	2	7.5	32-48	6-10	3
Excretion (%)	Urine 87	Urine 30	Urine 58	Urine 70 Feces 20	Urine >80 Feces <17
Plasma half-life (hr)		30	32-48	6	5 EM 22 PM
Time to steady-state concentration (d)	3	ND	6-8	3	5 (EM) 22 (PM)

ND, not determined.

the patient be closely monitored and the dosage of the drug be tapered gradually to reduce the risk of withdrawal symptoms. Although venlafaxine is a weak inhibitor of CYP2D6, variability has been observed in the pharmacokinetic parameters of venlafaxine in patients with hepatic or renal function impairment. As a precaution, elderly patients taking venlafaxine concurrently with a drug that has a narrow therapeutic index and also is metabolized by CYP2D6 should be carefully monitored. Concurrent use of CYP3A4 inhibitors with venlafaxine has been shown to interfere with its metabolism and clearance. Similar to the other antidepressants that block 5-HT reuptake, venlafaxine may interact pharmacodynamically to cause toxic levels of 5-HT to accumulate, leading to the 5-HT syndrome.

DESVENLAFAXINE. Desvenlafaxine (ODV) is the main active CYP2D6 metabolite of venlafaxine (Fig. 11.45). Similar to venlafaxine, ODV is an SNRI and has been approved for use in the US and Canada as an antidepressant, but not approved for use in the European market. Non–FDA approved (off-label) use is as a nonhormonal-based vasomotor (hot flashes) treatment for menopause. The European Union has not approved desvenlafaxine for any indication because, in relation to its parent, venlafaxine, desvenlafaxine seemed to be less effective with no advantages in terms of safety and tolerability. Since venlafaxine is already approved for the treatment of MDD and is almost entirely transformed into ODV, it would be expected that efficacy and safety of ODV in the treatment of MDD would be very similar to that of venlafaxine. ODV is approximately 10-fold more potent at inhibiting 5-HT reuptake than NE reuptake. When most normal metabolizers take venlafaxine, ~ 70% of the parent drug is metabolized into ODV, so the effects are very similar. Side effects for ODV include nausea (most common 30%-50% vs. placebo 9%-11%) and the most common reason for discontinuation. Other adverse reactions were dizziness, insomnia, sweating, constipation, somnolence, decreased appetite, priapism, night terrors, anxiety, and delayed ejaculation, which are consistent with those of other SNRIs. Suicidal risk was significant in some patients in each study.

Structure-Activity Relationships for the Phenoxyphenylpropylamines

(±)-NISOXETINE. Nisoxetine (Fig. 11.43) was the initial phenoxyphenylpropylamine synthesized in the Lilly research laboratories during the early 1970s from the rearrangement of an oxygen atom in diphenyhydramine, a diphenylmethoxyethylamine, to a phenoxyphenylpropylamine (Fig. 11.43). Nisoxetine was discovered to be a potent and very selective SNRI, with little affinity for other receptors. It underwent clinical studies as an alternative to Lilly's best-selling antidepressant, nortriptyline, but without the adverse effects associated with the TCAs. It was never marketed, however, because of a greater interest in developing its 4-trifluoromethyl analogue, fluoxetine, an SSRI.

The type and position of the ring substitution plays a critical role in the mechanism of action for these phenoxyphenylpropyamines (see Table 11.12 for structure-activity relationships of the phenoxypropylamines). The unsubstituted molecule is a weak SSRI. However, 2-substitution into the phenoxy ring (except for the 2-trifluoromethyl) yields compounds with high potency and selectivity for blocking NE reuptake, whereas the 4-substitution results in compounds having potent SSRI activity, with the 4-trifluormethyl group (fluoxetine) being the most potent and selective for SERT.[216,217] The substantial changes in transporter selectivity for NET and SERT and the differences in affinity are more likely attributed to the bulky 2-(*ortho*)-substituted groups, which restricts the flexibility of the aromatic rings, thereby enhancing alignment of the hydrogen-bond acceptor group (the methoxy) with a donor group on the binding site on NET for NE that is not available for the 5-HT binding site. The *R*-isomer of nisoxetine has 20 times greater affinity than its *S*-isomer for NET. The NET K_i for nisoxetine is 0.8 nM and is 40 times more selective for NET than for SERT. Its tertiary amine is approximately 100 times less effective at inhibiting NET. Increasing the size of the methylamino with ethyl or larger alkyl groups eliminates all activity. The 2- and 4-analogues exhibited weak effects on neuronal uptake of DA and lack affinity for other neuroreceptors at therapeutic concentrations. Substituting the 2-methoxy with the isosteric 2-methylthio (thionisoxetine) produced a more potent SNRI (K_i = 0.2 nM for the *R*-enantiomer at NET) and 600 times more selective for NET than for SERT. Thionisoxetine is approximately 10 times more potent than nisoxetine at inhibiting NET, and unlike nisoxetine, it reduces food consumption in rodents and has been studied for the treatment of obesity and eating disorders. Substitution of the phenoxy group with a naphthyloxy group and the phenyl ring with the isosteric thienyl (thiophene) group results in a drug with mixed inhibition of NE and SERT (i.e., duloxetine) (Fig. 11.43).

R(-)-ATOMOXETINE. *R*(−)-atomoxetine, 2-methylphenoxyphenylpropylamine, was marketed in 2003 as a "nonstimulant" treatment for ADHD in both adults and children.[226] The 2-methyl substitution (c.f., nisoxetine) (Fig. 11.43) confers selectivity for inhibiting NE reuptake (Fig. 11.30).[190,191,216] The *R*-enantiomer is 10 times more potent than the *S*-enantiomer as a NET reuptake inhibitor. Atomoxetine has a low propensity for anticholinergic and adverse cardiovascular effects.

Pharmacokinetics. Atomoxetine is well absorbed from the GI tract and cleared primarily by metabolism, with the majority of the dose being excreted into the urine. Atomoxetine is metabolized primarily by CYP2D6 to its major active metabolite, 4-hydroxyatomoxetine, which is eliminated as its glucuronide (Fig. 11.46). Peak plasma concentrations of atomoxetine occur 1-2 hours after oral administration. Significant differences are seen in the elimination half-life between normal metabolizers, extensive metabolizers, and poor metabolizers (Table 11.7). Atomoxetine exhibited an elimination half-life of 3-6 hours for normal and extensive metabolizers and 17-21 hours for poor metabolizers.[227] CYP2C19 is the other enzyme primarily responsible for the formation of its minor metabolite N-desmethylatomoxetine.[227]

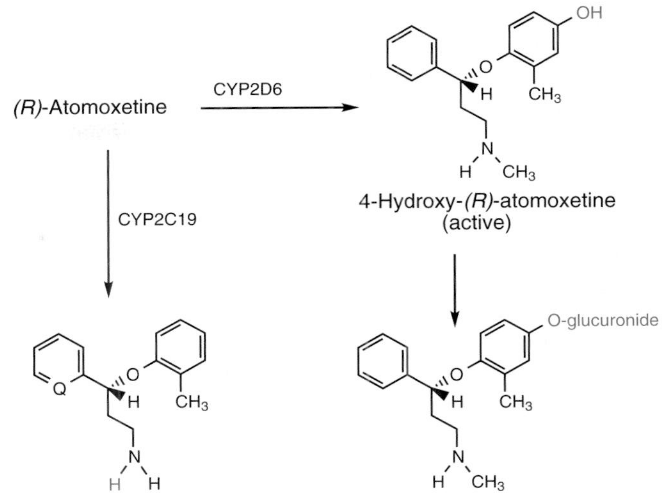

(R)-Atomoxetine

CYP2D6

CYP2C19

4-Hydroxy-(R)-atomoxetine (active)

O-glucuronide

Figure 11.46 Metabolism of atomoxetine.

Adverse Effects. At therapeutic doses, no serious drug-related adverse effects have been encountered. Adverse effects have included modest increases in diastolic blood pressure and heart rate, anorexia, weight loss, somnolence, dizziness, nausea, dry mouth, and skin rash.

Therapeutic Uses. Atomoxetine is used as a safe and well-tolerated "nonstimulant" treatment of ADHD in both adults and children. Among children and adolescents aged 8-18 years, atomoxetine was superior to placebo in reducing symptoms of ADHD and in improving social and family functioning symptoms. Oral atomoxetine is promoted as an alternative to conventional ADHD therapy with methylphenidate, dextroamphetamine, and pemoline (see section below on ADHD medications). It also can be a replacement for bupropion or for TCAs. Onset of action is approximately 7 days.

MILNACIPRAN. (±)-Milnacipran is the *cis*-aminomethyl derivative of phenylcyclopropanecarboxamide (Fig. 11.44) that acts as an SNRI. It is structurally different from the other SNRIs and currently is only available in Europe as a racemic mixture, with both enantiomers exhibiting antidepressant activity. It is marketed in the United States as 1*S*,2*R*-levomilnacipran. Substituting the aminomethyl group of levomilnacipran with an aminopropyl gives a milnacipran homologue that exhibits antidepressant activity as a potent NMDA receptor antagonist. A glutamate hypothesis is being investigated as an alternative mechanism of depression (see the subsection on NMDA antagonists).

LEVOMILNACIPRAN. Recently, levomilnacipran (LVM) (1*S*,2*R*)-milnacipran was approved by the US FDA for the treatment of MDD.[228] It is the levo enantiomer of the racemic drug, milnacipran (Fig. 11.44), which is approved for the treatment of MDD in Europe and Japan and for fibromyalgia in the USA. Levomilnacipran has been developed solely as a sustained-release formulation (once per day). Preclinical studies have found that LVM is a more potent inhibitor of NE and 5-HT (50 and 13 times, respectively) than the less active enantiomer (*1R, 2S*).[229] Furthermore, it has a better pharmacokinetic profile than its enantiomer, having a longer elimination half-life with a higher maximal concentration (Table 11.13). LVM binds with high affinity to human 5-HT and NE transporters (K_i = 11 and 91 nM, respectively). It inhibits 5-HT and NE reuptake (IC_{50} = 16-19 and 11 nM, respectively). LVM does not bind to any other receptors, ion channels, or transporters, including serotonergic (5-HT $_{1-7}$), α- and β adrenergic, muscarinic, or histaminergic receptors and Ca^{2+}, Na^+, K^+, or Cl^- channels to a significant degree. LVM does not inhibit MAO. Furthermore, LVM does not prolong the QTc interval to a clinically relevant extent. Thus, LVM is a dual neurotransmitter reuptake inhibitor of NE and 5-HT.

LVM is fairly well tolerated, with the most common adverse events being nausea, headache, dry mouth, and constipation. Adverse events were not dose-related except for urinary hesitancy and erectile dysfunction. LVM was not toxic to the liver and did not cause clinically significant QTc prolongation. LVM is a relatively safe alternative antidepressant treatment with minimal drug-drug interactions.

Pharmacokinetics. The pharmacokinetics of LVM follows linear dynamics with a half-life of approximately 12 hours and a time to peak concentration of 32-48 hours.[230,231] Absorption is not affected by food intake, and the drug is 22% bound to protein. Metabolism is primarily through CYP3A4, which can contribute to potential drug-drug interactions if the concomitant drug is a strong inhibitor of cytochrome 3A4, such as ketoconazole, clarithromycin, or ritonavir.[231] Therefore, in these situations, a dose adjustment is recommended. Excretion of LVM is predominantly via the kidney. LVM should not be used in patients with end-stage renal disease.

Levomilnacipran has a high oral bioavailability of 92% and a low plasma protein binding of 22%. It is metabolized in the liver by the CYP3A4 by N-deethylation to norlevomilnacipran, thereby making the medication susceptible to grapefruit-drug interactions. The drug has an elimination half-life of approximately 12 hours, allowing for once-daily administration. LVM is excreted in urine.

DULOXETINE. Duloxetine (Fig. 11.44) has been approved for the treatment of depression and diabetic peripheral neuropathic pain, but not for stress urinary incontinence or fibromyalgia. It is manufactured and marketed by Eli Lilly and Company. It is another analogue in the line of fluoxetine-based products from Lilly, in which the phenyl and phenoxy groups of fluoxetine have been respectively replaced with the benzene isostere, thiophene, and a naphthyloxy group (previously described under fluoxetine). Duloxetine exhibits dual inhibition with high affinity for the SERT and NET, with a nine times preferential inhibition of the SERT.[232] Duloxetine appears to be a more potent in vitro blocker of SERT and NET than venlafaxine. In humans, duloxetine has a low affinity for the other neuroreceptors, suggesting low incidence of unwanted adverse effects.

Duloxetine appears to be fairly well absorbed after oral doses, with peak plasma levels in 6-10 hours and linear pharmacokinetics (Table 11.13).[232] The drug is extensively metabolized in the liver to active metabolites, with 72% of an oral dose primarily excreted in the urine as conjugated metabolites and up to 15% appearing in the feces. Its elimination half-life, time to steady-state blood levels, and mean volume of distribution are shown in Table 11.13.

N-demethylation to an active metabolite (CYP2D6) and hydroxylation of the naphthyl ring (CYP1A2) at either the 4-, 5-, or 6-positions are the main metabolic pathways for duloxetine. Its metabolites are primarily excreted into the urine as glucuronide, sulfate, and O-methylated conjugation products (Fig. 11.47). The major metabolites found in plasma also were found in the urine. Preclinical data for 4-hydroxyduloxetine suggest it has a similar pharmacological profile to duloxetine, with selective inhibition of SERT but less activity at NET.

Adverse effects have included insomnia, somnolence, headache, nausea, diarrhea, and dry mouth. Mild withdrawal symptoms on abrupt discontinuation have been described in studies with healthy subjects.[233]

Duloxetine is a moderately potent CYP2D6 inhibitor (intermediate between paroxetine and sertraline). Thus, duloxetine should be used with caution when CYP2D6 substrates and inhibitors are coadministered.

DA and Norepinephrine Reuptake Inhibitor (DNRIs)

BUPROPION. Bupropion is an arylisopropylaminoketone that is structurally related to the phenylisopropylamine CNS stimulant, methamphetamine and the phenylisopropylaminoketone, cathinone (a constituent in khat), and the anorexiant, diethylpropion (Fig. 11.48). Although structurally similar to the CNS stimulants, bupropion exhibits distinctively different pharmacologic and therapeutic effects mostly because of its metabolites. The absence of the tricyclic ring system in bupropion results in a better adverse-effect profile

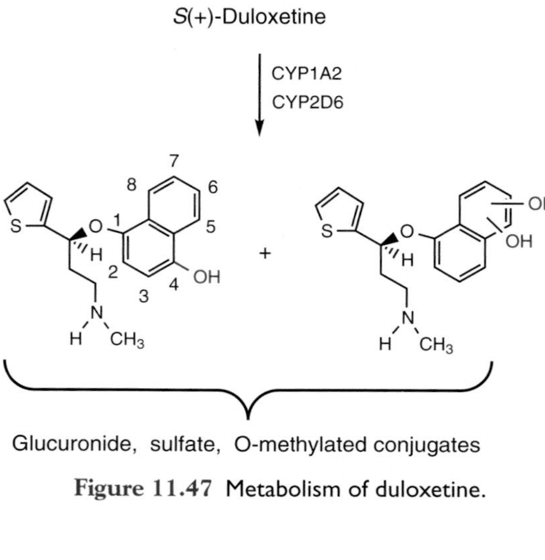

S(+)-Duloxetine
CYP1A2
CYP2D6
Glucuronide, sulfate, O-methylated conjugates

Figure 11.47 Metabolism of duloxetine.

than with the TCAs. The tertiary butyl group in bupropion prevents its N-dealkylation to metabolites that could possess sympathomimetic and/or anorexigenic properties.

Wellbutrin and Zyban (an aid in smoking cessation treatment) are trade name products for bupropion.[234] Therefore, the potential exists for an overdose toxicity in a patient receiving multiple brand name and generic prescriptions containing bupropion for the treatment of depression, smoking cessation, and other off-label uses.

Mechanism of Action. The mechanism of antidepressant action for bupropion is more complex because of its metabolism to its three principal metabolites (Fig. 11.48). These metabolites contribute to its antidepressant mechanism of action, because their accumulated plasma concentrations are higher than those of bupropion, with a longer duration of action.[235] Bupropion appears to be a selective, albeit weak, DAT inhibitor, but also acts as an SNRI (Table 11.14)—and may be a DA and NE releaser. A potential, additional mechanism of action for bupropion is as a noncompetitive antagonist of several neuronal nAChRs—studies have shown at high μM concentrations, bupropion can inhibit nAChRs. Whether this is clinically relevant is still debatable (as is its reported high μM negative allosteric modulatory activity at 5-HT_3 receptors). The neuronal nAChRs are ligand-gated ion channels of the CNS that regulate synaptic activity from both pre- and postsynaptic sites. Bupropion blocks noncompetitively the activation of $\alpha_3\beta_2$, $\alpha_4\beta_2$, and α_7 neuronal nAChRs and is approximately 5 and 12 times more effective in blocking activation of $\alpha_3\beta_2$ and $\alpha_4\beta_2$ (the brain nicotine binding site) than α_7 receptors. Bupropion, however, at high concentration failed to displace nicotine from the $\alpha_4\beta_2$ receptors, suggesting it binds an allosteric site. Bupropion inhibition of $\alpha_3\beta_2$ and $\alpha_4\beta_2$ ion channel receptors on neuronal nAChRs involves initial binding to the ion channels in the resting state, decreasing the probability of the ion channels opening and further interaction with a binding domain in the ion channel shared with the tricyclic antidepressants.[235] Bupropion does not exhibit clinically significant anticholinergic (muscarinic), antihistaminic, α_1-adrenergic blocking activity or MAO inhibition.

Bupropion reduces the discomfort and craving associated with smoking cessation, which suggests that the principal mode of action by bupropion as an aid in smoking cessation is on the withdrawal symptoms following smoking cessation.[234] The efficacy of bupropion in smoking cessation does not appear to depend on the presence of depression. The current presumed mechanism of action of bupropion involves modulation of dopaminergic and noradrenergic systems that have been implicated in addiction, by increasing extracellular CNS DA concentrations, most likely as a result of its inhibition of DA and noradrenaline reuptake transporters[234] (Table 11.4). As nicotine CNS concentrations drop with smoking cessation, the firing rates of noradrenergic neurons increase, which may be the basis for the withdrawal symptoms. During withdrawal, bupropion and its active metabolite, hydroxybupropion, reduce the firing rates of these noradrenergic neurons in a dose-dependent manner, attenuating the symptoms of smoking cessation—the exact mechanisms underlying these effects are unknown. Bupropion's ability to block nicotinic receptors also may prevent relapse by attenuating the reinforcing properties of nicotine.[184]

Bupropion is extensively metabolized in humans with its three major hydroxylated metabolites reaching plasma levels higher than those of bupropion itself. These hydroxylated metabolites share many of the

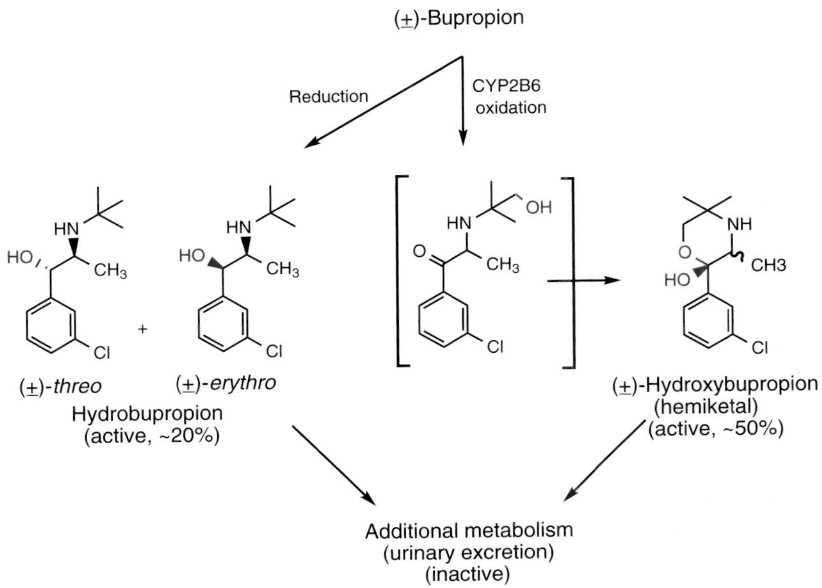

Figure 11.48 Metabolism of bupropion.

Table 11.14 Pharmacokinetics of the DA and NE Reuptake Inhibitors (DNRIs) and Serotonin Receptor Modulators (SMSs)

Parameters	Bupropion	Trazodone	Mirtazapine	Levomilnan-cipran	Vilazodone	Vortioxetine
Oral bioavailability (%)	5-20	65 (60-70)	~50	92	72	75
Lipophilicity (Log $D_{7.4}$)	2.88	2.59	2.40	−1.09	ND	3.37
Protein binding (%)	80	90-95	85	22	98	98
Volume of distribution (L/kg)	19-21	0.84 (0.5-1.2)	107	387-473		2,600
Elimination half-life (hr)	21 (14-24) ~20 (S,S)-hydroxy	7 (4-9)	16-40	12	25	66
Cytochrome P450 major isoform	2B6	3A4	3A4 and 2D6	3A4	3A4	2D6, 3A4/5
Major active metabolites	(S,S)-Hydroxyl	m-Chloro-phenylpip-erazine	None	None	None	None
Peak plasma concentration (hr)	2-3 8 (S,S)-hydroxy	1-2	2	6-8	4-5	7-11
Excretion (%)	Urine 87 Feces 10	Urine 70-75 Feces 25-30	Urine 75 Feces 15	Urine 58	Urine >90 Feces 2	Urine 60
Plasma half-life (hr)	3-4 20 (S,S)-hydroxy	6 (4-8)	2			
Time to steady-state concentration (d)	5-8 (S,S)-hydroxy	3-7	5			

pharmacological properties of bupropion, so they can play a greater role in attenuating the withdrawal and relapse by which bupropion exerts its activity in smoking cessation.[235,236]

Pharmacokinetics. Bupropion is absorbed from the gastrointestinal tract, with a low oral bioavailability as a result of first-pass metabolism. The pharmacokinetic properties of bupropion are shown in Table 11.14. Food does not appear to substantially affect its peak plasma concentration or AUC. Following oral administration, peak plasma concentrations usually are achieved within 2 hours for bupropion and 3 hours for sustained-released bupropion products, followed by a biphasic decline for bupropion. Plasma concentrations are dose-proportional (linear pharmacokinetics) following single doses of 100-250 mg/d. The fraction of a dose excreted unmetabolized was less than 1%.

Bupropion hydroxylation of the tert-butyl group to hydroxypropion intermediate which cyclizes to a phenylmorpholinol metabolite is mediated exclusively by CYP2B6.[235,237] Other metabolites include reduction of the aminoketone to amino-alcohol isomers, *threo*-hydrobupropion and *erythro*-hydrobupropion (Fig. 11.48). Further oxidation of the bupropion side chain results in the formation of *m*-chlorobenzoic acid, which is eliminated in the urine as its glycine conjugate. Hydroxybupropion is approximately 50% as potent as bupropion, whereas *threo*-hydrobupropion and *erythro*-hydrobupropion have 20% of the potency of bupropion. Peak plasma concentrations for hydroxybupropion are approximately 20 times the peak level of the parent drug at steady state, with an elimination half-life of approximately 20 hours. Thus, CYP2B6-catalyzed bupropion hydroxylation is a clinically important bioactivation and elimination pathway. The times to peak concentrations for the *erythro*-hydrobupropion and *threo*-hydrobupropion metabolites are similar to that of the hydroxybupropion metabolite. The plasma levels of the *erythro*-hydrobupropion correlate with several side effects, such as insomnia and dry mouth. Their elimination half-lives, however, are longer (~33 and 37 hr, respectively) and steady-state AUCs are 1.5 and 7.0 times that of bupropion, respectively. The hepatic clearance in patients with liver disease was increased from 19 to 29 hours. The median observed T_{max} was 19 hours for hydroxybupropion and 31 hours for *threo*/*erythro*-hydrobupropion. The mean half-lives for hydroxybupropion and *threo/erythro*-hydrobupropion were increased by five and two times, respectively, in patients with severe hepatic cirrhosis compared with healthy volunteers. Bupropion and its metabolites are distributed into breast milk.

In geriatric patients, the apparent half-life of hydroxybupropion averaged approximately 34 hours. Reduction in renal or hepatic function may affect elimination of the major metabolites because these compounds are moderately polar and are likely to be metabolized further or conjugated in the liver before urinary excretion.

The pharmacokinetic parameters for bupropion and hydroxybupropion did not differ between smokers and nonsmokers, but adolescent females exhibited increased AUCs and volume of distribution (normalized to body weight) and a longer elimination half-life than do males. No differences in clearance between males and females, however, were observed.[235,236]

Drug Interactions. Inhibition studies with the SSRIs and bupropion suggest that bupropion is a potent CYP2D6 inhibitor.[236] Bupropion hydroxylation was strongly inhibited by, in the following order, paroxetine > fluvoxamine > sertraline > desmethylsertraline > norfluoxetine > fluoxetine and only weakly inhibited by venlafaxine, ODV, citalopram, and desmethylcitalopram. The inhibition of bupropion hydroxylation in vitro by SSRIs suggests the potential for clinical drug interactions. Therefore, coadministration of drugs that inhibit CYP2D6 warrants careful monitoring. Because of its selective inhibition of DAT, pharmacodynamic interactions with DA agonists (e.g., levodopa) and antagonists should be anticipated. Coadministration of bupropion with drugs that lower the seizure threshold should be avoided because of the risk of serious seizures.

Drugs that affect metabolism by CYP2B6 (e.g., methadone, nicotine, and cyclophosphamide) also have the potential to interact with bupropion.

Therapeutic Uses. Besides being used to treat depression, bupropion aids in the cessation of smoking. The efficacy of bupropion in smoking cessation is comparable to that of nicotine replacement therapy and should be considered as a second-line treatment in smoking cessation.[184,236] It possesses a broad spectrum of infrequent adverse effects, however, with potential drug metabolism interactions with TCAs, β-adrenergic blocking drugs, and class Ic antiarrhythmics.

Serotonin Receptor Modulators and Stimulator (SMSs)

A serotonin modulator and stimulator (SMS), sometimes referred to more simply as a 5-HT modulator (regulator), is a type of drug with multiple pharmacologic modes of action at receptor sites specific to the 5-HT neurotransmitter system. SMSs simultaneously regulates one or more 5-HT receptors and inhibits the reuptake of 5-HT.

SMSs are a distinct class of atypical antidepressants used to treat MDD. SMSs have several modes of interaction with the various serotonin receptors in the brain and simultaneously modulate one or more 5-HT receptors and inhibit the reuptake of 5-HT. There are many different subtypes of 5-HT receptors. There being at least 14 unique, genetically encoded 5-HT receptors currently known. A few 5-HT receptors appear to be involved in the antidepressant effects of SSRIs. A drug which combines the actions of SSRI, 5-HT_{1A} partial agonism, 5-HT_{2A} antagonism, and 5-HT_7 receptor antagonism could prove more effective than pure SSRIs.

SMS describes the mechanism of action of the serotonergic antidepressant vortioxetine, which acts as an SSRI, agonist at the 5-HT_{1A} receptor, and antagonist at the 5-HT_3 and 5-HT_7 receptors. Drugs in this class of antidepressants include trazodone, vilazodone, and vortioxetine. Serious adverse effects of SMSs include hepatic failure and should be used with precaution in patients with cardiac abnormalities. Patients should be monitored for suicidal thinking and behavior. There is also risk of hypotension and of abnormal bleeding.

General Mechanism of Action. SMSs are a class of antidepressants that modulate the concentration of 5-HT in the brain and directly impact 5-HT receptor cellular signaling. A neuromodulator functions as a "volume control in the brain and nervous system," regulating the other neurotransmitters through its receptors in the brain in response to external stimuli. The serotonergic system modulates a large number of physiological events, such as cognition, emotion, temperature regulation, sleep, learning and memory, motor behavior, sexual function, hormonal secretions, and immune activity and is implicated in stress, anxiety, aggressiveness, and depression disorders. Of the various types of 5-HT receptors mediating serotonergic activity, the 5-$HT_{1\text{-type}}$ receptors play an important role in modulating the serotonergic system. Many of these receptors are autoreceptors localized on serotonergic presynaptic nerve terminals, where they inhibit the release of 5-HT and its biosynthesis; they also inhibit the release of other neurotransmitters, such as ACh, GABA, and NE. Excessive amounts of 5-HT in the brain may cause relaxation, sedation, and a decrease in sexual drive; inadequate amounts of 5-HT can lead to psychiatric disorders. Therefore, the SMSs exert their antidepressant effects by mechanisms involving complicated interactions between several neurotransmitter systems. Specific examples include drugs acting as dual 5-HT antagonists/5-HT reuptake inhibitors (SARI; trazodone and vilazodone) and drugs acting as α_2 adrenergic antagonists, 5-HT_2 and 5-HT_3 antagonists (NaSSA; mirtazapine). Chronic antidepressant treatment with SARIs and NaSSAs modulate receptor expression in a manner that is not clearly mapped mechanistically to treatment effects.

Arylpiperazine Antidepressants. In order to avoid benzodiazepine's undesirable side effects, a third-generation anxiolytic agent, buspirone, the focus of the arylpiperazine group of antianxiety agents, was introduced as a new class of mood-regulating agents. Arylpiperazine derivatives possess 5-HT_{1A} receptor partial agonist activity and are known as serotonin modulators—however, most also have significant activity at multiple other targets (e.g., see aripiprazole above, in antipsychotics section). Clinical and preclinical studies support the efficacy of 5-HT_{1A} receptor partial agonists as anxiolytics and potentially antipsychotics (see above, regarding negative symptoms of psychosis). The mechanisms of action underlying the activity of arylpiperazines are currently unknown. There is speculation that efficacy might be due to the activation of postsynaptic 5-HT_{1A} receptors, although 5-HT_{1A} receptor agonists can also activate autoreceptors which diminish the release of 5-HT—there is also development underway of compounds that selectively target pre- versus postsynaptic 5-HT_{1A} receptors. The arylpiperazine derivatives have no sedative and muscle relaxant effects, but they have a rather weak anxiolytic action and a slow onset of action.

Most compounds described below, with 5-HT_{1A} activity, are readily absorbed but are also rapidly eliminated, thereby often producing either suboptimal therapeutic responses at low doses, or cumbersome adverse effects at higher doses. Extended-release formulations allow once-daily dosing regimens, thus avoiding sharp peak plasma concentrations. This improves compliance and permits the use of higher dosages, which may be associated with enhanced efficacy and better tolerability relative to the immediate-release formulations.

Trazodone. Trazodone is a phenylpiperazine-triazolopyridine antidepressant that is structurally unrelated to most of the other antidepressant classes (Fig. 11.49). It acts as a mixed 5-HT receptor antagonist and 5-HT reuptake inhibitor.[237]

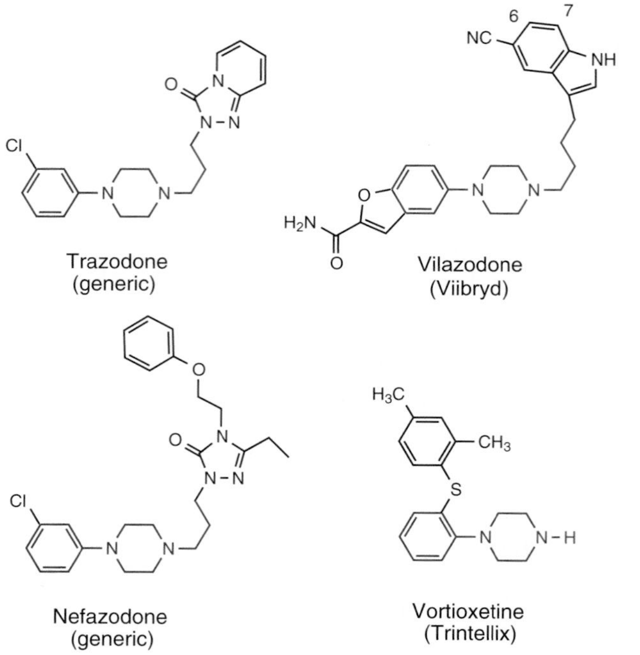

Mechanism of Action. Although the exact mechanism of action is unknown, trazodone acts as an antagonist at 5-HT_{2A} receptors and is a weak inhibitor of 5-HT reuptake at the presynaptic neuronal membrane, potentiating the synaptic effects of 5-HT. It also has off-target activity at α1 and α2 receptors. Its mechanism of action is complicated by the presence of its metabolite, *m*-chlorophenylpiperazine (Fig. 11.50), which is a 5-HT_{2C} agonist.[238] At therapeutic dosages, trazodone does not appear to affect the reuptake of DA or NE within the CNS. It has little anticholinergic activity and is relatively devoid of toxic cardiovascular effects. Long-term administration of trazodone decreases the number of postsynaptic serotonergic (i.e., 5-HT_2) and β-adrenergic binding sites in the brains of animals, decreasing the sensitivity of adenylyl cyclase to stimulation by β-adrenergic agonists. It has been suggested that postsynaptic serotonergic receptor modification is mainly responsible for the antidepressant action observed during long-term administration of trazodone.[238] Trazodone does not inhibit MAO and, unlike amphetamine-like drugs, does not stimulate the CNS.

Trazodone is rapidly and almost completely absorbed from the gastrointestinal tract following oral administration, with an oral bioavailability of approximately 65% (Table 11.14).[239] Peak plasma concentrations of trazodone occur approximately 1 hour after oral administration when

Trazodone (generic)

Vilazodone (Viibryd)

Nefazodone (generic)

Vortioxetine (Trintellix)

Figure 11.49 Serotonin receptor modulators.

taken on an empty stomach or 2 hours when taken with food. At steady state, its plasma concentrations exhibit wide interpatient variation.

Trazodone is extensively metabolized in the liver by N-dealkylation to its primary circulating active metabolite, *m*-chlorophenylpiperazine, which subsequently undergoes aromatic hydroxylation to *p*-hydroxy-*m*-chlorophenylpiperazine (Fig. 11.50).[239] In vitro studies indicate that CYP3A4 is the major isoform involved in the production of *m*-chlorophenylpiperazine from trazodone (and CYP2D6 to a lesser extent). 4′-Hydroxy-*m*-chlorophenylpiperazine and oxotriazolopyridinepropionic acid (the major metabolite excreted in urine) are conjugated with glucuronic acid. Less than 1% of a dose is excreted unmetabolized. *m*-chlorophenylpiperazine is 4′-hydroxylated by CYP2D6. *m*-chlorophenylpiperazine is of significant interest because of its 5-HT_2 activities that may contribute to trazodone antidepressant action.[239]

Trazodone therapy has been associated with several cases of idiosyncratic hepatotoxicity. Although the mechanism of hepatotoxicity remains unknown, the generation of an iminoquinone, an epoxide reactive metabolite, or both may play a role in the initiation of trazodone-mediated hepatotoxicity (Fig. 11.50).[240-242] Studies have shown that the bioactivation of trazodone involves, first, aromatic hydroxylation of the 3-chlorophenyl ring, followed by its oxidation to a reactive iminoquinone intermediate, which then reacts with glutathione, or oxidation of the triazolopyridinone ring to an electrophilic epoxide and ring opening by either a nucleophile or to generate the corresponding hydrated trazodone-nucleophile conjugate or the stable diol metabolite, respectively.[241,242] The pathway involving trazodone bioactivation to the iminoquinone also has been observed with many para-hydroxyanilines (e.g., acetaminophen). The reactive intermediates

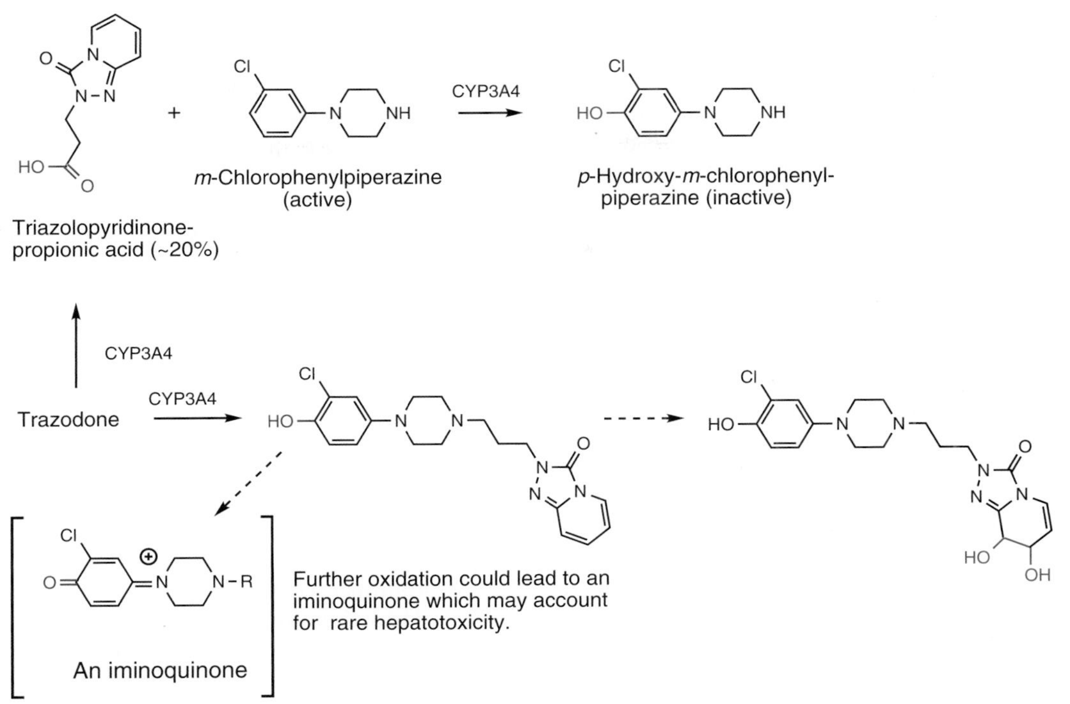

Figure 11.50 Metabolism of trazodone.

consume the available glutathione, allowing the reactive intermediate to react with hepatic tissue leading to liver damage.

Unlike the TCAs, trazodone does not block the fast sodium channels and, thus, does not have significant arrhythmic activity. Compared with the SSRIs, it has a lesser tendency to cause drug-induced male sexual dysfunction as a side effect. Although trazodone displays α_1-adrenergic blocking activity, hypotension is relatively uncommon. Signs of overdose toxicity include nausea, vomiting, and decreased level of consciousness. Trazodone produces a significant amount of sedation in normal and mentally depressed patients (principally from its central α_1-adrenergic blocking activity and antihistamine action).

Drug Interactions. Trazodone possesses serotonergic activity; therefore, the possibility of developing 5-HT syndrome should be considered in patients who are receiving trazodone and other SSRIs or serotonergic drugs concurrently. When trazodone is used concurrently with drugs metabolized by CYP3A4, caution should be used to avoid excessive sedation. Trazodone can cause hypotension, including orthostatic hypotension and syncope; concomitant administration of antihypertensive therapy may require a reduction in dosage of the antihypertensive agent.

The possibility of drug-drug interactions with trazodone and other substrates, inducers, and/or inhibitors of CYP3A4 exists.[239]

Therapeutic Uses. Trazodone is used primarily in the treatment of depression. The drug also has shown some efficacy in the treatment of benzodiazepine or alcohol dependence, diabetic neuropathy, and panic disorders.

NEFAZODONE

Nefazodone is an arylpiperazine antidepressant structurally related to trazodone, but it differs pharmacologically from trazodone, the SSRIs, the MAOIs, and the TCAs (Fig. 11.25). When compared with trazodone, nefazodone displays approximately twice the affinity potency for SERT. Nefazodone therapy, however, was associated with life-threatening cases of idiosyncratic hepatotoxicity, and as a result, nefazodone was withdrawn from both the North American and European markets in 2003. The mechanism of hepatotoxicity remains unknown, but nefazodone, being structurally similar to trazodone (Fig. 11.24), is metabolized to *p*-hydroxynefazodone, *m*-chlorophenylpiperazine, and phenoxyethyltriazoledione. In turn, *p*-hydroxynefazodone is thought to be oxidized to an iminoquinone and/or an epoxide reactive metabolite, which may play a role in the initiation of nefazodone-mediated hepatotoxicity.

Vilazodone. Vilazodone is a arylpiperazine-2-benzofurancarboxamide antidepressant that is structurally related to trazodone (Fig. 11.49).

Mechanism of Action. The mechanism of the antidepressant effect of vilazodone is not fully understood but could be related to its enhancement of CNS serotonergic activity through selective inhibition of 5-HT reuptake.[249] In addition, vilazodone is also a partial agonist at 5-HT_{1A} receptors, and thus may be considered an SMS. Vilazodone binds with high affinity to the 5-HT reuptake site (K_i = 0.1 nM), but not to the

NE (K_i = 56 nM) or DA (K_i = 37 nM) reuptake sites. Vilazodone is a potent and selective inhibitor of 5-HT reuptake (IC_{50} = 1.6 nM) (Fig. 11.30). As a 5-HT_{1A} receptor partial agonist, it potently, but partially activates 5-HT_{1A} receptors (IC_{50} = 2.1 nM; E_{MAX} ~60%)). Vilazodone does not prolong the QTc interval as do the TCAs and is below the threshold for clinical concern. Clinical trials of vilazodone showed significant antidepressant efficacy with a relatively rapid onset of effect of 1 week, unlike other antidepressants. The 1-week onset of its antidepressant action has been linked to its combined SERT inhibition and partial agonist action at the 5-HT_{1A} receptor.[244,245]

Pharmacokinetics. The antidepressant activity for vilazodone activity is due primarily to the parent drug. Vilazodone exhibits dose-proportional linear pharmacokinetics, and steady-state is achieved in about 3 days.[246] Elimination of vilazodone is primarily by hepatic metabolism with a terminal half-life of approximately 25 hours (Table 11.14). Peak plasma concentrations (T_{max}) occur at 4-5 hours after oral administration. The absolute bioavailability of vilazodone is 72% with food. Food (high fat or light meal) increases the C_{max} of vilazodone by approximately 147%-160%, and AUC increases by approximately 64%-85%. Vilazodone is widely distributed and approximately 96%-99% protein-bound. Vilazodone is extensively metabolized by CYP3A4 to 6-hydroxyvilazodone (inactive metabolite) with minor contributions from CYP2C19 and CYP2D6.[246-248] Only 1% of the oral dose is recovered in the urine and 2% recovered in the feces as unchanged vilazodone. In vitro studies indicate that vilazodone is unlikely to inhibit or induce the metabolism of other CYP (except for CYP2C8) substrates and does not alter the pharmacokinetics of CYP2C19, 2D6, and 3A4 substrates.[247] Renal impairment or mild or moderate hepatic impairment does not affect the clearance of vilazodone, thus no dose adjustment is required.[247,248] Coadministration of vilazodone with ethanol or with a proton pump inhibitor (e.g., pantoprazole) does not affect the rate or extent of vilazodone absorption. Vilazodone is excreted into the milk of lactating rats, but the effect on lactation and nursing in humans is unknown. Breast feeding in women treated with vilazodone should be considered only if the potential benefit outweighs the potential risk to the child. A pharmacokinetic study in elderly (>65 yr old) versus young (24-55 yr old) subjects demonstrated that the pharmacokinetics was generally similar between the two age groups. No dose adjustment is recommended on the basis of age. Greater sensitivity of some older individuals to vilazodone cannot be ruled out. After adjustment for body weight, the systemic exposures between males and females are similar.[248]

Adverse Effects. The most commonly observed adverse reactions in vilazodone-treated MDD patients with an incidence greater than 5% were diarrhea, nausea, vomiting, and insomnia. Sexual dysfunction was minimal with vilazodone. As with all antidepressants, use vilazodone cautiously in patients with a history or family history of bipolar disorder, mania, or hypomania. Vilazodone has safety risks associated with the induction of suicidal thoughts in young adults, adolescents, and children (a boxed warning).

Drug Interactions. The risk of using vilazodone in combination with other CNS-active drugs has not been evaluated. Because of potential interactions with MAOIs, vilazodone should not be prescribed concomitantly with an MAOI or within 14 days of discontinuing or starting an MAOI. Based on the drug's mechanism of action and the potential for 5-HT toxicity (serotonin syndrome), caution is advised when coadministered with other drugs that may affect the serotonergic neurotransmitter systems (e.g., MAOI, SSRIs, SNRIs, triptans, buspirone, tramadol, and tryptophan products). Because 5-HT release by platelets plays an important role in hemostasis, concurrent use of an nonsteroidal anti-inflammatory drug or aspirin with vilazodone may potentiate the risk of abnormal bleeding. Altered anticoagulant effects, including increased bleeding, have been reported when SSRIs and SNRIs are coadministered with warfarin. Thus, patients receiving warfarin therapy should be carefully monitored when vilazodone is initiated or discontinued. Concomitant use of vilazodone and strong/moderate inhibitors of CYP3A4 (e.g., ketoconazole) can increase vilazodone plasma concentrations by approximately 50%, requiring a dosage adjustment. No dose adjustment is recommended when coadministered with mild inhibitors of CYP3A4 (e.g., cimetidine). Concomitant use of vilazodone with inducers of CYP3A4 has the potential to reduce vilazodone plasma levels. Concomitant administration of vilazodone with inhibitors of CYP2C19 and CYP2D6 is not expected to alter its plasma concentration. These isoforms are minor elimination pathways in the metabolism of vilazodone. Coadministration of vilazodone with substrates for CYP1A2, CYP2C9, CYP3A4, or CYP2D6 is unlikely to result in clinically significant changes in the concentrations of the CYP substrates. Vilazodone coadministration with mephenytoin results in a small (11%) increase in mephenytoin biotransformation, suggestive of a minor induction of CYP2C19. In vitro studies have shown that vilazodone is a moderate inhibitor of CYP2C19 and CYP2D6. In vitro studies suggest that vilazodone may inhibit the biotransformation of substrates of CYP2C8, thus coadministration of vilazodone with a CYP2C8 substrate may lead to an increase in the plasma concentration of the CYP2C8 substrate. Chronic administration of vilazodone is unlikely to induce the metabolism of drugs metabolized by CYP1A1, 1A2, 2A6, 2B6, 2C9, 2C19, 2D6, 2E1, 3A4/5. Because vilazodone is highly bound to plasma protein, administration to a patient taking another drug that is highly protein bound may cause increased free concentrations of the other drug.[247,248]

Vortioxetine. Vortioxetine is an arylpiperazine that was FDA approved in 2013 for the treatment of adults with MDD. Vortioxetine is classified as a SMS. It has a multimodal mechanism of action toward the 5-HT neurotransmitter system whereby it simultaneously modulates one or more 5-HT receptors and inhibits the reuptake of 5-HT (Fig. 11.51).

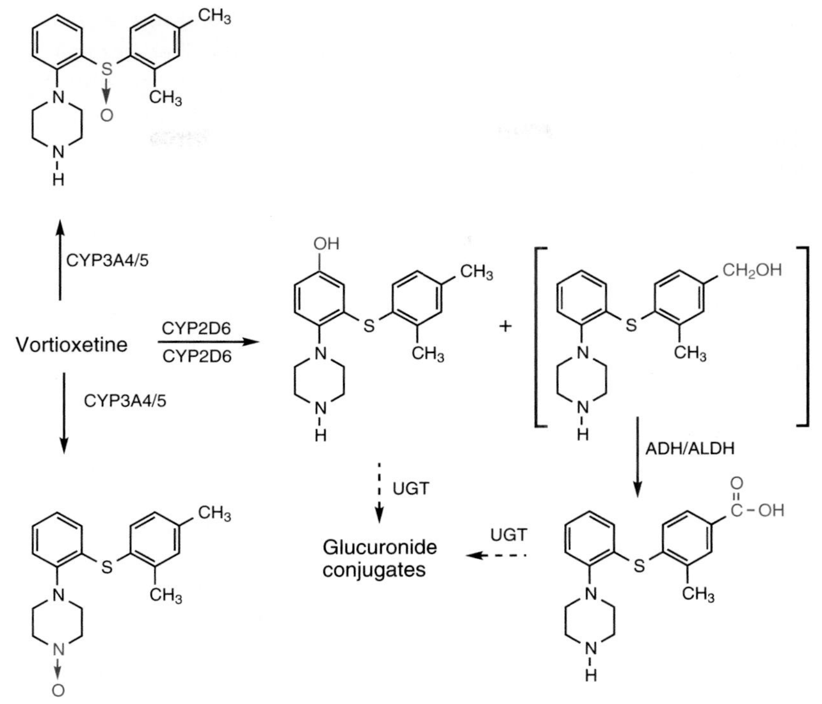

Figure 11.51 Metabolism of vortioxetine

Mechanism of Action. Its mechanism of action is not fully understood, but it inhibits SERT (K_i = 1.6 nM, IC_{50} = 5.4 nM), has lower activity at NET (K_i = 113 nM), and has very low activity at DAT (K_i > 1,000 nM). Vortioxetine displays high affinity for 5-HT_3 (K_i = 3.7 nM), moderate affinity for 5-HT_{1A} (K_i = 15 nM), 5-HT_7 (K_i = 19 nM), 5-HT_{1D} (K_i = 54 nM), and 5-HT_{1B} (K_i = 33 nM) receptors and is a 5-HT_3, 5-HT_{1D}, and 5-HT_7 receptor antagonist, 5-HT_{1B} receptor partial agonist, and 5-HT_{1A} receptor agonist.[249,250,251] Animal studies suggest that vortioxetine increases extracellular levels of several neurotransmitters in several neural systems in the brain associated with depression, including the prefrontal cortex and hippocampus. Vortioxetine can be discontinued 1 week before complete discontinuation.[250,252]

Drug Interactions. Since vortioxetine is an agonist and antagonist of multiple 5-HT receptors, potential interactions may occur with other medications that alter the serotonergic system. There is an increased risk of serotonin syndrome when vortioxetine is used in combination with other serotonergic agents. Medications that should be avoided because of the increased risk of serotonin syndrome when combined with vortioxetine include SNRIs, SSRIs, TCAs, triptans, MAOIs, lithium, and antipsychotic agents. St. John's wort and dextromethorphan, common over-the-counter medications, should also be avoided because of their serotonergic effects. Vortioxetine has been known to cause abnormal bleeding with nonsteroidal anti-inflammatory drugs, warfarin, and aspirin, and patients should watch for signs and symptoms of abnormal bleeding.[251,252]

Pharmacokinetics. Vortioxetine is extensively metabolized by CYP2D6 and with CYP3A4/5, CYP2C19, and CYP2C9 and subsequent glucuronic acid conjugation, also contributing to its metabolism (Fig. 11.51, Table 11.14). CYP2D6 hydroxylates vortioxetine into its phenolic inactive metabolite and hydroxylates the arylmethyl group to hydroxymethyl followed by alcohol and aldehyde dehydrogenase (ADH/ALDH) oxidation to the carboxylic acid metabolite. Since vortioxetine primarily goes through CYP2D6, the probability of interactions with CYP2D6 inhibitors and inducers affecting its concentration is high. The half-life of vortioxetine is approximately 66 hours and is primarily eliminated in urine (59%) and feces (26%), with a negligible amount of unchanged vortioxetine in the urine. Drug interactions involve inhibitors and inducers of CYP2D6. The dose of vortioxetine should be reduced by half when it is combined with strong CYP2D6 inhibitors, and the dose of vortioxetine should be increased if strong CYP2D6 inducers are used for 14 days or longer (up to three times the maximum recommended dose can be used with strong CYP2D6 inducers). After oral administration, vortioxetine is absorbed from the gastrointestinal tract and exhibits peak plasma concentrations in about 7-11 hours. Its oral bioavailability is 75%. Consumption of food does not affect its bioavailability, and taking vortioxetine with food has not been shown to increase its C_{max}. The steady-state concentration is achieved in about 2 weeks. Vortioxetine has a linear and dose-proportional pharmacokinetic profile with single daily dosing of 2.5-60 mg.[250]

Therapeutic Effects. In clinical trials, 10 mg vortioxetine significantly alleviated depressive symptoms, compared to placebo, after 8 weeks of treatment. All doses of vortioxetine showed reductions in antidepressant scores by week 2 and week 8, but 10 mg demonstrated better efficacy, suggesting a potential dose effect. In addition, all doses were statistically superior to placebo in regard to response rates, as well as remission rates.

MIRTAZAPINE. Mirtazapine is a pyrazinopyridobenazepine antidepressant that is an isostere of the antidepressant mianserin[253] (Fig. 11.52). A seemingly simple isosteric replacement of an aromatic methine group (CH) in mianserin with a nitrogen to give a pyridine ring (mirtazapine) has profound effects on the physicochemical properties, pharmacokinetics, mechanisms of action, and antidepressant activities (Table 11.15). Profound differences between receptor affinity and transporter affinity, pharmacokinetics, regioselectivity in the formation of metabolites, and toxicity are observed for mianserin and mirtazapine and their antidepressant mechanisms of action.[253] The pyridine ring increases the polarity of the molecule and decreases the measured partition coefficient and the basicity. Mianserin is a potent inhibitor of NET, whereas mirtazapine has negligible effects on the inhibition of NET and SERT (K_i >4,600 and >10,000 nM respectively).

Mianserin is currently marketed in Europe as an antidepressant. Mianserin has not been approved by the FDA for use in the United States because of its serious adverse effects of agranulocytosis and leukopenia. Mirtazapine has not exhibited this adverse effect.

Mechanism of Action. Mirtazapine is a NaSSA that antagonizes central presynaptic α_2 adrenergic autoreceptors (K_i = 20 nM)[254] and α_2-adrenergic heteroreceptors on both NE and 5-HT presynaptic axons, and potently antagonizes postsynaptic 5-HT_2 and 5-HT_3 receptors (K_i = 6.3 and 8 nM) (Fig. 11.27). It shows no significant

Mirtazapine → Desmethylmirtazapine + 8-Hydroxymirtazapine (weak activity)

Mirtazapine → Mirtazapine-N-oxide

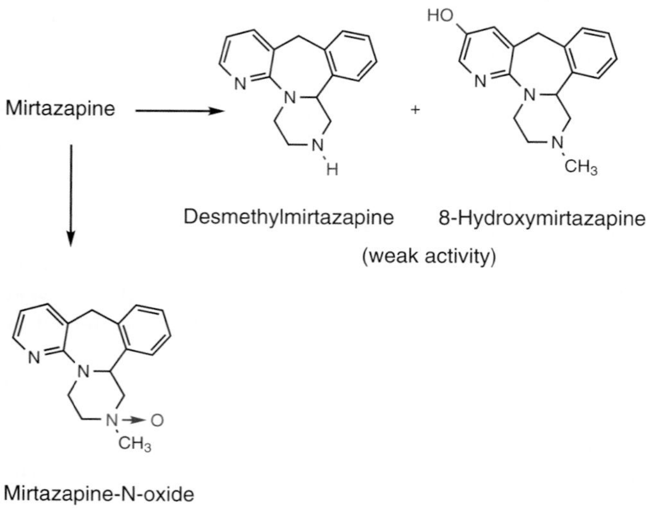

Figure 11.52 Metabolism of mirtazapine.

Table 11.15 Physicochemical Properties of Mirtazapine and Mianserin

Properties	Mirtazapine	Mianserin
pK_a	7.1	7.4
Lipophilicity (Log $D_{7.4}$)	2.72	3.17
Polarity	2.63 debye	0.82 debye
NET affinity (pK_i)	5.8	7.1
5-HT release	Yes	No

affinity for 5-HT_{1A} or 5-HT_{1B} receptors (K_i > 4,000 nM), and likewise, does not have significant affinity for any of the monoamine transporters. Mirtazapine increases NE and 5-HT release, likely via its activity at α2 receptors. Mirtazapine is extensively metabolized in the liver. CYP1A2, CYP2D6, and CYP3A4 are mainly responsible for its metabolism. Steady-state concentrations are reached after 4 days in adults and 6 days in the elderly. In vitro studies suggest that mirtazapine is unlikely to cause clinically significant drug-drug interactions. Dry mouth, sedation, and increases in appetite and body weight are the most common adverse effects. In contrast to the SSRIs, mirtazapine has no sexual side effects. In clinical depression, its efficacy is comparable to that of amitriptyline, clomipramine, doxepin, fluoxetine, paroxetine, citalopram, or venlafaxine. It seems to be safe and effective during long-term use. It displays some anticholinergic properties and it produces sedative effects because of potent histamine H_1 receptor antagonism and orthostatic hypotension (because of moderate antagonism at peripheral α_1-adrenergic receptors).

The pharmacokinetics for mirtazepine is shown in Table 11.15. Mirtazapine absorption is rapid and complete, with a bioavailability of approximately 50% as a result of first-pass metabolism. The rate and extent of mirtazapine absorption are minimally affected by food. Dose and plasma levels are linearly related over a dose range of 15-80 mg. The elimination half-life of the (−)-enantiomer is approximately twice that of the (+)-enantiomer. In females of all ages, the elimination half-life is significantly longer than in males (mean half-life, 37 vs. 26 hr).[255]

Following oral administration, mirtazapine undergoes first-pass metabolism by N-demethylation and ring hydroxylation to its 8-hydroxy metabolite, followed by O-glucuronide conjugation.[255] In vitro studies indicate that CYP2D6 and CYP1A2 are involved in the formation of the 8-hydroxy metabolite and that CYP3A4 is responsible for the formation of the N-desmethyl and N-oxide metabolites (Fig. 11.52). The 8-hydroxy and N-desmethyl metabolites possess weak pharmacological activity, but their plasma levels are very low and, thus, are unlikely to contribute to the antidepressant action of mirtazapine. Clearance for mirtazapine may decrease in patients with hepatic or renal impairment, increasing its plasma concentrations. Therefore, it should be used with caution in these patients. In vitro studies have shown mirtazapine to be a weak inhibitor of CYP1A2, CYP2D6, and CYP3A4.

Monoamine Oxidase Inhibitors

The discovery of MAOIs resulted from a search for derivatives of isoniazid (isonicotinic acid hydrazide) (Fig. 11.53) with antitubercular activity. During clinical trials with this hydrazine derivative, a rather consistent beneficial effect of mood elevation was noted in depressed patients with tuberculosis.[256] Although no longer used clinically, iproniazid (Fig. 11.53), the first derivative to be synthesized, was found to be hepatotoxic at dosage levels required for antitubercular and antidepressant activity. The antidepressant activity of iproniazid, however, prompted a search for other MAOIs, which resulted in the synthesis of hydrazine and nonhydrazine MAOIs that were relatively less toxic than iproniazid.

The MAOIs can be classified as hydrazines (e.g., phenelzine) and nonhydrazines (e.g., tranylcypromine), which can block the oxidative deamination of naturally occurring monoamines. MAOIs can also be classified according to their ability to selectively inhibit MAO-A or MAO-B (nonselective inhibitors). The currently available MAOI antidepressants, phenelzine and tranylcypromine, (Fig. 11.53) are considered to be irreversible inhibitors of both MAO-A and MAO-B. The mechanism of antidepressant action of the MAOIs suggests that an increase in free 5-HT and NE and/or alterations in other amine concentrations within the CNS are mainly responsible for their antidepressant effect.

Mechanisms of Action Common to MAOIs

An enzyme found mainly in nerve tissue and in the liver and lungs, MAO catalyzes the oxidative deamination of various amines, including epinephrine, NE, DA, and 5-HT. At least two isoforms of MAO exist, MAO-A and MAO-B, with differences in substrate preference, inhibitor specificity, and tissue distribution. The MAO-A substrates include 5-HT and the MAO-B substrates include phenylethylamine. Tyramine, epinephrine, NE, and DA are substrates for both MAO-A and MAO-B. The cloning of MAO-A and MAO-B has demonstrated unequivocally that these enzymes consist of different amino acid sequences and also has provided insight regarding their structure, regulation, and function.[256] Both MAO-A and MAO-B knockout mice exhibit distinct differences in neurotransmitter metabolism and behavior. The MAO-A knockout mice have elevated brain levels of 5-HT, NE, and DA and they manifest aggressive behavior. Low activity of MAO-A in human males is also associated with aggressive behavior, and deletion of MAO-A in human males is associated with severe intellectual disabilities and autistic behaviors. In contrast, MAO-B knockout mice do not exhibit aggression and only levels of phenylethylamine are increased. Both MAO-A and MAO-B knockout mice show increased reactivity to stress.[256]

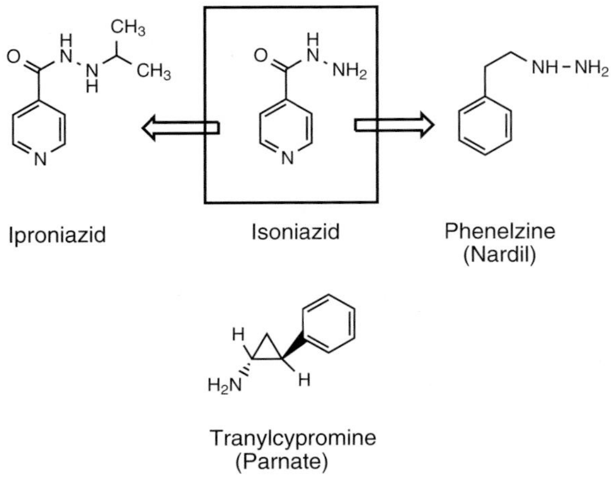

Figure 11.53 MAOI antidepressants.

The pharmacological effects of MAOIs are cumulative. A latent period of a few days to several months may occur before the onset of the antidepressant action and effects may persist for up to 3 weeks following discontinuance of therapy.

Adverse Effects Common to MAOIs

Common side effects for the nonselective MAOIs include sleeping difficulties, daytime insomnia, agitation, dizziness on standing that results in fainting (orthostatic hypotension), dry mouth, tremor (slight shake of muscles of arms and hands), syncope, palpitations, tachycardia, dizziness, headache, confusion, weakness, overstimulation including increased anxiety, constipation, gastrointestinal disturbances, edema, dry mouth, weight gain, and sexual disturbances.

Drug Interactions Common to MAOIs

Hypertensive crises with MAOIs have occurred in patients following ingestion of foods containing significant amounts of tyramine. In general, patients taking MAOIs should avoid protein foods that have undergone breakdown by aging, fermentation, pickling, smoking, or bacterial contamination. Some of the common foods to avoid are shown in Table 11.16. Excessive amounts of caffeine also reportedly may precipitate hypertensive crisis. Similarly, patients should not take sympathomimetic drugs (e.g., amphetamines, methylphenidate, epinephrine). The combination of MAOIs and tryptophan has been reported to cause neurological and behavioral toxicities including disorientation, confusion, amnesia, delirium, agitation, in addition to several other effects. Serious reactions can also occur when MAOIs are taken with serotonergic drugs.

The MAOIs interfere with the hepatic metabolism of many prescription and nonprescription (over-the-counter) drugs and may potentiate the actions of their pharmacological effects (i.e., cold decongestants, sympathomimetic amines, general anesthetics, barbiturates, and morphine).

Table 11.16 Foods to Be Avoided due to Potential Monoamine Oxidase Inhibitor-Food Interactions

Cheeses	Cheddar	**Meats**	Chicken livers
	Camembert		Genoa salami
	Stilton		Hard salami
	Processed cheese		Pepperoni
	Sour cream		Lebanon bologna
Spirits	Alcohol should be avoided	**Fruit**	Figs (over-ripe/canned)
			Raisins
			Overripe bananas
Fish	Pickled herring	**Dairy product**	Yogurt
	Anchovies	**Vegetable products**	Yeast extract
	Caviar		Pods-broad beans
Miscellaneous	Shrimp paste		Bean curd
	Chocolate		Soy sauce
	Meat tender-izers (papaya)		Avocado

Therapeutic Uses Common to MAOIs

The MAOIs are indicated in patients with atypical (exogenous) depression and in some patients who are unresponsive to other antidepressive therapy. They rarely are a drug of first choice. Unlabeled uses have included bulimia (having characteristics of atypical depression), treatment of cocaine addiction (phenelzine), night terrors, posttraumatic stress disorder, migraines resistant to other therapies, seasonal affective disorder (30 mg/d), and treatment of some panic disorders.

A list of information that should be transmitted to the patient concerning use of MAOIs is shown in Table 11.17.

Nonselective MAOI Antidepressants

PHENELZINE. Phenelzine is a hydrazine MAOI (Fig. 11.53). Its mechanism of action is the prolonged, irreversible inhibition of MAO-A and MAO-B. Phenelzine has been used with some success in the management of bulimia nervosa. The MAOIs, however, are potentially dangerous in patients with binge eating and purging behaviors, and the American Psychiatric Association states that MAOIs should be used with caution in the management of bulimia nervosa.

Limited information is available regarding MAOI pharmacokinetics of phenelzine (Table 11.18). Phenelzine appears to be well absorbed following oral administration; however, maximal inhibition of MAO occurs within 5-10 days. Acetylation of phenelzine to its inactive acetylated metabolite appears to be a minor metabolic pathway.[257] Phenelzine is a substrate as well as an inhibitor of MAO, and major identified metabolites of phenelzine include phenylacetic acid and *p*-hydroxyphenylacetic acid. Phenelzine also elevates brain GABA levels, probably via its β-phenylethylamine metabolite. The clinical effects of phenelzine may continue for up to 2 weeks after discontinuation of therapy. Phenelzine is excreted in the urine mostly as its N-acetyl metabolite.[257] Interindividual variability in plasma concentrations have been observed among patients who are either slow or fast acetylators. Slow acetylators of hydrazine MAOIs may yield exaggerated adverse effects

Table 11.17 Common Information for Patients Taking Monoamine Oxidase Inhibitors (MAOIs)

Patient Information	Recommendation
Discontinuance of therapy or dose adjustment	Consult physician
Adding medication (prescription/over-the-counter)	Consult physician
Tyramine-containing foods and over-the-counter products	Avoid
Drowsiness, blurred vision	Avoid driving or performing tasks requiring alertness or coordination
Dizziness, weakness, fainting	Arise from sitting position slowly
Alcohol use	Avoid alcohol
Onset of action	Effects may be delayed for a few weeks
Severe headache, palpitation, tachycardia, sense of constriction in throat or chest, sweating, stiff neck, nausea or vomiting	Consult physician
New physician or dentist	Inform practitioner of MAOI use

after standard dosing. If adverse neurological reactions occur during phenelzine therapy, phenelzine-induced pyridoxine deficiency should be considered. Pyridoxine supplementation can correct the deficiency while allowing continuance of phenelzine therapy.

TRANYLCYPROMINE. Tranylcypromine is a nonhydrazine, irreversible MAOI antidepressant agent that was designed as the cyclopropyl analogue of amphetamine (Fig. 11.53). Instead of exhibiting amphetamine-like stimulation, its mechanism of action is nonselective, irreversible inhibition of MAO. Its onset of antidepressant action is more rapid than for phenelzine. Tranylcypromine is well absorbed following oral administration (Table 11.18). Metabolism occurs via aromatic ring hydroxylation and N-acetylation. It is a competitive inhibitor of CYP2C19 and CYP2D6 and a noncompetitive inhibitor of CYP2C9.[257] Most metabolism studies suggest that tranylcypromine is not metabolized to amphetamine contrary to debate. Maximal MAO inhibition, however, occurs within 5-10 days. The gastrointestinal absorption of the tranylcypromine shows interindividual variation and may be biphasic in some individuals, achieving an initial peak within approximately 1 hour and a secondary peak within 2-3 hours. It has been suggested that this apparent biphasic absorption in some individuals may represent different absorption rates. Following discontinuance of tranylcypromine, the drug is excreted within 24 hours. On withdrawal of tranylcypromine, MAO activity is recovered in 3-5 days (possibly in up to 10 d). Concentrations of urinary tryptamine, an indicator of MAO-A inhibition return to normal, however, within 72-120 hours.

Mood Stabilizers

Mood stabilizers have acute and long-term effects and, at a minimum, are prophylactic for manic or depressive disorders. Lithium is the classic mood stabilizer and exhibits significant effects on mania and depression but may be augmented or substituted by some antiepileptic drugs. The biochemical basis for mood stabilizer therapies or the molecular origins of bipolar disorder is unknown. Lithium can reduce excitatory (glutamate) and increase inhibitory (GABA) neurotransmission. Lithium ions directly inhibit two signal transduction pathways. It suppresses inositol trisphosphate signaling through depletion of intracellular myo-inositol (lithium blocks inositol monophosphatase, which is necessary to produce myo-inositol) and inhibits glycogen synthase kinase-3, a multifunctional protein kinase. A number of glycogen synthase kinase-3 substrates are involved in neuronal function and organization and, therefore, present plausible targets for manic-depression. Despite these intriguing observations, it remains unclear how changes in inositol trisphosphate signaling underlie the origins of bipolar disorder.[258]

Myo-inositol, a naturally occurring isomer of glucose, is a key intermediate of the phosphatidylinositol signaling pathway, a second messenger system used by many GPCRs, including noradrenergic, serotonergic, and cholinergic receptors. It has been suggested that lithium might treat mania via its reduction of myo-inositol levels, which would indirectly desensitize hyperactive receptors.[259] Valproic acid and carbamazepine are antiepileptic drugs with mood-stabilizing properties that also inhibit inositol trisphosphate signaling.

Table 11.18 Pharmacokinetics of the Monoamine Oxidase Inhibitors (MAOIs)

Parameters	Phenelzine (Nardil)	Tranylcypromine (Parnate)
Oral bioavailability (%)	NA	~50
Lipophilicity (Log $D_{7.4}$)	0.51	0.46
Protein binding (%)		NA
Volume of distribution (L/kg)	NA	1.1-5.7
Elimination half-life (hr)	NA	79
Peak plasma concentration (hr)	2-3	1.5 (0.7-3.5)
Excretion route	Urine	Urine 62
		Feces

NA, not available.

Paroxetine —CYP2D6→ *o*-Quinoid metabolite of paroxetine

Paroxetine

Lithium

Lithium (from the Greek word *lithos*, meaning "stone") is a monovalent cation that competes with sodium, potassium, calcium, and magnesium ions at intracellular binding sites; at sugar phosphatases; at protein surfaces; at carrier binding sites; and at transport sites. Because of its small ionic size, lithium ion (Li^+) readily passes through sodium channels of cellular membranes and high concentrations can block the narrow potassium channels during impulse conduction. In the 1870s, claims for the healthful effects of Li^+ fueled the markets for products such as Lithia Beer and Lithia Springs Mineral Water. [In 1887, analysis of Lithia Springs Mineral Water proved the water to be rich not only in Li^+ but also in potassium, calcium, magnesium, fluoride, and other essential trace minerals.] In 1890, the Lithia Springs Sanitorium (Georgia) was established using natural lithium water to treat alcoholism, opium addiction, and compulsive behavior, even though manic depression had not been identified as a form of mental illness until the early 1900s.

Lithium's mood-stabilizing properties were revitalized in the 1940s when an Australian physician, John Cade, hypothesized that a toxin in the blood was responsible for bipolar illness. Believing that uric acid would protect individuals from this toxin, he began studying the effects of a mixture of uric acid and Li^+ in rats. Lithium carbonate was used to dissolve the uric acid. He observed a calming effect of this combination on the rats and subsequently determined that the Li^+, rather than the uric acid, was responsible for this calming effect. He then speculated that lithium might be useful in humans as a mood attenuator, subsequently administered lithium to a sample of patients with bipolar disorder and discovered that Li^+ not only decreased the symptoms of mania but also prevented the recurrence of both depression and mania when taken regularly by these patients. After a decade of clinical trials, the FDA approved lithium for treatment of mania in 1970.[259,260]

Lithium carbonate (Eskalith) is the most commonly used salt of lithium to treat manic depression. Lithium carbonate dosage forms are labeled in mg and mEq/dosage unit, and lithium citrate (Lithobid) is labeled as mg equivalent to lithium carbonate and mEq/dosage unit. Lithium is effectively used to control and prevent manic episodes in 70%-80% of those with bipolar disorder as well as to treat other forms of depression. Those who respond to lithium for depression often are those who have not responded to TCAs after several weeks of treatment. When giving lithium in addition to their antidepressants, some of these people have shown significant improvement.

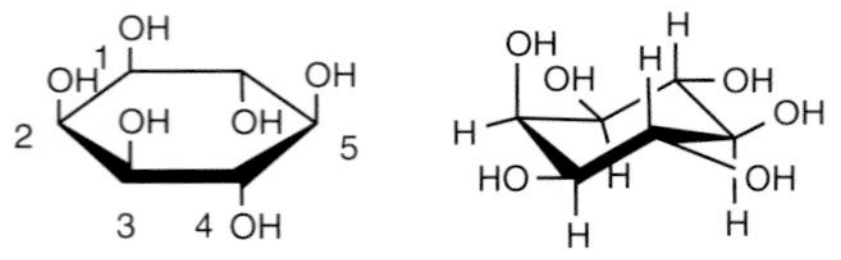

myo - Inositol

MECHANISM OF ACTION. Lithium therapy for disorders is believed to be effective because of its ability to reduce signal transduction through the phosphatidylinositol signaling pathway (Fig. 11.54).[259,260] In this pathway, the second messengers diacylglycerol and inositol 1,4,5-trisphosphate are produced from the enzymatic hydrolysis of phosphatidylinositol-4,5-bisphosphate (a membrane phospholipid) by the receptor-mediated activation of the membrane-bound, phosphatidylinositol-specific phospholipase C. The second messenger activity for inositol 1,4,5-trisphosphate is terminated by its hydrolysis in three steps by inositol monophosphatases to inactive myo-inositol, thus completing the signaling pathway. To recharge the signaling pathway, myo-inositol must be recycled back to phosphatidylinositol bisphosphate by inositol phospholipid–synthesizing enzymes in the CNS, because myo-inositol is unable to cross the blood-brain barrier in sufficient concentrations to maintain the signaling pathway. By uncompetitive inhibition of inositol phosphatases in the signaling pathway, the therapeutic plasma concentrations of lithium ion deplete the pool of myo-inositol available for the resynthesis of phosphatidylinositol-4,5-bisphosphate, ultimately decreasing its cellular levels and, thereby, reducing the enzymatic formation of the second messengers. Thus, Li^+ restores the balance among aberrant signaling pathways in critical regions of the brain.

The clinical efficacy of lithium in the prophylaxis of recurrent affective episodes in bipolar disorder is characterized by a lag in onset and remains for weeks to months after discontinuation. Thus, the long-term therapeutic effect of lithium likely requires neuroplastic changes involving alterations in gene expression. Protein kinase C and glycogen synthase kinase-3 signal transduction pathways are perturbed by chronic lithium at therapeutically relevant concentrations and have been implicated in modulating synaptic function in nerve terminals.[260]

PHARMACOKINETICS. The absorption of Li^+ is rapid and complete within 6-8 hours. The absorption rate of slow-release capsules is slower and the total amount of Li^+ absorbed is lower than with other dosage forms. Li^+ is not protein bound. The elimination half-life for elderly patients (39 hr) is longer than that for adult patients (24 hr), which in turn is longer than that for adolescent patients (18 hr). The time to peak serum concentration for lithium carbonate is dependent on the dosage form (tablets, 1-3 hr; extended tab, 4 hr; slow release, 3 hr). Steady-state serum concentrations are reached in 4 days, with the desirable dose targeted to give a maintenance Li^+ plasma concentration range of 0.6-1.2 mEq/L, with a level of 0.5 mEq/L for elderly patients. The risk of bipolar recurrence was approximately threefold greater for patients with Li^+ dosages that gave plasma concentrations of 0.4-0.6 mEq/L. Adverse reactions are frequent at therapeutic doses and adherence is a big problem. Toxic reactions are rare at serum Li^+ levels of less than 1.5 mEq/L. Mild to moderate toxic reactions may occur at levels from 1.5 to 2.5 mEq/L and severe reactions may be seen at levels from 2.0 to 2.5 mEq/L, depending on individual response. The onset of therapeutic action for clinical improvement is 1-3 weeks. Renal elimination of Li^{+1} is 95%, with 80% actively reabsorbed in the proximal tubule. The rate of Li^+ urinary excretion decreases with age. Fecal elimination is less than 1%.

DRUG INTERACTIONS. Lithium pharmacokinetics may be influenced by a number of factors, including age. Elderly patients require lower doses of Li^+ to achieve serum concentrations similar to those observed in younger adults as a result of reduced volume of distribution and reduced renal clearance. Li^+ clearance decreases as the glomerular

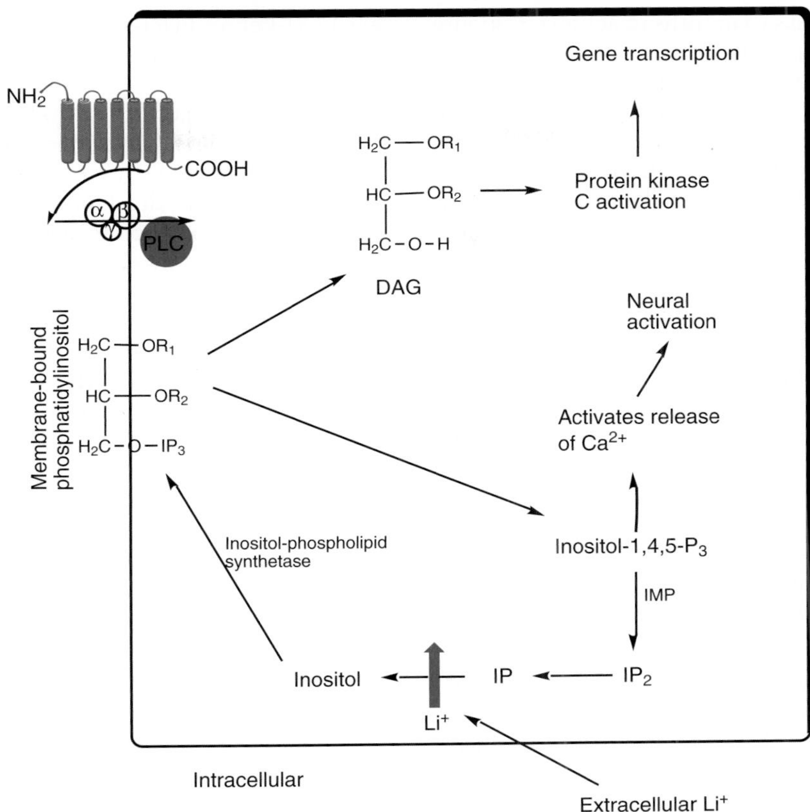

Figure 11.54 Intracellular phosphatidylinositol signaling pathway and site of action for lithium. Phospholipase (PLC) is a membrane-bound enzyme. *DAG*, diacylglyceride; *IMP*, inositol monophosphatase; *IP*, inositol monophosphate.

filtration rate decreases with increasing age. Reduced Li^+ clearance is expected in patients with hypertension, congestive heart failure, or renal dysfunction. Larger Li^+ maintenance doses are required in obese compared with nonobese patients. The most clinically significant pharmacokinetic drug interactions associated with lithium involve drugs that are commonly used in the elderly and that can increase serum Li^+ concentrations. People who are taking lithium should consult their physician before taking the following drugs: acetazolamide, antihypertensives, angiotensin-converting enzyme inhibitors, nonsteroidal anti-inflammatory drugs, calcium channel blockers, carbamazepine, thiazide diuretics, hydroxyzine, muscle relaxants, neuroleptics, table salt, baking powder, tetracycline, TCAs, MAOIs, and caffeine. The tolerability of lithium is lower in elderly patients. Lithium toxicity can occur in the elderly at concentrations considered to be therapeutic in the general adult populations. Serum concentrations of Li^+ ion need to be markedly reduced in the elderly population—and particularly so in the very old and frail.

Adverse Effects. Common side effects of Li^+ include nausea, loss of appetite, and mild diarrhea, which usually taper off within first few weeks. Dizziness and hand tremors also have been reported. Increased production of urine and excessive thirst are two common side effects that usually are not serious problems, but patients with kidney disease should not be given Li^{+1}. Taking the day's dosage of Li^+ at bedtime also seems to help with the problem of increased urination. Other side effects of Li^+ include weight gain, hypothyroidism, increased white blood cell count, skin rashes, and birth defects.[259,260]

While on Li^+, a patient's blood level must be closely monitored. If the blood level of Li^+ is too low, the patient's symptoms will not be relieved. If the blood level of lithium ion is too high, there is a danger of a toxic reaction including impairments in kidney function.

Therapeutic Uses. For many years, lithium has been the treatment of choice for bipolar disorder because it can be effective in smoothing out the mood swings common to this condition. Its use must be carefully monitored, however, because the range between an effective and a toxic dose is small.

Nonmonoaminergic Antidepressants

N-Methyl-D-Aspartate Receptor Antagonists

In spite of intensive research, the problem of treating antidepressant-resistant patients and that existing treatments for MDD usually take weeks to months to achieve response and remission of their depression has not yet been solved. The past decade has seen a steady accumulation of evidence supporting a role for the excitatory amino acid neurotransmitter, glutamate, and many of its receptors, most notably mGluR1/5, α-amino-3-hydroxy-5-methyl-4-isoxazolepropionic acid (AMPA), and NMDA, in depression and antidepressant activity.[261,262] Antagonists of mGluR1 and mGluR5 receptors, as well as PAMs of AMPA receptors, show antidepressant-like activity in a variety of preclinical models. Furthermore, evidence implicates disturbances in glutamate metabolism, NMDA and mGluR1/5 receptors in depression and suicidality.

cis-1-Phenyl-2-[1-aminopropyl]-N,N-diethylcyclopropanecarboxamide, an NMDA receptor antagonist and homologue of milnacipran, produces sustained relief from depressive symptoms. Several studies have shown that chronic antidepressant treatment can modulate NMDA receptor expression and function. Preclinical studies with this and other NMDA receptor antagonists have demonstrated their potential antidepressant properties.[262]

KETAMINE. Ketamine acts primarily as a noncompetitive NMDA receptor antagonist, but many studies purport additional pharmacodynamic effects. In addition to its dissociative anesthetic effects, it shows properties of being a rapid-acting antidepressant. (*S*)-ketamine or (*S*)-(+)-ketamine (esketamine) is approximately twice as potent as an anesthetic as (±)-ketamine (ketalar).[263] It is eliminated from the human body more quickly than *R*(−)-ketamine (arketamine) and (±)-ketamine. In studies in mice, the rapid antidepressant effect of arketamine was greater and lasted longer than that of esketamine or the metabolite (2*R*,6*R*)-hydroxynorketamine (HNK); though, no human clinical trial has compared the antidepressant efficacy of esketamine and arketamine, or the antidepressant actions of arketamine.[263,264]

Esketamine has an affinity for the PCP binding site of the NMDA receptor three to four times greater than that of arketamine. Esketamine was introduced for medical use in Germany in 1997 and was subsequently marketed in other countries. Esketamine nasal spray approved by the FDA (in conjunction with an oral antidepressant), for the treatment of treatment-resistant depression in 2019, provided the first new mechanism of action in 30 years to treat this debilitating mental illness. Esketamine nasal spray will be self-administered by patients under the supervision of health care professionals.[265]

KETAMINE PHARMACOKINETICS. (*R*,*S*)-Ketamine ((*R*,*S*)-ket) is extensively metabolized[266,267] involving enantioselective N-demethylation to (*R*,*S*)-norketamine (*R*,*S*)-norket) by human liver microsomes (HLM) and confirmed by expressed CYPs (Fig. 11.55). The N-demethylation of (*S*)-ket to (*S*)-norket is greater than that of (*R*)-ket to (*R*)-norket. The CYPs associated with the metabolic N-demethylation of (*R*,*S*)-ket to (*R*,*S*)-norket are primarily 2B6 with some contribution of CYP2A6 and CYP3A4/5. Expressed studies with (*S*)-ket and (*R*)-ket suggest that CYP3A4/5 plays a greater role in the metabolic clearance of (*R*)-ket than (*S*)-ket.

(*R*,*S*)-norket is further transformed regio- and enantioselectively into a series of diastereomeric HNK metabolites arising from hydroxylation of the cyclohexanone ring at the C6, C5, and C4 positions, with (*S*)-hydroxylation being preferred at these positions. (*R*,*S*)-norket hydroxylation is enantioselective and regioselective with (*S*)-norket preferentially converted to (2*S*,6*S*) and (2*S*,6*R*)-HNK (2a, Fig. 11.55) and to (2*R*,6*S*)-and (2*R*,6*R*)-HNK diastereomer (2b). The CYP isoforms associated with the regio- and enantioselective 6-hydroxylation of (*R*,*S*)-norket have demonstrated that the *S*-hydroxylation is mediated primarily by CYP2B6 and CYP2A6.

The enantioselective hydroxylation of (*S*)-ket predominates relative to (*R*)-ket. Thus, the primary HK diastereomeric metabolite from the HLM incubation of (*R*,*S*)-ket is (2*S*,6*S*)-HK and (2*R*,6*S*) HK, respectively (1a,1b). With expressed enzymes, (*R*)- and (*S*)-ket were hydroxylated into the HK diastereomers with the formation of (2*R*,6*S*)-HK diastereomer (1b) slightly favored relative to the (2*S*,6*R*)-HK diastereomer (1a). The expressed CYP isoforms associated with the regio- and enantioselective 6- hydroxylation of (*R*,*S*)-ket have demonstrated that the 6*S*-hydroxylation is primarily mediated by CYP2B6 and CYP2A6, and minor contribution from CYP3A4/5. Regio hydroxylation at the 6 position is the preferred site of hydroxylation because of C-H activation by the adjacent 1-ketone group. The HK diastereomers are further transformed by N-demethylation into the corresponding HNK diastereomers, 2a and 2b. The 4-HNK and 5-HNK diastereomers are found in minor amounts which indicate that the incubation of (*R*,*S*)-ket with HLMs also produced phenolic metabolites.

The rates of formation of 1a and 1b diastereomers with expressed CYP3A4/5 suggest their greater role in the metabolic clearance of (*R*)-ket than (*S*)-ket. The formation of 1a,1b is enantioselective with the hydroxylation of (*S*)-ket predominating relative to (*R*)-ket and that the reaction is enantiospecific producing primarily an *S*-configuration at the C6 carbinol. Thus, the primary HK metabolite from the expressed incubation of (*S*)-ket with 2B6 is (2*S*,6*S*)-HK (1a). (*R*,*S*)-ket was hydroxylated into the HNK diastereomers, 2a and 2b, with the formation of (2*R*,6*S*)-HNK slightly favored relative to the (2*S*,6*R*)-HNK diasteromer.

(*R*,*S*)-ket is also transformed into the enantiomeric 5,6-dehydroketamine ((*R*,*S*)-DHK), and the expressed results suggest that DHK is derived from 5-HK produced by CYP2B6-mediated hydroxylation at the C5 position on the cyclohexanone ring of (*R*,*S*)-ket. The primary isoform associated with the formation of the phenolic metabolite from (*R*,*S*)-ket was CYP2C9, while FMO appeared to be the major factor in the formation of this metabolite from (*S*)-ket.

The metabolic transformations observed in the in vitro HLM studies are consistent with the metabolism and

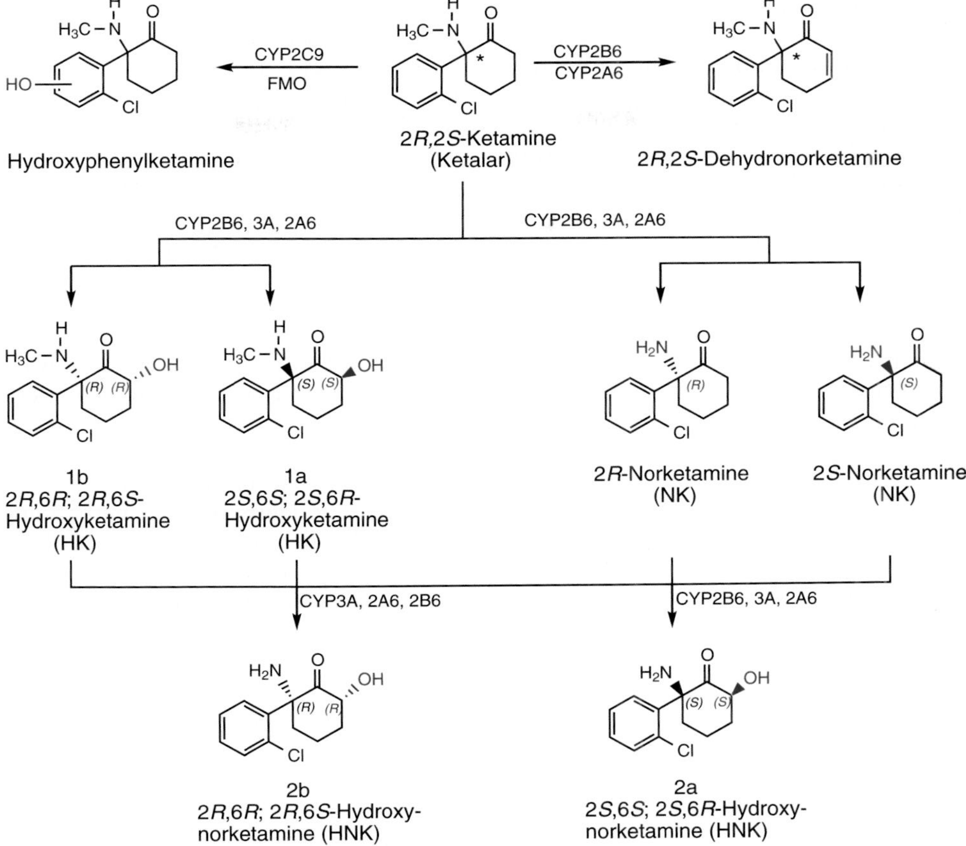

Figure 11.55 Metabolism of ketamine.

disposition of (*R*,*S*)-ket determined in clinical studies. (*R*,*S*)-ket, (*R*,*S*)-norket, and (*R*,*S*)-DHNK were identified in plasma samples obtained from patients receiving (*R*,*S*)-ket, and all of the major metabolites of (*R*,*S*)-ket were identified in urine samples from a single 50 mg oral dose of (*R*,*S*)-ket.

The most typical route of administration is via IV infusion, which rapidly attains maximum plasma concentrations 5-30 minutes after administration. Oral bioavailability of (±)-ketamine is 16%-29%, with peak concentration levels of the drug occurring within 20-120 minutes because of extensive first-pass hepatic metabolism. Oral bioavailability of (*S*)-(+)-ketamine is 8%-11% with greater first-pass metabolism. Intranasal bioavailability is 45%-50%. Oral bioavailability of (2*S*,6*S*)-HNK was estimated to be 46.3% in rats and mice; the oral bioavailability of (2*R*,6*R*)-HNK is estimated to be approximately 50%

(±)-Ketamine is rapidly distributed into the brain, with protein binding of approximately 50%, resulting in a large steady-state volume of distribution (Vd = 3-5 L/kg). A single IV bolus administration of an anesthetic dose of (±)-ketamine in humans (2 mg/kg) leads to equal plasma concentrations of (*S*)-ketamine and (*R*)-ketamine 1 minute post-administration. Although plasma levels of (±)-ketamine are below detectable limits within 1 day following an IV antidepressant dose (40-minute infusion), circulating levels of *2R,6R- and 2S,6S*-HNK were observed for up to 3 days after (±)-ketamine infusion in patients diagnosed with bipolar depression. Norketamine was detectable for up to 14 in the urine of children.[263-265] A short elimination half-life (155-158 min) was demonstrated for both (*S*)-ketamine and (*R*)-ketamine. Elimination of (±)-ketamine is primarily performed by the kidneys. The majority of the drug (80%) is excreted as glucuronide conjugates of HK and HNK in urine and bile. In adult humans, the IV terminal plasma half-life was 186 minutes and intramuscular half-life was 155 minutes.

Utility of Ketamine's Hydroxynorketamine Metabolites as Drug Treatments[266]. It has been reported that metabolism of ketamine is necessary for its full antidepressant action in mice. Specific metabolites (2*S*,6*S*)-HNK, and (2*R*,6*R*)-HNK, derived from the metabolism of (*S*)-ketamine and (*R*)-ketamine, respectively, do not bind to or inhibit the NMDA receptor at antidepressant-relevant concentrations, but exert antidepressant behavioral effects similar to those observed following administration of ketamine itself. These observations challenge the NMDA receptor inhibition hypothesis of ketamine's antidepressant actions. In addition, (2*R*,6*R*)-HNK exerts antidepressant effects without the sensory dissociation, ataxia, and abuse liability of ketamine in animal tests.

The recent findings that ketamine metabolites may be involved in the antidepressant actions of ketamine suggest the possible use of these metabolites in the treatment of depression and open new paths for investigating their role in other brain disorders.[266] This may provide a framework for a novel ketamine metabolite paradigm, which posits clinically relevant effects dependent upon metabolic conversion of ketamine, but not dependent on NMDA receptor inhibition. Nevertheless, future studies are needed to support the contention that NMDA receptor inhibition is not required for the effectiveness of ketamine's metabolites as fast-acting antidepressants and to identify the underlying mechanism of action of these metabolites.

Herbal Therapy

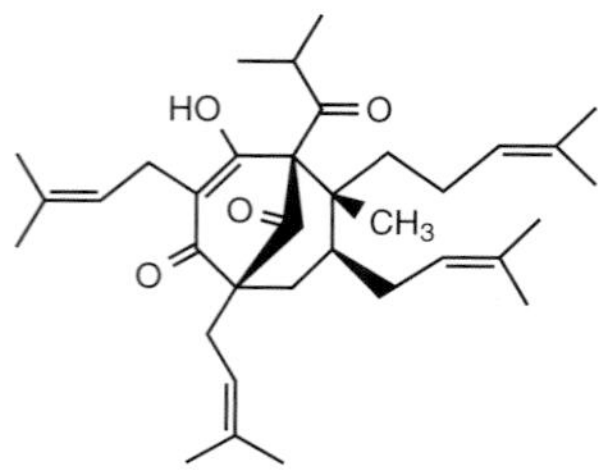

HO O O CH3 O

Hyperforin

In the past few years, much interest has been generated regarding the use of herbs in the treatment of both depression and anxiety.[268] Recent studies, however, have revealed potentially fatal interactions between herbal remedies and traditional drugs.

St. John's wort (*Hypericum perforatum*), an herb used extensively in the treatment of mild to moderate depression in Europe, aroused interest in the United States.[269] A bushy, low-growing plant covered with yellow flowers in summer, St. John's wort has been used for centuries in many folk and herbal remedies. The scientific studies that have been conducted regarding its use have been short-term, however, and have used several different doses. Preclinical studies report that high doses of extracts from St. John's wort increase DA and 5-HT levels in the frontal cortex.

Ingestion of St John's wort increases the expression (i.e., upregulation) of intestinal P-glycoprotein and of CYP3A4 in the liver and intestine, which impairs the absorption and stimulates the metabolism of other CYP3A4 substrates (e.g., the protease inhibitors indinavir and nevirapine, oral contraceptives, and TCAs [e.g., amitriptyline]), resulting in their subtherapeutic plasma levels.[115] Hyperforin, the principal component in St. John's wort (2%-4% in the fresh herb), contributes to the induction of CYP3A4. Some studies suggest that it not only inhibits the neuronal reuptake of 5-HT, and DA but also inhibits GABA and L-glutamate uptake. This broad-spectrum effect is obtained by an elevation of the intracellular sodium ion concentration, probably resulting from activation of sodium conductive pathways not yet finally identified but most likely to be ion channels.[269] Hypericin, the other component in St. John's wort, also may exhibit inhibitor action on key neuroreceptors and may be responsible for the phototoxicity/photosensitivity of St. John's wort.

The National Institutes of Health conducted a double-blind, 3-year study in patients with MDD with moderate severity using St. John's wort and sertraline. This study did not support the use of St. John's wort in the treatment of MDD, but a possible role for St. John's wort in the treatment of milder forms of depression was suggested. Health care providers should alert their patients about potential drug interactions with St. John's Wort. Some other frequently used herbal supplements that have not been evaluated in large-scale clinical trials are ephedra, ginkgo biloba, echinacea, and ginseng. Any herbal supplement should be taken only after consultation with the physician or other health care provider.

Mechanisms underlying the efficacy of ECT are unclear, but likely involve modulation of several neurotransmitter systems.

Drugs Used to Treat Alzheimer's Dementia

I don't remember your name, but I do know you're someone I love.

Alzheimer's patient

Introduction

As a rule, disease is a universally unwelcomed reality of life, but a few diagnoses pack an emotional (and potentially financial) punch that deeply impacts not only patients, but also their loved ones for years or decades to come. Alzheimer's dementia (AD) is such a diagnosis. According to the Alzheimer's Association,[271] in 2018 almost 6 million U.S. citizens were living with this diagnosis and being cared for by an estimated 16 million unpaid providers. It was the sixth leading cause of death and cost the U.S. health care system approximately $277 billion (with 22% being "out of pocket" expense), a figure predicted to increase to $1.1 trillion by 2050 as patient numbers rise to over 14 million.

Etiology

AD accounts for 60%-80% of all dementia,[272,273] with the vast majority of these cases being sporadic (SAD) versus the 1%-2% caused by genetic mutation.[274] While SAD can involve predisposing genetic factors (specifically one or more apolipoprotein E ε4 alleles), mutation-driven AD is associated with genetic alterations in amyloid precursor protein (APP) or presenilin (PS1 or PS2).[274] Known as familial Alzheimer's dementia (FAD), this aggressive form of the disease commonly presents earlier in life and progresses more rapidly than SAD. Both forms are pathologically characterized by the deposition of extracellular plaques or soluble oligomers composed of amyloid-beta peptide (Aβ), as well as the formation of intracellular neurofibrillary tangles made up of an atypical protein kinase–generated hyperphosphorylated tau protein (p-tau) that is normally associated with microtubular assembly.[272,274]

In healthy individuals, soluble α-helical peptides that promote neuronal survival are produced via cleavage of APP by α- or β-secretases. In contrast, AD patients produce insoluble Aβ through sequential cleavage of APP by β- and γ-secretase, producing aberrant proteins with an unnatural β-sheet structure. Aβ is self-propagating, as the circulating protein stimulates further production in other cells it encounters, with subsequent neurotoxicity and neuronal death.[275] Disappointingly, γ-secretase inhibitors developed as novel anti-Alzheimer's therapy yielded poor results in clinical trials and, in some cases, increased skin cancer risk.[274]

Sustained cytosolic Ca^{2+} signaling pathway derangement, which precedes the formation of Aβ plaques and p-tau tangles, has been hypothesized to potentially play a causative role in disease development.[274] Ca^{2+} dyshomeostasis within lysosomes, mitochondria, and endoplasmic reticulum may be the most impactful to AD pathogenesis, although much research remains to be conducted before a clear understanding of clinical relevance is gained.

Pathology and Approaches to Treatment

The preclinical or silent phase of AD can be as long as 20 years, during which time visible cognitive changes are nonexistent or mild (prodromal AD). The first overt symptoms generally arise from entorhinal cortex and hippocampal neuronal atrophy that results in short-term memory loss, an inability to recall familiar names, places and/or events, and a depressed and/or apathetic affect. Attention, concentration, planning, problem-solving, and completing tasks become impaired. Other symptoms include language problems, such as recalling words, and declines in vocabulary, speech, and writing. Judgment also becomes impaired, and patients often start to withdraw from social engagements. As the disease progresses, patients experience more profound cognitive and communicative dysfunctions, confusion, behavioral and personality changes, and may ultimately lose the ability to walk and/or swallow.[271] A total of five drugs have received FDA approval to treat Alzheimer's symptoms, and one (tacrine) was discontinued in 2013 due to an unacceptable hepatotoxicity risk. Despite the clinical development and testing of hundreds of potential candidates, the last symptom-targeting drug currently available (memantine) was approved in 2003.[273]

Without a defined path to cure, disease management is aimed primarily at attenuating symptoms and slowing progression, with much effort focused on prevention.[272] Primary prevention strategies seek to minimize disease acquisition risk through healthy diet and lifestyle choices, fostering cardiovascular health, and encouraging ongoing educational enrichment and mental stimulation. Secondary prevention seeks to forestall disease progression before significant loss of cognitive function; strategies including nutritional guidance, exercise, social and mental engagement, and cardiovascular risk factor management are being studied.

Chemical entities that complement and/or synergize with secondary prevention strategies to provide a sustained arrest in disease progression are now drawing the scientific attention of medicinal chemists involved in anti-Alzheimer's drug design and development programs.[273] Known as disease-modifying treatments (DMTs), these neuroprotective agents target processes including Aβ plaque and p-tau toxicity, chronic neuroinflammatory and oxidative damage, and mitochondrial and myelination dysfunction with the ultimate goal of preserving cells and synapses.[276] Others are calling for research that sheds critical light on the "proximal origin" of the disorder so that drugs that selectively home in on rational targets can be made available.[274] There is hope that novel and effective treatment strategies, including stem cell therapy,[275] immunotherapy,[277] molecular chaperones,[277] and nutraceuticals,[278,279] will emerge from these efforts to help those diagnosed with AD live longer and more highly functional lives. Health economic modeling of promising new therapies should ensure large study populations are followed throughout the entire AD pathological continuum so that short-term findings can better predict long-term outcomes.[273]

Pharmacotherapy

Figure 11.56 provides the structures of the four anti-AD drugs currently marketed in the United States, three structurally distinct acetylcholinesterase (AChE) inhibitors (donepezil, galantamine, rivastigmine) and one N-methyl-D-aspartate (NMDA) receptor antagonist (memantine).

The neurotransmitter acetylcholine (ACh) is critical to cognition, and inhibiting the esterase that inactivates it is one approach to elevating the significantly diminished levels of functional transmitter in central cholinergic neurons in the basal forebrain of AD patients.[279,280] AChE inhibitors are generally recommended in the early stages of the disease when patients are exhibiting mild-moderate symptoms.[274,280] Other approaches to augmenting ACh in cognitively impaired brains have been tried (specifically ACh precursors and synthetic muscarinic agonists) but they were not successful, primarily due to challenging pharmacokinetic and/or adverse effect profiles.[280] As the disease progresses, patients are subject to neuronal destruction via the overstimulation of NMDA receptors by the excitatory neurotransmitter glutamate. NMDA receptors are intimately involved in learning and memory, and by antagonizing these receptors, memantine blocks glutamate-induced excitotoxicity in patients with moderate-severe disease.[274,279]

Selected pharmacokinetic parameters of these four agents are provided in Table 11.19.[281] All are administered orally in immediate or extended release formulations, and rivastigmine is also available in a transdermal patch dosage form.

Acetylcholinesterase Inhibitors

AChE's catalytic site contains a Ser203 residue activated for nucleophilic attack at ACh's electrophilic carbonyl carbon through an intramolecular association with a His447 and Glu334 (residue numbers for the human enzyme).[282,283] Although contained within a deeply recessed active site,

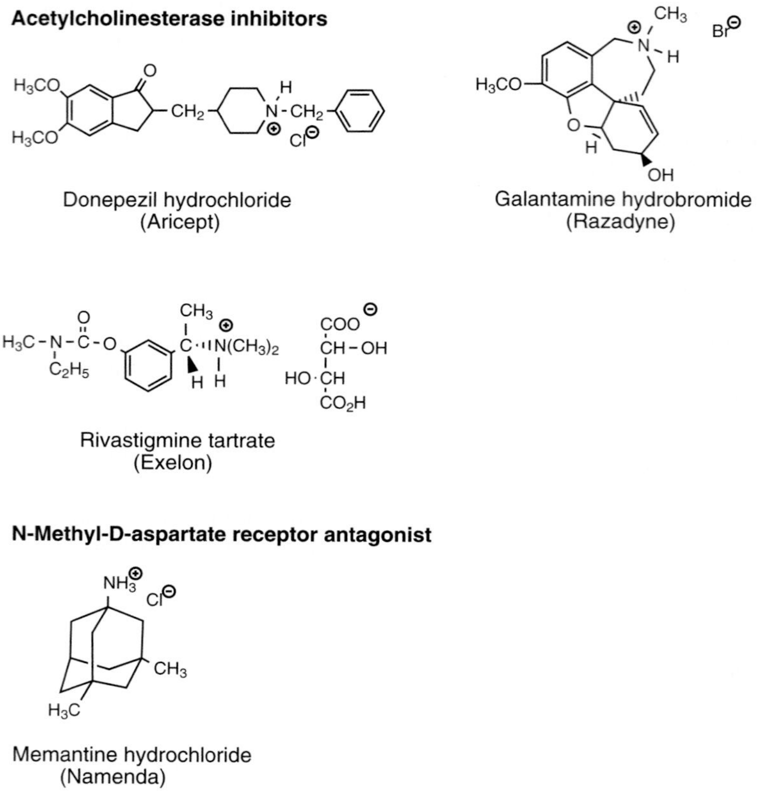

Acetylcholinesterase inhibitors

Donepezil hydrochloride (Aricept)

Galantamine hydrobromide (Razadyne)

Rivastigmine tartrate (Exelon)

N-Methyl-D-aspartate receptor antagonist

Memantine hydrochloride (Namenda)

Figure 11.56 Drugs currently available to treat Alzheimer's dementia.

this catalytic triad is a powerful hydrolyzing "machine," cleaving up to 25,000 ACh molecules per second.[282] Other domains that appropriately orient and hold ACh in place include: (1) an anionic domain which, despite its name, has only aromatic residues that anchor the onium head of ACh through cation-π, interactions, (2) an acyl pocket containing sterically restricting Phe residues that ensure no choline esters larger than ACh can enter, and (3) an oxyanion hole with Gly and Ala residues and one structured water molecule that facilitates enzyme-substrate binding, as well as the tetrahedral hydrolytic transition state.[283]

As noted above, tacrine, the first cholinesterase inhibitor to be marketed in the United States, was discontinued due to reversible hepatotoxicity that was viewed as intolerable when safer options became available. In addition to elevating central levels of ACh, AChE inhibitors also block the cytotoxicity-promoting action of AChE on Aβ aggregation and p-tau hyperphosphorylation, thus decreasing the formation of destructive plaques and neurofibrillary tangles.[279] AChE inhibitors can modestly improve cognition and the ability to engage in the activities of daily living (ADL), but only about 30%-40% of patients respond and the duration of therapeutic benefit is generally limited to 2 years or less.[280] While there is currently no clearly defined way to identify responders prior to therapy, apolipoprotein E ε4 carrier status has been associated with a lack of responsiveness, as this allele appears to thwart compensatory hippocampal cholinergic sprouting in lesion-induced mammalian brain damage designed to mimic early AD.[280]

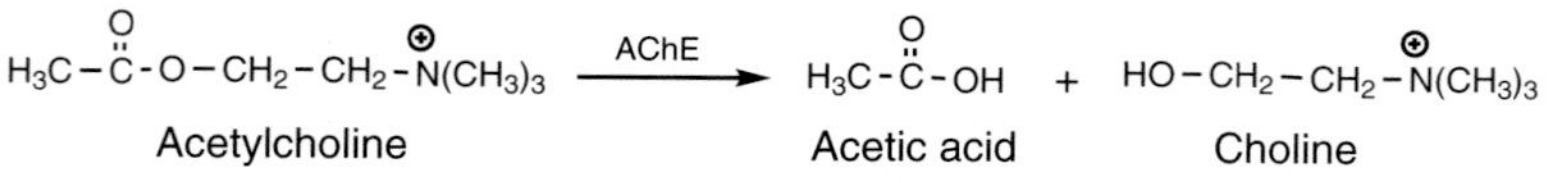

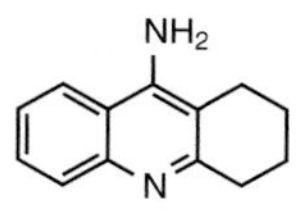

$$H_3C-\overset{O}{\overset{\|}{C}}-O-CH_2-CH_2-\overset{\oplus}{N}(CH_3)_3 \xrightarrow{AChE} H_3C-\overset{O}{\overset{\|}{C}}-OH + HO-CH_2-CH_2-\overset{\oplus}{N}(CH_3)_3$$

Acetylcholine — Acetic acid — Choline

AChEhydrolysis

Tacrine (Cognex)

While no longer considered the "be all and end all" of AD pharmacotherapy, cholinergic augmentation through

AChE inhibition is still proposed to have an important place at the therapeutic table due to its neuroprotective and compensatory neuronal plasticity benefits.[280] Research into the development of new inhibitors is ongoing, and four goals have been recommended to advance therapeutic efficacy: (1) ability to bind to both the catalytic and peripheral sites of the esterase, (2) ability to inhibit both synaptic, membrane-bound AChE and the more ubiquitous, nonspecific and glial-based butyrylcholinesterase (BuChE), which may take over for AChE when the latter enzyme is specifically inhibited, (3) targeted delivery to/activity in the basal forebrain, and (4) attention to the impact/timing of ACh release on presynaptic autoreceptor stimulation (which inhibits further release) and the ability to respond to postsynaptic phasic cholinergic signaling.[280] Combination therapies that couple AChE inhibitors with anti-amyloid, antioxidant and/or anti-inflammatory agents (among others) are also being actively explored, as is the development of highly selective and centrally active M_1 muscarinic receptor agonists that could serve as DMTs.

SPECIFIC DRUGS

Donepezil Hydrochloride. Donepezil was the second AChE inhibitor approved for use in AD and is currently the oldest such drug clinically available. It is chemically classified as a 2-benzylpiperidine-indenone, and structure-activity studies have confirmed that both the basic benzylpiperidine moiety and the indenone C1 carbonyl are essential. Expansion of the cyclopentenone component of the indenone ring to six- or seven-membered systems diminished activity. The aromatic methoxy groups at indenone C5 and C6 increase activity over 25-fold compared to the unsubstituted derivative, and the activity provided by the methylene spacer between rings is second only to propylene. While marketed as the racemic mixture, AChE inhibiting activity resides exclusively in the *R* isomer.[282]

Donepezil binding to the AChE active site is reversible, highly selective (minimal BuChE inhibition occurs), and predominantly noncompetitive. Key interactions with AChE isolated from *Torpedo californica* (electric eel) are shown in Figure 11.57. The essential cationic piperidine nitrogen anchors to Asp72, as well as to Phe330 and Tyr121, the latter bridged through a water molecule. Trp residues engage in affinity-enhancing π-π interactions with both aromatic systems, and another molecule of water links the two methoxy oxygen atoms to anionic Glu185. The carbonyl oxygen serves an orientation function to permit edge-on π-π stacking with Phe331 and Phe290. Three Gly residues and Ser200, again working through water molecules, interface with the aromatic segment of the benzyl moiety.[282] The bound drug is believed to inhibit both the formation of the endogenous enzyme-substrate (ACh) complex and the hydrolysis of any neurotransmitter that finds its way into the catalytic pocket.

In addition to binding at the enzyme's active site, donepezil also interacts within a peripheral anionic site adjacent to the recessed catalytic gorge, which inhibits other nonhydrolytic enzyme functions.[283,284] Aβ is known to bind to this peripheral site, and inhibiting its association with the enzyme protects cholinergic neurons from complex-induced cytotoxicity, as well as minimizes AChE-induced fibrillation of the amyloid protein. Some have postulated neuroprotective effects for donepezil independent of AChE inhibition (including protection against Aβ- and glutamate-induced cell destruction, ischemia, and hippocampal atrophy) that might qualify it as a DMT.[284] Further research on the potentially multifaceted clinical mechanism of donepezil in early to late stage AD is warranted.

As noted in Table 11.19, donepezil is vulnerable to CYP-catalyzed metabolism and is excreted primarily via the kidneys. Only about 15% of the dose found in urine is in parent drug form. CYP2D6 and CYP3A4 are both involved in donepezil biotransformation, and blood levels can be significantly impacted by 2D6 phenotype. The active *R* isomer is metabolized more readily than the inactive *S* enantiomer,[282] but clinically relevant interactions with coadministered drugs are fairly rare due to the generally slow rate of metabolic transformation. However, strong CYP3A4 inhibitors, such as conazole antifungal agents, can significantly elevate serum levels of the drug.

The most prevalent donepezil metabolite (M1) is the 6-phenol (11% of the administered dose), which is essentially equally active with donepezil.[282,285] A minor *p*-hydroxybenzyl metabolite[286] (M3) also exhibits activity on a

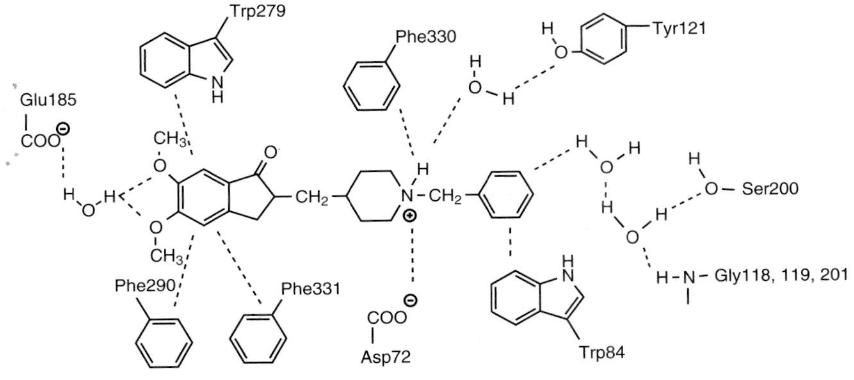

Trp279
Phe330
Tyr121
Glu185
Ser200
Gly118, 119, 201
Phe290
Phe331
Asp72
Trp84

Figure 11.57 Binding interactions between *Torpedo californica* acetylcholinesterase and donepezil.

Table 11.19 Selected Pharmacokinetic Parameters of Anti-Alzheimer's Drugs[a]

Drug	$T_{1/2}$ (hr)	T_{max} (hr)	Protein Binding (%)	Metabolism	Renal Excretion (%)
Donepezil	70	3-8 (dose dependent)	96	CYP2D6, CYP3A4, glucuronidation	57
Galantamine	7	1 (IR); 4.5-5 (ER)	18	O-demethylation (CYP2D6), N-oxidation (CYP3A4)	20
Rivastigmine	1.5; 3 (TD)	1; 8-16 (TD)	40	Hydrolysis, N-methylation, sulfonation (non-CYP)	97
Memantine	60-80	3-7 (IR); 9-12 (ER)	45	Hepatic (non-CYP)	74

[a]Orally administered unless otherwise noted.

par with the parent drug. The most common phase 1 metabolic reactions, or those that produce an active metabolite, are shown in Figure 11.58.[282,287] Glucuronidation (M1, M2) or sulfonation (M3) of phenolic metabolites is known to occur prior to excretion.[282]

Donepezil is marketed as 5, 10, and 23 mg tablets. The two lower doses are also available in a disintegrating tablet formulation that may be particularly helpful in patients who are losing the ability to swallow safely, and the 23 mg tablet is film coated. The 5 and 10 mg doses are reserved for patients with mild-moderate cognitive symptoms, and inhibition of AChE runs between 20% and 40%.[282] The 23 mg dose provides a significantly increased C_{max} and more persistently high serum levels, making it useful in more advanced disease. The therapeutic value of the 23 mg dose was initially questioned, as disease severity as measured by several markers (including the Mini-Mental State Examination, or MMSE) was not noticeably improved over the lower doses. Interestingly, the actions of the 23 mg dose cannot be duplicated by simply taking more doses of the 5 or 10 mg tablets.

Patients should be slowly and carefully titrated to their optimum dosage, and it is recommended that the 23 mg dose not be started until the patient has shown success on lower doses for 3-4 months. The most commonly observed adverse effects are those associated with elevated cholinergic activity, including bradycardia, nausea, vomiting, and diarrhea, as well as muscle cramping and vertigo.[282] Adverse effects are dose-dependent,[288] and providers and caregivers should work collaboratively when assessing relative risks and benefits of ongoing therapy.

Galantamine Hydrobromide. Galantamine, an alkaloid found in bulbs and flowers of plants of the genus *Galanthus*, has enjoyed therapeutic use in several neuromuscular-related pathologies, including myasthenia gravis and residual poliomyelitis.[283] Its ability to concentrate in the central nervous system and impact cholinergic systems made it a natural for investigation in the treatment of AD, and it received FDA approval in 2001 for use in mild-moderate disease.

Galantamine's selective, competitive, and reversible binding to AChE involves the catalytic and acyl pockets,

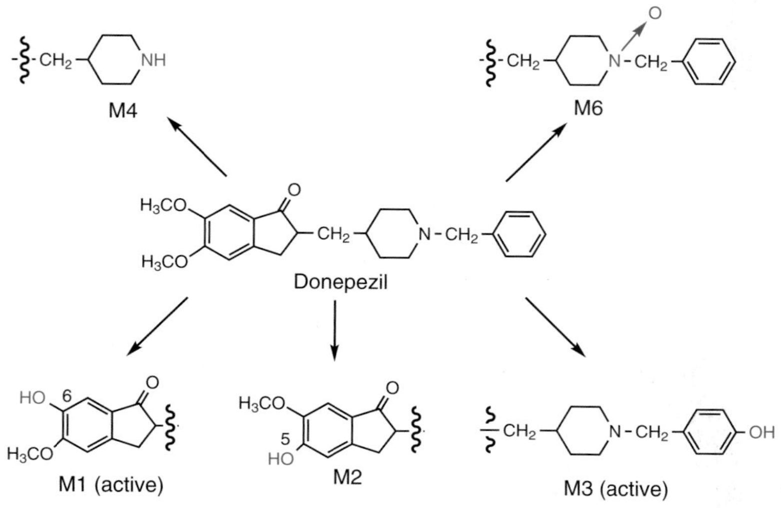

Figure 11.58 Major CYP2D6- and CYP3A4-catalyzed phase I metabolism of donepezil.

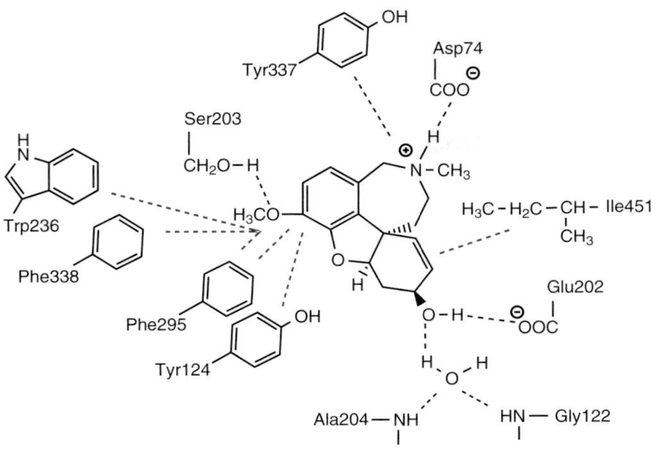

Figure 11.59 Binding interactions between human acetylcholinesterase and galantamine. Hydrophobic interactions are shown in red.

as well as the adjacent peripheral anionic site (Fig. 11.59). Hydrogen and hydrophobic interactions predominate, but an important cation-π bond between the protonated amine and Tyr337 mimics the interaction of the onium head of endogenous ACh with the enzyme. Molecular docking studies performed with N-aralkyl-modified analogues document that affinity for the peripheral anionic site increases significantly due to π-π stacking interactions with Tyr341 (not shown).[283] Studies in animal models have demonstrated the ability of galantamine to promote Aβ clearance and microglial phagocytosis.[288] The drug is known to uniquely modulate nicotinic cholinergic receptors through allosteric binding, leading to increased intracellular Ca^{2+}, augmented release of ACh and NE from central synapses, and potentially enhanced cognition.[288,289] Despite this, the clinical relevance of nicotinic receptor involvement in anticholinergic AD drug action has been recently called into question.[280]

Galantamine absorption is complete and minimally impacted by food. Like donepezil, it is vulnerable to CYP2D6 and CYP3A4 metabolism, which generates O-dealkylated and N-oxide metabolites, respectively (Fig. 11.60).[289] Unlike donepezil, neither metabolite retains therapeutic activity. Approximately 75% of a dose will be biotransformed, and both the parent drug and metabolites can undergo glucuronidation prior to renal excretion. CYP2D6 phenotype impacts the generation of the O-desmethyl metabolite, but dosage adjustments in poor 2D6 metabolizers are not required.[289] Likewise, drug-drug interactions (DDIs) based on metabolic vulnerabilities are of only minor clinical concern, although strong inhibitors of these isoforms should be used with appropriate caution.[281,289]

A meta-analysis of galantamine efficacy in AD showed cognition enhancement when compared to placebo and, with long-term use, improvement in performance of ADL.[290] It has been shown to be an acceptable alternative for mild-moderate AD patients who are nonresponsive to donepezil therapy[291] and is available in tablet, extended-release capsule, and oral solution dosage forms. The daily maintenance dose ranges from 16 to 24 mg administered once (extended release) or in two divided doses (immediate release) in a 24-hour period, most commonly with meals. Initial doses are half the lower maintenance dose, and 4 weeks should elapse between dose escalations. Adverse effects that can prompt drug discontinuation are primarily gastrointestinal in nature (nausea, vomiting, diarrhea), vertigo, and urinary tract infection.[289,290] More serious adverse effects include dermatological toxicity, including Stevens-Johnson syndrome, and arrhythmia (bradycardia, AV block). Additive effects with coadministered drugs that prolong the QT interval can lead to potentially fatal arrhythmia, including torsades de pointes.

Rivastigmine Tartrate. Unlike the other cholinesterase inhibitors used in AD, S(−)-rivastigmine stereoselectively inhibits both AChE and BuChE in the CNS, which is advantageous in patients experiencing disease-associated loss of AChE.[292] Rivastigmine acts through the slow carbamylation of the catalytic site Ser residue of both cholinesterases, destroying its ability to act as a hydrolytic nucleophile on the endogenous ACh substrate.[293] The carbamylation reaction with hAChE Ser203 is shown in Figure 11.61; the reaction with BuChE is analogous, although this enzyme is known to have a less constrained active site cavity.[293] After

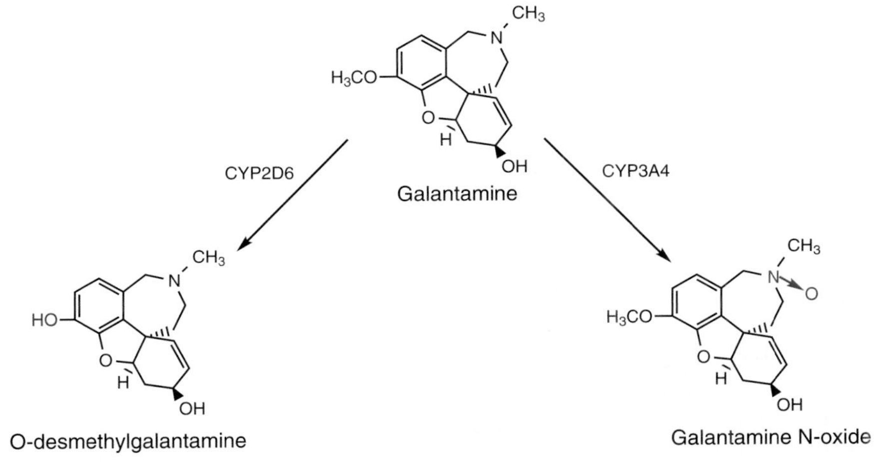

Figure 11.60 CYP2D6- and CYP3A4-catalyzed phase I metabolism of galantamine.

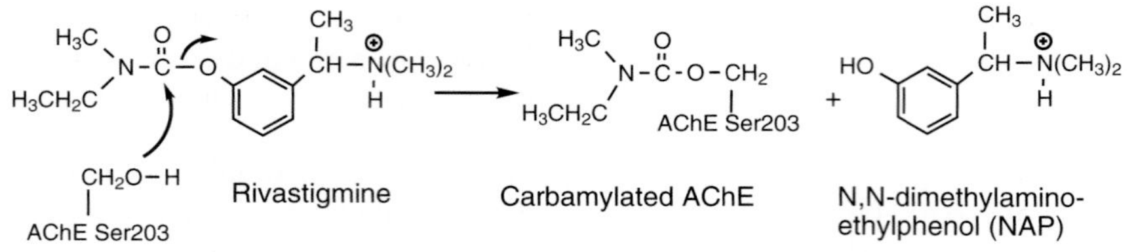

Figure 11.61 Rivastigmine carbamylation of acetylcholinesterase.

carbamylation, the normal interaction of the other two catalytic triad residues, His and Glu, is sterically disrupted by rivastigmine's N-ethyl moiety and/or the displaced 3-[1-(N,N-dimethylamino)ethyl]phenol (NAP). This hinders the positioning of the water molecule needed to liberate the carbamylated esterase,[293,294] with the result being a prolonged "pseudoirreversible" inhibition of the enzyme that persists for 10 hours or longer. Enzyme inhibition is enhanced by the displaced NAP, as it is believed to be captured within the anionic domain of the esterase.

Imaging studies have demonstrated that patients responding to rivastigmine show enhanced hippocampal metabolism and metabolic activity in memory-related areas of the brain compared to nonresponders. In patients with likely AD, BuChE inhibition in cerebral spinal fluid was associated with improvement in attentiveness and memory more so than AChE inhibition, and these clinical benefits persisted for up to 6 months of therapy.[295] BuChE containing an A539T mutation (known as a K-variant) shows a 30% decrease in hydrolytic efficacy compared to the wild-type enzyme, and patients expressing this polymorph experience less aggressive disease progression and respond less vigorously to rivastigmine.[295] Meta-analyses on the relative value of rivastigmine in AD compared to donepezil and galantamine are mixed, but the risk of gastrointestinal adverse effects is generally highest for oral rivastigmine.[296]

Rivastigmine metabolism is straightforward and involves hydrolytic cleavage of the carbamate with possible N-demethylation and/or phase 2 sulfonation of the resultant NAP metabolite (Fig. 11.62).[297] The relative lack of CYP involvement in biotransformation, along with a low affinity for serum protein, translates to a decreased risk of DDIs in a highly vulnerable population.[298] Oral absorption from the capsule formulation is rapid and complete within an hour. The initial dose is 1.5 mg administered twice daily with meals and can be gradually increased up to a maximum of 12 mg daily as long as there is a 2-week interval between dosing elevations.

As noted above, gastrointestinal distress, coupled with difficulty swallowing and/or challenges in achieving optimal plasma concentrations, can compromise patient well-being and may result in drug discontinuation. This therapeutic reality prompted the development of a transdermal patch formulation of rivastigmine.[298,299] Drug release is controlled through an acrylic polymer mixture, and the silicone matrix against the skin optimizes patch adherence while minimizing trauma on removal (important in the often fragile skin of elders).[298] Rivastigmine patches can deliver 4.6, 9.5, or 13.3 mg of drug per 24 hours. The 9.5 mg daily dose has been shown to lower C_{max} while prolonging T_{max} compared to the maximum oral dose (6 mg capsules taken twice daily) without compromising overall drug exposure, thus improving pharmacokinetic stability and overall tolerability.[298-300] Efficacy is dose-dependent, with the 13.3 mg transdermal dose providing greater therapeutic benefit than the 4.6 mg daily dose relative to cognition, ADL, and overall function.[295] A minimum of 4 weeks on a lower dose should precede dose escalation. The adverse effect profile (including weight loss) is significantly decreased compared to the capsule formulation, with some studies showing gastrointestinal distress with the 9.5 mg/d dose on par with placebo.[299,300] The short 3 hour elimination half-life ensures that serum levels will fall quickly if the patch must be removed in an emergency.[299]

Rivastigmine bioavailability from the patch formulation is highest when applied to the upper back, upper arm, or chest.[299,300] While skin reactions are possible, they can be minimized by site rotation and do not generally result in therapy discontinuation.[298,299] Convenience/compliance advantages for the patch include simplified

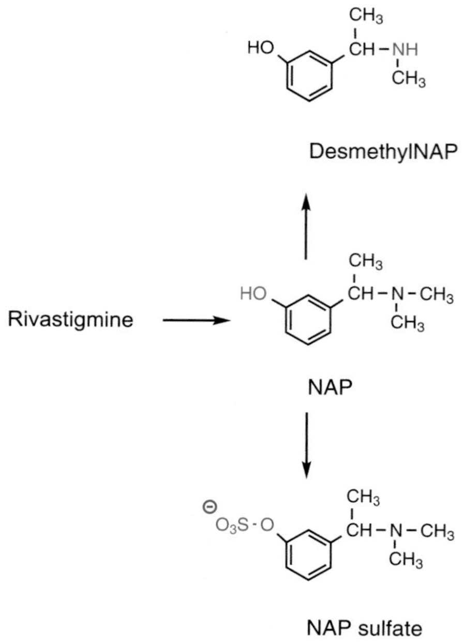

Figure 11.62 Metabolism of rivastigmine.

once-daily administration without regard to meals and readily visible confirmation of medication adherence for caregivers.[299]

Rivastigmine is the only anti-Alzheimer's cholinesterase inhibitor approved for use in Parkinson's disease dementia. It has also shown value in the symptomatic treatment of dementia resulting from subcortical vascular insufficiency.[295]

N-Methyl-D-Aspartate Antagonists

The fact that augmentation of central cholinergic activity does not, in and of itself, permanently halt the progression of AD exemplifies the multifaceted pathology of this disease. Glutamate is another neurotransmitter linked to neurophysiologic health and cognition that has provided a novel avenue for dementia drug development, as levels of glutamate are known to be elevated in AD.[301]

NMDA Receptors, Excitotoxicity, and Uncompetitive Receptor Antagonism. NMDA receptors are ligand-gated ion channels. When stimulated by the excitatory neurotransmitter glutamate or an exogenous agonist, they depolarize and liberate a bound regulatory Mg^{2+} ion, which opens the channel to allow for an influx of Ca^{2+} and Na^{+} into the postsynaptic neuron. The liberation of Mg^{2+} and the short-term opening of the channel is associated with synaptic plasticity in the hippocampus (the central seat of episodic memory) and improves the ability to learn, think, and remember.[279,301] Overstimulation of NMDA receptors by moderately (but chronically) elevated levels of glutamate or neuronal insult by Aβ results in a situation termed excitotoxicity. Excitotoxicity damages neurons secondary to excessively high levels of intracellular Ca^{2+} and the free radicals and other neurotoxins that are subsequently generated.[301,302] Overexcited neurons become highly depolarized, and the increasing intraneuronal positive charge repels Mg^{2+} and inhibits its normal involvement with the ion channel, maintaining a persistently open state that negatively impacts cognition.[302] NMDA hyperactivity also stimulates the hyperphosphorylation of p-tau, promoting the formation of neurofibrillary tangles. The interconnectedness of glutamate, NMDA receptors, Aβ (particularly soluble oligomers of the amyloid protein), and p-tau has been described in the literature.[303]

The uncompetitive blockade of NMDA receptors by compounds like memantine antagonizes only excessive overstimulation by glutamate, leaving homeostatic stimulation unaffected. It does this through low-affinity binding to the receptor-associated Ca^{2+} channel in its open state, with minimal retention in the channel during its closed state. This keeps Ca^{2+} concentrations in check and improves cognition in moderate-advanced disease without the risk of adverse effects that a complete and total receptor block could induce (e.g., dissociation, excessive sedation, hallucinations).[302]

An important distinction between uncompetitive and noncompetitive receptor antagonism is the former's requirement for a receptor activated by an agonist. An uncompetitive NMDA receptor antagonist must gain access to the ion channel after it is opened by glutamate, and this requires that the channel stay open long enough for it to enter (longer than homeostatic opening). This is why the antagonist shows greater efficacy when levels of glutamate are high (pathologic) as opposed to low (homeostatic). The antagonist should not bind too tightly or work too aggressively when the receptor is only minimally activated, but it should spend a longer time in the channel than the endogenous Mg^{2+} gatekeeper.[302] To paraphrase a famous line in a familiar children's story, the "dwell time" in the channel should not be too long (homeostatic antagonism) or too short (ineffective excitotoxicity blockade), but "just right."

Memantine Hydrochloride. Memantine blocks glutamate-induced excitotoxicity by binding close to the Mg^{2+} site within the NMDA-associated ion channel. It gains access to this site through its protonated amine, and the two bridgehead CH_3 groups help retain it in situ for the appropriate amount of time. Since it blocks neurodegeneration from the overstimulation of NMDA receptors by glutamate, it is considered a neuroprotective agent and, therefore, has DMT characteristics.[301,302]

Randomized controlled trials on efficacy and therapeutic value have produced conflicting results: safe and effective versus a high risk for adverse effects. However, a meta-analysis with well-defined inclusion criteria published in 2015 found evidence of significant benefits to cognition, ADL, mental state, and the clinician's global impression of status, primarily due to memantine's ability to retard mental and functional decline in patients with moderate to severe disease.[304] Approximately 4,100 AD patients from 13 double-blinded placebo-controlled trials were included in the analysis, and the investigators determined that the only troublesome or serious adverse effect more likely with memantine compared to placebo was somnolence. These outcomes were confirmed in a 2017 meta-analysis conducted by others.[305]

Memantine is available in immediate-release tablets and extended-release capsules. The immediate-release medication is started at 5 mg daily and slowly titrated upward on a weekly basis in 5 mg increments to a maximum of 20 mg/d. The same approach is taken with the extended-release formulation, only the starting and maximum doses are 7 and 28 mg/d, respectively. An oral 2 mg/mL solution is also commercially available. Absorption of memantine is complete and food-independent. Patients with an alkaline urine may show higher than normal serum levels of drug and should be monitored for adverse effects. In addition to drowsiness, dizziness may be a problem for some patients but, overall, drug discontinuation rates are comparable to placebo.[306] Metabolism is CYP-independent and none of the three primary metabolites are active (Fig. 11.63).

Memantine/Donepezil Combination Therapy. Combination NMDA/AChE antagonist therapy has been proposed to be beneficial, as glutamateric terminal

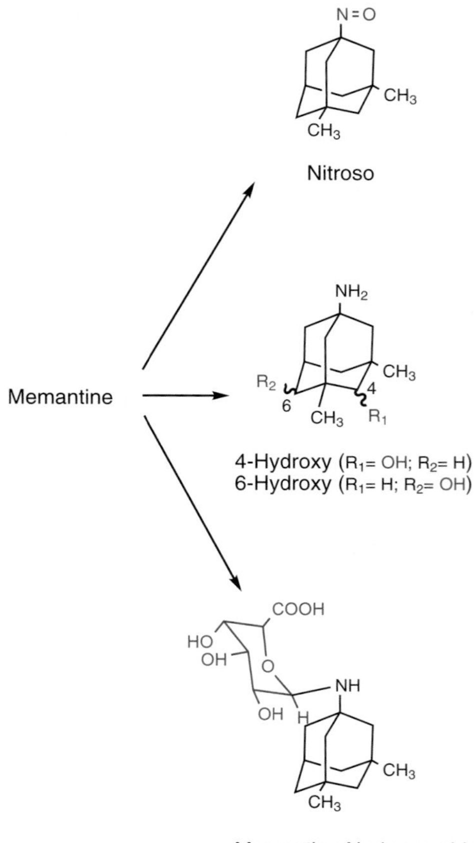

Figure 11.63 Metabolism of memantine.

reorganization occurs in brain regions that exhibit cholinergic plasticity.[280] Additional evidence of the interconnectedness of these two neurotransmitter systems has been documented.[307] Specifically, glutamatergic neurons interact directly with cholinergic neurons in several areas of the brain, including the hippocampus, and it has been proposed that NMDA receptor activation stimulates the release of ACh from neurons in the basal forebrain. Glutamate-induced excitotoxicity and accompanying neuronal cell death takes a toll on cholinergic neurons in cerebral cortex, and inhibition of that destructive process can protect cholinergic receptors and synaptic AChE.

In short, both cholinergic and NMDA-related dysfunction underpin AD pathology, and the distinct mechanisms of action of the inhibitors of these two systems are complementary with regard to positive impacts on learning, memory, cognitive function, and emotional well-being. NMDA antagonists may have more pronounced benefits on agitation and delusional thinking, while AChE inhibitors can more positively impact anxious and depressive behaviors and apathetic affect, so combining the two can allow for a broader approach to therapeutic intervention. Preclinical studies have documented the value of combination NMDA/AChE antagonist therapy over monotherapy with either type of agent.[307]

A memantine/donepezil combination product is marketed as Namzaric and intended for use in patients with moderate-severe AD previously stabilized on 10 mg donepezil.[308] The extended-release capsules contain 10 mg of donepezil hydrochloride and 7, 14, 21, or 28 mg of memantine hydrochloride. While the combination product is more costly than monotherapy ($449 per month vs. $330 per month for both drugs administered separately), it has been reported that the overall economic savings is higher with the combination product due to a 4-month delay in admission to a skilled care facility.[308] A pharmacoeconomic study of AD therapy options (including memantine/donepezil combination therapy) that evaluated 38 articles containing economic models was published in 2018, but several limitations, including the prevalence of industry-funded studies in the data set, compromised data evaluation.[309]

Importantly, combining memantine and donepezil into a single dosage form does not significantly alter the efficacy of either drug, nor the adverse effect profile or discontinuation rate compared to monotherapy with either agent.[306-308] There are several potential advantages to the combination product, including: (1) improved adherence to therapeutic regimens, (2) decreased caregiver burden related to medication administration, and (3) the ability to sprinkle the contents of the capsule on applesauce for safer consumption in patients with swallowing difficulties.[308] In the opinion of some, the combination product represents first-line therapy for moderate-severe AD, with memantine monotherapy as the second-line approach.[306]

Drugs Used to Treat Attention-Deficit Hyperactivity Disorder (ADHD)

Attention-Deficit Hyperactivity Disorder

Children, adolescents, and adults who demonstrate a pattern of inattention, impulsivity, and hyperactivity are diagnosed with attention-deficit hyperactivity disorder (ADHD). ADHD is considered to be a neurodevelopmental condition which often significantly impairs functioning and places children at an elevated risk for a variety of adverse outcomes. The *Diagnostic and Statistical Manual of Mental Disorders*, Fifth Edition (DSM-5) identifies diagnostic criteria for ADHD as two main subtypes: (1) inattention and (2) hyperactivity/impulsivity and allows for combined criteria for (1) and (2) along with the stipulation that several symptoms were present prior to age 12.[1,310] Although ADHD is most often thought of as an affliction of children and adolescents, there is now a body of evidence that suggests it also occurs in adults.[311]

Patients exhibit deficits in attention to detail, do not follow instructions, show poor organization, and make careless mistakes at or fail to complete work. Patients show inattention while playing, because they are easily side-tracked and have difficulty listening to others. Also, people with ADHD often are forgetful and misplace things frequently. Hyperactivity-impulsivity symptoms include a general increase in psychomotor behavior, akin to a bee constantly flying from one place to another. People with ADHD often fidget their hands and feet and squirm regularly, i.e., they do not seem to be able to sit still. Excessive talking and interrupting are also common.

An accurate prevalence of ADHD is difficult to determine, as there remains debate in the medical literature about whether or not the disorder is overdiagnosed. The prevalence of ADHD in children and adolescents aged 4-17 years is reported to be 11% (6.4 million) with inattentive subtype predominating. The prevalence of diagnosed ADHD in children increased 28% from 2007 to 2011, and the percent of all children 2-17 years of age in the U.S. taking ADHD medication was 5.2% in 2016. There is a higher incidence in males with the male:female ratio ranging from 2:1 to 9:1.[310,312,313]

It is generally believed that ADHD might be an inherited disorder; however, environmental factors can play a significant role in the etiology.[314,315] Numerous studies have identified genes involved in ADHD. To date these studies implicate several genes with dopamine 4/5 receptor genes (DRD4, DRD5), the dopamine transporter gene (DAT1), the dopamine beta hydroxylase gene (DBH), and the noradrenergic adrenoceptor alpha 2 gene (ADRA2A) being studied the most.[315,316] A great deal more research is needed to identify and confirm the link between genetics and ADHD.

Treatment of ADHD

Therapy for ADHD generally requires a combination of pharmacological and nonpharmacological therapeutic approaches. The nonpharmacological treatment, often referred to as psychosocial intervention, consists of family therapy and cognitive behavioral therapy. The key to success with this type of therapy is to educate against the stigma of ADHD, enhance academic organization, modify behavior in the classroom and at home and develop social skills. A healthy balanced diet is always recommended, although diet is not directly related to ADHD behaviors.[317]

Pharmacological Treatment of ADHD

In 1937, Charles Bradley, a Rhode Island pediatrician, treated "problem" children with benzedrine (amphetamine sulfate) for headache complaints and discovered that this CNS stimulant had a profound positive effect on their behavior.[318] Ever since, the phenylethylamine stimulants amphetamine, methylphenidate, and their analogues have been the drugs of choice for the treatment of ADHD.[319] These stimulants work by mimicking the structures of DA and NE and modulate their release, reuptake, and signaling within the brain. This leads to an increased concentration of DA and NE within the synaptic cleft and has led to the theory that ADHD is a disorder of DA and NE release in the striatal and prefrontal areas of the brain.[320] This theory is perhaps an oversimplification since ADHD may be complicated with comorbidities such as anxiety disorder, major depression, autism spectrum disorder, or Tourette's disorder which implies a more complicated etiology.[321] The overall objective of therapy is to see improvement in core ADHD symptoms of inattention, hyperactivity, and impulsivity. Although psychosocial therapy is recommended along with medication, studies have not shown significant improvements of outcomes over medication alone.[317]

In addition to CNS stimulants, there are second-line drugs which are used in ADHD treatment. These drugs are discussed in detail elsewhere in the text (Chapters 11,15 & 16) and are listed in Table 11.20. They include the SNRI atomoxetine, the α-adrenergic agonist antihypertensives (e.g., clonidine and guanfacine), and several antidepressants (e.g., the tricyclic antidepressant imipramine and bupropion).

Specific Stimulant Drugs for ADHD

AMPHETAMINE SALTS. The stimulant mechanism action of amphetamine derives from its structural similarity to the neurotransmitters, DA and NE, and to a lesser extent to 5-HT since it has the arylethylamine moiety in common. It competes with reuptake by their transporters DAT (dopamine transporter), NET (norepinephrine transporter), and SERT (5-HT transporter) in the striatum and prefrontal cortex. In addition, amphetamine inhibits translocation of DA and NE from the cytosol into storage vesicles in the neuron by inhibiting the vesicular monoamine transporter 2 (VMAT2). Through this type of competition, amphetamine actually overloads the transporters and causes a reversal of their action and pumps DA and NE out of the neurons into the synapse.[322,323]

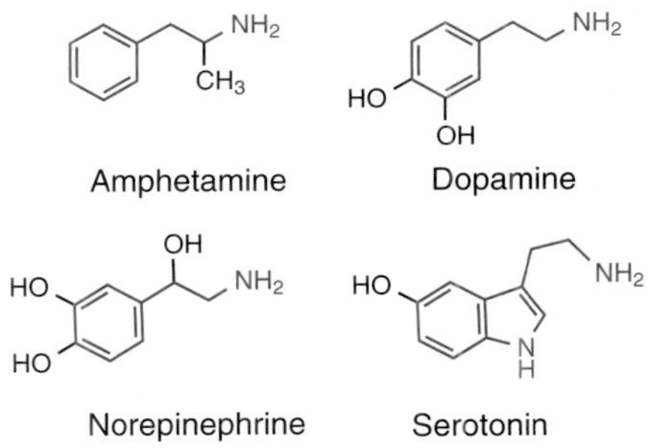

NH_2 CH_3 Amphetamine

HO OH NH_2 Dopamine

OH HO HO NH_2 Norepinephrine

HO NH_2 N H Serotonin

ADHD Neurotransmitters

Since amphetamine has a chiral center (Fig. 11.64), it exists in the dextro (D-) and levo (L-) enantiomeric forms. The D-amphetamine is the more potent form (~4X) and has been marketed as such since the early 1940s. However, it has subsequently been determined that both enantiomers are effective in treating ADHD, but the only current use of the L-amphetamine is in the mixed enantiomers/salts product (Adderall, Table 11.21) which consists of a 3:1 enantiomer mixture of D-amphetamine:L-amphetamine. The D-amphetamine is a more potent DA releaser;

Table 11.20 Nonstimulant Drugs for ADHD Treatment

Drug	Structure	Mechanism of Action	Indication	Detailed Discussion Chapter
Atomoxetine	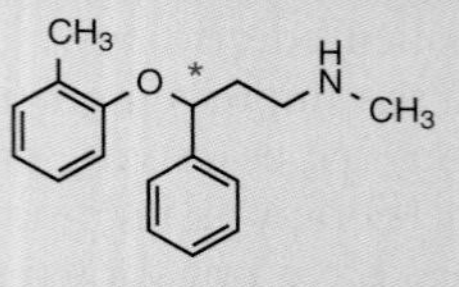	SNRI	ADHD +/− enuresis, TIC disorder, anxiety, oppositionality + ADHD	11
Bupropion	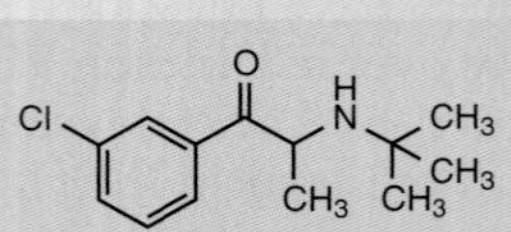	Antidepressant DNRI	ADHD +/− depression Anxiety disorder, obsessive compulsive disorder (OCD)	11
Clonidine	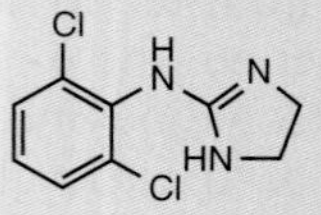	Antihypertensive Central α2-agonist	Tourette's syndrome, aggression, self-abuse, oppositionality + ADHD	15 and 16
Guanfacine	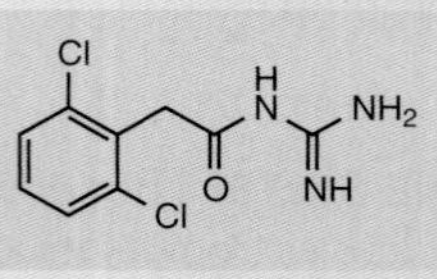	Antihypertensive Central α2-agonist	Tourette's syndrome, aggression, self-abuse, oppositionality + ADHD	15 and 16
Imipramine	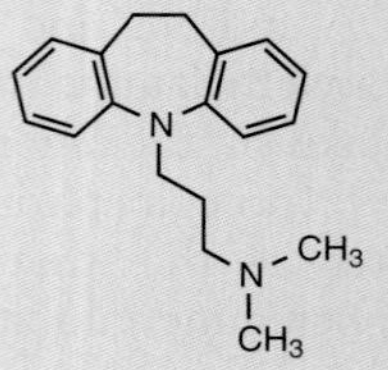	Tricyclic Antidepressant (TCA)	ADHD +/- enuresis, TIC disorder, anxiety diorder, oppositionality + ADHD	11

DNRI, dopamine/norepinephrine reuptake inhibitor; NSRI, norepinephrine/serotonin reuptake inhibitor; SNRI, selective norepinephrine reuptake inhibitor.

however, the L-amphetamine is equal or more potent as a releaser of NE. In addition, the L-isomer in the 3:1 mixture appears to prolong the efflux of DA presumably due to modulation of the L-isomer on the effect of the D-isomer on the DAT.[323]

Amphetamine is metabolized by oxidative deamination to benzoic acid via a CYP2C isoform pathway and to 4-hydroxynorephedrine by 2D6 and dopamine β-hydroxylase (Fig. 11.65). The benzoic acid is excreted in the urine as the hippuric acid conjugate and 4-hydroxynorephedrine is excreted as either the glucuronide or sulfate conjugates. Amphetamine is 30%-40% excreted unchanged, and the pH of the urine has an effect on its elimination. Alkaline urine decreases its elimination, whereas acidic urine increases its urinary elimination.[324]

Amphetamine is available in a variety of formulations including immediate-release (IR) tablets as well as a number of extended-release formulations (Table 11.21). Orally administered IR amphetamine is rapidly absorbed and has high bioavailability. IR formulations demonstrate dose-proportional pharmacokinetics with a T_{max} of 2-3 hours and age dependent $t_{1/2}$ from 7 to 10 hours. Body weight has an inverse effect on amphetamine's maximum concentration and systemic exposure. As body weight decreases volume of distribution, clearance and half-life increases.[325]

Amphetamine has a high abuse potential and all marketed products come with a boxed warning to that effect. The common adverse effects of amphetamine include decreased appetite, weight loss, insomnia, headache and irritability, and jitteriness. The less common adverse effects are dysphoria, a Zombie-like state, priapism, hypertension, and psychosis especially with prolonged use. Dose adjustment usually moderates these effects.[310,326]

Lisdexamfetamine is the first amphetamine prodrug approved for the treatment of ADHD. Structurally it is the lysine amide derivative of D-amphetamine (Fig. 11.64) and as such it is unlikely to cross the blood-brain barrier. Lisdexamphetamine is metabolized in red blood cells to D-amphetamine by amide hydrolysis. The hydrolysis is a rate-limited process and as such, the release of D-amphetamine is slowed compared with IR D-amphetamine. The AUC values were equal; however, the C_{max} was lower by 50% and the time to C_{max} was doubled. This pharmacokinetic effect produced a gradual and sustained increase of striatal DA and a much slower decline as compared to IR D-amphetamine resulting in a longer duration of action (8-14 hr). Lisdexamfetamine is eliminated via the urine, 42% as amphetamine metabolites, 2% unchanged lisdexamfetamine, and 25% as the hippuric acid conjugate.[323,327] As a pro-drug for D-amphetamine, lisdexamfetamine has the same box warning and adverse-effect profile as amphetamine. In 2016, lisdexamfetamine (dimesylate, Vyvanse) also was approved by the FDA to treat binge-eating disorder.

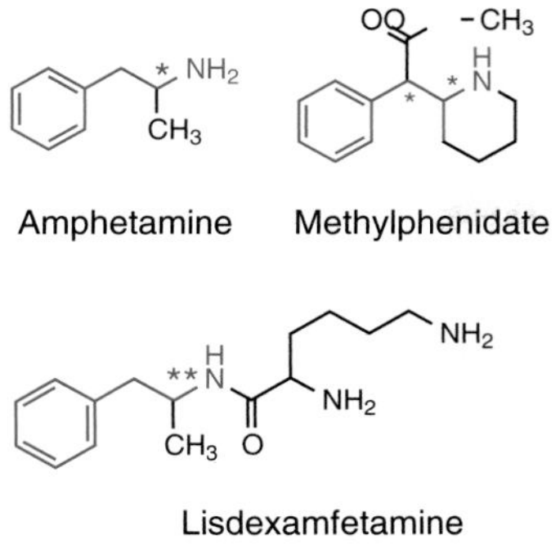

Amphetamine Methylphenidate

Lisdexamfetamine

Figure 11.64 Structures of stimulant drugs used to treat ADHD. Common phenylethylamine moiety outlined in red.

METHYLPHENIDATE. Methylphenidate was the leading stimulant for ADHD treatment since its marketing (as Ritalin) in 1955, but the use of amphetamine salts (Adderall) advanced to nearly equal use since its introduction in 1996. Methylphenidate is an analogue of amphetamine which contains the phenylethylamine pharmacophore buried inside a methylphenyl(piperidinyl)acetate moiety (Fig. 11.64). Its mechanism of action is similar to amphetamine in that it increases DA and NE by inhibition of DAT, NET, and redistribution of VMAT2 in the striatum and prefrontal cortex of the brain. However, MPH also has affinity and agonist activity at both the $5\text{-}HT_{1A}$ and α^2-adenergic receptors. The clinical importance of this is not clearly understood.[316]

Table 11.21 Stimulant Medications for the Treatment of ADHD

Medication	Product Name	Formulation	DOA (hr)	Recommended Dose
Methylphenidate	Ritalin	Short-acting tablet	3-5	5-10 mg/bid to tid
	Ritalin-SR	Intermediate/WM	8	20-30 mg/bid
	Ritalin LA	Long-acting/SODAS	8-12	10-60 mg/qdam
	Concerta	Long-acting/OROS	12	18-36 mg/qdam
	Metadate ER	Intermediate-acting/WM	8	10-20 mg/bid to tid
	Metadate CD	Long-acting/CD	12	20-60 mg/qdam
	Methylin	Short-acting tablet	3-4	5-60 mg/bid
	Methylin CT	Short-acting chewable	3-4	5-60 mg/bid
	Daytrana Patch	Transdermal	12	10-30 mg/qdam
	Equasym XL	Long-acting/CD/DC	8	
	QuilliChew ER	Short-acting chewable	3-4	20-60 mg/qdam
	Quillivant XR	Oral suspension	8-12	20-60 mg/qdam
	Aptensio XR	Long-acting/SRB	3-12	10-60 mg/qdam
Dexmethylphenidate	Focalin	Short-acting tablet	3-4	2.5-10 mg/bid to tid
	Focalin XR	Intermediate-acting/MSRP	6-8	5-20 mg/qdam
Dextroamphetamine (D-amphetamine)	Dexedrine	Intermediate-acting spansules	8	5-40 mg/bid
D:L amphetamine 1:1	Evekeo	Short acting	3-4	2.5-40 mg/bid to tid
D:L amphetamine 3.2:1	Dyanavel XR	Long-acting oral suspension	12	5-20 mg/qdam
D:L amphetamine 3:1	Adzenys XR-ODT	Long-acting/ODT	10-12	3.1-18.8 mg/qdam
Lisdexamfetamine	Vyvanse	Long-acting amphetamine prodrug	12	30-70 mg/qdam
Dextroamphetamine 3:1 *D/L* amphetamine salts	Adderall	Intermediate-acting	4-6	5 mg bid Increase to 40 mg max
	Adderall XR	Long-acting/SRB	12	5-30 mg/qdam

bid, twice a day; CD, controlled delivery; DC, diffucaps; MC, methyl cellulose base; MSPR, mechanical sustained release preparation; ODT, oral disintegrating tablet; OROS, osmotic release oral system; qdam, once a day in the morning; SODAS, spheroidal oral drug absorption system; SRB, sustained release beads; tid, three times a day; WM, wax matrix.

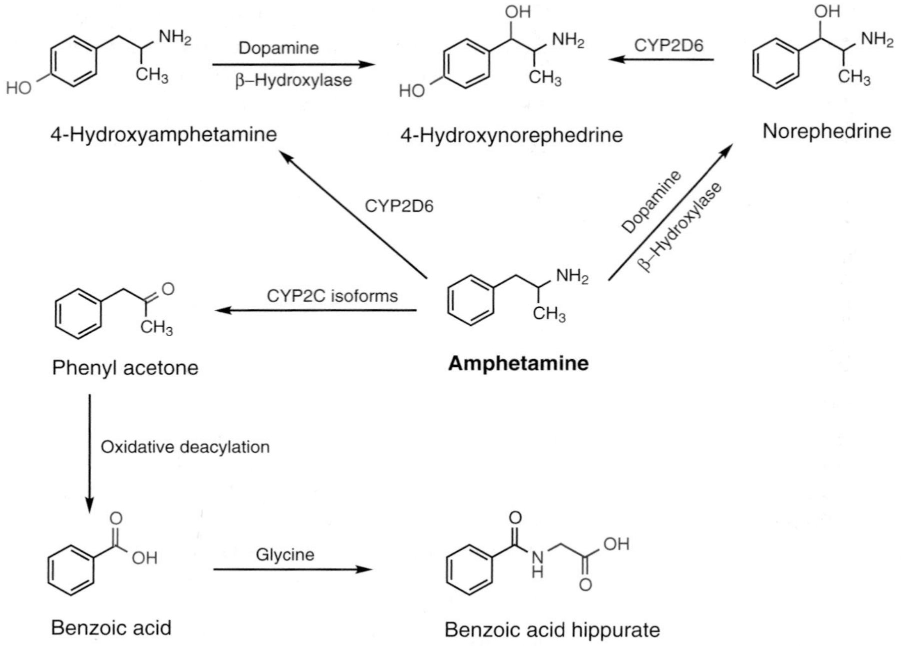

Figure 11.65 Metabolism of amphetamine.

Methylphenidate has two chiral centers and therefore there are four possible isomers (two sets of enantiomer pairs), *D/L-threo* and *D/L-erythro*-methylphenidate. Only the racemic mixture of the *D/L-threo*-methylphenidate is used clinically since the *D/L*-erythro pair has greater side effects. The clinical effect of *D/L*-threo-methylphenidate is attributed to the *D*-enantiomer since the L-enantiomer had no stimulant effect when administered by itself; subsequently a *D*-threo-methylphenidate formulation has become available (Table 11.21).[328,329]

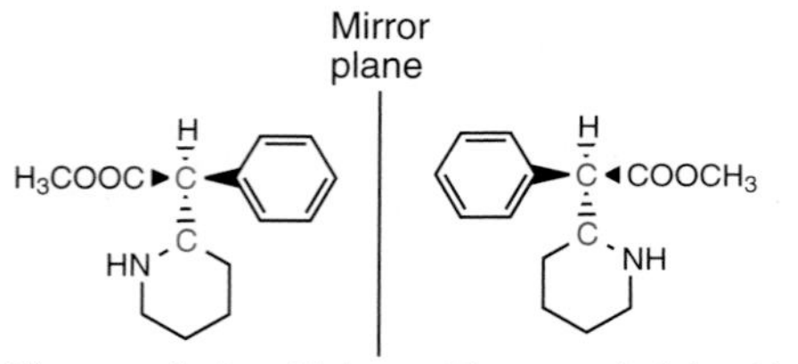

MPH stereo

The absolute oral bioavailability of methylphenidate is only ~30% due to presystemic metabolism. Studies have shown that D/L-methylphenidate is metabolized by ester hydrolysis by a carboxylesterase 1A1 and the hydrolysis is stereoselective. This enzyme is present in the stomach and liver and shows a preference for L-threo-methylphenidate. Consequently, plasma concentration of the D-threo-enantiomer after an oral dose of the racemic mixture is higher than that of the L-threo-enantiomer. The product of methylphenidate metabolism is D/L-ritalinic acid (α-2-phenyl-2-piperidyl acetic acid) formed by the ester hydrolysis of the acetic acid ester.[330] Methylphenidate is well absorbed orally and after extensive first-pass metabolism peak plasma levels occur within 2 hours after oral administration of IR formulations. Protein binding is low (10%-30%) and apparent distribution volume after IV dosing is ~ 6 L/kg. Excretion is via the kidneys with 78%-97% as metabolites (primarily ritalinic acid) and only minor amounts of unchanged methylphenidate and a small amount appearing in the feces. The excretion half-life varies from 2.5 to 7 hours depending on the formulation.[331]

The adverse effects of methylphenidate are analogous to those seen with amphetamine: overstimulation of the CNS, including insomnia, night terrors, nervousness, restlessness, euphoria and irritability. Often these effects can be followed by fatigue and depression. Other effects include dry mouth, anorexia, gastrointestinal disturbances (e.g., abdominal cramps), headache, dizziness, and sweats. Tachycardia, myocardial infarction, altered libido, and impotence can be seen in adults with ADHD. There is an abuse potential with methylphenidate, and the FDA has issued a boxed warning to that effect. [332]

ACKNOWLEDGMENT

The authors wish to acknowledge the work of Victoria F. Roche, PhD, and S. William Zito, PhD, for contributing subsections of text to the chapter.

Structure Challenge

The structures of six drugs from this chapter are provided. Use your knowledge of drug chemistry to identify which would be the most appropriate to recommend for each patient described below.

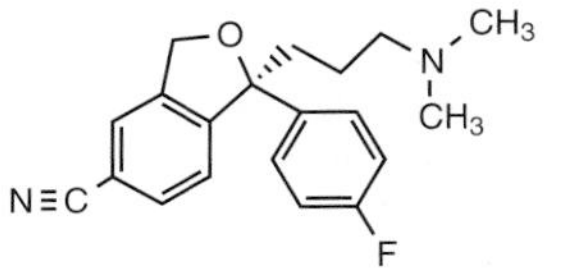

A 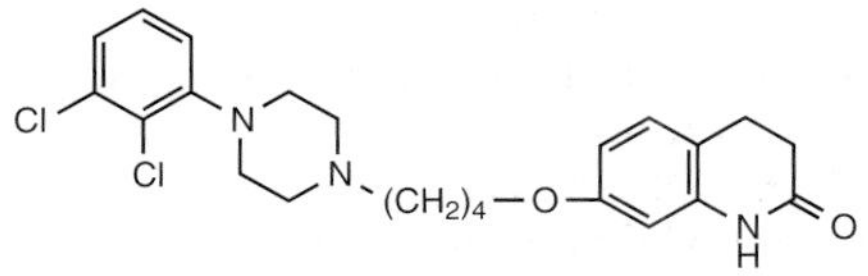 B 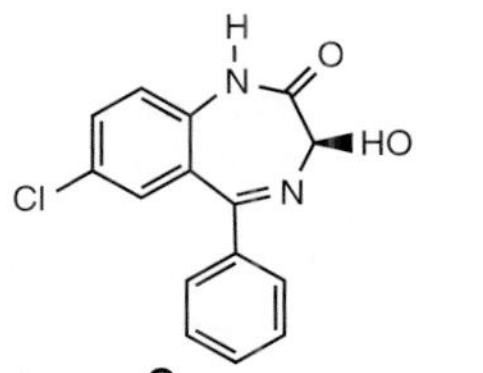 C

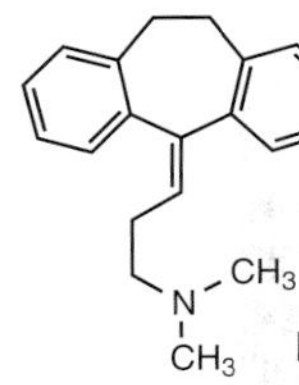

D 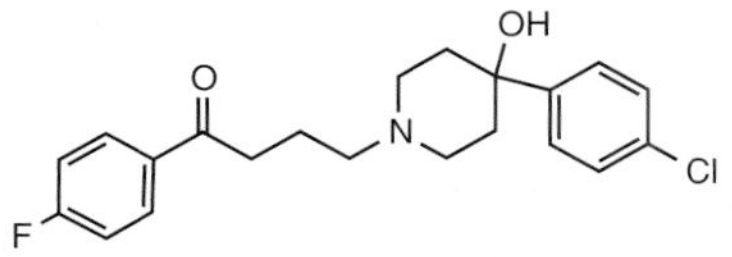 E 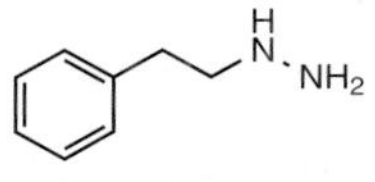 F

1. An Alzheimer's patient who is taking rivastigmine but who also suffers from depression.
2. An Alzheimer's patient who is taking rivastigmine, but who also has paranoia and delusions.
3. An Alzheimer's patient who is taking rivastigmine, but who also displays agitation and restlessness that interferes with sleep.
4. Which antidepressant drug should be avoided in an Alzheimer's patient on rivastigmine due to its prominent antimuscarinic receptor activity?
5. Which antidepressant drug would be most problematic in a depressed patient with hypertension?

Structure Challenge answers found immediately after References.

REFERENCES

1. American Psychiatric Association; DSM-5 Task Force. *Diagnostic and Statistical Manual of Mental Disorders: DSM-5*. 5th ed. Washington, DC: American Psychiatric Association; 2013.
2. Moreno-Kustner B, Martin C, Pastor L. Prevalence of psychotic disorders and its association with methodological issues. A systematic review and meta-analyses. *PLoS One*. 2018;13(4):e0195687.
3. McGrath JJ, Saha S, Al-Hamzawi A, et al. Psychotic experiences in the general population: a cross-national analysis based on 31,261 respondents from 18 countries. *JAMA Psychiatry*. 2015;72(7):697-705.
4. Chong HY, Teoh SL, Wu DB, Kotirum S, Chiou CF, Chaiyakunapruk N. Global economic burden of schizophrenia: a systematic review. *Neuropsychiatr Dis Treat*. 2016;12:357-373.
5. Kessler RC, Petukhova M, Sampson NA, Zaslavsky AM, Wittchen HU. Twelve-month and lifetime prevalence and lifetime morbid risk of anxiety and mood disorders in the United States. *Int J Methods Psychiatr Res*. 2012;21(3):169-184.
6. Kraepelin E, Barclay RM, Robertson GM. *Dementia Præcox and Paraphrenia*. Edinburgh: E & S Livingstone; 1919.
7. Bleuler E. *Dementia Praecox*. New York: International Universities Press; 1950.
8. Tandon R, Gaebel W, Barch DM, et al. Definition and description of schizophrenia in the DSM-5. *Schizophr Res*. 2013;150(1):3-10.
9. Schneider K. *Clinical Psychopathology*. New York: Grune & Stratton; 1959.
10. Barch DM, Bustillo J, Gaebel W, et al. Logic and justification for dimensional assessment of symptoms and related clinical phenomena in psychosis: relevance to DSM-5. *Schizophr Res*. 2013;150(1):15-20.
11. Hilker R, Helenius D, Fagerlund B, et al. Heritability of schizophrenia and schizophrenia spectrum based on the Nationwide Danish twin register. *Biol Psychiatry*. 2018;83(6):492-498.
12. O'Tuathaigh CM, Desbonnet L, Moran PM, Waddington JL. Susceptibility genes for schizophrenia: mutant models, endophenotypes and psychobiology. *Curr Top Behav Neurosci*. 2012;12:209-250.
13. Schizophrenia Working Group of the Psychiatric Genomics C. Biological insights from 108 schizophrenia-associated genetic loci. *Nature*. 2014;511(7510):421-427.
14. Genovese G, Fromer M, Stahl EA, et al. Increased burden of ultra-rare protein-altering variants among 4,877 individuals with schizophrenia. *Nat Neurosci*. 2016;19(11):1433-1441.
15. Skene NG, Bryois J, Bakken TE, et al. Genetic identification of brain cell types underlying schizophrenia. *Nat Genet*. 2018;50(6):825-833.
16. Wray NR, Ripke S, Mattheisen M, et al. Genome-wide association analyses identify 44 risk variants and refine the genetic architecture of major depression. *Nat Genet*. 2018;50(5):668-681.
17. Duncan LE, Ratanatharathorn A, Aiello AE, et al. Largest GWAS of PTSD (N=20 070) yields genetic overlap with schizophrenia and sex differences in heritability. *Mol Psychiatry*. 2018;23(3):666-673.

18. Cross-Disorder Group of the Psychiatric Genomics C. Identification of risk loci with shared effects on five major psychiatric disorders: a genome-wide analysis. *Lancet*. 2013;381(9875):1371-1379.
19. Anttila V, Bulik-Sullivan B, Finucane HK, et al. Analysis of shared heritability in common disorders of the brain. *Science*. 2018;360(6395).
20. Howes OD, McCutcheon R. Inflammation and the neural diathesis-stress hypothesis of schizophrenia: a reconceptualization. *Transl Psychiatry*. 2017;7(2):e1024.
21. Howes OD, Kapur S. The dopamine hypothesis of schizophrenia: version III–the final common pathway. *Schizophr Bull*. 2009;35(3):549-562.
22. Moghaddam B, Javitt D. From revolution to evolution: the glutamate hypothesis of schizophrenia and its implication for treatment. *Neuropsychopharmacology*. 2012;37(1):4-15.
23. Poels EM, Kegeles LS, Kantrowitz JT, et al. Imaging glutamate in schizophrenia: review of findings and implications for drug discovery. *Mol Psychiatry*. 2014;19(1):20-29.
24. Carlsson A, Lindqvist M. Effect of chlorpromazine or haloperidol on formation of 3methoxytyramine and Normetanephrine in mouse brain. *Acta Pharmacol Toxicol (Copenh)*. 1963;20:140-144.
25. Howes O, Bose S, Turkheimer F, et al. Progressive increase in striatal dopamine synthesis capacity as patients develop psychosis: a PET study. *Mol Psychiatry*. 2011;16(9):885-886.
26. Snyder SH. *Drugs and the Brain*. New York: Scientific American Books: Distributed by W.H. Freeman; 1986.
27. Heinz A, Knable MB, Weinberger DR. Dopamine D2 receptor imaging and neuroleptic drug response. *J Clin Psychiatry*. 1996;57(suppl 11):84-88; discussion 89-93.
28. Kenakin T, Christopoulos A. Measurements of ligand bias and functional affinity. *Nat Rev Drug Discov*. 2013;12(6):483.
29. Kenakin T. Inverse, protean, and ligand-selective agonism: matters of receptor conformation. *FASEB J*. 2001;15(3):598-611.
30. Liu Y, Canal CE, Cordova-Sintjago TC, Zhu W, Booth RG. Mutagenesis analysis reveals distinct amino acids of the human serotonin 5-HT2C receptor underlying the pharmacology of distinct ligands. *ACS Chem Neurosci*. 2017;8(1):28-39.
31. Mottola DM, Kilts JD, Lewis MM, et al. Functional selectivity of dopamine receptor agonists. I. Selective activation of postsynaptic dopamine D2 receptors linked to adenylate cyclase. *J Pharmacol Exp Ther*. 2002;301(3):1166-1178.
32. Chen X, McCorvy JD, Fischer MG, et al. Discovery of G protein-biased D2 dopamine receptor partial agonists. *J Med Chem*. 2016;59(23):10601-10618.
33. Lovenberg TW, Brewster WK, Mottola DM, et al. Dihydrexidine, a novel selective high potency full dopamine D-1 receptor agonist. *Eur J Pharmacol*. 1989;166(1):111-113.
34. Cervenka S. PET radioligands for the dopamine D1-receptor: application in psychiatric disorders. *Neurosci Lett*. 2019;691:26-34.
35. Arnsten AFT, Girgis RR, Gray DL, Mailman RB. Novel dopamine therapeutics for cognitive deficits in schizophrenia. *Biol Psychiatry*. 2017;81(1):67-77.
36. Sokoloff P, Le Foll B. The dopamine D3 receptor, a quarter century later. *Eur J Neurosci*. 2017;45(1):2-19.
37. Bitter I, Groc M, Delsol C, et al. Efficacy of F17464, a new preferential D3 antagonist in a placebo-controlled phase 2 study of patients with an acute exacerbation of schizophrenia. *Eur Psychiatry*. 2017;41:S387.
38. Lindsley CW, Hopkins CR. Return of D4 dopamine receptor antagonists in drug discovery. *J Med Chem*. 2017;60(17):7233-7243.
39. Mohr P, Decker M, Enzensperger C, Lehmann J. Dopamine/serotonin receptor ligands. 12(1): SAR studies on hexahydro-dibenz[d,g]azecines lead to 4-chloro-7-methyl-5,6,7,8,9,14-hexahydrodibenz[d,g]azecin-3-ol, the first picomolar D5-selective dopamine-receptor antagonist. *J Med Chem*. 2006;49(6):2110-2116.
40. Arbilla S, Langer SZ. Stereoselectivity of presynaptic autoreceptors modulating dopamine release. *Eur J Pharmacol*. 1981;76(4):345-351.
41. Booth RG, Baldessarini RJ, Kula NS, Gao Y, Zong R, Neumeyer JL. Presynaptic inhibition of dopamine synthesis in rat striatal tissue by enantiomeric mono- and dihydroxyaporphines. *Mol Pharmacol*. 1990;38(1):92-101.
42. Lieberman JA, Stroup TS. The NIMH-CATIE schizophrenia study: what did we learn? *Am J Psychiatry*. 2011;168(8):770-775.
43. Leucht S, Cipriani A, Spineli L, et al. Comparative efficacy and tolerability of 15 antipsychotic drugs in schizophrenia: a multiple-treatments meta-analysis. *Lancet*. 2013;382(9896):951-962.
44. Haddad PM, Das A, Keyhani S, Chaudhry IB. Antipsychotic drugs and extrapyramidal side effects in first episode psychosis: a systematic review of head-head comparisons. *J Psychopharmacol*. 2012;26(5 suppl):15-26.
45. Roth BL, Lopez E, Patel S, Kroeze WK. The multiplicity of serotonin receptors: uselessly diverse molecules or an embarrassment of riches? *Neuroscientist*. 2000;6(4):252-262.
46. Canal CE. Serotonergic psychedelics: experimental approaches for assessing mechanisms of action. *Handb Exp Pharmacol*. 2018;252:227-260.
47. Nichols DE. Psychedelics. *Pharmacol Rev*. 2016;68(2):264-355.
48. Canal CE, Murnane KS. The serotonin 5-HT2C receptor and the non-addictive nature of classic hallucinogens. *J Psychopharmacol*. 2017;31(1):127-143.
49. Weiner DM, Burstein ES, Nash N, et al. 5-hydroxytryptamine2A receptor inverse agonists as antipsychotics. *J Pharmacol Exp Ther*. 2001;299(1):268-276.
50. Vanover KE, Weiner DM, Makhay M, et al. Pharmacological and behavioral profile of N-(4-fluorophenylmethyl)-N-(1-methylpiperidin-4-yl)-N'-(4-(2-methylpropyloxy)phen ylmethyl) carbamide (2R,3R)-dihydroxybutanedioate (2:1) (ACP-103), a novel 5-hydroxytryptamine(2A) receptor inverse agonist. *J Pharmacol Exp Ther*. 2006;317(2):910-918.
51. Cummings J, Isaacson S, Mills R, et al. Pimavanserin for patients with Parkinson's disease psychosis: a randomised, placebo-controlled phase 3 trial. *Lancet*. 2014;383(9916):533-540.
52. Choksi NY, Nix WB, Wyrick SD, Booth RG. A novel phenylaminotetralin (PAT) recognizes histamine H1 receptors and stimulates dopamine synthesis in vivo in rat brain. *Brain Res*. 2000;852(1):151-160.
53. Johnson EA, Tsai CE, Shahan YH, Azzaro AJ. Serotonin 5-HT1A receptors mediate inhibition of tyrosine hydroxylation in rat striatum. *J Pharmacol Exp Ther*. 1993;266(1):133-141.
54. Pogorelov VM, Rodriguiz RM, Cheng J, et al. 5-HT2C agonists modulate schizophrenia-like behaviors in mice. *Neuropsychopharmacology*. 2017;42(11):2163-2177.
55. Perez XA, Bordia T, Quik M. The striatal cholinergic system in L-dopa-induced dyskinesias. *J Neural Transm (Vienna)*. 2018;125(8):1251-1262.
56. Canal CE, Morgan D, Felsing D, et al. A novel aminotetralin-type serotonin (5-HT) 2C receptor-specific agonist and 5-HT2A competitive antagonist/5-HT2B inverse agonist with preclinical efficacy for psychoses. *J Pharmacol Exp Ther*. 2014;349(2):310-318.
57. Casey AB, Canal CE. Classics in chemical neuroscience: aripiprazole. *ACS Chem Neurosci*. 2017;8(6):1135-1146.
58. Katritch V, Cherezov V, Stevens RC. Structure-function of the G protein-coupled receptor superfamily. *Annu Rev Pharmacol Toxicol*. 2013;53:531-556.
59. Chien EY, Liu W, Zhao Q, et al. Structure of the human dopamine D3 receptor in complex with a D2/D3 selective antagonist. *Science*. 2010;330(6007):1091-1095.
60. Juncal-Ruiz M, Ramirez-Bonilla M, Gomez-Arnau J, et al. Incidence and risk factors of acute akathisia in 493 individuals with first episode non-affective psychosis: a 6-week randomised study of antipsychotic treatment. *Psychopharmacology*. 2017;234(17):2563-2570.
61. Hauser RA, Factor SA, Marder SR, et al. KINECT 3: a phase 3 randomized, double-blind, placebo-controlled trial of valbenazine for tardive dyskinesia. *Am J Psychiatry*. 2017;174(5):476-484.
62. Sykes DA, Moore H, Stott L, et al. Extrapyramidal side effects of antipsychotics are linked to their association kinetics at dopamine D2 receptors. *Nat Commun*. 2017;8(1):763.
63. Snyder SH, Greenberg D, Yamumura HI. Antischizophrenic drugs: affinity for muscarinic cholinergic receptor sites in the brain predicts extrapyramidal effects. *J Psychiatr Res*. 1974;11:91-95.

64. Reynolds GP, Kirk SL. Metabolic side effects of antipsychotic drug treatment–pharmacological mechanisms. *Pharmacol Ther.* 2010;125(1):169-179.
65. Kroeze WK, Hufeisen SJ, Popadak BA, et al. H1-histamine receptor affinity predicts short-term weight gain for typical and atypical antipsychotic drugs. *Neuropsychopharmacology.* 2003;28(3):519-526.
66. Lord CC, Wyler SC, Wan R, et al. The atypical antipsychotic olanzapine causes weight gain by targeting serotonin receptor 2C. *J Clin Invest.* 2017;127(9):3402-3406.
67. Zhang Y, Liu Y, Su Y, et al. The metabolic side effects of 12 antipsychotic drugs used for the treatment of schizophrenia on glucose: a network meta-analysis. *BMC Psychiatry.* 2017;17(1):373.
68. Ungar G, Parrot JL, Bovet D. The inhibition of the effects of histamine on the isolated intestine of the Guinea pig by some sympathicolytic and sympathicomimetic substances. *Cr Soc Biol.* 1937;124:445-446.
69. Laborit H, Huguenard P, Alluaume R. A new vegetative stabilizer; 4560 R.P.. *Presse Med.* 1952;60(10):206-208.
70. Delay J, Deniker P, Harl J. Utilization therapeutique psychiatrique d'une phenothiazine d'action centrale elective. *Ann Med Psychol (Paris).* 1952;110:112-117.
71. Lopez-Munoz F, Alamo C, Cuenca E, Shen WW, Clervoy P, Rubio G. History of the discovery and clinical introduction of chlorpromazine. *Ann Clin Psychiatry.* 2005;17(3):113-135.
72. Horn AS, Snyder SH. Chlorpromazine and dopamine: conformational similarities that correlate with the antischizophrenic activity of phenothiazine drugs. *Proc Natl Acad Sci USA.* 1971;68(10):2325-2328.
73. Janssen PA. The evolution of the butyrophenones, haloperidol and trifluperidol, from meperidine-like 4-phenylpiperidines. *Int Rev Neurobiol.* 1965;8:221-263.
74. Murray M. Role of CYP pharmacogenetics and drug-drug interactions in the efficacy and safety of atypical and other antipsychotic agents. *J Pharm Pharmacol.* 2006;58(7):871-885.
75. Subramanyam B, Pond SM, Eyles DW, Whiteford HA, Fouda HG, Castagnoli N Jr. Identification of potentially neurotoxic pyridinium metabolite in the urine of schizophrenic patients treated with haloperidol. *Biochem Biophys Res Commun.* 1991;181(2):573-578.
76. Halliday GM, Pond SM, Cartwright H, McRitchie DA, Castagnoli N Jr, Van der Schyf CJ. Clinical and neuropathological abnormalities in baboons treated with HPTP, the tetrahydropyridine analog of haloperidol. *Exp Neurol.* 1999;158(1):155-163.
77. Igarashi K, Matsubara K, Kasuya F, Fukui M, Idzu T, Castagnoli N Jr. Effect of a pyridinium metabolite derived from haloperidol on the activities of striatal tyrosine hydroxylase in freely moving rats. *Neurosci Lett.* 1996;214(2-3):183-186.
78. Rollema H, Skolnik M, D'Engelbronner J, Igarashi K, Usuki E, Castagnoli N Jr. MPP(+)-like neurotoxicity of a pyridinium metabolite derived from haloperidol: in vivo microdialysis and in vitro mitochondrial studies. *J Pharmacol Exp Ther.* 1994;268(1):380-387.
79. Ulrich S, Sandmann U, Genz A. Serum concentrations of haloperidol pyridinium metabolites and the relationship with tardive dyskinesia and parkinsonism: a cross-section study in psychiatric patients. *Pharmacopsychiatry.* 2005;38(4):171-177.
80. Mailman RB, Murthy V. Third generation antipsychotic drugs: partial agonism or receptor functional selectivity? *Curr Pharm Des.* 2010;16(5):488-501.
81. Gründer G, Hippius H, Carlsson A. The "atypicality" of antipsychotics: a concept re-examined and re-defined. *Nature Reviews Drug Discovery.* 2009;8:197.
82. Wenthur CJ, Lindsley CW. Classics in chemical neuroscience: clozapine. *ACS Chem Neurosci.* 2013;4(7):1018-1025.
83. Goldstein JI, Jarskog LF, Hilliard C, et al. Clozapine-induced agranulocytosis is associated with rare HLA-DQB1 and HLA-B alleles. *Nat Commun.* 2014;5:4757.
84. Schmid CL, Streicher JM, Meltzer HY, Bohn LM. Clozapine acts as an agonist at serotonin 2A receptors to counter MK-801-induced behaviors through a betaarrestin2-independent activation of Akt. *Neuropsychopharmacology.* 2014;39(8):1902-1913.
85. Wu Y, Blichowski M, Daskalakis ZJ, et al. Evidence that clozapine directly interacts on the GABAB receptor. *Neuroreport.* 2011;22(13):637-641.
86. Schwieler L, Linderholm KR, Nilsson-Todd LK, Erhardt S, Engberg G. Clozapine interacts with the glycine site of the NMDA receptor: electrophysiological studies of dopamine neurons in the rat ventral tegmental area. *Life Sci.* 2008;83(5-6):170-175.
87. Sur C, Mallorga PJ, Wittmann M, et al. N-desmethylclozapine, an allosteric agonist at muscarinic 1 receptor, potentiates N-methyl-D-aspartate receptor activity. *Proc Natl Acad Sci USA.* 2003;100(23):13674-13679.
88. Gigout S, Wierschke S, Dehnicke C, Deisz RA. Different pharmacology of N-desmethylclozapine at human and rat M2 and M 4 mAChRs in neocortex. *Naunyn Schmiedebergs Arch Pharmacol.* 2015;388(5):487-496.
89. Raedler TJ, Hinkelmann K, Wiedemann K. Variability of the in vivo metabolism of clozapine. *Clin Neuropharmacol.* 2008;31(6):347-352.
90. Vainer JL, Chouinard G. Interaction between caffeine and clozapine. *J Clin Psychopharmacol.* 1994;14(4):284-285.
91. Desai HD, Seabolt J, Jann MW. Smoking in patients receiving psychotropic medications: a pharmacokinetic perspective. *CNS Drugs.* 2001;15(6):469-494.
92. Haring C, Meise U, Humpel C, Saria A, Fleischhacker WW, Hinterhuber H. Dose-related plasma levels of clozapine: influence of smoking behaviour, sex and age. *Psychopharmacology (Berl).* 1989;99(suppl 1):S38-S40.
93. Urichuk L, Prior TI, Dursun S, Baker G. Metabolism of atypical antipsychotics: involvement of cytochrome p450 enzymes and relevance for drug-drug interactions. *Curr Drug Metab.* 2008;9(5):410-418.
94. Kassahun K, Mattiuz E, Nyhart E Jr, et al. Disposition and biotransformation of the antipsychotic agent olanzapine in humans. *Drug Metab Dispos.* 1997;25(1):81-93.
95. DeVane CL, Nemeroff CB. Clinical pharmacokinetics of quetiapine: an atypical antipsychotic. *Clin Pharmacokinet.* 2001;40(7):509-522.
96. Jensen NH, Rodriguiz RM, Caron MG, Wetsel WC, Rothman RB, Roth BL. N-desalkylquetiapine, a potent norepinephrine reuptake inhibitor and partial 5-HT1A agonist, as a putative mediator of quetiapine's antidepressant activity. *Neuropsychopharmacology.* 2008;33(10):2303-2312.
97. Shahid M, Walker GB, Zorn SH, Wong EH. Asenapine: a novel psychopharmacologic agent with a unique human receptor signature. *J Psychopharmacol.* 2009;23(1):65-73.
98. Yasui-Furukori N, Hidestrand M, Spina E, Facciola G, Scordo MG, Tybring G. Different enantioselective 9-hydroxylation of risperidone by the two human CYP2D6 and CYP3A4 enzymes. *Drug Metab Dispos.* 2001;29(10):1263-1268.
99. Subramanian N, Kalkman HO. Receptor profile of P88-8991 and P95-12113, metabolites of the novel antipsychotic iloperidone. *Prog Neuro-psychopharmacol Biol Psychiatry.* 2002;26(3):553-560.
100. Newman-Tancredi A, Gavaudan S, Conte C, et al. Agonist and antagonist actions of antipsychotic agents at 5-HT1A receptors: a [35S]GTPgammaS binding study. *Eur J Pharmacol.* 1998;355(2-3):245-256.
101. Hirose T, Uwahodo Y, Yamada S, et al. Mechanism of action of aripiprazole predicts clinical efficacy and a favourable side-effect profile. *J Psychopharmacol.* 2004;18(3):375-383.
102. Shapiro DA, Renock S, Arrington E, et al. Aripiprazole, a novel atypical antipsychotic drug with a unique and robust pharmacology. *Neuropsychopharmacology.* 2003;28(8):1400-1411.
103. Lawler CP, Prioleau C, Lewis MM, et al. Interactions of the novel antipsychotic aripiprazole (OPC-14597) with dopamine and serotonin receptor subtypes. *Neuropsychopharmacology.* 1999;20(6):612-627.
104. Genaro-Mattos TC, Tallman KA, Allen LB, et al. Dichlorophenyl piperazines, including a recently-approved atypical antipsychotic, are potent inhibitors of DHCR7, the last enzyme in cholesterol biosynthesis. *Toxicol Appl Pharmacol.* 2018;349:21-28.

105. Maeda K, Sugino H, Akazawa H, et al. Brexpiprazole I: in vitro and in vivo characterization of a novel serotonin-dopamine activity modulator. *J Pharmacol Exp Ther*. 2014;350(3):589-604.
106. Nemeth G, Laszlovszky I, Czobor P, et al. Cariprazine versus risperidone monotherapy for treatment of predominant negative symptoms in patients with schizophrenia: a randomised, double-blind, controlled trial. *Lancet*. 2017;389(10074):1103-1113.
107. Girgis RR, Slifstein M, D'Souza D, et al. Preferential binding to dopamine D3 over D2 receptors by cariprazine in patients with schizophrenia using PET with the D3/D2 receptor ligand [(11)C]-(+)-PHNO. *Psychopharmacology (Berl)*. 2016;233(19-20):3503-3512.
108. Choi YK, Adham N, Kiss B, Gyertyan I, Tarazi FI. Long-term effects of cariprazine exposure on dopamine receptor subtypes. *CNS Spectr*. 2014;19(3):268-277.
109. Choi YK, Adham N, Kiss B, Gyertyan I, Tarazi FI. Long-term effects of aripiprazole exposure on monoaminergic and glutamatergic receptor subtypes: comparison with cariprazine. *CNS Spectr*. 2017;22(6):484-494.
110. Earley W, Durgam S, Lu K, Laszlovszky I, Debelle M, Kane JM. Safety and tolerability of cariprazine in patients with acute exacerbation of schizophrenia: a pooled analysis of four phase II/III randomized, double-blind, placebo-controlled studies. *Int Clin Psychopharmacol*. 2017;32(6):319-328.
111. Rohde M, N MR, Hakansson AE, et al. Biological conversion of aripiprazole lauroxil – an N-acyloxymethyl aripiprazole prodrug. *Results Pharma Sci*. 2014;4:19-25.
112. O'Brien CF, Jimenez R, Hauser RA, et al. NBI-98854, a selective monoamine transport inhibitor for the treatment of tardive dyskinesia: a randomized, double-blind, placebo-controlled study. *Mov Disord*. 2015;30(12):1681-1687.
113. Anderson KE, Stamler D, Davis MD, et al. Deutetrabenazine for treatment of involuntary movements in patients with tardive dyskinesia (AIM-TD): a double-blind, randomised, placebo-controlled, phase 3 trial. *Lancet Psychiatry*. 2017;4(8):595-604.
114. Ballard C, Banister C, Khan Z, et al. Evaluation of the safety, tolerability, and efficacy of pimavanserin versus placebo in patients with Alzheimer's disease psychosis: a phase 2, randomised, placebo-controlled, double-blind study. *Lancet Neurol*. 2018;17(3):213-222.
115. Campbell-Sills L, Simmons AN, Lovero KL, Rochlin AA, Paulus MP, Stein MB. Functioning of neural systems supporting emotion regulation in anxiety-prone individuals. *Neuroimage*. 2011;54(1):689-696.
116. Martin EI, Ressler KJ, Binder E, Nemeroff CB. The neurobiology of anxiety disorders: brain imaging, genetics, and psychoneuroendocrinology. *Clin Lab Med*. 2010;30(4):865-891.
117. Nordahl TE, Semple WE, Gross M, et al. Cerebral glucose metabolic differences in patients with panic disorder. *Neuropsychopharmacology*. 1990;3(4):261-272.
118. Beutel ME, Stark R, Pan H, Silbersweig D, Dietrich S. Changes of brain activation pre- post short-term psychodynamic inpatient psychotherapy: an fMRI study of panic disorder patients. *Psychiatry Res*. 2010;184(2):96-104.
119. Rauch SL, Savage CR, Alpert NM, et al. A positron emission tomographic study of simple phobic symptom provocation. *Arch Gen Psychiatry*. 1995;52(1):20-28.
120. Caseras X, Mataix-Cols D, Trasovares MV, et al. Dynamics of brain responses to phobic-related stimulation in specific phobia subtypes. *Eur J Neurosci*. 2010;32(8):1414-1422.
121. Gershenfeld HK, Philibert RA, Boehm GW. Looking forward in geriatric anxiety and depression: implications of basic science for the future. *Am J Geriatr Psychiatry*. 2005;13(12):1027-1040.
122. Cheung A, Mayes T, Levitt A, et al. Anxiety as a predictor of treatment outcome in children and adolescents with depression. *J Child Adol Psychop*. 2010;20(3):211-216.
123. Olsen RW, Sieghart W. International Union of Pharmacology. LXX. Subtypes of gamma-aminobutyric acid(A) receptors: classification on the basis of subunit composition, pharmacology, and function. Update. *Pharmacol Rev*. 2008;60(3):243-260.
124. Cutting GR, Lu L, O'Hara BF, et al. Cloning of the gamma-aminobutyric acid (GABA) rho 1 cDNA: a GABA receptor subunit highly expressed in the retina. *Proc Natl Acad Sci USA*. 1991;88(7):2673-2677.
125. Schofield PR, Darlison MG, Fujita N, et al. Sequence and functional expression of the GABA A receptor shows a ligand-gated receptor super-family. *Nature*. 1987;328(6127):221-227.
126. Wisden W, Laurie DJ, Monyer H, Seeburg PH. The distribution of 13 GABAA receptor subunit mRNAs in the rat brain. I. Telencephalon, diencephalon, mesencephalon. *J Neurosci*. 1992;12(3):1040-1062.
127. Zhu S, Noviello CM, Teng J, Walsh RM Jr, Kim JJ, Hibbs RE. Structure of a human synaptic GABAA receptor. *Nature*. 2018;559(7712):67-72.
128. Sanger DJ, Benavides J, Perrault G, et al. Recent developments in the behavioral pharmacology of benzodiazepine (omega) receptors: evidence for the functional significance of receptor subtypes. *Neurosci Biobehav Rev*. 1994;18(3):355-372.
129. Sieghart W. Anxioselective anxiolytics: additional perspective. *Trends Pharmacol Sci*. 2013;34(3):145-146.
130. Frangaj A, Fan QR. Structural biology of GABAB receptor. *Neuropharmacology*. 2018;136(pt A):68-79.
131. Kaupmann K, Malitschek B, Schuler V, et al. GABA(B)-receptor subtypes assemble into functional heteromeric complexes. *Nature*. 1998;396(6712):683-687.
132. Couve A, Filippov AK, Connolly CN, Bettler B, Brown DA, Moss SJ. Intracellular retention of recombinant GABA(B) receptors. *J Biol Chem*. 1998;273(41):26361-26367.
133. Jones KA, Borowsky B, Tamm JA, et al. GABA(B) receptors function as a heteromeric assembly of the subunits GABA(B)R1 and GABA(B)R2. *Nature*. 1998;396(6712):674-679.
134. White JH, Wise A, Main MJ, et al. Heterodimerization is required for the formation of a functional GABA(B) receptor. *Nature*. 1998;396(6712):679-682.
135. Stewart GD, Comps-Agrar L, Norskov-Lauritsen LB, Pin JP, Kniazeff J. Allosteric interactions between GABA(B1) subunits control orthosteric binding sites occupancy within GABA(B) oligomers. *Neuropharmacology*. 2018;136:92-101.
136. Geng Y, Bush M, Mosyak L, Wang F, Fan QR. Structural mechanism of ligand activation in human GABA(B) receptor. *Nature*. 2013;504(7479):254-259.
137. Pin JP, Galvez T, Prezeau L. Evolution, structure, and activation mechanism of family 3/C G-protein-coupled receptors. *Pharmacol Ther*. 2003;98(3):325-354.
138. Berry-Kravis E, Hagerman R, Visootsak J, et al. Arbaclofen in fragile X syndrome: results of phase 3 trials. *J Neurodev Disord*. 2017;9:3.
139. Veenstra-VanderWeele J, Cook EH, King BH, et al. Arbaclofen in children and adolescents with autism spectrum disorder: a randomized, controlled, phase 2 trial. *Neuropsychopharmacology*. 2017;42(7):1390-1398.
140. Ertzgaard P, Campo C, Calabrese A. Efficacy and safety of oral baclofen in the management of spasticity: a rationale for intrathecal baclofen. *J Rehabil Med*. 2017;49(3):193-203.
141. Brown KM, Roy KK, Hockerman GH, Doerksen RJ, Colby DA. Activation of the gamma-aminobutyric acid type B (GABA(B)) receptor by agonists and positive allosteric modulators. *J Med Chem*. 2015;58(16):6336-6347.
142. Kumar K, Sharma S, Kumar P, Deshmukh R. Therapeutic potential of GABA(B) receptor ligands in drug addiction, anxiety, depression and other CNS disorders. *Pharmacol Biochem Behav*. 2013;110:174-184.
143. Lal R, Sukbuntherng J, Tai EH, et al. Arbaclofen placarbil, a novel R-baclofen prodrug: improved absorption, distribution, metabolism, and elimination properties compared with R-baclofen. *J Pharmacol Exp Ther*. 2009;330(3):911-921.
144. Garattini S, Mussini E, Randall LO. *The Benzodiazepines*. New York: Raven Press; 1973.

145. Sternbach LH. The benzodiazepine story. *J Med Chem.* 1979;22(1):1-7.
146. Randall LO, Schallek W, Heise GA, Keith EF, Bagdon RE. The psychosedative properties of methaminodiazepoxide. *J Pharmacol Exp Ther.* 1960;129:163-171.
147. Randall LO, Scheckel CL, Banziger RF. Pharmacology of the metabolites of chlordiazepoxide and diazepam. *Curr Ther Res Clin Exp.* 1965;7(9):590-606.
148. Braestrup C, Nielsen M, Olsen CE. Urinary and brain beta-carboline-3-carboxylates as potent inhibitors of brain benzodiazepine receptors. *P Natl Acad Sci-Biol.* 1980;77(4):2288-2292.
149. Cole BJ, Hillmann M, Seidelmann D, Klewer M, Jones GH. Effects of benzodiazepine receptor partial inverse agonists in the elevated plus-maze test of anxiety in the rat. *Psychopharmacology.* 1995;121(1):118-126.
150. Braestrup C, Schmiechen R, Neef G, Nielsen M, Petersen EN. Interaction of convulsive ligands with benzodiazepine receptors. *Science.* 1982;216(4551):1241-1243.
151. Haefely W, Kyburz E, Gerecke M, al. e. *Recent advances in the molecular pharmacology of benzodiazepine receptors and the structure-activity relationships of these agonists and antagonists.* In: *Advances in Drug Research.* Vol 14. London: Academic Press; 1985:166-322.
152. Hunkeler W, Mohler H, Pieri L, et al. Selective antagonists of benzodiazepines. *Nature.* 1981;290(5806):514-516.
153. Mohler H, Richards JG. Agonist and antagonist benzodiazepine receptor interaction in vitro. *Nature.* 1981;294(5843):763-765.
154. Wieland HA, Luddens H, Seeburg PH. A single histidine in gaba-a receptors is essential for benzodiazepine agonist binding. *J Biol Chem.* 1992;267(3):1426-1429.
155. Rowlett JK, Platt DM, Lelas S, Atack JR, Dawson GR. Different GABAA receptor subtypes mediate the anxiolytic, abuse-related, and motor effects of benzodiazepine-like drugs in primates. *Proc Natl Acad Sci USA.* 2005;102(3):915-920.
156. Blount JF, Fryer RI, Gilman NW, Todaro LJ. Quinazolines and 1,4-benzodiazepines. 92. Conformational recognition of the receptor by 1,4-benzodiazepines. *Mol Pharmacol.* 1983;24(3): 425-428.
157. Sunjic V, Lisini A, Sega A, Kovac T, Kajfez F, Ruscic B. Conformation of 7-chloro-5-phenyl-D5-3(S)-Methyldihydro-1,4-Benzodiazepin-2-One in solution. *J Heterocyclic Chem.* 1979;16(4):757-761.
158. Olkkola KT, Ahonen J. Midazolam and other benzodiazepines. *Handb Exp Pharmacol.* 2008(182):335-360.
159. Gerecke M. Chemical structure and properties of midazolam compared with other benzodiazepines. *Br J Clin Pharmacol.* 1983;16(suppl 1):11S-16S.
160. Davies M, Newell JG, Derry JM, Martin IL, Dunn SM. Characterization of the interaction of zopiclone with gamma-aminobutyric acid type A receptors. *Mol Pharmacol.* 2000;58(4):756-762.
161. Rosenberg R, Caron J, Roth T, Amato D. An assessment of the efficacy and safety of eszopiclone in the treatment of transient insomnia in healthy adults. *Sleep Med.* 2005;6(1):15-22.
162. Herrmann WM, Kubicki ST, Boden S, Eich FX, Attali P, Coquelin JP. Pilot controlled double-blind study of the hypnotic effects of zolpidem in patients with chronic 'learned' insomnia: psychometric and polysomnographic evaluation. *J Int Med Res.* 1993;21(6):306-322.
163. Auta J, Costa E, Davis JM, Guidotti A. Imidazenil: an antagonist of the sedative but not the anticonvulsant action of diazepam. *Neuropharmacology.* 2005;49(3):425-429.
164. Basile AS, Lippa AS, Skolnick P. Anxioselective anxiolytics: can less be more? *Eur J Pharmacol.* 2004;500(1-3):441-451.
165. National Institute of Mental Health. *Depression: What You Need to Know.* Depression (NIH Publication No. 15-3561). Bethesda, MD: U.S. Government Printing Office. National Institutes of Health Publication; 2015:2000.
166. *Real Men; Real Depression*: National Institutes of Health Publication; 2003:03-4972.
167. Manji HK, Lenox RH. Signaling: cellular insights into the pathophysiology of bipolar disorder. *Biol Psychiatry.* 2000;48: 518-530.
168. Schüle C, Nothdurfter C, Rupprecht R. The role of allopregnanolone in depression and anxiety. *Prog Neurobiol.* 2014;113:79-87.
169. Osborne LM, Gispen F, Sanyal A, et al. Lower allopregnanolone during pregnancy predicts postpartum depression: an exploratory study. *Psychoneuroendocrinology.* 2017;79:116–121.
170. Kanes S, Colquhoun H, Gunduz-Bruce H, et al. Brexanolone (SAGE-547 injection) in post-partum depression: a randomised controlled trial. *Lancet.* 2017;390:480-489.
171. Meltzer-Brody S, Colquhoun H, Riesenberg R, et al. Brexanolone injection in post-partum depression: two multicentre, double-blind, randomised, placebo-controlled, phase 3 trials. *Lancet.* 2018;392:1058-1070.
172. Bäckström T, Bixo M, Johansson M, et al. Allopregnanolone and mood disorders. *Prog Neurobiol.* 2014;113:88-94.
173. Hellgren C, Åkerud H, Skalkidou A, et al. Low serum allopregnanolone is associated with symptoms of depression in late pregnancy. *Neuropsychobiology.* 2014;69(3):147-153.
174. Schiller CE, Schmidt PJ, Rubinow DR. Allopregnanolone as a mediator of affective switching in reproductive mood disorders. *Psychopharmacology (Berl).* 2014;231:3557-3567.
175. Moret C, Briley M. The importance of norepinephrine in depression. *Neuropsychiatr Dis Treat.* 2011;7(suppl 1):9-13.
176. Delgado PL, Moreno FA. Role of norepinephrine in depression. *J Clin Psychiatry.* 2000;61(suppl 1):5-12.
177. Duman RS, Heninger GR, Nestler EJ. A molecular and cellular theory of depression. *Arch Gen Psychiatry.* 1997;54:597-606.
178. Schildkraut JJ, Klerman GL, Hammond R, et al. Excretion of 3-methoxy-mandelic acid (VMA) in depressed patients treated with antidepressant drugs. *J Psychiatr Res.* 1965;2:257-266.
179. Janowsky DS, Davis JM. Adrenergic-cholinergic balance in affective disorders. *Psychopharmacol Bull.* 1978;14(4):58-60.
180. van Praag HK, Korf J. Endogenous depression with and without disturbance of 5-hydroxytryptamine metabolism: a biochemical classification? *Psychopharmacology.* 1971;19:148-152.
181. Coppen A, Prange AJ Jr, Whybrow PC, et al. Abnormalities of indoleamines in affective disorders. *Arch Gen Psychiat.* 1972;26:474-478.
182. Lenox RH, Frazer A. Mechanism of action of antidepressants and mood stabilizers. In: Davis KL, Charney D, Coyle JT, et al, eds. *Neuropsychopharmacology: The Fifth Generation of Progress.* Baltimore: Lippincott Williams & Wilkins; 2002;1139-1164.
183. Brown AS, Gershon S. DA and depression. *J Neural Transm.* 1993;91:75-109.
184. Shytle RD, Silver AA, Lukas RJ, et al. Nicotinic acetylcholine receptors as targets for antidepressants. *Mol Psychiatry.* 2002;7:525-535.
185. Kuhn R. Uber die behandlung depressives zustande mit einem iminobenzylderivat (G 22,355). *Schweiz Med Wschr.* 1957;87:1135-1140.
186. Loomer HP, Saunders JC, Kline NS. A clinical and pharmacodynamic evaluation of iproniazid as a psychic energizer. *Psychiatr Res Rep Am Psychiatr Assoc.* 1957;8:129-141.
187. Baldessarini RJ. Drug therapy of depression and anxiety disorders. In: Brunton LL, Lazo JS, Parker KL, eds. *Goodman & Gilman's the Pharmacological Basis of Therapeutics.* 11th ed. New York: McGraw-Hill; 2006:429-460.
188. Hogberg T, Ulff B, Renyi AL, et al. Synthesis of pyridylallylamines related to zimelidine and their inhibition of neuronal monoamine uptake. *J Med Chem.* 1981;24:1499-1507.
189. Ogren SO, Ross SB, Hall H, et al. The pharmacology of zimelidine: a 5-HT selective reuptake inhibitor. *Acta Psychiatr Scand Suppl.* 1981;290:127-151.
190. Wong DT, Bymaster FP, Horng JS, et al. A new selective inhibitor for uptake of serotonin into synaptosomes of rat brain: 3-(p-trifluoromethylphenoxy). N-methyl-3-phenylpropylamine. *J Pharmacol Exp Ther.* 1975;193:804-811.

191. Wong DT, Bymaster FP, Engleman EA. Prozac (Fluoxetine, Lilly 110140), the first selective serotonin uptake inhibitor and an antidepressant drug: twenty years since its first publication. *Life Sci.* 1995;57:411-441.
192. Skolnick P, Popik P, Janowsky A, et al. "Broad spectrum" antidepressants: is more better for the treatment of depression? *Life Sci.* 2003;73:3175-3179.
193. Torres GE, Gainetdinov RR, Caron MG. Plasma membrane monoamine transporters: structure, regulation and function. *Nat Rev Neurosci.* 2003;4:13-25.
194. Owens MJ, Morgan WN, Plott SJ, et al. Neurotransmitter receptor and transporter binding profile of antidepressants and their metabolites. *J Pharmacol Exp Ther.* 1997;283:1305-1322.
195. Sanchez C, Hyttel J. Comparison of the effects of antidepressants and their metabolites on reuptake of biogenic amines and on receptor binding. *Cell Mol Neurobiol.* 1999;19:467-489.
196. Cipriani A, Furukawa TA, Salanti G, et al. Comparative efficacy and acceptability of 21 antidepressant drugs for the acute treatment of adults with major depressive disorder: a systematic review and network meta-analysis. *Lancet.* 2018;391:1357-1366.
197. Brunello N, Mendlewicz J, Kasper S, et al. The role of noradrenaline and selective noradrenaline reuptake inhibition in depression. *Eur Neuropsychopharmacol.* 2002;12:461-475.
198. Mandrioli R, Protti M, Mercolini L. New-generation, non-SSRI antidepressants: therapeutic drug monitoring and pharmacological interactions. Part 1: SNRIs, SMSs, SARIs. *Curr Med Chem.* 2018;25:772-792.
199. Kelder J, Funke C, De Boer T, et al. A comparison of the physicochemical and biological properties of mirtazapine and mianserin. *J Pharm Pharmacol.* 1997;49:403-411.
200. Baker GB, Prior TI. Stereochemistry and drug efficacy and development: relevance of chirality to antidepressant and antipsychotic drugs. *Ann Med.* 2002;34:537-543.
201. Budău M, Hancu G, Rusu A, et al. Chirality of modern antidepressants: an overview. *Adv Pharm Bull.* 2017;7:495-500.
202. Norregaard L, Gether U. The monoamine neurotransmitter transporters: structure, conformational changes and molecular gating. *Curr Opin Drug Discov Dev.* 2001;4:591-601.
203. Casarotto MG, Craik DJ. Ring flexibility within tricyclic antidepressant drugs. *J Pharm Sci.* 2001;90:713-719.
204. Venkatakrishnan K, Von Moltke LL, Greenblatt DJ. Human drug metabolism and the cytochromes P450: application and relevance of in vitro models. *J Clin Pharmacol.* 2001;41:1149-1179.
205. Yan JH, Hubbard JW, McKay G, et al. Absolute bioavailability and stereoselective pharmacokinetics of doxepin. *Xenobiotica.* 2002;32:615-623.
206. Haritos VS, Ghabrial H, Ahokas JT, et al. Role of cytochrome P450 2D6 (CYP2D6) in the stereospecific metabolism of E- and Z-doxepin. *Pharmacogenetics.* 2000;10:591-603.
207. Eap CB, Bender S, Gastpar M, et al. Steady-state plasma levels of the enantiomers of trimipramine and of its metabolites in CYP2D6-, CYP2C19- and CYP3A4/5-phenotyped patients. *Ther Drug Monit.* 2000;22:209-214.
208. Kirchheiner J, Muller G, Meineke I, et al. Effects of polymorphisms in CYP2D6, CYP2C9 and CYP2C19 on trimipramine pharmacokinetics. *J Clin Psychopharmacol.* 2003;23:459-466.
209. Eriksson E. Antidepressant drugs: does it matter if they inhibit the reuptake of noradrenaline or serotonin? *Acta Psychiatr Scand Suppl.* 2000;402:12-17.
210. Olivier B, Soudjin W, van Wijngaarden I. Serotonin, DA and norepinephrine transporters in the CNS and their inhibitors. In: Jucker E, ed. *Progress in Drug Research.* Vol 54. Basel, Switzerland: Birkhäuser-Verlag; 2000:59-120.
211. Cowen PJ. Serotonin hypothesis. In: Feighner JP, Boyer WR, eds. *Selective Serotonin Reuptake Inhibitors.* 2nd ed. 1996;63-86.
212. SHPreskorn. Clinical Pharmacology of SSRIs. 1st ed. Available at http://www.preskorn.com. Accessed December 8, 2018.
213. Preskorn SH. Clinically relevant pharmacology of selective serotonin reuptake inhibitors. An overview with emphasis on pharmacokinetics and effects on oxidative drug metabolism. *Clin Pharmacokinet.* 1997;32(suppl 1):1-19.
214. Hyttel J. Pharmacological characterization of selective serotonin reuptake inhibitors (SSRIs). *Int Clin Psychopharmacol.* 1994;9(suppl 1):19-26.
215. Bordet R, Thomas P, Dupuis B. Effect of pindolol on onset of action of paroxetine in the treatment of major depression: intermediate analysis of a double-blind, placebo-controlled trial. Reseau de Recherche et d'Experimentation Psychopharmacologique. *Am J Psychiatr.* 1998;155:1346-1351.
216. Wong DT, Threlkeld PG, Robertson DW. Affinities of fluoxetine, its enantiomers and other inhibitors of serotonin uptake for subtypes of serotonin receptors. *Neuropsychopharmacology.* 1991;5:43-47.
217. Wong DT, Bymaster FP, Reid LR, et al. Norfluoxetine enantiomers as inhibitors of serotonin uptake in rat brain. *Neuropsychopharmacology.* 1993;8:337-344.
218. Bertelsen KM, Venkatakrishnan K, Von Moltke LL, et al. Apparent mechanism-based inhibition of human CYP2D6 in vitro by paroxetine: comparison with fluoxetine and quinidine. *Drug Metab Dispos.* 2003;31:289-293.
219. Nakajima M, Suzuki M, Yamaji R, et al. Isoform selective inhibition and inactivation of human cytochrome P450s by methylenedioxyphenyl compounds. *Xenobiotica.* 1999;29:1191-1202.
220. Bolton JL, Acay NM, Vukomanovic V. Evidence that 4-allyl-o-quinones spontaneously rearrange to their more electrophilic quinone methides: potential bioactivation mechanism for the hepatocarcinogen safrole. *Chem Res Toxicol.* 1994;7:443-450.
221. Sanchez C, Bogeso KP, Ebert B, et al. Escitalopram versus citalopram: the surprising role of the R-enantiomer. *Psychopharmacology.* 2004;174:163-176.
222. Owens MJ, Knight DL, Nemeroff CB. Second-generation SSRIs: human monoamine transporter binding profile of escitalopram and R-fluoxetine. *Biol Psychiatry.* 2001;50:345-350.
223. Obach RS, Cox LM, Tremaine LM. Sertraline is metabolized by multiple cytochrome P450 enzymes, monoamine oxidases and glucuronyl transferase in human; an in vitro study. *Drug Met Disposition.* 2005;33:262-270.
224. Wong DT, Bymaster FP. Dual serotonin and noradrenaline uptake inhibitor class of antidepressants potential for greater efficacy or just hype? *Prog Drug Res.* 2002;58:169-222.
225. Bymaster FP, Dreshfield-Ahmad LJ, Threlkeld PG, et al. Comparative affinity of duloxetine and venlafaxine for serotonin and norepinephrine transporters in vitro and in vivo, human serotonin receptor subtypes and other neuronal receptors. *Neuropsychopharmacology.* 2001;25:871-880.
226. Zerbe RL, Rowe H, Enas GG, et al. Clinical pharmacology of atomoxetine, a potential antidepressant. *J Pharmacol Exp Ther.* 1985;232:139-143.
227. Sauer JM, Ponsler GD, Mattiuz EL, et al. Disposition and metabolic fate of atomoxetine hydrochloride: the role of CYP2D6 in human disposition and metabolism. *Drug Metab Dispos.* 2003;31:98-107.
228. Asnis GM, Henderson MA. Levomilnacipran for the treatment of major depressive disorder: a review. *Neuropsychiatr Dis Treat.* 2015;11:125-135.
229. Vaishnavi SN, Nemeroff CB, Plott SJ, et al. Milnacipran: a comparative analysis of human monoamine uptake and transporter binding affinity. *Biol Psychiatry.* 2004;55:320-322.
230. Chen L, Greenberg WM, Gommoll C, et al. Levomilnacipran pharmacokinetics in healthy volunteers versus patients with major depressive disorder and implications for norepinephrine and serotonin reuptake inhibition. *Clin Ther.* 2015;37(9):2059-2070.
231. Brunner V, Maynadier B, Chen L, et al. Disposition and metabolism of [14C]-levomilnacipran, a serotonin and norepinephrine reuptake inhibitor, in humans, monkeys, and rats. *Drug Des Devel Ther.* 2015;9:3199-3215.

232. Lantz RJ, Gillespie TA, Rash TJ, et al. Metabolism, excretion and pharmacokinetics of duloxetine in healthy human subjects. *Drug Metab Dispos.* 2003;31:1142-1150.
233. Jensen TS, Madsen CS, Finnerup NB. Pharmacology and treatment of neuropathic pains. *Curr Opin Neurol.* 2009;22:467-474.
234. Warner C, Shoaib M. How does bupropion work as a smoking cessation aid? *Addict Biol.* 2005;10:219-231.
235. Coles R, Kharasch ED. Stereoselective metabolism of bupropion by cytochrome P4502B6 (CYP2B6) and human liver microsomes. *Pharm Res.* 2008;25:1405-1411.
236. Hesse LM, Venkatakrishnan K, Court MH, et al. CYP2B6 mediates the in vitro hydroxylation of bupropion: potential drug interactions with other antidepressants. *Drug Metab Dispos.* 2000;28:1176-1183.
237. Bryant SG, Ereshefsky L. Antidepressant properties of trazodone. *Clin Pharm.* 1982;15:406-417.
238. Stahl SM. Mechanism of action of trazodone: a multifunctional drug. *CNS Spectr.* 2009;14:536-546.
239. Karhu D, Gossen ER, Mostert A, Cronjé T, Fradette C. Safety, tolerability, and pharmacokinetics of once-daily trazodone extended-release caplets in healthy subjects. *Int J Clin Pharmacol Ther.* 2011;49:730-743.
240. Wen B, Ma L, Rodrigues AD, Zhu M. Detection of novel reactive metabolites of trazodone: evidence for CYP2D6-mediated bioactivation of m-chlorophenylpiperazine. *J Chromatogr B Analyt Technol Biomed Life Sci.* 2008;871:44-54.
241. Boulton DW, Miller LF, Miller RL. Pharmacokinetics of trazodone and its major metabolite m-chlorophenylpiperazine in plasma and brain of rats. *Drug Metab Dispos.* 2008;36:841-850.
242. Rotzinger S, Fang J, Baker GB. Trazodone is metabolized to m-chlorophenylpiperazine by CYP3A4 from human sources. *Drug Metab Dispos.* 1998;26:572-575.
243. Iranikhah M, Wensel TM, Thomason AR. Vilazodone for the treatment of major depressive disorder. *Pharmacotherapy.* 2012;32(10):958-965.
244. Reinhold JA, Mandos LA, Lohoff FW, Rickels K. Evidence for the use of vilazodone in the treatment of major depressive disorder. *Expert Opin Pharmacother.* 2012;13:2215-2224.
245. McCormack PL. Vilazodone: a review in major depressive disorder in adults. *Drugs.* 2015 Nov;75(16):1915-1923.
246. El-Bagary R, Hashem H, Fouad M, Tarek S.UPLC-MS-MS method for the determination of vilazodone in human plasma: application to a pharmacokinetic study. *J Chromatogr Sci.* 2016;54:1365-1372.
247. Shi L, Wang J, Xu S, Lu Y. Efficacy and tolerability of vilazodone for major depressive disorder: evidence from phase III/IV randomized controlled trials. *Drug Des Devel Ther.* 2016;25(10):3899-3907.
248. Stuivenga M, Giltay EJ, Cools O, et al. Evaluation of vilazodone for the treatment of depressive and anxiety disorders. *Expert Opin Pharmacother.* 2018;26:1-10.
249. Connolly KR, Thase ME. Vortioxetine: a new treatment for major depressive disorder. *Expert Opin Pharmacother.* 2016;17:421-431.
250. Chen G, Højer AM, Areberg J, Nomikos G. Vortioxetine: clinical pharmacokinetics and drug interactions. *Clin Pharmacokinet.* 2018;57:673-686.
251. Chen G, Nomikos GG, Affinito J, et al. Effects of intrinsic factors on the clinical pharmacokinetics of vortioxetine. *Clin Pharmacol Drug Dev.* 2018;7:880-888.
252. Greenblatt DJ, Harmatz JS, Chow CR. Vortioxetine disposition in obesity: potential implications for patient safety. *J Clin Psychopharmacol.* 2018;38:172-179.
253. Benjamin S1, Doraiswamy PM. Review of the use of mirtazapine in the treatment of depression. *Expert Opin Pharmacother.* 2011;12:1623–1632.
254. Thompson C. Mirtazapine versus selective serotonin reuptake inhibitors. *J Clin Psychiatry.* 1999;60(suppl 17):18-22.
255. Stormer E, von Moltke LL, Shader RI, et al. Metabolism of the antidepressant mirtazapine in vitro: contribution of cytochromes P-450 1A2, 2D6 and 3A4. *Drug Metab Dispos.* 2000;28:1168-1175.
256. Shih JC, Chen K, Ridd MJ. MAO: from genes to behavior. *Annu Rev Neurosci.* 1999;22:197-217.
257. Baker GB, Urichuk LJ, McKenna KF, et al. Metabolism of monoamine oxidase inhibitors. *Cell Mol Neurobiol.* 1999;19:411-426.
258. Harwood AJ. Neurodevelopment and mood stabilizers. *Curr Mol Med.* 2003;3:472-482.
259. Berridge MJ. The Albert Lasker Medical Awards. Inositol trisphosphate, calcium, lithium and cell signaling. *JAMA.* 1989;262:1834-1841.
260. Lenox RH, Wang L. Molecular basis of lithium action: integration of lithium-responsive signaling and gene expression networks. *Mol Psychiatry.* 2003;8:135-144.
261. Skolnick P, Popik P, Trullas R. Glutamate-based antidepressants: 20 years on. *Trends Pharmacol Sci.* 2009;30:563-569.
262. Ono S, Ogawa K, Yamashita K, et al. Conformational analysis of the NMDA receptor antagonist (1S,2R)-1-phenyl-2-[S-1-aminopropyl]-N,N-diethylcyclopropanecarboxamide (PPDC) designed by a novel conformational restriction method based on the structural feature of cyclopropane ring. *Chem Pharm Bull (Tokyo).* 2002;50:966-968.
263. Zanos P, Gould TD. Mechanisms of ketamine action as an antidepressant. *Mol Psychiatry.* 2018;23:801-811.
264. Zanos P, Thompson SM, Duman RS, et al. Convergent mechanisms underlying rapid antidepressant action. *CNS Drugs.* 2018;32:197-227.
265. Zanos P, Gould TD. Intracellular signaling pathways involved in (S)- and (R)-Ketamine antidepressant actions. *Biol Psychiatry.* 2018;83:2-4.
266. Zanos P, Moaddel R, Morris PJ, et al. Ketamine and ketamine metabolite pharmacology: insights into therapeutic mechanisms. *Pharmacol Rev.* 2018;70:621-660.
267. Desta Z, Moaddel, Ogburn ET, et al. Stereoseleective and regioselective hydroxylation of ketamine and norketamine. *Xenobiotica.* 2012;42:1076-1087.
268. Ioannides C. Pharmacokinetic interactions between herbal remedies and medicinal drugs. *Xenobiotica.* 2002;32:451-478.
269. Muller WE, Singer A, Wonnemann M. Hyperforin—antidepressant activity by a novel mechanism of action. *Pharmacopsychiatry.* 2001;34(suppl 1):S98-S102.
270. Christopher EJ. Electroconvulsive therapy in the medically ill. *Curr Psychiatry Rep.* 2003;5:225-230.
271. 2010 Alzheimer's Disease Facts and Figures *Alzheimer's Association.* Available at https://www.alz.org/media/HomeOffice/Facts%20and%20Figures/facts-and-figures.pdf. Accessed November 26, 2018.
272. Crous-Bou M, Miguillon C, Gramunt N, et al. Alzheimer's disease prevention: from risk factors to early intervention. *Alzheimers Res Ther.* 2017;9. doi:10.1186/s13195-017-0297-z.
273. Gustavsson A, Green C, Jones RW, et al. Current issues and future research priorities for health economic modelling across the full continuum of Alzheimer's disease. *Alzheimers Dement.* 2017;13:312-321.
274. Tong BC-K, Wu AJ, Li M, et al. Calcium signaling in Alzheimer's disease and therapies. *BBA-Mol Cell Res.* 2018;1865:1745-1760.
275. Lee JH, Oh I-H, Lim HK. Stem cell therapy: a prospective treatment for Alzheimer's disease. *Psychiatry Investig.* 2015;13:583-589.
276. Cummings J, Fox N. Defining disease modifying therapy for Alzheimer's disease. *J Prev Alzheimers Dis.* 2017;4:109-115.
277. Graham WV, Bonito-Oliva A, Sakmar TP. Update on Alzheimer's disease therapy and prevention strategies. *Annu Rev Med.* 2017;68:413-430.
278. Sadhukhan P, Saha S, Dutta S, et al. Nutraceuticals: an emerging therapeutic approach against the pathogenesis of Alzheimer's disease. *Pharmacol Res.* 2018;129:100-114.
279. Anand A, Patience AA, Sharma N, et al. The present and future of pharmacotherapy of Alzheimer's disease: a comprehensive review. *Eur J Pharmacol.* 2017;815:365-375.

280. Douchamps F, Mathis C. A second wind for the cholinergic system in Alzheimer's therapy. *Behav Pharmacol* 2017;28. doi:10.1097/FBP.0000000000000300.
281. *Facts & Comparisons [database online]*. St. Louis, MO: Wolters Kluwer Health, Inc.; March, 2005.
282. Brewster JT II, Dell'Acqua S, Thach DQ, et al. Classics in chemical neuroscience development: donepezil. *ACS Chem Neurosci*. 2018. doi:10.1021/acschemneuro.8b00517.
283. Atanasova M, Yordanov N, Dimitrov I, et al. Molecular docking study on galantamine derivatives as cholinesterase inhibitors. *Mol Inf*. 2015;34:394-403.
284. Kim AH, Kandiah N, Hsu J-L, et al. Beyond symptomatic effects: potential of donepezil as a neuroprotective agent and disease modifier in Alzheimer's disease. *Br J Pharmacol*. 2017;174:4224-4232.
285. Mano Y, Hotta K, Kusano K. Simultaneous determination of donepezil and its three major metabolites in human plasma using LC-MS-MS. *J Chromato Sci*. 2016;54:1328-1335.
286. Matsui K, Mashima M, Nagai Y, et al. Absorption, distribution, metabolism and excretion of donepezil (Aricept) after a single oral administration to rat. *Drug Metab Dispos*. 1990;27:1046-1414.
287. Meier-Davis SR, Murgasova R, Toole C, et al. Comparison of metabolism of donepezil in rat, mini-pig, and human, following oral and transdermal administration, and in an in vitro model of human epidermis. *Drug Metab Toxicol*. 2012;3:doi:10.4172/2157–7609.1000129.
288. Adlimoghaddam A, Neuendorff M, Roy B, et al. A review of clinical treatment considerations of donepezil in severe Alzheimer's disease. *CNS Neurosci Ther*. 2018;24:876-888.
289. Farlow MR. Clinical pharmacokinetics of galantamine. *Clin Pharmacokinet*. 2003;42:1383-1392.
290. Jiang D, Yang X, Li M, et al. Efficacy and safety of galantamine treatment for patients with Alzheimer's disease: a meta-analysis of randomized controlled trials. *J Neural Transm*. 2015;122: 1157-1166.
291. Hwang T-Y, Ahn I-S, Kim S, et al. Efficacy of galantamine on cognition in mild-to-moderate Alzheimer's dementia after failure to respond to donepezil. *Psychiatry Investig*. 2016;13:341-348.
292. Wang L, Wang Y, Tian Y, et al. Design, synthesis, biological evaluation, and molecular modeling studies of chalcone-rivastigmine hybrids as cholinesterase inhibitors. *Biorg Med Chem*. 2017;25:360-371.
293. Bar-On P, Millard CB, Harel M, et al. Kinetic and structural studies on the interaction of cholinesterases with the anti-Alzheimer's drug rivastigmine. *Biochem*. 2002;41:3555-3564.
294. Bolognesi ML, Bartolini M, Cavalli A, et al. Design, synthesis, and biological evaluation of conformationally restricted rivastigmine analogues. *J Med Chem*. 2004;47:5945-5952.
295. Kandiah N, Pai M-C, Senanarong V, et al. Rivastigmine: the advantage of dual inhibition of acetylcholinesterase and butyrylcholinesterase and its role in subcortical vascular dementia and Parkinson's disease dementia. *Clin Interv Aging*. 2017;12:697-707.
296. Hansen RA, Gartlehner G, Webb AP, et al. Efficacy and safety of donepezil, galantamine, and rivastigmine for the treatment of Alzheimer's disease: a systematic review and meta-analysis. *Clin Interv Aging*. 2008;3:211-225.
297. Williams BR, Nazarians A, Gill MA. A review of rivastigmine: a reversible cholinesterase inhibitor. *Clin Ther*. 2003;25:1634-1653.
298. Sadowsky CH, Micca JL, Grossberg GT, et al. Rigastigmine from capsule to patch: therapeutic advances in the management of Alzheimer's disease and Parkinson's disease dementia. *Prim Care Companion CNS Disord*. 2014;16. doi:10.4088/PCC.14r01654.
299. Emre M, Bernabei R, Blesa R, et al. Drug profile: transdermal rivastigmine patch in the treatment of Alzheimer disease. *CNS Neurosci Ther*. 2010;16:246-253.
300. Kurz A, Farlow M, Lefevre G. Pharmacokinetics of a novel transdermal rivastigmine patch for the treatment of Alzheimer's disease: a review. *Int J Clin Pract*. 2009;63:799-805.
301. Molinuevo JL, Llado A, Rami L. Memantine: targeting glutamate excitotoxicity in Alzheimer's disease and other dementias. *Am J Alzheimers Dis Other Demen*. 2005;20:77-85.
302. Lipton SA. The molecular basis of memantine action in Alzheimer's disease and other neurologic disorders: low-affinity, uncompetitive antagonism. *Curr Alzheimer Res*. 2005;2:155-165.
303. Danysz W, Parsons CG. Alzheimer's disease, β-amyloid, glutamate, NMDA receptors and memantine – searching for the connections. *Br J Pharmacol*. 2012;167:324-352.
304. Jiang J, Jiang H. Efficacy and adverse effects of memantine treatment for Alzheimer's disease from randomized controlled trials. *Neurol Sci*. 2015;36:1633-1641.
305. Kishi T, Matsunaga S, Oya K, et al. Memantine for Alzheimer's disease: an updated systematic review and meta-analysis. *J Alzheimers Dis*. 2017;60:401-425.
306. Matsunaga S, Kishi T, Normura I, et al. The efficacy and safety of memantine for the treatment of Alzheimer's disease. *Exp Opin Drug Saf*. 2018;17:1053-1061.
307. Parsons CG, Danysz W, Dekundy A, et al. Memantine and cholinesterase inhibitors: complementary mechanisms in the treatment of Alzheimer's disease. *Neurotox Res*. 2013;24:358-369.
308. Calhoun A, King C, Khoury R, et al. An evaluation of memantine ER + donepezil for the treatment of Alzheimer's disease. *Exp Opin Pharmacother*. 2018;15:1711-1717.
309. Ebrahem AS, Oremus M. A pharmacoeconomic evaluation of cholinesterase inhibitors and memantine in the treatment of Alzheimer's disease. *Exp Opin Pharmacother*. 2018;19:1245-1259.
310. Sparrow EP, Erhardt D. *Essentials of ADHD Assessment for Children and Adolescents*. John Wiley & Sons; 2014.
311. Surman C, Biederman J, Spencer T, et al. Understanding deficient emotional self-regulation in adults with attention deficit hyperactivity disorder: a controlled study. *Atten Defici Hyperact Disord*. 2013;5:273-281.
312. Willcutt EG. The prevalence of DSM-IV attention-deficit/hyperactivity disorder: a meta-analytic review. *Neurotherapeutics*. 2012;9:490-499.
313. Visser SN, Danielson ML, Bitsko RH, et al. Trends in the parent-report of health care provider-diagnosed and medicated attention-deficit/hyperactivity disorder: United States, 2003–2011. *J Am Acad Child Adolesc Psychiatry*. 2014;53:34-46.e2.
314. Sciberras E., Mulraney M., Silva D., Coghill D. Prenatal risk factors and the etiology of ADHD-review of existing evidence. *Curr Psychiatry Rep*. 2017;19:1.
315. Gallo EF, Posner J. Moving towards causality in attention-deficit hyperactivity disorder: overview of neural and genetic mechanisms. *Lancet Psychiatry*. 2016;3:555-567.
316. Faraone SV. The pharmacology of amphetamine and methylphenidate: relevance to the neurobiology of attention-deficit/hyperactivity disorder and other psychiatric comorbidities. *Neurosci Biobehav Rev*. 2018;87:255-270.
317. Harvard Health P. Diet and Attention Deficit Hyperactivity Disorder. Harvard Health. Available at https://www.health.harvard.edu/newsletter_article/Diet-and-attention-deficit-hyperactivity-disorder. Accessed November 8, 2018.
318. Strohl MP. Bradley's benzedrine studies on children with behavioral disorders. *Yale J Biol Med*. 2011;84:27-33.
319. Sharma A., Couture J. A review of the pathophysiology, etiology, and treatment of attention-deficit hyperactivity disorder (ADHD). *Ann Pharmacother*. 2014;48:209-225.
320. Levy F, Swanson JM. Timing, space and ADHD: the dopamine theory revisited. *Aust N Z J Psychiatry*. 2001;35:504-511.
321. Austerman J. ADHD and behavioral disorders: assessment, management, and an update from DSM-5. *Cleve Clin J Med*. 2015;82:S2-S7.
322. Wang KH, Penmatsa A, Gouaux E. Neurotransmitter and psychostimulant recognition by the dopamine transporter. *Nature*. 2015;521:322-327.
323. Heal DJ, Smith SL, Gosden J, Nutt DJ. Amphetamine, past and present – a pharmacological and clinical perspective. *J Psychopharmacol Oxf Engl*. 2013;27:479-496.
324. Yamada H., Shiiyama S, Soejima-Ohkuma T, et al. Deamination of amphetamines by cytochromes P450: studies on substrate specificity and regioselectivity with microsomes and purified CYP2C subfamily isozymes. *J Toxicol Sci*. 1997;22:65-73.

325. Markowitz JS, Patrick KS. The clinical pharmacokinetics of amphetamines utilized in the treatment of attention-deficit/hyperactivity disorder. *J Child Adolesc. Psychopharmacol.* 2017;27:678-689.
326. Cortese S, Holtmann M, Banaschewski T, et al. Practitioner review: current best practice in the management of adverse events during treatment with ADHD medications in children and adolescents: practitioner review: management of AEs with ADHD medications. *J Child Psychol Psychiatry*. 2013;54:227-246.
327. Dopheide JA, Pliszka SR. Attention-deficit–hyperactivity disorder: an update. *Pharmacotherapy*. 2009;29:656-679.
328. Markowitz JS, Straughn AB, Patrick KS. Advances in the pharmacotherapy of attention-deficit-hyperactivity disorder: focus on methylphenidate formulations. *Pharmacotherapy*. 2003;23:1281-1299.
329. Markowitz JS, Patrick KS. Differential pharmacokinetics and pharmacodynamics of methylphenidate enantiomers: does chirality matter? *J Clin Psychopharmacol*. 2008;28:S54-S61.
330. Sun Z, Murry DJ, Sanghani SP, et al. Methylphenidate is stereoselectively hydrolyzed by human carboxylesterase CES1A1. *J Pharmacol Exp Ther*. 2004;310:469-476.
331. Cortese S, D'Acunto G, Konofal E, Masi G, Vitiello B. New formulations of methylphenidate for the treatment of attention-deficit/hyperactivity disorder: pharmacokinetics, efficacy, and tolerability. *CNS Drugs*. 2017;31:149-160.
332. Golmirzaei J, Mahboobi H, Yazdanparast M, et al. Psychopharmacology of attention-deficit hyperactivity disorder: effects and side effects. *Curr Pharm Des*. 2016;22:590-594.

Structure Challenge Answers

1-A; 2-B; 3-C; 4-D; 5-F.

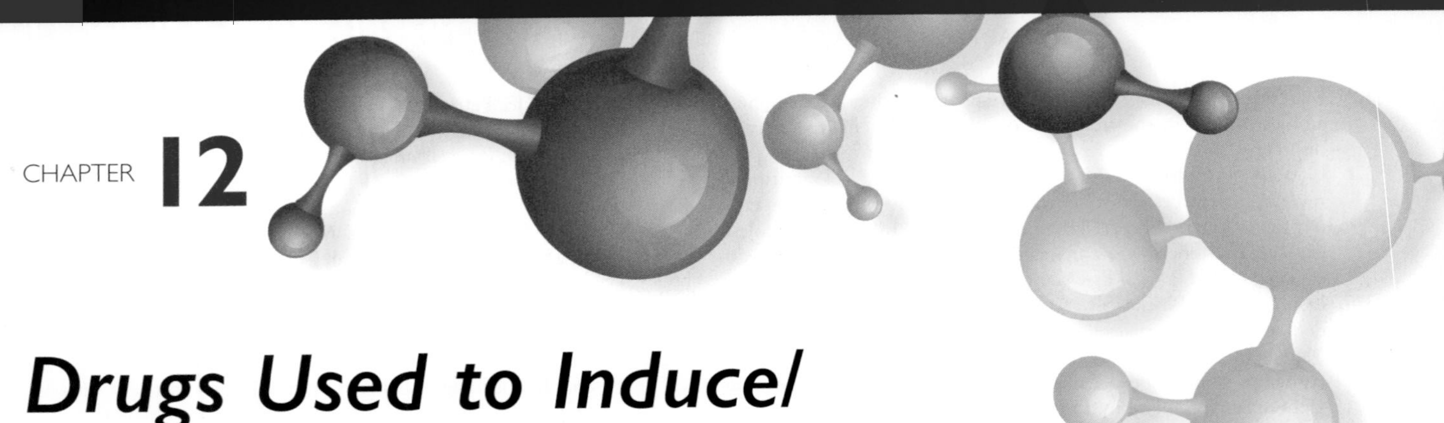

CHAPTER 12

Drugs Used to Induce/ Support Sedation or Anesthesia

Nader H. Moniri

Drugs covered in this chapter:

AGENTS THAT INDUCE OR PROMOTE SEDATION AND SLEEP:

BARBITURATES:
- Amobarbital
- Butabarbital
- Pentobarbital
- Phenobarbital
- Secobarbital

BENZODIAZEPINE SEDATIVE-HYPNOTICS:
- Estazolam
- Flurazepam
- Quazepam
- Temazepam
- Triazolam

NONBENZODIAZEPINE SEDATIVE-HYPNOTICS:
- Zolpidem
- Zaleplon
- Eszopiclone

MELATONIN RECEPTOR AGONISTS:
- Ramelteon

OREXIN RECEPTOR ANTAGONISTS:
- Suvorexant

HISTAMINE H1 RECEPTOR ANTAGONISTS:
- Diphenhydramine
- Doxylamine
- Doxepin

AGENTS THAT INDUCE OR PROMOTE GENERAL ANESTHESIA:

THIOBARBITURATES:
- Thiopental
- Thiamylal

INHALED ANESTHETICS:
- Nitrous oxide
- Isoflurane
- Sevoflurane
- Enflurane
- Desflurane

INTRAVENOUS ANESTHETICS:
- Propofol
- Etomidate
- Ketamine

NEUROMUSCULAR JUNCTION BLOCKING AGENTS:
- Succinylcholine
- *d*-Tubocurarine
- Pancuronium
- Vecuronium
- Rocuronium
- Atracurium
- Cisatracurium

Abbreviations

ACh acetylcholine
AMP adenosine monophosphate
AMPA α-amino-3-hydroxy-5-methyl-4-isoxazolepropionic acid
BZ benzodiazepine
Bz1R Bz_1 receptor
Bz2R Bz_2 receptor
CHO Chinese hamster ovary cells
CNS central nervous system
CYP cytochrome P-450
DEA US Drug Enforcement Agency
DORA dual orexin receptor antagonist
EEG electroencephalograph
FDA U.S. Food and Drug Administration
GA general anesthetic
$GABA_A$ γ-aminobutyric acid-A receptor
GPCR G protein–coupled receptor
IM intramuscular
IV intravenous
MT melatonin
MT1R Melatonin1 Receptor
MT2R Melatonin2 receptor
nAChR nicotinic acetylcholine receptor
NE norepinephrine
NMDA-R N-methyl-*D*-aspartate receptor

Abbreviations—Continued

NMJ neuromuscular junction
OXR orexin receptor
OX1R oxrein$_1$ receptor
OX2R oxrein$_2$ receptor
PKA cyclic AMP-dependent protein kinase
REM rapid eye movement
SAR structure-activity relationship
SCN suprachiasmatic nucleus
SORA orexin receptor antagonist
TMH transmembrane helix
TMN tuberomammillary nucleus

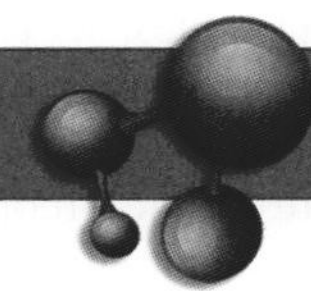

CLINICAL SIGNIFICANCE

Susan W. Miller, PharmD

Following the diagnosis of insomnia, several options exist for its management. These include nonpharmacological therapies such as stimulus control and effective sleep hygiene, in addition to pharmacological therapies with differing mechanisms of action. Options for pharmacological management of insomnia include older agents such as barbiturate and benzodiazepine sedative-hypnotics, as well as over-the-counter (OTC) histamine H$_1$ receptor antagonists. As a result of off-target and adverse effects, these agents are least preferred for treatment of insomnia and have led to the recent marketing of nonbenzodiazepine sedative-hypnotics, orexin receptor (OXR) antagonists, and melatonin receptor agonists, with a more favorable overall safety profile.

The medicinal chemistry of the agents used to treat insomnia plays an especially important role in allowing the clinician to understand the molecular interactions of the agent with the specific central nervous system (CNS) target that is responsible for inducing sedation and sleep. Since the desired effects of sedative-hypnotics should ideally be eliminated by morning, attention to the chemistry of these agents allows the clinician to understand the basis for their pharmacokinetics, which dictates how long the agents take to induce sleep as well as the duration of sleep time that they promote. Knowledge of structure-activity relationships (SAR) and medicinal chemistry also allows the clinician to predict metabolism of the agents in order to minimize drug-drug interactions and residual next-day side effects that may result from improper metabolic breakdown of sleep-inducing drugs.

Although barbiturates promote beneficial effects on the time it takes to fall asleep and on total sleep time, these agents have poor metabolic profiles and can also cause tolerance and, as a result, have largely fallen out of favor as primary sedative-hypnotics. Although all of the benzodiazepines are capable of producing sedative-hypnotic effects, the short-acting agents approved by the U.S. Food and Drug Administration (FDA) for use as sedative-hypnotics all share chemical features that ensure that their pharmacokinetics and metabolism are appropriate for use as nighttime sleep agents, with decreased risk for next-day effects. The nonbenzodiazepine sedative-hypnotics have comparable efficacy to the benzodiazepines in improving sleep patterns and, owing to their enhanced chemical affinity for α_1-containing benzodiazepine receptors, can be selectively used to reduce sleep latency, nighttime awakenings, and/or total sleep time. Newer classes of agents such as OXR antagonists and melatonin receptor agonists are becoming increasingly prescribed for the management of insomnia due to enhanced sleep and safety profiles.

Taken together, mechanism of action, pharmacokinetics, and metabolism can all be informed by drug chemistry and SARs and are factors that should be considered in order to appropriately optimize each unique insomnia patient's drug regimen.

Objectives

The general objective of this chapter is to provide the reader with an in-depth understanding of the molecular and chemical basis of agents that produce or promote sedation-hypnosis, as well as loss of consciousness and sensation leading to general anesthesia. The first half of the chapter covers the neuronal regulation of sleep/wake cycles and stages of sleep, followed by the neurobiological targets of sedative-hypnotic agents and SARs, pharmacodynamics, and pharmacokinetics of agents used to treat sleep disorders. The second half of the chapter covers the neurobiology of general anesthesia, the molecular targets of general anesthetics (GAs), and SARs, pharmacodynamics, and pharmacokinetics of agents used to induce or maintain general anesthesia.

AGENTS THAT INDUCE OR PROMOTE SEDATION AND SLEEP

Neurobiology of Sleep

Sleep is a reversible process that is typified by sensory and motor inactivity as well as reduced cortical responses to external stimuli. This process is distinct from complete states of unconsciousness (e.g., general anesthesia or coma), in which decreased cortical activity is unresponsive to all external stimuli. In human physiology, sleep/wake cycles are regulated to a large degree by endogenous circadian rhythms as well as homeostatic mechanisms, which in turn are governed by a myriad of neuronal pathways. Critical experiments performed in felines in the late 1940s demonstrated that impairment of the reticular formation within the brainstem triggered behavioral and electroencephalographic (EEG) activity consistent with comalike states, suggesting that this area of the brain was involved in regulating sleep and wakefulness.[1] This was contrary to observations that showed that felines with lesions of ascending sensory neurons distal to the reticular formation displayed no impairment to wakefulness or sleep, indicating that sleep/wake regulation by the reticular formation was not dependent on sensory neurons which leave it.[2] Further experiments showed that the reticular formation contained a high density of afferent input and that direct stimulation of the reticular formation facilitated wakefulness.[3] Taken together, these key observations suggested that sleep and wakefulness were likely controlled by factors within the reticular formation and that this structure behaves as a relay center that transmits afferent input to the cortex.

These and other pioneering studies led to the ascending reticular activating system (ARAS) hypothesis of sleep/wake regulation and subsequent identification of ARAS function as being critical in modification of sleep/wake transitions. Many decades of ensuing research on sleep/wake responses of the ARAS have revealed that projections to and from various nuclei within the brainstem can modulate ARAS activity in order to facilitate wakefulness and sleep. These include serotonergic neurons of the raphe nucleus within the reticular formation itself; cholinergic neurons of the pedunculopontine tegmentum and noradrenergic neurons of the locus coeruleus, within the pons; as well as dopaminergic neurons of the substantia nigra and ventral tegmental areas of the midbrain. These structures themselves are regulated in a highly orchestrated manner primarily by the excitatory neurotransmitter glutamate and the inhibitory neurotransmitter γ-aminobutyric acid (GABA) to regulate their respective activities.

In addition to the cell structures that make up the brainstem ARAS, there are additional populations of highly specialized cells that modulate sleep/wakefulness, either independently or in concert with cells of the ARAS. For example, stimulation of the tuberomammillary nucleus (TMN) within the posterior hypothalamus facilitates wakefulness and arousal, and these cells are predominantly active only during wakeful periods.[4] TMN-mediated regulation of wakefulness is dependent on histaminergic neurons that densely project into the cortex as well as other wake-promoting structures within the brainstem.[5] The firing rate of these cortical-projecting histaminergic TMN neurons decreases upon sleep and increases upon arousal, while lesioning of histaminergic neurons within the TMN promotes sleep.[6-8] Biochemically, the release of histamine from these neurons is increased upon and during wakefulness and is under the control of glutaminergic-stimulatory and GABAergic-inhibitory circuits.[9,10] Studies with histamine receptor knockout mice as well as in vivo pharmacological studies have established that the TMN effects of histamine on wakefulness and sleep are mediated primarily by histamine H_1 G protein–coupled receptors (GPCRs; see Chapter 6).

While the posterior hypothalamic TMN is involved in regulating arousal, the anterior hypothalamus, specifically the suprachiasmatic nucleus (SCN), is involved in induction of sleep. Studies have shown that lesions of the posterior hypothalamus (e.g., TMN) induce sleepfulness, while lesions of the anterior hypothalamus are associated with wakefulness.[11] Decades of further work have established that the SCN is critical for the maintenance of circadian rhythms, in essence, behaving as the brain's endogenous master clock, thereby regulating sleep/wake cycles and synchronizing circadian phase timings with other brain structures. Importantly, the SCN receives visual input from the retina via the retinohypothalamic tract, and this key connection serves to synchronize circadian rhythms to daylight.[12] The firing rate of SCN neurons is strongly correlated with day/night cycles, which serve to establish an approximate 24-hour circadian rhythm. While the SCN is largely under the control of glutaminergic and GABAergic neurons, which originate in the preoptic nucleus, it also works in concert with the pineal gland to regulate circadian rhythms.[13] As such, inhibitory GABAergic outflow from SCN neurons to the pineal is enhanced during the daylight hours and declines proportionally to decreases in daylight. Light-sensitive neurons from the SCN project to the hypothalamic paraventricular nuclei and through the lateral horn of the spinal cord primarily by way of vasopressin and GABAergic neurons. The signal is then relayed to the pineal gland through noradrenergic ganglionic sympathetic fibers that directly innervate the pineal gland. Hence, during periods of light, GABA output is elevated, which inhibits the release of norepinephrine (NE) at the pineal gland. In contrast, during periods of darkness the inhibitory GABAergic outflow from the SCN is reduced, resulting in increased levels of NE released at the level of the pineal gland.[12] Here, NE acts primarily through pineal β_1- and α_{1B}-adrenergic receptors to stimulate a rapid and profound (ca. 10-fold) synthesis and release of melatonin, another key regulator of circadian rhythms and the sleep/wake cycle, into the bloodstream.[14]

The synthesis of melatonin occurs within the pineal gland, where the amino acid L-tryptophan is converted to serotonin, which is subsequently acetylated to yield N-acetylserotonin by the enzyme arylalkylamine N-acetyltransferase (AA-NAT). N-acetylserotonin is converted to melatonin by the enzyme hydroxyindole O-methyltransferase (HIOMT) (Fig. 12.1). The activity of AA-NAT is greatly influenced by β_1-adrenergic receptors that are activated upon the release of NE via the SCN circuit described above. β_1-Receptor–mediated increases in intracellular cyclic AMP stimulate AA-NAT expression, and it also increases PKA-mediated phosphorylation of AA-NAT, which stabilizes and activates the enzyme.[15] The rhythm of AA-NAT activity is thus correspondingly coupled to light exposure, as increases in light lead to decreases in AA-NAT activity. Activity of AA-NAT can also be effectively abolished by lesions of the SCN, further demonstrating that melatonin synthesis is dependent on retinohypothalamic input.[16] Once synthesized, melatonin diffuses into capillary blood vessels and rapidly reaches all tissues of the body, where it can agonize its cognate GPCRs, MT1R and MT2R, leading to various physiological responses. With specific regard to sleep, melatonin has profound effects in the SCN, where it agonizes MT1R to mediate the acute inhibition of SCN neurons, thereby promoting sleep. Additionally, agonism of MT2R in the SCN is associated with the phase-shifting effects on circadian rhythms.

In addition, orexinergic neurons within the lateral hypothalamus receive an abundance of afferent input from emotional, physiological, and environmental stimuli that

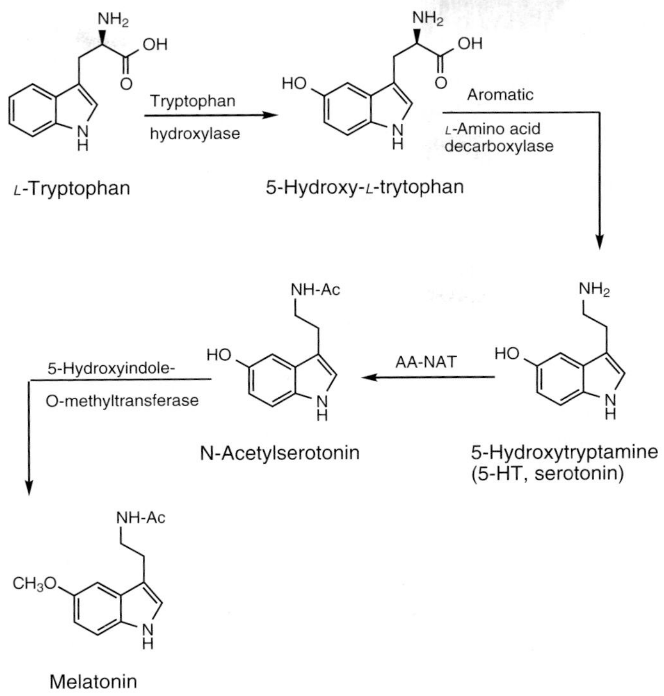

Figure 12.1 Biosynthesis of melatonin. *AA-NAT*, arylalkylamine N-acetyltransferase.

regulate the synthesis and secretion of the excitatory neuropeptides orexin-A and orexin-B, also referred to as hypocretins.[17-19] In turn, these orexinergic neuronal projections innervate all of the brain regions noted above to promote wakefulness and arousal, including the dorsal raphe nucleus, locus coeruleus, TMN, and cortex.[20] Release of the orexins into synapses at these sites activates two separate GPCRs, OX1R and OX2R, which together modulate the activities of the orexin neuropeptides.[19] Specifically, agonism of postsynaptic OX1R/OX2R by orexins facilitates depolarization and subsequent activity of postsynaptic neurons that promote wakefulness and arousal via excitatory neurotransmission toward the complement of wake-promoting brain regions.[21]

Human Sleep Cycles

The EEG has afforded researchers the ability to assess the electrical activity of the brain during the course of sleep, and these findings have revealed the presence of distinct EEG activity, which correlates to five stages of sleep. These stages, which cycle throughout the night, include four non-REM (rapid eye movement) stages, often referred to as "quiet sleep," as well a single stage of REM sleep, referred to as "active sleep." Non-REM sleep stages correlate to periods of low metabolic rate and low neuronal activity; hence brain activity and EEG events are "quiet". In non-REM sleep, heart rate and blood pressure are also reduced due to an increase in parasympathetic nervous system activity coupled with a decrease in sympathetic outflow. As a result of these autonomic reflexes, non-REM sleep also causes pupillary constriction, which diminishes the amount of light that is allowed to enter the retina.[22]

The initial period of sleep is stage 1, which lasts only a brief period of time (5-15 min) and represents the period of transitioning from wakefulness to sleep. While EEG activity in awake humans mainly consists of high-frequency (15-25 Hz) alpha-wave events, the progression to stage 1 sleep results in the emergence of slower theta waves with lower frequency (4-10 Hz) as the individual progresses to the light or drowsy sleep characterized by stage 1. In stage 2 sleep, which often lasts 15-20 minutes, background theta waves continue but are periodically interrupted by characteristic sleep spindles, which are short bursts of higher frequency (12-15 Hz) EEG events. Stage 2 of the sleep cycle is still considered a light sleep; however, skeletal muscle activity is decreased in this stage compared to the transitionary stage 1. Stages 3 and 4, often referred to as slow-wave sleep, are characterized by the appearance of higher amplitude, slower frequency (0.5-4 Hz) delta waves that occur less often in stage 3 and more often in stage 4. Both of these stages represent deep sleep, as the characteristic delta-activity is least similar to arousal state alpha-activity. If awakened in this stage of sleep, an individual will likely be confused and disoriented.[23]

The fifth stage of sleep is referred to as REM sleep and is characterized by increases in eye movement, respiration rate, and brain activity. EEG changes in REM sleep include high-voltage firing spikes that originate in the pons, lateral geniculate nucleus, and occipital cortex, and these spikes are correlated with bursts of REMs associated with this stage of sleep.[24] The increased brain activity in REM sleep is consistent with an increase in dreaming as well as an increase in metabolic rate, thus the naming convention "active sleep"; yet, it is inversely proportional to skeletal muscle tonicity, which effectively paralyzes skeletal movements.

The sleep stages are normally cycled every 90-100 minutes throughout the night, and it is important to note that sleep does not necessarily advance sequentially through the five stages. Healthy adults typically enter sleep through a progression through the stages, with the first REM stage occurring after 75-90 minutes of non-REM sleep and a typical return to stage 2 or 3 sleep thereafter. As sleep progresses over the course of a night, the amount of time spent in REM sleep increases such that, over a typical 8 hours sleep cycle, approximately 55%-60% of sleep time is spent in stages 1-2 (light sleep), 20% in stages 3-4 (deep sleep), and 20%-25% in stage 5 (REM sleep).

Pharmacological Targets of Sedative-Hypnotic Agents

As described above, there are many physiological and biochemical factors that can influence the various stages of sleep, and as such, numerous targets for pharmacological intervention have arisen. In fact, nearly every neurotransmitter system in the mammalian brain, including adenosinergic, serotonergic, dopaminergic, adrenergic, histaminergic, and cholinergic systems, has at one time or another been associated with induction of sleep or wakefulness. Despite this wide breadth of potential biochemical targets, the development of sedative-hypnotic agents has primarily focused on (1) agents that cause CNS depression via agonism of $GABA_A$ receptors and (2) agents that modulate hypothalamic histaminergic, melatonergic, or orexinergic systems which, as described above, regulate sleep and arousal. This section will focus on chemical perspectives toward SARs, pharmacodynamics, and pharmacokinetics of these agents, including barbiturates, benzodiazepines, and non-benzodiazepine $GABA_A$ agonists, as well as melatonin receptor agonists and histamine H1 and OXR antagonists.

$GABA_A$ Receptors

γ-Aminobutyric acid (GABA) is the major inhibitory neurotransmitter in the mammalian CNS and is critical in balancing neuronal excitation. GABA is widely distributed throughout the CNS and can be in found at concentrations up to 1000-fold (high μM to low mM) greater than that of monoaminergic neurotransmitters in various CNS nuclei. GABA-induced physiological functions are mediated by at least two distinct classes of membrane-bound receptors, ionotropic $GABA_A$ receptors and metabotropic $GABA_B$ receptors. $GABA_B$ receptors belong to the second messenger–linked GPCR superfamily and share homology with metabotropic glutamate receptors. Meanwhile, $GABA_A$ receptors are ligand-gated ion channels that modulate conductance of chloride ions (Cl^-) through the cell membrane upon binding of GABA. The activation of $GABA_A$ receptors on excitable neurons leads to membrane hyperpolarization, facilitating an increase in the firing threshold potential and consequently reducing the likelihood of generating a neuronal action potential. Hence, agonism of $GABA_A$ receptors leads to neuronal inhibition and CNS depression. Not surprisingly, $GABA_A$ receptors are important targets for treatment of a variety of CNS disorders in which CNS depression provides a therapeutic benefit, including anxiety (see Chapter 11), convulsions and seizures (see Chapter 13), sleep disorders, and anesthesia. In this regard, drugs that increase $GABA_A$–mediated Cl^- flux (e.g., $GABA_A$ agonists) provide anxiolytic, anticonvulsant, sedative-hypnotic, and anesthetic activity, while agents that block the Cl^- channel (e.g., picrotoxin) can lead to convulsions and heightened states of awareness and arousal.

The $GABA_A$ receptor-channel complex is related to the nicotinic acetylcholine receptor (nAChR) superfamily, which also includes the strychnine-sensitive glycine receptors and serotonin $5\text{-}HT_3$ receptors. In the human brain, $GABA_A$ complexes are formed by oligomerization of individual subunits that produce heteropentomeric complexes consisting of α, β, γ, δ, ε, or ρ subunits that assemble a ligand-gated channel with a central pore that allows for the conductance of Cl^- (Fig. 12.2).[25] Moreover, the α, β, and γ subunits of $GABA_A$ receptors are expressed as distinct alternatively spliced variants (e.g., $\alpha_{[1-6]}$, $\beta_{[1-3]}$, $\gamma_{[1-3]}$). Functional channels typically require multiple α and β subunits in combination with another subunit, allowing for tremendous diversity in the makeup of the channels (Fig. 12.2). The distribution of various $GABA_A$ receptors vary according to the subtype combinations. The $\alpha_1\beta_2\gamma_2$, $\alpha_2\beta_3\gamma_2$, and $\alpha_3\beta_3\gamma_2$ subtypes are the most abundant receptors, accounting for nearly 80% of $GABA_A$ receptors in the mammalian brain.[25] The α_1 subunit is the most widely expressed, while α_4, α_5, and α_6 subunits are restricted to localized neuronal populations.[25] Two distinct GABA binding sites are formed at the two α and β subunit interfaces, while the binding sites for GABA-modulating drugs such as barbiturates and benzodiazepines (BZ) are at allosteric sites (Fig. 12.2). Upon binding of barbiturates or benzodiazepines to their respective allosteric sites on the $GABA_A$ receptor, alterations in the conductance of Cl^- occur as described for each class of agent below.

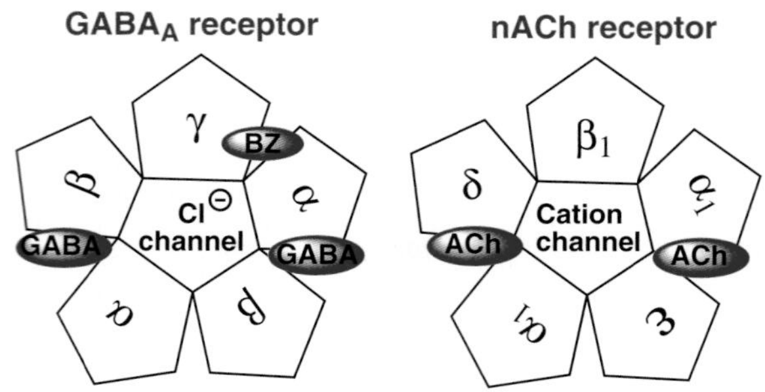

Figure 12.2 The pentameric assembly of γ-aminobutyric acid-A ($GABA_A$) receptors (left) and neuromuscular αβδε nicotinic acetylcholine receptors (nAChR) (right), whose monomers assemble to form the ion channel at the center. The GABA and benzodiazepine (BZ) binding sites of a distinct αβγ-type $GABA_A$ receptor are noted (left). The two acetylcholine (ACh) binding sites on the αβδε nAChR are noted (right).

BARBITURATES. Barbiturates are potent CNS depressants with sedative-hypnotic, anesthetic, and anticonvulsant activity and were widely considered sedative-hypnotic agents of choice until the marketing of benzodiazepines in the late 1960s. Barbiturates played a crucial role in our understanding of $GABA_A$ receptor function, and while there are special instances which call for barbiturate use, they have largely been replaced as sedative-hypnotic agents by other agents due to safety concerns, including tolerance, dependence, potential for abuse, as well as a relatively low toxicity threshold that can lead to overdosage and poisoning. Currently, there are five barbiturates approved by the FDA for use as sedative-hypnotics: amobarbital, butabarbital, pentobarbital, phenobarbital, and secobarbital.

Barbiturate Mechanism of Action. Upon binding of GABA to the $GABA_A$ receptor, the Cl^- conductance channel opens in bursts of approximately 1, 5, and 10 msec of duration, followed by brief periods of closure. Channel opening increases in frequency and duration upon increases in GABA concentrations. Binding of barbiturates to their $GABA_A$ binding site causes an increase in the binding of GABA to the receptor, enhancing the actions of GABA and leading to prolongation of the longest-duration open state.[26] While the exact site of barbiturate binding on $GABA_A$ receptors remains elusive, the barbiturate binding site does not seem to require specific subunits, and it is distinct from both of the better characterized GABA and BZ binding sites. Indeed, using related bacterial receptor orthologs, it was recently shown that barbiturates bind deep within the central ion channel pore.[27] Higher therapeutic concentrations of barbiturates can also enhance the binding of benzodiazepines, while supratherapeutic concentrations of barbiturates can cause opening of the channel independently of GABA, although the clinical importance of this response has not been widely studied.[28]

Notably, in addition to their augmentation of $GABA_A$ responses, the physiological effects of higher concentrations of barbiturates can also be mediated by kainite-sensitive AMPA glutamate receptors, as well as voltage-gated Na^+ and Ca^{+2} channels.

Pharmacological Effects of Barbiturates. Barbiturates act as reversible inhibitors of virtually all excitable neurons and can produce dose-dependent CNS depression that ranges in effect from weak sedation to general anesthesia. With regard to their effects on sleep, barbiturates significantly decrease the time it takes to fall asleep, known as sleep latency, increase the total time of sleep, and decrease occurrences of nighttime awakenings. Because of these effects, barbiturates significantly impair psychomotor abilities and also decrease memory as well as cognitive performance. Additionally, barbiturates can cause physical dependence, and sudden withdrawal of these agents can lead to serious neuropsychiatric symptoms as well as convulsions of excitable tissue, an effect that can facilitate seizures and respiratory spasms. Long-term use of barbiturates has also been shown to lead to tolerance, in which higher doses of the agent are needed to achieve the same therapeutic endpoints (e.g., sleep) previously obtained with a lower dose. Since these agents have relatively narrow safety margins, higher doses due to tolerance can lead to toxicity. Due to these concerns, the use of barbiturates in treatment of insomnia has been virtually discontinued, and when these agents are used for treatment of insomnia, they are used in special cases and/or restricted to only short-term use. Other, older barbiturate-like drugs (e.g., chloral hydrate, glutethimide, and ethylchlorvynol) also act on the $GABA_A$ receptor to produce sedative-hypnotic effects but have fallen out of favor due to numerous adverse effects. These agents have been reviewed in previous editions of this text.

Structure-Activity Relationships of Barbiturates. Barbiturates are derivatives of a cylized ureide of malonic acid, commonly referred to as barbituric acid (2,4,6-trioxyhexahydropyrimidine) (Fig. 12.3), which is itself devoid of sedative-hypnotic, anesthetic, anxiolytic, and anticonvulsant activity. As shown in Figure 12.3, barbituric acid can undergo pH-dependent keto-enol tautomerization through transfer of either an imino hydrogen or methylene hydrogen to a carbonyl oxygen. This tautomerization is based on a fairly acidic enol ($pK_a \sim 4$) at the 2-position that is stabilized in either molecular form based on the acidity of the solution. Empirical and computational studies have demonstrated that the tricarbonyl form is the most stable in aqueous solutions, while the 4,6-dialcohol tautomeric forms are the least stable.[29,30] While barbituric acid itself lacks pharmacological activity, addition of 5,5-disubstituents to the barbituric backbone yields compounds with potent sedative-hypnotic, anesthetic, anxiolytic, and anticonvulsant activity. Termed barbiturates, the 5,5-disubstituted barbituric acids all possess a high degree of lipophilicity and, as weak acids, can be easily converted to sodium salts by treatment with sodium hydroxide.

Despite the fact that thousands of barbiturate-like compounds have been synthesized, the 5,5-disubstituted barbituric acid backbone is the primary pharmacophore required for sedative-hypnotic and anesthetic activity, and efforts to further derivatize this backbone leads to a general loss in these activities. These efforts show that amide formation at either of the 1,3-diazine nitrogen atoms decreases hypnotic activity. While substitution of these nitrogens with aliphatic carbons retained anticonvulsant effects, it led to only weak hypnotic activity for N-methylated substituents, and this activity was lost upon increases in chain length and/or bulk.[31,32] Likewise, esterification of the 5-position substituents (e.g., 5-phenyl, 5-methylester) yielded agents with analgesic activity but only weak hypnotic effects.[33] While early work on barbiturate derivatization demonstrated the importance of the 5-position substitutions on CNS-depressant activity, the inclusion of polar functional groups at C_5 resulted in compounds that were fully devoid of sedative-hypnotic, anesthetic, or anticonvulsant activity.[34]

There are currently five barbiturates approved by the FDA for short-term sedative-hypnotic use and treatment of insomnia (Fig. 12.4). Structurally, pharmacological activity is imparted to all five compounds due to the lipophilic disubstitutions at the 5-position (e.g., 5^a and 5^b, Table 12.1). The first commercially marketed barbiturate, barbital, contained identical 5,5-diethyl substituents, and as such, a plane of symmetry. However, many clinically useful barbiturates contain distinct 5,5-disubstitutions and substituted nitrogens that form an asymmetric chiral center at C_5 and/

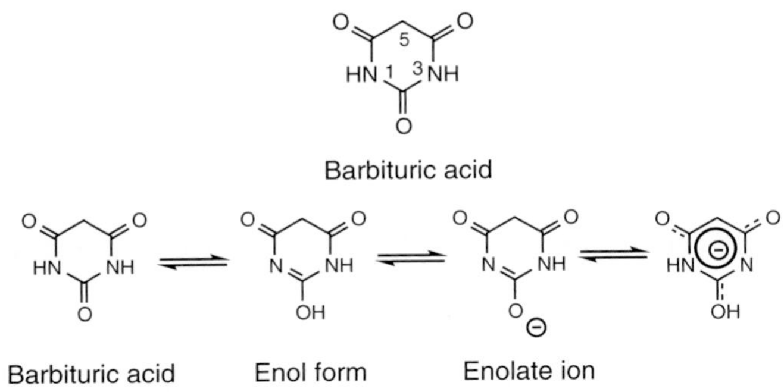

Barbituric acid

Barbituric acid　Enol form　Enolate ion

Figure 12.3 The structure of barbituric acid (top) and tautomerization of barbituric acid (bottom).

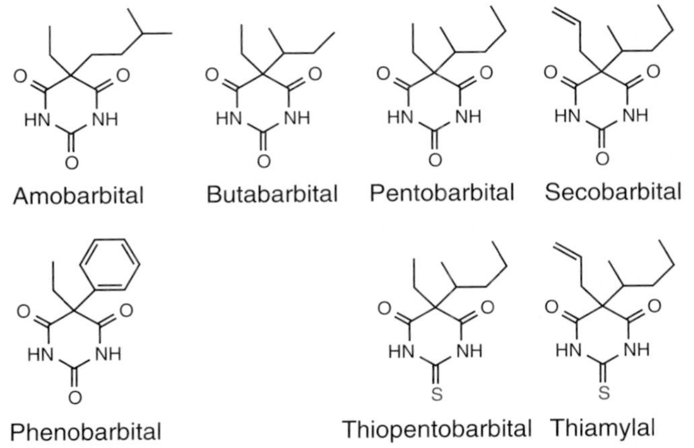

Amobarbital　Butabarbital　Pentobarbital　Secobarbital

Phenobarbital　Thiopentobarbital　Thiamylal

Figure 12.4 The barbiturates that are indicated for sedative-hypnotic use and the anesthetic-acting thiobarbiturates underneath their respective oxybarbiturate congeners.

Table 12.1 Pharmacokinetic Parameters of Barbiturates Approved for Sedative-Hypnotic Use

Barbiturate	R_1[a]	R_2[b]	Log P	Onset Time (min)[d]	Duration of Action (hr)[d]	Classification
Pentobarbital	C_2H_5	$-CH(CH_3)CH_2CH_2CH_3$	2.10[a]	10-15	3-4	Short-acting
Secobarbital	$CH_2=CHCH_2-$	$-CH(CH_3)CH_2CH_2CH_3$	2.36[b]	10-15	3-4	Short-acting
Amobarbital	C_2H_5	$-CH_2CH_2CH(CH_3)_2$	2.07[c]	45-60	6-8	Intermediate-acting
Butabarbital	C_2H_5	$-CH(CH_3)CH_2CH_3$	1.60[b]	45-60	6-8	Intermediate-acting
Phenobarbital	C_2H_5	phenyl	1.46[b]	30-60	10-16	Long-acting

[a]From Freese, IE, Levin, BC, Pearce, R, et al. Correlation between the growth inhibitory effects, partition coefficients and teratogenic effects of lipophilic acids. *Teratology*. 1979;20:413-444.

[b]Average determinations from Slater, B, McCormack, A, Avdeef, A, et al. Comparison of partition coefficients determined by HPLC and potentiometric methods to literature values. *J Pharm Sci*. 1994;83:1280-1283.

[c]From Kakemi, K, Arita, T, Hori, R, et al. Absorption and excretion of drugs. XXXI. On the relationship between partition coefficients and chemical structures of barbituric acid derivatives. *Chem Pharm Bull*. 1967;15:1705-1712.

[d]On oral administration

or within one of the 5-position alkyl chains. While barbiturates are dispensed as racemic mixtures, *L*-stereoisomers typically have twice the potency of the respective *D*-stereoisomers, consistent with observations that demonstrate stereoselectivity of $GABA_A$ receptors. With the exception of secobarbital, which contains an allylic group at 5^a, the remaining agents contain ethyl substitutions at this position (Fig. 12.4, Table 12.1). Differences in these sedative-hypnotic barbiturates occur at the 5^b position, where substitutions can affect the potency, rate of onset, and duration of action of the various congeners.

The activity of these agents is strongly influenced by the lipophilicity of both substituents at the 5-position. As the number of carbon atoms at the 5^b position increases, the lipophilicity of the barbiturate will also increase such that comparative predictions on activity and time to onset can be made. For example, pentobarbital is more potent and has faster onset compared to butabarbital, which contains one less methylene group and is thus less lipophilic (Fig. 12.4, Table 12.1). Although the lipophilicity of the molecule greatly influences its ability to cross the blood-brain barrier, leading to potency and effecting the time of onset (see below), too high a degree of lipophilicity will offset the required hydrophilicity that is necessary for dissolution and solubility of the compound in aqueous fluids. Hence, a limit to lipophilicity is reached and pharmacological activity will begin to decrease if this threshold is surpassed. A somewhat paradoxical situation exists in the case of phenobarbital (Fig. 12.4, Table 12.1), which contains a 5^b-phenyl substitution that on first look appears to increase lipophilicity of the molecule, due to the six carbons and increased π-electron density afforded by the aromatic ring. However, the high electron density of phenobarbital stabilizes the formation of the more hydrophilic enolate anion due to the tautomerization process described above. Because of this electronic effect, phenobarbital exhibits a higher degree of hydrophilicity compared to the other barbiturates, as demonstrated by its lower log P (Table 12.1). The consequence of this is lower sedative-hypnotic potency and a longer time of onset.

A final note regarding the SAR of barbiturates is more critical in the role of this class as anesthetic agents. Specifically, modification of the C_2 oxygen of the barbiturate backbone with the larger sulfur atom yields thiobarbiturate derivatives with increased lipophilicity, faster time of onset, and shorter duration of action compared to the oxy-derivatives. For example, thiobarbital and thiamylal have much faster onset and shorter durations than their respective oxy-congeners, pentobarbital and secobarbital, respectively (Fig. 12.4). Thus, thiobarbiturates have specialized roles as anesthetics, as described in further detail in the anesthetic section below.

Pharmacokinetics and Metabolism of Barbiturates. The barbiturate salts approved for use as sedative-hypnotics are rapidly and completely absorbed following oral ingestion, in contrast to the free acids which are absorbed at a much slower rate. The time of onset and duration of action is also significantly influenced by the lipophilicity of the individual agent as well as the route of administration. The five sedative-hypnotic barbiturates described here are all highly lipophilic, with corresponding log P values above 1.5 compared to barbital, which has a log P of 0.65 (Table 12.1).[35] Given the high proportion of cardiac output that is directed toward the brain, more lipophilic barbiturates are more rapidly distributed to the CNS and will have a faster time of onset. As with other CNS-acting agents, the time of onset is also dependent on the route of administration, with intravenous (IV) administration being the fastest and having near immediate effects, followed by intramuscular (IM) administration, which leads to faster brain distribution than the 10-60 minutes typical of orally administered sedative-hypnotics (Table 12.1).

While the lipophilic nature of barbiturates coupled with the high cardiac output to the brain dictates a rapid CNS distribution leading to fast time of onset, lipophilicity also facilitates the relatively short duration of action of these agents due to redistribution from the brain to other body compartments upon equilibration. This redistribution (e.g., to muscle or adipose tissue) is the major mechanism that contributes to the loss of sedative-hypnotic and anesthetic activity of these agents. Durations of 3-8 hours define the short- and intermediate-acting agents, while phenobarbital, due to the electronic influence described above, has the lowest lipophilicity and, therefore, the longest (10-16 hr) duration of action (Table 12.1). Since lipophilicity and route of administration can affect both time to onset and duration of action of barbiturates, these factors will influence a particular barbiturate's place in therapy. The anticonvulsant barbiturates are typically less lipophilic (e.g., phenobarbital) and correspondingly have slow onset and long durations upon oral dosing, while the sedative-hypnotic agents described here are typically administered orally to achieve an optimum balance between achievement of sleep onset and duration. In contrast, anesthesia-inducing barbiturates such as thiamylal are termed ultrashort acting due to their extremely high lipophilicity (log P > 3), which confers immediate onset and very short durations upon IV injection.

While loss of barbiturate sedative-hypnotic activity occurs primarily due to redistribution, the agents are also metabolically transformed. Metabolism of barbiturates is dependent on their individual degrees of lipid solubility: the more lipophilic compounds generally have greater hepatic penetration and, hence, undergo greater metabolic transformation. It is important to understand that metabolism of barbiturates leads to metabolites that lack a high degree of lipophilicity, and as a result, lack sedative-hypnotic activity. To achieve loss of lipophilicity, barbiturates are typically converted to phase 2 glucuronide or sulfate conjugates that are strongly ionized and, therefore, hydrophilic and will allow for renal excretion of the agents. The most important pathway of barbiturate metabolism is oxidation or removal of the substituents at the 5-position (Fig. 12.5). These phase 1 oxidation transformants are typically alcohols or phenols in the case of phenobarbital, which can appear in the urine as either free or conjugated metabolites, the latter as a result of further phase 2 reactions with glucuronic acid or sulfate. The formed alcohols can also be further oxidized to yield ketones or carboxylic acid metabolites, which can be excreted freely or also conjugated (Fig. 12.5). Although not as significant as the route described above, oxidative desulfuration of thiobarbiturates can also occur, leading to more hydrophilic oxybarbiturates. Oxybarbiturate metabolites of thiamylal and thiobarbital are subsequently oxidized by the phase 1 and phase 2 reactions as described above (Fig. 12.5).

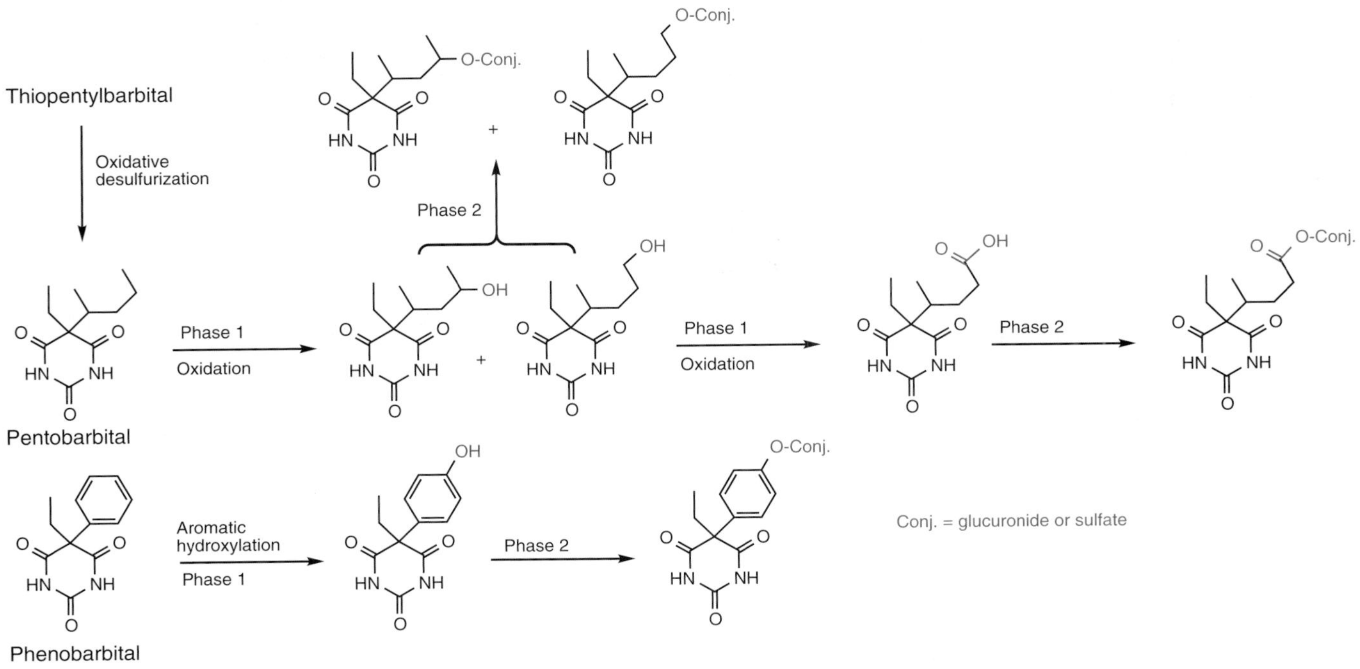

Figure 12.5 Major routes of metabolism of barbiturates. Thiobarbital and pentobarbital are used as examples to describe metabolism of alkyl thio- and oxybarbiturates, while phenobarbital is used as an example to describe metabolism of aromatic barbiturates.

BENZODIAZEPINES. As with the barbiturates, benzodiazepines modulate the function of $GABA_A$ receptors leading to neuronal hyperpolarization and CNS depressant effects. In contrast to the barbiturate binding site of $GABA_A$ receptors, the benzodiazepine binding site has been well characterized and is known to be formed by the interface of α and γ subunits. Not surprisingly, $GABA_A$ receptors lacking the γ subunit (e.g., $\alpha_6\beta\delta$) are completely insensitive to all benzodiazepines. Additionally, it has been shown that isoforms of the α subunit have differential BZ binding affinities, with the α_1 subunit–containing receptors (often termed Bz_1 receptors) having high benzodiazepine affinity and the α_2, α_3, and α_5 subunit–containing receptors (often termed Bz_2 receptors) having moderate affinity. Furthermore, some combinations that include α_4 or α_6 subunits are completely insensitive to benzodiazepine agonists, even in the presence of an appropriate γ subunit.[25]

Binding of benzodiazepines to the allosteric BZ-binding site can produce agonist, partial agonist, inverse agonist, or antagonist physiological responses. Benzodiazepine agonists are used clinically as sedative-hypnotic agents as well as for the treatment of anxiety and convulsant disorders, in accordance with their ability to allosterically augment GABA-mediated inhibitory Cl^- conductance through the $GABA_A$ channel. Specifically, binding of benzodiazepines to the BZ site leads to increases in the binding on-rate and affinity of one GABA molecule to the first GABA-binding site of the receptor.[33] The increased affinity and rate of binding of GABA correlate with an increase in the frequency of the open-channel bursts.[33] It is important to distinguish that benzodiazepines increase the frequency of channel opening, while barbiturates increase the duration of the open channel, and, as such, the two classes of agents have distinct molecular effects on the $GABA_A$ receptor. Furthermore, unlike barbiturates, benzodiazepines lack any effects in the absence of GABA. The reader is referred to Chapter 11 (mental/behavioral disorders) for more detailed descriptions of benzodiazepine receptor binding and function.

Pharmacological Effects of Benzodiazepines. All benzodiazepines are capable of producing sedative-hypnotic effects; however, currently only five shorter acting benzodiazepine agents are approved by the FDA for use as sedative-hypnotics: estazolam, flurazepam, quazepam, temazepam, and triazolam. Residual hypnosis as well as psychomotor and cognitive inhibition are common side effects associated with their use. All of these agents are agonists of the BZ-site of $GABA_A$ receptors containing α and γ subunits. Physiologically, they significantly reduce sleep latency and the number and duration of nighttime awakenings, resulting in an increase in total sleep time. The clinical use of these agents as sedative-hypnotics is not free from adverse effects, which are primarily manifested as excessive residual next-day sleepiness, tolerance upon long-term use, and withdrawal upon discontinuation. Another clinically important effect is the ability of BZs to produce a high degree of anterograde amnesia, in which recent events are not transferred to long-term memory.[36]

Structure-Activity Relationships of Benzodiazepines The SARs of benzodiazepines are described in detail in Chapter 11. Regarding the SAR of sedative-hypnotic BZs, all five agents contain the 5-phenyl-1,4-benzodiazepine-2-one backbone required for $GABA_A$ activity, and all include an electronegative 7-position chlorosubstitution on ring A (see Chapter 11 and Fig. 12.6). Similarly, all contain a pendant 5-phenyl ring (ring C), which is required for in vivo agonism and can be substituted with *o*-electronegative halogens to increase lipophilicity, as is the case with flurazepam, quazepam, temazepam, and triazolam. Importantly, *p*-substitution on ring C leads to inactive benzodiazepines, suggesting that steric restrictions are important at this site. Of note, several benzodiazepines, including estazolam are metabolized at the C-ring *p* (4′) position, leading to inactivation of the agent. The major structural differences, which impart distinct pharmacokinetic properties to the sedative-hypnotic BZs are located within ring B, the major site of metabolic transformation of these agents. The structural features of ring B that contribute to metabolic vulnerability are discussed below.

Pharmacokinetics and Metabolism of Benzodiazepines Benzodiazepine agents, like the barbiturates, are lipophilic and can be easily absorbed upon oral ingestion and rapidly distributed to the brain. Among the oral benzodiazepine formulations specifically indicated for the treatment of insomnia, flurazepam is absorbed most rapidly, achieving mean peak plasma concentrations

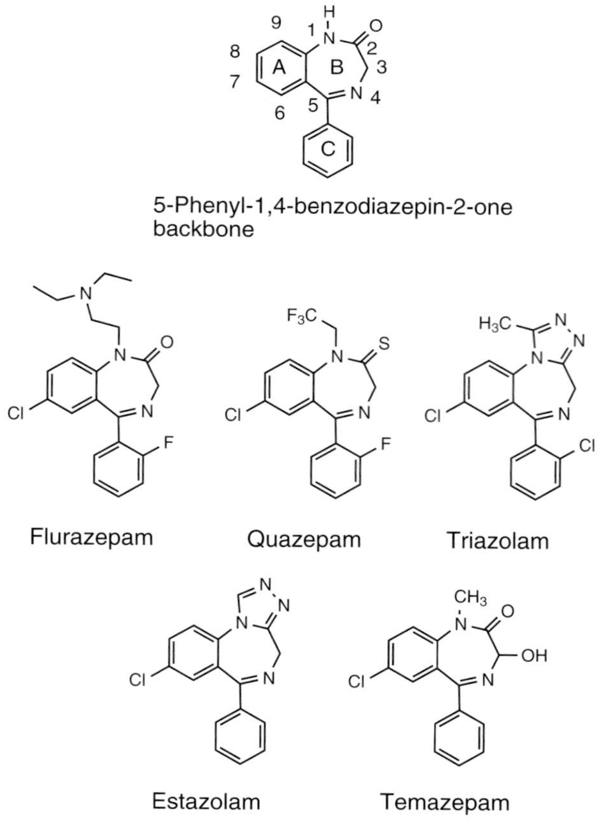

5-Phenyl-1,4-benzodiazepin-2-one backbone

Flurazepam Quazepam Triazolam

Estazolam Temazepam

Figure 12.6 The benzodiazepine backbone and the benzodiazepines that are indicated for sedative-hypnotic use.

Table 12.2 Pharmacokinetic Parameters of Benzodiazepines Approved for Sedative-Hypnotic Use

	Flurazepam	Quazepam	Estazolam	Triazolam	Temazepam
Log P[a]	2.35	4.03	3.51	2.42	2.19
Time to peak concentration (hr)	0.5-1.0	ca. 2	0.5-6.0	<2	1.2-1.6
Parent elimination half-life (hr)	ca. 2	39	10-24	1.5-5.5	0.4-0.6
Major metabolites (half-life, hr)	N1-desethyl-(47-100, active) N1-hydroxyethy-(2-4, active)	2-Oxo-(40, active) N-desalkyl(73, active)	4′-Hydroxy- 4-Hydroxy- 2-Oxo (all inactive)	α-hydroxy-(50%-100% active) 4-hydroxy-(inactive)	O-Glucuronides (Major) Oxazepam (Minor)
Predominant CYP isoforms involved	3A4	3A4/2C9	3A4	3A4	

[a]From Sangster Research Laboratories LOGKOW database.

within 0.5-1.0 hours. Temazepam and triazolam reach mean peak plasma concentrations within 0.5-2.0 hours, while estazolam and quazepam take longer (Table 12.2).

The sedative-hypnotic duration and side effect potential of benzodiazepines are greatly influenced by metabolism of the parent agent and the activity of resulting metabolites. Flurazepam has an elimination half-life of approximately 2 hours and is primarily metabolized by cytochrome P450-3A4 mediated N-dealkylation and hydroxylation yielding active N1-desethyl and N1-hydroxyethyl metabolites with elimination half-lives of 47-100 and 2-4 hours, respectively (Fig. 12.7, Table 12.2).[37] Following a single 30 mg dose, the N1-hydroxyethyl metabolite is undetectable in the plasma after 24 hours. On the contrary, levels of N1-desethylflurazepam are 5- to 6-fold higher after 7 days of administration than they are following 24 hours, suggesting buildup of this active metabolite. Conjugation of N1-hydroxyethylflurazepam in phase 2 reactions allows for urinary excretion, and this conjugate is the major urinary metabolite, accounting for up to 55% of a single dose (Fig. 12.7). The long half-life of these metabolites explains the clinical findings that flurazepam exhibits faster sleep latency and decreases in total wake time following several days of use and also why it is still efficacious for one to two nights following discontinuation of the parent drug. These observations are especially important in elderly populations, in whom the elimination half-life of N1-desethylflurazepam is significantly higher, upward of 160 hours.

Quazepam is metabolized by CYP3A4 to yield 2-oxoquazepam, which is subsequently N-dealkylated to N-desalkyl-2-oxoquazepam (Fig. 12.7).[38] Both of these metabolites are pharmacologically active and have long durations, with mean plasma elimination half-lives of 40 and 73 hours, respectively (Table 12.2).[38] Both 2-oxoquazepam and N-desalkyl-2-oxoquazepam can be further hydroxylated at the 3-position yielding 3-hydroxy-2-oxoquazepam and 3-hydroxy-N-desalkyl-2-oxoquazepam, respectively. These hydroxylated metabolites are inactive and can be O-glucuronidated and excreted readily in the urine (Fig. 12.7). As a consequence of the slow elimination of multiple active metabolites of both flurazepam and quazepam, residual hypnotic effects, including excessive daytime drowsiness and over-sedation as well as cognitive decline and confusion, are common and clinically relevant adverse effects.

These problems led to the development of newer triazolobenzodiazepines, such as estazolam and triazolam, with high $GABA_A$ receptor affinity and relatively shorter durations. The 1,4-triazolo ring of these congeners prevents oxidative metabolism typical of the benzodiazepines, which in the case of flurazepam and quazepam results in formation of active metabolites with long elimination half-lives. The presence of the fused fourth ring of these agents also changes the numbering convention, such that numbering priority proceeds around the triazole ring (Fig. 12.8). Estazolam has a longer elimination half-life (10-24 hr) compared to flurazepam, but this agent is primarily metabolized by CYP3A4 yielding 4′-hydroxyestazolam as a major metabolite and 1-oxoestazolam as a minor metabolite (Fig. 12.8, Table 12.2). Additionally, a 4′-hydroxyestazolam metabolite has been identified in humans and is also detected in the urine at high levels.[39] While these metabolites have weak pharmacological activity, three important factors prevent them from contributing to any significant sedative-hypnotic effects. The first is the low affinities of the metabolites for the $GABA_A$ receptor. In particular, 4′-hydroxestazolam is sterically hindered from optimal $GABA_A$ binding, consistent with SAR findings described above showing that *p*-substitutions of ring C lead to decreased potency. The second factor that impedes the activity of estazolam metabolites is their decreased lipophilicity compared to the parent drug. This decrease facilitates the final factor, which is that the circulating metabolites are found in low concentrations due to direct

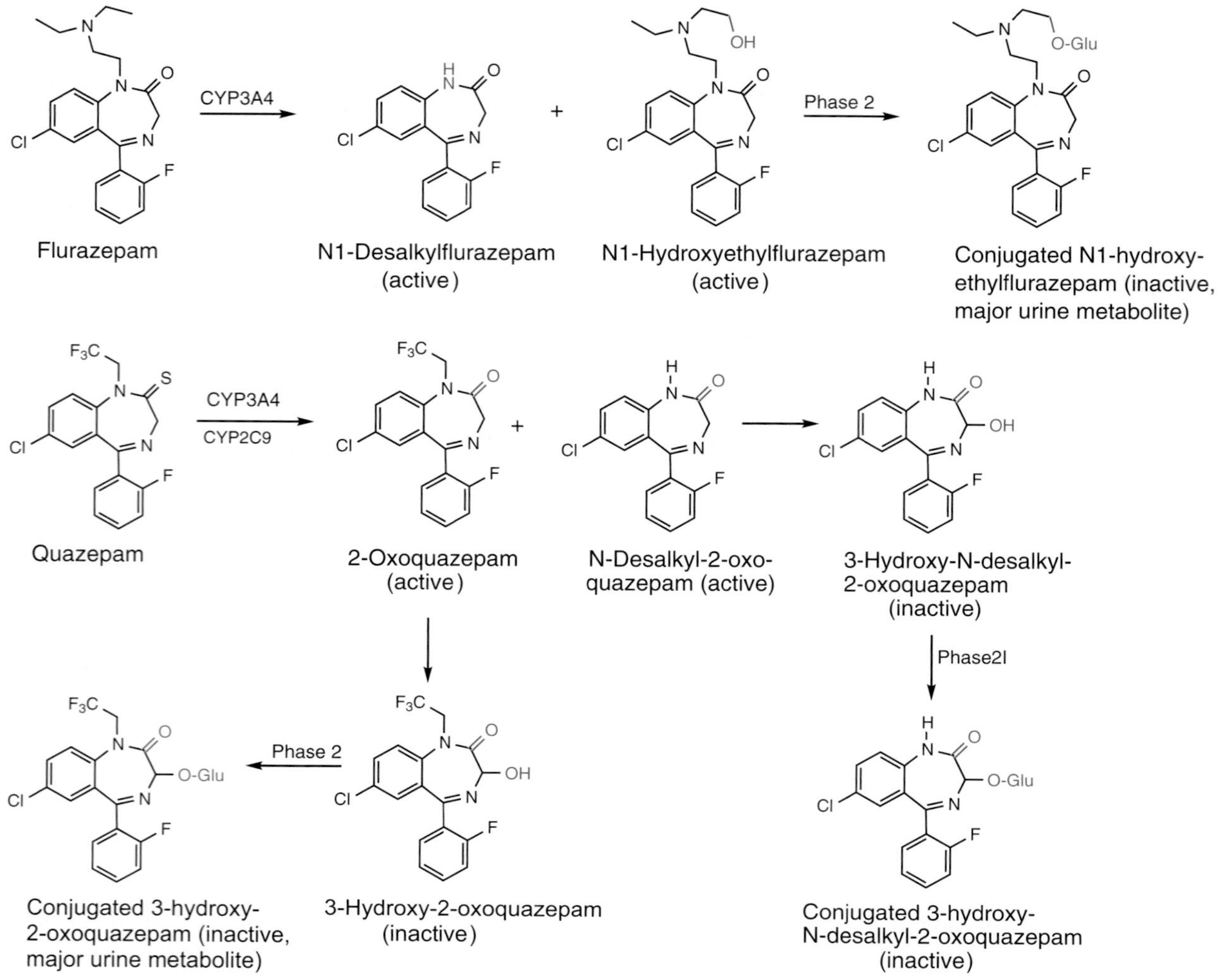

Figure 12.7 Metabolism of flurazepam and quazepam leads to formation of multiple long-acting active metabolites.

excretion of the hydrophilic free metabolites or their rapid O-glucuronidation to highly ionized and readily excreted conjugates (Fig. 12.8).

Triazolam has a short duration of approximately 4 hours and is metabolized in humans to six metabolites, one of which, α-hydroxytriazolam, has been shown to retain 50%-100% of the potency of the parent compound. While only small amounts of the parent drug are found in the urine, glucuronides of α-hydroxytriazolam as well as 4-hydroxytriazolam are the principal metabolites found in the urine, and these account for approximately 80% of triazolam excretion (Fig. 12.9).[40] There is no evidence of accumulation of triazolam metabolites, and the clinical effects of the active α-hydroxytriazolam are unclear, as this metabolite has been detected in the plasma primarily in its glucuronidated form. Taken together, the relatively short half-life of the parent, coupled with the urinary excretion of glucuronidated metabolites, affords triazolam a relatively short duration of action compared with other benzodiazepines.

Temazepam is unique among the sedative-hypnotic benzodiazepines in that it contains a 3-hydroxy group and, as such, the agent circumvents phase 1 oxidation reactions prior to conjugation and excretion. The O-glucuronide of temazepam accounts for greater than 90% of all metabolites recovered in man, and this feature affords a 0.4-0.6 hour elimination half-life and rapid excretion of the parent, while also providing the additional benefit of bypassing oxidative hepatic metabolism (Fig. 12.9).[41] In a secondary pathway, temazepam can also be N-demethylated to N-desmethyltemezepam, which itself is marketed as oxazepam. Oxazepam is further metabolized by phase 2 conjugation, yielding the O-glucuronide of oxazepam or N-desmethyltemazepam (Fig. 12.9).[41] Importantly, these metabolites are also formed independent of CYP450 isoforms and are rapidly excreted in the urine, with half-lives of approximately 2 hours.[41] Due to the rapid excretion of the phase 2 conjugates of temazepam, the metabolism of the parent drug serves as the rate-limiting step in the termination of the sedative-hypnotic effect.

Adverse Effects of Benzodiazepines. Benzodiazepines are used as sedative-hypnotic agents, as well as general muscle relaxants, anxiolytics, and anticonvulsants; however, as mentioned previously, their use can be confounded by presentation of undesirable side effects. While death by benzodiazepine overdose is rare and typically only results as a consequence of concomitant use with other CNS

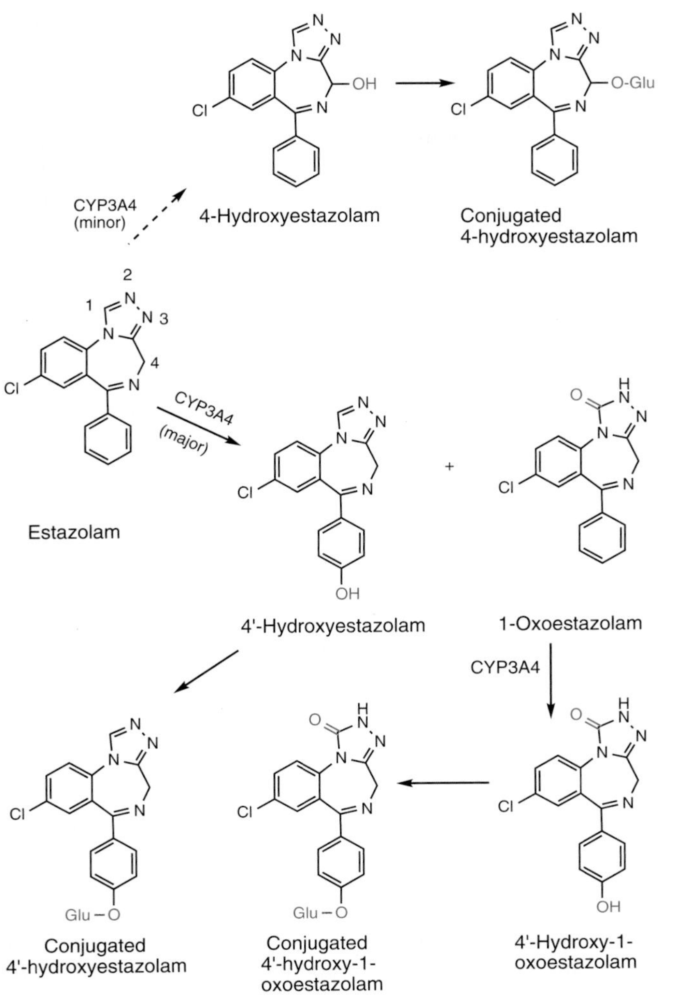

Figure 12.8 Metabolism of estazolam.

depressants, these agents are not free from adverse side effects and toxicities. Nearly all benzodiazepines have been reported to cause dose-dependent alterations in behavior, specifically, bizarre uninhibited and confused behaviors. The propensity of benzodiazepines to cause tolerance and their potential for physical dependence and abuse also limits their use. Additionally, misuse of short-acting hypnotic benzodiazepines such as flunitrazepam (Rohypnol) has had profound social and medicolegal implications due to their use as "date-rape" or "robbery" drugs. This illicit use is based on the ability to produce rapid hypnosis in combination with anterograde amnesia. In addition to cognitive effects, benzodiazepines may also exhibit respiratory depressant effects depending on the dose and the duration, and as such, they are contraindicated in patients with pulmonary conditions or sleep apnea. These factors contributed to the development of non-benzodiazepine sedative-hypnotics devoid of many of the adverse effects induced by classical benzodiazepines.

NONBENZODIAZEPINE GABA$_A$ AGONISTS. Due to advances in molecular biology, genetics, and pharmacology in the late 1980s to early 1990s, numerous lines of evidence demonstrated that different GABA$_A$ receptor subtypes may bring about distinct functions depending on their localization in the brain. Future work revealed that α_2, α_3, and α_5 subtype–containing GABA$_A$ receptors (Bz$_2$) play critical roles in the anxiolytic, anticonvulsant, muscle-relaxant, and cognitive-impairment properties of classical benzodiazepines, while modulation of the α_1-containing GABA$_A$ receptor subtypes (Bz$_1$) was shown to be the key to benzodiazepine-induced sedation and hypnosis.[42-46] Importantly, these findings revealed that it could be feasible to design functionally selective drugs that act as selective agonists at specific GABA$_A$ subtypes to yield the appropriate

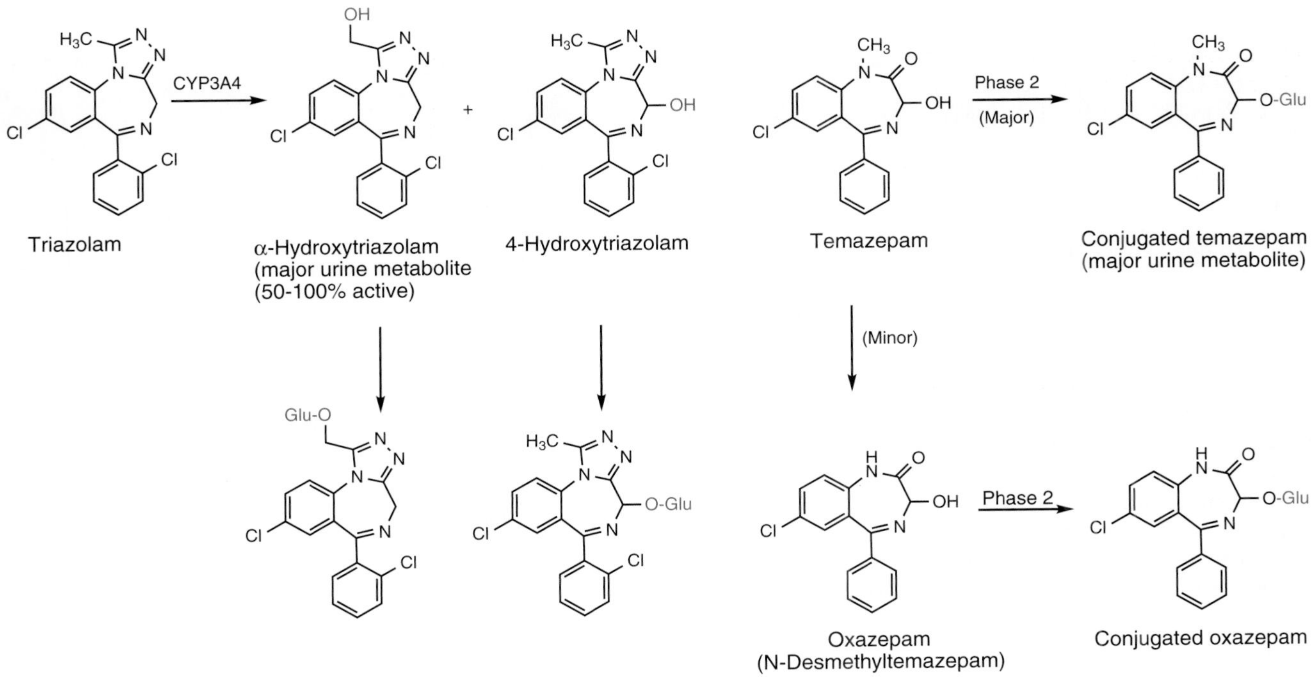

Figure 12.9 Metabolism of triazolam and temazepam.

pharmacotherapeutic outcomes. For example, selective α_2- or α_3-acting agents could have anxiolytic properties while being devoid of sedative effects, whereas selective α_1-acting agents would behave specifically as sedative-hypnotic agents. While classical benzodiazepines described here and in Chapter 11 are nonselective and demonstrate sedative-hypnotic as well as anxiolytic and other effects, the discovery of novel nonbenzodiazepine compounds with a high degree of selectivity for α_1 subtype–expressing $GABA_A$ receptors allowed for the specific use of these agents as sedative-hypnotics. Currently, three structurally distinct nonbenzodiazepines, zolpidem, eszopiclone, and zaleplon, which are often referred to as the Z-drugs, are approved in the U.S. for treatment of insomnia, and several other investigational agents are in various stages of clinical trials.

Zolpidem.

H_3C N N O CH_3 N CH_3 CH_3

Zolpidem is an imidazopyridine that is a highly selective agonist of the α_1 subunit–expressing $GABA_A$ receptors (Bz_1), demonstrating five- and ten-fold greater affinity for α_1 versus α_2 and α_3 subtypes, respectively.[47] Similar to the benzodiazepines, zolpidem lacks appreciable affinity for α_4 and α_5 receptors.[47] Of the three marketed nonbenzodiazepine drugs, zolpidem also has the greatest functional potency at potentiating GABA currents.[48] The hypnotic effects of zolpidem parallel those seen for temazepam and triazolam, but based on its selective pharmacological profile, zolpidem demonstrates weaker anxiolytic, anticonvulsant, and muscle-relaxant effects compared to the classical benzodiazepines. Zolpidem has been shown to significantly improve sleep latency and prolong the duration of sleep in healthy volunteers as well as in patients with insomnia. Studies that compare the sleep outcomes of zolpidem with those of benzodiazepines have generally revealed comparable onset and sleep durations, while also showing that zolpidem leads to significantly fewer nighttime awakenings and, at the same time, being free from residual morning sedation, confusion, or memory impairment.[48-52] Further studies demonstrated that zolpidem exhibits significant improvements with regard to sleep latency as well as subjective accounts of sleep quality compared to benzodiazepines. Extensive review of trial data, which compare sleep outcomes of zolpidem to various benzodiazepines, shows that zolpidem is comparable or superior to various benzodiazepines with respect to sleep outcomes.[53-55]

Zolpidem is currently available in the U.S. in multiple formulations including immediate or controlled release oral tablets, as well as sublingual tablets and an oral spray. Oral administration leads to bioavailability of approximately 70% and peak maximal plasma concentrations within 1.6 hours, while the sublingual formulation peaks at 35-75 minutes (Table 12.3). While plasma concentrations of zolpidem begin to decrease at approximately 2 hours following administration of the immediate-release formulation, the extended-release formulation produces a more sustained peak plasma concentration that results in higher plasma concentrations over an 8 hour period. Direct comparison of the two formulations shows that plasma concentration profiles are generally identical for 2 hours following administration, after which decreases in blood levels are seen with the immediate release formulation. The controlled-release formulation allows for this peak blood level to be extended for approximately 1-2 additional hours, allowing for correspondingly sustained blood levels

Table 12.3 Pharmacokinetic Parameters of Nonbenzodiazepines Approved for Sedative-Hypnotic Use

	Zolpidem	Eszopiclone	Zaleplon
Log P	2.31	−0.34	1.23
Time to peak concentration (hr)	Immediate release—1.6[a]/1.6[b] Controlled release—1.5[c] Oral spray—0.25 Sublingual—0.5-1.0	1	1
Parent elimination half-life (mean, hr)	Immediate release—2.5[a]/ 2.6[b] Controlled release—2.6[c]	6.5	1
Major metabolites (half-life, hr)	None active	N-oxide (inactive) N-desmethyl (active, lower affinity)	None active
Predominant CYP isoforms involved	3A4 (major) 2C9, 1A2, and 2D6 (minor)	1A2 3A4	3A4 (minor)

[a]5 mg tablets.
[b]10 mg tablets.
[c]12.5 mg tablets.

throughout the night. Administration of the agent with food doubles the time required to reach peak and lowers the peak concentration by 30%. Accumulation of zolpidem does not seem to occur upon repeated exposure, regardless of the formulation. In addition, an available zolpidem oral spray formulation is distinguished by the fact that it allows for significantly faster time of onset of approximately 15 minutes (Table 12.3) and, as such, is clinically useful for patients with difficulties in achieving sleep initiation.

Structure-Activity Relationships of Zolpidem. There have been a great deal of medicinal-chemical efforts to define the SARs of zolpidem and to characterize interaction of the agent with the Bz_1 receptor. Anzini and colleagues have integrated these models using the structurally similar, but non–α_1-selective, imidazopyridine anxiolytic agent alpidem.[56] Based on these results, they have described a freely rotating aromatic ring region (FRAR), an electron-rich region (ERR), an antiplanar region (APR), and a planar aromatic region (PAR) (Fig. 12.10), which contribute to the binding of alpidem to benzodiazepine receptors. Studies on each of these regions have demonstrated that the replacement of alpidem's electronegative chloro groups at both the FRAR and PAR with methyl groups, as in zolpidem, does not affect receptor binding affinity but significantly increases the selectivity for α_1-subtype receptors.[57]

Further studies on the ERR have shown that conversion of either of imidazopyridine's H-bond–accepting imidazole nitrogen atoms to a hydrogen donor (i.e., indole nitrogen) leads to complete loss of selectivity for α_1-subtype $GABA_A$ receptors, suggesting an interaction of this H-bonding H-acceptor with the $GABA_A$ receptor.[56] The importance of the ERR is also demonstrated by studies that convert the imidazole of zolpidem to its azaisostere congener. This simple change does not affect binding to α_1 subtype receptors but decreases binding to α_2 and α_3 such that potency at these subtypes is negligible, similar to that seen for the α_5 subtype.[58]

The APR has also been shown to be critical in facilitating binding to $GABA_A$ receptors by allowing for hydrogen bonding interactions. Molecular modeling studies have shown that the APR carbonyl group of zolpidem can hydrogen bond to Ser204 or near Thr206/Gly207 within the backbone of loop C of α_1 subunits, as well as to Arg194 within loop F of γ_2 subunits, which form $\alpha_1\gamma_2$ complexes.[59] Finally, the APR also contributes to binding selectivity and affinity, as sterically hindered bulky amide nitrogen substitutions show decreased binding to α_1-subtype receptors. This study also identifies three additional α_1 and three additional γ_2 residues that are within 5 Å of zolpidem upon molecular docking simulations, suggesting that other hydrogen bonding or salt bridge interactions can occur within the ligand-binding domain.

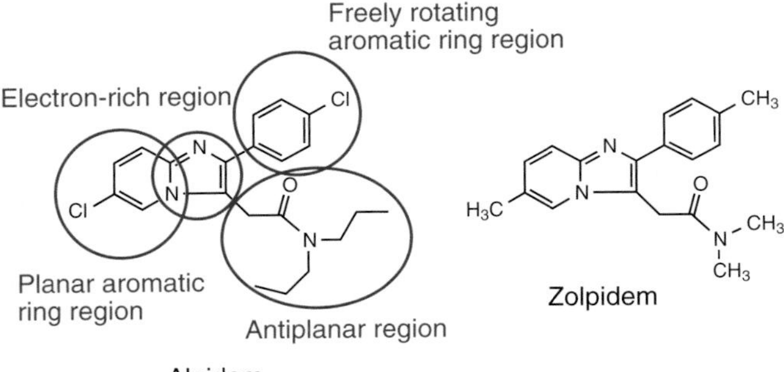

Figure 12.10 Structures of alpidem and zolpidem.

Metabolism of Zolpidem. Zolpidem is rapidly eliminated with a mean half-life of approximately 2.5 hours (Table 12.3). Repeated doses do not seem to accumulate, and elimination of the parent is achieved through extensive metabolism with only trace amounts of unchanged drug being found in urine or feces.[60] In humans, zolpidem can be oxidatively metabolized to yield four metabolites, MII, MIV, MX, and MXI, all of which lack pharmacological activity. As shown in Figure 12.11, the major metabolite is formed by CYP3A4-mediated hydroxylation of the *p*-tolyl methyl group yielding MIII, which is subsequently oxidized to the corresponding carboxylic acid, MI, by alcohol dehydrogenase.[61] The MI metabolite is the principal metabolite found in human urine, accounting for approximately 70%-85% of the administered dose. CYP1A2, CYP2C9, and CYP2D6 can also metabolize a minor proportion of zolpidem to the MIII metabolite (Fig. 12.11).[61,62]

Similarly, microsomal enzyme-mediated hydroxylation of the *p*-methyl substituent on the imidazopyridine backbone can also occur, leading to formation of metabolite MIV. As with formation of MIII, this occurs primarily via CYP3A4, with more minor contributions through either CYP1A2 or CYP2 isoforms. The MIV metabolite can be further oxidized to the corresponding carboxylic acid MII, accounting for approximately 10% of the administered dose.[61,62] Since expression of CYP1A2 and CYP2D6 in human liver is generally significantly less than that of CYP3A4, the clinical contribution of these enzymes in transformation of zolpidem to MIII and MIV is expected to be minor, and it is now well accepted that CYP3A4 plays the clinically more significant role.

More recent studies have confirmed these suspicions and demonstrated that the contribution of CYP enzymes to zolpidem metabolism is greatest for CYP3A4 (61%), followed by CYP2C9 (22%), CYP1A2 (14%), and less than 3% for CYP2D6.[62] Since MIII and MIV are not detectable in human urine or feces, but rather, the respective carboxylic acids MI and MII are, it was proposed that rapid formation of these secondary metabolites occurs. Indeed, studies in rodents have demonstrated that the conversion of the alcohol metabolites to their corresponding acids occurs very rapidly and requires a nonmicrosomal enzyme, perhaps alcohol dehydrogenase.[63] Finally, as shown in Figure 12.11, CYP3A4-mediated aromatic and side chain oxidation of zolpidem can lead to formation of the minor metabolites MX and MXI, respectively.

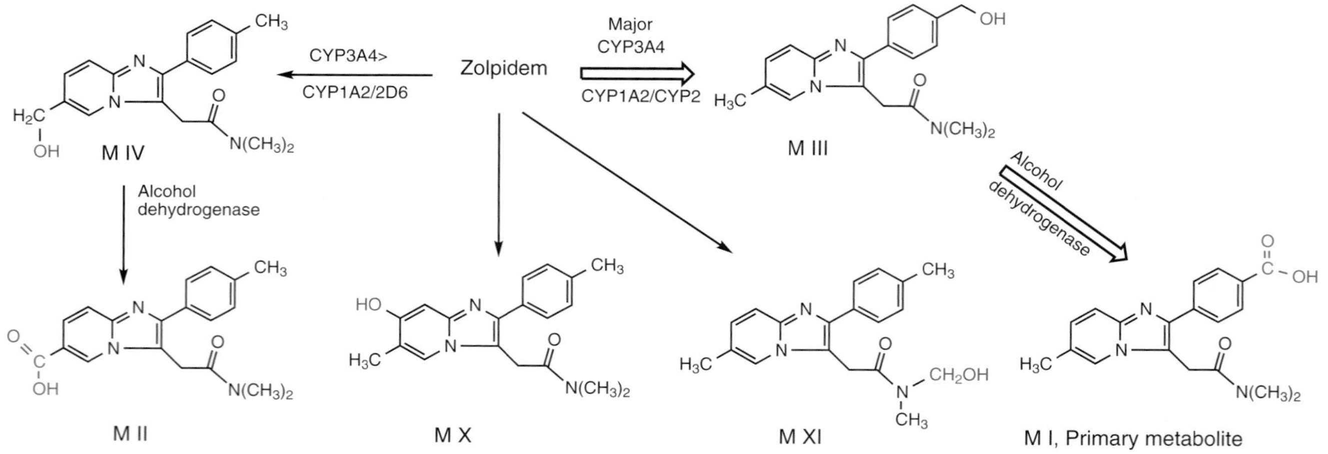

Figure 12.11 Metabolism of zolpidem.

In elderly populations, dose adjustments must be made to account for the 50% increase in elimination half-life of the drug.[64] Similarly, in patients with hepatic dysfunction, the plasma concentration of zolpidem doubles, with an increase in elimination half-life to a mean of 10 hours. There has been recent interest in the likelihood of differential gender-based metabolism of zolpidem based on the ability of circulating free testosterone to increase CYP3A4 activity.[64,65] Given this correlation, women are likely to have higher plasma concentrations of zolpidem and, as such, may be more likely to have higher degrees of zolpidem-mediated adverse effects.[66] For this reason, the dose given to women is 50% of that given to men.

Eszopiclone.

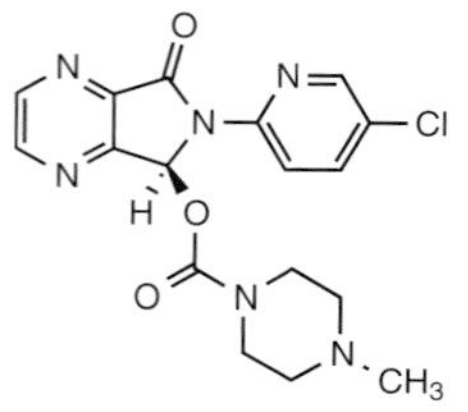

Eszopiclone, a pyrrolopyrazine cyclopyrrolone, is the active (S)-enantiomer of zopiclone, a racemic mixture that is no longer marketed in the U.S. Compared to zopiclone, eszopiclone significantly improves sleep latency and sleep maintenance and increases the time spent in stage III and IV sleep. It is distinguished by the fact that its approval is not limited to short-term utilization and that it has no potential for development of tolerance or abuse. Several trials have demonstrated that hypnotic efficacy is maintained and eszopiclone is well tolerated upon chronic dosing up to 12 months.[67] In contrast to the racemic zopiclone, eszopiclone is devoid of substantial residual next-day sedative and cognitive effects. Unlike zolpidem, eszopiclone is not subtype selective. However, despite this lack of selectivity, it does not behave as a classical benzodiazepine with respect to its pharmacodynamics and pharmacological activity (see SAR section below). Eszopiclone binds with higher affinity to α_1 receptors but also has appreciable affinity for α_3 subunits and thus has hypnotic as well as other CNS activities. The affinity for α_1-subtype receptors is less than the other marketed nonbenzodiazepine agonists.

Eszopiclone is rapidly absorbed following oral administration, and peak plasma concentrations are reached within 1 hour. The elimination half-life of 6.5 hours is the longest of the nonbenzodiazepine hypnotics (Table 12.3). Similar to zolpidem, eszopiclone does not accumulate following repeated administration, and administration after a high-fat meal delays the time to peak plasma concentration by 1 hour and decreases this concentration by over 20%.[68] Eszopiclone dosing in the elderly must also be adjusted to account for 41% greater drug levels and a significantly longer half-life of 9 hours. Similar dose adjustments must be made in patients with liver dysfunction, as total exposure to eszopiclone increases 2-fold at the 2 mg dose, although the time to peak concentration and the concentration itself were unaffected.[68]

Structure-Activity Relationships of Eszopiclone. Eszopiclone exhibits 50-fold greater binding affinity for $GABA_A$ receptors than does the (R)-enantiomer. This leads to significant improvement in GABA agonist potency, but more importantly, enantiomeric separation of the (S)-enantiomer seems to reduce adverse effects such as residual sedation seen with racemic zopiclone, despite the fact that the racemic mixture has a shorter half-life (5.0 vs. 6.5 hr). Racemization of one enantiomer to the other does not occur in mammals in vivo.

While SAR studies for cyclopyrrolones have not been performed to a great degree, it is known that this subclass recognizes a distinct site of the $GABA_A$ receptor complex that is allosteric to the recognition site for classical BZs.[69] The regional distribution and specificity of sites labeled by radiolabeled cyclopyrrolones are similar to those labeled by classical benzodiazepine ligands, suggesting that the cyclopyrrolone binding site resides on the BZ site of the $GABA_A$ complex.[69] However, unlike classical benzodiazepine agonists, binding of cyclopyrrolones is not affected by GABA or barbiturates. Furthermore, radioreceptor displacement binding studies revealed a noncompetitive interaction of cyclopyrrolones at sites labeled by classical benzodiazepines, whereas displacement of radiolabeled cyclopyrrolones by classical benzodiazepines occurred competitively, validating that cyclopyrrolones recognize a site on the BZ receptor complex that is allosteric to the recognition site of classical BZs.[69] Others have suggested that perhaps cyclopyrrolones can interact with one of multiple BZ binding sites on the $GABA_A$ receptor and, in doing so, cause allosteric changes in ligand affinity at the remaining sites. In this manner, eszopiclone could be thought to act in a positive cooperative binding manner with respect to itself.[70]

With regard to binding within the ligand recognition site, molecular modeling and mutagenesis studies have shown that eszopiclone is within 4 Å of many amino acid residues within the GABA-BZ complex binding pocket, and such proximity allows anchoring and stabilization by multiple hydrogen bonding interactions with Arg144, Tyr209, Tyr159, and various other residues.[59] These studies also revealed that the structural requirements for eszopiclone binding are different than that for zolpidem, and these differences may account for the lack of selectivity of eszopiclone.[59]

Metabolism of eszopiclone. Eszopiclone is metabolized extensively by CYP3A4 and CYP1A2 isozymes that yield the primary metabolites (S)-N-desmethylzopiclone and (S)-N-oxidezopiclone, respectively. The oxide metabolite is inactive while N-desmethyleszopiclone exhibits lower potency and affinity at $GABA_A$ receptors and therefore has only very weak hypnotic activity compared to the parent (Fig. 12.12). Interestingly, due to its lower affinity and lack of subtype selectivity, together with its weak sedative effects, this metabolite has been investigated as an novel anxiolytic agent.[71] Only small amounts (<7%) of unchanged eszopiclone are excreted in the urine, and greater than 75% of a dose is excreted via this route as inactive transformants of the two primary metabolites.

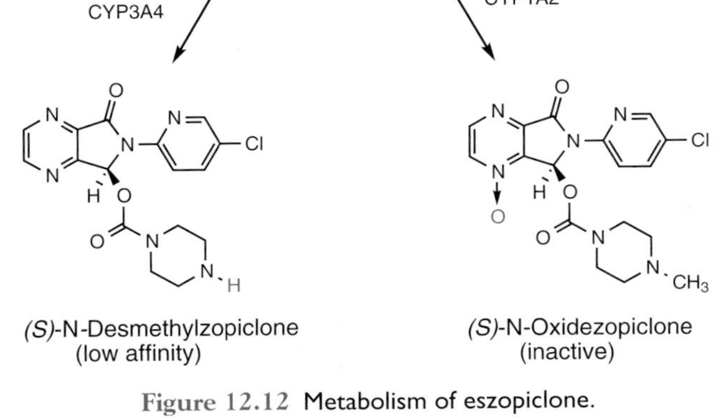

Eszopiclone

CYP3A4 CYP1A2

(S)-N-Desmethylzopiclone (low affinity)

(S)-N-Oxidezopiclone (inactive)

Figure 12.12 Metabolism of eszopiclone.

Zaleplon.

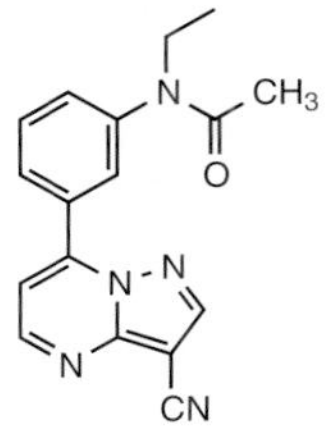

Zaleplon, a pyrazolopyrimidine, is a hypnotic agent that has a pharmacological profile similar to zolpidem but is primarily distinguished by its extremely rapid onset and short half-life. Similar to zolpidem, zaleplon has greater affinity at the α_1- versus α_2- and α_3-containing receptors, albeit with one-third to one-half the potency of zolpidem.[72] Unlike zolpidem, which does not recognize α_5-containing receptors with any appreciable affinity, zaleplon is able to potentiate the effects of GABA at α_5-containing receptors; however, its affinity for these receptors is approximately 15-fold less than that for α_1-containing receptors.[72] Thus, zaleplon is considered an α_1-selective GABA modulator, which lacks the classical benzodiazepine effects on non–sleep-related physiology.

The distinguishing features which afford zaleplon a unique place in the therapy of insomnia are its rapid rate of onset combined with its relatively fast rate of excretion. Oral administration of zaleplon leads to a peak plasma concentration in less than 1 hour, regardless of dose, the fastest of the nonbenzodiazepines.[73] While zaleplon is completely absorbed following oral administration, it is subject to first-pass metabolism, leading to an absolute bioavailability of 30% (Table 12.3).[73] As with zolpidem and eszopiclone, administration with heavy meals, particularly high-fat foods, delays the time to peak plasma concentration to 3 hours and reduces the peak plasma concentration by 35%.[74,75] Following oral administration, zaleplon is rapidly eliminated with a mean elimination half-life of 1 hour, an effect that is delayed significantly in patients with hepatic dysfunction. Taken together, these pharmacokinetic properties facilitate the rapid-onset and short-duration hypnotic effects.[74,75]

Clinically, zaleplon is distinguished by its ability to significantly reduce sleep latency for up to five weeks compared to placebo, an effect that can be contributed to its rapid onset.[75,76] However, numerous clinical trials have failed to consistently show that a 5 or 10 mg nightly dose of zaleplon significantly improves sleep duration, decreases the number of awakenings, or improves overall sleep quality compared with placebo. This is likely due to the short half-life of the agent, which precludes hypnotic effects throughout the night. Higher nightly doses of zaleplon (20 mg) do significantly improve both sleep latency and duration, but effects on total sleep quality and number of awakenings compared to placebo have been inconsistent in clinical trials at this dose.[75] Tolerance and withdrawal effects have not been reported during short-term treatment (up to 5 weeks), and the agent also seems to be free from rebound insomnia and residual next-day sedative effects, similar to other nonbenzodiazepine hypnotics.[76] As a result of these effects, zaleplon is approved only for patients with difficulties falling asleep; however, an extended-release formulation, which could improve sleep maintenance and duration, has been under development for some time.

Structure-Activity Relationships of Zaleplon. Unlike zolpidem and eszopiclone, extensive studies that examine the SARs of zaleplon with regard to binding potency and interaction within the binding pocket have not been performed. However, there have been numerous studies comparing the binding and function of zaleplon to the closely related compound indiplon (Fig. 12.13), allowing for deduction of SAR from pharmacological results. These studies show that zaleplon exhibits approximately 7- and 10-fold greater selectivity for α_1- over α_3- and α_5-containing $GABA_A$ receptors, respectively, whereas indiplon demonstrates only 1.6- and 4-fold selectivity.[77] Importantly, indiplon has 3-, 12-, and 7-fold higher affinity at α_1-, α_3-, and α_5-containing receptors, respectively, than does zaleplon. Further work has demonstrated that indiplon is greater than 100-fold more potent than zaleplon at potentiating GABA currents through α_1-containing receptors but is also 46- and 25-fold more potent at doing so through α_3- and α_5-containing receptors, respectively.[48,77] This work suggests that the thiophene-2-carbonyl moiety of indiplon (Fig. 12.13) drives higher binding affinity and thus potency but decreases overall selectivity for one subtype over another. Meanwhile, zaleplon contains only a cyano group at this position, suggesting that electronic rather than steric factors influence selectivity.

Metabolism of Zaleplon. As described above, zaleplon is subject to significant first-pass metabolism that accounts for its low oral bioavailability. Following oral administration of the agent in humans, less than 0.1% of the drug is recovered unchanged in the urine. Animal studies have demonstrated distinct interspecies variability in the metabolism of orally administered zaleplon due to differences in the activity of hepatic aldehyde oxidase, which is the principle metabolic enzyme responsible for the transformation of zaleplon.[78] In rodents and canines, which have decreased expression and activity of aldehyde oxidase, zaleplon is predominantly metabolized by CYP3A4 to N-desethylzaleplon, with only minor oxidation by aldehyde oxidase to yield 5-oxozaleplon. In humans, these metabolic routes are interchanged due to greater activity of aldehyde oxidase, and as a result, the major metabolite is 5-oxozaleplon, while CYP3A4-mediated transformation, yielding N-desethylzaleplon, is a minor route (Fig. 12.13). Both primary metabolites are inactive and, once formed, can either be directly eliminated in the urine or oxidized further and excreted as a glucuronide conjugate. In addition, the N-desethylzaleplon metabolite can be rapidly converted, presumably also via aldehyde oxidase, to 5-oxo-N-desethylzaleplon (Fig. 12.13).[74] Following oral administration of radiolabeled zaleplon to healthy volunteers, 70% of the dose was recovered in the urine within two days, almost exclusively as the two primary metabolites or their O-glucuronide conjugates (Fig. 12.13).[74] The 5-oxozaleplon metabolite also predominates in the feces, where over 15% of an administered dose can be found within six days.[74]

The nonbenzodiazepines represent major advancements in treatment of insomnia. They are highly effective hypnotic agents with negligible residual daytime drowsiness and are generally free from the psychomotor and cognitive side effects of classical benzodiazepines. Despite their primary use at nighttime and their relatively short half-lives, these agents are also not completely devoid of adverse side effects. Recently, there has been an increase in reported occurrences of nonbenzodiazepine-induced sleepwalking and associated amnesic sleep-related complex behaviors such as sleep driving, sleep eating, sleep cooking, sleep talking, and sleep sex.[79-87] These effects have been reported at therapeutic as well as supratherapeutic doses and are potentiated by alcohol consumption. Importantly, patients

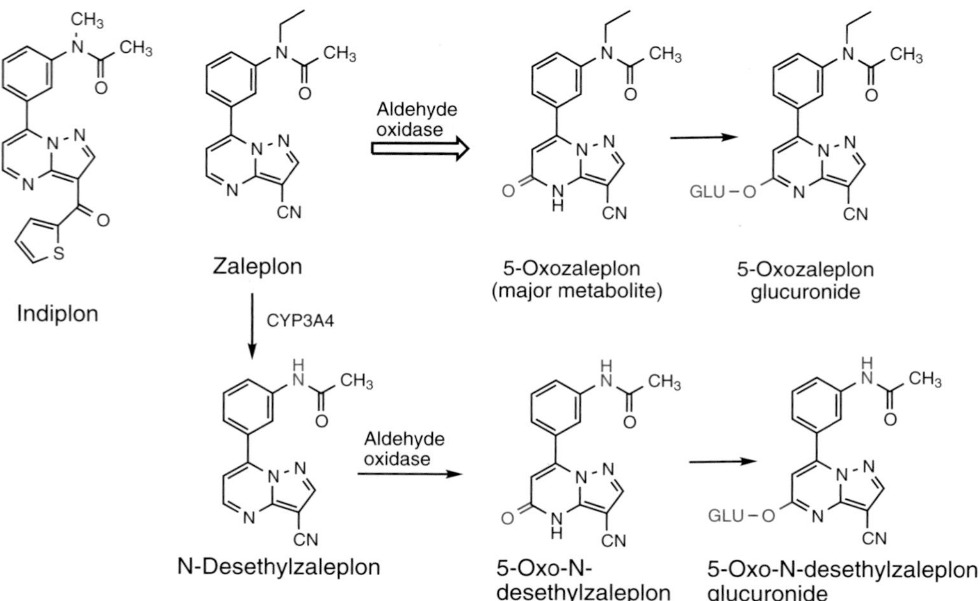

Figure 12.13 Structures of zaleplon and indiplon and metabolism of zaleplon.

do not have any recall or memory of these events. While these unintended effects are rare, they are potentially very serious, as they can affect social, emotional, and physical health and pose risks for fatal incidents.

MELATONIN RECEPTOR AGONISTS. As described previously, melatonin is a neurohormone that is primarily synthesized in the pineal gland from its precursor, serotonin (Fig. 12.1). Since melatonin synthesis is concurrent with sleep, the increase in endogenous nighttime melatonin levels correlates with the onset of sleepiness. The sleep-promoting and circadian effects of melatonin are due to agonism of both MT_1 and MT_2 receptors (MT1R, MT2R), both of which are present in very high density (~ 4 fmol/mg protein) within the SCN.[88] Agonism of SCN MT1R directly facilitates inhibition of SCN neuron firing, promoting sleep, while activation of SCN MT2R effects the circadian rhythm settings related to the central clock.[89,90]

Melatonin itself is a poor chemotherapeutic agent due to its poor absorption and low oral bioavailability of less than 10%, as well as its ubiquitous effects on sleep and circadian rhythms. Moreover, because melatonin is a supplement that is unregulated by the FDA, preparations vary in their purity and concentration and, as a result, poor sleep outcomes are often encountered. The significant effects of MT receptor agonism on sleep, coupled with the relatively poor nature of melatonin as a drug, prompted intense medicinal-chemical efforts to develop novel small molecule congeners of melatonin that behave as potent agonists of MT receptors. These efforts led to the successful launch of the first-in-class melatonin receptor agonist (*S*)-ramelteon, which has an excellent sleep and safety profile.

Structure-Activity Relationships of Melatonin Receptor Agonists. SARs for melatonin and its congeners have been reviewed at length.[91-96] Early studies demonstrated that the indole backbone of melatonin was not required for activity as long as it was replaced by an aromatic isostere as in ramelteon (which contains an indane) or as in other MTR agonists such as tasimelteon and agomelatine (Fig. 12.14).[94] It has been proposed that the importance of the aromatic ring system is to offer an optimum distance between the amide side chain at position-3 and the 5-methoxy substituent.[95,96] The aromatic

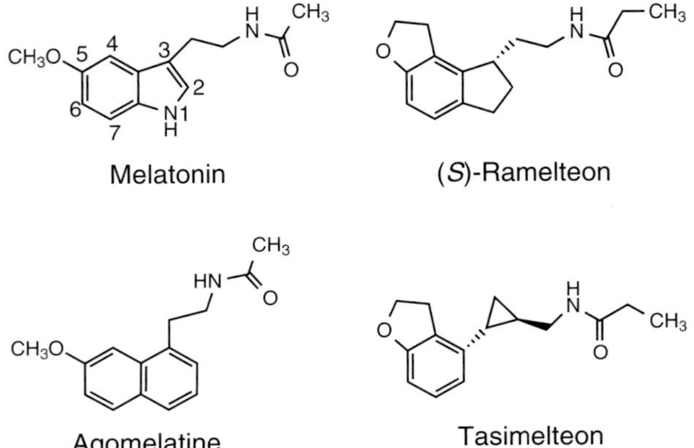

Figure 12.14 Structures of melatonin and the melatonin receptor agonists (*S*)-ramelteon, agomelatine, and tasimelteon.

moiety has also been suggested to interact with aromatic receptor residues within the binding pocket through π-π stacking.[95,96] While the aromatic portion contributes to spacing and likely π-π-interactions, the 3-position amide and the 5-methoxy side chains are responsible for binding and functional activation of the receptors by interacting with two proposed binding pockets.

The amide group is critical for agonist activity at both MT receptors and is thought to interact with key serine (Ser110 and Ser114) and asparagine (Asn175) residues in transmembrane helix (TMH) III of MT_1 and TMH IV of TM2, respectively.[97] Meanwhile, the 5-methoxy moiety is critical for functional effects. It has been proposed that the methoxy oxygen interacts with His195 and His208 within TMH VI of MT1R and MT2R, respectively.[96,98] Movement of the methoxy group to the 4-, 6-, or 7-positions significantly decreases functional activity, suggesting that distance to these conserved histidine residues is critical in maintaining binding affinity and functional activity.[92] Additionally, Val192, which is located nearly one turn above His195 within the ligand-binding domain, has been shown to be involved in binding the methyl component of the methoxy group.[96]

Finally, the binding pocket of MTRs is highly stereoselective, an important feature that must be considered for drug design. As a consequence of the three-dimensional requirements of binding to MT receptors, ramelteon (discussed below) is dispensed as the enantiomerically pure (*S*)-enantiomer, which has 500-fold greater affinity for MT_1 than does (*R*)-ramelteon.

Ramelteon.

(*S*)-Ramelteon selectively binds to both MT1R and MT2R, recognizing the human receptors with extremely high affinity of 14 and 112 pM (picomolar), respectively. This represents an 8- to 10-fold greater affinity for MT1R compared to MT2R, and 6-fold greater affinity than melatonin for MT1R.[99] The high potency and slight preference for MT1R correlate to the ability of the drug to primarily reduce sleep latency, as opposed to influenceing regulation of phase—circadian rhythms.

With regard to functional pharmacology, in Chinese hamster ovary (CHO) cells ectopically expressing the human MT1R and MT2R, ramelteon was 4- and 17-fold more potent at inhibiting cyclic AMP production compared to melatonin, respectively, consistent with observations that demonstrate coupling of MT receptors to $G\alpha_{i/o}$ proteins.[99] Moreover, ramelteon does not have any appreciable affinity for a third physiologically relevant melatonin binding site known as MT3R, which is a melatonin-sensitive quinine reductase not involved in sleep/wake functions.[100,101] Taken together, the absence of binding to brain receptors other than MT1R/MT2R, along with its potent activity at these melatonin receptors, makes ramelteon an efficacious sleep-inducing agent that is free from many of the CNS side effects common to other sedative-hypnotics.

Animal studies demonstrate that ramelteon significantly decreases wakefulness and increases both short wave and REM sleep compared with placebo.[100-102] In clinical trials, no effects on short wave sleep have been noted, but the agent leads to significant decreases in sleep latency and increases in total sleep duration over a five week period compared to placebo.[103-105] Importantly, ramelteon, consistent with its melatonin receptor–related mechanism which is free of endogenous GABAergic signaling, does not produce residual next-day sedation or decreases in psychomotor function.[104] Likewise, due to its unique mechanism, ramelteon does not hinder learning, cognition, and memory like the benzodiazepine agents do. It also lacks the potential for abuse, does not lead to tolerance, and poses no risk of withdrawal or rebound insomnia upon discontinuation.[103-106] One potential adverse effect, which can be predicted for melatonin receptor agonists, is based on the ability of melatonin to influence prolactin and testosterone levels via agonism of MT_1 and MT_2 receptors located within endocrine and reproductive tissue. Similarly, ramelteon has been reported to affect mean free and total testosterone levels.[100] Further studies are necessary to gauge the clinical consequences, if any, that exogenous melatonin receptor agonists have on endocrine and reproductive function. In summary, from a sleep-therapy standpoint, melatonin receptor agonists such as ramelteon have highly efficacious hypnotic effects while being free of many of the cognitive and residual effects common to $GABA_A$–modulating agents.

Metabolism of Ramelteon. (S)-Ramelteon is rapidly absorbed following oral administration, and mean peak plasma concentrations are achieved at 0.75 hours. In a study in healthy volunteers who were administered radiolabeled ramelteon, 84% of recovered radioactivity was found in the urine and 4% in the feces, suggesting that at least 84% of the drug was absorbed. However, ramelteon is subject to extensive first-pass metabolism leading to an absolute oral bioavailability of only approximately 2%.[107] Ramelteon has a short elimination half-life of 1-2.5 hours, and once-nightly dosing does not lead to accumulation of the drug. The time to peak plasma concentration was delayed by 45 minutes upon administration with food, and the peak plasma concentrations were decreased by 22% in this case.[107]

Ramelteon is primarily metabolized by oxidation in phase 1 reactions, with secondary metabolites being excreted as glucuronide conjugates.[108] Hepatic CYP1A2 is the major isoform responsible for transformation (49%), while CYP2C19 (42%) and CYP3A4 (8.6%) isoforms are also contributors to ramelteon metabolism in the liver. In contrast, in the intestines, only CYP3A4 contributes to transformation.[109] The major metabolite of ramelteon in humans is the hydroxylated propionamide MII metabolite (Fig. 12.15), which is active, has a 2-5 hour half-life, and has 20- to 100-fold greater systemic exposure than the parent, suggesting slower removal from the circulation.[107,108] Moreover, this metabolite has one-fifth to one-tenth the binding affinity of the parent for human MT_1 and MT_2 receptors and shows potent hypnotic effects in animals, suggesting that it may contribute to the sedative-hypnotic effects of ramelteon.[92] In addition to the MII metabolite, ramelteon can be oxidized to the ring-opened MI metabolite or transformed to a carboxy-metabolite, MIII (Fig. 12.15), both of which are inactive. Biotransformation of the MII and MIII metabolites by sequential oxidation can lead to formation of MIV. The rank order of prevalence of the four metabolites in human serum is MII, MIV, MI, and MIII, and all three of the hydroxylated metabolites can be excreted as glucuronide conjugates (Fig. 12.15).

Importantly, ramelteon is also subject to significant drug interactions upon coadministration with the antidepressant fluvoxamine, the fluoroquinolone antibiotic ciprofloxin, or the OTC H_2-antagonist cimetidine, which are all relatively strong CYP1A2 inhibitors. Coadministration of any of these agents with ramelteon significantly increases the total systemic exposure of ramelteon (greater than 100-fold in the case of fluvoxamine) and should be avoided.

OREXIN RECEPTOR ANTAGONISTS. As described previously, the hypothalamic neuropeptides orexin-A and orexin-B activate their cognate GPCRs, OX1R and OX2R, to depolarize and excite downstream neurons in order to promote arousal and alertness. Hypothalamic orexin neurons are highly active during wakefulness and quiesce during all

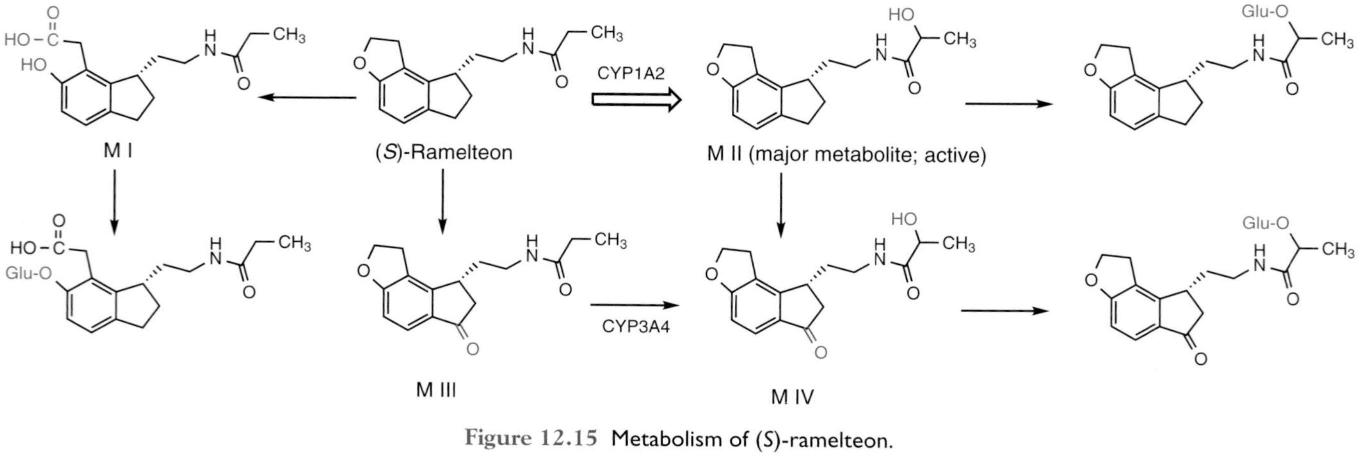

Figure 12.15 Metabolism of (S)-ramelteon.

stages of sleep, which correlates with heightened levels of orexin-A during wake periods that fall significantly during sleep.[110-112] The discovery that disturbances in orexinergic function are linked to the pathophysiology of narcolepsy, coupled with evidence linking loss of function mutations of OX2R to heritable narcolepsy in animals, demonstrates the critical role of OXRs in regulating vigilance and arousal.[113,114]

Consistent with these observations, exogenous administration of orexins in mammals increases wakefulness, decreases REM and non-REM sleep, and increases locomotor activity.[115,116] On the contrary, antagonism of the orexin GPCRs facilitates hyperpolarization of postsynaptic neurons, which promotes drowsiness and somnolence. Using genetic knockout models coupled to approaches that utilize selective single- or dual-OXR antagonists (i.e., SORA and DORA, respectively), it has become evident that arousal is principally regulated by the OX2R, while both OXRs are involved in modulating vigilance states within the sleep/wake architecture.[117] In addition, dual OXR knockout animals exhibit the most pronounced sleep phenotype compared to single OXR knockouts, and when compared to SORA, DORA provide enhanced in vivo and clinical sleep efficacy. Consequently, recent drug discovery efforts have led to development of DORA for clinical therapy of insomnia.

Almorexant (structure shown below) was one of the first DORA to be assessed clinically for the treatment of insomnia and proved to be effective at increasing total sleep time and decreasing sleep latency, including time to induction of REM sleep. This is consistent with its reported low nanomolar affinity for both OXR (IC_{50}'s of 13 and 8 nM for OX1R and OX2R, respectively).[118-120] Unlike zolpidem, almorexant lacked sedative-hypnotic effects in OX1R/OX2R knockout mice and had no effects on next-day motor function or muscle relaxation.[118,121] In clinical trials, almorexant improved measures of sleep efficiency and showed minimal residual next-day impairments to motor function or cognition in insomniac patients; however, development of this agent was halted in late 2011 due to undisclosed reasons.

Suvorexant. In 2014, the FDA approved Suvorexant, developed by Merck & Co. as MK-4305, as the first DORA for clinical use for the treatment of insomnia. Suvorexant (Fig. 12.16) has high binding affinity of 0.55 and 0.35 nM for OX1R and OX2R, respectively. This translates to 50 and 56 nM functional potency, as determined by the ability to inhibit orexin-mediated Ca^{+2}-mobilization in clonal CHO expression systems.[122] In an off-target screen of 170 enzymes, receptors, and ion channels, suvorexant displays a noteworthy >10,000-fold

A

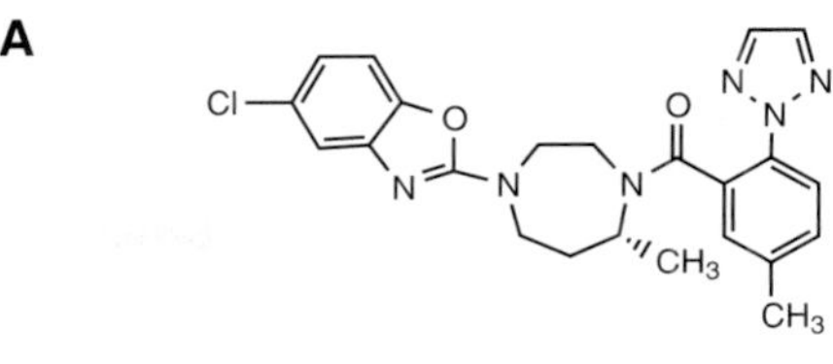

(*R*)-Suvorexant

B

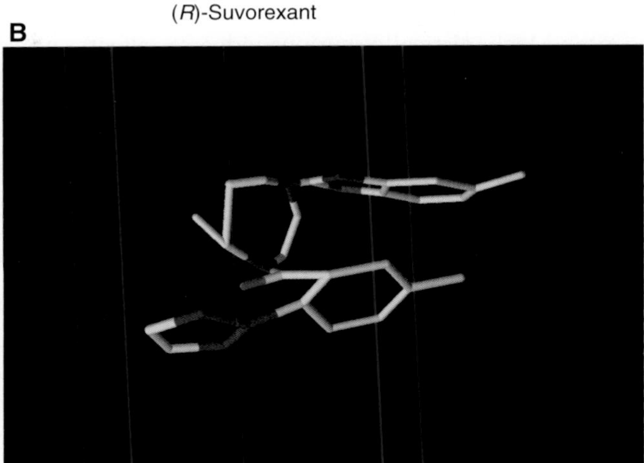

Figure 12.16 Structure of (*R*)-suvorexant (A) and its horseshoe-oriented preferred binding configuration (B).

selectivity for the OXR, an effect that alleviates concerns regarding ancillary target profiles.[122]

Pharmacokinetically, suvorexant has moderate passive brain permeability owing to a high degree of lipophilicity (log P = 3.6) and is not a substrate for *P*-glycoprotein efflux from the brain.[122] In animals, suvorexant significantly increased REM sleep and delta-stage activity (stage 4 sleep) and induced corresponding decreases in wake time, with analogous receptor occupancy of greater than 90%.[122]

In human clinical trials of durations ranging from one month to over one year, suvorexant was dose-dependently superior to placebo in regard to time to sleep onset and time to onset of REM sleep.[123-126] Furthermore, suvorexant increased total sleep time and decreased number and time of awakenings compared to placebo.[123-126] It was also demonstrated to be effective in reducing time to sleep onset and total sleep time in elderly patients with insomnia.[126,127] Together, these clinical data demonstrate that suvorexant is effective for both latency and maintenance of sleep.

In clinical trials, as would be expected given the indicated use of the agent, the most common adverse effect of suvorexant was somnolence, which was dose dependent.[128] Interestingly, the incidence of somnolence was significantly higher in females (8%) than in males (3%), suggesting that gender-based metabolism plays a role in metabolic breakdown of suvorexant. Gender-specific metabolism was also seen with zolpidem (see above). Residual somnolence, drowsiness and general CNS-depressant effects may persist for several days following discontinuation of suvorexant. Of note, this effect led to a clinically meaningful next-morning impaired driving performance, and consequently, patients on suvorexant should be warned about residual next-day impairments to mental alertness.

Given its unique mechanism of action, suvorexant would be predicted to have a distinct adverse effect profile compared to other sedative-hypnotic agents. After somnolence, the next most frequently occurring adverse effects were headache, abnormal dreams, and dry mouth, which while occurring in a dose-dependent manner in suvorexant-treated patients[128] are common to many CNS-acting agents. Mechanistically curious adverse effects noted in clinical trials included a significant dose-dependent increase in serum cholesterol, which became apparent after 4 weeks of treatment, as well as a dose-dependent increase in suicidal ideation.[128] Overall, the adverse effects in elderly patients were consistent with those observed in nonelderly patients, and the long-term (i.e., up to 1 year) adverse effects were consistent with those observed in the first three months of suvorexant treatment.

Finally, although there was no evidence for physical dependence or withdrawal symptoms after discontinuation, an abuse liability study in a small sampling of recreational drug users showed that suvorexant was similar to zolpidem in producing subjective drug-desirableness, lending to its categorization as a DEA Schedule IV controlled substance.

Structure-Activity Relationships of Suvorexant. Suvorexant (Fig. 12.16) was derived from high-throughput screening efforts that identified diazepane-based compounds as novel high-affinity antagonists of both OXRs and which promoted sleep in rodents.[122] The early diazepane derivatives contained chloro-benzisothiazole or quinazoline ring substituents relative to the central 1,4-diazepane ring; however, compounds with these substituents yielded poor in vivo bioavailabilities in rats and canines as a consequence of first-pass metabolism and heightened clearance rates.[122] Assessment of these metabolites revealed oxidation of both the central diazepane ring as well as the quinazoline substituent, prompting synthetic efforts to modify the quinazoline ring in order to prevent rapid oxidation and clearance. Halogenation of the 6-position of the quinazoline ring improved OX1R/OX2R affinities and also reduced clearance of the agent, leading to enhanced bioavailability. Replacement of the entire quinazoline ring with a 5-chloro-benzoxazole ring, as seen with suvorexant, resulted in additional decreases in clearance, increasing bioavailability and preserving affinity for both OXRs.[122] Suvorexant is dispensed as the enantiomerically resolved (7*R*)-isomer (as shown in Fig. 12.16), which has 10- to 20-fold greater functional potency at both OXRs compared to the (*S*)-enantiomer.[122]

The crystal structure of the human OX2 receptor bound to suvorexant was recently resolved to a resolution of 2.5 Å and sheds a great degree of insight into the atomic interactions of the antagonist with the receptor.[129] As shown in Figure 12.17A, suvorexant is accessible to the OX2R binding pocket via a solvent accessible channel that is enclosed by amino acid residues from TMH II, VI, VI, and VII, as well as a β-hairpin turn from extracellular loop 2.[129] As shown by early SAR studies,[122] the early 1,4-disubstituted diazepane OX1R/OX2R antagonists, including suvorexant, exhibited hindered rotations about the C-N bond between the central diazepane and the quinazoline rings, a structural feature that facilitates U-shaped, or horseshoelike, conformations of the outer heterocyclic ring systems. This allows for an unusual intramolecular π-π stacking between the aromatic *p*-toluene and benzoxazole moieties (see Fig. 12.16).[122] These early observations were confirmed in the crystal structure, revealing that suvorexant rests in the ligand-binding pocket of OX2R in a horseshoe configuration (Fig. 12.17C), due to a boat conformation of the diazepane ring and intramolecular π-π stacking of the aromatic benzoxazole and *p*-toluamide functional groups.

As shown in Figure 12.17B and C, suvorexant makes contact with all OX2R TMH except for TMH I. A hydrogen bond exists between Asn324 in TMH VI and the carbonyl group of the suvorexant amide, while a water molecule that is centrally located 2.85 Å from the amide and 2.92 Å from His350 in TMH VII coordinates additional hydrogen bond interactions; and together, these form a water-bridge between these polar functional groups to the agent (Fig. 12.17). The aromatic functionality of His350 is also responsible to contributing to π-π stacking with the aromatic *p*-toluene moiety of suvorexant, while neighboring Tyr317 contributes to π-π stacking with the triazole moiety (Fig. 12.17). Additionally, van der Waals interactions occur between Phe227 and the (*R*)-oriented methyldiazepane ring, which is itself in boat conformation due to the horseshoe orientation noted above. Meanwhile, the chlorobenzoxazole moiety is stabilized via interactions with Ile130 and Pro131 in TMH III and Ala110 and Thr111 in TMH II (Fig. 12.17).[129]

Metabolism and Pharmacokinetics of Suvorexant. Maximal suvorexant plasma concentrations are obtained within 2 hours after oral administration under fasting conditions, an effect that is delayed to 3.5 hours if administered with a high-fat meal.[128] Given a mean elimination half-life of 12.3 hours (range of 9-15 hr), it is reasonable to expect some residual next-day drowsiness.[130] Indeed, in phase III trials, patients on the 40 mg dose had 12-hour plasma concentrations equivalent to the Tmax observed in patients taking the 20 mg dose. Therefore, the nightly dose should not exceed 20 mg.

As shown in Figure 12.18, in man, suvorexant is metabolized primarily by CYP3A4 with an additional minor contribution from CYP2C19.[130] Following single oral dose administration of radioactive suvorexant to healthy human volunteers, 66% of the dose is recovered in the feces while 23% is recovered in the urine, with the majority (82%) of the dose being excreted in 6 days.[130] The major proposed metabolites of suvorexant found in the urine include the carboxylic acid M4 and its glucuronide conjugate M19, which account for 4.1% and 5.3% of the administered dose, respectively (Fig. 12.18).[130] Glucuronide conjugates of metabolites M8, M10A, and M9, yielding M3, M12, and M11, respectively, accounted for the remaining urinary metabolites. These phase 2 conjugates were respectively responsible for 3.8%, 2.7%, and 1.4% of the total dose. No other metabolites nor the parent drug was localized to the urine. As seen in the urine, the major metabolite accounted for in the feces was the carboxylic acid M4,

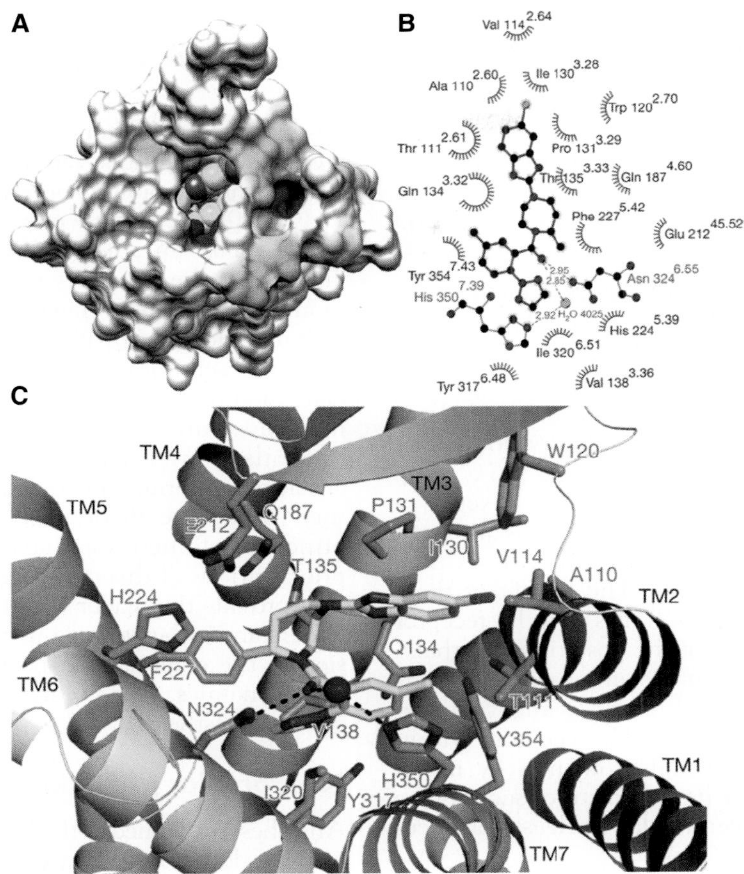

Figure 12.17 Crystallographic interactions of suvorexant with the human orexin-2 receptor. (A) Accessibility of suvorexant to the OX2R binding pocket via a solvent accessible channel. (B and C) Suverexant interactions with amino acids in TMH II-VII of the OX2R binding pocket. Reprinted by permission from Macmillan Publishers Ltd: *Nature*. March 12, 2015;519:247-250.

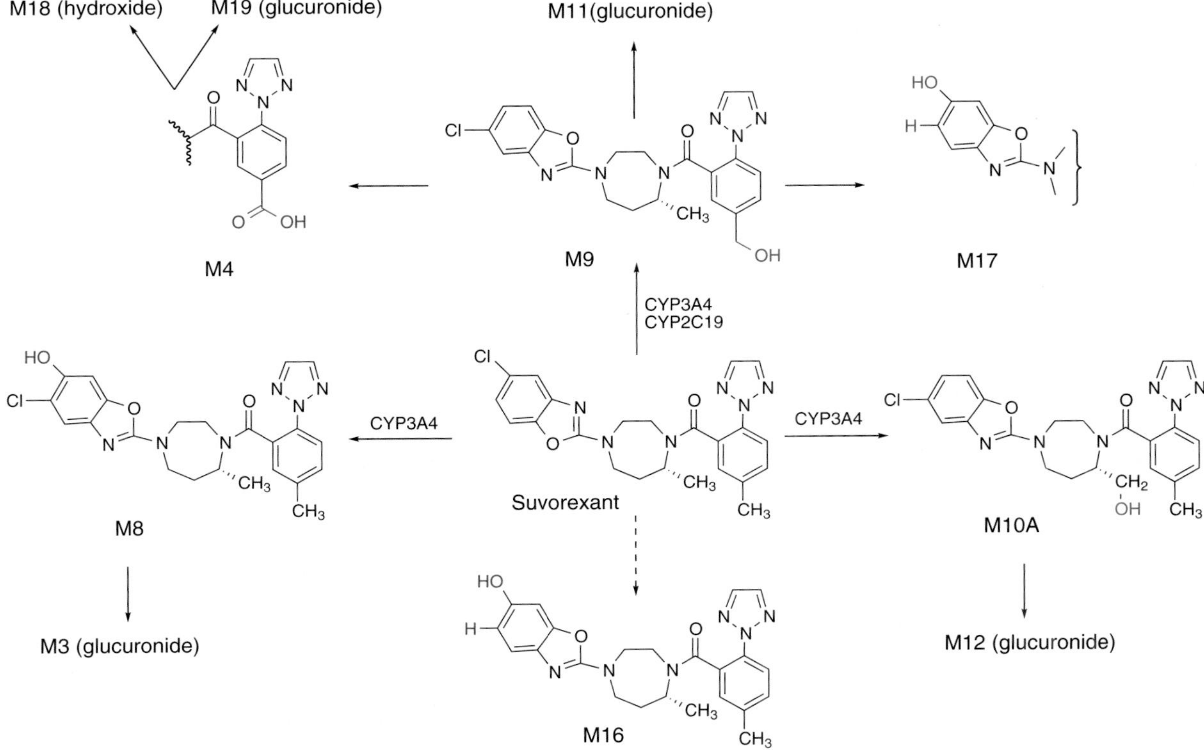

Figure 12.18 Metabolism of suvorexant.

which accounted for 17% of the total dose. Further oxidation of M4 to M18 represented 10.6%, while oxidation of the *p*-toluene to the alcohol M9 and oxidation of the methyldiazepan to the alcohol M10A each represented 9% of the dose. Given the role of CYP3A4 and CYP2C19 on suvorexant metabolism, analysis of CYP inhibitory properties revealed that the agent weakly inhibits both P450 enzymes, with IC50's of 4.0 and 4.0 μM, respectively.[130]

HISTAMINE H_1 RECEPTOR ANTAGONISTS. The first generation of ethanolamine ether histamine H_1 receptor antagonists (i.e., antihistamines) that cross the blood-brain barrier are used for acute insomnia due to their sedation-promoting side effects. In particular, diphenhydramine and doxylamine, both high-affinity (low-nanomolar) H_1 receptor antagonists, are sold as OTC sleep aids. Recently, the tricyclic antidepressant doxepin, a potent subnanomolar-affinity H_1 antagonist, has also been approved for treatment of insomnia at lower doses than that used for depression (Silenor). The benefit of these agents for treatment of insomnia comes from H_1 receptor antagonism within the TMN of the posterior hypothalamus, where the normal release of histamine during the day causes arousal, and its decreased release at night reduces arousal responses. Antagonism of H_1 receptors within the TMN promotes sedation and drowsiness by inhibiting TMN outflow to other brain structures such as the dorsal raphe nucleus, paraventricular nucleus, and locus coeruleus.

Overall, antihistamines bring about increased drowsiness and sedation with marginal beneficial effects on sleep latency and total sleep time. There is very little in the way of rigorous clinical trial data that support their sedative-hypnotic efficacy, and to the contrary, some results reveal that these agents disrupt sleep architecture by delaying the onset to, and duration of, REM sleep. Regardless, these drugs are utilized heavily as sedative-hypnotics, and in the case of diphenhydramine and doxylamine, patients are able to readily self-medicate due to the ease in their availability.

While diphenhydramine, doxylamine, and doxepin also exhibit antimuscarinic activity, leading to corresponding side effects such as dry mouth, urinary retention, and blurred vision, a major side effect of these agents is excessive daytime drowsiness and residual next-day sedation. These next-day effects can lead to impaired cognition and performance and are attributed to the relatively long half-lives. Finally, nightly use of first generation antihistamines as sleep-aids has been associated with tolerance to the hypnotic effect with long-term use.

AGENTS THAT INDUCE OR MAINTAIN GENERAL ANESTHESIA

Historic records document the use of a myriad of natural products, including a variety of herbs, as well as wines, vapors, and the opium poppy for use in anesthesia. In the early 1500s, the first use of ether was documented to provide a robust anesthetic effect in animals, while in the late 1700s, the discovery of nitrous oxide (N_2O), commonly referred to as "laughing gas", led to observations that it could "destroy physical pain". Based on these and similar observations, in the mid-1800s Georgia physician and pharmacist Crawford Long pioneered the use of inhaled sulfuric ether as an anesthetic, which gave rise to efforts to investigate novel anesthetics such as diethyl ether, chloroform, and cocaine going into the 20th century. While the theoretical considerations and kinetic principles of anesthesia have been covered in depth in prior editions of this text, the aim of the current section is to provide the reader with the neurochemical basis for understanding anesthesia as well as an in depth discussion of the chemical perspectives regarding SAR, pharmacodynamics, and pharmacokinetics of agents used for general anesthesia.

Neurobiology of Anesthesia

Anesthesia is defined as the loss of feeling or sensation, and can, but does not necessary have to be coupled to concurrent loss of consciousness. Drug-induced anesthesia typically refers to either the systemic administration of agents that promote loss of sensation and consciousness through CNS depression (i.e., general anesthesia) or, alternatively, regional administration of agents that promote loss of sensation by inhibiting local sensory neurotransmission in a given tissue (i.e., local anesthesia). In addition, sedative-hypnotics, analgesics, and neuromuscular blocking agents can induce or potentiate anesthesia and are routinely utilized clinically for such use.

While sleep is characterized by diminished consciousness that is responsive to external stimuli, general anesthesia is typified by the complete loss of consciousness that is not responsive to external stimuli. Importantly, induction of general anesthesia is also characterized by amnesia, analgesia, and temporary paralysis of muscles, allowing for its utility in clinical diagnostic procedures as well as surgical and operative procedures. Based on current understanding of the effects of anesthetics in consciousness, the induction of general anesthesia and the emergence from it back toward conscious states is driven primarily by acetylcholine (ACh) neurons within the thalamus. The

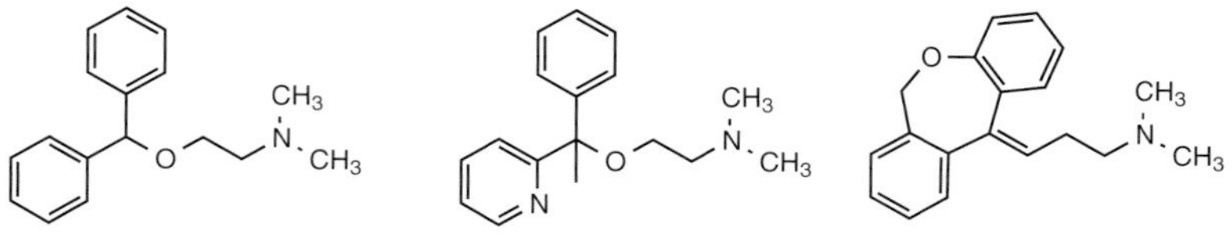

Diphenhydramine Doxylamine Doxepin

same glutamatergic, GABAergic, and orexinergic neurons within the reticular formation, thalamus, and hypothalamus noted above as being responsible for sedative/hypnotic effects are also involved. Upon induction of anesthesia with certain agents, cerebral blood flow and brain glucose metabolism are drastically affected within the thalamus,[131-133] suggesting that this region of the brain is greatly influenced by GAs. Certain anesthetics have also been shown to influence brain metabolism in a manner that is directly proportional to density of GABA receptor expression within a given brain region, such that higher levels of GABA receptors in thalamus may be responsible for the reduced metabolism seen in that region upon induction. Since the thalamus behaves as a relay center for ascending and descending processing to and from the cortex, the thalamo-cortical axis is a major regulator of anesthetic-induced unconsciousness.[134,135] Indeed, it is typically well-accepted that GAs induce unconsciousness by inhibiting the high-frequency pulses of arousal sensing information through the thalamo-cortical and reticulo-thalamo-cortical ascending arousal structures.[136-138] Mechanistically, this is thought to occur primarily via four pharmacological targets, modulation of which facilitates hyperpolarization of neurons that are responsible for arousal, awareness, and conscious states. These four targets include (1) $GABA_A$ receptors, activation of which enhances inhibitory neurotransmission; (2) NMDA receptors (NMDA-R), antagonism of which inhibits excitatory neurotransmission; (3) nicotinic-ACh receptors (nAChR), antagonism of which inhibits excitatory neurotransmission; and (4) two-pore domain K^+ channels (e.g., K2P channels) that modulate background K^+ currents, agonism of which directly hyperpolarizes neurons. As will be described here, GAs will function through one or more of these routes to inactivate brain regions, resulting in CNS depression and loss of consciousness.

In contrast to GA where loss of sensory perception is coupled with unconsciousness, local anesthesia causes a reversible loss of sensory perception with no effect on central arousal state. These agents are administered topically or by injection directly into localized areas. The local administration of these agents causes the loss of propagation of the action potential in peripheral nerve fibers, thereby blocking nerve conductance that transmits sensory and nociceptive information from the localized area to the brain. Local anesthetics, which are discussed in detail in Chapter 15 of this text, block nerve conductance by binding to specific sites on voltage-gated Na^+ channels on excitable nerves, thereby preventing the passage of Na^+ and interfering with the action potential that is required for excitability.

Stages of General Anesthesia

The early works that characterized the inhaled effects of diethyl ether led to Arthur Guedel's classification of the stages of anesthesia in the late 1930s. In the first stage, referred to as *analgesia*, the patient experiences mild thalamo-cortical depression leading to pain relief without amnesia. In the second stage, referred to as *excitement*, CNS depression deepens, particularly within reticulo-thalamic centers, and the patient may appear excitable or even delirious but is fully amnesic. Here, respiration, cardiac chronotropy, and blood pressure may increase and involuntary muscle activity could occur. The ideal anesthetic agent should produce very little time in the first two stages, and increased concentrations of the GA can shorten time in these stages. Stage III, referred to as *surgical anesthesia*, begins with normalization of unconscious respiration and chronotropy and extends to four distinct planes as the depth of anesthesia increases. These planes include cessation of ocular activity, paralysis of the intercostal muscles, dilation of pupils, and the loss of muscle tone. If the depth of anesthesia is allowed to increase, the paralysis of the diaphragm and respiratory function, known as *apnea*, ensues in stage IV, which is indicative of severe depression of vasomotor medullary activity in the brainstem. Under the careful observation of the anesthesiologist, stages I to II should occur as rapidly as possible while stage IV should never occur.

General Anesthetics

Clinically Useful Inhalation Agents

The gaseous GA agents include the volatile fluorinated hydrocarbons isoflurane, sevoflurane, desflurane, and enflurane, which along with the nonvolatile gas nitrous oxide (N_2O), make up the family of clinically useful inhalation agents that are administered under the care of the anesthesiologist (Fig. 12.19). The concentration of inhaled anesthetics is carefully controlled by the anesthesiologist in order to maximize the anesthetic effect while ensuring proper emergence from it. The volatile

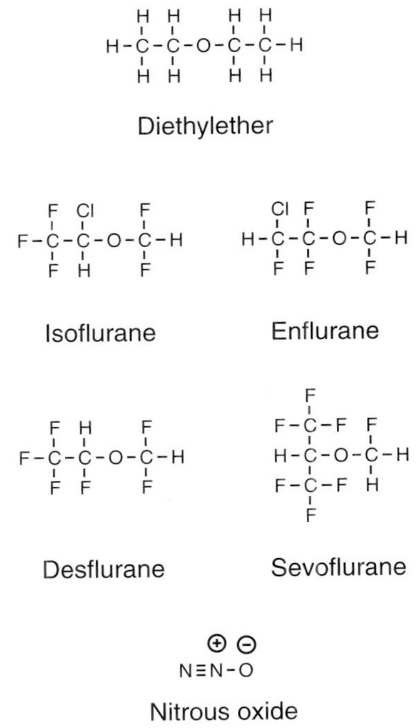

Diethylether

Isoflurane

Enflurane

Desflurane

Sevoflurane

Nitrous oxide

Figure 12.19 Structures of inhaled general anesthetics.

anesthetics are vaporized prior to inhalation with O_2, whereas N_2O can be inhaled directly as a gas mixed with O_2. Upon inhalation, the concentration of anesthetic in the bronchiolar alveoli reaches equilibrium with that in the inspired gas mixture. Transfer from the alveolar space to the blood proceeds quickly, as the partial pressure (tension) in the alveoli is in equilibrium with the blood. Subsequent passage to the brain and other tissue moves toward equilibrium of the partial pressures in each compartment based on the solubility and physiochemical characteristics of each individual agent (Table 12.4). Since the partial pressure of the inhaled anesthetic equilibrates throughout the body in this manner, the alveolar concentration of the agent is reflective of the amount in the brain.

Solubility of the inhaled anesthetics is defined by the partition coefficient, the ratio of the concentration of the dissolved gas in the blood or tissue to the concentration in the gaseous phase at equilibrium (i.e., blood/gas or blood/tissue partition coefficient, respectively) (Table 12.4). Due to lipophilicity, the solubility of the anesthetic in the blood will differ from that in the tissue, and the partition coefficient plays an essential role of the kinetics of these agents. While the fluorinated agents, all derived from diethyl ether (Fig. 12.19), all have high degrees of lipophilicity, before significant amounts of the anesthetic enter the brain from the blood, the latter must be saturated with the anesthetic. The blood-tissue/gas partition coefficients explain the ability of the agent to partition within a given target at equilibrium, when the partial pressures of the agent will be the same. For example, the blood/gas partition coefficient of isoflurane is 1.4, and at equilibrium, the concentration in the blood will be 1.4-fold the concentration in the alveolar space. Therefore, the blood/gas partition coefficient and the brain/blood partition coefficient play meaningful roles in anesthetic effects. Practically, this implies that agents that have higher blood/gas coefficients will have longer times to saturate the blood compartment before the partial pressure rises enough to induce anesthesia in the brain. As a consequence, these agents have longer anesthesia induction onset times. In general, agents with higher partition coefficients have higher lipophilicity and higher blood solubility, meaning that more anesthetic will need to be dissolved to saturate the blood in order to reach the brain, yielding a slower induction.

Given that the rate of inhaled anesthetic induction is not dependent on absorption of the drug, but rather, primarily on the relative partial pressure in each compartment, the rate of emergence from anesthesia is correlated to the induction rate, such that agents with high blood solubility and slow induction will also exhibit slow recovery and emergence from anesthesia. In contrast, agents with low blood solubility and lower blood/gas partition coefficients will quickly saturate the blood and then rapidly enter the brain for a quick inductive effect, as well as faster emergence and recovery from the anesthetic effect. In addition to this important physiochemical characteristic, induction of anesthesia can be modulated by other factors including concentration, ventilation, and cardiac output, the latter of which is inversely correlated to induction. Greater levels of cardiac output will remove more anesthetic from the gas phase via the greater blood flow to the lungs.

Blood/gas partition coefficients for the inhaled anesthetics are in the rank order of enflurane > isoflurane > sevoflurane > nitrous oxide ≥ desflurane, as shown in Table 12.4.[139] Since the initial alveolar concentration of inhaled agent drives blood and brain permeation, the potency of inhaled anesthetics is measured as the minimum alveolar concentration (MAC). MAC is defined as the concentration of vapor (as a percentage of 1 atmosphere in the alveoli) required to prevent motor responses in 50% of adult patients subjected to a standardized surgical stimulus. Importantly, MAC values assume that equilibrium between the gas/alveoli/blood/brain compartments has been reached, and a variety of patient factors including body temperature, acidosis, blood pressure, pregnancy, and age can alter MAC. Nonetheless, a lower MAC value denotes a more potent anesthetic effect. The rank order of potencies for the anesthetics discussed here in 100% oxygen, as MAC_{50}, is isoflurane > enflurane > sevoflurane > desflurane > nitrous oxide (Table 12.4).[139] Additionally, the coadministration of nitrous oxide with a volatile anesthetic is additive; in general, a 1% increase in nitrous oxide allows for a similar percentage reduction in the MAC of the volatile anesthetic.[140,141]

Mechanism of Action of Inhaled Anesthetics

In the early 1900s, Meyer and Overton noted a strong correlation between the potency of volatile anesthetics and their lipophilicity and, based on this, theorized that these agents act nonspecifically on protein targets or on lipid components of CNS cells.[142] However, other highly lipophilic agents, lipid disruptors, and membrane modulators lack anesthetic capabilities, suggesting that other mechanisms are at play. The pharmacological characterization of the effects of the agents on a variety of CNS-acting ion channels, along with the structural diversity of the different types of inhaled anesthetics that have been used over the years, now supports the concept that a myriad of mechanisms are utilized by inhaled GAs to promote anesthesia. Indeed, the now-accepted mechanism of these agents is based on their ability to modulate a diverse assortment of CNS ion channels including all of the "cysteine loop" neurotransmitter receptors, which include $GABA_A$, nACh, $5\text{-}HT_3$, and glycine receptors, as well as the excitatory glutaminergic NMDA and AMPA receptors.[143-145] The known in vitro and in vivo pharmacological effects of the halogenated agents and nitrous oxide on these receptors are summarized in Table 12.4. The volatile agents are known to inhibit voltage-gated Na^+ channels in addition to nAChR, NMDA, AMPA, and $5\text{-}HT_3$ receptors, while at the same time enhancing the activity of $GABA_A$, two-pore domain K^+ channels, and glycine receptors.[146-161] Modulation of these ion channels facilitates membrane hyperpolarization and decreases synaptic neuronal excitability. On the contrary, nitrous oxide has only weak activity at potentiating $GABA_A$ and glycine receptor currents but can activate two-pore K^+ channels and also inhibits nAChR and NMDA-R flux.

Table 12.4 Partition Coefficients, Minimum Alveolar Concentrations (MACs), and Ion Channel Modulation of Clinically Utilized Inhaled Anesthetics[a]

Anesthetic	Blood/Gas Partition Coefficient	MAC[b] (Vol %)		Ion Channel Modulation[c]							
		$- N_2O$	$+ N_2O$	$GABA_A$	Glycine	nAChR	$5\text{-}HT_3$	NMDA	AMPA	K^+	Na^+
Isoflurane	1.4	1.15	0.50	+++	+++	–––	–	––	––	++	–
Enflurane	1.91	1.68	0.60	+++	+++	–––	–	––	––	++	–
Sevoflurane	0.63	1.71	0.66	+++	+++	–––	–	––	––	++	–
Desflurane	0.42	6.0	2.83	+++	+++	–––	–	––	––	++	–
Nitrous oxide	0.47	104	–	Weak	Weak	––	Weak	––	None	+	None

[a]Adapted from Refs. [146-161].

[b]Minimum alveolar concentration.

[c]Modulatory activity is indicated by + for agonism and – for antagonism. The number of symbols correlates to the degree of either activity at the given site of action.

CHEMICAL CONSIDERATIONS AND STRUCTURE-ACTIVITY RELATIONSHIPS OF INHALED ANESTHETICS. The volatile inhaled anesthetics are derived from the structure of diethyl ether (Fig. 12.19). Replacement of diethyl ether's hydrogen groups with fluorine atoms preserves the steric features of the small hydrogen atom while greatly enhancing lipophilicity of the fluorinated congeners. This effect also lowers the boiling point, decreases flammability and toxicity, and increases stability. Halothane, an older agent described in previous editions of this text, is a halogenated alkane; however, this structural backbone was associated with cardiac arrhythmias. On the contrary, an ether backbone reduces the likelihood of this effect 4-fold, and hence the clinically useful agents of today are based on the halogenated methyl ethyl ether backbone.

Given these considerations, one would speculate that SARs for this family of anesthetics would be easily concluded. On the contrary, no definitive SAR exist for these agents that allow for accurate predictions of anesthetic activity, other than that at least one hydrogen is necessary for anesthetic effect. In this regard, full halogenation of the agents shown in Figure 12.19 results in loss of anesthetic effect and promotes convulsant effects, suggesting that the role of electron withdrawing groups, coupled with heightened lipophilicity, mediate vastly different effects on excitatory versus inhibitory neurotransmission.[162] All of the clinically useful fluorinated anesthetics contain a chiral carbon and hence exist as (+) and (−) enantiomers, although all of the commercially available formulations contain racemic mixtures. Early work with enantiomerically resolved isoflurane showed that (+)-isoflurane was more effective at inducing anesthesia compared to the (−) enantiomer. This observation correlated with in vitro studies that show that the (+) enantiomer has twofold the efficacy of the (−) enantiomer in potentiating K^+-efflux and inhibiting nAChR.[163,164] Similarly, (+)-isoflurane is significantly more potent that (−)-isoflurane in potentiating effects at $GABA_A$ receptors.[165,166] Such results argue further against the Meyer and Overton theory and, given the known stereoselective requirements of ion channels and receptors, further support modulation of these channels by inhaled anesthetics as part of their mechanisms of action.

PROPERTIES AND METABOLISM OF INDIVIDUAL INHALED ANESTHETIC AGENTS

Enflurane. Enflurane, 2-chloro-1,1,2-trifluoroethyl-difluoromethyl ether, was introduced clinically in the 1960s and, of the inhaled GAs discussed here, has a higher relative solubility in the blood (blood/gas partition coefficient of 1.91). This property facilitates slower induction of, and emergence from, anesthesia compared to agents with lower blood/gas partition coefficients. Inhalation of 2%-4.5% enflurane produces surgical analgesia in 7-10 minutes after a single dose, while recovery occurs within 5 minutes following discontinuation.[167,168] Between 80% and 90% of the inhaled dose is expired unchanged, while CYP2E1 metabolizes approximately 10% yielding the oxidized metabolite that is subsequently excreted in the urine (Fig. 12.20) along with inorganic fluoride anion (F^-).[169,170] A marked distinction of enflurane compared to its more nephrotoxic congener methoxyflurane, which is no longer commonly used clinically, is the relatively lower release of F^-. While methoxyflurane yielded high levels of F^-, which persisted for days after dosing and facilitated nephrotoxicity, normal clinical use of enflurane yields peak plasma F^- concentrations that are below 25 μmol 4 hours following anesthesia and further decrease by 50% within 31 hours. Greater than 95% of the F^- is excreted readily after termination of anesthesia[169,170], significantly decreasing the comparative clinical incidence of toxicity.

Isoflurane. Isoflurane, 1-chloro-2,2,2-trifluoroethyl difluromethly ether, is a structural isomer of enflurane, which has a blood/gas partition coefficient that is intermediate compared to enflurane and the highly insoluble sevoflurane and desflurane. Given this property, 3% isoflurane induction time is in the 7-12 minutes range and single-dose recovery times are within the 10-20 minutes range. Since isoflurane has a pungent odor, too rapid rates of inhalation administration may produce unpleasant or adverse effects such as cough, laryngospasm, or inadvertent breath-holding. Greater than 99% of inhaled isoflurane is expired unchanged from the lungs. Isoflurane is unique compared to sevoflurane and enflurane, given that it is fairly resistant to human metabolism, with less than 0.5% of the agent being biotransformed by the liver to yield trifluoroacetic acid and F^- (Fig. 12.20).[171]

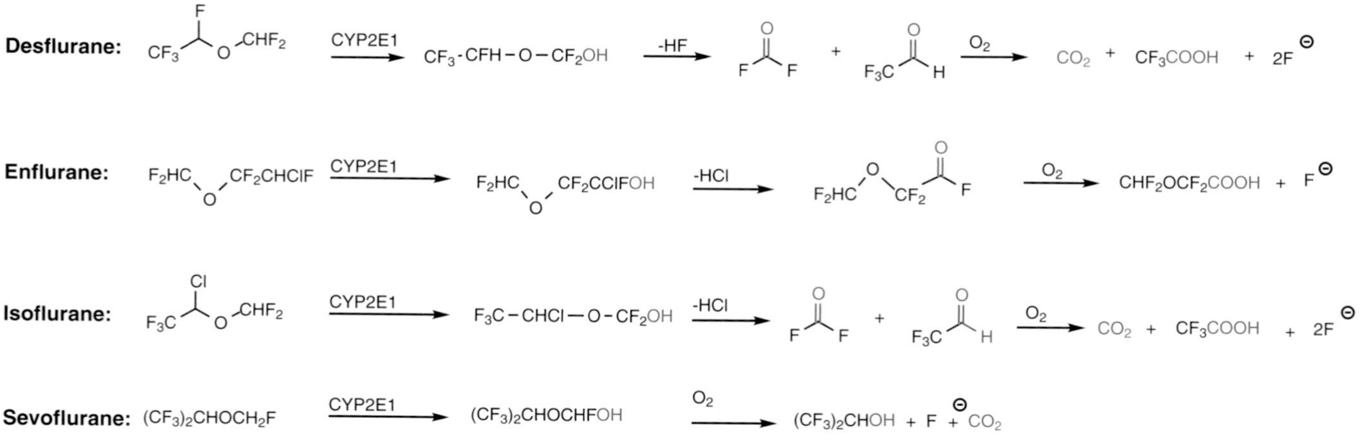

Desflurane: $CF_3CHFOCHF_2$ —CYP2E1→ CF_3-CFH−O−CF_2OH —-HF→ $F_2C{=}O$ + F_3C–CHO —O_2→ CO_2 + CF_3COOH + $2F^{\ominus}$

Enflurane: F_2HC–O–CF_2CHClF —CYP2E1→ F_2HC–O–$CF_2CClFOH$ —-HCl→ F_2HC–O–CF_2–C(=O)F —O_2→ CHF_2OCF_2COOH + $F^{\ominus}$

Isoflurane: F_3C–CHCl–O–CHF_2 —CYP2E1→ F_3C−CHCl−O−CF_2OH —-HCl→ $F_2C{=}O$ + F_3C–CHO —O_2→ CO_2 + CF_3COOH + $2F^{\ominus}$

Sevoflurane: $(CF_3)_2CHOCH_2F$ —CYP2E1→ $(CF_3)_2CHOCHFOH$ —O_2→ $(CF_3)_2CHOH$ + $F^{\ominus}$ + CO_2

Figure 12.20 Metabolism of volatile inhaled general anesthetics.

Sevoflurane. Sevoflurane, fluoromethyl 2,2,2-trifluoro-l-(trifluoromethyl) ethyl ether is an isopropyl ether with a significantly lower blood/gas partition coefficient (0.63) compared to enflurane or isoflurane, allowing for rapid induction of anesthesia and rapid recovery following discontinuation from inhalation. Inhalation anesthesia induction times are achieved in 1-2 minutes, and single-dose emergence is slightly shorter than that of isoflurane, ranging from 4-10 minutes.[172,173] Based on this profile, sevoflurane is widely used in outpatient surgical and pediatric care settings. Approximately 40% of inhaled sevoflurane is excreted unchanged in expired air, while hepatic CYP2E1 is responsible for oxidative defluorination of 3%-5% of the inspired agent. The remainder is likely metabolized by unknown extrahepatic mechanisms yielding hexafluoroisopropanol and F^- (Fig. 12.20).[174-176] As blood concentrations of sevoflurane approach 0.6 mM, F^- levels that result from this biotransformation can exceed 50 μM, which is potentially nephrotoxic. However, this is greatly dose and time dependent, and serum levels of fluoride rapidly decrease following discontinuation. For example, 3% sevoflurane exposure for 1 hour causes a peak of 22 μM of F^- load in blood, decreasing to 4 μM after 24 hours.[174-176]

Desflurane Desflurane, 1,2,2,2-tetrafluoroethyl-difluoromethyl ether, differs from isoflurane by a single atom fluoro- for chlorosubstitution. However, this effect is significant, as it decreases blood solubility substantially (blood/gas partition coefficient of 1.4 for isoflurane vs. 0.42 for desflurane), distinguishing desflurane as the least soluble of the volatile GAs. This single-atom change also significantly decreases the boiling point (48.5°C for isoflurane and 22.8°C for desflurane), while greatly increasing the room temperature vapor pressure of desflurane (669 mm Hg) compared to isoflurane (238 mm Hg). These physical properties make desflurane incompatible with conventional vaporizers at room temperatures, as inconceivable gas flow would be required to deliver clinically meaningful doses. As a consequence, desflurane is delivered via specially designed vaporizers that can be heated to 39°C to facilitate vaporization. Nonetheless, due to its low blood solubility, desflurane is characterized by very rapid induction and emergence compared to the other volatile GAs. Inhalation anesthesia induction times are achieved in 1-2 minutes, and single-dose emergence occurs within 5-6 minutes.[177,178] Similar to isoflurane, desflurane is resistant to human biotransformation, with greater than 99% being recoverable from expired air. Less than 0.02% of the dose is converted, presumably via hepatic oxidation like isoflurane, to F^- and trifluoroacetic acid, neither of which are readily detectible in urine (Fig. 12.20).[179,180]

Nitrous Oxide Historically referred to as "laughing gas", nitrous oxide (N_2O) has very a low blood/gas partition coefficient (0.47), allowing for rapid induction. However, with a MAC of 105%, it is incapable of producing surgical anesthesia when used alone. Hence, when used as monotherapy, it is most efficacious in instances where full surgical anesthesia is not necessary, for example, in dental procedures or as an adjuvant to local anesthesia. The relatively low anesthetic potency of nitrous oxide monotherapy may be ancillary to its strong analgesic and weak muscle relaxant properties. Most commonly, nitrous oxide is used in combination with other GAs, where it synergizes the anesthetic effects allowing for reductions in the concentration of the other agent required to produce the desired anesthetic response.

Although the exact mechanism of nitrous oxide–mediated analgesia remains elusive, in vivo positron emission tomography (PET) imaging reveals decreases in pain-induced activation of thalamo-cortical brain regions as described above, suggesting that the effects of nitrous oxide may be similar to that of the volatile GAs. Pharmacologically, nitrous oxide has been postulated to exert its effects through blockade of nAChR and NMDA channels, as well as via activation of two-pore K^+ channels. However, it is very likely that other mechanisms are also involved.[148-159]

Nitrous oxide is rapidly and nearly fully eliminated unchanged from expired air, with minor excretion from the skin. Major toxicities associated with nitrous oxide use include cardiac arrhythmia and the N_2O-induced irreversible oxidation of the cobalt atom of vitamin B_{12}. In the latter case, the gas converts the monovalent cobalt form of vitamin B_{12} (Co^+) to the divalent form that is incapable of acting as a cofactor for the enzyme methionine synthetase, which is itself critical for nucleic acid synthesis and neurotransmission and specifically for the synthesis of myelin. Methionine synthetase activity is reduced in a small percentage of patients after acute inhalation of N_2O and can be restored only upon de novo translation of the enzyme. This effect has possible consequences related to vitamin B_{12}-dependent effects such as erythropoiesis, anemia, and myelosuppression.

Clinically Useful Parenteral Agents

The clinically useful parenteral agents are small molecules characterized by high lipophilicity, allowing for a high degree of partitioning into the well-perfused tissue (such as the brain) within a single cycle of blood circulation following IV administration. As described with the highly lipophilic barbiturate agents above, time-dependent redistribution from the CNS to less well-perfused or less lipophilic tissues greatly influences the kinetics of these agents. The IV agents discussed here, which include the barbiturates thiopental and thiamylal, as well as propofol, ketamine, and etomidate, have a faster rate of anesthetic action than the inhaled GAs and, as a consequence, are utilized greatly in the induction of anesthesia.

THIOPENTAL AND THIAMYLAL.

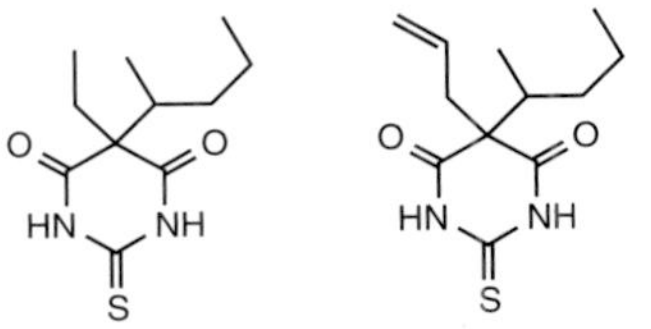

Thiopentobarbital Thiamylal

As described in the sedative-hypnotic section above, the oxybarbiturates thiopental (thiopentylbarbital) and thiamylal contain 2-position sulfur atoms within the barbiturate backbone. This increases lipophilicity and allows for ultrarapid anesthetic effects compared to their 2-oxy congeners, due to rapid penetration to the brain that typically occurs within 10-20 seconds. The effects are rapidly lost within 5-7 minutes of a bolus dose due to redistribution from the CNS into the muscle, adipose, and other less lipophilic tissues. While the effects of single bolus dose thiobarbiturates are short acting, continuous infusion or multiple administrations can lead to long-lasting unconsciousness because of a change from first-order to zero-order kinetics with slow biotransformation and elimination (Fig. 12.5). This may be particularly problematic in patients with hepatic or renal dysfunction or in pregnant mothers induced for caesarian section.[181,182] In this regard, the approximate 1.5-3.0 mL/kg/min clearance rate of thiopental is the slowest amongst the injectable GAs and can cause prolonged unconsciousness if not used acutely.[181,182] Thiobarbiturate mechanisms of action, SARs, and metabolism are described with sedative-hypnotic agents above.

Similarly, adverse effects of thiobarbitals mimic those seen with their oxy-congeners and can include hypotension, decreases in cardiac inotropy, and respiratory depression. As described above, since barbiturates tautomerize and are active in the enolate form (Fig. 12.3), they are formulated in alkaline solutions. Mixing these agents with other drugs in more acidic solutions inhibits tautomerization and shifts the equilibrium, stabilizing the inactive barbituric acid form. Hence, when used for anesthesia, barbiturates are administered first and should clear the tubing prior to administration of other IV agents.

PROPOFOL.

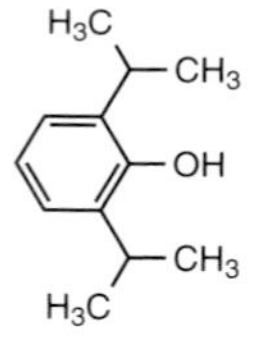

Propofol, 2,6-diisopropylphenol is a very popular GA that is commonly used in surgical and diagnostic procedures. Propofol exerts its anesthetic action via modulation of neuronal $GABA_A$ receptors. Specifically, propofol significantly decreases the dissociation rate of the endogenous neurotransmitter from the receptor, thereby enhancing GABA binding. This effect facilitates Cl^- flux, postsynaptic hyperpolarization, and CNS depression, similar to that described for other GABAergic agents above. Propofol has synergistic effects with other GABAergics, for example, benzodiazepines and barbiturates, enhancing their effects. In addition, propofol inhibits presynaptic GABA uptake and may also influence GABA release in addition to modulation of glycine, nACh, and NMDA receptors.[183]

Structure-Activity Relationships of Propofol. SARs of early 2,6-dialkylphenols revealed that the anesthetic potencies and kinetics are strongly correlated to the lipophilicity and steric bulk/localization of the substitutions.[184] As a class, mono-*o*-substituted alkyl phenols showed only moderate hypnotic/anesthetic effects with poor therapeutic ratios, while mono-*p*-substituted phenols, like the parent phenol compound, proved to be toxic, yielding high degrees of respiratory depression. Similarly, compounds with *m*-alkyl substitutions or di-, tri-, or tetrasubstitutions that included a *m*-position alkyl displayed poor anesthetic properties.

Meanwhile, propofol-like 2,6-disubstituted alkyl derivatives with linear ethyl, *n*-propyl, or *n*-butyl groups displayed moderate anesthetic properties with slow induction and increased durations as the chain lengths increased. A further series of 2-*n*-alkyl, 6-*sec*-alkyl substitutions further increased anesthetic potency until the total number of carbons in the substituents reached 8, while cyclohexyl substitution decreased potency. Interestingly, 2,6-di-sec substituted alkyl congeners yielded highest anesthetic potencies as long as the total number of carbons did not exceed 6 and the substitutions were acyclic. Similarly, anesthetic kinetics were rapid and sleep times were short when the total carbons were less than 7, while induction became slow and recovery prolonged when the total number of carbons in the substituents surpassed 8. Of congeners within the 2,6-di-sec substituted alkyl series, 2,6-diisopropyl (i.e., propofol) was noted to have exceptional characteristics denoted by a smooth and rapid induction and recovery, as well as a short but useful duration.[184]

Pharmacokinetics and Metabolism of Propofol. Propofol has pharmacokinetic properties that are similar to thiobarbitals and, yet, has distinct and important differences. Like the thiobarbitals, it is a highly lipophilic agent that produces rapid CNS effects with a fast blood-brain equilibrium half-life of 3 minutes and rapid redistribution from the CNS after a single bolus dose.[185] This property allows for onset within a single circulation time and recovery periods of 3-8 minutes depending on the dose.[186] However, unlike thiobarbitals, propofol has a very high rate of clearance of 25-50 mL/kg/min, a roughly 10-fold faster rate than thiopental, and this characteristic allows for much faster recovery when administered in multiple doses or upon infusion.[187]

Propofol is metabolized rapidly via hepatic CYP2B6-mediated biotransformation to 4-hydroxy propofol (2,6-diisopropyl-1,4-hydroquinone) followed by conjugation of either the 1- or 4-position hydroxy with glucuronic acid or sulfate, accounting for approximately 60% of the urinary detectible dose. Direct phase 2 conjugation of the parent accounts for the remainder of the major metabolites found in the urine (Fig. 12.21).[188-190] Less than 0.3% of the parent drug is recovered unchanged in the urine, and the recovery of metabolites is comparable in male and female patients, consistent with the observation that clinical pharmacokinetics of propofol exhibit no gender-based differences.

Due to its very poor water solubility, propofol is formulated in a 10 mg/mL emulsion with 10% (w/v) soybean oil, 1.2% egg phosphatide, and 2.25% glycerol, a formulation that can support bacterial growth and, as such, requires the use of strict aseptic technique. Owing to this poor aqueous solubility, the phosphate ester prodrug fospropofol, which contains a 1-hydroxy phosphate and avoids the need for the emulsion formulation, is also available in the U.S. The effects of fospropofol are entirely due to its conversion to

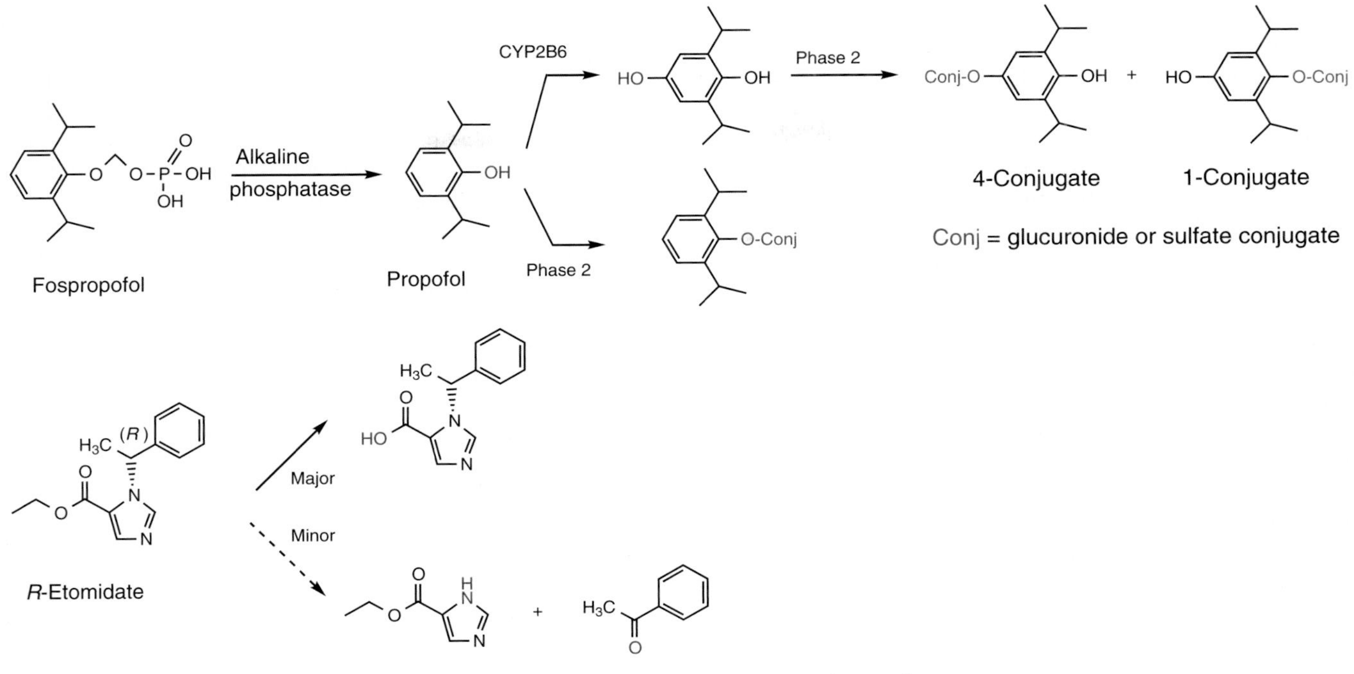

Figure 12.21 Metabolism of propofol and etomidate.

propofol by serum alkaline phosphatases. Due to this need for bioactivation, the onset of fospropofol is significantly slower (4-12 min) and the anesthetic effect is prolonged (5-18 min) compared to propofol. Given these changes in pharmacokinetics, the clinical utility of fospropofol is inferior to other agents. Detailed discussions of fospropofol can be found in previous editions of this text.

ADVERSE EFFECTS OF PROPOFOL. Propofol can reduce blood pressure and respiration to a greater degree than the thiobarbiturates and can also cause bradycardia and decreased cardiac output. The effects on blood pressure are mediated by vasodilation and decreased peripheral resistance secondary to reductions in sympathetic nervous system tone. Upward of 60% of patients report injection-site pain.

ETOMIDATE.

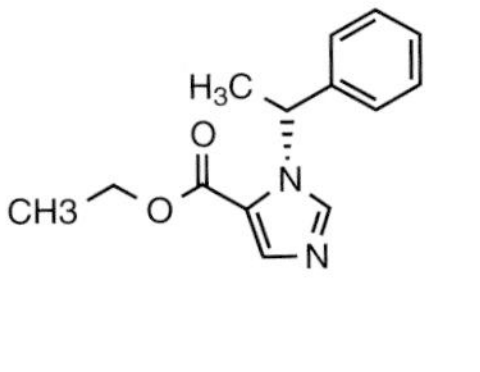

Etomidate, ethyl 3-(1-phenylethyl)imidazole-4-carboxylate, is a phenyl-substituted carboxylated imidazole that was initially developed as part of a novel series of antifungal agents and is primarily used as an induction anesthetic owing to its ultrarapid hypnotic onset and short duration of action. Distinct from propofol, etomidate seems to exert its hypnotic and anesthetic effects exclusively via modulation of $GABA_A$ receptors and, more specifically, $GABA_A$ receptors that contain the β_2 or β_3 subunits.[191] At clinically relevant concentrations of etomidate, the agent potentiates the binding of GABA to $GABA_A$ receptors, an effect that causes postsynaptic hyperpolarization. At higher concentrations, etomidate directly and allosterically agonizes $GABA_A$ receptors in the absence of GABA.[192]

Structure-Activity Relationships of Etomidate. Stereoselectivity is a critical aspect of etomidate's ability to either potentiate the binding of GABA to the $GABA_A$ receptor or directly stimulate the receptor. The *R*-(+)-enantiomer is 10- to 20-fold more potent at modulating these activities compared to the *L*-(-)-enantiomer, and as such, the clinically used agent contains the resolved *R*-(+)-enantiomer (Fig. 12.21). SARs of the series of 1-(1-substituted)-imidazole-5-carboxylic acid esters showed that these agents exhibited extremely potent hypnotic effects with short durations.[193] The nature of the imidazole nitrogen substituent is critical to hypnotic/anesthetic effect, and a one-carbon distance between the aryl substitution and nitrogen affords greatest hypnotic/anesthetic effects. Branching at the opposite end of the α-carbon also affected potency, with alkyl substituents having the greatest activity, especially smaller methyl substitutions.[193] Anesthetic activity was completely lost if the side chain was lengthened to two carbons, if the α-carbon was unbranched, or if the aryl group was directly attached to the imidazole nitrogen.[193] An ester moiety at the 4-position was essential for anesthetic effects, as corresponding carboxylic acids lacked activity. However, the absolute nature of the ester substitution allowed for variability, as methyl, ethyl, *n*-propyl, or isopropyl substituents all provided high activity. Of the series, etomidate, which contains an ethyl ester and phenylethyl-imidazole substitution provided the ideal safety ratio, which takes into account the hypnotic activity and toxicity.

Pharmacokinetics and Metabolism of Etomidate. After a single IV injection, (*R*)-etomidate induces anesthesia with an onset time on the order of 10-20 seconds and emergence from anesthesia in 2-10 minutes, depending on the dose used.[194,195] While the duration of anesthetic action is somewhat limited by redistribution of the agent out of the brain into other compartments, biotransformation of etomidate occurs rapidly due to plasma and hepatic hydrolysis of the ester, which is the primary driver of the limited duration. As noted above, the SAR requirement for an ester group to retain anesthetic activity signifies that the carboxylic acid metabolite formed upon hydrolysis of the ester is inactive (Fig. 12.21). Oxidative metabolism of etomidate can also produce benzoic acid, and together, these metabolites account for the urinary (75%) and biliary (25%) excretion of etomidate (Fig. 12.21).[196,197] Etomidate also provides effective anesthesia upon rectal administration, although the onset of action is significantly delayed (ca. 5 min).

Adverse Effects of Etomidate. Although a major advantage of etomidate compared to other agents is the decreased incidence of cardiovascular and respiratory adverse effects, etomidate does precipitate other adverse activities. Nearly 40% of patients exhibit pain at the site of injection, and over 25% demonstrate involuntary movements that are directly due to GABAergic disinhibition within the basal ganglia. Consistent with its initial envisioned use as an antifungal agent intended to disrupt fungal steroidogenesis, etomidate also has high inhibitory affinity for the adrenocortical enzyme 11β-hydroxylase, which is intricately involved in adrenal cortisol synthesis. As a consequence, prolonged use of etomidate strongly inhibits adrenal gland function and profoundly suppresses cortisol in a manner that is unresponsive to ACTH, an effect that occurs at the level of the adrenal cortex itself.

KETAMINE.

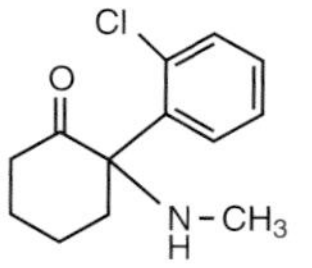

Ketamine, 2-(*o*-chlorophenyl)-2-methylaminocyclohexanone, is a structural derivative of the abused dissociative drug phencyclidine (i.e., PCP or "angel dust"). Phencyclidine was initially used as an anesthetic; however, patients often emerged into lengthy states of delirium, prompting efforts to modify the structure to optimize anesthetic effects with a lesser degree psychogenic disturbances. These efforts led to the discovery of ketamine, an agent with pronounced anesthetic and analgesic effects and a lower propensity to induce psychiatric effects compared to phencyclidine. As a consequence of its similarities to phencyclidine, ketamine is the only IV GA that produces dissociative anesthesia, which is characterized by analgesia, catatonia, catalepsy, and amnesia. This is distinct from other GAs, as the patient's eyes could remain open and they may breathe spontaneously.

As opposed to the GABAergic-acting agents that disrupt thalamo-cortical and reticulo-thalamo-cortical brain activity, the resulting anesthesia is thought to be due to thalamo-neocortical and limbic system disruption secondary to direct antagonism of excitatory glutamate NMDA receptors. Other results suggest that ketamine may also function indirectly by modulation of opioid, norepinephrine, serotonin, and ACh neurotransmission. Together, these activities prevent ascending brain pathways from perceiving pain or auditory/visual sensations, producing a disconnected cataleptic state with amnesia and analgesia, with minimal depression of respiration.[198] Based on this unique dissociative mechanism, emergence from analgesia can be accompanied by reactions that include confused mental state, hallucination, dreamlike states, and delirium, which typically can last a few hours.

Structure-Activity Relationships of Ketamine. A chiral center within the cyclohexanone ring affords two optical isomers of ketamine, *R*-(-)- and *S*-(+)-, both of which are included in the commercial preparation of the agent. However, in animals, *S*-(+)-ketamine has a significantly greater therapeutic index than the racemate or the *R*-(-)-enantiomer, and exhibits 3- and 1.5-fold more analgesic and hypnotic potency as the *R*-(-)-enantiomer.[199] These observations extend to human studies where *S*-(+)-ketamine produces more effective anesthesia than the racemate or *R*-(-)-ketamine, and also produced less of the ketamine-emergence reactions described above. Moreover, patients anesthetized with *R*-(-)-ketamine were more agitated that those induced with the racemate or *S*-(+)-ketamine. When compared to phencyclidine, ketamine has a lower calculated log P and only a slightly lower affinity for human recombinant NMDA receptors. Heterocyclic substitution of the cyclohexanone ring results in significant loss of antagonistic activity and lipophilicity, while substitution of the second *o*-position of this ring also lowers activity.[200] Previous SAR studies on phencyclidine derivatives have shown that agents with electron-withdrawing substituents on the aromatic ring, such as the halogen on ketamine, decrease psychotropic effects, while N-alkyl substitution increases the hypnotic potency.

Pharmacokinetics and Metabolism of Ketamine. The analgesic effects of ketamine occur at much lower doses than those required for anesthesia (40-200 ng/mL vs. 1500 to >2000 ng/mL). A single IV injection of ketamine in this range induces anesthesia within 30-40 seconds, while an IM dose provides a slower onset time of 3-4 minutes.[201] Ketamine is also clinically useful following oral, nasal, rectal, or epidural administration. The duration of action following a single IV dose is 5-10 minutes, with longer recovery times upon IM (12-25 min), nasal (45-60 min), or epidural (>240 min) administration.[202,203] Like the other agents described here, duration is limited by the redistribution of ketamine from the brain to the muscle and peripheral tissues over time.[203]

The activity of ketamine is also regulated by its extensive hepatic metabolism, which is thought to play an important role in its therapeutic utilization. Oral ketamine is subject to significant first-pass metabolism leading to 15% bioavailability. As shown in Figure 12.22, CYP2B6 is the primary enzyme required for in vitro and clinically meaningful biotransformation of ketamine enantiomers, with the 2A6, 3A4, and 3A5 isoforms also playing minor roles.[204-209] As shown, both *R*-(-)- and *S*-(+)-ketamine are N-demethylated to the primary major metabolite *R*-(-)- and *S*-(+)-norketamine, respectively. Norketamine is an active circulating metabolite with approximately one-third the

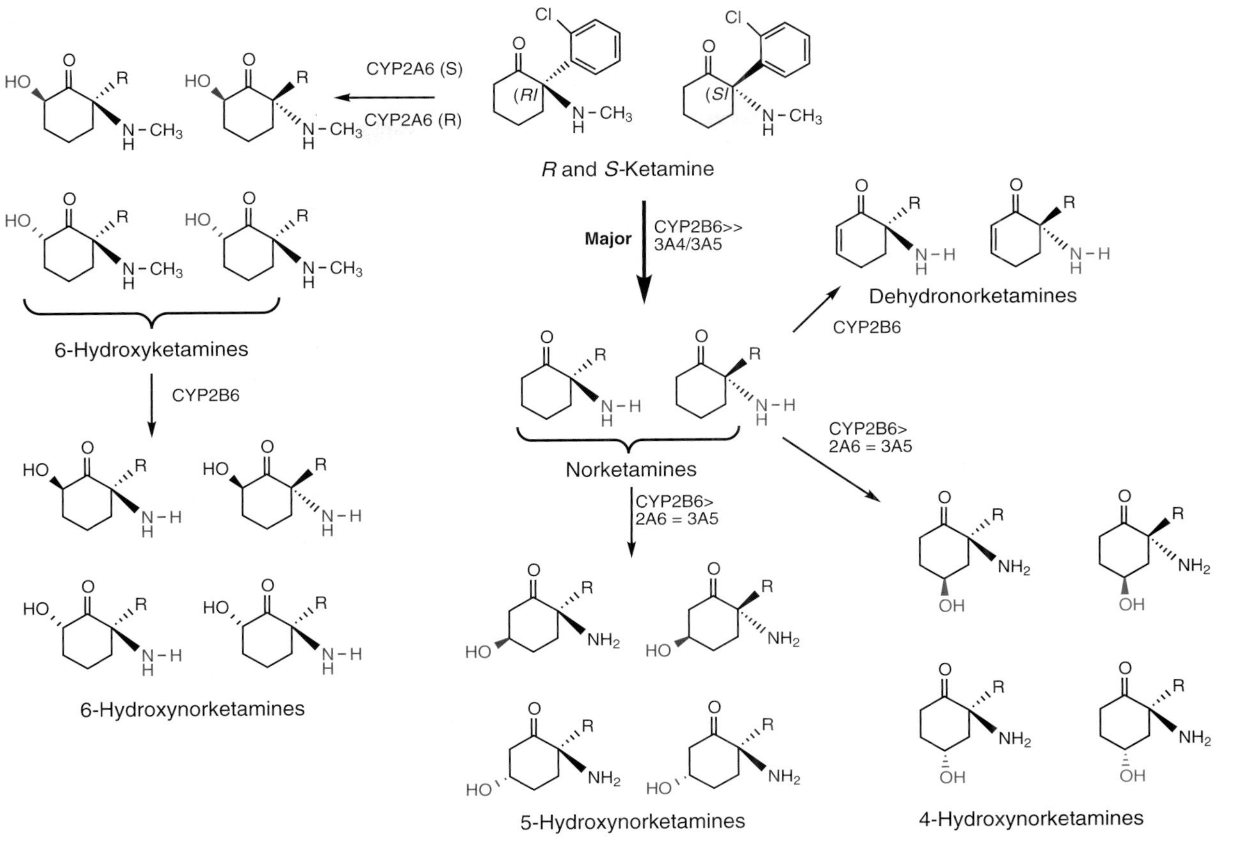

Figure 12.22 Metabolism of ketamine.

analgesic and anesthetic potency of the respective parent enantiomer and is the primary basis for the use of oral ketamine to provide analgesia and anesthesia. Peak concentrations of norketamine appear in 60 and 75 minutes following an oral or IM dose, respectively.[210] The primary norketamine metabolites can be further biotransformed to the respective enantiomers of dehydronorketamine or to three pairs of hydroxylated norketamine diastereomers via *o*-, *m*-, or *p*-hydroxylation to 4-, 5-, or 6-hydroxynorketamine, respectively (Fig. 12.22). Ketamine can also be metabolized to hydroxyketamine, which is not abundant in human circulation, as it is further N-demethylated to 6-hydroxynorketamine (Fig. 12.22). After IV administration of ketamine, the major circulating human metabolites are *R*-(-)- and *S*-(+)-norketamine, (2*S*,6*S*;2*R*,6*R*)-6-hydroxynorketamine, (2*S*,5*R*;2*R*,5*S*)- 5-hydroxynorketamine, and *R*-(-)- and *S*-(+)-dehydronorketamine.[204-209] The majority of the dose is excreted by the kidneys as either the hydroxylated metabolites or their conjugates, while less than 4% is excreted unchanged or as norketamine.[198]

Adverse Effects of Ketamine. As a dissociative anesthetic, ketamine has unique properties and induces adverse effects that are distinct from other IV anesthetics. In this regard, ketamine exhibits sympathomimetic activity that increase both blood pressure and cardiac chronotropy and output. This effect can also produce heightened salivation and elevated muscle tone. Similarly, it can increase cerebral blood flow, cerebral metabolic rate, and intracranial pressure. Taken together, these effects are precisely in opposition to those seen with the other IV agents. Due to its unique mechanism, psychiatric effects upon emergence from anesthesia (i.e., emergence delirium), which are characterized by vivid and unpleasant dreams, out-of-body experiences, hallucinations, confusion, and agitation, occur in a high percentage of patients (12%-50%).

Neuromuscular Blocking Agents

Neuromuscular blocking agents promote muscle relaxation, and as a result, their primary therapeutic utility is as an adjuvant to GA. The muscle relaxant effects of these agents afford reductions in the depth requirement for GAs and allows for optimization of induction and recovery times. This allows for intracavitary operative procedures such as abdominal or thoracic surgeries, as well as placement of devices into muscle-laden organs; for example, tracheal intubation or insertion of ventilation tubes within the airway. When used systemically, the fast-twitching smaller muscles (e.g., ocular and facial muscles) are affected first, followed by the muscles of the neck, abdomen, and limbs, and finally the larger intercostal muscles and diaphragm. The recovery from paralysis typically occurs in the reverse order.

Mechanism of Action of Neuromuscular Blocking Agents

All neuromuscular blockers act via inhibition of propagation of the action potential at the neuromuscular junction (NMJ), which serves as a distinct synapse that allows for the transmission of electrical impulses from nerves to muscle cells at the motor end plate. At this site, the depolarization of "presynaptic" parasympathetic neurons at the NMJ facilitates the voltage- and Ca^{+2}-dependent release of ACh into the synaptic cleft. Within this synapse, ACh rapidly binds to and stimulates postsynaptic nicotinic ACh receptors (nAChR) on the muscle cell end plate. Once activated by ACh, these ligand-gated nAChR modulate the robust influx of Na^+ and smaller relative efflux of K^+, within the muscle cells of the end plate, leading to a muscle action potential.

The nACh receptors (Fig. 12.2) are similar to the heteropentameric $GABA_A$ receptors previously described. Human adult motor end plates specifically express high levels of postsynaptic nAChRs that contain $\alpha_1\beta_1\varepsilon\delta$ subunits that assemble in a 2:1:1:1 ratio to give rise to the postsynaptic ligand-gated cation channel (Fig. 12.2). Also, similar to $GABA_A$ receptors, postsynaptic $\alpha_1\beta_1\varepsilon\delta$-containing nAChR are comprised of two distinct clusters of anionic amino acids that form two separate ACh binding sites: a high-affinity site formed by one $\alpha_1\delta$ interface and a low-affinity site formed by another $\alpha_1\varepsilon$ interface. Upon binding of ACh to the high-affinity site, conformational changes allow for positive cooperative binding of another ACh molecule to the low-affinity site, and together, these drive further conformational changes that allow for Na^+/K^+ antitransport through the pore. In addition to these postsynaptic receptors, neuronal nAChR consisting of $\alpha_3\beta_2$ subunits act as presynaptic ACh autoreceptors that further promote the release of ACh in a positive-feedback manner, thereby further increasing release of the neurotransmitter into the NMJ.

Upon neuronal release of ACh and subsequent agonism of $\alpha_1\beta_1\varepsilon\delta$ nAChRs, the resulting Na^+ influx and K^+ efflux in the postsynaptic muscle cells cause the local motor end plate membrane potential to change. This change is directly correlated to the magnitude of nAChR activity and leads to activation and opening of voltage-gated Na^+ channels on the motor end plate. The high density of Na^+ channels here amplifies the membrane potential signal and produces the electrical gradient that facilitates an action potential and subsequent generation of muscle contraction. The effects of ACh within the NMJ are tightly regulated by acetylcholinesterase (AChE), which rapidly degrades the neurotransmitter and resets the motor end plate.

The neuromuscular blocking agents can be divided into two subclasses, depolarizing and nondepolarizing, based on their differing abilities to modulate this normal NMJ transmission. The only depolarizing NMJ blocking agents used clinically is succinylcholine (Fig. 12.23), which consists of two molecules of ACh linked endwise. In this paradoxical mechanism, succinylcholine binds to postsynaptic nAChRs to profoundly depolarize the motor end plate, as ACh itself does. Since the succinylcholine molecule is intrinsically more resistant to hydrolysis than ACh, the effects are prolonged and more intensified, leading to repeated muscle contractions manifesting as fasciculations due to the vast activation of nAChRs. As a consequence of this overexcitation of the motor end plate, the requirement for repolarization of the membrane that must exist to elicit the next contraction does not occur and the muscle tone effectively becomes flaccidly paralyzed. This phenomenon is referred to as phase I depolarizing block, and inhibition of AChE at this stage in the process further promotes succinylcholine-mediated paralysis. Upon continued activity of succinylcholine at the NMJ, the nAChR become desensitized and refractory to the effects of the agent, while at the same time, repolarization is occurring as normal primarily due to end plate Na^+/K^+-ATPase activity. Despite the repolarization, upon desensitization of nAChRs, Na^+ channels on the NMJ become inactivated through mechanisms that remain elusive, and this combination of inhibited Na^+ flux effectively paralyzes the muscle cells. This is referred to as phase II depolarizing block, and these effects can be reversed by inhibition of AChE, which allows ACh to compete with the succinylcholine for the nAChR.

In contrast to this depolarizing mechanism, the second subclass of NMJ blocking agents, which include all other FDA-approved agents, behave as nondepolarizing competitive antagonists of ACh binding for both pre- and postsynaptic nAChRs. Unlike succinylcholine, these agents do not possess intrinsic receptor modulating activity; rather, they inhibit muscle contraction by directly competing with ACh for the dianionic receptor binding sites. As a consequence of this mechanism, it can be inferred that structurally, these agents will possess dicationic pharmacophores (see below). Inhibition of binding of ACh to postsynaptic nAChR by these agents facilitates flaccid paralysis of musculature without producing depolarization of the motor end plate and lessens the amount of anesthetic required for surgical procedures. Nondepolarizing NMJ blocking agents also inhibit ACh binding to neuronal nAChR, thereby inhibiting the positive-feedback role of the autoreceptor. This effectively decreases additional synaptic ACh release and further promotes NMJ blockade.

Structure-Activity Relationships of Neuromuscular Blocking Agents

The historical use of NMJ blocking agents can be dated to the 1500s, where South American natives utilized crude extracts of the climbing vine *Chondrodendron tomentosum* to construct "poisoned" arrows with which they hunted animals. These poisoned arrows, termed "ourare" (i.e., curare) by the indigenous population, effectively asphyxiated the prey once injected into the animal, yet ingestion of the meat of the animal did no harm. Pioneering experiments by Claude Bernard in the 1850s led to the recognition that these extracts acted at a site between a nerve and the skeletal muscle, now known as the NMJ. In the late 1800s, curare extracts were found to contain a variety of quaternary ammonium–containing alkaloids, and in the 1930s, Henry Dale demonstrated that ACh acted at the NMJ and that curare blocked this activity. In 1935, Harold King was the first to isolate and publish the chemical structure of one of the active curare

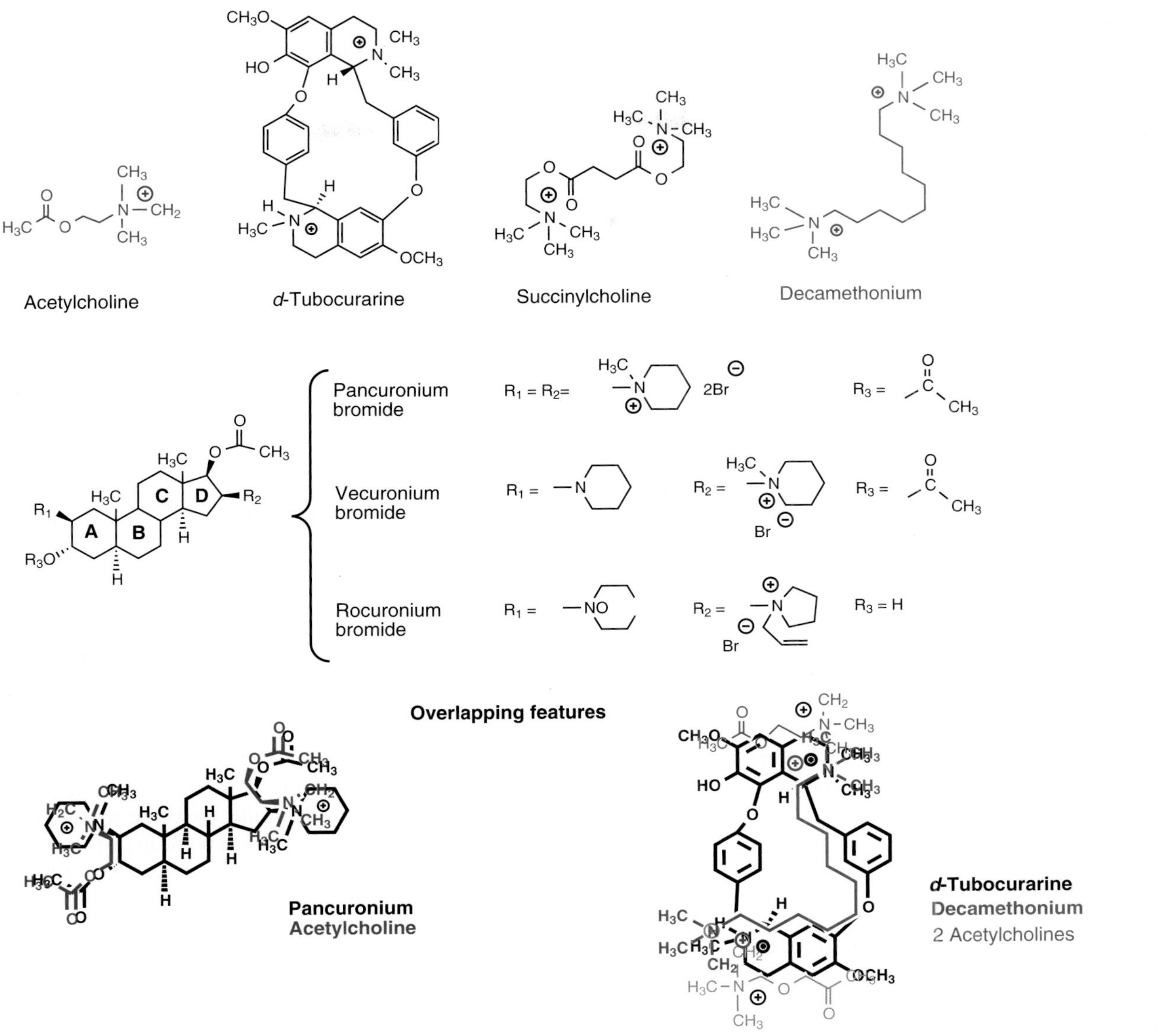

Figure 12.23 Structures of acetylcholine, succinylcholine, *d*-tubocurarine, and the aminosteroid neuromuscular blocking agents. Overlapping features are shown for pancuronium/acetylcholine and *d*-tubocararine, acetylcholine, and decamethonium.

alkaloids, which he called tubocurarine. Importantly, in this published work, King described that the structure of the active *d*-tubocurarine contained two quaternary nitrogen functional groups (i.e., bisquaternary amine),[211] and this discovery prompted development of derivatives of *d*-tubocurarine, such as decamethonium, as novel NMJ blockers based on the requirement for bisquaternary ammonium nitrogens.

It was not until 35 years after King's initial report that it was found that the structure of *d*-tubocurarine actually contained a single quaternary ammonium functional group in addition to a tertiary amine functional group (Fig. 12.23). At physiological pH, the tertiary nitrogen is primarily ionized, so overall, King's assessment of two positively charged centers holds true to form. Nonetheless, the bisquaternary ammonium–based structure served as the basis for development of many of the agents used clinically today. Since these agents all contain bis-ionizable nitrogen groups, they are poorly permeable through cell membranes and are hence not orally available, requiring direct IV or IM injection. This structural feature also explains why animals that were injected with curare arrows could be eaten with no harm to the consumer.

In addition to activation of nAChRs, acetylcholine nonselectively stimulates muscarinic GPCRs (mAChR), and previous studies have demonstrated that the distance from the center of the quaternary nitrogen to the van der Waals radius of the carbonyl oxygen of ACh is critical to selectivity for agonism of mAChR versus nAChR. In this regard, an N-O distance of 4.4 Å was proposed to yield muscarinic selectivity, while a distance of 5.9 Å would yield nicotinic activity.[212] This difference implies that nAChRs are receptive to larger agents with greater distance between the ionized amine and H-bond donor oxy groups.

The depolarizing agents such as decamethonium and succinylcholine provided much of the acquired knowledge of NMJ blocking agent SAR. As shown in Figure 12.23, these two agents typify the family of bismethonium-containing compounds that contain two bulky nitrogen-containing heads separated by a distinct number of atoms. The positively charged dicationic nitrogen groups play critical roles by binding to the two anionic ACh binding sites of the nAChRs The bismethonium NMJ blocking agents contain the general structure of $(H_3C)_3N^+-(CH_2)_n-N^+(CH_3)_3$ and display nicotinic agonistic activity when n is equal to either 5-12 or 18 carbons. The optimal depolarizing neuromuscular blockade occurs when n = 10, which approximates to the 5.9 Å optimal distance for nAChR agonism by ACh. Bismethonium agents with 5-6 carbons are also effective as ACh ganglionic blockers, while agents with long carbon chains (e.g., 18 or longer) regain neuromuscular blocking activity but become nondepolarizing.[213] While the SAR requirements of succinylcholine and decamethonium are in agreement with those of the nondepolarizing agent *d*-tubocurarine, which also has 10 atoms that span between the two cationic nitrogens (Fig. 12.23 overlay), it is well accepted that, like ACh, a single succinylcholine molecule exists in its lowest energy conformation in a bent arrangement (as shown in Fig. 12.23), which cannot span both anionic sites of the nAChR. Rather, two molecules of succinylcholine act individually on each anionic site of a single nAChR to modulate channel activity.[214] In contrast, the nondepolarizing agents such as *d*-tubocurarine that contain bis-nitrogen groups allow for simultaneous engagement of both anionic ACh-binding sites of a single nAChR by each individual molecule, which spans the channel.[214]

In addition to *d*-tubocurarine, aminosteroid-, and tetrahydroisoquinoline-based agents function as competitive antagonists of nAChRs with a greater degree of clinical utility as highly efficacious nondepolarizing NMJ blocking agents. The clinically useful agents that make up the aminosteroid subfamily discussed here include pancuronium, vecuronium, and rocuronium, while tetrahydroisoqunolines are typified by atracurium and cisatracurium. The androstane-derived aminosteroids that contained monoquaternary ammonium salts were first noted to possess weak NMJ blocking activity in the 1960s. These early derivatives included ACh-likeness in the form of A-ring acetyl esters linked to the monoquaternary ammonium group (Fig. 12.23). Addition of a similar D-ring ACh mimic, as in pancuronium, facilitated markedly enhanced NMJ blocking activity (Fig. 12.23). As shown in Figure 12.23, pancuronium contains identical bisquaternary piperidinium substitutions (R_1 and R_2) and bisacetyloxy moieties that overlay identically with that of the structure of ACh. Meanwhile, the androstane backbone provides a rigid and bulky structural base to uphold a critical three-dimensional geometry.

In this regard, the A-ring ACh mimic is maintained in a *trans*-orientation, with the ionized ammonium in an upward β-position in reference to the plane of the androstane backbone, while the acetoxy moiety is oriented in a downward α-position (Fig. 12.23). Single crystal X-ray diffraction studies on pancuronium demonstrate that the A-ring is held in a twisted-boat orientation that mimics the binding of ACh to the high-affinity anionic binding site of the nAChR.[215] On the eastern face of the molecule, the D-ring has a cis-orientation with both the quaternary ammonium and the acetoxy groups facing in the upward β-position relative to the androstane backbone (Fig. 12.23). Due to the critical role of the ionized nitrogen groups in binding to nAChR, SAR studies show that the highest potency steroid-based NMJ blocking agents have at least one quaternary ammonium, which in addition to a second tertiary nitrogen is capable of being ionized on the D-ring. Abiding to the structural mimicry of ACh, diacetate ester substitutions have greater potency than dipropionate esters, which were more potent than dipivalate or dibenzoate esters. Finally, N-alkyl substitution on the heterocyclic rings (R_1 and R_2, Fig. 12.23) affects potency with methyl providing optimal potency, followed by allyl substituents.[216]

In comparison to pancuronium, vecuronium contains a nonmethylated (nor) A-ring piperidine substitution (Fig. 12.23), hence the initial marketing under the brand name of Norcuron. This tertiary amine substitution preserves potency but markedly alters the pharmacokinetics and side effect potential as described below and, perhaps more significantly, provides structural insight that the quaternary substitution at the D-ring is likely more important than that of the A-ring. Similar to vecuronium, rocuronium loses the quaternary functional group at the R_1 position of the A-ring but also loses the acetoxy ester moiety at R_3, in essence, losing its ACh-likeness on the western face (i.e., A-ring) of the molecule (Fig. 12.23). As can be expected, this change imparts nearly 10-fold less potency to rocuronium compared to the other two steroid-based agents but produces a favorable pharmacokinetic profile, as discussed below.

The final grouping of NMJ blocking agents discussed here are the tetrahydroisoquinolines, of which, atracurium and cisatracurium are utilized clinically to a high degree. These compounds were rationally designed to be nonsteroidal, nondepolarizing NMJ blocking agents that could be biodegraded in vivo in a manner independent of hepatic or renal transformation. The structural similarity of atracurium to ACh is readily apparent, with the former having a long and flexible diester-containing chain that connects two quaternary onium heads, (Fig. 12.24), both of which engage the two anionic ACh binding sites of the nAChR. Importantly, the ester linkage of atracurium is reversed from that of ACh. This two atom separation between the quaternary nitrogen and the ester carbonyl readily allows for pH- and temperature-dependent elimination of the α-β carbons from the quaternary nitrogen in a process termed Hofmann elimination, which, along with ester hydrolysis, provides the basis for organ-independent breakdown of these agents (see metabolism discussion below). Atracurium contains four chiral centers (denoted by asterisks in Fig. 12.24) that give rise to 16 enantiomers. However, since a plane of symmetry exists

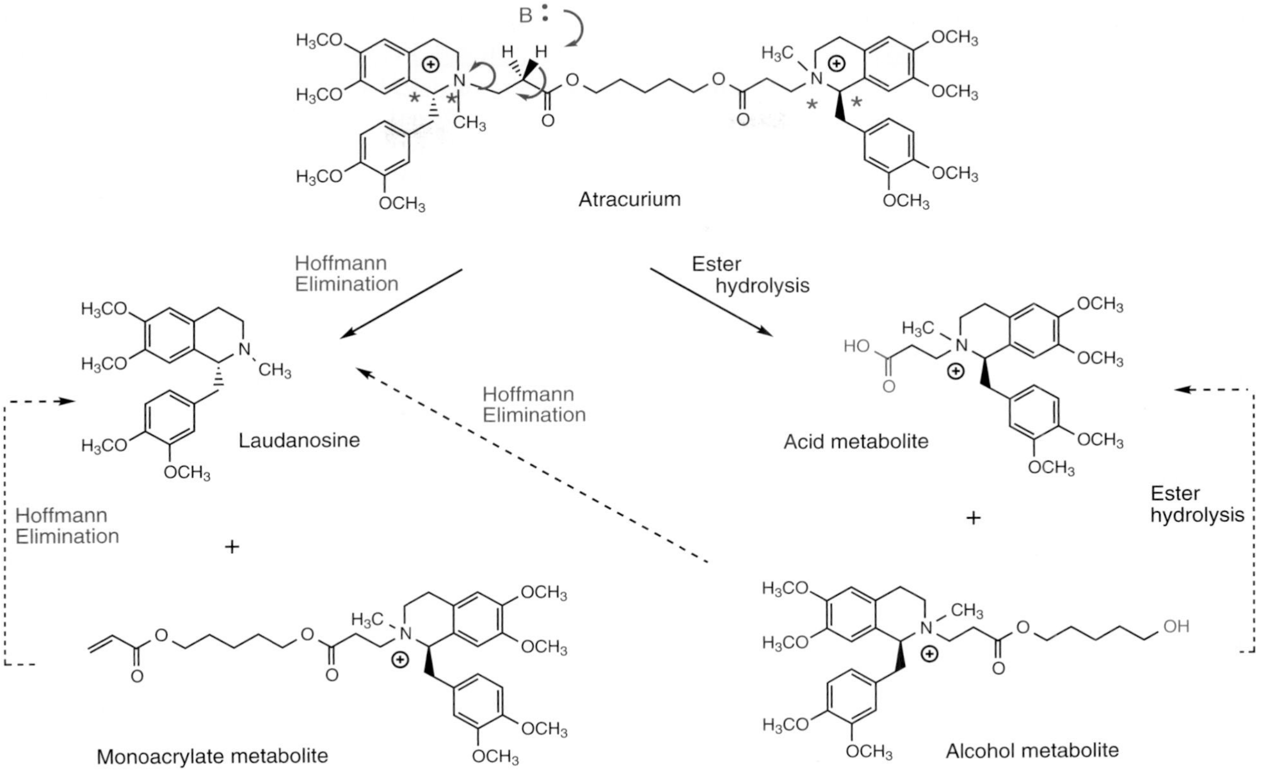

Figure 12.24 Structure of atracurium and organ-independent metabolism of atracurium.

between the two ester moieties, the commercial product contains 6 meso structures and 10 optically distinct active enantiomers. Only 6 of the 10 stereoisomers have NMJ blocking activity, and of these, the *cis*-(1*R*, 2*R*, 1′*R*, 2′*R*) absolute isomer, which is commercialized as cisatracurium, is approximately 4-fold more potent than atracurium and is devoid of atracurium's side effects.

Adverse Effects of Neuromuscular Blocking Agents

Many of the adverse effects of NMJ blocking agents are outcomes directly related to their mechanism or durations of actions, for example, prolonged muscle relaxation, paralysis, or myalgia. However, other serious reactions can occur, including apnea due to paralysis of respiratory muscles and cardiovascular effects due to direct ganglionic blockade or secondary to histamine release. Succinylcholine, atracurium, and especially *d*-tubocurarine, but not so much the steroid-based agents or cisatracurium, can directly stimulate mast cells to facilitate the release of histamine, which can cause clinically manifested complications such as hypotension, bronchospasm, and hypersecretion. The depolarizing agents, prototyped by succinylcholine, can also release K^+ leading to hyperkalemia and cardiovascular and muscular issues, including rhabdomyolysis. Pancuronium can produce vagolytic effects, putatively via blockage of cardiovascular mAChRs, that can give rise to serious cardiovascular effects including hypertension, tachycardia, and increased cardiac output. The newer steroid-based agents, including vecuronium and rocuronium, provide a greater degree of cardiostability and are relatively free from these effects. Atracurium is associated with hypotension, tachycardia, and flushing, while cisatracurium is relatively free from these adverse reactions.

Pharmacokinetics and Metabolism of Neuromuscular Blocking Agents

The pharmacokinetic profiles of the NMJ blocking agents are summarized in Table 12.5. Succinylcholine produces neuromuscular blockade within 30-60 seconds of IV administration and within 1-4 minutes of IM administration. The duration of action for these routes is 6-10 minutes and 15-20 minutes, respectively.[217] Unlike ACh, succinylcholine is fairly resistant to breakdown by AChE but is readily hydrolyzed by plasma pseudocholinesterases, including butyrylcholinesterase, yielding succinylmonocholine, which is itself 20- to 50-fold less active as an NMJ blocker than the parent drug.[218] 70% of a bolus dose of succinylcholine is degraded to succinylmonocholine within 1 minute, and the metabolite is then further degraded to succinic acid and choline (Fig. 12.25).

Tubocurarine provides NMJ blockade within 2 minutes of an IV dose and within 10-25 minutes of an IM dose. Following a single IV dose, paralysis usually lasts 20-30 minutes, but the duration of blockade depends on the number of doses used and the overall depth of anesthesia, often lasting 60-120 minutes. Most of the drug is

Table 12.5 Classification and Pharmacokinetics of Neuromuscular Junction Blocking Agents

Agent	Structural Classification	Mechanism	Time to Peak (min)	Single-Dose Duration of Action (min)	Elimination	Distinct Effects
Succinyl-choline	Diacetylcholine ester	Depolarizing Ultrashort acting	0.5-1 (IV) 1-4 (IM)	6-10 (IV) 15-20 (IM)	Hydrolysis by plasma pseudocho-linesterases	Histamine release K^+ release
d-Tubocu-rarine	Isoquinoline alkaloid	Nondepolarizing Long acting	1-2 (IV) 10-25 (IM)	20-120	Renal (88%-90%) Biliary (10%-12%)	Histamine release CV effects
Pancuronium	Androstane—amino-steroid	Nondepolarizing Long acting	2-3 (IV)	45-60 (IV)	Renal (69%) Hepatic (25%)	CV effects Hepatic effects
Vecuronium	Androstane—amino-steroid	Nondepolarizing Intermediate acting	2-5 (IV)	30-40 (IV)	Renal (15%) Biliary (50%) Hepatic (33%)	Cardioselective, lacks CV effects of others
Rocuronium	Androstane—amino-steroid	Nondepolarizing Intermediate acting	0.8-2 (IV)	22-40 (IV)	Renal (33%) Biliary (67%)	Cardioselective, lacks CV effects of others
Atracurium	Tetrahydroisoquinoline	Nondepolarizing Intermediate acting	2-3 (IV)	60-70 (IV)	Hofmann elimination Ester hydrolysis	Flushing, hypotension
Cisatracurium	Tetrahydroisoquinoline	Nondepolarizing Intermediate acting	2-8 (IM)	42-90 (IV)	Hofmann elimination Ester hydrolysis	

CV, cardiovascular; IM, intramuscular; IV, intravenous.

excreted unchanged by the kidneys within 24 hours, while 10%-12% can be excreted in the bile, which also contains a small percentage (ca. 1%) of N-demethylated metabolite (Fig. 12.25).[219]

For the steroid-based agents, peak blockade for pancuronium, vecuronium, and rocuronium occurs within 2-3, 2-5, and 0.8-2 minutes, respectively. The duration of action of a single IV dose of each agent is 45-60, 30-40, and 22-40 minutes, respectively. Notably, the loss of the quaternizing methyl in vecuronium is directly responsible for reduction of the duration by a third of that seen with pancuronium. Similarly, the loss of ACh-likeness at the A-ring of rocuronium decreases the time to onset and the duration of action of this agent compared to the androstane-steroid agents.

The majority of a pancuronium dose (69%) is excreted unchanged in the urine after 24 hours, while 25% is hepatically metabolized to an active 3-desacetyl (3-OH-containing) metabolite that is excreted in the urine. The remainder appears in the urine as 17-desacetyl or 3,17-desacetyl metabolites (Fig. 12.26).[220] For vecuronium, approximately 15% of an administered dose is recovered unchanged in the urine while nearly 50% is excreted in the bile and 33% is metabolized hepatically to 3-desacetyl-, 17-desacetyl-, or 3,17-descetyl-vecuronium metabolites, all of which have activity as NMJ blocking agents (Fig. 12.26). Accumulation of the 3-desacetylvecuronium metabolite in critically ill patients may be associated with prolonged neuromuscular blockade in those receiving long-term therapies.[221-223] The major route of elimination of rocuronium is via biliary excretion, with approximately one-third of a dose also being excreted unchanged in the urine. Hepatic metabolism accounts for the formation of an inactive 17-desacetyl metabolite with no clinical relevance (Fig. 12.26).[224,225]

Atracurium and cisatracurium are fast-onset NMJ blocking agents with peak blockade occurring within 2-3 and 2-8 minutes of IV injection, respectively. Single dose durations via this route are 60-70 and 42-90 minutes, respectively. These agents are not metabolized by organ-based transformation, but rather, as discussed in the SAR section above, via Hofmann elimination and ester hydrolysis in the blood. The base-catalyzed

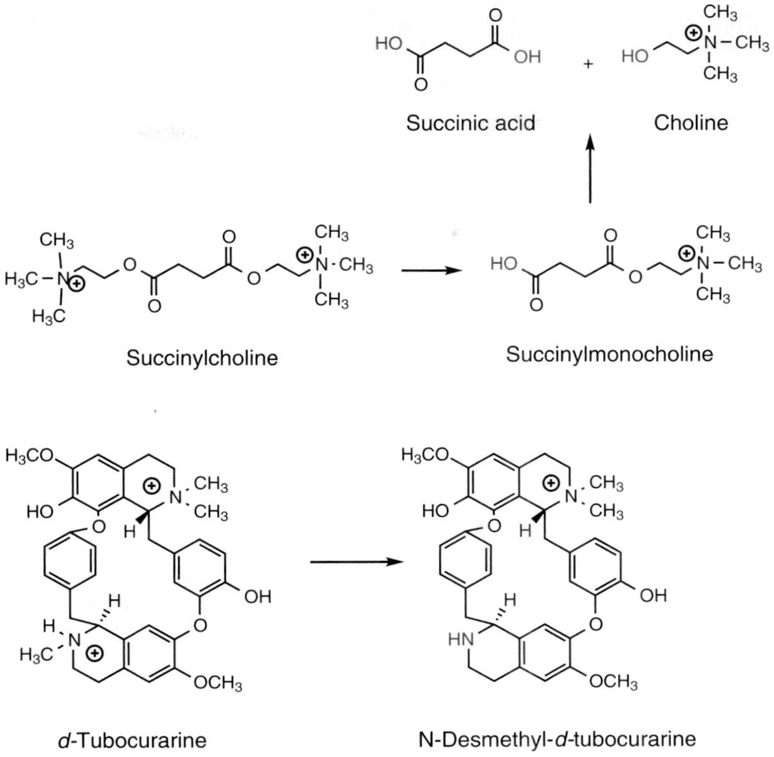

Succinic acid + Choline

Succinylcholine → Succinylmonocholine

d-Tubocurarine → N-Desmethyl-*d*-tubocurarine

Figure 12.25 Metabolism of succinylcholine and *d*-tubocurarine.

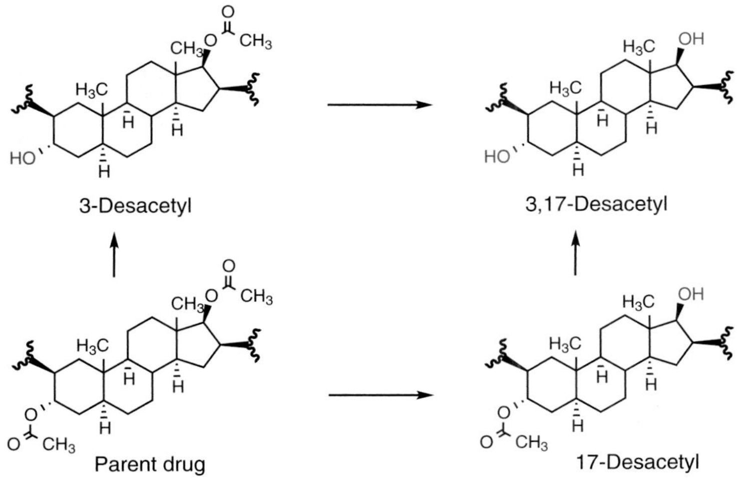

3-Desacetyl → 3,17-Desacetyl

Parent drug → 17-Desacetyl

Figure 12.26 Metabolism of pancuronium, vecuronium, and rocuronium.

Hofmann elimination of atracurium coupled with ester hydrolysis is illustrated in Figure 12.24 and leads to formation of laudanosine, a quaternary monoacrylate, a monoquaternary carboxylic acid, and a dialcohol, all of which are inactive. At physiological temperature and pH, base-mediated abstraction of one of the α-hydrogens respective to the ester carbonyl facilitates bond movements that, together with the ionized nitrogen, weakens its adjacent bonds, allows for the fissure of the molecule at the β-carbon respective to the ester carbonyl (Fig. 12.24). This forms laudanosine and the monoacrylate metabolite, which itself can undergo Hofmann elimination to yield laudanosine (Fig. 12.24). At the same time, ester hydrolysis of atracurium in plasma can lead to the formation of the acid and the alcohol metabolites, the latter of which can undergo further ester hydrolysis to the acid metabolite or Hofmann elimination to yield laudanosine.[226,227] This biodegradative pathway also holds true for cisatracurium and together, due to this independence on hepatic or renal biotransformation, atracurium and cisatracurium are especially useful in patients with liver or kidney dysfunction.

Clinical Scenario

Susan W. Miller, PharmD, Nader H. Moniri, PhD

SCENARIO

WK, a 78-year-old white female, presents to the ambulatory care clinic for a medication therapy management (MTM) consult prior to her appointment for her annual assessment with her primary care provider. WK is accompanied by her daughter, with whom she lives. WK's medical problems (and medications) are type 2 diabetes (glipizide 5 mg po QD), hypertension (verapamil SR 180 mg po QD), depression (fluvoxamine 100 mg po Q HS), and osteoporosis (alendronate 70 mg po once weekly, and calcium citrate 200 mg/vitamin D 250 IU 2 tabs po BID). WK's problems have been controlled with a hemoglobin A_{1C} stable at 6.8% and a blood pressure at 126/78 mm Hg, but at today's visit, she reports of her inability to get a good night's rest over the last four months. WK's daughter reports that WK has begun to experience some memory loss, specifically in recalling familiar names and in misplacing items around the house and that about three months prior, she had purchased a nonprescription analgesic product with "PM" (at nighttime) in the label to help her mother get a restful sleep. WK takes one caplet of the product prior to bedtime on a regular basis and reports that she sleeps well but is often drowsy in the morning after awakening.

OUTCOME

Following review and assessment of the medications and related problems, the pharmacist's recommendations are to discontinue the use of the nonprescription sleep aid (possibly contributing to the mild cognitive dysfunction and residual next-day sedation) and initiate therapy for the insomnia with ramelteon dosed at 8 mg po 30 minutes prior to bedtime and discontinue the fluvoxamine due to the potential drug interaction with ramelteon through CYP1A2 inhibition and prescribe sertraline 50 mg po QD for the depression. WK should continue to monitor her diabetes and hypertension as she has and return for a follow-up visit in three months to assess the efficacy of the new therapies. No changes are suggested for the diabetes or hypertension therapies at this time.

Chemical Analysis found immediately after References.

REFERENCES

1. Moruzzi G, Magoun HW. Brain stem reticular formation and activation of the EEG. *Electroencephalogr Clin Neurophysiol.* 1949;1:455-473.
2. Lindsley DB, Schreiner LH, Knowles WB, et al. Behavioral and EEG changes following chronic brain stem lesions in the cat. *Electroencephalogr Clin Neurophysiol.* 1950;2:483-498.
3. Maghoun HW. Caudal and cephalic influences of the brain stem reticular formation. *Physiol Rev.* 1950;30:459-474.
4. Lu J, Greco MA. Sleep circuitry and the hypnotic mechanism of GABA drugs. *J Clin Sleep Med.* 2006;2:S10-S26.
5. Panula P, Pirvola U, Auvinen S, et al. Histamine immunoreactive nerve fibers in the rat brain. *Neuroscience.* 1989;28:585-610.
6. Takahashi K, Lin JS, Sakai K. Neuronal activity of histaminergic tuberomammillary neurons during wake-sleep states in the mouse. *J Neurosci.* 2006;26:10292-10298.
7. Reiner PB, McGeer EG. Electrophysiological properties of cortically projecting histamine neurons of the rat hypothalamus. *Neurosci Lett.* 1987;73:43-47.
8. Lin JS, Jouvet M. Evidence for histaminergic arousal mechanisms in the hypothalamus of cat. *Neuropharmacology.* 1988;27:111-122.
9. Mochizuki T, Yamatodani A, Okakura K, et al. Circadian rhythm of histamine release from the hypothalamus of freely moving rats. *Physiol Behav.* 1992;51:391-394.
10. Lin JS, Sakai K, Vanni-Mercier G, et al. A critical role of the posterior hypothalamus in the mechanisms of wakefulness determined by microinjection of muscimol in freely moving rats. *Brain Res.* 1989;479:225-240.
11. Nauta WH. Hypothalamic regulation of sleep in rats. *J Neurophysiol.* 1946;9:285-316.
12. Moore RY. Retinohypothalamic projection in mammals: a comparative study. *Brain Res.* 1973;49:403-409.
13. Kalsbeek A, Cutrera RA, Van Heerikhuize JJ, et al. GABA release from suprachiasmatic nucleus terminals is necessary for the light-induced inhibition of nocturnal melatonin release in the rat. *Neuroscience.* 1999;91:453-461.
14. Roseboom PH, Coon SL, Baler R, et al. Melatonin synthesis: analysis of the more than 150-fold nocturnal increase in serotonin N-acetyltransferase messenger ribonucleic acid in the rat pineal gland. *Endocrinology.* 1996;13:3033-3045.
15. Ganguly S, Weller JL, Ho A, et al. Melatonin synthesis: 14-3-3-dependent activation and inhibition of arylalkylamine N-acetyltransferase mediated by phosphoserine-205. *Proc Natl Acad Sci USA.* 2005;102:1222-1227.
16. Klein DC, Moore RY. Pineal N-acetyltransferase and hydroxyindole-O-methyltransferase: control by the retinohypothalamic tract and the suprachiasmatic nucleus. *Brain Res.* 1979;174:245-262.
17. Yoshida K, McCormack S, España RA, et al. Afferents to the orexin neurons of the rat brain. *J Comp Neurol.* 2006;494:845-61.
18. de Lecea L, Kilduff TS, Peyron C, et al. The hypocretins: hypothalamus-specific peptides with neuroexcitatory activity. *Proc Natl Acad Sci USA.* 1998;95:322-327.
19. Sakurai T, Amemiya A, Ishii M, et al. Orexins and orexin receptors: a family of hypothalamic neuropeptides and G protein-coupled receptors that regulate feeding behavior. *Cell.* 1998;92:573-585.
20. Saper CB, Scammell TE, Lu J. Hypothalamic regulation of sleep and circadian rhythms. *Nature.* 2005;437:1257-1263.
21. van den Pol AN, Gao XB, Obrietan K, et al. Presynaptic and postsynaptic actions and modulation of neuroendocrine neurons by a new hypothalamic peptide, hypocretin/orexin. *J Neurosci.* 1998;18:7962-7971.
22. Steriade M. Acetylcholine systems and rhythmic activities during the waking-sleep cycle. *Prog Brain Res.* 2004;145:179-196.
23. Datta S. Cellular and chemical neuroscience of mammalian sleep. *Sleep Med.* 2010;11:431-440.

24. Datta S. Cellular basis of pontine ponto-geniculo-occipital wave generation and modulation. *Cell Mol Neurobiol.* 1997;17:341-365.
25. McKernan RM, Whiting PJ. Which GABAA-receptor subtypes really occur in the brain? *Trends Neurosci.* 1996;19:139-143.
26. Macdonald RL, Rogers CJ, Twyman RE. Barbiturate regulation of kinetic properties of the GABAA receptor channel of mouse spinal neurones in culture. *J Physiol.* 1989;417:483-500.
27. Fourati Z, Ruza RR, Laverty D, et al. Barbiturates bind in the GLIC ion channel pore and cause inhibition by stabilizing a closed state. *J Biol Chem.* 2017;292:1550-1558.
28. Akaike N, Maruyama T, Tokutomi N. Kinetic properties of the pentobarbitone-gated chloride current in frog sensory neurones. *J Physiol.* 1987;394:85-98.
29. Vida JA, Hooker ML, Samour CM. Anticonvulsants. 4. Metharbital and phenobarbital derivatives. *J Med Chem.* 1973;16:1378-1381.
30. Vida JA, Samour CM, O'Dea MH, et al. Analgesics. 2. Selected 5-substituted 5-(1-phenylethyl)barbituric acids. *J Med Chem.* 1974;17:1194-1197.
31. Blicke FH, Cox RH, eds. *Medicinal Chemistry*; vol. 4. New York: Wiley; 1959.
32. Basak SC, Harriss DK, Magnuson VR. Comparative study of lipophilicity versus topological molecular descriptors in biological correlations. *J Pharm Sci.* 1984;73:429-437.
33. Lavoie AM, Twyman RE. Direct evidence for diazepam modulation of GABAA receptor microscopic affinity. *Neuropharmacology.* 1996;35:1383-1392.
34. Twyman RE, Rogers CJ, Macdonald RL. Differential regulation of gammaaminobutyric acid receptor channels by diazepam and phenobarbital. *Ann Neurol.* 1989;25:213-220.
35. Windholz M, ed. *The Merck Index.* 9th ed. Rahway, NJ: Merck & Co.; 1976.
36. Mejo SL. Anterograde amnesia linked to benzodiazepines. *Nurse Pract.* 1992;17:49-50.
37. Clatworthy AJ, Jones LV, Whitehouse MJ. The gas chromatography mass spectrometry of the major metabolites of flurazepam. *Biomed Mass Spectrom.* 1977;4:248-254.
38. Zampaglione N, Hilbert JM, Ning J, et al. Disposition and metabolic fate of 14C-quazepam in man. *Drug Metab Dispos.* 1985;13:25-29.
39. Miura M, Otani K, Ohkubo T. Identification of human cytochrome P450 enzymes involved in the formation of 4-hydroxyestazolam from estazolam. *Xenobiotica.* 2005;35:455-465.
40. Eberts FS Jr, Philopoulos Y, Reineke LM, et al. Triazolam disposition. *Clin Pharmacol Ther.* 1981;29:81-93.
41. Schwarz HJ. Pharmacokinetics and metabolism of temazepam in man and several animal species. *Br J Clin Pharmacol.* 1979;8:23S-29S.
42. Sanger DJ, Benavides J, Perrault G, et al. Recent developments in the behavioral pharmacology of benzodiazepine (omega) receptors: evidence for the functional significance of receptor subtypes. *Neurosci Biobehav Rev.* 1994;18:355-372.
43. McKernan RM, Rosahl TW, Reynolds DS, et al. Sedative but not anxiolytic properties of benzodiazepines are mediated by the GABA(A) receptor alpha1 subtype. *Nat Neurosci.* 2000;3:587-592.
44. Löw K, Crestani F, Keist R, et al. Molecular and neuronal substrate for the selective attenuation of anxiety. *Science.* 2000;290:131-134.
45. Collinson N, Kuenzi FM, Jarolimek W, et al. Enhanced learning and memory and altered GABAergic synaptic transmission in mice lacking the alpha 5 subunit of the GABAA receptor. *J Neurosci.* 2002;22:5572-5580.
46. Crestani F, Keist R, Fritschy JM, et al. Trace fear conditioning involves hippocampal alpha5 GABA(A) receptors. *Proc Natl Acad Sci USA.* 2002;99:8980-8985.
47. Smith AJ, Alder L, Silk J, et al. Effect of alpha subunit on allosteric modulation of ion channel function in stably expressed human recombinant gamma-aminobutyric acid(A) receptors determined using (36)Cl ion flux. *Mol Pharmacol.* 2001;59:1108-1118.
48. Petroski RE, Pomeroy JE, Das R, et al. Indiplon is a high-affinity positive allosteric modulator with selectivity for alpha1 subunit-containing GABAA receptors. *J Pharmacol Exp Ther.* 2006;317:369-377.
49. Frattola L, Maggioni M, Cesana B, et al. Double blind comparison of zolpidem 20 mg versus flunitrazepam 2 mg in insomniac in-patients. *Drugs Exp Clin Res.* 1990;16:371-376.
50. Bensimon G, Foret J, Warot D, et al. Daytime wakefulness following a bedtime oral dose of zolpidem 20 mg, flunitrazepam 2 mg and placebo. *Br J Clin Pharmacol.* 1990;30:463-469.
51. Declerck AC, Ruwe F, O'Hanlon JF, et al. Effects of zolpidem and flunitrazepam on nocturnal sleep of women subjectively complaining of insomnia. *Psychopharmacology* 1992;106:497-501.
52. Roger M, Attali P, Coquelin JP. Multicenter, double-blind, controlled comparison of zolpidem and triazolam in elderly patients with insomnia. *Clin Ther.* 1993;15:127-136.
53. Priest R, Terzano M, Parrino L, et al. Efficacy of zolpidem in insomnia. *Eur Psychiatry.* 1997;12S:5-14.
54. Kerkhof G, Van Vianen BG, Kamphuisen HC. A comparison of zolpidem and temazepam in psychophysiological insomniacs. *Eur Neuropsychopharmacol.* 1996;6:155-156.
55. Holm KJ, Goa KL. Zolpidem: an update of its pharmacology, therapeutic efficacy and tolerability in the treatment of insomnia. *Drugs.* 2000;59:865-889.
56. Anzini M, Cappelli A, Vomero S, et al. Molecular basis of peripheral vs central benzodiazepine receptor selectivity in a new class of peripheral benzodiazepine receptor ligands related to alpidem. *J Med Chem.* 1996;39:4275-4284.
57. Trapani G, Franco M, Ricciardi L, et al. Synthesis and binding affinity of 2-phenylimidazo[1,2-alpha]pyridine derivatives for both central and peripheral benzodiazepine receptors. A new series of high-affinity and selective ligands for the peripheral type. *J Med Chem.* 1997;40:3109-3118.
58. Selleri S, Bruni F, Costagli C, et al. A novel selective GABA(A) alpha1 receptor agonist displaying sedative and anxiolytic-like properties in rodents. *J Med Chem.* 2005;48:6756-6760.
59. Hanson SM, Morlock EV, Satyshur KA, et al. Structural requirements for eszopiclone and zolpidem binding to the gamma-aminobutyric acid type-A (GABAA) receptor are different. *J Med Chem.* 2008;51:7243-7252.
60. Sauvantet JP, Langer SZ, Morselli PL, eds. *Imidazopyridines in Sleep Disorders.* New York: Raven Press; 1988.
61. Pichard L, Gillet G, Bonfils C, et al. Oxidative metabolism of zolpidem by human liver cytochrome P450S. *Drug Metab Dispos.* 1995;23:1253-1262.
62. Von Moltke LL, Greenblatt DJ, Granda BW, et al. Zolpidem metabolism in vitro: responsible cytochromes, chemical inhibitors, and in vivo correlations. *Br J Clin Pharmacol.* 1999;48:89-97.
63. Gillet G, Thénot JP, Morselli PL. *In vitro and in vivo metabolism of zolpidem in three animal species and in man. Proc 3rd Intl ISSX Meeting, Amsterdam, the Netherlands*; 1991:153.
64. Olubodun JO, Ochs HR, von Moltke LL, et al. Pharmacokinetic properties of zolpidem in elderly and young adults: possible modulation by testosterone in men. *Br J Clin Pharmacol.* 2003;56:297-304.
65. Nakamura H, Nakasa H, Ishii I, et al. Effects of endogenous steroids on CYP3A4-mediated drug metabolism by human liver microsomes. *Drug Metab Dispos.* 2002;30:534-540.
66. Cubala WJ, Landowski J, Wichowicz HM. Zolpidem abuse, dependence and withdrawal syndrome: sex as susceptibility factor for adverse effects. *Br J Clin Pharmacol.* 2008;65:444-445.
67. Hair PI, McCormack PL, Curran MP. Eszopiclone: a review of its use in the treatment of insomnia. *Drugs.* 2008;68:1415-1434.
68. *Lunesta (Eszopiclone) Tablets 1 mg, 2 mg, 3 mg: US Prescribing Information.* Marlborough, MA: Sepracor, Inc.;January 2009.
69. Trifiletti RR, Snyder SH. Anxiolytic cyclopyrrolones zopiclone and suriclone bind to a novel site linked allosterically to benzodiazepine receptors. *Mol Pharmacol.* 1984;26:458-469.

70. Sieghart W. Structure and pharmacology of gamma-aminobutyric acid-A receptor subtypes. *Pharmacol Rev*. 1995;47:181-234.
71. Carlson JN, Haskew R, Wacker J, et al. Sedative and anxiolytic effects of zopiclone's enantiomers and metabolite. *Eur J Pharmacol*. 2001;415:181-189.
72. Sanna E, Busonero F, Talani G, et al. Comparison of the effects of zaleplon, zolpidem, and triazolam at various GABA(A) receptor subtypes. *Eur J Pharmacol*. 2002;451:103-110.
73. Rosen AS, Fournié P, Darwish M, et al. Zaleplon pharmacokinetics and absolute bioavailability. *Biopharm Drug Dispos*. 1999;20:171-175.
74. *Sonata (zaleplon) capsules 5 mg, 10 mg: US prescribing information*. Bristol, TN: King Pharmaceuticals, Inc., March 2006.
75. Dooley M, Plosker GL. Zaleplon: a review of its use in the treatment of insomnia. *Drugs*. 2000;60:413-445.
76. Walsh JK, Vogel GW, Scharf M, et al. A five week, polysomnographic assessment of zaleplon 10 mg for the treatment of primary insomnia. *Sleep Med*. 2000;1:41-49.
77. Wegner F, Deuther-Conrad W, Scheunemann M, et al. GABAA receptor pharmacology of fluorinated derivatives of the novel sedative-hypnotic pyrazolopyrimidine indiplon. *Eur J Pharmacol*. 2008;580:1-11.
78. Kawashima K, Hosoi K, Naruke T, et al. Aldehyde oxidase-dependent marked species difference in hepatic metabolism of the sedative-hypnotic, zaleplon, between monkeys and rats. *Drug Metab Dispos*. 1999;27:422-428.
79. Dolder CR, Nelson MH. Hypnosedative-induced complex behaviours: incidence, mechanisms and management. *CNS Drugs*. 2008;22:1021-1036.
80. Hoque R, Chesson AL Jr. Zolpidem-induced sleepwalking, sleep related eating disorder, and sleep-driving: fluorine-18-flourodeoxyglucose positron emission tomography analysis, and a literature review of other unexpected clinical effects of zolpidem. *J Clin Sleep Med*. 2009;5:471-476.
81. Tsai JH, Yang P, Chen CC, et al. Zolpidem-induced amnesia and somnambulism: rare occurrences? *Eur Neuropsychopharmacol*. 2009;19:74-76.
82. Siddiqui F, Osuna E, Chokroverty S. Writing emails as part of sleepwalking after increase in zolpidem. *Sleep Med*. 2009;10:262-264.
83. Doane JA, Dalpiaz AS. Zolpidem-induced sleep-driving. *Am J Med*. 2008;121:e5.
84. Sansone RA, Sansone LA. Zolpidem, somnambulism, and nocturnal eating. *Gen Hosp Psychiatry*. 2008;30:90-91.
85. Iruela LM. Zolpidem and sleepwalking. *J Clin Psychopharmacol*. 1995;15:223.
86. Ferentinos P, Paparrigopoulos T. Zopiclone and sleepwalking. *Int J Neuropsychopharmacol*. 2009;12:141-142.
87. Liskow B, Pikalov A. Zaleplon overdose associated with sleepwalking and complex behavior. *J Am Acad Child Adolesc Psychiatry*. 2004;43:927-928.
88. Gauer F, Masson-Pevet M, Stehle J, et al. Daily variations in melatonin receptor density of rat pars tuberalis and suprachiasmatic nuclei are distinctly regulated. *Brain Res*. 1994;641:92-98.
89. Liu C, Weaver DR, Jin X, et al. Molecular dissection of two distinct actions of melatonin on the suprachiasmatic circadian clock. *Neuron*. 1997;19:91-102.
90. Dubocovich ML, Yun K, Al-Ghoul WM, et al. Selective MT2 melatonin receptor antagonists block melatonin-mediated phase advances of circadian rhythms. *FASEB J*. 1998;12:1211-1220.
91. Mor M, Plazzi PV, Spadoni G, et al. *Melatonin*. *Curr Med Chem*. 1999;6:501-518.
92. Spadoni G, Mor M, Tarzia G. Structure-affinity relationships of indole-based melatonin analogs. *Biol Signals Recept*. 1999;8:15-23.
93. Rivara S, Mor M, Bedini A, et al. Melatonin receptor agonists: SAR and applications to the treatment of sleep-wake disorders. *Curr Top Med Chem*. 2008;8:954-968.
94. Yous S, Andrieux J, Howell HE, et al. Novel naphthalenic ligands with high affinity for the melatonin receptor. *J Med Chem*. 1992;35:1484-1486.
95. Sugden D, Davidson K, Hough KA, et al. Melatonin, melatonin receptors and melanophores: a moving story. *Pigment Cell Res*. 2004;17:454-460.
96. Dubocovich ML, Delagrange P, Krause DN, et al. International union of basic and clinical pharmacology. LXXV. Nomenclature, classification, and pharmacology of G protein-coupled melatonin receptors. *Pharmacol Rev*. 2010;62:343-380.
97. Farce A, Chugunov AO, Logé C, et al. Homology modeling of MT1 and MT2 receptors. *Eur J Med Chem*. 2008;43:1926-1944.
98. Gerdin MJ, Mseeh F, Dubocovich ML. Mutagenesis studies of the human MT2 melatonin receptor. *Biochem Pharmacol*. 2003;66:315-320.
99. Kato K, Hirai K, Nishiyama K, et al. Neurochemical properties of ramelteon (TAK-375), a selective MT1/MT2 receptor agonist. *Neuropharmacology*. 2005;48:301-310.
100. Miyamoto M, Nishikawa H, Doken Y, et al. The sleep-promoting action of ramelteon (TAK-375) in freely moving cats. *Sleep*. 2004;27:1319-1325.
101. Nosjean O, Ferro M, Coge F, et al. Identification of the melatonin-binding site MT3 as the quinone reductase 2. *J Biol Chem*. 2000;275: 31311-31317.
102. Yukuhiro N, Kimura H, Nishikawa H, et al. Effects of ramelteon (TAK-375) on nocturnal sleep in freely moving monkeys. *Brain Res*. 2004;1027:59-66.
103. Mini L, Wang-Weigand S, Zhang J. Ramelteon 8 mg/d versus placebo in patients with chronic insomnia: post hoc analysis of a 5-week trial using 50% or greater reduction in latency to persistent sleep as a measure of treatment effect. *Clin Ther*. 2008;30:1316-1323.
104. Roth T, Stubbs C, Walsh JK. Ramelteon (TAK-375), a selective MT1/MT2-receptor agonist, reduces latency to persistent sleep in a model of transient insomnia related to a novel sleep environment. *Sleep*. 2005;28:303-307.
105. Erman M, Seiden D, Zammit G, et al. An efficacy, safety, and dose-response study of Ramelteon in patients with chronic primary insomnia. *Sleep Med*. 2006;7:17-24.
106. Griffiths RR, Johnson MW. Relative abuse liability of hypnotic drugs: a conceptual framework and algorithm for differentiating among compounds. *J Clin Psychiatry*. 2005;66:31-41.
107. *Rozarem (Ramelteon) Tablets 8 mg: US Prescribing Information*. Deerfield, IL: Takeda Pharmaceuticals America, Inc.; October 2008.
108. Karim A, Tolbert D, Cao C. Disposition kinetics and tolerance of escalating single doses of ramelteon, a high-affinity MT1 and MT2 melatonin receptor agonist indicated for treatment of insomnia. *J Clin Pharmacol*. 2006;46:140-148.
109. Obach RS, Ryder TF. Metabolism of ramelteon in human liver microsomes and correlation with the effect of fluvoxamine on ramelteon pharmacokinetics. *Drug Metab Dispos*. 2010;38:1381-1391.
110. Lee MG, Hassani OK, Jones BE. Discharge of identified orexin/hypocretin neurons across the sleep-waking cycle. *J Neurosci*. 2005, 25:6716-6720.
111. Takahashi K, Lin JS, Sakai K. Neuronal activity of orexin and non-orexin waking-active neurons during wake-sleep states in the mouse. *Neuroscience*. 2008, 153:860-870.
112. Mileykovskiy BY, Kiyashchenko LI, Siegel JM. Behavioral correlates of activity in identified hypocretin/orexin neurons. *Neuron*. 2005;46:787-798.
113. Lin L, Faraco J, Li R, Kadotani H, et al. The sleep disorder canine narcolepsy is caused by a mutation in the hypocretin (orexin) receptor 2 gene. *Cell*. 1999; 98:365-376.
114. Aldrich MS, Reynolds PR. Narcolepsy and the hypocretin receptor 2 gene. *Neuron*. 1999;23:625-626.
115. Hagan JJ, Leslie RA, Patel S, et al. Orexin A activates locus coeruleus cell firing and increases arousal in the rat. *Proc Natl Acad Sci USA*. 1999;96:10911-10916.
116. España RA, Plahn S, Berridge CW. Circadian-dependent and circadian-independent behavioral actions of hypocretin/orexin. *Brain Res*. 2002, 943:224-236.

117. Gotter AL, Webber AL, Coleman PJ, et al. International union of basic and clinical pharmacology. LXXXVI. Orexin receptor function, nomenclature and pharmacology. *Pharmacol Rev.* 2012;64:389-420.
118. Mang GM, Dürst T, Bürki H, et al. The dual orexin receptor antagonist almorexant induces sleep and decreases orexin-induced locomotion by blocking orexin 2 receptors. *Sleep.* 2012;35: 1625-1635.
119. Hoever P, de Haas SL, Dorffner G, et al. Orexin receptor antagonism: an ascending multiple-dose study with almorexant. *J Psychopharmacol.* 2012;26:1071-1080.
120. Brisbare-Roch C, Dingemanse J, Koberstein R, et al. Promotion of sleep by targeting the orexin system in rats, dogs and humans. *Nat Med.* 2007;13:150-155.
121. Steiner MA, Lecourt H, Strasser DS, et al. Differential effects of the dual orexin receptor antagonist almorexant and the GABA(A)-α1 receptor modulator zolpidem, alone or combined with ethanol, on motor performance in the rat. *Neuropsychopharmacology.* 2011; 36:848-856.
122. Cox CD, Breslin MJ, Whitman DB, et al. Discovery of the dual orexin receptor antagonist [(7R)-4-(5-chloro-1,3-benzoxazol-2-yl)-7-methyl-1,4-diazepan-1-yl][5-methyl-2-(2H-1,2,3-triazol-2-yl)phenyl]methanone (MK-4305) for the treatment of insomnia. *J Med Chem.* 2010;53:5320-5332.
123. Michelson D, Snyder E, Paradis E, et al. Safety and efficacy of suvorexant during 1-year treatment of insomnia with subsequent abrupt treatment discontinuation: a phase 3 randomised, double-blind, placebo-controlled trial. *Lancet Neurol.* 2014;13:461-471.
124. Herring WJ, Snyder E, Budd K, et al. Orexin receptor antagonism for treatment of insomnia: a randomized clinical trial of suvorexant. *Neurology.* 2012;79:2265-2274.
125. Herring WJ, Connor KM, Ivgy-May N, et al. Suvorexant in patients with insomnia: results from two 3-month randomized controlled clinical trials. *Biol Psychiatry.* 2016; 79:136-148.
126. Herring WJ, Connor KM, Snyder E, et al. Suvorexant in elderly patients with insomnia: pooled analyses of data from phase III randomized controlled clinical trials. *Am J Geriatr Psychiatry.* 2017;25:791-802.
127. Herring WJ, Connor KM, Snyder E, et al. Suvorexant in patients with insomnia: pooled analyses of three-month data from phase-3 randomized controlled clinical trials. *J Clin Sleep Med.* 2016;12:1215-1225.
128. *Belsomra® (Suvarexant) Tablets 10 mg, 20 mg, 40 mg: US Prescribing Information.* Whitehouse Station, NJ: Merck & Co, Inc.; May 2016.
129. Yin J, Mobarec JC, Kolb P, Rosenbaum DM. Crystal structure of the human OX2 orexin receptor bound to the insomnia drug suvorexant. *Nature.* 2015;519:247-250.
130. Cui D, Cabalu T, Yee KL, et al. In vitro and in vivo characterisation of the metabolism and disposition of suvorexant in humans. *Xenobiotica.* 2016;46:882-895.
131. Alkire MT, Miller J. General anesthesia and the neural correlates of consciousness. *Prog Brain Res.* 2005;150:229-244.
132. Heinke W, Schwarzbauer C. In vivo imaging of anaesthetic action in humans: approaches with positron emission tomography (PET) and functional magnetic resonance imaging (fMRI). *Br J Anaesth.* 2002;89:112-122.
133. Alkire MT, Haier RJ. Correlating in vivo anaesthetic effects with ex vivo receptor density data supports a GABAergic mechanism of action for propofol, but not for isoflurane. *Br J Anaesth.* 2001;86:618-626.
134. Alkire MT, Haier RJ, Fallon JH. Toward a unified theory of narcosis: brain imaging evidence for a thalamocortical switch as the neurophysiologic basis of anesthetic-induced unconsciousness. *Conscious Cogn.* 2000;9:370-386.
135. Hentschke H, Schwarz C, Antkowiak B. Neocortex is the major target of sedative concentrations of volatile anaesthetics: strong depression of firing rates and increase of GABAA receptor-mediated inhibition. *Eur J Neurosci.* 2005;21:93-102.
136. French JD, Livingston RB, Hernandez-Peon R. Cortical influences upon the arousal mechanism. *Trans Am Neurol Assoc.* 1953;3:57-58.
137. Nicoll RA, Madison DV. General anesthetics hyperpolarize neurons in the vertebrate central nervous system. *Science.* 1982;217:1055-1057.
138. Dringenberg HC, Olmstead MC. Integrated contributions of basal forebrain and thalamus to neocortical activation elicited by pedunculopontine tegmental stimulation in urethane-anesthetized rats. *Neuroscience.* 2003;119:839-853.
139. Torri G. Inhalation anesthetics: a review. *Minerva Anestesiol.* 2010;76:215-228.
140. Di Fazio CA, Brown RE, Ball CG, et al. Additive effects of anesthetics and theories of anesthesia. *Anesthesiology.* 1972;36:57-63.
141. Torri G, Damia G, Fabiani ML. Effect of nitrous oxide on the anaesthetic requirement of enflurane. *Br J Anaesth.* 1974;46:468-72.
142. Meyer H. Zur Theorie der Alkoholnarkose. *Arch Exp Pathol Pharmakol.* 1899;42:109-118.
143. Mennerick S, Jevtovic-Todorovic V, Todorovic SM, et al. Effect of nitrous oxide on excitatory and inhibitory synaptic transmission in hippocampal cultures. *J Neurosci.* 1998;18:9716-9726.
144. Narahashi T, Aistrup GL, Lindstrom JM, et al. Ion channel modulation as the basis for general anesthesia. *Toxicol Lett.* 1998;100:185-191.
145. Franks NP, Lieb WR. Which molecular targets are most relevant to general anaesthesia? *Toxicol Lett.* 1998;100:1-8.
146. Olsen RW. The molecular mechanism of action of general anesthetics: structural aspects of interactions with GABAA receptors. *Toxicol Lett.* 1998;100:193-201.
147. Harrison NL, Kugler JL, Jones MV, et al. Positive modulation of human gamma-aminobutyric acid type A and glycine receptors by the inhalation anesthetic isoflurane. *Mol Pharmacol.* 1993;44:628-632.
148. Flood P, Role LW. Neuronal nicotinic acetylcholine receptor modulation by general anesthetics. *Toxicol Lett.* 1998;100:149-153.
149. Mascia MP, Machu TK, Harris RA. Enhancement of homomeric glycine receptor function by long-chain alcohols and anaesthetics. *Br J Pharmacol.* 1996;119:1331-1336.
150. Violet JM, Downie DL, Nakisa RC, et al. Differential sensitivities of mammalian neuronal and muscle nicotinic acetylcholine receptors to general anesthetics. *Anesthesiology.* 1997; 86:866-874.
151. Dilger JP, Vidal AM, Mody HI, Liu Y. Evidence for direct actions of general anesthetics on an ion channel protein: a new look at a unified mechanism of action. *Anesthesiology.* 1994; 81:431-442.
152. Raines DE, Claycomb RJ, Scheller M, Forman SA. Nonhalogenated alkane anesthetics fail to potentiate agonist actions on two ligand-gated ion channels. *Anesthesiology.* 2001; 95:470-477.
153. Dilger JP, Vidal AM, Mody HI, Liu Y. Evidence for direct actions of general anesthetics on an ion channel protein: a new look at a unified mechanism of action. *Anesthesiology.* 1994; 81:431-442.
154. Kendig JJ. In vitro networks: subcortical mechanisms of anaesthetic action. *Br J Anaesth.* 2002;89:91-101.
155. Jenkins A, Franks NP, Lieb WR. Actions of general anaesthetics on 5-HT3 receptors in N1E-115 neuroblastoma cells. *Br J Pharmacol.* 1996;117:1507-1515.
156. Perouansky M, Baranov D, Salman M, Yaari Y. Effects of halothane on glutamate receptor-mediated excitatory postsynaptic currents: a patch-clamp study in adult mouse hippocampal slices. *Anesthesiology.* 1995;83:109-119.
157. Lin LH, Chen LL, Harris RA. Enflurane inhibits NMDA, AMPA, and kainate-induced currents in Xenopus oocytes expressing mouse and human brain mRNA. *FASEB J.* 1993; 7:479-485.
158. Kohro S, Hogan QH, Nakae Y, et al. Anesthetic effects on mitochondrial ATP-sensitive K channel. *Anesthesiology.* 2001;95:1435-1440.
159. Huneke R, Jungling E, Skasa M, et al. Effects of the anesthetic gases xenon, halothane, and isoflurane on calcium and potassium currents in human atrial cardiomyocytes. *Anesthesiology.* 2001;95:999-1006.

160. Yost CS. Potassium channels: basic aspects, functional roles, and medical significance. *Anesthesiology*. 1999;90:1186-1203.
161. Patel AJ, Honore E, Lesage F, et al. Inhalational anesthetics activate two-pore-domain background K+ channels. *Nat Neurosci*. 1999;2:422-426.
162. Terrell RC. The invention and development of enflurane, isoflurane, sevoflurane and desflurane. *Anesthesiology*. 2008;108:531-533.
163. Lysko GS, Robinson JL, Casto R, Ferrone RA. The stereospecific effects of isoflurane isomers in vivo. *Eur J Pharmacol*. 1994;263: 25-9.
164. Franks NP, Lieb WR.What is the molecular nature of general anaesthetic target sights. *Trends Pharmacol Sci*. 1987;8:169-174.
165. Moody EJ, Harris BD, Skolnick P. Stereospecific actions of the inhalation anesthetic isoflurane at the GABAA receptor complex. *Brain Res*. 1993;615:101-106.
166. Harris B, Moody EJ, Basile T, Skolnick P. Volatile anesthetics bidirectionally and stereospecifically modulate ligand binding to GABA receptors. *Eur J Pharmacol*. 1994;267:269-274.
167. *Ethrane(R), Enflurane. US Prescribing Information*. Liberty Corner, NJ, USA: Ohmeda Pharmaceuticals; 1995.
168. Black GW, Johnston HML, Scott MG. Clinical impressions of enflurane. *Br J Anaesth*. 1977;49:857-880.
169. Hitt BA, Mazze RI, Beppu WJ, et al. Enflurane metabolism in rats and man. *J Pharmacol Exp Ther*. 1977;203:193-202.
170. Imbenotte M, Erb F, Goldstein P, et al. Halothane and enflurane metabolite elimination during anaesthesia in man. *Eur J Anaesthesiol*. 1987;4:175-182.
171. Holaday DA, Fiserova-Bergerova V, Latto IP, Zumbiel MA. Resistance of isoflurane to biotransformation in man. *Anesthesiology*. 1975;43:325-332.
172. Quinn AC, Newman PJ, Hall GM, Grounds RM. Sevoflurane anaesthesia for major intra-abdominal surgery. *Anaesthesia*. 1994 49:567-571.
173. Frink EJ Jr, Malan P, Atlas M, et al. Clinical comparison of sevoflurane and isoflurane in healthy patients. *Anesth Analg*. 1992;74:241-245.
174. Kharasch ED, Thummel KE. Identification of cytochrome P450 2E1 as the predominant enzyme catalyzing human liver microsomal defluorination of sevoflurane, isoflurane, and methoxyflurane. *Anesthesiology*. 1993;79:795-807.
175. Van Obbergh LJ, Verbeeck RK, Michel I, et al. Extrahepatic metabolism of sevoflurane in children undergoing orthoptic liver transplantation. *Anesthesiology*. 2000;92:683-686.
176. Jiaxiang NI, Sato N, Fujii K, Yuge O. Urinary excretion of hexafluoroisopropanol glucuronide and fluoride in patients after sevoflurane anaesthesia. *J Pharm Pharmacol*. 1993; 45:67-69.
177. Van Hemelrijck J, Smith I, White PF. Use of desflurane for outpatient anesthesia: a comparison with propofol and nitrous oxide. *Anesthesiology*. 1991;75:197-203.
178. Wrigley SR, Fairfield JE, Jones RM, Black AE. Induction and recovery characteristics of desflurane in day case patients: a comparison with propofol. *Anaesthesia*. 1991;46:615-622.
179. Smiley RM, Ornstein E, Pantuck EJ, et al. Metabolism of desflurane and isoflurane to fluoride ion in surgical patients. *Can J Anaesth*. 1991;38:965-968.
180. Jones RM, Koblin DD, Cashman JN, et al. Biotransformation and hepato-renal function in volunteers after exposure to desflurane (I-653). *Br J Anaesth*. 1990; 64:482-487.
181. White PF. Clinical uses of intravenous anesthetic and analgesic infusions. *Anesth Analg*. 1989;68:161-171.
182. Swerdlow BN, Holley FO. Intravenous anaesthetic agents: pharmacokinetic-pharmacodynamic relationships. *Clin Pharmacokinet*. 1987;12:79-110.
183. Trapani G, Altomare C, Liso G, et al. Propofol in anesthesia. Mechanism of action, structure-activity relationships, and drug delivery. *Curr Med Chem*. 2000;7:249-271.
184. James R, Glen JB. Synthesis, biological evaluation, and preliminary structure-activity considerations of a series of alkylphenols as intravenous anesthetic agents. *J Med Chem*. 1980;23:1350-1357.
185. Schuttler J, Schwilden H, & Stoeckel H. Pharmacokinetic-dynamic modelling of diprivan. *Anesthesiology*. 1986;65:A549.
186. Adam HK, Kay B, Douglas EJ. Blood disoprofol levels in anaesthetised patients. *Anaesthesia*. 1982;37:536-540.
187. *Diprivan(R), Propofol US Prescribing Information*. Lake Zurich, IL, USA: Fresenius Kabi USA, LLC; 2014.
188. Oda Y, Hamaoka N, Hiroi T, et al. Involvement of human liver cytochrome P4502B6 in the metabolism of propofol. *Br J Clin Pharmacol*. 2001;51:281-285.
189. Sneyd JR, Simons PJ, Wright B. Use of proton nmr spectroscopy to measure propofol metabolites in the urine of the female Caucasian patient. *Xenobiotica*. 1994;24:1021-1028.
190. Simons PJ, Cockshott ID, Douglas EJ, et al. Disposition in male volunteers of a subanaesthetic intravenous dose of an oil in water emulsion of 14C-propofol. *Xenobiotica*. 1988;18:429-440.
191. Sanna E, Murgia A, Casula A, Biggio G. Differential subunit dependence of the actions of the general anesthetics alphaxalone and etomidate at gamma-aminobutyric acid type A receptors expressed in Xenopus laevis oocytes. *Mol Pharmacol*. 1997;51:484-490.
192. Rüsch D, Zhong H, Forman SA. Gating allosterism at a single class of etomidate sites on alpha1beta2gamma2L GABA A receptors accounts for both direct activation and agonist modulation. *J Biol Chem*. 2004;279:20982-20989.
193. Godefroi EF, Janssen PAJ, Van der Eycken CAM, et al. DL-(1-arylalkyl)imidazole-5-carboxylate esters. A novel type of hypnotic agents. *J Med Chem*. 1965;56:220-223.
194. Tornetta FJ, Song S, Smoyer AD. Etomidate: a pharmacologic profile of a new hypnotic. *J Am Assoc Nurse Anesthetists*. 1980;48:517-525.
195. Morgan M, Lumley J, Whitwam JG. Etomidate, a new water-soluble nonbarbiturate intravenous induction agent. *Lancet*. 1975;1:955-956.
196. Fragen RJ, Caldwell N, Brunner EA. Clinical use of etomidate for anesthesia induction: a preliminary report. *Anesth Analg*. 1976;55:730-733.
197. Gooding JM, Corssen G: Etomidate: an ultrashort-acting nonbarbiturate agent for anesthesia induction. *Anesth Analg*. 1976;55:286-288.
198. White PF, Way WL, Trevor AJ. Ketamine - its pharmacology and therapeutic uses. *Anesthesiology*. 1982;56:119-136.
199. Marietta MP, WAY WL, Castagnoli N Jr, Trevor AJ. On the pharmacology of the ketamine enantiomorphs in the rat. *J Pharmacol Exp Ther*. 1977;202:157-165.
200. Zarantonello P, Bettini E, Paio A, et al. Novel analogues of ketamine and phencyclidine as NMDA receptor antagonists. *Bioorg Med Chem Lett*. 2011;21:2059-2063.
201. *Ketalar(R), Ketamine Hydrochloride. US Prescribing Information*. Bristol, TN, USA: Monarch Pharmaceuticals, Inc.; 1998.
202. Grant IS, Nimmo WS, Clements JA. Pharmacokinetics and analgesic effects of IM and oral ketamine. *Br J Anaesth*. 1981;53:805-810.
203. Kreter B. Ketamine as an anesthetic agent for interventional radiology. *Semin Intervent Radiol*. 1987;4:183-188.
204. Desta Z, Moaddel R, Ogburn ET, et al. Stereoselective and regiospecific hydroxylation of ketamine and norketamine. *Xenobiotica*. 2012;42:1076-1087.
205. Kharasch ED, Herrmann S, Labroo R. Ketamine as a probe for medetomidine stereoisomer inhibition of human liver microsomal drug metabolism.. *Anesthesiology*. 1992;77: 1208-1214.
206. Yanagihara Y, Kariya S, Ohtani M, et al. Involvement of CYP2B6 in N-demethylation of ketamine in human liver microsomes. *Drug Metab Dispos*. 2001;29:887-890.
207. Portmann S, Kwan HY, Theurillat R, et al. Enantioselective capillary electrophoresis for identification and characterization of human cytochrome P450 enzymes which metabolize ketamine and norketamine in vitro. *J Chromatogr A*. 2010;1217:7942-7948.
208. Hijazi Y, Boulieu R. Contribution of CYP3A4, CYP2B6, and CYP2C9 isoforms to N-demethylation of ketamine in human liver microsomes. *Drug Metab Dispos*. 2002;30:853-858.

209. Li Y, Coller JK, Hutchinson MR, et al. The CYP2B6*6 allele significantly alters the N-demethylation of ketamine enantiomers in vitro. *Drug Metab Dispos*. 2013;41:1264-1272.
210. Grant IS, Nimmo WS, Clements JA. Pharmacokinetics and analgesic effects of IM and oral ketamine. *Br J Anaesth*. 1981;53:805-810.
211. King H. Curare alkaloids. Part 1: tubocurarine. *J Chem Soc*. 1935;5:1381-1389.
212. Beers WH, Reich E. Structure and activity of acetylcholine. *Nature*. 1970;22: 917-922.
213. Paton WDM, Zaimis EJ. The pharmacological actions of polymethylene bistrimethylammonium salts. *Br J Pharmacol*. 1949;4381-4400.
214. Lee C. Structure, conformation, and action of neuromuscular blocking drugs. *Br J Anaesth*. 2001;87:755-769.
215. Savage DS, Cameron AF, Ferguson G, et al. Molecular structure of pancuronium bromide (3α,17β-diacetoxy-2β,16β-dipiperidino-5α-androstane dimethobromide), a neuromuscular blocking agent. Crystal and molecular structure of the water: methylene chloride solvate. *J Chem Soc B*. 1971;410-415.
216. Buckett WR, Hewett CL, Savage DS. Pancuronium bromide and other steroidal neuromuscular blocking agents containing acetylcholine fragments. *J Med Chem*. 1973; 16:1116-1124.
217. Donati F, Bevan JC, Devan DR. Neuromuscular blocking drugs in anaesthesia. *Can Anaesth Soc J*. 1984;31:324-335.
218. Thompson MA. Muscle relaxant drugs. *Br J Hosp Med*. 1980;23:164-179.
219. Ramzan MI, Somogyi AA, Walker JS, et al. Clinical pharmacokinetics of the nondepolarizing muscle relaxants. *Clin Pharmacokinet*. 1981;6:25-60.
220. Agoston S, Vermeer GA, Kertsten UW, Meijer DK. The fate of pancuronium in man. *Anaesthesist*. 1975;24:13-16. Acta Anaesthesiol Scand. 1973;17:267-75.
221. Hilgenberg JC. Comparison of the pharmacology of vecuronium and atracurium with that of other currently available muscle relaxants. *Anesth Analg*. 1983;62:524-531.
222. Segredo V, Matthay MA, Sharma ML, et al. Prolonged neuromuscular blockade after long-term administration of vecuronium in two critically ill patients. *Anesthesiology*. 1990;72:566-570.
223. Watling SM, Dasta JF. Prolonged paralysis in intensive care unit patients after the use of neuromuscular blocking agents: a review of the literature. *Crit Car Med*. 1994;22:884-893.
224. Wierda JMKH, Kleef UW, Lambalk LM, et al. The pharmacodynamics and pharmacokinetics of Org 9426, a new non-depolarizing neuromuscular blocking agent, in patients anaesthetized with nitrous oxide, halothane and fentanyl. *Can J Anaesth*. 1991;38:430-435.
225. Agoston S, Vandenbrom RHG, Wierda JMKH. Clinical pharmacokinetics of neuromuscular blocking drugs. *Clin Pharmacokinet*. 1992;22:94-115.
226. Basta SJ, Ali HH, Savarese JJ, et al. Clinical pharmacology of atracurium besylate (BW 33A): A new non-depolarizing muscle relaxant. *Anesth Analg*. 1982; 61:723-729.
227. Stenlake JB, Waigh RD, Urwin J, et al. Atracurium: conception and inception. *Br J Anaesth*. 1983;55:3S-10S.

Clinical Scenario

SEDATIVE HYPNOTICS

Susan W. Miller, PharmD, Nader H. Moniri, PhD

CHEMICAL ANALYSIS

WK has been having difficulty sleeping and does not feel well-rested. Her daughter reveals that she has been self-medicating with a "PM" (at night time) OTC product at unknown frequencies for the last 3 months. These products typically contain histamine H1 receptor antagonists such as diphenhydramine or doxylamine, which act to inhibit the arousal centers of the hypothalamus in order to promote sedation. While these agents may be useful for inducing acute drowsiness, they may in fact disturb REM sleep, leading to poor sleep quality and significant next-day grogginess. With time, patients can also become tolerant to the sedative effects. Importantly, due to their tertiary amine functional groups, H_1R antagonists also have high antagonistic affinity for muscarinic acetylcholine receptors, leading to adverse effects such as dry mouth, tachycardia, and cognitive dysfunction, including memory loss. WK's daughter describes such memory loss, which could be an adverse effect associated with this off-target mechanism.

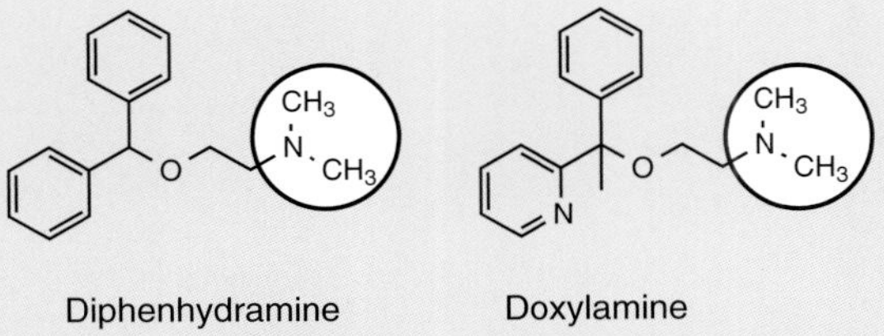

Diphenhydramine Doxylamine

Ramelteon is a structural mimic of melatonin and potently stimulates the MT_1 and MT_2 melatonin receptors with an affinity of 14 and 112 pM (picomolar), respectively. Agonism of the MT_1 receptor is primarily involved in induction and maintenance of sleep, while agonism of the MT_2 receptor primarily influences circadian rhythms. Melatonin contains an indole ring system that provides optimum distance between the amide side chain at position-3 and the 5-methoxy substituent, both of which are required to engage amino acid residues on MT_1/MT_2 to elicit functional responses. SARs for ramelteon reveal that isosteric replacement of melatonin's indole for an indane preserves functional activity. The 5-methoxy group of melatonin is

(continued)

Clinical Scenario—Continued

converted to a ring-closed furan, allowing for H-bonding with residues within TMH VI of the MT_1/MT_2 receptors, an effect that directly increases the affinity of the agent for the receptors. Since the binding pocket of melatonin receptors is highly stereoselective, ramelteon is dispensed as the enantiomerically pure (*S*)-enantiomer, which has 500-fold greater affinity for MT_1 than (*R*)-ramelteon.

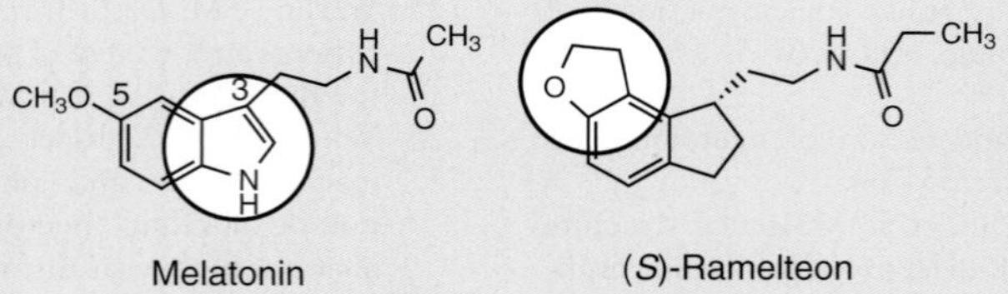

Melatonin

(*S*)-Ramelteon

The elimination of ramelteon's sedative-hypnotic effects occurs through hepatic metabolism to inactive glucuronate conjugates, which arise primarily via CYP1A2 and also via CYP2C19 and CYP3A4. WK has been taking the SSRI fluvoxamine, a strong CYP1A2 inhibitor, for depression. Inhibition of CYP1A2 by fluvoxamine would be expected to inhibit metabolism of ramelteon, leading to heightened systemic levels of the agent and pronounced sedative-hypnotic effects into the next day. Since CYP1A2 is also responsible for metabolism of caffeine, including that obtained in trace amounts from dietary sources, inhibition of this effect by fluvoxamine could also contribute to undesirable nighttime CNS stimulation and insomnia.

Initiation of ramelteon and sertraline, coupled with discontinuation of the "PM" (at night time) sleep product and fluvoxamine, should lead to more favorable sleep outcomes for WK. Finally, since alendronate, like all bisphosphonates, chelates calcium, it is also important to counsel the patient that she should take her weekly oral dose of alendronate at least 1 hour before eating her first food and taking her calcium citrate supplement on that day.

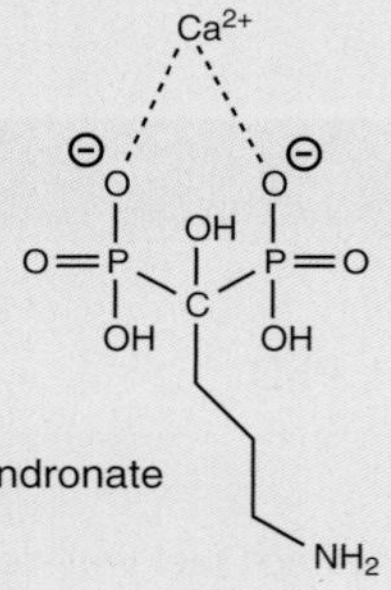

Ca^{2+}-chelated alendronate

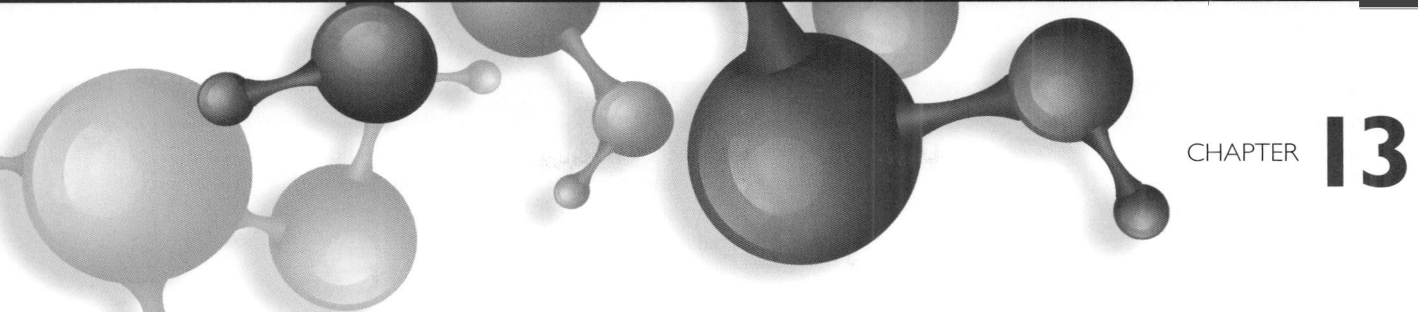

CHAPTER 13

Drugs Used to Treat Seizure Disorders

Christopher W. Cunningham

Drugs covered in this chapter:

VOLTAGE-GATED SODIUM CHANNEL BLOCKERS:
- Carbamazepine
- Eslicarbazepine acetate
- Fosphenytoin
- Lacosamide
- Lamotrigine
- Oxcarbazepine
- Phenytoin
- Rufinamide

VOLTAGE-GATED CALCIUM CHANNEL BLOCKERS:
- Ethosuximide
- Gabapentin
- Pregabalin

GABA MODULATORS:
- Clobazam
- Clonazepam
- Clorazepate
- Diazepam
- Lorazepam
- Midazolam
- Phenobarbital
- Primidone
- Tiagabine
- Vigabatrin

GLUTAMATE ANTAGONISTS:
- Brivaracetam
- Levetiracetam
- Perampanel

MULTIMODAL AEDs:
- Felbamate
- Topiramate
- Valproic acid
- Zonisamide

Abbreviations

ADH alcohol dehydrogenase
AED antiepileptic drug
AKR arylketone reductase
AMPAR α-amino-3-hydroxy-5-methyl-4-isoxazolepropionic acid receptor
AUC area under the dose-response curve
BDNF brain-derived neurotrophic factor
BZR benzodiazepine receptor
CA carbonic anhydrase
Ca_V voltage-gated calcium channels
CB1R, CB2R cannabinoid receptors 1 and 2
CBD cannabidiol
CBDV cannabidivarin
CBZ carbamazepine
CBZ-E **CBZ**-10,11-epoxide
CBZ-IQ **CBZ**-iminoquinone
cLogP cLogP calculated from Advanced Chemical Development, Toronto, Canada, 2018.
CRMP2 collapsin response mediator protein 2
DDI drug-drug interaction
DHFR dihydrofolate reductase
EAAC-1 excitatory amino acid carrier-1
EEG electroencephalography
ESL eslicarbazepine acetate
GABA γ-aminobutyric acid
GABA-T GABA transaminase
GAD glutamate decarboxylase
GAT1 GABA transporter 1
GEFS+ generalized epilepsy with febrile seizures plus
GIT gastrointestinal tract
HVA high voltage-activated
ILAE International League Against Epilepsy
IM intramuscular
IV intravenous
KR kainate receptor
LAT system L amino acid transporter
mTOR mammalian target of rapamycin
Na_V voltage-gated sodium channels
NDA new drug application
NDMC N-desmethylclobazam
NMDAR N-methyl-D-aspartate receptor
OXC oxcarbazepine
PAM positive allosteric modulator
PEMA phenylethylmalonamide
P-gp P-glycoprotein

Abbreviations—Continued

PK pharmacokinetics
SHARE Support, Help, and Resources for Epilepsy Program
SV2 synaptic vesicle 2
TEN toxic epidermal necrosis
Δ^9-THC Δ^9-tetrahydrocannabinol
TPSA topological polar surface area
TSC tuberous sclerosis complex
UGT UDP-glucuronosyltransferase
VPA valproic acid

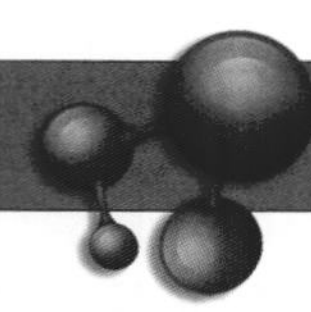

CLINICAL SIGNIFICANCE

Ernest S. Stremski, MD, MBA

The National Health Interview Survey of 2015 estimates the incidence of epilepsy in the US population as being 1.2%, affecting approximately 3 million adults and one-half million children.[1] Epilepsy is a chronic disorder characterized by unprovoked and unpredictable onset of seizures. Seizures themselves are a sudden surge of electrical activity in the brain. This electrical excitation, be it localized or generalized, results in uncontrolled neuron depolarization that is able to be captured by electroencephalogram (EEG) testing. The physical manifestation of a seizure, known as a convulsion, can affect any part of the body and often includes altered consciousness and vital sign instability with muscular rigidity or hypotonia. Characterizing the seizure by type, brain location, frequency, and EEG findings can be used by the clinical neurologist in determining the need for initiation, and proper selection, of an antiepileptic drug (AED) regimen.

Despite variability in drug classes, the AEDs minimize neuron excitation. AEDs may stop a seizure in process or be prophylaxis against recurrent seizures. Mechanisms of action of existing AEDs include preventing sodium or calcium ion influx into neurons, enhancing GABA-mediated neuron inhibition, or preventing glutamate effect on neuron excitation. Targets of the AEDs include ion channels, metabolic enzymes, and proteins of presynaptic vesicles. Knowing the structure-activity relationships between AEDs and their target has been the predominant method of identifying similar in-class AEDs. Discovering the underlying pathophysiologic alterations of neurons can aid in the design of new and novel AEDs to manage refractory epilepsy, defined as failure of AEDs to adequately control seizure occurrence. In addition, as seizures are a disturbance in the electrical balance between neurons of the brain, the existing and future AEDs must be capable of crossing the blood-brain barrier. The interaction of AEDs with *P*-glycoprotein and similar brain transporter proteins must also be taken into account when screening for and developing AEDs.

While the treatment options for ongoing seizure is well-defined, selection of an AED regimen for seizure prophylaxis is a more complex process. Many options exist and the drug's mechanism of action must best fit the underlying pathophysiologic disturbance. Expanded use of an individual's pharmacogenetic data is guiding AED decision-making by assessing metabolizer status of key enzymes (CYP2C9), risks of adverse complications based on HLA antigen presence (Stevens-Johnson syndrome), and potential for drug resistance due to efflux pumps (ABCB1). Many AEDs are known to be human teratogens, further affecting AED decision-making as such drugs must be avoided in pregnancy.

Living with epilepsy is not only challenging but carries a risk of increased mortality. Minimizing seizure frequency and duration may minimize that risk while providing enhanced quality of life. Optimal management should involve a multidisciplinary team approach at an epilepsy program to address both pharmaceutical and nonpharmaceutical approaches to treatment. Understanding how the structure of an AED may enhance that molecule's mechanism of action, or provide a more favorable kinetic property, can be an essential means to optimize pharmaceutical therapy of epilepsy.

OVERVIEW OF SEIZURE DISORDERS

Epileptic seizures were documented over 4000 years ago in early Babylonian and Hebrew writings. The work of Hippocrates, *On the Sacred Disease* (400 BC), was the first to characterize epileptic seizures as a treatable medical disorder and not a product of spiritual origin. To this point, seizure disorders were seen as a divine affliction handed down by the gods; the remedies including the avoidance of "unwholesome" foods and shunning black robes that are "expressive of death." Instead, Hippocrates proposed, seizures are a result of a hereditary dysregulation of the patient's brain. This is largely seen as a turning point in medicine: if seizures are due to an affliction in the brain, then they might be treatable with the proper medication.[2]

A seminal publication on the modern treatments of seizure disorders at the time was written by British epileptologist William Aldren Turner in 1907. His book, *Epilepsy—A Study of the Idiopathic Disease*, outlined a patient-centered approach to treating epileptic seizures that focused on the use of medications to stop active seizures and prophylactic treatments, control of diet, stress management, and also surgery to prevent future seizures. Turner considered bromide salts, first reported in the mid-1800s in London,[3] as the treatment of choice for treating patients with uncontrolled epilepsy. His studies concluded that bromide therapy was effective in 50% of his patients, with long-term remission in 23.5%; however, use of chronic, high-dose bromides resulted in "bromism," which, he remarked, "is characterized by a blunting of the intellectual faculties, impairment of the memory, and the production of a dull and apathetic state."[4] The use of bromides continued into the early 20th century when small-molecule antiepileptic drugs, phenobarbital (phenobarbitone) and phenytoin, emerged as rivals with improved outcomes in the 1920s-1930s.

The period between 1938 and 1958 saw the approval of 14 antiepileptic drugs (AEDs) by the U.S. Food and Drug Administration (FDA). The first-in-class medications were discovered largely through serendipitous findings in animal seizure models, and combinations of these medications were often more effective at preventing seizures than one drug alone. More effective second-generation AEDs were developed in the 1950s-1970s that operate simultaneously through multiple mechanisms of action and can be used as monotherapy. The third-generation AEDs were developed using modern drug discovery and medicinal chemistry techniques to avoid the side effects of first- and second-generation agents. Despite the many advances that have been made, modern AED therapy still suffers from some of the same side effects that Dr. Turner observed in his bromide patients: somnolence, memory impairment, and cognitive slowing hinder patient satisfaction and compliance. Newer medications that operate through novel, nonion channel inhibitory mechanisms may provide therapeutic benefits absent these adverse cognitive effects.

Epilepsy affects 2.2-3 million Americans and more than 65 million people worldwide. An estimated 1 in 26 people in the United States will develop epilepsy at some point in their lives, making epilepsy the fourth most common neurological disorder. Recent estimates put the costs of treating seizure disorders around $15.5 billion USD. This figure does not include the intangible adverse impact of seizure disorders on patients' quality of life.[5]

What Are Seizures?

Definitions for epileptic seizures and epilepsy are available from The International League Against Epilepsy (ILAE). An epileptic seizure is "a transient occurrence of signs and/or symptoms due to abnormal excessive or synchronous neuronal activity in the brain."[6] A hallmark of this neuronal activity is the rapid firing of electrical impulses caused by uncontrolled ion channel gating. These electrical impulses are monitored using electroencephalography (EEG). EEG measures the fluctuation of electronic current throughout the brain using noninvasive electrodes attached to the skin. Analysis of EEG readouts helps clinicians diagnose epilepsy and seizure disorders: for example, diagnosis of Lennox-Gastaut syndrome is aided by EEGs that show a definitive pattern of slow, sharp waves and paroxysmal fast activity.[7] When a patient experiences a single seizure for 5 or more minutes, or two seizures within 5 minutes, they are said to be experiencing status epilepticus.

The ILAE defines epilepsy as "a disorder of the brain characterized by an enduring predisposition to generate epileptic seizures and by the neurobiologic, cognitive, psychological, and societal consequences of this condition." These definitions clarify that a patient must experience at least one epileptic seizure in order to be diagnosed with epilepsy. Seizures may be either symptomatic—meaning the underlying cause for the seizure is known—or idiopathic. For example, symptomatic seizures may result from brain lesions, cortical malformations, or tumors, whereas the mechanisms causing idiopathic seizures are unknown. Differentiating between classifications of seizures and epilepsy disorders is critical to providing optimal patient care. For example, patients with Dravet syndrome—a symptomatic seizure disorder—should not be administered lamotrigine and carbamazepine, as these the AEDs may exacerbate seizures in these patients.[8,9]

Types of Seizures

Seizure types are classified based on three key parameters: (1) onset of action; (2) the level of consciousness in the patient; and (3) whether motor symptoms are observed. Recently, the ILAE has come up with new guidelines that clarify these seizure types (Table 13.1).[10] These guidelines were developed, in part, to be easier to understand and to permit classification of previously difficult-to-classify seizure types. These guidelines may also permit targeted selection of the appropriate medications to treat different disease states. Throughout this section, we will refer to the historically used terms; their modern counterparts can also be found in Table 13.1.

Table 13.1 Classification of Seizure Types

Onset (ILAE 2017)[a]	Examples
Partial-Onset (Focal)	
Simple (aware)	
Complex (impaired-awareness)	
Motor onset	Automatisms, atonic, clonic, epileptic spasms, hyperkinetic, myoclonic, tonic
Nonmotor onset	Autonomic, behavior arrest, cognitive, emotional, sensory
Generalized Onset	
Motor onset	Tonic-clonic or grand mal seizures, myoclonic, atonic, epileptic spasms
Nonmotor onset	Absence or petit mal seizures, myoclonic
Unknown Onset	
Motor onset	Epileptic spasms, tonic-clonic
Nonmotor onset	Behavior arrest

Based on Fisher RS, Cross JH, French JA, et al. Operational classification of seizure types by the International League against epilepsy: position paper of the ILAE Commission for classification and terminology. *Epilepsia.* 2017;58(4):522-530.

[a]Modern terms proposed by the ILAE in 2017.

Seizures are first classified by their region of onset, if it is known. Partial seizures are then classified according to the level of consciousness of the patient. All seizures are classified according to whether abnormal motor function is present (motor onset) or absent (non-motor onset).

Seizures are first classified by the degree of localization of onset in the brain. Seizures that are generalized originate simultaneously throughout the cortex in two or more of the frontal, temporal, parietal, and occipital lobes. Focal seizures (partial seizures) are those that are localized initially in a single region. A distinguishing factor between generalized and partial seizures is whether patients experience physical responses throughout the whole body as opposed to only a single region. For example, a patient experiencing visual disturbances without cognitive impairment may be experiencing a seizure localized within the occipital lobe. Seizures where the region of onset was missed or is obscured would be considered unknown onset seizures.

Partial or focal seizures can be further subdivided by the patient's level of awareness during the event. A seizure is considered simple or aware when a patient is conscious and maintains memory during the seizure; conversely, a seizure is classified as complex or impaired awareness if any of these features is lost at any point during the event. The new terminology for a simple partial seizure is "focal aware seizure," and a complex partial seizure can be considered a "focal impaired awareness seizure." Simple partial seizures are the most common form of seizure in adults. When describing a seizure event, the patient's level of awareness may not be communicated, particularly if it is either not known or not applicable. For example, impaired awareness may not be able to be communicated explicitly in a patient experiencing a generalized seizure.

Seizures can be further categorized as motor or nonmotor onset based on the most prominent observed effects. A motor seizure is one that causes the patient to experience motor disturbances, whereas a seizure that does not cause motor disturbances is considered a nonmotor or absence seizure. Tonic motor seizures cause an increase in muscle tone which results in sudden muscle stiffening. The muscles that are affected are related to the localization of the seizure: for example, a seizure that results in sudden stiffening of only a single region of the body would be considered a partial or focal tonic seizure, whereas seizures that affect the whole body tonus would be considered a generalized tonic seizure. A clonic seizure is one that causes the patient's muscles to contract and relax rapidly (a "clonus"). As with tonic seizures, clonic seizures can be either generalized or partial. A patient who experiences tonic effects followed by clonic effects is experiencing a tonic-clonic seizure, sometimes referred to as grand mal. The duration of the clonus in a tonic-clonic seizure can last several minutes. Myoclonic seizures are those that affect a single muscle or a group of muscles and result in brief spasms that last on the order of seconds. Myoclonic seizures typically affect both sides of the body simultaneously. Absence seizures were previously called petit mal seizures. Absence seizures are characterized by a brief loss of consciousness and return to normal function without subsequent lethargy.

Epilepsy Syndromes

The ILAE defines an epilepsy syndrome as "a group of clinical entities that are reliably identified by a cluster of electroclinical characteristics."[11] Epilepsy syndromes are classified by the type of seizures experienced, their frequency, and the patient population affected. Not all epilepsy syndromes may be treated using AEDs; for example, seizures from benign rolandic epilepsy generally remit spontaneously before adulthood, and AEDs may not provide much added benefit.[12]

Dravet syndrome in infants younger than 1 year of age often begins as severe febrile seizures, which are seizures precipitated by hyperthermia. These seizures progress to myoclonic or tonic-clonic seizures and may precipitate developmental delay. In 70%-85% of cases, Dravet syndrome is associated with a missense mutation in the *SNC1A* gene encoding the voltage-gated sodium channel 1α subunit ($Na_V1.1$) that causes a loss-of-function phenotype.[13,14] Patients with Dravet syndrome should not be treated with Na_V channel blockers that may exacerbate the pathology inherent in this phenotype.

Lennox-Gastaut syndrome is a childhood-onset epilepsy syndrome that is characterized by (1) tonic, atonic, and atypical absence seizures; (2) cognitive and behavioral abnormalities; (3) EEGs with generalized or diffuse slow spikes and waves, and generalized paroxysmal fast activity. Comorbidities, such as autism, cognitive, and behavioral delays, are common. Treatment of Lennox-Gastaut syndrome is challenging: over 90% of children with Lennox-Gastaut syndrome have drug-resistant epilepsy, and patients may experience additive side effects from the use of multiple medications.[15] When traditional pharmacologic treatments are ineffective, patients may experience benefits from a ketogenic diet.[16] Surgical options include the use of vagal nerve stimulation and corpus callostomy, wherein the corpus callosum is severed to block the spread of generalized seizures from one brain hemisphere to the other.[17]

West syndrome, more generally termed epileptic spasms or infantile spasms, is a rare seizure disorder in infants and young children that is characterized by three symptoms: myoclonic convulsions ("lightning attacks") that affect the whole body; sudden convulsions of neck muscles that cause the chin to jerk toward the chest ("nodding attacks"); sudden flexor spasms of the trunk and contraction of the legs and arms ("jackknife or Salaam attacks"). Most cases of West syndrome are symptomatic, rather than idiopathic. The most common cause of West syndrome is tuberous sclerosis complex (TSC), a genetic condition associated with benign tumors that precipitate seizures. Targeted therapies to treat TSC, and possibly West syndrome, are in development.

Physiologic Mechanisms Involved in Seizures

Seizures are the result of uncontrolled, asynchronous neuronal firing. Although the source(s) of this uncontrolled signaling can differ between seizure disorders and epileptic syndromes, all pharmacologic treatments modulate excitatory and inhibitory neurotransmission. Most classes of AEDs block seizures through one of three general mechanisms: (1) direct modulation of ion channels involved in neuronal depolarization; (2) inhibition of excitatory neurotransmission; (3) enhancement of inhibitory neurotransmission. A visual representation of the pharmacologic targets of AEDs can be found in Figure 13.1.

As described in more detail in Chapter 8, neurons maintain a resting potential of −70 mV. This polarized state is normally maintained by ion channels that regulate the

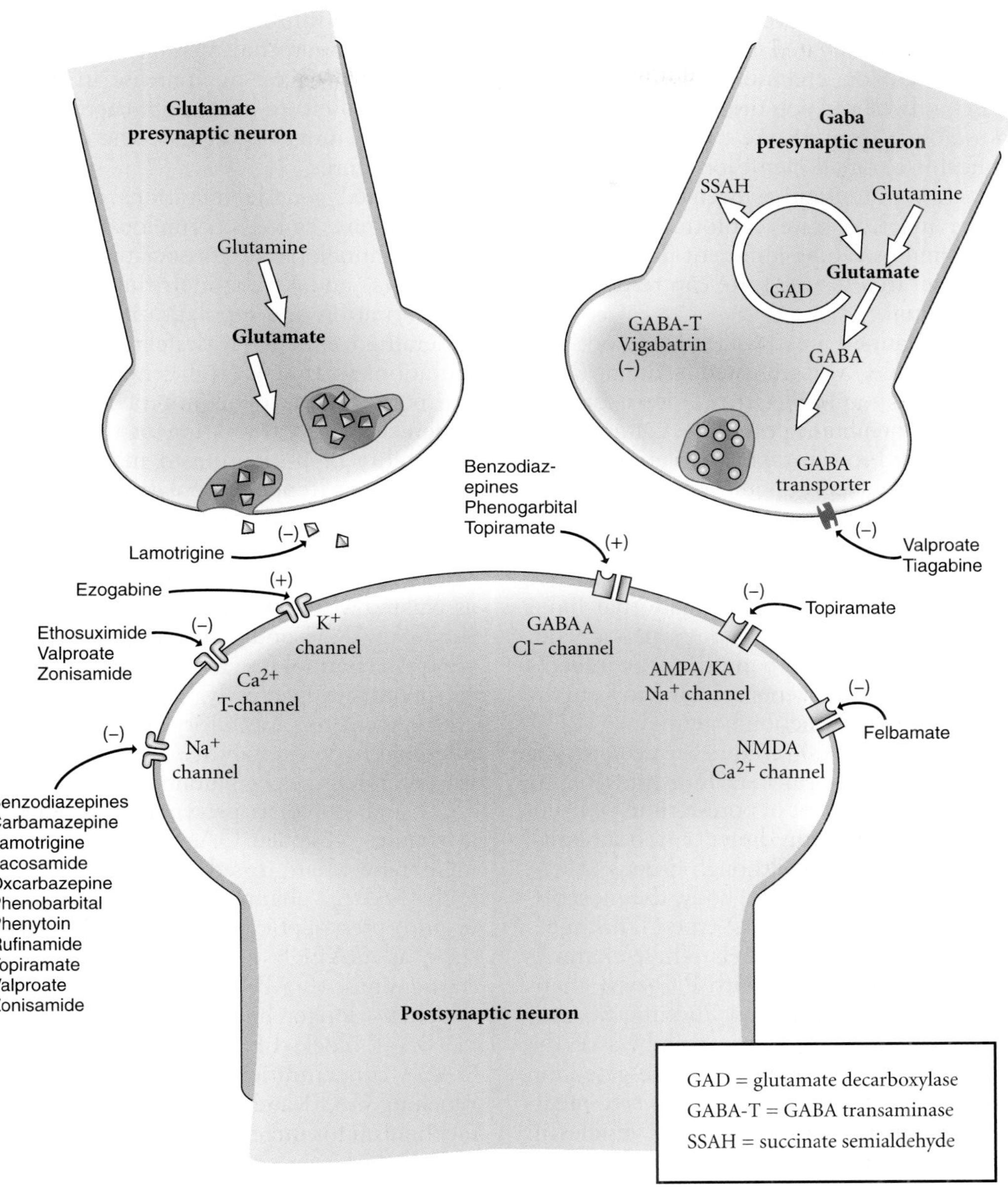

Figure 13.1 A summary of the sites of action for the antiepileptic drugs. Adapted from Taylor CP. Mechanisms of new antiepileptic drugs. In: Delgado-Escueta AV, Wilson WA, Olsen RW, et al, eds. *Jasper's Basic Mechanisms of the Epilepsies*. 3rd ed. Philadelphia: Lippincott Williams & Wilkins; 1999:1012-1027. Advances in Neurology; vol. 79; with permission.

movement of anions and cations across the cellular membrane. Channel opening that permits the influx of positively charged metal ions—sodium (Na^+), potassium (K^+), calcium (Ca^{2+})—causes cellular depolarization. Once the membrane potential is approximately −55 mV, it is said to have reached the threshold potential. Reaching threshold potential triggers a rapid depolarization phase that initiates an action potential at approximately +40 mV. After depolarization, a repolarization phase occurs, returning the membrane potential to a hyperpolarized state below −70 mV (approximately −80 mV). Hyperpolarization is reached when ion channels open to permit efflux of Na^+ or K^+ or influx of chloride (Cl^-) ions.

Ion channels activated by neurotransmitters are considered ligand-gated ion channels. Once released to the synapse, excitatory neurotransmitters like glutamate and aspartate activate ion channels such as α-amino-3-hydroxy-5-methyl-4-isoxazolepropionic acid receptors (AMPARs), N-methyl-D-aspartate receptors (NMDARs), and kainate receptors (KRs). These channels facilitate the influx of Na^+ and Ca^{2+} ions that leads to cellular depolarization. Thus, AMPAR, NMDAR, and KR blockers are able to attenuate uncontrolled neuronal firing associated with epilepsy. Following ion channel activation, excess glutamate and aspartate is taken up into presynaptic cells by excitatory amino acid transporters (EAACs), notably EAAC-1. In contrast, binding of the inhibitory neurotransmitter γ-aminobutyric acid (GABA) to the $GABA_A$ ion channel causes a conformational change that permits influx of Cl^-. This causes cellular hyperpolarization that makes the neuron less capable of firing. Positive allosteric modulators of $GABA_A$ channels block seizures by lowering the membrane potential of the cell.

Ion channels that are responsive to changes in membrane potential and not activated by neurotransmitters are called voltage-gated ion channels. A voltage-gated channel that senses a threshold potential will change conformation from a closed, resting state to an open, active state that is permeable to small metal ions (e.g., Na^+, K^+, Ca^{2+}). Once the action potential has been reached, these channels adopt an inactive state conformation that is unresponsive to a stimulus. This is different from a resting state in that a channel in a resting state can respond to a suitable electric potential.

Voltage-gated ion channels are classified based on ionic permeability: for example, voltage-gated sodium (Na_V) channels are exclusively permeable to Na^+ ions. Because they respond quickly to membrane potentials, voltage-gated ion channels are involved in the rapid depolarization and repolarization phases of the action potential. Once threshold potential is reached, postsynaptic Na_V channels open to permit the influx of Na^+ ions, causing neuronal depolarization. Reaching the action potential triggers two events: first, Na_V channels close, adopting an inactive state that limits Na^+ influx and depolarization. Then, postsynaptic voltage-gated potassium channels open, permitting the influx of K^+ ions into the cell. These two events combine to form the rapid repolarization phase of the action potential.

Voltage-gated calcium (Ca_V) channels mediate the release of excitatory neurotransmitters from presynaptic vesicles. The Ca_V channels consist of pore-forming $\alpha 1$ subunits, an extracellular glycoprotein dimer of $\alpha 2\delta$ subunits, and an intracellular β subunit.[18] Although dozens of Ca_V channels are expressed throughout the body, the most relevant to epileptic disorders are the P/Q-type ("Purkinje") channels and N-type ("neural") channels. These channels are expressed throughout the brain, with P/Q-type channels located in high concentrations on Purkinje neurons in the cerebellum. These channels are members of the high voltage-activated (HVA) family of voltage-gated ion channels. A critical role of HVA Ca_V channels is to mediate the release of glutamate from presynaptic vesicles in response to a high-voltage action potential, thereby propagating a signal. Thus, agents that inhibit glutamate release would decrease neuronal signaling by reducing excitatory neurotransmission. Low voltage-activated Ca_V channels are also known as T-type ("transient") or Ca_V3. T-type Ca_V channels can open at lower membrane potential and have smaller, shorter conductance. Hyperfunction of Ca_V3 channels contributes specifically to absence seizures.

Presynaptic vesicles respond to intracellular Ca^{2+} by releasing excitatory neurotransmitters. The synaptic vesicle 2 (SV2) family of membrane glycoproteins consists of three isoforms (SV2A, SV2B, SV2C) that are expressed on vesicular membranes throughout the brain. Of these, SV2A is the most widely expressed on glutamatergic and GABAergic vesicles. SV2A regulates the response of vesicles to an increase in intracellular Ca^{2+} mediated by presynaptic Ca^{2+} ion channels. Because SV2A is expressed on both excitatory and inhibitory vesicles, regulation of protein expression and function is critical to maintaining proper neuronal excitability. For example, both genetic knockout animals and overexpressing SV2A animals show a proconvulsant phenotype, perhaps due to decreased inhibitory neurotransmission and increased excitatory neurotransmission, respectively.[19,20] Animal studies also suggest an increase in SV2A expression in response to seizure kindling[21]; therefore, agents that control SV2A function regulate the neuronal hyperactivity during seizures.

Inherited genetic mutations that affect ion channel function are called channelopathies.[22] The most common channelopathies associated with seizure disorders affect Na^+ and K^+ channels that are involved in the fast depolarization and repolarization phases, respectively. In generalized epilepsy with febrile seizures plus (GEFS+), mutations in the *SCN1A* gene result in modifications of the pore-forming α-subunit of $Na_V1.1$ that can lead to hyperexcitability. Mutation of the *SCN1B* gene impairs the ability of β-subunits to inactivate $Na_V\beta 1$ channels, causing an extended depolarization phase.[23,24] Mutations to voltage-gated potassium channel genes *KCNQ2* and *KCNQ3* are associated with benign neonatal epilepsy disorders.[25-28] Genetic disruption of GABAergic signaling is associated with human idiopathic epilepsies. Mutations to the *GABARA1* and *GABARG2* genes result in impaired $GABA_A$ channel function due to modifications of $\alpha 1$ and $\gamma 2$ subunits, respectively.[29-31]

Augmenting inhibitory neurotransmission dampens neuronal hyperexcitability. Glutamate is converted to the inhibitory GABA by glutamate decarboxylase (GAD; Fig. 13.2) and stored in presynaptic vesicles. In response to a stimulus, vesicular GABA is transported to the axonal membrane where it is drawn into the synapse to interact with $GABA_A$ channels. Synaptic GABA is then taken up into presynaptic cells by GABA transporters (GATs), such as GAT1.[32] Degradation of GABA by GABA-transaminase (GABA-T) results in succinic semialdehyde, which no longer binds $GABA_A$ channels. Inhibitors of GABA-T block this process, thereby increasing synaptic GABA concentrations and inhibitory neurotransmission. Blocking GAT1 and preventing cellular uptake is another mechanism for increasing synaptic GABA.

Polypharmacy and polypharmacology are important topics when discussing AEDs. Polypharmacy is the concomitant use of multiple medications, generally agreed to be approximately five or more. In treating patients with seizures, particularly those with seizures that are refractory to AED monotherapy, many patients will be prescribed multiple AEDs. Polypharmacology describes the situation where a single agent operates through multiple mechanisms of action. For example, valproic acid produces anticonvulsant actions through binding to glutamatergic, GABAergic, and even monoamine neurotransmitter targets (e.g., dopamine, serotonin). Although a single "magic bullet" medication may be the most desirable from

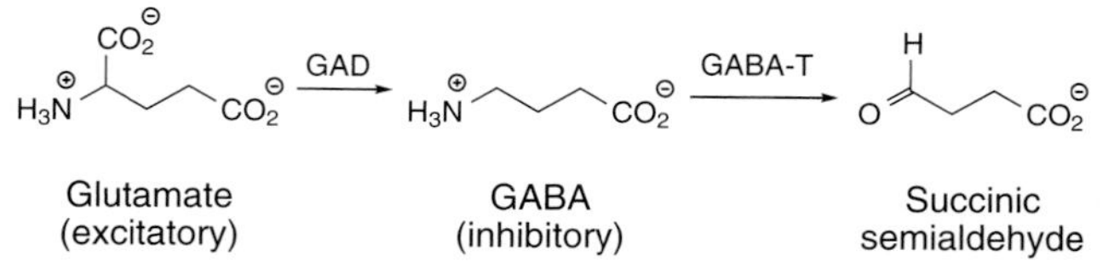

Glutamate (excitatory) —GAD→ GABA (inhibitory) —GABA-T→ Succinic semialdehyde

Figure 13.2 Regulation of glutamate and GABA. *GAD*, glutamate decarboxylase; *GABA-T*, GABA-transaminase.

a patient compliance and tolerance perspective, in many cases a rational polytherapeutic approach may lead to optimal outcomes. In this approach, two AEDs with complementary, synergistic mechanisms of action may be used in combination to best control seizures.[33]

CHEMISTRY OF COMMONLY USED ANTIEPILEPTIC DRUGS

Over 20 AEDs are available to treat seizure disorders, and the most commonly used AEDs covered in this chapter are described in Table 13.2. Health care providers may rationally combine medications that operate through synergistic mechanisms of action to afford optimal outcomes. A visual representation of the therapeutic applications of AEDs can be found in Figure 13.3.

Many AEDs are enzyme inducers, which can lead to clinically relevant drug-drug interactions (DDIs) by inducing the transcription of cytochromes P450 (CYP450s) and UDP-glucuronosyltransferases (UGTs) that are involved in metabolism and clearance of AEDs and non-AEDs. Because AEDs are frequently given in combination, it is important to understand how inducing and noninducing AEDs interact across drug classes.

Voltage-Gated Sodium Channel Modulators

Iminostilbenes

One of the oldest and most widely used classes of antiepileptic drugs is the iminostilbenes. Since the approval of carbamazepine (CBZ) in 1968, two additional iminostilbenes have reached the market, namely oxcarbazepine (OXC) and *S*(+)-licarbazepine (eslicarbazepine; Fig. 13.4).

RECEPTOR BINDING/MOA. Iminostilbenes bind to the intracellular surface of the inactive state of Na_V channels, preventing transition to the resting state. The inactive state is therefore unable to respond when the hyperactive neuron reaches threshold. By preferentially stabilizing the inactive state of Na_V, iminostilbenes have some selectivity for hyperfunctioning neurons compared to normal neuronal signaling; however, this selectivity is

Table 13.2 Mechanisms of Action of AEDs

Generic Name	Trade Name[a]	Approval (Year)[b]	Generation	Pharmacologic Targets[c]
Voltage-Gated Sodium Channel Blockers				
Phenytoin sodium	Dilantin	1953	First	Na_V
Carbamazepine	Tegretol	1968	First	Na_V
Oxcarbazepine	Trileptal	1990	Second	Na_V
Lamotrigine	Lamictal	1994	Second	Na_V, Ca_V1-3, DHFR
Fosphenytoin sodium	Cerebyx	1996	Second	Na_V
Lacosamide	Vimpat	2008	Third	Na_V(slow), CRMP2
Rufinamide	Banzel	2008	Third	Na_V1.1, Na_V1.6
Eslicarbazepine acetate	Aptiom	2013	Third	Na_V
Voltage-Gated Calcium Channel Blockers				
Ethosuximide	Zarontin	1958	First	Ca_V3
Gabapentin	Neurontin	1993	Second	$Ca_V(\alpha2\delta)$
Pregabalin	Lyrica	2005	Third	$Ca_V(\alpha2\delta)$
GABA Modulators				
Phenobarbital	Luminal	1912	First	$GABA_A$-PAM
Primidone	Mysoline	1954	First	$GABA_A$-PAM
Diazepam	Valium	1963	First	$GABA_A$-BZR
Clonazepam	Klonopin	1964	First	$GABA_A$-BZR
Midazolam	Versed	1976	First	$GABA_A$-BZR
Lorazepam	Ativan	1977	First	$GABA_A$-BZR
Clorazepate	Tranxene	1987	Second	$GABA_A$-BZR

(continued)

Table 13.2 Mechanisms of Action of AEDs (Continued)

Generic Name	Trade Name[a]	Approval (Year)[b]	Generation	Pharmacologic Targets[c]
Tiagabine	Gabitril	1997	Second	GAT-1
Vigabatrin	Sabril	2009	Third	GABA-T
Clobazam	Onfi	2011	Third	$GABA_A$-BZR
Glutamate Antagonists				
Levetiracetam	Keppra	1999	Second	SV2A
Brivaracetam	Briviact	2016	Third	SV2A
Perampanel	Fycompa	2016	Third	AMPAR
AEDs with Multiple Mechanisms of Action				
Valproic acid	Depakene, Depakote, Depacon	1976	First	GABA-T, Na_V, NMDAR, DA, 5-HT
Felbamate	Felbatol	1993	Second	$GABA_A$, Na_V, NMDAR
Topiramate	Topamax	1996	Second	Na_V, Ca_V, GABA, AMPAR, CA-II, CA-IV
Zonisamide	Zonegran	2000	Second	Na_V, Ca_V3, DA, EAAC, GAT-1, CA

[a]FDA-approved trade name.
[b]Year of FDA approval.
[c]See abbreviations section at the beginning of this chapter.

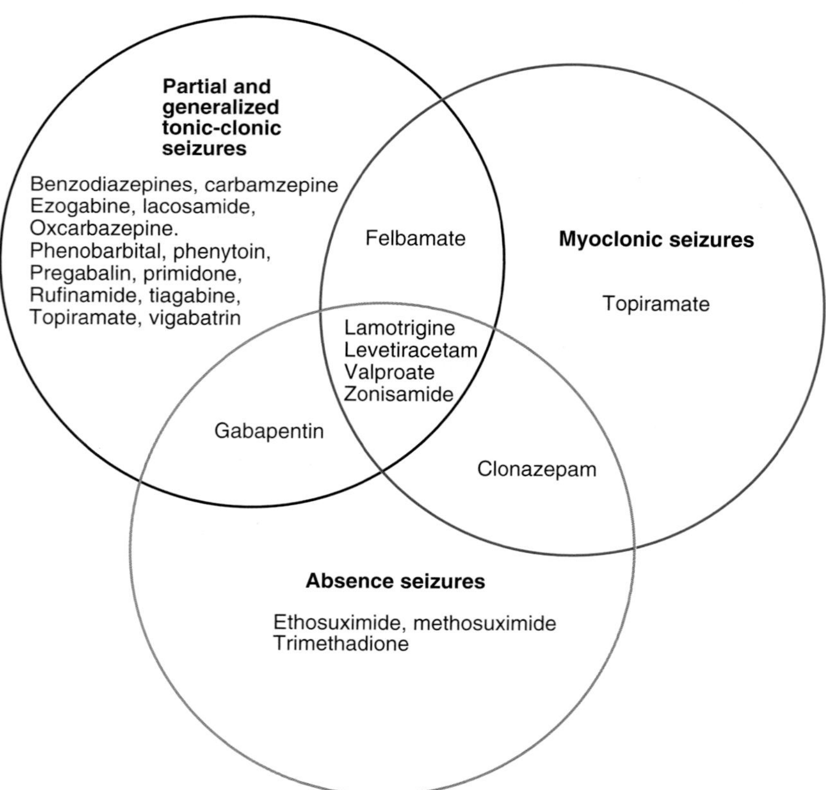

Figure 13.3 The antiseizure drugs used in treatment of the various seizures.

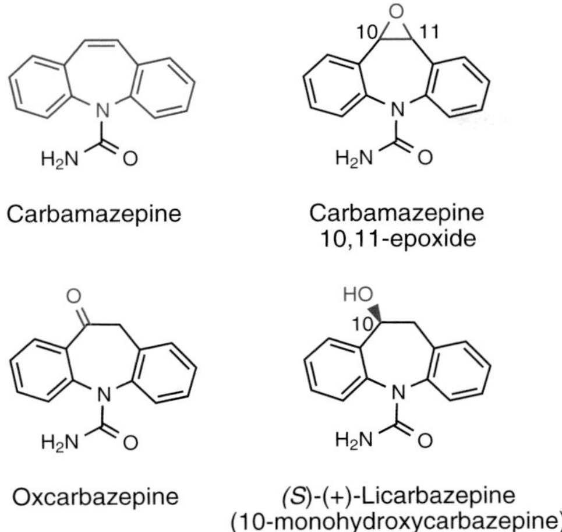

Figure 13.4 Iminostilbenes.

lost at higher doses of the older drugs, CBZ and OXC. These agents have a slow onset and long duration of anticonvulsant action.

SAR. Iminostilbenes consist of a dibenzazepine core functional moiety that resembles the tricyclic pharmacophore of chlorpromazine and other tricyclic antidepressants (Chapter 11). In fact, CBZ produces similar anticholinergic side effects as these medications. The drug retains activity when the ethylene group connecting the two aromatic rings is metabolically oxidized (Fig. 13.5). The dibenzazepine nitrogen is functionalized by a terminal urea group. This urea must be unsubstituted: alkylation here leads to a dramatic loss of anticonvulsant activity.

Physicochemical and pharmacokinetic properties of iminostilbene antiseizure agents are provided in Table 13.3.

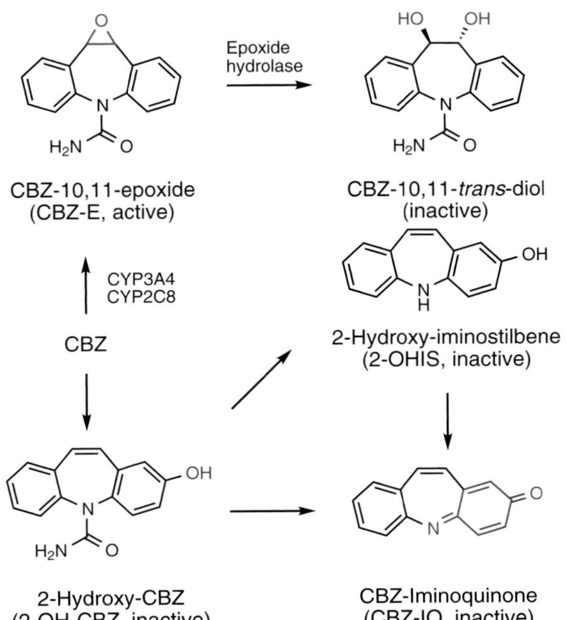

Figure 13.5 Bioactivation pathways for carbamazepine. Reactive portions of intermediates shown in red.

Table 13.3 Physicochemical and Pharmacokinetic Properties of Iminostilbenes

	CBZ	OXC	ESL[a]
clogP	2.67	1.44	0.93
Solubility (mg/mL)	0.018	0.16	0.11
TPSA (Å)	43.33	63.4	72.63
f (%)[b]	85-90	>95	>95
$t_{1/2}$ (hr)	26.2[b] 12.3[c] 8.2[d]	1-5[e] 7-20[f]	9
t_{max} (hr)	3-8	1-3	1-4
Protein binding (%)	75	37-40	30
V_d (L/kg)	0.79-1.86	0.3-0.8	0.65-0.85
Metabolized by:	CYP3A4 CYP2C8	AKR UGT	Esterases AKR
Inducer of:	CYP1A2 CYP2B6 CYP2C9 CYP3A4 UGTs P-gp	CYP3A4 CYP3A5	CYP3A4
Inhibitor of:	none	CYP2C19	CYP2C19

[a]Active (S)-licarbazepine metabolite.
[b]After a single dose.
[c]After repeated doses.
[d]When taken with other AEDs
[e]Parent drug.
[f]Active monohydroxy derivative (MHD) metabolite.
AKR, arylketone reductase; CBZ, carbamazepine; ESL, eslicarbazepine acetate; F, oral bioavailability; OXC, oxcarbazepine; TPSA, topologic polar surface area; UGT, UDP-glucuronosyltransferase; V_d, volume of distribution.

CARBAMAZEPINE (TEGRETOL). CBZ was one of the first AEDs discovered and developed entirely by the pharmaceutical industry. Initially designed as an antidepressant and antipsychotic, CBZ is one of the most commonly prescribed AEDs and is considered the gold standard against which new AED medications are compared. CBZ is indicated for complex partial and generalized tonic-clonic seizures but is inactive against absence seizures. CBZ is on the World Health Organization's 20th List of Essential Medicines.

Metabolism. The major route of metabolism of CBZ is CYP3A4 and CYP2C8 oxidation of the stilbene to the active metabolite, CBZ-10,11-epoxide (CBZ-E), followed by hydrolytic cleavage to the *trans*-diol by epoxide hydrolase (Fig. 13.5). A minor route of biotransformation is oxidation of the 2-position to produce 2-hydroxy-CBZ (2-OH-CBZ). Secondary oxidation of 2-OH-CBZ removes the urea to produce the pharmacologically inactive 2-hydroxyiminostilbene (2-OHIS), which can be converted to the iminoquinone (CBZ-IQ). CBZ-IQ may also be produced directly from 2-OH-CBZ. Some intermediates are reactive and can cause toxicities at high concentrations: for example, CBZ-E and CBZ-IQ form covalent adducts with CYP3A4 and other nucleophiles in vivo. The iminoquinone of CBZ-IQ consists of two Michael acceptors that are highly electrophilic and reactive with cell nucleophiles. The epoxide has been associated with ataxic gait in certain patients, and both reactive products may contribute to idiosyncratic toxicities.[34-36]

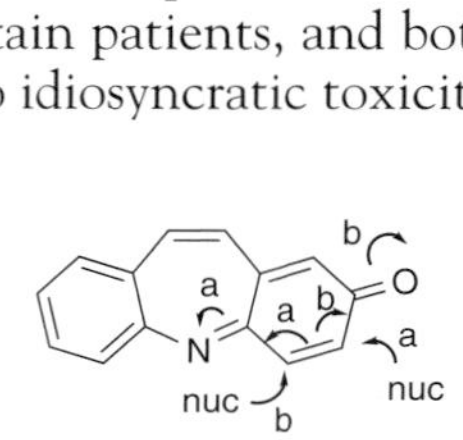

CBZ-IQ

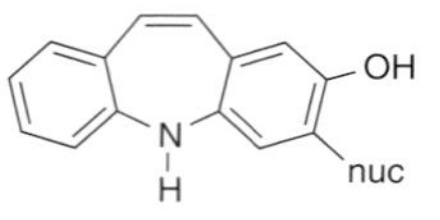

Nucleophilic attack a

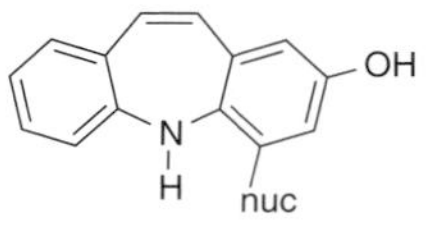

Nucleophilic attack b

The inductive effect of CBZ on CYP3A4 stimulates its own metabolism (i.e., metabolic autoinduction). Because CBZ is metabolized by CYP3A4 and induces its metabolic activity, repeated administration of CBZ results in increasingly faster clearance. In practice, this means that the dose of CBZ must be increased in patients over time to maintain therapeutic plasma levels.

Physicochemical Properties. The clogP of CBZ is approximately 2.67 and the topological polar surface area (TPSA) is 46.33Å. CBZ contains no ionizable functional groups and, as a result, is practically insoluble in water (17.7 μg/mL).

Pharmacokinetics. Tablet, capsule, and suspension formulations of CBZ are available in the United States. Dissolution of CBZ from tablets is slow, therefore absorption is unpredictable. Absorption of CBZ from the suspension is faster than that of the immediate-release (IR) tablet; thus, when substituting the suspension for the IR tablet, the dosing interval should be shortened without changing the daily dose. The IR tablet formulation has high apparent bioavailability (f_{app} 85%-90%) and the t_{max} is 3-8 hours. Plasma protein binding is approximately 75%, and V_d is 0.79-1.86 L/kg.[37] Approximately 97% of CBZ is metabolized, leaving little parent drug excreted unchanged. Elimination of CBZ and metabolites is largely renal (~70%). A pharmacokinetics study in 1985 found that the single dose $t_{1/2}$ is 26.2 hours; this was much lower in patients on CBZ monotherapy ($t_{1/2}$ 12.3 hours) and in patients taking CBZ concomitantly with other AEDs ($t_{1/2}$ 8.2 hours). Enhanced CBZ elimination means lower circulating plasma levels in these patients.[38] CBZ is a possible P-glycoprotein (P-gp) substrate.[39]

Specific Adverse Events and DDIs. Toxic epidermal necrosis (TEN) and Stevens-Johnson syndrome are rare, but serious, side effects of CBZ. The incidence is greater in patients with the *HLA-B*1502* gene variant, found almost exclusively in patients of Chinese ancestry. The risk of aplastic anemia and agranulocytosis is low, although patients should be monitored for cardiac and hepatic toxicities.[40] When coadministered with valproic acid, plasma protein binding of CBZ is reduced, causing increased free plasma fractions.[41] CBZ is an inducer of CYP1A2, CYP2B6, CYP2C9, and CYP3A4, the latter of which is the primary enzyme responsible for CBZ metabolism. Thus, coadministration of CBZ with antiepileptic drugs metabolized by these enzymes will enhance their metabolism and increase clearance. Metabolism of CBZ is also impacted by other enzyme-inducing AEDs, including phenytoin and phenobarbital: these drugs increase CBZ-E/CBZ ratio when coadministered.[42]

During pregnancy, CBZ-E/CBZ ratio is increased and CBZ and CBZ-diol plasma levels are decreased. This is a result of CYP upregulation and epoxide hydrolase downregulation. CBZ and CBZ-E cross the placental barrier and are found in breast milk; daily exposure is approximately 2-5 mg, doses sufficiently low to minimize concern when breastfeeding.[43] CBZ significantly decreases AUCs of the oral contraceptives norethisterone and ethinylestradiol by approximately 50%, increasing the risk of unplanned pregnancy unless other contraceptive methods are employed.

OXCARBAZEPINE (TRILEPTAL). Originally developed alongside CBZ in the 1960s, OXC was approved for clinical use as monotherapy or adjunctive therapy for partial seizures in adults and children in 1990. This makes OXC a second-generation AED. Though OXC and CBZ are structurally similar and act through similar MOAs, the safety and tolerability profile of OXC offers some clinical advantages over CBZ.

Metabolism. OXC is rapidly oxidized into a mixture of (*R*)- and (*S*)-monohydroxy derivatives (MHDs, also known as licarbazepine) by hepatic arylketone reductase (AKR) (Fig. 13.6). This is a largely stereoselective reduction, as the ratio of (*S*)- to (*R*)-MHD is approximately 80:20. In healthy volunteers, it was found that circulating

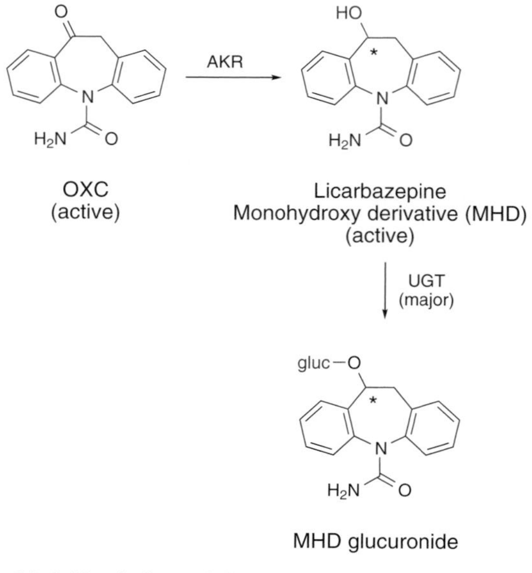

OXC (active) → AKR → Licarbazepine Monohydroxy derivative (MHD) (active) → UGT (major) → MHD glucuronide

Figure 13.6 Metabolism of OXC. *AKR*, arylketone reductase; *UGT*, UDP-glucuronosyltransferase (*chiral center).

levels of the active MHD metabolites were approximately 6-fold higher than OXC.[44] Glucuronidation of the resulting alcohols is the major phase 2 metabolic pathway. Unlike CBZ, OXC is not metabolized into CBZ-E and CBZ-10,11-*trans*-diol metabolites, the entities responsible for CBZ-induced neurotoxicities[45] and hepatic enzyme induction,[46] respectively.

Physicochemical Properties. Like CBZ, OXC contains no ionizable functional groups and is practically insoluble in water. The clogP is 1.44 and the TPSA is 63.4. Compared to CBZ, OXC is slightly more hydrophilic and polar than CBZ due to the ketone at C5. Though OXC is more hydrophilic and polar than CBZ, aqueous solubility remains low due to a lack of ionizable functional groups.

Pharmacokinetics. OXC is rapidly and completely absorbed, reaching peak concentrations within 1-3 hours. The mixture of active MHD metabolites reaches peak concentration within 2-4 hours post dose at steady state.[46] Though the AUC and C_{max} for OXC was increased when taken with food, this has negligible impact on therapeutic dosing. Calculation of the V_d of OXC is difficult because OXC is rapidly and completely metabolized. The apparent V_d of the MHD metabolites is 0.3-0.8 L/kg, with low plasma protein binding (37%-40%).[47] OXC exhibits first-order linear kinetics: $t_{1/2}$ of OXC is 1-5 hours, and $t_{1/2}$ for MHD is between 7-20 hours on oral administration. Elimination of oral OXC is mostly renal (96%), with an OXC:MHD:MHD-glucuronide ratio of approximately <1%:27%:49%.[46] Several studies estimate renal clearance in healthy volunteers is approximately 21 mL/min, which increases in elderly patients with impaired renal function. OXC is a P-gp substrate.[39]

Specific Adverse Events and DDIs. Because OXC is not a CYP substrate and, therefore, is not biotransformed to the same reactive metabolites as CBZ, tolerability of OXC is generally improved. Specifically, fewer allergic reactions and psychomotor impairments have been reported.[48] Pharmacokinetic DDIs are less pronounced for OXC compared to CBZ.[47] Only CYP3A4 and CYP3A5 are induced by OXC, compared to the pan-induction by CBZ. This is clinically relevant in that metabolic autoinduction does not occur, meaning that therapeutic dose does not need to be increased with long-term use. Coadministration with hormonal contraceptives still causes plasma levels of ethinylestradiol and progestins to decrease. OXC is an inhibitor of CYP2C19, suggesting that DDIs are possible when high doses of OXC are coadministered with AEDs phenytoin and phenobarbital, both of which are substrates of this isoform.[47]

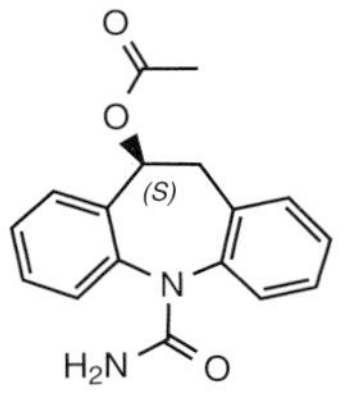

Eslicarbazepine acetate
(Aptiom)

ESLICARBAZEPINE ACETATE (APTIOM). Eslicarbazepine acetate (ESL) is a third-generation AED approved in 2013 as an add-on medication for the treatment of partial seizures. The activity of ESL is similar to other iminostilbenes in that they are structurally related and operate through the same mechanism of action, yet ESL possesses fewer toxic side effects due to a unique receptor binding profile. ESL derives its name as the acetate ester of the (*S*)-enantiomer of licarbazepine, which, as noted above, is another name for the OXC monohydroxy derivative metabolites (MHDs).

Receptor Binding/MOA. Like CBZ and OXC, ESL and its active metabolites stabilize the inactivated state of Na_V channels, thereby preventing transition to the resting state. Unlike CBZ and OXC, ESL has lower affinity for the resting state of Na_V channels; thus, ESL is expected to be more selective for rapidly firing neurons over those firing at normal, baseline levels. This means ESL is expected to produce less toxic side effects compared to other agents in this class.[49]

SAR. ESL was designed to be a prodrug of (*S*)-licarbazepine, an active MHD product of OXC metabolism (Fig. 13.6). A series of racemic aliphatic and aromatic O-esters was synthesized and evaluated for neuroprotection in a rat seizure model and a rotarod test to determine motor toxicity.[50] The greatest neuroprotection occurred with the O-acetate. Extending the ester alkyl chain to ethyl and propyl led to progressively lower antiepileptic potency. When tested for neurotoxicity, ESL was found to be two to three times less toxic than CBZ and OXC when given by intraperitoneal injection, resulting in a wider therapeutic window.

Metabolism. ESL is rapidly metabolized by hepatic esterases to the active metabolite, (*S*)-licarbazepine. This is the (*S*)-enantiomer of the same active MHD metabolite discussed earlier for OXC; thus, the metabolic fate of ESL metabolites is the same for these two agents. A minor redox biotransformation is catalyzed by AKR, which oxidatively converts (*S*)-licarbazepine to OXC that is then reduced back to enantiomeric licarbazepine, as shown in Figure 13.6.

Physicochemical Properties. Like the other iminostilbines, ESL contains no ionizable functional groups at physiologic pH. ESL is moderately more lipophilic than OXC, with clogP of 0.93. The polar ester functional group affords ESL a TPSA of 72.63. Less than 1 mg/mL is soluble in water.

Pharmacokinetics. ESL is readily absorbed following oral administration and undergoes rapid first-pass hydrolytic metabolism to the active (*S*)-licarbazepine by liver esterases. Food does not affect absorption. The drug is bound to plasma protein (~30%) and blood cells (~46%). Ninety two percent of administered ESL is eliminated in the urine as (*S*)-licarbazepine (67%) and (*S*)-licarbazepine-O-glucuronide (33%), along with other metabolites (8%). The half-life for (*S*)-licarbazepine is approximately 9 hours.[51] ESL is a probable P-gp substrate.[39]

Specific Adverse Events and DDIs. Adverse effects are generally mild and consist of somnolence, vomiting, diplopia, headaches, and dizziness. Adverse effects are dose-related, and increased doses may augment the risk of depression and suicidal thoughts and behavior occasionally

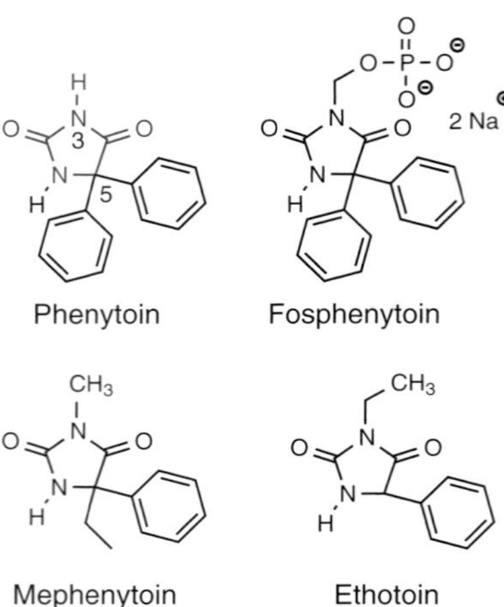

Figure 13.7 Hydantoins. The pharmacophore is shown in red.

seen with antiepileptic drugs in general. The extent of CYP induction is considerably lower compared to CBZ. The parent drug ESL does not induce major CYP isoforms, although the (*S*)-licarbazepine MHD metabolite does induce CYP3A4. This can reduce plasma levels of ethinylestradiol and progestin hormonal contraceptives. Both ESL and MHD are inhibitors of CYP2C19 and enhance blood plasma levels of phenytoin and phenobarbital.[52]

Hydantoins

The hydantoins have been used as AEDs since the mid-1950s. The antiepileptic efficacy of the first hydantoin to be discovered, phenytoin (Fig. 13.7), resulted from a rational search of structurally related analogues of phenobarbital that do not cause sedation. Several hydantoin analogues have been developed since, including fosphenytoin, mephenytoin, and ethotoin.

RECEPTOR BINDING/MOA. Like iminostilbenes, hydantoins inhibit Na_V channels. In fact, the pharmacologic actions of hydantoins—slow onset and long duration of action—so closely resemble those of other Na_V blockers that it is proposed that they all share a similar molecular mechanism of action.[53] As shown in Figure 13.8, the two aromatic rings of phenytoin occupy a similar chemical space as the two aromatic rings of the Na^+ channel blockers CBZ and lamotrigine. Molecular modeling using a Na_V homology model suggests that hydantoins, like iminostilbenes and lamotrigine, are capable of binding to a lipophilic domain containing Tyr1771 and Phe1764.[54] In this model, the imide NH of phenytoin (bolded in Fig. 13.8) engages in a unique hydrogen bond with the π-electrons of the Phe side chain.

SAR. Hydantoins contain a common five-membered core called a ureide. The term ureide is derived from the functional groups "urea" and "imide." The imide nitrogen (position 3, Fig. 13.7) of phenytoin bears a weakly acidic proton with a p*K*a of approximately 8-9. The conjugate base form is resonance-stabilized by the two adjacent carbonyl groups. The acidic character of the imide is nonessential, as the imide nitrogen can also be alkylated (mephenytoin, ethotoin) and retain activity. Another critical element to the hydantoin pharmacophore is the presence of one to two unsubstituted phenyl rings on position 5. Substitution on even one phenyl ring, such as addition of a *p*-fluorine, results in a substantial loss of activity.[55,56]

Physicochemical and pharmacokinetic properties of N_{av} antiseizure agents, including hydantoins, are provided in Table 13.4.

PHENYTOIN SODIUM (DILANTIN). Phenytoin was the first hydantoin discovered that effectively suppresses electrically induced convulsions in animals.[57,58] In fact, the name phenytoin is derived from the common name of its chemical structure, which is a 5,5-diphenylhydantoin. An analogue of phenobarbital and an AED with potent sedative/hypnotic activity, phenytoin was found to be anticonvulsant absent sedative effects.[59] At the time of its discovery, phenytoin was the most potent, nonsedating anticonvulsant available. Oral dosage forms of phenytoin are approved to treat tonic-clonic and focal seizures, and fast-acting injectable formulations of phenytoin sodium are available to treat status epilepticus. Phenytoin is on the World Health Organization's 20th List of Essential Medicines.

Metabolism. Phenytoin is metabolized extensively (>95%) by CYP2C9 and CYP2C19 to the *p*-phenol metabolite, 5-(4′-hydroxyphenyl)-5-phenylhydantoin (HPPH), and to a lesser extent to the corresponding catechol (Fig. 13.9). The first step in oxidation occurs through the formation of an arene oxide intermediate. This epoxide is highly reactive to proteins, including the CYP enzymes responsible for its formation. Formation of covalent protein adducts is one possible mechanism underlying phenytoin toxicity.[60] Further oxidation of HPPH to the phenytoin catechol can be catalyzed by a number of CYP

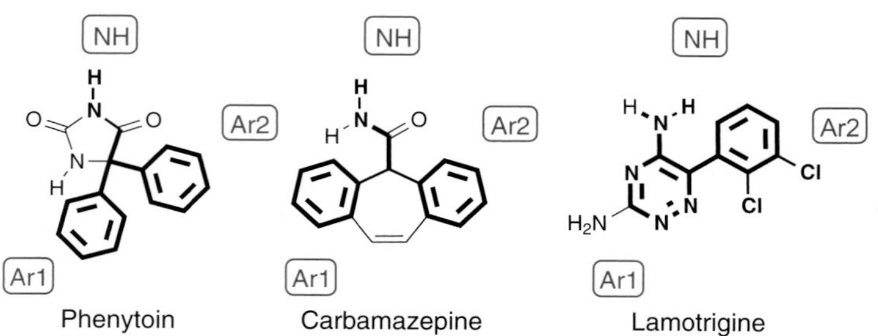

Figure 13.8 Proposed common binding mode within the Na_V channel for phenytoin, carbazepine, and lamotrigine. Ar1 and Ar2 on each agent may interact with F978, L1465, I1469, and Y1771, and the bolded NH is proposed to engage in an orthogonal π-dipole interaction with F1771.

Table 13.4 Physicochemical and Pharmacokinetic Properties of Na_V Blockers

	PHT	FPHT	LTG	LAC	RFM
clogP	2.52	0.47	−0.19	0.90	0.05
Solubility (mg/mL)	0.02 (free acid) 3 (Na^+ salt)	142	0.17	20.1	0.03
TPSA (Å)	58.2	116.17	89.12	67.43	73.8
f (%)	70-100	100[a]	>98	100	80-85
$t_{1/2}$ (hr)	15-22	<0.2	25-30	12-16	6-10
t_{max} (hr)	1.5-3	3	1.4-4.8	0.5-4	4-6
Protein binding (%)	95	95-99	55	<15	26-34
V_d (L/kg)	0.7-0.8	0.04-0.13	0.9-1.3	0.6	0.8-1.2
Metabolized by:	CYP2C9 CYP2C19	Phosphatases	UGT1A4	CYP2C19	CEs
Inducer of:	CYP3A4 CYP2C9	CYP3A4[b] CYP2C9	None	None	CYP3A4
Inhibitor of:	None	None	None	None	None

[a]Bioavailability of phenytoin after biotransformation.
[b]Based on conversion to phenytoin.
CE, carboxyesterase; F, oral bioavailability; FPHT, fosphenytoin; LAC, lacosamide; LTG, lamotrigine; PHT, phenytoin; RFM, rufinamide; TPSA, topologic polar surface area; V_d, volume of distribution.

isoforms, with CYP2C19 potentially playing a key role. The catechol is subjected to further oxidation to the *o*-quinone, which is capable of direct oxidation of DNA.[61] This second mechanism of oxidative toxicity may also contribute to the toxicologic profile of phenytoin.[62,63] Conversion of phenytoin and HPPH into innocuous metabolites by UGTs is a protective mechanism against toxicity.[64]

Physicochemical Properties. Phenytoin is weakly acidic (pKa 8.3). With a clogP of 2.52, it is lipopophilic and poorly water soluble (20-30 μg/mL).[65] While the sodium salt is substantially more soluble in water (3 mg/mL), it is still considered to be of low aqueous solubility. The polar surface area is 58.2 Å and is readily able to enter the brain.

Pharmacokinetics. Oral capsule, tablet, and suspensions show high bioavailability (70%-100%) and high plasma protein binding (90%). In adults, V_d is approximately 0.7-0.8 L/kg and C_{max} is reached between 1.5-3 hours. The elimination $t_{1/2}$ of phenytoin ranges from 15-22 hours following repeated dosing of a standard 300 mg oral dose. Phenytoin is a substrate for P-gp.[39]

Phenytoin demonstrates nonlinear pharmacokinetics. From a therapeutic perspective, this means that higher doses cause saturation of metabolizing enzymes and a decrease in elimination rate. Once metabolic saturation has been reached, a small increase in phenytoin dose can cause a large increase in drug plasma levels. Furthermore,

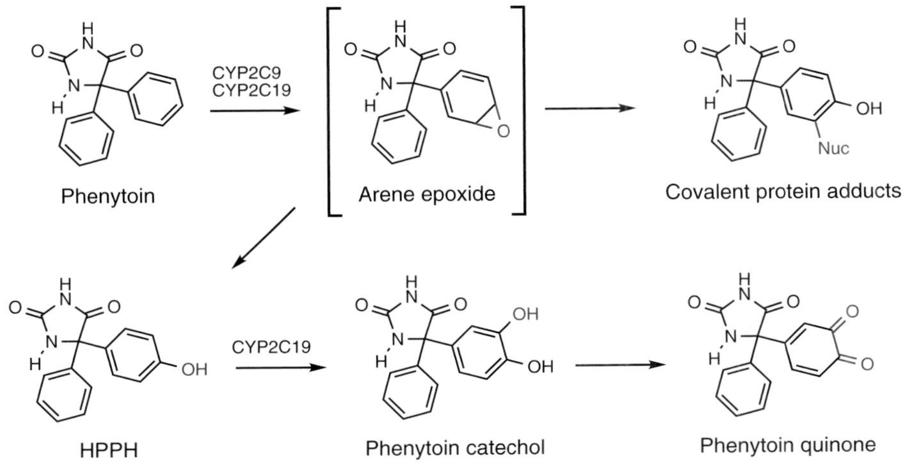

Figure 13.9 Phase I metabolism of phenytoin. *Nuc*, nucleophile.

there is wide interpatient variability in phenytoin metabolism and elimination, as discussed above. For these reasons, phenytoin therapeutic drug monitoring (TDM) is clinically important, especially so in patients with hepatic or renal dysfunction.

Specific Adverse Events and DDIs. Severe toxicities associated with unintentional phenytoin poisoning include Stevens-Johnson syndrome and TEN, both of which can be life-threatening. A rare disorder called purple glove syndrome can occur in elderly patients taking high doses of phenytoin. This is characterized by localized pain, swelling, and a blue-purple discoloration of the skin proximal to the injection of intravenous (IV) phenytoin. In extreme cases, the skin will become necrotic and may require excision. Fetal hydantoin syndrome is the collection of teratogenic effects in children of mothers administered phenytoin during pregnancy. Children are born with microcephaly and limb and cardiac birth defects and often experience cognitive and developmental delays. Due to poor solubility in aqueous solution, injectable phenytoin formulations contain propylene glycol and ethanol that may contribute to cardiac toxicities. These toxicities are rare with ingested phenytoin.

Phenytoin has a narrow therapeutic window; thus, coadministration with other agents that enhance absorption and distribution, or inhibit metabolism and elimination, will potentially cause an increase in toxicities. Because phenytoin has high plasma protein binding (90%), coadministration with other highly bound agents, or in patients with renal impairment, free (unbound) drug levels will be enhanced to potentially toxic levels. Enzyme-inducing AEDs, such as CBZ and OXC, enhance phenytoin metabolism, shortening duration. Phenytoin induces CYP2C9 and CYP3A4. This can significantly impact the clearance of coadministered agents, including certain AEDs and hormonal contraceptives.

Other Important Aspects of Drug Chemistry. Although phenytoin sodium is available as an injectable formulation to treat status epilepticus, significant issues arise on injection. As discussed earlier, phenytoin and phenytoin sodium are poorly aqueous-soluble. Phenytoin sodium is formulated in pH 12 buffer containing 40% propylene glycol/10% ethanol to facilitate solubility and dissolution. Precipitation of active drug following IV administration can cause significant soft tissue pain and irritation to the local venous environment. Intramuscular (IM) injection also produces intense pain due to precipitation of the drug in muscle. Furthermore, rapid injection of phenytoin sodium can result in severe, life-threatening hypotension.

FOSPHENYTOIN SODIUM (CEREBYX). Due to the clinical success of phenytoin in treating seizures, and the significant adverse effect profile associated with the injectable formulation, development began in the early 1980s to develop an aqueous-soluble prodrug of phenytoin. The result of a decade of research was fosphenytoin sodium (Cerebyx; Fig. 13.7), a second-generation AED approved in 1996 to treat convulsive status epilepticus.

Metabolism. Fosphenytoin sodium is rapidly and completely metabolized by phosphatases to 3-hydroxymethylphenytoin. This 3-hydroxymethyl intermediate is chemically unstable and rapidly degrades to release the active phenytoin and a formaldehyde byproduct. The rate of metabolic conversion to phenytoin is on the order of 8-10 minutes. Unchanged fosphenytoin is not detected in urine samples. Metabolism of phenytoin then occurs as described above (Fig. 13.9).

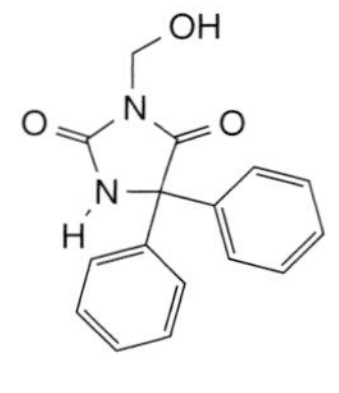

3-Hydroxymethylphenytoin

Physicochemical Properties. Fosphenytoin sodium is over 4400 times more aqueous-soluble than phenytoin (142 mg/mL vs. 0.02 mg/mL).[65] The phosphate ester prodrug has an acidic pKa (1.46) and is formulated as the disodium salt. The polar surface area of the prodrug is 116.17 Å, which would suggest poor central bioavailability; however, rapid bioactivation produces phenytoin which, with a polar surface area of only 58.2 Å, is readily able to cross the blood-brain barrier (BBB).

Pharmacokinetics. The bioavailability of fosphenytoin's active metabolite, phenytoin, is nearly 100% following IM injection based on the AUC of IV phenytoin.[66] When given orally, the phenytoin AUC for fosphenytoin sodium solution is indistinguishable from oral phenytoin.[67] Compared to IV phenytoin, administration of IM fosphenytoin sodium results in a lower C_{max} (8.92 ± 0.35 vs. 5.68 ± 0.20 μg/mL, respectively) and higher t_{max} (0.32 ± 0.03 vs. 3.13 ± 0.23 hr, respectively).[68] This may be due to the poor aqueous solubility of phenytoin suspension interfering with bioavailability.[67] Due to high polarity and plasma protein binding, phosphenytoin has an apparent V_d of approximately 0.04-0.13 L/kg.[69] Fosphenytoin clearance ranges from 12.9 to 22.8 L/hr as a function of dose and infusion rate, with higher doses leading to higher unbound fraction and enhanced clearance.[69]

Specific Adverse Events and DDIs. The adverse event profile of fosphenytoin is similar to that of phenytoin. A statistically relevant observation in clinical trials is that fewer patients experience injection-site pain with fosphenytoin sodium (6%) compared to phenytoin sodium (25%).[70]

Miscellaneous Na_V Channel Modulators

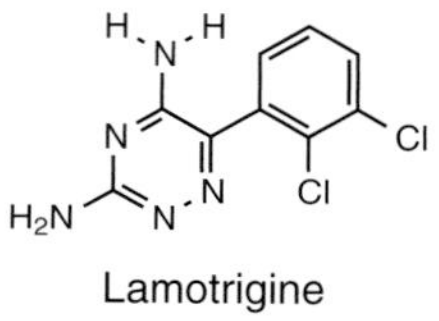

Lamotrigine

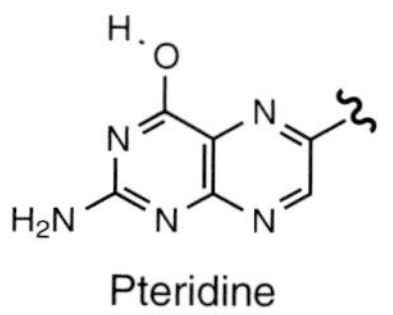

Pteridine (enol tautomer)

LAMOTRIGINE (LAMICTAL). Lamotrigine was approved in 1994 as adjunctive therapy for partial seizures, Lennox-Gastaut syndrome, and primary generalized tonic-clonic seizures in adults and pediatric patients over 2 years of age. Lamotrigine is also approved for conversion to monotherapy for adults with partial seizures who are receiving another single AED.

Receptor Binding/MOA. Lamotrigine works similarly to CBZ and phenytoin as an inhibitor of presynaptic fast Na_V channels. Evidence supports additional anticonvulsant mechanisms, including blockade of L-, N-, and P/Q/R-type Ca_V channels that may lead to a broader spectrum of anticonvulsant activity. Lamotrigine is an inhibitor of dihydrofolate reductase. This does not impact anticonvulsant activity but may contribute to a unique adverse effect profile.

SAR. Lamotrigine is a 1,2,4-triazine, the only approved AED with this structural core. The central hypothesis that led to the discovery of lamotrigine was that, because other AEDs known in the 1960s (phenytoin and phenobarbital) caused folate deficiency, perhaps anticonvulsant activity was directly related to folate antagonism. Wellcome Research Laboratories studied several series of N-heterocycles that mimic the pteridine ring system of folic acid and found that BW430C, later known as lamotrigine, produced strong anticonvulsant effects with weak antifolate activity.[71]

Metabolism. Lamotrigine is extensively metabolized to pharmacologically inactive products. The major metabolite is the N2-glucuronide (LMG-N2-G; Fig. 13.10), which accounts for 75%-90% of the dose. A minor route of metabolism results in generation of an arene epoxide intermediate that is highly reactive to biologic nucleophiles such as reduced glutathione (GSH). Reaction of GSH with this arene oxide may result in a lamotrigine-GSH adduct, which could be responsible for the AED hypersensitivity reactions seen in some patients.[72]

Physicochemical Properties. The 1-amino substituent of lamotrigine is weakly basic, with pKa = 5.87. This means that over 90% of the drug will be in the uncharged conjugate base state at physiologic pH. Lamotrigine is very slightly soluble in water (0.17 mg/mL). The physicochemical properties are in line with properties suggestive of high CNS bioavailability (clogP = −0.19, TPSA = 89.12 Å).

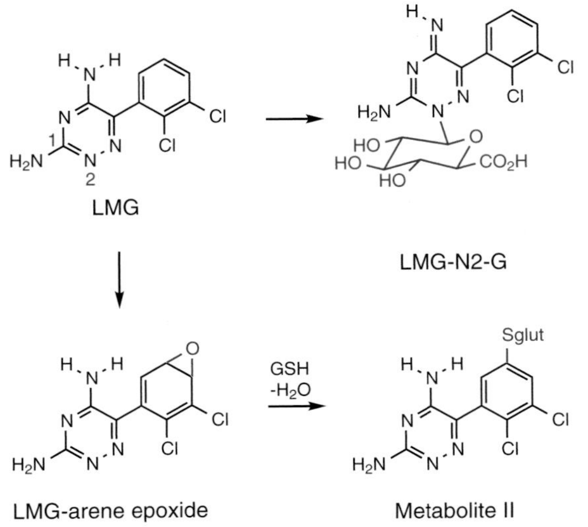

Pharmacokinetics. Lamotrigine is rapidly and completely absorbed on oral administration (absolute bioavailability >98%) with negligible first-pass metabolism. Food does not impact absorption and t_{max} is reached between 1.4-4.8 hours. The estimated V_d range is 0.9-1.3 L/kg and is not altered in patients with epilepsy compared to healthy volunteers. Lamotrigine is not extensively bound to plasma proteins (55%). The major route of inactivation is through N2-glucuronidation (Fig. 13.10). Elimination is largely renal (94%) and consists of 10% unchanged drug, 85% glucuronides, and around 5% other minor metabolites (e.g., GSH conjugate). The elimination $t_{1/2}$ in patients taking only lamotrigine ranges from 25-30 hours over single and multiple doses. Apparent plasma clearance is 0.44-0.58 mL/min/kg. Patients with renal and hepatic insufficiency have significantly increased $t_{1/2}$ and lowered plasma clearance. Lamotrigine is a P-gp substrate.[39]

Specific Adverse Events and DDIs. Serious adverse events related to AED hypersensitivity syndrome may be seen, especially when coadministered with valproic acid. The development of myoclonus after 2-3 years of treatment has also been reported.[73] Other common side effects include somnolence, headache, dizziness, diplopia, ataxia, and nausea. Concomitantly administered AEDs that induce UGT enzymes cause a significant decrease in blood plasma levels of lamotrigine. Valproate significantly reduces lamotrigine clearance by inhibiting UGT; thus, the dose of lamotrigine should be reduced to avoid toxicities. Coadministration with the oral contraceptive ethinylestradiol increased apparent clearance of lamotrigine by 2-fold, but the AED did not impact ethinylestradiol pharmacokinetics.[74] In contrast to estrogens, progestins have no effect on lamotrigine pharmacokinetics. While lamotrigine itself has no effect on the plasma levels of coadministered ethinylestradiol, it does impact the clearance of progestins.

LMG

LMG-N2-G

LMG-arene epoxide

GSH
$-H_2O$

Metabolite II

Figure 13.10 Metabolism of lamotrigine. *GSH*, glutathione; *glut*, glutathione.

LACOSAMIDE (VIMPAT). Lacosamide is a third-generation AED approved by the FDA in 2008 as an adjuvant for partial-onset seizures in adults. The deceptively simple amino acid structure of lacosamide belies a complex mechanism of action that remains incompletely understood. Lacosamide has an improved safety profile over older Na_V channel blockers, with minimal DDIs or induction of metabolic enzymes.

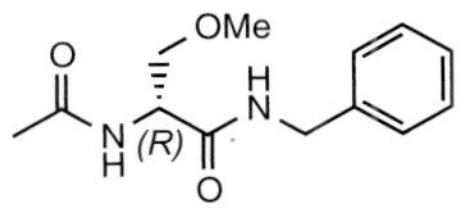

(*R*)-Lacosamide

Receptor Binding/MOA. Lacosamide has a multimodal mechanism of action. First, lacosamide inhibits hyperexcitability through enhanced slow inactivation of

Na_V channels. This is different from CBZ and phenytoin, which modify fast inactivation of Na_V channels. This distinct mechanism of Na_V blockade suggests that lacosamide may potentially be effective as an adjuvant for patients with drug-resistant epilepsy.[75,76]

A second lacosamide mechanism that may contribute to its antiepileptic effects involves the intracellular phosphoprotein collapsin response mediator protein 2 (CRMP2).[77] CRMP2 is involved in neuronal differentiation and axonal outgrowth induced by brain-derived neurotrophic factor (BDNF). Since CRMP2 function is dysregulated in treatment-resistant epilepsy patients compared to controls,[78] there is a potentially unique neuroprotective mechanism of lacosamide in treating refractory epilepsy disorders.[79]

SAR. Lacosamide can be considered a "functionalized amino acid" because of a simple substituted amino acid backbone. Since the discovery that N-acetyl-D, L-alanine benzyl amide was effective in animal models of epilepsy, extensive SAR studies showed several key trends that led to the development of lacosamide. First, there is a stereochemical preference for (*R*)- over (*S*)-enantiomers, with a eudismic (*R*)/(*S*) ratio of approximately 10. Second, there is a preference for heteroatoms separated from the amino acid backbone by a single carbon atom; in lacosamide, the methyl ether assumes this role. Substitution of this side chain with heteroaromatic groups—particularly 2-furyl, 2-pyrrolyl, or 2-pyridinyl that possesses the properly spaced heteroatom—also maintains activity. The N-acetamide can be replaced by a *t*-butyl amide with a modest loss of potency, but other modifications are not tolerated. The benzyl group is also required for activity and is modestly sensitive to substitution.[80,81]

Metabolism. Compared to Na^+ channel blockers described previously, lacosamide is relatively stable to metabolism. Approximately 40% of the parent drug is excreted unchanged, and 30% is eliminated as the inactive O-desmethyl metabolite. The rest of the dose is excreted as presently unidentified polar metabolites. The enzyme primarily responsible for this metabolism is CYP2C19.

Physicochemical Properties. Lacosamide solubility in phosphate-buffered saline at pH 7.5 is 20.1 mg/mL.[79] As an amino acid derivative, lacosamide is modestly polar with a clogP of approximately 0.90. The TPSA of lacosamide is 67.43 Å, which is appropriate for high central bioavailability.

Pharmacokinetics. Lacosamide displays linear pharmacokinetics. The drug is rapidly and completely absorbed (100%) following oral administration, with t_{max} 0.5-4 hours after dose. Peak plasma concentrations (C_{max}) rise proportionately with increasing dose: in a phase I trial in healthy volunteers, C_{max} following a single 400 mg dose was 8.7 ± 1.8 μg/mL and 14.3 ± 2.3 μg/mL after a 600 mg dose.[82] Lacosamide has low (<15%) plasma protein binding and the V_d is 0.6 L/kg.[83] The elimination $t_{1/2}$ is approximately 3 hours in otherwise healthy patients, which increases with severe renal impairment. Renal excretion accounts for around 95% of lacosamide elimination, which should also be monitored in renally impaired patients.[82] An intravenous form of lacosamide is available for refractory status epilepticus.[84]

Specific Adverse Events and DDIs. Compared to other AEDs, lacosamide is generally well-tolerated with few serious adverse effects. In preclinical animal studies, ataxia and reduced motility were mild and dose-limiting. A particular advantage of lacosamide over other AEDs like phenytoin, valproate, and zonisamide is the lack of teratogenic effects.[79] Emerging evidence suggests patients with cardiac risk factors should be monitored when taking lacosamide because of its effect on modulating slow inactivation of Na^+ channels in cardiac cells.[85]

Preclinical evaluation of lacosamide revealed no induction of five CYP isoforms (1A2, 2B6, 2C9, 2C19, 3A4) in human hepatocytes, and only weak inhibition of a panel of 10 CYPs at concentrations 30-fold higher than therapeutic plasma levels.[79] Thus, there are few clinically relevant DDIs to consider with lacosamide.

Other Important Aspects of Drug Chemistry. Like many AEDs, lacosamide is also effective in certain pain conditions, for example, neuropathic pain.[86] Lacosamide is a DEA Schedule V drug.

RUFINAMIDE (BANZEL). Rufinamide was FDA-approved in 2008 as an adjuvant agent to treat children over 4 years of age and adults with Lennox-Gastaut syndrome. More recent evidence suggests rufinamide may also be effective as an add-on for treating refractory partial seizures.[87] As a third-generation AED, rufinamide operates through a unique mechanism of action that may aid in treating refractory seizures, and its pharmacokinetic properties suggest enhanced safety and tolerability compared to older agents.

F N N N F NH2 O

Rufinamide
(CGP 33,101)

Receptor Binding/MOA. Like the AEDs described earlier, the mechanism of action of rufinamide includes inhibition of Na_V channels. Unlike other Na_V inhibitors, however, rufinamide appears to selectively alter $Na_V1.1$ and $Na_V1.6$ channel activation. Rufinamide prolongs Na_V channel time in the inactive state by slowing the recovery from inactivation.

SAR. Rufinamide is the sole member of a class of N-benzyltriazole-based AEDs. Little is definitively understood about the SAR of this class. The benzyl ring is substituted at the 2,6 (*ortho*) positions with fluorines. These fluorine atoms are not hard-and-fast requirements, however, as defluorinated analogues maintain inhibitory efficacy at $Na_V1.1$ channels.[88] The central triazole core is substituted at the 4-position by a terminal carboxamide group. This amide group appears to be essential for activity, as the carboxylic acid metabolite (Fig. 13.11) and a synthetic alcohol derivative are both inactive at Na_V channels.[88]

Metabolism. Rufinamide is biotransformed into an inactive carboxylic acid metabolite by human carboxyesterase-1 (hCE-1; Fig. 13.11). Other minor metabolites found in urine appear to be acyl glucuronides of this acid metabolite.[89]

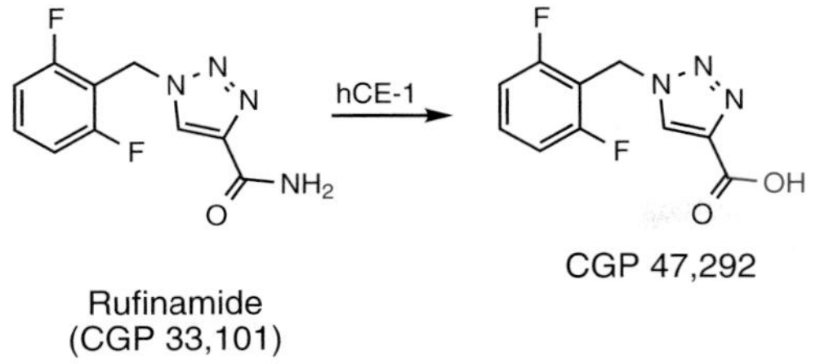

hCE-1

Rufinamide (CGP 33,101)

CGP 47,292

Figure 13.11 Rufinamide (CGP 33,101) and its inactive carboxylic acid metabolite. *hCE-1*, human carboxyesterase-1.

Physicochemical Properties. Rufinamide is a chemically neutral small molecule, with clogP 0.05 and TPSA 73.8 Å. Rufinamide is practically insoluble in aqueous solution (31 μg/mL) and is very slightly soluble in ethanol (440 μg/mL).[90]

Pharmacokinetics. Oral bioavailability of rufinamide is 80%-85%, which is enhanced when taken with food. Rufinamide has low (26%-34%) plasma protein binding, and t_{max} 4-6 hours. The V_d is 0.8-1.2 L/kg. The $t_{1/2}$ for rufinamide is 6-10 hours, which is not altered by renal impairment. Only ~2% of parent drug is excreted in urine. Elimination of rufinamide follows nonlinear Michaelis-Menten kinetics.

Specific Adverse Events and DDIs. Rufinamide is generally well-tolerated in children and adults. An analysis from clinical trials found that the most common side effects in children were somnolence, vomiting, and headache, which can be limited by slowing the increase in dose.[91] Another trial found that rufinamide causes no cognitive impairment over a range of therapeutic doses.[92] Children can also experience higher incidence of rash and AED hypersensitivity syndrome, which both subside on discontinuation.[93]

Though rufinamide does not inhibit major CYP isoforms at therapeutic doses, significant DDIs are possible, particularly in younger patients. Induction of CYP3A4 may be responsible for the observed increase in metabolism of midazolam, ethinylestradiol, and progestins that are metabolized by this isoform. Rufinamide has no effect on the plasma concentrations of valproate, topiramate, or olanzapine and may decrease plasma levels of CBZ and lamotrigine and increase levels of phenobarbital and phenytoin. Valproate increases plasma concentrations of rufinamide, possibly through inhibition of hCE-1. Phenobarbital, primidone, and phenytoin modestly decrease plasma levels of rufinamide through unknown mechanisms.[94]

Voltage-Gated Calcium Channel Modulators

Gabapentinoids

The most successful class of voltage-gated calcium (Ca_V) channel modulators are actually structural analogues of GABA, known as gabapentinoids (Fig. 13.12). Owing to the serendipity of drug discovery, both agents were initially designed to mimic GABA binding to GABAergic targets: in the case of gabapentin, the idea was to develop a more lipophilic and bioavailable $GABA_A$ receptor agonist, and pregabalin was designed as a GABA-T inhibitor. Instead, both compounds are potent blockers of HVA Ca_V channels.

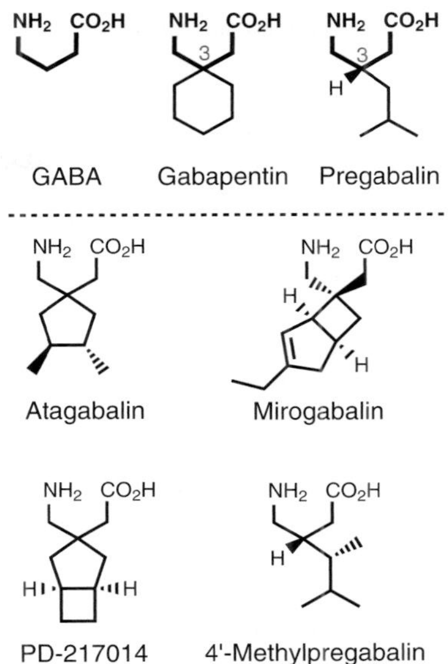

Figure 13.12 Structures of gabapentinoid Ca_V channel blockers (top). The GABA backbone is shown in bold. Analogues of gabapentin and pregabalin that are in various stages of development are shown (bottom).

RECEPTOR BINDING/MOA. The gabapentinoids bind to the α2δ subunit of Ca_V channels. The α2δ subunit is a membrane glycoprotein with a large extracellular domain that couples to Ca_V α1 pore-forming subunits.[95] In the absence of a cocrystal structure, site-directed mutagenesis studies suggest that gabapentin and pregabalin bind to a conserved Arg217 of α2δ-1 and α2δ-2 isoforms, presumably through an ion/ion interaction with the carboxylic acid group.[96,97] Both gabapentin and pregabalin modulate HVA Ca_V channel gating, causing a net reduction in glutamate release.[98] By attenuating the release of this excitatory neurotransmitter, gabapentinoids reduce excessive hyperactivity associated with seizures.

A second critical target of gabapentinoids is the system L amino acid transporter (LAT). As amino acids, gabapentinoids are poorly permeable by passive diffusion and must be taken up by a facilitated transport mechanism. The LAT family recognizes dietary amino acids like leucine, isoleucine, valine, and phenylalanine. The close structural similarity between the gabapentinoids and dietary amino acids is responsible for active uptake by LAT.

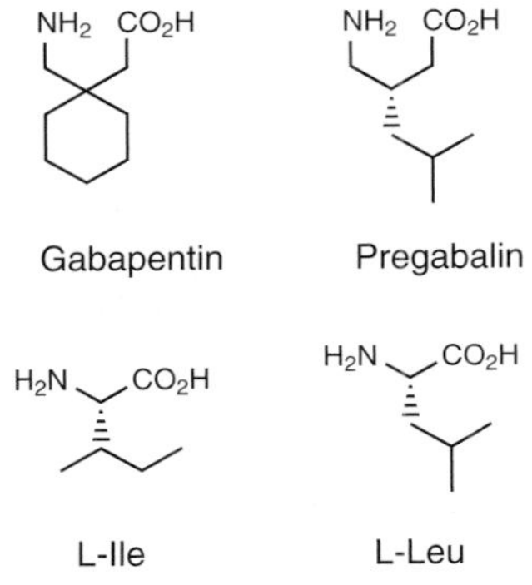

Gabapentin Pregabalin

L-Ile L-Leu

SAR. Gabapentin and pregabalin contain a GABA amino acid core (Fig. 13.12). The pharmacophore for this class of AEDs consists of (1) a weakly acidic carboxylic acid or bioisostere; (2) cyclic or acyclic hydrocarbons attached to the 3-position; (3) a weakly basic primary amine. For gabapentin, the 3-position alkyl modification is a cyclohexane ring: careful inspection of the structure shows that this is a molecule of GABA modified by the addition of five carbons to form the cyclohexane moiety. This is the basis for the name, gabapentin. Alternate cycloalkyl analogues have been shown to produce even more potent antiepileptic activity than the parent in vitro and are currently under development. For example, atagabalin (a "gababutin") demonstrates more potent α2δ inhibitory effects in vitro, though limited LAT-mediated transport limits its clinical efficacy in vivo. Other agents, such as mirogabalin, PD-217014, and 4′-methylpregabalin are also efficacious at α2δ sites and are in development as novel analgesics.

Physicochemical and pharmacokinetic properties of Ca_V blockers are provided in Table 13.5.

METABOLISM. Gabapentin and pregabalin are not appreciably metabolized. This means no meaningful drug/drug interactions are expected, and dose adjustments from metabolically compromised patients are likewise unnecessary.

Table 13.5 Physicochemical and Pharmacokinetic Properties of Ca_V Blockers

	GBP	PGB	ETX
clogP	1.19	1.12	0.38
Solubility (mg/mL)	10	>30	39.2
TPSA (Å)	63.32	63.32	46.17
f (%)	80	>90	90-95
$t_{1/2}$ (hr)	5-7	6.3	30-40 (children) 40-60 (adults)
t_{max} (hr)	3.3-3.5	0.6 (fasted) 2-3 (with food)	1-4
Protein binding (%)	None	None	None
V_d (L/kg)	0.8	0.5	0.7
Metabolized by:	None	None	CYP3A
Inducer of:	None	None	None
Inhibitor of:	None	None	None

ETX, ethosuximide; f, oral bioavailability; GBP, gabapentin; PGB, pregabalin; TPSA, topologic polar surface area; V_d, volume of distribution.

GABAPENTIN (NEURONTIN). Gabapentin was FDA-approved in 1993 as adjunctive treatment of partial seizures and is also approved to treat postherpetic neuralgia. Gabapentin is available in capsules, tables, and oral solution.

Physicochemical Properties. Gabapentin has both weakly acidic and weakly basic functional groups, making it an zwitterionic compound. The p*K*a of the carboxylic acid is 3.7 and the p*K*a of the primary amine is 10.7, meaning gabapentin predominately exists in a charged, zwitterionic state at pH 7. Gabapentin is highly water soluble (10 mg/mL) with a clogP of 1.19 at pH 7.4.[99]

Pharmacokinetics:. The zwitterionic nature of gabapentin suggests poor passive permeability across cell membranes. As introduced earlier, LAT type 1 (LAT-1) contributes to the high systemic bioavailability of gabapentin. At high doses, gabapentin overwhelms LAT-1, resulting in dose-limited absorption.[100] This corresponds to a sizable difference in oral bioavailability between low doses (80%, 100 mg every 8 hr) and high doses (27%, 1600 mg every 8 hr).[101] Peak plasma concentrations (C_{max}) of approximately 3-3.5 μg/mL occur at t_{max} of 3.3-3.5 hours. There is a modest effect of food, which causes ~10% increase in C_{max} and AUC.[102] Due to high aqueous solubility, hydrophilicity, and low plasma protein binding, gabapentin has a V_d of 0.8 L/kg, similar to total body water. Gabapentin $t_{1/2}$ ranges from 5 to 7 hours. Gabapentin is renally excreted, and doses must be monitored in renally compromised patients accordingly. Gabapentin is a possible P-gp substrate.[39]

Specific Adverse Events and DDIs. Gabapentin, at therapeutic concentrations, neither inhibits nor induces major CYP isoforms, which is suggestive of a safer DDI profile compared to other AEDs. Dizziness and somnolence are the most frequent adverse effects, which are dose-dependent and reversible.[103]

Due to an active uptake mechanism within the gastrointestinal tract (GIT), agents that prolong gastric transit time may enhance gabapentin bioavailability. For example, coadministration with the mu opioid receptor agonist morphine causes a 50% increase in bioavailability of a 600 mg dose of gabapentin.[104] Cimetidine, which is also excreted through a renal elimination route, reduces gabapentin clearance by approximately 12%.[105]

PREGABALIN (LYRICA). Pregabalin was approved in 2005 as adjunctive treatment of partial-onset seizures. Pregabalin is also approved to treat neuropathic pain, generalized anxiety disorder, and fibromyalgia. Pregabalin is available in oral capsule and suspension formulations. A controlled-release formulation, Lyrica-CR, is approved to treat diabetic peripheral neuropathy and postherpetic neuralgia; however, it has not been tested in seizure disorders.

Physicochemical Properties. Pregabalin is an zwitterionic GABA analogue with weakly acidic and basic functional groups. The p*K*a of the carboxylic acid is 4.2 and the p*K*a of the basic amine is 10.6. Pregabalin is highly soluble in water (>30 mg/mL).

Pharmacokinetics. Like gabapentin, the zwitterionic pregabalin is actively transported by LAT transporters. A key difference between the absorption of these two agents is that pregabalin is a substrate of multiple LAT transporters, not just LAT-1. This means the absorption of pregabalin is linear and approximately threefold greater than gabapentin. Peak plasma concentrations for a single dose during a fasted state are reached within an hour (t_{max} 0.6 hr), which can rise to 2-3 hours with food.[101] Pregabalin is not plasma protein bound and has V_d 0.5 L/kg. The $t_{1/2}$ of pregabalin in healthy patients is 6.3 hours. A population pharmacokinetic study showed that patients with creatinine clearance of 100 mL/min had pregabalin clearance of 70 mL/min, indicative of renal resorption.[101]

Specific Adverse Events and DDIs. Pregabalin has few adverse events or clinically relevant DDIs. Dizziness and somnolence are common side effects and are dose-limited. Pregabalin does not induce or inhibit major CYP isoforms.

Other Important Aspects of Drug Chemistry. Pregabalin is a Schedule V drug.

Succinimides and Oxazolidinediones (Fig. 13.13)

Older classes of Ca_V blockers that are structurally related to the ureides are the succinimides and oxazolidinediones. Following the success of phenytoin, these agents were originally developed in the 1940-1950s to be safer seizure-reducing analogues of phenobarbital. The oxazolidinediones trimethadione and paramethadione were the first of this series to show efficacy at treating absence seizures, although severe toxicities, including hemeralopia and agranulocytosis, limited their therapeutic use. As a serendipitous discovery, the succinimide ethosuximide (Zarontin) emerged in 1958 with an alternate mechanism of action and a better safety profile when compared to both phenobarbital and phenytoin. As such, ethosuximide is clinically effective at treating absence seizures, where these other AEDs are not.

RECEPTOR BINDING/MOA. In contrast to α2δ subunits of HVA currents that modulate neurotransmitter release, T-type Ca_V channels (Ca_V3) are responsible for "low-threshold Ca^{2+} spikes." These channels are located in the thalamus and cause bursting and intrinsic oscillations that are hallmarks of generalized absence seizures. Succinimides block firing of several Ca_V3 channel types, including α1G ($Ca_V3.1$), α1H ($Ca_V3.2$), and α1I ($Ca_V3.3$). The mechanism of Ca_V3 channel blockade appears to include both blockade of the open (activated) state of the channel as well as preferential blockade of inactivated channels.[106]

SAR. Like phenytoin, oxazolidinediones and succinimides share a similar pharmacophore: (1) a 5-membered heterocyclic ring system containing an imide and (2) an sp^3-hybridized carbon containing up to two hydrocarbon groups, only one of which may be aromatic (Fig. 13.13). A key difference in the pharmacophore responsible for the divergent pharmacodynamics of these classes is the lack of a *gem*-diphenyl substituent that is posited to be required for Na_V blockade (Fig. 13.8). The Ca_V-selective oxazolidinediones and succinimides do not have this group and are thus inactive at Na_V channels. Another point of differentiation between the classes can be found at position 3. The hydantoins have a nitrogen atom at this position, which is exchanged for an oxygen (oxazolidinediones) or a carbon (succinimides) atom. Although this modification has little impact on pharmacodynamics, there are modest differences in pharmacokinetics between these classes. Both N-methyl and N-desmethyl succinimide metabolites are pharmacologically active.

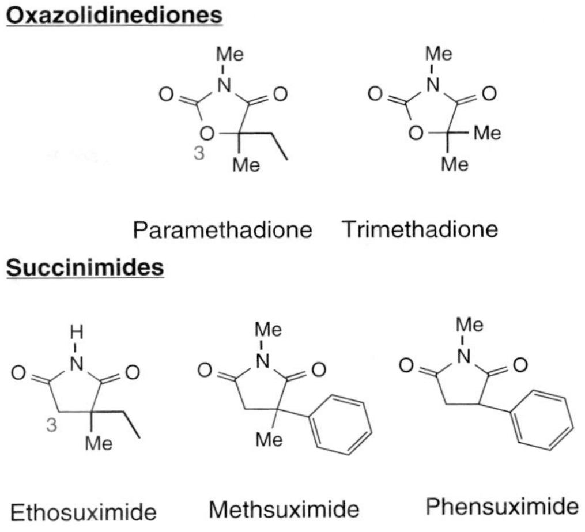

Oxazolidinediones

Paramethadione Trimethadione

Succinimides

Ethosuximide Methsuximide Phensuximide

Figure 13.13 Oxazolidinediones and succinimides.

ETHOSUXIMIDE (ZARONTIN)

Metabolism. Ethosuximide is metabolized by both phase 1 and phase 2 mechanisms to inactive metabolites. As shown in Figure 13.14, the major route of elimination is ω-1 oxidation of the 2-ethyl group (40%-60% of the administered dose). Since ethosuximide is administered as a racemic mixture of (2*R*) and (2*S*) isomers, the resulting 2-(1-hydroxyethyl) metabolites are generated as a mixture of four diastereomeric products. The same is true when the ring itself is oxidized at the 3-position (3-hydroxylation, 7%-8%). This metabolic route is not possible in the hydantoin series. A minor route of metabolism is oxidation of the terminal carbon of the 2-ethyl substituent to give 2-(2-hydroxyethyl)succinimide. This product can be oxidized further to the terminal carboxylic acid metabolite. These phase 1 metabolic pathways are mediated selectively by CYP3A isoforms. Glucuronidation of these hydroxylated metabolites is a major metabolic route, accounting for 20%-40% of the administered dose of ethosuximide.[107,108]

Physicochemical Properties. The *gem*-dialkyl-substituted carbon of ethosuximide is a chiral center. No significant differences in pharmacologic activity have been reported for (*R*)- and (*S*)-enantiomers, and ethosuximide is administered as the racemate. Like phenytoin, the imide of ethosuximide is weakly acidic with a p*Ka* of 9.3.

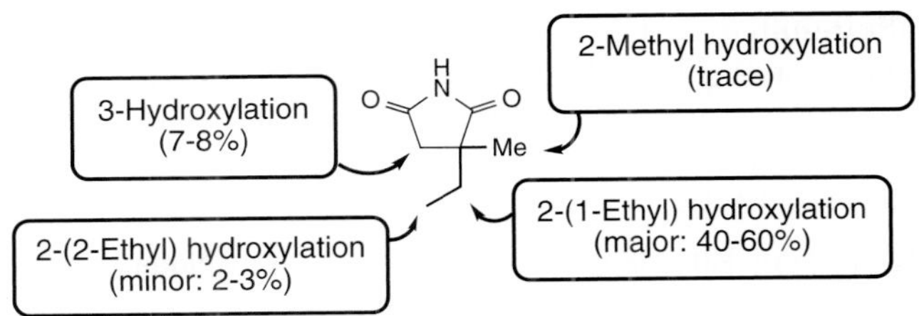

Figure 13.14 Sites of metabolic inactivation of ethosuximide.

Ethosuximide is more hydrophilic than phenytoin (clogP 0.38 compared to 2.52) and is also more water soluble (39.2 mg/mL). The TPSA is 46.17 Å and is freely centrally bioavailable.

Pharmacokinetics. Ethosuximide has high oral bioavailability (90%-95%), reaching maximum concentration at t_{max} 1-3 hours. The syrup formulation is absorbed faster than capsules, though the AUCs are similar. Ethosuximide is not bound to plasma proteins and has V_d of 0.7 L/kg. This suggests few DDIs when coadministered with plasma-bound AEDs. The $t_{1/2}$ is approximately 40-60 hours in adults and 30-40 hours in children, meaning once-daily dosing is appropriate. In light of the substantial effect of CYP3A metabolism on the pharmacokinetic profile of ethosuximide, $t_{1/2}$ may increase in patients with hepatic impairment. Elimination follows first-order kinetics. Clearance is 0.01 L/kg/hr in adults and 0.016-0.013 L/kg/hr in children.[109-111] Ethosuximide is unlikely to be a P-gp substrate.[39]

Specific Adverse Events and DDIs. Like other AEDs, ethosuximide can cause somnolence, headache, and dizziness. Confusion, sleep disturbances, depression, and aggression can be behavioral consequences of ethosuximide use.[112] Episodes of psychotic behavior have been reported that are resolved on discontinuation.[113]

Unlike other first-generation AEDs, ethosuximide does not induce CYPs or UGT enzymes. One report showed a significant decrease in serum concentration of valproic acid.[114] Due to extensive hepatic metabolism by CYP3A enzymes, there is a significant decrease in ethosuximide plasma concentrations when coadministered with CYP-inducing AEDs, e.g., carbamazepine, phenytoin, and phenobarbital.[115] Likewise, care should be taken when administering ethosuximide with other CYP3A inhibitors, which may increase drug plasma levels.

Modulators of GABA Signaling

The first clinically used AEDs, the barbiturates, produce potent sedative/hypnotic effects through inhibitory mechanisms. We now understand that GABA is the predominant inhibitory neurotransmitter system in the brain, and extensive research into the mechanisms behind GABAergic signaling has revealed many therapeutic targets for treating epilepsy disorders.

Barbiturates

The discovery of the anticonvulsant properties of the sedative-hypnotic phenobarbital arguably began the era of development of pharmacotherapies to treat seizure disorders. Attempts to separate the anticonvulsant properties from sedation, hypnosis, and abuse potential of phenobarbital resulted in the hydantoins, succinimides, and oxazolidinediones. The sedative-hypnotic effects of barbiturates are discussed in more detail in Chapter 12; here, we will focus on the properties of barbiturates that afford anticonvulsant activity.

RECEPTOR BINDING/MOA. At clinically relevant doses, barbiturates (Fig. 13.15) are positive allosteric modulators of $GABA_A$ channels. Barbiturates increase the amount of time the channel stays open when bound by GABA but have no effect on the frequency of channel opening. At high doses, barbiturates can act as $GABA_A$ agonists in the absence of GABA. Barbiturates also inhibit AMPA and kainate receptors (glutamate receptors), nicotinic receptors, and at higher doses, P/Q-type Ca_V channels and glutamate release. The exact binding site for barbiturates on $GABA_A$ channels is not fully understood, though evidence suggests β subunits are involved.[116]

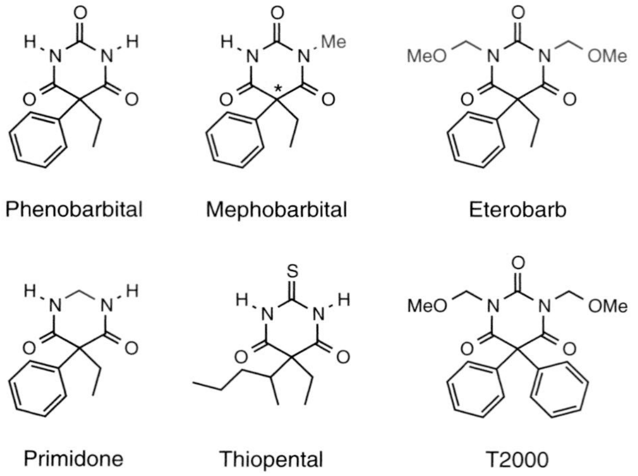

Phenobarbital Mephobarbital Eterobarb

Primidone Thiopental T2000

Figure 13.15 Anticonvulsant barbiturates. Labile portions of analogues that are metabolized to phenobarbital are shown in red (* = chiral center).

SAR. Barbiturates are characterized by their barbituric acid core, a six-membered ring system consisting of alternating imide carbonyl and nitrogen atoms (Fig. 13.16, R1 = R2 = H). To be pharmacologically active, barbituric acid must be *gem*-disubstituted at position 5 (R1=R2 = alkyl or aryl). Most barbiturates are substituted with an ethyl group (R1 = ethyl), and the nature of R2 substitution determines the onset and duration of action, and consequently the indication. For example, when R2 = phenyl (phenobarbital), the low lipophilicity (clogP = 1.67) means less drug is distributed to peripheral tissues than more lipophilic drugs such as the ultra-short-acting thiopental (R2 = *sec*-pentyl,

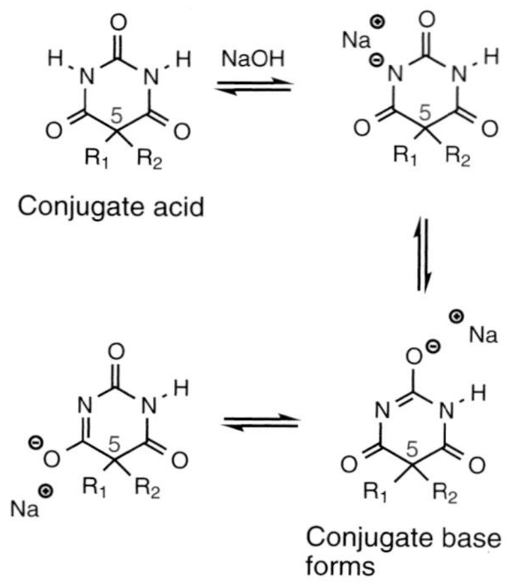

NaOH

Conjugate acid

Conjugate base forms

Figure 13.16 Conjugate acid and base forms of barbiturates.

clogP 2.99). Long-acting hydrophilic barbiturates are useful as AEDs due to infrequent dosing. Alkylation of the imide nitrogen atoms is a prodrug strategy for enhancing duration of action and avoiding reinforcing effects that can cause abuse. To be fully active AEDs, both imides must be secondary, which requires dealkylation of tertiary imide prodrugs. This is the rationale behind the design of mephobarbital, metharbital, eterobarb, and the investigational drug T2000: the delayed onset of action reduces the rapid rewarding effects.

PHYSICOCHEMICAL PROPERTIES. Barbituric acids are weakly acidic (p*K*a 7.4). In the presence of weak base such as sodium hydroxide, the imide is deprotonated to one of three conjugate base forms (Fig. 13.16). The sodium salt of the conjugate base is much more water soluble than the protonated free conjugate acid form and is therefore available for parenteral injection. Long-acting anticonvulsant barbiturates are generally more hydrophilic (clogP approximately 0.5) than shorter-acting derivatives used for anesthetic and sedative-hypnotic purposes. Double-prodrugs like eterobarb and T2000 are neutral until metabolized into their active barbituric acid–derived products.

Physicochemical and pharmacokinetic properties of barbiturate antiseizure agents are provided in Table 13.6.

PHENOBARBITAL (LUMINAL). Phenobarbital is one of the first clinically used anticonvulsants, and its use has been consistent through the past century. Its high effectiveness and low cost make phenobarbital a reasonable treatment option in situations where alternatives are cost-prohibitive. Its common modern use is in tonic-clonic and partial

Table 13.6 Physicochemical and Pharmacokinetic Properties of Barbiturates and Benzodiazepines

	PBT	PRM	CLB	CLO	CZM	DZP	LZP	MDZ
clogP	1.67	0.40	1.69	2.90	2.34	2.91	2.47	3.93
Solubility (mg/mL)	1[a] 1000[b]	0.6	0.18	0.02	0.01	0.005	0.08	>5 (HCl salt)
TPSA (Å)	75.27	58.20	40.62	78.76	87.28	32.67	61.69	27.96
f (%)	>90	100	87	90	>95	>90	100 (IM)	>90 (IM) 75-80 (oromucosal)
$t_{1/2}$ (hr)	>48[c] >120[d]	10	24	30-100	17-56	48[e] ~100[f]	14	3-4
t_{max} (hr)	0.5-4	1.5-3	0.5-2	1-3	1-4	0.5-1	3	0.5-1
Protein binding (%)	50	20-30	90	98	85	98	>90	98
V_d (L/kg)	0.7	0.4-1.0	1.31	0.8-1.0	1.5-4.4	0.8-1.0	1.3	5.3
Metabolized by:	CYP2C9 CYP2C19	CYPs[g]	CYP2C19 CYP3A4	CYP3A4[h]	CYP3A4	CYP2C19 CYP3A4	UGTs	CYP3A4
Inducer of:	CYP2C9 CYP2C19 CYP3A4	CYP2C9 CYP2C19 CYP3A4 UGTs	CYP3A4	None	None	None	None	None
Inhibitor of:	None	None	CYP2D6 CYP2C19[i] UGTs[i]	None	None	None		None

[a]Free acid.
[b]Na^+ salt.
[c]In children.
[d]In adults.
[e]Initial distribution phase.
[f]Active metabolite, nordiazepam.
[g]Isoform(s) unknown.
[h]Clorazepate is chemically unstable to acid and converted to nordiazepam, which is metabolized by CYP3A4.
[i]NDMC metabolite.
CLB, clobazam; CLO, clorazepate; CZM, clonazepam; DZP, diazepam; f, oral bioavailability; IM, intramuscular; LZP, lorazepam; MZD, midazolam; PBT, phenobarbital; PRM, primidone; TPSA, topologic polar surface area; V_d, volume of distribution.

seizures. Originally developed and approved in 1912 as a sedative/hypnotic, its anticonvulsant activity was discovered serendipitously by Alfred Hauptmann to help his epileptic patients—and therefore himself—sleep through the night. He found that one dose of Luminal blocked their seizures in addition to helping them sleep. This discovery led to phenobarbital usurping bromides as the treatment of choice for seizures, causing a revolution in AED treatment.[4] Phenobarbital is on the World Health Organization's 20th List of Essential Medicines.

Physicochemical Properties. Phenobarbital has a clogP of 1.67 and TPSA of 75.27 Å. The free acid is only slightly soluble in water (1 mg/mL), whereas the sodium salt is very water-soluble (1000 mg/mL).

Metabolism. The phenyl ring of phenobarbital is oxidized to the arene oxide intermediate II (Fig. 13.17), which undergoes an NIH shift to the inactive *p*-phenol. The particular isoform(s) responsible for this transformation remain unexplored, but the reaction may be catalyzed in part by CYP2C9.[117]

Pharmacokinetics. Phenobarbital bioavailability is greater than 90% when given orally in tablet or elixir form. The low clogP of phenobarbital (1.67) contributes to low plasma protein binding of approximately 50%. Thus, clinically relevant DDIs due to plasma protein binding are not anticipated. The V_d of phenobarbital is 0.7 L/kg. Approximately 20% of phenobarbital dose is eliminated unchanged in urine through a first-order process. Clearance in children (Cl = 4 mL/kg/hr) is faster when compared to adults (Cl = 4 mL/kg/hr) and the elderly (3 mL/kg/hr). Consequently, the $t_{1/2}$ in children (2.5 d) and adults (5 d) permits once-daily dosing.[118] Therapeutic drug monitoring should be undertaken for patients with renal and kidney disease. Phenobarbital is a substrate and inducer of CYP2C9 and has autoinducing properties. Phenobarbital is a P-gp substrate.[39]

Specific Adverse Events and DDIs. As a sedative/hypnotic, phenobarbital causes severe somnolence at higher doses, as well as disrupts memory and cognition. Maternal use of phenobarbital during pregnancy and exposure to phenobarbital during the first 3 years of life are associated with increased risk of cognitive and intelligence deficits.[119,120]

Phenobarbital is an inducer of CYP2C9, CYP2C19, CYP3A4, and UGT enzymes, which is responsible for many DDIs with other AEDs and non-anticonvulsants, such as hormonal contraceptives. Thus, care should be taken when using phenobarbital with other CYP substrates in polydrug therapy. Additionally, the use of other enzyme-inducing AEDs impacts phenobarbital clearance, underscoring the point that therapeutic drug monitoring is critical when using this agent.[121]

Other Important Aspects of Drug Chemistry. Phenobarbital is a Schedule IV controlled substance.

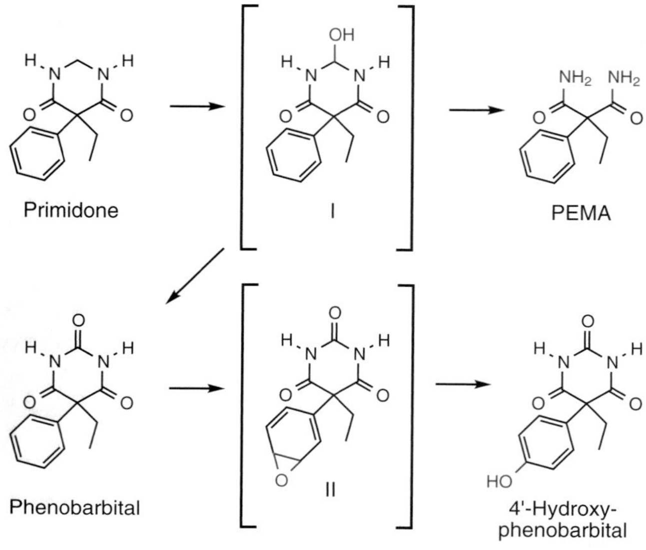

PRIMIDONE (MYSOLINE). Primidone was FDA approved in 1954 and is used to treat generalized seizures. Primidone is a prodrug of phenobarbital and is not entirely understood whether the anticonvulsant properties of primidone are due exclusively to metabolism to phenobarbital in vivo, or whether the parent drug contributes to the pharmacologic profile.

Metabolism. Primidone is metabolized to phenobarbital through an oxidized intermediate I (Fig.13.17). This step is CYP-dependent, although the identities of the responsible isoforms are unknown. Intermediate I can also undergo hydrolysis to phenylethylmalonamide (PEMA). Whether PEMA contributes to the anticonvulsant effects of primidone is controversial, although evidence suggests it does not. The ratio of phenobarbital:PEMA is approximately 1:2.5.

Physicochemical Properties. Primidone is technically not a barbituric acid derivative, although it is a prodrug of phenobarbital. Instead of a barbituric acid core, primidone contains two uncharged amides within a six-membered ring. Primidone is poorly water-soluble (0.6 mg/mL) and, unlike barbiturates, is not weakly acidic and, therefore, cannot be formulated as the sodium salt. Primidone has a clogP of 0.40 and a TPSA of 58.2 Å.

Pharmacokinetics. It is important to consider that primidone is metabolized to phenobarbital; thus, phenobarbital contributes to the observed clinical effects of primidone. Primidone is nearly completely absorbed on oral administration, with t_{max} occurring within 1.5-3 hours. The V_d is approximately 0.4-1 L/kg and plasma protein binding is low (20%-30%). Hepatic metabolism accounts for approximately 60% of the elimination of primidone, with the remaining 40% of the unchanged parent drug found in urine. Around 25% of the dose is excreted as PEMA. Phenobarbital (2%) and *p*-OH-phenobarbital (2%) are minor metabolites, as are *p*-OH-phenobarbital conjugates. Clearance of PEMA is significantly lower in the elderly owing to the renal elimination of this metabolite.[122]

Specific Adverse Events and DDIs. Side effects of primidone are similar to other barbiturates, though generally milder. Like phenobarbital and phenytoin, primidone is associated with osteoporosis and osteopenia. Primidone, like its phenobarbital metabolite, is a CYP and UGT inducer, thereby impacting the clearance of coadministered CYP and UGT substrates.

Figure 13.17 Metabolism of primidone and phenobarbital. *PEMA*, phenylethylmalonamide.

Other Important Aspects of Drug Chemistry. Though primidone is metabolized to phenobarbital in vivo, it is not a scheduled substance.

Benzodiazepines

The serendipitous discovery by Leo Sternbach in the 1950s that the benzodiazepine, chlordiazepoxide, is active against seizures and anxiety disorders quickly proved to be revolutionary. This important class of agents is discussed in greater detail elsewhere in this book (Chapter 12); this section will focus on the features of benzodiazepines that are important for their antiepileptic mechanisms of action (Fig. 13.18). The benzodiazepines most frequently used to treat epilepsy disorders are clonazepam (Klonopin), diazepam (Valium, Diastat), chlorazepate (Tranxene), lorazepam (Ativan), midazolam (Versed), and the newest agent, clobazam (Onfi). Midazolam (buccal, oromucosal solution) and diazepam (rectal gel) are special formulations that can be used in emergency situations to treat status epilepticus. Diazepam, lorazepam, and midazolam are on the World Health Organization's 20th List of Essential Medicines.

RECEPTOR BINDING/MOA. Like barbiturates, benzodiazepines augment $GABA_A$ channel signaling through an allosteric mechanism; however, benzodiazepines bind $GABA_A$ via a different binding site that increases the frequency of channel opening when bound by GABA. The allosteric binding sites are flanked by α and γ subunits on pentameric $GABA_A$ ion channels. When bound by ligands, these "benzodiazepine receptors" (BZRs) permit a conformational change in the channel that promotes enhanced channel opening in the presence of GABA. Of the six cloned and characterized α subunits, only α4 and α6 are insensitive to classical benzodiazepines and thus are not responsible for their antiepileptic mechanism. All currently available benzodiazepines are nonselective positive allosteric modulators of α1-3 and α5. Reported $GABA_A$ channelopathies contribute to seizure disorders through mutations of γ2 subunits that reduce channel signaling.[30,31]

Clonazepam
Clobazam
Diazepam
Clorazepate
Lorazepam
Midazolam

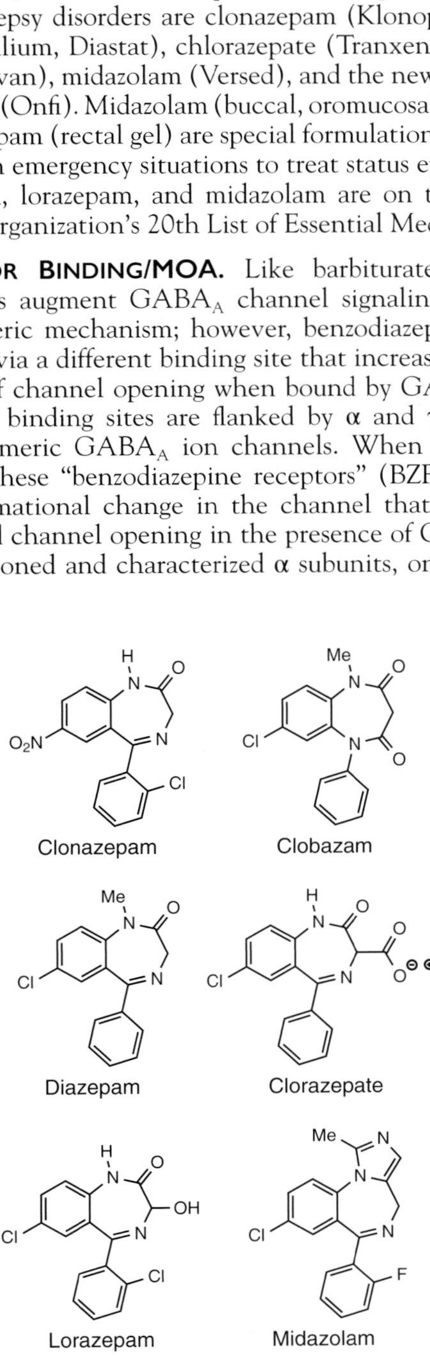

Figure 13.18 Benzodiazepines used to treat seizures.

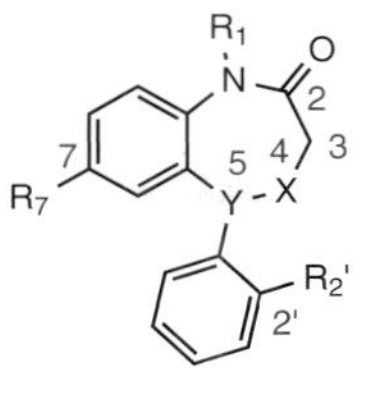

Series A:

R_1:	short, linear alkyl groups, H = optimal.
2:	branched alkyl = inactivating.
3.	HBA required.
4,5:	oxidation (OH) is tolerated. rigidity needed.
7:	X-Y: N=C or (C=O)-N.
2':	EWG increases antiepileptic potency. Halogens tolerated.

Series B:

R:	H or Me tolerated.
X:	H, F, or Cl.
Y:	CH (imidazole) or N (triazole).
4:	oxidation (OH) is not tolerated.

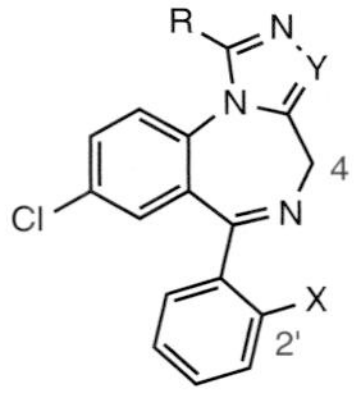

Figure 13.19 SAR for anticonvulsant benzodiazepines. *EWG*, electron-withdrawing group; *HBA*, hydrogen bond acceptor.

SAR. Figure 13.19 shows the SAR of benzodiazepines in the "azepam" (Series A) and "azolam" (Series B) series. In Series A, short-chain N-alkyl groups are tolerated at position 1 (R1), as is the nonalkylated 2° amide. Position 2 must have a hydrogen bond–accepting carbonyl or bioisostere. Position 3 can be unsubstituted or oxidized to a secondary alcohol. Chlorazepate, which has an exocyclic carboxylate group at the 3-position, is a prodrug that is converted to the active metabolite through decarboxylation. Most benzodiazepines have an imine in the 4,5-position, though the newest anticonvulsant benzodiazepine, clobazam, has an amide. The role of this structural region is to maintain rigidity in the diazepine ring. Electron-withdrawing groups at position 7 enhance antiepileptic activity, as well as sedative and hypnotic effects. Halogens at the 2′ position are also tolerated and add to the sedative actions of the molecule.

METABOLISM. Clonazepam, diazepam, and clorazepate are N-dealkylated by CYP3A4 into active N-desmethyl metabolites II (Fig. 13.20). Clorazepate is chemically unstable in acid and is converted to N-desmethyldiazepam (II, R1 = H, R7 = Cl, R2' = H) in the acidic environment of the stomach. Intermediates of type II can be oxidized further at position 3 into active 3-hydroxy metabolites (III) by CYP3A4, or inactivated to 9-hydroxy (IV) or 4′-hydroxy (V) metabolites. Oxidized metabolites III–V can be glucuronidated by UGT enzymes prior to elimination.

PHYSICOCHEMICAL PROPERTIES. Benzodiazepines of the "azepam" class generally have poor aqueous solubility (<1 mg/mL) and can be given orally or by injection. Injection of aqueous-insoluble benzodiazepines requires the use of propylene glycol, which can cause local pain. Clorazepate is an exception: the chemically unstable

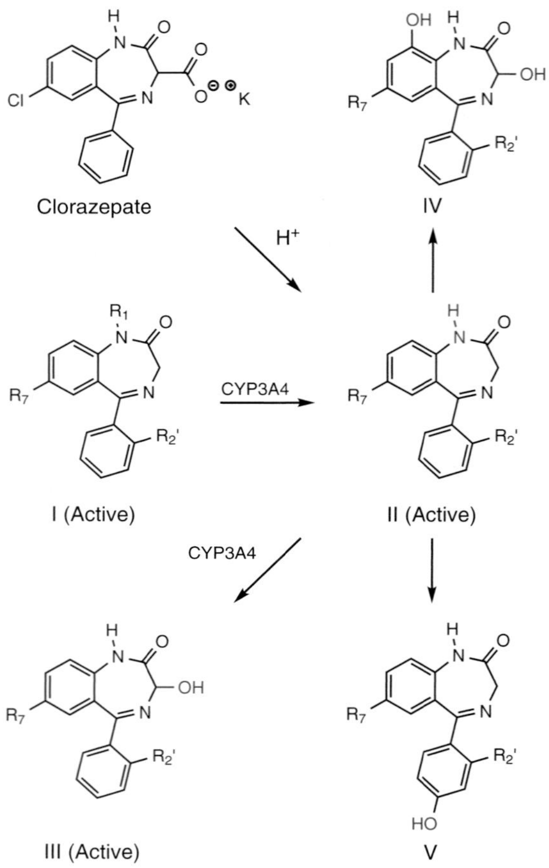

Figure 13.20 Metabolism of clonazepam, diazepam, and clorazepate. Clonazepam: R1 = H, R7 = NO_2, R2' = Cl. Diazepam: R1 = Me, R7 = Cl, R2' = H. Site of metabolism shown in red. Oxidized metabolites III-V can be metabolized further into inactive glucuronide conjugates.

carboxylic acid prodrug is formulated as the disodium salt. Benzodiazepines are modestly lipophilic, with clogP values ranging from 1.69 (clobazam) to 2.91 (diazepam). The TPSA of benzodiazepines ranges from 32.67 Å (diazepam) to 93.27 Å (clonazepam). The 7-nitro substituent of clonazepam likely contributes to this higher value.

Physicochemical and pharmacokinetic properties of benzodiazepine antiseizure agents are provided in Table 13.6.

SPECIFIC ADVERSE EVENTS AND DDIS. Tolerance to benzodiazepines can develop quickly, leading to decreased effectiveness with continued use. Abrupt discontinuation of benzodiazepines can lower seizure threshold, leading to increased risk of convulsions. Benzodiazepines are sedative-hypnotics, thus sedation and memory impairment are common side effects that may be undesirable when treating seizure disorders. Benzodiazepines used as AEDs can cause life-threatening respiratory events and excessive sedation, so their use should be monitored in emergency settings. Respiratory depression is exacerbated by opioids, meaning that benzodiazepine doses should be lowered when given concomitantly.

OTHER IMPORTANT ASPECTS OF DRUG CHEMISTRY. Benzodiazepines carry abuse and dependence potential and are thus on the Schedule IV list.

LORAZEPAM (ATIVAN). Lorazepam is a first-generation AED that has sedative hypnotic and antiepileptic properties. Though tablet formulations are prescribed to treat anxiety and sleeping disorders, injectable formulations of lorazepam are available as treatments for status epilepticus. Lorazepam is on the WHO List of Essential Medicines.

Metabolism. The 3-hydroxyl group of lorazepam is extensively metabolized through phase 2 processes by UGT enzymes from the UGT1A and UGT2B subfamilies. The resulting lorazepam-3-O-glucuronide is pharmacologically inactive. This is in contrast to the metabolites of other "azepams" used as AEDs that can be biotransformed through phase 1 mechanisms to pharmacologically active products.

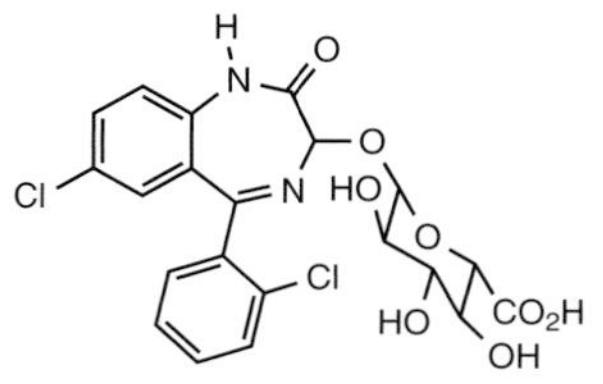

Lorazepam-3-O-glucuronide

Pharmacokinetics. Pharmacokinetic parameters are similar for IV or IM administration of lorazepam. Bioavailability is high (100%) on IM administration. Maximal concentrations are slightly lower for IM (C_{max} = 48 ng/mL) compared to IV (C_{max} = 90 ng/mL). Lorazepam is lipophilic (clogP = 2.47) and plasma protein bound (90%). Maximal concentrations are reached within 3 hours, similar to other "azepam" benzodiazepines; the terminal half-life of lorazepam is shorter than that of clonazepam and diazepam ($t_{1/2}$ = 14 hr). The V_d (1.3 L/kg) and Cl (1.1 ± 0.4 mL/min/kg) are similar to other benzodiazepines. The hepatic metabolite lorazepam-3-O-glucuronide undergoes enterohepatic recycling and is eliminated by the kidneys. Renal impairment significantly impacts half-life and clearance: patients with renal dysfunction or under hemodialysis experience 55%-125% increase in $t_{1/2}$ and 75%-90% decrease in clearance compared to healthy controls.[123]

Specific Adverse Events and DDIs. Lorazepam should not be used in pregnant women in the first trimester except for in life-threatening situations due to the potential to produce fetal abnormalities. Both lorazepam and lorazepam-3-O-glucuronide have been found in umbilical cord blood. Poor aqueous solubility (<0.1 mg/mL) requires formulation in benzyl alcohol that can cause hypotension and other toxicities in neonates and preterm infants. Use of lorazepam in these patients should be minimized.

Coadministration of lorazepam with valproic acid causes a significant decrease in formation of the 3-O-glucuronide metabolite due to competition with UGT enzymes. The dose of lorazepam should be lowered in patients taking valproic acid as a prophylactic treatment for seizures. Women on hormonal contraception experience a significant increase in metabolic clearance of lorazepam; doses of lorazepam need to be increased in these patients. Lorazepam is unlikely to be a P-gp substrate.

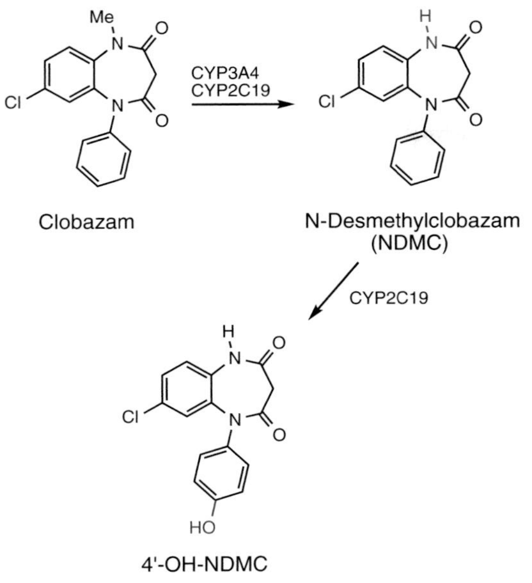

Figure 13.21 Metabolism of clobazam.

CLOBAZAM (ONFI). Clobazam is a structurally unique benzodiazepine in that it contains a 1,5-diazepine ring instead of a 1,4-diazepine. Originally developed in the 1970s as an anxiolytic, clobazam was FDA-approved in 2011 for the adjunctive treatment of Lennox-Gastaut syndrome in patients over 2 years of age. It is also used as an adjuvant to treat refractory seizures. Clobazam is available in tablet and suspension forms.

Metabolism. Hepatic metabolism of clobazam is afforded through CYP3A4 and CYP2C19. Both enzymes are implicated in the generation of the active metabolite, N-desmethylclobazam (NDMC; Fig. 13.21), although the higher expression of CYP3A4 in the liver suggests this isoform is most clinically relevant. Conversion of NDMC to the inactive 4′-OH-NDMC is mediated by CYP2C19. Though NDMC has preferential affinity for α2-containing $GABA_A$ channels, this does not impact its antiepileptic profile.[124]

Pharmacokinetics. Clobazam is rapidly and extensively absorbed when given orally. Peak concentrations are reached between 0.5 and 2 hours after a single dose, which increases on multiple dosing. Food has no effect on C_{max}, AUC, or t_{max}. The apparent V_d of clobazam is approximately 1.31 L/kg. Clobazam and NDMC are highly protein bound (89%-90% and 70%, respectively). Elimination is primarily renal, although only approximately 2% of clobazam is recovered unchanged in urine. The most prevalent urinary metabolites are NDMC and its conjugates (94%). Circulating concentrations of NDMC are three to five times higher than the parent drug. The elimination $t_{1/2}$ is 24 hours. Clearance of clobazam is significantly impaired in elderly patients, although renal and hepatic impairment has a small effect on pharmacokinetics.[125]

Specific Adverse Events and DDIs. Like all benzodiazepines, excessive somnolence and lethargy are frequent side effects. Patients who are CYP2C19 poor metabolizers may have trouble clearing NDMC, leading to artificially high plasma levels of active drug. Coadministration of clobazam with CYP-inducing AEDs accelerates clobazam metabolism to NDMC and 4′-OH-NDMC. Furthermore, coadministration with a CYP2C19 inhibitor like felbamate inhibits the clearance of NDMC, causing an increase in plasma concentrations of this active metabolite. Such combinations may cause toxicities.[126,127] Clobazam is a weak CYP3A4 inducer and CYP2D6 inhibitor. NDMC is a weak inhibitor of CYP2C9 and several UGT isoforms.[125] The CYP3A4 inducing effect of clobazam may contribute to a loss of contraceptive efficacy.

MIDAZOLAM (VERSED). Midazolam plays an important role in treating seizure disorders as an emergency medication to treat status epilepticus. The unique chemical and pharmacokinetic properties of midazolam are perfect for oromucosal absorption, effective distribution, and rapid metabolism. In this way, emergency personnel may treat patients who are unable to receive intravenous injections, and the sedative effects will subside in relatively short order.

Physicochemical Properties. As an "azolam" benzodiazepine, the physicochemical properties of midazolam are quite different from classical, "azepam" benzodiazepines. The 2-position of the fused imidazole is weakly basic, with a pKa of 6.15. This means midazolam may be formulated as the hydrochloride salt (Fig. 13.22), which has higher aqueous solubility (>5 mg/mL). In acidic solutions (pH 3.3), the diazepine ring is in equilibrium between ring-closed states (80%-85%) and hydrolyzed ring-open states (15%-20%). This means midazolam has two conjugate acid forms (CA1, CA2; Fig. 13.22). In the bloodstream (pH 7.4), the dihydrochloride (CA2) shifts its equilibrium back to the ring-closed free base state, which has a clogP

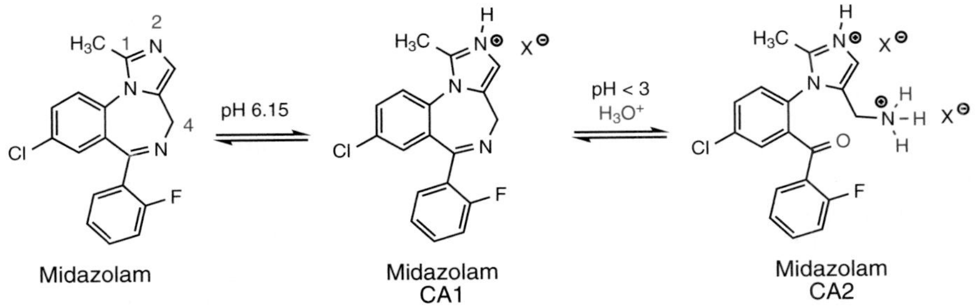

Figure 13.22 Equilibrium between charged conjugate acid (CA) states of midazolam. In aqueous buffer (pH 3.3), the CA1:CA2 ratio is approximately 80:20.

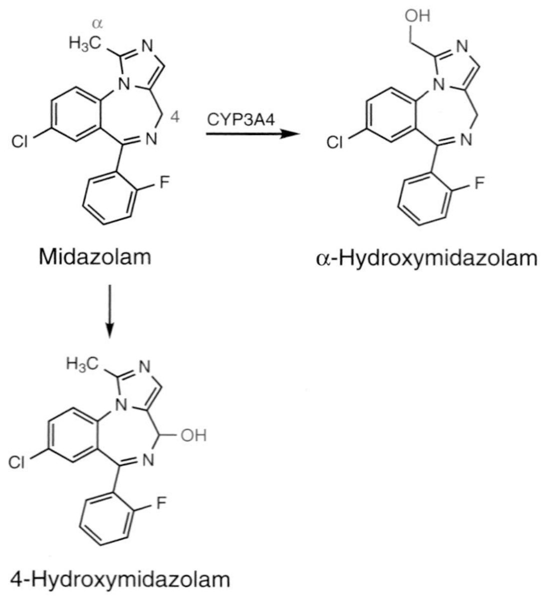

Figure 13.23 Metabolism of midazolam.

of 3.93 and TPSA of 27.96 Å. These properties make midazolam highly BBB-penetrating, with a fast onset of antiepileptic action.[128]

Metabolism. Midazolam is rapidly metabolized to inactive products. The major route of inactivation is CYP3A4-mediated oxidation of the α-carbon on position 1 of the imidazole ring (Fig. 13.23). This is responsible for the short duration of antiepileptic and sedative action. The α-OH-midazolam metabolite is conjugated and eliminated as the glucuronide. A minor route of metabolism is oxidation at the 4-position, analogous to the 3-position of classical "azepams." Unlike 3- hydroxylated azepam metabolites, 4-OH-midazolam is inactive.[128]

Pharmacokinetics. Approximately 75%-80% of oromucosal midazolam hydrochloride is absorbed with a t_{max} within 30 minutes in children. Midazolam is lipophilic, highly protein bound (98%), and extensively distributed (V_d 5.3 L/kg). Midazolam is 60% metabolized by hepatic oxidation (CYP3A4) to inactive metabolites. The major metabolite is α-hydroxymidazolam and its glucuronide conjugate. This metabolite is more prevalent in children than adults. Plasma clearance in children is 30 mL/kg/min, which is increased in hepatically impaired patients. The elimination $t_{1/2}$ of oromucosal midazolam is around 200 minutes. Renal impairment does not impact clearance.

Specific Adverse Events and DDIs. Midazolam can cause life-threatening respiratory depression and arrest in adults, children, and neonates. Thus, patients should be monitored for labored breathing when given midazolam and other benzodiazepines. Reversal of benzodiazepine overdose is achieved with the $GABA_A$ antagonist, flumazenil. Importantly, flumazenil will only reverse the effects of benzodiazepines, and not other concomitantly administered AEDs. Midazolam can cross the placental barrier and enter human milk.

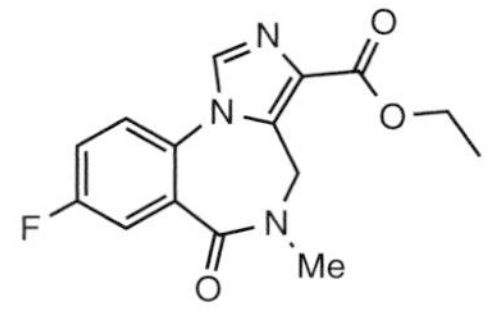

Inhibitors of GABA Uptake and Metabolism

Physicochemical and pharmacokinetic properties of GABA modulators are provided in Table 13.7.

TIAGABINE (GABITRIL). Tiagabine is a structurally unique AED that was FDA-approved in 1997 as an adjunctive agent to treat partial seizures in patients over age 12. Tiagabine is the first agent approved that inhibits GABA uptake as its primary mechanism of action.

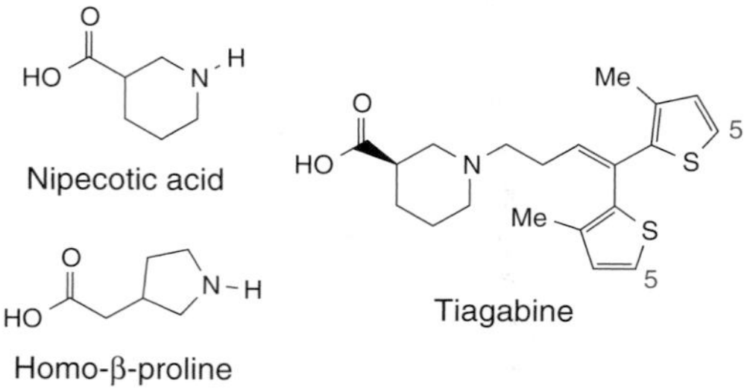

Receptor Binding/MOA. Tiagabine is a selective inhibitor of GAT-1, the most abundant isoform of the GAT family. Little is known definitively about the molecular mechanisms by which tiagabine binds GAT-1. Homology modeling suggests the carboxylate anion engages a sodium ion in the GAT-1 active site, and the protonated amine engages in an ion/dipole bond with the backbone carbonyl of Phe294. The diaryl tail group engages a hydrophobic cleft stabilized by π-stacking with Tyr140.[129]

SAR. Tiagabine emerged from the observation that two conformationally constrained GABA analogues, nipecotic acid and homo-β-proline, were GABA uptake inhibitors in vitro that were BBB-impermeable in vivo. The BBB permeability of the lead nipecotic acid was improved by enhancing the lipophilicity, ultimately resulting in tiagabine.[130] The basic amine and carboxylic acid are required for GAT-1 binding (see above), and the lipophilic tail enhances GAT-1 affinity and CNS bioavailability.

Metabolism. Tiagabine is extensively metabolized by CYP3A oxidation. The primary sites of oxidation are the equivalent 5-positions on the thiophene rings. These 5-oxo-thiophene metabolites are pharmacologically inert. Glucuronide conjugates are also common, though their exact structures remain to be determined.[131]

Physicochemical Properties. Tiagabine possesses both weakly acidic (p*K*a 4.14) and basic (p*K*a 9.26) functional groups. Thus, tiagabine carries a molecular charge across the pH scale. The hydrochloride salt is sparingly soluble in water (11 mg/mL) and the TPSA is 40.54 Å.

Table 13.7 Physicochemical and Pharmacokinetic Properties of Glutamate and GABA Modulators

	TGB	VGB	LEV	BRV	PER
clogP	5.69	−0.10	−0.67	0.88	3.70
Solubility (mg/mL)	11 (HCl salt)	55.1	>40	>40	<0.01
TPSA (Å)	40.54	63.32	63.40	63.40	56.46
f (%)[b]	95	>90	99	100	100
$t_{1/2}$ (hr)	7-9		6-8	7-8	105
t_{max} (hr)	0.75[a] 2[b]	0.5-1.0[a] 2[b]	1.3	1.0	1.0
Protein binding (%)	96	None	None	17	95
V_d (L/kg)	1.0	1.0-1.1	0.5-0.7	0.5	0.6-0.7
Metabolized by:	CYP3A4,5	None	Hydrolysis	CYP2C8	CYP3A4
Inducer of:	None	None	None	None	None
Inhibitor of:	None	None	None	Epoxide hydrolase	CYP2C8

[a]Fasting.

[b]With high-fat meal.

BRV, brivaracetam; F, oral bioavailability; LEV, levetiracetam; PER, perampanel; TGB, tiagabine; TPSA, topologic polar surface area; V_d, volume of distribution; VGB, vigabatrin.

Pharmacokinetics. Tiagabine is rapidly and nearly completely absorbed (95%), exhibiting a linear pharmacokinetic profile. The t_{max} occurs around 45 minutes, which is extended to 2.5 hours when given with a high-fat meal. The extent of absorption (AUC) is not affected by food. Two peaks can be found in the plasma profile curve of tiagabine, suggestive of enterohepatic recycling. Tiagabine is highly bound to plasma proteins (96%) and has a V_d of 1 L/kg. Tiagabine is heavily metabolized, with only 2% of the parent drug eliminated unchanged. Elimination of metabolites occurs in the urine (25%) and feces (63%). Tiagabine $t_{1/2}$ (7-9 hr) and clearance (109 mL/min) is impacted by concomitantly administered CYP-inducing AEDs. No dose adjustments are needed for patients with renal impairment, though those with hepatic insufficiency should see dose reductions.[131]

Specific Adverse Events and DDIs. Nonepileptic patients may experience new-onset seizures and status epilepticus while taking tiagabine. Since tiagabine is frequently given as an adjuvant with enzyme-inducing drugs, the dose should be decreased if given alone or in noninduced patients. Enzyme-inducing AEDs increase clearance by about 60% and valproate reduces plasma protein binding by approximately 2%, leading to a 40% increase in blood plasma levels of tiagabine. Tiagabine is not an inducer of CYP or UGT enzymes.

VIGABATRIN (SABRIL). Vigabatrin was approved by the FDA in 2009 as monotherapy in the treatment of infantile spasms, spasms due to West syndrome, and generalized tonic-clonic seizures. It is approved to treat refractory complex partial seizures in adults over age 10. It is a mechanism-based "suicide-inhibitor," and perhaps the first AED that was rationally designed.

Receptor Binding/MOA. Vigabatrin is a first-in-class inhibitor of GABA-transaminase (GABA-T), an enzyme that catalyzes the breakdown of GABA into inactive succinic semialdehyde (Fig. 13.24). The mechanism by which GABA-T converts the primary amine into an aldehyde is shown in Figure 13.24A. In the first step, GABA reacts with pyridoxamine-5′-phosphate (PLP) to form Schiff base I. An active site lysine (Lys329) within GABA-T removes a proton α to the iminium, forming a second unstable aldimine intermediate II. Hydrolysis of II forms pyridoxamie-5′-phosphate (PAP) and releases succinic semialdehyde (SSA). PAP can then be converted back to PLP by converting α-ketoglutarate to glutamate. The action of vigabatrin is shown in Figure 13.24B. Like GABA, vigabatrin reacts with PAP to form aldimine III, and then Lys329 removes the α-proton, forming enimine IV. Regeneration of the conjugate base of Lys329 affords imine V. Here, the vinyl group is susceptible to nucleophilic Michael attack by Lys329, resulting in product VI that has covalently bound the substrate, enzyme, and cofactor, permanently inactivating GABA-T.[132]

SAR. Vigabatrin is also known as γ-vinyl-GABA (GVG). In fact, the name "vigabatrin" arises from the fact that it is a vinyl GABA-transaminase inhibitor. The simple addition of a vinyl group to the γ-carbon is key to the mechanism of covalent binding (see above). If this alkene were not exactly one carbon removed from the γ-amine, vigabatrin would not covalently bind GABA-T. Conformationally constrained GVG analogues are in development, which orient this double bond toward the lysine. Such agents are designed to be much more potent irreversible GABA-T inhibitors.

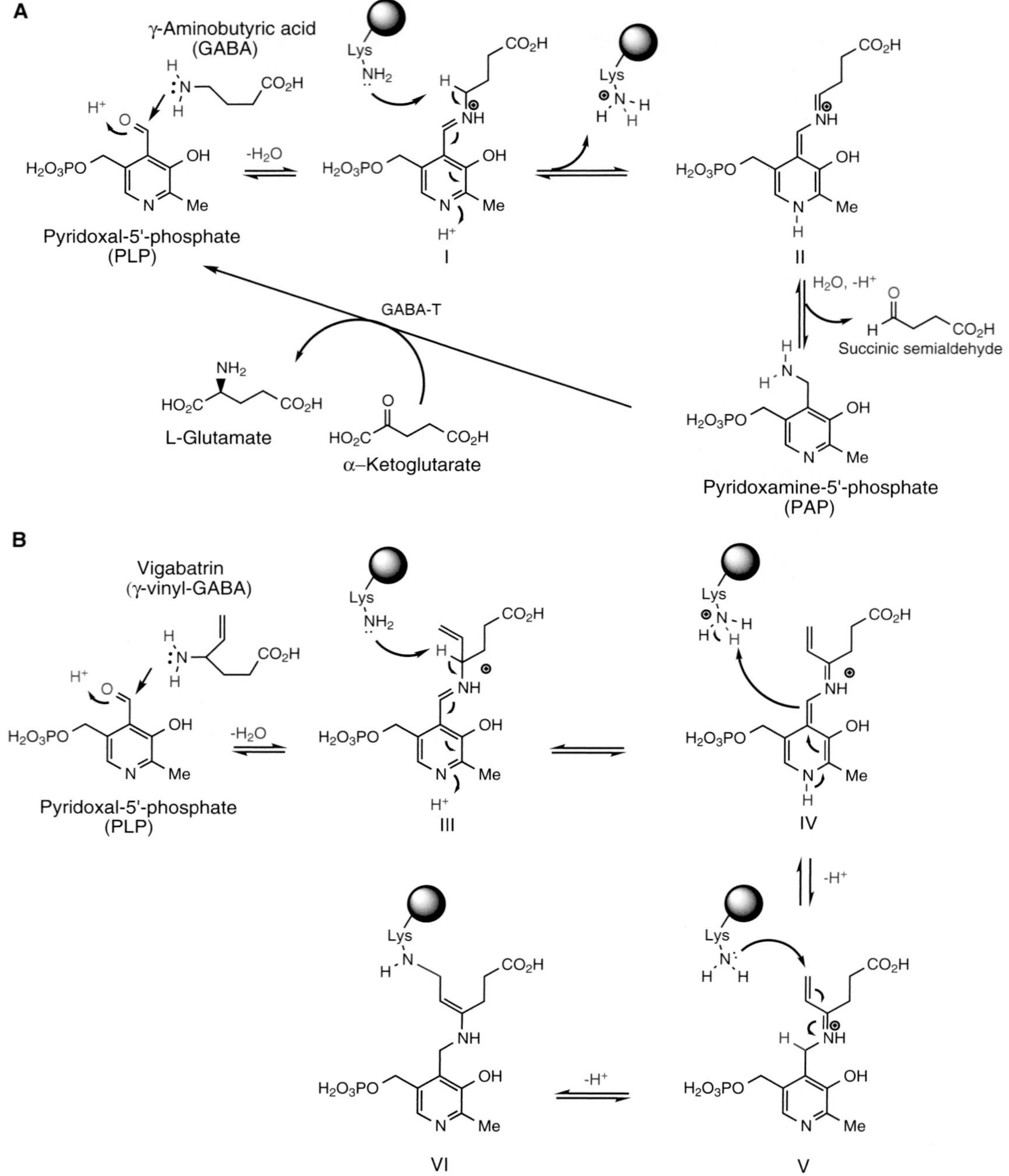

Figure 13.24 Mechanism of covalent inhibition of GABA-T. A, Mechanism of GABA-T metabolism of GABA. B, The role of the vinyl group of vigabatrin in covalent alkylation of the active site lysine.

Metabolism. Like other GABA analogues, vigabatrin is not extensively metabolized.

Physicochemical Properties. Vigabatrin contains both acidic (p*K*a 4.61) and basic (p*K*a 9.91) functional groups. An amino acid, vigabatrin is zwitterionic and soluble in aqueous solution (55.1 mg/mL) and can be administered as an oral solution or tablet. Vigabatrin is hydrophilic, with clogP −0.10.

Pharmacokinetics. Vigabatrin displays linear pharmacokinetics over single and repeated doses between 0.5 and 4 g. Vigabatrin is fully absorbed following oral administration with t_{max} reached within 0.5-1 hour. The effect of food is a 33% decrease in C_{max} and an increase of $t_{1/2}$ to approximately 2 hours, with no significant change in AUC. Vigabatrin is not bound to plasma proteins and has V_d = 1.0-1.1 L/kg. Elimination is renal and age-dependent: $t_{1/2}$(infants, 0.5-2 yr) = 5.7 hours, $t_{1/2}$(children, 10-16 yr) = 9.5 hours, $t_{1/2}$(adults) = 10.5 hours. This translates to substantial differences in clearance: Cl(infants) = 2.4 L/hr, Cl(children) = 5.8 L/hr, Cl(adults) = 7 L/hr. Dose adjustment in renally impaired patients should be taken into consideration, as the AUC increases substantially in these patients and may cause toxicities.[133] Unlike gabapentin and pregabalin, vigabatrin is not known to be transported by

LAT-1; however, evidence suggests alternate amino acid transporters contribute to oral bioavailability.[134] Vigabatrin is unlikely to be a P-gp substrate.[39]

Specific Adverse Events and DDIs. The potential for producing severe, permanent visual field defects (VFDs) led to a Black Box warning for vigabatrin. The estimated prevalence of vigabatrin-induced VFD is 15%-31% in infants, 15% in children, and 25%-50% in adults. AED-induced VFD is specific to vigabatrin, although the exact mechanism is unknown.[135] Due to this severe side effect, vigabatrin is only available through the Support, Help and Resources for Epilepsy (SHARE) program. As part of SHARE, patients are routinely tested for evidence of vision loss and potential markers for future toxicities.

Vigabatrin is a selective inducer of CYP2C9. This does not require dose adjustments with other coadministered AEDs, although clearance of non-AED CYP2C9 substrates may be impacted.

Other Important Aspects of Drug Chemistry. Initial studies performed in rats[136] and human subjects[137] support the efficacy of vigabatrin in treating cocaine and methamphetamine addiction disorders, although subsequent clinical trials were less impressive.

Inhibitors of Glutamate Signaling

Physicochemical and pharmacokinetic properties of glutamate modulators are provided in Table 13.7.

BRIVARACETAM (BRIVIACT) AND LEVETIRACETAM (KEPPRA)

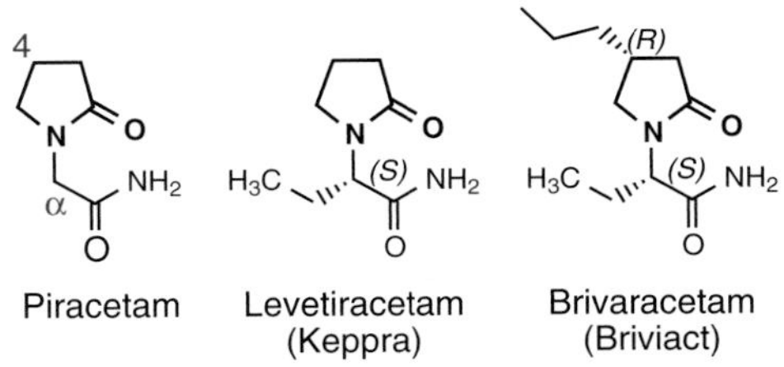

4 N O NH2 α O Piracetam; H3C N O (S) NH2 O Levetiracetam (Keppra); (R) H3C N O (S) NH2 O Brivaracetam (Briviact)

Brivaracetam has been approved by the FDA as an adjunct for the treatment of partial-onset seizures. Brivaracetam and the structurally related levetiracetam are members of the racetam class characterized by an N-substituted pyrrolidinone core. Animal studies suggest that brivaracetam is more potent and has a broader spectrum of activity when compared to levetiracetam.

Receptor Binding/MOA. Brivaracetam and levetiracetam are ligands for the synaptic vesicle protein SV2A, which appears to account for antiseizure activity by protecting against epileptiform responses. Brivaracetam binds SV2A with an affinity approximately 10× that of levetiracetam. In addition, brivarecetam inhibits voltage-gated sodium currents and reversibly blocks the effects of inhibitory GABA and glycine receptors on currents.

SAR. Piracetam is a nootropic that was shown to produce modest anticonvulsant effects in animal models.

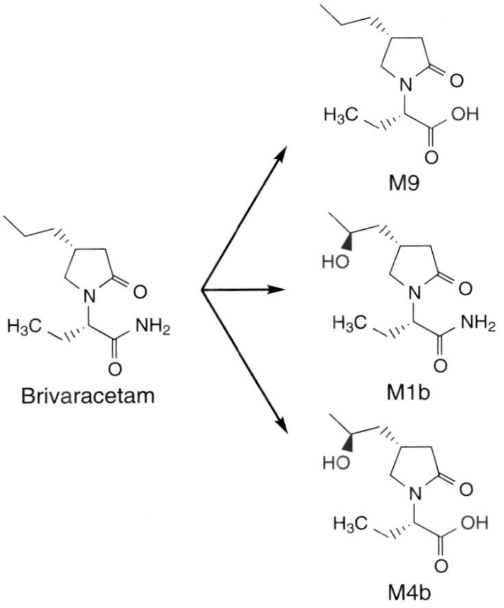

Brivaracetam → M9; M1b; M4b

Figure 13.25 Metabolism of brivaracetam.

Addition of an ethyl group to the α-carbon of piracetam (etiracetam) enhanced this activity, and isolation of the enantiomers showed that the (*S*)-*levo* isomer (levetiracetam) is over 1000× more potent than the (*R*)-*dextro* isomer. An unsubstituted carboxamide group is required for activity, as is a cyclic pyrrolidinone. Addition of unbranched alkyl groups to position 4 are also tolerated, with *n*-propyl (brivaracetam) being the most potent.

Metabolism. Brivaracetam was the main product identified in the plasma, while metabolites M9, M1b, and M4b accounted for 34.2, 15.9, and 15.2% of the administered dose, respectively (Fig. 13.25). Approximately 8.6% of the parent drug was recovered in the urine. The hydrolysis products M9 and M4b are associated with amide hydrolases, while the major oxidizing enzyme is CYP2C8.[138] Unlike brivaracetam, levetiracetam is not extensively metabolized.[139] Approximately 34% of the dose is metabolized, with the major inactive metabolite (LO57) generated by a hydrolytic mechanism.

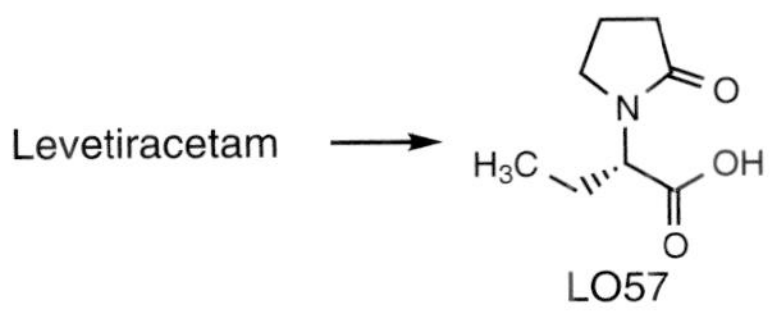

Levetiracetam → LO57

Physicochemical Properties. Brivaracetam and levetiracetam contain two amide functional groups and are net neutral molecules. Racetams are relatively hydrophilic molecules, with log $D_{pH7.4}$ in the range of −0.64 (levetiracetam) to 1.04 (brivaracetam).[140] Levetiracetam and brivaracetam are therefore highly soluble in aqueous solutions and are considered BCS class I substances. The TPSA for both agents is 63.4 Å, which is well within ranges suggestive of high brain permeability.[141]

Pharmacokinetics. Brivaracetam is rapidly absorbed and has an elimination $t_{1/2}$ of 7-8 hours. The drug is poorly bound to plasma protein (~17%). Brivaracetam and its metabolites are excreted primarily in the urine. Absorption of levetiracetam is rapid (t_{max} 1.3 hr) and not impacted by food. Levetiracetam is not bound to plasma proteins and has V_d of 0.5-0.7 L/kg. Elimination is primarily renal; thus, elderly patients and those with compromised creatinine clearance may need dosage adjustment. Levetiracetam is a probable P-gp substrate.[39]

Specific Adverse Events and DDIs. The most common adverse effects consist of nausea, vomiting, dizziness, and drowsiness. Brivaracetam has no effect on plasma levels of CBZ; however, plasma levels of the reactive epoxide metabolite, CBZ-E, are increased due to inhibition of epoxide hydrolase by brivaracetam. Enzyme induction by CBZ enhances clearance of brivaracetam.[142]

Other Important Aspects of Drug Chemistry. Brivaracetam is on the Schedule V list, and levetiracetam is not scheduled.

Miscellaneous Glutamate Antagonists

PERAMPANEL (FYCOMPA)

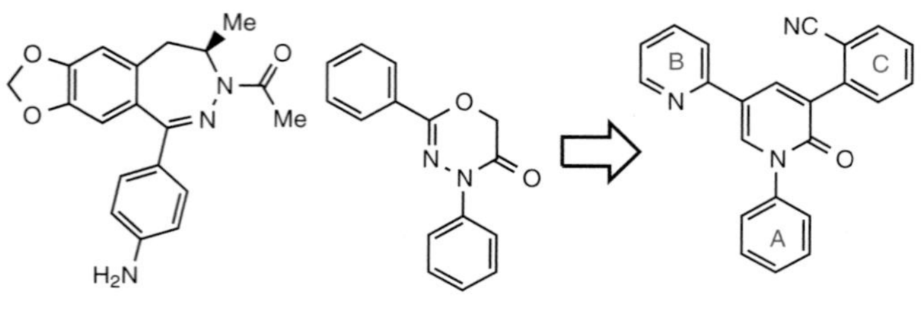

Talampanel HTS hit Perampanel

Perampanel is the only approved AED that works through an AMPAR-blocking mechanism. It is approved as adjunctive treatment for partial-onset seizures, with or without secondarily generalized seizures, in patients 12 years of age and older. Compared to talampanel, an earlier AMPAR blocker in development, perampanel has a long duration of action that permits once-daily dosing.

Receptor Binding/MOA. Perampanel is a selective, noncompetitive antagonist of AMPARs. As a noncompetitive agonist, it is expected that perampanel will produce less sedation compared to competitive antagonists.

SAR. Four aromatic rings are required for potent noncompetitive AMPAR binding. Introduction of basic groups is tolerated by rings B and C. Electron-withdrawing substitutions on ring A at the *o*-position enhance affinity 5-fold. Bioisosteres for the aromatic phenyl rings, for example, thiophene, are generally not tolerated. The AMPAR binding site is generally not tolerant of charged or sterically demanding functional groups.[143]

Metabolism. Over 15 metabolites of perampanel have been isolated in urine and feces. Over 60% of the dose is metabolized to oxidized products on rings A and C (M7, M13, M14). Metabolite M7 arises from hydrolytic ring-opening of arene oxide intermediate M19 (Fig. 13.26). The pyridine ring-opened metabolite M2 is generated by a ring-contraction/rearrangement (M6). Metabolism is mediated primarily by CYP3A4 and CYP3A5.[144]

Physicochemical Properties. Perampanel is a sparingly soluble triaryl pyridone. The pyridine is weakly basic, with p*K*a of 4.0. The calculated clogP is 3.70 and TPSA is 56.46 Å.

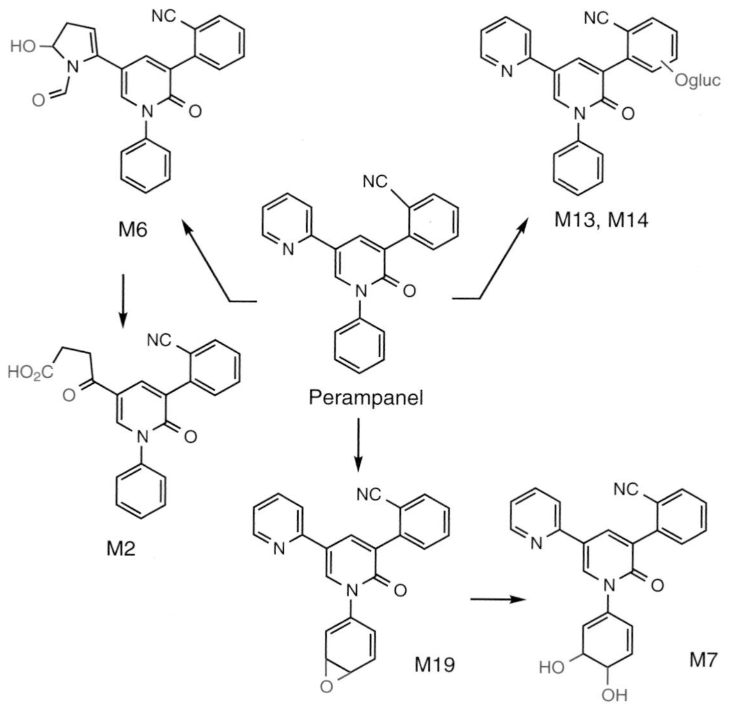

Figure 13.26 Metabolic profile of perampanel.

Table 13.8 Physicochemical and Pharmacokinetic Properties of Multimodal AEDs

	FBM	TPM	VPA	ZNS
clogP	1.20	2.97	2.72	−0.16
Solubility (mg/mL)	0.7	9.8	1.3 (free acid) 50 (Na^+ salt)	0.8
TPSA (Å)	104.64	115.54	37.3	81.75
f (%)[b]	>90	80	100	100
$t_{1/2}$ (hr)	20-23	21	9-18	63[a] 105[b]
t_{max} (hr)	3-5	1-2	2-3 (IR) 5-10 (SR)	2-6
Protein binding (%)	<25	15-41	>90	40
V_d (L/kg)	0.8	0.8-0.55[c]	0.13-0.19	1.45
Metabolized by:	Esterases ADH CYP3A4 CYP2E1	CYP3A4	UGTs CYP2C9 CYP2A6 CYP2B6	CYP3A4
Inducer of:	None	CYP3A4	None	None
Inhibitor of:	CYP2C19	CYP2C19	Epoxide hydrolase	None

[a]In plasma.
[b]In erythrocytes.
[c]V_d is inversely related to dose.
F, oral bioavailability; FBM, felbamate; IR, immediate release; SR, sustained release; TPM, topiramate; TPSA, topologic polar surface area; UGT, UDP-glucuronosyltransferase; V_d, volume of distribution; VPA, valproic acid; ZNS, zonisamide.

Pharmacokinetics. Perampanel follows linear kinetics. Perampanel is readily absorbed from the GIT (~100%), with no significant first-pass metabolism. The t_{max} is approximately 1 hour, which is delayed by a high-fat meal (2-3 hr). Though C_{max} is also lowered by 28%-40%, food does not affect AUC. Perampanel is highly protein bound (95%) to both albumin and α-1-acid glycoprotein. Perampanel is metabolized 90% by liver enzymes of the CYP3A family; patients with hepatic impairment will have substantially increased AUC and elimination $t_{1/2}$ compared to healthy cohorts. Clearance is approximately 0.6-0.7 L/hr, which is not affected by age. The elimination $t_{1/2}$ is highly variable among patients, with a mean of 105 hours. No dose adjustments are required for patients with mild-to-moderate renal impairment.

Specific Adverse Events and DDIs. Perampanel carries a Black Box warning indicating that severe behavioral reactions, such as aggression, hostility, irritability, and homicidal ideation, should be monitored. Like other AEDs, drowsiness and somnolence are frequent side effects. Perampanel is a weak inhibitor of CYP2C8 at high concentrations (30 μmol/L) and a substrate of CYP3A4. Perampanel does not induce CYP or UGT isoforms and has few clinically relevant DDIs with other AEDs. Coadministration with enzyme-inducing AEDs (CBZ, OXC, phenytoin) decreases perampanel AUC by 50%. Ketoconazole, a significant CYP3A4 inhibitor, was found to increase perampanel AUC values by approximately 20%.

Other Important Aspects of Drug Chemistry. Perampanel is a C-III-controlled substance. Subjective assessments in phase III clinical trials reported that some patients (<1%) reported feeling drunk and euphoric while taking perampanel. A recent study comparing perampanel with alprazolam and ketamine reports similar subjective, "drug liking" effects for all three agents at supratherapeutic doses.[145]

Multimodal AEDs

Physicochemical and pharmacokinetic properties of multimodal AEDs are provided in Table 13.8.

FELBAMATE (FELBATOL). Felbamate was approved in 1993 as a treatment for refractory partial seizures and Lennox-Gastaut syndrome and is available in tablet and oral suspension dosage forms. Despite excellent efficacy in treating difficult disease states, the severe idiosyncratic toxicity profile led to a Black Box warning and massive drop in its use.

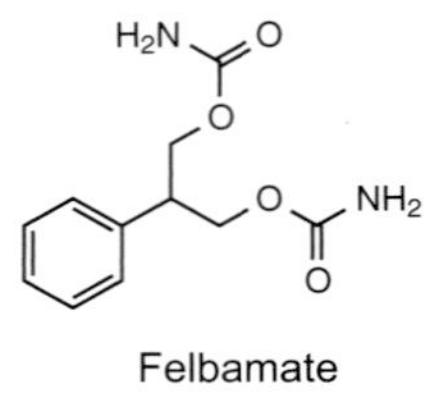

Felbamate

Receptor Binding/MOA. The mechanism of action of felbamate is poorly understood and controversial. Evidence suggests felbamate potentiates GABA currents via $GABA_A$ channels, inhibits Na_V channels, and inhibits NMDARs. Binding is thought to occur through interactions with NR2B and NR1 subunits of NMDARs.[146]

SAR. The biscarbamates possess skeletal muscle relaxant effects in addition to antiseizure activity. A comprehensive SAR study showed that the 2-position (Fig. 13.27) is tolerant of diverse alkyl substitutions to maintain antiseizure activity. Disubstitution at this position, for example, with two alkyl or aromatic groups, generally enhances muscle relaxant activity. The most potent anticonvulsant effects were found with the mono-phenyl substitution (felbamate). Importantly, the EC_{50} for anticonvulsant activity is over 40-fold lower than the EC_{50} for muscle relaxant effects. Anticonvulsant potency is reduced and muscle relaxant activity increased on carbamate hydrolysis (monocarbamoyl felbamate, MCF; Fig. 13.27).

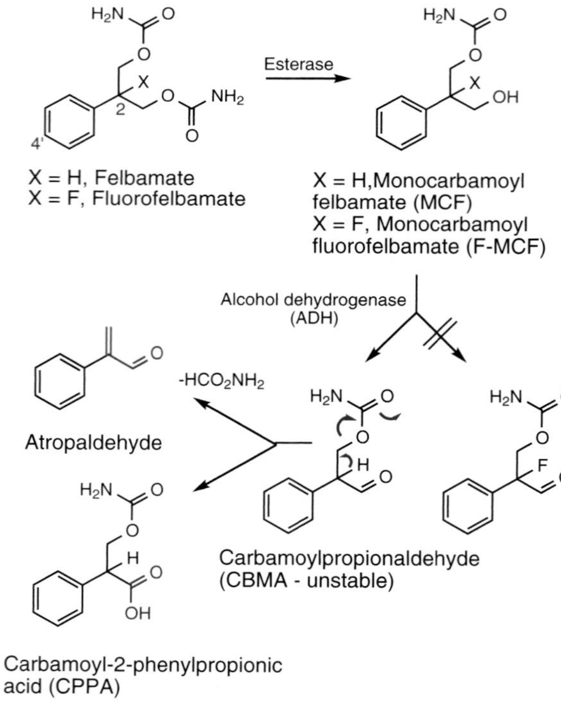

X = H, Felbamate
X = F, Fluorofelbamate

Esterase

X = H, Monocarbamoyl felbamate (MCF)
X = F, Monocarbamoyl fluorofelbamate (F-MCF)

Alcohol dehydrogenase (ADH)

Atropaldehyde

$-HCO_2NH_2$

Carbamoylpropionaldehyde (CBMA - unstable)

Carbamoyl-2-phenylpropionic acid (CPPA)

Figure 13.27 Metabolism of felbamate that leads to the generation of toxic metabolite atropaldehyde. Fluorofelbamate is not converted to atropaldehyde. ADH, alcohol dehydrogenase; CBMA, carbamoylpropionaldehyde; CPPA, 3-carbamoyl-2-phenylpropionic acid; MCF, mono-carbamoyl felbamate.

Metabolism. Felbamate metabolism is shown in Figure 13.27. Esterase hydrolysis of one carbamate produces MCF. The resulting alcohol is a substrate for alcohol dehydrogenase (ADH), which oxidizes the alcohol to an aldehyde (carbamoylpropionaldehyde, CBMA). Chemical instability of CBMA results in the loss of carbamic acid and the formation of atropaldehyde, a highly reactive product that has acrolein-like toxicity in vivo. The analogue 2-fluorofelbamate was designed as a safer alternative that is a weak ADH substrate and, therefore, is not metabolized to atropaldehyde.[147] The 2- and 4′-positions of felbamate are also prone to oxidation by CYP3A4 and CYP2E1 to the alcohol or phenol, respectively.

Physicochemical Properties. Felbamate is available in tablet, capsule, and suspension formulations. The structure consists of a 1,3-propanediol core with a single phenyl substitution at position 2. The terminal alcohols are modified as unsubstituted carbamates. Felbamate is uncharged under normal physiologic conditions and has no ionizable functional groups. The clogP is approximately 1.20 and the TPSA is 104.64 Å. Despite this high polar surface area, felbamate readily penetrates into the CNS. Felbamate has poor aqueous solubility (<1 mg/mL).

Pharmacokinetics. Felbamate follows linear pharmacokinetics. Over 90% of it is absorbed on oral administration and the absorption is not impacted by food. Felbamate shows weak plasma protein binding (<25% to albumin) and a V_d of 0.8 L/kg. The brain:plasma ratio is approximately 1.8:1, meaning high penetration into the CNS. The terminal $t_{1/2}$ is 20-23 hours, and clearance is 26-30 mL/hr/kg in healthy patients. Renally impaired patients show a 40%-50% reduction in total body clearance and an increase in $t_{1/2}$ of 9-15 hours. Approximately 50% of the parent drug is eliminated unchanged, and 10% is eliminated as the 2- or 4′-hydroxy metabolites. The carboxylic acid metabolite, 3-carbamoyl-2-phenylpropionic acid (CPPA), accounts for roughly 10% of the metabolites isolated in urine. The remainder (30%) is excreted as glucuronide conjugates.[148] Felbamate is a possible P-gp substrate.[39]

Specific Adverse Events and DDIs. Idiosyncratic toxicities are common in patients taking felbamate, particularly aplastic anemia and hepatotoxicity. These are likely due to the generation of the highly reactive atropaldehyde in vivo.[149] Felbamate is an inhibitor of CYP2C19, which influences phenytoin clearance but is not an inducer of any enzyme. Enzyme-inducing AEDs increase felbamate clearance.

TOPIRAMATE (TOPAMAX). Topiramate was originally designed as an antidiabetic drug, although its powerful anticonvulsant activity was seen as much more promising. Topiramate was FDA-approved in 1996 as monotherapy or adjunctive therapy in patients over 2 years of age with partial-onset or primary generalized tonic-clonic seizures, and as adjunctive therapy in treating Lennox-Gastaut syndrome. It can also be used as prophylactic treatment of migraines. Topiramate is available as a tablet or sprinkle capsules. It was heralded for its powerful antiepileptic effects, but a poor side effect profile remains a considerable drawback.

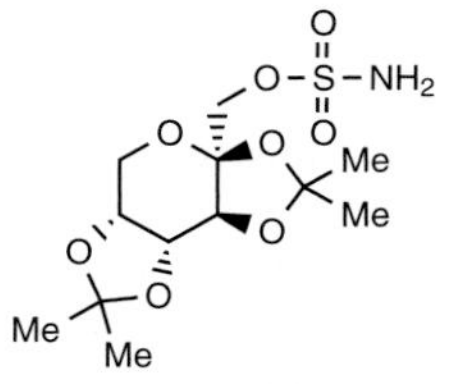

Topiramate

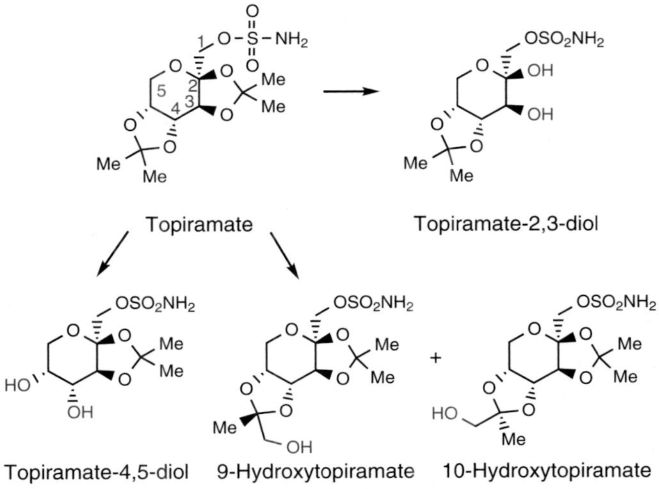

Topiramate → Topiramate-2,3-diol

Topiramate-4,5-diol 9-Hydroxytopiramate 10-Hydroxytopiramate

Figure 13.28 Metabolism of topiramate.

Receptor Binding/MOA. Topiramate produces antiepileptic effects through multiple mechanisms: (1) blockade of voltage-gated Na_V channels and HVA Ca_V channels; (2) augmentation of $GABA_A$ channel activity; (3) inhibition of AMPA/kainate receptors; (4) inhibition of carbonic anhydrase isoforms II and IV (CA-II, CA-IV). It is thought that the broad efficacy of topiramate in treating seizures and its considerable side-effect profile are related to its multiple mechanisms of action.

SAR. Topiramate is a unique pharmacologic agent: the core of the molecule is a simple sugar, fructose, which is modified at the 1-position by a sulfamate functional group. The hydroxyl groups attached to the central pyran ring are connected by acetonide ethers (2,3- and 4,5-acetonide). Extensive SAR studies indicated a eudismic ratio of 1.5 in favor of the (*S*)-enantiomer found in topiramate. The unmodified sulfamate group is required for activity, as is a linking group between the oxygen atoms at the 4,5-position. Replacement of the 4,5-acetonide with a sulfate is approximately as active as the parent.[150]

Metabolism. Topiramate is not extensively metabolized. The major metabolites arise from hydrolysis of the 2,3- and 4,5-acetonide groups and result in inactive products. A second route of oxidative metabolism is ω-oxidation at the acetonide carbons at positions 9 and 10 (Fig. 13.28). The CYP isoforms responsible for the oxidation of topiramate are unknown, although CYP3A4 may be involved (see Specific Adverse Events and DDIs). Some glucuronide metabolites have also been observed.

Physicochemical Properties. The sulfamate group is weakly acidic, pKa = 8.66. Topiramate is relatively hydrophilic and polar compared to other AEDs, with clogP = 2.97 and TPSA = 115.54 Å. These values are outside of typically accepted ranges for agents with high passive CNS permeability. Topiramate is soluble in water (9.8 mg/mL).

Pharmacokinetics. Topiramate is rapidly and completely absorbed with t_{max} = 2 hours following an oral dose. Pharmacokinetics is linear over a therapeutic dose range. The V_d is inversely related to dose: 0.8-0.55 L/kg between 100 and 1200 mg. V_d for female patients is approximately 50% of the values found in males. The mean plasma elimination $t_{1/2}$ is 21 hours, meaning steady state concentration is reached within 4 days. Topiramate is modestly protein-bound (15%-41%). Coadministration with valproate decreased topiramate protein binding by 13%-23%. Approximately 70% of the oral dose is eliminated unchanged in urine, and only 5% of the administered dose is excreted as one of six oxidized and conjugated metabolites. Oral plasma clearance is approximately 23-30 mL/min. Animal studies suggest renal tubule reabsorption is possible with topiramate. Dose reduction may be necessary in elderly patients or those with renal impairment.[151] Topiramate is a possible P-gp substrate.[39]

SPECIFIC ADVERSE EVENTS AND DDIS. Cases of metabolic acidosis have been reported for topiramate. This is likely caused by inhibition of CA-II and CA-IV. Other significant adverse events include paresthesia, weight loss, difficulty with concentration and memory, and depression. The severity of adverse events is responsible for nearly one-third of patients discontinuing treatment.[151] Coadministration with enzyme-inducing AEDs (phenytoin, carbamazepine, phenobarbital) has a significant enhancing effect on topiramate clearance. Coadministration with valproate causes a modest, clinically insignificant decrease in topiramate clearance. Lamotrigine and topiramate can be coadministered without incident.[152] When given in high doses, topiramate is an inducer of CYP3A4, which may be responsible for increased clearance of ethinylestradiol and other CYP3A4 substrates.[153]

VALPROIC ACID. Valproic acid (VPA; Depakene), divalproex sodium (Depakote), and valproate sodium (Depacon) are indicated for monotherapy and adjunctive therapy of complex partial seizures and simple and complex absence seizures. In 1976, valproate was initially approved only for treatment of absence seizures. Divalproex sodium is a mixture of valproate sodium and its conjugate acid, VPA. It is available in many dosage forms, including tablets and capsules, syrup, and intravenous injection. VPA was discovered serendipitously in France in 1962: it was being used as a delivery solvent for a series of experimental tranquilizers when it was discovered that the solvent itself had exceptional anticonvulsant action.[154] VPA is on the World Health Organization's 20th List of Essential Medicines.

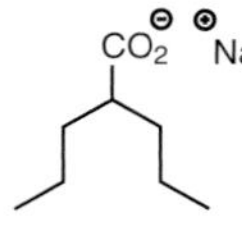

Sodium valproate

Receptor Binding/MOA. Although the molecular mechanism or mechanisms are unknown, VPA produces anticonvulsant effects through inhibitory and excitatory mechanisms: enhancement of GABA synthesis and release and inhibition of the release of β-hydroxybutyric acid, an excitatory neurotransmitter. The enhanced levels of synaptic GABA may be due to inhibition of GABA-T. VPA may also block NMDAR signaling and Na_V channels. Dopaminergic and serotonergic neurotransmission is also altered by VPA, though the exact mechanisms are unknown.[155]

SAR. When administered as the sodium salt, the drug dissipates rapidly in weakly acidic solution, generating the uncharged conjugate acid (VPA). A carboxylic acid or amide bioisostere and two alkyl chains are required for activity. Anticonvulsant activity is directly associated with lipophilicity, with increasing alkyl chain length and branching generally resulting in more potent agents. Adding rigidity to the chains, for example, through introducing a double bond, modestly lowers activity.

Metabolism. VPA is extensively metabolized by phase 1 and phase 2 mechanisms (Fig. 13.29). The principle metabolite (50%) is the carboxylic acid conjugate VPA glucuronide. This is mediated by several UGT isoforms. Oxidation occurs primarily at the 3- and 5-positions to produce the respective alcohols. This occurs primarily in the mitochondria (~40%) by several CYP isoforms (~10%).[156] Dehydration of these intermediates results in Δ^2- and Δ^4-VPA, respectively. Conjugation of Δ^4-VPA by coenzyme A produces the intermediate Δ^4-VPA-SCoA, which is rapidly metabolized to $\Delta^{2,4}$-VPA-SCoA. The α,β,γ,δ-unsaturated carbonyl group is extremely reactive to Michael attack by endogenous nucleophiles, including plasma proteins, enzymes, and glutathione.[157] This is likely responsible for the toxicity profile of VPA.

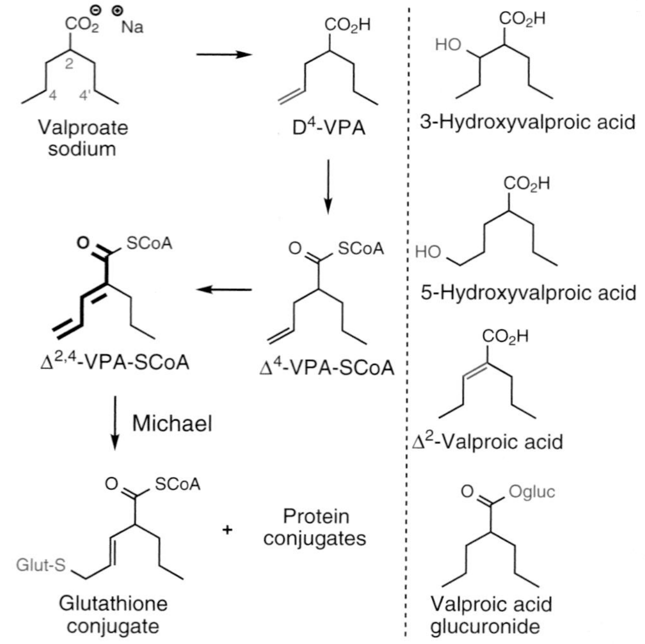

Figure 13.29 Metabolism of valproate. *Left:* mechanism by which ω-oxidation to Δ^4-valproate-SCoA (Δ^4-VPA-S-coenzyme A) leads to hepatotoxic metabolites. The electrophilic α,β,γ,δ-unsaturated Michael acceptor portion of $\Delta^{2,4}$-valproate-SCoA ($\Delta^{2,4}$-VPA-S-coenzyme A) is shown in bold. *Right:* Nontoxic phase I and phase 2 metabolites. *GSH*, glutathione.

Physicochemical Properties. VPA is an amphiphilic, branched, short-chain fatty acid derivative. The clogP is 2.72 and the TPSA is 37.3 Å. VPA is slightly soluble in water in its conjugate free acid form (solubility = 1.3 mg/mL), which is greatly enhanced by formulation as the sodium salt (valproate sodium solubility = 50 mg/mL).

Pharmacokinetics. VPA dose/concentration relationships are nonlinear due to saturable plasma protein binding. VPA is almost completely bioavailable on oral administration, although formulation and route of delivery play a role in t_{max}. The t_{max} for non–enteric coated or immediate-release formulations is reached within 2-3 hours; this rises to 5-10 hours for sustained release formulations. VPA is >90% albumin-bound, with V_d between 0.13 and 0.19 L/kg and brain:plasma ratio between 0.1 and 0.5. Active transport mechanisms, specifically anion exchange uptake transporters in the BBB, aid central bioavailability. Due to impaired plasma protein binding, elderly patients may need a reduction in dose. The $t_{1/2}$ of valproic acid is between 9 and 18 hours, which drops to 5-12 when taken with enzyme-inducing AEDs. VPA is extensively metabolized by multiple CYP isoforms, including CYP2C9, CYP2A6, and CYP2C19, and less than 3% is excreted unchanged in urine. Mean clearance for multiple day dosing ranges from 6.67-8.20 mL/hr/kg to 500-1500 mg/d[158] VPA is a possible P-gp substrate.[39]

Specific Adverse Events and DDIs. Hepatotoxicity and pancreatitis due to the generation of a toxic metabolite is severe and can be life-threatening. VPA can also cause birth defects, and this should be considered when given to women of childbearing age. Platelet counts should be monitored for thrombocytopenia. As with many AEDs, suicidal ideation and somnolence are possible and should be monitored.[159]

Enzyme-inducing AEDs (iminostilbenes, hydantoins, barbiturates) significantly enhance VPA metabolism and clearance. VPA is not an enzyme-inducer, though clinically important increases in plasma concentrations of phenobarbital and lamotrigine are known to occur. Inhibition of epoxide hydrolase may increase CBZ-mediated toxicities by blocking metabolism of the intermediate CBZ-10,11-epoxide (Fig. 13.5). Other plasma protein-bound AEDs may be displaced by valproate, for example, phenytoin.[155]

ZONISAMIDE (ZONEGRAN). Like lamotrigine, zonisamide produces antiepileptic effects through inhibition of voltage-gated ion channels, Na_V and Ca_V. In contast to lamotrigine, evidence suggests zonisamide has effects on multiple neurotransmitter systems that may contribute to a wider spectrum of anticonvulsant activity. Zonisamide capsules are indicated as adjunctive therapy in treating partial seizures in adults, and the drug is effective in treating complex partial seizures, generalized tonic-clonic seizures, myoclonic seizures, and Lennox-Gastaut syndrome. Used in Japan and Korea since 1990, zonisamide was first approved in the United States in 2000.

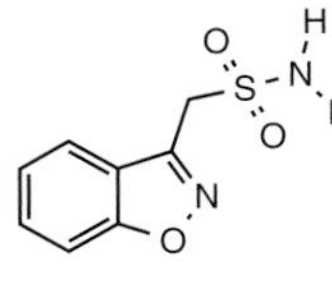

Zonisamide

Receptor Binding/MOA. Available evidence indicates that zonisamide binds and stabilizes inactivated Na_V channels, slowing recovery from inactivation. Zonisamide also inhibits T-type $Ca_V3.2$ channels and glutamate release, though the magnitude of this effect suggests that it only partially contributes to the anticonvulsant mechanism of action. Zonisamide modulates dopaminergic signaling and may also affect free radical scavenging. Evidence shows that chronic zonisamide causes upregulation of excitatory amino acid carrier-1 (EAAC-1) and downregulation of GAT-1. This is expected to decrease synaptic glutamate levels and increase synaptic GABA availability.[160] Although zonisamide contains a sulfonamide function that resembles the sulfonamide class of CA inhibitors, zonisamide is a very weak CA inhibitor.

SAR. Detailed SAR of zonisamide at multiple targets is lacking. An early SAR study showed that sulfonamide N-alkylation by one or two short-chain (e.g., methyl, ethyl) groups was tolerated, although longer chain derivatives were inactive. The fact that N,N-dialkylation was tolerated suggests an acidic group is not a rigid requirement in this region. Halogen substitution of the aromatic ring enhances anticonvulsant and neurotoxic potency, resulting in a net drop in therapeutic index.

Metabolism. Zonisamide is subject to extensive CYP-mediated oxidation, reduction, and acetylation (Fig. 13.30). The major route of metabolism is reduction of the benzoxazole heterocyclic ring to a short-lived, ring-opened imine intermediate that rapidly decomposes to 2-(sulfamoylacetyl)-phenol (2-SMAP). This is catalyzed by CYP3A4. Glucuronide conjugation produces metabolite M3 (12.6%). Acetylation (M8, 7.7%) and conjugation (M6, 7.6%) are minor metabolic pathways.[161]

Physicochemical Properties. Zonisamide is the only AED with a benzisoxazole core. Like other CA inhibitors, zonisamide has a weakly acidic primary sulfonamide group (pKa = 10.2). Zonisamide is relatively hydrophilic, with calculated clogP = −0.16, and it has a modestly high TPSA (81.75 Å). In spite of this, zonisamide has high central bioavailability. Zonisamide is only slightly soluble in aqueous solution (0.80 mg/mL).

Pharmacokinetics. Zonisamide is rapidly and completely absorbed, with peak plasma concentrations reached in 2-6 hours. Food modestly delays t_{max} (4-6 hr), but AUC is unaffected. Zonisamide is extensively concentrated in plasma erythrocytes, likely due to the affinity of zonisamide for CA enzymes. Absorption is linear until high concentrations (800 mg) saturate erythrocyte binding. Apparent V_d is 1.45 L/kg and plasma protein binding is modest at around 40%. Approximately 60% of the oral dose is found unchanged in urine, and major metabolites are glucuronide conjugates of 2-SMAP (metabolite M3; Fig. 13.30). Plasma $t_{1/2}$ is 63 hours and the elimination $t_{1/2}$ in red blood cells is approximately 105 hours. Plasma clearance during monotherapy is 0.30-0.35 mL/min/kg, which is increased to 0.50 mL/min/kg when taken with enzyme-inducing AEDs. In patients with renal damage (CrCl <20 mL/min), renal clearance dropped from 3.5 to 2.23 mL/min and AUC rose 35%. Doses should be decreased in these patients. There is no effect of age on zonisamide pharmacokinetics. Zonisamide is unlikely to be a P-gp substrate.[39]

Specific Adverse Events and DDIs. Zonisamide is a sulfonamide and should not be given to patients with sulfonamide allergies, as this could lead to life-threatening reactions (e.g., Stevens-Johnson syndrome, TEN). Thus, discontinuation of zonisamide should be considered if a rash is observed. Oligohidrosis (deficient sweat production) and hyperthermia in pediatric patients are also potentially life-threatening side effects of zonisamide

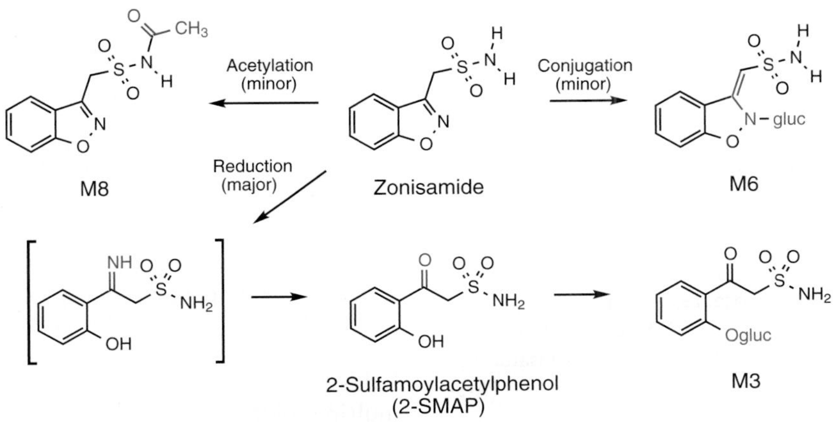

M8 — Acetylation (minor) — Zonisamide — Conjugation (minor) — M6

Reduction (major)

2-Sulfamoylacetylphenol (2-SMAP) — M3

Figure 13.30 Metabolism of zonisamide.

Afinitor (Everolimus)

Valnoctamide (R = Me) (Valpromide, R = H)

Fenfluramine (ZX008)

Acetazolamide

Diacomit (Stiripentol)

Cenobamate (YKP3089)

Retigabine

Figure 13.31 Antiepileptic drugs in the pipeline.

therapy. Women of child-bearing age should be aware of teratogenic effects and fetal abnormalities when taking zonisamide. Psychiatric (depression, psychosis) and psychomotor slowing (difficulty concentrating, speech and language problems) are cognitive adverse events. Somnolence and fatigue are also common.[162]

Zonisamide does not induce metabolic enzymes. When taken with enzyme-inducing AEDs, the $t_{1/2}$ falls to 27 hours (phenytoin), 38 hours (phenobarbital, CBZ), and 46 hours (valproate). Plasma protein binding is not affected by other AEDs.

AEDs IN THE PIPELINE

The quest continues for the discovery of efficacious AEDs with an optimal adverse effect profile. Development of prodrugs of existing AEDs resulted in the approval of ESL in 2013. This approach is also applied to the development of primary amides, valproamide and valnoctamide (Fig. 13.31), which are hydrolyzed to their corresponding carboxylic acid analogues in vivo. Although less teratogenic effects have been observed in preclinical trials, their development is currently limited by potent epoxide hydrolase inhibition, which can cause toxic accumulation of CBZ-10,11-epoxide when taken with CBZ.

Repurposing of existing FDA-approved medications as syndrome-specific AEDs is an approach that has much potential.

- Everolimus (Afinitor), an inhibitor of the mammalian target of rapamycin (mTOR), significantly reduced seizures in patients with treatment-resistant tuberous sclerosis complex (TSC), a rare genetic disorder that causes seizures arising from benign tumor growth in the brain. Because upregulation of mTOR is a hallmark of TSC, this represents a unique mechanism-based approach to epilepsy treatment.
- Clinical trials of low-dose fenfluramine, once infamously used as an anorectic agent with phentermine (Fen-Phen), have shown promise in treating patients with Dravet syndrome. Though the exact anticonvulsant mechanism remains to be elucidated, fenfluramine is a known serotonin-releasing agent.[163]
- The CA inhibitor acetazolamide blocks seizures through an incompletely understood mechanism that may be related to acidosis. More discussion of CA as a therapeutic target can be found in Chapter 16.
- As of 2017, stiripentol (Diacomit) is an approved AED in European markets, Canada, and Japan, but not in the United States. The mechanism of action includes augmentation of GABAergic signaling, and is a safe and effective agent for treating Dravet syndrome.[164]
- Retigabine (Potiga), a mechanistically unique KCNQ K^+ channel opener, was FDA-approved in 2011 and removed from the market in 2017.

PHYTOCANNABINOIDS AS ANTISEIZURE DRUGS

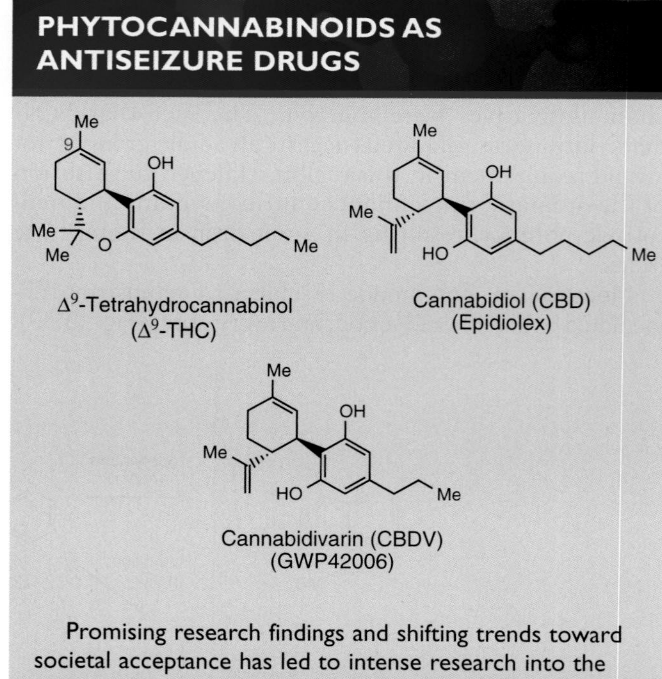

Promising research findings and shifting trends toward societal acceptance has led to intense research into the anticonvulsant potential of phytocannabinoids isolated from *Cannabis sativa* and *Cannabis indica*. Reports of cannabis use to treat convulsive disorders originate as far back as 2900 BC in Sumerian and Arabic texts. Following a medical trip to India, British surgeon William O'Shaughnessy wrote in

1843 about the efficacy of cannabis in treating epilepsy. In the years since, unsupervised use of medical cannabis preparations has been documented in many anecdotal reports regarding safety and efficacy in treating rare and severe epilepsies in children and adults. Reviews conducted by the American Academy of Neurology and Cochrane Database conclude that medical cannabis is of "unknown efficacy" to treat epilepsy[165,166]; nonetheless, clinical trials of phytocannabinoids—agents of plant-based origin that engage cannabinoid receptors, CB1R and CB2R—are currently under way to clarify these unknowns.[167]

Perhaps the most well-known of the phytocannabinoids is Δ^9-tetrahydrocannabinol (Δ^9-THC). A CB1R partial agonist, Δ^9-THC is primarily responsible for the psychomotor and reinforcing effects of cannabis. Δ^9-THC produced an anticonvulsive effect in over 60% of animal seizure model studies, although another 32% showed no significant effect. Comparatively, the nonpsychoactive phytocannabinoids cannabidiol (CBD) and cannabidivarin (CBDV) were effective in 80% of 41 animal seizure model studies.[167] Owing to their lipophilicity ($clogP_{CBD}$ 7.03, $clogP_{CBDV}$ 5.97), CBD and CBDV are formulated as oral solutions in sesame oil.

The pharmacologic targets of CBD are numerous and include TRP channels, 5-HT_{1A} receptors, T-type Ca_V channels, and GPR55. Unlike Δ^9-THC, CBD is not an agonist at CB1R or CB2R; in fact, recent studies suggest CBD may act as a CB1R negative allosteric modulator.[168] This means CBD is free from the psychoactive effects of Δ^9-THC and thus is a potentially safer therapeutic option. The efficacy of CBD was recently demonstrated in a clinical trial of 214 children with drug-resistant Dravet syndrome,[169] and in 2017 a New Drug Application (NDA) was submitted to the FDA for CBD (Epidiolex, GW Pharmaceuticals) for the treatment of Dravet and Lennox-Gastaut syndromes. On June 25, 2018, Epidiolex was approved by the FDA to treat seizures associated with these severe diseases. This is significant because Epidiolex is the first FDA-approved medication containing a purified agent from cannabis plant material and is also the first approved drug for the treatment of patients with Dravet syndrome.

The structurally related CBDV differs from CBD only by a shortening of the 4′-alkyl chain from pentyl to propyl. Similar to CBD, CBDV produces only weak effects at CB1R and CB2R and stronger actions at TRP channels and GPR55. CBDV is anticonvulsant with minimal behavioral effects in animal models and is in phase II clinical trials for epilepsy under the identifier GWP42006. The volume of natural and synthetic analogues of CBD and CBDV[170] suggest a long future for phytocannabinoid-derived treatments for epilepsy.

Structure Challenge

The structures of 10 AEDs are shown below (A-J). Use your understanding of SAR and MOA to match the appropriate medication or medications for each question. Note that an AED may be used more than once, or not at all.

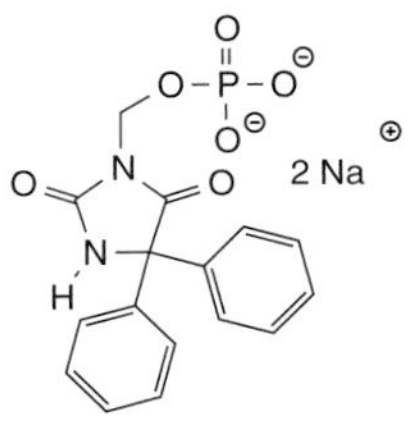

A 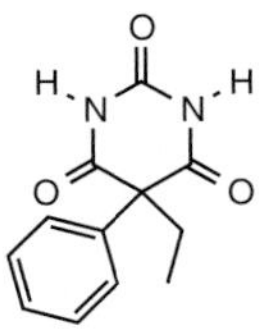 B 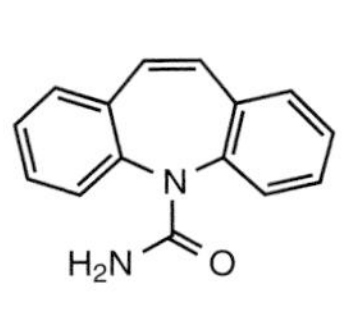 C 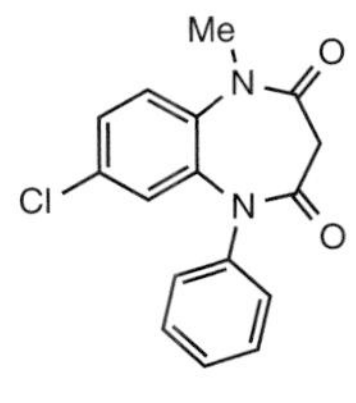 D 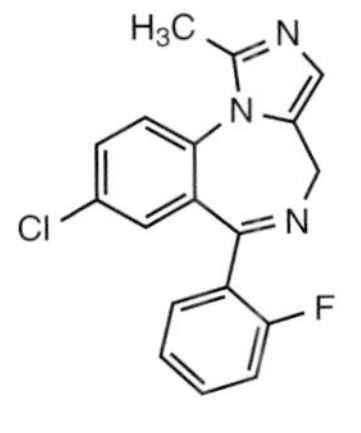 E

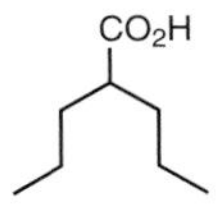

F 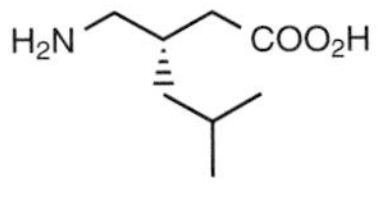 G 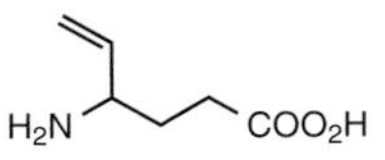 H 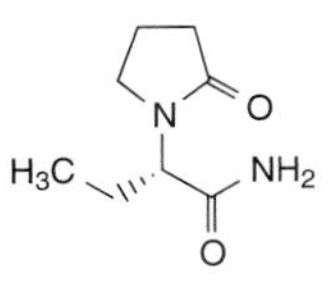 I 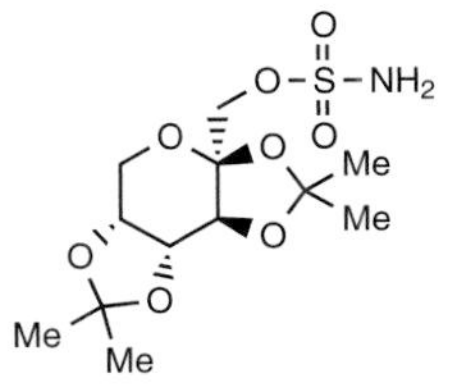 J

1. A short-acting benzodiazepine to treating status epilepticus: ____, and a longer-acting benzodiazepine suitable for daily seizure prophylaxis: ____.
2. A water-soluble prodrug that generates an active AED on injection: ____.
3. An AED that blocks seizures through covalent modification of GABA-T: ____.
4. Four compounds whose AED activities are understood to include direct binding to $GABA_A$ ion channels: ____, ____, ____, ____.

Structure Challenge—*Continued*

5. An AED that can cause toxic acidosis through inhibition of carbonic anhydrase: ____.
6. AEDs are often administered in combination, and many influence the pharmacokinetic profile of coadministered drugs. Fill in the table below, indicating whether the AEDs on the left cause an increase (+), decrease (−), or no change (±) on the metabolism of those on the top. Refer to the text or other resources, if necessary.

	A	B	C	D	E	F	G	H	I	J
Drug Name:										
A										
B										
C										
D										
E										
F										
G										
H										
I										
J										

Structure Challenge answers found immediately after References.

REFERENCES

1. Zack MM, Kobau R. National and state estimates of the numbers of adults and children with active epilepsy – United States, 2015. *MMWR Morb Mortal Wkly Rep*. 2017;66:821-825.
2. Stevenson DC. Hippocrates: On the Sacred Disease. The Internet Classics Archive. http://classics.mit.edu/Hippocrates/sacred.html. Accessed 27 December 2017.
3. Friedlander WJ. *History of Modern Epilepsy: The Beginning, 1865-1914*. Westport: Greenwood Press; 2001.
4. Shorvon SD. Drug treatment of epilepsy in the century of the ILAE: the first 50 years, 1909-1958. *Epilepsia*. 2009;50:69-92.
5. Institute of Medicine (IOM). *Epilepsy across the Spectrum: Promoting Health and Understanding*. Washington, DC: The National Academies Press; 2012.
6. Fisher RS, van Emde Boas W, Blume W, et al. Epileptic seizures and epilepsy: definitions proposed by the International League against epilepsy (ILAE) and the International Bureau for epilepsy (IBE). *Epilepsia*. 2005;46:470-472.
7. Liang JG, Lee D, Youn SE, et al. Electroencephalography network effects of corpus callosotomy in patients with Lennox-Gastaut syndrome. *Front Neurol*. 2017;8:456.
8. Genton P. When antiepileptic drugs aggravate epilepsy. *Brain Dev*. 2000;22:75-80.
9. Ceulemans B, Boel M, Claes L, et al. Severe myoclonic epilepsy in infancy: toward an optimal treatment. *J Child Neurol*. 2004;19:516-521.
10. Fisher RS, Cross JH, French JA, et al. Operational classification of seizure types by the International League against epilepsy: position paper of the ILAE Commission for classification and terminology. *Epilepsia*. 2017;58:522-530.
11. Berg AT, Berkovic SF, Brodie MJ, et al. Revised terminology and concepts for organization of seizures and epilepsies: report of the ILAE Commission on Classification and Terminology, 2005-2009. *Epilepsia*. 2010;51:676-685.
12. Guerrini R, Pellacani S. Benign childhood focal epilepsies. *Epilepsia*. 2012;53:9-18.
13. Wu YW, Sullivan J, McDaniel SS, et al. Incidence of Dravet syndrome in a US population. *Pediatrics*. 2015;136:e1310-e1315.
14. Yu FH, Mantegazza M, Westenbroek RE, et al. Reduced sodium current in GABAergic interneurons in a mouse model of severe myoclonic epilepsy in infancy. *Nat Neurosci*. 2006;9:1142-1149.
15. Ostendorf AP, Ng YT. Treatment-resistant Lennox-Gastaut syndrome: therapeutic trends, challenges and future directions. *Neuropsychiatr Dis Treat*. 2017;13:1131-1140.
16. Hartman AL, Gasior M, Vining EP, Rogawski MA. The neuropharmacology of the ketogenic diet. *Pediatr Neurol*. 2007;36:281-292.
17. Lancman G, Virk M, Shao H, et al. Vagus nerve stimulation vs. corpus callosotomy in the treatment of Lennox-Gastaut syndrome: a meta-analysis. *Seizure*. 2013;22:3-8.
18. Catterall WA. Voltage-gated calcium channels. *Cold Spring Harb Perspect Biol*. 2011;3:a003947.
19. Venkatesan K, Alix P, Marquet A, et al. Altered balance between excitatory and inhibitory inputs onto CA1 pyramidal neurons from SV2A-deficient but not SV2B-deficient mice. *J Neurosci Res*. 2012;90:2317-2327.
20. Nowack A, Malarkey EB, Yao J, et al. Levetiracetam reverses synaptic deficits produced by overexpression of SV2A. *PLoS One*. 2011;6:e29560.
21. Winden KD, Karsten SL, Bragin A, et al. A systems level, functional genomics analysis of chronic epilepsy. *PLoS One*. 2011;6:e20763.

22. Hess EJ. Migraines in mice? *Cell*. 1996;87:1149-1151.
23. Wallace RH, Wang DW, Singh R, et al. Febrile seizures and generalized epilepsy associated with a mutation in the Na^+-channel beta1 subunit gene SCN1B. *Nat Genet*. 1998;19:366-370.
24. Sugawara T, Mazaki-Miyazaki E, Ito M, et al. Nav1.1 mutations cause febrile seizures associated with afebrile partial seizures. *Neurology*. 2001;57:703-705.
25. Biervert C, Schroeder BC, Kubisch C, et al. A potassium channel mutation in neonatal human epilepsy. *Science*. 1998;279: 403-406.
26. Singh NA, Charlier C, Stauffer D, et al. A novel potassium channel gene, KCNQ2, is mutated in an inherited epilepsy of newborns. *Nat Genet*. 1998;18:25-29.
27. Charlier C, Singh NA, Ryan SG, et al. A pore mutation in a novel KQT-like potassium channel gene in an idiopathic epilepsy family. *Nat Genet*. 1998;18:53-55.
28. Dedek K, Kunath B, Kananura C, et al. Myokymia and neonatal epilepsy caused by a mutation in the voltage sensor of the KCNQ2 K^+ channel. *Proc Natl Acad Sci USA*. 2001;98:12272-12277.
29. Cossette P, Liu L, Brisebois K, et al. Mutation of GABRA1 in an autosomal dominant form of juvenile myoclonic epilepsy. *Nat Genet*. 2002;31:184-189.
30. Wallace RH, Marini C, Petrou S, et al. Mutant GABA(A) receptor gamma2-subunit in childhood absence epilepsy and febrile seizures. *Nat Genet*. 2001;28:49-52.
31. Baulac S, Huberfeld G, Gourfinkel-An I, et al. First genetic evidence of GABA(A) receptor dysfunction in epilepsy: a mutation in the gamma2-subunit gene. *Nat Genet*. 2001;28:46-48.
32. Sarup A, Larsson OM, Schousboe A. GABA transporters and GABA-transaminase as drug targets. *Curr Drug Targets CNS Neurol Disord*. 2003;2:269-277.
33. Brodie MJ, Sills GJ. Combining antiepileptic drugs–rational polytherapy? *Seizure*. 2011;20:369-375.
34. Pearce RE, Uetrecht JP, Leeder JS. Pathways of carbamazepine bioactivation in vitro: II. The role of human cytochrome P450 enzymes in the formation of 2-hydroxyiminostilbene. *Drug Metab Dispos*. 2005;33:1819-1826.
35. Pearce RE, Lu W, Wang Y, et al. Pathways of carbamazepine bioactivation in vitro. III. The role of human cytochrome P450 enzymes in the formation of 2,3-dihydroxycarbamazepine. *Drug Metab Dispos*. 2008;36:1637-1649.
36. Lu W, Uetrecht JP. Peroxidase-mediated bioactivation of hydroxylated metabolites of carbamazepine and phenytoin. *Drug Metab Dispos*. 2008;36:1624-1636.
37. Bertilsson L. Clinical pharmacokinetics of carbamazepine. *Clin Pharmacokinet*. 1978;3:128-143.
38. Eichelbaum M, Tomson T, Tybring G, Bertilsson L. Carbamazepine metabolism in man. Induction and pharmacogenetic aspects. *Clin Pharmacokinet*. 1985;10:80-90.
39. Zhang C, Kwan P, Zuo Z, Baum L. The transport of antiepileptic drugs by P-glycoprotein. *Adv Drug Deliv Rev*. 2012;64:930-942.
40. FDA Product Information: Tegretol (Carbamazepine). https://www.accessdata.fda.gov/drugsatfda_docs/label/2009/016608s101,018281s048lbl.pdf. Accessed 16 November 2017.
41. Mattson GF, Mattson RH, Cramer JA. Interaction between valproic acid and carbamazepine: an in vitro study of protein binding. *Ther Drug Monit*. 1982;4:181-184.
42. Bertilsson L, Tomson T. Clinical pharmacokinetics and pharmacological effects of carbamazepine and carbamazepine-10,11-epoxide. An update. *Clin Pharmacokinet*. 1986;11:177-198.
43. Froescher W, Eichelbaum M, Niesen M, Dietrich K, Rausch P. Carbamazepine levels in breast milk. *Ther Drug Monit*. 1984;6:266-271.
44. Larkin JG, McKee PJ, Forrest G, et al. Lack of enzyme induction with oxcarbazepine (600 mg daily) in healthy subjects. *Br J Clin Pharmacol*. 1991;31:65-71.
45. Patsalos PN, Stephenson TJ, Krishna S, et al. Side-effects induced by carbamazepine-10,11-epoxide. *Lancet*. 1985;2:496.
46. Lloyd P, Flesch G, Dieterle W. Clinical pharmacology and pharmacokinetics of oxcarbazepine. *Epilepsia*. 1994;35:S10-S13.
47. May TW, Korn-Merker E, Rambeck B. Clinical pharmacokinetics of oxcarbazepine. *Clin Pharmacokinet*. 2003;42:1023-1042.
48. Dam M, Ekberg R, Loyning Y, Waltimo O, Jakobsen K. A double-blind study comparing oxcarbazepine and carbamazepine in patients with newly diagnosed, previously untreated epilepsy. *Epilepsy Res*. 1989;3:70-76.
49. Almeida L, Soares-da-Silva P. Eslicarbazepine acetate (BIA 2-093). *Neurotherapeutics*. 2007;4:88-96.
50. Benes J, Parada A, Figueiredo AA, et al. Anticonvulsant and sodium channel-blocking properties of novel 10,11-dihydro-5H-dibenz[b,f]azepine-5-carboxamide derivatives. *J Med Chem*. 1999;42:2582-2587.
51. Bialer M, Soares-da-Silva P. Pharmacokinetics and drug interactions of eslicarbazepine acetate. *Epilepsia*. 2012;53:935-946.
52. Brown ME, El-Mallakh RS. Role of eslicarbazepine in the treatment of epilepsy in adult patients with partial-onset seizures. *Ther Clin Risk Man*. 2010;6:103-109.
53. Kuo CC. A common anticonvulsant binding site for phenytoin, carbamazepine, and lamotrigine in neuronal Na^+ channels. *Mol Pharmacol*. 1998;54:712-721.
54. Lipkind GM, Fozzard HA. Molecular model of anticonvulsant drug binding to the voltage-gated sodium channel inner pore. *Mol Pharmacol*. 2010, 78:631-638.
55. Poupaert JH, Adline J, Claesen MH, et al. Stereochemical aspects of the metabolism of 5-(4'-fluorophenyl)-5-phenylhydantoin in the rat. *J Med Chem*. 1979;22:1140-1142.
56. Nelson WL, Kwon YG, Marshall GL, et al. Fluorinated phenytoin anticonvulsant analogs. *J Pharm Sci*. 1979;68:115-117.
57. Friedlander WJ. Putnam, Merritt, and the discovery of Dilantin. *Epilepsia*. 1986;27:S1-S20.
58. Glazko AJ. Addendum to "Putnam, Merritt, and the discovery of Dilantin". *Epilepsia*. 1987;28:87-88.
59. Putnam TJ, Merritt HH. Experimental determination of the anticonvulsant properties of some phenyl derivatives. *Science*. 1937;85:525-526.
60. Spielberg SP, Gordon GB, Blake DA, et al. Predisposition to phenytoin hepatotoxicity assessed in vitro. *N Engl J Med*. 1981;305:722-727.
61. Winn LM, Wells PG. Phenytoin-initiated DNA oxidation in murine embryo culture, and embryo protection by the antioxidative enzymes superoxide dismutase and catalase: evidence for reactive oxygen species-mediated DNA oxidation in the molecular mechanism of phenytoin teratogenicity. *Mol Pharmacol*. 1995;48: 112-120.
62. Munns AJ, De Voss JJ, Hooper WD, et al. Bioactivation of phenytoin by human cytochrome P450: characterization of the mechanism and targets of covalent adduct formation. *Chem Res Toxicol*. 1997;10:1049-1058.
63. Cuttle L, Munns AJ, Hogg NA, et al. Phenytoin metabolism by human cytochrome P450: involvement of P450 3A and 2C forms in secondary metabolism and drug-protein adduct formation. *Drug Metab Dispos*. 2000;28:945-950.
64. Kim PM, Winn LM, Parman T, Wells PG. UDP-glucuronosyltransferase-mediated protection against in vitro DNA oxidation and micronucleus formation initiated by phenytoin and its embryotoxic metabolite 5-(p-hydroxyphenyl)-5-phenylhydantoin. *J Pharmacol Exp Ther*. 1997;280:200-209.
65. Varia SA, Schuller S, Sloan KB, Stella VJ. Phenytoin prodrugs III: water-soluble prodrugs for oral and/or parenteral use. *J Pharm Sci*. 1984;73:1068-1073.
66. Browne TR, Davoudi H, Donn KH, et al. Bioavailability of ACC-9653 (phenytoin prodrug). *Epilepsia*. 1989;30:S27-S32.

67. Burstein AH, Cox DS, Mistry B, Eddington ND. Phenytoin pharmacokinetics following oral administration of phenytoin suspension and fosphenytoin solution to rats. *Epilepsy Res.* 1999;34:129-133.
68. Boucher BA. Fosphenytoin: a novel phenytoin prodrug. *Pharmacotherapy.* 1996;16:777-791.
69. Fischer JH, Patel TV, Fischer PA. Fosphenytoin: clinical pharmacokinetics and comparative advantages in the acute treatment of seizures. *Clin Pharmacokinet.* 2003;42:33-58.
70. Boucher BA, Feler CA, Dean JC, et al. The safety, tolerability, and pharmacokinetics of fosphenytoin after intramuscular and intravenous administration in neurosurgery patients. *Pharmacotherapy.* 1996;16:638-645.
71. Cohen AF, Ashby L, Crowley D, et al. Lamotrigine (BW430C), a potential anticonvulsant. Effects on the central nervous system in comparison with phenytoin and diazepam. *Br J Clin Pharmacol.* 1985;20:619-629.
72. Maggs JL, Naisbitt DJ, Tettey JN, et al. Metabolism of lamotrigine to a reactive arene oxide intermediate. *Chem Res Toxicol.* 2000;13:1075-1081.
73. Janszky J, Rasonyi G, Halasz P, et al. Disabling erratic myoclonus during lamotrigine therapy with high serum level–report of two cases. *Clin Neuropharmacol.* 2000;23:86-89.
74. FDA Prescribing Information: Lamictal (Lamotrigine). https://www.accessdata.fda.gov/drugsatfda_docs/label/2006/020241s10s21s25s26s27, 020764s3s14s18s19s20lbl.pdf. Accessed 29 December 2017.
75. Chung SS. Lacosamide: new adjunctive treatment option for partial-onset seizures. *Expert Opin Pharmacother.* 2010;11:1595-1602.
76. Casas-Fernandez C, Martinez-Bermejo A, Rufo-Campos M, et al. Efficacy and tolerability of lacosamide in the concomitant treatment of 130 patients under 16 years of age with refractory epilepsy: a prospective, open-label, observational, multicenter study in Spain. *Drugs R D.* 2012;12:187-197.
77. Wilson SM, Khanna R. Specific binding of lacosamide to collapsin response mediator protein 2 (CRMP2) and direct impairment of its canonical function: implications for the therapeutic potential of lacosamide. *Mol Neurobiol.* 2015;51:599-609.
78. Czech T, Yang JW, Csaszar E, et al. Reduction of hippocampal collapsin response mediated protein-2 in patients with mesial temporal lobe epilepsy. *Neurochem Res.* 2004;29:2189-2196.
79. Beyreuther BK, Freitag J, Heers C, et al. Lacosamide: a review of preclinical properties. *CNS Drug Rev.* 2007;13:21-42.
80. Conley JD, Kohn H. Functionalized DL-amino acid derivatives. Potent new agents for the treatment of epilepsy. *J Med Chem.* 1987;30:567-574.
81. Kohn H, Sawhney KN, LeGall P, et al. Preparation and anticonvulsant activity of a series of functionalized alpha-aromatic and alpha-heteroaromatic amino acids. *J Med Chem.* 1990;33:919-926.
82. Cawello W, Fuhr U, Hering U, et al. Impact of impaired renal function on the pharmacokinetics of the antiepileptic drug lacosamide. *Clin Pharmacokinet.* 2013;52:897-906.
83. FDA Full Prescribing Information, Vimpat(R) (Lacosamide). Reference ID: 3294138. https://www.accessdata.fda.gov/drugsatfda_docs/label/2013/022253s024, 022254s018, 022255s010lbl.pdf. Accessed 22 December 2017.
84. Tilz C, Resch R, Hofer T, Eggers C. Successful treatment for refractory convulsive status epilepticus by non-parenteral lacosamide. *Epilepsia.* 2010;51:316-317.
85. DeGiorgio AC, Desso TE, Lee L, DeGiorgio CM. Ventricular tachycardia associated with lacosamide co-medication in drug-resistant epilepsy. *Epilepsy Behav Case Rep.* 2013;1:26-28.
86. McCleane G, Koch B, Rauschkolb C. Does SPM 927 have an analgesic effect in human neuropathic pain? An open label study. *Neurosci Lett.* 2003;352:117-120.
87. Brodie MJ, Rosenfeld WE, Vazquez B, et al. Rufinamide for the adjunctive treatment of partial seizures in adults and adolescents: a randomized placebo-controlled trial. *Epilepsia.* 2009;50(8):1899-1909.
88. Gilchrist J, Dutton S, Diaz-Bustamante M, et al. Nav1.1 modulation by a novel triazole compound attenuates epileptic seizures in rodents. *ACS Chem Biol.* 2014;9:1204-1212.
89. FDA Prescribing Information for Banzel (Rufinamide). https://www.accessdata.fda.gov/drugsatfda_docs/label/2008/021911lbl.pdf. Accessed 22 December 2017.
90. CDER FDA Center for Drug Evaluation Research Review of Environmental Assessment for Inovelon Oral Tablets, NDA 21-911. https://www.accessdata.fda.gov/drugsatfda_docs/nda/2008/021911s000_EA.pdf. Accessed 22 December 2017.
91. Wheless JW, Conry J, Krauss G, et al. Safety and tolerability of rufinamide in children with epilepsy: a pooled analysis of 7 clinical studies. *J Child Neurol.* 2009;24:1520-1525.
92. Aldenkamp AP, Alpherts WC. The effect of the new antiepileptic drug rufinamide on cognitive functions. *Epilepsia.* 2006;47:1153-1159.
93. Chu-Shore CJ, Thiele EA. New drugs for pediatric epilepsy. *Semin Pediatr Neurol.* 2010;17:214-223.
94. Perucca E, Cloyd J, Critchley D, Fuseau E. Rufinamide: clinical pharmacokinetics and concentration-response relationships in patients with epilepsy. *Epilepsia.* 2008;49:1123-1141.
95. Dolphin AC. The alpha2delta subunits of voltage-gated calcium channels. *Biochim Biophys Acta.* 2013;1828:1541-1549.
96. Wang M, Offord J, Oxender DL, Su TZ. Structural requirement of the calcium-channel subunit alpha2delta for gabapentin binding. *Biochem J.* 1999;342:313-320.
97. Bian F, Li Z, Offord J, et al. Calcium channel alpha2-delta type 1 subunit is the major binding protein for pregabalin in neocortex, hippocampus, amygdala, and spinal cord: an ex vivo autoradiographic study in alpha2-delta type 1 genetically modified mice. *Brain Res.* 2006;1075:68-80.
98. Dooley DJ, Mieske CA, Borosky SA. Inhibition of K(+)-evoked glutamate release from rat neocortical and hippocampal slices by gabapentin. *Neurosci Lett.* 2000;280:107-110.
99. FDA Approved Labeling Information for Neurontin(R) (Gabapentin). https://www.accessdata.fda.gov/drugsatfda_docs/label/2011/020235s050, 020882s035, 021129s033lbl.pdf. Accessed 26 December 2017.
100. Stewart BH, Kugler AR, Thompson PR, Bockbrader HN. A saturable transport mechanism in the intestinal absorption of gabapentin is the underlying cause of the lack of proportionality between increasing dose and drug levels in plasma. *Pharm Res.* 1993;10:276-281.
101. Bockbrader HN, Wesche D, Miller R, et al. A comparison of the pharmacokinetics and pharmacodynamics of pregabalin and gabapentin. *Clin Pharmacokinet.* 2010;49:661-669.
102. Bockbrader HN, Radulovic LL, Posvar EL, et al. Clinical pharmacokinetics of pregabalin in healthy volunteers. *J Clin Pharmacol.* 2010;50:941-950.
103. Eisenberg E, River Y, Shifrin A, Krivoy N. Antiepileptic drugs in the treatment of neuropathic pain. *Drugs.* 2007;67:1265-1289.
104. Eckhardt K, Ammon S, Hofmann U, et al. Gabapentin enhances the analgesic effect of morphine in healthy volunteers. *Anesth Analg.* 2000;91:185-191.
105. Radulovic LL, Turck D, von Hodenberg A, et al. Disposition of gabapentin (neurontin) in mice, rats, dogs, and monkeys. *Drug Metab Dispos.* 1995;23:441-448.
106. Gomora JC, Daud AN, Weiergraber M, Perez-Reyes E. Block of cloned human T-type calcium channels by succinimide antiepileptic drugs. *Mol Pharmacol.* 2001;60:1121-1132.
107. Horning MG, Stratton C, Nowlin J, et al. Metabolism of 2-ethyl-2-methylsuccinimide (ethosuximide) in the rat and human. *Drug Metab Dispos.* 1973;1:569-576.
108. Sarver JG, Bachmann KA, Zhu D, Klis WA. Ethosuximide is primarily metabolized by CYP3A when incubated with isolated rat liver microsomes. *Drug Metab Dispos.* 1998;26:78-82.
109. Eadie MJ, Tyrer JH, Smith GA, McKauge L. Pharmacokinetics of drugs used for petit mal 'absence' epilepsy. *Clin Exp Neurol.* 1977;14:172-183.

110. Vajda FJ, Eadie MJ. The clinical pharmacology of traditional antiepileptic drugs. *Epileptic Disord.* 2014;16:395-408.
111. Buchanan RA, Fernandez L, Kinkel AW. Absorption and elimination of ethosuximide in children. *J Clin Pharmacol J New Drugs.* 1969;9:393-398.
112. Nadkarni S, Devinsky O. Psychotropic effects of antiepileptic drugs. *Epilepsy Curr.* 2005;5:176-181.
113. Landolt H. Serial electroencephalographic investigations during psychotic episodes in epileptic patients and during schizophrenic attacks. In: de Haas L, ed. *Lectures on Epilepsy.* Vol. 3. New York: Elsevier; 1958: 91-133.
114. Salke-Kellermann RA, May T, Boenigk HE. Influence of ethosuximide on valproic acid serum concentrations. *Epilepsy Res.* 1997;26:345-349.
115. Warren JW, Benmaman JD, Wannamaker BB, Levy RH. Kinetics of a carbamazepine-ethosuximide interaction. *Clin Pharmacol Ther.* 1980;28:646-651.
116. Greenfield LJ. Molecular mechanisms of antiseizure drug activity at GABAA receptors. *Seizure.* 2013;22:589-600.
117. Pacifici GM. Clinical pharmacology of phenobarbital in neonates: effects, metabolism and pharmacokinetics. *Curr Pediatr Rev.* 2016;12:48-54.
118. Messina S, Battino D, Croci D, et al. Phenobarbital pharmacokinetics in old age: a case-matched evaluation based on therapeutic drug monitoring data. *Epilepsia.* 2005;46:372-377.
119. Reinisch JM, Sanders SA, Mortensen EL, Rubin DB. In utero exposure to phenobarbital and intelligence deficits in adult men. *JAMA.* 1995;274:1518-1525.
120. Farwell JR, Lee YJ, Hirtz DG, et al. Phenobarbital for febrile seizures–effects on intelligence and on seizure recurrence. *N Engl J Med.* 1990;322:364-369.
121. Lambie DG, Johnson RH. The effects of phenytoin on phenobarbitone and primidone metabolism. *J Neurol Neurosurg Psychiatry.* 1981;44:148-151.
122. Martines C, Gatti G, Sasso E, et al. The disposition of primidone in elderly patients. *Br J Clin Pharmacol.* 1990;30:607-611.
123. FDA Prescribing Information for Ativan (Lorazepam). https://www.accessdata.fda.gov/drugsatfda_docs/label/2017/018140s041s042lbl.pdf. Accessed 21 April 2018.
124. Ralvenius WT, Acuna MA, Benke D, et al. The clobazam metabolite N-desmethyl clobazam is an alpha2 preferring benzodiazepine with an improved therapeutic window for antihyperalgesia. *Neuropharmacology.* 2016;109:366-375.
125. FDA Prescribing Information for Onfi (Clobazam). https://www.accessdata.fda.gov/drugsatfda_docs/label/2016/203993s005lbl.pdf. Accessed 29 December 2017).
126. Contin M, Riva R, Albani F, Baruzzi AA. Effect of felbamate on clobazam and its metabolite kinetics in patients with epilepsy. *Ther Drug Monit.* 1999;21:604-608.
127. Giraud C, Tran A, Rey E, et al. In vitro characterization of clobazam metabolism by recombinant cytochrome P450 enzymes: importance of CYP2C19. *Drug Metab Dispos.* 2004;32:1279-1286.
128. Gerecke M. Chemical structure and properties of midazolam compared with other benzodiazepines. *Br J Clin Pharmacol.* 1983;16:11S-16S.
129. Jurik A, Zdrazil B, Holy M, et al. A binding mode hypothesis of tiagabine confirms liothyronine effect on gamma-aminobutyric acid transporter 1 (GAT1). *J Med Chem.* 2015;58:2149-2158.
130. Andersen KE, Braestrup C, Gronwald FC, et al. The synthesis of novel GABA uptake inhibitors. 1. Elucidation of the structure-activity studies leading to the choice of (R)-1-[4,4-bis(3-methyl-2-thienyl)-3-butenyl]-3-piperidinecarboxylic acid (tiagabine) as an anticonvulsant drug candidate. *J Med Chem.* 1993;36:1716-1725.
131. FDA Prescribing Information for Gabitril (Tiagabine). https://www.accessdata.fda.gov/drugsatfda_docs/label/2009/020646s016lbl.pdf. Accessed 29 December 2017.
132. Nanavati SM, Silverman RB. Mechanisms of inactivation of gamma-aminobutyric acid aminotransferase by the antiepilepsy drug gamma-vinyl GABA (vigabatrin). *J Am Chem Soc.* 1991;113:9341-9349.
133. FDA Prescribing Information for Vigabatrin (Sabril). https://www.accessdata.fda.gov/drugsatfda_docs/label/2013/020427s010s011s012,022006s011s012s013lbl.pdf. Accessed 30 December 2017.
134. Abbot EL, Grenade DS, Kennedy DJ, et al. Vigabatrin transport across the human intestinal epithelial (Caco-2) brush-border membrane is via the H^+ -coupled amino-acid transporter hPAT1. *Br J Pharmacol.* 2006;147:298-306.
135. Hawker MJ, Astbury NJ. The ocular side effects of vigabatrin (Sabril): information and guidance for screening. *Eye (Lond).* 2008;22:1097-1098.
136. Kushner SA, Dewey SL, Kornetsky C. The irreversible gamma-aminobutyric acid (GABA) transaminase inhibitor gamma-vinyl-GABA blocks cocaine self-administration in rats. *J Pharmacol Exp Ther.* 1999;290:797-802.
137. Brodie JD, Case BG, Figueroa E, et al. Randomized, double-blind, placebo-controlled trial of vigabatrin for the treatment of cocaine dependence in Mexican parolees. *Am J Psychiatry.* 2009;166:1269-1277.
138. Sargentini-Maier ML, Espie P, Coquette A, Stockis A. Pharmacokinetics and metabolism of 14C-brivaracetam, a novel SV2A ligand, in healthy subjects. *Drug Metab Dispos.* 2008;36:36-45.
139. Patsalos PN. Clinical pharmacokinetics of levetiracetam. *Clin Pharmacokinet.* 2004;43:707-724.
140. Nicolas JM, Hannestad J, Holden D, et al. Brivaracetam, a selective high-affinity synaptic vesicle protein 2A (SV2A) ligand with preclinical evidence of high brain permeability and fast onset of action. *Epilepsia.* 2016;57:201-209.
141. Rankovic Z. CNS drug design: balancing physicochemical properties for optimal brain exposure. *J Med Chem.* 2015;58:2584-2608.
142. Stockis A, Chanteux H, Rosa M, Rolan P. Brivaracetam and carbamazepine interaction in healthy subjects and in vitro. *Epilepsy Res.* 2015;113:19-27.
143. Hibi S, Ueno K, Nagato S, et al. Discovery of 2-(2-oxo-1-phenyl-5-pyridin-2-yl-1,2-dihydropyridin-3-yl)benzonitrile (perampanel): a novel, noncompetitive alpha-amino-3-hydroxy-5-methyl-4-isoxazolepropanoic acid (AMPA) receptor antagonist. *J Med Chem.* 2012;55:10584-10600.
144. Patsalos PN. The clinical pharmacology profile of the new antiepileptic drug perampanel: a novel noncompetitive AMPA receptor antagonist. *Epilepsia.* 2015;56:12-27.
145. Hawkins KL, Gidal BE. When adverse effects are seen as desirable: abuse potential of the newer generation antiepileptic drugs. *Epilepsy Behav.* 2017;77:62-72.
146. Chang HR, Kuo CC. Molecular determinants of the anticonvulsant felbamate binding site in the N-methyl-D-aspartate receptor. *J Med Chem.* 2008;51:1534-1545.
147. Parker RJ, Hartman NR, Roecklein BA, et al. Stability and comparative metabolism of selected felbamate metabolites and postulated fluorofelbamate metabolites by postmitochondrial suspensions. *Chem Res Toxicol.* 2005;18:1842-1848.
148. Dieckhaus CM, Thompson CD, Roller SG, Macdonald TL. Mechanisms of idiosyncratic drug reactions: the case of felbamate. *Chem Biol Interact.* 2002;142:99-117.
149. Popovic M, Nierkens S, Pieters R, Uetrecht J. Investigating the role of 2-phenylpropenal in felbamate-induced idiosyncratic drug reactions. *Chem Res Toxicol.* 2004;17:1568-1576.
150. Maryanoff BE, Costanzo MJ, Nortey SO, et al. Structure-activity studies on anticonvulsant sugar sulfamates related to topiramate. Enhanced potency with cyclic sulfate derivatives. *J Med Chem.* 1998;41:1315-1343.
151. FDA Prescribing information: Topamax (topiramate). https://www.accessdata.fda.gov/drugsatfda_docs/label/2009/020505s038s039,020844s032s034lbl.pdf. Accessed 29 December 2017.
152. Britzi M, Perucca E, Soback S, et al. Pharmacokinetic and metabolic investigation of topiramate disposition in healthy subjects in the absence and in the presence of enzyme induction by carbamazepine. *Epilepsia.* 2005;46:378-384.

153. Nallani SC, Glauser TA, Hariparsad N, et al. Dose-dependent induction of cytochrome P450 (CYP) 3A4 and activation of pregnane X receptor by topiramate. *Epilepsia*. 2003;44:1521-1528.
154. Shorvon SD. Drug treatment of epilepsy in the century of the ILAE: the second 50 years, 1959-2009. *Epilepsia*. 2009;50:93-130.
155. Perucca E. Pharmacological and therapeutic properties of valproate: a summary after 35 years of clinical experience. *CNS Drugs*. 2002;16:695-714.
156. Ghodke-Puranik Y, Thorn CF, Lamba JK, et al. Valproic acid pathway: pharmacokinetics and pharmacodynamics. *Pharmacogenet Genomics*. 2013;23:236-241.
157. Kassahun K, Farrell K, Abbott F. Identification and characterization of the glutathione and N-acetylcysteine conjugates of (E)-2-propyl-2,4-pentadienoic acid, a toxic metabolite of valproic acid, in rats and humans. *Drug Metab Dispos*. 1991;19:525-535.
158. Bowdle AT, Patel IH, Levy RH, Wilensky AJ. Valproic acid dosage and plasma protein binding and clearance. *Clin Pharmacol Ther*. 1980;28:486-492.
159. FDA Prescribing Information for Depakote (divalproex sodium). https://www.accessdata.fda.gov/drugsatfda_docs/label/2011/018723s037lbl.pdf. Accessed 29 December 2017.
160. Ueda Y, Doi T, Tokumaru J, Willmore LJ. Effect of zonisamide on molecular regulation of glutamate and GABA transporter proteins during epileptogenesis in rats with hippocampal seizures. *Brain Res*. 2003;116:1-6.
161. Stiff DD, Zemaitis MA. Metabolism of the anticonvulsant agent zonisamide in the rat. *Drug Metab Dispos*. 1990;18:888-894.
162. FDA Prescribing Information: Zonegran (zonisamide). https://www.accessdata.fda.gov/drugsatfda_docs/label/2003/20789scm001_zonegran_lbl.pdf. Accessed 27 December 2017.
163. Schoonjans AS, Lagae L, Ceulemans B. Low-dose fenfluramine in the treatment of neurologic disorders: experience in Dravet syndrome. *Ther Adv Neurol Disord*. 2015;8:328-338.
164. Wirrell EC, Laux L, Franz DN, et al. Stiripentol in Dravet syndrome: results of a retrospective US study. *Epilepsia*. 2013;54:1595-1604.
165. Koppel BS, Brust JC, Fife T, et al. Systematic review: efficacy and safety of medical marijuana in selected neurologic disorders: report of the Guideline Development Subcommittee of the American Academy of Neurology. *Neurology*. 2014;82:1556-1563.
166. Gloss D, Vickrey B. Cannabinoids for epilepsy. *Cochrane Database Syst Rev*. 2014;:CD009270.
167. Rosenberg EC, Tsien RW, Whalley BJ, Devinsky O. Cannabinoids and epilepsy. *Neurotherapeutics*. 2015;12:747-768.
168. Laprairie RB, Bagher AM, Kelly ME, Denovan-Wright EM. Cannabidiol is a negative allosteric modulator of the cannabinoid CB1 receptor. *Br J Pharmacol*. 2015;172:4790-4805.
169. Devinsky O, Cross JH, Laux L, et al; and Cannabidiol in Dravet syndrome study Group. Trail of cannabidiol for drug-resistant seizures in the Dravet syndrome. *N Engl J Med*. 2017;376:2011-2020.
170. Morales P, Reggio PH, Jagerovic N. An overview on medicinal chemistry of synthetic and natural derivatives of cannabidiol. *Front Pharmacol*. 2017;8:422.

Structure Challenge Answers

1. **E, D**; 2. **A**; 3. **H**; 4. **B, D, E, J**; 5. **J.**

	A	B	C	D	E	F	G	H	I	J
Drug Name:	Fosphenytoin	Phenobarbital	Carbamazepine	Clobazam	Midazolam	Valproic acid	Pregabalin	Vigabatrin	Levetiracetam	Topiramate
A	±	+	+	+	+	+	±	±	±	+
B	+	±	+	+	+	+	±	±	±	+
C	+	+	+	+	+	+	±	±	±	+
D	±	±	±	±	±	±	±	±	±	±
E	–	–	–	±	±	±	±	±	±	±
F	±[1]	–	±[1,2]	–	±[1]	±	±	±	±	±/–
G	±	±	±	±	±	±	±	±	±	±
H	±	±	±	±	±	±	±	±	±	±
I	±	±	±	±	±	±	±	±	±	±
J	±	±	+[3]	+[3]	+[3]	±	±	±	±	±

Significant displacement from plasma proteins can cause increase in free (unbound) plasma levels.
Inhibits metabolism of reactive epoxide metabolite.
At high doses.

SECTION 2
Drugs Impacting Pain Perception

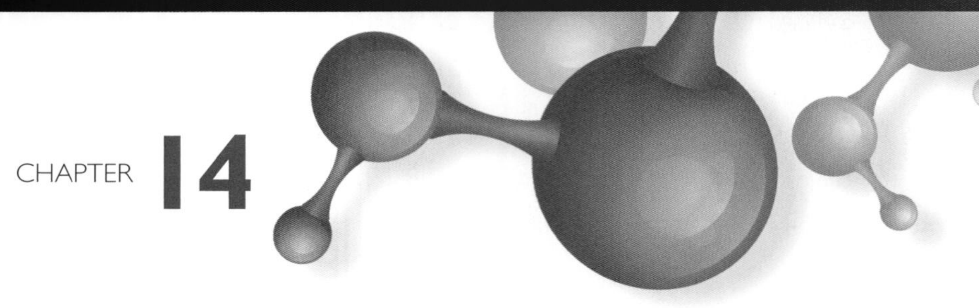

CHAPTER 14

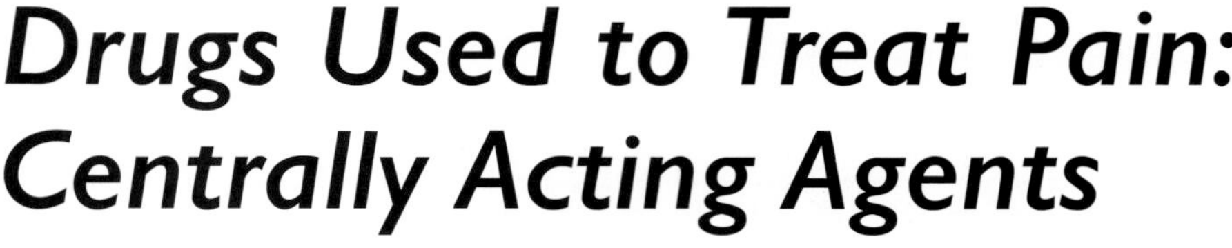

Drugs Used to Treat Pain: Centrally Acting Agents

Victoria F. Roche and Edward B. Roche

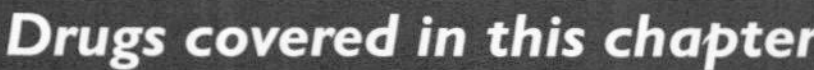

Drugs covered in this chapter

OPIOID ANALGESICS

PHENANTHRENE-BASED RIGID μ AGONISTS
- Buprenorphine
- Codeine
- Hydrocodone
- Hydromorphone
- Levorphanol
- Morphine
- Oxycodone
- Oxymorphone

PHENANTHRENE-BASED RIGID κ AGONISTS/μ ANTAGONISTS
- Butorphanol
- Nalbuphine
- Pentazocine

FLEXIBLE μ AGONISTS
- Alfentanil
- Fentanyl
- Meperidine
- Methadone
- Remifentanil
- Sufentanil
- Tapentadol (dual action)
- Tramadol (dual action)

OPIOID ANTAGONISTS
- Methylnaltrexone bromide
- Naloxegol
- Naloxone
- Naltrexone

OPIOID-BASED ANTIDIARRHEALS
- Difenoxin
- Diphenoxylate
- Loperamide

NEUROPATHIC ANALGESICS

FIRST-LINE AGENTS
- Amitriptyline
- Desipramine
- Duloxetine
- Gabapentin
- Nortriptyline
- Pregabalin

SECOND-LINE AGENTS
- Capsaicin
- Lidocaine

ANTIMIGRAINE DRUGS

TRIPTANS
- Almotriptan
- Eletriptan
- Frovatriptan
- Naratriptan
- Rizatriptan
- Sumatriptan
- Zolmitriptan

Abbreviations

ACE angiotensin converting enzyme
ADF abuse-deterrent formulation
AMPA α-amino-3-hydroxy-5-methyl-4-isoxazolepropionic acid
ALDH aldehyde dehydrogenase
BBB blood-brain barrier
cAMP cyclic adenosine monophosphate
CGRP calcitonin gene–related peptide
CNS central nervous system
EM extensive metabolizer
FDA U.S. Food and Drug Administration
GABA γ-aminobutyric acid
GI gastrointestinal
GPCR G-protein coupled receptor
5-HT serotonin
IM intramuscular
IM intermediate metabolizer
IV intravenous
MAO monoamine oxidase
MCT-1 monocarboxylate transporter-1
NE norepinephrine
NMDA N-methyl-D-aspartate
NSAIDs nonsteroidal anti-inflammatory drugs

Abbreviations—Continued

OIC opioid-induced constipation
ORL 1 opioid receptor-like 1
OTC over the counter
PAMORA peripherally acting μ-opioid receptor antagonists
PAPS 3′-phosphoadenosine-5′-phosphosulfate
PCP primary care physicians
P-gp P-glycoprotein
PM poor metabolizer
REMS Risk Evaluation and Mitigation Strategy
Rx prescription
SAMHSA Substance Abuse and Mental Health Services Administration
SAR structure-activity relationships
SNP single nucleotide polymorphism
SSRI selective serotonin reuptake inhibitor
TCA tricyclic antidepressant
TIRF transmucosal immediate release fentanyl
TRPV1 transient receptor potential vanilloid 1
UGT UDP-glucuronosyltransferase
UM ultrarapid metabolizer

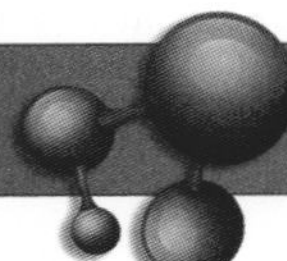

CLINICAL SIGNIFICANCE

Amy M. Pick

The management of pain is extremely complex. The therapeutic approach includes a thorough patient assessment with the clinician determining acute or chronic pain. Chronic pain can be further divided into two physiologically distinct pain pathways, nociceptive or neuropathic. This distinction is important when selecting the appropriate pain medication, as opioid agonists are an option for nociceptive pain; however, they have limited evidence in the management of neuropathic pain.

Generally, opioid agonists should be reserved for the management of acute and severe pain. The opioid agonists' structure-activity relationships (SAR) in the management of nociceptive pain is well defined, allowing the pharmacist to tailor therapy to an individual's pain relief needs while taking vulnerability to hallmark adverse effects into account. Analgesia primarily occurs via activation of the opioid μ receptors in the central and peripheral nervous systems. In addition to dependence and addiction, the opioid's central mechanisms are also responsible for many adverse effects such as mental clouding, somnolence, and respiratory depression. The opioid's peripheral mechanisms cause delayed peristalsis, leading to constipation, and pruritus.

While acute pain may be effectively managed with the use of opioid agonists, the treatment of chronic pain continues to remain a challenge for clinicians. Studies regarding opioids in the management of chronic pain have limited and mixed results, suggesting the use of alternative classes of medications, such as anticonvulsants. One welcomed class is the centrally acting triptans ($5\text{-HT}_{1B/1D}$ agonists) where they have demonstrated efficacy in the management of migraines. There are numerous triptans commercially available and key differences are in their pharmacokinetics properties. Changes in the chemical structure in the newer generation triptans improve the oral bioavailability of the medication and the higher lipophilicity increases the penetration into the blood-brain barrier. The appropriate selection of the triptan depends not only on their chemically dependent pharmacokinetic and physicochemical properties but also on the patient's response to treatment and the adverse effect profile.

The excessive prescribing of opioids for pain indications with insufficient evidence is one of many factors implicated in the opioid epidemic. Numerous organizations are addressing the prescription drug opioid crisis and urging clinicians to be prudent in the prescribing of opioids. The future of pain management will likely depend on a holistic approach, incorporating alternative pain medications, as demonstrated by the triptans for migraine treatment.

PAIN

"The greatest evil is physical pain"

St. Augustine

While not everyone would agree with St. Augustine's sweeping characterization, most people will go to great lengths to avoid physical pain. Pain is defined as an unpleasant sensory and emotional experience associated with actual or potential tissue damage, or described in terms of such damage.[1,2] Pain is part of the body's defense system, is designed to protect against more serious injury (i.e., a "necessary evil"), and usually resolves once the offensive stimulus is removed and healing is complete. However, some pain persists well after offending injuries have healed and/or arises in the absence of any detectable stimulus.[3]

Regardless of how it presents, serious pain can be disabling, demoralizing, and destructive to a person's quality of life. Reflecting this importance to well-being, in 1995 the President of the American Pain Society, Dr. James Campbell, proposed that pain be considered the fifth vital sign to raise awareness among health care providers on the need to adequately treat it.[4] However, some have questioned whether pain management has advanced as a result of this characterization.[5] Although supporting the goal of pain assessment in all patients, the fifth vital sign concept was never formally endorsed by the Joint Commission.[6] In 2016, the American Medical Association House of Delegates voted that it be eliminated from professional standards based on concerns related, at least in part, to reimbursement.[7] A possible link between the fifth vital sign view and increases in opioid prescribing has been raised in the literature, as has the critical need for expanded medical education on pain assessment and management.[8,9]

The intensity, character, and tolerability of each person's pain are subjective and, thus, challenging to assess objectively. Differences in pain prevalence, perception, tolerance thresholds, and/or management are associated with, among other factors, age, economic status, race/ethnicity, genetics, and sex. To account for variability in perception, standardized pain scales, such as the Wong-Baker FACES Pain Rating Scale,[10] are commonly used to clue providers on patients' pain intensity. They are also used to evaluate the effectiveness of therapy, although some would criticize these scales for their simplicity. Differences and/or disparities in pain perception, coping, and treatment based on a patient's race/ethnicity are claimed to have psychosocial components. Research and professional education designed to address current inequities in quality pain care have been advocated.[11]

The economic toll of pain in the United States has been estimated at $634 billion, including the cost of treatment and the impact of lost productivity.[8,12] A recent 13-year retrospective study on pain prevalence in a U.S. adult population of over 6.5 million persons documented that a mean of 2.68 distinct pain diagnoses commonly occur in individual patients.[12] Back pain was cited as the most prevalent diagnosis. Over half (58%) of the pain patients in the study population were females, and they suffered more than males from complex regional pain syndrome, limb pain, and back pain. Geographical differences in specific pain diagnoses were also uncovered. Pain prevalence spikes over the study period were hypothesized to be linked to improved awareness of pain as a manageable disease and changes in insurance coverage and coding.

Pathophysiology of Pain

Pain is categorized pathophysiologically as nociceptive, neuropathic, or due to sensory hypersensitivity.

Nociceptive Pain

Nociceptive pain is due to trauma, inflammation, or other injury occurring in nonneural tissue. It is mediated through nociceptors located in the skin, bone, connective tissue, muscle, and viscera.[13] Nociceptive pain is often described with adjectives such as tender, dull, aching, throbbing, or cramping[3] and usually responds to nonsteroidal anti-inflammatory drugs (NSAIDs) and opioids.

The nociceptive pain mechanism is highly complex.[2,13] Tissue damage in the periphery depolarizes neuronal membranes and releases chemical mediators such as prostaglandins, bradykinin, serotonin, substance P, and histamine, which stimulate nociceptors. The ensuing action potential travels along afferent neurons, designated as C fibers and Aδ fibers, to receptors at the dorsal horn of the spinal cord. There the excitatory amino acid glutamate is released and stimulates α-amino-3-hydroxy-5-methyl-4-isoxazolepropionic acid (AMPA) receptors on secondary neurons. A surge of released glutamate allows activation of N-methyl-D-aspartate (NMDA) receptors normally inhibited by Mg^{+2}, leading to central sensitization. Pain perception is due to the transmission of the nociceptive message from the thalamus to the somatosensory cortex, parietal lobe, frontal lobe, and limbic system.

Aδ fibers are thinly myelinated and transmit the action potentials more rapidly (~20 m/s) than unmyelinated C fibers (~2 m/s). Aδ axons associated with acute pain mediate the reflex process that results in avoidance of the noxious stimuli (e.g., pulling away from a hot surface or sharp implement). The more slowly conducting C fibers are responsible for the longer-lasting pain that follows acute injury.

Neuropathic Pain

Neuropathic pain involves damage to peripheral or central neurons. Peripheral neuropathic pain is commonly associated with diseases such as diabetes, polio, herpes zoster virus (shingles), cancer, and some cancer chemotherapies. Central neuropathic pain can be experienced by patients who have suffered a stroke or spinal cord injury.[3]

Excitatory impulses are repeatedly transmitted in neuropathic pain, leading to sensitization of peripheral nociceptors, hyperexcitability of central neurons, and ultimately to structural and/or functional changes in these neurons. The result can be recurrent or continuous abnormal responses to painful stimuli, including hyperalgesia (excessive response), hypoalgesia (attenuated response) and/or paresthesia or dysesthesia (annoying or more intensely unpleasant sensations, respectively).[13,14]

Adjectives commonly used to describe neuropathic pain include tingling, shock-like, pins and needles, burning, and stabbing.[3] Patients living with neuropathic pain are also at higher risk for anxiety, depression, and sleep disturbances compared to the general population and are known to have a lower health-related quality of life.[14]

Sensory Hypersensitivity

Sensory hypersensitivity can be thought of as neuropathic pain without identifiable nerve damage.[3,14] Sustained functional disruption of central neurons is believed to result in lowered pain thresholds and an augmentation of pain impulses. Generalized hypersensitivity of central neurons can also lead to exaggerated responses to other environmental stimuli, such as light, sounds, and/or smells. The pathophysiological mechanisms of these two categories of pain are believed to be very similar, and they respond to similar therapeutic interventions (e.g., α2δ ligands, tricyclic antidepressants [TCAs], and serotonin [5-HT] or norepinephrine [NE] reuptake inhibitors). Opioids, of use primarily in nociceptive pain, are third-line therapy in neuropathic pain and contraindicated in sensory hypersensitivity.

Fibromyalgia, chronic fatigue syndrome, and restless leg syndrome are examples of disorders resulting in sensory hypersensitivity-related pain. Patients can present with complaints of widely disseminated pain, hyperalgesia, allodynia (pain in response to nonpainful stimuli), fatigue, and disorders in cognition and/or mood.

Acute Pain

Acute pain is defined as the normal and predictable physiologic response to an identifiable noxious stimulus, such as surgery, trauma, inflammation, or short-term illness.[1,8] Acute pain results from nociceptor activation at the site of tissue damage and is viewed as adaptive since it attenuates activities that would exacerbate the pain-inducing pathology and/or jeopardize healing.[15] Acute pain is typically self-limiting and resolves over days to weeks, but it can persist for months or longer as healing occurs. It can also be episodic, as in the case of migraine headaches or dysmenorrhea, and is classified "breakthrough" when it manifests during a period of otherwise controlled pain.

Approaches to therapeutic management of acute pain often involve an "analgesic ladder" of drugs known to be effective in nociceptive pain. Peripheral agents such as local anesthetics, NSAIDS, and/or acetaminophen are considered first-line therapy, with central analgesics (opioids) of increasing potency added if pain intensifies or persists.[16] An overview of systematic reviews of the efficacy of nonprescription pain medications in treating acute postoperative pain was published in 2015.[17] Physical pain can be complicated by psychological, emotional, social, cultural, and spiritual elements,[15,16] which reinforces the wisdom of introducing nonpharmacological approaches to pain management, as appropriate.

While often viewed as straightforward and "simpler" than chronic pain, Radnovich et al.[15] argue that acute pain is complex, dynamic, and highly variable in its manifestations. There is significant potential for negative patient care outcomes if acute pain is inadequately treated, including longer hospitalizations; compromised cardiac, pulmonary, and immunological functioning; and risk of progression to chronic pain situations. Therefore, acute pain warrants comprehensive and multidimensional assessments to guide holistic therapy and minimize risk of inadequate management due to patient-provider miscommunications or assumptions.[15,18]

Chronic Pain

Chronic pain persists at least 3-6 months after an initiating stimulus has resolved. Chronic pain can be related to degenerative disease such as rheumatoid arthritis, and it can be a lifelong phenomenon. It has been referred to as maladaptive since it has no protective purpose and serves no recognizably useful function.[15] Recent studies have estimated chronic pain prevalence in the U.S. at 10%-30%,[19-21] impacting over 100 million people.[21,22] It carries a significant public health and economic burden.[3,23]

Chronic pain is commonly of mixed pathophysiologic mechanism (nociceptive, neuropathic, sensory hypersensitivity) with approximately 20% arising from neuropathic origins.[24] While the literature often distinguishes chronic malignant pain from noncancer-related chronic pain due to the complexity of cancer's etiology, pathology, and level of patient care, the underlying physiological processes may be the same.[3,25]

Chronic pain that is predominantly nociceptive is routinely treated with peripheral and/or central analgesics. As with acute pain, a therapeutic ladder is recommended that initiates pharmacotherapy with peripheral agents (NSAIDs, acetaminophen) and moves to opioids only if/when truly warranted.[3] As noted earlier, chronic pain with a significant neuropathic component is commonly treated with antiepileptic $\alpha 2\delta$ ligands (gabapentin, pregabalin), antidepressants (venlafaxine, imipramine), local anesthetics (lidocaine), or central analgesics (tramadol, tapentadol), but only 40%-60% of patients may see significant benefits.[24] Surgical or other invasive procedures, such as deep brain stimulation, may be employed if indicated by the etiology and/or if noninvasive pain control strategies prove insufficient. Enzymes that regulate neuronal function and impact glial activation are currently being investigated as potential targets for the development of novel therapies to treat chronic pain.[24,26,27]

In addition to conventional pharmacologic therapies, patients living with chronic pain often seek alternative treatments such as chiropractic adjustments, acupuncture, traditional Chinese medicine, cognitive behavior therapy (e.g., relaxation, hypnosis), massage, and, more recently, virtual reality therapy.[28] Chronic pain induces pathophysiologic changes in the central nervous system that negatively impact body, mind, and spirit,[29] and it can rob patients of a sense of control over their well-being. Delgado et al.[22] suggest that the use of alternative therapies may allow patients to play a proactive and empowering role in their own holistic healing. Stanos et al.[3] reinforce the importance of individualized treatment that incorporates nonpharmacologic therapies deemed appropriate after a rigorous physiologic and psychosocial assessment. They also emphasize the importance of an interprofessional team approach (including pharmacists) to the treatment of chronic pain.

Similarly, Peppin et al.[20] have commented on the traditionally linear approach to chronic pain therapy that adopts an opioid-focused model of care delivered, in large measure, by primary care physicians (PCPs). They advocate for a nonlinear "complexity model" of personalized collaborative care involving PCPs and pain specialists, who stratify patient care needs after an extensive and multifaceted pain evaluation that includes things such as medical comorbidities, body mass index, history of sleep disorders/head trauma/tobacco use, education/employment status, social support, and risk for medication abuse/diversion.

Opioid Analgesics and Antagonists

> "Oh! just, subtle, and mighty opium! That to the hearts of poor and rich alike, for the wounds that will never heal, and for 'the pangs that tempt the spirit to rebel,' bringest an assuaging balm"
>
> *Thomas de Quincey, Confessions of an English Opium Eater*

The juice (*opium* in Greek) or latex from the unripe seed pods of the poppy *Papaver somniferum* is among the oldest recorded medication used by humans and may have been employed as a tonic as early as 3500 BC. In 1803, the pharmacist Friedrich Surtürner isolated an alkaloid from opium he named morphine, after Morpheus, the Greek god of dreams. Structural modifications of morphine and two other morphine-like alkaloids found in the opium poppy, codeine and thebaine, provide us with many of the most commonly used (and, in some cases, abused) opioids on the world market today.

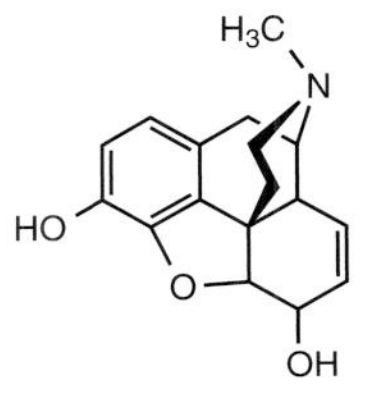

H_3C N HO O OH

Morphine

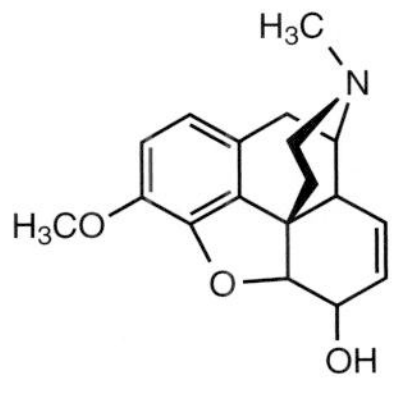

H_3C N H_3CO O OH

Codeine

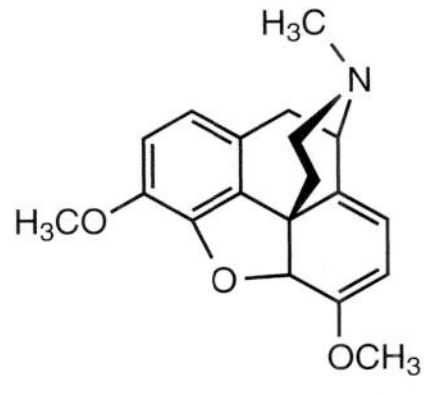

H_3C N H_3CO O OCH_3

Thebaine

Endogenous Opioid Peptides

Alkaloidal and synthetic opioids in common therapeutic use mimic the action of three major endogenous peptides, two enkephalins[30] (pentapeptides), and β-endorphin[31] (31 residues). Endogenous opioids exert a receptor-dependent analgesic action at spinal and supraspinal sites by inhibiting neurotransmitter or neuromodulator action on afferent pain-signaling neurons in the dorsal horn of the spinal cord and on interconnecting neuronal pathways for pain signals within the brain. While several opioid receptor subtypes have been identified, two are associated with the analgesic response of natural/synthetic opioid agonists used clinically, mu (μ) receptors and kappa (κ) receptors. Early hopes of harnessing the analgesic action of opioid peptides as "natural" pain-relieving drugs have not been realized due to their short half-lives, along with delivery and distribution challenges. No opioid peptide is currently marketed.

The N-terminal sequence Tyr-Gly-Gly-Phe is common to all opioid peptides, and the fifth residue in most is either Leu or Met. The two enkephalins differ only in which fifth C-terminal residue they contain. The protonated amine, aromatic ring, and phenolic hydroxyl group of the Tyr residue, along with the aromatic ring of the Phe moiety, are important in holding these peptides to opioid receptors. The two Gly residues, at a minimum, promote activity by maintaining the proper distance between the aromatic residues. One additional opioid peptide that bears mentioning is dynorphin.[32] Dynorphin peptides are larger than the enkephalins, and two Arg resides at positions 6 and 7 are believed to confer selectivity for κ opioid receptors over μ receptors.

Tyr-Gly-Gly-Phe-Met
Met-enkephalin

Tyr-Gly-Gly-Phe-Leu
Leu-Enkephalin

Tyr-Gly-Gly-Phe-Leu-Arg-Arg-Ile
Dynorphin$^{1\text{-}8}$

Opioid Receptors

Centrally, μ receptors are found in abundance in the arcuate nucleus, periaqueductal gray, and thalamic areas of the brain, while κ receptor density is highest in the dorsal horn and substantia gelatinosa of the spinal cord. They are both coupled to $G_{i/o}$ proteins (see Chapter 6, G Protein-Coupled Receptors) and mediate analgesia through the activation of ATP-gated K^+ channels and the inhibition of voltage-gated Ca^{+2} channels, leading to decreases in intracellular Ca^{+2}.[33] Levels of cAMP also decrease, and it is the compensatory upregulation of adenylyl cyclase that leads to the tolerance and dependence phenomena associated with the chronic use of opioid analgesics.[34]

Opioid receptors are also found in the periphery. The ability of many opioid analgesics to inhibit gastrointestinal (GI) motility by stimulating intestinal μ receptors is well known and has spawned a new generation of therapeutic agents to treat opioid-induced constipation (OIC).

Table 14.1 Adverse Effects of Opioid Agonists

μ Agonists	κ Agonists
Sedation	Sedation
Nausea and vomiting	Dysphoria
Constipation[a]	Diuresis
Miosis[a]	Increase in cardiac workload (excluding nalbuphine)
Respiratory depression	Respiratory depression
Euphoria	
Tolerance and dependence	

[a]No tolerance to these adverse reactions

Kappa opioid receptors have been identified in cardiac tissue,[35] and some κ agonists can induce cardiopulmonary toxicity. Opioids acting at peripheral κ receptors may have value in attenuating inflammatory visceral pain.[36]

The array of adverse effects elicited by opioid analgesics is receptor dependent (Table 14.1), which historically advanced the assumption that separation of the desired analgesic effect from use-limiting activities was impossible. However, it is now recognized that biochemical events occurring downstream of opioid receptor activation may hold the key to the development of safer central analgesics. β-Arrestin-2 is a regulatory protein known to desensitize μ opioid receptors through recruitment to the Ser375-phosphorylated receptor. The result is an inhibition of μ agonist-receptor coupling and, eventually, receptor internalization. If β-arrestin-2's normal engagement secondary to receptor phosphorylation is blocked, μ agonist analgesia via G protein-coupled receptor (GPCR) mechanisms is enhanced, while the adverse effects of constipation, respiratory depression, severe nausea, and tolerance (but not dependence) are attenuated.[33,34,37,38] Molecules that can stimulate the μ receptor without recruitment of β-arrestin proteins (termed "biased ligands") have the potential to provide potent pain relief without the serious and use-limiting effects associated with μ agonists. One such agent, TRV130, is currently in clinical development,[37] and another, PZM21,[38] may lead to the development of even more selective μ receptor–biased ligands.

Of potential clinical interest is the fact that individuals with the single nucleotide polymorphism (SNP) 118A>G in the gene coding for the μ receptor have reduced expression of this protein and, as a result, higher μ agonist dosing requirements. While this has been claimed to be of questionable importance in the general population, many Asian populations carry this modified gene with a frequency three to four times that of Caucasians (40%-50% vs. 10%). Some hypothesize the 118A>G SNP to be the biggest contributing factor to the attenuated response to opioids observed in some patients of Asian ancestry.[39]

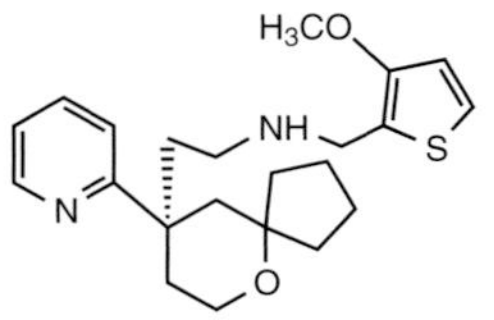

H_3CO NH S N O TRV130

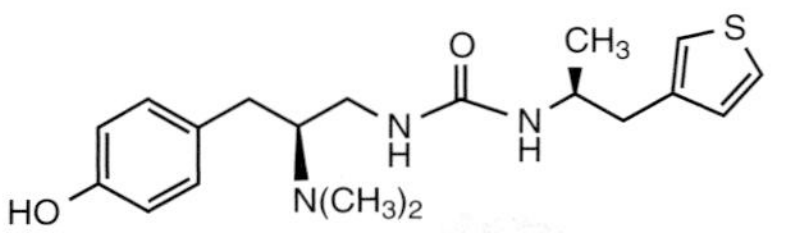

HO O CH_3 S N H N H $N(CH_3)_2$ PZM21

Tolerance and Dependence

Tolerance is the situation where an increasingly larger dose of drug is required to produce the same degree of biologic response that had previously been obtained with a lower dose. As additional molecules of adenylyl are synthesized in response to $G_{i/o}$-mediated inhibition, higher doses of agonist are required to inhibit both original and new enzyme populations. If the agonist used on a chronic basis is suddenly withdrawn, the inhibition of adenylyl cyclase abruptly stops and all enzymes begin producing cAMP. The significantly elevated cAMP concentrations are believed responsible for the physiologic symptoms of opioid withdrawal.

Euphoria and Dysphoria

The ability of μ agonists to induce a profound euphoria is well known. The agonist-induced decrease in cAMP inhibits the release of the inhibitory neurotransmitter γ-aminobutyric acid (GABA) from the ventral tegmental area, which is upstream of the nucleus accumbens. The nucleus accumbens is the brain's self-reward or pleasure center and is activated by dopamine. GABA normally inhibits dopamine release from this cerebral "candy land," so the decrease in GABA levels induced by μ-receptor stimulation enhances dopamine release from these terminals. The subsequent elevation in dopamine receptor stimulation in the nucleus accumbens is perceived as a feeling of intense well-being or euphoria. Euphoria is the psychological driver behind opioid addiction.

In contrast, κ agonists have the potential to induce dysphoria, a feeling of intense discomfort. Stimulation of κ receptors in the nucleus accumbens results in a direct inhibitory effect on presynaptic dopaminergic neurons, resulting in a decrease in dopamine and an attenuation of pleasure-related responses that translates as dysphoria.

Clinical Use

Opioid analgesics are the therapeutic mainstay in the treatment of moderate to severe pain, and there is no question that they are effective. U.S. citizens paid \$7.4 billion for prescription opioids in 2012, with insurers (including Medicare and Medicaid) covering 82% of the cost; a dramatic shift from primarily (53%) patient-financed medication purchases in 1999.[40]

While routinely used in chronic pain situations, long-term efficacy of opioids is compromised by the use-limiting adverse effects noted above and by the induction of tolerance to their antinociceptive effects. Significant drug interactions with opioid analgesic as a class occur with other CNS depressants (including alcohol) and agents that impact the rate of biotransformation. The latter may be particularly important for O-methylated opioid prodrugs, which depend on the highly polymorphic CYP2D6 for activation.

Other indications for lower potency opioids include cough and diarrhea, the latter of which takes advantage of the constipating effect of μ agonists. Centrally active opioid antagonists are used predominantly to reverse or prevent life-threatening overdose, while peripherally restricted antagonists can treat OIC without precipitating withdrawal.

A recent study examined beliefs and attitudes on opioid analgesic use among a small sample of primary care physicians in the U.S. (high use) and Japan (low use) and found that differences in health systems, regulations, provider education, and cultural mind-sets likely impacted the 26-fold prescribing difference for six high potency opioids.[41] The drive to alleviate suffering and to secure patient satisfaction with their care plan impacted opioid prescribing patterns in both physician cohorts. A more robust retrospective study of 377,345 Medicare patients treated in (and discharged from) U.S. emergency rooms between 2008 and 2011 identified a wide variability in opioid prescribing patterns among emergency care physicians, with patients treated by "high-intensity prescribers" significantly more likely to remain on long-term opioid therapy.[42] A retrospective study of opioid use in U.S. pediatric care settings over the course of 1 year found that 43.5% of over 8000 inpatients 18 years or younger were prescribed an opioid, and that 75% of these were treated for less than 5 days (i.e., acute therapy).[43] Cancer, followed by cardiac disorders, was the most common diagnosis in pediatric patients receiving opioids for longer than 1 month.

The relationship between legitimate chronic opioid use and abuse is a significant public health concern. Using a system dynamics approach, Schmidt et al.[44] identified twelve data gaps that must be bridged to better understand the use and potential misuse of prescribed opioids, including incidence/diagnosis rate/opioid use in treating nonmalignant chronic pain, the fraction of opioid prescriptions diverted for nonmedical use, and the "thwart rate" of prescription forgery and "doctor shopping" to secure multiple prescriptions for opioids-of-choice. Recommendations for expanding current data collection efforts to address these knowledge gaps were provided. Kattan et al.[45] described the positive impact of an opioid public health detailing initiative to health care providers in Staten Island, NY, on knowledge of sound opioid prescribing practices and prescribing rate. They recommended their successful approach be expanded to other communities and jurisdictions. Given that opioid-dependent people can also experience painful illnesses or surgical interventions requiring potent analgesia, Raub and Vettese[46] have offered an evidence-based review and clinician's guide on the use of opioids in this patient population.

Clearly, there is a continuing need for a scientific approach to the use of these powerful molecules; one that mitigates risk while allowing patients in significant pain access to provider-monitored pharmacotherapy that can give them a better quality of life. The importance of a collaborative patient-provider partnership in assuring the appropriate use of opioid analgesics cannot be overstated.

Opioid Addiction

Addiction has been defined as "a primary, chronic neurobiologic disease with genetic, psychosocial and environmental factors influencing its development and manifestations."[47] It has a strong psychosocial and genetic component, leading to drug craving and drug-seeking behavior in the absence of pain, destructive behavior patterns, and compulsive use in the face of negative mental and/or social consequences. The risk of addiction in patients with chronic pain on opioids has been estimated at 3.3%, with genetic predisposition possibly accounting for 40%-60% of that risk,[48] but some claim data around addiction risk in patients with chronic pain are inconsistent.[49]

Prescription opioids are a major source of the drugs misused, abused, and diverted in the U.S.[50] More than 259 million opioid prescriptions were written in 2012, and the number has increased 3- to 4-fold since 1999. Despite comprising only 4.6% of the global population, U.S. citizens consume 81% of the world's oxycodone, and the consumption of the international supply of hydrocodone has been as pegged as high as 99%. The economic burden of opioid abuse and misuse, born extensively by payers, has been documented by many.[49,51,52]

The National Safety Council has determined that 80% of heroin abusers started their addiction journey with prescription opioids,[53] and opioid overdose claims approximately one U.S. life every 36 minutes.[41] Zhou et al.[40] noted the coincidental rise in opioid-induced mortality with the increase in opioid prescribing secondary to more relaxed views on the use of opioids to treat chronic nonmalignant pain, along with widespread marketing efforts by opioid manufacturers. In response, some states have enacted legislation to limit the number of opioids, the length of initial treatment, and/or the doses physicians can prescribe. In early 2018, the makers of controlled-release OxyContin, an oxycodone product with a high misuse/abuse potential, voluntarily cut their sales force by more than half and halted the active marketing of the analgesic to physicians.

Overdose deaths from prescription opioids have leveled off since 2011, as deaths from fatal administrations of heroin and illicitly produced fentanyl and its more potent analogues (e.g., carfentanil) have risen.[54] The number of opioid overdose deaths quadrupled between 1999 and 2013[40] and continues to escalate, with the U.S. Attorney General estimating 60,000 overdose deaths in 2016.[55] Not all victims of opioid overdose are intentional abusers. Near deaths from fentanyl exposure have occurred in law enforcement officers who accidently came in contact with trace amounts of powdered drug in the course of their work. In 2017, a 10-year-old Miami boy is known to have died from fentanyl exposure presumably after accidently coming in contact with discarded drug on his way home from a neighborhood swimming pool.

Some states are now making the rapid-acting opioid antagonist naloxone (autoinjector and nasal spray) available to law enforcement, librarians, high school staff, and/or family and caregivers of addicted individuals. Naloxone administered by IM, subcutaneous, or intranasal routes reverses life-threatening overdose within minutes. Pharmacists have a vital role to play in educating these first responders and the public at large on the safe and effective use of this life-saving drug.

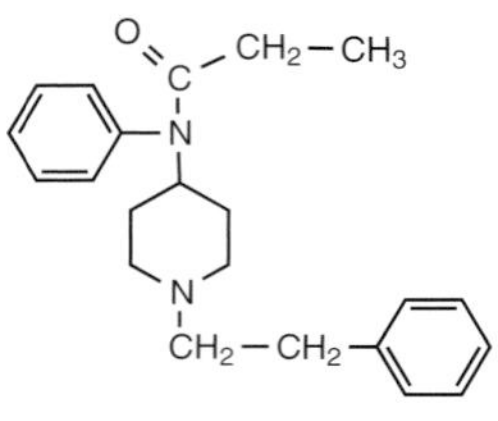

Fentanyl

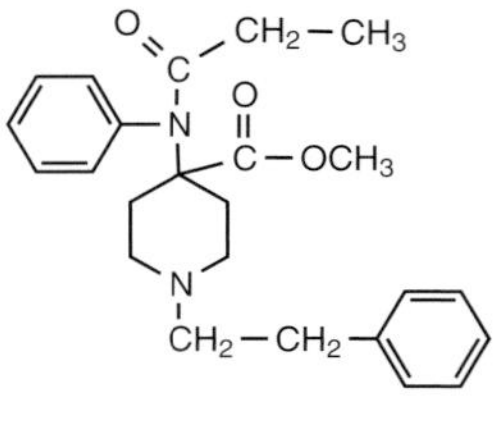

Carfentanil

The U.S. opioid epidemic was officially declared a national public health emergency in October 2017, which stopped short of the national emergency status that would have deployed additional federal resources to combat it. Those interested in reading more about the national approach to the U.S. opioid crisis are directed to the references cited.[56-59]

Opioid Chemistry

Opioid Receptor Binding

Residues important to the high-affinity binding of opioid ligands to μ and κ receptors have been identified, and crystal structures of both receptors have been determined.[60,61] The μ receptor is dimeric, with parallel receptor proteins closely associated through transmembrane helices 5 and 6. The ligand binding pocket is spacious, shallow, and open to the extracellular surface, which helps explain the fast dissociation rates of high-affinity ligands and the ease with which agonists can be displaced by antagonists. The κ receptor also exhibits parallel dimerism, and the ligand binding pocket is large and fairly narrow.

Opioid receptors bind only the levorotatory (−) isomers of chiral opioids, although exceptions are known in selected flexible opioid structures (e.g., tramadol).[62,63] The dextrorotatory (+) isomers of phenanthrene-based rigid opioids do not bind to these receptors; however, both (+) and (−) isomers of several μ agonists are potent antitussives. For example, millions of people purchase OTC dextromethorphan (e.g., Robitussin DM) to control cough. While this pure (+) isomer does not stimulate opioid receptors in therapeutic doses, its levorotatory enantiomer, called levomethorphan, is a potent, full μ-receptor agonist which, if marketed, would require a prescription.

Table 14.2 identifies proposed μ receptor binding residues for phenanthrene-based and flexible opioids, and corresponding κ residues where appropriate.[60,61,64-66] The majority of marketed opioid analgesics and antagonists bind preferentially to the μ receptor, and a graphic of the rigid opioid agonist oxymorphone binding with proposed μ receptor residues is provided in Figure 14.1. In some cases, the binding interactions are facilitated by receptor-associated water molecules. A similar graphic depicting the flexible opioid fentanyl interacting at the μ receptor is provided in Figure 14.2.[65,66]

Table 14.2 Proposed Opioid Binding Residues of μ and κ Receptors[60,61,64-66]

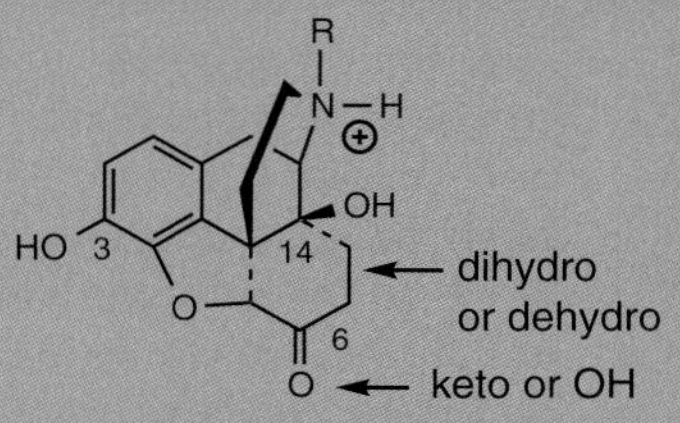

Phenanthrene-based opioid

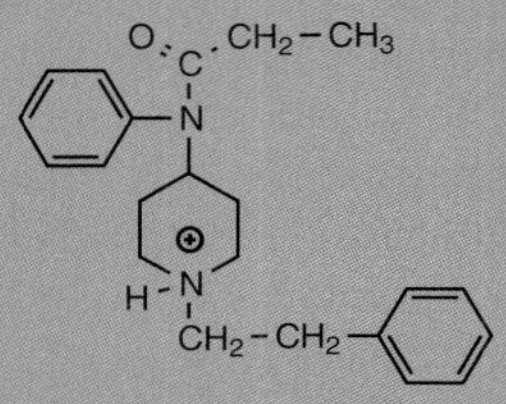

Flexible opioid

Opioid Functional Group	μ Receptor Residue	κ Receptor Residue	Binding Interaction
Phenanthrene-Based			
Cationic amine	Asp147	Asp138	Ionic bond
C3-OH	His297	His291, Tyr139	H-bond
Aromatic A ring	Trp293		Pi stacking
C6-OH or keto	Asn230, Tyr326	Leu224	H-bond
C14-OH	Tyr148	Tyr139, Glu297	H-bond
Piperidine carbons	Ile322, other aliphatic residues		Hydrophobic
Flexible (Fentanyls)			
Cationic amine	Asp147		Ionic
Propanamide N-phenyl	His319, Trp283		Pi stacking
Propanamide oxygen	Lys233		Ion-dipole
Propanamide carbons	Trp318, Asn230		Hydrophobic
Piperidine carbons	Tyr148		Hydrophobic
Phenethyl (CH_2-CH_2)	Tyr326		Hydrophobic
Phenethyl (phenyl)	His297		Pi stacking/ donor-acceptor

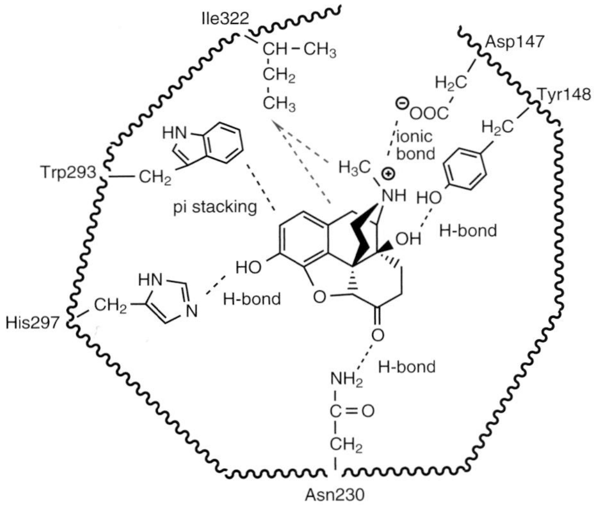

Figure 14.1 Proposed binding of oxymorphone at the μ opioid receptor (hydrophobic bonding represented in red).

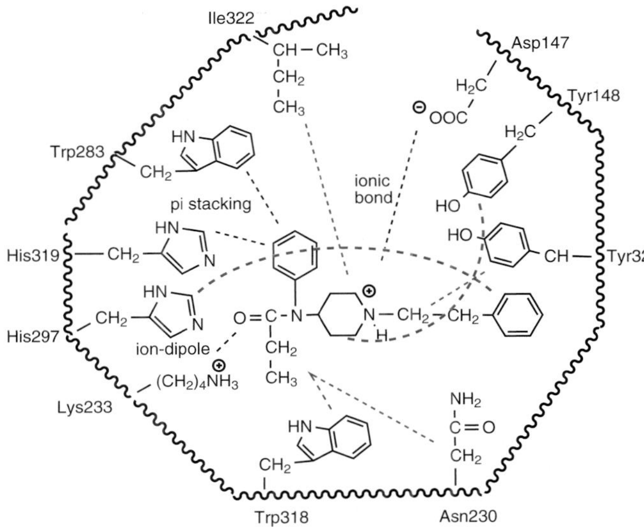

Figure 14.2 Proposed binding of fentanyl at the μ opioid receptor (hydrophobic bonding represented in red).

Stereochemistry

Morphine, the prototypical opioid agonist, is a pentacyclic structure with five asymmetric centers. The rings are commonly designated by letters A-E. Rings A and D are joined at C_{13} and by C_{10}, forming the 4-phenylpiperidine moiety that is commonly considered the pharmacophore of opioid ligands. Naturally occurring levorotatory (-) morphine has the 5*R*,6*S*,9*R*,13*S*,14*R* absolute configuration, which is the most active isomeric form at μ-opioid receptors.

(-)-Morphine with 4-phenylpiperidine pharmacophore highlighted

Pentacyclic opioids are referred to as morphine analogues. Tetracyclic opioids that are missing ring E are called morphinans, morphinans missing C ring carbons 6 and 7 are referred to as benzazocines or benzomorphans, and orvinols are morphine analogues with a bicyclic C ring. Ring C of morphines is forced into a pseudoboat conformation by the 7,8-double bond and the restraining E ring. Activity will increase if structural changes allow the C ring to assume the more stable chair conformation. The B/C ring fusion in naturally occurring (-)-morphine is *cis*, placing rings B and C at right angles to one another. This gives morphine a decidedly nonplanar T-shaped conformation. The 14R (B/C *cis*) configuration is indicated in two-dimensional drawings by a C14β substituent (in front of the plane of the paper). An α substituent at C14 (indicated by a dotted line) would denote 14S stereochemistry and the more planar B/C *trans* ring fusion.

Because the absolute configuration at C14 influences molecular conformation and degree of fit at the receptor surface, it is not surprising that analgesic activity is also impacted. In pentacyclic morphines, the B/C *cis* fused system is 10-fold more potent than the B/C *trans* system. In contrast, B/C *cis* morphinans are about 2-fold less active than B/C *trans* isomers. Only the B/C *cis* form of rigid opioids is marketed.

In phenanthrene-based rigid opioids, the A ring is held in an axial orientation relative to ring D, which forces a π-stacking (van der Waals) interaction with the μ-opioid receptor Trp293 residue that normally binds Tyr1 of the enkephalins.[65] For that reason, the aromatic A ring of rigid opioids requires a phenolic hydroxyl group to elicit analgetic action. If the orientation of the A ring can become equatorial to ring D (which occurs in more flexible meperidine and anilidopiperidine-based opioids) the phenyl ring will bind to a different aromatic residue (e.g., the μ receptor Trp283) that normally binds enkephalin Phe4.[65] In that case, a phenolic OH is a binding liability.

Structure-Activity Relationships of Opioid Agonists and Antagonists

The opioid agonists and antagonists molecules marketed in the U.S. have not changed over the past several years, and opioid structure-activity relationships (SAR) have been well established. The majority of these agents are rigid phenanthrene-based structures (Figs. 14.3-14.5), which include the natural alkaloids morphine and codeine and their synthetic analogues. Interest in the discovery of new alkaloidal analgesics and antagonists, including novel analogues of old standards, is ongoing. Close to 200 papers on this drug discovery focus area were published between 2000 and 2013.[67]

The nonphenanthrene-based flexible opioid agonists on the U.S. market include meperidine (a 4-substituted N-methyl-4-phenylpiperidine), the straight chain analgesic methadone, four anilidopiperidine structures known collectively as fentanyl analogues, and two dual action opioids that elicit analgesia through μ receptor stimulation and inhibition of neurotransmitter reuptake (Fig. 14.6.). Recent SAR studies on this general class of analgesics have been focused on the fentanyl analogues[68,69] and dual-action agents.[70]

PHENANTHRENE-BASED RIGID OPIOIDS

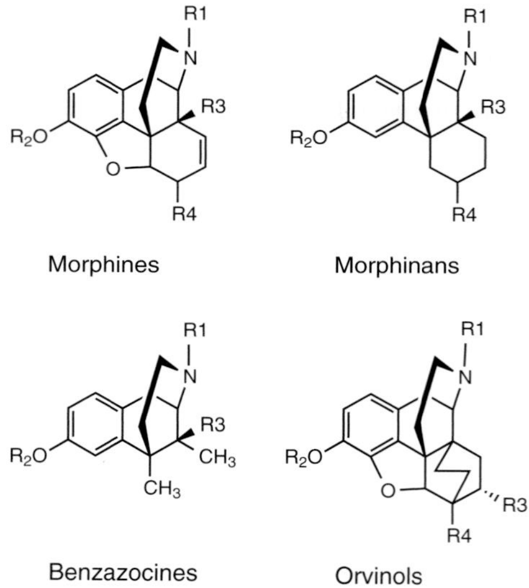

R1. A basic amine is an essential feature of all opioids because, in cationic conjugate acid form, it forms an essential electrostatic bond with the Asp residue conserved in all GPCRs. With the exception of dezocine, an opioid agonist no longer available in the U.S., only tertiary amines provide clinically significant central opioid agonist or antagonist activity.

Dezocine

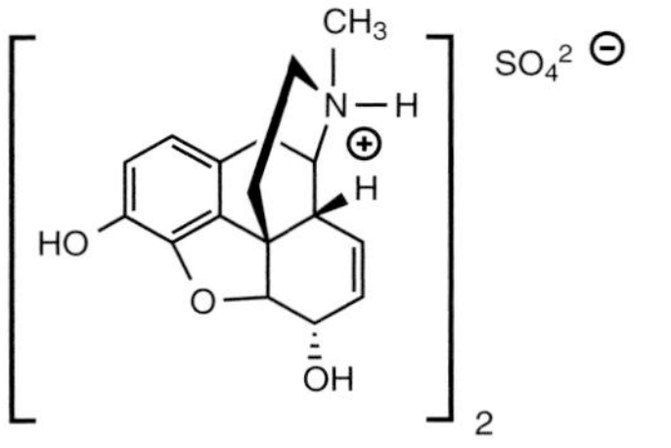

Morphine sulfate

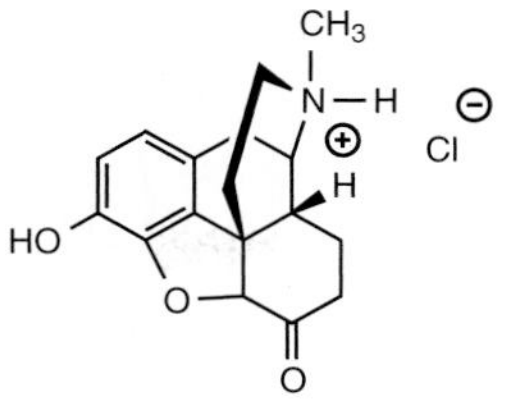

Hydromorphone hydrochloride (Dilaudid)

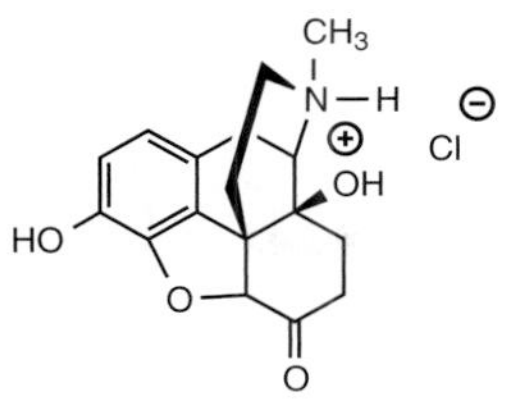

Oxymorphone hydrochloride (Opana)

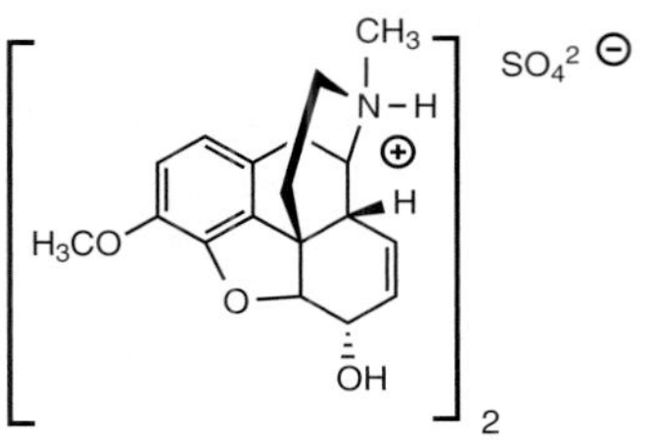

Codeine sulfate

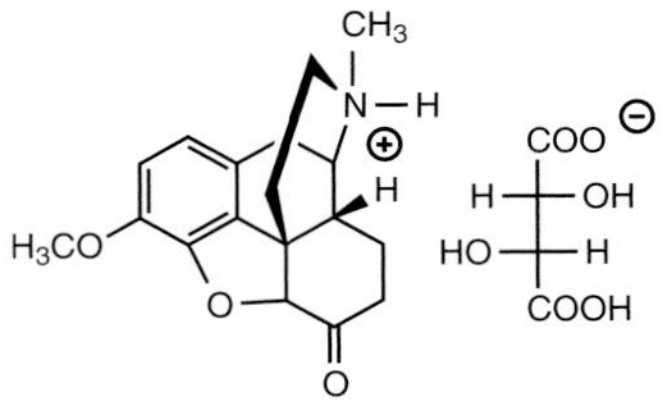

Hydrocodone bitartrate

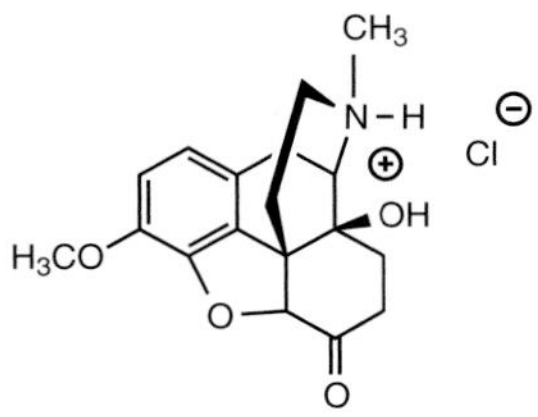

Oxycodone hydrochloride (Roxicodone)

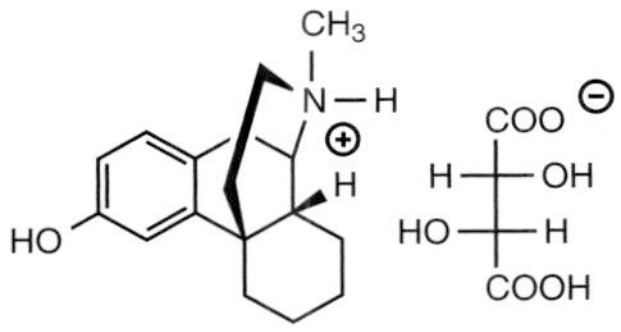

Levorphanol tartrate (Levo-Dromeran)

Partial μ agonist

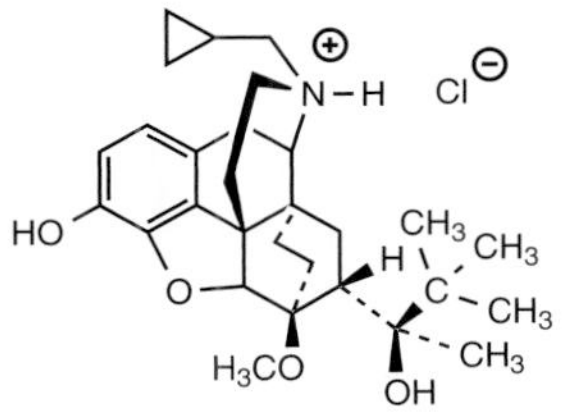

Buprenorphine hydrochloride (Buprenex)

Figure 14.3 Rigid μ agonists.

The most common nitrogen substituent found on tertiary μ-selective rigid opioid agonists, as well as on the flexible opioids meperidine and methadone, is CH_3. This group interacts hydrophobically with μ-receptor residues, including Trp293 and Tyr326 for the rigid structures.[70] An aralkyl substituent (e.g., phenethyl) would significantly enhance μ-receptor affinity and CNS distribution, but no such substituent is currently found on any marketed rigid opioid.

Extending the length of R1 to three carbons or its equivalent and incorporating an area of high electron density two atoms away from the nitrogen shifts the μ-receptor activity profile from agonist to antagonist. The antagonist site on the μ receptor has been proposed to be a narrow, primarily hydrophobic cleft formed between the side chains of Asp, Met, Tyr, Ile, and Gly residues.[65] Tyr326 and Trp293 have also been suggested as antagonist substituent binding residues.[60] Some authors caution that ligand-induced conformational changes in receptor proteins can obscure or otherwise complicate the binding specifics.[71]

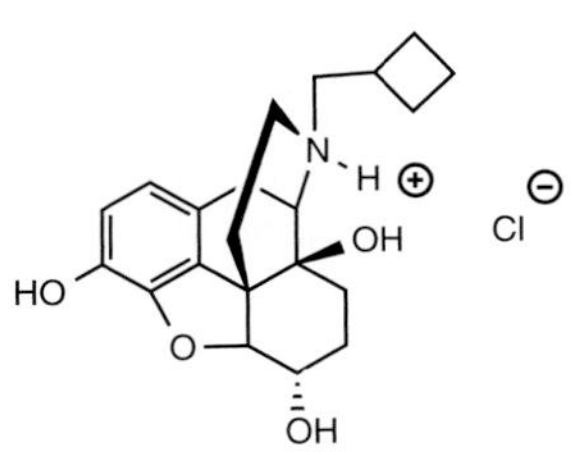

If the moiety providing the high electron density is a double bond (R1 = allyl) or a highly strained cyclopropane ring (R1 = cyclopropylmethyl), μ antagonist activity predominates. If found on a pentacyclic structural framework containing a 14β-OH group and a 7,8-dihydro-6-one C ring, allyl and cyclopropylmethyl substituents provide a pure opioid antagonist. Pure antagonists have their highest affinity for the μ receptor but, in higher doses, will block other opioid receptor subtypes too. They provide no analgesic action at any receptor at any dose. In other rigid systems, these two nitrogen substituents can provide κ agonism, but only in doses much higher than those needed to elicit μ antagonism. Strong dysphoria at these higher doses precludes their use as analgesics, and no such drugs are marketed.

If ring strain is eased (R1 = cyclobutylmethyl) or if the allyl moiety is converted to dimethylallyl, κ agonism (analgesia) becomes the therapeutically predominant action. The action at μ receptors will be either partial agonism (tetracyclic or tricyclic structure) or antagonism (pentacyclic structure). While often potent, the level of μ antagonism exhibited by N-cyclobutylmethyl opioids will always be lower than that of their allyl or cyclopropylmethyl counterparts because of a less-than-optimal fit within (and affinity for) the antagonist receptor cleft. However, because clinically significant partial μ agonism or antagonism will always accompany κ agonism, analgesics with cyclobutylmethyl or dimethylallyl nitrogen substituents will precipitate withdrawal in patients dependent

Nalbuphine hydrochloride (Nubain)

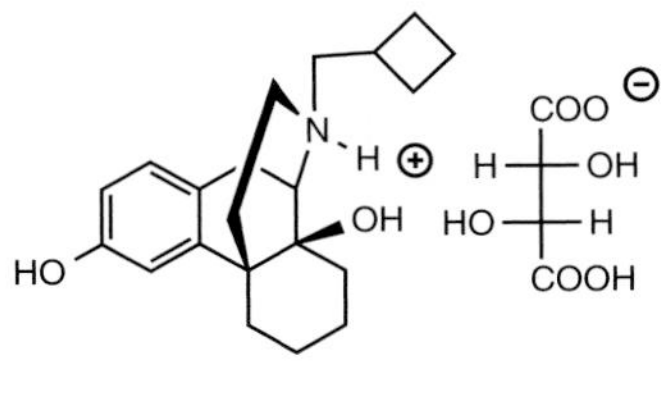

Butorphanol tartrate (Stadol)

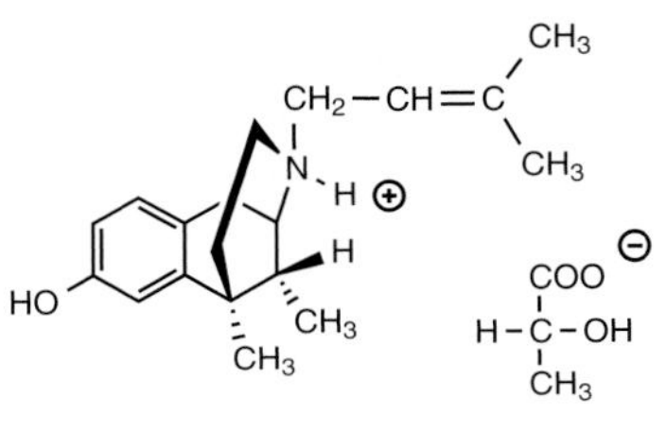

Pentazocine lactate (Talwin)

Figure 14.4 Rigid κ agonists/μ antagonists.

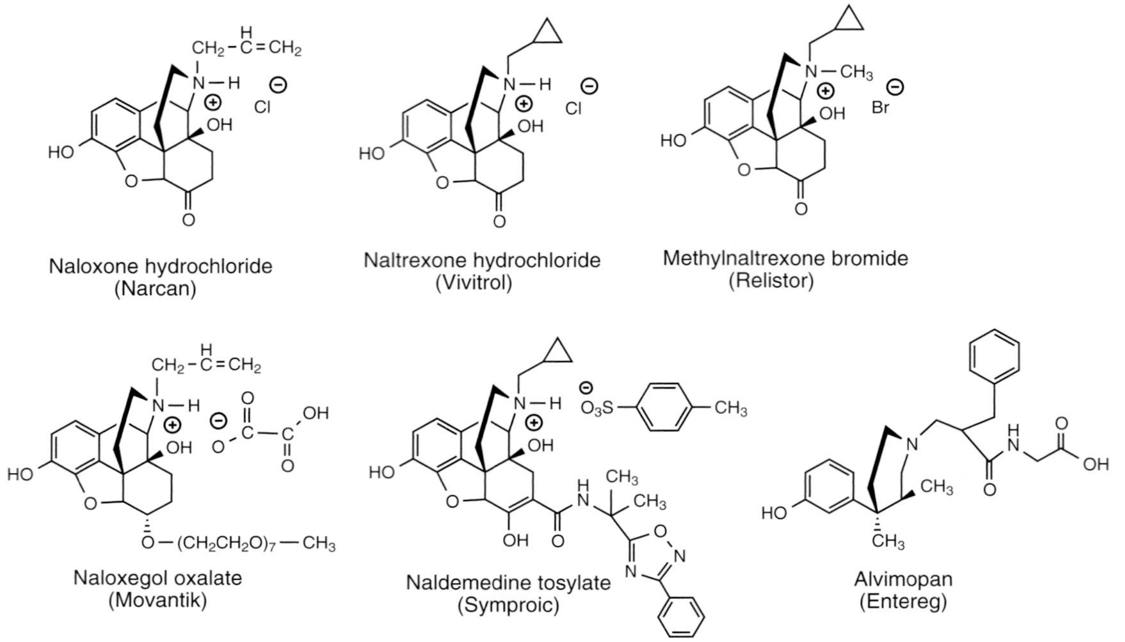

Naloxone hydrochloride (Narcan)
Naltrexone hydrochloride (Vivitrol)
Methylnaltrexone bromide (Relistor)
Naloxegol oxalate (Movantik)
Naldemedine tosylate (Symproic)
Alvimopan (Entereg)

Figure 14.5 Rigid opioid antagonists.

on N-methyl- or N-aralkyl-substituted full μ analgesics. In other words, these two chemically distinct classes of pain-relieving opioids are not cross tolerant.

R2. A phenolic hydroxyl group or a methoxy ether will be found at C3 of all marketed phenanthrene-based rigid opioids. The phenol is required for H-bonding at μ and κ receptors, so the methoxy ethers (codeine analogues) are prodrugs. CYP2D6 O-dealkylation of these methoxy groups is activating, but it is a somewhat sluggish reaction. For example, only about 5%-10% of a dose of the codeine will be activated to morphine.[72] Poor CYP2D6 metabolizers (PM) may not realize the full impact of codeine-based analgesics,[73,74] although this generalized presumption in patients with "real" pain has recently been called into question.[39] Conversely, patients of the ultrarapid metabolizer (UM) phenotype have more than three functional copies of the gene that codes for CYP2D6 and would be at risk for life-threatening toxicity from CNS/respiratory depression if given standard doses of methoxylated

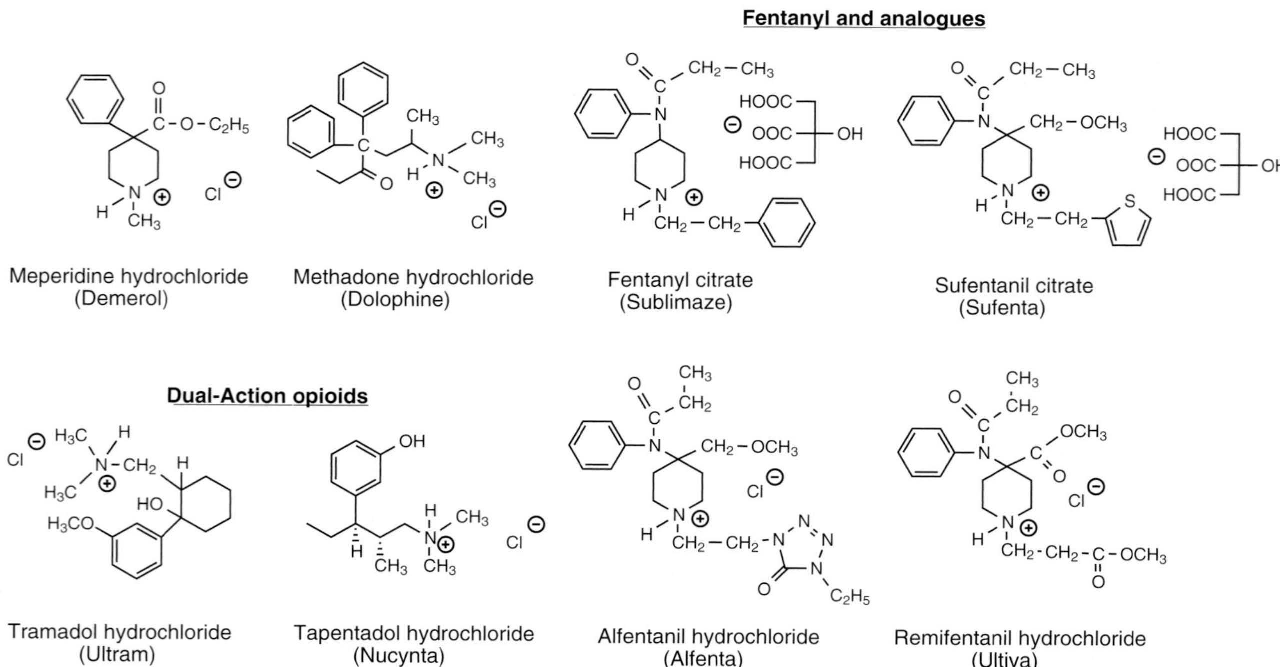

Figure 14.6 Flexible μ agonists.

opioids.[72-74] The tragic deaths of neonates who breastfed from lactating UM mothers administered standard doses of codeine have been documented.[39]

When present, the phenolic OH group will be vulnerable to inactivating prehepatic GI and first-pass (liver) phase 2 metabolism.[74] Premature conjugation with glucuronic acid (catalyzed by UGT2B7)[39] or 3′-phosphoadenosine-5′-phosphosulfate (PAPS) significantly compromises the oral bioavailability of many phenolic opioids. Phenols also undergo in vitro oxidation to therapeutically inactive quinones. Phenolic drugs, including active opioids, should always be protected from light, base, and oxygen in the air or, over time, they can decompose.

R3. Rigid opioids currently on the market have either a 14β-H or OH moiety, which provides a B/C *cis* or equivalent configuration. The polar 14β-OH slows penetration of the blood-brain barrier (BBB), but the negative impact this would have on analgesic potency is more than overridden by a significant increase in receptor affinity. Hydrogen bonds have been proposed between the 14β-OH and μ and κ receptor Tyr or Glu residues, respectively.[65] Overall, a 2- to 3-fold increase in opioid activity is achieved through the addition of a 14β-OH. There is a decrease in antitussive (cough suppression) action[75] and 14β-OH opioids are not used for this therapeutic purpose.

R4. The impact of the C6 substituent of rigid opioids on pharmacologic action is tied to the presence or absence of the 7,8-double bond. The 6α-OH found in naturally occurring morphine and codeine is believed to engage in a hydrogen bond with a μ-receptor Asn residue,[65] but the bond formed is not strong. Despite the loss of this drug-receptor interaction, removal of the 6-OH group results in an approximate 10-fold increase in activity due to a significant increase in molecular lipophilicity. If the 6α-OH is oxidized to an α,β-unsaturated ketone, the H-bonding role of the 6-substituent converts from H-donor to H-acceptor. In the inflexible pseudoboat C ring ensured by the 7,8-olefin, a marked decrease in receptor affinity occurs, and activity decreases 3-fold. However, if the 7,8-double bond is reduced, the C ring becomes significantly more flexible and can properly position the H-accepting C6 ketone for high-affinity receptor binding. A 6-fold gain in analgesic potency is achieved by changing C ring structure from the natural 7,8-dehydro-6α-ol to 7,8-dihydro-6-one. Antitussive action also increases approximately 4-fold.[75]

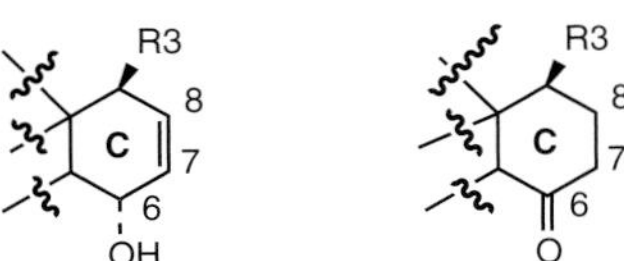

7,8-Dehydro-6α-ol 7,8-Dihydro-6-one

The 6α-OH group of morphine and codeine is associated with mast cell degranulation and histamine release, which can lead to an allergic-like response involving hypotension, intense pruritus, and rash.[76] The mechanism involves activation of protein kinase A and inositol triphosphate kinase, which not only releases histamine but also stimulates the production of proinflammatory chemokines in mast cells.[77] Pruritus induced via this mechanism is not reversed by opioid antagonists.[77,78] A μ receptor-linked pruritus mechanism, which can be reversed with low-dose antagonists, has also been proposed.[78] The pruritus associated with opioids increases significantly with intravenous (IV) and/or epidural administration.[78] This adverse effect is particularly intense with codeine, and as a result, parenteral administration of this analgesic is generally not recommended. Pruritus and hypotension are not generally observed with 6-keto or 6-desoxy opioids,[78,79] and the risk of nausea may also be lowered. Kappa agonists, which have inherent μ antagonist action, do not induce pruritus.[78]

FLEXIBLE OPIOIDS: ANILIDOPIPERIDINES. The anilidopiperidine analgesics, commonly known as the fentanyls, are the only class of flexible opioids with more than two members (Fig. 14.6). The crystal structure of fentanyl has confirmed a chair conformation of the piperidine ring and the equatorial conformation of the 4-phenylpropanamide moiety.[65] In that conformation the phenyl ring may interact with the μ receptor residue that normally binds Phe4 of enkephalin, and no phenolic OH group is incorporated into their structures. Vardanyan and Hruby[68] have proposed that the anilidopiperidine opioids are pharmacophorically unrelated to the phenanthrene-based opioids (4-phenylpiperidine pharmacophore), claiming that the N-arylethyl moiety might be the structural driver in directing μ receptor binding. Anilidopiperidine opioids are highly lipophilic molecules that distribute rapidly across the BBB, resulting in a fast and potent, albeit short-lived, analgesic response.[69]

While no 3-substituted anilidopiperine analgesics are currently marketed, it bears mentioning that a 3-CH_3 substituent increases μ receptor affinity and analgesic activity. Stereochemistry is critical, with the *cis* isomers being six to eight times as active as the *trans*, and the *cis* (+) isomer being approximately 120-fold more potent than its (−) enantiomer.[68,69] The synthesis of myriad fentanyl analogues has added significantly to our understanding of anilidopiperidine SAR.[68]

cis-(+)-3-Methylfentanyl

Anilidopiperidine pharmacophore

R1. With few exceptions, the SAR of the nitrogen substituent of all flexible opioids essentially parallels that of the rigid phenanthrene-based analgesics. While the N-CH_3 substituent of meperidine and methadone provides anticipated selective μ agonism, the N-CH_3 analogue of fentanyl is surprisingly inactive.[68] However, N-aralkyl substituents promote potent, selective μ agonism regardless of the class of opioids under discussion. The aralkyl substituents (e.g., R1 = phenethyl, thienylethyl) of fentanyl and sufentanil promote a very fast penetration of the BBB and a very high affinity at μ receptors through hydrophobic and π-stacking interactions. This results in an analgesic activity that runs between 80- and 800-fold that of morphine. The substantial lipophilicity of these aralkyl substituents contributes to the very high calculated/experimental log P values of fentanyl (4.12/4.05) and sufentanil (3.4/3.95).[80]

Replacing the lipophilic phenyl or thienyl ring found in fentanyl and sufentanil, respectively, with the polar tetrazolinone system found in alfentanil (calculated/experimental log P = 2.2/2.16)[80] produces some complex but predictable changes in in vivo drug behavior. One might logically expect the decrease in molecular lipophilicity to translate to a more sluggish journey across the BBB. However, this strongly electron-withdrawing ring system decreases the pK_a of the piperidino nitrogen atom to 6.5 compared to 8.4 for fentanyl's basic nitrogen atom,[81] which significantly decreases the ratio of ionized to unionized conjugate forms in the bloodstream. Contrary to what would be expected from a simple comparison of log P values, the lower pK_a of alfentanil allows for a faster penetration of the BBB. However, this depressed ionized:unionized ratio is maintained at the receptor surface, which means less cationic drug is available for essential ion-ion anchoring with the μ receptor Asp147. Therefore, despite a positive CNS distribution profile, the potency of alfentanil decreases to 25-fold that of morphine because of a lower μ-receptor affinity.

The electron-withdrawing ester moiety at R1 of remifentanil is required for activity. This group drops amine pK_a to 7.1, increasing the fraction of unionized drug in the blood compared to N-CH_3 analogues fentanyl and sufentanil. CNS penetration is facilitated and the onset of action is very fast. The fact that the amine pK_a is higher than alfentanil translates to a higher percentage of cationic drug at the receptor surface (33% vs. 11%) and augmented receptor affinity. However, inactivating hydrolysis is rapid, leading to an exceptionally brief (3-10 min) duration of action appropriate for the induction or maintenance of anesthesia.

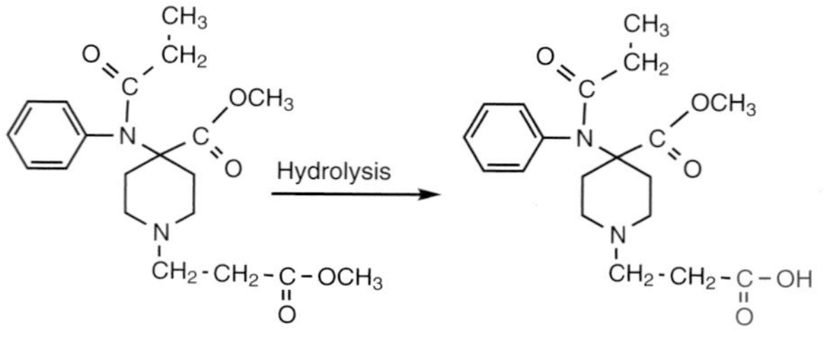

Hydrolysis

Remifentanil (active)

Remifentanil acid (inactive)

Conversion of μ agonist to μ antagonist in flexible opioids cannot be accomplished by the straightforward amine substitution approach found in the phenanthrene-based structural series.[68] The allyl and cyclopropylmethyl amine substituents that provided such potent μ antagonism in rigid opioids attenuate agonist action in these flexible structures, and they will not be encountered.

R2. The axial methoxymethyl moiety at C4 of the piperidine ring of sufentanil and alfentanil is lipophilic and contributes to their rapid distribution to central sites of action. It also promotes high-affinity binding at the μ-receptor surface.[68,69] A similar spike in μ affinity is realized with a 4-methylcarboxylate moiety (e.g., carfentanil, lofentanil).

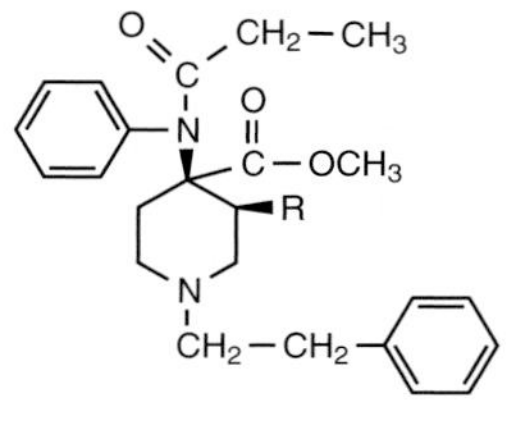

R = H: Carfentanil
R = CH_3: Lofentanil

FLEXIBLE OPIOIDS: DUAL ACTION AGENTS. Inhibiting central monoamine reuptake in descending nociceptive pathways has been shown to alleviate chronic pain. While both NE and 5-HT have a mechanistic role to play,[82] NE reuptake inhibition appears to provide the stronger analgetic response.[83]

Tapentadol and tramadol (Fig. 14.6) both inhibit central NE reuptake to about the same extent, but the former drug, administered as the pure 1*R*,2*R*-(-) isomer, does so selectively. Complicating its therapeutic activity profile, tramadol is marketed as a racemic mixture of *cis* isomers, each of which targets a different neurotransmitter. 1*S*,2*S*-(-)-Tramadol inhibits the reuptake of NE while the 1*R*,2*R*-(+) enantiomer blocks 5-HT reuptake.[84]

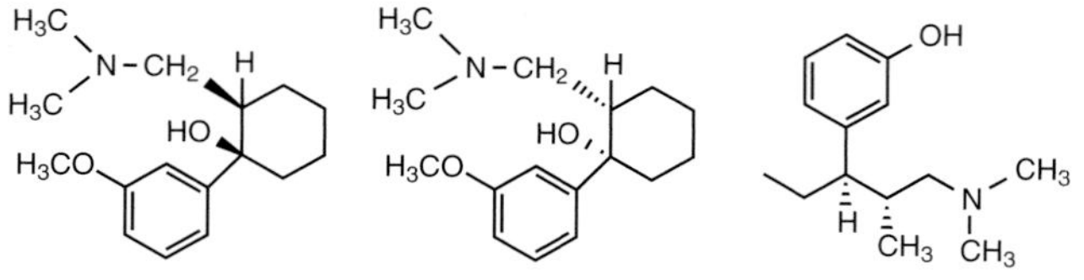

1*R*,2*R*-(+)-Tramadol 1*S*,2*S*-(-)-Tramadol 1*R*,2*R*-(-)-Tapentadol

Both tapentadol and tramadol also elicit analgesia through μ receptor agonism that synergizes with the pain relief gained through inhibition of neurotransmitter reuptake. Phenolic (-)-tapentadol, a rationally designed drug that is the more potent analgesic of the two, is active intact. Similar to codeine-based analgesics, tramadol's aromatic methoxy group must be O-dealkylated by the highly polymorphic CYP2D6 before significant μ receptor binding can occur, and only the (+) isomer generates a clinically active μ agonist. CYP3A4 may play a secondary role in tramadol O-dealkylation.[84] Since neurotransmitter reuptake activity resides primarily in the parent tramadol structure, the mechanism by which this drug provides analgesia shifts as O-dealkylation progresses.[83] In addition to selective NE reuptake, the time-independent mechanism of tapentadol's analgetic action is viewed as a distinct therapeutic advantage. The chemical and mechanistic distinctions of tramadol and tapentadol are summarized in Table 14.3.

The dimethylamino moiety is an essential feature for both analgetic mechanisms of tramadol and tapentadol. Tapentadol is missing tramadol's 3° alcohol, as drug development studies documented replacement with hydrogen (or fluorine) enhanced μ receptor affinity. While the binding affinity of tapentadol to the human μ receptor is almost 50-fold less than the (+)-phenol metabolite of tramadol, the opioid agonist potency of tapentadol is higher due to a more favorable CNS distribution profile.[84] Its μ agonist activity is commonly compared against morphine or oxycodone.

Shen et al.[70] have confirmed that the active phenolic metabolite of (+)-tramadol binds to the μ receptor in a manner similar to morphine. Molecular docking studies indicate that ion-ion anchoring to Asp147, hydrophobic bonding of N-substituents with Trp293 and Tyr326, and H-bonding of the phenolic OH with His297 occur with both structures.

The metabolic pathways of tramadol and tapentadol have been recently reviewed.[85] While tapentadol's metabolism is straightforward and yields six metabolites, the more complex biotransformation of racemic tramadol yields 26 metabolites; 14 phase 1 and 12 phase 2 metabolites are generated, with glucuronidation predominating over sulfonation.

Common Metabolic Reactions

The common metabolic pathways of opioids are predictable from their structure. Many μ agonists have an N-methyl group that can be dealkylated by CYP3A4.[86] From a therapeutic standpoint, normetabolites have limited clinical relevance due to a decrease in distribution-enhancing lipophilicity and the loss of an agonist-promoting hydrophobic interaction with the receptor.

In contrast, CYP2D6-mediated O-dealkylation of the aryl methoxy group of codeine analogues (Fig. 14.7) and tramadol are required to generate the phenolic OH group essential for μ-receptor binding. As noted previously, patients deficient in this activating enzyme may show an attenuated response to these prodrug analgesics. Within the U.S., the incidence of CYP2D6 PM phenotype has been estimated at approximately 10%.[74] Although the *CYP2D6*3* and *CYP2D6*4* alleles common in Caucasian PMs are present in only 1% or less of persons of Asian ancestry, the *CYP2D6*10* allele associated with reduced CYP2D6 catalytic capability (intermediate metabolizer (IM) phenotype) is found in up to 50% of Asians.[87-89] Approximately 1%-2% of the U.S. population is of the UM phenotype, but the incidence rises to up to 28% in individuals of Arab, Ethiopian, and North African descent.[72,74]

Table 14.3 Chemical and Mechanistic Properties of Tramadol and Tapentadol

	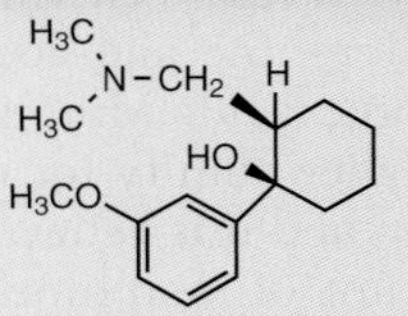 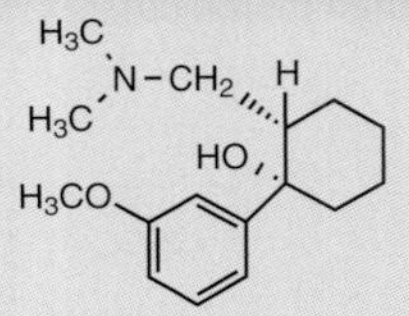 1*R*,2*R*-(+)-Tramadol / 1*S*,2*S*-(-)-Tramadol	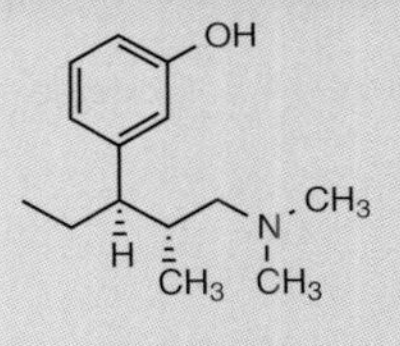 1*R*,2*R*-(-)-Tapentadol
Aliphatic structure	Cyclic	Open chain
Marketed as	Racemic mixture of *cis* isomers	Single isomer
Neurotransmitter reuptake profile	Serotonin and norepinephrine (1*S*,2*S*)	Norepinephrine
Prodrug opioid?	Yes: activated by CYP2D6-catalyzed O-dealkylation	No: active intact
μ agonist isomer	Dextrorotatory	Levorotatory
μ agonist potency	Weak	Weak-moderate (1.5-4 x tramadol)
Analgesic mechanism	Time dependent: neurotransmitter reuptake (parent drug) decreases as μ agonism ((+)-phenol metabolite) increases	Time independent: neurotransmitter reuptake and μ agonism provided by parent drug
Inactivating metabolism	CYP3A4/CYP2B6-catalyzed N-dealkylation; glucuronic acid or sulfate conjugation	CYP2C-catalyzed N-dealkylation (13%), glucuronic acid (55%) or sulfate (15%) conjugation
Abuse potential	C-IV	C-II

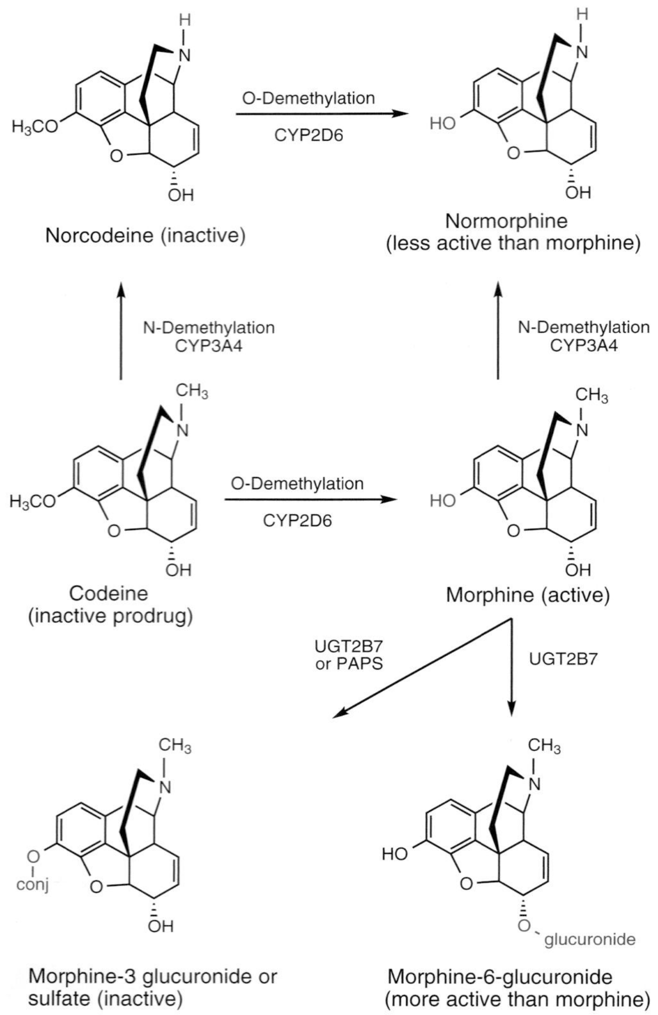

Norcodeine (inactive) — O-Demethylation, CYP2D6 → Normorphine (less active than morphine)

Codeine (inactive prodrug) — N-Demethylation, CYP3A4 → Norcodeine (inactive)

Morphine (active) — N-Demethylation, CYP3A4 → Normorphine

Codeine (inactive prodrug) — O-Demethylation, CYP2D6 → Morphine (active)

Morphine (active) — UGT2B7 or PAPS → Morphine-3 glucuronide or sulfate (inactive)

Morphine (active) — UGT2B7 → Morphine-6-glucuronide (more active than morphine)

Figure 14.7 Codeine metabolism.

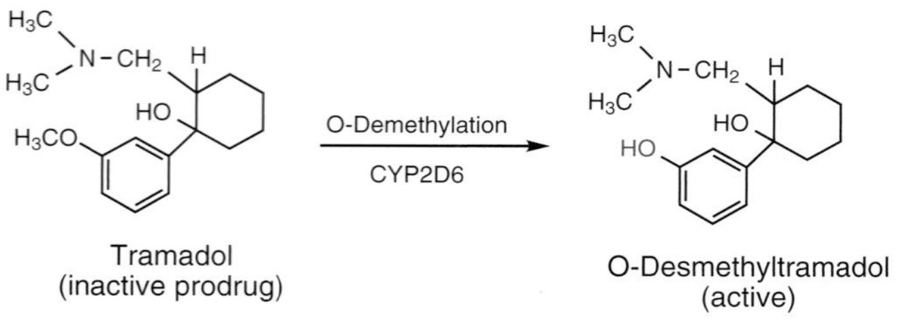

Tramadol (inactive prodrug) — O-Demethylation, CYP2D6 → O-Desmethyltramadol (active)

Tramadol activation.

Heroin — Hydrolysis → 6-Monoacetylmorphine (6-MAM, active) — Hydrolysis → Morphine (active)

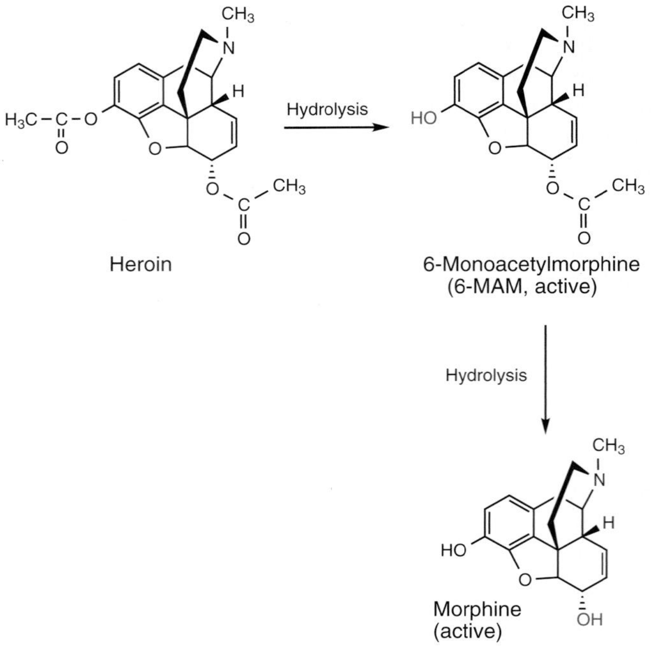

Figure 14.8 Heroin metabolism.

While no clinically marketed opioid analgesic has a C3-ester, the need for metabolic liberation of the phenol would still hold true. For example, the 3-acetate ester of heroin is readily hydrolyzed in the CNS to generate the analgesically active monoacetylmorphine (Fig. 14.8). The 6-acetate ester is slower to cleave because its carbonyl carbon is less electrophilic due to a lack of resonance delocalization of electron density, but it will eventually succumb to hydrolysis to produce morphine.

Opioids are also subject to phase 2 metabolism prior to excretion. Phenols conjugate with either glucuronic acid or PAPS, and both glucuronide and sulfate conjugates are found in the urine of patients taking most opioids. These conjugates, like most, are inactive, and phase 2 conjugation in the GI tract impacts the oral bioavailability of many phenolic opioids (Table 14.4). Those administered by mouth must be given in doses higher than one would administer parenterally, and/or they are formulated to promote rapid absorption and limit exposure to intestinal transferase enzymes. Alcohols like those found at C6 of morphine and codeine can also conjugate with glucuronic acid. Morphine's C6 glucuronide actually has a higher affinity for the μ receptors than the free alcohol,[90] and it is believed to be responsible for a significant amount of morphine's and codeine's analgesic action.[86] Glucuronidation at both C3 and C6 is catalyzed by UGT2B7.

The metabolic pathway of codeine (Fig. 14.7) is illuminating in that it contains essentially all of the aforementioned biotransformations and includes reactions that are analgetically activating, inactivating, attenuating, and augmenting.

Physicochemical and Pharmacokinetic Properties

As GPCR ligands, opioids have a tertiary amine that will be predominantly cationic at pH 7.4. Amine pK_a values range from 6.5 (alfentanil) to 9.4 (tramadol). Phenolic opioids are sensitive to in vitro oxidation and must be protected from light, air, and elevated pH. As drugs with a central mechanism of action, opioid agonists and antagonists are generally highly lipophilic structures capable of penetrating the BBB. Only morphine, the most polar opioid, has a predicted log P value less than 1.0. As noted earlier, the analgetic action of chiral opioids is highly stereoselective, with the (-) isomer being the clinically active form for all but tramadol.

Table 14.4 Selected Physicochemical and Pharmacokinetics Properties of Opioid Analgesics and Antagonists

Opioid Analgesic: Rigid Phenanthrene-Based	Log P (Calc)	Oral Bioavailability (%)	Extended-Release Dosage Form Available?	Protein Binding (%)
Buprenorphine	4.53	NA 31 (sl)	No	96
Butorphanol	3.65	5-17 60-70 (nas)	No	80
Codeine	1.2	90	Yes	7-25
Hydrocodone	2.13	–	Yes	19-45
Hydromorphone	1.69	24	Yes	19
Levorphanol	3.29	Low	No	40
Morphine	0.99	30	Yes	30-40
Oxycodone	1.04	60-87	Yes	45
Oxymorphone	1.26	10	Yes	8-19
Nalbuphine	2.0	NA 81-83 (im) 76-79 (sc)	No	Little appreciable binding
Pentazocine	4.44	Low	No	
Opioid Analgesic: Flexible				
Alfentanil	2.2	NA	No	92
Fentanyl	4.12	50 (buccal) 92 (td)	No	80-85
Meperidine	2.9	50-60	No	60-80
Methadone	4.14	36-100	No	85-90
Remifentanil	1.75	NA	No	70
Sufentanil	3.4	NA	No	91-93
Tapentadol	3.47	32	Yes	20
Tramadol	2.71	75	Yes	20
Opioid Antagonist				
Naloxone	1.47	NA	No	10
Naltrexone	2.07	5-40	Yes	21
Methylnaltrexone bromide	0.59	Low (approx. 2%)	No	11-15
Naloxegol	1.73	–	No	4.2

Opioid Analgesic: Rigid Phenanthrene-Based	Onset (min) of Analgesia (po unless noted)	$T_{1/2}$ (hr)	Duration of Action (hr)	Excretion (%)	T_{max} (hr) (po unless noted)
Buprenorphine	15 (im)	2.2 (iv) 37 (sl)	≥6 (im)	10-30 renal 70 fecal	0.67-3.5 (sl) 1 (im) 72 (td)
Butorphanol	≤15	18	3-4 (im, iv) 4-5 (nas)	70-80 renal 15 fecal	0.5-1 (im, iv) 1-2 (nas)

(continued)

Table 14.4 Selected Physicochemical and Pharmacokinetics Properties of Opioid Analgesics and Antagonists (Continued)

Opioid Analgesic: Rigid Phenanthrene-Based	Onset (min) of Analgesia (po unless noted)	$T_{1/2}$ (hr)	Duration of Action (hr)	Excretion (%)	T_{max} (hr) (po unless noted)
Codeine	30-60	2.5-3.5	4-6	90 renal	1-1.5
Hydrocodone	60	1.5-3	3-4	26 renal	2
Hydromorphone	15-30	2-3	3-4	Primarily renal	0.5-1
Levorphanol	10-60	11-16	≤8	Primarily renal	1
Morphine	30 5-10 (iv)	2-4	3-5	90 renal 7-10 fecal	0.5
Oxycodone	10-15	2-4	3-6	80 renal	0.5-1
Oxymorphone	5-10 (im, sc, iv)	7-9 (po)	3–6 (im, sc, iv)	49 renal	–
Nalbuphine	2-3 (iv) <15 (sc, im)	5	3-6	Primarily fecal 7 renal	1 (sc, im)
Pentazocine	15-30 (sc, im)	2-3	4-6	Primarily renal	0.25-1 (sc, im)
Opioid Analgesic: Flexible					
Alfentanil	2-3 iv	1.5-2	0.5-1	Primarily renal	15 min (im)
Fentanyl	<1 iv 7-8 (im) 6 hr (td) 5-15 (buc, sl, nas)	2-4 (iv) 20-27 (td)	72 (td) 0.5-1 (iv) 1-2 (im)	75 renal 9 fecal	0.25-8 (buc, sl, nas) 20-72 (td)
Meperidine	10-15 (im, sc)	2.5-4	2-4 (po, sc, im) 2-3 (iv)	Primarily renal	2 1 (im, sc)
Methadone	30-60 10-20 (im, sc, iv)	8-59	4-8	Primarily renal	1-2 (im, sc) 3-5 d (continuous po)
Remifentanil	1-3 (iv)	<0.33	0.05-0.17 (iv)	Primarily renal	<0.080 (iv)
Sufentanil	1-3 iv	2.7	0.5 (iv) 1.7 (epidural)	Primarily renal	
Tapentadol	32	4	4-6	99 renal	1.25
Tramadol	60-75	6-8	4-6	90 renal 10 fecal	2
Opioid Antagonist					
Naloxone	2-5 (im, sc, nas)	0.5-1.5 (im, sc, iv) 2 (nas)	0.5-2	40 renal (<6h)	0.25 (im, sc) 0.33-0.5 (nas)
Naltrexone	–	4 5-10 d (im)	24-72 4 wk (im)	53–79 renal 5-10 fecal	1 2 (im, 1st phase) 48-72 (im, second phase)
Methylnaltrexone bromide	–	15 (po)	–	44-45 renal 17 fecal	1.5 (po) 0.5 (sc)
Naloxegol	–	6-11	–	16 renal 68 fecal	<2 hr

Data from *Drug Bank*. Available at https://www.drugbank.ca/. Accessed 9/30/2017; *Drug Facts and Comparisons. Facts & Comparisons [Database Online]*. In: Louis S., ed. MO: Wolters Kluwer Health, Inc.; March 2005; and *Lexicomp Online® Lexi-drugs® Hudson*. Ohio: Lexi-Comp, Inc.

buc, buccal; im, intramuscular; iv, intravenous; nas, intranasal; po, oral; sc, subcutaneous; sl, sublingual; td, transdermal; $T_{1/2}$, elimination half-life; T_{max}, time to peak plasma concentration.

Many opioid pharmaceuticals are administered only by parenteral, buccal, sublingual, or transdermal routes due to inactivating prehepatic or first pass metabolism. Those able to be given by mouth are usually given in doses higher than would be administered by injection. Extended duration dosage forms are available for many agents, although concerns about their potential for abuse and fatal misuse have prompted the removal of some from the marketplace (e.g., Opana ER).

Key physicochemical and pharmacokinetic properties of marketed opioid agonists and antagonists are provided in Table 14.4.[80,91,92]

Phenanthrene-Based Rigid μ Agonists (Fig. 14.3)

The opioid agonists discussed below are those that currently enjoy the most widespread clinical use.

MORPHINE SULFATE. Morphine is the prototypical opioid agonist, and all synthetic multicyclic analgesics are based on the morphine nucleus to some degree. The presence of the N-CH_3 substituent, phenolic hydroxyl, and B/C *cis* configuration assure potent and selective μ agonism. Despite being well absorbed from the GI tract, morphine has very poor oral bioavailability due to extensive prehepatic and first-pass metabolism to inactive 3-glucuronide and 3-sulfate conjugates. The C3 glucuronide undergoes extensive enterohepatic cycling, so if oral administration is required, large initial doses must be given followed by lower maintenance doses. At 0.99, morphine's log P is low, and opioids of higher lipophilicity exhibit better oral bioavailability, as well as a faster onset of analgesic action (Table 14.4). Polar and metabolically vulnerable morphine is generally considered 3- to 6-fold more active by parenteral routes than by the oral route.

Approximately 5% of a dose of morphine is metabolized by CYP3A4-mediated N-dealkylation to normorphine[93] which, at 1/20 the activity of the parent drug, is not clinically relevant. Inactivation is primarily a result of C3 glucuronidation by UGT2B7 (57%), with sulfonation taking on a minor conjugating role. Glucuronidation of the C6-OH (5%-10%) by the same UGT isoform provides a highly active metabolite.[94,95] The potency ratio between morphine and morphine-6-glucuronide in humans has been estimated between 1:2 and 1:3,[95,96] and the metabolite is believed to account for up to 85% of morphine's analgesic action.[97] Polar morphine-6-glucuronide has a log P of 0.13,[80] and it passively crosses the BBB with some difficulty. Along with morphine, it is a substrate for central P-glycoprotein (P-gp) efflux proteins.[93,98] To facilitate entry into the CNS, the molecule can hide its polar groups through folding[95] and active transport mechanisms are being investigated, but more work is needed to fully elucidate how these powerful analgesics reach central receptors.[98] The 6-glucuronide can accumulate in patients with renal failure or poor renal function (e.g., elderly),[94,95] increasing the risk of inadvertent overdose. A small study found that morphine-6-glucuronide did not induce the pruritus associated with the free 6α-OH group of morphine and codeine.[99] Phase 2 clinical trials have demonstrated efficacy of morphine-6-glucuronide in the treatment of postoperative pain. Compared to morphine, morphine-6-glucuronide provides long-lasting (12-24 hr) analgesia with a significantly slower onset of action and fewer and/or less severe adverse effects.[95,96]

Morphine is one of the safest opioids to use to treat the pain of myocardial infarction, unstable angina, and other ischemic disorders because of its positive hemodynamic effects.[100] Its negative chronotropic effect and venous and arterial vasodilation result in a decrease in myocardial oxygen demand. Morphine decreases blood pressure secondary to histamine release, an activity linked to the 6α-OH group and must be used with caution in patients with hypovolemia.

Extreme caution is advised with the use of all opioids in patients with head trauma because opioids can increase intracranial pressure, which in turn can exacerbate respiratory depression. Inhibition of cough reflex, however, is a valuable action in this situation because it helps keep intracranial pressure within defined limits. Morphine lacks the 14β-OH group that attenuates cough suppression and, along with fentanyl, it is the opioid most commonly used to treat pain in patients with head injury.[101] On a precautionary note, inflammation associated with head injury may downregulate efflux proteins such as P-gp and multidrug-resistant protein, resulting in an accumulation of morphine and the active 6-glucuronide in cerebral tissue.[102]

Morphine is available in a variety of dosage forms, including solution for injection, liposomal injection, oral solution, tablets, extended-release tablets and capsules, suppositories, and patient-controlled intramuscular administration devices. Extended-release morphine is marketed under the names of Kadian, Avinza MS Contin, Oramorph, MorphaBond ER, and Arymo ER. Extended-release formulations of any opioid should only be administered to opioid-tolerant patients. Oral dosage forms must be swallowed whole and not chewed, crushed, or dissolved in liquid. If patients have difficulty swallowing, the pellets in some extended-release capsules may be sprinkled on food (e.g., applesauce) and swallowed without chewing.

Some extended-release oral formulations have been designed to thwart morphine misuse and/or abuse. For example, MorphaBond ER contains inactive ingredients that produce physical and chemical barriers to product adulteration. The extended-release tablet cannot be easily cut, crushed, or broken. If an attempt is made to isolate morphine from the tablet by extraction, a viscous solution is formed that cannot be easily injected or inhaled.[103] Another abuse-deterring product is Embeda, a capsule which contains morphine sulfate in combination with the opioid antagonist naltrexone hydrochloride. This trade name refers to the fact that a core of naltrexone is embedded in a pellet of extended-release morphine. A variety of strengths is available, but the mg-to-mg ratio of agonist-to-antagonist is consistently held at 25:1. If the capsule or its contents was crushed and the active constituents extracted for IV injection, the naltrexone hydrochloride would be extracted along with the morphine salt. If injected, the antagonist would bind to opioid receptors, thereby blocking any euphoric responses an abuser might be seeking. Fortunately, morphine-induced hemodynamic responses would also be blocked, at least to some extent. If a patient tolerant to opioids is injected this illicit formulation, a naltrexone-induced withdrawal syndrome would most certainly be precipitated.

All extended-release opioids are for use only when continuous long-term analgesia requiring "around the clock" opioid agonist therapy is warranted. Patients taking this and all extended-release products must not be opioid-naïve, or potentially fatal respiratory depression could result. The consumption of alcohol while on opioid agonists is never advised, but it could prove fatal when taking extended-release capsules because alcohol can promote rapid capsule dissolution in the GI tract. Consuming alcohol and/or other CNS depressants (e.g, benzodiazepines) with opioids, regardless of formulation, can increase the risk of respiratory depression, excessive sedation, coma, and death. Some patients will experience an allergic-like reaction to morphine (attributed to the free 6α-OH) while others may be hypersensitive to the phenanthrene structural moiety.[104] Hypersensitive patients may react to all rigid opioid agonists, regardless of whether they contain a 6α-OH group.

The 7,8-dihydromorphine analogue that is also missing the furan and C6-oxygen atoms is marketed as levorphanol (Table 14.5). While more potent and longer acting than morphine, this tetracyclic μ agonist is used less commonly in the clinic than pentacyclic opioids.

HYDROMORPHONE HYDROCHLORIDE AND OXYMORPHONE HYDROCHLORIDE. Hydromorphone differs in structure from morphine only in the area of ring C. The 7,8-dihydro-6-one structural motif adds flexibility to the system and permits a more efficacious H-bond between the 6-keto moiety and the μ receptor. The increase in analgesic action arising from this single structural modification has been estimated at 4- to 7-fold by the oral route.[105] As μ receptor–elicited analgesia and side effects such as respiratory depression and constipation go hand-in-hand, the risk of toxicity with hydromorphone as compared to morphine also increases. Hydromorphone is metabolized primarily by C3 glucuronidation, but a small amount undergoes reduction of the 6-keto group to isomeric alcohols.[106]

Hydromorphone 6-hydroxy metabolites

A Cochrane Review of the use of hydromorphone in cancer pain, including pain that disrupts sleep, revealed efficacy similar to other μ agonists like morphine and oxycodone but concluded that more comprehensive studies were needed to positively document relative value in this patient population.[107] A recent retrospective study on inpatient deaths due to hydromorphone or morphine underscores the importance of vigilance against errors in prescribing, dispensing, administration, and monitoring.[108]

Hydromorphone hydrochloride is available as a solution for intramuscular (IM) or IV injection, rectal suppositories, tablets, liquid for oral administration, and abuse-deterrent extended-release tablets (Exalgo). Exalgo tablets are resistant to crushing and product extraction

Table 14.5 Clinically Important Information on Less Commonly Prescribed Opioids

Opioid	Pharmacodynamics	Analgesic Potency (x Morphine)	Dosage Forms	Schedule	Precipitate Withdrawal in μ Agonist–Dependent Patient?
Levorphanol	Full μ agonist	4-8	Tab	C-II	No
Nalbuphine	κ agonist/partial μ antagonist	0.5-1	Sol for inj	Rx	Yes
Butorphanol	κ agonist/partial μ agonist	5-7	Sol for inj, nas	C-IV	Yes
Pentazocine	κ agonist/partial μ agonist	0.16-0.33	Sol for inj, tab (with naloxone)	C-IV	Yes
Meperidine	Full μ agonist	0.1	Tab, sol for inj, po sol	C-II	No
Sufentanil	Full μ agonist	600-900	Sol for inj	C-II	No
Remifentanil	Full μ agonist	≥80	Sol for inj	C-II	No
Tapentadol	Full μ agonist	0.4-1	Tab, ER tab	C-II	No

ER, extended-release; inj, injection; nas, intranasal; po, oral; sol, solution; tab, tablets.

and, like all extended-release opioids, are reserved for use in patients tolerant to and dependent on μ agonists who require high-potency pain management on a chronic basis. As with morphine, boxed warnings caution patients and providers on hydromorphone's potential for abuse/addiction, profound respiratory depression, and life-threating interactions if coadministered with other CNS depressants.

Oxymorphone's 14β-OH group increases analgesic action approximately 3- to 4-fold over hydromorphone due to an increase in μ-receptor affinity. It is considered approximately 10 times more potent than morphine,[109,110] and its metabolic pathway mirrors that of hydromorphone. Since only a small amount is reduced to the isomeric 6-oxymorphol metabolites, it can be used in patients sensitive to the histamine-releasing action of the 6α-OH opioids codeine and morphine.[110] As oxymorphone is not metabolized by CYP enzymes, there is essentially no risk for CYP-related drug-drug interactions.

Oxymorphone is commercially available as a solution for injection, tablets, and, until recently, abuse-deterrent extended-release tablets (Opana ER). The abuse-deterrent formulation (ADF) chemical strategy for this potent opioid is claimed to be the same as that used for an abuse-deterrent formulation of oxycodone (OxyContin). However, a study involving over 12,000 individuals with an opioid abuse disorder showed that, while abuse via insufflation (snorting) decreased with both ADF drugs, abuse by IV injection decreased only for oxycodone while a trend toward increased oxymorphone misuse was observed.[111] In mid-2017 the U.S. Food and Drug Administration (FDA) recommended that sales of Opana ER be suspended due to "dangerous unintended consequences" as a result of its high potential for misuse/abuse. Within a month, the manufacturer voluntarily withdrew the product from the market.

CODEINE SULFATE, HYDROCODONE BITARTRATE, AND OXYCODONE HYDROCHLORIDE. Codeine, hydrocodone, and oxycodone are the 3-methoxy analogues of morphine, hydromorphone, and oxymorphone, respectively, and they have the same potency relationship to one another as their parent structures demonstrated. All are prodrugs that must undergo CYP2D6-mediated activation to the phenol required for high-affinity binding to μ receptors.

Unlike morphine, CYP3A4-mediated N-dealkylation plays a major role in oxycodone metabolism. Noroxycodone represents 23% of oxycodone urinary metabolites, while 2D6-generated oxymorphone represents only 11%.[112] Although N-dealkylation is not as prominent, these two reactions are also the major phase 1 biotransformation processes for hydrocodone and, to a lesser extent, codeine.[91,113] In contrast to hydrocodone and oxycodone, glucuronidation comprises a major component (70%) of codeine metabolism (Fig. 14.9).

A clinical guideline on the use of codeine in patients of varying CYP2D6 phenotypes has been published,[114] and hydrocodone analgesia has also been assumed to be linked to this genetic profile.[113] Interestingly, 2D6 genotype is reported to be relatively unimportant to the analgesic response to oxycodone, despite having the predicted impact on the extent of O-dealkylation.[112,115] The risk of drug-drug interactions involving oxycodone is also claimed to be less significant with CYP2D6 inducers and inhibitors than with modifiers of CYP3A4 activity. Codeine's diminished risk of CYP-related interactions (particularly CYP3A4) is related to its strong metabolic reliance on glucuronidation, although CYP3A4 inhibition can complicate the codeine response picture when coupled with other factors, such as CYP2D6 genotype.[114]

All three drugs are available as single agent products. Although the potency of each is about 10- to 12-fold lower than its phenolic counterpart, oral bioavailability is greatly enhanced (Table 14.4). They are efficacious analgesics that are generally well tolerated. Codeine and oxycodone are available as immediate-release tablets and as a solution for injection. As previously noted, the risk of a severe pseudoallergic reaction to parenterally administered codeine phosphate is high due to the presence of the 6α-OH group. Very little reduction to 6-OH metabolites occurs with hydrocodone (3%)[91] or oxycodone (10%),[112] so the risk of significant histamine release is slight.

All three codeine-based opioids are also formulated with peripheral analgesics acetaminophen, ibuprofen, or aspirin. These combination analgesics attack pain on both central and peripheral mechanistic fronts and allow lower doses of each potentially toxic drug to be utilized. Codeine and hydrocodone are found in combination with a variety of antihistamines, adrenergic agonist decongestants, and expectorants for use in treating cold symptoms that include serious cough. The attenuating impact of the 14β-OH group of oxycodone on cough suppression, along with the fact that protracted cough requiring opioid therapy is best treated with lower-potency agents, explains the lack of similar oxycodone-containing combination products.

Oxycodone was one of the first μ agonist analgesics to be made available in controlled-release tablet form (OxyContin). There was much focus in the literature and lay press on the potential for misuse/abuse of this drug when it was first released, leading to the development of the ADFs in use today. Abuse-deterrent extended-release tablets and capsules are the only single agent hydrocodone dosage forms available, and they too generated controversy at the national level before they came to market. The risk:benefit of extended-release hydrocodone (misuse: abuse liability vs. long-acting analgesia without fear of acetaminophen-induced heptatoxicity with chronic use), along with the pros and cons of various extended-release formulations, has been described in the literature.[113]

In April 2017 the FDA issued a special Safety Alert cautioning against administering codeine (and tramadol) to children younger than 12 years due to a high risk of excessive sedation and respiratory depression leading to death.[116] In 2010, codeine or oxycodone use in elderly patients for longer than 6 months was reported to increase the risk of serious or fatal cardiovascular events and to increase all-cause mortality when used for more than 30 days.[117] While this observation has been questioned by others, the call for additional research into this potentially serious and relatively unique cardiovascular health risk is clearly warranted.[118]

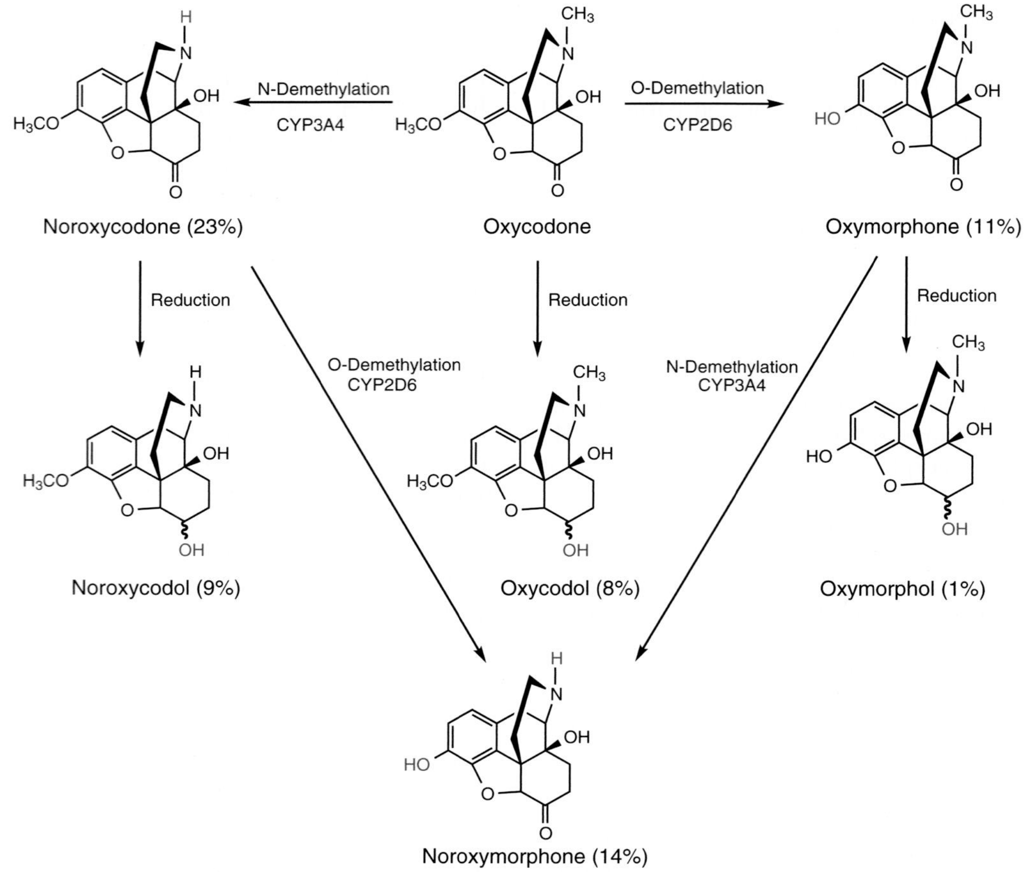

Figure 14.9 Oxycodone metabolism.

BUPRENORPHINE HYDROCHLORIDE. This structurally distinct opioid has an equally unique and interesting SAR.[119,120] Despite the presence of the N-cyclopropylmethyl group that normally promotes therapeutically useful μ antagonist action, buprenorphine is a very potent partial μ agonist. As a partial agonist, its intrinsic activity at μ receptors is less than maximal, and pharmacological actions eventually hit a ceiling as doses are increased. This significantly limits toxicity, including respiratory depression, physical dependence, and abuse potential.[121]

Estimates of buprenorphine's analgesic potency in comparison to morphine have ranged between 30 and 115:1, depending on the route of buprenorphine administration.[122,123] Buprenorphine's superior potency is attributed to high lipophilicity that facilitates concentration in the CNS and a very high affinity for μ receptors secondary to additional hydrophobic and hydrogen bonding capabilities of the C7 side chain. Buprenorphine also antagonizes κ receptors[124] and stimulates the opioid receptor-like 1 (ORL 1) protein, which some claim may help minimize hyperalgesia, dysphoria, and the development of tolerance.[122,123]

The μ-receptor binding of buprenorphine is strong enough to be classified as pseudoirreversible,[124] which provides an exceptionally long half-life of 37 hours and permits once-daily dosing. Slow dissociation from μ receptors minimizes withdrawal symptoms even if the drug is abruptly discontinued.[122,125] Any discomfort a patient experiences after abrupt withdrawal of buprenorphine normally occurs 5-14 days after the last dose. The downside of pseudoirreversible binding is that it is difficult to reverse receptor-mediated side effects, such as respiratory depression.[126] While less common or severe than that induced by full μ agonists, this adverse effect can be clinically significant, and it can take up to 10-fold the normal dose of naloxone to reverse. Buprenorphine-induced respiratory depression can outlast naloxone's duration of action, and a regimen of 2-3 mg of naloxone followed by a 4 mg/hr continuous infusion has been shown to restore normal breathing in respiratory-depressed patients within an hour. Kinetic models to explain this clinical observation have been published.[124] As with all opioids, the risk of potentially fatal respiratory depression increases significantly if other CNS depressants, including alcohol, are coadministered.

Buprenorphine undergoes significant first-pass metabolism. The CYP3A4-generated N-dealkylated metabolite norbuprenorphine retains analgesic activity, albeit 40-fold lower than the parent drug. Both buprenorphine and its nor metabolite are glucuronidated at C3 prior to fecal excretion.[123,127] The buprenorphine parent structure can be hepatotoxic in high doses secondary to inhibition of mitochondrial respiration and subsequent adenosine triphosphate depletion,[128] and the nor metabolite is believed responsible for buprenorphine-related respiratory depression.[123] Blood levels of norbuprenorphine are normally less than 10% of the parent drug,[123] but the buprenorphine dose may need to be adjusted if coadministered with CYP3A4 substrates or inhibitors.

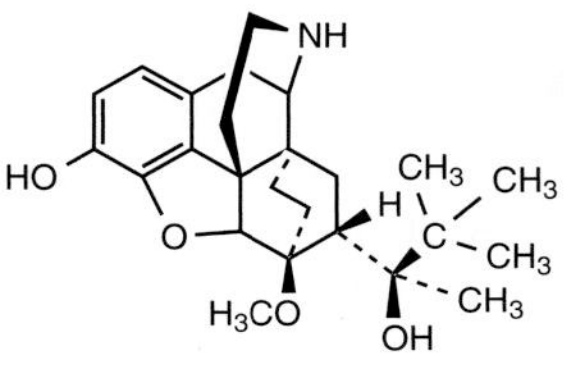

Norbuprenorphine

While pharmacologically classified as a partial μ agonist, buprenorphine has demonstrated full clinical efficacy in a large number of clinical trials evaluating relief of postoperative and cancer-related pain.[129] It is also viewed as effective in treating chronic noncancer pain[130] and, while additional studies are needed, it may have value in neuropathic pain.[123,131,132] Buprenorphine's relatively low risk of respiratory depression, constipation, and tolerance are considered therapeutic positives.[122] Additional reasons some have advocated for its use as a "frontline analgesic" include relative safety in the elderly and patients with renal failure, minimal impact on gonadal function, and lack of significant cardiotoxicity and immunosuppression.[123]

Buprenorphine is commonly administered sublingually (2 and 8 mg tablets), buccally (75-900 μg film) or via injection (0.3 mg/mL) to avoid inactivating conjugation in the gut and on first pass. The relative bioavailabilities of the sublingual and buccal formulations are 30%-50% and 28%, respectively.[123] Plasma levels of buprenorphine peak in 1.5 (sublingual) and 3 (buccal) hours, and consumption of liquids can lower blood levels from the buccal film by up to 37%. A transdermal patch formulation of buprenorphine (Butrans) is available in strengths ranging from 5-20 μg/hr. Steady-state concentrations are achieved in 72 hours, and patches are changed weekly. The previously described precaution on using extended-release opioids only in opioid-tolerant patients also applies to transdermal buprenorphine. In addition, patients must avoid exposing the applied patch to heat, as the release of drug from the patch matrix is temperature dependent and exposure to active drug can increase up to 55%.[91]

In addition to its use as an analgesic, buprenorphine is also employed in opioid addiction recovery. In 2 mg doses, buprenorphine blocks the euphoric effects of heroin. It has been shown to be as active as 30 mg of methadone in addiction treatment programs and is considered a safer alternative due to lower risks of overdose,[133] cardiovascular toxicity,[123] and drug-drug interactions.[121] Treatment programs generally range from 6 months to over 2 years. Patients initiating replacement therapy with buprenorphine must be opioid-free for at least 12 hours.[121] Either under the direct supervision of their physician or at home, the patient enters the preliminary phase of opioid withdrawal before the first dose of buprenorphine is administered. The partial μ agonism will suppress withdrawal symptoms, but it would have precipitated active withdrawal if the patient had been under the influence of opioids at the time of buprenorphine induction.

Buprenorphine induction is followed by the stabilization (dose optimization) and maintenance phases of therapy. If a recovering patient relapses (common in the first years of abstinence) and increases the buprenorphine dose in an attempt achieve euphoria, he or she will hit the partial agonist activity plateau and the attempt to abuse will be thwarted. When the time comes, the patient can be withdrawn from buprenorphine with few, if any, withdrawal symptoms due to its slow dissociation from the receptors and slow disappearance from the body. The patient's receptors essentially wean themselves off of the drug.[134]

A variety of formulations are available to deliver buprenorphine to patients in addiction recovery programs. As noted earlier, buprenorphine alone is marketed in 2 and 8 mg sublingual tablets (Subutex), and a 74.2 mg subcutaneous implant (Probuphine) is available for use in patients who have achieved success on a transmucosal formulation for a minimum of 3 months.[91] The "match stick sized" implants provide stable buprenorphine serum concentrations for 6 months (steady state achieved within 1 mo), and essentially eliminate concern relative to patient adherence and drug diversion or intentional/accidental misuse.[121] Interestingly, buprenorphine implants have been shown to significantly decrease cocaine use in opioid-dependent patients.[121] In November, 2017, the FDA approved a once-monthly injectable extended-release formulation of buprenorphine (Sublocade) for patients previously treated with transmucosally delivered drug for a minimum of 7 days. Sublocade utilizes the Atrigel Delivery System and is provided in prefilled syringes. After subcutaneous administration by health care providers, the delivery system forms a solid depot under the skin which releases active buprenorphine as the depot degrades. If the drug were to be injected IV, the mass formed would likely occlude vessels or form a mobile embolus, either of which could prove fatal. While the drug will not be dispensed directly to patients, the need for patient education is clear.

While buprenorphine's partial μ agonism attenuates abuse liability, diversion and misuse can still occur.[135] Dosage forms combining buprenorphine with the opioid antagonist naloxone, most commonly in a 4:1 mg:mg ratio, were designed to block euphoria if drug is extracted from the sublingual tablets or buccal film and injected IV. Naloxone has limited activity by the transmucosal route and does not interfere with buprenorphine actions when the combination product is used as prescribed.

The addition of buprenorphine to opioid addiction recovery therapeutic options is significant in that it allows recovering patients to receive care from the hands of their own physicians and pharmacists, environments that can be less emotionally stressful than a methadone clinic.[136] Once appropriately trained through the Substance Abuse and Mental Health Services Administration (SAMHSA), physicians may insert implants or dispense a small supply of buprenorphine (with or without naloxone) to patients in their office. Pharmacists can then dispense the combination product for long-term treatment. Patients in the maintenance phase of therapy require weekly-monthly monitoring, providing opportunities for interprofessional physician-pharmacist collaboration to promote positive patient care outcomes over the duration of recovery.[137] While buprenorphine is more expensive than methadone, the economic and quality-of-life costs to patients over the prolonged time course of recovery may actually be less due to, among other things, fewer office visits.[121,138] Expansion of buprenorphine use in addiction recovery will require greater patient access to SAMHSA-waivered physicians (especially problematic in rural areas), supportive insurance plans and reimbursement rates, interprofessional collaboration (including addiction specialists and counselors), and provider/patient education.[136]

ETORPHINE AND DIPRENORPHINE

Predictably, replacing the N-cyclopropylmethyl substituent of buprenorphine with a methyl group provides a full μ agonist. The N-methylated analogue that has also replaced the t-butyl group within the C7 side chain with n-propyl and oxidized the 6,14-endoethano bridge to endoetheno is known as etorphine. Etorphine has an analgesic potency estimated at up to 200-fold that of morphine in humans for reasons related to superior receptor affinity and central distribution properties. Although never marketed for human use in the U.S., etorphine has been widely used in veterinary medicine and as an immobilizer to permit the safe capture and/or handling of zoo animals and large game. Marketed alone or in combination with the sedative antiemetic acetylpromazine, etorphine has enjoyed the descriptive trade names of Captivon and Immobilon, respectively. Buprenorphine can also be converted into a potent and pure opioid antagonist (diprenorphine) simply by replacing the t-butyl moiety on the C7 side chain with methyl.

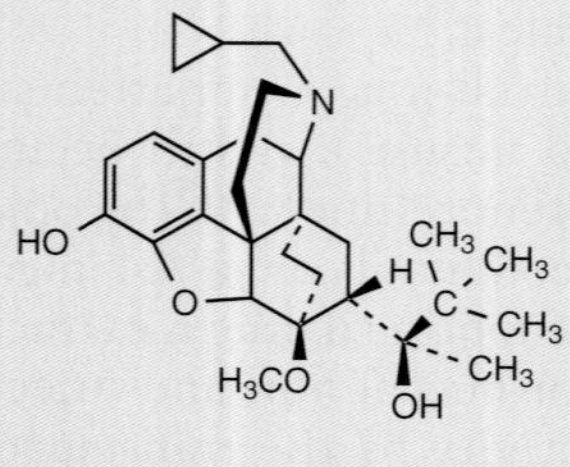

Buprenorphine

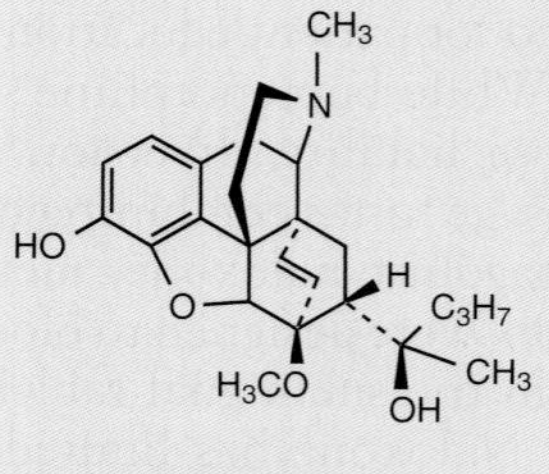

Etorphine

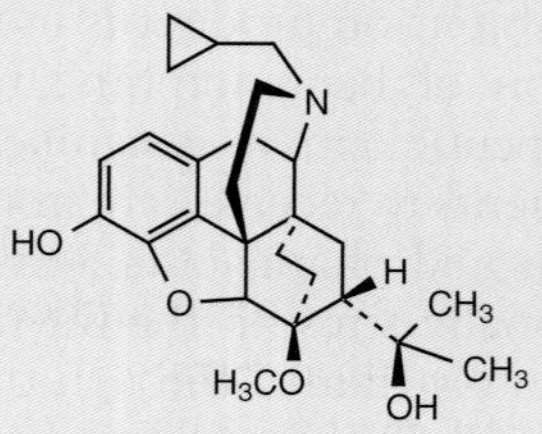

Diprenorphine

Phenanthrene-Based Rigid κ Agonists (Fig. 14.4)

NALBUPHINE HYDROCHLORIDE, BUTORPHANOL TARTRATE, AND PENTAZOCINE LACTATE. Replacing μ agonist-directing amine substituents with cyclobutylmethyl (nalbuphine, butorphanol) or dimethylallyl (pentazocine) results in clinically useful κ receptor-mediated analgesia. In analgesic doses, these structures also exhibit partial μ agonism (butorphanol, pentazocine) or partial μ antagonism (nalbuphine), and all will precipitate a withdrawal episode if administered to patients dependent on full μ agonists. They are less commonly utilized for pain control than the rigid μ agonists discussed above, possibly because of the risk of drug-induced dysphoria, particularly with pentazocine and butorphanol. Other κ-associated adverse effects include diuresis and sedation, but the risk of respiratory depression, constipation, euphoria, and addiction is lower than for μ agonists. Kappa agonist analgesics are generally more effective and/or longer acting in women, particularly when used in dental pain, and some studies have demonstrated an anti-analgesic effect in men.[139-141]

All three κ analgesics undergo significant first pass metabolism, and only pentazocine is available in an oral dosage form. Pentazocine tablets contain naloxone in a 100:1 mg:mg ratio to discourage misuse/abuse by drug extraction and IV injection. The major phase 1 metabolites of each κ agonist are shown below, and clinically relevant information is provided in Table 14.5.

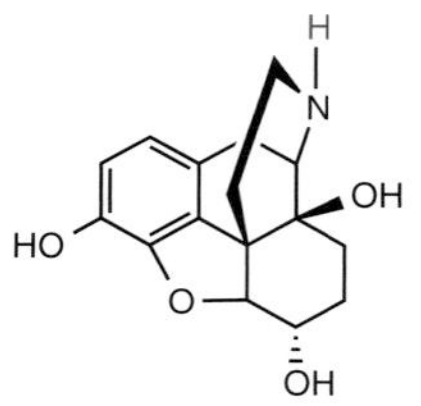

Nornalbuphine

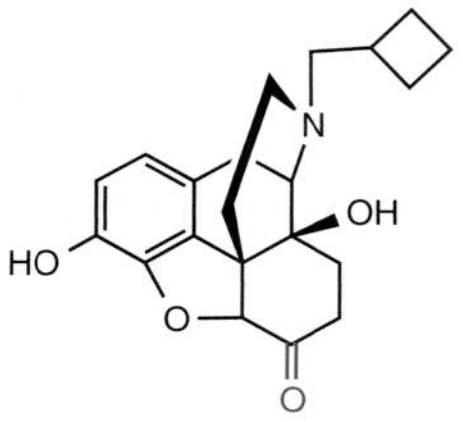

6-Ketonalbuphine

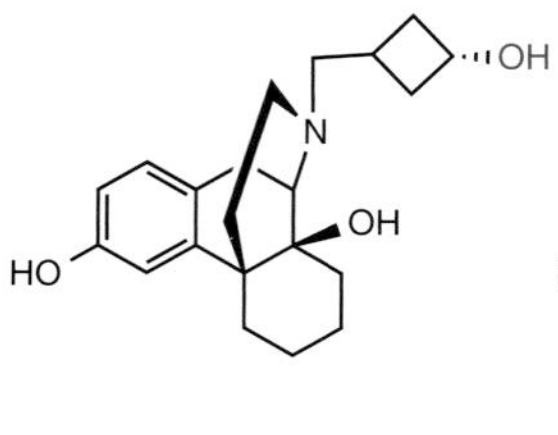

Trans-3'-hydroxybutorphanol

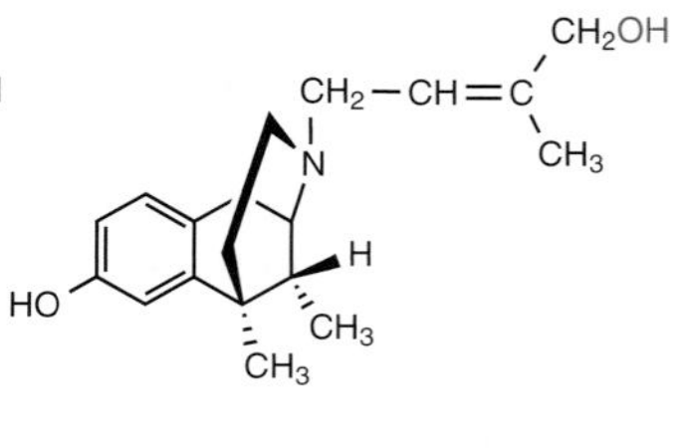

Hydroxypentazocine

Major metabolites of κ agonist analgesics.

Flexible Opioid Agonists (Fig. 14.6)

The flexible opioids, including the dual-action agents, are all μ agonists. The anilidopiperine analgesics fentanyl and alfentanil, along with the dual-action analgesic tramadol, enjoy the most widespread use within this major structural class for the treatment of pain and/or as adjuncts to anesthesia. Methadone is used predominantly in opioid addiction recovery.

Meperidine has fallen out of favor due to its serious adverse effect profile, which includes histamine release, serotonin syndrome, and neurotoxicity leading to seizures, the latter attributed to the nor metabolite. As noted previously, the newest marketed opioid, tapentadol, has several mechanistic advantages over tramadol, but is not yet as commonly employed in the clinic. Meperidine and tapentadol, along with sufentanil (a more lipophilic, faster/shorter-acting adjunct to anesthesia than the parent fentanyl), are included in Table 14.5. A transdermal patch formulation of sufentanil, originally in clinical trials, has been discontinued by the manufacturer.

FENTANYL BASE AND FENTANYL CITRATE SALT. Fentanyl is a very sedative and euphoria-inducing analgesic with a potency approximately 75-100 times morphine. The high activity of anilidopiperidines is due, in part, to their very high lipophilicity, which allows them to quickly penetrate the BBB and concentrate in the CNS. Because they leave the brain quickly too, their duration of analgesic action is short (30-60 min for fentanyl). Fentanyl citrate and its analogues are commonly administered IV as adjuncts to anesthesia (e.g., Sublimaze), but all formulations carry the risk of potentially fatal respiratory depression and other common μ opioid adverse effects.

Intranasal, transdermal, and transmucosal formulations of fentanyl are available to treat chronic pain, including the pain of cancer. The metered-dose nasal spray (Lazanda) provides rapid delivery of solubilized fentanyl citrate that is readily absorbed in the highly vascularized nasal passages. Intranasal fentanyl bioavailability is close to 70%, serum levels peak within 15 minutes, and the approximately 1 hour half-life is shorter than with IV or transmucosal formulations. It is fast acting, easy to use, and well tolerated in adults and pediatric populations.[142,143]

The transdermal patch formulation (Duragesic) releases fentanyl free base to maintain therapeutic blood levels for 72 hours, providing a convenient and reliable mechanism for patients with chronic pain to achieve analgesia at home. Strengths ranging from 12.5-100 μg/hr are available. Great care must be taken when disposing of used patches so that opioid naïve individuals do not accidently come in contact with residual drug. Serious toxicity or death can result, with children at particularly high risk. As with transdermal formulations of other high-potency opioids, exposure of Duragesic patches to external heat accelerates drug release and absorption and can have fatal consequences.

An iontophoretic transdermal dosage form (Ionsys) is available to manage acute postoperative pain for a maximum of 72 hours while patients are hospitalized. The system is preprogrammed to deliver a 40 μg dose of fentanyl hydrochloride in a patient-controlled, needle-free, electrical current–driven process. Patients are limited to six activations per hour, and devices are changed after 24 hours or 80 activations, whichever comes first.[144] The system is placed on the upper outer arm or chest, as studies have shown drug absorption to be optimal from these sites.[144]

Transmucosal formulations of fentanyl in a wide range of strengths are often used to treat chronic and/or breakthrough pain in opioid-tolerant patients and in pediatric burn patients undergoing painful cleansings and dressing changes. A sublingual tablet containing fentanyl citrate (Abstral) is placed under the deepest sublingual area, disintegrating to release particles that cling to the mucosal surface, which facilitates absorption. A sublingual liquid formulation (Subsys) delivers fentanyl base. Fentanyl base is also incorporated into a buccal soluble film (Onsolis, revised formation anticipated in early 2018). Fifty-one percent of the dose is rapidly absorbed across buccal membranes, with another 20% absorbed more slowly from the intestines after swallowing.[145] Doses should be administered no more often than four times per day, with doses separated by a minimum of 2 hours. Compared to the film, about half as much drug (25% of the dose) is absorbed buccally from the immediate-release fentanyl citrate "lozenge on a handle" formulation (Actiq),[146] with additional drug slowly absorbed from the GI tract.

Effervescent buccal tablets (Fentora) contain fentanyl citrate, citric acid, sodium bicarbonate, and sodium carbonate. When placed at the back of the mouth between the cheek and gum, the citric acid drops salivary pH to a minimum of 5.0, producing soluble protonated fentanyl. The tablet generally dissolves within 15-25 minutes. The dissolved citric acid reacts with sodium bicarbonate and sodium carbonate to generate sodium citrate and carbonic acid (H_2CO_3), which dissociates to CO_2 and H_2O. As CO_2 is expired, citric acid is consumed and salivary pH rises to 9-10. This shifts the fentanyl equilibrium to favor lipophilic fentanyl free base, which is readily absorbed across buccal membranes.[147] The absolute bioavailability is 65%, which represents a 30% greater fentanyl exposure compared to the buccal lozenge. If there is a need to switch a patient from the lozenge to the effervescent tablet, the dose should be cut by 25%-50% to avoid life-threatening toxicity.

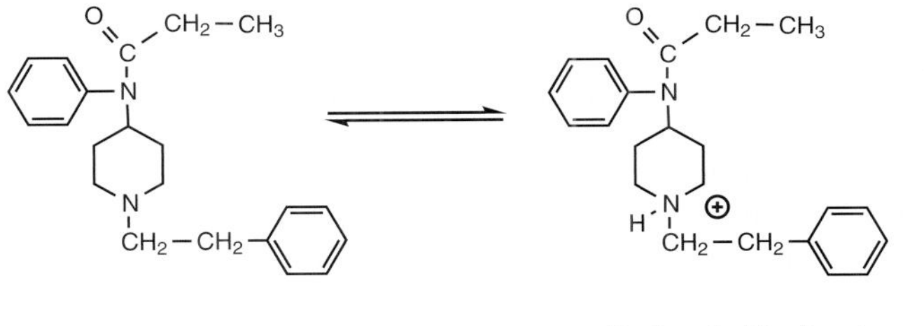

Fentanyl free base (predominates at pH > 8.4) | Protonated fentanyl (predominates at pH < 8.4)

Fentanyl acid-base equilibrium.

All transdermal and transmucosal dosage forms carry a boxed warning related to unintentional overdose, toxicity, and intentional abuse. The FDA requires transmucosal immediate-release fentanyl (TIRF) products be prescribed only by practitioners enrolled in and certified by the Risk Evaluation and Mitigation Strategy (TIRF REMS) program. This program carries strict responsibilities for provider education, patient and/or caregiver counseling, and the establishment of formal care agreements with each patient being treated. Prescribers must re-enroll in the TIRF REMS program on a biannual basis.

Fentanyl is extensively biotransformed via CYP3A4-mediated N-dealkylation to an inactive metabolite, and practitioners must be alert to the risk for potency-enhancing (CYP3A4 inhibitors or competitors) or attenuating (CYP3A4 inducers) interactions. Anilidopiperidines do not release histamine like meperidine and 6α-hydroxylated multicyclics do, and there is no risk of histamine-mediated allergic responses when fentanyl is administered IV. The fentanyl adverse reaction of greatest concern is respiratory depression. This potentially fatal reaction is persistent and can outlast the action of antagonists used to reverse it. The risk is significantly lower with sufentanil and alfentanil, as respiratory depression generally occurs only at doses higher than those needed to relieve pain or support anesthesia.

ALFENTANIL HYDROCHLORIDE. Alfentanil is the least potent of the currently marketed anilidopiperidine opioids, but it distributes and redistributes across the BBB more rapidly than either fentanyl or sufentanil. Analgesic action begins within 5 minutes of IV administration and lasts between 0.5-1 hour. It is commonly administered to patients undergoing very short surgical or medical procedures requiring anesthesia/sedation (e.g., colonoscopy). More recently, it has found use in attenuating pain during bedside burn dressing changes in patients with noncompromised respiration.[148]

METHADONE HYDROCHLORIDE. Methadone is one of only three marketed opioid analgesics that do not contain a piperidine ring. The N-methyl substituent accurately predicts its μ agonist activity profile, and the activity-attenuating impact of ketone reduction supports a receptor binding role for the C3 carbonyl oxygen. There is some evidence to suggest that methadone may function as a β-arrestin-biased μ agonist.[149] While most commonly associated with use in addiction recovery (methadone maintenance), its use as an analgesic is on the rise.[150,151] Despite its complex pharmacological and pharmacokinetic profile, it may be of value in patients who are nonresponsive to other opioids. The hydrochloride salt is marketed as an injectable solution and in a variety of oral dosage forms.

Methadone's lone chiral center, C6, equates to the C9 of morphine. While marketed as the racemic mixture, the *R*(-) isomer is responsible for methadone's opioid analgesic action. The *S*(+) enantiomer antagonizes the NMDA receptor[152] which, although of potential benefit in neuropathic and opioid-resistant pain, may also be responsible for methadone's potentially serious cardiovascular toxicities such as a prolonged QT interval and torsades de pointes.[153] The analgesic activity of methadone is shorter than its 1-2 day elimination half-life would suggest, and it can induce respiratory depression that outlasts the analgesic phase. Methadone's naturally long half-life is due in part to the generation of several active metabolites (Fig. 14.10), and it can be significantly increased in basified urine. Deaths from cardiac arrhythmia and respiratory depression have been noted, particularly as the drug is being introduced and/or the dose titrated. Dosing more frequently than once daily can allow drug accumulation, which sets the stage for serious and/or potentially fatal toxicity.

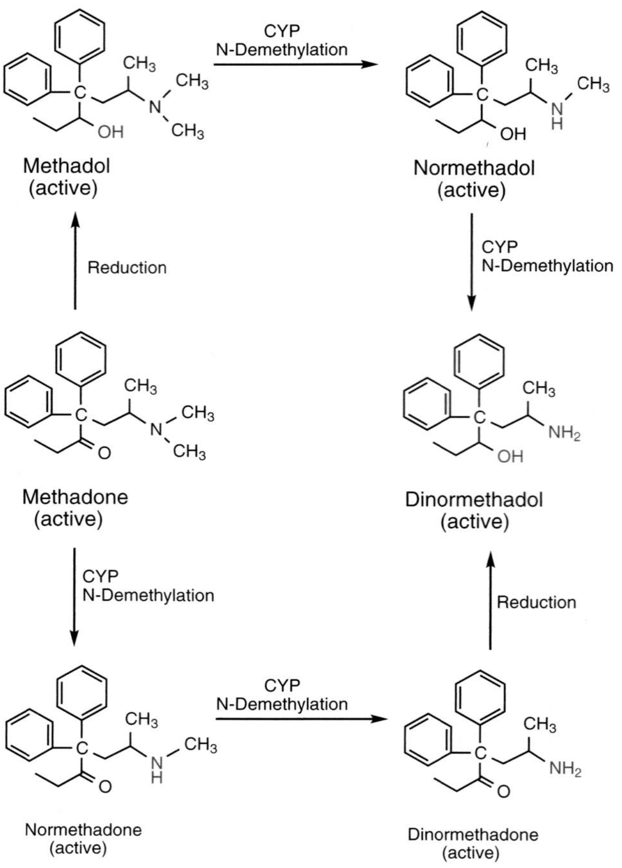

Figure 14.10 Methadone metabolism.

A recent review of methadone metabolism and transport has called into question the long-held belief in the pivotal role of CYP3A4 in methadone N-demethylation. Kharasch[150] summarized studies that demonstrated no impact of this isoform on single-dose methadone metabolism and clearance, and stated that methadone is not a CYP3A4 substrate. Rather, evidence was provided that identified CYP2B6 as the preferential methadone dealkylating isoform and confirmed previous understanding of its stereoselective action [*S*(+) > *R*(-)]. Evaluation of methadone plasma levels in patients of varying 2B6 genotype documented elevated concentrations in PMs (*CYP2B6**6*) compared to EMs (*CYP2B6**1*), with the lowest concentrations of parent drug coming from UMs (*CYP2B6**4*). The metabolic autoinduction known to occur over the first weeks of methadone therapy was attributed to CYP2B6 upregulation. Kharasch referred to the continued reference to CYP3A4-catalyzed methadone metabolism in literature and tertiary drug information resources as "CYP3A inertia." Because of the risk of serious/fatal cardiac and respiratory toxicity, pharmacists should be vigilant with regard to monitoring for metabolism-related interactions with CYP competitors, inhibitors, and inducers.

The N-dealkylated metabolites of methadone (but not methadol) can cyclize to form inactive pyrrolidine-based structures that are found in the urine of patients on methadone (Fig. 14.11). These compounds are commonly known as EDDP and EDMP, which are acronyms for their

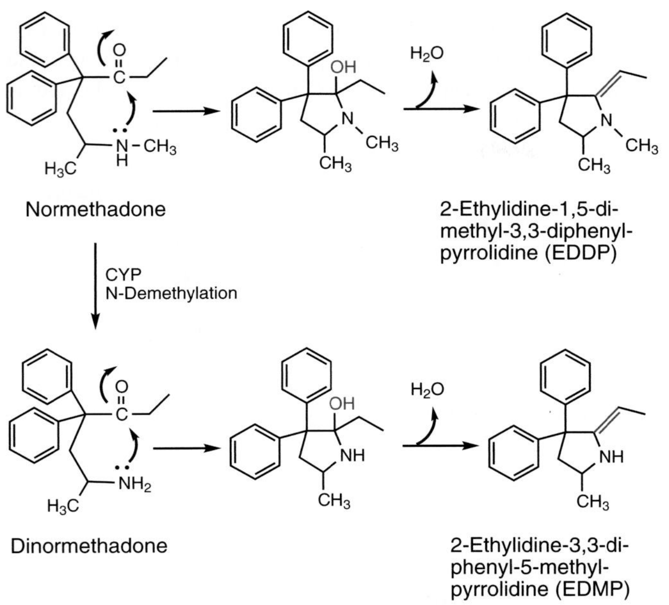

Figure 14.11 Formation of EDDP and EDMP.

chemical names. Methadone is incapable of generating a cyclic pyrrolidine metabolite because the N,N-dimethyl substitution pattern of the parent drug provides steric hindrance to nucleophilic attack by the unionized amine at the electrophilic carbonyl carbon. EDDP, and to a lesser extent EDMP, has recently been shown to be mechanism-based inhibitors of CYP2C19.[154] EDDP has an elimination half-life of 40-48 hours.

As previously noted, methadone has found its greatest use in addiction recovery programs. Its high oral bioavailability, long duration of action, daily dosing regimen, slow tolerance development, and relative lack of physical dependence are definitely advantages in its use as a heroin (or other potent μ agonist) substitute. Unlike buprenorphine, methadone used in addiction recovery is administered in strictly regulated federal- and state-licensed methadone clinics, commonly under direct supervision. The drug is administered in water or an acidic juice to ensure solubility and avoid unintended buccal absorption of unionized drug. If buccal absorption is required (e.g., patients with swallowing disorders), a basified solution can be held in the mouth for 2.5 minutes before expectorating.

Patients receiving methadone maintenance therapy are titrated upward from an initial 20-30 mg daily dose to a maintenance daily dose that is most commonly 80-120 mg.[134] Therapy usually continues over 1 to 2 (or more) years. Compliance can be tracked by quantifying urinary levels of EDDP and calculating the EDDP:urine creatinine ratio. This analytical technique provides results related to the consumed quantity of methadone that are independent of patient hydration status and resistant to attempts to adulterate the sample with agents like soap, bleach, or methadone itself.[155] When the time is right to discontinue methadone, any withdrawal symptoms experienced will generally be mild due to the prolonged duration of action of the drug and active metabolites. However, the patient will still be both tolerant to and dependent on methadone, which, unlike buprenorphine, is not a pseudoirreversible μ agonist. Therefore, the protocol for medically supervised drug discontinuation involves a "stair-step" dose-attenuation process, with reductions of less than 10% of the maintenance dose taking place no sooner than every 10-14 days.

TRAMADOL HYDROCHLORIDE. The dual mechanism of tramadol's analgesic action is complex and time-dependent.[156] Over time, as the parent isomers are O-dealkylated to phenolic metabolites, the μ-receptor agonist component of activity increases while the monoamine reuptake inhibition mechanism decreases. The μ receptor affinity of the (+) phenol is 300 times that of the parent drug and is the clinically relevant opioid entity.[109] As in codeine analogues, CYP2D6 catalyzes the O-dealkylation reaction, and patients deficient in this isoform will either not experience the μ agonist component of tramadol's action or require dosage increases of up to 30%.[109] Inactivating glucuronide or sulfate conjugation of the phenol will occur prior to urinary excretion. CYP3A4 and CYP2B6 catalyze inactivating N-dealkylation to secondary and primary amine metabolites.[109]

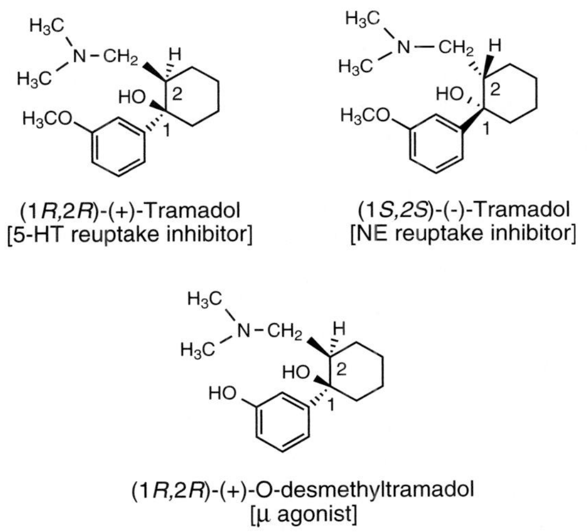

Tramadol isomers and active metabolite.

Since the (+) 1*R*,2*R* isomer of tramadol inhibits 5-HT reuptake, it has the potential to induce or exacerbate serotonin syndrome, a potentially life-threatening condition.[157] The symptoms of serotonin syndrome include neuromuscular hyperactivity with loss of coordination, cardiovascular and pulmonary distress, and cognitive dysfunction. Patients at greatest risk include those of advanced age and/or on high-dose therapy, coadministration of SSRI antidepressants or CYP2D6 inhibitors, and CYD2D6 PM phenotype.[157-159] Tramadol is not recommended in suicidal patients due to the elevation of central 5-HT.

Tramadol also carries a risk of seizure, especially in patients taking drugs that increase central levels of monoamines or whose seizure threshold is otherwise reduced. Seizures have been documented in doses as low as 200 mg (which is close to the maintenance dose of 50-100 mg) and generally occur within 6 hours of drug ingestion. Tramadol generally induces less respiratory depression, constipation, and abuse liability than other opioids, but withdrawal symptoms have been noted upon abrupt discontinuation. Life-threatening respiratory depression risk is increased in patients of CYP2D6 UM phenotype[160] and in children under 12. As a result, the FDA issued a safety alert in April 2017 restricting tramadol use in preteen patients. GI distress and sedation are the most commonly reported adverse effects.[109]

Tramadol is available in immediate-release tablets (Ultram), administered every 4-6 hours, and extended-release tablets (Ultram ER) and capsules (ConZip), administered once daily. Kits for compounding tramadol into a suspension (Synapryn FusePaq) or cream (EnovaRx) formulation are also marketed. Tramadol has demonstrated efficacy in chronic pain of moderate intensity, including low back pain and the pain of rheumatoid arthritis. Although further studies are needed, the drug may have a place in the treatment of premature ejaculation.[161]

Opioid Antagonists (Fig. 14.5)

NALOXONE HYDROCHLORIDE AND NALTREXONE HYDROCHLORIDE. Two pure opioid antagonists are marketed to reverse the central actions of opioid agonists, although they antagonize peripheral opioid receptors with equal ease. They both have a classic antagonist-directing amine substituent on a pentacyclic scaffold and contain the requisite 14β-OH and the 7,8-dihydro-6-one C ring. With a four-carbon N-cyclopropylmethyl substituent, naltrexone is twice as potent as the allyl-substituted naloxone, presumably due to enhanced distribution to central sites of action.

As noted above, each antagonist is incorporated into selected oral dosage forms of potent μ agonists to thwart misuse and abuse by agonist extraction and IV or intranasal administration. Either antagonist can rescue patients from life-threatening opioid overdose, but only naloxone carries that indication. Naloxone undergoes inactivating N-dealkylation, stereospecific reduction to 6α-naloxol, and glucuronide conjugation in the gut and liver and is only used via nonparenteral routes. In selected states, naloxone hydrochloride autoinjector (Evzio) and nasal spray (Narcan) formulations are being made available to first responders, teachers, family, and others likely to come into contact with individuals experiencing life-threatening overdose ("buddy-administration"), as well as to opioid-dependent persons for self-injection. Naloxone is also marketed in solution for IV or IM administration in the clinical setting.

In contrast, naltrexone has sufficient bioavailability (5%-40%) for oral administration, which enhances its utility in outpatient opioid dependence and alcoholism recovery programs. It is available in 50 mg tablets and as a suspension for IM injection. Patients should be opioid free for 7-10 days prior to initiating relapse prophylaxis therapy. Naltrexone's major metabolite is 6β-naltrexol.

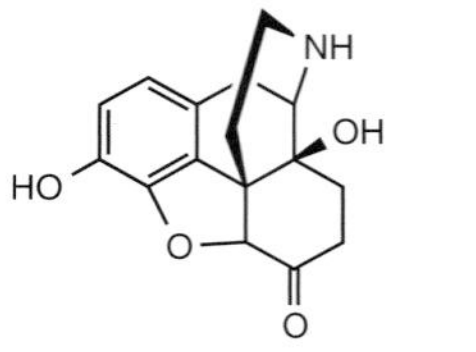

7,8-Dihydro-14β-hydroxy-normorphinone

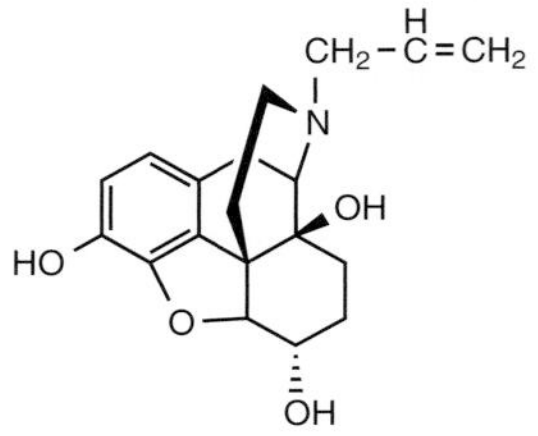

6α-Naloxol

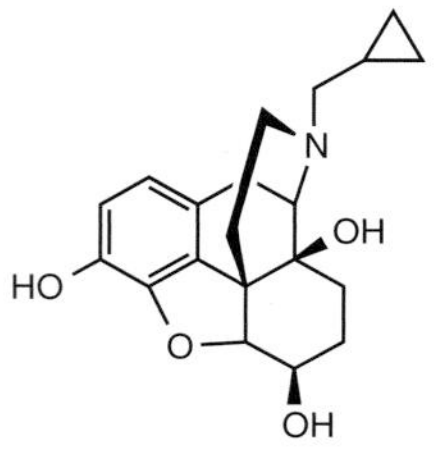

6β-Naltrexol

Naloxone and naltrexone metabolites.

In synergistic combination with a sustained-release formulation of the atypical antidepressant bupropion, sustained-release naltrexone is finding use in the treatment of obesity in adult populations. A review of clinical efficacy and safety data for this combination product (Contrave), along with a summary of pharmacodynamic and kinetic profiles of each agent, was recently published.[162] Preliminary data also indicate a potential role for low-dose naltrexone (4.5 mg/d) in inducing remission in Crohn's disease, possibly by stimulating production of Met-enkephalin which attenuates cell proliferation through a receptor-mediated process.[163,164]

METHYLNALTREXONE BROMIDE, NALOXEGOL OXALATE, NALDEMEDINE TOSYLATE, AND ALVIMOPAN. Unlike centrally acting naloxone and naltrexone, the quaternary methyl bromide salt of naltrexone (Relistor), naloxegol (PEGylated naloxol, Movantik), naldemedine (Symproic), and Alvimopan (Entereg) were designed to work as prokinetic agents in the gut to reverse the intractable constipation that is a hallmark of long-term μ opioid use. OIC impacts up to 40% of patients on chronic opioid therapy (some sources claim up to 90%), with elderly and cancer patients at higher risk. Tolerance to this adverse effect does not develop. OIC has a very negative impact on quality of life and can limit the dose of opioid prescribed to manage pain.[165] These peripherally selective antagonists will displace agonist from intestinal μ receptors and restore GI motility and bowel tone. Since none of these drugs penetrates the BBB to any significant extent (and, particularly in the case of naloxegol, is actively ejected from the CNS by P-gp efflux),[166] they will not precipitate a withdrawal episode in opioid-dependent patients suffering from OIC. Review articles on the action, efficacy, and safety of peripherally acting μ-opioid receptor antagonists (PAMORAs) have recently been published.[166,167]

Opioid antagonist therapy for OIC is recommended when dietary and activity-related modifications and maintenance laxatives have been less than optimally effective in restoring bowel function. Abdominal pain is the most common adverse effect, and patients with bowel obstructions should not receive these drugs until the blockage has been fully resolved. Laxatives should be discontinued for at least 3 days while antagonist therapy is established. They can then be reintroduced if the antagonist does not produce satisfactory results.

Methylnaltrexone bromide[167,168] is administered orally (450 mg daily) or by subcutaneous injection. In seriously ill patients, the subcutaneous dose is based on patient weight and initiated on an every-other-day schedule. If warranted, the frequency can be increased to a maximum of once daily. OIC associated with chronic noncancer pain is often treated orally or with a daily 12 mg injection. The permanently water-soluble drug is excreted in urine and feces primarily in unchanged form. The biotransformation that does occur involves reduction of the 6-keto group to isomeric alcohols and phenol sulfonation, so CYP-related drug-drug interactions are of little concern.

Naloxegol is dosed at 25 mg once daily, although 12.5 mg daily can be administered to patients with significant renal dysfunction or who do not tolerate the higher dose. The drug should be taken 1-2 hours before the morning meal to ensure an empty stomach. As naloxegol is N- and O-dealkylated by CYP3A4 prior to predominantly fecal elimination, coadministration with CYP substrates, inducers, or inhibitors (including grapefruit juice) should be avoided or undertaken only with great care. Coadministration of strong P-gp inhibitors significantly increases naloxegol plasma levels, potentially leading to attenuated analgesia and withdrawal symptoms.[166]

Naldemedine[169] has many properties in common with naloxegol, including CYP3A4-catalyzed N-dealkylation to a secondary amine metabolite, which is active. Coadministration of CYP3A4 competitors or inhibitors can increase the risk of adverse effects, and grapefruit juice should be avoided. C3-glucuronidation is minor, but a significant fraction undergoes amide hydrolysis in the gut to produce naldemedine carboxylic acid. Like naloxegol, naldemedine has affinity for P-gp, but its significantly higher binding to serum proteins (94% vs. 4%), along with the relatively polar C7 side chain, limits BBB penetration. Still, careful monitoring for adverse effects is warranted if P-gp inhibitors are coadministered. Unlike naloxegol, there is no requirement for administration on an empty stomach, and the drug and its metabolites are excreted primarily in urine (57%) compared to feces (35%).

Alvimopan is an orally administered benzazocine derivative that hydrolyzes via the action of gut flora to provide an active carboxylic acid derivative. Bioavailability is low (6%) and the polarity of both the parent drug and the carboxylic acid "metabolite" keep the structure from crossing the BBB. There is minimal hepatic metabolism, and the drug is excreted primarily by secretion into the bile.[170] This PAMORA is administered exclusively in the inpatient setting to treat postsurgical ileus. Institutions providing the drug must be registered with the Entereg Access Support Education (E.A.S.E.) program, which assures that providers are appropriately instructed on its actions and use restrictions. Patients receive one dose prior to surgery and up to 14 additional doses administered twice daily for a maximum of 7 days. The use of alvimopan accelerates bowel function recovery without antagonizing opioid analgesia and can result in shorter hospital stays.[171]

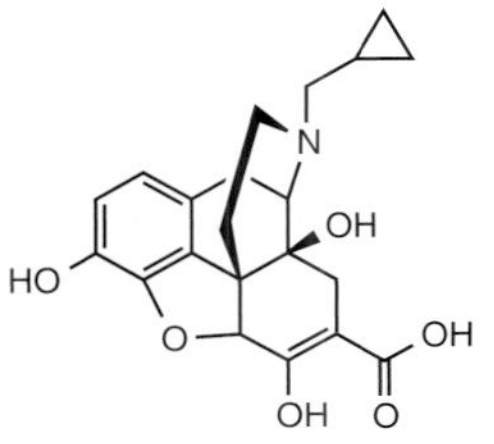

Naldemedine carboxylic acid

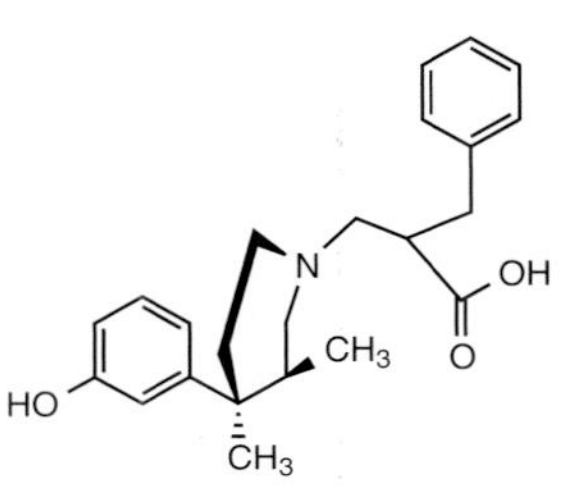

Alvimopan carboxylic acid

Opioid-Based Antidiarrheals (Fig. 14.12)

"You've probably been asked to care about things like HIV/AIDS or TB or measles, but diarrhea kills more children than all those three things put together. It's a very potent weapon of mass destruction."

Rose George

As previously discussed, OIC is one of the most discomforting and, at times, serious complications of opioid analgesic use. However, medicinal chemists, following the old adage "When life hands you lemons, make lemonade," have modified the structure of the flexible μ agonist meperidine to limit BBB penetration without compromising GI mobility inhibition.[172] Two orally administered peripherally selective μ agonists, diphenoxylate and loperamide, have enjoyed significant therapeutic use as antidiarrheals for years.

Diphenoxylate Hydrochloride

Diphenoxylate (Lomotil) bears a close resemblance to the parent meperidine structure (Fig. 14.6). The only chemical difference between the two compounds is the nature of the amine substituent; meperidine has the prototypical μ agonist-directing methyl group while

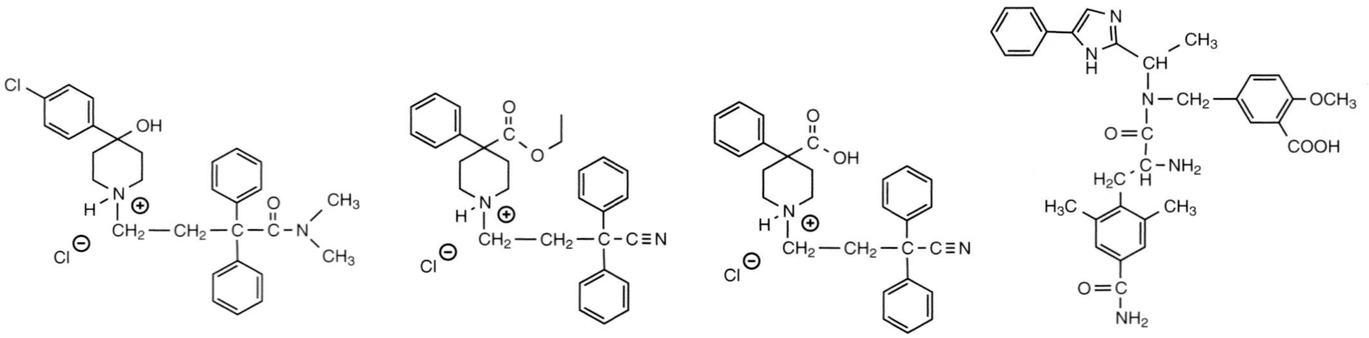

Loperamide hydrochloride (Imodium) | Diphenoxylate hydrochloride (Lomotil) | Difenoxin hydrochloride (Motofen) | Eluxadoline (Viberzi)

More commonly used | **Less commonly used**

Figure 14.12 Opioid-based antidiarrheals.

diphenoxylate has a more complex 3,3,-diphenyl-3-cyanopropyl functional group. The ethylcarboxylate ester is readily cleaved by plasma esterases, yielding a carboxylic acid metabolite that is approximately five times as active as diphenoxylate as an antidiarrheal. The zwitterionic metabolite, which is marketed as difenoxin, does not readily distribute into the CNS in therapeutic doses. In higher doses, the chemical reluctance to cross the BBB is overcome, and central μ receptors can be stimulated.

For reasons both therapeutic (anticholinergic) and abuse related, diphenoxylate and difenoxin are only available in combination with atropine sulfate. If a potential abuser attempts to extract the antidiarrheal agent with the intent to inject and abuse, the atropine will be extracted and injected too, leading to nausea, weakness, sedation, and annoying peripheral effects such as dry mouth, blurred vision, and urinary retention. The diphenoxylate combination product is a Schedule V drug, indicating that there is a slight potential for abuse and/or addiction, whereas the difenoxin combination product is classified as Schedule IV (a medically useful drug with a low potential for abuse and/or addiction). If used alone, these antidiarrheals would be classified as Schedule II agents, indicating that they have a significant potential for abuse and/or addiction without the atropine "safety net."

Loperamide Hydrochloride

Loperamide is a nonhydrolyzable amide analogue of meperidine that is available OTC (Imodium) for the treatment of diarrhea. Meperidine's ethylcarboxylate ester has been replaced by a tertiary hydroxyl group, and the phenyl ring has been chlorinated at the para position. The amine substituent is reminiscent of that incorporated into diphenoxylate, although a dimethylamide moiety has replaced the nitrile. While the highly lipophilic drug (log P_{calc} 4.44) acts as a full μ-receptor agonist in the gut, it lacks central μ agonist action due to very low oral bioavailability and extensive P-gp-mediated exclusion from the CNS.[173,174] In contrast to diphenoxylate (which is not a P-gp substrate)[175] loperamide was assumed to have no potential for abuse, which allowed it to be available without a prescription.[176] In addition to and/or in concert with its μ agonist action, loperamide's GI motility inhibition has been linked to the μ agonist–mediated release of 5-HT[177] and calcium channel antagonism.[178]

N-Demethylation of loperamide's tertiary amide is catalyzed by CYP3A4 and CYP2C8.[179] While few interactions with CYP3A4 substrates have been reported, clinically relevant interactions are known to occur with P-gp inducers (decreased serum concentrations) and inhibitors (increased serum concentrations). Significant first-pass metabolism minimizes oral bioavailability. Desmethylloperamide, the major metabolite, does not bind to μ receptors and is inactive as an antidiarrheal.

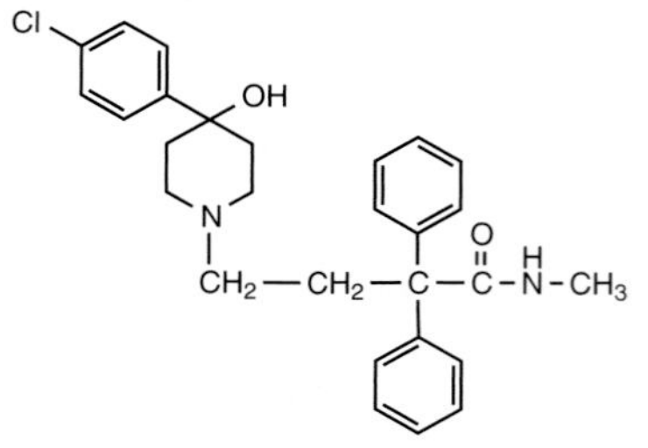

Desmethylloperamide

Loperamide has been compared favorably to diphenoxylate with regard to potency, duration and specificity of action, and safety margin.[172] However, the misuse/abuse of this drug, termed the "poor man's methadone" because of its ready availability and low cost, is currently on the rise. A retrospective review of loperamide toxicity reports issued at the bedside by physicians or nurses to the San Diego division of the California Poison Control System noted a sharp uptick in calls in 2014-2015, concurrent with the availability of Internet-disseminated instructions on methods of loperamide abuse.[180] When taken in doses 40-100 times the recommended maximum dose of 8 (OTC) to 16 (Rx) mg per day, loperamide can saturate P-gp, cross the BBB, and induce euphoria or attenuate withdrawal symptoms.[174] The drug is cardiotoxic when taken chronically at these high doses. Prolonged QTc interval, widened QRS complex, ventricular tachycardia, torsades de pointes, heart block, and sudden cardiac death have all been documented. Interference with myocardial Na^+/K^+ channel conductivity, including blockade of the hERG K^+ channel, has been proposed as a possible arrhythmogenic mechanism.[174,181] Symptoms can persist for as long as 4-5 days, and treatment sometimes requires an overdrive pacemaker in addition to drugs like lidocaine, amiodarone, isoproterenol, and metoprolol. In 2016 the FDA issued a warning about the risk of potentially fatal cardiotoxicity due to loperamide misuse/abuse.

Eluxadoline

While not currently as commonly used as diphenoxylate and loperamide, eluxadoline (Viberzi) is being heavily advertised for use in irritable bowel syndrome with diarrhea. Eluxadoline has a complex opioid receptor profile, with μ and κ agonist and δ antagonist actions, and it acts directly in the GI tract to inhibit motility and ease discomfort. Administration with food decreases T_{max} from 2 to 1.5 hours, although a high-fat meal cuts C_{max} in half.[91] The standard dose is 75-100 mg twice daily. Eluxadoline is a substrate and an inhibitor of the hepatic OATP1B1 carrier protein, and the lower dose is used if coadministered with other drugs also known to inhibit this transporter.

Eluxadoline is 81% protein bound and excreted primarily in feces. The complete metabolic pathway has not been determined, but glucuronic acid conjugation of the carboxylic acid moiety is believed to occur. Adverse effects are predominantly GI-related and include nausea, abdominal pain, and constipation. Therapy should be discontinued if severe constipation develops.

Drugs Used to Treat Neuropathic Pain

"We may not look sick, but turn our bodies inside out and they would tell different stories."

Wade Sutherland

It has been estimated that 25% of the U.S. population suffers from neuropathic pain, which represents an enormous public health burden.[182] Most of this pain is peripheral in origin, arising from injury, trauma (including surgical trauma), or disease such as diabetes or polio, with the remainder arising from CNS disorders such as Parkinson's disease, multiple sclerosis, and phantom limb pain. Individual differences in pain perception, along with mechanism-related complexity and varied concurrent pain sensations, complicate the diagnosis of this pervasive type of pain despite the availability of a variety of validated screening and assessment tools.[14,183,184] However, an accurate diagnosis is critical, since many OTC analgesics that patients might independently gravitate to from past experience in treating nociceptive pain are ineffective in neuropathic pain.

The Neuropathic Pain Special Interest Group of the International Association for the Study of Pain has developed evidence-based guidelines to assist practitioners in approaching therapy,[185] and a review of neuropathic pain management from etiology to contemporary approaches to treatment has recently been published.[14] Treatment options include pharmacotherapy and procedures such as spinal cord stimulation, radiotherapy, nerve block, and neurofeedback. Levels of proinflammatory cytokines are known to be elevated during times of pain flare and may potentially serve as biomarkers to assist in the evaluation of various therapeutic interventions.[182]

A number of drugs and natural products have been tested in neuropathic pain, including rigid and flexible opioids, cannabinoids, angiotensin receptor blockers, dynorphin A, Botulinum toxin A, and ziconotide. Currently, only a few selected anticonvulsants (pregabalin, gabapentin), 5-HT and/or NE reuptake inhibitors (duloxetine), and TCAs (amitriptyline, nortriptyline, desipramine) are considered first-line therapy.[14,186] The topically applied local anesthetic lidocaine and the chili pepper extract capsaicin are second-line drugs for this indication (Fig. 14.13).[14,186-188]

DRUGS LESS COMMONLY USED TO TREAT NEUROPATHIC PAIN

- Carbamazepine
- Lacosamide
- Oxcarbazepine
- Tramadol
- Venlafaxine
- Metanex

Pregabalin and Gabapentin

Pregabalin (Lyrica) and gabapentin (Neurontin) are anticonvulsant ligands of the α_2-δ subunit of central voltage-gated calcium channels, and they inhibit the release of several excitatory neurotransmitters, including glutamate and substance P. Immediate-release formations are dosed twice (pregabalin) or three times (gabapentin) daily, with the standard daily dose of gabapentin between three and six times that of pregabalin.

Pregabalin has demonstrated efficacy in a wide variety of peripheral and central neuropathic pathologies, including fibromyalgia, diabetic peripheral neuropathy, postherpetic neuralgia, and pain resulting from neuromas and spinal cord injury. It is well absorbed orally and follows linear pharmacokinetics. Its metabolism in humans is negligible, leading to 90% being recovered in urine as unchanged zwitterionic drug. The N-methylated derivative, the major

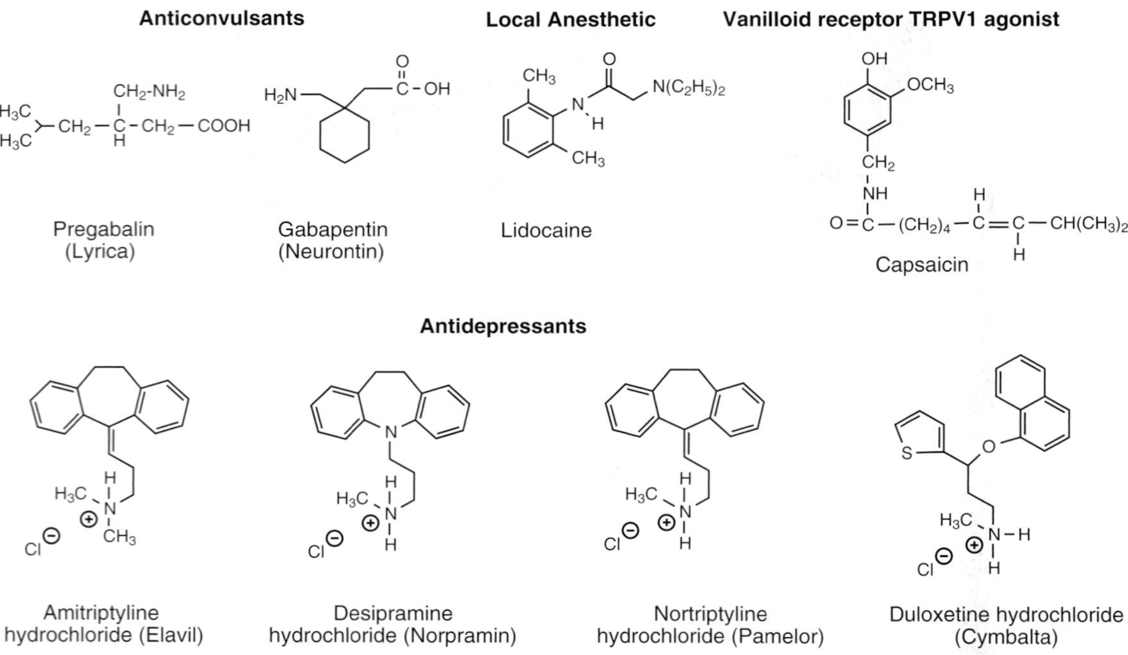

Figure 14.13 Drugs most commonly used to treat neuropathic pain.

metabolite, accounts for only 0.9% of the dose. The lack of interaction with metabolizing enzymes and the absence of protein binding leads to essentially no drug-drug interactions. However, synergism with other CNS depressants may be noted. Among the more concerning adverse effects are suicide ideation, angio- and peripheral edema, thrombocytopenia, vision disturbances, and myopathy secondary to elevated creatine kinase.[91]

Similar to pregabalin, zwitterionic gabapentin has negligible protein binding (<3%) and is metabolism-resistant. The entire dose is renally excreted as unchanged drug. Unlike pregabalin, its use is restricted to postherpetic neuralgia, and the pharmacokinetics of the immediate-release formulation are nonlinear. Due to a saturable L-amino acid transport-facilitated absorption process, oral bioavailability decreases as the dose increases. Gabapentin enacarbil, an extended-release prodrug preparation, is marketed as Horizant, which is also actively absorbed via monocarboxylate transporter-1 (MCT-1). Hydrolysis to the active gabapentin metabolite is predominantly intestinal, and the time to peak serum concentrations is essentially twice that of the immediate-release formulation (3 vs. 6 hr). Gabapentin extended-release tablets (Gralise), oral solutions, suspensions, and cream formulations are also available. Adverse effects shared with pregabalin include sedation, vertigo, vision disturbances, impaired thinking, and edema leading to weight gain.

Gabapentin enacarbil

Duloxetine Hydrochloride

Duloxetine hydrochloride (Cymbalta) is dosed at 60 mg once daily in diabetic neuropathy and titrated to no more than 60 mg daily after a 7-day initial regimen of 30 mg daily in fibromyalgia. Gradual dose increases can also be employed in diabetic peripheral neuropathy patients if tolerance is an issue. Its relatively early onset of pain relief (typically within the first week) is in contrast to the 2-3 weeks it may take to elicit a sustained antidepressant effect. However, the dual action is viewed as particularly beneficial in patients with these comorbidities.[188]

Duloxetine is over 90% protein bound and extensively metabolized by the highly polymorphic CYP2D6 (N-demethylation) and CYP1A2 (aromatic hydroxylation), leading to a high risk of drug-drug interactions. CYP1A2 is induced by cigarette smoke, and smokers experience a 33% decrease in duloxetine bioavailability.[91] Nausea, sedation, and constipation are among the most common adverse effects. Morning administration may help attenuate any negative impact on sleep quality.[14,188]

Tricyclic Antidepressants

Secondary TCAs (e.g., desipramine, nortriptyline) selectively inhibit NE reuptake, while tertiary TCAs (e.g., amitriptyline) inhibit the reuptake of 5-HT in parent form, and NE once N-monodealkylated by CYP2D6. Numerous studies have confirmed the efficacy of TCAs in the treatment of neuropathic pain, particularly diabetic peripheral neuropathy and postherpetic neuralgia, although it can take up to 8 weeks for the maximum benefit to be realized.[187] TCA-induced analgesia is independent of the antidepressant effect but, as with duloxetine, these agents are frequently used in depressed patients suffering with neuropathic pain. The marked anticholinergic actions associated with tertiary TCAs, including their cardiovascular adverse effects, have led to a preference for the secondary amine derivatives. This is particularly true in elderly patients at risk for falls and fractures, mental confusion or hallucinations, vision impairment, heart block and/or sedation. While daily doses of 25-150 mg are allowed, the risk of sudden death is minimized if doses are kept to less than 100 mg/d[187]

Lidocaine and Capsaicin

The local anesthetic lidocaine (Lidoderm) and the transient receptor potential vanilloid 1TRPV1 agonist capsaicin (Qutenza) are topical agents available in patch form for the treatment of localized peripheral neuropathic pain.[14,186,189] While the body of evidence for the efficacy of 8% capsaicin is stronger than for 5% lidocaine, the higher safety margin of the latter has kept it in the second-line therapeutic category.

Lidocaine inhibits nerve conduction by blocking voltage-gated sodium channels and it is used in postherpetic neuralgia. Up to three patches (the maximum daily dose) may be applied to painful intact skin and left in place for 12 hours. Approximately 3% of the dose reaches the general circulation. A study of lidocaine metabolism in healthy human skin documents the formation of the monoethylglycine xylidide (MEGX) metabolite in quantities less than 12.8% of the amount of drug found in skin after a 2 hour exposure to 5 mg/cm^2 of 5% lidocaine.[190]

Monoethylglycine xylidide (MEGX)

The capsaicin patch is indicated in general neuropathic pain and is thought to work by calming ("defunctionalizing") hyperactive cutaneous nerve endings. Up to four patches can be applied to intact skin at the most painful sites and left on for up to an hour. The head and face should be avoided, and 3 months should elapse between applications. The major adverse effect is burning at the site of application, but pretreatment with a topical anesthetic can ease the discomfort. Patients taking ACE inhibitors may notice an increase in drug-induced cough.[188] A 0.075% cream formulation is available for off-label use in painful diabetic peripheral neuropathy and, to be effective, should be applied four times daily on a chronic basis.

ANTIMIGRAINE DRUGS

"Migraines...the only time when taking a hammer to your own skull seems like an appropriate solution."

CoyoteRed

Migraine impacts over 14% of the U.S. population, approximately 35 million people, with females suffering from the disorder more commonly than males.[191,192] Presentation includes throbbing headache that is often unilateral and which can last from hours to days, environmental sensitivity (e.g, light, sound, odors, activity), and nausea and/or vomiting.[193] In approximately 20%-30% of migraine sufferers (called migraineurs), headache is preceded by an aura (most commonly lines and shapes in the visual field, but also sensory tingling and numbness) that persists for up to an hour. Between 10% and 20% of patients experience a 1- to 2-day prodrome phase characterized by specific behaviors (e.g. irritability), feelings (e.g., depression), or conditions (e.g., constipation). In addition to symptoms, the frequency of migraine "attacks" also informs the diagnosis; headache on at least half the days in a month for 3 months, with at least 8 of those days being "migraine-like", warrants a diagnosis of chronic migraine.[193] The chronically episodic and often incapacitating symptoms of migraine interfere with school, employment, and social engagement. Migraine presents a serious economic and public health burden and is considered one of the 40 most disabling conditions in the world.[194-196]

Migraine Pathology

The pathology of migraine headache is complex, genetically rooted, and believed to involve dysfunction in the trigeminal innervation of cranial vasculature impacting parasympathetic outflow.[194] Activation of central and peripheral trigeminal nociceptive pathways is also evident. As intracranial extracerebral vessels dilate, blood volume increases with each heartbeat, leading to pulsating pain. Inflammatory neuropeptides such as calcitonin gene–related peptide (CGRP) and substance P are released, augmenting pain and stimulating hallmark symptoms of nausea/vomiting and aversion to light. Nitric oxide may also play a role in pain induction.

Migraine Prophylaxis

Prevention of migraine headaches often involves dietary/activity/sleep-related lifestyle modifications, headache trigger management, and nonpharmacologic interventions such as deep breathing, biofeedback, and cognitive behavior modification. If needed, certain nonselective/selective β_1 receptor blockers or antiseizure agents can be prescribed, but side effects can be use-limiting (Fig. 14.14). Interestingly, central accumulation is not required for β-blocker therapeutic efficacy.[194] OnabotulinumtoxinA (Botox) is a better-tolerated approach to migraine prophylaxis despite the need for administration by multiple facial IM injections. Newer strategies under investigation to prevent or abort migraine headaches include antagonism of CGRP and glutamate receptors, stimulation of adenosine A_1 and nociception ORL 1 receptors, inhibition of nitric oxide synthase, and transcranial magnetic and/or vagal nerve stimulation.[193,195,197,198]

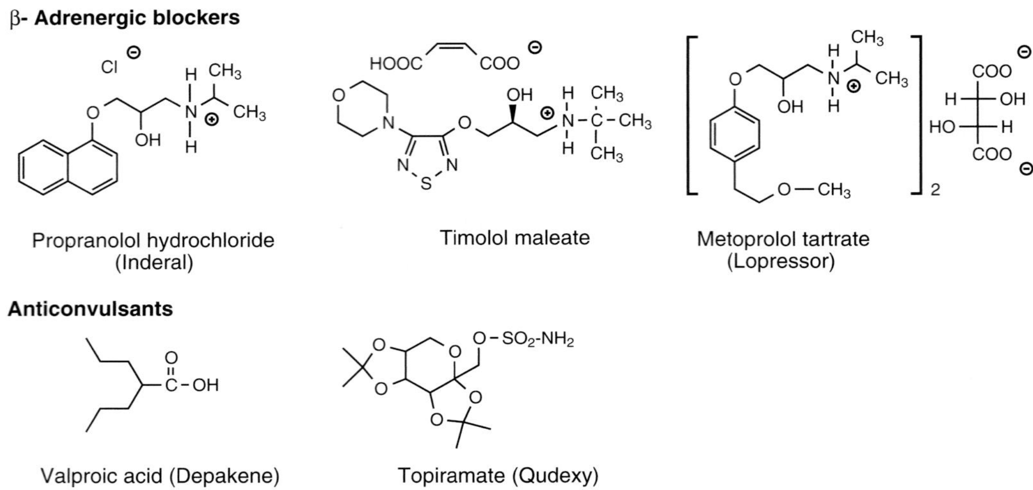

Figure 14.14 Drugs used to prevent migraine headache.

Pharmacotherapy of Active Migraine

Many receptor types and subtypes have been associated with migraine pathology and pharmacotherapy, but the 5-$HT_{1B/1D}$ target has received the most focused drug development attention. When stimulated, these two closely related subtypes induce constriction of cranial vessels (1B) and inhibit trigeminal vascular activity, inflammatory neuropeptide release, and nociception (1D).[194,199] Ergotamine and dihydroergotamine were among the first nonselective 5-$HT_{1B/1D}$ agonists used in the treatment of acute migraine. While still commercially available, their significant adverse effect profile (including nausea, rebound headache and risk of cerebral ischemia if coadministered with CYP3A4 inhibitors), inconsistent pharmacokinetic behavior, and inferior therapeutic effect compared to the more highly 5$HT_{1B/1D}$-selective triptans have relegated them to second-line agents.

Ergotamine Dihydroergotamine

Ergot derivatives.

Triptans (Fig. 14.15)

OTC NSAID or acetaminophen use is common in the attempt to abort an active migraine headache, but the centrally active 5-$HT_{1B/1D}$ agonists known collectively as the triptans are the mainstay of prescription migraine pharmacotherapy. Opioids are not used to treat migraine pain and can actually accelerate the progression from episodic to chronic migraine.[200]

Triptans have been in clinical use for over 25 years, and they have a well-recognized effect on pain relief and function, and thus on patient quality of life. However, some studies have shown that an initial incomplete or inconsistent response to a prescribed triptan, coupled with problematic adverse effects, can cause up to 60% of patients to not refill their medication. Up to 9% switch immediately to a different triptan, rather than persisting with the original drug for the recommended number of trials.[201] The importance of detailed and descriptive medical and pain histories, along with patient-provider discussion of preferred dosage forms and education on clinical expectations, is paramount to arriving expediently at the optimal therapeutic approach for each migraine patient.

MECHANISM AND PHARMACOKINETICS. All seven marketed triptans act by constricting intracranial extracerebral vessels, attenuating neuroinflammation, and inhibiting the release of neurotransmitters at trigeminal nociceptive terminals. While their mechanism is identical, they differ significantly in their pharmacokinetic properties (Table 14.6).[196,199] The triptans have calculated log P values ranging from 1.17 (sumatriptan) to 3.84 (eletriptan). Oral bioavailability also varies widely, and nasal spray formulations are available for some products on the lower end of the scale. Gastric emptying slows during active migraine attacks, which can delay drug absorption. Therapeutic action generally begins within 2 hours of oral administration, and elimination half-lives are commonly in the 2- to 4-hour range. Serum levels can be elevated in patients with significant hepatic or renal dysfunction.

In general, the higher the bioavailability and the faster the penetration of the BBB, the more beneficial the therapeutic action. However, patients nonresponsive to one triptan might be robust responders to

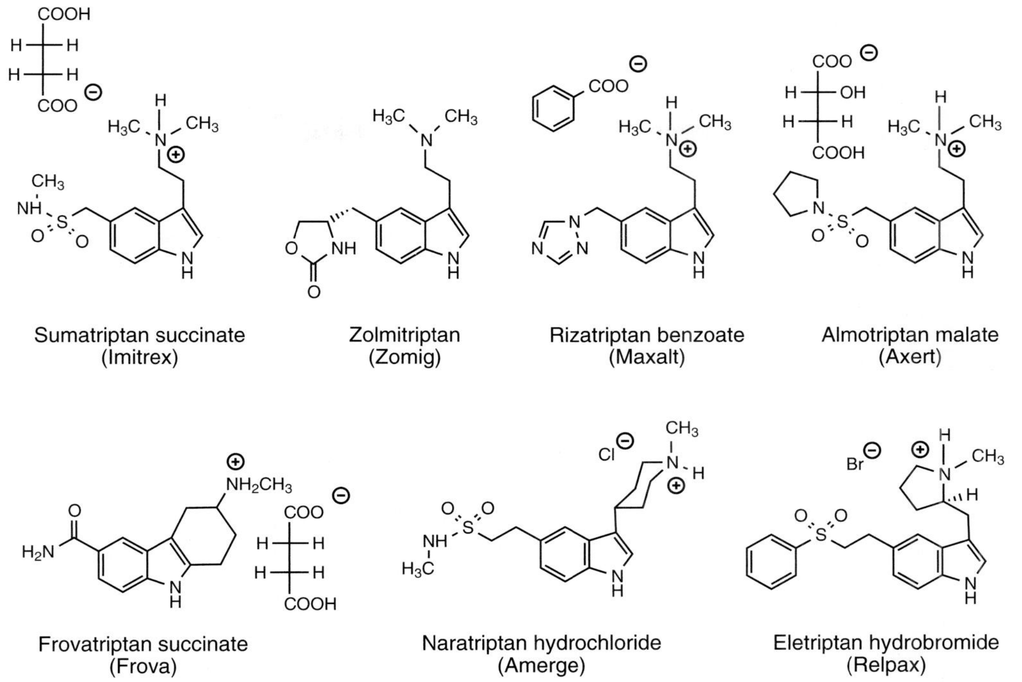

Sumatriptan succinate (Imitrex)

Zolmitriptan (Zomig)

Rizatriptan benzoate (Maxalt)

Almotriptan malate (Axert)

Frovatriptan succinate (Frova)

Naratriptan hydrochloride (Amerge)

Eletriptan hydrobromide (Relpax)

Figure 14.15 Triptan antimigraine agents.

another depending on the individual patient's constellation of symptoms and the pharmacokinetic advantages of the effective agent.[202] Treatment should begin when pain intensity is low, and doses titrated until efficacy is achieved or the maximum allowed dose is reached. If therapy is delayed until central trigeminal sensitization has occurred (signaled by cutaneous allodynia), triptan therapy can become ineffective.[196] Approximately 25%-35% of migraineurs get no relief from triptans, and 60% of those who do not respond to NSAIDs fall into the triptan-resistant category. Although in the early stages, pharmacogenomics studies hope to eventually identify genes related to disease susceptibility and etiology so that more rational and individualized approaches to pharmacotherapy can be implemented.[203]

CHEMISTRY. All triptan antimigraine agents contain the indolethylamine moiety that allows access to 5-HT receptors. In naratriptan, three carbons separate the indole ring from the terminal amine, but the distance is shortened by incorporating the amine into a piperidine ring. All triptans are tertiary amines except frovatriptan, which is secondary. Amine substituents are limited in size to methyl, presumably to restrict steric hindrance to electrostatic interaction of the protonated amine at G protein-coupled $5\text{-HT}_{1B/1D}$ receptors.

The 5-phenol of the serotonin moiety is replaced by a more metabolically stable polar functional group such as an amide (frovatriptan), secondary or tertiary sulfonamide (sumatriptan, almotriptan, naratriptan), sulfone (eletriptan), or heterocyclic ring (zolmitriptan, rizatriptan). In all cases but sumatriptan, the polar moiety is separated from the indole ring by one to two carbon atoms.

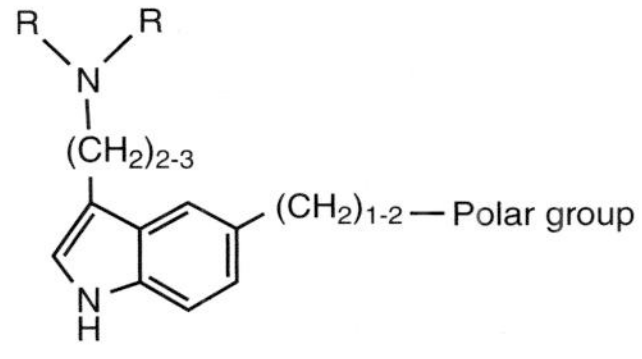

Triptan pharmacophore (R most commonly alkyl)

METABOLISM (FIGS. 14.16-14.18)[204-210]

Common metabolic reactions of the triptans include N-dealkylation of the terminal amine and/or deamination by MAO-A. The aldehyde generated by MAO can be either oxidized to the indoleacetic acid or reduced to the indole ethyl alcohol by aldehyde dehydrogenase (ALDH). Some triptans are oxidized by flavin monooxygenase (FMO) to inactive N-oxides.

The isoforms involved in CYP-vulnerable triptan metabolism vary and include 2D6 (almotriptan), 1A2 (frovatriptan, zolmitriptan), and 3A4 (naratriptan, almotriptan, and eletriptan). The desmethyl metabolites of rizatriptan, zolmitriptan, eletriptan, and frovatripan are active. Desmethylrizatriptan is approximately equipotent with rizatriptan, and desmethylzolmitriptan's activity is between two and six times that of the parent drug. The 50% longer half-life of desmethylzolmitriptan likely contributes to its augmented potency.[196,208] Desmethyleletriptan has a half-life and time to maximum plasma concentration (T_{max}) similar to its parent drug, but the peak concentrations are about 3-fold lower. Desmethylfrovatriptan binds to target receptors with approximately one-third the affinity of its parent, but has a 3-fold longer half-life.[196]

Table 14.6 Triptan Pharmacokinetics

Parameters	Sumatriptan	Zolmitriptan	Naratriptan	Rizatriptan	Almotriptan	Frovatriptan	Eletriptan
Trade name	Imitrex	Zomig	Amerge	Maxalt	Axert	Frova	Relpax
Log P (calc)	1.17	2.25	2.16	1.67	2.04	1.2	3.84
Oral Bioavailability (%)	15 17-19 (nas) 97 (sc)	40 102 (nas compared to po)	74	45	70	20-30[a]	50
Protein binding (%)	14-21	25	28-31	14	35	15	85
Volume of distribution (po unless noted)	2.7 L/kg 50 L (sc)	7 L/kg 8.4 L/kg (nas)	170 L	110-140 L[a]	180-200 L	3-4.2 L/kg	138 L
$T_{1/2}$ (hr) (po unless noted)	2 1.8 (nas) 2 (sc)	3 3 (nas)	6	2-3	3-5	26-30	4
Major phase I metabolites (%)	Indoleacetic acid	N-Desmethyl (act)	Hepatic: 50%	Indole acetic acid	Indole acetic acid	N-Desmethyl (act)	N-Desmethyl (act)
		Indole ethyl alcohol		N-Desmethyl (act)	GABA	N-Ac-desmethyl	
		Indole acetic acid		6-OH	N-Desmethyl		
Metabolizing enzymes	MAO-A	CYP1A2	CYP3A4 and other isoforms	MAO-A	CYP3A4/CYP2D6	CYP1A2	CYP3A4
		MAO-A	MAO-A		MAO-A		

Excretion (%)	60 renal 40 fecal (3-22 unchanged drug)	60 renal 30 fecal (8 unchanged drug)	30 renal 15 fecal (50 unchanged drug)	82 renal 12 fecal (14 unchanged drug)	75 renal 13 fecal (~53 unchanged drug)	32 renal 62 fecal	90 renal <10 fecal (<20 unchanged drug)
T_{max} (hr) (po unless noted)	2-2.5 0.75-1.5 (nas) 0.2 (sc)	1.5[b] 3 (dt) 3 (nas)	2-3[b]	1-1.5 1.6-2.5 (dt)	1-3	2-4	1.5-2[b]
C_{max} (mg/L) (po)	54	10[a]	12.6[a]	19.8[a]	49.5	4.2-7.0[a]	246[b]
% Pain relief [c] at 2 hr (at 4 hr) (po unless noted)	56-67 (71) 72-74 (nas) 80 (sc)	62-65 (70-75)	40 (60-68)	67-77	70	38 (68)	77
Initial dosage range (mg) (po unless noted)	25-100 5-20 (nas) 6 (sc)	1.25-5 2.5 (nas)	1-2.5	5-10	6.25-12.5	2.5-5	20-40
Maximum p.o. dose (mg/24 hr)	200	10	5	30	25	7.5	80

Data from *Drug Bank*. Available at https://www.drugbank.ca/. Accessed 9/30/2017; *Drug Facts and Comparisons. Facts & Comparisons [Database Online]*. In: Louis S, ed. MO: Wolters Kluwer Health, Inc.; March 2005; Burch R, Loder S, Loder E, et al. The prevalence and burden of migraine and severe headache in the United States: updated statistics from government health surveillance studies. *Headache*. 2015;55:21-34; and Weatherall M. The diagnosis and treatment of chronic migraine. *Ther Adv Chronic Dis*. 2015;6:115-123.

[a]Gender dependent (women > men).

[b]Increased during active migraine.

[c]Compared to placebo.

act, active; C_{max}, peak plasma concentration after po administration; dt, disintegrating tablets; nas, intranasal; po, oral; sc, subcutaneous; $T_{1/2}$, elimination half-life; T_{max}, time to peak plasma concentration.

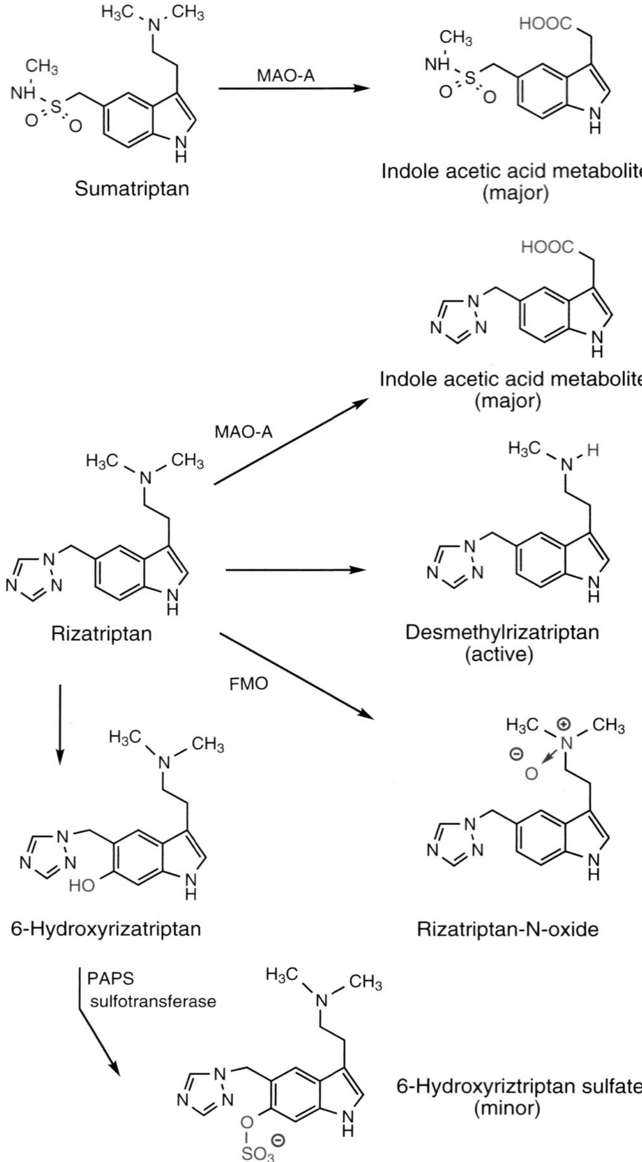

Figure 14.16 Sumatriptan and rizatriptan metabolism.

Sumatriptan, almotriptan, and naratriptan have no active metabolites, which is one proposed reason for their lower incidence of central adverse effects.

Adverse Effects. While they have no affinity for 5-HT_{2A} receptors that mediate the majority of 5-HT-linked coronary vasoconstriction, triptans can bind to the small 1B subtype reserve in that tissue and have the potential to constrict coronary vessels.[211] While serious cardiac events are uncommon, triptans should be avoided in patients with known or suspected ischemic or vasoactive coronary artery disease. To minimize the risk of synergistic vasoconstriction, patients should be restricted to a single triptan, and triptans and ergot derivatives should not be coadministered in the same 24-hour period.[212]

Molecular lipophilicity of triptans and their active metabolites has been positively correlated with risk of CNS adverse effects, including drowsiness, dizziness, and cognition or sensory disturbances. This is of clinical importance since the fear of CNS toxicity is known to prompt decisions to delay therapy, leading to prolonged pain and patient disengagement from social or work-related activities.[196] Nausea and dry mouth can also occur with triptan use.

TRIPTAN DRUG-DRUG INTERACTIONS

- Ergot derivatives
  - Augmented ergot-induced vasoconstriction
- 5-HT_3 antagonist antiemetics
  - Serotonin syndrome
- Opioid analgesics
  - Serotonin syndrome
- Antipsychotic drugs
  - Serotonin syndrome and/or neuroleptic malignant syndrome
- Metoclopramide
  - Serotonin syndrome and/or neuroleptic malignant syndrome
- Droxidopa
  - Augmented droxidopa-induced hypertension
- CYP3A4 inhibitors
  - Strong: Elevated eletriptan and almotriptan serum levels
  - Moderate: Elevated eletriptan serum levels
- MAO inhibitors
  - Elevated sumatriptan, zolmitriptan, rizatriptan, and almotriptan serum levels

Specific Drugs

Sumatriptan Succinate. Sumatriptan was the first triptan to be marketed, and it stands alone in the "first generation" class of triptan antimigraine drugs. It has one of the lowest lipophilicities of the triptans, and its activity is predominantly peripheral.[199] It is marketed in a variety of dosage forms, including tablets, nasal solution, nasal exhale powder (Onzetra Xsail), solution for subcutaneous injection, subcutaneous auto-injector (Imitrex StatDose, Zembrace SymTouch), and jet-injector (Sumavel DosePro). A combination product with the NSAID naproxen sodium is marketed in tablet form as Treximet.

Subcutaneous administration provides faster and more efficacious pain-relieving action than tablets and is useful in patients whose pain is escalating or who are nauseated. However, the injection formulation is associated with an elevated risk of usually short-lived adverse effects such as dizziness, sensory disturbances, chest/throat tightness, and shortness of breath. Likewise, the nasal spray relieves pain more quickly than the tablets, but patients can experience recurrent headache at the 2-hour pain relief benchmark, as well as an unpleasant taste.[212] Regardless of formulation, the dose can be repeated no sooner than

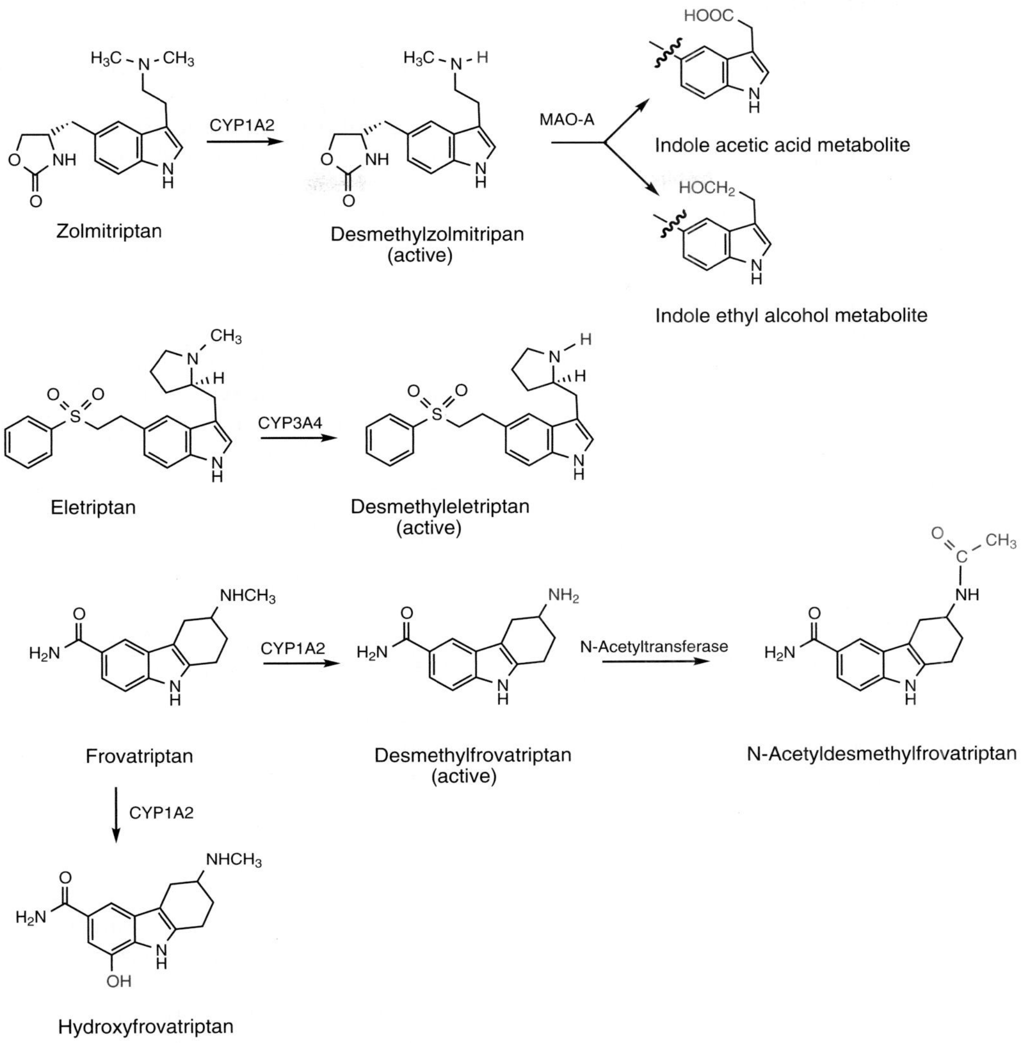

Zolmitriptan → (CYP1A2) → Desmethylzolmitripan (active) → (MAO-A) → Indole acetic acid metabolite; Indole ethyl alcohol metabolite

Eletriptan → (CYP3A4) → Desmethyleletriptan (active)

Frovatriptan → (CYP1A2) → Desmethylfrovatriptan (active) → (N-Acetyltransferase) → N-Acetyldesmethylfrovatriptan

Frovatriptan → (CYP1A2) → Hydroxyfrovatriptan

Figure 14.17 Zolmitriptan, eletriptan and frovatriptan metabolism.

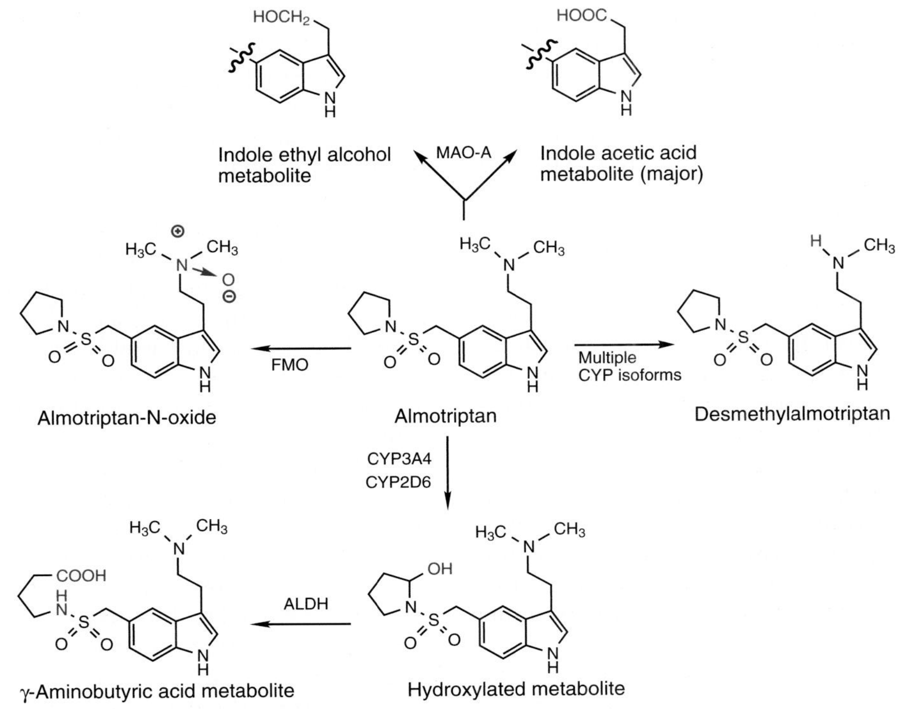

Almotriptan → (MAO-A) → Indole ethyl alcohol metabolite; Indole acetic acid metabolite (major)

Almotriptan → (FMO) → Almotriptan-N-oxide

Almotriptan → (Multiple CYP isoforms) → Desmethylalmotriptan

Almotriptan → (CYP3A4, CYP2D6) → Hydroxylated metabolite → (ALDH) → γ-Aminobutyric acid metabolite

Figure 14.18 Almotriptan metabolism.

2 hours (oral, nasal) or 1 hour (injection) after the initial dose, but the maximum allowed dose should not be exceeded (Table 14.6).

Zolmitriptan. Zolmitriptan was designed to improve upon sumatriptan's fairly low oral bioavailability. Its higher lipophilicity promotes absorption from the GI tract and penetration of the BBB, although clinical efficacy of the two triptans is essentially equivalent. The ability of a second dose of zolmitriptan to address unresolved headache pain 2 hours postadministration led to the establishment of a secondary (4 hour) endpoint for evaluating clinical efficacy, and it is uniquely effective when a second dose is taken for persistent headache.[212] As noted previously, the N-desmethyl metabolite has an activity between two and six times that of the parent drug with a 50% longer half-life. Females may show higher mean serum concentrations of zolmitriptan compared to males.[91] The use of oral contraceptives increases maximum serum concentrations by 30% while delaying time to peak concentrations by 30 minutes.[199]

Zolmitriptan is one of two triptans available in a disintegrating tablet formulation (rizatriptan is the other). Absorption is intestinal (not buccal), but nauseated patients may appreciate not having to swallow a tablet, plus it can be taken when water is not immediately at hand. The nasal spray formulation has similar advantages and disadvantages as sumatriptan's intranasal dosage form.[212]

Naratriptan Hydrochloride. Naratriptan's relative low incidence of adverse effects has caused it to be termed the "gentle triptan" by some.[212] Available only in tablet form, it has the highest oral bioavailability of any marketed triptan and a longer half-life than all but frovatriptan. Still, its single-dose efficacy is among the lowest of the triptan antimigraine drugs, but the risk of recurrent headache is also lower compared to zolmitriptan or sumatriptan. The time to peak serum concentration is delayed to 3-4 hours during acute migraine episodes, leading to enhanced pain relief at 4 hours (60%-68%) versus 2 hours (40%). Similar to zolmitriptan, serum levels are about 1.5 times higher in women compared to men, and oral contraceptive use contributes to this by decreasing clearance by 26%. The fact that smoking increases clearance by 30% lends support to the concept of CYP1A2 being involved in naratriptan metabolism.[199]

Rizatriptan Benzoate. As noted above, rizatriptan is available in oral disintegrating tablets as well as traditional tablets. Its onset of action is among the fastest, and elimination half-life among the shortest, of currently marketed triptans. It has the highest 2-hour clinical efficacy and is able to sustain a pain-free state up through 24 hours. The low (45%) bioavailability is due to significant first-pass metabolism, with the equally active desmethyl metabolite being formed to a relatively minor extent (14%). Serum levels of both the parent drug and active metabolite increase dramatically in the presence of MAO inhibitors and substrates, requiring dose reductions when coadministration cannot be avoided.[199]

While the drug is known to accumulate in rodent breast milk, rizatriptan has been assigned a Briggs category rating of Probably Compatible, indicating that available data suggest no significant risk to nursing infants. All other triptans received the same rating with the exception of sumatriptan, which was classified as Compatible (safe) despite being excreted into human milk.[213] Still, given the low protein-binding potential of triptans, coupled with their moderate half-lives and fairly low molecular weights, care and counseling is warranted when prescribing these drugs for breast-feeding women.

Almotriptan Malate. Almotriptan is lipophilic and rapidly absorbed from the GI tract. Marketed in tablet form, two-thirds of the dose is delivered to the bloodstream within 1 hour postadministration, and patients can begin to experience relief within 30 minutes.[199,212] It is well tolerated, but drug-drug interactions are possible with agents that impact the availability and activity of CYP3A4 and CYP2D6 (especially strong CYP3A4 inhibitors) and MAO-A. The adverse effect profile is mild, with dizziness and drowsiness being the most commonly observed effects.

Frovatriptan Succinate. Frovatriptan has a lipophilicity, oral bioavailability, and protein binding profile very similar to sumatriptan. While its onset of action is relatively sluggish, its half-life is extended approximately 15-fold compared to sumatriptan, regardless of dose or route of administration. This allows it to have its major impact on pain relief at the 4-hour (vs. 2-hr) efficacy benchmark. Frovatriptan has the highest affinity for 5-HT_{1B} receptors of all triptans and demonstrates selectivity for cerebral, as opposed to coronary, vessels, making it safer to use in patients with coronary artery disease.[199] Appropriate caution, counseling and monitoring, however, is always warranted.

Like eletriptan, frovatriptan is not metabolized by MAO-A and can be more safely administered with drugs that are MAO-A substrates or inhibitors. It is a recommended agent for the treatment of migraine headaches triggered by menstruation.[193]

Eletriptan Hydrobromide. Eletriptan is a cyclized N-methylpyrrolidine analogue of sumatriptan. In this constrained conformation, affinity for 5-HT_{1D} receptors rises to the highest level of all triptans, and its affinity for the 1B subtype is second only to frovatriptan.[199] It is the most lipophilic triptan and rapidly reaches peak plasma concentrations that are higher by severalfold than any other drug in the class (Table 14.6). Like frovatriptin, it is effective in treating menstruation-related migraine, and its efficacy is not impacted by the concomitant use of oral contraceptives.[199]

Eletriptan is marketed only in tablet form. The adverse effect risk appears to be dose-related and includes nausea, dizziness, drowsiness, and general weakness. It carries the highest risk of toxicity when coadministered with CYP3A4 substrates or inhibitors, although some studies have shown the adverse effect profile insignificantly impacted by CYP3A4 activity modulators.[212]

Structure Challenge

The structures of 10 drugs discussed in this chapter are provided. Use your knowledge of drug chemistry to identify the agent that would be most appropriate for use in each patient care situation described below.

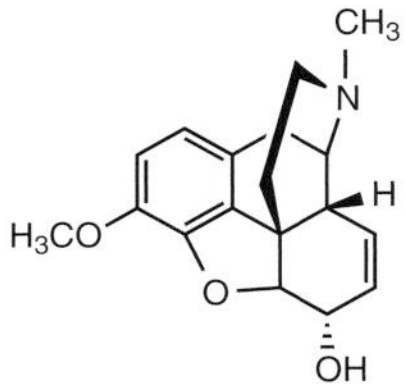

1 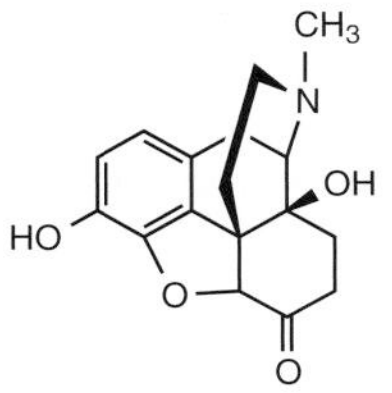 2 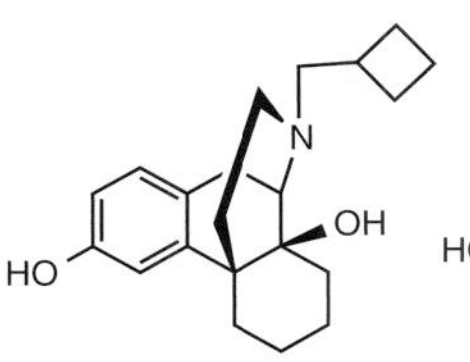 3 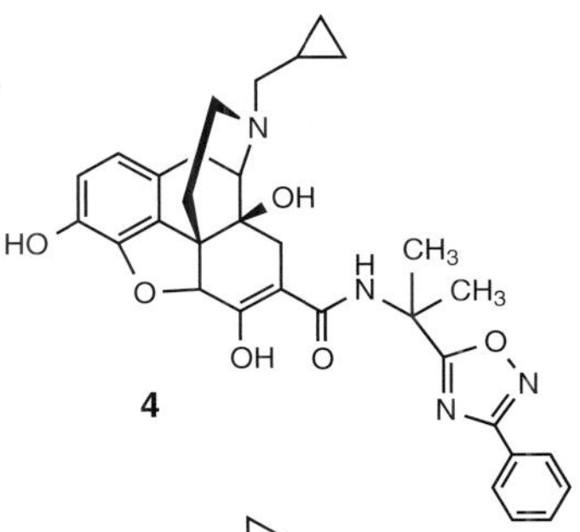 4

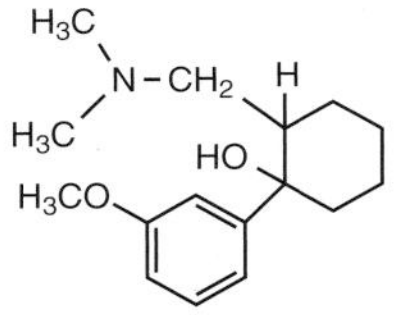

5 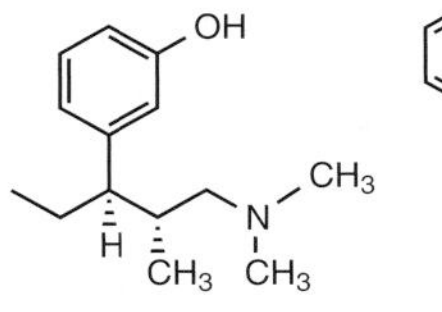 6 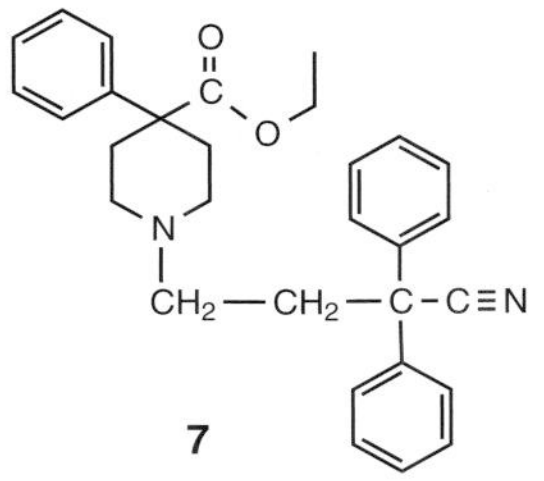 7 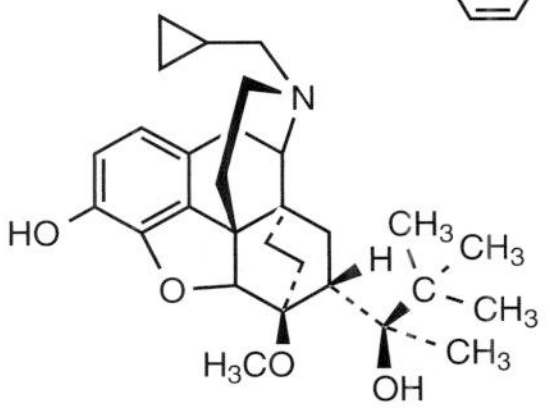 8

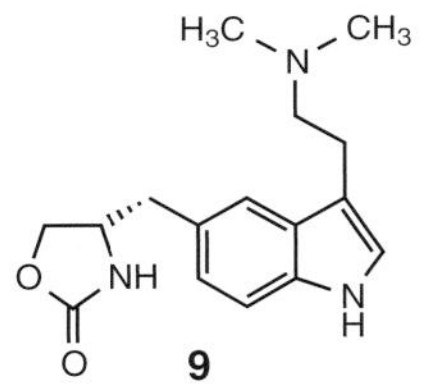

9 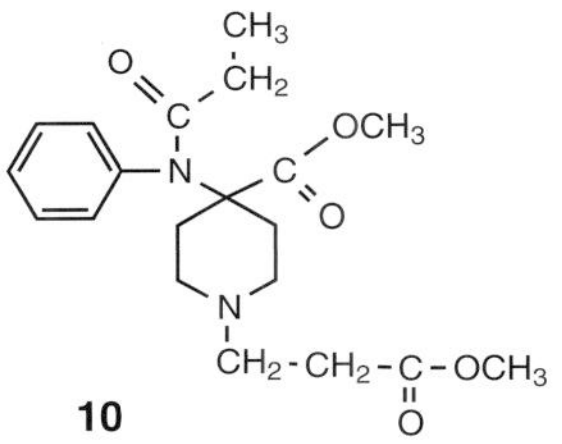 10

A. An active heroin addict, newly committed to recovery, who is in her physician's office ready to take the first step. # ___

B. A survivor of a serious motorcycle crash in need of strong pain control. This patient has a recent history of oxycodone (μ agonist) abuse after having being prescribed that medication 3 years ago for postsurgical pain, but he is now "clean." # ___

C. A surgical patient about to be administered anesthesia. # ___

D. A known 2D6 PM being prescribed a dual-acting analgesic for debilitating acute pain. # ___

E. A patient with migraine attempting to abort a disabling headache. # ___

F. A patient with cancer on chronic opioid therapy who needs relief from opioid-induced constipation. # ___

G. A patient with pertussis in need of a strong antitussive to relieve the disease's intractable cough. # ___

H. An international traveler who is experiencing severe diarrhea after eating tainted food. # ___

Structure Challenge answers found immediately after References.

REFERENCES

1. Merskey H, Bogduk N. *Classification of Chronic Pain*. 2nd ed. Seattle: International Association for the Study of Pain Press; 2004:209-214.
2. Griffen R, Woolf C, eds. *Pharmacology of Analgesia*. 2nd ed. Philadelphia: Lippcott Williams & Wilkins; 2008. Golan D, Tashjian A, Armstrong E, et al, eds. *Principles of Pharmacology: The Physiologic Basis of Drug Therapy*.
3. Stanos S, Brodsky M, Argoff C, et al. Rethinking chronic pain in a primary care setting. *Postgrad Med*. 2016;128:502-515.
4. Campbell J. APS presidential address. *J Pain*. 1996;5:85-88.
5. Mularski R, White-Chu F, Overbay D, et al. Measuring pain as the 5th vital sign does not improve quality of pain management. *J Gen Int Med*. 2006;21:607-612.
6. Joint Commission Statement on Pain Management. Available at https://www.jointcommission.org/joint_commission_statement_on_pain_management/. Accessed 7/30/2017.

7. http://www.painmed.org/membercenter/2016-ama-hod-annual-meeting/. Accessed 7/30/2017.
8. Institute of Medicine. *Relieving Pain in America; a Blueprint for Transforming Prevention, Care, Education and Research*. Washington, DC: The National Academies Press (US); 2011.
9. Morone N, Weiner D. Pain as the 5th vital sign: exposing the vital need for pain education. *Clin Ther*. 2013;35:1728-1732.
10. Wong-Baker FACES Foundation. Available at http://wongbakerfaces.org. Accessed 7/30/2017.
11. Tait R, Chibnall T. Racial/ethnic disparities in the assessment and treatment of pain. *Am Psychologist*. 2014;69:131-141.
12. Murphy K, Han J, Yang S, et al. Prevalence of specific types of pain diagnoses in a sample of United States adults. *Pain Phys*. 2017;20:E247-E268.
13. Fornasari D. Pain mechanisms in patients with chronic pain. *Clin Drug Invest*. 2012;32:45-52.
14. McCarberg B, D'Arcy Y, Parsons B, et al. Neuropathic pain: a narrative review of etiology, assessment, diagnosis and treatment for primary care providers. *Curr Med Res Opin*. 2017;33:1361-1369 (and references therein).
15. Radnovich R, Chapman C, Gudin J, et al. Acute pain: effective management requires comprehensive assessment. *Postgrad Med*. 2014;126:59-72.
16. Tawfic Q, Faris A. Acute pain service: past present and future. *Pain Manag*. 2015;5:47-58.
17. Moore R, Wiffen P, Derry S, et al. Non-prescription (OTC) oral analgesics for acute pain – an overview of Cochrane reviews. *Cochrane Database Syst Rev*. 2015;11:1-30.
18. Gordon D. Acute pain assessment tools: let us move beyond simple pain ratings. *Curr Opin*. 2015;28:565-569.
19. Henschke N, Kamper S, Maher C. The epidemiology and economic consequences of pain. *Mayo Clinic Proc*. 2015;90:139-147.
20. Peppin J, Cheatle M, Kirsh K, et al. The complexity model: a novel approach to improve chronic pain care. *Pain Med*. 2015;16:653-666.
21. Trang T, Al-Hasani R, Salvemini D, et al. Pain and poppies: the good, the bad and the ugly of opioid analgesics. *J Neurosci*. 2015;35:13879-13888.
22. Delgado R, York A, Lee C, et al. Assessing the quality, efficacy and effectiveness of the current evidence base of active self-care complementary and integrative medicine therapies for the management of chronic pain: a rapid evidence assessment of the literature. *Pain Med*. 2014;15:S9-S20.
23. Zidarov D, Visca R, Gogovor A, et al. Performance and quality indicators for the management of non-cancer chronic pain: a scoping review protocol. *BMJ Open*. 2016;6:e010487.
24. Lisi L, Aceto P, Navarra P, et al. mTOR kinase: a possible pharmacological target in the management of chronic pain. *Biomed Res Int*. 2015;2015:394257.
25. Turk D. Remember the distinction between malignant and benign pain? Well forget it. *Clin J Pain*. 2002;18:75-76.
26. Sun R, Zhang W, Bo J, et al. Spinal activation of alpha7-nicotinic acetylcholine receptor attenuates posttraumatic stress disorder chronic pain via suppression of glial activation. *Neuroscience*. 2016;344:243-254.
27. Loo L, Wright B, Zylka M. Lipid kinases as therapeutic targets for chronic pain. *Pain*. 2015;156(suppl 1):S2-S10.
28. Jones T, Moore T, Choo J. The impact of virtual reality on chronic pain. *PLoS One*. 2016;11:e0167523.
29. Pain Management Task Force Final Report: Providing a standardized DoD and VHA vision and approach to pain management to optimize the care for warriors and their families. Available at https://permanent.access.gpo.gov/gpo60064/Pain-Management-Task-Force.pdf. Accessed 8/1/2017.
30. Hughes J, Smith T, Kosterlitz H, et al. Identification of two related pentapeptides from the brain with potent opiate agonist activity. *Nature*. 1975;258:577-579.
31. Li C, Lemaire S, Yamashiro D, et al. The synthesis and opiate activity of β-endorphin. *Biochem Biophys Res Commun*. 1976;71:19-25.
32. Goldstein A, Tachibana SL, Lowney LI, et al. Procaine pituitary dynorphin: complete amino acid sequence of the biologically active heptadecapeptide. *Proc Natl Acad Sci*. 1979;76:6666-6670.
33. DeWire S, Yamashita D, Rominger D, et al. A G protein-biased ligand at the mu opioid receptor is potently analgesic with reduced gastrointestinal and respiratory dysfunction compared with morphine. *J Pharmacol Exp Ther*. 2013;344:708-717.
34. Bohn L, Gainetdinov P, Lin F-T, et al. Mu opioid receptor desensitization by beta-arrestin-2 determines morphine tolerance but not dependence. *Nature*. 2000;408:720-723.
35. Lendeckel U, Muller C, Rocken C, et al. Expression of opioid subtypes and their ligands in fibrillating human atria. *PACE*. 2005;28:S275-S279.
36. Riviere P-M. Peripheral kappa opioid agonists for visceral pain. *Br J Pharmacol*. 2004;141:1331-1334.
37. Soergel DS, Subach RA, Burnham N, et al. Biased agonism of the mu-opioid receptor by TRV130 increases analgesia and reduces on-target adverse effects versus morphine: a randomized double-blind, placebo-controlled, crossover study in heathy volunteers. *Pain*. 2014;155:1829-1835.
38. Manglik A, Lin H, Aryal D, et al. Structure-based discovery of opioid analgesics with reduced side effects. *Nature*. 2016;537:185-190.
39. Somogyi A, Coller J, Barratt D. Pharmacogenetics of opioid response. *Clin Pharmacol Ther*. 2015;97:125-127.
40. Zhou C, Florence C, Dowell D. Payments for opioids shifted substantially to public and private insurers while consumer spending on these medications declined, 1999-2012. *Health Aff*. 2016;35:824-831.
41. Onishi E, Kobayashi T, Dexter E, et al. Comparison of opioid prescribing patterns in the United States and Japan: primary care physicians' attitudes and perceptions. *J Am Board Fam Med*. 2017;30:248-254.
42. Barnett M, Olenski A, Jena A. Opioid-prescribing patterns of emergency physicians and risk of long term use. *New Eng J Med*. 2017;376:663-673.
43. Walco G, Gove N, Phillips J, et al. Opioid analgesics administered for pain in the inpatient pediatric setting. *J Pain*. 2017;18:1270-1276.
44. Schmidt T, Haddox J, Nielsen A, et al. Key data gaps regarding the public health issues associated with opioid analgesics. *J Behav Health Serv Res*. 2015;42:540-553.
45. Kattan J, Tuazon E, Paone D, et al. Public health detailing-A successful strategy to promote judicious opioid analgesic prescribing. *Am J Pub Health*. 2016;106:1430-1438.
46. Raub J, Vettese T. Acute pain management in hospitalized adult patients with opioid dependence: a narrative review and guide for clinicians. *J Hosp Med*. 2017;12:371-379.
47. Definitions related to the use of opioids for the treatment of pain. Available at https://www.asam.org/docs/default-source/public-policy-statements/1opioid-definitions-consensus-2-011.pdf. Accessed 8/15/2017.
48. Jan S. Introduction: landscape of opioid dependence. *J Manag Care Pharm*. 2010;16:S4-S8.
49. Lipman A, Webster L. The economic impact of opioid use in the management of chronic nonmalignant pain. *J Manag Care Spec Pharm*. 2015;21:891-899.
50. 2015 *National Survey on Drug Use and Health: Detailed Tables*. Available at https://www.samhsa.gov/data/sites/default/files/NSDUH-DetTabs-2015/NSDUH-DetTabs-2015/NSDUH-DetTabs-2015.pdf. Accessed 8/12/2017.
51. Oderda G, Lake J, Rudell K, et al. Economic burden of prescription opioid misuse and abuse: a systematic review. *J Pain Palliat Care Pharmacother*. 2015;29:388-400.
52. Kirson N, Scarpati L, Enloe C, et al. The economic burden of opioid abuse: updated findings. *J Manag Care Spec Pharm*. 2017;23:427-445.
53. Prescription Nation 2016: Addressing America's Drug Epidemic. Available at http://www.nsc.org/RxDrugOverdoseDocuments/Prescription-Nation-2016-American-Drug-Epidemic.pdf. Accessed 8/12/2017.
54. National Vital Statistics System, Mortality. Available at https://wonder.cdc.gov/. Accessed 8/13/2017.

55. Sessions on the opioid epidemic: 'Treatment cannot be our only policy'. Business Insider. Available at http://www.businessinsider.com/ap-sessions-drug-overdoses-the-top-lethal-issue-in-the-us-2017-8. Accessed 8/31/2017.
56. Volkow N, Collins F. The role of science in addressing the opioid crisis. *New Eng J Med*. 2017;377:391-394.
57. Volkow N. NIH's efforts to reduce the opioid epidemic. Available at https://acd.od.nih.gov/documents/presentations/06092017Volkow.pdf. Accessed 8/15/2017.
58. Secretary Price Announces HHS Strategy for Fighting Opioid Crisis. Available at https://www.hhs.gov/about/leadership/secretary/speeches/2017-speeches/secretary-price-announces-hhs-strategy-for-fighting-opioid-crisis/index.html. Accessed 8/15/2017.
59. Opioid Crisis. Available at https://www.drugabuse.gov/drugs-abuse/opioids/opioid-crisis. Accessed 8/15/2017.
60. Manglik A, Kruse A, Kobilka T, et al. Crystal structure of the mu opioid receptor bound to a morphinan antagonist. *Nature*. 2012;485:321-326.
61. Wu H, Wacker D, Mileni M, et al. Structure of the human kappa opioid receptor in complex with JDTic. *Nature*. 2012;485:327-332.
62. Klotz U. Tramadol – the impact of its pharmacokinetic and pharmacodynamic properties on the clinical management of pain. *Arzneim-Forsch Drug Res*. 2003;53:681-687.
63. Okulicz-Koraryn I, Leppert W, Mikolajczak P, et al. Analgesic effect of tramadol in combination with adjuvant drugs: an experimental study in rats. *Pharmacol Rep*. 2013;91:7-11.
64. Cong X, Campomanes P, Kless A, et al. Structural determinants for the binding of morphinan agonists to the mu-opioid receptor. *PLoS One*. 2015;10:e0135998.
65. Pogozheva I, Lomize A, Mosberg H. Opioid receptor three-dimensional structures from distance geometry calculations with hydrogen bonding constraints. *Biophys J*. 1998;75:612-634.
66. Dosen-Micovic L, Ivanovic M, Micovic V. Steric interactions and the activity of fentanyl analogs at the mu opioid receptor. *Bioorg Med Chem*. 2006;14:2887-2895.
67. Radulovic N, Blagojevic P, Randjelovic P, et al. The last decade of antinociceptive alkaloids: structure, synthesis, mechanism of action and prospect. *Curr Top Med Chem*. 2013;13:2134-2170.
68. Vardanyan R, Hruby V. Fentanyl-related compounds and derivatives: current status and future prospects for pharmaceutical applications. *Future Med Chem*. 2014;6:385-412.
69. Vuckovic S, Prostran M, Ivanovic M, et al. Fentanyl analogs: structure-activity relationship study. *Curr Med Chem*. 2009;16:2468-2474.
70. Shen Q, Qian Y, Xu X, et al. Design, synthesis and biological evaluation of N-phenylalkyl-substitutetd tramadol derivaties as novel mu opioid receptor ligands. *Acta Pharmacol Sin*. 2015;36:887-894.
71. Cui X, Yeliseev A, Liu R. Ligand interaction, binding site and G-protein activation of the mu opioid receptor. *Eur J Pharmacol*. 2013;702:309-315.
72. Hudak M. Codeine Pharmacogenetics as a proof of concept for pediatric precision medicine. *Pediatrics*. 2016;138:e320161359.
73. St. Sauver J, Olson J, RogerVL, et al. CYP2D6 phenotypes are associated with adverse outcomes related to opioid medication. *Pharmacogenomics Pers Med*. 2017;10:217-227.
74. Gammal R, Crews K, Haidar C, et al. Pharmacogenetics for safe codeine use in Sickle Cell disease. *Pediatrics*. 2016;138:e20153479.
75. Homsi J, Walsh D, Nelson K. Important drugs for cough in advanced cancer. *Support Care Cancer*. 2001;9:565-574.
76. Voorhorst R, Sparreboom S. Four cases of recurrent pseudo-scarlet fever caused by phenathrene alkaloids with a 6-hydroxy group (codeine and morphine). *Ann Allergy*. 1980;44:116-120.
77. Sheen C, Schleimer R, Kulka M. Codeine induces mast cell chemokine and cytokine production: involvement of G-protein activation. *Allergy*. 2007;62:532-538.
78. Golembiewski J. Opioid-induced pruritus. *J Perianesth Nurs*. 2013;28:247-249.
79. Katcher J, Walsh D. Opioid-induced itching: morphine sulfate and hydromorphone hydrochloride. *J Pain Symptom Manage*. 1999;17:70-72.
80. Drug Bank. Available at https://www.drugbank.ca/. Accessed 9/30/2017.
81. Williams D. pKa values for some drugs and miscellaneous organic acids and bases. In: Lemke T, Williams D, Roche V, et al, eds. *Foye's Principles of Medicinal Chemistry*. 7th ed. Philadelphia: Lippincott Williams & Wilkin; 2103:1469-1477.
82. Nossaman V, Ramadhyani U, Kadowitz P, et al. Advances in perioperative pain: use of medications with dual analgesic mechanisms, tramadol and taptentadol. *Anesthesiology Clin*. 2010;28:647-666.
83. Guay D. Is tapentadol an advantage on tramadol? *Consult Pharm*. 2009;24:833-840.
84. Raffa R, Buschmann H, Christoph T, et al. Mechanistic and functional differentiation of tapentadol and tramadol. *Expert Opin Pharmacother*. 2012;13:1437-1449.
85. Barbosa J, Faria J, Queiros O, et al. Comparative metabolism of tramadol and tapentadol: a toxicological perspective. *Drug Metab Rev*. 2017;48:577-592.
86. Coller JK, Christrup LL, Somogyi AA. Role of active metabolites in the use of opioids. *Eur J Clin Pharmacol*. 2009;65:121-139.
87. Bernard S, Neville K, Nguyen A, et al. Interethnic differences in genetic polymorphisms of CYP2D6 in the U.S. population: clinical implications. *Oncologist*. 2006;11:126-135.
88. Matsui A, Azuma J, Witcher J, et al. Pharmacokinetics, safety and tolerability of atomoxetine and effect of CYP2D6*10/*10 genotype in healthy Japanese men. *J Clin Pharmacol*. 2012;52:388-403.
89. Zhou S-F. Polymorphism of human cytochrome P450 2D6 and its clinical significance. Part 1. *Clin Pharmacokinet*. 2009;48:689-723.
90. Mazák K, Noszál B, Hosztafi S. Physicochemical and pharmacological characterization of permanently charged opioids. *Curr Med Chem*. 2017;24(33):3633-3648.
91. *Drug Facts and Comparisons. Facts & Comparisons [Database Online]*. In: Louis S, ed. MO: Wolters Kluwer Health, Inc.; March 2005.
92. *Lexicomp Online® Lexi-drugs® Hudson*. Ohio: Lexi-Comp, Inc.
93. Sverrisdottir E, Lund T, Olesen A, et al. A review of morphine and morphine-6-glucuronide's pharmacokinetic-pharmacodynamic relationships in experimental and clinical pain. *Eur J Pharm Sci*. 2015;74:45-62.
94. Klimas R, Milus G. Morphine-6-glucuronide is responsible for the analgesic effect after morphine administration: a quantitative review of morphine, morphine-6-glucuronide, and morphine-3-glucuronide. *Br J Anaesth*. 2014;113:935-944.
95. van Dorp E, Morariu A, Dahan A. Morphine-6-glucuronide: potency and safety compared with morphine. *Exp Opin Pharmacother*. 2008;9:1955-1961.
96. van Dorp E, Romberg R, Sarton E, et al. Morphine-6-glucuronide: morphine's successor for postoperative pain relief? *Anesth Analg*. 2006;102:1789-1797.
97. Hand C, Blunnie W, ClaffeyLP, et al. Potential analgesic contribution from morphine-6-glucuronide in CSF. *Lancet*. 1987;2:1207-1208.
98. De Gregori S, De Gregori M, Ranzani G, et al. Morphine metabolism, transport and brain disposition. *Metab Brain Dis*. 2012;27:1-5.
99. Hannah M, Peat S, Knibb A, et al. Disposition of morphine-6-glucuronide and morphine in healthy volunteers. *Br J Anaesth*. 1991;66:103-107.
100. Kou V, Nassisi D. Unstable angina and non-ST segment myocardial infarction: an evidence-based approach to management. *Mt Sinai J Med*. 2006;449-468.
101. Hocker S, Fogelson J, Rabinstein A. Refractory intracranial hypertension due to fentanyl administration following closed head injury. *Front Neurol*. 2013;4.
102. Roberts D, Goralski K, Renton K, et al. Effect of acute inflammatory brain injury on the accumulation of morphine and morphine 3- and 6-glucuronide in the human brain. *Crit Care Med*. 2009;37:2767-2774.
103. New medical devices. *Pharm Therap*. 2015;40:716-774.
104. Saljoughian M. Opioids: allergy vs. pseudoallergy. *US Pharm*. 2006;7:HS-5-HS-9.
105. Palliative Care: Opioid Conversion/Equivalency Table. Stanford School of Medicine. Available at https://palliative.stanford.edu/opioid-conversion/equivalency-table/. Accessed 10/18/17.

106. Cone E, Darwin W, Buchwald W, et al. Oxymorphone metabolism and urinary excretion in human, rat, Guinea pig, rabbit and dog. *Drug Metab Dispos*. 1983;11:446-450.
107. Bao Y, Hou W, Kong X, et al. Hydromorphone for cancer pain. *Cochrane Database Syst Rev*. 2016;10:1-45.
108. Lowe A, Hamilton M, Greenall J, et al. *Can Med Assoc J Open*. 2017;5:E184-E189.
109. Vadivelu N, Chang D, Helander E, et al. Ketorolac, oxymorphone, tapentadol and tramadol: a comprehensive review. *Anesthesiol Clin*. 2017;35:e1-e20.
110. Vadivelu N, Maria M, Jolly S, et al. Clinical applications of oxymorphone. *J Opioid Manag*. 2103;9:439-452.
111. Cicero T, Ellis M, Kasper Z. A tale of 2 ADFs: differences in the effectiveness of abuse-deterrent formations of oxymorphone and oxycodone extended-release drugs. *Pain*. 2016;157.
112. Olkkola K, Kontinen V, Saari T. Does the pharmacology of oxycodone justify its increasing use as an analgesic? *Trends Pharmacol Sci*. 2013;23:206-214.
113. Krashin D, Murinova N, Trescot A. Extended-release hydrocodone – gift or curse? *J Pain Res*. 2013;6:53-57.
114. Madadi P, Amstutz U, Rieder M, et al. Clinical practice guideline: CYP2D6 genotyping for safe and efficacious codeine therapy. *J Popul Ther Clin Pharmacol*. 2013;20:e369-396.
115. Andreassen T, Eftedal I, Kelpstad P, et al. Do CYP2D6 genotypes reflect oxycodone requirements for cancer patients treated for cancer apin? A cross-sectional multi-centre study. *Eur J Clin Pharmacol*. 2012;68:55-64.
116. Gardiner S, Chang A, Marchant J, et al. Codeine versus placebo in chronic cough in children. *Cochrane Database Syst Rev*. 2016;7:1-23.
117. Soloman D, Rassen J, Glynn R, et al. The comparative safety of opioids of nonmalignant pain in older adults. *Arch Intern Med*. 2010;170:1979-1986.
118. Becker W, O'Connor P. The safety concerns of opioid analgesics in the elderly: new data raise new concerns. *Arch Intern Med*. 2010;170:1986-1988.
119. Heel R, Brogden R, Speight T, et al. Buprenorphine: a review of its pharmacological properties and therapeutic efficacy. *Drugs Aging*. 1979;17:81-110.
120. Jasinski D, Pevnick J, Griffith J. Human pharmacology and abuse potential of the analgesic bupenorphine. *Arch Gen Psych*. 1978;35:501-516.
121. Barnwal P, Das S, Mondal S, et al. Probuphine (buprenorphine implant): a promising candidate in opioid dependence. *Ther Adv Psychopharmacol*. 2017;7:119-134.
122. Cote J, Montgomery L. Sublingual buprenorphine as an analgesic in chronic pain: a systematic review. *Pain Med*. 2014;15:1171-1178.
123. Davis M. Twelve reasons for considering buprenorphine as a frontline analgesic in the management of pain. *J Support Oncol*. 2012;10:209-219.
124. Dahan A, Aarts L, Smith T. Incidence, reversal and prevention of opioid-induced respiratory depression. *Anesthesiology*. 2010;112:226-238.
125. Fudala P, Jaffe J, Dax E, et al. Use of buprenorphine in the treatment of opioid addiction II. Physiologic and behavior effects of daily and alternate day administration and abrupt withdrawal. *Clin Pharmacol Ther*. 1990;47:525-534.
126. Gal T. Naloxone reversal of buprenorphine-induced respiratory depression. *Clin Pharmacol Ther*. 1989;66-71.
127. Kobayashi K, Yamamoto T, Chiba K, et al. Human buprenorphine N-dealkylation is catalyzed by cytochrome P450 3A4. *Drug Metab Dispos*. 1998;26:818-821.
128. Berson A, Fau D, Fornacciari R, et al. Mechanisms for experimental buprenorphine hepatotoxicity: major role of mitochondria dysfunction versus metabolic activation. *J Hepatol*. 2001;34:261-269.
129. Raffa R, Haidery M, Huang H-M, et al. The clinical analgesic efficacy of buprenorphine. *J Clin Pharm Ther*. 2014;39:577-583.
130. CADTH. Buprenorphine for chronic pain: a review of the clinical effectiveness. 2017:1-22.
131. Wiffin P, Derry S, Moore T, et al. Buprenorphine for neuropathic pain in adults. *Cochrane Database of Syst Rev*. 2015;9:1-2.
132. Hans G. Buprenorphine – a review of its role in neuropathic pain. *J Opioid Manag*. 2007;3:195-206.
133. Kahan M, Srivastava A, Ordean A, et al. Buprenophine: new treatment of opioid addiction in primary care. *Can Fam Phys*. 2011;57:281-289.
134. Nicholls L, Bragaw L, Ruetsch C. Opioid dependence: treatment and guidelines. *J Manag Care Pharm*. 2010;16:S14-S21.
135. Lofwall M, Walsh S. A review of buprenorphine diversion and misuse: the current evidence base and experiences from around the world. *J Addict Med*. 2014;8:315-326.
136. Murphy S, Fishman P, McPherson S, et al. Determinants of buprenorphine treatment for opioid dependence. *J Subst Abuse Treat*. 2014;46:315-319.
137. DiPaula B, Menachery E. Physician-pharmacist collaborative care model for buprenorphine-maintained opioid-dependent patients. *J Am Pharm Assoc*. 2015;55:187-192.
138. Barnett P. Comparison of costs and utilization among buprenorphine and methadone patients. *Addiction*. 2009;104:982-992.
139. Rasakham K, Liu-Chen L-Y. Sex difference in kappa opioid pharmacology. *Life Sci*. 2011;88:2-16.
140. Vijay A, Wang S, Worhunsky P, et al. PET imaging reveals sex differences in kappa opioid receptor availability in humans, in vivo. *Am J Nucl Med Mol Imaging*. 2016;6:205-214.
141. Gear R, Miaskowski C, Gordon N, et al. Kappa-opioids produce significantly greater analgesia in women than in men. *Nat Med*. 1996;2:1248-1250.
142. Prommer E, Thompson L. Intranasal fentanyl for pain control: current status with a focus on patient considerations. *Patient Prefer Adherence*. 2011;5.
143. Rodriguez D, Urrutia G, Escobar Y, et al. Efficacy and safety of oral or nasal fentanyl for treatment of breakthrough pain in cancer patients: a systematic review. *J Pain Palliat Care Pharmacother*. 2015;29:228-246.
144. Scott L. Fentanyl iontophoretic transdermal system: a review in acute postoperative pain. *Clin Drug Invest*. 2016;36:321-330.
145. Garnock-Jones K. Fentanyl buccal soluble film: a review in breakthrough cancer pain. *Clin Drug Invest*. 2016;36:413-419.
146. Blasco A, Berzosa M, Iranzo V, et al. Update in cancer pain. *Cancer Chemother Rev*. 2009;4:95-109.
147. Durfee S, Messina J, Khankari R. Fentanyl effervescent buccal tablets: enhanced buccal absorption. *Am J Drug Deliv*. 2006;4:1-5.
148. Fontaine M, Latarjet J, Payre J, et al. Feasibility of monomodal analgesia with IV alfentanil during burn dressing changes at bedside (in spontaneously breathing non-intubated patients). *Burns*. 2017;43:337-342.
149. Doi S, Tomohisa M, Uzawa N, et al. Characterization of methadone as a beta-arrestin-biased mu-opoiod receptor agonist. *Molec Pain*. 2016;12:1-9.
150. Kharasch E. Current concepts in methadone metabolism and transport. *Clin Phamacol Drug Devel*. 2017;6:125-134.
151. Elefritz J, Murphy C, Papadimos T, et al. Methadone analgesia in the critically ill. *J Crit Care*. 2016;34:84-88.
152. Moryl N, Tamasdan C, Tarcatu D, et al. A phase I study of D-methadone in patients with chronic pain. *J Opioid Manag*. 2016;12:47-55.
153. Romero J, Baldinger S, Goodman-Meza D, et al. Drug-induced torsades de pointes in an underserved urban population. Methadone: is there therapeutic equipoise. *J Interv Card Electrophysiol*. 2016;45:37-45.
154. Wenjie J, Bies R, Kamden L, et al. Methadone: a substrate and mechanism-based inhibitor of CYP2C19 (Aromatase). *Drug Metab Dispos*. 2010;38:1308-1313.
155. Larson M, Richards T. Quantification of a methadone metabolite (EDDP) in urine: assessment of compliance. *Clin Med Res*. 2009;7:134-141.
156. Grond S, Sablotzki A. Clinical pharmacology of tramadol. *J Pharmacol Exp Ther*. 2004;43:879-923.
157. Beakley B, Kaye A, Kaye A. Tramadol pharmacology, side efects, and serotonin syndrome: a review. *Pain Phys*. 2015;18:395-400.

158. Park S, Wackernah R, Stimmel G. Serotonin syndrome: is it a reason to avoid the use of tramadol with antidepressants? *J Pharm Pract*. 2014;27:71-78.
159. Miotto K, Cho A, Khali M, et al. Trends in tramadol: pharmacology, metabolism and misuse. *Anesth Clin Pharmacol*. 2017;124:44-51.
160. Editors "Weak" opioid analgesics codeine, dihydrocodeine and tramadol: no less risky than morphine. *Prescrire Intern*. 2016;25:45-51.
161. Kirby E, Carson C, Coward R. Tramadol for the management of premature ejaculation: a timely systematic review. *Int J Impot Res*. 2015;27:121-127.
162. Saunders K, Igel L, Aronne L. An update on naltrexone/bupropion extended release in the treatment of obesity. *Expert Opin Pharmacother*. 2016;17:2235-2242.
163. Segal D, Macdonald J, Chande N. Low dose naltrexone for induction of remission in Crohn's disease. *Cochrane Database Syst Rev*. 2014;21:1-21.
164. Ludwig M, Zagon I, McLaughlin P. Serum [Met^5]-enkephalin levels are reduced in multiple sclerosis and restored by low-dose naltrexone. *Exp Biol Med*. 2017;242:1524-1533.
165. Prichard D, Norton C, Bharucha A. Management of opioid-induced constipation. *Br J Nurs*. 2016;25:S4-S11.
166. Garnock-Jones K. Naloxegol: a review of its use in patients with opioid-induced constipation. *Drugs*. 2015;75:419-425.
167. Siemens W, Becker G. Methylnaltrexone for opioid-induced constipation: review and meta-analysis for objective plus subjective efficacy and safety outcomes. *Ther Clin Risk Manag*. 2016;12: 401-412.
168. Bader S, Jaroslawski K, Blum H, et al. Opioid-induced constipation in advanced illness: safety and efficacy of methylnaltrexone bromide. *Clin Med Insights Oncol*. 2011;5:201-211.
169. Baker D. Formulary drug review: Naldemedine. *Hosp Pharm*. 2017;52:464-468.
170. Erowele G. Alvimopan (Entereg), a peripherally acting mu-opioid receptor antagonist for postoperative ileus. *Pharm Therap*. 2008;33:574-583.
171. Xu L-L, Zhou X-Q, Yi P-S, et al. Alvimopan combined with enhanced recovery strategy for managing postoperative ileus after open abdominal surgery: a systematic review and meta-analysis. *J Surg Res*. 2016;203.
172. Niemegeers C, McGuireJL, Heykants J, et al. Dissociation between opiate-like and antidiarrheal activities of antidiarrheal drugs. *J Pharmacol Exp Ther*. 1979;210:327-333.
173. Sadeque A, Wandel C, He H, et al. Increased drug delivery to the brain by P-glycoprotein inhibition. *Clin Pharmacol Ther*. 2000;68:231-237.
174. Akel T, Bekheit S. Loperamide toxicity: "A brief review". *Ann Noninvasive Electrocardiol*. 2017;e12505:1-4.
175. Crowe A, Wong P. Potential roles of P-gp and calcium channels in loperamide and diphenoxylate transport. *Toxicol Appl Pharmacol*. 2003;193:127-137.
176. Baker D. Loperamide: a pharmacological review. *Rev Gastroenterol Disord*. 2007;7(suppl 3):S11-S18.
177. De Luca A, Coupar I. Difenoxin and loperamide: studies on possible mechanisms of intestinal antisecretory action. *Naunyn-Schmiedeberg's Arch Pharmacol*. 1993;347:231-237.
178. Reynolds I, Gould R, Snyder S. Loperamide: blockade of calcium channels as a mechanism for antidiarrheal effects. *J Pharmacol Exp Ther*. 1984;231:628-632.
179. Kim K-A, Chung J, Jung D-H, et al. Identification of cytochrome P450 isoforms involved in the metabolism of loperamide in human liver microsomes. *Eur J Clin Pharmacol*. 2004;60:575-581.
180. Lasoff D, Koh C, Corbett B, et al. Loperamide trends in abuse and misuse over 13 years: 2002-2015. *Pharmacother*. 2017;37:249-253.
181. Salama A, Levin Y, Jha P, et al. Ventricular fibrillation due to overdose of loperamide, the "poor man's methadone". *J Community Hosp Intern Med Perspect*. 2017;7:222-226.
182. Nwagwu C, Sarris C, Tao Y-X, et al. Biomarkers for chronic neuropathic pain and their potential application in spinal cord stimulatin: a review. *Transl Perioper Pain Med*. 2016;1:33-38.
183. CADTH. Diagnostic methods for neuropathic pain: a review of diagnostic accuracy. 2015:1-11.
184. Morgan K, Anghelescu D. A review of adult and pediatric neuropathic pain assessment tools. *Clin J Pan*. 2017;33:844-452.
185. O'Connor A, Dworkin R. Treatment of neuropathic pain: an overview of recent guidelines. *Am J Med*. 2009;122:S22-S32.
186. Finnerup N, Attal N, Haroutounian S, et al. Pharmacotherapy for neuropathic pain in adults: a systematic review and meta-analysis. *Lancet Neurol*. 2015;14:162-173.
187. Kerstman E, Ahn S, Battu S, et al. Neuopathic pain. In: Barnes M, Good D, eds. *Handbook of Clinical Neurology*. Vol. 110. Amsterdam, The Netherlands: Elsevier BV; 2013:175-187.
188. Mendlik M, Uritsky T. Treatment of neuropathic pain. *Curr Treat Options Neurol*. 2015;17.
189. Binder A, Baron R. The pharmacological therapy of chronic neuropathic pain. *Dtsch Arztebl Int*. 2016;113:616-626.
190. Rolsted K, Benfeldt E, Kissmeyer A-M, et al. Cutaneous in vivo metabolism of topical lidocaine formulation in human skin. *Skin Pharmacol Physiol*. 2009;22:124-127.
191. Stewart W, Lipton R, Celentano D, et al. Prevalence of migrane headache in the United States. Relation to age, income, race, and other sociodemographic factors. *J Am Med Assoc*. 1992;267:64-69.
192. Burch R, Loder S, Loder E, et al. The prevalence and burden of migraine and severe headache in the United States: updated statistics from government health surveillance studies. *Headache*. 2015;55:21-34.
193. Antonaci F, Ghiotto N, Wu S, et al. Recent advances in migraine therapy. *Springerplus*. 2016;5:673-686.
194. Mehrotra S, Gupta S, Chan K, et al. Current and prospective pharmacological targets in relation to antimigraine action. *Naunyn-Schmiedelbergs Arch Pharmacol*. 2008;378:371-394.
195. Weatherall M. The diagnosis and treatment of chronic migraine. *Ther Adv Chronic Dis*. 2015;6:115-123.
196. Dodick D, Martin V. Triptans and CNS side effects: pharmacokinetic and metabolic mechanisms. *Cephalalgia*. 2004;24:417-424.
197. Goadsby P. Post-triptan era for the treatment of acute migraine. *Curr Pain Headache Rep*. 2004;8:393-398.
198. Rapoport A, Bigal M. Migraine preventative therapy: current and emerging treatment options. *Neurol Sci*. 2005;26:S111-S120.
199. Jhee S, Shiovitz T, Crawford A, et al. Pharmacokinetics and pharmacodynamics of the triptan antimigraine agents. *Clin Pharmacokinet*. 2001;40:189-205.
200. Bigal M, Ferrari M, Silberstein S, et al. Migraine in the triptan era: lessons from epidemiology, pathophysiology and clinical sciences. *Headache*. 2009;49:S21-S33.
201. Messali A, Yang M, Gillard P, et al. Treatment persistence and switching in triptan users: a systematic literature review. *Headache*. 2014;54:1120-1130.
202. Rapoport A, Tepper S, Sheftell F, et al. Which triptan for which patient? *Neurol Sci*. 2006;27:S123-S129.
203. Johnson M, Fernandez F, Colson N, et al. A pharmacogenomic evaluation of migraine therapy. *Exp Opin Pharmacother*. 2007;8:1821-1835.
204. Vyas K, Halpin R, Geer L. Disposition and pharmacokinetics of the antimigraine drug, rizatriptan, in humans. *Drug Metab Dispos*. 2000;28:89-95.
205. Buchan P, Keywood C, Wade A, et al. Clinical pharmacokinetics of frovatriptan. *Headache*. 2002;42(suppl 2):S54-S62.
206. Wild M, McKillop D, Butters C. Determination of the human cytochrome P450 isoforms involved in the metabolism of zolmitriptan. *Xenobiotica*. 1999;29:847-857.
207. Dixon C, Park G, Tarbit M. Characterization of the enzyme responsible for the metabolism of sumtriptan in human liver. *Biochem Pharmacol*. 1994;47:1253-1257.
208. Yu A-M. Indolealkylamines: biotransformations and potential drug-drug interactions. *AAPS J*. 2008;10:242-253.
209. Evans D, O'Connor D, Lake B, et al. Eletriptan metabolism by human hepatic CYP450 enzymes and transport by human P-glycoprotein. *Drug Metab Dispos*. 2003;31:861-869.

210. Salva M, Jansat J, Martinez-Tobed A, et al. Identification of human liver enzymes involved in the metabolism of the antimigraine agent almotriptan. *Drug Metab Dispos*. 2003;31:404-411.
211. Bigal M, Krymchantowski A, Ho T. Migraine in the tripan era. *Arq Neuropsiquiatr*. 2009;67:559-569.
212. Rapoport A, Tepper S, Bigal M, et al. The triptan formulations: how to match patients and products. *CNS Drugs*. 2003;17:431-447.
213. Hutchingson S, Marmura M, Calhoun A, et al. Use of common migraine treatments in breast-feeding women: a summary of recommendations. *Headache*. 2013;53:614-627.

Structure Challenge Answers

A-8, B-3, C-10, D-6, E-9, F-4, G-1, H-7.

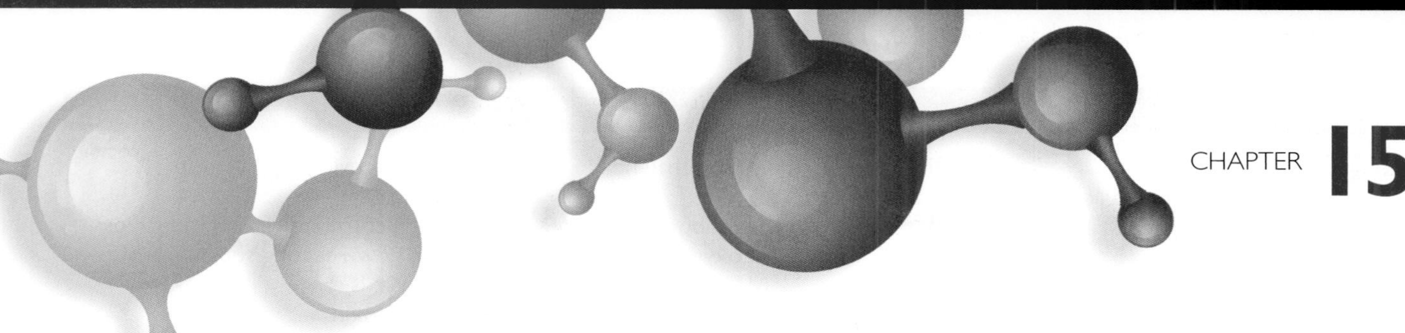

CHAPTER 15

Drugs Used to Treat Pain: Peripherally Acting Agents

E. Jeffrey North

Drugs covered in this chapter:

ANTIPYRETIC ANALGESICS
- Acetaminophen

ANTI-INFLAMMATORY ANALGESICS
- Aspirin and other salicylates
- Bromfenac
- Diclofenac
- Diflunisal
- Etodolac
- Fenoprofen
- Flurbiprofen
- Ibuprofen
- Indomethacin
- Ketoprofen
- Ketorolac
- Meclofenamic acid
- Mefenamic acid
- Meloxicam
- Nabumetone
- Naproxen
- Nepafenac
- Oxaprozin
- Piroxicam
- Sulindac
- Tolmetin

COX-2 INHIBITORS
- Celecoxib

MONOCLONAL ANTIBODIES FOR RHEUMATOID ARTHRITIS
- Adalimumab
- Basiliximab
- Brodalumab
- Canakinumab
- Certolizumab
- Golimumab
- Infliximab
- Ixekizumab
- Reslizumab
- Rilonacept
- Rituximab
- Secukinumab
- Siltuximab
- Tocilizumab
- Ustekinumab
- Vedolizumab

DISEASE-MODIFYING DRUGS FOR ARTHRITIS
- Abatacept
- Apremilast
- Anakinra
- Etanercept
- Gold salts
- Hydroxychloroquine
- Leflunomide
- Methotrexate
- Sulfasalazine

DRUGS FOR THE TREATMENT OF GOUT
- Allopurinol
- Colchicine
- Lesinurad
- Febuxostat
- Pegloticase
- Probenecid

LOCAL ANESTHETICS
- Articaine
- Benzocaine
- Bupivacaine
- Chloroprocaine
- Dibucaine
- Mepivacaine
- Lidocaine
- Prilocaine
- Procaine
- Ropivacaine
- Tetracaine

Abbreviations

APC antigen-presenting cell
5-ASA 5-aminosalicylic acid
AUC area under the plasma concentration curve
BTX batrachotoxin
CHO Chinese hamster ovary
C_{max} maximum plasma concentration
C_{min} minimum plasma concentration
CNS central nervous system
COX cyclooxygenase
CTLA-4 cytotoxic T-lymphocyte antigen-4
CYP cytochrome P450
DAG diacylglycerol
DMARD disease-modifying antirheumatic drug
ED_{50} median effective dose
EEG electroencephalograph
EMLA Eutectic Mixture of a Local Anesthetic
FAAH fatty acid amide hydrolase
FDA U.S. Food and Drug Administration
GABA γ-aminobutyric acid

Abbreviations—Continued

GI gastrointestinal
GPCR G protein–coupled receptor
HPETE hydroperoxy-eicosatetraenoic acid
IC_{90} 90% of maximal inhibitory concentration
ID_{50} half maximal inhibitory concentration
Ig immunoglobulin
IL interleukin
IM intramuscular
IV intravenous
JAK Janus-activated kinase
LT leukotriene
6MNA 6-methoxynaphthalene-2-acetic acid
MAb monoclonal antibody
mPEG monomethoxypoly(ethylene glycol)
Na/K-ATPase sodium-potassium adenosine triphosphatase
NO nitric oxide
NMDA N-methyl-D-aspartate
NF-κB nuclear factor-κB
NSAID nonsteroidal anti-inflammatory drug
OTC over the counter
PABA *p*-aminobenzoic acid
PCP phencyclidine
PEG polyethylene glycol
PG prostaglandin
SAR structure-activity relationships
SRS-A slow-reacting substance of anaphylaxis
STX saxitoxin
TTX tetrodotoxin
T_{max} time to maximum serum concentration
TNF tumor necrosis factor
TNFR tumor necrosis factor receptor
TX thromboxane
UMP uridine monophosphate

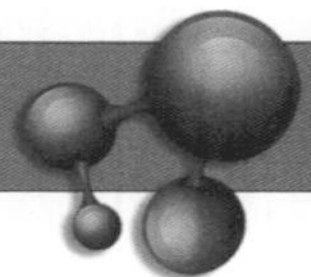

CLINICAL SIGNIFICANCE

Amy M. Pick, PharmD, BCOP

The nonsteroidal anti-inflammatory drugs (NSAIDs) are one of the oldest and most widely utilized classes of medications. Both prescription and over-the-counter NSAIDs are commercially available and are frequently used in the treatment of pain, fever, and inflammation. While NSAIDs are a chemically heterogeneous class of drugs, they share a similar mechanism of action by inhibiting the cyclooxygenase (COX) enzymes responsible for prostaglandin synthesis in the arachidonic acid pathway. There are at least three recognized COX isoforms, with the inhibition of COX-1 and COX-2 being clinically relevant. Most NSAIDs are nonselective and inhibit varying degrees of COX-1 and COX-2. However, many newer NSAIDs predominantly inhibit the COX-2 isoenzyme with celecoxib being the only commercially available COX-2 selective inhibitor.

Changes in the NSAIDs' molecular structure can affect the ratio of COX-1 to COX-2 inhibition, clinical response, and adverse effect profile. Although NSAIDs are commonly prescribed medications, as a class they are associated with serious adverse effects including gastrointestinal bleeding, cardiovascular events, and nephrotoxicity. The inhibition of COX-1 affects gastric prostaglandin synthesis and thromboxane formation by platelets, increasing the risk of gastrointestinal bleeds. The COX-2 selective inhibitors were developed to reduce the GI adverse effects by avoiding COX-1 inhibition. The inhibition of COX-2, however, may affect renal physiology and increase cardiovascular disease without concomitant COX-1 inhibition. Patients should be instructed to use the lowest effective dose and shortest duration to reduce the likelihood of experiencing an adverse event.

The clinician should be mindful of clinically significant drug-drug interactions (DDIs) with NSAIDs. Concomitant administration of low-dose aspirin and other reversibly acting NSAIDs may negate the structure-dependent irreversible antiplatelet effects of aspirin when used for cardiovascular protection. Clinicians should recommend a change in medications or give low-dose aspirin 2 hours prior to other NSAIDs. NSAIDs in combination with selective serotonin-reuptake inhibitors (SSRIs) may increase the risk of bleeding and gastrointestinal effects. NSAIDs may attenuate the antihypertensive effects of diuretics, angiotensin-converting enzymes inhibitors (ACE-inhibitors), and angiotensin receptor blockers (ARBs) or may worsen or cause patients to develop renal failure. Practitioners should assess the risk of DDI's adverse effect reactions for all over-the-counter and prescription NSAIDs.

NSAIDs will continue to remain an important class of drugs in the management of pain, fever, and inflammation. An understanding of the chemical features underlying the pharmacokinetic and pharmacodynamic variability of these drugs will allow clinicians to select the best NSAID for the patient.

INTRODUCTION

Pain management is an essential part of a health care team's responsibility for patient well-being in operative, postoperative, emergency, and acute and chronic disease situations (see Chapter 14 for an overview of pain and its management). Chemotherapeutic pain relief can occur through central (Chapter 14) or peripheral mechanisms of action. This chapter will focus on drugs that elicit pain relief in the periphery. These drugs include antipyretic analgesics, nonsteroidal anti-inflammatory drugs (NSAIDs), small molecule and monoclonal antibody (MAb) therapies for rheumatoid arthritis, and local anesthetic agents.

INFLAMMATION

Inflammation is a normal and essential response to any noxious stimulus that threatens the host and can vary from a localized to a generalized response.[1] One of the primary mechanisms for an inflammatory event is the release of proinflammatory chemical mediators (e.g., histamine, serotonin, leucokinins, slow-reacting substance of anaphylaxis [SRS-A], lysosomal enzymes, lymphokinins, and prostaglandins [PGs]). The most common sources of these chemical mediators include neutrophils, basophils, mast cells, platelets, macrophages, and lymphocytes. Currently available drugs relieve the painful symptoms of the disease but are not considered curative.

The anti-inflammatory drugs discussed in this chapter act by modulating any one of several mechanisms, including immunologic processes, activation of complement system, cellular activities such as phagocytosis, interference with the formation and release of the chemical mediators of inflammation, or stabilization of lysosomal membranes.

Role of Chemical Mediators in Inflammation

As indicated previously, a number of chemical mediators have been postulated to have important roles in the inflammatory process. Before 1971, the proposal by T.Y. Shen that the NSAIDs exert their effects by interacting with a hypothetical anti-inflammatory receptor was widely accepted.[2,3]

In 1971, J.R. Vane published a classic paper in which he reported that some NSAIDs, including aspirin, inhibited the biosynthesis of PGs from arachidonic acid.[4] This theory has become the most widely accepted mechanism of action of NSAIDs. Vane's hypothesis was subsequently modified, and it was proposed that the earlier anti-inflammatory receptor model actually described the active site of the key enzyme in PG biosynthesis (i.e., PG cyclooxygenase).[5]

Prostaglandins, Thromboxanes, Prostacyclin, and Leukotrienes

PROSTAGLANDINS. PGs are eicosanoids which are a group of autocoids that also include thromboxanes, prostacyclin, and leukotrienes. PGs are naturally occurring products produced in mammalian tissue. They are found throughout the body and, through the activation of specific G protein–coupled receptors (GPCRs), possess many pharmacological properties impacting the cardiovascular system, platelets, inflammation, smooth muscle, central nervous system, and endocrine system. As we will see later, the inhibition of PG biosynthesis is the primary mechanism of NSAID-mediated anti-inflammatory activity.

Prostaglandin Structure. PGs are 20-carbon cyclopentano-fatty acid derivatives produced from polyunsaturated fatty acids. The general structure of the PGs is shown in Figure 15.1. All naturally occurring PGs have a 15α-hydroxy group and a *trans* double bond at C13. The chain containing the carboxylic acid group is the α-chain, and the chain substituted with the 15α-hydroxyl group is

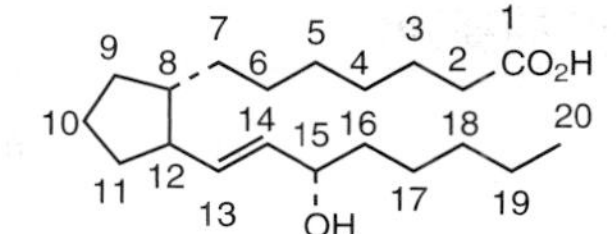

Figure 15.1 General structure of the prostaglandins.

labeled the β-chain. The PGs are classified by the capital letters A, B, C, D, E, F, G, H, and I (e.g., PGA, PGB, PGC) depending on the nature and stereochemistry of oxygen substituents at the 9- and 11-positions. For example, members of the PGE series possess a keto function at C9 and an α-hydroxy group at C11, whereas members of the PGF series possess α-hydroxy groups at both of these positions. The number of double bonds in the side chains connected to the cyclopentane ring is designated by subscripts 1, 2, or 3. The subscript 2 indicates an additional *cis* double bond between C5 and C6 and the subscript 3 indicates a third double bond (C17-18) of *cis* stereochemistry. Members of the PGG and PGH series are cycloendoperoxide intermediates in the biosynthesis of PGs and contain a peroxide group bridging the C9 and C11 carbons as depicted in Figure 15.2.

Prostaglandin Biosynthesis. PGs are derived biosynthetically from unsaturated fatty acid precursors (Fig. 15.2). The number of double bonds contained in the naturally occurring PGs reflects the nature of the biosynthetic precursors. The most common of these fatty acids in humans is arachidonic acid which is derived from dietary linoleic acid or is ingested from the diet and esterified to phospholipids (primarily phosphatidylethanolamine or phosphatidylcholine) in cell membranes.[6]

The primary source of arachidonic acid is stored as acyl chains in membrane glycerophospholipids. Liberation of free arachidonic acid can occur through a variety of enzymatic reactions (Fig. 15.2). When activated by various initiating factors that interact with membrane receptors coupled to guanine nucleotide–binding regulatory proteins (G proteins; see Chapter 6), phospholipase A2 catalyzes the hydrolysis of the two acyl chains from the glycerol backbone of the phospholipid. Other phospholipases (e.g., phospholipase C [PLC]) also play a role. PLC hydrolyzes the phosphodiester bond forming 1,2-diacylglycerides from phospholipids with the subsequent release of arachidonic acid by the actions of mono- and diacylglyceride lipases.[7] An inflammation-mediating polypeptide produced by leukocytes, interleukin-1, increases phospholipase activity and, thus, arachidonic acid release.

Once arachidonic acid is released, arachidonic acid cyclooxygenase (PG endoperoxide synthase, COX) produces PGs, along with thromboxanes and prostacyclin. Alternatively, arachidonic acid is susceptible to lipoxygenase activity to produce leukotrienes.

Cyclooxygenases. Cyclooxygenase (COX) in the presence of oxygen and heme first produces the cyclic endoperoxide PGG_2 from arachidonic acid, and then, through its peroxidase activity, PGH_2. Both PGG_2 and PGH_2 are chemically unstable due to the reactive peroxide group and decompose rapidly (half-life of 5 min) to generate more persistent PGs (Fig. 15.2). PGE_2 is a proinflammatory

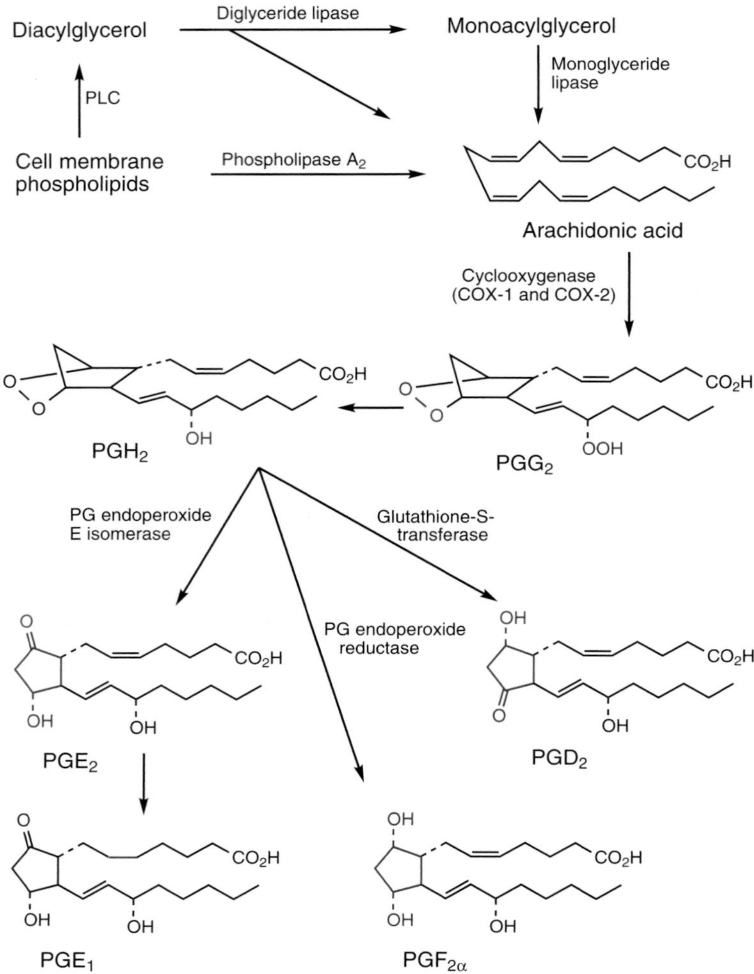

Figure 15.2 Biosynthesis of prostaglandins from arachidonic acid.

PG formed by the action of PGE isomerase and PGD_2 by the actions of isomerases or glutathione-S-transferase on PGH_2, whereas proinflammatory $PGF_{2\alpha}$ is formed from PGH_2 via an endoperoxide reductase system (Fig. 15.2). Interestingly, PGE_1 is a reduced form of PGE_2 and possesses GI cytoprotective properties (discussed further below in the Prostaglandin Effects on Gastrointestinal Tract section). The biological target for NSAIDs is COX, where they inhibit PG biosynthesis to prevent inflammation.

Three isoforms of COX have been identified: COX-1, COX-2, and COX-3. COX was first purified in 1976.[8] Interestingly, COX-2 expression is inducible by cytokines and growth factors.[9-13] Attenuated COX-1 proteins have been identified; however, their clinical impact is yet to be determined.[14] The primary mechanism by which NSAIDS are believed to produce their pharmacologic effects is attributed to inhibition of the COX-1 and COX-2 enzymes. Both isoforms carry out the same two reactions in the PG biosynthetic pathway: the double dioxygenation of arachidonic acid to PGG_2 at the cyclooxygenase active site and the subsequent reduction to PGH_2 at the peroxidase site.[15] Analgesic/antipyretic drugs selectively target COX-3; thus inhibition of COX-3 can represent a primary mechanism by which acetaminophen decreases pain and fever.[14]

Both human COX-1 and COX-2 are quite similar in structure and almost identical in length, varying from 599 (COX-1) to 604 (COX-2) amino acids.[16,17] Both isoforms possess molecular masses of 70-74 kDa and contain just over 600 amino acids, with an approximately 60% homology within the same species.[18,19] The active site cavities of COX-1 and COX-2 are illustrated in Figure 15.3.[17] Residues that form the substrate binding and catalytic sites, and residues immediately adjacent to those sites, are essentially identical with two minor (but very important) exceptions. The Ile at positions 434 and 523 in COX-1 is exchanged for Val in COX-2. The smaller size of Val434 and Val523 in COX-2 allows inhibitor access to an allosteric pocket adjacent to the active site, whereas the longer side chain of Ile in COX-1 sterically blocks inhibitor access. The available space in the binding pocket of COX-2 is 20%-25% larger than that of the COX-1 binding site because of the replacement of the smaller Val434 and Val523 residues in COX-2 for the larger Ile434 and Ile523 residues in COX-1 and, thus, is the basis for COX-2 selectivity. Large inhibitors that utilize this extra space are essentially too big to fit in the COX-1 site, making them COX-2 selective.

COX-2 lacks a sequence of 17 amino acids at the N-terminus and has an additional 18 amino acids at the

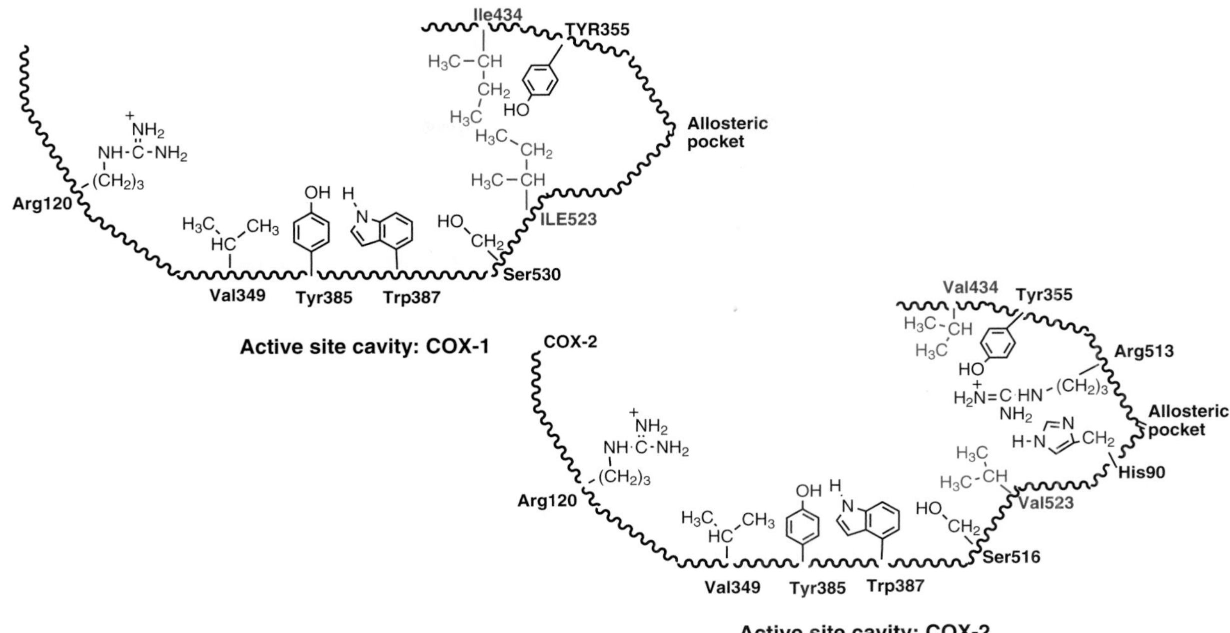

Figure 15.3 **Representations of COX-1 and COX-2 active sites.** Reprinted from Roche VF. A receptor-grounded approach to teaching nonsteroidal anti-inflammatory drug chemistry and structure-activity relationships. *Am J Pharm Educ.* 2009;73(8):143, with permission.

C-terminus. The sequence differences cause a disparity in the numbering systems of the two isoforms such that the Ser residue essential for aspirin's irreversible action in COX-1 is Ser530, whereas in COX-2, the equivalent Ser residue is Ser516 (COX inhibition by aspirin is discussed in detail below).

From a therapeutic standpoint, the major difference between COX-1 and COX-2 lies in physiologic function rather than in structure. Little COX-2 is present in resting cells, but its expression can be induced at sites of inflammation by cytokines in vascular smooth muscle, fibroblasts, and epithelial cells. COX-1 functions to produce PGs that are involved in normal homeostatic cellular activity, and COX-2 produces PGs at inflammatory sites.[20] Inducible COX-2 linked to inflammatory cell types and tissues is believed to be the target enzyme in the treatment of inflammatory disorders by NSAIDs. Most NSAIDs inhibit both COX-1 and COX-2 with varying degrees of selectivity and are termed nonselective. Selective COX-2 inhibitors can attenuate (but not eliminate) COX-1–related adverse effects commonly associated with NSAIDs, such as gastric and renal effects.

Prostaglandin Effects on Gastrointestinal Tract. One of the primary adverse effects of nonselective NSAIDs is GI disturbances, which is due to the reduction of specific PGs in the GI tract. Some PGs appear to have a major cytoprotective role in maintaining the integrity of gastric mucosa. More specifically, PGE_1 exerts a protective effect on gastroduodenal mucosa by stimulating secretion of an alkaline mucus and bicarbonate ion and by maintaining or increasing mucosal blood flow. Interestingly, PGE_1 production in the GI tract is primarily mediated through COX-1. Thus, inhibition of PG biosynthesis in the GI tract is unfavorable because it can cause disruption of mucosal integrity, resulting in GI distress including peptic ulcer disease that is commonly associated with the use of NSAIDs.

Prostanoid Receptors. The existence of distinct PG receptors can explain the broad spectrum of action displayed by the PGs.[21,22] PGs exert their various effects by activating GPCRs. Ten members of the prostanoid receptor family have been identified (DP1-2, EP1-4, FP, IP1-2, and TP). The nomenclature of these receptors is based on the affinity displayed by natural PGs, prostacyclin, or thromboxanes at each receptor type. Thus, EP receptors are those receptors for which the PGEs have high affinity, FP receptors are those for PGFs, DP receptors are those for PGDs, IP receptors are those for PGI2, and TP receptors are those for thromboxane (TX) A2. These receptors are coupled through G proteins to effector mechanisms that include stimulation of adenylyl cyclase and, thus increased cyclic adenosine monophosphate (cAMP) levels and phospholipase C, which results in increased levels of intracellular inositol-1,4,5-triphosphate (IP_3) and diacylglycerol (DAG) in the membrane. Three distinct receptors for leukotrienes have been identified as well.

Nonprostanoid Products of the Arachidonic Acid Pathway

Thromboxane and Prostacyclin. In addition to forming the various PGs, nonprostanoids can also be formed from PGH_2, as illustrated in Figure 15.4. Thromboxane synthase acts on PGH_2 to produce TXA_2, whereas prostacyclin synthase converts PGH_2 to prostacyclin (PGI_2), both of which possess short biologic half-lives. A potent vasoconstrictor and inducer of platelet aggregation, TXA_2 has a biologic half-life of approximately 30 seconds, being rapidly and nonenzymatically converted to the more stable, but inactive, TXB_2. Prostacyclin, a potent hypotensive and

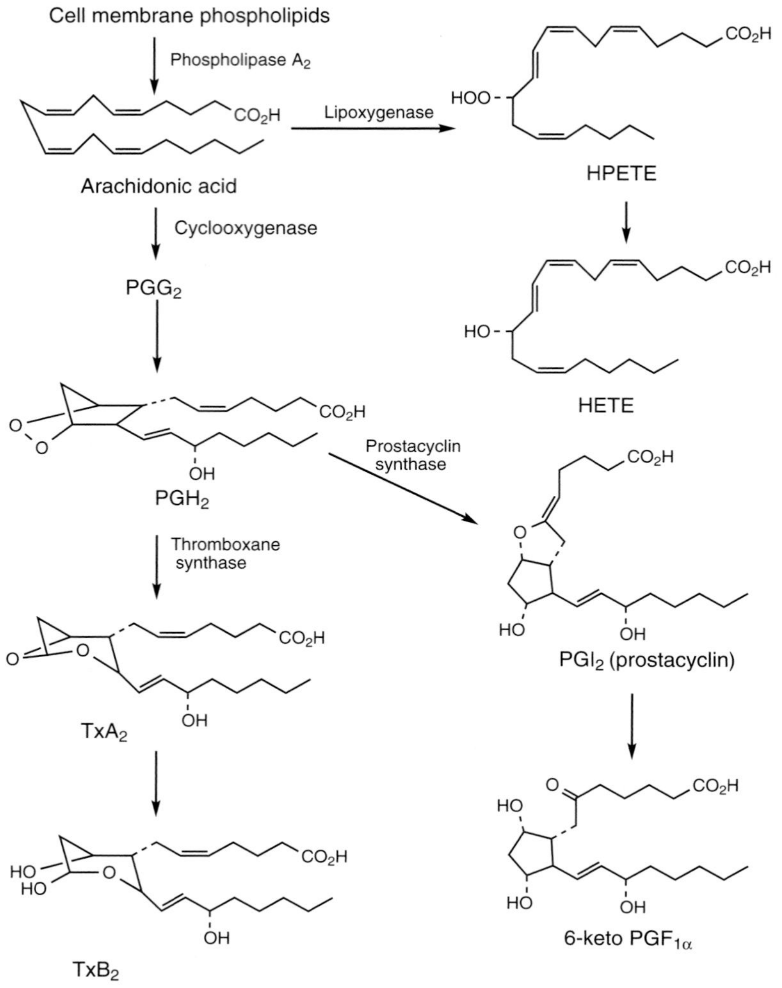

Figure 15.4 Biosynthesis of thromboxanes, prostacyclin, and leukotrienes.

inhibitor of platelet aggregation, has a half-life of approximately 3 minutes and is nonenzymatically converted to 6-keto-$PGF_{1\alpha}$. Platelets contain primarily thromboxane synthase, whereas endothelial cells contain primarily prostacyclin synthase. Considerable research efforts are being expended in the development of stable prostacyclin analogues and thromboxane antagonists as cardiovascular drugs. The pharmacologic effects of some PGs, TXA_2, and prostacyclin are summarized in Table 15.1.

Leukotrienes. Upon NSAID therapy, where COX enzymes are inhibited, arachidonic acid is now forced to be metabolized by lipoxygenase enzymes. Lipoxygenases are a group of enzymes that oxidize polyunsaturated fatty acids possessing two *cis* double bonds separated by a methylene group to produce lipid hydroperoxides.[23] Arachidonic acid is thus metabolized by lipoxygenase enzymes to a number of hydroperoxy-eicosatetraenoic acid (HPETE) derivatives. Lipoxygenases differ in the position at which they peroxidize arachidonic acid and in their tissue specificity. For example, platelets possess only a 12-lipoxygenase, whereas leukocytes possess both a 12-lipoxygenase and a 5-lipoxygenase.[24] Leukotrienes are products of the 5-lipoxygenase pathway and are divided into two major classes: hydroxylated eicosatetraenoic acids (LTs), represented by

Table 15.1 Pharmacologic Properties of Prostaglandins, Thromboxane, and Prostacyclin

	PGE_2	$PGF_{2\alpha}$	PGI_2	TXA_2
Uterus	Oxytocic dilation	Oxytocic constriction		
Bronchi	Dilation	Constriction		Constriction
Platelets			Proaggregatory	Antiaggregatory
Blood vessels	Dilation	Constriction	Dilation	Constriction

LTB_4, and peptidoleukotrienes (pLTs), such as LTC_4, LTD_4, and LTE_4. 5-Lipoxygenase will produce leukotrienes from 5-HPETE, as shown in Figure 15.5.

LTA synthase converts 5-HPETE to an unstable epoxide called LTA4 that can be converted by LTA hydrolase to the leukotriene LTB_4 or by glutathione-S-transferase to LTC_4. Other cysteinyl leukotrienes (e.g., LTD_4, LTE_4, and LTF_4) can then be formed from LTC_4 by the removal of glutamic acid and glycine and then reconjugated with glutamic acid. The cysteinyl leukotrienes produce airway edema, smooth muscle constriction, and altered cellular activity associated with the inflammatory process, all of which are associated with the pathophysiology of asthma (Chapter 28). Cysteinyl leukotrienes activate at least two receptors, designated as CysLT1 and CysLT2. A long-recognized mediator of inflammation, SRS-A, is primarily a mixture of leukotrienes LTC_4 and LTD_4.

The physiological role of LTB_4 is a potent chemotactic agent for polymorphonuclear leukocytes, causing the accumulation of leukocytes at inflammation sites.[25] Both LTC_4 and LTD_4 are potent hypotensives and bronchoconstrictors and are the leukotrienes responsible for NSAID-induced asthmatic responses.

General GI Considerations for NSAID Therapy

NSAIDs do have some use-limiting adverse effects including GI, renal, and cardiovascular toxicities. However, GI toxicity remains the most common adverse effect observed with chronic NSAID users. GI toxicities include dyspepsia, abdominal pain, heartburn, gastric erosion leading to wall perforation, peptic ulcer formation, bleeding, and diarrhea. These gastric ailments are attributed to one or two arms of the dual insult mechanism (Fig. 15.6). Nearly all NSAIDs are weak acids with pK_a values of approximately 3, making them poorly soluble in gastric fluid, which has a pH of ~1.5. The primary insult is committed when pieces of insoluble NSAID lodge in gastric mucosa, resulting in direct tissue damage. The secondary insult is committed through reduction in cytoprotective PG concentrations in the GI tract, which is primarily mediated through COX-1 inhibition. The secondary insult is a significant reason for the development of COX-2 selective inhibitors; however, they are accompanied by significant cardiotoxic liabilities (discussed below).

Arachidonic acid → (5-Lipoxygenase) → 5-HPETE → (LTA synthetase) → LTA_4 → (LTA hydrolase) → LTB_4; LTA_4 → (Glutathione-S-transferase) → LTC_4, LTD_4, LTE_4, or LTF_4

Figure 15.5 Biosynthesis of leukotrienes.

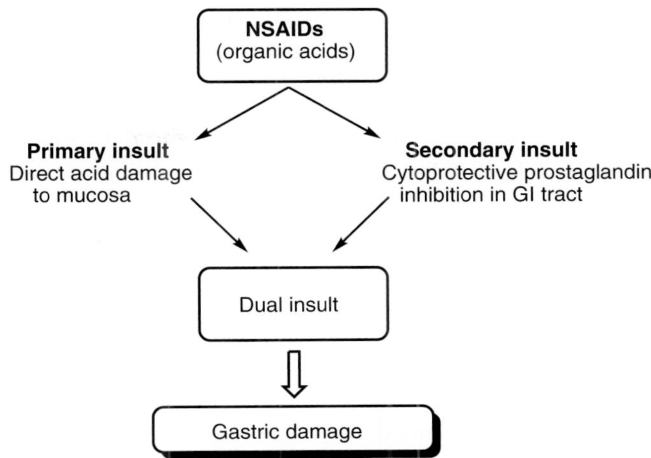

Figure 15.6 NSAID-induced production of gastric damage by a dual-insult mechanism.

Therapeutic Classifications

Antipyretic Analgesics

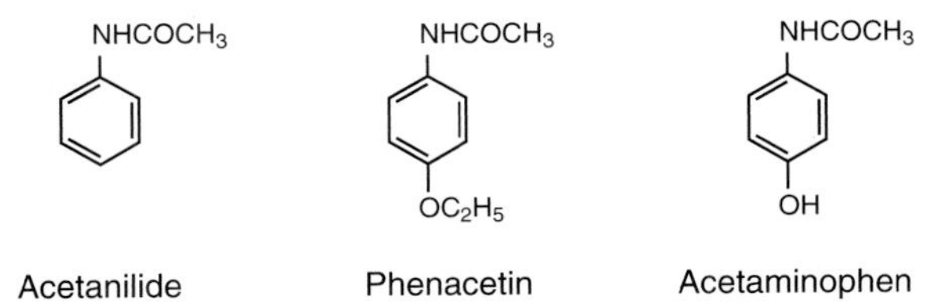

Mechanism of Action

Drugs included in this class possess analgesic and antipyretic actions but lack anti-inflammatory effects. Antipyretics interfere with pyrogenic factors that produce fever, but they do not appear to lower body temperature in afebrile subjects. It had been historically accepted that the antipyretics exert their actions within the central nervous system (CNS), primarily at the hypothalamic thermoregulatory center. Endogenous leukocytic pyrogens can be released from cells that have been activated by various stimuli, and antipyretics can act by (1) inhibiting the activation of these cells by an exogenous pyrogen or (2) inhibiting the release of endogenous leukocytic pyrogens from the cells once they have been activated by the exogenous pyrogen. Substantial evidence exists suggesting a central antipyretic mechanism, an antagonism that can result from either a direct competition of a pyrogen and the antipyretic agent at CNS receptors or an inhibition of PG synthesis in the CNS.[26,27]

Despite the extensive use of acetaminophen, the mechanism of action is not fully clear.[28] Acetaminophen can inhibit pain impulses by exerting a depressant effect on peripheral receptors, and an antagonistic effect on the actions of bradykinin can also play a role. The antipyretic effects might not result from inhibition of release of endogenous pyrogen from leukocytes but, rather, from inhibiting its action on hypothalamic thermoregulatory centers. As noted earlier, the fact that acetaminophen is an effective antipyretic/analgesic, but an ineffective anti-inflammatory agent, may be explained by its greater inhibition of PG biosynthesis via inhibition of the COX-3 isoform (a splice variant of COX-1) in the CNS compared with that in the periphery.

The ability of selected analgesic/antipyretic drugs to inhibit COX-1, COX-2, and COX-3 is shown in Table 15.2.[14]

Structure-Activity Relationships

The structure-activity relationships of *p*-aminophenol derivatives have been widely studied. Based on the comparative toxicity of acetanilide and acetaminophen, aminophenols are less toxic than the corresponding aniline derivatives, although *p*-aminophenol itself is too toxic for therapeutic purposes. Etherification of the phenolic function with methyl or propyl groups produces derivatives with more side effects than ethyl groups. Substituents on the nitrogen atom that reduce basicity reduce activity unless that substituent is metabolically labile (e.g., acetyl). Amides derived from aromatic acids (e.g., N-phenylbenzamide) are less active or inactive.

Acetaminophen

Acetaminophen is indicated for use as an antipyretic/analgesic and may be particularly useful in individuals displaying an allergy or sensitivity to aspirin. It is weakly acidic (phenolic $pK_a = 9.51$) and not extensively bound to plasma proteins (18%-25%).[29] It does not possess anti-inflammatory activity; however, it will produce analgesia in a wide variety of arthritic and musculoskeletal disorders. It is available in various formulations, including suppositories, tablets, capsules, granules, and solutions. The usual adult dose is 325-650 mg every 4-6 hours. Doses greater than 2.6 g/d are not recommended for long-term therapy because of potential hepatotoxicity. Acetaminophen, unlike aspirin, is stable in aqueous solution, making liquid formulations readily available, which is particularly advantageous in pediatric patients. Because acetaminophen is water insoluble, liquid formulations are prepared with solvents such as propylene glycol to keep acetaminophen in solution; otherwise, the formulation is administered as a suspension.

Table 15.2 Potency (IC_{50}, μM) of Selected NSAIDs for the COX Enzymes

Drug	COX-1	COX-2	COX-3
Acetaminophen	>1,000	>1,000	460
Phenacetin	>1,000	>1,000	102
Aspirin	10	>1,000	3.1
Diclofenac	0.035	0.041	0.008
Ibuprofen	2.4	5.7	0.24
Indomethacin	0.010	0.66	0.016

METABOLISM AND TOXICITY. The metabolism of acetaminophen is illustrated in Figure 15.7.[30] Both acetanilide and phenacetin are metabolized to acetaminophen. Additionally, both undergo hydrolysis to yield aniline derivatives that produce significant methemoglobinemia and hemolytic anemia (either directly or through conversion to hydroxylamines), which resulted in their removal from the US market. Acetaminophen undergoes rapid first-pass metabolism in the GI tract primarily by conjugation reactions, with the O-sulfate being the primary metabolite in children and the O-glucuronide being the primary metabolite in adults.

It has been known for more than 40 years that CYP450-mediated metabolism is responsible for the hepatotoxicity of acetaminophen.[31] A minor, but significant, product of acetaminophen is N-hydroxyamide produced by CYP2E1 and CYP3A4.[32] CYP2E1 is the rate-limiting enzyme that initiates the cascade of events leading to acetaminophen hepatotoxicity; in the absence of this enzyme toxicity will only be apparent at high concentrations.[32] The N-hydroxyamide metabolite is converted to a reactive toxic metabolite, an acetimidoquinone (N-acetyl-*p*-benzoquinoneimine, or NAPQI) that has been suggested to produce the nephrotoxicity and hepatotoxicity associated with acetaminophen and phenacetin.[33,34] Normally, this iminoquinone is detoxified by conjugation with hepatic glutathione. In cases of ingestion of large doses or overdoses of acetaminophen, however, hepatic stores of glutathione can be depleted by more than 70%, allowing the electrophilic quinone to react with nearby nucleophilic functional groups, primarily thiol (-SH) groups, on hepatic proteins, resulting in the formation of covalent adducts that produce hepatic necrosis. Both CYP2E1 and CYP3A4 are induced by the ingestion of alcohol, accounting for the increase in acetaminophen toxicity, especially among alcoholics, observed upon the concomitant consumption of alcoholic beverages and acetaminophen.[35]

Various sulfhydryl-containing compounds were found to be useful as antidotes to acetaminophen overdose. The most useful is N-acetylcysteine (Mucomyst, Acetadote), a thiol-containing reagent which serves as a substitute for the endogenous and depleted glutathione and competes with hepatic protein thiols for reaction with the electrophilic and toxic NAPQI. N-acetylcysteine is also a cysteine prodrug, thereby enhancing hepatic glutathione stores.[36,37]

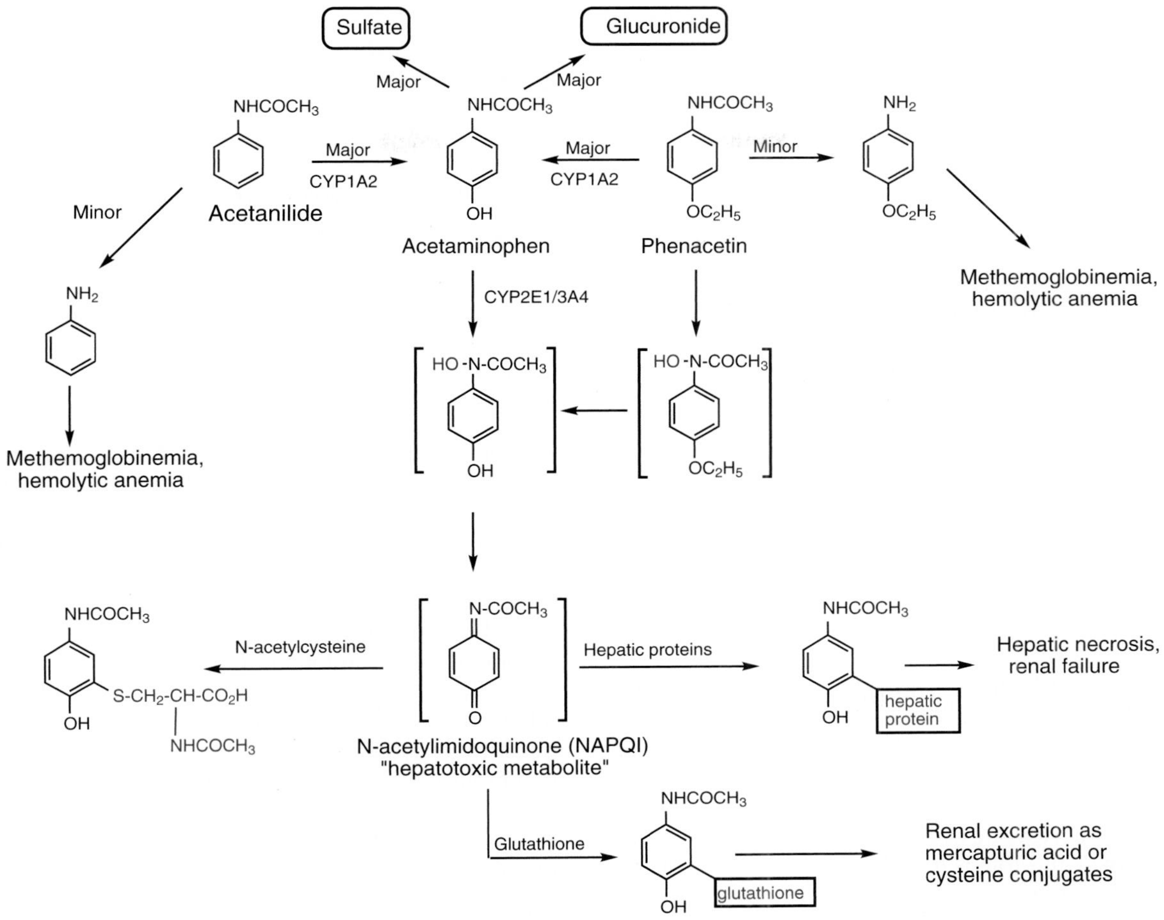

Figure 15.7 Metabolism of acetaminophen.

DRUG INTERACTIONS. Hepatic necrosis develops at much lower doses of acetaminophen in some heavy drinkers than would be expected, perhaps because of the induction of the CYP2E1 system, depletion of glutathione stores, or aberrations in the primary sulfate and glucuronide conjugation pathways.[30] Interactions with warfarin, dicumarol, anisindione, and diphenadione have been suggested. The mechanism of these interactions has not been fully elucidated but may be associated with competition for plasma protein binding sites. Acetaminophen is weakly bound to plasma proteins and can also interfere with the enzymes involved in vitamin K–dependent coagulation factor synthesis. Chemical incompatibilities have also been reported based on hydrolysis by strong acids or bases or by phenolic oxidation in the presence of oxidizing agents. Acetaminophen forms "sticky" mixtures with diphenhydramine HCl and discolors under humid conditions in the presence of caffeine or codeine phosphate, two drugs with which it is commonly used in combination.

Anti-inflammatory Drugs

Salicylate-based Therapeutics

Salicylates are one of the oldest classes of drugs in history. Their use dates back to the 5th century BC where Hippocrates prescribed chewing willow bark, a natural source for salicylic acid, for pain relief. Salicylates have many therapeutic actions including antipyretic, analgesic, and anti-inflammatory properties. The most prevalent and widely used salicylate is aspirin, and its medical use began in 1899 and continues to gain therapeutic utility today. For example, recent studies have shown aspirin's ability to help prevent cardiovascular disease[38] and colorectal cancer.[39] However, the salicylates target COX-1 preferentially; thus many undesirable side effects stem from GI disturbances. There are many marketed salicylate products; however, many of them have reduced clinical use. Thus the salicylates discussed in this section will be restricted to commonly used salicylate-based therapeutic agents.

MECHANISM OF ACTION. Salicylate-based NSAIDs exhibit their pain relief primarily through the inhibition of COX enzymes, thereby blocking PG biosynthesis. This class is generally more active against COX-1 over COX-2 as exemplified in Table 15.2 for aspirin. The salicylate-based NSAIDs, except for aspirin, are competitive inhibitors, blocking COX-mediated oxidation of arachidonic acid. Aspirin is a suicide- or mechanism-based COX inhibitor, meaning it reacts with and covalently modifies the enzyme by acetylating Ser530 in COX-1 and Ser516 in COX-2 (Fig. 15.8). Acetylation of COX-1 renders it inactive;

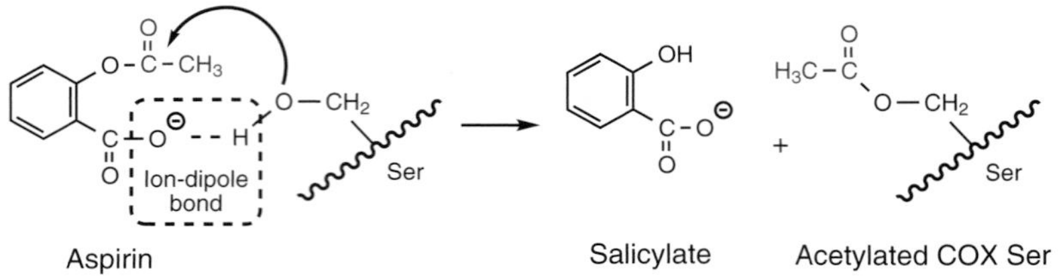

Aspirin — Salicylate — Acetylated COX Ser

Figure 15.8 Acetylation of COX Ser by aspirin.

however, acetylation of COX-2 converts it to more of a lipoxygenase where it can still produce the monooxygenated product 15(*R*)-hydroxyeicosatetraenoic acid.[18]

STRUCTURE-ACTIVITY RELATIONSHIPS

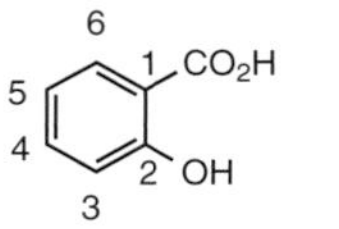

Salicylic acid

Salicylic acid is a 2-hydroxybenzoic acid and comprises the core requirements for all salicylate analogues. The carboxylic acid functional group at position 1 has a pK_a ~3; thus, at physiological pH it is highly ionized. This is important, as the resultant carboxylate anion (except for aspirin) makes a key ion-ion bond with Arg120 in COX active sites. For aspirin, the carboxylate's role is to reduce the pK_a of the active site Ser residue, resulting in its increased nucleophilicity for attack on the acetoxy carbonyl carbon (Fig. 15.8). The phenolic hydroxy group at the 2-position, whether free or acetylated, is also important for anti-inflammatory activity as hydroxy substitutions at the 3- and 4-positions are inactive. The addition of a second conjugated aromatic ring to the salicylate phenyl ring increases anti-inflammatory activity, as the resultant analogue makes more effective van der Waals and hydrophobic interactions with Tyr348, Val349, Tyr385, and Trp387.

ABSORPTION AND METABOLISM. Most salicylates are rapidly and effectively absorbed after oral administration. The rate of absorption and the extent of oral bioavailability are dependent on a number of factors, including formulation, gastric pH, food in the stomach, gastric emptying time, the presence of buffering agents or antacids, and particle size.[40] Salicylates are weak acids (aspirin pK_a = 3.5) and highly unionized in the stomach; thus solubility in gastric fluid is poor. This is one of the primary reasons for GI distress of the salicylates. Absorption takes place primarily from the small intestine because of better drug dissolution, where unionized molecules can passively diffuse across the gut wall.

The major metabolic routes of salicylic acid are illustrated in Figure 15.9 and have been extensively reviewed.[41] The initial route of metabolism for aspirin is conversion to salicylic acid, which can be excreted in the urine as the free acid (10%) or undergo conjugation with glycine or glucuronic acid.[42] The major metabolite is the glycine conjugate (75%), with glucuronide ethers and esters accounting for 15% of metabolites.[42] In addition, microsomal aromatic hydroxylation of salicylic acid also occurs, albeit to a limited extent.

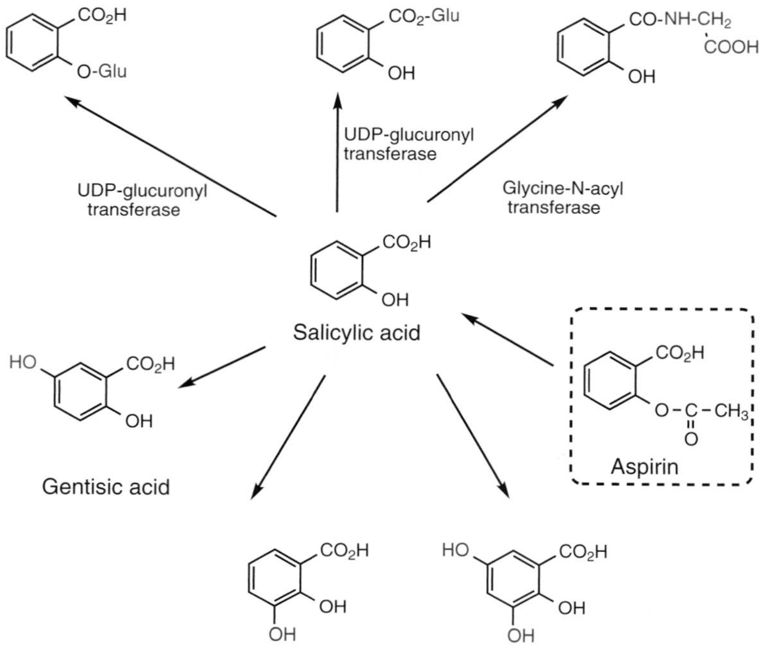

UDP-glucuronyl transferase — UDP-glucuronyl transferase — Glycine-N-acyl transferase — Salicylic acid — Gentisic acid — Aspirin

Figure 15.9 Metabolism of salicylic acid derivatives (Glu = glucuronide conjugate).

ADVERSE EFFECTS. Although the rate of salicylate poisoning has declined, salicylates still account for a significant percentage of all accidental poisonings in the United States.[43] The most commonly observed side effects associated with the use of salicylates relate to disturbances of the GI tract, including nausea, vomiting, epigastric discomfort, aggravation of peptic ulcers, gastric ulcerations, erosive gastritis, and GI hemorrhage. These adverse effects typically occur in individuals on high doses of aspirin. The incidence of these side effects is rarer at low doses, but a single dose of aspirin can cause GI distress in 5% of individuals. Salicylate-induced GI distress is typically mediated by the dual insult (Fig. 15.6) and/or inhibition of platelet aggregation, which promotes bleeding.

Reye syndrome is an acute and potentially fatal condition that can follow influenza and chickenpox infections in children from infancy to their late teens, with the majority of cases occurring between the ages of 5 and 14 years.[44] It is characterized by symptoms including sudden vomiting, violent headaches, and unusual behavior in children who appear to be recovering from a viral infection. Reye syndrome is a rare disease and incidence rates are largely unknown since reporting to the CDC is not mandated; however, ≤2 cases per year have been reported since 1994.[44] The vast majority (>90%) of children diagnosed with Reye syndrome were on aspirin therapy while afflicted with their viral infection. Based on these statistics, the FDA has mandated that aspirin and other salicylates be labeled with a warning against their use in children younger than 16 years with influenza, chickenpox, or other flu-like illness. Acetaminophen is suggested to be the drug of choice in children with these conditions.

COMMONLY USED SALICYLATE-BASED THERAPEUTICS. The structures of the commonly used salicylate-based therapeutics are presented in Figure 15.10. The physicochemical and pharmacokinetic properties of all NSAIDs, including aspirin, are provided in Table 15.3.

Aspirin. Acetylsalicylic acid, or aspirin, is indicated for the relief of minor aches and mild to moderate pain, arthritis and related arthritic conditions, to reduce the risk of transient ischemic attacks, myocardial infarction prophylaxis, and as a platelet aggregation inhibitor. Aspirin contains the acetoxy functional group; therefore it is able to irreversibly acetylate the COX active site Ser residue. This is especially important for aspirin's action as a platelet aggregation inhibitor. Platelets utilize COX-1 to produce TXA_2 (a pro-aggregatory prostanoid), and since platelets cannot produce new COX-1 protein because they do not have any DNA biosynthetic machinery, acetylation of COX-1 Ser leads to prolonged inhibitory action. Patients should take care not to take another nonselective NSAID for pain concurrently with low-dose "heart healthy" aspirin, as the other NSAID would compete for COX-1 active site residues, leading to ineffective COX-1 inhibition in platelets. The acetoxy group is responsible for aspirin's short duration of action since it is susceptible to plasma esterase–catalyzed hydrolysis. Aspirin is stable in a dry environment; however, it can be hydrolyzed to salicylic acid and acetic acid under humid or moist conditions or when exposed to basic media. Salicylic acid contains a typically light-sensitive phenol functional group, which commonly degrade to provide inactive colored quinones. Thus, if an aspirin medication smells like vinegar (acetic acid; CH_3COOH) or has discolored, it has degraded and should be discarded. Aspirin is available in a large number of dosage forms and strengths as tablets, suppositories, capsules, enteric-coated tablets, and buffered tablets.

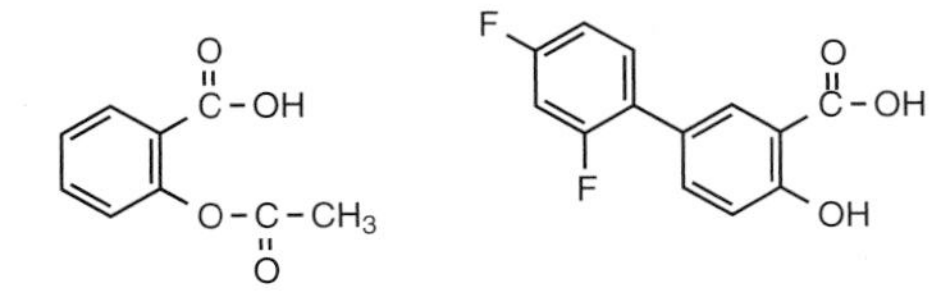

Drug Interactions. Aspirin is widely and routinely used for many clinically relevant reasons; therefore it is not surprising that many concerning drug-drug interactions have been observed. Aspirin is highly bound to plasma proteins (Table 15.3)[45]; therefore competition for plasma protein binding sites with other drugs is a concern. The interaction of salicylates with oral anticoagulants (e.g., warfarin) represents one of the most widely documented and clinically significant drug interactions reported to date.[46] The plasma concentration of free anticoagulant increases in the presence of salicylates through one of two mechanisms: (1) the salicylate may simply block expected anticoagulant plasma protein binding or (2) the salicylate may displace bound anticoagulant. These pharmacokinetic implications may require a reduced dose of anticoagulant. These interactions are also evident with other nonsalicylated NSAIDs, and coadministration can increase the incidence and severity of GI distress. Ingestion of alcohol also exacerbates salicylate-induced gastric bleeding.[47]

Diflunisal (Dolobid). Diflunisal is indicated for mild to moderate pain, rheumatoid arthritis, and osteoarthritis. Interestingly, diflunisal was recently reported to have antimicrobial properties against *Francisella tularensis*, supporting the notion of its potential to be repurposed for as an antitularemia agent.[48] Diflunisal is a 5-(2,4-difluorophenyl)-2-hydroxybenzoic acid and lacks the reactive acetoxy group seen in aspirin; therefore, it is a competitive and reversible inhibitor of the COX enzymes. It is more potent than aspirin because of the second conjugated phenyl ring on the 5-position of the salicylic acid moiety that can make more effective van der Waals and hydrophobic interactions with COX aromatic and hydrophobic residues. The two fluorine atoms play important roles in increasing potency and duration of action. The *o*-fluoro is a potency driver because its proximity to the salicylic acid H atoms at positions 4 and 6 forces the two aromatic rings to assume a non-coplanar orientation. It is rapidly and completely absorbed on oral administration.[49] The *p*-fluorine atom increases duration of action because it blocks phase 1 oxidative metabolism. The metabolism of diflunisal occurs primarily through phase 2 conjugation, and it is excreted

Acetylsalicylic acid

Diflunisal (Dolobid)

Figure 15.10 Commonly used salicylate-based NSAIDs.

Table 15.3 Pharmacokinetic and Physicochemical Properties of NSAIDs

Drug	Anti-Inflammatory Dose (mg)	Onset (Duration) of Action	Peak Plasma Levels (hr)	Protein Binding (%)	Biotransformation	Elimination Half-Life (hr)	pK_a
Aspirin	3,200-6,000	ND	2	90	Plasma hydrolysis and hepatic	<30 min	3.5
Diclofenac (Voltaren)	100-200	30 min (~8 hr)	1.5-2.5	99	Hepatic; first-pass metabolism: 3A4	1-2	4.0
Diflunisal (Dolobid)	500-1,000	1 hr (8-12 hr)	2-3	99	Hepatic	8-12	3.3
Etodolac (Lodine)	800-1,200	30 min (4-6 hr)	1-2	99	Hepatic: 2C9	6-7	4.7
Fenoprofen calcium (Nalfon)	1,200-2,400	NR	2	99	Hepatic: 2C9	3	4.5
Flurbiprofen (Ansaid)	200-300	NR	1.5	99	Hepatic: 2C9	6 (2-12)	4.2
Ibuprofen (Motrin, Advil)	1,200-3,200	30 min (4-6 hr)	2	99	Hepatic; first-pass metabolism: 2C9, 2C19	~2	4.4
Indomethacin (Indocin)	75-150	2-4 hr (2-3 d)	2-3	97	Hepatic: 2C9	5 (3-11)	4.5
Ketoprofen (Orudis)	150-300	NR	0.5-2	99	Hepatic: 2C9, 3A4	~2	5.9
Meclofenamate sodium (Meclomen)	200-400	1 hr (4-6 hr)	4.0	99	Hepatic: 2C9	2-3	NR
Mefenamic acid (Ponstel)	1,000	NR	2-4	79	Hepatic: 2C9	2	4.2
Meloxicam (Mobic)	7.5-15	NR	4-5	99	Hepatic 2C9	15-20	1.1, 4.2
Nabumetone[a] (Relafen)	1,500-2,000	NR	2.5 (1-8) 6MNA	99[b]	Hepatic; first-pass metabolism to 6MNA	6MNA, 23	Neutral
Naproxen (Naprosyn, Anaprox)	500-1,000	NR	2-4	99	Hepatic: 3A4, 1A2	13	4.2
Oxaprozin (Daypro)	1,200	NR	3-5	99	Hepatic: 2C9	25	4.3
Piroxicam (Feldene)	20	2-4 hr (24 hr)	2	99	Hepatic: 2C9	50	1.8, 5.1

Table 15.3 Pharmacokinetic and Physicochemical Properties of NSAIDs (Continued)

Drug	Anti-Inflammatory Dose (mg)	Onset (Duration) of Action	Peak Plasma Levels (hr)	Protein Binding (%)	Biotrans-formation	Elimination Half-Life (hr)	pK_a
Sulindac[a] (Clinoril)	400	NR	2-4	93	Hepatic; sulfide metabolite active	50	4.5
Tolmetin (Tolectin)	1,200	NR	<1	99	Hepatic	5	3.5

[a] Prodrug.
[b] Protein binding data is for the active 6-MNA metabolite.
6MNA, 6-methoxynaphthalene-2-acetic acid; ND, not determined; NR, not reported.

in the urine primarily as glucuronide ester and ether conjugates.[50] The most frequently reported side effects include disturbances of the GI system (e.g., nausea, dyspepsia, and diarrhea), dermatologic reactions, and CNS effects (e.g., dizziness and headache). Lastly, it does not have any effect on platelet aggregation.

Arylalkanoic Acids

GENERAL STRUCTURE-ACTIVITY RELATIONSHIPS

$$AR-\overset{R}{\underset{\alpha}{CH}}-\overset{O}{\overset{\|}{C}}-OH$$

R = H, CH_3 or alkyl
AR = aryl or heteroaryl

Arylalkanoic acid

These general structure-activity relationships (SAR) that apply to all arylalkanoic acids will be discussed here, and specific SAR or exceptions to these general rules will be presented below for each drug or drug class.

The arylalkanoic acids class of NSAIDs structurally comprise an aromatic ring attached to a carboxylic acid group primarily through a one or two carbon saturated chain. The bridging carbon is termed the α-carbon and can accommodate a methyl group substituent. If there is no substituent (i.e., R = H), then the compounds are identified as the arylacetic acid class. When the α-carbon is substituted with a methyl group, the resulting α-methyl acetic acid, or aryl-propionic acid, analogues have been given the class name "profens" by the U.S. Adopted Names Council. If all other structural features are identical, the arylpropionic acid class has improved activity over the arylacetic acid class. Groups larger than methyl decrease activity.

Introduction of a methyl group makes the α-carbon a chiral center. For chiral NSAIDs, the S enantiomer is the active isomer. Activity increases with the addition of a second conjugated aromatic ring. Introduction of aromatic substituents that increase non-coplanarity of the two rings also enhances activity by optimizing the van der Waals and hydrophobic interactions with COX aromatic and aliphatic residues.

ARYL- AND HETEROARYLACETIC ACIDS. The structures of the aryl- and heteroarylacetic acid derivatives ("fenacs") and the aryl- and heteroarylpropionic acids ("profens") clinically available are presented in Figure 15.11.

Indomethacin. Indomethacin is an indoleacetic acid and is indicated for moderate to severe rheumatoid arthritis, ankylosing spondylitis, osteoarthritis, joint-related bursitis and tendinitis, and acute gouty arthritis.[51] There is a reconstituted IV injectable formulation available to close a hemodynamically significant patent ductus arteriosus in premature infants. Indomethacin possesses both antipyretic and anti-inflammatory activity.

Structure-Activity Relationships. The carboxylic acid group is essential for activity as, when ionized, it will make a required ion-ion bond with Arg120 in COX active sites. Increasing or decreasing the carbon chain between the carboxylic acid and the indole ring reduces activity. Replacement of the carboxyl group with other acidic functionalities decreases activity. Anti-inflammatory activity typically increases as the acidity of the carboxylic acid increases. Amide analogues are inactive due to significantly reduced acidity. Methylation of the α-carbon increases activity; however, the resulting chiral center must be in the S configuration. Aracylation of the indole nitrogen is important for activity, as the carbonyl linker between the indole- and phenyl-ring is sp2 hybridized which maintains π electron conjugation. If this carbonyl was reduced to a methylene, activity would significantly reduce. N-benzoyl derivatives substituted in the *p*-position with lipophilic groups including fluoro, chloro, trifluoromethyl, or thiomethyl are the most active. Aqueous solutions of indomethacin, which contains the *p*-chlorobenzoyl group, are not stable because of the ease of hydrolysis of this group.

The 2-methyl group plays two important roles in indomethacin's activity. First, it is believed to contribute to indomethacin's time-dependent pseudoirreversible inhibition of COX enzymes by sliding into a small hydrophobic pocket.[52] Interestingly, conversion of the 2-methyl to 2-trifluoromethyl increases COX-2 selectivity.[53] Second, it creates enough steric bulk to push the N-*p*-chlorobenzoyl group *cis* to the methoxybenzo component of the indole system, which is the more active conformation. After this

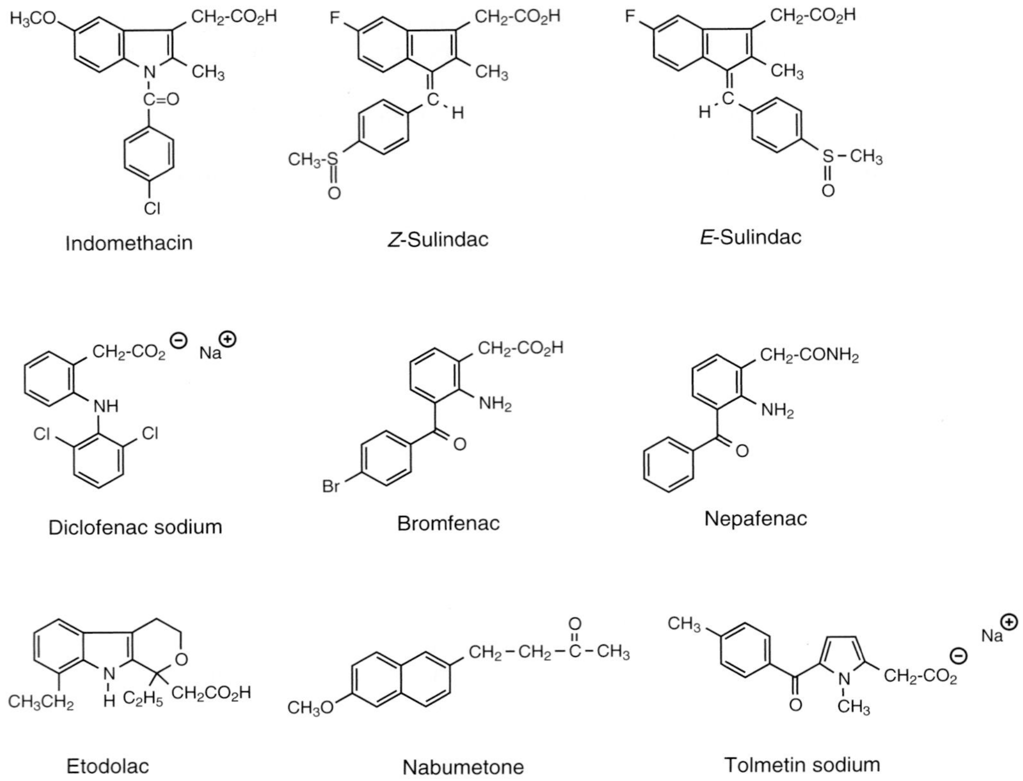

Figure 15.11 Aryl- and heteroarylacetic acid derivatives.

happens, one of the *o*-hydrogen atoms on the phenyl ring clashes with the C7-hydrogen on the indole ring, increasing the non-coplanarity of the two aromatic rings. These conformations are represented as follows:

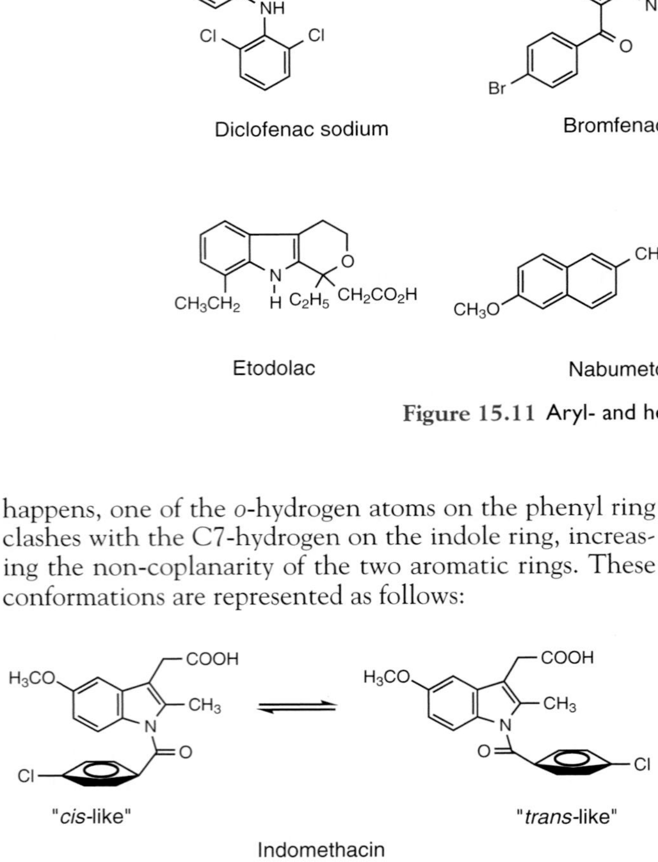

The 5-position of the indole ring can accommodate a variety of both electron-donating and electron-withdrawing substituents including methoxy, fluoro, dimethylamino, methyl, allyloxy, and acetyl, all of which are more active than the unsubstituted indole ring. The presence of an indole nitrogen is not essential for activity because the corresponding 1-benzylidenylindene analogues (e.g., sulindac) are active.

Absorption and Metabolism. Indomethacin's 2-methyl and *p*-chloro groups are lipophilic substituents that increase membrane permeability; thus absorption of indomethacin occurs rapidly on oral administration.[54] The metabolism of indomethacin is shown in Figure 15.12. The 5-position is susceptible to CYP-mediated hydroxylation. The 5-methoxy group on indomethacin increases duration of action since the CYP2C9-mediated O-dealkylation reaction is slow. Approximately 50% of a single dose is 5-O-demethylated by CYP2C9 and 10% is conjugated with glucuronic acid.[54,55] Glucuronide conjugates are formed with the carboxylic acid (forming the ester conjugate) and the 5-hydroxy indole (forming the ether conjugate). Amidase or esterase enzymes hydrolyze indomethacin to N-deacylated metabolites. All of indomethacin's metabolites are inactive.

Adverse Effects. Similar to all other acidic non-selective NSAIDs, indomethacin is highly bound to plasma proteins.[54,56] Interestingly, despite the high degree of plasma protein binding, indomethacin does not suffer from drug/drug interactions through displacement of other drugs from plasma protein binding sites. A large number of individuals taking indomethacin, especially those over the age of 70, experience undesirable effects of the GI tract, CNS, and ears. As with other arylalkanoic acids, administration of indomethacin with food or milk decreases GI side effects.

Sulindac. Sulindac is indicated for acute and long-term treatment of osteoarthritis, rheumatoid arthritis, ankylosing spondylitis, and acute gouty arthritis. Sulindac is essentially a sulfinyl-containing prodrug analogue of indomethacin with reduced side effects commonly associated with indomethacin, particularly GI irritation. In anti-inflammatory and antipyretic assays, it is only about half as potent as indomethacin but is equipotent in analgesic assays.

Structure-Activity Relationships. Sulindac is an indene-based arylalkanoic acid where an sp2 hybridized carbon

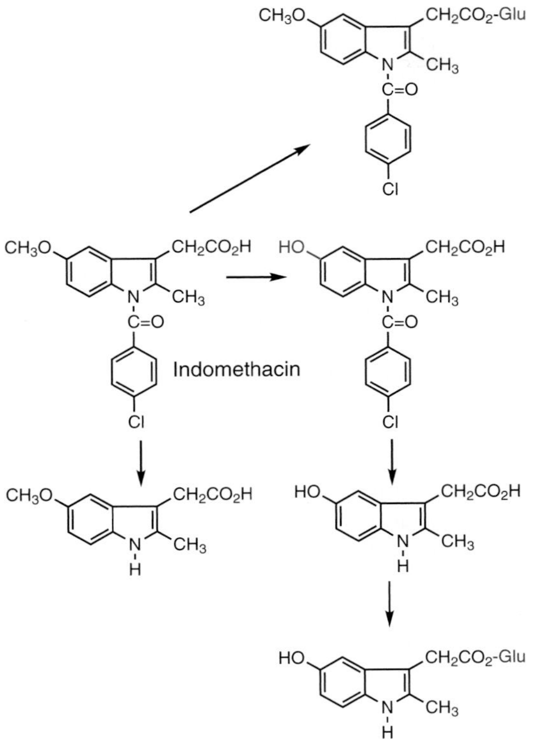

Figure 15.12 Metabolism of indomethacin (Glu = glucuronide).

has replaced the indole nitrogen on indomethacin. Indene analogues achieve activity with benzylidene, where the carbonyl linker seen in indomethacin is replaced with an sp2 hybridized carbon that is doubly bonded to the sp2 hybridized C3 carbon on indene. This is another important SAR point, as this sp2 hybridized linker maintains conjugation between the aromatic indene and phenyl rings. The benzylidene group substituted with a *p*-chloro group was active; however, it suffered from poor aqueous solubility. Indene analogue potency increased with a 5-fluoro group over the 5-methoxy seen in indomethacin. The *cis* conformation (*Z* isomer) of the benzylidene group relative to the phenyl ring in the indene ring is significantly more potent than the corresponding *E* isomer (Fig. 15.11). This *cis* relationship of the phenyl substituent to the aromatic ring bearing the fluoro substituent is similar to the proposed active conformation of indomethacin, suggesting that both indomethacin and sulindac assume similar conformations in the COX active site. The 4-methylsulfinyl (or 4-methylsulfoxide) group on the benzylidene group is the reason why sulindac is a prodrug. The reduced methylsulfide is the active anti-inflammatory agent and the oxidized methylsulfone is inactive.

Absorption and Metabolism. Sulindac is well absorbed on oral administration and, being acidic, is highly bound to serum proteins. It is recommended that sulindac be administered with food. As stated above, sulindac is a prodrug and metabolism has a major role in its pharmacological and therapeutic actions.[57] Sulindac is absorbed as the inactive sulfoxide, which is not an inhibitor of COX enzymes. Therefore, in the GI tract, there is no reduction in gastric PGs. Since some PGs exert a protective effect in the GI tract, the lack of inhibition by sulindac reduces GI distress compared to other NSAIDs that are active intact. Once sulindac enters the general circulation, it is reduced to the active sulfide, which is the active inhibitor of COX enzymes (Fig. 15.13). The reduction of sulindac is reversible and mediated through CYP or flavin-containing monooxygenase (FMO) enzymes, and the cyclic redox reactions extend duration of action, mimicking a slow and sustained release of active drug. Sulindac is irreversibly inactivated by CYP/FMO oxidation to the sulfone. A minor metabolite results from hydroxylation of the methyl group at the 2-position on the indene ring, a reaction comparable to benzylic hydroxylation. Despite the fact that the sulfide metabolite is the primary activation product and is found in high concentration in human plasma, it is not found in human urine, perhaps because of its high degree of protein binding and/or oxidation to the sulfone via ubiquitous cytosolic enzymes. The major excretion product is the sulfone metabolite and its glucuronide conjugate (Fig. 15.13).

Adverse Effects. The toxicity of sulindac, especially in the GI tract, is lower than that observed for indomethacin and many other NSAIDs, but the spectrum of adverse reactions is very similar. The most frequent side effects reported are associated with irritation of the GI tract, although these effects are generally mild. Even though sulindac is inactive in the GI tract, it still contains a carboxylic acid functional group and violates the first arm of the dual insult (direct irritation). Effects on the CNS are less common, and dermatologic reactions are infrequently encountered.

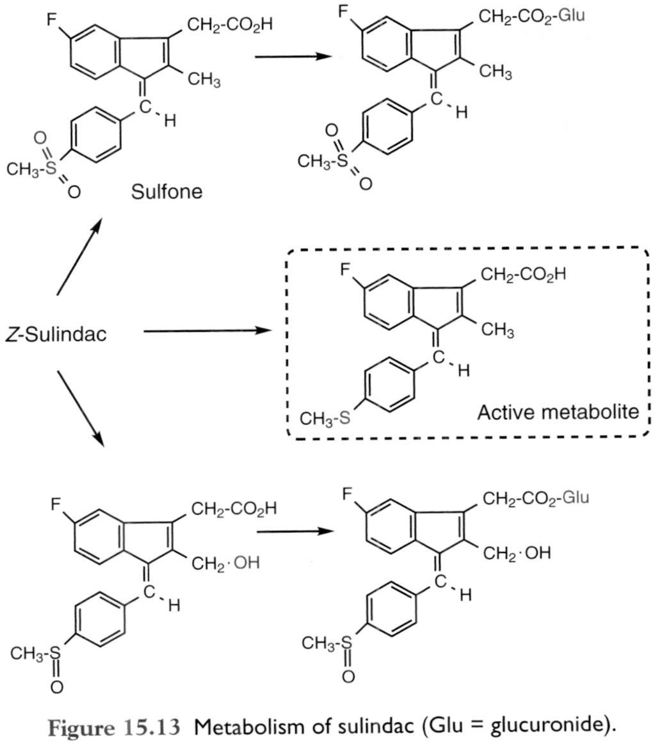

Figure 15.13 Metabolism of sulindac (Glu = glucuronide).

Tolmetin Sodium. Tolmetin sodium is indicated for the treatment of rheumatoid arthritis, juvenile rheumatoid arthritis, and osteoarthritis. In addition to PG inhibition, tolmetin also inhibits polymorph migration and decreases capillary permeability. Tolmetin has more inhibitory activity against COX-1 over COX-2; thus most adverse effects are due to GI issues. Its anti-inflammatory activity is less than that of indomethacin.

Structure-Activity Relationships. Tolmetin is an analogue of indomethacin, possessing a pyrrole ring instead of the indole ring. Replacement of the 5-*p*-toluoyl group with a *p*-chlorobenzoyl moiety produced little effect on activity.[58] Substitution of the *p*-methyl group of tolmetin with a *p*-chloro group blocked oxidative metabolism, increasing duration of action to approximately 24 hours. This *p*-chloro compound was marketed in 1980 as zomepirac, an analgesic that was removed from the market in 1983 because of severe anaphylactic reactions. Contrary to the general SAR rules discussed above for the arylalkanoic acids, methylation of the α-carbon reduces activity.

Absorption and Metabolism. Tolmetin sodium is rapidly and almost completely absorbed on oral administration.[59] It has a relatively short plasma half-life due to extensive first-pass metabolism of the benzylic methyl group to the primary alcohol, which is subsequently oxidized to the inactive dicarboxylic acid through subsequent reactions with alcohol dehydrogenase followed by aldehyde dehydrogenase (Fig. 15.14).[60] The free acid is highly bound to plasma proteins, and excretion of tolmetin and its metabolites occurs primarily in the urine. Approximately 15%-20% of an administered dose is excreted unchanged, and 10% is excreted as the glucuronide ester conjugate of the parent drug. Ester conjugates of the dicarboxylic acid metabolite account for the majority of the remaining administered drug.

Diclofenac Sodium. Diclofenac sodium is one of the most widely used NSAID globally and is indicated for the treatment of rheumatoid arthritis, osteoarthritis, ankylosing spondylitis, and mild to moderate pain. In addition, diclofenac is often administered to patients with tuberculosis for inflammation and has been shown to synergize with streptomycin against *Mycobacterium tuberculosis*, the causative pathogen for tuberculosis.[61] Diclofenac is a phenylacetic acid substituted at the 2-position with a 2,6-dichloroanilino group and displays anti-inflammatory, analgesic, and antipyretic properties. It is twice as potent as indomethacin as an antiflammatory agent and 450 times as potent as aspirin. As an analgesic, it is 6 times more potent than indomethacin and 40 times as potent as aspirin. As an antipyretic, it is twice as potent as indomethacin and more than 350 times as potent as aspirin. Diclofenac is unique among NSAIDs in that it possesses three putative mechanisms of action: (1) inhibition of the COX system, resulting in a decreased production of PGs and thromboxanes; (2) inhibition of the lipoxygenase pathway, resulting in decreased production of leukotrienes, particularly the proinflammatory LKB4; and (3) inhibition of arachidonic acid release and stimulation of its reuptake, resulting in a reduction of arachidonic acid availability.[62]

Structure-Activity Relationships. Diclofenac is a bioisostere of salicylic acid where the 2-hydroxyl group on salicylic acid has been replaced with an -NH- group. This nitrogen atom adopts an sp2 hybridization, which maintains conjugation between the two aromatic rings. The two *o*-chloro groups are significant potency boosters, which is a primary reason for its high anti-inflammatory potency (estimated at 3-1,000 times most other NSAIDs). The two *o*-chloro groups sterically hinder the C3-hydrogen and the carboxylic acid group on the phenylacetic acid moiety, forcing a non-coplanar conformation between the halogenated phenyl ring and the phenyl acetic acid portion, thus optimizing binding to the active site of the COX.[63] They also add to the lipophilicity of the compound, which promotes passive penetration into inflamed tissue.

Absorption and Metabolism. Diclofenac is rapidly and completely absorbed on oral administration.[64] The free acid (pK_a = 4.0) is highly bound to serum proteins.[65] Only 50%-60% of an oral dose is bioavailable due to extensive hepatic metabolism (Fig. 15.15). This is primarily due to the high lipophilicity and open *p*-positions. The major CYP3A4-catalyzed metabolite is the 4′-hydroxy derivative and accounts for 20%-30% of the excreted dose, whereas the 5-hydroxy, 3′-hydroxy, and

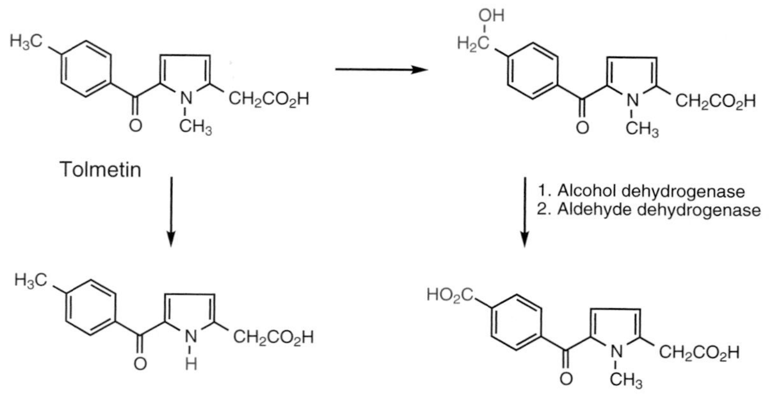

Figure 15.14 Metabolism of tolmetin.

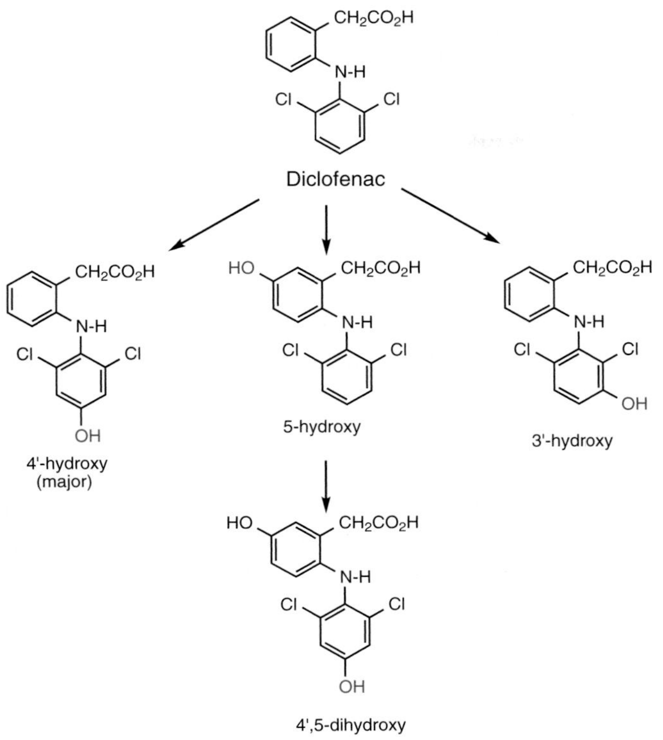

Diclofenac
4'-hydroxy (major)
5-hydroxy
3'-hydroxy
4',5-dihydroxy

Figure 15.15 Metabolism of diclofenac.

4′,5-dihydroxy metabolites are catalyzed by CYP2C9 and account for 10%-20% of the excreted dose.[66] Phase 2 conjugation yield sulfate conjugates, which is unusual as most other NSAIDs are excreted as glucuronide conjugate.

Diclofenac can also produce a hepatotoxic quinonimine metabolite similar to that reported in the metabolism of acetaminophen.[67] The formation and reactivity of the quinonimine metabolite is shown in Figure 15.16. The 4′-hydroxy metabolite formed under normal CYP3A4

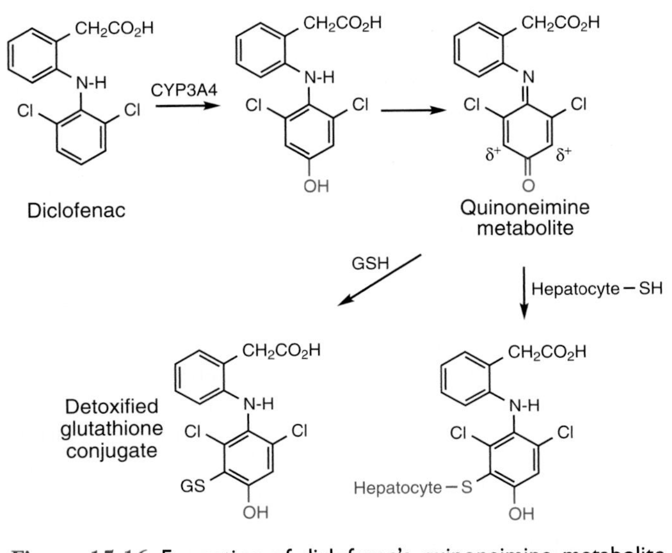

Diclofenac
CYP3A4
Quinoneimine metabolite
GSH
Hepatocyte – SH
Detoxified glutathione conjugate

Figure 15.16 Formation of diclofenac's quinoneimine metabolite and reactions with GSH and hepatocyte Cys.

oxidation can undergo further oxidation to the reactive and toxic quinonimine metabolite. The carbons on the quinonimine at the 3′- and 5′-positions are highly electrophilic (δ+) and will nonspecifically react with nearby nucleophiles. The quinonimine is normally inactivated via conjugation with glutathione but, if GSH levels are depleted, can induce chemically predictable hepatotoxicity. Nucleophilic Cys residues on liver hepatocytes will attack the electrophilic quinonimine metabolite, leaving them irreversibly alkylated. This is particularly important because diclofenac is currently the only NSAID capable of active transport into the liver mediated through the OATP1B3 transporter protein.[68] Therefore it is important that patients taking diclofenac have their liver function monitored regularly.

Bromfenac. Bromfenac is indicated for the treatment of postoperative inflammation and reduction of ocular pain in patients who have undergone cataract extraction. Bromfenac is a phenylacetic acid substituted with a 2-amino group and 3-(4-bromobenzoyl) group. The carbonyl linker, similar to indomethacin, maintains conjugation between the two aromatic rings. The 4-bromo group is more lipophilic than chlorine or fluorine and helps with penetration into lipophilic ocular tissue. It is available as a 0.09% ophthalmic solution for once-daily dosing. An oral formulation of bromfenac was removed from the market due to significant toxicity (primarily hepatic) and fatalities.[69]

Nepafenac. Similar to bromfenac, nepafenac is indicated for the treatment of pain and inflammation after ocular surgery. It is available in either a 0.1% (Nevanac) or 0.3% (Ilevro) eye drop solution and is commonly prescribed for use three times per day. Nepafenac lacks the required carboxylic acid functional group that other NSAIDs use to form the essential ion-ion bond with Arg120 in COX-1 and COX-2; thus nepafenac is a prodrug. The nonionizable amide functional group promotes drug penetration through the cornea compared to ophthalmic solutions of ketorolac (discussed below) or bromfenac.[70] It is converted from the amide to the active carboxylic acid by ocular hydrolases after corneal penetration. Ophthalmic nepafenac, compared to ophthalmic ketorolac, seems to be a more effective pain reliever in patients following cataract surgery.[71]

Etodolac. Etodolac, a pyranocarboxylic acid, is indicated for the acute and long-term treatment of osteoarthritis and the management of pain. It also has an antipyretic action. SAR studies evaluating a number of analogues found that the etodolac structure provided the most effective anti-inflammatory activity with the best margin of safety.[72,73] Although not strictly an arylacetic acid derivative (there is a two-carbon separation between the carboxylic acid and heteroaromatic ring), the drug still possesses structural characteristics similar to those of the heteroarylacetic acids and is classified as such here. The structures below illustrate how the relative position of the essential carboxylic acid and aromatic moieties found in true arylacetic acids can be retained in etodolac.

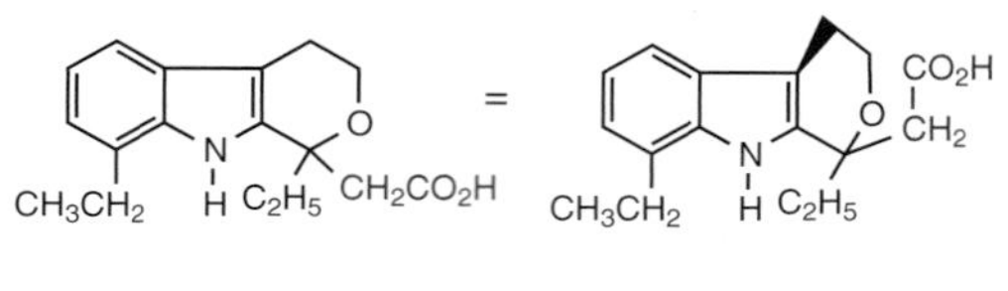

Etodolac stereochemistry

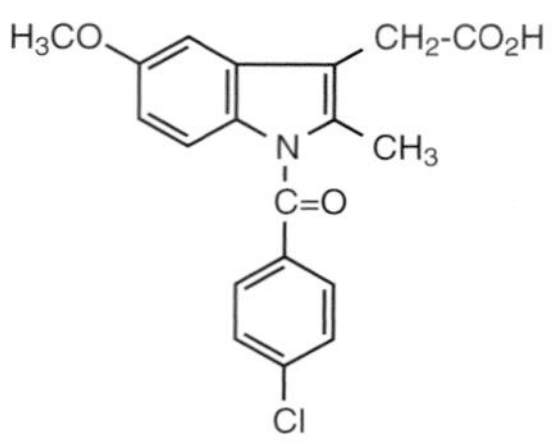

Etodolac is marketed as a racemic mixture, and as expected only the S-(+)-enantiomer possesses the anti-inflammatory activity. With regard to its anti-inflammatory actions, etodolac is approximately 50 times more active than aspirin, 3 times more potent than sulindac, and one-third as active as indomethacin. Etodoloc is a COX-2 preferential inhibitor; therefore, it produces less GI bleeding than other active NSAIDs due to a lower incidence of gastric PG biosynthesis inhibition, a COX-1 action.

Absorption and Metabolism. Etodolac is rapidly absorbed following oral administration and is highly bound to plasma proteins.[72] The penetration of etodolac into synovial fluid is greater than or equal to that of other NSAIDs; only diclofenac appears to provide greater penetration. Phase 1 metabolism of etodolac yields three hydroxylated metabolites (Fig. 15.17). Phase 2 glucuronide conjugates form at the resultant hydroxy groups before urinary excretion. All metabolites of etodolac are inactive.[74] Metabolism appears to be the same in the elderly as in the general population, so no dosage adjustment appears necessary.

Nabumetone. Nabumetone is indicated for the acute and chronic treatment of osteoarthritis and rheumatoid arthritis. However, studies have linked nabumetone use to an increased risk of acute pancreatitis.[75] Nabumetone is a nonacidic prodrug, making it quite a unique NSAID. It is rapidly metabolized after absorption to form a major active metabolite, 6-methoxynaphthaleneacetic acid (6MNA; Fig. 15.16). Since nabumetone is nonacidic, it does not induce the primary insult (direct GI mucosal damage). An additional benefit to nabumetone's action is that it is not metabolized to the active metabolite until after absorption; therefore, nabumetone does not engage in the secondary insult (COX-1 inhibition in GI tract). The net result is

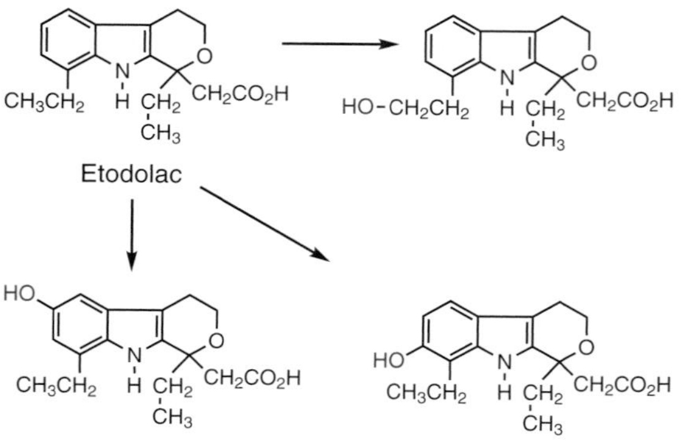

Figure 15.17 Metabolism of etodolac.

that gastric side effects of nabumetone are reduced. Once the parent drug enters the circulatory system, however, it is metabolized to the active 6MNA metabolite, which is an effective inhibitor of COX enzymes.

Structure-Activity Relationships. Alkylation of the butanone side chain with either methyl or ethyl groups reduced anti-inflammatory activity. Removal of the methoxy group at the 6-position reduced activity, but replacement of the methoxy with a methyl or chloro group resulted in active compounds.[76] In contrast, replacement of the methoxy with hydroxy, acetoxy, or N-methylcarbamoyl, or positional isomers of the methoxy group at the 2- or 4-positions, reduced activity.[76] 6MNA is closely related to naproxen structurally (discussion on naproxen below), differing only by the lack of an α-methyl group. Interestingly, the ketone precursor 4-(6-methoxy-2-naphthyl)pentan-2-one that would be expected to produce naproxen as a metabolite via a metabolic mechanism similar to that which produces 6-MNA was inactive in chronic models of inflammation.

Absorption and Metabolism. Nabumetone is absorbed primarily from the duodenum. Milk and food increase the rate of absorption and the bioavailability of the active metabolite.[77] Higher plasma levels of the active metabolite were seen in elderly patients.[78] Nabumetone undergoes rapid and extensive metabolism in the liver, with a mean absolute bioavailability of the active metabolite of 38% (Fig. 15.18). The 6-MNA metabolite is formed via β-oxidase catalysis. O-dealkylation of the 6-methoxy group is mediated through CYP2C9. However, this reaction is sluggish; thus nabumetone's duration of action is extended over most other NSAIDs, affording once-a-day dosing. Metabolites where the carbonyl has been reduced to the secondary alcohol are inactive.

ARYL- AND HETEROARYLPROPIONIC ACIDS. Members of this class represent the most widely used NSAIDs because several members of the class are available OTC. The introduction of the α-methyl group in the carboxylic acid side chain results in a chiral carbon atom and thus the existence of enantiomers, with oxaprozin being the sole exception. The structures of aryl- and heteroarylpropionic acid derivatives are shown in Figure 15.19.

Ibuprofen. Ibuprofen is available as a nonprescription (OTC) drug and is indicated for the relief of the signs and symptoms of rheumatoid arthritis and osteoarthritis, the relief of mild to moderate pain, the reduction of fever, and the treatment of dysmenorrhea. It is marketed as the racemic mixture, although biologic activity resides almost exclusively in the S-(+)-isomer. Ibuprofen is more potent than aspirin but less potent than indomethacin in

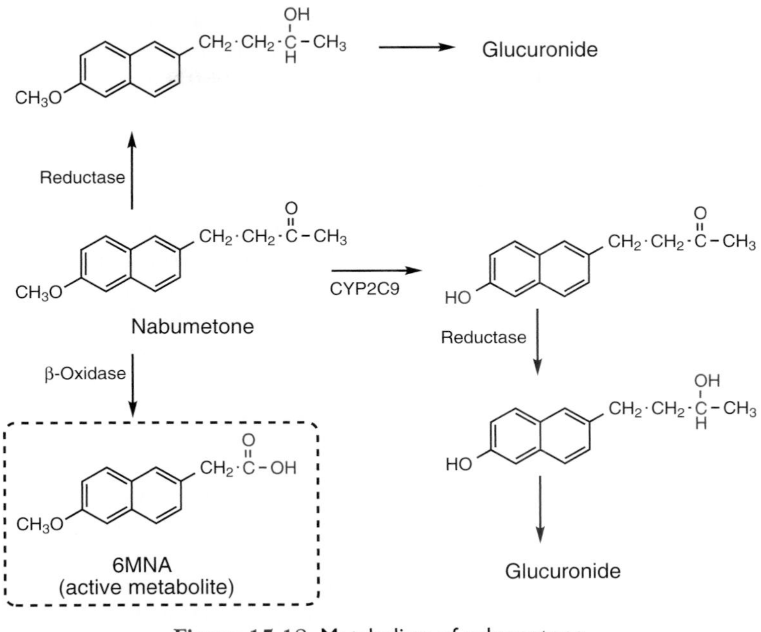

Figure 15.18 Metabolism of nabumetone.

anti-inflammatory and PG biosynthesis inhibition assays, and it produces moderate degrees of gastric irritation. Ibuprofen has been linked to cardiovascular toxicities and caution should be taken when administering to patients with existing cardiovascular disease or risk factors including hypertension.[79-81]

Structure-Activity Relationships. Ibuprofen has only one aromatic ring; thus its potency and anti-inflammatory activity is lower than that of other NSAIDs that contain two conjugated aromatic moieties. The 4-isobutyl group is hydrophobic and compensates to some extent for the lack of the second conjugated aromatic ring. The substitution of an α-methyl group on the alkanoic acid portion of arylacetic acid NSAIDs enhances anti-inflammatory actions and reduces many side effects.[82] The α-methyl group creates a chiral center and, as with many other chiral NSAIDs that are marketed as a racemic mixture, the *S*-(+)-enantiomer of ibuprofen possesses greater anti-inflammatory activity than the *R*-(−)-isomer.

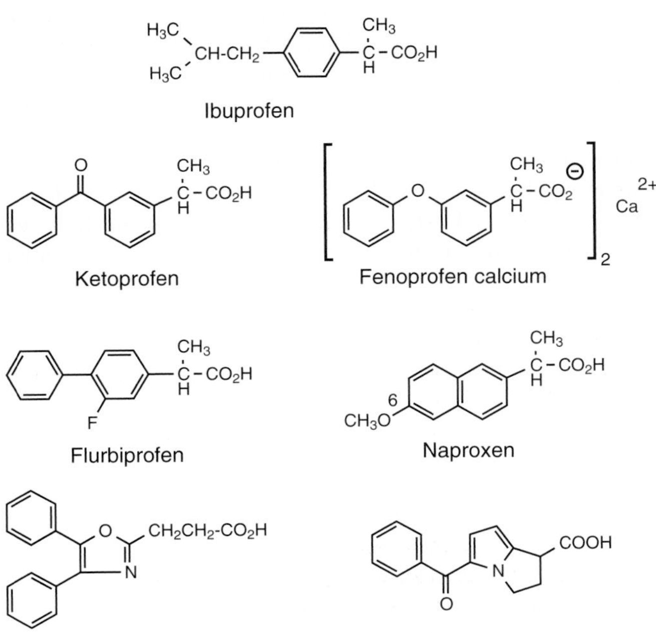

Figure 15.19 Aryl- and heteroarylpropionic acid derivatives.

Absorption and Metabolism. Ibuprofen is rapidly absorbed on oral administration.[83] As with most acidic NSAIDs, ibuprofen is extensively bound to plasma proteins; however, displacement interactions do not seem to be clinically significant.[84,85] Ibuprofen is metabolized rapidly to many inactive metabolites, explaining why it has a short duration of action requiring dosing every 4-6 hours. Ibuprofen is nearly completely excreted in the urine as either unchanged drug or oxidative metabolites within 24 hours after administration (Fig. 15.20).[85]

Metabolism by CYP2C9 (90%) and CYP2C19 (10%) involves primarily ω-1 and ω-oxidation of the *p*-isobutyl side chain, followed by oxidation of the primary alcohol via sequential reactions with alcohol dehydrogenase and aldehyde dehydrogenase to the corresponding carboxylic acid.[86] When ibuprofen is administered as the individual enantiomers, the major metabolite isolated is the *S*-(+)-enantiomer regardless of the configuration of the starting enantiomer. The inactive *R*-(−)-enantiomer is completely inverted to the active *S*-(+)-enantiomer in vivo via a reaction also requiring CoASH, accounting for the observation that the two enantiomers are bioequivalent.[87] This is a metabolic phenomenon that has been also observed for other arylpropionic acids, such as ketoprofen, benoxaprofen, fenoprofen, and naproxen.[88]

Fenoprofen Calcium. Fenoprofen calcium is indicated for treatment of rheumatoid arthritis and osteoarthritis and for the relief of mild to moderate pain. The calcium salt is less hygroscopic than other salts with other cations

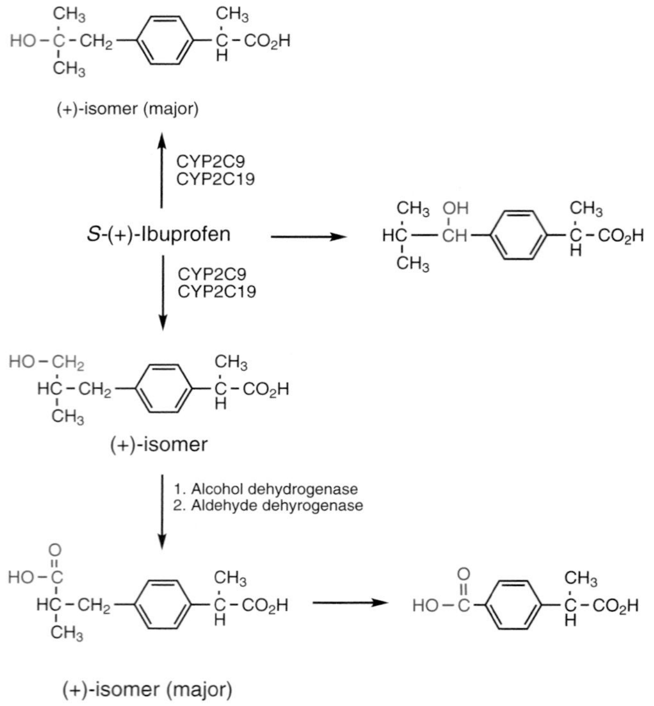

Figure 15.20 Metabolism of ibuprofen.

and therefore easier to formulate into solid dosage forms. Fenoprofen is less potent in anti-inflammatory assays than many other NSAIDs. As an inhibitor of PG biosynthesis, it is much less potent than indomethacin, more potent than aspirin, and about equipotent with ibuprofen. Fenoprofen also possesses analgesic and antipyretic activity. It possesses other pharmacologic properties, such as inhibition of phagocytic and complement functions and stabilization of lysosomal membranes. Fenoprofen is marketed as a racemic mixture, because chiral interconversion ensures the active *S*-(+) isomer will be generated from the *R*-(−) enantiomer in vivo.

Structure-Activity Relationships. Placing the phenoxy group in the *o*- or *p*-position of the arylpropionic acid ring markedly decreases activity. Replacement of the oxygen bridge between the two aromatic rings with a carbonyl group results in a marketed analogue (ketoprofen) with superior potency, presumably through the carbonyl's ability to better enable a non-coplanar conformation between the two rings.

Absorption and Metabolism. Fenoprofen is readily absorbed on oral administration and is highly plasma protein bound.[89] It is susceptible to rapid CYP2C9-mediated oxidation at the *p*-position of the phenolyl ring (Fig. 15.21). Phase 2 glucuronide conjugation reactions occur with the carboxylic acid or the newly added *p*-phenolic hydroxyl group.[90]

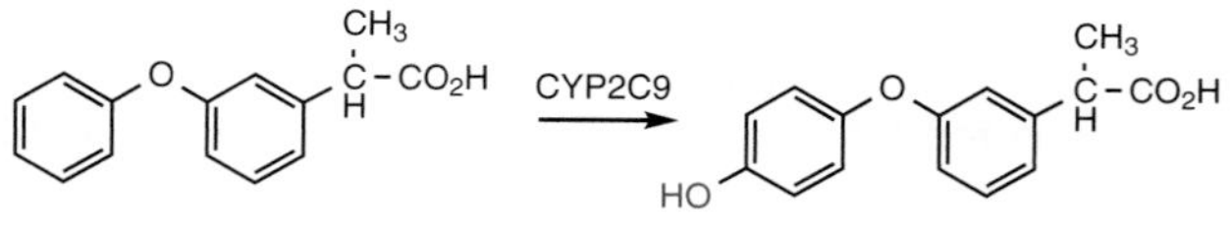

Figure 15.21 Metabolism of fenoprofen.

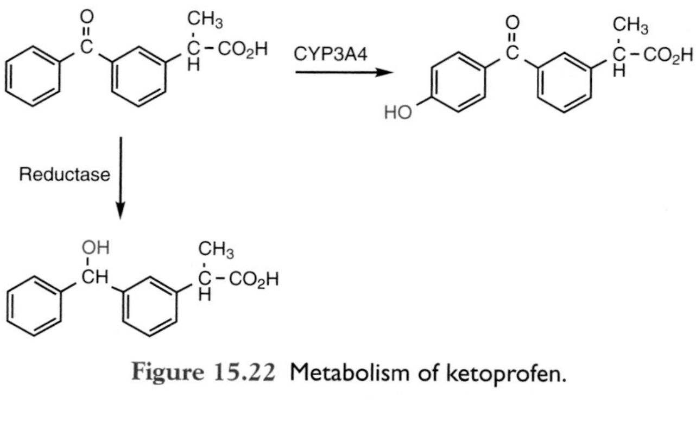

Ketoprofen. Ketoprofen is marketed as the racemic mix and is indicated for the long-term management of rheumatoid arthritis and osteoarthritis, for mild to moderate pain, and for primary dysmenorrhea.[91] It is less potent than indomethacin as an anti-inflammatory agent and an analgesic; however, its ability to produce gastric lesions is effectively equivalent.[92] Ketoprofen is an arylpropionic acid substituted at the *m*-position with a benzoyl group. The ketone linker is sp2 hybridized and maintains conjugation between the two aromatic rings.

Absorption and Metabolism. Ketoprofen is rapidly and nearly completely absorbed on oral administration, reaching peak plasma levels within 0.5-2 hours.[93] It is highly plasma protein bound despite a lower acidity than other NSAIDs (pK_a = 5.9).[94] It is metabolized by CYP3A4 and CYP2C9-catalyzed *p*-hydroxylation of the benzoyl ring, and reduction of the keto function (Fig. 15.22). Phase 2 conjugation reactions occur at the carboxylic acid, forming glucuronide ester conjugates. There are no known active metabolites of ketoprofen, and its vulnerability to metabolic inactivation results in a short half-life of 2-4 hours after administration of the immediate release tablet. Drug interactions may occur with drugs that are metabolized via CYP2C9, as ketoprofen is a known inhibitor of that enzyme.

Naproxen. Naproxen is indicated for the treatment of rheumatoid arthritis, osteoarthritis, juvenile arthritis, ankylosing spondylitis, tendinitis, bursitis, acute gout, and primary dysmenorrhea and for the relief of mild to moderate pain. It is marketed as the pure *S*-(+)-enantiomer. Naproxen contains two fused benzene rings (naphthalene), which is considered a single aromatic moiety; therefore naproxen's potency is relatively low compared to other NSAIDs that have two distinct conjugated aromatic rings.

Structure-Activity Relationships. In a series of substituted 2-naphthylacetic acids, substitution in the 6-position led to maximum anti-inflammatory activity. Small lipophilic groups such as chloro, methylsulfide, and difluoromethoxy were active analogues, with methoxy being the most potent.[95] Larger groups were found to be less active.[95] Removal of the α-methyl group from the acetic acid side chain reduced activity. Prodrug mimics of naproxen that replaced the carboxylic acid group with functional groups capable of being metabolized to the carboxylic acid function (e.g., methyl ester, aldehyde, or hydroxymethyl) led to retention of activity. Not surprising, the *S*-(+)-isomer

Figure 15.22 Metabolism of ketoprofen.

is the more potent enantiomer. Naproxen is the only arylalkanoic acid NSAID currently marketed as the optically pure *S* enantiomer.

Absorption and Metabolism. Naproxen is almost completely absorbed following oral administration.[96] Like most of the acidic NSAIDs, it is highly bound to plasma proteins. Approximately 70% of an administered dose is eliminated as either unchanged drug (60%) or conjugates of unchanged drug (10%).[97] The remainder is slowly O-dealkylated to the 6-O-desmethyl metabolite by either CYP2C9 or CYP1A2. Similar to nabumetone, this slow inactivating metabolic reaction accounts for naproxen's extended duration of action, allowing for twice-a-day dosing. Phase 2 glucuronide conjugation of the demethylated metabolite occurs.[98] Like most of the arylalkanoic acids, the most common side effects associated with the use of naproxen are irritation to the GI tract and CNS disturbances.

Flurbiprofen. Flurbiprofen is indicated for the acute or long-term treatment of rheumatoid arthritis and osteoarthritis and is also available in ophthalmic solution for the inhibition of intraoperative miosis induced by PGs in cataract surgery. Unlike other members of this class, there is no *R*- to *S*-isomerization observed in humans, although isomerization has been observed in mice.[99,100] The brand name for flurbiprofen is Ansaid, which stands for Another NSAID. The second aromatic ring is not fused to the arylpropionic acid phenyl ring, and thus is a distinct second conjugated ring, making flurbiprofen more potent over NSAIDs with only one aromatic ring. The 3-fluro group promotes the non-coplanarity of the two aromatic rings, further increasing potency. Lastly, similar to indomethacin's 2-methyl group, the 3-fluoro group is thought to promote a time-dependent conformational change in COX enzymes when bound, leading to pseudoirreversible inhibition.[15]

Absorption and Metabolism. Flurbiprofen is well absorbed after oral administration, with peak plasma levels being attained within 1.5 hours.[101,102] Food alters the rate of absorption, but not the extent of its bioavailability. It is extensively bound to plasma proteins and has a short plasma half-life.[103,104] Flurbiprofen experiences interesting metabolic patterns (Fig. 15.23), with 40%-47% converted to the *p*-hydroxy metabolite, 5% to the *m,p*-dihydroxy (catechol) metabolite, 20%-30% to the *m*-hydroxy-*p*-methoxy metabolite, and the remaining 20%-25% of the drug being excreted unchanged.[104] Metabolism is extensive, with 60%-70% of flurbiprofen and its metabolites being excreted as sulfate and glucuronide conjugates. None of these metabolites demonstrates significant anti-inflammatory activity.

Ketorolac Tromethamine. Ketorolac is a pyrroleacetic acid where the α-methyl group is bonded to the N-methyl group, forming a pyrrolidine ring. It is indicated as a peripheral analgesic for short-term use and for the relief of ocular itching caused by seasonal allergies. Ketorolac exhibits anti-inflammatory and antipyretic activity as well. Ketorolac also exhibits analgesic activity similar to morphine, and with the concern about the overuse of opioids and the potential for addiction, ketorolac is viable alternative to opioid therapy, primarily in the inpatient setting.[105] Although the analgesic effect is achieved within 10 minutes of injection, peak analgesia lags behind peak plasma levels by 45-90 minutes. As with the other acidic NSAIDs, ketorolac is highly plasma protein bound.[106] Ketorolac is rapidly metabolized by CYP2C9 to its *p*-hydroxy derivative and to conjugates that are excreted primarily in the urine.[106] Concomitant use of aspirin or other NSAIDs is contraindicated due to an increased risk of serious toxicity (hemorrhage, renal toxicity, cardiotoxicity). Along with other NSAIDs, this drug carries boxed warnings for GI ulceration/perforation and potentially fatal thromboembolic events. To reduce its GI and kidney toxicities, ketorolac use should be limited to 5 days.

Oxaprozin. Oxaprozin is marketed for acute and long-term use in the management of osteoarthritis and rheumatoid arthritis. Oxaprozin is a unique arylpropionic acid where the "propyl" group is linear as opposed to the traditional branched chain with an α-methyl group. Oxaprozin is well absorbed after oral administration, but maximum plasma concentrations are not reached until 3-5 hours following ingestion, which is longer than most other NSAIDs. Oxaprozin is an anti-inflammatory agent possessing a rapid onset of action and a significantly extended duration of action. Oxaprozin, aspirin, ibuprofen, indomethacin, naproxen, and sulindac have comparable efficacy in the treatment of rheumatoid arthritis, whereas oxaprozin, aspirin, naproxen, and piroxicam have comparable efficacy in osteoarthritis. It is highly bound to plasma proteins, is highly lipophilic, yet undergoes little first-pass metabolism. Metabolism is via hepatic microsomal oxidation and glucuronidation. Two hydroxylated phenolic

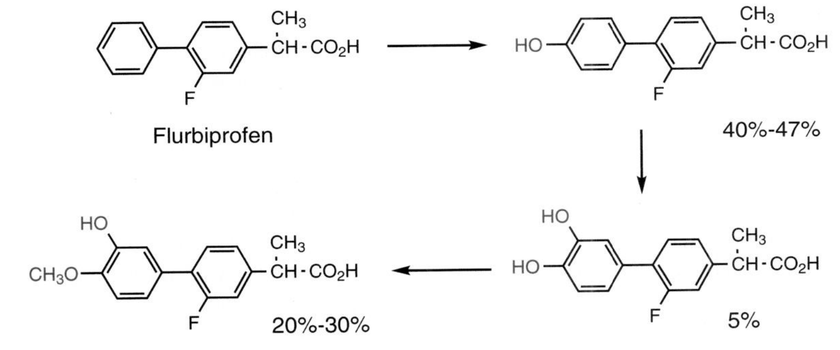

Figure 15.23 Metabolism of flurbiprofen.

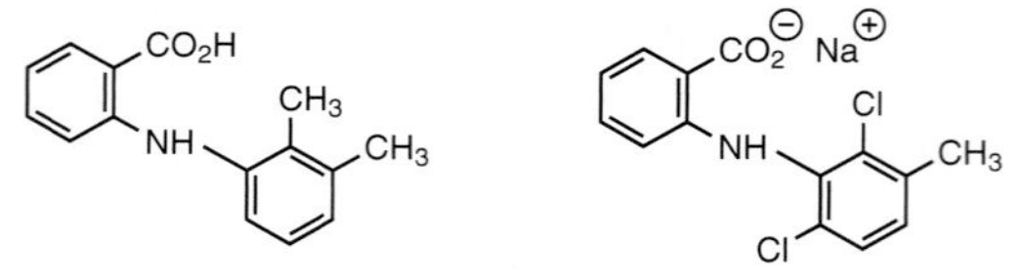

Mefenamic acid (Ponstel) Meclofenamate sodium

Figure 15.24 N-arylanthranilic acids (fenamic acids).

metabolites that are produced (<5%) have been shown to possess anti-inflammatory activity but do not appear to contribute significantly to the overall pharmacologic activity of oxaprozin.[107] Oxaprozin's minimal metabolic profile and long elimination half-life that ranges from 26 to 92 hours enables once-daily dosing.[107] Administration with food appears to delay absorption but not bioavailability. Oxoprozin can induce phototoxicity in patients exposed to sunlight, producing rash.

N-ARYLANTHRANILIC ACIDS (FENAMIC ACIDS). The anthranilic acid class of NSAIDs are bioisosteres of the salicylic acid class, where an –NH– has replaced the -OH of salicylic acid. Additionally, they could be considered structural analogues of the phenylacetic acid derivative, diclofenac (Fig. 15.11). The fenamic acids possess little advantage over the salicylates with respect to their anti-inflammatory and analgesic properties, and this has diminished interest in their large-scale development relative to the arylalkanoic acids. The structures of the fenamic acids are shown in Figure 15.24.

The fenamic acids share a number of pharmacologic properties with the other NSAIDs. They were shown to block PG biosynthesis primarily through the inhibition of COX enzymes, which is their primary mechanism of therapeutic action.[108,109] Their chemical structures fit the NSAID general SAR, where they have an acidic functional group connected to an aromatic ring along with an additional conjugated aromatic ring.[2] Interestingly, fenamic acid NSAIDs, including mefenamic acid, have shown promise for Alzheimer's disease in animal models through a mechanism of action independent of COX inhibition.[110] Side effects are those primarily associated with GI disturbances, some CNS effects, skin rashes, and transient hepatic and renal abnormalities.

General Structure-Activity Relationships

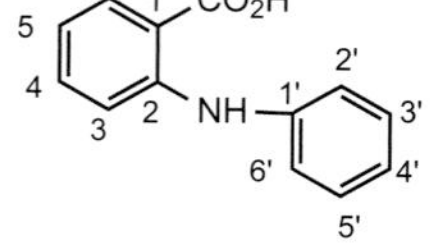

Fenamate numbering

The benzoic acid portion of the fenamic acid structure is essential for activity, as the carboxylic acid group makes an essential ion-ion bond with the COX active site Arg120. Replacement of the carboxylic acid function with the isosteric tetrazole moiety has little effect on activity. The *o*-anilino group increases COX binding capabilities, as the second conjugated ring makes more effective van der Waals and hydrophobic interactions in the COX active sites. Substituents on the anilino ring that promote noncoplanarity with the benzoic acid ring enhance binding at this site and, thus, activity. This can account for the enhanced anti-inflammatory activity of meclofenamic acid, which has two large *o*-substituents forcing this ring out of the plane of the anthranilic acid ring. Meclofenamic acid (conjugate acid of meclofenamate sodium) possesses 25 times greater anti-inflammatory activity than mefenamic acid, likely attributable to both steric and lipophilicity-related parameters of the aromatic chloro substituents of the former. The NH-moiety of anthranilic acid appears to be essential for activity, as replacement of the NH function with oxygen, methylene (CH_2), sulfur, sulfone (SO_2), N-CH_3, or acetamide (N-$COCH_3$) functionalities significantly reduces activity.[111] The *o*-substituted anilino group is critical for activity, as *m*- and *p*- substitutions are inactive.

Drug Interactions. The fenamic acid class of acidic NSAIDs are highly plasma protein bound, and significant drug interactions can occur with other highly plasma protein bound drugs. The most common interactions reported are those of mefenamic acid and meclofenamic acid with oral anticoagulants, potentially requiring a reduction in anticoagulant dose.[112]

Specific Drugs

Mefenamic Acid. Mefanamic acid is indicated for the short-term relief of moderate pain and for primary dysmenorrhea. It is the only fenamic acid derivative that produces analgesia centrally and peripherally.

Mefenamic acid is absorbed rapidly following oral administration. It is highly bound to plasma proteins and has a short plasma half-life which can be explained by the rapid inactivating metabolic pathway. Mefenamic acid does have an open *p*-position on the anilino ring which is usually a vulnerable site for CYP-mediated oxidation. However, benzylic methyl groups are also a metabolic liability and mefenamic acid has two of them. Phase 1 metabolism occurs through CYP2C9-mediated regioselective oxidation of the least hindered 3′-methyl group to the primary alcohol with subsequent oxidation to the carboxylic acid. Phase 2 glucuronidation occurs at the carboxylic acid of the parent or its metabolites. Urinary excretion accounts for approximately 50%-55% of an administered dose, with unchanged drug accounting for 6%, the 3′-hydroxymethyl metabolite (primarily as the glucuronide) accounting for 25%, and the remaining 20% as the dicarboxylic acid (of which 30% is the glucuronide conjugate) (Fig. 15.25).[113] Only the primary alcohol metabolite is active; however, the therapeutic action may be irrelevant due to quick inactivating cytosolic oxidation.

Meclofenamate Sodium. Meclofenamate sodium is indicated for the relief of mild to moderate pain, the acute and chronic treatment of rheumatoid arthritis and osteoarthritis, the treatment of primary dysmenorrhea, and the treatment of idiopathic, heavy menstrual blood loss. Meclofenamate sodium is a tri-substituted fenamic acid, where the two *o*-chloro groups provide significant steric bulk that greatly enhance the non-coplanarity of the two aromatic rings. This contributes to its ~25-fold potency increase over mefenamic acid. Meclofenamate sodium is rapidly and

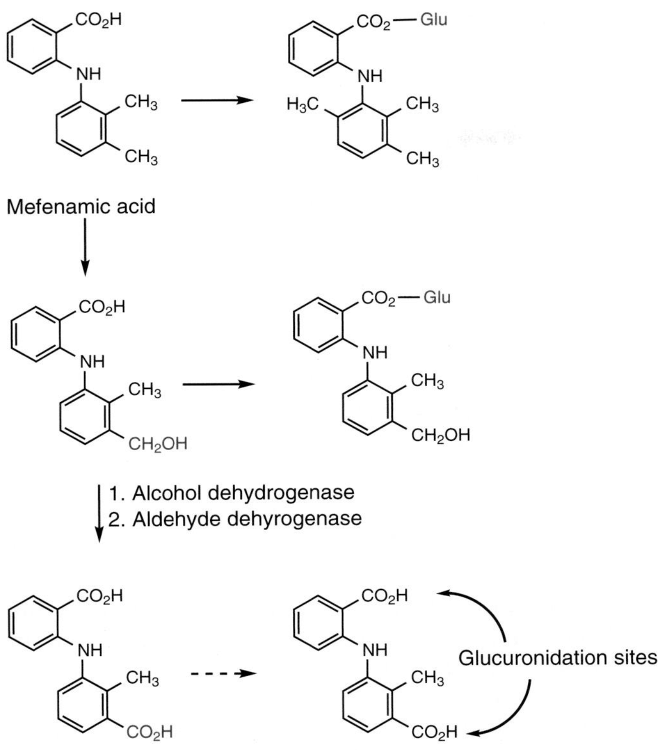

Figure 15.25 Metabolism of mefenamic acid (Glu = glucuronide).

almost completely absorbed following oral administration.[114] It is highly bound to plasma proteins and has a short plasma half-life. Meclofenamate sodium has a similar metabolic profile to mefenamic acid, where the benzylic methyl is oxidized rapidly by CYP2C9 to the primary alcohol (Fig. 15.26). In addition, meclofenamate sodium is also susceptible to *p*-hydroxylation and dehalogenation reactions that result in the removal of one of the *o*-chloro groups. Phase 2 glucuronidation occurs at the carboxylic acid of the parent drug and its metabolites. Urinary excretion of the parent and metabolites accounts for approximately 75% of the administered dose. The major metabolite is the product of 3′-methyl oxidation, which has been shown to possess anti-inflammatory activity. Although the *p*-hydroxy metabolite is minor, the fact that it could generate an electrophilic quinoneimine (similar to that generated from diclofenac) may help explain its hepatotoxicity.

OXICAMS. The enolic acid class of NSAIDs has been termed "oxicams" by the U.S. Adopted Name Council to describe the series of 4-hydroxy-1,2-benzothiazine carboxamides that possess anti-inflammatory and analgesic properties.

General Structure-Activity Relationships. Given the general structure shown below, the cyclic sulfonamide must be tertiary and optimum activity was observed when R_1 was methyl. The carboxamide substituent, R, is optimal with an aryl or heteroaryl substituent. Alkyl substituents for R are less active.

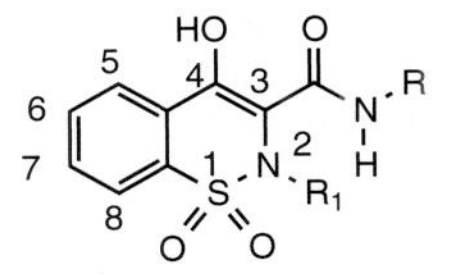

Oxicams have an acidic enol functional group with pK_a values in the range of 4-6. The acidic nature of the enol is attributed to stabilization of the enolate anion (conjugate base of enolic acid) by (1) an intramolecular ion-dipole bond (shown in structure A) and (2) the extended resonance as illustrated in the figure at the top of the next page in resonance hybrid A and hybrid B.[115] This explains the observation that secondary carboxamides are more potent than the corresponding tertiary derivatives, because no N–H bond would be available to enhance the stabilization of the enolate anion in the latter.

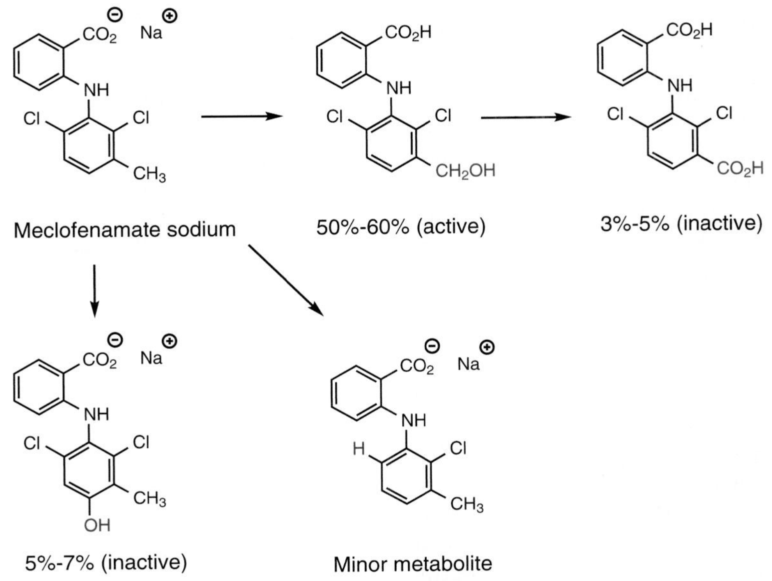

Figure 15.26 Metabolism of meclofenamate sodium.

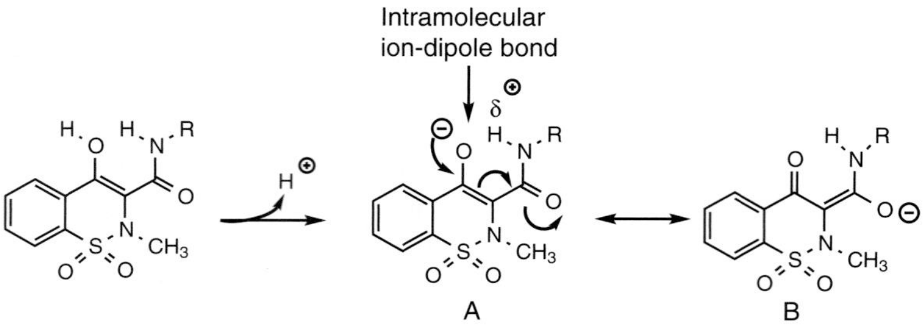

Piroxicam enolate stabilization

The optimal substituents on the secondary carboxamide group are heteroaromatics such as 2-pyridyl (piroxicam), 2-thiazolyl (meloxicam), or 3-(5-methyl) isoxazolyl ring system substituents. In addition to possessing anti-inflammatory activity equal to or greater than indomethacin, the heteroaryl carboxamides also possess longer plasma half-lives, providing less frequent dosing regimens.

Drug Interactions. A number of reports of therapeutically significant interactions of oxicams with other drugs have appeared. Concurrent administration of aspirin has been shown to reduce oxicam plasma levels by approximately 20%, whereas anticoagulant effects can be potentiated, presumably as a result of plasma protein displacement.[116,117]

Specific Drugs

Piroxicam. Piroxicam is indicated for long-term use in rheumatoid arthritis and osteoarthritis. It is readily absorbed on oral administration, reaching peak plasma levels in approximately 2 hours.[118] Food does not markedly affect the bioavailability of piroxicam. Despite being a very weak acid ($pK_a = 6.3$), it is highly bound to plasma proteins (99%) similar to other NSAIDs.[119] Piroxicam possesses an extended plasma half-life (38 hours), making single daily dosing possible. It possesses COX-1 preferential inhibitory activity; therefore GI distress can be problematic.

Metabolism. Piroxicam is extensively metabolized, with less than 5% of an administered dose being excreted unchanged. The major metabolites result from CYP2C9 hydroxylation at C5 of the pyridine ring followed by glucuronidation (Fig. 15.27).[120] Aromatic hydroxylation at several positions on the aromatic benzothiazine ring also occurs.[121] Other novel metabolic reactions occur, including ring contraction following amide hydrolysis and decarboxylation, which yields saccharin.[121] All the known metabolites of piroxicam are inactive.

Meloxicam. Meloxicam is indicated for the treatment of osteoarthritis. Meloxicam is an analogue of piroxicam where the 2-pyridyl ring has been replaced with a 5-methylthiazolyl ring. Despite having such similar structural features to piroxicam, meloxicam is a COX-2 preferential inhibitor having approximately two times more COX-2 inhibitory activity over other non-COX-2 selective NSAIDs.[122,123] Due to meloxicam being COX-2 preferential, it carries a lower risk of GI disturbances. Meloxicam is readily absorbed when administered orally and is highly bound to plasma proteins.[124]

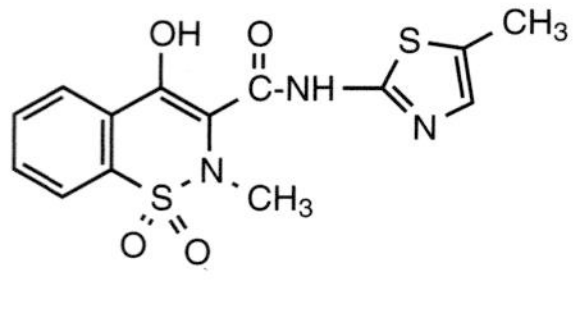

Meloxicam

Metabolism. Meloxicam is extensively metabolized in the liver, primarily by CYP2C9 and, to a lesser extent, by CYP3A4.[125] The 5-methyl group on the thiazole ring is akin to a benzylic carbon and is highly susceptible to CYP oxidation. Oxidation of the thiazole methyl to the primary alcohol is catalyzed by CYP2C9/CYP3A4. The primary alcohol metabolite then undergoes subsequent oxidation reactions to the carboxylic acid.[125] All metabolites are inactive.[125] The metabolism of meloxicam is shown in Figure 15.28.

Gastroenteropathy Induced by Nonselective COX-Inhibiting NSAIDs

The effectiveness and popularity of the NSAIDs make this one of the most commonly used classes of therapeutic entities. As emphasized several times in this chapter, most

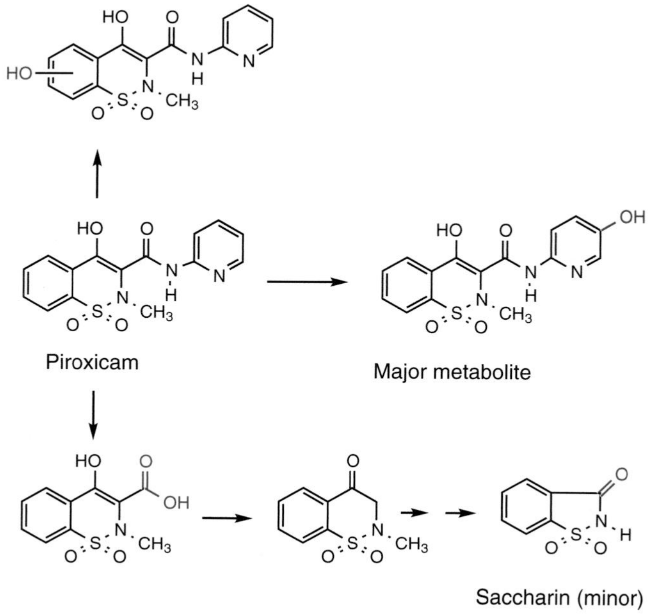

Figure 15.27 Metabolism of piroxicam.

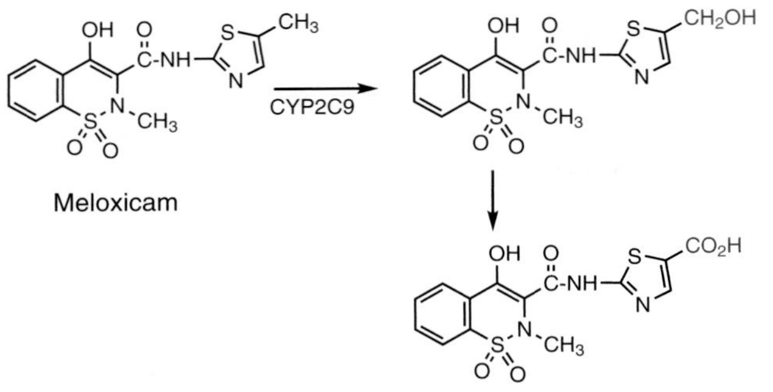

Figure 15.28 Metabolism of meloxicam.

NSAIDs are nonselective COX-1 and COX-2 inhibitors and may exhibit damaging effects to gastric and intestinal mucosa, resulting in erosion, ulcers, and GI bleeding, and these represent the major adverse reactions to the use of NSAIDs.[126]

Normally, the stomach protects itself from the harmful effects of hydrochloric acid and pepsin by a number of protective mechanisms referred to as the gastric mucosal barrier, which consists of epithelial cells, the mucous and bicarbonate layer, and mucosal blood flow. Gastric mucosa is actually a gel consisting of polymers of glycoprotein, which limit the diffusion of hydrogen ions. These polymers reduce the rate at which hydrogen ions (produced in the lumen) and bicarbonate ions (secreted by the mucosa) mix; thus, a pH gradient is created across the mucus layer. Normally, gastric mucosal cells are rapidly repaired when they are damaged by factors such as food, ethanol, or acute ingestion of NSAIDs. Among the cytoprotective mechanisms is the ability of PGs of the PGE series, particularly PGE_1, to increase the secretion of bicarbonate ion and mucus and to maintain mucosal blood flow. The PGs also decrease acid secretion, permitting the gastric mucosal barrier to remain intact.

The use of exogenously administered PGE_1 to reduce NSAID-induced gastric damage is limited by the fact that it is ineffective orally and degrades rapidly on parenteral administration, primarily by oxidation of the secondary 15-hydroxy group. To overcome these limitations, misoprostol was introduced as a PG prodrug analogue in which oral activity was achieved by administering the drug as the methyl ester. The methyl ester must be hydrolyzed by esterases before misoprostol is active. In comparison to PGE_1, the hydroxy group has been moved from C15 to C16. The 16-hydroxy group is now tertiary, which prevents it from being oxidized to the inactive ketone.

Misoprostol was introduced in 1989 as a mixture of C16-stereoisomers for the prevention of NSAID-induced gastric ulcers (but not duodenal ulcers) in patients at high risk of complications from a gastric ulcer, particularly the elderly and patients with concomitant debilitating disease and in individuals with a history of gastric ulcers. However, misoprostol should be used with caution, as it is an abortifacient and should not be given to pregnant women who want to remain pregnant. Another approach to preventing GI distress is the administration of proton pump inhibitors, which stop the active secretion of acid into the gastric lumen (Chapter 26), in combination with an NSAID.[127]

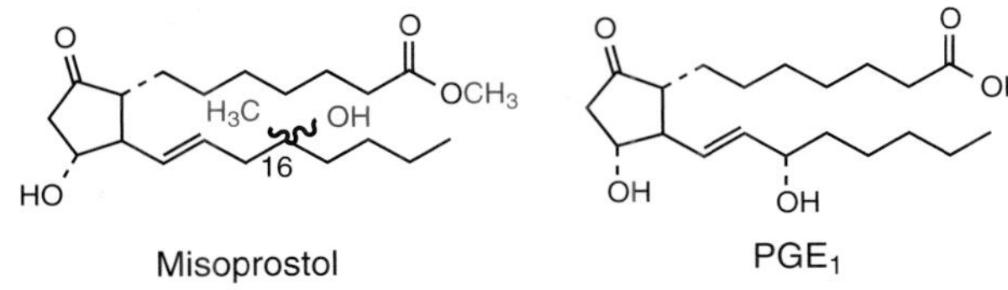

Selective COX-2 Inhibitors

Since COX-2 is inducible in inflammatory events and COX-1 is homeostatic and produces cytoprotective PGs, a COX-2 selective inhibitor would, in theory, be an active anti-inflammatory agent with significantly reduced GI toxicity. Selectivity for COX-2 over COX-1 can be achieved through structures that are large enough to be rejected by the sterically restricted COX-1 active site, but which can still bind within the allosteric binding pocket that serves as a secondary site of enzyme inhibition. The allosteric domain in COX-2 is accessible because it has two Val gatekeeper residues flanking the active site cavity that are smaller than the corresponding Ile residues found on COX-1.

Several selective COX-2 inhibitors reached the US market (celecoxib, rofecoxib, lumiracoxib, and valdecoxib), but safety risks and cardiovascular side effects led to the voluntary removal of all except celecoxib (the first to be marketed and the least COX-2 selective of them all). The development of other selective COX-2 inhibitors, such as parecoxib and etoricoxib, has been halted (Fig. 15.29). To explain why the least COX-2 selective agent was the only one to survive, it is important to note that, while COX-1 is found in platelets and is involved in the biosynthesis of the vasoconstrictive and pro-aggregatory thromboxane A_2, COX-2 is the enzyme that catalyzes the biosynthesis of the vasodilating and anti-aggregatory prostacyclin (PGI_2) in the vessel wall. Therefore, the more COX-2 selective an inhibitor, the higher the TXA_2/PGI_2 ratio and the greater the risk for platelet aggregation–facilitated cardiovascular damage. Rofecoxib was the first COX-2 selective NSAID pulled from the U.S. market (soon followed by valdecoxib and, later, lumiracoxib) due to the very real risk of potentially fatal myocardial infarction, stroke, and other serious cardiovascular pathologies.[128] Patients with underlying cardiovascular disease are most vulnerable to these toxicities, and the elderly are at increased risk for all serious NSAID adverse events, including those induced by COX-2 selective inhibitors. An excellent review of the various chemical classes of selective COX-2 inhibitors has been published.[128]

Perhaps as interesting as the role that COX-2 selective inhibitors have played in reducing the incidence of GI side effects caused by NSAIDs are the reports of other potential therapeutic uses for this new class of drugs, including in Alzheimer's disease and carcinomas of various types.

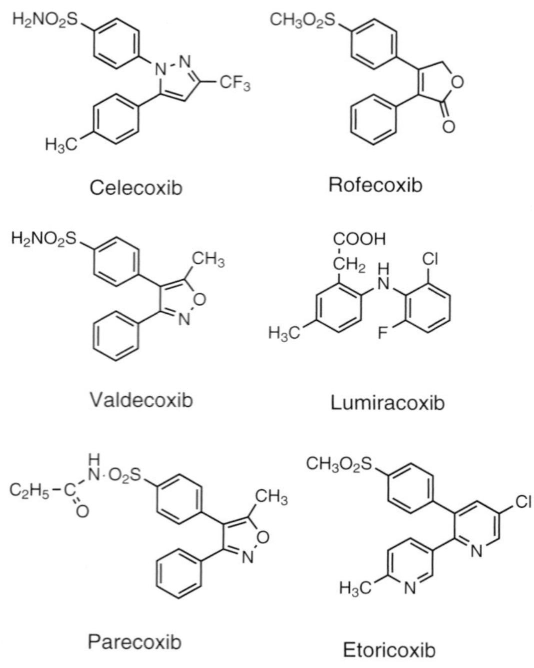

Figure 15.29 Selective COX-2 inhibitors.

Epidemiologic studies suggest a significant reduction in the risk for colon cancer in patients regularly taking aspirin.[39] Additionally, NSAIDs have been reported to reduce the growth rate of polyps in the colon of humans, as well as the incidence of colonic tumors in animals. The expression of COX-2 appears to be significantly upregulated in carcinoma of the colon. The effectiveness of NSAIDs in the prevention and treatment of other cancers, such as prostate cancer and mammary carcinoma, has been reported as well.[129] This effectiveness is more noticeable among COX-2 selective drugs, as this is the isoform upregulated in pathological conditions; however, the potential for this drug class is not certain, as clinical trials have yielded mixed results.[130,131]

SPECIFIC DRUGS

Celecoxib (Celebrex). Celecoxib was the first NSAID to be marketed as a truly selective COX-2 inhibitor. Celecoxib is indicated for the relief of osteoarthritis and rheumatoid arthritis and to reduce the number of adenomatous colorectal polyps in familial adenomatous polyposis as an adjunct to usual care. Celecoxib is well absorbed from the GI tract, with peak plasma concentrations normally being attained within 3 hours of administration.[132] Celecoxib is excreted in the urine and feces primarily as inactive metabolites, with less than 3% of an administered dose being excreted as unchanged drug.[133] Metabolism occurs primarily in the liver by CYP2C9 and involves hydroxylation of the benzylic 4-methyl group to the primary alcohol, which is subsequently oxidized to the corresponding inactive carboxylic acid, the major metabolite (73% of the administered dose) (Fig. 15.30).[134] The carboxylic acid can conjugate with glucuronic acid to form a minor phase 2 metabolite. None of the metabolites are active. Drug interactions are a concern for other drugs metabolized by CYP2D6, as celecoxib inhibits this isoform.

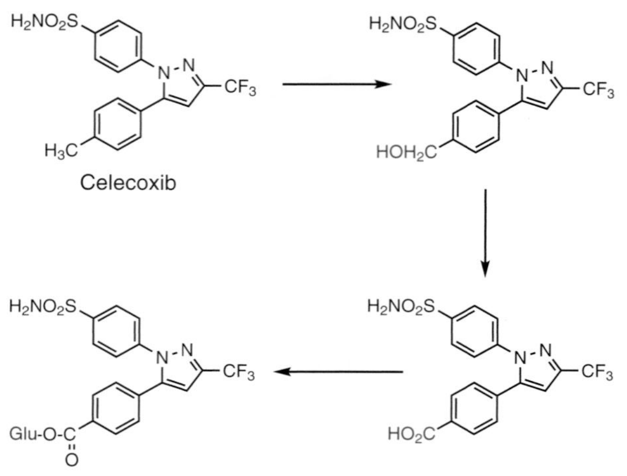

Figure 15.30 Metabolism of celecoxib.

Celecoxib is at least as effective as naproxen in the symptomatic management of osteoarthritis, and at least as effective as naproxen and diclofenac in the symptomatic treatment of rheumatoid arthritis, while being less likely to cause adverse GI effects. Unlike aspirin, celecoxib does not exhibit antiplatelet activity (a COX-1 mediated activity), but concomitant administration of aspirin and celecoxib in an effort to secure the cardiovascular benefits of nonselective COX inhibitors can increase the incidence of GI side effects. Another notable potential drug interaction with celecoxib is its ability to reduce the blood pressure response to angiotensin-converting enzyme inhibitors, an effect it shares with other NSAIDs. A more detailed discussion of the chemical, pharmacologic, pharmacokinetic, and clinical aspects of celecoxib is available.[135]

DISEASE-MODIFYING ANTIRHEUMATIC DRUGS

Disease-modifying antirheumatic drugs (DMARDs) differ from the previously discussed NSAIDs in that they retard or halt the underlying disease progression, limiting the amount of joint damage that occurs in rheumatoid arthritis while lacking the anti-inflammatory and analgesic effects observed with NSAIDs. Although both NSAIDs and DMARDs improve symptoms of active rheumatoid arthritis, only DMARDs have been shown to alter the disease course. DMARDs should be considered for chronic rheumatic disease and are generally slow acting, taking as long as 3 months to experience a therapeutic benefit. Therefore, DMARDs are routinely used with an NSAID or a corticosteroid, as the latter improves the immediate symptoms and limits inflammation while the DMARD affects the disease itself. Interestingly, taking DMARDs at early stages in the development of rheumatoid arthritis has been shown to be especially important to slow the disease and to save the joints and other tissues from permanent damage.[136,137]

The DMARDS can be divided into two general categories: synthetic DMARDS, which can be taken orally, and biologic DMARDS, which are given by IV infusion or subcutaneously. Both classes target and inactivate cell proteins (cytokines) and T lymphocytes (T cells) from causing irreversible joint inflammation.

Synthetic Disease-Modifying Antirheumatic Drugs

Gold Compounds

MECHANISM OF ACTION. The biochemical and pharmacologic properties shared by gold compounds are quite diverse. The mechanism by which they produce their antirheumatic actions has not been totally determined. Several hypotheses were advanced, and ultimately discarded or fell out of favor. Specifically:

- *Antimicrobial activity*—Gold compounds do not consistently inhibit microbial growth in vitro while inhibiting the arthritic process independent of microbial origins.
- *Immunosuppression*—While enzymatic pro-inflammatory mediators released as a result of the immune response can be inhibited, no direct effect on either immediate or delayed cellular responses is evident to suggest any immunosuppressive mechanism.
- *Macroglobulin aggregation*—Gold compounds may inhibit the aggregation of macroglobulins, leading to immune complex formation, thus slowing connective tissue degradation; however, this has not been widely accepted as the primary mechanism of action.
- *Collagen reactivity reduction*—Interaction with collagen fibrils and, thus, reduction of collagen reactivity that alters the course of the arthritic process has been also postulated, but not yet fully accepted.

The most widely accepted mechanism of antiarthritic action for gold compounds is inhibition of lysosomal enzymes, the release of which promotes the inflammatory response. The lysosomal enzymes glucuronidase, acid phosphatase, collagenase, and acid hydrolases are inhibited by these agents, putatively through stable and reversible gold-thiol interactions.

Specific mechanistic observations have been made relative to specific gold compounds. Gold sodium thiosulfate is a potent uncoupler of oxidative phosphorylation. Gold sodium thiomalate is a fairly effective inhibitor of PG biosynthesis in vitro, but the relationship of this effect to the antiarthritic actions of gold compounds has not been clarified. More recent studies suggest that auranofin suppressed the TLR4-mediated activation of the transcription factors by nuclear factor-κB (NF-κB) and IRF3, thus preventing the expression of cytokines and COX-2.[138] Previously it was shown that zinc is a necessary component of NF-κB for DNA binding and that gold ion can block this binding by oxidizing CYS residues associated with zinc.[139] Auranofin has also been shown to decrease tumor necrosis factor (TNF)-α–induced NF-κB activation, suggesting that effective inhibitors of NF-κB can be useful immunosuppressive and anti-inflammatory agents.[140]

ADVERSE EFFECTS. Toxic side effects have been associated with the use of gold compounds, with the incidence of reported adverse reactions in patients on chrysotherapy (aurotherapy or treatment with gold salts) being as high as 55%. Serious toxicity occurs in 5%-10% of reported cases. The most common adverse reactions include dermatitis (e.g., erythema, papular, vesicular, and exfoliative dermatitis), mouth lesions (e.g., stomatitis preceded by a metallic taste and gingivitis), pulmonary disorders (e.g., interstitial pneumonitis), nephritis (e.g., albuminuria and glomerulitis), and hematologic disorders (e.g., thrombocytopenic purpura, hypoplastic and/or aplastic anemia, and eosinophilia; blood dyscrasias are rare in incidence but can be severe). Less commonly reported reactions are GI disturbances (e.g., nausea, anorexia, and diarrhea), ocular toxicity (e.g., keratitis with inflammation and ulceration of the cornea and subepithelial deposition of gold in the cornea), and hepatitis. In those cases in which severe toxicity occurs, excretion of gold can be markedly enhanced by the administration of chelating agents, the two most common of which are dimercaprol (British Anti-Lewisite) and penicillamine. Glucocorticoids also suppress the symptoms of gold toxicity, and the concomitant administration of dimercaprol and corticosteroids has been recommended in cases of severe gold intoxication.

SH HO SH
Dimercaprol

O HS OH NH2
Penicillamine

GENERAL STRUCTURE-ACTIVITY RELATIONSHIPS. Despite the longevity that gold compounds have enjoyed over the last century, the SAR of gold compounds is limited. Monovalent gold (aurous ion [Au^+]) is more effective than trivalent gold (auric ion [Au^{3+}]). Only compounds with aurous ions attached to a sulfur-containing ligand are active (Fig. 15.31). Substituents attached to the aurous ion are typically polar and designed to enhance water solubility and primarily impact tissue distribution and excretion. Aurous ion is short-lived in solution, being rapidly converted to metallic gold or auric ion. Aqueous solutions decompose on standing at room temperature, posing a stability problem for gold compounds formulated as injections (aurothioglucose and gold sodium thiomalate).

In order to increase solution-phase aurous ion stability, complexation of Au^+ with phosphine ligands, such as triethylphosphine (Fig. 15.31), has been employed. Triethylphosphine stabilizes the reduced valence state and results in both nonionic complexes that are soluble in organic solvents and enhanced oral bioavailability. Phosphine compounds lacking an aurous ion are ineffective in arthritic assays; however, compared to other groups bound to gold, the phosphine ligand in the gold coordination complexes appears to play a role in promoting antiarthritic activity. The structures of the three therapeutically available gold compounds in the United States are shown in Figure 15.31.

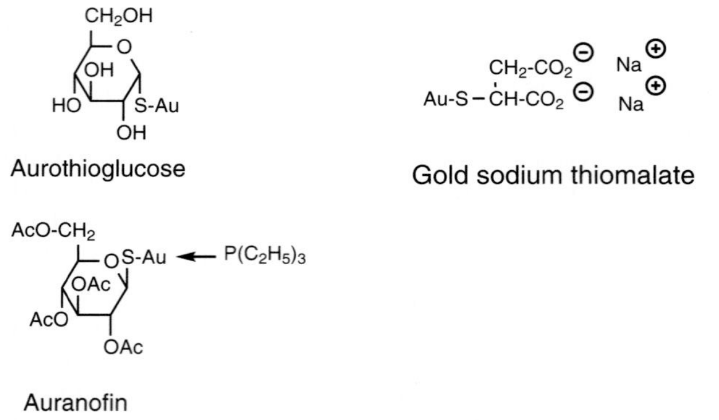

Aurothioglucose

Gold sodium thiomalate

Auranofin

Figure 15.31 Gold compounds as disease-modifying antirheumatic drugs (DMARDs).

ABSORPTION AND METABOLISM. Gold compounds are rapidly absorbed following IM injection and the gold is widely distributed in the body. The highest concentrations are found in the reticuloendothelial system and in adrenal and renal cortices. They are also highly bound to plasma proteins.[141] Binding of gold from orally administered agents to red blood cells is higher than that of injectable gold.[142] Gold accumulates in inflamed joints, where high levels persist for at least 20 days after injection. Although gold is excreted primarily in the urine, the bulk of injected gold is retained. Gold can be found in the urine months after therapy has been discontinued.

DRUG INTERACTIONS. The only significant drug interactions reported for gold compounds are concurrent administration of drugs that decrease excretion of gold compounds, leading to blood dyscrasias (most notably the antimalarial and immunosuppressive drugs).

SPECIFIC DRUGS

Gold Sodium Thiomalate. Gold sodium thiomalate is indicated as an anti-inflammatory agent in the treatment of rheumatoid arthritis. Gold thiomalate inhibits glucosamine-6-phosphate synthase, a rate-limiting step involved in the mucopolysaccharide biosynthesic pathway. Gold sodium thiomalate (actually a mixture of mono- and disodium salts of gold thiomalic acid) is highly water soluble and is available as a light-sensitive aqueous solution of pH 5.8-6.5. The gold content is approximately 50%. It is administered as an IM injection and is not orally bioavailable.

Aurothioglucose. Aurothioglucose is indicated for the adjunctive treatment of adult and juvenile rheumatoid arthritis when other anti-inflammatory agents have been ineffective. It is a glucose analogue where the α-hydroxy group at the 1-position is substituted with an aurothio group, making it highly water soluble. However, aqueous solutions are unstable and decompose; therefore, it is available as a suspension in sesame oil for IM injection. The gold content is approximately 50%. It is highly bound to plasma proteins (95%), and peak plasma levels are achieved within 2-6 hours. The half-life ranges from 3 to 27 days, but following successive weekly doses, the half-life increases to 14-40 days after the third dose. The therapeutic effect does not correlate with serum plasma gold levels but appears to depend on total accumulated gold.

Auranofin. Auranofin is indicated for use in adults with active rheumatoid arthritis who have not responded sufficiently to one or more NSAIDs. It is an analogue of aurothioglucose where all the hydroxy groups have been acetylated and the aurothio group at the 1-position has been epimerized to the β-configuration. The increased lipophilicity of auranofin makes it orally effective, and it is the first orally bioavailable gold compound used to treat rheumatoid arthritis. Auranofin contains approximately 29% gold. Daily oral doses produce a rapid increase in kidney and blood gold levels for the first 3 days of treatment, with a more gradual increase on subsequent administration. Oral absorption is not complete, as plasma gold levels after oral administration are lower than those attained with parenteral gold compounds. The major route of excretion is via the urine. Auranofin can produce fewer adverse reactions than parenteral gold compounds, but its therapeutic efficacy can also be less.

Aminoquinolines

HYDROXYCHLOROQUINE SULFATE. Hydroxychloroquine sulfate, a 4-aminoquinoline, is indicated for the treatment of rheumatoid arthritis, lupus erythematosus, and malaria. While the nonhydroxylated analogue chloroquine was discontinued for use in the treatment of rheumatoid arthritis due to corneal and renal toxicities, hydroxychloroquine, being less toxic, is still indicated for this use. The mechanism of antirheumatic action is currently unknown; however, it is largely accepted that it accumulates in and stabilizes lysosomes.

Hydroxychloroquine sulfate is highly water soluble and is readily absorbed on oral administration, reaching peak plasma levels within 1-3 hours. It concentrates in organs such as the liver, spleen, kidneys, heart, lung, and brain, thereby prolonging elimination. Hydroxychloroquine is metabolized by N-dealkylation of the tertiary amine, followed by oxidative deamination of the resulting primary amine to the carboxylic acid derivative. In addition to possessing mild corneal and renal toxicity, hydroxychloroquine can also cause CNS, neuromuscular, GI, and hematologic side effects.

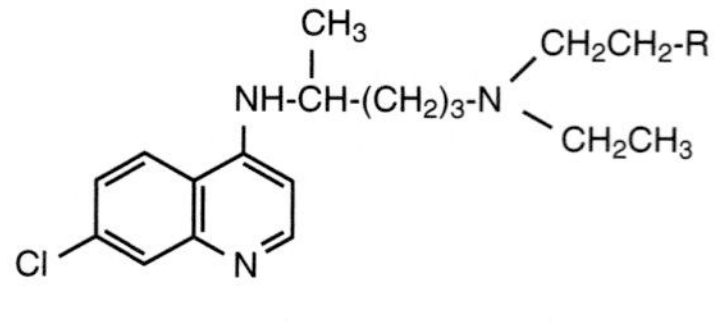

Chloroquine (R = H)
Hydroxychloroquine (R = OH)

Immunosuppressants

Several substances that suppress the immune system have been explored as antirheumatic drugs because the etiology of rheumatoid arthritis can involve a destructive immune response. Thus, unlike drugs previously discussed, immunosuppressive drugs can act at the steps involved in the pathogenesis of the inflammatory disorders. As a group, however, these drugs (shown in Fig. 15.32) are cytotoxic, as evidenced by their initial development as anticancer agents.

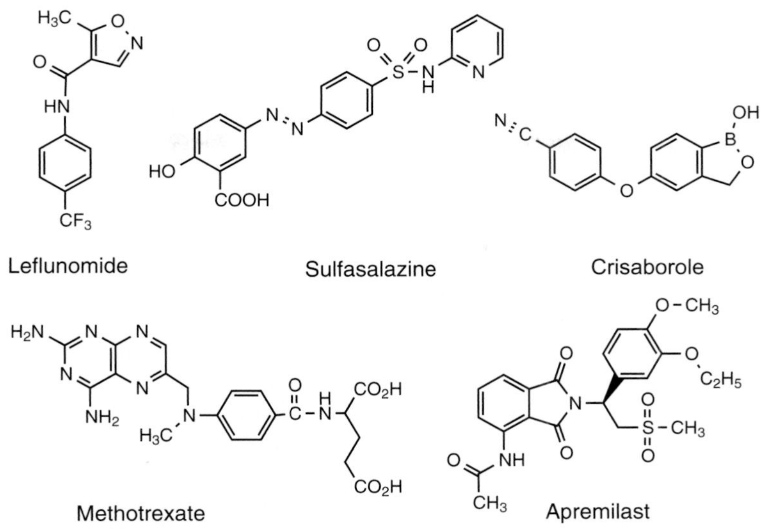

Leflunomide Sulfasalazine Crisaborole

Methotrexate Apremilast

Figure 15.32 DMARD immunosuppressants.

SPECIFIC DRUGS

Leflunomide. Leflunomide is a DMARD used for the management of rheumatoid arthritis. It retards structural damage associated with arthritis in adults who have moderate to severe active rheumatoid arthritis.

Leflunomide is a prodrug that is rapidly and almost completely metabolized (half-life < 60 min) after oral administration to teriflunomide (Fig. 15.33). Teriflunomide is formed from hepatic and GI-mediated isoxazole ring opening to an α-cyanoenol. The C3-H of the isoxazole ring is essential for ring opening.

The mechanism of action of leflunomide is through teriflunomide's ability to inhibit the pyrimidine biosynthetic pathway, specifically inhibiting dihydroorotate dehydrogenase. Inhibition of the pyrimidine biosynthetic pathway results in decreasing DNA and RNA nitrogen-containing bases, and arresting the B-cell and T-cell proliferation cycles and production of antibodies (Fig. 15.34). It is the reduction of B-cell concentrations that downregulates the immune process.

At high therapeutic doses, leflunomide inhibits protein tyrosine kinases. Leflunomide is administered orally as a single daily dose without regard to meals. Therapy can be initiated with a loading dosage given for 3 days, followed by the usual maintenance dose. It undergoes primarily enterohepatic circulation, extending its duration of action.

Methotrexate. Methotrexate (Fig. 15.32) is an antifolate approved for the treatment of severe active rheumatoid arthritis in adults who are intolerant to, or have had an insufficient response to, first-line therapy. There are many putative mechanisms of action for the antirheumatic activity of methotrexate.[143] Similar to leflunomide, methotrexate blocks the pyrimidine biosynthetic pathway and the proliferation of B-cells by interfering with DNA synthesis, repair, and replication. It accomplishes this by pseudoirreversibly inhibiting dihydrofolate reductase. An additional action implicated in methotrexate's antirheumatic activity is the inhibition of the production of polyamines that can be responsible for inducing tissue damage and the activation of NF-κB. Methotrexate is well absorbed after oral administration, and oral bioavailability is approximately 60%, where food can delay absorption and reduce peak serum concentrations. Methotrexate is approximately 50% bound to plasma proteins.

Approximately 10%-20% of a dose of methotrexate is metabolized to active polyglutamated and 7-hydroxylated metabolites.[144] Some prehepatic metabolism occurs in the GI tract after oral administration. Methotrexate is actively transported by the human organic anion transporter (hOAT3) into the urine and is excreted primarily unchanged. Its elimination half-life is 3-10 hours.

Life-threatening drug interactions are known to occur between methotrexate and NSAIDs, probenecid, and penicillin G. These drugs inhibit hOAT3-mediated active transport of methotrexate into the urine. Thus, patients with rheumatoid arthritis should not take NSAIDs while taking methotrexate. Methotrexate therapy requires

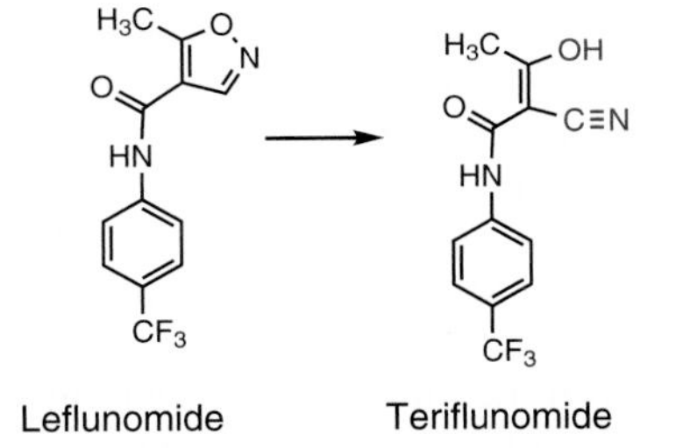

Leflunomide Teriflunomide

Figure 15.33 Metabolism of leflunomide.

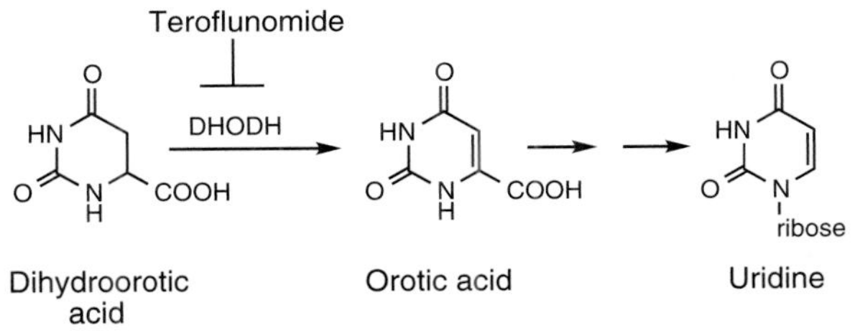

Teroflunomide DHODH

Dihydroorotic acid Orotic acid Uridine

Figure 15.34 Dihydroorotate dehydrogenase (DHODH) pathway.

monitoring of liver enzymes and is contraindicated in those with hepatic disease and in women who are pregnant or considering pregnancy.

Sulfasalazine (Azulfidine). Sulfasalazine is used for the treatment of mild to moderate ulcerative colitis, as adjunct therapy in the treatment of severe ulcerative colitis, for the treatment of Crohn's disease, and for the treatment of rheumatoid arthritis or ankylosing spondylitis. Sulfasalazine is a prodrug that is hydrolyzed by colonic bacteria into 5-aminosalicylic acid (5-ASA; mesalamine) and sulfapyridine (Fig. 15.35). Some controversy exists regarding which of these two products is responsible for the activity of sulfasalazine. 5-ASA, like aspirin, is an inhibitor of PG biosynthesis and is known to have therapeutic benefit. However, it is not clear whether sulfapyridine adds any further benefit since it is the metabolite that is more extensively absorbed. It was shown to inhibit purine biosynthesis by inhibiting 5-aminoimidazole-4-carboxamisoribonucleotide transformylase and to enhance adenosine release, enhancing the ability of adenosine to decrease inflammation by binding to A2 adenosine receptors on inflammatory cells.[145] Sulfasalazine and/or its metabolites have been shown to inhibit the release of inflammatory cytokines and TNFα. In the colon, the products created by the breakdown of sulfasalazine work as anti-inflammatory agents for treating colon inflammation. The beneficial effect of sulfasalazine is believed to result from a local effect on the bowel, although there can also be a beneficial systemic immunosuppressant effect.

Following oral administration, sulfasalazine is poorly absorbed, with approximately 20% reaching the systemic circulation. The remainder of the ingested dose is metabolized by colonic bacteria as shown in Figure 15.35. Most of the sulfapyridine metabolized from sulfasalazine (60%-80%) is absorbed from the colon, compared with approximately 25% of the metabolically generated 5-ASA. Protein binding is approximately 99% for sulfasalazine, approximately 50% for sulfapyridine, and approximately 43% for 5-ASA. The absorbed sulfapyridine is acetylated and hydroxylated in the liver, followed by conjugation with glucuronic acid. 5-ASA undergoes N-acetylation in the intestinal mucosal wall and the liver. The elimination half-life is 5-10 hours for sulfasalazine and 6-14 hours for sulfapyridine, depending on acetylator status of the patient, and 0.6-1.4 hours for 5-ASA. Time to peak serum concentration is 1.5-6 hours for oral sulfasalazine and 9-24 hours for oral sulfapyridine; for enteric-coated tablets, time to peak serum concentration is 3-12 hours for sulfasalazine and 12-24 hours for sulfapyridine. Approximately 5% of sulfapyridine and approximately 67% of 5-ASA are eliminated in the feces, and 75%-91% of sulfasalazine and sulfapyridine metabolites are excreted in urine within 3 days, depending on the dosage form used. 5-ASA is excreted in urine mostly in acetylated form. Contraindications include hypersensitivity to sulfonamide antibiotics, salicylates, intestinal or urinary obstruction, and porphyria.

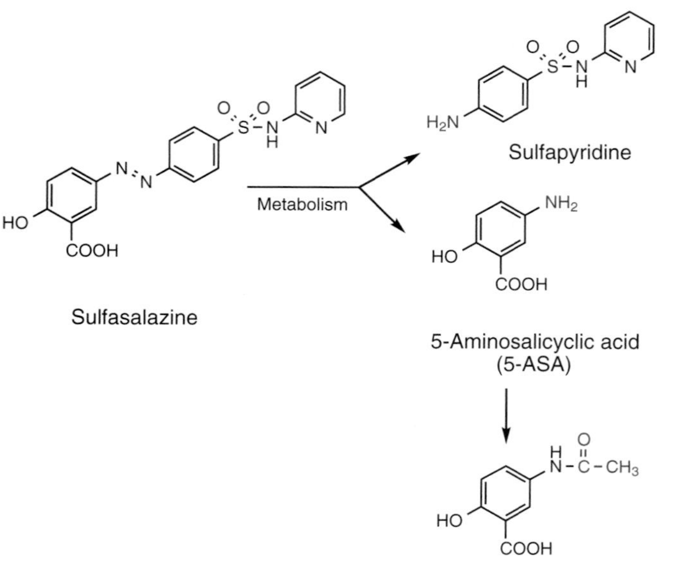

Figure 15.35 Metabolism of sulfasalazine.

Apremilast (Otezla). Apremilast (Fig. 15.32) is a phthalimide analogue approved for treatment of active psoriatic arthritis or plaque psoriasis and which is being tested for a number of additional inflammatory conditions such as ankylosing spondylitis, Behcet's disease, and rheumatoid arthritis.[146,147] The treatment of psoriatic arthritis (PsA) normally calls for the use of costly biologicals, which are administered via injection. The advent of an orally active low molecular weight drug is highly desirable.

A variety of inflammatory mediators are associated with the onset of psoriasis. These include TNF, a number of interleukins (ILs), interferon γ (IFNγ), vascular endothelial growth factor (VEGF), and several chemokines (CXCL). The most recent therapeutic approach to attenuating the inflammatory impact of these mediators has been to inhibit the hydrolysis of cyclic cAMP. The concentration of cAMP is regulated by adenylyl cyclases (synthesis) and phosphodiesterase (PDE) (degradation); therefore inhibition of cAMP hydrolysis translates to inhibition of PDE.

Apremilast is an orally active PDE4 inhibitory drug, which does not show selectivity for any particular PDE4 receptor subclass.[148] Among the PDEs, the PDE4 isoforms are found within immune cells such as lymphocytes, granulocytes, and cells of the monocyte/macrophage system. Important PDEs within immune cells are PDE4A, B, and D. Unfortunately, nonspecific inhibitors of PDE4 cause significant adverse events, including diarrhea by binding to intestinal ion channels and stimulating chloride ion secretion into the small intestine, and emesis. Headache, a runny and/or stuffy nose, upper respiratory tract infections, and abdominal pain may also be experienced.

Apremilast is rapidly absorbed following oral administration and exhibits a long half-life (~8 hr). The T_{max} occurs at approximately 2.5 hours. Apremilast is extensively metabolized to a wide variety of products, and only 7% of the drug is excreted unchanged. It is primarily inactivated through CYP3A4-mediated O-dealkylation of the methoxy group, forming metabolite M3, followed by glucuronide conjugation to give M12 (Fig. 15.36).[149] Apremilast should not be administered to patients taking CYP3A4 inducers, as this results in significantly reduced serum concentrations. The addition of ketoconazole to the regimen results in a significant increase in the AUC, also suggesting

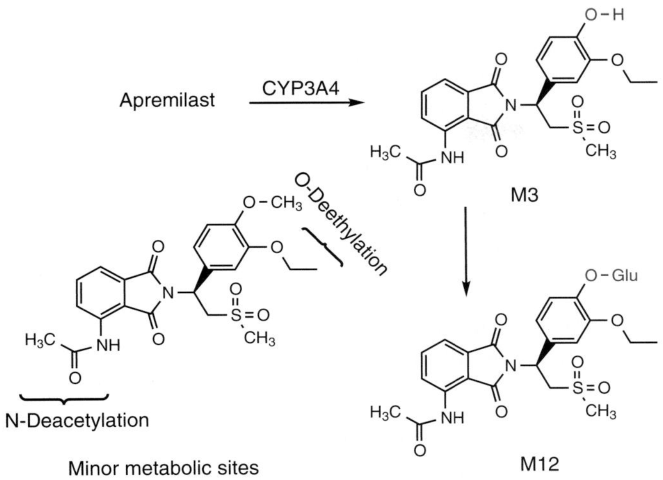

Figure 15.36 Metabolism of apremilast.

CYP3A4/5 as the metabolizing enzyme. Minor metabolites include those generated through O-deethylation, N-deacetylation, and additional aromatic hydroxylation reactions. The majority of the metabolites are found in the urine and all are inactive.

Crisaborole (Eucrisa). Crisaborole is an immunosuppressant approved for the treatment of atopic dermatitis and has also completed phase 2 clinical trials for the treatment of psoriasis.[150] Atopic dermatitis is commonly associated with an increased level of phosphodiesterase 4B activity which, in turn, leads to increased levels of TNFα, IL-12, and IL-23. The disease is characterized by the symptoms of severe pruritus and skin barrier disruption. Crisaborole contains a boron atom, which is typically not seen in pharmaceuticals; however, it is essential for its activity and also promotes skin penetration. Crisaborole is structurally similar to the topical antifungal agent, tavaborole. The most common adverse effect consists of pain at the site of application.

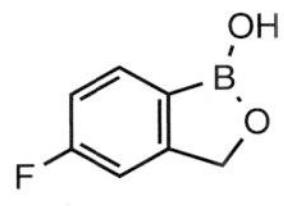

Tavaborole

Crisaborole is an inhibitor of PDE4 and, as such, results in decreased levels of TNFα and various ILs (Fig. 15.37).[151] As with apremilast, inhibition of PDE4 by crisaborole leads to increased levels of cAMP[151] but, unlike apremilast, it has been shown to exhibit selectivity toward isoforms A and B of the PDE4 enzyme. More specifically, the boron atom binds in a tetrahedral configuration to bimetal ions in the catalytic site of the PDE4B enzyme.[152] In so doing, crisaborole, through the hydrated boron atom, appears to be taking the normal binding site that the phosphate in cAMP would occupy, which spares the cyclic nucleotide from hydrolytic destruction.[152]

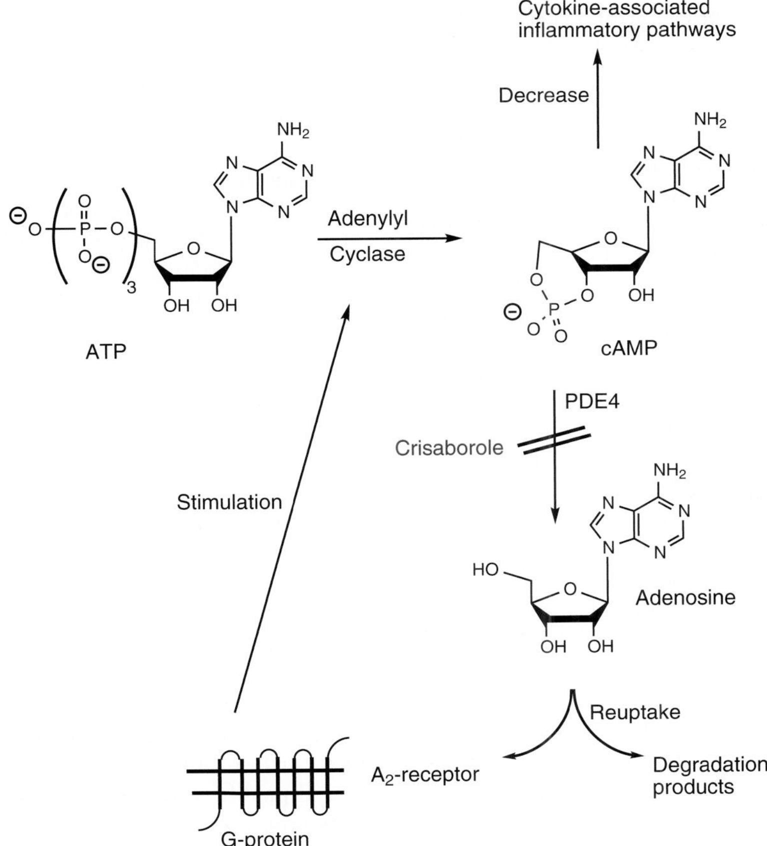

Figure 15.37 Mechanism of action for crisaborole.

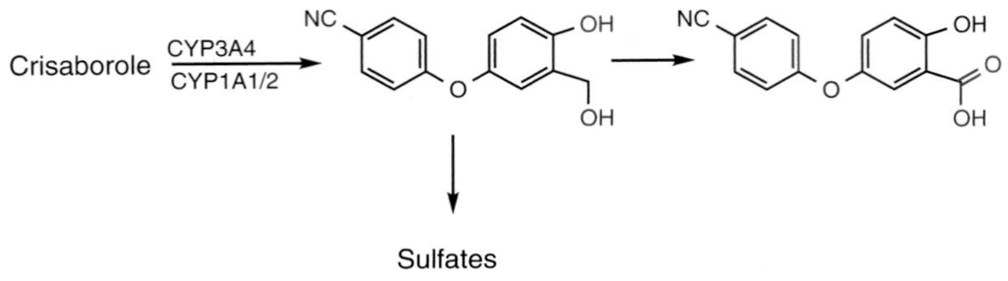

Crisaborole —CYP3A4, CYP1A1/2→ [NC–C6H4–O–C6H3(OH)(CH2OH)] → [NC–C6H4–O–C6H3(OH)(COOH)]; ↓ Sulfates

Figure 15.38 Metabolism of crisaborole.

Crisaborole is available as a 2% ointment and is used topically. The drug is absorbed following topical administration (~25%), extensively metabolized to inactive metabolites (Fig. 15.38), and excreted via the urine. The major CYP3A4- and 1A1/2-generated metabolite results from oxidative deboronation followed by hydrolysis of crisaborole, yielding 5-(4-cyanophenoxy)-2-hydroxyl benzyl alcohol. The primary alcohol is then further oxidized to the carboxylic acid. The drug is highly bound to plasma protein.

Biologic Disease-Modifying Antirheumatic Drugs

Interleukin-1 Receptor Antagonist

ANAKINRA (KINERET). Anakinra is approved for use in adults with moderate to severe active rheumatoid arthritis and in whom conventional DMARD therapy was ineffective, and it can be used in combination with methotrexate.[153] Anakinra is a recombinant, nonglycosylated form of the human IL-1 receptor antagonist (IL-1Rα) that neutralizes the inflammatory activity of the pro-inflammatory IL-1 cytokine by competing with IL-1 for binding to its IL-1 type 1 receptor (IL-1R1). IL-1R1 activation leads to increases in the formation of nitric oxide, PGE_2, and collagenase in synovial cells, resulting in cartilage degradation and stimulation of bone resorption. IL-1R1 receptor activity is regulated by the endogenous antagonist IL-1Rα. Synovial fluid has increased concentrations of IL-1 in rheumatoid synovium, resulting imbalance between IL-1 and IL-1Rα leading to rheumatic progression. The levels of the naturally occurring IL-lRα in synovium and synovial fluid from rheumatoid arthritic patients are insufficient to compete with the elevated amount of locally produced IL-1; therefore exogenous anakinra (IL-1Rα analogue) can be administered to effectively neutralize the proinflammatory activity of IL-1 through competitive inhibition of IL-1RI.

Anakinra consists of 153 amino acids and has a molecular weight of 17.3 kDa. It is produced by recombinant DNA technology using an *Escherichia coli* bacterial expression system and differs from native human IL-1Rα by the addition of a single Met residue at its amino terminus.

Anakinra is administered subcutaneously on a once-daily basis, and its elimination half-life ranges from 4 to 6 hours. Some potential side effects include injection site reactions, decreased white blood cell counts, headache, and an increase in upper respiratory infections. There can be a slightly higher rate of respiratory infections in people who have asthma or chronic obstructive pulmonary disease. Persons with an active infection are advised not to use anakinra.

Interleukin-6 Receptor Antagonist

TOCILIZUMAB (ACTEMRA). Tocilizumab is approved for use in adults with moderate to severe active rheumatoid arthritis, cytokine release syndromes, and giant cell arteritis. It can be used in combination with methotrexate and is an alternative therapy for rheumatic patients not responding to TNFα blockers (discussed below). Tocilizumab is a recombinant humanized antihuman monoclonal antibody that binds to and inhibits solubilized and membrane-bound IL-6 receptors.[154] IL-6 is the endogenous pro-inflammatory agonist for the IL-6 receptors. Tocilizumab is a member of the IgG1κ subclass with a typical H2L2 (two heavy and two light chains) polypeptide structure. Each light chain consists of 214 amino acids, whereas the heavy chain contains 448 residues. The four polypeptide chains are linked by disulfide bonds both intra- and intermolecularly. It has a molecular weight of approximately 148 kDa.

Tocilizumab's dosing regimen is either 4 or 8 mg/kg IV every 4 weeks. Steady-state is reached following the first administration for C_{max} and AUC, respectively, and after 16 weeks for C_{min}. The half-life is concentration dependent and is 11 days for the 4 mg/kg dose and 13 days for the 8 mg/kg dose. The total dose should not exceed 800 mg per infusion. The most frequently observed adverse effects are upper respiratory tract infection, headache, hypertension, increased alanine transaminase activity, and nasopharyngitis.

Costimulation Modulators

Two signals are required to activate a T-cell response to an antigen, and the process is referred to as costimulation. Costimulation activation is shown in Figure 15.39. The two signals for the costimulation process are:

1. An unactivated antigen-presenting cell (APC) "presents" an antigen complex that is recognized by the T-cell receptor.
2. A costimulatory ligand, such as B7, that interacts with CD28 on the T-cell surface to form a B7-CD28 complex and which is also presented by the APC

If only process 1 above happens, the T cell does not respond and becomes unreactive and nonresponsive to any further antigenic stimuli. If both processes occur, T-cell proliferation and differentiation in response to the antigenic stimulus is initiated and T cell binding proinflammatory cytokines are released, further enhancing its

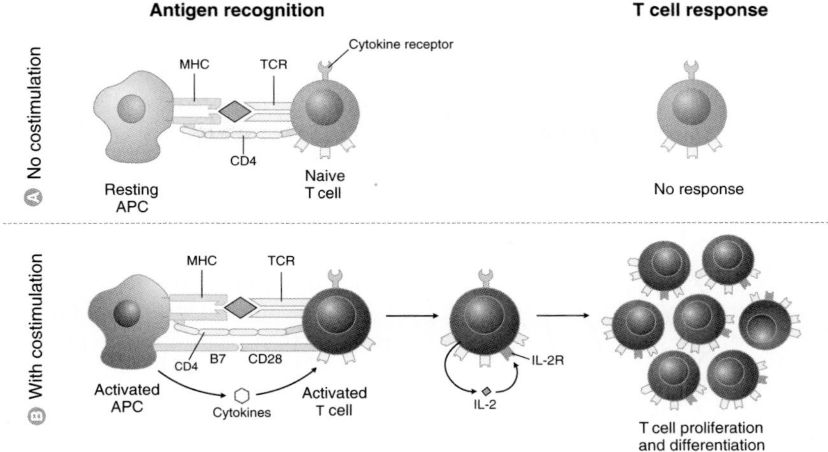

Figure 15.39 Costimulation in the T-cell activation pathway.

activation. T-cell costimulation activation is regulated by T-lymphocyte antigen 4 (CTLA-4) which is also expressed on the T-cell surface and is upregulated on T-cell activation. B7 ligands on the surface of APCs now have a choice on where to bind on the surface of T-cells, CD28 or CTLA-4. The B7 ligands bind with a greater affinity to CTLA-4 than to CD28, preventing delivery of the costimulatory signal. This built-in limit prevents T-cell activation from spiraling out of control.

ABATACEPT (ORENCIA). As described above, the costimulatory process ends with a B7-CD28 complex between the APC and the T-cell, resulting in T-cell activation and the subsequent proliferation and release of proinflammatory cytokines. Abatacept, a costimulation modulator acting through reduced T-cell activation, was designed to inhibit this process and is an alternative for rheumatic patients who have failed on TNF blockers (discussed below).[155] Abatacept is a novel chimeric CTLA-4–IgG1 fused protein created from the fusion of the extracellular domain of the mouse CTLA-4 with the modified heavy-chain constant region of human IgG1. It acts like an antibody, where the extracellular portion binds with high affinity to B7 ligands and prevents them from interacting with CD28 on activated T-cells. This inhibits the costimulatory process, suppresses T-cell proliferation and release of proinflammatory cytokines, and slows bone and cartilage damages while relieving rheumatic symptoms.

Abatacept is administered monthly by IV infusion. Side effects can include headache, nausea, and mild infections such as upper respiratory tract infections. Serious infections, such as pneumonia, can occur. There is some concern that blocking of the suppressive signal from B7 to CTLA-4 can have a negative effect on regulatory T cells and thus, eventually, promote autoimmunity.

Cytokine Inhibitors

T-cells are activated as described above, and therefore they multiply and release cytokines that promote the destruction of tissues surrounding the joints and cause the signs and symptoms of rheumatoid arthritis.[156] This section describes antirheumatic therapeutics that act downstream from T-cell activation, inhibiting cytokine activity.

TUMOR NECROSIS FACTOR BLOCKERS. Upon T-cell activation, the expression of the cytokines, IL-1, IL-6, and TNFα by the rheumatoid synovium is upregulated leading to rheumatoid arthritis disease progression. More specifically, TNFα is a proinflammatory cytokine that has a major role in the pathologic inflammatory process of rheumatoid arthritis. As TNFα concentrations increase in joints, it leads to joint inflammation and ultimately, joint destruction. Therefore, rendering TNFα inactive has become an effective therapy for rheumatoid arthritis, as well as ankylosing spondylitis and psoriatic arthritis.[145]

Two effective approaches have been developed to decrease TNFα activity.

1. Soluble TNF receptor (TNFR) decoys that bind present TNFα (etanercept)
2. Anti-TNFα antibodies that bind to TNFα, preventing it from activating TNFRs (infliximab, adalimumab, golimumab, certolizumab)

These actions help to reduce pain, morning stiffness, and tender or swollen joints, usually within 1 or 2 weeks after treatment begins. TNF blockers work synergistically with methotrexate, and the two drugs are often coadministered. Common adverse effects include blood disorders, lymphoma, demyelinating diseases, and increased risk of infection. Because TNF is also important for host defense against infections, the effects of long-term use on toxicity may be problematic.

Structural illustrations of the anti-TNF agents etanercept, infliximab, adalimumab, golimumab, and certolizumab are provided in Figure 15.40. For a comprehensive review of biologic DMARD drug, please see the recent publication by Combe et al.[157]

Etanercept (Enbrel). Etanercept is used for the treatment of rheumatoid arthritis in patients who have not adequately responded to one or more of the synthetic DMARDs. It can also be used in psoriatic arthritis and ankylosing spondylitis.

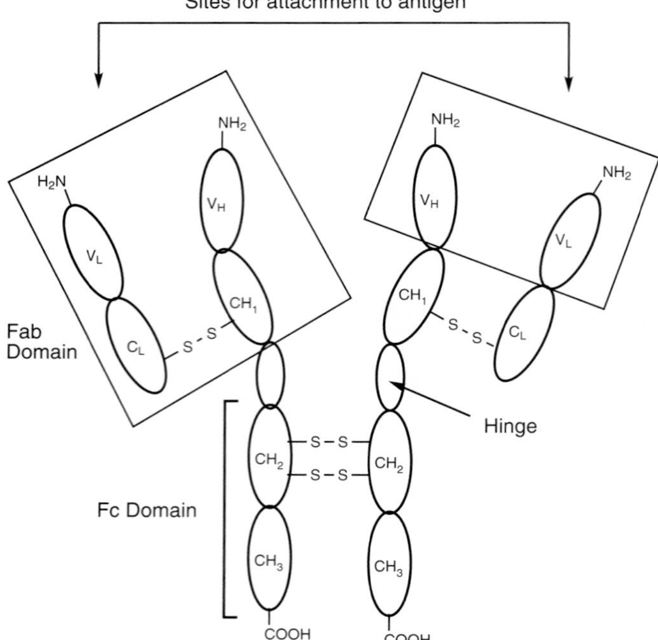

Figure 15.40 Anti-tumor necrosis factor (TNF) agents. Etanercept is the extracellular portion of the human TNF receptor fused to the Fc domain of human immunoglobulin (Ig) G1. Infliximab is a partially humanized monoclonal antibody against TNFα. The Fv domains are derived from mouse antihuman sequences, whereas the Fc domain is composed of human IgG1 sequence. Adalimumab is fully humanized antibody to human TNFa (Fv and Fc derived from human sequences). Golimumab is a fully humanized antibody. Certolizumab has a human Fab domain and no Fc domain. The Fc domain for certolizumab is replaced with PEG.

Etanercept is a dimeric soluble form of p75 TNFR and acts as a decoy receptor capable of binding to two TNFα molecules in the circulation, rendering them unavailable for binding to the TNFR. It consists of the extracellular ligand binding portion of the 75-kDa human TNFR fused to the Fc portion of human immunoglobulin (Ig) G1. The Fc component of etanercept contains the CH_2 domain, the CH_3 domain, and the hinge region, but not the CH_1 domain of IgG1. It consists of 934 amino acids and has an apparent molecular weight of approximately 150 kDa, requiring specific disulfide bridging for optimal activity.[158] Etanercept also binds TNFβ. Some concern exists because of reports that etanercept can cause serious infections and could have contributed to the deaths of several patients using the drug. A review of the clinical utility of etanercept is available.[159]

Etanercept is available as a powder to be reconstituted for injection. Dosing can be once (50 mg/dose) or twice (25 mg/dose) a week. Patients may experience irritation at the injection site.

Infliximab (Remicade). Infliximab is indicated for the treatment of rheumatoid arthritis in combination with methotrexate and to induce remission in moderate to severe Crohn's disease patients who have not responded to conventional therapy. It can also be used to treat psoriatic arthritis and ulcerative colitis. Infliximab is a chimeric IgG1κ monoclonal antibody to human TNFα, blocking its ability to bind TNFRs. The Fv domain of the mouse antibody responsible for recognizing TNFα is combined with a human Fc domain of IgG1 (IgG1κ). This fused protein has been "humanized" and has increased immunostability with a lower risk of degradation by the host's immune system. Infliximab has an approximate molecular weight of 149 kDa. It blocks TNFα activity by binding both the transmembrane and soluble forms of TNFα. It does not bind to TNFβ (lymphotoxin A), a related cytokine that uses the same receptors as TNFα and, thus, is more specific in its action than etanercept. Cells expressing transmembrane TNFα bound by infliximab can be lysed.

Infliximab is supplied as a lyophilized powder to be formulated for IV infusion in sterile water. The solution should be used immediately after reconstitution, as the product does not contain antibacterial preservatives. The volume of distribution at steady-state is independent of dose. The terminal half-life of infliximab is 8.0-9.5 days, which is sufficiently long enough to allow dosing every 6-8 weeks. No systemic accumulation of infliximab occurred on continued repeated treatment at 4- or 8-week intervals.

Long-term use can be associated with the development of anti-infliximab antibodies, an effect that does not appear when it is used in combination with methotrexate. Warnings associated with the use of infliximab include risks of autoimmunity, infections, hypersensitivity reactions, and worsening congestive heart failure. Reviews and reports of the properties and use of infliximab are available.[160,161]

Adalimumab (Humira). Adalimumab is a recombinant human IgG1 monoclonal antibody targeted for human TNFα. It is fully humanized and comprises human-derived, heavy- and light-chain variable regions (Fab) and human IgG1κ constant regions. It consists of 1,330 amino acids and has a molecular weight of approximately 148 kDa. Adalimumab has the same mechanism of action as infliximab; however, since it is a fully humanized IgG1 monoclonal antibody, there is increased immune-stability and lessened chance for degradation by the immune system. In addition, similar to infliximab, adalimumab does not bind or inactivate TNFβ. It is supplied in single-use, prefilled, glass syringes as a sterile, preservative-free, colorless solution for biweekly subcutaneous administration. Irritation at the site of injection may occur. The pharmacokinetics of adalimumab are linear over the dose range of 0.5-10.0 mg/kg following a single IV dose. The mean elimination half-life is approximately 2 weeks.

Golimumab (Symponi). Golimumab is a human IgG1k monoclonal antibody specific for human TNFα. It is an alternative to etanercept, adalimumab, and infliximab for the treatment of rheumatoid arthritis. Golimumab weighs approximately 150-151 kDa[162] and binds to both the soluble and transmembrane forms of human TNFα, with high affinity.[155] The advantage golimumab possesses over other anti-TNFα agents is the once-monthly subcutaneous dosing.

The average terminal half-life of golimumab is 2 weeks. Subcutaneous dosing every 4 weeks leads to steady-state serum concentrations by week 12. Its metabolic pathway is unknown. The most frequent adverse effects are upper respiratory tract infection, sore throat, and nasopharyngitis. Serious infections can occur, along with lymphomas and other malignancies. Labeling includes a boxed warning that alerts patients to the risk of tuberculosis and invasive fungal infections.

Certolizumab Pegol (Cimzia). Certolizumab is a monoclonal antibody directed against TNFα.[163] It selectively inhibits TNFα over lymphotoxin A (TNFβ). Certolizumab is composed of a humanized anti-TNFα antibody Fab' fragment, which is linked to polyethylene glycol (PEG). The purpose of linking the antibody to PEG (pegolate) is to (1) reduce the immunogenicity of the antibody, (2) increase the circulating half-life of the antibody which expands the dosing range to once every 4 weeks, rather than the every 2 week regimen common with non-pegylated MAbs, and (3) enhance TNFα targeting. The Fab' fragment is composed of a light chain with 214 amino acid residues and a heavy chain with 229 amino acids. The antibody lacks an Fc portion and thus binds to only TNFα without having to bind to the cell surface receptors for antibodies. One of the major advantages of certolizumab over the other monoclonal antibodies directed against TNFα is its lower cost.

Subcutaneous and single IV dosing studies of certolizumab demonstrate predictable and linear dose-related plasma concentrations. Metabolism of the Fab' fragment is unknown, whereas the PEG moiety is excreted in the urine. The major adverse effects are mild and include rash and upper respiratory and urinary tract infections.

B LYMPHOCYTE BLOCKER

Rituximab (Rituxan). Rituximab, in combination with methotrexate, can reduce signs and symptoms of rheumatoid arthritis in adult patients with moderate to severe disease who have had an inadequate response to one or more TNF blockers. Rituximab is a genetically engineered, fused mouse/human anti-CD40 MAb that targets B lymphocytes by binding specifically to the CD20 antigen, a protein found on the surface of B cells at certain stages in the life cycle. Rituximab is composed of two heavy chains of 451 amino acids and two light chains of 213 amino acids with an approximate molecular weight of 145 kDa. Its binding affinity for the CD20 antigen is approximately 8.0 nM. The mouse light- and heavy-chain Fab domains of rituximab, which bind to the CD20 antigen on B cells, are linked to the human Fc domains of IgG1κ. Once the rituximab molecule attaches to the B cells, it initiates B-cell lysis, inducing rapid and profound depletion of peripheral B cells, with patients showing near-complete B-cell depletion within 2 weeks after receiving the first dose of rituximab.

Rituximab is a sterile, clear, colorless, preservative-free, liquid concentrate formulated for IV administration. It is given as two 1,000-mg IV infusions separated by 2 weeks. Adverse effects include hypersensitivity and flu-like symptoms such as fever, chills, and nausea. Patients experiencing significant hypersensitivity can show bronchospasm, hypotension, myocardial infarction, and ventricular fibrillation that can be fatal. Interested readers are referred to published reviews on the clinical applications of rituximab.[164,165]

DRUGS USED TO TREAT GOUT

Pathophysiology

Gout is an acute or chronic form of inflammatory arthritis characterized by significant joint pain, tenderness, redness, and swelling. It is the most common inflammatory arthritis in men, with the incidence in Black males almost twice that of White males. The major factors that can precipitate gout include lifestyle, genetics, and medications. Lifestyle factors include high meat and seafood diet, emotional stress, physical trauma, and excessive alcohol intake. Medications such as diuretics, β-blockers, and even aspirin have also been attributed to gout attacks. Gout is also associated with an increased risk of kidney stones.[166]

Gout results from elevated levels of uric acid in the blood with subsequent accumulation of needle-like crystals of monosodium urate monohydrate within the joints, synovial fluid, and periarticular tissue. The formation of uric acid from adenine and guanine is illustrated in Figure 15.41. Xanthine is a common metabolic product formed from either adenine or guanine. Adenine deaminase converts the 6-amino group of adenine to a 6-hydroxy group, forming hypoxanthine. Xanthine oxidase then oxidizes hypoxanthine at the 2-position, yielding xanthine. Uric acid is subsequently formed by the oxidation of xanthine by the enzyme xanthine oxidase. Finally, uric acid is metabolized by uricase, forming allantoin with subsequent hydrolysis to provide urea and glyoxylic acid.

Uric acid is a weak acid with two pK_a values (5.7 and 10.3), and at physiologic pH it exists primarily as the urate monoanion. Uric acid has low water solubility (~6 mg/100 mL); however, the urate monoanion is approximately 50 times more soluble in aqueous media. When levels of uric acid in the body increase, the solubility limits of urate monoanion are exceeded and precipitation of sodium urate from the resulting supersaturated solution

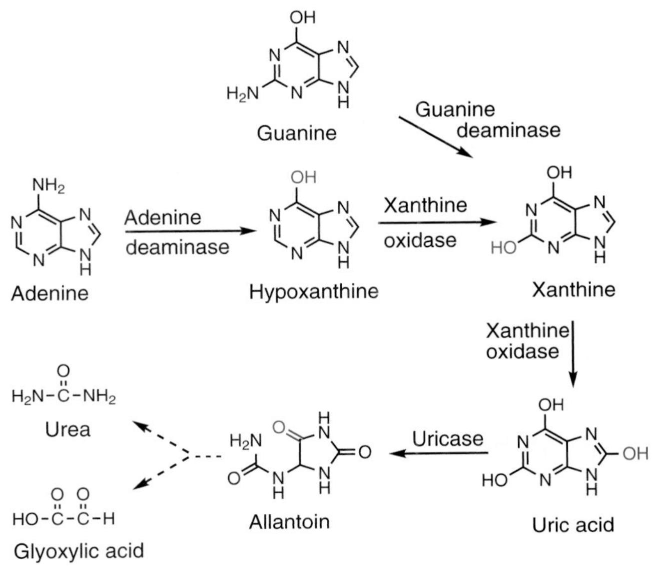

Figure 15.41 Formation of uric acid, urea, and glyoxylic acid from purines.

causes deposits of urate crystals. It is the formation of these urate crystals in joints and connective tissue that initiate attacks of gouty arthritis.

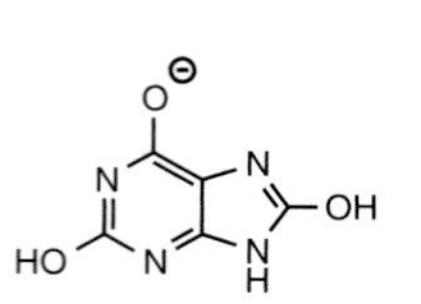

Urate monoanion

Blood levels of urate monoanion are maintained by a careful balance between its formation and excretion. The kidney has a dominant role in urate elimination, excreting about 70% of the daily urate production. Excretion of urate requires the urate anion transporter (URAT1) located in renal proximal tubule cells, which also has a central role in urate homeostasis. The URAT1 is targeted by uricosuric and antiuricosuric agents that affect urate excretion.

The structures of the drugs used to treat gout are shown in Figure 15.42.

Treatment of Acute Gout

The management of gout has been approached with the following therapeutic strategies: (1) control of acute attacks with drugs that reduce inflammation caused by the deposition of urate crystals and (2) control of chronic gout by increasing the rate of uric acid excretion and halting the biosynthesis of uric acid by inhibiting the enzyme xanthine oxidase. Treatment of acute gout includes NSAIDs such as indomethacin or naproxen (see previous NSAID discussion) colchicine, and glucocorticoids. The choice of an NSAID is usually based on the side effect profile.

Colchicine

Colchicine is a natural product obtained from various species of *Colchicum*, primarily *Colchicum autumnale* L, and is used in the prophylaxis and treatment of acute gout. It darkens on exposure to light and possesses moderate water solubility.

Colchicine does not alter serum levels of uric acid; however, it does appear to retard the inflammation attributed to the deposition of urate crystals. Colchicine's mechanism of action is multifaceted and essentially reduces pro-inflammatory mechanisms while increasing anti-inflammatory chemical mediators. A comprehensive review of colchicine's mechanism of action as it relates to the treatment of gout has been published.[167] The FDA approved the first single-ingredient oral colchicine formulation, Colcrys, for the treatment of acute gout flares in 2010. The drug is also approved for the treatment of familial Mediterranean fever.[168] Because colchicine does not lower serum urate levels, it is beneficial to combine it with a uricosuric agent, most commonly probenecid.

ABSORPTION AND METABOLISM. Colchicine is absorbed on oral administration, with peak plasma levels being attained within 0.5-2 hours after dosing. Plasma protein binding is only 31%. It concentrates primarily in the GI tract, liver, kidney, and spleen and is excreted primarily in the feces, with only 20% of an oral dose being excreted in the urine. It is retained in the body for considerable periods of time, being detected in the urine and leukocytes for 9-10 days following a single dose. This is partially attributed to colchicine being recycled in bile through enterohepatic circulation. Metabolism occurs primarily in the liver via CYP3A4, with the major metabolite being the amine resulting from hydrolysis of the acetamide.

ADVERSE EFFECTS. Colchicine can produce bone marrow depression with long-term therapy resulting in thrombocytopenia or aplastic anemia. At maximum dose levels, GI disturbances (e.g., nausea, diarrhea, and abdominal pain) can occur. Acute toxicity is characterized by GI distress, including severe diarrhea resulting in excessive fluid loss, respiratory depression, and kidney damage. Treatment normally involves measures that prevent shock, as well as morphine and atropine administration to diminish abdominal pain. A number of drug interactions have been reported. In general, the actions of colchicine are potentiated by alkalinizing substances and inhibited by acidifying agents, consistent with its mechanism of action of increasing the pH of synovial fluid. Responses to CNS depressants and to sympathomimetic drugs appear to be enhanced. Clinical tests can be affected; most notably, elevated alkaline phosphatase and serum glutamate oxaloacetate transaminase values, and decreased thrombocyte values. Because colchicine is a P-gp and CYP3A4 substrate, life-threatening drug interactions have been reported as a result of significant increases in colchicine plasma levels in patients treated with P-gp and strong CYP3A4 inhibitors.

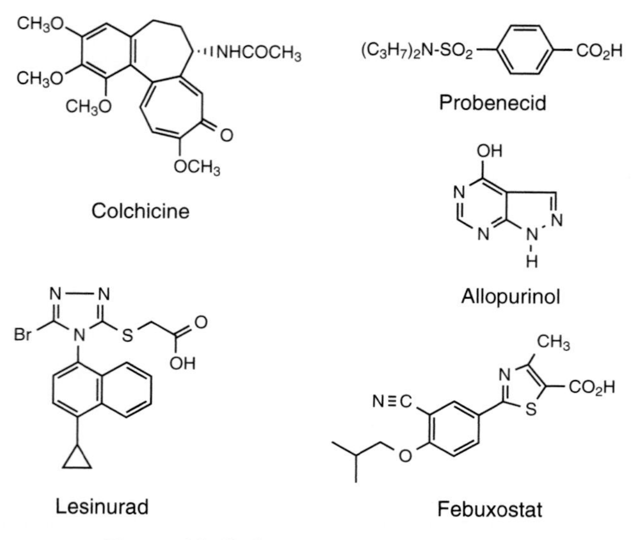

Colchicine Probenecid Allopurinol Lesinurad Febuxostat

Figure 15.42 Agents used to control gout.

Treatment of Chronic Gout

Drugs That Increase Uric Acid Secretion

PROBENECID. Probenecid is insoluble in water and acidic solutions but is soluble in alkaline solutions buffered to pH 7.4. Probenecid promotes the excretion of uric acid by inhibiting the URAT1 transporter, which decreases the reabsorption of uric acid in the proximal tubules and promoting its excretion. With the increase in uric acid excretion, blood concentrations decrease, leading urate depositions to decrease due to enhanced solubilization. Probenecid is an N-dialkylsulfamyl benzoate, and increased uric acid excretion occurs with smaller N-alkyl substituents.

Probenecid is essentially completely absorbed from the GI tract on oral administration, with peak plasma levels observed within 2-4 hours. Like most acidic compounds that are highly ionized at physiologic pH, probenecid (pK_a = 3.4) is extensively plasma protein bound (93%-99%). It is extensively metabolized, with only 5%-10% excreted unchanged. The metabolic reactions of probenecid are shown in Figure 15.43. The primary phase 1 metabolites result from N-dealkylation and ω-oxidation of the *n*-propyl side chain, followed by subsequent oxidation of the resulting primary alcohol to the carboxylic acid via sequential alcohol dehydrogenase and aldehyde dehydrogenase enzymatic reactions. Phase 2 reactions include glycine conjugation with the carboxylic acids. All metabolites retain uricosuric activity. The primary route of elimination of probenecid and its metabolites is the urine.

Probenecid is well tolerated with few adverse reactions. The primary side effects are mild GI irritation and hypersensitivity reactions. Despite the high degree of plasma protein binding, displacement interactions with other drugs bound to plasma proteins do not appear to occur to any significant extent, although other drug interactions have been reported. For example, salicylates can block the uricosuric effects of probenecid. Probenecid can block the tubular secretion of penicillin, aminosalicylic acid, methotrexate, sulfonamides, dapsone, sulfonylureas, naproxen, indomethacin, rifampin, and sulfinpyrazone, yielding higher plasma concentrations for these drugs.

LESINURAD. Similar to probenecid, lesinurad is a URAT1 inhibitor, leading to reduced renal reabsorption and increased urinary excretion of uric acid. When used with a uric acid biosynthesis inhibitor (e.g., allopurinol or febuxostat), the combination offers a dual mechanism of action in reducing uric acid concentrations in patients diagnosed with gout. Lesinurad also inhibits organic anion transporter (OAT) 4 but does not affect OAT1 or OAT3.

Lesinurad is readily absorbed following oral administration (absolute bioavailability of ~100%). The drug is highly bound to plasma proteins (>98%) and has an elimination half-life of ~5 hours. The drug and metabolites are excreted in both the urine (63%) and feces (32%).

Lesinurad is reported to exist as a nearly 50:50 mixture of atropisomers 1 and 2 (presumably those shown below). While there are no chiral centers in lesinurad, the isomers arise due to the restricted rotation about triazole N1-naphthylene bond. The two atropisomers have a different half-life, with atropisomer 1 $t_{1/2}$ of approximately 3.8 hours and the more slowly biotransformed atropisomer 2 $t_{1/2}$ of approximately 6.2 hours.

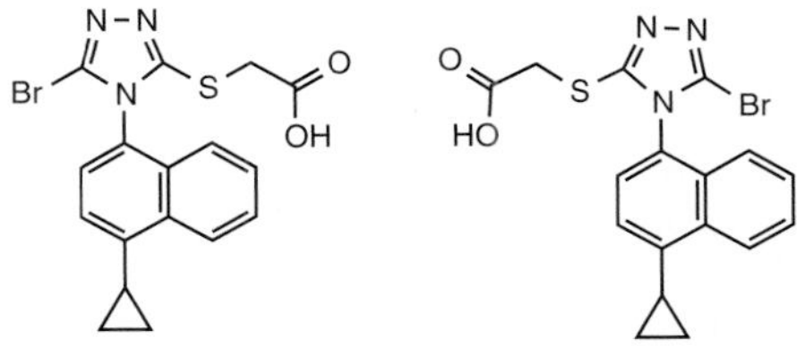

1 2

Atropisomers of Lesinurad

Lesinurad undergoes extensive oxidative metabolism by CYP2C9 leading to inactive metabolites M4 (24.8%) and M3 (18.9%) (Fig. 15.44). M4 is reported to arise from M3c. A number of additional metabolites are also reported

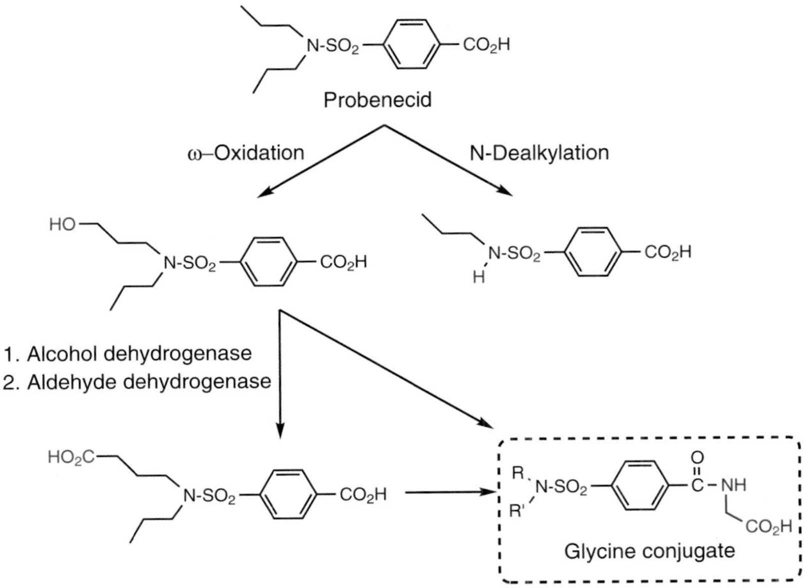

Probenecid

ω–Oxidation

N-Dealkylation

1. Alcohol dehydrogenase
2. Aldehyde dehydrogenase

Glycine conjugate

Figure 15.43 Metabolism of probenecid.

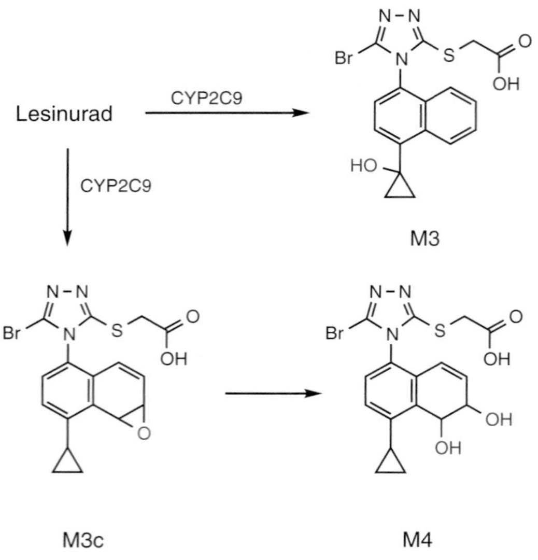

Figure 15.44 Metabolism of lesinurad.

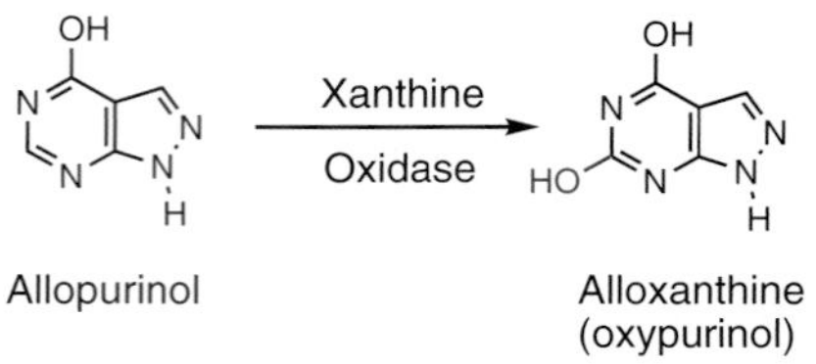

Figure 15.45 Metabolism of allopurinol.

but are present in low quantities. Lesinurad is reported to exhibit potential drug-drug interactions with CYP2C9 inhibitors.

Lesinurad is contraindicated in patients with severe renal impairment, end stage renal disease, kidney transplant patients, or patients on dialysis. Common adverse effects consist of headache, influenza, increased blood creatinine, and gastroesophageal reflux disease. A boxed warning cautions of an increased risk for acute kidney failure, especially when not used with a xanthine oxidase inhibitor.

Drugs That Decrease Uric Acid Formation

ALLOPURINOL

Mechanism of Action. Allopurinol is effective for chronic gout and acts through inhibition of the uric acid biosynthetic pathway. Specifically, allopurinol is a xanthine mimic and a competitive inhibitor of xanthine oxidase. It is a purine analogue where the pyrimidine ring is fused to a pyrazole ring instead of imidazole and the 6-position has been oxidized. Allopurinol has an affinity for xanthine oxidase that is 15-20 times higher than that of the endogenous substrate xanthine. Therefore, when allopurinol is administered, xanthine and hypoxanthine are elevated in the urine and uric acid levels decrease. When this happens, plasma urate monoanion concentrations decrease and urate crystal deposits dissolve, eliminating the primary cause of gout.

Absorption and Metabolism. Allopurinol is well absorbed on oral administration, with peak plasma concentrations appearing within 1 hour. Decreases in uric acid plasma levels can be observed within 24-48 hours. Allopurinol is metabolized via C2 oxidation (Fig. 15.45). The major oxidative metabolite, alloxanthine or oxypurinol, has a much longer half-life than the parent drug (18-30 vs. 2-3 hr) and is also an inhibitor of xanthine oxidase. Thus, the extended plasma half-life of alloxanthine leads to once-a-day dosing. Allopurinol and alloxanthine are not bound to plasma proteins. Their excretion occurs primarily in the urine, with approximately 20% of a dose being excreted in the feces.

Adverse Effects. The primary adverse effects of allopurinol are GI distress (nausea, vomiting, and diarrhea) and dermatological allergic reactions (typically skin rash). Luckily, these symptoms tend to disappear when the medication is discontinued. Allopurinol can also initiate attacks of acute gouty arthritis during the early stages of therapy due to the release of tissue uric acid, requiring the concomitant administration of colchicine and an NSAID. Drug interactions can occur with xanthine oxidase competitors, some of which are therapeutically beneficial. For example, the oxidation of 6-mercaptopurine, an antineoplastic agent used to treat acute lymphoblastic anemia, is inhibited, permitting a reduction in the therapeutic dose of the toxic anticancer agent. Allopurinol also has an inhibitory effect on hepatic microsomal enzymes and can prolong the half-lives of vulnerable drugs that normally are metabolized and inactivated by these enzymes. As might be anticipated, this effect is quite variable. The incidence of ampicillin-related skin rashes increases with the concurrent administration of allopurinol.

Allopurinol is indicated for the treatment of primary and secondary gout and for the treatment of patients with recurrent calcium oxalate calculi. Recently, a fixed combination of lesinurad and allopurinol (Duzallo) has been approved for the treatment of hyperuricemia in gout patients.

FEBUXOSTAT. Febuxostat is the first nonpurine selective inhibitor of xanthine oxidase. It is indicated for the chronic management of hyperuricemia in patients with gout and for patients who cannot tolerate allopurinol. Febuxostat is a noncompetitive inhibitor of both the oxidized and reduced forms of xanthine oxidase, thereby inhibiting the oxidation of the endogenous substrates hypoxanthine and xanthine.[169,170] Therefore, similar to allopurinol, plasma uric acid levels are attenuated. Since febuxostat is a nonpurine analogue, it does not inhibit enzymes involved in purine (or pyrimidine) metabolism, resulting in fewer adverse events compared to allopurinol.

Absorption and Metabolism. Febuxostat is well absorbed on oral administration, with peak plasma concentrations appearing within 1.5 hours and a half-life of 5-8 hours. Phase 1 oxidative metabolism of febuxostat is primarily mediated by CYP1A1, generating the O-dealkylated and ω-1 hydroxy products (Fig. 15.46).[171] CYP2C9 is responsible for oxidation of the ω carbon of the isobutyl group. Phase 2 metabolic reactions are catalyzed by glucuronosyltransferase enzymes, including UGT1A1, UGT1A3, UGT1A9, and UGT2B7, forming the glucuronide ester through either carboxylic acid.[171,172] Excretion of febuxostat, as various metabolites and their conjugates,

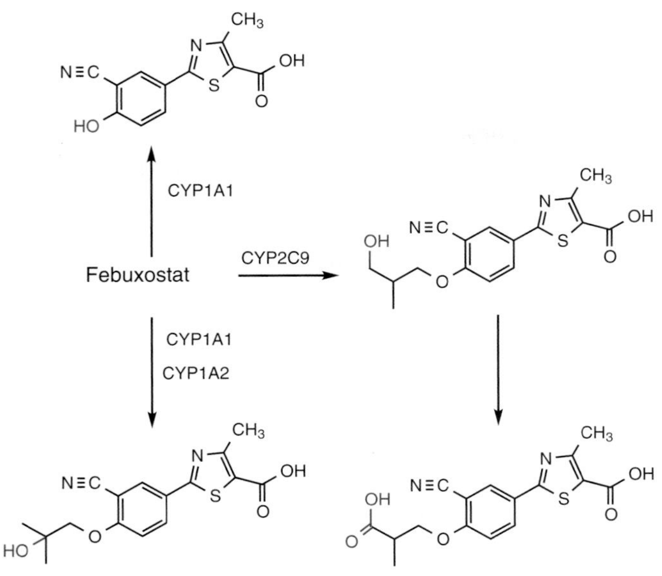

Figure 15.46 Metabolism of febuxostat.

occurs primarily in the urine (49%) and feces (45%). From an administered dose, only 3% and 12% are recovered as unchanged drug in urine and feces, respectively.

Adverse Effects. The major adverse effects of febuxistat include GI distress, liver function abnormalities, and headache. Cardiovascular safety is concurrently monitored as there is evidence of increased myocardial infarction and stroke.[173] Similar to allopurinol, initial dosing can initiate gout flares and may require the concomitant administration of an NSAID or colchicine. Drug interactions include those drugs that are also metabolized by xanthine oxidase, such as azathioprine, mercaptopurine, and theophylline. A review of the clinical properties of febuxostat as a treatment option for chronic gout has been published.[174]

Drugs Acting by Enhancing the Degradation of Uric Acid

PEGLOTICASE. Pegloticase is indicated for the treatment of chronic gout in patients in whom traditional small-molecule therapy has failed. Pegloticase is a recombinant porcine-like uricase that enhances the elimination of uric acid by converting it to allantoin (Fig. 15.41). Pegloticase is a uric acid–specific enzyme that consists of recombinant modified mammalian uricase produced by a genetically modified strain of *E. coli* and then covalently joined to monomethoxypoly(ethylene glycol) (mPEG). The cDNA coding for uricase was derived from mammalian sequences, and each uricase subunit is approximately 34 kDa. The average molecular weight of pegloticase (tetrameric enzyme conjugated to mPEG) is approximately 540 kDa.

Adverse Effects. The recommended dose of pegloticase is 8 mg administered IV every 2 weeks. After administration, common adverse effects are GI distress, allergic reaction (sore throat, runny nose, hives), and new gout flares. Prior to beginning the infusion, premedication with antihistamines and corticosteroids is recommended to prevent infusion reactions and possible anaphylaxis, which are thought to result from cytokine release. To counter new gout flares that can occur, NSAIDs and/or colchicine should be started at least 1 week prior to pegloticase therapy.

LOCAL ANESTHETICS

Anesthesia is a medically and chemically induced loss of sensation with or without loss of consciousness. There are generally three accepted forms of anesthetics including general, sedation, and local. Although various mechanisms of action are attributed to anesthetics, they all produce their action by inhibiting neurons.

Local anesthetic agents are drugs that, when given either topically or administered directly into a localized area, produce a state of local anesthesia by reversibly blocking nerve conductance that transmits the sensations of pain from this localized area to the brain. Conductance occurs when sodium ions (Na^+) pass through the pores of Na^+ ion channels. Local anesthetics bind to specific sites on the Na^+ ion channel and inhibit its function. The anesthesia produced by local anesthetics is without loss of consciousness or impairment of vital central cardiorespiratory functions.

The Discovery of Local Anesthetics

As with many drugs in the era of rational drug design, the initial leads for the design of clinically useful local anesthetics originated from natural sources. In 1860 A. Niemann obtained a crystalline alkaloid from coca leaves to which he gave the name cocaine, and who noted the anesthetic effect on the tongue (Fig. 15.47). In 1884, the first successful surgical use of cocaine was performed by C. Koller, and this discovery led to the rapid development of new local anesthetic agents and anesthetic techniques.[175]

Cocaine dependence (or addiction) is psychological dependency on the regular use of cocaine.

Although the structure of cocaine was not known until 1924, many attempts were made to prepare new analogues that lacked its addicting liability and other therapeutic shortcomings, such as allergic reactions,

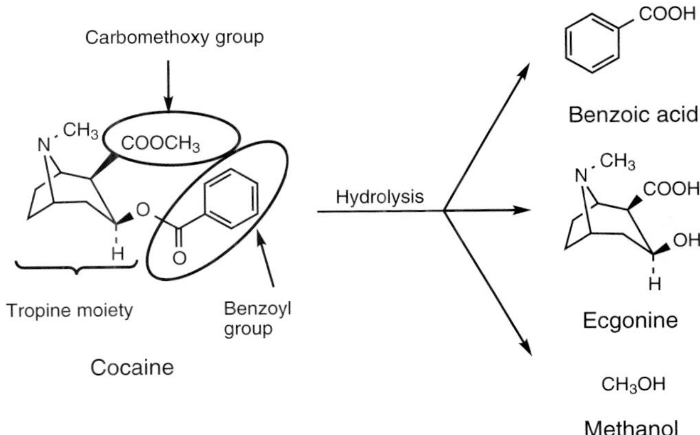

Figure 15.47 Cocaine and its hydrolysis products.

tissue irritations, and poor stability in aqueous solution. For example, cocaine is easily decomposed to hydrolysis products ecgonine and benzoic acid, when the solution is sterilized (Fig. 15.47).

When the chemical structure of ecgonine became known, the preparation of active compounds containing the ecgonine nucleus accelerated. It was soon realized that a variety of benzoyl esters of amino alcohols, including benzoyltropine, exhibited strong local anesthetic properties without any of cocaine's addiction liability. Thus, removal of the methyl ester group at the 2-position from cocaine abolished its addiction liability. This discovery eventually led to the discovery of procaine, which then became the local anesthetic prototype for nearly half a century, due to its lower toxicity.

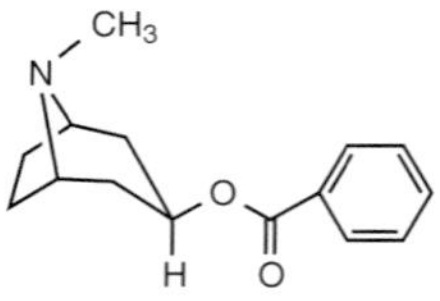

Benzoyltropine

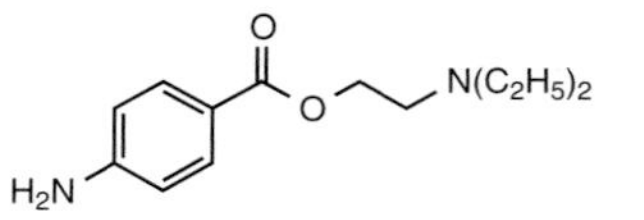

Procaine

Although procaine did enjoy many years of first-line local anesthetic use, it did have some liabilities, including low potency and a short duration. To address these therapeutic shortcomings, tetracaine was discovered and remains the most potent, long-acting, ester-type local anesthetic agent, which is used by injection in spinal anesthesia and also found in some topical combination products.

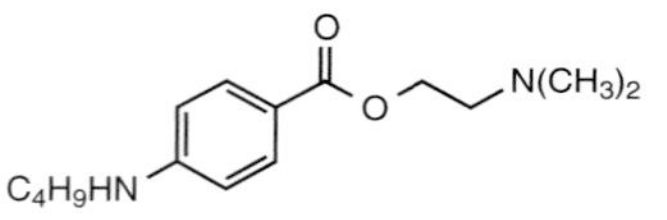

Tetracaine

The serendipitous discovery of the local anesthetic activity of another natural alkaloidal product, isogramine, in 1935 by H. von Euler and H. Erdtman was the next major turning point in the development of clinically useful local anesthetic agents. This observation led to the synthesis of lidocaine (Xylocaine) by N. Löfgren in 1946; lidocaine was the first nonirritating, amide-type local anesthetic agent with good local anesthetic properties, yet less prone to allergenic reactions than procaine analogues, and was found to be stable in aqueous solution due to its amide functionality. Structurally, lidocaine can be viewed as an open-chain bioisosteric analogue of isogramine.

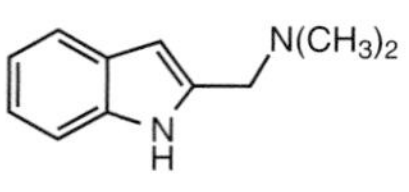

Isogramine

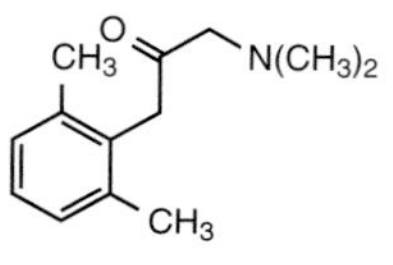

Lidocaine

Characteristics of an Ideal Local Anesthetic

The ideal local anesthetic should produce reversible blockade of sensory neurons with a minimal effect on the motor neurons. It also should possess a rapid onset, have a sufficient duration of action for the completion of surgical procedures without any systemic toxicity, and be easily sterilized and not inordinately expensive (Table 15.4). There is opportunity for an improved local anesthetic with regard to its selective actions on the Na^+ ion channels. Additional leads for the design of ideal local anesthetics could also come from a more systematic metabolic and toxicity study of currently available agents.

Therapeutic Considerations for Using Local Anesthetic Drugs

Since the discovery of cocaine in 1880 as a surgical local anesthetic, several thousand new compounds have been tested and found to produce anesthesia by blocking nerve conductance. Among these agents, approximately 20 are currently clinically available in the United States as local anesthetic preparations (Table 15.5). Figure 15.48 provides the chemical structures of the agents in common use.

Pharmaceutical Preparations

Local anesthetic agents generally are prepared in various dosage forms: aqueous solutions for parenteral injection, and creams and ointments for topical applications. Thus, chemical stability and aqueous solubility become primary factors in the preparations of suitable pharmaceutical dosage forms. Compounds containing an amide linkage are ideal as they have greater chemical hydrolytic stability than do the esters. In this regard, an aqueous solution of an amino ester–type local anesthetic is more likely to hydrolyze under normal conditions of use and cannot withstand heat sterilization as a result of base-catalyzed hydrolysis of the ester.

Table 15.4 Characteristics of the Ideal Local Anesthetic Agent
Produces a reversible blockade
Selective for sensory neurons with no effect on motor neurons
Rapid onset
Sufficient duration of action
Chemically stable when sterilized
No systemic toxicity
Wide margin of safety
Compatible with other coadministered drugs
Absence of adverse effects
Inexpensive

Table 15.5 Clinically Available Local Anesthetics

Generic Name	Trade Name	Recommended Application
Articaine	Septocaine, Septanest	Parenteral (dental)
Benzocaine	Americaine, Anbesol, Benzodent, Orajel, Oratect, Rid-A-Pain, Hurricaine	Topical
Bupivacaine	Marcaine, Sensorcaine	Parenteral
Chloroprocaine	Nesacaine	Parenteral
Cocaine	Cocaine Topical	Topical
Dibucaine	Nupercainal, Cinchocaine	Topical
Lidocaine	Xylocaine, L-Caine, DermaFlex, Dilocaine, Lidoject, Lignocaine, Octocaine	Parenteral, topical
Mepivacaine	Carbocaine, Polocaine, Isocaine	Parenteral, topical
Prilocaine	Citanest	Parenteral, topical
Procaine	Novocain	Parenteral
Proparacaine	Proxymetacaine	Topical
Ropivacaine	Naropin	Parenteral
Tetracaine	Pontocaine, Amethocaine, Prax	Parenteral, topical

Local anesthetic activity usually increases with increasing lipid solubility, although this is inversely related to water solubility and suitable parenteral dosage forms may not be possible. For this reason, a suitable parenteral dosage form might not be available for these agents because of poor water solubility under acceptable conditions. For example, benzocaine, which contains an anilino amine and is not basic enough for salt formation, is insoluble in water at pH values used in parenteral dosage forms. Protonation of the anilino amine in benzocaine results in a conjugate acid with a pK_a of 2.78, which is far too acidic for use by injection. For this reason, benzocaine is used mostly in creams or ointments to provide topical anesthesia.

The only commonly accepted organic additives to local anesthetics are vasoconstrictors, such as epinephrine and levonordefrin (α-methylnorepinephrine). These compounds often increase the frequency of successful anesthesia and, to a limited degree, increase the duration of activity by reducing the rate of drug loss from the injection site by constricting arterioles that supply blood to the area of the injection. The effect of these vasoconstrictors is less pronounced if they are injected in an area that has profuse venous drainage but is remote from an arterial supply.

Administration of a local anesthetic in a carbonic acid–carbon dioxide aqueous solution, rather than the usual solution of a hydrochloride salt, appreciably improves the time to onset and the duration of action without causing increased local or systemic toxicity. Carbon dioxide is believed to potentiate the action of local anesthetics by initial indirect depression of the axon, followed by diffusion trapping of the active form of the local anesthetic within the nerve.

A Eutectic Mixture of a Local Anesthetic (EMLA) cream containing 2.5% lidocaine and 2.5% prilocaine (or etidocaine) is used for the topical application through the keratinized layer of the intact skin to provide dermal or epidermal analgesia. This mode of administration allows the use of higher concentrations of local anesthetic with minimal local irritation and lower systemic toxicity. The use of EMLA creams, especially those containing prilocaine, on mucous membranes is not recommended, however, because of the faster absorption of the drugs and, therefore, the increasing risk of systemic toxicity, such as methemoglobinemia.[176]

Toxicity and Adverse Effects

The toxicity of local anesthetics seem to be related to their actions on other excitable membrane proteins, such as in the Na^+ and K^+ channels in the heart, the nicotinic acetylcholine receptors in the neuromuscular junctions, and the nerve cells in the CNS. In general, neuromuscular junctions and the CNS are more susceptible than the cardiovascular system to the toxic effects of local anesthetics. The actions on skeletal muscles tend to be transient and reversible, whereas the CNS side effects can be more deleterious. The primary effect of the toxicity seems to be convulsions, followed by severe CNS depression, particularly of the respiratory and cardiovascular centers. This can be related to an initial depression of inhibitory neurons, such as GABAergic systems, causing convulsions, followed by depression of other neurons, leading to general depression of the CNS.

The amino amide–type local anesthetics (lidocaine derivatives) are, in general, more likely to produce CNS side effects than the amino ester–type compounds (procaine analogue). However, it should be noted that the toxic effects observed depend heavily on the route and site of administration, as well as on the lipid solubility and metabolic stability of a given local anesthetic molecule. For example, most amide-type local anesthetics are first degraded via N-dealkylation by hepatic enzymes (discussed below). Unlike lidocaine, however, the initial metabolic degradation of prilocaine in humans is hydrolysis of the amide linkage to give *o*-toluidine and N-propylalanine. Formation of *o*-toluidine and its metabolites can cause methemoglobinemia in some patients.[176]

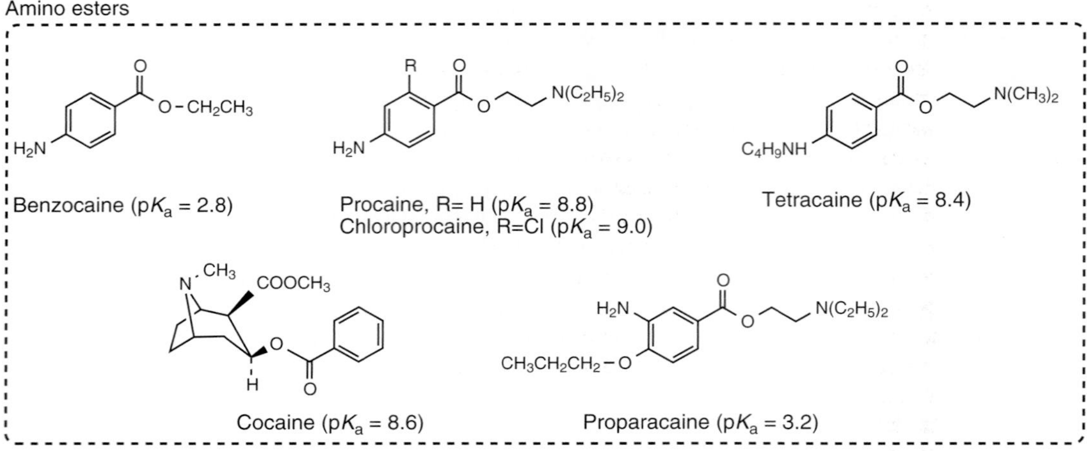

Amino amides

Lidocaine (pK_a = 7.8)

Prilocaine (pK_a = 7.9)

Mepivacaine, R= CH_3 (pK_a = 7.6)
Bupivacaine, R= n-C_4H_9 (pK_a = 8.1)

Ropivacaine (pK_a = 8.2)

Articaine (pK_a = 7.8)

Dibucaine (pK_a = 8.8)

Figure 15.48 Commonly used local anesthetics.

o-Toluidine

Allergic reactions to local anesthetics, although rare, are known to occur exclusively with *p*-aminobenzoic acid (PABA) ester–type local anesthetics.[177] This may be attributed increased concentrations of PABA since it is formed upon ester hydrolysis. However, the preservatives, such as methylparaben, used in the preparation of amide-type local anesthetics are metabolized to the PABA analogue *p*-hydroxybenzoic acid. Thus, patients who are allergic to amino ester–type local anesthetics should be treated with a preservative-free amino amide–type local anesthetic.

PABA *p*-Hydroxy benzoic acid

Amide-type local anesthetics (e.g., procainamide and lidocaine) also possess antiarrhythmic activity when given parenterally and at subanesthetic doses (see Chapter 16). Although this action is likely an extension of their effects on Na^+ channels in cardiac tissues, some evidence suggests an alternative mechanism of action with respect to the modulation of channel receptors binding sites for these compounds.[178,179]

Chemical and Pharmacodynamic Aspects of Local Anesthetics

Mechanism of Action

Local anesthetics act by decreasing the excitability of nerve cells without affecting the resting potential. Because the action potential, or the ability of nerve cells to be excited, is associated with the movement of Na^+ across the nerve membranes, anything that interferes with the movement of these ions will interfere with cell excitability. For this reason, many hypotheses have been suggested to explain how local anesthetics regulate the changes in Na^+ permeability that underlie the nerve impulse. These hypotheses include direct action on ion channels that interfere with ionic fluxes and interaction with phospholipids and calcium that reduces membrane flexibility and responsiveness to changes in electrical fields. The nonspecific membrane actions of local anesthetics can be easily ruled out, because most clinically useful agents, in contrast to general anesthetics, possess a defined SAR. At much higher drug concentrations, local anesthetics also bind and block K^+ channels.

Structure-Activity Relationships

Figure 15.48 shows the two major classes of marketed local anesthetics: amino esters (procaine analogues) and amino amides (lidocaine analogues). Most of the clinically useful local anesthetics are basic tertiary amines with pK_a values of 7.0-9.0. Thus, under physiologic conditions, both protonated forms (cationic) and the molecular (unionized) forms are available for binding to the channel proteins. The ratio between the protonated [HB^+] and the unionized molecules [B] can be easily calculated based on the pH of the medium and the pK_a of the drug molecule by the Henderson-Hasselbalch equation: $pH - pK_a = \log [B]/[HB^+]$. The effect of pH changes on the potency of local anesthetics has been extensively investigated.[180]

It is the protonated conjugate [HB^+] capable of selective binding to and inhibiting Na^+ channels. For this reason, any structural modifications that significantly alter the lipid solubility, pK_a, and rate/extent of metabolic inactivation have a pronounced effect on the ability of a drug molecule to reach or interact with the hypothetical binding sites, thus modifying its local anesthetic properties.

LIPOPHILIC PORTION. The lipophilic portion of the molecule is essential for local anesthetic activity. For most of the clinically useful local anesthetics, this portion of the molecule consists of an aromatic group directly attached to either a carbonyl function (the amino ester series) or through an –NH– group (the amino amide series) (Fig. 15.49). Lipophilic aromatic rings incorporated into the amino ester series that have *o*- or *p*- (or both) electron donating groups typically as amino or alkoxy groups increase potency. The aromatic rings incorporated into the amino amide series are routinely disubstituted at the *o*-position with methyl groups, but may be monosubstituted. The lipophilic aromatic rings appear to play an important role in the binding of local anesthetics to the channel proteins.

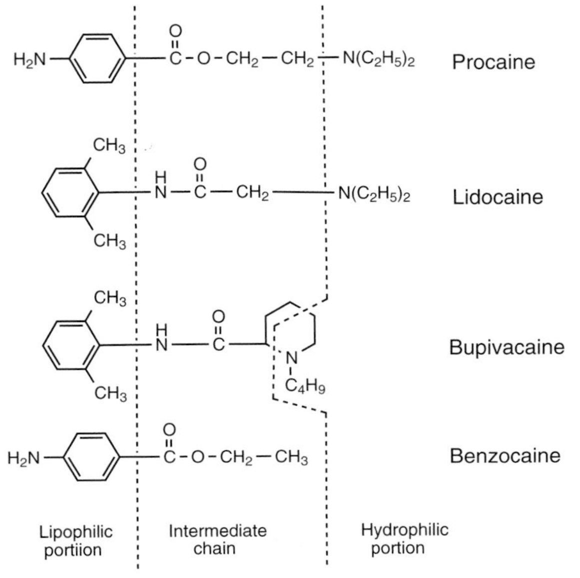

Figure 15.49 Structure-activity relationship comparison of local anesthetics.

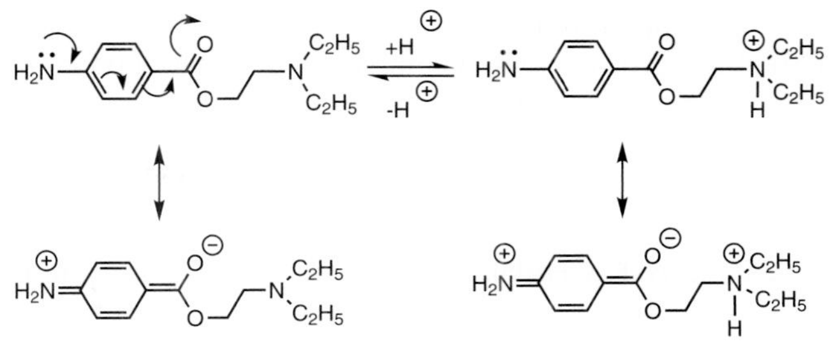

Figure 15.50 Resonance hybrid structures of procaine.

As illustrated in Figure 15.50, resonance is expected to give rise to a zwitterionic resonance hybrid. Neither drawn resonance hybrid of procaine in Figure 15.50 can accurately represent the structure of procaine, as the actual structure is a combination of all resonance hybrids whether protonated or not. This is also true for procaine when it interacts with the local anesthetic binding site; however, the greater the resemblance to the zwitterionic form, the greater the affinity for the binding site. Thus, addition of any aromatic substitution that can enhance the formation of the zwitterionic form through electron donation will produce more potent local anesthetic agents. Electron-withdrawing groups, such as nitro (—NO_2), hinder the formation of the zwitterion and, thus, reduce the local anesthetic activity.

Insertion of a methylene group between the aromatic moiety and the carbonyl function, as shown below in the procaine analogue, blocks extended electron delocalization and prohibits the formation of the zwitterionic form with a resonance hybrid where the negative charge localizes on the carbonyl oxygen. Therefore, this procaine analogue has greatly reduced anesthetic potency. When an amino or an alkoxy group is attached to the *m*-position of the aromatic ring no resonance delocalization of their electrons can localize at the carbonyl oxygen. The addition of this function only increases (alkoxy group) or decreases (amino group) the lipophilicity of the molecule, where increased lipophilicity increases potency.

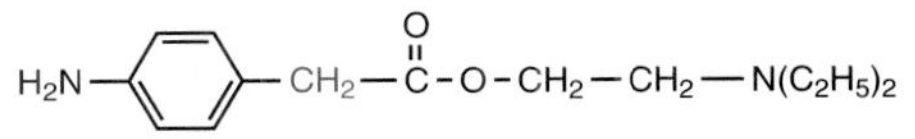

Procaine analog

Tetracaine is approximately 50-fold more potent than procaine. Experimentally, this increase in potency cannot be correlated solely with the 2,500-fold increase of lipid solubility by the n-butyl group (Log $D_{pH\ 7.4} = 2.73$ vs. procaine Log $D_{pH\ 7.4} = -0.32$). Perhaps part of this activity potentiation can be attributed to the electron-releasing property of the n-butyl group via the positive inductive effect, which indirectly enhances the electron density of the *p*-amino group. This, in turn increases electron donation through resonance to the carbonyl oxygen, promoting the formation of zwitterion for optimal interaction with the binding site proteins.

In the amino amides (lidocaine analogues), the *o,o*-dimethyl groups offer steric and electronic (positive induction) protection from amide hydrolysis, increasing duration of action. The shorter duration of action, however, observed with chloroprocaine when compared with that of procaine can be explained by the negative inductive effect of the *o*-chloro group, which pulls the electron density away from the carbonyl function, thus making it more susceptible to nucleophilic attack by the plasma esterases.

INTERMEDIATE CHAIN. The intermediate chain almost always contains a short alkyl segment of one to three carbons linked to the aromatic ring via several possible functional groups. The nature of this intermediate chain determines the chemical stability of the drug, which directly influences the duration of action and relative toxicity. In general, amino amides are more resistant to metabolic hydrolysis than the amino esters and, thus, have a longer duration of action. The placement of small alkyl groups (i.e., branching), especially around the ester function or the amide function, also hinders esterase- or amidase-catalyzed hydrolysis, prolonging the duration of action. It should be mentioned, however, that prolonging the duration of action of a compound usually increases its systemic toxicities unless it is more selective toward the voltage-gated Na^+ channel, as in the case of the levorotatory isomer of bupivacaine (levobupivacaine).[181,182]

HYDROPHILIC PORTION. Most clinically useful local anesthetics have a tertiary alkylamine, which readily forms water-soluble salts with organic and inorganic acids, and this portion is commonly considered to be the hydrophilic portion of the molecule (Fig. 15.49). The necessity of this portion of the molecule for amino ester–type local anesthetics remains a matter of debate. The strongest opposition for requiring a basic amino group for local anesthetic action comes from the observation that benzocaine, which lacks the basic aliphatic amine function, has potent local anesthetic activity. For this reason, it is often suggested that the tertiary amine function in procaine analogues is needed only for the formation of water-soluble salts suitable for pharmaceutical preparations. With the understanding of the voltage-activated Na^+ channel it is logical that the cations produced by protonation of the tertiary amine group are also required for binding in the voltage-gated Na^+ channels.

The hydrophilic group in most of the clinically useful drugs can be in the form of a secondary or tertiary alkylamine or part of a nitrogen heterocycle (Fig. 15.49). As mentioned earlier, most of the clinically useful local anesthetics have pK_a values of 7.0-9.0. The effects of an alkyl substituent on the pK_a depend on the size, length, and hydrophobicity of the group; and thus, it is difficult to see a clear SAR among these structures. It is generally accepted that local anesthetics with higher lipid solubility and lower pK_a values appear to exhibit more rapid onset of action through more effective tissue penetration and lower toxicity.

Stereochemistry

A number of clinically used local anesthetics contain a chiral center (i.e., bupivacaine, mepivacaine, and prilocaine); however, the effect of optically pure isomers on isolated nerve preparations revealed a lack of stereospecificity. In a few cases (e.g., prilocaine, bupivacaine), however, small differences in the total pharmacologic profile of optical isomers have been noted when administered in vivo.[183-185]

The stereochemistry of the local anesthetics, however, plays an important role in their observed toxicity and pharmacokinetic properties. For example, ropivacaine, the only optically active local anesthetic currently being marketed, has considerably lower cardiac toxicities than its closest structural analogue, bupivacaine.[186] Since ropivacaine is marketed as the pure *S*-(−) isomer, the observed cardiac toxicity of racemic bupivacaine has been attributed to the *R*-(+)-bupivacaine enantiomer.[183-185] Furthermore, the degree of separation between motor and sensory blockade is more apparent with ropivacaine relative to bupivacaine at a lower end of the dosage scale.[187]

Metabolism of Local Anesthetics

The amino ester–type local anesthetics are rapidly hydrolyzed by plasma esterase, which is widely distributed in body tissues. Compounds that either inhibit or compete with local anesthetics for access to esterase will prolong local anesthetic activity and/or toxicity. Another potential drug interaction with clinical significance is between benzocaine and sulfonamides because benzocaine is hydrolyzed to PABA, which can antagonize the antibacterial activity of sulfonamides.

The amino amide–type local anesthetics, however, are metabolized primarily in the liver, involving CYP1A2 isozymes.[188] A general metabolic scheme for lidocaine is shown in Figure 15.51.

Lidocaine is N-dealkylated via CYP1A2 to the monoethylglycinexylidide metabolite. This reaction occurs again leading to the primary amine (glycinexylidide). In addition, the monoethylglycinexylidide can also undergo amide hydrolysis forming 2,6-xylidine. The metabolite 2,6-xylidine can then undergo aromatic or benzylic oxidation ending with either phenol- or carboxylic acid–based metabolites. These are then susceptible to phase 2 metabolic conjugation reactions. Although the exact

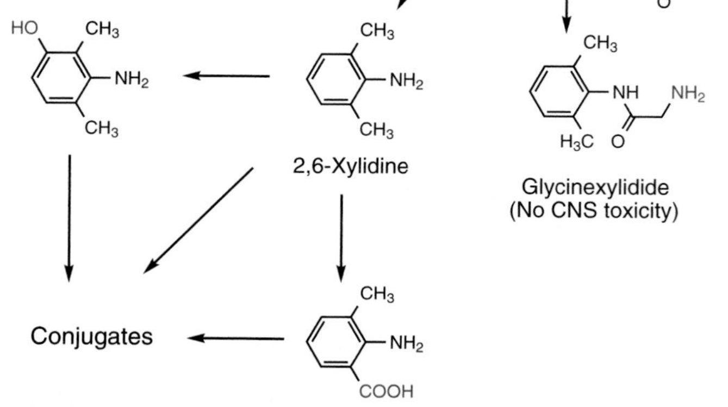

Lidocaine
CNS toxicities

N-dealkylation
(CYP1A2)

Monoethylglycinexylidide
(CNS toxicities)

2,6-Xylidine

Glycinexylidide
(No CNS toxicity)

Conjugates

Figure 15.51 Metabolic scheme for lidocaine.

mechanism for the CNS toxicity of lidocaine remains unclear, the metabolic studies of lidocaine provide some insight for future studies. Of all the metabolites of lidocaine, only monoethylglycinexylidide (and not glycinexylidide) contributes to some of the CNS side effects of lidocaine.

Common Agents Used for Local Anesthesia

Local anesthetics are widely used in many primary care settings. Techniques for their administration in these settings include topical application, local infiltration, field block, and peripheral nerve block. Their use can be maximized by an understanding of their potencies, durations of action, routes of administration, and pharmacokinetic and side effect profiles. The generic name, trade name, and recommended application are given in Table 15.5, and the chemical structures of these agents can be found in Figure 15.48.

Articaine

Articaine has been widely used in dentistry due to its quick onset and short duration of action. The structure differs from the structures of all other amino amide–type local anesthetics in that it contains a thiophene ring instead of a benzene ring and a unique methyl ester group. Both of these groups make articaine more lipophilic and, thus, makes it easier to cross membranes to reach sodium channel binding sites.

Articaine's local anesthetic potency is approximately 1.5-fold that of lidocaine, that can primarily be attributed to the increase in lipophilicity and plasma protein binding (76%) properties. The carbomethoxy ester is hydrolyzed primarily by plasma esterases and, therefore, articaine has a much shorter duration of action than lidocaine (i.e., only approximately one-fourth that of lidocaine). The hydrolysis product, articainic acid, is eliminated either unchanged (75%) or as its glucuronides (25%). Compared with other short-acting, amino amide–type local anesthetics, such as mepivacaine, lidocaine, or prilocaine, articaine is said to be a much safer drug for regional anesthesia.[189,190]

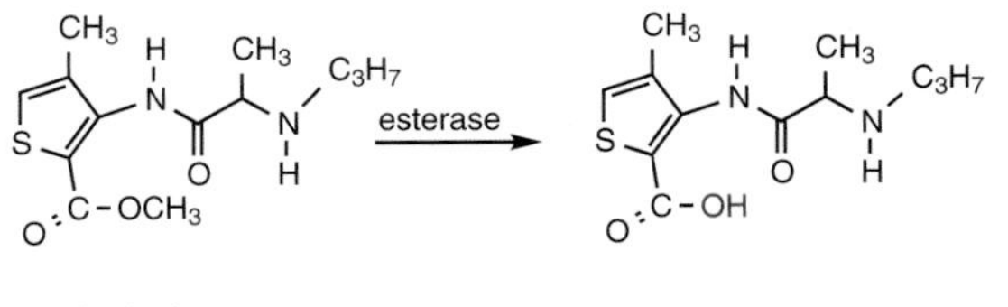

Articaine —esterase→ Articainic acid

Articaine hydrolysis

Benzocaine

Benzocaine is used topically alone or in combination with menthol or phenol in nonprescription dosage forms such as gels, creams, ointments, lotions, aerosols, and lozenges to relieve pain or irritation caused by such conditions as sunburn, insect bites, toothache, teething, cold sores or canker sores in or around the mouth, and fever blisters. Benzocaine is a lipophilic local anesthetic agent with a short duration of action.

Bupivacaine —CYP1A2→ (3-hydroxy product); —Amide hydrolysis→; —CYP3A4→

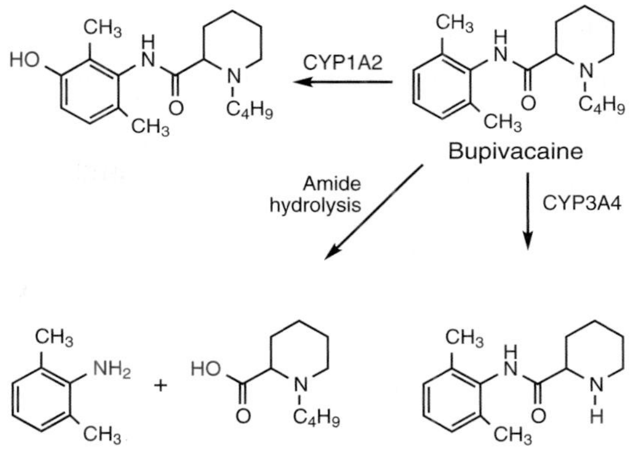

Figure 15.52 Metabolism of bupivacaine.

Like most amino ester–type local anesthetics, it is easily hydrolyzed by plasma esterase. Benzocaine has a low pK_a and is primarily unionized at physiological pH. Therefore, when administered topically to abraded skin, it can easily cross membranes into the systemic circulation to cause systemic toxicities. Furthermore, being a PABA derivative, it has similar allergenic properties to procaine and is contraindicated with sulfonamide antibacterial agents.

Bupivacaine

Bupivacaine hydrochloride is a racemic mixture of the *S*-(−)- and *R*-(+)-enantiomers. Bupivacaine has higher lipid solubility ($\log D_{pH\ 7.4}$ = 2.54) and a much decreased rate of hepatic degradation compared with lidocaine, leading to an extended duration of action. For this reason bupivacaine has significantly greater tendency than lidocaine to produce cardiotoxicity. Because of its greater affinity for voltage-gated Na^+ channels, the *R*-(+)-enantiomer confers greater cardiotoxicity than racemic bupivacaine.

Possible pathways for metabolism of bupivacaine include CYP1A2 aromatic 3-hydroxylation, CYP3A4 N-dealkylation, and to a minor extent, the amide hydrolysis (Fig. 15.52). Only the N-dealkylated product, however, has been identified in urine after epidural or spinal anesthesia.

Chloroprocaine

Chloroprocaine is a very short-acting, amino ester–type local anesthetic used to provide regional anesthesia by infiltration as well as by peripheral and central nerve block, including lumbar and caudal epidural blocks.[191,192] The presence of a chlorine atom ortho to the carbonyl of the ester function increases its lipophilicity. Its rate of hydrolysis by plasma esterase is at least threefold that of procaine and benzocaine due to an enhancement of the electrophilic character of the carbonyl carbon. Like PABA, the hydrolysis product of chloroprocaine is 4-amino-2-chlorobenzoic acid, which also inhibits the action of sulfonamides. Therefore, its use with sulfonamides should be avoided.

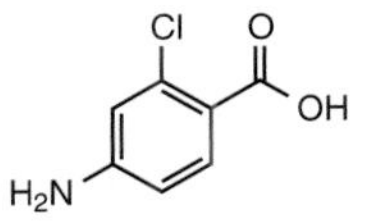

4-Amino-2-chlorobenzoic acid

Lidocaine

Lidocaine is the most commonly used amino amide–type local anesthetic. Lidocaine is very lipid soluble ($logD_{pH\ 7.4} = 2.26$) and, thus, has a more rapid onset and a longer duration of action than most amino ester–type local anesthetics, such as procaine and tetracaine. It can be administered parenterally (with or without epinephrine) or topically either alone or in combination with prilocaine as a eutectic mixture that is very popular with pediatric patients.

Adverse effects of the CNS are the most frequently observed systemic toxicities of lidocaine. The initial manifestations are restlessness, vertigo, tinnitus, and slurred speech. Eventually, seizures, followed by CNS depression with a cessation of convulsions and the onset of unconsciousness and respiratory depression or cardiac arrest, can occur. This biphasic effect occurs because local anesthetics initially block the inhibitory GABAergic pathways, resulting in stimulation, and eventually block both inhibitory and excitatory pathways (i.e., block the Na^+ channels associated with the NMDA receptors, resulting in overall CNS inhibition).[193]

Lidocaine is extensively metabolized in the liver by CYP3A4 N-dealkylation and aromatic hydroxylation catalyzed by CYP1A2 (Fig. 15.51). Lidocaine also possesses a weak inhibitory activity toward the CYP1A2 isozymes and, therefore, can interfere with metabolism of other medications.[194]

Mepivacaine

Mepivacaine hydrochloride is an amino amide–type local anesthetic agent widely used to provide regional analgesia and anesthesia by local infiltration, peripheral nerve block, and epidural and caudal blocks. The pharmacologic and toxicologic profile of mepivacaine is quite similar to that of lidocaine, except that mepivacaine is less lipophilic ($logD_{pH\ 7.4} = 1.95$), has a slightly longer duration of action, and lacks the vasodilator activity of lidocaine. For this reason, it serves as an alternate choice for lidocaine when addition of epinephrine is not recommended (e.g., in patients with hypertensive vascular disease).

Mepivacaine undergoes extensive hepatic metabolism similar to bupivacaine. Phase 1 metabolism of mepivacaine is catalyzed by CYP3A4 and CYP1A2, with only a small percentage of the administered dosage (<10%) being excreted unchanged in the urine. The major metabolic biotransformations of mepivacaine are N-dealkylation (to give the N-demethylated compound 2′,6′-pipecoloxylidide) and aromatic hydroxylations. These metabolites are excreted as their corresponding glucuronides.

Ropivacaine

S(−)-Ropivacaine hydrochloride is the first optically active, amino amide–type local anesthetic marketed. It combines the anesthetic potency and long duration of action of racemic bupivacaine with a side effect profile intermediate between those of bupivacaine and lidocaine. Although ropivacaine has a pK_a nearly identical to that of bupivacaine, it is two- to threefold less lipid soluble and has a smaller volume of distribution, a greater clearance, and a shorter elimination half-life than bupivacaine in humans.

The metabolism of ropivacaine in humans is mediated by hepatic CYP1A2 and, to a minor extent, by CYP3A4.[195] The major metabolite is 3-hydroxyropivacaine, and the minor metabolite is *S*-2′,6′-pipecoloxylidide (an N-dealkylated product).

Structure Challenge

NSAIDs structure challenge. Evaluate the NSAID structures drawn below and identify which would be the most appropriate for each numbered description.

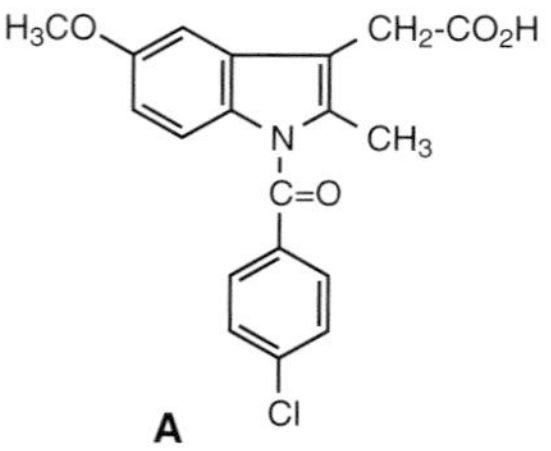

A 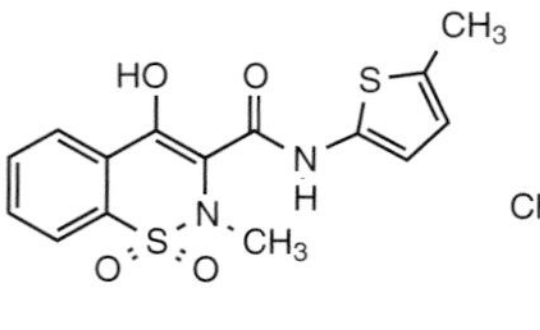 B 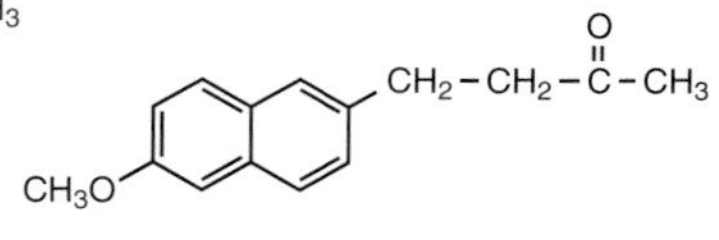 C

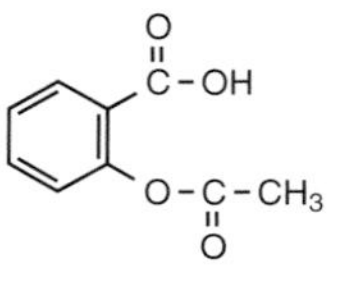

D 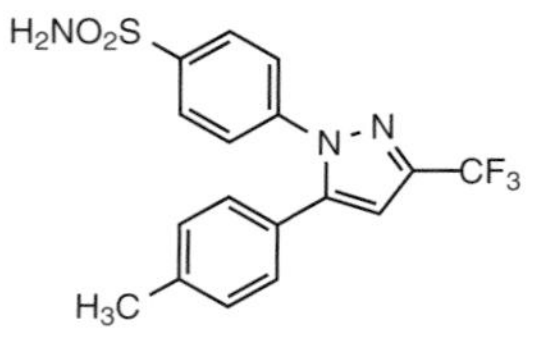 E 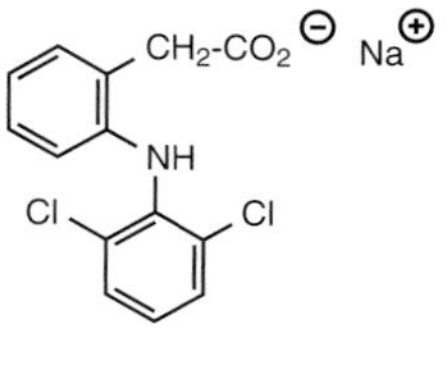 F

Structure Challenge—Continued

1. Which two NSAIDs have the highest propensity for cardiovascular toxicity?
2. Which NSAID is a prodrug? What is the structural basis for your answer?
3. Which NSAID has the highest propensity for hepatic toxicity?
4. Regarding NSAID B, what is the ionizable functional group?
5. Which three NSAIDs have the highest propensity for GI toxicity? What is the structural or pharmacological basis for your answer?

Structure Challenge answers found immediately after References.

ACKNOWLEDGMENTS

The author wishes to acknowledge the work of the late Ronald Borne, PhD, and Mark Levi, PhD, Timothy J. Maher, PhD, and Norman Wilson, PhD, who authored a significant component of the content used within this chapter in a previous edition of this text.

REFERENCES

1. Hamor GH. Non-steroidal anti-inflammatory drugs. In: Foye WO, ed. *Principles of Medicinal Chemistry*. 3rd ed. Philadelphia, PA: Lea & Febiger; 1989:503-530.
2. Shen TY. Anti-inflammatory agents. *Top Med Chem*. 1967;1:29-38.
3. Vane JR. Inhibition of prostaglandin synthesis as a mechanism of action for aspirin-like drugs. *Nat New Biol*. 1971;231(25):232-235.
4. Gund P, Shen TY. A model for the prostaglandin synthetase cyclo-oxygenation site and its inhibition by antiinflammatory arylacetic acids. *J Med Chem*. 1977;20(9):1146-1152.
5. Campbell WB. Lipid-derived autacoids: eicosanoids and platelet-activating factor. In: Gilman AG, Rall TW, Nies AS, et al, eds. *Goodman and Gilman's the Pharmacological Basis of Therapeutics*. New York: Pergamon Press; 1990:600-601.
6. von Euler US. On the specific vaso-dilating and plain muscle stimulating substances from accessory genital glands in man and certain animals (prostaglandin and vesiglandin). *J Physiol*. 1936;88(2):213-234.
7. Miyamoto T, Ogino N, Yamamoto S, et al. Purification of prostaglandin endoperoxide synthetase from bovine vesicular gland microsomes. *J Biol Chem*. 1976;251(9):2629-2636.
8. Hla T, Neilson K. Human cyclooxygenase-2 cDNA. *Proc Natl Acad Sci USA*. 1992;89(16):7384-7388.
9. Jones DA, Carlton DP, McIntyre TM, et al. Molecular cloning of human prostaglandin endoperoxide synthase type II and demonstration of expression in response to cytokines. *J Biol Chem*. 1993;268(12):9049-9054.
10. Kennedy BP, Chan CC, Culp SA, et al. Cloning and expression of rat prostaglandin endoperoxide synthase (cyclooxygenase)-2 cDNA. *Biochem Biophys Res Commun*. 1993;197(2):494-500.
11. Kujubu DA, Fletcher BS, Varnum BC, et al. TIS10, a phorbol ester tumor promoter-inducible mRNA from Swiss 3T3 cells, encodes a novel prostaglandin synthase/cyclooxygenase homologue. *J Biol Chem*. 1991;266(20):12866-12872.
12. Xie WL, Chipman JG, Robertson DL, et al. Expression of a mitogen-responsive gene encoding prostaglandin synthase is regulated by mRNA splicing. *Proc Natl Acad Sci USA*. 1991; 88(7):2692-2696.
13. Chandrasekharan NV, Dai H, Roos KL, et al. COX-3, a cyclooxygenase-1 variant inhibited by acetaminophen and other analgesic/antipyretic drugs: cloning, structure, and expression. *Proc Natl Acad Sci USA*. 2002;99(21):13926-13931.
14. Blobaum AL, Marnett LJ. Structural and functional basis of cyclooxygenase inhibition. *J Med Chem*. 2007;50(7):1425-1441.
15. Flower RJ. The development of COX2 inhibitors. *Nat Rev Drug Discov*. 2003;2:179-191.
16. Roche VF. A receptor-grounded approach to teaching nonsteroidal antiinflammatory drug chemistry and structure-activity relationships. *Am J Pharm Educ*. 2009;73(8):143.
17. Chang HW, Jahng Y. Selective cyclooxygenase-2 inhibitors as anti-inflammatory agents. *Eur J Med Chem*. 1998;8:48-79.
18. Vane JR, Bakhle YS, Botting YM. Cyclooxygenases 1 and 2. *Annu Rev Pharmacol Toxicol*. 1998;38:97-120.
19. Botting JH. Nonsteroidal anti-inflammatory agents. *Drugs Today*. 1999;35:225-235.
20. Hata AN, Breyer RM. Pharmacology and signaling of prostaglandin receptors: multiple roles in inflammation and immune modulation. *Pharmacol Ther*. 2004;103(2):147-166.
21. Tsuboi K, Sugimoto Y, Ichikawa A. Prostanoid receptor subtypes. *Prostaglandins Other Lipid Mediat*. 2002;68-69:535-556.
22. Smyth EM, Burke A, Fitzgerald GA. Lipid-derived autocoids: eicosanoids and platelet-activating factor. In: Brunton LI, Lazo JS, Parker KI, eds. *Goodman and Gilman's the Pharmacological Basis of Therapeutics*. 11th ed. New York: Pergamon Press; 2006:653-670.
23. Okazaki T, Sagawa N, Okita JR, et al. Diacylglycerol metabolism and arachidonic acid release in human fetal membranes and decidua vera. *J Biol Chem*. 1981;256(14):7316-7321.
24. Rubin P, Mollison KW. Pharmacotherapy of diseases mediated by 5-lipoxygenase pathway eicosanoids. *Prostaglandins Other Lipid Mediat*. 2007;83(3):188-197.
25. Clark WG. Mechanisms of antipyretic action. *Gen Pharmacol*. 1979;10(2):71-77.
26. Aronoff DM, Neilson EG. Antipyretics: mechanisms of action and clinical use in fever suppression. *Am J Med*. 2001;111(4):304-315.
27. Graham GC, Scott RF. Mechanism of action of paracetamol. *Am J Ther*. 2005;12:46.
28. Forrest JA, Clements JA, Prescott LF. Clinical pharmacokinetics of paracetamol. *Clin Pharmacokinet*. 1982;7(2):93-107.
29. Kunkel DB. *Emergency Medicine*. Basel: Geigy Pharmaceuticals; 1985.
30. Mitchell JR, Jollow DJ, Potter WZ, et al. Acetaminophen-induced hepatic necrosis. I. Role of drug metabolism. *J Pharmacol Exp Ther*. 1973;187(1):185-194.
31. McGill MR, Jaeschke H. Metabolism and disposition of acetaminophen: recent advances in relation to hepatotoxicity and diagnosis. *Pharm Res*. 2013;30(9):2174-2187.
32. Calder IC, Creek MJ, Williams PJ, et al. N-hydroxylation of *p*-acetophenetidide as a factor in nephrotoxicity. *J Med Chem*. 1973;16(5):499-502.
33. Yan M, Huo Y, Yin S, et al. Mechanisms of acetaminophen-induced liver injury and its implications for therapeutic interventions. *Redox Biol*. 2018;17:274-283.
34. Sinclair J, Jeffery E, Wrighton S, et al. Alcohol-mediated increases in acetaminophen hepatotoxicity: role of CYP2E and CYP3A. *Biochem Pharmacol*. 1998;55(10):1557-1565.

35. Buckpitt AR, Rollins DE, Mitchell JR. Varying effects of sulfhydryl nucleophiles on acetaminophen oxidation and sulfhydryl adduct formation. *Biochem Pharmacol*. 1979;28(19):2941-2946.
36. Atkuri KR, Mantovani JJ, Herzenberg LA, et al. N-Acetylcysteine–a safe antidote for cysteine/glutathione deficiency. *Curr Opin Pharmacol*. 2007;7(4):355-359.
37. Capodanno D, Angiolillo DJ. Aspirin for primary prevention of cardiovascular disease. *Lancet*. 2018;392(10152):988-990.
38. Garcia-Albeniz X, Chan AT. Aspirin for the prevention of colorectal cancer. *Best Pract Res Clin Gastroenterol*. 2011;25(4-5):461-472.
39. Verbeeck RK, Blackburn JL, Loewen GR. Clinical pharmacokinetics of non-steroidal anti-inflammatory drugs. *Clin Pharmacokinet*. 1983;8(4):297-331.
40. Davison C. Salicylate metabolism in man. *Ann N Y Acad Sci*. 1971;179:249-268.
41. Hutt AJ, Caldwell J, Smith RL. The metabolism of aspirin in man: a population study. *Xenobiotica*. 1986;16(3):239-249.
42. Gummin DD, Mowry JB, Spyker DA, et al. 2016 Annual report of the American association of Poison control centers' National Poison data system (NPDS): 34th Annual report. *Clin Toxicol (Phila)*. 2017;55(10):1072-1252.
43. Chapman J, Arnold JK. *Reye Syndrome*. StatsPearls Publishing; 2018. Available at: https://www.ncbi.nlm.nih.gov/books/NBK526101/. Accessed December 20, 2018.
44. Ghahramani P, Rowland-Yeo K, Yeo WW, et al. Protein binding of aspirin and salicylate measured by in vivo ultrafiltration. *Clin Pharmacol Ther*. 1998;63(3):285-295.
45. Chan TY. Adverse interactions between warfarin and nonsteroidal antiinflammatory drugs: mechanisms, clinical significance, and avoidance. *Ann Pharmacother*. 1995;29(12):1274-1283.
46. Goulston K, Cooke AR. Alcohol, aspirin, and gastrointestinal bleeding. *Br Med J*. 1968;4(5632):664-665.
47. Jayamani E, Tharmalingam N, Rajamuthiah R, et al. Characterization of a Francisella tularensis-Caenorhabditis elegans Pathosystem for the evaluation of therapeutic compounds. *Antimicrob Agents Chemother*. 2017;61(9).
48. Nuernberg B, Koehler G, Brune K. Pharmacokinetics of diflunisal in patients. *Clin Pharmacokinet*. 1991;20(1):81-89.
49. Verbeeck R, Tjandramaga TB, Mullie A, et al. Biotransformation of diflunisal and renal excretion of its glucuronides in renal insufficiency. *Br J Clin Pharmacol*. 1979;7(3):273-282.
50. Sylvia L. The pharmacology of indomethacin. *Headache*. 2016;56(2):436-446.
51. Prusakiewicz JJ, Felts AS, Mackenzie BS, et al. Molecular basis of the time-dependent inhibition of cyclooxygenases by indomethacin. *Biochemistry*. 2004;43(49):15439-15445.
52. Blobaum AL, Uddin MJ, Felts AS, et al. The 2'-trifluoromethyl Analogue of indomethacin is a potent and selective COX-2 inhibitor. *ACS Med Chem Lett*. 2013;4(5):486-490.
53. Helleberg L. Clinical pharmacokinetics of indomethacin. *Clin Pharmacokinet*. 1981;6(4):245-258.
54. Vree TB, van den Biggelaar-Martea M, Verwey-van Wissen CP. Determination of indomethacin, its metabolites and their glucuronides in human plasma and urine by means of direct gradient high-performance liquid chromatographic analysis. Preliminary pharmacokinetics and effect of probenecid. *J Chromatogr*. 1993;616(2):271-282.
55. Alvan G, Orme M, Bertilsson L, et al. Pharmacokinetics of indomethacin. *Clin Pharmacol Ther*. 1975;18(3):364-373.
56. Davies NM, Watson MS. Clinical pharmacokinetics of sulindac. A dynamic old drug. *Clin Pharmacokinet*. 1997;32(6):437-459.
57. Taylor RJ Jr, Salata JJ. Inhibition of prostaglandin synthetase by tolmetin (Tolectin, McN-2559), a new non-steroidal anti-inflammatory agent. *Biochem Pharmacol*. 1976;25(22):2479-2484.
58. Selley ML, Glass J, Triggs EJ, et al. Pharmacokinetic studies of tolmetin in man. *Clin Pharmacol Ther*. 1975;17(5):599-605.
59. Sumner DD, Dayton PG, Cucinell SA, et al. Metabolism of tolmetin in rat, monkey, and man. *Drug Metab Dispos*. 1975;3(4):283-286.
60. Dutta NK, Mazumdar K, Dastidar SG, et al. Activity of diclofenac used alone and in combination with streptomycin against Mycobacterium tuberculosis in mice. *Int J Antimicrob Agents*. 2007;30(4):336-340.
61. Gan TJ. Diclofenac: an update on its mechanism of action and safety profile. *Curr Med Res Opin*. 2010;26(7):1715-1731.
62. Moser P, Sallmann A, Wiesenberg I. Synthesis and quantitative structure-activity relationships of diclofenac analogues. *J Med Chem*. 1990;33(9):2358-2368.
63. Davies NM, Anderson KE. Clinical pharmacokinetics of diclofenac. Therapeutic insights and pitfalls. *Clin Pharmacokinet*. 1997;33(3):184-213.
64. Chan KK, Vyas KH, Brandt KD. In vitro protein binding of diclofenac sodium in plasma and synovial fluid. *J Pharm Sci*. 1987;76(2):105-108.
65. Tang W. The metabolism of diclofenac–enzymology and toxicology perspectives. *Curr Drug Metab*. 2003;4(4):319-329.
66. Poon GK, Chen Q, Teffera Y, et al. Bioactivation of diclofenac via benzoquinone imine intermediates-identification of urinary mercapturic acid derivatives in rats and humans. *Drug Metabo Dispos*. 2001;29(12):1608-1613.
67. Kindla J, Muller F, Mieth M, et al. Influence of non-steroidal anti-inflammatory drugs on organic anion transporting polypeptide (OATP) 1B1- and OATP1B3-mediated drug transport. *Drug Metab Dispos*. 2011;39(6):1047-1053.
68. Hunter EB, Johnston PE, Tanner G, et al. Bromfenac (Duract)-associated hepatic failure requiring liver transplantation. *Am J Gastroenterol*. 1999;94(8):2299-2301.
69. Walters T, Raizman M, Ernest P, et al. In vivo pharmacokinetics and in vitro pharmacodynamics of nepafenac, amfenac, ketorolac, and bromfenac. *J Cataract Refract Surg*. 2007;33(9):1539-1545.
70. Zhao X, Xia S, Wang E, et al. Comparison of the efficacy and patients' tolerability of Nepafenac and Ketorolac in the treatment of ocular inflammation following cataract surgery: a meta-analysis of randomized controlled trials. *PLoS One*. 2017;12(3):e0173254.
71. Brocks DR, Jamali F. Etodolac clinical pharmacokinetics. *Clin Pharmacokinet*. 1994;26(4):259-274.
72. Martel RR, Demerson CA, Humber LG, et al. Etodolic acid and related compounds. Chemistry and antiinflammatory actions of some potent di- and trisubstituted 1, 3, 4, 9-tetrahydropyrano[3, 4-b]indole-1-acetic acids. *J Med Chem*. 1976;19(3):391-395.
73. Humber LG. Etodolac: the chemistry, pharmacology, metabolic disposition, and clinical profile of a novel anti-inflammatory pyranocarboxylic acid. *Med Res Rev*. 1987;7(1):1-28.
74. Hung SC, Liao KF, Hung HC, et al. Nabumetone use and risk of acute pancreatitis in a case-control study. *Pancreatology*. 2016;16(3):353-357.
75. Goudie AC, Gaster LM, Lake AW, et al. 4-(6-Methoxy-2-naphthyl)butan-2-one and related analogues, a novel structural class of anti-inflammatory compounds. *J Med Chem*. 1978;21(12):1260-1264.
76. Hyneck ML. An overview of the clinical pharmacokinetics of nabumetone. *J Rheumatol Suppl*. 1992;36:20-24.
77. Davies NM. Clinical pharmacokinetics of nabumetone. The dawn of selective cyclo-oxygenase-2 inhibition? *Clin Pharmacokinet*. 1997;33(6):404-416.
78. Arfe A, Scotti L, Varas-Lorenzo C, et al. Non-steroidal anti-inflammatory drugs and risk of heart failure in four European countries: nested case-control study. *BMJ*. 2016;354:i4857.
79. Wen YC, Hsiao FY, Chan KA, et al. Acute respiratory infection and use of nonsteroidal anti-inflammatory drugs on risk of acute myocardial infarction: a Nationwide case-crossover study. *J Infect Dis*. 2017;215(4):503-509.
80. Bally M, Dendukuri N, Rich B, et al. Risk of acute myocardial infarction with NSAIDs in real world use: bayesian meta-analysis of individual patient data. *BMJ*. 2017;357:j1909.
81. Goldkind L, Laine L. A systematic review of NSAIDs withdrawn from the market due to hepatotoxicity: lessons learned from the bromfenac experience. *Pharmacoepidemiol Drug Saf*. 2006;15(4):213-220.

82. Davies NM. Clinical pharmacokinetics of ibuprofen. The first 30 years. *Clin Pharmacokinet.* 1998;34(2):101-154.
83. Aarons L, Grennan DM, Siddiqui M. The binding of ibuprofen to plasma proteins. *Eur J Clin Pharmacol.* 1983;25(6):815-818.
84. Bushra R, Aslam N. An overview of clinical pharmacology of ibuprofen. *Oman Med J.* 2010;25(3):155-1661.
85. Kepp DR, Sidelmann UG, Hansen SH. Isolation and characterization of major phase I and II metabolites of ibuprofen. *Pharm Res.* 1997;14(5):676-680.
86. Rudy AC, Knight PM, Brater DC, et al. Stereoselective metabolism of ibuprofen in humans: administration of R-, S- and racemic ibuprofen. *J Pharmacol Exp Ther.* 1991;259(3):1133-1139.
87. Hutt AJ, Caldwell J. The metabolic chiral inversion of 2-arylpropionic acids–a novel route with pharmacological consequences. *J Pharm Pharmacol.* 1983;35(11):693-704.
88. Nash JF, Bechtol LD, Bunde CA, et al. Linear pharmacokinetics of orally administered fenoprofen calcium. *J Pharm Sci.* 1979;68(9):1087-1090.
89. Rubin A, Warrick P, Wolen RL, et al. Physiological disposition of fenoprofen in man. 3. Metabolism and protein binding of fenoprofen. *J Pharmacol Exp Ther.* 1972;183(2):449-457.
90. Farge D, Messer MN, Moutonnier C. (3-benzoylphenyl) alkanoic acids. US Patent 3,641,127. 1972.
91. Ueno K, Kubo S, Tagawa H, et al. 6,11-Dihydro-11-oxodibenz [b,e] oxepinacetic acids with potent antiinflammatory activity. *J Med Chem.* 1976;19(7):941-946.
92. Jamali F, Brocks DR. Clinical pharmacokinetics of ketoprofen and its enantiomers. *Clin Pharmacokinet.* 1990;19(3):197-217.
93. Hayball PJ, Nation RL, Bochner F, et al. Plasma protein binding of ketoprofen enantiomers in man: method development and its application. *Chirality.* 1991;3(6):460-466.
94. Harrison IT, Lewis B, Nelson P, et al. Nonsteroidal antiinflammatory agents. I. 6-substituted 2-naphthylacetic acids. *J Med Chem.* 1970;13(2):203-205.
95. Davies NM, Anderson KE. Clinical pharmacokinetics of naproxen. *Clin Pharmacokinet.* 1997;32(4):268-293.
96. Segre EJ. Naproxen metabolism in man. *J Clin Pharmacol.* 1975;15(4 pt 2):316-323.
97. Miners JO, Coulter S, Tukey RH, et al. Cytochromes P450, 1A2, and 2C9 are responsible for the human hepatic O-demethylation of R- and S-naproxen. *Biochem Pharmacol.* 1996;51(8):1003-1008.
98. Geisslinger G, Lotsch J, Menzel S, et al. Stereoselective disposition of flurbiprofen in healthy subjects following administration of the single enantiomers. *Br J Clin Pharmacol.* 1994;37(4):392-394.
99. Menzel-Soglowek S, Geisslinger G, Beck WS, et al. Variability of inversion of (R)-flurbiprofen in different species. *J Pharm Sci.* 1992;81(9):888-891.
100. Davies NM. Clinical pharmacokinetics of flurbiprofen and its enantiomers. *Clin Pharmacokinet.* 1995;28(2):100-114.
101. Kaiser DG, Brooks CD, Lomen PL. Pharmacokinetics of flurbiprofen. *Am J Med.* 1986;80(3a):10-15.
102. Szpunar GJ, Albert KS, Wagner JG. Pharmacokinetics of flurbiprofen in man. II. Plasma protein binding. *Res Commun Chem Pathol Pharmacol.* 1989;64(1):17-30.
103. Risdall PC, Adams SS, Crampton EL, et al. The disposition and metabolism of flurbiprofen in several species including man. *Xenobiotica.* 1978;8(11):691-703.
104. Marzuillo P, Calligaris L, Amoroso S, et al. Narrative review shows that the short-term use of ketorolac is safe and effective in the management of moderate-to-severe pain in children. *Acta Paediatr.* 2018;107(4):560-567.
105. Brocks DR, Jamali F. Clinical pharmacokinetics of ketorolac tromethamine. *Clin Pharmacokinet.* 1992;23(6):415-427.
106. Davies NM. Clinical pharmacokinetics of oxaprozin. *Clin Pharmacokinet.* 1998;35(6):425-436.
107. Scherrer RA. Introduction of the chemistry of antiinflammatory and antiarthritic agents. In: Scherrer RA, Whitehouse MW, eds. *Anti-Inflammatory Agents.* Vol 1. New York: Academic Press; 1974:35-55.
108. Scherrer RA. Aryl- and heteroarylcarboxylic acids. In: Scherrer RA, Whitehouse MW, eds. *Anti-Inflammatory Agents.* Vol 1. New York: Academic Press; 1974:56-74.
109. Daniels MJ, Rivers-Auty J, Schilling T, et al. Fenamate NSAIDs inhibit the NLRP3 inflammasome and protect against Alzheimer's disease in rodent models. *Nat Commun.* 2016;7:12504.
110. Brannigan LH, Hodge RB, Field L. Biologically oriented organic sulfur chemistry. 14. Antiinflammatory properties of some aryl sulfides, sulfoxides, and sulfones. *J Med Chem.* 1976;19(6):798-802.
111. Diana FJ, Veronich K, Kapoor AL. Binding of nonsteroidal anti-inflammatory agents and their effect on binding of racemic warfarin and its enantiomers to human serum albumin. *J Pharm Sci.* 1989;78(3):195-199.
112. Sato J, Yamane Y, Ito K, et al. Structures of mefenamic acid metabolites from human urine. *Biol Pharm Bull.* 1993;16(8):811-812.
113. Koup JR, Tucker E, Thomas DJ, et al. A single and multiple dose pharmacokinetic and metabolism study of meclofenamate sodium. *Biopharm Drug Dispos.* 1990;11(1):1-15.
114. Lombardino JG, Wiseman EH. Piroxicam and other antiinflammatory oxicams. *Med Res Rev.* 1982;2:127-152.
115. Wells PS, Holbrook AM, Crowther NR, et al. Interactions of warfarin with drugs and food. *Ann Intern Med.* 1994;121(9):676-683.
116. Olkkola KT, Brunetto AV, Mattila MJ. Pharmacokinetics of oxicam nonsteroidal anti-inflammatory agents. *Clin Pharmacokinet.* 1994;26(2):107-120.
117. Verbeeck RK, Richardson CJ, Blocka KL. Clinical pharmacokinetics of piroxicam. *J Rheumatol.* 1986;13(4):789-796.
118. Trnavska Z, Trnavsky K. Plasma protein binding and interaction studies with piroxicam. *Naunyn Schmiedebergs Arch Pharmacol.* 1984;327(1):81-85.
119. Saganuwan SA. In vivo piroxicam metabolites: possible source for synthesis of central nervous system (CNS) acting depressants. *Cent Nerv Syst Agents Med Chem.* 2017;17(3):172-177.
120. Hobbs DC, Twomey TM. Metabolism of piroxicam by laboratory animals. *Drug Metab Dispos.* 1981;9(2):114-118.
121. Panara MR, Renda G, Sciulli MG, et al. Dose-dependent inhibition of platelet cyclooxygenase-1 and monocyte cyclooxygenase-2 by meloxicam in healthy subjects. *J Pharmacol Exp Ther.* 1999;290(1):276-280.
122. Fleischmann R, Iqbal I, Slobodin G. Meloxicam. *Expert Opin Pharmacother.* 2002;3(10):1501-1512.
123. Turck D, Roth W, Busch U. A review of the clinical pharmacokinetics of meloxicam. *Br J Rheumatol.* 1996;35(suppl 1):13-16.
124. Chesne C, Guyomard C, Guillouzo A, et al. Metabolism of Meloxicam in human liver involves cytochromes P4502C9 and 3A4. *Xenobiotica.* 1998;28(1):1-13.
125. Laine L. The gastrointestinal effects of nonselective NSAIDs and COX-2-selective inhibitors. *Semin Arthritis Rheum.* 2002;32(3 suppl 1):25-32.
126. Yuan JQ, Tsoi KK, Yang M, et al. Systematic review with network meta-analysis: comparative effectiveness and safety of strategies for preventing NSAID-associated gastrointestinal toxicity. *Aliment Pharmacol Ther.* 2016;43(12):1262-1275.
127. Zarghi A, Arfaei S. Selective COX-2 inhibitors: a review of their structure-activity relationships. *Iran J Pharm Res.* Fall 2011;10(4):655-683.
128. Zhao X, Xu Z, Li H. NSAIDs use and reduced metastasis in cancer patients: results from a meta-analysis. *Sci Rep.* 2017;7(1):1875.
129. Dai P, Li J, Ma XP, et al. Efficacy and safety of COX-2 inhibitors for advanced non-small-cell lung cancer with chemotherapy: a meta-analysis. *OncoTargets Ther.* 2018;11:721-730.
130. Liu B, Qu L, Yan S. Cyclooxygenase-2 promotes tumor growth and suppresses tumor immunity. *Cancer Cell Int.* 2015;15:106.
131. Davies NM, McLachlan AJ, Day RO, et al. Clinical pharmacokinetics and pharmacodynamics of celecoxib: a selective cyclo-oxygenase-2 inhibitor. *Clin Pharmacokinet.* 2000;38(3):225-242.
132. Gong L, Thorn CF, Bertagnolli MM, et al. Celecoxib pathways: pharmacokinetics and pharmacodynamics. *Pharmacogenet Genomics.* 2012;22(4):310-318.

133. Sandberg M, Yasar U, Stromberg P, et al. Oxidation of celecoxib by polymorphic cytochrome P450 2C9 and alcohol dehydrogenase. *Br J Clin Pharmacol.* 2002;54(4):423-429.
134. Penning TD, Talley JJ, Bertenshaw SR, et al. Synthesis and biological evaluation of the 1,5-diarylpyrazole class of cyclooxygenase-2 inhibitors: identification of 4-[5-(4-methylphenyl)-3-(trifluoromethyl)-1H-pyrazol-1-yl]benze nesulfonamide (SC-58635, celecoxib). *J Med Chem.* 1997;40(9):1347-1365.
135. Demoruelle MK, Deane KD. Treatment strategies in early rheumatoid arthritis and prevention of rheumatoid arthritis. *Curr Rheumatol Rep.* 2012;14(5):472-480.
136. McEvoy GK. *American Hospital Formulary Service Drug Information 2011*; 2017. Accessed November 2, 2017.
137. Korpela M, Laasonen L, Hannonen P, et al. Retardation of joint damage in patients with early rheumatoid arthritis by initial aggressive treatment with disease-modifying antirheumatic drugs: five-year experience from the FIN-RACo study. *Arthritis Rheum.* 2004;50(7):2072-2081.
138. Youn HS, Lee JY, Saitoh SI, et al. Auranofin, as an anti-rheumatic gold compound, suppresses LPS-induced homodimerization of TLR4. *Biochem Biophys Res Commun.* 2006;350(4):866-871.
139. Yang JP, Merin JP, Nakano T, et al. Inhibition of the DNA-binding activity of NF-kappa B by gold compounds in vitro. *Febs Lett.* 1995;361(1):89-96.
140. Blocka KL, Paulus HE, Furst DE. Clinical pharmacokinetics of oral and injectable gold compounds. *Clin Pharmacokinet.* 1986;11(2):133-143.
141. Capparelli EV, Bricker-Ford R, Rogers MJ, et al. Phase I clinical trial results of auranofin, a novel Antiparasitic agent. *Antimicrob Agents Chemother.* 2017;61(1).
142. Brown PM, Pratt AG, Isaacs JD. Mechanism of action of methotrexate in rheumatoid arthritis, and the search for biomarkers. *Nat Rev Rheumatol.* 2016;12(12):731-742.
143. Kremer JM, Galivan J, Streckfuss A, et al. Methotrexate metabolism analysis in blood and liver of rheumatoid arthritis patients. Association with hepatic folate deficiency and formation of polyglutamates. *Arthritis Rheum.* 1986;29(7):832-835.
144. Flanagan ME, Blumenkopf TA, Brissette WH, et al. Discovery of CP-690,550: a potent and selective Janus kinase (JAK) inhibitor for the treatment of autoimmune diseases and organ transplant rejection. *J Med Chem.* 2010;53(24):8468-8484.
145. Palfreeman AC, McNamee KE, McCann FE. New developments in the management of psoriasis and psoriatic arthritis: a focus on apremilast. *Drug Des Devel Ther.* 2013;7:201-210.
146. Wittmann M, Helliwell PS. Phosphodiesterase 4 inhibition in the treatment of psoriasis, psoriatic arthritis and other chronic inflammatory diseases. *Dermatol Ther.* 2013;3(1):1-15.
147. Schafer P. Apremilast mechanism of action and application to psoriasis and psoriatic arthritis. *Biochem Pharmacol.* 15 2012;83(12):1583-1590.
148. Hoffmann M, Kumar G, Schafer P, et al. Disposition, metabolism and mass balance of [(14)C]apremilast following oral administration. *Xenobiotica.* 2011;41(12):1063-1075.
149. Zane LT, Chanda S, Jarnagin K, et al. Crisaborole and its potential role in treating atopic dermatitis: overview of early clinical studies. *Immunotherapy.* 2016;8(8):853-866.
150. Moustafa F, Feldman SR. A review of phosphodiesterase-inhibition and the potential role for phosphodiesterase 4-inhibitors in clinical dermatology. *Dermatol Online J.* 2014;20(5):22608.
151. Freund YR, Akama T, Alley MR, et al. Boron-based phosphodiesterase inhibitors show novel binding of boron to PDE4 bimetal center. *Febs Lett.* 2012;586(19):3410-3414.
152. Singh JA, Hossain A, Tanjong Ghogomu E, et al. Biologics or tofacitinib for rheumatoid arthritis in incomplete responders to methotrexate or other traditional disease-modifying anti-rheumatic drugs: a systematic review and network meta-analysis. *Cochrane Database Syst Rev.* 2016(5):CD012183.
153. Oldfield V, Dhillon S, Plosker GL. Tocilizumab: a review of its use in the management of rheumatoid arthritis. *Drugs.* 2009;69(5):609-632.
154. Shealy DJ, Cai A, Staquet K, et al. Characterization of golimumab, a human monoclonal antibody specific for human tumor necrosis factor alpha. *MAbs.* 2010;2(4):428-439.
155. Gadangi P, Longaker M, Naime D, et al. The anti-inflammatory mechanism of sulfasalazine is related to adenosine release at inflamed sites. *J Immunol.* 1996;156(5):1937-1941.
156. Combe B, Lula S, Boone C, et al. Effects of biologic disease-modifying anti-rheumatic drugs on the radiographic progression of rheumatoid arthritis: a systematic literature review. *Clin Exp Rheumatol.* 2018;36(4):658-667.
157. Lamanna WC, Mayer RE, Rupprechter A, et al. The structure-function relationship of disulfide bonds in etanercept. *Sci Rep.* 2017;7(1):3951.
158. Scott LJ. Etanercept: a review of its use in autoimmune inflammatory diseases. *Drugs.* 2014;74(12):1379-1410.
159. Naguwa SM. Tumor necrosis factor inhibitor therapy for rheumatoid arthritis. *Ann N Y Acad Sci.* 2005;1051:709-715.
160. Perdriger A. Infliximab in the treatment of rheumatoid arthritis. *Biologics.* 2009;3:183-191.
161. McCluggage LK, Scholtz JM. Golimumab: a tumor necrosis factor alpha inhibitor for the treatment of rheumatoid arthritis. *Ann Pharmacother.* 2010;44(1):135-144.
162. Kaushik VV, Moots RJ. CDP-870 (certolizumab) in rheumatoid arthritis. *Expert Opin Biol Ther.* 2005;5(4):601-606.
163. King KM, Younes A. Rituximab: review and clinical applications focusing on non-Hodgkin's lymphoma. *Expert Opin Biol Ther.* 2001;1(2):177-186.
164. Schioppo T, Ingegnoli F. Current perspective on rituximab in rheumatic diseases. *Drug Des Devel Ther.* 2017;11:2891-2904.
165. Ferrari P, Bonny O. [Diagnosis and prevention of uric acid stones]. *Ther Umsch.* 2004;61(9):571-574.
166. Leung YY, Yao Hui LL, Kraus VB. Colchicine–Update on mechanisms of action and therapeutic uses. *Semin Arthritis Rheum.* 2015;45(3):341-350.
167. Portincasa P. Colchicine, biologic agents and more for the treatment of familial mediterranean fever. The old, the new, and the rare. *Curr Med Chem.* 2016;23(1):60-86.
168. Bruce SP. Febuxostat: a selective xanthine oxidase inhibitor for the treatment of hyperuricemia and gout. *Ann Pharmacother.* 2006;40(12):2187-2194.
169. Stamp LK, O'Donnell JL, Chapman PT. Emerging therapies in the long-term management of hyperuricaemia and gout. *Intern Med J.* 2007;37(4):258-266.
170. Grabowski BA, Khosravan R, Vernillet L, et al. Metabolism and excretion of [14C] febuxostat, a novel nonpurine selective inhibitor of xanthine oxidase, in healthy male subjects. *J Clin Pharmacol.* 2011;51(2):189-201.
171. Mukoyoshi M, Nishimura S, Hoshide S, et al. In vitro drug-drug interaction studies with febuxostat, a novel non-purine selective inhibitor of xanthine oxidase: plasma protein binding, identification of metabolic enzymes and cytochrome P450 inhibition. *Xenobiotica.* 2008;38(5):496-510.
172. White WB, Saag KG, Becker MA, et al. Cardiovascular safety of febuxostat or allopurinol in patients with gout. *N Engl J Med.* 2018;378(13):1200-1210.
173. Frampton JE. Febuxostat: a review of its use in the treatment of hyperuricaemia in patients with gout. *Drugs.* 2015;75(4):427-438.
174. Liljestrand G. The historical development of local anesthesia in local anesthetics. In: Lechat P, ed. *International Encyclopedia of Pharmacology and Therapeutics.* Oxford: Pergamon Press; 1971:1-38.
175. Arthur GR. Pharmacokinetics of local anesthetics. In: Strichartz GR, ed. *Local Anesthetics Handbook of Experimental Pharmacology.* Vol 81. Berlin: Springer; 1987:165-186.

176. Eggleston ST, Lush LW. Understanding allergic reactions to local anesthetics. *Ann Pharmacother.* 1996;30(7-8):851-857.
177. Bean BP, Cohen CJ, Tsien RW. Lidocaine block of cardiac sodium channels. *J Gen Physiol.* 1983;81(5):613-642.
178. Makielski JC, Sheets MF, Hanck DA, et al. Sodium current in voltage clamped internally perfused canine cardiac Purkinje cells. *Biophys J.* 1987;52(1):1-11.
179. Narahashi T, Frazier DT. Site of action and active form of local anesthetics. *Neurosci Res.* 1971;4:65-99.
180. Mather LE, Chang DH. Cardiotoxicity with modern local anaesthetics: is there a safer choice? *Drugs.* 2001;61(3):333-342.
181. Rood JP, Coulthard P, Snowdon AT, et al. Safety and efficacy of levobupivacaine for postoperative pain relief after the surgical removal of impacted third molars: a comparison with lignocaine and adrenaline. *Br J Oral Maxillofac Surg.* 2002;40(6):491-496.
182. Rutten AJ, Mather LE, McLean CF. Cardiovascular effects and regional clearances of i.v. bupivacaine in sheep: enantiomeric analysis. *Br J Anaesth.* 1991;67(3):247-256.
183. Denson DD, Behbehani MM, Gregg RV. Enantiomer-specific effects of an intravenously administered arrhythmogenic dose of bupivacaine on neurons of the nucleus tractus solitarius and the cardiovascular system in the anesthetized rat. *Reg Anesth.* 1992;17(6):311-316.
184. Rutten AJ, Mather LE, McLean CF, et al. Tissue distribution of bupivacaine enantiomers in sheep. *Chirality.* 1993;5(7):485-491.
185. McClure JH. Ropivacaine. *Br J Anaesth.* 1996;76(2):300-307.
186. Markham A, Faulds D. Ropivacaine. A review of its pharmacology and therapeutic use in regional anaesthesia. *Drugs.* 1996;52(3):429-449.
187. Imaoka S, Enomoto K, Oda Y, et al. Lidocaine metabolism by human cytochrome P-450s purified from hepatic microsomes: comparison of those with rat hepatic cytochrome P-450s. *J Pharmacol Exp Ther.* 1990;255(3):1385-1391.
188. Shirvani A, Shamszadeh S, Eghbal MJ, et al. Effect of preoperative oral analgesics on pulpal anesthesia in patients with irreversible pulpitis-a systematic review and meta-analysis. *Clin Oral Investig.* 2017;21(1):43-52.
189. Tong HJ, Alzahrani FS, Sim YF, et al. Anaesthetic efficacy of articaine versus lidocaine in children's dentistry: a systematic review and meta-analysis. *Int J Paediatr Dent.* 2018;28(4):347-360.
190. Goldblum E, Atchabahian A. The use of 2-chloroprocaine for spinal anaesthesia. *Acta Anaesthesiol Scand.* 2013;57(5):545-552.
191. Forster JG, Rosenberg PH, Harilainen A, et al. Chloroprocaine 40 mg produces shorter spinal block than articaine 40 mg in day-case knee arthroscopy patients. *Acta Anaesthesiol Scand.* 2013;57(7):911-919.
192. Castaneda-Castellanos DR, Nikonorov I, Kallen RG, et al. Lidocaine stabilizes the open state of CNS voltage-dependent sodium channels. *Brain Res Mol Brain Res.* 2002;99(2):102-113.
193. Wei X, Dai R, Zhai S, et al. Inhibition of human liver cytochrome P-450 1A2 by the class IB antiarrhythmics mexiletine, lidocaine, and tocainide. *J Pharmacol Exp Ther.* 1999;289(2):853-858.
194. Arlander E, Ekstrom G, Alm C, et al. Metabolism of ropivacaine in humans is mediated by CYP1A2 and to a minor extent by CYP3A4: an interaction study with fluvoxamine and ketoconazole as in vivo inhibitors. *Clin Pharmacol Ther.* 1998;64(5):484-491.

Structure Challenge Answers

1. B and E
2. C. Nabumetone lacks an acidic functional group required for making and ion-ion bond with COX active site Arg. Nabumetone is activated by β-oxidase.
3. F
4. The enol
5. A, D, and F. All three of these NSAIDs commit the dual insult for GI distress. They all have an acidic functional group (primary insult) and they are all active NSAIDs and will inhibit COX-1 in the GI tract, reducing the cytoprotective PGE_1 concentrations.

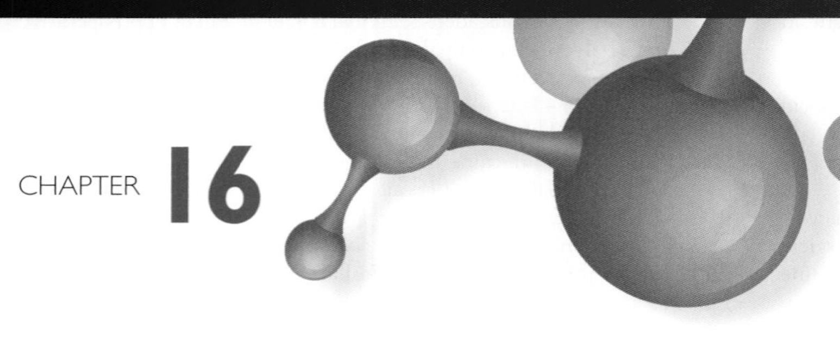

CHAPTER 16

Drugs Used to Treat Cardiac Disorders

Raghunandan Yendapally and Helmut B. Gottlieb

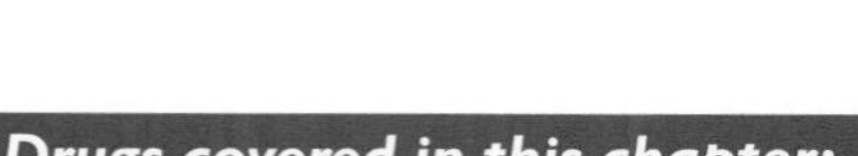

Drugs covered in this chapter:

ANTIANGINAL AGENTS

NITRATES AND NITRITES
- Nitroglycerin
- Amyl nitrite
- Pentaerythrityl tetranitrate
- Isosorbide dinitrate and mononitrate

CALCIUM CHANNEL BLOCKERS
- Amlodipine
- Diltiazem
- Nifedipine
- Nicardipine
- Verapamil

β-BLOCKERS
- Atenolol
- Bisoprolol
- Carvedilol
- Esmolol
- Metoprolol
- Propranolol

SODIUM CHANNEL BLOCKER
- Ranolazine

I_F INHIBITOR
- Ivabradine

DRUGS USED TO TREAT HEART FAILURE

CARDIAC GLYCOSIDES POSITIVE INOTROPIC AGENTS
- Digoxin
- Digitoxin

NONGLYCOSIDIC POSITIVE INOTROPIC AGENTS
- Dobutamine
- Dopamine
- Inamrinone
- Milrinone

NITRATE VASODILATORS
- Nitroglycerin
- Isosorbide dinitrate and mononitrate
- Isosorbide dinitrate in combination with hydralazine

NEPRILYSIN INHIBITOR/ARB
- Sacubitril/valsartan

ANTIARRHYTHMIC AGENTS

CLASS IA
- Procainamide
- Quinidine
- Disopyramide

CLASS IB
- Lidocaine
- Tocainide
- Mexiletine
- Phenytoin

CLASS IC
- Flecainide
- Propafenone

CLASS II
- Esmolol

CLASS III
- Sotalol
- Amiodarone
- Dronedarone
- Dofetilide
- Ibutilide

CLASS IV
- Verapamil
- Diltiazem

MISCELLANEOUS AGENTS
- Adenosine
- Magnesium Sulfate

Abbreviations

1,2-GDN 1,2-glyceryl dinitrate
1,3-GDN 1,3-glyceryl dinitrate
1,4-DHPs 1,4-dihydropyridines
AAD antiarrhythmic drug
ACC American College of Cardiology
ACE angiotensin-converting enzyme
AHA American Heart Association
AP action potential
ARB angiotensin II receptor blocker
ATP adenosine triphosphate
AV atrioventricular
AUC area under curve
BBB blood-brain barrier
CAD coronary artery disease
CCB calcium channel blocker
cAMP cyclic adenosine monophosphate
cGMP cyclic guanosine 3′,5′-monophosphate
CHF congestive heart failure
CNS central nervous system
CYP cytochrome P450
DCI dichloroisoproterenol
DHP dihydropyridine
Digoxin-Fab digoxin-specific antibody fragments
ECG electrocardiogram
FDA Food and Drug Administration
GFR glomerular filtration rate
HH hydralazine hydrazone
IBW ideal body weight
IHD ischemic heart disease
IV intravenous
MAO monoamine oxidase
MEGX monoethylglycinexylidide
mtALDH mitochondrial aldehyde dehydrogenase
NAcHPZ N-acetylhydrazinophthalazinone
NEP neprilysin
NTG nitroglycerin
NYHA New York Heart Association
NO nitric oxide
NO_2^- nitrite anion
PDE phosphodiesterase
PNS parasympathetic nervous system
PEDN pentaerythrityl dinitrate
PEMN pentaerythrityl mononitrate
PETN/PENT/PENTA/TEN pentaerythrityl tetranitrate
PETriN pentaerithrityl trinitrate
PZ phthalazinone
RAAS renin-angiotensin-aldosterone system
ROS radical reactive oxygen species
SA sinoatrial
sGC soluble guanylyl cyclase
SNS sympathetic nervous system
SNO S-nitrosothiol
TP triazolophthalazine

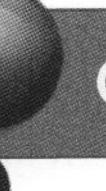

CLINICAL SIGNIFICANCE

Bethany A. Kalich, PharmD, BCPS-AQ Cardiology

Physicochemical, pharmacokinetic, and pharmacodynamic properties may predict potential clinical benefits in therapies for cardiovascular disorders, including ischemic heart disease, heart failure, and arrhythmias. Some therapies improve quality of life by relieving symptoms, while others improve cardiac function, further reducing the risk of cardiovascular death. The focus of guideline-directed therapy and management is to recommend therapeutic regimens that provide clinical benefit while minimizing risk of harm. A stepwise approach to the management of angina in patients with stable ischemic heart disease begins with the use of sublingual nitroglycerin and β-blocker therapy. Sublingual nitroglycerine has a quick onset of action and avoids hepatic first-pass metabolism. Addition or substitution of a calcium channel blocker and/or long-acting nitrate may be recommended to improve symptoms. Though therapies may lead to reductions in heart rate, this does not always result in improvements in outcomes such as cardiovascular death or myocardial infarction, as is the case with ivabradine. Understanding the mechanism of proposed benefit is essential to applying evidence-based concepts to patient care.

Heart failure is a syndrome in which the heart is unable to provide sufficient supply of blood to meet the demands of the body. The renin-angiotensin-aldosterone system (RAAS) and the sympathetic nervous system (SNS) inhibition are proposed to improve outcomes in patient with heart failure. Angiotensin-converting enzyme (ACE) inhibitors and angiotensin receptor blockers (ARB) have long been a standard of care for improving heart failure outcomes. Combining an ARB with a neprilysin inhibitor, sacubitril, resulted in a combination drug therapy that demonstrated superiority over the ACE inhibitor, enalapril, for heart failure outcomes. Sacubitril is a prodrug that is metabolized to sacubitrilat, which prevents the breakdown of natriuretic peptide. Understanding the potential benefit of a drug therapy to preserve the body's endogenous natriuretic peptide resulted in a paradigm shift in the management of heart failure therapy. Again, understanding the mechanism of proposed benefit is essential to applying evidence-based concepts to patient care.

Medicinal chemical properties are essential to understanding the differences in therapeutic effects between various antiarrhythmic drug (AAD) therapies. In patients with coronary artery disease (CAD), use of flecainide, resulted in increased rates of arrhythmia related death, leading many providers to avoid most class I AAD therapies in patients with CAD. Class III AAD therapies are broadly effective in the conversion and maintenance of normal sinus rhythm for patients with atrial fibrillation; however, selection of therapy is often guided by adverse drug reaction profile. For example, each of the class III AAD therapies, by nature of the mechanism of action, prolong the QT interval of the electrocardiogram (ECG), though the risk of the life-threatening arrhythmia, torsades de points. However, the prolongation varies greatly, with ibutilide and dofetilide being greatest, followed by sotalol and the least being amiodarone. Amiodarone is a unique, highly lipophilic molecule that is well distributed to organs such as adipose tissue, lungs, and liver and may cause toxic side effects. Clear understanding of the medicinal chemical properties guiding pharmacokinetic and pharmacodynamics effects of these AAD therapies is essential to providing evidence-based clinical care that optimizes the appropriateness, efficacy, safety, and adherence of therapeutic regimens.

DRUGS FOR THE TREATMENT OF ANGINA

Ischemic Heart Disease

According to the Center for Disease Control, cardiovascular disease is the number one cause of death in the United States. More than half of the deaths are caused by heart disease, and coronary artery disease (CAD) is the most frequent type of heart disease. Because of its prevalence, CAD is one of the costliest chronic diseases for both men and women, racial, and ethnic groups. With the aging of the "baby boom" population, it is predicted that the health care cost, mortality and morbidity rate associated with CAD will continue to rise. Although our understanding and treatment of CAD has improved over the last few years, these efforts have been insufficient to slow down or reverse the epidemic trend.

One of the most common manifestations of CAD is ischemic heart disease (IHD), also known as angina pectoris. IHD is manifested as asymptomatic (silent IHD) or symptomatic chest pain.[1] In both cases, it is caused by the buildup of atherosclerotic plaques in the coronary arteries, or by the disruption and rupture of atherosclerotic plaque's protective fibrous cap. Increase in plaque buildup leads to a reduction in the coronary artery lumen radius, which results in a decrease of blood flow to certain areas of the heart. In contrast, rupture of the plaque's cap leads to thrombosis, which can completely occlude the coronary blood vessel. A thrombus can also be dislodged and travel within the blood vessels, which is known as an embolus. Eventually an embolus can lodge within a small blood vessel and completely block the blood supply, resulting in an embolism. Thus, if an embolism occurs in the coronary arteries, it can deprive the myocardium of essential blood flow, which is essential for the maintenance of healthy tissue. As such, angina pectoris occurs when there is an imbalance between the amount of oxygenated blood being delivered to the heart (supply) versus the amount of blood required by the heart to maintain its required metabolic needs (demand).[2] It is widely accepted that decreased blood delivery, either by partial or total occlusion, to coronary arteries will lead to myocardial ischemia with consequent damage or death of the myocardial tissue. These effects can contribute to an increase in mortality and morbidity, as well as the development of other cardiovascular diseases discussed in this chapter (heart failure and arrhythmias). Ischemic heart disease is typically divided into three major classes.[1,3,4]

1. Stable IHD is caused by the partial blockade or narrowing of the coronary artery. In these patients, exertion typically causes an increase in the demand with no significant change in the supply of oxygenated blood. Resting and drug therapy typically resolve the chest pain within a few minutes. Drug therapy for most patients includes agents that decrease the workload of the heart and thus decreasing the frequency of angina attacks. Drugs that cause vasodilation to increase the delivery of blood to the ischemic site may also be utilized. Finally, drugs such as statins and aspirin are useful in maintaining the supply of blood flow and are indicated for patients with other comorbidities.
2. Unstable IHD is caused by the rupture of atherosclerotic plaques which lead to thrombosis and embolism. In this case, aggressive drug therapy and surgical procedures may be required to resolve and prevent further myocardium damage. Prophylactic therapy is aimed at reducing the clot formations or increasing the plaque cap stability.
3. Coronary artery vasospasm, aka Prinzmetal or variant angina is triggered by the quivering of the coronary smooth muscle and can occur in both atherosclerotic and nonatherosclerotic coronary arteries. However, patients with variant angina are typically younger and do not have many IHD risk factors. Drug therapy is aimed at producing vasodilation at the coronary artery and restoring blood flow.

There are several factors that can affect the myocardial oxygen demand. The primary site of action is the heart itself, which is modulated by the parasympathetic nervous system (PNS) and sympathetic nervous system (SNS).[5] Under exercise conditions, the SNS, via the release of norepinephrine, activates β-adrenergic receptors. Activation of these receptors produces an increase in heart rate, which is determined by the diastolic filling time and strength of myocardial contraction. Both responses lead to an increase in the demand for oxygen. In addition, increase in intramyocardial wall tension can also increase the need for oxygen. Among the factors that can change wall tension are the preload, afterload, and wall thickness.[6] Preload, also known as diastolic pressure, is directly related to the volume of blood in the left ventricle at the end of diastole. Preload is typically affected by venous smooth muscle tension and urine output. The higher the preload is, the harder the ventricles must work in order to pump blood out. Afterload, also known as systolic pressure, is determined by the arterial smooth muscle resistance against which the heart must pump to open the valves and eject blood into the main circulation. Similar to the preload, the higher the afterload, the higher the oxygen demand. Finally, the ventricular wall thickness can also play a role. The thicker the ventricular wall is, the more oxygen it will require to maintain normal function. In contrast, myocardial oxygen supply can be affected by perfusion pressure, hemoglobin-dependent oxygen-carrying capacity, and coronary blood flow. In patients with advanced atherosclerotic plaque buildup or who have experienced a myocardium ischemia, there is development or growth of new blood vessels. This phenomenon is known as collateral blood flow, which is a compensatory mechanism designed to bypass the narrowed coronary blood vessel and reestablish blood flow.[7] The severity or extent of CAD can be determined by several tests including electrocardiogram, cardiac stress test, and angiography. In patients who are experiencing severe chest pain, emergency physicians may check laboratory biomarkers to differentiate between stable and unstable IHD. The most common biomarkers are cardiac troponin, creatine kinase, creatine kinase-MB, and lactate dehydrogenase.

As such, drugs used to treat CAD and IHD diseases are designed to decrease the workload of the heart, thus decreasing the demand (Table 16.1). Alternatively, drugs that increase the supply of blood by inducing coronary vasodilation may also be used (Table 16.1). Drugs that decrease the progression of atherosclerotic plaque buildup or thrombus formation may be beneficial a well (Chapters 18 and 19).

Mechanism of Action of Antianginal Agents

ORGANIC NITRATES. NTG, isosorbide dinitrate, and isosorbide mononitrate are the three most commonly used drugs in this class. These drugs have several routes of administration and can be used in combination with other drug classes to decrease the demand and in some cases to increase the supply of blood to the ischemic heart. Organic nitrates have very similar pharmacodynamic properties, which is the release of NO upon metabolism. NO easily dissolves across bilayer membranes, and it works in the

Table 16.1 Pharmacological Summary of Drugs Used to Treat IHD

Drug Class		Drug Name	Mechanism of Action	Primary Site of Action	Pharmacological Effect	IHD Effect
Organic Nitrates		Nitroglycerin, isosorbide dinitrate, isosorbide mononitrate	NO donor	Arteries, veins, and coronary arteries	Decrease preload and afterload	Decrease workload and increase blood supply
CCBs	Dihydropyridine CCBs	Amlodipine, nifedipine, nicardipine, etc.	L-type Ca^{2+} channel	Arteries and coronary arteries	Decrease afterload	Decrease workload and increase blood supply
	Nondihydropyridine CCBs	Verapamil, diltiazem	L-type Ca^{2+} channel	Arteries, heart and coronary arteries	Decreases heart rate and afterload	Decrease workload and increase blood supply
β-blockers	Selective β_1-blockers	Metoprolol, atenolol, etc.	Selective β_1-adrenergic receptor antagonist	Heart	Decreases heart rate and myocardial contractile force	Decrease workload
	Nonselective β-blockers	Propranolol, etc.	Nonselective β_1- and β_2-adrenergic receptor antagonist	Heart	Decreases heart rate and myocardial contractile force	Decrease workload
	Mixed α- and β-blockers	Carvedilol labetalol	Nonselective β_1-, β_2-, and α_1-adrenergic receptor antagonist	Heart, arteries, and veins	Decreases heart rate, myocardial contractile force, afterload, and preload	Decrease workload
Late Na^+ channel blocker		Ranolazine	Late Na^+ channel blocker	Heart	Prevents Ca^{2+} overload	Prevents worsening of ischemic effects
I_f channel antagonist		Ivabradine	I_f channel antagonist	Heart	Bradycardia	Decrease workload

CCBs, calcium channel blockers; IHD, ischemic heart disease; NO, Nitric Oxide.

cytoplasm of smooth muscles of blood vessels. It couples with sGC and activates the enzyme leading to an increased production of cyclic guanosine 3′,5′-monophosphate (cGMP), which is a second messenger that is responsible for the dephosphorylation of myosin light chain kinase and smooth muscle relaxation.[8] At lower doses, the primary site of action of organic nitrates is the venous smooth muscle and coronary arteries (Table 16.1). By increasing the levels of cGMP in these tissues, drugs such as NTG can decrease preload and consequently decrease ventricular wall tension. These two effects ultimately lead to a decreased workload of the heart. By producing vasodilation in the coronary arteries, it may also increase coronary blood flow and thus increases the supply of oxygenated blood.[9] In variant angina patients, NTG via its vasodilatory properties can also relieve the coronary vasospasm. At higher doses, it becomes less site specific, and it can also vasodilate arterial smooth muscle. These drugs have a quick onset of action and may cause a marked decrease in arterial pressure. This sudden decrease in afterload will decrease the baroreceptor tone and increase SNS output to the heart, which may be counterproductive, since activation of β-adrenergic receptors in the heart increases the workload of the heart. This is typically not a problem since β-blockers are first-line drug therapy for IHD, and it would prevent this baroreceptor-mediated reflex tachycardia.

CALCIUM CHANNEL BLOCKERS. Calcium channel blockers (CCBs) are used to treat several cardiovascular diseases including hypertension, IHD, and arrhythmias. CCBs are broadly divided into two groups, i.e., the dihydropyridines (DHPs) and nondihydropyridines.[10] The DHPs are composed of several drugs including amlodipine, nifedipine, nicardipine, and others. Nondihydropyridine analogs include verapamil and diltiazem. Both groups of drugs have affinity for the L-type Ca^{2+} channels that are present in the arterial smooth muscle, and they block/prevent the influx of Ca^{2+} into the smooth muscle, thereby relaxing vascular smooth muscle.[11] Therefore, CCBs decrease afterload and consequently the workload of the heart. These drugs are also believed to produce coronary vasodilation which may increase the supply of oxygenated blood or decrease the quivering associated with variant angina. Among the CCBs, it is accepted that drugs belonging to the DHP class are more potent than nondihydropyridines with respect to their vasodilatory effects but little to no net effect on heart. In addition to their effects on the arterial and coronary smooth muscle, verapamil and diltiazem can also bind to voltage dependent L-type Ca^{2+} channels in the atrioventricular (AV) node and decrease the slope of phase 0.[12] This results in a slowing down of AV node conduction, which is reflected as a prolongation of the PR interval in the electrocardiogram (ECG) (see corresponding subsection in antiarrhythmic drugs).[13] As a result, heart rate is reduced which in turn reduces the myocardial oxygen requirement. When comparing the effects that CCBs evoke in the myocardium, verapamil and diltiazem produce the greatest reduction in the heart rate when compared to the DHP drugs but are weaker vasodilators.

β-BLOCKERS. β-blockers are one of the oldest and most widely prescribed medications used to treat several types of cardiovascular diseases.[14] There are several β-blockers available in the United States and their pharmacological response is dependent on the drug-receptor affinity and selectivity.[15] At normal therapeutic doses, cardioselective β-blockers such as atenolol, metoprolol, bisoprolol, and nebivolol are more selective toward the β_1-adrenergic receptor subtype. Other drugs like propranolol antagonize both β_1- and β_2-adrenergic receptors. Drugs like carvedilol and labetalol are mixed adrenergic antagonists that not only block β_1- and β_2-receptors but also block α_1-adrenergic receptors.[16] In addition, some research suggest that certain β-blockers can produce antioxidant effects, improve NO release, and act as partial agonists at the β_2-adrenergic receptors.[17] β_1-receptors are one of the major receptors expressed in the heart that are involved in its function. Because all β-blockers have affinity for the β_1-receptor, this class of drugs inhibit the binding of norepinephrine and epinephrine causing slow heart rate and decreased myocardium contractile force and myocardium rate of relaxation. As such, β-blockers are utilized in IHD to decrease the workload of the heart. β_1-receptors are also present in the juxtaglomerular cells of the kidney and activation of these receptors can produce an increase in renin secretion.[18] Renin is the rate-limiting enzyme involved in the production of angiotensin II, a powerful vasoconstrictor. Thus, β-blockers may decrease the secretion of renin, which would decrease plasma levels of angiotensin II and potentially decrease preload and afterload. Although β_2 appears to be the predominant receptor subtype in the central nervous system (CNS), β_1-selective drugs can also produce CNS side effects. Activation of β-adrenergic receptors in the brain has been associated with increased sympathetic activity. Thus, β-blockers may produce additional beneficial effects via a decrease in SNS tone to the heart and vasculature. α_1-adrenergic receptors are primarily expressed in the eye, brain, and arterial and venous blood vessels. Activation of the α_1-receptors by the SNS is one of the major pathways in which the body controls blood pressure. Certain β-blockers such as carvedilol and labetalol can also antagonize α_1-adrenergic receptors, which reduces the workload of the heart by decreasing the preload and afterload.[19]

RANOLAZINE (RANEXA). Ranolazine's anti-ischemic mechanism of action is primarily associated with its ability to block the late inward sodium channel.[20] Under normal physiological conditions, these late sodium channels are mostly closed. The Na^+/K^+ ATPase and Na^+/Ca^{2+} exchangers are involved in the reestablishment of ion balance homeostasis which promotes relaxation of the left ventricle.[21] During hypoxic/ischemic events, there is an increase in the production of metabolites and reactive oxygen species by the myocytes that triggers an increase in the opening of late inward sodium channels. This increase in intracellular sodium concentration causes a reversal of the Na^+/Ca^{2+} exchanger and consequently increases intracellular Ca^{2+} overload as an attempt to restore blood flow to the ischemic site. Unfortunately, increase in Ca^{2+} binding to contractile elements aggravates the ischemia by increasing left ventricle wall tension, ATP consumption, and diastolic contractile dysfunction. At optimum therapeutic dose, ranolazine prevents cardiac overload by decreasing myocardial Ca^{2+} overload during ischemia without major changes in heart rate or blood pressure.[20] In animal models, ranolazine has also been shown to block the delayed rectifier potassium channels and inhibit fatty acid oxidation.[22] Although these alternative mechanisms of action may provide additional pathways to decrease ischemia angina, its effect in humans is still not determined.

IVABRADINE (CORLANOR). Ivabradine decreases the workload of the heart by decreasing heart rate, which increases diastolic perfusion time. It is an antagonist at the I_f channel, which is the primary channel responsible for the spontaneous diastolic depolarization, also known as the pacemaker current.[21] This channel was first named as the "funny current."[23] It allows sodium influx which increases the slope of the sinoatrial node, which then makes the membrane potential less negative and allows for the opening of voltage-gated ion channels. I_f channels are one of the major determinants of automaticity and heart rate. Ivabradine decreases the heart rate by dose-dependent selective inhibition of the I_f channel, which decreases the slope of depolarization, and produces a prolongation of sinus node recovery time. It is a novel approach to decrease the heart rate and differs from β-blockers by not affecting the myocardial contractile force or atrioventricular conduction. In addition to being used for angina, ivabradine has also been approved by the FDA for use in heart failure patients.

Chemistry of Nitrates and Nitrites

Nitroglycerin (NTG) or glyceryl trinitrate (Fig. 16.1) is a synthetic molecule that was discovered by an Italian scientist Ascanio Sobrero in 1846 by reacting glycerol with the classical nitration mixture (nitric and sulfuric acid).[24] He not only observed its uncontrolled explosive properties, but when tasted in small quantities, he noted its headache-causing properties.[25] Subsequently, Alfred Nobel by combining NTG with kieselguhr developed dynamite, which is an explosive under controlled conditions.[24] This has led to the success of the Nobel family and eventually much of his wealth was used in the establishment of the renowned Nobel Prize that has been awarded since 1901.[25,26]

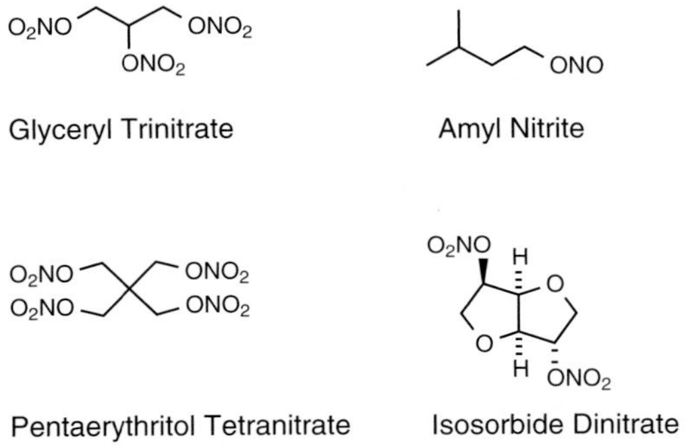

The medicinal properties of amyl nitrite (Fig. 16.1) for the treatment of angina were documented in 1867 by British physician, Thomas Lauder Brunton.[27] In the following decade, it was largely replaced by NTG because of the ease of administration and long duration of action.[28] In fact, in 1890, Alfred Nobel's physician prescribed him NTG for the treatment of his heart disease.[29]

NTG is a prodrug (Fig. 16.2).[30] It is primarily bioactivated in smooth muscles by undergoing complex metabolic reactions and is converted to nitric oxide (NO) or a related compound S-nitrosothiol (SNO) intermediate.[31] Recently, a few scientists have questioned whether NTG effect on smooth muscle relaxation is actually dependent on the generation of free NO or not.[32] There are several hypotheses that have been put forward regarding the activation of NTG including enzymatic (e.g., glutathione S-transferase, cytochrome P450 [CYP]–related enzymes) and nonenzymatic (e.g., cellular thiol compounds) activation.[9] NTG metabolic activation primarily takes place by the enzyme mitochondrial aldehyde dehydrogenase (mtALDH), a novel reductase mechanism.[31] Human mtALDH contains two cysteine thiols in the active site and NTG serves as a substrate and is converted to 1,2-glyceryl dinitrate (1,2-GDN).[33]

Pentaerythrityl tetranitrate (PETN) (Fig. 16.1) is similar to NTG and is synthesized by nitration of the polyalcohol pentaerythritol instead of glycerol.[34] PETN appears more spherical in shape than the glycerol backbone of NTG.[35] PETN contains a central carbon which in turn is attached to four groups of $-CH_2$-ONO_2.[35] The application of pentaerythritol tetranitrate for the treatment of angina is limited in the United States but is widely used in the Europe.[36] Pentaerythrityl tetranitrate is abbreviated as PETN but is also referred to as PENT, PENTA, and TEN. It is also used as an explosive for military purposes.[35]

Isosorbide (Fig. 16.1) is a bicyclic sugar derivative that is prepared by the dehydration of sorbitol. Chemically, isosorbide mono- and dinitrate are nitrate ester derivatives of isosorbide.[35] The nitrate attached to the sugar largely reduces the explosive properties, which makes it a more stable compound.[35] The difference in number of nitrate groups (mono- and dinitrate) results in pharmacokinetic differences.

Figure 16.1 Organic nitrates and nitrites.

PHARMACEUTICAL PREPARATIONS. NTG is available in various formulations. It is administered orally in the form of extended-release capsules, translingual spray, sublingual powder, and tablets; topically in the form of ointment, transdermal patch; and parenterally in the form of IV infusion. Isosorbide mono- and dinitrate are available as oral immediate- and extended-release formulations. Isosorbide dinitrate is also available as a sublingual formulation. PETN is available as an oral formulation.

PHARMACOKINETICS. The onset of action of IV NTG formulation is immediate and is rapid for the sublingual tablet and translingual spray (2 min). The onset of action

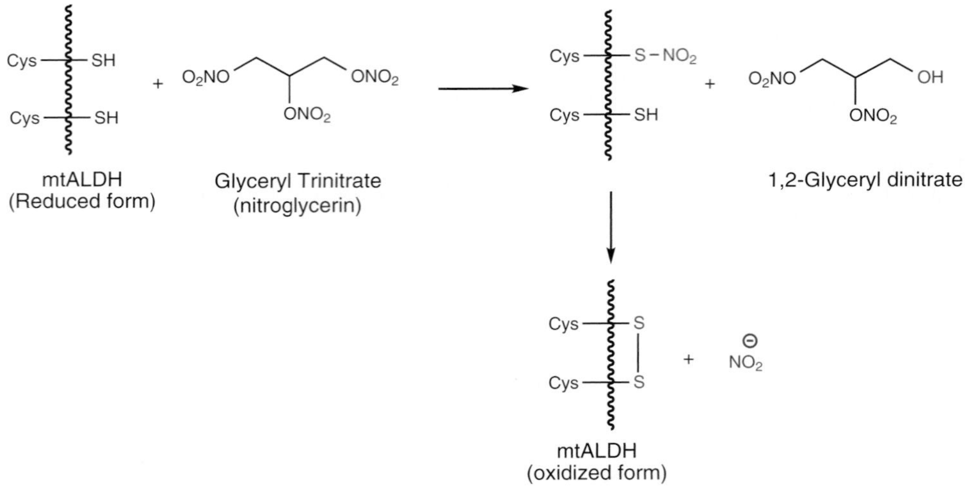

Figure 16.2 Activation of glyceryl trinitrate.

is not immediate for topical (15-30 min), extended-release capsule (60 min), and transdermal patch (about 30 min).[37] Therefore, for acute anginal attacks, IV, or sublingual formulations are appropriate choices of treatment when compared to other routes.

The duration of action of IV NTG formulation is about 3-5 minutes and sublingual tablet is about 25 minutes. Whereas, extended-release capsule (4-8 hr), transdermal patch (10-12 hr), and topical (about 7 hr) preparations have a longer duration of action making these formulations suitable for a sustained effect.[37]

The plasma kinetics of NTG is highly variable due to intra- and interindividual differences.[38] When administered by IV infusion, NTG was shown to have a high apparent volume of distribution of approximately 3 L/kg and a short plasma half-life of about 3 minutes.[38]

NTG is metabolized in systemic vasculature, liver, lungs, kidneys, and erythrocytes. The amount and extent of metabolites formed is also dependent on the route of administration. For example, the IV, sublingual, and transdermal routes of administration avoid first-pass metabolism and have higher bioavailability than orally administered capsules. Irrespective of the route of administration, the amount of metabolites formed far exceeds the intact NTG indicating extensive metabolism.[39] NTG is metabolized to 1,2-glyceryl dinitrate (1,2-GDN), 1,3-glyceryl dinitrate (1,3-GDN), NO, and SNO.[31] However, 1,2-GDN is the major metabolite in the vascular smooth muscle cells and NO is generated via an obligate intermediate nitrite ion (Fig. 16.2).[31] Dinitrates of NTG can further be metabolized by denitration into 1-glyceryl mononitrate, 2-glyceryl mononitrate, and subsequently to glycerol.[39] Dinitrate and mononitrate NTG may also undergo glucuronide conjugation.[40] Pharmacokinetics of pentaerythrityl tetranitrate is different from NTG. When administered orally, PETN is metabolized to pentaerythrityl dinitrate (PEDN), pentaerythrityl mononitrate (PEMN), and not much of pentaerithrityl trinitrate (PETriN) is observed.[35,41]

When administered orally, isosorbide dinitrate is rapidly absorbed. It has only about 30% bioavailability because of extensive first-pass metabolism in the liver.[42,43] Isosorbide dinitrate is distributed rapidly and primarily metabolized by denitration to 2-isosorbide mononitrate (about 25%) and 5-isosorbide mononitrate (about 75%).[42,43] The half-life elimination of oral, sublingual, and IV isosorbide dinitrate is about 30, 9, and 5 minutes, respectively.[42,43] To the contrary, its metabolites 2-isosorbide mononitrate and 5-isosorbide mononitrate have longer elimination half-lives of about 2 and 5 hours, respectively.[42,43] Majority of isosorbide metabolites are eliminated in the urine.

The orally administered isosorbide mononitrate is rapidly and completely absorbed with a bioavailability close to 100%.[42] It is metabolized by conjugation and denitration to isosorbide and sorbitol, which are predominantly eliminated renally.

ADVERSE EFFECTS. Headache due to the vasodilation of blood vessels in the brain is the most common side effect associated with NTG, especially with the longer duration of action formulations. Other side effects include hypotension associated with syncope, nausea, and vomiting.

NITRATE TOLERANCE. The major limitation of chronic administration of organic nitrates is tolerance, which results in decreased antianginal efficacy because of desensitization of blood vessels.[31] NTG tolerance is partly due to the impaired bioactivation and the loss of function of mtALDH function.[31] NTG tolerance is also attributed to its ability to generate free radical reactive oxygen species (ROS) by the endothelium, which are capable of oxidizing membrane lipids.[36] On the contrary, PETN is not associated with an increase in ROS and does not cause tolerance.[36]

DRUG-DRUG INTERACTIONS. Organic nitrates may have significant drug interactions and have profound hypotensive effects with other vasodilators. Riociguat and phosphodiesterase-5 (PDE5) inhibitors must be avoided in combination with organic nitrates. Riociguat used for the treatment of pulmonary hypertension is a direct activator of the soluble guanylyl cyclase (sGC) enzyme.[44] In addition, it can also sensitize the sGC to the endogenous NO which is produced by the activation of the NO synthase enzyme. In contrast, PDE5 inhibitors such as sildenafil block the PDE5 enzyme, which is involved in the breakdown of cGMP.[45] Concurrent use of NTG with either one of these drugs may lead to marked increase in cGMP and a severe drop in blood pressure. On the contrary, concurrent administration of vasoconstrictor agents such as ergot alkaloids (e.g., ergotamine) may lead to a decreased antianginal efficacy of NTG.

Chemistry of Calcium Channel Blockers

The clinically available DHPs and non-DHP calcium channel blockers act on L-type or long-lasting channels; however, the structural diversity of these compounds emphasizes the importance of their specificities in cardiac tissues and arteriolar vasculature.[46] Since clinically available DHPs contain hydrogens at 1 and 4 positions on the DHP ring, they are specifically referred as 1,4-dihydropyridines (1,4-DHPs). Several 1,4-DHPs are also found effective in the treatment of hypertension (refer to Chapter 17).[47] The 1,4-DHPs that are primarily used in the management of angina include amlodipine, nifedipine, and nicardipine (Fig. 16.3). The nondihydropyridines can further be divided into phenyl alkylamine derivative (verapamil), benzothiazepine derivative (diltiazem), and diaminopropanol ether derivative (bepridil). Currently, verapamil and diltiazem are the only nondihydropyridines that are clinically available in the United States (Fig. 16.4). Verapamil is the first calcium channel blocker that was discovered based on the structure of papaverine, one of the important constituents of opium poppy alkaloids.[48] Verapamil was first synthesized as D365 (Iproveratril) by Dr. Ferdinand Dengel at the German pharmaceutical company Knoll AG, and in the early 1960s, its coronary vasodilatory properties and antiarrhythmic properties were discovered.[48,49]

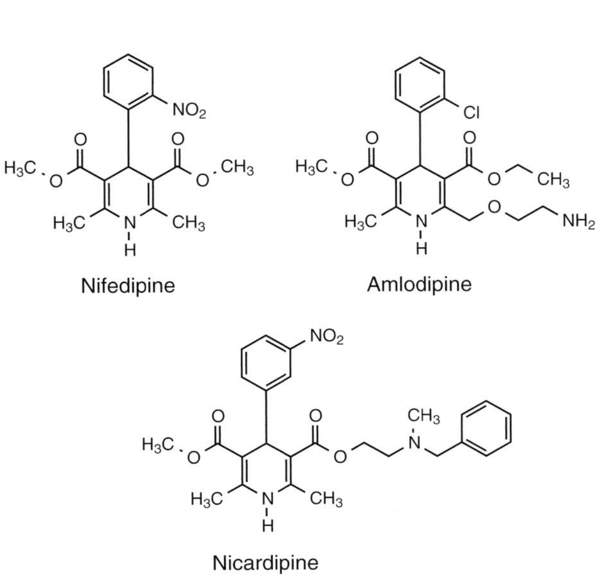

Nifedipine

Amlodipine

Nicardipine

Figure 16.3 1,4-Dihydropyridine calcium channel blockers.

Verapamil

Diltiazem

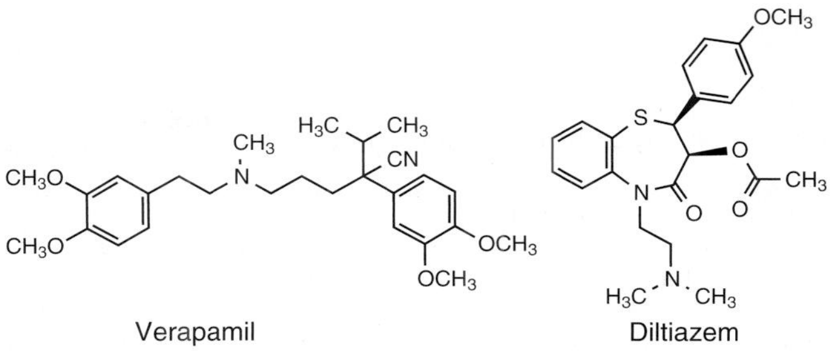

Figure 16.4 Nondihydropyridine calcium channel blockers.

1,4-DIHYDROPYRIDINES. Nifedipine is the prototype molecule in the 1,4-DHP class of calcium channel blocker and was discovered in the early 1970s.[50] Nifedipine is a symmetrical 1,4-DHP in which both esters (methyl ester) at C-3 and C-5, as well as substitutions at C-2 and C-6 (methyl group), are identical. Nifedipine is light sensitive and undergoes decomposition into a pyridine analog and a nitroso pyridine analog.[51]

The replacement of the 1,4-DHP ring with other rings leads to compounds with reduced or loss of activity indicating the importance of the ring for optimal activity.[52] The 1,4-DHP ring adopts a boat confirmation.[52] The hydrogen attached to the nitrogen in the 1,4 DHP ring forms hydrogen bonding with tyrosine in the receptor.[52] Replacement of the hydrogen with other groups and oxidation of the nitrogen is detrimental for its activity.[52] The presence of C-3 and C-5 ester groups on the 1,4-DHP ring is required for optimal activity. The C-4 is attached to an *ortho* and/or *meta* electron-withdrawing phenyl ring.[52] The *ortho* and/or *meta* derivatives are considered to be critical for activity because they lock the phenyl ring perpendicular to the 1,4-DHP ring.[52] Nifedipine contains an *ortho*-nitrophenyl group, amlodipine contains an *ortho*-chlorophenyl group, and nicardipine contains a *meta*-nitrophenyl group (Fig. 16.3).

Nicardipine and amlodipine have distinguishable physiochemical properties among the 1,4-DHP derivatives.[53] Amlodipine besylate and nifedipine hydrochloride salt forms have good aqueous solubility. Amlodipine has an amino-ethoxy methyl side chain, and nicardipine has an N-benzyl-N-methylamino side chain (Fig. 16.3). Therefore, at physiological pH, they exist as ionized forms which have higher hydrophilicity than their unionized forms.[53]

NONDIHYDROPYRIDINES. Verapamil contains a basic tertiary nitrogen and is marketed as the hydrochloride salt. It contains one chiral center, but it is administered as a racemic mixture of *S*-enantiomer and *R*-enantiomer. The *S*(−)-isomer of verapamil is about 10-20 times more potent than the *R*(+)-isomer as a vasodilator.[54] However, the *R*-isomer is less cardiotoxic than the *S*-isomer.[54] The clinically available diltiazem is a (+)-*cis* isomer and has two chiral centers 2*S*, 3*S* configuration.[55] The (−)-*cis* enantiomer 2*R*, 3*R* does not have vasodilatory properties. The *trans* diastereomers (2*R*, 3*S* and 2*S*, 3*R*) have weak activity.[55] Therefore, stereochemistry has an absolute impact on the pharmacological activity of diltiazem.[55]

PHARMACEUTICAL PREPARATIONS. Although several nicardipine formulations are clinically available, only the oral immediate-release formulation is used in the treatment of chronic stable angina.[56] Whereas, oral sustained release products and IV nicardipine are clinically used in the management of hypertension along with the oral immediate-release formulation.[56] The oral formulation of verapamil and diltiazem are used in the treatment of angina, and IV formulations are used in supraventricular tachycardias.[56]

PHARMACOKINETICS. The bioavailability of orally administered nifedipine is about 45%-70%.[57] Nifedipine is highly protein bound (>95%), primarily to albumin.[58] Nifedipine undergoes significant first-pass metabolism in the liver and intestine.[57] It is primarily oxidized by CYP3A4 to pyridine which is further metabolized into acid metabolites by ester hydrolysis.[57,59] Nifedipine immediate-release formulation has a half-life elimination of 2 hours, and it reaches the maximum blood concentration in about 30 minutes.[60] Whereas, the controlled-release formulation of nifedipine has a half-life elimination of 7 hours and time to reach the maximum blood concentration is 1.6-4 hours.[60] About 60%-80% of orally administered nifedipine is eliminated in the urine predominantly as metabolites with the remaining drug eliminated in feces.[61] In patients with liver cirrhosis, there is an increased bioavailability and reduced systemic clearance of nifedipine necessitating the need for adjustment of doses.[62] Nifedipine pharmacokinetic parameters may be affected by the genetic differences. For example, South Asians have a lower systemic clearance than Caucasians, and as a result nicardipine its half-life is significantly longer in South Asians.[57]

Nicardipine is completely and rapidly absorbed after an oral administration.[63] However, the bioavailability is moderately low (35%) because of extensive first-pass metabolism.[63] The bioavailability of nicardipine is further decreased when food is consumed before or along with the nicardipine.[63] The bioavailability is further dependent on the dose because of saturable presystemic effect.[63] Nicardipine undergoes extensive serum protein binding (>95%).[64] It binds to albumin, lipoproteins, and erythrocytes.[64] Nicardipine has a half-life elimination of 1-4 hours, and the maximum blood concentration is achieved in 0.5-2 hours.[60] It is predominantly metabolized in the liver.[63] Apart from the oxidation of the 1,4-DHP ring to pyridine, the N-benzyl side chain also undergoes debenzylation which is further metabolized.[63] Glucuronide conjugates are also identified in the urine.[63] About 60% (primarily in the form of metabolites) of nicardipine is eliminated in the urine and 25% is eliminated in feces.[65]

Amlodipine has unique pharmacokinetic properties because of its high degree of ionization.[53] Food does not have an effect on the bioavailability of amlodipine, and the estimated bioavailability is about 64%-90%.[66] Amlodipine has a large volume of distribution of about 21 L/kg and a high degree of protein binding of about 98%.[53] Among 1,4-DHPs, amlodipine has the highest half-life elimination of 35-50 hours, and time to reach the maximum blood concentration is 6-12 hours.[60] Amlodipine once-daily dosing is effective for the treatment of angina pectoris owing to its slow clearance.[60] Amlodipine does not undergo extensive first-pass metabolism; however, it does undergo significant metabolism in the liver.[53] CYP3A4 plays a major role in metabolizing the 1,4-DHP ring of amlodipine to its oxidized pyridine metabolite.[67] It can further undergo metabolism via O-demethylation, O-dealkylation, and oxidative deamination.[67] The elimination half-life of amlodipine is significantly prolonged in patients with hepatic cirrhosis ($t_{1/2}$ is about 60 hr) leading to a greater accumulation.[68] About 60% of the administered amlodipine is eliminated in the urine predominantly in the form of metabolites.[69] In elderly patients, amlodipine has a prolonged elimination half-life because of decreased clearance and may require adjustment of doses.[68]

Verapamil is well absorbed orally.[70] However, the bioavailability is only 10%-35% because of extensive hepatic first-pass metabolism.[70,71] Verapamil is extensively bound to proteins (about 90%).[72] Verapamil undergoes stereoselective metabolism and the *S*-enantiomer is metabolized at a faster rate than the *R*-enantiomer.[73,74] Verapamil undergoes N-demethylation catalyzed extensively by CYP3A4 and CYP3A5 to norverapamil.[74] Verapamil and norverapamil further undergoes O-demethylation by CYP2C8.[74] Norverapamil has about 20% cardiovascular activity when compared to verapamil. The immediate-release formulation of verapamil has an elimination half-life of about 3-10 hours, but is extended up to 17 hours during chronic administration.[75] Norverapamil has a longer elimination half-life than verapamil.[75] About 70% of the administered verapamil is eliminated in the urine and 16% is eliminated in feces, primarily as metabolites.

The absolute bioavailability of diltiazem is 40%-50%.[76] The volume of distribution of diltiazem is 8-14 L/kg.[76] About 80% of the diltiazem is protein bound with significant interindividual differences.[77] It is primarily bound to lipoproteins and α_1-acid glycoprotein.[77] Diltiazem undergoes extensive metabolism and less than 5% of the drug is eliminated unchanged.[78] Diltiazem primarily undergoes O-deacetylation by esterases to desacetyldiltiazem and N-demethylation by CYP3A4 to N-monodesmethyl diltiazem.[78,79] Diltiazem also undergoes O-demethylation by CYP2D6.[80] The desacetyldiltiazem and N-monodesmethyl diltiazem are pharmacologically active vasodilators; therefore, the activity is due to the intact drug and its active metabolites.[78] Diltiazem and its N-monodesmethyl and N,N-didesmethyl metabolites are CYP3A4 inhibitors.[79] The half-life elimination of immediate- and extended-release formulations are 3-4.5 and 4-9 hours, respectively.[56,77] During chronic oral administration, N-monodesmethyl diltiazem accumulates to a greater extent than desacetyldiltiazem.[81] During chronic therapy, accumulation of diltiazem metabolites leads to the decreased elimination of diltiazem.[79]

ADVERSE EFFECTS. The most common side effects of calcium channel blockers are related to their vasodilatory abilities on smooth muscle vasculature. As such, patients may complain of dizziness, fatigue, headache, constipation, and flushing. Because of their potency, some patients may experience peripheral edema and palpitations with dihydropyridines. This is most likely caused by the baroreceptor-mediated increase in sympathetic tone to the venous system and heart. Gastrointestinal side effects are also observed. Verapamil frequently produces gingival hyperplasia and constipation.

DRUG-DRUG INTERACTIONS. Calcium channel blockers are contraindicated in patients with heart failure because of the risk of developing pulmonary edema. Because β-blockers are first-line therapy for most of the heart failure patients, concurrent administration of β-blockers with verapamil or diltiazem may lead to severe bradycardia and potential heart block.

Simvastatin used in the treatment of hypercholesterolemia is predominantly metabolized by CYP3A4 enzyme. Amlodipine coadministration may increase the plasma concentrations of simvastatin, but it is a safer option than verapamil and diltiazem.[82] Verapamil is a potent CYP3A4 inhibitor and coadministration of verapamil with other drugs that are metabolized by CYP3A4 may lead to altered drug concentrations.[83] For instance, verapamil is shown to increase the plasma concentrations of simvastatin by about 3-fold and increase the adverse effects of statins such as rhabdomyolysis.[83] Therefore, simvastatin doses should be adjusted and appropriately monitored when combined with verapamil.[83]

Rifamycin antibiotic, a potent CY3A4 inducer, may increase metabolism and systemic elimination of calcium channel blockers, thereby diminishing their therapeutic effects.[84] To the contrary, azole antifungal agents such as itraconazole are potent CYP3A4 inhibitors and may decrease the metabolism and enhance the plasma concentrations of calcium channel blockers.[85] Itraconazole may further potentiate negative inotropic effects associated with verapamil and diltiazem.[56] Grapefruit juice is a known CYP3A4 and CYP3A5 inhibitor.[86] It predominantly inhibits the CYPs in the intestine with a minor effect on hepatic CYP enzymes.[86] Among DHPs, amlodipine and nifedipine are less affected by grapefruit juice because their oral bioavailability is greater than other DHPs.[86] However, the blood levels of these two drugs may still be increased by about 15%-30% when coadministered with the grapefruit juice.[86] Therefore, caution and monitoring is essential when calcium channel blockers are coadministered with grapefruit juice.

Verapamil is a substrate and inducer of P-glycoprotein.[87] Coadministration of verapamil with digoxin, a P-glycoprotein substrate, may decrease renal tubular elimination and increase plasma concentrations of digoxin.[88] Since this can lead to deleterious effects of digoxin, the dose of digoxin should be reduced when given in combination with verapamil.[89] Verapamil may inhibit the P-glycoprotein in the blood-brain barrier (BBB) and thereby prevent the efflux of drugs.[90] This may be a disadvantage and may lead to unwanted toxic drug-drug interactions in some cases. For instance, verapamil being a P-glycoprotein inhibitor may have the potential to increase antidiarrheal loperamide (P-glycoprotein substrate) concentrations in the BBB, which may lead to loperamide unwanted opioid CNS side effects such as respiratory depression.[91] Verapamil and diltiazem may also precipitate the neurotoxic side effects associated with anticonvulsants such as carbamazepine and phenytoin.[92,93] Therefore, the combination should either be avoided or patients must carefully be monitored.

Development of β-blockers

Catecholamines such as norepinephrine and epinephrine are synthesized from the amino acid L-tyrosine.[94] Tyrosine is in turn obtained from the diet and biosynthesized from the amino acid L-phenylalanine catalyzed by the enzyme tyrosine hydroxylase.[94] Catecholamines bind and intrinsically activate G-protein–coupled α- and β-adrenergic receptors (discussed in Chapter 6).

Isoproterenol, a synthetic catecholamine is a potent β-adrenergic agonist. In the 1950s, the 3,4 dihydroxy groups in isoproterenol were replaced with the dichloro group to afford dichloroisoprenaline or dichloroisoproterenol (DCI) (Fig. 16.5).[95] DCI was shown to inhibit adrenergic effects of epinephrine and isoproterenol.[95] However, DCI was not a clinically useful β-blocker because of its potent intrinsic sympathomimetic activity.[96] In 1962, Sir James Black et al., noted that the development of β-blockers free of intrinsic sympathomimetic activity could potentially be valuable for the treatment of angina and tachycardias.[96] The 3,4 dichloro phenyl ring in DCI was replaced with the naphthyl ring to afford pronethalol (Nethalide, Alderlin) (Fig. 16.5).[96] However, pronethalol had serious unpleasant side effects.[97] In mice, pronethalol induced malignant tumors, primarily thymic and lymphosarcomata.[97] Pronethalol also has intrinsic sympathomimetic activity, albeit not as potent as DCI.[97] Sir James Black et al., continued further research to discover newer drug molecules with decreased toxicity. The important breakthrough was achieved by introducing the oxymethylene (-OCH_2) group between the aryl (naphthyl) ring and ethanolamine to yield aryloxypropanolamine.[97] This modification resulted in the discovery of propranolol (Fig. 16.5), a prototype β-blocker which was devoid of carcinogenic properties

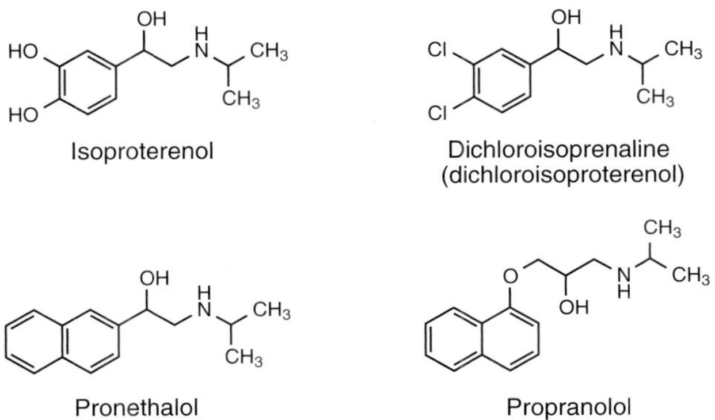

Figure 16.5 Development of β-adrenergic antagonists.

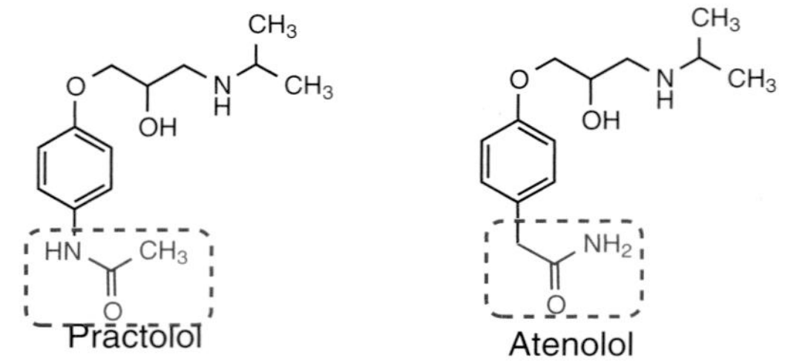

Practolol

Atenolol

Figure 16.6 Development of selective β-1 adrenergic antagonists.

and the intrinsic sympathomimetic activity possessed by pronethalol.[97] In 1988, Sir James Black received the Nobel Prize in Physiology or Medicine for his contribution to the "important principles for drug treatment."[98]

The classification of β-receptors into β_1 and β_2 was first reported in 1967 by Lands et al.[99] This has paved the way for the classification of β-blockers into nonselective β-blockers antagonizing both β_1- and β_2-receptors and cardioselective β-blockers that specifically antagonize β_1-receptors at low doses.[100] Selective β_1-blockers may have better safety profile in patients with bronchospasm than nonselective β-blockers.[100] Practolol (Fig. 16.6) was the first clinically available selective β_1-blocker but was later withdrawn from clinical use because of adverse oculomucocutaneous syndrome such as vision loss, fibrous or plastic peritonitis, mucosal and nasal ulceration, otitis media, and rashes.[100,101] Practolol is a phenyloxypropanolamine containing N-acetamide (-$NHCOCH_3$) at the *para* position (Fig. 16.5). It possibly undergoes deacetylation to yield an aromatic amine which may be responsible for its untoward side effects.[102] Replacement of the acetamide -$NHCOCH_3$ with -CH_2CONH_2 at the *para* position led to the discovery of atenolol (Fig. 16.5). Unlike practolol, atenolol did not possess severe oculomucocutaneous side effects.[101]

Today, several selective and nonselective β-blockers are available worldwide for the treatment of hypertension (clinical use of β-blockers to treat hypertensive disorders is discussed in Chapter 17), angina, heart failure, arrhythmias, and glaucoma. All clinically available β-blockers end with the suffix -lol; nonselective β-blockers include carteolol, nadolol, penbutolol, pindolol, propranolol, sotalol, and timolol (Fig. 16.7). Selective β_1-blockers include acebutolol, atenolol, betaxolol, bisoprolol, esmolol, metoprolol, and nebivolol (Fig. 16.8). Labetalol and carvedilol are mixed adrenergic antagonists blocking both α_1- and β-adrenergic receptors (Fig. 16.7).[100]

STRUCTURAL PROPERTIES OF β-BLOCKERS. The chemical features of clinically available β-blockers are as follows:[103]

1. At least one aromatic and/or heteroaromatic ring system.[103] They are devoid of catechol functional groups.
2. The aromatic/heteroaromatic ring is in turn attached to an alkyl side chain containing a chiral secondary hydroxyl group and an amine.[103] The amine group is either attached to an isopropyl or a tertiary butyl group with few exceptions.
3. Many of the β-blockers are aryloxypropanolamine derivatives. Exceptions include sotalol, which is an arylethanolamine derivative containing a sulfonamide group at the *para* position.

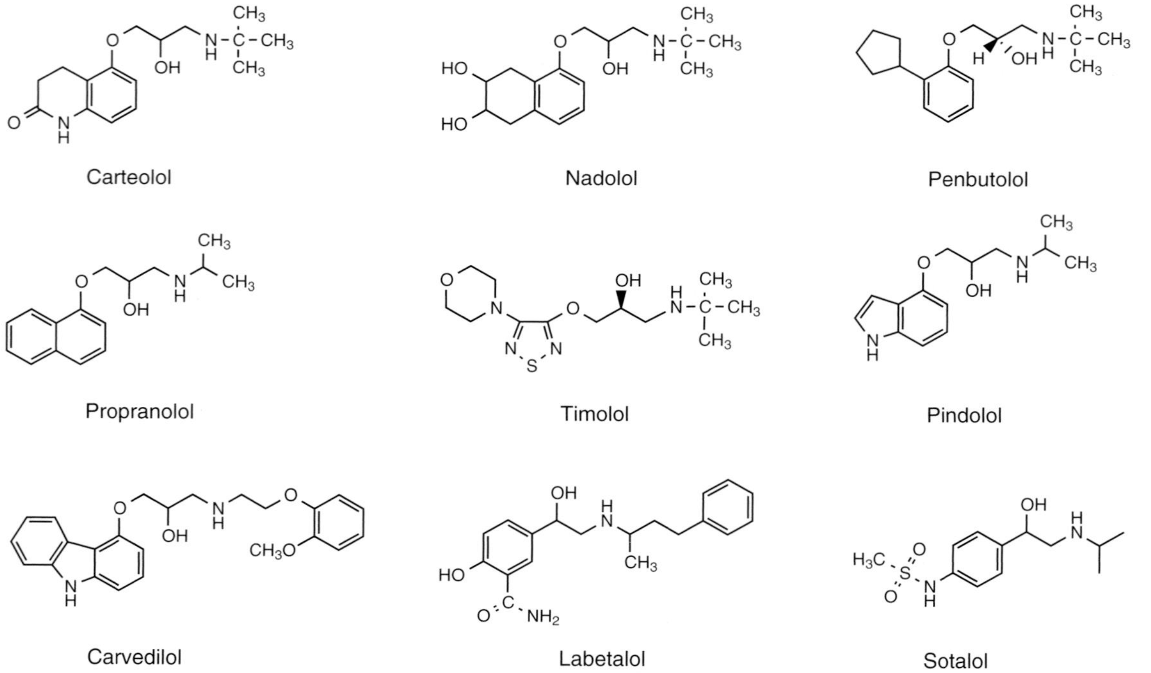

Carteolol

Nadolol

Penbutolol

Propranolol

Timolol

Pindolol

Carvedilol

Labetalol

Sotalol

Figure 16.7 Nonselective β-adrenergic antagonists.

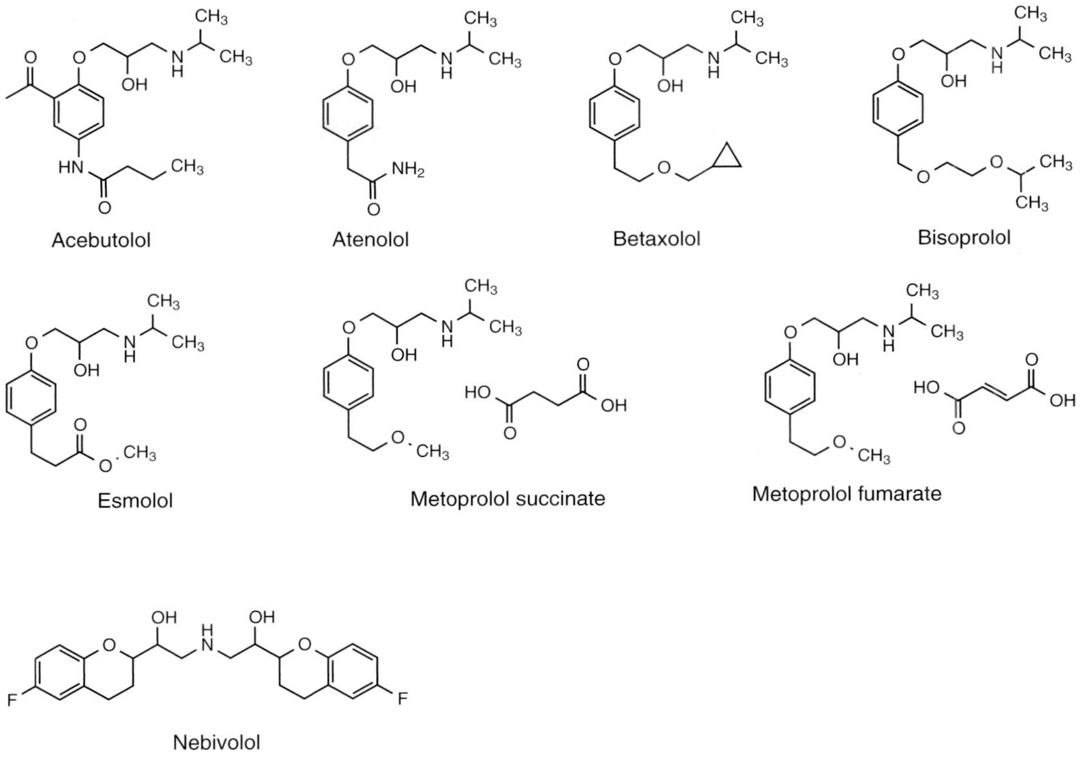

Figure 16.8 Selective β-1 adrenergic antagonists.

4. Majority of the clinically available selective β_1-blockers are phenyloxypropanolamine derivatives containing substitutions at the *para* position.
5. Due to the presence of oxymethylene (-OCH_2) group in aryloxypropanolamine, the *S*-enantiomer of aryloxypropanolamine side chain occupy similar space in the β-receptor as the *R*-enantiomer side chain of arylethanolamine. In general, in β-blockers with one chiral center, the *S*(−)-enantiomer has better β-receptor binding affinity than the *R*(+)-enantiomer.[103]
6. Majority of β-blockers are clinically administered as a racemic mixture. Exceptions include timolol which is only available as *S*(−)-timolol.[103]

β-blockers based on their partition coefficient can be classified into lipophilic and hydrophilic β-blockers. This may account for the pharmacokinetic differences between β-blockers. For example, a lipophilic β-blocker such as propranolol has a higher partition coefficient (Log P = 2.65; cLog P = 2.75)[104] because of the hydrocarbon naphthyl ring system, and as a result, it has a greater ability to penetrate the BBB. To the contrary, hydrophilic β-blockers such as atenolol containing a polar acetamide group (Log P = 0.5; cLog P = -0.1)[104] are less likely to cross the CNS.[105] Lipophilic β-blockers undergo extensive hepatic metabolism leading to shorter half-lives than the hydrophilic β-blockers which are minimally metabolized by the liver.[106]

Propranolol. Propranolol (Fig. 16.7), a lipophilic nonselective β-blocker is almost completely absorbed after oral administration.[107] However, the bioavailability is poor (about 25%) because of extensive hepatic metabolism.[108] Protein-rich food may increase its bioavailability.[109] The *S*(−)-propranolol is about 100 times more potent than the *R*(+)-propranolol.[110] It is well distributed to various tissues, and about 90% of the drug is protein bound.[107] The volume of distribution of propranolol is about 6 L/kg.[108] The naphthyl ring in propranolol is hydroxylated at the 4 and 5 position predominantly by CYP2D6 and undergoes N-desisopropylation by CYP1A2.[111] The 4-hydroxy propranolol metabolite possesses potent β-blocking properties similar to propanol and is also a weak CYP2D6 inhibitor.[112] Propranolol is also metabolized by glucuronidation.[110] Propranolol is predominantly excreted in the urine as metabolites, and only <1% is eliminated as the intact drug.[113] Since propranolol crosses the BBB it may cause depression.[114] However, it is CNS effects may be beneficial in patients with anxiety.[115] Propranolol is also used as a prophylactic agent in migraine.[116]

Propranolol is available as oral conventional propranolol hydrochloride (Inderal) and extended-release capsules (Inderal XL, Inderal LA). The extended-release formulation takes a longer time for dissolution and releases the drug in a controlled and predictable manner when compared to conventional formulation.[117] In extended-release formulation the bioavailability is lower, time to attain peak plasma levels is longer, and the peak plasma levels are lower than the conventional formulation.[117,118] The elimination half-life of conventional propranolol is about 3-6 hours and requires multiple dosing.[107] Whereas, the elimination half-life of extended-release formulation is significantly longer (8-11 hr).[118] The extended-release capsule constantly maintains the plasma concentrations for 24 hours, which allows for once-daily dosing and thereby improves patient compliance.[118]

Atenolol. Atenolol (Tenormin) (Fig. 16.8) is a hydrophilic selective β_1-blocker and is incompletely absorbed after oral administration.[119] The oral bioavailability is about 50%, and the peak plasma levels are attained in 2-4 hours.[119] Atenolol is not significantly bound to plasma proteins (3%-5%).[120] While the majority of β-blockers undergo metabolism, atenolol is not significantly metabolized.[121] Only 5%-10% of the drug is metabolized in the liver.[119] About 50% of the orally administered drug is eliminated unchanged by the kidneys and remaining in feces.[121] After IV administration, about 85% of atenolol is eliminated unchanged in the urine.[122] The elimination half-life is about 6-9 hours and is increased in patients with renal impairment.[119]

Metoprolol Tartrate and Succinate. Metoprolol (Fig. 16.8) is a moderately lipophilic (Log P = 1.72; cLog P = 1.48)[104] selective β_1-blocker. Chemically, it is a phenyloxypropanolamine containing methyloxyethyl substitution (ether moiety) at the *para* position (Fig. 16.8). It is sold as the tartrate and succinate dicarboxylate salt forms. Metoprolol tartrate (Lopressor) is an immediate-release and a short-acting formulation dosed twice daily.[123] Metoprolol succinate (Metoprolol Succinate ER, Toprol XL) (Fig. 16.8) is an extended-release formulation that provides consistent β-blocking properties for over 24 hours allowing once-daily administration.[124] Metoprolol succinate was shown to reduce the relative risk of mortality and provides substantial morbidity benefits in patients with heart failure.[124] Orally administered metoprolol is well absorbed in the intestine, but the bioavailability is only about 50% because it undergoes extensive first-pass hepatic metabolism.[125] The bioavailability may be enhanced when taken with food and during chronic administration.[125] In patients with hepatic cirrhosis because of decreased first-pass metabolism, bioavailability may be increased.[125] Approximately 15% of metoprolol is bound to plasma proteins.[126] Metoprolol is metabolized via hydroxylation to α-hydroxymetoprolol and O-dealkylation to yield a primary alcohol, which is further oxidized to the carboxylic acid metabolite.[127,128] Metoprolol is predominantly metabolized by CYP2D6 and exhibits genetic polymorphism.[129] The elimination half-life of metoprolol in extensive and poor CYP2D6 metabolizers is about 3.1 and 7.2 hours, respectively.[130] The peak plasma concentrations of metoprolol is about 3-fold higher in poor CYP2D6 metabolizers than extensive metabolizers.[130] Consequently, poor CYP2D6 individuals may be associated with a greater risk of metoprolol adverse effects.[131] It is predominantly excreted as metabolites in the urine.[125] In patients with impaired renal function, metabolites may accumulate in the body for a longer time.[125]

Bisoprolol. Bisoprolol (Zebeta) is a moderately lipophilic (Log P = 1.94; cLog P = 1.79)[104] selective β_1-blocker containing an ether substitution (Fig. 16.8). It is sold as the fumarate salt. It exhibits relatively small inter- and intraindividual variability with predictable pharmacokinetics.[132] The orally administered bisoprolol is well absorbed, and the bioavailability is about 90%.[132] About 30% of the drug is protein bound. It undergoes moderate first-pass metabolism and is primarily metabolized by CYP3A4 and CYP2D6 to inactive metabolites.[132,133] The plasma half-life is relatively long (about 10-11 hr) allowing for once-daily dosing.[132] Bisoprolol is eliminated renally and hepatically in similar proportions.[132]

Carvedilol. Carvedilol (Coreg) is a weakly basic (pK_a = 7.8) lipophilic (Log P = 2.68; cLog P = 3.28)[104] blocker antagonizing α_1-, β_1-, and β_2-receptors (Fig. 16.7).[134,135] Carvedilol prevents reflex tachycardia by acting as a potent competitive antagonist at β_1- and β_2-receptors.[136] Carvedilol vasodilatory properties are due to α_1-adrenoceptor blockade.[136] At high concentrations, carvedilol acts as a calcium channel antagonist and in cutaneous circulation it increases blood flow.[136] It contains one chiral center but sold as a racemic mixture consisting of *S*(−)-enantiomer and *R*(+)-enantiomer.[137,138] Carvedilol contains a unique tricyclic heterocyclic ring system known as carbazole. Carbazole contains a central five-membered heteroaromatic ring system, which is in turn fused to two phenyl rings on the either side. The β-blocking properties of carvedilol are about 10 times more potent than the α-blocking properties.[137] The *S*(−)-enantiomer is almost exclusively responsible for its β-blocking properties; whereas, both *S*(−)- and *R*(+)-enantiomers equally block α_1-receptors.[137]

After oral administration carvedilol is rapidly absorbed and undergoes extensive hepatic first-pass metabolism.[137] The absolute oral bioavailability is about 25%.[139] The peak plasma concentration is achieved in about 1-2 hours.[137,139] The absorption is delayed when taken with food.[137] It undergoes extensive protein binding (>98%) and primarily bound to albumin.[134] The volume of distribution is about 115L.[134] Carvedilol undergoes both phase-I and phase-II metabolic reactions.[139] Carvedilol phase-I reactions involve aromatic ring hydroxylation and side chain cleavage.[139] The hydroxylated and demethylated carvedilol also have activity.[134] Specifically, the 4′-hydroxyphenyl metabolite of carvedilol is a more potent β-blocker, by about 13-fold, than carvedilol.[134] Phase-II reaction occurs predominantly by glucuronidation.[139] Carvedilol display stereoselective drug disposition.[138] In poor CYP2D6 metabolizers the plasma concentrations of *R*-carvedilol is significantly greater than extensive metabolizers.[138] However, the plasma concentrations of *S*-carvedilol is similar in both poor and extensive metabolizers. Therefore, poor CYP2D6 metabolizers may have significant α-blockade.[138] Other CYP enzymes that are involved in the metabolism of carvedilol include CYP2C9, CYP1A2, and CYP3A4.[140] The majority of carvedilol is eliminated as metabolites. About 60% is eliminated in feces.[139] Only 2% of the intact drug and 16% as metabolites are eliminated in the urine.[141]

DRUG INTERACTIONS. The drug interactions associated with β-blockers are pharmacodynamic or pharmacokinetic interactions.[142] Pharmacodynamic interactions are attributed to the mechanism of action of administered drugs, while pharmacokinetic interactions are attributed to alterations of drug metabolizing enzymes such as CYP enzymes and transporters such as MDR1 (P-glycoprotein).[142]

Diphenhydramine, a first-generation antihistamine, inhibits CYP2D6 metabolism of metoprolol in extensive metabolizers.[143] This will potentiate the adverse effects of metoprolol such as prolonged negative chronotropic and inotropic effects.[143] Therefore, CYP2D6 inhibitors (e.g., quinidine, paroxetine, fluoxetine) may increase the plasma concentrations of CYP2D6 β-blocker substrates.[144,145] Carvedilol is a potent inhibitor of P-glycoprotein and increases plasma digoxin levels.[89,146] Bisoprolol also significantly inhibits P-glycoprotein, whereas, atenolol, metoprolol, and sotalol are not P-glycoprotein inhibitors.[89,147] Carvedilol is also a P-glycoprotein substrate and coadministration with rifampin leads to significantly decreased carvedilol serum concentrations.[148]

ADVERSE EFFECTS. The side effects associated with β-blockers include atrioventricular blockade, bradycardia, hypotension, gastrointestinal disturbances, and pruritic rash.[149] Pulmonary side effects such as bronchitis and bronchospasm are associated with all β-blockers. However, cardiovascular selectivity may be achieved with small doses of selective β_1-blockers.[149] Nonselective β-blockers are contraindicated in patients with a history of reactive airway disease, e.g., asthma. Lipophilic β-blockers have a greater ability to cause CNS disturbances such as insomnia, dreams, hallucinations, and depression.[149] Some of the β-blockers may cause a rare oculomucocutaneous reaction.[149] β_2-adrenergic receptors play a significant role in insulin release and gluconeogenesis. Nonselective β-blockers are also contraindicated in patients with insulin-dependent (type 1) diabetes. Nonselective β-blockers can slow down the recovery of insulin-induced hypoglycemia and block/mask most of these signs of hypoglycemia with the exception of sweating. Patients should also avoid sudden discontinuation of β-blockers because of the risk for hypertensive crises caused by the receptor upregulation.

Chemistry of Ranolazine

Ranolazine is a newer antianginal agent that was approved by the United States FDA in 2006.[150] Chemically it is N-(2,6-dimethylphenyl)-2-(4-(2-hydroxy-3-(2-methoxyphenoxy)propyl)piperazin-1-yl)acetamide.[150] It contains a chiral center but is synthesized and sold as a racemic mixture.[151] Ranolazine immediate-release capsule and oral solution have a short elimination half-life, which had subsequently led to the development of an extended-release formulation which allows for twice-daily dosing.[151]

PHARMACOKINETICS. Ranolazine has an absolute oral bioavailability of 35%-50%. The amount and extent of ranolazine absorption from an extended-release formulation is not significantly affected by food.[151] Approximately 60% of the drug is protein bound.[151] Ranolazine is extensively metabolized in the liver by CYP3A4 and is a minor substrate for CYP2D6.[151] Ranolazine undergoes methyl hydroxylation on one end of the aromatic ring and both the aromatic rings are metabolized by hydroxylation.[152] The amide group attached to the aromatic ring undergoes amide hydrolysis to yield a piperazine carboxylic acid metabolite and 2,6-dimethyl aniline.[152] It undergoes N-dealkylation metabolic reactions at the either side of the piperazine ring system.[152] It is metabolized by O-dearylation and O-demethylation at the methoxy phenoxy end. Nitrogens on the piperazine ring can directly undergo N-oxidation.[152] Ranolazine also directly undergoes glucuronidation and several of its metabolites are further metabolized by glucuronidation and sulfation.[152,153] The half-life elimination of immediate- and extended-release ranolazine is about 2 and 7 hours, respectively.[151] Approximately 75% of ranolazine and its metabolites are excreted in the urine and less than 5% of the intact drug is excreted unchanged.[151] The plasma concentration of ranolazine is increased in patients with renal impairment.[151] Heart failure and diabetes mellitus does not significantly alter pharmacokinetic parameters of ranolazine.[151] Ranolazine peak plasma concentration is increased in patients with cirrhosis. Therefore, ranolazine is contraindicated in liver cirrhotic patients.

DRUG-DRUG INTERACTIONS. Ranolazine is a weak CYP3A4 inhibitor and increases simvastatin plasma concentrations by about 2-fold.[151] Ranolazine is a P-glycoprotein inhibitor and increases plasma digoxin concentrations.[151] Concurrent administration of other CYP3A4 inhibitors such as ketoconazole increases ranolazine concentration by about 4-fold, and verapamil increases ranolazine concentration by about 2-fold.[151] Since ranolazine is only a minor substrate for CYP2D6, concurrent administration of other drugs which are CYP2D6 inhibitors have a minor effect on ranolazine plasma concentrations.[151]

ADVERSE EFFECTS. The most common adverse effects associated with ranolazine include nausea, dizziness, headache, and constipation.[154] Ranolazine prolongs the QT interval and may potentially contribute to torsade de pointes, a unique form of polymorphic ventricular tachycardia.[155]

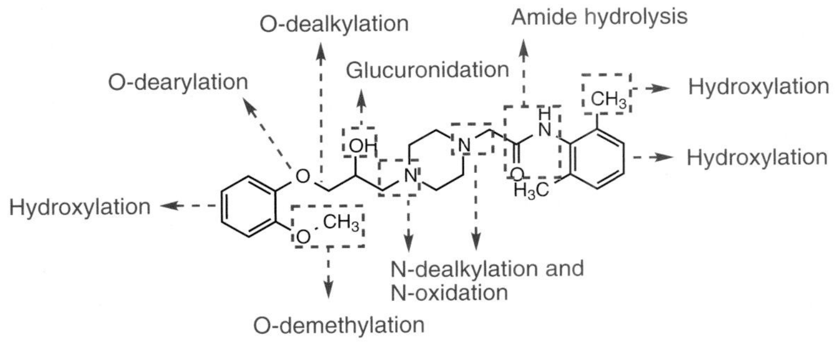

Chemistry of Ivabradine

Scientists at the Servier Research Institute screened various compounds to reduce the heart rate.[156] In that screen, they identified two potent classes of molecules benzocyclobutane and indane derivatives.[156] However, indane derivatives prolong the action potential duration.[156] Ivabradine is an optically pure S-isomer of a benzocyclobutane analog (Fig. 16.9).[156]

PHARMACOKINETICS. Ivabradine is completely absorbed, but the absolute oral bioavailability is about 40% due to extensive intestinal and hepatic first-pass metabolism by CYP3A4.[157] The peak plasma levels are achieved in about 1 hour after the oral administration under fasting conditions.[157] Even though food delays the absorption of ivabradine, it enhances the plasma level by about 20%-40%.[157] Ivabradine is about 70% bound to plasm proteins. Ivabradine undergoes N-demethylation by CYP3A4 to form desmethyl ivabradine, which may further be metabolized (Fig. 16.9).[157] Both ivabradine and desmethyl metabolite have equal potency.[157] The half-life elimination of ivabradine is about 6 hours. Ivabradine is excreted in feces and urine.[157]

DRUG-DRUG INTERACTIONS. Since ivabradine is metabolized by CYP3A4, drug-drug interactions may occur with CYP3A4 inhibitors and inducers.[158] Carbamazepine which is an anticonvulsant drug and a CYP3A4 inducer increases the first-pass metabolism of ivabradine and decreases plasma concentrations and AUC by about 5-fold.[159] Phenytoin used in the treatment of epilepsy is a potent CYP3A4 inducer, which significantly decreases the plasma concentrations and bioavailability of ivabradine.[158] Therefore, coadministration of ivabradine with CYP3A4 inducers may lead to reduced biological response. Potent CYP3A4 inhibitors such as itraconazole and clarithromycin may increase the plasma concentrations of ivabradine leading to increased toxic side effects.[157]

TOXIC EFFECTS. Even though toxic effects are extremely rare, ivabradine has the potential to cause sinus bradycardia. Ivabradine should be avoided in patients with sick sinus syndrome because it acts on the sinus node.[160]

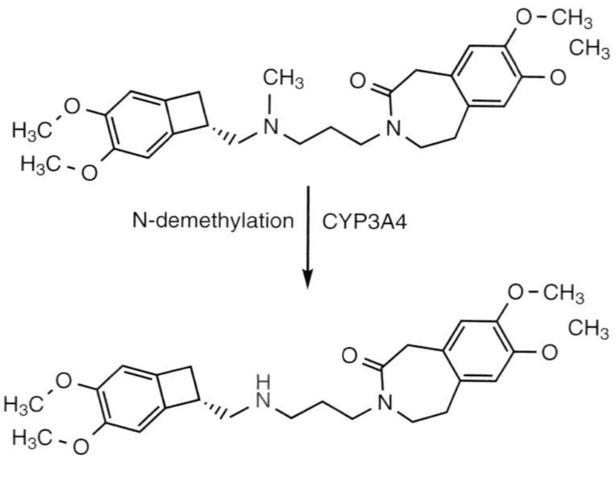

Figure 16.9 Metabolism of ivabradine.

Ivabradine can prolong the QT interval, but by itself may not cause torsades.[160] However, ivabradine should not be coadministered with other agents that can cause the QT prolongation and/or agents that lower the heart rate.[160] Ivabradine binds to the I(h) channels in the eye, and at high doses, it leads to changes in the electroretinogram.[160] In about 15% patients, it resulted in mild to moderate visual disturbances.[160]

DRUGS FOR THE TREATMENT OF HEART FAILURE

Heart Failure

According to the American Heart Association (AHA), chronic heart failure (CHF) affects over five million Americans and more than 800,000 new cases are diagnosed each year.[161] CHF is a debilitating disease with a high rate of morbidity and mortality. The five-year prognosis for patients with CHF is either a heart transplant or mortality of 50%. CHF is a complex disease that involves several neuronal and humoral pathways. It is characterized by the body's inability to maintain its normal metabolic needs, which is caused by the functional or structural loss of viable myocardial cells. This can occur over a long (chronic) or short (acute) period. There are several comorbidities that cause CHF, but the most common causes are ischemic heart disease, hypertension, myocardial infarction, and diabetes. Heart failure is classified by the New York Heart Association (NYHA) into four classes: I, II, III, and IV. Patients in class I are the least severe and do not present any limitations or symptoms. Classes II and III are described as patients who are comfortable at rest but demonstrate symptoms at different degrees of physical activity. In contrast, patients in class IV are the most severe with symptoms at rest and are unable to carry out any physical activities without symptoms. In addition to the NYHA, the American College of Cardiology (ACC) and the AHA have developed a system that focuses on the progression of the disease. In this system, patients are classified by stages A through D. Stage A being patients with high risk for developing heart failure. Stage B is associated with patients with structural damage but do not demonstrate symptoms. Stage C patients have had or are currently showing structural heart disease and have symptoms. Patients in stage D have end-stage heart disease and require aggressive therapy.

From a physiological standpoint, heart failure can be divided into left ventricle heart failure or right ventricle heart failure. It can also be further divided into diastolic heart failure (the heart cannot relax and fill the ventricle properly) or systolic heart failure (cannot contract and eject blood properly). The major purpose of the circulation is to move blood forward and perfuse organs and tissues. However, if the heart cannot relax or contract properly, blood starts to accumulate in the ventricles and/or move backward. This movement of blood backward will lead to accumulation of fluids and edema. Right ventricle failure typically leads to peripheral edema as observed by swelling of the ankles. Left ventricle failure produces accumulation of fluid in the lungs. As a result of fluid overload, patients will present with signs and symptoms that are usually characterized by shortness of breath, increased fatigue, edema, nausea, lack of appetite, and arrhythmias.[162]

Under normal physiological tone, the cardiac output (4-8 L/min) is defined as the product of heart rate times stroke volume. Stroke volume is directly affected by three factors: myocyte contractile force, preload (left ventricle end-diastolic pressure), and afterload (systolic pressure). The relationship between the stroke volume and left ventricle filling pressure (LVFP) is represented by the Frank-Starling curve (FS) (Fig. 16.10).[163] Under normal physiological conditions, the stroke volume is directly proportional to LVFP and/or myocardium contractile force. As a result, the stroke volume increases as the LVFP increases and/or myocardium contractile force. In contrast, the stroke volume is indirectly proportional to afterload. Stroke volume decreases as systemic vascular resistance increases because it requires greater workload for the heart to compensate for this increase in arterial pressure.[164] The FS curve relationship can be subdivided into four quadrants. The FS curve in healthy individuals is typically in quadrant I with enough room for compensation. If the preload is further increased, the LVFP would exceed the normal range (10-15 mm Hg), and the stroke volume would plateau and extend into quadrant II. In this case, patients would become congested and show symptoms of edema. If contractile force is markedly reduced or the afterload is too high, patients may fall under quadrant III. This would lead to poor organ perfusion and possible organ damage. Patients who fall into quadrant IV are decompensated and would demonstrate symptoms of both poor organ perfusion and congestion. This FS curve reflects severe, stage IV CHF. In these patients, the FS curve plateaus much faster at a lower volume. Drugs used in the treatment of CHF are designed to modify preload, afterload, and contractility as a therapeutic approach to increase stroke volume, decrease edema, and perfuse organs.[165]

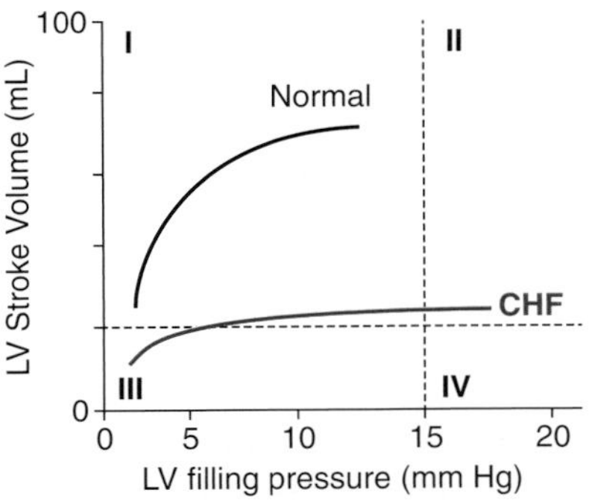

Figure 16.10 Frank-Starling curve.

Mechanism of Action of Drugs Used to Treat Heart Failure

Glyosidic Positive Inotropic Agents

Digoxin and digitoxin are potent and selective antagonists at the $3Na^+/2K^+$-ATPase pump.[166] The Na^+/K^+-ATPase is one of the major pumps involved in the reestablishment of ion homeostasis in the myocyte.[167] Digoxin binds to the Na^+/K^+-ATPase pump and blocks its ability to efficiently move Na^+ out and K^+ into the cell leading to an increase in intracellular Na^+ concentrations. This in turn causes the reversal of the Na^+/Ca^{2+} exchanger leading to an increase in intracellular Ca^{2+} levels, which contributes to an increase in contractile force and consequently stroke volume. Digoxin has not been shown to decrease mortality, but it improves the quality of life.[168]

Nonglycosidic Positive Inotropic Agents

PHOSPHODIESTERASE INHIBITORS. Phosphodiesterases (PDEs) are a group of intracellular enzymes that catalyze the breakdown of cyclic adenosine monophosphate (cAMP) and cyclic guanosine monophosphate (cGMP) and are distributed ubiquitously throughout the human body.[169,170] Eleven different isoenzymes (PDE 1-11) have been identified.[170] The PDE3 isoenzyme is mainly responsible for cleaving cAMP to AMP.[171] Inhibition of PDE3 leads to a decreased degradation and increased intracellular cAMP and thereby increases the myocardium contraction.[171] Therefore, PDE3 inhibitors are therapeutically used for the short-term treatment of CHF.[169] PDE4 inhibitors are being investigated for their use in inflammatory airway diseases.[169] PDE5 inhibitors such as sildenafil citrate are used in the treatment of erectile dysfunction.[169]

Milrinone is a PDE3 antagonist with lower affinity for other PDE isoenzyme subtypes. Its major sites of action are the heart and vasculature. By blocking the PDE3 in the heart, milrinone increases intracellular levels of cAMP and Ca^{2+}-mediated increase in inotropic contractile force.[172] Although the benefit of increased contractile force appears to be useful in the short-term, milrinone increases the workload of the heart and the risk for arrhythmias in the long term, which may increase mortality. In addition to its effects in the heart, milrinone also increases the levels of cAMP in the vasculature. Increase of cAMP in the arteries and veins leads to a reduction in afterload and preload, respectively. These two effects are believed to be beneficial since it decreases the myocardium oxygen demand. This class of drugs can be used for the short-term support of critically ill chronic heart failure patients.[173] However, patients who have ischemia appear to present with prolonged hospitalization and have an increase in mortality compared to nonischemic patients.[174]

DOPAMINE AND DOBUTAMINE. Both dopamine and dobutamine increase myocardium contractile force by activating β_1-adrenergic receptors.[175,176] These receptors are coupled to Gs G-protein, which leads to increased levels of cAMP and consequently Ca^{2+} ions. Dobutamine not only increases the force of contraction (inotropic), but also the speed of contraction (chronotropic). At low to moderate therapeutic doses, the effects on the heart are predominant with the effects on β_2 (vasodilator) offsetting the effects of the α_1-receptors(vasoconstriction). At higher infusion doses, dobutamine's effect on the α_1-receptors starts to predominate over its β_2 effect, which leads to an increase in blood pressure. The chronotropic effects also become more predominant and increase the risk for arrhythmias and angina pectoris. In contrast to dobutamine, dopamine at lower doses has higher affinity for the D_1- and D_2 dopamine receptors.[177] Activation of D_1 evokes primarily renal and mesenteric vasodilation via an increase in cAMP. The effects on the renal vasculature may increase the glomerular filtration rate (GFR) and benefit certain patients. At moderate doses, dopamine begins to bind and activate β_1-adrenergic receptors in the heart and produce an increase in the contractile force and heart rate. This effect is in addition to its renal effects. At higher doses, it becomes less selective and begins to bind and activate α_1-adrenergic receptors, which causes an increase in systemic vascular resistance. The increase in blood pressure will increase afterload and oxygen demand.

Nitrate Vasodilators

Refer to the antianginal agents section for the mechanism of action of organic nitrates.

ISOSORBIDE DINITRATE IN COMBINATION WITH HYDRALAZINE. The specific mechanism of action by which hydralazine produces its effect is not clear. However, it has been established that hydralazine is a potent vasodilator of arterial smooth muscle and decreases the afterload.[178] It is not usually used as monotherapy because of the compensatory effects it can evoke, including baroreflex-mediated tachycardia and water retention. In heart failure, hydralazine is used in combination with isosorbide dinitrate (BiDil) resulting in a better outcomes than with either drug alone.[179] This is due to the fact that hydralazine decreases the workload of the heart by decreasing afterload, while low doses of nitrates favor vasodilation of the venous system, thus decreasing preload. As a result, the stroke volume is improved. BiDil has also been shown to be more beneficial to African Americans who are resistant to angiotensin-converting enzyme (ACE) inhibitors.[179] Depending on the patients genetics, sex, dose, and race, there is a risk for the development of drug-induced lupus syndrome and other autoimmune reactions.[180]

Other Vasodilators

The three β-blockers approved by the FDA for the treatment of CHF include metoprolol succinate, bisoprolol, and carvedilol. All three have been shown to decrease mortality and morbidity. At therapeutic doses, bisoprolol and metoprolol are selective to the β_1-adrenergic receptors. In contrast, carvedilol is a nonselective β_1-, β_2-, and α_1-adrenergic receptor antagonist. Patients who are starting on these drugs should begin with the lowest doses and titrate their way up. Initial therapy with β-blockers in heart failure patients causes a major decrease in cardiac output. However, by blocking the β_1-adrenergic receptor in the heart over the long term, patients not only improve their ejection fraction, but also decrease mortality.

In addition to β-blockers, drugs affecting the renin-angiotensin-aldosterone system have also been shown to be beneficial in heart failure patients. Both ACE inhibitors and angiotensin receptor blockers (ARB) decrease preload and afterload. ACE inhibitors block the conversion of angiotensin I into angiotensin II and, consequently, decrease the activation of angiotensin type I receptor (AT1) by angiotensin II.[181] In addition, ACE inhibitors also decrease the breakdown of bradykinin. The increase in bradykinin plasma levels has been associated with the vasodilatory properties of ACE inhibitors. It is also accepted that by blocking the conversion of angiotensin I into angiotensin II, ACE inhibitors redirect the pathway and increase the production of angiotensin 1-7, which has been proposed to oppose the effects of angiotensin II. In contrast to ACE inhibitors, ARBs have a high affinity for the angiotensin AT1 receptor. Both ACE inhibitors and ARBs decrease cardiovascular remodeling and mortality. The specific drugs in these two classes, detailed mechanism of action, and side effects are further discussed in Chapter 17. However, both ACE inhibitors and ARBs cause similar side effects, including hypotension, hyperkalemia, increase in serum creatinine, and potential fetus damage.

Diuretics, in particular loop diuretics, have also been shown to decrease volume overload in CHF patients. Furosemide is the prototypical drug, and it decreases preload by blocking the $Na^+/K^+/2Cl^-$ transporter in the ascending loop of Henle. Although these drugs do not decrease mortality, they can decrease the symptoms associated with hypervolemia and decrease edema. Providers should be careful using these drugs since they may cause electrolyte imbalance and dehydration (refer to Chapter 17).

Neprilysin Inhibitor/ARB: Sacubitril/Valsartan (Entresto)

This is the first drug of its kind in this combination.[182] Valsartan is an ARB that acts primarily by blocking the activation of AT1 receptors. Valsartan is approved as part of CHF therapy by the FDA for patients who cannot tolerate ACE inhibitors. Sacubitril is rapidly metabolized to sacubitrilat, a neprilysin endopeptidase (NEP) antagonist. NEP is involved in the breakdown of atrium natriuretic peptide (ANP), which belongs to a family of peptides that are released by the atria in response to an increase in preload and consequently atrial pressure via stretch-sensitive ion channels.[183] Once in the circulation, this peptide has natriuretic, diuretic, and vasodilatory properties. However, it has a short half-life and is readily metabolized in the liver, lung, and kidneys by the NEP enzyme. By blocking the NEP enzyme, sacubitril prolongs the half-life of ANP and increases its circulating plasma levels. When combined with valsartan, it further decreases preload and afterload in the heart failure patients.

Chemistry of the Cardiac Glycosides

In ancient times, cardiac glycosides were applied to arrows and were used as poisons in human warfare.[184] In 1785, William Withering, a physician and botanist, described the medical uses of the foxglove plant (*Digitalis purpurea*) in "*An account of the foxglove, and some of its medical uses: with practical remarks on dropsy, and other diseases*."[185] Reports indicate that even though the foxglove plant was used for many centuries for various purposes, it was Withering who paved the way for the standard use of cardiac glycosides in modern practice.[186] Sydney Smith, in 1930, isolated the active ingredient digoxin from *Digitalis lanata*.[187] Cardiac glycosides are composed of carbohydrates and steroids. The steroid portion is commonly referred to as aglycone or genin and the carbohydrate portion as glycone.[188] The carbohydrate units are linked to one another as well as to the steroid template by glycosidic bonds.

AGLYCONES. The steroid template contains fused A, B, C, and D rings which in turn are fused to an unsaturated lactone ring at C-17 in a β configuration.[184] Cardiac glycosides can be classified into cardenolides and bufadienolides based on the aglycone portion.[184] Cardenolides contain a five-membered α, β unsaturated lactone (butyrolactone), and the steroid template (including the lactone ring) is composed of 23 carbon atoms.[189] In contrast, bufadienolides contain a six-membered unsaturated lactone (α-pyrone) ring, and the steroid template (including the lactone ring) is composed of 24 carbon atoms.[189] The cardiac glycosides commonly occur in plants, and the sources of important cardiac glycosides include the leaves of *Digitalis purpurea* and *Digitalis lanata* and the seeds of *Stropanthus kombe* and *Stropanthus gratus*.[189] The major aglycones in *Digitalis* species include digitoxigenin, gitoxigenin, digoxigenin, and gitaligenin; whereas, *Stropanthus* species include stropanthidin and ouabagenin (Fig. 16.11).[189] The therapeutically used cardiac glycoside preparations are primarily obtained from the *Digitalis* species. In nature, some animals also contain cardiac glycosides, such as the venom glands in the skin of toads contain bufadienolides.[189]

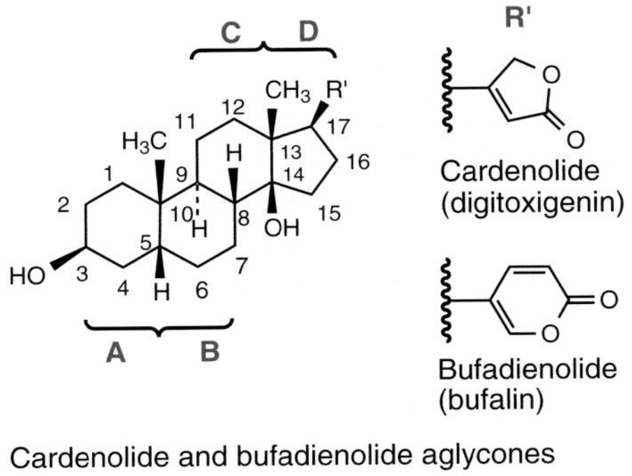

Cardenolide and bufadienolide aglycones

GLYCONES. The sugar portion of the cardiac glycoside contains one or more units typically attached at the 3-position of the steroid. The commonly occurring sugars in

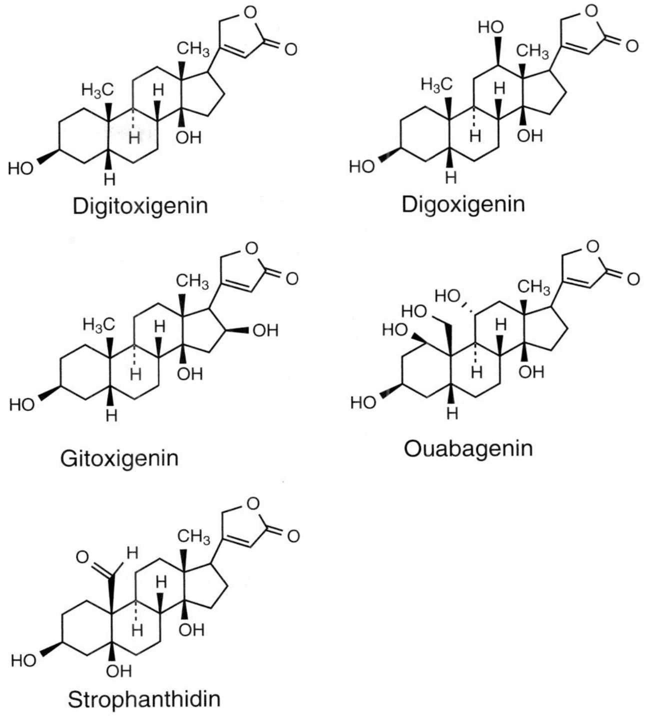

Figure 16.11 Cardenolide aglycones.

Digitalis species include glucose, 3-acteyl digitoxose, and/or digitoxose; whereas, *Stropanthus* species include glucose, cymarose, and/or rhamnose (Fig. 16.12). The presence of side chains such as the 3-acetyl groups affects the physicochemical and pharmacokinetic properties of molecules. The sugars are predominantly linked to one another by the β (1 → 4) glycosidic bonds.

The two commonly used cardiac glycoside preparations include digoxin and digitoxin. In the United States, digoxin is the only approved cardia glycoside for therapeutic use. Digoxin contains the aglycone digoxigenin and three units of digitoxose sugars; whereas, digitoxin contains the aglycone digitoxigenin and three units of digitoxose sugars.[189] In digoxigenin, digitoxigenin, and stropanthidin-based cardenolides, rings A-B, B-C, and C-D have *cis*, *trans*, and *cis* configurations, respectively (Fig. 16.11). Because of this specific fusion of rings, the steroid template acquires a characteristic bent shape, as opposed to a flat shape.[184]

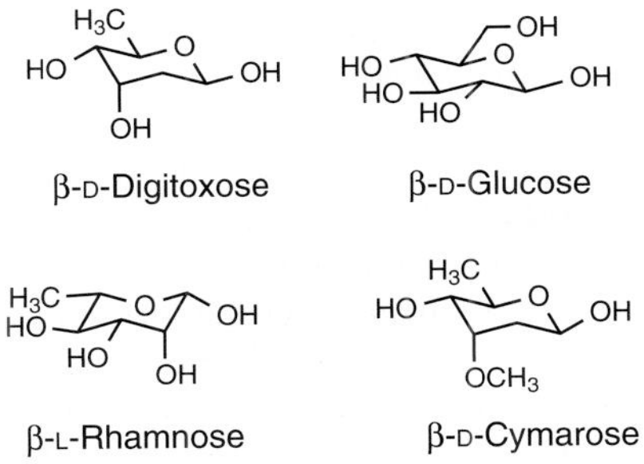

Figure 16.12 Selected sugars found in naturally occurring cardiac glycosides.

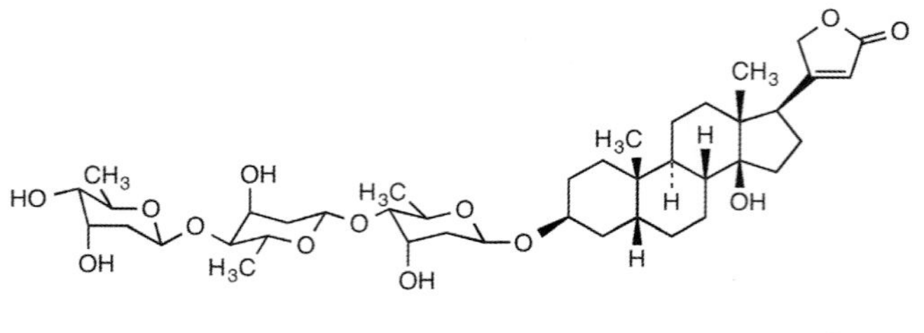

Digitoxin

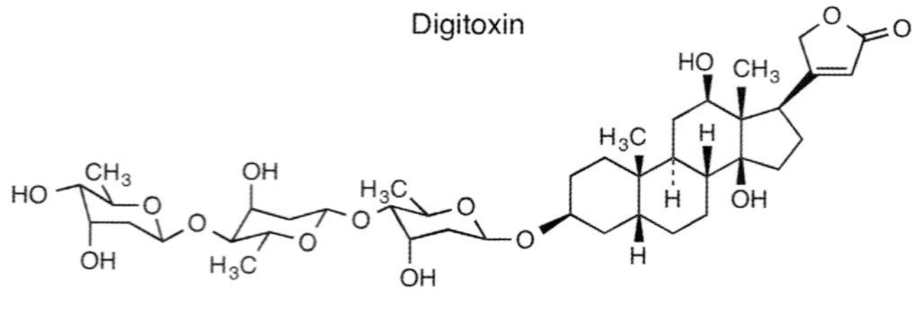

Digoxin

STRUCTURAL REQUIREMENTS FOR CARDIOTONIC ACTIVITY. The Na^+/K^+-ATPase contains both α and β subunits; the α subunit exists in α_1, α_2, α_3, and α_4 isoforms, and the β subunit exists in β_1, β_2, and β_3 isoforms.[190] The α_2 isoform is primarily present in skeletal, smooth, and cardiac muscle and is believed to be an important target of the cardiac glycosides.[191]

IMPORTANCE OF SUGARS. The number of sugars attached to the steroid template appears to play a key role in its cardiotonic properties.[191,192] Tridigitoxosyl digoxigenin (digoxin) is more active than didigitoxosyl digoxigenin, which in turn is more active than monodigitoxosyl digoxigenin. On the contrary, tetradigitoxosyl digoxigenin is less active than digoxin (tridigitoxosyl digoxigenin). This indicates that three sugars in digoxin are optimal for the cardiotonic activity, and the hydrophilic pocket present in the enzyme can accommodate three sugars, but four sugars are detrimental for the inhibitory activity.[166] Although the sugar portion of the glycoside is not absolutely essential, it is required for optimal cardiotonic activity.[191,192] Digoxigenin (only the steroid component of digoxin) has some cardiotonic properties, but its activity is significantly lower than monodigitoxosyl digoxigenin.[191,192]

IMPORTANCE OF THE STEROID NUCLEUS. The specific fusion of the steroid rings seems to be very critical for the activity. For example, digitoxigenin, which has an A-B cis configuration, has 35 times higher binding affinity than Uzarigenin, which has an A-B *trans* configuration.[192] Introduction of polar head groups on the steroid template such as the hydroxyl group may reduce the activity.[192] For example, 16-hydroxy digitoxin (gitoxin) has about a 7-fold lower binding affinity than digitoxin.[192] Further, it was recently shown that digoxin's steroid concave surface (α-surface) interacts with the hydrophobic surface by nonpolar interactions.[166] Digoxin and digitoxin are both potent molecules. Digoxin has a hydroxy group at the 12-position on the steroid nucleus making it slightly more hydrophilic than digitoxin, which is also one of the primary reasons for their pharmacokinetic differences.

IMPORTANCE OF THE LACTONE. The unsaturated lactone ring is optimal for activity. If the carbon-carbon double bond is reduced in the lactone ring, the biding affinity is tremendously diminished.[192] The lactone ring fits into the hydrophobic pocket which most likely leads to the cationic-binding site occupied by Mg^{2+} or K^+.[166] The lack of the lactone ring may lead to compounds with some cardiotonic properties. For example, investigations of synthetic compounds in which the C-17 β lactone ring has been replaced with basic moieties such as guanylhydrazone and O-aminoalkyloximes androstane diol derivatives led to compounds with Na^+/K^+-ATPase inhibitory activity.[193,194] Overall, the cardiotonic properties of the cardiac glycosides are affected by the degree/type of glycosylation, the type of substituents/configuration of the steroid rings, and the size and degree of unsaturation of the lactone ring.[166]

Pharmacokinetics of Drugs Used to Treat Cardiac Heart Failure

About 70%-80% of the orally administered digoxin is primarily absorbed in the small intestine.[195] Digoxin absorption is dependent on the type of oral formulation. Approximately 70% is absorbed when given in the form of tablets and 80% absorbed in the form of elixir.[196] The discontinued Lanoxicaps capsules of digoxin have an oral bioavailability up to 100%.[197] Digoxin reaches a steady state concentration in about 5-7 days.[198] It has a high volume of distribution (7 L/kg)[195] and is highly bound to skeletal muscles, heart, and kidneys.[195] Only about 20%-30% of digoxin is bound to serum albumin.[195] Digoxin is similarly distributed in healthy individuals and obese individuals, when the ideal body weight (IBW) that is represented by the lean body mass is considered in obese individuals.[199] Therefore, in obese individuals digoxin dosages are calculated based on the IBW rather than the total body weight, which includes the adipose tissue.[199] From the structural perspective, since the sugar portion of the digoxin contributes to its hydrophilic nature, it is not well distributed into lipophilic adipose tissue.[200] The volume of distribution is decreased in patients with impaired renal function, requiring dose reduction.[201] The apparent volume of distribution in infants is higher than in adults.[202] Digoxin when administered to pregnant women rapidly crosses the placental barrier and is equally distributed in maternal and fetal blood.[203]

Digoxin is primarily eliminated by the kidneys (about 70%), predominantly as unchanged drug. Approximately 25%-30% of digoxin is eliminated by the hepatic and biliary routes, but the enterohepatic circulation is of less significance.[195,196] In the body, digoxin is hydrolyzed to digoxigenin bisdigitoxoside, digoxigenin monodigitoxoside, and digoxigenin. In about 10% of the patient population, the lactone ring on the digoxin is reduced by gastrointestinal bacteria to dihydrodigoxin, a cardio inactive metabolite.[204] Further, administration of antibiotics such as tetracycline or erythromycin to these individuals leads to an increased serum digoxin concentration, which indicates that any alteration of the gut flora may affect the absorption of digitalis.[204] The half-life elimination of digoxin in healthy volunteers is approximately 40 hours.[195] The major route of elimination is by glomerular filtration and to a lesser extent by tubular secretion and tubular reabsorption.[195] P-glycoprotein is involved in tubular secretion of digoxin.[205] In elderly patients, digoxin has a longer half-life and increased blood concentration, which can be attributed to reduced body size and decreased urinary elimination.[206] Thus, the dosage of digoxin needs to be appropriately adjusted. It was observed that in patients with hypothyroidism, serum digoxin concentrations were at higher levels and in hyperthyroidism patients' digoxin serum concentrations were at lower levels, which correlated with changes in the GFR and digoxin serum half-life.[207] Patients with hyperthyroidism also have higher digoxin clearances.[208]

Digitoxin has a long plasma half-life ranging from 5 to 7 days and requires 35 days to attain a plateau.[198] Digitoxin is less dependent on renal function than digoxin and about 50% of digitoxin is eliminated renally.[198,209] Digitoxin is metabolized by hydrolysis to digitoxigenin bisdigitoxoside, digitoxigenin monodigitoxoside, and digitoxigenin.[210,211] Digitoxin minimally undergoes hydroxylation at C-12 of the aglycone to form digoxin.[210]

Toxicity

Digoxin and other cardiac glycosides have a narrow therapeutic window and within this window they are therapeutically effective.[212] Therefore, even slight variations in digoxin's blood concentrations may lead to either toxic concentrations or subtherapeutic concentrations.[212] Increased digoxin serum levels >2 ng/mL is commonly associated with its toxicity.[213] Therefore, patients need to be carefully monitored for acute and chronic toxicity.[214] Digoxin toxicity includes gastrointestinal disturbances such as nausea, vomiting, anorexia, abdominal pain, and diarrhea; neuropsychiatric symptoms such as headache, delirium, hallucinations, convulsions, and drowsiness; yellow or green vision disturbances; and cardiac disorders such as dysrhythmias and ventricular tachycardia.[214,215] Digoxin binding to Na^+/K^+-ATPase is inhibited by high levels of potassium. Therefore, hyperkalemia decreases digoxin activity and hypokalemia increases its toxicity.[216]

Drug Interactions

Several drugs alter digoxin absorption, distribution, and elimination.[217] Digoxin is a well-known substrate for intestinal and renal P-glycoprotein.[218] Since P-glycoprotein is a multidrug efflux transporter, medications that are P-glycoprotein inhibitors can reduce efflux of digoxin in the intestine and/or decrease the elimination of digoxin by the kidneys leading to increased plasma digoxin levels causing digoxin toxicity.[218,219] In contrast, P-glycoprotein inducers decrease plasma digoxin levels by an opposing mechanism and as a result digoxin may not reach therapeutic levels.[218,219] In vitro studies show that quinidine is a substrate for P-glycoprotein and a strong inhibitor of digoxin efflux transport.[220] Coadministration of quinidine with digoxin increases digoxin's rate and extent of absorption, resulting in a 2-fold rise in its serum concentration.[221] Further, the renal clearance of digoxin is reduced by 51% with an increase in its mean elimination half-life (up to 72 hr).[222,223] Concomitant administration of verapamil, a P-glycoprotein inhibitor, leads to noncompetitive inhibition of digoxin's transport.[224] Verapamil reduces the total clearance of digoxin by 35% and increases its half-life by about 30%.[225,226] The antiarrhythmic agent amiodarone, a P-glycoprotein inhibitor, increases the plasma concentration and AUC of digoxin.[227] This interaction may be sustained for several months potentiating its toxicity.[227] Cyclosporine inhibits renal tubular secretion and thereby increases digoxin's serum concentration by 50%.[228]

Rifampin, an intestinal P-glycoprotein inducer, decreases digoxin's oral bioavailability by about 30% and plasma levels up to 58%.[229] However, administration of rifampin does not significantly affect renal clearance and terminal half-life of digoxin.[229] Cholestyramine, a bile acid–binding sequestering resin used in reducing cholesterol levels, decreases digoxin's serum concentration and half-life probably by interfering with enterohepatic recycling and thereby leading to enhanced elimination of digoxin.[230] Antacids, such as magnesium carbonate and magnesium trisilicate decrease the absorption of digoxin.[231] Macrolide antibiotics, especially clarithromycin, are associated with a high risk of digoxin toxicity.[219]

Drugs that decrease or increase potassium plasma levels should be avoided or used with caution. Loop (e.g., furosemide) and thiazide (e.g., hydrochlorothiazide) diuretics can cause hypokalemia, which may lead to an increased distribution of digoxin to its target receptor site resulting in an increased risk of toxicity. In contrast, potassium sparing diuretics such as spironolactone can cause hyperkalemia that may lead to a diminished therapeutic effect of digoxin.

Digoxin-Immune Fab (Digibind)

In acute and chronic digoxin poisoning, digoxin-specific antibody fragments (DigiFab) is the effective choice of treatment.[232] DigiFab has a stronger affinity to digoxin than the affinity of digoxin toward its target receptor and biological membranes.[233] The administration of DigiFab results in binding of free digoxin molecules to form a DigiFab-digoxin complex, and this shifts the equilibrium of digoxin bound to receptors.[233] Eventually, DigiFab-digoxin complexes are eliminated resulting in reduced digoxin levels in the body and decreased toxic effects.[233,234] DigiFab has an elimination half-life of about 16-20 hours and its clearance can be reduced up to 75% in patients with renal failure.[234]

Nonglycosidic Positive Inotropic Agents

Phosphodiesterase3 Inhibitors: Inamrinone and Milrinone

Milrinone and inamrinone are bipyridine derivatives (Fig. 16.13). Inamrinone was the first PDE3 bipyridine derivative approved for the treatment of CHF.[235] It was initially referred to as amrinone, but its name was later changed to inamrinone. The elimination half-life of IV inamrinone is up to 4 hours in healthy individuals.[236] In 2011, production

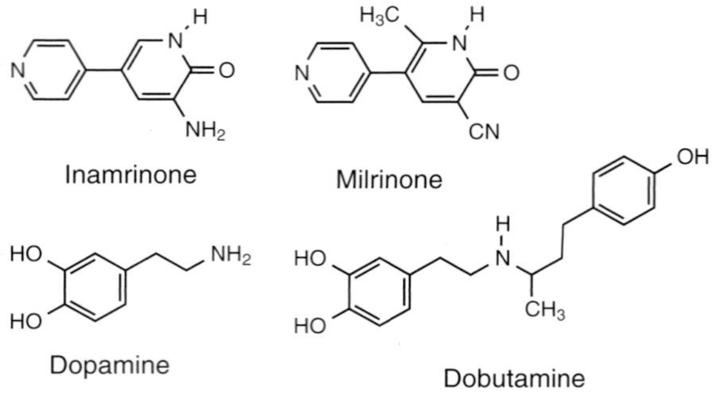

Figure 16.13 Nonglycosidic positive inotropic agents.

of the inamrinone lactate injection in the United States was discontinued by its manufacturer Bedford laboratories. Inamrinone is largely replaced with a less toxic and more specific PDE3 inhibitor milrinone.[235] In fact, milrinone has direct vasodilatory properties and is about 10-75 times a more potent ionotropic agent than inamrinone.[237]

An oral preparation of milrinone is not available in the United States. The prolonged administration of oral milrinone led to increased morbidity and mortality in severe chronic heart failure patients limiting its use.[238] Milrinone is only administered by IV in the form of its water-soluble lactate salt.[239] Milrinone has a quick onset of action of about 15 minutes and approximately 70% of the drug is protein bound.[171] In adults, milrinone has an apparent volume of distribution 0.4-0.5 L/kg.[240] The half-life elimination of milrinone is about 2 hours. However, the half-life elimination can be extended up to 20 hours in patients undergoing continuous veno-venous hemofiltration.[241] The majority of milrinone (about 83%) is excreted unchanged renally. Metabolism of milrinone includes glucuronide conjugation. Milrinone doses should be adjusted in patients with moderate or severe kidney disease.[242]

Inamrinone may be associated with the increased risk of thrombocytopenia, which is usually not the case with milrinone.[235] Patients who are taking milrinone or inamrinone should be monitored for hepatic and renal functions.[235] Overdoses of PDE3 inhibitors may lead to hypotension and reflex tachycardia.[235] Since there is an increased risk of mortality with PDE3 inhibitors in patients with chronic heart failure, long-term treatment of PDE3 inhibitors should be avoided.[243] Milrinone is chemically incompatible with the loop diuretic furosemide and combining these two in admixture results in precipitation.[244] Therefore, they should be administered separately.[244]

DOPAMINE. Dopamine (Fig. 16.13) is an endogenous catecholamine that is biosynthesized from the amino acid L-tyrosine. Dopamine affects both the renal and cardiovascular functions but only has a limited utility in the cardiogenic circulatory failure.[245] Dopamine plasma concentration, distribution, and metabolism are highly variable because of intra- and interindividual differences.[246] Unlike PDE3 inhibitors, half-life elimination of catecholamines dopamine and dobutamine are in minutes.[171] When dopamine is administered exogenously, its agonistic activity at various receptors is dose and concentration dependent.[245] Dopamine metabolism is complex and undergoes both phase I and phase II metabolic reactions. Since dopamine undergoes quick metabolism, it is only administered through IV infusion. The free base dopamine is formulated in the form of water soluble hydrochloride salt for IV infusion. The primary amine group in dopamine is oxidized by monoamine oxidase (MAO) to 3,4-dihydroxyphenylacetaldehyde (DOPAL). DOPAL further undergoes oxidation by aldehyde dehydrogenase to carboxylic metabolite (3,4-Dihydroxyphenylacetic acid [DOPAC]) and reduction by alcohol dehydrogenase to an alcohol (3,4-dihydroxyphenylethanol [DOPET]).[247] Further, catechol-O-methyltransferase (COMT) catalyzes 3-O-methylation of DOPAC to form homovanillic acid (HVA).[247] Dopamine is also directly metabolized by COMT to 3-methoxy tyramine, which is subsequently metabolized by MAO to 3-methoxy-4-hydroxyphenyl acetaldehyde.[247] Aldehyde metabolite further undergoes oxidation to carboxylic acid metabolite HVA.[247] Dopamine also undergoes sulfation and glucuronidation.[247] The major excretion products of dopamine include dopamine conjugates, its metabolites HVA, DOPAC, and their glucuronide and sulfate conjugates.[247]

DOBUTAMINE. Dobutamine is a catecholamine that is synthetically produced in the laboratory. Dobutamine contains a secondary amine and a sec-butyl side chain that in turn is attached to a phenol (Fig. 16.13). Dobutamine was developed in the early 1970s as part of structure-activity relationship studies of isoproterenol and dopamine.[248] Dobutamine contains a chiral center but is clinically sold as a racemic mixture (±). The (+) enantiomer of dopamine is a potent α_1-adrenergic antagonist and the (−) enantiomer is a potent α_1-adrenergic agonist.[249] Both isomers are β-adrenergic agonists, but the (+)-isomer is much more potent than the (−) isomer.[249]

Like dopamine, dobutamine is administered by IV infusion and undergoes rapid metabolism. Dobutamine is formulated as the water-soluble hydrochloride salt and contains an antioxidant, sodium metabisulfite. Since it contains a sulfite in its formulation, it may trigger hypersensitive reactions such as rash and eosinophilia.[250] Dobutamine has a quick onset of action. Steady-state concentration is achieved within 10 minutes and the half-life elimination is about 2 minutes.[251] Dobutamine is predominantly metabolized by COMT to 3-O-methyldobutamine.[252] Dobutamine is excreted as dobutamine sulfate, 3-O-methyldobutamine, and 3-O-methyldobutamine sulfate conjugates.[252] Unlike dopamine, dobutamine appears not to be a substrate of MAO.[253] Its resistance to MAO metabolism is probably due to the bulky sec-butyl phenolic ring attached to the amine side chain.

Nitrate Vasodilators

Nitroglycerin, isosorbide dinitrate, and mononitrate are used in the heart failure (refer to the section on drugs for the treatment of angina). In addition, the fixed dose of isosorbide dinitrate in combination with hydralazine is used as an adjunct therapy in patients with heart failure.[254] Hydralazine is also used as an antihypertensive agent (Chapter 17). Chemically, hydralazine is a

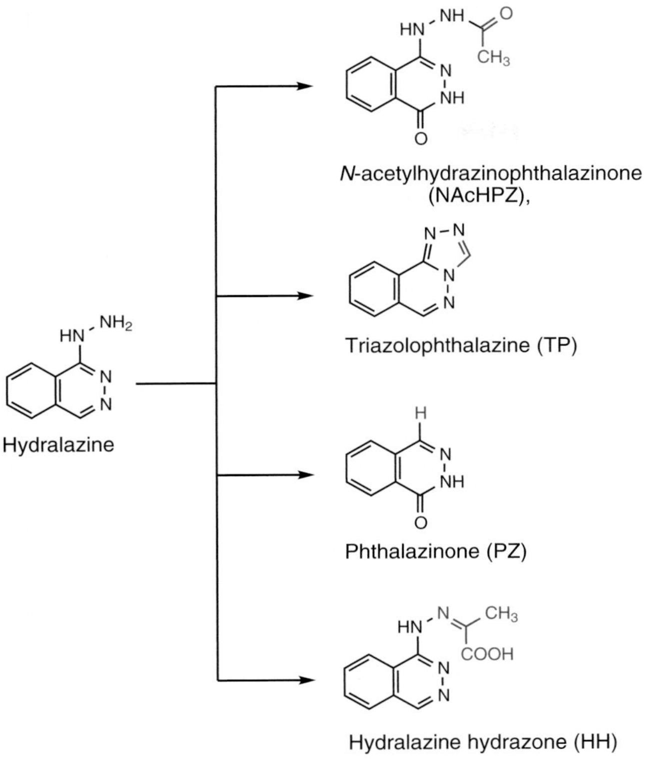

Figure 16.14 Metabolism of hydralazine.

hydrazine derivative containing a phthalazine ring (Fig. 16.14).[255] The bioavailability of hydralazine in patients with heart failure for a single dose is about 10%-26%.[256] Patients who are slow acetylators tend to have a higher percentage of bioavailability than fast acetylators probably due to lower first-pass metabolism. Increasing the dose and repeated administration of hydralazine increases its plasma concentration due to saturable first pass metabolism.[256] Hydralazine reaches peak plasma concentration in 1 hour, and the elimination half-life is about 4 hours but is longer in slow acetylators.[256] Hydralazine undergoes extensive metabolism and several metabolites including N-acetylhydrazinophthalazinone (NAcHPZ), triazolophthalazine (TP), phthalazinone (PZ), and hydralazine hydrazone (HH) are eliminated in the urine (Fig. 16.14).[257] The patient's acetylator phenotype influences hydralazine metabolism.[257] Slow acetylators are more prone to lupus syndrome than the rapid acetylators due to greater accumulation of non-acetylated metabolites.[257] Slow acetylators eliminate lower amounts of NAcHPZ and TP, but more of PZ and HH than the rapid acetylators.[257] The common side effects of this combination include headache, dizziness, nausea, and hypotension.[256]

Neprilysin Inhibitor/ARB: Sacubitril/Valsartan

The combination of sacubitril and valsartan (Entresto) was approved by the FDA in 2015.[258] It was reviewed under the FDA's priority review program and was granted the fast track designation to reduce the risk associated with heart failure.[258] Sacubitril and valsartan are present in equal ratios in Entresto. Sacubitril is an ethyl ester prodrug, which undergoes rapid enzymatic hydrolysis to yield an active dicarboxylic metabolite (sacubitrilat or LBQ 657) (Fig. 16.15).[259] Sacubitril and its metabolite (LBQ 657) are biphenyl derivatives containing two chiral centers (*R*, *S* isomer). The enantiomer (*S*, *R*) and diastereomers (*S*, *S* and *R*, *R*) of LBQ 657 are less active indicating the importance of stereospecificity on its biological activity.[260] Researchers at the Novartis Institutes for BioMedical Research Inc., studied the crystal structure of LBQ 657 with Neprilysin (NEP), a zinc-dependent peptidase.[261] LBQ 657 interacts by reversible non-covalent interactions with NEP.[261] This study reveals several key interactions (Fig. 16.16)[261]:

1. The negatively charged oxygen on the carboxylate interacts with the zinc ion by ionic interactions.
2. The second carboxylate interacts with the Arg102 and Arg110 side chains by ionic interactions.
3. The amide backbone interacts with the side chains of Asn542 and Arg717 via hydrogen bonding.
4. The biphenyl ring and the methyl group fits into the hydrophobic binding pockets.

Chemically, valsartan contains a biphenyl ring and two acidic functional groups i.e., a tetrazole ring (pK_a = 4.73) and a carboxylic acid (pK_a = 3.9).[262] Valsartan at physiological pH exists predominantly in ionized form.[262] It is a unique ARB (refer to Chapter 17) containing an acylated valine amino acid.[263] It has a chiral center and is the (*S*)-isomer. Unlike sacubitril, valsartan does not require bioactivation and undergoes minimal metabolism to hydroxy valsartan.[264]

The sacubitril/valsartan combination has good aqueous solubility (>100 mg/mL).[265] Sacubitril has high permeability and the bioavailability is predicted to be about 60%.[266] Although the absorption of valsartan in Entresto is decreased with the food, it is not clinically significant. Therefore, it can be administered with or without food.[264] The peak plasma concentrations of sacubitril, LBQ 657, and valsartan are achieved in 0.5, 2.5, and 2 hours, respectively.[267] Sacubitril, LBQ 657, and valsartan have

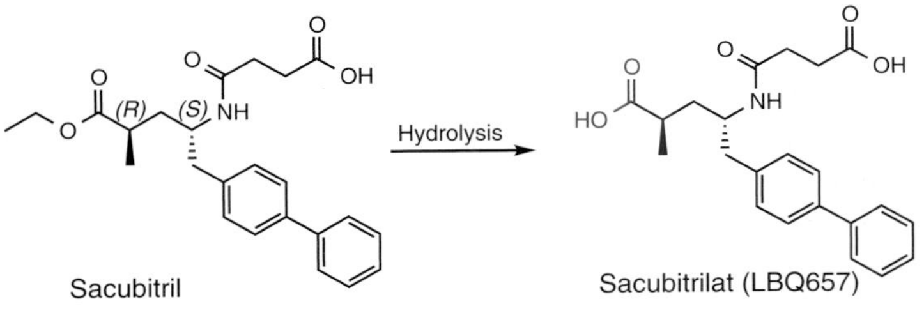

Figure 16.15 Metabolism of sacubitril.

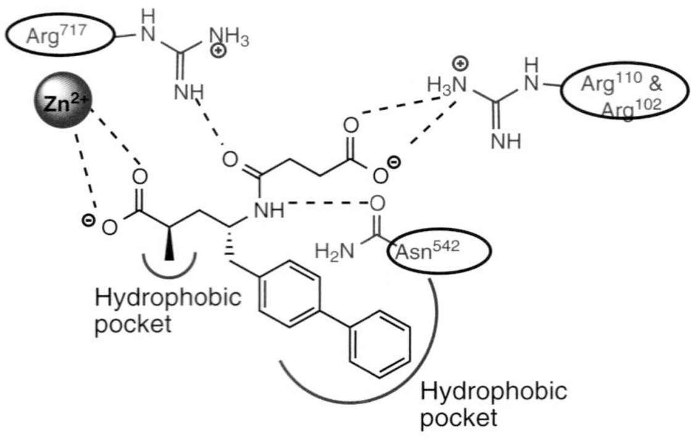

Figure 16.16 Sacubitrilat (LBQ657) binding to neprilysin.

high plasma protein binding (94%-97%).[264,266] Hepatic carboxylesterase-1 rapidly metabolizes oral sacubitril to LBQ 657.[268,269] Interindividual variability in metabolic activation of sacubitril is attributed to genetic variants in carboxylesterase-1.[269] The plasma half-lives are about 4, 18, and 14 hours for sacubitril, LBQ 657, and valsartan, respectively.[267] About 86% of sacubitril is eliminated as LBQ 657 in the urine and feces.[268] About 86% of valsartan and its metabolites are eliminated in the feces.[264] In patients with moderate and severe renal impairment the AUC of sacubitrilat is increased. Therefore, doses should be adjusted accordingly.[266] Sacubitril/valsartan should not be combined with nonsteroidal anti-inflammatory drugs because of the increased risk of renal failure.[264] In vitro studies indicate that sacubitril and LBQ 657 may not significantly inhibit or induce CYP enzymes to potentially cause clinically relevant CYP mediated drug-drug interactions.[268] The use of sacubitril/valsartan is contraindicated in patients with a previous history of angioedema related to the use of ARB or ACE inhibitors.[264] Concomitant use with potassium-sparing diuretics is contraindicated because it may lead to increased potassium levels.[264] The common side effects include hypotension, hyperkalemia, cough, dizziness, elevated creatinine levels, and renal failure.[182,264]

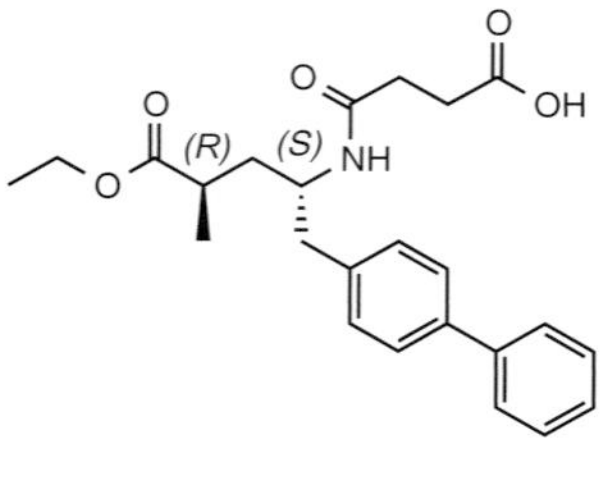

Sacubitril

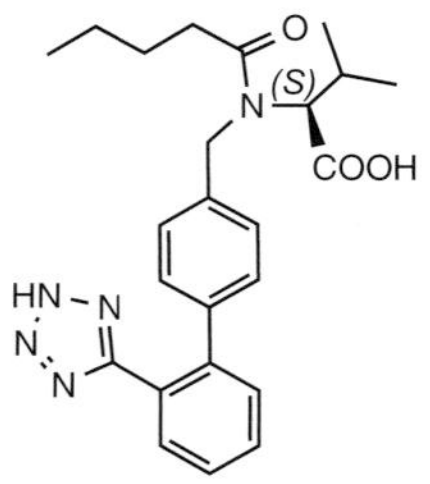

Valsartan

Drugs for the Treatment of Cardiac Arrhythmia

Arrhythmias

Arrhythmias typically describe a change or the creation of an abnormal rate, and/or rhythm related to an action potential (AP) propagation in the heart.[270] Drugs described in this section modulate the function of receptors involved in electrical impulses and/or myocyte contractile function. In order for the heart to function properly, an AP is generated and transmitted through the myocytes throughout the myocardial conduction system. This occurs by a coordinated and synchronized opening and closing of unique ion channels, which allows certain positive ions to influx or outflow from the cells.[271] These APs are repeated during every heart beat (normal range; 60-100 beats/min) in which cardiac cells undergo depolarization and repolarization. The type of ion channel and the direction of ion flow determine the shape and speed of the AP. Under normal situations, an AP starts in the sinoatrial node (SA node), which is the automatic focus or "pace maker" of the heart. The SA node's AP is spread through the atrial myocytes rejoining at the AV node, and then conducting down through the ventricles via the bundle of His, the left and right bundle branch system, and the Purkinje fibers. When all these APs are measured together, the electrical impulse on the electrocardiogram (ECG) is generated. Because the ECG reflects the time required for an AP to travel over an area of the heart, only atrial (P wave), ventricle depolarization (QRS complex), and ventricular repolarization (T wave) are observed (Fig. 16.17).[272] The SA and AV nodes are too small to register in the ECG. However, the automaticity of these nodes can be determined by measuring how often a P wave occurs and how long it takes to go from the P wave to the QRS (PR interval). The smaller these intervals are, the faster the heart rate will occur.[273] For simplicity, the AP occurring in the SA node and ventricle will be discussed.

The SA and AV nodes express I_f channels which passively open and are modulated by the autonomic nervous system.[274] Although the SA node can depolarize spontaneously, it is typically under the influence of the sympathetic and parasympathetic nervous systems. Thus, the autonomic nervous system can speed up or slow down the rate of depolarization, increasing or decreasing heart rate. I_f channels allow Na^+, which is high outside of the cells, to follow its electrochemical gradient and move inside the cell. The influx of Na^+ makes the cell membrane potential more positive and eventually causes the opening of voltage gated T-type Ca^{2+} channels, which leads to the influx of Ca^{2+} into the myocyte until it reaches the threshold (Phase 4). At this point, voltage-gated L-type Ca^{2+} channels open and the SA node depolarizes (Phase 0) (Fig. 16.18). Calcium is the depolarizing ion in the SA and AV node, but this Ca^{2+}

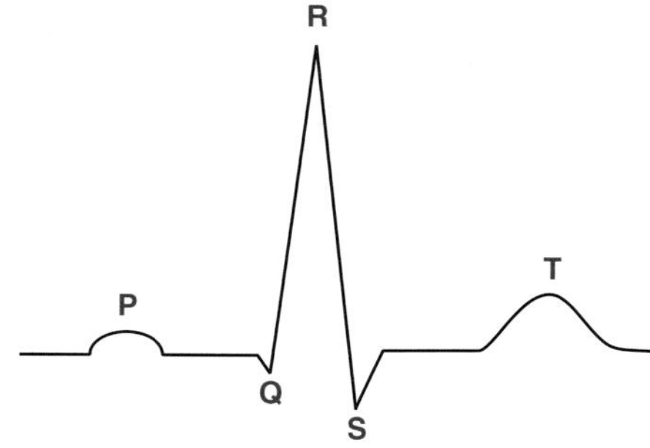

Figure 16.17 Depiction of electrocardiography recording.

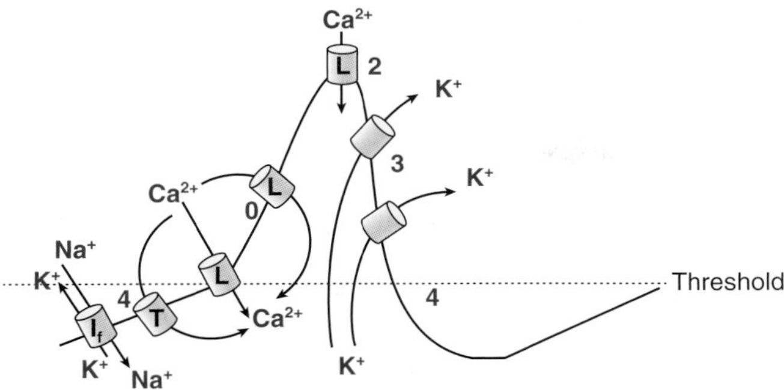

Figure 16.18 Depiction of cardiac action potential from a sinoatrial node.

current and the slope it creates are slower. Since it takes a little longer to depolarize, the SA and AV nodes are commonly referred to as slow AP. As it starts to reach its peak, voltage-gated potassium channels start to open and allow the movement of K^+ from inside of the cell to the outside. This is the beginning of the repolarization process (phases 2 and 3). It is important to note that I_f channels are not selective Na^+ channels, and it also allows other ions to cross, but the function of these channels determines the rate of depolarization. From the SA node, the AP travels to the atrial myocytes producing the depolarization and contraction of the atrium. The AP reaches the AV node, which follows a very similar pattern of depolarization and repolarization as the SA node. Once the AP travels through the AV node and other fast AP tissues, it reaches the ventricular myocytes.

In the ventricles, Na^+ is the major depolarizing ion (phase 0) (Fig. 16.19). As the tissue reaches the threshold, Na^+ channels move from the resting (closed) state to the active (open) state. The opening of these channels allows the influx of Na^+, which is responsible for the upstroke. During phase 1, Na^+ channels change their conformational state into the inactive mode, and Na^+ no longer can enter the cells. During phases 1 and 2, Ca^{2+} channels open; consequently, the entry of Ca^{2+} produces the ventricle contraction, and the blood is pumped out of the ventricle into the main circulation. During phases 1, 2, and 3, K^+ channels open and that is the beginning of the repolarization process.[272] During these phases, Na^+ channels move from the inactive state into the resting state. The conformational state of the Na^+ channels defines the refractory period, which can be characterized into two

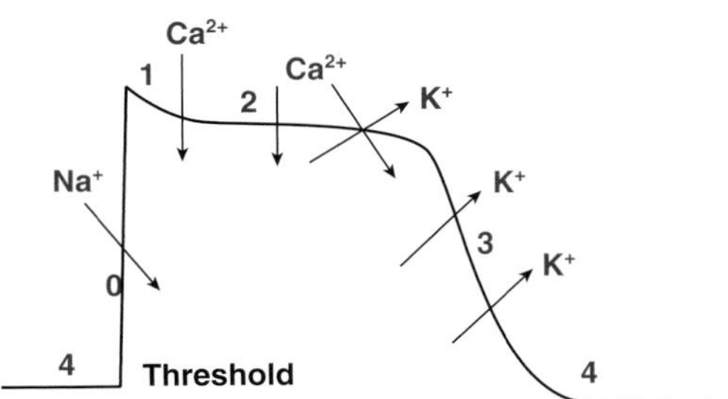

Figure 16.19 Depiction of cardiac action potential from a ventricle.

groups, absolute and relative refractory periods. During the absolute refractory period, an AP cannot be created because the majority of Na^+ channels are present in the inactive state. In contrast, during the relative refractory period (which typically begins during phase 3), a smaller AP maybe elicited depending how many Na^+ channels are present in the resting state. During phase 4, most of the sodium channels are restored to the resting states.

As described above, arrhythmias occur when there is a perturbation in ion channel function that affects either the creation and/or propagation of the AP. This can result from high sympathetic input, myocardium infarction, and congenital defects.[275] Drugs in this class are used to either change the rate or the rhythm by altering the flow of specific ions.[181] Antiarrhythmic drugs are classified based on the Vaughan-Williams classification.[276]

Mechanism of Action of Antiarrhythmic Drugs

Class I Antiarrhythmic Drugs: Sodium Channel Blockers

All drugs in this class have affinity for the Na^+ channels present in the fast AP tissue and decrease the influx of Na^+.[277] However, they differ in their selectivity, onset, and offset times.

CLASS IA ANTIARRHYTHMIC DRUGS. Drugs belonging to class 1A have an intermediate onset and offset binding which can affect the myocardium AP during resting and arrhythmic states.[278] Procainamide, by blocking Na^+ channels, decreases the speed of conduction through the fast AP tissues (e.g., ventricle) and increases the threshold. This can be observed on the ECG as a widening of the QRS complex. In addition, by also blocking the K^+ channels there is a prolongation of the AP duration and an increase in the refractory period. This is observed by a prolongation of the QT interval.[279] The next drug in this class is quinidine, which has a more complex pharmacological profile. In addition to blocking Na^+ channels, it also can bind and antagonize K^+ channels and α_1-adrenergic receptors. At higher doses, it may also block L-type Ca^{2+} channels. It produces greater hypotensive effects than procainamide due to the blockade of α_1-receptors with a variable effect on the heart rate. Because its lacks receptor selectivity, quinidine produces a wide spectrum of side effects. The most concerning side effect is the marked prolongation of the QT interval. Disopyramide is another drug in this class, and it has affinity for the Na^+ channels. The (S)-enantiomer can also bind and block K^+ channels. One of the major differences between disopyramide and the other drugs in this class is its pronounced antimuscarinic effects. In similar fashion to the other two, it widens the QRS and prolongs the QT intervals. By blocking the muscarinic (M_2) receptor in the heart, it will increase the heart rate as reflected by the shortening of the PR interval. It also may cause dry mouth and constipation associated with the blockade of the muscarinic system.

CLASS IB ANTIARRHYTHMIC DRUGS. Lidocaine, mexiletine, and phenytoin belong to class IB, and they have fast onset and fast offset kinetics. These drugs produce most of their effects when the heart is undergoing an arrhythmia or ischemic event. These selective Na^+ channel blockers primarily widen the QRS complex with little to no significant effect on the PR and QT intervals. Lidocaine's preferred route of administration is intravenous and mexiletine can be given orally.[280]

CLASS IC ANTIARRHYTHMIC DRUGS. Class IC drugs have slow onset/offset kinetics. Flecainide and propafenone are the two drugs in this class. These drugs have high affinity for the Na^+ channels and will produce marked tonic blockade, which will lead to a decrease in automaticity, widening of the QRS, and increase in AP durations. Flecainide also blocks K^+ channels, which is reflected as a prolongation of the QT interval and refractory period.[281] In addition, flecainide also blocks Ca^{2+} channels, thus decreasing the heart rate and prolonging the PR interval. Propafenone lacks affinity for the K^+ and Ca^{2+} channels, but it antagonizes β_1-adrenergic receptors. This results in a decrease of SA node automaticity and slowing down of the heart rate that is reflected as a prolongation of the PR interval.[282]

CLASS II ANTIARRHYTHMIC DRUGS: β-ADRENERGIC BLOCKERS. Class II drugs are composed of β-blockers.[276] β_1-adrenergic receptors are one of the most prominent receptors in the heart and are directly modulated by the sympathetic nervous system. By blocking the ability of norepinephrine from binding and activating β_1-receptors, these drugs produce a significant decrease in SA and AV nodes automaticity, which is reflected as a prolongation of the PR interval. The drugs in this class differ primarily on their selectivity (e.g., metoprolol is a β_1-selective antagonist vs. propranolol is a nonselective β_1- and β_2-antagonist).

CLASS III ANTIARRHYTHMIC DRUGS: POTASSIUM CHANNEL BLOCKERS. Class III drugs are primarily K^+ channel antagonists. The drugs in this class include amiodarone, dronedarone, sotalol, dofetilide, and ibutilide.[283] Because all these drugs block the outflow of K^+, they tend to prolong the refractory period and AP duration. This is observed as a prolongation of the QT interval. Although there are K^+ channels on the SA and AV node, these drugs have affinity directed toward the K^+ channels present on the fast AP tissues.

Amiodarone is one of the most commonly used drugs in this class. In addition to blocking K^+ channels, it can also block Na^+ (widening of the QRS), Ca^{2+} (prolongation of the PR interval), α_1 (hypotension) and β_1-adrenergic receptors (sinus bradycardia).[284] Amiodarone has serious side effects, which increase with time. Dronedarone was developed to circumvent these side effects. In vitro studies suggest that dronedarone can bind and antagonize Na^+, K^+, and Ca^{2+} channels. It also has affinity for the α_1- and β_1-adrenergic receptors. However, clinical studies do not support improved efficacy for dronedarone when compared to amiodarone.

Sotalol is a K^+ channel blocker with affinity for the β-receptors.[285] As such, it prolongs both the QT and PR intervals. Ibutilide and dofetilide are selective K^+ channel antagonists and these drugs will prolong the QT interval with minimal effect on the PR or QRS complex.

CLASS IV ANTIARRHYTHMIC DRUGS: CALCIUM CHANNEL BLOCKERS. Class IV drugs belong to the class of nondihydropyridine Ca^{2+} channel blockers, verapamil and diltiazem.[10] These drugs have the greatest affinity for the L-type Ca^{2+} channel blockers present on the SA and AV nodes. By decreasing the influx of Ca^{2+}, these two drugs decrease the slope of phase 0 and prolong the refractory period of the SA and AV nodes.[286] This is reflected by a decrease in the heart rate and prolongation of the PR interval, thus taking longer for the AP to travel from the atrial myocardium to the ventricle.

MISCELLANEOUS AGENTS. In addition to the drugs described above, digoxin, adenosine, and magnesium may be used in the inpatient setting. Magnesium has been shown to be useful in terminating an ongoing torsade de pointes, but the exact mechanism of action is not fully understood.[287] Digoxin, in addition to its inotropic effects, enhances parasympathetic tone. This vagotonic effect decreases the heart rate, which is observed as a prolongation of the PR interval. This appears to be an indirect effect of digoxin that is not associated with the blockade of Na^+/K^+-ATPase. Adenosine is an endogenous nucleoside that binds to its own receptor. It works in a similar fashion to acetylcholine and appears to slow AP currents in the SA and AV nodes.

Physicochemical Properties, Pharmacokinetics, and Drug Interactions of Antiarrhythmic Drugs

Class I Antiarrhythmic Drugs: Sodium Channel Blockers

CLASS IA ANTIARRHYTHMIC DRUGS

Quinidine. Quinidine (dextrorotatory [+]) and quinine (levorotatory [–]) are naturally occurring alkaloids that are isolated from the bark of the cinchona tree.[288] Quinidine (Fig. 16.20) is therapeutically used as an antiarrhythmic agent; whereas, quinine is used an antimalarial agent.[288] Quinidine and quinine each contain four chiral centers, and are diastereomers of one another. Chemically, quinidine contains a bicyclic amine known as quinuclidine and a methoxy quinoline ring. The quinoline and quinuclidine rings are linked by a hydroxy methylene group. Quinuclidine is further connected to a vinyl group. The quinuclidine tertiary aliphatic nitrogen is more basic (pK_a = 8.4) than the quinoline aromatic nitrogen (pK_a = 4.2).[289] As a result, quinidine can be converted into water-soluble salts by reacting with acids. Commercially, quinidine is available as quinidine sulfate and gluconate salt forms as immediate- and extended-release oral formulations. Quinidine gluconate is also available in an IV formulation. Quinidine sulfate and gluconate have 83% and 62% of quinidine base, respectively.[290] Since the two salt forms have different quinidine percentages, they are not directly interchangeable.[290] Quinidine formulations may contain dihydroquinidine as a common impurity.[291]

Oral quinidine is rapidly absorbed. It is moderately metabolized by hepatic first-pass metabolism and has a bioavailability of about 70%-80%.[292] The apparent volume of distribution is about 2.4 L/kg.[293] Quinidine has high protein binding (70%-95%). It primarily binds to α_1-acid glycoprotein and serum albumin.[294] About 60%-85% of quinidine is metabolized in the liver.[294] It is primarily metabolized by CYP3A4 into an active metabolite (3S)-3-hydroxy-quinidine.[295] Other metabolites of quinidine include quinidine N-oxide and dihydroquinidine.[295] About 15%-40% of intact quinidine is excreted renally.[294] Quinidine has an elimination half-life of about 7 hours.[294] Age and disease states affect the clearance of quinidine. In elderly patients, quinidine clearance is reduced and half-life elimination is prolonged (about 10 hr) which can lead to toxic side effects unless doses are adjusted accordingly.[293] The amount of serum albumin and α_1-acid glycoprotein is lower in patients with liver failure resulting in an increase in unbound quinidine fraction and volume of distribution.[296] In patients with hepatic cirrhosis, the half-life elimination is significantly increased (about 9 hr).[293] In patients with congestive heart failure, the volume of distribution of quinidine is decreased because of elevated levels of plasma proteins and the total drug clearance is also reduced because of reduced unbound concentrations.[290,297] However, the average half-life of quinidine in CHF patients is similar to normal individuals.[297]

Quinidine is a substrate and a strong inhibitor of P-glycoprotein.[220] P-glycoprotein mediated inhibition of quinidine leads to decreased digoxin elimination and increased plasma levels.[220] Quinidine is also a potent inhibitor of CYP2D6.[298] Concurrent administration of quinidine with CYP2D6 substrates, such as metoprolol may lead to a significant increase in metoprolol concentrations and half-life.[144] Quinidine and its metabolites may cause the QT prolongation leading to potentially toxic torsade de pointes in about 1%-3% of patients.[299] The combination of amiodarone and quinidine can have cumulative toxic side effects by enhancing the QT interval.[300] The adverse effects associated with quinidine include gastrointestinal disturbances, fever, hepatic dysfunction, leukopenia, cinchonism, hemolytic anemia, and cardiac arrhythmias.[301] Quinidine can also cause hypokalemia and decreased heart rate.[299]

Procainamide. Procainamide (Fig. 16.20) is a bioisostere of procaine. Procaine, a local anesthetic agent, was used by cardiologists as an alternative to quinidine during World War II.[302] However, the clinical application of procaine as a cardiovascular agent is limited due to its rapid metabolism by esterases and high incidence of CNS side effects.[302] The ester group of procaine was later replaced with an amide functionality to produce procainamide, which is more resistant to hydrolysis by esterases. Procainamide, because of its lower lipophilicity, has fewer incidences of CNS side effects.[302]

Procainamide is rapidly and completely absorbed after oral administration. The oral bioavailability is about 75%-95%.[303] It reaches peak plasma concentrations in about 1-2 hours.[303] The oral form of procainamide is not available in the United States and is only administered intravenously. Procainamide's volume of distribution is about 2 L/kg, and only 15% is bound to plasma proteins.[303] The half-life elimination of procainamide is about 3 hours and is longer in patients with the renal impairment.[303] Procainamide undergoes hepatic metabolism by N-acetyltransferase-II to N-acetylprocainamide, a major metabolite with similar pharmacological effects comparable to those of procainamide.[303] The acetylation metabolism of procainamide is genetically determined and is dependent on the rapid or slow acetylation phenotypes.[304] Chronic oral administration of procainamide is associated with systemic lupus–like syndrome.[305] In slow acetylators, the rate at which procainamide induces antinuclear antibodies and lupus syndrome is much faster and more frequent than rapid acetylators indicating the unacetylated procainamide is responsible for its side effect.[305] The *para*-amino group on procainamide undergoes oxidation to hydroxylamine and nitro derivatives, which are responsible for hypersensitive reactions.[306] Procainamide is also metabolized to N-hydroxyprocainamide by CYP2D6.[307] Ethnic background may play an important role in determining the dose and systemic lupus–like side effect.[308] In Caucasian and African American populations about 50% are rapid acetylators, in Japanese and Eskimo populations about 80%-90% are rapid acetylators, whereas in Egyptians and certain Jewish populations ≤20% are rapid acetylators.[308] About 50% of the intact procainamide and majority of its metabolites are eliminated renally by glomerular filtration and active tubular secretion.[303] The plasma concentration of procainamide and N-acetylprocainamide is significantly increased in patients with impaired renal function because of reduced elimination.[309]

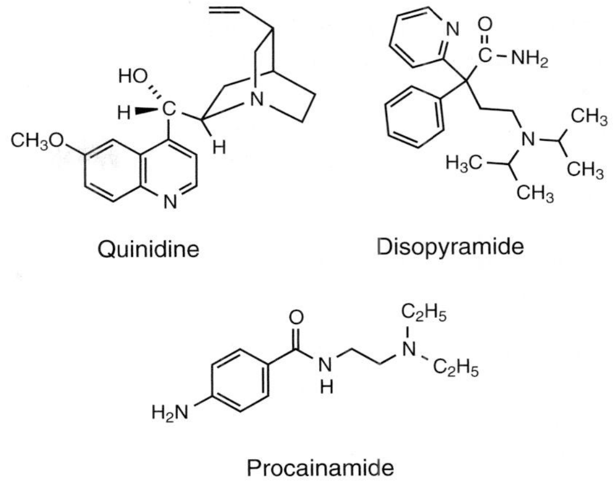

Quinidine

Disopyramide

Procainamide

Figure 16.20 Class IA antiarrhythmic agents.

Drugs interfering with the tubular secretion of procainamide may potentially have significant drug-drug interactions.[308] Fluoroquinolone antibacterials, such as ciprofloxacin and levofloxacin significantly decrease renal clearance of procainamide and N-acetylprocainamide.[310] Cimetidine, a histamine H_2 receptor antagonist, is shown to decrease the clearance, increase the plasma levels, and enhance adverse effects of procainamide. Therefore, either of these combinations should be avoided or doses should be adjusted accordingly and side effects carefully monitored.[311]

The adverse effects associated with procainamide include gastrointestinal upset, fever, bradycardia and hypotension.[312] Procainamide increases the risk of developing torsade de pointes.

Disopyramide. Disopyramide (Fig. 16.20) is a unique molecule containing a chiral carbon that is linked to a pyridine ring, phenyl ring, an amide, and an alky diisopropyl amine. It is commercially sold as a racemic mixture. The tertiary amine is converted into salts, such as phosphate, to improve water solubility.

Disopyramide is available as immediate- and controlled-release formulations.[313] The controlled-release formulation of disopyramide provides more constant pharmacological effects and lower interdose variation in unbound drug levels than the immediate-release formulation.[313] The oral bioavailability of disopyramide is about 85%.[314] It reaches peak plasma concentrations in about 0.5-3 hours.[315] Disopyramide has a unique and complex protein binding pattern that is dependent on the concentration of the drug and exhibits stereoselectivity because the *S*(+)-disopyramide is more highly protein bound than the *R*(−)-disopyramide.[316] Disopyramide is primarily bound (70%) to α_1-acid glycoprotein with high affinity.[317,318] About 5% of disopyramide is bound to albumin with low affinity.[317] Disopyramide, when administered orally, does not undergo significant first-pass metabolism.[315] About 55% of the drug is excreted unchanged primarily by the kidneys.[318] Disopyramide is metabolized in the liver by CYP3A4 N-dealkylation to mono-N-desisopropyldisopyramide, which is pharmacologically active.[318,319] Disopyramide has an elimination half-life of about 7 hours.[315] In patients with renal impairment, the levels of disopyramide and mono-N-desisopropyldisopyramide are increased.[320]

Concurrent administration of disopyramide with CYP3A4 inhibitors such as macrolide antibiotics can significantly enhance the plasma levels of disopyramide and could potentially cause ventricular tachycardia.[321,322] Disopyramide can potentially cause anticholinergic side effects such as nausea, dry mouth (xerostomia), abdominal discomfort, constipation, and urinary urgency and retention.[323] Disopyramide in combination with other anticholinergic agents such as ipratropium and tiotropium should be avoided. Disopyramide can have negative inotropic actions and may reduce the contractions of the heart.[324]

CLASS IB ANTIARRHYTHMIC DRUGS

Lidocaine. Lidocaine (Fig. 16.21) was synthesized in the early 1940s.[325] Over the years, lidocaine has been used as a local anesthetic agent similar to procaine. It is antiarrhythmic activity effect was first reported in 1950.[325] Lidocaine is widely used in the treatment of ventricular arrhythmias. Structurally, lidocaine contains 2,6-dimethylphenyl attached to N-acetamide linked to a diethylamine functionality (Fig. 16.21).[325] The tertiary amine is weakly basic ($pK_a = 8$).[325]

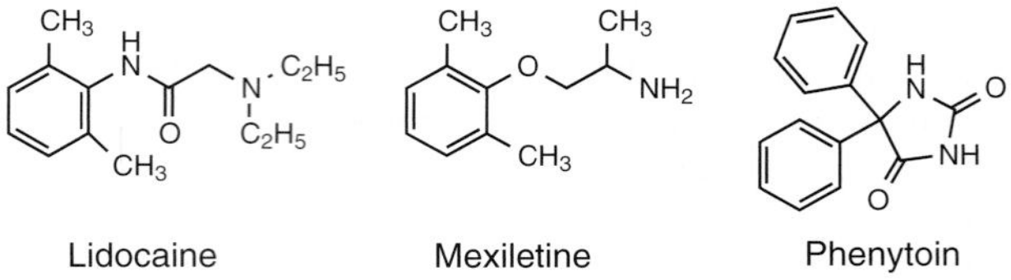

Lidocaine Mexiletine Phenytoin

Figure 16.21 Class IB antiarrhythmic agents.

The oral bioavailability is about 35%.[326] When administered orally, lidocaine undergoes extensive hepatic first-pass metabolism and does not attain sufficient plasma levels to have antiarrhythmic effects.[326] Therefore, lidocaine is usually administered intravenously for its antiarrhythmic effects.[326] Lidocaine is highly protein bound (60%-80%) to α_1-acid glycoprotein, and alteration of this glycoprotein concentration results in either decreased or increased protein binding.[327] Lidocaine's protein binding is variable and is dependent on inter- and intraindividual differences.[327] The volume of distribution is about 1.5 L/kg.[326,328] The liver is the primary site of metabolism, and the hepatic blood flow is very important for clearance of lidocaine because of its high hepatic extraction ratio.[325] The major metabolic pathway of lidocaine is by N-deethylation to yield monoethylglycinexylidide (MEGX), a pharmacologically active metabolite.[325] CYP1A2 and CYP3A4 are the two important isoforms that are responsible for metabolism of lidocaine.[329] The amide moiety in MEGX undergoes hydrolysis to yield 2,6-xylidine (2,6-dimethyl aniline) and N-ethylglycine (amino acid).[325] Up to 10% of lidocaine is excreted unchanged in the urine.[325] Since lidocaine is a weak base, alkalization of the urine may decrease its clearance, and acidification of the urine may increase its clearance.[325] Lidocaine has a plasma half-life of about 1.5 hours.[326] Elderly patients may have a prolonged half-life when compared to young individuals.[330] In patients with hepatic failure lidocaine metabolism is impaired, resulting in reduced plasma clearance and increased half-life (≥5 hr).[331] In patients with heart failure, lidocaine's clearance and volume of distribution are significantly reduced and doses must be reduced accordingly.[331] The side effects of lidocaine and its metabolites are concentration dependent.[332] Common side effects are CNS effects, which include dizziness, drowsiness, and euphoria.[332] At therapeutic levels it can cause seizures, confusion, agitation, and psychosis.[332] At higher concentrations, it can cause cardiovascular side effects such as hypotension, atrioventricular block, and circulatory collapse.[332]

The concurrent administration of antidepressant fluvoxamine, a strong CYP1A2 inhibitor, significantly reduces the metabolism of lidocaine in patients with normal liver function.[333] Therefore, caution must be taken when lidocaine is administered with other CYP1A2 inhibitors. Erythromycin, a CYP3A4 inhibitor, is shown to modestly decrease the clearance of lidocaine and increase the levels of MEGX possibly by inhibiting its further metabolism.[334] Amiodarone, another CYP3A4 inhibitor, decreases the systemic clearance and increases the plasma levels of lidocaine.[335] Concurrent administration of cimetidine may decrease the clearance of lidocaine and may increase its plasma levels because of decreased hepatic blood flow.[336]

Mexiletine. Mexiletine (Fig. 16.21) was originally developed as an anticonvulsant agent, but its cardiac properties were quickly observed and thereafter clinically used as an antiarrhythmic agent.[337] The amide bond in lidocaine is replaced with the ether function to make it metabolically more resistant to hydrolysis (Fig. 16.21). Mexiletine contains a chiral center and is sold as a racemic mixture.

Mexiletine is weakly basic (pK_a = 8.5) and primarily exists in the ionized state (hydrophilic form) in the stomach and unionized state (lipophilic form) in the intestine.[337] Therefore, most of the absorption takes place in the small intestine.[337] Orally administered mexiletine is rapidly and almost completely absorbed with a bioavailability of about 80%-90%.[280] It undergoes minimal first-pass hepatic metabolism.[280] About 70% of mexiletine is bound to plasma proteins (albumin and α_1-acid glycoprotein).[337] The volume of distribution ranges from 5 to 9 L/kg and is distributed to the heart, liver, and brain.[337] Mexiletine undergoes extensive metabolism in the liver into several metabolites.[337] The primary metabolic routes of mexiletine are hydroxylation of primary amine to N-hydroxymexiletine, *para* or *meta* aromatic hydroxylation, hydroxylation of the methyl group on the aromatic ring to hydroxymethylmexiletine and glucuronide conjugation.[337] CYP1A2 catalyzes the formation of N-hydroxymexiletine and CYP2D6 predominantly catalyzes the formation of hydroxymethylmexiletine and *para/meta* hydroxymexiletine.[337] Genetic polymorphisms of CYP2D6 influence the metabolism of mexiletine based on whether the individual is a poor or extensive metabolizer.[337] The clearance of hydroxymethylmexiletine and *para* and *meta* hydroxymexiletine were all decreased in poor metabolizers compared to extensive metabolizers.[337,338] The elimination half-life of mexiletine is about 10 hours and is prolonged in patients with hepatic failure, congestive heart failure, and myocardial infarction.[339] The plasma concentration of mexiletine varies significantly with pH and extreme pH values may lead to either decreased efficacy or increased risk of adverse effects.[340] Acidic urinary pH would significantly favor the elimination of mexiletine resulting in decreased plasma concentrations.[340] In contrast, an increase in the urinary pH would decrease its elimination.[340]

Atropine decreases and metoclopramide enhances the rate of mexiletine absorption.[341] The time to reach the maximum plasma concentration of mexiletine is slightly increased by concurrent administration with antacids due to a delay in gastric emptying.[342] Concurrent administration of mexiletine with theophylline, a CYP1A2 substrate, increases the serum concentration of theophylline by about 2-fold, but mexiletine serum concentration is unaffected.[343] H_2-receptor antagonists, such as cimetidine may slightly prolong the absorption and decrease the plasma concentration of mexiletine.[344] Strong CYP2D6 inhibitors (e.g., quinidine) and CYP1A2 inhibitors may decrease the metabolism of mexiletine.[337,345] The common side effects associated with mexiletine include gastrointestinal disturbances and CNS side effects such as dizziness, nervousness, and insomnia.[339]

Phenytoin. Chemically, phenytoin (Fig. 16.21) is 5,5-diphenylhydantoin. It was discovered in 1936, and its clinical efficacy was established in 1937.[346] Since then it is widely used as an antiepileptic drug. The use of phenytoin as an antiarrhythmic drug is not officially approved. Phenytoin is a weakly acidic drug and has poor solubility. Therefore, it is usually administered as a sodium salt.[347] Phenytoin is administered either orally or intravenously.[348] Approximately 90% of phenytoin is bound to plasma proteins.[347] However, in patients with chronic kidney disease, phenytoin protein binding is significantly reduced, which may lead to increased free (unbound) concentrations of the drug.[349] The drugs that displace phenytoin from plasma protein binding sites such as valproic acid may increase the unbound fraction of phenytoin.[350]

Phenytoin is predominantly metabolized via hydroxylation by various CYP enzymes to 5-hydroxylated metabolite.[351] CYP2C19 is the major metabolizing enzyme of phenytoin. Phenytoin metabolism is nonlinear, and metabolizing enzymes are saturated at therapeutic doses leading to an increase in phenytoin concentrations and toxicity.[352] The mean elimination half-life is about 22 hours.[353] Phenytoin and its metabolites are excreted into bile and undergo reabsorption from the gastrointestinal tract and eventually eliminated renally by glomerular filtration and tubular secretion.[353]

Co-administration of phenytoin with CYP2C19 inhibitors leads to an increased phenytoin plasma level and toxicity.[354] Poor CYP2C9 metabolizers are associated with reduced clearance and an increased phenytoin level in the body and serious adverse effects.[355]

CLASS IC ANTIARRHYTHMIC DRUGS

Flecainide (Tambocor). Flecainide (Fig. 16.22) is therapeutically used in maintaining the sinus rhythm in patients with atrial flutter.[356] Flecainide has a local anesthetic effect and is drastically different from class IA or IB agents.[356] Flecainide is a bis-trifluoroethoxy benzamide derivative and sold as an acetate salt. It is well absorbed orally and the bioavailability is about 70%.[357] Food does not significantly affect the rate and extent of absorption.[357] Only about 40% of flecainide is bound to plasma proteins and the volume of distribution is 5-6 L/kg.[358] The plasma half-life of flecainide is 13-16 hours.[358] Flecainide is predominantly metabolized by CYP2D6 into two major metabolites.[358] It undergoes dealkylation to *meta*-O-dealkylated metabolites, which further undergo oxidation.[359] Flecainide metabolites do not have significant activity.[358] Pharmacokinetics of flecainide are influenced by genetic differences.[360] Poor and intermediate CYP2D6 metabolizers have reduced flecainide clearance.[360] About 86% of flecainide and its metabolites are eliminated renally and only

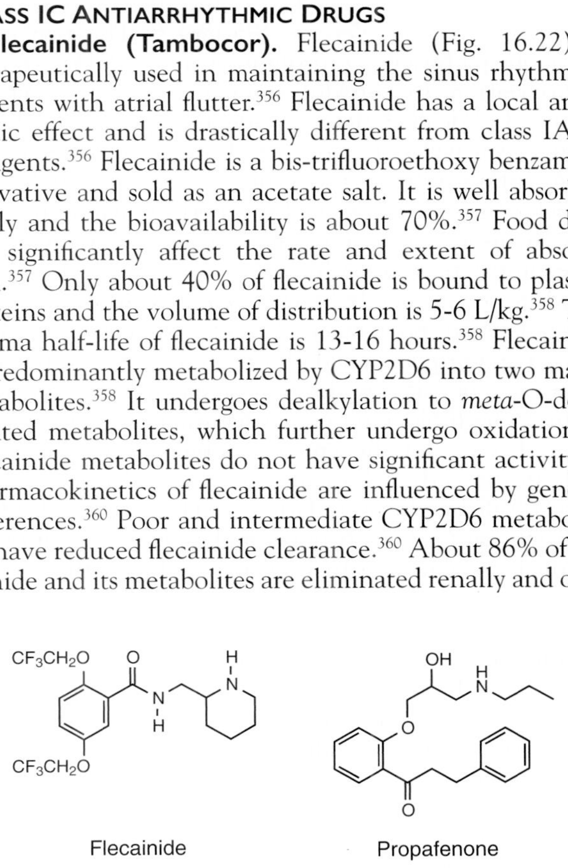

CF_3CH_2O ... Flecainide

Propafenone

Figure 16.22 Class IC antiarrhythmic agents.

about 5% are eliminated in the feces.[358] Renal elimination of flecainide is by both glomerular filtration and tubular secretion.[357] Flecainide's rate of elimination is possibly reduced with age.[358] Flecainide has a good safety profile, but it has proarrhythmic effects and may cause supraventricular proarrhythmia.[356] The less serious side effects of flecainide include headache, diarrhea, and nausea.[356] Concurrent administration of flecainide with digoxin or propranolol significantly prolongs the ECG PR interval.[361]

Propafenone. Propafenone contains a chiral center and is administered as a racemic mixture of *S*(+)- and *R*(−)-propafenone (Fig. 16.22).[362] Both enantiomers of propafenone have an equal antiarrhythmic effect as sodium channel blockers, but the *S*(+)-isomer is primarily responsible for its β_1-blocking properties.[363] It contains a phenyloxypropanolamine group, which is structurally similar to some of the β_1-adrenergic antagonists.[363] Since it contains a weakly basic secondary amine, it is converted to the hydrochloride salt for improved water solubility.

Greater than 90% of propafenone is absorbed after oral administration.[362] Propafenone undergoes extensive first-pass metabolism and the bioavailability varies from 5% to 50%.[362] Food may increase its bioavailability.[364] Peak plasma concentrations are reached in about 2 hours, and the amount of the drug that reaches the systemic circulation is dependent on the concentration.[362,365] Majority of propafenone is bound to α_1-acid glycoprotein.[366] Propafenone is distributed to the heart, liver, and lungs and the apparent volume of distribution is 2.5-4 L/kg.[367] *R*(−)-propafenone (92.4%) is slightly less protein bound than the *S*(+) propafenone (95.1%).[368] The two major metabolic pathways of propafenone are CYP2D6 catalyzed hydroxylation to 5-hydroxypropafenone and CYP3A4 catalyzed N-dealkylation to N-depropylpropafenone.[369,370] Both hydroxylated and N-dealkylated metabolites have antiarrhythmic properties.[371] The metabolism of propafenone is influenced by genetic polymorphisms.[372] Individuals who are extensive metabolizers rapidly metabolize propafenone to 5-hydroxypropafenone when compared to poor metabolizers.[373] Approximately, 10% of Caucasians are poor metabolizers.[362] At high doses, both extensive and poor metabolizers are prone to β-blocking properties, but at low doses poor metabolizers are more prone to its β-blocking properties than extensive-metabolizers because of the greater accumulation of propafenone in the body.[372] Propafenone also undergoes phase II metabolism by glucuronidation.[374] The mean half-life of propafenone is about 6 hours and is subject to inter-individual variability.[375] In poor metabolizers, the half-life elimination is 3.4-7.6 hours and in extensive metabolizers it is 9-25 hours.[376] Propafenone exhibits stereoselectivity in elimination. Long-term administration of propafenone results in enhanced β-blocking properties and increased *S*(+)-propafenone concentrations due to faster rate elimination of the *R*(−)-isomer.[377]

Concurrent administration of propafenone with digoxin significantly increases digoxin's plasma concentrations and reduces digoxin's clearance.[378] Propafenone impairs warfarin's metabolism and increases its plasma concentration by about 38% and this may lead to an enhanced anticoagulant effect.[379] Propafenone when administered along with the CY2D6 substrate metoprolol, enhances metoprolol concentrations 2- to 5-fold.[380] In extensive metabolizers, coadministration of quinidine, a potent CYP2D6 inhibitor, increases propafenone plasma concentrations more than two times and decreases its clearance and metabolism to 5-hydroxypropafenone.[381]

The most common adverse effects of propafenone include cardiovascular side effects such as aggravation of arrhythmia, induction or worsening of congestive heart failure, conduction abnormalities; gastrointestinal disturbances, and CNS side effects. The side effects are commonly observed during chronic therapy and at high doses (900 mg d or higher).[382]

CLASS II ANTIARRHYTHMIC DRUGS: β-ADRENERGIC BLOCKERS. Refer to the antianginal section for chemical structures and pharmacokinetic properties of β-blockers.

Esmolol. Esmolol (Brevibloc) is an ultrashort-acting selective β-blocker (Fig. 16.23) making it an effective agent for acute critical care settings.[383] It is only administered by the IV route. The *para* ester substituent is required for its β-blocking activity.[383] The onset of action is attained in about 2 minutes and in 5 minutes about 90% of the steady-state β-blockade is achieved.[384] The ester group is rapidly hydrolyzed by red blood cells esterases into a carboxylic acid metabolite and methanol.[383,384] The carboxylic acid metabolite is essentially inactive and methanol levels are in the normal endogenous range.[384] The elimination half-life is about 10 minutes.[385] The therapeutic effect of esmolol quickly dissipates in 30 minutes after its discontinuation.[385]

CLASS III ANTIARRHYTHMIC DRUGS: POTASSIUM CHANNEL BLOCKERS.

Sotalol. Sotalol (Betapace) (Fig. 16.24) is a phenyl-hydroxyethyl-isopropylamine *para*-methane sulfonamide.[386] Sotalol contains a chiral center and is sold as a racemic mixture of D(+)-sotalol and L(−)-sotalol.[387] Both enantiomers have potassium channel blocking (class III) properties.[387] In addition, the L(−) sotalol is 30-60 times more potent as a β-blocker (class II) than D(+)-sotalol.[387]

Sotalol is administered by oral and intravenous routes. It is rapidly and completely absorbed after oral administration.[388] The bioavailability is 90%-100% indicating minimal or no fast-pass metabolism.[388] The bioavailability is reduced by about 20% in the presence of food.[388] The peak plasma concentrations are attained rapidly in about 2-4 hours.[388] Sotalol is not significantly bound to plasma proteins and is well distributed to the lungs, liver, and

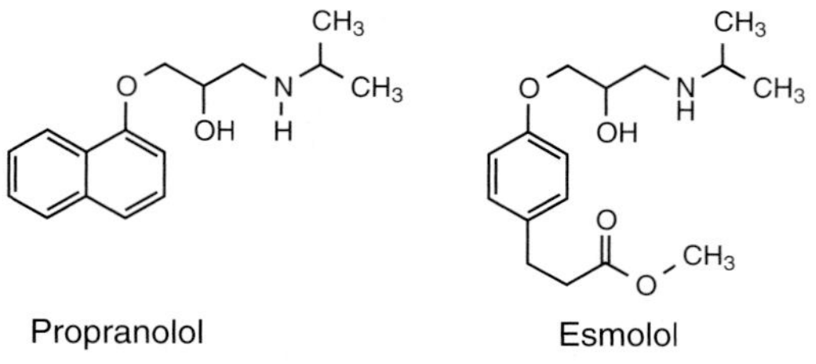

Figure 16.23 Class II antiarrhythmic agents.

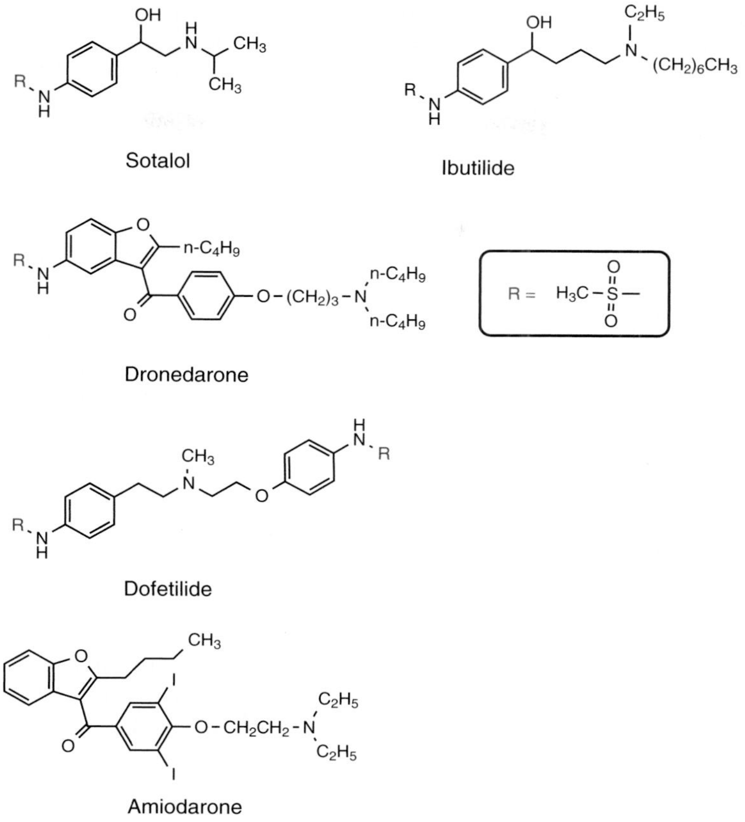

Figure 16.24 Class III antiarrhythmic agents.

kidneys with an apparent volume of distribution of 1.2-2.4 L/kg.[387,388] It is hydrophilic in nature and not well distributed to the CNS.[388] Sotalol's metabolism is insignificant and about 80%-90% of the unchanged drug is eliminated in the urine.[387,388] In patients with renal impairment, sotalol doses should be adjusted accordingly.[387] Both D(+)- and L(−)-sotalol are eliminated equally in the urine.[388] The elimination half-life is in the range of 10-20 hours.[388]

Since sotalol does not undergo any significant metabolism, drug interactions associated with CYP inducers or inhibitors appears to be less likely.[389] However, several pharmacodynamic drug-drug interactions can occur.[389] Concurrent administration of sotalol with antacids such as magnesium hydroxide, decreases sotalol's oral absorption and plasma levels, and this interaction can be avoided by administering at a 2 hour interval space.[390] Sotalol may prolong the QT interval, syncope, and ventricular tachycardia.[391] Concurrent administration with other class IA or III antiarrhythmic agents have a combined effect on QT prolongation potentiating the possibility of torsade de pointes.[389] Sotalol may worsen bradycardia associated with digoxin when given in combination.[392] Sotalol should be used with caution with diuretics that cause hypokalemia since hypokalemia is a risk factor for prolonged QT interval.[391]

Amiodarone. Amiodarone (Fig. 16.24) is a highly lipophilic (Log P: 7.78) diiodinated benzofuran derivative.[393] The iodine content is 39.3% in amiodarone free base.[393] Amiodarone is a weakly basic molecule (pK_a is 7.0)[394] and is converted into its hydrochloride salt to improve water solubility.

The oral absorption of amiodarone is erratic and incomplete and the bioavailability is 22%-86%.[393] Because of its high lipophilicity, it is sequestered in many body parts including adipose tissue, liver, lungs, skin, and skeletal muscle.[393,395] Amiodarone has a high volume of distribution (66 L/kg), and about 96% of the drug is protein bound.[393,395] Orally administered amiodarone has a slow onset and offset of action.[395] The plasma half-life of a single oral dose of amiodarone is about 3-80 hours, but after withdrawal of chronic administration the half-life can be as long as 100 days.[393] The onset of action after a single IV administration is within 30 minutes.[393] However, after oral administration there is a delay of about 2-21 days to observe its complete therapeutic effects.[393] The duration of action could last up to 1 month even after withdrawing amiodarone.[393] The majority of the drug undergoes metabolism, and only about 1% of the drug is eliminated unchanged in the urine.[393] Amiodarone is hepatically metabolized by CYP3A4 catalyzed N-deethylation to desethylamiodarone, a major metabolite.[396] Desethylamiodarone is pharmacologically active and has a similar elimination half-life as amiodarone.[395] Minor metabolites include bis-N-desethylamiodarone and deiodinated metabolites.[395] Since amiodarone undergoes negligible renal elimination, dosage needs not be reduced in patients with renal impairment.[395]

Amiodarone and its metabolite, desethylamiodarone are CYP2C9, CYP2D6, and CYP3A4 inhibitors.[397] Amiodarone inhibits the metabolism of warfarin and thereby increases its plasma levels and anticoagulant effect.[393] Concurrent administration of cholestyramine, a bile acid sequestrant, with amiodarone decreases the enterohepatic circulation of amiodarone and enhances its elimination.[398] Amiodarone also has calcium channel blocking properties and when combined with CCBs it may have additive effects.[389,399] Amiodarone when combined with diltiazem could lead to sinus arrest and hypotension.[400] Amiodarone decreases cyclosporine clearance by more than 50% probably by inhibiting CYP3A4 in the gastrointestinal mucosa.[389,401]

The common adverse effects of amiodarone are gastrointestinal side effects, most commonly constipation; ocular disturbances related to the formation of corneal microdeposits; neuromotor effects in the form of tremor, ataxia, and sleeplessness; photosensitivity in the form of sunburn, erythema, and swelling.[402,403] Amiodarone may cause a rise in hepatic enzymes, hypothyroidism, and hyperthyroidism.[402] It also has the potential to cause pulmonary fibrosis.[402] Side effects are dose dependent, and chronic administration may increase its propensity to cause adverse reactions.[402,403]

Dronedarone. Dronedarone (Fig. 16.24) is a noniodinated benzofuran derivative of amiodarone that was approved by the United States FDA in 2009.[404] It was designed to reduce the toxic side effects associated with chronic amiodarone therapy.[405] The lack of the iodine atoms, and the addition of the methanesulfonyl group makes dronedarone (Log P: 5.2) more hydrophilic in nature than amiodarone (Log P: 7.78).[405]

Orally administered dronedarone is well absorbed (70%-94%). However, it has poor bioavailability (15%) because it undergoes extensive first-pass metabolism primarily by hepatic CYP3A4.[406,407] Food increases its bioavailability 2- to 3-fold, and a high fat meal can increase the bioavailability to 3- to 4.5-fold.[407] Relatively, dronedarone has a low tissue distribution and a shorter half-life than amiodarone.[405] Dronedarone is well tolerated and side effects include bradycardia, QT-interval prolongation; gastrointestinal disturbances such as nausea, diarrhea and vomiting; skin related events such as rash; and may increase serum creatinine.[405,408] Unlike amiodarone, dronedarone has a better side effect profile and does not significantly increase thyroid abnormalities and pulmonary disorders.[408]

Ibutilide. Ibutilide (Fig. 16.24) is structurally similar to sotalol and is another methanesulfonamide derivative.[409] It contains hydroxy butyl and heptyl side chains.[410] Ibutilide is more effective than sotalol in terminating atrial fibrillation or atrial flutter.[411] Ibutilide is sold as the fumarate salt and has good water solubility (>100 mg/mL) at a pH less than 7.[410,412] Although ibutilide has a chiral center, it is sold as a racemic mixture since both the enantiomers have similar pharmacokinetic properties.[410] Ibutilide undergoes extensive first-pass metabolism making it unsuitable for long-term oral administration.[409] Therefore, ibutilide is administered via intravenous infusion.[409] About 40% of the administered ibutilide is bound to plasma proteins.[412] Ibutilide is extensively distributed with a large volume of distribution of about 11 L/kg and patients have high interindividual variability.[410,412] Ibutilide is metabolized by hepatic enzymes into eight metabolites.[412] The heptyl side chain undergoes omega-oxidation and subsequently β-oxidation.[412] The metabolites are inactive, except the omega-hydroxyl metabolite which showed in vitro activity in the rabbit myocardium model.[412] However, this metabolite is only 10% of the circulating plasma levels indicating the activity is largely from the intact ibutilide and not from its metabolites.[412] It has high systemic plasma clearance and is also rapidly cleared from the body.[410] The average half-life elimination is about 6 hours.[410,412] About 82% of ibutilide is excreted in the urine and 18% in feces.[410,412]

Since ibutilide is not metabolized by CYP3A4 and CYP2D6, agents affecting these enzymes do not have drug-drug interactions.[412] Other cardiovascular drug such as calcium channel blockers, β-blockers or digoxin do not affect the safety and efficacy of ibutilide.[412] Ibutilide is associated with the risk of polymorphic ventricular tachycardia.[413] Ibutilide may prolong the QT interval and torsade de pointes.[413] Therefore, it should not be used with other drugs that significantly prolong the QT interval.

Dofetilide. Dofetilide is a bis-methanesulfonamide (Fig. 16.24) derivative and is a highly selective potassium channel blocker when compared to sotalol and amiodarone.[414] Dofetilide is well absorbed with an absolute oral bioavailability >90%.[415] After oral administration, the time to reach maximum plasma concentrations is about 2-3 hours.[415,416] About 60%-70% of dofetilide is protein bound and the volume of distribution is about 3 L/kg. In vitro studies show that dofetilide is metabolized by CYP3A4. It predominantly undergoes N-demethylation to form the N-desmethyl metabolite.[417] It is also metabolized by N-oxidation to form the N-oxide, which has weak Class I antiarrhythmic properties.[417] Its biological response is largely due to unchanged dofetilide and metabolites are either inactive or do not have significant activity.[417] The elimination half-life is approximately 10 hours.[418] Dofetilide is primarily eliminated renally (80%) and the majority of the drug is eliminated unchanged. Concurrent administration with other drugs that significantly interfere with renal elimination should be avoided.[418,419] For example, hydrochlorothiazide and triamterene significantly increase the plasma concentrations of dofetilide and must be avoided.[418] Coadministration of dofetilide with verapamil or organic cation transporter inhibitors such as cimetidine must also be avoided because they increase dofetilide plasma concentrations.[418]

Dofetilide prolongs the QT interval duration and is proportional to the plasma concentration of the drug.[415] Torsade de pointes ventricular tachycardia is the significant adverse side effect associated with dofetilide.[419] Patients with renal impairment and decreased creatinine clearance will experience an increased plasma concentration of dofetilide. Therefore, the dose must be adjusted according to the creatinine clearance and must be avoided in patients with severe renal impairment (creatinine clearance <20 mL/min).[418]

CLASS IV ANTIARRHYTHMIC DRUGS: CALCIUM CHANNEL BLOCKERS. Nondihydropyridines calcium channel blockers i.e., verapamil and diltiazem comprise class IV agents (Fig. 16.4). Refer to the antianginal section for chemical structures and pharmacokinetic properties.

MISCELLANEOUS AGENTS. Adenosine is a naturally occurring purine nucleoside composed of adenine base and ribose sugar. Adenosine monophosphate undergoes dephosphorylation to adenine and inorganic phosphate. Adenosine is used as a drug in treating supraventricular tachycardias.[420] Adenosine is administered by rapid intravenous bolus and is quickly metabolized by erythrocytes and vascular endothelium.[420] The clinical effects of adenosine last for about 20 seconds and it has an ultra-short-acting half-life up to 10 seconds.[420] After administration, the effectiveness is typically observed between 10 and 20 seconds and is dependent on the dose, cardiac output, and speed of administration.[420] Dipyridamole, a PDE3 enzyme inhibitor, decreases the metabolism and increases adenosine concentrations and thereby potentiating its effects.[421] Therefore, the adenosine dose should be lowered when administered with dipyridamole and should be used with extreme caution.[420] Methylxanthines such as theophylline and caffeine act as adenosine receptor antagonists primarily at the A_1 receptors.[422,423] Thus, in the presence of methylxanthine derivatives adenosine may have reduced pharmacological effect.[420] The most common side effects with adenosine include flushing due to coronary vasodilation, acute dyspnea due to transient bronchoconstriction and carotid body chemoreceptor activation.[420] Although rare, adenosine has significant proarrhythmic effects.[420]

Magnesium sulfate may be indicated in the treatment of torsade de pointes.[424] However, oral magnesium preparations do not have any effect as an antiarrhythmic agent.[424]

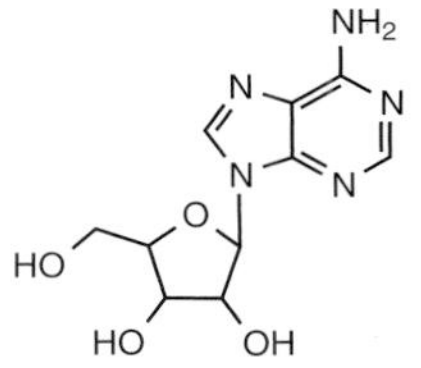

Adenosine

Structure Challenge

Antiarrhythmic structure challenge: Evaluate the antiarrhythmic structures drawn below and identify the correct description associated with each of the drug.

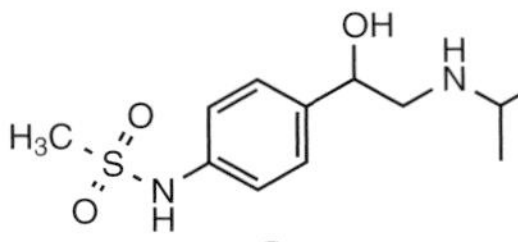

a

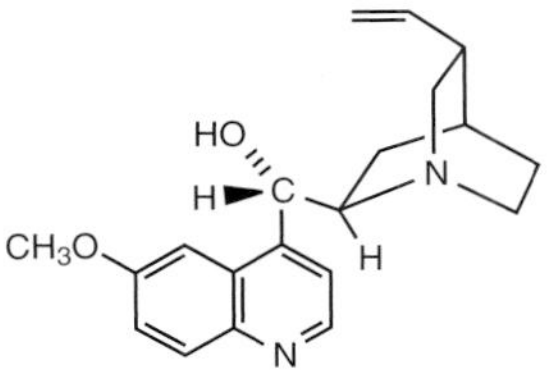

b

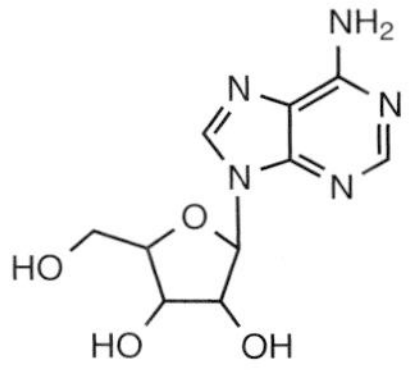

c

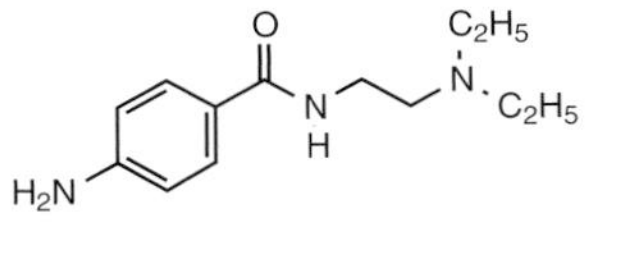

d

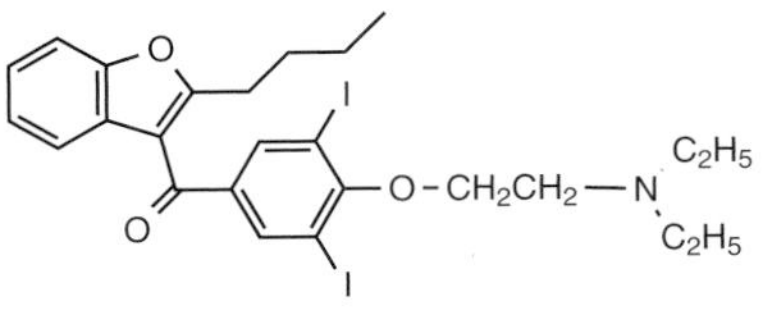

e

1. Rapid intravenous bolus for treating supraventricular tachycardias
2. Slow acetylators are more prone to lupus syndrome
3. Potassium channel opener with β-blocker properties
4. Potential to cause pulmonary fibrosis and hypo- or hyperthyroidism
5. May cause cinchonism and hemolytic anemia

Structure Challenge answers found immediately after References.

ACKNOWLEDGMENTS

The authors wish to acknowledge the work of Griffith RK, PhD, and Mehanna AS, PhD, who authored content used within this chapter in a previous edition of this text.

REFERENCES

1. Ford TJ, Corcoran D, Berry C. Stable coronary syndromes: pathophysiology, diagnostic advances and therapeutic need. *Heart*. 2018;104:284-292.
2. Radico F, Cicchitti V, Zimarino M, et al. Angina pectoris and myocardial ischemia in the absence of obstructive coronary artery disease: practical considerations for diagnostic tests. *JACC Cardiovasc Interv*. 2014;7:453-463.
3. Braunwald E, Morrow DA. Unstable angina: is it time for a requiem? *Circulation*. 2013;127:2452-2457.
4. Ong P, Aziz A, Hansen HS, et al. Structural and functional coronary artery abnormalities in patients with vasospastic angina pectoris. *Circ J*. 2015;79:1431-1438.
5. Meyrelles SS, Mill JG, Cabral AM, et al. Cardiac baroreflex properties in myocardial infarcted rats. *J Auton Nerv Syst*. 1996;60:163-168.
6. Norton JM. Toward consistent definitions for preload and afterload. *Adv Physiol Educ*. 2001;25:53-61.
7. Ginsberg MD. Expanding the concept of neuroprotection for acute ischemic stroke: the pivotal roles of reperfusion and the collateral circulation. *Prog Neurobiol*. 2016;145-146:46-77.
8. Ferreira JC, Mochly-Rosen D. Nitroglycerin use in myocardial infarction patients. *Circ J*. 2012;76:15-21.
9. Mayer B, Beretta M. The enigma of nitroglycerin bioactivation and nitrate tolerance: news, views and troubles. *Br J Pharmacol*. 2008;155:170-184.
10. Godfraind T. Discovery and development of calcium channel blockers. *Front Pharmacol*. 2017;8:286.
11. Godfraind T. Calcium channel blockers in cardiovascular pharmacotherapy. *J Cardiovasc Pharmacol Ther*. 2014;19:501-515.
12. Diness JG, Bentzen BH, Sorensen US, et al. Role of calcium-activated potassium channels in atrial fibrillation pathophysiology and therapy. *J Cardiovasc Pharmacol*. 2015;66:441-448.
13. Elliott WJ, Ram CV. Calcium channel blockers. *J Clin Hypertens (Greenwich)*. 2011;13:687-689.
14. Wallukat G. The beta-adrenergic receptors. *Herz*. 2002;27:683-690.
15. Smith C, Teitler M. Beta-blocker selectivity at cloned human beta 1- and beta 2-adrenergic receptors. *Cardiovasc Drugs Ther*. 1999;13:123-126.
16. Prichard BN, Richards DA. Comparison of labetalol with other anti-hypertensive drugs. *Br J Clin Pharmacol*. 1982;13:41S-47S.
17. Gupta S, Wright HM. Nebivolol: a highly selective beta1-adrenergic receptor blocker that causes vasodilation by increasing nitric oxide. *Cardiovasc Ther*. 2008;26:189-202.
18. Blumenfeld JD, Sealey JE, Mann SJ, et al. Beta-adrenergic receptor blockade as a therapeutic approach for suppressing the renin-angiotensin-aldosterone system in normotensive and hypertensive subjects. *Am J Hypertens*. 1999;12:451-459.
19. Schnabel P, Maack C, Mies F, et al. Binding properties of beta-blockers at recombinant beta1-, beta2-, and beta3-adrenoceptors. *J Cardiovasc Pharmacol*. 2000;36:466-471.
20. Wimmer NJ, Stone PH. Anti-anginal and anti-ischemic effects of late sodium current inhibition. *Cardiovasc Drugs Ther*. 2013;27:69-77.
21. Mason PK, DiMarco JP. New pharmacological agents for arrhythmias. *Circ Arrhythm Electrophysiol*. 2009;2:588-597.
22. Schram G, Zhang L, Derakhchan K, et al. Ranolazine: ion-channel-blocking actions and in vivo electrophysiological effects. *Br J Pharmacol*. 2004;142:1300-1308.
23. DiFrancesco D. The role of the funny current in pacemaker activity. *Circ Res*. 2010;106:434-446.
24. Nitroglycerine and Dynamite. http://www.Nobelprize.Org/alfred_nobel/biographical/articles/life-work/nitrodyn.html.
25. Marsh N, Marsh A. A short history of nitroglycerine and nitric oxide in pharmacology and physiology. *Clin Exp Pharmacol Physiol*. 2000;27:313-319.
26. Alfred Nobel's Will. http://www.Nobelprize.Org/alfred_nobel/will/.
27. Brunton TL. On the use of nitrite of amyl in angina pectoris. *Lancet*. 1867;2:97-98.
28. Nossaman VE, Nossaman BD, Kadowitz PJ. Nitrates and nitrites in the treatment of ischemic cardiac disease. *Cardiol Rev*. 2010;18:190-197.
29. Alfred Nobel's Health and His Interest in Medicine by Nils Ringertz. http://www.Nobelprize.Org/alfred_nobel/biographical/articles/ringertz/.
30. Elkayam U, Bitar F, Akhter MW, et al. Intravenous nitroglycerin in the treatment of decompensated heart failure: potential benefits and limitations. *J Cardiovasc Pharmacol Ther*. 2004;9:227-241.
31. Chen Z, Zhang J, Stamler JS. Identification of the enzymatic mechanism of nitroglycerin bioactivation. *Proc Natl Acad Sci USA*. 2002;99:8306-8311.
32. Kleschyov AL, Oelze M, Daiber A, et al. Does nitric oxide mediate the vasodilator activity of nitroglycerin? *Circ Res*. 2003;93:e104-e112.
33. Klemenska E, Beresewicz A. Bioactivation of organic nitrates and the mechanism of nitrate tolerance. *Cardiol J*. 2009;16:11-19.
34. Munzel T, Meinertz T, Tebbe U, et al. Efficacy of the long-acting nitro vasodilator pentaerithrityl tetranitrate in patients with chronic stable angina pectoris receiving anti-anginal background therapy with beta-blockers: a 12-week, randomized, double-blind, placebo-controlled trial. *Eur Heart J*. 2014;35:895-903.
35. Daiber A, Munzel T. Organic nitrate therapy, nitrate tolerance, and nitrate-induced endothelial dysfunction: emphasis on redox biology and oxidative stress. *Antioxid Redox Signal*. 2015;23:899-942.
36. Jurt U, Gori T, Ravandi A, et al. Differential effects of pentaerythritol tetranitrate and nitroglycerin on the development of tolerance and evidence of lipid peroxidation: a human in vivo study. *J Am Coll Cardiol*. 2001;38:854-859.
37. Lexicomp. http://online.Lexi.Com/lco/action/doc/retrieve/docid/patch_f/7377#f_pharmacology-and-pharmacokinetics.
38. McNiff EF, Yacobi A, Young-Chang FM, et al. Nitroglycerin pharmacokinetics after intravenous infusion in normal subjects. *J Pharm Sci*. 1981;70:1054-1058.
39. Hashimoto S, Kobayashi A. Clinical pharmacokinetics and pharmacodynamics of glyceryl trinitrate and its metabolites. *Clin Pharmacokinet*. 2003;42:205-221.
40. Hodgson JR, Lee CC. Trinitroglycerol metabolism: denitration and glucuronide formation in the rat. *Toxicol Appl Pharmacol*. 1975;34:449-455.
41. Neurath GB, Dunger M. Blood levels of the metabolites of glyceryl trinitrate and pentaerythritol tetranitrate after administration of a two-step preparation. *Arzneimittelforschung*. 1977;27:416-419.
42. Straehl P, Galeazzi RL. Isosorbide dinitrate bioavailability, kinetics, and metabolism. *Clin Pharmacol Ther*. 1985;38:140-149.
43. Sporl-Radun S, Betzien G, Kaufmann B, et al. Effects and pharmacokinetics of isosorbide dinitrate in normal man. *Eur J Clin Pharmacol*. 1980;18:237-244.
44. Ghofrani HA, Humbert M, Langleben D, et al. Riociguat: mode of action and clinical development in pulmonary hypertension. *Chest*. 2017;151:468-480.
45. Kloner RA. Novel phosphodiesterase type 5 inhibitors: assessing hemodynamic effects and safety parameters. *Clin Cardiol*. 2004;27:I20-I25.
46. Triggle DJ. Calcium-channel drugs: structure-function relationships and selectivity of action. *J Cardiovasc Pharmacol*. 1991;18(suppl 10):S1-S6.
47. Scholz H. Pharmacological aspects of calcium channel blockers. *Cardiovasc Drugs Ther*. 1997;10(suppl 3):869-872.

48. Davies MK, Hollman A. The opium poppy, morphine, and verapamil. *Heart*. 2002;88:3.
49. Melville KI, Shister HE, Huq S. Iproveratril: experimental data on coronary dilatation and antiarrhythmic action. *Can Med Assoc J*. 1964;90:761-770.
50. Vater W, Kroneberg G, Hoffmeister F, et al. Pharmacology of 4-(2′-nitrophenyl)-2,6-dimethyl-1,4-dihydropyridine-3,5-dicarboxylic acid dimethyl ester (nifedipine, bay a 1040). *Arzneimittelforschung*. 1972;22:1-14.
51. Shamsipur M, Hemmateenejad B, Akhond M, et al. A study of the photo-degradation kinetics of nifedipine by multivariate curve resolution analysis. *J Pharm Biomed Anal*. 2003;31:1013-1019.
52. Shaldam MA, Eman MH, Esmat A, El-Moselhy TF. 1,4-dihydropyridine calcium channel blockers: homology modeling of the receptor and assessment of structure activity relationship. *Med Chem*. 2014;2014:1-14.
53. Meredith PA, Elliott HL. Clinical pharmacokinetics of amlodipine. *Clin Pharmacokinet*. 1992;22:22-31.
54. Nguyen LA, He H, Pham-Huy C. Chiral drugs: an overview. *Int J Biomed Sci*. 2006;2:85-100.
55. Ishii K, Minato K, Nakai H, Sato T. Simultaneous assay of four stereoisomers of diltiazem hydrochloride. Application to in vitro chiral inversion studies. *Chromatographia*. 1995;41.
56. Lexicomp. https://online.Lexi.Com/lco/action/home.
57. Rashid TJ, Martin U, Clarke H, et al. Factors affecting the absolute bioavailability of nifedipine. *Br J Clin Pharmacol*. 1995;40:51-58.
58. Otto J, Lesko LJ. Protein binding of nifedipine. *J Pharm Pharmacol*. 1986;38:399-400.
59. Renwick AG, Robertson DR, Macklin B, et al. The pharmacokinetics of oral nifedipine–a population study. *Br J Clin Pharmacol*. 1988;25:701-708.
60. Wang JG, Kario K, Lau T, et al. Use of dihydropyridine calcium channel blockers in the management of hypertension in eastern Asians: a scientific statement from the Asian Pacific Heart Association. *Hypertens Res*. 2011;34:423-430.
61. Food and Drug Administration. https://www.Accessdata.Fda.Gov/drugsatfda_docs/label/2011/020198s023lbl.Pdf.
62. Kleinbloesem CH, van Harten J, Wilson JP, et al. Nifedipine: kinetics and hemodynamic effects in patients with liver cirrhosis after intravenous and oral administration. *Clin Pharmacol Ther*. 1986;40:21-28.
63. Graham DJ, Dow RJ, Hall DJ, et al. The metabolism and pharmacokinetics of nicardipine hydrochloride in man. *Br J Clin Pharmacol*. 1985;20(suppl 1):23S-28S.
64. Urien S, Albengres E, Comte A, et al. Plasma protein binding and erythrocyte partitioning of nicardipine in vitro. *J Cardiovasc Pharmacol*. 1985;7:891-898.
65. Food and Drug Administration. https://www.Accessdata.Fda.Gov/drugsatfda_docs/label/2016/020005s014lbl.Pdf.
66. Judd E, Jaimes EA. Aliskiren, amlodipine and hydrochlorothiazide triple combination for hypertension. *Expert Rev Cardiovasc Ther*. 2012;10:293-303.
67. Zhu Y, Wang F, Li Q, et al. Amlodipine metabolism in human liver microsomes and roles of CYP3A4/5 in the dihydropyridine dehydrogenation. *Drug Metab Dispos*. 2014;42:245-249.
68. Abernethy DR. The pharmacokinetic profile of amlodipine. *Am Heart J*. 1989;118:1100-1103.
69. Beresford AP, McGibney D, Humphrey MJ, et al. Metabolism and kinetics of amlodipine in man. *Xenobiotica*. 1988;18:245-254.
70. Echizen H, Eichelbaum M. Clinical pharmacokinetics of verapamil, nifedipine and diltiazem. *Clin Pharmacokinet*. 1986;11:425-449.
71. Eichelbaum M, Ende M, Remberg G, et al. The metabolism of DL-[14C]verapamil in man. *Drug Metab Dispos*. 1979;7:145-148.
72. Keefe DL, Yee YG, Kates RE. Verapamil protein binding in patients and in normal subjects. *Clin Pharmacol Ther*. 1981;29:21-26.
73. Vogelgesang B, Echizen H, Schmidt E, et al. Stereoselective first-pass metabolism of highly cleared drugs: studies of the bioavailability of l- and d-verapamil examined with a stable isotope technique. *Br J Clin Pharmacol*. 1984;18:733-740.
74. Tracy TS, Korzekwa KR, Gonzalez FJ, et al. Cytochrome p450 isoforms involved in metabolism of the enantiomers of verapamil and norverapamil. *Br J Clin Pharmacol*. 1999;47:545-552.
75. Schwartz JB, Keefe DL, Kirsten E, et al. Prolongation of verapamil elimination kinetics during chronic oral administration. *Am Heart J*. 1982;104:198-203.
76. Ochs HR, Knuchel M. Pharmacokinetics and absolute bioavailability of diltiazem in humans. *Klin Wochenschr*. 1984;62:303-306.
77. Hermann P, Rodger SD, Remones G, et al. Pharmacokinetics of diltiazem after intravenous and oral administration. *Eur J Clin Pharmacol*. 1983;24:349-352.
78. Yeung PK, Prescott C, Haddad C, et al. Pharmacokinetics and metabolism of diltiazem in healthy males and females following a single oral dose. *Eur J Drug Metab Pharmacokinet*. 1993;18:199-206.
79. Sutton D, Butler AM, Nadin L, et al. Role of CYP3A4 in human hepatic diltiazem n-demethylation: inhibition of CYP3A4 activity by oxidized diltiazem metabolites. *J Pharmacol Exp Ther*. 1997;282:294-300.
80. Molden E, Johansen PW, Boe GH, et al. Pharmacokinetics of diltiazem and its metabolites in relation to CYP2D6 genotype. *Clin Pharmacol Ther*. 2002;72:333-342.
81. Montamat SC, Abernethy DR. N-monodesmethyldiltiazem is the predominant metabolite of diltiazem in the plasma of young and elderly hypertensives. *Br J Clin Pharmacol*. 1987;24:185-189.
82. Nishio S, Watanabe H, Kosuge K, et al. Interaction between amlodipine and simvastatin in patients with hypercholesterolemia and hypertension. *Hypertens Res*. 2005;28:223-227.
83. Kantola T, Kivisto KT, Neuvonen PJ. Erythromycin and verapamil considerably increase serum simvastatin and simvastatin acid concentrations. *Clin Pharmacol Ther*. 1998;64:177-182.
84. Yoshimoto H, Takahashi M, Saima S. Influence of rifampicin on antihypertensive effects of dihydropiridine calcium-channel blockers in four elderly patients. *Nihon Ronen Igakkai Zasshi*. 1996;33:692-696.
85. Jalava KM, Olkkola KT, Neuvonen PJ. Itraconazole greatly increases plasma concentrations and effects of felodipine. *Clin Pharmacol Ther*. 1997;61:410-415.
86. Sica DA. Interaction of grapefruit juice and calcium channel blockers. *Am J Hypertens*. 2006;19:768-773.
87. Kim RB. Drugs as p-glycoprotein substrates, inhibitors, and inducers. *Drug Metab Rev*. 2002;34:47-54.
88. Verschraagen M, Koks CH, Schellens JH, et al. P-glycoprotein system as a determinant of drug interactions: the case of digoxin-verapamil. *Pharmacol Res*. 1999;40:301-306.
89. Wessler JD, Grip LT, Mendell J, et al. The p-glycoprotein transport system and cardiovascular drugs. *J Am Coll Cardiol*. 2013;61:2495-2502.
90. Summers MA, Moore JL, McAuley JW. Use of verapamil as a potential p-glycoprotein inhibitor in a patient with refractory epilepsy. *Ann Pharmacother*. 2004;38:1631-1634.
91. Sadeque AJ, Wandel C, He H, et al. Increased drug delivery to the brain by p-glycoprotein inhibition. *Clin Pharmacol Ther*. 2000;68:231-237.
92. Bahls FH, Ozuna J, Ritchie DE. Interactions between calcium channel blockers and the anticonvulsants carbamazepine and phenytoin. *Neurology*. 1991;41:740-742.
93. Brodie MJ, MacPhee GJ. Carbamazepine neurotoxicity precipitated by diltiazem. *Br Med J (Clin Res Ed)*. 1986;292:1170-1171.
94. Flatmark T. Catecholamine biosynthesis and physiological regulation in neuroendocrine cells. *Acta Physiol Scand*. 2000;168:1-17.
95. Powell CE, Slater IH. Blocking of inhibitory adrenergic receptors by a dichloro analog of isoproterenol. *J Pharmacol Exp Ther*. 1958;122:480-488.
96. Black JW, Stephenson JS. Pharmacology of a new adrenergic beta-receptor-blocking compound (nethalide). *Lancet*. 1962;2:311-314.
97. Black JW, Duncan WA, Shanks RG. Comparison of some properties of pronethalol and propranolol. *Br J Pharmacol Chemother*. 1965;25:577-591.

98. The Nobel Prize in Physiology or Medicine. https://www.Nobelprize.Org/nobel_prizes/medicine/laureates/1988/press.Html.
99. Lands AM, Arnold A, McAuliff JP, et al. Differentiation of receptor systems activated by sympathomimetic amines. *Nature*. 1967;214:597-598.
100. Frishman WH. A historical perspective on the development of β-adrenergic blockers. *J Clin Hypertens*. 2007;9:19-27.
101. Wright P. Untoward effects associated with practolol administration: oculomucocutaneous syndrome. *Br Med J*. 1975;1:595-598.
102. Wall-Manning HJ. Problems with practolol. *Drugs*. 1975;10:336-341.
103. Mehvar R, Brocks DR. Stereospecific pharmacokinetics and pharmacodynamics of beta-adrenergic blockers in humans. *J Pharm Pharm Sci*. 2001;4:185-200.
104. Log P and cLog P Reported Using Perkinelmer Chemdraw 16.0.
105. McAinsh J, Cruickshank JM. Beta-blockers and central nervous system side effects. *Pharmacol Ther*. 1990;46:163-197.
106. Poirier L, Tobe SW. Contemporary use of beta-blockers: clinical relevance of subclassification. *Can J Cardiol*. 2014;30:S9-S15.
107. Shand DG. Pharmacokinetics of propranolol: a review. *Postgrad Med J*. 1976;52(suppl 4):22-25.
108. Borgström L, Johansson CG, Larsson H, et al. Pharmacokinetics of propranolol. *J Pharmacokinet Biopharm*. 1981;9:419-429.
109. Liedholm H, Wahlin-Boll E, Melander A. Mechanisms and variations in the food effect on propranolol bioavailability. *Eur J Clin Pharmacol*. 1990;38:469-475.
110. Silber B, Riegelman S. Stereospecific assay for (−)- and (+)-propranolol in human and dog plasma. *J Pharmacol Exp Ther*. 1980;215:643-648.
111. Masubuchi Y, Hosokawa S, Horie T, et al. Cytochrome p450 isozymes involved in propranolol metabolism in human liver microsomes. The role of cyp2d6 as ring-hydroxylase and cyp1a2 as n-desisopropylase. *Drug Metab Dispos*. 1994;22:909-915.
112. Rowland K, Yeo WW, Ellis SW, et al. Inhibition of cyp2d6 activity by treatment with propranolol and the role of 4-hydroxy propranolol. *Br J Clin Pharmacol*. 1994;38:9-14.
113. Food and Drug Administration. https://www.Accessdata.Fda.Gov/drugsatfda_docs/label/2011/016418s080, 016762s017, 017683s008lbl.Pdf.
114. Patten SB. Propranolol and depression: evidence from the antihypertensive trials. *Can J Psychiatry*. 1990;35:257-259.
115. Suzman MM. Propranolol in the treatment of anxiety. *Postgrad Med J*. 1976;52(suppl 4):168-174.
116. Garza I, Swanson JW. Prophylaxis of migraine. *Neuropsychiatr Dis Treat*. 2006;2:281-291.
117. McAinsh J, Baber NS, Smith R, et al. Pharmacokinetic and pharmacodynamic studies with long-acting propranolol. *Br J Clin Pharmacol*. 1978;6:115-121.
118. Nace GS, Wood AJ. Pharmacokinetics of long acting propranolol. Implications for therapeutic use. *Clin Pharmacokinet*. 1987;13:51-64.
119. Kirch W, Gorg KG. Clinical pharmacokinetics of atenolol–a review. *Eur J Drug Metab Pharmacokinet*. 1982;7:81-91.
120. Barber HE, Hawksworth GM, Kitteringham NR, et al. Protein binding of atenolol and propranolol to human serum albumin and in human plasma [proceedings]. *Br J Clin Pharmacol*. 1978;6:446P-447P.
121. Reeves PR, McAinsh J, McIntosh DA, et al. Metabolism of atenolol in man. *Xenobiotica*. 1978;8:313-320.
122. Food and Drug Administration. https://www.Accessdata.Fda.Gov/drugsatfda_docs/label/2011/018240s031lbl.Pdf.
123. Kukin ML, Mannino MM, Freudenberger RS, et al. Hemodynamic comparison of twice daily metoprolol tartrate with once daily metoprolol succinate in congestive heart failure. *J Am Coll Cardiol*. 2000;35:45-50.
124. Tangeman HJ, Patterson JH. Extended-release metoprolol succinate in chronic heart failure. *Ann Pharmacother*. 2003;37:701-710.
125. Regårdh CG, Johnsson G. Clinical pharmacokinetics of metoprolol. *Clin Pharmacokinet*. 1980;5:557-569.
126. Rigby JW, Scott AK, Hawksworth GM, et al. A comparison of the pharmacokinetics of atenolol, metoprolol, oxprenolol and propranolol in elderly hypertensive and young healthy subjects. *Br J Clin Pharmacol*. 1985;20:327-331.
127. McGourty JC, Silas JH, Lennard MS, et al. Metoprolol metabolism and debrisoquine oxidation polymorphism–population and family studies. *Br J Clin Pharmacol*. 1985;20:555-566.
128. Quarterman CP, Kendall MJ, Jack DB. The effect of age on the pharmacokinetics of metoprolol and its metabolites. *Br J Clin Pharmacol*. 1981;11:287-294.
129. Rau T, Heide R, Bergmann K, et al. Effect of the cyp2d6 genotype on metoprolol metabolism persists during long-term treatment. *Pharmacogenetics*. 2002;12:465-472.
130. Blake CM, Kharasch ED, Schwab M, et al. A meta-analysis of cyp2d6 metabolizer phenotype and metoprolol pharmacokinetics. *Clin Pharmacol Ther*. 2013;94:394-399.
131. Wuttke H, Rau T, Heide R, et al. Increased frequency of cytochrome P450 2D6 poor metabolizers among patients with metoprolol-associated adverse effects. *Clin Pharmacol Ther*. 2002;72:429-437.
132. Leopold G. Balanced pharmacokinetics and metabolism of bisoprolol. *J Cardiovasc Pharmacol*. 1986;8(suppl 11):S16-S20.
133. Zisaki A, Miskovic L, Hatzimanikatis V. Antihypertensive drugs metabolism: an update to pharmacokinetic profiles and computational approaches. *Curr Pharm Des*. 2015;21:806-822.
134. Food and Drug Administration. https://www.Accessdata.Fda.Gov/drugsatfda_docs/label/2005/020297s013lbl.Pdf.
135. Hamed R, Awadallah A, Sunoqrot S, et al. Ph-dependent solubility and dissolution behavior of carvedilol–case example of a weakly basic BCS class II drug. *AAPS PharmSciTech*. 2016;17:418-426.
136. Ruffolo RR, Gellai M, Hieble JP, et al. The pharmacology of carvedilol. *Eur J Clin Pharmacol*. 1990;38(suppl 2):S82-S88.
137. Morgan T. Clinical pharmacokinetics and pharmacodynamics of carvedilol. *Clin Pharmacokinet*. 1994;26:335-346.
138. Zhou HH, Wood AJ. Stereoselective disposition of carvedilol is determined by CYP2D6. *Clin Pharmacol Ther*. 1995;57:518-524.
139. Neugebauer G, Akpan W, von Mollendorff E, et al. Pharmacokinetics and disposition of carvedilol in humans. *J Cardiovasc Pharmacol*. 1987;10(suppl 11):S85-S88.
140. Oldham HG, Clarke SE. In vitro identification of the human cytochrome P450 enzymes involved in the metabolism of R(+)- and S(−)-carvedilol. *Drug Metab Dispos*. 1997;25:970-977.
141. Gehr TW, Tenero DM, Boyle DA, et al. The pharmacokinetics of carvedilol and its metabolites after single and multiple dose oral administration in patients with hypertension and renal insufficiency. *Eur J Clin Pharmacol*. 1999;55:269-277.
142. Brodde OE, Kroemer HK. Drug-drug interactions of beta-adrenoceptor blockers. *Arzneimittelforschung*. 2003;53:814-822.
143. Hamelin BA, Bouayad A, Methot J, et al. Significant interaction between the nonprescription antihistamine diphenhydramine and the CYP2D6 substrate metoprolol in healthy men with high or low CYP2D6 activity. *Clin Pharmacol Ther*. 2000;67:466-477.
144. Johnson JA, Burlew BS. Metoprolol metabolism via cytochrome P4502D6 in ethnic populations. *Drug Metab Dispos*. 1996;24:350-355.
145. Molden E, Spigset O. Interactions between metoprolol and antidepressants. *Tidsskr Nor Laegeforen*. 2011;131:1777-1779.
146. Kakumoto M, Sakaeda T, Takara K, et al. Effects of carvedilol on MDR1-mediated multidrug resistance: comparison with verapamil. *Cancer Sci*. 2003;94:81-86.
147. Bachmakov I, Werner U, Endress B, et al. Characterization of beta-adrenoceptor antagonists as substrates and inhibitors of the drug transporter p-glycoprotein. *Fundam Clin Pharmacol*. 2006;20:273-282.
148. Giessmann T, Modess C, Hecker U, et al. CYP2D6 genotype and induction of intestinal drug transporters by rifampin predict presystemic clearance of carvedilol in healthy subjects. *Clin Pharmacol Ther*. 2004;75:213-222.
149. Frishman WH. Beta-adrenergic receptor blockers. Adverse effects and drug interactions. *Hypertension*. 1988;11:II21-II29.

150. Abrams J, Jones CA, Kirkpatrick P. Ranolazine. *Nat Rev Drug Discov*. 2006;5:453-454.
151. Jerling M. Clinical pharmacokinetics of ranolazine. *Clin Pharmacokinet*. 2006;45:469-491.
152. Jerling M, Huan BL, Leung K, et al. Studies to investigate the pharmacokinetic interactions between ranolazine and ketoconazole, diltiazem, or simvastatin during combined administration in healthy subjects. *J Clin Pharmacol*. 2005;45:422-433.
153. Penman AD, Eadie J, Herron WJ, et al. The characterization of the metabolites of ranolazine in man by liquid chromatography mass spectrometry. *Rapid Commun Mass Spectrom*. 1995;9:1418-1430.
154. Morrow DA, Scirica BM, Karwatowska-Prokopczuk E, et al. Effects of ranolazine on recurrent cardiovascular events in patients with non-st-elevation acute coronary syndromes: the merlin-timi 36 randomized trial. *JAMA*. 2007;297:1775-1783.
155. Liu Z, Williams RB, Rosen BD. The potential contribution of ranolazine to torsade de pointe. *J Cardiovasc Dis Res*. 2013;4:187-190.
156. Vilaine JP. The discovery of the selective I(f) current inhibitor ivabradine. A new therapeutic approach to ischemic heart disease. *Pharmacol Res*. 2006;53:424-434.
157. Amgen Inc. Corlanor (ivabradine) prescribing information. http://pi.Amgen.Com/~/media/amgen/repositorysites/pi-amgen-com/corlanor/corlanor_pi.Pdf.
158. Vlase L, Popa A, Neag M, et al. Pharmacokinetic interaction between ivabradine and phenytoin in healthy subjects. *Clin Drug Investig*. 2012;32:533-538.
159. Vlase L, Neag M, Popa A, et al. Pharmacokinetic interaction between ivabradine and carbamazepine in healthy volunteers. *J Clin Pharm Ther*. 2011;36:225-229.
160. Savelieva I, Camm AJ. Novel if current inhibitor ivabradine: safety considerations. *Adv Cardiol*. 2006;43:79-96.
161. Mozaffarian D, Benjamin EJ, Go AS, et al. Heart disease and stroke statistics–2015 update: a report from the american heart association. *Circulation*. 2015;131:e29-e322.
162. Toschi-Dias E, Rondon M, Cogliati C, et al. Contribution of autonomic reflexes to the hyperadrenergic state in heart failure. *Front Neurosci*. 2017;11:162.
163. Kobirumaki-Shimozawa F, Inoue T, Shintani SA, et al. Cardiac thin filament regulation and the frank-starling mechanism. *J Physiol Sci*. 2014;64:221-232.
164. Sequeira V, van der Velden J. Historical perspective on heart function: the frank-starling law. *Biophys Rev*. 2015;7:421-447.
165. LaCombe P, Lappin SL. *Physiology, Cardiovascular, Starling Relationships*; 2018.
166. Laursen M, Gregersen JL, Yatime L, et al. Structures and characterization of digoxin- and bufalin-bound Na+, K+-ATPase compared with the ouabain-bound complex. *Proc Natl Acad Sci USA*. 2015;112:1755-1760.
167. Tian J, Xie ZJ. The Na-K-ATPase and calcium-signaling microdomains. *Physiology (Bethesda)*. 2008;23:205-211.
168. Konstantinou DM, Karvounis H, Giannakoulas G. Digoxin in heart failure with a reduced ejection fraction: a risk factor or a risk marker. *Cardiology*. 2016;134:311-319.
169. Boswell-Smith V, Spina D, Page CP. Phosphodiesterase inhibitors. *Br J Pharmacol*. 2006;147(suppl 1):S252-S257.
170. Lugnier C. Cyclic nucleotide phosphodiesterase (PDE) superfamily: a new target for the development of specific therapeutic agents. *Pharmacol Ther*. 2006;109:366-398.
171. Lehtonen LA, Antila S, Pentikainen PJ. Pharmacokinetics and pharmacodynamics of intravenous inotropic agents. *Clin Pharmacokinet*. 2004;43:187-203.
172. Teerlink JR. A novel approach to improve cardiac performance: cardiac myosin activators. *Heart Fail Rev*. 2009;14:289-298.
173. Koster G, Bekema HJ, Wetterslev J, et al. Milrinone for cardiac dysfunction in critically ill adult patients: a systematic review of randomised clinical trials with meta-analysis and trial sequential analysis. *Intensive Care Med*. 2016;42:1322-1335.
174. Felker GM, Benza RL, Chandler AB, et al. Heart failure etiology and response to milrinone in decompensated heart failure: results from the OPTIME-CHF study. *J Am Coll Cardiol*. 2003;41:997-1003.
175. Tuttle RR, Hillmann CC, Toomey RE. Differential beta adrenergic sensitivity of atrial and ventricular tissue assessed by chronotropic, inotropic, and cyclic amp responses to isoprenaline and dobutamine. *Cardiovasc Res*. 1976;10:452-458.
176. Ruffolo RR. The pharmacology of dobutamine. *Am J Med Sci*. 1987;294:244-248.
177. Clark D, Hjorth S, Carlsson A. Dopamine-receptor agonists: mechanisms underlying autoreceptor selectivity. I. Review of the evidence. *J Neural Transm*. 1985;62:1-52.
178. Gerber JG, Freed CR, Nies AS. Antihypertensive pharmacology. *West J Med*. 1980;132:430-439.
179. Cole RT, Kalogeropoulos AP, Georgiopoulou VV, et al. Hydralazine and isosorbide dinitrate in heart failure: historical perspective, mechanisms, and future directions. *Circulation*. 2011;123:2414-2422.
180. Ramsay LE, Cameron HA. The lupus syndrome induced by hydralazine. *Br Med J (Clin Res Ed)*. 1984;289:1310-1311.
181. Roden DM. Antiarrhythmic drugs: from mechanisms to clinical practice. *Heart*. 2000;84:339-346.
182. Fala L. Entresto (sacubitril/valsartan): first-in-class angiotensin receptor neprilysin inhibitor fda approved for patients with heart failure. *Am Health Drug Benefits*. 2015;8:330-334.
183. Volpe M, Carnovali M, Mastromarino V. The natriuretic peptides system in the pathophysiology of heart failure: from molecular basis to treatment. *Clin Sci (Lond)*. 2016;130:57-77.
184. Agrawal AA, Petschenka G, Bingham RA, et al. Toxic cardenolides: chemical ecology and coevolution of specialized plant-herbivore interactions. *New Phytol*. 2012;194:28-45.
185. Withering W. *An Account of the Foxglove and Some of Its Medical Uses With Practical Remarks on Dropsy and Other Diseases*. London: G.G.J. and J. Robinson; 1785.
186. Wilkins MR, Kendall MJ, Wade OL. William withering and digitalis, 1785 to 1985. *Br Med J*. 1985;290:7-8.
187. Smith S. Digoxin, a new digitalis glycoside. *J Chem Soc*. 1930:508-510.
188. Patel S. Plant-derived cardiac glycosides: role in heart ailments and cancer management. *Biomed Pharmacother*. 2016;84:1036-1041.
189. Hollman A. Plants and cardiac glycosides. *Br Heart J*. 1985;54:258-261.
190. Blanco G, Mercer RW. Isozymes of the na-k-atpase: heterogeneity in structure, diversity in function. *Am J Physiol*. 1998;275:F633-F650.
191. Katz A, Lifshitz Y, Bab-Dinitz E, et al. Selectivity of digitalis glycosides for isoforms of human Na,K-ATPase. *J Biol Chem*. 2010;285:19582-19592.
192. Erdmann E. Influence of cardiac glycosides on their receptor. In: Greef K, ed. *Cardiac Glycosides: Part I: Experimental Pharmacology*. Vol 56. Berlin: Springer-Verlag; 1981:337-380.
193. Cerri A, Serra F, Ferrari P, et al. Synthesis, cardiotonic activity, and structure-activity relationships of 17 beta-guanylhydrazone derivatives of 5 beta-androstane-3 beta, 14 beta-diol acting on the Na+,K(+)-ATPase receptor. *J Med Chem*. 1997;40:3484-3488.
194. Cerri A, Almirante N, Barassi P, et al. 17beta-o-aminoalkyloximes of 5beta-androstane-3beta,14beta-diol with digitalis-like activity: synthesis, cardiotonic activity, structure-activity relationships, and molecular modeling of the Na(+),K(+)-ATPase receptor. *J Med Chem*. 2000;43:2332-2349.
195. Iisalo E. Clinical pharmacokinetics of digoxin. *Clin Pharmacokinet*. 1977;2:1-16.
196. Aronson JK. Clinical pharmacokinetics of digoxin 1980. *Clin Pharmacokinet*. 1980;5:137-149.
197. Food and Drug Administration. https://www.Accessdata.Fda.Gov/scripts/cder/daf/index.Cfm?Event=overview.Process&applno=018118.

198. Marcus FI. Digitalis pharmacokinetics and metabolism. *Am J Med.* 1975;58:452-459.
199. Abernethy DR, Greenblatt DJ, Smith TW. Digoxin disposition in obesity: clinical pharmacokinetic investigation. *Am Heart J.* 1981;102:740-744.
200. Noviasky J, Darko W, Akajabor D, et al. Digoxin. In: Cohen H, ed. *Casebook in Clinical Pharmacokinetics and Drug Dosing.* New York, NY: McGraw-Hill Education; 2015.
201. Cheng JW, Charland SL, Shaw LM, et al. Is the volume of distribution of digoxin reduced in patients with renal dysfunction? Determining digoxin pharmacokinetics by fluorescence polarization immunoassay. *Pharmacotherapy.* 1997;17:584-590.
202. Bendayan R, McKenzie MW. Digoxin pharmacokinetics and dosage requirements in pediatric patients. *Clin Pharm.* 1983;2:224-235.
203. Soyka LF. Digoxin: placental transfer, effects on the fetus, and therapeutic use in the newborn. *Clin Perinatol.* 1975;2:23-35.
204. Lindenbaum J, Rund DG, Butler VP, et al. Inactivation of digoxin by the gut flora: reversal by antibiotic therapy. *N Engl J Med.* 1981;305:789-794.
205. Ito S, Woodland C, Harper PA, et al. P-glycoprotein-mediated renal tubular secretion of digoxin: the toxicological significance of the urine-blood barrier model. *Life Sci.* 1993;53:PL25-PL31.
206. Ewy GA, Kapadia GG, Yao L, et al. Digoxin metabolism in the elderly. *Circulation.* 1969;39:449-453.
207. Croxson MS, Ibbertson HK. Serum digoxin in patients with thyroid disease. *Br Med J.* 1975;3:566-568.
208. Bauer LA. *Digoxin. Applied Clinical Pharmacokinetics.* 3rd ed. New York, NY: McGraw-Hill Medical; 2015.
209. Kramer P. Digitalis pharmacokinetics and therapy with respect to impaired renal function. *Klin Wochenschr.* 1977;55:1-11.
210. Santos SR, Kirch W, Ohnhaus EE. Simultaneous analysis of digitoxin and its clinically relevant metabolites using high-performance liquid chromatography and radioimmunoassay. *J Chromatogr.* 1987;419:155-164.
211. Nokhodian A, Santos SR, Kirch W. Digitoxin and its metabolites in patients with liver cirrhosis. *Eur J Drug Metab Pharmacokinet.* 1993;18:207-213.
212. Currie GM, Wheat JM, Kiat H. Pharmacokinetic considerations for digoxin in older people. *Open Cardiovasc Med J.* 2011;5:130-135.
213. Dec GW. Digoxin remains useful in the management of chronic heart failure. *Med Clin North Am.* 2003;87:317-337.
214. Ehle M, Patel C, Giugliano RP. Digoxin: clinical highlights: a review of digoxin and its use in contemporary medicine. *Crit Pathw Cardiol.* 2011;10:93-98.
215. MacLeod-Glover N, Mink M, Yarema M, et al. Digoxin toxicity: case for retiring its use in elderly patients? *Can Fam Physician.* 2016;62:223-228.
216. Dawson AH, Buckley NA. Digoxin. *Medicine.* 2016;44:158-159.
217. Hooymans PM, Merkus FW. Current status of cardiac glycoside drug interactions. *Clin Pharm.* 1985;4:404-413.
218. de Lannoy IA, Silverman M. The MDR1 gene product, p-glycoprotein, mediates the transport of the cardiac glycoside, digoxin. *Biochem Biophys Res Commun.* 1992;189:551-557.
219. Gomes T, Mamdani MM, Juurlink DN. Macrolide-induced digoxin toxicity: a population-based study. *Clin Pharmacol Ther.* 2009;86:383-386.
220. Fromm MF, Kim RB, Stein CM, et al. Inhibition of p-glycoprotein-mediated drug transport: a unifying mechanism to explain the interaction between digoxin and quinidine [seecomments]. *Circulation.* 1999;99:552-557.
221. Bigger JT, Leahey EB. Quinidine and digoxin. An important interaction. *Drugs.* 1982;24:229-239.
222. Schenck-Gustafsson K, Dahlqvist R. Pharmacokinetics of digoxin in patients subjected to the quinidine-digoxin interaction. *Br J Clin Pharmacol.* 1981;11:181-186.
223. Pedersen KE, Christiansen BD, Klitgaard NA, et al. Effect of quinidine on digoxin bioavailability. *Eur J Clin Pharmacol.* 1983;24:41-47.
224. Ledwitch KV, Barnes RW, Roberts AG. Unravelling the complex drug-drug interactions of the cardiovascular drugs, verapamil and digoxin, with p-glycoprotein. *Biosci Rep.* 2016;36.
225. Ledwitch KV, Roberts AG. Cardiovascular ion channel inhibitor drug-drug interactions with p-glycoprotein. *AAPS J.* 2017;19:409-420.
226. Pedersen KE, Dorph-Pedersen A, Hvidt S, et al. Digoxin-verapamil interaction. *Clin Pharmacol Ther.* 1981;30:311-316.
227. Robinson K, Johnston A, Walker S, et al. The digoxin-amiodarone interaction. *Cardiovasc Drugs Ther.* 1989;3:25-28.
228. Okamura N, Hirai M, Tanigawara Y, et al. Digoxin-cyclosporin a interaction: modulation of the multidrug transporter p-glycoprotein in the kidney. *J Pharmacol Exp Ther.* 1993;266:1614-1619.
229. Greiner B, Eichelbaum M, Fritz P, et al. The role of intestinal p-glycoprotein in the interaction of digoxin and rifampin. *J Clin Invest.* 1999;104:147-153.
230. Hall WH, Shappell SD, Doherty JE. Effect of cholestyramine on digoxin absorption and excretion in man. *Am J Cardiol.* 1977;39:213-216.
231. McElnay JC, Harron DW, D'Arcy PF, et al. Interaction of digoxin with antacid constituents. *Br Med J.* 1978;1:1554.
232. Chan BS, Buckley NA. Digoxin-specific antibody fragments in the treatment of digoxin toxicity. *Clin Toxicol (Phila).* 2014;52:824-836.
233. Digifab Prescribing Information. http://www.Digifab.Us/download/digifab_package_insert.pdf.
234. Ujhelyi MR, Robert S. Pharmacokinetic aspects of digoxin-specific Fab therapy in the management of digitalis toxicity. *Clin Pharmacokinet.* 1995;28:483-493.
235. Erdman r A. Phosphodiesterase inhibitors. In: Dart CR, ed. *Medical Toxicology.*3rd ed. Philadelphia: Lippincott Williams & Wilkins; 2004:706-710.
236. Levy JH, Bailey JM. Amrinone: pharmacokinetics and pharmacodynamics. *J Cardiothorac Anesth.* 1989;3:10-14.
237. Young RA, Ward A. Milrinone. A preliminary review of its pharmacological properties and therapeutic use. *Drugs.* 1988;36:158-192.
238. Packer M, Carver JR, Rodeheffer RJ, et al. Effect of oral milrinone on mortality in severe chronic heart failure. The promise study research group. *N Engl J Med.* 1991;325:1468-1475.
239. Shipley JB, Tolman D, Hastillo A, et al. Milrinone: basic and clinical pharmacology and acute and chronic management. *Am J Med Sci.* 1996;311:286-291.
240. Edelson J, Stroshane R, Benziger DP, et al. Pharmacokinetics of the bipyridines amrinone and milrinone. *Circulation.* 1986;73:III145-III152.
241. Taniguchi T, Shibata K, Saito S, et al. Pharmacokinetics of milrinone in patients with congestive heart failure during continuous venovenous hemofiltration. *Intensive Care Med.* 2000;26:1089-1093.
242. Woolfrey SG, Hegbrant J, Thysell H, et al. Dose regimen adjustment for milrinone in congestive heart failure patients with moderate and severe renal failure. *J Pharm Pharmacol.* 1995;47:651-655.
243. Amsallem E, Kasparian C, Haddour G, et al. Phosphodiesterase III inhibitors for heart failure. *Cochrane Database Syst Rev.* 2005;(1):CD002230.
244. Riley CM. Stability of milrinone and digoxin, furosemide, procainamide hydrochloride, propranolol hydrochloride, quinidine gluconate, or verapamil hydrochloride in 5% dextrose injection. *Am J Hosp Pharm.* 1988;45:2079-2091.
245. Maron BA, Rocco TP. Pharmacotherapy of congestive heart failure. In: Brunton LL, Chabner BA, Knollmann BC, eds. *Goodman & Gilman's: The Pharmacological Basis of Therapeutics.* 12th ed. New York, NY: McGraw-Hill Education; 2011.
246. MacGregor DA, Smith TE, Prielipp RC, et al. Pharmacokinetics of dopamine in healthy male subjects. *Anesthesiology.* 2000;92:338-346.
247. Meiser J, Weindl D, Hiller K. Complexity of dopamine metabolism. *Cell Commun Signal.* 2013;11:34.

248. Tuttle RR, Mills J. Dobutamine: development of a new catecholamine to selectively increase cardiac contractility. *Circ Res*. 1975;36:185-196.
249. Ruffolo RR, Spradlin TA, Pollock GD, et al. Alpha and beta adrenergic effects of the stereoisomers of dobutamine. *J Pharmacol Exp Ther*. 1981;219:447-452.
250. Kang SY, Lee JW, Park DE, et al. Hypereosinophilia with rash to dobutamine infusion; sulfite hypersensitivity diagnosed by in vitro stimulation assays. *Allergol Int*. 2016;65:477-480.
251. Hilal-Dandan R, Brunton LL. *Adrenergic Agonists and Antagonists. Goodman and Gilman's Manual of Pharmacology and Therapeutics*. 2nd ed. New York, NY: McGraw-Hill Education; 2016.
252. Yan M, Webster LT, Blumer JL. 3-O-methyldobutamine, a major metabolite of dobutamine in humans. *Drug Metab Dispos*. 2002;30:519-524.
253. Yan M, Webster LT, Blumer JL. Kinetic interactions of dopamine and dobutamine with human catechol-O-methyltransferase and monoamine oxidase in vitro. *J Pharmacol Exp Ther*. 2002;301:315-321.
254. Taylor AL, Ziesche S, Yancy C, et al. Combination of isosorbide dinitrate and hydralazine in blacks with heart failure. *N Engl J Med*. 2004;351:2049-2057.
255. Reece PA. Hydralazine and related compounds: chemistry, metabolism, and mode of action. *Med Res Rev*. 1981;1:73-96.
256. Arbor Pharmaceuticals, LLC. Bidil (Isosorbide Dinitrate and Hydralazine Hydrochloride) Tablet Prescribing Information.
257. Facchini V, Timbrell JA. Further evidence for an acetylator phenotype difference in the metabolism of hydralazine in man. *Br J Clin Pharmacol*. 1981;11:345-351.
258. Food and Drug Administration. https://www.Fda.Gov/newsevents/newsroom/pressannouncements/ucm453845.Htm.
259. Gu J, Noe A, Chandra P, et al. Pharmacokinetics and pharmacodynamics of LCZ696, a novel dual-acting angiotensin receptor-neprilysin inhibitor (ARNi). *J Clin Pharmacol*. 2010;50:401-414.
260. Ksander GM, Ghai RD, deJesus R, et al. Dicarboxylic acid dipeptide neutral endopeptidase inhibitors. *J Med Chem*. 1995;38:1689-1700.
261. Schiering N, D'Arcy A, Villard F, et al. Structure of neprilysin in complex with the active metabolite of sacubitril. *Sci Rep*. 2016;6:27909.
262. Flesch G, Muller P, Lloyd P. Absolute bioavailability and pharmacokinetics of valsartan, an angiotensin ii receptor antagonist, in man. *Eur J Clin Pharmacol*. 1997;52:115-120.
263. Criscione L, de Gasparo M, Buhlmayer P, et al. Pharmacological profile of valsartan: a potent, orally active, nonpeptide antagonist of the angiotensin ii at1-receptor subtype. *Br J Pharmacol*. 1993;110:761-771.
264. Novartis Pharmaceuticals Corporation. Entresto (Sacubitril and Valsartan) Prescribing Information.
265. Feng L, Karpinski PH, Sutton P, et al. LCZ696: a dual-acting sodium supramolecular complex. *Tetrahedron Lett*. 2012;53(3):275-276.
266. Ayalasomayajula S, Langenickel T, Pal P, et al. Clinical pharmacokinetics of sacubitril/valsartan (LCZ696): a novel angiotensin receptor-neprilysin inhibitor. *Clin Pharmacokinet*. 2017;56(12):1461-1478.
267. Kobalava Z, Kotovskaya Y, Averkov O, et al. Pharmacodynamic and pharmacokinetic profiles of sacubitril/valsartan (LCZ696) in patients with heart failure and reduced ejection fraction. *Cardiovasc Ther*. 2016;34:191-198.
268. Flarakos J, Du Y, Bedman T, et al. Disposition and metabolism of [(14)C] sacubitril/valsartan (formerly LCZ696) an angiotensin receptor neprilysin inhibitor, in healthy subjects. *Xenobiotica*. 2016;46:986-1000.
269. Shi J, Wang X, Nguyen J, et al. Sacubitril is selectively activated by carboxylesterase 1 (ces1) in the liver and the activation is affected by ces1 genetic variation. *Drug Metab Dispos*. 2016;44:554-559.
270. Antzelevitch C, Burashnikov A. Overview of basic mechanisms of cardiac arrhythmia. *Card Electrophysiol Clin*. 2011;3:23-45.
271. Klabunde RE. Cardiac electrophysiology: normal and ischemic ionic currents and the ECG. *Adv Physiol Educ*. 2017;41:29-37.
272. Glitsch HG. Electrophysiology of the sodium-potassium-atpase in cardiac cells. *Physiol Rev*. 2001;81:1791-1826.
273. Wright SH. Generation of resting membrane potential. *Adv Physiol Educ*. 2004;28:139-142.
274. Bartos DC, Grandi E, Ripplinger CM. Ion channels in the heart. *Compr Physiol*. 2015;5:1423-1464.
275. Schmitt N, Grunnet M, Olesen SP. Cardiac potassium channel subtypes: new roles in repolarization and arrhythmia. *Physiol Rev*. 2014;94:609-653.
276. King GS, McGuigan JJ. Antiarrhythmic medications. 2018.
277. Grant AO, Starmer CF, Strauss HC. Antiarrhythmic drug action. Blockade of the inward sodium current. *Circ Res*. 1984;55:427-439.
278. Sheets MF, Fozzard HA, Lipkind GM, et al. Sodium channel molecular conformations and antiarrhythmic drug affinity. *Trends Cardiovasc Med*. 2010;20:16-21.
279. Cubeddu LX. QT prolongation and fatal arrhythmias: a review of clinical implications and effects of drugs. *Am J Ther*. 2003;10:452-457.
280. Manolis AS, Deering TF, Cameron J, et al. Mexiletine: pharmacology and therapeutic use. *Clin Cardiol*. 1990;13:349-359.
281. Salvage SC, Chandrasekharan KH, Jeevaratnam K, et al. Multiple targets for flecainide action: implications for cardiac arrhythmogenesis. *Br J Pharmacol*. 2017;175(8):1260-1278.
282. Bryson HM, Palmer KJ, Langtry HD, et al. Propafenone. A reappraisal of its pharmacology, pharmacokinetics and therapeutic use in cardiac arrhythmias. *Drugs*. 1993;45:85-130.
283. Naccarelli GV, Wolbrette DL, Khan M, et al. Old and new antiarrhythmic drugs for converting and maintaining sinus rhythm in atrial fibrillation: comparative efficacy and results of trials. *Am J Cardiol*. 2003;91:15D-26D.
284. Singh BN. Antiarrhythmic actions of amiodarone: a profile of a paradoxical agent. *Am J Cardiol*. 1996;78:41-53.
285. Anderson JL, Prystowsky EN. Sotalol: an important new antiarrhythmic. *Am Heart J*. 1999;137:388-409.
286. Singh B. A fourth class of anti-dysrhythmic action? Effect of verapamil and ouabain toxicity, on atrial and ventricular intracellular potentials, and on other features of cardiac function. *Cardiovasc Res*. 2000;45:39-42.
287. Thomas SH, Behr ER. Pharmacological treatment of acquired qt prolongation and torsades de pointes. *Br J Clin Pharmacol*. 2016;81:420-427.
288. Weinreb SM. Chemistry. Synthetic lessons from quinine. *Nature*. 2001;411:429, 431.
289. Warhurst DC, Craig JC, Adagu IS, et al. The relationship of physico-chemical properties and structure to the differential antiplasmodial activity of the cinchona alkaloids. *Malar J*. 2003;2:26.
290. Bauer LA. *Quinidine. Applied clinical pharmacokinetics*. 3rd ed. New York, NY: McGraw-Hill Medical; 2015.
291. Ueda CT, Williamson BJ, Dzindzio BS. Disposition kinetics of dihydroquinidine following quinidine administration. *Res Commun Chem Pathol Pharmacol*. 1976;14:215-225.
292. Ueda CT, Williamson BJ, Dzindzio BS. Absolute quinidine bioavailability. *Clin Pharmacol Ther*. 1976;20:260-265.
293. Ochs HR, Greenblatt DJ, Woo E, et al. Reduced quinidine clearance in elderly persons. *Am J Cardiol*. 1978;42:481-485.
294. Ochs HR, Greenblatt DJ, Woo E. Clinical pharmacokinetics of quinidine. *Clin Pharmacokinet*. 1980;5:150-168.
295. Nielsen F, Nielsen KK, Brosen K. Determination of quinidine, dihydroquinidine, (3S)-3-hydroxyquinidine and quinidine N-oxide in plasma and urine by high-performance liquid chromatography. *J Chromatogr B Biomed Appl*. 1994;660:103-110.
296. Mihaly GW, Ching MS, Klejn MB, et al. Differences in the binding of quinine and quinidine to plasma proteins. *Br J Clin Pharmacol*. 1987;24:769-774.
297. Ueda CT, Dzindzio BS. Quinidine kinetics in congestive heart failure. *Clin Pharmacol Ther*. 1978;23:158-164.
298. McLaughlin LA, Paine MJ, Kemp CA, et al. Why is quinidine an inhibitor of cytochrome P450 2D6? The role of key active-site residues in quinidine binding. *J Biol Chem*. 2005;280:38617-38624.

299. Roden DM, Thompson KA, Hoffman BF, et al. Clinical features and basic mechanisms of quinidine-induced arrhythmias. *J Am Coll Cardiol*. 1986;8:73A-78A.
300. Tartini R, Kappenberger L, Steinbrunn W, et al. Dangerous interaction between amiodarone and quinidine. *Lancet*. 1982;1:1327-1329.
301. Cohen IS, Jick H, Cohen SI. Adverse reactions to quinidine in hospitalized patients: findings based on data from the boston collaborative drug surveillance program. *Prog Cardiovasc Dis*. 1977;20:151-163.
302. Sneader W. *In Drug Discovery: A History*. West Sussex, England: John Wiley and Sons, Ltd.; 2005.
303. Karlsson E. Clinical pharmacokinetics of procainamide. *Clin Pharmacokinet*. 1978;3:97-107.
304. Giardina EG. Procainamide: clinical pharmacology and efficacy against ventricular arrhythmias. *Ann NY Acad Sci*. 1984;432:177-188.
305. Woosley RL, Drayer DE, Reidenberg MM, et al. Effect of acetylator phenotype on the rate at which procainamide induces antinuclear antibodies and the lupus syndrome. *N Engl J Med*. 1978;298:1157-1159.
306. Uetrecht JP, Sweetman BJ, Woosley RL, et al. Metabolism of procainamide to a hydroxylamine by rat and human hepatic microsomes. *Drug Metab Dispos*. 1984;12:77-81.
307. Lessard E, Fortin A, Belanger PM, et al. Role of CYP2D6 in the n-hydroxylation of procainamide. *Pharmacogenetics*. 1997;7:381-390.
308. Bauer LA. *Procainamide/N-acetyl procainamide*. *Applied clinical pharmacokinetics*. 3rd ed. New York, NY: McGraw-Hill Medical; 2015.
309. Drayer DE, Lowenthal DT, Woosley RL, et al. Cumulation of N-acetylprocainamide, an active metabolite of procainamide, in patients with impaired renal function. *Clin Pharmacol Ther*. 1977;22:63-69.
310. Bauer LA, Black DJ, Lill JS, et al. Levofloxacin and ciprofloxacin decrease procainamide and N-acetylprocainamide renal clearances. *Antimicrob Agents Chemother*. 2005;49:1649-1651.
311. Bauer LA, Black D, Gensler A. Procainamide-cimetidine drug interaction in elderly male patients. *J Am Geriatr Soc*. 1990;38:467-469.
312. Lawson DH, Jick H. Adverse reactions to procainamide. *Br J Clin Pharmacol*. 1977;4:507-511.
313. Davies RF, Siddoway LA, Shaw L, et al. Immediate- versus controlled-release disopyramide: importance of saturable binding. *Clin Pharmacol Ther*. 1993;54:16-22.
314. Lima JJ, Haughey DB, Leier CV. Disopyramide pharmacokinetics and bioavailability following the simultaneous administration of disopyramide and 14C-disopyramide. *J Pharmacokinet Biopharm*. 1984;12:289-313.
315. Siddoway LA, Woosley RL. Clinical pharmacokinetics of disopyramide. *Clin Pharmacokinet*. 1986;11:214-222.
316. Lima JJ, Boudoulas H, Shields BJ. Stereoselective pharmacokinetics of disopyramide enantiomers in man. *Drug Metab Dispos*. 1985;13:572-577.
317. Lima JJ, Boudoulas H, Blanford M. Concentration-dependence of disopyramide binding to plasma protein and its influence on kinetics and dynamics. *J Pharmacol Exp Ther*. 1981;219:741-747.
318. Bredesen JE, Kierulf P. Relationship between alpha 1-acid glycoprotein and plasma binding of disopyramide and mono-n-dealkyldisopyramide. *Br J Clin Pharmacol*. 1984;18:779-784.
319. Echizen H, Tanizaki M, Tatsuno J, et al. Identification of cyp3a4 as the enzyme involved in the mono-n-dealkylation of disopyramide enantiomers in humans. *Drug Metab Dispos*. 2000;28:937-944.
320. Aitio ML. Plasma concentrations and protein binding of disopyramide and mono-n-dealkyldisopyramide during chronic oral disopyramide therapy. *Br J Clin Pharmacol*. 1981;11:369-375.
321. Granowitz EV, Tabor KJ, Kirchhoffer JB. Potentially fatal interaction between azithromycin and disopyramide. *Pacing Clin Electrophysiol*. 2000;23:1433-1435.
322. Hayashi Y, Ikeda U, Hashimoto T, et al. Torsades de pointes ventricular tachycardia induced by clarithromycin and disopyramide in the presence of hypokalemia. *Pacing Clin Electrophysiol*. 1999;22:672-674.
323. Teichman S. The anticholinergic side effects of disopyramide and controlled-release disopyramide. *Angiology*. 1985;36:767-771.
324. Di Bianco R, Gottdiener JS, Singh SN, et al. A review of the effects of disopyramide phosphate on left ventricular function and the peripheral circulation. *Angiology*. 1987;38:174-183.
325. Collinsworth KA, Kalman SM, Harrison DC. The clinical pharmacology of lidocaine as an antiarrhythymic drug. *Circulation*. 1974;50:1217-1230.
326. Boyes RN, Scott DB, Jebson PJ, et al. Pharmacokinetics of lidocaine in man. *Clin Pharmacol Ther*. 1971;12:105-116.
327. Routledge PA, Barchowsky A, Bjornsson TD, et al. Lidocaine plasma protein binding. *Clin Pharmacol Ther*. 1980;27:347-351.
328. Abernethy DR, Greenblatt DJ. Lidocaine disposition in obesity. *Am J Cardiol*. 1984;53:1183-1186.
329. Wang JS, Backman JT, Taavitsainen P, et al. Involvement of CYP1A2 AND CYP3A4 in lidocaine N-deethylation and 3-hydroxylation in humans. *Drug Metab Dispos*. 2000;28:959-965.
330. Nation RL, Triggs EJ, Selig M. Lignocaine kinetics in cardiac patients and aged subjects. *Br J Clin Pharmacol*. 1977;4:439-448.
331. Thomson PD, Melmon KL, Richardson JA, et al. Lidocaine pharmacokinetics in advanced heart failure, liver disease, and renal failure in humans. *Ann Intern Med*. 1973;78:499-508.
332. Bauer LA. Chapter 7. Lidocaine. In: Bauer LA, ed. *Applied Clinical Pharmacokinetics*. 2nd ed. New York, NY: The McGraw-Hill Companies; 2008.
333. Orlando R, Piccoli P, De Martin S, et al. Cytochrome P450 1A2 is a major determinant of lidocaine metabolism in vivo: effects of liver function. *Clin Pharmacol Ther*. 2004;75:80-88.
334. Orlando R, Piccoli P, De Martin S, et al. Effect of the CYP3A4 inhibitor erythromycin on the pharmacokinetics of lignocaine and its pharmacologically active metabolites in subjects with normal and impaired liver function. *Br J Clin Pharmacol*. 2003;55:86-93.
335. Ha HR, Candinas R, Stieger B, et al. Interaction between amiodarone and lidocaine. *J Cardiovasc Pharmacol*. 1996;28:533-539.
336. Knapp AB, Maguire W, Keren G, et al. The cimetidine-lidocaine interaction. *Ann Intern Med*. 1983;98:174-177.
337. Labbe L, Turgeon J. Clinical pharmacokinetics of mexiletine. *Clin Pharmacokinet*. 1999;37:361-384.
338. Turgeon J, Fiset C, Giguere R, et al. Influence of debrisoquine phenotype and of quinidine on mexiletine disposition in man. *J Pharmacol Exp Ther*. 1991;259:789-798.
339. Fenster PE, Comess KA. Pharmacology and clinical use of mexiletine. *Pharmacotherapy*. 1986;6:1-9.
340. Johnston A, Burgess CD, Warrington SJ, et al. The effect of spontaneous changes in urinary ph on mexiletine plasma concentrations and excretion during chronic administration to healthy volunteers. *Br J Clin Pharmacol*. 1979;8:349-352.
341. Wing LM, Meffin PJ, Grygiel JJ, et al. The effect of metoclopramide and atropine on the absorption of orally administered mexiletine. *Br J Clin Pharmacol*. 1980;9:505-509.
342. Herzog P, Holtermuller KH, Kasper W, et al. Absorption of mexiletine after treatment with gastric antacids. *Br J Clin Pharmacol*. 1982;14:746-747.
343. Ueno K, Miyai K, Seki T, et al. Interaction between theophylline and mexiletine. *DICP*. 1990;24:471-472.
344. Klein A, Sami M, Selinger K. Mexiletine kinetics in healthy subjects taking cimetidine. *Clin Pharmacol Ther*. 1985;37:669-673.
345. Broly F, Vandamme N, Caron J, et al. Single-dose quinidine treatment inhibits mexiletine oxidation in extensive metabolizers of debrisoquine. *Life Sci*. 1991;48:PL123-PL128.
346. Anderson RJ. The little compound that could: how phenytoin changed drug discovery and development. *Mol Interv*. 2009;9:208-214.
347. Richens A. Clinical pharmacokinetics of phenytoin. *Clin Pharmacokinet*. 1979;4:153-169.

348. Eddy JD, Singh SP. Treatment of cardiac arrhythmias with phenytoin. *Br Med J*. 1969;4:270-273.
349. Vanholder R, Van Landschoot N, De Smet R, et al. Drug protein binding in chronic renal failure: evaluation of nine drugs. *Kidney Int*. 1988;33:996-1004.
350. Perucca E, Hebdige S, Frigo GM, et al. Interaction between phenytoin and valproic acid: plasma protein binding and metabolic effects. *Clin Pharmacol Ther*. 1980;28:779-789.
351. Cuttle L, Munns AJ, Hogg NA, et al. Phenytoin metabolism by human cytochrome P450: involvement of P450 3A and 2C forms in secondary metabolism and drug-protein adduct formation. *Drug Metab Dispos*. 2000;28:945-950.
352. Aronson JK, Hardman M, Reynolds DJ. ABC of monitoring drug therapy. Phenytoin. *BMJ*. 1992;305:1215-1218.
353. Food and Drug Administration. https://www.Accessdata.Fda.Gov/drugsatfda_docs/label/2009/084349s060lbl.Pdf.
354. Desta Z, Zhao X, Shin JG, et al. Clinical significance of the cytochrome P450 2C19 genetic polymorphism. *Clin Pharmacokinet*. 2002;41:913-958.
355. Franco V, Perucca E. CYP2C9 polymorphisms and phenytoin metabolism: implications for adverse effects. *Expert Opin Drug Metab Toxicol*. 2015;11:1269-1279.
356. Aliot E, Capucci A, Crijns HJ, et al. Twenty-five years in the making: flecainide is safe and effective for the management of atrial fibrillation. *Europace*. 2011;13:161-173.
357. Tjandra-Maga TB, Verbesselt R, Van Hecken A, et al. Flecainide: single and multiple oral dose kinetics, absolute bioavailability and effect of food and antacid in man. *Br J Clin Pharmacol*. 1986;22:309-316.
358. Conard GJ, Ober RE. Metabolism of flecainide. *Am J Cardiol*. 1984;53:41B-51B.
359. McQuinn RL, Quarfoth GJ, Johnson JD, et al. Biotransformation and elimination of 14C-flecainide acetate in humans. *Drug Metab Dispos*. 1984;12:414-420.
360. Doki K, Homma M, Kuga K, et al. Effect of CYP2D6 genotype on flecainide pharmacokinetics in Japanese patients with supraventricular tachyarrhythmia. *Eur J Clin Pharmacol*. 2006;62:919-926.
361. Lewis GP, Holtzman JL. Interaction of flecainide with digoxin and propranolol. *Am J Cardiol*. 1984;53:52B-57B.
362. Hii JT, Duff HJ, Burgess ED. Clinical pharmacokinetics of propafenone. *Clin Pharmacokinet*. 1991;21:1-10.
363. Stoschitzky K, Klein W, Stark G, et al. Different stereoselective effects of (R)- and (S)-propafenone: clinical pharmacologic, electrophysiologic, and radioligand binding studies. *Clin Pharmacol Ther*. 1990;47:740-746.
364. Axelson JE, Chan GL, Kirsten EB, et al. Food increases the bioavailability of propafenone. *Br J Clin Pharmacol*. 1987;23:735-741.
365. Hollmann M, Brode E, Hotz D, et al. Investigations on the pharmacokinetics of propafenone in man. *Arzneimittelforschung*. 1983;33:763-770.
366. Oravcova J, Lindner W, Szalay P, et al. Interaction of propafenone enantiomers with human alpha 1-acid glycoprotein. *Chirality*. 1991;3:30-34.
367. Funck-Brentano C, Kroemer HK, Lee JT, et al. Propafenone. *N Engl J Med*. 1990;322:518-525.
368. Brode E, Muller-Peltzer H, Hollmann M. Comparative pharmacokinetics and clinical pharmacology of propafenone enantiomers after oral administration to man. *Methods Find Exp Clin Pharmacol*. 1988;10:717-727.
369. Cai WM, Chen B, Cai MH, et al. The influence of CYP2D6 activity on the kinetics of propafenone enantiomers in Chinese subjects. *Br J Clin Pharmacol*. 1999;47:553-556.
370. Jazwinska-Tarnawska E, Orzechowska-Juzwenko K, Niewinski P, et al. The influence of CYP2D6 polymorphism on the antiarrhythmic efficacy of propafenone in patients with paroxysmal atrial fibrillation during 3 months propafenone prophylactic treatment. *Int J Clin Pharmacol Ther*. 2001;39:288-292.
371. Thompson KA, Iansmith DH, Siddoway LA, et al. Potent electrophysiologic effects of the major metabolites of propafenone in canine purkinje fibers. *J Pharmacol Exp Ther*. 1988;244:950-955.
372. Lee JT, Kroemer HK, Silberstein DJ, et al. The role of genetically determined polymorphic drug metabolism in the beta-blockade produced by propafenone. *N Engl J Med*. 1990;322:1764-1768.
373. Kroemer HK, Mikus G, Kronbach T, et al. In vitro characterization of the human cytochrome P-450 involved in polymorphic oxidation of propafenone. *Clin Pharmacol Ther*. 1989;45:28-33.
374. Fromm MF, Botsch S, Heinkele G, et al. Influence of renal function on the steady-state pharmacokinetics of the antiarrhythmic propafenone and its phase I and phase II metabolites. *Eur J Clin Pharmacol*. 1995;48:279-283.
375. Connolly SJ, Kates RE, Lebsack CS, et al. Clinical pharmacology of propafenone. *Circulation*. 1983;68:589-596.
376. Siddoway LA, Thompson KA, McAllister CB, et al. Polymorphism of propafenone metabolism and disposition in man: clinical and pharmacokinetic consequences. *Circulation*. 1987;75:785-791.
377. Kroemer HK, Funck-Brentano C, Silberstein DJ, et al. Stereoselective disposition and pharmacologic activity of propafenone enantiomers. *Circulation*. 1989;79:1068-1076.
378. Calvo MV, Martin-Suarez A, Martin Luengo C, et al. Interaction between digoxin and propafenone. *Ther Drug Monit*. 1989;11:10-15.
379. Kates RE, Yee YG, Kirsten EB. Interaction between warfarin and propafenone in healthy volunteer subjects. *Clin Pharmacol Ther*. 1987;42:305-311.
380. Wagner F, Kalusche D, Trenk D, et al. Drug interaction between propafenone and metoprolol. *Br J Clin Pharmacol*. 1987;24:213-220.
381. Funck-Brentano C, Kroemer HK, Pavlou H, et al. Genetically-determined interaction between propafenone and low dose quinidine: role of active metabolites in modulating net drug effect. *Br J Clin Pharmacol*. 1989;27:435-444.
382. Ravid S, Podrid PJ, Novrit B. Safety of long-term propafenone therapy for cardiac arrhythmia – experience with 774 patients. *J Electrophysiol*. 1987;1:580-590.
383. Reynolds RD, Gorczynski RJ, Quon CY. Pharmacology and pharmacokinetics of esmolol. *J Clin Pharmacol*. 1986;26(suppl A):A3-A14.
384. Wiest D. Esmolol. A review of its therapeutic efficacy and pharmacokinetic characteristics. *Clin Pharmacokinet*. 1995;28:190-202.
385. Turlapaty P, Laddu A, Murthy VS, et al. Esmolol: a titratable short-acting intravenous beta blocker for acute critical care settings. *Am Heart J*. 1987;114:866-885.
386. Lish PM, Weikel JH, Dungan KW. Pharmacological and toxicological properties of two new beta-adrenergic receptor antagonists. *J Pharmacol Exp Ther*. 1965;149:161-173.
387. Funck-Brentano C. Pharmacokinetic and pharmacodynamic profiles of d-sotalol and d,l-sotalol. *Eur Heart J*. 1993;(14 suppl H):30-35.
388. Hanyok JJ. Clinical pharmacokinetics of sotalol. *Am J Cardiol*. 1993;72:19A-26A.
389. Yamreudeewong W, DeBisschop M, Martin LG, et al. Potentially significant drug interactions of class III antiarrhythmic drugs. *Drug Saf*. 2003;26:421-438.
390. Laer S, Neumann J, Scholz H. Interaction between sotalol and an antacid preparation. *Br J Clin Pharmacol*. 1997;43:269-272.
391. McKibbin JK, Pocock WA, Barlow JB, et al. Sotalol, hypokalaemia, syncope, and torsade de pointes. *Br Heart J*. 1984;51:157-162.
392. Singh S, Saini RK, DiMarco J, et al. Efficacy and safety of sotalol in digitalized patients with chronic atrial fibrillation. The sotalol study group. *Am J Cardiol*. 1991;68:1227-1230.
393. Latini R, Tognoni G, Kates RE. Clinical pharmacokinetics of amiodarone. *Clin Pharmacokinet*. 1984;9:136-156.
394. Bonati M, Gaspari F, D'Aranno V, et al. Physicochemical and analytical characteristics of amiodarone. *J Pharm Sci*. 1984;73:829-831.
395. Singh BN. Amiodarone: the expanding antiarrhythmic role and how to follow a patient on chronic therapy. *Clin Cardiol*. 1997;20:608-618.
396. Trivier JM, Libersa C, Belloc C, et al. Amiodarone N-deethylation in human liver microsomes: involvement of cytochrome P450 3A enzymes (first report). *Life Sci*. 1993;52:PL91-PL96.

397. Ohyama K, Nakajima M, Suzuki M, et al. Inhibitory effects of amiodarone and its n-deethylated metabolite on human cytochrome P450 activities: prediction of in vivo drug interactions. *Br J Clin Pharmacol*. 2000;49:244-253.
398. Nitsch J, Luderitz B. Acceleration of amiodarone elimination by cholestyramine. *Dtsch Med Wochenschr*. 1986;111:1241-1244.
399. Wagner JA, Weisman HF, Levine JH, et al. Differential effects of amiodarone and desethylamiodarone on calcium antagonist receptors. *J Cardiovasc Pharmacol*. 1990;15:501-507.
400. Lee TH, Friedman PL, Goldman L, et al. Sinus arrest and hypotension with combined amiodarone-diltiazem therapy. *Am Heart J*. 1985;109:163-164.
401. Nicolau DP, Uber WE, Crumbley AJ, et al. Amiodarone-cyclosporine interaction in a heart transplant patient. *J Heart Lung Transplant*. 1992;11:564-568.
402. Harris L, McKenna WJ, Rowland E, et al. Side effects and possible contraindications of amiodarone use. *Am Heart J*. 1983;106:916-923.
403. Greene HL, Graham EL, Werner JA, et al. Toxic and therapeutic effects of amiodarone in the treatment of cardiac arrhythmias. *J Am Coll Cardiol*. 1983;2:1114-1128.
404. Baroletti S, Catella J, Ehle M, et al. Dronedarone: a review of characteristics and clinical data. *Crit Pathw Cardiol*. 2010;9:94-101.
405. Garcia D, Cheng-Lai A. Dronedarone: a new antiarrhythmic agent for the treatment of atrial fibrillation. *Cardiol Rev*. 2009;17:230-234.
406. Patel C, Yan GX, Kowey PR. Dronedarone. *Circulation*. 2009;120:636-644.
407. Dorian P. Clinical pharmacology of dronedarone: implications for the therapy of atrial fibrillation. *J Cardiovasc Pharmacol Ther*. 2010;15:15S-18S.
408. Hohnloser SH, Crijns HJ, van Eickels M, et al. Effect of dronedarone on cardiovascular events in atrial fibrillation. *N Engl J Med*. 2009;360:668-678.
409. Murray KT. Ibutilide. *Circulation*. 1998;97:493-497.
410. Pharmacia and Upjohn Company LLC. Corvert (Ibutilide Fumarate Injection) Prescribing Information.
411. Vos MA, Golitsyn SR, Stangl K, et al. Superiority of ibutilide (a new class iii agent) over dl-sotalol in converting atrial flutter and atrial fibrillation. The ibutilide/sotalol comparator study group. *Heart*. 1998;79:568-575.
412. Cropp JS, Antal EG, Talbert RL. Ibutilide: a new class iii antiarrhythmic agent. *Pharmacotherapy*. 1997;17:1-9.
413. Stambler BS, Wood MA, Ellenbogen KA, et al. Efficacy and safety of repeated intravenous doses of ibutilide for rapid conversion of atrial flutter or fibrillation. Ibutilide repeat dose study investigators. *Circulation*. 1996;94:1613-1621.
414. Gwilt M, Arrowsmith JE, Blackburn KJ, et al. UK-68,798: a novel, potent and highly selective class III antiarrhythmic agent which blocks potassium channels in cardiac cells. *J Pharmacol Exp Ther*. 1991;256:318-324.
415. Le Coz F, Funck-Brentano C, Morell T, et al. Pharmacokinetic and pharmacodynamic modeling of the effects of oral and intravenous administrations of dofetilide on ventricular repolarization. *Clin Pharmacol Ther*. 1995;57:533-542.
416. Allen MJ, Nichols DJ, Oliver SD. The pharmacokinetics and pharmacodynamics of oral dofetilide after twice daily and three times daily dosing. *Br J Clin Pharmacol*. 2000;50:247-253.
417. Walker DK, Alabaster CT, Congrave GS, et al. Significance of metabolism in the disposition and action of the antidysrhythmic drug, dofetilide. In vitro studies and correlation with in vivo data. *Drug Metab Dispos*. 1996;24:447-455.
418. Pfizer Inc. Tikosyn (dofetilide capsule) prescribing information. http://labeling.Pfizer.Com/showlabeling.Aspx?Id=639.
419. Torp-Pedersen C, Brendorp B, Kober L. Dofetilide: a class iii anti-arrhythmic drug for the treatment of atrial fibrillation. *Expert Opin Investig Drugs*. 2000;9:2695-2704.
420. Wilbur SL, Marchlinski FE. Adenosine as an antiarrhythmic agent. *Am J Cardiol*. 1997;79:30-37.
421. Stafford A. Potentiation of adenosine and the adenine nucleotides by dipyridamole. *Br J Pharmacol Chemother*. 1966;28:218-227.
422. Biaggioni I, Paul S, Puckett A, et al. Caffeine and theophylline as adenosine receptor antagonists in humans. *J Pharmacol Exp Ther*. 1991;258:588-593.
423. Bertolet BD, Belardinelli L, Avasarala K, et al. Differential antagonism of cardiac actions of adenosine by theophylline. *Cardiovasc Res*. 1996;32:839-845.
424. Brugada P. Magnesium: an antiarrhythmic drug, but only against very specific arrhythmias. *Eur Heart J*. 2000;21:1116.

Structure Challenge Answers

1-C, 2-D, 3-A, 4-E, 5-B

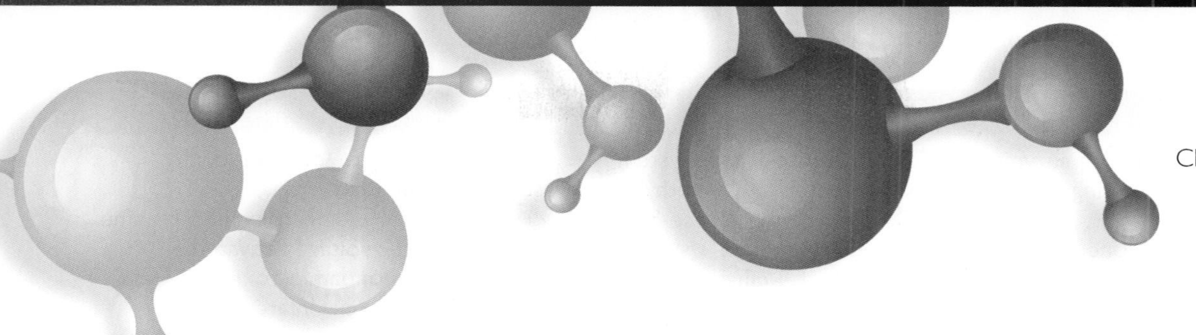

CHAPTER 17

Drugs Used to Treat Hypertensive/Hypotensive Disorders

Peter J. Harvison and Marc W. Harrold

Drugs covered in this chapter[a]:

OSMOTIC DIURETICS
- Mannitol
- Sorbitol

CARBONIC ANHYDRASE INHIBITORS
- Acetazolamide
- Brinzolamide/dorzolamide
- Methazolamide

THIAZIDE DIURETICS
- Bendroflumethiazide
- Chlorothiazide
- Hydrochlorothiazide
- Hydroflumethiazide
- Methyclothiazide

THIAZIDE-LIKE DIURETICS
- Chlorthalidone
- Indapamide
- Metolazone

LOOP DIURETICS
- Bumetanide
- Ethacrynic acid
- Furosemide
- Torsemide

ALDOSTERONE ANTAGONISTS (MINERALOCORTICOID RECEPTOR ANTAGONISTS)
- Eplerenone
- Spironolactone

POTASSIUM-SPARING DIURETICS
- Amiloride
- Triamterene

ANGIOTENSIN-CONVERTING ENZYME INHIBITORS
- Benazepril
- Captopril
- Enalapril
- Fosinopril
- Lisinopril
- Moexipril
- Perindopril
- Quinapril
- Ramipril
- *Spirapril*
- Trandolapril

ANGIOTENSIN II RECEPTOR BLOCKERS
- Azilsartan
- Candesartan
- Eprosartan
- Irbesartan
- Losartan
- Olmesartan
- Telmisartan
- Valsartan

RENIN INHIBITOR
- Aliskiren

CALCIUM CHANNEL BLOCKERS
- Amlodipine
- Clevidipine
- Diltiazem
- Felodipine
- Nicardipine
- Nifedipine
- Nimodipine
- Nisoldipine
- Verapamil

β-NONSELECTIVE BLOCKERS
- Carteolol
- Levobunolol
- Nadolol
- Penbutolol
- Pindolol
- Propranolol
- Timolol

β_1-SELECTIVE BLOCKERS
- Acebutolol
- Atenolol
- Betaxolol
- Bisoprolol
- Esmolol
- Metoprolol
- Nebivolol

α_1-BLOCKERS
- Prazosin
- Doxazosin
- Terazosin

MIXED α-/β-BLOCKERS
- Carvedilol
- Labetalol

α_2-AGONISTS
- Methyldopa
- Clonidine
- *Moxonidine*
- *Rilmenidine*
- Guanabenz
- Guanfacine

α_1-AGONISTS
- Metaraminol
- Methoxamine
- Phenylephrine

VASODILATORS
- Hydralazine
- Minoxidil
- Diazoxide

NITRODILATOR
- Sodium nitroprusside

[a]Drugs listed include those that are available inside and outside of the United States; drugs available outside of the United States are shown in italics.

Abbreviations

ACE angiotensin-converting enzyme
ACEI angiotensin-converting enzyme inhibitor
ADH antidiuretic hormone, vasopressin
ADHD attention-deficit hyperactivity disorder
ARB angiotensin receptor blocker
AT_1 angiotensin II subtype 1 receptor
AT_2 angiotensin II subtype 2 receptor
AT-II angiotensin II
ATP adenosine triphosphate
AV atrioventricular
BB β-blocker
BPF bradykinin-potentiating factor
CaM calmodulin
cAMP cyclic adenosine monophosphate
cGMP cyclic guanosine monophosphate
CCB calcium channel blocker
CNS central nervous system
COMT catechol-O-methyltransferase
COX-2 cyclooxygenase-2
DAG diacylglycerol
1,4-DHPs 1,4-dihydropyridines
ENaC epithelial sodium channel
eNOS endothelial nitric oxide synthase
ET endothelin
FDA U.S. Food and Drug Administration
GFR glomerular filtration rate
GI gastrointestinal
HVA high-voltage activated
IC_{50} half maximal inhibitory concentration
iNOS inducible nitric oxide synthase
IP_3 inositol triphosphate
ISA intrinsic sympathomimetic activity
IV intravenous
JNC8 Eighth Joint National Committee
L-DOPA L-dihydroxyphenylalanine
LVA low-voltage activated
MAO monoamine oxidase
MI myocardial infarction
MLCK myosin light-chain kinase
MR mineralocorticoid receptor
NMDA N-methyl-D-aspartate
nNOS neuronal nitric oxide synthase
NO nitric oxide
NOS nitric oxide synthase
PVD peripheral vascular disease
PIP_2 phosphatidylinositol
PKC protein kinase C
PLC phospholipase C
PSVT paroxysmal supraventricular tachycardia
SAR structure-activity relationship
SR sarcoplasmic reticulum
VSM vascular smooth muscle

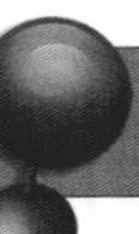

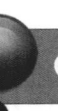

CLINICAL SIGNIFICANCE

DRUGS USED TO TREAT HYPERTENSIVE/HYPOTENSIVE DISORDERS

Michael W. Perry, PharmD, BCPS, BCCCP

In clinical practice, hypertension is a frequent finding among patients and is well established as a risk factor for cardiovascular disease and stroke.[1] Traditionally, clinicians have used a combination of dietary changes, exercise, weight loss, and then pharmacologic therapy to treat patients diagnosed with hypertension to a blood pressure goal that is less than 140/90 mm Hg. The Systolic Blood Pressure Intervention Trial (SPRINT) was recently completed and showed that targeting a systolic blood pressure less than 120 mm Hg may result in fewer cardiovascular disease events and a reduction in mortality when compared with systolic blood pressure less than 140 mm Hg.[1] As clinical practice shifts toward lower target blood pressure, clinicians are likely to require multiple medications from several different classes to manage the blood pressure of a hypertensive patient. The patients on these medications will need to be closely monitored for compliance, efficacy, and adverse effects.

Clinicians opting to initiate pharmacologic therapy will need to select a medication from over 60 different agents across over 18 different drug classes. The abundance of antihypertensive medications is due in part to the use of medicinal chemistry to develop and improve agents within a drug class. Modification of the chemical structure of a medication has led to the development of agents with specific purposes. The use of prodrugs and the alterations of drug structures have allowed for the optimization of oral absorption, routes of administration, duration of action, and specific therapeutic uses. Within the angiotensin-converting enzyme (ACE) inhibitor class, the SAR and structural modifications of captopril led to the development of more potent and longer lasting agents such as lisinopril. These structural changes have led to improved patient compliance by introducing once daily dosing of the ACE inhibitors and decreasing adverse effects (skin rashes and dysgeusia) related to the sulfhydryl group. Several structural changes to spironolactone, including the addition of an 9α,11α-epoxy group, led to the development of eplerenone, which is an effective diuretic, but has less sexual side effects when compared with spironolactone. New medications will continue to come to market and will likely be the result of structural modifications of existing medications.

Cardiovascular disease remains a leading cause of morbidity and mortality worldwide.[1] Improved compliance with an antihypertensive regimen will aid in the prevention of myocardial infarction, heart failure, kidney disease, and stroke. There are numerous antihypertensive agents to select from for an initial medication regimen. Clinicians with the knowledge of the medicinal chemistry and history of antihypertensive medications will be able to improve patient outcomes by improving compliance, reducing adverse effects, and maintaining patients below their target blood pressures.

CARDIOVASCULAR HYPERTENSION

Overview

Hypertension is the most common cardiovascular disease and is the major risk factor for coronary artery disease, heart failure, stroke, and renal failure. Approximately 85.7 million adult (age greater than or equal to 20 years) Americans (44.9 million women and 40.8 million men) have a systolic or diastolic blood pressure ≥140/90 mm Hg, and the incidence of this disease increases with age in both sexes.[1]

The importance of controlling blood pressure is well documented,[1] although the rates of awareness, treatment, and control of hypertension have not risen as expected in the National Health and Nutrition Examination Survey.[2] This survey showed that 68% of Americans are aware that they have high blood pressure but that only 53% are receiving treatment and only 27% have their blood pressure under control. Since 1976, there has been a significant improvement in the rates of awareness, treatment, and control of hypertension; however, since 1990, whatever progress had been achieved has now reached a plateau.[2] Although the age-adjusted death rates from stroke and coronary heart disease during this period have fallen by 59% and 53%, respectively, their rates of decline also appear to have reached a plateau.[2] These troubling trends should awaken clinicians to be more aggressive in the treatment of patients with hypertension.

When the decision to initiate hypertensive therapy is made, physicians often are presented with the dilemma of which of more than 80 antihypertensive products, representing more than seven different drug classes, to use for their patients (Table 17.1).[1,3] The factors that can affect the outcomes from the treatment of hypertension, including potential adverse effects, clinically significant drug-drug interactions (especially when so many different drug classes are involved), patient compliance, affordability, risk/benefit ratios, and dosing frequency, must be considered.[3] Having considered these factors, the health care provider (clinician or pharmacist) arrives at an appropriate choice of antihypertensive drug.[3] Once the patient is stabilized with an antihypertensive medication, some of these issues need to be reevaluated. Patients should be continually asked about side effects because many of the antihypertensive drugs possess side effects that the patient cannot tolerate.[1] This problem and the cost of drug therapy can affect compliance to drug therapy especially for the elderly and those on fixed incomes.[4]

Drug therapy in the management of hypertension must be individualized and adjusted based on coexisting risk factors, including the degree of blood pressure elevation, severity of the disease (e.g., presence of target organ damage), presence of underlying cardiovascular or other risk factors, response to therapy (single or multiple drugs), and tolerance to drug-induced adverse effects.[1,3] Antihypertensive therapy is generally reserved for patients who fail to respond to nondrug therapies along with lifestyle modifications, such as diet including sodium restriction and adequate potassium intake, regular aerobic physical activity, moderation of alcohol consumption, and weight reduction.[3]

Table 17.1 Classification of Antihypertensive Activity According to Mechanism of Action

Drug Class	Drug Subclass
Diuretics	1. Osmotic diuretics 2. Carbonic anhydrase inhibitors 3. Thiazide diuretics 4. Thiazide-like diuretics 5. Loop diuretics 6. Aldosterone antagonists 7. Potassium-sparing diuretics
Angiotensin-converting enzyme inhibitors	
Angiotensin II receptor blockers	
Renin inhibitor	
Calcium channel blockers	
Sympatholytic drugs	1. β-Adrenergic receptor blockers 2. α_1-Adrenergic receptor blockers 3. Mixed α-/β-adrenergic receptor blockers 4. α_1-Adrenergic receptor agonists 5. α_2-Adrenergic receptor agonists
Vasodilators	1. Arterial 2. Arterial and venous

It is not surprising that compliance with antihypertensive therapy can be as low as 40% when one considers that the patient, if he or she has other chronic diseases, can be taking as many as 10 different drugs and up to 40 tablets or capsules per day.[4] To achieve better compliance requires educating the patient and simplifying the drug regimen by reducing the number of drugs being taken.

Hypertension in pregnancy presents a formidable therapeutic challenge and requires comprehensive management with close monitoring for both maternal and fetal welfare.[5] Mechanisms involved with pregnancy-related hypertension include a hyperadrenergic state, plasma volume reduction, reduction in uteroplacental perfusion, hormonal control of vascular reactivity, and prostacyclin deficiency and can result from or activate the mechanisms that elevate blood pressure. Effective blood pressure control for pregnancy-related hypertension can often be achieved with methyldopa (recommended), β-blockers (BBs), or mixed α-/β-blockers (dual combination of α- and β-blocker activity). The vasodilating agent hydralazine is used to treat hypertensive emergencies associated with eclampsia.[1,6] The presence or development of proteinuria (preeclampsia) in a hypertensive pregnant woman implies a major increase in risk to the fetus and warrants immediate admission to a hospital for specialist management.[5]

Patients with diabetes mellitus have a much higher rate of hypertension than would be expected in the general population. Regardless of the antihypertensive agent used, a reduction in blood pressure helps to prevent or reduce diabetic microvascular and macrovascular complications, such as blindness and kidney failure. Angiotensin-converting enzyme (ACE) inhibitors (ACEIs) and angiotensin receptor blockers (ARBs) are considered first-line therapy in patients with diabetes and hypertension because of their well-established renal protective effects. Most diabetic patients with hypertension require combination therapy with low-dose diuretics and BBs to achieve optimal blood pressure goals.

Combination Antihypertensive Therapy

It is well documented that monotherapy adequately controls hypertension only in approximately 50% of patients.[7,8] Therefore, a large percentage of patients will require at least a combination of two drugs to control their blood pressure and symptoms of hypertension. By combining different antihypertensive drug classes in low doses, their different mechanisms of action result in synergistic blood pressure lowering as well as in minimizing the adverse effects and improving compliance issues.[1,8] For example, the addition of a low-dose thiazide diuretic dramatically increases the response rates to methyldopa, ACEIs, and BBs without producing the undesirable side effects. In the latest guidelines for treatment of hypertension, the Joint National Committee for Prevention, Detection, Evaluation, and Treatment of High Blood Pressure (JNC8), clinicians are encouraged to begin initially with thiazide-type diuretics, angiotensin-converting enzyme inhibitors (ACEIs), angiotensin receptor blockers (ARBs), or calcium channel blockers (CCBs) in hypertensive patients without compelling risk factors (Table 17.2). These drug classes have been shown to decrease morbidity and mortality in long-term clinical trials.[2] Other antihypertensive drugs (including stage 1 agents) are considered in patients with compelling risk factors, such as heart disease, clinical manifestations of cardiovascular diseases or diabetes (Table 17.2). In patients with compelling risk factors for cardiovascular disease, treatment should be more aggressive, with the goal of reducing blood pressure to less than 130/80 mm Hg (Table 17.3). These recommendations reflect the current awareness of the importance of addressing other cardiovascular conditions aside from just lowering the blood pressure.

DIURETICS

Overview

Diuretics are chemicals that increase the rate of urine formation.[9] Diuretic usage leads to increased excretion of electrolytes (especially sodium and chloride ions) and water from the body by increasing the urine flow rate, without affecting protein, vitamin, glucose, or amino acid reabsorption. These pharmacological properties have led to the use of diuretics in the treatment of edematous conditions resulting from a variety of causes (e.g., congestive heart failure, nephrotic syndrome, and chronic liver disease) and in the management of hypertension. Diuretic drugs also are useful as the sole agent or as adjunct therapy in the treatment of a wide range of other clinical conditions, including hypercalcemia, diabetes insipidus, acute mountain sickness, primary hyperaldosteronism, and glaucoma.

The primary target organ for diuretics is the kidney, where these drugs interfere with the reabsorption of sodium and other ions from the lumina of the nephrons, which are the functional units of the kidney. The amount

Table 17.2 Initial Drug Choices (JNC8)

Without compelling risk factors		**With compelling risk factors**
Blood pressure goal, <120/80 mm Hg		Blood pressure goal, <130/80 mm Hg
Stage 1 hypertension	**Stage 2 hypertension**	**Compelling risk factors include**
SBP 130-139 or DBP 80-89 mm Hg	SBP ≥140 or DBP ≥90 mm Hg	Heart failure After myocardial infarction High coronary disease risk Diabetes Chronic kidney disease Recurrent stroke prevention
Monotherapy with first-line drugs (thiazide-type diuretics, ACEIs, ARBs or CCBs) or combinations to achieve blood pressure goal	Two first-line drugs (thiazide-type diuretics, ACEIs, ARBs or CCBs) in different classes	Drugs for compelling indications: Stage 1 drugs and other antihypertensive drugs
Not at Blood Pressure Goal		
Optimize stage 2 drug treatment, or add additional classes of antihypertensive drugs until blood pressure goal is achieved		

ACEI, angiotensin-converting enzyme inhibitor; ARB, angiotensin receptor blocker; CCB, calcium channel blocker; DBP, diastolic blood pressure; SBP, systolic blood pressure.

Table 17.3 Risk Factors for Cardiovascular Disease

Correctable	Noncorrectable
Cigarette smoking	Age >60 yr
Hypertension	Sex (men and postmenopausal women)
Elevated cholesterol	Family history of cardiovascular disease or stroke (women <65 yr, men <55 yr)
Reduced HDL (high-density lipoprotein) cholesterol	
Diabetes mellitus	
Obesity	Target organ damage
HDL	

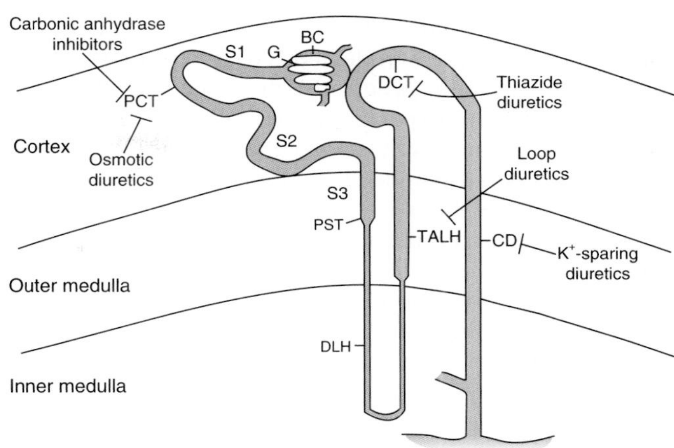

Figure 17.1 The nephron. BC, Bowman's capsule; CD, collecting duct; DCT, distal convoluted tubule; DLH, descending limb of the Loop of Henle; G, glomerulus; PCT, proximal convoluted tubule; PST, proximal straight tubule; TALH, thick ascending limb of the loop of Henle.

of ions and accompanying water that are excreted as urine following administration of a diuretic, however, is determined by many factors, including the chemical structure of the diuretic, the site or sites of action of the agent, the salt intake of the patient, and the amount of extracellular fluid present. In addition to the direct effect of diuretics to impair solute and water reabsorption from the nephron, diuretics also can trigger compensatory physiological events that have an impact on either the magnitude or the duration of the diuretic response. Thus, it is important to be aware of the normal mechanisms of urine formation and renal control mechanisms to understand clearly the ability of chemicals to induce diuresis.

Normal Physiology of Urine Formation

Two important functions of the kidney are (1) to maintain a homeostatic balance of electrolytes and water and (2) to excrete water-soluble end products of metabolism. The kidney accomplishes these functions through the formation of urine by the nephrons (Fig. 17.1). Each kidney contains approximately one million nephrons and is capable of forming urine independently. The nephrons are composed of a specialized capillary bed called the glomerulus and a long tubule divided anatomically and functionally into the proximal tubule, loop of Henle, and distal tubule. Each component of the nephron contributes to the normal functioning of the kidney in a unique manner; thus, all are targets for different classes of diuretic agents.

Urine formation begins with the filtration of blood at the glomerulus. Approximately 1,200 mL of blood per minute flows through both kidneys and reaches the nephron by way of afferent arterioles. Approximately 20% of the blood entering the glomerulus is filtered into Bowman's capsule to form the glomerular filtrate. The glomerular filtrate is composed of blood components with a molecular weight less than that of albumin (~69,000 Da) and not bound to plasma proteins. The glomerular filtration rate (GFR) averages 125 mL/min in humans but can vary widely even in normal functional states.

The glomerular filtrate leaves the Bowman's capsule and enters the proximal convoluted tubule (S1, S2 segments, Fig. 17.1), where the majority (50%-60%) of filtered sodium is reabsorbed osmotically. Sodium reabsorption is coupled electrogenetically with the reabsorption of glucose, phosphate, and amino acids and nonelectrogenetically with bicarbonate reabsorption. Glucose and amino acids are completely reabsorbed in this portion of the nephron, whereas phosphate reabsorption is between 80% and 90% complete. The early proximal convoluted tubule also is the primary site of bicarbonate reabsorption (80%-90%), a process that is mainly sodium dependent and coupled to hydrogen ion secretion. The reabsorption of sodium and bicarbonate is facilitated by the enzyme carbonic anhydrase, which is present in proximal tubular cells and catalyzes the formation of carbonic acid from water and carbon dioxide. The carbonic acid provides the hydrogen ion, which drives the reabsorption of sodium bicarbonate. Chloride ions are reabsorbed passively in the proximal tubule, where they follow actively transported sodium ions into tubular cells.

The reabsorption of electrolytes and water also occurs isosmotically in the proximal straight tubule or pars recta (S3 segment, Fig. 17.1). By the end of the straight segment, between 65% and 70% of water and sodium, chloride, and calcium ions; 80%-90% of bicarbonate and phosphate; and essentially 100% of glucose, amino acids, vitamins, and protein have been reabsorbed from the glomerular filtrate. The proximal tubule also is the site for active secretion of weakly acidic and weakly basic organic compounds. Thus, many of the diuretics can enter luminal fluid not only by filtration at the glomerulus but also by active secretion.

The descending limb of the loop of Henle is impermeable to ions, but water can freely move from the luminal fluid into the surrounding medullary interstitium, where the higher osmolality draws water into the interstitial space and concentrates luminal fluid. Luminal fluid continues to concentrate as it descends to the deepest portion of the loop of Henle, where the fluid becomes the most concentrated. The hypertonic luminal fluid next enters the water-impermeable, thick ascending limb of the loop of Henle. In this segment of the nephron, approximately 20%-25% of the filtered sodium and chloride ions are reabsorbed via a cotransport system ($Na^+/K^+/2Cl^-$) on the luminal membrane. Reabsorption of sodium and chloride in the medullary portion of the thick ascending limb is important for maintaining the medullary interstitial concentration gradient. Reabsorption of sodium chloride in the cortical component of the thick ascending limb of the loop of Henle and the early distal convoluted tubule contributes to urinary dilution, and as a result, these two nephron sections sometimes are called the cortical diluting segment of the nephron.

Luminal fluid leaving the early distal tubule next passes through the late distal tubule and cortical collecting tubule (collecting duct), where sodium is reabsorbed in exchange for hydrogen and potassium ions. This process is partially controlled by mineralocorticoids (e.g., aldosterone) and accounts for the reabsorption of between 2 and 3% of filtered sodium ions. Although the reabsorption of sodium ions from these segments of the nephron is not large, this sodium/potassium/hydrogen ion exchange system determines the final acidity and potassium content of urine. Several factors, however, can influence the activity of this exchange system, including the amount of sodium ions delivered to these segments, the status of the acid-base balance in the body, and the levels of circulating aldosterone.

The urine formed during this process represents only approximately 1%-2% of the original glomerular filtrate, with more than 98% of electrolytes and water filtered at the glomerulus being reabsorbed during passage through the nephron. Thus, a change in urine output of only 1%-2% could double urine volume. Urine leaves the kidney through the ureters and travels to the bladder, where it is stored until urination removes it from the body.

Normal Regulation of Urine Formation

The body contains several control mechanisms that regulate the volume and contents of urine. These systems are activated by changes in solute or water content of the body, by changes in systemic or renal blood pressure, and by a variety of other stimuli. Activation of one or more of these systems by diuretic drugs can modify the effectiveness of these drugs to produce their therapeutic response and may require additional therapeutic measures to ensure a maximal response.

The kidney can respond to changes in the GFR through the action of specialized distal tubular epithelial cells called the macula densa. These cells are in close contact with the glomerular apparatus of the same nephron and detect changes in the rate of urine flow and luminal sodium chloride concentration. An increase in the urine flow rate at this site (as can occur with the use of some diuretics) activates the macula densa cells to communicate with the granular cells and vascular segments of the juxtaglomerular apparatus. Stimulation of the juxtaglomerular apparatus causes renin to be released, which leads to the formation of angiotensin II and subsequent renal vasoconstriction. Renal vasoconstriction leads to a decrease in GFR and, possibly, a decrease in the effectiveness of the diuretic. Renin release also can be stimulated by factors other than diuretics, including decreased renal perfusion pressure, increased sympathetic tone, and decreased blood volume.

Another important regulatory mechanism for urine formation is antidiuretic hormone (ADH), also known as vasopressin, which is released from the posterior pituitary in response to reduced blood pressure and elevated plasma osmolality. In the kidney, ADH acts on the collecting tubule to increase water permeability and reabsorption. As a result, the urine becomes more concentrated, and water is conserved in the presence of ADH.

Role of Fluid Volume in Hypertension and Other Cardiovascular Disorders

The diuretic drugs are used primarily to treat two medically important conditions, edema and hypertension.[10–13] Both conditions are common, although some patients exhibit refractory disease states that require additional modification of the drug regimen to include alternative diuretics or the addition of nondiuretic drugs. Edema (excessive extracellular fluid) normally results from disease of the heart, kidney, or liver. Decreased cardiac function (e.g., congestive heart disease) can result in decreased perfusion of all organs (e.g., kidney) and limbs and an accumulation of edema fluid in the extremities, particularly around the ankles and in the hands. Left-sided heart failure can lead to the development of acute pulmonary edema, which is a medical emergency. Right-sided heart failure shifts extracellular fluid volume from the arterial circulation to the venous circulation, which leads to general edema formation.

Kidney dysfunction can lead to edema formation because of decreased formation of urine and the subsequent imbalance of water and electrolyte (e.g., sodium ion) homeostasis. Retention of salt and water results in an expansion of the extracellular fluid volume and edema formation. Thus, when salt intake exceeds salt excretion, edema can form. Edema formation also is associated with deceased protein levels in blood, as seen in nephrotic syndrome and liver disease. Cirrhosis of the liver leads to increased lymph in the space of Disse. Eventually, the increased lymph volume results in movement of fluid into the peritoneal cavity and ascites develops.

Patients with hypertension are at increased risk for developing cardiovascular disease. One key element in controlling blood pressure is sodium ion, and early antihypertensive effects of diuretics are related to increased salt and water excretion. Additionally, however, diuretics have long-term effects resulting in decreased vascular resistance that contribute to blood pressure control. Although effects on vascular calcium-activated potassium channels have been proposed as contributing to the chronic antihypertensive effects of thiazide diuretics, the exact mechanisms of long-term effects remain to be determined.

Diuretics also are useful in treating a number of other conditions including increased cranial (trauma or surgery) or intraocular (glaucoma) pressure (e.g., osmotic diuretics), diabetes insipidus (e.g., thiazides), hypercalcemia (e.g., loop diuretics), acute mountain sickness (e.g., carbonic anhydrase inhibitors), primary hyperaldosteronism (e.g., aldosterone antagonists), and osteoporosis (e.g., thiazides).

General Therapeutic Approaches

Diuretic drugs may be administered acutely or chronically to treat edematous states. When immediate action to reduce edema (e.g., acute pulmonary edema) is needed, intravenous administration of a loop diuretic is often the approach of choice. Thiazide or loop diuretics normally are administered orally to treat nonemergency edematous states. The magnitude of the diuretic response is directly proportional to the amount of edema fluid that is present. As the volume of edema decreases, so does the magnitude of the diuretic response with each dose. If concern exists about diuretic-induced hypokalemia developing, then a potassium supplement or potassium-sparing diuretic may be added to the drug regimen. The development of hypokalemia is particularly important for patients with congestive heart failure who also are taking cardiac glycosides, such as digoxin. Digoxin has a narrow therapeutic index, and developing hypokalemia can potentiate digitalis-induced cardiac effects with potentially fatal results.

Diuretic drugs (thiazide and loop diuretics) are administered orally to help control blood pressure in the treatment of hypertension. Diuretics often are the first drugs used to treat hypertension, and they also may be added to other drug therapies used to control blood pressure with beneficial effects.

Diuretics have also been used illicitly by some athletes for "sport doping."[14] This is a consequence of the drugs' ability to quickly produce weight loss (via increased excretion of water) and masking of urine contents (via dilution of other drugs or metabolites that might be present in the urine). Furosemide, triamterene, and hydrochlorothiazide are the most commonly used diuretics for sport doping, as they are eliminated rapidly and are therefore more difficult to detect in urine samples taken at later time points after use. Another consideration is that some diuretics can degrade in urine samples; for example, thiazides may hydrolyze to aminobenzenedisulfonamide derivatives.[15] Use of diuretics by athletes without a documented therapeutic need has been banned since 1988, and routine monitoring for these drugs and their degradation products is commonplace. A list of banned drugs, including diuretics, is maintained and updated by the International Olympic Committee and the World Anti-Doping Agency.

Diuretic Drug Classes

History

Compounds that increase the urine flow rate have been known for centuries. One of the earliest substances known to induce diuresis is water, an inhibitor of ADH release. Calomel (mercurous chloride) was used as early as the 16th century as a diuretic, but because of poor absorption from the gastrointestinal tract and toxicity, calomel was replaced clinically by the organomercurials (e.g., chlormerodrin). The organomercurials represented the first group of highly efficacious diuretics available for clinical use. The need to administer these drugs parenterally, the possibility of tolerance, and their potential toxicity, however, soon led to the search for newer, less toxic diuretics. Today, the organomercurials are no longer used as diuretics, but their discovery began the search for many of the diuretics used today. Other compounds previously used as diuretics include the acid-forming salts (ammonium chloride) and methylxanthines (theophylline).

Diuretic Classification

Diuretics are classified (Table 17.4) by their chemical class (thiazides), mechanism of action (carbonic anhydrase inhibitors and osmotics), site of action (loop diuretics), or effects on urine contents (potassium-sparing diuretics). These drugs vary widely in their efficacy (i.e., their ability to increase the rate of urine formation) and their site of action within the nephron. Efficacy often is measured as the ability of the diuretic to increase the excretion of sodium ions filtered at the glomerulus (i.e., the filtered load of sodium) and should not be confused with potency, which is the amount of the diuretic required to produce a specific diuretic response.

Efficacy is determined, in part, by the site of action of the diuretic. Drugs (e.g., carbonic anhydrase inhibitors) that act primarily on the proximal convoluted tubule to induce diuresis are weak diuretics because of the ability of the nephron to reabsorb a significant portion of the luminal contents in latter portions of the nephron. Likewise, drugs (potassium-sparing diuretics) that act at the more distal segments of the nephron are weak diuretics because most of the glomerular filtrate has already been reabsorbed in the proximal tubule and ascending limb of the loop of Henle before reaching the distal tubule. Thus, the most efficacious diuretics discovered so far, the high-ceiling or loop diuretics, interfere with sodium chloride reabsorption at the ascending limb of the loop of Henle, which is situated after the proximal tubule but before the distal portions of the nephron and collecting tubule (Fig. 17.1).

Osmotic Diuretics

Therapeutic Role of Osmotic Diuretics

Osmotic diuretics are not frequently used in medicine today except in the prophylaxis of acute renal failure, in which these drugs inhibit water reabsorption and maintain urine flow. They also may be helpful in maintaining urine flow in cases where urinary output is diminished because of severe bleeding or traumatic surgical experiences. The osmotic diuretics also have been used to acutely reduce increased intracranial or intraocular pressure.

Mannitol is the most commonly used osmotic diuretic and is administered intravenously in solutions of 5%-50%

Table 17.4 Diuretics: Sites and Mechanisms of Action

Diuretic Class	Site of Action	Mechanism of Action
Osmotics	Proximal tubule	Osmotic effects decrease sodium and water reabsorption
	Loop of Henle	Increases medullary blood flow to decrease medullary hypertonicity and reduce sodium and water reabsorption
	Collecting tubule	Sodium and water reabsorption decreases because of reduced medullary hypertonicity and elevated urinary flow rate
Carbonic anhydrase inhibitors	Proximal convoluted tubule	Inhibition of renal carbonic anhydrase decreases sodium bicarbonate reabsorption
Thiazides and thiazide-like	Cortical portion of the thick ascending limb of loop of Henle and distal tubule	Inhibition of Na^+/Cl^- symporter
Loop or high ceiling	Thick ascending limb of the loop of Henle	Inhibition of the luminal $Na^+/K^+/2Cl^-$ transport system
Potassium sparing	Distal tubule and collecting duct	Inhibition of sodium and water reabsorption by competitive inhibition of aldosterone (spironolactone) or blockade of sodium channel at the luminal membrane (triamterene and amiloride)

at a rate of administration that is adjusted to maintain the urinary output at 30-50 mL/hr.[16] Sorbitol, a close structural analog of mannitol (see below), is used as a hyperosmotic laxative for the treatment of constipation.

Pharmacology Overview of Osmotic Diuretics

MECHANISM OF ACTION. Osmotic diuretics are low-molecular-weight compounds that are freely filtered through the Bowman's capsule.[16] Once in the renal tubule, osmotic diuretics have limited reabsorption because of their high-water solubility. When administered as a hypertonic (hyperosmolar) solution, these agents increase intraluminal osmotic pressure, causing water to pass from the body into the tubule. As the osmotic agent and associated water are not reabsorbed from the nephron, a diuretic effect is observed. Osmotic diuretics increase the volume of urine and the excretion of water and almost all electrolytes.

COMMON ADVERSE EFFECTS. Osmotic diuretics induce few adverse effects, but expansion of the extracellular fluid volume can occur, which limits their use in treating ordinary edemas. Alteration of blood sodium levels can be seen, and these drugs should not be used in anuric or unresponsive patients. If cranial bleeding is present, mannitol should not be used.

COMMON INTERACTIONS. Mannitol may interfere with lithium therapy by increasing urinary elimination of that drug.

Medicinal Chemistry of Osmotic Diuretics

RECEPTOR BINDING, SAR, AND PHYSICOCHEMICAL PROPERTIES. These drugs do not interact with a receptor and exert their diuretic or laxative activity via an osmotic effect. Mannitol and sorbitol are highly water-soluble sugar alcohols and differ from each other only in the stereochemical orientation of the hydroxyl group on carbon atom 2.

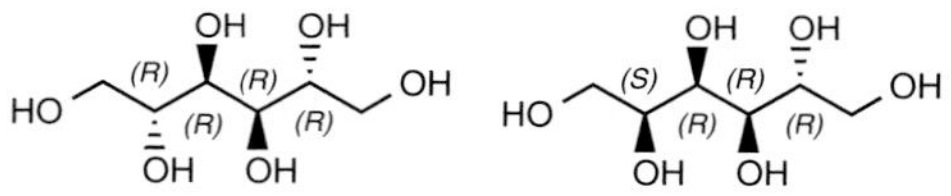

Mannitol Sorbitol

PHARMACOKINETIC PROPERTIES AND METABOLISM. Due to their polarity, mannitol and sorbitol have poor oral bioavailability and are administered intravenously or rectally. They undergo limited hepatic metabolism and are excreted mostly as unchanged parent drugs (see Table 17.5 for mannitol's pharmacokinetic properties). Sorbitol is metabolized by intestinal bacteria.

Carbonic Anhydrase Inhibitors

Therapeutic Role of Carbonic Anhydrase Inhibitors

Carbonic anhydrase inhibitors are not currently used in the management of hypertension. Their most common therapeutic role is in the treatment of glaucoma, in which they inhibit carbonic anhydrase in the eye, reduce the rate of aqueous humor formation, and consequently reduce intraocular pressure.[17] These compounds also have found some limited use in the treatment of absence seizures, to alkalinize the urine, to treat familial periodic paralysis, to reduce metabolic alkalosis, and, prophylactically, to reduce acute mountain sickness.

Table 17.5 Pharmacologic and Pharmacokinetic Properties of the Nonthiazide Diuretics

Drug	Trade Name	Relative Potency	Oral Absorption (%)	Peak Plasma	Half-Life	Duration of Effect	Elimination
Osmotic Diuretics							
Mannitol			<20	1-3 hr IV	0.5-1.5 hr	6-8 hr	Urine, as parent drug
Carbonic Anhydrase Inhibitors							
Acetazolamide	Diamox		>90	1-3 hr	6-9 hr	8-12 hr	Urine (major), as parent drug (70%-100%)
Methazolamide	Neptazane		>90	NA	~14 hr	10-18 hr	Urine, as parent drug (~25%) and metabolites
Brinzolamide	Azopt		topical use only (eye)	NA	~111 d*	8-12 hr	Urine, as parent drug (major)
Dorzolamide	Truspot		topical use only (eye)	NA	4 mo*	8-12 hr	Urine, as parent drug (major)
Loop Diuretics							
Furosemide	Lasix	1	11-90[a]	4-5 hr	0.5-4 hr (>3 hr)[b]	6-8 hr	Urine/feces, as parent drug (60%-70%) and metabolites
Bumetamide	Bumex	40	80-100	<2 hr	1-1.5 hr (>3 hr)[b]	5-6 hr	Urine (major), as parent drug (~50%) and ~5 metabolites
Torsemide	Demadex	3	80-100	1-2 hr	0.8-4 hr	6-8 hr	Urine/feces (2:8), as parent drug
Ethacrynic acid	Edecrin	0.7	>90	2 hr	0.5-1 hr	6-8 hr	Urine/feces, as parent drug (30%-60%) and mercapturic acid
Mineralocorticoid Receptor Antagonists							
Spironolactone	Aldactone	20-40	>90[c]	1-2 hr	1-3 hr (parent drug)	2-3 d	Urine/feces, as active metabolite(s)

(continued)

Table 17.5 Pharmacologic and Pharmacokinetic Properties of the Nonthiazide Diuretics (Continued)

Drug	Trade Name	Relative Potency	Oral Absorption (%)	Peak Plasma	Half-Life	Duration of Effect	Elimination
Eplenerone	Inspra	1	70	1.5 hr	4-6 hr	NA	Urine/feces (2:1), as metabolites (>95%)
Potassium-Sparing Diuretics							
Amiloride	Midamor	1	~50[a]	3-4 hr	6-9 hr normal (21 hr)[b]	24 hr	Urine/feces (5:4), as parent drug
Triamterene	Dyrenium	0.1	>70	2-4 hr	2-3 hr	Can be 24 hr or greater	Urine, as parent drug and metabolites

Data from AHFS Drug Information (2010), American Society of Health-System Pharmacists; Lexicomp Online (2011), Lexicomp, Inc.; Facts and Comparisons (2010), Wolters Kluwer Health.
[a]Food affects bioavailability.
[b]In patients with renal insufficiency.
[c]Formulation affects bioavailability.
*Strongly bound to red blood cells.
NA, data not available.

With prolonged use of the carbonic anhydrase inhibitor diuretics, the urine becomes more alkaline and the blood becomes more acidic. When acidosis occurs, the carbonic anhydrase inhibitors lose their effectiveness as diuretics. They remain ineffective until normal acid-base balance in the body has been regained.

Acetazolamide, a thiadiazole derivative, was the first carbonic anhydrase inhibitors to be used as an orally effective diuretic, with a therapeutic effect that lasts ca. 8-12 hours (Table 17.5).

Pharmacology Overview of Carbonic Anhydrase Inhibitors

MECHANISM OF ACTION. In 1937, it was proposed that the normal acidification of urine was caused by secretion of hydrogen ions by the tubular cells of the kidney. These ions were provided by the action of the enzyme carbonic anhydrase, which catalyzes the formation of carbonic acid (H_2CO_3) from carbon dioxide and water.

$$CO_2 + H_2O \xrightleftharpoons{\text{carbonic anhydrase}} H_2CO_3 \rightleftharpoons H^{\oplus} + HCO_3^{\ominus}$$

It also was observed that sulfanilamide rendered the urine of dogs alkaline because of the inhibition of carbonic anhydrase. This inhibition of carbonic anhydrase resulted in a lesser exchange of hydrogen ions for sodium ions in the kidney tubule. Sodium ions, along with bicarbonate ions, and associated water molecules were then excreted, and a diuretic effect was noted.

Carbonic anhydrase inhibitors induce diuresis by inhibiting the formation of carbonic acid within proximal (proximal convoluted tubule; S2) and distal tubular cells to limit the number of hydrogen ions available to promote sodium reabsorption. For a diuretic response to be observed, more than 99% of the carbonic anhydrase must be inhibited. Although carbonic anhydrase activity in the proximal tubule regulates the reabsorption of approximately 20%-25% of the filtered load of sodium, the carbonic anhydrase inhibitors are not highly efficacious diuretics. An increased excretion of only 2%-5% of the filtered load of sodium is seen with carbonic anhydrase inhibitors because of increased reabsorption of sodium ions by the ascending limb of the loop of Henle and more distal nephron segments.

COMMON ADVERSE EFFECTS. The carbonic anhydrase inhibitors generally do not produce serious side effects. However, monitoring for electrolyte disturbances may be necessary. Symptoms resulting from adverse effects on the gastrointestinal tract (nausea, vomiting, etc.), nervous system (sedation, headache, etc.) and kidneys (formation of stones) have been reported. Although they contain sulfonamide groups, hypersensitivity reactions with other sulfonamide-containing drugs are not common. As noted above, these drugs can produce metabolic acidosis.

COMMON INTERACTIONS. Carbonic anhydrase inhibitors may increase elimination of lithium and consequently decrease the therapeutic activity of this drug.

As they alkalinize urine, carbonic anhydrase inhibitors may decrease elimination of basic drugs. This occurs because the higher pH shifts the equilibrium to the ionized conjugate acid, which is less extensively reabsorbed from the renal tubular fluid than the nonionized base.

Medicinal Chemistry of Carbonic Anhydrase Inhibitors

RECEPTOR BINDING, SAR, AND PHYSICOCHEMICAL PROPERTIES. Sulfanilamide inhibits carbonic anhydrase; however, the large doses required for inhibition and the side effects associated with this compound prompted a search for more effective carbonic anhydrase inhibitors as diuretics. This led to the discovery that the sulfonamide portion of an active diuretic molecule could not be monosubstituted or disubstituted.[18,19] As a result, it was reasoned that a more acidic sulfonamide would bind more tightly to the carbonic anhydrase enzyme. Synthesis of more highly acidic sulfonamides produced compounds with activities greater than 2,500-fold that of sulfanilamide. Acetazolamide was introduced in 1953 as an orally effective diuretic drug. Methazolamide is a close structural analog of acetazolamide in which one of the active hydrogens in the thiadiazole ring has been replaced by a methyl group. This decreases polarity of the compound and permits a greater penetration into the ocular fluid, where it acts as a carbonic anhydrase inhibitor, reducing intraocular pressure.

Brinzolamide and dorzolamide contain ionizable amino groups and are the result of efforts to develop water-soluble compounds that retain sufficient lipophilicity to penetrate the cornea.[11] They are only indicated for topical eye administration in glaucoma patients.

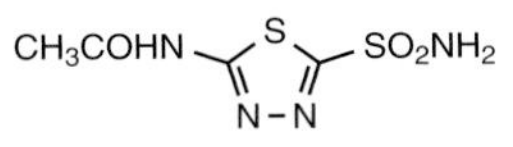

CH_3COHN S SO_2NH_2 N–N

Acetazolamide

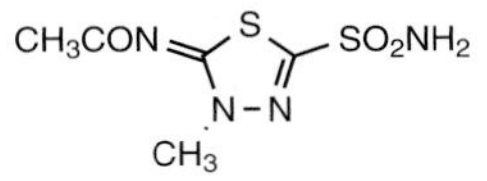

CH_3CON S SO_2NH_2 N–N CH_3

Methazolamide

$NHCH_2CH_3$ SO_2NH_2 H_3C S O S O

Dorzolamide

$NHCH_2CH_3$ SO_2NH_2 $CH_3O(CH_2)_3$ S O S O

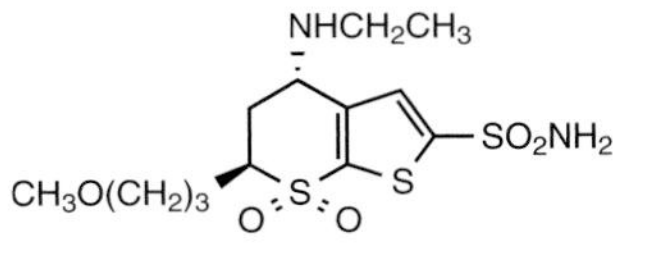

Brinzolamide

PHARMACOKINETIC PROPERTIES AND METABOLISM. The pharmacokinetic properties of the carbonic anhydrase inhibitors are summarized in Table 17.5. These drugs are administered orally or topically to the cornea (for ocular use) and are eliminated in urine predominantly as unchanged parent compounds.

Thiazide Diuretics

Therapeutic Role of Thiazide Diuretics

Thiazide and thiazide-like (see next section) diuretics are a mainstay in the treatment of hypertension.[20,21] Interestingly, increasing doses of thiazides correlates with an increase in adverse effects, but not diuretic activity. Consequently, the doses currently used are lower than when these drugs first came into clinical use. They are also used to treat edemas caused by cardiac decompensation as well as in hepatic or renal disease. Their effect may be attributed to a reduction in blood volume and a direct relaxation of vascular smooth muscle. The thiazide diuretics are administered once a day or in divided daily doses. Some have a duration of action that permits administration of a dose every other day. They are used in monotherapy and in combination with other antihypertensive drugs, including ACE inhibitors, ARBs, and β-blockers.[21] The specific structures for the thiazide diuretics, relative activities, and inhibitory potencies are summarized in Table 17.6.

Pharmacology Overview of Thiazide Diuretics

MECHANISM OF ACTION. Further study of the benzene disulfonamide derivatives was undertaken to find more efficacious carbonic anhydrase inhibitors. These studies provided some compounds with a high degree of diuretic activity. Chloro and amino substitution gave compounds with increased activity, but these compounds were weak carbonic anhydrase inhibitors. When the amino group was acylated, an unexpected ring closure took place. These compounds possessed a diuretic activity independent of the carbonic anhydrase inhibitory activity, and a new series of diuretics called the benzothiadiazines (thiazides) was discovered.[20]

These diuretics are actively secreted in the proximal tubule and are carried to the loop of Henle and to the distal tubule. The major site of action of these compounds is in the distal convoluted tubule, where these drugs compete for the chloride binding site of the Na^+/Cl^- symporter and inhibit the reabsorption of sodium and chloride ions. For this reason, they are referred to as saluretics. They also inhibit the reabsorption of potassium and bicarbonate ions, but to a lesser degree.

COMMON ADVERSE EFFECTS. Thiazide diuretics may induce several adverse effects, including hypersensitivity reactions, gastric irritation, nausea, and electrolyte imbalances, such as hyponatremia, hypokalemia, hypomagnesemia, hypochloremic alkalosis, hypercalcemia, and hyperuricemia. Individuals who exhibit hypersensitivity reactions to one thiazide are likely to have a hypersensitivity reaction to other thiazides and sulfamoyl-containing diuretics (e.g., thiazide-like and some high-ceiling diuretics). Potassium and magnesium supplements may be administered to treat hypokalemia or hypomagnesemia, but their use is not always indicated. These supplements usually are administered as potassium chloride, potassium gluconate, potassium citrate, magnesium oxide, or magnesium lactate. The salts are administered as solutions, tablets, or timed-release tablets. Potassium-sparing diuretics (e.g., triamterene or amiloride) also may be used to prevent hypokalemia. Combination preparation of hydrochlorothiazide or a potassium-sparing diuretic is available (e.g., Dyazide and moduretic).

Long-term use of thiazide diuretics also may result in decreased glucose tolerance and increased blood lipid (low-density lipoprotein cholesterol, total cholesterol, and total triglyceride) content.

COMMON INTERACTIONS. As noted above, the thiazides may be used in combination with ACE inhibitors

Table 17.6 Pharmacological and Pharmacokinetic Properties of the Thiazide Diuretics

Thiazides: Structure I   Thiazides: Structure II

Generic Name	Trade Name	Structure	Relative Potency[a]	Carbonic Anhydrase Inhibition[b]	Bioavailability	Peak Plasma	Half-Life	Duration of Effect	Elimination
Bendroflumethiazide	Naturetin	Structure II: R_1 = benzyl; R_2 = CF_3; R_3 = H	1.8	3×10^{-4} M	>90%	4 hr	8.5 hr	6-12 hr	Urine, as parent drug
Chlorothiazide	Diuril	Structure I: R_1 = H	0.8	2×10^{-6} M	<25%	4 hr	0.75-2 hr	12-16 hr	Urine, as parent drug
Hydrochlorothiazide	HydroDiuril Esidrix	Structure II: R_1 = H; R_2 = Cl; R_3 = H	1.4	2×10^{-5} M	>80%	4-6 hr	6-15 hr	12-16 hr	Urine, as parent drug
Hydroflumethiazide	Saluron Diucardin	Structure II: R_1 = H; R_2 = CF_3; R_3 = H	1.3	2×10^{-4} M	Inc	3-4 hr	17 hr	18-24 hr	Urine, as parent drug and metabolites
Methyclothiazide	Aquatensen	Structure II: R_1 = CH_2Cl; R2 = Cl; R3 = CH_3	1.8		Var	6 hr	NA	>24 hr	Urine, as parent drug

Data from AHFS Drug Information (2010), American Society of Health-System Pharmacists; Lexicomp Online (2011), Lexicomp, Inc.; Facts and Comparisons (2010), Wolters Kluwer Health.

[a]The numerical values refer to potency ratios (in humans) with the natriuretic response to that of a standard dose of meralluride, which is given a value of one.

[b]50% inhibition of carbonic anhydrase in vitro.

Inc., incomplete absorption; *NA*, data not available; *Var*, variables absorption.

or ARBs to achieve an enhanced antihypertensive effect. However, it may be necessary to monitor blood pressure or adjust doses to avoid hypotension.[21] Potentiation of antihypertensive activity can also be seen with other drugs, such as barbiturates, MAO inhibitors, and tricyclic antidepressants.

Nonsteroidal anti-inflammatory drugs (NSAIDs) can cause retention of sodium ions, which may antagonize the therapeutic effects of the thiazides.[12,21] Glucocorticoid-induced hyperkalemia can also exert an antagonistic effect. Oral thiazides should be taken one hour before or four hours after cholestyramine or colestipol (bile acid sequestrants) to avoid a decrease in absorption and consequent reduction in diuretic activity.

Thiazides can enhance toxicity of other drugs,[21] including digitalis (increased risk of cardiac arrhythmias and ventricular tachycardia), lithium (decreased renal excretion of lithium resulting in increased toxicity), and allopurinol (increased allergic response).

Medicinal Chemistry of Thiazide Diuretics

RECEPTOR BINDING, SAR, AND PHYSICOCHEMICAL PROPERTIES. Although these compounds inhibit carbonic anhydrase (Table 17.6), there is no correlation of this activity with their saluretic effect. In fact, their diuretic activity is due to an effect on the Na^+/Cl^- symporter in the distal convoluted tubule.

Thiazide diuretics are weakly acidic compounds, with a common benzothiadiazine 1,1-dioxide nucleus.

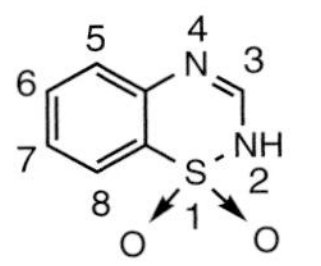

5 4 N 3 6 NH 7 S 2 8 1 O O

Chlorothiazide is the simplest member of this series, with pK_a values of 6.7 and 9.5. The hydrogen atom at the N-2 is the most acidic because of the electron-withdrawing effects of the neighboring sulfone group. The sulfonamide group that is substituted at C-7 provides an additional point of acidity in the molecule but is less acidic than the N-2 proton. These acidic protons make possible the formation of a water-soluble sodium salt that can be used for intravenous administration of the diuretics.

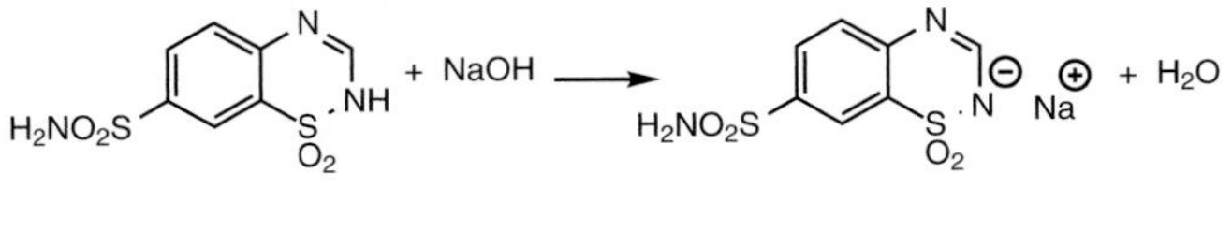

H_2NO_2S–(chlorothiazide, NH, O_2) + NaOH → H_2NO_2S–(N⊖ Na⊕, O_2) + H_2O

An electron-withdrawing group is necessary at position 6 for diuretic activity. Little diuretic activity is seen with a hydrogen atom at position 6, whereas compounds with either chloro (e.g., chlorothiazide, hydrochlorothiazide, and methyclothiazide) or trifluoromethyl (e.g., bendroflumethiazide and hydroflumethiazide) substituents are highly active.[19–21] The trifluoromethyl-substituted diuretics are more lipid soluble and have a longer duration of action than their chloro-substituted analogs. When electron-releasing groups, such as methyl or methoxyl, are placed at position 6, the diuretic activity is markedly reduced.

Replacement or removal of the sulfonamide group at position 7 yields compounds with little or no diuretic activity. Saturation of the double bond to give a 3,4-dihydro derivative (cf. chlorothiazide and hydrochlorothiazide) produces a diuretic that is 10-fold more active than the unsaturated derivative. Substitution with a lipophilic group at position 3 gives a marked increase in the diuretic potency. Haloalkyl, aralkyl, or thioether substitution increases the lipid solubility of the molecule and yields compounds with a longer duration of action. Alkyl substitution on the 2-N position also decreases the polarity and increases the duration of diuretic action (Table 17.6).

PHARMACOKINETIC PROPERTIES AND METABOLISM. The pharmacokinetic properties of the thiazide diuretics are summarized in Table 17.6. Several of these compounds are rapidly absorbed orally and can show their diuretic effect within an hour. These drugs are highly bound to plasma proteins and therefore are primarily cleared from the circulation via renal tubular secretion.[21] Thiazides are not extensively metabolized and are primarily excreted unchanged in the urine.

Thiazide-Like Diuretics

Therapeutic Role of Thiazide-Like Diuretics

This is a structurally diverse group of sulfonamide-containing compounds that are derivatives of quinazolin-4-one, phthalimidine, or indoline. In spite of their dissimilar structures and lack of a benzothiadiazine ring, these drugs have the same mechanism of action and similar therapeutic activities and adverse effects as the thiazide diuretics.[21]

However, in contrast to thiazide diuretics, metolazone (2.5-20 mg given as a single oral dose) may be effective as a diuretic when the GFR falls below 40 mL/min. In addition, chlorthalidone has a long duration of action (48-72 hr). For example, although metolazone is administered daily, chlorthalidone may be administered in doses of 25-100 mg three times a week. Uses of indapamide include the treatment of essential hypertension and edema resulting from congestive heart failure. Like metolazone, indapamide is an effective diuretic drug when the GFR is below 40 mL/min. The duration of action is approximately 24 hours, with the normal oral adult dosage starting at 2.5 mg given each morning. The dose may be increased to 5.0 mg/d, but doses beyond this level do not appear to provide additional results.

Pharmacology Overview of Thiazide-Like Diuretics

MECHANISM OF ACTION. These drugs have the same mechanism of action as the thiazide diuretics.

COMMON ADVERSE EFFECTS. Side effects for the thiazide-like diuretics are similar to those of the thiazides.

COMMON INTERACTIONS. These drugs have the same interactions as the thiazide diuretics.

Medicinal Chemistry of Thiazide-Like Diuretics

RECEPTOR BINDING, SAR, AND PHYSICOCHEMICAL PROPERTIES. The quinazolin-4-one molecule has been structurally modified in a manner similar to the modification of the thiazide diuretics. Metolazone (pK_a = 9.7) is an example of this class of drug (Table 17.7). The structural difference between the quinazolinone and thiazide diuretics is the replacement of the 4-sulfone group (—SO_2—) in the former with a 4-keto group (—CO—) in the latter. Because of their similar structures, it is not surprising that the quinazolin-4-ones have a diuretic effect similar to that of the thiazides.

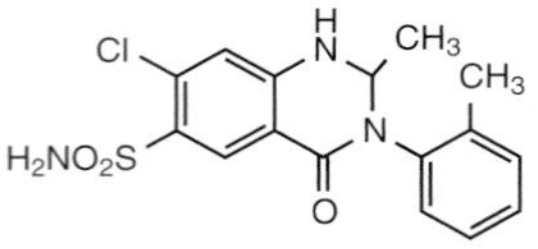

Metolazone

Chlorthalidone (pK_a = 9.4) is an example of a diuretic in this class of compounds that bears a structural analogy to the quinazolin-4-ones (Table 17.7). This compound may be named as a 1-oxo-isoindoline or a phthalimidine. Although the molecule exists primarily in the phthalimidine form, the ring may be opened to form a benzophenone derivative. The benzophenone form illustrates the relationship to the quinazolin-4-one series of diuretics.

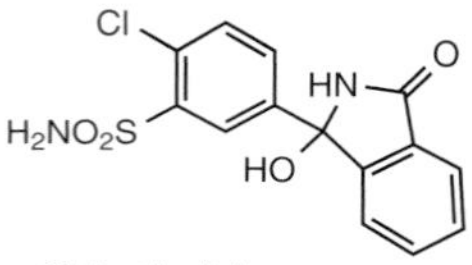

Chlorthalidone (Thalitone)

The prototypic indoline diuretic is indapamide, which was reported as a diuretic in 1984. Indapamide contains a polar chlorobenzamide moiety and a nonpolar lipophilic methylindoline group. In contrast to the thiazides, indapamide does not contain a thiazide ring, and only one sulfonamide group is present within the molecular structure of this drug (pK_a = 8.8).

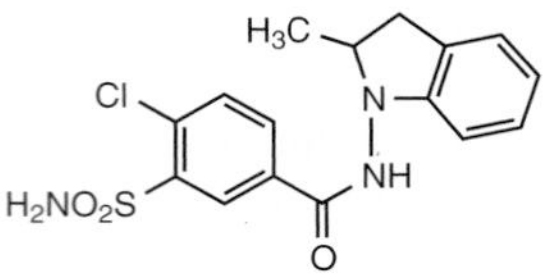

Indapamide

PHARMACOKINETIC PROPERTIES AND METABOLISM. The pharmacokinetic properties for the thiazide-like diuretics are listed in Table 17.7.

Chlorthalidone binds extensively to plasma proteins, as well as carbonic anhydrase in erythrocytes, and consequently has a long duration of action, up to 72 hours.[21] When chlorthalidone is formulated with the excipient povidone, the product, Thalitone, has greater bioavailability (>90%) and reaches peak plasma concentrations in a shorter time.

Like chlorthalidone, metolazone binds to plasma proteins and carbonic anhydrase in erythrocytes and has a long duration of action, 12-24 hours.[21] Metolazone has a bioavailability of 65% (Zaroxolyn) and a prolonged onset to reach peak plasma concentrations of action ranging from 8 to 12 hours.

Indapamide is rapidly and completely absorbed from the gastrointestinal tract and reaches its peak plasma level in 2-3 hours, with a duration of action of up to 36 hours.[21] This prolonged effect is associated with its extensive binding to carbonic anhydrase in the erythrocytes. It exhibits biphasic kinetics, with a half-life of 14-18 hours and an elimination half-life of 24 hours. Indapamide is extensively metabolized (60%-70%), with several of the metabolites being shown in Figure 17.2.[22,23] In vitro studies support aromatic hydroxylation as a metabolic route. Less than 10% of the drug is excreted unchanged, while the remaining 20%-30% is eliminated via enterohepatic recycling.

Table 17.7 Pharmacokinetic Properties for the Thiazide-Like Diuretics

Generic Name	Trade Name	Bioavailability	Peak Plasma	Half-Life	Duration	Elimination
Chlorthalidone	Hygroton Thalitone[a]	Var/Inc	4 hr	35-50 hr[b]	48-72 hr	Urine, as parent drug (50%-65%)
Indapamide	Lozol	>90%	2-3 hr	14-18 hr	24-36 hr	Urine/feces (6:2), as parent drug (70%) and metabolites
Metolazone	Zaroxylon	<65%	8-12 hr	14 hr	12-24 hr	Urine/feces (8:2), as parent drug (>70%)

Data from AHFS Drug Information (2010), American Society of Health-System Pharmacists; Lexicomp Online (2011), Lexicomp, Inc.; Facts and Comparisons (2010), Wolters Kluwer Health.

[a]Not interchangeable with similar drug.

[b]Strongly bound to red blood cells.

Inc, incomplete absorption; *NA,* data not available; *Var,* variable absorption.

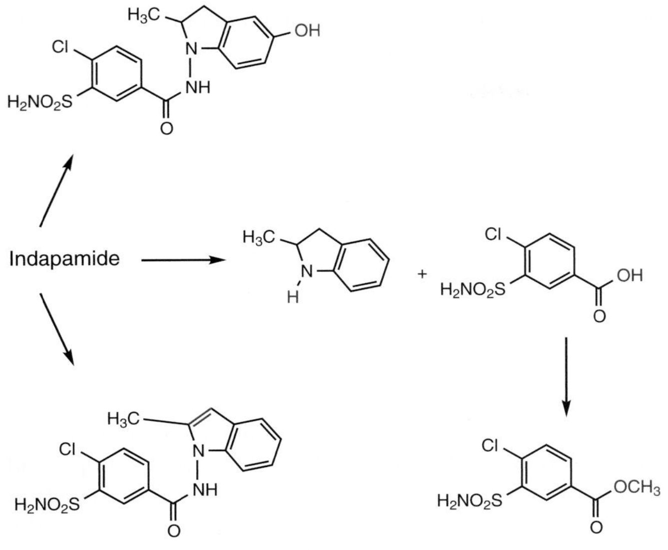

Figure 17.2 Metabolism of indapamide.

High-Ceiling or Loop Diuretics

Therapeutic Role of High-Ceiling or Loop Diuretics

This class of drugs is characterized more by its pharmacological similarities than by its chemical similarities.[24,25] Examples include furosemide, bumetanide, torsemide, and ethacrynic acid. These drugs produce a peak diuresis much greater than that observed with the other commonly used diuretics, hence the name high-ceiling diuretics. Their diuretic effect appears in approximately 30 minutes and lasts for approximately 6 hours. However, the loop diuretics are less effective in treating hypertension than thiazide diuretics. As they have a different mechanism of action, they may be used in combination with other diuretics for improved antihypertensive effects.

Furosemide has a saluretic effect 8- to 10-fold that of the thiazide diuretics; however, it has a shorter duration of action (~6-8 hr). It can cause a marked excretion of sodium, chloride, potassium, calcium, magnesium, and bicarbonate ions, with as much as 25% of the filtered load of sodium excreted in response to initial treatment. It is effective for the treatment of edemas connected with cardiac, hepatic, and renal sites.

Bumetanide has a duration of action of approximately 4 hours. The dose of bumetanide is 0.5-2 mg/d given as a single dose. Like other high-ceiling diuretics, torsemide exerts its effect in the ascending limb of the loop of Henle to promote the excretion of sodium, potassium, chloride, calcium, and magnesium ions and water. An additional effect on the peritubular side at chloride channels may enhance the luminal effects of torsemide. In contrast to furosemide and bumetanide, however, torsemide does not act at the proximal tubule and, therefore, does not increase phosphate or bicarbonate excretion.

Another major class of high-ceiling diuretics are the phenoxyacetic acid derivatives, of which ethacrynic acid is the prototypical agent. These compounds were developed at about the same time as furosemide but were designed to act mechanistically like the organomercurials (i.e., via inhibition of sulfhydryl-containing enzymes involved in solute reabsorption). Ethacrynic acid is the only loop diuretic which is not a sulfonamide derivative and may be useful in patients who are allergic to sulfonamides.

Pharmacology Overview of High-Ceiling or Loop Diuretics

MECHANISM OF ACTION. The main site of action for the high-ceiling (loop) diuretics is believed to be on the thick ascending limb of the loop of Henle, where they inhibit the luminal $Na^+/K^+/2Cl^-$ symporter. Additional effects on the proximal and distal tubules also are possible. High-ceiling diuretics are characterized by a quick onset and short duration of activity.[24,25]

The mechanism of action of ethacrynic acid appears to be more complex than the simple Michael addition of the α,β-unsubstituted ketone of the drug to enzyme sulfhydryl groups. When the double bond of ethacrynic acid is reduced, the resulting compound is still active, although the diuretic activity is diminished. The sulfhydryl groups of the enzyme would not be expected to add to the drug molecule in the absence of the α,β-unsaturated ketone.

COMMON ADVERSE EFFECTS. Clinical toxicity of furosemide and other loop diuretics primarily involves abnormalities of fluid and electrolyte balance. As with the thiazide diuretics, hypokalemia is an important adverse effect that can be prevented or treated with potassium supplements or coadministration of potassium-sparing diuretics. Increased calcium ion excretion can be a problem for postmenopausal osteopenic women, and furosemide generally should not be used in these individuals. Hyperuricemia, glucose intolerance, increased serum lipid levels, ototoxicity, and gastrointestinal side effects might be observed as well. Hypersensitivity reactions also are possible with furosemide (a sulfonamide-based drug), and cross-reactivity with other sulfonamide containing drugs is possible. The adverse effects of bumetanide and torsemide are similar to those induced by furosemide. In patients with cirrhosis and ascites, torsemide should be used with caution.

Toxicity induced by ethacrynic acid is similar to that induced by furosemide and bumetanide. Ethacrynic acid is not widely used as a diuretic because it also induces a greater incidence of ototoxicity and more serious gastrointestinal effects than furosemide or bumetanide.

COMMON INTERACTIONS. The loop diuretics exhibit many of the same interactions with other drugs as occurs with the thiazides.[25] For example, hypotension may result when they are used in combination with ACE inhibitors or ARBs, and their activity may be antagonized by NSAIDs and glucocorticoids.

Loop diuretics may alter the pharmacokinetics of the anticoagulant warfarin by displacing this highly protein-bound drug from its binding sites on serum albumin; this interaction may necessitate a dosage reduction for warfarin.[25]

Kidney damage may be increased when the loop diuretics are used together with other nephrotoxic drugs including aminoglycosides and NSAIDs. The combination of a loop diuretic and the anticancer drug cisplatin may increase the risk of nephrotoxicity and ototoxicity in patients receiving both drugs.[25]

Medicinal Chemistry of High-Ceiling or Loop Diuretics

RECEPTOR BINDING, SAR, AND PHYSICOCHEMICAL PROPERTIES. High-ceiling diuretics exert their diuretic effects via inhibition of $Na^+/K^+/2Cl^-$ symporter in the thick ascending limb of the loop of Henle.

Research on 5-sulfamoylanthranilic acids at the Hoechst Laboratories in Germany showed them to be effective diuretics.[19] The most active of a series of variously substituted derivatives was furosemide.

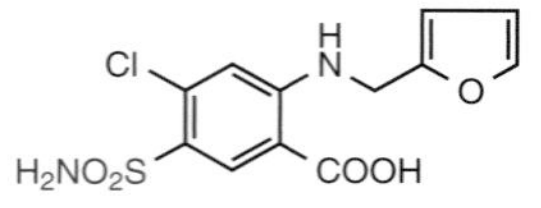

Furosemide

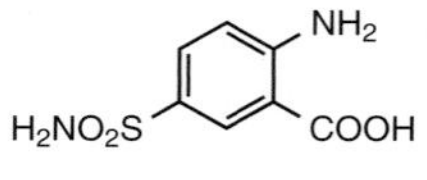

5-Sulfamoyl-anthranilic acid

Chlorine and sulfonamide substituents are also found in other diuretics. Because the molecule possesses a free carboxyl group, furosemide is a stronger acid than the thiazide diuretics ($pK_a = 3.9$). This drug is excreted primarily unchanged.[26] A small amount of metabolism, however, can take place on the furan ring, which is substituted on the aromatic amino group (see Table 17.5 for its other pharmacokinetic properties).

In bumetanide, a phenoxy group has replaced the customary chloro or trifluoromethyl substituents seen in other diuretic molecules.[27] The phenoxy group is an electron-withdrawing group similar to the chloro or trifluoromethyl substituents. The amine group customarily seen at position 6 has been moved to position 5. These minor variations from furosemide produced a compound with a mode of action similar to that of furosemide, but with a marked increase in diuretic potency. The short duration of activity is similar, but the compound is approximately 50-fold more potent. Replacement of the phenoxy group at position 4 with a C_6H_5NH- or C_6H_5S- group also gives compounds with a favorable activity. When the butyl group on the C-5 amine is replaced with a furanylmethyl group, such as in furosemide, however, the results are not favorable.

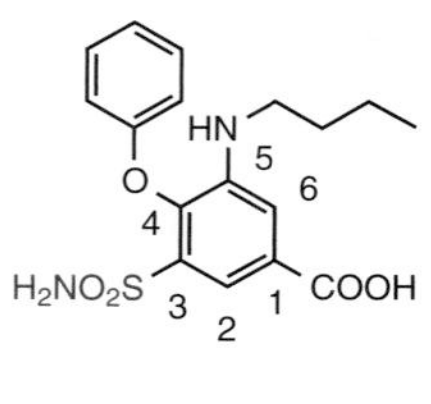

Bumetanide

Further modification of furosemide-like structures led to the development of torsemide.[28] Instead of the sulfonamide group found in furosemide and bumetanide, torsemide contains a sulfonylurea moiety.

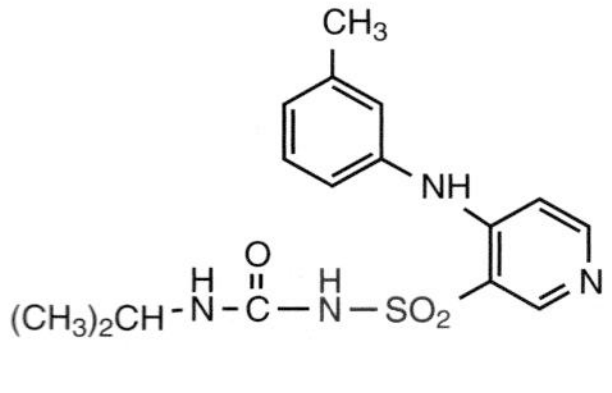

Torsemide

Optimal diuretic activity was obtained when an oxyacetic acid group was positioned para to an α,β-unsaturated carbonyl (or other sulfhydryl-reactive group) and chloro or methyl groups were placed at the 2- or 3-position of the phenyl ring.[29] In addition, hydrogen atoms on the terminal alkene carbon also provided maximum reactivity. Thus, a molecule with a weakly acidic group to direct the drug to the kidney and an alkylating moiety to react with sulfhydryl groups and lipophilic groups seemed to provide the best combination for a diuretic in this class. These features led to the development of ethacrynic acid as the prototypic agent in this class.

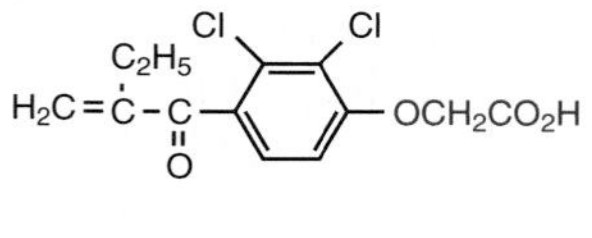

Ethacrynic acid

PHARMACOKINETIC PROPERTIES AND METABOLISM. The pharmacokinetic properties for the loop diuretics are listed in Table 17.5. Furosemide is orally effective but may be used parenterally when a prompter diuretic effect is desired, such as in the treatment of acute pulmonary edema. The dosage of furosemide, 20-80 mg/d, may be given in divided doses because of the short duration of action of the drug and carefully increased up to a maximum of 600 mg/d. Bumetanide exhibits similar pharmacokinetics to furosemide. Both drugs are eliminated in urine and feces (furosemide) as a mixture of parent compounds and metabolites.

The oral bioavailability of torsemide is very good (~80%) and absorption is not affected by the presence of food in the gastrointestinal tract.[28] Peak diuresis is observed 1-2 hours following oral or intravenous administration, with a duration of action of approximately 6 hours (Table 17.5). Torsemide is indicated for the treatment of edema resulting from congestive heart failure and for the treatment of hypertension. In contrast to furosemide and bumetanide, torsemide is eliminated predominantly as unmetabolized parent drug.

Oral administration of ethacrynic acid results in diuresis within 1 hour and a duration of action of 6-8 hours. This drug is eliminated renally and hepatically as parent compound and metabolites, including a mercapturic acid derivative.

Mineralocorticoid Receptor Antagonists

Therapeutic Role of Mineralocorticoid Receptor Antagonists

The adrenal cortex secretes a potent mineralocorticoid called aldosterone, which promotes salt and water retention and potassium and hydrogen ion excretion. Aldosterone exerts its biological effects through binding to the mineralocorticoid receptor (MR), a nuclear transcription factor.[30]

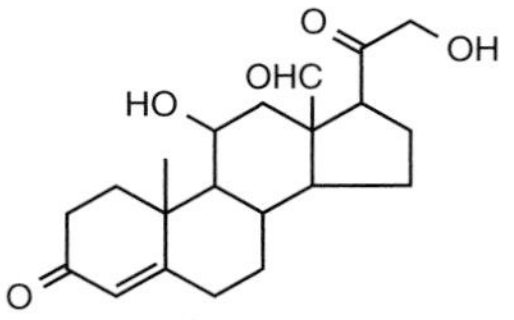

Aldosterone (aldol from)

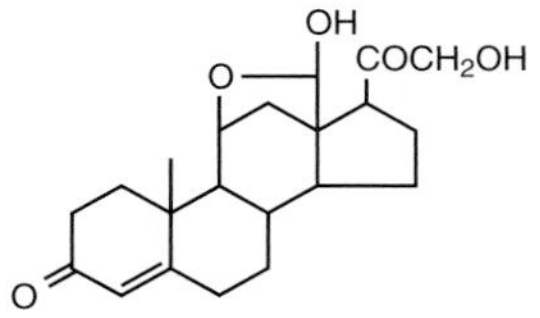

Aldosterone (hemiacetal form)

Other mineralocorticoids influence the electrolytic balance of the body, but aldosterone is the most potent. Its ability to cause increased reabsorption of sodium and chloride ion and increased potassium ion excretion is approximately 3,000-fold that of hydrocortisone. A substance that antagonizes the effects of aldosterone could conceivably be a good diuretic drug. Spironolactone and eplerenone are examples of such antagonists. These drugs are also classified as potassium-sparing diuretics. The pharmacological properties of spironolactone and eplerenone are summarized in Table 17.5.

Spironolactone is useful in treating edema resulting from primary hyperaldosteronism and refractory edema associated with secondary hyperaldosteronism. Spironolactone is the drug of choice for treating edema resulting from cirrhosis of the liver. The dose of spironolactone is 100 mg/d given in single or divided doses. Another use of spironolactone is coadministration with a potassium-depleting diuretic (e.g., a thiazide or loop diuretic) to prevent or treat diuretic-induced hypokalemia. However, it should not be combined with potassium-sparing diuretics (e.g., triamterene or amiloride). Spironolactone can be administered in a fixed-dose combination with hydrochlorothiazide for this purpose, but optimal individualization of the dose of each drug is recommended.

Eplerenone came out of efforts to develop spironolactone analogs with reduced adverse effects.[31,32] Like spironolactone, eplerenone is used alone or with other diuretics for the treatment of hypertension or left ventricular systolic dysfunction and congestive heart failure after myocardial infarction. Single daily oral doses are 25-50 mg.

Pharmacology Overview of Mineralocorticoid Receptor Antagonists

MECHANISM OF ACTION. Spironolactone and eplerenone competitively inhibit aldosterone binding to the MR,[30] thereby interfering with reabsorption of sodium and chloride ions and the associated water. The most important renal site of the MR receptors, and hence the primary site of action of spironolactone and eplerenone, is in the late distal convoluted tubule and collecting system (collecting duct).

COMMON ADVERSE EFFECTS. The primary concern with the use of spironolactone is the development of hyperkalemia, which can be fatal. Spironolactone may cause hypersensitivity reactions, gastrointestinal disturbances, and peptic ulcer. Sexual side effects (i.e., gynecomastia, decreased libido, and impotence) can also occur and are due to nonselective binding of spironolactone to the androgen receptor (AR), glucocorticoid receptor (GR), or progesterone receptor (PR). It also has been implicated in tumor production during chronic toxicity studies in rats, but human risk has not been documented.

Hyperkalemia is also a serious and potentially fatal side effect with eplenerone. However; in contrast to spironolactone, eplenerone has limited or no inhibitory effects on AR, GR, and PR and is therefore a more selective aldosterone antagonist.[31,32] Consequently, it has fewer sexual side effects.

COMMON INTERACTIONS. The MR antagonists can produce additive effects when combined with other antihypertensive drugs.[25] As seen with other diuretics, NSAIDs, and glucocorticoids may exert antagonistic effects. Hyperkalemia may result if MR antagonists are used in combination with other drugs (e.g., ACE inhibitors, ARBs, β-blockers, etc.) that elevate blood potassium levels.

Eplerenone is extensively metabolized by CYP3A4 (see below). Combination with inhibitors (e.g., ketoconazole or erythromycin) of this CYP isozyme may therefore alter eplerenone metabolism and pharmacokinetics.[25]

Medicinal Chemistry of Mineralocorticoid Receptor Antagonists

RECEPTOR BINDING, SAR, AND PHYSICOCHEMICAL PROPERTIES. MR antagonist activity is dependent on the presence of a γ-lactone ring on C-17 and a substituent on C-7 in spironolactone and structurally related compounds.[33,34] Interaction of C-7-unsubstituted agonists, such as aldosterone, with a methionine residue in the MR ligand binding domain is important for receptor activation and subsequent transcription. However, this interaction is sterically hindered by C-7 substituents on aldosterone antagonists, thereby leaving MR in an inactive conformation.[33,34]

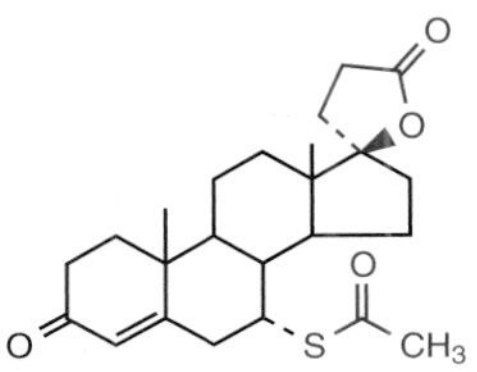

Spironolactone

In addition to the lactone ring and C-7 substituent (in this case an acetyl group) that are important for MR antagonism, eplerenone has a 9α,11α-epoxy group as part of its structure. Like spironolactone, it binds to the MR and is an aldosterone antagonist. However, it has a 20- to 40-fold lower affinity for the MR than spironolactone (see Table 17.5).[31] This reduced binding is believed to be due to the epoxy group.[35,36] Nevertheless, eplerenone is an effective diuretic and has certain therapeutic advantages over spironolactone.

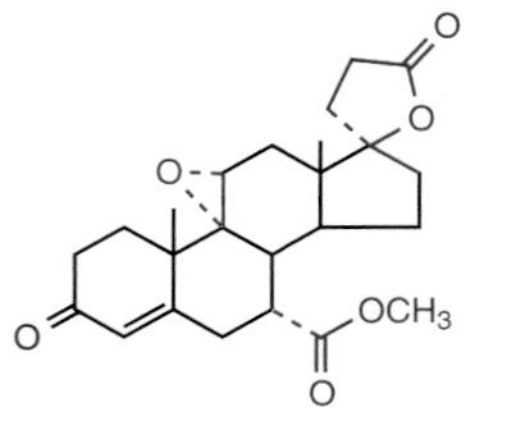

PHARMACOKINETIC PROPERTIES AND METABOLISM. The pharmacokinetic properties of spironolactone and eplerenone are summarized in Table 17.5. On oral administration, approximately 90% of the dose of spironolactone is absorbed and is significantly metabolized during its first passage through the liver to its major active metabolite, canrenone, which is interconvertible with its canrenoate anion (Fig. 17.3).[37,38] Canrenone is an antagonist to aldosterone and exists in equilibrium with its ring-opened form, canrenoate.

The canrenoate anion is not therapeutically active but acts as an aldosterone antagonist because of its conversion back to canrenone, which exists in the lactone form. Canrenone has been suggested to be the active form of spironolactone as an aldosterone antagonist. The formation of canrenone, however, cannot fully account for the total activity of spironolactone.[37,38] Both canrenone and potassium canrenoate are used as diuretics in other countries, but they are not available in the United States.

Eplerenone has good (~70%) oral bioavailability and, unlike spironolactone, only undergoes limited first pass metabolism (Table 17.5). Absorption is not affected by the presence of food in the GI tract. In plasma, it is about 50% bound to plasma α_1-acid glycoprotein. Eplerenone has a half-life of approximately 5 hours and undergoes extensive metabolism by hepatic CYP3A4 to inactive metabolites (Fig. 17.4).[39] Elimination occurs in the urine and feces.

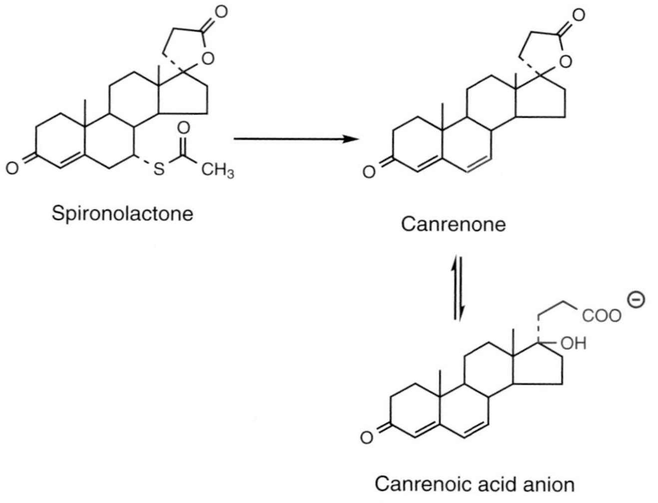

Potassium-Sparing Diuretics

Therapeutic Role of Potassium-Sparing Diuretics

Two drugs in this class of diuretics are triamterene and amiloride (Table 17.5), which are derivatives of pteridine and aminopyrazine, respectively. Individually, amiloride and triamterene exert a mild diuretic effect and are usually used in combination with other diuretic agents.

Triamterene is useful in combination with a thiazide or loop diuretic in the treatment of edema or hypertension. Liddle syndrome, which is due to an inherited mutation in the epithelial sodium channel (ENaC) leading to increased activity of the receptor, also may be treated with a sodium channel blocking drug, such as triamterene or amiloride. Triamterene is administered initially in doses of 100 mg twice a day. A maintenance dose for each patient should be individually determined. This dose may vary from 100 mg a day to as low as 100 mg every other day.

Like triamterene, amiloride combined with a thiazide or loop diuretic is used to treat edema or hypertension. Aerosolized amiloride has shown some benefit in improving mucociliary clearance in patients with cystic fibrosis.

Pharmacology Overview of Potassium-Sparing Diuretics

MECHANISM OF ACTION. In vitro experiments have shown that triamterene and amiloride exert a diuretic effect by blocking an ENaC in principal cells of the late distal convoluted tubule and collecting duct.[40,41] Both drugs

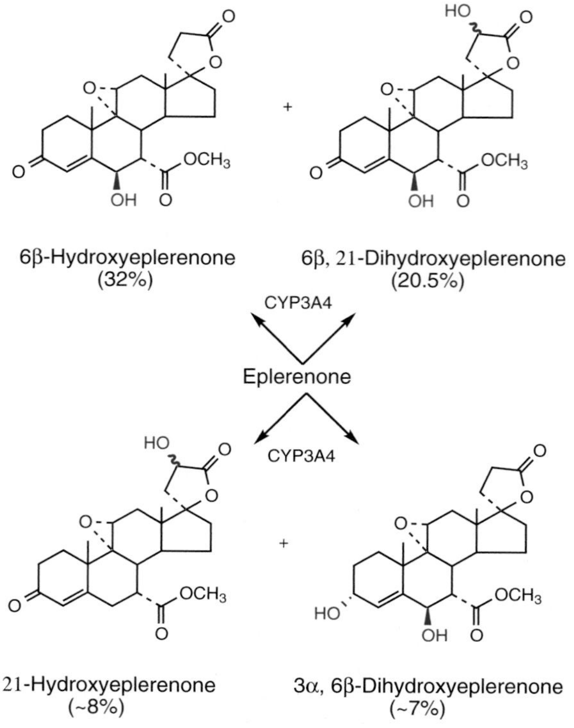

Spironolactone

Canrenone

Canrenoic acid anion

Figure 17.3 Metabolic conversion of spironolactone to canrenone.

6β-Hydroxyeplerenone (32%)

6β, 21-Dihydroxyeplerenone (20.5%)

CYP3A4

Eplerenone

CYP3A4

21-Hydroxyeplerenone (~8%)

3α, 6β-Dihydroxyeplerenone (~7%)

Figure 17.4 Major metabolic products formed from eplerenone.

are weak organic bases and inhibit ENaC in a voltage- and pH-dependent manner. Inhibition occurs because amiloride and triamterene bind to negatively charged regions of the sodium channel in the ENaC. The greater potency (approximately 100-fold in vitro) of amiloride is probably due to the fact that it is a stronger base (pK_a = 8.7) and is therefore more extensively protonated at physiological pH than triamterene (pK_a = 6.2). Sodium channel inhibitors block the reabsorption of sodium ion and inhibit the secretion of potassium ion. The net result is increased sodium and chloride ion excretion in the urine and almost no potassium excretion. Consequently, amiloride and triamterene can be used to offset the effect of other diuretics that result in loss of potassium.

COMMON ADVERSE EFFECTS. The most serious side effect associated with the use of triamterene is hyperkalemia. For this reason, potassium supplements are contraindicated, and serum potassium levels should be checked regularly. Triamterene also is used in combination with hydrochlorothiazide. Here, the hypokalemic effect of the hydrochlorothiazide counters the hyperkalemic effect of the triamterene. Other side effects that are seen with the use of triamterene are nausea, vomiting, and headache. Amiloride can produce similar side effects as triamterene, including hyperkalemia.

COMMON INTERACTIONS. Hypotension can result if amiloride or triamterene are used in combination with other diuretics and other antihypertensive agents.[25]

Medicinal Chemistry of the Potassium-Sparing Diuretics

RECEPTOR BINDING, SAR, AND PHYSICOCHEMICAL PROPERTIES. Pteridine ring–containing compounds have a marked potential for influencing biological processes. Early screening of pteridine derivatives revealed that 2,4-diamino-6,7-dimethylpteridine had diuretic activity.

Pteridine   Triamterene

Structural modifications of the pteridine nucleus led to the development of triamterene. Further alterations of the triamterene structure are not usually beneficial in terms of diuretic activity. Activity is retained if an amine group is replaced with a lower alkylamine group. Introduction of a para-methyl group on the phenyl ring decreases the activity by approximately half. Introduction of a para-hydroxyl group on the phenyl ring yields a compound that is essentially inactive as a diuretic.

Amiloride is an aminopyrazine structurally related to triamterene as an open-chain analog.

PHARMACOKINETIC PROPERTIES AND METABOLISM. Triamterene is more than 70% absorbed on oral administration (see Table 17.5 for its other pharmacokinetic properties). The diuretic effect occurs rapidly (~30 min) and reaches a peak plasma concentration in 2-4 hours, with a duration of action of more than 24 hours. This drug is extensively metabolized to 4′-hydroxytriamterene, which subsequently undergoes sulfation (Fig. 17.5). Both metabolites are still active as diuretics and, along with the parent drug triamterene, are excreted in the urine.[42]

Oral amiloride is approximately 50% absorbed (see Table 17.5 for its other pharmacokinetic properties), with a duration of action of up to about 24 hours, which is slightly shorter than that of triamterene. Although triamterene is extensively metabolized, approximately 50% of amiloride is excreted unchanged. Renal impairment can increase its elimination half-life. The dose of amiloride is 5-10 mg per day. Amiloride also is combined with hydrochlorothiazide in a fixed-dose combination.

THE RENIN-ANGIOTENSIN PATHWAY

Overview

The renin-angiotensin system is a complex, highly regulated pathway that is integral in the regulation of blood volume, electrolyte balance, and arterial blood pressure. It consists of two main enzymes, renin and angiotensin-converting enzyme (ACE), the primary purpose of which is to release angiotensin II from its endogenous precursor, angiotensinogen (Fig. 17.6). Angiotensin II is a potent vasoconstrictor that affects peripheral resistance, renal function, and cardiovascular structure.[43]

Historically, the renin-angiotensin system dates back to 1898, when Tiegerstedt and Bergman demonstrated the existence of a pressor substance in crude kidney extracts. A little more than 40 years later, two independent research groups discovered that this pressor substance, which had previously been named renin, actually was an enzyme and that the true pressor substance was a peptide formed by the catalytic action of renin. This peptide pressor substance initially was assigned two different names, angiotonin and hypertensin; however, these names eventually were combined to produce the current designation, angiotensin. In the 1950s, it was discovered that angiotensin exists as both an inactive

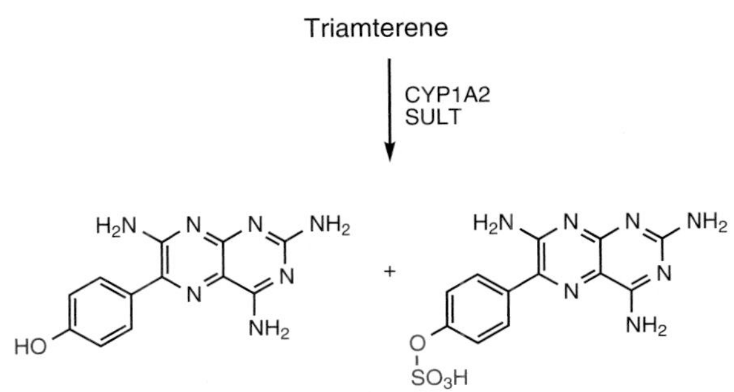

Figure 17.5 Metabolism of triamterene. Coloration indicates site of metabolism.

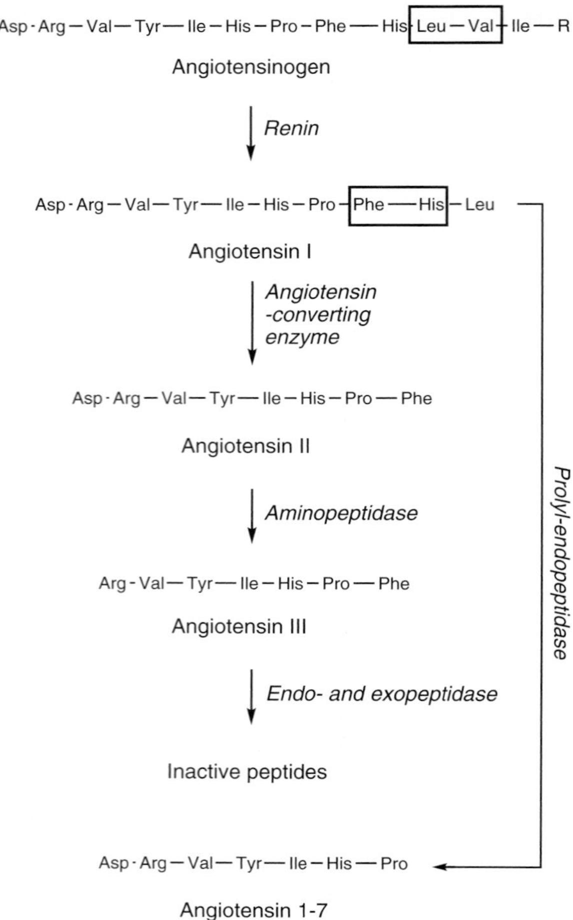

Figure 17.6 Schematic representation of the renin-angiotensin pathway. The labile peptide bonds of angiotensinogen and angiotensin I are highlighted.

decapeptide, angiotensin I, and an active octapeptide, angiotensin II, and that the conversion of angiotensin I to angiotensin II is catalyzed by an enzyme distinct from renin.[44]

Angiotensinogen is an α_2-globulin with a molecular weight of 58,000-61,000 Da. It contains 452 amino acids, is abundant in the plasma, and is continually synthesized and secreted by the liver. A number of hormones, including glucocorticoids, thyroid hormone, and angiotensin II, stimulate its synthesis. The most important portion of this biomoleule is the N-terminus, specifically the Leu10-Val11 bond. This bond is cleaved by renin and produces the decapeptide angiotensin I. The Phe8-His9 peptide bond of angiotensin I is then cleaved by ACE to produce the octapeptide angiotensin II. Aminopeptidase can further convert angiotensin II to the active heptapeptide angiotensin III by removing the N-terminal arginine residue. Further actions of carboxypeptidases, aminopeptidases, and endopeptidases result in the formation of inactive peptide fragments. An additional peptide can be formed by the action of a prolyl-endopeptidase on angiotensin I. Cleavage of the Pro7-Phe8 bond of angiotensin I produces a heptapeptide known as angiotensin 1-7.[44]

Normal Actions of the Renin-Angiotensin Pathway

Renin is an aspartyl protease that determines the rate of angiotensin II production and is a much more specific enzyme than ACE. Its primary function is to cleave the leucine-valine bond at residues 10 and 11 of angiotensinogen. The stimulation of renin release is controlled very closely by hemodynamic, neurogenic, and humoral signals (Fig. 17.7). Hemodynamic signals involve the renal juxtaglomerular cells. These cells are sensitive to the hemodynamic stretch of the afferent glomerular arteriole. An increase in the stretch implies a raised blood pressure and results in a reduced release of renin, whereas a decrease in the stretch increases renin secretion. Additionally, these cells also are sensitive to NaCl flux across the adjacent macula densa. Increases in NaCl flux across the macula densa inhibit renin release but decreases in the flux stimulate release. Furthermore, neurogenic enhancement of renin release occurs via activation of β_1 receptors. Finally, a variety of hormonal signals influence the release of renin. Somatostatin, atrial natriuretic factor, and angiotensin II inhibit renin release, whereas vasoactive intestinal peptide, parathyroid hormone, and glucagon stimulate renin release.[45]

In contrast, ACE, also known as kininase II, is a zinc protease that is under minimal physiologic control. It is not a rate-limiting step in the generation of angiotensin II and is a relatively nonspecific dipeptidyl carboxypeptidase that requires only a tripeptide sequence as a substrate. The only structural feature required by ACE is that the penultimate amino acid in the peptide substrate cannot be proline. For this reason, angiotensin II, which contains a proline

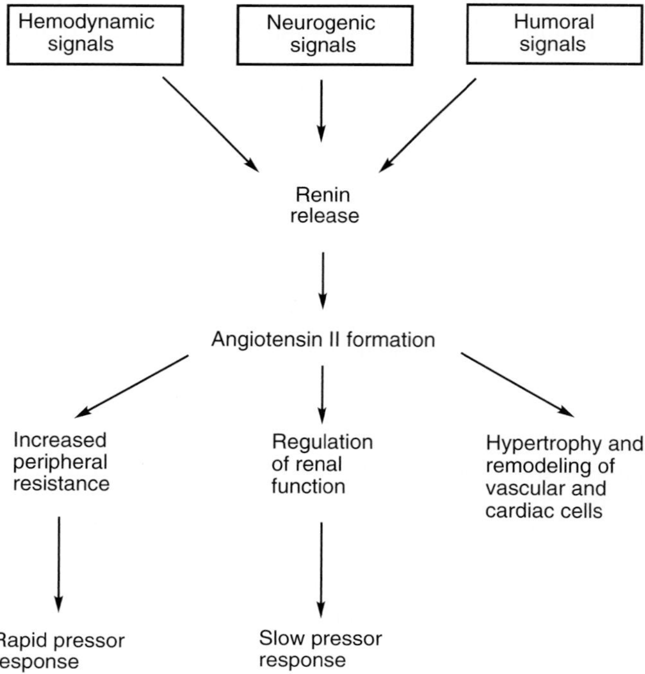

Figure 17.7 Summary of the factors involved in renin release and the effects mediated by angiotensin II.

in the penultimate position, is not further metabolized by ACE. The lack of specificity and control exhibited by ACE results in its involvement in the bradykinin pathway (Fig. 17.8). Bradykinin is a nonapeptide that acts locally to produce pain, cause vasodilation, increase vascular permeability, stimulate prostaglandin synthesis, and cause bronchoconstriction. Similar to angiotensin II, bradykinin is produced by proteolytic cleavage of a precursor peptide. Cleavage of kininogens by the protease kallikrein produces a decapeptide known as either kallidin or lysyl-bradykinin. Subsequent cleavage of the N-terminal lysine by aminopeptidase produces bradykinin. The degradation of bradykinin to inactive peptides occurs through the actions of ACE. Thus, ACE not only produces a potent vasoconstrictor but also inactivates a potent vasodilator.[43,45,46]

Angiotensin II is the dominant peptide produced by the renin-angiotensin pathway (Fig. 17.7). It is a potent vasoconstrictor that increases total peripheral resistance through a variety of mechanisms: direct vasoconstriction, enhancement of both catecholamine release and neurotransmission within the peripheral nervous system, and increased sympathetic discharge. The result of all these actions is a rapid pressor response. Additionally, angiotensin II causes a slow pressor response, resulting in long-term stabilization of arterial blood pressure. This long-term effect is accomplished by the regulation of renal function. Angiotensin II directly increases sodium reabsorption in the proximal tubule. It also alters renal hemodynamics and causes the release of aldosterone from the adrenal cortex. Finally, angiotensin II causes the hypertrophy and remodeling of both vascular and cardiac cells through a variety of hemodynamic and nonhemodynamic effects.[43]

The secondary peptides, angiotensin III and angiotensin 1-7, can contribute to the overall effects of the renin-angiotensin pathway. Angiotensin III is equipotent with angiotensin II in stimulating aldosterone secretion; however, it is only 10%-25% as potent in increasing blood pressure. In contrast, angiotensin 1-7 does not cause either aldosterone secretion or vasoconstriction, but it does have potent effects that are distinct from those of angiotensin II. Similar to angiotensin II, angiotensin 1-7 causes neuronal excitation and vasopressin release. Additionally, it enhances the production of prostaglandins

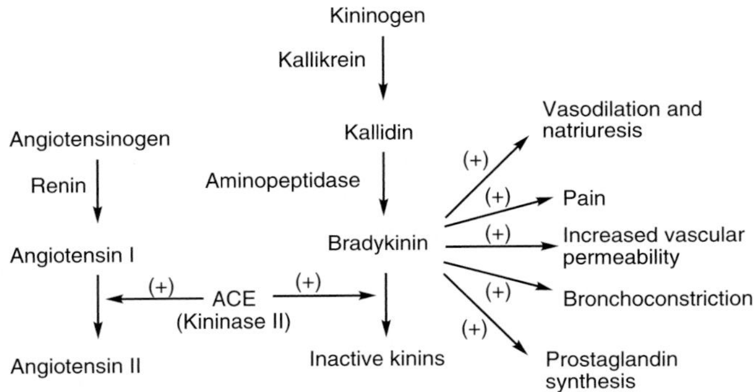

Figure 17.8 Schematic representation of the bradykinin pathway and its relationship to angiotensin-converting enzyme (ACE) and the renin-angiotensin pathway.

via a receptor-mediated process that does not involve an increase in intracellular calcium levels. It has been proposed to be important in the modulation of cell-to-cell interactions in cardiovascular and neural tissues.[47]

Role of Renin-Angiotensin Pathway in Hypertension and Other Cardiovascular Disorders

Abnormalities in the renin-angiotensin pathway (e.g., excessive release of renin and overproduction of angiotensin II) can contribute to hypertension through the rapid and slow pressor responses previously described. In addition, high levels of angiotensin II can cause or exacerbate heart failure, a disorder in which the heart is unable to supply blood at a rate sufficient to meet the demands of the body. Similar to hypertension, this pathophysiologic state can occur via a variety of mechanisms. Any pathophysiologic event that causes either systolic or diastolic dysfunction will result in heart failure. Systolic dysfunction, or decreased contractility, can be caused by dilated cardiomyopathies, ventricular hypertrophy, or a reduction in muscle mass. Diastolic dysfunction, or restriction in ventricular filling, can be caused by increased ventricular stiffness, mitral or tricuspid valve stenosis, or pericardial disease. Both ventricular hypertrophy and myocardial ischemia can contribute to increased ventricular stiffness. Angiotensin II causes and/or exacerbates heart failure by increasing systemic vascular resistance, promoting sodium retention, stimulating aldosterone release, and stimulating ventricular hypertrophy and remodeling.[48] Heart failure affects approximately six million Americans and is the most common hospital discharge diagnosis in patients older than 65 years. From an economic standpoint, heart failure expenditures approach or exceed approximately $40 billion dollars on an annual basis.[49]

Development of Drugs to Block the Actions of the Renin-Angiotensin Pathway

A more in-depth discussion of the development of ACE inhibitors, ARBs, and renin inhibitors can be found in the 7th edition of *Foye's*.[50]

Development of Angiotensin-Converting Enzyme Inhibitors

Cushman, Ondetti, and coworkers developed a hypothetical model of the binding site of ACE that lead to the development of captopril, the first FDA-approved ACE inhibitor.[51–53] Their model was based upon the enzymatic actions of ACE, the actions of several naturally occurring peptides, and the similarities between ACE and pancreatic carboxypeptidases. The original peptides were isolated from the venom of the South American pit viper *Bothrops jararaca* and contained a proline residue at their carboxylate terminus.[54,55] These peptides were shown to inhibit ACE and potentiate the actions of bradykinin.

Carboxypeptidase A, like ACE, is a zinc-containing exopeptidase. The binding of a substrate to carboxypeptidase

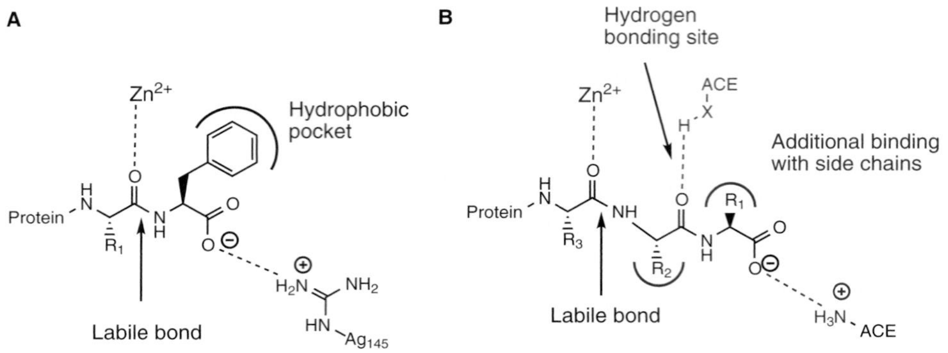

Figure 17.9 A model of substrate binding to carboxypeptidase A (A) and angiotensin-converting enzyme (ACE) (B). ACE substrate binding sites are highlighted in red.

A involves three major interactions (Fig. 17.9A): (1) an ionic interaction between the negatively charged carboxylate terminus and the positively charged Arg145 on the enzyme, (2) van der Waals interactions between a hydrophobic pocket in the enzyme and the side chains of C-terminal aromatic or nonpolar residues, and (3) a complexation between a zinc atom and the labile peptide bond. The zinc atom helps to polarize the carbonyl bond and to stabilize the negatively charged tetrahedral intermediate that results.[56] The binding of substrates to ACE was proposed to involve similar interactions with three specific differences (Fig. 17.9B). First, because ACE cleaves dipeptides instead of single amino acids, the position of the zinc atom was assumed to be located two amino acids away from the cationic center for it to be adjacent to the labile peptide bond. Second, ACE does not show specificity for C-terminal hydrophobic amino acids; however, it was proposed that the side chains, R_1 and R_2, of ACE substrates could contribute to the overall binding affinity. Finally, as the C-terminal peptide bond is nonlabile (i.e., not cleaved), it was assumed to provide hydrogen bonding between the substrate and ACE.

Using this model and the knowledge that D-2-benzylsuccinic acid was an extremely potent inhibitor of carboxypeptidase A, Cushman, Ondetti, and coworkers sequentially examined succinyl L-proline analogs (Fig. 17.10). Due to the fact that proline was present as the C-terminal amino acid in a number of potent, inhibitory snake venom peptides, it was used instead of leucine, the C-terminal amino acid present in angiotensin I. One of the most important alterations to succinyl-L-proline was the replacement of the succinyl carboxylate with a sulfhydryl group. The further addition of a methyl group yielded captopril. Captopril is a dipeptide mimic and a competitive inhibitor of ACE. It has a K_i value of 1.7 nmol/L and was the first ACE inhibitor to be marketed.

The sulfhydryl group of captopril proved to be responsible not only for the excellent inhibitory activity of the drug but also for the two most common side effects, skin rashes, and taste disturbances (e.g., metallic taste and loss of taste). These side effects usually subsided on dosage reduction or discontinuation of captopril. They were attributed to the presence of the sulfhydryl group because similar effects had been observed with penicillamine, a sulfhydryl-containing agent used to treat Wilson disease and rheumatoid arthritis.[57,58]

Researchers at Merck[59] sought to develop drugs that lacked the sulfhydryl group of captopril yet maintained some ability to chelate zinc. Their investigations lead to the development of dicarboxylate inhibitors that have the general structure shown below.

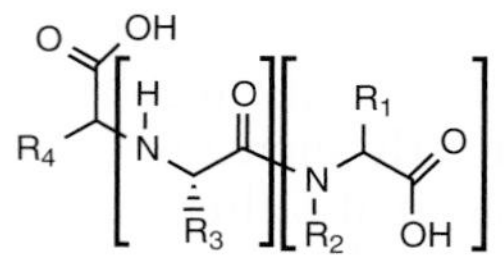

C B A

These are tripeptide substrate analogs in which the C-terminal (A) and penultimate (B) amino acids are retained but the third amino acid is isosterically replaced by a substituted N-carboxymethyl group (C). Similar to the results seen in the development of captopril, C-terminal proline analogs provided optimum activity. The use of a methyl group at R_3 (i.e., B = Ala) and a phenylethyl group at R_4 resulted in enalaprilat. In comparing the activity of captopril and enalaprilat, it was found that enalaprilat, with a K_i of 0.2 nmol/L, was approximately 10-fold more potent than captopril. Despite its excellent intravenous (IV) activity, enalaprilat has very poor oral bioavailability. Esterification of enalaprilat produced enalapril, a drug

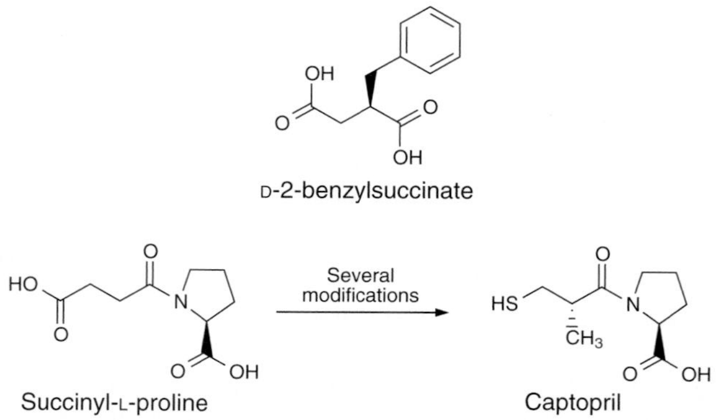

Figure 17.10 Development of captopril from succinyl-L-proline.

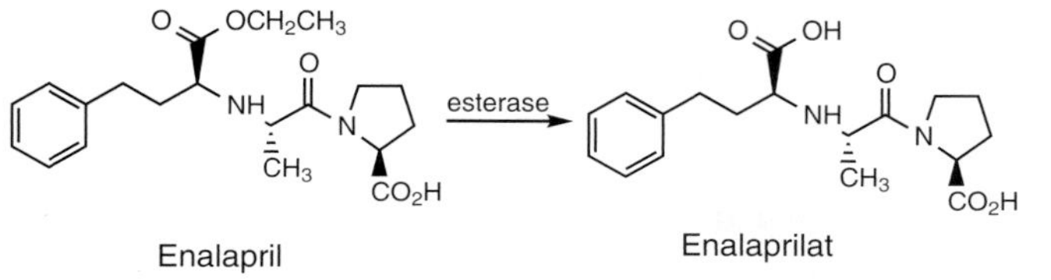

Enalapril → (esterase) → Enalaprilat

Figure 17.11 Bioactivation of enalapril to enalaprilat.

with superior oral bioavailability (Fig. 17.11). The success of enalapril and enalaprilat lead to the development of eight additional dicarboxylate inhibitors.

The search for ACE inhibitors that lacked the sulfhydryl group also led to the investigation of phosphorous-containing compounds.[60] The phosphinic acid shown in Figure 17.12 is capable of binding to ACE in a manner similar to enalaprilat. The interaction of the zinc atom with the phosphinic acid is similar to that seen with sulfhydryl and carboxylate groups. Additionally, this compound is capable of forming the ionic, hydrogen, and hydrophobic bonds similar to those seen with enalaprilat and other dicarboxylate analogs. Modification of the proline ring resulted in fosinoprilat, a drug that has a higher inhibitory activity than captopril.

Development of Angiotensin II Receptor Blockers

From an historical perspective, the angiotensin II receptor was the initial target for developing drugs that could inhibit the renin-angiotensin pathway. Efforts to develop angiotensin II receptor antagonists began in the early 1970s and focused on peptide-based analogs of the natural agonist. While peptide analogs demonstrated the ability to reduce blood pressure, these compounds lacked oral bioavailability and expressed unwanted partial agonist activity. The use of peptide mimetics circumvented these inherent problems and lead to the development of losartan, the first nonpeptide angiotensin II receptor blocker (ARB).[43,61] Two 1982 patent publications described the antihypertensive effects of a series of imidazole-5-acetic acid analogs. Exemplified by S-8038 (Fig. 17.13), these analogs were found to selectively block the angiotensin II receptor without producing any unwanted agonist activity. A computerized molecular modeling overlap of angiotensin II with the structure of S-8308 revealed three common structural features: The ionized carboxylate of S-8308 correlated with the C-terminal carboxylate of angiotensin II, the imidazole ring of S-8308 correlated with the imidazole side chain of the His6 residue, and the n-butyl group of S-8308 correlated with the hydrocarbon side chain of the Ile5 residue (Fig. 17.13). The benzyl group of S-8308 was proposed to lie in the direction of the N-terminus of angiotensin II; however, it was not believed to have any significant receptor interactions.

From S-8308, a number of molecular modifications were carried out in an attempt to improve receptor binding and lipid solubility, with the latter being important to assure adequate oral absorption. These changes resulted in losartan, a drug with high receptor affinity (IC_{50} = 0.019 μmol/L) and oral activity (Fig. 17.14). Seven additional ARBs have been approved for therapeutic use.

Development of Renin Inhibitors

In 1957, Skeggs et al. reported the activities of a purified amino acid sequence that could function as a renin substrate and proposed that the inhibition of renin would be beneficial in the treatment of hypertension.[62] Renin is a very specific enzyme that recognizes the Pro7-Phe8-His9-Leu10-Val11-Ile12-His13-Asn14 octapeptide sequence of angiotensinogen. Initial attempts to design renin inhibitors focused upon peptide analogs designed to mimic portions or all of this sequence. Many of these analogs, exemplified by compound A in Figure 17.15, showed effective inhibition of renin; however, susceptibility to proteolytic cleavage, poor or absent oral bioavailability, and short durations of action limited the therapeutic utility of these peptidic agents. Sequential structural modifications produced peptide-based compounds with the ability to mimic the transition state of angiotensinogen cleavage. Compounds such as zankiren (Fig. 17.15) possessed improved potency, favorable lipid solubility, and better oral bioavailability as compared to their predecessors. Unfortunately, the cost of synthetic preparation coupled with the success of newly approved ARBs temporarily curtailed commercial interest in this area. Success was finally obtained when the peptide backbone was abandoned and replaced with a nonpeptidic template. This template was used in the development of aliskiren (Fig. 17.15), the first nonpeptide, low-molecular-weight, orally active, transition-state renin inhibitor.[63–65]

Therapeutic Role of Drugs That Block the Renin-Angiotensin Pathway

All ACE inhibitors, ARBs, and aliskiren, a renin inhibitor, are approved for the treatment of hypertension. In addition, specific ACE inhibitors and ARBs have also been approved for heart failure, left ventricular dysfunction (either after myocardial infarction [MI] or asymptomatic),

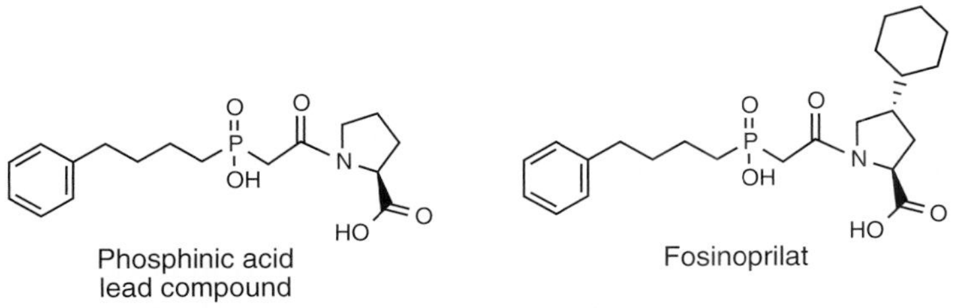

Phosphinic acid lead compound   Fosinoprilat

Figure 17.12 Structures of a phosphinic acid lead compound and fosinoprilat.

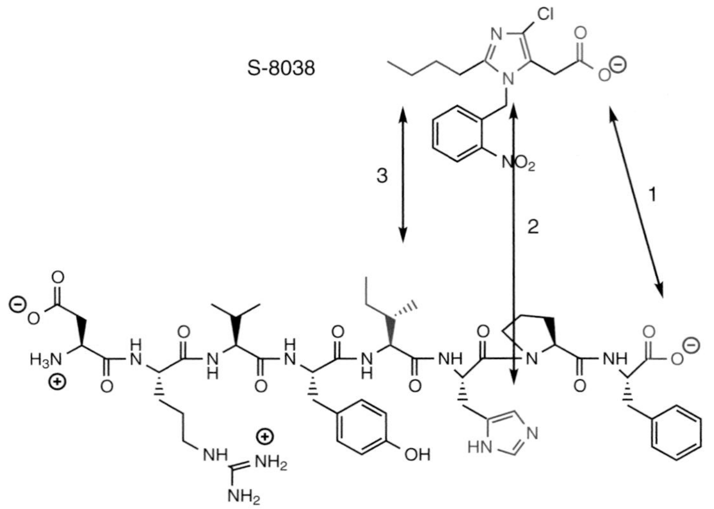

Figure 17.13 **Structural comparison of S-8308, an imidazole-5-acetic acid analog, with angiotensin II.** Adapted from Timmermans PB, Wong PC, Chiu AT, et al. Angiotensin II receptors and angiotensin II receptor antagonists. *Pharmacol Rev.* 1993;45:205-213, with permission.

improved survival after MI, stable coronary heart disease, diabetic nephropathy, and reduction of the risk of MI, stroke, and death from cardiovascular causes. Although all ACE inhibitors and ARBs block the action of angiotensin II, the approved indications differ among the currently available drugs.[66,67] These drugs can be used either individually or in combination with other classes of drugs.

According to the 2014 report from the Eighth Joint National Committee (JNC8), ACE inhibitors and angiotension II receptor blockers (ARBs), along with thiazide-type diuretics and calcium blockers, are recommended for the treatment of hypertension in the general nonblack population. Additionally, ACE inhibitors and ARBs are recommended as either initial or add-on therapy for hypertension in patients of age 18 years or older with chronic kidney disease.[68] Arterial and venous dilation seen with ACE inhibitors not only lowers blood pressure but also has favorable effects on both preload and afterload in patients with heart failure. According to the American College of Cardiology/American Heart Association Task Force on Clinical Practice Guidelines, ACE inhibitors and ARBs are recommended for patients with chronic heart failure with reduced ejection fraction.[69] The ability of ACE inhibitors to cause regression of left ventricular hypertrophy has been demonstrated to reduce the incidence of further heart disease in patients with hypertension. The use of ACE inhibitors and ARBs in patients with MI is based

Figure 17.14 The development of losartan from S-8308.

on their ability to decrease mortality by preventing postinfarction left ventricular hypertrophy and heart failure. Both ACE inhibitors and ARBs are beneficial to patients with impaired left ventricular systolic impairment regardless of the presence of observable symptoms due to their ability to block the vascular and cardiac hypertrophy and remodeling caused by angiotensin II. Finally, ACE inhibitors and ARBs also have been reported to slow the progression of diabetic nephropathy and, thus, are preferred agents in the treatment of hypertension in patients with diabetes.[43,48,70]

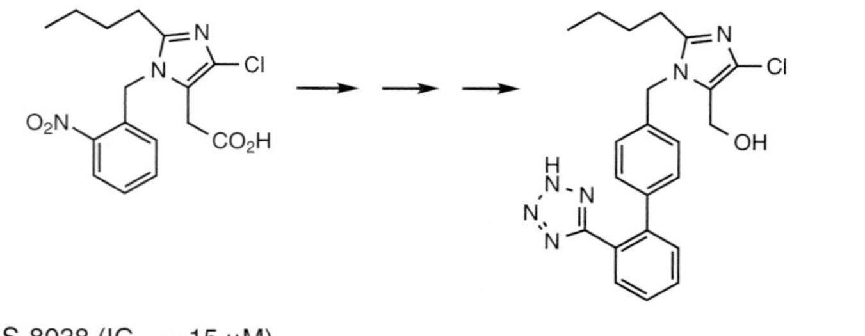

UNLABELED USES OF DRUGS THAT BLOCK THE RENIN-ANGIOTENSIN PATHWAY

Hypertensive crises, renovascular hypertension, neonatal and childhood hypertension, stroke prevention, migraine prophylaxis, nondiabetic nephropathy, chronic kidney disease, scleroderma renal crisis, Raynaud phenomenon, and Bartter syndrome.[66,67]

Pharmacology Overview of Drugs That Block the Renin-Angiotensin Pathway

Mechanisms of Action

ANGIOTENSIN-CONVERTING ENZYME INHIBITORS. The ACE inhibitors attenuate the effects of the renin-angiotensin system by inhibiting the conversion of angiotensin I to angiotensin II (Fig. 17.6). They also inhibit the conversion of (des-Asp1) angiotensin I to angiotensin III; however, this action has only a minor role in the overall cardiovascular effects of these drugs. They are selective in that they do not directly interfere with any other components of the renin-angiotensin system; however, they do cause other effects that are unrelated to the decrease in angiotensin II

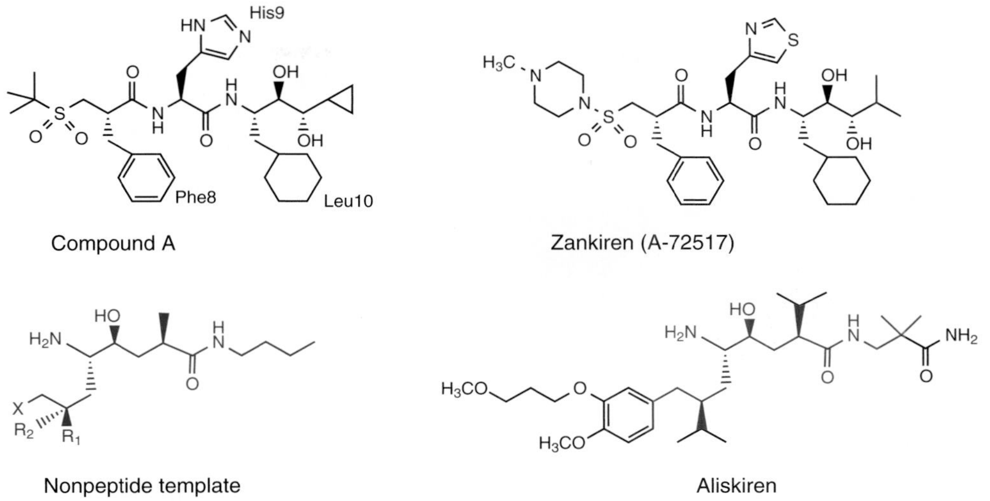

Compound A

Zankiren (A-72517)

Nonpeptide template

Aliskiren

Figure 17.15 Aliskiren and predecessor compounds.

concentration. Inhibitors of ACE increase bradykinin levels that, in turn, stimulate prostaglandin biosynthesis (Fig. 17.8). Both of these endogenous compounds have been proposed to contribute to the overall action of ACE inhibitors. Additionally, decreased angiotensin II levels increase the release of renin and the production of angiotensin I. Because ACE is inhibited, angiotensin I is shunted toward the production of angiotensin 1-7 and other peptides. The contribution of these peptides to the overall effect of ACE inhibitors is unknown.[43]

ANGIOTENSIN II RECEPTOR BLOCKERS. The angiotensin II receptor exists in at least two subtypes: type 1 (AT_1) and type 2 (AT_2). The AT_1 receptors are located in the brain, neuronal, vascular, renal, hepatic, adrenal, and myocardial tissues and mediate the cardiovascular, renal, and central nervous system (CNS) effects of angiotensin II. All currently available ARBs are 10,000-fold more selective for the AT_1 receptor subtype and act as competitive antagonists at this site. In terms of relative affinity for the AT_1 receptor, azilsartan, candesartan, and olmesartan have the greatest affinity; irbesartan and eprosartan have a somewhat lower affinity; and telmisartan, valsartan, and losartan have the lowest affinity. All ARBs prevent and reverse all of the known effects of angiotensin II, including rapid and slow pressor responses, stimulatory effects on the peripheral sympathetic nervous system, CNS effects, release of catecholamines, secretion of aldosterone, direct and indirect renal effects, and all growth-promoting effects. The function of the AT_2 receptors is not as well characterized; however, they have been proposed to mediate a variety of growth, development, and differentiation processes.[43,71]

RENIN INHIBITORS. Aliskiren is currently the only FDA-approved renin inhibitor. It directly inhibits renin, thereby preventing the formation of angiotensin I and angiotensin II. As previously mentioned, this is the rate-limiting step in this pathway and is highly regulated by hemodynamic, neurogenic, and humoral signals. Studies have shown that there are two potential advantages of inhibiting this enzyme as compared to inhibiting ACE or using an ARB.[63,72] Inhibition of the renin-angiotensin pathway through any of these mechanisms has been shown to cause a compensatory increase in renin concentration; however, unlike ACE inhibitors and ARBs, the ability of renin inhibitors to directly bind to the enzyme blocks the increase in plasma renin activity seen with ACE inhibitors and ARBs. Additionally, alternate pathways, such as the chymostatin-sensitive pathway present in the heart, can convert angiotensin I to angiotensin II. While this alternate pathway could affect the efficacy of ACE inhibitors, it would not alter the effects of direct renin inhibition.

Common Adverse Effects

The most prevalent or significant side effects of drugs affecting the renin-angiotensin pathway have been highlighted.[43,66,67,72–74] Some adverse effects can be attributed to specific functional groups within individual agents, whereas others can be directly related to the mechanism of action of this class of drugs. The higher incidence of maculopapular rashes and taste disturbances observed among those using captopril have been linked to the presence of the sulfhydryl group in this drug. All drugs affecting the renin-angiotensin pathway can cause hypotension and hyperkalemia. Hypotension results from an extension of the desired physiologic effect, whereas hyperkalemia results from a decrease in aldosterone secretion secondary to a decrease in angiotensin II production. A dry cough is by far the most prevalent and bothersome side effect seen with the use of ACE inhibitors. It is seen in 5%-20% of patients, usually is not dose related, and apparently results from the lack of selectivity of this class of drugs. As previously discussed, ACE inhibitors also prevent the breakdown of bradykinin (Fig. 17.8), and because bradykinin stimulates prostaglandin synthesis, prostaglandin levels also increase. The increased levels of both bradykinin and prostaglandin have been proposed to be responsible for the cough.[73] Bradykinin accumulation has also been linked to angioedema. This adverse drug reaction is rare and occurs at a higher incidence in black patients as compared to nonblack patients. ACE inhibitors should be immediately discontinued if angioedema occurs. The dry cough and angioedema are notably absent with ARBs and aliskiren. This is because these drugs are more specific in their action and do not affect the levels of bradykinin or prostaglandins.

ADVERSE EFFECTS OF DRUGS THAT BLOCK THE RENIN-ANGIOTENSIN PATHWAY

Common to ACE inhibitors, ARBs, and Aliskiren: Hypotension, hyperkalemia, headache, dizziness, fatigue, dyspepsia, diarrhea, and abdominal pain.

ACE inhibitors: Cough, rash, taste disturbances, angioedema, nausea, vomiting, acute renal failure, neutropenia, proteinuria, and angioedema.

ARBs: Upper respiratory tract infections, myalgia, back pain, pharyngitis, and rhinitis.

Aliskiren: Gastroesophageal reflux, and rash.

The use of ACE inhibitors, ARBs, and aliskiren during pregnancy is contraindicated. These drugs are not teratogenic during the first trimester, but administration during the second and third trimester is associated with an increased incidence of fetal morbidity and mortality. All of these drugs can be used in women of childbearing age; however, they should be discontinued as soon as pregnancy is confirmed.

Common Interactions

Common drug interactions are listed in Table 17.8. Due to the ability to block aldosterone, all of these drugs have interactions with potassium preparations and potassium sparring diuretics. Nonsteroidal anti-inflammatory drugs may alter the response to antihypertensive because of inhibition of vasodilatory prostaglandins. Studies have shown that indomethacin, naproxen, and piroxicam have a greater propensity for causing this interaction. Rifampin, because of its ability to induce CYP3A4, can decrease the plasma levels of losartan and its active metabolite, EXP-3174.

Table 17.8 Drug Interactions for ACE Inhibitors, ARBs, and Aliskiren

Drug	Offending Drug or Drug Class	Result of Interaction
Allopurinol	Captopril	Increased risk of hypersensitivity
Antacids	ACE Inhibitors	Decreased bioavailability of ACE inhibitor (more likely with captopril and fosinopril)
Capsaicin	ACE Inhibitors	Exacerbation of cough
Digoxin	ACE inhibitors and ARBs	Impaired excretion of digoxin and increased digoxin levels
Diuretics	All	Potential excessive reduction in blood pressure; the effects of loop diuretics may be reduced
Drospirenone	All	Elevated serum potassium levels
Iron salts	Captopril	Reduction of captopril levels unless administration is separated by at least 2 hr
K^+ preparations or K^+-sparing diuretics	All	Elevated serum potassium levels
Lithium	All	Increased serum lithium levels
NSAIDs	All	Decreased hypotensive effects
P-glycoprotein inhibitors (e.g., atorvastatin, cyclosporine, ketoconazole)	Aliskiren	Increased aliskiren levels
Phenothiazides	ACE Inhibitors	Increased pharmacologic effects of ACE inhibitor
Probenecid	Captopril	Decreased clearance and increased blood levels of captopril
Rifampin	Enalapril and losartan	Decreased plasma levels of enalapril and losartan
Tetracycline	Quinapril	Decreased absorption of tetracycline (may result from high magnesium content of quinapril tablets)

ACE, angiotensin-converting enzyme; *ARB*, angiotensin receptor blocker; *NSAIDs*, nonsteroidal anti-inflammatory drugs.

Medicinal Chemistry of Angiotensin-Converting Enzyme Inhibitors

Receptor Binding and SAR

With the exception of captopril, all ACE inhibitors mimic the Phe8—His9—Leu10 tripeptide sequence seen at the carboxylic acid end of angiotensin I. As ACE is a relatively nonspecific dipeptidyl carboxypeptidase, the side chains of His9 and Leu10 are replaced by alanine and either proline or proline analogs, respectively. A comparison of the transition state of angiotensin I hydrolysis by ACE and the binding of enalaprilat is shown in Figure 17.16. The structure of enalaprilat and all dicarboxylate-containing ACE inhibitors have a tetrahedral carbon atom in place of the labile peptide. Additionally, the carboxylic acid attached to this tetrahedral carbon atom can chelate with the enzyme-bound zinc, while the carboxylic acid of the proline analog can form an ionic bond with either a lysine or arginine residue on ACE. The nonlabile peptide bond between the alanine and proline analog can form a hydrogen bond with ACE, while the phenylethyl group mimics the hydrophobic side chain of Phe8 that is present in angiotensin I. All of these binding interactions closely resemble the binding of angiotensin I to ACE.

Captopril and fosinoprilat exhibit similar binding to ACE with a few structural changes (Fig. 17.17). Captopril is a dipeptide mimic or His9—Leu10. Its structure does not contain the tetrahedral carbon atom or the phenylethyl group seen in enalaprilat; however, the sulfhydryl group is superior to the carboxylic acid in binding to the zinc atom. Fosinoprilat is capable of binding to ACE in a manner similar to enalaprilat. The interaction of the zinc atom with the phosphinic acid is similar to that seen with sulfhydryl group of captopril and carboxylate group seen with enalaprilat. The phosphinic acid is able to more truly mimic the ionized, tetrahedral intermediate of peptide hydrolysis. The spacing of the functional groups in fosinoprilat is slightly different than enalaprilat; however, it is able to mimic the side chains of Phe8 and Leu10.

While the carboxylic acid of enalaprilat is required to bind to the zinc atom, the overall oral bioavailability this drug is poor. The two carboxylate groups and the secondary amine present within the structure of enalaprilat will be primarily ionized in the small intestine and will contribute to its low lipophilicity and poor bioavailability. As previously discussed, the conversion of enalaprilat to an ester prodrug, enalapril, produced a drug with superior oral bioavailability (Fig. 17.11). Interestingly, the ester prodrug has a significant effect on the pK_a of the secondary amine of enalapril. The adjacent ester forms a hydrogen bond with the secondary amine and decreases its pK_a to 5.49. Thus, in the small intestine, the secondary amine will be primarily unionized, and zwitterion formation with the proline carboxylic acid will not occur. This adds to the overall enhanced lipid solubility of enalapril.[75,76] Bioactivation by hepatic esterases (Fig. 17.11) has been suggested as the most probable mechanism for the conversion of the prodrug enalapril to the active drug enalaprilat formation.[77,78]

Similar to the enalaprilat, the phosphinic acid present within the structure of fosinoprilat contributed to low lipophilicity and poor oral activity. The prodrug fosinopril contains an (acyloxy)alkyl group that allows better lipid solubility and improved bioavailability.[60] Bioactivation via esterase activity in the intestinal wall and liver produces fosinopril (Fig. 17.18).

Eight other dicarboxylate-containing ACE inhibitors (Table 17.9) have been approved for various therapeutic indications; however, spirapril has never been marketed. Lisinopril is chemically unique in two respects. First, it contains the basic amino acid lysine (R_1 = $CH_2CH_2CH_2CH_2NH_2$) instead of the standard nonpolar alanine (R = CH_3) residue. Second, it does not require bioactivation, because neither of the carboxylic acid groups are esterified (i.e., R_2 = H). Lisinopril was developed at the same time as enalapril. Despite the addition of another ionizable group, the oral absorption of lisinopril was found to be superior to that of enalaprilat but less than that of enalapril. In vitro studies of enalaprilat and lisinopril showed lisinopril to be slightly more potent than enalaprilat.[77,78]

The major structural difference among the remaining dicarboxylate-containing ACE inhibitors is in the ring of the C-terminal amino acid. As previously mentioned, proline was the C-terminal amino acid on the naturally occurring snake venom peptides used to develop ACE inhibitors. Attempts to replace it with other amino acids

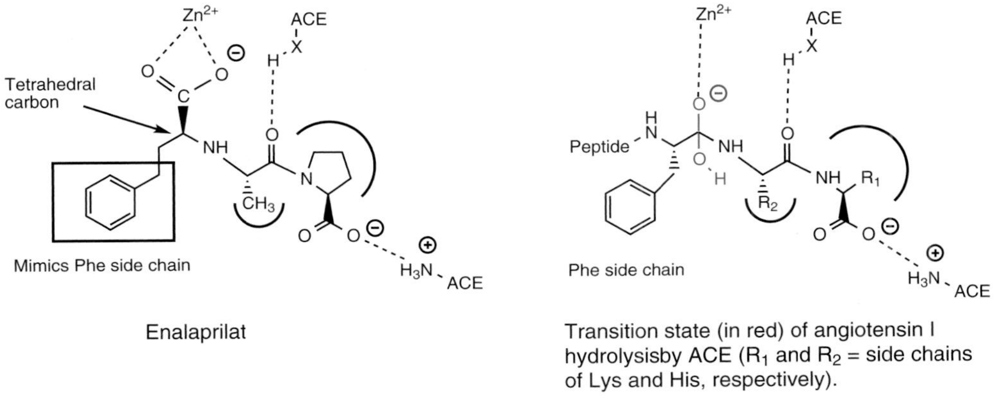

Tetrahedral carbon

Mimics Phe side chain

Enalaprilat

Phe side chain

Transition state (in red) of angiotensin I hydrolysisby ACE (R_1 and R_2 = side chains of Lys and His, respectively).

Figure 17.16 A comparison of enalaprilat and the transition state of angiotensin I hydrolysis by angiotensin-converting enzyme (ACE).

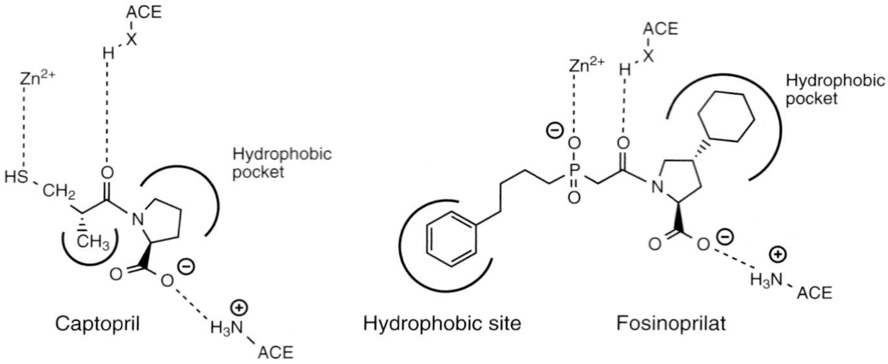

Figure 17.17 The binding of captopril and fosinoprilat to angiotensin-converting enzyme (ACE).

were not successful; however, structural variations of proline with larger hydrophobic ring systems enhanced binding. In general, the varied ring systems seen in benazepril, moexipril, perindopril, quinapril, ramipril, spirapril, and trandolapril provide enhanced binding and potency as compared to enalapril and lisinopril (the two original drugs from this sub-class). The larger hydrophobic ring systems also lead to differences in absorption, plasma protein binding, elimination, onset of action, duration of action, and dosing among the drugs.

A summary of the SAR for ACE inhibitors is provided in Table 17.10. ACE is a stereoselective drug target. Because currently approved ACE inhibitors act as either di- or tripeptide substrate analog, they must contain a stereochemistry that is consistent with the L-amino acids present in the natural substrates. This was established very early in the development of ACE inhibitors when compounds with carboxyl-terminal D-amino acids were discovered to be very poor inhibitors.[79] Later work by Patchett et al.[59] reinforced this idea. They reported a 100- to 1,000-fold loss in inhibitor activity whenever the configuration of either the carboxylate or the R_1 substituent (Table 17.9) was altered. The *S,S,S*-configuration seen in enalapril and other dicarboxylate inhibitors meets the previously stated criteria and provides for optimum enzyme inhibition.

Physiocochemical Properties

Captopril and fosinopril are acidic drugs, but all other ACE inhibitors are amphoteric. The carboxylic acid attached to the N-ring is a common structural feature in all ACE inhibitors. It has a pK_a in the range of 2.5-3.5 and will be primarily ionized at physiologic pH. As discussed earlier with enalapril, the pK_a and ionization of the secondary amine in the dicarboxylate series depend on whether the adjacent functional group is in the prodrug or active form. In the prodrug form, the amine is adjacent to an ester, is less basic, and is primarily un-ionized at physiologic pH. Following bioactivation, the amine is adjacent to an ionized carboxylic acid that enhances both the basicity (pK_a = 8.02) and ionization of the amine. Similarly, the basic nitrogen enhances the acidity of the adjacent carboxylic acid such that it usually has a lower pK_a than the carboxylic acid attached to the N-ring. As an example, the pK_a values of the two carboxylic acids in enalaprilat are 3.39 and 2.30. These values correspond to the carboxylic acid on the N-ring and the carboxylic acid adjacent to the amine, respectively. The analogous values for these functional groups in lisinopril are 3.3 and 1.7.[76]

The calculated log P values[76] along with other pharmacokinetic parameters for the ACE inhibitors are shown in Table 17.11. With three notable exceptions, captopril, enalaprilat, and lisinopril, all of the drugs possess good lipid solubility. Drugs that contain hydrophobic bicyclic ring systems are more lipid soluble than those that contain proline. A comparison of the log P values of benazepril, fosinopril, moexipril, perindopril, quinapril, ramipril, spirapril, and trandolapril to those for captopril and enalapril illustrates this fact. As previously discussed, enalaprilat is much more hydrophilic than its ester prodrug and is currently the only ACE inhibitor marked for IV administration. In terms of solubility, lisinopril is an interesting drug in that it is the most hydrophilic inhibitor, yet unlike

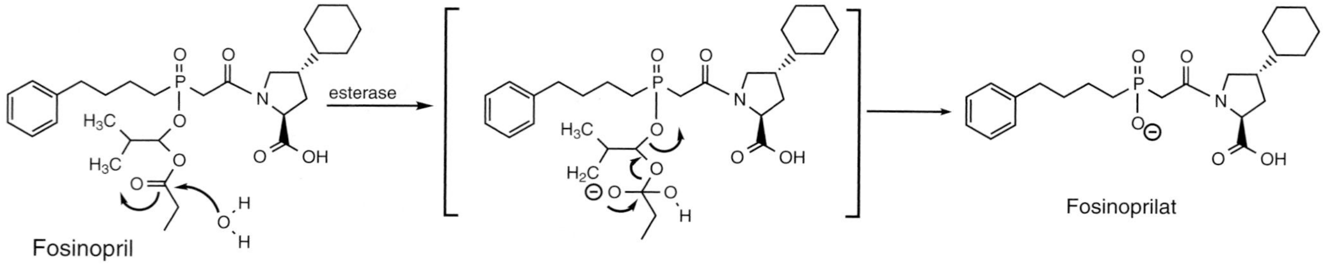

Figure 17.18 Bioactivation of fosinopril.

Table 17.9 Additional Dicarboxylate-Containing Angiotensin-Converting Enzyme Inhibitors

General Structure:

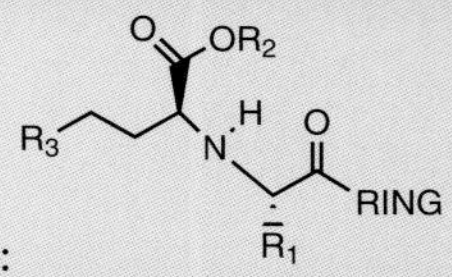

Benazepril

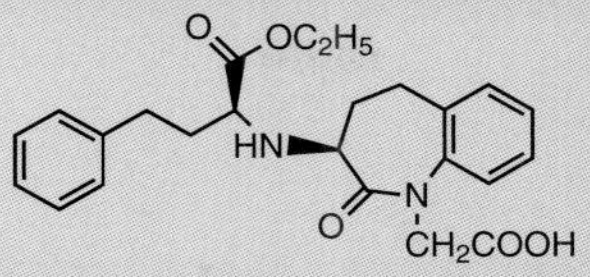

Compounds	Ring	R_1	R_2	R_3
Lisinopril	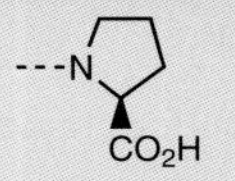	$(CH_2)_4NH_2$	H	
Moexipril	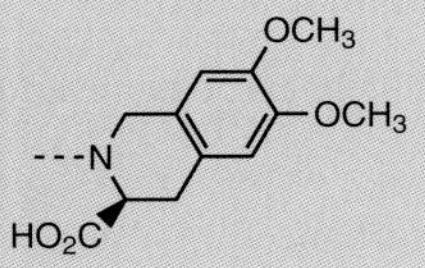	CH_3	CH_2CH_3	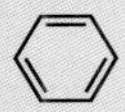
Perindopril	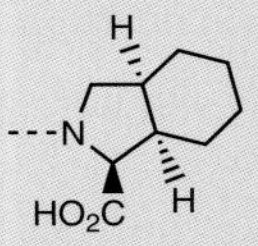	CH_3	CH_2CH_3	CH_3
Quinapril	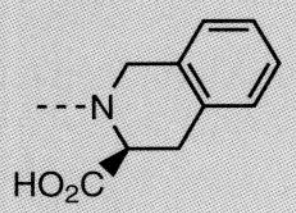	CH_3	CH_2CH_3	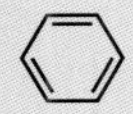
Ramipril	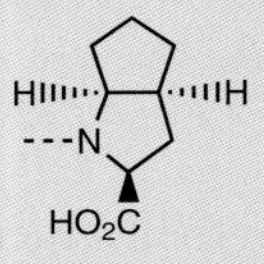	CH_3	CH_2CH_3	
Spirapril	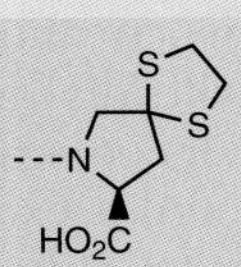	CH_3	CH_2CH_3	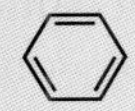
Trandolapril	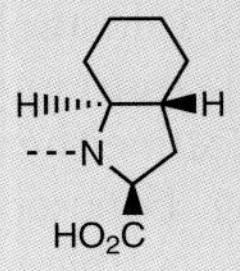	CH_3	CH_2CH_3	

enalaprilat, it is orally active. One possible explanation for this phenomenon is that in the duodenum, lisinopril will exist as a di-zwitterion in which the ionized groups can internally bind to one another. In this manner, lisinopril may be able to pass through the lipid bilayer with an overall net neutral charge.

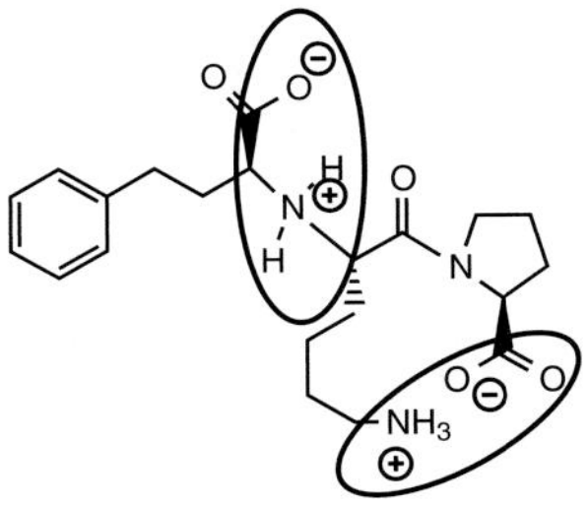

Pharmacokinetic Properties

The pharmacokinetic parameters and dosing information for ACE inhibitors are summarized in Tables 17.11 and 17.12, respectively.[43,66,67,74] The oral bioavailability of this class of drugs ranges from 13% to 95%. Differences in both lipid solubility and first-pass metabolism are most likely responsible for this wide variation. Both parameters should be considered when comparing any two or more drugs. With the exceptions of enalapril and lisinopril, the concurrent administration with food adversely affects the oral absorption of ACE inhibitors. Product literature specifically instructs that captopril should be taken 1 hour before meals and that moexipril should be taken in the fasting state. Although not specifically stated, similar instructions also should benefit patients taking an ACE inhibitor whose absorption is affected by food.

Table 17.10 Structure-Activity Relationships of Angiotensin-Converting Enzyme (ACE) Inhibitors

Zn^{2+} binding groups

Ph–$(CH_2)_n$–[Zn^{2+} binding group]–CH(X)–C(=O)–N-ring

A: HS-CH_2—

B: —CH(CO_2H)–NH—

C: —P(OH)(=O)—

a. The N-ring must contain a carboxylic acid to mimic the C-terminal carboxylate of ACE substrates.
b. Large hydrophobic heterocyclic rings (i.e., the N-ring) increase potency and alter pharmacokinetic parameters.
c. The zinc-binding groups can be either sulfhydryl (A), a carboxylic acid (B), or a phosphinic acid (C).
d. The sulfhydryl group shows superior binding to zinc (the side chain mimicking the Phe in carboxylate and phosphinic acid compounds partially compensates for the lack of a sulfhydryl group).
e. Sulfhydryl-containing compounds produce high incidence of skin rash and taste disturbances.
f. Sulfhydryl-containing compounds can form dimers and disulfides, which may shorten duration of action.
g. Compounds that bind to zinc through either a carboxylate or phosphinate mimic the peptide hydrolysis transition state and enhance binding.
h. Esterification of the carboxylate or phosphinate produces an orally bioavailable prodrug.
i. X is usually methyl to mimic the side chain of alanine. Within the dicarboxylate series, when X equals n-butylamine (lysine side chain), this produces a compound that does not require prodrug for oral activity.
j. Optimum activity occurs when stereochemistry of inhibitor is consistent with L-amino acid stereochemistry present in normal substrates.

The extent of protein binding also exhibits wide variability among the different drugs. The data suggest that this variation has some correlation with the calculated log P values for the drugs (Table 17.11). Three of the more lipophilic drugs—fosinopril, quinapril, and benazepril—exhibit protein binding of greater than 90%, whereas three of the least lipophilic drugs—lisinopril, enalapril, and captopril—exhibit much lower protein binding.

Renal elimination is the primary route of elimination for most ACE inhibitors. With the exceptions of fosinopril and spirapril, altered renal function significantly diminishes the plasma clearance of ACE inhibitors, including those that are eliminated primarily by the feces. Therefore, the dosage of most ACE inhibitors should be reduced in patients with renal impairment.[43]

With one exception, all ACE inhibitors have a similar onset of action, duration of action, and dosing interval. Captopril has a more rapid onset of action; however, it also has a shorter duration and requires a more frequent dosing interval than any of the other drugs. When oral dosing is inappropriate, enalaprilat can be used IV. The normal dose administered to hypertensive patients is 0.625-1.25 mg every 6 hours. The dose usually is administered over 5 minutes and may be titrated up to 5 mg IV every 6 hours.

Metabolism

Lisinopril and enalaprilat are excreted unchanged, whereas all other ACE inhibitors undergo some degree of metabolic transformation.[43,66,67,74] As previously discussed and illustrated (Figs. 17.11 and 17.18), all dicarboxylate and phosphonate prodrugs must undergo bioactivation via hepatic esterases. Additionally, based on their structural features, specific drugs can undergo metabolic inactivation via various pathways (Fig. 17.19). Because of its sulfhydryl group, captopril is subject to oxidative dimerization or conjugation. Approximately 40%-50% of a dose of captopril is excreted unchanged, whereas the remainder is excreted as either a disulfide dimer or a captopril-cysteine disulfide. Glucuronide conjugation has been reported for benazepril, fosinopril, quinapril, and ramipril. This conjugation can occur either with the parent prodrug or with the activated drug. Benazepril, with the N-substituted glycine, is especially susceptible to this reaction because of a decrease in steric hindrance. For all ACE inhibitors, except benazepril, the carbon atom directly adjacent to the carboxylic acid is part of a ring system and provides some steric hindrance to conjugation. The unsubstituted methylene group (i.e., –CH_2–) of benazepril provides less steric hindrance and, thus, facilitates conjugation. Moexipril, perindopril, and ramipril can undergo cyclization to produce diketopiperazines. This cyclization can occur with either the parent or active forms of the drugs.

Medicinal Chemistry of Angiotensin II Receptor Blockers

Receptor Binding and SAR

Angiotensin II receptor blockers have structural features that mimic the side chains of the amino acids present within the structure of angiotensin II as illustrated with losartan in Figure 17.20. All other ARBs, with the exception of eprosartan, are biphenyl analogs of losartan,

Table 17.11 Pharmacokinetic Parameters of Angiotensin-Converting Enzyme (ACE) Inhibitors

Drug	Calculated Log P	Oral Bioavailability (%)	Effect of Food on Absorption	Active Metabolite	Protein Binding (%)	Onset of Action (hr)	Duration of Action (hr)	Major Route(s) of Elimination
Benazepril	5.50	37	Slows Absorption	Benazeprilat	>95	1	24	Renal (primary) Biliary (secondary)
Captopril	0.27	60-75	Reduced	NA	25-30	0.25-0.50	6-12	Renal
Enalapril	2.43	60	None	Enalaprilat	50-60	1	24	Renal/fecal
Enalaprilat	1.54	NA	NA	NA	—	0.25	6	Renal
Fosinopril	6.09	36	Slows absorption	Fosinoprilat	95	1	24	Renal (50%) Hepatic (50%)
Lisinopril	1.19	25-30	None	NA	25	1	24	Renal
Moexipril	4.06	13	Reduced	Moexiprilat	50	1	24	Fecal (primary) Renal (secondary)
Perindopril	3.36	65-95	Reduced	Perindoprilat	60-80	1	24	Renal
Quinapril	4.32	60	Reduced	Quinaprilat	97	1	24	Renal
Ramipril	3.41	50-60	Slows absorption	Ramiprilat	73	1-2	24	Renal (60%) Fecal (40%)
Spirapril	3.16	50	—	Spiraprilat	—	1	24	Renal (50%) Hepatic (50%)
Trandolapril	3.97	70	Slows Absorption	Trandolaprilat	80	0.5-1.0	24	Fecal (primary) Renal (secondary)

NA, not applicable; —, data not available.

Table 17.12 Dosing Information for Orally Available ACE Inhibitors

Generic Name	Trade Name(s)	Approved Indications	Dosing Range (Treatment of Hypertension)	Maximum Daily Dose	Dose Reduction With Renal Dysfunction	Available Tablet Strengths (mg)
Benazepril	Lotensin	Hypertension	40 mg once daily or b.i.d.	80 mg	Yes	5, 10, 20, 40
Captopril	Capoten (n/a)	Hypertension, heart failure, left ventricular dysfunction (post-MI), diabetic nephropathy	25-150 mg b.i.d. or t.i.d.	450 mg	Yes	12.5, 25, 50, 100
Enalapril	Vasotec	Hypertension, heart failure	2.5-40 mg once daily or b.i.d.	40 mg	Yes	2.5, 5, 10, 20
Fosinopril	Monopril	Hypertension, heart failure	10-40 mg once daily	80 mg	No	10, 20, 40
Lisinopril	Prinivil, Zestril	Hypertension, heart failure, improve survival post-MI	10-40 mg once daily	80 mg	Yes	2.5, 5, 10, 20, 30, 40
Moexipril	Univasc (n/a)	Hypertension	7.5-30 mg once daily or b.i.d.	30 mg	Yes	7.5, 15
Perindopril	Aceon	Hypertension, stable CAD	4-8 mg once daily or b.i.d.	16 mg	Yes	2, 4, 8
Quinapril	Accupril	Hypertension, heart failure	10-80 mg once daily or b.i.d.	80 mg	Yes	5, 10, 20, 40
Ramipril	Altace	Hypertension, heart failure (post-MI), reduce risk of MI, stroke, and death from cardiovascular causes	2.5-20 mg once daily or b.i.d.	20 mg	Yes	1.25, 2.5, 5, 10
Trandolapril	Mavik (n/a)	Hypertension, heart failure (post-MI), left ventricular dysfunction (post-MI)	1-4 mg once daily	8 mg	Yes	1, 2, 4

b.i.d., twice a day; *CAD*, coronary artery disease; *MI*, myocardial infarction; *n/a*, no longer available; *t.i.d.*, three times a day.

and all ARBs have similar structural features and binding abilities (Fig. 17.21). Azilsartan medoxomil, candesartan cilexetil, and olmesartan medoxomil are prodrugs that are rapidly and completely hydrolyzed to their respective carboxylic acids.

In terms of SAR, all commercially available ARBs are analogs of the following general structure:

Acidic group

Acid groups: $-CO_2H$

A B C

1. The "acidic group" is thought to mimic either the Tyr4 phenol or the Asp1 carboxylate of angiotensin II. Groups capable of such a role include the carboxylic acid (A), a phenyl tetrazole or isostere (B), or a phenyl carboxylate (C).
2. In the biphenyl series, the tetrazole and carboxylate groups must be in the ortho position for optimal activity (the tetrazole group is superior in terms of metabolic stability, lipophilicity, and oral bioavailability).
3. The n-butyl group of the model compound provides hydrophobic binding and, most likely, mimics the side chain of Ile5 of angiotensin II. As seen with azilsartan, candesartan, telmisartan, and olmesartan, this n-butyl group can be replaced with either an ethyl ether or an n-propyl group.

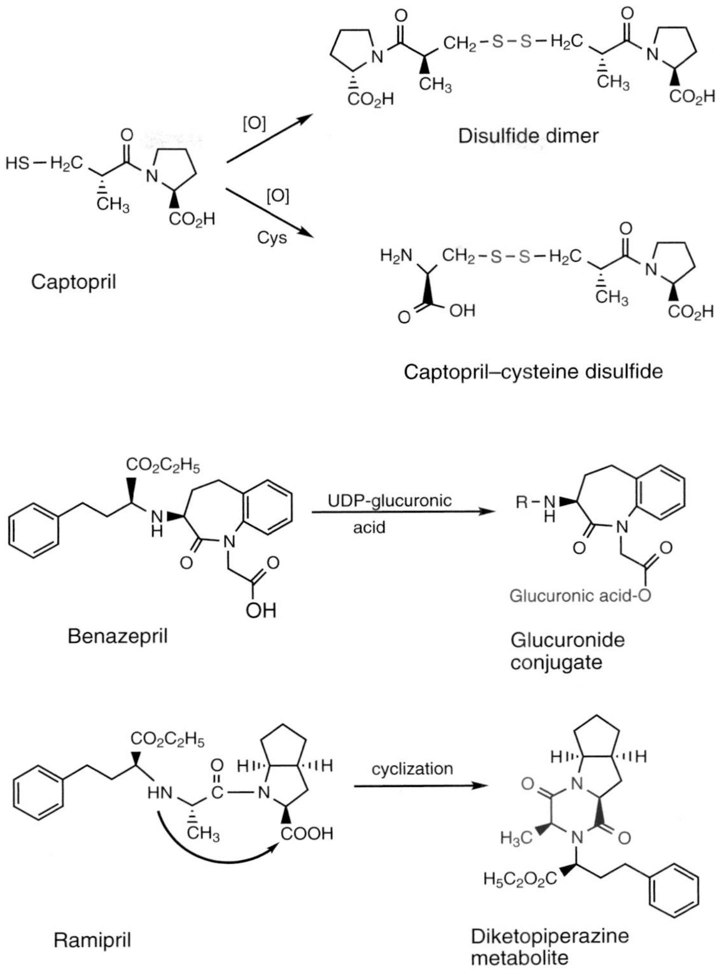

Figure 17.19 Metabolic routes of angiotensin-converting enzyme (ACE) inhibitors.

4. The imidazole ring or an isosteric equivalent is required to mimic the His6 side chain of angiotensin II.
5. Substitution can vary at the "R" position. A variety of R groups, including a carboxylic acid, a hydroxymethyl group, a ketone, or a benzimidazole ring, are present in currently available ARBs and are thought to interact with the AT_1 receptor through either ionic, ion-dipole, or dipole-dipole bonds. The thienyl ring present within the structure of eposartan isosterically mimics the Phe8 phenyl ring of angiotensin II.

Physiocochemical Properties

All ARBs are acidic drugs. The tetrazole ring present within the structures of losartan, valsartan, irbesartan, candesartan, and olmesartan has a pK_a of approximately 6 and will be at least 90% ionized at physiologic pH. The 5-oxo-1,2,4-oxadiazole ring present in azilsartan is a tetrazole isostere and has a similar pK_a value. The carboxylic acids found on valsartan, candesartan, olmesartan, telmisartan, azilsartan, and eprosartan have pK_a values in the range of 3-4 and also will be primarily ionized. Currently, available agents have adequate, but not excellent, lipid solubility. As previously mentioned, the tetrazole group is more lipophilic than a carboxylic acid. Additionally, the four nitrogen atoms present in the tetrazole ring can create a greater charge distribution than that available for a carboxylic acid. These properties have been proposed to be responsible for the enhanced binding and bioavailability of the tetrazole-containing drugs.[80] Similar to ACE inhibitors, the stereochemistry of valsartan is consistent with the L-amino acids in the natural agonist.

Pharmacokinetic Properties

The pharmacokinetic parameters and dosing information for angiotensin receptor antagonists are summarized in Tables 17.13 and 17.14, respectively.[66,67,74] With the exception of azilsartan medoxomil (60%), irbesartan (60%-80%) and, possibly, telmisartan (42%-58%), all of these drugs have low, but adequate, oral bioavailability (15%-33%). Given the fact that most of the drugs are excreted unchanged, the most probable reasons for the low bioavailability are poor lipid solubility and incomplete absorption. The effect of food on the absorption of losartan, eprosartan, valsartan, and eprosartan is to reduce absorption; however, this effect has been deemed to be clinically insignificant; thus, these drugs can be taken either with or without food.

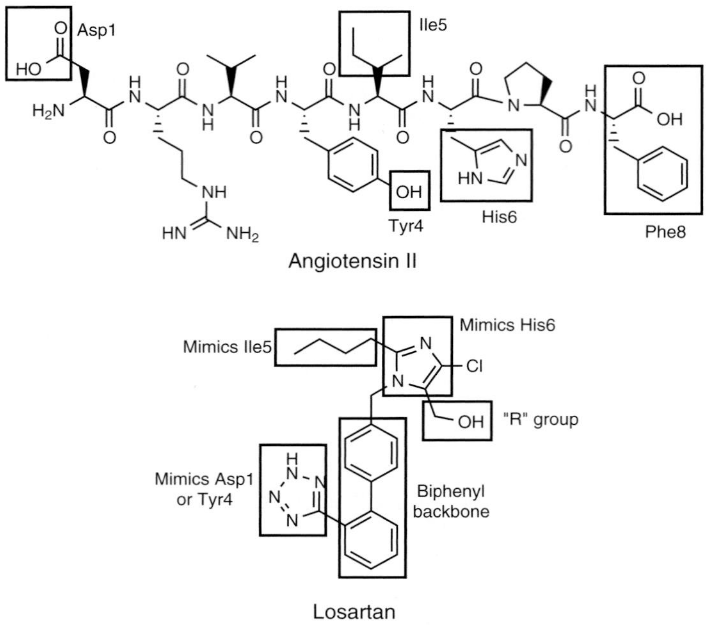

Asp1 Ile5 Tyr4 His6 Phe8

Angiotensin II

Mimics Ile5 Mimics His6 "R" group Mimics Asp1 or Tyr4 Biphenyl backbone

Losartan

Figure 17.20 Structural similarities between angiotensin II and losartan.

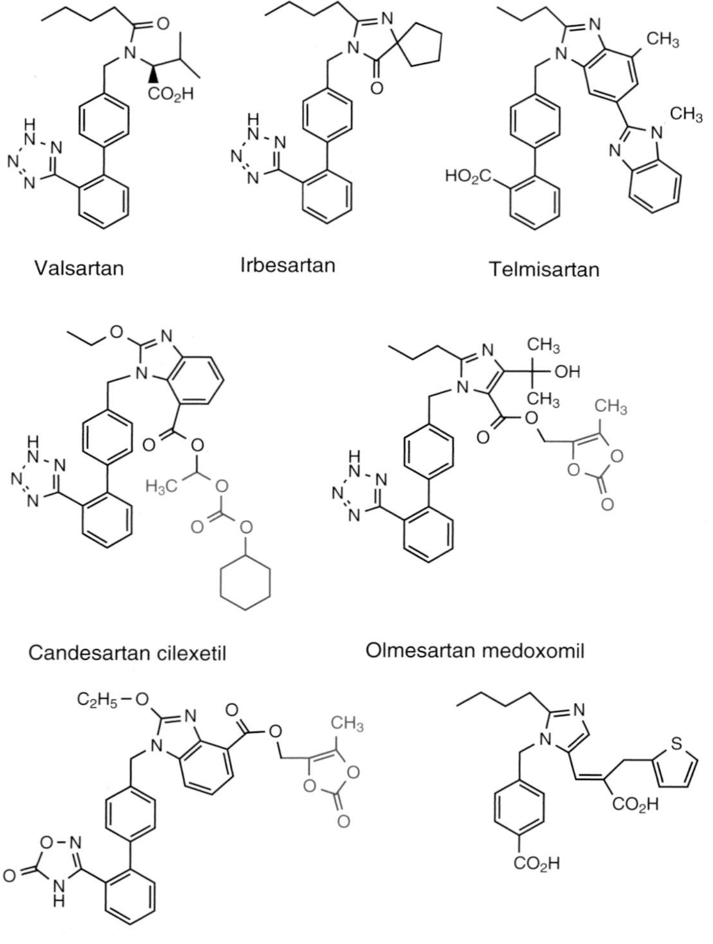

Figure 17.21 Structures of angiotensin II receptor blockers. The highlighted portions of candesartan cilexetil, olmesartan medoxomil, and azilsartan medoxomil are hydrolyzed via esterases to produce their respective active carboxylate metabolites.

Table 17.13 Pharmacokinetic Parameters of Angiotensin II Receptor Blockers

Drug	Oral Bioavailability (%)	Active Metabolite	Protein Binding (%)	Time to Peak Plasma Concentration (hr)	Elimination Half-Life (hr)	Major Route(s) of Elimination
Azilsartan Medoxomil	60	Azilsartan	99	1.5-3.0	11	Fecal (55%) Renal (42%)
Candesartan Cilexetil	15	Candesartan	99	3-4	9	Fecal (67%) Renal (33%)
Eprosartan	15	None	98	1-2	5-9	Fecal (90%) Renal (10%)
Irbesartan	60-80	None	90	1.5-2.0	11-15	Fecal (80%) Renal (20%)
Losartan	33	EXP-3174	98.7 (losartan)	1 (losartan)	1.5-2.0 (losartan)	Fecal (60%)
			99.8 (EXP-3174)	3-4 (EXP-3174)	6-9 (EXP-3174)	Renal (35%)
Olmesartan Medoxomil	26	Olmesartan	99	1.5-3.0	10-15	Fecal (35%-50%) Renal (50%-65%)
Telmisartan	42-58	None	100	5	24	Fecal (97%)
Valsartan	25	None	95	2-4	6	Fecal (83%) Renal (13%)

All of the drugs have similar onsets, are highly protein bound, have elimination half-lives that allow once- or twice-daily dosing, and with the exception of olmesartan, are primarily eliminated via the fecal route. Candesartan and telmisartan appear to require a slightly longer time to reach peak plasma concentrations.

Metabolism

Approximately 14% of a dose of losartan is oxidized by the isozymes CYP2C9 and CYP3A4 to produce EXP-3174, a noncompetitive AT_1 receptor antagonist that is 10- to 40-fold more potent than losartan (Fig. 17.22). The overall cardiovascular effects seen with losartan result from the combined actions of the parent drug and the active metabolite; thus, losartan should not be considered to be a prodrug.[43] As previously mentioned, azilsartan medoxomil, candesartan cilexetil, and olmesartan medoxomil are prodrugs that are rapidly and completely hydrolyzed to azilsartan, candesartan, and olmesartan, respectively, in the intestinal wall. These active metabolites have the highest renal elimination within this drug class.

None of the other drugs in this class are converted to active metabolites. All of these drugs are primarily (80%) excreted unchanged. Approximately 20% of valsartan is metabolized to inactive compounds via mechanisms that do not appear to involve the CYP450 system. The primary circulating metabolites for irbesartan, telmisartan and eprosartan, are inactive glucuronide conjugates. A small amount of irbesartan is oxidized by CYP2C9; however, irbesartan does not substantially induce or inhibit the CYP450 enzymes normally involved in drug metabolism.[43,66,67,74] Azilsartan is primarily metabolized by CYP2C9 to an inactive O-dealkyated metabolite. Losartan and telmisartan are the only two drugs in this class that require initial dose reductions in patients with hepatic impairment. Because of significantly increased plasma concentration, patients with impaired hepatic function or biliary obstructive disorders should avoid the use of telmisartan.

Medicinal Chemistry of Aliskiren

Receptor Binding and SAR

Renin is an aspartyl protease that uses two aspartic acid residues to cleave angiotensinogen between the Leu10 and Val11 peptide bond. As shown in Figure 17.23, the structure of aliskiren contains two isopropyl groups that are capable of mimicking the side chains of these two amino acids, while the secondary hydroxyl group is able to mimic the transition state of peptide hydrolysis. The spacing of the two isopropyl groups is longer than the natural substrate; however, it has been proposed that these two groups occupy the P_1 and P_1' binding sites of angiotensinogen. Additionally, the ether side chain has been proposed to occupy a subpocket of the enzyme. Its flexible nature has been proposed to enhance binding through hydrogen bonds (oxygen atom) and van der Waals interactions (carbon atoms).[81,82]

Table 17.14 Dosing Information for Angiotensin II Receptor Blockers

Generic Name	Trade Name(s)	Approved Indications	Dosing Range (Treatment of Hypertension)	Maximum Daily Dose	Initial Dose Reduction With Hepatic Dysfunction	Dose Reduction With Renal Dysfunction	Available Tablet Strengths (mg)
Azilsartan Medoxomil	Edarbi	Hypertension	40-80 mg once daily	80 mg	No	No	40, 80
Candesartan Cilexetil	Atacand	Hypertension, heart failure	8-32 mg once daily	32 mg	No	Only with severe impairment	4, 8, 16, 32
Eprosartan	Teveten (n/a)	Hypertension	400-800 mg once daily or b.i.d.	900 mg	No	Decrease maximum daily dose to 600 mg	600
Irbesartan	Avapro	Hypertension, nephropathy in type 2 diabetics	150-300 mg once daily	300 mg	No	No	75, 150, 300
Losartan	Cozaar	Hypertension, nephropathy in type 2 diabetics, stroke prevention in hypertensive patients with left ventricular hypertrophy	25-100 mg once daily or b.i.d.	100 mg	Yes (reduce to 25 mg once daily)	Adults, no Children, yes	25, 50, 100
Olmesartan Medoxomil	Benicar	Hypertension	20-40 mg once daily	40 mg	No	No	5, 20, 40
Telmisartan	Micardis	Hypertension, cardiovascular risk reduction of MI and stroke	40-80 mg once daily	80 mg	Yes (reduce to 20 mg once daily)	No	20, 40, 80
Valsartan	Diovan	Hypertension, heart failure, post-MI in patients with left ventricular failure or dysfunction	80-320 mg once daily	320 mg	No	No	40, 80, 160, 320

b.i.d., twice a day; *MI*, myocardial infarction; *n/a*, no longer available.

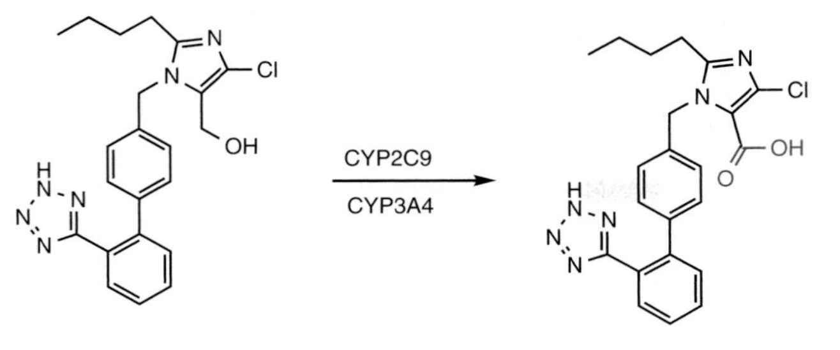

Losartan → (CYP2C9, CYP3A4) → EXP-3174

Figure 17.22 The metabolic conversion of losartan to EXP-3174 by cytochrome P450 isozymes.

Physiocochemical Properties

Aliskiren is a basic drug and is marketed as its hemifumarate salt. The calculated log P value for the unionized form of aliskiren is 4.32[76]; however, its salt form is highly water soluble. Aliskiren contains four chiral centers and is marketed as the pure 2S, 4S, 5S, 7S enantiomer.[74]

Pharmacokinetic Properties

Aliskiren is poorly absorbed and has a bioavailability of approximately 2.5%. Following oral administration, peak plasma concentrations are reached within 1-3 hours, and steady-state blood concentration is reached within 7-8 days. The normal, initial dose of aliskiren is 150 mg once daily. This may be increased to 300 mg once daily in patients whose blood pressure is not adequately controlled. The antihypertensive effects are usually attained within 2 weeks. High-fat meals have been shown to significantly decrease absorption, and patients are encouraged to establish a fixed/routine time to take aliskiren. No adjustment in dose is required for elderly patients or those with renal impairment or hepatic insufficiency. Caution, however, should be used in dosing patients with severe renal impairment.[66,67,72]

Metabolism

Approximately 90% of aliskiren is eliminated unchanged in the feces. Due to its poor bioavailability, the extent of systemic metabolism is unclear; however, clearance through the hepatobiliary tract appears to be the primary route of elimination. While metabolism is a minor pathway, the two major metabolites of aliskiren are an O-demethylated alcohol derivative and a carboxylic acid derivative. The primary metabolizing enzyme is CYP3A4. Aliskiren has not been shown to either inhibit or induce any of the CYP450 isoenzymes.[66,67,74]

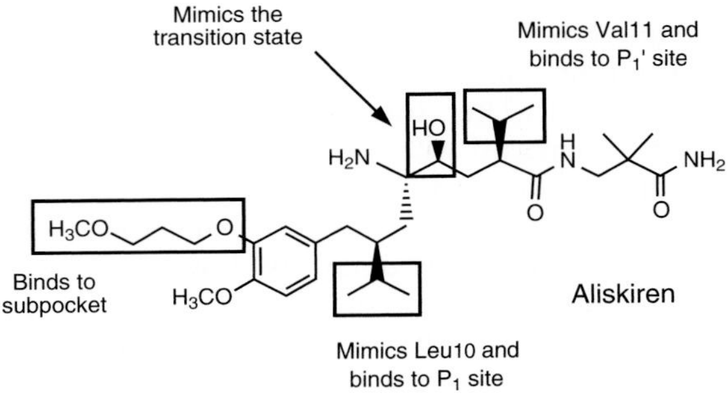

Figure 17.23 Binding interactions of aliskiren with renin.

Calcium Channel Blockers

Overview

Calcium is a key component of the excitation-contraction coupling process that occurs within the cardiovascular system. It acts as a cellular messenger to link internal or external excitation with cellular response. Increased cytosolic concentrations of Ca^{2+} result in the binding of Ca^{2+} to a regulatory protein, either troponin C in cardiac and skeletal muscle or calmodulin in vascular smooth muscle. This initial binding of Ca^{2+} uncovers myosin binding sites on the actin molecule, and subsequent interactions between actin and myosin result in muscle contraction. All of these events are reversed once the cytosolic concentration of Ca^{2+} decreases. In this situation, Ca^{2+} binding to troponin C or calmodulin is diminished or removed, myosin-binding sites are concealed, actin and myosin can no longer interact, and muscle contraction ceases.[83,84]

Normal Mechanisms of Calcium Movement and Storage

The regulation of cytosolic calcium levels occurs via specific influx, efflux, and sequestering mechanisms (Fig. 17.24). The influx of calcium can occur through receptor-operated channels (site 1), the Na^+/Ca^{2+} exchange process (site 2), "leak" pathways (site 3), and potential-dependent channels (site 4). Influx via either receptor-operated or voltage-dependent channels has been proposed to be the major entry pathway for Ca^{2+}. Receptor-operated channels have been defined as those associated with cellular membrane receptors and activated by specific agonist-receptor interactions. In contrast, potential-dependent channels,

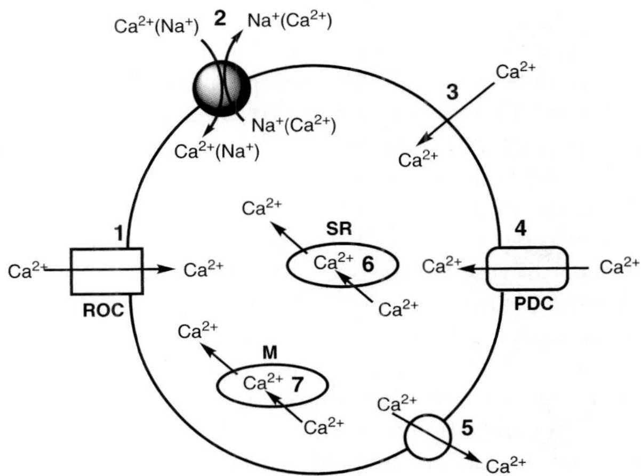

Figure 17.24 Cellular mechanisms for the influx, efflux, and sequestering of Ca^{2+}. *M*, mitochondria; *PDC*, potential-dependent Ca^{2+} channels; *ROC*, receptor-operated Ca^{2+} channels; *SR*, sarcoplasmic reticulum.

also known as voltage-dependent or voltage-gated calcium channels, have been defined as those activated by membrane depolarization. The Na^+/Ca^{2+} exchange process can promote either influx or efflux, because the direction of Ca^{2+} movement depends on the relative intracellular and extracellular ratios of Na^+ and Ca^{2+}. The "leak" pathways, which include unstimulated Ca^{2+} entry as well as entry during the fast inward Na^+ phase of an action potential, play only a minor role in calcium influx.

Efflux can occur through either an adenosine triphosphate–driven membrane pump (site 5) or via the Na^+/Ca^{2+} exchange process previously mentioned (site 2). In addition to these influx and efflux mechanisms, the sarcoplasmic reticulum (site 6) and the mitochondria (site 7) function as internal storage/release sites. These storage sites work in concert with the influx and efflux processes to assure that cytosolic calcium levels are appropriate for cellular needs. Although influx and release processes are essential for excitation-contraction coupling, efflux and sequestering processes are equally important for terminating the contractile process and for protecting the cell from the deleterious effects of Ca^{2+} overload.[85,86]

Role of Calcium and Potential-Dependent Calcium Channels in Hypertension and Other Cardiovascular Disorders

The movement of calcium underlies the basic excitation-contraction coupling process; therefore, vascular tone and contraction are primarily determined by the availability of calcium from extracellular or intracellular sources. Potential-dependent Ca^{2+} channels are important in regulating the influx of Ca^{2+}, causing vasoconstriction, and regulating blood pressure. Inhibition of Ca^{2+} flow through these channels results in both vasodilation and decreased cellular response to contractile stimuli. Arterial smooth muscle is more sensitive to this action than venous smooth muscle. Additionally, coronary and cerebral arterial vessels are more sensitive than other arterial beds.[86,87]

The term "ischemic heart disease," or coronary heart disease, encompasses a variety of syndromes. These include angina pectoris, silent myocardial ischemia, acute coronary insufficiency, and MI. According to the American Heart Association, coronary heart disease is the leading cause of deaths attributable to cardiovascular disease in the United States, and cardiovascular disease is the leading global cause of death, accounting for more than 17.3 million deaths per year in 2013. In 2010, the estimated global cost of cardiovascular disease was $863 billion.[88]

Angina pectoris is a clinical manifestation that results from coronary atherosclerotic heart disease. It is characterized by a severe constricting pain in the chest that often radiates to the left shoulder, the left arm, or the back. Clinically, angina pectoris can be classified as either exertional, variant, or unstable. Exertional angina, otherwise known as stable angina or exercise-induced angina, is the most common form and results from an imbalance between myocardial oxygen supply and demand. Variant angina, otherwise known as Prinzmetal angina, results from the vasospasm of large, surface coronary vessels or branches. Unstable angina is the most difficult to treat and may occur as a result of advanced atherosclerosis and coronary vasospasm.[89]

Excitation-contraction coupling in the heart is different from that in vascular smooth muscle in that a portion of the inward current is carried by Na^+ through the fast channel. In the sinoatrial and atrioventricular (AV) nodes, however, depolarization depends primarily on the movement of Ca^{2+} through the slow channel. Attenuation of this Ca^{2+} movement produces a negative inotropic effect and decreased conduction through the AV node. This latter effect is especially useful in treating paroxysmal supraventricular tachycardia (PSVT), an arrhythmia primarily caused by AV nodal reentry and AV reentry.[87]

Development of Calcium Channel Blockers

Drugs that are capable of blocking the calcium channel can be grouped into one of three chemical classifications (Fig. 17.25), each of which produces a distinct pharmacologic profile: 1,4-dihydropyridines (1,4-DHPs; e.g., nifedipine), phenylalkylamines (e.g., verapamil), and benzothiazepines (e.g., diltiazem). The majority of calcium channel blockers are 1,4-DHPs, and a detailed description of the SAR for this chemical class is provided below. In contrast, verapamil and diltiazem are the lone representatives of their chemical classes.

Identification of drugs that could block the inward movement of Ca^{2+} through slow cardiac channels occurred in the early 1960s. Verapamil and other phenylalkylamines were shown to possess negative inotropic and chronotropic effects that were distinct from other coronary vasodilators. Further investigations revealed that these agents mimicked the cardiac effects of Ca^{2+} withdrawal: They reduced contractile force without affecting the action potential. The effects of these drugs could be reversed by the addition of Ca^{2+}, thus suggesting that the negative inotropic effect was linked to an inhibition of excitation-contraction coupling. Subsequently, derivatives of verapamil, as well as other chemical classes of drugs (including the benzothiazepine, diltiazem), were shown to competitively block Ca^{2+} movement through the slow channel and, thus, alter the cardiac action potential. Therefore, calcium channel blockers are also known as slow channel blockers, calcium entry blockers, and calcium antagonists.[85,87]

The development of dihydropyridines can be traced back to an 1882 paper in which Hantzsch described their utility as intermediates in the synthesis of substituted pyridines. Fifty years later, interest in this chemical class of compounds increased when it was discovered that a 1,4-DHP ring was responsible for the "hydrogen-transfer" properties of the coenzyme NADH. Numerous biochemical studies followed this discovery; however, it was not until the early 1970s that the pharmacologic properties of 1,4-DHPs were fully investigated. Loev and coworkers at Smith, Klein & French laboratories investigated the activities of "Hantzsch-type" compounds. As shown in

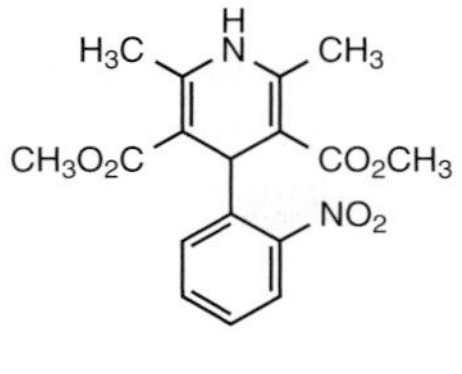

Nifedipine
(a 1,4-dihydropyridine)

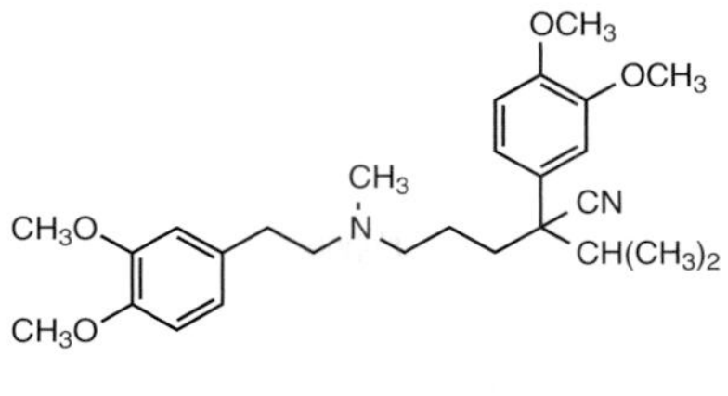

Verapamil
(a phenylalkylamine)

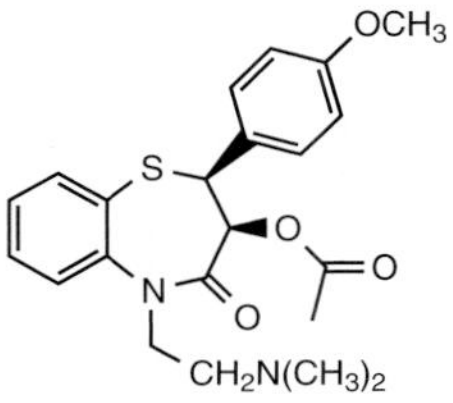

Diltiazem
(a benzothiazepine)

Figure 17.25 Chemical classes of calcium channel blockers.

Figure 17.26, the Hantzsch reaction produced a symmetrical compound in which both the esters (i.e., CO_2R_2) and the C2 and C6 substituents (i.e., CH_3) are identical with each other. Structural requirements necessary for activity were identified by sequentially modifying the C4 substituent (i.e., the R_1 group), the C3- and C5-esters (i.e., the R_2 groups), the C2- and C6-alkyl groups, and the N1-H substituent. The initial drug to emerge from these efforts was nifedipine.[90–93]

Therapeutic Role of Calcium Channel Blockers

Calcium channel blockers have been approved for the treatment of hypertension, angina pectoris, subarachnoid hemorrhage, and specific types of arrhythmias.[66,67] All calcium channel blockers cause vasodilation and decrease peripheral resistance. With the exceptions of nimodipine, all are approved to treat hypertension. According to the 2014 report from the Eighth Joint National Committee (JNC8), calcium channel blockers are recommended as first-line treatment of hypertension in general black and nonblack populations. Studies have indicated that immediate-release formulations of short-acting calcium channel blockers, especially nifedipine, can cause an abrupt vasodilation that can result in MI. As a result, only the sustained-release formulations of nifedipine and diltiazem should be used in the treatment of essential hypertension.[94] Due to its short duration of action, clevidipine is approved for the parenteral treatments of perioperative hypertension, hypertensive urgency, and hypertensive emergency. Five of the 10 drugs are approved for the treatment of angina pectoris. Verapamil is the most versatile agent in that it is indicated for all three types of angina: vasospastic, chronic stable, and unstable. Amlodipine, nifedipine, and diltiazem are indicated for both vasospastic and chronic stable angina, whereas nicardipine is indicated only for chronic stable angina. Nimodipine is unique in that it has a greater effect on cerebral arteries than on other arteries. As a result, nimodipine is indicated for the improvement of neurologic deficits caused by spasm following subarachnoid hemorrhage from ruptured congenital intracranial aneurysms in patients otherwise in good neurologic condition after the episode. Verapamil and diltiazem are pharmacologically different from the 1,4-DHPs in that they block sinus and AV nodal conduction. As a result, IV formulations of verapamil and diltiazem are indicated for the treatment of atrial fibrillation, atrial flutter, and PSVT. Verapamil also can be used orally, either alone (for prophylaxis of repetitive PSVT) or in combination with digoxin (for atrial flutter or atrial fibrillation).

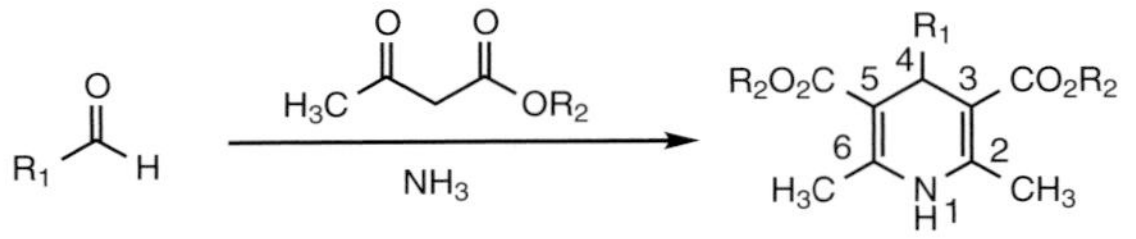

General structure for
1,4-dihydropyridines

Figure 17.26 Synthesis of 1,4-dihydropyridines (1,4-DHPs) using the Hantzsch reaction.

UNLABELED USES OF CALCIUM CHANNEL BLOCKERS

Migraine headache, pulmonary hypertension, preterm labor, cardiomyopathy, acute MI, claudication, mania, peripheral vascular disease, diabetic neuropathy, and pulmonary edema associated with altitude sickness.

Pharmacology Overview of Calcium Channel Blockers

Mechanisms of Action

Calcium channel blockers exert their effects through interaction with potential-dependent channels. To date, six functional subclasses, or types, of potential-dependent Ca^{2+} channels have been identified: T, L, N, P, Q, and R. These types differ in location and function and can be divided into two major groups: low-voltage–activated (LVA) channels and high-voltage–activated (HVA) channels. Of the six types, only the T (transient, tiny) channel can be rapidly activated and inactivated with small changes in the cell membrane potential. It is thus designated as an LVA channel. All of the other types of channels require a larger depolarization and are thus designated as HVA channels. The L (long-lasting, large) channel is the site of action for currently available calcium channel blockers and, therefore, has been extensively studied. It is located in skeletal, cardiac, and smooth muscle and, thus, is highly involved in organ and vessel contraction within the cardiovascular system. The N channel is found in neuronal tissue and exhibits kinetics and inhibitory sensitivity distinct from both L and T channels. The functions, sensitivities, and properties of the other three types of channels are not as well known. The P channel has been named for its presence in the Purkinje cells, whereas the Q and R channels have been characterized by their abilities to bind to certain polypeptide toxins.[87,95,96]

The L channel is a pentameric complex consisting of α_1, α_2, β, γ, and δ polypeptides (Fig. 17.27). The α_1 subunit is a transmembrane-spanning protein that consists of four domains that functions as the pore-forming subunit. The α_1 subunit also contains binding sites for all the currently available calcium channel blockers. The other four subunits surround the α_1 portion of the channel and contribute to the overall hydrophobicity of the pentamer. This hydrophobicity is important in that it allows the channel to be embedded in the cell membrane. Additionally, the α_2, δ, and β subunits modulate the α_1 subunit. Other types of potential-dependent channels are similar to the L channel. They all have a central α_1 subunit; however, molecular cloning studies have revealed that there are at least six α_1 genes: α_{1S}, α_{1A}, α_{1B}, α_{1C}, α_{1D}, and α_{1E}. Three of these genes, α_{1S}, α_{1C}, and α_{1D}, have been associated with L channels. The L channels found in skeletal muscle result from the α_{1S} gene; those in the heart, aorta, lung, and fibroblast result from the α_{1C} gene; and those in endocrine tissue result from the α_{1D} gene. Both α_{1C} and α_{1D} are used for L channels in the brain. Thus, there are some differences among the L channels located in different organs and tissues. Additionally, differences in α_1 genes and differences among the other subunits are responsible for the variations seen among the other five types of potential-dependent channels. As an example, the N channel lacks the γ subunit and contains an α_1 subunit derived from the α_{1B} gene.[87,95]

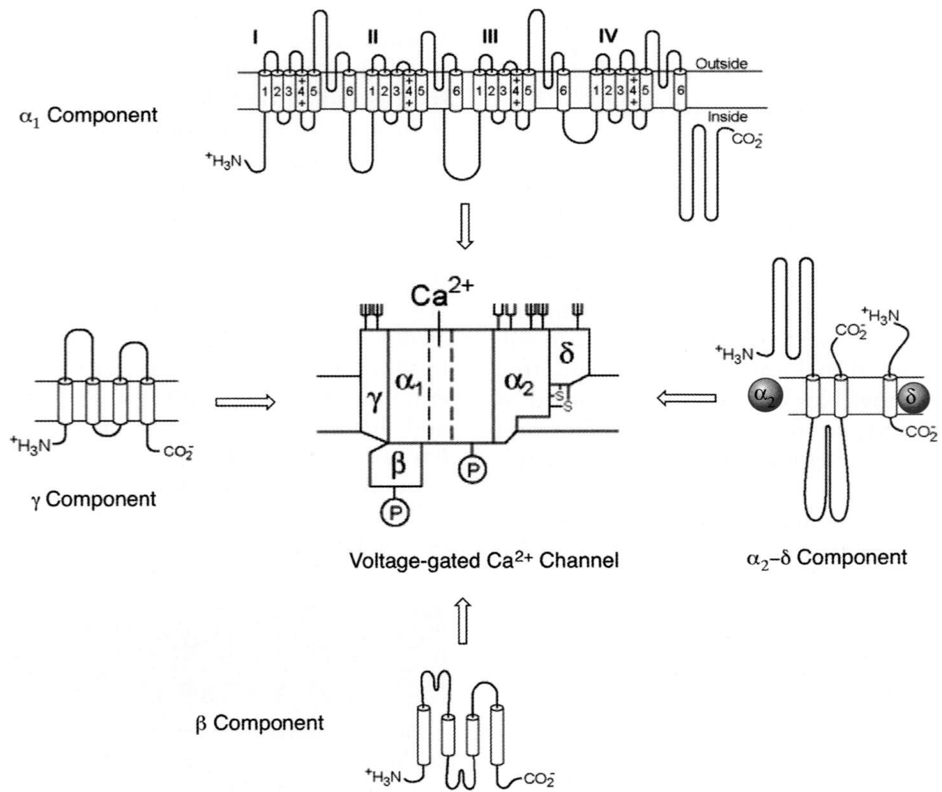

Figure 17.27 Representation of the structure of the voltage-gated Ca^{2+} channel (L channel) composed of several subunits—α_1, α_2-δ, β, γ—organized as depicted in the central area.

Table 17.15 Actions of Calcium Channel Blockers and Interactions Among Their Receptor Sites

Calcium Channel Blocker	Effect on Ca^{2+} Channel	Allosteric Effect on the Binding of		
		Verapamil	Diltiazem	1,4-Dihydropyridines
Verapamil	Antagonist; blocks channel	NA	Inhibits	Inhibits
Diltiazem	Antagonist; blocks channel	Inhibits	NA	Enhances
1,4-Dihydropyridines	Antagonist/agonist; can either block or open channel	Inhibits	Enhances	NA

NA, not applicable.

Calcium channel blockers bind to specific receptor sites located within the central α_1 subunit of L-type, potential-dependent channels and prevent the influx of calcium into the cell. Three distinct, but allosterically interacting, receptors have been identified for verapamil, diltiazem, and the 1,4-DHPs. As shown in Table 17.15, the binding of verapamil to its receptor inhibits the binding of both diltiazem and the 1,4-DHPs to their respective receptors. Likewise, the binding of either diltiazem or the 1,4-DHPs inhibits the binding of verapamil. In contrast, diltiazem and the 1,4-DHPs mutually enhance the binding of each other.[90]

Potential-dependent channels can exist in one of three conformations: a resting state, which can be stimulated by membrane depolarization; an open state, which allows the Ca^{2+} to enter; and an inactive state, which is refractory to further depolarization. Calcium channel blockers have been shown to be more effective when membrane depolarization is either longer, more intense, or more frequent. This use dependency suggests that these drugs preferentially interact with their receptors when the Ca^{2+} channel is in either the open or inactive state. This state dependence is not identical for all classes of Ca^{2+} channel blockers and, in combination with the different binding sites, allosteric interactions, basicity, and solubility, may be responsible for the pharmacologic differences among verapamil, diltiazem, and the 1,4-DHPs. A summary of these differences is provided in Table 17.16. The 1,4-DHPs are primarily vasodilators, whereas verapamil and diltiazem have both vasodilator and cardiodepressant actions. The increased heart rate seen with the 1,4-DHPs results from a reflex mechanism that tries to overcome the vasodilation and subsequent drop in blood pressure caused by these drugs. In contrast, the compensatory mechanism does not occur to the same extent with either verapamil or diltiazem. This difference is the result of the ability of verapamil and diltiazem to block AV nodal conductance and the increased ability of 1,4-DHPs to activate the baroreceptor reflex. Ultimately, these pharmacologic differences are reflected in the clinical use of these agents.[86,89,90]

Common Adverse Effects

The most prevalent or significant side effects of calcium channel blockers are listed below.[66,67,86,87,89] In most instances, these side effects do not cause long-term complications, and they often resolve with time or dosage adjustments. Many of these effects are simply extensions of the pharmacologic effects of this class of drugs. Excessive vasodilation results in edema, flushing, hypotension, nasal congestion, headache, and dizziness. Additionally, the palpitations, chest pain, and tachycardia seen with 1,4-DHPs are a result of sympathetic responses to the vasodilatory effects of this chemical class. The use of a β-blocker in combination with a 1,4-DHP can minimize these compensatory effects and can be very useful in treating hypertension. Verapamil and diltiazem can cause bradycardia and AV block because of their ability to depress AV nodal conduction. Because of risks associated with additive cardiodepressive effects, they should not be used in combination with β-blockers. Clevidipine is formulated as an oil-in-water emulsion that contains soybean oil, glycerin, and purified egg yolk phospholipids. As a result, this drug is contraindicated in patients with egg hypersensitivity or soya lecithin hypersensitivity. Additionally, the emulsion used in this formulation can aggravate preexisting disorders of lipid metabolism.

Table 17.16 Similarities and Differences Among 1,4-Dihydropyridines (DHPs), Verapamil, and Diltiazem

Cardiovascular Effect	1,4-DHPs	Verapamil and Diltiazem
Peripheral vasodilation	Increase	Increase
Blood pressure	Decrease	Decrease
Heart rate	Increase	Decrease or no effect
Atrioventricular node conduction	No effect	Decrease
Contractility	No effect or moderate increase	Decrease

ADVERSE EFFECTS OF CALCIUM CHANNEL BLOCKERS

Edema, flushing, hypotension, nasal congestion, palpitations, chest pain, tachycardia, headache, fatigue, dizziness, rash, nausea, abdominal pain, constipation, diarrhea, vomiting, shortness of breath, weakness, bradycardia, and AV block.

Common Interactions

Drug interactions for calcium channel blockers[66,67] are listed in Table 17.17.

Medicinal Chemistry of Calcium Channel Blockers

Receptor Binding and SAR

The general and specific structures of the 1,4-DHPs are shown in Table 17.18. Based upon the importance of several structural features, the following SAR statements can be made regarding this class of drugs.

1. A substituted phenyl ring at the C4 position optimizes activity (heteroaromatic rings, such as pyridine, produce similar therapeutic effects but are not used because of observed animal toxicity), and C4 substitution with a small nonplanar alkyl or cycloalkyl group decreases activity.

Table 17.17 Drug Interactions for Calcium Channel Blockers

Drug	Calcium Blocker(s)	Result of Interaction
α_1-Blockers (prazosin, terazosin)	Verapamil	Increased prazosin and terazosin levels
Amiodarone	Diltiazem, verapamil	Increased bradycardia and cardiotoxicity; decreased cardiac output
Aspirin	Verapamil	Increased incidence of bruising
Azole antifungals	Felodipine, isradipine, nifedipine, nisoldipine	Increased serum concentrations of the calcium channel blockers
Barbiturates	Felodipine, nifedipine, verapamil	Decreased pharmacologic effects of the calcium channel blockers
β-Blockers	All	Coadministration may cause additive or synergistic effects; increased cardiodepressant effects (more extensive with verapamil and diltiazem); inhibition of β-blocker metabolism by diltiazem, isradipine, nicardipine, nifedipine, and verapamil
Buspirone	Diltiazem, verapamil	Increase buspirone levels
Carbamazepine, oxcarbazepine	Felodipine, diltiazem, verapamil	Carbamazepine and oxcarbazepine decrease felodipine levels; verapamil and diltiazem increase carbamazepine levels
Cimetidine	All	Increased 1,4-DHP levels
Cyclosporine	Felodipine, nicardipine, nifedipine, diltiazem, verapamil	Increased cyclosporine levels when used with all of these except for nifedipine; cyclosporine increases felodipine and nifedipine levels
CYP3A4 inhibitors	All	Potentially can increase the plasma levels of calcium channel blockers
Digoxin	Nifedipine, diltiazem, verapamil	Increased digoxin levels
Disopyramide, flecainide	Verapamil	Additive cardiodepressant effects
Dofetilide	Verapamil	Increased dofetilide levels
Doxorubicin	Verapamil	Increased doxorubicin levels
Erythromycin, clarithromycin	All	Increased 1,4-DHP levels and increased toxicity
Fentanyl	All	Severe hypotension and/or bradycardia

Table 17.17 Drug Interactions for Calcium Channel Blockers (Continued)

Drug	Calcium Blocker(s)	Result of Interaction
General anesthetics	All	Potentiation of the cardiac effects and vascular dilation associated with anesthetics
HMG-CoA reductase inhibitors	Diltiazem, verapamil	Increase levels of HMG-CoA reductase inhibitor
Imipramine	Diltiazem, verapamil	Increased imipramine levels
Lithium	Diltiazem, verapamil	Decreased lithium levels with verapamil; neuro-toxicity with diltiazem
Drug	Calcium blocker(s)	Result of interaction
Lovastatin	Isradipine	Decreased effects of lovastatin
Melatonin	All	Decreased therapeutic effects of calcium channel blockers
Methylprednisolone	Diltiazem, verapamil	Increased methylprednisolone levels
Midazolam, triazolam	Diltiazem, verapamil	Increased effects of these benzodiazepines
Moricizine	Diltiazem	Increased moricizine levels; decreased diltiazem levels
Phenobarbital	All	Decreased bioavailability of calcium channel blocker
Phenytoin	All	Decreased effectiveness of calcium channel blocker due to induction of metabolism
Quinidine	Diltiazem, nifedipine, nisoldipine, verapamil	Variable responses: quinidine decreases AUC of nisoldipine but increases actions of nifedipine; diltiazem and verapamil increase the effects of quinidine; nifedipine decreases quinidine levels and actions
Rifampin	Diltiazem, isradipine, nicardipine, nifedip-ine, verapamil	Decreased levels of calcium channel blocker
Sirolimus, tacrolimus	Diltiazem, nifedipine, verapamil	Increased sirolimus and tacrolimus levels
St. John's wort	Nifedipine	Decreased nifedipine levels (St.John's wort most likely increases the metabolism of all calcium channel blockers)
Theophylline	Diltiazem, verapamil	Increased theophylline levels and toxicity
Valproic acid	Nimodipine	Increased nimodipine levels
Vecuronium	Verapamil	Increased vecuronium levels
Vincristine	Nifedipine	Increased vincristine levels

AUC, area under the curve; *HMG-CoA*, 3-hydroxy-3-methyl-glutaryl-coenzyme A.

2. Phenyl ring substitution (X) is important for size and position rather than for electronic nature. Drugs with ortho or meta substitutions possess optimal activity, whereas those that are unsubstituted or that contain a para substitution show a significant decrease in activity. Despite the fact that all commercially available 1,4-DHPs have electron-withdrawing ortho and/or meta substituents, this is not an absolute requirement. Drugs with electron-donating groups at these same positions also have demonstrated good activity. The importance of the ortho and meta substituents is to provide sufficient bulk to "lock" the conformation of the 1,4-DHP such that the C4 aromatic ring is perpendicular to the 1,4-DHP ring (Fig. 17.28). This perpendicular conformation has been proposed to be essential for the activity of the 1,4-DHPs.
3. The 1,4-DHP ring is essential for activity. Substitution at the N1 position or the use of oxidized (piperidine) or reduced (pyridine) ring systems greatly decreases or abolishes activity.

Table 17.18 Structures of the 1,4-Dihydropyridine Ca^{2+} Channel Blockers

General Structure:

Isradipine:

Compounds	R_1	R_2	R_3	X
Amlodipine	$CH_2O(CH_2)_2NH_2$	$CO_2CH_2CH_3$	CO_2CH_3	2-Cl
Clevidipine	CH_3	$CO_2CH_2O\text{-}C(=O)\text{-}nC_3H_7$	CO_2CH_3	2,3-Cl_2
Felodipine	CH_3	$CO_2CH_2CH_3$	CO_2CH_3	2,3-Cl_2
Nicardipine	CH_3	$CO_2(CH_2)_2\text{-}N(CH_3)\text{-}H_2C\text{-}C_6H_5$	CO_2CH_3	3-NO_2
Nifedipine	CH_3	CO_2CH_3	CO_2CH_3	2-NO_2
Nimodipine	CH_3	$CO_2CH_2CH_2OCH_3$	$CO_2CH(CH_3)CH_3$	3-NO_2
Nisoldipine	CH_3	$CO_2CH_2CH(CH_3)_2$	CO_2CH_3	2-NO_2

4. Ester groups at the C3 and C5 positions optimize activity. Other electron-withdrawing groups show decreased antagonist activity and may even show agonist activity. For example, the replacement of the C3 ester of isradipine with a NO_2 group produces a calcium channel activator or agonist. Thus, the term "calcium channel modulators" is a more appropriate classification for the 1,4-DHPs.
5. When the esters at C-3 and C5 are nonidentical, the C4 carbon becomes chiral, and stereoselectivity between the enantiomers is observed. Additionally, evidence suggests that the C3 and C5 positions of the dihydropyridine ring are not equivalent positions. Crystal structures of nifedipine, a symmetrical 1,4-DHP, have shown that the C3 carbonyl is synplanar to the C2-C3 bond but that the C_5 carbonyl is antiperiplanar to the C5-C6 bond (Fig. 17.29). Asymmetrical drugs have shown enhanced selectivity for specific blood vessels and were preferentially developed. Nifedipine, the first 1,4-DHP to be marketed, is the only symmetrical drug in this chemical class.

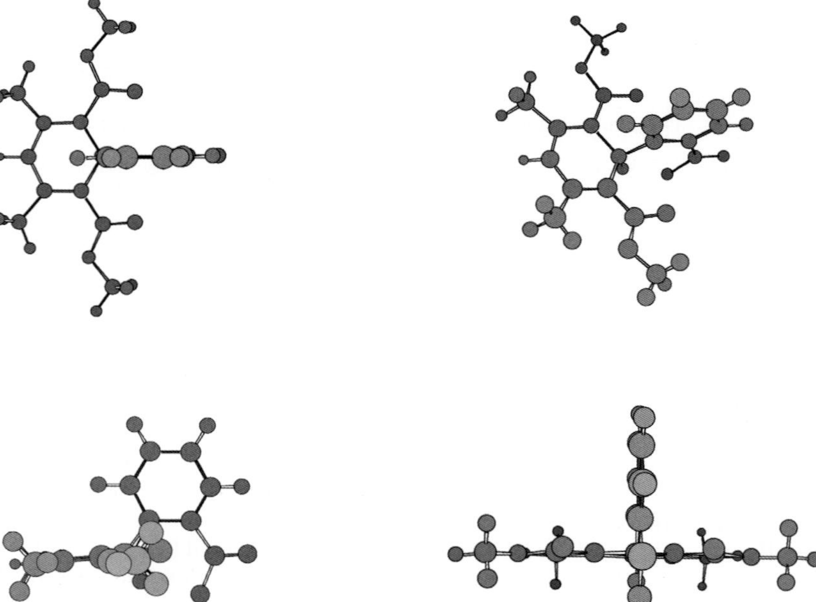

Figure 17.28 Molecular models of nifedipine. The ortho-nitro group of nifedipine provides steric bulk and ensures that the required perpendicular nature of the phenyl and dihydropyridine rings is maintained.

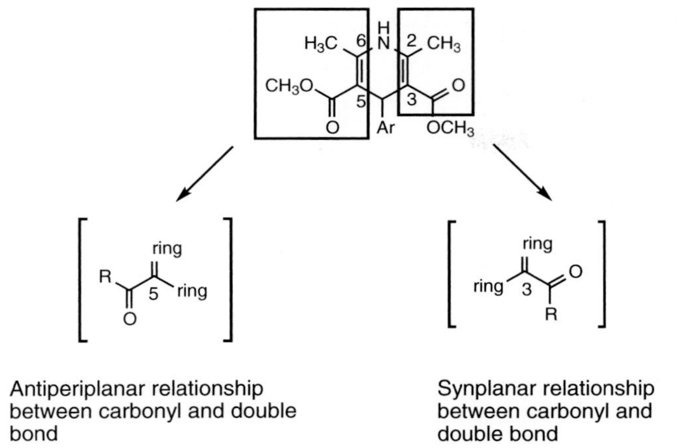

Antiperiplanar relationship between carbonyl and double bond

Synplanar relationship between carbonyl and double bond

Figure 17.29 Conformation of the C3 and C5 esters of nifedipine (Ar = 2-nitrophenyl). The C3 carbonyl is synplanar to the C2-C3 bond, and the C5 carbonyl is antiperiplanar to the C5-C6 bond.

6. With the exception of amlodipine, all 1,4-DHPs have C2 and C6 methyl groups. The enhanced potency of amlodipine (vs. nifedipine) suggests that the 1,4-DHP receptor can tolerate larger substituents at this position and that enhanced activity can be obtained by altering these groups.

Physiocochemical Properties

A comparison of the acid-base properties of verapamil, diltiazem, and the 1,4-DHPs reveals that all of these drugs are basic; however, the 1,4-DHPs are considerably less basic than verapamil and diltiazem. Verapamil and diltiazem both contain tertiary amines with pK_a values of 8.9 and 7.7, respectively.[76] In contrast, the nitrogen atom of the 1,4-DHP ring is part of a conjugated carbamate. Its electrons are involved in resonance delocalization and are much less available for protonation. Thus, at physiologic pH, verapamil and diltiazem are primarily ionized, whereas the 1,4-DHPs are primarily un-ionized. There are two exceptions to this. Amlodipine and nicardipine contain basic amine groups as part of the side chains connected to the 1,4-DHP ring. Although the 1,4-DHP ring of these drugs is un-ionized, the side chain amines will be primarily ionized at physiologic pH. Because ionic attraction often is the initial interaction between a drug and its receptor, the differences in basicity between the 1,4-DHP ring and the tertiary amines of verapamil and diltiazem are consistent with the previously noted fact that the binding site for the 1,4-DHPs is distinct from those for verapamil and diltiazem.

The calculated log P values for the calcium channel blockers are listed in Table 17.19.[76,97] As evidenced by the data, all of these drugs possess good lipid solubility and, hence, excellent oral absorption (not shown in Table 17.19). Within the 1,4-DHP class, enhanced lipid solubility occurs in drugs that contain either larger ester groups or disubstituted phenyl rings. A comparison of the log P values of nifedipine and nisoldipine illustrates this fact. It should be noted that the calculated log P values listed in Table 17.16 are for the un-ionized drugs. These values significantly decrease for the ionized forms of amlodipine, nicardipine, verapamil, and diltiazem such that the latter three agents possess sufficient water solubility to be used both orally and parenterally.

All calcium channel blockers, with the exception of nifedipine, contain at least one chiral center; however, they are all marketed as their racemic mixtures. As previously noted, 1,4-DHPs with asymmetrically substituted esters exhibit stereoselectivity between the enantiomers. Additionally, the *S*-(-)-enantiomers of verapamil and other phenylalkylamines are more potent than the *R*-(+)-enantiomers. Very few SAR studies are available for diltiazem; however, the *cis* arrangement of the acetyl ester and the substituted phenyl ring is required for activity.[90]

Pharmacokinetic Properties

The pharmacokinetic parameters and oral dosing information for calcium channel blockers are summarized in Tables 17.19 and 17.20, respectively.[66,67,74] The primary differences among the drugs are their onsets of action, half-lives, and oral bioavailability. All calcium channel blockers have excellent oral absorption; however, because they also are subject to rapid first-pass metabolism in the liver, the actual oral bioavailability of these drugs varies considerably depending on the extent of metabolism. All of these drugs are highly plasma protein bound and primarily eliminated as inactive metabolites in the urine. Because of extensive hepatic transformation, calcium channel blockers should be used cautiously in patients with hepatic disease. Recommendations for these patients include dosage reductions, careful titrations, and close therapeutic monitoring. Diltiazem and verapamil also require dosage adjustments in patients with renal dysfunction, because renal impairment can significantly increase the concentrations of the active metabolites of these drugs. Dosage adjustments usually are not required for the other eight drugs, because seven of them produce inactive metabolites and nisoldipine produces active metabolites with significantly lower activity.

Immediate-release and sustained-release (or extended-release) formulations vary from one drug to another and are summarized in Table 17.20. Additionally, clevidipine, nicardipine, verapamil, and diltiazem are available as parenteral preparations. Unlike immediate-release tablets and capsules, sustained-release (or extended-release) formulations cannot be chewed or crushed because this may lead to an immediate, rather than a sustained, release of the compound. This effect not only will decrease the duration of the dose but also could produce an overdose and subsequent toxicities in the patient. Parenteral preparations of nicardipine and verapamil are incompatible with IV solutions containing sodium bicarbonate. In each case, sodium bicarbonate increases the pH of the solution, resulting in the precipitation of the calcium channel blocker. Although this interaction is not listed for diltiazem, it is reasonable to assume that a similar interaction may occur. Additionally, nicardipine is incompatible with lactated Ringer's solution, and verapamil will precipitate in solutions having a pH greater than or equal to 6.[66,67]

Table 17.19 Pharmacokinetic Parameters of Calcium Channel Blockers

Drug	Calculated Log P	Oral Bioavailability (%)	Effect of Food on Absorption	Active Metabolite	Protein Binding (%)	T_{max} (hr)	Elimination Half-Life (hr)	Major Route(s) of Elimination
1,4-Dihydropyridines								
Amlodipine	2.76	64-90	None	None	93-97	6-12	35-50	Renal (60%) Fecal (20%-25%)
Clevidipine	2.96	NA	NA	None	>99	2-4 (min)	0.15	Renal (63%-74%) Fecal (7%-22%)
Felodipine	4.69	10-25	Increase	None	>99	2.5-5.0	11-16	Renal (70%) Fecal (10%)
Isradipine	3.19	15-24	Reduced rate, same extent	None	95	7-18 (CR)	8	Renal (60%-65%) Fecal (25%-30%)
Nicardipine	4.27	35	Reduced	None	>95	0.5-2.0 (IR) 1-4 (SR)	2-4	Renal (60%) Fecal (35%)
Nifedipine	2.40	45-70 86 (SR)	None	None	92-98	0.5 (IR) 6 (SR)	2-5 (IR) 7 (SR)	Renal (60%-80%) Biliary/fecal (15%)
Nimodipine	3.14	13	Reduced	None	>95	1	8-9	Renal
Nisoldipine	3.86	5	High-fat meal increases immediate release but lowers overall amount	Hydroxylated analog	>99	6-12	7-12	Renal (70%-75%) Fecal (6%-12%)
Phenalkylamines								
Verapamil	3.53	20-35	Reduced (SR form only)	Norverapamil	90	1-2 (IR) 7-11 (SR) 0.1-0.2 (IV)	3-7 (IR) 12 (SR)	Renal (70%) Fecal (16%)
Benzothiazepines								
Diltiazem	3.55	40-60	None	Deacetyldiltiazem	70-80	2-4 (IR) 6-14 (SR)	3.0-4.5 (IR) 4.0-9.5 (SR) 3.4 (IV)	Renal (35%) Fecal (60%-65%)

CR, controlled-release product; *IR*, immediate-release product; *IV*, intravenous administration; *NA*, not applicable; *SR*, sustained-release product; T_{max}, time to maximum blood concentration.

Table 17.20 Oral Dosing Information for Calcium Channel Blockers

Generic Name	Brand Name(s)	Approved Indications	Normal Dosing Range	Maximum Daily Dose	Precautions With Hepatic Dysfunction	Available Tablet or Capsule Strengths (mg)
1,4-Dihydropyridines						
Amlodipine	Norvasc	Angina (V, CS), hypertension	5-10 mg once daily	10 mg	Reduce dosage	2.5, 5, 10
Clevidipine	Cleviprex	Hypertension	4-6 mg/hr IV	32 mg/hr IV	None	25 mg/50 mL emulsified suspension
Felodipine	Plendil (n/a)	Hypertension	2.5-10.0 mg once daily	10 mg	Reduce dosage	ER: 2.5, 5, 10
Isradipine	DynaCirc (n/a)	Hypertension	2.5-10.0 mg b.i.d.	20 mg	Titrate dosage	2.5, 5
Nicardipine	Cardene, Cardene IV	Angina (CS), hypertension	20-40 mg t.i.d. (SR: 30-60 mg b.i.d.) (IV: 5-15 mg/hr)	120 mg	Titrate dosage	20, 30 (ER: 30, 45) (IV: 2.5 mg/mL)
Nifedipine	Procardia, Adalat	Angina (V, CS), hypertension	10-20 mg t.i.d. (SR: 30-60 mg once a day)	180 mg (SR: 90 mg)	Reduce dosage	10, 20 (ER: 30, 60, 90)
Nimodipine	Nimotop	Subarachnoid hemorrhage	60 mg every 4 hr for 21 d	360 mg	Reduce dosage	30 (30 mg/10 mL oral suspension)
Nisoldipine	Sular	Hypertension	17-34 mg once daily	34 mg	Closely monitor blood pressure	ER: 8.5, 17, 20, 25.5, 30, 34, 40
Phenylalkylamines						
Verapamil	Calan, Isoptin, Verelan	Angina (V, CS, U), hypertension, atrial fibrillation/flutter, PSVT	80-120 mg t.i.d. or q.i.d. (SR: 180-480 mg once daily or b.i.d.)	480 mg	Reduce dosage	40, 80, 120 (SR: 100, 120, 180, 200, 240, 300, 360) (IV: 2.5 mg/mL)
Benzothiazepines						
Diltiazem	Cardizem, Cartia, Dilt-CD, Dilt-XR, Diltzac, Matzim, Taztia, Tiazac	Angina (V, CS), hypertension, atrial fibrillation/flutter, PSVT	30-120 mg t.i.d. or q.i.d. (SR: 120-480 mg once daily)	480 mg (SR: 540 mg)	Reduce dosage	30, 60, 90, 120 (SR: 60, 90, 120, 180, 240, 300, 360, 420) (IV: 5 mg/mL)

b.i.d., twice a day; *CR*, controlled release; *CS*, chronic stable angina; *ER*, extended release; *IV*, intravenous; *n/a*, no longer available; *PSVT*, paroxysmal supraventricular tachycardia; *q.i.d.*, four times a day; *SR*, sustained release; *t.i.d.*, three times a day; *U*, unstable angina; *V*, vasospastic angina.

Metabolism

With the exception of clevidipine, all calcium channel blockers undergo extensive first-pass metabolism in the liver and are substrates for the CYP3A4 isozyme.[66,74] Additionally, several of these drugs can inhibit CYP3A4. Clevidipine was designed to have an ultra-short duration of action. Upon IV infusion, clevidipine exerts its antihypertensive actions within 2-4 minutes. Rapid ester hydrolysis (Fig. 17.30) inactivates the drug and allows it to be used in patients with either renal or hepatic dysfunction without any dosage adjustments.[66] All other 1,4-DHPs are oxidatively metabolized to a variety of inactive compounds. In

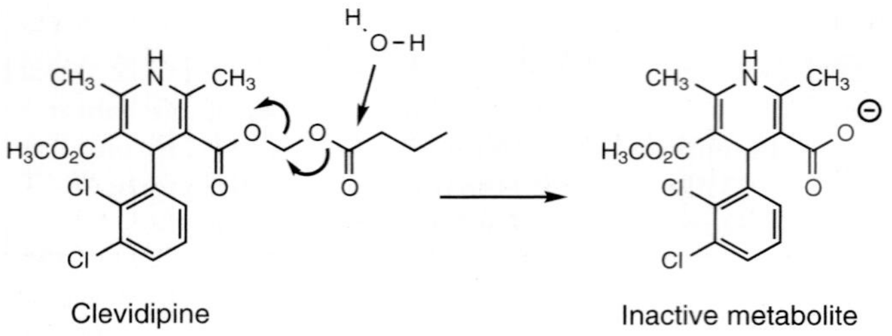

Clevidipine Inactive metabolite

Figure 17.30 In vivo metabolic hydrolysis of clevidipine to an inactive metabolite.

many cases, the dihydropyridine ring is initially oxidized to an inactive pyridine analog (Fig. 17.31). These initial metabolites are then further transformed by hydrolysis, conjugation, and additional oxidation pathways. Nisoldipine is also subject to these processes; however, hydroxylation of its isobutyl ester produces a metabolite that retains 10% of the activity of the parent compound. In addition to the drug-drug interactions listed in Table 17.14, an interesting drug-food interaction occurs with the 1,4-DHPs and grapefruit juice.[98] Coadministration of 1,4-DHPs with grapefruit juice produces an increase systemic concentration of the 1,4-DHPs. The mechanism of this interaction appears to result from inhibition of intestinal CYP450 by flavonoids and furanocoumarins specifically found in grapefruit juice. It has been proposed that limiting daily intake to either an 8-oz. glass of grapefruit juice or half of a fresh grapefruit would likely avoid significant drug interactions with most CYP3A4-metabolized drugs.[99]

Verapamil is primarily converted to an N-demethylated metabolite, norverapamil, which retains approximately 20% of the pharmacologic activity of verapamil and can reach or exceed the steady-state plasma levels of verapamil. Interestingly, the more active *S*-(-)-isomer undergoes more extensive first-pass hepatic metabolism than does the less active *R*-(+)-isomer. This is important to note, because when given IV, verapamil prolongs the PR interval of the electrocardiogram to a greater extent than when it is given orally.[100] This is because the preferential metabolism of the more active enantiomer does not occur with parenteral administration. Diltiazem is primarily hydrolyzed to deacetyldiltiazem. This metabolite retains 25%-50% of the coronary vasodilatory effects of diltiazem and is present in the plasma at levels of 10%-45% of the parent compound.

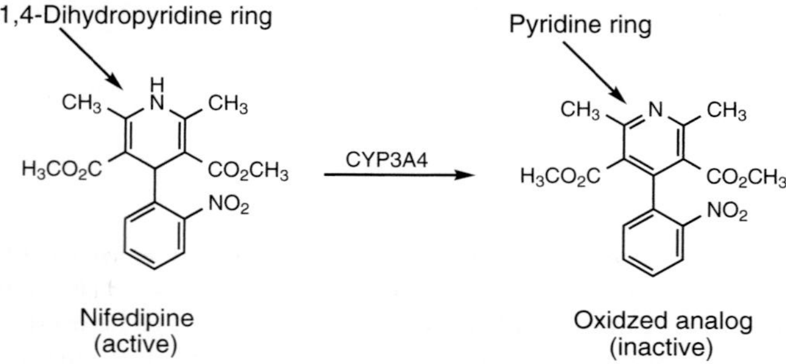

Figure 17.31 Oxidation of the 1,4-dihydropyridine ring of nifedipine.

Central and Peripheral Sympatholytics and Vasodilators

Background

Arterial pressure is the product of cardiac output and peripheral vascular resistance and, therefore, can be lowered by decreasing or inhibiting either or both of these physiologic responses.[87,101] This section will discuss antihypertensives that are classified as either sympatholytics (i.e., having a central or peripheral mechanism of action) or vasodilators. These classes of drugs are less commonly used today because of the higher incidence of side effects associated with inhibition of the sympathetic nervous system (sympathoinhibition) or vasodilation. In many instances, they have been replaced because of availability of newer and more effective antihypertensive drugs with fewer side effects, such as ACEIs and ARBs.

Overview of Vascular Tone

Before beginning the discussion of the sympatholytics and vasodilators, it is important to review the nature of vascular tone. The term "vascular tone" refers to the degree of constriction experienced by a blood vessel relative to its maximally dilated state. All resistance (arteries) and capacitance (venous) vessels under basal conditions exhibit some degree of smooth muscle contraction, which determines the diameter and, hence, the tone of the vessel.[101]

Basal vascular tone varies among organs. Those organs having a large vasodilatory capacity (e.g., myocardium, skeletal muscle, skin, and splanchnic circulation) have high vascular tone, whereas organs having relatively low vasodilatory capacity (e.g., cerebral and renal circulations) have low vascular tone. Vascular tone is determined by many different competing vasoconstrictor and vasodilator influences acting on the blood vessel. Influences such as sympathetic nerves and circulating angiotensin II regulate arterial blood pressure by increasing vascular tone (i.e., vasoconstriction). On the other hand, mechanisms for local blood flow regulation within an organ include endothelial factors (e.g., nitric oxide [NO] and endothelin [ET]) or local hormones/chemical substances (e.g., prostanoids, thromboxanes, histamine, and bradykinin) that can either increase or decrease tone. The mechanisms by which the above influences either constrict or relax blood vessels involve a variety of signal transduction mechanisms that, ultimately, influence the interaction between actin and myosin in the smooth muscle.

Overview of the Regulation of Vascular Smooth Muscle Contraction and Relaxation

The contractile characteristics and the mechanisms that cause contraction of vascular smooth muscle (VSM) are very different from those of cardiac muscle.[101] The VSM undergoes slow, sustained, tonic contractions, whereas cardiac muscle contractions are rapid and of relatively short duration (a few hundred milliseconds). Although VSM contains actin and myosin, it does not have the regulatory protein troponin, as is found in the heart. Furthermore, the arrangement of actin and myosin in VSM is not organized into distinct bands, as it is in cardiac muscle. This is not to imply that the contractile proteins of VSM are disorganized and not well developed. Actually, they are highly organized and well suited for their role in maintaining tonic contractions and reducing lumen diameter.

Contraction of the VSM can be initiated by mechanical, electrical, and chemical stimuli. Passive stretching of VSM can cause contraction that originates from the smooth muscle itself and, therefore, is termed a "myogenic response." Electrical depolarization of the VSM cell membrane also elicits contraction, most likely by opening voltage-dependent calcium channels (L-type calcium channels) and causing an influx (increase) in the intracellular concentration of calcium ion. Finally, a number of chemical stimuli, such as norepinephrine, angiotensin II, vasopressin, endothelin-1, and thromboxane A_2, can cause contraction. Each of these substances binds to specific receptors on the VSM cell (or to receptors on the endothelium adjacent to the VSM), which then leads to VSM contraction. The mechanism of contraction involves different signal transduction pathways, all of which converge to increase intracellular Ca^{2+}.

The mechanism by which an increase in intracellular Ca^{2+} stimulates VSM contraction is illustrated in the left panel of Figure 17.32.

An increase in free intracellular Ca^{2+} results from either increased flux of Ca^{2+} into the VSM cell through calcium channels or by release of Ca^{2+} from intracellular stores of the sarcoplasmic reticulum (SR). The SR is an internal membrane system within the VSM that functions as the major regulator of Ca^{2+} for managing VSM contractility and relaxation. The SR releases Ca^{2+} during contraction, and the released free intracellular Ca^{2+} binds to a special calcium binding protein called calmodulin (CaM), which in turn activates myosin light-chain kinase (MLCK), an enzyme that phosphorylates the myosin light chains by means of adenosine triphosphate (ATP). Phosphorylation of the myosin light chain leads to actin-myosin cross-bridge formation between the myosin heads and the actin filaments and, hence, VSM contraction. Dephosphorylation of the phosphorylated myosin light chain by myosin light-chain phosphorylase yields myosin light chain, which results in relaxation of the VSM. The concentration of intracellular Ca^{2+} depends on the balance between the Ca^{2+} that enters the VSM cells, the Ca^{2+} released by the SR, and the removal of Ca^{2+} either transported by an ATP-dependent calcium pump back into SR where the Ca^{2+} is resequestered or removed from the VSM cell to the external environment by an ATP-dependent calcium pump or by the sodium-calcium exchanger.

The activation of the calcium second messenger system by hormones, neurotransmitters, local mediators, and sensory stimuli is very important in regulating VSM contraction. Several signal transduction mechanisms modulate intracellular calcium concentration and, therefore, the state of vascular tone. These calcium second messenger systems are the phosphatidylinositol (PIP_2)/G_q protein–coupled pathway, the cyclic adenosine monophosphate (cAMP)/G_s protein–coupled pathway, and the NO/cyclic guanosine monophosphate (cGMP) pathway.

The PIP_2 pathway in VSM is similar to that found in the heart (Fig. 17.33). The VSM membrane is lined with specific receptors for norepinephrine (α_1-adrenoceptors),

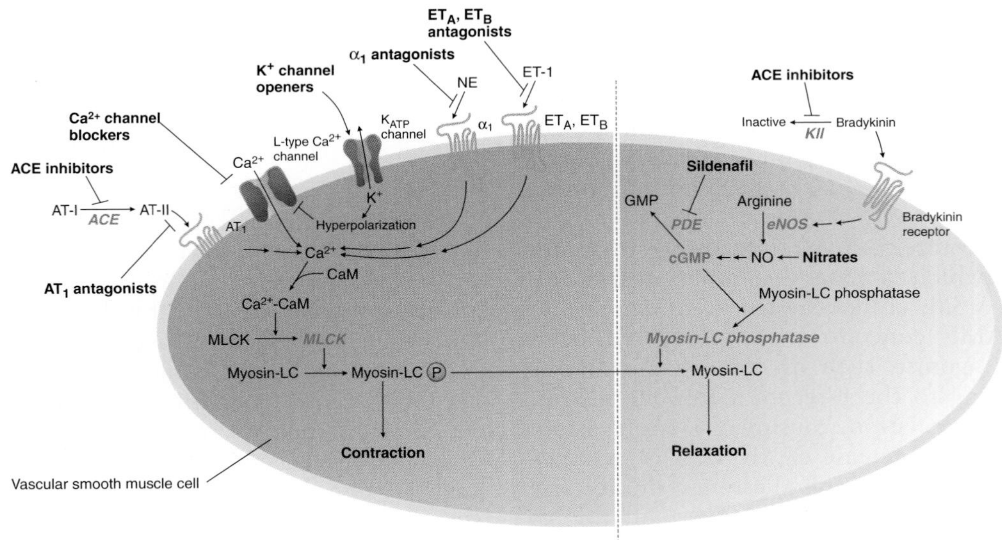

Figure 17.32 Calcium second messenger mechanism of vascular smooth muscle contraction and relaxation and sites of action of the peripheral and centrally acting sympatholytics and vasodilators. *ACE*, angiotensin-converting enzyme; *AT*, angiotensin; *CaM*, calmodulin; *ET-1*, endothelin peptide; *ET*$_A$ and *ET*$_B$, endothelin receptors; *eNOS*, endothelial nitric oxide synthase; *KII*, kininase II or ACE; *MLCK*, myosin light chain kinase; *PDE*, phosphodiesterase. From Yeh DC, Michel T. Pharmacology of vascular tone. In: Golan DE, Tashjian A, Armstrong E, et al., eds. *Principles of Pharmacology: The Pathophysiologic Basis of Drug Therapy*, 2nd ed. Baltimore, MD: Wolters Kluwer/Lippincott Williams & Wilkins; 2008:367-385, with permission.

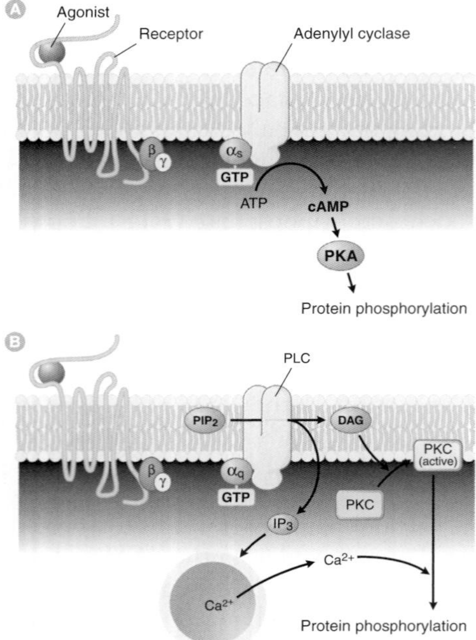

Figure 17.33 **The mechanism of activation of the cyclic adenosine monophosphate (cAMP)/G_s protein–coupled pathway and the phospholipase C/phosphatidylinositol (PIP_2) pathway in vascular smooth muscle.** ***DAG*, diacylglycerol; *IP_3*, inositol triphosphate; *PKA*, protein kinase A.** From Yeh DC, Michel T. Pharmacology of vascular tone. In: Golan DE, Tashjian A, Armstrong E, et al., eds. *Principles of Pharmacology: The Pathophysiologic Basis of Drug Therapy*, 2nd ed. Baltimore, MD: Wolters Kluwer/Lippincott Williams & Wilkins; 2008:367-385, with permission.

angiotensin II (AT-II), or endothelin-1 (ET-1, which binds one of two receptors ET_A or ET_B), that stimulate G_q protein, activating phospholipase C (PLC) and resulting in the formation of inositol triphosphate (IP_3) from PIP_2 in the membrane. Then, IP_3 stimulates the SR to release calcium, which in turn activates the phosphorylation of myosin light chain, causing contraction. The formation of diacylglycerol (DAG) activates protein kinase C (PKC), which also contributes to VSM contraction via protein phosphorylation.

The cAMP/G_s protein–coupled pathway stimulates adenylyl cyclase, which catalyzes the formation of cAMP (Fig. 17.33). In VSM, unlike the heart, an increase in intracellular cAMP concentrations stimulated by a β_2-adrenoceptor agonist, such as epinephrine or isoproterenol, binding to the β-receptor inhibits myosin light-chain phosphorylation, causing VSM relaxation. Therefore, drugs that increase cAMP (e.g., β_2-adrenoceptor agonists, PDE3 phosphodiesterase inhibitors) cause vasodilation. On the other hand, stimulation of G_i protein inhibits cyclase.

A third mechanism that is also very important in regulating VSM tone is the NO/cGMP pathway (Fig. 17.32, right panel). The formation of NO in the endothelium activates guanylyl cyclase, which causes increased formation of cGMP and vasodilation. The precise mechanisms by which cGMP relaxes VSM is unclear; however, cGMP can activate a cGMP-dependent PKC, inhibit calcium entry into the VSM, activate K^+ channels, and decrease IP_3.

Sympatholytics

Adrenergic Drugs

Adrenergic drugs are a broad class of agents employed in the treatment of disorders of widely varying severity. Adrenergic drugs include popular prescription drugs, such as albuterol for asthma and atenolol for hypertension, as well as many common over-the-counter cold remedies, such as the nasal decongestant pseudoephedrine.

Adrenergic drugs act on effector cells through adrenoceptors that normally are activated by the neurotransmitter norepinephrine (noradrenaline), or they can act on the neurons that release the neurotransmitter. The term "adrenergic" stems from the discovery early in the 20th century that administration of the hormone adrenaline (epinephrine) had specific effects on selected organs and tissues similar to the effects produced by stimulation of the sympathetic (adrenergic) nervous system. For a number of years, adrenaline was thought to be the neurotransmitter in the sympathetic nervous system, but it was also recognized that the effects of administered epinephrine were not quite identical to those of sympathetic stimulation. Finally, in the 1940s, norepinephrine was identified as the true neurotransmitter at the terminus of the sympathetic nervous system.[102,103] Adrenoceptors are widely located in various organs and tissues as well as on neurons of both the peripheral nervous system and central nervous system (CNS).

OH
HO NHR
HO

Norepinephrins, R = H
Epinephrine, R = CH_3

Norepinephrine and epinephrine are members of a class of pharmacologically active substances known as catecholamines because they contain within their structures both an amine and an *ortho*-dihydroxybenzene moiety, which is known by the common chemical name of catechol.

Neurons at the terminus of an adrenergic neuron fiber release norepinephrine to influence the target tissue through binding to receptors on cells of the tissue or organ. The cells bearing the receptors are called effector cells, because they produce the effect seen by adrenergic stimulation.

Norepinephrine has limited clinical application because of the nonselective nature of its action, which causes both vasoconstriction and cardiac stimulation. In addition, it must be given intravenously because it has no oral activity (poor oral bioavailability) due to its rapid metabolism by intestinal and liver catechol O-methyltransferase (COMT) and monoamine oxidase (MAO), 3′-O-glucuronidation/

sulfation in the intestine, and low lipophilicity. Rapid metabolism by MAO and COMT limits its duration of action to only 1 or 2 minutes, even when given by infusion. The drug is used to counteract various hypotensive crises, because its α-activity raises blood pressure, and as an adjunct treatment in cardiac arrest, where its β-activity stimulates the heart.

Epinephrine is far more widely used clinically than norepinephrine, although it also lacks oral activity for the same reasons as norepinephrine. Epinephrine, like norepinephrine, is used to treat hypotensive crises and, because of its greater β-activity, to stimulate the heart in cardiac arrest. The β_2-activity of epinephrine leads to its administration intravenously and in inhalers to relieve bronchoconstriction in asthma and to its application in inhibiting uterine contractions. Because it has significant α-activity, epinephrine has been used in nasal decongestants. Constriction of dilated blood vessels in mucous membranes shrinks the membranes and reduces nasal congestion, although significant rebound congestion can limit its utility.

Characterization of Adrenergic Receptor Subtypes

The discovery of subclasses of adrenergic receptors and the ability of relatively small-molecule drugs to stimulate differentially or block these receptors represented a major advance in several areas of pharmacotherapeutics. Adrenergic receptors were subclassified by Ahlquist[104] in 1948 into α- and β-adrenoreceptor classes according to their responses to different adrenergic receptor agonists, principally norepinephrine, epinephrine, and isoproterenol. These catecholamines can stimulate α-adrenoceptors in the following descending order of potency: epinephrine > norepinephrine > isoproterenol. In contrast, β-adrenoceptors are stimulated in the following descending order of potency: isoproterenol > epinephrine > norepinephrine.

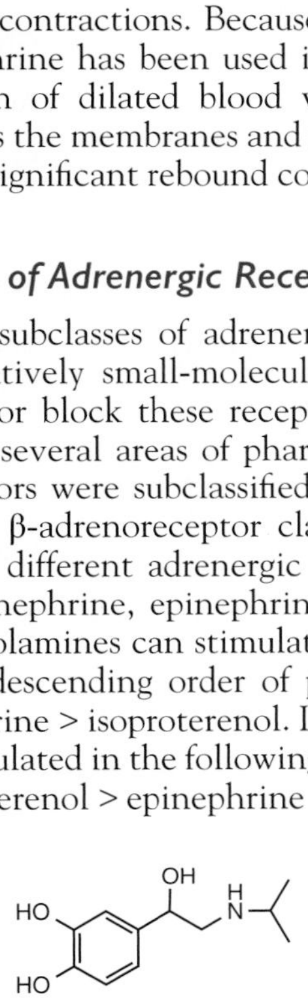

Isoproterenol

In the years since Ahlquist's original classification, additional small-molecule agonists and antagonists have been used to allow further subclassification of α- and β-receptors into the α_1 and α_2 subtypes of α-receptors and the β_1, β_2, and β_3 subtypes of β-adrenoceptors. The powerful tools of molecular biology have been used to clone, sequence, and identify even more subtypes of α-receptors for a total of six. Currently, three types of α_1-adrenoceptors, called α_{1A}, α_{1B}, and α_{1D}, are known. (There is no α_{1C} because identification of a supposed α_{1C} was found to be incorrect.) Currently, three subtypes of α_2, known as α_{2A}, α_{2B}, and α_{2C}, are also known.[105] The data derived from molecular biology provide a wealth of information on the structures and biochemical properties of both α- and β-receptors. Intensive research continues in this area, and the coming years can provide evidence of additional subtypes of both α- and β-receptors. At this time, however, only the α_1-, α_2-, β_1-, and β_2-receptor subtypes are sufficiently well differentiated by their small-molecule binding characteristics to be clinically significant in pharmacotherapeutics, although therapeutic agents acting selectively on β_3-adrenoceptors to induce fat catabolism could become available in the near future.[106]

Therapeutic Relevance of Adrenergic Receptor Subtypes

The clinical utility of receptor-selective drugs becomes obvious when one considers the adrenoreceptor subtypes and effector responses of only a few organs and tissues innervated by the sympathetic nervous system. The major adrenoceptor subtypes are listed in Table 17.21. For example, the predominant response to adrenergic stimulation of smooth muscle of the peripheral vasculature is constriction causing a rise in blood pressure. Because this response is mediated through α_1-receptors, an α_1-antagonist would be expected to cause relaxation of the blood vessels and a drop in blood pressure with clear implications for treating hypertension. The presence of α_1-adrenoceptors in the prostate gland also leads to the use of α_1-antagonists in treating benign prostatic hyperplasia. The principal therapeutic uses of adrenergic agonists and antagonists are shown in Table 17.22. A smaller number of β_2-receptors on vascular smooth muscle mediate arterial dilation, particularly to skeletal muscle, and a few antihypertensives act through stimulation of these β_2-receptors. Adrenergic stimulation of the lungs causes smooth muscle relaxation and bronchodilation mediated through β_2-receptors. Drugs acting as β_2-agonists are useful for alleviating respiratory distress in persons with asthma or other obstructive pulmonary diseases. Activation of β_2-receptors in the uterus also causes muscle relaxation, and so some β_2-agonists are used to inhibit uterine contractions in premature labor. Adrenergic stimulation of the heart causes an increase in rate and force of contraction, which is mediated primarily by β_1-receptors. Drugs with β_1-blocking activity slow the heart rate and decrease the force of contraction. These drugs have utility in treating hypertension, angina, and certain cardiac arrhythmias.

Peripherally Acting Sympatholytics

β-ADRENERGIC RECEPTOR BLOCKERS

Therapeutic Overview of β-Adrenergic Receptor Blockers. β-Blockers (BBs) decrease arterial blood pressure by reducing cardiac output.[6,101,107] Many forms of hypertension are associated with an increase in blood volume and cardiac output. Therefore, reducing cardiac output by β-blockade can be an effective treatment for hypertension, especially when used in conjunction with a diuretic. Hypertension in some patients is caused by emotional stress, which causes enhanced sympathetic activity. BBs are very effective in these patients and are especially useful in treating hypertension caused by a pheochromocytoma, which results in elevated circulating catecholamines. BBs have an additional benefit as a treatment for hypertension in that they inhibit the

Table 17.21 Selected Tissue Responses to Stimulation of Adrenoceptor Subtypes

Organ or Tissue	Major Receptor Type	Response
Arterioles, vascular bed	α_1, α_2	Constriction
Skeletal muscle	β_2	Dilation
Eye (radial muscle)	α_1	Contraction (papillary dilation)
Heart	β_1	Increased rate and force
Lungs	β_2	Relaxation (bronchodilation)
Liver	α_1, β_2	Increased gluconeogenesis and glycogenolysis
Fat cells	α_1, β_3	Lipolysis
Uterus (pregnant)	α_1	Contraction
	β_2	Relaxation
Intestine	α_1, β_2	Decreased motility

release of renin by the kidneys (the release of which is partly regulated by β_1-adrenoceptors in the kidney). Decreasing circulating plasma renin leads to a decrease in angiotensin II and aldosterone, which enhances renal loss of sodium and water and further diminishes arterial pressure. Acute treatment with a BB is not very effective in reducing arterial pressure because of a compensatory increase in systemic vascular resistance. This can occur because of the baroreceptor reflexes working in conjunction with the removal of β_2 vasodilatory influences that normally offset, to a small degree, α-adrenergic–mediated vascular tone. Chronic treatment with BB lowers arterial pressure more than acute treatment, possibly, because of reduced renin release and effects of β-blockade on central and peripheral nervous systems.

Several of the nonselective BBs are also used to reduce intraocular pressure in the treatment of glaucoma. These include carteolol (Occupress), levobunolol (Betagan), and timolol (Timoptic).

The selection of oral BBs as monotherapy for stage 1 or 2 hypertension without compelling risk factors (Table 17.2) is based on several factors, including their cardioselectivity and preexisting conditions, ISA, lipophilicity, metabolism, and adverse effects (exception is esmolol) (Table 17.23). Esmolol is a very short-acting cardioselective β_1-blocker administered by infusion because of its rapid hydrolysis by plasma esterases to a rapidly excreted zwitterionic metabolite (plasma half-life, 9 min). After the discontinuation of esmolol infusion, blood pressure returns to preexisting conditions in approximately 30 minutes.

Table 17.22 Principal Therapeutic Uses of Adrenergic Agonists and Antagonists

Adrenoceptor	Drug Action	Therapeutic Uses
α_1	Agonists	Shock, hypotension (to raise blood pressure)
		Nasal decongestants
	Antagonists	Antihypertensives
		Benign prostatic hyperplasia
α_2	Agonists	Antihypertensives
		Glaucoma
		Analgesia
		Sedatives
β_1	Antagonists	Antihypertensives
		Antiarrhythmics
β_2	Agonists	Bronchodilators (asthma and chronic obstructive pulmonary disorder)
		Glaucoma
β_3	Agonists	Weight loss (investigational drugs)

The elderly hypertensive patient (age, ≥65 yr) cannot tolerate or respond to these drugs because of their mechanism of lowering cardiac output and increasing systemic vascular resistance.[108]

Pharmacology Overview of β-Adrenergic Receptor Blockers

Mechanism of Action. The VSMs are lined with β_2-adrenoceptors that normally are activated by norepinephrine released from sympathetic adrenergic nerves or by circulating epinephrine. These receptors, like those in the heart, are coupled to a G_s protein, which stimulates the formation of cAMP. Although increased cAMP enhances cardiac contraction, with VSM an increase in cAMP leads to smooth muscle relaxation (Fig. 17.33). Therefore, increases in intracellular cAMP caused by β_2-agonists inhibit MLCK, thereby producing less contractile force (i.e., promoting relaxation). Inhibition of cardiac β_1- and β_2-adrenoceptors reduces the contractility of the myocardium (negative inotropic), decreasing heart rate (negative chronotropic), blocking sympathetic outflow from the central nervous system (CNS), and suppressing renin release.[87]

BBs are drugs that bind to β-adrenoceptors and, thereby, block the binding of norepinephrine and epinephrine to these receptors, causing inhibition of normal sympathetic effects. Therefore, BBs are sympatholytic drugs. Some

Table 17.23 Pharmacologic/Pharmacokinetic Properties of Antihypertensive β-Adrenergic Blocking Agents

Drug	Adrenergic Receptor Blocking Activity	Membrane-Stabilizing Activity	Intrinsic Sympathomimetic Activity	Lipophilicity[e] (log D at pH 7.4)	Extent of Absorption (%)	Absolute Oral Bioavailability (%)	Half-Life (hr)	Protein Binding (%)	Metabolism/ Excretion
Acebutolol (Sectral)	β_1[a]	+	+	0.09	90	20-60	3-4	26	Hepatic; renal excretion 30%-40%, nonrenal excretion 50%-60% (bile)
Atenolol (Tenormin)	β_1[a]	0	0	2.01	50	50-60	6-9	5-16	~50% excreted unchanged in feces
Betaxolol (Kerlone)	β_1[a]	0	0	2.4	~100	89	14-22	50	Hepatic; >80% recovered in urine, 15% unchanged
Bisoprolol (Zebeta)	β_1[a]	0	0	2.2	≥0	80	9-12	30	~50% excreted unchanged in urine, remainder as inactive metabolites; <2% excreted in feces
Esmolol (Brevibloc)	β_1[a]	0	0	1.7	NA	NA	0.15	55	Rapid metabolism by esterases in cytosol of red blood cells
Metoprolol (Lopressor)	β_1[a]	0[b]	0	0.24	95	40-50	3-7	12	Hepatic; renal excretion, <5% unchanged
Metoprolol, LA			—	—	77	—			

(continued)

Table 17.23 Pharmacologic/Pharmacokinetic Properties of Antihypertensive β-Adrenergic Blocking Agents (Continued)

Drug	Adrenergic Receptor Blocking Activity	Membrane-Stabilizing Activity	Intrinsic Sympathomimetic Activity	Lipophilicity[e] (log D at pH 7.4)	Extent of Absorption (%)	Absolute Oral Bioavailability (%)	Half-Life (hr)	Protein Binding (%)	Metabolism/Excretion
Nebivolol (Bystolic)	β_1[a]	0	0	2.34	NA	12-fast metabolizers 96-poor metabolizers	12-19	98	Hepatic; glucuronidation, N-dealkylation and oxidation by CYP2D6 Renal: 38%-67%; <1% renal unchanged; fecal 13%-44%
Carteolol (Cartrol, Ocupress)	β_1 β_2	0	+ +	−1.56	80	85	6	23-30	50%-70% excreted unchanged in urine
Levobunolol (Betagan)	β_1 β_2	0	0	0.19	NA	NA	NA	NA	Ophthalmic
Nadolol (Corgard)	β_1 β_2	0	0	1.43	30	30-50	20-24	30	Urine, unchanged
Penbutolol (Levatol)	β_1 β_2	0	+	2.06	~100	>90	5	80-98	Hepatic (conjugation, oxidation); renal excretion of metabolites (17% as conjugate)
Pindolol (Visken)	β_1 β_2	+	+ + +	−0.36	95	>90	3-4[c]	40	Urinary excretion of metabolites (60%-65%) and unchanged drug (35%-40%)

Propranolol (Inderal)	$\beta_1\ \beta_2$	+ +	0	1.41	90	30	3-5	90	Hepatic; <1% excreted unchanged in urine
Propranolol, LA						9-18	8-11		
Timolol (Blocadren, Timoptic)	$\beta_1\ \beta_2$	0	0	0.03	90	75	4	10	Hepatic; urinary excretion of metabolites and unchanged drug
Labetalol[d] (Normodyne)	$\beta_1\ \beta_2\ \alpha_1$	0	0	1.08	100	30-40	5.5-8.0	50	55%-60% excreted in urine as conjugates or unchanged drug
Carvedilol (Coreg)	$\beta_1\ \beta_2\ \alpha_1$	0	0	3.53	>90	25-35	7-10	98	

Adapted from Drug Facts and Comparison 2000; with permission.
[a]Inhibits β_2-receptors (bronchial and vascular) at higher doses.
[b]Detectable only at doses much greater than required for β-blockade.
[c]In elderly hypertensive patients with normal renal function; half-life variable, 7-15 hr.
[d]Not labetalol monograph.
[e]Measured logD at pH 7.4 from Avdeef A. *Absorption and Drug Development*. Hoboken, NJ: Wiley-Interscience, 2003:59-66.
NA, not applicable (available as intravenous only); 0, none; +, low; + +, moderate; + + +, high.

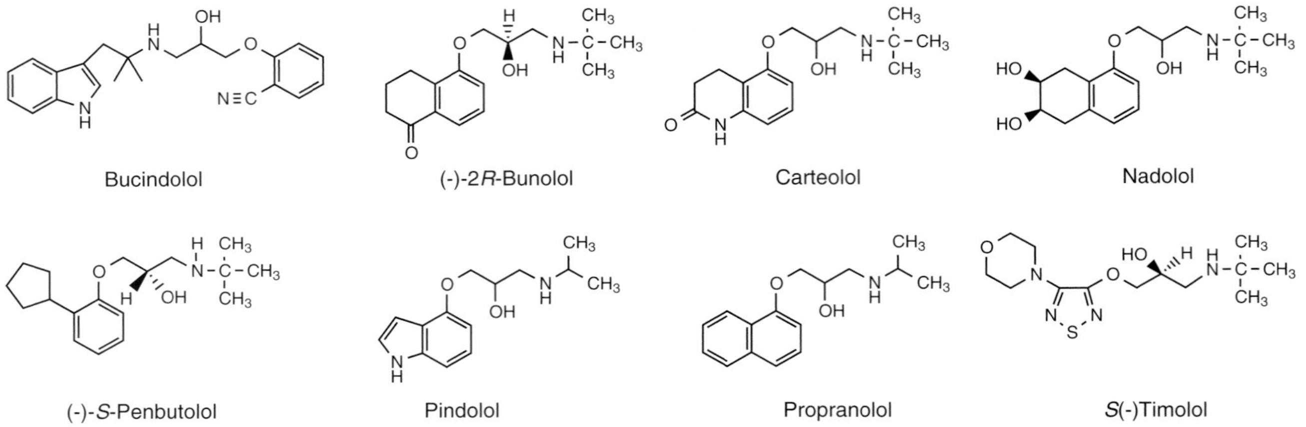

Figure 17.34 Nonselective β-adrenergic blockers.

BBs, when they bind to the β-adrenoceptor, partially activate the receptor while preventing norepinephrine from binding to the receptor. These partial agonists therefore provide some "background" of sympathetic activity while preventing normal and enhanced sympathetic activity. These particular BBs (partial agonists) are said to possess intrinsic sympathomimetic activity (ISA). Some BBs also possess what is referred to as membrane-stabilizing activity. This effect is similar to the membrane-stabilizing activity of sodium channel blockers that represent class I antiarrhythmics.

The first generation of BBs were nonselective, meaning that they blocked both β_1- and β_2-adrenoceptors (Fig. 17.34). Second-generation BBs are more cardioselective because they are relatively selective for β_1-adrenoceptors (Fig. 17.35). Note that this relative selectivity can be lost at higher drug doses. Finally, the third-generation BBs are drugs that also possess vasodilator actions through blockade of vascular α-adrenoceptors (mixed α_1-/β_1-adrenergic blockers) (see Fig. 17.36). Their structure-activity relationship, pharmacokinetics, and metabolism are presented in Table 17.23. In addition to uncomplicated hypertension, they can also be used as monotherapy in the treatment of angina, arrhythmias, mitral valve prolapse, myocardial infarction, migraine headaches, performance anxiety, excessive sympathetic tone, or "thyroid storm" in hyperthyroidism.[6]

Common Adverse Effects. Common adverse effects for the BBs include decreased exercise tolerance, cold extremities, depression, sleep disturbance, and impotence, although these side effects can be less severe with the β_1-selective blockers, such as metoprolol, atenolol, or bisoprolol.[109] The use of lipid-soluble BBs, such as propranolol (Table 17.23), has been associated with more CNS side effects, such as dizziness, confusion, or depression.[6,101] These side effects can be avoided, however, with the use of hydrophilic drugs, such as nadolol or atenolol. The use of β_1-selective drugs also helps to minimize adverse effects associated with β_2-blockade, including suppression of insulin release and increasing the chances for bronchospasms (asthma).[6,101] It is important to emphasize that none of the BBs, including the cardioselective ones, are cardiospecific. At high doses, these cardioselective BBs can still adversely affect asthma, peripheral vascular disease, and diabetes.[6,101] Nonselective BB are contraindicated in patients with bronchospastic disease (asthma), and β_1-selective blockers should be used

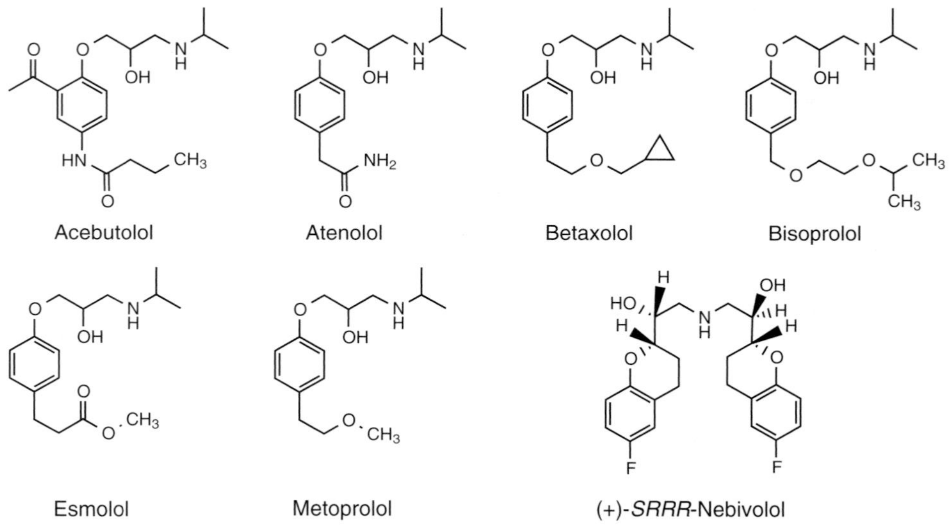

Figure 17.35 β_1-Selective adrenergic blockers.

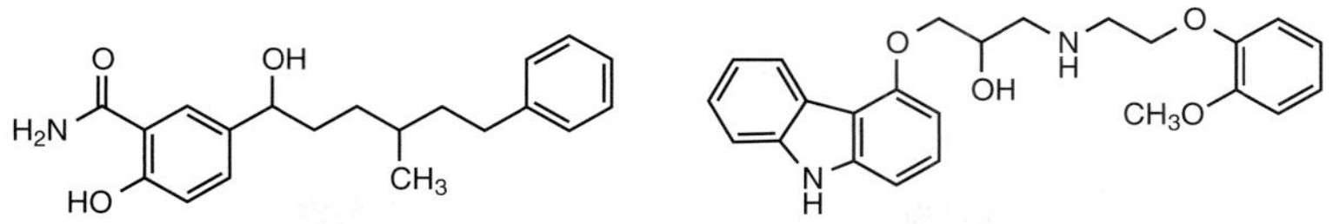

Labetalol

Carvedilol (Coreg)

Figure 17.36 Mixed α-/β-selective adrenergic blockers.

with caution in these patients. BBs with ISA, such as acebutolol, pindolol, carteolol, or penbutolol (Table 17.23), partially stimulate the β-receptor while also blocking it.[110] The proposed advantages of BBs with ISA over those without ISA include less cardiodepression and resting bradycardia as well as neutral effects on lipid and glucose metabolism. Neither cardioselectivity nor ISA, however, influences the efficacy of BBs in lowering blood pressure.[6]

Common Interactions. Table 17.24 summarizes common drug-drug interactions for the β-adrenergic receptor blockers.

Medicinal Chemistry of β-Adrenergic Receptor Blockers

Receptor Binding, SAR, and Physicochemical Properties. In the 1950s, dichloroisoproterenol, a derivative of isoproterenol in which the catechol hydroxyls had been replaced by chlorines, was discovered to be a β-antagonist that blocked the effects of sympathomimetic amines on bronchodilation, uterine relaxation, and heart stimulation.[111] Although dichloroisoproterenol had no clinical utility, replacement of the 3,4-dichloro substituents with a carbon bridge to form a naphthylethanolamine derivative did afford a clinical candidate, pronethalol, which was introduced in 1962 only to be withdrawn in 1963 because of tumor induction in animal tests.

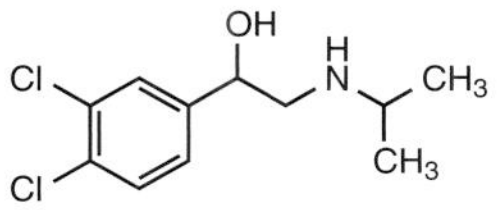

Dichloroisoproterenol

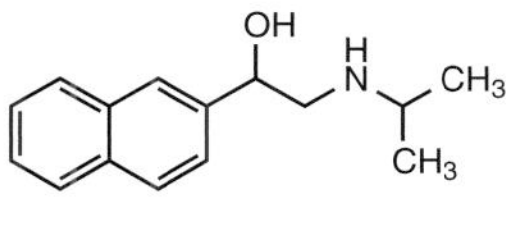

Pronethalol

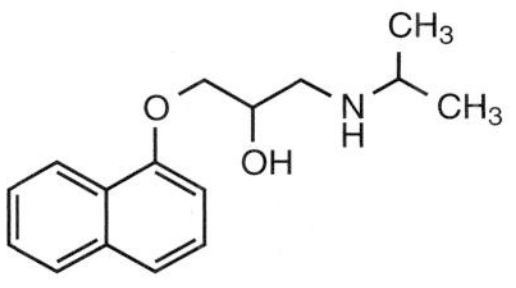

Propranolol

Shortly thereafter, a major innovation in drug development for the β-adrenergic antagonists was introduced when it was discovered that an oxymethylene bridge, OCH_2, could be inserted into the arylethanolamine

Table 17.24 Common Drug Interactions for Adrenergic Drugs

Drug Class	Interactions
β-Adrenergic receptor blockers	Other antihypertensive agents may produce additive effects Nonsteroidal anti-inflammatory drugs (NSAIDs) may reduce antihypertensive activity Use with some cardiovascular agents may adversely impact atrioventricular (AV) or sinoatrial (SA) node conduction Activity of metoprolol and other β-blockers that are metabolized by CYP2D6 may be altered by inhibitors of this isozyme
α-/β-Adrenergic receptor blockers	Other antihypertensive agents may produce additive effects Activity of carvedilol and other α-/β-blockers that are metabolized by CYP2D6 may be altered by inhibitors of this isozyme
α_1-Adrenergic receptor blockers	Other antihypertensive agents may produce additive effects Displacement of prazosin from plasma proteins by other drugs is possible
α_2-Adrenergic receptor agonists	Other antihypertensive agents may produce additive effects Levodopa may enhance the antihypertensive activity of methyldopa Oral iron (ferrous salts) may reduce absorption of methyldopa from the gastrointestinal tract Tricyclic antidepressants may antagonize antihypertensive activity of clonidine Metabolism of guanfacine may be increased by microsomal enzyme inducers
α_1-Adrenergic receptor agonists	Possible increase in activity when phenylephrine is used with monoamine oxidase (MAO) inhibitors
Vasodilators	Other antihypertensive agents may produce additive effects Diazoxide may displace other drugs that are highly bound to plasma proteins

Data from AHFS Drug Information (2018), American Society of Health-System Pharmacists.

structure of pronethalol to afford propranolol, an aryloxypropanolamine and the first clinically successful β-blocker. Note that along with the introduction of the oxymethylene bridge, the side chain has been moved from C2 of the naphthyl group to the C1 position. In general, the aryloxypropanolamines are more potent β-blockers than the corresponding arylethanolamines, and most of the β-blockers currently being used clinically are aryloxypropanolamines. β-Blockers have found wide use in treating hypertension and certain types of glaucoma.

Initially, it might appear that lengthening the side chain would prevent appropriate binding of the required functional groups to the same receptor site. Molecular models, however, show that the side chains of aryloxypropanolamines can adopt a conformation that places the hydroxyl and amine groups into approximately the same position in space (Fig. 17.37). Although the simple two-dimensional drawing in Figure 17.37 exaggerates the true degree of overlap, elaborate molecular modeling studies confirm that the aryloxypropanolamine side chain can adopt a low-energy conformation that permits close overlap with the arylethanolamine side chain.[112]

A factor that sometimes causes confusion when comparing the structures of arylethanolamines with aryloxypropanolamines is the stereochemical nomenclature of the side-chain carbon bearing the hydroxyl group. For maximum effectiveness in receptor binding, the hydroxy group must occupy the same region in space as it does for the phenylethanolamine agonists in the *R* absolute configuration. Because of the insertion of an oxygen atom in the side chain of the aryloxypropanolamines, the Cahn-Ingold-Prelog priority of the substituents around the asymmetric carbon changes, and the isomer with the required special arrangement now has the *S* absolute configuration. This is an effect of the nomenclature rules; the groups still have the same spatial arrangements (Fig. 17.38).

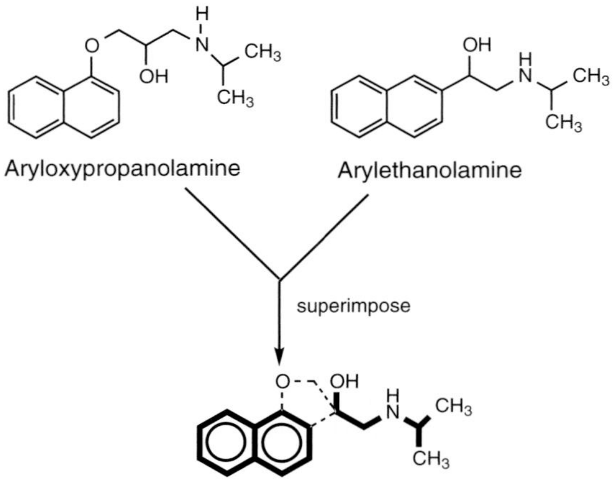

Figure 17.37 Overlap of aryloxypropanolamines and arylethanolamines. The structures of prototype β-antagonists propranolol and pronethalol can be superimposed so the critical functional groups occupy the same approximate regions in space, as indicated by the bold lines in the superimposed drawings. The dotted lines are those parts that do not overlap but are not necessary to receptor binding.

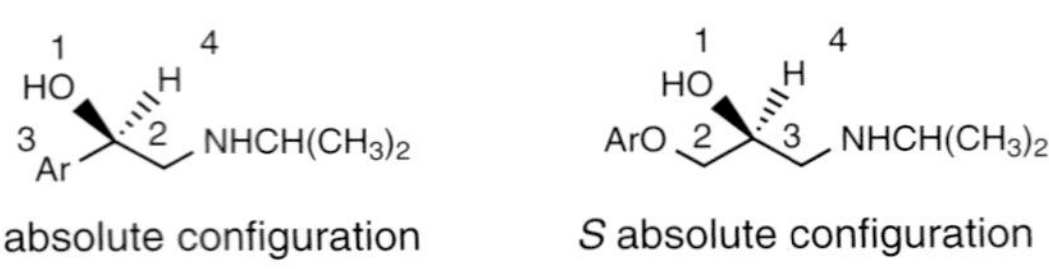

Figure 17.38 Stereochemical nomenclature for arylethanolamines versus aryloxypropanolamines. The relative positions in space of the four functional groups are the same in the two structures; however, one is designated *R* and the other *S*. This is because the introduction of an oxygen atom into the side chain of the aryloxypropanolamine changes the priority of two of the groups used in the nomenclature assignment.

Unlike the conventional cardioselective β_1-receptor blockers, nebivolol also exhibits NO-potentiating vasodilatory effect for the treatment of hypertension. Chemically, it is a mixture of stereoisomers (+)-nebivolol ([+]-*SRRR* nebivolol) and (−)-nebivolol ([−]-*RSSS* nebivolol) that differs chemically and pharmacologically from other BBs. The selective β_1-blocking effect is determined almost exclusively by the (+)-stereoisomer. The combination of (+)-nebivolol and (−)-nebivolol acts synergistically to produce a cardiovascular profile that differs noticeably from that of conventional BBs with respect to enhanced blood pressure reduction at lower doses. The drug is highly cardioselective at low doses, but at higher doses, it loses its cardioselectivity and blocks both β_1- and β_2-receptors. The (−)-stereoisomer has minimal effect on systolic and diastolic blood pressure. Nebivolol is unique among the conventional BBs by stimulating endothelial NO synthesis, thereby producing a sustained vasodilation in VSM, which results in decreased peripheral resistance and blood pressure. The (−)-stereoisomer indirectly increases NO availability by the inhibition of endothelial NO synthase, thereby reducing NO inactivation. Neither nebivolol nor its stereoisomers show any intrinsic sympathomimetic activity, without the undesirable BB effects, such as a decrease in cardiac output.

Pharmacokinetic Properties and Metabolism. Details about the pharmacokinetic parameters and metabolism of the β-blockers are provided in Table 17.23. Esmolol is the methyl ester of a carboxylic acid, which makes it susceptible to hydrolysis by serum esterases. The acid metabolite generated by hydrolysis is essentially inactive and readily excreted as its zwitterion. For this reason, esmolol has a half-life of approximately 8 minutes and is used to control supraventricular tachycardia during surgery when a short-acting β_1-adrenergic antagonist is desirable.

Another physicochemical parameter with some clinical correlation is the relative lipophilicity of different agents. Propranolol is by far the most lipophilic of the available β-blockers, and it enters the CNS far better than the less lipophilic agents, such as atenolol or nadolol. Lipophilicity as measured by octanol-water partitioning also correlates with the primary site of clearance, as seen in Table 17.23. The more lipophilic drugs are primarily cleared by the liver, whereas the more hydrophilic agents are cleared by the kidney. This could influence the choice of agents in cases of renal failure or liver disease. Several of the β-blockers must be dose adjusted in patients with impaired renal function.

Nebivolol is not cardioselective when taken by patients who are poor CYP2D6 metabolizers of nebivolol (and other drugs). As many as 1 in 10 whites and even more blacks are poor CYP2D6 metabolizers and therefore would not likely benefit from nebivolol's cardioselectivity.

α_1-ADRENERGIC RECEPTOR BLOCKERS

Therapeutic Overview of α_1-Adrenergic Receptor Blockers. α_1-Blockers are effective agents for the initial management of hypertension and are especially advantageous for older men who also suffer from symptomatic benign prostatic hyperplasia.[6,113] Prazosin, the first known selective α_1-blocker, was discovered in the late 1960s[114] and is now one of a small group of selective α_1-antagonists that includes other quinoxaline antihypertensives such as terazosin and doxazosin. They have been shown to be as effective as other major classes of antihypertensives in lowering blood pressure in equivalent doses. α_1-Blockers possess a characteristic "first-dose" effect, which means that orthostatic hypotension frequently occurs with the first few doses of the drug. This side effect can be minimized by slowly increasing the dose and by administering the first few doses at bedtime.

Pharmacology Overview of α_1-Adrenergic Receptor Blockers

Mechanism of Action. These drugs block the effect of sympathetic nerves on blood vessels by selectively binding to α_1-adrenoceptors located on the VSM (Fig. 17.32), which then stimulate the G_q protein, activating smooth muscle contraction through the IP_3 signal transduction pathway. Most of these drugs act as competitive antagonists by competing with the binding of norepinephrine to α_1-adrenergic receptors on VSM. Some α-blockers are noncompetitive (e.g., phenoxybenzamine, which greatly prolongs their action. Prejunctional α_2-adrenoceptors located on the sympathetic nerve terminals serve as a negative feedback mechanism for norepinephrine release.

α-Blockers dilate both arteries and veins because both vessel types are innervated by sympathetic adrenergic nerves. The vasodilator effect is more pronounced, however, in the arterial resistance vessels. Because most blood vessels have some degree of sympathetic tone under basal conditions, these drugs are effective dilators. They are even more effective under conditions of elevated sympathetic activity (e.g., during stress) or during pathologic increases in circulating catecholamines caused by an adrenal gland tumor (pheochromocytoma).[87] α_2-Adrenoceptors are also abundant in the smooth muscle of the bladder neck and prostate and, when inhibited, cause relaxation of the bladder muscle, increasing urinary flow rates and the relief of benign prostatic hyperplasia.

Common Adverse Effects. The most common side effects are related directly to α_1-adrenoceptor blockade. These side effects include dizziness, orthostatic hypotension (because of loss of reflex vasoconstriction on standing), nasal congestion (because of dilation of nasal mucosal arterioles), headache, and reflex tachycardia (especially with nonselective α-blockers). Fluid retention is also a problem that can be rectified by use of a diuretic in conjunction with the α_1-blocker. α-Blockers have not been shown to be beneficial in heart failure or angina and should not be used in these conditions.

Common Interactions. Common drug-drug interactions for the α_1-adrenergic receptor blockers are summarized in Table 17.24.

Medicinal Chemistry of α_1-Adrenergic Receptor Blockers

Receptor Binding, SAR, and Physicochemical Properties. The structures for the available α_1-receptor blockers are shown in Figure 17.39. These include prazosin (log $D_{7.4}$ = 1.70), doxazosin (log $D_{7.4}$ = 1.97) and terazosin (log $D_{7.4}$ = 2.13). Prazosin, doxazosin, and terazosin contain a 4-amino-6,7-dimethoxyquinazoline ring system attached to a piperazine ring.

Pharmacokinetic Properties and Metabolism. Important structural differences between these drugs are the heterocyclic acyl groups attached to the second nitrogen of the piperazine or the propyl chain. The differences in these groups afford dramatic differences in some of the pharmacokinetic properties of these agents (Table 17.25). For example, reduction of the furan ring for prazosin to the tetrahydrofuran ring of terazosin increases its duration of action by altering its rate of metabolism. Some of the important clinical parameters of the quinazolines are shown in Table 17.25.

MIXED α-/β-ADRENERGIC RECEPTOR BLOCKERS

Therapeutic Overview of Mixed α-/β-Adrenergic Receptor Blockers. Monotherapy with these mixed-acting antihypertensive drugs reduces blood pressure as effectively as other major antihypertensives and their combinations.[115–117] Selection of mixed α-/β-blockers is recommended for management of hypertension when the stage 2 family of drugs cannot be used alone or when a compelling indication (Table 17.2) is present that requires the use of a specific drug. Both drugs effectively lower blood pressure in essential and renal hypertension. Carvedilol is also effective in ischemic heart disease.

Pharmacology Overview of Mixed α-/β-Adrenergic Receptor Blockers

Mechanism of Action. The mixed α-/β-receptor blocking properties in the same molecule confer some advantages in the lowering of blood pressure. Vasodilation via

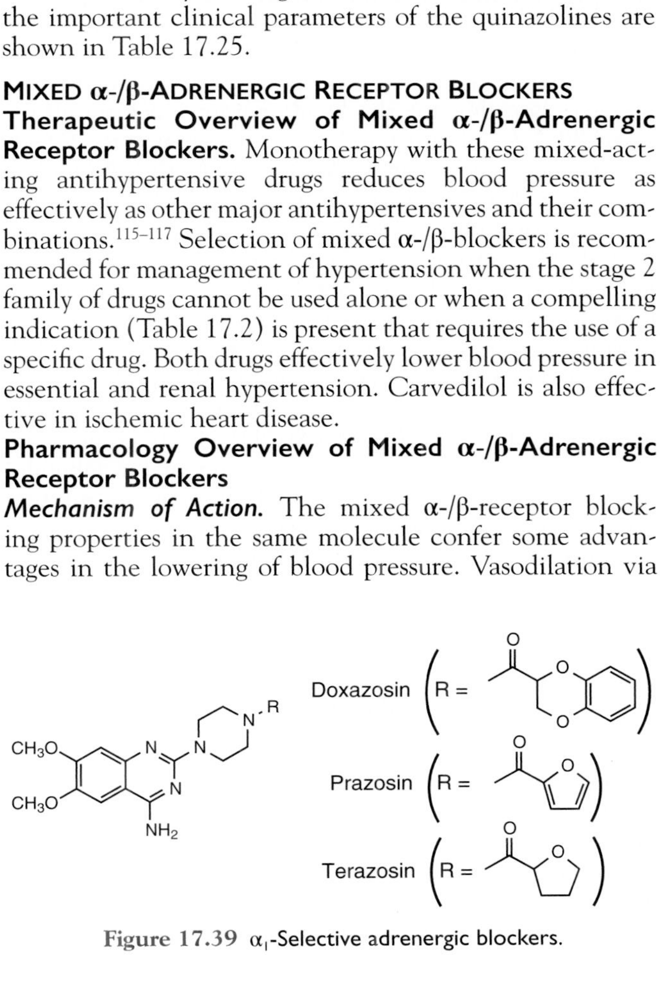

Doxazosin (R = ...)
Prazosin (R = ...)
Terazosin (R = ...)

Figure 17.39 α_1-Selective adrenergic blockers.

Table 17.25 Selected Clinical Parameters of α_1-Adrenergic Antagonists

Drug	Trade Name	cLog P/log $D_{pH\ 7.0}$	Half-Life (hr)	Duration of Action (hr)	Bioavailability (%)
Prazosin	Minipres	−1.1/−1.3[a]	2-3	4-6	45-65
Terazosin	Hytrin	−1.0/−1.0[a]	12	>18	90
Doxazosin	Cardura	0.7/0.5[a]	22	18-36	65

[a]Chemical Abstracts, American Chemical Society, calculated using Advanced Chemistry Development (ACD/Labs) Software V8.19 for Solaris (1994-2011 ACD/Labs).

α_1-blockade lowers peripheral vascular resistance to maintain cardiac output, thus preventing bradycardia more effectively when compared to BBs.[117] β-Blockade helps to avoid the reflex tachycardia sometimes observed with the other vasodilators listed later in this chapter.

Common Adverse Effects. Any adverse effects are usually related to β_1- or α_1-blockade. The β effects are usually less bothersome because the α_1-blockade reduces the effects of β-blockade.

Common Interactions. Table 17.24 summarizes common drug-drug interactions for the mixed α-/β-adrenergic receptor blockers.

Medicinal Chemistry of Mixed α-/β-Adrenergic Receptor Blockers

Receptor Binding, SAR, and Physicochemical Properties. Carvedilol[115] and labetalol[116] are the currently available mixed α-/β-receptor blockers (Fig. 17.36). The α-methyl substituent attached to the N-arylalkyl group appears to be responsible for the α-adrenergic blocking effect. Carvedilol is administered as its racemate; its *S*-(−)-enantiomer is both an α- and nonselective β-blocker, whereas its *R*-(+)-enantiomer is an α_1-blocker. Labetalol possesses two chiral centers and, therefore, is administered as a mixture of four stereoisomers, of which *R*(CH_3),*R*(OH) is the active β-blocker diastereomer with minimal α_1-blocking activity and the *S*(CH_3),*R*(OH) diastereomer is predominantly an α_1-blocker. The *R*,*R* diastereomer is also known as dilevalol, which was not approved by the FDA because of hepatotoxicity. The *S*(CH_3),*S*(OH) and *R*(CH_3),*S*(OH) diastereomers are both inactive. The comparative potency for labetalol reflects the fact that 25% of the diastereomeric mixture is the active *R*,*R*-diastereomer. The β-blocking activity of labetalol is approximately 1.5-fold that of its α_1-blocking activity. Carvedilol has an estimated β-blocking activity 10- to 100-fold its α_1-blocking activity.

Pharmacokinetic Properties and Metabolism. The pharmacokinetic properties and metabolism of carvedilol and labetalol are summarized in Table 17.23.

α_1-ADRENERGIC RECEPTOR AGONISTS

Therapeutic Overview of α_1-Adrenergic Receptor Agonists. Examples of drugs in this class include metaraminol, methoxamine, and phenylephrine. Their α_1-agonist activity makes them strong vasoconstrictors, and their primary systemic use is limited to treating hypotension during surgery or severe hypotension accompanying shock.

Pharmacology Overview of α_1-Adrenergic Receptor Agonists

Mechanism of Action. Metaraminol, methoxamine, and phenylephrine are selective agonists for α_1-receptors in the peripheral vasculature and have minimal cardiac stimulatory properties.

Common Adverse Effects. Table 17.26 lists common adverse effects for the α_1-adrenergic receptor agonist phenylephrine.

Common Interactions. Common drug-drug interactions for the α_1-adrenergic receptor agonists are summarized in Table 17.24.

Medicinal Chemistry of α_1-Adrenergic Receptor Agonists

Receptor Binding, SAR, and Physicochemical Properties. The aromatic ring substitution pattern in phenylethanolamines is an important structural factor in adrenergic receptor selectivity. In compounds with only 3′-OH substituents, such as phenylephrine and metaraminol, activity is reduced at α_1 sites but almost eliminated at β sites, thus affording selective α_1-agonists. Indication that α_1 sites have a wide range of substituent tolerance for agonist activity is shown by the 2′,5′-dimethoxy substitution pattern of methoxamine.

Phenylephrine Metaraminol Methoxamine

Pharmacokinetics and Metabolism. Because they are not substrates for catechol-O-methyltransferase (COMT), the duration of action for the α_1-agonists is significantly longer than that of norepinephrine. Methoxamine is bioactivated by 5′-O-demethylation to an active 5′-phenolic metabolite. The β-blocking activity of methoxamine, which is seen at high concentrations, affords some use in treating tachycardia. Phenylephrine, which is also a selective α_1-agonist, is used similarly to metaraminol and methoxamine for hypotension. It also has widespread use as a nonprescription nasal decongestant in both oral and topical preparations. However, its oral bioavailability is less than 10% because of its hydrophilic properties and intestinal 3′-O-glucuronidation/sulfation.

Table 17.26 Common Adverse Effects for Some Drugs Used in the Treatment of Hypertensive/Hypotensive Disorders.

Drug Class	Interactions
α_1-Adrenergic receptor agonists	Systemic use of phenylephrine can be associated with a number of side effects impacting the cardiovascular system (e.g., bradycardia, vasoconstriction that may decrease blood flow to tissues, etc.) and the central nervous system (e.g., dizziness, anxiety, etc.). Sensitive patients may exhibit allergic reactions (potentially severe) to sodium metabisulfite, a preservative that is added to some parenteral preparations of phenylephrine.
Vasodilators (direct-acting)	Common sites for adverse effects associated with hydralazine include the cardiovascular system (e.g., tachycardia) and the central nervous system (CNS) (e.g., headache). An autoimmune syndrome, resembling systemic lupus erythematosus (SLE) has been reported in patients using hydralazine. This is characterized by the presence of antinuclear antibodies in the circulation and can negatively impact multiple organs in the body. The incidence of this condition is more common with higher doses of the drug and may correlate with a patient's acetylator status (see below). Hydralazine has been shown to be mutagenic in bacterial assays, carcinogenic in mice, and teratogenic in some laboratory animal species.
Vasodilators (potassium channel openers)	Heart palpitations and increased heart rate can occur in patients who are taking diazoxide Chronic use of diazoxide has been associated with CNS effects (extrapyramidal effects), an hyperglycemia, which may be severe Diazoxide has been shown to be teratogenic in rabbits Retention of water and sodium has been shown to occur with both diazoxide and minoxidil Minoxidil is commonly associated with tachycardia in patients. Severe cardiac effects have also been noted, and patients receiving this drug should be closely monitored. Increased hair growth has been observed with minoxidil, and the drug has been marketed for this purpose to treat hair loss under the trade name Rogaine

Data from AHFS Drug Information (2018), American Society of Health-System Pharmacists

Centrally Acting Sympatholytics

α_2-ADRENERGIC RECEPTOR AGONISTS

Therapeutic Overview of α_2-Adrenergic Receptor Agonists. The sympathetic adrenergic nervous system plays a major role in the regulation of arterial pressure. Activation of these nerves to the heart increases the heart rate (positive chronotropy), contractility (positive inotropy), and velocity of electrical impulse conduction (positive chronotropy). Within the medulla are located preganglionic sympathetic excitatory neurons, which travel from the spinal cord to the ganglia. They have significant basal activity, which generates a level of sympathetic tone to the heart and vasculature even under basal conditions. The sympathetic neurons within the medulla receive input from other neurons within the medulla, and together, these neuronal systems regulate sympathetic (and parasympathetic) outflow to the heart and vasculature. Sympatholytic drugs can block this sympathetic adrenergic system on three different levels. First, peripheral sympatholytic drugs, such as α-adrenoceptor and β-adrenoceptor antagonists, block the influence of norepinephrine at the effector organ (heart or blood vessel). Second, there are ganglionic blockers that block impulse transmission at the sympathetic ganglia. Third, centrally acting sympatholytic drugs block sympathetic activity within the brain. Centrally acting sympatholytics block sympathetic activity by binding to and activating α_2-adrenoceptors, which reduces sympathetic outflow to the heart, thereby decreasing cardiac output by decreasing heart rate and contractility. Reduced sympathetic output to the vasculature decreases sympathetic vascular tone, which causes vasodilation and reduced systemic vascular resistance, which in turn decreases arterial pressure.

Methyldopa is used in the management of moderate to severe hypertension and is reserved for patients who fail to achieve blood pressure goals with stage 2 drugs.[6,101] Methyldopa is also coadministered with diuretics and other classes of antihypertensive drugs, permitting a reduction in the dosage of each drug and minimizing adverse effects while maintaining blood pressure control. Methyldopa has been used in the management of hypertension during pregnancy without apparent substantial adverse effects on the fetus and also for the management of pregnancy-induced hypertension (i.e., preeclampsia).[5] Intravenous methyldopate can be used for the management of hypertension when parenteral hypotensive therapy is necessary. Because of its slow onset of action, however, other agents, such as sodium nitroprusside, are preferred when a parenteral hypotensive agent is employed for hypertensive emergencies.

HO, HO, COOH, H_2N, CH_3

Methyldopa

Clonidine, guanabenz, and guanfacine (Fig. 17.40) are used in the management of mild to moderate hypertension

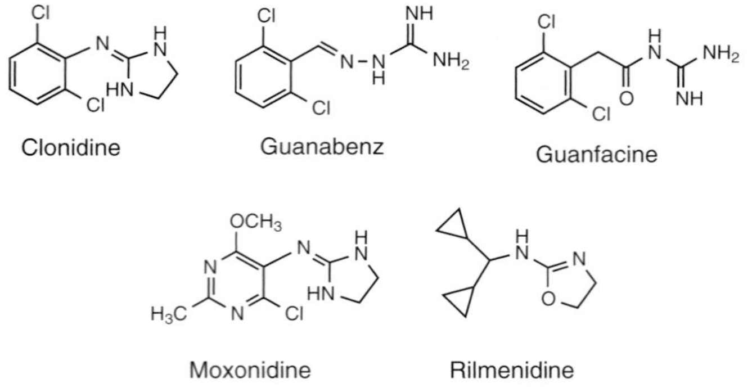

Figure 17.40 Centrally acting sympatholytics.

or when stage 2 drugs have been ineffective in achieving blood pressure goals.[6,101] They have been used as monotherapy or to achieve lower dosages in combination with other classes of antihypertensive agents. The centrally acting sympatholytics are generally reserved for patients who fail to respond to therapy with a stage 1 drug (e.g., diuretics, β-adrenergic blocking agents, ACEIs, or ARBs). Clonidine, guanabenz, and guanfacine can be used in combination with diuretics and other stage 1 hypotensive agents, permitting a reduction in the dosage of each drug, which minimizes adverse effects while maintaining blood pressure control. Geriatric patients, however, cannot tolerate the adverse cognitive effects of these sympatholytics. All three drugs reduce blood pressure to essentially the same extent in both supine and standing patients; thus, orthostatic effects are mild and infrequently encountered. Exercise does not appear to affect the blood pressure response to guanabenz and guanfacine in patients with hypertension. Plasma renin activity can be unchanged or reduced during long-term therapy with these drugs.

Clonidine is administered twice a day for the management of mild to moderate hypertension in those patients not achieving the blood pressure goal with stage 2 drugs.[6] Transdermal clonidine has also been successfully substituted for oral clonidine in some patients with mild to moderate hypertension whose compliance with a daily dosing regimen can be a problem.[118] When administered by epidural infusion, clonidine is used as adjunct therapy in combination with opiates for the management of severe cancer pain not relieved by opiate analgesics alone. Other nonhypertensive uses for clonidine include the prophylaxis of migraine headaches, the treatment of severe dysmenorrhea, menopausal flushing, rapid detoxification in the management of opiate withdrawal in opiate-dependent individuals, in conjunction with benzodiazepines for the management of alcohol withdrawal, and for the treatment of tremors associated with the adverse effects of methylphenidate in patients with attention-deficit hyperactivity disorder (ADHD). Clonidine has been used to reduce intraocular pressure in the treatment of open-angle and secondary glaucoma. Clonidine, a nonstimulant drug, is also used in reducing the symptoms of ADHD and bipolar disorders, whose mechanism of action is thought to regulate norepinephrine release from the locus ceruleus, part of the brain stem involved with physiologic responses to stress and panic. Clonidine can also reduce symptoms of aggression as with patients with bipolar disorders and reduce the insomnia associated with CNS stimulants such as methylphenidate. Once stabilized, children on larger doses can be switched to the transdermal clonidine patch.

The therapeutic applications for guanabenz are similar to those of clonidine and other α_2-adrenergic agonists. One advantage for guanabenz is its once-a-day dosing schedule. Guanabenz has been used in diabetic patients with hypertension without adverse effect on the control of or therapy for diabetes, and it has been effective in hypertensive patients with chronic obstructive pulmonary disease, including asthma, chronic bronchitis, or emphysema. Guanabenz has been used alone or in combination with naltrexone in the management of opiate withdrawal in patients physically dependent on opiates and undergoing detoxification. Guanabenz has also been used as an analgesic in a limited number of patients with chronic pain.

The therapeutic applications for guanfacine are similar to those of the other centrally acting α_2-adrenergic agonists and methyldopa.[6,119] It has been effective as monotherapy in the treatment of patients with mild to moderate hypertension. One advantage for guanfacine is its once-a-day dosing schedule. The use of diuretics to prevent accumulation of fluid can allow a reduction in the dosage for guanfacine. Somnolence and sedation were commonly reported adverse events in clinical trials. The most common adverse events associated with guanfacine treatment include somnolence/sedation, abdominal pain, dizziness, hypotension/decreased blood pressure, dry mouth, and constipation.

Guanfacine extended-release tablets (Intuniv) have been FDA approved for the nonstimulant treatment of ADHD in children and adolescents of age 6-17 years. Although the mechanism of action for treatment of ADHD is unknown, guanfacine is thought to directly bind to postsynaptic α_2-adrenoceptors in the prefrontal cortex of the brain, an area of the brain that has been linked to ADHD. Stimulation of these adrenoceptors is theorized to strengthen working memory, reduce susceptibility to distraction, improve attention regulation, improve behavioral inhibition, and enhance impulse control. Guanfacine treatment can cause decreases in blood pressure and heart rate, which can lead to syncope. This drug should be used with caution in ADHD patients with a history of hypotension, heart block, bradycardia, cardiovascular disease, syncope, orthostatic hypotension, or dehydration and should be used with caution in patients being treated concomitantly with antihypertensive agents or other drugs that reduce blood pressure or heart rate or increase the risk of syncope. Guanfacine extended-release tablets should not be crushed, chewed, or broken before they are swallowed and not substituted for immediate-release tablets. ADHD patients should be reevaluated periodically for the long-term usefulness of this drug. When ADHD therapy with guanfacine is discontinued, the dose should be tapered over a period of 7 days.

Pharmacology Overview of α_2-Adrenergic Receptor Agonists

Mechanism of Action. The central mechanism for the antihypertensive activity of the prodrug methyldopa is not caused by its inhibition of norepinephrine biosynthesis but, rather, by its metabolism in the CNS to α-methylnorepinephrine, an α_2-adrenergic agonist (Fig. 17.41).[87] Other more powerful inhibitors of aromatic L-amino acid decarboxylase (e.g., carbidopa) have proven to be clinically useful, but not as antihypertensives. Rather, these agents are used to inhibit the metabolism of exogenous L-DOPA administered in the treatment of Parkinson disease.

The mechanism of the central hypotensive action for methyldopa is attributed to its transport into the CNS via an aromatic amino acid transport mechanism, where it is decarboxylated and hydroxylated into α-methylnorepinephrine (Fig. 17.41).[87] This active metabolite of methyldopa decreases total peripheral resistance, with little change in cardiac output and heart rate, through its stimulation of central inhibitory α_2-adrenoceptors. A reduction of plasma renin activity can also contribute to the hypotensive action of methyldopa. Postural hypotension and sodium and water retention are also effects related to a reduction in blood pressure. If a diuretic is not administered concurrently with methyldopa, tolerance to the antihypertensive effect of the methyldopa during prolonged therapy can result.

The overall mechanism of action for the centrally active sympatholytics, clonidine, guanabenz, and guanfacine, appears to be stimulation of α_2-adrenoceptors and specific binding to nonadrenergic imidazoline I_1 receptors in the CNS (mainly in the medulla oblongata), causing inhibition of sympathetic output (sympathoinhibition).[120,121] This effect results in reduced peripheral and renovascular resistance and leads to a decrease in systolic and diastolic blood pressure. Through the use of imidazoline and α_2-adrenergic antagonists, specific I_1 receptors have recently been characterized in CNS control of blood pressure.[122] The I_1 receptors are pharmacologically distinct from α_2-receptors, because they are not activated by catecholamines but characterized by their high affinity for 2-iminoimidazolines (or 2-aminoimidazolines) and low affinity for guanidines.[122] Thus, the central hypotensive action for clonidine, other 2-aminoimidazolines, and structurally related compounds needs both the I_1 and α_2-adrenoceptors to produce their central sympatholytic response.[121] Because of this discovery, a new generation of centrally acting antihypertensive agents selective for the I_1 receptor has been developed and includes moxonidine (a pyrimidinyl aminoimidazoline) and rilmenidine (an alkylaminooxazoline) (Fig. 17.40). Rilmenidine and moxonidine are both highly selective for the I_1 receptor while having low affinity for α_2-adrenoceptors, and both control blood pressure effectively without the adverse effects associated with binding to α_2-receptors (e.g., sedation, bradycardia, and mental depression).[121] Clonidine appears to be more selective for α_2-adrenoceptors than for I_1 receptors.

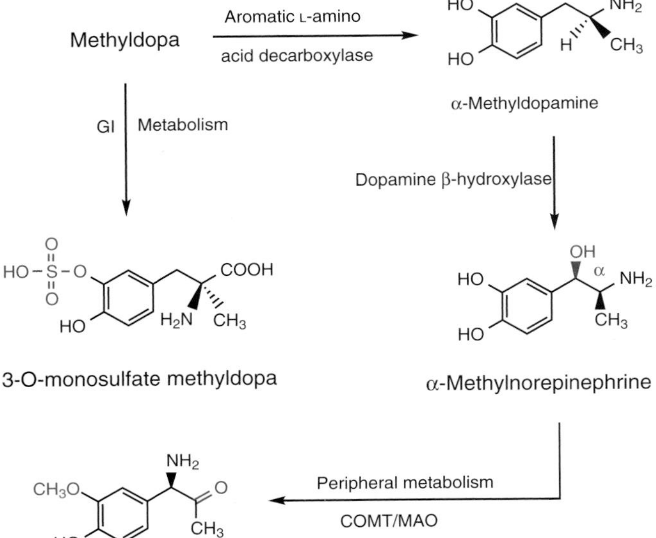

Figure 17.41 Metabolism of methyldopa. *COMT*, catechol-O-methyltransferase; *MAO*, monoamine oxidase.

In addition to its central stimulation of I_1 receptors and α_2-adrenoceptors,[121,122] clonidine (as well as other α_2-adrenergic agonists), when administered epidurally, produces analgesia by stimulation of spinal α_2-adrenoceptors, inhibiting sympathetically mediated pain pathways that are activated by nociceptive stimuli, thus preventing transmission of pain signals to the brain.[87] The administration of clonidine, while blocking opiate withdrawal, causes sympathetic inhibition and reduction in arterial pressure. The actions of clonidine on morphine pain response and withdrawal are most likely mediated by its ability to block NMDA receptor channels. Analgesia resulting from clonidine therapy is not antagonized by opiate antagonists. Activation of α_2-adrenoceptors also apparently stimulates acetylcholine release and inhibits the release of substance P, an inflammatory neuropeptide.

Common Adverse Effects. The most common adverse effect for methyldopa is drowsiness, which occurs within the first 48-72 hours of therapy and can disappear with continued administration of the drug.[6] Sedation commonly recurs when its dosage is increased. A decrease in mental acuity, including impaired ability to concentrate, lapses of memory, and difficulty in performing simple calculations, can occur and usually necessitates withdrawal of the drug. Patients should be warned that methyldopa can impair their ability to perform activities requiring mental alertness or physical coordination (e.g., operating machinery or driving a motor vehicle). Nightmares, mental depression, orthostatic hypotension, and symptoms of cerebrovascular insufficiency can occur during methyldopa therapy and are indications for dosage reduction. Orthostatic hypotension can be less pronounced with methyldopa than with guanethidine but can be more severe than with reserpine, clonidine, hydralazine, propranolol, or thiazide diuretics. Nasal congestion commonly occurs in patients receiving methyldopa. Positive direct antiglobulin (Coombs') test results have been reported in approximately 10%-20% of patients receiving methyldopa, usually after 6-12 months of therapy. This phenomenon is dose related. Methyldopa should be used with caution in patients with a history of previous liver disease or dysfunction, and it should be stopped if unexplained drug-induced fever and jaundice occur. These effects commonly occur within 3 weeks after initiation of treatment.

Dosage forms of methyldopa and methyldopate can contain sulfites, which can cause allergic-type reactions, including anaphylaxis and life-threatening or less severe asthmatic episodes. These allergic reactions are observed more frequently in asthmatic than in nonasthmatic individuals. Methyldopa is contraindicated in patients receiving MAO inhibitors.

Overall, the frequency of adverse effects produced by clonidine, guanabenz, and guanfacine are similar and appear to be dose related.[6] Drowsiness, tiredness, dizziness, weakness, bradycardia, headache, and dry mouth are common adverse effects for patients receiving clonidine, guanabenz, and guanfacine. The sedative effect for these centrally acting sympatholytics can result from their central α_2-agonist activity. The dry mouth induced by these drugs can result from a combination of central and peripheral α_2-adrenoceptor mechanisms, and the decreased salivation can involve inhibition of cholinergic transmission via stimulation of peripheral α_2-adrenoceptors. Orthostatic hypotension does not appear to be a significant problem with these drugs, because there appears to be little difference between supine and standing systolic and diastolic blood pressures in most patients. Other adverse effects include increased urinary frequency (nocturia), urinary retention, sexual dysfunction (e.g., decreased libido, erectile dysfunction, and impotence), nasal congestion, tinnitus, blurred vision, and dry eyes. These symptoms most often occur within the first few weeks of therapy and tend to diminish with continued therapy, or they can be relieved by a reduction in dosage. Although adverse effects of these drugs are generally not severe, discontinuance of therapy has been necessary in some patients because of intolerable sedation or dry mouth. Sodium and fluid retention can be avoided or relieved by administration of a diuretic.

Adverse effects occurring with transdermal clonidine generally appear to be similar to those occurring with oral therapy.[118,123] They have been mild and have tended to diminish with continued treatment. Hypotension has occurred in patients receiving clonidine by epidural infusion as adjunct therapy with epidural morphine for the treatment of cancer pain. With the transdermal system, localized skin reactions, such as erythema and pruritus, have occurred in some patients. The use of clonidine and methylphenidate in combination for managing ADHD can adversely affect cardiac conduction and increase risk for arrhythmias. ADHD patients need to be closely monitored and screened for a patient or family history of rhythm disturbances, and periodic monitoring of blood pressure, heart rate, and rhythm is recommended. Within 2-3 hours following the abrupt withdrawal of oral clonidine therapy, a rapid increase in systolic and diastolic blood pressures occurs, and blood pressures can exceed pretreatment levels. Associated with the clonidine withdrawal syndrome, the symptoms observed include nervousness, agitation, restlessness, anxiety, insomnia, headache, sweating, palpitations, increased heart rate, tremor, and increased salivation. The exact mechanism of the withdrawal syndrome following discontinuance of α_2-adrenergic agonists has not been determined but can involve increased concentrations of circulating catecholamines, increased sensitivity of adrenoceptors, enhanced renin-angiotensin system activity, decreased vagal function, failure of autoregulation of cerebral blood flow, and failure of central α_2-adrenoceptor mechanisms to regulate sympathetic outflow from the CNS.[6] The clonidine withdrawal syndrome is more pronounced after abrupt cessation of long-term therapy and with administration of high oral dosages (>1.2 mg daily). Withdrawal symptoms have been reported following discontinuance of transdermal therapy or when absorption of the drug is impaired because of dermatologic changes (e.g., contact dermatitis) under the transdermal system. Epidural clonidine can prolong the duration of the pharmacologic effects, including both sensory and motor blockade, of epidural local anesthetics.

Overall, the frequency of adverse effects produced by guanabenz is similar to that produced by clonidine and the other α_2-adrenergic agonists, but the incidence is lower.[6,124] As with the other centrally active sympatholytics (e.g., clonidine), abrupt withdrawal of guanabenz can result in rebound hypertension, but the withdrawal syndrome symptoms appear to be less severe.

Although the frequency of troublesome adverse effects produced by guanfacine is similar to that produced by clonidine and the other centrally acting sympatholytics, their incidence and severity are lower with guanfacine.[6,119] Unlike clonidine, abrupt discontinuation of guanfacine rarely results in rebound hypertension. When a withdrawal syndrome has occurred, its onset was slower and its symptoms less severe than the syndrome observed with clonidine.

Common Interactions. Table 17.24 summarizes common drug-drug interactions for the α_2-adrenergic receptor agonists. More detailed information follows.

A pharmacokinetic-based interaction occurs where oral iron preparations (ferrous salts) can interfere with the absorption of methyldopa from the gastrointestinal tract, reducing its systemic bioavailability.

The hypotensive actions for clonidine, guanabenz, and guanfacine can be additive with, or can potentiate the action of, other CNS depressants, such as opiates or other analgesics, barbiturates or other sedatives, anesthetics, or alcohol.[6] Coadministration of opiate analgesics with clonidine can also potentiate the hypotensive effects of clonidine. Tricyclic antidepressants (i.e., imipramine and desipramine) have reportedly inhibited the hypotensive effect of clonidine, guanabenz, and guanfacine, and the increase in blood pressure usually occurs during the second week of tricyclic antidepressant therapy. Dosage should be increased to adequately control hypertension if necessary. Sudden withdrawal of clonidine, guanabenz, and guanfacine can result in an excess of circulating catecholamines; therefore, caution should be exercised in concomitant use of drugs that affect the metabolism or tissue uptake of these amines (MAO inhibitors or tricyclic antidepressants, respectively). Because clonidine, guanabenz, and guanfacine can produce bradycardia, the possibility of additive effects should be considered if these drugs are given concomitantly with other drugs, such as hypotensive drugs or cardiac glycosides.

Medicinal Chemistry of α_2-Adrenergic Receptor Agonists

Receptor Binding, SAR, and Physicochemical Properties. Methyldopa is structurally and chemically related to L-dihydroxyphenylalanine (L-DOPA) and the catecholamines. To increase its water solubility for parenteral administration, the zwitterion methyldopa is esterified and converted to its hydrochloride salt, methyldopate ethyl ester hydrochloride (referred to as methyldopate). Methyldopate ester hydrochloride is used to prepare parenteral solutions of methyldopa, having a pH in the range of 3.5-6.0. Methyldopa is unstable in the presence of oxidizing agents (i.e., air), alkaline pH, and light. Being related to the catecholamines, which are subject to air oxidation, metabisulfite/sulfite can be added to dosage formulations to prevent oxidation. Some patients, especially those with asthma, can exhibit sulfite-related hypersensitivity reactions. Methyldopate hydrochloride injection has been reported to be physically incompatible with drugs that are poorly soluble in an acidic medium (e.g., sodium salts of barbiturates and sulfonamides) and with drugs that are acid labile. Incompatibility depends on several factors (e.g., concentrations of the drugs, specific diluents used, resulting pH, and temperature).

Clonidine is an aryl-2-aminoimidazoline (Fig. 17.40) that is more selective for α_2-adrenoceptors than for I_1 receptors in producing its hypotensive effect. It is available as oral tablets, injection, or a transdermal system. Clonidine was originally synthesized as a vasoconstricting nasal decongestant but, in early clinical trials, was found to have dramatic hypotensive effects—in contrast to all expectations for a vasoconstrictor.[125] Subsequent pharmacologic investigations showed that clonidine not only has some α_1-agonist (vasoconstrictive) properties in the periphery but also is a powerful α_2-adrenergic agonist and exhibits specific binding to nonadrenergic imidazoline binding sites in the CNS (mainly in the medulla oblongata), causing inhibition of sympathetic output (sympathoinhibition). Because of its peripheral activity on extraneuronal vascular postsynaptic α_{2B}-receptors,[126] initial doses of clonidine can produce a transient vasoconstriction and an increase in blood pressure that is soon overcome by vasodilation as clonidine penetrates the blood-brain barrier and interacts with CNS α_{2A}-receptors.

Clonidine has lipophilic ortho-dichloro substituents on the phenyl ring, and the uncharged form of clonidine exists as a pair of tautomers as shown.

Guanidino moiety

Clonidine

The pK_a of clonidine is 8.3 and it is approximately 80% ionized at physiologic pH. Its experimental log $D_{pH\ 7.4}$ = 1.03. The positive charge is shared through resonance by all three nitrogens of the guanidino group. Steric crowding by the bulky ortho-chlorine groups does not permit a coplanar conformation of the two rings, as shown.

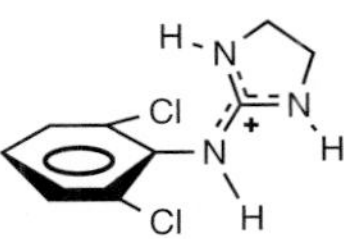

Protonated clonidine

After the discovery of clonidine, extensive research into the SAR of central α_2-agonists showed that the imidazoline ring was not necessary for activity in this class but that the phenyl ring required at least one ortho chlorine or methyl group. Two clinically useful antihypertensive agents resulting from this effort are guanabenz and guanfacine.

Guanabenz, a centrally active hypotensive agent, is pharmacologically related to clonidine but differs structurally from clonidine by the presence of an aminoguanidine side chain rather than an aminoimidazoline ring (Fig. 17.40). Guanabenz (pK_a = 8.1; log $D_{7.4}$ = 2.42) occurs largely (~80%) in the nonionized, lipid-soluble base form. Guanabenz can be given as a single daily dose administered at bedtime to minimize adverse effects.

Guanfacine, a phenylacetyl guanidine derivative (pK_a = 7.1; log $D_{7.4}$ = 1.52) (Fig. 17.40), is a centrally acting sympatholytic that is more selective for α_2-adrenoceptors than is clonidine. Its mechanism of action is similar to clonidine and is an effective alternative to that of the other centrally acting antihypertensive drugs. Although guanfacine is 5- to 20-fold less potent than clonidine on a weight basis, comparable blood pressure–lowering effects have been achieved when the two drugs were given in equipotent dosages. Its relatively long elimination half-life permits a once-a-day dosing schedule. Guanfacine activates peripheral α_2-adrenoceptors because a transient increase in blood pressure is observed in normotensive, but not in hypertensive, patients.

Pharmacokinetics and Metabolism. Methyldopa is an α_2-agonist acting in the CNS via its active metabolite, α-methylnorepinephrine (Fig. 17.41).[127] Methyldopa is transported across the blood-brain barrier, where it is decarboxylated by aromatic L-amino acid decarboxylase in the brain to α-methyldopamine, which is then stereospecifically hydroxylated to 1*R*,2*S*-α-methylnorepinephrine. This stereoisomer is a selective α_2-agonist and acts as an antihypertensive agent much like clonidine to inhibit sympathetic neural output from the CNS, thus lowering blood pressure. α-Methylnorepinephrine and α-methyldopamine do not cross the blood-brain barrier because of their hydrophilicity.

Originally synthesized as a norepinephrine biosynthesis inhibitor, methyldopa was thought to act through a combination of inhibition of norepinephrine biosynthesis through DOPA decarboxylase inhibition and metabolic decarboxylation to generate α-methylnorepinephrine. The latter was thought to replace norepinephrine in the nerve terminal and, when released, to have less intrinsic activity than the natural neurotransmitter. This latter mechanism is an example of the concept of a false neurotransmitter.

The oral bioavailability of methyldopa ranges from 20% to 50% and varies among individuals. Optimum blood pressure response occurs in 12-24 hours in most patients. After withdrawal of the drug, blood pressure returns to pretreatment levels within 24-48 hours. Methyldopa and its metabolites are weakly bound to plasma proteins. Although 95% of a dose of methyldopa is eliminated in hypertensive patients with normal renal function, with a plasma half-life of approximately 2 hours, in patients with impaired renal function, the half-life is doubled to approximately 3-4 hours, with about 50% of it excreted. Orally administered methyldopa undergoes presystemic first-pass metabolism in the gastrointestinal (GI) tract to its 3-O-monosulfate metabolite (Fig. 17.41). Sulfate conjugation occurs to a greater extent when the drug is given orally than when it is given intravenously (IV). Its rate of sulfate conjugation is decreased in patients with renal insufficiency. Methyldopa is excreted in urine as its mono-O-sulfate conjugate. Any peripherally decarboxylated α-methylnorepinephrine is metabolized by catechol-O-methyltransferase (COMT) and monoamine oxidase (MAO) (Fig. 17.41).

Methyldopate is slowly hydrolyzed in the body to form methyldopa. The hypotensive effect of IV methyldopate begins in 4-6 hours and lasts 10-16 hours.

Clonidine has an oral bioavailability of more than 90%, with a log $D_{7.4}$ of 1.82. It is well absorbed when applied topically to the eye and is well absorbed percutaneously following topical application of a transdermal system to the arm or chest.[118,123,128] Following application of a clonidine transdermal patch, therapeutic plasma concentrations are attained within 2-3 days. Studies have indicated that release of clonidine from the patch averages from 50% to 70% after 7 days of wear. Plasma clonidine concentrations attained with the transdermal systems are generally similar to twice-daily oral dosing regimens of the drug. Percutaneous absorption of the drug from the upper arm or chest is similar, but less drug is absorbed from the thigh.[123] Replacement of the transdermal system at a different site at weekly intervals continuously maintains therapeutic plasma clonidine concentrations. After discontinuance of transdermal therapy, therapeutic plasma drug concentrations persist for approximately 8 hours and then decline slowly over several days; over this time period, blood pressure returns gradually to pretreatment levels.

Blood pressure begins to decrease within 30-60 minutes after an oral dose of clonidine, with the maximum decrease in approximately 2-4 hours.[6] The hypotensive effect lasts up to 8 hours. Following epidural administration of a single bolus dose of clonidine, it is rapidly absorbed into the systemic circulation and into cerebrospinal fluid (CSF), with maximal analgesia within 30-60 minutes. Although the CSF is not the presumed site of action of clonidine-mediated analgesia, the drug appears to diffuse rapidly from the CSF to the dorsal horn of the spinal cord. After oral administration, clonidine appears to be well distributed throughout the body, with the lowest concentration in the brain. Clonidine is approximately 20%-40% bound to plasma proteins, and it crosses the placenta. The plasma half-life of clonidine is 6-20 hours in patients with normal renal function and 18-41 hours in patients with impaired renal function. Clonidine is metabolized in the liver to its inactive major metabolite 4-hydroxyclonidine and its glucuronide and sulfate conjugates (10%-20%) (Fig. 17.42). In humans, 40%-60% of an oral or IV dose of clonidine is excreted in urine as unchanged drug within 24 hours. Approximately 85% of a single dose is excreted within 72 hours, with 20% of the dose excreted in feces, probably via enterohepatic circulation.

The effective oral dose range for rilmenidine is 1-3 mg, with a dose-dependent duration of action of 10-20 hours. Moxonidine is administered once a day at a dose range of 0.2-0.4 mg. The oral bioavailability of moxonidine in humans is greater than 90%, with approximately 40%-50% of the oral dose excreted unmetabolized in the urine.[129,130] The principal route of metabolism for moxonidine is oxidation of the 2-methyl group in the pyrimidine ring to 2-hydroxymethyl and 2-carboxylic acid derivative as well as the formation of corresponding glucuronides. After an oral dose of moxonidine, peak hypotensive effects occur within 2 hours, with an elimination half-life of greater than 8 hours.[130,131] Rilmenidine is readily absorbed from the GI tract, with an oral bioavailability greater than 95%. It is poorly metabolized and is excreted unchanged in the urine, with an elimination half-life of 8 hours.[132,133] After IV or oral administration of these drugs in normotensive patients, an initial hypertensive response to the drug occurs that is caused by activation of the peripheral α_2-adrenoceptors and the resulting vasoconstriction. This response is not observed, however, in patients with hypertension.

The oral bioavailability of guanabenz is 70%-80%. After an oral dose, the hypotensive effect of guanabenz begins within 1 hour, peaks within 2-7 hours, and is diminished within 6-8 hours. It has an elimination half-life averaging 4-14 hours. The blood pressure response can persist for at least 12 hours. After IV dosing, guanabenz is distributed into the CNS, with brain concentrations 3-70 times higher than concurrent plasma concentrations. Guanabenz is approximately 90% bound to plasma proteins. In patients

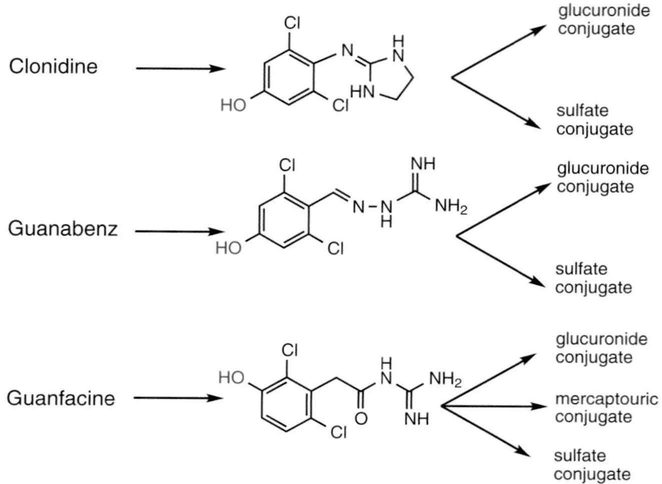

Figure 17.42 Metabolites formed from clonidine, guanabenz, and guanfacine.

with hepatic or renal impairment, its elimination half-life can be prolonged.

Guanabenz is metabolized principally by hydroxylation to its inactive metabolite, 4-hydroxyguanabenz, which is eliminated in the urine as its glucuronide (major) and sulfate conjugates (Fig. 17.42). Guanabenz and its inactive metabolites are excreted principally in urine, with approximately 70%-80% of its oral dose excreted in urine within 24 hours and approximately 10%-30% excreted in feces via enterohepatic cycling. Approximately 40% of an oral dose of guanabenz is excreted in urine as 4-hydroxyguanabenz and its glucuronide, and less than 5% is excreted unchanged. The remainder is excreted as unidentified metabolites and their conjugates.

The pharmacokinetic properties for guanfacine differ from those of clonidine, guanabenz, and α-methyldopa.[119,134,135] At pH 7.4, guanfacine is predominately (67%) in the nonionized, lipid-soluble base form, which accounts for its high oral bioavailability (>80%). Following an oral dose, peak plasma concentrations occur in 1-4 hours, with a relatively long elimination half-life of 14-23 hours. The maximum blood pressure response occurs in 8-12 hours after oral administration and is maintained up to 36 hours after its discontinuation. After IV dosing, guanfacine achieves the highest concentrations in liver and kidney, with low concentrations in the brain. Guanfacine is 64% bound to plasma proteins. In patients with hepatic or renal impairment, its elimination half-life can be prolonged.

Guanfacine is metabolized principally by hepatic hydroxylation to its inactive metabolite, 3-hydroxyguanfacine (20%), which is eliminated in the urine as its glucuronide (30%), sulfate (8%), or mercapturic acid conjugate (10%), and 24%-37% is excreted as unchanged guanfacine (Fig. 17.42). Its nearly complete bioavailability suggests no evidence of any first-pass effect. Guanfacine and its inactive metabolites are excreted principally in urine, with approximately 80% of its oral dose excreted in urine within 48 hours.

Vasodilators

Overview

Vasodilator drugs relax the smooth muscle in blood vessels, which causes the vessels to dilate.[101] Dilation of arterial vessels leads to a reduction in systemic vascular resistance, which leads to a fall in arterial blood pressure. Dilation of venous vessels decreases venous blood pressure.

Arterial dilator drugs are used to treat systemic and pulmonary hypertension, heart failure, and angina. They reduce arterial pressure by decreasing systemic vascular resistance, thereby reducing the afterload on the left ventricle and enhancing stroke volume and cardiac output. They also decrease the oxygen demand of the heart and, thereby, improve the oxygen supply/demand ratio. The primary functions of venous dilators in treating cardiovascular hypertension include reduction in venous pressure, thus reducing preload on the heart and decreasing cardiac output and capillary fluid filtration and edema formation (a decrease in capillary hydrostatic pressure). Therefore, venous dilators sometimes are used in the treatment of heart failure along with other drugs, because they help to reduce pulmonary and/or systemic edema that results from heart failure.

There are three potential drawbacks in the use of vasodilators: First, vasodilators can lead to a baroreceptor-mediated reflex stimulation of the heart (increased heart rate and inotropy) from systemic vasodilation and arterial pressure reduction. Second, they can impair the normal baroreceptor-mediated reflex vasoconstriction when a person stands up, which can lead to orthostatic hypotension and syncope on standing. Third, they can lead to renal retention of sodium and water, increasing blood volume and cardiac output.

Vasodilator drugs are classified either based on their site of action (arterial vs. venous) or, more commonly, by their primary mechanism of action.

Direct-Acting Vasodilators

THERAPEUTIC OVERVIEW OF DIRECT-ACTING VASODILATORS. Hydralazine, the only drug in this class, is used in the management of moderate to severe hypertension.[6] It is reserved for patients with compelling indications and who fail to respond adequately to a stage 2 antihypertensive regimen. This drug is recommended for use in conjunction with cardiac glycosides and other vasodilators for the short-term treatment of severe congestive heart failure. Patients who engage in potentially hazardous activities, such as operating machinery or driving motor vehicles, should be warned about possible faintness, dizziness, or weakness. Hydralazine should be used with caution in patients with cerebrovascular accidents or with severe renal damage.

NHNH$_2$ N N

Hydralazine

Parenteral hydralazine can be used for the management of severe hypertension when the drug cannot be given orally or when blood pressure must be lowered immediately. Other agents (e.g., sodium nitroprusside) are preferred for the management of severe hypertension or hypersensitive emergencies when a parenteral hypotensive agent is employed.

PHARMACOLOGY OF DIRECT-ACTING VASODILATORS

Mechanism of Action. Hydralazine does not fit neatly into the other mechanistic classes of vasodilators, in part, because its mechanism of action is not entirely clear. It seems to have multiple, direct effects on the VSM. First, it causes smooth muscle hyperpolarization, quite likely through the opening of K^+ channels. Activation therefore increases the efflux of potassium ions from the cells, causing hyperpolarization of VSM cells and, thus, prolonging the opening of the potassium channel and sustaining a greater vasodilation on arterioles than on veins.[87] It can also inhibit the second messenger, IP_3-induced release of calcium from the smooth muscle SR (the PIP_2 signal transduction pathway) (Fig. 17.33). Finally, hydralazine stimulates the formation of NO by the vascular endothelium, leading to cGMP-mediated vasodilation (Fig. 17.32). The arterial vasodilator action of hydralazine reduces systemic vascular resistance and arterial pressure. Diastolic blood pressure is usually decreased more than systolic pressure. The hydralazine-induced decrease in blood pressure and peripheral resistance causes a reflex response, which is accompanied by increased heart rate, cardiac output, and stroke volume and an increase in plasma renin activity. It has no direct effect on the heart.[6] This reflex response could offset the hypotensive effect of arteriolar dilation, limiting its antihypertensive effectiveness. Hydralazine also causes sodium and water retention and expansion of plasma volume, which could develop tolerance to its antihypertensive effect during prolonged therapy. Thus, coadministration of a diuretic improves the therapeutic outcome.

Common Adverse Effects. Examples of adverse effects associated with the use of hydralazine are summarized in Table 17.26.

Common Interactions. The coadministration of hydralazine with diuretics and other hypotensive drugs can have a synergistic effect, resulting in a marked decrease in blood pressure.

MEDICINAL CHEMISTRY OF DIRECT-ACTING VASODILATORS

Receptor Binding, SAR and Physicochemical Properties. Hydralazine, a phthalazine-substituted hydrazine antihypertensive drug with a pK_a of 7.3 and log $D_{7.4}$ of 0.52, is highly specific for arterial vessels, producing its vasodilation by a couple of different mechanisms.

Pharmacokinetic Properties and Metabolism. Hydralazine is well absorbed from the GI tract and is metabolized in the GI mucosa (prehepatic systemic metabolism) and in the liver by acetylation, hydroxylation, and conjugation with glucuronic acid (Fig. 17.43).[6,87] Little of the hydralazine dose is excreted unchanged while most of the dose appears as metabolites in the urine which are without significant therapeutic activity. A small amount of hydralazine is reportedly converted to a hydrazone, most likely with vitamin B_6 (pyridoxine), which can be responsible for some its neurotoxic effects. Following the oral administration of hydralazine, its antihypertensive effect begins in 20-30 minutes and lasts 2-4 hours. The plasma half-life of hydralazine is generally 2-4 hours but, in some patients, can be up to 8 hours (i.e., slow acetylators). In slow acetylator patients or those with impaired renal function, the plasma concentrations for hydralazine are increased and, possibly, prolonged. Approximately 85% of hydralazine in the blood is bound to plasma proteins following administration of usual doses.

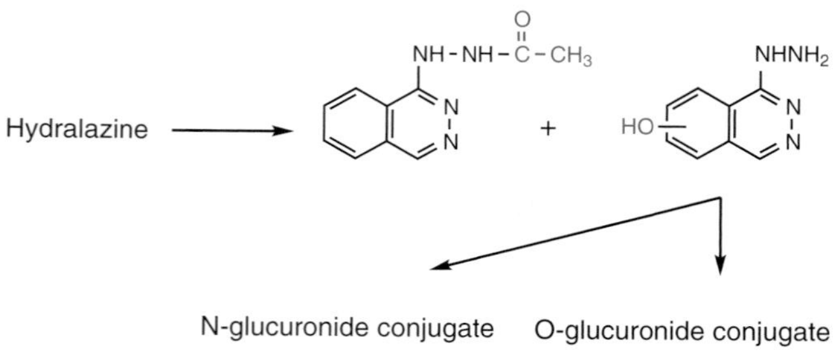

First-pass acetylation in the GI mucosa and liver is related to genetic acetylator phenotype. Acetylation phenotype is an important determinant of the plasma concentrations of hydralazine when the same dose of hydralazine is administered orally. Slow acetylators have an autosomal recessive trait that results in a relative deficiency of the hepatic enzyme N-acetyl transferase, thus prolonging the elimination half-life of hydralazine. This population of hypertensive patients will require an adjustment in dose to reduce the increased overactive response. Approximately 50% of African Americans and whites and the majority of American Indians, Eskimos, and Asians are rapid acetylators of hydralazine. This population of patients will have subtherapeutic plasma concentrations of hydralazine because of its rapid metabolism to inactive metabolites and shorter elimination times. Patients with hydralazine-induced systemic lupus erythematosus frequently are slow acetylators.[87]

Figure 17.43 Metabolism of hydralazine.

Potassium Channel Openers

THERAPEUTIC OVERVIEW OF POTASSIUM CHANNEL OPENERS. The two drugs in this class are minoxidil and diazoxide. Being effective arterial dilators, potassium-channel openers are used in the treatment of hypertension. However, these drugs are not first-line therapy for hypertension because of their side effects; therefore, they are relegated to treating refractory, severe hypertension. They are generally used in conjunction with a BB and a diuretic to attenuate the reflex tachycardia and retention of sodium and fluid, respectively.

Minoxidil is used in the management of severe hypertension. It is reserved for resistant cases of hypertension that have not been managed with maximal therapeutic dosages of a diuretic and two other hypotensive drugs or for patients who have failed to respond adequately with hydralazine. To minimize sodium retention and increased plasma volume, minoxidil must be used in conjunction with a diuretic. A BB must be given before beginning minoxidil therapy and should be continued during minoxidil therapy to minimize minoxidil-induced tachycardia and increased myocardial workload. Minoxidil is also used topically to stimulate regrowth of hair in patients with androgenic alopecia (male pattern alopecia, hereditary alopecia, or common male baldness) or alopecia areata.

Intravenous diazoxide has been used in hypertensive crises for emergency lowering of blood pressure when a prompt and urgent decrease in diastolic pressure is required in adults with severe nonmalignant and malignant hypertension and in children with acute severe hypertension.[6] However, other IV hypotensive agents are preferred for the management of hypertensive crises. Diazoxide is intended for short-term use in hospitalized patients only. Although diazoxide has also been administered orally for the management of hypertension, its hyperglycemic and sodium-retaining effects make it unsuitable for chronic therapy. Diazoxide is also administered orally in the management of hypoglycemia caused by hyperinsulinism associated with inoperable islet cell adenoma or carcinoma or extrapancreatic malignancy in adults.

PHARMACOLOGY OVERVIEW OF POTASSIUM CHANNEL OPENERS

Mechanism of Action. Potassium channel openers are drugs that activate (i.e., open) ATP-sensitive K^+ channels in the VSM (Fig. 17.32).[136] By opening these potassium channels, there is increased efflux of potassium ions from the cells, causing hyperpolarization of VSM, which closes the voltage-gated calcium channels and, thereby, decreases intracellular calcium. With less calcium available to combine with calmodulin, there is less activation of MLCK and phosphorylation of myosin light chains. This leads to relaxation and vasodilation. Because small arteries and arterioles normally have a high degree of smooth muscle tone, these drugs are particularly effective in dilating these resistance vessels, decreasing systemic vascular resistance, and lowering arterial pressure. The fall in arterial pressure leads to reflex cardiac stimulation (baroreceptor-mediated tachycardia).

Minoxidil, as its active metabolite minoxidil O-sulfate, prolongs the opening of the potassium channel, sustaining greater vasodilation on arterioles than on veins. The drug decreases blood pressure in both the supine and standing positions, and there is no orthostatic hypotension. Associated with the decrease in peripheral resistance and blood pressure is a reflex response that is accompanied by increased heart rate, cardiac output, and stroke volume, which can be attenuated by the coadministration of a BB.[6] Along with this decrease in peripheral resistance is increased plasma renin activity and sodium and water retention, which can result in expansion of fluid volume, edema, and congestive heart failure. The sodium- and water-retaining effects of minoxidil can be reversed by coadministration of a diuretic. When minoxidil is used in conjunction with a β-adrenergic blocker, pulmonary artery pressure remains essentially unchanged.

Diazoxide reduces peripheral vascular resistance and blood pressure by a direct vasodilating effect on the VSM with a mechanism similar to that described for minoxidil by activating (opening) the ATP-modulated potassium channel.[137] Thus, diazoxide prolongs the opening of the potassium channel, sustaining greater vasodilation on arterioles than on veins.[87] The greatest hypotensive effect is observed in patients with malignant hypertension. Although oral or slow IV administration of diazoxide can produce a sustained fall in blood pressure, rapid IV administration is required for maximum hypotensive effects, especially in patients with malignant hypertension.[6] Diazoxide-induced decreases in blood pressure and peripheral vascular resistance are accompanied by a reflex response, resulting in an increased heart rate, cardiac output, and left ventricular ejection rate. In contrast to the thiazide diuretics, diazoxide causes sodium and water retention and decreased urinary output, which can result in expansion of plasma and extracellular fluid volume, edema, and congestive heart failure, especially during prolonged administration.

Diazoxide increases blood glucose concentration (diazoxide-induced hyperglycemia) by several different mechanisms: by inhibiting pancreatic insulin secretion, by stimulating release of catecholamines, or by increasing hepatic release of glucose.[6,87] The precise mechanism of inhibition of insulin release has not been elucidated but, possibly, can result from an effect of diazoxide on cell-membrane potassium channels and calcium flux.

Common Adverse Effects. Common adverse effects for the potassium channel openers, diazoxide and minoxidil, are listed in Table 17.26.

Common Interactions. When minoxidil is administered with diuretics or other hypotensive drugs, the hypotensive effect of minoxidil increases, and concurrent use can cause profound orthostatic hypotensive effects.

MEDICINAL CHEMISTRY OF POTASSIUM CHANNEL OPENERS

Receptor Binding, SAR, and Physicochemical Properties. Minoxidil is the N-oxide of a piperidinopyrimidine hypotensive agent with a pK_a 4.6 and log $D_{7.4}$ of 0.62. Diazoxide is a nondiuretic hypotensive and hyperglycemic agent that is structurally related to the thiazide diuretics. Being a sulfonamide with a pK_a of 8.5 and log $D_{7.4}$ of 1.28, it can be solubilized in alkaline solutions (pH of injection is 11.6). Solutions or oral suspension of diazoxide are unstable to light and will darken when exposed to light. Such dosage forms should be protected from light, heat, and freezing. Darkened solutions can be subpotent and should not be used.

Pharmacokinetic Properties and Metabolism. Minoxidil is not an active hypotensive drug until it is metabolized by hepatic thermolabile phenol sulfotransferase (SULT1A1) to minoxidil N-O-sulfate.[87] Plasma concentrations for minoxidil sulfate peak within 1 hour and then decline rapidly. Following an oral dose of minoxidil, its hypotensive effect begins in 30 minutes, is maximal in 2-8 hours, and persists for approximately 2-5 days. The delayed onset of the hypotensive effect for minoxidil is attributed to its metabolism to its active metabolite. The drug is not bound to plasma proteins. The major metabolite for minoxidil is its N-O-glucuronide, which unlike the sulfate metabolite, is inactive as a hypotensive agent. Approximately 10%-20% of an oral dose of minoxidil is metabolized to its active metabolite, minoxidil O-sulfate, and approximately 20% of minoxidil is excreted unchanged.

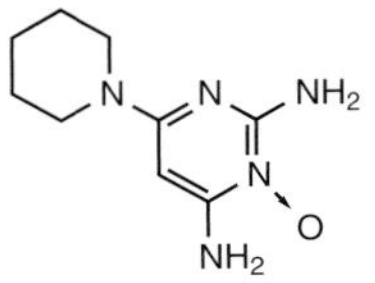

Minoxidil 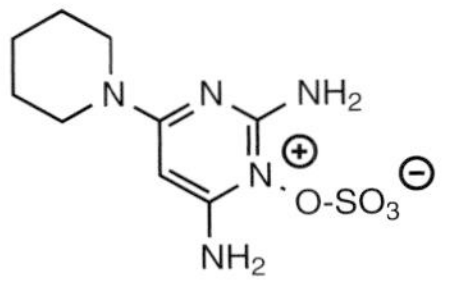 Minoxidil N-O-sulfate 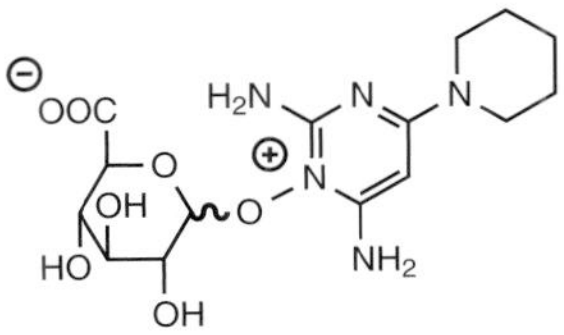 Minoxidil N-O-glucuronide

After rapid IV administration, diazoxide produces a prompt reduction in blood pressure, with maximum hypotensive effects occurring within 5 minutes.[6] The duration of its hypotensive effect varies from 3 to 12 hours, but ranges from 30 minutes to 72 hours have been observed. The elimination half-life of diazoxide following a single oral or IV dose has been reported to range from 21 to 45 hours in adults with normal renal function. In patients with renal impairment, the half-life is prolonged. Approximately 90% of the diazoxide in the blood is bound to plasma proteins. Approximately 20%-50% of diazoxide is eliminated unchanged in the urine, along with its major metabolites, resulting from the oxidation of the 3-methyl group to its 3-hydroxymethyl- and 3-carboxyl-metabolites.

Cl, O, O, S, NH, N, CH_3 —Metabolism→ Cl, O, O, S, NH, N, CH_2OH → Cl, O, O, S, NH, N, CO_2H

Diazoxide

Nitrodilators

THERAPEUTIC OVERVIEW OF NITRODILATORS. Intravenous sodium nitroprusside is used as an infusion for hypertensive crises and emergencies.[6] The drug is consistently effective in the management of hypertensive emergencies, irrespective of etiology, and can be useful even when other drugs have failed. It can be used in the management of acute congestive heart failure.

PHARMACOLOGY OF NITRODILATORS

Mechanism of Action. Nitric oxide (NO), a molecule produced by many cells in the body, has several important actions. NO is a highly reactive gas that participates in many chemical reactions. It is one of the nitrogen oxides ("NOx") in automobile exhaust and plays a major role in the formation of photochemical smog, but NO has also many physiologic functions. It is synthesized within cells by an enzyme NO synthase (NOS). There are three isoenzymes, neuronal NOS (nNOS or NOS-1), inducible NOS (iNOS or NOS-2) found in macrophages, and endothelial NOS (eNOS or NOS-3) found in the endothelial cells that line the lumen of blood vessels. Whereas the levels of nNOS and eNOS are relatively steady, expression of iNOS genes awaits an appropriate stimulus. All types of NOS produce NO from arginine with the aid of molecular oxygen and NADPH. Because NO diffuses freely across cell membranes, there are many other molecules with which it can interact, and NO is quickly consumed close to where it is synthesized. Thus, NO affects only cells adjacent to its point of synthesis. NO relaxes the smooth muscle in the walls of the arterioles. At each systole, the endothelial cells that line the blood vessels release a puff of NO, which diffuses into the underlying smooth muscle cells, causing them to relax and, thus, to permit the surge of blood to pass through easily. The signaling functions of NO begin with its binding to protein receptors on or in the cell, triggering the formation of cGMP from soluble guanylyl cyclase (Fig. 17.32). Mice in which the genes for the NOS found in endothelial cells (eNOS) have been "knocked out" suffer from hypertension. Nitroglycerin, which is often prescribed to reduce the pain of angina, does so by generating NO, which relaxes venous walls and arterioles, improving the oxygen supply/demand ratio (see Chapter 16). NO also inhibits the aggregation of platelets and, thus, keeps inappropriate clotting from interfering with blood flow. Other actions on smooth muscle include penile erection and peristalsis aided by the relaxing effect of NO on the smooth muscle in intestinal walls. NO also inhibits the contractility of the smooth muscle wall of the uterus, but at birth, the production of NO decreases, allowing contractions to occur. Nitroglycerin has helped some women who were at risk of giving birth prematurely to carry their baby to full term. The NO from iNOS inhibits inflammation in blood vessels by blocking the release of mediators of inflammation from the endothelial cells, macrophages, and T lymphocytes. NO produced by iNOS has also been shown to S-nitrosylate cyclooxygenase-2 (COX-2), increasing its activity, and drugs that prevent this interaction could work synergistically with the nonsteroidal anti-inflammatory drugs inhibiting COX-2. NO affects hormonal secretion from several endocrine glands. Hemoglobin transports NO at the same time that it carries oxygen, and when it unloads oxygen in the tissues, it also unloads NO. Fireflies use NO to turn on their flashers.

Since the dawn of recorded human history, nitrates have been used to preserve meat from bacterial spoilage. Harmless bacteria in our throat convert nitrates in our food into nitrites. When the nitrites reach the stomach, the acidic gastric juice (pH ~1.4) generates NO from these nitrites, killing almost all the bacteria that have been swallowed in our food.

In the cardiovascular system, NO is produced primarily by vascular endothelial cells. This endothelial-derived NO has several important functions, including relaxing VSM (vasodilation), inhibiting platelet aggregation (antithrombotic), and inhibiting leukocyte-endothelial interactions (anti-inflammatory). These actions involve NO-stimulated formation of cGMP (Fig. 17.32). Nitrodilator are drugs that mimic the actions of endogenous NO by releasing NO or forming NO within tissues. These drugs act directly on the VSM to cause relaxation and, therefore, serve as endothelial-independent vasodilators.

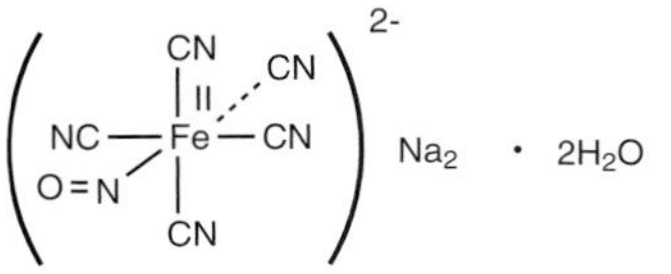

Sodium nitroprusside

There are two basic types of nitrodilators: those that release NO spontaneously (e.g., sodium nitroprusside) and those that require an enzyme activation to form NO (organic nitrates). Sodium nitroprusside is a direct-acting vasodilator on VSM, producing its vasodilation by the release of NO. Since 1929, it has been known as a rapidly acting hypotensive agent when administered as an infusion. It is chemically and structurally unrelated to other available hypotensive agents.

Common Adverse Effects. The most clinically important adverse effects of sodium nitroprusside are profound hypotension and the accumulation of cyanide and thiocyanate.[6] Thiocyanate can accumulate in the blood of patients receiving sodium nitroprusside therapy, especially in those with impaired renal function. Thiocyanate is mildly neurotoxic at serum concentrations of 60 μg/mL and can be life-threatening at concentrations of 200 μg/mL. Other adverse effects of thiocyanate include inhibition of both the uptake and binding of iodine, producing symptoms of hypothyroidism.

Sodium nitroprusside can bind to vitamin B_{12}, interfering with its distribution and metabolism, and it should be used with caution in patients having low plasma vitamin B_{12} concentrations. Use of this drug can result in the formation of methemoglobin (which contains ferric iron in its heme groups), an oxidized form of hemoglobin that cannot bind or transport oxygen, in erythrocytes.

Common Interactions. The hypotensive effect of sodium nitroprusside is augmented by concomitant use of other hypotensive agents and is not blocked by adrenergic blocking agents. It has no direct effect on the myocardium, but it can exert a direct coronary vasodilator effect on VSM. When sodium nitroprusside is administered to hypertensive patients, a slight increase in heart rate commonly occurs, and cardiac output is usually decreased slightly. Moderate doses of sodium nitroprusside in patients with hypertension produce renal vasodilation without an appreciable increase in renal blood flow or decrease in glomerular filtration.[6]

MEDICINAL CHEMISTRY OF NITRODILATORS

Receptor Binding, SAR and Physicochemical Properties. The potency of sodium nitroprusside is expressed in terms of the dihydrated drug. When reconstituted with 5% dextrose injection, sodium nitroprusside solutions are reddish-brown in color, with a pH of 3.5-6.0. Its crystals and solutions are sensitive and unstable to light and should be protected from extremes of light and heat. The exposure of sodium nitroprusside solutions to light causes deterioration, which can be evidenced by a change from a reddish-brown to a green to a blue color, indicating a rearrangement of the nitroso to the inactive isonitro form. Sodium nitroprusside solutions in glass bottles undergo approximately 20% degradation within 4 hours when exposed to fluorescent light and even more rapid degradation in plastic bags. Sodium nitroprusside solutions should be protected from light by wrapping the container with aluminum foil or other opaque material. When adequately protected from light, reconstituted solutions are stable for 24 hours. Trace metals, such as iron and copper, can catalyze the degradation of nitroprusside solutions, releasing cyanide. Any change in color for the nitroprusside solutions is an indication of degradation, and the solution should be discarded. No other drug or preservative should be added to stabilize sodium nitroprusside infusions.

Pharmacokinetic Properties and Metabolism. Intravenous infusion of sodium nitroprusside produces an almost immediate reduction in blood pressure. Blood pressure begins to rise immediately when the infusion is slowed or stopped and returns to pretreatment levels within 1-10 minutes.

Sodium nitroprusside is not an active hypotensive drug until metabolized to its active metabolite, NO, the mechanism of action of which has been previously described (Fig. 17.32). Studies with sodium nitroprusside suggest that it releases NO by its interaction with glutathione or with sulfhydryl groups in the erythrocytes and tissues to form a *S*-nitrosothiol intermediate, which spontaneously produces NO, which in turn freely diffuses into the VSM, thereby increasing intracellular cGMP concentration.[6,87] NO also activates K^+ channels, which leads to hyperpolarization and relaxation.

Sodium nitroprusside undergoes a redox reaction that releases cyanide.[6,87] The cyanide that is produced is rapidly converted into thiocyanate in the liver by the enzyme thiosulfate sulfotransferase (rhodanase) and is excreted in the urine.[6,87] The rate-limiting step in the conversion of cyanide to thiocyanate is the availability of sulfur donors, especially thiosulfate. Toxic symptoms of thiocyanate begin to appear at plasma thiocyanate concentrations of 50-100 μg/mL. The elimination half-life of thiocyanate is 2.7-7.0 days when renal function is normal but longer in patients with impaired renal function.

ACKNOWLEDGMENTS

The authors wish to acknowledge the work of Robert K. Griffiths, Gary O. Rankin, and David A. Williams, who authored content used within this chapter in a previous edition of this text.

Clinical Scenario

Michael W. Perry, PharmD, BCPS, BCCCP

SCENARIO

VT is a 54-year-old black male who has a history of uncontrolled hypertension, medication noncompliance, dyslipidemia, and active smoking (5 packs per year history). He presents to the hospital with a blood pressure of 200/120 mm Hg and sudden onset of chest pain. He has not been taking his medications because he does not ever "feel" like his blood pressure is elevated and never remembers to take his medications. His primary care physician prescribed him topical clonidine, but he never filled the medication due to the cost.

Allergies:

Lisinopril (dry cough)

Current Medications:

Clonidine 0.2 mg/24 hour patch apply topically to arm once weekly
Isosorbide Dinitrate 10 mg by mouth t.i.d.
Hydralazine 100 mg by mouth t.i.d.
Simvastatin 40 mg by mouth daily
Nicotine patch 14 mg topically daily

While being evaluated in the emergency room he is found to have a type B aortic dissection. A cardiothoracic surgeon wants to start the patient on a continuous infusion of a short-acting intravenous β-receptor blockers and a short-acting intravenous dihydropyridine calcium channel blocker. What agents would be appropriate to recommend for the initial intravenous therapy?

OUTCOME

An aortic dissection is a tear in the lining of the aorta and is a serious consequence of uncontrolled hypertension. The initial management of a type B aortic dissection is strict blood pressure control with continuous infusions of short-acting antihypertensive medications. In order to prevent the dissection from enlarging, a β-blocker may be administered first to slow the heart rate and blunt any reflex tachycardia caused by other antihypertensive medications used to control the blood pressure. Intravenous dihydropyridine calcium channel blockers are commonly used with β-receptor blockers to maintain the blood pressure and heart rate within the specified parameters.

Esmolol and labetalol are both able to be administered as an intravenous continuous infusion. While both of these agents are β-receptor blockers, differences in their structures lead to vastly different pharmacokinetic and pharmacodynamic effects. Esmolol is a β_1-selective agent that has an extremely short half-life. This allows clinicians to quickly titrate the infusion rate up and down to quickly control the patient's heart rate. While esmolol is excellent at lowering the heart rate, its overall antihypertensive effects are less than labetalol. Labetalol is a mixed α-/β-receptor blocker, which allows for additional blood pressure lowering effects due to vasodilation via α_1-blockade. Labetalol has a longer half-life than esmolol, which does not allow for as rapid of a titration when compared with esmolol. Labetalol is also available as an oral medication that may facilitate the transition from intravenous to oral antihypertensive. Esmolol does not have an oral formulation.

Similar to the relationship between labetalol and esmolol, nicardipine and clevidipine, while both are intravenous dihydropyridine calcium channel blockers, have different pharmacokinetic profiles. Clevidipine has an ultra-short half-life that allows the infusion to be titrated every 90 seconds to achieve a goal blood pressure. The half-life of nicardipine is longer than clevidipine but can still be titrated every 5-15 minutes to the desired blood pressure target. The chemical structures also factor into the administration of the medications. Due to the pH of a nicardipine infusion, it can be irritating to veins. Nicardipine should be administered via a central line to avoid venous irritation. If a central line is not available, the nicardipine must be diluted in a larger volume. Clevidipine is formulated in a lipid emulsion, which can be administered via a central or peripheral intravenous line. Unfortunately, the lipid emulsion makes clevidipine susceptible to contamination with bacteria and fungus. A bottle of clevidipine must be discarded 12 hours after it is opened. Availability of an oral formulation may facilitate the transition from an intravenous antihypertensive to oral therapy. Clevidipine does not have an oral formulation. An oral dosage form of nicardipine is available, but it is dosed every eight hours, which may decrease compliance.

Overall, patients requiring continuous infusions of antihypertensive medications will require close hemodynamic monitoring. This will allow the health care team to make quick adjustments to the medication dosing in response to rapidly changing vital signs and clinical status. Labetalol would be a reasonable choice to start in this patient, as it provides both heart rate lowering effects via β_1-receptor blockade and vasodilation via α_1-blockade. If the patient's blood pressure is still not under control, nicardipine may be added to the antihypertensive regimen to provide additional vasodilation via calcium channel blockade. Eventually, the patient could be transitioned to an oral labetalol formulation and a once daily oral dihydropyridine calcium channel blocker, such as amlodipine.

Chemical Analysis found immediately after References.

REFERENCES

1. Benjamin EJ, Blaha MJ, Chiuve SE, et al. Heart disease and stroke statistics – 2017 update: a report from the American Heart Association. *Circulation*. 2017;135:e146-e603.
2. Weibert RT. Hypertension. In: Herfindal ET, Gourley DR, eds. *Textbook of Therapeutics: Drug and Disease Management*. 7th ed. Baltimore, MD: Lippincott Williams & Wilkins; 2000: 795-824.
3. James PA, Oparil S, Carter BL, et al. evidence-based guideline for the management of high blood pressure in adults: report from the panel members appointed to the Eighth Joint National Committee (JNC 8). *JAMA*. 2014;311:(5):507-520.
4. Brown MJ, Haydock S. Pathoetiology, epidemiology and diagnosis of hypertension. *Drugs*. 2000;59(suppl 2):1-12.
5. Sibai B. Treatment of hypertension in pregnant women. *N Engl J Med*. 1996;335:257-265.
6. McEvoy GK, ed. *AHFS 2000 Drug Information*. Bethesda, MD: American Society of Health-System Pharmacists; 2000:1658-1726.
7. Kaplan NM. Combination therapy for systemic hypertension. *Am J Cardiol*. 1995;76:595-597.
8. Abernethy DR. Pharmacological properties of combination therapies for hypertension. *Am J Hypertens*. 1997;10:13S-16S.
9. Reilly RF, Jackson EK. Regulation of renal function and vascular volume. In: Brunton LL, Chabner BA, Knollmann BC, eds. *Goodman and Gilman's the Pharmacological Basis of Therapeutics*. 12th ed. New York: McGraw-Hill; 2011:671-719.
10. Padilla MCA, Armas-Hernandez MJ, Hernandez RH, et al. Update of diuretics in the treatment of hypertension. *Am J Ther* 2007;14:154-160.
11. Supuran CT. Diuretics: from classical carbonic anhydrase inhibitors to novel applications of the sulfonamides. *Curr Pharm Des*. 2008;14:641-648.
12. Ernst ME, Moser M. Use of diuretics in patients with hypertension. *N Engl J Med*. 2009;361:2153-2164.
13. Ernst ME, Gordon JA. Diuretic therapy: key aspects in hypertension and renal disease. *J Nephrol*. 2010;23:487-493.
14. Cadwallader AB, de la Torre X, Tieri A, et al. The abuse of diuretics as performance-enhancing drugs and masking agents in sport doping: pharmacology, toxicology and analysis. *Brit J Pharmacol*. 2010;161:1-16.
15. Deventer K, Baele G, Van Eenoo P, et al. Stability of selected chlorinated thiazide diuretics. *J Pharm Biomed Anal*. 2009;49:519-524.
16. Nissenson AR, Weston RE, Kleeman CR. Mannitol. *West J Med*. 1979;131:277-284.
17. Mincione F, Menabuoni L, Supuran CT. Clinical applications of carbonic anhydrase inhibitors in ophthalmology. In: Supuran CT, Scozzafava A, Conway J, eds. *Carbonic Anhydrase Its Inhibitors and Activators*. Boca Raton: CRC Press; 2004:243-254.
18. Sprague JM. The chemistry of diuretics. *Ann NY Acad Sci*. 1958;71:328-342.
19. Maren TH. Relations between structure and biological activity of sulfonamides. *Annu Rev Pharmacol Toxicol*. 1976;16:309-327.
20. Fitzgerald D. Trails of discovery. A cornerstone of cardiovascular therapy: the thiazide diuretics. *Dialogues Cardiovasc Med*. 2005;10:175-182.
21. Tamargo J, Segura J, Ruilope LM. Diuretics in the treatment of hypertension. Part 1: thiazide and thiazide-like diuretics. *Expert Opin Pharmacother*. 2014;15:527-547.
22. Campbell DB, Taylor AR, Hopkins YW, et al. Pharmacokinetics and metabolism of indapamide: a review. *Curr Med Res Opin*. 1977;5(suppl S1):13-24.
23. Sun H, Moore C, Dansette PM, et al. Dehydrogenation of the indoline-containing drug 4-chloro-N-(2-methyl-1-indolinyl)-3-sulfamoylbenzamide (Indapamide) by CYP3A4: correlation with in silico predictions. *Drug Metab Dispos*. 2009;37:672-684.
24. Wargo KA, Banta WM. A comprehensive review of the loop diuretics: should furosemide be first line? *Ann Pharmacother*. 2009;43:1836-1847.
25. Tamargo J, Segura J, Ruilope LM. Diuretics in the treatment of hypertension. Part 2: loop diuretics and potassium-sparing agents. *Expert Opin Pharmacother*. 2014;15:605-621.
26. Beermann B, Dalen E, Lindstrom B et al. On the fate of furosemide in man. *Eur J Clin Pharmacol*. 1975;9:57-61.
27. Feit PW. Bumetanide – the way to its chemical structure. *J Clin Pharmacol*. 1981;21:531-536.
28. Blose JS, Adams KF, Patterson JH. Torsemide: a pyridine-sulfonylurea loop diuretic. *Ann Pharmacother*. 1995;29:396-402.
29. Koechel DA. Ethacrynic acid and related diuretics: relationship of structure to beneficial and detrimental actions. *Annu Rev Pharmacol Toxicol*. 1981;21:265-293.
30. Fogerson FM, Brennan FE, Fuller PJ. Mineralocorticoid receptor binding, structure and function. *Mol Cell Endocrinol*. 2004;217:203-212.
31. Garthwaite SM, McMahon EG. The evolution of aldosterone antagonists. *Mol Cell Endocrinol*. 2004;217:27-31.
32. Craft J. Eplerenone (Inspra), a new aldosterone antagonist for the treatment of systemic hypertension and heart failure. *Proc (Bayl Univ Med Cent)*. 2004;17:217-220.
33. Fagart J, Seguin C, Pinon GM, et al. The Met852 residue is a key organizer of the ligand-binding cavity of the human mineralocorticoid receptor. *Mol Pharmacol*. 2005;67:1714-1722.
34. Huyet J, Pinon GM, Fay MR et al. Structural basis of spironolactone recognition by the mineralocorticoid receptor. *Mol Pharmacol*. 2007;72:563-571.
35. de Gasparo M, Joss U, Ramjoue HP, et al. Three new epoxy-spironolactone derivatives: characterization in vivo and in vitro. *J Pharmacol Exp Ther*. 1987;240:650-656.
36. Rogerson FM, Yao Y, Smith BJ, et al. Differences in the determinants of eplerenone, spironolactone and aldosterone binding to the mineralocorticoid receptor. *Clin Exp Pharmacol Physiol*. 2004;31:704-709.
37. Ramsay L, Shelton J, Harrison I, et al. Spironolactone and potassium canrenoate in normal man. *Clin Pharmacol Ther*. 1976;20:167-177.
38. Overdiek HW, Merkus FW. The metabolism and biopharmaceutics of spironolactone in man. *Drug Metab Drug Interact*. 1987;5:273-302.
39. Cook CS, Berry LM, Bible RH, et al. Pharmacokinetics and metabolism of [^{14}C]eplerenone after oral administration to humans. *Drug Metab Dispos*. 2003;31:1448-1455.
40. Canessa CM, Schild L, Buell G, et al. Amiloride-sensitive epithelial Na^+ channel is made of three homologous subunits. *Nature*. 1994;367:463-467.
41. Busch AE, Suessbrich H, Kunzelmann K, et al. Blockade of epithelial Na^+ channels by triamterenes – underlying mechanisms and molecular basis. *Pflugers Arch Eur J Physiol*. 1996;432:760-766.
42. Fuhr U, Kober S, Zaigler M, et al. Rate-limiting biotransformation of triamterene is mediated by CYP1A2. *Int J Clin Pharmacol Ther*. 2005;43:327-334.
43. Hilal-Dandan R. Renin and angiotensin. In: Brunton LL, Chabner BA, Knollman BC, eds. *Goodman & Gilman's the Pharmacological Basis of Therapeutics*. 12th ed. New York: McGraw-Hill; 2011:721-744.
44. Skeggs L. Historical overview of the renin-angiotensin system. In: Doyle AE, Bearn AG, eds. *Hypertension and the Angiotensin System: Therapeutic Approaches*. New York: Raven Press; 1984:31-45.
45. Vallotton MB. The renin-angiotensin system. *Trends Pharmacol Sci*. 1987;8:69-74.
46. Skidgel RA, Kaplan AP, Erdos EG. Histamine, bradykinin, and their antagonists. In: Brunton LL, Chabner BA, Knollman BC, eds. *Goodman & Gilman's the Pharmacological Basis of Therapeutics*. 12th ed. New York: McGraw-Hill; 2011:911-935.
47. Ferrario CM, Brosnihan KB, Diz DI, et al. Angiotensin-(1–7): a new hormone of the angiotensin system. *Hypertension*. 1991;18(5 suppl):126-133.
48. Parker RB, Nappi JM, Cavallari LH. Chronic heart failure. In: Dipiro JT, Talbert RL, Yee GC, et al, eds. *Pharmacotherapy: A Pathophysiologic Approach*. 9th ed. New York: McGraw-Hill; 2014:85-122.

49. Agarwal SK, Chambless LE, Ballantyne CM, et al. Prediction of incident heart failure in general practice: the Atherosclerosis Risk in Communities (ARIC) study. *Circ Heart Fail.* 2012;5:422-429.
50. Harrold M. In: Lemke TL, Williams DA, Roche VF, Zito SW, eds. *Foye's Principles of Medicinal Chemistry.* 7th ed. Philadelphia: Wolters Kluwer/Lippincott Williams & Wilkins; 2013:747-780.
51. Ondetti MA, Rubin B, Cushman DW. Design of specific inhibitors of angiotensin-converting enzyme: new class of orally active antihypertensive agents. *Science.* 1977;196:441-444.
52. Cushman DW, Cheung HS, Sabo EF, et al. Design of potent competitive inhibitors of angiotensin-converting enzyme. Carboxyalkanoyl and mercaptoalkanoyl amino acids. *Biochemistry.* 1977;16:5484-5491.
53. Ondetti MA, Cushman DW. Enzymes of the renin-angiotensin system and their inhibitors. *Annu Rev Biochem.* 1982;51:283-308.
54. Ferreira SH, Bartelt DC, Lewis LJ. Isolation of bradykinin-potentiating peptides from Bothrops jararaca venom. *Biochemistry.* 1970;9:2583-2593.
55. Bakhle YS. Conversion of angiotensin I to angiotensin II by cell-free extracts of dog lung. *Nature.* 1968;220:919-921.
56. Stryer L. *Biochemistry.* 4th ed. New York: Freeman and Company; 1995:218-222.
57. Klaassen CD. Heavy metals and heavy-metal antagonists. Brunton L, Lazo J, Parker K, et al, eds. *Goodman & Gilman's the Pharmacological Basis of Therapeutics.* 11th ed. New York: McGraw-Hill; 2006:1753-1775.
58. Atkinson AB, Robertson JIS. Captopril in the treatment of clinical hypertension and cardiac failure. *Lancet.* 1979;2:836-839.
59. Patchett AA, Harris E, Tristram EW, et al. A new class of angiotensin-converting enzyme inhibitors. *Nature.* 1980;288:280-283.
60. Krapcho J, Turk C, Cushman DW, et al. Angiotensin-converting enzyme inhibitors. Mercaptan, carboxyalkyl dipeptide, and phosphinic acid inhibitors incorporating 4-substituted prolines. *J Med Chem.* 1988;31:1148-1160.
61. Timmermans PB, Wong PC, Chiu AT, et al. Angiotensin II receptors and angiotensin II receptor antagonists. *Pharmacol Rev.* 1993;45:205-213.
62. Skeggs L, Kahn JR, Lentz K, et al. Preparation, purification and amino acid sequence of a polypeptide renin substrate. *J Exp Med.* 1957;106:439-453.
63. Sepehrdad R, Frishman WH, Steier C, et al. Direct inhibition of renin as a cardiovascular pharmacotherapy: focus on aliskiren. *Cardiol Rev.* 2007;15:242-256.
64. Maibaum J, Stutz S, Goschke R, et al. Structural modification of the P2' position of 2,7-dialkyl-substituted 5(S)-amino-4(S)-hydroxy-8-phenyl-octanecarboxamides: the discovery of aliskiren, a potent nonpeptide human renin inhibitor active after once daily dosing in marmosets. *J Med Chem.* 2007;50:4832-4844.
65. Fisher NDL, Hollenberg NK. Renin inhibition: what are the therapeutic opportunities? *J Am Soc Nephrol.* 2005;16:592-599.
66. Clinical Pharmacology Online. Gold Standard Elsevier, 2017. Available at: http://clinicalpharmacology.com. Accessed October 2017.
67. Facts & Comparisons eAnswers. St. Louis, MO: Wolters Kluwer Health. Available at: http://www.wolterskluwercdi.com/facts-comparisons-online. Accessed October 2017.
68. James PA, Oparil S, Carter BL, et.al. 2014 evidence-based guideline for the management of high blood pressure in adults. *JAMA.* 2014;311(5):507-520.
69. Yancy CW, Jessup M, Bozkurt B, et al. 2017 ACC/AHA/HFSA focused update of the 2013 ACCF/AHA guideline for the management of heart failure. *Circulation.* 2017;136:e137-e161.
70. Saseen JJ, MacLaughlin EJ. Hypertension. In: Dipiro JT, Talbert RL, Yee GC, et al, eds. *Pharmacotherapy: A Pathophysiologic Approach.* 9th ed. New York: McGraw-Hill; 2014:49-84.
71. Bauer JH, Reams GP. The angiotensin II type 1 receptor antagonists: a new class of antihypertensive drugs. *Arch Intern Med.* 1995;155:1361-1368.
72. Aliskiren (Tekturna) for hypertension. *Med Lett Drugs Ther.* 2007;49:29-31.
73. Lacourciere Y, Brunner H, Irwin R, et al. Effects of modulators of the renin-angiotensin-aldosterone system on cough. Losartan Cough Study Group. *J Hypertens.* 1994;12:1387-1393.
74. Micromedex Solutions. Truven Health Analytics. Available at https://truvenhealth.com/products/micromedex. Accessed October 2017.
75. Gringauz A. *Introduction to Medicinal Chemistry.* New York: Wiley; 1997:450-461.
76. SciFindeer. Calculated Using Advanced Chemistry Development (ACD/Lab) Software V8.14 for Solaris (1994–2005 ACD/Lab) (V8.19 Used for Perindolpril).
77. Gross DM, Sweet CS, Ulm EH, et al. Effect of N-[(S)-1-carboxy-3-phenylpropyl]-L-Ala-L-Pro and its ethyl ester (MK-421) on angiotensin converting enzyme in vitro and angiotensin I pressor responses in vivo. *J Pharmacol Exp Ther.* 1981;216:552-557.
78. Ulm EH, Hichens M, Gomez HJ, et al. Enalapril maleate and a lysine analogue (MK-521): disposition in man. *Br J Clin Pharmacol.* 1982;14:357-362.
79. Oparil S, Koerner T, Tregear GW, et al. Substrate requirements for angiotensin I conversion in vivo and in vitro. *Circ Res.* 1973;32:415-423.
80. Carini DJ, Duncia JV, Aldrich PE, et al. Nonpeptide angiotensin II receptor antagonists: the discovery of a series of N-(biphenylylmethyl)imidazoles as potent, orally active antihypertensives. *J Med Chem.* 1991;35:2525-2547.
81. Lunney EA, Hamilton HW, Hodges JC, et al. Analyses of ligand binding in five endothiapepsin crystal complexes and their use in the design and evaluation of novel renin inhibitors. *J Med Chem.* 1993;36:3809-3820.
82. Matter H, Scheiper B, Steinhagen H, et al. Structure-based design and optimization of potent renin inhibitors on 5- or 7-azaindole-scaffolds. *Bio Med Chem Lett.* 2011;21:5487-5492.
83. Cutler SJ. Cardiovascular agents. In: Block JH, Beale JM, eds. *Wilson and Gisvold's Textbook of Organic Medicinal and Pharmaceutical ChemistrAliskiren (Tekturna) for Hypertensiony.* 12th ed. Philadelphia: Lippincott Williams & Wilkins; 2011:617-665.
84. Silverthorn DU. *Human Physiology: An Integrated Approach.* Upper Saddle River, NJ: Prentice Hall; 1998:325-361.
85. Janis RA, Triggle DJ. New developments in Ca^{2+} channel antagonists. *J Med Chem.* 1983;26:775-785.
86. Swamy VC, Triggle DJ. Calcium channel blockers. In: Craig CR, Stitzel RE, eds. *Modern Pharmacology with Clinical Applications.* 5th ed. Boston: Little, Brown; 1997:229-234.
87. Michel T, Hoffman BB. Treatment of myocardial ischemia and hypertension. In: Brunton LL, Chabner BA, Knollman BC, eds. *Goodman & Gilman's the Pharmacological Basis of Therapeutics,* 12th ed. New York: McGraw-Hill; 2011:745-788.
88. American Heart Association. Heart Disease and Stroke Statistics 2017 At-a-Glance. Available at: http://www.heart.org/HEARTORG/General/Heart-and-Stroke-Association-Statistics_UCM_319064_SubHomePage.jsp. Accessed October 2017.
89. Vaghy PL. Calcium antagonists. In: Brody TM, Larner J, Minneman KP, et al, eds. *Human Pharmacology: Molecular to Clinical,* 2nd ed. St. Louis: Mosby; 1994:203-213.
90. Triggle DJ. Drugs acting on ion channels and membranes. In: Hansch C, Sammes PG, Taylor JB, eds. *Comprehensive Medicinal Chemistry.* Vol. 3. Oxford, UK: Pergamon Press; 1990:1047-1099.
91. Loev B, Ehrreich SJ, Tedeschi RE. Dihydropyridines with potent hypotensive activity prepared by the Hantzsch reaction. *J Pharm Pharmacol.* 1972;24:917-918.
92. Loev B, Goodman MM, Snader KM, et al. "Hantzsch-type" dihydropyridine hypotensive agents. *J Med Chem.* 1974;17:956-965.
93. Triggle AM, Shefter E, Triggle DJ. Crystal structures of calcium channel antagonists: 2,6-dimethyl-3,5-dicarbomethoxy-4-[2-nitro, 3-cyano-, 4-(dimethylamino)-, and 2,3,4,5,6-pentafluorophenyl]-1,4-dihydropyridine. *J Med Chem.* 1980;23:1442-1445.

94. Safety of calcium-channel blockers. *Med Lett Drugs Ther.* 1997;39:13-14.
95. Varadi G, Mori Y, Mikala G, et al. Molecular determinants of Ca^{2+} channel function and drug action. *Trends Pharmacol Sci.* 1995;16:43-49.
96. Gilmore J, Dell C, Bowman D, et al. Neuronal calcium channels. *Annu Rep Med Chem.* 1995;30:51-60.
97. Calculated Using ChemBioDraw Ultra Software V12.0 (1986–2009), Cambridge Soft, http://www.cambridgesoft.com.
98. Bailey DG, Arnold JMO, Spence JD. Grapefruit juice and drugs: how significant is the interaction? *Clin Pharmacokinet.* 1994;26:91-98.
99. Drug interactions with grapefruit juice. *Med Lett Drugs Ther.* 2004;46:2-4.
100. Sampson KJ, Kass RS. Anti-arrhythmic drugs. In: Brunton LL, Chabner BA, Knollman BC, eds. *Goodman & Gilman's the Pharmacological Basis of Therapeutics*. 12th ed. New York: McGraw-Hill; 2011:815-848.
101. Yeh D, Michel T. Pharmacology of vascular tone. In: Goan DE, Tashjian A, Armstrong E, et al, eds. *Principles of Pharmacology: The Pathophysiologic Basis of Drug Therapy*. Baltimore, MD: Lippincott Williams & Wilkins; 2004:317-330.
102. Von Euler US. Synthesis, uptake, and storage of catecholamines in adrenergic nerves: the effect of drugs. In: Blaschko H, Marshall E, eds. *Catecholamines*. New York: Springer; 1972:186-230.
103. Griffith RK. Adrenergics and adrenergic-blocking drugs. In: Abraham DJ, ed. *Burger's Medicinal Chemistry and Drug Discovery*. Hoboken, NJ: John Wiley and Sons; 2003:1-37.
104. Ahlquist RP. A study of the adrenotropic receptors. *Am J Physiol.* 1948;153:586-600.
105. Harrison JK, Pearson WR, Lynch KR. Molecular characterization of α_1- and α_2-adrenoceptors. *Trends Pharmacol Sci.* 1991;12:62-67.
106. De Souza CJ, Burkey BF. β_3-Adrenoceptor agonists as anti-diabetic and antiobesity drugs in humans. *Curr Pharm Des.* 2001;7:1433-1449.
107. Robertson JIS. State-of-the-art review: β-blockade and the treatment of hypertension. *Drugs.* 1983;25(suppl 2):5-11.
108. Freis ED, Papademetriou V. Current drug treatment and treatment patterns with antihypertensive drugs. *Drugs.* 1996;52:1-16.
109. Husserl FE, Messerli FH. Adverse effects of antihypertensive drugs. *Drugs.* 1981;22:188-210.
110. Goldberg M, Fenster PE. Clinical significance of intrinsic sympathomimetic activity of beta blockers. *Drug Therapy.* 1991:35-43.
111. Moran NC. New adrenergic blocking drugs: their pharmacological, biochemical, and clinical actions. *Ann NY Acad Sci.* 1967;139:545-548.
112. Jen T, Frazee JS, Schwartz MS, et al. Adrenergic agents. 8. Synthesis and β-adrenergic agonist activity of some 3-*tert*-butylamino-2-(substituted phenyl)-1-propanols. *J Med Chem.* 1977;20:1263-1268.
113. Cauffield JS, Gums JG, Curry RW. Alpha blockers: a reassessment of their role in therapy. *Am Fam Physician.* 1996;54:263-270.
114. Scriabine A, Constantine JW, Hess HJ, et al. Pharmacological studies with some new antihypertensive aminoquinazolines. *Experientia.* 1968;24:1150-1151.
115. Dunn CJ, Lea AP, Wagstaff AJ. Carvedilol. A reappraisal of its pharmacological properties and therapeutic use in cardiovascular disorders. *Drugs.* 1997;54:161-185.
116. Goa KL, Benfield P, Sorkin EM. Labetalol: a reappraisal of its pharmacology, pharmacokinetics and therapeutic use in hypertension and ischemic heart disease. *Drugs.* 1989;37:583-627.
117. Van Zwieten PA. An overview of the pharmacodynamic properties and therapeutic potential of combined α- and β-adrenoreceptor antagonists. *Drugs.* 1993;45:509-517.
118. Fujimura A, Ebihara A, Ohashi K-I, et al. Comparison of the pharmacokinetics, pharmacodynamics and safety of oral (Catapres) and transdermal (M-5041T) clonidine in healthy subjects. *J Clin Pharmacol.* 1994;34:260-265.
119. Cornish LA. Guanfacine hydrochloride. A centrally acting antihypertensive agent. *Clin Pharm.* 1988;7:187-197.
120. Bousquet P, Feldman J. Drugs acting on imidazoline receptors. A review of their pharmacology, their use in blood pressure control and their potential interest in cardioprotection. *Drugs.* 1999;58:799-812.
121. Piletz JE, Regunathan S, Ernsberger P. Agmatine and imidazolines: their novel receptors and enzymes. *Ann NY Acad Sci.* 2003;1009-1043.
122. Dardonville C, Rozas I. Imidazoline binding sites and their ligands: an overview of the different chemical structures. *Med Res Rev.* 2004;24:639-661.
123. Ebihara A, Fujimura A, Ohashi K-I, et al. Influence of application site of a new transdermal clonidine M-5041T on its pharmacokinetics and pharmacodynamics in healthy subjects. *J Clin Pharmacol.* 1993;33:1188-1191.
124. Holmes B, Brogden RN, Heel RC, et al. Guanabenz. A review of its pharmacodynamic properties and therapeutic efficacy in hypertension. *Drugs.* 1983;26:212-225.
125. Kobinger W. Central α-adrenergic systems as targets for hypotensive drugs. *Rev Physiol Biochem Pharmacol.* 1978;81:39-100.
126. Kanagy NL. α_2-Adrenergic receptor signaling in hypertension. *Clin Sci (Lond).* 2005;109:431-437.
127. Skerjanec A, Campbell NRC, Robertson S, et al. Pharmacokinetics and presystemic gut metabolism of methyldopa in healthy human subjects. *J Clin Pharmacol.* 1995;35:275-280.
128. Langley MS, Heel RC. Transdermal clonidine. A preliminary review of its pharmacodynamic properties and therapeutic efficacy. *Drugs.* 1988;35:123-142.
129. Ziegler D, Haxhiu MA, Kaan EC, et al. Pharmacology of moxonidine, an I_1–imidazoline receptor agonist. *J Cardiovascular Pharmacol.* 1996;27(suppl 3):S26-S37.
130. Theodor R, Weimann HJ, Weber W, et al. Absolute bioavailability of moxonidine. *Eur J Drug Metab Pharmacokinet.* 1991;16:153-159.
131. Chrisp P, Faulds D. Moxonidine: a review of its pharmacology and therapeutic use in essential hypertension. *Drugs.* 1992;44:993-1012.
132. Genissel P, Bromet N, Fourtillan JB, et al. Pharmacokinetics of rilmenidine in healthy subjects. *Am J Cardiol.* 1988;61:47D-53D.
133. Genissel P, Bromet N. Pharmacokinetics of rilmenidine. *Am J Med.* 1989;87:8S-23S.
134. Sorkin EM, Heel RC. Guanfacine: a review of its pharmacodynamic and pharmacokinetic properties and therapeutic efficacy in the treatment of hypertension. *Drugs.* 1986;31:301-336.
135. Carchman SH, Crowe JT, Wright GJ. The bioavailability and pharmacokinetics of guanfacine after oral and intravenous administration to healthy volunteers. *J Clin Pharmacol.* 1987;27:762-767.
136. Duty S, Weston AH. Potassium channel openers. Pharmacological effects and future uses. *Drugs.* 1990;40:785-791.
137. Campese VM. Minoxidil: a review of its pharmacological properties and therapeutic use. *Drugs.* 1981;22:257-278.

Clinical Scenario

Michael W. Perry, PharmD, BCPS, BCCCP

CHEMICAL ANALYSIS

Esmolol is unique from all other selective β_1 receptor blockers in that its structure contains an ester functional group located *para* to the required oxypropanolamine group. Similar to atenolol and other selective β_1 receptor, the *para* side chain contains hydrogen bonding groups not present in nonselective β blockers. Additionally, the isopropyl chain connected to the secondary amine is optimal for β_1 receptor binding. The ester allows for rapid hydrolysis by plasma esterases, resulting in a very short duration of action ($t_{½}$ ~ 9 min) and the need for continuous IV infusion. As stated above, this chemical feature is clinically useful in allowing for rapid changes in infusion rate and the control of the patient's heart rate. The resulting metabolite contains a carboxylic acid, is unable to form the same bonds as the original ester, and is inactive.

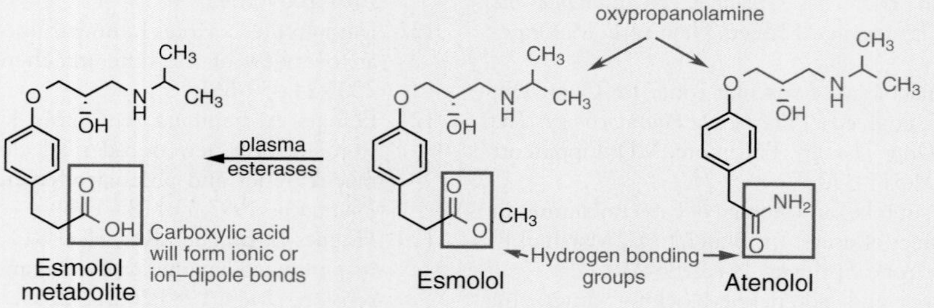

oxypropanolamine
plasma esterases
Carboxylic acid will form ionic or ion–dipole bonds
Esmolol metabolite
Esmolol
Hydrogen bonding groups
Atenolol

Similar to esmolol, clevidipine is the only 1,4-DHP that contains an easily accessible, isolated ester on one of its side chains. The presence of this ester allows for rapid hydrolysis by plasm esterases ($t_{½}$ = 2-4 min) and rapid titration to achieve the desired blood pressure. Analogous to esmolol, the resulting metabolite is inactive due to the presence of a carboxylic acid in a receptor-binding region that lacks the ability to form ionic or ion-dipole bonds with this functional group. As discussed earlier in this chapter, the nitrogen atom of the 1,4-DHPs is part of a conjugated carbamate in which its electrons are involved in resonance delocalization. As such, this nitrogen atom is weakly basic and not ionized. In comparing the structures and the calculated log P values (Table 17.19) of clevidipine (log P = 2.96) and nicardipine (log P = 4.27), it is found that nicardipine is more lipid soluble despite the presence of a tertiary amine. This is primarily due to the presence of the adjacent aromatic ring. In addition to its lipid solubility, this ring imparts some steric hindrance to ionization of the tertiary amine (pK_a = 8.2). Both of these drugs are highly lipid soluble and require special formulations in order to allow for parenteral administration. Acidification of the IV solution for nicardipine (pH = 3.7-4.7) ensures higher ionization of the tertiary amine and increases the ability to concentrate it as an IV formulation. Unfortunately, this formulation can cause venous irritation as noted above. The structure of clevidpine does not contain a basic amine; hence, the drug is not ionized at physiological pH, has poor dissolution characteristics, and must be formulated as a lipid emulsion.

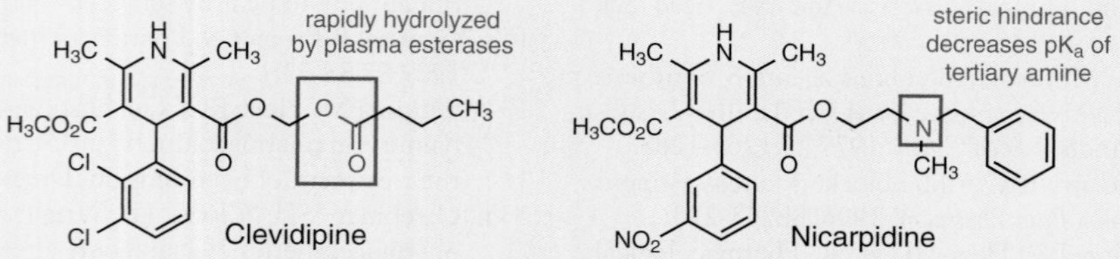

rapidly hydrolyzed by plasma esterases
Clevidipine
steric hindrance decreases pK_a of tertiary amine
Nicarpidine

A few final comments regarding VT's antihypertensive medications. When he arrived at the hospital, he stated that he was prescribed both clonidine and hydralazine and that he was allergic to lisinopril (dry cough). According to current guidelines, neither clonidine nor hydralazine is recommended as either first- or second-line therapy. During the course of his hospital stay, VT has been prescribed a calcium channel blocker and β receptor blocker due to his overall presentation and therapeutic needs. As described in this chapter, VT's dry cough is not the result of an allergic reaction but is due to the inhibition of bradykinin breakdown by lisinopril. Lisinopril, as well as all ACEIs, inhibit kininase II and enhance the levels of both bradykinin and prostaglandins (Fig. 17.8). These two biomolecules have been proposed to be responsible for the dry cough. If VT's hypertension is not managed by oral labetalol formulation and a 1,4-DHP, such as amlodipine, the addition of an ARB could be considered, as they block the renin-angiotensin pathway without interfering with bradykinin metabolism.

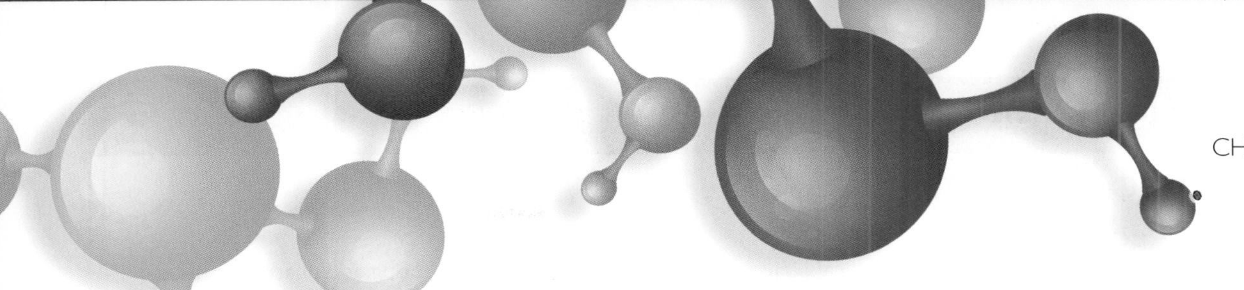

CHAPTER 18

Drugs Used to Treat Coagulation Disorders

Anand Sridhar

Drugs covered in this chapter:

WARFARIN

HEPARINS
- High molecular weight heparin
- Low molecular weight heparin
- Dalteparin
- Enoxaparin
- Fondaparinux

DIRECT THROMBIN INHIBITORS
- Argatroban
- Bivalirudin
- Desirudin
- Dabigatran etexilate
- Idarucizumab (Praxbind; for dabigatran reversal)

ANTIFACTOR XA INHIBITORS
- Apixaban
- Betrixaban
- Edoxaban
- Rivaroxaban
- Andexanet alfa (Andexxa; for factor Xa inhibitor reversal)

ANTIPLATELET DRUGS
- Abciximab
- Aspirin
- Cilostazol
- Clopidogrel
- Dipyridamole
- Eptifibatide
- Prasugrel
- Ticagrelor
- Ticlopidine
- Tirofiban

THROMBIN RECEPTOR (PAR-1) AGONISTS
- Vorapaxar

OLIGONUCLEOTIDES
- Defibrotide

THROMBOLYTIC DRUGS
- Alteplase
- Reteplase
- Streptokinase
- Tenecteplase

COAGULANTS
- Protamine
- Vitamin K

THROMBOPOIETIN RECEPTOR AGONISTS
- Eltrombopag
- Romiplostim

ANTIFIBRINOLYTIC AGENTS
- Tranexamic acid
- ε-Aminocaproic acid

Abbreviations

ADP adenosine diphosphate
aPTT activated partial thromboplastin time
ATP adenosine triphosphate
a-Xa U antifactor Xa units
cAMP cyclic adenosine monophosphate
COX cyclooxygenase
CYP cytochrome P450
DTI direct thrombin inhibitor
DVT deep vein thrombosis
FDA U.S. Food and Drug Administration
FXa activated factor X
GP glycoprotein
HIT heparin-induced thrombocytopenia
5-HT serotonin
HTB 2-hydroxy-4-trifluoromethylbenzoic acid
IC_{50} half maximal inhibitory concentration
INR international normalized ratio
ITP idiopathic thrombocytopenia purpura
KH_2 vitamin K hydroquinone
LMWH low molecular weight heparin
MI myocardial infarction
NSAID nonsteroidal anti-inflammatory drug
PAI-1 plasminogen activator inhibitor 1
PAR-1 protease-activated receptor 1
PDE phosphodiesterase
PE pulmonary embolism
PF4 platelet factor 4
PGI_2 prostacyclin
PT prothrombin time
TF tissue factor
TFPI tissue factor pathway inhibitor
tPA tissue-type plasminogen activator
TXA_2 thromboxane A_2
USP U.S. Pharmacopeia
V_d volume of distribution
VKORC1 vitamin K 2,3-epoxide reductase complex 1
VTE venous thromboembolism
vWF von Willebrand factor

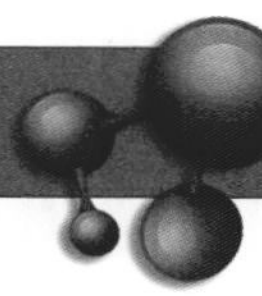

CLINICAL SIGNIFICANCE

ANTICOAGULANTS

Dr. Kathryn A. Connor, BCPS, BCNSP

Anticoagulants are among the highest-risk drugs in clinical pharmacy and require frequent monitoring and pharmacist intervention, across multiple practice settings. Other health care providers and patients will rely on the pharmacy clinician's knowledge of medicinal chemistry principles and pharmacology of the anticoagulants to facilitate safe and effective treatment for vulnerable patients. However, it can be challenging to balance the risks-versus-benefits of anticoagulant use in complex patients, e.g., those who have both active clot burden and risk for bleeding, those with organ dysfunction, for patients who will accept certain anticoagulants but not others, and in emergent reversal and perioperative anticoagulation situations. It is critical for pharmacists to understand the principles of the clotting cascade, clot formation and lysis, and how specific drugs affect these processes. Clinicians must apply their knowledge of anticoagulant mechanisms of action, pharmacokinetics and pharmacodynamics, and structure-activity relationships in caring for individual patients to optimize care in preventing and managing thrombogenesis. For example, when considering pharmacologic thrombolysis options, it can be clinically advantageous that tenectaplase has higher fibrin specificity and a longer half-life than alteplase and can be given as a single dose. In the hospital, unfractionated heparin is commonly used over low-molecular weight heparin (LMWH) for venous thromboembolism (VTE) prophylaxis in patients who are at a higher risk of bleeding, as unfractionated heparin has a shorter half-life and is more reversible with protamine. Pharmacists will also be expected to provide education on and appropriately integrate newly approved drugs into day-to-day clinical practice, e.g., idarucizumab (a newer drug that is FDA-approved for dabigatran reversal) and andexanet alfa (FDA-approved to reverse apixaban or rivaroxaban), along with a multitude of older agents, such as warfarin, aspirin, clopidogrel, and unfractionated heparin.

Clinical Scenario

Kathryn A. Connor, PharmD, BCPS, Anand Sridhar, PhD

SCENARIO

RC is a 64-year-old man who is admitted to the medical ICU for a COPD exacerbation. His platelet count is 275,000/mm^3 on admission, and he is started on prophylactic subcutaneous unfractionated heparin for VTE prophylaxis. Seven days later, his platelet count has decreased to 108,000/mm^3. He has normal renal and hepatic function. The ICU provider is concerned for heparin-induced thrombocytopenia (HIT) and discusses the likelihood of a HIT diagnosis with the multidisciplinary team. It is decided that the clinical suspicion of HIT is intermediate to high, and additional laboratory testing should be ordered to help diagnosis HIT. Additional recommendations include (1) that heparin administration be stopped and (2) an alternative anticoagulant agent that has no cross-reactivity with heparin should be started.

OUTCOME

The hematology team was consulted to help manage HIT in this critically ill patient. Commonly used alternative anticoagulant options for the management of HIT include bivalirudin, argatroban, and fondaparinux. The patient was started on bivalirudin, a direct thrombin inhibitor, at 0.15 mg/kg/hr via IV infusion and the rate was adjusted to maintain a therapeutic aPTT. Two days later the HIT diagnostic laboratory results were finalized, and it is indicated that the patient likely has HIT. Bivalirudin was continued, and the patient recovered from his COPD exacerbation. His platelet count slowly increased to above 200,000/mm^3. The patient was transitioned to warfarin, which was continued for 4 weeks. The patient was discharged to home and did not suffer any thrombotic or bleeding complications.

Chemical Analysis found immediately after References.

Venous thromboembolism (VTE) is a vascular disorder that affects approximately half a million individuals in the US annually. VTE is defined as deep vein thrombosis (DVT) or pulmonary embolism (PE), or a combination of both. DVT progresses to PE in 600,000 of these patients, and results in the death of 200,000 from PE. Furthermore, nearly a third of patients with extensive DVT are also likely to develop postphlebitic syndrome. Thus, VTE is a growing public health concern in the United States due to its high morbidity and mortality.[1] The etiology of VTE is still unclear but is believed to be multifactorial in nature. Identified risk factors include genetic elements (e.g., family history, antithrombin deficiency), acquired conditions (e.g., advanced age, obesity), and transiently acquired risk factors (e.g., hospitalization, immobilization, surgery). The prevention and treatment of VTE involves the use of different classes of anticoagulant drugs.[2]

The discovery of the medical effects of heparin led to the development of orally active anticoagulants for prophylaxis in VTE and other thrombotic disorders.[3] The narrow therapeutic indices of warfarin and coumarins, alongside frequent drug monitoring and dose adjustment aspects, make this class of drugs challenging to work with.[4,5] Thus, further development of novel anticoagulation agents with targeted specificity on the coagulation cascade, accompanied by predictable ADME profiles, and with minimal continuous monitoring requirements is still required for treating platelet disorders.[6-8]

Thrombolytics are drugs that dissolve the newly formed thrombi in conditions such as DVT, PE, or myocardial infarction (MI). However, these agents are contraindicated with many other therapeutic agents as they may cause internal bleeding.

A variety of pathologic and toxicologic conditions can result in excessive bleeding from inadequate coagulation. Depending on the etiology and severity of the hemorrhagic episode, specific coagulants that induce blood coagulation are therapeutically used to prevent excessive bleeding.

Disease States Requiring Antithrombotic Therapy

In Western society, thrombotic conditions are the major cause of morbidity and mortality. It is believed that these disorders will be the leading cause of death worldwide within two decades.[9,10] As would be expected from the gravity of thrombotic disorders, many of the conditions involve the major vasculature, heart, brain, and lungs.

In the heart, a thrombotic condition may be involved in the disease state of acute MI, valvular heart disease, unstable angina, and atrial fibrillation. Surgical procedures, such as percutaneous transluminal coronary angioplasty and prosthetic heart valve replacement, may also lead to thrombotic conditions. Other thrombotic conditions involving the vasculature include VTE, primary and secondary prevention of arterial thromboembolism, and peripheral vascular disease. PE and cerebrovascular accidents are the most significant conditions affecting the lungs and the brain. Anticoagulation therapy is indicated for these conditions.

Venous Thromboembolism and Pulmonary Embolism

VTE occurs when erythrocytes, leukocytes, platelets, and fibrin coagulate to form a clot (thrombus) within an intact cardiovascular system.[11] A patient undergoing orthopedic surgery incurs the greatest risk for VTE.[2,12] PE results when a portion of a thrombus arising from VTE detaches itself from the blood vessel, travels in the blood, and lodges within the pulmonary arteries. Thus, the proper detection and treatment of VTE and PE is critical. Improper management can lead to recurrent VTE and postthrombotic syndrome, characterized by persistent pain, swelling, skin discoloration, ulceration, and necrosis of the affected tissue.[9,13]

Atrial Fibrillation

Atrial fibrillation is a common cardiac arrhythmia, found in more than 2.5 million Americans. It is one of the leading risk factors for ischemic stroke for individuals over the age of 50 years.[14-16] Atrial fibrillation is more prevalent in males than in females, with the median age of afflicted patients being 72 years. For patients with atrial fibrillation, effective treatment includes the modification of lifestyle and management of risk factors (e.g., hypertension, obesity), alongside the use of cardiovascular drugs such as anticoagulants and antiarrhythmic agents.[17,18]

Pathophysiology of Thrombogenesis

Arterial thrombosis usually occurs in medium-sized vessels that become thrombogenic due to surface lesions resulting from atherosclerosis.[6,19] Arterial thrombosis involves a platelet-rich clot, while venous thrombosis is caused by blood pooling (stasis), ineffective activation of the coagulation cascade, or vascular trauma (e.g., surgery). The latter is known as Virchow's triad.[11] Venous thrombi are usually rich in fibrin and contain fewer platelets than arterial thrombi. A dislodged clot that floats in the vasculature is termed an embolus. Both thrombi and emboli are dangerous as they can occlude blood vessels and deprive tissues of oxygen and key nutrients. As such, arterial thrombi cause serious conditions through localized occlusive ischemia, whereas venous thrombi give rise to pleural embolic complications.

Biochemical Mechanism of Blood Coagulation: The Coagulation Cascade

The formation of a blood clot happens through a cascade of biochemical reactions that sequentially modify specific plasma factors, from their inactive to activated forms (Fig. 18.1).

Coagulation is initiated by tissue factor (TF; thromboplastin), a small molecular weight glycoprotein that initiates the TF pathway (also known as the extrinsic pathway).[5,6] The TF glycoprotein is expressed on the surface of macrophages and is a major initiating factor of arterial thrombogenesis. As shown in Figure 18.1, TF binds and activates factor VII to form the TF-VIIa activated complex. The TF-VIIa complex activates two factors, *viz.*, factor X (extrinsic pathway) and factor IX (intrinsic pathway). This results in the formation of the corresponding activated factors, factor Xa and factor IXa, respectively.

Initiation of the contact activation pathway (also known as the intrinsic pathway) arises from the sequential transformation of factors XII, XI, and IX to their active forms. In the presence of calcium ions, factor IXa binds to factor VIIIa on the surface of activated platelets. This results in an intrinsic factor Xase complex, which promotes the conversion of factor X to factor Xa. Thus, factor Xa is a common node of the two pathways.

The coagulation cascade is unique in that the activated form of a specific factor catalyzes the activation of the next factor in the cascade. The final steps in the coagulation cascade involve the activation of factor

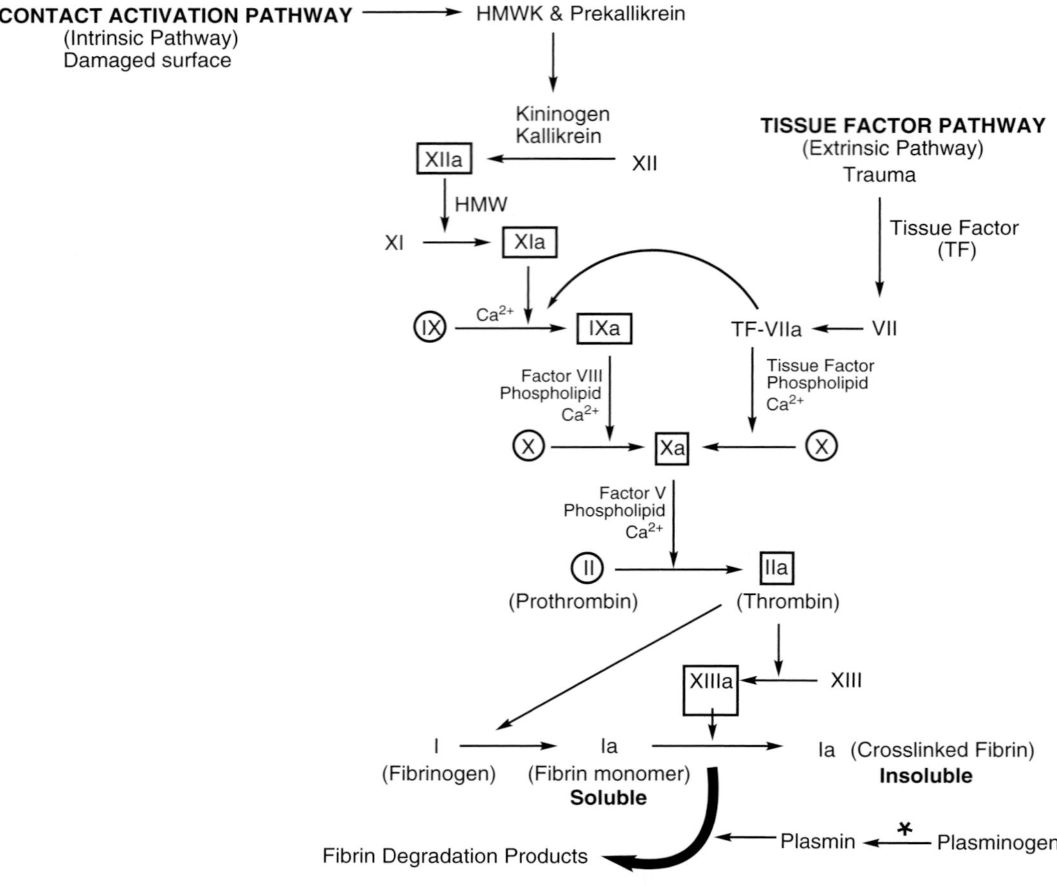

Figure 18.1 The coagulation cascade. *Circled factors* are those inhibited by warfarin-like drugs; *boxed factors* are those affected by heparin. The * indicates the site of action of thrombolytic drugs, such as streptokinase and urokinase.

II (prothrombin) to liberate factor IIa (thrombin; Fig. 18.2) via the prothrombinase complex (factors Va and Xa). Furthermore, thrombin catalyzes the conversion of fibrinogen to soluble fibrin, which turns insoluble by the action of XIIIa. Factor XIIIa is a transamidase that catalyzes the formation of cross-linked isopeptide bonds between the lysine and glutamine side chains (Fig. 18.3). The contact activation pathway helps maintain homeostasis.

Strategies for Regulating Coagulation

The regulation of coagulation occurs at several levels.[5,13] These levels include TF pathway inhibitors (TFPIs), antithrombin, and the protein C pathways. The design of many new anticoagulant drugs is directed at enhancing either endogenous anticoagulant or fibrinolytic mechanisms.

TFPIs modulate factor VIIa/TF catalytic activity by a two-step process, which results in the inhibition of the

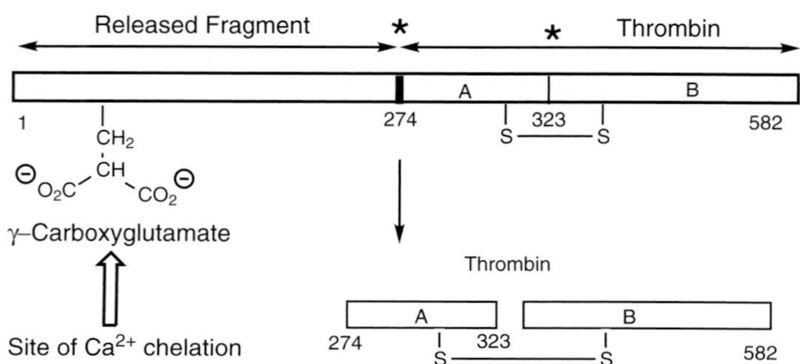

Figure 18.2 Structure of prothrombin. Thrombin is liberated through the cleavage of the Arg274-Thr275 and Arg323-Ile324 peptide bonds (indicated by the *red stars*). The γ-carboxyglutamate residues are in the released N-terminal portion of prothrombin and are not part of thrombin. The A and B chains of thrombin are joined by a disulfide bond.

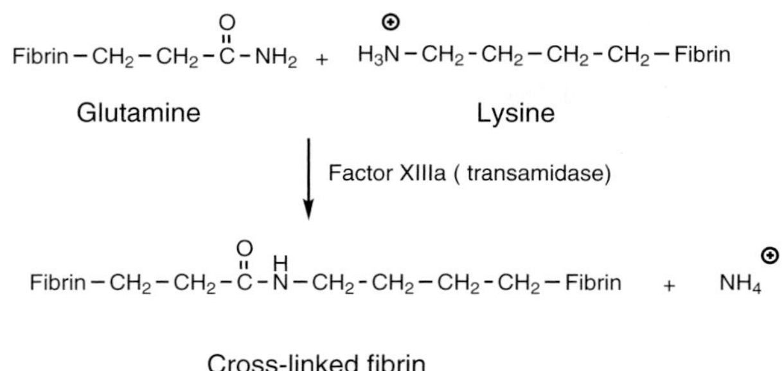

Figure 18.3 Cross-linking of soluble fibrin monomers (factor Ia) through the activity of factor XIIIa, a transamidase enzyme.

extrinsic pathway.[20] First, a TFPI molecule binds and inactivates factor Xa by forming the TFPI-Xa complex. In the next step, this TFPI-Xa/complex binds to factor VIIa within the TF-VIIa complex to modulate its catalytic activity. Additionally, TFPI potentiates the effect of heparins. The injection of either unfractionated heparin or low molecular weight heparins (LMWHs) provides increased local concentrations of TFPIs at sites of tissue damage and ongoing thrombosis, and reduces coagulation.[21] When TFPI concentrations are low, the propagation of coagulation will continue.[13]

Antithrombin is a potent inhibitor of thrombin and factors IXa and Xa. It also has inhibitory actions on other clotting factors, such as the TF-VIIa complex. Antithrombin action is enhanced more than 2,000-fold in the presence of heparin and is reduced in the absence of heparin.[5] Although heparin is not naturally found in the blood, the vascular endothelium is rich in heparan sulfate. Heparan sulfate contains the antithrombin-binding pentasaccharide sequence of heparin. Fondaparinux affects coagulation by inactivating factor Xa, which results in the inhibition of thrombin formation.[5,13] Direct thrombin inhibitors (DTIs; e.g., hirudin, argatroban) work by inhibiting both clot-bound thrombin and free thrombin, which prevents fibrin formation in the final step of the coagulation cascade.[5,13]

Thrombomodulin is a thrombin receptor found in the endothelium. In the protein C pathway, thrombin binds to thrombomodulin. The resulting conformational change converts thrombin into a potent activator of protein C, a vitamin K–dependent protein. Activated protein C consequently degrades and inactivates factors Va and VIIa, which in turn reduces thrombus formation.[22,23]

General Approaches to Anticoagulant Therapy

Overview

Current therapeutic agents target only a few specific areas within the coagulation cascade to effect anticoagulation. The factors governing the selection of an appropriate anticoagulant include patient-specific factors, underlying diagnosis of the disease state, location of the clot, and ultimate goal of the therapeutic intervention. If the therapeutic goal is to dissolve an existing clot, then the activation of plasminogen with the thrombolytic agent is the conventional approach. If the therapeutic goal is the prevention of thrombus formation, then the inhibition of an activated factor higher up in the cascade (with heparin and other oral anticoagulants) is the most appropriate strategy.

Some key properties of an ideal anticoagulant are rapid onset of action, a wide therapeutic window, reproducible pharmacokinetic/pharmacodynamic properties, and no drug-drug or drug-food interactions, and it needs little to no monitoring.[6,13]

Laboratory Assessment and Monitoring

Anticoagulant dosing requires an optimal balance between reducing the morbidity and mortality associated with the underlying thrombotic condition and managing the risk of serious hemorrhage from therapeutic anticoagulation. The consequences of either inadequate or excessive anticoagulation are potentially life-threatening. Therefore, patients on anticoagulant medications (e.g., warfarin and unfractionated heparin) are monitored closely with specific clinical laboratory assays. A baseline assessment of the patient's coagulation features is performed before initiating anticoagulant therapy. This allows detection of any existing coagulation factor deficiencies, vascular abnormalities, liver or kidney insufficiency, or platelet deficiency. Any of these would be deleterious if anticoagulant therapy was instituted without obtaining a baseline.

For monitoring oral anticoagulant therapy (e.g., vitamin K antagonists), prothrombin time (PT) is measured to assess the activity of vitamin K–dependent clotting factors (II, VII, IX, and X).[24,25] The PT is particularly sensitive to factor VII, which is not of great clinical significance by itself, but serves as a marker for the ability of the liver to synthesize proteins, or of the extent of vitamin K depletion from warfarin therapy. The PT assay measures the time taken for a clot formation in citrated plasma, after the addition of tissue thromboplastin and calcium. In normal (warfarin-free) plasma, this takes 10-13 seconds.[24,25] Clinical laboratories report PT results in terms of international normalized ratios (INRs), to account for the variance in commercially available thromboplastin. Patients on warfarin therapy are maintained with an INR of 2.0-3.0. At the initiation of warfarin therapy, daily PTs are performed. Subsequently, drug dosage is adjusted and the length of time between PT assessments can be weekly, and once optimized, even bimonthly.

Heparin directly deactivates clotting factors II and X. Heparin therapy is monitored based on the aPTT (activated partial thromboplastin time) assay which monitors factors II and X as well as several others.[24,25] Deficiencies of clotting factors that affect the aPTT result can be of little clinical significance (e.g., prekallikrein and factor XII), of potential clinical significance (e.g., factor XI), or of great clinical significance (e.g., factors VIII and IX and the hemophilic factors). In the aPTT assay, a surface activator, such as elegiac acid, kaolin, or silica, is used to activate the intrinsic pathway. When this agent comes in contact with citrated plasma in the presence of calcium and phospholipid, a clot begins to form. The phospholipid potentiates the intrinsic pathway without activating factor VII, resulting in "partial activation." In normal (nonheparinized) plasma, the average aPTT result is 25-45 seconds. A therapeutic aPTT in a patient receiving heparin is 70-140 seconds, a comparative threefold increase. In vivo, the platelet membrane is the source of several clotting factors and is the site of many coagulation reactions of the intrinsic pathway.

Many other laboratory assays are used to assess function at various points within the clotting cascade. Quantitative levels of fibrinogen and fibrin degradation products are used to assess the extent of the effects of conditions such as acute inflammation, disseminated intravascular coagulation, and severe liver disease. The specific clotting factors in which a given patient may be deficient also can be determined using various mixing studies.[24-26] These assessments are specialized and are performed much less frequently than the PT and aPTT.

ORAL ANTICOAGULANTS

There are two different chemical classes of orally active anticoagulants, *viz.*, coumarin derivatives and 1,3-indandiones. The discovery of bovine hemorrhaging from consuming sweet clover hay and other subsequent findings eventually led to the isolation of dicoumarol (bishydroxycoumarin) in 1934, followed by use in humans in 1954 as the first orally active anticoagulant drug.[26]

Coumarin Derivatives

Warfarin and other vitamin K antagonists have been the mainstay of oral anticoagulant therapy for more than 50 years.[5] Although their effectiveness in the prophylaxis of thrombotic disorders has been established through many well-designed clinical trials, their use in clinical practice is challenging because of their narrow therapeutic index, potential for drug-drug/drug-food interactions, and patient variability including genetic polymorphisms (CYP2C9, VKORC1) that require close assessment and drug monitoring.[25,27,28]

Mechanism of Action

Vitamin K antagonists produce their effect on blood coagulation by interfering with the cyclic interconversion of vitamin K and vitamin K 2,3-epoxide (Fig. 18.4).[29] Vitamin K is an essential cofactor necessary for the posttranslational carboxylation of the glutamic acid residues on the N-terminal portions of the specific clotting factors (II, VII, IX, and X) and anticoagulant proteins, such as protein C.[22] This γ-glutamyl carboxylation results in a new amino acid, γ-carboxyglutamate, which causes a conformational change to proteins by chelation of calcium ion. The resulting modified tertiary structure facilitates the activation of four vitamin K–dependent clotting factors, which then bind to the negatively charged phospholipid membranes during the coagulation cascade.

γ-Glutamyl carboxylase enables the carboxylation of vitamin K–dependent coagulation factors. This proceeds through the oxidation of the hydroquinone isomer of vitamin K (KH_2) to vitamin K 2,3-epoxide, in the presence of molecular oxygen, and carbon dioxide as cofactors. The return of the epoxide to the active hydroquinone KH_2 is the result of a two-step reduction. In the first step, the epoxide is reduced to the quinone, by vitamin K 2,3-epoxide reductase complex 1 (VKORC1), in the presence of NADH.[30] This quinone intermediate is then further reduced back to KH_2 by vitamin K quinone reductase. The warfarin-like anticoagulants (i.e., vitamin K antagonists) exert their anticoagulant activity through the inhibition of VKORC1 and, possibly, through inhibition of vitamin K quinone reductase, which in turn inhibits activation of the four affected coagulation factors. Unlike heparin, and as a direct result of their mechanism of action, the vitamin K antagonists only inhibit blood coagulation in vivo.

Structure-Activity Relationship of Coumarin Derivatives

All of the coumarin derivatives (Fig. 18.5) are water-insoluble lactones. Structure-activity relationship requirements revolve around the substitution of the lactone ring, particularly the 3- and 4-positions. Although coumarin is neutral, the clinically available derivatives are weakly acidic as a result of 4-hydroxy substitution, which enables the formation of water-soluble sodium salts. Furthermore, warfarin can exist in solution as two diastereomeric cyclic hemiketals, in addition to its open-chain isomer (Fig. 18.5). These hemiketal conformers may be the active conformers, as they resemble the active hemiketal of vitamin K.[31]

Pharmacokinetics

The substituents at the 3-position affect significantly the pharmacokinetic and toxicologic properties of warfarin and its derivatives (Table 18.1).[32] Dicoumarol has modest GI absorption, causes GI discomfort, and is rarely used. Today, the only coumarin used in the United States is warfarin, but phenprocoumon and acenocoumarol are used in Europe.

Warfarin

Warfarin sodium is rapidly and completely absorbed (~100% bioavailability) following oral or parenteral administration. Upon initiation of therapy, peak plasma concentrations occur at 180 minutes. However, warfarin's anticoagulant effects are delayed as it is first preceded by the clearance of certain clotting factors, such as factor V (~5 hr) and factor II (~48-72 hr). The concomitant depletion of protein C levels results in an initial period of elevated coagulability, followed by the desired anticoagulation state.[24,27,33]

Warfarin is highly plasma-protein bound (95%-99%) and is susceptible to warfarin-protein-drug interaction. Warfarin toxicity can manifest when another drug displaces the bound warfarin, resulting in possible hemorrhage caused by elevated levels of free warfarin. High degree of plasma-protein-bound warfarin results in low volume of distribution and extended plasma half-life.[24,27,33]

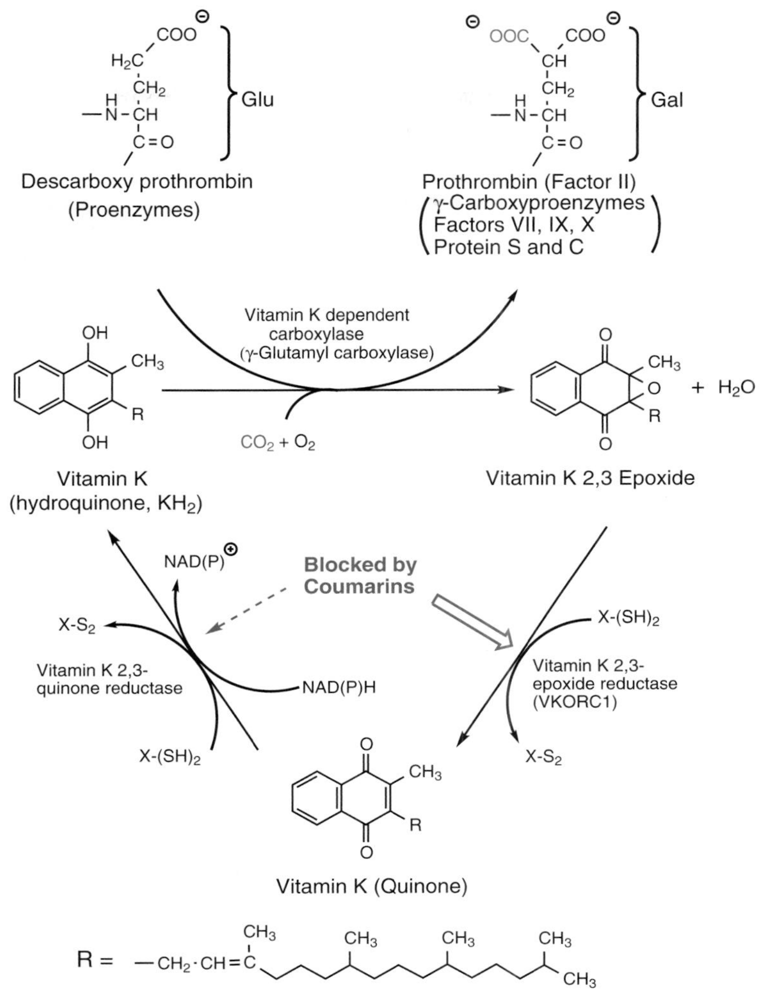

Figure 18.4 Redox cycling of vitamin K in the activation of blood clotting, which involves conversion of glutamate residues to γ-carboxyglutamates.

"SUPERWARFARIN" RODENTICIDES

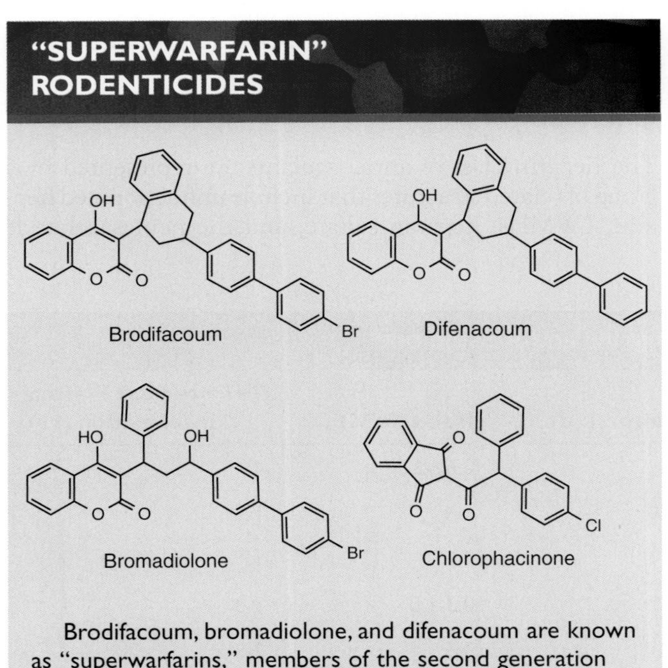

Brodifacoum, bromadiolone, and difenacoum are known as "superwarfarins," members of the second generation of anticoagulant rodenticides developed to combat rodent resistance to warfarin.[34]

Brodifacoum is readily available over the counter in hardware stores and supermarkets, and it is marketed under numerous trade names in North America, Europe, Australia, and New Zealand. Human ingestion of brodifacoum typically is accidental in children but intentional in adults in order to commit suicide.[35] In cases when large quantities are ingested, severe and potentially fatal hemorrhaging can result. Brodifacoum exhibits its anticoagulant effects by inhibiting vitamin K epoxide reductase. Despite the similarity in mechanism of action between brodifacoum and warfarin, brodifacoum is at least fivefold more potent, has a volume of distribution about sixfold greater, and has a half-life that is ninefold longer (24.2 d) than warfarin.[34,36-38] Consequently, vitamin K therapy may be needed for many weeks after the ingestion of a superwarfarin rodenticide.[38]

The clinically used preparation of warfarin is racemic, but the (*S*)- and (*R*)-enantiomers are not equipotent in anticoagulant activity. (*S*)-Warfarin is at least fourfold more potent than (*R*)-warfarin. Several stereoselective drug interactions can be used to explain the difference in the activities and metabolism of the two warfarin enantiomers. In the case of

Figure 18.5 Chemical structures of coumarin and coumarin-derived drugs.

acenocoumarol, the (*R*)-isomer is responsible for the majority of its activity. Similar stereochemical properties have been noted for the other asymmetric coumarins (Fig. 18.5).

Hepatic CYP2C9 is responsible for metabolizing (*S*)-warfarin and other coumarin derivatives to the 6- and 7-hydroxywarfarins as the major inactive metabolites. Hepatic CYP3A4, CYP1A2, and CYP2C19 isozymes inactivate (*R*)-warfarin to give 4′-, 6-, and 8-hydroxywarfarins, respectively.[39] The ketone on the C-3 side chain is reduced to a pair of pharmacologically active, diastereomeric 2′-hydroxywarfarins (Fig. 18.6), but this is to a lesser extent compared to hepatic oxidation. Individuals with compromised hepatic function are at greater risk for warfarin toxicity, secondary to diminished clearance. Additionally, individuals with VKORC1 and CYP2C9 variants may require a lower maintenance dose of warfarin to avoid serious bleeding complications.[40] Many of the drug-drug interactions are associated with changes to warfarin metabolism as a result of CYP2C9 induction or inhibition. Additional drugs and conditions also have profound effects on warfarin therapy. A partial list of these factors is shown in Table 18.2.[32]

INDANDIONES

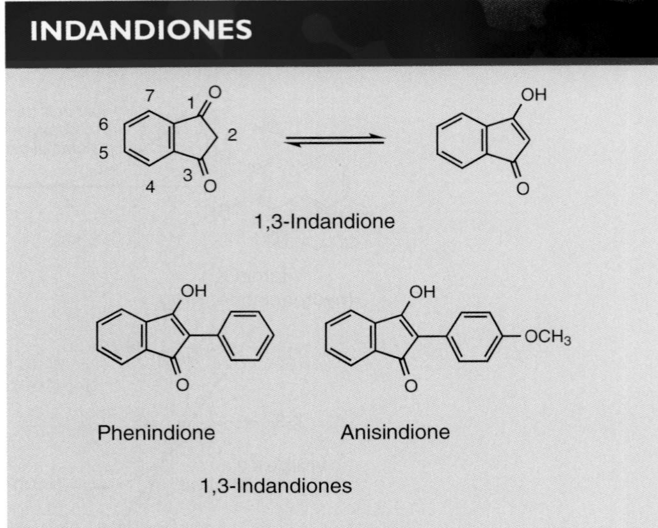

Phenindione and anisindione belong to the class of indan-1,3-dione derivatives, a group of orally active anticoagulants similar to the coumarins. Patients who are allergic to warfarin will experience cross-sensitivity with anisindione and other indandione anticoagulants due to structural similarity.[41] The pharmacokinetic properties also are similar to those of the coumarins (Table 18.1; Fig. 18.5). These agents possess significant renal and hepatic toxicities which preclude their clinical use. Most of the indandione drugs are marketed as potent rodenticides.

HEPARIN-BASED ANTICOAGULANTS

Chemistry

The heparin class of anticoagulants are represented by a group of related structures that include unfractionated heparin, LWMHs, heparan sulfate, and the pentasaccharide

Table 18.1 Pharmacokinetic Properties of the Coumarins and Anisindione

Drug	Trade Name	Onset (hr)	Duration (d)	Half-Life (d)	Time to Peak Plasma Concentration (hr)
Warfarin	Coumadin	1.5-3.0	2-5	0.62-2.5	4
Dicoumarol		1-5	2-10	1-4	1-9
Phenprocoumon	Marcumar[a]	24-48	7-14	5-6	
Acenocoumarol	Sinthrome[a]		2	0.3-1.0	1-3
Anisindione	Miradon	~6	1-3	3-5	2-3

[a]Not available in the United States but available in Europe.

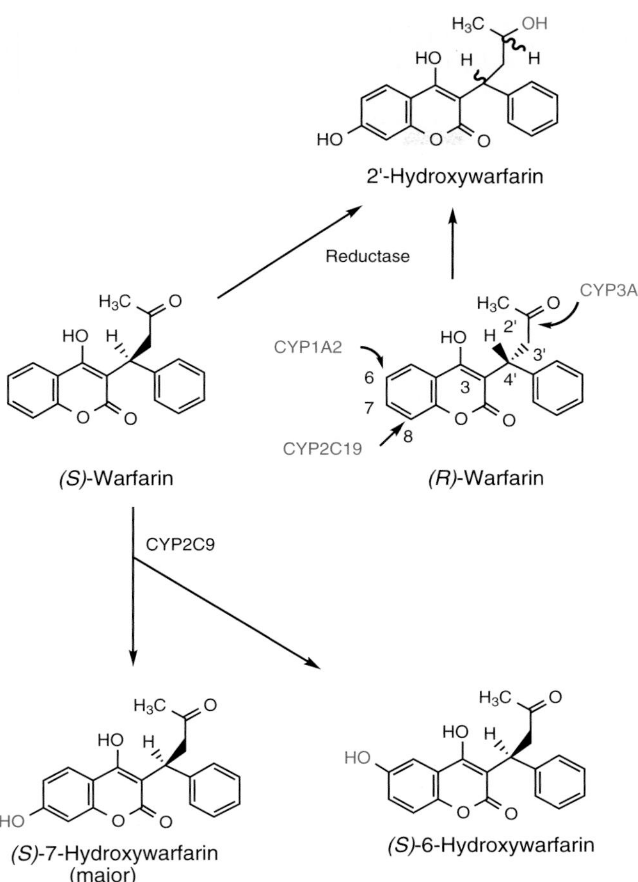

Figure 18.6 Metabolism of warfarin.

drug, fondaparinux. Heparin is composed of a heterogeneous mixture of straight-chain, sulfated, and negatively charged mucopolysaccharides (MW: 5-30 kDa) isolated from bovine lung or porcine intestinal mucosa. Heparin (heparinic acid) is an acidic molecule analogous to chondroitin and hyaluronic acid. The polysaccharide polymer chains of heparin are composed of two alternating sugar units, N-acetyl-D-glucosamine and uronic acid (either D-glucuronic or L-iduronic), linked by α, 1 → 4 bonds (Fig. 18.7).[39]

Heparin is a glycosaminoglycan synthesized from UDP-sugar precursors as a polymer of alternating D-glucuronic acid and N-acetyl-D-glucosamine and is stored in mast cells. About 10-15 glycosoaminoglycan chains (each 200-300 monosaccharide units) are attached to a core protein to create the heparin molecule (MW: 750-1,000 kDa). Prior to binding to antithrombin, the proteoglycan structure must undergo multiple chemical modifications such as O-sulfation and N-sulfation of the D-glucosamine residues at carbons 6 and 2, respectively; O-sulfation of the D-glucuronic acid at carbon 2; epimerization of the D-glucuronic acid at carbon 5 to form L-iduronic acid; O-sulfation at carbon 2 of the L-iduronic acid; N-deacetylation of the glucosamine; and O-sulfation of the glucosamine at position 3.[39] None of these reactions goes to completion, resulting in structurally diverse polysaccharide chains.[42-44] Degradation of the heparin proteoglycan by an endo-β-glucuronidase present in mast cell granules releases active 5- to 30-kd polysaccharide chains.

At physiologic pH, heparin exists primarily as polysulfate anions; therefore, it is usually administered as a salt. In clinical use, standard heparin is usually the sodium salt, but calcium heparin is also effective. However, lithium heparin is used in blood sample collection tubes to prevent clotting of the blood samples in vitro but not in vivo. Heparin salts possess aqueous solubility, which is useful for parenteral administration. Heparin may be administered intravenously or subcutaneously, but not orally, as it is degraded by gastric acid. Intramuscular injection of heparin is not recommended, as it is associated with a high risk of hematoma formation.

Mechanism of Action

Heparin acts at multiple sites in the coagulation cascade.[39] It binds to circulating antithrombin (AT-III; serine protease) through ionic bonding between the sulfate and carboxylate anions in the pentasaccharide chain of heparin, and the arginine and lysine cations in antithrombin III.[45,46] This potentiates the antithrombin III–mediated inhibition of factor IIa (thrombin-Pathway 1) and factor Xa (Pathway 2) (which also activates factor II) (Fig. 18.8), of the coagulation cascade (Fig. 18.1).[46,47] In doing so, antithrombin III forms a stable complex with factor II and factor Xa complex in a 1:1 ratio, which is accelerated more than 2,000-fold by the catalytic action of heparin.[46] This is explained by the conformational change induced as a result of heparin binding to AT-III, which increases the exposure of its active sites, and increasing the interaction with protease substrates, such as factor IIa and factor Xa. Furthermore, the ability of heparin to expose the active sites of antithrombin III is positively correlated to the large molecular size of heparin. Thus, with smaller molecules like LMWH and fondaparinux, the binding of antithrombin to thrombin is diminished, making these drugs become more selective (see LMWH and fondaparinux). The formation of the antithrombin-protease complex results in the release of bound heparin, which can then catalyze the formation of additional antithrombin-protease complexes (Fig. 18.8).[47] Additionally, heparin exerts effects on activator inhibitor, protein C inhibitor, and TFPI and negatively affects coagulation.[22,23]

Pharmacokinetics

The pharmacokinetic profiles of heparin and LMWHs are very different. After subcutaneous injection, only 30% of heparin is absorbed, while 90% of LMWH is systemically absorbed.[40,48] The high, nonspecific binding affinity of heparin to various protein receptors, including platelets, platelet factor 4 (PF4), and macrophages, is explained by the high negative-charge density of heparin.[44] Heparin's nonspecific binding to PF4 may account for heparin's narrow therapeutic window as well as heparin-induced thrombocytopenia (HIT), which is a major limitation

Table 18.2 Factors Affecting Warfarin Therapy

Potentiate Anticoagulation Drugs		Antagonize Anticoagulation Drugs
Acetaminophen	Miconazole	Alcohol (chronic abuse)
Alcohol/ethanol (acute intoxication)	Nalidixic acid	Aminoglycosides
Allopurinol	Naproxen	Antacid
Amiodarone	Omeprazole	Antihistamines
Anabolic and androgenic steroids	Oral hypoglycemics	Barbiturates
Aspirin	Pentoxifylline	Carbamazepine
Bromelains	Phenylbutazone	Chlordiazepoxide
Cephalosporins	Phenytoin	Cholestyramine
Chenodiol	Piroxicam	Colestipol
Chloral hydrate	Propafenone	Corticosteroids
Cimetidine	Propranolol	Dextrothyroxine
Clofibrate	Quinidine, quinine	Griseofulvin
Chlorpropamide	Sulfamethoxazole-trimethoprim	Haloperidol
Cotrimoxazole	Sulfinpyrazone	Meprobamate
Dextran	Sulfonylureas	Nafcillin
Diazoxide	Sulindac	Oral contraceptives
Diflunisal	Tamoxifen	Penicillins (large doses)
Disulfiram	Thyroxine	Phenytoin
Erythromycin	Ticlopidine	Pyrimidone
Ethacrynic acid	Tolmetin	Rifampin
Fenoprofen	Tricyclic antidepressants	Sucralfate
Fluconazole		Trazodone
Glucagon	**Other Factors:**	Vitamin K (large doses)
Heparin	Fever	
Ibuprofen	Stress	**Other Factors:**
Indomethacin	Congestive heart failure	High–vitamin K diet: spinach, cheddar cheese, cabbage
Inhalation anesthetics	Radioactive compounds	Edema
Isoniazid	Diarrhea	Hypothyroidism
Ketoconazole	Cancer	Nephrotic syndrome
Lovastatin	X-rays	
Mefenamic acid	Hyperthyroidism	
Metronidazole	Hepatic dysfunction	

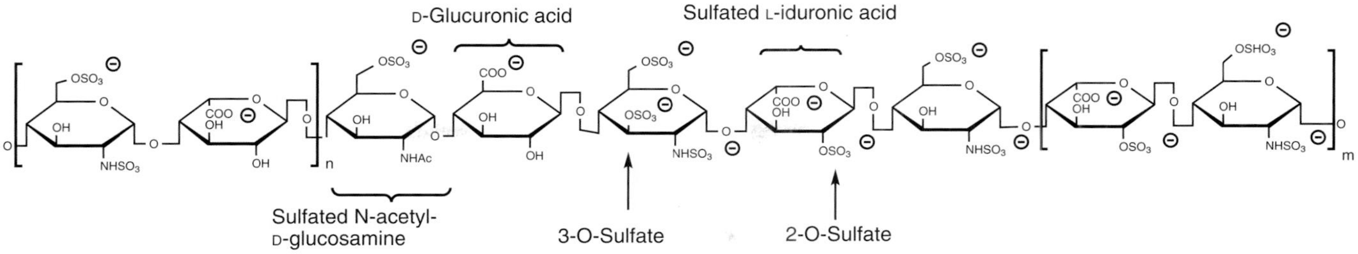

Figure 18.7 Chemical structure of heparin polymer.

of heparin therapy.[26,46] These affinities are quite low, in the case of LMWHs, resulting in several benefits. The favorable absorption kinetics and low protein binding affinity of the LMWHs result in a greater bioavailability compared with heparin. The lowered affinity of LMWHs for PF4 seems to correlate with a reduced incidence of HIT.[44] Heparin is subject to fast zero-order metabolism in the liver, followed by slower first-order clearance from the kidneys.[49] The LMWHs are renal cleared and follow first-order kinetics. This makes the clearance of LMWHs more predictable as well as resulting in a prolonged half-life. Finally, the incidence of heparin-mediated osteoporosis is diminished significantly when LMWHs are used, as opposed to heparin.

Metabolism

The metabolic fate of the heparin and LMWH is the same, irrespective of molecular weight. The distribution of the compounds is limited primarily to the circulation, but heparins also are taken up by the reticuloendothelial system.[50] Once this uptake occurs, rapid depolymerization and desulfation follows, resulting in inactive products. These inactive metabolites are excreted in urine with some of the parent compound.[50] Because of the depolymerization of heparin in the liver and ultimate renal elimination of both metabolites and parent drug, half-life is prolonged in patients with hepatic or renal dysfunction.

Specific Heparin Drugs

High Molecular Weight Heparin (Unfractionated Heparin)

Standard heparin is unfractionated and contains mucopolysaccharides ranging in molecular weight from 5 to 30 kDa (mean: ~15 kDa) and is referred to as high molecular weight heparin (Table 18.3). This group of compounds has a very high affinity for antithrombin III and causes significant in vivo anticoagulant effects. Because heparin is a heterogeneous mixture of polysaccharides with different affinities for the target receptor, dosing based on milligrams of drug is inappropriate (i.e., there frequently is a limited correlation between the concentration of heparin given and the anticoagulant effect produced). Therefore, heparin is dosed in terms of standardized activity units that must be established by bioassay. One U.S. Pharmacopeia (USP) unit for heparin is the quantity of heparin required to prevent 1.0 mL of citrated sheep blood from clotting for 1 hour after the addition of 0.2 mL of 1% calcium chloride. Commercially available heparin sodium USP must contain at least 120 USP units per milligram. Heparin therapy typically is monitored by the aPTT assay. A therapeutic aPTT is represented by a clotting time in the assay that is 1.5- to 2.5-fold the normal mean aPTT.[51] Monitoring therapy with laboratory testing is critical.

Low Molecular Weight Heparins

In the past two decades, an increased interest has surfaced in a group of compounds known as LMWHs.[49] The LMWHs typically are in the 4-6 kDa molecular weight range and are isolated as fractions from heparin using gel filtration chromatography or differential precipitation with ethanol.[46] The LMWHs have favorable pharmacokinetic and pharmacodynamic profiles, in comparison with standard heparins (Table 18.3).[52,53] The mechanism of action of LMWHs is similar to conventional heparin, but the binding of LMWHs is more selective. In other words, LMWHs have more targeted activity against activated factor Xa (Pathway 2) and less against activated factor IIa (thrombin) (Pathway 1) (Fig. 18.8). While LMWHs still possess the exact and specific pentasaccharide sequence needed for binding and potentiating the antithrombin III–mediated inhibition of activated factor Xa, most of the LMWH-antithrombin III complex is of insufficient length to bind and inhibit factor Xa and thrombin at the same time.[52] Thus, although all LMWHs inactivate factor Xa (Pathway 1), only 25%-50% of these molecules also inactivate thrombin (Pathway 2).[49] This factor selectivity is defined as a higher factor Xa:thrombin (anti-Xa:anti-IIa) activity ratio. And although standard (unfractionated) heparin has an anti-Xa:anti-IIa ratio of 1:1, the same ratio in the LMWHs varies from 2:1 to 4:1 (Table 18.3).[49]

Two LWMHs, enoxaparin and dalteparin (Table 18.3), are commercially available in the United States. Both compounds are indicated for perioperative thromboembolism prevention for specific abdominal and orthopedic surgeries. Enoxaparin and dalteparin are also approved for use, in combination with aspirin, for the prophylaxis of ischemic complications of unstable angina and non–Q-wave MI.[54] Enoxaparin is also used in therapy for DVT with or without concomitant PE.[54,55] Because of the increased homogeneity

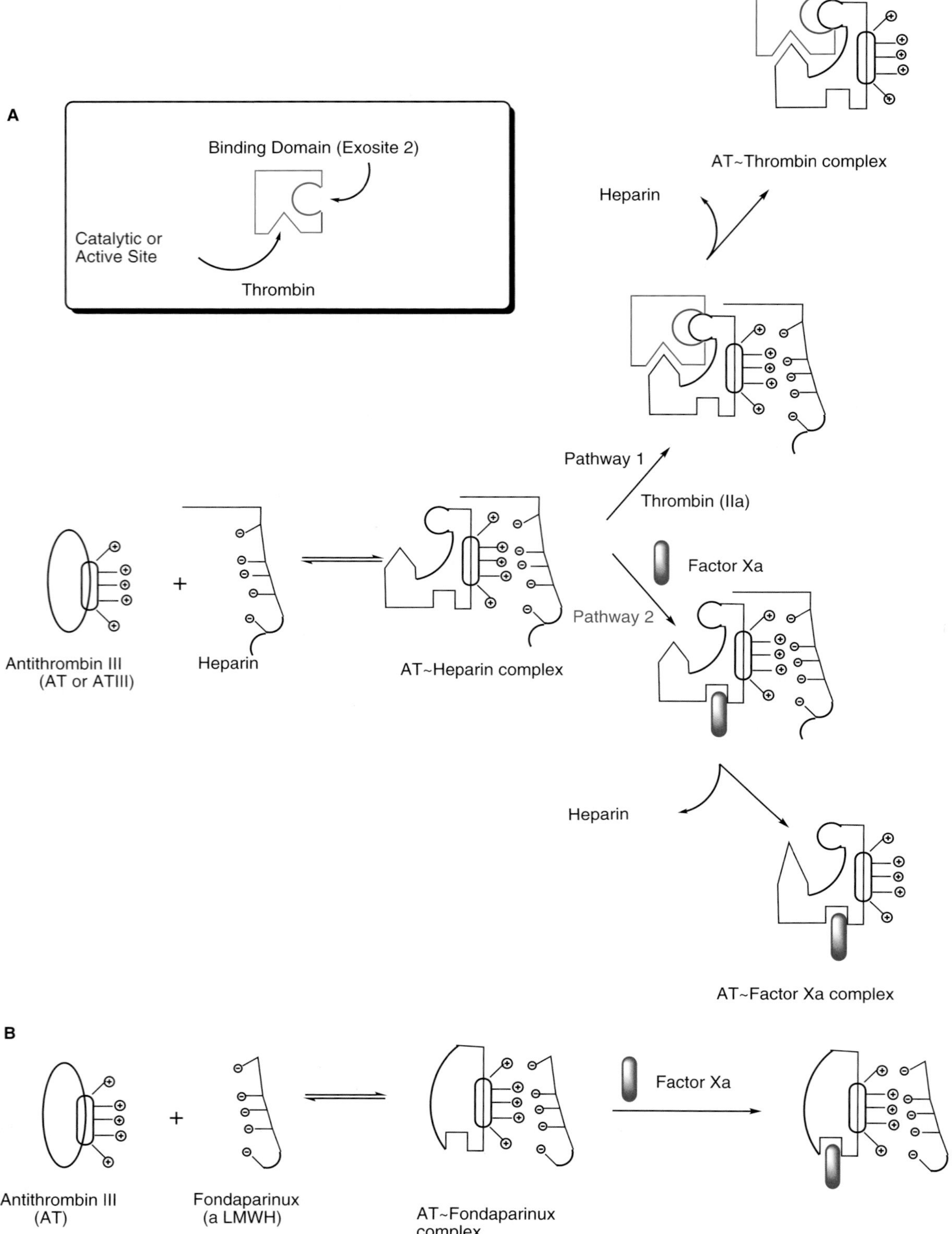

Figure 18.8 Schematic representation of catalytic role of the heparin-based drugs in promoting (A) antithrombin-factor Xa and antithrombin-thrombin complexes and (B) antithrombin-fondaparinux complex.

of enoxaparin compared to heparin, dosing of enoxaparin is based on drug weight rather than in USP units. A typical dosing scheme for enoxaparin is the administration of 1 mg/kg once or twice daily. In the case of dalteparin, dosage is based on antifactor Xa units (a-Xa U). Dalteparin is given as a once-daily subcutaneous injection at a dose of 2,500-5,000 a-Xa U. LMWHs have limited anticoagulant effect on in vitro clotting assays, such as the aPTT, and have highly predictable dose-response relationships, which reduces the need for monitoring.[49,52]

Table 18.3 Properties of Heparin Derivatives

Drug	Trade Name	Dosing	Molecular Weight (Da)	Binding Ratio
Unfractionated heparin				
Heparin		bid, tid	5-30	1:1
Low molecular weight heparins				
Dalteparin	Fragmin	qd	3-8	2.2:1
Enoxaparin	Lovenox	qd, bid	3.5-5.5	2.7-3.9:1
Pentasaccharide				
Fondaparinux	Arixtra	qd	1.728	Xa only

bid, twice a day; *qd*, every day; *tid*, three times a day.

Fondaparinux (Arixtra)

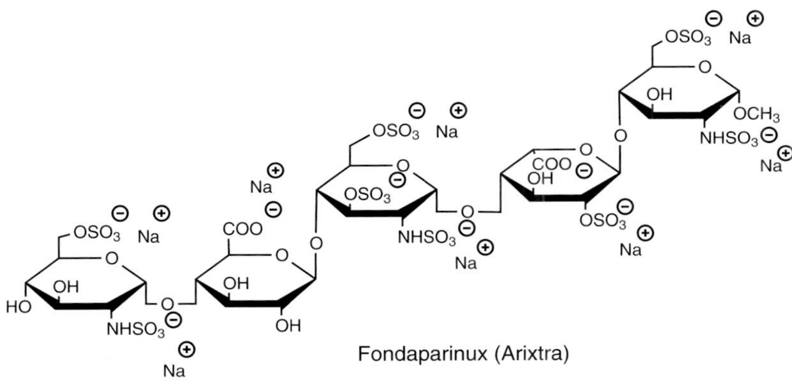

Fondaparinux (Arixtra)

Fondaparinux is a synthetic, highly sulfonated pentasaccharide, designed on the basis of the active site of heparin.[56] It binds specifically to and activates antithrombin III, demonstrating a refinement of fondaparinux over the heparin structure.[57,58] The immediate advantage of fondaparinux is that as a synthetic drug, its composition is steady, resulting in improved pharmacokinetics and a more selective anticoagulant action. It is chemically related to the LMWH and offers significant advantages over heparin.[59]

MECHANISM OF ACTION. Fondaparinux is a specific, indirect inhibitor of activated factor Xa, via its activation of antithrombin (Fig. 18.8). Fondaparinux has strategically located sulfonates that bind to antithrombin, based on the heparin template. Its shorter saccharide chain length results in nonbinding to thrombin, compared to the longer chains (seen in heparin and LMWH) which favor thrombin binding. The highly sulfated heparins exhibit nonselective binding to additional proteins, which results in reduced bioavailability and significant variation in activity (Table 18.3).

PHARMACOKINETICS. Fondaparinux is administered via subcutaneous (SC) injection with a single daily dose and shows complete absorption. The bioavailability of fondaparinux is reported to be 100% when administered SC. The drug is highly bound to antithrombin III (~94%), with no significant binding to other plasma proteins. It does not require routine coagulation monitoring as it has a predictable anticoagulant effect.[60] The drug is excreted in the urine unchanged within 72 hours in patients with normal renal function. Fondaparinux has an elimination half-life of 17 hours.

THERAPEUTIC APPLICATION. Fondaparinux is the first selective factor Xa inhibitor that was approved for the prophylaxis of DVT, which may occur in patients undergoing hip fracture surgery or hip or knee replacement surgery.[61] The most common side effect is major and minor bleeding, and the patient must be carefully monitored because its anticoagulant effect cannot be neutralized by protamine sulfate.[62] The drug is contraindicated for use during spinal anesthesia or spinal puncture to avoid the development of blood clots in the spine. Fondaparinux is 100% bioavailable, with little or no protein binding, and does not appear to cause thrombocytopenia, a known side of heparin therapy.[61,63]

DIRECT THROMBIN INHIBITORS

In recent years, many new anticoagulants that target almost every step in the coagulation pathway have been developed.[62] This has been enabled by deeper understanding of

Table 18.4 Direct Thrombin Inhibitors

Drugs	Trade Name	Route of Administration	Site of Binding	Reversibility	Route of Excretion	Protein Binding
Desirudin	Iprivask	SC	CS, exosite-I	Irreversible	Kidney	0
Bivalirudin	Angiomax Generic	IV	CS, exosite-I	Reversible	Kidney	0
Argatroban	Generic	IV	CS	Reversible	Hepatobiliary	54%
Dabigatran etexilate	Pradaxa	PO	CS	Reversible	Hepatobiliary	35%

CS, catalytic site; *IV*, intravenous; *PO*, oral; *SC*, subcutaneous.

coagulation cascade, targeted structure-based drug design strategies, and the availability of recombinant technologies. DTIs (e.g., desirudin, bivalirudin, argatroban, and dabigatran etexilate) have been approved for clinical use in recent years (Table 18.4).

Discovery and Design of Direct Thrombin Inhibitors

Hirudin, the lead compound for the design of DTIs, is a 65-mer protein, originally isolated from the salivary glands of the medicinal leech, *Hirudo medicinalis*.[64] Hirudin has potent and specific inhibitory effects on thrombin through the formation of a 1:1 complex with the clotting factor. The anticoagulant activity of hirudin appears to be located at its anionic C-terminus. Several clinical studies have compared hirudin and its analog, hirulog, against heparin in the treatment of several thrombotic disorders. In many cases, hirudin seems to be more efficacious and the responses are more predictable. Some of the studies have also shown a lower incidence of bleeding complications with hirudin as compared to heparin. Hirudin is produced by recombinant technology, and many hirulogs continue to be explored.[65,66] The emergence of orally active DTIs may simplify the prevention and treatment of various thromboembolic disorders.[67–69]

Mechanism of Action

DTIs bind directly and reversibly to the active site of factor IIa (thrombin) and inactivate both free thrombin and fibrin-bound thrombin (Fig. 18.9). Unlike the heparin class, these inhibitors do not require activated AT-III for anticoagulant activity. Additionally, DTIs are superior to heparin in that they inhibit only factor IIa, while heparin indirectly inhibits multiple factors (IIa, IXa, Xa, XIa, and XIIa).[70] There are three distinct domains where DTIs bind and oppose the action of thrombin: the active site (or catalytic site, CS) as well as two additional exosites.[71] Exosite-1 acts as a binding dock for substrates such as fibrin. This site orients the appropriate peptide bonds in the active site for its biotransformation. Exosite-2 is also known as the heparin-binding domain. Bivalent DTIs, such as desirudin and bivalirudin, block thrombin at the

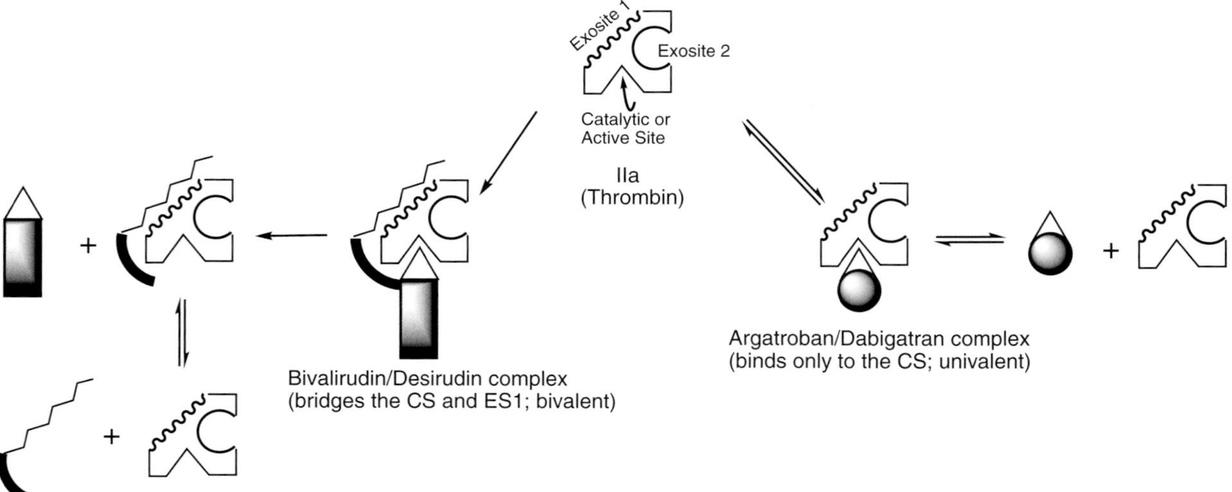

Figure 18.9 Schematic representation of the reaction of direct thrombin inhibitors (bivalirudin, desirudin, argatroban, dabigatran) with thrombin.

active site and exosite-1, whereas argatroban and dabigatran are univalent DTIs and, thus, binds only to the active site of thrombin.

Recombinant Hirudin Derivatives

Desirudin (Iprivask)

Desirudin is a synthetic recombinant hirudin derivative approved for the treatment of HIT and of HIT with thrombotic syndrome.[72-74] The N-terminal amino acids in desirudin are Val-1 and Val-2, and Tyr-63 is nonsulfated. The secondary structure includes disulfide bridges between cysteine residues (shown as gray bonds in Fig. 18.10).

Desirudin is a bivalent DTI that binds to both the active site and exosite-1 of thrombin. The result of this binding is that it creates a nearly irreversible inhibition of thrombin. Desirudin inhibits both soluble thrombin and fibrin-bound thrombin.[70,75]

Desirudin is administered subcutaneously twice daily (Table 18.2).[73,76] It is cleared renally and excreted 50% unchanged.

Bivalirudin (Angiomax)

Bivalirudin (Fig. 18.10) is a synthetic, 20–amino acid peptide (MW: 2180.18 Da) and has been approved for use in patients with unstable angina undergoing percutaneous coronary intervention.[77]

Bivalirudin is a rapid-onset, short-acting DTI that binds to both the active site and the exosite-1 of thrombin. Bivalirudin is a reversible inhibitor of both free thrombin and fibrin-bound thrombin. In the active site, bound bivalirudin undergoes cleavage at N-terminal proline-4, to release the portion of the drug that is bound to the active site. The carboxyl-terminal portion of bivalirudin dissociates from thrombin to regenerate free thrombin (Fig. 18.11).[78]

Bivalirudin is administered via intravenous bolus injection, followed by continuous infusion (Table 18.4). The drug exhibits a rapid onset and a short duration of action. Bivalirudin is eliminated by renal excretion. It has been suggested that dosage adjustments be made in patients with severe renal impairment and in patients undergoing dialysis. Approximately 30% is eliminated unchanged along with proteolytic cleavage products. Because of the reversible nature of bivalirudin, the drug exhibits less risk of bleeding than other antithrombotics. There have been no reported cases of antibody formation to bivalirudin.[79]

Argatroban (Argatroban)

Argatroban (Fig. 18.10) has been approved for the prophylaxis and treatment of thrombosis in patients with HIT.[80] Argatroban is a peptidomimetic that binds selectively to the active site of thrombin as a univalent competitive DTI. It is a reversible inhibitor of both free thrombin and clot-bound thrombin. (*S*)-isomer of Argatroban is approximately twice as potent as the (*R*)-isomer.[81] Argatroban is available as a 64:36 mixture of diastereomers [21-(*R*) and 21-(*S*)].

PHARMACOKINETICS. Argatroban is administered subcutaneously because of the low lipophilicity of the drug. The drug is bound to plasma protein and is metabolized via CYP3A4/5 to the aromatized metabolite and the two hydroxylated metabolites (Fig. 18.12). The M-1 metabolite retains 20%-30% of the antithrombotic activity. Coadministration of argatroban with inhibitors of CYP3A4 does not appear to produce clinically significant effects. Argatroban is fecally eliminated via biliary secretion.[82]

Dabigatran Etexilate (Pradaxa)

Dabigatran etexilate (Fig. 18.10) is an orally active DTI used for the prevention of stroke and blood clots in individuals with atrial fibrillation. Dabigatran etexilate is a non-peptidomimetic prodrug that is biotransformed to dabigatran (Fig. 18.13), a reversible, basic, benzimidazole DTI that binds and inactivates both free and fibrin-bound thrombins.[83,84] The drug is also available in the European Union and Canada, where it is approved for treatment of VTE in patients undergoing hip or knee replacement surgery, and it is being studied for treatment of DVT and PE.

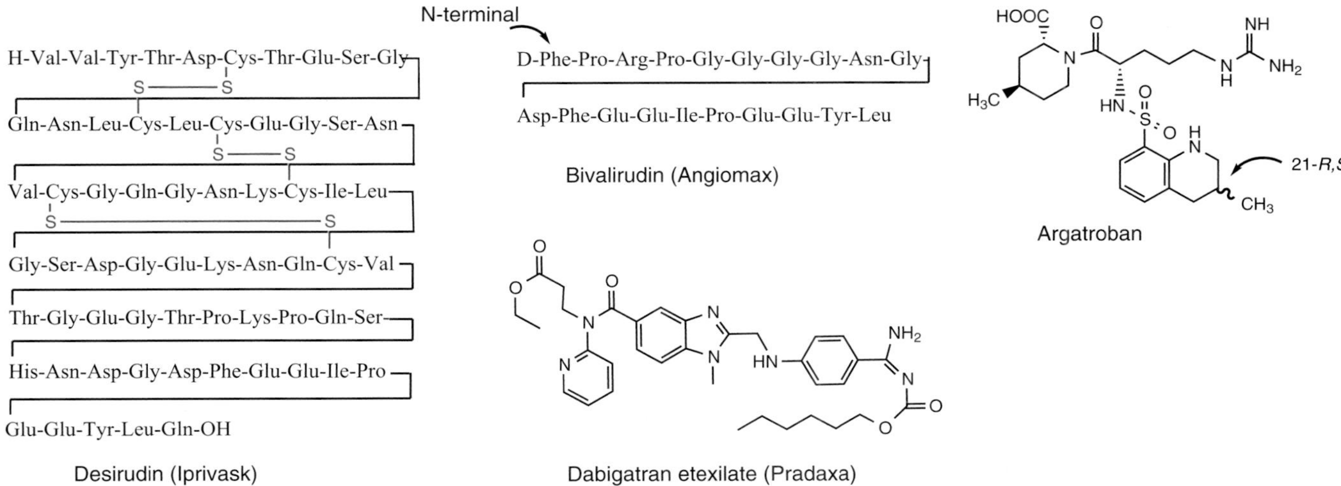

Figure 18.10 Structures of the direct thrombin inhibitors. Disulfide bonds in desirudin are shown in red.

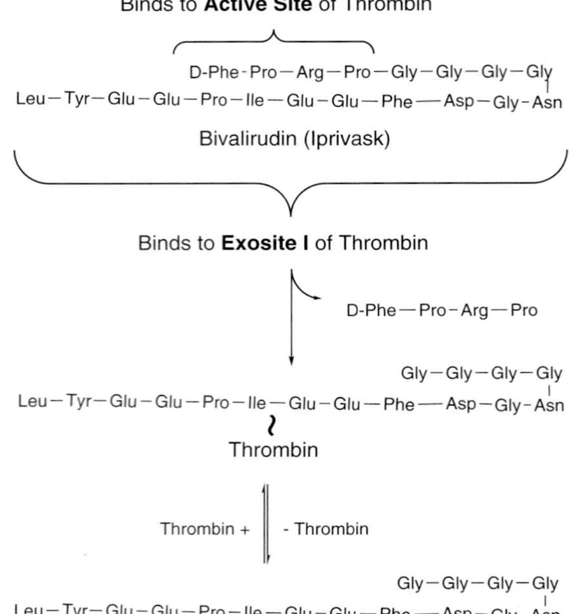

Figure 18.11 Bivalirudin binding sites to thrombin and release from thrombin.

PHARMACOKINETICS. Dabigatran etexilate (formulated as the mesylate salt) has a rapid onset of action, reaching maximum plasma concentrations within 30-120 minutes after oral administration. Dabigatran etexilate is also converted to dabigatran by esterase action (Fig. 18.13).[84,85] Very little dabigatran etexilate or the intermediate metabolites (BIBR0951-1087) are detectable in plasma. Dabigatran is a hydrophilic molecule, due to the charged amidine moiety that forms at physiologic and gastric pH, the latter impairing oral absorption. Dabigatran etexilate has a low bioavailability (~6.5%), which is offset by the administration of a large dose (75-150 mg twice a day). Up to 80% of dabigatran is eliminated unchanged in the kidneys with the remainder excreted in acylglucuronide form.[85] Due to dabigatran's rapid onset and rapid offset, the drug does not require coagulation monitoring, conferring a major advantage in anticoagulant therapy. However, the drug is reported to produce a significant increase in risk of major gastrointestinal bleeding.

IDARUCIZUMAB (PRAXBIND)

In 2015, the FDA approved idarucizumab (Praxbind) for the reversal of anticoagulant effects of dabigatran. This humanized monoclonal antibody is effective for dabigatran reversal among patients who have uncontrolled bleeding or will be undergoing urgent surgery.[86] Idarucizumab binds reversibly to free and thrombin-bound dabigatran as well as the acylglucuronide metabolite of dabigatran. The drug is effective in reversing effects of dabigatran in 88%-98% of patients.

Pharmacokinetic Properties

Idarucizumab is administered intravenously. The drug is rapidly eliminated with a half-life of 47 minutes. The route of elimination appears to be the urine (~32%).[87] The drug is likely metabolized by peptide hydrolysis. The most common adverse effects include headache, hypokalemia, delirium, constipation, pyrexia, and pneumonia. Deaths were reported in 20% of the patients studied, but this may have been the result of coexisting illnesses.

ANTIFACTOR Xa INHIBITORS

Small-molecule inhibitors that specifically target thrombin or activated factor X (FXa) for VTE, atrial fibrillation, and other thrombotic diseases have been discovered.[84,88]

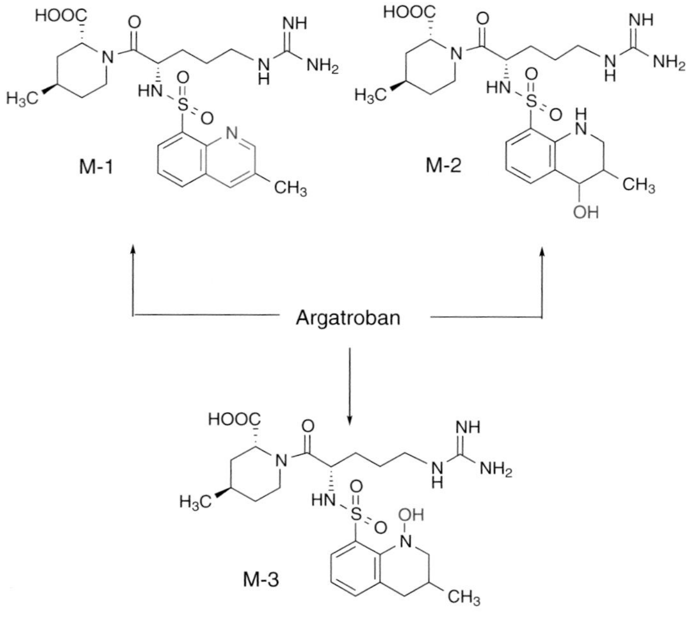

Figure 18.12 Metabolism of argatroban.

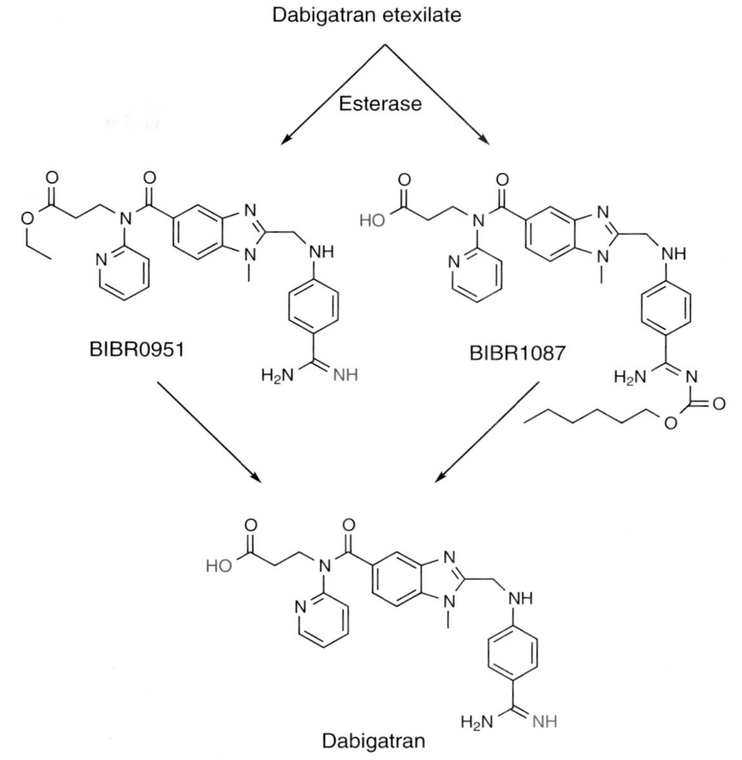

Figure 18.13 Metabolic activation of dabigatran etexilate to dabigatran.

The drugs of this class are apixaban, betrixaban, edoxaban, and rivaroxaban (Fig. 18.14).

Mechanism of Action

Factor Xa inhibitors act on factor Xa, which is a converging point of the intrinsic and extrinsic coagulation pathways (Fig. 18.1). These agents are orally active, highly selective molecules capable of inhibiting both the free and the clot-bound form of FXa. The prothrombinase complex comprises factors Va, Xa, prothrombin (free thrombin), and calcium ions. Inhibition of thrombin formation results in the activation of platelets, without interfering with existing thrombin levels, which improves drug safety.

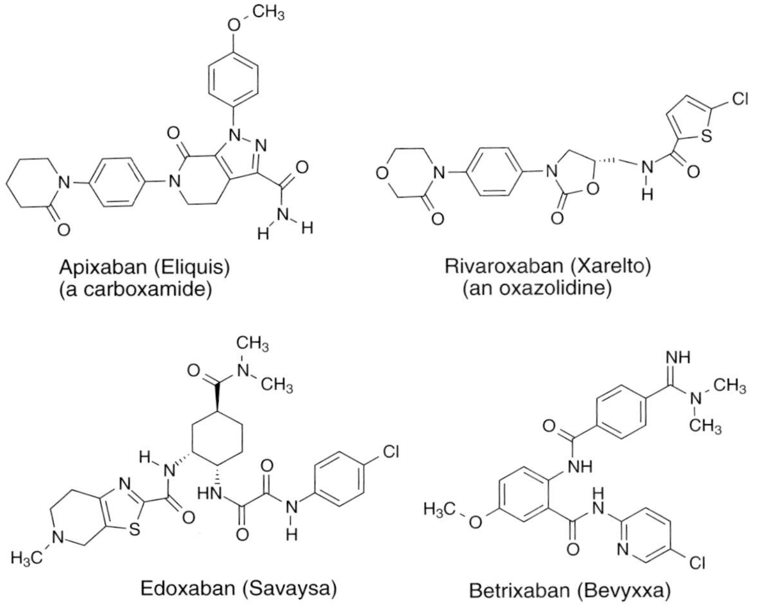

Figure 18.14 Antifactor Xa inhibitors.

Structure-Activity Relationship

The X-ray crystal structure of rivaroxaban-complexed human factor Xa helps explain the structural requirements of FXa inhibitors. High affinity accrues from two types of intermolecular interactions: the critical hydrogen bonding interactions of the oxazolidine carbonyl and chlorothiophene carboxamide with Gly-219, and the hydrophobic interactions with the amino acids lining the S1 and S4 pockets of factor Xa. The intermolecular interactions of FXa inhibitors within the active site are depicted in Figure 18.15. The hydrophobic interactions due to the morpholinone results in superior activity, when compared to morpholine, piperazine, or pyrolidinone. Additional structural requirements for activity are outlined in Figure 18.16.

Metabolism and Pharmacokinetics

Rivaroxaban (Xarelto) was the first orally active, anti-factor Xa inhibitor (Fig. 18.14) with the most published clinical trials data showing similar efficacy and safety to enoxaparin in preventing VTE in major orthopedic surgery.[85,89,90] Rivaroxaban is a highly selective and reversible inhibitor of direct factor Xa (K_i = 0.4 nmol/L) that binds to the active site of both free and prothrombinase-bound factor Xa. It is rapidly absorbed, reaching maximum plasma concentrations 3 hours after oral administration, and has a half-life of 5-9 hours. The drug is a substrate for CYP3A4/2J2 resulting in several hydroxylation products (Fig. 18.17).

Apixaban (Eliquis) is the second selective and potent oral direct Xa inhibitor (K_i = 0.8 nmol/L) that exhibits a superior risk-to-benefit ratio with respect to bleeding than enoxaparin (Fig. 18.14).[14,91,92] It is well absorbed after oral administration, reaching peak plasma levels in about 3 hours with a half-life of 12 hours. Metabolic profile studies have shown that apixaban is the major drug-related component in plasma, urine, and feces in humans, with the O-desmethylapixaban sulfate as a stable, water-soluble inactive metabolite (Fig. 18.17).[93] Apixaban is susceptible to drug interactions, as it is a substrate for CYP3A4, CYP1A2, and P-glycoprotein. 63% of this drug is eliminated fecally, while 27% is cleared in the urine. Renal function has no impact on the plasma concentration of this drug, so there are no renal dose adjustments recommended for VTE treatment, which makes it an appealing option.[93]

Edoxaban (Savaysa) is an anthranilamide-based direct factor Xa inhibitor (Fig. 18.14). It is rapidly absorbed and its bioavailability (62%) is not altered by the presence of food. Rapid absorption allows for peak plasma levels to be achieved within 1-2 hours following dose administration. 55% of the drug is protein bound and the drug has a large volume of distribution (>300 L). The half-life of the drug is 10-14 hours, and 70% of a dose of edoxaban is eliminated primarily unchanged (Fig. 18.17).[94] Studies have shown that patients with low body weight (<60 kg), moderate or severe kidney dysfunction, or coadministration of P-glycoprotein inhibitors will require their edoxaban

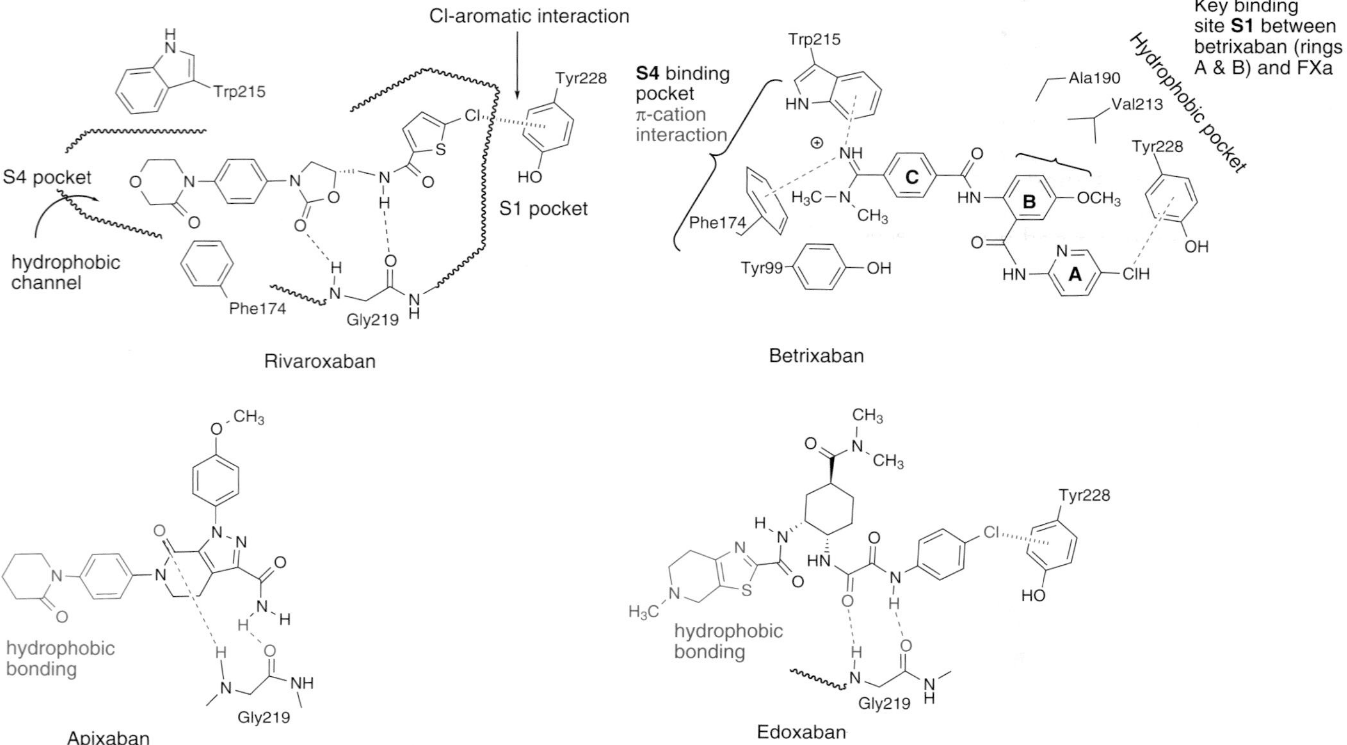

Figure 18.15 Binding sites of rivaroxaban and betrixaban to human FXa and potential binding sites in apixaban and edoxaban.

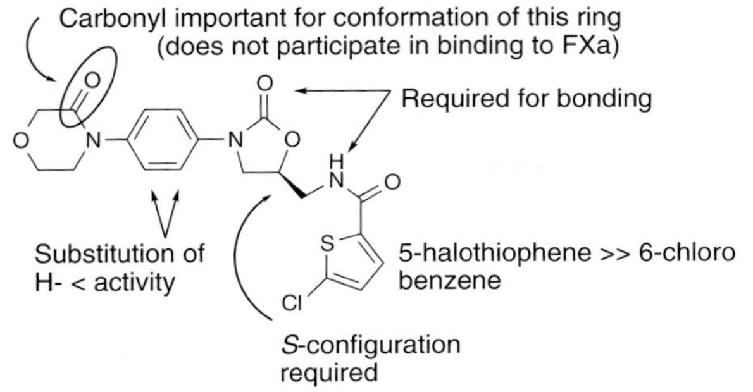

Figure 18.16 Structure-activity relationship requirements for the direct factor Xa inhibitor rivaroxaban and related analogs.

dose to be decreased 50%.[95] Edoxaban is a P-glycoprotein substrate.

Betrixaban (Bevyxxa) is an oral factor Xa inhibitor that inhibits free factor Xa and prothrombinase activity resulting in anticoagulant action (Fig. 18.14). When taken orally, betrixaban has modest oral bioavailability (34%) and is ideally taken on an empty stomach. Peak plasma concentrations were achieved within 3-4 hours, with 60% plasma protein binding. Betrixaban has a half-life of 19-27 hours. The drug is metabolized by non-CYP450 hydrolysis and <1% is metabolized by CYP450s (Fig. 18.17). It is excreted unchanged in the bile and has low renal excretion.[96] Betrixaban is also a substrate of P-glycoprotein.

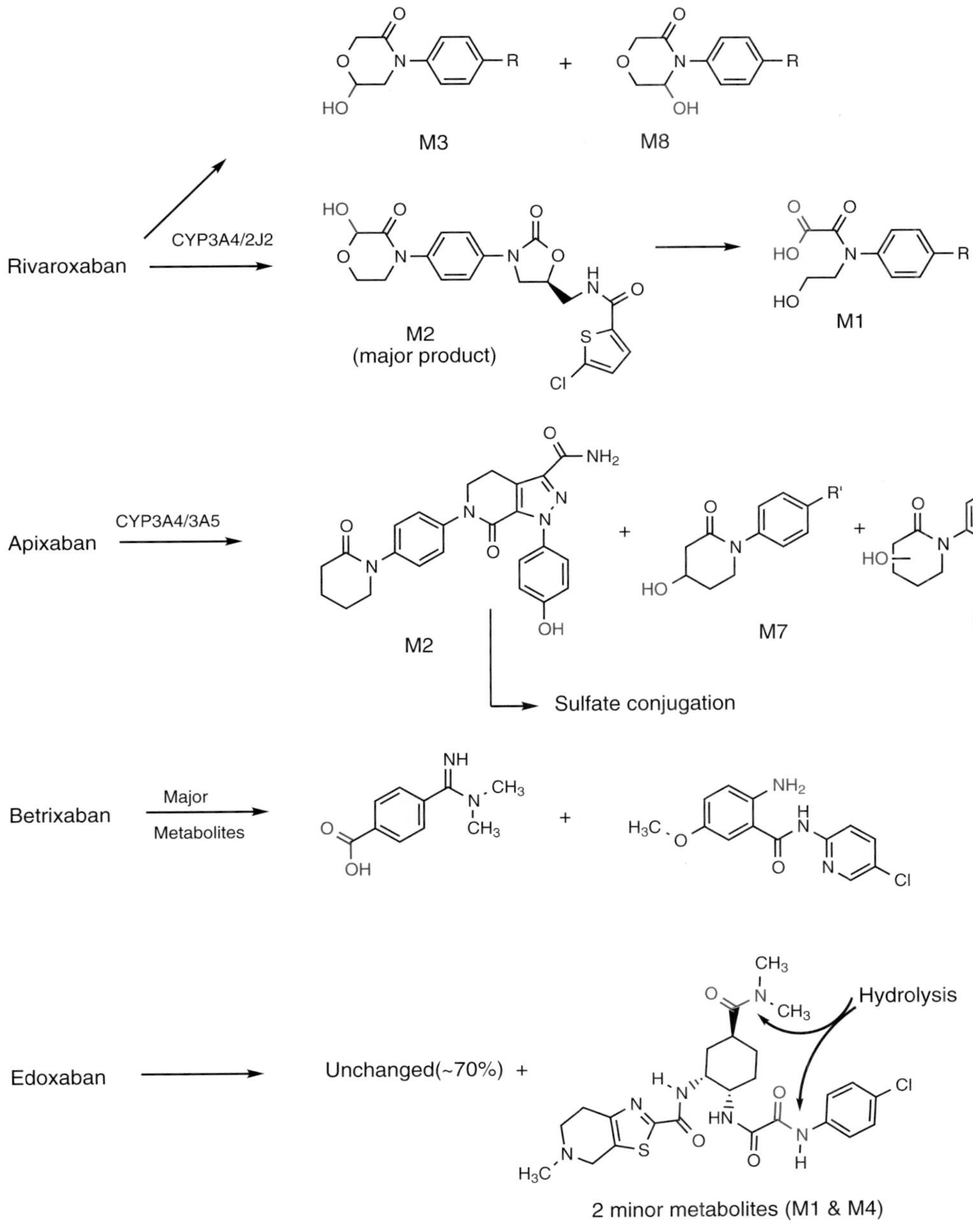

Figure 18.17 Metabolic products formed from rivaroxaban, apixaban, betrixaban, and edoxaban.

ANDEXANET ALFA (ANDEXXA)

Andexanet alfa (Andexxa) is a recombinant coagulation factor Xa approved in May 2018 to reverse anticoagulation when faced with the life-threatening or uncontrolled bleeding actions of rivaroxaban and apixaban. It has not been shown to be effective for other factor Xa inhibitors. Andexanet alfa is given intravenously (initial bolus, followed by infusion), and recommended dosing is based upon the last dose of the factor Xa inhibitor (either rivaroxaban or apixaban).

The active ingredient of andexxanet alfa is a genetically modified variant of human Factor Xa. In this protein, the active site serine is replaced with alanine. This renders it unable to cleave and activate prothrombin. The γ-carboxyglutamic acid (Gla) domain was removed to eliminate the protein's ability to assemble into the prothrombinase complex. These features combine to remove the potential anticoagulant effects of factor Xa inhibitors.[97]

ANTIPLATELET DRUGS

Antiplatelet drugs work by inhibiting platelet activation via different mechanisms that affect blood coagulation and subsequent thrombus formation.[98,99] The major role of antiplatelet drugs is in the prevention of ischemic complications in patients with coronary diseases.[98,100,101] They also are effective in combination with moderate-intensity anticoagulants for patients with atrial fibrillation.

Pathophysiology of Arterial Thrombosis

The central role of platelets in thrombus formation and potential sites for drug interventions are depicted in Figure 18.18.[99,100] Normal endothelial cells in the vascular wall synthesize and release prostacyclin (PGI_2), enabling the conversion of adenosine triphosphate (ATP) to cyclic adenosine monophosphate (cAMP), thus preventing platelet aggregation and degranulation. In the case of an injury to the vascular wall, glycoprotein (GP) receptors bind von Willebrand factor (vWF) and collagen from the exposed subendothelial surface, resulting in platelet activation. The GPIIb/IIIa receptors (also known as the fibrinogen receptor or integrin αIIbβ3 receptor) then mediate the final step of platelet aggregation by binding to fibrinogen or vWF, causing platelets to cross-link and form aggregates.

The adherent platelets degranulate and release additional aggregating substances, such as thromboxane A_2 (TXA_2), serotonin (5-HT), thrombin, and adenosine diphosphate (ADP). These substances serve as secondary chemical messengers to recruit more platelets to the site of vascular injury and, thereby, amplify

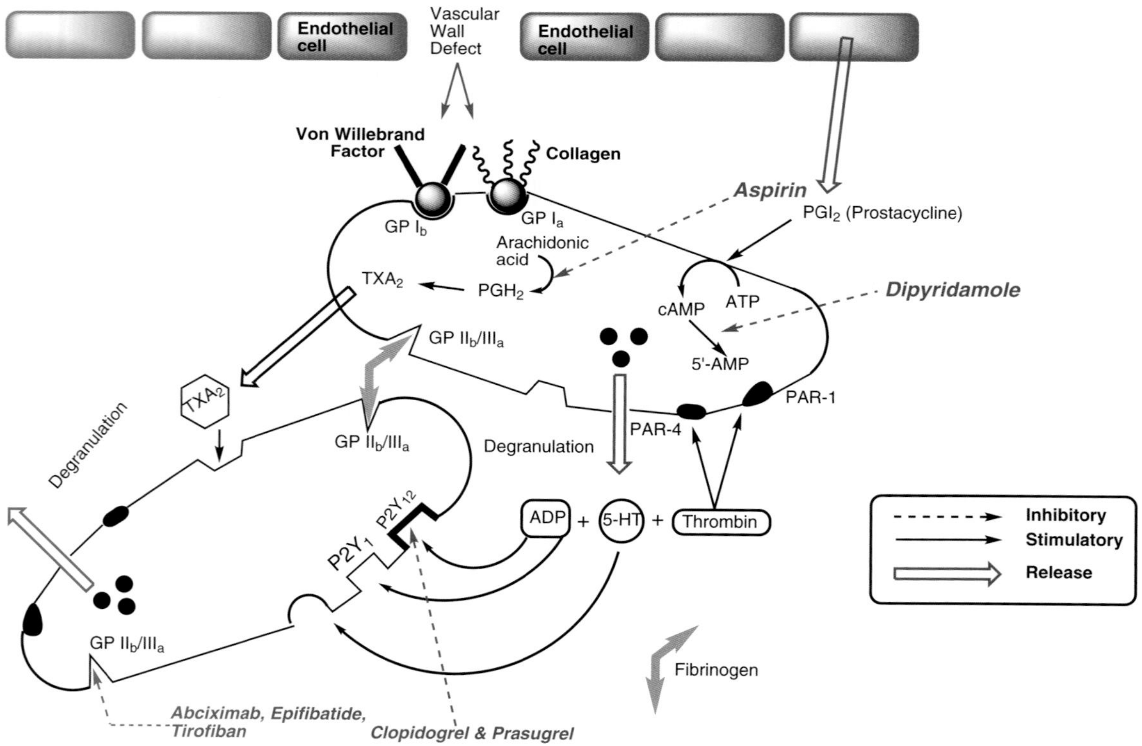

Figure 18.18 Scheme describing platelet activation as it relates to blood clot formation. The thrombus is formed at the site of a damaged wall in the vasculature. Normal endothelial cells in vascular wall provide prostacyclin, which stimulates the conversion of adenosine triphosphate (ATP) to cAMP, preventing platelet aggregation. In injury, glycoprotein (GP) receptors bind substances such as von Willebrand factor and collagen, activating the platelet. The GPIIb/IIIa receptors cross-link platelets via fibrinogen binding. As the platelet degranulates, additional aggregating substances including TXA_2, serotonin (5-HT), and adenosine diphosphate (ADP) are released. ADP by binding to P2Y1 and P2Y12 promote and sustain platelet aggregation, respectively. Also shown, in italics, are the drugs and sites of inhibition of platelet aggregation.

platelet aggregation.[99,100] For example, thrombin production releases ADP, which is a potent inducer of platelet aggregation and stimulates prostaglandin synthesis from arachidonic acid in the platelet. The prostaglandins synthesized, PGI_2 and TXA_2, have opposite effects on thrombogenesis. PGI_2 is synthesized in the walls of the vasculature and inhibits thrombus formation. Conversely, TXA_2, which is synthesized in the platelets, induces vasoconstriction and thrombogenesis. Serotonin, which also is released from the platelets, has similar and additive effects to those of TXA_2.

This rapid platelet aggregation and thrombus formation at the site of vascular injury is the main mechanism of hemostasis (stoppage of bleeding, a normal process of wound healing). When platelets are activated on the ruptured atherosclerotic plaques or in regions of restricted blood flow, it can lead to thromboembolic complications that contribute to MI or ischemic stroke.

Mechanism of Action of Antiplatelet Drugs

Antiplatelet drugs, such as aspirin, dipyridamole, and ticlopidine, exert their actions by affecting only the secondary platelet aggregation pathways.[101,102] For example, aspirin inhibits the biosynthesis of TXA_2 in the platelets by irreversibly and permanently inactivating cyclooxygenase (COX)-1 through covalent acetylation of a key serine residue. A cumulative inactivation effect occurs on platelets with long-term aspirin therapy in doses as low as 30 mg/d, because platelets do not synthesize new COX enzyme.[98] Therefore, the effects of aspirin lasts for the lifetime of the platelet (7-10 d). Dipyridamole interrupts platelet function by inhibiting phosphodiesterase, which results in the increased cellular concentration of cAMP (Fig. 18.18). Dipyridamole may also stimulate PGI_2 release and inhibit TXA_2 formation. Ticlopidine, clopidogrel, and prasugrel selectively inhibit ADP-induced platelet aggregation with no direct action on prostaglandin production. New and more selective antiplatelet drugs, such as thrombin receptor antagonists, protease-activated receptor 1 (PAR-1) antagonists, integrin αIIbβ3 receptor antagonists (GPIIb/IIIa blockers), thromboxane synthase inhibitors, and TXA_2 receptor antagonists, have been developed for anticoagulant therapy.[102] Recent trials with the PAR-1 antagonists have indicated that these agents may provide a better overall platelet inhibition without the liability of increased bleeding when used with aspirin or clopidogrel.[100]

COX-1 Inhibitors

TXA_2 is a potent vasoconstrictor and an inducer of platelet aggregation. Thus, the inhibition of TXA_2 synthesis will block platelet aggregation. Aspirin and related analogs exhibit their effectiveness as antiplatelet aggregating agents through the COX-TXA_2 pathway.

Aspirin

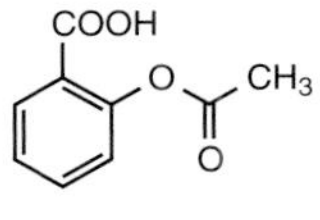

Aspirin

Aspirin is a well-established antiplatelet drug in the treatment of atherothrombotic vascular disease.[13,98,99,101] Aspirin works by acetylating (Fig. 18.19) and irreversibly deactivating platelet cyclooxygenase (COX-1), and its effect lasts the life of the platelet. Aspirin also has been shown to have other antithrombotic effects that are unrelated to its action on COX-1.[101] These include the dose-dependent inhibition of platelet function, the enhancement of fibrinolysis, and the attenuation of blood coagulation.

Aspirin is rapidly absorbed in the stomach and quickly degraded by plasma cholinesterase (half-life, 15-20 min). A once-daily dose of 50-100 mg of aspirin, colloquially known as a "baby aspirin," is sufficient to completely, and irreversibly, inactivate platelet COX-1.[98,101] Higher doses of aspirin are needed for anti-inflammatory and analgesic actions, but also can result in significant internal bleeding and upper gastrointestinal irritations.

In recent years, the term "aspirin resistance" has been used to describe those situations wherein the use of aspirin is unable to protect a patient from thrombotic complications, or to produce an anticipated effect on one or more in vitro tests of platelet function.[98,101,103] One plausible explanation for aspirin-resistant TXA_2 biosynthesis is the transient expression of COX-2 in newly formed platelets.[104] Many other clinical, pharmacodynamic, biologic, and genetic factors, such as drug interactions, alternative pathways for platelet activation, and genetic polymorphism or mutations of the COX-1 gene, may be involved.[105]

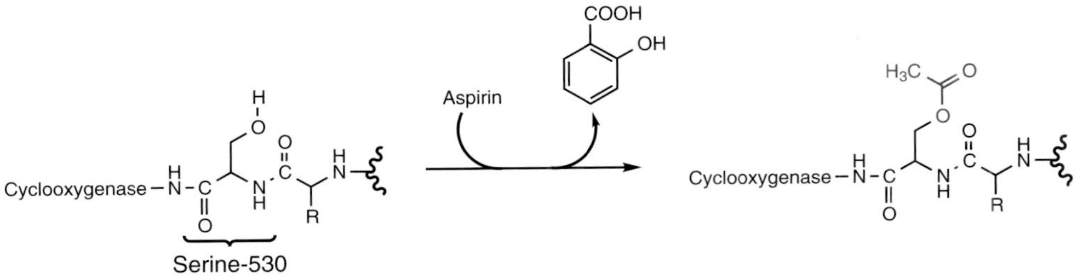

Figure 18.19 Irreversible acetylation of serine-530 in cyclooxygenase-1 by aspirin.

Phosphodiesterase Inhibitors

Phosphodiesterase-3 (PDE3) is an enzyme responsible for the degradation of cAMP to AMP in platelets and blood vessels. Selective cAMP PDE3 inhibitors, such as dipyridamole and cilostazol (Fig. 18.20), inhibit the degradation of cAMP. The resulting increase in the cellular concentration of cAMP promotes increased levels of protein kinase A and causes the inhibition of platelet aggregation.[106]

Dipyridamole (Aggrenox)

Dipyridamole (Fig. 18.20) is a pyrimido-pyrimidine derivative with vasodilatory and antiplatelet properties. Dipyridamole exerts its antiplatelet function by increasing cellular concentrations of cAMP by inhibiting cyclic nucleotide PDE3. It also blocks adenosine uptake, which acts on adenosine A_2 receptors to stimulate platelet adenylyl cyclase. Less common uses for this drug include the inhibition of embolization from prosthetic heart valves when used in combination with warfarin (the only currently recommended use) and the reduction of thrombosis in patients with thrombotic disease when combined with aspirin. Dipyridamole has little benefit in the treatment of thrombotic conditions as a stand-alone drug.[101,107]

Cilostazol (Pletaal)

Cilostazol (Fig. 18.20) is a potent orally active antiplatelet drug approved for the treatment of intermittent claudication (a peripheral artery disease resulting from blockage of blood vessels in the limbs). Cilostazol exhibits greater selectivity than dipyridamole as an inhibitor of PDE3A (Fig. 18.21).[107] The drug does not affect the other PDE isoforms (PDEs 1, 2, or 4). Cilostazol reversibly inhibits platelet aggregation that may be induced by specific stimuli, such as thrombin, ADP, collagen, or stress from exercise.[106,108] Additionally, cilostazol inhibits adenosine uptake, leading to increased activity of adenosine at A_1 and A_2 receptors. Adenosine's action on A_2 receptors in platelets increases cAMP levels, which leads to decreased platelet aggregation.[109]

METABOLISM AND PHARMACOKINETICS. Cilostazol is rapidly absorbed after oral administration, particularly with a high-fat meal, which greatly increases its bioavailability to approximately 90%. It is extensively metabolized in the liver by CYP450 enzymes. The most important ones appear to be CYP3A4 and, to a lesser extent, CYP2C19, with an elimination half-life of approximately 11-13 hours.[110] Among the various metabolites produced (11 metabolites are known), the two major and pharmacologically active metabolites are 3,4-dehydrocilostazol and 4′-*trans*-hydroxycilostazol (Fig. 18.22). Studies indicate that the concomitant administration of cilostazol with CYP3A inhibitors can greatly increase cilostazol blood concentrations, and a dose reduction may be required.[110,111] Similar results are seen when CYP2C19 is inhibited, which leads to the decreased formation of 4′-*trans*-hydroxycilostazol and accompanying increases in 3,4-dehydrocilostazol and the native drug.[110]

Platelet P2Y Purinergic Receptor Antagonists

ADP plays a pivotal role in platelet activation and platelet aggregation.[8,98] The purinergic G protein–coupled P2Y receptors are targets of ADP. There are three nucleotide receptors: P2X1, a cation channel receptor activated by ATP, and the purinergic receptors P2Y1 and P2Y12, both of which are activated by ADP. Initial binding of ADP to the purinergic P2Y1 receptor (373–amino acid protein) induces changes in platelet shape, elevates intracellular calcium mobilization, and initiates platelet aggregation. Subsequent binding of ADP to the other purinergic receptor, P2Y12 (342 amino acids) leads to inhibition of adenylate cyclase and, thereby, decreasing cellular cAMP levels.[112] The result of this series of events is sustained platelet aggregation. The antithrombotic drugs ticlopidine, clopidogrel, and prasugrel are irreversible antagonists of the P2Y12 purinergic receptor, while ticagrelor and is a reversible antagonist (Fig. 18.23).[113,114] The pharmacological and clinical relevance of P2Y12 antagonists has been extensively reviewed.[114-116]

Irreversible Inhibitors of P2Y12 Receptors

Ticlopidine, clopidogrel, and prasugrel inhibit platelet aggregation, prolong bleeding time, and delay clot retraction.[116] They belong to the thienopyridine class and are prescribed for reduction of MI and stroke, for treatment of peripheral arterial disease, and in combination with aspirin for acute coronary syndromes. This last indication appears to result from the fact that both aspirin and the thienopyridines block major amplification pathways, leading to platelet aggregation and, consequently, producing

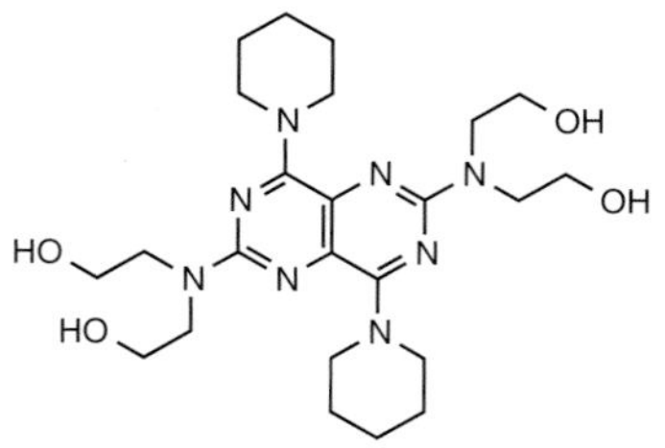

Dipyridamole
(Aggrenox, Persantine)

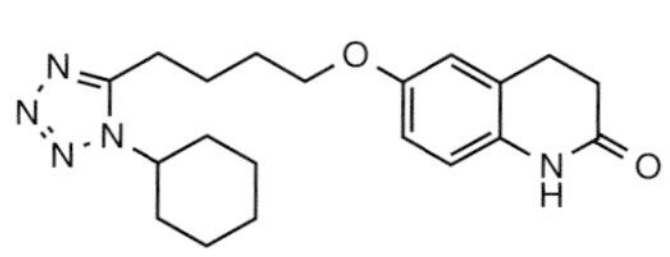

Cilostazol
(Pletal)

Figure 18.20 Chemical structures of phosphodiesterase inhibitors.

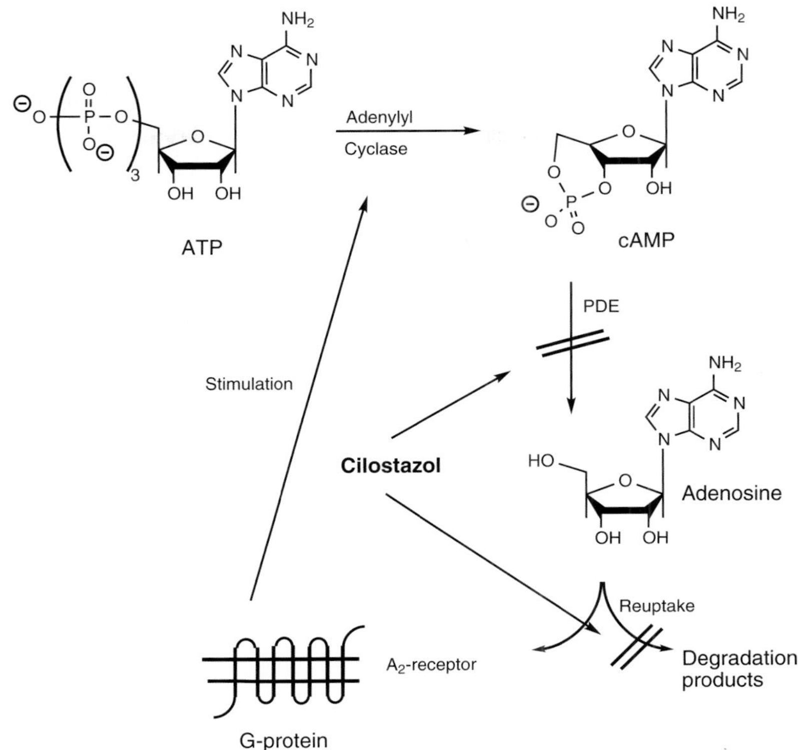

Figure 18.21 Sites of action of cilostazol, blocking phosphodiesterase 3A (PDE) and adenosine uptake, leading to increased levels of cyclic adenosine monophosphate (cAMP) directly by inhibition of cAMP breakdown and indirectly through adenosine binding to adenosine 2 receptors (A_2-receptor), which, through G protein coupling, stimulate adenylyl cyclase.

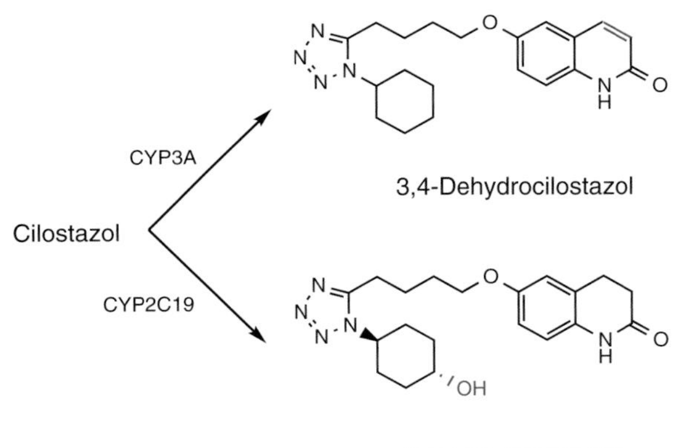

Figure 18.22 Metabolism of cilostazol.

enhanced effectiveness. Ticlopidine has safety concerns in that in a small population (1%-2%), it can induce potentially fatal neutropenia or thrombocytopenic purpura. These same side effects are rare with clopidogrel, and therefore, ticlopidine has been largely replaced with clopidogrel.[117]

Prasugrel is approved for treatment of acute coronary syndrome when managed with percutaneous coronary intervention.[118-120] The drug has also been shown to reduce the rate of thrombotic cardiovascular events in unstable angina and some forms of MI. Prasugrel is similar to clopidogrel and ticlopidine in the prevention of platelet aggregation.

Mechanism of Action Through Metabolism

The thienopyridine class exhibits a selective inhibition of ADP-induced platelet aggregation. The actions of ticlopidine, clopidogrel, and prasugrel appears to be irreversible since antiplatelet activity persists for 7-10 days after the discontinuation of therapy (Fig. 18.24).[121] The possible irreversible inhibition of P2Y12 may be explained by the observation that ticlopidine is not effective in inhibiting platelet aggregation in vitro when compared to the in vivo effect of the drug on the platelets of patients taking ticlopidine. Ticlopidine and clopidogrel are rapidly absorbed and extensively oxidized by the action of CYP450 enzymes, particularly CYP3A4 and CYP2B6 (Fig. 18.25). (S)-clopidogrel is oxidatively transformed to the thiolactone, which undergoes hydrolysis. The resulting free thiol forms a covalent disulfide bond with critical cysteine residues (Cys97, Cys175) in the active site of P2Y12 and prevents the binding of endogenous agonists.[122-124] With ticlopidine, oxidative activation occurs, but additional metabolites that are formed include dihydrothienopyridinium (M5) and thienodihydropyridinium (M6). These short-lived cationic metabolites may be responsible for the toxic adverse reactions.[125]

Prasugrel is a prodrug that is activated to form an irreversible inhibitor of P2Y12 receptors. Unlike (S)-clopidogrel, prasugrel's initial activation involves hydrolysis of the pendant ester. The resulting thiolactone is further hydrolyzed to reveal the reactive thiol (R-138727), which

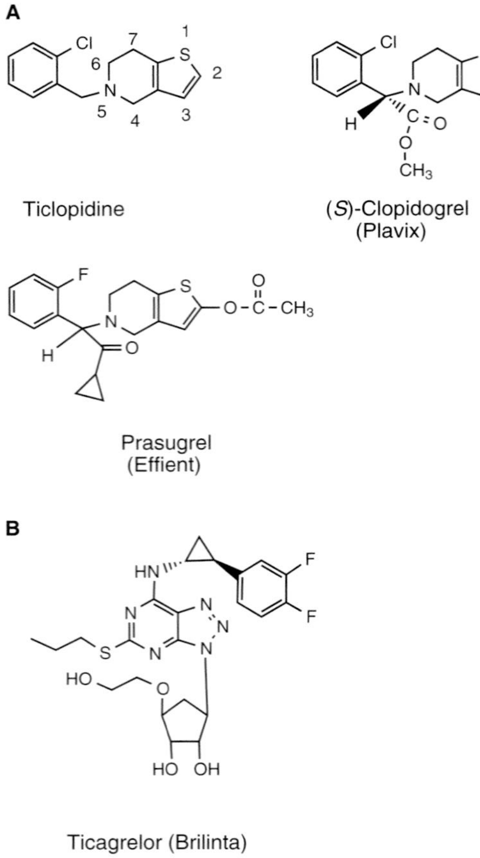

A

Ticlopidine

(*S*)-Clopidogrel (Plavix)

Prasugrel (Effient)

B

Ticagrelor (Brilinta)

Figure 18.23 2PY12 inhibitors. A, Irreversible inhibitors. B, Reversible inhibitor.

forms a covalent disulfide bridge with Cys97 and Cys175 of P2Y12.[124] As a result, P2Y12 is irreversibly inhibited.[116,126-128] The secondary fate of R-138727 is its inactivation via S-methylation (Fig. 18.25), which effectively prevents it from forming disulfide bridges. Additional minor metabolites formed through CYP-catalyzed reactions have been isolated.

Pharmacokinetics

All three drugs are rapidly absorbed following oral administration and are highly bound to plasma protein (~98%). Clopidogrel can be administered with or without food and it exhibits a $t_{1/2}$ of ~6 hours. The drug and its metabolites are excreted nearly equally in both urine and feces. Prasugrel reaches peak plasma concentration of R-138727 within 30 minutes. High-fat diets may slow the time to reach maximum plasma concentration, and it is recommended that the drug be taken on an empty stomach. Prasugrel is excreted as the inactive metabolite through both urine (68%) and fecal routes (27%). Prasugrel is commonly used in combination with aspirin and is reported to be more effective than clopidogrel in treatment of unstable angina or MI. Prasugrel has a higher rate of major bleeding and life-threatening bleeding than clopidogrel.[129] Even though prasugrel has a faster onset and reduced interpatient variability compared with clopidogrel, it appears to have a higher rate of bleeding incidences than clopidogrel. This underscored the need to discover reversible inhibitors of P2Y12 to overcome these issues.

Reversible Inhibitor of P2Y12: Ticagrelor (Fig. 18.23)

Mechanism of Action

Ticagrelor (Brilinta) is a cyclopentyltriazolopyrimidine that exerts antiplatelet aggregative effects by reversibly inhibiting the P2Y12 receptor.[130,131] The drug is metabolized in the plasma by CYP3A4 and 3A5 to form an equipotent, active metabolite AR-C124910XX (Fig. 18.26).[132] The metabolism is extensive with a number of metabolites identified in the urine. The major urinary metabolite results from N-dealkylation.

Pharmacokinetics

Ticagrelor is rapidly absorbed, with a median time to peak concentration (T_{max}) of 2-3 hours after multiple twice/day oral dosing. Mean elimination half-lives of ticagrelor and

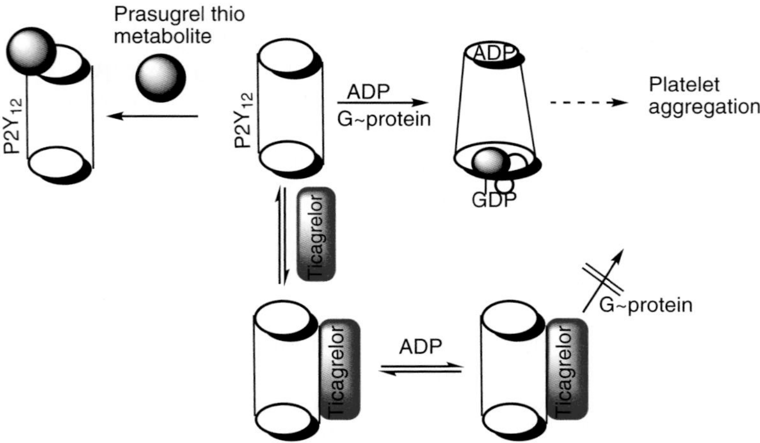

Figure 18.24 Scheme describing platelet aggregation resulting from ADP binding to the P2Y12 receptor, conformational changes in the receptor, and G protein coupling. This process can be inhibited irreversibly by the thio metabolite of prasugrel binding near the ADP binding site or reversibly by ticagrelor binding to a remote site resulting in blocking conformational changes to the receptor.

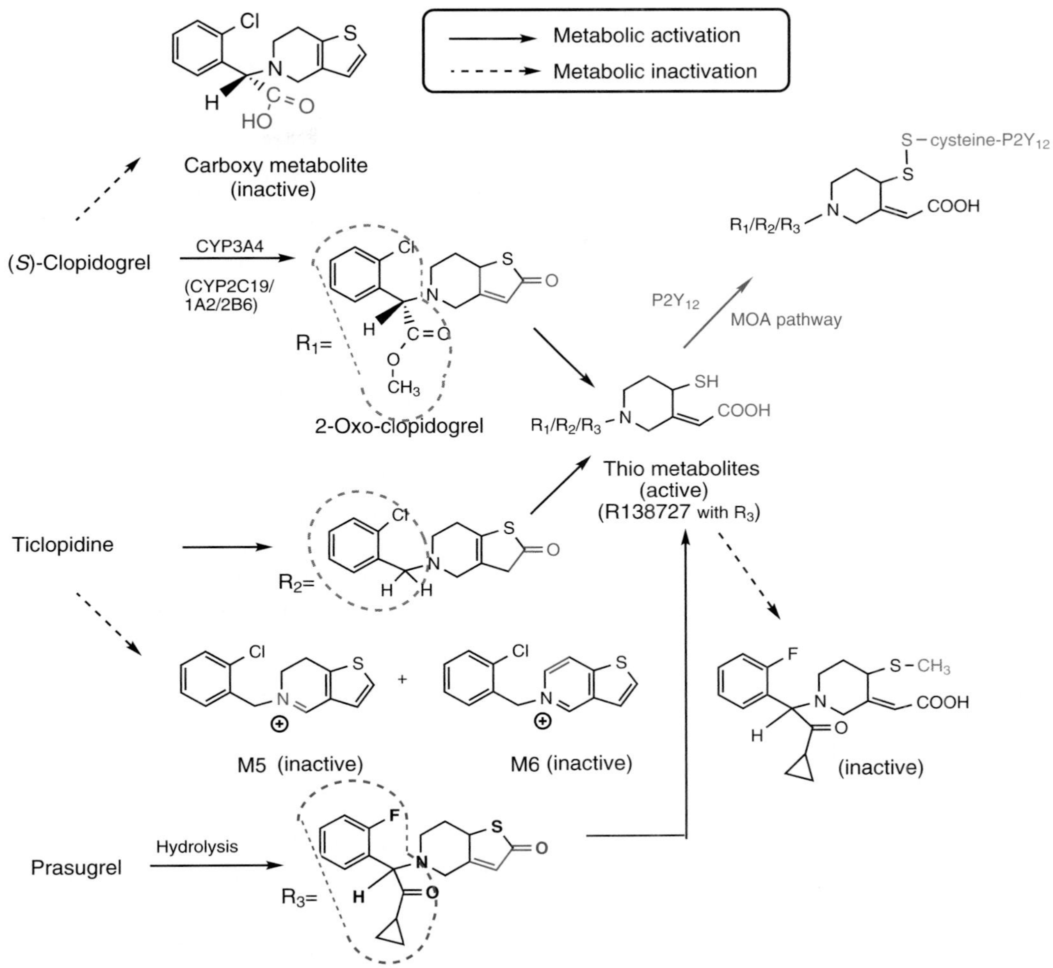

Figure 18.25 Metabolism of clopidogrel, ticlopidine, and prasugrel. The thio metabolites react irreversibly with P2Y12.

the active metabolite were 8.1 and 9.9 hour, respectively. Ticagrelor is eliminated in the feces (58%) and in the urine (27%).[133] Levels of unchanged drug and metabolites were <0.05% in the urine, which suggests compatibility of use in patients with renal impairment. Ticagrelor is indicated to reduce the rate of cardiovascular death, MI, and stroke in patients with acute coronary syndrome (ACS) or a history of MI.[116,131,134,135] For the first year following acute coronary syndrome, ticagrelor is found to be superior to clopidogrel.

Glycoprotein GPIIb/IIIa Receptor Antagonists

Glycoprotein IIb/IIIa receptors are a group of integrins that are expressed on the surface of platelets (Fig. 18.18). The binding of adhesive proteins, such as fibronectin and vWF, to these integrins is a Ca^{2+}-dependent process and involves a γ-dodecapeptide and the specific tripeptide sequence of arginine, glycine, and aspartic acid (RGD sequence). The RGD motif of fibronectin enables its binding to two

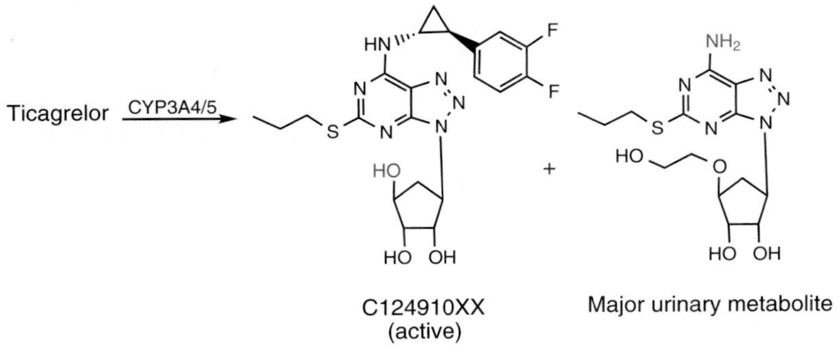

Figure 18.26 Metabolism of ticagrelor.

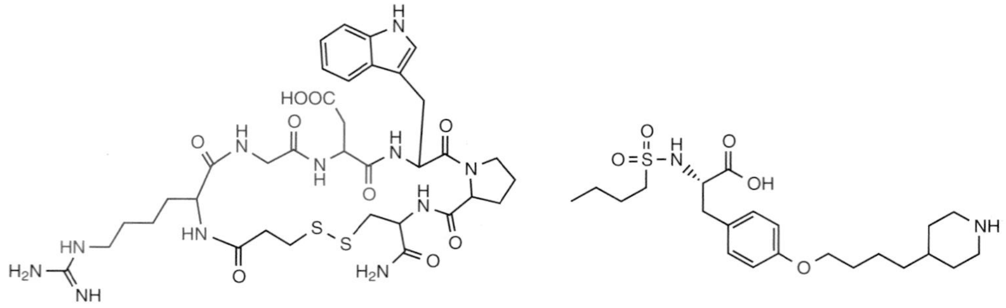

Figure 18.27 GPIIb/IIIa receptor antagonists eptifibatide and tirofiban.

GPIIb/IIIa receptors, creating a cross-link, and eventually results in platelet aggregation. Antagonists of the GPIIb/IIIa receptor antagonists are a new class of antithrombotic agents that impair platelet aggregation by competing for binding with fibrinogen.[98,136,137] These agents have demonstrated comprehensive inhibition of platelet aggregation when compared to the standard combination of aspirin and heparin.[134] The drugs that are classified as GPIIb/IIIa receptor antagonists are abciximab, a monoclonal antibody against the GPIIb/IIIa receptor, and the small molecules, eptifibatide and tirofiban (Fig. 18.27).[138,139]

The GPIIb/IIIa receptor antagonists are indicated in therapy for unstable angina, non–Q-wave MI, and percutaneous coronary procedures. Like other antithrombotic agents, the main concern associated with GPIIb/IIIa receptor antagonists is excessive bleeding. Additionally, these drugs have been suggested to possibly increase the risk of thrombocytopenia.[101,140] Although many orally active GPIIb/IIIa receptor antagonists have been prepared and evaluated, their clinical efficacy in the treatment of patients with acute unstable angina and in those undergoing angioplasty has not been fully proven.[138]

Abciximab (ReoPro)

Abciximab is a chimeric human-mouse 7E3 Fab that has a high binding affinity at the GPIIb/IIIa receptor and is widely studied in patients undergoing percutaneous coronary intervention.[141,142] For an adult patient, the usual dosing scheme is 0.25 mg/kg as an intravenous bolus given 10-60 minutes before percutaneous coronary intervention, followed by the continuous infusion of 0.125 μg/kg/min for 12 hours, to a maximum of 10 μg/kg. The elimination of abciximab is biphasic. The initial phase has a half-life of 10 minutes, whereas the second phase has a half-life of 30 minutes, which results from platelet binding. Platelet function returns to normal within 48 hours after infusion, even though abciximab stays bound to circulating platelets for about 2 weeks (Table 18.6).[143,144]

Eptifibatide (Integrilin)

Eptifibatide (Fig. 18.27) is derived from rattlesnake venom and contains the Lys-Gly-Asp (KGD) sequence along with synthetic peptides containing either Arg-Gly-Asp (RGD), derived from barbourin,[145] and peptidomimetic and nonpeptide RGD mimetics that compete against fibrinogen, vWF, and fibronectin via occupancy of the receptor.[101] Fibrinogen, vWF, and fibronectin contain the natural RGD sequence making them natural ligands for the GPIIb/IIIa receptor.

MECHANISM OF ACTION. Eptifibatide is a cyclic hexapeptide composed of six amino acids and one mercaptopropionyl residue, which is connected to the cysteine via a disulfide linkage. The Lys-Gly-Asp (KDG) component of eptifibatide targets the GPIIb/IIIa receptor, with low binding affinity as indicated by the rapid dissociation constant (Table 18.5). Therefore, eptifibatide is a reversible, parenterally administered antagonist of platelet aggregation.

METABOLISM AND CLINICAL IMPORTANCE. Eptifibatide is eliminated primarily through the kidney in the form of eptifibatide and deaminated eptifibatide. The clinical importance of eptifibatide and its benefits in comparison with

Table 18.5 Pharmacokinetic Properties of Antifactor Xa Inhibitors

Drugs	Bioavailability (%)	Protein Binding (%)	$T_{1/2}$ (hr)	Maximum Plasma Concentration (hr)	K_i (nmol/L)
Apixaban	~87%	92-95	12	3	0.8
Betrixaban	34%	~50	19-27	3-4	
Edoxaban	62%	55	10-14	1-2	
Rivaroxaban	>80%	60	5-9	3	0.4

other therapeutic agents used in the treatment of acute coronary syndromes and percutaneous coronary intervention have recently been reviewed by Curran and Keating.[146]

Tirofiban Hydrochloride (Aggrastat)

MECHANISM OF ACTION. Tirofiban (Fig. 18.27) is a member of a new class of antithrombotic agents known as the "fibans" as they act as fibrinogen receptor antagonists. Tirofiban is a nonpeptide antagonist that structurally mimics the RGD loop of disintegrin (isolated from snake venom) using an optimized tyrosine residue. The location of the carboxylic acid and amine functional groups in the fibans is identical to the distance between the same functional groups within the RGD loop of disintegrin. Consequently, fibans effectively prevent the binding of fibrinogen to the GPIIb/IIIa receptor in a reversible manner.

CLINICAL IMPORTANCE. Tirofiban has a rapid dissociation constant, which explains the reversibility (Table 18.6). Tirofiban is parenterally administered. It has modest binding affinity for the GPIIb/IIIa receptor and exhibits a reduced risk of bleeding because of its shorter biologic half-life compared to abciximab.[147] The clinical use of tirofiban in ST elevation for MI is effective and has an acceptable safety profile.[147,148]

Pathophysiology of Arterial Thrombosis

The central role of platelets in thrombus formation and potential sites for drug interventions are depicted in Fig. 18.18.[99,100] Normal endothelial cells in the vascular wall synthesize and release prostacyclin (PGI_2), enabling the conversion of ATP to cAMP, thus preventing platelet aggregation and degranulation. In the case of an injury to the vascular wall, glycoprotein (GP) receptors bind vWF and collagen from the exposed subendothelial surface, resulting in platelet activation. The GPIIb/IIIa receptors (also known as the fibrinogen receptor or integrin $\alpha IIb\beta 3$ receptor) then mediate the final step of platelet aggregation by binding to fibrinogen or vWF, causing platelets to cross-link and form aggregates.

The adherent platelets degranulate and release additional aggregating substances, such as thromboxane A_2 (TXA_2), serotonin (5-HT), thrombin, and adenosine diphosphate (ADP). These substances serve as secondary chemical messengers to recruit more platelets to the site of vascular injury and, thereby, amplify platelet aggregation.[99,100] For example, thrombin production releases ADP, which is a potent inducer of platelet aggregation and stimulates prostaglandin synthesis from arachidonic acid in the platelet. The prostaglandins synthesized, PGI_2 and TXA_2, have opposite effects on thrombogenesis. PGI_2 is synthesized in the walls of the vasculature and inhibits thrombus formation. Conversely, TXA_2, which is synthesized in the platelets, induces vasoconstriction and thrombogenesis. Serotonin, which also is released from the platelets, has similar and additive effects to those of TXA_2.

This rapid platelet aggregation and thrombus formation at the site of vascular injury is the main mechanism of hemostasis (stoppage of bleeding, a normal process of wound healing). When platelets are activated on the ruptured atherosclerotic plaques or in regions of restricted blood flow, it can lead to thromboembolic complications that contribute to MI or ischemic stroke.

Protease-Activated Receptor 1

PARs are glycoprotein-coupled receptors (GPCRs). Four PARs (PARs 1-4) have been identified, of which PAR-1 and PAR-4 are present on the platelet surface. These receptors are involved in the process of α-thrombin–initiated platelet aggregation. Thrombin is a serine protease that binds to PAR-1, resulting in the scission between Arg41 and Ser42 of the N-terminus exo-membrane 7-transmembrane-spanning GPCR. The released N-terminal serine then binds to the serine binding site on loop II of the GPCR to initiate platelet aggregation (Fig. 18.28).

Mechanism of Action

Vorapaxar (Zontivity) is a potent, highly selective, reversible, himbacine-based PAR-1 antagonist of thrombin binding to PAR-1 blocking Step 1 in the thrombin-mediated platelet aggregation (Fig. 18.29) process shown in Figure 18.28.

Pharmacokinetics

Vorapaxar is rapidly absorbed following oral administration and has ~100% bioavailability. The drug is highly bound (>99%) to plasma proteins. The drug has a long half-life (159-311 hr), suggesting that its release from PAR-1 is quite slow. Vorapaxar is metabolized by CYP3A4 to the primary metabolite (M19) and minor amounts of M20 at a slow rate (Fig. 18.30). Elimination via biliary and gastrointestinal routes by CYP3A4 isozymes is at a very

Table 18.6 Pharmacokinetic Properties of the Glycoprotein IIb/IIIa Receptor Antagonists

Drug	Trade Name	Route of Administration	Molecular Weight (Da)	Dissociation Constant (nmol/L)	Plasma Half-Life (hr)	Protein Binding (%)
Abciximab	ReoPro	IV	47,615	5	72	
Eptifibatide	Integrilin	IV	800	120	4	25
Tirofiban	Aggrastat	IV	495	15	3-4	65

IV, intravenous; *hr*, hours.

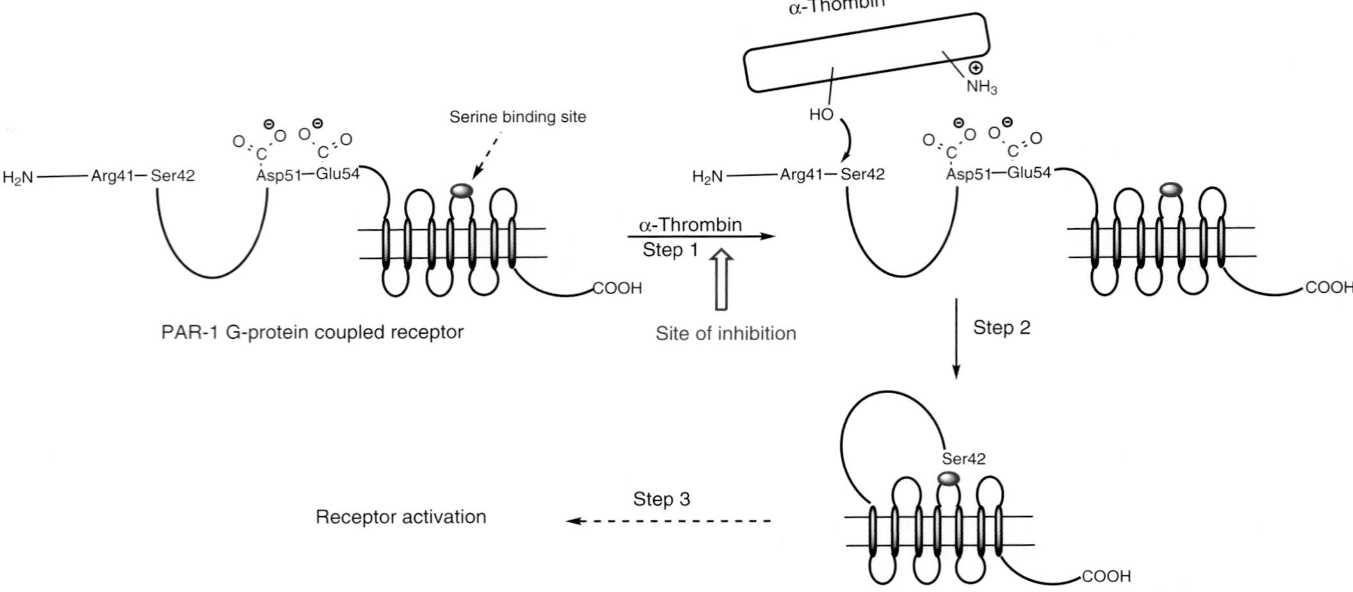

Figure 18.28 Activation of platelet aggregation via thrombin. The thrombin binds to the PAR-1 receptor as shown in Step 1 through ionic binding involving a charge portion of amino acids 51-56 in the PAR-1, while the serine protease portion of thrombin catalyzes the hydrolysis at arginine-41/serine-42. The tethered serine-42 then binds to a portion of exomembrane loop II of the GPCR shown in Step 2 which initiates platelet aggregation as shown in Step 3. Vorapaxar is a reversible competitive inhibitor of thrombin receptor–activation peptide, thus selectively blocking platelet aggregation.

slow rate.[149] The drug is eliminated in the feces (58%) and urine (25%). CYP3A4 inhibitors and inducers can significantly affect plasma levels of vorapaxar. Therefore, this may require dose adjustment in the presence of CY3A4 inhibitors or inducers.

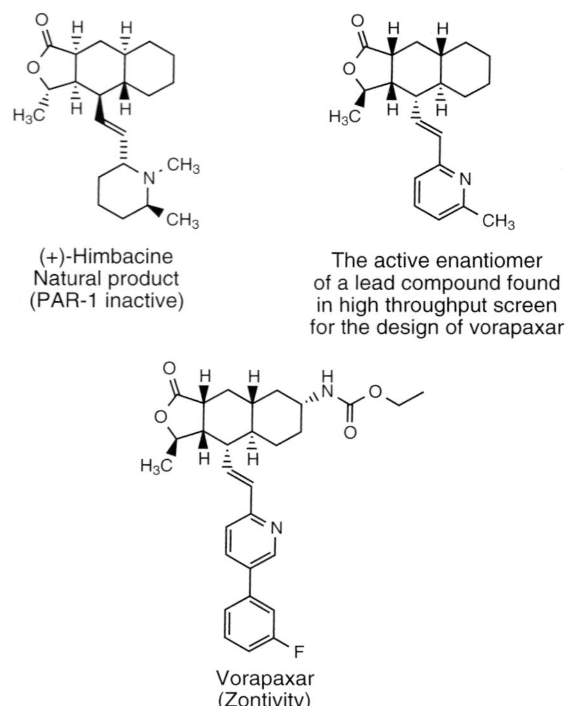

Figure 18.29 Structures of compounds leading to the design of the PAR-1 receptor antagonist vorapaxar.

Clinical Applications

Vorapaxar is well tolerated in patients undergoing nonurgent percutaneous coronary intervention.[149,150] It has been demonstrated in clinical trials that vorapaxar improves ischemic outcomes without significantly increasing the bleeding liability, compared to prasugrel.[98,100,102] Vorapaxar has been approved for use in reducing the risk of MI, stroke, or cardiovascular death in patients with a previous MI or peripheral

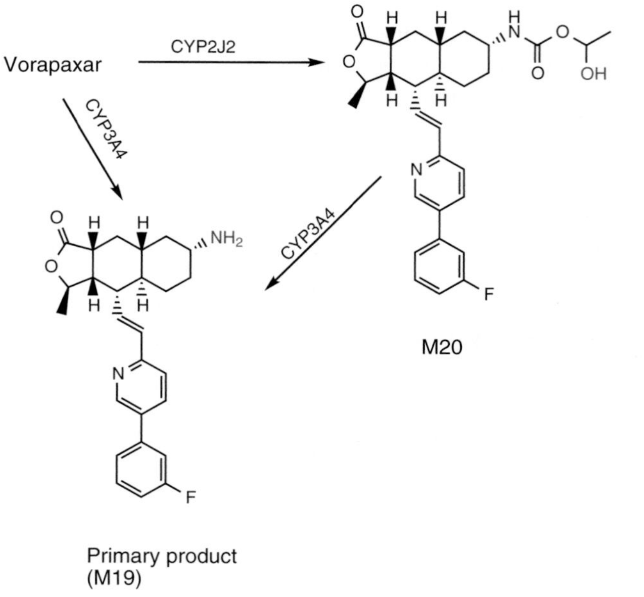

Figure 18.30 Vorapaxar metabolism

artery disease.[151] The drug is also used in combination with aspirin or clopidogrel for optimal therapeutic management.

Oligonucleotide Anticoagulant

Defibrotide (Defitelio)

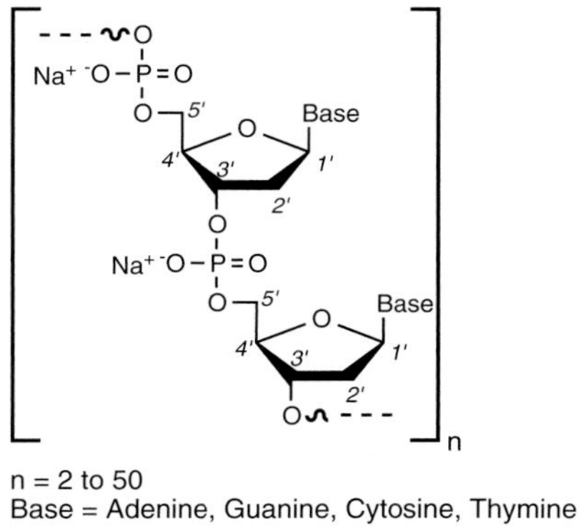

n = 2 to 50
Base = Adenine, Guanine, Cytosine, Thymine

Defibrotide (Defitelio)

Defibrotide is a single-stranded DNA oligonucleotide 9-80 phosphodiester units (9-80-mer) with an average of 50-mer (MW: 16.5 + 2.5 kDa) units. The drug is derived from the cow lung or porcine mucosa.[152]

MECHANISM OF ACTION. The mechanism of action is not fully clear. Defibrotide has been shown to improve the enzymatic activity of plasmin to hydrolyze fibrin. When evaluated against a human microvascular endothelial cell line, defibrotide caused the increased expression of thrombomodulin and tissue-type plasminogen activator (tPA) and a reduction in the expression of plasminogen activator inhibitor 1 (PAI-1) and vWF. This resulted in the overall decrease in endothelial cell activation and increase in cell-mediated breakdown of fibrin. It acts as an anticoagulant as it helps dissolve blood clots by a combination of multiple mechanisms that involve increasing levels of PGI2, E2, and prostacyclin.[153]

Pharmacokinetics

Defibrotide is reported to be effective via orally, IM, or IV routes of administration. Under IV conditions, peak plasma levels are reached at the end of the infusion. Drug bioavailability orally is 58%-70% with a half-life of less than 2 hours and therefore must be given two to four times a day. The exact pathway of degradation is unclear, but since defibrotide is a polynucleotide, it is believed to be rapidly degraded by enzymes (e.g., nucleases, deaminases, phosphorylases). Defibrotide is metabolized to 2′-deoxyribose and purine and pyrimidine bases, and these are eliminated by urinary excretion. Side effects include increased bleeding and bruising, nausea, vomiting, heartburn, and low blood pressure.

THERAPEUTIC APPLICATIONS. Defibrotide is approved for treatment of severe hepatic venoocclusive disease (VOD) after hematopoietic stem cell transplantation (HSCT) in adult and pediatric populations. VOD is a complication associated with stem cell transplantation and is often fatal (>80% mortality). VOD results in multiorgan dysfunction and may include kidney, lung, and heart dysfunction.[152] The drug is also indicated off-label for other conditions such as peripheral obliterative arterial disease, thrombophlebitis, and Raynaud's disease. The concomitant use of defibrotide with anticoagulants or fibrinolytics may increase the risk of hemorrhage.

THROMBOLYTIC DRUGS

The use of thrombolytic agents in the rapid and early application of reperfusion therapy has significantly improved the outcomes of conditions such as PE, DVT, arterial thrombosis, acute MI, and peripheral vascular thromboembolism.[154]

The first-generation of thrombolytic drugs were approved in the 1980s, with subsequent improvements emerging as second- and third-generation drugs. Thus, thrombolytic therapy is a part of the treatment modality for patients with acute MI or stroke.[154,155] A recent editorial suggests that the use of thrombolytics for the treatment of stroke may not be effective and may actually result in brain hemorrhage.

Mechanism of Action

Newly formed blood clots are dissolved by the protease action of plasmin, which digests fibrin (see coagulation cascade, Fig. 18.1). A lack of substrate specificity of plasmin is evident in that it degrades fibrin clots as well as some plasma proteins and coagulation factors.

Plasmin is produced from the inactive proenzyme plasminogen by the action of plasminogen activators, such as tissue-type plasminogen activator (tPA) that is released from the vascular endothelium. The cleavage of a single peptide bond of plasminogen by a group of trypsin-like serine proteases results in the activation. Endogenously, plasmin activity is regulated by two specific inactivators, known as tPA inhibitors 1 and 2. Plasmin cannot be used directly as a drug because of the presence of naturally occurring plasmin antagonists in plasma. Thrombolytic drugs, such as streptokinase and alteplase, act as plasminogen activators that enable the formation of active plasmin.

First-Generation Thrombolytic Agents

Streptokinase (Streptase)

Streptokinase is an exocellular protein produced by several strains of β-hemolytic streptococci. It is the only thrombolytic drug approved by the FDA for peripheral vascular disease.[156] While it has been approved for treatment of MI, it has since been replaced with improved fibrin-specific agents.[157] It is also a drug of choice for thrombolytic therapy owing to its cost-effectiveness.

MECHANISM OF ACTION. Streptokinase is a protein purified from group C β-hemolytic streptococci bacteria. Streptokinase contains a single polypeptide chain of 414–amino acid residues with a molecular weight of 47 kDa.[156]

To become active, inactive streptokinase binds with plasminogen to form an activator complex (1:1 complex). This complex then acts to convert uncomplexed plasminogen to the active fibrinolytic enzyme, plasmin. The streptokinase/plasminogen complex not only degrades fibrin clots but also catalyzes the breakdown of fibrinogen and factors V and VII.[156] As a result, streptokinase is considered a fibrin-nonspecific drug.

PHARMACOKINETICS. Unfortunately, the half-life of the activator complex is less than 30 minutes, which frequently is too short to fully degrade a thrombus. Anistreplase (APSAC; Eminase) is a 1:1 streptokinase/lysine-plasminogen complex that has been acylated with an anisoyl group at the active site serine within the lysine-plasminogen. Anistreplase complexes with fibrin, resulting in the slow cleavage of the anisoyl group. This exposes the active site of fibrin and results in its degradation. The prodrug nature of anistreplase exhibits an improved pharmacokinetic profile, with anistreplase acting as a semiselective lytic agent at the clot site. The inactivity of the circulating anistreplase also allows this drug to be given as a very rapid intravenous infusion (typically, 30 units over 3-5 min). Tissue reperfusion following anistreplase therapy compares favorably to streptokinase because of the extended half-life (90 min).

SIDE EFFECTS. Streptokinase is associated with significant hypersensitivity reactions. Individuals who have had a streptococcal infection may have developed circulating antistreptococcal antibodies. These antibodies frequently are active against streptokinase, a foreign protein. The response of streptokinase to these antibodies can vary widely, from the inactivation of the fibrinolytic properties of the protein to rash, fever, and rarely, anaphylaxis. Significant allergic reactions to streptokinase occur in approximately 3% of patients.

Second-Generation Thrombolytic Agents

Alteplase (Activase)

Alteplase is a serine protease and an unmodified human tPA. It has a low affinity for free plasminogen but a very high affinity for fibrin-bound plasminogen (Fig. 18.31). This makes alteplase a fibrin-specific agent, unlike streptokinase which acts on free plasminogen. Alteplase has a greater specificity for older clots compared with newer clots, relative to streptokinase. At low doses, alteplase is quite selective for degrading fibrin without the simultaneous breakdown of other proteins, such as fibrinogen. However, at therapeutically useful doses, alteplase activates some

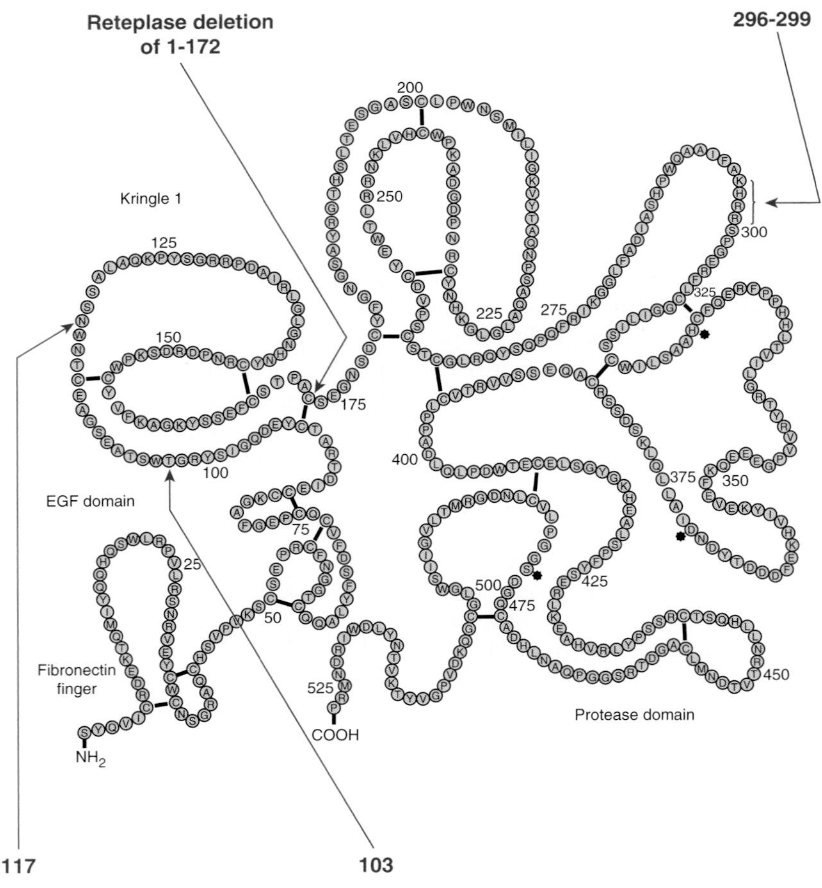

Figure 18.31 Schematic diagram of alteplase, reteplase (removal of amino acids 1-172), and tenecteplase in which threonine (T) at position 103 is replaced with asparagines, asparagine (N) at position 117 is replaced with glutamine, and lysine (K)-histidine-arginine-asparagine at positions 296-299 are replaced with four alanines. Adapted with permission from Nordt TK, Bode C. Thrombolysis: newer thrombolytic agents and their role in clinical medicine. *Heart*. 2003;89:1358-1362.

free plasminogen which can cause hemorrhage. The half-life of alteplase is very short (~5 min), necessitating its administration as a 15 mg intravenous bolus, followed by a 85 mg intravenous infusion over 90 minutes, or as 60 mg infused over the first hour, with the remaining 40 mg given at a rate of 20 mg/hr.

Third-Generation Thrombolytic Agents

The third-generation of thrombolytic agents are derived from structural modifications of the basic plasminogen activators (tPA or other tPA of animal origins) using technologies such as mutations, conjugation with monoclonal antibodies, or hybridization with another thrombolytic agent. Agents in this class include reteplase and tenecteplase.

Reteplase (Retavase)

Reteplase is a recombinant deletion mutant of human tPA lacking its finger, epidermal growth factor, kringle 1 domain, and carbohydrate side chain (Fig. 18.31).[158] As a highly fibrin-specific thrombolytic agent, reteplase is missing the first 172 amino acids that are present in alteplase and has 355 amino acids with a molecular weight of 39 kDa.[159] With the removal of the finger kringle 1 domain, reteplase binding to fibrin is reduced from that of alteplase, and reteplase has reduced fibrin selectivity. In addition, the structural modification reduces hepatic elimination, leading to a longer half-life (reteplase, 14-18 min compared to alteplase, 3-4 min). Reteplase is approved for use in acute MI and is administered as a double bolus of 10 U every 30 minutes.

Tenecteplase (TNKase)

Tenecteplase is composed of 527 amino acids with 17 disulfide bridges. It differs structurally from alteplase by three point mutations (Fig. 18.31). The mutations were bioengineered to occur at amino acid 103, where threonine (T) is replaced by asparagine (N); at amino acid 117, where asparagine (N) is replaced by glutamine (E); and at amino acids 296-299, where the lysine-histidine-arginine-arginine (KHRR) sequence is replaced with four alanine residues (AAAA). Thus, the name TNK is derived from the original amino acid that underwent mutation. The replacement of these amino acids along with their attached carbohydrate side chains results in a prolonged half-life (~17 min) and allows a single bolus application.[155] These point-mutations also increase the binding of tenecteplase to PAI-1 by 80-fold, thereby improving activity. Finally, tenecteplase shows a 15-fold higher specificity for fibrin. The drug is eliminated via hepatic mechanisms.

TOXICITY OF ANTITHROMBOTICS AND THROMBOLYTICS

Antithrombotic Toxicity

Warfarin exhibits its anticoagulation effects by preventing γ-carboxylation of specific glutamate residues necessary for vitamin K–dependent coagulation (Fig. 18.4). However, γ-carboxyglutamate proteins are not unique to coagulation factors and are also synthesized in the bone. Expectedly, warfarin inhibits the effects of vitamin K on osteoblast development. It has been suggested that this is the mechanism responsible for bone abnormalities in neonates born to mothers who were treated with warfarin while pregnant.[160] However, there is no evidence to suggest that bone metabolism or development is affected by warfarin when the drug is administered to children or adults. Because of the mechanism of action of these warfarin-like drugs, the management of their toxicity is based on vitamin K therapy (see "Coagulants," later in this chapter).

Unlike warfarin, heparin is safe for anticoagulant therapy during pregnancy.[160] Heparin does not cross the placental barrier and has shown no tendency to induce fetal damage, unlike warfarin which is known to cause serious fetal malformations. Furthermore, heparin does not increase fetal mortality or prematurity. However, to minimize the risk of postpartum hemorrhage, it is recommended that heparin therapy be withdrawn 24 hours before delivery.

Despite its safety in pregnancy, several potential problems are associated with heparin therapy. Heparins (HMWHs and LMWHs) are isolated from animal sources, which may result in antigenic hypersensitivity. Heparin competitively binds many other plasma proteins such as vitronectin and PF4 in addition to the antithrombin, which results in the inactivation of the heparin as an anticoagulating agent.[44] This may be the reason for heparin resistance and for a serious condition known as heparin-induced thrombocytopenia (HIT). Typically, this condition occurs 7-14 days after initiation of heparin therapy, but it may occur earlier in some patients who have had previous exposures to heparin. In these cases, heparin-induced platelet aggregation occurs and may result in the production of antiplatelet antibodies. Development of this condition necessitates the termination of heparin therapy and the institution of antiplatelet drugs or oral anticoagulants. The thrombocytopenia usually is reversible upon withdrawal of heparin. Mild increases in liver function tests frequently are associated with heparin therapy. Long-term use of full therapeutic doses of heparin (>20,000 U/d for 3-6 mo) has been associated with osteoporosis, and spontaneous vertebral fractures have been infrequently reported.[44] Hemorrhagic complications of heparin therapy are managed, in part, with the specific antagonist protamine sulfate (for further discussion, please refer to the section on "Coagulants").[44]

Thrombolytic Toxicities

The toxicity of anticoagulant drugs is of immense concern, as it may lead to hemorrhage or other drug-specific toxicities. The lack of specificity of plasmin results in the degradation of many plasma proteins, including several coagulation factors and the anticoagulating factor, activated protein C, in addition to fibrin. Thus, most thrombolytic drugs not only attack pathologic clots but also exert their actions on any other site of compromised vascular integrity. The dissolution of necessary clots results in the principal side effect of thrombolytic therapy, hemorrhage. Its action on the activated protein C also may be responsible for its neurovascular toxicities.[161]

Multiple studies have examined the incidence of life-threatening hemorrhage (i.e., intracranial hemorrhage) with the various thrombolytic medications. These studies indicate that the rate of significant hemorrhagic complication is essentially the same (0.1%-0.7%) regardless of the specific therapeutic agent used. Supportive care is indicated in cases of thrombolytic toxicity. No specific antagonist exists to manage thrombolytic medication–induced hemorrhage, but antifibrinolytic drugs, such as ε-aminocaproic acid and tranexamic acid, often are used.

COAGULANTS

A variety of pathologic and toxicologic conditions can result in excessive bleeding from inadequate coagulation. Depending on the etiology and severity of the hemorrhagic episode, several possible blood coagulation inducers may be employed.

Vitamin K

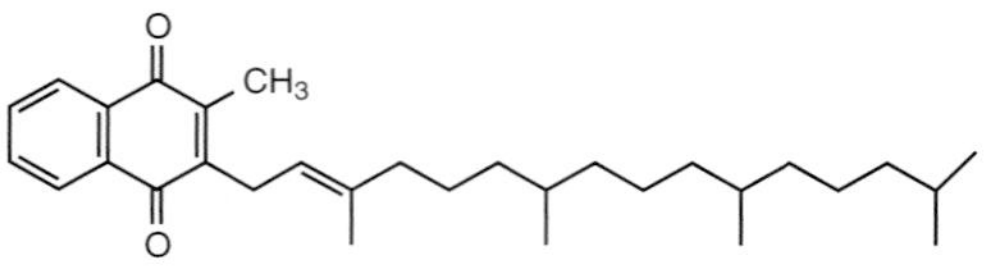

Vitamin K_1

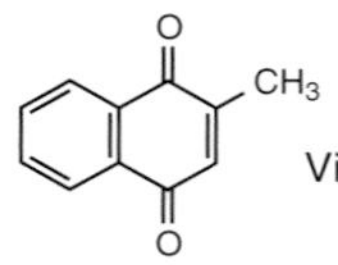

Vitamin K_3

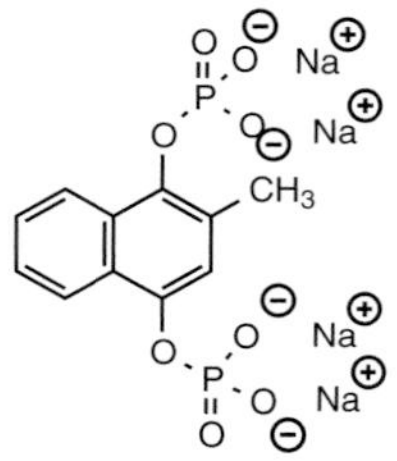

Vitamin K_4

Orally active anticoagulants, such as warfarin and the indandiones, act through interruption of the normal actions of vitamin K. Therefore, it is reasonable to assume that vitamin K should be effective in the treatment of bleeding induced by these agents.[154] Vitamin K_1 (phytonadione, Mephyton) is the fat-soluble form of vitamin K most often used therapeutically. Vitamin K_1 is safe for use in infants, pregnant women, and patients with glucose-6-phosphate deficiency. Furthermore, phytonadione has greater lipid solubility, has a faster onset of action, and requires smaller doses than vitamin K_3 (menadione) or vitamin K_4 (menadiol sodium diphosphate). Vitamins K_3 and K_4 are absorbed from the small intestine.[154] However, they produce hyperbilirubinemia and kernicterus in neonates as well as hemolysis in neonates and glucose-6-phosphate–deficient patients. Only vitamin K_1 is the appropriate therapy for bleeding associated with warfarin and superwarfarin poisoning. Vitamin K_2 is not used therapeutically.

Vitamin K_1 is effective at inducing coagulation when administered orally or parenterally. Although the oral route is preferred, it is not always practical in a patient who is critically hemorrhaging. The other routes of administration (SC, IM, IV), though used clinically, have significant potential drawbacks. Larger doses (e.g., volume >5 mL) are not appropriate for subcutaneous administration, and intramuscular injection generally is avoided in patients who are at risk for significant hematoma formation (e.g., hemophiliacs). Intravenous dosing of vitamin K has been associated with severe anaphylactic reactions, and even death.

The half-life of vitamin K_1 is 1.7 hours via the intravenous route, and 3-5 hours via the oral route. When given orally, vitamin K_1 is absorbed directly from the proximal small intestine in an energy-dependent and saturable process involving the presence of bile salts. These kinetic features argue for administration of vitamin K in smaller divided doses rather than a larger, single, daily dose. The typical starting point for adults with drug-induced hypoprothrombinemia is 2.5-10 mg of vitamin K_1 orally, repeating in 12-48 hours if needed. In cases of ingestion of long-acting superwarfarin rodenticides (e.g., brodifacoum), therapy may be 125 mg/d for weeks or months. Practically speaking, because vitamin K_1 is dispensed as 5 mg tablets, superwarfarin-poisoned patients may require 10-30 tablets every 6 hours.

Because of the short half-life of vitamin K_1, dosing must be repeated two to four times per day for the duration of treatment. Furthermore, regardless of the route of administration, coagulant effects are not evident for up to 24 hours. Because of this delay in onset, severe acute hemorrhage is better managed initially with intravenous infusion of fresh-frozen plasma, followed by vitamin K therapy.

Protamine

Mechanism of Action

Protamine sulfate has been approved in the United States as a specific antagonist to heparin since 1968.[7] Protamines are an arginine-rich, highly basic group of simple proteins derived from salmon sperm. The highly acidic heparin polysaccharides exhibit their anticoagulant activity through binding to antithrombin III. Because of the basicity of protamine, heparin has an increased affinity for protamine relative to antithrombin III. Due to its high binding affinity, protamine induces the dissociation of the heparin/antithrombin III complex. If protamine is administered in the absence of heparin, it can have marked effects on coagulation. Protamine is not completely selective for heparin and, in vivo, also interacts with fibrinogen, platelets, and other plasma proteins causing anticoagulation. For this reason, the minimal amount of protamine necessary to antagonize heparin-associated bleeding should be used (usually 1 mg of protamine intravenously for every 100 U of heparin remaining in the patient).

Side Effects

Anaphylaxis also has been associated with the use of protamine. Although development of protamine anaphylaxis is not limited to diabetics, those patients with diabetes who have used protamine-containing insulin (NPH or protamine zinc) do have a slightly increased risk of anaphylaxis. Some less common reactions to protamine include pulmonary vasoconstriction, hypotension, and thrombus formation.

Thrombopoietin Receptor Agonists

Chronic idiopathic thrombocytopenia purpura (ITP), unlike HIT, is an autoimmune disorder characterized by persistent thrombocytopenia involving antibody-mediated platelet destruction and decreased platelet production, which may lead to life-threatening bleeding.[162,163] The disease is characterized by platelet counts of less than 30,000 platelets/μL (normal platelet count: ~150,000-450,000 platelets/μL). Successful treatment is indicated by platelet counts of 200,000 platelets/μL. The diagnosis and management of this autoimmune disorder is a challenge to clinicians because the pathophysiology of ITP is understood poorly.[162,164] Recent evidence supports the coexistence of antibody-induced megakaryocyte abnormalities that impair proliferation and differentiation of megakaryocytes, decreased platelet formation, and subsequent platelet release in ITP patients.[164]

Romiplostim and eltrombopag are two thrombopoietin receptor agonists that have recently been approved for the short-term treatment of thrombocytopenia in patients with chronic ITP.[165,166] These drugs work by binding to the transmembrane domain of the human thrombopoietin receptor (c-Mp1) on the platelet surface as well as megakaryocytes and megakaryocyte precursor cells, thereby activating multiple signaling pathways, including tyrosine phosphorylation of c-Mp1, Janus kinase 2, and signal transduction and activation of transcription, which results in an increase in the synthesis of new platelets.[165,167]

Romiplostim (Nplate)

Romiplostim is an F_c-peptide fusion protein analog of thrombopoietin with a molecular weight of 59 kDa that is administered subcutaneously in a dose range of 3-15 μg/kg/wk, based on the patient's platelet count.[165,168] It was approved in 2003 by the FDA as an orphan drug and subsequently in 2008 for long-term treatment of adult chronic ITP, especially in relapsed postsplenectomy patients.[168] The serum half-life of romiplostim ranges from 1 to 34 days (median 3.5 d) following subcutaneous injection.

Eltrombopag (Promacta)

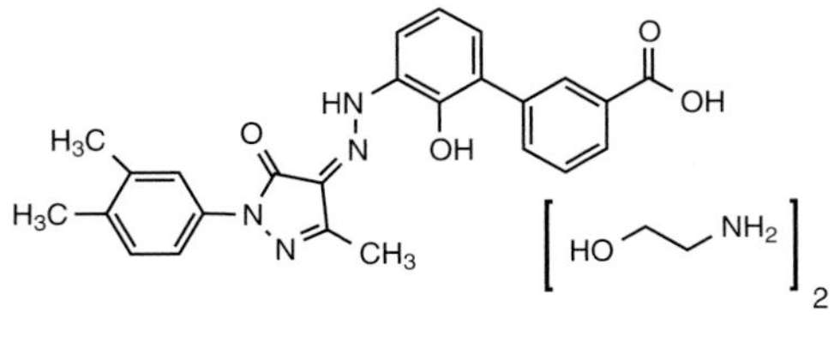

Eltrombopag

Eltrombopag is indicated for the treatment of thrombocytopenia in patients with chronic immune ITP. It is an orally active small molecular weight agonist of the thrombopoietin receptor, approved in 2008.[166,169,170]

Eltrombopag is rapidly absorbed, reaching maximum plasma concentrations in 3-6 hours and is highly bound to plasma protein (~99%). Coadministration of eltrombopag with heavy metals found in antacids results in reduced (~70%) systemic exposure, whereas the fat content of food does not affect eltrombopag absorption. Therefore, the drug should be administered on an empty stomach.

Pharmacokinetics

Eltrombopag is metabolized in the liver, although only minor CYP-catalyzed oxidation is reported, and some glucuronidation also occurs. The half-life of eltrombopag is approximately 26-35 hours, with elimination occurring through the feces (~59%) and urine (~31%). Eltrombopag can cause hepatotoxicity, and patients must have liver function tests done every 2 weeks during initial drug therapy and monthly after establishment of a maintenance dose.

Antifibrinolytic Agents

Mechanism of Action

Plasmin binds to fibrin through a lysine binding site to activate the final stages of fibrinolysis (Fig. 18.1). Control of a variety of fibrinolytic states can be achieved using different synthetic antifibrinolytic agents, such as tranexamic acid (Cyklokapron) and ε-aminocaproic acid (Amicar) that completely inhibit plasminogen activation. ε-Aminocaproic acid, a lysine analog, and tranexamic acid have a high affinity for the five lysine binding sites of plasminogen, which effectively competes and prevents the binding of plasmin to fibrin.

$H_2N-CH_2-CH_2-CH_2-CH_2-CH_2-COOH$

ε-Aminocaproic acid

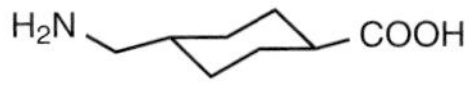

Tranexamic acid

$H_2N-CH_2-CH_2-CH_2-CH_2-CH(NH_2)-COOH$

Lysine

Pharmacokinetics

Both ε-aminocaproic acid and tranexamic acid are readily absorbed when administered orally. They also can be given intravenously, although significant hypotension can result if the infusion is given too quickly. Elimination of the drugs is primarily renal, with little metabolism taking place. The half-lives of ε-aminocaproic acid and tranexamic acid are each approximately 2 hours.

Therapeutic Use

These drugs find clinical utility in settings such as prevention of relapse of bleeding in intracranial hemorrhages, as adjunct therapy in hemophiliacs, and treatment of bleeding following fibrinolytic therapy. In most bleeding conditions, ε-aminocaproic acid therapy has not been shown to be of significant benefit. In recent trials, tranexamic acid was found to reduce red cell transfusion better than ε-aminocaproic acid or placebo in patients undergoing liver transplantation.[171]

Side Effects

The major risk associated with ε-aminocaproic or tranexamic acid therapy is intravascular thrombosis as a direct result of the inhibition of plasminogen activator. Additional possible complications include hypotension, abdominal discomfort, and in some cases, myopathy and muscle necrosis.

Plasma Fractions

Spontaneous bleeding can result from dysfunction or deficiencies of specific coagulation factors. A list of coagulation factors and deficiency states is shown in Table 18.7.

Spontaneous bleeding usually occurs when the activity of coagulation factors falls below 5% of normal. Typically, these deficiencies are the result of a chronic disease state, such as von Willebrand disease or hemophilia. Management of an acute hemorrhagic event in a coagulation factor–deficient patient includes administration of the appropriate factors in concentrated form. The most common inherited clotting factor deficiencies involve factor VIII (classic hemophilia A) and factor IX (hemophilia B or Christmas disease).

Two forms of factor VIII concentrate are clinically available: cryoprecipitate and lyophilized factor VIII concentrate. Cryoprecipitate is a factor VIII–rich plasma protein fraction prepared from whole blood that also contains approximately 300 mg of fibrinogen per unit. Immediately before infusion, the required number of cryoprecipitate units are thawed in a sterile saline/citrate solution and pooled. The lyophilized factor VIII concentrates are prepared from large plasma pools and also are rich in fibrinogen. Lyophilized factor VIII concentrates are not useful in therapy for von Willebrand disease, because during the extraction and lyophilization process, the polymeric

Table 18.7 Clotting Factors

Factor	Common Name	Deficiency State	Source	Half-Life of Infused Factor (d)	Target for Action of
I	Fibrinogen	Afibrinogenemia, defibrination syndrome	Liver	4	
II	Prothrombin	Prothrombin deficiency	Liver (requires vitamin K)	3	Heparin (IIa), warfarin (synthesis)
III	Tissue thromboplastin, thrombokinase, tissue factor		Liver (may require vitamin K)		
IV	Calcium (Ca^{2+})				
V	Proaccelerin, labile factor	Factor V deficiency	Liver	1	
VI	Deleted factor				
VII	Proconvertin, stable factor	Factor VII deficiency	Liver (requires vitamin K)	0.25	Heparin (VIIa); warfarin (synthesis)
VIII	Antihemophilic A factor (AHF), antihemophilic globulin (AHG)	Hemophilia A (classic) von Willebrand disease	Liver	0.5 Unknown	
IX	Antihemophilic B factor, plasma thromboplastin component (PTC), Christmas factor	Hemophilia B (Christmas disease)	Liver (requires vitamin K)	1	Heparin (IXa); warfarin (synthesis)

Table 18.7 Clotting Factors (Continued)

Factor	Common Name	Deficiency State	Source	Half-Life of Infused Factor (d)	Target for Action of
X	Stuart or Stuart-Prower factor	Stuart-Prower defect	Liver (requires vitamin K)	1.5	Heparin (IXa); warfarin (synthesis)
XI	Plasma thrombo-plastin antecedent (PTA)	PTA deficiency	Unknown	3	
XII	Hageman factor, contact factor	Hageman defect	Unknown	Unknown	
XIII	Fibrin-stabilizing factor, fibrinase	Fibrin-stabilizing factor deficiency	Unknown	6	
	Fletcher factor, prekallikrein factor		Liver		
	Fitzgerald factor, high molecular weight kininogen		Liver		
Antithrombin III; proteins C and S; plasminogen		Antithrombin III deficiency		3	Warfarin (synthesis); thrombolytic enzymes; aminocaproic acid

structure of factor VIII in the vW protein that supports platelet adhesion is destroyed, rendering the preparation inactive. Because of the pooling of blood from multiple donors in the preparation of lyophilized factor VIII concentrates, it is considered safer to use the cryoprecipipate isolated from a single donor.

The major concern associated with the use of concentrated clotting factors is the risk of viral transmission (primarily HIV and hepatitis B). This fear has somewhat attenuated the use of concentrated plasma fractions, even in diseases such as hemophilia. Ultrapure factor VIII concentrates produced using recombinant DNA technology have been approved for use. Frequently, however, the expense of these recombinant agents is the reason why the more traditional plasma isolates are used despite the possibility of viral transmission.

Lyophilized preparations of prothrombin, factor IX, and factor X also are available. The manufacturing process involves plasma extraction with solvents and detergents that renders the preparations virally inactive but still able to activate clotting factors. To prevent excessive thrombus formation in these situations, heparin often is added to the therapeutic regimen.

At times, a hemorrhagic event is possible, but the patient does not require immediate coagulation therapy. For example, if a patient with mild hemophilia A needs to have a dental extraction performed, the potential for hemorrhage exists. In these cases, it is possible to increase the activity of the endogenous factor VIII through pretreatment with desmopressin acetate. This preoperative measure may alleviate the need for clotting factor replacement.

REFERENCES

1. Beckman MG, Hooper WC, Critchley SE, et al. Venous thromboembolism. *Am J Prev Med.* 2009;38:S495-S501.
2. Geerts WH, Bergqvist D, Pineo GF, et al. Prevention of venous thromboembolism. *Chest.* 2008;133:381S-453S.
3. Kakkar VV, Spindler J, Flute PT, et al. Efficacy of low doses of heparin in prevention of deep-vein thrombosis after major surgery. *Lancet.* 1972;300:101-106.
4. Blanchard E, Ansell J. Extended anticoagulation therapy for the primary and secondary prevention of venous thromboembolism. *Drugs.* 2005;65:303-311.
5. Ruff CT, Braunwald E. Review: will warfarin ever be replaced? *J Cardiovas Pharmacol Ther.* 2010;15:210-219.
6. Weitz JI, Hirsh J, Samama MM. New anticoagulant drugs. *Chest.* 2004;126:265S-286S.
7. Bates SM, Weitz JI. The status of new anticoagulants. *Br J Haematol.* 2006;134:3-19.
8. Garcia D, Libby E, Crowther MA. The new oral anticoagulants. *Blood.* 2009;115:15-20.
9. Weitz J. Emerging anticoagulants for the treatment of venous thromboembolism. *Thromb Haemostasis.* 2006;96:274-284.
10. Gross PL, Weitz JI. New anticoagulants for treatment of venous thromboembolism. *Arterioscler Thromb Vasc Biol.* 2008; 28:380-386.

11. Kyrle PA, Eichinger S. Deep vein thrombosis. *Lancet.* 2005;365:1163-1174.
12. Geerts WH, Pineo GF, Heit JA, et al. Prevention of venous thromboembolism. *Chest.* 2004;126:338S-400S.
13. Weitz JI, Hirsh J, Samama MM. New antithrombotic drugs. *Chest.* 2008;133:234S-256S.
14. Turpie AGG. New oral anticoagulants in atrial fibrillation. *Eur Heart J.* 2007;29:155-165.
15. Nutescu EA, Helgason CM. Concomitant drug, dietary, and lifestyle issues in patients with atrial fibrillation receiving anticoagulation therapy for stroke prophylaxis. *Curr Treat Options Cardiovasc Med.* 2005;7:241-250.
16. Lane DA, Lip GYH. Atrial fibrillation and mortality: the impact of antithrombotic therapy. *Eur Heart J.* 2010;31:2075-2076.
17. Prystowsky EN, Padanilam BJ, Fogel RI. Treatment of atrial fibrillation. *JAMA.* 2015;314:278-288.
18. Nguyen T, Jolly U, Sidhu K, et al. Atrial fibrillation management: evaluating rate vs rhythm control. *Expert Rev Cardiovasc Ther.* 2016;14:713-724.
19. Khrenov A. Coagulation pathways in atherothrombosis. *Trends Cardiovasc Med.* 2002;12:317-324.
20. Broze GJ. Tissue factor pathway inhibitor: structure-function. *Front Biosci.* 2012;17:262
21. Sandset PM, Bendz B, Hansen J-B. Physiological function of tissue factor pathway inhibitor and interaction with heparins. *Pathophysiol Haemost Thromb.* 2000;30:48-56.
22. Esmon CT. The protein C pathway. *Chest.* 2003;124:26S-32S.
23. Mosnier LO, Zlokovic BV, Griffin JH. The cytoprotective protein C pathway. *Blood.* 2007;109:3161-3172.
24. Ansell J, Hirsh J, Poller L, et al. The pharmacology and management of the vitamin K antagonists. *Chest.* 2004;126:204S-233S.
25. Jones M. Evaluation of the pattern of treatment, level of anticoagulation control, and outcome of treatment with warfarin in patients with non-valvar atrial fibrillation: a record linkage study in a large British population. *Heart.* 2005;91:472-477.
26. O'Reilly RA. Vitamin K and the oral anticoagulant drugs. *Annu Rev Med.* 1976;27:245-261.
27. Ansell J, Hirsh J, Hylek E, et al. Pharmacology and management of the vitamin K antagonists. *Chest.* 2008;133:160S-198S.
28. Le Cam-Duchez V, Frétigny M, Cailleux N, et al. Algorithms using clinical and genetic data (CYP2C9, VKORC1) are relevant to predict warfarin dose in patients with different INR targets. *Thromb Res.* 2010;126:e235-e237.
29. Hirsh J, Dalen JE, Anderson DR, et al. Oral anticoagulants: mechanism of action, clinical effectiveness, and optimal therapeutic range. *Chest.* 2001;119:8S-21S.
30. Wajih N, Sane DC, Hutson SM, et al. Engineering of a recombinant vitamin K-dependent γ-carboxylation system with enhanced γ-carboxyglutamic acid forming capacity. *J Biol Chem.* 2005;280:10540-10547.
31. Valente EJ, Lingafelter EC, Porter WR, et al. Structure of warfarin in solution. *J Med Chem.* 1977;20:1489-1493.
32. Information D. *USP DI Volume 1 Drug Information for the Healthcare Professional.* 16th ed. Thomson PDR, Micromedex; 1998.
33. Ansell J, Hirsh J, Dalen J, et al. Managing oral anticoagulant therapy. *Chest.* 2001;119:22S-38S.
34. Hollinger BR. Case management and plasma half-life in a case of brodifacoum poisoning. *Arch Intern Med.* 1993;153:1925-1928.
35. Palmer RB, Alakija P, Cde Baca JE, et al. Fatal brodifacoum rodenticide poisoning: autopsy and toxicologic findings. *J Forensic Sci.* 1999;44:14566J.
36. Bachmann KA, Sullivan TJ. Dispositional and pharmacodynamic characteristics of brodifacoum in warfarin-sensitive rats. *Pharmacology.* 1983;27:281-288.
37. Redfern R, Gill JE, Hadler MR. Laboratory evaluation of WBA 8119 as a rodenticide for use against warfarin-resistant and non-resistant rats and mice. *J Hyg (Lond).* 1976;77:419-426.
38. Laposata M, Van Cott EM, Lev MH. Case 1-2007. *N Engl J Med.* 2007;356:174-182.
39. Linhardt RJ. 2003 Claude S. Hudson award address in carbohydrate chemistry. Heparin: structure and activity. *J Med Chem.* 2003;46:2551-2564.
40. Pasmant E, de Beauvoir C, Plessier A, et al. VKORC1 and CYP2C9 genetic polymorphisms in hepatic or portal vein thrombosis. *Thromb Res.* 2010;126:e134-e136.
41. Spyropoulos AC, Hayth KA, Jenkins P. Anticoagulation with anisindione in a patient with a warfarin-induced skin eruption. *Pharmacotherapy.* 2003;23:533-536.
42. Codee JDC, Overkleeft HS, van der Marel GA, et al. The synthesis of well-defined heparin and heparan sulfate fragments. *ChemInform.* 2005;36:317-326.
43. Codée JDC, Overkleeft HS, van der Marel GA, et al. The synthesis of well-defined heparin and heparan sulfate fragments. *Drug Discov Today Technol.* 2004;1:317-326.
44. Hirsh J, Raschke R. Heparin and low-molecular-weight heparin. *Chest.* 2004;126:188S-203S.
45. Jin L, Abrahams JP, Skinner R, et al. The anticoagulant activation of antithrombin by heparin. *Proc Natl Acad Sci USA.* 1997;94:14683-14688.
46. Desai UR. New antithrombin-based anticoagulants. *Med Res Rev.* 2003;24:151-181.
47. de Kort M, Buijsman RC, van Boeckel CAA. Synthetic heparin derivatives as new anticoagulant drugs. *Drug Discov Today.* 2005;10:769-779.
48. Weitz JI. Low-molecular-weight heparins. *N Engl J Med.* 1997;337:688-699.
49. Hovanessian HC. New-generation anticoagulants: the low molecular weight heparins. *Ann Emerg Med.* 1999;34:768-779.
50. Hastedt M. *R. C. Baselt (ed.): Disposition of Toxic Drugs and Chemicals in Man, 10th edition*; 2015:147-147.
51. Brookoff D. Hematologic evaluation. In: Flomenbaum N, Goldfrank L, Jacobson A, eds. *Emergency Diagnostic Testing.* 2nd ed. St. Louis, MO: Mosby; 1995.
52. Kakkar AK. Low- and ultra-low-molecular-weight heparins. *Best Pract Res Clin Haematol.* 2004;17:77-87.
53. Louzada ML, Majeed H, Wells PS. Efficacy of low- molecular-weight- heparin versus vitamin K antagonists for long term treatment of cancer-associated venous thromboembolism in adults: a systematic review of randomized controlled trials. *Thromb Res.* 2009;123:837-844.
54. Siddiqui MAA, Wagstaff AJ. Enoxaparin. *Drugs.* 2005;65:1025-1036.
55. Sinnaeve P, Van de Werf F. Enoxaparin and fibrinolysis: ExTRACTing prognosis from bleeding complications. *Eur Heart J.* 2010;31:2077-2079.
56. Bauer KA. Fondaparinux: a new synthetic and selective inhibitor of Factor Xa. *Best Pract Res Clin Haematol.* 2004;17:89-104.
57. Koopman MMW, Buller HR. Short- and long-acting synthetic pentasaccharides. *J Intern Med.* 2003;254:335-342.
58. Petitou M, Duchaussoy P, Jaurand G, et al. Synthesis and pharmacological properties of a close analogue of an antithrombotic pentasaccharide (SR 90107A/ORG 31540). *J Med Chem.* 1997;40:1600-1607.
59. Nutescu EA, Helgason CM. Evolving concepts in the treatment of venous thromboembolism: the role of factor Xa inhibitors. *Pharmacotherapy.* 2004;24:82S-87S.
60. Hawkins D. Limitations of traditional anticoagulants. *Pharmacotherapy.* 2004;24:62S-65S.
61. Cheng JWM. Fondaparinux: a new antithrombotic agent. *Clin Ther.* 2002;24:1757-1769.
62. Hirsh J, O'Donnell M, Eikelboom JW. Beyond unfractionated heparin and warfarin: current and future advances. *Circulation.* 2007;116:552-560.
63. Dager WE, Andersen J, Nutescu E. Special considerations with fondaparinux therapy: heparin-induced thrombocytopenia and wound healing. *Pharmacotherapy.* 2004;24:88S-94S.
64. Johnson PH. Hirudin: clinical potential of a thrombin inhibitor. *Annu Rev Med.* 1994;45:165-177.

65. Krstenansky JL, Owen TJ, Yates MT, et al. Design, synthesis and antithrombin activity for conformationally restricted analogs of peptide anticoagulants based on the C-terminal region of the leech peptide, hirudin. *Biochim Biophys Acta*. 1988;957:53-59.
66. Maraganore JM, Bourdon P, Jablonski J, et al. Design and characterization of hirulogs: a novel class of bivalent peptide inhibitors of thrombin. *Biochemistry*. 1990;29:7095-7101.
67. Agnelli G. Clinical potential of oral direct thrombin inhibitors in the prevention and treatment of venous thromboembolism. *Drugs*. 2004;64:47-52.
68. Haas S. Oral direct thrombin inhibition. *Drugs*. 2004;64:7-16.
69. Nutescu EA, Shapiro NL, Chevalier A. New anticoagulant agents: direct thrombin inhibitors. *Clin Geriatr Med*. 2006;22:33-56.
70. Di Nisio M, Middeldorp S, Büller HR. Direct thrombin inhibitors. *N Engl J Med*. 2005;353:1028-1040.
71. Ayala Y, Cera ED. Molecular recognition by thrombin. Role of the slows→fast transition, site-specific ion binding energetics and thermodynamic mapping of structural components. *J Mol Biol*. 1994;235:733-746.
72. Greinacher A, Lubenow N. Recombinant hirudin in clinical practice: focus on lepirudin. *Circulation*. 2001;103:1479-1484.
73. Matheson AJ, Goa KL. Desirudin: a review of its use in the management of thrombotic disorders. *Drugs*. 2000;60:679-700.
74. Eikelboom JW, French J. Management of patients with acute coronary syndromes. *Drugs*. 2002;62:1839-1852.
75. Hirsh J. Current anticoagulant therapy—unmet clinical needs. *Thromb Res*. 2003;109:S1-S8.
76. Levy JH. Novel intravenous antithrombins. *Am Heart J*. 2001;141:1043-1047.
77. Caron MF, McKendall GR. Bivalirudin in percutaneous coronary intervention. *Am J Health Syst Pharm*. 2003;60:1841.
78. Warkentin TE. Bivalent direct thrombin inhibitors: hirudin and bivalirudin. *Best Pract Res Clin Haematol*. 2004;17:105-125.
79. Curran MP. Bivalirudin: in patients with acute coronary syndromes: planned for urgent or early intervention. *Drugs*. 2010; 70:909-918.
80. Saugel B, Phillip V, Moessmer G, et al. Argatroban therapy for heparin-induced thrombocytopenia in ICU patients with multiple organ dysfunction syndrome: a retrospective study. *Crit Care*. 2010;14:R90.
81. Nagashima H. Studies on the different modes of action of the anticoagulant protease inhibitors DX-9065a and argatroban. *J Biol Chem*. 2002;277:50439-50444.
82. Hauptmann J. Pharmacokinetics of an emerging new class of anticoagulant/antithrombotic drugs. *Eur J Clin Pharmacol*. 2001;57:751-758.
83. Baetz BE, Spinler SA. Dabigatran etexilate: an oral direct thrombin inhibitor for prophylaxis and treatment of thromboembolic diseases. *Pharmacotherapy*. 2008;28:1354-1373.
84. Eriksson BI, Quinlan DJ, Weitz JI. Comparative pharmacodynamics and pharmacokinetics of oral direct thrombin and factor Xa inhibitors in development. *Clin Pharmacokinet*. 2009;48:1-22.
85. Blech S, Ebner T, Ludwig-Schwellinger E, et al. The metabolism and disposition of the oral direct thrombin inhibitor, dabigatran, in humans. *Drug Metab Dispos*. 2007;36:386-399.
86. Pollack CVJ, Reilly PA, van Ryn J, et al. Idarucizumab for dabigatran reversal—full cohort analysis. *N Engl J Med*. 2017;377:431-441.
87. Glund S, Stangier J, van Ryn J, et al. Effect of age and renal function on idarucizumab pharmacokinetics and idarucizumab-mediated reversal of dabigatran anticoagulant activity in a randomized, double-blind, crossover phase Ib study. *Clin Pharmacokinet*. 2017;56:41-54.
88. Garcia DA, Crowther MA, Ageno W. *The Direct Oral Anticoagulants*. *Practical Hemostasis and Thrombosis*: John Wiley & Sons Ltd.; 2016:253-268.
89. Morell J, Sullivan B, Khalabuda M, et al. Role of orally available antagonists of factor Xa in the treatment and prevention of thromboembolic disease: focus on rivaroxaban. *J Clin Pharmacol*. 2010;50:986-1000.
90. Imberti D, Dall'Asta C, Pierfranceschi MG. Oral factor Xa inhibitors for thromboprophylaxis in major orthopedic surgery: a review. *Intern Emerg Med*. 2009;4:471-477.
91. Lassen MR, Raskob GE, Gallus A, et al. Apixaban versus enoxaparin for thromboprophylaxis after knee replacement (ADVANCE-2): a randomised double-blind trial. *Lancet*. 2010;375:807-815.
92. Turpie AGG. Oral, direct factor Xa inhibitors in development for the prevention and treatment of thromboembolic diseases. *Arterioscler Thromb Vasc Biol*. 2007;27:1238-1247.
93. Raghavan N, Frost CE, Yu Z, et al. Apixaban metabolism and pharmacokinetics after oral administration to humans. *Drug Metab Dispos*. 2008;37:74-81.
94. Nutescu EA, Burnett A, Fanikos J, et al. Pharmacology of anticoagulants used in the treatment of venous thromboembolism. *J Thromb Thrombolysis*. 2016;41:15-31.
95. Giugliano RP, Ruff CT, Braunwald E, et al. Edoxaban versus warfarin in patients with atrial fibrillation. *N Engl J Med*. 2013;369:2093-2104.
96. Connolly SJ, Eikelboom J, Dorian P, et al. Betrixaban compared with warfarin in patients with atrial fibrillation: results of a phase 2, randomized, dose-ranging study (Explore-Xa). *Eur Heart J*. 2013;34:1498-1505.
97. Connolly SJ, Milling TJ, Eikelboom JW, et al. Andexanet alfa for acute major bleeding associated with factor Xa inhibitors. *N Engl J Med*. 2016;375:1131-1141.
98. Coccheri S. Antiplatelet drugs – do we need new options? *Drugs*. 2010;70:887-908.
99. Davì G, Patrono C. Platelet activation and atherothrombosis. *N Engl J Med*. 2007;357:2482-2494.
100. Leonardi S, Tricoci P, Becker RC. Thrombin receptor antagonists for the treatment of atherothrombosis. *Drugs*. 2010;70: 1771-1783.
101. Patrono C, Baigent C, Hirsh J, et al. Antiplatelet drugs. *Chest*. 2008;133:199S-233S.
102. Angiolillo DJ, Capodanno D, Goto S. Platelet thrombin receptor antagonism and atherothrombosis. *Eur Heart J*. 2009;31:17-28.
103. Sztriha LK, Sas K, Vecsei L. Aspirin resistance in stroke: 2004. *J Neurol Sci*. 2005;229-230:163-169.
104. Rocca B, Secchiero P, Ciabattoni G, et al. Cyclooxygenase-2 expression is induced during human megakaryopoiesis and characterizes newly formed platelets. *Proc Natl Acad Sci USA*. 2002;99:7634-7639.
105. Mason PJ, Jacobs AK, Freedman JE. Aspirin resistance and atherothrombotic disease. *J Am Coll Cardiol*. 2005;46:986-993.
106. Lee S-W, Park S-W, Hong M-K, et al. Comparison of cilostazol and clopidogrel after successful coronary stenting. *Am J Cardiol*. 2005;95:859-862.
107. Diener H-C, Bogousslavsky J, Brass LM, et al. Aspirin and clopidogrel compared with clopidogrel alone after recent ischaemic stroke or transient ischaemic attack in high-risk patients (MATCH): randomised, double-blind, placebo-controlled trial. *Lancet*. 2004;364:331-337.
108. Ahn JC, Song WH, Kwon JA, et al. Effects of cilostazol on platelet activation in coronary stenting patients who already treated with aspirin and clopidogrel. *Korean J Intern Med*. 2004;19:230-236.
109. Schror K. The pharmacology of cilostazol. *Diabetes Obes Metab*. 2002;4:S14-S19.
110. Suri A, Forbes WP, Bramer SL. Effects of CYP3A inhibition on the metabolism of cilostazol. *Clin Pharmacokinet*. 1999;37:61-68.
111. Suri A, Bramer SL. Effect of omeprazole on the metabolism of cilostazol. *Clin Pharmacokinet*. 1999;37:53-59.
112. Nguyen TA, Diodati JG, Pharand C. Resistance to clopidogrel: a review of the evidence. *J Am Coll Cardiol*. 2005;45:1157-1164.
113. Gachet C. The platelet P2 receptors as molecular targets for old and new antiplatelet drugs. *Pharmacol Ther*. 2005;108:180-192.
114. van Giezen JJJ. Optimizing platelet inhibition. *Eur Heart J Suppl*. 2008;10:D23-D29.
115. Gachet C. P2 receptors, platelet function and pharmacological implications. *Thromb Haemostasis*. 2008;99:466-472.

116. Wallentin L. P2Y12 inhibitors: differences in properties and mechanisms of action and potential consequences for clinical use. *Eur Heart J*. 2009;30:1964-1977.
117. Dorsam RT, Murugappan S, Ding Z, et al. Clopidogrel: interactions with the P2Y12 receptor and clinical relevance. *Hematology*. 2003;8:359-365.
118. Duggan ST, Keating GM. Prasugrel: a review of its use in patients with acute coronary syndromes undergoing percutaneous coronary intervention. *Drugs*. 2009;69:1707-1726.
119. Jakubowski JA, Winters KJ, Naganuma H, et al. Prasugrel: a novel thienopyridine antiplatelet agent. A review of preclinical and clinical studies and the mechanistic basis for its distinct antiplatelet profile. *Cardiovasc Drug Rev*. 2007;25:357-374.
120. Wiviott SD. Randomized comparison of prasugrel (CS-747, LY640315), a novel thienopyridine P2Y12 antagonist, with clopidogrel in percutaneous coronary intervention: results of the joint utilization of medications to block platelets optimally (JUMBO)-TIMI 26 trial. *Circulation*. 2005;111:3366-3373.
121. Cattaneo M. *Platelet Receptors and Drug Targets*: John Wiley & Sons Ltd.; 2014.
122. Ding Z. Inactivation of the human P2Y12 receptor by thiol reagents requires interaction with both extracellular cysteine residues, Cys17 and Cys270. *Blood*. 2003;101:3908-3914.
123. Savi P, Zachayus JL, Delesque-Touchard N, et al. The active metabolite of clopidogrel disrupts P2Y12 receptor oligomers and partitions them out of lipid rafts. *Proc Natl Acad Sci USA*. 2006;103:11069-11074.
124. Algaier I, Jakubowski JA, Asai F, et al. Interaction of the active metabolite of prasugrel, R-138727, with cysteine 97 and cysteine 175 of the human P2Y12 receptor. *J Thromb Haemost*. 2008;6:1908-1914.
125. Dalvie DK. Characterization of novel dihydrothienopyridinium and thienopyridinium metabolites of ticlopidine in vitro: role of peroxidases, cytochromes p450, and monoamine oxidases. *Drug Metab Dispos*. 2004;32:49-57.
126. Farid NA, Kurihara A, Wrighton SA. Metabolism and disposition of the thienopyridine antiplatelet drugs ticlopidine, clopidogrel, and prasugrel in humans. *J Clin Pharmacol*. 2010;50:126-142.
127. Farid NA, Smith RL, Gillespie TA, et al. The disposition of prasugrel, a novel thienopyridine, in humans. *Drug Metab Dispos*. 2007;35:1096-1104.
128. Nishiya Y, Hagihara K, Ito T, et al. Mechanism-based inhibition of human cytochrome P450 2B6 by ticlopidine, clopidogrel, and the thiolactone metabolite of prasugrel. *Drug Metab Dispos*. 2008;37:589-593.
129. Veverka A, Hammer JM. Prasugrel: a new thienopyridine inhibitor. *J Pharm Pract*. 2009;22:158-165.
130. Moser M, Bode C. Antiplatelet therapy for atherothrombotic disease: how can we improve the outcomes? *J Thromb Thrombolysis*. 2010;30:240-249.
131. Oliphant C, Doby J, Blade C, et al. Emerging P2Y12 receptor antagonists: role in coronary artery disease. *Curr Vasc Pharm*. 2010;8:93-101.
132. Dobesh PP, Oestreich JH. Ticagrelor: pharmacokinetics, pharmacodynamics, clinical efficacy, and safety. *Pharmacotherapy*. 2014;34:1077-1090.
133. Teng R, Oliver S, Hayes MA, et al. Absorption, distribution, metabolism, and excretion of ticagrelor in healthy subjects. *Drug Metab Dispos*. 2010;38:1514-1521.
134. Dovlatova NL, Jakubowski JA, Sugidachi A, et al. The reversible P2Y12 antagonist cangrelor influences the ability of the active metabolites of clopidogrel and prasugrel to produce irreversible inhibition of platelet function. *J Thromb Haemost*. 2008;6:1153-1159.
135. Anderson SD, Shah NK, Yim J, et al. Efficacy and safety of ticagrelor: a reversible P2Y12 receptor antagonist. *Ann Pharmacother*. 2010;44:524-537.
136. Berger PB. The glycoprotein IIb/IIIa inhibitor wars. *J Am Coll Cardiol*. 2010;56:476-478.
137. Proimos G. Platelet aggregation inhibition with glycoprotein IIb–IIIa inhibitors. *J Thromb Thrombolysis*. 2001;11:99-110.
138. Mousa SA. Antiplatelet therapies: from aspirin to GPIIb/IIIa-receptor antagonists and beyond. *Drug Discov Today*. 1999;4:552-561.
139. Hashemzadeh M, Furukawa M, Goldsberry S, et al. Chemical structures and mode of action of intravenous glycoprotein IIb/IIIa receptor blockers: a review. *Exp Clin Cardiol*. 2008;13:192-197.
140. Moliterno DJ, Ziada KM. The safety and efficacy of glycoprotein IIb/IIIa inhibitors for primary angioplasty. *J Am Coll Cardiol*. 2008;51:536-537.
141. Vergara-Jimenez J, Tricoci P. Safety and efficacy of abciximab as an adjunct to percutaneous coronary intervention. *Vasc Health Risk Manag*. 2010;6:39-45.
142. Reverter JC, Béguin S, Kessels H, et al. Inhibition of platelet-mediated, tissue factor-induced thrombin generation by the mouse/human chimeric 7E3 antibody. Potential implications for the effect of c7E3 Fab treatment on acute thrombosis and "clinical restenosis". *J Clin Investig*. 1996;98:863-874.
143. Genetta TB, Mauro VF. Abciximab: a new antiaggregant used in angioplasty. *Ann Pharmacother*. 1996;30:251-257.
144. Tam SH, Sassoli PM, Jordan RE, et al. Abciximab (ReoPro, chimeric 7E3 Fab) demonstrates equivalent affinity and functional blockade of glycoprotein IIb/IIIa and v 3 integrins. *Circulation*. 1998;98:1085-1091.
145. Brooks PC, Clark RA, Cheresh DA. Requirement of vascular integrin alpha v beta 3 for angiogenesis. *Science*. 1994;264(5158):569.
146. Curran MP, Keating GM. Eptifibatide. *Drugs*. 2005;65:2009-2035.
147. van't Hof AWJ, Valgimigli M. Defining the role of platelet glycoprotein receptor inhibitors in STEMI. *Drugs*. 2009;69:85-100.
148. Juwana YB, Suryapranata H, Ottervanger JP, et al. Tirofiban for myocardial infarction. *Expert Opin Pharmacother*. 2010;11:861-866.
149. Becker RC, Moliterno DJ, Jennings LK, et al. Safety and tolerability of SCH 530348 in patients undergoing non-urgent percutaneous coronary intervention: a randomised, double-blind, placebo-controlled phase II study. *Lancet*. 2009;373:919-928.
150. Chackalamannil S, Wang Y, Greenlee WJ, et al. Discovery of a novel, orally active himbacine-based thrombin receptor antagonist (SCH 530348) with potent antiplatelet activity. *J Med Chem*. 2008;51:3061-3064.
151. Magnani G, Bonaca MP, Braunwald E, et al. Efficacy and safety of vorapaxar as approved for clinical use in the United States. *J Am Heart Assoc*. 2015;4:1-9.
152. Kornblum N, Ayyanar K, Benimetskaya L, et al. Defibrotide, a polydisperse mixture of single-stranded phosphodiester oligonucleotides with lifesaving activity in severe hepatic veno-occlusive disease: clinical outcomes and potential mechanisms of action. *Oligonucleotides*. 2006;16:105-114.
153. Pescador R, Capuzzi L, Mantovani M, et al. Defibrotide: properties and clinical use of an old/new drug. *Vasc Pharmacol*. 2013;59:1-10.
154. Gresele P, Agnelli G. Novel approaches to the treatment of thrombosis. *Trends Pharmacol Sci*. 2002;23:25-32.
155. Baruah DB, Dash RN, Chaudhari MR, et al. Plasminogen activators: a comparison. *Vasc Pharmacol*. 2006;44:1-9.
156. Banerjee A, Chisti Y, Banerjee UC. Streptokinase—a clinically useful thrombolytic agent. *Biotechnol Adv*. 2004;22:287-307.
157. Perler B. Thrombolytic therapies:the current state of affairsThrombolytic therapies:the current state of affairsThrombolytic therapies:the current state of affairs. *J Endovasc Ther*. 2005;12:224-232.
158. Nordt TK. Thrombolysis: newer thrombolytic agents and their role in clinical medicine. *Heart*. 2003;89:1358-1362.
159. Antman EM. *Braunwald's Heart Disease: A Textbook of Cardiovascular Medicine*. 10th ed. Mann DL, Zipes DP, Libby P, et al, eds. Philadelphia, PA: Elsevier/Saunders; 2015.
160. Bates SM, Greer IA, Hirsh J, et al. Use of antithrombotic agents during pregnancy. *Chest*. 2004;126:627S-644S.
161. Liu D, Cheng T, Guo H, et al. Tissue plasminogen activator neurovascular toxicity is controlled by activated protein C. *Nat Med*. 2004;10:1379-1383.

162. Rank A. Management of chronic immune thrombocytopenic purpura: targeting insufficient megakaryopoiesis as a novel therapeutic principle. *Biologics*. 2010;4:139-145.
163. Schwartz RS. Immune thrombocytopenic purpura—from agony to agonist. *N Engl J Med*. 2007;357:2299-2301.
164. Pruemer J. Epidemiology, pathophysiology, and initial management of chronic immune thrombocytopenic purpura. *Am J Health Syst Pharm*. 2009;66:S4-S10.
165. Frampton JE, Lyseng-Williamson KA. Romiplostim. *Drugs*. 2009;69:307-317.
166. Garnock-Jones KP. Eltrombopag. *Drugs*. 2011;71:1333-1353.
167. Burzynski J. New options after first-line therapy for chronic immune thrombocytopenic purpura. *Am J Health Syst Pharm*. 2009;66:S11-S21.
168. Bussel JB, Kuter DJ, George JN, et al. AMG 531, a thrombopoiesis-stimulating protein, for chronic ITP. *N Engl J Med*. 2006;355:1672-1681.
169. Garnock-Jones KP, Keam SJ. Eltrombopag. *Drugs*. 2009;69:567-576.
170. Rice L. Treatment of immune thrombocytopenic purpura: focus on eltrombopag. *Biologics*. 2009:151.
171. Dalmau A, Sabaté A, Acosta F, et al. Tranexamic acid reduces red cell transfusion better than ε-aminocaproic acid or placebo in liver transplantation. *Anesth Analg*. 2000;91:29-34.

Clinical Scenario

CHEMICAL ANALYSIS

Anand Sridhar, PhD

The use of anticoagulant agents, such as heparin, is indicated for VTE and PE. Heparin binds to antithrombin III, causing a conformational change to the protein and potentiating its action. As a result, dissolution of the clot is accompanied by a significant reduction of platelet levels. Heparin-induced thrombocytopenia (HIT) was confirmed by laboratory results.

Direct thrombin inhibitors such as bivalirudin, argatroban, and fondaparinux are indicated for HIT. In this case, bivaluridin was chosen by the clinical team. Unlike heparin, bivaluridin binds to thrombin (Fig. 18.11), but not to AT-III. In the absence of AT-III inhibition, downstream platelet activation is impaired. The mechanism of action of bivaluridin explains the associated increase of platelet levels to above 200,000/mm^3. Thus, bivaluridin is an excellent choice as a heparin alternative for treating HIT.

The patient was transitioned shortly after to warfarin for 4 weeks. Warfarin works on the external cascade by inhibiting vitamin K epoxide reductase. This prevents the carboxylation of vitamin K–dependent coagulation factors (factors II, VII, IX, and X) and renders them unable to bind calcium ions. The decreased activity of these factors has to be considered as the warfarin dosage is adjusted. It is also to be noted that this management happens under clinical supervision, and the patient was subsequently discharged without further complications. The combined actions of these medications provide comprehensive management of pulmonary embolism.

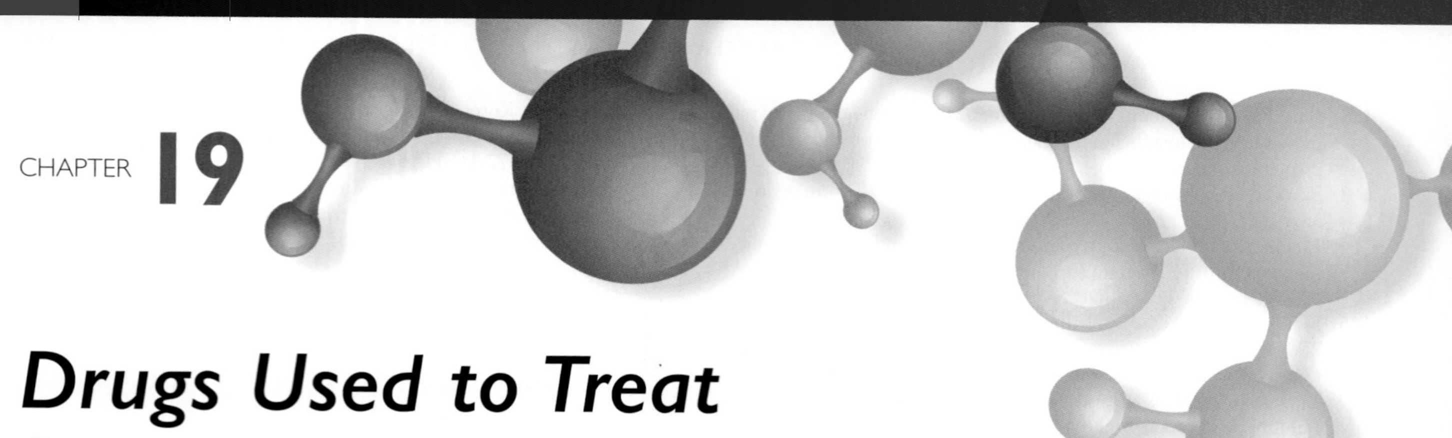

CHAPTER 19

Drugs Used to Treat Dyslipidemic Disorders

Marc W. Harrold

Drugs covered in this chapter[a]:

- Alirocumab
- Atorvastatin
- *Bezafibrate*
- Cholestyramine
- *Ciprofibrate*
- *Clofibric acid*
- Colesevelam
- Colestipol
- Evolocumab
- Ezetimibe
- Fenofibric acid
- Fluvastatin
- Gemfibrozil
- Lomitapide
- Lovastatin
- Mipomersen
- Nicotinic acid/niacin
- Pitavastatin
- Pravastatin
- Rosuvastatin
- Simvastatin

[a]Drugs listed include those available inside and outside of the United States; drugs available outside of the United States are shown in italics.

Abbreviations

ACAT acyl CoA-cholesterol acyltransferase
ALT alanine transaminase
Apo apolipoprotein
ASCHD atherosclerotic cardiovascular disease
AST aspartate transaminase
CETP cholesterol ester transfer protein
CHD coronary heart disease
CoA coenzyme A
FDA U.S. Food and Drug Administration
GERD gastroesophageal reflux disorder
HDL high-density lipoprotein
HMG 3-hydroxy-3-methylglutaryl
HMGRIs HMG-CoA reductase inhibitors
HeFH heterozygous familial hypercholesterolemia
HoFH homozygous familial hypercholesterolemia
IDL intermediate-density lipoprotein
LDL low-density lipoprotein
MI myocardial infarction
MTTP microsomal triglyceride transport protein
NAD^+ nicotinamide adenine dinucleotide
$NADP^+$ nicotinamide adenine dinucleotide phosphate
PPAR peroxisome proliferator-activated receptor
SAR structure-activity relationship
RCT reverse cholesterol transport
VLDL very-low-density lipoprotein

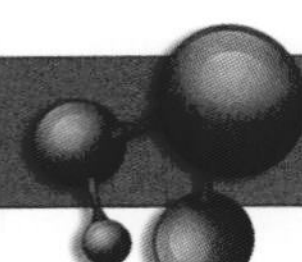

CLINICAL SIGNIFICANCE

Michael W. Perry, PharmD, BCPS, BCCCP

Numerous studies show a positive correlation between elevated blood cholesterol and the development of cardiovascular disease.[1-3] According to the Center for Disease Control and Prevention, cardiovascular disease is the leading cause of death in the United States.[4] The World Health Organization estimates that ischemic heart disease and stroke are the most frequent causes of death globally, with a combined 15 million deaths in 2015.[5] The development of medications to lower blood cholesterol levels has been essential in the prevention and treatment of cardiovascular disease.

Along with diet modification, early strategies to lower blood cholesterol focus around the use of bile acid sequestrants, nicotinic acids, and the fibrates. Medications in these classes are effective at lowering blood cholesterol, but the effects are modest and come with adverse effects, inconvenient dosing frequencies, and drug interactions. The use of these therapies have decreased due to the development of the HMG-CoA reductase class of lipid-lowering medications, commonly known as the statins.

The most current guidelines from the American College of Cardiology/American Heart Association, National Lipid Association, and the European Society of Cardiology/European Atherosclerosis Society recommend the use of statins medications as the first-line agent to treat dyslipidemia.[6-8] Statin medications have significant LDL-lowering effects, improve clinical outcomes, anti-inflammatory properties, and other pleiotropic effects. To obtain these benefits, clinicians often must use high-intensity statin dosing strategies. Using high doses of statins are not without risks, as these medications have known adverse effects and drug interactions.

Statin intolerance from muscle-related symptoms is one of the leading causes of early discontinuation of therapy.[9-11] Patients that cannot tolerate taking a statin will be without the known benefits of this drug class. Hydrophilic statins must enter hepatocytes via transporters, whereas more lipophilic statins diffuse nonselectively into hepatic and extrahepatic tissues, such as muscle.[12] Changing a patient from a mild to high lipophilic statin to a more hydrophilic statin may have less symptoms of muscle pain and weakness. Lipid solubility can have an effect on half-life and duration of action. Dosing of a statin intermittently (i.e., two to three times per week) may reduce adverse effects but requires an agent with a longer half-life.[10,11] The addition of ezetimide or a PCSK9 inhibitor to the highest dose of statin tolerated may also be an effective strategy to lower LDL and obtain some benefit of the statin therapy.[8,13] Clinicians with knowledge and understanding of the medicinal chemistry of the statin class are able to make therapy changes to allow patient to better tolerate statin therapy.

THE CHEMISTRY AND BIOCHEMISTRY OF PLASMA LIPIDS

The major lipids found in the bloodstream are cholesterol, cholesterol esters, triglycerides, and phospholipids. An abnormal concentration of one or more of these endogenous compounds is known as dyslipidemia. Since most abnormalities cause an increase in these endogenous lipids, the term hyperlipidemia is often used. Dyslipidemia/hyperlipidemia has been strongly associated with atherosclerotic lesions and coronary heart disease (CHD).[14,15] Prior to discussing lipoproteins, their role in cardiovascular disease, and drugs to decrease their concentrations, it is essential to review the biochemistry and normal physiological functions of cholesterol, triglycerides, and phospholipids.

Synthesis and Degradation of Cholesterol

Cholesterol is a C27 steroid that serves as an important component of all cell membranes and is the precursor for androgens, estrogens, progesterone, and adrenocorticoids (Fig. 19.1). It is synthesized from acetyl coenzyme A (Acetyl CoA), as shown in Figure 19.2.[16,17] The first stage of the biosynthesis is the formation of isopentenyl pyrophosphate from three acetyl CoA molecules.

The conversion of 3-hydroxy-3-methylglutaryl (HMG)-CoA to mevalonic acid is especially important, because it is a primary control site for cholesterol biosynthesis. This reaction is catalyzed by HMG-CoA reductase and reduces the thioester of HMG-CoA to a primary hydroxyl group. The second stage involves the coupling of six isopentenyl pyrophosphate molecules to form squalene. Initially, three isopentenyl pyrophosphate molecules are condensed to form farnesyl pyrophosphate, a C15 intermediate. Two farnesyl pyrophosphate molecules are then combined using a similar type of reaction. The next stage involves the cyclization of squalene to lanosterol. This process involves an initial epoxidation of squalene, followed by a subsequent cyclization requiring a concerted flow of four pairs of electrons and the migration of two methyl groups. The final stage involves the conversion of lanosterol to cholesterol. This process removes three methyl groups from lanosterol, reduces the side-chain double bond, moves the other double bond within the ring structure, and requires approximately 20 steps.

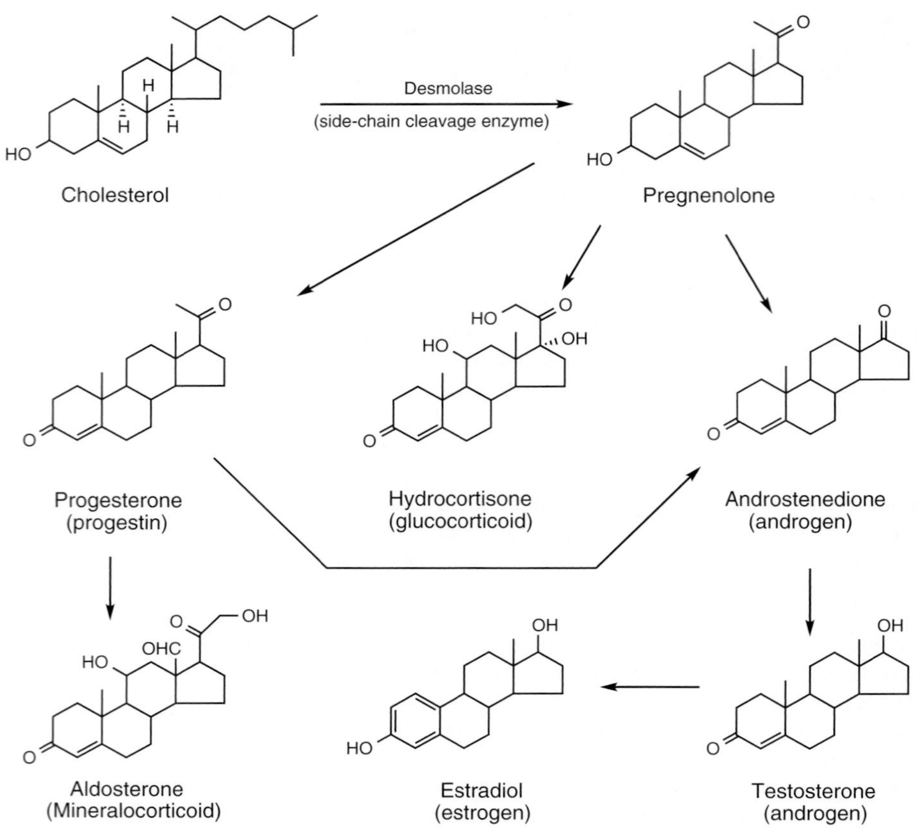

Figure 19.1 Cholesterol's role as a key intermediate in the biosynthesis of endogenous steroids.

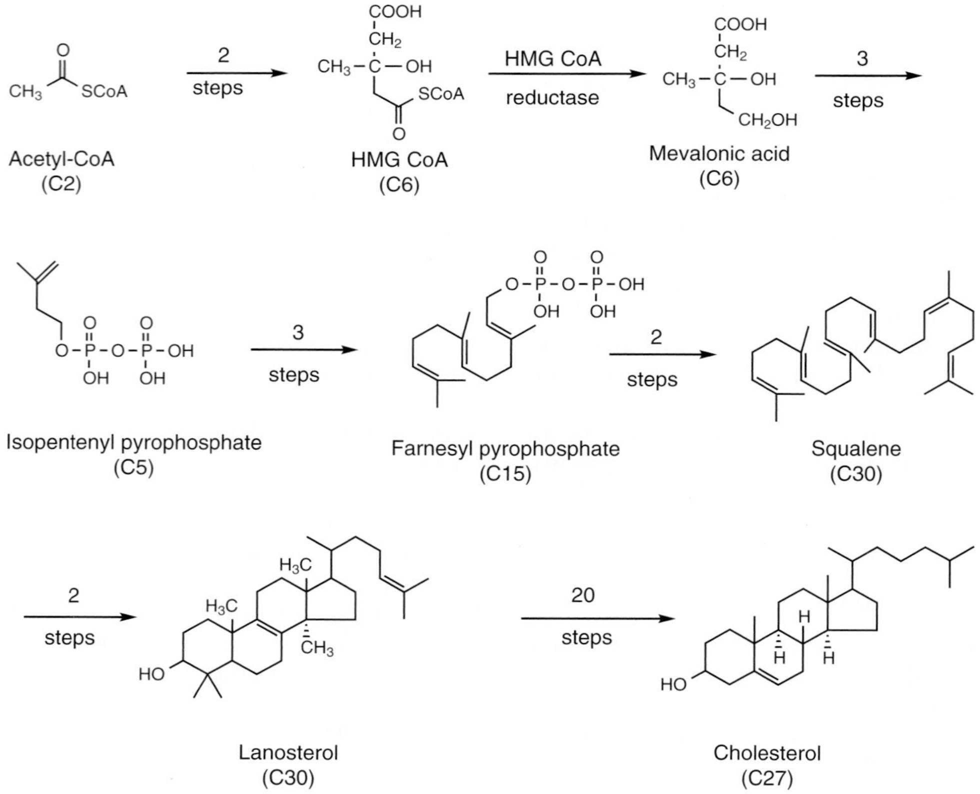

CH_3 SCoA — 2 steps → COOH CH_2 CH_3–C–OH SCoA — HMG CoA reductase → COOH CH_2 CH_3–C–OH CH_2OH — 3 steps →

Acetyl-CoA (C2) HMG CoA (C6) Mevalonic acid (C6)

O-P-O-P-OH OH OH — 3 steps → O-P-O-P-OH OH OH — 2 steps →

Isopentenyl pyrophosphate (C5) Farnesyl pyrophosphate (C15) Squalene (C30)

— 2 steps → H_3C H_3C CH_3 HO — 20 steps → H H H HO

Lanosterol (C30) Cholesterol (C27)

Figure 19.2 The biosynthesis of cholesterol.

SQUALENE SYNTHASE:, A POTENTIAL DRUG TARGET

Inhibitors of squalene synthase, the enzyme responsible for catalyzing the two-step conversion of two molecules of farnesyl pyrophosphate to squalene, continue to be investigated as antihyperlipidemic agents. Squalene synthase catalyzes the first committed step in sterol biosynthesis and offers some potential advantages over HMG-CoA reductase as a drug target. The latter group of drugs inhibits cholesterol synthesis at an early stage of the pathway and, thus, lacks specificity. Mevalonic acid, the immediate product of HMG-CoA reductase, is a common intermediate in the biosynthesis of other isoprenoids, such as ubiquinone (an electron carrier in oxidative phosphorylation), dolichol (a compound involved in oligosaccharide synthesis), and farnesylated proteins (the farnesyl portion targets the protein to cell membrane as opposed to the cytosol). Inhibitors of squalene synthase target an enzyme involved in a later stage of cholesterol biosynthesis and could potentially accomplish the same desired outcomes as currently available agents without interfering with the biosynthesis of other essential, nonsteroidal compounds. Numerous classes of drug molecules have been investigated over the past two decades; however, despite the ability of some of these compounds to effectively inhibit squalene synthase and produce a marked decrease in serum cholesterol, none of them have been approved or marketed. Additional analogues and other structural classes continue to be investigated and, ultimately, may produce alternatives to currently available therapy.[18-20]

Cholesterol is enzymatically transformed by two different pathways. As illustrated in Figure 19.1, cholesterol can be oxidatively cleaved by the enzyme desmolase (side chain–cleaving enzyme). The resulting compound, pregnenolone, serves as the common intermediate in the biosynthesis of all other endogenous steroids. Cholesterol also can be converted to bile acids and bile salts (Fig. 19.3). This pathway represents the most important mechanism for cholesterol catabolism. The enzyme 7α-hydroxylase catalyzes the initial, rate-limiting step in this metabolic pathway and, thus, is the key control enzyme for this pathway. Cholic acid and its derivatives are primarily (99%) conjugated with either glycine (75%) or taurine (24%). Bile salts, such as glycocholate, are surface-active agents that act as anionic detergents.

The bile salts are synthesized in the liver, stored in the gallbladder, and released into the small intestine, where they emulsify dietary lipids and fat-soluble vitamins. This solubilization promotes the absorption of these dietary compounds through the intestinal mucosa. Bile salts are predominantly reabsorbed through enterohepatic circulation and returned to the liver, where they exert a negative feedback control on 7α-hydroxylase and, thus, regulate any subsequent conversion of cholesterol.[16,21]

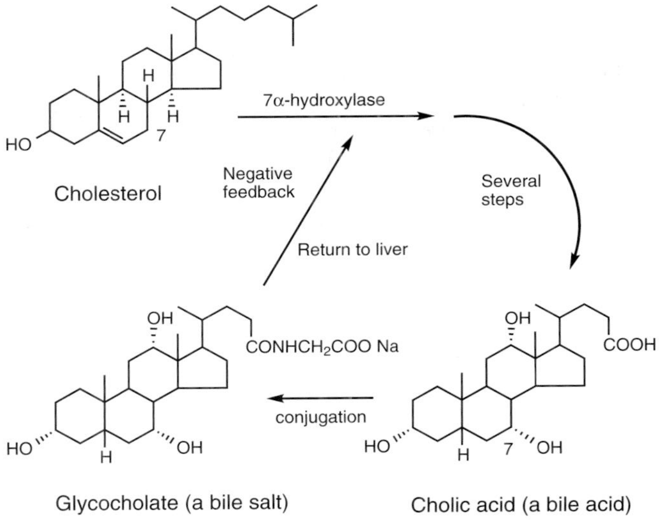

Figure 19.3 The conversion of cholesterol to bile acids and bile salts.

The terms "bile acid" and "bile salt" refer to the un-ionized and ionized forms, respectively, of these compounds. For illustrative purposes only, Figure 19.3 shows cholic acid as an un-ionized bile acid and glycocholate as an ionized bile salt (as the sodium salt). At physiologic and intestinal pH values, both compounds would exist almost exclusively in their ionized forms.

Overview of Triglycerides

Triglycerides (or, more appropriately, triacylglycerols) are highly concentrated stores of metabolic energy. They are formed from glycerol-3-phosphate and acylated CoA (Fig. 19.4) and accumulate primarily in the cytosol of adipose cells. When required for energy production, triglycerides are hydrolyzed by lipase enzymes to liberate free fatty acids that are then subjected to β-oxidation, the citric acid cycle, and oxidative phosphorylation.

Lipoproteins and Transport of Cholesterol and Triglycerides

Cholesterol and triglycerides are freely soluble in organic solvents, such as isopropanol, chloroform, and diethyl ether, but are relatively insoluble in aqueous, physiologic fluids. To be transported within the blood, these lipids are solubilized through association with macromolecular aggregates known as lipoproteins. Each lipoprotein is associated with additional proteins, known as apolipoproteins, on their outer surface. These apolipoproteins provide structural support and stability, bind to cellular receptors, and act as cofactors for enzymes involved in lipoprotein metabolism. The compositions and primary functions of the six major lipoproteins are listed in Table 19.1.[21,22]

Lipoprotein nomenclature is based on the mode of separation. When preparative ultracentrifugation is used, lipoproteins are separated according to their

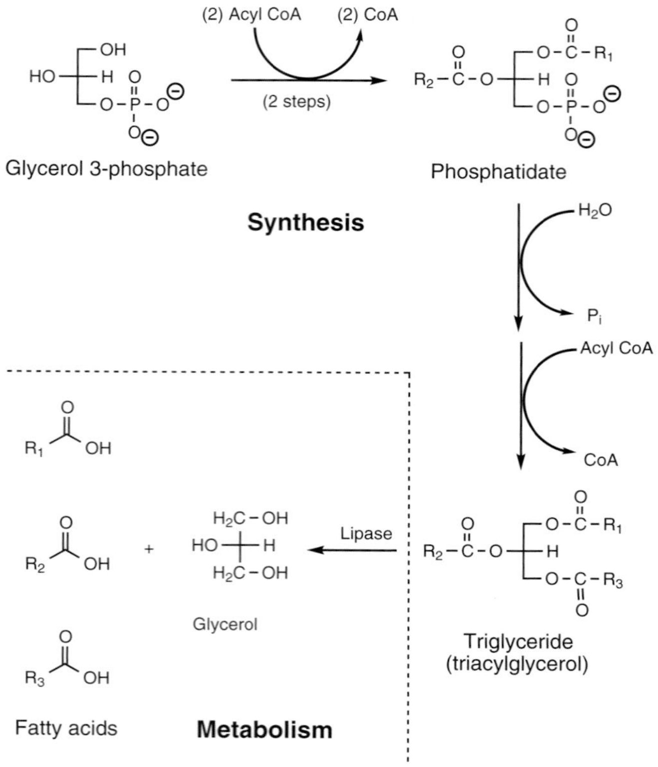

Figure 19.4 The biosynthesis and metabolism of triglycerides.

density and identified as very-low-density lipoproteins (VLDLs), intermediate-density lipoproteins (IDLs), low-density lipoproteins (LDLs), and high-density lipoproteins (HDLs). When electrophoresis is used in the separation, lipoproteins are designated as pre-β, β, and α. The IDLs are mainly found in the pre-β fraction as a second electrophoretic band and are currently believed to be an intermediate lipoprotein in the catabolism of VLDL to LDL. Chylomicron remnants and IDLs may show similar electrophoretic and ultracentrifugation separation characteristics. In general, VLDL, LDL, and HDL correspond to pre-β, β, and α lipoprotein, respectively.

The interrelationship among the lipoproteins is shown in Figure 19.5.[22,23] As illustrated, the pathway can be divided into exogenous (dietary intake) and endogenous (synthetic) components. The exogenous pathway begins after the ingestion of a fat-containing meal or snack. Dietary lipids are absorbed in the form of cholesterol and fatty acids, with fatty acids being the predominant lipid. The fatty acids are then re-esterified within the intestinal mucosal cells and, along with the cholesterol, are incorporated into chylomicrons, the largest lipoprotein. During circulation, chylomicrons are degraded into remnants by the action of lipoprotein lipase, a plasma membrane enzyme located on capillary endothelial cells in adipose and muscle tissue. The interaction of chylomicrons with

Table 19.1 Classification and Characteristics of Major Plasma Lipoproteins

Classification	Composition	Major Apolipoproteins	Primary Function(s)
Chylomicrons	Triglycerides 80%-95%, free cholesterol 1%-3%, cholesterol esters 2%-4%, phospholipids 3%-9%, apoproteins 1%-2%	apoA-I, apoA-IV, apoB-48, apoC-I, apoC-II, apoC-III	Transport dietary triglycerides to adipose tissue and muscle for hydrolysis by lipoprotein lipase
Chylomicron remnants	Primarily composed of dietary cholesterol esters	apoB-48, apoE	Transport dietary cholesterol to liver for receptor-mediated endocytosis
VLDL	Triglycerides 50%-65%, free cholesterol 4%-8%, cholesterol esters 16%-22%, phospholipids 15%-20%, apoproteins 6%-10%	apoB-100, apoE, apoC-I, apoC-II, apoC-III	Transport endogenous triglycerides to adipose tissue and muscle for hydrolysis by lipoprotein lipase
IDL	Intermediate between VLDL and LDL	apoB-100, apoE, apoC-II, apoC-III	Transport endogenous cholesterol for either conversion to LDL or receptor-mediated endocytosis by the liver
LDL	Triglycerides 4%-8%, free cholesterol 6%-8%, cholesterol esters 45%-50%, phospholipids 18%-24%, apoproteins 18%-22%	apoB-100	Transport endogenous cholesterol for receptor-mediated endocytosis by either the liver or extrahepatic tissues
HDL	Triglycerides 2%-7%, free cholesterol 3%-5%, cholesterol esters 15%-20%, phospholipids 26%-32%, apoproteins 45%-55%	apoA-I, apoA-II, apoE, apoC-I, apoC-II, apoC-III	Removal of cholesterol from extrahepatic tissues via transfer of cholesterol esters to IDL and LDL

apo, apolipoprotein; HDL, high-density lipoprotein; IDL, intermediate-density lipoprotein; LDL, low-density lipoprotein; VLDL, very-low-density lipoprotein.

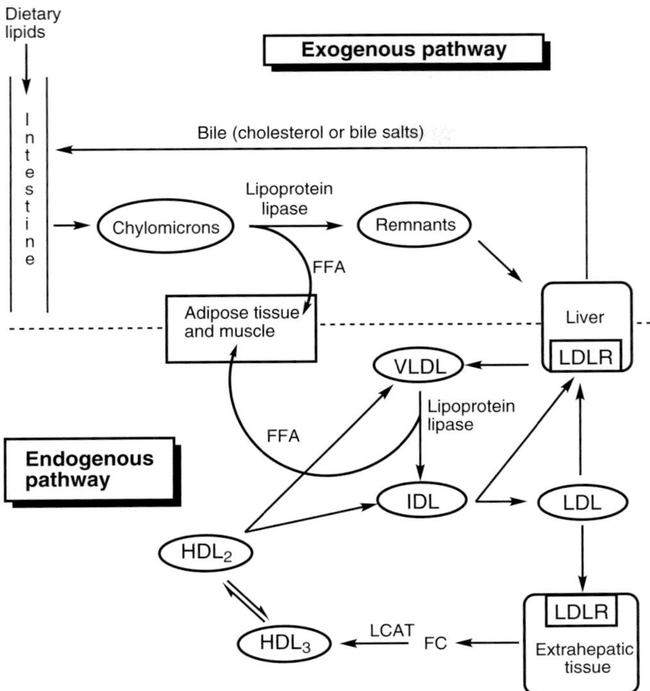

Figure 19.5 Endogenous and exogenous pathways for lipid transport and metabolism. *FC*, free unesterified cholesterol; *FFA*, free fatty acids; *LCAT*, lecithin-cholesterol acyltransferase; *LDLR*, low-density lipoprotein receptor.

lipoprotein lipase requires apolipoprotein (apo) C-II. The absence of either the enzyme or the apolipoprotein can lead to hypertriglyceridemia and pancreatitis. The liberated free acids are then available for either storage or energy generation by these tissues. The remnants are predominantly cleared from the plasma by liver parenchymal cells via recognition of the apoE portion of the carrier.

The endogenous pathway begins in the liver with the formation of VLDL. Similar to chylomicrons, triglycerides are present in a higher concentration than either cholesterol or cholesterol esters; however, the concentration difference between these lipids is much less than that seen in chylomicrons. The metabolism of VLDL also is similar to that of chylomicrons in that lipoprotein lipase reduces the triglyceride content of VLDL and increases the availability of free fatty acids to the muscle and adipose tissue. The resulting lipoprotein, IDL, either can be further metabolized to LDL or can be transported to the liver for receptor-mediated endocytosis. This latter effect involves an interaction of the LDL receptor with the apolipoproteins, apoB-100 and apoE, on IDL. The amount of IDL delivered to the liver is approximately the same as that converted to LDL. The half-life of IDL is relatively short as compared to that of LDL and, thus, accounts for only a small portion of total plasma cholesterol. In contrast, LDL accounts for approximately two-thirds of total plasma cholesterol and serves as the primary source of cholesterol for both hepatic and extrahepatic cells. As with IDL, the uptake of LDL by these cells is mediated by a receptor interaction with the apoB-100 on LDL. The number of LDL receptors on the cell surface mediates regulation of cellular LDL uptake. Cells requiring increased amounts of cholesterol will increase the biosynthesis of LDL receptors. Conversely, it has been demonstrated that increased hepatic concentrations of cholesterol will inhibit both HMG-CoA reductase as well as the production of LDL receptors. As previously discussed, hepatic cholesterol can be converted to bile acids and bile salts and reenter the endogenous pathway through the bile and enterohepatic circulation.

Synthesized in the liver and intestine, HDL initially exists as a dense, phospholipid disk composed primarily of apoA-I. The primary function of HDL is to act as a scavenger to remove cholesterol from extrahepatic cells and to facilitate its transport back to the liver. Nascent HDL accepts free, unesterified cholesterol. A plasma enzyme, lecithin-cholesterol acyltransferase, then esterifies the cholesterol. This process allows the resulting cholesterol esters to move from the surface to the core and results in the production of spherical HDL_3 particles. As cholesterol content is added, HDL_3 is converted to HDL_2, which is larger and less dense than HDL_3. The ultimate return of cholesterol from HDL_2 to the liver is known as reverse cholesterol transport and is accomplished via an intermediate transfer of cholesterol esters from HDL_2 to either VLDL or IDL. This process regenerates spherical HDL_3 molecules that can recirculate and acquire excess cholesterol from other tissues. In this manner, HDL serves to prevent the accumulation of cholesterol in arterial cell walls and other tissue and may serve as the basis for its cardioprotective properties.[22,23]

THERAPEUTIC OVERVIEW

Diseases and Disorders Caused by Hyperlipidemias

Atherosclerosis, which is named from the Greek terms for "gruel" (*athere*) and "hardening" (*sclerosis*), is the underlying cause of CHD. It is a gradual process in which an initial accumulation of lipids in the arterial intima leads to thickening of the arterial wall, plaque formation, thrombosis, and occlusion.[14,24,25] The involvement of LDL cholesterol in this process is shown in Figure 19.6. Within the extracellular space of the intima, LDL is more susceptible to oxidative metabolism, because it is no longer protected by plasma antioxidants. This metabolism alters the properties of LDL such that it is readily scavenged by macrophages. Unlike normal LDL, the uptake of oxidized LDL is not regulated; thus, macrophage cells can readily become engorged with oxidized LDL. Subsequent metabolism produces free cholesterol, which either can be released into the plasma or reesterified by the enzyme acyl CoA-cholesterol acyltransferase (ACAT). Cholesterol released into plasma can be scavenged by HDL_3 and returned to the liver, thus preventing

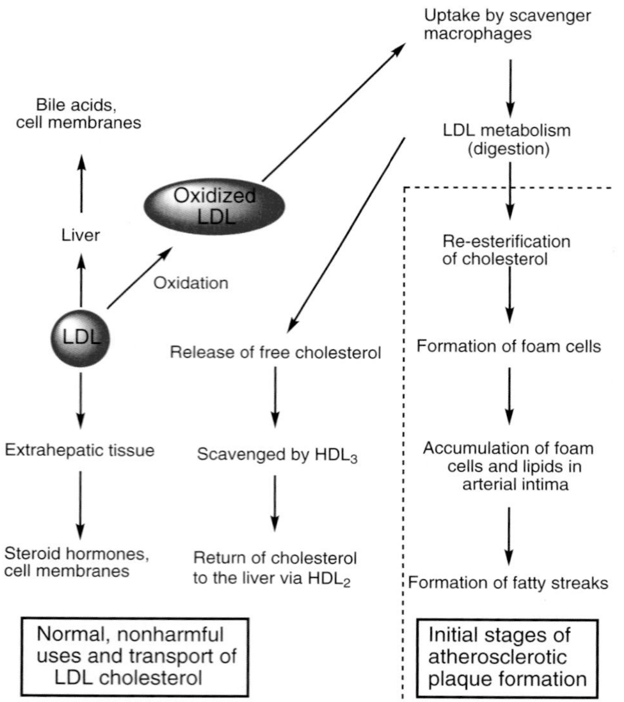

Figure 19.6 The role of LDL cholesterol in the development of atherosclerotic plaques and the cardioprotective role of HDL. The oxidation of LDL occurs within the extracellular space of the intima.

any accumulation or damage. In this manner, HDL acts as a cardioprotective agent, because high concentrations of reesterified cholesterol can morphologically change macrophages into foam cells. Accumulation of lipid-engorged foam cells in the arterial intima results in the formation of fatty streaks, the initial lesion of atherosclerosis. Later, the deposition of lipoproteins, cholesterol, and phospholipids causes the formation of softer, larger plaques. Associated with this lipid deposition is the proliferation of arterial smooth muscle cells into the intima and the laying down of collagen, elastin, and glycosaminoglycans, leading to fibrous plaques. Ultimately, the surface of the plaque deteriorates, and an atheromatous ulcer is formed with a fibrous matrix, accumulation of necrotic tissue, and appearance of cholesterol and cholesterol ester crystals. A complicated lesion also shows calcification and hemorrhage with the formation of organized mural thrombi. Thrombosis results from changes in the arterial walls and in the blood-clotting mechanism.

Elevated plasma triglyceride levels can contribute to atherosclerosis and CHD in mixed hyperlipoproteinemias, whereas pure hypertriglyceridemias are primarily associated with pancreatitis and show little to no relationship to CHD.[21,22]

Classification of Hyperlipoproteinemias

Hyperlipoproteinemia can be divided into primary and secondary disorders. Primary disorders are the result of genetic deficiencies or mutations, whereas secondary disorders are the result of other conditions or diseases. Secondary hyperlipoproteinemia has been associated with diabetes mellitus, hypothyroidism, renal disease, liver disease, alcoholism, and certain drugs.[14,21,22]

In 1967, Fredrickson et al.[23] classified primary hyperlipoproteinemias into six phenotypes (I, IIa, IIb, III, IV, and V) based on which lipoproteins and lipids were elevated. Current literature and practice, however, appear to favor the more descriptive classifications and subclassifications listed in Table 19.2. Primary disorders are currently classified as those that primarily cause hypercholesterolemia, those that primarily cause hypertriglyceridemia, and those that cause a mixed elevation of both cholesterol and triglycerides. Subclassifications are based on the specific biochemical defect responsible for the disorder. Classifications developed by Fredrickson have been included in Table 19.2

Table 19.2 Characteristics of the Major Primary Hyperlipoproteinemias

Current Classification	Biochemical Defect	Elevated Lipoproteins	Previous Classification
Hypercholesterolemias			
Familial hypercholesterolemia	Deficiency of LDL receptors	LDL	IIa
Familial defective apoB-100	Mutant apoB-100	LDL	IIa
Polygenic hypercholesterolemia	Unknown	LDL	IIa
Hypertriglyceridemias			
Familial hypertriglyceridemia	Unknown	VLDL	IV
Familial lipoprotein lipase deficiency	Deficiency of lipoprotein lipase	Chylomicrons, VLDL	I (chylomicron elevation only), V
Familial apoC-II deficiency	Deficiency of apoC-II	Chylomicrons, VLDL	I (chylomicron elevation only), V
Mixed hypercholesterolemia and hypertriglyceridemia			
Familial combined hyperlipidemia	Unknown	VLDL, LDL	IIb
Dysbetalipoproteinemia	Presence of $apoE_2$ isoforms	VLDL, IDL	III

apo, apolipoprotein; IDL, intermediate-density lipoprotein; LDL, low-density lipoprotein; VLDL, very-low-density lipoprotein.

under the heading *Previous Classification* for comparative and reference purposes.

As shown in Table 19.2, some disorders are well characterized, whereas others are not.[14,21,22] Familial hypercholesterolemia is caused by a deficiency of LDL receptors. This results in a decreased uptake of IDL and LDL by hepatic and extrahepatic tissues and an elevation in plasma LDL levels. The homozygous form of this disorder is rare but results in extremely high LDL levels and early morbidity and mortality because of the total lack of LDL receptors. A related disorder, familial defective apoB-100, also results in elevated LDL levels but is caused by a genetic mutation rather than a deficiency. Alteration of apoB-100 decreases the affinity of LDL for the LDL receptor and thus hinders normal uptake and metabolism. Elevations in chylomicron levels can result from a deficiency of either lipoprotein lipase or apoC-II. These deficiencies cause decreased or impaired triglyceride hydrolysis and result in a massive accumulation of chylomicrons in the plasma. Dysbetalipoproteinemia results from the presence of an altered form of apoE and is the only mixed hyperlipoproteinemia with a known cause. Proper catabolism of chylomicron and VLDL remnants requires apoE. The presence of a binding-defective form of apoE, known as $apoE_2$, results in elevated levels of VLDL and IDL triglyceride and cholesterol levels.

Prevalence and Public Health Burden of CHD

According to a 2017 report, CHD, which includes acute myocardial infarction, ischemic heart disease, and angina pectoris, affects approximately 16.5 million Americans 20 years of age or older and is the leading cause of mortality in the United States.[26] The overall prevalence of CHD in this age group is 6.3%, with the prevalence being higher in males (7.4%) than it is in females (5.3%). On the basis of the Framingham Heart Study, greater than 50% of all cardiovascular events occurring in patients 75 years old or less are due to CHD. In 2014, CHD was responsible for slightly less than 364,500 deaths, and an underlying cause of one in every seven deaths. From a positive perspective, the percentage of US adults with a 10-year predicted atherosclerotic cardiovascular disease (ASCVD) greater than 20% has decreased from 13% in 1999 to 2000 to 9.4% in 2011 to 2012. Risk factors associated with CHD include hypertension, cigarette smoking, elevated plasma cholesterol levels, physical inactivity, diabetes, and obesity.[27,28]

Economic Impact of Therapy

Current guidelines for lowering plasma LDL-cholesterol focus on the use of HMG-CoA-reductase inhibitors, commonly known as statins, and other dietary and pharmacological/chemical classes of drugs, commonly known as nonstatin therapy.[8,15] These guidelines define four patient population groups that would benefit from the use of statins as well as other factors that need to be considered. These include adherence, lifestyle, the control of other risk factors, the balance between risks and benefits of using a statin, the patient's preference for one medication over another, the total LDL reduction that is set as the patient's goal, and patient monitoring. Current drug options beyond statin therapy include ezetimibe (an inhibitor of dietary cholesterol), bile acid sequestrants, proprotein convertase subtilisin/kexin type 9 (PCSK9) inhibitors, niacin (for HDL elevation), mipomersen (a microsomal triglyceride transfer protein inhibitor), and lomitapide (an apoB-100 protein translation inhibitor).

Additionally, fibrates are useful for lowering triglyceride levels, reducing the risk of pancreatitis, and increasing HDL levels.[29] The estimated cost of myocardial infarction (MI) and CHD is approximately $22 billion dollars based on discharge diagnoses in 2011. This includes hospitalization costs, the costs of physician and other health service providers, and overall drug prescription costs. These costs are projected to gradually increase by 100% by the year 2030.[26]

As such, the selection of appropriate therapy based on desired patient outcomes plays a key role in the pharmacotherapy of treating risk factors such as dyslipidemia.

HMG-CoA Reductase Inhibitors

The development and use of HMGRIs began in 1976 with the discovery of mevastatin, a lactone containing prodrug. Originally named compactin, this fungal metabolite was isolated from two different species of *Penicillium*. Its hydrolyzed metabolite demonstrated potent, competitive inhibition of HMG-CoA reductase with an affinity that was 10,000-fold greater than that of the substrate HMG-CoA.[30] Several years later, a structurally similar compound known as mevinolin was isolated from *Monascus ruber* and *Aspergillus terreus*. Mevinolin was later renamed lovastatin and its hydrolyzed metabolite was shown to be more than twofold more potent than mevastatin (Fig. 19.7). Clinical trials of mevastatin were halted after reports of altered intestinal morphology in dogs[31]; however, lovastatin received approval by the U.S. Food and Drug Administration (FDA) in 1987, representing the first HMGRI to be available in the United States for therapeutic use.

All HMGRIs are approved for the treatment of primary hypercholesterolemia and mixed dyslipidemia as shown in Table 19.3. Additional indications for this class of drugs include primary dysbetalipoproteinemia, hypertriglyceridemia, homozygous familial hyperlipidemia, and primary and secondary prevention of cardiovascular events (e.g., myocardial infarction, stroke). At their highest approved doses, atorvastatin and rosuvastatin have been shown to be the most effective drugs at lowering LDL cholesterol levels.[29]

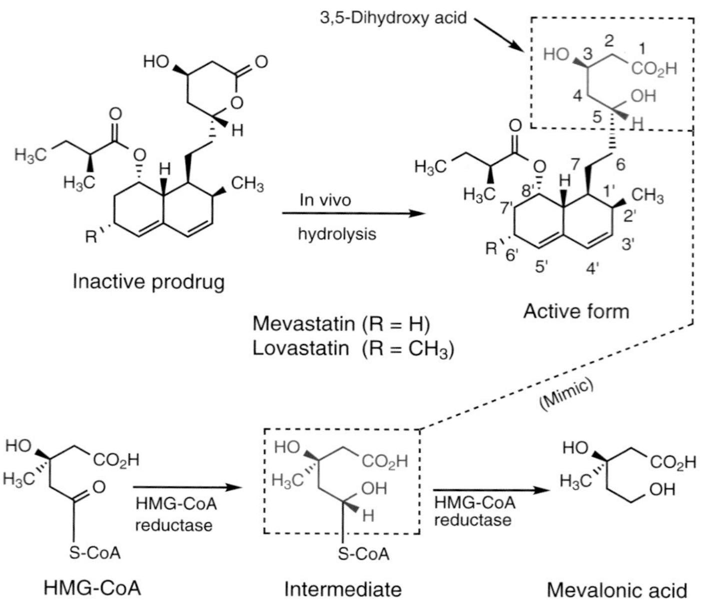

Figure 19.7 Mechanism of action of mevastatin and lovastatin. Hydrolysis of these prodrugs produces a 3,5-dihydroxy acid that mimics the tetrahedral intermediate produced by HMG-CoA reductase.

Table 19.3 Approved Therapeutics Conditions for HMG-CoA Reductase Inhibitors

Therapeutics Condition	Atorvastatin	Fluvastatin	Lovastatin	Pitavastatin	Pravastatin	Rosuvastatin	Simvastatin
Primary hypercholesterolemia	√	√	√	√	√	√	√
Primary dysbetalipoproteinemia	√				√	√	√
Mixed dyslipidemia	√	√	√	√	√	√	√
Hypertriglyceridemia	√			√	√	√	√
Homozygous familial hyperlipidemia	√					√	√
Primary prevention of cardiovascular events	√		√		√	√	√
Secondary prevention of cardiovascular events	√	√	√		√	√	√

Mechanism of Action

Inhibitors of HMG-CoA reductase lower plasma cholesterol levels by three related mechanisms: inhibition of cholesterol biosynthesis, enhancement of receptor-mediated LDL uptake, and reduction of VLDL precursors.[32,33] HMG-CoA reductase is the rate-limiting step in cholesterol biosynthesis. Competitive inhibition of this enzyme causes an initial decrease in hepatic cholesterol. Compensatory mechanisms result in an enhanced expression of both HMG-CoA reductase and LDL receptors. The net result of all these effects is a slight to modest decrease in cholesterol synthesis, a significant increase in receptor-mediated LDL uptake, and an overall lowering of plasma LDL levels. Evidence to support the theory that enhanced LDL receptor expression is the primary mechanism for lowering LDL levels comes from the fact that most statins do not lower LDL levels in patients who are unable to produce LDL receptors (i.e., homozygous familial hypercholesterolemia). The increased number of LDL receptors also may increase the direct removal of VLDL and IDL. Because these lipoproteins are precursors to LDL, this action may contribute to the overall lowering of plasma LDL cholesterol. Finally, all HMGRIs can produce a modest (8%-12%) increase in HDL.[32]

Atorvastatin, rosuvastatin, and simvastatin appear to have some effects beyond those seen with the other HMGRIs. These compounds have been shown to decrease plasma LDL levels in patients with homozygous familial hypercholesterolemia, an effect that is proposed to result from their ability to produce a more significant decrease in the hepatic production of LDL cholesterol. Additionally, atorvastatin and rosuvastatin can produce a significant lowering in plasma triglycerides. In the case of atorvastatin, this effect has been attributed to its ability to produce an enhanced removal of triglyceride-rich VLDL.[29,34,35]

A number of additional cardioprotective effects, other than lowering LDL cholesterol, are thought to be associated with HMGRIs. HMGRIs cause an upregulation of nitric oxide synthetase expression resulting in vasodilation and improved endothelial function, and they have been postulated to stabilize plaques, provide an anti-inflammatory effect, reduce the susceptibility of LDL to oxidation, and reduce platelet aggregation.[21]

Common Adverse Effects

The most prevalent or significant side effects of HMGRIs are highlighted in the box entitled Adverse Effects of HMGRIs.[21,32,33] In general, this class of drugs is well tolerated. Gastrointestinal disturbances are the most common complaint; however, these and other adverse reactions tend to be mild and transient. Elevations in hepatic transaminase levels can occur with all HMGRIs. These increases usually occur shortly after the initiation of therapy and resolve after the discontinuation of medication. In a small percentage of patients, these levels can increase to more than threefold the upper limit of normal. Current guidelines require that liver function tests be performed prior to starting HMGRI therapy and, if there is a clinical indication, during therapy. Routine monitoring is not required or recommended based on the facts that serious hepatic injury is rare and that routine monitoring has not been shown to detect or prevent hepatic injury. Approximately 5%-10% of patients will experience mild increases in creatine phosphokinase levels; however, less than 1% will develop symptoms of myalgia and myopathy (e.g., fever, muscle aches or cramps, and unusual tiredness or weakness). Tests for creatine phosphokinase levels should be performed in patients reporting muscle complaints. Rhabdomyolysis (i.e., massive muscle necrosis with secondary acute renal failure) has occurred, but this is rare.

ADVERSE EFFECTS OF HMGRIs

Abdominal pain, arthralgia, chest pain, constipation, diarrhea, dyspepsia, elevated hepatic enzymes, flatulence, headache, muscle cramps, myalgia, myopathy, nausea, rhabdomyolysis, rhinitis, sinusitis, and vomiting.

Common Interactions

A list of common drug and food interactions is provided in Table 19.4.[32-35] As discussed later in this section, most HMGRIs are metabolized by CYP3A4; therefore, other drugs that inhibit or induce this isozyme will increase or decrease the levels of HMGRIs, respectively. Inhibition of CYP3A4 may increase the risk of myopathy and rhabdomyolysis; therefore, specific dosage reductions are suggested whenever an HMGRI is used in combination with a CYP3A4 inhibitor. If used in combination with bile acid sequestrants, HMGRIs should be administered at least 1 hour prior or 4-6 hours after the bile acid sequestrant to avoid decreased absorption. Inhibitors of HMG-CoA reductase are contraindicated in pregnancy. Fetal development requires cholesterol as a precursor for the synthesis of steroids and cell membranes; thus, inhibition of its synthesis may cause fetal harm. Additionally, HMGRIs are excreted in breast milk and should not be used by nursing mothers.

Receptor Binding and SAR

Mevastatin and lovastatin served as lead compounds in the development of additional HMGRIs. The only structural difference between lovastatin and mevastatin was the presence of a methyl group at the 6′ position of the bicyclic ring of lovastatin. As illustrated in Figure 19.7, mevastatin and lovastatin can bind very tightly with HMG-CoA reductase, because their hydrolyzed lactones mimic the tetrahedral intermediate produced by the reductase enzyme.[21]

Table 19.4 Drug Interactions for HMG-CoA Reductase Inhibitors (HMGRIs)

Drug	HMGRIs	Result of Interaction
Amiodarone	Lovastatin, simvastatin	Increased risk of myopathy
Antacids	Atorvastatin, rosuvastatin	Decreased levels of atorvastatin, rosuvastatin; no change in plasma LDL reduction; administer rosuvastatin at least 2 hr after antacid
Azole antifungal agents	All	Increased risk of severe myopathy or rhabdomyolysis; increased plasma levels of atorvastatin, lovastatin, and simvastatin because of inhibition of CYP3A4; additive decreases in concentrations or activity of endogenous steroid hormones
Bile acid sequestrants	All	Decreased bioavailability of HMGRI if administration is not adequately spaced
Cimetidine	Fluvastatin	Increase in plasma fluvastatin levels
Cyclosporine	All	Increased risk of severe myopathy or rhabdomyolysis
Danazol	Lovastatin	Increased risk of severe myopathy or rhabdomyolysis
Digoxin	Atorvastatin, fluvastatin, simvastatin	Slight elevation in plasma concentrations of digoxin
Diltiazem	Atorvastatin, lovastatin, simvastatin	Increased risk of severe myopathy
Erythromycin, clarithromycin	All	Increased risk of severe myopathy or rhabdomyolysis; increased plasma levels of atorvastatin, lovastatin, and simvastatin because of inhibition of CYP3A4
Ethanol	Fluvastatin, lovastatin	Increased risk of hepatotoxicity
Fibrates	All	Increased risk of severe myopathy or rhabdomyolysis
Grapefruit juice	Atorvastatin, lovastatin, simvastatin	Elevated plasma levels of the HMGRIs and increased risk of myopathy
HIV protease inhibitors	Atorvastatin, lovastatin, pitavastatin, simvastatin	Elevated plasma levels of the HMGRIs and increased risk of myopathy
Isradipine	Lovastatin	Increased clearance of lovastatin and its metabolites
Itraconazole	Pitavastatin	Decreased plasma levels of pitavastatin
Niacin	All	Increased risk of severe myopathy or rhabdomyolysis
Omeprazole	Fluvastatin	Increase in plasma fluvastatin levels
Oral contraceptives	Atorvastatin, rosuvastatin	Increased plasma concentrations of norethindrone and ethinyl estradiol
Phenytoin	Fluvastatin	Increased plasma concentrations of both compounds because of CYP2C9 interaction
Ranitidine	Fluvastatin	Increase in plasma fluvastatin levels
Rifampin	Fluvastatin, pitavastatin	Increased plasma clearance of fluvastatin
Ritonavir, saquinavir	Pravastatin	Decreased plasma levels of pravastatin
Spironolactone	All	Additive decreases in concentrations or activity of endogenous steroid hormones
St. John's wort	Lovastatin, simvastatin	Decreased HMGRI plasma levels
Warfarin	Fluvastatin, lovastatin, rosuvastatin, simvastatin	Anticoagulant effect of warfarin may be increased

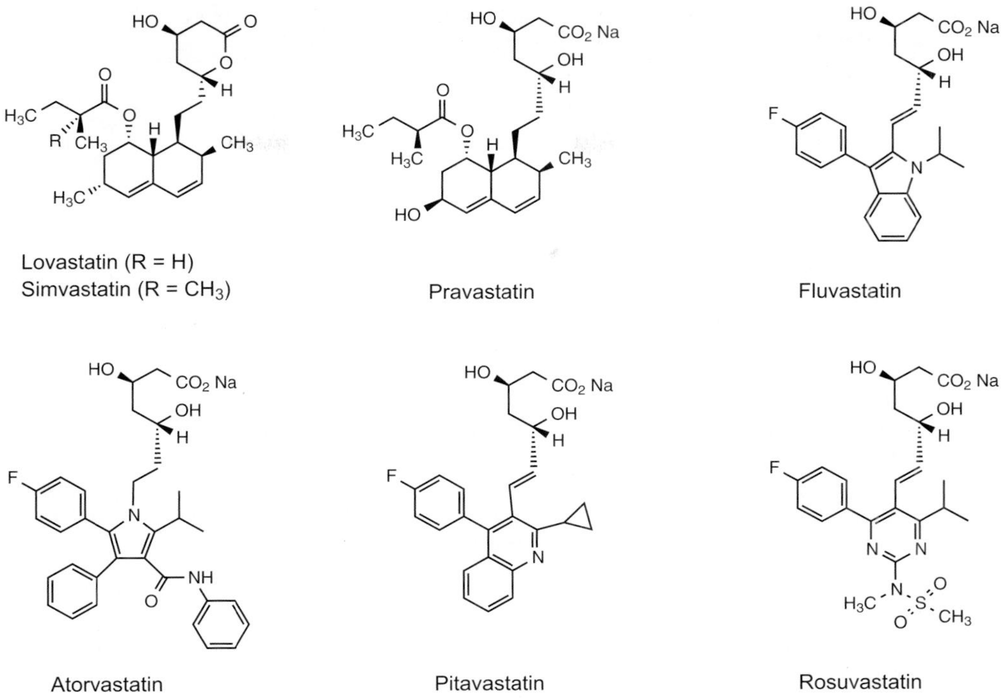

Lovastatin (R = H)
Simvastatin (R = CH_3)

Pravastatin

Fluvastatin

Atorvastatin

Pitavastatin

Rosuvastatin

Figure 19.8 Commercially available HMG-CoA reductase inhibitors.

Studies published in 1985 confirmed this theory and established that the bicyclic portions of these compounds bind to the CoA site of the enzyme.[36]

Initial research published by Merck Pharmaceuticals examined alterations of the lactone and bicyclic rings as well as the ethylene bridge between them. The results demonstrated that the activity of HMGRIs is sensitive to the stereochemistry of the lactone ring, the ability of the lactone ring to be hydrolyzed, and the length of bridge connecting the two ring systems. Additionally, it was found that the bicyclic ring could be replaced with other lipophilic rings and that the size and shape of these other ring systems were important to the overall activity of the compounds.[37]

Minor modifications of the bicyclic ring and side-chain ester of lovastatin produced simvastatin and pravastatin (Fig. 19.8). Pravastatin, a ring-opened dihydroxy acid with a 6′α-hydroxyl group, is much more hydrophilic than either lovastatin or simvastatin. Proposed advantages of this enhanced hydrophilicity are minimal penetration into the lipophilic membranes of peripheral cells, better selectivity for hepatic tissues, and a reduction in the incidence of side effects seen with lovastatin and simvastatin.[38,39]

The replacement of the bicyclic ring with various substituted, aromatic ring systems led to the development of atorvastatin, fluvastatin, pitavastatin, and rosuvastatin (Fig. 19.8). The initial rationale centered on a desire to simplify the structures of mevastatin and lovastatin. The 2,4-dichlorophenyl analogue (compound A) was one of the first compounds to demonstrate that this type of substitution was possible; however, compound A was considerably less potent than mevastatin. Subsequent research investigated a variety of aromatic substitutions and heterocyclic ring systems to optimize HMGRI activity. The substituted pyrrole (compound B) retained 30% of the activity of mevastatin[40] and was a key intermediate in the development of atorvastatin. The 4-fluorophenyl and isopropyl (or cyclopropane) substitutions found in compound B also are seen in the indole, quinoline, and pyrimidine ring systems of fluvastatin, pitavastatin, and rosuvastatin, respectively, and most likely represent the optimum substitutions at their respective positions. The design of all four of these compounds included the ring-opened dihydroxy acid functionality first seen in pravastatin.

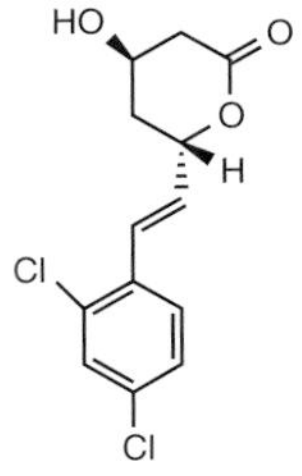

Compound A

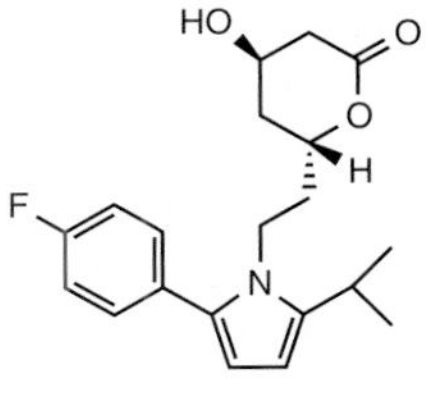

Compound B

A summary of the structure-activity relationships (SARs) for HMGRIs is presented in Table 19.5. The structures of all HMGRIs contain a 7-substituted-3,5-dihydroxyheptanoic acid which is required for activity. Additionally, this class of drugs can be subclassified based on their lower ring. Drugs structurally related to the

Table 19.5 Structure-Activity Relationship of HMG-CoA Reductase Inhibitors

	7-Substituted-3,5-dihydroxyheptanoic acid (Ring system) — Ring A — Ring B
Common for all HGMIs	1. The 3,5-dihydroxycarboxylate is essential for inhibitory activity. Drugs containing a lactone are prodrugs requiring in vivo hydrolysis. 2. The absolute stereochemistry of the 3- and 5-hydroxyl groups must be the same as that found in mevastatin and lovastatin. 3. Altering the two-carbon distance between C5 and the ring system diminishes or fails to improve activity. 4. A double bond between C6 and C7 can either increase or decrease activity. The ethyl group provides optimal activity for compounds containing ring A and some heterocyclic rings (e.g., pyrrole ring of atorvastatin). The ethenyl group is optimal for compounds with other ring systems, including the indole, quinoline, and pyrimidine rings seen in fluvastatin, pitavastatin, and rosuvastatin, respectively.
Ring A subclass	1. The decalin ring is essential for anchoring the drug to the enzyme active site. Replacement with a cyclohexane ring resulted in a 10,000-fold decrease in activity. 2. Stereochemistry of the ester side chain is not important for activity; however, conversion of this ester to an ether results in a decrease in activity. 3. Methyl substitution at the R2 position increases activity (i.e., simvastatin is more potent than lovastatin). 4. β-Hydroxyl group substitution at the R1 position enhances hydrophilicity and may provide some cellular specificity.
Ring B subclass	1. Substituents W, X, Y, and Z can be either carbon or nitrogen; n is equal to either zero or one (i.e., five- or six-member heterocyclic). 2. The para-fluorophenyl cannot be coplanar with the central aromatic ring. (Structural restraints to cause coplanarity have resulted in a loss of activity.) 3. R substitution with aryl groups, hydrocarbon chains, amides, or sulfonamides enhances lipophilicity and inhibitory activity.

natural products mevastatin and lovastatin have structural features common to ring A, whereas those that are completely synthetic have structural features common to ring B.[37,39-47]

Physiocochemical Properties

In their active forms, all HMGRIs contain a carboxylic acid. This functional group is required for inhibitory activity, has a pKa in the range of 2.5-3.5, and will be primarily ionized at physiologic pH. Lovastatin and simvastatin are neutral, lactone prodrugs and should be classified as nonelectrolytes. Pravastatin, fluvastatin, and atorvastatin can be classified as acidic drugs. The nitrogen atoms in the indole and pyrrole rings of fluvastatin and atorvastatin, respectively, are aromatic nitrogens that are not ionizable. This is because the lone pair electrons of these atoms are involved in maintaining the aromaticity of their respective rings and are not available to bind protons. Pitavastatin and rosuvastatin are amphoteric compounds; however, their quinoline and pyrimidine rings are weakly basic and will be primarily un-ionized at physiologic pH.

The calculated log P values for the HMGRIs are shown in Table 19.6. Although some variation exists among the values for lovastatin, pravastatin, and simvastatin, the general trends are the same, regardless of what program was used to calculate the values. Atorvastatin, fluvastatin, pitavastatin, and the prodrugs lovastatin and simvastatin have a much higher lipid solubility than either pravastatin and rosuvastatin. Hydrolysis of the lactone ring for the two prodrugs produces a 3,5-dihydroxycarboxylate which significantly improves water solubility.

The HMG-CoA reductase enzyme is stereoselective. The 3*R*, 5*R* stereochemistry seen in the active forms of mevastatin and lovastatin (Fig. 19.6) is required for inhibitory activity and is present in all other HMGRIs. The stereochemistry of substituents on the bicyclic rings of lovastatin, simvastatin, and pravastatin is less crucial to activity, as described in Table 19.5.

Metabolism

Lovastatin and simvastatin are inactive prodrugs that must undergo in vivo hydrolysis to produce their effects (Fig. 19.7). The active forms of these two drugs as well

Table 19.6 Pharmacokinetic Parameters of HMG-CoA Reductase Inhibitors

Drug	Calculated log P[a]	Oral Bioavailability (%)	Active Metabolite(s)	Protein Binding (%)	Time to Peak Concentration (hr)	Elimination Half-Life (hr)	Major Route(s) of Elimination
Atorvastatin	4.13	12-14	*ortho*- and *para*- hydroxylated	98	1-2	14-19	Biliary/fecal (>90%) Renal (<2%)
Fluvastatin	3.62	20-30	None	98	0.5-1.0	1	Biliary/fecal (95%) Renal (5%)
Lovastatin	4.07 (4.04)[a]	5	3,5-Dihydroxy acid	>95	2	3-4	Fecal (83%) Renal (10%)
Pravastatin	1.44 (0.5)[b]	17	None	43-55	1.0-1.5	2-3	Fecal (70%) Renal (20%)
Pitavastatin	3.45	51	None	>99	1	12	Fecal (79%) Renal (15%)
Rosuvastatin	0.42	20	N-Desmethyl	88	3-5	19-20	Fecal (90%) Renal (10%)
Simvastatin	4.42 (4.2)[b]	5	3,5-Dihydroxy acid	95	4	3	Fecal (60%) Renal (13%)

[a]A commercial program was used for calculated values.[64]
[b]Calculated using the CLOG program.[40]

as most HMGRIs undergo extensive first-pass metabolism.[32,34,35,48] The CYP3A4 isozyme is responsible for the oxidative metabolism of atorvastatin, lovastatin, and simvastatin. In the case of atorvastatin, the *ortho*- and *para*-hydroxylated metabolites are equiactive with the parent compound and contribute significantly to the overall activity of the drug (Table 19.6). Rosuvastatin is metabolized to a limited extent by CYP2C9 to form an N-desmethyl metabolite that can contribute to activity, but is sevenfold less potent. Approximately 90% of rosuvastatin is excreted unchanged. In contrast, the activity of lovastatin and simvastatin resides primarily in the initial hydrolysis product (i.e., further oxidation decreases activity). Fluvastatin is metabolized by the CYP2C9 and CYP3A4 isozymes to active hydroxylated metabolites; however, these metabolites do not circulate systemically and do not contribute to the overall activity. Pravastatin also undergoes oxidative metabolism, but the resulting metabolites retain only minimal activity and are not significant. Neither pitavastatin, pravastatin, nor rosuvastatin is metabolized by CYP3A4; therefore, these drugs are potentially advantageous for patients who must take concurrent medication that alters the activity of this isozyme. Pitavastatin is primarily metabolized by CYP2CP and undergoes lactonization to an inactive compound.

Pharmacokinetic Properties

The pharmacokinetic parameters and dosing information for HMGRIs are summarized in Tables 19.6 and 19.7,[21,22,29,32-34,48-50] respectively. With a few exceptions, these drugs have similar onsets of action, durations of action, dosing intervals, and plasma protein binding.

Despite the ability to attain a peak plasma concentration in 1-4 hours, HMGRIs require approximately 2 weeks to demonstrate an initial lowering of plasma cholesterol. Peak reductions of plasma cholesterol occur after 4-6 weeks of therapy for most compounds. Studies with atorvastatin, however, indicate that it may only need 2 weeks to produce its peak reduction. Atorvastatin and rosuvastatin also are unique in that they have much longer durations of action than the other compounds. With the exception of pravastatin, which is one of the more hydrophilic drugs in this class, most HMGRIs bind extensively to plasma proteins.

Because of first-pass metabolism, the oral bioavailability of this class of drugs generally is low and does not reflect the actual absorption of the individual drugs. For example, 60%-80% of a dose of simvastatin is orally absorbed, but only 5% is available to produce an effect. The same is true with fluvastatin, pravastatin, and lovastatin, which have oral absorptions of 90%, 34%, and 35%, respectively, but much lower bioavailabilities. Pitavastatin has the highest oral bioavailability in this class of compounds (Table 19.6). With the exception of lovastatin, the concurrent administration of food does not affect the overall therapeutic effects of HMGRIs. Lovastatin should always be administered with food to maximize oral bioavailability. Failure to do this results in a 33% decrease in plasma concentrations. In general, HMGRIs should be administered in the evening or at bedtime to counteract the peak cholesterol synthesis, which occurs in the early morning hours. Exceptions to this are atorvastatin and rosuvastatin, which because of their long half-lives are equally effective regardless of when they are administered. The primary route of elimination of these compounds is through the feces. Because of extensive

Table 19.7 Dosing Information for HMG-CoA Reductase Inhibitors

Generic Name	Brand Name(s)	Dosing Range	Maximum Daily Dose	Dose Reduction with Renal Dysfunction	Tablet Strengths (mg)
Atorvastatin	Lipitor	10-80 mg once daily	80 mg	No	10, 20, 40, 80
Fluvastatin	Lescol Lescol XL	20-80 mg once daily or b.i.d.	80 mg	Caution in severe impairment	20, 40, 80 (XR)
Lovastatin	Mevacor (N/A) Altoprev (XR)	10-80 mg once daily or b.i.d.	80 mg (60 mg if XR) (20 mg with fibrate)	Only with severe impairment	10, 20, 40, 20 (XR), 40 (XR), 60 (XR)
Pitavastatin	Livalo	1-4 mg once daily	40 mg	Yes	1, 2, 4
Pravastatin	Pravachol	10-80 mg once daily	80 mg	Yes	10, 20, 40, 80
Rosuvastatin	Crestor	5-40 mg once daily	40 mg (10 mg with fibrate)	Only with severe impairment	5, 10, 20, 40
Simvastatin	Zocor FloLipid	5-40 mg once daily	80 mg (10 mg with fibrate; 20 mg with lomitapide)	Only with severe impairment	5, 10, 20, 40, 80 (20 mg/5 mL; 40 mg/5 mL suspension)

b.i.d., twice a day; N/A, no longer available; XR, extended release.

hepatic transformation and the ability to elevate hepatic enzymes, HMGRIs are contraindicated in patients with active hepatic disease or unexplained persistent elevations in serum aminotransferase concentrations. Dosage reductions in patients with renal dysfunction depend on the individual drug. Atorvastatin, which has minimal renal excretion, requires no dosage reduction and may be the best agent for patients with renal disorders. Fluvastatin, rosuvastatin, and simvastatin require dosage reductions only in cases of severe renal impairment and are better choices than lovastatin, pitavastatin, and pravastatin, which require dosage reductions in mild or moderate impairment.

CHOLESTEROL ABSORPTION INHIBITOR

Mechanism of Action

Ezetimibe (*Zetia*), currently the only drug to act via this mechanism, lowers plasma cholesterol levels by inhibiting the absorption of cholesterol at the brush border of the small intestine.[29,32] Specifically, ezetimibe binds to the sterol transporter, Niemann-Pick C1-Like 1 (NPC1L1). This transporter is located in the epithelial cells of small intestine and is required for the intestinal uptake of cholesterol and phytosterols.[51] Ezetimibe appears to be selective in its actions in that it does not interfere with the absorption of triglycerides, lipid-soluble vitamins, or other nutrients. The decreased absorption of cholesterol eventually leads to enhanced receptor-mediated LDL uptake similar to that seen with HMGRIs. When used as monotherapy, the decreased absorption of cholesterol causes a compensatory increase in cholesterol biosynthesis; however, it is insufficient to override the overall LDL-lowering effects of ezetimibe.

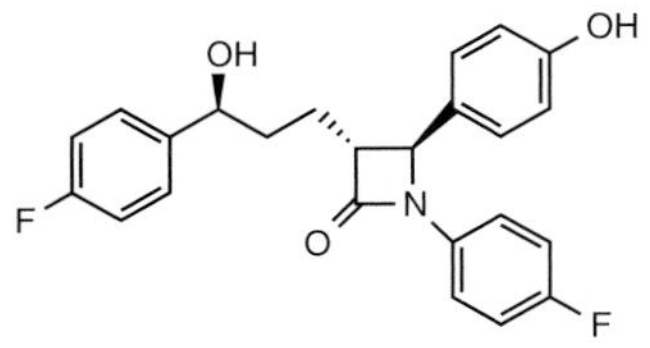

OH OH F O N F

Ezetimibe

Common Adverse Effects and Drug Interactions

Ezetimibe generally is well tolerated. The most common adverse effects are abdominal pain, diarrhea, back pain, cough, pharyngitis, sinusitis, fatigue, and viral infection. More serious adverse effects, such as rhabdomyolysis, hepatitis, pancreatitis, and thrombocytopenia, have been reported. Whenever ezetimibe is used in combination with an HMGRI, the incidence of myopathy or rhabdomyolysis does not increase above that seen with HMGRI monotherapy.[32,33]

Drug interactions for ezetimibe are listed in Table 19.8.

Table 19.8 Drug Interactions for Ezetimibe

Drug	Result of Interaction
Antacid	Aluminum and magnesium-containing antacids decrease the maximum plasma concentration of ezetimibe
Bile acid sequestrants	Decreased bioavailability of ezetimibe if administration is not adequately spaced
Cyclosporine	Increased ezetimibe concentration
Fibrates	Increased ezetimibe concentration and possible increased risk of cholelithiasis. With the exception of fenofibrate, concomitant use is not recommended

Receptor Binding and SAR

The 1,4-diaryl-β-lactam ring is essential for the binding of ezetimibe to NPC1L1. Hydrolysis of this ring or the use of larger lactam rings produce inactive compounds. It has been proposed that this ring primarily serves as a scaffold to orient the two aromatic rings and the aliphatic chain. The phenolic and aliphatic hydroxyl groups enhance activity; although a *para*-methoxy group has also been shown to be active. The hydrophilic nature of these two functional groups are important for helping ezetimibe localize in the small intestine. The *para*-fluoro group prevents aromatic oxidation and thus prolongs the duration of action.[52,53]

Physicochemical Properties

Ezetimibe is a crystalline powder that is practically insoluble in water but is freely soluble in ethanol and other organic solvents. Its calculated log P value is 3.50.[49] The phenol present in ezetimibe allows this compound to be classified as an acidic compound; however, the phenol has a pKa of 9.72 and is predominantly un-ionized at physiologic pH.

Metabolism

After oral administration, ezetimibe is rapidly and extensively metabolized in the intestinal wall and the liver to its active metabolite, a corresponding phenol glucuronide (Fig. 19.9). This glucuronide is excreted in the bile back to its active site. A small amount (<5%) of ezetimibe undergoes oxidation to convert the benzylic hydroxyl group to a ketone; however, ezetimibe does not appear to exert any significant effect on the activity of CYP450 enzymes.[32,48,51]

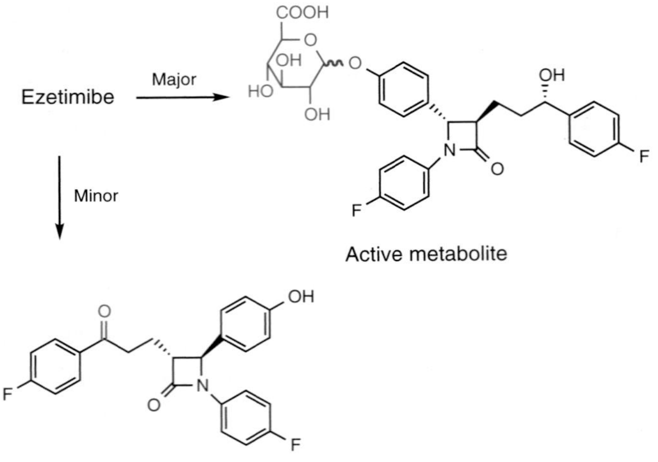

Figure 19.9 Metabolism of ezetimibe to its active and inactive metabolites.

Pharmacokinetic Properties

Ezetimibe is administered orally; however, its absolute bioavailability cannot be determined because of its aqueous insolubility and the lack of an injectable formulation. Based on its area under the curve values, the oral absorption ranges from 35%-60%. Mean peak concentrations of the active glucuronidated metabolite are reached within 1-2 hours. Both ezetimibe and its glucuronide conjugate are extensively bound (>90%) to plasma proteins. The relative plasma concentrations of ezetimibe and its glucuronide conjugate range from 10% to 20% and from 80% to 90%, respectively. Both compounds have a long half-life of approximately 22 hours. The coadministration of food with ezetimibe has no effect on the extent of absorption. The normal dose of ezetimibe is 10 mg once daily. Dosage reduction for patients with renal impairment, intermittent hemodialysis, or mild hepatic impairment is not necessary. Because of insufficient data, the use of ezetimibe is not recommended in patients with moderate to severe hepatic impairment.[32,33,48]

BILE ACID SEQUESTRANTS

Cholestyramine (*Questran, Prevalite*) was originally developed in the 1960s to treat pruritus secondary to elevated plasma concentrations of bile acids in patients with cholestasis. Its ability to bind (i.e., to hold or to sequester) bile acids and to increase their fecal elimination was subsequently shown to produce beneficial effects in lowering serum cholesterol levels.

Mechanism of Action

Cholestyramine, colestipol (*Colestid*), and colesevelam (*WelChol*) lower plasma LDL levels by indirectly increasing the rate at which LDL is cleared from the bloodstream. Under normal circumstances, approximately 97% of bile acids are reabsorbed into the enterohepatic circulation. As previously discussed, bile acids are returned to the liver where they regulate their own production. Bile acid sequestrants are not orally absorbed but, rather, act locally within the gastrointestinal tract to interrupt this process. They bind the two major bile acids, glycocholic acid and taurocholic acid, and greatly increase their fecal excretion. As a result, decreased concentrations of these compounds are returned to the liver. This removes the feedback inhibition of 7α-hydroxylase and increases the hepatic conversion of cholesterol to bile acids (Fig. 19.3). The decrease in hepatic cholesterol concentrations causes an increased expression of LDL receptors and an increased hepatic uptake of plasma LDL similar to that previously described for HMGRIs and ezetimibe. Compensatory responses also lead to the induction of HMG-CoA reductase and increased biosynthesis of cholesterol; however, similar to ezetimibe, these effects are insufficient to counteract the decrease in plasma LDL. The combination use of a bile acid sequestrant with an HMGRI will counter this compensatory response and provide and additive effect in lowering LDL cholesterol.[21,32,54,55]

The decreased return of bile acids to the liver also will produce an increase in triglyceride synthesis and a transient rise in VLDL levels; however, the increased expression of LDL receptors will eventually return VLDL levels to predrug levels. One exception to this is seen in patients with preexisting hypertriglyceridemia. For these patients, the increase in LDL receptors is inadequate to counter the rise in VLDL levels.[21]

Common Adverse Effects

Because bile acid sequestrants are not orally absorbed, they produce minimal systemic side effects and, thus, are one of the safest drugs to use for hypercholesterolemia. Constipation is by far the most frequent patient complaint. Increasing dietary fiber or using bulk-producing laxatives, such as psyllium, often can minimize this adverse effect. Other gastrointestinal symptoms include bloating, heartburn, nausea, eructation, and abdominal discomfort. These adverse effects usually dissipate with continued use; however, the possibility of fecal impaction requires that extreme caution be used in patients with preexisting constipation.[29,32]

Common Drug Interactions

Because of their mechanism of action, bile acid sequestrants can potentially bind with and decrease the oral absorption of almost any other drug. Because these drugs contain numerous positive charges, they are much more likely to bind to acidic compounds than to basic compounds or nonelectrolytes. This is not an absolute, however, because cholestyramine and colestipol have been reported to decrease the oral absorption of propranolol (a base) and the lipid-soluble vitamins A, D, E, and K (nonelectrolytes). As a result, the current recommendation is that all other oral medication should be administered at least 1 hour before or 4 hours after cholestyramine and colestipol. Colesevelam seems to be less likely to interfere with the absorption of concurrently administered drugs; however, drugs that have not been studied in combination with colesevelam should be spaced similar to cholestyramine and colestipol.[21,32]

Receptor Binding and SAR

Cholestyramine, colestipol, and colesevelam (Fig. 19.10) do not bind to specific receptors but rather to negatively charged atoms or functional groups present on drug molecules or biomolecules. Since they can selectively bind and exchange negatively charged atoms and molecules, they are chemically classified as anion-exchange resins. The selectivity comes from the fact that these positively charged resins do not bind equally to all anions. For example, the chloride ion of cholestyramine can be displaced by, or exchanged with, other anions (e.g., bile acids) that have a greater affinity for the positively charged functional groups on the resin.

All three of these drugs are large polycationic polymers. Cholestyramine is a copolymer consisting primarily of polystyrene, divinylbenzene, and approximately 4 mEq of fixed quaternary ammonium groups per gram of dry resin. Colestipol is a copolymer of tetraethylenepentamine and epichlorohydrin and is commercially marked as its hydrochloride salt. The key functional groups on colestipol are the basic secondary and tertiary amines.

Colesevelam is a more diverse polymer containing four different basic and/or quaternary fragments; however, similar to colestipol, epichlorohydrin acts to cross link these fragments. The key structural feature of all three of these polymers is the presence of multiple basic or quaternary functional groups that can bind to negatively charged atoms or functional groups.[19,32]

Physiocochemical Properties

All bile acid sequestrants are large, hygroscopic, water-insoluble resins. The molecular weight of cholestyramine is reported to be greater than 1,000,000 daltons; however, no specific molecular weight has

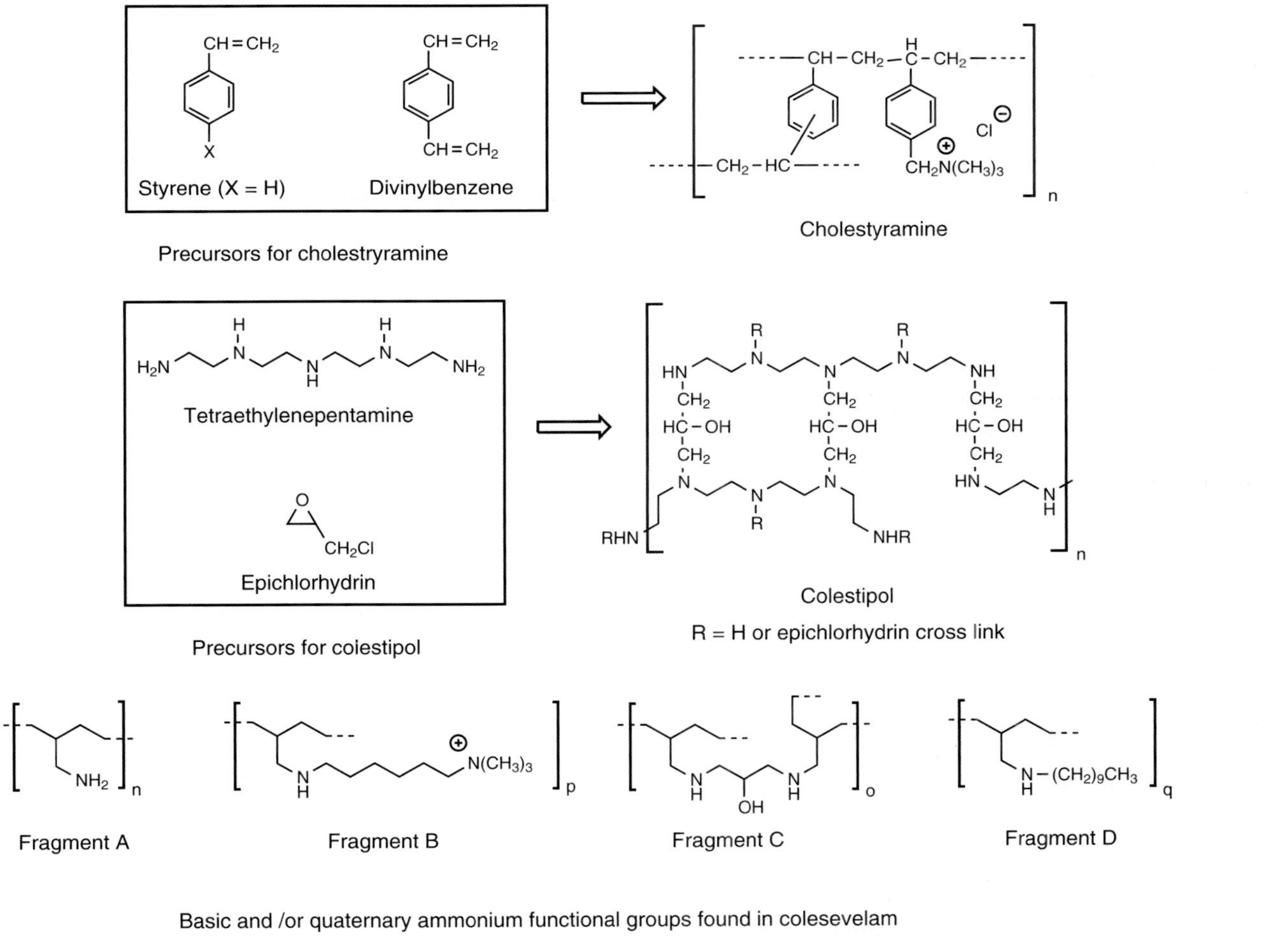

Styrene (X = H) Divinylbenzene

Precursors for cholestryramine

Cholestyramine

Tetraethylenepentamine

Epichlorhydrin

Precursors for colestipol

Colestipol

R = H or epichlorhydrin cross link

Fragment A Fragment B Fragment C Fragment D

Basic and /or quaternary ammonium functional groups found in colesevelam

Figure 19.10 Structures of cholestyramine, colestipol, and precursors for these polymeric resins. Also included are the basic and quaternary functional groups found on colesevelam. Note that cholestyramine will contain a fraction of unsubstituted aromatic rings (i.e., those that are neither cross-linked nor contain a quaternary ammonium group).

been assigned to either colestipol or colesevelam. Cholestyramine contains a large number of quaternary ammonium groups and has multiple permanent positive charges. Colestipol contains a large number of secondary and tertiary amines, whereas colesevelam contains quaternary ammonium groups as well as primary and secondary amines. Normal pKa values for the amines range from 9.0 to 10.5; thus, all of these groups should be primarily ionized at intestinal pH.

Metabolism and Pharmacokinetic Properties

Cholestyramine, colestipol, and colesevelam are not orally absorbed and are not metabolized by gastrointestinal enzymes. They are excreted in the feces as an insoluble complex with bile acids. Their onset of action occurs within 24-48 hours; however, it may take up to 1 month to achieve peak response.[21,32,48] Cholestyramine is available as a powder that is mixed with water, juice, or other noncarbonated beverages to create a slurry to drink. Colestipol is available as either granules or 1-g tablets. The granules should be taken in a manner similar to that described for the cholestyramine powder. Colesevelam is available as a 625-mg tablet and a 3.75-g powder for suspension. Both formulations should be taken with a meal.

Proprotein Convertase Subtilisin/Kexin Type 9 Inhibitors

The hepatic enzyme, proprotein convertase subtilisin/kexin type 9 (PCSK9), is involved in cholesterol homeostasis. The binding of this enzyme to LDL receptors leads to their degradation and an overall increase in plasma LDL levels. Alirocumab (*Pradulent*) and evolocumab (*Repatha*) are human monoclonal IgG antibodies that bind to PCSK9 and inhibits its action. Both drugs have been approved for treatment of hypercholesterolemia in individuals with severe forms of hereditary high cholesterol who cannot tolerate or who do not exhibit sufficient LDL lowering by HGMRIs.

Mechanism of Action

The normal function of circulating PCSK9 is to bind to LDL receptors located on the surface or hepatocytes. Internalization of the resulting complex leads to LDL receptor destruction and the inability of the liver to remove LDL from the plasma. This in turn increases plasma LDL cholesterol. While this regulatory function is crucial for maintaining normal plasma LDL levels in healthy patients, it can contribute to hypercholesterolemia in other patients. Both alirocumab and evolocumab inhibit the binding of PCSK9 to LDL receptors, thus increasing the number of functional LDL receptors available to clear plasma LDL and lower LDL cholesterol.[29,56-58]

Common Adverse Effects and Drug Interactions

Both drugs are well tolerated but can cause injection-site reactions, muscle aches, rash, and itching. Flu-like symptoms, nasopharyngitis, allergic skin reactions, and cognitive effects (i.e., confusion, dementia, and memory impairment) may also occur. To date, there are no reported drug interactions with either alirocumab or evolocumab.

Receptor Binding and SAR

Similar to other antibodies, alirocumab and evolocumab are composed of two heavy chains linked through disulfide bonds to two light chains. The two heavy chains are also linked together through a disulfide bond. The fragment antigen binding (Fab) regions on both of these drugs have complementary binding areas that allow the antibodies to bind to a specific site on PCSK9 and thus prevent it from binding to LDL receptors.

Physicochemical and Pharmacokinetic Properties

Both alirocumab and evolocumab are human monoclonal antibodies, a specialized type of proteins. The molecular weights of these drugs are approximately 146 and 144 kDa, respectively. Neither of these drugs are orally active and must be administered subcutaneously (SC). They require approximately 3-7 days to achieve peak serum concentrations.

Due to their peptidic nature, metabolism occurs via degradation to smaller peptides and amino acids.

Nicotinic Acid (Niacin)

The history of nicotinic acid (niacin) began in 1867, when it was first synthesized by oxidation of nicotine. The name niacin was derived later from the words ***ni**cotinic **ac**id* and *vitam**in*** in an effort to avoid confusing nicotinic acid and nicotinamide with nicotine. Although the terms "niacin" and "nicotinic acid" are used interchangeably, only the more chemically descriptive term, "nicotinic acid," will be used in the following discussions.

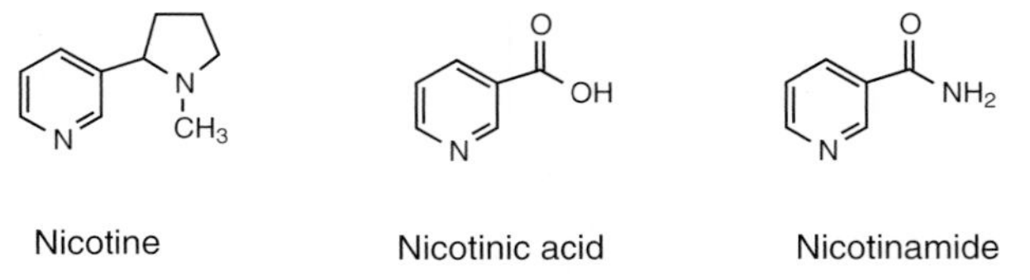

Nicotine   Nicotinic acid   Nicotinamide

Nicotinic acid is a vitamin that is an essential structural component of nicotinamide adenine dinucleotide (NAD^+) and nicotinamide adenine dinucleotide phosphate ($NADH^+$), two cofactors involved in electron transport and intermediary metabolism.[59] In 1955, Altschul et al. observed that high doses of nicotinic acid lowered cholesterol levels in humans, an activity unrelated to its properties as a vitamin.[60]

Mechanism of Action

Nicotinic acid exerts a variety of effects on lipoprotein metabolism.[21,54,61] One of its most important actions is the inhibition of lipolysis in adipose tissue. Impaired lipolysis decreases the mobilization of free fatty acids, thus reducing their plasma levels and their delivery to the liver.

In turn, this decreases hepatic triglyceride synthesis and results in a decreased production of VLDL. Enhanced clearance of VLDL through stimulation of lipoprotein lipase also has been proposed to contribute to the reduction of plasma VLDL levels. Because LDL is derived from VLDL (Fig. 19.5), the decreased production of VLDL ultimately leads to a decrease in LDL levels. The sequential nature of this process has been clinically demonstrated. The reduction in triglyceride levels occurs within several hours after initiation of nicotinic acid therapy, whereas the reduction in cholesterol does not occur until after several days of therapy. Nicotinic acid also increases HDL levels due to a reduction in the clearance of apoA-I, an essential component of HDL. Nicotinic acid does not have any effects on cholesterol catabolism or biosynthesis.

Common Adverse Effects and Drug Interactions

The most common (and, often, dose-limiting) side effects of nicotinic acid are cutaneous vasodilation (flushing and pruritus) and gastrointestinal intolerance, which may occur in 20%-50% of treated patients. Flushing and pruritus are prostaglandin-mediated effects and may be prevented by taking aspirin or indomethacin prior to nicotinic acid. Gastrointestinal side effects, such as flatulence, nausea, vomiting, and diarrhea, can be minimized if nicotinic acid is taken either with or immediately after meals. All of these effects can be minimized by slowly titrating the dose of nicotinic acid. Hepatic dysfunction is one of the more serious complications of high-dose nicotinic acid. Plasma AST, ALT, lactate dehydrogenase, and alkaline phosphatase levels often are elevated but usually return to normal when therapy is either adjusted or discontinued.[8,32,33]

Drug interactions for nicotinic acid are listed in Table 19.9.

Table 19.9 Drug Interactions for Nicotinic Acid

Drug	Result of Interaction
Adrenergic blocking agents	Enhanced vasodilation and postural hypotension
Bile acid sequestrants	Decreased bioavailability of nicotinic acid if administration is not adequately spaced
Ethanol	Potential enhanced hepatotoxicity and excessive peripheral or cutaneous vasodilation
HMG-CoA reductase inhibitors	Increased risk of myopathy and rhabdomyolysis
Vasodilating agents (calcium channel blockers, epoprostenol, nitrates)	Enhanced cutaneous vasodilation

Receptor Binding and SAR

The actions of nicotinic acid on lipolysis have been suggested to be due its ability to bind to a G protein–coupled receptor. The carboxylic acid is essential in providing either an ionic bond or an ion-dipole bond. Conversion of the carboxylic acid to an amide, as seen with nicotinamide, results in an inactive compound. The pyridine ring can interact with the receptor through hydrogen bond formation (as the acceptor), van der Waals interactions, and charge-transfer interactions. Structural changes to nicotinic acid result in loss of activity.[62,63]

Physicochemical Properties

Nicotinic acid (niacin) is a stable, nonhygroscopic, white, crystalline powder. Its carboxylic acid has a pKa of 4.76 and, thus, is predominantly ionized at physiologic pH. The pyridine nitrogen is a very weak base (pKa = 2.0) and, therefore, primarily exists in the un-ionized form. Nicotinic acid is freely soluble in alkaline solutions and has a measured log P of −0.20 at pH 6.0.[64]

Metabolism

Nicotinic acid is a B-complex vitamin that is converted to nicotinamide, NAD^+, and $NADP^+$. The latter two biomolecules are coenzymes and are required for oxidation/reduction reactions in a variety of biochemical pathways. Additionally, nicotinic acid is metabolized to a number of inactive compounds, including nicotinuric acid and N-methylated derivatives. Normal biochemical regulation and feedback prevent large doses of nicotinic acid from producing excess quantities of NAD^+ and $NADP^+$. Thus, small doses of nicotinic acid, such as those used for dietary supplementation, will be primarily excreted as metabolites, whereas large doses, such as those used for the treatment of hyperlipoproteinemia, will be primarily excreted unchanged by the kidney.[32]

Pharmacokinetic Properties

Nicotinic acid is readily absorbed. Peripheral vasodilation is seen within 20 minutes, and peak plasma concentrations occur within 45 minutes. The half-life of the compound is approximately 1 hour, thus necessitating frequent dosing or an extended-release formulation. Extended-release tablets produce peripheral vasodilation within 1 hour, reach peak plasma concentrations within 4-5 hours, and have a duration of 8-10 hours.

Dosing of nicotinic acid should be titrated to minimize adverse effects. An initial dose of 50-100 mg three times a day often is used with immediate-release tablets. The dose then is gradually increased by 50-100 mg every 3-14 days, up to a maximum of 6 g/d, as tolerated. Therapeutic monitoring to assess efficacy and prevent toxicity is essential until a stable and effective dose is reached. Similar dosing escalations are available for extended-release products, with doses normally starting at 500 mg once daily at bedtime.[21,32,33]

FIBRATES

The use of this class of drugs to treat hyperlipoproteinemias can be traced back to 1962 and thus predates the use of most of the other drugs in this chapter. The name of this class of drugs is an acronym for ethyl *p*-chloro**ph**enoxy**i**so**b**uty**rate**, the chemical name of clofibrate (Fig. 19.11). Clofibrate was approved for therapeutic use in 1967 and was initially a widely prescribed drug. Results from a 1978 World Health Organization trial changed the acceptance of clofibrate and dramatically decreased its use. These trials indicated that despite a 9% lowering of cholesterol, patients taking clofibrate showed no reduction of cardiovascular events and actually had an increase in overall mortality.[21] Although clofibrate is no longer available in the United States, it has served as the prototype for the design of safer and more effective fibrates. Structural modifications, focused primarily on ring substitutions and the addition of spacer groups, have produced a number of active drugs (Fig. 19.11). Gemfibrozil and fenofibrate are currently available in the United States; ciprofibrate and bezafibrate are used in other countries.

Mechanism of Action

Overall, fibrates decrease plasma triglyceride levels much more dramatically than they decrease plasma cholesterol levels. They significantly decrease VLDL levels, cause a moderate increase in HDL levels, and have variable effects on LDL concentrations. As an example of this latter point, gemfibrozil will raise LDL levels in patients with hypertriglyceridemia but lower LDL levels in patients with normal triglyceride levels. The exact mechanisms for these actions have not been fully elucidated; however, studies have shown that this class of compounds can produce a variety of beneficial effects on lipoprotein metabolism. It has been proposed that these effects are mediated through the activation of peroxisome proliferator-activated receptors (PPARs) and an alteration of gene expression. Specifically, fibrates bind to PPARα.[21,32,65]

Decreases in plasma VLDL levels primarily result from the ability of these drugs to stimulate the activity of lipoprotein lipase, the enzyme responsible for removing triglycerides from plasma VLDL (Fig. 19.5). Additionally, fibrates can lower VLDL levels through PPARα-mediated stimulation of fatty acid oxidation, inhibition of triglyceride synthesis, and reduced expression of apoC-III. This latter effect enhances the action of lipoprotein lipase because apoC-III normally serves as an inhibitor of this enzyme. Favorable effects on HDL levels appear to be related to increased transcription of apoA-I and apoA-II as well as a decreased activity of cholesteryl ester transfer protein.

All fibrates accelerate the turnover and removal of cholesterol from the liver. This increases the biliary secretion of cholesterol, enhances its fecal excretion, and may cause cholelithiasis (i.e., gallstone formation).

Common Adverse Effects and Drug Interactions

The most prevalent or significant side effects caused by the fibrates are highlighted in the box entitled Adverse

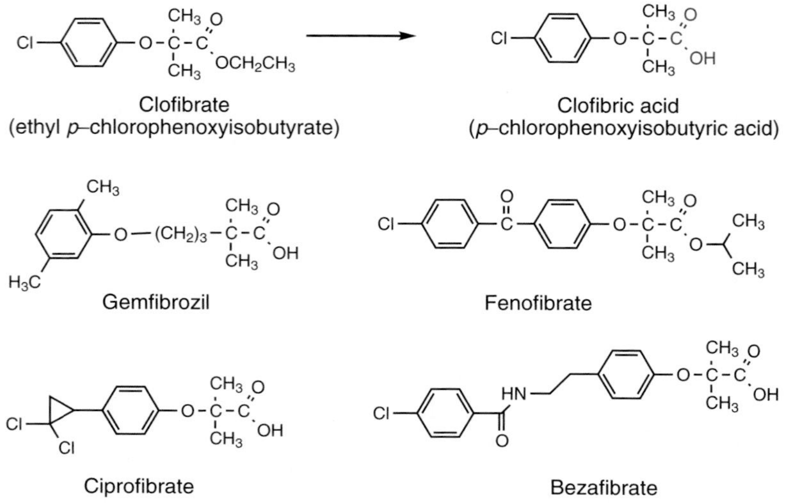

Clofibrate
(ethyl *p*-chlorophenoxyisobutyrate)

Clofibric acid
(*p*-chlorophenoxyisobutyric acid)

Gemfibrozil

Fenofibrate

Ciprofibrate

Bezafibrate

Figure 19.11 Bioactivation of clofibrate and chemical structures of other fibrates.

Effects of Fibrates.[21,32,33] Overall, fibrates are usually well tolerated. Gastrointestinal complaints are the most common but do not usually cause discontinuation of therapy. In general, gemfibrozil and fenofibrate appear to be less problematic than the original compound, clofibrate. In fact, many of the concerns regarding fibrate therapy are based on the effects of clofibrate and the results of a 1978 clinical trial in which patients taking clofibrate had a significantly higher morbidity and mortality from causes other than CHD. These causes included malignancy, gallbladder disease, pancreatitis, and postcholecystectomy complications. Studies with gemfibrozil and fenofibrate have not shown similar increases; however, because all fibrates have similar pharmacologic actions, cautions and contraindications generally are applied to the entire drug class. Similar to HMGRIs, fibrates can cause myopathy, myositis, and rhabdomyolysis. Although rare, the risk of these serious effects increases when these two classes of agents are used together. Fibrates also cause increases in plasma aspartate transaminase (AST), alanine transaminase (ALT), and creatine phosphokinase levels.

Drug interactions for fibrates are listed in Table 19.10.

ADVERSE EFFECTS OF FIBRATES

Abdominal pain, dyspepsia, nausea, vomiting, diarrhea, constipation, cholestasis, jaundice, cholelithiasis, pancreatitis, headache, dizziness, drowsiness, blurred vision, mental depression, impotence, decreased libido, myopathy, myositis, rhabdomyolysis, anemia, leukopenia, eosinophilia, pruritus, and rash

Receptor Binding and SAR

All fibrates are analogues of phenoxyisobutyric acid. A structure of this pharmacophore as well as a summary of the SAR for this class of drugs is shown in Figure 19.12. Fibrates bind to PPARα via an ion-dipole bond with a tyrosine residue. Fenofibrate, which contains an ester, is a prodrug and requires in vivo hydrolysis in order to be active. The isobutyric acid group is essential for activity; however, PPARα has some flexibility and will accommodate a spacer up to three carbon atoms between the isobutyric acid and the phenoxy ring, as seen with gemfibrozil. This spacer enhances lipid solubility and allows gemfibrozil to be absorbed through the gastrointestinal membrane without the need of an ester prodrug. Substitution at the para position of the aromatic ring with a chloro group or a chlorine-containing cyclopropyl ring produces compounds with significantly longer half-lives.

Physicochemical Properties

As noted above, a carboxylic acid is a required structural feature for fibrate binding and activity. The pKa of this functional group on clofibric acid is reported to be 3.5, and thus, it will be primarily ionized at physiologic pH.[49] The pKa and ionization values of gemfibrozil, fenofibric acid, and other fibrates can reasonably be assumed to be similar. Fenofibrate is a neutral, ester prodrug and can be classified as nonelectrolyte, while gemfibrozil can be classified as an acidic drug. The calculated log P values for fenofibrate and gemfibrozil are shown in Table 19.11.[64] Both drugs are highly lipid soluble even though gemfibrozil contains a water-soluble carboxylic acid. This can be partially explained by examining the π

Table 19.10 Drug Interactions for Fibrates

Drug	Fibrate	Result of Interaction
Antidiabetic agents	All	Increased hypoglycemic effect through increased sensitivity and decreased glucagon secretion
Bexarotene	Gemfibrozil	Increased bexarotene plasma concentrations
Bile acid sequestrants	All	Decreased bioavailability of fibrate if administration is not adequately spaced
Cyclosporine	Fenofibrate	Increased potential for nephrotoxicity
Ezetimibe	All	Increased ezetimibe concentration and possible increased risk of cholelithiasis; concomitant use is not recommended
HMG-CoA reductase inhibitors	All	Increased risk of severe myopathy or rhabdomyolysis
Oral anticoagulants	All	Increased hypoprothrombinemic effect
Repaglinide	Gemfibrozil	Increased repaglinide plasma concentrations
Ursodiol	All	Increased hepatic cholesterol secretion, which may increase the possibility of gallstone formation and counteract the effectiveness of ursodiol

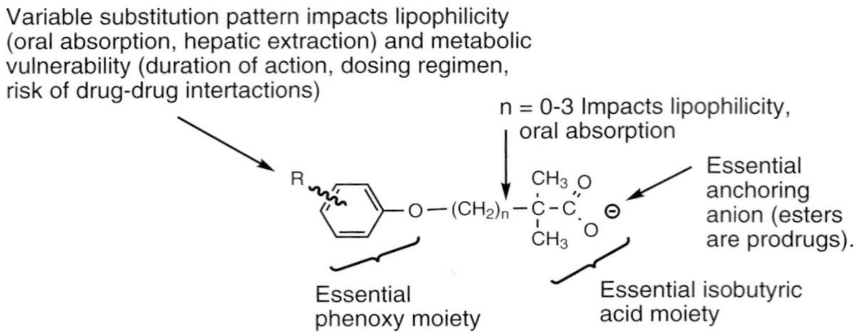

Figure 19.12 Fibrate pharmacophore and summary of SAR.

values for the substituents on fenofibrate and gemfibrozil.[66] The 2,5-dimethyl ring in gemfibrozil is predicted to be much more hydrophobic than the 4-chloro ring of fenofibrate. Additionally, the propyl bridge seen in gemfibrozil, but not in fenofibrate, significantly adds to its hydrophobicity. The isopropyl ester as well as the additional aromatic ring account for the enhanced lipid solubility of fenofibrate. All currently available fibrates are achiral molecules and not subject to stereochemical concerns.

Metabolism

The metabolic pathways of gemfibrozil and fenofibrate are shown in Figure 19.13. Oxidation of the aromatic methyl groups of gemfibrozil by CYP3A4, alcohol dehydrogenase, and aldehyde dehydrogenase produces inactive hydroxymethyl and carboxylic acid analogues. These functional groups can be further metabolized by conjugation with glucuronic acid. Fenofibrate is a prodrug that undergoes rapid hydrolysis to produce fenofibric acid. This active metabolite can then be conjugated with glucuronic acid, similar to gemfibrozil. The *para*-chloro group of fenofibric acid deactivates the ring from aromatic oxidation. Both drugs are primarily excreted as glucuronide conjugates in the urine. While oxidation of gemfibrozil requires the CYP3A4 isozyme, it can be conjugated and eliminated either with or without oxidation. As such, drug interactions with gemfibrozil and other drugs affecting the CYP3A4 system are less important here than with other drug classes.

Pharmacokinetic Properties

The pharmacokinetic properties for fenofibrate and gemfibrozil are summarized in Table 19.11.[21,32,33,48,65] The prodrug, fenofibrate, requires a longer time to reach peak concentrations compared with gemfibrozil. Because of differences in aromatic substitution, fenofibrate also has a much longer half-life than gemfibrozil. The 2,5-dimethyl substitution in gemfibrozil is much more susceptible to oxidative metabolism than the *para*-chloro group present in fenofibrate. Changes in lipid levels are not seen immediately, and up to 2 months may be required to reach maximal clinical effects and to determine the overall clinical efficacy. Fenofibrate and gemfibrozil have excellent bioavailability and are extensively bound to plasma proteins. Because food can significantly enhance their oral absorption, these drugs should be taken either with or just before meals. Renal elimination is the primary route through which these drugs are excreted from the body. Patients with mild renal dysfunction often can be managed with minor dosage adjustments, whereas those with severe impairment or renal failure may have to discontinue its use.

POTENTIAL DRUG TARGETS: ACAT AND CEPT

Inhibitors of ACAT have been investigated as cholesterol-lowering or antiatherosclerotic agents. In addition to its role in foam cell formation, ACAT also is required for esterification of cholesterol in intestinal mucosal cells and for synthesis of cholesterol esters in hepatic VLDL formation. Thus, ACAT inhibitors have the potential of providing three beneficial effects in patients with hypercholesterolemia: decreased cholesterol absorption, decreased hepatic VLDL synthesis, and decreased foam cell formation. To date, the development of ACAT inhibitors has been hampered by toxicity profiles and the inability to provide effective cholesterol reduction in human patients. Interestingly, the most effective compound in these studies turned out to be an azetidinone derivative that blocked cholesterol absorption through binding to the sterol transporter, NPC1L1 instead of ACAT. Further structural modification of this lead compound produced ezetimibe.[67,68]

Cholesterol ester transfer protein (CETP) interacts with HDL, LDL, and VLDL to mediate the transfer of cholesterol esters from HDL (primarily HDL_2) to LDL and VLDL while balancing this exchange in a 1:1 fashion with a transfer of triglycerides from LDL and VLDL to HDL. The end result of this process is a higher concentration of LDL cholesterol and a lower concentration of HDL cholesterol. It has been postulated that CETP inhibitors would produce a therapeutic benefit due to their ability to prevent these transfers and favorably increase HDL cholesterol and lower LDL cholesterol. The initial development of potent CETP inhibitors proved to be challenging due to the nonenzymatic nature of a transport protein, the lack of a transition state and/or tightly bound intermediates, and the lack of potent natural and synthetic inhibitors. A number of chemical classes of compounds have been investigated over the years; however, despite some success in clinical trials, no drug has yet been approved. In a recent development, Merck decided not to pursue an FDA filing for anacetrapib, its most promising CETP inhibitor. The company decided that while anacetrapib met its primary clinical objective, the compound provided only a small improvement, was unable to show superiority in secondary endpoints, and still possessed safety concerns. The future of this drug target is currently in question.[68-70]

Anacetrapib

Orphan Drugs for the Treatment of Homozygous Familial Hypercholesterolemia

Homozygous familial hypercholesterolemia (HoFH) results from genetic mutations of the LDL receptor in both parents. Patients with HoFH can develop severed hypercholesterolemia within the first two decades of life and can develop accelerated atherosclerosis and coronary heart disease. The overall prevalence of HoFH is one case in a million individuals. In comparison, the overall prevalence of heterozygous familial hypercholesterolemia (HeFH) is one case in 500 individuals.[71]

Lomitapide and mipomersen have been approved for the treatment of this rare genetic disorder. According to current therapeutic guidelines, these drugs are indicated for patients with HoHF who have a baseline LDL-C ≥190 mg/dL and who have had an inadequate response to statins with or without ezetimibe and PCSK9 inhibitors. Both drugs are currently available only through a Risk Evaluation and Mitigation Strategy (REMS) program.[8,29]

Lomitapide

Mechanism of Action

Lomitapide exerts its mechanism of action by inhibiting the microsomal triglyceride transport protein (MTTP) located in the lumen of the endoplasmic reticulum. This prevents the assembly of apoB-containing lipoproteins (i.e., VLDL and LDL) in both hepatocytes and enterocytes. The overall result of these actions is an initial decrease in the synthesis of chylomicrons and VLDL and an ultimate reduction in plasma LDL cholesterol.[32,72]

Lomitapide (Juxtapid)

Common Adverse Effects and Drug Interactions

The most commonly seen adverse effects of lomitapide involve the gastrointestinal tract and include abdominal discomfort, abdominal distension, abdominal pain, constipation, diarrhea, flatulence, gastroenteritis, gastroesophageal reflux disorder (GERD), nausea, and vomiting. The most serious adverse effect is an increased risk of hepatotoxicity.

Lomitapide normally undergoes oxidative metabolism by CYP3A4. Inhibitors of this isozyme will increase the plasma concentrations of lomitapide. Because of this, concurrent use of lomitapide with strong or moderate inhibitors of CYP3A4 is contraindicated. A 50% dosage reduction is required if lomitapide is used in combination with a weak CYP3A4 inhibitor. Patients taking this drug should also avoid grapefruit juice.[32,72]

Table 19.11 Pharmacokinetic Parameters of Fibrates

Drug	Calculated log P	Oral Bioavailability (%)	Active Metabolite	Protein Binding (%)	Time to Peak Concentration (hr)	Elimination Half-Life (hr)	Major Route(s) of Elimination
Fenofibrate	5.24	60-90	Fenofibric acid	99	4-8	20-22	Renal (60%-90%) Fecal (5%-25%)
Gemfibrozil	3.9	>90	None	99	1-2	1.5	Renal (70%) Fecal (6%)

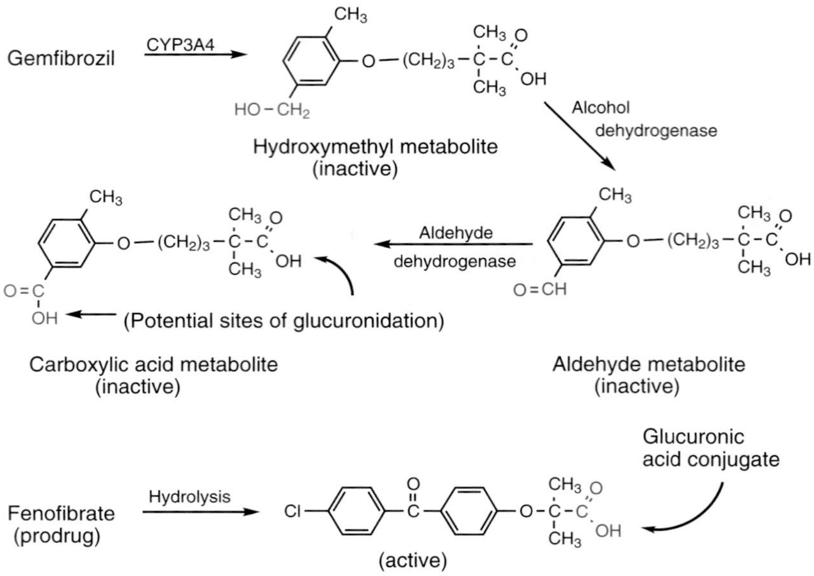

Figure 19.13 Metabolic pathways for gemfibrozil and fenofibrate.

Physicochemical Properties

The structure of lomitapide contains a basic tertiary amine that will be primarily ionized at all physiological environments. Overall, lomitapide is highly lipid soluble and over 99% is bound to plasma proteins.

Metabolism and Pharmacokinetic Properties

Due to its high lipid solubility, lomitapide is extensively metabolized in the liver via a variety of oxidations followed by glucuronide conjugation. The primary metabolic route is N-dealkylation of the piperidine ring. This essentially breaks the molecule in half and renders the drug inactive. Lomitapide is administered orally; however, it has a very low bioavailability (~7%). This is due to its high lipid solubility. While it can easily pass through lipid-soluble membranes, it has a lower ability to initially dissolve in the GI tract.[32,72]

Mipomersen

Mechanism of Action

Mipomersen is a stable oligonucleotide that contains a modified DNA sequence that is complementary to the coding region of the mRNA for apoB-100. This complementary, or antisense, nature allows it to bind to the mRNA and create a 20-nucleotide hybrid DNA/mRNA sequence. This results in RNase-H-mediated degradation of the mRNA and an inhibition of the production of the apoB-100 protein required for the synthesis of both LDL and VLDL.[32,73]

Common Adverse Effects and Drug Interactions

Injection site reactions, including erythema, pain, hematoma, pruritus, swelling, discoloration, and rash are the most common adverse effects seen with mipomersen. Approximately 85% of patients will experience one or more of these reactions. Other common adverse effects include elevations in serum ALT levels, flu-like symptoms, headache, and nausea. The most serious adverse effect is an increased risk of hepatotoxicity. To date, no clinically relevant drug interactions have been reported; however, caution should be exercised when using mipomersen in combination with other medications known to have potential for hepatotoxicity.[32,73]

Receptor Binding and SAR

The 20 nucleotides present within the structure of mipomersen form hydrogen bonds consistent with Watson-Crick pairing with a specific, complementary sequence in the mRNA for apoB-100. The isosteric replacement of phosphate oxygen atoms with sulfur atoms increases the chemical stability of the oligonucleotide, while the 2′-O-(2-methoxyethyl) groups present on the terminal five nucleotides at the 5′ and 3′ ends inhibit nuclease action. These two chemical alterations enhance the duration of action.[73]

Metabolism and Physicochemical and Pharmacokinetic Properties

The phosphorothioate groups that link the nucleotides are acidic in nature and allow for the formation of sodium salts. Mipomersen is administered once weekly as a SC injection. The estimated bioavailability ranges from 54% to 78% and the elimination half-life is 1-2 months. It is greater than 90% plasma protein bound. Metabolism of mipomersen involves endonuclease activity to produce shorter oligonucleotides that are further metabolized by exonucleases. Additionally, mipomersen is eliminated renally.[32,73]

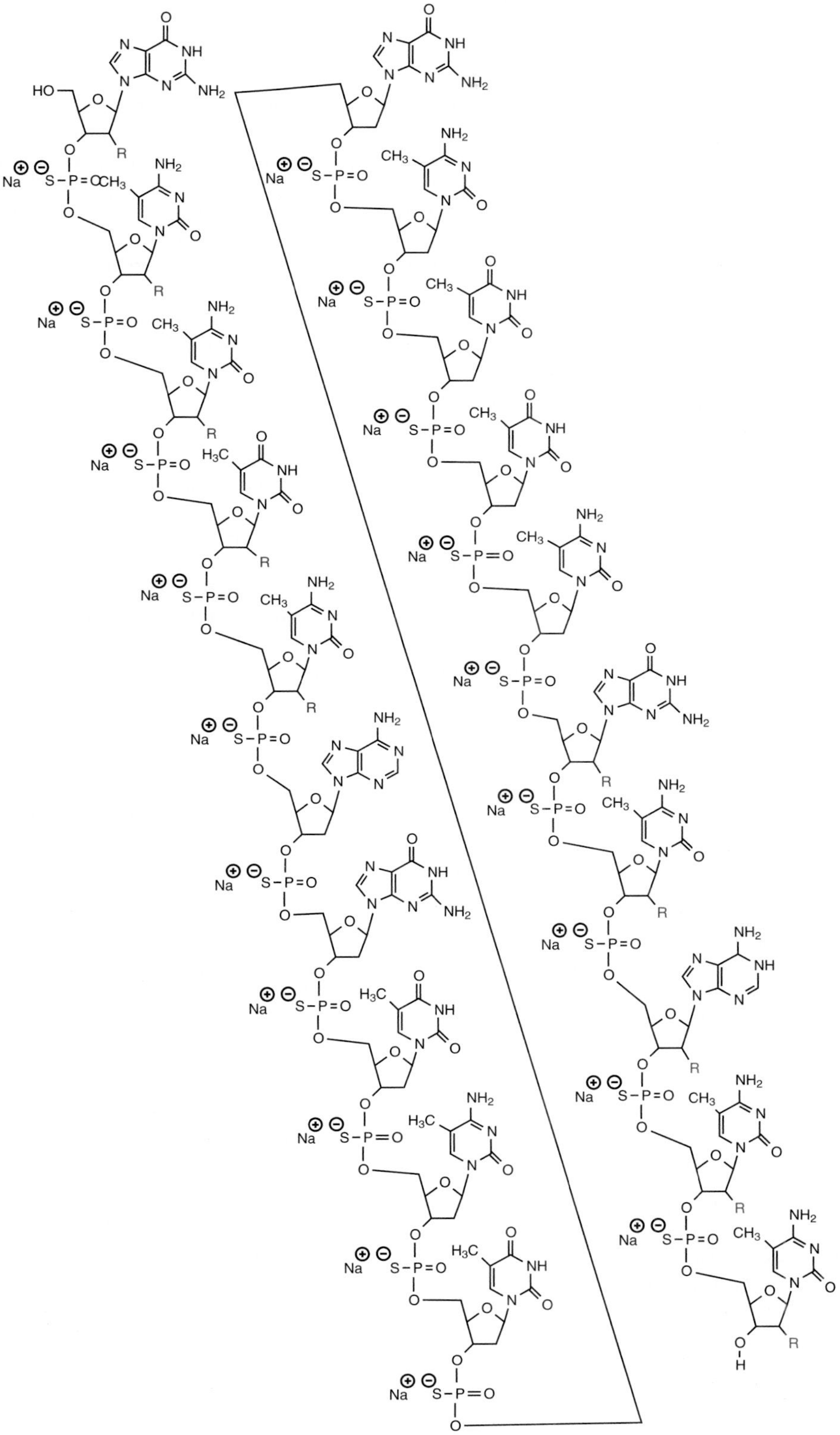

Mipomersen sodium

R = [wavy bond]–O–CH₂CH₂–O–CH₃

Clinical Scenario

Michael W. Perry, PharmD, BCPS, BCCCP

SCENARIO

BT is a 41-year-old Caucasian male who has a history of uncontrolled hypertension (current blood pressure 150/85 mm Hg), dyslipidemia, and active smoking (5 packs per year history). His physician had started him on appropriate diet and lifestyle modifications, but they were unsuccessful in controlling his dyslipidemia. He was then started on simvastatin 20 mg by mouth daily, which did provide a slight 10% lowering of his LDL-C. The dose of simvastatin was increased to 40 mg by mouth daily to achieve a greater LDL-C lowering effect. After 6 weeks of treatment, his most recent lab values indicated his LDL-C is back to baseline. The patient reports that he began to have muscle pain and weakness shortly after the dose of simvastatin was increased. The patient stopped taking the simvastatin and the muscular adverse effects went away. BT's current medications are:

Aspirin 81 mg by mouth daily; lisinopril 20 mg by mouth daily; simvastatin 40 mg by mouth daily (not taking); nicotine patch 14 mg topically daily. The physician wants to continue the patient on statin therapy for the cardiovascular benefits, but wants to avoid the muscular adverse effects. What recommendations can be made to help achieve the optimal clinical outcomes in this patient and avoid adverse drug effects?

OUTCOME

The physician has a few options to maintain this patient on statin therapy and minimize the risk, statin-related adverse effects. If the patient is agreeable, the patient can be rechallenged with simvastatin to ensure that it was the cause of the myopathies. If it is determined that the simvastatin is no longer an option, the patient may be initiated on a less lipophilic agent such as pravastatin or rosuvastatin. These agents may be less likely to diffuse into extrahepatic tissues and therefore less likely to cause myopathies. If the patient does not tolerate daily dosing of statin therapy, alternate day dosing may be attempted with atorvastatin or rosuvastatin, which have longer half-lives. It would also be appropriate to place the patient on a lower but tolerable dose of statin, and add on a nonstatin agent such as ezetimide or a PCSK9 inhibitor. The overall goal is to provide the patient with a medication regimen that is safe and effective at lowering the patient's cholesterol levels and preventing cardiovascular disease.

Chemical Analysis found immediately after References.

REFERENCES

1. Stamler J, Vaccaro O, Neaton JD, et al. Diabetes, other risk factors, and 12-yr cardiovascular mortality for men screened in the multiple risk factor intervention trial. *Diabetes Care*. 1993;16:434-444.
2. Chen Z, Peto R, Collins R, et al. Serum cholesterol concentration and coronary heart disease in population with low cholesterol concentrations. *BMJ*. 1991;303:276-282.
3. Prospective Studies Collaboration. Blood cholesterol and vascular mortality by age, sex, and blood pressure: a meta-analysis of individual data from 61 prospective studies with 55,000 vascular deaths. *Lancet*. 2007;370:1829-1839.
4. Centers for Disease Control and Prevention. National Center for Health Statistics. Multiple Cause of Death 1999-2016 on *CDC WONDER* Online Database, Released December, 2017. Data are From the Multiple Cause of Death Files, 1999-2016, as Compiled From Data Provided by the 57 Vital Statistics Jurisdictions Through the Vital Statistics Cooperative Program. Available at http://wonder.cdc.gov/mcd-icd10.html on 31 January 2018.
5. *Global Health Estimates 2015: Deaths by Cause, Age, Sex, by Country and by Region, 2000-2015*. Geneva: World Health Organization; 2016. Available at http://www.who.int/healthinfo/global_burden_disease/estimates/en/index1.html.
6. Jacobson TA, Ito MK, Maki KC, et al. National lipid association recommendations for patient-centered management of dyslipidemia: Part 1—full report. *J Clin Lipidol*. 2015;9(2):129-169.
7. Catapano AL, Reiner Z, De Backer G, et al. European society of cardiology. European atherosclerosis society ESC/EAS guidelines for the management of dyslipidaemias the task force for the management of dyslipidaemias of the European society of cardiology (ESC) and the European atherosclerosis society (EAS). *Atherosclerosis*. 2011;217(1):3-46.
8. Lloyd-Jones DM, Morris PB, Ballantyne CM et al. 2017 focused update of the 2016 ACC expert consensus decision pathway on the role of non-statin therapies for LDL-cholesterol lowering in the management of atherosclerotic cardiovascular disease risk. *J Am Coll Cardiol*. 2017;70(14):1785-1822.
9. Zhang H, Plutzky J, Skentzos S, et al. Discontinuation of statins in routine care settings: a cohort study. *Ann Intern Med*. 2013;158:526-534.
10. Bitzur R, Cohen H, Kamari Y, et al. Intolerance to statins: mechanisms and management. *Diabetes Care*. 2013;36(2):S325-S330.
11. Pirillo A, Catapano AL. Statin intolerance: diagnosis and remedies. *Curr Cardiol Rep*. 2015;17(5):17-27.
12. Neuvonen PJ, Niemi M, Backman JT. Drug interactions with lipid-lowering drugs: mechanisms and clinical relevance. *Clin Pharmacol Ther*. 2006;80:565-581.
13. Orringer CE, Jacobson TA, Saseen JJ, et al. National lipid association updated recommendations on the use of pcsk9 inhibitors. *J Clin Lipidol*. 2017;11:880-890.
14. Ginsberg HN, Goldberg IJ. Disorders of lipoprotein metabolism. In: Fauci AS, Braunwald E, Isselbacher KJ, et al, eds. *Harrison's Principles of Internal Medicine*. 14th ed. New York: McGraw-Hill; 1998:2138-2149.
15. Stone NH, Robinson J, Lichtenstein AH, et al. *ACC/AHA Guideline on the Treatment of Blood Cholesterol to Reduce Atherosclerotic Cardiovascular Risk in Adults*; 2013. Available at https://doi.org/10.1161/01.cir.0000437738.63853.7a. Accessed November 2017.
16. Berg JM, Tymoczko JL, Stryer L. *Biochemistry*. 5th ed. New York: Freeman & Company; 2002:715-743.
17. Nelson DL, Cox MM. *Lehninger Principles of Biochemistry*. 7th ed. New York: W.H. Freeman; 2017:811-858.

18. Kourounakis AP, Charitos C, Rekka EA, et al. Lipid-lowering (hetero)aromatic tetrahydro-1,4-oxazine derivatives with antioxidant and squalene synthase inhibitory activity. *J Med Chem.* 2008;51:5861-5865.
19. Chan C, Andreotti D, Cox B, et al. The squalestatins: decarboxy and 4-deoxy analogues as potent squalene synthase inhibitors. *J Med Chem.* 1996;39:207-216.
20. Miki T, Kori M, Mabuchi H, et al. Synthesis of novel 4,1-benzoxazepine derivatives as squalene synthase inhibitors and their inhibition of cholesterol synthesis. *J Med Chem.* 2002;45:4571-4580.
21. Bersot TP. Drug therapy for hypercholesterolemia and dyslipidemia. In: Brunton L, Chabner B, Knollman B, eds. *Goodman & Gilman's the Pharmacological Basis of Therapeutics.* 12th ed. New York: McGraw-Hill; 2011:877-908.
22. Talbert RL. Hyperlipidemia. In: Dipiro JT, Talbert RL, Yee GC, et al, eds. *Pharmacotherapy: A Pathophysiologic Approach.* 9th ed. New York: McGraw-Hill; 2014:291-317.
23. Fredrickson DS, Levy RI, Lees RS. Fat transport in lipoproteins—an integrated approach to mechanisms and disorders. *N Engl J Med.* 1967;276:34-42.
24. Libby P. Atherosclerosis. In: Fauci AS, Braunwald E, Isselbacher KJ, et al, eds. *Harrison's Principles of Internal Medicine.* 14th ed. New York: McGraw Hill; 1998:1345-1352.
25. Sliskovic DR, White AD. Therapeutic potential of ACAT inhibitors as lipid lowering and antiatherosclerotic agents. *Trends Pharmacol Sci.* 1991;12:194-199.
26. Benjamin EJ, Blaha MJ, Chiuve SE, et al. *Heart Disease and Stroke Statistics—2017 Update; a Report From the American Heart Association.* Available at http://circ.ahajournals.org/content/136/10/e196. Accessed November 2017.
27. Ford ES, Will JC, Mercado CI, et al. Trends in predicted risk for atherosclerotic cardiovascular disease using the pooled cohort risk equations among US adults from 1999 to 2012. *JAMA Intern Med.* 2015;175:299-302.
28. Thom T, Kannel WB, Silbershatz H, D'Agostino RB. Cardiovascular diseases in the United States and prevention approaches. In: Fuster V, Alexander R, Schlant R, O'Rourke R, Roberts R, Sonnenblick E, eds. *Hurst's the Heart.* 10th ed. New York, NY: McGraw-Hill; 2001:3-7.
29. Lipid-lowering drugs. *Med Lett.* 2016;58:133-140.
30. Heathcock CH, Hadley CR, Rosen T, et al. Total synthesis and biological evaluation of structural analogues of compactin and dihydromevinolin. *J Med Chem.* 1987;30:1858-1873.
31. Cutler SJ, Cocolas GH. Cardiovascular agents. In: Block JH, Beale JM, eds. *Wilson and Gisvold's Textbook of Organic Medicinal and Pharmaceutical Chemistry.* 11th ed. Philadelphia, PA: Lippincott Williams & Wilkins; 2004:657-663.
32. *Clinical Pharmacology Online. Gold Standard Elsevier*; 2017. Available at http://clinicalpharmacology.com. Accessed November 2017.
33. *Facts & Comparisons eAnswers.* St. Louis, MO: Wolters Kluwer Health. Available at http://www.wolterskluwercdi.com/facts-comparisons-online. Accessed November 2017.
34. Atorvastatin—a new lipid-lowering drug. *Med Lett Drugs Ther.* 1997;39:29-31.
35. Rosuvastatin—a new lipid-lowering drug. *Med Lett Drugs Ther.* 2003;45:81-83.
36. Adams JL, Metcalf BW. *Therapeutic consequences of the inhibition of sterol metabolism.* In: Hansch C, Sammes PG, Taylor JB, eds. *Comprehensive Medicinal Chemistry.* Vol. 2. Oxford, UK: Permagon Press; 1990:333-363.
37. Stokker GE, Hoffman WF, Alberts AW, et al. 3-Hydroxy-3-methylglutaryl–coenzyme A reductase inhibitors. 1. Structural modification of 5-substituted 3,5-dihydroxypentanoic acids and their lactone derivatives. *J Med Chem.* 1985;28:347-358.
38. Sliskovic DR, Blankley CJ, Krause BR, et al. Inhibitors of cholesterol biosynthesis. 6. *trans*-5-[2-(-N-heteroaryl-3,5-disubstituted-pyrazol-4-yl)ethyl/ethenyl]tetrahydro-4-hydroxy-2H- pyran-2-ones. *J Med Chem.* 1992;35:2095-2103.
39. Bone EA, Davidson AH, Lewis CN, et al. Synthesis and biological evaluation of dihydroeptastatin, a novel inhibitor of 3-hydroxy-3-methylglutaryl–coenzyme A reductase. *J Med Chem.* 1992;35:3388-3393.
40. Roth BD, Ortwine DF, Hoefle ML, et al. Inhibitors of cholesterol biosynthesis. 1. *trans*-6-(2- pyrrol-1-ylethyl)-4-hydroxypyran-2-ones, a novel series of HMG-CoA reductase inhibitors. 1. Effects of structural modifications at the 2-and 5-positions of the pyrrole nucleus. *J Med Chem.* 1990;33:21-31.
41. Hoffman WF, Alberts AW, Cragoe EJ, et al. 3-Hydroxy-3-methylglutaryl–coenzyme A reductase inhibitors. 2. Structural modification of 7-(substituted aryl)-3,5-dihydroxy-6- heptenoic acids and their lactone derivatives. *J Med Chem.* 1986;29:159-169.
42. Stokker GE, Alberts AW, Anderson PS, et al. 3-Hydroxy-3-methylglutaryl-coenzyme A reductase inhibitors. 3. 7-(3,5-Disubstituted [1,1'-biphenyl]-2-yl)-3,5-dihydroxy-6-heptenoic acids and their lactone derivatives. *J Med Chem.* 1986;29:170-181.
43. Heathcock CH, Davis BR, Hadley CR. Synthesis and biological evaluation of a monocyclic, fully functional analogue of compactin. *J Med Chem.* 1989;32:197-202.
44. Lee TJ, Holtz WJ, Smith RL, et al. 3-Hydroxy-3-methylglutaryl–coenzyme A reductase inhibitors. 8. Side chain ether analogues of lovastatin. *J Med Chem.* 1991;34:2474-2477.
45. Hoffman WF, Alberts AW, Anderson PS, et al. 3-Hydroxy-3-methylglutaryl-coenzyme A reductase inhibitors. 4. Side chain ester derivatives of mevinolin. *J Med Chem.* 1986;29:849-852.
46. Stokker GE, Alberts AW, Gilfillan JL, et al. 3-Hydroxy-3-methylglutaryl–coenzyme A reductase inhibitors. 5. 6-(Fluoren-9-yl)- and 6-(fluoren-9-ylidenyl)-3,5-dihydroxyhexanoic acids and their lactone derivatives. *J Med Chem.* 1986;29:852-855.
47. Procopiou PA, Draper CD, Hutson JL, et al. Inhibitors of cholesterol biosynthesis. 2. 3,5- dihydroxy-7-(N-pyrrolyl)-6-heptenoates, a novel series of HMG-CoA reductase inhibitors. *J Med Chem.* 1993;36:3658-3662.
48. Micromedex Solutions. Truven Health Analytics. Available at http://truvenhealth.com/products/micromedex/navitem/footermicromedex. Accessed January 2018.
49. Craig PN. Drug compendium. In: Hansch C, Sammes PG, Taylor JB, eds. *Comprehensive Medicinal Chemistry.* Vol. 6. Oxford, UK: Permagon Press; 1990:237-991.
50. Zocor (Simvastatin) Product Literature. *Merck.* 1999-2015. Available at https://www.merck.com/product/usa/pi_circulars/z/zocor/zocor_pi.pdf.
51. Kosoglou T, Statkevich P, Johnson-Levonas AO, et al. Ezetimibe: a review of its metabolism, pharmacokinetics, and drug interactions. *Clin Pharmacokinet.* 2005;44:467-494.
52. Clader JW, Burnett DA, Caplen MA, et al. 2-Azetidinone cholesterol absorption inhibitor: structure-activity relationship on the heterocyclic nucleus. *J Med Chem.* 1996;39:3684-3693.
53. Rosenblum SB, Huynh T, Afonso A, et al. Discovery of l-(4-fluorophenyl)-(3P)-[3-(4- fluorophenyl)-(35)-hydroxypropyl]-(45)-(4-hydroxyphenyl)-2-azetidinone (SCH 58235): a designed, potent, orally active inhibitor of cholesterol absorption. *J Med Chem.* 1998;41:973-980.
54. Cendella RJ. *Cholesterol and hypocholesterolemic drugs.* In: Craig CR, Stitzel RE, eds. *Modern Pharmacology With Clinical Applications.* 5th ed. Boston: Little, Brown & Co; 1997:279-289.
55. Brown MS, Goldstein JL. A receptor-mediated pathway for cholesterol homeostasis. *Science.* 1986;232:34-47.
56. Praluent (Alirocumab) Prescribing Information. *Regeneron Pharmaceuticals, Inc.*; 2017. Available at http://products.sanofi.us/praluent/praluent.pdf.
57. Repatha (Evolocumab) Prescribing Information. *Amgen Inc.*; 2017. Available at https://pi.amgen.com/~/media/amgen/repositorysites/pi-amgen-com/repatha/repatha_pi_hcp_english.pdf.
58. Kuhnast S, van der Hoorn JWA, Pieterman EJ, et al. Alirocumab inhibits atherosclerosis, improves the plaque morphology, and enhances the effects of a statin. *J Lipid Res.* 2014;55:2103-2112.

59. Nelson DL, Cox MM. *Lehninger Principles of Biochemistry*. 7th ed. New York: W.H. Freeman; 2017:522-525.
60. Altschul R, Hoffer A, Stephen JD. Influence of nicotinic acid on serum cholesterol in man. *Arch Biochem*. 1955;54:558-559.
61. Drood JM, Zimetbaum PJ, Frishman WH. Nicotinic acid for the treatment of hyperlipoproteinemia. *J Clin Pharmacol*. 1991;31:641-650.
62. Zhang Y, Schmidt RJ, Foxworthy P, et al. Niacin mediates lipolysis in adipose tissue through its G-protein coupled receptor HM74A. *Biochem Biophys Res Com*. 2005;334:729-732.
63. DiPalma J, Thayer WS. Use of niacin as a drug. *Annu Rev Nutr*. 1991;11:169-187.
64. 2010. *Obtained from Advanced Chemistry Development, Inc*. Available at http://www.acdlabs.com.
65. Hussar DA. New drugs of 1998. *J Am Pharm Assoc*. 1999;39:170-172.
66. Hansch C, Leo A. *Substituent Constants for Correlation Analysis in Chemistry and Biology*. New York: Wiley; 1979:49-54.
67. Roth B. ACAT inhibitors: evolution from cholesterol-absorption inhibitors to antiatherosclerotic agents. *Drug Discov Today*. 1998;3:19-25.
68. Edmondson SE, Weber AE, Elliot J. *Cardiovascular and metabolic diseases: 50 years of progress*. In: Desai MC, ed. *2015 Medicinal Chemistry Reviews*. Vol. 50. Washington, DC: American Chemical Society; 2015:83-116.
69. Sikorski JA. Oral cholesteryl ester transfer protein (CETP) inhibitors: a potential new approach for treating coronary artery disease. *J Med Chem*. 2006;49:1-22.
70. Cannon CP, Shah S, Dansky HM, et al. Safety of anacetrapib in patients with or at high risk for coronary heart disease. *N Engl J Med*. 2010;363:2406-2415.
71. Raul FJ, Santos RD. Homozygous familial hypercholesterolemia: current perspectives on diagnosis and treatment. *Atherosclerosis*. 2012;223:262-268.
72. Juxtapib (Lomitapide) Prescribing Information. *Aegerion Pharmaceuticals*; 2016. Available at http://www.juxtapidpro.com/prescribing-information.
73. Kynamro (Mipomersen) Prescribing Information. *Genzyme Corporation*; 2016. Available at http://www.kynamro.com/media/pdfs/Kynamro_Prescribing_information.pdf.

Clinical Scenario

Michael W. Perry, PharmD, BCPS, BCCCP

CHEMICAL ANALYSIS

In evaluating the structures of simvastatin and pravastatin, it is seen that there are three structural differences. First, simvastatin has a lactone ring that must be hydrolyzed in vivo, while pravastatin has a 3,5-dihydroxypentanoic acid chain. Second, the decalin ring system of simvastatin contains two methyl groups, while the decalin ring system of pravastatin contains one methyl group and one hydroxyl group. Finally, the ester side chain of simvastatin contains an extra methyl group, as compared to the hydrogen atom of pravastatin. In each of these comparisons, it is found that pravastatin contains a functional group that is more water soluble than the functional group in simvastatin. These differences account for the fact that simvastatin (log P = 4.42) is much more lipid soluble than pravastatin (log P = 1.44) and therefore less likely to diffuse into extrahepatic tissues and cause myopathies.

Difference 1 Difference 3 Difference 2

Simvastatin

Difference 1 Difference 2

Pravastatin

Atorvastatin and rosuvastatin have longer durations of action than other HMGRIs. For atorvastatin, its prolonged duration of action can be attributed to the fact that its *ortho*-hydroxyl and *para*-hydroxyl metabolites are equiactive as atorvastatin, and for rosuvastatin, its prolonged duration of action can be attributed to its decreased lipophilicity and minimal metabolism. Both of these drugs have the ability to provide a more extensive lowering of plasma LDL due in part to their ability to form key hydrogen bonds within the active site of HMGR using their amide (atorvastatin) and sulfonamide (rosuvastatin) groups. In comparing these two drugs, the structure of atorvastatin (log P = 4.13) contains two additional aromatic rings. Additionally, the pyrimidine ring present within the structure of rosuvastain (log P = 0.42) is more basic than the pyrrole ring of atorvastatin. Similar to the above comparison, these differences account for the differences in lipophilicity and potential to cause myopathy among these two drugs.

Atorvastatin

* = site of hydroxylated metabolites

Rosuvastatin

SECTION 4

Drugs Impacting Hormonal Systems

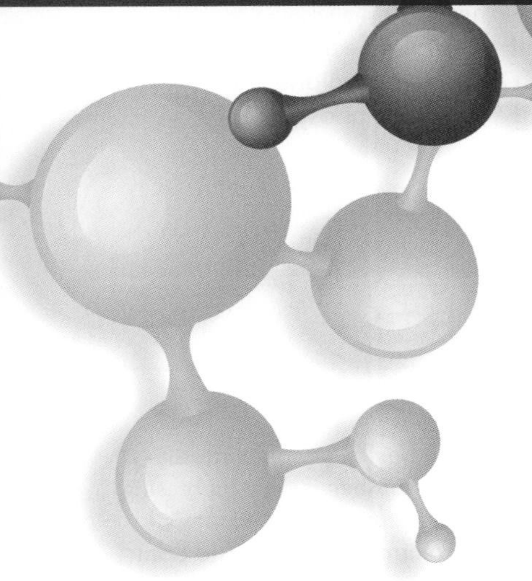

CHAPTER 20

Drugs Used to Treat Diabetic Disorders

S. William Zito

Drugs covered in this chapter:

INSULINS
- Aspart
- Degludec
- Determir
- Glargine
- Concentrated glargine
- Glulisine
- Human insulin
  - Regular insulin U100/U500
  - NPH
  - Inhaled
- Lispro
- Ultralente

SULFONYLUREAS
- Acetohexamide
- Chlorpropamide
- Glimepiride
- Glipizide
- Glyburide (also known as glibenclamide)
- Tolazamide
- Tolbutamide

MEGLITINIDES
- Nateglinide
- Repaglinide

BIGUANIDES
- Metformin

THIAZOLIDINEDIONES
- Pioglitazone
- Rosiglitazone
- Troglitazone

α–GLUCOSIDASE INHIBITORS
- Acarbose
- Miglitol
- Voglibose

GLP-1 AGONISTS
- Albiglutide
- Dulaglutide
- Exenatide
- Liraglutide
- Lixisenatide
- Semaglutide

DIPEPTIDYL PEPTIDASE IV INHIBITORS
- Alogliptin
- Linagliptin
- Saxagliptin
- Sitagliptin
- Vildagliptin

AMYLIN AGONISTS
- Pramlintide

SODIUM GLUCOSE COTRANSPORTER-2 INHIBITORS
- Canagliflozin
- Dapagliflozin
- Empagliflozin
- Ertugliflozin

DOPAMINE AGONIST
- Bromocriptine

BILE ACID SEQUESTRANT
- Colesevelam

Abbreviations

ADA American Diabetes Association
ADP adenosine diphosphate
AGE advanced glycation end product
Arg arginine
Asp aspartate
ATP adenosine triphosphate
DAG diacylglycerol
DPP-IV dipeptidyl peptidase-IV
FDA U.S. Food and Drug Administration
FFA free fatty acid
FPG fasting plasma glucose
GAPDH glyceraldehyde-3-phosphate dehydrogenase
GIP glucose-dependent insulinotropic polypeptide
GLP-1 glucagon-like peptide-1
Glu glutamate
GLUT facilitative glucose transporter
Gly glycine
HbA1c hemoglobin A1c

Abbreviations—Continued

HLA human leukocyte antigen
IRS insulin receptor substrate
IU international unit of enzyme activity
Lys lysine
NPH neutral protamine Hagedorn
OGTT oral glucose tolerance test
PARP poly(ADP-ribose) polymerase
PKC phosphokinase C
PPAR peroxisome proliferator-activated receptor
PTP protein tyrosine phosphatase
Ser serine
SGLT sodium-glucose cotransporters
SUR sulfonylurea receptor
Thr threonine
TNF-α tumor necrosis factor-α
TZD thiazolidinedione
UPD uridine diphosphate

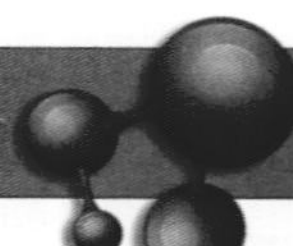

CLINICAL SIGNIFICANCE

Emily Ambizas, PharmD

Diabetes is a common metabolic disorder that has become a global public health concern. The number of people with diabetes has quadrupled since the 1980s, now affecting more than 400 million people worldwide. This number is only increasing with rising levels of obesity and sedentary lifestyles. If left untreated, diabetes can lead to blindness, neuropathies, kidney disease, cardiovascular disease, and stroke. Most people with diabetes have type 2, with only approximately 10% of the population diagnosed with type 1. Type 1 diabetes is a result of pancreatic B cell destruction leading to absolute insulin deficiency, while type 2 diabetes is associated with insufficient insulin production and/or increased insulin resistance.

Over the years, many pharmacological agents have been developed to help manage the diabetic patient, targeting the many different pathophysiologic defects in diabetes. Understanding the structure-activity relationships and physicochemical and biopharmaceutical properties of these various agents has led to the development of more effective and safer medications. By modifying the insulin molecule and adjusting the solubility, we now have insulins with different durations of action allowing for the easier control of blood glucose levels with less incidences of hypoglycemia.

Secretagogues, such as sulfonylureas and meglitinides, increase the production of pancreatic insulin. The first sulfonylurea was introduced in 1956, and since then structural changes have led to the development of second and third generation agents, as well the meglitinides. These changes allowed for enhanced potency, longer duration of action, and a better adverse effect profile. Similarly, in 1918, guanidine was found to lower blood glucose in animals but was considered too toxic for human use, causing GI effects, shortness of breath, and increased muscle contractility.

With the addition of another guanidine structure the biguanides were discovered. With a few structural differences, metformin proved to be better tolerated with a more favorable adverse effect profile when compared to the other biguanides such as phenformin.

In 2005, the first new class of diabetic agents were introduced, the incretin mimetics. The intestinal hormone glucagon-like peptide-1 (GLP-1) was known to play a role in glucose regulation but has a very short half-life in the plasma, making it unsuitable as a drug. With a few chemical modifications, agents have been developed that are more resistant to degradation by the dipeptidyl peptidase-4 (DPP-4) enzyme.

More recently, the sodium-dependent glucose cotransporter 2 (SGLT2) located in the proximal portion of the renal tubule has shown to be a promising new target for the management of diabetes. Ninety percent of glucose reabsorption occurs at this site. The naturally occurring compound phlorizin, which is found in plants, is an SGLT inhibitor. It has been known to induce glucosuria but cannot be used as a pharmacologic agent due to various drawbacks. With modifications to the structure-activity relationship, our newest agents to the market were discovered, SGLT2 inhibitors, with improved SGLT2 selectivity and enhanced stability allowing for oral administration.

Despite the plethora of agents available for the management of diabetes, there is still a need for medications with improved efficacies and adverse effect profiles. A clear understanding of the structure-activity relationship and structural modifications will help in achieving this goal.

DIABETES MELLITUS: HISTORICAL PERSPECTIVES

Diabetes mellitus is a metabolic disorder characterized by hyperglycemia where the patient experiences polyuria (frequent urination), polydipsia (extreme thirst), and polyphagia (constant hunger). Physicians have been documenting the signs and symptoms of diabetes for thousands of years. The first description of the symptoms of diabetes is attributed to Hesy-Ra, an Egyptian physician in 1552 BC, in the Ebers Papyrus. Chinese, Greek, and Arab physicians have also described a disease that is characterized by frequent urination and caused emaciation. Aretaeus of Cappadocia in the second century AD provided the first accurate description and coined the term diabetes, which means "siphon" or to "run through" in Greek. Galen, also in the second century, described the disease as "diarrhea urinosa" and "dipsakos" (disease of thirst). The term "mellitus" (Latin for honey or sweet) was added to the disease name in the 17th century by Thomas Willis to describe the sweet taste of the urine and to distinguish it from a similar polyuric disease, diabetes insipidus, where the urine was tasteless (insipid). Glucose was identified in the urine of diabetics in 1776 by Mathew Dobson, and glycogen, a polysaccharide in the liver, was identified in 1875 by Claude Bernard.

The role of the pancreas in diabetes was discovered by the experiments of Oskar Minkowski who, in 1889, noted that when the pancreas was removed from a dog, the animal developed all the signs and symptoms of diabetes.[1-4] Small clusters of ductless cells on the pancreas were identified in 1869 by Paul Langerhans, and in 1902 the work of Eugene Opie clearly linked these ductless cells, which by then were called the islets of Langerhans, to diabetes. Although a hypothetical secretion of the islet cells was postulated and called insulin (from insula, or island), it took the work of Frederick Banting, Charles Best, and John Macloud to isolate insulin and use it as a diabetes medication. In 1923, Banting and Macloud shared the Nobel Prize in medicine, and Banting subsequently shared his prize with Best.[5] Insulin was identified as a protein by Frederick Sanger and Hans Tuppy, who defined its amino acid sequence in 1951.[6,7] The total synthesis of active insulin was accomplished by Katsoyannis et al. in 1963.[8] Small, nonprotein molecules for the treatment of diabetes were developed from the discovery by Janbon et al. in 1942 that sulfonamide 3-(*p*-aminobenzenesulfonamide)-5-isopropylthiadiazole) (IPTD) induced hypoglycemia.[9]

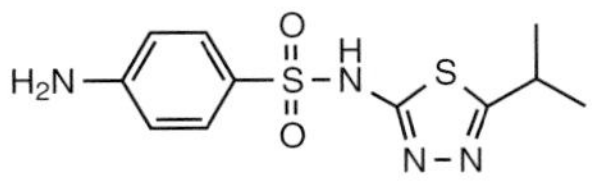

IPTD

Types of Diabetes

Diabetes can be classified into four major types; type 1 diabetes, type 2 diabetes, gestational diabetes, and specific types of diabetes, including maturity-onset diabetes of youth (MODY), diabetes secondary to other disease states, and drug- or chemically induced diabetes.[10,11] Type 1 diabetes was formerly called insulin-dependent diabetes mellitus (IDDM) or juvenile-onset diabetes. It occurs in 5%-10% of patients[12] and is largely recognized as an autoimmune disease, whereby the β-cells are destroyed by the body's own antibodies. Since the pancreas can no longer produce insulin, type 1 diabetics have an absolute requirement for exogenous insulin.[11]

Type 2 diabetes (non–insulin-dependent diabetes mellitus [NIDDM] or adult-onset diabetes) accounts for 90%-95% of adult cases of diabetes. Type 2 diabetes slowly progresses from a state where the patient develops insulin resistance to a state where the pancreas loses its ability to produce enough insulin to compensate for the insulin resistance of peripheral tissues. Insulin resistance is the state where tissues do not utilize insulin properly. Insulin resistance is associated with a number of physiological risk factors (hyperinsulinemia, hypertension, dyslipidemia, hypercoagulation, proinflammatory state, and abdominal obesity) and most commonly referred to as "the metabolic syndrome." Nondiabetic patients with metabolic syndrome (Table 20.1) are at high risk for the development of type 2 diabetes, which then gives that patient a 2 to 4-fold greater risk of developing coronary heart disease (CHD) and stroke.[13,14] In addition, outcomes of type 2 diabetes are strongly associated with race, ethnicity, and social determinants of health.[15,16]

Gestational diabetes is diagnosed during pregnancy. It occurs more often in obese women who have a family history of diabetes and/or are a member of a high-risk ethnic group (African American, Hispanic/Latina, Asian/Pacific Islander, and American Indian). Gestational diabetes requires treatment to control the hyperglycemia and avoid complications to the infant. Most women return to normal blood glucose levels postpartum; however, there is increased risk of developing diabetes within the next 10 years.[17]

Maturity-onset diabetes of youth (MODY) is characterized by faulty secretion of insulin, is rare (<5% of type 2), and is associated with a number of genetic defects of β-cell function. These defects are inherited and occur at six loci identified on chromosomes 20q, 7p, 12q, 13q, 17q,

Table 20.1 American Heart Association Definition of Metabolic Syndrome[13]

Central Obesity	Waist circumference race and gender specific US male: >40 inches US female: >35 inches Plus any <u>two</u> of the following:
Triglycerides	≥150 mg/dL or if under treatment for this dyslipidemia
HDL cholesterol	Males: <40 mg/dL Females: <50 mg/dL or if under treatment for this dyslipidemia
Blood pressure	≥130/85 mm Hg or if under treatment for hypertension
Fasting plasma glucose	≥100 mg/dL or previously diagnosed type 2 diabetes

HDL, high-density lipoprotein.

and 2q.[11] This form of diabetes is the result of impaired secretion of insulin, and there is no evidence that insulin action on tissue targets is decreased.

Diagnosis of Diabetes

The American Diabetes Association (ADA) has established four criteria for the diagnosis of diabetes.

1. A fasting plasma glucose (FPG) ≥126 mg/dL. Fasting is defined as no caloric intake for at least 8 hours prior to the assessment.
2. A 2 hour plasma glucose (PG) ≥200 mg/dL during an oral glucose tolerance test (OGTT). The test should be performed as described by the World Health Organization (WHO),[18] using a glucose load containing the equivalent of 75 g anhydrous glucose dissolved in water.
3. In patients with overt symptoms of hyperglycemia (polyphagia, polyuria, polydipsia, weight loss), a random plasma glucose of ≥200 mg/dL.
4. A hemoglobin A_{1c} (HbA_{1c}) of ≥6.5%.

In addition, the ADA has recognized a prediabetic state for patients who are at risk of developing diabetes. The criteria include an FPG 100-125 mg/dL, referred to as impaired fasting glucose (IFG), a 2-hour OGTT of 140-199 mg/dL, referred to as impaired glucose tolerance (IGT), and/or an A_{1c} of 5.7%-6.4%. The A_{1c} is perhaps the most accurate indicator of glucose because it reflects plasma glucose levels over the previous 2-3 months and is now accepted as the ideal standard for assessing glycemic control.[17,19]

Epidemiology

Diabetes is a global health problem. More than 400 million people worldwide have diabetes. It is predicted that by the year 2040 more than 640 million people will have diabetes.[20] In 2015, diabetes was the seventh leading cause of death in the United States. The most recent data from the American Diabetes Association (ADA) report that 30.3 million children and adults have diabetes, of which 1.25 million are diagnosed with type 1 diabetes. The number of diabetic Americans aged 65 years and older is approximately 12 million. The ADA also predicts 1.5 million new cases of diabetes (both type 1 and type 2) will be diagnosed each year. In 2015, 84.1 million Americans aged 18 years and older had prediabetes. Relatively few diabetics (~0.24%) are under the age of 20 years, with the majority having type 1 diabetes.

There are race and ethnic differences in the prevalence of diabetes in adults. Figure 20.1 shows that American Indians and Native Alaskans have the highest prevalence (15.1%) followed closely by non-Hispanic blacks (12.7%). Hispanics, which include Cubans, Mexican Americans, Central and South Americans, and Puerto Ricans, are similar in prevalence to non-Hispanic blacks (12.1%). The prevalence of diabetes in Asian Americans is 8.0% while non-Hispanic whites have a prevalence of 7.4%.

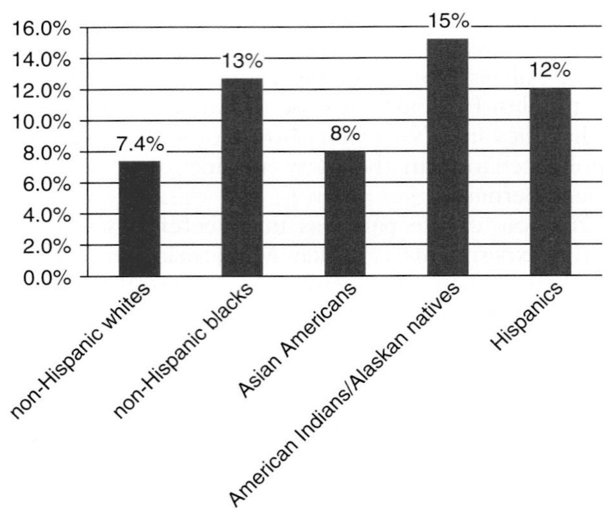

Figure 20.1 Prevalence of diabetes in US adults by race/ethnicity—2015.

The risk of death for people with diabetes is twice that for people without the disease.[17] However, diabetes is not likely to be reported as an official cause of death, since death is more likely to be attributed to one of the many complications associated with diabetes, such as heart disease, hypertension, kidney disease, and nervous system disease.

Biochemistry of Diabetes

Regulation of Glucose Homeostasis

Glucose is the primary source of cellular energy, and plasma glucose concentration is, therefore, tightly controlled between 65 and 104 mg/dL. Glucose homeostasis is maintained by a number of hormones, the most important being insulin and glucagon. Insulin is secreted by pancreatic β-cells when blood glucose concentration rises. It reduces glucose levels either by inhibiting hepatic glucose production (glycogenolysis and gluconeogenesis) or by increasing glucose uptake into the liver, muscle, and fat tissue. Glucagon is secreted by pancreatic α-cells in response to low concentrations of glucose. It acts principally on the liver and antagonizes the effects of insulin by increasing glycogenolysis and gluconeogenesis. In addition to glucagon, hydrocortisone and catecholamines also raise plasma glucose levels.

Other hormones also function in maintaining normal plasma glucose levels. These include amylin, glucagon-like peptide-1 (GLP-1), and glucose-dependent insulinotropic polypeptide (GIP). Amylin is actually cosecreted with insulin from β-cells and functions in slowing gastric emptying, which enhances glucose absorption following a meal. GLP-1 and GIP are incretins or gut-derived factors, which have a multitude of effects, primarily promoting the synthesis and secretion of insulin from β-cells.[21]

It is surprising that such an essential nutrient as glucose is not freely absorbed from the intestines or by cells that require it for energy. Instead, glucose must be transported across membranes by glucose transporters. The glucose transporters are a family of membrane-bound glycoproteins divided into two main types; sodium-glucose cotransporters (SGLT) and facilitative glucose transporters (GLUTS). The SGLT1-type is expressed in the absorptive epithelial cells of the intestines and transports glucose against its concentration gradient. SGLT1 is composed of 664 amino acids arranged into 14-transmembranes helices, and both the N- and C-terminals face the extracellular fluid. The SGLT2-type is expressed in the brush border membrane of the kidney and is the major transporter involved in the reabsorption of glucose from the glomerular filtrate. There are as many as six SGLTs found in a variety of tissues, including the liver, brain, lung, and heart.[22]

In contrast to the SGLTs, the GLUT family of transporters is sodium independent and composed of 12 membrane-spanning α-helices connected through extracellular hydrophilic loops. Their N- and C-terminals are located on the cytoplasmic side of the cell membrane. Helices 7, 8, and 11 are believed to form an aqueous pore providing a channel for substrate passage. Mammalian cells have 12 GLUT transporters (GLUTs 1-12). GLUTs 1, 3, and 4 have D-glucose specificity while GLUTs 2 and 5 have specificity for fructose. The GLUT4 transporter is by far the most abundant type, is expressed in adipose tissue and muscle (heart, smooth, and skeletal), and is responsible for insulin-stimulated transport of glucose.[23] Figure 20.2 depicts the GLUT transporter, showing the 12 trans helices and the aqueous pocket, as well as the glycosylation site.

When insulin binds to its receptor on sensitive cells, it sets off a complicated cascade of events involving both phosphatidylinositol-3-kinase (PI3K) and protein kinase Akt or protein kinase B (Akt or PKB) pathways that results in the release of GLUT 4 from storage vesicles and its translocation to the cell membrane (Fig. 20.3). The insulin receptor is a transmembrane glycoprotein composed of two α-subunits and two β-subunits linked by disulfide bonds.[24] The α-subunits contain the insulin binding site and are located extracellularly. The β-subunits contain a tyrosine kinase enzyme that is activated by insulin binding–induced autophosphorylation. When insulin binds to the receptor's two α-subunits, it enables a conformational change that allows for ATP binding to the β-subunit's intracellular domain. ATP binding initiates receptor autophosphorylation that, in turn, enables the

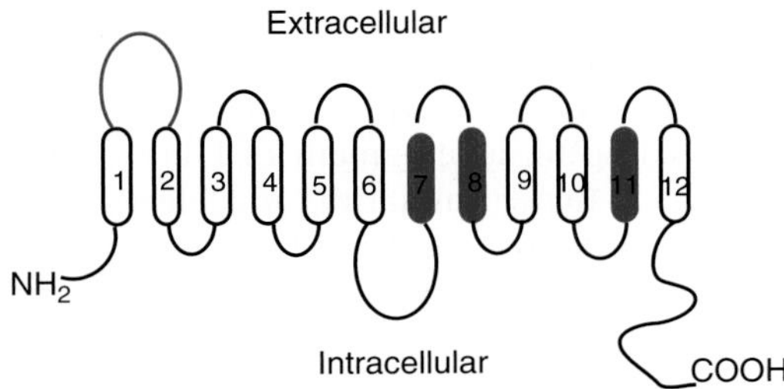

Figure 20.2 Schematic of the GLUT receptor showing the membrane-spanning α-helices (1-12). Helices 7, 8, and 11 (red) are believed to form the hydrophilic channel. The extracellular loop between helices 1 and 2 is the location of glycosylation.

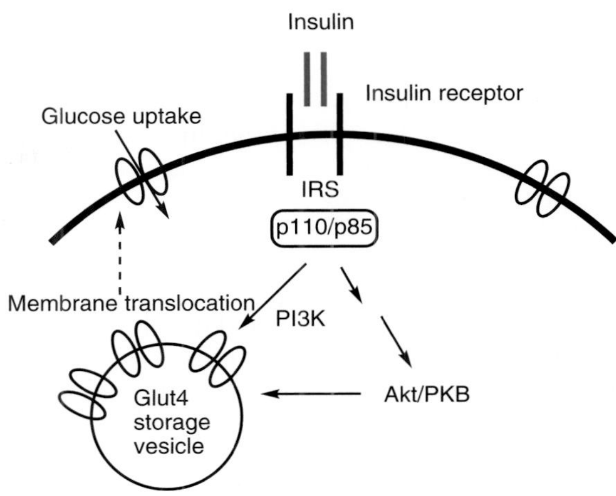

Figure 20.3 Overview of the insulin signaling pathway leading to translocation of the GLUT4 transporter from storage vesicles. *Akt*, protein kinase Akt; *IRS*, insulin receptor substrates; *PKB*, protein kinase B; *p110*, catalytic subunit of PI3K; *p85*, regulatory subunit of PI3K; *PI3K*, phosphatidylinositol-3-kinase.

receptor's tyrosine kinase to phosphorylate insulin receptor substrates (IRS). The IRS family of proteins consists of four closely related members (IRS-1 to 4) and a related homolog, Gab-1. These IRS proteins act as intracellular messengers that begin the cascade of events that result in the translocation of GLUT 4 to the cell surface, as well as other processes necessary for cell survival.[25]

Pathogenesis of Diabetes

Type I Diabetes

It is well established that type 1 diabetes results from immunological destruction of the insulin-producing β-cells of the pancreas. However, it is now understood that type 1 diabetes involves interplay between genetic susceptibility and certain external triggers such as viruses (mumps, Cosackie B4, enteroviruses), environmental toxins (nitrosamines), or foods (cow's milk proteins, cereals, gluten). Genetic susceptibility to type 1 diabetes is linked to two genes found on chromosome 6. These genes code for the production of human lymphocyte antigens (HLAs) DR3 and DR4. Most, but not all, patients with type 1 diabetes express both of these antigens. Interestingly, patients who carry the antigen-producing *HLA-DQA1*0102* or *HLA-DQB1*0602* genes are actually resistant to type 1 diabetes. HLA complex polymorphic alleles are responsible for 40%-50% of the genetic risk of type 1 diabetes development. The insulin gene (*Ins-VNTR*, *IDDM 2*) polymorphisms on chromosome 11 and the cytotoxic T lymphocyte–associated antigen-4 gene (*CTLA-4*) on chromosome 2 are responsible for 15% of the genetic predisposition. Type 1 diabetes is characterized by a long preclinical period marked by the presence of immune markers such as circulating antibodies, islet cell antibodies, and insulin autoantibodies. It is not known when the interplay between genetic susceptibility and environmental factors combine to develop the full-blown disease with the resulting absolute insulin deficiency.[26,27]

Type 2 Diabetes

The pathogenesis of type 2 diabetes is complex but typically begins with insulin resistance at target organs such as the liver, muscle, and adipose tissue. In order to compensate, there is initially an increase in insulin production. This hyperinsulinemic state is only temporary, and over time, insulin secretion diminishes due to progressive β-cell deterioration. The combined effect of insulin resistance and β-cell dysfunction results in a diminished capacity to limit hepatic glucose production and the ability to take up and utilize glucose in muscle and adipose tissue.

Insulin resistance is a complex pathological state that typifies the metabolic syndrome and is likely caused by a number of defects along the insulin signaling cascade. Other factors include increased concentrations of free-fatty acids (FFAs), tumor necrosis factor-α (TNF-α), and the hormone resistin.[28] The increase in plasma FFAs produces insulin resistance by inhibiting glucose uptake and glycolysis in skeletal muscle. It also increases hepatic gluconeogenesis. Both TNF-α and resistin are produced by adipose tissue in greater amounts in obese diabetic individuals. TNF-α impairs insulin action while resistin is known to antagonize the effects of insulin.

Increased hepatic glucose production in type 2 diabetes is attributed to both hepatic insulin resistance and increased glucagon levels. β-cells can compensate for insulin resistance by secreting more insulin. The hyperinsulinemic state is only temporary, since β-cells cannot produce the insulin levels required to maintain normal plasma glucose levels. Impaired insulin secretion and increased glucagon contribute to continued hepatic glucose output, resulting in elevated fasting blood glucose levels. When insulin resistance can no longer be overcome, transition to type 2 diabetes occurs.[29]

Hyperglycemia can be caused by a number of other mechanisms. Some patients have abnormal hormone levels including elevated glucagon, somatostatin, growth hormone, hydrocortisone, and epinephrine. Of special importance for the treatment of diabetes is the effect of certain drugs on plasma glucose levels. Table 20.2 lists some common drugs that alter plasma glucose levels.[30]

Table 20.2 Drugs That Alter Plasma Glucose Levels

Drugs That Increase Plasma Glucose	Drugs That Decrease Plasma Glucose
Acetazolamide	Alcohol (ethanol)
Birth control pills	Anabolic steroids
Atypical antipsychotics: clozapine, olanzapine, risperidone	ACE inhibitors
β-adrenergic blockers	Chloramphenicol
Caffeine	Clofibrate
Calcium channel blockers	Coumadin when coadministered with oral hypoglycemic agents
Clonidine	Gatifloxin
Diuretics: thiazides>loop>K-sparing	MAO inhibitors
Glucocorticoids	Saquinavir
Niacin	
Phenytoin	
Rifampin	
Thyroid hormones	

ACE, angiotensin-converting enzyme; MAO, monoamine oxidase.

Diabetic Complications

The hyperglycemia so characteristic of diabetes is the result of defects in insulin secretion and/or insulin action, but is also accompanied by impaired fat, carbohydrate, and protein metabolism that progressively leads to chronic microvascular, macrovascular, and neuropathic complications.[31]

All types of diabetics constantly battle to control their chronic hyperglycemia. If high levels of plasma glucose are uncontrolled or poorly controlled, it will result in the development of both acute and chronic pathologies. The short-term effects are usually those symptoms generally associated with type 1 diabetics, such as polydipsia, polyuria, polyphagia, blurred vision, urinary tract infections, weight loss, and fatigue. Although these acute effects are relatively minor, they can lead to two rather serious complications: diabetic ketoacidosis (DKA) and a hyperosmolar hyperglycemic state (HHS).

DKA can be life-threatening. Insulin blocks the action of lipases that hydrolyze stored fats to FFAs. In the diabetic with diminished or no insulin, the increased serum levels of free fatty acids are oxidized to acetone, acetoacetic acid, and β-hydroxybutyric acid, presumably to make up for lack of glucose for oxidative energy (glycolysis). These keto acids can be metabolized, but in prolonged periods of insulin deficiency, the body cannot keep up with their production and ketoacidosis occurs. Decreased insulin levels also allow unchecked glucagon activity to increase plasma glucose by gluconeogenesis and glycogenolysis. The lowering of plasma pH by keto acids, along with hyperglycemia, leads to symptoms of ketoacidosis—vomiting, dehydration, hyperventilation, confusion, and possibly coma and death.

When plasma glucose levels become higher than 600 mg/dL, increased amounts of glucose are excreted in the urine, leading to development of HHS characterized by dehydration, hyperosmolarity, and electrolyte imbalance. HHS symptoms include tachycardia, dry skin, and orthostatic hypotension which, if not treated, can lead to death in as many as 30% of those afflicted.[21]

The long-term effects of diabetes are serious and often not detected until they become overt. Both microvascular and macrovascular effects occur. The microvascular pathologies involve the retina, renal glomerulus, and peripheral nerves, and as a consequence, diabetes is a leading cause of blindness, end-stage renal disease, and painful neuropathies. The macrovascular effects involve arteries that supply the heart, brain, and lower extremities. Therefore diabetics have a much higher risk of cardiovascular disease, including atherosclerosis, myocardial infarct, stoke, and limb amputation.[32,33]

The essential question is as follows: how does diabetes result in so many diverse microvascular and macrovascular pathologies? The answer centers around four main molecular mechanisms, all related to the diabetic hyperglycemic state and all seemingly associated with the overproduction of superoxide radical anion by the mitochondrial electron transport chain. The four biochemical mechanisms are increased polyol pathway flux; increased advanced glycation end-product (AGE) formation; activation of protein kinase C (PKC) isoforms; and increased hexosamine pathway flux.[34,35]

The polyol pathway (Fig. 20.4) involves the reduction of aldehydes generated by reactive oxygen species (ROS) to inactive alcohols and glucose to sorbitol by the enzyme aldose reductase. Aldose reductase is a cytosolic oxidoreductase that utilizes NADPH. The sorbitol produced is oxidized by sorbitol dehydrogenase to fructose using NAD^+ as cofactor. When glucose levels are high, the activation of the polyol pathway can deplete reduced glutathione (GSH) leading to cellular oxidative stress. The effect of the polyol pathway flux is implicated in the formation of cataracts, as well as development of peripheral neuropathies.[36]

Increased levels of AGEs have been found in both retinal blood vessels and renal glomeruli. They arise from intracellular hyperglycemia by the autoxidation of glucose to glyoxal and the subsequent formation of 3-deoxyglucosone and the dephosphorylation of glyceraldehyde-3 phosphate and dihydroxyacetone phosphate to methylglyoxal (Fig. 20.5). These products are often referred to as dicarbonyls, and they react with amino groups of Lys and Arg and the thiol group of Cys to form AGEs. AGEs damage vascular cells and also alter several cellular functions, including gene expression in endothelial cells and macrophages.[37]

Activation of the family of protein kinase C (PKC) enzymes is brought about by the secondary messenger diacylglycerol (DAG). In hyperglycemic cells, DAG is increased by de novo synthesis involving reduction of dihydroxyacetone phosphate to glycerol-3-phosphate

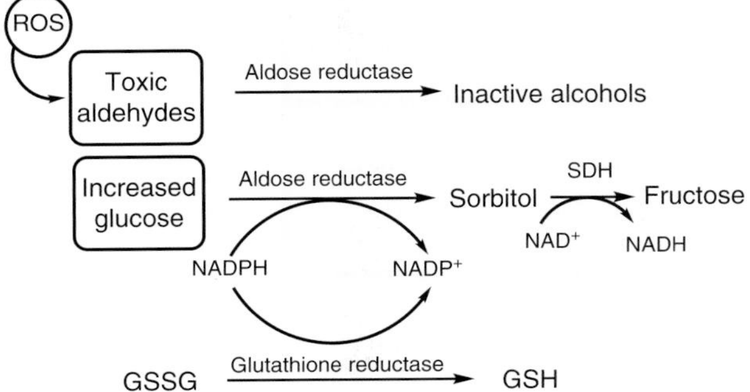

Figure 20.4 The polyol pathway showing the role of aldose reductase in reducing toxic aldehydes and glucose to sorbitol. *GSH*, reduced glutathione; *ROS*, reactive oxygen species; *SHD*, sorbitol dehydrogenase.

Figure 20.5 Formation of advanced glycation end products (AGEs) precursors, glyoxal, 3-deoxyglucosone, and methylglyoxal.

followed by stepwise acylation. PKCs may also be activated indirectly through ligation of AGE receptors and increased activity of the polyol pathway.[35] When increased in cells, PKC is involved in a significant number of biochemical pathways leading to blood flow abnormalities, vascular permeability and angiogenesis, capillary and vascular occlusion, proinflammatory gene expression, and ROS elevation (see Table. 20.3). Elevated levels of PKCs, primarily the α- and β-isoforms, have been found in the retina and renal glomeruli of diabetic animals, as well as in cultured vascular cells.[38]

When intracellular glucose levels are in excess, it gets shunted into the hexosamine pathway. In this pathway, fructose-6-phosphate is converted to glucosamine-6-phosphate and then to UDP-N-acetylglucosamine by the rate limiting enzyme glutamine:fructose-6-phosphate

Table 20.3 Pathological Consequences of Protein Kinase C Activation

Factor Effected	Pathology
↓ eNOS (endothelial nitric oxide synthase)	Blood flow abnormalities
↑ ET-1 (endothelin-1)	Blood flow abnormalities
↑ VEGF (vascular endothelial growth factor)	Vascular permeability and angiogenesis
↑ Collagen	Capillary occlusion
↑ Fibronectin	Capillary occlusion
↑ PAI-1 (plasminogen activator inhibitor-1)	↓ Fibrinolysis and vascular occlusion
↑ NF-κB (nuclear factor κ-light-chain–enhancer of activated B cells)	Proinflammatory gene expression
↑ NAD(P)H oxidases	Increased ROS and multiple effects

ROS, reactive oxygen species.

amidotransferase (GFAT). UDP-N-acetylglucosamine is added to intracellular protein Ser and Thr residues by O-linked N-acetylglucosamine transferase (OGT). Since both phosphorylation and OGT acylation compete for the same substrates, the two processes may compete for sites. The increased donation of N-acetylglucosamine to Ser and Thr residues on transcription factors leads to alterations in both gene expression and protein function that, together, contribute to the pathologies of diabetic complications.

Each of the four different pathogenic mechanisms responsible for diabetic micro/macrovascular complications is activated by a single hyperglycemic event—overproduction of superoxide by the mitochondrial electron transport chain.[35] It is now believed that the overproduction of superoxide activates the four pathogenic pathways (Fig. 20.6). Excess superoxide inhibits the glycolytic enzyme glyceraldehyde-3-phosphate dehydrogenase (GAPDH) through its effect on poly(ADP-ribose) polymerase (PARP). This inhibition causes intermediate metabolites of glycolysis to accumulate. Thus, the inhibition of the conversion of glyceraldehyde-3-phosphate to 1, 3-diphosphoglycerate results in increased amounts of dihydroxyacetone phosphate (DHAP) which, in turn, increase the formation of diacylglycerol (DAG), the intracellular activator of PKC. The increase in DAG also results in the formation of methylglyoxal, the main precursor to AGEs. Earlier in the glycolytic chain, increased levels of fructose-6-phosphate are shunted into the hexosamine pathway, producing UDP-N-acetylglucosamine which, in turn, forms O-linked glycoproteins that affect transcription. Finally, increased amounts of glucose are diverted through the polyol pathway that consumes NADPH and depletes GSH. It was originally thought that superoxide itself directly inhibited GAPDH; however, further investigations revealed that GAPDH is actually inhibited by poly(ADP-ribose) polymerase (PARP). PARP is a DNA repair enzyme found in the nucleus. PARP is activated in response to DNA single strand breaks caused by superoxide radicals. Once activated, PARP splits NAD^+ into nicotinic acid and ADP-ribose. PARP then makes polymers of ADP-ribose, which accumulate on GAPDH, inhibiting its activity.[34,39]

Therapeutic Approaches to the Treatment of Diabetes

Diabetes is a complex chronic disease with no cure. Therefore, therapy is directed at controlling hyperglycemia, as well as toward the reduction of the symptoms and morbidities associated with microvascular and macrovascular complications. Early diagnosis and aggressive maintenance of euglycemia will go a long way to moderate the microvascular pathologies.[40,41] However, reduction of the risk for macrovascular pathologies requires management of cardiovascular risk factors, such as smoking cessation, treatment for dyslipidemia, control of hypertension, and antiplatelet therapy. The ADA[42] recommends that appropriate medical care for the diabetic include setting goals for glycemia, as well as for therapeutic lifestyle changes (diet and exercise) along with control of blood pressure, plasma lipids, and the use of appropriate medications.[43]

Glycemic control assessment involves two primary techniques, patient self-monitoring, and measurement of hemogobin A1C (HbA_{1c}). A1C is perhaps the most accurate indicator of glucose load because it reflects plasma glucose levels over the previous 2-3 months and is accepted as the gold standard for assessing glycemic control. A1C is formed by the glycosylation of hemoglobin's amino terminal Val residue. This endogenous substance has a half-life equivalent to that of an erythrocyte. The UK Prospective Diabetes Study and the Diabetes Control

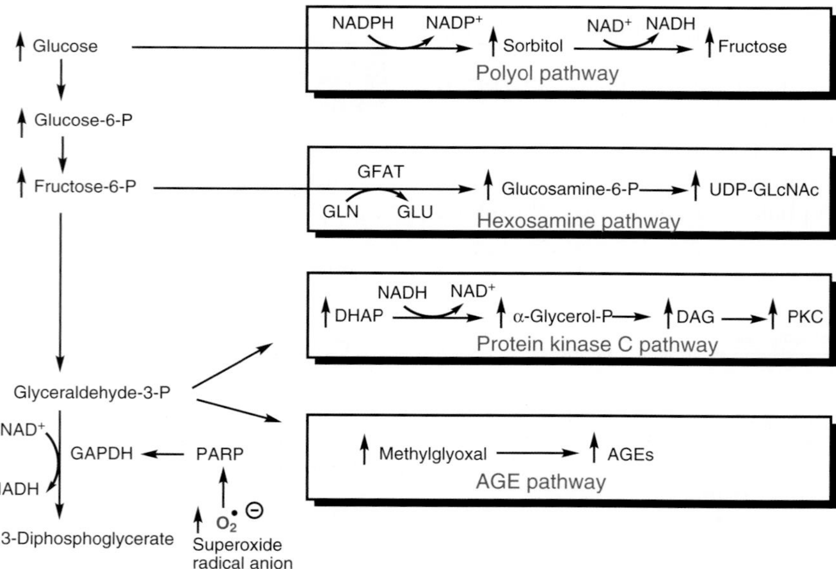

Figure 20.6 The role of hyperglycemia-induced mitochondrial excess superoxide in activation of the four pathways involved in diabetic microvascular and macrovascular damage. *AGEs*, advanced glycation end products; *DAG*, diacylglycerol; *DHAP*, dihydroxyacetone phosphate; *GAPDH*, glyceraldehyde-3-P dehydrogenase; *GFAT*, glut-amine:fructose-6-P amidotransferase; *GLN*, glutamine; *GLcNAc*, N-acetylglucosamine; *PARP*, poly(ADP-ribose)polymerase; *PKC*, protein kinase C.

and Complications Trial/Epidemiology of Diabetes Interventions and Complications Study (DCCT/EDIC) have established that if a patient's A1C is maintained below 7%, the development and progression of neuropathy, nephropathy, retinopathy, and cardiovascular disease in type 1 or 2 patients can be significantly decreased.[31,44]

Pharmacologic treatment for type 1 diabetics requires intensive insulin therapy. The large number of short- and long-acting insulin analogues allows for the use of multiple doses of basal, as well as, prandial insulin. Therefore the patient can match their dose of prandial insulin to carbohydrate intake, premeal plasma glucose, and anticipated physical activity level. The most common side effect of insulin use is the risk of severe hypoglycemia; however, the development of both quick-acting and long-acting insulin analogues has moderated this adverse effect while maintaining equal A1C lowering.[26]

Medical treatment of the type 2 diabetic requires management of hyperglycemia, as measured by the patient's A1C (target <7%). Along with lifestyle interventions, the array of different classes of hypoglycemic drugs offers the provider many different treatment options. Obesity and sedentary lifestyle are the major risk factors for diabetes; therefore, weight loss, dietary changes, and increased physical activity levels should be the initial approach to treating the type 2 diabetic. As a matter of fact, morbidly obese patients who have undergone weight loss surgery and who have maintained at least a 40 lb weight loss over 5 years effectively show no evidence of disease.[45] When diet and exercise are insufficient to maintain the patient's A1C below 7%, it then becomes necessary to initiate blood glucose–lowering medications. In addition to insulin, there are several classes of oral hypoglycemic agents available. They include the insulin secretagogues (sulfonylureas, meglitinides), biguanides (metformin), insulin sensitizers (TZD, glitazones), α-glucosidase inhibitors, glucagon-like peptide 1 analogues (GLP-1), dipeptidyl peptidase-IV (DPP-IV) inhibitors, amylin agonist, and sodium-glucose cotransporter 2 inhibitors (SGLT2).

It is currently recommended to begin medication therapy with metformin along with lifestyle interventions (Fig. 20.7). If this therapy fails to maintain or sustain glucose levels, then another medication should be added, usually one of the other oral hypoglycemic agents. Insulin (intermediate- or long-acting) is indicated for patients who have trouble decreasing their A1C level below 8.5%.

If lifestyle, metformin, and one of the other oral hypoglycemic agents do not result in achievement of target glycemia, the next step is to add a third oral hypoglycemic agent or basal insulin. If insulin is initiated, this usually consists of injections of a short- or rapid-acting insulin analogue given before meals. At this stage, insulin secretagogues (sulfonylureas or meglitinides) should be terminated since they are not considered to be synergistic. The choice of added oral hypoglycemic agents for dual or triple therapy is made based on patient preference, as well as patient, disease, and drug characteristics. The goal is to reduce blood glucose levels while minimizing adverse effects, especially hypoglycemia. The use of amylin agonists and α-glucosidase inhibitors is generally reserved for those patients who cannot tolerate the first-line drugs because they do not have equivalent glucose-lowering ability, they are relatively expensive, and there are limited clinical data demonstrating effectiveness.[46]

Therapeutic Classes of Drugs Used to Treat Diabetes

Insulin

Insulin was isolated in crystalline form by John Jacob Abel in 1926 which was only 5 years after it was isolated from

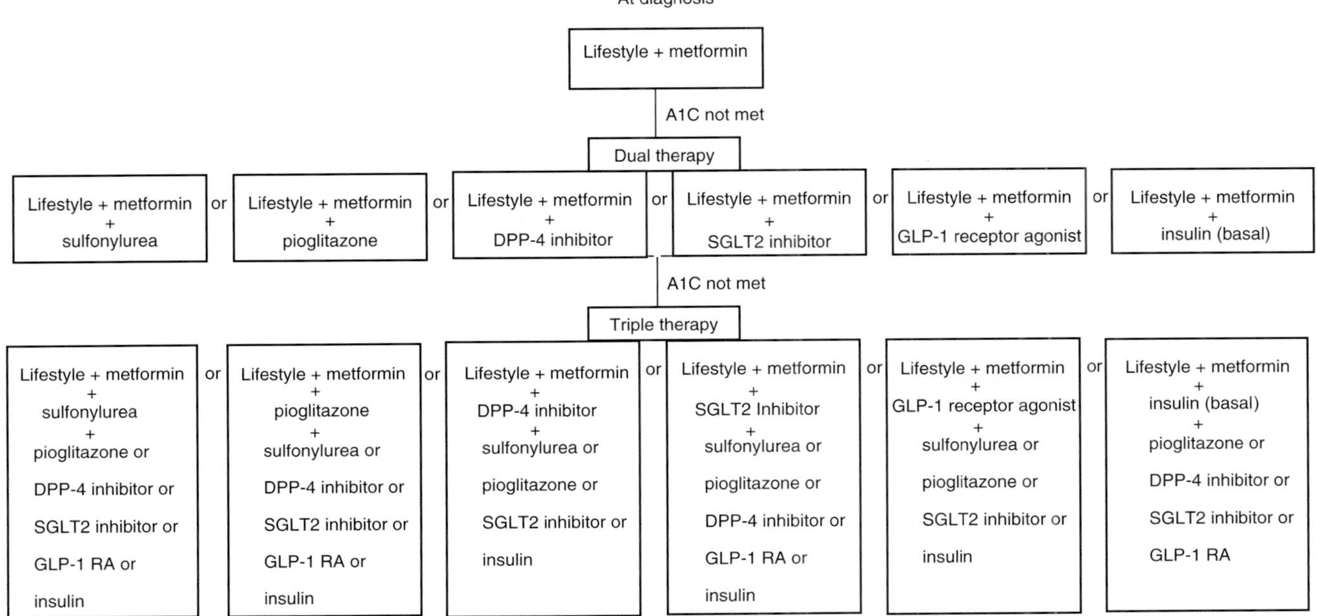

Figure 20.7 Decision tree for the management of type 2 diabetes. Lifestyle management is reinforced at every stage, and A1C is recommended to be less than 7%. Adapted from American Diabetes Association Standards of Care[46].

canine pancreas by Banting, Best, Collip, and Macleod. As noted previously, Banting and Macleod received the 1923 Nobel Prize for their work and Banting announced that he would share his prize with Best; Macleod did the same with Collip. In 1958, Sanger received the Nobel Prize for the determination of the amino acid sequence of insulin, and Dorothy Hodgkin received the Nobel Prize in 1964 for determining its three-dimensional structure. The development of an immunoassay for insulin by Solomon Berson and Rosalyn Yallow in 1960 earned Yallow the Nobel Prize in 1977 after Berson's death. Clearly, the awarding of so many Nobel Prizes points to the importance of insulin-related research throughout the 20th century.[47]

The insulin molecule is composed of two polypeptide chains (A and B) linked together by two disulfide bonds. There is an additional intramolecular disulfide bond in chain A. The A chain contains 21 amino acid residues and the B chain has 30 amino acids, giving a molecular weight of 5734 daltons. Insulin is biosynthesized in the β-cells of the pancreas from preproinsulin, a 110 amino acid chain with a molecular weight of 12,000 daltons. Preproinsulin is cleaved in the endoplasmic reticulum, losing a 24–amino acid unit from the N-terminus. The product is called proinsulin (MW 9000), which folds to form the disulfide bonds and undergoes further proteolytic modification in the Golgi apparatus, losing four basic amino acids (ArgB31, ArgB32, LysA64, ArgA65) and releasing a 31–amino acid connector C-chain by the action of prohormone convertases PC 1 and 2 (Fig. 20.8).

The biologically active form of insulin is the monomer; however, in solution, insulin can exist as a dimer and hexamer. The hexamer is formed by coordination with two zinc ions and is believed to be the storage form in the granules of the β-cells. When released from the granules, the hexamer is diluted in the plasma to nanomolar concentrations and dissociates into monomers. Secretion of insulin is primarily regulated by glucose, but many other nutrients and hormones also play a role. Amino acids, fatty acids, and ketone bodies promote the secretion of insulin. On the other hand, stimulation of

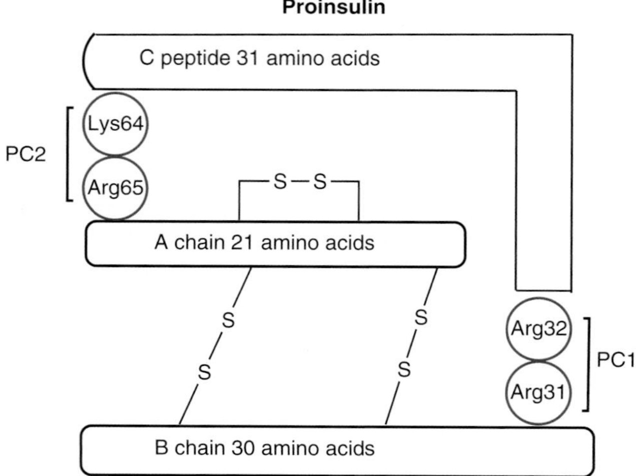

Figure 20.8 Structure of proinsulin. Prohormone convertases (PC1 and 2) cleave dipeptides (red) to form insulin.

α^2-adrenergic receptors on the β-cells inhibits secretion while β^2-adrenergic receptor stimulation and vagal nerve stimulation enhance the release of insulin. It follows that any physiological condition that activates the sympathetic nervous system causes a decrease in the secretion of insulin via stimulation of the α^2-adrenergic receptors and an increased secretion of insulin by the β^2-adrenergic receptors. Such conditions include exercise, hypothermia, surgery, hypoxia, and of course hypoglycemia. In addition, α^2-adrenergic receptor antagonists will be expected to increase basal insulin levels while β^2-adrenergic receptor blockers will decrease them.[48]

Insulin secretion results from the metabolism of glucose in the pancreatic β-cells. Glucose enters the β-cell facilitated by GLUT-2 transport, is phosphorylated to glucose-6-phosphate by a specific isoform of glucokinase, and enters glycolysis, ultimately generating ATP. The increase in ATP changes the ratio of ATP to adenosine diphosphate (ADP) and prevents an ATP-sensitive K^+ channel from functioning, which in turn leads to depolarization of the β cells. This prompts activation of a voltage-gated calcium channel, and calcium flows into the β cells. The elevated intracellular calcium concentration causes activation of phospholipases A_2 and C and increased levels of inositol triphosphate (IP_3), an intracellular second messenger. IP_3 facilitates additional release of calcium into the cytosol, and concentrations of calcium are now sufficiently high to promote insulin secretion from the β-cells. The ATP-sensitive K^+ channel is an octameric heterocomplex consisting of four pore-forming inwardly rectifying K^+ channel subunits (Kir6.2) and four regulatory sulfonylurea receptor subunits (SUR1). ATP binding to Kir6.2 closes the channel. Binding of sulfonylureas and the meglitinides to SUR1 also closes the channel, whereas binding of ADP to SUR1 opens the channel.[49] Therefore, sulfonylurea binding to SUR1 causes the same effect as an increase in the ATP/ADP ratio—closing the channel which leads to the depolarization of the β-cell membrane and the ultimate secretion of insulin (Fig. 20.9).

Fifty percent of the insulin secreted from the pancreas is degraded in the liver and never reaches the general circulation. Hepatic degradation of insulin is the result of the action of a thiol metalloproteinase, which may also be involved in the degradation of glucagon. Insulin is internalized into the hepatocyte by receptor-mediated endocytosis and stored along with its receptor in small vesicles termed endosomes. Insulin is filtered by the renal glomeruli and can then be reabsorbed and degraded by the tubules. Insulin is also degraded at the cell surface of insulin-sensitive tissues.[48]

The primary target cells for insulin are the liver, muscle, and adipocytes. Insulin interacts with amino acid residues of the α-subunit of its receptor via key amino acid residues on both the A and B chains. Table 20.4 shows that the N-terminus and C-terminus of the A and B chains are involved in receptor binding.[48] Insulin binding to its receptor activates a series of intracellular events that lead to translocation of the GLUT4 transporter to the cell surface. The details of this process have previously been described (Fig. 20.3).

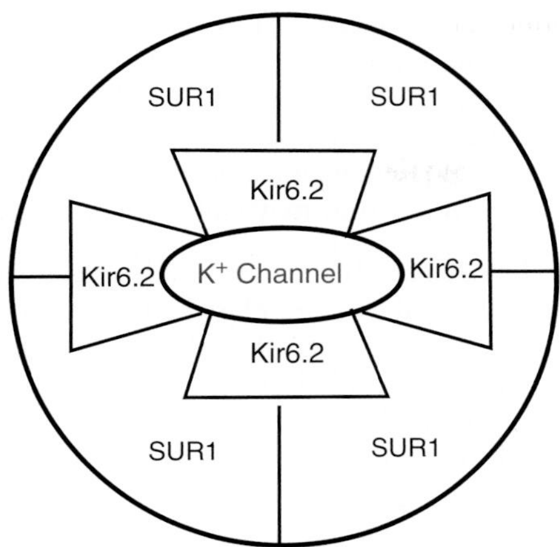

Figure 20.9 Idealized topographical view of the ATP-sensitive potassium channel showing four pore-forming inwardly rectifying potassium subunits (Kir6.2) surrounded by four regulatory sulfonylurea receptor subunits (SUR1).

SOURCES AND STABILITY OF INSULIN. Historically, patients only had the option of administering either bovine-based or porcine-based insulins. They were viable alternatives to human insulin because the amino acid sequence homology between these species was superb. However, with the availability of biosynthetic and semisynthetic human insulin and its analogues, these sources have fallen into disuse. Human insulin is the least antigenic of the available insulins and tends to be more soluble than nonhuman insulin. Human insulin and insulin analogues are formed by recombinant DNA techniques carried out by inserting the human or a modified human gene for proinsulin into *Escherichia coli* or yeast. Upon fermentation, these genetically altered organisms produce proinsulin, which is harvested and enzymatically altered to produce insulin. Human insulin is also produced semisynthetically by enzymatic transpeptidation of pork insulin, which alters position 30 of the B chain with the substitution of Thr for Ala.[21]

Only the insulin monomer is able to interact with insulin receptors, and native insulin exists as a monomer only at low, physiological concentrations (<0.1 μM). Insulin dimerizes at the higher concentrations (0.6 mM) found in pharmaceutical preparations. At neutral pH and in the presence of zinc ions, hexamers will form. These zinc-associated hexamers are also the storage forms of insulin in β cells. At concentrations greater than 0.2 mM, hexamers form even in the absence of zinc ions. The monomeric form of insulin is the only readily absorbable form, so when insulin is administered subcutaneously (SC) at concentrations wherein dimers and hexamers exist, it is absorbed significantly more slowly.[48]

Table 20.4 Interactions of Insulin Amino Acid Residues With the Insulin Receptor

Chain	N-Terminus	C-Terminus
A	Gly A1, Glu A4, Gln A5	Tyr A19, Asn A21
B	Val B12	Tyr B16, Gly B23, Phe B24, Phe B25, Tyr B26

The importance of zinc ions for stabilizing insulin preparations has been known since the first reported crystallization of insulin in their presence in 1934. Presently, all pharmaceutical preparations are either solutions of zinc insulin or suspensions of insoluble forms of zinc insulin. A longer-acting and more stable form of insulin is protamine zinc insulin, which is prepared by precipitating insulin in the presence of zinc ions and protamine, a basic protein. This precipitate is known to contain two zinc ions per insulin hexamer. A somewhat shorter-acting and more useful preparation is neutral protamine Hagedorn (NPH) insulin, which includes *m*-cresol as a preservative. Six *m*-cresol molecules occupy cavities in the hexamer involving the B1-B8 helix formed by the presence of the *m*-cresol. Later, it was reported that when small additional amounts of zinc ions were added to hexameric two-zinc insulin in neutral acetate buffer, insulin could be made to crystallize in several forms with varying rates of dissolution in water. Thus, the slowly soluble lente insulin is a two-zinc insulin, and the crystalline, more slowly soluble ultralente insulin is a four-zinc form.

Fibrils (partially unfolded insulin) are viscous or insoluble insulin precipitates. Shielding of hydrophobic domains is the principal driving force for the aggregation. Further studies revealed that when the exposed hydrophobic domain (A2, A3, B11, and B15) interacts with the normally buried aliphatic residues (A13, B6, B14, and B18) in the hexameric structure, fibrils form. Insulin fibrils do not resuspend on shaking; thus, they are pharmaceutically inactive. Insulin fibril formation is particularly important with the advent of infusion pumps to deliver insulin. In these devices, insulin is exposed to elevated temperatures, the presence of hydrophobic surfaces, and shear forces—all factors that increase insulin's tendency to aggregate. These problems can be overcome if the insulin is prepared with phosphate buffer or other additives. Another physical stability problem associated with insulin is adsorption to tubing and other surfaces. This normally occurs if the insulin concentration is less than 5 international units (IU)/mL (0.03 mM), and it can be prevented by adding albumin to the dosage form if a dilute insulin solution must be used.[48]

There also are chemical instability issues associated with insulin. For many years, the only rapid-acting form of insulin was a solution of zinc insulin held at pH 2-3. If this insulin is stored at 4°C, deamidation of the Asn at A21 occurs at a rate of 1%-2% per month. The C-terminal Asn, under acidic conditions, undergoes cyclization to the anhydride which, in turn, can react with water, leading to deamidation. The anhydride also can react with the N-terminal Phe of another chain to yield a cross-linked molecule. If stored at 25°C, the inactive deamidated derivative constitutes 90% of the total protein after 6 months (Fig. 20.10).

If insulin is stored at neutral pH, a different reaction may occur. Deamidation occurs on the Asn at B3, and the products, the aspartate- and isoaspartate-containing insulins, are equiactive with native insulin (Fig. 20.10).

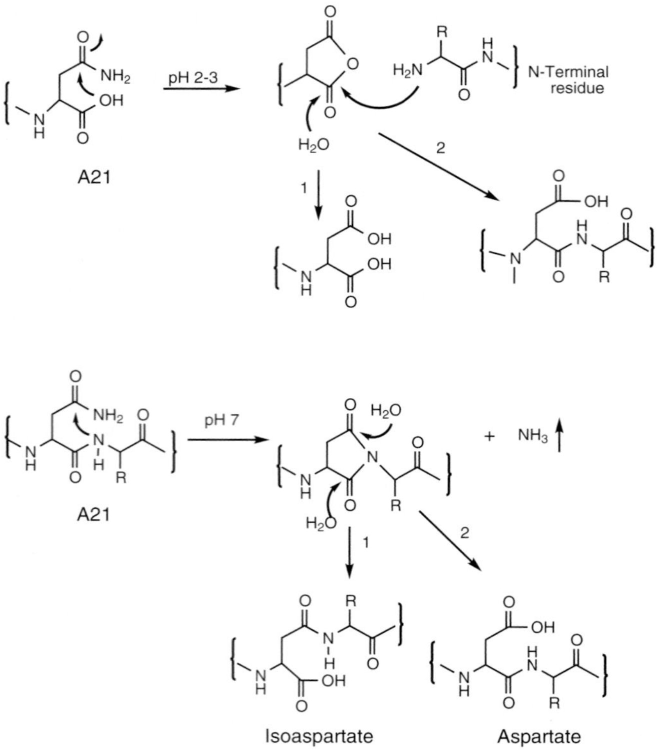

Figure 20.10 Chemical degradation of insulin.

More problematic transformations are possible, including chain cleavage between A8 Thr and A9 Ser and covalent cross-linking, either with a second insulin chain or with protamine, if present. These processes are relatively slow compared to the deamidations, but they have the potential of leading to products that may cause allergic reactions.[48]

TYPES OF INSULIN. The insulin analogues available for the treatment of diabetes are classified according to their rate of onset and duration of action. Structure-activity relationship studies revealed that variations in or addition/removal of amino acid residues from the C-terminus of the B chain could influence the rate of dimer formation while not drastically changing the biological activity. Inhibiting dimer formation can allow for rapid-acting insulin. Thus, the various insulin analogues that have been developed have substitutions in, or additions to, the C-terminus of the B chain starting at residue B28. The resulting analogues have either a faster onset or a longer duration of action relative to native insulin. These analogues are all produced by recombinant DNA technology using a modified DNA template. The available insulin preparations are summarized in Table 20.5.

Rapid-acting insulin analogues include insulin lispro, aspart, and glulisine. All have changes made to the amino acid residues in the C-terminus of the B chain (Table 20.6). In insulin lispro, the B29 Lys is switched with B28

Table 20.5 Classification, Appearance, and Pharmacokinetic Properties of Insulin Preparations

Type	Appearance	Onset (hr)	Peak (hr)	Duration (hr)
Rapid-acting				
Lispro	Clear	<0.25	0.5-1.5	3-4
Aspart	Clear	<0.25	0.5-1.5	3-4
Glulisine	Clear	<0.25	0.5-1.5	3-4
Short-acting				
Human insulin	Clear	0.5-1	2-3	4-6
Intermediate-acting				
Lente	Cloudy	2-4	6-12	18-26
NPH	Cloudy	2-4	4-12	18-26
Long-acting				
Ultralente	Cloudy	4-8	10-30	>36
Glargine	Clear	1-4	5-24	20-24
Detemir	Cloudy	1-4	5-24	20-24
Ultralong-acting				
Degludec	Clear	0.5-1.5	NA	>48

NPH, neutral protamine Hagedorn.

Pro, whereas in insulin aspart the B28 Pro is changed to an Asp. Glulisine's B3 Val is changed to a Lys, and its B29 Lys is changed to a Glu. These modifications, as previously stated, result in insulin analogues that do not form dimers in solution and dissociate immediately into monomers, producing a very quick onset of action. Pharmacodynamically, lispro, aspart, and glulisine bind as well to insulin receptors as human insulin and have a low mitogenic potency. Mitogenic activity is the ability of insulin to induce cell division and is believed to be associated with insulin's binding to insulin-like growth factor receptors (IGFs I and II).[50] Lispro, aspart, and glulisine have an onset of action within 15 minutes, a peak activity at 30-90 minutes, and a duration of 3-4 hours (Table 20.5).

Regular human insulin is the prototype of short-acting insulin. It has an onset of action within 30-60 minutes, reaches its peak effect 2-3 hours after injection, and has a duration ranging 4-6 hours. Its slow onset inconveniently requires it to be administered 30-60 minutes before meals, but this property is retained with intravenous administration, making regular insulin a good choice for intravenous treatment of diabetics.

Intermediate-acting insulin is prepared by adding stoichiometric amounts of protamine to regular insulin to form a poorly soluble insulin-protamine complex. The complex is known as neutral protamine Hagedorn insulin (NPH). NPH insulin has an onset of action of 2-4 hours, peak effect at 4-12 hours, and duration of 18-26 hours after injection. However, most patients get little effect after 13-15 hours.[51] Another way to prepare intermediate-acting insulin is to combine regular insulin and zinc in an acetate buffer to form a crystalline complex that dissolves slowly in subcutaneous fluids. This product is termed insulin lente, and it has a similar onset, peak effect, and duration of action as NPH insulin.

The first long-acting insulin analogue to be introduced to the market was insulin glargine. This analogue results from the replacement of A21 Asn by Gly and the addition of two Arg amino acids to the C-terminus of the B chain (Table 20.6). The resulting analogue has an isoelectric point close to 7, which results in its precipitation on SC injection. Slow dissolution from the site of injection results in an onset of 1-4 hours, a peak between 5 and 24 hours, and a duration of 20-24 hours that represents a fairly constant release of insulin glargine over 24 hours. It has been demonstrated to be comparable or slightly better than NPH insulin at maintaining or reducing A1C levels without nocturnal hypoglycemia.[52]

Insulin ultralente is a long-acting insulin which is a four-zinc acetate crystalline product with an even slower dissolution rate than the two-zinc acetate insulin lente. Insulin detemir is another long-acting analogue. This analogue results from N-acylation of the B29 Lys with the 14-carbon myristic acid (Table 20.6). The fatty acid side chain binds to plasma albumin to produce a depot, resulting in a longer duration of action. It has approximately the same duration of action as insulin glargine when administered in equivalent doses.

Insulin degludec is an ultra-long-acting insulin that can be administered daily or three times a week and is comparable to glargine and detemir in onset and duration of action. Insulin degludec results from the removal of B30 Glu, N-acylation of B29 Lys with L-γ-Glu that is acylated with hexadecanedioic acid. The long duration of action of insulin degludec is believed to be due to the combination of (1) the formation of soluble multihexamer assemblies upon SC administration which slowly release monomers and (2) hexadecandioic acid side chain binding to plasma albumin to produce a depot.[53] An important difference between glargine, ultralente, and determir is that glargine is a clear solution, whereas the others are cloudy. This may be a problem for patients who rely on the physical appearance of their insulin to distinguish NPH, lente, and ultralente from regular, lispro, aspart, glulisine, glargine, or degludec, which are all clear (Table 20.5).

Table 20.6 Insulin Analogues

Generic Name	Brand Name	Change in a Chain	Change in B Chain
Lispro	Humalog	None	B28 Pro → Lys B29 Lys → Pro
Aspart	Novolog	None	B28 Pro → Asp
Glulisine	Apidra	None	B3 Val → Lys B29 Lys → Glu
Glargine	Lantus	A21 Asn → Gly	Add: B31 Arg and B32 Arg
Detemir	Levemir	None	Remove: B30 Thr Add: C14 fatty acid to B29 Lys
Degludec	Tresiba	None	Remove: B30 Thr Acylate B29 Lys with hexadecandioic acid via a γ-L-glutamic acid linker.

Different types of insulin may be premixed and are usually prescribed for patients needing a simple insulin treatment plan (Table 20.7). The benefit of using premixed insulin is that rapid-acting and long-acting insulin can be administered at the same time and can be given twice a day, usually at breakfast and supper. The drawback of using such a regimen is that, to be effective, the amount of carbohydrate to be eaten at each meal is preset. This works best for patients who can follow strict adherence to a consistent schedule of meals and activity and who are able to follow a prescribed diet.[54]

Sulfonylureas

The discovery sulfonylureas as antidiabetic agents resulted from research conducted in 1942 that noted the hypoglycemic effect of sulfonamides used to treat typhoid fever.[55] Subsequent investigations revealed that modifying the sulfonamide antibacterial agents with a urea moiety resulted in sulfonylureas with significant hypoglycemic effects, and the first generation oral hypoglycemic drugs were born. These agents include tolbutamide, chlorpropamide, tolazamide, and acetohexamide (Fig. 20.11).

The mechanism of action of all the sulfonylureas is to stimulate the release of insulin from the β-cells of the pancreas. These cells metabolize glucose in the mitochondria to produce ATP, which increases the intracellular ratio of ATP/ADP, resulting in the closure of the ATP-sensitive K^+ channel on the plasma membrane. Closure of this channel triggers the opening of voltage-sensitive Ca^{2+} channels leading to rapid influx of Ca^{2+}. Increased intracellular Ca^{2+} causes an alteration in the cytoskeleton and stimulates translocation of insulin-containing granules to the plasma membrane, allowing the exocytotic release of insulin.[56]

The ATP-sensitive K^+ channel is an octameric heterocomplex consisting of two units of the binding site for both sulfonylureas and ATP, designated as the sulfonylurea receptor type 1 (SUR1) and an inwardly rectifying K^+ channel (Kir6.2) (see Fig. 20.9). The SUR1 subunits consist of 3 transmembrane domains (TMD 0, 1, and 2), an intracellular loop (L0) and 2 nucleotide binding domains (NBD1 and 2). The NDB1 is adjacent to the TMD1, and the NBD2 is adjacent to the TMD2 (Fig. 20.12).[57]

The ATP-sensitive K^+ channels are not only found in the plasma membrane of β-cells of the pancreas but also in the vasculature (SUR2B) and the cardiac myocytes (SUR2A). The binding of sulfonylureas to vascular and cardiac SURs, like the binding to the β-cell receptors, has a number of physiologic consequences. In cardiac myocytes, sulfonylurea binding to SUR2B prevents the opening of these channels that, in turn, prevents the reduction of Ca^{2+} influx that results in myocardial cell death. In vascular cells, blocking SUR2B by sulfonylureas increases smooth muscle tone, resulting in decreased blood flow. Both these effects are detrimental to the heart during an ischemic attack.[58] Furthermore, inhibition of SUR2A in the heart prevents ischemic preconditioning. Ischemic preconditioning reduces the size of an infarct and protects against repeated ischemic episodes.[59]

The first generation sulfonylureas structurally differ in the chemical nature of the small lipophilic substituent on the *p*-position of the phenyl ring (R_1 of the pharmacophore, see Fig. 20.11) and the lipophilic alkyl or cycloalkyl

Table 20.7 Combination Antidiabetic Medications

Oral Hypoglycemics	Brand Name	Insulin Combinations	Brand Name
Ertugliflozin/sitagliptin	Steglujan	Insulin glargine/lixisenatide	Soliqua
Dapagliflozin/saxagliptin	Qtern	Insulin degludec/liraglutide	Xultophy
Empagliflozin/linagliptin	Glyxambi	Insulin aspart/insulin degludec	Ryzodeg
Empagliflozin/metformin	Synjardy	70% Insulin aspart protamine + 30% insulin aspart	NovoLog 70/30
Canagliflozin/metformin	Invokamet	75% Insulin lispro protamine + 50% insulin lispro	Humalog 75/25
Pioglitazone/glimepiride	Duetact	50% Insulin lispro protamine + 50% insulin lispro	Humalog 50/50
Linagliptin/metformin	Janumet	70% NPH + 30% regular insulin	Humulin 70/30
Linagliptin/metformin XR	Jentadueto		
Sitagliptin/simvastatin	Juvisync		
Saxagliptin/metformin XR	Kombiglyze XR		
Repaglinide/metformin	Prandimet		
Pioglitazone/metformin	ACTOplus met		
Rosiglitazone/metformin	Avandamet		

NPH, neutral protamine Hagedorn.

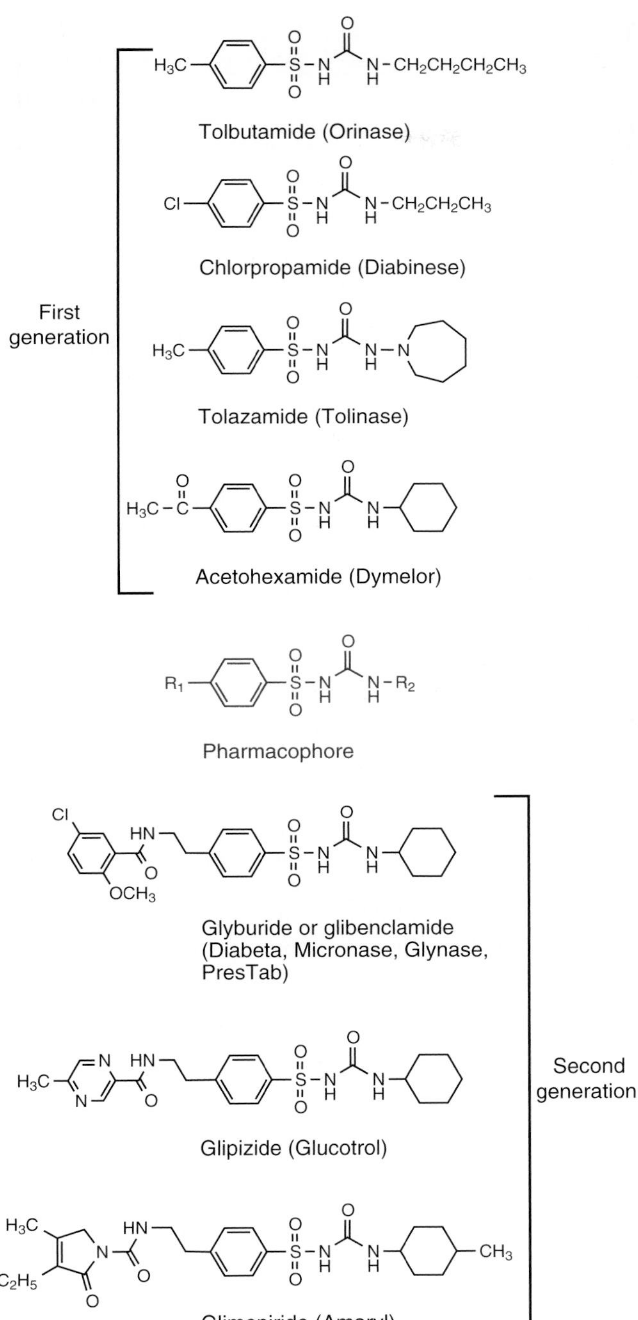

Figure 20.11 First and second generation sulfonylurea oral hypoglycemics.

substituent on the non–sulfonyl-attached urea nitrogen (R_2 of the pharmacophore). However, these structural modifications do little to increase their binding efficiency to the ATP-sensitive K^+ channel; thus, they all require relatively high doses to achieve effectiveness, which increases the potential for adverse events. In addition, the plasma half-life of these first generation sulfonylureas is fairly long (5-36 hrs), which also increases their potential for adverse effects.

The second generation sulfonylureas developed out of research efforts intended to design hypoglycemic agents

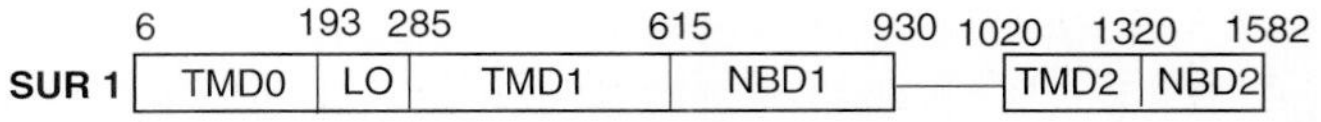

Figure 20.12 A schematic diagram of the sulfonylurea receptor subunits (SUR1) polypeptide. Numbers indicate residue numbers at the beginning and end of the domain.

with increased potency, a more rapid onset, shorter plasma half-lives, and longer durations of action. Thus, glyburide (also known as glibenclamide), glipizide, and glimepiride are 50-100 times more active than first generation molecules, with plasma half-lives of 1-4 hours and durations of action up to 24 hours. This enhancement of activity is the result of strong binding affinity to the ATP-sensitive K^+ channel associated with the larger *p*-(β-arylcarboxyamidoethyl) group which replaces the small lipophilic *p*-substituents found in the first generation agents (Fig. 20.11). Sulfonylurea binding to the SUR1 subunit is coordinated by the inner helices of the TMD1 and TMD2 domains. Figure 20.13 visualizes the current understanding of the binding of glyburide. The important residues on TDM2 are Asp1245, Thr1242, and Arg1246 and 1300; those on TMD1 are Tyr377 and Asp437.[57]

SULFONYLUREA PHARMACOKINETICS AND METABOLISM. Sulfonylureas are highly protein bound, primarily to albumin, which leads to a large volume of distribution (~0.2 L/kg) (Table 20.8). Food can delay the absorption of these drugs but does not typically affect bioavailability. Metabolism takes place in the liver, and the metabolites are renally excreted.

Glipizide and glyburide are extensively metabolized (Fig. 20.14) to less active or inactive metabolites. Glipizide metabolites are excreted primarily in the urine, whereas glyburide's metabolites are excreted equally in the urine and bile.

Glimepiride is metabolized in the liver, primarily by CYP2C9, to the active metabolite M-1 (Fig. 20.15). It is then further metabolized by cytosolic dehydrogenases to the inactive metabolite M-2.

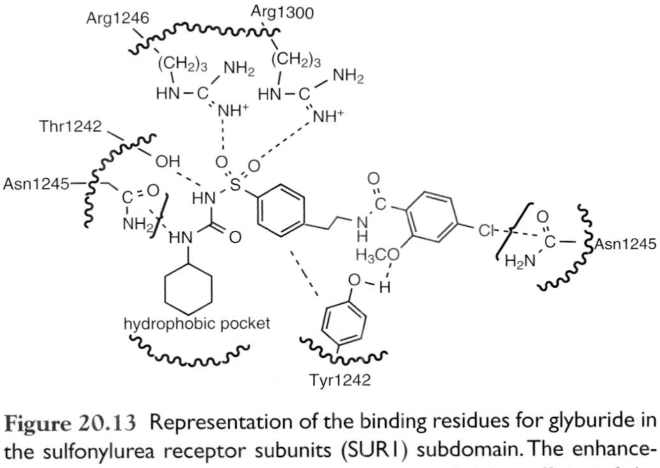

Figure 20.13 Representation of the binding residues for glyburide in the sulfonylurea receptor subunits (SUR1) subdomain. The enhancement of its activity is attributed to the strong binding affinity of the *p*-(arylcarboxyamidoethyl) group (in red) to Asn1245 and Tyr1242.

Table 20.8 Pharmacokinetic Properties of the First-Line Sulfonylureas

Sulfonylurea	Equivalent Dose (mg)	Serum Protein Binding (%)	Half-Life (hr)	Duration (hr)	Renal Excretion (%)
Glyburide	5	99	1.5-3.0	Up to 24	50
Glipizide	5	92-97	4	Up to 24	68
Glimepiride	2	99	2-3	Up to 24	40

Meglitinides

Meglitinide is the prototype structure that defines this class of insulin secretagogues. It is the benzoic acid derivative of the nonsulfonylurea moiety of glyburide, i.e., the *p*-(β-arylcarboxyamidoethyl group (Fig. 20.16). These agents exert their effects by inducing closure of the ATP-sensitive K^+ channel found on the plasma membrane of the pancreatic β-cells.[60,61]

REPAGLINIDE. Repaglinide is an analogue of meglitinide containing additional substituents (*m*-ethoxy, isobutyl and piperidine ring) added to the basic benzoic acid structure. The aromatic chloro and methoxy groups of meglitinide have been eliminated, and the amide moiety has been transposed. Repaglinide stimulates insulin secretion by binding to three different receptors on the β-cells; one is the SUR1 and the other two receptors have yet to be completely characterized.[60] Repaglinide is not tissue specific and binds well to SUR1, SUR2A, and SUR2B found on cardiac and smooth muscle cells, therefore conferring extrapancreatic effects in much the same way as sulfonylureas do.[62]

Repaglinide has a rapid onset and short duration of action compared to other hypoglycemic drugs. It is not associated with the prolonged hyperinsulinemia seen with the sulfonylureas, and possibly for this reason, it produces fewer side effects, including weight gain and potentially dangerous hypoglycemia. Repaglinide is at least 5-fold more potent than glyburide on intravenous administration and nearly 10-fold more active on oral administration.

NATEGLINIDE. Nateglinide is a phenylalanine analogue of meglitinide where the benzoic acid carboxylate group is transposed to the α-carbon of the N-ethyl side chain, creating the amino acid functionality. Nateglinide binds selectively to the SUR1 on β-cells and has a much lower affinity for cardiac and skeletal muscles.[63] It is a chiral molecule synthesized as the *S*(+)-isomer with traces of the *R*(-)-isomer as an impurity. The *S*(+)-isomer is 100-fold more potent than the *R*(-)-isomer. Nateglinide is a rapidly absorbed insulin secretagogue that has a mechanism of action similar to that of repaglinide, with effects appearing within 20 minutes following oral dosing. Bioavailability is 73%, and it is 98% protein bound, primarily to albumin. Nateglinide is tissue selective, with low affinity for cardiac

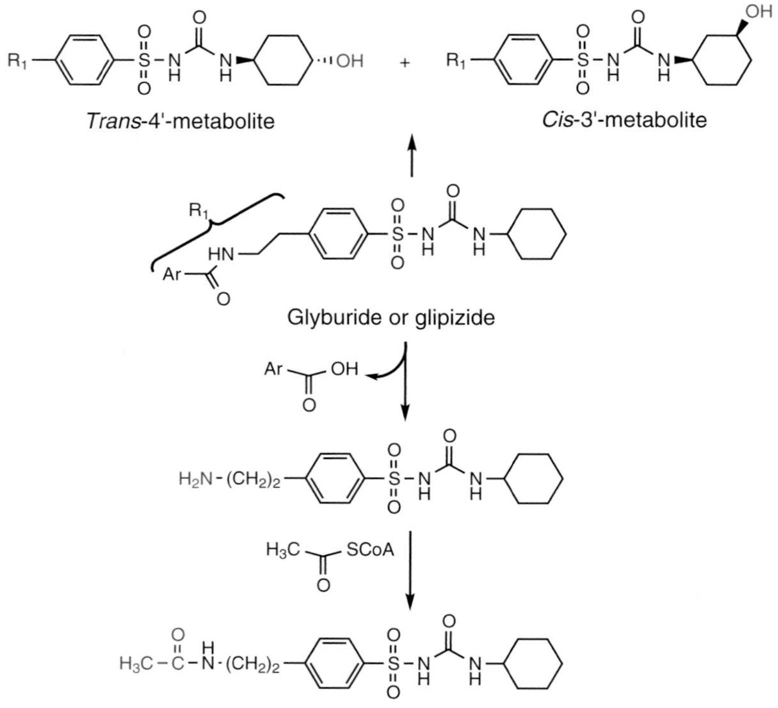

Figure 20.14 Metabolism of glyburide and glipizide.

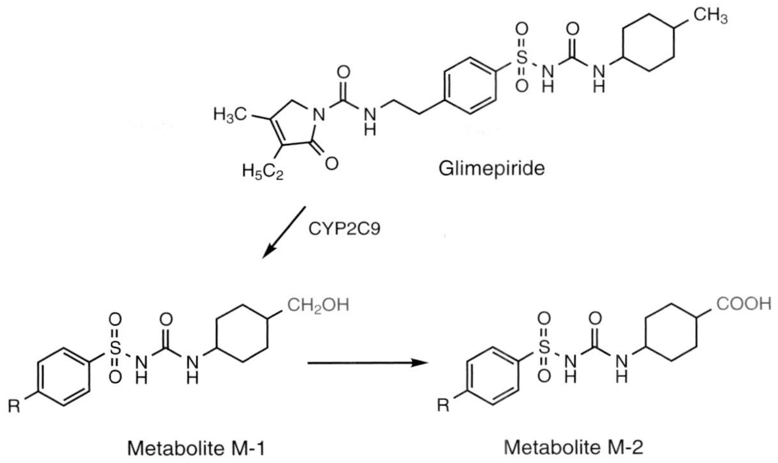

Figure 20.15 Metabolism of glimepiride.

and skeletal muscles.[64] It is metabolized in the liver, with 16% being excreted unchanged in the urine. The major metabolites are hydroxyl derivatives (CYP2C9, 70%; CYP3A4, 30%) that are further conjugated to glucuronides (Fig. 20.17). The drug has an elimination half-life of 1.5 hours.

It has been shown by molecular modeling studies that there is a similar conformation between the sulfonylurea hypoglycemics, glyburide and glimepiride, and the meglitinides, which might be important in the interaction of these drugs with the SUR1 on the β-cells. Specifically, these agents display a common U-shape formed by the hydrophobic interaction between the cyclic structures located at the ends of these molecules and a peptide bond at the bottom of the U. Moreover, the inactive analogues of the meglitinides, including the inactive enantiomer of repaglinide, are unable to adopt this U-shape and thus cannot bind effectively to the SUR1.[65]

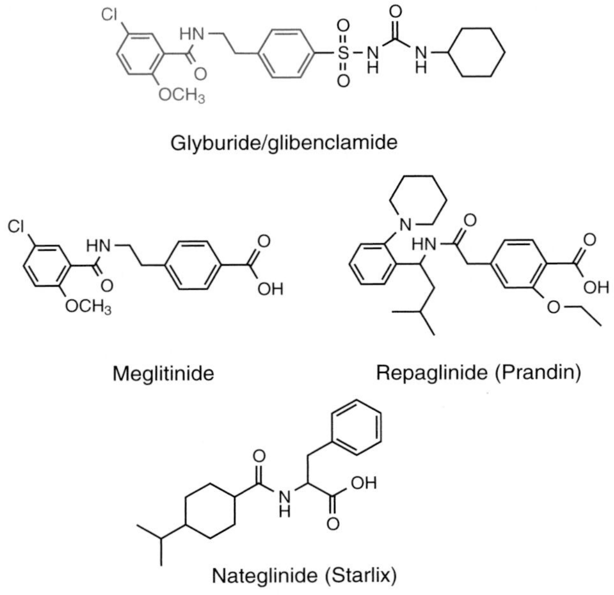

Figure 20.16 The meglitinide hypoglycemic agents.

Biguanides

The use of biguanides can be traced back to medieval times. The plant *Galega officinalis* was not only traditionally used for promoting perspiration during plague epidemics and as a galactogogue in milk-producing farm animals (e.g., cows), but it was also prescribed for the relief of frequent urination associated with diabetes. G. *officinalis* has several common names, including Goat's rue, French lilac, and Italian fitch. This plant contains active compounds such as galegine (isoamylene guanidine), which were shown to have blood glucose–lowering effects.[69] The hypoglycemic properties of the plant ultimately led to the synthesis of the biguanide compounds. The biguanides are chemically represented by the linkage of two guanidine groups with different side chains. Despite the toxicity associated with guanidine, the biguanides were shown to exert beneficial effects and quickly became available therapeutic agents for diabetes in the 1950s.

Oral hypoglycemic agents from the biguanide chemical class primarily act by reducing hepatic glucose production and by enhancing insulin sensitivity. The mechanism of action of the biguanides is primarily to reduce hepatic glucose output by decreasing gluconeogenesis and stimulating glycolysis. In addition, they affect anabolic pathways such as lipid and cholesterol biosynthesis. These metabolic actions are related to inhibition of the mitochondrial respiratory chain complex I, as well as activation of the AMP-activated protein kinase (AMPK) pathway. The biguanides target the mitochondria, where they reduce complex I of the electron transport chain. This results in a reduction in oxidative phosphorylation and, ultimately, a reduction in the synthesis of ATP, which causes AMP levels to rise. Increasing AMP activates AMPK and inhibits cyclic AMP-protein kinase A (cAMP-PKA) and fructose-1,6-bisphosphatase, all resulting in the inhibition of gluconeogenesis.[66] In addition, the activation of AMPK-dependent phosphorylation blocks the breakdown of fatty acids.

Insulin secretion is not directly affected by the biguanides, so they do not cause hypoglycemia. Importantly, biguanides do not induce weight gain, which is very

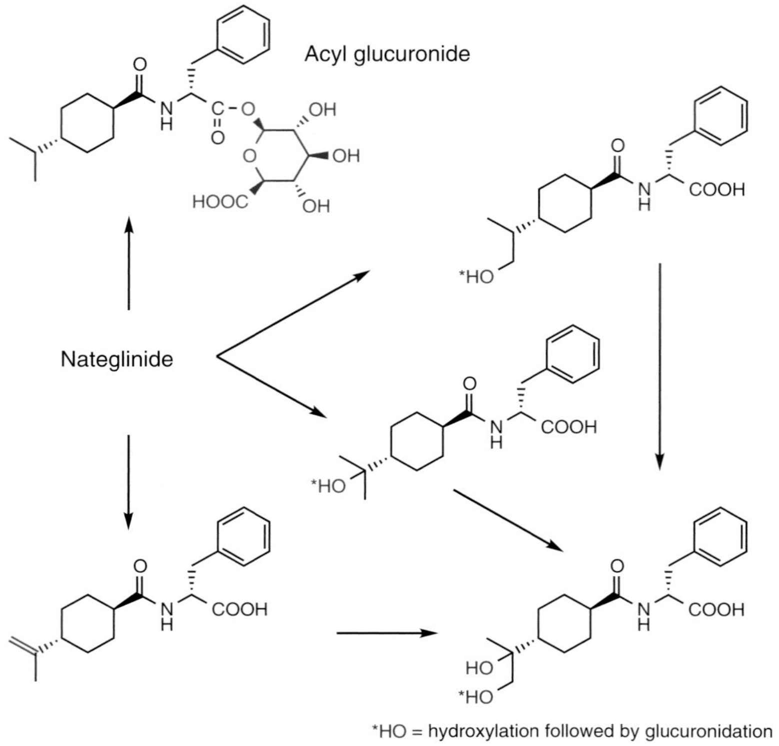

Figure 20.17 Urinary metabolites of nateglinide.

beneficial for insulin-resistant obese patients.[67] They are also considered to have antihypertriglyceridemic effects and to possess vasoprotective properties, important actions in treating cardiovascular complications.[68]

Approved in 1995, metformin is currently the only available biguanide in the United States and is considered to be the first-line treatment for type 2 diabetes. It is widely used as monotherapy or in combination with other oral antidiabetic agents.[41]

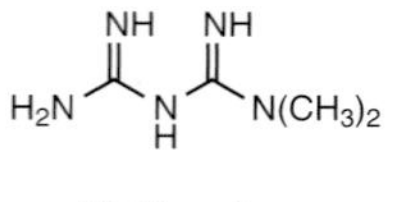

Metformin is quickly absorbed from the small intestine. Bioavailability ranges from 50% to 60%, and the drug is not protein bound. Peak plasma concentrations occur at approximately 2 hours. The drug is widely distributed in the body and accumulates in the wall of the small intestine. This depot of drug serves to maintain plasma concentrations, but also may contribute to drug-induced gastrointestinal (GI) distress, lactic acidosis, and diarrhea, the latter of which can be minimized by food intake.[70]

Metformin is excreted in the urine via tubular excretion as unmetabolized drug, and it has a half-life of approximately 2-5 hours; therefore, renal impairment as well as hepatic disease are contraindications for the drug. Since metformin is not metabolized in the liver, drug-drug interactions through the inhibition of metformin transporters (OCTs and MATEs) are clinically relevant. Genetic polymorphisms in these transporter genes are also likely to have a direct impact on metformin pharmacokinetics and variability in drug responses. Recent drug-drug interaction studies suggest that proton-pump inhibitors inhibit metformin uptake in vitro by inhibiting organic cation transporting (OCT) proteins OCT1, OCT2, and OCT3. Oral antidiabetic drugs repaglinide and rosiglitazone also inhibited OCT1-mediated metformin transport in vitro. The H_2 blocker cimetidine is associated with reduced renal tubular secretion and increased systemic exposure to metformin when the drugs are coadministered. Inhibition of MATEs, but not OCT2, is the likely mechanism underlying the drug-drug interaction with cimetidine in renal elimination. A recent study suggests the potential for a transporter-mediated drug-drug interaction between metformin and specific tyrosine kinase inhibitors (e.g. imatinib, nilotinib, gefitinib, and erlotinib; see Chapter 33), which may have clinical implications in the disposition, efficacy, and toxicity of metformin.[71]

As noted above, metformin may induce lactic acidosis if not taken in proper doses. Nevertheless, metformin is not recommended for type 2 diabetic patients who are inclined toward metabolic ketoacidosis induced by certain conditions, including hepatic disease, heart failure, respiratory disease, hypoxemia, severe infection, alcohol abuse, or renal disease.[72]

Peroxisome Proliferator Activated Receptor (PPAR) Agonists (Insulin Sensitizers)

Activators of PPARs in the treatment of insulin resistance and type 2 diabetes mellitus is a much sought after target, since PPARs are central regulators of lipid and carbohydrate metabolism and inflammatory pathways and help maintain homeostasis. They belong to the nuclear hormone receptor superfamily of ligand-activated transcription factors and are closely related to steroid, retinoid, and thyroid hormone receptors (Chapter 7). This receptor family is comprised of three members: PPARα, δ, and γ. PPARδ is ubiquitously present in tissues of adult mammals, whereas the α subtype is abundantly present in tissues catalyzing lipid oxidation, which includes the liver, kidney, and heart. PPARγ is primarily expressed in adipose tissue, where it helps control lipid differentiation.[73]

The thiazolidenediones (TZD) are classic examples of PPARγ agonists and are commonly referred to as the "glitazones." These agents were developed when clofibric acid analogues (Chapter 19) were being screened for antihyperglycemic and lipid-lowering activity. Although initially the mechanism of action of the TZDs was unclear, it was soon discovered that they enhanced adipocyte differentiation by activation of the nuclear hormone receptor superfamily, PPAR. Upon binding to PPAR, an endogenous or exogenous ligand induces a conformational change in the receptor, thus stabilizing the interaction with the retinoid X receptor which, in turn, results in the stimulation of transcription by target genes. The endogenous ligand(s) for PPARγ have not been identified; however, studies suggest that certain arachidonic acid metabolites and long chain unsaturated fatty acids, such as linoleic acid, may be the intrinsic agonists (Fig. 20.18).[73]

PPARγ agonists, such as the glitazones, act by increasing the sensitivity of cells to insulin. The glitazones also decrease both systemic fatty acid production and fatty acid uptake, which contributes to increased sensitization of cells to insulin. Patients with type 2 diabetes are known to have high triglyceride and low HDL levels. The glitazones increase the lipolysis of triglycerides in VLDLs and, as a result, increase HDL levels. They also increase LDL levels, particularity in patients and this could be a major drawback to the use of these drugs.[74,75]

PPARγ activation improves glucose uptake by skeletal muscle and, at the same time, reduces glucose production by slowing gluconeogenesis. Hence, these drugs improve metabolism of glucose not only in diabetic patients but also in obese individuals who have impaired glucose tolerance.[73] As mentioned earlier, the first PPARγ agonists to be introduced were the glitazones. The pharmacophore responsible for activity is the thiazolidinedione moiety outlined in red in Figure 20.18. A phenyl ring attached to the thiazolidinone ring via a methylene group is essential for activity and, in many instances, a saturated linker is found to be more potent than the unsaturated counterpart.

The first generation TZDs include pioglitazone, rosiglitazone, and ciglitazone (Fig. 20.18). The rationale used for the development of these agents was the fact that the structure of troglitazone (the first drug in this class to be marketed) includes the structure of α-tocopherol, an antioxidant that retards the oxidation of LDLs.[76] However, due to severe hepatoxicity and cardiovascular effects, troglitazone and rosiglitazone have been withdrawn, leaving pioglitazone as the only clinically used drug in the TZD family.[74,77] The metabolism of pioglitazone has been studied in rats and dogs and has led to the discovery of up to eight metabolic products. These products result from oxidation at either carbon adjacent to the pyridine ring and are found as various conjugates in the urine and bile (Fig. 20.19). Metabolites M-1, M-2, and M-3 appear to contribute to the biological activity of pioglitazone.

Recently, dual PPARα/γ agonists have become much sought after targets, and many research groups are actively involved in synthesizing these bioactive compounds as novel antidiabetic agents. The combined activation of PPARα and PPARγ is believed to induce complementary and synergistic action on lipid metabolism, insulin sensitivity, and inflammation control, possibly circumventing or reducing the side effects of PPARγ. To date there are no PPARα/γ agonists approved for use in the United States.

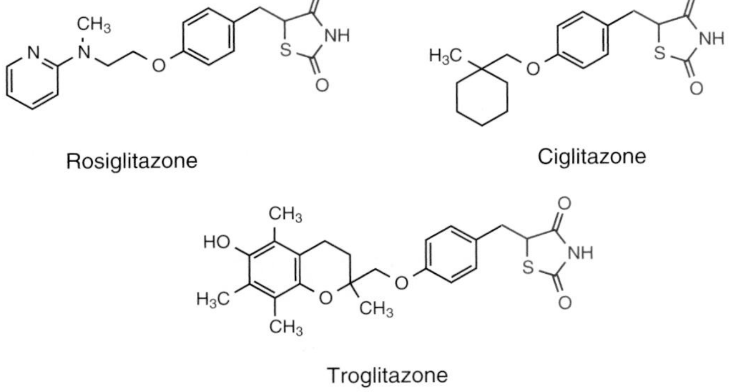

Linoleic acid

Pioglitazone

Rosiglitazone

Ciglitazone

Troglitazone

Figure 20.18 Linoleic acid and thiazolidinedione (outlined in red) PPARγ agonists (glitazones).

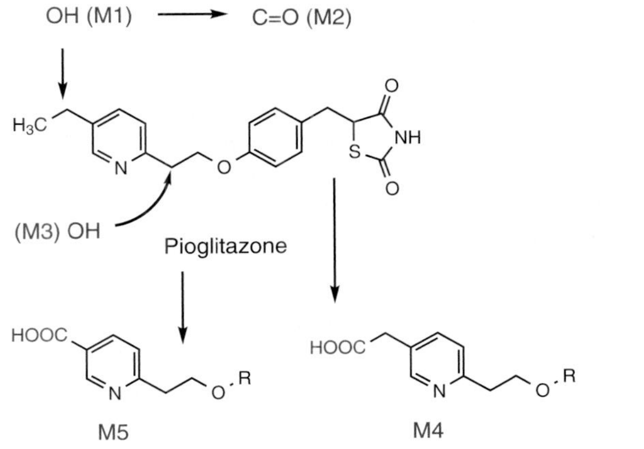

OH (M1) → C=O (M2)

(M3) OH

Pioglitazone

M5

M4

Figure 20.19 Metabolism of pioglitazone.

However, saroglitazar is an approved drug in India for the treatment of type 2 diabetes and triglyceridemia in patients whose dyslipidemia is not controlled by statin therapy.[78]

Saroglitazar

Acarbose

Voglibose

Miglitol

Figure 20.20 Clinically useful α-glucosidase inhibitors.

α-Glucosidase Inhibitors

α-Amylase and α-glucosidase are key enzymes responsible for the metabolism of carbohydrates. The salivary and pancreatic α-amylases are responsible for the breakdown of complex polysaccharides into oligo- and disaccharides, preparing them for intestinal absorption. α-Glucosidase, which consists of maltase, sucrase, isomaltase, and glucoamylase, is a membrane-bound enzyme present in the brush border of the small intestine and is in relatively high concentrations in the proximal part of the jejunum. This enzyme catalyzes the conversion of the disaccharides sucrose and maltose into glucose. The resulting monosaccharides are then absorbed by the enterocytes of the jejunum and enter systemic circulation, as well as various biochemical pathways for the production of energy.[79] Thus, inhibiting α-glucosidase will delay carbohydrate absorption in the gut by moving undigested disaccharides into the distal sections of the small intestine and colon. The result is the prevention of glucose production, thereby reducing postprandial hyperglycemia. All known α-glucosidase inhibitors act locally and are excreted unchanged in the feces, obviating metabolic drug interactions.[80]

ACARBOSE. The α-glucosidase inhibitors were first introduced in 1996 with the drug acarbose (Fig. 20.20).[81] It is an oligosaccharide obtained from *Actinomyces utahensis* and is the drug of choice in this category. It is a competitive inhibitor of the α-glucosidase enzyme, with a high affinity for sucrase and a lesser affinity for glucoamylase and pancreatic α-amylase in humans.[82] When used in monotherapy, there is no risk of hypoglycemia and weight gain, as seen with the first and second generation sulfonylureas. However, GI irritation, bloating, and flatulence caused by fermentation of undigested sugars in the large bowel by intestinal microflora are some drawbacks common to all α-glucosidase inhibitors.[79] These side effects can be minimized to a certain extent by gradual dose titration and the right combination therapy with other orally active hypoglycemic drugs.

VOGLIBOSE AND MIGLITOL. Voglibose and miglitol are other α-glucosidase inhibitors in clinical use for the management of diabetes. α-Glucosidase inhibitors reduce postprandial hyperglycemia to a lesser extent as compared to other oral antidiabetic agents, and clinical trials with acarbose have shown that the reduction in A1C levels is 0.5%-1% when compared to placebo.[81] These agents are therefore seldom used as monotherapy and frequently find use in combination therapy, especially with sulfonylureas.[82] Apart from diabetes, their use can be extended to the treatment of glycosphingolipid lysosomal storage disease and HIV infections and in the management of certain tumors.[83,84]

Glucagon-Like Peptide 1 (GLP-1) Agonists and Dipeptidyl Peptidase IV (DPP-IV) Inhibitors

Glucagon-like peptide 1 (GLP-1) is a 36 amino acid peptide secreted by L-cells of the gut in response to a meal. It exerts control over glucose levels by promoting insulin secretion in a glucose-dependent manner.[85] The role of GLP-1 was first proposed based on the observation that the amount of insulin secreted following an oral glucose dose exceeded that of an equivalent glucose dose administered intravenously in both diabetic and nondiabetic individuals.[86] This observation was termed the incretin effect and is the result of two gut hormones, GLP-1 and glucose-dependent insulinotropic polypeptide (GIP).[87] GLP-1 secretion from L-cells is similar to that of glucose-induced insulin secretion from pancreatic β-cells. Metabolism of glucose in the intestinal L-cells leads to closure of ATP-linked K^+ channels resulting in depolarization of the membrane and entry of Ca^{2+} that leads to the secretion of GLP-1.[88] With an in vivo half-life of 1-2 minutes, GLP-1 is rapidly metabolized by an aminopeptidase enzyme, dipeptidyl peptidase-IV (DPP-IV), yielding an inactive peptide that is two amino acids shorter.[89,90] It follows that GLP-1 agonists or DDP-IV inhibitors would be effective agents to control blood glucose levels in diabetic patients.

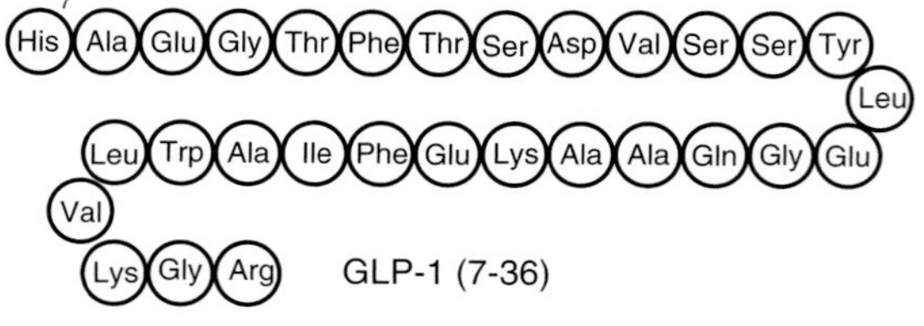

GLP-1 ANALOGUES. GLP-1 is deactivated by DPP-IV, which removes a dipeptide from the N-terminus. One of the principle reasons why GLP-1 is so susceptible to DPP-IV is because it contains an Ala in the penultimate N-terminal position. Substitution at this position gives analogues with increased stability. Indeed, substitution of the Ala with Thr ($t_{1/2}$ = 197 min), Gly ($t_{1/2}$ = 159 min), Ser ($t_{1/2}$ = 174 min), or α-aminoisobutyric acid (AiB) each gave analogues that are more stable in vitro than GLP-1 ($t_{1/2}$ = 28 min) under the same conditions.[91] In fact, the AiB analogue exhibited no degradation even after 6 hours. While such analogues are found to be more stable to DPP-IV in vitro, the in vivo half-life is increased only from 1-2 to 3-4 minutes, and this is attributed to rapid elimination by the kidneys. Interestingly, these analogues still retained binding affinity to the GLP-1 receptor, with the AiB analogue almost twice as potent as GLP-1.

More useful in vivo analogues, therefore, required both DPP-IV resistance and decreased renal elimination. This was achieved with the introduction of the GLP-1 analogue exenatide as a parenteral therapy into the market in April 2005. Exenatide is a 39-amino acid peptide analogue of GLP-1 (7-36) isolated from the saliva of the gila monster (*Heloderma suspectum*). It is a GLP-1 receptor agonist resistant to the action of DPP-IV. It has a Gly instead of Ala in the penultimate N-terminal position, is 53% homologous to human GLP-1, and has an in vivo half-life of approximately 3 hours.

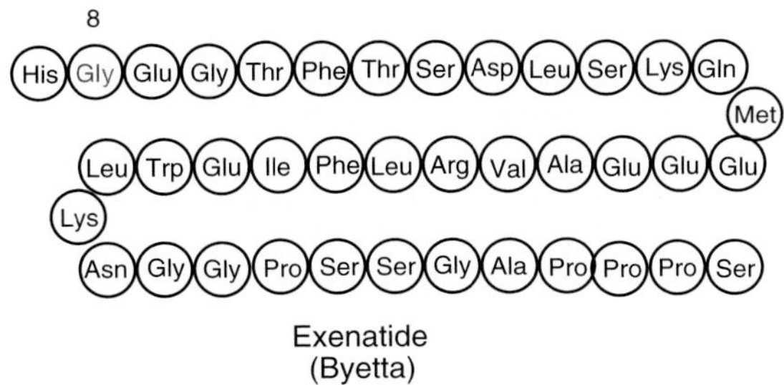

Exenatide
(Byetta)

Exenatide has been shown to reduce A1C levels in sulfonylurea treated patients with type 2 diabetes and is associated with weight loss.[92] This weight loss is probably due to a decrease in appetite. In *db/db* mice, it increased β-cell mass and delayed the onset of diabetes, indicating that it may even have a prophylactic use.[93]

CURRENTLY MARKETED GLP-1 ANALOGUES

Liraglutide. Liraglutide, which represents amino acid residues 7-37 of GLP-1, was developed from a series of acylated GLP-1 (7-37) derivatives. Several positions of GLP-1 were substituted with different acyl moieties ranging in length from 12-18 carbons. The C16 derivative α-L-glutamoyl-(N-α-hexadecanoyl)-Lys26 Arg34-GLP-1 (liraglutide) was found to have the best combination of albumin binding to retard renal elimination and DPP-IV degradation resistance (due to the replacement of Lys34 with Arg34).[94,95] This analogue of GLP-1 (7-37) has multiple actions in addition to reduction of hyperglycemia, including suppression of inappropriate glucagon secretion, slowing of gastric emptying, and enhancement of β-cell function and mass.[96] Liraglutide was FDA approved for marketing under the name Victoza in 2010. However, because of a possible link to the production of thyroid C-cell tumors, the product label has a black box warning with the recommendation that it be used only in patients for whom the potential benefits outweigh the potential risk.[97]

Liraglutide
(Victoza)

Dulaglutide. Dulaglutide is a fusion protein that is prepared by fusing two identical GLP-1 (7-37) analogues (Gly8, Glu22, Gly36) to a modified IgG4 Fc fragment. The linker is a small peptide joined to the dimer via disulfide bonds.[98] The IgG4 moiety acts to decrease both renal clearance and antigen-antibody formation. It has ~90% amino acid homogeneity to human GLP-1 (7-39).[99]

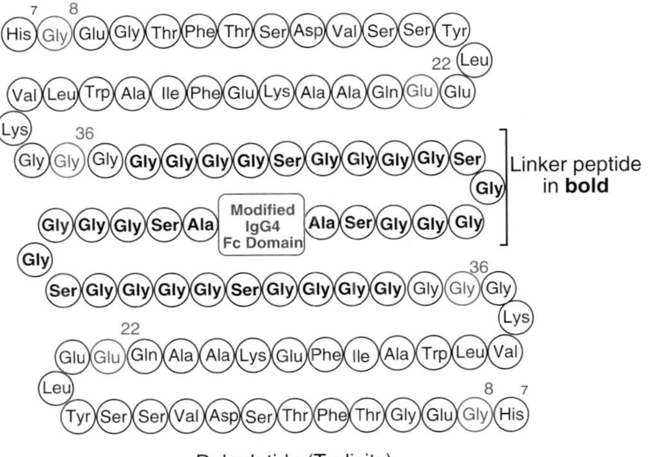

Dulaglutide (Trulicity)

Dulaglutide is administered SC and is slowly absorbed. It attains peak plasma concentration in about 48 hours and steady state at 2-4 weeks. It is administered on a weekly basis and has a half-life of ~5 days. As monotherapy, it has a slightly greater reduction in A1C as compared to metformin, with about the same degree of body weight loss and GI distress. Dulaglutide is metabolized by proteases and not significantly eliminated renally. However, it is not recommended for use by patients with severe kidney dysfunction (GFR <30 mL/min).[98]

Albiglutide. Albiglutide is composed of a tandem dimer of an analogue of human GLP-1 (7-37)–Gly8. This construct inhibits DPP-IV metabolism and is covalently bonded to recombinant human albumin. The albumin serves as a carrier protein and substantially reduces renal clearance.[98]

Albiglutide (Tanzeum)

Albiglutide has 97% amino acid homology with human GLP-1. It has a half-life of 6-8 days allowing for weekly SC administration. In monotherapy versus placebo, it lowered A1C by 1.4% without significant change in body weight. Albiglutide is metabolized by endogenous proteases, and its use is cautioned in patients with compromised renal function (<50 mL/min). Albiglutide has been compared to sitagliptin (discussed below), pioglitazone, liraglutide, and basal insulin in trials. In those trials albiglutide displayed a modest decrease in A1C or was noninferior to comparators.[100]

Lixisenatide. Lixisenitide was approved in the United States in July 2016. Structurally it is a modified version of exenatide, with one amino acid deleted (Pro38) and a string of six Lys residues added to the Ser at the carboxylic acid terminus. This modification extends the half-life to about 2-5 hours and allows for once to twice daily SC administration.

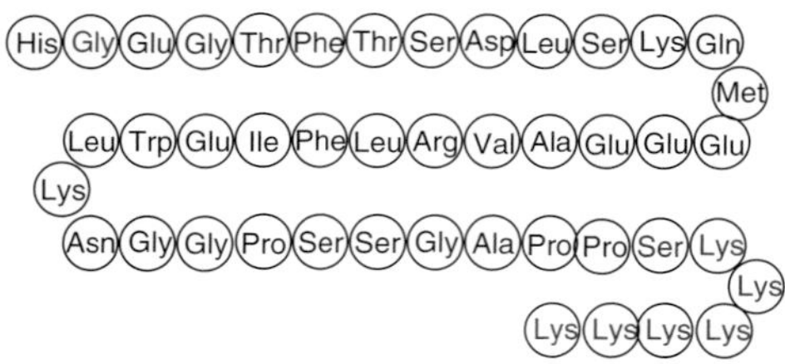

Lixisenatide (Adlyxin)

Lixisenitide has only about 50% amino acid homology to human GLP-1 (7-37). In monotherapy, lixisenitide showed modest A1C decreases (−1.0% to −0.7%), and body weight loss was also minimal (range −0.4 to −0.2 kg). Compared to basal insulin, lixisenitide patients experienced less symptomatic hypoglycemia and experienced greater body weight loss. Lixisenitide undergoes renal elimination but is reabsorbed in the tubules and then degraded by plasma proteases. Patients develop antibodies against this peptide (50%-60%), and severe hypersensitivity reactions have been observed.[98]

Semaglutide. Semaglutide is a long-acting human GLP-l analogue ([Aib8, Arg34]-hGLP-1). The amino-terminal sequence substitutes Ala8 for AiB8 which allows for resistance to DPP IV degradation. In addition, Lys26 is derivatized with a C18 fatty diacid using an ADO-linker (8-amino-3,6-dioxooctanoic acid) bridged via a glutamic acid moiety. Semaglutide has a 94% amino acid homology to hGLP-1.[101]

Semaglutide (Ozempic)

As was seen with liraglutide, the fatty acid side chain enhances affinity for albumin; however, in this case the affinity is 3-fold greater. Therefore, semaglutide exhibits an extremely long half-life of ~165 hours enabling once weekly SC dosing. A once weekly oral tablet has been developed by coformulating the peptide with sodium N-(8-[2-hydoxybenzoyl amino] caprylate) (SNAC), which acts as a transcellular carrier across GI enterocytes by increasing solubility through higher local pH and decreasing proteolysis. Semaglutide is slowly metabolized by proteolytic cleavage of the peptide backbone and β-oxidation of the fatty acid side chain. Only ~3% is excreted unchanged in the urine.[101]

DPP-IV INHIBITORS. The major problem with GLP-1 analogues is their need for SC administration, which may limit patient compliance. Also, GLP-1 analogues, as with any peptide drug, have the potential to be immunogenic. This therefore stimulated the search for small molecule inhibitors of DPP-IV.

DPP-IV is a serine protease that exists in both a membrane-bound and a plasma-soluble form. It is a proline-specific aminopeptidase responsible for the degradation of a number of biologically important peptides other than GLP-1 and GIP. DPP-IV belongs to a family of dipeptidyl peptidase enzymes which include DPP's VI-X, fibroblast protein-a (FAP), acylaminoacyl carboxypeptidase (APP), prolyl carboxypeptidase (PCP), and quiescent cell proline dipeptidase (QPP).[102] Since the clinical importance of these other prolyl peptidases has not been established, it is important that inhibitors have specificity for DPP-IV.

There are currently five DPP-IV inhibitors commercially available; sitagliptin, vildagliptin, saxagliptin, linaglitin, and alogliptin. The development of many structural variants has led to the understanding that there is an absolute requirement for a basic amino function in the position equivalent to the penultimate amino acid (Ala) in GLP-1. Most active inhibitors are peptide derivatives of α-aminoacylpyrrolidines or α-aminoacylthiazolidines, which also take advantage of the enzyme's high preference for Pro binding. The most active inhibitors also have an electrophilic group in the 2-position of the pyrrolidine or thiazolidine ring. The most common group is cyano and is present in vildagliptin, saxagliptin, and alogliptin (Fig. 20.21).

Sitagliptin has a piperazine ring fused to a pyrazole in place of the pyrorolidine ring making it a triazole ring, but it still contains the α-amino acyl moiety and the amide bond. Linagliptin contains a xanthine ring as the central pharmacophore. Alogliptin contains the 2,4-pyrimidine pharmacophore with the essential amino group on the piperidine ring.

All DPP-IV inhibitors bind inside a hydrophobic pocket of DDP-IV made up of Arg125, Glu205, Glu206, Tyr547, Tyr662, Tyr666, Ser630, and Phe357. Their binding residues, however, differ depending upon their pharmacophore and the specific moieties attached. Saxagliptin, vildagliptin, and alogliptin contain the cyano group that most likely forms a reversible covalent amidate with the enzyme Ser630, resulting in the deactivation of DPP-IV.[103,104] Figure 20.22 depicts a proposed mechanism for the amidate formation.

All inhibitors bind through ionic interaction with Glu205 and Glu206. The xanthine pharmacophore of linagliptin has a C8 aminopiperidine and an N7 butynyl substituent for binding to the DPP-IV catalytic site. The aminopiperidine's primary amino group occupies the recognition site for the amino terminus of GLP-1, and hydrogen bonds with the aforementioned Glu residues. The xanthine is held in place by π stacking with Tyr547. The N7 butynyl group interacts hydrophobically with Tyr662, Ser630, and Tyr666, and the quinazoline ring interacts by π-stacking with the aromatic ring of Trp629.[103]

Sitagliptin. Sitagliptin was approved by the FDA in 2006 for the treatment of type 2 diabetes, either as monotherapy or in combination with metformin, TDZs, or sulfonylureas. Sitagliptin has good oral bioavailability (87%) with no effect from food. It is protein bound only to about 37%, and 80% is excreted unchanged in the urine. It is important to have high specificity for DPP-IV, as inhibition of DPP-VIII and DPP-IX has been shown to cause severe toxicity in animal studies including alopecia,

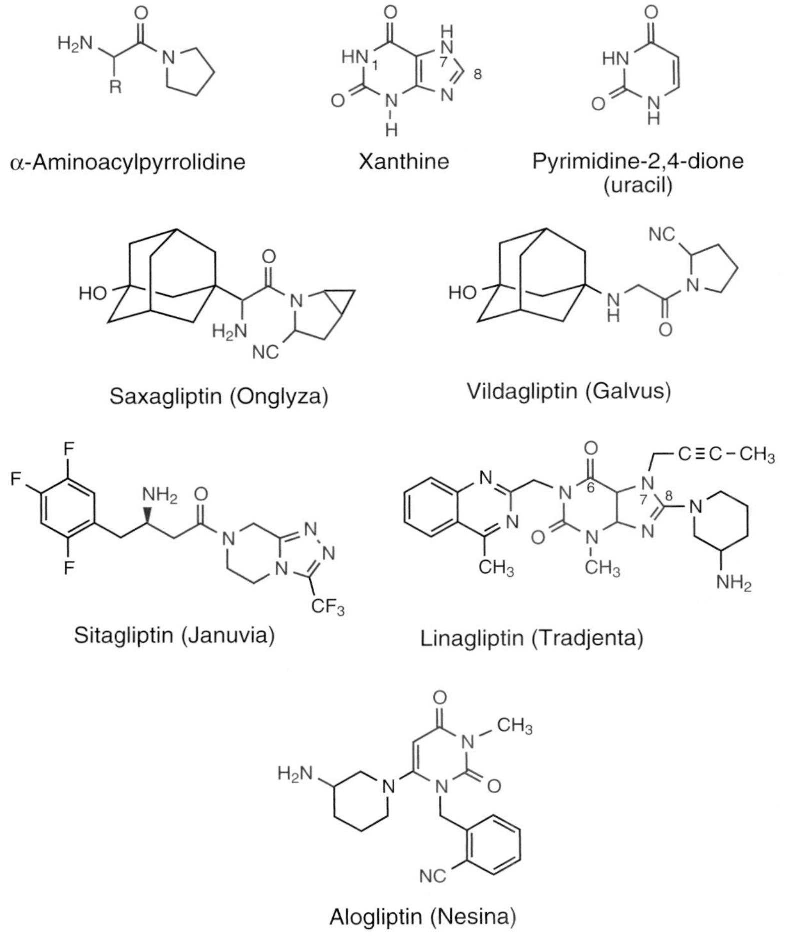

α-Aminoacylpyrrolidine

Xanthine

Pyrimidine-2,4-dione (uracil)

Saxagliptin (Onglyza)

Vildagliptin (Galvus)

Sitagliptin (Januvia)

Linagliptin (Tradjenta)

Alogliptin (Nesina)

Figure 20.21 α-Aminoacylpyrrolidine, xanthine and uracil pharmacophores, and currently available DPP-IV inhibitors.

thrombocytopenia, splenomegaly, and death. The selectivity of sitagliptin for DPP-IV compared to DPP-VIII and IX is >2600-fold. Sitagliptin has no effect on glucose levels in healthy patients; however, it reduces A1C about 0.6%-0.9% in type 2 diabetics. Sitagliptin has a number of side effects, including upper respiratory tract infection, nasopharyngitis, and headache. Patients experience nausea if the drug is taken with metformin, leg swelling when taken with TDZs, and hypoglycemia when administered with a sulfonylurea. There have also been reports of anaphylaxis, angioedema, and rashes, although a causal link has not been established.[105]

Vildagliptin. Vildagliptin was approved in 2008 by the European Medicines Agency for use in the European Union (EU), but the manufacturer has withdrawn its intent to submit it for FDA approval since the FDA demanded additional clinical data assuring that the skin lesions and kidney impairment observed in animal studies were not seen in humans. Due to these adverse events, vildagliptin is not a first-line treatment for diabetes. In phase III clinical trials, vildagliptin showed good oral bioavailability (85%) and low protein binding (9.3%) and was 21% excreted unchanged in the urine. It has a high specificity for DPP-IV compared to DPP-VIII and IX that ranges from 32- to 250-fold. In clinical trials, no patients discontinued medication because of adverse effects, which are similar to sitaglipin (upper respiratory tract infections, diarrhea, nausea, and hypoglycemia).[105]

Saxagliptin. The FDA approved saxagliptin in 2009. It is 10 times more potent as an inhibitor of DPP-IV than either vildagliptin or sitagliptin. It shows a higher specificity for DPP-IV compared to DPP-VIII and IX (400 and 75-fold, respectively). Trials using doses of 2.5-10 mg have shown reductions of A1C of 0.5%-0.8% with no significant weight gain. Saxagliptin was well tolerated with side effects equivalent to placebo and a very low incidence of hypoglycemia.[105] Saxagliptin is metabolized by CYP3A4 to 5-hydroxy saxagliptin that is half as potent as the parent drug. Therefore, the patient should be monitored when CYP3A4 inhibitors or inducers are coadministered.

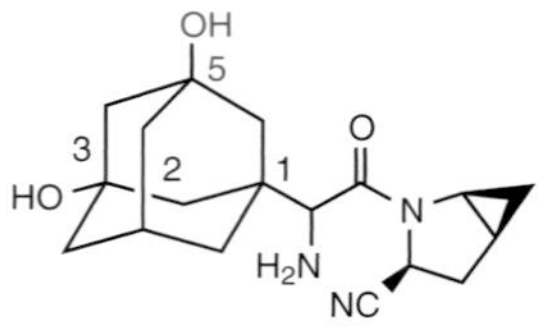

5-Hydroxysaxagliptin

Linagliptin. Linaglitin was approved by the FDA in 2011 as an oral treatment for type 2 diabetes, either as stand-alone medication or in combination with other therapies. Linagliptin should not be prescribed for patients with diabetic ketoacidosis. Its most common adverse effects are upper respiratory tract infections, stuffy nose, sore throat, muscle pain, and headache. Linagliptin has a high selectivity for DPP-IV over other isoforms of DPP, especially DPP-VIII and DPP-IX. Linagliptin inhibits DDP-IV activity by more than 80% over 24 hours. Linagliptin binds extensively to plasma proteins and is not significantly metabolized. Approximately 85% of the drug excreted unchanged via the feces.[106]

Alogliptin. Alogliptin contains the 2,4-pyrimidinedione pharmacophore with the essential basic amino group on the piperidine ring and the cyano group on the benzyl substituent. The piperidine amino interacts with the Glu205 and Glu206, whereas the pyrimidinedione interacts by π-stacking with Tyr547. The cyano moiety most likely binds to Ser630 in a manner similar to saxagliptin (Fig. 20.22). In addition, the cyanobenzyl group reportedly π-stacks with Tyr662.[103]

Alogliptin was approved by the FDA in 2013 as a stand-alone medication or in combination with metformin or pioglitazone. When used in combination with metformin, there can be an induction of lactic acidosis. When combined with pioglitazone, there is a warning that it may exacerbate congestive heart failure. A single oral dose is well absorbed with a T_{max} of 1-2 hours and a bioavailability of 63%. In clinical trials, it was well tolerated with no dose-limiting toxicity. Alogliptin is eliminated via the kidney, with 60%-71% of the drug excreted unchanged. Metabolism is a minor elimination pathway, with two minor metabolites M-I and M-II (Fig. 20.23).[107]

The most common adverse reactions (>4%) of patients treated with alogliptin were nasopharyngitis (4.4%), headache (4.2%), and upper respiratory tract infection (4.2%). When in combination with metformin the most common adverse reactions (≥4%) were upper respiratory tract infection (8%), nasopharyngitis (6.8%), diarrhea (5.5%), hypertension (5.5%), headache (5.3%), back pain (4.3%), and urinary tract infection (4.2%). In combination with pioglitazone the most common adverse effects (>4) were nasopharyngitis (4.9%), back pain (4.2%), and upper respiratory tract infection (4.1%).[108]

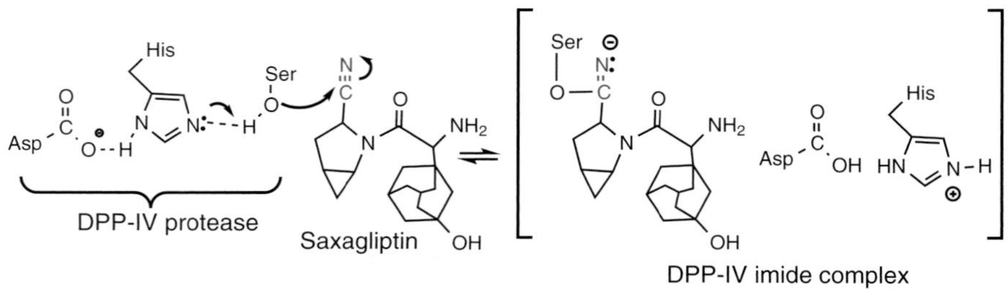

Figure 20.22 Proposed mechanism of reversible inhibition of DPP-IV by saxagliptin.

Figure 20.23 Structures of alogliptin and its metabolites M-I (N-demethylated) and M-II (N-acetylated).

Table 20.9 summarizes the pharmacokinetic parameters of the DPP-IV inhibitors, as well as the key metabolic indications. Bioavailability ranges from 30% to 90%, with only linagliptin having significant protein binding.

Amylin Agonists

Amylin is a hormone that consists of a single chain of 37 amino acids. It is released from pancreatic β-cells, is cosecreted with insulin, and is primarily involved in controlling postprandial glucose levels. Amylin, like insulin, shows similar fasting and postprandial patterns in healthy individuals by a variety of mechanisms, including, delayed gastric emptying and suppression of glucagon secretion (not normalized by insulin alone), which leads to a suppression of endogenous glucose output from the liver.[109] Amylin also regulates food intake by modulating the appetite center of the brain. The observation that amylin was deficient in both type 1 and type 2 diabetics stimulated research and development of amylin analogues that would be able to control postprandial glucose levels by (1) modulation of gastric emptying, (2) prevention of postprandial rise in glucagon, and (3) inhibition of caloric intake and potential weight gain. Amylin itself is unsuitable as a drug because it aggregates and is insoluble in solution, which encouraged the development of chemical analogues.[110]

PRAMLINTIDE. Pramlintide is a chemical analogue of amylin designed for enhanced water solubility and reduced aggregation liability by replacement of Ala25, Ser28, and Ser29 of the amylin peptide chain with Pro residues.[111] The SQ administration of 15 mg of the drug shows an optimum peak effect within 20 minutes, thus permitting the drug to be used before meals. Pramlintide has a duration of action of 150 minutes, no significant accumulation liability with repetitive administration, and a renal clearance rate of 1-2 L/min. The drug is primarily metabolized in the kidneys, with an elimination half-life of 30-50 minutes, and should be used with caution in patients with compromised renal function. Pramlintide is used together with insulin for those who are unable to achieve their target postprandial blood sugars on insulin alone.[112,113] Pramlintide delays gastric emptying, suppresses glucagon release, and has a central nervous system anorectic effect via unknown mechanisms. The nucleus accumbens and dorsal vagal complex of the brain have been shown to contain the amylin receptor that may be involved in the central effects of this hormone. Because of the wide differences between the pH of pramlintide and insulin products (4.0 vs. 7.8, respectively), concurrent mixing within the same syringe is not recommended. To avoid severe hypoglycemia with initial drug titration, only short or rapid insulin dosage forms should be used together with pramlintide. In this case, the dose of insulin should be reduced by 50%.[114]

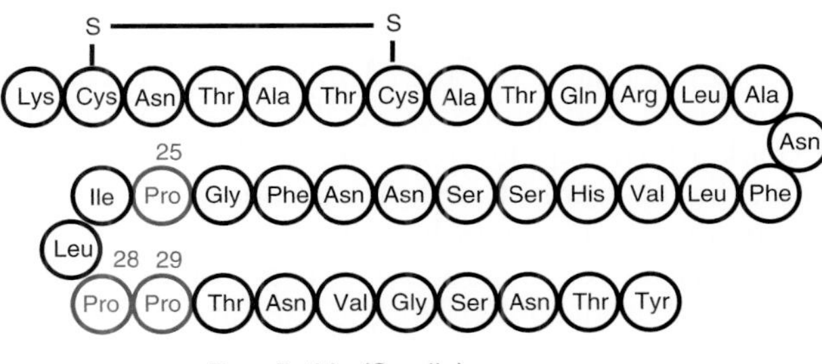

Pramlintide (Symlin)

Sodium Glucose Cotransporter Inhibitors (SGLT2 Inhibitors)

The kidney plays an important role in glucose homeostasis. All plasma glucose is filtered into the renal tubules and must be reabsorbed into the plasma. The nephrons reabsorb all filtered glucose through two types of sodium-glucose cotransporters (SGLT1 and SGLT2) unless the plasma glucose reaches a threshold of approximately 180 mg/dL. In the diabetic, plasma glucose often reaches levels above that threshold, and the urine will then contain glucose. This is called glycosuria, and it is a classic sign of diabetes. As a matter of fact, increased excretion of glucose upregulates SGLTs, enhancing, in a negative way, the plasma levels of glucose by as much as 20% in the diabetic patient.[115]

There are several SGLT transporters; however, the major types are SGLT1 and SGLT2. SGLT2 is expressed in the epithelial cells of the brush border of S1 and S2 segments of the renal tubule. SGLT1 is expressed primarily in the small intestines. SGLT2 reabsorbs 80%-90% of filtered glucose, whereas the remainder is reabsorbed by SGLT1 in the small intestines. It follows that inhibiting SGLT2 reabsorption of glucose can provide a reduction of hyperglycemia in the diabetic. SGLT2 is a transmembrane protein consisting of 672 amino acids arranged in 14 transmembrane (TM) α-helices. TMs 4-7 and TMs 10-13 form a hydrophilic cavity that is involved in glucose (and other substrate) binding and transport. Glucose and the natural inhibitor phlorizin (Fig. 20.24) bind to Thr156 and Lys157 in TM 4.[116,117]

Table 20.9 Selected Pharmacokinetic Parameters of Dipeptidyl Peptidase-IV (DPP-IV) Inhibitors

Inhibitor	Bioavailability	Protein Binding	Metabolism
Sitagliptin (Januvia)	87%	38%	No significant metabolism. 79% excreted unchanged in urine; remainder in feces
Linagliptin (Tradjenta)	30%	70-80%	No significant metabolism. 90% excreted unchanged; 80% in feces; remainder in urine
Saxagliptin (Onglyza)	67%	<10%	50% of absorbed dose metabolized by CYP3A4 yielding an active metabolite
Valdagliptin (Galvus)	90%	<10%	No significant metabolism. Elimination half-life of ~90 min
Alogliptin (Nesina)	63%	NS	Minimal metabolism (10-20%) to inactive metabolites. 63% excreted unchanged in urine

The development of SGLT2 inhibitors was based on the discovery that phlorizin, a glycoside isolated from the bark of the apple tree, increased the amount of glucose in the urine. It was not a good drug candidate since it was quickly hydrolyzed by β-glucosidases in the GI tract. However, it served as a basis for the development of stable glycosides for the inhibition of SGLT2. Phlorizin's aglycone moiety is a 2,4,6-trihydroxyphenyl with a phenyl propanone moiety at position one and the glycoside as a substituent on the 6-hydroxy group. The challenge was to develop structures that were not easily hydrolyzed by β-glucosidases in the gut. This was accomplished by changing the O-glycoside linkage to a C-glycoside linkage, providing the gliflozin pharmacophore. The aglycone portion of this pharmacophore consists of an aryl moiety linked to a benzyl group (Fig. 20.24). To date, there are four SGLT2 inhibitors approved for the treatment of type 2 diabetes: canagliflozin, dapagliflozin, empagliflozin, and ertugliflozin (Fig. 20.24). Collectively, they are called the "gliflozins."[118]

CANAGLIFLOZIN. Canagliflozin was approved by the FDA in 2013. It has a 65% bioavalability with a T_{max} of 1-2 hours. It is highly bound to plasma protein (99%). The $t_{1/2}$ is between 10.6 and 13 hours depending on the dose. Its elimination via the feces consists of 41.5% unchanged, 7%

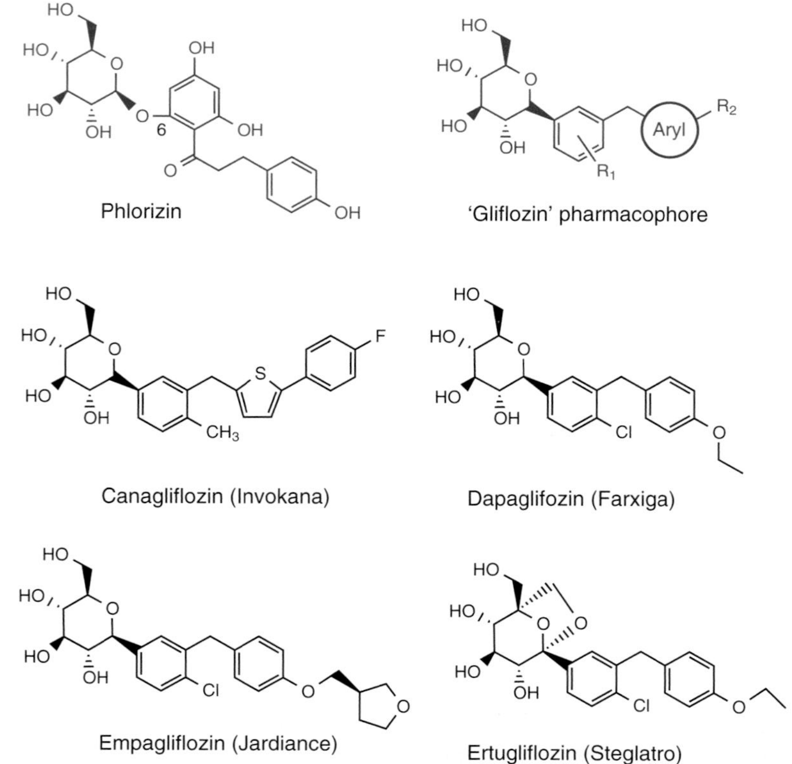

Figure 20.24 Structures of phlorizin, gliflozin pharmacophore, and currently marketed SGLT2 inhibitors.

as a hydroxylated metabolite, and 3.2% as O-glucuronides (Fig. 20.25). Canagliflozin is also eliminated in the urine (30.5%) as O-glucuronide with <1% as unchanged drug. It is metabolized by both UGT1A9 (uridine glucuronyltransferase) and UGT2B4. In addition, it is metabolized to a minor degree by CYP3A4.[119] It is available in tablet and extended release tablets for monotherapy, as well as in fixed combination with metformin hydrochloride.[120]

DAPAGLIFLOZIN. Dapagliflozin was approved by the FDA in 2014. It binds well to plasma proteins (91%) and has an 80% bioavailability with a T_{max} of 1-2 hours. Its mean plasma half-life is 12.9 hours with a 118 L volume of distribution. Dapagliflozin is extensively metabolized, with 73.7% recovered in excretia (72.0% in urine and 1.65% in feces). Metabolic routes included glucuronidation (UGT1A9), dealkylation, and oxidation at various positions to produce desmethyldapagliflozin glucuronides. The major metabolite is 3-O-glucuronide (60.7%), which is eliminated via the kidney. The 2-O-glucuronide was the only other urinary metabolite (Fig. 20.25). As with canagliflozin, dapagliflozin is available in fixed combination tablets with metformin hydrochloride. In 2017, the FDA approved a fixed combination of dapagliflozin with saxaglitin.[120,121]

EMPAGLIFLOZIN. Also in 2014, the FDA approved emagliflozin for the treatment of type 2 diabetes as either monotherapy or in combination with other oral hypoglycemic drugs. It has good selectivity for the SGLT2 receptor (>2500-fold compared to SGLT1). Empagliflozin is 86% protein bound with 60% oral bioavailability. Its mean plasma half-life is 13.1 hours with renal excretion as three major glucuronides (2-O-, 3-O- and 6-O-glucuronide). Glucuronidation occurs via a number of UGTs, including UGT2B7, UGT1A3, UGT1A8, and UGT1A9 (Fig. 20.25). Administered radioactive empagliflozin was recovered in the feces (41% unchanged) and the urine (54%) with about half the radioactivity in the urine as unmetabolized drug.[122] Empagliflozin is also approved for use in fixed combination with metformin and linagliptin.[120]

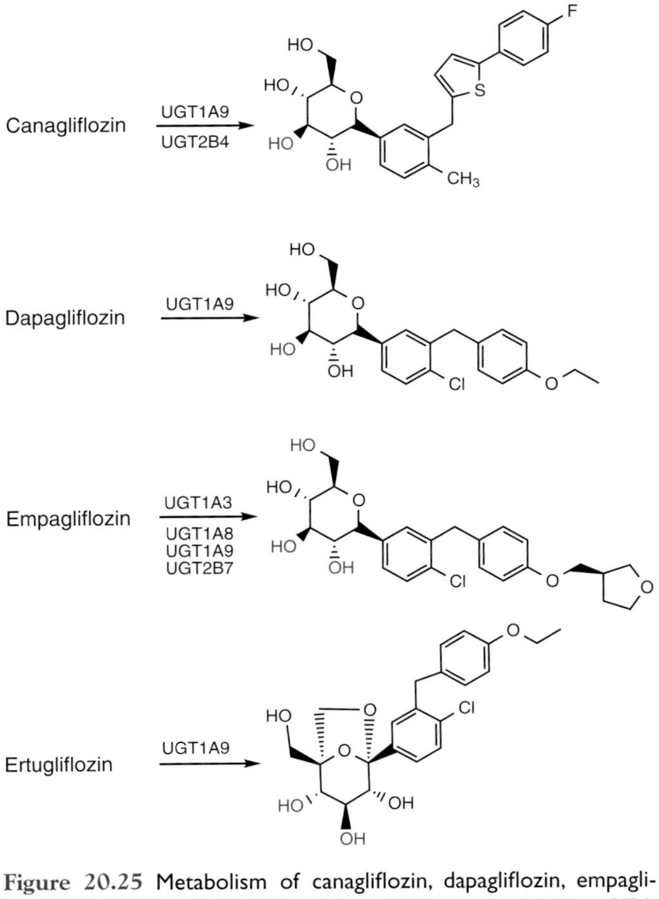

Figure 20.25 Metabolism of canagliflozin, dapagliflozin, empagliflozin, and ertugliflozin by uridine glucuronyltransferases (UGTs). Hydroxyl groups in red denote sites for glucuronidation.

ERTUGLIFLOZIN. The newest glifozin to enter the market is ertugliflozin. The FDA approved it in late 2017 for use as monotherapy and as a fixed dose combination with both metformin and sitagliptin. Ertugliflozin is a new structural class of SGLT2 inhibitors incorporating a unique dioxa-bicyclo[3.2.1]octane ring system (Fig. 20.24). It is highly selective for the SGLT2 receptor (>2000-fold compared to SGLT1) and comparable to empaglifozin in its SGLT2 inhibiting action. It demonstrates good concentration-dependent glycosuria after oral administration. Plasma levels peak one hour after the administration of a single oral dose with an elimination half-life of 17 hours, making once daily dosing possible. It is 94% bound to plasma protein and, like the other gliflozins, is metabolized by glucuronidation of the hydroxyl groups on the sugar moiety. The two predominant glucuronides are 4-O-glucuronide and 3-O-glucuronide, generated by UGT1A9 (Fig. 20.25). The oxidative pathway through CYP isoforms plays a minor role, yielding monohydroxylated metabolites and a desethyl ertugliflozin.[118]

THE ROLE OF SGLT2 INHIBITORS IN THE TREATMENT OF TYPE 2 DIABETES. Clinical data have shown that SGLT2 inhibitors are effective as monotherapy. Metformin is the drug of choice for treating diabetics who cannot reduce their A1C <7 with diet, weight loss, and exercise (Fig. 20.7). This relegates the monotherapy role of the SGLT2 inhibitors for patients who cannot tolerate metformin. SGLT2 inhibitors are also effective as an add-on to any of the other oral hypoglycemics and insulin. When administered once daily, they are well tolerated and do not have any relevant drug-drug interactions. They have a unique mechanism of action since they are insulin independent, which not only promotes reduction in plasma glucose but also contributes to weight loss, an improvement in blood pressure, and a low risk of hypoglycemia. This makes them a good choice as an add-on medication for treating obese and/or hypertensive type 2 diabetics. Since the SGLT2 drugs are relatively new to the clinical arena, the data on long-term safety are lacking. Therefore, as their use increases, postmarket surveillance will increase our knowledge in this area.[123]

Miscellaneous Drugs for the Treatment of Type 2 Diabetes

BROMOCRYPTINE. Bromocriptine is a dopamine D_2 receptor agonist. It is a structural analogue of ergotamine

(Fig. 20.26), and it is primarily used to treat Parkinson's disease (Chapter 10). It has a unique mechanism for the treatment of type 2 diabetes since it does not have a specific receptor that mediates its action on glucose and lipid metabolism. Bromocriptine's mechanism of action is believed to augment low hypothalamic dopamine levels and inhibit excessive sympathetic tone within the central nervous system. This reduction results in a decrease in postprandial plasma glucose levels due to enhanced suppression of hepatic glucose production (glycogenolysis).

Bromocriptine is administered as the mesylate salt. It is rapidly absorbed within 30 minutes, and its maximum plasma concentration is reached in 60 minutes. Food delays absorption, and there is extensive first-pass metabolism, with only 5%-10% of the oral dose being bioavailable. It is highly protein bound with an elimination half-life of about 6 hours. It is metabolized in the liver to 20-30 metabolites, and 98% of the oral dose is excreted via the bilary route. Adverse effects are common and dose related. Weakness, depression, and hypotension are frequently observed, along with nausea, vomiting, and diarrhea. Bromocriptine has major drug-drug interacts with 68 drugs, and most importantly, its effect is additive when used in conjunction with antihypertensive agents.[124]

Bile Acid Sequestrants (BAS). Colesevalam was found to improve plasma glucose control in data from clinical trials for lipid lowering in type 2 diabetics with hypercholesterolemia. The exact mechanism on how colesevelam regulates plasma glucose levels is not clearly understood. It is postulated that colesevelam has effects on the farnesoid X receptor (FXR or BAS receptor) that may ultimately reduce endogenous glucose production. The FXR is a nuclear receptor found in the liver and intestines. The bile acids are natural ligands for FXR. When activated, FXR translocates to the cell's nucleus, forms a dimer (RXR), and binds to hormone response elements on the DNA. This causes either increases or decreases in gene expression (Chapter 7). Colesevelam may also affect the secretion of incretin hormones GLP-1 and GIP, as levels were found to increase in patients administered 1.5 g/d.

Ergotamine

Bromocriptine

Figure 20.26 Comparison of the structure of bromocriptine to the ergot alkaloid ergotamine. Differences highlighted in red.

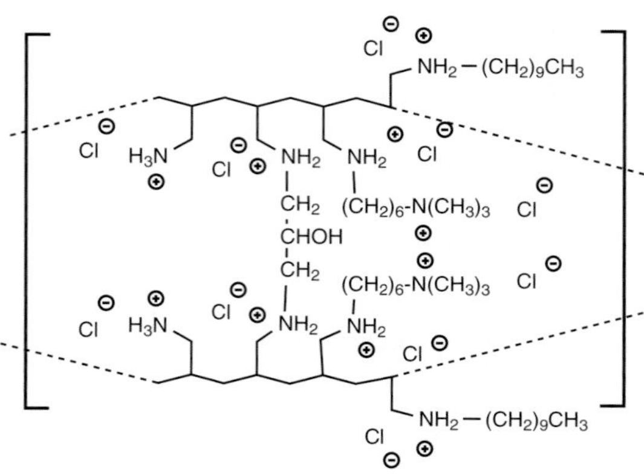

Colesevelam

In patients with type 2 diabetes, colesevlam consistently reduced A1C by ~0.4% when coadministered to patients taking metformin, sulfonylureas, or insulin.[125]

Drugs in Development

Protein Tyrosine Phosphatase 1B (PTP1B) Inhibitors. Protein tyrosine phosphatase 1B (PTP1B) and its potential role in the treatment of type 2 diabetes was first discovered in 1999 in mice lacking the PTP1B gene. Studies using the PTP1B knockout mice demonstrated enhanced sensitivity to insulin due to prolonged phosphorylation of the insulin receptor (IR). A lack of PTP1B activity is also associated with increased glucose clearance in both glucose and insulin tolerance tests, as well as a decrease in plasma insulin levels. In addition, mice lacking the *PTP1B* gene were resistant to weight gain when placed on a high-fat diet, and no increase in total plasma triglycerides or cholesterol levels were detected.[126,127] Since then, PTP1B has become an attractive, novel drug target for the development of potent and selective inhibitors for the treatment of both type 2 diabetes and obesity.[128,129]

The PTPs belong to a superfamily of enzymes that catalyze protein tyrosine dephosphorylation. The importance of this class of enzymes is that they act as modulators in various signal transduction pathways.[130] There are currently 38 PTPs, and as the name suggests, they target proteins containing phosphotyrosine (pTyr). PTPs also have dual specificity and recognize proteins that contain phosphothreonine (pThr), phosphoserine (pSer), as well as pTyr residues.[129,130]

PTP1B belongs to the subclass of classical pTyr-specific PTPs. It is universally expressed and is found in insulin-targeted tissues including the liver, muscle, and fat. PTP1B plays an important role in the regulation of signal transduction networks. These signaling pathways are regulated by protein tyrosine kinases (PTKs) that catalyze the tyrosine phosphorylation cascade, a major posttranslational modification process utilized by cells. In order to counterbalance the kinases, the PTPs are responsible for dephosphorylation processes that control the rate and duration of a particular response. Therefore, both the PTKs and PTPs are equally important in signaling pathways, and an imbalance or defective operation of these networks can cause abnormal Tyr phosphorylation. The consequence is often seen by the development of human diseases.[131]

Type 2 diabetics have an inability to propagate the insulin signaling pathway, which results in insulin resistance.[127,131] One possible explanation for insulin resistance would be abnormalities of the insulin signaling events downstream from the receptor. In the complex insulin signaling pathway, PTP1B participates by dephosphorylating the Tyr residues on the activated β subunit of the insulin receptor (IR), as well as dephosphorylating the IRSs.[132] PTP1B acts as a negative regulator in the insulin signal transduction pathway[133]; in fact, an overexpression of PTP1B has been shown to cause a decrease in the insulin-stimulated pathway and thus contributes to diabetes and obesity. Inhibition of PTP1B activity would prove to be advantageous in augmenting insulin-initiated signaling events; therefore, there is interest in development of PTP1B inhibitors as a potential treatment for type 2 diabetes.

Numerous PTP1B inhibitors have been synthesized with the hope of developing treatments for type 2 diabetes and obesity. Figure 20.27 shows the variety of chemical structures of some PTP1B inhibitors in development.[132] Designing effective PTP1B inhibitors poses multiple challenges to drug development. The first and major challenge is that, in order to design selective active site–directed compounds, they must mimic the negatively charged pTyr residues. Highly charged molecules rarely make good drug candidates, primarily, because they demonstrate inferior pharmacokinetics and are poorly absorbed and distributed in the body. Fortunately, research has discovered that the active site of PTP1B contains subpockets (allosteric sites) that can be targeted for inhibitor development. This has led to the concept known as bidentate ligand binding, which aims to design inhibitors that bind to both the active site and a unique adjacent peripheral site. The bioavailability issue has been addressed either by charge reduction, increasing the molecule's hydrophobicity, or by targeting the subpocket sites only.[130]

The development of PTP1B inhibitors continues to be an active area of research. Although, as far as we know, there are no compounds in clinical trials, it is most likely that effective PTP1B-selective inhibitors with improved pharmacokinetics will be developed in the near future.[134]

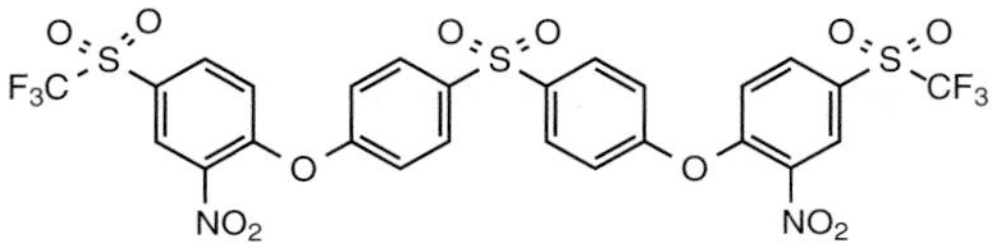

Trifluoromethyl sulfonyl derivatives (IC_{50}=400nM)

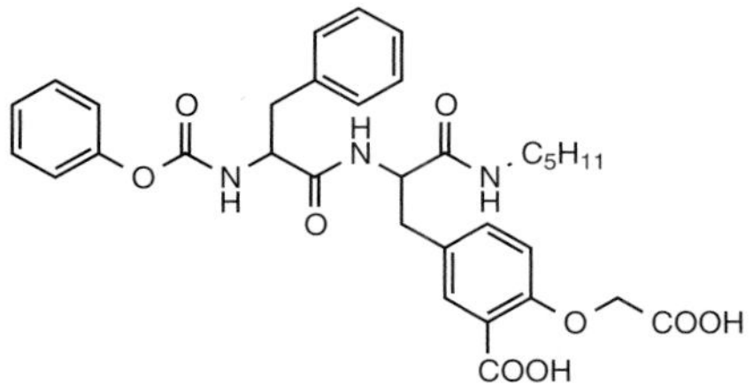

3'-Carboxy-4'-(O-carboxymethyl)tyrosine derivative (Ki = 870nM)

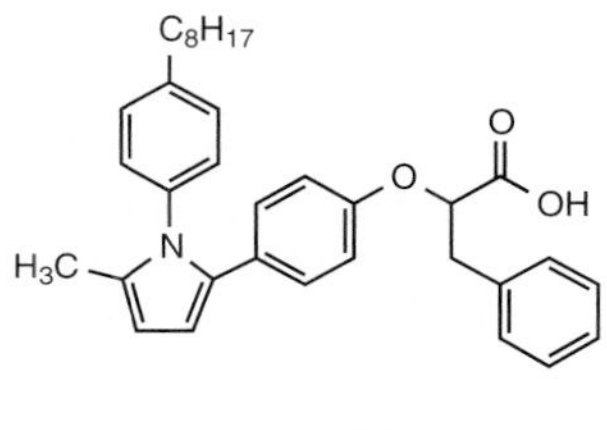

Pyrrole phenoxy proprionic acid derivative (IC_{50}=90nM)

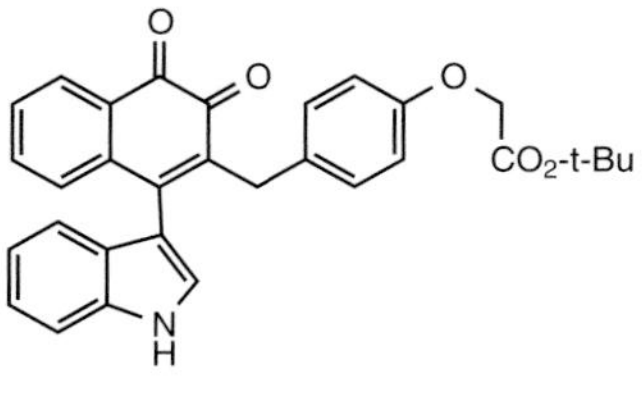

1,2-Naphthoquinone derivative (IC_{50}=650nM)

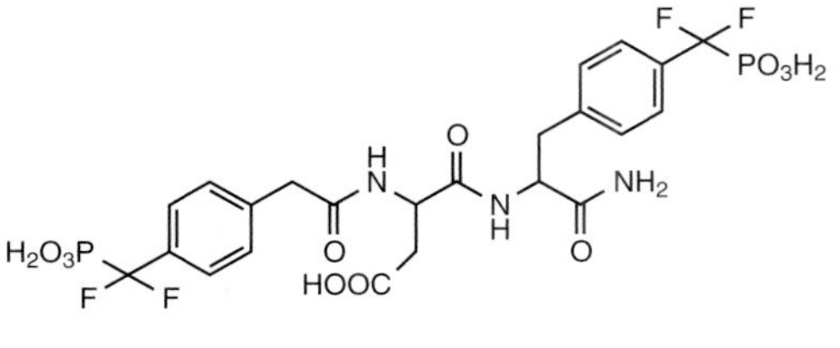

4'-Phosphonyldifluoromethyl-phenylalanine derivative (Ki=2.4nM)

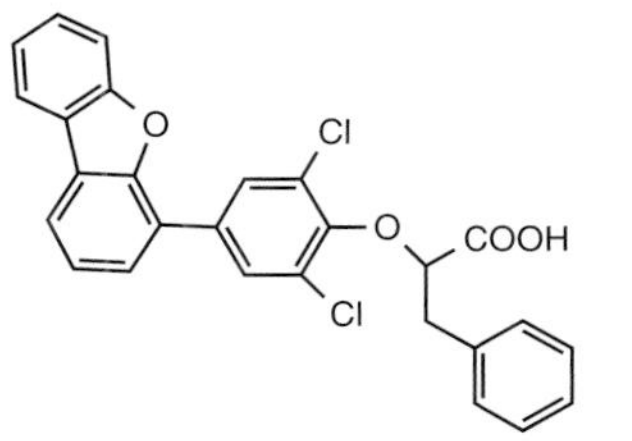

4-Dichlorophenyloxy-dibenzofuran derivative (IC_{50}=14uM)

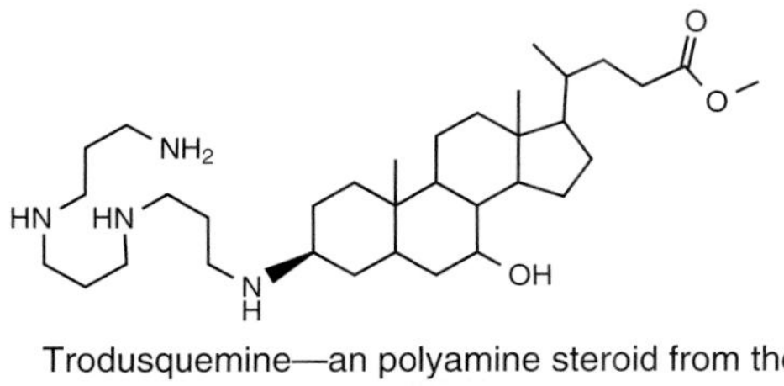

Trodusquemine—an polyamine steroid from the dogfish shark

Figure 20.27 Structures of some PTP1B inhibitors in development.[134]

Structure Challenge

Use your knowledge of drug pharmacophores presented in this chapter to identify the agent that would be most appropriate for use in each patient situation given below.

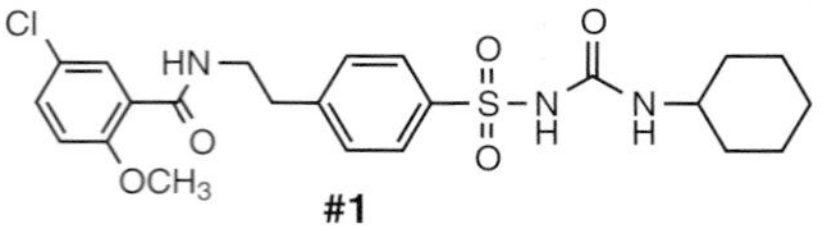

#1 #2 #3

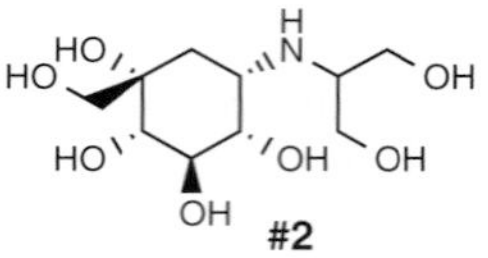

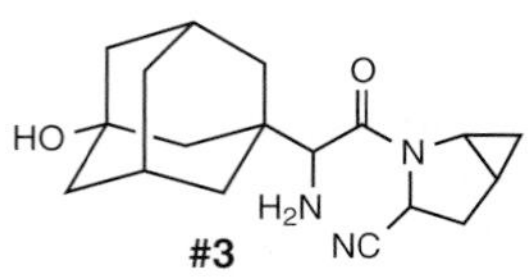

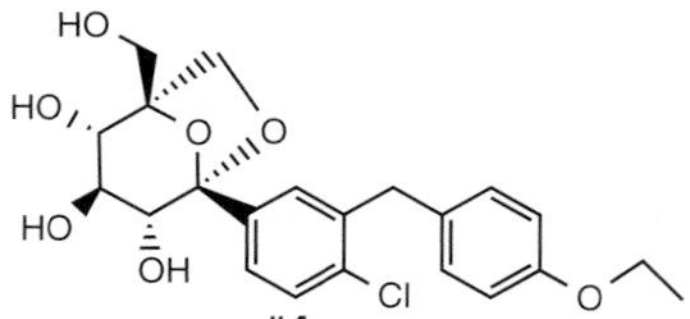

#4 #5

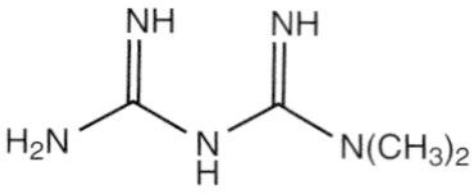

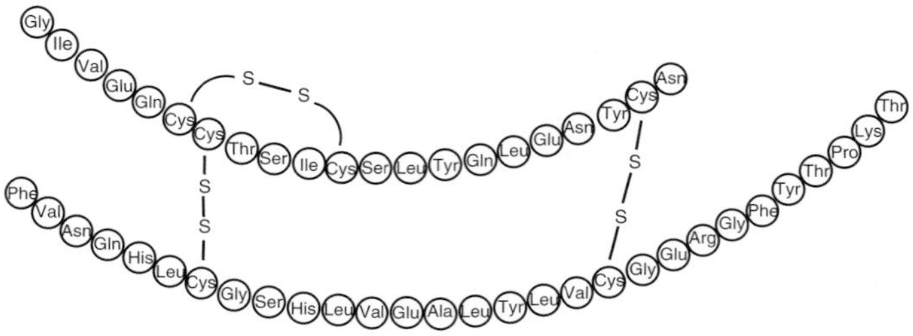

#6

A. A newly diagnosed patient with type 2 diabetes advised to make lifestyle changes would most likely be prescribed with which structure?

B. A patient is unable to decrease his or her A1C below 8.5 with lifestyle changes and metformin. Which structure would be added to his or her drug regimen?

C. Which structure could be added as triple therapy for a patient who is unable to decrease A1C below 7 with current therapy that includes metformin and a DPP IV inhibitor?

D. A patient who is on metformin needs a second oral hypoglycemic, but cannot tolerate pioglitazone, sulfonylureas, DPP IV inhibitors, and SGLT2 inhibitors. Which structure could be used?

E. A patient requires a third oral hypoglycemic added to his or her regimen of metformin and a GLP-1 agonist, but is reluctant to start injecting insulin. Which structure would be contraindicated?

F. Which of the above structures is the only class of oral hypoglycemics that can be a third addition to a therapeutic regimen no matter which combination of dual therapy the patient is on?

Structure challenge answers found immediately after References.

REFERENCES

1. Loriaux DL. Diabetes and the Ebers Papyrus: 1552 B.C. *The Endocrinologist*. 2006;16:55-56.
2. Karamanou M, Protogerou A, Tsoucalas G, et al. Milestones in the history of diabetes mellitus: the main contributors. *World J Diabetes*. 2016;7:1-7.
3. Carpenter S, Rigaud M, Barile M, et al. Possibly having to do with diabetes mellitus. *Annandale Hudson NY Bard Coll*. 2006;22.
4. Farmer L. Notes on the history of diabetes mellitus. *Bull NY Acad Med*. 1952;28:408-416.
5. Karamitsos DT. The story of Insulin discovery. *Diabetes Res Clin Pract*. 2011;93:S2-S8.
6. Sanger F, Tuppy H. The amino-acid sequence in the phenylalanyl chain of insulin. 1. The identification of lower peptides from partial hydrolysates. *Biochem J*. 1951;49:463-481.
7. Sanger F, Tuppy H. The amino-acid sequence in the phenylalanyl chain of insulin. 2. The investigation of peptides from enzymic hydrolysates. *Biochem J*. 1951;49:481-490.
8. Katsoyannis PG, Tometsko A, Fukuda K. Insulin peptides. IX. The synthesis of the A-chain of insulin and its combination with natural B-chain to generate insulin activity. *J Am Chem Soc*. 1963;85:2863-2865.
9. Auguste L. The hypoglycemic sulfonamides: history and development of the problem from 1942 to 1955. *Ann NY Acad Sci*. 2007;71:4-11.
10. IDF Diabetes Atlas. http://www.diabetesatlas.org/. Accessed 28 March 2018.
11. Triplitt CL, Repas T, Alvarez C. Chapter 74 diabetes mellitus. In: *Pharmacotherapy: A Pathophysiologic Approach*. New York, NY: McGraw-Hill Education; 2017. accesspharmacy.mhmedical.com/content.aspx?aid=1148576724.

12. Menke A, Orchard TJ, Imperatore G, et al. The prevalence of type 1 diabetes in the United States. *Epidemiol Camb Mass.* 2013;24:773-774.
13. Symptoms and Diagnosis of Metabolic Syndrome. http://www.heart.org/HEARTORG/Conditions/More/MetabolicSyndrome/Symptoms-and-Diagnosis-of-Metabolic-Syndrome_UCM_301925_Article.jsp#.Wrvpda3_mi4. Accessed 28 March 2018.
14. Huang PL. A comprehensive definition for metabolic syndrome. *Dis Model Mech.* 2009;2:231-237.
15. Morigny M, Houssier M, Mouisel E, et al. Adipocyte lipolysis and insulin resistance. *Biochimie.* 2016;125:259-266.
16. Walker R, William JS, Egede LE. Influence of race, ethnicity and social determinants of health on diabetes outcomes. *Am J Med Sci.* 2016;351:366-373.
17. Centers for Disease Control and Prevention. *National Diabetes Fact Sheet: National Estimates and General Information on Diabetes and Prediabetes in the United States*; 2011:12.
18. WHO. WHO | About Diabetes. http://www.who.int/diabetes/action_online/basics/en/index2.html. Accessed 28 March 2018.
19. American Diabetes Association. Classification and diagnosis of diabetes. *Diabetes Care.* 2017;40:S11-S24.
20. Marin-Penalver JJ, Martin-Timon I, Sevillano-Collantes C. Update on the treatment of type 2 diabetes mellitus. *World J Diabetes.* 2016;7:354-395.
21. Helms R, Quan DJ, Herfindal ET, et al. *Textbook of Therapeutics. Drug and Disease Management.* 8th ed. Lippincott Williams & Wilkins; 2006.
22. Yamazaki Y, Harada S, Tokuyama S. Sodium–glucose transporter as a novel therapeutic target in disease. *Eur J Pharmacol.* 2018;822:25-31.
23. Mueckler M, Thorens B. The SLC2 (GLUT) family of membrane transporters. *Mol Aspects Med.* 2013;34:121-138.
24. Kido Y, Nakae J, Accili D. Clinical review 125: the insulin receptor and its cellular targets. *J Clin Endocrinol Metab.* 2001;86:972-979.
25. Haeusler RA, McGraw TE, Accili D. Biochemical and cellular properties of insulin receptor signalling. *Nat Rev Mol Cell Biol.* 2018;19:31-44.
26. Atkinson MA, Eisenbart GS. Type 1 diabetes: new perspectives on disease pathogenesis and treatment. *Lancet.* 2001;358:221-229.
27. Paschou SA, Papadopoulou-Marketou N, Chrousos GP, et al. On type 1 diabetes mellitus pathogenesis. *Endocr Connect.* 2017;7:R38-R46.
28. Moneva MH, Dagogo-Jack S. Multiple drug targets in the management of type 2 diabetes. *Curr Drug Targets.* 2002;3:203-221.
29. Curtis T, Alison W, Elaine C. Incretin mimetics and dipeptidyl peptidase-IV inhibitors: potential new therapies for type 2 diabetes mellitus. *Pharmacother J Hum Pharmacol Drug Ther.* 2012;26:360-374.
30. 390 Drugs That Can Affect Blood Glucose Levels: Cause Hyperglycemia, Hypoglycemia, or Mask Hypoglycemia. Diabetes In Control. A Free Weekly Diabetes Newsletter for Medical Professionals; 2018. http://www.diabetesincontrol.com/drugs-that-can-affect-blood-glucose-levels/. Accessed 29 March 2018.
31. Nathan DM, DCCT/EDIC Research Group. The diabetes control and complications trial/epidemiology of diabetes interventions and complications study at 30 years: overview. *Diabetes Care.* 2014;37:9-16.
32. American Diabetes Association. Cardiovascular disease and risk management. *Diabetes Care.* 2017;40:S75-S87.
33. American Diabetes Association. Microvascular complications. *Diabetes Care.* 2017;40:S88-S98.
34. Brownlee M. The pathological implications of protein glycation. *Clin Investig Med Med Clin Exp.* 1995;18:275-281.
35. Brownlee M. Biochemistry and molecular cell biology of diabetic complications. *Nature.* 2001;414:813-820.
36. Lee AY, Chung SS. Contributions of polyol pathway to oxidative stress in diabetic cataract. *FASEB J.* 1999;13:23-30.
37. Degenhardt TP, Thorpe SR, Baynes JW. Chemical modification of proteins by methylglyoxal. *Cell Mol Biol Noisy.* 1998;44:1139-1145.
38. Xia P, Inoguchi T, Kern TS, et al. Characterization of the mechanism for the chronic activation of diacylglycerol-protein kinase C pathway in diabetes and hypergalactosemia. *Diabetes.* 1994;43:1122-1129.
39. Brownlee M. The pathobiology of diabetic complications: a unifying mechanism. *Diabetes.* 2005;54:1615-1625.
40. Bergenstal RM, Bailey CJ, Kendall DM. Type 2 diabetes: assessing the relative risks and benefits of glucose-lowering medications. *Am J Med.* 2010;123:374. e9-18.
41. Qaseem A, Barry MJ, Humphrey LL, et al. Oral pharmacologic treatment of type 2 diabetes mellitus: a clinical practice guideline update from the American College of physicians. *Ann Intern Med.* 2017;166: 279-290.
42. American Diabetes Association. Glycemic targets: standards of medical care in diabetes—2018. *Diabetes Care.* 2018;41:S55-S64.
43. American Diabetes Association. Lifestyle management: standards of medical care in diabetes—2018. *Diabetes Care.* 2018;41:S38-S50.
44. Fox CS, Golden SH, Anderson C, et al. Update on prevention of cardiovascular disease in adults with type 2 diabetes mellitus in light of recent evidence: a scientific statement from the American heart association and the American diabetes association. *Diabetes Care.* 2015;38:1777-1803.
45. Pontiroli AE, Folli F, Paganelli M, et al. Laparoscopic gastric banding prevents type 2 diabetes and arterial hypertension and induces their remission in morbid obesity: a 4-year case-controlled study. *Diabetes Care.* 2005;28:2703-2709.
46. American Diabetes Association. Pharmacologic approaches to glycemic treatment. *Diabetes Care.* 2017;40:S64-S74.
47. Kahn CR, Roth J. Berson, Yalow, and the JCI: the agony and the ecstasy. *J Clin Invest.* 2004;114:1051-1054.
48. Weiss M, Steiner DF, Philipson LH. Insulin biosynthesis, secretion, structure, and structure-activity relationships. In: De Groot LJ, Chrousos G, Dungan K, et al, eds. *Endotext.* South Dartmouth, MA: MDText.com, Inc.; 2000. http://www.ncbi.nlm.nih.gov/books/NBK279029/. Accessed 30 March 2018.
49. Aguilar-Bryan L, Clement JP, Gonzalez G, et al. Toward understanding the assembly and structure of KATP channels. *Physiol Rev.* 1998;78:227-245.
50. Ish-Shalom D, Christoffersen CT, Vorwerk P, et al. Mitogenic properties of insulin and insulin analogues mediated by the insulin receptor. *Diabetologia.* 1997;40:S25-S31.
51. Peyrot M, Bailey TS, Childs BP, et al. Strategies for implementing effective mealtime insulin therapy in type 2 diabetes. *Curr Med Res Opin.* 2018;34(6):1153-1162.
52. Insulin Analogues | NEJM. New England Journal of Medicine. http://www.nejm.org/doi/pdf/10.1056/NEJMra040832. Accessed 6 April 2018.
53. Jonassen I, Havelund S, Hoeg-Jensen T, et al. Design of the novel protraction mechanism of insulin degludec, an ultra-long-acting basal insulin. *Pharm Res.* 2012;29:2104-2114.
54. Zinman B, Fulcher G, Rao PV, et al. Insulin degludec, an ultra-long-acting basal insulin, once a day or three times a week versus insulin glargine once a day in patients with type 2 diabetes: a 16-week, randomised, open-label, phase 2 trial. *Lancet Lond Engl.* 2011;377:924-931.
55. Loubatières-Mariani M-M. The discovery of hypoglycemic sulfonamides. *J Soc Biol.* 2007;201:121-125.
56. Meglasson MD, Matschinsky FM. Pancreatic islet glucose metabolism and regulation of insulin secretion. *Diabetes Metab Rev.* 1986;2:163-214.
57. Martin GM, Kandasamy B, DiMaio F, et al. Anti-diabetic drug binding site in K channels revealed by Cryo-EM. *eLife.* 2017;6:e31054. doi:10.7554/eLife.31054.
58. Thisted H, Johnsen SP, Rungby J. Sulfonylureas and the risk of myocardial infarction. *Metab Clin Exp.* 2006;55:S16-S19.

59. Downey JM. An explanation for the reported observation that ATP dependent potassium channel openers mimic preconditioning. *Cardiovasc Res*. 1993;27:1565.
60. Malaisse WJ. Stimulation of insulin release by non-sulfonylurea hypoglycemic agents: the meglitinide family. *Horm Metab Res*. 1995;27:263-266.
61. Malaisse WJ. Pharmacology of the meglitinide analogs: new treatment options for type 2 diabetes mellitus. *Treat Endocrinol*. 2003;2:401-414.
62. Proks P, Reimann F, Green N, et al. Sulfonylurea stimulation of insulin secretion. *Diabetes NY*. 2002;51:S368-S376.
63. Chachin M, Yamada M, Fujita A, et al. Nateglinide, a D-phenylalanine derivative lacking either a sulfonylurea or benzamido moiety, specifically inhibits pancreatic beta-cell-type K(ATP) channels. *J Pharmacol Exp Ther*. 2003;304:1025-1032.
64. Weaver ML, Orwig BA, Rodriguez LC, et al. Pharmacokinetics and metabolism of nateglinide in humans. *Drug Metab Dispos*. 2001;29:415-421.
65. Lins L, Brasseur R, Malaisse WJ. Conformational analysis of non-sulfonylurea hypoglycemic agents of the meglitinide family. *Biochem Pharmacol*. 1995;50:1879-1884.
66. Adak T, Samadi A, Unal AU, et al. A reappraisal on metformin. *Regul Toxicol Pharmacol*. 2018;92:324-332.
67. Augusti KT, Sunil NP, Abraham A, et al. A comparative study on the effects of diet and exercise, metformin and metformin+pioglitazone treatment on NIDDM patients. *Indian J Clin Biochem*. 2007;22:65-69.
68. Bailey CJ. Biguanides and NIDDM. *Diabetes Care*. 1992;15:755-772.
69. Witters LA. The blooming of the French lilac. *J Clin Invest*. 2001;108:1105-1107.
70. Bolen S, Feldman L, Vassy J, et al. Systematic review: comparative effectiveness and safety of oral medications for type 2 diabetes mellitus. *Ann Intern Med*. 2007;147:386-399.
71. Gong L, Goswami S, Giacomini KM, et al. Metformin pathways: pharmacokinetics and pharmacodynamics. *Pharmacogenet Genomics*. 2012;22:820-827.
72. Weisberg LS. Lactic acidosis in a patient with type 2 diabetes mellitus. *Clin J Am Soc Nephrol*. 2015;10:1476-1483.
73. Monsalve FA, Pyarasani RD, Delgado-Lopez F, et al. Peroxisome proliferator-activated receptor targets for the treatment of metabolic diseases. *Mediators Inflamm*. 2013;2013:549627. doi:10.1155/2013/549627.
74. Schwartz S, Raskin P, Fonseca V, et al. Effect of troglitazone in insulin-treated patients with type II diabetes mellitus. Troglitazone and exogenous insulin study group. *N Engl J Med*. 1998;338:861-866.
75. Suter SL, Nolan JJ, Wallace P, et al. Metabolic effects of new oral hypoglycemic agent CS-045 in NIDDM subjects. *Diabetes Care*. 1992;15:193-203.
76. Parker JC. Troglitazone: the discovery and development of a novel therapy for the treatment of type 2 diabetes mellitus. *Adv Drug Deliv Rev*. 2002;54:1173-1197.
77. Yokoi T. Troglitazone. *Handb Exp Pharmacol*. 2010;(196):419-435.
78. Agrawal R. The first approved agent in the Glitazar's class: saroglitazar. *Curr Drug Targets*. 2014;15:151-155.
79. Cheng AY, Josse RG. Intestinal absorption inhibitors for type 2 diabetes mellitus: prevention and treatment. *Drug Discov Today Ther Strateg*. 2004;1:201-206.
80. Bell DSH. Type 2 diabetes mellitus: what is the optimal treatment regimen? *Am J Med*. 2004;116:23S-29S.
81. Inzucchi SE. Oral antihyperglycemic therapy for type 2 diabetes: scientific review. *JAMA*. 2002;287:360-372.
82. Emilien G, Maloteaux JM, Ponchon M. Pharmacological management of diabetes: recent progress and future perspective in daily drug treatment. *Pharmacol Ther*. 1999;81:37-51.
83. Borges de Melo E, Gomes AS, Carvalho I. α- and β-Glucosidase inhibitors: chemical structure and biological activity. *Tetrahedron*. 2006;62:10277-10302.
84. Platt FM, Butters TD. Substrate deprivation: a new therapeutic approach for the glycosphingolipid lysosomal storage diseases. *Expert Rev Mol Med*. 2000;2:1-17.
85. Holst JJ, Orskov C, Nielsen OV, et al. Truncated glucagon-like peptide I, an insulin-releasing hormone from the distal gut. *FEBS Lett*. 1987;211:169-174.
86. Perley MJ, Kipnis DM. Plasma insulin responses to oral and intravenous glucose: studies in normal and diabetic sujbjects. *J Clin Invest*. 1967;46:1954-1962.
87. Dupre J, Ross SA, Watson D, et al. Stimulation of insulin secretion by gastric inhibitory polypeptide in man. *J Clin Endocrinol Metab*. 1973;37:826-828.
88. Reimann F, Gribble FM. Glucose-sensing in glucagon-like peptide-1-secreting cells. *Diabetes*. 2002;51:2757-2763.
89. Deacon CF, Johnsen AH, Holst JJ. Degradation of glucagon-like peptide-1 by human plasma in vitro yields an N-terminally truncated peptide that is a major endogenous metabolite in vivo. *J Clin Endocrinol Metab*. 1995;80:952-957.
90. Mentlein R, Gallwitz B, Schmidt WE. Dipeptidyl-peptidase IV hydrolyses gastric inhibitory polypeptide, glucagon-like peptide-1(7-36)amide, peptide histidine methionine and is responsible for their degradation in human serum. *Eur J Biochem*. 1993;214:829-835.
91. Deacon CF, Knudsen LB, Madsen K, et al. Dipeptidyl peptidase IV resistant analogues of glucagon-like peptide-1 which have extended metabolic stability and improved biological activity. *Diabetologia*. 1998;41:271-278.
92. Buse JB, Henry RR, Han J, et al. Effects of exenatide (exendin-4) on glycemic control over 30 weeks in sulfonylurea-treated patients with type 2 diabetes. *Diabetes Care*. 2004;27:2628-2635.
93. Wang Q, Brubaker PL. Glucagon-like peptide-1 treatment delays the onset of diabetes in 8 week-old db/db mice. *Diabetologia*. 2002;45:1263-1273.
94. Elbrønd B, Jakobsen G, Larsen S, et al. Pharmacokinetics, pharmacodynamics, safety, and tolerability of a single-dose of NN2211, a long-acting glucagon-like peptide 1 derivative, in healthy male subjects. *Diabetes Care*. 2002;25:1398-1404.
95. Knudsen LB. Glucagon-like peptide-1: the basis of a new class of treatment for type 2 diabetes. *J Med Chem*. 2004;47:4128-4134.
96. Sturis J, Gotfredsen CF, Rømer J, et al. GLP-1 derivative liraglutide in rats with beta-cell deficiencies: influence of metabolic state on beta-cell mass dynamics. *Br J Pharmacol*. 2003;140:123-132.
97. Victoza-Product-Monograph.pdf. http://www.novonordisk.ca/content/dam/Canada/AFFILIATE/www-novonordisk-ca/OurProducts/PDF/victoza-product-monograph.pdf. Accessed 6 April 2018.
98. Lovshin JA. Glucagon-like Peptide-1 receptor agonists: a class update for treating type 2 diabetes. *Can J Diabetes*. 2017;41:524-535.
99. Glaesner W, Vick AM, Millican R, et al. Engineering and characterization of the long-acting glucagon-like peptide-1 analogue LY2189265, an Fc fusion protein. *Diabetes Metab Res Rev*. 2010;26:287-296.
100. Pratley RE, Nauck MA, Barnett AH, et al. Once-weekly albiglutide versus once-daily liraglutide in patients with type 2 diabetes inadequately controlled on oral drugs (HARMONY 7): a randomised, open-label, multicentre, non-inferiority phase 3 study. *Lancet Diabetes Endocrinol*. 2014;2:289-297.
101. Jensen L, Helleberg H, Roffel A, et al. Absorption, metabolism and excretion of the GLP-1 analogue semaglutide in humans and nonclinical species. *Eur J Pharm Sci*. 2017;104:31-41.
102. Rosenblum JS, Kozarich JW. Prolyl peptidases: a serine protease subfamily with high potential for drug discovery. *Curr Opin Chem Biol*. 2003;7:496-504.
103. Arulmozhiraja S, Matsuo N, Ishitsubo E, et al. Comparative binding analysis of dipeptidyl peptidase IV (DPP-4) with antidiabetic drugs – an Ab initio fragment molecular orbital study. *PLoS One*. 2016;11:e0166275.

104. Metzler WJ, Yanchunas J, Weigelt C, et al. Involvement of DPP-IV catalytic residues in enzyme–saxagliptin complex formation. *Protein Sci*. 2008;17:240-250.
105. Tahrani AA, Piya MK, Kennedy A, et al. Glycaemic control in type 2 diabetes: targets and new therapies. *Pharmacol Ther*. 2010;125:328-361.
106. Blech S, Ludwig-Schwellinger E, Gräfe-Mody EU, et al. The metabolism and disposition of the oral dipeptidyl peptidase-4 inhibitor, linagliptin, in humans. *Drug Metab Dispos*. 2010;38:667-678.
107. Christopher R, Covington P, Davenport, et al. Pharmacokinetics, pharmacodynamics, and tolerability of single increasing doses of the dipeptidyl peptidase-4 inhibitor alogliptin in healthy male subjects. *Clin Ther*. 2008;30:513-527.
108. FDA Advisory Committee Reviews Takeda's Alogliptin EXAMINE Cardiovascular Safety Outcomes Trial. https://www.takeda.com/newsroom/newsreleases/2015/fda-advisory-committee-reviews-takedas-alogliptin-examine–cardiovascular-safety-outcomes-trial/. Accessed 7 April 2018.
109. Ryan GJ, Jobe LJ, Martin R. Pramlintide in the treatment of type 1 and type 2 diabetes mellitus. *Clin Ther*. 2005;27:1500-1512.
110. Kruger DF, Gloster MA. Pramlintide for the treatment of insulin-requiring diabetes mellitus: rationale and review of clinical data. *Drugs*. 2004;64:1419-1432.
111. Heptulla RA, Rodriguez LM, Bomgaars L, et al. The role of amylin and glucagon in the dampening of glycemic excursions in children with type 1 diabetes. *Diabetes*. 2005;54:1100-1107.
112. Owen SK. Amylin replacement therapy in patients with insulin-requiring type 2 diabetes. *Diabetes Educ*. 2006;32:105S-110S.
113. Pullman J, Darsow T, Frias JP. Pramlintide in the management of insulin-using patients with type 2 and type 1 diabetes. *Vasc Health Risk Manag*. 2006;2:203-212.
114. Singh-Franco D, Robles G, Gazze D. Pramlintide acetate injection for the treatment of type 1 and type 2 diabetes mellitus. *Clin Ther*. 2007;29:535-562.
115. DeFronzo RA, Davidson JA, Del Prato S. The role of the kidneys in glucose homeostasis: a new path towards normalizing glycaemia. *Diabetes Obes Metab*. 2012;14:5-14.
116. Turk E, Wright EM. Membrane topology motifs in the SGLT cotransporter family. *J Membr Biol*. 1997;159:1-20.
117. Reja M, Kinne RK. Identification of phlorizin binding domains in sodium-glucose cotransporter family: SGLT1 as a unique model system. *Biochimie*. 2015;115:187-193.
118. Cinti F, Moffa S, Impronta F, et al. Spotlight on ertugliflozin and its potential in the treatment of type 2 diabetes: evidence to date. *Drug Des Devel Ther*. 2017;11:2905-2919.
119. Kalra S. Sodium glucose co-transporter-2 (SGLT2) inhibitors: a review of their basic and clinical pharmacology. *Diabetes Ther*. 2014;5:355-366.
120. Orange Book: Approved Drug Products with Therapeutic Equivalence Evaluations. https://www.accessdata.fda.gov/scripts/cder/ob/search_product.cfm. Accessed 10 April 2018.
121. Kasichayanula S, Liu X, LaCreta F, et al. Clinical pharmacokinetics and pharmacodynamics of dapagliflozin, a selective inhibitor of sodium-glucose co-transporter type 2. *Clin Pharmacokinet*. 2014;53:17-27.
122. Mondick J, Riggs M, Kaspers S, et al. Population pharmacokinetic-pharmacodynamic analysis to characterize the effect of empagliflozin on renal glucose threshold in patients with type 1 diabetes mellitus. *J Clin Pharmacol*. 2018;58:640-649. doi:10.1002/jcph.1051.
123. Solini A. Role of SGLT2 inhibitors in the treatment of type 2 diabetes mellitus. *Acta Diabetol Heidelb*. 2016;53:863-870.
124. DeFronzo RA. Bromocriptine: a sympatholytic, D2-dopamine agonist for the treatment of type 2 diabetes. *Diabetes Care*. 2011;34:789-794.
125. Handelsman Y. Role of bile acid sequestrants in the treatment of type 2 diabetes. *Diabetes Care*. 2011;34:S244-S250.
126. Rotella DP. Novel 'second-generation' approaches for the control of type 2 diabetes. *J Med Chem*. 2004;47:4111-4112.
127. Montalibet J, Kennedy B. Therapeutic strategies for targeting PTP1B in diabetes. *Drug Discov Today Ther Strateg*. 2005;2:129-135.
128. Tamrakar AK, Maurya CK, Rai AK. PTP1B inhibitors for type 2 diabetes treatment: a patent review (2011-2014). *Expert Opin Ther Pat*. 2014;24:1101-1115.
129. Koren S, Fantus IG. Inhibition of the protein tyrosine phosphatase PTP1B: potential therapy for obesity, insulin resistance and type-2 diabetes mellitus. *Best Pract Res Clin Endocrinol Metab*. 2007;21:621-640.
130. Zhang ZY. Protein tyrosine phosphatases: prospects for therapeutics. *Curr Opin Chem Biol*. 2001;5:416-423.
131. Saltiel AR, Kahn CR. Insulin signalling and the regulation of glucose and lipid metabolism. *Nature*. 2001;414:799-806.
132. Hooft van Huijsduijnen R, Bombrun A, Swinnen D. Selecting protein tyrosine phosphatases as drug targets. *Drug Discov Today*. 2002;7:1013-1019.
133. Patankar SJ, Jurs PC. Classification of inhibitors of protein tyrosine phosphatase 1B using molecular structure based descriptors. *J Chem Inf Comput Sci*. 2003;43:885-899.
134. Krishnan N, Konidaris KF, Gasser G, et al. A potent, selective, and orally bioavailable inhibitor of the protein-tyrosine phosphatase PTP1B improves insulin and leptin signaling in animal models. *J Biol Chem*. 2018;293:1517-1525.

Structure Challenge Answers

A-5; B-6; C-1; D-2; E-3; F-4.

CHAPTER 21

Drugs Used to Treat Inflammatory and Corticosteroid Deficiency Disorders

Michael L. Mohler, Ramesh Narayanan, and James T. Dalton

Drugs covered in this chapter:

GLUCOCORTICOSTEROIDS
- Betamethasone
- Dexamethasone
- Deflazacort
- Fludrocortisone
- Hydrocortisone and derivatives
- Methylprednisolone
- Prednisolone
- Prednisone
- Triamcinolone

GLUCOCORTICOSTEROIDS USED TOPICALLY OR FOR INHALATION
- Alclometasone dipropionate
- Amcinonide
- Beclomethasone dipropionate
- Budesonide
- Ciclesonide
- Clobetasol propionate
- Clocortolone pivalate
- Desonide
- Desoximetasone
- Diflorasone diacetate
- Flunisolide
- Fluocinolone acetonide
- Fluocinonide
- Fluorometholone
- Flurandrenolide
- Fluticasone propionate
- Halcinonide
- Halobetasol propionate
- Mometasone furoate
- Prednicarbate
- Triamcinolone acetonide

MINERALOCORTICOSTEROIDS
- Aldosterone
- 11-Desoxycorticosterone

ADRENOCORTICOID ANTAGONISTS
- Mifepristone
- Ulipristal
- Spironolactone
- Eplerenone
- Aminoglutethimide
- Metyrapone
- Trilostane

Abbreviations

17-BMP beclomethasone 17α-monopropionate
21-BMP beclomethasone 21-monopropionate
21-desDFZ 21-desacetyldeflazacort
11β-HSD1 type 1 11β-hydroxysteroid dehydrogenase
11β-HSD2 type 2 11β-hydroxysteroid dehydrogenase
17βHSD3 17β-hydroxysteroid dehydrogenase type 3
3β-HSD 5-ene-3β-hydroxysteroid dehydrogenase
ACTH adrenocorticotropic hormone
AKR1C3 aldoketoreductase type 1C3
AUC area under the plasma concentration over time curve
BDP beclomethasone dipropionate
cAMP cyclic adenosine monophosphate
CoA coactivator
CFC chlorofluorocarbon
COPD chronic obstructive pulmonary disease
CRF corticotropin-releasing factor
CYP11B2 11β-hydroxylase
CYP17 17α-hydroxylase
CYP21 21-hydroxylase
des-CIC desisobutyrylciclesonide
DHEA dehydroepiandrosterone
DHT dihydrotestosterone
DMD Duchenne muscular dystrophy
DPI dry powder inhaler
EDS exhalation delivery system
GI gastrointestinal
GR glucocorticoid receptor
HFA hydrofluoroalkane
HPA hypothalamic-pituitary-adrenal

Abbreviations—Continued

HRE hormone-responsive element
HSP heat shock protein
IL interleukin
IM intramuscular
IV intravenous
LABA long-acting β-adrenergic agonist
MR mineralocorticoid receptor
SAR structure-activity relationship
scc side chain cleavage
SGRM selective glucocorticoid receptor modulator
StAR steroidogenic acute regulatory protein

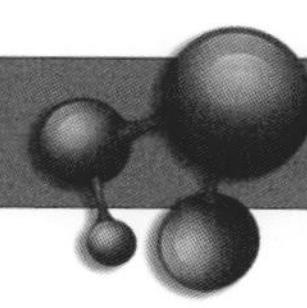

CLINICAL SIGNIFICANCE

Trisha D. Wells, PharmD

Corticosteroids are used regularly to treat a multitude of disorders and diseases. Treatments range from oral and parenteral therapies for various treatments, including hormone therapy and rheumatologic disorders, to inhaled steroids for respiratory conditions and topical steroids for allergies and dermatologic ailments. These corticosteroid therapies work very well for their intended purposes, and patients benefit greatly from their actions. The negative aspects to these therapies are their side effect profile and potential to cause long-term effects, such as diabetes and Cushing's syndrome when used for longer periods of time.

Prescribers and pharmacists alike must understand the different corticosteroid options available, their chemical structures, and subsequent actions on the body to be able to decide which options are best for the treatment needed. Usually the lowest effective dose used for the shortest effective time is the prudent use for many of these corticosteroid therapies. With a greater understanding of the properties of these medications, pharmacists and physicians can make the best informed decisions regarding appropriate route, administration, and duration of therapy for their patients while causing the least amount of adverse effects and interactions.

INTRODUCTION

The adrenal glands are flattened, caplike structures located above the kidneys. The inner core (medulla) of the gland secretes catecholamines, whereas the shell (cortex) of the gland synthesizes steroid hormones known as the adrenocorticoids. The adrenocorticoid steroids include the glucocorticoids, which regulate carbohydrate, lipid, and protein metabolism, and the mineralocorticoids, which influence salt balance and water retention. A third class of steroids produced by the adrenal glands is called the adrenal androgens, which have weak androgenic activity in men and women and can serve as precursors to the sex hormones, estrogens and androgens.

The adrenocorticoids and sex hormones have much in common. All are steroids; consequently, the rules that define their structures, chemistry, and nomenclature are the same. The rings of these biochemically dynamic and physiologically active compounds have a similar stereochemical relationship. Changes in the geometry of the ring junctures usually result in inactive compounds regardless of the biologic category of the steroid. Similar chemical groups are used to render some of these agents water soluble or active when taken orally or to modify their absorption.

In addition, the adrenocorticoids and the sex hormones, which include the estrogens, progestins, and androgens, are mainly biosynthesized from cholesterol, which in turn is synthesized from acetyl-coenzyme A. Cholesterol and steroid hormone catabolism takes place primarily in the liver. Although the products found in the urine and feces depend on the hormone undergoing catabolism, many of the metabolic reactions are similar for these compounds. For example, reduction of double bonds at positions 4 and 5 or 5 and 6, epimerization of 3α-hydroxyl groups, reduction of 3-keto groups to the 3α-hydroxyl function, and oxidative removal of side chains are transformations common to these agents.

The adrenocorticoids have many clinical uses. Glucocorticoids and mineralocorticoids may be used for the treatment of endocrine disorders such as adrenal insufficiency (hypoadrenalism), which results from failure of the adrenal glands to synthesize adequate amounts of the hormones. Major pharmacologic uses of glucocorticoids include the treatment of rheumatoid diseases and acute exacerbations of diseases of the gastrointestinal, nervous, or respiratory systems, symptomatic relief from asthma and allergic conditions, topical application for various dermatologic and ophthalmic diseases, and treatment of various hematologic disorders and cancers. Toxicities arise when corticosteroids are used for longer than brief periods, and toxic effects can include glucocorticoid-induced adrenocortical insufficiency, glucocorticoid-induced osteoporosis and diabetes, and generalized protein depletion. Knowledge of the numerous steroid products, structure-activity relationships, and available dosage forms is necessary in order to maximize the benefits of these drugs for patients and minimize troublesome toxicities.

Despite the similarities in chemical structures and stereochemistry, each class of steroids demonstrates unique and distinctively pleotropic biologic activities. Minor structural modifications to the steroid nucleus, such as changes in or insertion of functional groups at different positions, cause marked changes in physiologic activity. The first part of this chapter focuses on the similarities among the steroids and reviews steroid nomenclature, stereochemistry, and general mechanism of action. The second portion of the chapter focuses on the adrenocorticoids and discusses the biosynthesis, metabolism, medicinal chemistry, pharmacology, and pharmacokinetics of endogenous steroid hormones, synthetic agonists, and synthetic antagonists.

STEROID NOMENCLATURE AND STRUCTURE

Steroids consist of four fused rings (A, B, C, and D) (Fig. 21.1). Chemically, these hydrocarbons are cyclopentanoperhydrophenanthrenes; they contain a five-membered cyclopentane (D) ring plus the three rings of phenanthrene. A perhydrophenanthrene (rings A, B, and C) is the completely saturated derivative of phenanthrene. The polycyclic hydrocarbon known as cholestane will be used to illustrate the numbering system for a steroid (Fig. 21.1). The term "cholestane" refers to a steroid with 27 carbons that includes a side chain of eight carbons at position 17. Numbering begins in ring A at C1 and proceeds around rings A and B to C10, then into ring C beginning with C11, and snakes around rings C and D to C17. The angular methyl groups are numbered 18 (attached to C13) and 19 (attached to C10). Steroid chemists often refer to the series of carbon–carbon bonds from C1-C19 as the steroid backbone or template (Fig. 21.1). The 17-side chain begins with C20, and the numbering finishes in sequential order.

Using the rigid planar representation for drawing the steroid structure (Fig. 21.2A), the basic steroid structure becomes a plane with two surfaces: The top or β surface is pointing out toward the reader, and the bottom or α surface is pointing away from the reader. Hydrogens or functional groups on the β side of the molecule are denoted by solid lines; those on the α side are designated by dotted lines. The 5α notation is used to denote the configuration of the hydrogen atom at C5, which is opposite from the C19 angular methyl group, making the A/B ring juncture *trans* (Fig. 21.2B). The C19 angular methyl group is assigned the β side of the molecule. Similarly, the configuration of the 8β and 9α hydrogens (not shown), and the 14α hydrogen and C18 angular methyl group, denotes *trans* fusion for rings B/C and C/D. The side chains at position 17 are always β unless indicated by dotted lines or in the nomenclature of the steroid (e.g., 17β or 17α).

Cholestane is derived from cholesterol and can be 5α as in sex steroids or 5β as in cholic acids, with the α and β designations referring to the configuration of the hydrogen atom at C5. Just as cyclohexane can be drawn in a chair conformation, the three-dimensional representation for 5α-cholestane is shown by the following conformational formula (Fig. 21.2B). Although cyclohexane may undergo a flip in conformation, steroids are rigid structures with their cyclohexane rings locked into chair conformations. This is because they generally have at least one *trans* fused ring system, and these rings must be diequatorial to each other. In other words, the phenanthrene rings A-C are rigidly held in chair conformations.

If one is aware that the angular methyl groups at positions 18 and 19 are β and have an axial orientation (i.e., perpendicular to the plane of the rings), the conformational orientation of the remaining bonds of a steroid can be easily assigned. For example, in 5α-cholestane, the C19 methyl group attached at position 10 is always β-axial (βa; on the β-face of the steroid and oriented at a 90° angle to the plane of the steroid); the two bonds at position 3 must be β-equatorial (βe; on the β-face of the steroid and oriented at a slight angle to the plane of the steroid) and

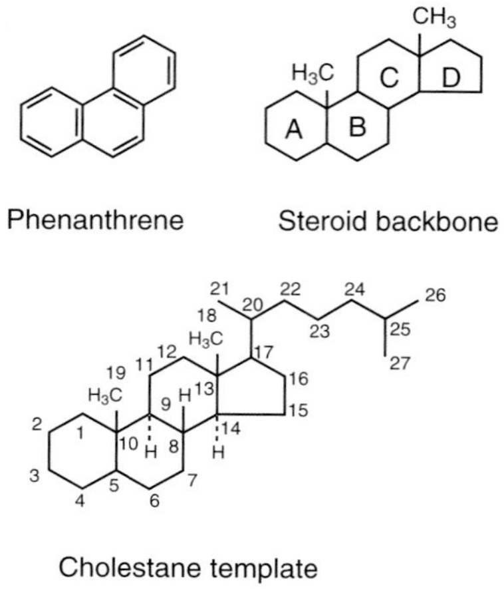

Figure 21.1 Basic steroid structure and numbering system.

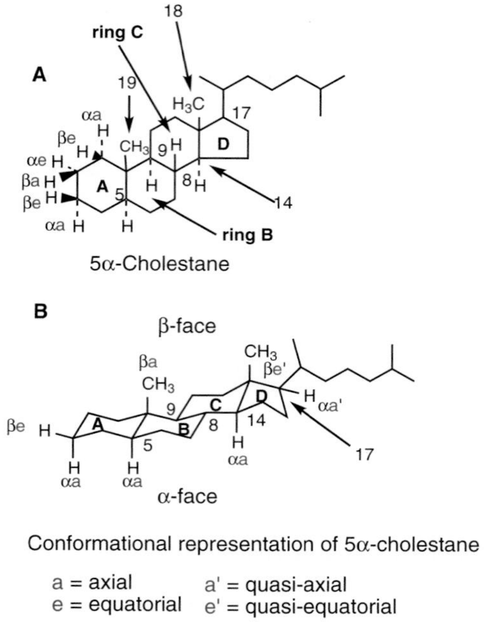

Figure 21.2 Planar (A) and conformational (B) structures of 5α-cholestane.

α-axial (αa), as indicated. The orientation of the remaining bonds on a steroid may be determined if one recalls that groups on a cyclohexane ring that are positioned on adjacent carbon atoms (vicinal, -C1H-C2H-) of the ring (i.e., 1,2 to each other) are *trans* if their relationship is 1,2-diaxial or 1,2-diequatorial and are *cis* if their relationship is 1,2-equatorial-axial.

The *cis* or *trans* relationship of the four rings may be expressed in terms of the steroid backbone. The compound 5α-cholestane (Fig. 21.2) is said to have a *trans-antitrans-antitrans* backbone. In this structure, all the fused rings have *trans* (diequatorial) stereochemistry; in other words, the A/B fused ring, the B/C fused ring, and the C/D fused ring are *trans*. The term *anti* is used in backbone notation to define the orientation of rings that are connected to each other and have a *trans*-type relationship. For example, the bond equatorial to ring B, at position 9, which forms part of ring C, is *anti* to the bond equatorial to ring B, at position 10, which forms part of ring A. 5β-Cholestane (Fig. 21.3) has a *cis-antitrans-antitrans* backbone in which the A/B rings are fused *cis*. The term *syn* is used in a similar fashion as *anti* to define a *cis*-type relationship. No natural steroids exist with a *syn*-type geometry, although such compounds can be chemically synthesized. Thus, the conventional drawing of the steroid nucleus is the natural configuration and does not show the hydrogens at 8β, 9α, or 14β positions. If the carbon at position 5 is saturated, the hydrogen is always drawn as either 5α or 5β. Also, the conventional drawing of a steroid molecule has the C18 and C19 methyl groups shown only as solid lines (no CH_3 drawn).

The stereochemistry of the rings markedly affects the biologic activity of a given class of steroids. Nearly all biologically active steroids have the cholestane-type backbone. For example, the active sex steroids are always the *trans*-configuration across the A-B ring system as seen in 5α-cholestane discussed below, while 5β-cholestanes, as seen in bile acids, are always inactive as sex steroids. In most of the important steroids discussed in this chapter, a double bond is present between positions 4 and 5 or 5 and 6; consequently, there is no *cis* or *trans* relationship between rings A and B. The symbol Δ is often used to designate a carbon–carbon double bond (C=C) in a steroid. If the C=C is between positions 4 and 5, the compound is referred to as a Δ^4-steroid. If the C=C bond is between positions 5 and 6, the compound is referred to as a Δ^5-steroid. If the C=C is between positions 5 and 10, the compound is designated a $\Delta^{5(10)}$-steroid.

Cholesterol (cholest-5-en-3α-ol) is a Δ^5-steroid or, more specifically, a Δ^5-sterol because it is an unsaturated alcohol (Fig. 21.4). Biologically active compounds include members of the 5α-pregnane, 5α-androstane, and 5α-estrane steroid classes (Fig. 21.4). Pregnanes are steroids with 21 carbon atoms. Androstanes contain 19 carbon atoms, and estranes contain 18 carbon atoms, with the C19 angular methyl group at C10 replaced by hydrogen. Numbering is the same as in 5α-cholestane.

The adrenocorticoids (adrenal cortex hormones) are pregnanes and are exemplified by the most potent endogenous glucocorticoid, cortisol (referred to hydrocortisone in medications), which is a 11β,17α,21-trihydroxypregn-4-ene-3,20-dione (Fig. 21.4). The most potent mineralocorticoid is aldosterone, which is a highly analogous pregnane that lacks the 17β-hydroxy and possesses an aldehyde functionality at C18 (Fig. 21.4). Progesterone (pregn-4-ene-3,20-dione), a female sex hormone synthesized by the corpus luteum, is also a pregnane analog. The male sex hormones (androgens) are based on the structure of 5α-androstane. Testosterone, an important and naturally occurring androgen, is named 17β-hydroxyandrost-4-en-3-one.

Dehydroepiandrosterone is the major adrenal androgen and is named 3β-hydroxyandrost-5-en-17-one (Fig. 21.4). The estrogens, exemplified by the major endogenous estrogen, 17β-estradiol, are female sex hormones synthesized by the Graafian follicle of the ovaries. These are estrane analogs containing an aromatic A ring. Although the A ring does not contain isolated C=C groups, these analogs are named as if the bonds were in the positions shown in 17β-estradiol. Hence, 17β-estradiol, a typical member of this class of drugs, is named estra-1,3,5(10)-triene-3,17β-diol. Other examples of steroid nomenclature are found throughout this chapter.

Aliphatic side chains at position 17 are always assumed to be β when cholestane or pregnane nomenclature is employed. Hence, the notation 17β need not be used when naming these compounds. If a pregnane has a 17α chain, however, this should be indicated in the nomenclature. Finally, the final "e" in the name for the parent steroid hydrocarbon is always dropped when it precedes a vowel, regardless of whether a number appears between

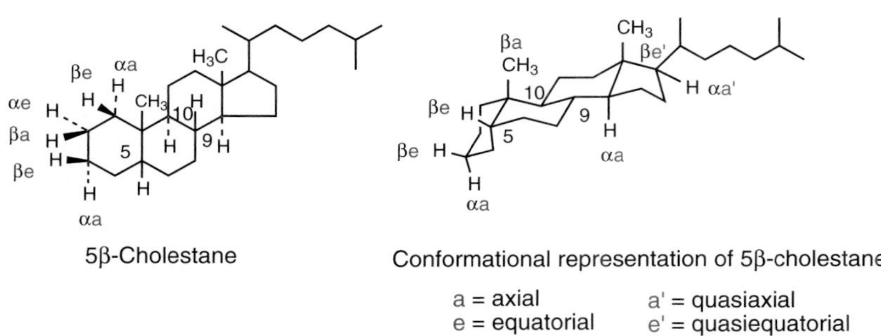

Figure 21.3 Planar and conformational structures of 5β-cholestane.

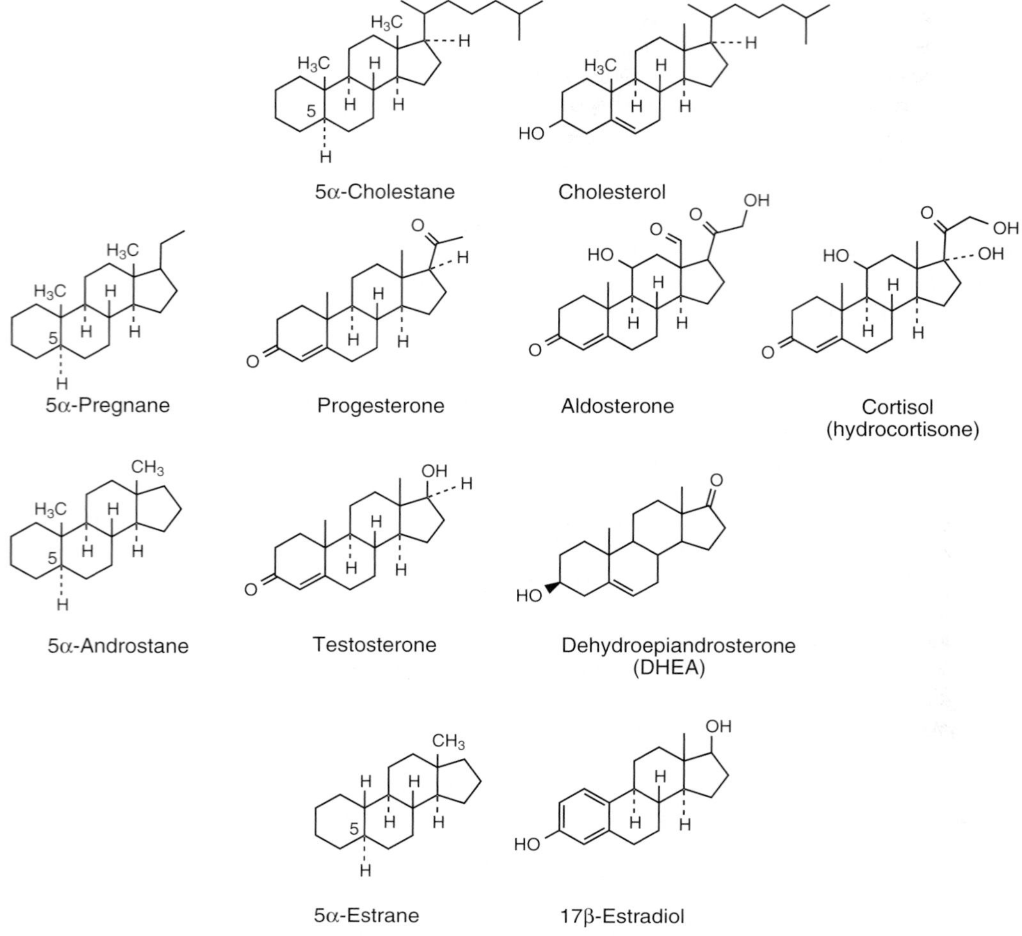

Figure 21.4 Steroid classes and corresponding natural hormones.

the two parts of the word (e.g., note the nomenclature for cholesterol and testosterone versus that for cortisol). For a more extensive discussion of steroid nomenclature, consult the literature.[1]

Mechanism of Steroid Hormone Action

In addition to their structural similarities, adrenocorticoids, estrogens, progestins, and androgens share a common mode of action. They are present in the body only in extremely low concentrations (e.g., 0.1-1.0 nmol/L), where they exert potent physiologic effects on sensitive tissues by binding with high affinity to intracellular receptors. Extensive research directed at elucidation of the general mechanism of steroid hormone action has revealed their molecular mechanism of action in great detail, and many reviews have appeared.[2-7] For details on steroid hormone action, the reader is referred to Chapter 7 (Intracellular Cytoplasmic/Nuclear Receptors).

Briefly, corticosteroids, similar to other steroidal hormones, enter cells by passive diffusion and bind to the ligand binding domain of glucocorticoid receptors (GR) and/or mineralocorticoid receptors (MR) which are present in target cells (Fig. 21.5). GR and MR in the absence of ligand are maintained in an inactive conformation by the heat shock proteins (HSPs) HSP70 and HSP90. Upon ligand binding, the GR and MR undergo conformational changes, which cause HSPs to dissociate. The steroid-bound receptor then enters the nucleus to bind to DNA in the regulatory regions of target genes. Several of these DNA elements, also called hormone response elements (HREs), share significant sequence homology that facilitates the binding of various receptors to the same DNA elements. For example, the gene metallothionein 2A (*MT2A*) can be induced by various hormone receptors binding to a promiscuous response element in the regulatory region of the gene.[8,9] The DNA-bound receptor recruits several coactivators (CoA; proteins that associate with the receptor to modulate transcription) and other general transcription factors (not shown) to propagate the transcription and translation of target genes. The varying degrees of corepressor dissociation and coactivator association that occur after ligand binding are thought to contribute to differences in the observed pharmacologic activity and tissue selectivity of agonists and antagonists for nuclear receptors and to be at least partially responsible

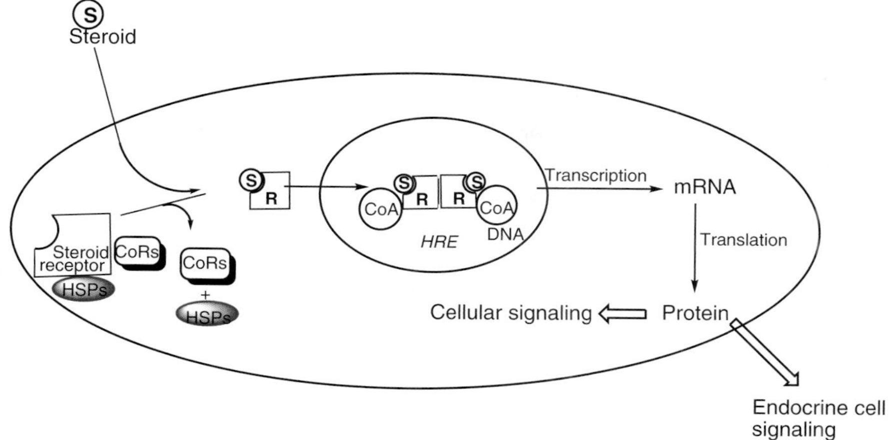

Figure 21.5 General steroid mechanism of action.

for the structure-activity relationships observed between different ligands. The proteins regulated by steroid receptors include enzymes, receptors, and secreted factors that subsequently result in the steroid hormonal response regulating cell function, growth, and differentiation and playing central roles in normal physiologic processes, as well as in many important diseases.

Steroid-receptor complexes have also demonstrated negative regulation of gene expression by interacting at negative response elements or by transrepression via direct or indirect protein-protein interactions with other known transcriptional proteins such as AP-1 and NFκB.[10,11] In fact, many of the important anti-inflammatory and immunosuppressive effects of corticosteroids are mediated through transrepression pathways, while some side effects (e.g., gluconeogenesis and bone loss) are mediated via transactivation, as described above. The transrepression mechanism can also be critical for crosstalk between signaling pathways within the cell and may have an important role in feedback systems. Additional evidence suggests that steroid receptors can activate transcription in the absence of hormone (ligand-independent activation), an effect that appears to depend on the phosphorylation of the receptor via crosstalk with membrane-bound adrenergic and/or growth factor receptors.[12] The interactions necessary for formation of the steroid-receptor complexes and subsequent activation or repression of gene transcription are complicated, involve multistage processes, and leave many unanswered questions. Lastly, nongenomic mechanisms involving cytosolic and/or membrane-bound steroid receptors have been identified to explain rapid onset actions of steroid hormones.[10]

History and Disease States

The importance of the adrenal glands was recognized long ago. Addison's disease, Cushing's disease, and Conn syndrome are pathologic conditions related to the adrenal cortex and the hormones produced by the gland. Addison's disease was named after Thomas Addison who, in 1855, described a syndrome in which the physiologic significance of the adrenal cortex was emphasized.[13] This disease results from decreased secretion of steroid hormones by the adrenal cortex and is characterized by extreme weakness, anorexia, anemia, nausea and vomiting, low blood pressure, hyperpigmentation of the skin, and mental depression. Addison's disease is a rare affliction that affects roughly 1 in 100,000 people and is seen equally in both sexes and in all age-groups.

Conditions of this type, usually referred to as hypoadrenalism, can result from several causes, including atrophy, destruction of the cortex by tuberculosis, or decreased secretion of adrenocorticotropin (adrenocorticotropic hormone [ACTH]) because of diseases of the anterior pituitary (adenohypophysis). Treatment of Addison's disease involves hormone replacement therapy.

Cushing's disease, or hyperadrenalism, on the other hand, can result from adrenal cortex tumors or increased production of ACTH caused by pituitary carcinoma. Cushing's syndrome is also rare, occurring in only 2-5 individuals for every 1 million people each year. Approximately 10% of newly diagnosed cases are observed in children and teenagers. Cushingoid refers to a constellation of symptoms associated with glucocorticoid excess including facial puffiness (moon facies), weight gain with truncal obesity but thin arms and legs, thin skin, and muscle weakness. While endogenous Cushing's syndrome is rare, iatrogenic or exogenous Cushing's syndrome arising from long-term and/or high-dose glucocorticoid therapy is common, emphasizing the need for judicious glucocorticoid selection and dosing.

Conn syndrome is caused by an inability of the adrenal cortex to carry out 17α-hydroxylation during the biosynthesis of the hormones from cholesterol. Consequently, the disease is characterized by a high secretory level of aldosterone, which lacks a 17α-hydroxyl functional group. Hypernatremia, polyuria, alkalosis, and hypertension, which are treatable via MR antagonism (e.g., using spironolactone, see below), are also observed.[14]

The importance of the adrenocorticoids is most dramatically observed in adrenalectomized animals. Glucocorticoid deficiency symptoms include an increase of urea in the blood, muscle weakness (asthenia), decreased liver glycogen, decreased insulin resistance, and lowered resistance to trauma (e.g., cold and mechanical or chemical shock).

Mineralocorticoid deficiency symptoms are also present, including electrolyte disturbances as potassium ions are retained and excretion of Na^+, Cl^-, and water is increased. Adrenalectomy in small animals causes death in a few days.

After Addison's observations in 1855, physiologists, pharmacologists, and chemists from many countries contributed to our understanding of adrenocorticoid structure and function. It was not until 1927, however, that J.M. Rogoff and G.N. Stewart found that extracts of adrenal glands, administered by intravenous (IV) injection, kept adrenalectomized dogs alive.

Since that discovery, similar experiments have been repeated many times. Originally, the biologic activity of the extract was thought to result from a single compound. Later, 47 compounds were isolated from such extracts, and some were highly active. Among the biologically active corticoids isolated (Fig. 21.6), cortisol, corticosterone, aldosterone, cortisone, 11-desoxycorticosterone (21-hydroxyprogesterone), 11-dehydrocorticosterone (11-keto,17α-desoxy-cortisol), and 17α-hydroxy-11-desoxycorticosterone were found to be most potent.[15] The biosynthesis of these steroids is described below.

BIOSYNTHESIS

Pregnenolone Formation and Conversion to Androgens and Estrogens

In the adrenal glands, cholesterol is converted by enzymatic side chain cleavage (scc) to pregnenolone, which serves as the biosynthetic precursor of the adrenocorticoids

Cortisol (hydrocortisone)

Cortisone

Corticosterone

11-Desoxycorticosterone or 21-hydroxyprogesterone

11-Dehydrocorticosterone

17α-Hydroxy-11-desoxycorticosterone

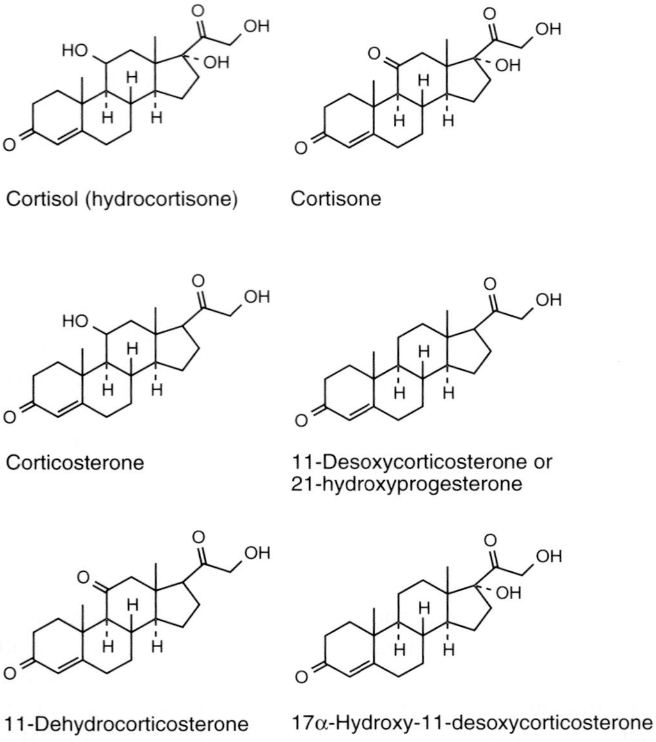

Figure 21.6 Biologically active corticoids.

Cholesterol

step a

O_2, NADPH

Cholest-5-ene-3β,22*R*-diol

O_2, NADPH step b

Pregnenolone

O_2, NADPH step c

Cholest-5-ene-3β,20*R*,22*R*-triol

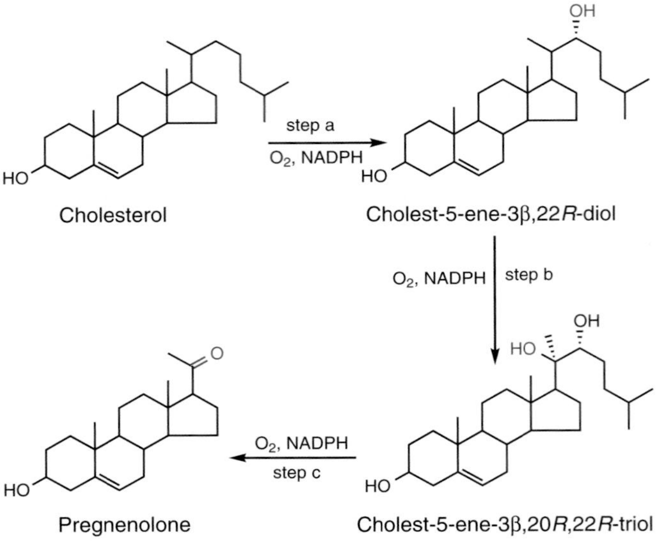

Figure 21.7 Biosynthesis of pregnenolone from cholesterol.

(Fig. 21.7). This biotransformation is performed by a mitochondrial cytochrome P450 enzyme complex. This enzyme complex found in the mitochondrial membrane consists of three proteins: CYP11A1 (also known as $P450_{SCC}$), adrenodoxin, and adrenodoxin reductase.[16] Defects in CYP11A1 lead to a lack of glucocorticoids, feminization, and hypertension. Three oxidation steps are involved in the conversion, and three moles of NADPH and molecular oxygen are consumed for each mole of cholesterol converted to pregnenolone. The first oxidation results in the formation of cholest-5-ene-3β,22*R*-diol (step a), followed by the second oxidation yielding cholest-5-ene-3β,20*R*,22*R*-triol (step b). The third oxidation step catalyzes the cleavage of the C20-C22 bond to produce pregnenolone (step c).

Pregnenolone serves as the common precursor in the formation of the adrenocorticoids and the sex steroid hormones. This C21 steroid is converted via enzymatic oxidations and isomerization of the double bond to a number of physiologically active C21 steroids, including the female sex hormone progesterone and the adrenocorticoids cortisol, corticosterone, and aldosterone (Fig. 21.8), as will be discussed below.

Androgen and estrogen biosynthesis requires oxidative cleavage of the pregnenolone two-carbon side chain and subsequent enzymatic oxidations and an isomerization leading to C19 steroids, including the androgens testosterone and dihydrotestosterone (see sex hormone pathway of Fig. 21.8). Specifically, 17α-hydroxylation of pregnenolone by 17α-hydroxylase produces 17α-hydroxypregnenolone (step b). Oxidative cleavage of the two-carbon side chain of 17α-hydroxypregnenolone by 17,20-lyase (step j) produces the adrenal androgen dehydroepiandrosterone (DHEA), which serves as the biosynthetic precursors to androgens and estrogens and is present at high serum concentrations as DHEA sulfate in men and women. 3β-HSD (5-ene-3β-hydroxysteroid dehydrogenase) oxidizes and isomerizes DHEA into androstenedione, which can be reduced to testosterone by testicular17βHSD3 (17β-hydroxysteroid dehydrogenase type 3). This reaction

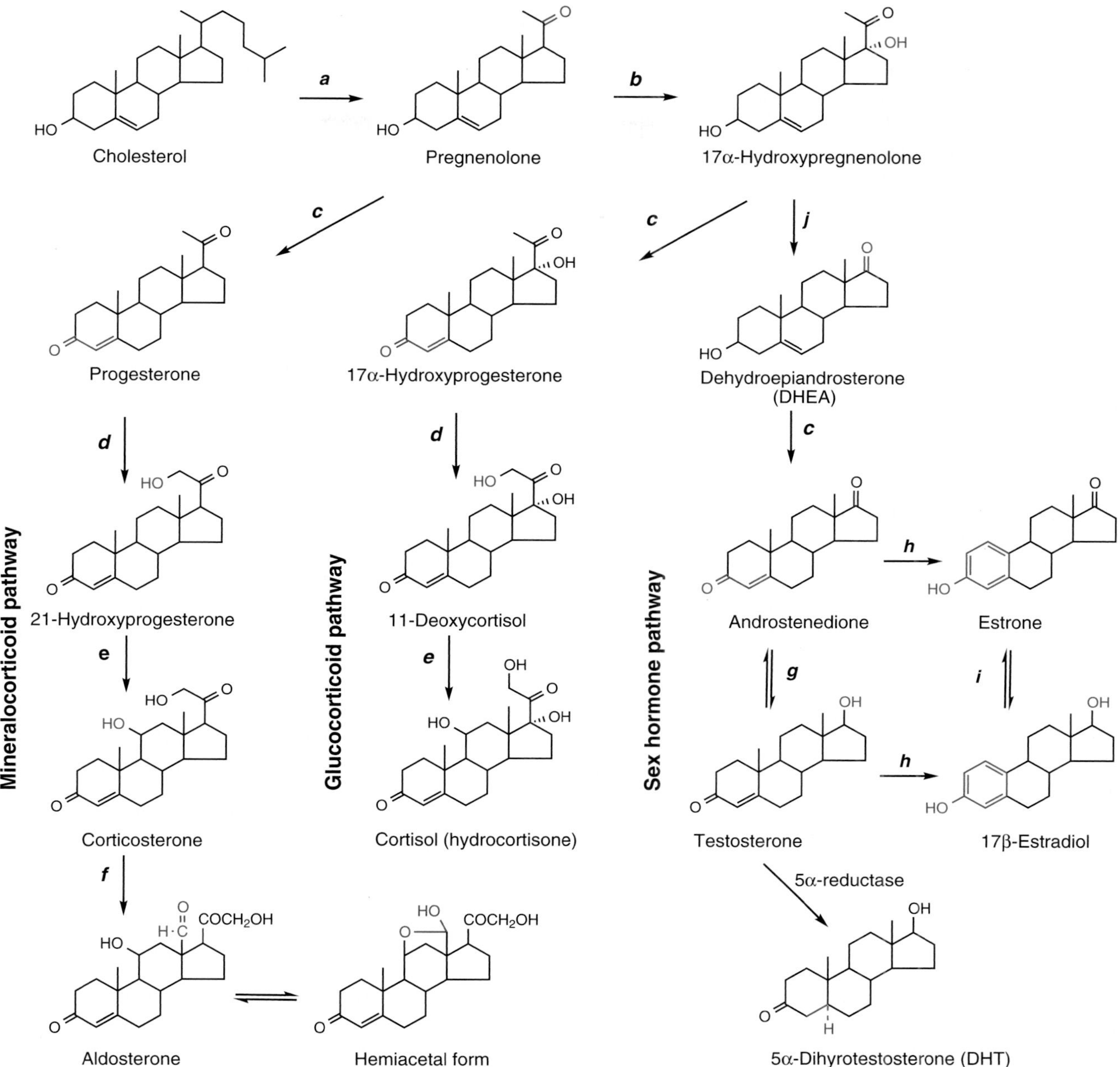

Figure 21.8 Biosynthesis of the adrenocorticoids and sex hormones from cholesterol.

is catalyzed in females and extratesticularly in males by aldoketoreductase type 1C3 (AKR1C3). Testosterone can be further activated in certain androgenic target tissues, such as skin and prostate, by 5α-reductase, which produces 5α-dihydrotestosterone (DHT), the most potent endogenous androgen.

The final group of steroids, the C18 female sex hormones, are derived from oxidative aromatization of the A ring of androgens to produce estrogens such as estrone and 17β-estradiol (step h of Fig. 21.8). This oxidative aromatization is performed by aromatase using either androstenedione or testosterone as substrates to produce estrone or 17β-estradiol. The latter is the most potent endogenous estrogen and can be deactivated by metabolism to the former by estradiol dehydrogenase (step i of Fig. 21.8). For further discussion of androgens, estrogens, and progestins (e.g., progesterone receptor ligands) see Chapter 24.

Pregnenolone to Glucocorticoids and Mineralocorticoids

The biosynthesis of the glucocorticoids and mineralocorticoids is regulated by independent mechanisms. The glucocorticoids, such as cortisol, are biosynthesized and released under the influence of peptide hormones secreted by the hypothalamus and anterior pituitary (adenohypophysis) to activate the adrenal cortex. This relay of activating biochemical events is known as the hypothalamic-pituitary-adrenal

(HPA) axis. Removal of the pituitary results in atrophy of the adrenal cortex and a marked decrease in the rate of glucocorticoid formation and secretion. On the other hand, the secretion of the mineralocorticoids, corticosterone, and aldosterone is under the influence of the octapeptide, angiotensin II. Angiotensin II is the active metabolite resulting from the renin (synthesized in the kidney)-catalyzed proteolytic hydrolysis of plasma angiotensinogen (synthesized in the liver) to angiotensin I (no known function) and subsequent proteolysis to angiotensin II. Mineralocorticoid regulation is almost independent of the HPA axis. Hypophysectomized animals have only slightly decreased or unchanged aldosterone levels. Consequently, the electrolyte balance remains nearly normal.

The peptide hormone in the anterior pituitary that influences glucocorticoid biosynthesis is ACTH, whereas the peptide hormone in the hypothalamus is corticotropin-releasing factor (CRF). The production of both ACTH and CRF is regulated by the central nervous system and by a negative corticoid feedback mechanism. CRF is released by the hypothalamus and is transported to the anterior pituitary, where it stimulates the release of ACTH into the bloodstream. ACTH is then transported to the adrenal glands, where it stimulates the biosynthesis and secretion of the glucocorticoids. The circulating levels of glucocorticoids act on the hypothalamus and anterior pituitary to regulate the release of both CRF and ACTH. As the levels of glucocorticoids rise, smaller amounts of CRF and ACTH are secreted, and a negative feedback is observed (HPA suppression). Stimuli, such as pain, noise, and emotional reactions, increase the secretion of CRF, ACTH, and consequently the glucocorticoids. Once the stimulus is alleviated or removed, the negative feedback mechanism inhibits further production and helps to return the body to a normal hormonal balance.[17,18]

ACTH acts at the adrenal gland by binding to a receptor protein on the surface of the adrenal cortex cell to stimulate the biosynthesis and secretion of glucocorticoids. The only steroid stored in the adrenal gland is cholesterol, which is found in the form of cholesterol esters sequestered in lipid droplets. ACTH stimulates the conversion of cholesterol esters to glucocorticoids by initiating a series of biochemical events through its surface receptor. The ACTH receptor protein is coupled to a G protein which has adenylate cyclase as its second messenger. Binding of ACTH to its receptor leads to activation of adenylate cyclase via the G protein. The result is an increase in intracellular cyclic adenosine monophosphate (cAMP) levels (see Chapter 6). One of the processes influenced by elevated cAMP levels is the activation of cholesterol esterase, which cleaves cholesterol esters and liberates free cholesterol. Another process is the rapid induction of steroidogenic acute regulatory protein, referred to as StAR, which transfers cholesterol into the mitochondrial membrane.

Free cholesterol is then converted within mitochondria to pregnenolone via the side-chain cleavage reaction described earlier (Fig. 21.7 and step a of Fig. 21.8). In overview, pregnenolone is converted to adrenocorticoids by a series of enzymatic oxidations and an isomerization of the double bond (see mineralocorticoid and glucocorticoid pathways of Fig. 21.8). The next several enzymatic steps in the biosynthesis of glucocorticoids (middle pathway of Fig. 21.8) occur in the endoplasmic reticulum of the adrenal cortex cell. Hydroxylation of pregnenolone at position 17 by the enzyme 17α-hydroxylase (CYP17) produces 17α-hydroxypregnenolone (step b). The 17α-hydroxyl group is important for adrenocorticoid hormone action, promoting glucocorticoid and diminishing mineralocorticoid activities. In one step, 17α-hydroxypregnenolone is oxidized to a 3-keto intermediate and isomerized to 17α-hydroxyprogesterone by the action of a single enzyme, 5-ene-3β-hydroxysteroid dehydrogenase (3β-HSD) (step c). Another hydroxylation occurs by the action of 21-hydroxylase (CYP21) to give rise to 11-deoxycortisol, which contains the physiologically important ketol ($-COCH_2OH$) side chain at the 17β position (step d). A lack of CYP21 prevents cortisol biosynthesis, diverting excess 17α-hydroxypregnenolone and 17α-hydroxyprogesterone into overproduction of C19 androgens. The final step in the biosynthesis of cortisol is catalyzed by the enzyme 11β-hydroxylase, a mitochondrial cytochrome P450 enzyme complex (CYP11B2). This last enzymatic step (step e) results in the formation of cortisol (hydrocortisone), the most potent endogenous glucocorticoid secreted by the adrenal cortex. Approximately 15-20 mg of cortisol is biosynthesized daily. Several reviews provide more detailed discussions about the enzymology and regulation of adrenal steroidogenesis.[16,18-21]

The pathway for the formation of the potent mineralocorticoid molecule aldosterone is similar to that for cortisol and uses several of the same enzymes (mineralocorticoid pathway of Fig. 21.8). The preferred pathway involves the conversion of pregnenolone to progesterone by 3β-HSD (step c). Hydroxylation at position 21 of progesterone by 21-hydroxylase results in 21-hydroxyprogesterone (also known as 11-desoxycorticosterone) (step d). Again, these first conversions occur in the endoplasmic reticulum of the cell, whereas the next enzymatic steps occur in the mitochondria. 11β-Hydroxylase (CYP11B2) catalyzes the conversion of 21-hydroxyprogesterone to corticosterone (step e), which exhibits mineralocorticoid activity. The final two oxidations involve hydroxylations at the C18 methyl group and are catalyzed by 18-hydroxylase (step f). Initially these reactions produce 18-hydroxycorticosterone (not shown) and then aldosterone, the most powerful endogenous mineralocorticoid secreted by the adrenal cortex. The aldehyde at C18 of aldosterone exists in equilibrium with its hemiacetal form.

METABOLISM

Cortisol (hormonally active) and cortisone (the relatively inactive metabolite of cortisol) are biochemically interconvertible by the enzyme 11β-hydroxysteroid dehydrogenase (Fig. 21.9). Two isozymes of 11β-hydroxysteroid dehydrogenase are present: type 1 11β-hydroxysteroid dehydrogenase (11β-HSD1), referred to as the "liver" isozyme, and type 2 11β-hydroxysteroid dehydrogenase (11β-HSD2), referred to as the "kidney" isozyme.[22-24] The

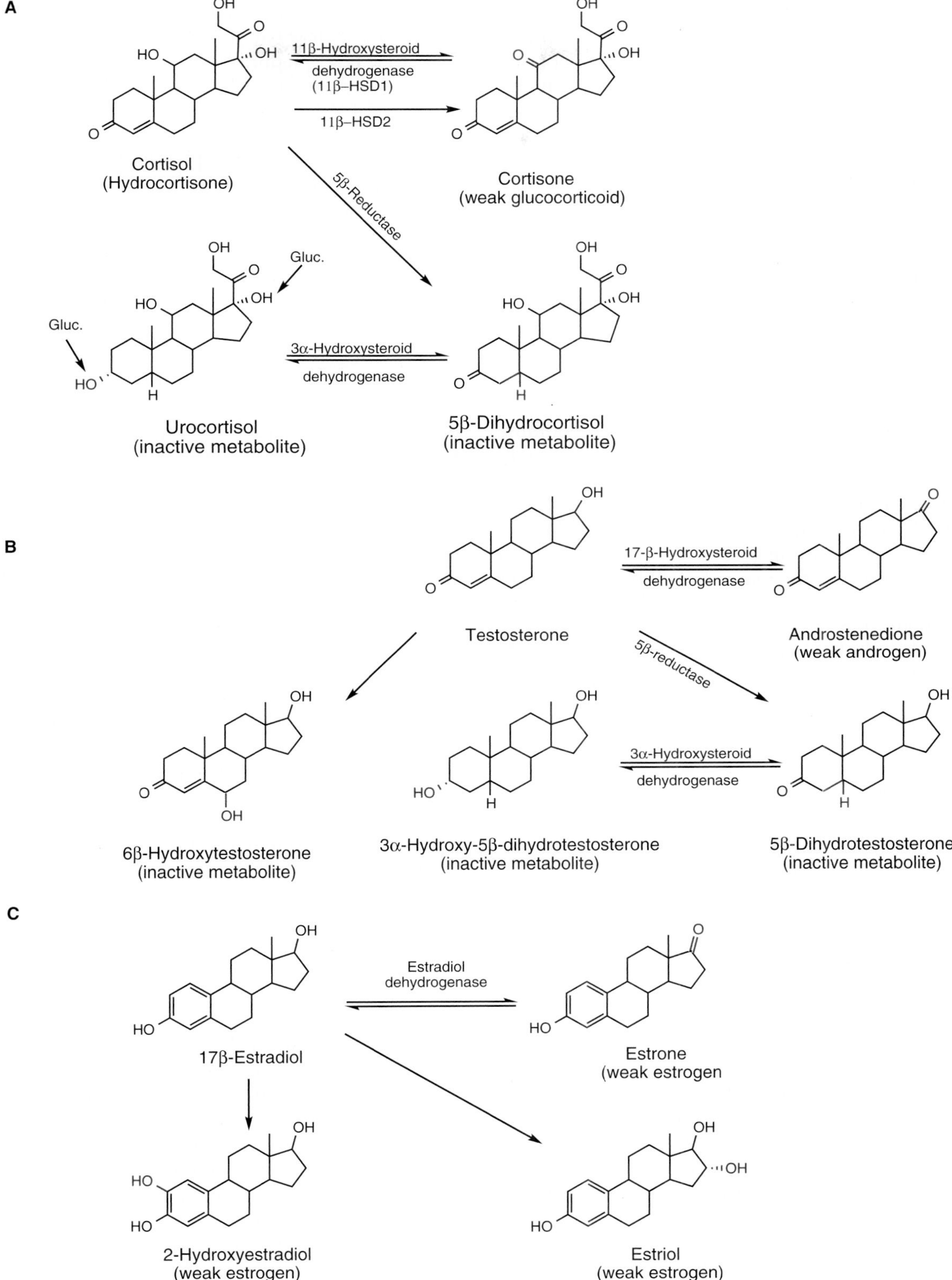

Figure 21.9 Major routes of inactivating metabolism for hydrocortisone (A), testosterone (B), and 17β-estradiol (C). Arrows from Gluc indicate the site of glucuronidation.

11β-HSD1 isozyme is a bidirectional enzyme, which readily interconverts cortisol and cortisone, and is found in many tissues in the body. This isozyme has an important role in the regulation of hepatic gluconeogenesis in the liver and in fat production in adipose tissues. By contrast, the 11β-HSD2 isozyme is unidirectional, catalyzing the 11β-dehydrogenation of cortisol to cortisone. 11β-HSD2 is present in the placenta and in the kidney, specifically the distal convoluted tubules and cortical collecting ducts in the kidney. The 11β-HSD2 isozyme has an important role in the rapid metabolism of cortisol, thus preventing cortisol from binding to the MRs present in the same kidney tissues. A deficiency of 11β-HSD2 is associated with the inherited genetic disease apparent mineralocorticoid excess syndrome, which is characterized by hypertension, excessive salt retention, and hypokalemia caused by the elevated cortisol levels in the kidney.

Cortisol is metabolized by the liver following administration by any route, with a half-life of approximately 1.0-1.5 hours.[25] Cortisol is mainly excreted in the urine as inactive O-glucuronide conjugates at 3 and 21 positions and minor O-sulfate conjugates of urocortisol, 5β-dihydrocortisol, and urocortisone (Fig. 21.9). The tetrahydro metabolite urocortisol is the major metabolite formed and has the 5β-pregnane geometry and 3α-hydroxyl function. The 5β configuration is the same ring geometry for bile acids (e.g., obeticholic acid, an agonist of farnesoid X receptor), a class of steroids devoid of adrenocorticoid or sex hormone activities. Several 5β metabolites of this type have been isolated.[26,27]

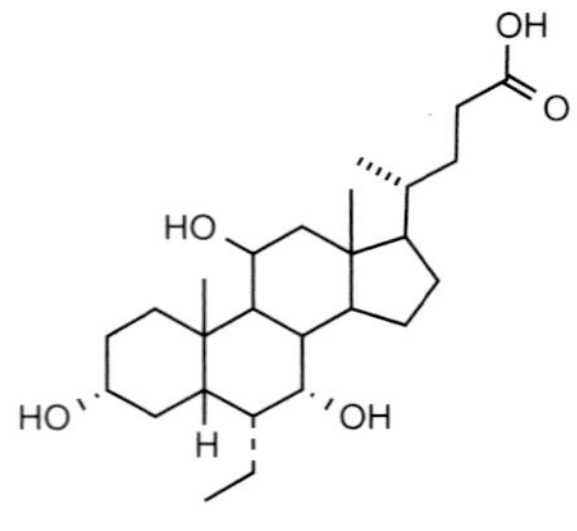

Obeticholic acid

All of the biologically active adrenocorticoids contain a ketone at the 3-position and a double bond in the 4,5-position. The formation of inactive 5β-metabolites from cortisol is characterized by reduction of the 4,5-double bond to a 5β geometry for rings A and B (a *cis* configuration) by 5β-reductase, which can be further reduced at the 3-ketone by 3α-hydroxysteroid dehydrogenase (3α-hydroxyl configuration) or 3β-hydroxysteroid dehydrogenase (3β-hydroxyl configuration). These reactions represent the major inactivating pathways of metabolism for the glucocorticoids and their endogenous counterparts. Urocortisol and urocortisone are named after cortisol and cortisone, respectively. Oxidation of the 11β-hydroxyl group of many glucocorticoids including cortisol, prednisolone, and methylprednisolone (but not dexamethasone and other 9α-fluorinated glucocorticoids) by 11β-HSD modulates the activities of these drugs in many tissues and limits their mineralocorticoid activity in the kidneys. Other routes of metabolism include the following: (1) 6β-hydroxylation (CYP3A4) and reduction of the 20-ketone (e.g., prednisolone) to form 20-hydroxyl analogs, (2) oxidation of the 17-ketol side chain to 17β-carboxylic acids, and (3) loss of the 17-ketol side chain, resulting in 11β-hydroxy-17-keto-C19 steroids with the geometry of either 5α-androstane or 5β-androstane.[18-21] In addition, some ring A aromatic adrenocorticoid metabolites that resemble the estrogens have been isolated.[28] Biliary and fecal excretion contributes little to the elimination of the adrenocorticoids. The rate of formation of 6β-hydroxycortisol is a biomarker for determining the level of HPA suppression and adrenal insufficiency.

Similarly, testosterone can be metabolically inactivated by 17βHSDs to androstenedione, a weak androgen, or reduced by 5β-reductases or 3α-hydroxysteroid dehydrogenases to inactive 5β-androstanes and/or 3α-hydroxy metabolites. It is important to note that 5β-dihydrotestosterone is inactive, while 5α-dihydrotestosterone (DHT) is the most potent endogenous androgen. 6β-Hydroxylation of testosterone by CYP3A4 in the liver is responsible for 75%-80% of cytochrome P450–mediated testosterone metabolism. Testosterone and its metabolites can also be substrates for direct conjugation via glucuronosyl transferase or sulfotransferase enzymes. Furthermore, androgens can be inactivated by aromatization of testosterone by aromatase to 17β-estradiol or estrone.

Inactivation of the most potent estrogen, 17β-estradiol, occurs primarily via conversion to less potent estrogens, estrone (17β-dehydrogenation), or estriol (16α-hydroxylation). Estriol is the major 17β-estradiol metabolite excreted in the urine. 17β-Estradiol and estrone are also metabolized by CYP enzymes in the liver to the catechol, 2-hydroxyestradiol. 17β-Estradiol and its metabolites are rapidly glucuronidated and/or sulfated and eliminated in the urine.

Physiologic Effects of Adrenocorticoids

Glucocorticoids

Corticosteroids influence all tissues of the body and produce numerous and varying effects in cells.[17] These steroids regulate carbohydrate, lipid, and protein biosynthesis and metabolism (glucocorticoid effects), and they influence water and electrolyte balance (mineralocorticoid effects). Hydrocortisone is the most potent glucocorticoid secreted by the adrenal gland, and aldosterone is the most potent endogenous mineralocorticoid. Both naturally occurring glucocorticoids and related semisynthetic analogs can be evaluated in terms of their ability to sustain life, to stimulate an increase in blood glucose concentrations and a deposition of liver glycogen, to decrease circulating eosinophils,[29] and to cause thymus involution in adrenalectomized animals.[30,31] In addition, corticosteroids can affect immune system functions, inflammatory responses, and cell growth.

The primary physiologic function of glucocorticoids is to maintain blood glucose levels and, thus, ensure glucose-dependent processes critical to life, particularly brain functions. Hydrocortisone and related steroids accomplish this by stimulating the formation of glucose, by diminishing glucose use by peripheral tissues, and by promoting glycogen synthesis in the liver to increase carbohydrate stores for later release of glucose. For glucose formation, glucocorticoids mobilize amino acids and promote amino acid metabolism and gluconeogenesis. These steroids, acting via the GR, induce the production of a variety of enzymes important for glucose formation. The synthesis of tyrosine aminotransferase increases within 30 minutes of glucocorticoid exposure.[32-34] This enzyme promotes the transfer of amino groups from tyrosine to α-ketoglutarate to form glutamate and hydroxyphenylpyruvate. Another amino acid–metabolizing enzyme induced rapidly by glucocorticoids is tryptophan oxidase.[35] This enzyme oxidizes tryptophan to formylkynurenine, which is subsequently converted to alanine. Alanine transaminase is also induced by glucocorticoids.[36] Alanine and, to a lesser extent, glutamate are important for gluconeogenesis in the liver.[37]

Several other enzymes important in gluconeogenesis and glycogen formation are elevated for several hours following glucocorticoid administration; these include glycogen synthetase, pyruvate kinase, phosphoenolpyruvate carboxykinase, and glucose-6-phosphate kinase.[17,38,39] The delayed increases in these enzymes suggest that their biosyntheses are not regulated directly by glucocorticoids. In peripheral tissues, glucocorticoid-induced inhibition of phosphofructokinase is observed.[40] This enzyme catalyzes the formation of D-fructose-1,6-diphosphate from D-fructose-6-phosphate during glycolysis. Inhibition of this enzyme decreases glucose utilization by peripheral tissues and results in maintenance of blood glucose levels. Reviews of the multiple effects of glucocorticoids on carbohydrate metabolism have been published.[17,40]

Additional effects of glucocorticoids in the body are preventing or minimizing inflammatory reactions and suppressing immune responses. These steroids interfere with both early events in inflammation (e.g., release of mediators, edema, and cellular infiltration) and later stages (e.g., capillary infiltration and collagen formation). Only a few of the mechanisms involved in glucocorticoid suppression of inflammation are known. Hydrocortisone will induce the production of lipocortin and related proteins by increasing gene expression through the GR.[41,42] Lipocortin inhibits the activity of phospholipase A_2, which liberates arachidonic acid and leads to the biosynthesis of eicosanoids (e.g., prostaglandins and leukotrienes).[43] Lipocortin also mediates the decreased production and release of platelet-activating factor,[44] and glucocorticoids can suppress the expression of interleukin (IL)-1, tumor necrosis factor, inducible nitric oxide synthase,[45-47] and other proinflammatory mediators. These eicosanoids and peptide factors are important as mediators in the inflammatory response. Some of these factors also have important roles in cellular infiltration and capillary permeability in the inflamed region. Suppression of the immune responses is mediated by inhibition of the synthesis and release of important mediators as well. In macrophages, glucocorticoids inhibit IL-1 synthesis and, thus, interfere with proliferation of B lymphocytes, which are important for antibody production.[38] Additionally, IL-1 is important for activation of resting T lymphocytes, which are important for cell-mediated immunity. The activated T cells produce IL-2, the biosynthesis of which is also reduced by glucocorticoids.[48]

Mineralocorticoids

The primary physiologic function of mineralocorticoids is to maintain electrolyte balance in the body by enhancing Na^+ reabsorption and increasing K^+ and H^+ secretion in the kidney. The mechanism of action of aldosterone involves binding of the steroid to the MR and initiation of gene transcription, mRNA biosynthesis, and cognate protein production.[39] A myriad of ligand-specific, tissue-specific, and gene-specific interactions of the MR with coactivator and corepressor proteins, as well as protein kinase signaling and other nongenomic mechanisms, work in concert to regulate electrolyte homeostasis and water balance.[48,49] Similar effects on cation transport are observed in a variety of secretory tissues, including the salivary glands, sweat glands, and mucosal tissues of the GI tract and the bladder. Aldosterone is the most potent endogenous mineralocorticoid. Deoxycorticosterone is approximately 20-fold less potent than aldosterone. Hydrocortisone exhibits weak mineralocorticoid activity in vivo because of rapid metabolism to cortisone by 11β-hydroxysteroid dehydrogenase.

SUMMARY OF STRUCTURE-ACTIVITY RELATIONSHIPS

The ring conformation and the absolute configuration of hydrocortisone and prednisolone illustrate the all-*trans* (B/C and C/D) backbone that is necessary for activity (Fig. 21.10).

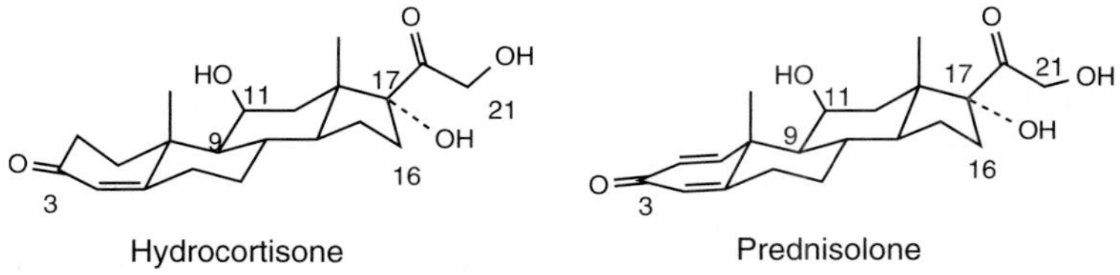

Figure 21.10 Absolute configuration of hydrocortisone and prednisolone.

Structural Biology of Adrenocorticoids

As previously pointed out, the adrenocorticoids are classified as either glucocorticoids, which activate the GR, affect intermediary metabolism, and are associated with inhibition of the inflammatory process, or mineralocorticoids activating the MR. In fact, most naturally occurring and semisynthetic analogs exhibit both of these actions. The conserved structural features of glucocorticoids (and mineralocorticoids) such as those present in the endogenous ligand hydrocortisone include Δ^4-keto, 11β-OH, 17α-OH, and 17β-ketol (20-ketone and 21-OH). Crystal structures of several glucocorticoids reveal a conserved array of polar interactions between the glucocorticoids and GR for each of these conserved features. Furthermore, they help to rationalize the importance of groups that have been added to the semisynthetic glucocorticoids to increase GR potency or selectivity over MR. All approved agents thus far are steroidal (i.e., derivatives of the endogenous agents); however, many nonsteroidal agents have been designed and optimized using these structure-based design techniques. Nonsteroidal agents are highly receptor selective and are generally not metabolized to cross-reactive agents.

As shown using the mometasone furoate:GR co-crystal (4e2j.pdb), the conserved polar interactions include the following: the binding of the Δ^4-3-ketone to the side chains of Gln570 and Arg611, the 11β-OH to the terminal amide of Asn564, 17α-OH group (present as furoate ester in mometasone furoate) to the side chains of Thr739 (not shown for simplicity) and Gln642, the 20-ketone of the 17β-ketol to the Asn564, and 21-OH (replaced by 21-Cl in mometasone furoate) of the ketol to Thr739 and Gln642 (Fig. 21.11, top panel).

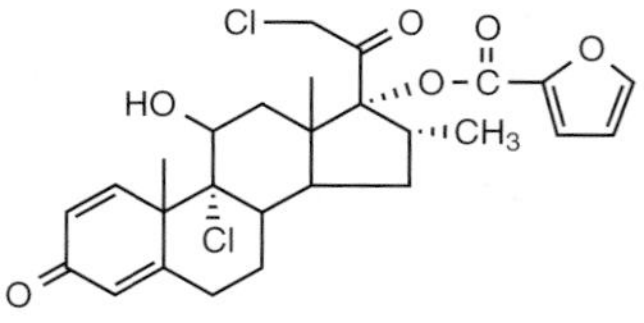

Mometasone furoate

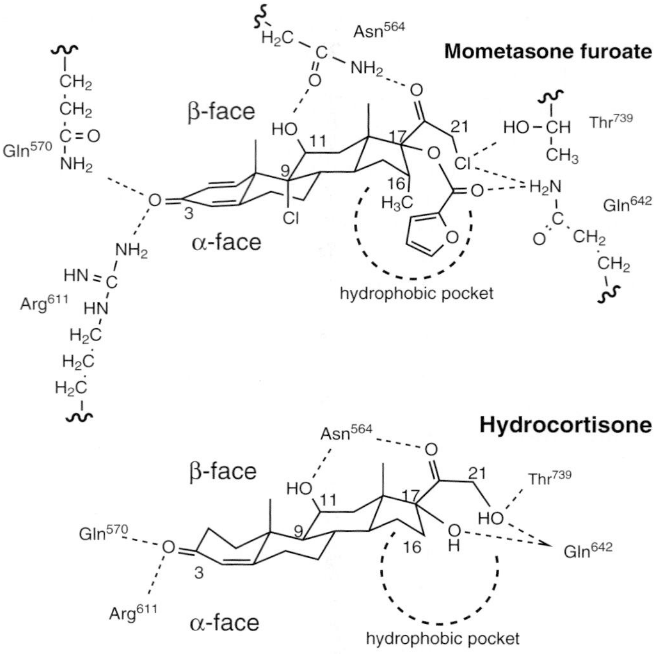

Furthermore, the crystal structures provide context for understanding the observed structure-activity relationship (SAR) of semisynthetic glucocorticoids. For example, it can be seen that the 9α-F/Cl groups inductively activate the hydrogen bond donation of the 11β-OH (all GR agonists). GR tolerates steric bulk on the α-face of the steroid nucleus, particularly at positions 16 and 17. The GR accommodates small groups such as the 16α-methyl of dexamethasone (a 16α-methyl glucocorticoid) and its synthetic derivatives (as discussed in the Topical Glucocorticoids section), as well as larger groups such as 16α-,17α-ethers of the triamcinolone (a 16α-OH glucocorticoid) and its synthetic derivatives (e.g., the 16α-,17α-acetonides; discussed in the Topical Glucocorticoids section) and 17α-esters like the 17α-propionate of betamethasone (a 16β-methyl glucocorticoid).

Mometasone furoate

Hydrocortisone

Figure 21.11 Interactions of mometasone furoate and hydrocortisone with glucocorticoid receptor.

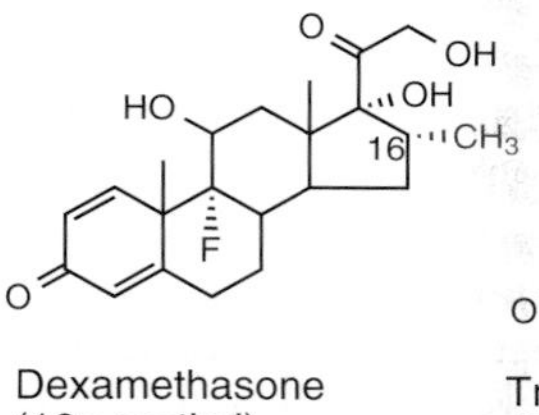

Dexamethasone (16α-methyl)

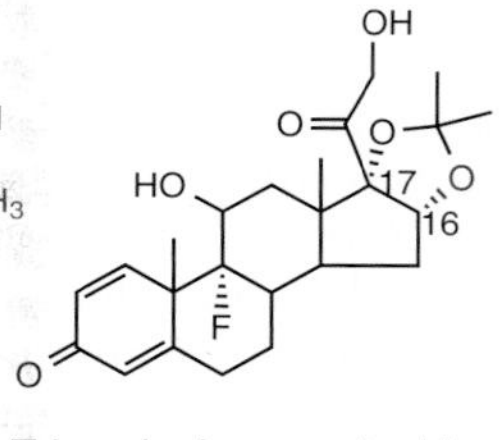

Triamcinolone acetonide (16α-hydroxy)

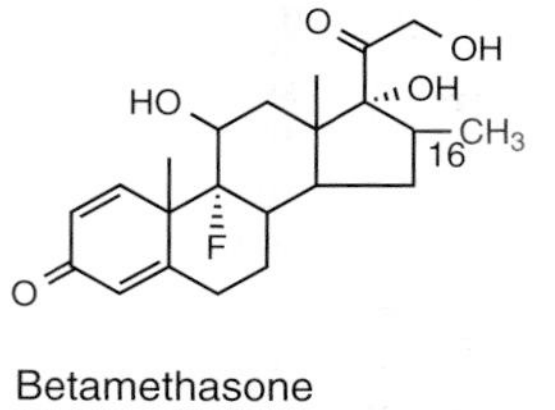

Betamethasone (16β-methyl)

The ether/ester oxygen atoms form polar interactions with the NH_2 of Gln642 of the GR side chain (Fig. 21.11 [top panel]), and the bulky aromatic or aliphatic substituents form hydrophobic interactions with a large hydrophobic pocket of GR lined by Phe, Ile, Cys, and Met side chains. Examples of bulky α-substituents accommodated by GR include the17α-furoate of mometasone, the 16α,17α-cyclopentylidenedioxy (ketal of cyclopentanone) of amcinonide, or the 16α,17α-acetal of cyclohexanecarboxaldehyde of ciclesonide (discussed in Topical Glucocorticoids section).

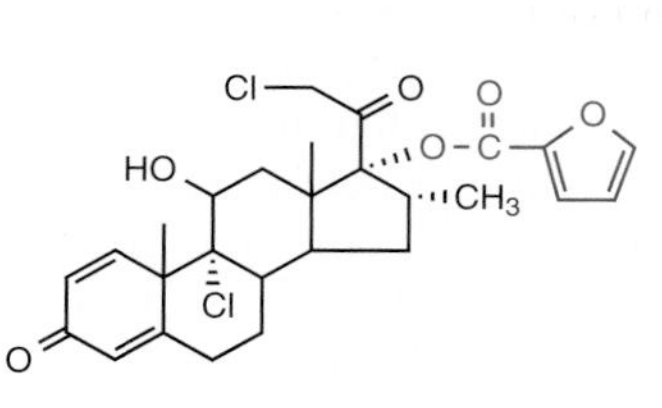

Mometasone furoate

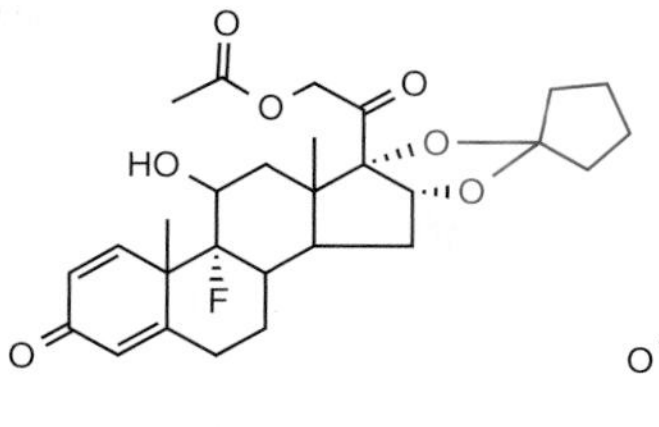

Amcinonide

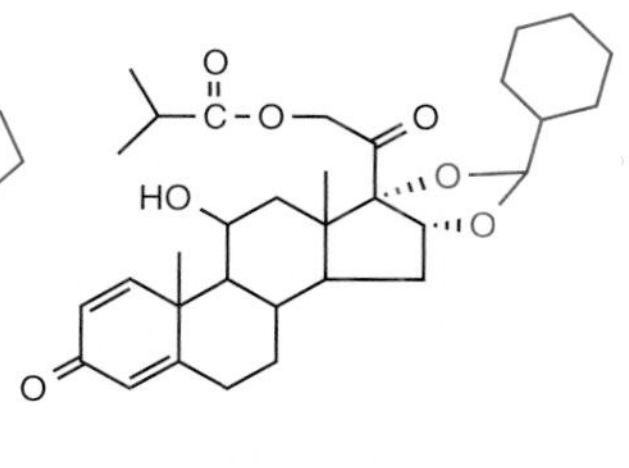

Ciclesonide

Derivation of the 21-OH to halogens (e.g., mometasone furoate) or esters (e.g., dexamethasone acetate) maintains the interactions with Thr739 or Gln642 of GR. Moreover, 16α- (e.g., mometasone furoate [shown]) and 16β-methyl (e.g., betamethasone) groups are well accommodated by the GR and enhance its activity.

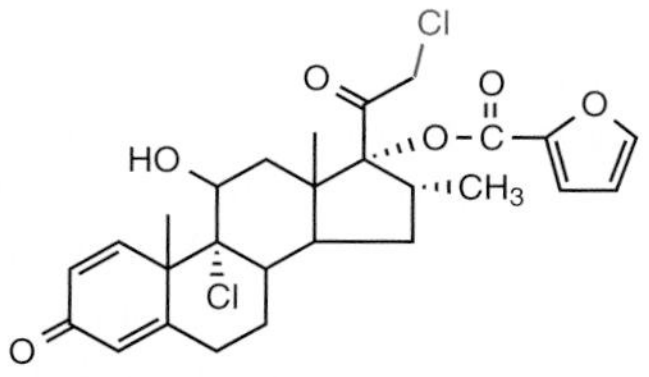

Mometasone furoate

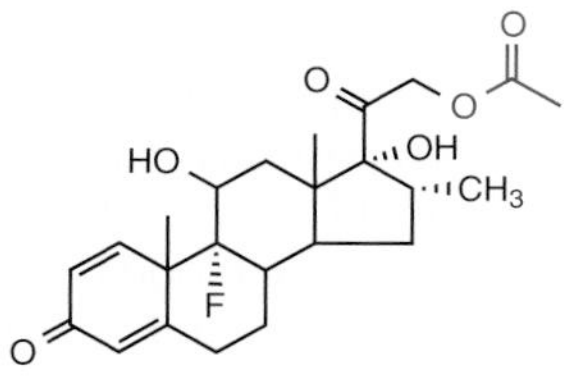

Dexamethasone acetate

The GR and MR are members of the nuclear hormone receptor family that also includes other steroid receptors such as androgen receptor, progesterone receptor, and estrogen receptor. The key polar interactions at position 3 (binds to Gln and Arg) and 17 (binds to Thr) are similar across the steroid receptor family. Unsurprisingly, many of the GR interactions described above are conserved between GR and MR, as shown by the crystal structure of dexamethasone bound to MR (4uda.pdb). For example, the Δ^4-3-ketone to Gln/Arg side chains interactions (i.e., Gln776 and Arg817 in MR) are maintained in MR, as are the 11β-OH to Asn770, 20-ketone to Asn770, and 21-OH to Thr945 (Fig. 21.12). Correspondingly, the 9α-F and 9α-Cl groups, which serve to inductively enhance the 11β-OH hydrogen bond to MR or GR, confer no MR selectivity (e.g., fludrocortisone vs. hydrocortisone as discussed in the Systemic Corticosteroids section). Similarly, the Δ^1 may enhance the Δ^4-3-ketone to Gln/Arg interaction with MR and GR and provides some GR selectivity (e.g., prednisolone vs. hydrocortisone as discussed in the Systemic Corticosteroids section). Similarly, 21-fluorination increases the activity at both GR and MR with little to no selectivity.

In contrast, the 16α-methylation of dexamethasone (and 16β-methylation of betamethasone) is poorly accommodated by MR, suggesting the inability of MR to form the hydrophobic pocket of GR. Lack of this α-face pocket and, importantly, the absence in MR of an analog to Gln642 explains the GR selectivity conferred by 16α-hydroxylation (e.g, triamcinolone; Fig. 21.12), 17α-hydroxylation (e.g., hydrocortisone vs. corticosterone), or 16α-,17α-acetals or ketals (e.g, triamcinolone acetonide as shown above). Moreover, 6α-methylation (e.g, methylprednisolone, as discussed in the Systemic Corticosteroids section) is not accommodated in MR, providing another basis for selectivity; however, halogenation is accommodated. The ability to predict interactions with GR and/or their contributions to GR activity is not the same across all substitution contexts. A more detailed SAR discussion is found in the section below.

Structure-Activity Relationships of Adrenocorticoids

17β-KETOL. The 17β-ketol ($-COCH_2OH$) side chain and the Δ^4-3-ketone functions are found in clinically used adrenocorticoids, and these groups contribute to the potency of these drugs (Figs. 21.11 and 21.12). Modifications of these groups result in derivatives that retain biologic activity. For example, replacement of the 21-OH group with fluorine increases glucocorticoid and sodium-retaining activities, whereas substitution with chlorine or bromine diminishes activity. Some compounds that do not contain the Δ^4-3-ketone system have appreciable activity. It has been suggested that this group makes only a minor contribution to the specificity of action by these drugs or to the steroid-receptor association constant.[50]

INTOLERANCE OF β-SUBSTITUENT BULK. Based on structure-activity studies, the C and D rings, involving positions 11, 12, 13, 16, 17, 18, 20, and 21, are more

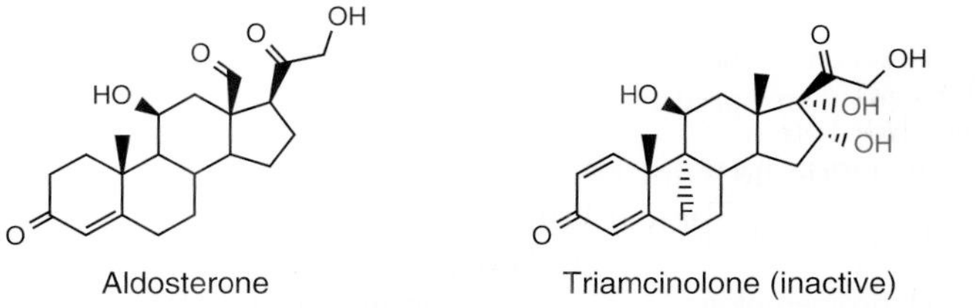

β-face

α-face

Triamcinolone (inactive)

intolerance of hydroxylation due to no polar analog to Gln^{642}

intolerance of hydroxy groups or steric bulk

Aldosterone

Triamcinolone (inactive)

Figure 21.12 Limited interactions of triamcinolone with mineralocorticoid receptor (MR). Red functional groups are not tolerated by MR, explaining lack of mineralocorticoid activity in triamcinolone and other glucocorticoids with similar substitution patterns.

important for receptor binding than the A and B rings. As a rule, insertion of bulky substituents on the β-side of the molecule abolishes glycogenic activity, whereas insertion on the α-side does not. As discussed above, it has been demonstrated that association of these steroids with receptors involves β-surfaces of rings C and D and the 17β-ketol side chain.[50] It is possible, however, that association with the unsubstituted α-surface of rings A, C, and D, as well as with the ketol side chain, is essential for sodium-retaining activity. Many functional groups, such as 17α-OH, 17α-CH_3, 16α-CH_3, 16β-CH_3, 16α-CH_3O, and 16α-OH substituents, abolish or reverse this activity in 11-desoxycorticosterone and 11-oxygenated steroids. Discussions of exceptions of these generalities are found in the literature.[50]

Although some steroids cause sodium retention, many have glucocorticoid and either sodium-retaining (MR agonist) or sodium-excreting action. Difficulties in correlating the structures of adrenocorticoids with biologic action are compounded by differences in assay methods, species variation, and mode of drug administration. For example, whereas liver glycogen and anti-inflammatory assays in the rat correlate well, some drugs show high anti-inflammatory action in the rat but little or no antirheumatic activity in humans. The 9α-F analog fludrocortisone acetate is more active than the 9α-Cl analog in terms of sodium retention in the dog; the reverse is true in the rat. Although 16α-methylation and 16β-methylation enhance glucocorticoid activity, anti-inflammatory action is increased disproportionately to glycogenic action in both series.

In humans, eosinopenic and hyperglycemic potencies are essentially the same. There is a close correlation in efficacy ratios derived from these tests and antirheumatic potency (Table 21.1). Because the eosinopenic-hyperglycemic activity and antirheumatic potency show excellent agreement, it has been suggested that these assays afford advantages in the preliminary estimation of anti-inflammatory potency.

Structure-activity studies of glucocorticoids have been carried out mainly in animals and are not necessarily applicable to clinical efficacy in man. Relative activity and dose correlations for some of the clinically useful drugs are discussed in the Systemic Corticosteroids section.

DOUBLE BONDS. Several other compounds have been studied in animals and used to derive structure-activity relationships. For example, insertion of a double bond between positions 1 and 2 in hydrocortisone increases glucocorticoid activity. The Δ^1-corticoids have a much longer half-life in the blood than hydrocortisone. Ring A is much more slowly metabolized, but it is oxidatively metabolized at other positions, especially the 6β position and the

Table 21.1 Biologic Potencies of Modified Adrenocorticoids in the Rat and Humans

		Potency Relative to Hydrocortisone (Cortisol)			
		Rat		Human	
Adrenocorticoid	Thymus Involution	Liver Glycogen Deposition	Eosinopenic Potency	Hyperglycemic Potency	Antirheumatic Potency
Corticosterone	–	0.8	0.06	0.06	<0.1
Prednisone	–	3	–	4	4
Prednisolone	2	3.9	4	4	4
Methylprednisolone	10	11	5	5	5
Triamcinolone	4	47	5	5	5
Paramethasone (6α-fluoro-16α-methylprednisolone)	–	150	12	12	11
Dexamethasone	56	265	28	28	29
Fludrocortisone acetate	6	9	8	8	10
Fluprednisolone (6α-fluoro-prednisolone)	6	81	9	9	10
Triamcinolone acetonide	33	242	3	3	3
Flurandrenolone	4	–	1	–	2
Fluorometholone	25	115	10	10	–
Fluocinolone	19	112	5	6	9

Data from Ringer I. Steroidal activity in experimental animals and man. In: Dorfman RI, ed. *Methods of Hormone Research*. Vol. 3, Part A. New York: Academic Press; 1964.

17β-ketol as discussed in the section entitled Prednisone, Prednisolone, and Its Derivatives (Δ^1). If, however, a double bond is inserted between positions 9 and 11 (no oxygen function at 11), a decrease in glucocorticoid activity is observed. Except for cortisone, which results in an analog with decreased glucocorticoid activity, a double bond inserted between position 6 and 7 generally produces no change in activity.[17]

α-METHYLATION. Insertion of an α-CH_3 group at positions 2 (in 11β-OH analogs), 6, and 16 increases glucocorticoid activity in animals. Again, insertion of a 2α-CH_3 group into the glucocorticoid almost completely prevents reduction of the Δ^4-3-ketone system in vivo and in vitro. Substitutions at positions 4α, 7α, 9α, 11α, and 21 decrease activity.

α-HYDROXYLATION. Although some analogs, such as 16α,17α-isopropylidinedioxy-6α-methylpregna-1,4-diene-3,20-dione, and the 1,2-dihydro derivative, are 11-desoxysteroids and biologically active, the hydrogen bond donating 11β-OH group of hydrocortisone has been demonstrated to be almost an essential drug-receptor interaction.[50] Cortisone, which contains an 11-keto function, is reduced in vivo to hydrocortisone. The drug 2α-methylhydrocortisone exhibits high glucocorticoid activity, probably because of steric hindrance by the methyl group to reductive inactivation at the 3-position (i.e., C=O → C-β-OH).[51-53] Insertion of α-OH groups into most other positions (e.g., 1, 6, 7, 9, 14, and 16) or reduction of the 20-ketone, however, decreases glucocorticoid activity, in part because of increased hydrophilicity.

The 9α-F group nearly prevents metabolic oxidation of the 11β-OH group to a ketone. Redox metabolism of Δ^4-3-ketone steroids is mainly restricted to the Δ^4-3-ketone, 6 and 16 positions, and 17β-ketol side chains, whereas for 9α-F Δ^4-3-ketone steroids, it is only the 6 and 16 positions and 17β-ketol side chains that are metabolized. Furthermore, the 9α-F group increases glucocorticoid affinity by an inductive effect, which increases the acidic dissociation constant of the 11β-OH group and, thereby, increases the ability of the drug to hydrogen bond to Asn564 of GR.

α-FLUORINATION. A 6α-F group also increases glucocorticoid activity, but it has less effect than the 9α-F function on sodium retention. Insertion of 2α-, 11α- (no OH group at 11), or 21-F groups decreases glucocorticoid activity. Of particular interest is a 12α-F group. When this function is inserted into corticosterone, which has no 17α-OH group, it potentiates activity to the same extent as a 9α-F group. However, although a 9α-F group potentiates activity in 16α,17α-dihydroxy steroids, a 12α-F group is inactivating. It has been proposed that intramolecular hydrogen bonding between the 12α-F and 17α-OH groups renders the analog inactive (Fig. 21.13). Conversion to the 16α,17α-isopropylidinedioxy (acetonide) derivative, which cannot hydrogen bond, restores biologic activity[54]; possibly by providing hydrogen bonding acceptors for the NH_2 of Gln642.

MINERALOCORTICOID RECEPTOR ACTIVATION. The mineralocorticoid activity of adrenocorticoids is another action of major significance. Many toxic side effects, making it necessary to withdraw steroid therapy in rheumatoid patients, are a result of this action. Some highly active, naturally occurring mineralocorticoids have no OH function in positions 11 and 17 (e.g., aldosterone in Fig. 21.12). In fact, OH groups in any position reduce the sodium-retaining activity of the adrenocorticoids.

9α-F, 9α-Cl, and 9α-Br substitution usually causes increased retention of urinary sodium with an order of activity of F > Cl > Br, but species differences do exist. For these reasons, such compounds are not used internally in the treatment of diseases such as rheumatoid arthritis. Insertion of a 16α-OH group into the molecule affects the sodium retention activity so markedly that it not only negates the effect of the 9α-F but also causes sodium excretion; see for example triamcinolone (Fig. 21.12) as discussed in the Systemic Corticosteroids section.

A double bond between positions 1 and 2 (Δ^1-corticoids) also reduces the sodium retention activity of the parent drug. However, this functional group contributes to the parent drug approximately one-fifth the sodium-excreting tendency of a 16α-OH group.[55]

The 12α-F, 2α-CH_3, and 9α-Cl substitutions contribute equally to sodium retention. A 21-OH group, found in all these drugs, contributes to this action to the same degree. Because 21-OH groups also contribute to glucocorticoid activity, it is easy to understand why it is difficult to develop compounds with only one major action.

A 2α-CH_3 group is approximately 3-fold, and a 21-F substituent 2-fold, as effective as unsaturation between positions 1 and 2 in reducing sodium retention. Other substituents reported to inhibit sodium retention include 16α-CH_3, 16β-CH_3, 16α-CH_3O, and 6α-Cl functions. A 17α-OH group, which is present in naturally occurring and semisynthetic analogs, reduces sodium retention to about the same extent as unsaturation between positions 1 and 2. Many of these effects can be rationalized in terms of GR versus MR structural biology (Figs. 21.11 and 21.12), as discussed above.

17α-ESTERS OR ETHERS VERSUS 21-ESTERS OR 21-HALOGENS. Conversion of the 17α-hydroxy to either a 17α-ester or an ether, as with 16α,17α-isopropylidinedioxy (acetonide), greatly enhances the anti-inflammatory potency and GR affinity. However, esterifying the 21-hydroxy group reduces activity and receptor affinity. On the other hand,

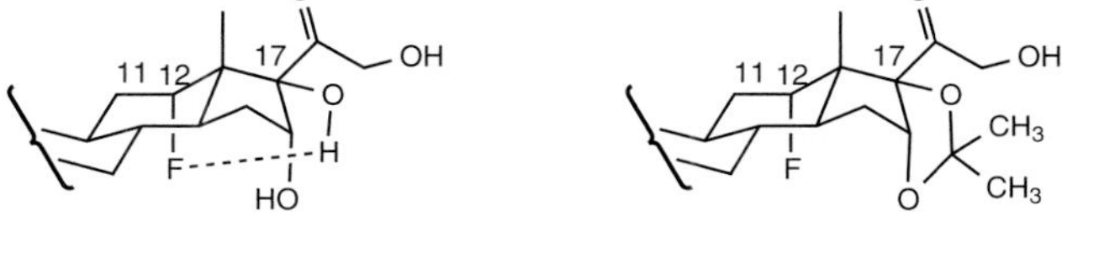

Figure 21.13 Role of intramolecular hydrogen bonding in adrenocorticoid activity.

21-halogens or 21-halomethylene groups greatly increase topical anti-inflammatory activity with no change or a decrease in mineralocorticoid activity. Perhaps a hydrogen bonding group at position 21 of the naturally occurring 17β-ketol enhances or retains mineralocorticoid receptor affinity, possibly through interaction with Thr945.

Pharmacologic Effects and Clinical Applications

In addition to their natural hormonal actions, the adrenocorticoids have many clinical uses. Glucocorticoids and mineralocorticoids can be used for the treatment of adrenal insufficiency (hypoadrenalism), which results from failure of the adrenal glands to synthesize adequate amounts of the hormones. Adrenocorticoids are also used to maintain patients who have had partial or complete removal of their adrenal glands or adenohypophysis (adrenalectomy and hypophysectomy, respectively).

Two major uses of glucocorticoids are in the treatment of rheumatoid diseases and allergic manifestations. Their use in the treatment of severe asthma is well documented, as is the utility of glucocorticoids in sepsis and acute respiratory distress syndrome.[56,57] They are effective in the treatment of rheumatoid arthritis, acute rheumatic fever, bursitis, spontaneous hypoglycemia in children, gout, rheumatoid carditis, sprue, allergy (including contact dermatitis), and other conditions. The treatment of chronic rheumatic diseases and allergic conditions with glucocorticoids is symptomatic and continuous. Symptoms return after withdrawal of the drug. Because the glucocorticoids can cross the placenta and distribute into milk, their use in pregnant women and new mothers warrants careful consideration of the glucocorticoid selected, route of administration, dose and duration of therapy, and potential effects on the child.

In addition, these drugs are moderately effective in the treatment of ulcerative colitis, dermatomyositis, periarteritis nodosa, idiopathic pulmonary fibrosis, idiopathic thrombocytopenic purpura, regional ileitis, acquired hemolytic anemia, nephrosis, cirrhotic ascites, neurodermatitis, and temporal arteritis. The newer analogs with medium- to high-potency rankings as discussed in the Topical Glucocorticoids section are effective topically in the treatment of psoriasis. Glucocorticoids can be combined with antibiotics to treat pneumonia, peritonitis, typhoid fever, and meningococcemia.

When dosages with equivalent antirheumatic potency are given to patients not previously treated with steroids, the Δ^1-corticoids prednisone and prednisolone promote the same pattern of initial improvement as hydrocortisone. Statistically significant improvements during the first few months of therapy have been similar with prednisone, prednisolone, and hydrocortisone. The results of longer-term therapy have been significantly better with the modified (Δ^1) compounds.

Satisfactory rheumatic control, lost after prolonged hydrocortisone therapy, may be regained in an appreciable number of patients by changing to prednisone, prednisolone, or other synthetic glucocorticoids. Of patients whose conditions deteriorate below adequate levels during hydrocortisone administration, nearly half reach their previous level of improvement using Δ^1-corticoids in doses slightly larger in terms of antirheumatic strength. With further prolongation of steroid therapy, improvement again wanes in some patients, but in other patients, such management is successful for longer than 2 years. In some instances, the improvement is attributed to increased effectiveness of the drug because of correction of salt and water retention; in other instances, there is no adequate explanation.

When these drugs are administered in doses that have similar antirheumatic strengths, the general incidence of adverse reactions with prednisone and prednisolone is about the same as that with hydrocortisone. The compounds differ, however, in their tendencies to induce specific side effects. The incidence and degree of salt and water retention and blood pressure elevation are less with the Δ^1-corticoids. Conversely, these analogs are more likely to promote digestive complaints, peptic ulcer, vasomotor symptoms, and cutaneous ecchymosis.

Although these analogs have unwanted side effects, most clinical investigators prefer the Δ^1-corticoids to hydrocortisone for rheumatoid patients who require steroid therapy. The reasons are that these drugs have a lower tendency to cause salt and water retention and potassium loss and that they restore improvement in a significant percentage of patients whose therapeutic control has been lost during hydrocortisone therapy.

Most importantly, glucocorticoids should not be withdrawn abruptly in cases of acute infections or severe stress, such as surgery or trauma. Myasthenia gravis, peptic ulcer, diabetes mellitus, hyperthyroidism, hypertension, psychological disturbances, pregnancy (first trimester), and infections may be aggravated by glucocorticoid administration. Hormone therapy is contraindicated in these conditions and should be used only with the utmost precaution.

Semisynthetic analogs exhibiting high mineralocorticoid activity are not employed in the treatment of rheumatic disorders because of toxic side effects resulting from a disturbance of electrolyte and water balance. Some newer synthetic steroids (Table 21.1) are relatively free of sodium-retaining activity. They can show other toxic manifestations, however, and eventually may need to be withdrawn.

Glucocorticoids are sometimes used in the treatment of scleroderma, discoid lupus, acute nephritis, osteoarthritis, acute hepatitis, hepatic coma, Hodgkin disease, multiple myeloma, lymphoid tumors, acute leukemia, and chronic lymphatic leukemia and to alleviate the side effects of chemotherapy and radiation therapy in nonhematologic malignancies. Glucocorticoids may be more or less effective in these diseases depending on the clinical condition.

Some modified compounds have been recommended for use when other analogs are no longer effective or when it is desirable to promote increased appetite and weight gain (e.g., wasting diseases). In contrast, triamcinolone can be used advantageously when salt and water retention (leading to hypertension or cardiac compensation) or excessive appetite and weight gain are problematic in corticosteroid therapy management.

Percutaneous absorption is one factor that must not be overlooked when applying potent anti-inflammatory agents with high mineralocorticoid activity to the skin. Sodium retention and edema occur in patients with dermatitis who apply as much as 75 mg of fludrocortisone acetate (i.e., 30 mL of a 0.25% lotion) to the skin in 24 hours. The relative rate of percutaneous absorption, administered as a cream in rats, was triamcinolone acetate ≥ hydrocortisone > dexamethasone. However, dexamethasone was deposited in skin longer than the other two drugs and hydrocortisone disappeared most rapidly.[58]

Topical Applications

Topical dermatologic products with a low potency ranking have a modest anti-inflammatory effect and are the safest for chronic application, as is discussed further in the Topical Glucocorticoids section. These products are also the safest products for use on the face, with occlusion, and in infants and young children. Those products with a medium potency ranking are used in moderate inflammatory dermatoses, such as chronic hand eczema and atopic eczema, and may be used for a limited duration on the face and intertriginous areas (areas where skin comes into contact with itself, such as the armpits, the groin, and beneath the breasts, which are more prone to infections and rashes because they are warm and often sweaty). High-potency preparations are used in more severe inflammatory dermatoses, such as severe eczema and psoriasis. They can be used for a limited duration and for longer periods in areas with thickened skin because of chronic conditions. High-potency preparations may also be used on the face and intertriginous areas, but only for a short treatment duration.

Very high–potency products are used primarily as an alternative to systemic corticosteroid therapy when local areas are involved. Examples of conditions for which very high–potency products frequently are used include thick, chronic lesions caused by psoriasis, lichen simplex chronicus, and discoid lupus erythematosus. They may be used for only a short duration of therapy and on small surface areas. Occlusive dressings should not be used with these products. It has been suggested that patients using a lotion or ointment containing these drugs be instructed to apply them sparingly and to spread them lightly over the affected areas. The extent and frequency of applications should be carefully considered. A lotion vehicle is more effective when treating a dermatitis, but a greater degree of percutaneous absorption occurs than when ointments are used.

Intranasal and Inhaled Applications

Pulmonary and nasal bioavailabilities are important determinants for the potential of an inhaled or nasally applied corticosteroid to cause systemic effects because the lung and nasal tissue provide an enormous surface area from which drug absorption can occur into the systemic circulation. The main areas of concern with regard to systemic effects include HPA axis suppression, change in bone mineral density and growth retardation in children, cataracts, and glaucoma. Systemic side effects depend on the dose, administration frequency, and the half-life of the drug, as well as time of day when administered and route of administration. Higher plasma corticosteroid concentrations and a longer half-life will produce greater systemic side effects.[59] The amount of an inhaled or nasal corticosteroid reaching the systemic circulation is the sum of the drug concentration available following absorption from the lungs/nasal mucosa and from the GI tract. The fraction deposited in the mouth will be swallowed, and the systemic availability will be determined by its absorption from the GI tract and the degree of first-pass metabolism.

Delivery devices can produce clinically significant differences in activity by altering the dose deposited in the lung (10%-25%) and, for orally absorbed drugs, the amount deposited in the oropharynx and swallowed (75%-90%). Clinical studies have shown the following relative potency differences: ciclesonide > mometasone furoate > fluticasone propionate > budesonide = beclomethasone dipropionate (BDP) > triamcinolone acetonide = flunisolide (see Inhaled and Intranasal Glucocorticoids section for structures and further discussion of these agents). Potency differences can be overcome by giving larger doses of the less potent drug, which increases risks from systemic effects. Adrenal suppression may be associated with high doses of inhaled corticosteroids (>1.5 or >0.75 mg/d for fluticasone propionate), although there is a considerable degree of interindividual susceptibility.

All currently used inhaled corticosteroids are rapidly cleared from the body but show varying levels of oral bioavailability, with fluticasone propionate having the lowest (as will be discussed). Following inhalation, there is also considerable variability in the rate of absorption from the lung; pulmonary residence times are greatest for fluticasone propionate and triamcinolone acetonide and shortest for budesonide and flunisolide. Adrenal suppression has been observed when intranasal fluticasone propionate was administered in doses of 200-4000 mcg daily for up to 12 months.

Adverse Effects

Although short-term administration of corticosteroids is unlikely to produce harmful effects, these drugs, when used for longer than brief periods, can produce a variety of devastating effects, including glucocorticoid-induced adrenocortical insufficiency, glucocorticoid-induced osteoporosis, and generalized protein depletion.[17] The duration of anti-inflammatory activity of glucocorticoids approximately equals the duration of HPA axis suppression. The durations of HPA axis suppression after a single oral dose of glucocorticoids in one study are shown in Table 21.2. When given for prolonged periods, glucocorticoids suppress the HPA axis, thereby decreasing secretion of endogenous corticosteroids and causing adrenal atrophy. Glucocorticoids inhibit ACTH production by the adenohypophysis, and in turn, this reduces endogenous glucocorticoid production. With time, atrophy of the adrenal glands takes place. The degree and duration of adrenocortical insufficiency produced by the synthetic glucocorticoids

Table 21.2 Effect of an Oral Single Dose on the Duration of Hypothalamic-Pituitary-Adrenal (HPA) Axis Suppression

Adrenocorticoid	Duration of Suppression (d)
Hydrocortisone (250 mg)	1.25-1.5
Cortisone (250 mg)	1.25-1.5
Methylprednisolone (40 mg)	1.25-1.5
Prednisone (50 mg)	1.25-1.5
Prednisolone (50 mg)	1.25-1.5
Triamcinolone (40 mg)	2.25
Dexamethasone (5 mg)	2.75
Betamethasone (6 mg)	3.25

is highly variable among patients and depends on the dose, frequency and time of administration, and duration of glucocorticoid therapy. This effect can be minimized by use of alternate-day therapy.

Patients who develop drug-induced adrenocortical insufficiency may require higher corticosteroid dosage when they are subjected to stress (e.g., infection, surgery, or trauma). In addition, acute adrenal insufficiency (even death) can occur if the drugs are withdrawn abruptly or if patients are transferred from systemic glucocorticoid therapy to oral inhalation therapy. Therefore, the drugs should be withdrawn very gradually following long-term therapy with pharmacologic doses. Adrenal suppression can persist up to 12 months in patients who receive large doses for prolonged periods. Until recovery occurs, patients may show signs and symptoms of adrenal insufficiency when they are subjected to stress and replacement therapy may be required. Because mineralocorticoid secretion can be impaired, sodium chloride or a mineralocorticoid also should be administered.

Although side effects and toxicities vary with the drug and, sometimes, with the patient, facial mooning, flushing, sweating, acne, thinning of the scalp hair, abdominal distention, and weight gain are observed with most glucocorticoids. Protein depletion (with osteoporosis and spontaneous fractures), myopathy (with weakness of muscles of the thighs, pelvis, and lower back), and aseptic necrosis of the hip and humerus are other side effects. These drugs can cause psychological disturbances, headache, vertigo, and peptic ulcer, and they can suppress growth in children.

Patients with well-controlled diabetes must be closely monitored and their insulin dosage increased if glycosuria or hyperglycemia ensues either during or following glucocorticoid administration. Patients should also be watched for signs of adrenocorticoid insufficiency after discontinuation of glucocorticoid therapy. Individuals with a history of tuberculosis should receive prophylactic doses of antituberculosis drugs.

Osteoporosis is one of the most serious adverse effects of long-term glucocorticoid therapy. Moderate- to high-dose glucocorticoid therapy is associated with loss of bone and an increased risk of fracture that is most rapid during the initial 6 months of therapy. These adverse effects of glucocorticoids appear to be both dose- and duration-dependent, with oral prednisone doses of 7.5 mg or more daily for 6 months or longer often resulting in clinically important bone loss and increased fracture risk. Bone loss has even been associated with oral inhalation of glucocorticoids and is of great concern in children. Most patients receiving long-term glucocorticoid therapy will develop some degree of bone loss, and more than 25% will develop osteoporotic fractures. Vertebral fractures have been reported in 11% of patients with asthma who are receiving systemic glucocorticoids for at least 1 year, and glucocorticoid-treated patients with rheumatoid arthritis are at increased risk of fractures of the hip, rib, spine, leg, ankle, and foot. Muscle wasting or weakness and atrophy of the protein matrix of the bone resulting in osteoporosis are manifestations of protein catabolism, which can occur during prolonged therapy with glucocorticoids. These adverse effects can be especially serious in debilitated patients, in geriatric populations, and in postmenopausal women who are especially prone to osteoporosis.

To minimize the risk of glucocorticoid-induced bone loss (osteoporosis) and in those with low mineral bone density, the smallest possible effective dose and duration should be used. Topical and inhaled preparations should be used whenever possible. The immunosuppressive effects of glucocorticoids increase the susceptibility to, and mask the symptoms of, infections and can result in activation of latent infection or exacerbation of intercurrent infections. The most common adverse effect of oral inhalation therapy with glucocorticoids is fungal infections of the mouth, the pharynx, and, occasionally, the larynx. The mineralocorticoid effects are less frequent with synthetic glucocorticoids (except fludrocortisone) than with hydrocortisone but may occur, especially when synthetic glucocorticoids are given in high doses for prolonged periods.

DEVELOPMENT OF ADRENOCORTICOID DRUGS

Systemic Corticosteroids

The route of administration depends on the disease being treated and the physicochemical, pharmacologic, and pharmacokinetic properties of the drug (Table 21.3). The clinically available adrenocorticoids may be administered by IV or IM injection, oral tablets or solutions, topical formulations, intra-articular or other local parenteral administration, and oral or nasal inhalation (Table 21.4). Several but not all of the corticosteroids are used clinically by the oral route, including betamethasone, budesonide, cortisone, deflazacort, dexamethasone, fludrocortisone, hydrocortisone, methylprednisolone, prednisolone, prednisone, and triamcinolone (Fig. 21.14 and Table 21.4). These corticosteroids are often described as short acting, intermediate acting, or long acting according to their biologic half-life and duration of action (Table 21.3). They are well-absorbed, undergo little first-pass

Table 21.3 Pharmacological and Pharmacokinetic Properties for Some Adrenocorticoids

		Potency Relative to Hydrocortisone			Half-Life (hr)		
Adrenocorticoid	Oral Glucocorticoid Dose[a] (mg)	Glucocorticoid Activity[b]	Mineralocorticoid Activity[c]	Protein Binding (%)[d]	Plasma	Biologic (Tissue)	Duration of Action (d)
Glucocorticoids							
Short-acting:							
Hydrocortisone	20	1	2+	>90	1.5-2.0	8-12	1.0-1.5
Cortisone	25	0.8	2+	>90	0.5	8-12	1.0-1.5
Intermediate-acting:							
Prednisone	5	3.5	1+	>90	3.4-3.8	18-36	1.0-1.5
Prednisolone	5	4	1+	>90	2.1-3.5	18-36	1.0-1.5
Methylprednisolone	5	5	0[e]	>90	>3.5	18-36	1.0-1.5
Triamcinolone	5	5	0[e]		2-5	18-36	1.0-1.5
Deflazacort	6	3	0[e]	40[f]			
Long-acting:							
Dexamethasone	0.75	20-30	0[e]	>90	3.0-4.5	36-54	2.8-3
Betamethasone	0.6	20-30	0[e]	>90	3-5	36-54	2.8-3
Mineralocorticoids							
Fludrocortisone	Not employed	10	10	<90	3.5	18-36	1-2
Aldosterone	Not employed	0.2	800				
11-Desoxycorticosterone	Not employed	0	40				
Corticosterone	IM	0.5	5				

[a]Based on the oral dose of an anti-inflammatory agent in rheumatoid arthritis.
[b]Anti-inflammatory, immunosuppressant, and metabolic effects.
[c]Sodium and water retention and potassium depletion effects.
[d]Hydrocortisone binds to transcortin (corticosteroid binding globulin [CBG]) and to albumin. Prednisone also binds to CBG, but betamethasone, dexamethasone, and tramcinolone do not.
[e]Although these glucocorticoids are considered not to have significant mineralocorticoid activity, hypokalemia and/or sodium and fluid retention may occur depending on the dosage, duration of use, and patient predisposition.
[f]Plasma protein binding for 21-desDFZ.

Table 21.4 Adrenocorticoids: Trade Names and Routes of Administration

Adrenocorticoid	Trade Name	PO	IV	IM or Local Injection	Inhaled or Intranasal	Topical
Alclometasone dipropionate						✓
Amcinonide						✓
Beclomethasone dipropionate (BDP)	Qnasl, Qvar				✓	
Beclomethasone dipropionate monohydrate	Beconase AQ				✓	
Betamethasone	Celestone	✓				
Betamethasone dipropionate	Diprolene, Diprolene AF, Maxivate					✓
Betamethasone sodium phosphate	Celestone Soluspan			✓		
Betamethasone valerate	BetaVal, Luxiq, Valisone					✓
Budesonide	Pulmicort TurbuHaler, Pulmicort Respules, Pulmicort Flexhaler, Rhinocort Allergy (OTC)[a]				✓	
Budesonide	Uceris[b], Entocort EC	✓				✓[b]
Ciclesonide	Alvesco, Omnaris, Zetonna				✓	
Clobetasol propionate	Clobex, Cormax, Embuline, Olux					✓
Clocortolone pivalate	Cloderm					✓
Cortisone acetate		✓		✓		
Deflazacort	Emflaza	✓				
Desonide	Desonate, Desowen, Verdeso					✓
Desoximetasone	Topicort					✓
Dexamethasone	Dexycu Kit[c], Maxidex[c], Ozurdex[c]	✓				✓[c]
Dexamethasone acetate	Dalalone, Dexasone			✓		
Dexamethasone sodium phosphate			✓	✓		✓[c]
Diflorasone diacetate	ApexiCon E					✓
Fludrocortisone acetate		✓				
Flunisolide	Aerospan HFA				✓	
Fluocinolone acetonide	Capex, Derma-Smoothe, Dermotic, Iluvien,[c] Retisert,[c] Synlar, Tri-Luma					✓
Fluocinonide	Lidex, Vanos					✓
Fluorometholone	FML					✓[c]
Fluorometholone acetate	Flarex					✓[c]
Flurandrenolide	Cordran					✓
Fluticasone furoate	Arnuity Ellipta, Veramyst				✓	
Fluticasone propionate	Cutivate, Flovent Diskus, Flovent HFA, Flonase Allergy Relief (OTC), Xhance				✓	✓

Table 21.4 Adrenocorticoids: Trade Names and Routes of Administration (Continued)

Adrenocorticoid	Trade Name	PO	IV	IM or Local Injection	Inhaled or Intranasal	Topical
Halcinonide	Halog					✓
Halobetasol propionate	Ultravate					✓
Hydrocortisone	Ala-Cort, Anusol HC, Colocort, Cortef, Texacort	✓				✓[b]
Hydrocortisone acetate	Cortiform, Micort HC, Pramosone, Proctofoam HC					✓[c]
Hydrocortisone buteprate	Pandel					✓
Hydrocortisone butyrate	Locoid					•
Hydrocortisone sodium phosphate			✓	✓		
Hydrocortisone sodium succinate	Solu-Cortef		✓	✓		
Hydrocortisone valerate						✓
Methylprednisolone	Medrol, Medrol Dose Pack	✓				
Methylprednisolone acetate	Depo-Medrol			✓		✓
Methylprednisolone sodium succinate	Solu-Medrol		✓	✓		
Mometasone furoate	Elocon					✓
Mometasone furoate	Nasonex, Asmanex HFA, Asmanex Twisthaler, Sinuva[d]				✓	✓
Prednicarbate	Dermatop					✓
Prednisolone	Delta-Cortef, Prelone	✓				
Prednisolone acetate	Omnipred, Predcor, Predalone	✓		✓		
Prednisolone acetate	Pred-Mild, Pred-Forte					✓[c]
Prednisolone sodium phosphate	Pediapred, Orapred ODT	✓		✓		✓[c]
Prednisone	Rayos	✓				
Triamcinolone acetonide		✓				
Triamcinolone acetonide	Kenalog, Triderm, Trianex, Delta-Tritex					✓
Triamcinolone acetonide	Allernaze, Nasacort Allergy (OTC), Nasacort AQ				✓	
Triamcinolone acetonide	Kenalog, Zilretta,[e] Triesence[c]			✓		
Triamcinolone diacetate				✓		
Triamcinolone hexacetonide	Aristospan			✓		

[a]Nasal spray is OTC. Aerosol has been discontinued.
[b]Rectal foam for ulcerative colitis.
[c]Ophthalmic formulation (drops, insert, injection, or ointment).
[d]Sinus insert.
[e]Intra-articular injectable extended-release suspension.
IM, intramuscular; IV, intravenous; PO, oral.

Table 21.5 Pharmacokinetics of Commonly Used Oral Adrenocorticoids

Adrenocorticoid	Bioavailability (%)	Half-Life (hr)	Protein Binding (%)	Volume Distribution (L/kg)	Log P (Experimental)	Clearance (mL/min/70 g)
Dexamethasone	78	3.0	90-95	0.2	1.83	260
Hydrocortisone	96	1.7	90	0.5	1.61	400
Methylprednisolone	90	2.3	90-95	1.5	1.76	430
Prednisone	80	3.6	~90	1.0	1.46	250
Prednisolone	82	2.8	90-95	0.7-1.5	1.62	60
Triamcinolone	23	2.96	~90	1.3	1.16	61

metabolism in the liver, and demonstrate oral bioavailabilities of 70%-80%, except for triamcinolone (Table 21.5). The larger volume of distribution for methylprednisolone compared to prednisolone is thought to result from a combination of increased lipophilicity, plasma and tissue protein binding, and better tissue penetration. Glucocorticoids vary in the extent to which they are bound to the plasma proteins albumin and corticosteroid-binding globulin (transcortin), but most are highly (>90%) bound (Table 21.5).

Hydrocortisone is extensively bound to plasma proteins, primarily to transcortin, with only 5%-10% of plasma hydrocortisone unbound. Prednisolone and methylprednisolone (but not the 9α-fluoro analogs betamethasone, dexamethasone, or triamcinolone) have a high affinity for transcortin and, thus, compete with hydrocortisone for this binding protein. The 9α-halo analogs bind primarily to albumin. As with other drugs, only the unbound fraction of the synthetic corticosteroids is biologically active. Glucocorticoids cross the placenta and can be distributed into milk.

The degree of systemic side effects is dose dependent, related to the half-life of the drug, frequency of administration, time of day when administered, and route of administration. In other words, the higher the plasma corticosteroid concentration and the longer the half-life, the greater the systemic side effects.[59]

Regardless of the route of administration, all synthetic adrenocorticoids are excreted from the body in a manner similar to the endogenous adrenocorticoids (i.e., they are metabolized in the liver and excreted into the urine primarily as glucuronide conjugates but also as sulfate conjugates).[60] In fact, hepatic oxidative metabolism rapidly converts many of the systemic and topical corticosteroids to inactive metabolites and, thus, serves to protect patients from the HPA axis–suppressive effects of these drugs on endogenous steroid production. The corticosteroids are metabolized in many tissues, including the liver, muscles, and red blood cells[18,20,61]; however, the liver metabolizes them most rapidly. The fact that many of the endogenous corticosteroids are rapidly metabolized by the liver precludes their administration by the oral route. Catabolic products can be isolated from the urine and bile and can be formed in tissue preparations in vitro.[62]

Specific Drugs (Fig. 21.14)

11-Desoxycorticosterone was the first naturally occurring corticoid to be synthesized. Before its isolation from the adrenal cortex, it was prepared by M. Steiger and T. Reichstein.[63] As a result of his synthesis of 11-desoxycorticosterone and other early work with corticoids, Reichstein later shared the Nobel Prize with E.C. Kendall, another chemist who was instrumental in carrying out early steroid syntheses, and with P.S. Hench, a rheumatologist who, in 1929, discovered that cortisone is effective in the treatment of rheumatoid arthritis. Kendall's basic research ultimately led to the synthesis of cortisone from naturally occurring bile acids.[63]

CORTISONE, HYDROCORTISONE, AND THEIR DERIVATIVES. After the synthesis of 11-desoxycorticosterone in 1937, all the corticoids were soon thereafter synthesized and their structures confirmed. The first synthesis of cortisone from methyl 3α-hydroxy-11-ketobisnorcholanate was reported by L.H. Sarett[64] in 1946. Earlier work of Kendall and coworkers involving its preparation from the methyl ester of desoxycholic acid was used in his research.[65] Later, several chemists, including Sarett,[66] Kendall, and M. Tishler, found ways to improve the yields and to decrease the labor involved in the multistep conversion of bile acids to cortisone acetate. In 1949, Merck sold limited quantities of this glucocorticoid to physicians at $200 per gram for treating rheumatoid arthritis. Subsequent improvements in the methods of synthesis reduced the price to $10 per gram by 1951. In 1955, Upjohn used an efficient process involving the synthesis of cortisone acetate from progesterone, with the latter steroid being prepared from diosgenin (a steroid sapogenin isolated from the tubers of the *Dioscorea* wild yam). This further reduced the price to $3.50 per gram.

Cortisone is administered orally or by intramuscular (IM) injection as its 21-acetate (cortisone acetate). Cortisone acetate or hydrocortisone (acetate) are usually the corticosteroids of choice for replacement therapy in patients with adrenocortical insufficiency because these drugs have both glucocorticoid and mineralocorticoid properties. Following oral administration, cortisone acetate and hydrocortisone acetate are completely and rapidly

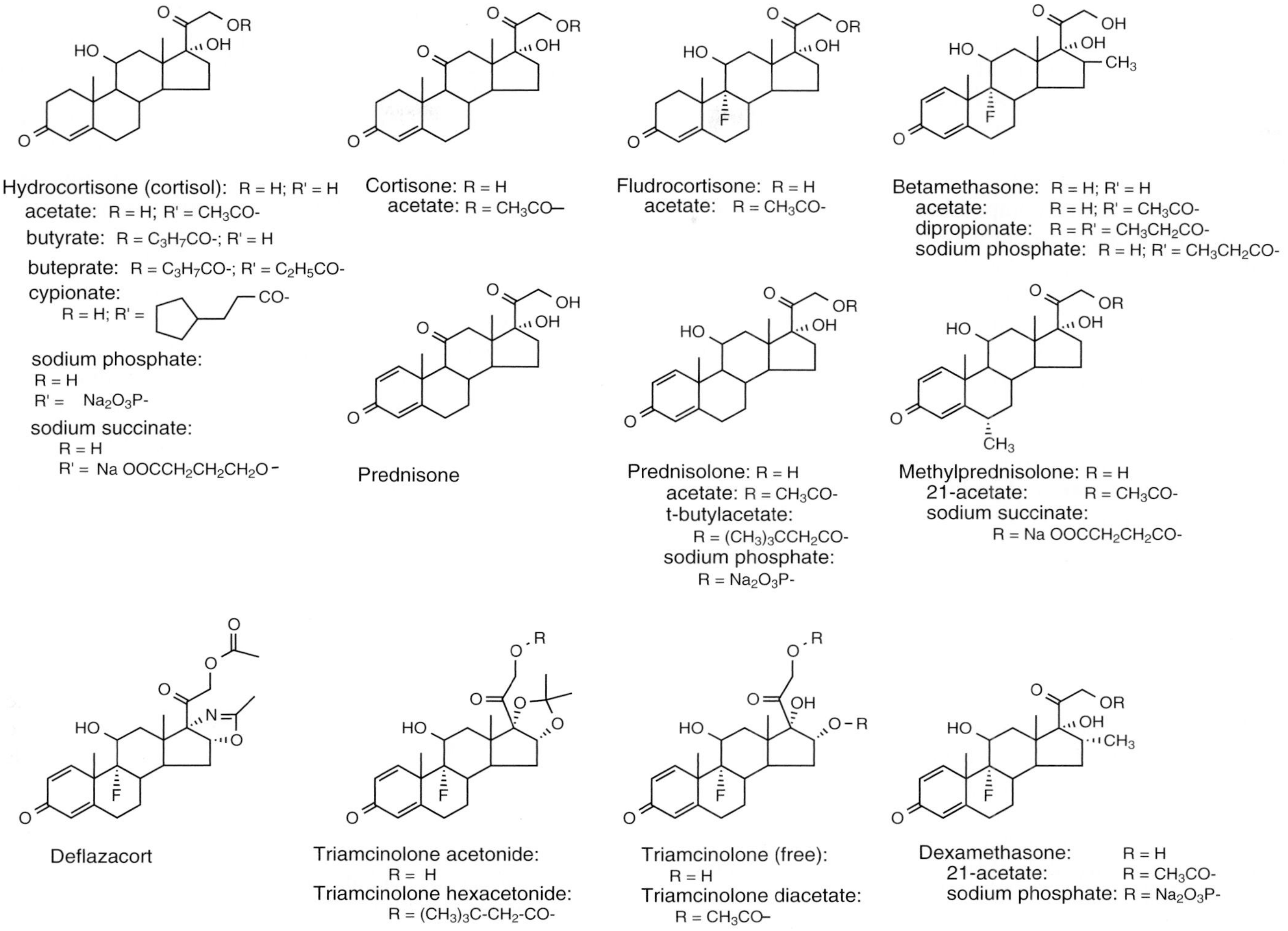

Hydrocortisone (cortisol): R = H; R' = H
acetate: R = H; R' = CH_3CO-
butyrate: R = C_3H_7CO-; R' = H
buteprate: R = C_3H_7CO-; R' = C_2H_5CO-
cypionate: R = H; R' = (cyclopentyl)CH_2CH_2CO-
sodium phosphate: R = H; R' = Na_2O_3P-
sodium succinate: R = H; R' = Na $OOCCH_2CH_2CH_2O$-

Cortisone: R = H
acetate: R = CH_3CO–

Fludrocortisone: R = H
acetate: R = CH_3CO-

Betamethasone: R = H; R' = H
acetate: R = H; R' = CH_3CO-
dipropionate: R = R' = CH_3CH_2CO-
sodium phosphate: R = H; R' = CH_3CH_2CO-

Prednisone

Prednisolone: R = H
acetate: R = CH_3CO-
t-butylacetate: R = $(CH_3)_3CCH_2CO$-
sodium phosphate: R = Na_2O_3P-

Methylprednisolone: R = H
21-acetate: R = CH_3CO-
sodium succinate: R = Na $OOCCH_2CH_2CO$-

Deflazacort

Triamcinolone acetonide: R = H
Triamcinolone hexacetonide: R = $(CH_3)_3C$-CH_2-CO-

Triamcinolone (free): R = H
Triamcinolone diacetate: R = CH_3CO–

Dexamethasone: R = H
21-acetate: R = CH_3CO-
sodium phosphate: R = Na_2O_3P-

Figure 21.14 Systemic corticosteroids.

deacetylated by first-pass esterase metabolism.[67] Much of the oral cortisone, however, is inactivated by oxidative metabolism (Fig. 21.9) before it can be converted to hydrocortisone in the liver.

The pharmacokinetics for hydrocortisone acetate is indistinguishable from that of orally administered hydrocortisone. Oral hydrocortisone is completely absorbed, with a bioavailability of greater than 95% and a half-life of 1-2 hours.[25] The metabolism of hydrocortisone (Fig. 21.9) has been previously described. Cortisone acetate is slowly absorbed from IM injection sites over a period of 24-48 hours and is reserved for patients who are unable to take the drug orally. The acetate ester derivative demonstrates increased stability and has a longer duration of action when administered by IM injection. Thus, smaller doses can be used. Similarly, hydrocortisone may be dispensed as its 21-acetate (hydrocortisone acetate), which is superior to cortisone acetate when injected intra-articularly. Systemic absorption of hydrocortisone acetate from intra-articular injection sites is usually complete within 24-48 hours. When administered intrarectally, hydrocortisone is poorly absorbed.[68,69]

Other ester derivatives that are available include the lipophilic hydrocortisone cypionate (21-[3-cyclopentylpropionate] ester), hydrocortisone butyrate (17α-butyrate ester), hydrocortisone buteprate (17α-butyrate, 21-propionate esters), and hydrocortisone valerate (17α-valerate ester), along with water soluble hydrocortisone sodium succinate (21-sodium succinate ester) and hydrocortisone sodium phosphate (the 21-sodium phosphate ester) (Fig. 21.14).

- The water-insoluble hydrocortisone cypionate is used orally in doses expressed in terms of hydrocortisone for slower absorption from the gastrointestinal (GI) tract.
- The water-insoluble butyrate, buteprate, and valerate esters are used topically.
- The extremely water-soluble 21-sodium succinate and 21-sodium phosphate esters are used for IV or IM injection in the management of emergency conditions that can be treated with anti-inflammatory steroids (e.g., adrenal crisis during surgery, shock). The phosphate ester is completely and rapidly metabolized by phosphatases, with a half-life of less than 5 minutes.[68] Peak hydrocortisone levels are reached in approximately 10 minutes. The sodium succinate ester is slowly and incompletely hydrolyzed, and peak hydrocortisone levels are attained in 30-45 minutes.[68]

After the introduction of cortisone (1948) and, later, hydrocortisone (1951) for the treatment of rheumatoid arthritis, many investigators began to search for superior agents having fewer side effects. When these drugs are used in doses necessary to suppress symptoms of rheumatoid arthritis, they also affect other metabolic processes. Side effects, such as excessive sodium retention and potassium excretion, negative nitrogen balance, increased gastric acidity, edema, and psychosis, are exaggerated manifestations of the normal metabolic functions of the hormones.

It was hoped that a compound with high glucocorticoid and low mineralocorticoid activity could be synthesized. Because it was recognized early from SAR that a carbonyl group at C3, a double bond between carbons 4 and 5, an oxygen (C=O or β-OH) at carbon 11, and a β-ketol side chain at position 17 are necessary for superior glucocorticoid activity, investigators began to synthesize analogs containing these functions. Additional groups were inserted into other positions of the basic steroid structure, with the expectation that these new substituents might modify the glucocorticoid and mineralocorticoid activities of the parent drugs.

FLUDROCORTISONE (9α-FLUORO). A 9α-bromo analog was prepared that had one-third the glucocorticoid activity of cortisone acetate.[51] Other halogens were introduced into the 9α-position, and it was soon observed that glucocorticoid activity is inversely proportional to the size of the halogen at carbon 9 due to diminishing electron withdrawing effects and increased steric hindrance with the larger halogens. The 9α-fluoro analog (fludrocortisone; Fig. 21.14) is approximately 11-fold more potent at GR and even more potent at MR than cortisone acetate (Table 21.3) due to inductive effects of the fluorine which enhance the ability of the 11β-OH to hydrogen bond with GR (Asn564) and MR (Asn770) and inhibition of metabolic oxidation to the less active 11-keto. Fludrocortisone is orally administered as its 21-acetate derivative. When tested clinically in patients with rheumatoid arthritis, it was found to be effective at approximately one-tenth the dose of cortisone acetate. Although glucocorticoid activity is increased 11-fold by insertion of the 9α-fluoro substituent, mineralocorticoid activity is increased 300- to 800-fold. Because of its intense sodium-retaining activity, fludrocortisone is contraindicated in all conditions except those that require a high degree of mineralocorticoid activity because it leads to edema.

Fludrocortisone acetate is used orally for mineralocorticoid replacement therapy in patients with adrenocortical insufficiency, such as Addison's disease. This drug, introduced in 1954, helped to provide the impetus for the synthesis and biologic evaluation of newer halogenated analogs.

PREDNISONE, PREDNISOLONE, AND THEIR DERIVATIVES (Δ^1). One year after the introduction of fludrocortisone, the Δ^1-corticoids were brought forth into clinical medicine. Investigators at Schering observed that the 1-dehydro derivatives of cortisone and hydrocortisone—namely, prednisone and prednisolone—are more potent antirheumatic and antiallergenic agents than the parent compounds and produced fewer undesirable side effects at lower doses. These compounds are known as Δ^1-corticoids because they contain an additional double bond between positions 1 and 2 (Fig. 21.14).

The Δ^1-corticoids were the first chemical innovation that led to the creation of modified compounds that could be prescribed for rheumatoid arthritis. Both prednisone and prednisolone were found to have adrenocortical activity as measured by eosinopenic response, liver glycogen decomposition, and thymus involution in adrenalectomized mice. In these tests, prednisone and prednisolone were found to be 3- to 4-fold more potent than cortisone and hydrocortisone. Antiphlogistic (anti-inflammatory) strengths in human subjects were similarly augmented, but their electrolyte activities were not proportionately increased (Table 21.3).

The increased potency reflects the effect of the change in geometry of ring A caused by the introduction of C1=C2 on GR affinity and altered pharmacokinetics (primarily metabolism). Although the remaining portions of the steroid are essentially unchanged (except for the less easily visualized molecular perturbations), the conformation of ring A changes from a chair, as in 5α-pregnan-3-one (structure A in Fig. 21.15), to a half-chair (pregn-4-en-3-one; B in Fig. 21.15) and to a flattened boat (pregna-1,4-dien-3-one; C in Fig. 21.15) on introduction of unsaturation.

The order of GR affinity is dexamethasone (10×) > triamcinolone (5×) > methylprednisolone (4×) > prednisolone (2×) > hydrocortisone (1×).[70] The GR binding affinity rank order can be rationalized from SAR observations.

- Addition of the Δ^1 to hydrocortisone to yield prednisolone doubles binding affinity due to A-ring geometry changes discussed above, which are likely to improve interaction with Gln570 and Arg611 of GR.
- Addition of 6α-methyl to prednisolone to yield methylprednisolone (Δ^1, 6α-CH_3) again doubles binding affinity (4× hydrocortisone) and provides GR selectivity. Additional benefits of Δ^1 and 6α-methyl groups include prevention of metabolism at the 3-keto and C6 positions.
- Addition of 9α-fluoro to hydrocortisone to yield fludrocortisone also enhances GR and MR affinity through inductive effects on the 11β-OH to enhance interactions with Asn564 (GR) and Asn770 (MR). Inactivating metabolism is also blocked.
- Addition of 16α-substitution provides GR selectivity due to the inability of MR to accommodate bulk or polar groups.

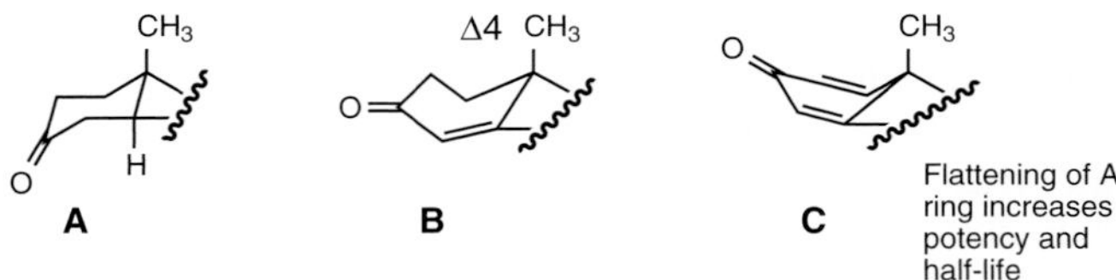

Figure 21.15 Ring A conformations for 5α-pregnan-3-one (A), for pregn-4-en-3-one (B), and for pregna-1,4-dien-3-one (C). All endogenous and some synthetic glucocorticoids are Δ^4 variants of 5α-pregnane; however, many higher potency glucocorticoids are also Δ^1 variants as depicted in (C) above.

- Addition of 9α-fluoro and 16α-OH to prednisolone (Δ^1) to yield triamcinolone more than doubles the GR affinity (5× hydrocortisone vs. 2× for prednisolone) due to an enhanced 11β-OH—Asn564 interaction and introduction of the 16α-OH—Gln642 interaction at the GR. The equivalent of Gln642 is unavailable in MR, explaining the greatly enhanced GR selectivity of triamcinolone relative to prednisolone.
- Changing the 16α-OH of triamcinolone (Δ^1, 9α-F, 16α-OH) to the 16α-methyl of dexamethasone (Δ^1, 9α-F, 16α-methyl) again doubles GR binding affinity (10× hydrocortisone vs. 5× for triamcinolone) due to favorable hydrophobic contacts of the 16α-methyl group within a hydrophobic pocket of GR that is not available in MR.
- The latter two molecules demonstrate that high GR affinity and high GR selectivity are possible through rational substitution of hydrocortisone.

Rank order of GR affinity:
Dexamethasone (10x) > triamcinolone (5x) > methylprednisolone (4x) > prednisolone (2x) > hydrocortisone (1x)

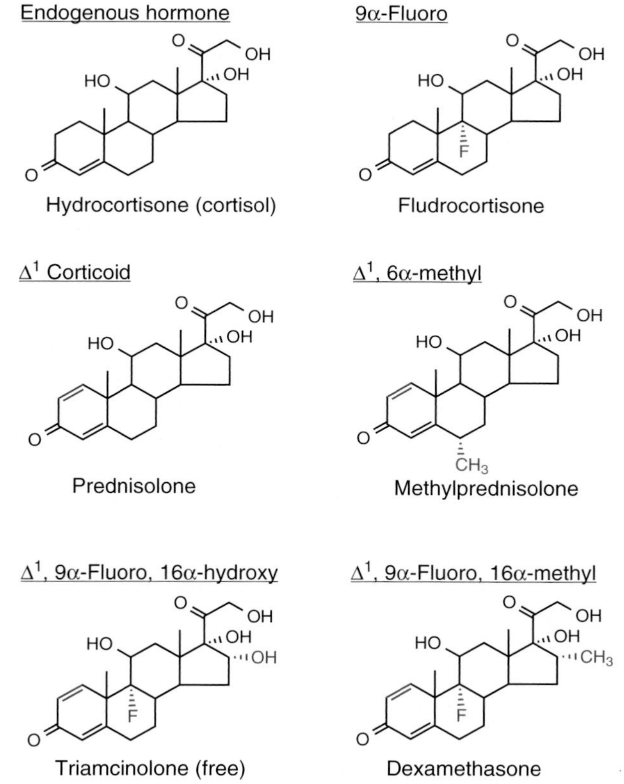

Endogenous hormone — Hydrocortisone (cortisol)

9α-Fluoro — Fludrocortisone

Δ^1 Corticoid — Prednisolone

Δ^1, 6α-methyl — Methylprednisolone

Δ^1, 9α-Fluoro, 16α-hydroxy — Triamcinolone (free)

Δ^1, 9α-Fluoro, 16α-methyl — Dexamethasone

When orally administered, prednisone and prednisolone are almost completely absorbed, with a bioavailability of greater than 80% (Table 21.5).[71,72] As with the relationship between cortisone and hydrocortisone, prednisone and prednisolone are also interconvertible by 11β-hydroxysteroid dehydrogenase type 1 (11β-HSD1) in the liver. For practical purposes, prednisone and prednisolone are equally potent and can be used interchangeably. Due to the higher GR affinity afforded by the flattened A-ring and metabolic stabilization of the 3-keto, when

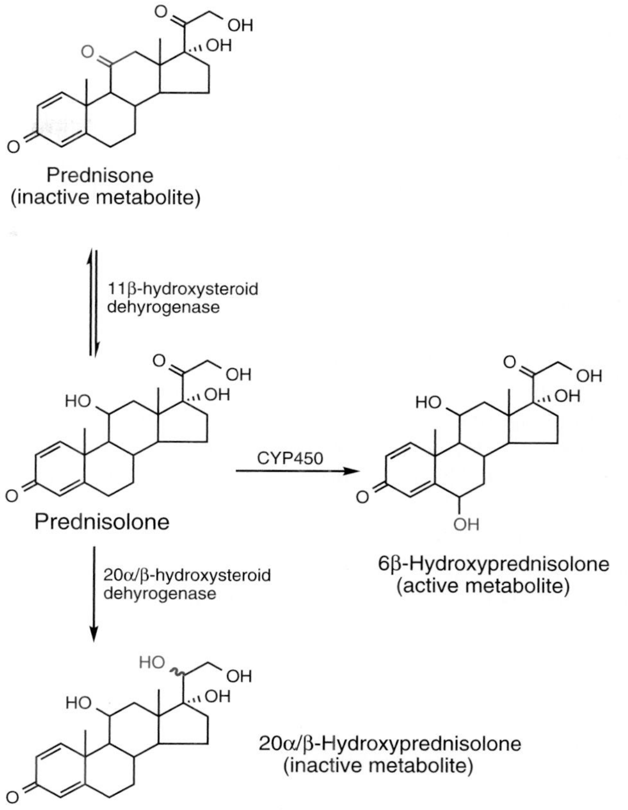

Prednisone (inactive metabolite)

11β-hydroxysteroid dehyrogenase

Prednisolone

CYP450

6β-Hydroxyprednisolone (active metabolite)

20α/β-hydroxysteroid dehyrogenase

20α/β-Hydroxyprednisolone (inactive metabolite)

Figure 21.16 Major routes of metabolism for prednisolone.

prednisone or prednisolone is used in the treatment of rheumatoid arthritis, smaller doses are required than with hydrocortisone. The usual dose is 5 mg two to four times a day.

Prednisolone is metabolized into a number of more hydrophilic and less active metabolites (Fig. 21.16), except that there is greatly decreased reduction of ring A compared with hydrocortisone due to the relatively stable 3-keto within this extended conjugated double bond system. The major metabolites (6β- and 20α/β-hydroxy) are primarily excreted as glucuronide conjugates in the urine.

Prednisolone acetate is available in suspension and ointment forms for external use. As with hydrocortisone, several other 21-esters of prednisolone are available. Prednisolone tebutate (*t*-butylacetate [3,3-dimethylbutyrate]) has been discontinued but was used in suspension form and by injection for the same reasons the 21-ester derivatives of hydrocortisone are currently employed. Prednisolone tebutate had a long duration of action because of low water solubility and a slow rate of hydrolysis.

Prednisolone sodium phosphate is the water-soluble sodium salt of the 21-phosphate ester. It has a half-life of less than 5 minutes because of rapid hydrolysis by phosphatases.[71-73] Peak plasma levels for prednisolone are attained in approximately 10 minutes following its administration by injection (usual dose of 20 mg IV or IM). Topically, one or two drops of a 0.5% solution may be used four to six times daily for its anti-inflammatory action in the eye.

As stated in the Pharmacologic Effects and Clinical Applications section, Δ^1-corticoids and hydrocortisone in equivalent antirheumatic doses promote the same pattern of initial improvement; however, the results of longer term therapy are more favorable with the Δ^1 and further modified synthetic corticoids. Studies indicate that the Δ^1-corticoids can be used continuously in patients with rheumatoid arthritis without undue GI distress. Although the Δ^1-corticoids are considered not to have significant mineralocorticoid activity, hypokalemia and sodium and fluid retention can occur depending on the dosage and duration of use.

METHYLPREDNISOLONE (6α-METHYL). Between 1953 and 1962, many derivatives of the Δ^1-corticoids and the halogen-containing analogs (especially 9α-fluorinated compounds) were synthesized, and some became useful clinical agents. Studies with methylcorticoids revealed 2α-methyl derivatives to be inactive, whereas the 2α-methyl-9α-fluoro analogs had potent mineralocorticoid activity.

Methylprednisolone (6α-methyl derivative of prednisolone) was synthesized in 1956 and introduced into clinical medicine (Fig. 21.14). Methylprednisolone is extensively metabolized, with approximately 10% recovered unchanged in urine.[74] The metabolic pathways include reduction of the C20 ketone, oxidation of 17β-ketol group to C21-COOH and C20-COOH, and 6β-hydroxylation (CYP3A4). Methylprednisolone potentiates glucocorticoid activity with negligible salt retention in short-term therapy (Table 21.3).[75]

In human subjects, the metabolic side effects did not differ appreciably from those of prednisolone. Its activities with respect to nitrogen excretion, ACTH suppression, and reduction of circulating eosinophils were similar to those of prednisolone. The sodium retention and potassium loss were slightly less than with prednisolone.[76]

Oral methylprednisolone (Medrol) is commonly used for its anti-inflammatory effects in chronic diseases such as arthritis, lupus, psoriasis, certain neoplasms, or conditions that affect the eyes, blood cells, intestines, or lung to relieve swelling, pain, and allergic-type reactions. It is also available as a dose pack (Medrol Dose Pak) for the treatment of acute asthmatic or allergic exacerbations. The dose pack provides a high initial dose needed to resolve the exacerbation and immediate tapering of this dose to avoid adrenal insufficiency crisis on discontinuation of therapy.

Methylprednisolone administered parenterally as the 21-acetate ester (Depo-Medrol) is rapidly cleaved to methylprednisolone. IM administration of 80-120 mg of methylprednisolone acetate to asthmatic patients provides systemic relief within 6-48 hours that persists for several days to two weeks. Intra-articular, soft tissue, or intralesional injection may provide acute local relief of symptoms of rheumatoid arthritis, acute gouty arthritis, or bursitis.

Methylprednisolone is administered IV as the water-soluble sodium salt of the 21-succinate ester. The succinate ester is slowly and incompletely hydrolyzed. Peak plasma levels for methylprednisolone are attained in approximately 30-60 minutes following IV administration, and approximately 15% of the IV dose is recovered unchanged in urine.[72,73] CYP3A4 inhibitors, such as the antifungals ketoconazole and itraconazole, can potentiate the effects of methylprednisolone, while CYP3A4 inducers may require methylprednisolone dose increases.

DEFLAZACORT (16α,17α-OXAZOLINE RING). Although prednisone and prednisolone demonstrate increased glucocorticoid potency, there was a need to improve the therapeutic index of these early Δ^1 corticoids. Addition of the five-membered 16α,17α-oxazoline ring of deflazacort (Fig. 21.14), reminiscent of the acetonide found in triamcinolone, produces an improved side effect profile, with deflazacort demonstrating bone-sparing and carbohydrate-sparing properties as compared to prednisone.[77-79] This is particularly important in long-term administration and/or in pediatric patients. Deflazacort was demonstrated to be effective against various rheumatoid diseases with similar potency as prednisolone, and on the merit of its lessened side effect profile, it was tested in various pediatric populations in the 1990s. It was first approved for use in Europe in 1985 but was not available in the United States until 2017, when it was approved for the treatment of Duchenne muscular dystrophy (DMD) in boys five years of age or older. DMD is a rare X-linked muscle wasting disease affecting exclusively young boys.

Deflazacort is rapidly and completely absorbed upon oral administration with a T_{max} of 1-2 hours. The 21-acetate of deflazacort is rapidly cleaved by plasma esterases to the active metabolite, 21-desacetyldeflazacort (21-desDFZ).[80] 21-DesDFZ is metabolized in the liver by CYP3A4 to inactive metabolites. The package insert recommends dose reductions of 1/3 if coadministered with moderate or strong CYP3A4 inhibitors and avoiding co-administration with moderate to strong CYP3A4 inducers. Urinary excretion, the primary route of elimination, is almost complete by 24 hours. Studies in children (5-11 years of age) and adolescents (11-16 years of age) demonstrated a higher C_{max} and systemic exposures in adolescents. Post hoc analysis of the phase III study in DMD demonstrated that deflazacort met its primary end point of increasing mean muscle strength at 12 weeks, an effect that was durable out to 52 weeks. Furthermore, deflazacort (but not prednisone) increased pulmonary function metrics. Side effects were similar to other corticosteroids and included facial puffiness, weight gain, increased appetite, upper respiratory tract infections, and central obesity. Deflazacort is available as an oral suspension (22.75 mg/mL) or oral tablet (6 mg, 18 mg, 30 mg, and 36 mg).

TRIAMCINOLONE (16α-HYDROXY). The original interest in 16α-hydroxycorticosteroids stemmed from their isolation from the urine of a boy with an adrenal tumor. The desire of chemists to synthesize these corticoids, and the hope that such analogs might have potent biologic activity, furthered their development.[81-83] Insertion of a 16α-hydroxy group into 9α-fluoroprednisolone resulted in triamcinolone, which has glucocorticoid activity equivalent to prednisolone but with decreased mineralocorticoid activity (Table 21.3). In fact, 16α-hydroxy analogs of natural corticoids retain glucocorticoid activity and have a considerably reduced mineralocorticoid activity. Thus, a natural extension of corticoid research involved examination of compounds containing a 9α-fluoro group, a double bond between positions 1 and 2, and a 16α-hydroxy group. Triamcinolone, introduced in 1958, combines the structural features of a Δ^1-corticoid and a 9α-fluoro corticoid plus a 16α-hydroxy group (Fig. 21.14). As mentioned previously, the 9α-fluoro group increases the anti-inflammatory potency through enhancement of hydrogen bonding between the 11β-OH and Asn564 and inhibition of oxidative metabolism at this site, but also markedly increases the mineralocorticoid potency. This is undesirable if the drug is to be used internally, for example, for the treatment of rheumatoid arthritis. However, by inserting a 16α-hydroxy group into the molecule, one decreases the mineralocorticoid activity due to the lack of a polar H bond accepting residue and/or steric hindrance in MR. These glucocorticoids actually can cause sodium excretion rather than sodium retention.

The lower-than-expected oral anti-inflammatory potency for triamcinolone (Table 21.3; only equipotent to prednisolone despite higher GR affinity) has been attributed to its low oral bioavailability (Table 21.5), in part because of increased hydrophilicity from the 16α-hydroxy group and first-pass metabolism, primarily to its 6β-hydroxy metabolite. Triamcinolone acetonide (16α,17α-acetal with acetone) is active intact and can be taken orally, injected, or topically applied via inhalation or creams/lotions, as discussed below. The 16α,17α-acetonide forms favorable hydrophobic interactions with hydrophobic pocket of GR, increasing affinity and improving GR selectivity. Triamcinolone diacetate (17,21-diacetate) and triamcinolone hexacetonide (16α,17α-acetonide-21-[3,3-dimethylbutyrate]) prodrug esters are administered IM or intra-articularly for a prolonged release of triamcinolone. Depending on route of administration, triamcinolone diacetate has a duration of action ranging from 1 to 8 weeks and triamcinolone hexacetonide has a duration of action of 3-4 weeks.[84,85]

On a weight-for-weight basis, the antirheumatic potency of triamcinolone is slightly greater than that of prednisolone (~20%) and approximately the same as that of methylprednisolone (Table 21.3). Initial improvement following administration of triamcinolone is similar to that noted with other compounds. Reports in the literature, however, indicate that the percentage of patients maintained satisfactorily for long periods has been distinctly smaller compared to prednisolone.

Although triamcinolone has an apparently decreased tendency to cause salt and water retention and edema and can even induce sodium and water diuresis, it causes other unwanted side effects, including anorexia, weight loss, muscle weakness, leg cramps, nausea, dizziness, and general malaise.[86] IM triamcinolone is reportedly effective and safe in the treatment of dermatoses. In combination with folic acid antagonists (e.g., methotrexate), it is effective in the treatment of psoriasis.[87,88]

DEXAMETHASONE (16α-METHYL). Research with 16-methyl–substituted corticoids was initiated in part because investigators hoped to stabilize the 17β-ketol side chain to metabolism in vivo and improve bioavailability. These studies led to the clinical development of dexamethasone, which combines the structural features of a Δ^1-corticoid and a 9α-fluoro corticoid plus a 16α-methyl group (Fig. 21.14). A 16α-methyl group decreases the reactivity of the 20-keto group to carbonyl reagents and increases the stability of the drug in human plasma in vitro.[89,90] Unlike 16α-hydroxylation, a methyl group increases the anti-inflammatory activity by increasing lipophilicity and, consequently, receptor affinity through bonding to lipophilic residues within a GR hydrophobic pocket. Like the 16α-hydroxyl group, the methyl group markedly reduces the salt-retaining properties of the corticosteroids (Table 21.3).[91-93] The activity of dexamethasone, as measured by glycogen deposition, is 20-fold greater than that of hydrocortisone. It has 5-fold higher anti-inflammatory activity than prednisolone. Clinical data indicate that this compound has seven times the antirheumatic potency of prednisolone and is roughly 30-fold more potent than hydrocortisone. Its pharmacokinetic parameters are presented in Table 21.5. Routes of metabolism for dexamethasone are similar to those for prednisolone, with the primary 6β-hydroxy metabolite being recovered in urine.[94]

Dexamethasone sodium phosphate is the water-soluble sodium salt of the 21-phosphate ester, with an IV half-life of less than 10 minutes because of rapid hydrolysis by plasma phosphatases.[94] Peak plasma levels for dexamethasone usually are attained in approximately 10-20 minutes following an IV administered dose. A similar reaction occurs when the phosphate ester is applied topically. Dexamethasone 21-acetate is a prodrug which is available as a suspension for IM injection. Dexamethasone is also administered by several other routes (Table 21.4) and is available in tablets, elixir, and ocular formulations.

In practical management of rheumatoid arthritis, 0.75 mg of oral dexamethasone promotes a therapeutic response equivalent to that from 4 mg of triamcinolone or methylprednisolone, 5 mg of prednisolone, and 20 mg of hydrocortisone. Clinical investigations with small groups of patients indicate that this compound could control patients who did not respond well to prednisolone. Over long periods, the improved status of some patients deteriorated.

In summarizing the biologic properties of this drug, it seems clear that, with doses of corresponding antirheumatic strength, this steroid has approximately the same tendency as prednisolone to produce facial mooning, acne, and nervous excitation. Peripheral edema is uncommon (7%) and mild. The more common and most objectionable side effects are excessive appetite and weight gain, abdominal bloating, and distention. The frequency and severity of these symptoms vary with the dose (1 mg maximum for females, and 1.5 mg maximum for males). The longer biologic half-life for dexamethasone significantly increases the potential for glucocorticoid-induced adrenal insufficiency (see Adverse Effects section).

The striking increase in potency does not confer a general therapeutic index on dexamethasone that is higher than that of prednisolone. Again, this drug probably is best employed as a special-purpose corticoid. It can be useful when other steroids are no longer effective or when increased appetite and weight gain are desirable. Its efficacy may be increased when it is used in combination with the H_1 antagonist cyproheptadine as an antiallergenic, antipyretic, and anti-inflammatory agent.[92]

BETAMETHASONE (16β-METHYL). Betamethasone, which differs from dexamethasone only in configuration of the 16-methyl group (Fig. 21.14), was made available for the treatment of rheumatic diseases and dermatologic disorders shortly after the introduction of dexamethasone.[95-98] This analog, which contains a 16β-methyl group, is as effective as dexamethasone or, perhaps, even slightly more active. Although this drug has been reported to be less toxic than other steroids, some clinical investigators suggest that it is best used for short-term therapy. Toxic side effects, such as increased appetite, weight gain, and facial mooning, occur with prolonged use. A 0.5 mg tablet of betamethasone is equivalent to a 5.0 mg tablet of prednisolone, which is on par with dexamethasone (Table 21.3). Dipropionate and sodium phosphate ester prodrugs are available for topical administration and injection, respectively, the latter in combination with betamethasone acetate (see Fig. 21.14 for substitution patterns).

Selective Glucocorticoid Receptor Modulators (SGRMs)

The long-term use of classical glucocorticoids is associated with severe adverse effects (see Adverse Effects section), including osteoporosis, hyperglycemia, muscle wasting, hypertension, and impaired wound healing. Improved glucocorticoids that demonstrate potent anti-inflammatory activity without these serious side effects would provide a significant therapeutic advance and are the focus of research efforts by the pharmaceutical industry. The molecular mechanism of the GR makes it a particularly suitable target for this effort. The majority of unwanted side effects of the glucocorticoids arise from the interaction of the GR with DNA (i.e., GR-mediated transcription), where the anti-inflammatory effects are mediated via protein-protein interactions between the GR and proinflammatory transcription factors (i.e., AP-1 and NFκB) that result in repression of the inflammatory response. A variety of GR modulators with the ability to repress inflammation, but with lesser ability to elicit GR-mediated transcription (dissociated glucocorticoids), have been reported.[99-104]

Early investigations indicate that a variety of different nonsteroidal pharmacophores (e.g., pentanamines, pyrazoles, and *trans*-decalins) bind with high affinity and selectivity to the GR. Importantly, some of these analogs demonstrate preferential ability to repress proinflammatory genes and a lesser ability to induce GR-mediated transcription. The mechanism(s) by which the SGRMs promote selective repression of inflammation without the transactivation activity has not been resolved beyond doubt.[101,105] Moreover, the ability to dissociate the activities of glucocorticoids in the clinic has proven to be difficult and dissociated glucocorticoids are still early in clinical investigation. Better understanding of GR may eventually allow the development of nonsteroidal ligands that are superior to synthetic steroidal glucocorticoids.

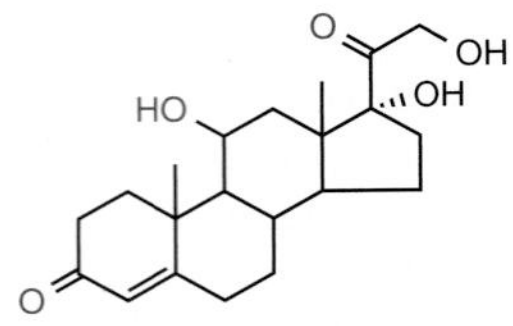

Hydrocortisone (cortisol)

Selected nonsteroidal glucocorticoids

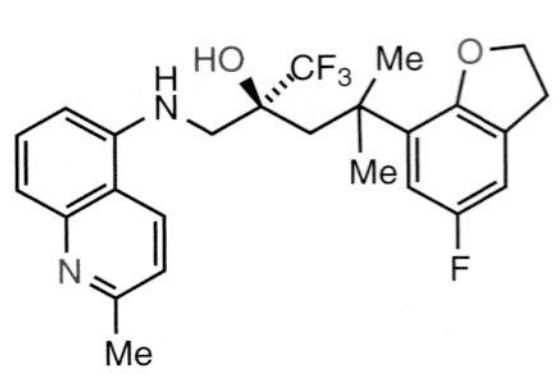

Mapracorat

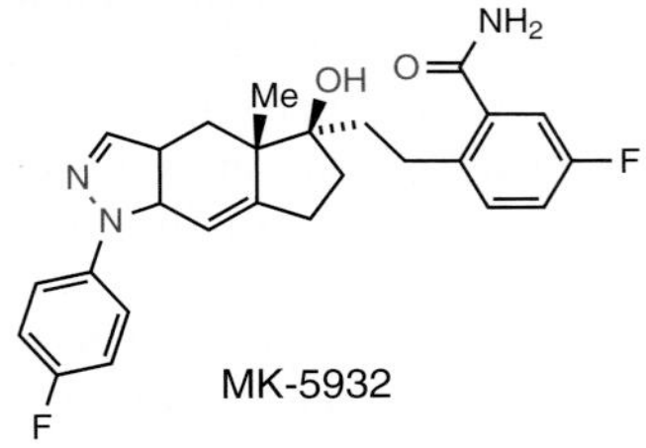

MK-5932

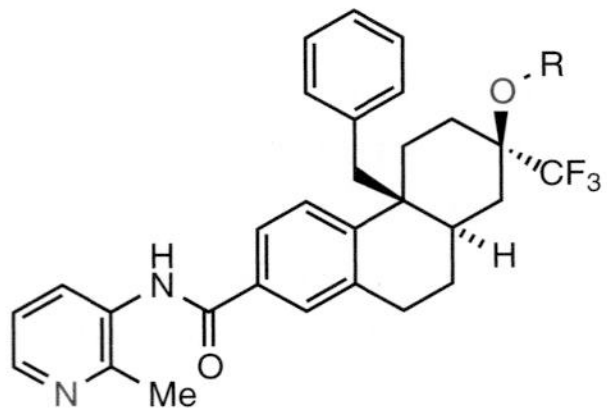

PF-802, R=H
Fosdagrocorat, R = phosphate

Topical Glucocorticoids (Fig. 21.17 and 21.18)

Topically applied glucocorticoids are also capable of being systemically absorbed, although to a much smaller extent than orally administered agents. The extent of absorption of topical adrenocorticoids is determined by several factors, including the type of cream or ointment, the condition of the skin to which it is being applied, and the use of occlusive dressings. Previous studies with halobetasol propionate (Fig. 21.17) showed that approximately 6% of the drug was systemically absorbed after topical application. Although this is a small fraction of the dose, the very high potency of halobetasol propionate contributed to its ability to cause mild adrenal suppression in some patients. The relative potency of the topical glucocorticoids is commonly determined using topical vasoconstriction assays and is dependent on the intrinsic activity of the drug, its concentration in the formulation, and the vehicle in which it is applied (Table 21.6).

Increased lipophilicity improves penetration through the stratum corneum and can be accomplished by introducing 6α, 7α, and/or 9α halogens, removing the 17α-hydroxy group (e.g., desoximetasone), masking 16α-, 17α-, or 21-hydroxy groups using cyclic ketals (e.g., acetonide) or esters (e.g., propionate), or replacing the 21-hydroxy

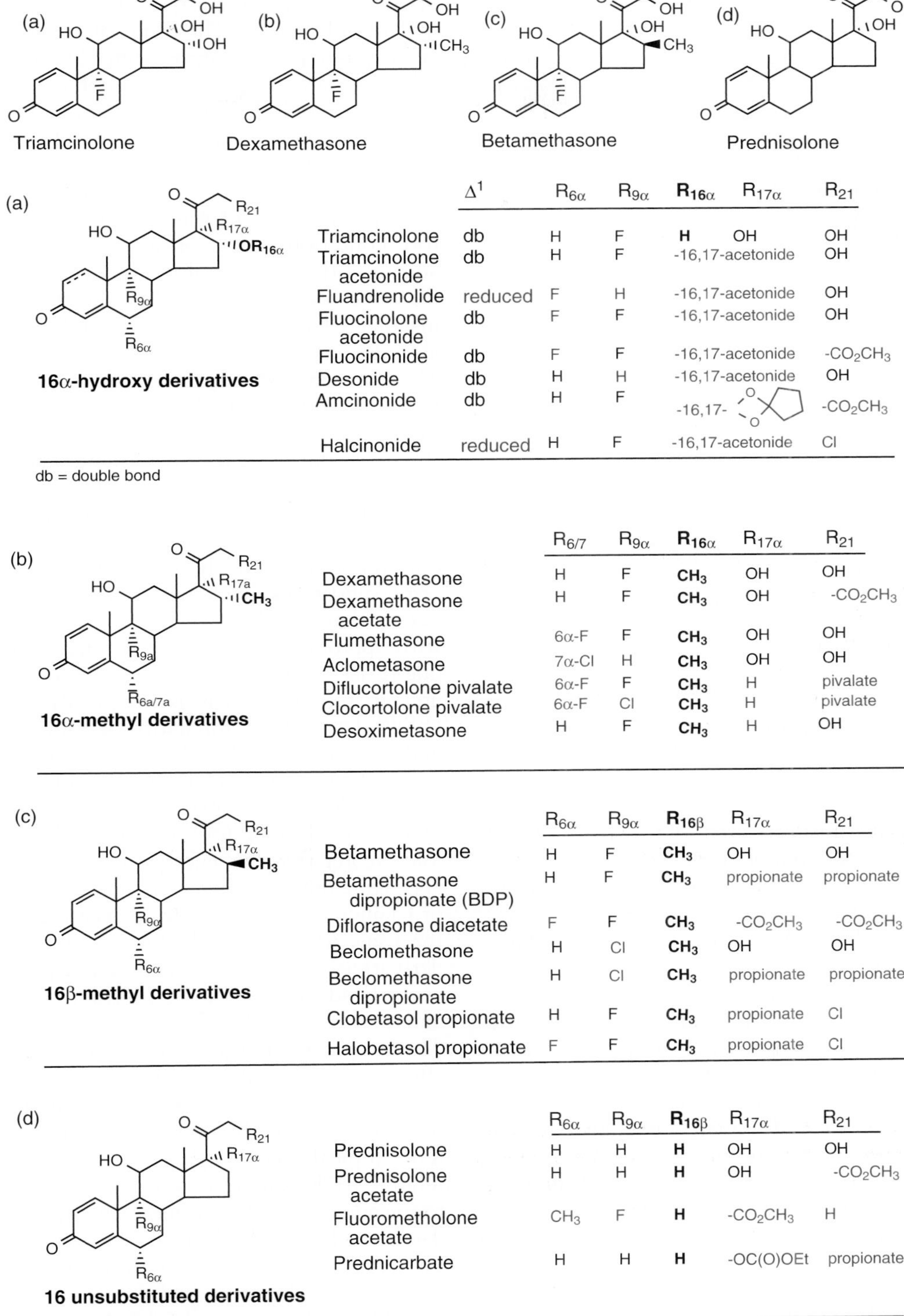

(a) 16α-hydroxy derivatives

	Δ^1	$R_{6\alpha}$	$R_{9\alpha}$	$R_{16\alpha}$	$R_{17\alpha}$	R_{21}
Triamcinolone	db	H	F	**H**	OH	OH
Triamcinolone acetonide	db	H	F	-16,17-acetonide		OH
Fluandrenolide	reduced	F	H	-16,17-acetonide		OH
Fluocinolone acetonide	db	F	F	-16,17-acetonide		OH
Fluocinonide	db	F	F	-16,17-acetonide		$-CO_2CH_3$
Desonide	db	H	H	-16,17-acetonide		OH
Amcinonide	db	H	F	-16,17- (cyclopentylidene dioxy)		$-CO_2CH_3$
Halcinonide	reduced	H	F	-16,17-acetonide		Cl

db = double bond

(b) 16α-methyl derivatives

	$R_{6/7}$	$R_{9\alpha}$	$R_{16\alpha}$	$R_{17\alpha}$	R_{21}
Dexamethasone	H	F	CH_3	OH	OH
Dexamethasone acetate	H	F	CH_3	OH	$-CO_2CH_3$
Flumethasone	6α-F	F	CH_3	OH	OH
Aclometasone	7α-Cl	H	CH_3	OH	OH
Diflucortolone pivalate	6α-F	F	CH_3	H	pivalate
Clocortolone pivalate	6α-F	Cl	CH_3	H	pivalate
Desoximetasone	H	F	CH_3	H	OH

(c) 16β-methyl derivatives

	$R_{6\alpha}$	$R_{9\alpha}$	$R_{16\beta}$	$R_{17\alpha}$	R_{21}
Betamethasone	H	F	CH_3	OH	OH
Betamethasone dipropionate (BDP)	H	F	CH_3	propionate	propionate
Diflorasone diacetate	F	F	CH_3	$-CO_2CH_3$	$-CO_2CH_3$
Beclomethasone	H	Cl	CH_3	OH	OH
Beclomethasone dipropionate	H	Cl	CH_3	propionate	propionate
Clobetasol propionate	H	F	CH_3	propionate	Cl
Halobetasol propionate	F	F	CH_3	propionate	Cl

(d) 16 unsubstituted derivatives

	$R_{6\alpha}$	$R_{9\alpha}$	$R_{16\beta}$	$R_{17\alpha}$	R_{21}
Prednisolone	H	H	**H**	OH	OH
Prednisolone acetate	H	H	**H**	OH	$-CO_2CH_3$
Fluorometholone acetate	CH_3	F	**H**	$-CO_2CH_3$	H
Prednicarbate	H	H	**H**	-OC(O)OEt	propionate

Figure 21.17 Topical corticosteroids.

group with a halogen, as will be discussed below.[106] Once absorbed through the skin, topical corticosteroids subject to metabolic pathways similar to the systemically administered corticosteroids. They are metabolized, primarily in the liver and are then excreted into the urine or in the bile.[107] The fact that circulating levels of the topical glucocorticoids are often extremely low, in some cases below the level of detection, does not reduce the risk for potential adverse effects from systemic exposure to topical corticosteroids. The structures for the glucocorticoids applied topically are shown in Fig. 21.17, and their relative potencies are shown in Table 21.6.

Structurally, the topical glucocorticoids can be segregated based on their 16-position substitution into derivatives of (1) triamcinolone (16α-hydroxyl); (2) dexamethasone (16α-methyl); (3) betamethasone (16β-methyl);

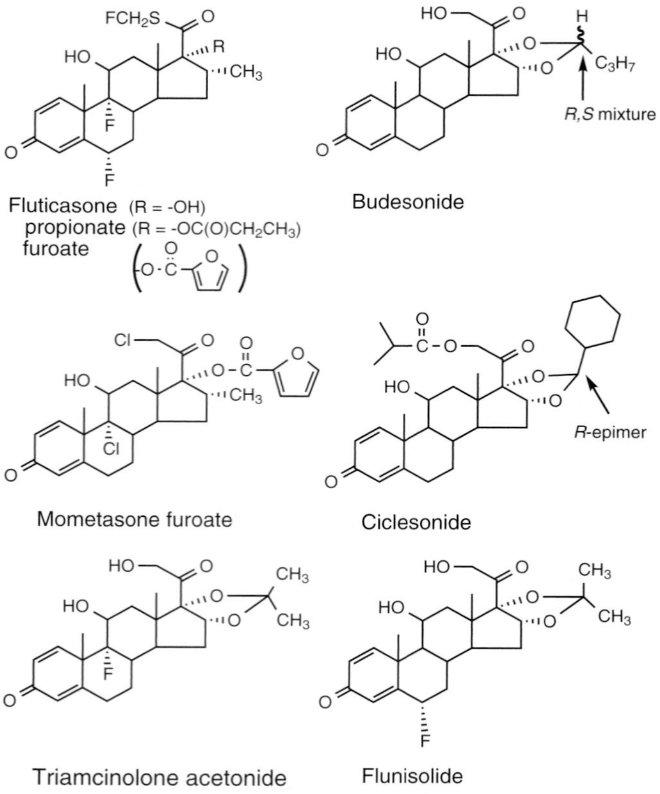

Figure 21.18 Inhaled and intranasal corticosteroids.

or (4) prednisolone (unsubstituted at the 16-position) (Fig. 21.17). These early template molecules have been modified at the 6, 7, 9, 16, 17, and 21 positions to generate many topical agents with a spectrum of topical potency rankings, allowing tailored glucocorticoid therapy via judicious selection of agents.

Topical dermatologic products with a low potency ranking have a modest anti-inflammatory effect and are safest for chronic application. Those products with a medium potency ranking are used in moderate inflammatory dermatoses of limited duration. High-potency preparations are used in more severe inflammatory dermatoses, but only for a short duration of treatment. Very high–potency products are used primarily as an alternative to systemic corticosteroid therapy when local areas are involved and for only a short duration of therapy and on small surface areas.

Several inhaled and intranasal corticosteroids shown in Fig. 21.18 are also available for topical administration and will be discussed in greater detail in the Inhaled and Intranasal Glucocorticoids section. An example is triamcinolone which is usually dispensed for topical use as its more potent and lipophilic 16α,17α-acetonide (Fig. 21.18). The acetonide is not cleaved and enhances GR affinity. It is effective in the treatment of psoriasis and other corticoid-sensitive dermatologic conditions. Topically, triamcinolone acetonide is a more potent derivative of triamcinolone and is approximately 8-fold more active than prednisolone. The side effects of the drug, however, have occurred with sufficient frequency to discourage its routine use for rheumatoid patients requiring steroid therapy. The drug can be employed advantageously as a special-purpose steroid for instances in which salt and water retention is a problem, e.g., from use of other corticoids, hypertension, or cardiac compensation, or when excessive appetite and weight gain are problems in management.

Triamcinolone acetonide suspension for intravitreal injection (Triesence) was approved for ocular inflammatory conditions unresponsive to topical corticosteroids, and recently intravitreal inserts of triamcinolone acetonide have been investigated in the treatment of diabetic macular edema (DME). An extended-release bioresorbable dexamethasone delivery system (Ozurdex in Table 21.4) and an extended-release nonbiosorbable fluocinolone acetonide insert (Iluvien in Table 21.4; see Fig. 21.17 for structure) have both achieved regulatory approval for the treatment of DME. All intravitreal corticosteroids are associated with risks of cataract progression, elevation of intraocular pressure, and endophthalmitis.[108]

Newer synthetic glucocorticoids have incorporated chlorine atoms onto the steroid molecule in place of fluorine substitutes. Beclomethasone, a 9α-chloro analog of betamethasone (Fig. 21.17), is a potent glucocorticoid with approximately half the potency of its fluoro analog due to less powerful electron withdrawing properties and greater steric bulk. It is used topically as its dipropionate (BDP) derivative in inhalation aerosol therapy for asthma and rhinitis (see Inhaled and Intranasal Glucocorticoids section) but not for treatment of steroid-responsive dermatoses.[109] The topical anti-inflammatory potency for BDP is approximately 5000-fold greater than hydrocortisone, 500-fold greater than betamethasone or dexamethasone, and approximately 5-fold greater than fluocinolone acetonide or triamcinolone acetonide, as measured by vasoconstrictor assay. Alclometasone, the 7α-chloro-9α-unsubstituted derivative of dexamethasone, is a low-potency topical glucocorticoid that contains a 7α-chloro group in the B-ring and is available as the 17α-,21-dipropionate[110] (Fig. 21.17). The low potency may partially result from weaker inductive effects of the 7α-chloro group on the 3-keto-Δ^4 functional group. Clocortolone pivalate is a dihalogenated analog related to dexamethasone and classified as a medium-potency topical agent (Fig. 21.17). The potency is enhanced relative to dexamethasone (Table 21.6) and is likely due to the addition of the 6α-fluoro and increased lipophilicity due to the lack of the 17α-OH. Desoximetasone is another 17α-dehydroxylated dexamethasone that is a high-potency topical glucocorticoid.

Additional mono- and difluorinated analogs for topical application include fluorometholone (a 6α-methyl-9α-fluoro-21-unsubstituted derivative of prednisolone for ophthalmic use; fluorometholone [17α-] acetate also used ophthalmically), flurandrenolide (a Δ^1 reduced, 6α-fluoro-9-unsubstituted-16α,17α-acetonide agent related to triamcinolone), fluocinolone acetonide (a 6α,9α-difluoro-16α,17α-acetonide related to triamcinolone), and fluocinonide (a 21-acetate ester of fluocinolone acetonide) (Fig. 21.17). These compounds are classified as high- to medium-potency anti-inflammatory agents depending on the concentration and vehicle used (Table 21.6). The

Table 21.6 Potency Ranking for Topical Corticosteroids

Potency Ranking	Topical Corticosteroids
I. Very high potency	Augmented[a] betamethasone dipropionate (lotion, ointment, and gel) Clobetasol propionate Diflorasone diacetate Halobetasol propionate
II. High potency	Amcinonide Augmented[a] betamethasone dipropionate (cream) Betamethasone dipropionate Betamethasone valerate Desoximetasone Diflorasone diacetate Fluocinolone acetonide Fluocinonide Halcinonide Triamcinolone acetonide
III. Medium potency	Betamethasone dipropionate Betamethasone valerate Clocortolone pivalate Fluocinolone acetonide Flurandrenolide Fluticasone propionate Hydrocortisone butyrate Hydrocortisone valerate Mometasone furoate Triamcinolone acetonide
IV. Low potency	Alclometasone dipropionate Desonide Dexamethasone Dexamethasone sodium phosphate Fluocinolone acetonide Hydrocortisone Hydrocortisone acetate Prednicarbate

[a]Augmented indicates the formulation is designed to penetrate the skin faster, making it more potent than (regular) betamethasone dipropionate.

The relative potency is based on the drug concentration, type of vehicle used, and the vasoconstrictor assay as a measure of topical anti-inflammatory activity.

acetonide (ketal) derivatives at the 16α,17α-position enhance GR affinity and lipophilicity to provide potent topical anti-inflammatory agents (Table 21.6).

Psoriasis is one of the few inflammatory dermatoses that has not responded to routine topical steroid therapy, but these more potent steroids appear to work if a special occlusive dressing is used. In this technique, a thin layer of cream or ointment containing flurandrenolide is applied to the individual patch of psoriasis. The area is then covered with an occlusive pliable plastic film which traps heat at the site of corticoid application and helps to drive the drug into the skin.

Clinical investigations show 0.05% flurandrenolide to be more effective than 1% hydrocortisone acetate and to have approximately the same activity as 0.1% triamcinolone acetonide. Some investigators believe that its greater activity results from an increased biologic half-life due to slower metabolism.

Clobetasol propionate, halcinonide, halobetasol propionate, and mometasone furoate are examples of 21-chlorocorticoids in which the 21-chloro group replaces the 21-hydroxyl group[111-114] (Figs. 21.17 and 21.18). Clobetasol propionate, the 21-chloro analog of betamethasone 17-propionate, is approximately 8-fold more active as topical anti-inflammatory agent than betamethasone 17α-valerate, the standard of comparison for topical vasoconstrictor/anti-inflammatory activity. Mometasone furoate, a 9α,21-dichloro derivative (see Inhaled and Intranasal Glucocorticoids section) related to betamethasone, is also approximately 8-fold more active than betamethasone 17α-valerate as a topical anti-inflammatory agent. Thus, substitution of a chlorine (or a fluorine) atom for the 21-hydroxyl group on the glucocorticoids greatly enhances topical anti-inflammatory activity.[112] Clobetasol propionate and halobetasol propionate are classified as very high–potency topical corticosteroid preparations (Table 21.6). HPA axis suppression has occurred following topical application of 2 g of the 0.05% clobetasol propionate ointment or cream (1 mg of clobetasol propionate total) daily. Because of its high potency and potential for causing adverse systemic effects during topical therapy, the usual dosage for very high–potency topical steroids should not be exceeded.

Fluticasone propionate is a betamethasone derivative which is similar to the 21-chlorocorticoids, except that it has a 17β-fluoromethylcarbothioate group instead of the 17β-ketol group (see Inhaled and Intranasal Glucocorticoids section) (Fig. 21.18). Although mometasone furoate and fluticasone propionate are very lipophilic and have the highest binding affinity for the GR when compared to triamcinolone acetonide and dexamethasone, their topical potency is listed as medium, in part because of their insolubility and poor dissolution into inflamed tissue.

Several nonfluorinated analogs of triamcinolone acetonide with the potency-enhancing cyclic ketal moieties are marketed, suggesting that halogens are not always necessary for topical activity. These nonfluorinated cyclic ketals include desonide (Fig. 21.17) and the cyclic acetal ciclesonide (Fig. 21.18). Furthermore, the potency of desonide (low potency) is greatly enhanced in its 9α-fluoro derivative, amcinonide (high potency), by the more lipophilic ketal of cyclopentanone (i.e., cyclopentylideneoxy) and 21-acetate groups. A recent addition to the nonhalogenated prednisolone derivatives is prednicarbate, a 17,21-diester (17α-ethylcarbonate-21-propionate) derivative of prednisolone (Fig. 21.17), which is used for the local treatment of corticoid-sensitive skin diseases.[115] Any prednicarbate that is absorbed systemically is readily metabolized by hydrolysis of the 21-ester to its primary and pharmacologically active metabolite, prednisolone-17-ethylcarbonate. This metabolite has a half-life of approximately 1-2 hours and is further metabolized by the liver to prednisolone. In vitro binding studies with the GR suggest that the ethyl carbonate metabolite has a receptor binding affinity comparable to that of dexamethasone.[115] The low systemic bioavailability for prednicarbate after dermal application has been attributed to its metabolism to less active prednisolone, which can be a factor for the low systemic side effects of prednicarbate.

Inhaled and Intranasal Glucocorticoids

The potent topical anti-inflammatory effect of glucocorticoids has made them the first-line therapy in controlling airway inflammation. It is generally accepted that the anti-inflammatory effects of approved (steroidal) glucocorticoids have not yet been separated from their adverse effects at the receptor level. Therefore, pulmonary and nasal pharmacokinetics become important determinants for the potential of an inhaled or nasally applied corticosteroid to cause systemic effects because the lung and nasal tissue provide an enormous surface area from which drug absorption can occur into the systemic circulation.[116,117] The main areas of concern with regard to drug-induced systemic effects include HPA axis suppression, change in bone mineral density and growth retardation in children, and cataracts and glaucoma in the elderly. The degree of systemic side effects increases proportionally to the area under the plasma concentration over time curve (AUC) of the corticosteroid. The AUC increases with longer half-life of the drug and higher dose and frequency of administration and depends on the route of administration and tissue penetration.[59] Thus, the focus of current research is to develop inhaled/intranasal corticosteroids combined with improved delivery devices that provide the following desirable pharmacokinetic qualities: a high degree of first-pass metabolism for the portion of the drug that enters the GI tract, short plasma half-life, lack of active metabolites, high affinity for the GR, and formulated to deliver the drug to the site of action and keep it there. These qualities determine the proportion of the drug that reaches the target cells, as well as the fraction of the dose that reaches the systemic circulation to produce side effects.

Modification of pharmacokinetics through structural alterations has provided several new steroids with a better GR affinity and therapeutic index and lower bioavailability than the older drugs (Fig. 21.18). The new inhaled/intranasal glucocorticoids, like mometasone furoate, budesonide, and fluticasone propionate, are more lipophilic than those used in oral and systemic therapy and have greater affinity for the GR than does dexamethasone as a consequence of their greater lipophilicity.[70] Several of the topical corticosteroids, such as mometasone furoate, BDP, triamcinolone acetonide, and flunisolide, were reintroduced as inhalation and intranasal dosage forms for treatment of respiratory diseases (e.g., asthma or rhinitis). Inhaled budesonide and flunisolide are readily absorbed from the airway mucosa into the blood and are rapidly biotransformed in the liver into inactive metabolites. Mometasone furoate and fluticasone propionate are very potent anti-inflammatory steroids with an oral bioavailability of less than 1%. Obviously, the risk of systemic side effects for these newer corticosteroids is greatly reduced when compared with the older glucocorticoids (e.g., dexamethasone).

BDP was discovered to be a prodrug cleaved by lung esterases, and this discovery led to the reexamination of other 17α-monoesters as the active form of the corticosteroid esters. The absorption of budesonide, fluticasone propionate, and BDP into the airway tissue was 25- to 130-fold greater than that for dexamethasone and hydrocortisone.[59] The GR affinity and the pharmacokinetic properties for the inhaled and intranasal corticosteroids are listed in Table 21.7.

Recently, multiple inhalation device technologies have been approved as nasal (e.g., Optinose® Exhalation Delivery System [EDS]) and lung (e.g., RespiClick® for β-adrenergic bronchodilator) formulations to improve drug delivery to the intended site of action, thereby providing the minimum effective dose to limit systemic (e.g., catabolism of muscle/bone) and local (e.g., oral or respiratory infections) side effects.[118,119] It is generally recognized that, when administered by oral inhalation, 10%-30% of a dose of the corticosteroid is deposited in the respiratory tract depending on type of inhaler (i.e., metered dose inhaler or dry powder inhaler [DPI]) and spacer used.[120,121] The remainder of the dose is deposited primarily in the mouth and throat to be swallowed into the GI tract, where the drug can be absorbed and metabolized or eliminated unchanged in the feces. Thus, systemic bioavailability of the inhaled/intranasal steroids is determined by the fraction of the dose absorbed from the lungs/nasal mucosa and the GI tract into systemic circulation and the degree of first-pass metabolism.

Although these corticosteroids are very lipid soluble, they display variable degrees of absorption from respiratory and GI tissues, in part because of dissolution problems. When systemically absorbed, they are capable of suppressing the HPA axis and adrenal function with high and chronic dosing regimens.[120,122] Although as much as 40% of the dose for the high-potency adrenocorticoids flunisolide, mometasone furoate, fluticasone propionate, or ciclesonide is absorbed into airway and nasal tissues during oral inhalation, the remainder of the drug is swallowed to undergo extensive first-pass metabolism in the liver to essentially inactive metabolites, with no apparent suppression effects on adrenal function with long-term therapy.

Lipophilicity can positively or negatively alter the pharmacokinetic and pharmacodynamic actions of the inhaled/intranasal steroids.[123] The lipophilic substituents attached to the corticosteroid nucleus can improve receptor affinity (Table 21.7), or they can affect pharmacokinetic properties, such as absorption, protein and tissue binding, distribution, and excretion. The inhaled/intranasal corticosteroids are inhaled as microcrystals and need sufficient water solubility to be dissolved in the nasal or lung epithelial tissue for local anti-inflammatory activity to occur. Lipophilicity, however, can delay their rate of dissolution into these tissues, which can be advantageous by prolonging their retention in these tissues, which affects their onset and duration in these tissues, or disadvantageous by facilitating their transport away from these tissues via mucociliary clearance before full dissolution could occur. The systemic steroids prednisolone and hydrocortisone are less effective as inhaled/intranasal steroids because of their higher water solubility and lower lipophilicity. For inhaled/intranasal steroids, there is a sharp drop in water solubility when the lipophilicity is high ($\log P \geq 4$ [$P = 10{,}000$]), which is the case for BDP, ciclesonide, fluticasone propionate, and mometasone furoate. High lipophilicity correlates well with low oral bioavailability and high protein binding (Table 21.7).

The first topical preparation for rhinitis was dexamethasone sodium phosphate (Decadron Turbinaire), which

Table 21.7 Pharmacokinetics of Inhaled and Intranasal Corticosteroids

Parameters	Beclomethasone Dipropionate (BDP)	Budesonide	Ciclesonide	Flunisolide[a]	Triamcinolone Acetonide	Fluticasone Propionate	Mometasone Furoate
GR binding affinity relative to dexamethasone[b]	0.4 13.5[c] (BMP)	9.4 11.2 (22R) 4.2 (22S)	12 (R-epimer) 1200[d] (R-epimer des-CIC)	1.8	3.6	18	25-27
CLog P[e]	4.3 3.2 (BMP)	2.9	5.3 3.9 (des-CIC)	2.4	2.2	3.8	4.1
Relative lipophilicity[f]	79,432 25,120 (BMP)	3,980	–	2,512	2,515	31,622	50,120
Pulmonary bioavailability	~20%[g]	~39%	~60% (des-CIC)	40%	25%[h]	~30% (aerosol)	<1% (aerosol)
Nasal bioavailability	~20%[g]	<20%	–	50%	25%[h]	13-16% (powder)	Not detectable (powder)
Oral bioavailability (systemic)	15-20%	~10%, oral	<1% parent and des-CIC	6-10%	23%	<2%	<1%
Protein binding	87% (transcortin & albumin)	85-90% (albumin)	99% <1% (des-CIC)	Moderate (transcortin & albumin)	68%[h] (albumin)	91% (albumin)	90%
Half-life	30 min IV 10 min inhaled 6.5 hr IV (BMP) 2-7 hr inhaled (BMP)	2-3 hr IV	1 hr 6-7 hr inhalation (des-CIC)	1-2 hr IV	1-2 hr IV 1-7 hr nasal 3.1 hr solution	~7.8 hr IV ~14 hr inhaled	4-6 hr IV Aerosol (not detectable) Inhaled (not detectable)
Metabolism	Lung and liver esterase, liver (CYP3A4) first pass	Liver (CYP3A) first pass	Liver (CYP3A) Lung esterase	Liver first pass	Liver first pass	Liver (CYP3A4) first pass	Liver
Onset of action	3-7 d	2-3 d	2-4 wk (Des-CIC)	3-7 d	4-7 d	2-3 d	7 hr
Excretion	Feces, urine 12-15%	~60% urine ~30% feces	<20% urine ~60% feces	~50% renal ~40% feces	~40% urine ~60% feces	80-90% feces <5% urine	50-90% feces 6-10% urine

Data from McEvoy GK, ed. *AHFS 2001 Drug Information*. Bethesda, MD: American Society of Health-System Pharmacists; 2001.

[a]Nasarel and Nasalide are not bioequivalent. Total absorption of Nasarel was 25% less, and the peak plasma concentration was 30% lower, than that of Nasalide. The clinical significance of this is likely to be small, however, because clinical efficacy is dependent on local effects on the nasal mucosa.

[b]Binding affinity to human glucocorticoid receptors in vitro relative to dexamethasone. Data from Kelly HW. Establishing a therapeutic index for the inhaled corticosteroids. Part 1: Pharmacokinetic pharmacodynamic comparison of the inhaled corticosteroids. *J Allergy Clin Immunol*. 1998;102:S36-S51.

[c]Beclomethasone diproprionate is converted in the liver to the more active beclomethasone 17-monophosphate (BMP).

[d]Ciclesonide is hydrolyzed into des-ciclesonide (des-CIC).

[e]Clog P values were calculated using ChemDraw Version 15.

[f]Measured from reverse-phase high-performance liquid chromatographic technique. Log k′ data from Brattsand R. *Eur Respir Rev*. 1997;7:356-361 were converted to antilogs. k′ values: water = 1, hydrocortisone = 794, prednisolone = 316, and dexamethasone = 400.

[g]Estimated for inhaled BDP aerosol.

[h]Data from oral inhalation administration.

BMP, beclomethasone 17-monopropionate; GR, glucocorticoid receptor; IV, intravenous.

was propelled by the chlorofluorocarbon Freon. The use of dexamethasone sodium phosphate inhalation aerosol is not recommended because of the potential for extensive systemic absorption and the long metabolic half-life for dexamethasone after absorption, resulting in an increased risk of adverse effects with usual inhalation doses. Following the oral inhalation of dexamethasone sodium phosphate, a cumulative dose of 1200 mcg/day will result in the systemic absorption of 400-600 mcg of dexamethasone, which is sufficient to cause HPA axis suppression. Dexamethasone sodium phosphate nasal aerosol delivers 100-mcg-per-metered spray. The total daily adult nasal dose is 1200 mcg.

Triamcinolone acetonide was frequently used by inhalation for the treatment of lung diseases (e.g., asthma) until 2010 but is no longer available as an inhalation aerosol. It was discontinued due to the chlorofluorocarbon (CFC) propellant ban but is still available as an aqueous nasal spray. Glucocorticoids are still commonly administrated as microcrystalline suspensions for pulmonary (inhalation aerosols or dry powders for inhalation) or nasal (aqueous solutions) delivery. Discontinuation of ozone-depleting CFC propellant inhalation products was complete by 2013. They were replaced by a variety of hydrofluoroalkane (HFA) propellant inhalation aerosols, aqueous nasal sprays, dry powder inhalers, or other novel delivery devices.

The discontinuation of CFC-based products accelerated the transfer of asthma patients from older inhaled agents such as triamcinolone, flunisalide, and beclomethasone (which are now largely nasal products for rhinitis or nasal polyps) to newer corticosteroids that are better optimized for inhalation therapy such as fluticasone, budesonide, ciclesonide, and mometasone. If monotherapy is ineffective for maintenance treatment, inhaled corticosteroids are commonly used as fixed combination products with long-acting β-adrenergic agonists (LABA) (see Chapters 28 and 35) such as fluticasone propionate/salmeterol, budesonide/formoterol, or mometasone furoate/formoterol combinations.

SPECIFIC DRUGS (FIG. 21.18)

Beclomethasone 17,21-Dipropionate (BDP). Beclomethasone dipropionate is used primarily as an inhalation aerosol therapy (e.g., the breath activated Qvar RediHaler) for asthma and rhinitis.[109] A breakthrough in the discovery of new inhalation corticosteroids with reduced risks from systemic absorption was that the 17α-monopropionate ester of beclomethasone (17-BMP) was more active than BDP and beclomethasone 21-monopropionate (21-BMP) esters.[124] Thus, BDP is a prodrug that is rapidly metabolized by esterases in the lung and other tissues to its more active metabolite, 17-BMP, which has 30-fold greater affinity for the GR than BDP due to the introduction of the 21-OH that may bind to Thr739 and Gln642 of GR. Furthermore, 17-BMP has approximately 14-fold greater GR affinity than dexamethasone (Table 21.7),[70] possibly due to polar interactions of 17α-propionate ester oxygens with Gln642 and hydrophobic interactions between the 17α-propionate side chain and 16β-methyl group with distinct regions of GR. 17-BMP is the first monoester to form because the 17α-propionate is more sterically hindered than the readily accessible 21-ester.

Whether orally administered or swallowed from inhalation, BDP undergoes rapid first-pass metabolism of the unhindered 21-ester via enzymatic hydrolysis in the liver or GI tract, primarily, to 17-BMP but more slowly to 21-BMP and to beclomethasone and other unidentified metabolites and polar conjugates.[125,126] The terminal half-life for 17-BMP is 6.5 hours. The portion of the inhaled dose of BDP that enters the lung is rapidly metabolized to 17-BMP in the respiratory tract before reaching systemic circulation, where it can be further metabolized by the liver. Following oral administration, BDP and its metabolites are excreted mainly in feces via biliary elimination, and 12%-15% of a 4-mg dose of BDP is excreted in urine as free and conjugated metabolites. The usual therapeutic dose (<1200 mcg/day) for BDP oral inhalation does not produce systemic glucocorticoid effects, probably because the drug is rapidly metabolized to less active metabolites. At doses greater than 1200 mcg/day, HPA axis suppression has been observed.

The BDP monohydrate nasal suspension is available as an aqueous microcrystalline suspension of BDP, which delivers 42-mcg-per-metered spray. The BDP nasal aerosol or inhalation aerosol consists of a microcrystalline suspension of BDP in HFA-134a (1,1,1,2-tetrafluoroethane) propellant, both of which deliver 40- or 80-mcg-per-metered spray. The total daily adult dose for BDP is 600 mcg from the nasal spray or nasal inhaler and 336-1000 mcg for the aerosol inhaler. Doses exceeding 2000 mcg/day need to be monitored for HPA axis suppression.

Flunisolide. Flunisolide (6α-fluoro) has high GR binding affinity, comparable to its fluorination position isomer, triamcinolone acetonide (9α-fluoro), but enhanced pulmonary and nasal bioavailabilities. When administered intranasally or by inhalation, flunisolide (Fig. 21.18) is rapidly absorbed from nasal or lung tissue (Table 21.7).[127] This corticosteroid is efficiently metabolized by the liver to inactive metabolites with no apparent effects on adrenal function with long-term therapy. Flunisolide that is swallowed undergoes extensive first-pass metabolism in the liver, while that which is absorbed directly from the nasopharyngeal mucosa or lung bypasses this initial metabolism.[128] It is not known if the drug undergoes metabolism in the GI tract. Flunisolide is rapidly hydroxylated by CYP3A4 at the 6β position, followed by elimination of the 6α-fluoro group to its more polar 6β-hydroxy metabolite, which attains plasma concentrations that usually are greater than those for flunisolide.[127,128]

Following IV administration of flunisolide, the 6β-hydroxy metabolite has 1/100 the potency of flunisolide and a plasma half-life of 3.9-4.6 hours. Flunisolide and its 6β-hydroxy metabolite are conjugated in the liver to inactive glucuronides and sulfates. After intranasal administrations of 100 mcg, the plasma levels for flunisolide were undetectable within 4 hours. The duration of its systemic effects is short because of its short half-life.

Flunisolide nasal solution (0.025%) is available in an aqueous solubilized form, which delivers 25 mcg per spray. The recommended starting dose for adults is two sprays in each nostril twice daily (200 mcg per day), with a maximum total daily dose of 400 mcg for adults. Flunisolide inhalation aerosol for pulmonary delivery is a microcrystalline suspension in a HFA propellant that delivers 80-mcg-per-metered spray from the built in spacer. The total daily adult inhalation dose for flunisolide is 1000 mcg. Doses exceeding 2000 mcg/day need to be monitored for HPA axis suppression.

Budesonide. Budesonide, another triamcinolone derivative, is a highly potent, nonhalogenated glucocorticoid intended for the local treatment of lung disease and rhinitis. It was designed to have a high ratio between local and systemic effects. Budesonide is composed of a 1:1 mixture of epimers of the 16,17-butylacetal, which creates a chiral center (Fig. 21.18).[129] The 22*R*-epimer binds to the GR with higher affinity than does the 22*S*-epimer (Table 21.7).[70] The butyl acetal chain provided the highest potency for the homologous acetal chains. Its rate of topical uptake into epithelial tissue is more than 100-fold faster than that of hydrocortisone and dexamethasone. Approximately 85% of the orally inhaled dose of budesonide undergoes extensive first-pass hepatic metabolism by CYP3A4 to its primary metabolites, 6β-hydroxybudesonide and 16α-hydroxyprednisolone, which have approximately 1/100 the potency of budesonide.[130,131] This is an important inactivation step in limiting the systemic effect of budesonide on adrenal suppression. Budesonide was metabolized 3- to 6-fold more rapidly than triamcinolone acetonide.

The pharmacokinetics of budesonide after inhalation, oral, and IV administration displayed a mean plasma half-life of 2.8 hours and a systemic bioavailability of approximately 10% after oral administration (Table 21.7).[131] Pulmonary bioavailability is less than 40% after inhalation (70%-75% after correction for the amounts of budesonide deposited in the inhalation device and oral cavity). No oxidative metabolism was observed in the lung. When given by inhalation, 32% of the dose is excreted in the urine as metabolites, 15% is excreted in the feces, and 41% remains in the mouthpiece of the inhaler. Following intranasal administration, very little of intranasal budesonide is absorbed from the nasal mucosa. Much of the intranasal dose (~60%) was swallowed, however, and remained in the GI tract to be excreted unchanged in the feces, whereas that fraction of the intranasal dose that was absorbed was extensively metabolized.

Inhaled budesonide, despite its lower lipophilicity, exhibits greater retention within the airways than other inhaled corticosteroids.[130,131] This unusual behavior for inhaled budesonide has been attributed to the subsequent formation of intracellular fatty acid esters of the 21-hydroxy group of budesonide in the airway and lung tissue.[132,133] Following inhalation, approximately 70%-80% of budesonide was reversibly esterified by free fatty acids in the airway tissue. These inactive esters behave like an intracellular depot drug by slowly regenerating free budesonide through hydrolysis. Thus, this reversible esterification prolongs the local anti-inflammatory action of budesonide in the airways and may contribute to the high efficacy and safety of budesonide in the treatment of mild asthma when inhaled once daily.

The systemic availability of budesonide in children was estimated to be 6.1% of the nominal dose, and the terminal half-life was 2.3 hours.[134,135] Approximately 6% of the nominal dose reached the systemic circulation of young children after inhalation of nebulized budesonide. This is approximately half the systemic availability found in healthy adults using the same nebulizer.

Budesonide powder for pulmonary inhalation uses micronized dry powder of budesonide only in a turboinhaler (DPI) inhalation-driven device that delivers 200 mcg per actuation. Another DPI device, the Flexhaler, delivers 1 mg of micronized formulation containing 90 or 180 mcg of micronized budesonide per actuation. The total daily adult dose for budesonide from the DPI is 200-800 mcg. Full benefit is attained in approximately 1-2 weeks. Budesonide ampules contain 0.25 mg/2 mL, 0.5 mg/ 2mL, and 1 mg/2 mL to be delivered as a sterile solution via a jet nebulizer. Budesonide nasal aerosol which is now available OTC is supplied as a micronized suspension of budesonide in an aqueous medium which delivers 32-mcg-per-metered spray. Budesonide inhalation aerosol delivers 80 or 160 mcg of budesonide in a fixed combination dose with the LABA formoterol (4.5 mcg) using an HFA propellant micronized formulation.

Ciclesonide. A third-generation nonhalogenated prednisolone analog approved in 2006 is ciclesonide (Fig 21.18). Ciclesonide is the 21-isobutyrate ester and the 16α,17α-acetal of the cyclohexanecarboxaldehyde analog of prednisolone. It is delivered as the *R*-epimer, which binds to the GR with high affinity (Table 21.7). The 21-isobutyrate ester and 16α,17α-acetal of cyclohexanecarboxaldehyde greatly enhance its lipid solubility. Ciclesonide is a prodrug that is converted locally in airways by carboxylesterases to produce the active metabolite, desisobutyrylciclesonide (des-CIC). With its free C21-OH available to bind (e.g., to Thr739), des-CIC has a 100-fold greater relative GR binding affinity than ciclesonide itself (relative GR binding affinities are 1200 and 12, respectively, and for dexamethasone, it is 100). If any ciclesonide or des-CIC enters the circulation, it is highly protein bound (99%) and undergoes extensive first-pass hepatic metabolism by CYP3A4 to 6β-hydroxy metabolites, resulting in very low systemic exposure. Clinical studies demonstrate that ciclesonide is effective as inhalation aerosol therapy for asthma and rhinitis.

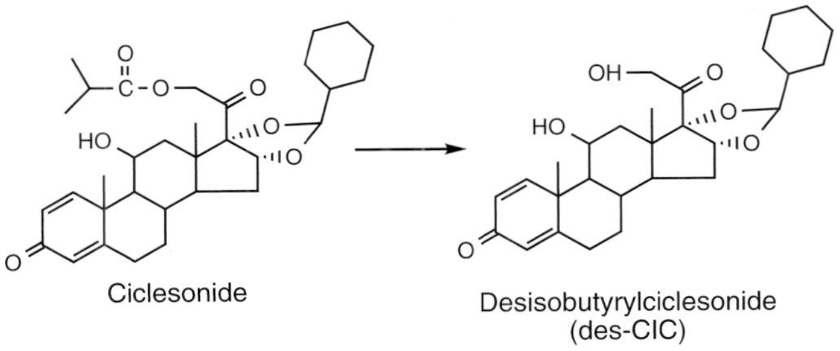

Ciclesonide

Desisobutyrylciclesonide (des-CIC)

Ciclesonide is supplied as an aqueous inhalation solution pump that dispenses 50 mcg per 70 μL spray for seasonal allergies or delivered in solution form via an HFA metered-dose inhaler with a once-daily dosing schedule, which facilitates asthmatic patient compliance. The total daily dose is 200 mcg for seasonal allergies and 80-160 mcg for asthma. In 2012, a new dry nasal aerosol spray was approved that delivers 37 mcg of ciclesonide with one spray per nostril daily.

Following inhalation administration, ciclesonide and des-CIC are not detected in the plasma. Ciclesonide has a half-life of less than 1 hour, and des-CIC has a half-life of 6-7 hours and an oral bioavailability of less than 1% due to extensive plasma protein binding (Table 21.7). Ciclesonide produces potent anti-inflammatory effects with an onset of action of approximately 2-4 weeks. It is extensively metabolized, with less than 20% of the administered dose recovered in the urine as des-CIC. The majority of the oral inhalation for ciclesonide is deposited in the airway passages and swallowed without absorption in the GI tract until eliminated in the feces (~60% of the administered dose is recovered in the feces). These results indicate that inhaled ciclesonide has negligible systemic bioavailability and is extensively metabolized, with reduced risk for causing systemic adrenal suppression effects.

Mometasone Furoate. The development of mometasone furoate resulted from the reexamination of the effect of 17α-ester functionalities on topical anti-inflammatory potency relative to the potent 17-benzoate ester of betamethasone. The structure-activity relationship study involved substitution of the 17-benzoate ester with heteroaromatic furoic, thienoic, and pyrrolic esters.[113,136] Of the numerous 17α-heteroaryl esters studied, the 2-furoate ester displayed the greatest increase in potency. Therefore, combining the 17α-(2-furoate) ester with the potency-enhancing effect of the 21-chloro group resulted in mometasone furoate (Fig. 21.18), which is 5- to 10-fold more potent and has a more rapid onset of action than the betamethasone benzoate ester.

Mometasone furoate was originally marketed as a topically applied corticosteroid, but because of its low systemic bioavailability, it was found to be more useful in the treatment of allergic disorders and lung diseases.[137] It has the greatest binding affinity for the GR (Table 21.7), followed by fluticasone propionate, budesonide, triamcinolone acetonide, and dexamethasone.[70] Mometasone furoate has strong local anti-inflammatory activity equivalent to that of fluticasone propionate. It has a quick onset of action relative to the other inhaled/intranasal steroids with the least systemic availability and, consequently, the fewest systemic side effects.

Mometasone furoate was detected in the plasma for up to 8 hours after administration of an inhaled aerosolized suspension, with an IV half-life of 4-6 hours (Table 21.7) and an oral bioavailability of less than 1% as compared to an intravenous dose. It is extensively metabolized with less than 10% of the administered dose recovered in the urine unchanged.[138] Among the polar metabolites (~80%) and their conjugates (42%) that were recovered were 6β-hydroxymometasone furoate and its 21-hydroxy metabolite. In contrast, following intranasal administration, its plasma concentrations were below the limit of quantification, and the systemic bioavailability by this route was estimated to be less than 1%. The majority of the intranasal dose for mometasone furoate is deposited in the nasal mucosa and swallowed without absorption in the GI tract until eliminated in the feces (~50%-90% of the intranasal dose is recovered in the feces). These results indicate that inhaled mometasone furoate has negligible systemic bioavailability and is extensively metabolized, with reduced risk for causing systemic adrenal suppression effects.

Mometasone furoate nasal suspension is supplied as an aqueous suspension with an atomizing pump that dispenses 50 mcg per metered spray. The total daily dose for mometasone furoate is 200 mcg. An inhalation powder (Twisthaler) or HFA-based inhalation aerosol delivers 100 mcg or 200 mcg of mometasone furoate with a daily dose of 100 mcg for children 4-11 years of age up to 400 mcg for adults. The inhalation aerosol comes as the same doses of mometasone in fixed combinations with LABA formeterol (5 mcg).

Fluticasone Propionate

Androstane-17β-carboxylates (R = $-OCH_2F$)
Androstane-17β-carbothioates (R = $-SCH_2F$)
X is acetate or propionate

Flumethasone

Fluticasone propionate

Fluticasone furoate

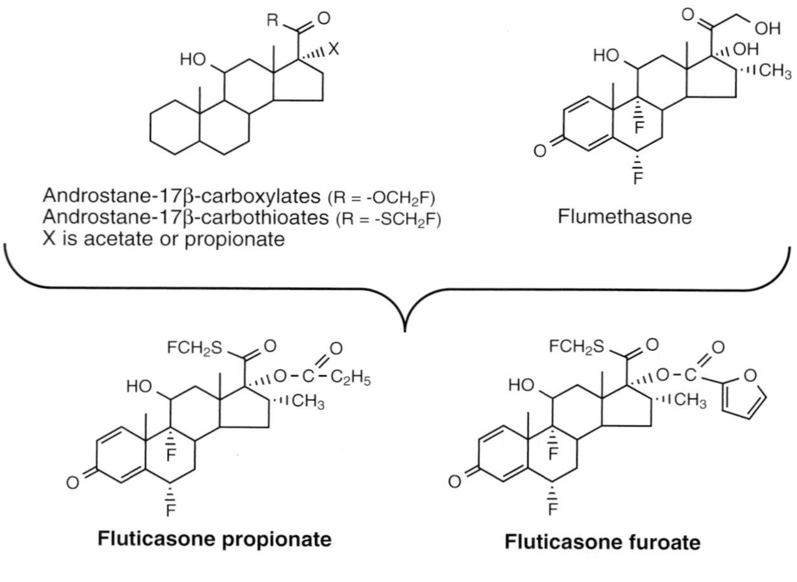

The discovery of fluticasone flowed from the investigation of the androstane 17α-hydroxyl-17β-carboxylates and 17α-hydroxyl-17β-carbothioates, which were designed to be metabolically susceptible to hydrolysis at the 17β position and to have a low systemic bioavailability to minimize systemic glucocorticoid-induced adrenal suppression. The androstane 17α-hydroxyl-17β-carboxylates lacked the 17-ketol group ($-COCH_2OH$) found in most of the systemic corticosteroids. When these 17β-carboxylates were esterified to their 17α/β-diesters, however, they proved to be extremely potent anti-inflammatory corticosteroids, whereas the parent carboxylic acids were inactive.[139] Thus, enzymatic hydrolysis of the 17-carboxylate ester function by intestinal or liver esterases would lead to formation of inactive metabolites. The greatest anti-inflammatory activity was observed with 17α-acetoxy and 17α-propionoxy groups and simple alkyl carboxylate esters, although the fluoromethyl esters showed the highest activity.

Superseding the androstane 17β-carboxylates were the corresponding 17β-carbothioates (thioesters) derived from flumethasone (i.e., Δ^1-6α,9α-difluoro-16α-methyl; Fig. 21.17). The 17β-fluoromethylcarbothioate, when combined with the 17α-propionoxy group, yielded fluticasone propionate (Fig. 21.18).[140] The androstane 17β-carbothioates proved not only to be very potent anti-inflammatory agents but also to exhibit weak HPA suppression in the rat. Both the androstane 17β-carboxylates and the androstane 17β-carbothioates are very lipophilic and exhibit minimal oral bioavailability and very low systemic activity after inhalation because of intestinal and hepatic enzymatic thioester hydrolysis to inactive metabolites, which have 1/2000 the activity of the parent molecule.[141]

Fluticasone propionate, a trifluorinated glucocorticoid based on the androstane 17β-carbothioate nucleus (Fig. 21.18), was designed to be metabolically susceptible to hydrolysis and to have a low systemic bioavailability to minimize the systemic effects on plasma hydrocortisone levels. Its susceptibility to metabolic hydrolysis is doubly enhanced by the combination of a thioester and the high electronegativity of the fluorine group. Fluticasone propionate is approximately as lipophilic as BDP, 8-fold more lipophilic than budesonide and 4-fold more lipophilic than triamcinolone acetonide (Table 21.7). It also displays high in vitro selectivity for the GR and a relative receptor affinity 1.5-fold that of 17-BMP and ciclesonide, about equal to mometasone furoate, 2-fold that of budesonide, 18-fold that of dexamethasone, 10-fold that of flunisolide, and 5-fold that of triamcinolone acetonide.[70] Its relatively tight binding reflects cumulative favorable effects to it substituents such as the inductive effect of the 9α-fluoro group on 11β-OH, the favorable hydrophobic pocket binding effects of the 16α-methyl and 17α-propionate groups, and the ability of the 17β-$FCH_2S(O)C$- group to maintain the hydrogen bonding interactions of the 17β-ketol with GR. The rate of association for fluticasone propionate with the receptor is faster, and the rate of dissociation is slower, than the other corticosteroids. The half-life of the fluticasone propionate active steroid-receptor complex is greater than 10 hours, compared with approximately 5 hours for budesonide, 7.5 hours for 17-BMP, and 4 hours for triamcinolone acetonide.[70]

After topical application to the nasal mucosa or after inhalation, fluticasone propionate produces potent anti-inflammatory effects, with an onset of action of approximately 2-3 days. The topical anti-inflammatory potency for fluticasone propionate is approximately equal to that for mometasone furoate, 13-fold greater than that for triamcinolone acetonide, 9-fold greater than that for fluocinolone acetonide, 3-fold greater than that for betamethasone 17-valerate, and 2-fold greater than that for BDP.[141] Because of its low systemic bioavailability when administered intranasally or by inhalation and nondetectability in plasma, most pharmacokinetic data for fluticasone propionate are based on IV or oral administration (Table 21.7). Its rate of topical uptake into epithelial tissue is more than 100-fold faster than that for hydrocortisone and dexamethasone but is similar to BDP and budesonide.

As a consequence of its high lipophilicity (Table 21.7), fluticasone propionate is very insoluble and, therefore, is poorly absorbed from the respiratory (10%-13%) and GI tracts following nasal inhalation of the drug.[142-144] The majority of the intranasal dose for fluticasone propionate is deposited in the nasal mucosa and swallowed into the GI tract until eliminated in the feces (~80%-90% of the intranasal dose is recovered metabolized and unchanged in the feces). After IV administration, fluticasone propionate displayed a systemic bioavailability of less than 2% and underwent extensive hydrolysis and CYP3A4 first-pass metabolism in the liver, with an elimination half-life of approximately 3 hours. Its primary hydrolysis product is 17β-carboxylate metabolite, which has 1/2000 the affinity for the GR and can be recovered from the urine along with other unidentified hydroxy metabolites and their conjugates.

Following oral administration of 1-40 mg, fluticasone propionate is poorly absorbed from the GI tract because of hydrolysis and its insolubility, with an oral bioavailability of less than 1%. Pulmonary bioavailability ranges between 16% and 30% depending on the inhalation device used, with an elimination half-life of approximately 14 hours, increasing its potential for drug accumulation with repeated dosing.[144] The long elimination half-life for fluticasone propionate results, in part, from its very high lipophilicity, very poor water solubility, and, consequently, slow dissolution into lung tissue. Some suppression of overnight hydrocortisone levels was reported with inhaled fluticasone propionate at higher doses (indicative of HPA axis suppression).[145]

Fluticasone propionate inhalation aerosol is available as a microcrystalline suspension of micronized fluticasone propionate in HFA propellant (Flovent HFA). Each actuation delivers 44, 110, or 220 mcg of fluticasone propionate from the mouthpiece. The recommended starting dose of fluticasone propionate aerosol is 88-220 mcg twice daily with the highest recommended dose of 440 mcg. Fluticasone propionate combined with the LABA salmeterol is also available as an HFA-based inhalation aerosol providing 45, 115, and 230 mcg each combined with 21 mcg of salmeterol.

Fluticasone propionate dry powder inhalers (DPI) deliver the corticosteroid alone (e.g., Flovent Diskus or ArmonAir RespiClick) or in fixed combinations with salmeterol (Advair Diskus or AirDuo RespiClick). DPIs come as Diskus plastic inhalers containing a foil blister strip. Each blister on the strip contains a white powder mix that delivers 50, 100, or 250 mcg (Flovent Diskus) per inhalation of micronized fluticasone propionate or 100, 250, or 500 mcg fluticasone proprionate and 72.5 mcg salmeterol xinafoate salt (equivalent to 50 mcg of salmeterol base) (Advair Diskus). The Diskus dose is 100-1000 mcg twice daily for patients 12 years of age and older. After the Diskus is activated, the powder is dispersed into the airstream created by the patient inhaling through the mouthpiece. The maximum recommended combination dose is 500/50 mcg twice daily. The RespiClick DPI formulations deliver the same active ingredients but involve resetting the dry powder dose via opening the mouthpiece cover until you hear a click. RespiClick allowed lowered daily doses of 110-464 mcg.

Fluticasone furoate, the 2-furoic acid ester of the 17α-hydroxyl group, is available as dry powder inhaler, alone (Arnuity Ellipta) or combined with another LABA vilanterol (Breo Ellipta). Fluticasone furoate nasal spray is also available (Veramyst). The furoate ester, like the propionate ester, is stable to metabolism, and neither is metabolized to fluticasone.[146] X-ray crystal structures demonstrate that the intact furoate side chain occupies a discrete pocket much more completely than the propionate side chain,[147] conferring fluticasone furoate with higher GR affinity and higher nasal and lung tissue affinity compared to fluticasone propionate.[148,149] The higher tissue affinity translates to enhanced lung residency and once-daily efficacy in asthma.[150] The superior properties of fluticasone furoate allow lowered daily dose for the nasal spray of 110 versus 200 mcg for the comparable aqueous fluticasone propionate nasal spray (Flonase). Care should be used to avoid abbreviating either fluticasone furoate or fluticasone propionate as fluticasone (Fig. 21.18).

Fluticasone propionate available as an antiallergic nasal spray further contains the histamine antagonist azelastine (Dymista). In addition to the aqueous formulation, a dry nasal fluticasone propionate (Xhance) is actuated by a pump spray into one nostril while simultaneously blowing into the mouthpiece. Recommended adult dosage is one or two sprays per nostril twice daily (total daily dose of 372-744 mcg).

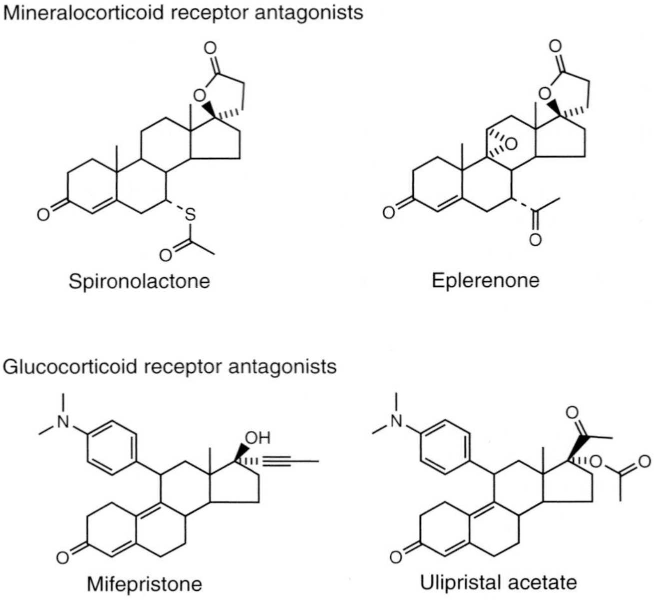

Mineralocorticoid receptor antagonists

Spironolactone

Eplerenone

Glucocorticoid receptor antagonists

Mifepristone

Ulipristal acetate

Figure 21.19 Adrenocorticoid receptor antagonists.

ADRENOCORTICOID ANTAGONISTS

Antagonists of adrenocorticoids include agents that compete for binding to steroid receptors (antiglucocorticoids or antimineralocorticoids) and inhibitors of adrenosteroid biosynthesis. The action of adrenal steroids can be blocked by antagonists that compete with the endogenous steroids for binding sites on their respective cytosolic receptor proteins (i.e., GR and MR). The antagonist-receptor complexes are unable to stimulate the production of new mRNA and cognate proteins in the target tissues and, thus, are unable to elicit the biologic responses of the hormone agonist. Spironolactone, eplerenone (Fig. 21.19), and related analogs bind to the mineralocorticoid receptor in the kidney and result in the diuretic response of increased Na^+ excretion and K^+ retention. The 3-keto-4-ene A ring is essential for this antagonistic activity, and the opening of the lactone ring dramatically reduces activity. The 7α-substituent increases both intrinsic activity and oral activity.[151,152] Progesterone has also shown antimineralocorticoid activity at 10^{-4} molar concentrations.

Receptor antagonists of glucocorticoids have been described that are derivatives of 19-nortestosterone.[153] Mifepristone, also referred to as RU-486 (Fig. 21.19), was originally developed as an antiprogestin but also exhibits very effective antagonism of glucocorticoids and was approved for Cushing's disease.[154] Ulipristal acetate is a weak antiglucocorticoid that has been approved as an abortifacient (antiprogestational agent) similar to mifepristone.

Several inhibitors of adrenocorticoid biosynthesis have been described, with the majority of nonsteroidal agents inhibiting one or more of the cytochrome P450 enzyme complexes involved in adrenosteroid biosynthesis (Fig. 21.20). Metyrapone reduces hydrocortisone biosynthesis by primarily inhibiting mitochondrial 11β-hydroxylase.[155,156] It also inhibits, to a lesser degree, 18-hydroxylase and side-chain cleavage. This agent is used to test pituitary-adrenal function and the ability of the pituitary to secrete ACTH.[156] Aminoglutethimide inhibits side-chain cleavage[156] and has been used as a medical adrenalectomy. Several azole antifungal drugs inhibit adrenocorticoid biosynthesis. Ketoconazole is one example of a potent inhibitor of fungal sterol biosynthesis at low concentrations; however, at higher doses, ketoconazole inhibits CYP3A4 in adrenosteroid

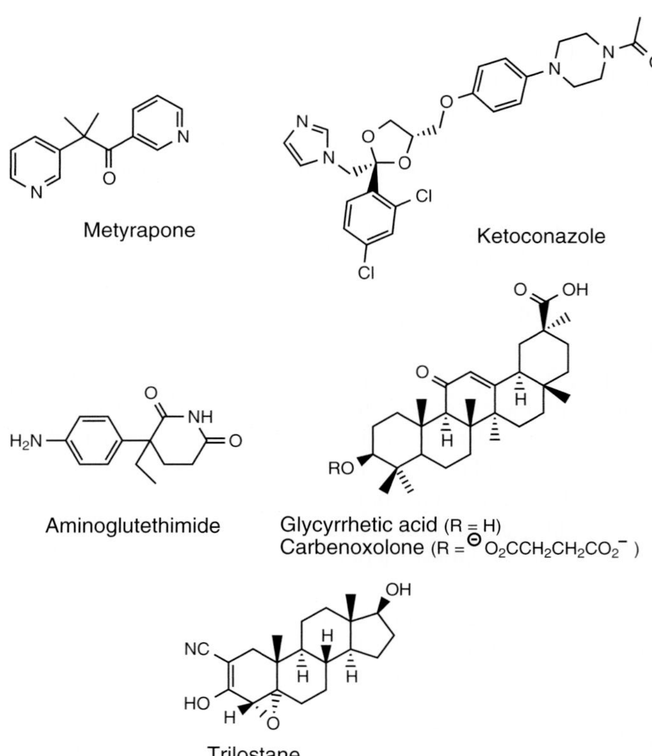

Figure 21.20 Inhibitors of adrenocorticoid biosynthesis.

biosynthesis.[157] Trilostane is a steroidal inhibitor of 3β-hydroxysteroid dehydrogenase[158] and has been used in the treatment of Cushing's syndrome.

Inhibition of the two 11β-hydroxysteroid dehydrogenase isozymes has been described. Excessive ingestion of licorice, an extract of the roots of *Glycyrrhiza glabra*, produces undesirable mineralocorticoid-like intoxication (hypertension, excessive salt retention, and hypokalemia). The active components of licorice, glycyrrhetic acid (Fig. 21.20), and carbenoxolone inhibit both 11β-HSD isozymes,[159] with the undesirable side effects resulting from inhibition of 11β-HSD2 in the kidney. Subtype selective and nonsteroidal 11β-HSD1[160,161] inhibitors are in clinical trials.[162] Such enzyme inhibitors may be useful in the treatment of metabolic syndrome, cardiovascular disease, or diabetes.[163]

ACKNOWLEDGMENTS

The authors wish to acknowledge the work of Duane D. Miller, PhD and Dr. Robert W. Brueggemeier, PhD who authored content used within this chapter in a previous edition of this text.

Structure Challenge

The structures of nine drugs discussed in this chapter are provided. Use your knowledge of drug chemistry to identify the agent that would be most appropriate for use in each patient care situation described below.

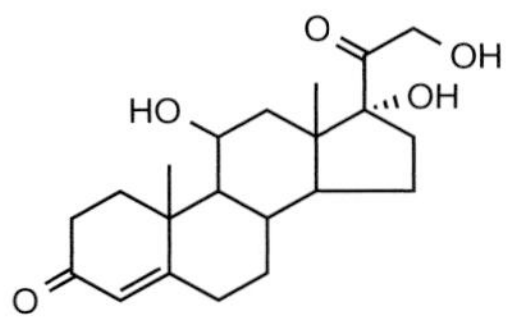

1.

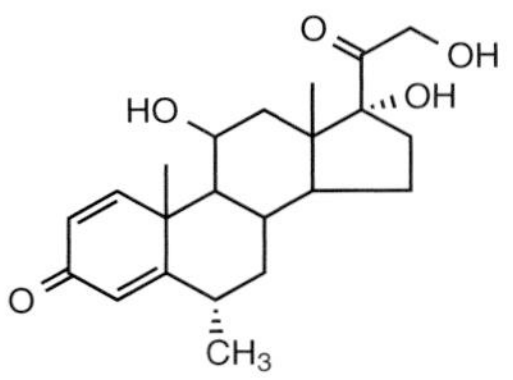

2.

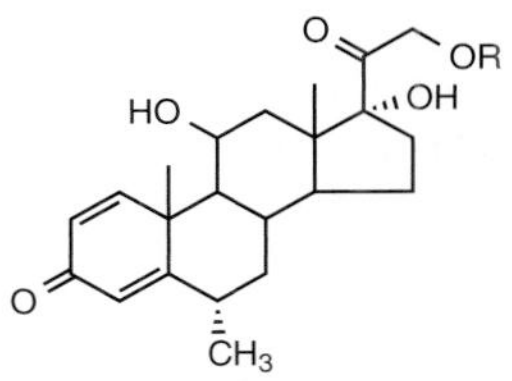

3. R = Na $OOCCH_2CH_2CO$- (sodium succinate)

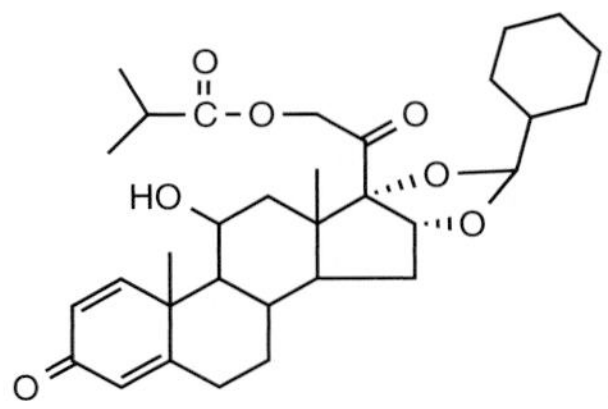

4.

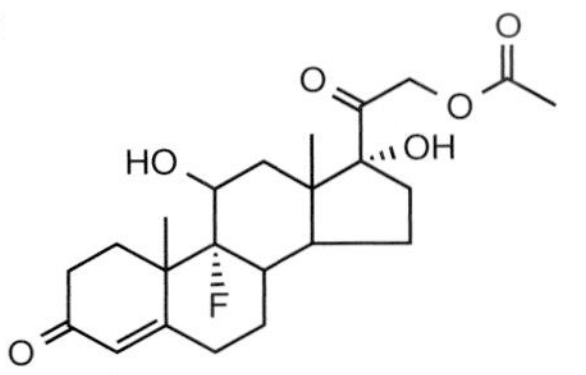

5.

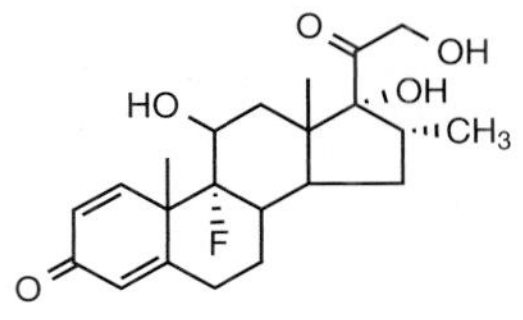

6.

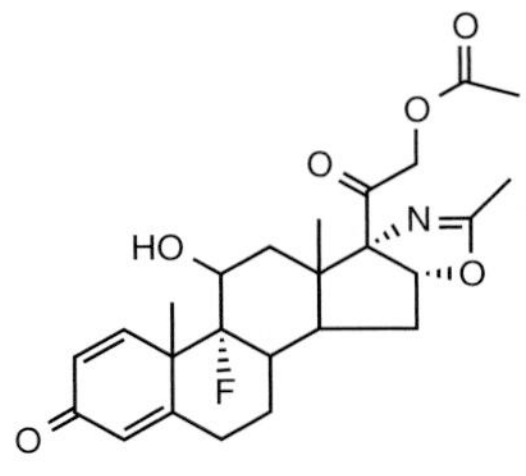

7.

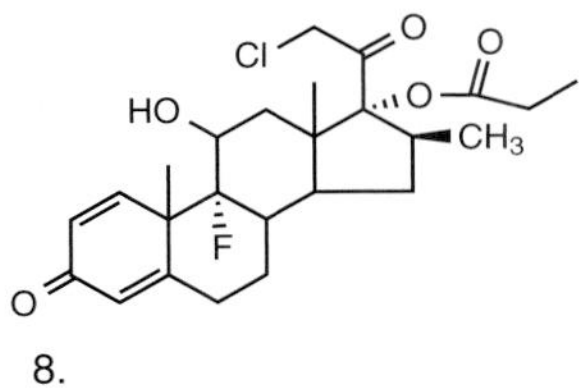

8.

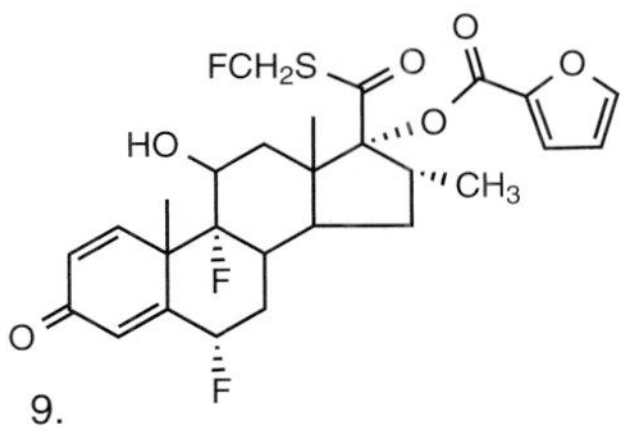

9.

A. A Duchenne muscular dystrophy patient (and parent) in his pediatrician's office looking for oral anti-inflammatory therapy with bone-sparing side effect profile. # ___

B. A pharmacist talking to a patient looking for an OTC cream to treat their mild poison ivy rash. # ___

C. An allergy patient having a severe acute exacerbation of their symptoms. Which short course oral medicine might be best for this patient? # ___

D. A hospital patient needing hormonal replacement therapy for Addison's disease. # ___

E. A hospital patient in surgery-associated adrenal insufficiency crisis due to sudden preoperative withdrawal of glucocorticoids (rapid onset glucocorticoid therapy). # ___

F. A patient at a clinic for a severe but small surface area contact dermatitis who wants to avoid oral "steroid" therapy. # ___

G. A diabetic patient diagnosed with diabetic macular edema seeking an extended-release bioresorbable ocular insert for DME. # ___

H. An asthmatic patient seeking once daily inhalation therapy (prodrug). # ___

I. An asthmatic patient seeking once daily inhalation therapy (not a prodrug). # ___

Structure Challenge answers found immediately after References.

REFERENCES

1. IUPAC-IUB Joint Commission on Biochemical Nomenclature (JCBN). The nomenclature of steroids. Recommendations 1989. *Eur J Biochem.* 1989;186:429-458.
2. Beato M. Gene regulation by steroid hormones. *Cell.* 1989;56: 335-344.
3. Carson-Jurica MA, Schrader WT, O'Malley BW. Steroid receptor family: structure and functions. *Endocr Rev.* 1990;11:201-220.
4. Evans RM. The steroid and thyroid hormone receptor superfamily. *Science.* 1988;240:889-895.
5. Ringold G. Steroid hormone action. In: Proceedings of the UCLA Symposium Park City, Utah, Januray 17-23, 1987; 1988.
6. Gustafsson JA, Carlstedt-Duke J, Poellinger L, et al. Biochemistry, molecular biology, and physiology of the glucocorticoid receptor. *Endocr Rev.* 1987;8:185-234.
7. O'Malley B. The steroid receptor superfamily: more excitement predicted for the future. *Mol Endocrinol.* 1990;4:363-369.
8. Narayanan R, Adigun AA, Edwards DP, et al. Cyclin-dependent kinase activity is required for progesterone receptor function: novel role for cyclin A/Cdk2 as a progesterone receptor coactivator. *Mol Cell Biol.* 2005;25:264-277.
9. Sato S, Shirakawa H, Tomita S, et al. The aryl hydrocarbon receptor and glucocorticoid receptor interact to activate human metallothionein 2A. *Toxicol Appl Pharmacol.* 2013;273:90-99.
10. Stahn C, Lowenberg M, Hommes DW, et al. Molecular mechanisms of glucocorticoid action and selective glucocorticoid receptor agonists. *Mol Cell Endocrinol.* 2007;275:71-78.
11. van der Laan S, Meijer OC. Pharmacology of glucocorticoids: beyond receptors. *Eur J Pharmacol.* 2008;585:483-491.
12. Eickelberg O, Roth M, Lorx R, et al. Ligand-independent activation of the glucocorticoid receptor by beta2-adrenergic receptor agonists in primary human lung fibroblasts and vascular smooth muscle cells. *J Biol Chem.* 1999;274:1005-1010.
13. Addison T. *On the Constitutional and Local Effects of Disease of the Suprarenal Capsules.* Birmingham, AL: Classics of Medicine Library; 1980.
14. Murison PJ. Hyperfunctioning adrenocortical diseases. *Med Clin North Am.* 1967;51:883-901.
15. Shoppee CW. *Chemistry of the Steroids.* London; 1964.
16. Simpson ER. Cholesterol side-chain cleavage, cytochrome P450, and the control of steroidogenesis. *Mol Cell Endocrinol.* 1979;13:213-227.
17. Schimmer BP, Parker KL. *Adrenocorticotropic Hormones.* New York: McGraw-Hill; 2001.
18. Simpson ER, Waterman MR. Regulation of the synthesis of steroidogenic enzymes in adrenal cortical cells by ACTH. *Annu Rev Physiol.* 1988;50:427-440.
19. Kremers P. Progesterone and pregnenolone 17 alpha-hydroxylase: substrate specificity and selective inhibition by 17 alpha-hydroxylated products. *J Steroid Biochem.* 1976;7:571-575.
20. Miller WL. Molecular biology of steroid hormone synthesis. *Endocr Rev.* 1988;9:295-318.
21. Miller WL, Auchus RJ. The molecular biology, biochemistry, and physiology of human steroidogenesis and its disorders. *Endocr Rev.* 2011;32:81-151.
22. Penning TM. Molecular endocrinology of hydroxysteroid dehydrogenases. *Endocr Rev.* 1997;18:281-305.
23. Tomlinson JW, Walker EA, Bujalska IJ, et al. 11beta-hydroxysteroid dehydrogenase type 1: a tissue-specific regulator of glucocorticoid response. *Endocr Rev.* 2004;25:831-866.
24. White PC, Mune T, Agarwal AK. 11 Beta-hydroxysteroid dehydrogenase and the syndrome of apparent mineralocorticoid excess. *Endocr Rev.* 1997;18:135-156.
25. Derendorf H, Mollmann H, Barth J, et al. Pharmacokinetics and oral bioavailability of hydrocortisone. *J Clin Pharmacol.* 1991;31:473-476.
26. Fukushima DK, Leeds NS, Bradlow HL, et al. The characterization of four new metabolites of adrenocortical hormones. *J Biol Chem.* 1955;212:449-460.
27. Romanoff LP, Morris CW, Welch P, et al. The metabolism of cortisol-4-C14 in young and elderly men. I. Secretion rate of cortisol and daily excretion of tetrahydrocortisol, allotetrahydrocortisol, tetrahydrocortisone and cortolone (20alpha and 20beta). *J Clin Endocrinol Metab.* 1961;21:1413-1425.
28. Chang E, Dao TL. Adrenal estrogens. II. Further characterizations of isolated urinary 11beta-hydroxyestradiol. *Biochim Biophys Acta.* 1962;57:609-612.
29. Speirs RS, Meyer RK. A method of assaying adrenal cortical hormones based on a decrease in the circulating eosinophil cells of adrenalectomized mice. *Endocrinology.* 1951;48:316-326.
30. Dorfman RI, Dorfman AS. The relative thymolytic activities of corticoids using the ovariectomized-adrenalectomized mouse. *Endocrinology.* 1961;69:283-291.
31. Ringler I, Brownfield R. The thymolytic activities of 16alpha, 17alpha ketals of triamcinolone. *Endocrinology.* 1960;66:900-902.
32. Kupfer D. Alteration in the magnitude of induction of tyrosine transaminase by glycocorticoids. The effects of phenobarbital, o,p'DDD and beta-diethylaminoethyl diphenylpropylacetate (SKF 525A). *Arch Biochem Biophys.* 1968;127:200-206.
33. Lee KL, Kenney FT. Induction of alanine transaminase by adrenal steroids in cultured hepatoma cells. *Biochem Biophys Res Commun.* 1970;40:469-475.
34. Sereni F, Kenney FT, Kretchmer N. Factors influencing the development of tyrosine-alpha-ketoglutarate transaminase activity in rat liver. *J Biol Chem.* 1959;234:609-612.
35. Feigelson P, Beato M, Colman P, et al. Studies on the hepatic glucocorticoid receptor and on the hormonal modulation of specific mRNA levels during enzyme induction. *Recent Prog Horm Res.* 1975;31:213-242.
36. Kenney F, Lee KL, Reel JR, et al. Regulation of tyrosine alpha-ketoglutarate transaminase in rat liver. IX. Studies of the mechanisms of hormonal inductions in cultured hepatoma cells. *J Biol Chem.* 1970;245:5806-5812.
37. Felig P, Pozefsky T, Marliss E, et al. Alanine: key role in gluconeogenesis. *Science.* 1970;167:1003-1004.
38. Landau BR. Adrenal steroids and carbohydrate metabolism. *Vitam Horm.* 1965;23:2-59.
39. McMahon M, Gerich J, Rizza R. Effects of glucocorticoids on carbohydrate metabolism. *Diabetes Metab Rev.* 1988;4:17-30.
40. Goulding NJ, Godolphin JL, Sharland PR, et al. Anti-inflammatory lipocortin 1 production by peripheral blood leucocytes in response to hydrocortisone. *Lancet.* 1990;335:1416-1418.
41. Peers SH, Smillie F, Elderfield AJ, et al. Glucocorticoid-and non-glucocorticoid induction of lipocortins (annexins) 1 and 2 in rat peritoneal leucocytes in vivo. *Br J Pharmacol.* 1993;108:66-72.
42. Solito E, Parente L. Modulation of phospholipase A2 activity in human fibroblasts. *Br J Pharmacol.* 1989;96:656-660.
43. Parente L, Flower RJ. Hydrocortisone and 'macrocortin' inhibit the zymosan-induced release of lyso-PAF from rat peritoneal leucocytes. *Life Sci.* 1985;36:1225-1231.
44. Beutler B, Cerami A. Cachectin: more than a tumor necrosis factor. *N Engl J Med.* 1987;316:379-385.
45. Goodwin JS, Atluru D, Sierakowski S, et al. Mechanism of action of glucocorticosteroids. Inhibition of T cell proliferation and interleukin 2 production by hydrocortisone is reversed by leukotriene B4. *J Clin Invest.* 1986;77:1244-1250.
46. Lew W, Oppenheim JJ, Matsushima K. Analysis of the suppression of IL-1 alpha and IL-1 beta production in human peripheral blood mononuclear adherent cells by a glucocorticoid hormone. *J Immunol.* 1988;140:1895-1902.
47. Radomski MW, Palmer RM, Moncada S. Glucocorticoids inhibit the expression of an inducible, but not the constitutive, nitric oxide synthase in vascular endothelial cells. *Proc Natl Acad Sci USA.* 1990;87:10043-10047.
48. Fuller PJ, Yang J, Young MJ. 30 years of the mineralocorticoid receptor: coregulators as mediators of mineralocorticoid receptor signalling diversity. *J Endocrinol.* 2017;234:T23-T34.
49. Harvey BJ, Thomas W. Aldosterone-induced protein kinase signalling and the control of electrolyte balance. *Steroids.* 2018;133:67-74.

50. Bush IE. Chemical and biological factors in the activity of adrenocortical steroids. *Pharmacol Rev*. 1962;14:317-445.
51. Bush IE, Mahesh VB. Metabolism of 11-oxygenated steroids. 2. 2-methyl steroids. *Biochem J*. 1959;71:718-742.
52. Dulin WE, Bowman BJ, Stafford RO. Effects of 2-methylation on glucocorticoid activity of various C-21 steroids. *Proc Soc Exp Biol Med*. 1957;94:303-305.
53. Glenn EM, Stafford RO, Lyster SC, et al. Relation between biological activity of hydrocortisone analogues and their rates of inactivation by rat liver enzyme systems. *Endocrinology*. 1957;61:128-142.
54. Fried J, Borman A. Synthetic derivatives of cortical hormones. *Vitam Horm*. 1958;16:303-374.
55. Funder JW, Feldman D, Highland E, et al. Molecular modifications of anti-aldosterone compounds: effects on affinity of spirolactones for renal aldosterone receptors. *Biochem Pharmacol*. 1974;23:1493-1501.
56. Meduri GU, Headley AS, Golden E, et al. Effect of prolonged methylprednisolone therapy in unresolving acute respiratory distress syndrome: a randomized controlled trial. *JAMA*. 1998;280:159-165.
57. Meduri GU, Kanangat S. Glucocorticoid treatment of sepsis and acute respiratory distress syndrome: time for a critical reappraisal. *Crit Care Med*. 1998;26:630-633.
58. Suzuki M. Percutaneous absorption and systemic distribution of corticosteroids. *Nihon Hifuka Gakkai Zasshi*. 1982;92:757-776.
59. Derendorf H, Hochhaus G, Meibohm B, et al. Pharmacokinetics and pharmacodynamics of inhaled corticosteroids. *J Allergy Clin Immunol*. 1998;101:S440-S446.
60. Gray CH, Green MA, Holness NJ, et al. Urinary metabolic products of prednisone and prednisolone. *J Endocrinol*. 1956;14:146-154.
61. Burton SD, Byers SO, Friedman M, et al. Hydrocortisone metabolism in the perfused isolated rat liver. *J Clin Endocrinol Metab*. 1957;17:111-115.
62. Glick JH. The isolation of two corticosteroids from cattle bile. *Endocrinology*. 1957;60:368-375.
63. Fieser LF, Fieser M. *Steroids*. New York: Reinhold Publishing Corporation; 1959.
64. Sarett LH. Partial synthesis of pregnene-4-triol-17(beta), 20(beta), 21-dione-3,11 and pregnene-4-diol-17(beta), 21-trione-3,11,20 monoacetate. *J Biol Chem*. 1946;162:601-631.
65. McKenzie BF, Mattox VR, Engel LL, et al. Steroids derived from bile acids: VI. an improved synthesis of methyl 3,8-epoxy-Δ11-cholenate from desoxycholic acid. *J Biol Chem*. 1948;173:271-281.
66. Sarett LH. Preparation of pregnane-17α,21-diol-3,11,20-trione acetate. *J Am Chem Soc*. 1949;71:2443-2444.
67. Heazelwood VJ, Galligan JP, Cannell GR, et al. Plasma cortisol delivery from oral cortisol and cortisone acetate: relative bioavailability. *Br J Clin Pharmacol*. 1984;17:55-59.
68. Lima JJ, Jusko WJ. Bioavailability of hydrocortisone retention enemas in relation to absorption kinetics. *Clin Pharmacol Ther*. 1980;28:262-269.
69. Mollmann H, Barth J, Mollmann C, et al. Pharmacokinetics and rectal bioavailability of hydrocortisone acetate. *J Pharm Sci*. 1991;80:835-836.
70. Smith CL, Kreutner W. In vitro glucocorticoid receptor binding and transcriptional activation by topically active glucocorticoids. *Arzneimittelforschung*. 1998;48:956-960.
71. Barth J, Damoiseaux M, Mollmann H, et al. Pharmacokinetics and pharmacodynamics of prednisolone after intravenous and oral administration. *Int J Clin Pharmacol Ther Toxicol*. 1992;30:317-324.
72. Rohatagi S, Barth J, Mollmann H, et al. Pharmacokinetics of methylprednisolone and prednisolone after single and multiple oral administration. *J Clin Pharmacol*. 1997;37:916-925.
73. Mollmann H, Rohdewald P, Barth J, et al. Pharmacokinetics and dose linearity testing of methylprednisolone phosphate. *Biopharm Drug Dispos*. 1989;10:453-464.
74. Vree TB, Verwey-van Wissen CP, Lagerwerf AJ, et al. Isolation and identification of the C6-hydroxy and C20-hydroxy metabolites and glucuronide conjugate of methylprednisolone by preparative high-performance liquid chromatography from urine of patients receiving high-dose pulse therapy. *J Chromatogr B Biomed Sci Appl*. 1999;726:157-168.
75. Spero GB, Thompson JL, Lincoln FH, et al. Adrenal hormones and related compounds. V. Fluorinated 6-methyl steroids. *J Am Chem Soc*. 1957;79:1515-1516.
76. Boland EW. Clinical comparison of the newer anti-inflammatory corticosteroids. *Ann Rheum Dis*. 1962;21:176-187.
77. Ganapati A, Ravindran R, David T, et al. Head to head comparison of adverse effects and efficacy between high dose deflazacort and high dose prednisolone in systemic lupus erythematosus: a prospective cohort study. *Lupus*. 2018:961203317751854.
78. Gonzalez-Perez O, Luquin S, Garcia-Estrada J, et al. Deflazacort: a glucocorticoid with few metabolic adverse effects but important immunosuppressive activity. *Adv Ther*. 2007;24:1052-1060.
79. Hahn BH, Pletscher LS, Muniain M. Immunosuppressive effects of deflazacort - a new glucocorticoid with bone-sparing and carbohydrate-sparing properties: comparison with prednisone. *J Rheumatol*. 1981;8:783-790.
80. Assandri A, Buniva G, Martinelli E, et al. Pharmacokinetics and metabolism of deflazacort in the rat, dog, monkey and man. *Adv Exp Med Biol*. 1984;171:9-23.
81. Hirschmann H, Hirschmann FB, Farrel GL. Partial synthesis of 16α,21-diacetoxyprogesterone. *J Am Chem Soc*. 1953;75:4862-4863.
82. Allen WS, Bernstein S. Steroidal cyclic ketals. XII.1 the preparation of Δ16-steroids. *J Am Chem Soc*. 1955;77:1028-1032.
83. Allen WS, Bernstein S. Steroidal cyclic ketals. XX.1 16-Hydroxylated steroids. III.2 the preparation of 16α-Hydroxyhydrocortisone and related compounds. *J Am Chem Soc*. 1956;78:1909-1913.
84. Hochhaus G, Portner M, Barth J, et al. Oral bioavailability of triamcinolone tablets and a triamcinolone diacetate suspension. *Pharm Res*. 1990;7:558-560.
85. Portner M, Mollmann H, Barth J, et al. Pharmacokinetics of triamcinolone following oral administration. *Arzneimittelforschung*. 1988;38:1838-1840.
86. Boland EW. The treatment of rheumatoid arthritis with adrenocorticosteroids and their synthetic analogues: an appraisal of certain developments of the past decade. *Ann N Y Acad Sci*. 1959;82:887-901.
87. Dobes WL. The use of folic acid antagonists and steroids in treatment of psoriasis. *South Med J*. 1963;56:187-192.
88. Weiner AL. Intramuscular triamcinolone diacetate therapy of dermatoses: preliminary report. *Antibiot Chemother (Northfield)*. 1962;12:360-366.
89. Arth GE, Johnston DBR, Fried J, et al. 16-methylated steroids I. 16α-methylated analogs of cortisone, a new group of anti-inflammatory steroids. *J Am Chem Soc*. 1958;80:3160-3161.
90. Oliveto EP, Rausser R, Weber L, et al. 16-alkylated corticoids. II. 9α-fluoro-16α-methylprednisolone 21-acetate1. *J Am Chem Soc*. 1958;80:4431.
91. Silber RH. The biology of anti-inflammatory steroids. *Ann N Y Acad Sci*. 1959;82:821-828.
92. Sperber PA. Cyproheptadine-dexamethasone combination in the treatment of pruritus. *Curr Ther Res Clin Exp*. 1962;4:70-74.
93. Tolksdorf S. Laboratory evaluation of anti-inflammatory steroids. *Ann N Y Acad Sci*. 1959;82:829-835.
94. Rohdewald P, Mollmann H, Barth J, et al. Pharmacokinetics of dexamethasone and its phosphate ester. *Biopharm Drug Dispos*. 1987;8:205-212.
95. Cohen A, Coldman J. Use of a new corticosteroid in rheumatoid arthritis. *Pa Med J*. 1962;65:347-350.
96. Cohen AI. Treatment of allergy with oral betamethasone in 141 patients. *Antibiot Chemother (Northfield)*. 1962;12:91-96.
97. Glyn JH, Fox DB. Preliminary clinical assessment of betamethasone. *Br Med J*. 1961;1:876-877.

98. Nierman MM. Management of steriod-responsive dermatologic disorders with betamethasone. *Clin Med (Northfield)*. 1962;69:1311-1320.
99. Buijsman RC, Hermkens PH, van Rijn RD, et al. Non-steroidal steroid receptor modulators. *Curr Med Chem*. 2005;12:1017-1075.
100. Cole TJ, Mollard R. Selective glucocorticoid receptor ligands. *Med Chem*. 2007;3:494-506.
101. De Bosscher K. Selective glucocorticoid receptor modulators. *J Steroid Biochem Mol Biol*. 2010;120:96-104.
102. Einstein M, Greenlee M, Rouen G, et al. Selective glucocorticoid receptor nonsteroidal ligands completely antagonize the dexamethasone mediated induction of enzymes involved in gluconeogenesis and glutamine metabolism. *J Steroid Biochem Mol Biol*. 2004;92:345-356.
103. Miner JN, Hong MH, Negro-Vilar A. New and improved glucocorticoid receptor ligands. *Expert Opin Investig Drugs*. 2005;14:1527-1545.
104. Mohler ML, He Y, Wu Z, et al. Dissociated non-steroidal glucocorticoids: tuning out untoward effects. *Expert Opin Ther Pat*. 2007;17:37-58.
105. Sundahl N, Bridelance J, Libert C, et al. Selective glucocorticoid receptor modulation: new directions with non-steroidal scaffolds. *Pharmacol Ther*. 2015;152:28-41.
106. Yohn JJ, Weston W. *Curr Probl Dermatol*. 1990;2:31-63.
107. Andersson P, Lihne M, Thalen A, et al. Effect of structural alterations on the biotransformation rate of glucocorticosteroids in rat and human liver. *Xenobiotica*. 1987;17:35-44.
108. Schwartz SG, Scott IU, Stewart MW, et al. Update on corticosteroids for diabetic macular edema. *Clin Ophthalmol*. 2016;10:1723-1730.
109. Brogden RN, Heel RC, Speight TM, et al. Beclomethasone dipropionate. A reappraisal of its pharmacodynamic properties and therapeutic efficacy after a decade of use in asthma and rhinitis. *Drugs*. 1984;28:99-126.
110. Green MJ, Berkenkopf J, Fernandez X, et al. Synthesis and structure-activity relationships in a novel series of topically active corticosteroids. *J Steroid Biochem*. 1979;11:61-66.
111. Asche H, Botta L, Rettig H, et al. Influence of formulation factors on the availability of drugs from topical preparations. *Pharm Acta Helv*. 1985;60:232-237.
112. Bodor N, Harget AJ, Phillips EW. Structure-activity relationships in the antiinflammatory steroids: a pattern-recognition approach. *J Med Chem*. 1983;26:318-328.
113. Popper TL, Gentles MJ, Kung TT, et al. Structure-activity relationships of a series of novel topical corticosteroids. *J Steroid Biochem*. 1987;27:837-843.
114. Shapiro EL, Gentles MJ, Tiberi RL, et al. 17-Heteroaroyl esters of corticosteroids. 2. 11 beta-Hydroxy series. *J Med Chem*. 1987;30:1581-1588.
115. Barth J, Lehr KH, Derendorf H, et al. Studies on the pharmacokinetics and metabolism of prednicarbate after cutaneous and oral administration. *Skin Pharmacol*. 1993;6:179-186.
116. Derendorf H. Pharmacokinetic and pharmacodynamic properties of inhaled corticosteroids in relation to efficacy and safety. *Respir Med*. 1997;91:22-28.
117. Kelly HW. Comparison of inhaled corticosteroids. *Ann Pharmacother*. 1998;32:220-232.
118. Vlckova I, Navratil P, Kana R, et al. Effective treatment of mild-to-moderate nasal polyposis with fluticasone delivered by a novel device. *Rhinology*. 2009;47:419-426.
119. Welch MJ. Pharmacokinetics, pharmacodynamics, and clinical efficacy of albuterol RespiClick(™) dry-powder inhaler in the treatment of asthma. *Expert Opin Drug Metab Toxicol*. 2016;12:1109-1119.
120. Shaw RJ. Inhaled corticosteroids for adult asthma: impact of formulation and delivery device on relative pharmacokinetics, efficacy and safety. *Respir Med*. 1999;93:149-160.
121. Wales D, Makker H, Kane J, et al. Systemic bioavailability and potency of high-dose inhaled corticosteroids: a comparison of four inhaler devices and three drugs in healthy adult volunteers. *Chest*. 1999;115:1278-1284.
122. Lipworth BJ. Systemic adverse effects of inhaled corticosteroid therapy: a systematic review and meta-analysis. *Arch Intern Med*. 1999;159:941-955.
123. Greiff L, Andersson M, Svensson C, et al. Effects of orally inhaled budesonide in seasonal allergic rhinitis. *Eur Respir J*. 1998;11:1268-1273.
124. Seale JP, Harrison LI. Effect of changing the fine particle mass of inhaled beclomethasone dipropionate on intrapulmonary deposition and pharmacokinetics. *Respir Med*. 1998;92(suppl A):9-15.
125. Harrison LI, Soria I, Cline AC, et al. Pharmacokinetic differences between chlorofluorocarbon and chlorofluorocarbon-free metered dose inhalers of beclomethasone dipropionate in adult asthmatics. *J Pharm Pharmacol*. 1999;51:1235-1240.
126. Lipworth BJ, Jackson CM. Pharmacokinetics of chlorofluorocarbon and hydrofluoroalkane metered-dose inhaler formulations of beclomethasone dipropionate. *Br J Clin Pharmacol*. 1999;48:866-868.
127. Mollmann H, Derendorf H, Barth J, et al. Pharmacokinetic/pharmacodynamic evaluation of systemic effects of flunisolide after inhalation. *J Clin Pharmacol*. 1997;37:893-903.
128. Dickens GR, Wermeling DP, Matheny CJ, et al. Pharmacokinetics of flunisolide administered via metered dose inhaler with and without a spacer device and following oral administration. *Ann Allergy Asthma Immunol*. 2000;84:528-532.
129. Thalen BA, Axelsson BI, Andersson PH, et al. 6 alpha-Fluoro- and 6 alpha,9 alpha-difluoro-11 beta,21-dihydroxy-16 alpha,17 alpha-propylmethylenedioxypregn-4-ene-3,20-dione: synthesis and evaluation of activity and kinetics of their C-22 epimers. *Steroids*. 1998;63:37-43.
130. Ryrfeldt A, Andersson P, Edsbacker S, et al. Pharmacokinetics and metabolism of budesonide, a selective glucocorticoid. *Eur J Respir Dis Suppl*. 1982;122:86-95.
131. Szefler SJ. Pharmacodynamics and pharmacokinetics of budesonide: a new nebulized corticosteroid. *J Allergy Clin Immunol*. 1999;104:175-183.
132. Miller-Larsson A, Jansson P, Runstrom A, et al. Prolonged airway activity and improved selectivity of budesonide possibly due to esterification. *Am J Respir Crit Care Med*. 2000;162:1455-1461.
133. Miller-Larsson A, Mattsson H, Hjertberg E, et al. Reversible fatty acid conjugation of budesonide. Novel mechanism for prolonged retention of topically applied steroid in airway tissue. *Drug Metab Dispos*. 1998;26:623-630.
134. Agertoft L, Andersen A, Weibull E, et al. Systemic availability and pharmacokinetics of nebulised budesonide in preschool children. *Arch Dis Child*. 1999;80:241-247.
135. Pedersen S, Steffensen G, Ekman I, et al. Pharmacokinetics of budesonide in children with asthma. *Eur J Clin Pharmacol*. 1987;31:579-582.
136. Shapiro EL, Gentles MJ, Tiberi RL, et al. Synthesis and structure-activity studies of corticosteroid 17-heterocyclic aromatic esters. 1. 9 alpha, 11 beta-dichloro series. *J Med Chem*. 1987;30:1068-1073.
137. Onrust SV, Lamb HM. Mometasone furoate. A review of its intranasal use in allergic rhinitis. *Drugs*. 1998;56:725-745.
138. Affrime MB, Cuss F, Padhi D, et al. Bioavailability and metabolism of mometasone furoate following administration by metered-dose and dry-powder inhalers in healthy human volunteers. *J Clin Pharmacol*. 2000;40:1227-1236.
139. Phillipps GH, Bailey EJ, Bain BM, et al. Synthesis and structure-activity relationships in a series of antiinflammatory corticosteroid analogues, halomethyl androstane-17 beta-carbothioates and -17 beta-carboselenoates. *J Med Chem*. 1994;37:3717-3729.
140. Harding SM. The human pharmacology of fluticasone propionate. *Respir Med*. 1990;84(suppl A):25-29.

141. Johnson M. Development of fluticasone propionate and comparison with other inhaled corticosteroids. *J Allergy Clin Immunol.* 1998;101:S434-S439.
142. Mackie AE, Ventresca GP, Fuller RW, et al. Pharmacokinetics of intravenous fluticasone propionate in healthy subjects. *Br J Clin Pharmacol.* 1996;41:539-542.
143. Mollmann H, Wagner M, Meibohm B, et al. Pharmacokinetic and pharmacodynamic evaluation of fluticasone propionate after inhaled administration. *Eur J Clin Pharmacol.* 1998;53:459-467.
144. Thorsson L, Dahlstrom K, Edsbacker S, et al. Pharmacokinetics and systemic effects of inhaled fluticasone propionate in healthy subjects. *Br J Clin Pharmacol.* 1997;43:155-161.
145. Rohatagi S, Bye A, Falcoz C, et al. Dynamic modeling of cortisol reduction after inhaled administration of fluticasone propionate. *J Clin Pharmacol.* 1996;36:938-941.
146. Biggadike K. Fluticasone furoate/fluticasone propionate - different drugs with different properties. *Clin Respir J.* 2011;5:183-184.
147. Biggadike K, Bledsoe RK, Hassell AM, et al. X-ray crystal structure of the novel enhanced-affinity glucocorticoid agonist fluticasone furoate in the glucocorticoid receptor-ligand binding domain. *J Med Chem.* 2008;51:3349-3352.
148. Salter M, Biggadike K, Matthews JL, et al. Pharmacological properties of the enhanced-affinity glucocorticoid fluticasone furoate in vitro and in an in vivo model of respiratory inflammatory disease. *Am J Physiol Lung Cell Mol Physiol.* 2007;293:L660-L667.
149. Valotis A, Hogger P. Human receptor kinetics and lung tissue retention of the enhanced-affinity glucocorticoid fluticasone furoate. *Respir Res.* 2007;8:54.
150. Allen A, Bareille PJ, Rousell VM. Fluticasone furoate, a novel inhaled corticosteroid, demonstrates prolonged lung absorption kinetics in man compared with inhaled fluticasone propionate. *Clin Pharmacokinet.* 2013;52:37-42.
151. Duval D, Durant S, Homo-Delarche F. Effect of antiglucocorticoids on dexamethasone-induced inhibition of uridine incorporation and cell lysis in isolated mouse thymocytes. *J Steroid Biochem.* 1984;20:283-287.
152. Peterfalvi M, Torelli V, Fournex R, et al. Importance of the lactonic ring in the activity of steroidal antialdosterones. *Biochem Pharmacol.* 1980;29:353-357.
153. Agarwal MK, Hainque B, Moustaid N, et al. Glucocorticoid antagonists. *FEBS Lett.* 1987;217:221-226.
154. Fleseriu M, Biller BM, Findling JW, et al. Mifepristone, a glucocorticoid receptor antagonist, produces clinical and metabolic benefits in patients with Cushing's syndrome. *J Clin Endocrinol Metab.* 2012;97:2039-2049.
155. Napoli JL, Counsell RE. New inhibitors of steroid 11beta-hydroxylase. Structure–activity relationship studies of metyrapone-like compounds. *J Med Chem.* 1977;20:762-766.
156. Shaw MA, Nicholls PJ, Smith HJ. Aminoglutethimide and ketoconazole: historical perspectives and future prospects. *J Steroid Biochem.* 1988;31:137-146.
157. Sonino N. The use of ketoconazole as an inhibitor of steroid production. *N Engl J Med.* 1987;317:812-818.
158. Potts GO, Creange JE, Hardomg HR, et al. Trilostane, an orally active inhibitor of steroid biosynthesis. *Steroids.* 1978;32:257-267.
159. Monder C, Stewart PM, Lakshmi V, et al. Licorice inhibits corticosteroid 11 beta-dehydrogenase of rat kidney and liver: in vivo and in vitro studies. *Endocrinology.* 1989;125:1046-1053.
160. Buhler H, Perschel FH, Fitzner R, et al. Endogenous inhibitors of 11 beta-OHSD: existence and possible significance. *Steroids.* 1994;59:131-135.
161. Diederich S, Grossmann C, Hanke B, et al. In the search for specific inhibitors of human 11beta-hydroxysteroid-dehydrogenases (11beta-HSDs): chenodeoxycholic acid selectively inhibits 11beta-HSD-I. *Eur J Endocrinol.* 2000;142:200-207.
162. Scott JS, Goldberg FW, Turnbull AV. Medicinal chemistry of inhibitors of 11beta-hydroxysteroid dehydrogenase type 1 (11beta-HSD1). *J Med Chem.* 2014;57:4466-4486.
163. Pereira CD, Azevedo I, Monteiro R, et al. 11beta-Hydroxysteroid dehydrogenase type 1: relevance of its modulation in the pathophysiology of obesity, the metabolic syndrome and type 2 diabetes mellitus. *Diabetes Obes Metab.* 2012;14:869-881.

Structure Challenge Answers

A-7, B-1, C-2, D-5, E-3, F-8, G-6, H-4, I-9.

CHAPTER 22

Drugs Used to Treat Thyroid Disorders

Ali R. Banijamali

Drugs covered in this chapter:

DRUGS FOR TREATMENT OF HYPOTHYROIDISM
- Levothyroxine
- Liothyronine
- Liotrix
- Thyroid gland products

DRUGS FOR TREATMENT OF HYPERTHYROIDISM
- Iodide
- Perchlorate
- Radioiodine
- 1-Methyl-2-mercaptoimidazole
- Propylthiouracil

Abbreviations

BMR basal metabolic rate
cAMP cyclic adenosine monophosphate
DIT diiodo-L-tyrosine
dT_4 dextrothyroxine
FAD flavin adenine dinucleotide
GRTH generalized resistance to thyroid hormone
HSA human serum albumin
$^{99m}TcO_4$ radioactive pertechnetate
MIT monoiodo-L-tyrosine
MMI 1-methyl-2-mercaptoimidazole
NADPH reduced form of nicotinamide adenine dinucleotide phosphate
NIS sodium/iodide symporter
PTU propylthiouracil
$rT_3$3 3′,5′-triiodo-L-thyronine (reverse T_3)
SAR structure-activity relationship
T_2 3,3′-diiodo-L-thyronine
T_3 Levo or L-triiodothyronine, Liothyronine
T_4 Levo or L-thyroxine
TBG thyroxine-binding globulin
Tg thyroglobulin
TPO thyroperoxidase
TRH thyroid-releasing hormone
TSH thyrotropin (thyroid-stimulating hormone)
TTR transthyretin
USP U.S. Pharmacopeia

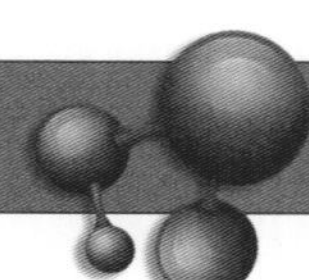

CLINICAL SIGNIFICANCE

Autumn Stewart, PharmD, BCACP

Differences in the activity profiles of available treatments for thyroid disorders make patient-specific drug selection extremely important. The development of synthetic thyroid hormones has significantly improved treatment of hypothyroidism by decreasing the variations in levothyroxine and liothyronine blood levels that often resulted from inconsistent bovine and porcine sources. Once-daily or once-weekly dosing, which has been associated with improved patient compliance, is another clinically significant benefit of synthetic T_4, resulting from its extended half-life. Knowledge of levothyroxine's pharmacokinetic profile has also prompted patient counseling efforts promoting premeal administration because of marked reduction in absorption when combined with meals. The understanding of structure-activity relationships also enabled the development of synthetic T_3 (liothyronine), the metabolically more active form of thyroid hormone with a much shorter duration of action. This is especially useful for patients with thyroid carcinoma who are to undergo radioiodine imaging and possible treatment. Because of a half-life of only 24 hours, liothyronine substitution enables more timely radioiodine imaging and treatment; as a result, patients experience less symptomatic hypothyroidism.

The study of medicinal chemistry has improved the treatment of thyroid disorders by reducing variability in plasma concentrations of T_3 and T_4 and by increasing the reliability of available monitoring methods. Accurate monitoring and therapy adjustments have resulted in fewer complications and increased quality of life among the millions of patients with thyroid disorders.

INTRODUCTION

The thyroid gland is a highly vascular, flat structure located at the upper portion of the trachea, just below the larynx. It is composed of two lateral lobes joined by an isthmus across the ventral surface of the trachea. The gland is the source of two fundamentally different types of hormones, thyroxine (T_4) and triiodothyronine (T_3). Both hormones are vital for normal growth and development and control essential functions, such as energy metabolism and protein synthesis.

The word thyroid, meaning shield-shaped, was introduced by Wharton in his description of the gland.[1] Like many before him, he attributed a solely cosmetic function to it because of the more frequent presence of enlarged glands in women, giving the throat region a more beautiful roundness. Later, however, it was observed that some characteristic symptoms for diseases always were accompanied by an obvious change in the size of the thyroid. This change was correctly interpreted as evidence that this structure plays a major role in normal body function.

An important step in the understanding of thyroid function was taken by Baumann,[2] who discovered that the thyroid gland was the only organ in mammals that had the capability to incorporate iodine into organic substances. That discovery was important in research concerning the phylogeny of the thyroid.

Major clues to the physiologic roles of thyroid hormones were provided when normal and abnormal thyroid functions were related to oxygen uptake[3] and when thyroid hormones were found to induce metamorphosis in tadpoles.[4] The first discovery led to investigations regarding the role of thyroid hormone in metabolism and calorigenesis, and the second inspired research concerning specific receptors as points of initiation of thyroid hormone expression. A patient lacking thyroid hormones may be treated with synthetic hormones or natural preparations. Better agents to treat hyperthyroidism are still being sought. Presently available drugs, other compounds affecting thyroid function, and current approaches in the search for new drugs are presented in this chapter within the context of thyroid biochemistry and physiology.

NORMAL BIOCHEMISTRY AND PHYSIOLOGY

Thyroid Follicular Cells

All vertebrates have a thyroid gland consisting of functional units, the follicles. The morphologic and functional characteristics of the follicles are essentially similar in all vertebrate groups.

The follicle is a spherical, cystlike structure approximately 300 μm in diameter, and it consists of a luminal cavity surrounded by a one-cell-deep layer of cells called follicular or acinar cells. The center of the follicles is filled with a gelatinous colloid, the main component of which is a glycoprotein called thyroglobulin. The follicular cells contain an extensive network of rough endoplasmic reticulum, a well-developed Golgi apparatus, and lysosomes of various sizes.[5] Thyroglobulin is synthesized in the rough endoplasmic reticulum of the follicular cells and transported by way of the Golgi complex to the apical membrane and then secreted into the follicle lumen.

The follicular cell contains two major assembly lines operating in opposite directions.[6] One line moves in an apical direction (toward the lumen of the cell) and produces thyroglobulin that is delivered to the follicle lumen; the other line begins at the apical cell surface (cell surface facing the lumen of the cell) with endocytosis of thyroglobulin and ends by delivering hormones at the basolateral cell membrane. Therefore, the follicular cell seems to fulfill the functions of secretory and absorptive cells simultaneously. In addition to the functions associated with these two lines, the follicle has the specific ability to metabolize iodine, comprising the accumulation of iodide, iodination of tryosyl residues in thyroglobulin, and coupling of the iodinated tyrosyls to form thyroid hormones.

Parafollicular cells, also called light cells or C cells, are located individually or in clusters between follicular cells but do not border on the colloid. These cells produce thyrocalcitonin, a peptide hormone involved in calcium homeostasis (see also Chapter 30). The extrafollicular space of the gland is occupied by blood vessels, capillaries, lymphatic vessels, and connective tissue.

Hormones of the Thyroid Gland

Thyroid hormones are essential for normal development, differentiation, growth, and metabolism of every cell in the body. Thyroid hormones are iodinated amino acids derived from L-tyrosine. They are synthesized in the thyroid gland and stored as amino acid residues of thyroglobulin. The first known biologically active iodine-containing compound of the thyroid gland was isolated from thyroid extracts and named L-thyroxine (T_4). Later, its structure was established as the 3,5,3′,5′-tetraiodo-L-thyronine (T_4) (Fig. 22.1), and its synthesis was accomplished. Twenty-five years later, with the availability of chromatographic techniques and radioactive iodine, researchers discovered another major thyroid hormone, 3,5,3′-triiodo-L-thyronine (T_3) (Fig. 22.1), which is derived mainly from T_4 deiodination by deiodinase enzymes outside the thyroid. The body is therefore able to use a dose of T_4 to produce its own T_3.

T_4 and T_3 play numerous and meaningful roles in regulating metabolism, growth, and development and in maintaining homeostasis. Their reactions and products influence carbohydrate metabolism, protein synthesis and breakdown, and cardiovascular, renal, and brain function. It is usually believed that these actions result from effects of thyroid hormones on protein synthesis.

The thyroid gland also contains two quantitatively important iodinated amino acids, diiodo-L-tyrosine (DIT) and monoiodo-L-tyrosine (MIT). In addition, there are small amounts of other iodothyronines, such as 3,3′-diiodo-L-thyronine (T_2) and 3,3′,5′-triiodo-L-thyronine (reverse T_3 [rT_3]). None of the latter compounds possesses any significant hormonal activity. Chemically, MIT is 3-iodo-L-tyrosine, and DIT is 3,5-diiodo-L-tyrosine. The

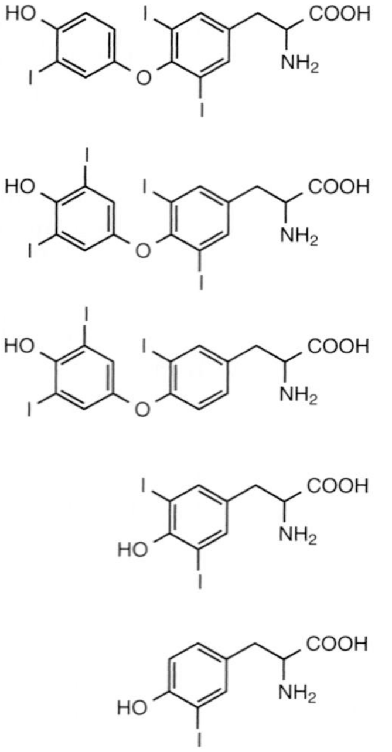

T3

T4

r-T3

DIT

MIT

Figure 22.1 Structure of the iodinated compounds of the thyroid gland.

coupling of the two outer rings of DIT or of one outer ring of DIT with that of MIT (each with the net loss of alanine) leads to the formation of the two major thyroid hormones, T_4 and T_3, respectively.

Thyroglobulin (Tg) is of special importance because it serves as the matrix for the synthesis of T_4 and T_3 and as the storage form of the hormones and iodide. Tg, a large glycoprotein with a molecular weight of 660,000 Da, accounts for about one-third of the weight of the thyroid gland. Tg carries an average of 6 tyrosyl residues as MIT, 5 residues as DIT, 0.3 residues as T_3, and 1 residue as T_4. From these values, it can be estimated that a 20-g thyroid stores roughly 10 μmol (7.8 mg) of T_4 and 3 μmol (2.0 mg) of T_3 and that the normal human thyroid gland contains enough potential T_4 to maintain a euthyroid state for 2 months without new synthesis. The structures of the iodinated compounds of the thyroid gland are shown in Figure 22.1.

Biosynthesis of Thyroid Hormones

The thyroid contains two hormones, L-thyroxine (T_4) and L-triiodothyronine (T_3). Iodine is an indispensable component of the thyroid hormones, comprising 65% of the weight of T_4 and 58% of the weight of T_3. The thyroid hormones are the only iodine-containing compounds with established physiologic significance in vertebrates. Ingested iodine is absorbed through the small intestine and transported in the plasma to the thyroid, where it is concentrated, oxidized, and then incorporated into Tg to form MIT and DIT and later T_4 and T_3. After a variable period of storage in thyroid follicles, Tg is subjected to proteolysis, and the released hormones are secreted into the circulation, where specific binding proteins carry them to target tissues.

The synthesis of the thyroid hormones, T_3 and T_4, is regulated by thyrotropin (also known as thyroid-stimulating hormone [TSH]), which stimulates the synthesis of Tg, thyroperoxidase (TPO), and hydrogen peroxide. The formation of the thyroid hormones depends on an exogenous supply of iodide. The thyroid gland is unique in that it is the only tissue of the body able to accumulate iodine in large quantities and incorporate it into hormones. Approximately 25% of the body's supply of iodide is located in the thyroid gland. The iodine atoms play a unique role in the conformational preferences for T_3 and T_4 because of their large steric bulkiness. The metabolism of iodine is so closely related to thyroid function that the two must be considered together. The formation of thyroid hormones involves the following complex sequence of events: (1) active uptake of iodide by the follicular cells, (2) oxidation of iodide and formation of iodotyrosyl residues of Tg, (3) formation of iodothyronines from iodotyrosines, (4) proteolysis of Tg and release of T_4 and T_3 into blood, and (5) conversion of T_4 to T_3. These processes are summarized in Figure 22.2.[7]

Active Uptake of Iodide by Follicular Cells

The first step in the synthesis of the thyroid hormones is the uptake of iodide from the blood by the thyroid gland. An adequate intake of iodide is essential for the synthesis of sufficient thyroid hormone. Ingested iodine is absorbed through the small intestine and transported in the plasma to the thyroid, where it is concentrated, oxidized, and then incorporated into Tg. Blood iodine is present in a steady state in which dietary iodide, iodide "leaked" from the thyroid gland, and reclaimed hormonal iodide provide the iodide input. Thyroid gland iodide uptake, renal elimination, and a small biliary excretion provide iodide loss. The thyroid gland regulates both the fraction of circulating iodide that it takes up and the amount of iodide that it leaks back into the circulation. A simplified scheme of iodide metabolism is shown in Figure 22.3.

The mechanism enabling the thyroid gland to concentrate blood iodide against a gradient into the follicular cell is the iodide pump (NIS, sodium/iodide symporter), which is regulated by TSH. Decreased stores of thyroid iodine enhance iodide uptake; conversely, dietary iodide can reverse this process. The iodide pump maintains a ratio of thyroid iodide to serum iodide (T:S ratio) of about 20:1 under basal conditions but of more than 100:1 in the hyperactive gland. Iodide uptake may be blocked by several inorganic ions, such as thiocyanate (SCN^-) and perchlorate. Because iodide uptake involves concurrent uptake of potassium, it can also be blocked by cardiac glycosides that inhibit potassium accumulation.

Oxidation of Iodide and Formation of Iodotyrosines

To serve as an iodinating agent, iodide must be oxidized to a higher oxidation state, a step that is hydrogen peroxide dependent and is catalyzed by TPO, a membrane-bound heme enzyme that utilizes hydrogen peroxide as the oxidant. In addition to catalyzing the oxidation of iodide,

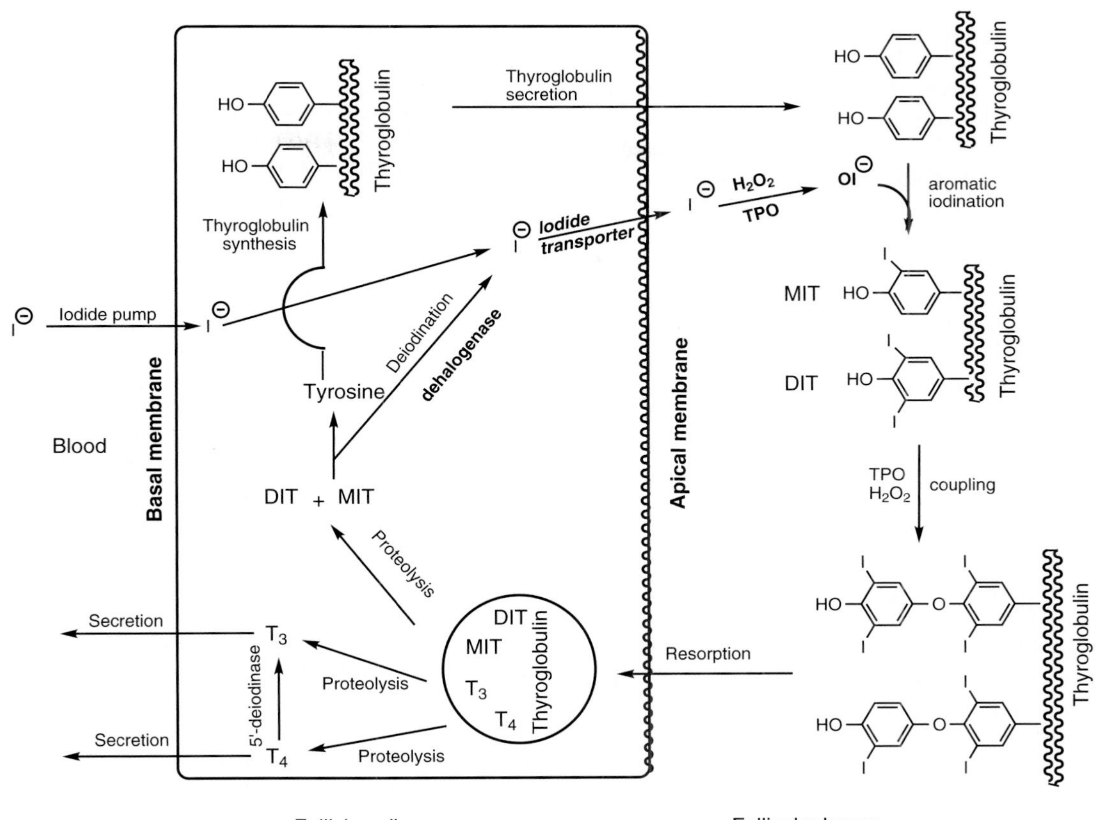

Figure 22.2 Summary of the major pathways for the biosynthesis and secretion of the thyroid hormones. When thyrotropin (TSH) binds to the TSH receptor at the basal membrane of the follicular cell, the biosynthesis of thyroglobulin (TG) is stimulated, as is that of thyroperoxidase (TPO) and the production of hydrogen peroxide. Noniodinated TG is synthesized by the rough endoplasmic reticulum of the follicular cell and secreted through the apical membrane of the follicular cell into the follicular lumen. Iodide enters the follicular cell by the iodide pump (NIS, sodium/iodide symporter) and is then transported into the follicular lumen. In the lumen, the iodide is oxidized by TPO-O (a π-cation radical intermediate formed from TPO and hydrogen peroxide) at the apical membrane to form hypoiodate anion (OI), followed by aromatic iodination of selected tyrosyl residues on TG to form diiodotyrosyl (DIT) and monoiodotyrosyl (MIT) residues. The tyrosyl ring of DIT couples with adjacent DIT and MIT residues with an ether linkage to form the outer ring of thyroxine (T_4) and of triiodothyronine (T_3), both of which remain attached to TG. Although shown as a sequential reaction, the iodination and coupling reactions occur simultaneously via TPO and hydrogen peroxide. Hydrogen peroxide is generated by an NADPH/FAD thyroid oxidase (THOX) at the apical membrane. Low plasma levels for T_4 cause the iodinated TG to be resorbed into the follicular cell, where complete proteolysis occurs by lysosomal protease to T_4, T_3, DIT, MIT, and noniodinated amino acids. Both T_4 and T_3 are secreted by the cell into the blood; T_4 is deiodinated to active T_3. Both DIT and MIT are recycled by a dehalogenase (or deiodinase) to free tyrosine and iodide, both of which are recycled back into iodinated thyroglobulin.

TPO is essential for the incorporation of iodide into tyrosine residues in Tg (aromatic iodination) and coupling of the iodotyrosyl residues from DIT to form T_4 and T_3. The activity of TPO is increased by TSH from increased synthesis of TPO.

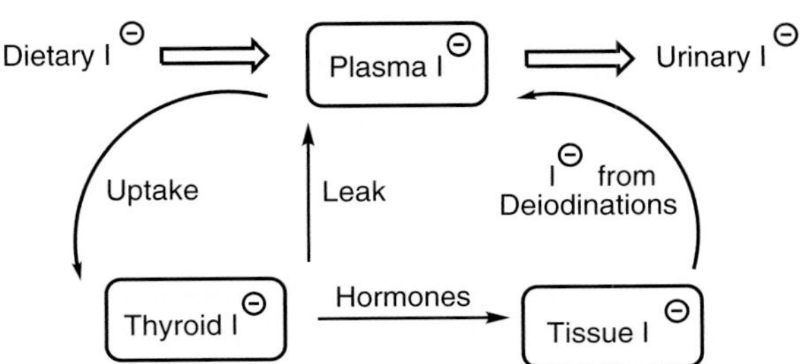

Figure 22.3 Simplified scheme of iodide metabolism.

The second step in the synthesis of the thyroid hormones is a concerted reaction at the apical membrane in which the iodide in the follicle lumen is oxidized by TPO in the presence of hydrogen peroxide to an active iodine species that, in turn, iodinates selected tyrosyl residues of Tg. Consistent with the conditions necessary for aromatic halogenation, the iodination of the tyrosyl residues requires the iodinating species to be in a higher oxidation state compared with the iodide anion. The iodinating species is thought to be hypoiodate (OI^-).[7] The two-electron oxidation of iodide to its hypoiodate reactive species is accomplished by TPO. Although the diiodotyrosyl residues constitute the major products, some MIT peptides are also produced. TSH stimulates the generation of hydrogen peroxide and, thus, the process of iodination.

Hydrogen peroxide is an essential and limiting factor in the oxidation of iodide, aromatic iodination of tyrosyl residues, and the coupling reaction. The hydrogen peroxide–generating system is localized at the apical membrane, and its generation involves the oxidation of the reduced form of nicotinamide adenine dinucleotide phosphate (NADPH) by an NADPH/flavin adenine dinucleotide (FAD) oxidase called thyroid oxidase. The reaction product of TPO with hydrogen peroxide is described as TPO-P, a π-cation radical, which generates hypoiodate. The generation of hydrogen peroxide is concentration controlled by iodide, which permits efficient hormone synthesis when iodide is scarce while avoiding excessive hormone synthesis when iodide is abundant. Deficient generation of hydrogen peroxide has been proposed as one explanation for goiter and decreased aromatic iodination in euthyroid patients. The in vitro addition of a hydrogen peroxide–generating system to thyroid homogenates or slices from these patients restored normal organification.

In the thyroid follicular cell, intracellular iodide taken up from blood is bound in organic form in a few minutes, so less than 1% of the total iodine of the gland is found as iodide. Therefore, inhibition of the iodide transport system requires blockade of organic binding. This can be achieved by the use of antithyroid drugs, of which n-propyl-6-thiouracil and 1-methyl-2-mercaptoimidazole (MMI) are the most potent.

Coupling of Iodotyrosine Residues

Coupling is also catalyzed by TPO at the apical membrane, and although shown in Figure 22.2 as sequential steps, they occur simultaneously. This coupling reaction takes place at Tg and involves the coupling of the two outer rings from DIT residues to become T_4, whereas the coupling of the outer ring from MIT with DIT results in the formation of T_3. During the coupling reaction as shown in Figure 22.2, a tyrosyl residue donates its iodinated phenyl group as a DIT radical to become the outer ring of the iodothyronine amino acid at an acceptor site, leaving dehydroalanine at the donor site. The location of the iodotyrosyl residues within Tg creates an optimal spatial alignment, facilitating the coupling reaction. These reactions are catalyzed by TPO and can be blocked by compounds such as thiourea, thiouracils, and sulfonamides.

Proteolysis of Thyroglobulin and Release of Iodothyronines

In response to demand for thyroid hormones, the release of thyroid hormones from Tg begins with the resorption of Tg via endocytosis into the follicular epithelial cells and its subsequent complete proteolysis by the lysosomal digestive enzymes of the follicular cells. Tg proteolysis yields MIT, DIT, T_3, and T_4. Although MIT and DIT are formed, they do not leave the thyroid but, instead, are selectively deiodinated to tyrosine and recycled into new Tg. The iodide is recycled into hypoiodate for subsequent iodination, conserving the essential nutrients for the thyroid gland. Both T_3 and T_4 are secreted by the cell into the circulation. A defect in the recyclization of MIT and DIT can lead to hypothyroidism and goiter by increasing their elimination in the urine.

Conversion of Thyroxine (T_4) to Triiodothyronine (T_3)

Although T_4 is by far the major thyroid hormone secreted by the thyroid (~8-10 times the rate of T_3), it is usually considered to be a prohormone. Because T_4 has a longer half-life, much higher levels of T_4 than of T_3 are in the circulation. The enzymatic conversion of T_4 to T_3 is an obligate step in the physiologic action of thyroid hormones in most extrathyroidal tissues. In the peripheral tissues, approximately 33% of the T_4 secreted undergoes 5′-deiodination to give T_3, and another 40% undergoes deiodination of the inner ring to yield the inactive material rT_3.[8] The 5′-deiodination of T_4 is a reductive process catalyzed by a group of enzymes named iodothyronine 5′deiodinases, referred to as 5′-deiodinases, and symbolized by 5′-D, which are found in a variety of cells. Approximately 80% of the T_3 is derived from circulating T_4.

Three types of 5′-deiodinases are currently known, and these are distinguished from each other primarily based on their location, substrate preference, and susceptibility to inhibitors. Type I 5′-deiodinase is found in liver and kidney and catalyzes both inner ring and outer ring deiodination (i.e., T_4 to T_3 and rT_3 to 3,3′-T_2). Type II 5′-deiodinase catalyzes mainly outer ring deiodination (i.e., T_4 to T_3 and T_3 to 3,3′-T_2) and is found in brain and the pituitary. Type III 5′-deiodinase is the principal source of rT_3 and is present in the brain, skin, and placenta.[9]

Transport of Thyroid Hormones

Transport in the Blood

Delivery of T_4 and T_3 from the thyroid gland through blood is primarily accomplished through serum carrier proteins that have varying affinities for the thyroid hormones. More than 99% of the circulating thyroid hormone is bound to plasma proteins but can be liberated rapidly for entry into cells. The thyroid hormone–binding proteins are comprised of thyroxine-binding globulin (TBG), transthyretin (TTR or thyroxine-binding prealbumin [TBPA]), human serum albumin (HSA), and lipoproteins. Their functions are most probably to ensure a constant supply of thyroid hormones to the cells and tissues by preventing urinary loss, protect the organism against abrupt changes in thyroid hormone production and degradation, protect against iodine deficiency, and target the amount of thyroid hormone delivery by ensuring a site-specific, enzymatic alteration of TBG. The binding proteins also appear to serve as an extrathyroidal storage site for thyroid hormones. This is probably necessary for constant and equal distribution among the tissues.

Thyroxine-Binding Globulin (TBG)

TBG carries the major part of both circulating T_4 and T_3 (as well as rT_3), and therefore, quantitative or qualitative abnormalities in TBG concentration have a high impact on total iodothyronine levels in serum. The protein is encoded by a single gene on the X chromosome and is produced and cleared by the liver. It has a single iodothyronine-binding site with higher affinity for T_4 compared to T_3. When TBG is fully saturated, it carries approximately

20 μg T_4/L. The TBG concentration in serum is between 11 and 21 mg/L (180-350 nM), present from the 12th week of fetal life and 1.5 times higher in newborns and children until 2-3 years of age. Estrogen has a marked effect on TBG by prolonging the biologic half-life from the normal 5 days, thus resulting in increased plasma concentrations of TBG and total thyroid hormones, whereas testosterone has the opposite effect.[10] In children and adolescents, this may have an implication in diseases with a severe sex hormone overproduction related to age, as well as oral contraceptive use and pregnancy in adolescent girls.

Transthyretin (TTR)

TTR (previously called thyroxine-binding prealbumin [TBPA]) binds only about 15%-20% of the circulating thyroid hormones and despite the 20-fold higher concentration of TTR in serum relative to that of TBG, it plays a lesser role in iodothyronine transport, thus dissociating from them more rapidly, and is responsible for much of the immediate delivery of T_4 and T_3. TTR is also the major thyroid hormone–binding protein in cerebrospinal fluid. It is synthesized in the liver and the choroid plexus and secreted into the blood and cerebrospinal fluid, respectively. Only 0.5% of the circulating TTR is occupied by T_4, and it has a rapid turnover ($t_{1/2}$ = 2 days) in plasma. Acquired abnormalities in TTR concentration associated with severe illness, nephrotic syndrome, liver disease, cystic fibrosis, hyperthyroidism, and protein-calorie malnutrition. However, changes in TTR concentrations have little effect on the serum concentrations of thyroid hormones.[10]

Human Serum Albumin (HSA)

HSA binds about 5% of the circulating T_4 and T_3. Its affinity for the hormones is even lower, and because HSA associates with a wide variety of substances, including a number of different hormones and drugs, the association between thyroid hormones and HSA can hardly be regarded as specific. Even marked fluctuations in serum HSA concentrations have no effect on thyroid hormone levels.

Lipoproteins

Lipoproteins transport a minor fraction of the circulating T_4 and to some extent T_3. The affinity for T_4-binding is similar to that of TTR. The binding site for thyroid hormones on apolipoprotein A1 is distinct from that which binds to cellular protein receptors.

Consequences of Abnormal Binding Protein Concentrations

Abnormalities of the thyroid hormone–binding proteins do not cause alterations in the metabolic state of the individual and do not result in thyroid disease. Thus, abnormal concentrations of these binding proteins, due to changed synthesis, degradation, or stability, result in maintaining normal free thyroid hormone concentrations.

Metabolism and Excretion

As discussed earlier, T_4 is considered to be a prohormone, and its peripheral metabolism occurs in two ways: outer ring deiodination by the enzyme 5′-D, which yields T_3, and inner ring deiodination by the enzyme 5-D, which yields rT_3, for which there is no known biologic function (Fig. 22.4). In humans, deiodination is the most important metabolic pathway of the hormone, not only because of its dual role in the activation and inactivation of T_4 but also in quantitative terms.

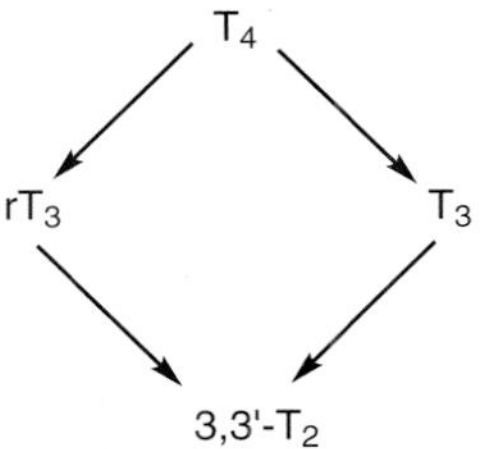

Figure 22.4 Deiodination of thyroxine (T_4).

A second pathway of thyroid hormone metabolism involves the conjugation of the phenolic hydroxyl group of the outer phenolic ring with sulfonate or glucuronic acid. These conjugation reactions occur primarily in the liver and to a lesser degree in the kidney and result in biotransformation of T_4 and T_3. The iodothyronine glucuronides are rapidly excreted in bile, but after hydrolysis in intestine by bacterial β-glucuronidases, at least part of the liberated iodothyronine is reabsorbed, constituting an enterohepatic cycle. In contrast, little iodothyronine sulfate appears as a rule in the bile or in the serum because the sulfate esters are rapidly deiodinated in the liver. Sulfonate conjugation is the primary step in irreversible deactivation of thyroid hormones. Thyroid hormones can also undergo deamination and decarboxylase reactions in the liver, resulting in the formation of so-called acetic acid analogs. These reactions occur at the alanine side chain of the inner tyrosyl ring. Although these analogs are thought to be metabolically active, little is known about the quantities produced or their contribution to hormone activity in humans. The reactions through which thyroid hormone is metabolized are summarized in Figure 22.5.

Physiologic Actions of Thyroid Hormones—Oxygen Consumption and Calorigenesis

The two most important actions of thyroid hormone are those related to oxygen consumption and those related to protein synthesis. A respiratory component of the action of thyroid hormones was first observed almost a century ago. Respiratory exchange was depressed in patients diagnosed as hypothyroid and increased in patients diagnosed as hyperthyroid.[3] The increase in respiration that follows the administration of thyroid hormone reflects an increase in metabolic rate, and thyroid function has, indeed, long been assessed by measuring the basal or resting metabolic rate (BMR), a test in which the oxygen consumed, as measured in an individual at rest, is used to calculate total-body energy production. The BMR of a hyperthyroid individual is above the normal range, or positive, and that of a hypothyroid individual is below the normal range, or negative.

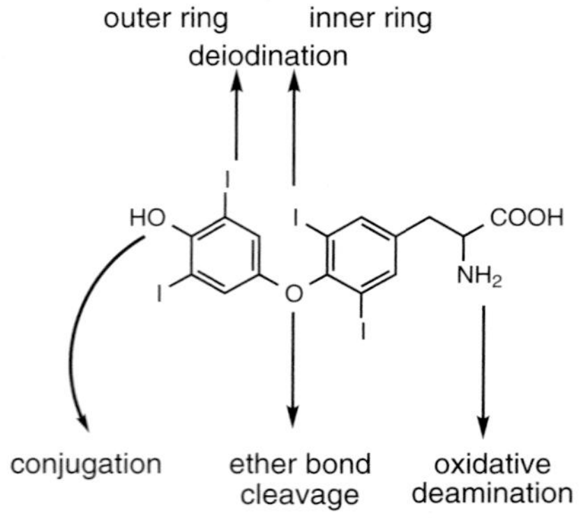

Figure 22.5 Metabolic pathways for thyroxine.

Because most of the energy produced by cellular respiration eventually appears as heat, an increase in cellular respiration necessarily leads to an increase in heat production (i.e., to a thermogenic or calorigenic effect). Thus, to the degree that thyroid hormones control BMR, they also control thermogenesis.[11]

Clinically, the inability to adjust to environmental temperature is symptomatic of departure from the euthyroid status. Patients with myxedema frequently have subnormal body temperature, have cold and dry skin, and tolerate cold poorly; the thyrotoxic patient, who compensates for excess heat production by sweating (warm, moist hands), does not easily tolerate a warm environment.

Thyroid hormones regulate the turnover of carbohydrates, lipids, and proteins. They promote glucose absorption, hepatic and renal gluconeogenesis, hepatic glycogenolysis, and glucose utilization in muscle and adipose tissue.[12] Thyroid hormones are anabolic when present at normal concentrations; they then stimulate the expression of many key enzymes of metabolism. Thyroid hormones at the levels present in hyperthyroidism are catabolic; they lead to the mobilization of tissue protein and, especially, of muscle tissue protein for gluconeogenetic processes.[13] Thus, the depletion of liver glycogen, the increased breakdown of lipids, and the negative nitrogen balance observed in hyperthyroidism represent toxic effects.

Differentiation and Protein Synthesis

In young mammals, thyroid hormone is necessary not only for general growth but also for proper differentiation of the central nervous system. A deficiency of thyroid hormone during the critical period when the developing human brain is sensitive to thyroid hormone results in an irreversible clinical entity termed cretinism, which is characterized by stunted growth and mental retardation. A great deal of attention has been devoted to the events taking place in the roughly 48-hour interval between the administration of thyroid hormone and the manifestation of certain effects caused by that administration. After Tata[14] had observed that the anabolic effects observed in rats given T_4 could be blocked by inhibitors of protein synthesis, further investigations led Tata and Widnell[15] to the conclusion that thyroid hormones were activating protein synthesis at the ribosomal level.

Control of Thyroid Hormone Biosynthesis

The primary role of thyroid is to produce thyroid hormones. The primary regulator of thyroid function and growth is the pituitary hormone TSH, a glycoprotein with a molecular weight of approximately 28,000 Da. The most important controller of TSH secretion is thyroid-releasing hormone (TRH). TRH is secreted by hypothalamic neurons into hypothalamic-hypophyseal portal blood and finds its receptors in the anterior pituitary, stimulating the secretion of TSH. TRH is three amino acids long (a tripeptide). Its basic sequence is *pyro*-glutamyl-histidine-proline amide. Secretion of TRH and, hence, TSH, is inhibited by high blood levels of thyroid hormones in a classical negative feedback loop.

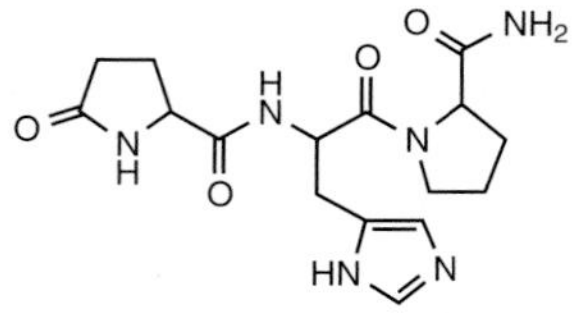

TRH

The amount of thyroid hormone circulating in body fluids and present in tissues remains fairly constant. Accounting for this constancy are the relatively long biologic half-life of the thyroid hormones, the regulation of gland activity by the pituitary-hypothalamic system, and the availability of iodide. Thyroid hormone research points toward T_3 as the more potent and active thyroid hormone than T_4; therefore, factors affecting peripheral T_3 formation by the 5′-D enzymes are highly relevant.

T_4 makes up the majority of thyroid hormone made by the thyroid gland; it is weaker and is considered to be a "reserve" form of hormone. T_4 is greater than 99.9% bound to plasma proteins and has a biologic half-life of 1 week, as compared to 1 day for the less firmly bound T_3. T_4 is converted into T_3, which is considered to be more potent or active, in peripheral tissues such as the liver, kidney, and intestines.

The biosynthesis and secretion of TSH is regulated by TRH and, thus, the quantity of thyroid hormone in circulation through feedback control. The ability of thyroid hormones to prevent the release of TSH is referred to as feedback regulation. The amount of iodide available to the gland for hormone synthesis is also an important regulator of thyroid function. The efficiency of the thyroid pump mechanism and the rate of Tg and TPO synthesis are all TSH dependent. In cases of iodide deficiency, the production of thyroid hormone is lowered, and TSH rises through the pituitary feedback mechanism previously described. The effect of the increased TSH is to produce more thyroid hormone by increasing efficiency of the iodide pump and increasing Tg and TPO synthesis. Thus, in iodide deficiency, there is an increased uptake of iodide[16] and larger MIT-to-DIT ratios, which lead to larger T_3-to-T_4 ratios. T_3 is the more rapidly acting hormone, mitigating the effect of iodide deficiency. When iodide deficiency is severe, a persistent rise in TSH is observed. This then results in thyroid gland growth.

In the presence of an excess of circulating iodide, the absolute amount of iodide taken up by the thyroid gland remains approximately constant, which is compensated by a decrease in the fraction of the total iodide taken up and an increase in the amount of iodide leaked from the thyroid gland. In addition, there may be a decrease in the formation of iodinated Tg residues and in the release of hormones from the gland. The decrease in the formation of iodinated Tg residues that occurs at excessive physiologic doses of iodide has been called the Wolff-Chaikoff block.[17] This block may be caused by an interaction of iodide with NADPH,[18] which depletes follicular NADPH and, in turn, depletes the hydrogen peroxide necessary for TPO activity. The decrease in hormone release occurs when iodide is given in pharmacologic (milligram) quantities; it may last for a few weeks.

The activity of deiodinases reflects thyroid status, general health, and food intake. In hypothyroidism, there is a decrease in hepatic 5′-D-I but an increase in 5′-D-II activity.[19] There is a decrease in T_3 and an increase in rT_3 after hepatic disease,[20] renal damage,[21] chronic illness,[22] and starvation,[23] indicating a decrease in the activity of the quantitatively more important 5′-D-I. An increase in deiodinase activity has been observed after overfeeding subjects or after administering a high-carbohydrate or high-fat diet[24] to experimental animals. The mechanism of deiodinase control is presumably intricate, but the inhibiting effects of propranolol on 5′-D-I[25] and of prazosin on the 5′-D-II of brown adipose tissue[26] infer the involvement of adrenergic components in the regulation. In addition, the rapid change in activity observed after asphyxia points toward a rapid, possibly cyclic adenosine monophosphate (cAMP)–related control.[27] A number of other factors have been shown to influence thyroid hormone secretion. In young children, exposure to a cold environment triggers TRH secretion, leading to enhanced thyroid hormone release. This makes sense considering the known ability of thyroid hormones to spark body heat production.

Diseases Involving the Thyroid Gland

Thyroid disease is associated with both inadequate production and overproduction of thyroid hormones from a variety of causes, and treatment typically involves the reversal of each respective state or targeting the causes. Both types of disease are relatively common afflictions of man and animals. Diet may influence the disease, and dietary supplementation may assist in the management of certain diseases involving the thyroid gland.[28,29]

Hypothyroidism

Hypothyroidism is the result of any condition that causes thyroid hormone deficiency. Two well-known examples include the following:

- Iodine deficiency: Iodide is required for production of thyroid hormones and without adequate iodine intake, thyroid hormones cannot be synthesized. Historically, this problem was seen particularly in areas with iodine-deficient soils, and frank iodine deficiency has been virtually eliminated by iodine supplementation of salt. In the case of iodide deficiency, the thyroid becomes inordinately large and is called a "goiter."
- Primary thyroid disease: Inflammatory diseases of the thyroid that destroy parts of the gland are clearly an important cause of hypothyroidism.
- Postpartum thyroid disease: There are a variety of thyroid conditions that may arise in the postpartum timeframe, and they may or may not be autoimmune in nature.[30] Postpartum thyroiditis may begin with a period of hyperthyroidism or thyrotoxicosis but is followed by hypothyroidism.

Hashimoto Disease

Hashimoto disease is an autoimmune disease in which the thyroid gland is gradually destroyed by a variety of cell- and antibody-mediated immune processes. Antibodies against thyroid peroxidase and/or Tg cause gradual destruction of follicles in the thyroid gland. Symptoms of Hashimoto thyroiditis include weight gain, depression, mania, sensitivity to heat and cold, paresthesia, fatigue, panic attacks, bradycardia, tachycardia, high cholesterol, reactive hypoglycemia, constipation, migraines, muscle weakness, cramps, memory loss, infertility, and hair loss. Hypothyroidism caused by Hashimoto thyroiditis is treated with thyroid hormone replacement agents such as levothyroxine or desiccated thyroid extract.

Goiter

An enlarged, palpable thyroid gland is referred to as a goiter. When insufficient thyroid hormone is liberated from the thyroid gland, the breakdown of the thyroid-pituitary-hypothalamic feedback mechanism results in the release of excess TSH and in the formation of a thyroid hypertrophy referred to as a nontoxic goiter. By contrast, if more thyroid hormone is produced and results in less TSH, this is known as toxic multinodular goiter (MNG). The gland enlarges as it tries to take up more iodine, leading to goiter. Endemic goiters are those that occur in a significant segment of a given population and are related to low dietary iodine.[31] Goiters are most frequently caused by inadequate intake of dietary iodide in regions not reached by iodide-providing sea mists and, occasionally, by the prolonged intake of goitrogens derived from plant sources or aquifers. This condition can be prevented with iodine supplements, and many industrialized countries now iodize salt. Goiters may or may not be associated with nodules (toxic or nontoxic).

A characteristic sign of hypothyroidism is a decrease in metabolic rate, with a reduction in calorigenic effect and defective thermoregulation. The elevated serum cholesterol level seen in hypothyroidism is the result of a decrease in cholesterol degradation that exceeds the decrease in cholesterol biosynthesis; it reflects a general slowdown in catabolic processes. Shared symptoms of hypothyroidism and cognitive disorders include fatigue, mental dullness, lethargy, and inattention. Treatment of hypothyroidism includes supplementation of T_4 with the goal of returning TSH levels to normal.

Nodules

Nodular thyroid disease is common, and prevalence is dependent on the method of detection and is identified through ultrasound, fine needle aspiration biopsy, and palpation on physical exam. Nuclear exams are reserved to identify rare nodules that cause hyperthyroidism. Molecular diagnostics and genetic testing is a growing area that is becoming helpful in the evaluation of nodules, especially when determining whether or not there is presence of cancer. Nodules may be solitary or multiple. A risk-based diagnostic and treatment approach includes a waiting period while monitoring TSH, thyroid hormone, surgery, or ablation depending on the level of concern or if nodules are present along with cancer.[32]

Cretinism

The most severe and devastating form of hypothyroidism is seen in young children with congenital thyroid deficiency. If that condition is not corrected by supplemental therapy soon after birth, the child will suffer from cretinism, a form of irreversible growth and mental retardation.

Myxedema

Common symptoms of hypothyroidism arising after early childhood include lethargy, fatigue, cold intolerance, weakness, hair loss, and reproductive failure. If these signs are severe, the clinical condition is called "myxedema."

Hyperthyroidism and Graves' Disease

The increased metabolic rate of hyperthyroidism results in symptoms opposite to those seen in hypothyroidism. Common signs of hyperthyroidism include nervousness, insomnia, high heart rate, eye disease, and anxiety. In most species, this condition is less common than hypothyroidism. In humans, the most common form of hyperthyroidism is Graves' disease, an autoimmune disease in which antibodies, formed by the immune system, bind to and activate the TSH receptor, leading to hypersecretion of thyroid hormones. Graves' disease is commonly treated with antithyroid drugs (e.g., PTU, MMI), which suppress synthesis of thyroid hormones (T_3 and T_4) from the thyroid gland primarily by interfering with iodination of Tg by thyroid peroxidase.

Generalized Resistance to Thyroid Hormone

Generalized resistance to thyroid hormone (GRTH) is a rare form of thyroid disorder and may be a heritable disorder characterized by reduced responsiveness of the pituitary and peripheral tissues to the action of thyroid hormones. Behavioral manifestations include hyperactivity, behavioral problems, and cognitive deficits.

Many have evaluated the association of GRTH to attention-deficit hyperactivity disorder and suggested that similar mechanistic pathways are shared between the two conditions.[33,34] In GRTH, T_4 fails to block TSH production, leading to excess levels of T_3 and T_4 with either normal or elevated levels of TSH. In conditions of an improperly functioning thyroid, thyroid hormones and TSH ratios are unregulated, producing symptoms that are characteristic of attention-deficit hyperactivity disorder.

Thyroid Cancer

Thyroid cancer is a disease in which malignant cells are found in the tissues of the thyroid gland. This disease is more common in women than in men. Four main types of cancer of the thyroid are differentiated based on how the cancer cells look under a microscope: papillary (75%-85% of cases),[35] follicular (10%-20% of cases), medullary (5%-8% of cases), and anaplastic (<5% of cases). Follicular and papillary carcinomas have the highest incidence in young women but have low mortality; they represent a different disease than anaplastic types or undifferentiated carcinomas, both of which occur among the older patients and have high death rates. Treatment of thyroid cancer is straightforward and effective.

THERAPEUTIC AGENTS

Thyroid Replacement Therapy

Thyroid hormone drugs are natural or synthetic preparations containing the sodium salt of T_4 known as levothyroxine (Synthroid, Levothroid, Levoxyl) or the sodium salt of T_3 known as liothyronine (Cytomel), or the natural combination of T_4 and T_3 (Armour Thyroid). Natural hormonal preparations include desiccated thyroid and Tg. Desiccated thyroid is derived from domesticated animals that are used for food by man (either beef or hog thyroid), and Tg is derived from thyroid glands of the hog. The U.S. Pharmacopeia (USP) has standardized the total iodine content of natural preparations. Thyroid USP contains no less than 0.17% and no more than 0.23% iodine, and Tg contains no less than 0.7% of organically bound iodine. Iodine content is only an indirect indicator of true hormonal biologic activity. Hormone replacement is the established therapy in the treatment of various forms of hypothyroidism, from the complete absence of thyroid function seen in myxedema to simple goiter and cretinism. A large number of organic and some inorganic compounds stimulate or prevent thyroid hormone formation by interfering with iodide uptake into follicular cells, inhibiting TPO, preventing thyroid hormone binding to plasma proteins, or acting as effectors of thyroid deiodinases. Some of the agents described in this section are of therapeutic or diagnostic value, some illustrate potential side effects of drugs, and some are experimental compounds designed to achieve unmet therapeutic goals or to define structural parameters necessary for thyroid hormone actions.

Dietary supplementation or the control of foods with goitregenic properties may also help in the management of certain conditions. Of note, there is a growing level of evidence supporting the maintenance of a physiological concentration of selenium[28] in a variety of hypothyroid conditions.

Thyroid hormone preparations belong to two categories: natural hormone preparations derived from animal thyroid and synthetic preparations.

Natural Thyroid Hormone Preparations (Armour Thyroid, Nature-Throid, Westhroid)

Natural preparations include desiccated thyroid and Tg. Desiccated thyroid and Tg are derived from thyroid glands of domesticated animals that are used for food by human. T_4, T_3, DIT, and MIT are released from the proteolytic activity of gastrointestinal enzymes. Potency is based on total iodine content or bioassay and is somewhat variable with different preparations.

Desiccated thyroid preparations (Thyroid USP) are essentially acetone powders of bovine or porcine thyroid glands compressed into oral tablets. A diluent is usually present because the preparations (especially those of porcine origin) commonly exceed the 0.17%-0.23% iodine content required by the USP. Because the iodine of desiccated thyroid is in the form of iodinated tyrosyl and thyronyl residues of the precipitated Tg, the preparation owes its efficacy to the hormones that eventually are liberated by intestinal proteases. In desiccated preparations, T_3 and T_4 may be present in a ratio of approximately the same as found in humans. Desiccated preparations are less expensive than synthetic hormones but have been shown to produce variable T_4/T_3 blood levels because of inconsistencies both between and within animal sources of the thyroid gland. Most comments regarding desiccated thyroid also apply to partially purified Tg because the two preparations differ in their total and relative amounts of T_4 and T_3.

Table 22.1 Some Properties and Pharmacokinetics for Levothyroxine and Liothyronine[a]

Parameters	L-Thyroxine	Liothyronine
Trade name	Synthroid, Levothroid, Levoxyl	Cytomel
pK_a(phenolic)	6.7	8.4
Oral bioavailability (%)	50-80[b]	95
Peak response	Several weeks (hypothyroid)	2-3 d (hypothyroid)
Duration of action	Several weeks (hypothyroid)	Several days (hypothyroid)
Protein binding (%)	99% (weakly)	Weakly bound
Time to peak concentration (hours)	2-4	1-2
Volume of distribution (L/kg)	8.7-9.7	41-45
Elimination half-life (days)	6-7 euthyroid 9-10 hypothyroid 3-4 hyperthyroid	1 euthyroid 1-2 hypothyroid 1 hyperthyroid
Excretion (%)	50 urine 50 feces	Urine

[a]Micromedex Healthcare Series; 2018. Available at https://www.micromedexsolutions.com/home/dispatch.
[b]Food decreases bioavailability.

Synthetic Thyroid Hormones

Synthetic, crystalline thyroid hormones are more uniformly absorbed than biologic preparations and contain more precisely measured amounts of active ingredient in their dosage forms. T_4, T_3, dT_4 (dextrothyroxine), and T_4–T_3 mixtures (Liotrix) are commonly used. Table 22.1 describes the pharmacokinetic properties for T_4 and T_3.

Levothyroxine Sodium (Synthroid, Levoxyl, Levothroid)

Because of its tight binding to plasma carrier proteins, synthetic crystalline levothyroxine (T_4) sodium salt has a slower onset of action than crystalline T_3 or a desiccated thyroid preparation. Its administration leads to a greater increase in serum T_4 but a lesser increase in serum T_3 compared with thyroid USP.[36] The availability of 11 different tablet strengths, ranging from 25 to 300 µg, allows individual dosing. T_4 treats hypothyroidism. It is also used to treat or prevent goiter, which can be caused by hormonal imbalances, radiation treatment, surgery, or cancer.

Liothyronine Sodium (Cytomel)

Liothyronine (T_3) sodium is a synthetic form of T_3. T_3 sodium is the therapy of choice when it is desirable to have a rapid onset or cessation of activity, such as in patients with heart disease.

Liotrix (Thyrolar)

The medication containing a mixture of the sodium salts of T_4 and T_3 in a 4:1 ratio by weight is called liotrix. Liotrix is used as replacement or supplemental therapy in patients with hypothyroidism. It works by supplying the thyroid hormones in the ratio they are normally produced by the body.

Vandetanib (Caprelsa)

Vandetanib has been approved for the treatment of unresectable locally advanced or metastatic medullary thyroid cancer (MTC). While papillary and follicular thyroid carcinomas represent the majority of thyroid cancers and are well treated with a low death rate, the same cannot be said for unresectable locally advanced or metastatic medullary thyroid cancer. MTC arising from C (parafollicular) cells has a mean survival time of 8.6 years and unresectable MTC is not effectively treated with common chemotherapeutic agents. Vandetanib is a newly developed drug which targets vascular endothelial growth factor receptor (VEGFR) and its proto-oncogene thus inhibiting angiogenesis and tumor growth.[37]

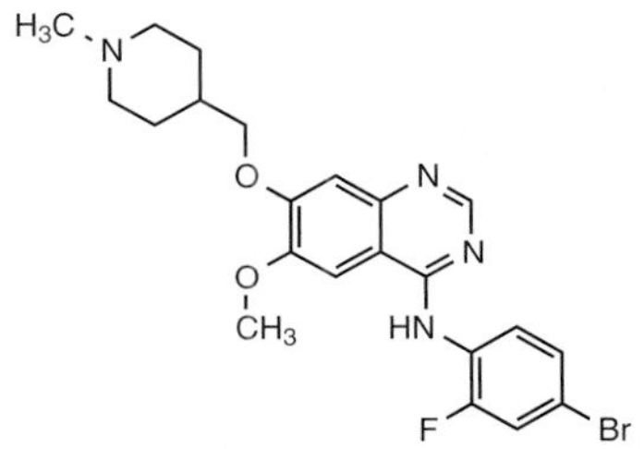

Vandetanib (Caprelsa)

Thyroid Imaging Agents

Radioiodine

All isotopes of iodine are rapidly taken up in thyroid follicles. So far, only the isotopes ^{131}I and ^{125}I have been used consistently. Isotope ^{131}I, which decays to ^{131}Xe mainly with the emission of a 0.6-meV β-particle and approximately 0.3-meV γ-rays, has a half-life of 8 days. Isotope ^{125}I, with a half-life of 60 days, decays to ^{125}Te by electron capture. The major component of its decay is 27-keV x-rays, and the minor component is a 35.5-keV γ-ray.

The γ-radiation emitted by ^{131}I can be detected by a suitably placed scintillation crystal. This is the basis for the diagnostic use of this isotope in iodine uptake and in thyroid-scanning procedures.

The absorption of ^{131}I β-radiation, which leads to the highly localized destruction of the thyroid follicles in which the isotope is taken up, has promoted radioiodine as a therapeutic alternative to surgical removal of the gland. Advantages of radioiodine therapy over surgery include the simplicity of the procedure, its applicability to patients who are poor surgical risks, and the avoidance of surgical complications, such as hypoparathyroidism. The development of late hypothyroidism[38] and the fear of chromosomal damage are arguments against the use of radioiodine in patients under 20 years of age and during pregnancy.

Radioiodine whole-body scan and serum Tg measurement are commonly used as the follow-up testing in patients with thyroid cancer. Both follow-up tests have limitations and are uncomfortable because they require a hypothyroid state. For thyroid cells to take up the labeled iodine, thyrotropin must be available, and for the pituitary to supply it, the body must be free of T_3 and T_4. This means that patients must completely stop taking medication for several weeks before the scan day. This results in a severe hypothyroidism, and approximately 25% of patients also produce antibodies against Tg, rendering the immunoassay useless. To make the follow-up tests easier, Thyrogen (thyrotropin alfa for injection), a recombinant human thyrotropin (rhTSH) produced in Chinese hamster ovary cells that stimulates the thyroid gland–like endogenous TSH to produce thyroid hormone is used. The effect of thyroid-stimulating hormone activation of thyroid cells is to increase uptake of radioiodine to allow scan detection or radioiodine killing of thyroid cells. TSH activation also leads to the release of thyroglobulin by thyroid cells. Thyroglobulin functions as a tumor marker that is detected in blood specimens. Thyrogen has been shown to significantly enhance the sensitivity of Tg testing in patients maintained on thyroid hormone therapy. It allows patients with thyroid cancer to avoid the debilitating effects of hypothyroidism when undergoing radioiodine imaging scans during diagnostic testing or as adjunctive treatment for radioiodine ablation.

Perchlorate and Pertechnetate

Perchlorates are the salts derived from perchloric acid ($HClO_4$). They occur both naturally and through manufacturing. They have been used as a medicine for more than 50 years to treat thyroid gland disorders. Perchlorate, which competitively inhibits the uptake of iodide, has been used in both diagnosis and treatment of thyroid disease. In continental Europe, perchlorate has been used for surgical preparation and in the long-term treatment of thyrotoxicosis. In the United States, the use of perchlorate was drastically curtailed after aplastic anemia and severe renal damage were reported following its use. The U.S. Environmental Protection Agency has issued substantial guidance and analysis concerning the impacts of perchlorate on the environment as well as drinking water.[39]

Radioactive pertechnetate $^{99m}TcO_4^-$ anion is an important radiopharmaceutical for the study and imaging of the thyroid gland, including its morphology, vascularity, and function. $^{99m}TcO_4^-$ is conveniently prepared from molybdenum-99, which decays with 87% probability to ^{99m}Tc. The advantages to $^{99m}TcO_4^-$ include its short half-life of 6 hours and the low radiation exposure to the patient. TcO_4- and iodide have a comparable charge/radius ratio and therefore are similarly incorporated into the thyroid gland. Pertechnetate anion ion is not incorporated into the Tg. Sodium pertechnetate cannot pass through the blood-brain barrier. $^{99m}TcO_4^-$ is renally eliminated for the first 3 days after being injected. After a scanning is performed, the patient is recommended to drink large amounts of water in order to expedite elimination of the radionuclide. In contrast to iodide and thiocyanate TcO_4 and perchlorate do not undergo intrathyroidal metabolism after they are trapped.

Antithyroid Drugs for the Treatment of Hyperthyroidism

Iodide

Inhibition of the release of thyroid hormone by iodide is the basis for its use in hyperthyroidism. Iodide decreases the vascularity of the enlarged thyroid gland and also lowers the elevated BMR. It has also been suggested that excess iodide might change the conformation of Tg, making the protein less susceptible to thyroidal proteolysis.[40]

With the use of antithyroid drugs, the role of iodide in hyperthyroidism has been relegated to that of preparation for thyroid surgery. Iodide, as Lugol's solution (Strong Iodine Solution USP) or as saturated potassium iodide solution, is administered for approximately 2 weeks to ensure decreased vascularity and firming of the gland. Iodism, a side effect of iodine administration, is apparently an allergic reaction characterized by dermatologic and common cold–like symptoms.[41]

Methimazole, Propylthiouricil,and Carbimazole

Thionamides are the major drugs for treatment of thyrotoxicosis and hyperthyroidism. These agents are potent inhibitors of TPO, which is responsible for the iodination of tyrosine residues of Tg and the coupling of iodotyrosine residues to form iodothyronines. These drugs have no effect on the iodide pump or on thyroid hormone release. The most clinically useful thionamides are thioureylenes, which are five- or six-membered heterocyclic derivatives of thiourea and include propylthiouracil (PTU) and thioimidazole 1-methyl-2-mercaptoimidazole (MMI, Tapazole). The uptake of these drugs into the thyroid gland is stimulated by TSH and inhibited by iodide.

PTU is widely used to treat patients with hyperthyroidism. In rare cases, this drug has been found to have severe toxic effects on the liver. The data on hepatotoxicity confirm the findings for agranulocytosis that low-dose MMI is safer than PTU and that MMI toxicity is more common in people older than 40 years. In contrast, PTU hepatotoxicity often occurs in younger patients. Most cases of hepatic injury occur in the first few months of drug therapy, as with agranulocytosis. The reason that MMI typically causes cholestatic hepatitis whereas PTU causes cytotoxic hepatitis remains unknown. In pregnancy, PTU is recommended in the first trimester due to less birth defects than methimazole, some physicians recommend switching to methimazole thereafter, including through nursing.[42,43]

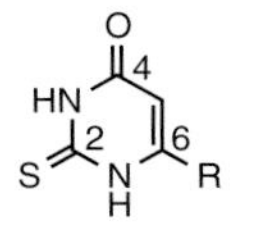

Thiouracil; R = H
Methylthiouracil; R = CH_3
Propylthiouracil (PTU); R = n-C_3H_7

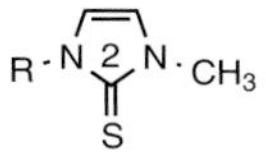

Methimazole(MMI, R = H)
Carbimazole (R = C_2H_5OCO)

The grouping R-CS-N- has been referred to as thioamide, thionamide, thiocarbamide, or if R is N, as it is in thiouracil, PTU, and MMI, it is called a thioureylene. This structure may exist in either the thioketo or thioenol tautomeric forms. The study of 6-alkylthiouracil showed maximal antithyroid activity with PTU. 6-Methylthiouracil has less than one-tenth the activity of PTU.

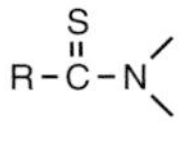

Thioamide

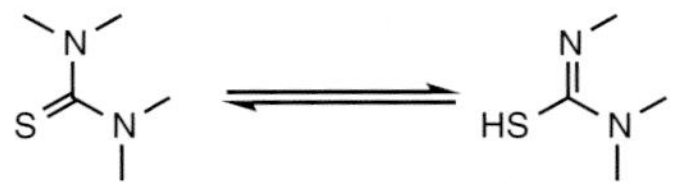

Thioketo   Thioenol (SH form)

Thioureylene tantomers

The ability of PTU to inhibit the enzyme 5′-D-I (i.e., the peripheral deiodination of T_4 to T_3, in addition to its intrathyroidal inhibition of thyroid hormone formation) has made PTU the drug of choice in the emergency treatment of thyroid storm.[44] Single doses of PTU in excess of 300 mg are capable of almost total blockage of peripheral T_3 production.[45]

A number of studies have defined the structure-activity relationships (SARs) of the thiouracils and other related compounds as inhibitors of outer ring deiodinase.[46] The C-2 thioketo/thioenol group and an unsubstituted N-1 position are essential for activity. The enolic hydroxyl group at C-4 in PTU and the presence of alkyl group at C-5 and C-6 enhance the inhibitory potency.

MMI has more TPO inhibitory activity and is longer acting than PTU but, in contrast to PTU, is not able to inhibit the peripheral deiodination of T_4, presumably because of the presence of the methyl group at N-1 position. The suggested maintenance dosages are 50-800 mg daily for PTU and 5-30 mg daily for MMI.

PHARMACOKINETICS. PTU is rapidly absorbed from the gastrointestinal tract, reaching peak serum levels after 1 hour. The bioavailability of 50%-80% may be due to incomplete absorption or a large first-pass effect in the liver. The volume of distribution approximates total-body water with accumulation in the thyroid gland. Most of an ingested dose of PTU is excreted by the kidney as the inactive glucuronide within 24 hours. In contrast, MMI is completely absorbed but at variable rates. It is readily accumulated by the thyroid gland and has a volume of distribution similar to that of PTU. Excretion is slower than with PTU; 65%-70% of a dose is recovered in the urine in 48 hours. The short plasma half-life of these agents (1.5 hr for PTU and 6 hr for MMI) has little influence on the duration of the antithyroid action or the dosing interval because both agents are accumulated by the thyroid gland. For PTU, giving the drug every 6-8 hours is reasonable since a single 100-mg dose can inhibit iodine organification by 60% for 7 hours. Since a single 30-mg dose of MMI exerts an antithyroid effect for longer than 24 hours, a single daily dose is effective in the management of mild to moderate hyperthyroidism. The two drugs differ in their binding to serum proteins. MMI is essentially free in serum, whereas 80%-90% of PTU is bound to albumin.

Efforts to improve the taste and decrease the rate of release of MMI led to the development of 1-carbethoxy-3-methylthioimidazole (carbimazole). Carbimazole, the prodrug derivative of MMI, gives rise to MMI in vivo and is used in the same dosage.

The side effects of thioamides include diarrhea, vomiting, jaundice, skin rashes, and, at times, sudden onset of agranulocytosis. There does not appear to be a great difference in toxicity among the compounds currently in use.

Antithyroid drugs are associated with a variety of minor side effects, as well as potentially life-threatening or even lethal complications. Side effects of MMI are dose related, whereas those of PTU are less clearly related to dose. This may favor use of low-dose MMI rather than PTU in the average patient with hyperthyroidism. Adverse reactions to the thioamides occur in 3%-12% of treated patients. Most reactions occur early, especially nausea and gastrointestinal distress. An altered sense of taste or smell may occur with MMI. The most common adverse effect is a maculopapular pruritic rash (4%-6%), at times accompanied by systemic signs such as fever.

Both PTU and MMI are concentrated several-fold by the thyroid gland and inhibit the iodination and coupling reactions of TPO. Taurog[47] described the thioureylenes as potent inhibitors of Tg iodination. He suggested that a thioureylene, such as PTU (PTU-SH), would irreversibly inhibit TPO-catalyzed iodination of Tg when the thioureylene-to-iodide ratio was high and reversibly when the PTU-SH-to-iodide ratio was low. In the course of the iodination reaction, the thioureylene PTU-SH would be oxidized,[48] possibly to a disulfide dimer, such as PTU-SS-PTU.

Iodination of tyrosyl residues resumes once oxidation of the drug to disulfide products occurs by either hypoiodate (OI^-) or an enzyme-hypoiodate complex (EOI^-). Under these conditions, the thioureylenes act as competitive inhibitors by competing with tyrosyls for hypoiodate. Conversely, at high drug concentrations, the thioureylenes are only partially oxidized, and the partially oxidized intermediate can presumably inactivate TPO by covalent binding of an oxidized form of the drug to the prosthetic heme group of TPO to prevent formation of the hydrogen peroxide-TPO complex. As a result, iodination is irreversibly blocked. Data obtained from rats fed an iodide-deficient diet are consistent with this in vitro model in that intrathyroidal metabolism of radiolabeled PTU and MMI is decreased.

Thioureylene drugs also effectively inhibit the coupling of the DIT/MIT residues on Tg to yield T_4 and T_3. This effect has been related to an alteration of the conformation of Tg brought on by the binding of the thioureylene to Tg (i.e., by the formation of a compound such as TPO-S-S-PTU).[49]

After the observation that PTU inhibited the peripheral deiodination of T_4,[44,50] attempts to relate deiodinase inhibitory activity to structural parameters were undertaken.[50] These studies emphasized the need for tautomerization to a thiol form and for the presence of a polar hydrogen on the nitrogen adjacent to the sulfur-bearing carbon. A study of the relation of chemical structure to 5′-D-I inhibitory activity related to similar studies of structural requirements for TPO inhibition could prove fruitful in the design of improved antithyroid drugs.

TOXICITY. Agranulocytosis is the most feared side effect of antithyroid drug therapy. Agranulocytosis (an absolute granulocyte count of $<500/mm^3$) occurred in 0.37% of patients receiving PTU and in 0.35% receiving MMI. Agranulocytosis must be distinguished from the transient, mild granulocytopenia (a granulocyte count of $<1,500/mm^3$) that occasionally occurs in patients with Graves' disease, in some patients of African descent, and occasionally in patients treated with antithyroid drugs. A baseline differential white blood cell count should be obtained before initiation of therapy.

Most cases of agranulocytosis occur within the first 90 days of treatment, but this complication can occur even a year or more after starting therapy. It is important to note that agranulocytosis can develop after a prior uneventful course of drug therapy, a finding that is important since renewed exposure to the drug frequently occurs when patients have a relapse and undergo a second course of antithyroid therapy. Agranulocytosis is thought to be autoimmune mediated, and antigranulocyte antibodies are shown by immunofluorescence and cytotoxicity assays. Agranulocytosis induced by PTU is evidence of a drug-dependent antibody reacting with granulocytes, monocytes, and hematopoietic progenitor cells. All patients should be instructed to discontinue the antithyroid drug and contact a physician immediately if fever or sore throat develops. Hepatotoxicity is another major side effect of antithyroid drugs. Estimates regarding the frequency of this condition are imprecise, but it probably ranges from 0.1% to 0.2%. The recognition of PTU-related hepatotoxicity may be difficult, since in up to 30% of patients with normal baseline aminotransferase levels who are treated with PTU, transient acute increases in those levels develop, ranging from 1.1 to 6 times the upper limit of normal levels, that resolve while therapy is continued. In addition, asymptomatic elevations in serum aminotransferase levels occur frequently in untreated patients with hyperthyroidism and are not predictive of further increases after the institution of PTU therapy.

Propylthiouracil-Induced Hepatotoxicity

Vasculitis is the third major toxic reaction seen with antithyroid drug treatment, more commonly found in connection with PTU than with MMI. Serologic evidence consistent with lupus erythematosus develops in some patients, fulfilling the criteria for drug-induced lupus. Antineutrophil cytoplasmic antibody–positive vasculitis has also been reported, especially in Asian patients treated with PTU. Most patients have perinuclear antineutrophil cytoplasmic antibodies, with a majority of them having antimyeloperoxidase antineutrophil cytoplasmic antibodies. It has been hypothesized that antithyroid drugs, especially PTU, can react with myeloperoxidase to form reactive intermediates that promote autoimmune inflammation. As a result of several cases of liver injury associated with propylthiouracil, the FDA issued a *Boxed Warning* in the package insert due to the severity of the cases, some of which were fatal. This was to ensure that health care professionals are aware of this risk and are vigilant for the signs and symptoms of hepatic toxicity. Of note, propylthyiouracil is associated with more serious liver injury than methimazole in both adults and pediatric patients.

Thyrotoxicosis

Hyperthyroidism is the term for overactive tissue within the thyroid gland causing an overproduction of thyroid hormones. Hyperthyroidism is thus a cause of thyrotoxicosis,[51] the clinical condition of increased thyroid hormones in the blood. It is important to note that hyperthyroidism and thyrotoxicosis are not synonymous. For instance, thyrotoxicosis could instead be caused by ingestion of exogenous thyroid hormone or inflammation of the thyroid gland, causing it to release its stores of thyroid hormones. Regardless, there are a variety of causes of thyrotoxicosis,[51] and symptoms of thyrotoxicosis include heat intolerance, palpitations, anxiety, fatigue, weight loss, and irregular menses in women and tremor. Because symptoms of thyrotoxicosis resemble those of adrenergic overstimulation, attempts to decrease such symptoms by adrenergic blockade have been undertaken. Reserpine and guanethidine, both of which are depleters of catecholamines, and propranolol, a β-blocking agent, have been used effectively to decrease the tachycardia, tremor, and anxiety of thyrotoxicosis. Because of its less serious side effects, propranolol has become the drug of choice in this adjunctive therapy. Reports of decreased T_3 plasma levels during propranolol treatment suggest that blocking of the peripheral deiodination of T_4 may contribute to the beneficial effects of propranolol. The use of propranolol as a preventive drug in acute thyrotoxicosis has been found to be beneficial by some investigators, but not by others. Hyperthyroidism has become a common and well-recognized disorder of middle-aged to older cats, and treatment with these antithyroid drugs has been equally effective in the long-term control of the feline hyperthyroidism.

Goitrogens and Drugs Affecting Thyroid Function

The presence of environmental goitrogens was suggested by the resistance of endemic goiters to iodine prophylaxis and iodide treatment in Italy and Colombia. In the past, endemic outbreaks of hypothyroidism have pointed toward calcium as a source of waterborne goitrogenicity, and it is presently believed that calcium is a weak goitrogen able to cause latent hypothyroidism to come to the surface.

Lithium salts have been used as safe adjuncts in the initial treatment of thyrotoxicosis.[52] Lithium is concentrated by the thyroid gland,[53] with a thyroid-to-serum ratio of more than 2:1, suggesting active transport. Lithium ion inhibits adenylyl cyclase, which forms cAMP. Formed in response to TSH, cAMP is a stimulator of the processes involved in thyroid hormone release from the gland. Inhibition of hormone secretion by lithium has proved to be a useful adjunct in treatment of hyperthyroidism.[54]

In view of the role of cysteine residues in the conformation of Tg, the mode of action of TPO, and the deiodination of T_4, the effect of sulfur-containing compounds on thyroid hormone formation is hardly surprising. Most naturally occurring sulfur compounds are derived from glucosinolates (formerly referred to as thioglucosides),[55] which are present in foods such as cabbage, turnip, mustard seed, salad greens, and radishes (most of these are from the genus *Brassica* or *Cruciferae*) as well as in the milk of cows grazing in areas containing *Brassica* weeds. Chemically, glucosinolates can give rise to many components, primarily to isothiocyanate (SCN^-) and lesser extent to thiocyanate (CNS-), isothiocyanate (SCN^-), nitriles (RCN), and thiooxazolidones. Thiocyanate is a large anion that competes with iodide for uptake by the thyroid gland; its goitrogenic effect can be reversed by iodide intake. Goitrin (5-*R*-vinyloxazolidine-2-thione) is a potent thyroid peroxidase inhibitor,[56] that reduces the production of thyroid hormones and is held to be the cause of a mild goiter endemic to Finland. In rats, goitrin is actively taken up by the thyroid gland and appears to inhibit the coupling of Tg diiodotyrosyl residues.[57] Many researchers, however, believe that the goitrogenic effects of *Brassica* result from the additive effects of all goitrogenic components present.

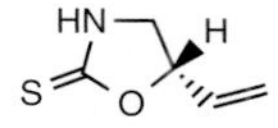

Goitrin

Other compounds affecting thyroid function include sulfonamides, anticoagulants, and oxygenated and iodinated aromatic compounds. The hypoglycemic agent carbutamide and the diuretic acetazolamide (Diamox) are examples of sulfonamides. Of the anticoagulants, heparin appears to interfere with the binding of T_4 to plasma transport proteins,[58] but warfarin (Coumadin) and dicoumarol are competitive inhibitors of the substrate T_4 or rT_3 in the 5′-D reaction, with a dissociation constant in the micromolar range.[59] Other oxygenated compounds affecting the 5′-D include resorcinol, long known to be a goitrogen, and phloretin, a dihydrochalocone with a half maximal inhibitory concentration of 4 mol/L.

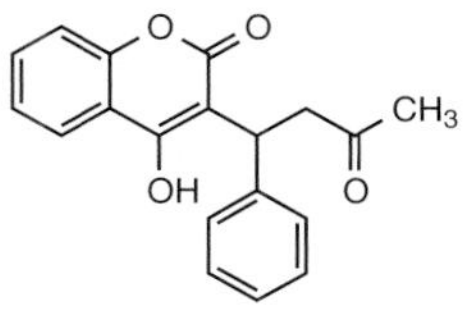

Warfarin

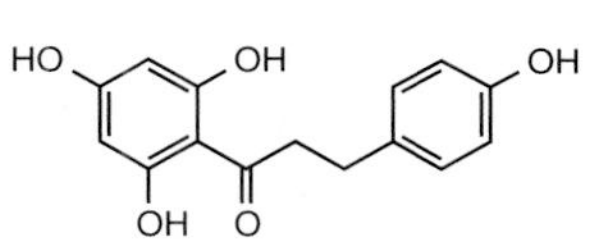

Phloretin

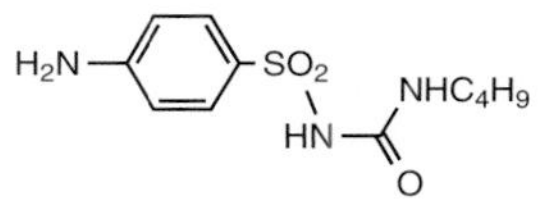

Carbutamide

The ability of oxidation products of 3,4-dihydroxycinnamic acid to prevent the binding of TSH to human thyroid membranes[60] suggests that other oxygenated phenols may interfere with thyroid hormone function in more than one way. Examples of iodinated drugs affecting thyroid function are the antiarrhythmic agent amiodarone and the radiocontrasting agent iopanoic acid. All of these compounds interfere with the peripheral deiodination of T_4 and are being tested as adjuncts in the treatment of hyperthyroidism.

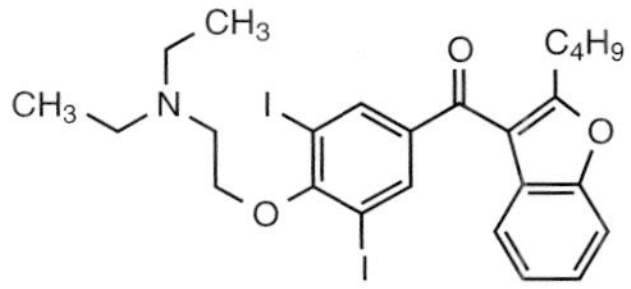

Amiodarone

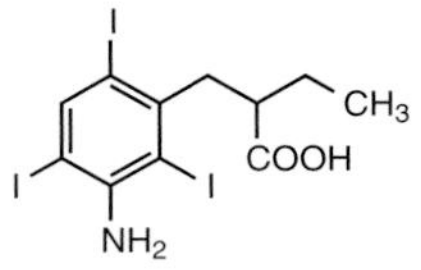

Iopanoic acid

The binding of thyroid hormones to plasma carrier proteins is affected by endogenous agents or by drugs that can change the concentration of these proteins or compete with thyroid hormones for binding sites. Examples of the first group are testosterone and related anabolic agents, which are able to decrease the concentration of T_4 binding globulin, and estrogens and related contraceptive agents, which are able to increase the concentration of T_4 binding globulin. Salicylates, diphenylhydantoin, and heparin are members of the large group competing with thyroid hormones for binding sites. Alterations in the binding of T_3 and T_4 are of no large physiologic consequence because the steady-state concentrations of free hormone are rapidly restored by homeostatic mechanisms. Knowledge regarding the presence of agents affecting thyroid hormone binding, however, is important for the interpretation of diagnostic tests assessing the presence of free or total hormone in plasma.

STRUCTURE-ACTIVITY RELATIONSHIPS OF THYROID ANALOGS

The synthesis and biologic evaluation of a wide variety of T_4 and T_3 analogs allowed a significant correlation of structural features with their relative importance in the production of hormonal responses. The key findings are summarized in Table 22.2. In general, only compounds with the appropriately substituted phenyl-X-phenyl nucleus (as depicted in the structure at the top of Table 22.2) have shown significant thyroid hormonal activities. Both single ring compounds such as DIT and a variety of its aliphatic and alicyclic ether derivatives showed no T_4-like activity in the rat antigoiter test,[61] the method most often used in determining thyromimetic activity in vivo.[62] The SARs are discussed in terms of single structural variations of T_4 in the (1) alanine side chain, (2) 3- and 5-positions of the inner ring, (3) bridging atom, (4) 3′- and 5′-positions of the outer ring, and (5) 4′-phenolic hydroxyl group.

Aliphatic Side Chain

The naturally occurring hormones are biosynthesized from L-tyrosine and possess the L-alanine side chain. The L-isomers of T_4 and T_3 (compounds 1 and 3 in Table 22.2) are more active than the D-isomers (compounds 2 and 4 in Table 22.2). The carboxylate ion and the number of atoms connecting it to the ring are more important for activity than is the intact zwitterionic alanine side chain. In the carboxylate series, the activity is maximum with the two-carbon acetic acid side chain (compounds 7 and 8) but decreases with either the shorter formic acid (compounds 5 and 6) or the longer propionic and butyric acid analogs (compounds 9-12). The ethylamine side chain analogs of T_4 and T_3 (compounds 13 and 14) are less active than the corresponding carboxylic acid analogs. In addition,

Table 22.2 Structure-Activity Relationships of Thyromimetics

Compound	R_1	R_3	R_5	X	$R_{3'}$	$R_{5'}$	$R_{4'}$	Antigoiter Activity[a]
1. L-T_4	L-Ala	I	I	O	I	I	OH	100
2. D-T_4	D-Ala	I	I	O	I	I	OH	17
3. L-T_3	L-Ala	I	I	O	I	H	OH	550
4. D-T_3	D-Ala	I	I	O	I	H	OH	41
5.	COOH	I	I	O	I	I	OH	0.1
6.	COOH	I	I	O	I	H	OH	0.4
7.	CH_2COOH	I	I	O	I	I	OH	50
8.	CH_2COOH	I	I	O	I	H	OH	36
9.	$(CH_2)_2COOH$	I	I	O	I	I	OH	15
10.	$(CH_2)_2COOH$	I	I	O	I	H	OH	20
11.	$(CH_2)_3COOH$	I	I	O	I	I	OH	4
12.	$(CH_2)_3COOH$	I	I	O	I	H	OH	5
13.	$(CH_2)_2NH_2$	I	I	O	I	I	OH	0.6
14.	$(CH_2)_2NH_2$	I	I	O	I	H	OH	6
15.	L-Ala	H	H	O	I	I	OH	<0.01
16.	L-Ala	H	H	O	I	H	OH	<0.01

Table 22.2 Structure-Activity Relationships of Thyromimetics (continued)

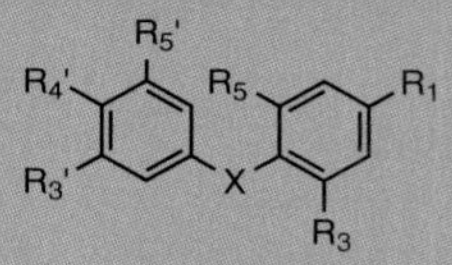

Compound	R_1	R_3	R_5	X	$R_{3'}$	$R_{5'}$	$R_{4'}$	Antigoiter Activity[a]
17.	DL-Ala	Br	Br	O	I	H	OH	93
18.	L-Ala	Br	Br	O	iPr	H	OH	166
19.	L-Ala	Me	Me	O	Me	H	OH	3
20.	L-Ala	Me	Me	O	iPr	H	OH	20
21.	DL-Ala	iPr	iPr	O	I	H	OH	0
22.	DL-Ala	sBu	sBU	O	I	H	OH	0
23.	DL-Ala	I	I	—	I	I	OH	0
24.	DL-Ala	I	I	S	I	H	OH	132
25.	DL-Ala	I	I	CH_2	I	H	OH	300
26.	L-Ala	I	I	O	H	H	OH	5
27.	L-Ala	I	I	O	OH	H	OH	1.5
28.	L-Ala	I	I	O	NO_2	H	OH	<1
29.	DL-Ala	I	I	O	F	H	OH	6
30.	L-Ala	I	I	O	Cl	H	OH	27
31.	DL-Ala	I	I	O	Br	H	OH	132
32.	L-Ala	I	I	O	Me	H	Oh	80
33.	L-Ala	I	I	O	Et	H	OH	517
34.	L-Ala	I	I	O	iPr	H	OH	786
35.	L-Ala	I	I	O	nPr	H	OH	200
36.	DL-Ala	I	I	O	Phe	H	OH	11
37.	DL-Ala	I	I	O	F	F	OH	2.3
38.	L-Ala	I	I	O	Cl	Cl	OH	21
39.	L-Ala	I	I	O	I	H	NH_2	<1.5
40.	DL-Ala	I	I	O	I	H	H	>150
41.	DL-Ala	I	I	O	CH_3	H	CH_3	0
42.	L-Ala	I	I	O	I	H	CH_3O	225

[a]See Ekins[73] and Ahmad et al.[74] In vivo activity in rats relative to L-T_4 = 100% or DL-T_4 = 100% for goiter prevention.

isomers of T_3 in which the alanine side chain is transposed with the 3-iodine or occupies the 2-position were inactive in the rat antigoiter test,[63] indicating a critical location for the side chain in the 1-position of the inner ring.

Alanine-Bearing Ring

The phenyl ring bearing the alanine side chain, called the inner ring or α-ring, is substituted with iodine in the 3- and 5-positions in T_4 and T_3. As shown in Table 22.2, removal of both iodine atoms from the inner ring to form 3′,5′-T_2 (compound 15) or 3′-T_1 (compound 16) produces analogs devoid of T_4-like activity, primarily, because of the loss of the perpendicular orientation of diphenyl ether conformation. Retention of activity observed on replacement of the 3- and 5-iodine atoms with bromine (compounds 17 and 18) implies that iodine does not play a unique role in thyroid hormone activity. Moreover, a broad range of hormone activity found with halogen-free analogs (compounds 19 and 20) indicates that a halogen atom is not essential for activity. In contrast to T_3, 3′-isopropyl-3,6-dimethyl-L-thyronine (compound 20) has the capacity to cross the placental membrane and exerts thyromimetic effects in the fetus after administration to the mother. This could prove to be useful in treating fetal thyroid hormone deficiencies or in stimulating lung development (by stimulating lung to synthesize special phospholipids [surfactant], which ensure sufficient functioning of the infant's lungs at birth) immediately before premature birth.[64] Substitution in the 3- and 5-positions by alkyl groups significantly larger and less symmetric than methyl groups, such as isopropyl and secondary butyl moieties, produces inactive analogs (compounds 21 and 22). These results show that 3,5-disubstitution by symmetric, lipophilic groups not exceeding the size of iodine is required for activity.

Bridging Atom

Several analogs have been synthesized in which the ether oxygen bridge has been removed or replaced by other atoms. The biphenyl analog of T_4 (compound 23 in Table 22.2), formed by removal of the oxygen bridge, is inactive in the rat antigoiter test. The linear biphenyl structure is a drastic change from the normal diphenyl ether conformation found in the naturally occurring hormones. Replacement of the bridging oxygen atom by sulfur (compound 24) or by a methylene group (compound 25) produces highly active analogs. This provides evidence against the Niemann quinoid theory, which postulates that the ability of a compound to form a quinoid structure in the phenolic ring is essential for thyromimetic activity, and emphasizes the importance of the three-dimensional structure and receptor fit of the hormones. Attempts to prepare amino- and carbonyl-bridged analogs of T_3 and T_4 have been unsuccessful.[65,66]

Phenolic Ring

The phenolic ring, also called the outer or β-ring, of the thyronine nucleus is required for hormonal activity. Variations in 3′- or 3′,5′-substituents on the phenolic ring have dramatic effects on biologic activity and affinity for the nuclear receptor. The unsubstituted parent structure of this series T_2 (compound 26 in Table 22.2) possesses low activity. Substitution at the 3′-position by polar hydroxyl or nitro groups (compounds 27 and 28) causes a decrease in activity as a consequence of both lowered lipophilicity and intramolecular hydrogen bonding with the 4′-hydroxyl.[67] Conversely, substitution by nonpolar halogen or alkyl groups results in an increase in activity in direct relation to the bulk and lipophilicity of the substituent—for example, F $<$ Cl $<$ Br $<$ I (compounds 29-31) and $CH_3 < CH_2CH_3 < CH(CH_3)_2$ (compounds 32-34). Although 3′-isopropylthyronine (compound 34) is the most potent analog known, being approximately 1.4 times as active as T_3, *n*-propylthyronine (compound 35) is only about one-fourth as active as isopropyl apparently because of its less compact structure. As the series is further ascended, activity decreases with a further reduction for the more bulky 3′-phenyl substituent (compound 36). Substitution in both 3′- and 5′-positions by the same halogen produces less active hormones (compounds 37 and 38) than the corresponding 3′-monosubstituted analogs (compounds 29 and 30). The decrease in activity has been explained as resulting from the increase in phenolic hydroxyl ionization and the resulting increase in binding to TBG (the primary carrier of thyroid hormones in human plasma).[68] In general, a second substituent adjacent to the phenolic hydroxyl (5′-position) reduces activity in direct proportion to its size.

Phenolic Hydroxyl Group

A weakly ionized phenolic hydroxyl group at the 4′-position is essential for optimum hormonal activity. Replacement of the 4′-hydroxyl with an amino group (compound 39 in Table 22.2) results in a substantial decrease in activity, presumably as a result of the weak hydrogen bonding ability of the latter group. The retention of activity observed with the 4′-unsubstituted compound (compound 40) provides direct evidence for metabolic 4′-hydroxylation as an activating step. Introduction of a 4′-substituent that cannot mimic the functional role of a phenolic group, such as a methyl group (compound 41), and that is not metabolically converted into a functional residue results in complete loss of hormonal activity. The thyromimetic activity of the 4′-methyl ether (compound 42) was ascribed to the ready metabolic cleavage to form an active 4′-hydroxyl analog. The pK_a of 4′-phenolic hydroxyl group is 6.7 for T_4 (90% ionized at pH 7.4) and 8.5 for T_3 (~10% ionized). The greater acidity for T_4 is reflective of its stronger affinity for plasma proteins and, consequently, of its longer plasma half-life.

Conformational Properties of Thyroid Hormones and Analogs

The importance of the diphenyl ether conformation for biologic activity was first proposed by Zenker and Jorgensen.[69,70] Through molecular models, they showed that a perpendicular orientation of the planes of the aromatic rings of 3,5-diiodothyronines would be favored to minimize interactions between the bulky 3,5-iodines and the 2′,6′-hydrogens. In this orientation, the 3′- and 5′-positions of the ring are not conformationally equivalent, and the 3′-iodine of T_3 could be oriented either distal (away from) or 5′ proximal (closer) to the side chain–bearing ring (Fig. 22.6). Because the activity of compounds such as 3′,5′-dimethyl-3,5-diiodothyronine had demonstrated that alkyl groups could replace the 3′- and 5′-iodine substituents, model compounds bearing alkyl groups in the 3′-position and alkyl or iodine substituents in the 5′-position (in addition to the blocking 2′-methyl group) were synthesized for biologic evaluation.[70]

Biologic evaluation of 2′,3′- and 2′,5′-substituted diiodothyronines[71] revealed that 3′-substitution was

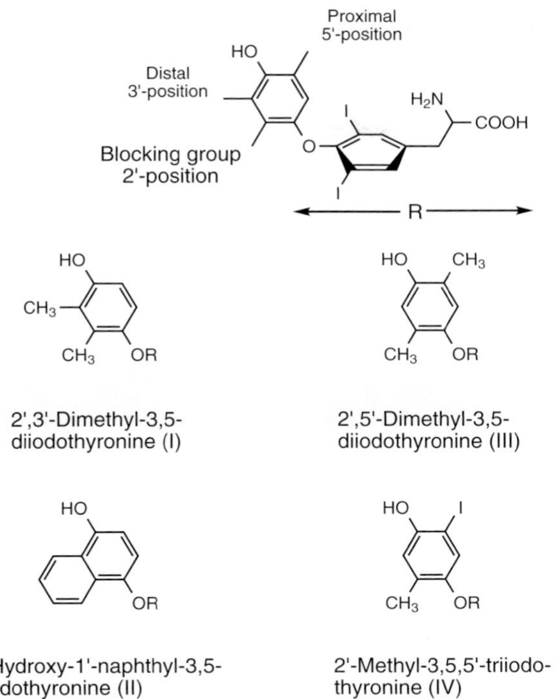

Figure 22.6 Structures of representative distal and proximal compounds.

favorable for thyromimetic activity but that 5′-substitution was not. The structures of representative distal analogs, 2′,3′-dimethyl-3,5-DL-diiodothyronine (compound I) and O-(4′-hydroxy-1′-naphthyl)-3,5-DL-diiodotyrosine (compound II), and of the proximal analogs, 2′,5′-dimethyl-3,5-DL-diiodothyronine (compound III) and 2′-methyl-3, 5,5′-DL-triiodothyronine (compound IV), are given in Figure 29.6. The effectiveness of these compounds in rat antigoiter assay[72] is presented in Table 22.3. These results clearly indicate that in 2′-blocked analogs, a distal 3′-substitution is favorable for thyromimetic activity, but a proximal 5′-substitution is not.

In addition to being perpendicular to the inner ring, the outer phenolic ring can adopt conformations relative to the alanine side chain, which would be *cis* or *trans*. In other words, the cisoid and transoid conformations result from the methine group in the alanine side chain being either *cis* or *trans* to the phenolic ring (Fig. 22.7). Although the bioactive conformation of the alanine side chain in thyroid hormone analogs has not yet been defined, these conformations appear to be similar in energy because both are found in thyroactive structures as determined by X-ray crystallography.[73] The synthesis of conformationally fixed cyclic or unsaturated analogs may allow evaluation of the bioactivity of the two conformers.

Table 22.3 Effectiveness of Distal and Proximal Compounds Antigoiter Assay

Compound[a]	Dose (mg/kg/d)	% T_4 Activity
I	0.025	50
II	0.013	>100
III	2.3	<1
IV	0.5	2

[a]See text for specific descriptions of compounds I to IV.

Transthyretin Receptor Model (TTR)

An additional tool in structural analysis and analog design has been TTR. TTR is a serum and cerebrospinal fluid carrier of T_4 and retinol. **TTR** is a transport protein in the serum and cerebrospinal fluid that carries the thyroid hormone thyroxine (T_4) and retinol-binding protein bound to retinol. This is how transthyretin gained its name: ***trans**ports **thy**roxine and **retin**ol*. The liver secretes transthyretin into the blood, and the choroid plexus secretes TTR into the cerebrospinal fluid. In cerebrospinal fluid TTR is the primary carrier of T_4. TTR also acts as a carrier of retinol (vitamin A) through its association with retinol-binding protein (RBP) in the blood and the CSF. TTR was originally called *prealbumin* because it ran faster than albumins on electrophoresis gels. TTR, a plasma protein, binds as much as 27% of plasma T_3.[74] The amino acid sequence of the TTR-T_3 binding site is known, and the protein has therefore served as a model, although admittedly an approximate model, for the T_3 receptor. The TTR model portrays the T_3 molecule as placed in an envelope near the axis of symmetry of the TTR dimer. In this envelope, hydrophobic residues, such as those of leucine, lysine, and alanine, are near pockets accommodating the 3,5,3′- and 5′-positions of T_3, whereas the hydrophilic groups of serine and threonine (hydrogen bonded to water) are between the 3′-substituent and the 4′-phenolic group. Taking this model into account, Ahmad et al.[75] suggested that 3′-acetyl-3,5-diiodothyronine might be a good analog or a good inhibitor of T_3 because the carbonyl group of the 3′ acetyl substituent would form a strong hydrogen bond with the 4′ phenolic hydrogen, thereby preventing its bonding with the hydrated residue of the putative receptor.

This compound, prepared by Benson et al.,[76] was found to be indistinguishable from T_3 in oxygen uptake and glycerophosphate activity tests and to be half as active as T_3 in displacing labeled T_3 from rat liver nuclei in specific in vivo conditions.

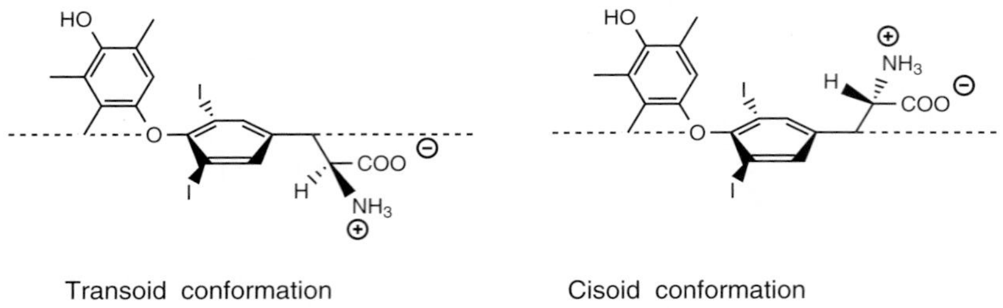

Figure 22.7 Side chain conformations of thyroid hormones: transoid (left) and cisoid (right).

Clinical Scenario

Gigi Shafai, PharmD

SCENARIO

HK, a 36-year-old otherwise healthy woman with no history of thyroid-related issues, presented with symptoms of extreme weight gain, fatigue, anxiety, and hair loss. Additionally, constipation and impaired memory were described. HK's family history includes thyroid fluctuations and thyroid carcinoma. Having recently delivered a baby, HK was attributing her fatigue to a return to work and/or sleepless nights with her newborn. However, a clinical workup documented a significantly elevated TSH (94 mIU/L; normal 0.04–5 mIU/L), a low free T_4 (<0.4 ng/dL, normal 0.9-1.8 ng/dL), along with a positive TPO antibody test. This was verified twice for confirmation of laboratory results. A diagnosis of severe hypothyroidism due to pregnancy was made, and levothyroxine replacement therapy was advised. The endocrinologist prescribed Synthroid at a dose of 125 μg per day, given weight-based dosing.

OUTCOME

After 1 month of receiving daily Synthroid, TSH trended down to 10.83 uIU/mL and after 2 months, the patient became euthyroid, with normal TSH of 0.09 ulu/mL and T4 1.5 ng/dL. Within 3 months, she was less fatigued and had lost 15 pounds. No adverse effects were noted with treatment. As part of long-term planning, the patient and physician then discussed incorporating a thyroid diet and implemented a total weekly dose reduction to the minimum necessary to maintain euthyroid status. HK is now maintained on Synthroid 125 μg 5 days weekly and has maintained euthyroid status.

Discuss the choices of approved thyroid hormone replacement brands and why Synthroid is the best choice in this case.

Chemical Analysis found immediately after References.

ACKNOWLEDGMENTS

The author wishes to acknowledge the contribution of Dr. Gigi Shafai to the writing of this chapter and thank Ariana Banijamali, a pharmacy student for reading the chapter and giving comments and insight from the prospective of a pharmacy student.

REFERENCES

1. Harington CR. Biochemical basis of thyroid function. *Lancet*. 1935;225:1261-1266.
2. Baumann E. Uber das normale vorkommen von jod in tierkorper. *Zeitschr Physiol Chem*. 1896;21:319.
3. Magnus-Levy A. Uber den respiratorischen gewechsel unter dem einfluss der thyroidea sowie unter verschiedenen pathologischen zustanden. *Berl Klin Wchnschr*. 1895;32:650.
4. Gudernatsch JF. Feeding experiments on tadpoles. *Arch Entw der Organismen*. 1912;35:457.
5. Nadler NJ. Thyroid anatomical features. In: Greer MA, Solomon DH, eds. *Handbook of Physiology, Sec 7*. Vol III. Washington, DC: American Physiological Society; 1974.
6. Ekholm R, Bjorkman U. Biochemistry of thyroid hormones. In: Martini L, ed. *The Thyroid Gland*. New York: Raven Press; 1990:83-125.
7. Taurog A. Hormone synthesis: thyroid iodine metabolism. In: Braverman L, Utiger R, eds. *Werner and Ingbar's the Thyroid: A Fundamental and Clinical Text*. 8th ed. Philadelphia, PA: Lippincott Williams & Wilkins; 2000:61-85.
8. Chopra IJ, Solomon DH, Chopra U, et al. Pathways of metabolism of thyroid hormones. *Recent Prog Horm Res*. 1978;34:521-567.
9. Visser TJ, Docter R, Krenning EP, et al. Regulation of thyroid hormone bioactivity. *Endocrinol Invest*. 1986;9(suppl 4):17-26.
10. Krassas GE, Rivkees SA, Kiess W, eds. Diseases of the thyroid in childhood and adolescence. *Pediatr Adolesc Med*. Vol 10. Basel: Karger; 2007:80-103.
11. Himms-Hagen J. Cellular thermogenesis. *Annu Rev Physiol*. 1976;38:315-351.
12. Muller MJ, Seitz HJ. Thyroid hormone action on intermediary metabolism. Part I: respiration, thermogenesis, and carbohydrate metabolism. *Klin Wochenschr*. 1984;62:11-18.
13. Muller MJ, Seitz HJ. Thyroid hormone action on intermediary metabolism. Part III Protein metabolism in hyper- and hypothyroidism. *Klin Wochenschr*. 1984;62:97-102.
14. Tata JR. Inhibition of the biological action of thyroid hormones by actinomycin D and puromycin. *Nature*. 1963;197:1167-1168.
15. Tata JR, Widnell CC. Ribonucleic acid synthesis during the early action of thyroid hormones. *Biochem J*. 1966;98:604-620.
16. Greenspan FS, Forsham PH. *Basic and Clinical Endocrinology*. Los Altos, CA: Lange Medical; 1983:141.

17. Wolff J, Chaikoff IL. Plasma inorganic iodide as homeostatic regulator of thyroid function. *J Biol Chem*. 1948;174:555-564.
18. Virion A, Michot JL, Deme D, et al. NADPH oxidation catalyzed by the peroxidase/H_2O_2 system. Iodide-mediated oxidation of NADPH to iodinated NADP. *Eur J Biochem*. 1985;148:239-248.
19. Leonard JL, Kaplan MM, Visser TJ, et al. Cerebral cortex responds rapidly to thyroid hormones. *Science*. 1981;214:571-573.
20. McConnon J, Row VV, Volpe R. The influence of liver damage in man on the distribution and disposal rates of thyroxine and triiodothyronine. *J Clin Endocrinol Metab*. 1972;34:144-153.
21. Lim VS, Fang VS, Katz AI, et al. Thyroid dysfunction in chronic renal failure. A study of the pituitary-thyroid axis and peripheral turnover kinetics of thyroxine and triiodothyronine. *J Clin Invest*. 1977;60:522-530.
22. Carter JN, Eastmen CJ, Corcoran JM, et al. Inhibition of conversion of thyroxine to triiodothyronine in patients with severe chronic illness. *Clin Endocrinol*. 1976;5:587-594.
23. Spaulding SW, Chopra IJ, Sherwin RS, et al. Effect of caloric restriction and dietary composition of serum T_3 and reverse T_3 in man. *J Clin Endocrinol Metab*. 1976;42:197-200.
24. Chacon MA, Tildon JT. Mode of death and post-mortem time effects on 3,3′,5-triiodothyronine levels—relevance to elevated post-mortem T_3 levels in SIDS. *Fed Proc*. 1984;43:866-868.
25. Heyma P, Larkins RG, Campbell DG. Inhibition by propranolol of 3,5,3′-triiodothyronine formation from thyroxine in isolated rat renal tubules: an effect independent of β-adrenergic blockade. *Endocrinology*. 1980;106:1437-1441.
26. Silva JE, Larsen PR. Adrenergic activation of triiodothyronime production in brown adipose tissue. *Nature*. 1983;305:712-713.
27. Zenker N, Chacon MA, Tildon JT. Mode of death effect on rat liver iodothyronine 5′-deiodinase activity: role of adenosine 3′,5′-monophosphate. *Life Sci*. 1984;35:2213-2217.
28. Ventura M, Melo M, Carrihlo F. Selenium and thyroid disease: from pathology to treatment. *Intl J Endocrinol*. 2017;2017:1297658.
29. Liontiris MI, Mazokopakis EE. A concise review of Hashimoto thyroiditis (HT) and the importance of iodine, selenium, vitamin D and gluten on the autoimmunity and dietary management of HT patients. Points that need more investigation. *Hell J Nucl Med*. 2017;20(1):51-56.
30. Di Bari F, Granese R, Vita R, Benvenga S. Autoimmune abnormalities of postpartum thyroid diseases. *Front Endocrinol (Lausanne)*. 2017;8:166.
31. Gaitan E, Nelson NC, Poole GV. Endemic goiter and endemic thyroid disorders. *World J Surg*. 1991;15(2):205-215.
32. Hagen B, Alexander E, Bible K, et al. 2015 American thyroid association management guidelines for adult patients with nThyroid nodules and diffrentiated thyroid cancer. *Thyroid*. 2016;26(1).
33. Weiss B, Landrian PJ. The developing brain and the environment: an introduction. *Environ Health Prospect*. 2000;108(suppl 3):373-374.
34. Hauser P, Zametkin AJ, Martinez P, et al. Attention-deficit hyperactivity disorder in people with generalized resistance to thyroid hormone. *N Engl J Med*. 1993;328:997-1001.
35. Mitchell RS, Kumar V, Abbas AK, et al. *Robbins Basic Pathology*. 8th ed. Philadelphia: Saunders; 2007.
36. Jackson IM, Cobb WE. Why does anyone still use desiccated thyroid USP? *Am J Med*. 1978;64:284-288.
37. Deshpande H, Marler V, Sosa JA. Clinical utility of vandetanib in the treatment of patients with advanced medullary thyroid cancer. *Onco Targets Ther*. 2011;4:209-215.
38. Pittman JA. In: Selenkow HA, Hoffman F, eds. *Diagnosis and Treatment of Common Thyroid Disease*. Amsterdam: Excerpta Medica; 1971:72-73.
39. Agency for Toxic Substances and Disease Registry, U.S. Department of Health and Human Services. *Draft Toxicological Profile for Perchlorates*. Washington, DC: U.S. Department of Health and Human Services; September 2005.
40. Lamas L, Ingbar SH. In: Robbins J, Braverman LE, eds. *Thyroid Research*. Amsterdam: Excerpta Medica; 1976:213.
41. Pittman JA. *Diagnosis and Treatment of Thyroid Disease*. Philadelphia, PA: FA Davis; 1963:48.
42. Hackmon R. The safety of methimazole and propylthiouracil in pregenancy: a systematic review. *J Obstet Gynaecol Can*. 2012;34(11):1077-1086.
43. Ross D. Patient Education: Anti Thyroid Drugs (Beyond the basics). UpToDate; 2017. Last updated: March 15, 2017.
44. Morreale de Escobar G, Escobar del Rey R. Extrathyroid effects of some antithyroid drugs and their metabolic consequences. *Rec Prog Horm Res*. 1967;23:87-137.
45. Cooper DS, Saxe VC, Meskell M, et al. Acute effects of PTU (PTU) on thyroidal iodide organification and peripheral iodothyronine deiodination: correlation with serum PTU levels measured by radioimmunoassay. *J Clin Endocrinol Metab*. 1982;54:101-107.
46. Visser TJ, van Overmeeren E, Fekkes D, et al. Inhibition of iodothyronine 5′-deiodinase by thioureylenes: structure–activity relationship. *FEBS Lett*. 1979;103:314-318.
47. Taurog A. The mechanism of action of the thioureylene antithyroid drugs. *Endocrinology*. 1976;98:1031-1046.
48. Nakashima T, Taurog A, Riesco G. Mechanism of action of thioureylene antithyroid drugs: factors affecting intrathyroidal metabolism of PTU and MMI in rats. *Endocrinology*. 1978;103:2187-2197.
49. Papapetrou PD, Mothon S, Alexander WD. Binding of the 35-S of 35-S-pro-pylthiouracil by follicular thyroglobulin in vivo and in vitro. *Acta Endocrinol*. 1975;79:248-258.
50. Chopra IJ, Chua Teco GN, Eisenberg JB, et al. Structure–activity relationships of inhibition of hepatic monodeiodination of thyroxine to 3,5,3′-triiodothyronine by thiouracil and related compounds. *Endocrinology*. 1982;110:163-168.
51. Pearce E. Diagnosis and management of thyrotoxicosis. *Br Med J*. 2006;332(7554):1369-1373.
52. Turner JG, Brownlie BE, Sadler WA, et al. An evaluation of lithium as an adjunct to carbimazole treatment in acute thyrotoxicosis. *Acta Endocrinol*. 1976;83:86-92.
53. Berens SC, Wolff J, Murphy DL. Lithium concentration by the thyroid. *Endocrinology*. 1970;87:1085-1087.
54. Temple R, Berman M, Robbins J, et al. The use of lithium in the treatment of thyrotoxicosis. *J Clin Invest*. 1972;51:2746-2756.
55. Tookey HL, Van Ettén CH, Daxenbichler ME. Glucosinolates. In: Liener IE, ed. *Toxic Constituents of Plant Foodstuffs*. New York: Academic Press; 1980:103-142.
56. Langer P, Michajlovskij N. Effect of naturally occurring goitrogens on thyroid peroxidase and influence of some compounds on iodide formation during the estimation. *Endocrinol Exp*. 1972;6:97-103.
57. Elfving S. Studies on the naturally occurring goitrogen 5-vinyl-2-thiooxazolidone. Metabolism and antithyroid effect in the rat. *Ann Clin Res*. 1980;12(suppl 28):7-47.
58. Tabachnick M, Hao YL, Korcek L. Effect of oleate, diphenylhydantoin, and heparin on the binding of ^{125}I-thyroxine to purified thyroxine-binding globulin. *J Clin Endocrinol Metab*. 1973;36:392-394.
59. Goswami A, Leonard JL, Rosenberg IN. Inhibition by coumadin anticoagulants of enzymatic outer ring monodeiodination of iodothyronine. *Biochem Biophys Res Commun*. 1982;104:1231-1238.
60. Auf'mkolk M, Amir SM, Kubota K, et al. The active principles of plant extracts with antithyrotropic activity: oxidation products of derivatives of 3,4-dihydroxycinnamic acid. *Endocrinology*. 1985;116:1677-1686.
61. Jorgensen EC, Lehman PA. Thyroxine analogues IV Synthesis of aliphatic and alicyclic ethers of 3,5-diiodo-DL-tyrosine. *J Org Chem*. 1961;26:894.
62. Mussett MV, Pitt-Rivers R. The physiologic activity of thyroxine and triiodothyronine analogs. *Metab Clin Exper*. 1957;6:18-25.
63. Jorgensen EC, Reid JAW. Thyroxine analogues XI Structural isomers of 3,5,3′-triiodo-DL-thyronine. *J Med Chem*. 1964;7:701-705.
64. Gluckman PD, Ballard PL, Kaplan SL, et al. Prolactin in umbilical cord blood and the respiratory distress syndrome. *J Pediatr*. 1978;93:1011-1014.

65. Tripp SL, Block FB, Barile G. Synthesis of methylene- and carbonyl-bridged analogues of iodothyronine and iodothyroacetic acids. *J Med Chem*. 1973;66:60-64.
66. Mukherjee R, Block P. Thyroxine analogues: synthesis and nuclear magnetic resonance spectral studies of diphenylamines. *J Chem Soc*. 1971;9:1596-1600.
67. Leeson PD, Ellis D, Emmett JC, et al. Thyroid hormone analogues. Synthesis of 3′-substituted 3,5-diiodo-L-thyronines and quantitative structure–activity studies of in vitro and in vivo thyromimetic activities in rat liver and heart. *J Med Chem*. 1988;31:37-54.
68. Jorgensen EC. Thyroid hormones and analogs II. Structure–activity relationships. In: Li CH, ed. *Hormonal Proteins and Peptides*. Vol 6. New York: Academic Press; 1978:107-204.
69. Malm J, Grover GJ. Thyroid hormones and thyromimetics. In: Abraham DJ, Rotella DP, eds. *Burger's Medicinal Chemistry*. Vol 4. 7th ed. New York: Wiley; 2010:189-222.
70. Zenker N, Jorgensen EC. Thyroxine analogues I Synthesis of 3,5-diiodi-4-(2′-alkylphenoxy)-DL-phenylalanine. *J Am Chem Soc*. 1959;81:4643-4647.
71. Jorgensen EC, Zenker N, Greenberg C, et al. Thyroxine analogues III Antigoitrogenic and calorigenic activity of some alkyl substituted analogues of thyroxine. *J Biol Chem*. 1960;235:1732-1737.
72. Jorgensen EC, Lehman PA, Greenberg C, et al. Thyroxine analogues VII Antigoitrogenic, calorigenic, and hypocholesteremic activities of same aliphatic, alicyclic, and aromatic ethers of 3,5-diiodotyrosine in the rat. *J Biol Chem*. 1962;237:3832-3838.
73. Cody V. Thyroid hormones: crystal structure, molecular conformation, binding, and structure-function relationships. *Rec Prog Horm Res*. 1978;34:437-475.
74. Ekins R. Methods for the measurement of free thyroid hormones. In: Ekins R, Faglia G, Pennisi F, et al, eds. *International Symposium on Free Thyroid Hormones*. Amsterdam: Excerpta Medica; 1979:7-29.
75. Ahmad P, Fyfe CA, Mellors A. Parachors in drug design. *Biochem Pharmacol*. 1975;24:1103-1110.
76. Benson MG, Ellis D, Emmett JC, et al. 3′-Acetyl-3,5-diiodo-L-thyronine: a novel highly active thyromimetic with low receptor affinity. *Biochem Pharmacol*. 1984;33:3143-3149.

Clinical Scenario

Gigi Shafai, PharmD

CHEMICAL ANALYSIS

Given the high TSH and the low free T_4 levels, thyroid hormone replacement therapy is necessary in this case. There are a variety of approved thyroid hormone replacement brands available, some of which are natural and others are synthetic.

Source	Brand	Hormones Included
Natural desiccated	Armour Thyroid	T_4 and T_3
Synthetic	Synthroid	T_4
Synthetic	Cytomel	T_3
Synthetic	Thyrolar	T_4 and T_3; 4:1 ratio

Desiccated preparations have been shown to produce variable T_4/T_3 blood levels because of inconsistencies both between and within animal sources of the thyroid gland. Synthetic hormones have more predictable pharmacokinetic and pharmacodynamic properties. Among the synthetic preparations, Synthroid contains T_4 alone, Cytomel contains only T_3, and Thyrolar contains a mixture of both T_4 and T_3.

Because the body converts T_4 to T_3, there is potential variability in pharmacodynamics when a mixture therapy is introduced. Therefore, mixture approach (T_4 and T_3 combined) is not the best choice for this patient. This ruled out Armour Thyroid and Thyrolar for treatment.

The half-life of T_4 is much longer than that of T_3 (1 wk vs. 1 day, respectively) and it also has a slower onset of action. Therefore, a synthetic preparation that contains T_4 is more desirable for chronic hypothyroidism than a preparation containing T_3. T_3, Cytomel is typically administered for acute thyroid emergencies given its rapid onset of action. In this case, the patient's hypothyroidism is not considered an emergency.

Synthroid is the drug of choice in this case since it has predictable pharmacokinetics and pharmacodynamics, it is not a mixture of hormones that might introduce variability, and it has a long half-life which is optimal for a chronic treatment of hypothyroidism.

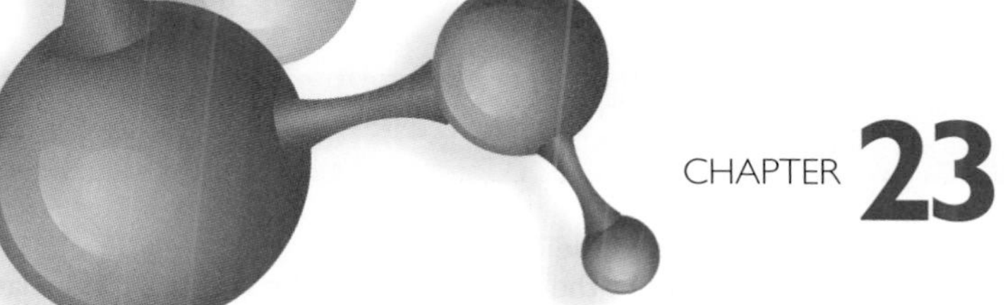

CHAPTER 23

Drugs Used to Treat Calcium-Dependent Disorders

Robin M. Zavod

Drugs covered in this chapter:

SELECTIVE ESTROGEN RECEPTOR MODULATORS
- Bazedoxifene acetate
- Raloxifene hydrochloride
- Tamoxifen

BISPHOSPHONATES
- Alendronate sodium
- Ibandronate sodium
- Pamidronate disodium
- Risedronate sodium
- Zoledronic acid

CALCITONIN

PTH ANALOGS
- Teriparatide
- Abaloparatide

MONOCLONAL ANTIBODY
- Denosumab

CALCIUM MIMETICS
- Cinacalcet hydrochloride
- Etelcalcetide

INORGANIC SALTS
- Calcium salts

Abbreviations

AF-2 activation factor-2
ATP adenosine triphosphate
BMD bone mineral density
cAMP cyclic adenosine monophosphate
CaSR calcium-sensing receptor
CYP450 cytochrome P-450
DIOP drug-induced osteoporosis
DNA deoxyribonucleic acid
ER estrogen receptor
ERE estrogen responding element
ERT estrogen replacement therapy
FPPS farnesyl pyrophosphate synthetase
FDA U.S. Food and Drug Administration
GPCR G protein–coupled receptor
IM intramuscular
IU international unit
IV intravenous
NFκB nuclear factor kappa-light-chain-enhancer of activated B cells
$1,25(OH)_2D_3$ 1,25-dihydroxycholecalciferol
$25(OH)D_3$ 25-hydroxycholecalciferol
OPGL osteoprotegerin ligand
PPARγ2 peroxisome proliferator-activated receptor γ2
PTH parathyroid hormone
PTHR1 parathyroid hormone receptor type 1
PTHrP parathyroid hormone related protein
RANKL receptor activator of nuclear factor-κB ligand
RRE raloxifene responding element
SAR structure-activity relationship
SC subcutaneous
SERM selective estrogen receptor modulator
TSEC tissue selective estrogen complex
UGT uridine diphosphate glucuronosyltransferase
WHI Women's Health Initiative

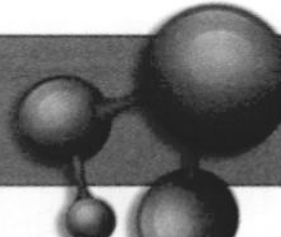

CLINICAL SIGNIFICANCE

Kathryn Neill, PharmD

As our knowledge about the development and risk factors associated with disruptions in calcium homeostasis has increased, so too have the modalities available to prevent and/or treat these disease processes. In general, disorders of calcium homeostasis involve the development of bone disease and/or alterations in serum calcium concentration. In the most basic sense, the development of bone disease is simply an inequity between bone breakdown and bone formation, which also may result in an altered serum calcium concentration. In addition to bone disease, disruptions in normal serum calcium concentrations may be related to an imbalance in calcium intake and renal calcium elimination. These disturbances can result from various factors, including increased activity of cells that cause bone breakdown, decreased activity of cells that form new bone, decreased absorption of calcium, or irregularities in levels of hormones that affect calcium absorption and influence cells involved in bone maintenance. An increased understanding of these physiologic pathways has led to the development of multiple classes of agents targeting the different mechanisms for evolution of these disease processes, including selective estrogen receptor modulators, bisphosphonates, parathyroid hormone analogs, calcium mimetics, and various calcium salts.

Application of the principles of medicinal chemistry has resulted in the formulation of agents with additional routes of administration, increased potency, and decreased frequency of dosing. These advances have increased the utility of these agents and improved the quality of life for countless individuals affected by calcium homeostasis disorders. Understanding the development of individual disease processes involved in disorders of calcium homeostasis (e.g., osteoporosis, osteopetrosis, hyperparathyroidism, Paget disease) and the pharmacodynamic effects of individual compounds used to treat these disorders is paramount for the practitioner making therapeutic decisions. Incorporation of these factors into the therapeutic plan is necessary to target the valued pharmacodynamic effects of these agents while minimizing unwanted or harmful effects. For example, the selection of raloxifene to treat osteoporosis in a patient with severe gastroesophageal reflux disease, as opposed to an oral bisphosphonate, which could increase the likelihood of developing erosive esophagitis. Finally, it is also important for the clinician to recognize the capacity of certain entities used to treat calcium disorders to be allergenic or more prone to produce adverse effects so that selection of the best agent for an individual patient is facilitated.

INTRODUCTION

Three primary hormones—calcitonin, parathyroid hormone, and vitamin D—control the homeostatic regulation of calcium and its principle counterion, inorganic phosphate. Homeostatic control of these ions is essential not only for the moderation of longitudinal bone growth and bone remodeling but also for blood coagulation, neuromuscular excitability, plasma membrane structure and function, muscle contraction, glycogen and adenosine triphosphate (ATP) metabolism, neurotransmitter/hormone secretion, and enzyme catalysis.[1] In an average 70-kg adult, approximately 1 kg of calcium is found, 99% of which is located in the bone. The principle calcium salt contained in the hydroxyapatite crystalline lattice of teeth and bones is $Ca_{10}(PO_4)_6(OH)_2$. Similarly, approximately 500-600 g of phosphate are present, 85% of which is found in the bone. The normal plasma concentration of calcium is approximately 4.5-5.7 mEq/L, 50% of which is protein bound. The remainder of the calcium is either complexed to corresponding counterions (46%) or exists in its ionized form (4%). It is only the ionized form of calcium that is tightly hormonally regulated (varies less than 5%-10%).[1,2] Because serum calcium concentrations fluctuate, so do the plasma levels of the hormones associated with calcium homeostasis. Serum phosphorous levels vary with age, diet, and hormonal status. The most common form of phosphate in the blood (pH 7.4) is HPO_4^{2-}

The bone is composed of two distinct tissue structures: cortical (compact) bone and trabecular (cancellous) bone.[3] Eighty percent of the skeleton is composed of cortical bone (e.g., long bones such as the humerus, radius, and ulna),[4,5] which is a relatively dense tissue (80%-90% calcified)[4] that provides structure and support.[3] Bone marrow cavities, flat bones, and the ends of long bones are all composed of trabecular bone, which is considerably more porous (5%-20% calcified).[4,5] To maintain healthy, well-mineralized bone, a continuous process of bone resorption (loss of ionic calcium from bone) and bone formation occurs along the bone surface. Cortical bone is remodeled at the rate of 3% per year, whereas 25% of trabecular bone, which has a considerably higher surface area, is remodeled annually.[3] In terms of calcium turnover in bone, approximately 500 mg are removed and replaced on a daily basis.

Both inorganic and organic components are present in the bone. The highly crystalline inorganic component is hydroxyapatite, and the collagen matrix comprises the major portion (90%) of the organic component. The collagen matrix serves as the foundation for hydroxyapatite mineralization. Osteocalcin and osteonectin are minor organic constituents that promote binding of hydroxyapatite and calcium to the collagen matrix and regulate the rate of bone mineralization, respectively.[5]

In general, peak bone mass occurs between 30 and 40 years of age[3] and is dependent on genetic factors as well as proper intake of calcium, maintenance of quality nutrition, and participation in weight-bearing exercise.[6] Thereafter, peak bone mass progressively declines at the rate of 0.3%-0.5% of cortical bone per year.[3] After menopause, bone loss is accelerated (2% per year in the spine)[6] for a period of 5-10 years because of the loss of estrogen. This can result in up to a 30% decrease in bone mineral density.

HORMONAL REGULATION OF SERUM CALCIUM LEVELS

There are complex interrelationships among the three hormones (parathyroid, calcitonin, and vitamin D) that control calcium homeostasis (serum concentrations of ionic calcium) and their target organs (bone, kidney, and intestine).[7] Figure 23.1 tracks the intake, utilization, and excretion of 1,000 mg calcium and the relative contributions of each of these three hormones. It is important to note that calcium homeostasis is achieved only if active vitamin D as well as sufficient levels of both parathyroid hormone (PTH) and calcitonin (CT) are present.

Calcitonin

S—S
Cys-Gly—Asn—Leu—Ser—Thr—Cys-Met—Leu—Gly—Thr—Tyr—Thr—Gln—Asp—Phe—Asn—Lys—Phe—His-Thr-Phe-Pro—ThrGln—Ala—Ile Gly—Val—Gly—Ala Pro-NH_2 (C=O amide)

Human calcitonin

Human calcitonin is a 32–amino acid peptide (molecular weight, 3,527 Da) biosynthesized in the parafollicular "C" cells found within the thyroid gland. This hormone contains a critical disulfide bridge between residues 1 and 7, with the entire amino acid sequence required for biologic activity. The carboxy-terminal residue is a proline amide. "Procalcitonin," a precursor peptide, has been identified and proposed to facilitate intracellular transport and secretion. Calcitonin is secreted in response to elevated serum calcium concentrations (>9 mg/100 mL) and serves to oppose the hormonal effects of parathyroid hormone. In response to a hypercalcemic state, increased calcitonin secretion drives serum calcium concentrations down via stimulation of urinary excretion of both calcium and phosphate, prevention of calcium resorption from the bone via inhibition of osteoclast activity, and inhibition of intestinal absorption of calcium. When serum calcium concentrations are low (hypocalcemia), the release of calcitonin is slowed.

Parathyroid Hormone

Parathyroid hormone (PTH) is biosynthesized as a 115–amino acid preprohormone in the rough endoplasmic reticulum of the parathyroid gland and is cleaved to the prohormone (90 amino acids) in the cisternal space of the reticulum (Fig. 23.2). The active hormone is finally produced (84 amino acids; molecular weight, 9,500 Da) in the Golgi complex and is stored in secretory granules in the parathyroid gland. This gland is exquisitely sensitive to serum calcium concentrations and is able to monitor these levels via calcium-sensing receptors (CaSR). These cell surface receptors help cells react to micromolar changes in the concentration of ionized calcium in the serum.[8] Binding of calcium to these receptors facilitates activation of phospholipase C and, ultimately, inhibition of parathyroid hormone (PTH) secretion. The relatively short-acting PTH is secreted from the parathyroid gland chief cells in response to a hypocalcemic state and serves to oppose

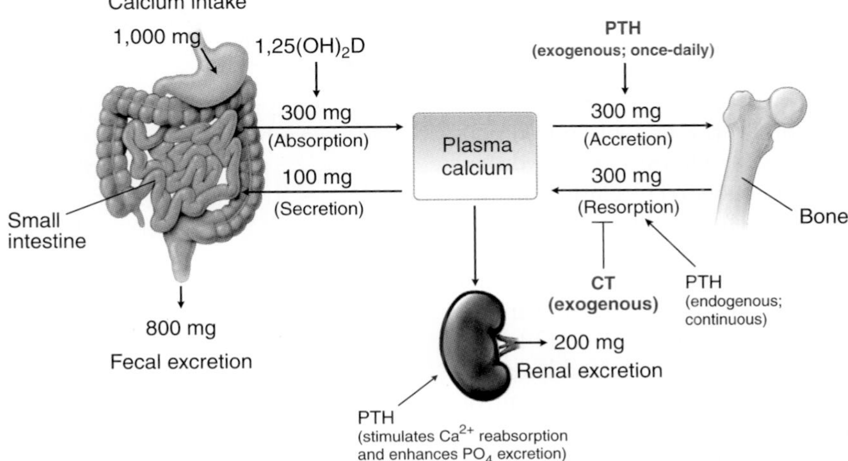

Figure 23.1 Calcium homeostasis; the fate of 1,000 mg of calcium. In a state of whole-body calcium balance, the fluxes of calcium include net uptake of 200 mg per day from the gastrointestinal (GI) tract and excretion of 200 mg per day by the kidneys. Calcitriol [$1,25(OH)_2D$] enhances absorption of Ca^{2+} from the GI tract. Continuous secretion of parathyroid hormone (PTH) increases bone formation and (even more) bone resorption and stimulates renal tubular reabsorption of calcium; both effects raise plasma Ca^{2+}. Exogenous calcitonin (CT) inhibits bone resorption. Adapted with permission from Slovik DM, Armstrong EJ. Pharmacology of bone mineral homeostasis. In: Golan DE, Armstrong EJ, Armstrong AW, eds. *Principles of Pharmacology: The Pathophysiologic Basis of Drug Therapy*. 4th ed. Philadelphia: Wolters Kluwer Health; 2017.

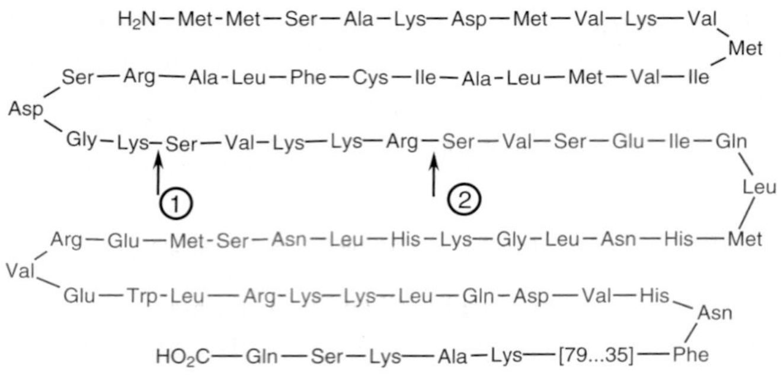

Figure 23.2 Preproparathyroid hormone is the 115–amino acid protein indicated above. Cleavage at site 1 gives rise to propara-thyroid hormone (89 amino acids) while cleavage at site 2 gives para-thyroid hormone (PTH, 84 amino acids). The protein shown in RED is teriparatide (34 amino acids).

the hormonal effects of calcitonin.[1] Unlike calcitonin, the biologic activity of PTH resides solely in residues 1-34 in the amino terminus.

PTH decreases renal excretion of calcium, indirectly stimulates intestinal absorption of calcium and, in combination with active vitamin D, promotes bone resorption. PTH stimulates bone resorption by several mechanisms: (1) transformation of osteoprogenitor cells into osteoclasts is stimulated in the presence of PTH, (2) PTH promotes the deep osteocytes to mobilize calcium from perilacunar bone, and (3) surface osteocytes are stimulated by PTH to increase the flow of calcium out of the bone. In addition, the secretion of PTH stimulates the biosynthesis, activation, and release of the third hormone associated with calcium homeostasis, vitamin D. When serum calcium concentrations are high, the release of PTH is inhibited.

Vitamin D

Derived from cholesterol, vitamin D is biosynthesized from its prohormone cholecalciferol (D_3), the product of solar ultraviolet irradiation of 7-dehydrocholesterol in the skin.[2] In 1966, it was first recognized that vitamin D must undergo activation via two oxidative metabolic steps (Fig. 23.3). The first oxidation to 25-hydroxycholecalciferol [25(OH) D_3: calcidiol; Rayaldee] occurs in the endoplasmic reticulum of the liver and is catalyzed by vitamin D 25-hydroxylase. This activation step is not regulated by plasma calcium concentrations. The major circulating form (10-80 μg/mL) is 25(OH)D_3, which also is the primary storage form of vitamin D.[2] In response to a hypocalcemic state and the secretion of PTH, a second oxidation step is activated in the mitochondria of the kidney, catalyzed by vitamin D 1α-hydroxylase.[2,9] The product of this reaction, 1,25-dihydroxycholecalciferol [1,25(OH)$_2$$D_3$: 1,25-calcitriol; Rocaltrol, Vectical is the active form of vitamin D. Its concentration in the blood is 1/500 that of its monohydroxylated precursor. The biosynthesis of vitamin D is tightly regulated based on the serum concentrations of calcium, phosphate, PTH, and active vitamin D.[2]

Sterol-specific cytoplasmic receptor proteins (vitamin D receptor) mediate the biologic action of vitamin D.[9] The active hormone is transported from the cytoplasm to the nucleus via the vitamin D receptor, and as a result of the interaction of the hormone with target genes, a variety of proteins are produced that stimulate the transport of calcium in each of the target tissues. Active vitamin D works in concert with PTH to enhance active intestinal absorption of calcium, to stimulate bone resorption, and to prohibit renal excretion of calcium.[2,9] If serum calcium or 1,25-calcitriol concentrations are elevated, then vitamin D 24-hydroxylase (in renal mitochondria) is activated to oxidize 25(OH)D_3 to inactive 24,25-dihydroxy-cholecalciferol and to further oxidize active vitamin D to the inactive 1,24,25-trihydroxylated derivative. Both the 1,24,25-trihydroxylated and the 24,25-dihydroxylated products have been found to suppress PTH secretion as well. Several factors have been identified in the regulation of the biosynthesis of vitamin D, including low phosphate concentrations (stimulatory) as well as pregnancy and lactation (stimulatory).

NORMAL PHYSIOLOGY

During growth periods in childhood and early adulthood, bone formation characteristically exceeds bone loss. In young adulthood, bone formation and bone resorption are nearly equal. After the age of 40 years, however, bone resorption is slightly greater than bone formation, and this results in a gradual decline in skeletal mass. Osteoblasts, osteoclasts, and osteocytes are the three types of cells that make up the bone remodeling unit or bone metabolizing unit and, therefore, are largely responsible for the bone remodeling process.[3,4]

The bone remodeling process is comprised of two opposing activities, bone resorption and bone formation.

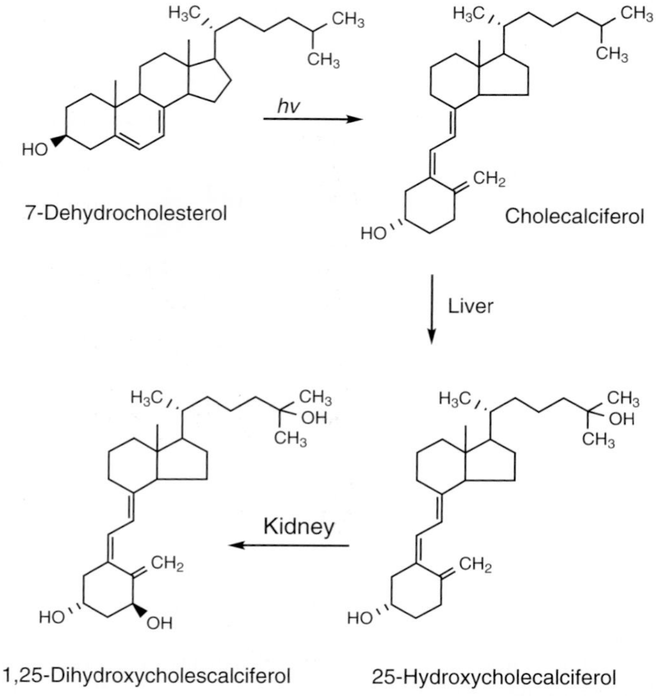

Figure 23.3 Bioactivation of vitamin D.

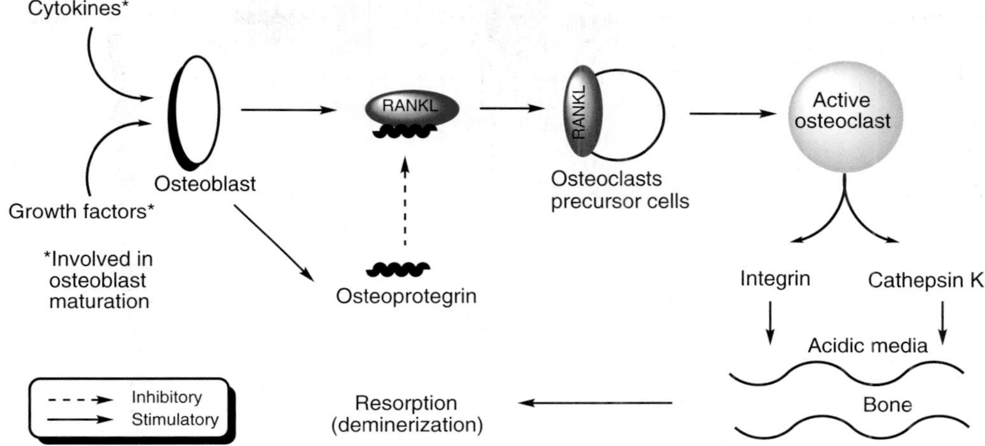

Figure 23.4 Bone resorption involving receptor activator of nuclear factor κB-ligand (RANKL).

Bone resorption is launched when osteocytes and those cells that line the bone surface release cytokines and growth factors (Fig. 23.4). These endogenous substances signal osteoblasts to release receptor activator of nuclear factor-κB ligand (RANK-ligand or RANKL).[10] This ligand interacts with and activates its receptor (RANK) found on (1) the surface of osteoclast precursor cells, which stimulates osteoclast differentiation, and (2) the surface of mature osteoclasts, which promotes activation.[10] Receptor activation regulates differentiation of the major skeletal cell types—osteoclasts, osteoblasts, osteocytes, and chondrocytes.

Osteoblasts, which are of mesenchymal origin and are formed in the bone marrow, stimulate bone formation.[6] In the maturation process, osteoblasts undergo multiple cell divisions and, in so doing, express the gene products that are needed to form the bone matrix or osteoid, as well as those products responsible for mineralization of that tissue.[3] It is in the rough endoplasmic reticulum that the biosynthesis of the bone matrix protein occurs.[4] Multiple endogenous substances are involved in osteoblast maturation, including many cytokines (interleukins and granulocyte-macrophage colony-stimulating factor), as well as hormones and growth factors.

Not only are osteoblasts involved in bone formation, but they also have a role in limiting bone resorption. Produced by osteoblasts, osteoprotegerin (OPG), a RANK receptor homolog, binds to RANKL and therefore prevents its interaction with its RANK receptors on the osteoclast.[10] As a result, osteoclast differentiation and bone resorption are inhibited.

Disease States Associated With Abnormal Calcium Homeostasis

Osteoporosis

Osteoporosis is a skeletal disease that is characterized by loss of bone mass as well as microarchitectural deterioration of the bone tissue. This disease is associated with increased bone fragility and susceptibility to fracture. It is a condition that is characterized not by inadequate bone formation but, rather, by a deficiency in the production of well-mineralized bone mass. Whereas no medical cause typically is evident in primary osteoporosis,[3] secondary osteoporosis classically stems from medical illness or medication use. There are two types of primary adult osteoporosis, type I, or postmenopausal, and type II, or senile (Table 23.1).[5,11,12] In type I primary osteoporosis, there is an accelerated rate of bone loss via enhanced resorption at the onset of menopause. In this form of the disease, the loss of trabecular bone is threefold greater than the loss of cortical bone. This disproportionate loss of bone mass is the primary cause of the vertebral crush fractures and the wrist and ankle fractures experienced by postmenopausal women. In type II primary osteoporosis, which is associated with aging, the degree of bone loss is similar in both trabecular and cortical bone and is caused by decreased bone formation by the osteoblasts.[5]

Drug- or disease-induced osteoporosis, otherwise known as secondary osteoporosis (Table 23.2), accounts for up to 30% of the cases of vertebral fractures reported annually. It can be caused by a variety of factors, including long-term suppression of osteoblast function, an inhibition of calcium absorption from the gut, altered vitamin D metabolism, or excessive loss of calcium in the urine.[13] Disease states or pharmacologic therapies that result in estrogen deficiency, hyperparathyroidism, hyperthyroidism, or hypogonadism have been correlated with the development of osteoporosis.[13,14] Drug-induced osteoporosis (DIOP) is associated with the use of glucocorticoids, thyroid hormone replacement, lithium, antiepileptic agents, selective serotonin reuptake inhibitors, proton pump inhibitors, thiazolidinediones, aromatase inhibitors, gonadotropin-releasing hormone agonists, and immunosuppressive therapy.[5,13-17] See Table 23.3 for a list of the drug-specific mechanisms associated with DIOP.[13]

After estrogen deficiency related to menopause, long-term therapy with glucocorticoids represents the most prevalent cause of DIOP. As much as 3%-27% of total bone loss can occur within the first 6-12 months of

Table 23.1 Classification of Osteoporosis

Etiology	Type I Primary (Postmenopausal) Increased Osteoclast Activity and Bone Resorption	Type II Primary (Senile) Decreased Osteoblast Activity and Bone Formation; Decreased Gastrointestinal Calcium Absorption	Type II (Secondary) Drug Therapies; Disease States
Typical age at diagnosis (years)	50-75	>70	Any age
Gender ratio (women:men)	6:1	2:1	1:1
Typical fracture site	Vertebrae, distal radius	Femur, neck, hip	Vertebrae, hip, extremities
Bone morphology	Decreased trabecular bone	Decreased trabecular and normal cortical bone	Decreases cortical bone
Rate of bone loss (per year)	2%-3%	0.3%-0.5%	Variable

From Hansen LB, Vondracek SF. Prevention and treatment of nonpostmenopausal osteoporosis. *Am J Health Syst Pharm*. 2004;61:2637-2656.

Table 23.2 Representative Causes of Secondary Osteoporosis

Gastrointestinal diseases	Anorexia nervosa, chronic liver disease, pancreatic disease, primary biliary cirrhosis, malabsorption syndromes (e.g., celiac disease, Crohn disease, gastric bypass, short bowel disease)
Nutritional excesses or deficiencies	Alcoholism, calcium deficiency, vitamin D inadequacy, protein deficiency, excess vitamin A, parenteral nutrition, high salt intake.
Endocrine-based diseases	Acromegaly, diabetes mellitus (types 1 and 2), disease-related elevated hormone levels (Cushing syndrome, hyperthyroidism, hyperparathyroidism), disease-related suppressed hormone levels (androgen insensitivity, athletic amenorrhea, premature menopause)
Genetic diseases	Cystic fibrosis, glycogen storage diseases, osteogenesis imperfecta, hemochromatosis, Gaucher disease, porphyria
Other disease states	Chronic obstructive pulmonary disease, hemophilia, myeloma, AIDS/HIV, end-stage renal disease, sarcoidosis, depression, multiple sclerosis, congestive heart failure
Drugs	Corticosteroids, aromatase inhibitors, thiazolidinediones, anticonvulsants, barbiturates, heparin, chemotherapeutic agents, lithium, proton pump inhibitors, selective serotonin reuptake inhibitors

From Cosman F, de Beur SJ, LeBoff MS, et al. Clinican's guide to prevention and treatment of osteoporosis. *Osteoporos Int*. 2014;25:2359-2381 and O'Connell MB, Borgelt LM, Bowles SK, et al. Drug-induced osteoporosis in the older adult. *Aging Health*. 2010;6:501-518.

Table 23.3 Mechanisms Related to Drug-Induced Osteoporosis

Drug Therapy	Proposed Mechanism Leading to Altered Bone Mineral Density (BMD)	Citations in Ref. 17 (14-17)
Aromatase inhibitors	Inhibit conversion of androgens to estrogen	62
Gonadotropin-releasing hormone agonists	Antiandrogenic effect on pituitary gland suppressing testosterone (results in hypogonadism)	70
Thyroid hormone replacement therapy	Increase in osteoclast activation and RANKL	81
Antipsychotic agents	Stimulation of prolactin secretion lowers estrogen and testosterone levels (results in hypogonadism)	99, 100
Lithium	Hyperparathyroidism	104-106
Thiazolidinediones	Decreases osteoblast differentiation and function via PPARγ activation	117-119
Loop diuretics	Enhances renal calcium excretion	15

glucocorticoid therapy.[13] From a mechanistic perspective, glucocorticoids cause an initial increase in bone resorption as a result of their ability to increase RANKL and macrophage colony-stimulating factor. This results in an increase in osteoclastogenesis and a decrease in osteoclast apoptosis. With the ability of the glucocorticoids to cause an increase in peroxisome proliferator-activated receptor γ2 [PPARγ(2)] signaling and a decrease in Wnt signaling protein, a decrease in osteoblast formation and function and an increase in osteoblast apoptosis result, and there is a decrease in bone formation.[18]

Vitamin D deficiency, as the cause of pseudohyperparathyroidism, is also a common cause of osteoporosis in elder individuals who are institutionalized and lack adequate sunlight exposure.[2] Many of the older antiepileptic agents induce cytochrome P45024A1 (CYP24A1) enzymes, which catalyze the conversion of vitamin D to inactive metabolites.[13] Additional risk factors associated with osteoporosis are presented in Table 23.4.

The National Osteoporosis Foundation estimates that 54 million United States adults over the age of 50 years suffer from either osteoporosis or low bone mass with an estimated 64.4 million affected by 2020 and 71.2 million by 2030.[19] Non-Hispanic African American and Mexican American adults are estimated to have much lower rates (0.5 and 0.6 million, respectively) of osteoporosis or low bone mass than non-Hispanic white adults (7.7 million).[20] The prevalence of this condition and poor adherence reports (70% of patients diagnosed as being at risk for osteoporosis and receiving drug therapy fail to continue therapy after one year) continues to position osteoporosis and low bone mass as significant health concerns in the United States.[10]

Table 23.4 Lifestyle and Genetic Risk Factors for Osteoporosis

Lifestyle Factors	Genetic Factors
Smoking	Female
Sedentary lifestyle/immobilization	Family history
Milk intolerance	Small frame
Excessive caffeine	Early menopause
Excessive alcohol	
Nulliparity	
Excessive thinness/weight loss	

From Cosman F, de Beur SJ, LeBoff MS, et al. Clinican's guide to prevention and treatment of osteoporosis. *Osteoporos Int.* 2014;25:2359-2381.

Osteopetrosis

Osteopetrosis, also known as marble bone disease, describes a group of heritable disorders that are centered on a defect in osteoclast-mediated bone resorption. There are four autosomal recessive forms and one autosomal dominant form of osteopetrosis.[21] It generally is characterized by abnormally dense, brittle bone and increased skeletal mass. Unlike osteoporosis, this disorder results from decreased osteoclast activity, which has an effect on both the shape and structure of the bone. In very extreme cases, the medullary cavity, which houses bone marrow, fills with new bone, and production of hematopoietic cells is hampered. Like osteoporosis, this disease can be detected radiographically and appears as though there is a "bone within a bone."

Hypocalcemia

Hypocalcemia can be caused by PTH deficiency, vitamin D deficiency, various pharmacologic agents, and miscellaneous disorders (Table 23.5).[22] A state of hypocalcemia will inhibit calcitonin release. This results in an elevation of PTH biosynthesis and release and indirectly causes an increase in the production of vitamin D. As a result, there is an increase in serum calcium concentrations. In the absence of calcitonin, osteoclast activity is unregulated; therefore, bone resorption is accelerated. Acute hypocalcemia is best treated with IV calcium gluconate, whereas chronic hypocalcemia is best remedied with oral calcium and vitamin D supplements.

Table 23.5 Causes of Hypocalcemia

PTH Deficiency	Vitamin D Deficiency	Drugs	Miscellaneous
Hypoparathyroidism	Nutritional deficiency	Chemotherapeutic agents	Osteoblastic metastases
Pseudohypoparathyroidism	Gastrointestinal malabsorption	Diuretics, furosemide	Phosphate infusion
Hypomagnesemia	Renal Failure Tubule disorders Nephrotic syndrome Hepatobiliary disease (decreases synthesis) Pancreatic disease (malabsorption) Anticonvulsant therapy (malabsorption, abnormal metabolism)	Inhibitors of bone resorption	Rapid infusion of citrate buffered plasma or blood or large amounts of albumin

Hypercalcemia

A state of hypercalcemia (Table 23.6) will promote calcitonin biosynthesis and release. As a result, PTH biosynthesis and its secretion are inhibited, as is the production of vitamin D. As a result, serum calcium concentrations decrease. In the presence of calcitonin, osteoclast activity is inhibited, so bone resorption is slowed. In acute cases of hypercalcemia, calcitonin is administered to reestablish calcium homeostasis. Hypercalcemia also can be treated with saline hydration, IV zolendronic acid or pamidronate, glucocorticoids, and denosumab (if refractory to zolendronic acid). Loop diuretics are reserved for patients with renal insufficiency or heart failure.

Hypoparathyroidism

Hypoparathyroidism is caused by decreased serum PTH concentrations. It is characterized by hypocalcemia, hyperphosphatemia, reduced levels of circulating vitamin D, and low serum calcium concentrations. Administration of intravenous (IV) calcium gluconate and PTH serves to acutely correct plasma calcium levels. Chronic oral administration of active vitamin D as well as calcium supplements has been effective in maintaining appropriate serum calcium concentrations.

Pseudohypoparathyroidism

In this disease state, levels of PTH are normal or even elevated; however, serum calcium concentrations are low. End-organ insensitivity to PTH has been proposed to be the cause of the hypocalcemic state. Treatment of this condition with calcium and vitamin D has proven to be successful.

Hyperparathyroidism

Increased levels of PTH lead to moderate to severe elevated serum calcium concentrations and, as a result, a significant loss of calcium from the bone.[2] Deposits of calcium salts in soft tissue, as well as formation of renal calculi, also can result from this hormonal imbalance. Treatment of this condition with salmon calcitonin, loop diuretics, or other classical treatments for hypercalcemia has been favorable. The vitamin D analog paricalcitol (Zemplar), which is used for both prevention and treatment of hyperparathyroidism secondary to chronic renal failure, has been shown to reduce PTH levels by an average of 30% after 6 weeks of treatment. Whereas paricalcitol is a fully active form of vitamin D, doxercalciferol requires activation by the liver.

Doxercalciferol (Hectoral) also is indicated for the treatment of secondary hyperparathyroidism. Treatment of secondary hyperparathyroidism with vitamin D therapy is problematic, however, because it often leads to hypercalcemia, hyperphosphatemia, or both because of increased intestinal absorption of both calcium and phosphorous.[23] In patients with chronic renal failure, CaSR agonists are able to limit progression of hyperparathyroidism and growth of the parathyroid gland.

Rickets and Osteomalacia

During the Industrial Revolution, there was widespread incidence of rickets in both children and adults, because inadequate exposure to sunlight prevented the biosynthesis of the precursor to active vitamin D in the skin. Both rickets and osteomalacia are metabolic bone diseases that are characterized by poor bone mineralization. Without adequate plasma levels of vitamin D and calcium, deposition of the calcium salts in the bone markedly decreases. Vitamin D supplementation (to improve intestinal absorption of calcium and mineralization of the bone) as well as oral calcium supplementation are required to treat these diseases once established. The incidence of rickets in the United States dropped dramatically through vitamin D–supplemented food programs. The increased use of milk substitutes (e.g., soy) and reduced exposure to sunlight has recently led to a rise in rickets in the Americas, Europe and the Middle East. Rickets due to calcium deficiency is still considered to be a worldwide health problem, especially in Africa and Asia.[24]

In addition to the classical environmental or nutritional cause of these diseases, both osteomalacia and rickets can have a pharmacologic origin as a result of chronic treatment with anticonvulsants (phenobarbital and phenytoin) or glucocorticoids. These agents interfere with intestinal absorption of calcium and, thereby, cause pseudohyperparathyroidism. As a result, an increase in bone turnover and a decrease in the formation of appropriately mineralized bone are observed. In these patients, treatment with vitamin D improves calcium absorption, ultimately enhancing mineralization of the bone.

Table 23.6 Calcium Homeostasis–Related Disorders

Type of Disorder	Treatment	Examples
Disorders leading to hypercalcemia	Fluids, low-calcium diet, sulfate, glucocorticoids, calcitonin, EDTA	Hyperparathyroidism Hypervitaminosis D Sarcoidosis Neoplasia Hyperthyroidism Immobilization Paget disease of the bone
Disorders of bone remodeling	Bisphosphonates, calcitonin, estrogen, calcium, fluoride, PTH + vitamin D	Osteoporosis

EDTA, ethylenediaminetetraacetic acid.

Table 23.7 Osteoporosis Treatment Selection Criteria

Patient Data	Alendronate	Risedronate	Raloxifene	Calcitonin	Teriparatide
PM women: (+) osteoporosis/(+) fracture	X	X	X	X	X
PM women: (+) osteoporosis/(-) fracture	X				
Men: (+) osteoporosis	X				X
Corticosteroid-induced osteoporosis	X		X		
(+) Esophageal or upper GI disorder	(-)	(-)	X	X	
(+) Vasomotor symptoms	X	X	(-)	X	
(+) Venous thromboembolic event	X	X	(-)	X	
(+) Vertebral compression fracture pain				X	

From Grese TA, Sluka JP, Bryant HU, et al. Benzopyran selective estrogen receptor modulators (SERMs): pharmacological effects and structural correlation with raloxifene. *Bioorg Med Chem Lett.* 1996;6:903-908.
X, recommended; (-) not recommended; GI, gastrointestinal; PM, postmenopausal.

Paget Disease of the Bone

Paget disease of the bone (Table 23.6) is characterized by excessive bone resorption, followed by replacement of the normally mineralized bone with soft, poorly mineralized tissue.[25] It has been determined that the osteoclasts have an abnormal structure, are hyperactive, and are present at elevated levels. Patients afflicted with this painful condition often suffer from multiple compression fractures. Administration of calcitonin and oral calcium and phosphate supplements had been the treatment of choice until the bisphosphonate risedronate sodium was approved by the U.S. Food and Drug Administration (FDA). Daily administration of risedronate sodium (see later discussion of bisphosphonates) results in a decreased rate of bone turnover and a decrease in the levels of serum alkaline phosphatase and urinary hydroxyproline, two biochemical markers of bone turnover.[4] A significant advantage to treatment with the bisphosphonates is long-term suppression of the disease. Calcium supplementation, which often is necessary in these patients, must be dosed separately from risedronate sodium because calcium- and aluminum- or magnesium-containing antacids interfere with absorption of the bisphosphonates.

DRUG THERAPIES USED TO TREAT OSTEOPOROSIS

Agents used in the treatment and prevention of osteoporosis are categorized as antiresorptive agents or bone-forming agents depending on their primary mechanism of action.[14,26] For most of the effective therapies, bone mass is observed to increase for the first few years of treatment. Eventually, however, all the pits or lacunae will be filled in with new bone, and no additional increase in bone mass will occur. Antiresorptive agents have been shown to increase bone mass by as much as 8%-9% at the lumbar spine and 3%-6% in the femoral neck. Once a diagnosis of osteoporosis and the likely cause has been established, it is important to consider both patient fracture history and general medical history when selecting the appropriate treatment for a given patient (Table 23.7).[5,27]

Antiresorptive Agents

Estrogen Analogs—Estrogen Replacement Therapy

MECHANISM OF ACTION. The precise mechanism by which estrogen prevents bone resorption has not been elucidated; however, it continues to be associated with inhibition of osteoclast activity. Limited evidence supports the presence of estrogen-specific receptors (present on osteoclasts) having a biochemical role in the regulation of bone remodeling.[11] Estrogen improves calcium absorption, promotes calcitonin biosynthesis, and increases the vitamin D receptors on osteoclasts. Although the primary mechanism of action remains unclear and its use is controversial at best, estrogen replacement therapy (i.e., 17β-estradiol, estrone sodium sulfate, or 17-ethinyl estradiol) has value in the treatment and prevention of osteoporosis.[5]

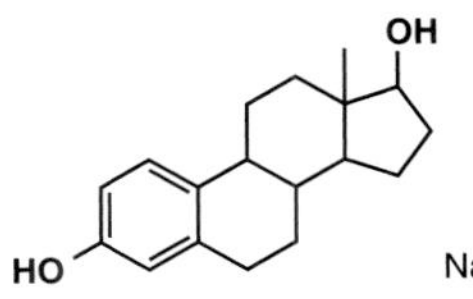

17β-estradiol

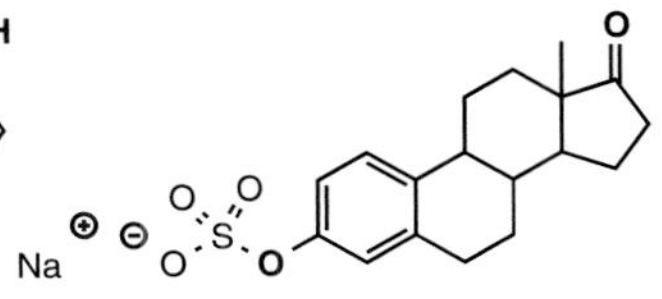

Estrone sodium sulfate

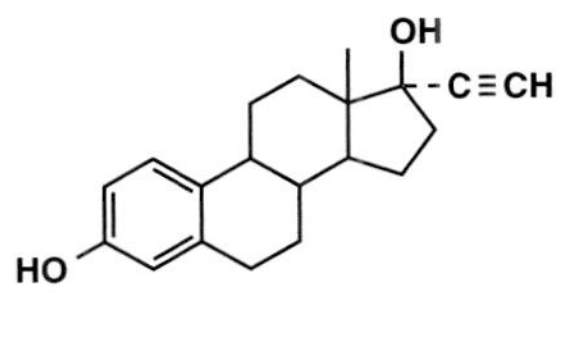

17-Ethinyl estradiol

In light of the findings of the Women's Health Initiative (WHI) study,[28] the FDA recommends the use of short-term hormone replacement therapy (estrogen and progestin) in the prevention of osteoporosis only in select cases. The pharmacokinetics of the estrogens is covered in detail in Chapter 24.

THERAPEUTIC EFFECTS. The WHI study reported that a five year course of treatment with hormone replacement therapy led to a 34% decrease of risk of clinical vertebral fracture and hip fractures and a 23% decrease in other types of osteoporetic fractures.[5] The minimum dose required and that which is considered to be standard therapy is 0.625 mg/d of conjugated estrogens (Premarin); however, a 0.3 mg/d dose of esterified estrogen (e.g., Menest) has been shown to be adequate for the prevention of osteoporosis.[5] Estrogen replacement therapy (ERT) is available in several types of formulations, including transdermal patches (e.g., 17β-estradiol: Alora, Climera, Estraderm, Menostar, Vivelle-Dot).

Initiated at the onset of menopause, this therapy also has favorable effects on serum cholesterol levels (reduces low-density lipoprotein and elevates high-density lipoprotein levels). Women taking ERT have found relief from hot flashes, vaginal dryness, and urinary stress incontinence.[26] It is recommended that the estrogen be combined with a progestin for those women with an intact uterus so as to decrease the risk of endometrial cancer.[11]

Selective Estrogen Receptor Modulators

TAMOXIFEN CITRATE AND RALOXIFENE HYDROCHLORIDE (EVISTA). Tamoxifen citrate, classified chemically as a triarylethylene, is a selective estrogen receptor modulator (SERM). As an antiestrogenic agent in breast tissue, it is indicated as adjuvant therapy in the treatment of axillary node–negative or –positive breast cancer following partial or full mastectomy. Raloxifene hydrochloride (Evista), a benzothiophene derivative, is a semi-rigid analog of tamoxifen (Fig. 23.5).

The two drugs are similar in that they both possess agonist activity in certain tissues (e.g., bone, cardiovascular) and antagonist activity in others (e.g., breast, uterus) (see Chapter 24).[26] Raloxifene hydrochloride, the first selective estrogen receptor modulator (SERM) approved for the prevention of osteoporosis in postmenopausal women, acts as an estrogen agonist on receptors in osteoblasts and osteoclasts but as an antagonist at breast and uterine estrogen receptors. This selective action means that this agent does not increase the risk of endometrial or breast cancer, as is the case with long-term tamoxifen therapy. Because this agent does not have a stimulatory effect at its receptors on most tissues, it does not prevent the hot flashes and other symptoms of menopause as estrogen does.[5,28]

Therapeutic Action. Raloxifene hydrochloride decreases the risk of vertebral fracture by 30% but has no bearing on nonvertebral or hip fractures. Long-term treatment with raloxifene hydrochloride has beneficial effects on breast cancer in high-risk patients; however it increases the risk of cardiovascular events.[29,30] Raloxifene hydrochloride has been shown to have a beneficial effect on lipid profiles.[29] Raloxifene hydrochloride should not be administered in combination with cholestyramine (decreased absorption), warfarin (prothrombin times and international normalized ratios must be monitored more closely), and those drugs that are highly protein bound, such as clofibrate, diazepam, ibuprofen, indomethacin, and naproxen.[31]

Structure-Activity Relationship. From a structural perspective, the only pure antiestrogens are 7α-substituted estrogens.[26] In the triarylethylene class of agents (e.g., tamoxifen), the phenol or phenoxy ring system is critical for interaction with the portion of the estrogen receptor (ER) protein referred to as the activation factor-2 (AF-2) region, because it mimics the essential C3 phenol group found in estrogen.[26] This interaction initiates a change in protein conformation to the form of the receptor able to interact with a specific deoxyribonucleic acid (DNA) sequence known as the estrogen responding element (ERE). As a result, activation of a specific group of genes occurs, and protein biosynthesis ensues. The orientation of the three aryl rings in a propeller type of arrangement also is important for tight receptor binding and biologic activity.[26] In raloxifene hydrochloride, the substituted benzothiophene ring mimics the estrogen A ring; however because of the presence of a semirigid, amine-containing side chain, raloxifene is unable to interact with AF-2.[32,33] As a result, interaction with ERE is prevented and antiestrogenic action is observed in reproductive tissues. The raloxifene hydrochloride-estrogen receptor (ER) complex, in concert with specific adapter proteins, is also able to interact with and activate a raloxifene responding element (RRE). Activation of this DNA sequence facilitates activation of another group of genes responsible for the production of proteins that allows for agonist action in nonreproductive tissues.[32,33]

Pharmacokinetics. Raloxifene hydrochloride is rapidly absorbed following oral administration, with an estimated 60% absorption, but it has a very low bioavailability

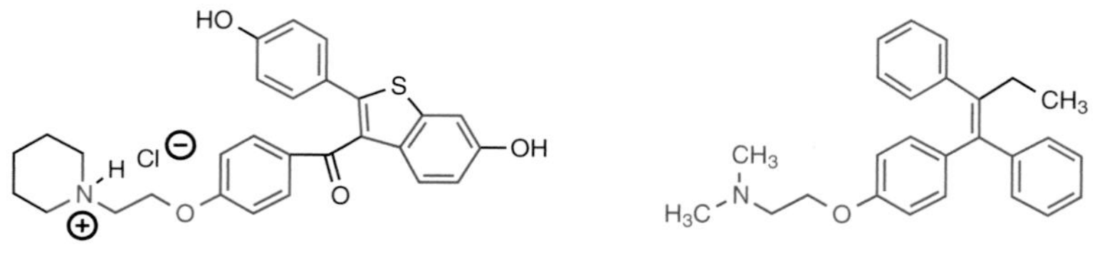

Raloxifene hydrochloride (Evista)

Tamoxifen (Nolvadex)

Figure 23.5 Structures of raloxifene and tamoxifen highlighting the structural similarity between the two drugs.

(2%), associated with extensive phase II metabolism. The metabolites are excreted via the bile, with potential enterohepatic recycling that could account for the interaction with cholestyramine. Supportive of the enterohepatic recycling is the half-life of 28 hours. Metabolism of raloxifene hydrochloride occurs to a great extent in the intestine and consists of glucuronide conjugation catalyzed by uridine diphosphate glucuronosyltransferase (UGT).[31] The UGT1A family is responsible for intestinal human metabolism, as shown in Figure 23.6. Efflux by intestinal cells of the resulting glucuronide occurs via P-glycoprotein and multidrug resistance–related protein. The combination of rapid metabolism and efflux can account for the low bioavailability. Raloxifene action is diminished when co-administered with warfarin.

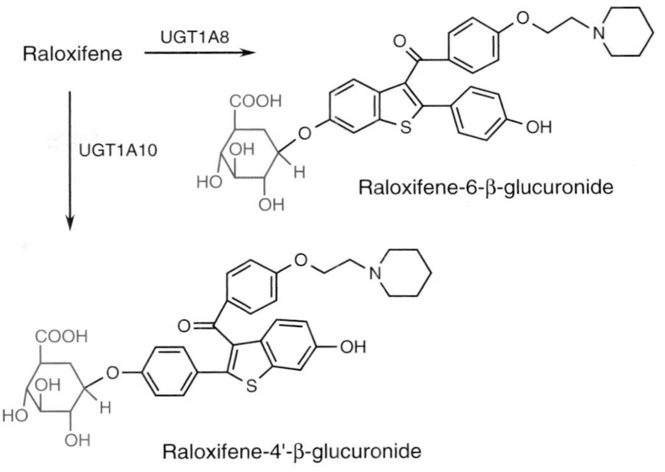

Figure 23.6 Metabolism of raloxifene.

BAZEDOXIFENE ACETATE. Bazedoxifene acetate is an indole-based third generation SERM that is used in combination with conjugate estrogens (Duavee) for the prevention of postmenopausal osteoporosis and for the treatment of moderate to severe vasomotor symptoms associated with menopause. It is recommended for patients who cannot or refuse to take bisphosphonates due to issues related to either tolerability or safety[34] who have an intact uterus. For those patients who anticipate the need for long term therapy, bazedoxifene may be an appropriate alternative to avoid the effects of long term bisphosphonate therapy.

Therapeutic Action. This combination of agents is referred to as a tissue selective estrogen complex (TSEC). It acts as an estrogen agonist at the bone and as an estrogen antagonist at the uterus and breast.[35] Bazedoxifene acetate displaces 17β-estradiol from ERs and has excellent binding affinity for the receptor itself (both ERα and ERβ). It is less ERα selective than raloxifene and exhibits 10-fold less affinity for ERα than 17β-estradiol. Unlike raloxifene hydrochloride, this agent does not cause hot flashes at the doses required to have a beneficial effect on bone.

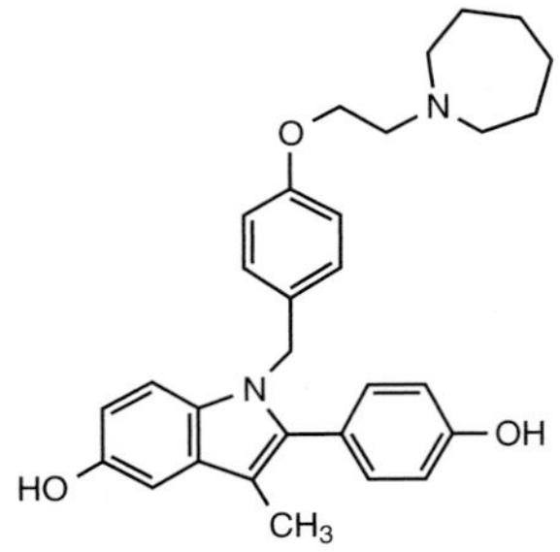

Pharmacokinetics. This combination agent can be administered orally (once daily) with or without meals. Calcium and vitamin D supplements are important adjunct therapy. Given that estrogens are at least partially metabolized by CYP3A4, this combination agent should not be given concurrently with inducers or inhibitors of this isoform. Glucuronidated metabolites have been isolated; therefore agents that induce UGT (e.g., rifampin, carbamazepine) should also be avoided.[35] This combination agent is eliminated via urinary and biliary routes and is not recommended in patients with renal or hepatic impairment. The primary adverse effects include muscle spasms, dizziness, nausea, diarrhea, dyspepsia, as well as neck and throat pain. Given the inclusion of an estrogen component, it is prudent to monitor for any signs or symptoms of cardiovascular effects.[35]

Bisphosphonates

MECHANISM OF ACTION. The bisphosphonates are synthetic in origin and are designed to mimic pyrophosphate, where the oxygen in P-O-P is replaced with a carbon atom to create a nonhydrolyzable backbone (Fig. 23.7).[36] Because pyrophosphate is a normal constituent of bone, these analogs selectively target the hydroxyapatite portion of the bone. Mechanistically the bisphosphonates can be split into two categories. The nonnitrogen bisphosphonates (e.g., clondronate) (Fig. 23.8) most closely mimic pyrophosphate and get incorporated into nonhydrolyzable ATP analogs via amino acyl tRNA synthetases. The resulting nonhydrolyzable nucleotides accumulate within osteoclasts and negatively impact their function. The nitrogen-containing bisphosphonates (e.g., alendronate, palmidronate, ibandronate) (Fig. 23.8) operate by a distinctly different mechanism. This is largely accomplished via inhibition of the mevalonate pathway (specifically farnesyl pyrophosphate synthetase, FPPS) and interferes with protein prenylation within osteoclasts, as well as via inhibition of ATP-dependent enzymes (impairing cellular energetics). By these mechanisms,

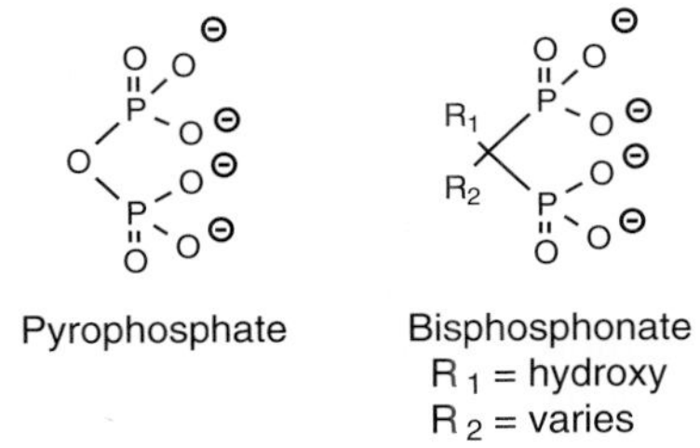

Figure 23.7 Bisphosphonate structure-activity relationships.

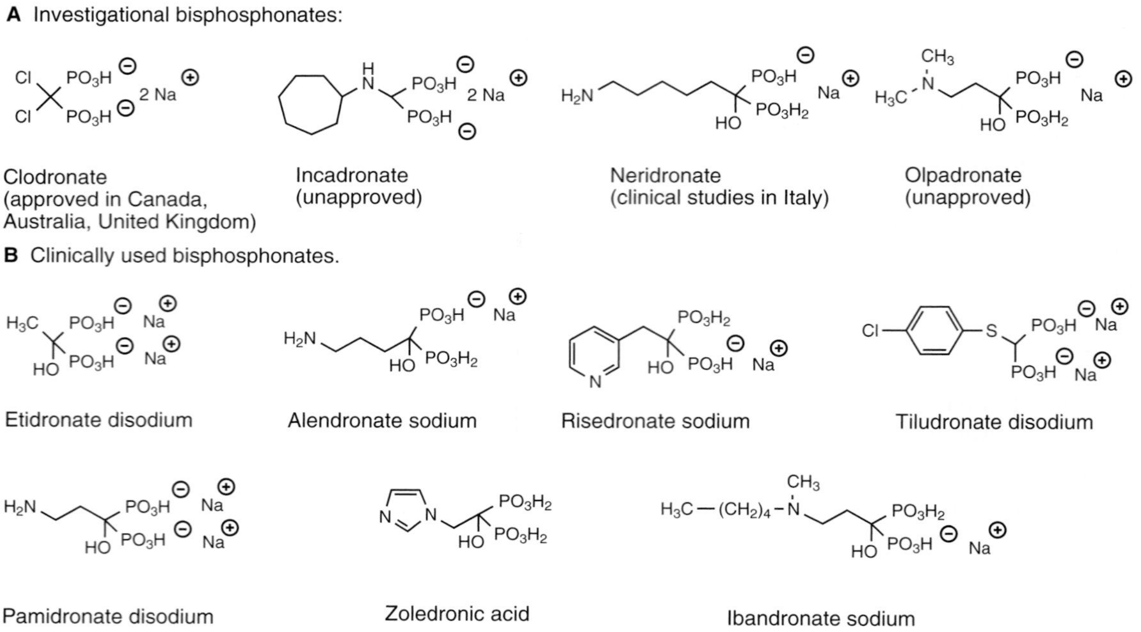

A Investigational bisphosphonates:

Clodronate (approved in Canada, Australia, United Kingdom)

Incadronate (unapproved)

Neridronate (clinical studies in Italy)

Olpadronate (unapproved)

B Clinically used bisphosphonates.

Etidronate disodium

Alendronate sodium

Risedronate sodium

Tiludronate disodium

Pamidronate disodium

Zoledronic acid

Ibandronate sodium

Figure 23.8 Bisphosphonates: investigational and clinically used.

the bisphosphonates are able to limit bone turnover and allow the osteoblasts to form well-mineralized bone without opposition.[36]

STRUCTURE-ACTIVITY RELATIONSHIPS. From a structural perspective, the nitrogen-containing bisphosphonates have been proposed to have specific molecular interactions with their biologic target for drug action farnesyl pyrophosphate synthetase (FPPS), and structure-activity relationships (SARs) have been elucidated. The central carbon of the geminal phosphonate has been substituted with a variety of functional groups to yield a large family of compounds with differing physicochemical and biologic properties.[37,38] The SAR studies (Fig. 23.7) have concluded that a hydroxyl substituent (R_1) maximizes the affinity of the agent for the hydroxyapatite as well as improves the antiresorptive character of the agent.[38] The bisphosphonate itself, as well as the hydroxyl group at R_1, should be included as critical SAR features due to their ability to act as a bone "hook."[38] Because structural variation of R_2 has a significant effect on potency, it can be surmised that R_2 interacts at an "active site" and participates in a specific molecular interaction within a carbocation binding site within the biological target.

The character of the R_2 substituent varies widely and clearly has a significant influence on the potency of this class of compounds (Fig. 23.8). The R_2 amino–substituted bisphosphonates (pamidronate disodium, alendronate sodium, and neridronate) are more potent than etidronate disodium and clodronate disodium (not available in the United States). The R_2 3-carbon amino linear chain for alendronate sodium is more potent than the R_2 2-carbon derivative pamidronate disodium and the R_2 6-carbon analog neridronate.[38] Alkylation of the amine functional group improves potency as is demonstrated by compounds with N substituted amino alkyls at R_2 (e.g., olpadronate, ibandronate sodium) and those that contain rings at R_2 (e.g., risedronate sodium, incadronate, tiludronate disodium, zoledronic acid). The third-generation analogs contain a basic heterocyclic side chain at R_2 tethered to the central carbon by a variety of linkages (potency: $NH > CH_2 > S > O$).[38]

PHARMACOKINETICS. To date, four generations of bisphosphonates have been developed for the treatment of osteoporosis (Fig. 23.8). Absorption of these agents from the gut is quite poor (1%-5%) because of their polar nature, and as a therapeutic class, they have limited cellular penetration.[39] A significant portion of the actual absorbed dose is taken up specifically by the bone within 4-6 hours, and the rest is exclusively excreted by the kidney. Uptake of these agents in the bone is concentrated in areas of the bone that are actively undergoing remodeling.[39] Between the selective uptake and the rapid rate of clearance, the bisphosphonates enjoy a short circulating half-life and very limited drug exposure to nontarget tissues.[37] Because the bisphosphonates are only released from the bone when the bone is resorbed, they have a tissue half-life of 1-10 years; however, these agents remain pharmacologically active only while they are exposed on bone resorption surfaces.[39]

SPECIFIC DRUGS

Alendronate Sodium (Fosamax). The second-generation agent alendronate sodium was the first bisphosphonate agent approved by the FDA for the prevention and treatment of osteoporosis and Paget disease of the bone and is 1,000-fold more potent than etidronate disodium (Fig. 23.8).[40,41] Alendronate sodium is also indicated for the treatment of glucocorticoid-induced osteoporosis. This derivative, when dosed continuously (5-10 mg/d for osteoporosis and 40 mg/d for Paget disease of the bone) and given with oral calcium supplements (500 mg/d), produced well-mineralized bone and significantly improved BMD (7% in the spine and 4% in the hip) within 18 months.[6] In addition, the vertebral fracture rate was shown to decrease by 47%. A side effect associated with alendronate sodium, chemical esophagitis, has been attributed to inadequate intake of water and lying down after taking the medication.[2] Specific patient instructions were developed to limit the incidence of upper gastrointestinal problems and include (1) taking the medication with 6-8 ounces of water on arising in the morning, (2) remaining in an upright position for at least 30 minutes after taking the medication, and (3) delaying drinking other liquids/eating for at least 30 minutes, if not 1-2 hours, to allow maximal absorption of the agent.[14] To enhance absorption, calcium supplements and any aluminum- or magnesium-containing antacids should be dosed separately from agents in this class. These agents are not recommended in patients with renal impairment (serum creatinine, <2.5 mg/dL), a history of esophageal disease, gastritis, or peptic ulcer.[5] In an attempt to address the inconvenience associated with tablet administration, a once-weekly, 70-mg buffered effervescent formulation of alendronate is available (Binosto).

Risedronate Sodium (Actonel). The third-generation agent risedronate sodium has been approved for both the prevention and treatment of osteoporosis (both postmenopausal and in men), Paget disease of the bone, and glucocorticoid-induced osteoporosis (Fig. 23.8).[40,42] Risedronate sodium is 1,000- to 5,000-fold more potent than etidronate disodium. At the end of an 18-month study, 53% of patients who took risedronate sodium for 2 months remained in remission, as compared to 14% of patients who took etidronate disodium, an earlier-generation bisphosphonate, for 6 months. Oral administration of this agent suffers from the same problems as that of other bisphosphonate agents. Risedronate sodium should not be given to patients with creatinine clearance of less than 30 mL/min. A once-weekly, delayed-release formulation (Atelvia) that can be taken immediately after breakfast with 4 oz. of water is available. Other oral formulations of risedronate sodium include tablets to be consumed daily (5 mg) and monthly (150 mg).

Ibandronate Sodium (Boniva). Ibandronate sodium is approved for the treatment and prevention of osteoporosis in postmenopausal women and has a mechanism of action that is identical to the other bisphosphonate agents (Fig. 23.8). Administered daily (2.5 mg), ibandronate sodium has been clinically shown to reduce the risk of vertebral fractures by 62%.[43] It has little to no effect on nonvertebral or hip fractures.[14] If administered on an intermittent basis (20 mg), it reduces the risk of vertebral fractures by 50%. Ibandronate sodium (2.5 mg daily), along with 500 mg of supplemental calcium, has been clinically shown to increase BMD in the hip (1.8%), femoral neck (2.0%), and lumbar spine (3.1%). A 150-mg formulation has been approved by the FDA for once-monthly administration as well as a 3-mg IV formulation for quarterly administration.

ADDITIONAL DOSAGE FORMS

A unique formulation of alendronate sodium, FOSAMAX PLUS D, includes 70 mg of alendronate sodium and 2,800 or 5,600 IU of vitamin D_3 (i.e., a 7-day supply of both the bisphosphonate and vitamin D). This formulation should not be used in patients with severe kidney disease or low serum calcium levels and should not be the only therapy used to correct a vitamin D deficiency.

Risedronate sodium with calcium carbonate (Actonel with Calcium) represents an additional type of packaging for this class of agents. It addresses the Surgeon General's Report on Bone Health and Osteoporosis, which states that treatments for osteoporosis need to be made simpler and more structured. Sold in units that contain a 1-month supply, each week of therapy includes a total of seven tablets, including one 35mg tablet of risedronate and six 500mg tablets of calcium carbonate.

The oral bioavailability of this agent is extremely poor (0.6%) and is adversely affected by the presence of food, beverages other than water, and other medications, including calcium or vitamin D supplements and antacids.[43] Because of the increased calcium content in mineral water, patients should not take this medication with this type of water. Drugs that inhibit gastric acid secretion (e.g., H_2 antagonists, proton pump inhibitors) actually promote ibandronate sodium absorption. Like the other agents in this therapeutic class, ibandronate sodium is not metabolized, and that which is not bound to the bone (40%-50% of the absorbed dose) is eliminated renally unchanged. It does not inhibit the CYP450 isozymes. This agent does not require any dosage adjustment for patients with hepatic impairment or mild to moderate renal impairment (creatinine clearance, >30 mL/min). Ibandronate sodium should not be prescribed for patients with severe renal impairment (creatinine clearance, <30 mL/min).[43]

Zoledronic Acid (Reclast; Zometa). Zoledronic acid is approved for the treatment of glucocorticoid-induced osteoporosis and prevention and treatment of postmenopausal osteoporosis, male osteoporosis, and Paget disease of the bone (Fig. 23.8). For the treatment of osteoporosis, zoledronic acid (Zometa) is formulated as a 5-mg, once-yearly IV infusion. The frequency of IV infusion decreases to 5 mg every 2 years for the prevention of osteoporosis. In order to prevent hypocalcemia, concomitant calcium (1,500 mg) and vitamin D (800-1,000 IU) intake and/or supplementation is recommended in patients being treated for osteoporosis. On the day of treatment, patients should drink at least two glasses of water and eat normally.

Osteonecrosis of the jaw has been reported in patients receiving IV bisphosphonate therapy.[44] The majority of the patients who developed osteonecrosis of the jaw were undergoing chemotherapy (typically for multiple myeloma, breast, prostate, or lung cancers), taking corticosteroids, and had undergone a dental procedure (e.g., tooth extraction). The FDA recommends that patients receive a thorough dental examination before initiation of IV bisphosphonate therapy and that they avoid invasive dental work during treatment.

There have also been reports of an increase in risk of atypical femur fracture in patients undergoing long-term bisphosphonate therapy.[45,46] In addition, an increase in the risk of developing esophageal cancer has surfaced in patients with approximately 5 years of oral bisphosphonate use. Because of these adverse effects, it is recommended that clinicians weigh the benefits against the potential risks.

The remaining bisphosphonates, pamidronate disodium and zoledronic acid, are approved for treatment of hypercalcemia of malignancy as well as other cancer conditions and will be discussed later in the chapter.

Calcitonin (Miacalcin)

Calcitonin (see earlier discussion in this chapter) has been approved for the treatment of postmenopausal osteoporosis, hypercalcemia of malignancy, and Paget disease of the bone. The calcitonin isolated from salmon is the preferred source, because it has greater receptor affinity and a longer half-life than the human hormone.[7]

STRUCTURE-ACTIVITY RELATIONSHIPS. Calcitonin is commercially available as synthetic calcitonin-salmon, which contains the same linear sequence of 32 amino acids, as occurs in natural calcitonin-salmon. Calcitonin-salmon differs structurally from human calcitonin at 16 of 32 amino acids (see Fig. 23.9 for primary structure differences between human and salmon calcitonin). A disulfide bond (Cys1-Cys7) is required for biological activity.

PHARMACOKINETICS. The pharmacologic activity of these calcitonins is the same, but calcitonin-salmon is approximately 50-fold more potent on a weight basis than human calcitonin with a longer duration of action. The duration of action for calcitonin salmon is 8-24 hours following intramuscular (IM) or subcutaneous (SC) administration and 0.5-12.0 hours following IV administration. The parenteral dose required for the treatment of osteoporosis is 100 IU/d.[47] The peptide hormone calcitonin-salmon is also available as a nasal spray.[6] The bioavailability of calcitonin-salmon nasal spray shows great variability (range, 0.3%-30.6% of an IM dose). It is absorbed rapidly from the nasal mucosa, with peak plasma concentrations appearing 30-40 minutes after nasal administration, compared with 16-25 minutes following parental dosing. Calcitonin-salmon is readily metabolized in the kidney, with an elimination half-life calculated at 43 minutes. As a result, the intranasal dose required is 200 IU/d.

THERAPEUTIC APPLICATION. Calcitonin therapy requires the concomitant oral administration of elemental calcium (500 mg/d, see Table 23.8). Clinical studies have shown that the combination of intranasal calcitonin-salmon (200 IU/d), oral calcium supplementation (>1,000 mg/d of elemental calcium), and vitamin D (400 IU/d) has decreased the rate of new fractures by more than 75% and has improved vertebral BMD by as much as 3% annually.[47] Calcitonin prevents the abnormal bone turnover characteristic of Paget disease of the bone and has antiresorptive activity. Side effects are significantly more pronounced when calcitonin-salmon is administered by injection and can include nausea, vomiting, anorexia, and flushing.[47] Because calcitonin-salmon is protein in nature, the possibility of a systemic allergic reaction should be considered, and appropriate measures for treatment of hypersensitivity reaction should be readily available. Although calcitonin-salmon does not cross the placenta, it may pass into breast milk. Calcitonin-salmon is a possible alternative to ERT; however, only limited evidence suggests that it has efficacy in women who already have fractures. Resistance to calcitonin-salmon can result from the development of neutralizing antibodies.[47]

In addition to its antiresorptive action via suppression of osteoclast activity, calcitonin-salmon exhibits a potent analgesic effect and has provided considerable relief to those patients suffering from the pain associated with Paget disease of the bone and osteoporosis. This analgesic effect is a result of calcitonin-stimulated endogenous opioid release. The potency of this analgesic effect has been demonstrated to be 30- to 50-fold

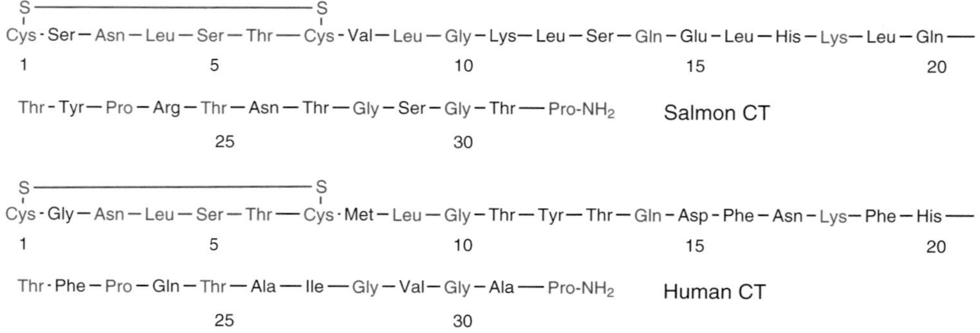

Figure 23.9 Primary structures of salmon and human calcitonin (CT). Similarities are highlighted in red.

Table 23.8 Percent of Elemental Calcium Content in Various Salts

Salt	Calcium (%)	Elemental Calcium (mg/tablet)
Calcium carbonate	40	
Tums (500 mg chewable)		200 mg
Os-Cal 500 (1,250 mg tablet)		500 mg
Viactive (1,250 mg chewable)		500 mg
Tribasic calcium phosphate	39 27 23	
Posture (1,565.2 mg tablets)		600 mg
Calcium citrate	21	
Citrical (950 mg tablets)		200 mg
Citrical Liquitab (2,376 mg effervescent tablets)		500 mg
Calcium lactate	13	
Generics (325 mg tablets)		42 mg
Generics (650 mg tablets)		84 mg
Calcium gluconate	9.3	
Generics (500 mg tablets)		46.5 mg
Generics (650 mg tablets)		60.4 mg
Calcium glubionate	6.5	
Neo-Calglucon (1.8 g/5 mL syrup)		115 mg/5 mL

From Haines ST, Caceres B, Yancey L. Alternatives to estrogen replacement therapy for preventing osteoporosis. *J Am Pharm Assoc.* 1996;NS36:707-715.

that of morphine in selected patients. Calcitonin is preferred over estrogen and the bisphosphonates when treatment of both osteoporosis and related bone pain is warranted.

Bone-Forming Agents

Teriparatide (Forteo)

Teriparatide is approved for the treatment of postmenopausal osteoporosis in patients who have a high risk of fracture, for the treatment of glucocorticoid-induced osteoporosis, and to increase bone mass in men with primary or hypogonadal osteoporosis who have a high risk of fracture.[48] Teriparatide is recombinant human PTH 1-34 (Fig. 23.2), the biologically active portion of the endogenously produced preprohormone. Unlike the bisphosphonates, which are classified as bone restorative agents, teriparatide is the first approved bone-forming agent.

MECHANISM OF ACTION. Teraparatide is an agonist at the parathyroid hormone type 1 receptor (PTHR1), a GPCR. Receptor activation leads to a prolonged response to the cAMP second messenger. This receptor is also activated by parathyroid hormone related peptide (PTHrP), however the cAMP response is much shorter.[49] Bone formation is possible because of the ability of this agent to increase the number of osteoblasts. Although teriparatide enhances the function of both osteoclasts and osteoblasts, the exposure incidence dictates its effect on the skeleton. If administered once daily or intermittently, teriparatide preferentially enhances osteoblastic function, and bone formation occurs. Continuous exposure to endogenous PTH may result in poor skeletal composition because of enhanced osteoclast-mediated bone resorption.[50] After 18 months of treatment, lumbar BMD increased up to 12% in postmenopausal women. After 10 months of treatment, 53% of men had an increase of 5% or greater in spine bone mineral density (BMD). The risk for developing new vertebral fractures was reduced by 65% after 18 months of treatment, and the number of nonvertebral fragility fractures was reduced by 35%.[51] There is limited evidence that teriparatide can regrow jaw bone that has been damaged by osteonecrosis and periodontitis.

PHARMACOKINETICS. Administered as a once-daily 20-μg SC injection in the thigh or abdominal wall, teriparatide is a clear, colorless liquid. Concurrent calcium (1,000 mg) and vitamin D (400 IU) supplementation is recommended. Teriparatide is rapidly absorbed, demonstrates 95% bioavailability, and is quickly eliminated via both hepatic and extrahepatic routes.[48] The half-life is 1 hour when administered SC. Metabolic studies have not been performed on teriparatide; however, the entire PTH preprohormone has been shown to undergo enzyme-mediated transformations in the liver. Dizziness, nausea, and leg cramps are the most commonly reported adverse side effects.[5]

Temporary increases in serum calcium levels occur following administration of teriparatide. As a result, this agent is contraindicated in patients who are predisposed to hypercalcemia. Teriparatide should not be prescribed to patients with Paget disease of the bone, children, young adults, women who are pregnant or nursing, and patients who have received skeletal radiation therapy.[5]

A black box warning from the FDA advises that treatment with teriparatide should be avoided in patients with an increased baseline risk for osteosarcoma and that treatment should not exceed 2 years in a patient's lifetime.[30]

Abaloparatide (Tymlos)

H-Ala-Val-Ser-Glu-His-Gln-Leu-Leu-His-Asp-Lys-Ser-Ile-Gln-Asp-Leu-Arg-Arg-Arg-Glu-Leu-

-Glu-Lys-Aib-Lys-Leu-His-Thr-Ala-NH_2

Abaloparatide

Abaloparatide was approved in April 2017 for the treatment of postmenopausal women with osteoporosis at high risk for fracture. It has been shown to reduce the risk of vertebral and nonvertebral fractures regardless of age, timeframe post menopause, prior fracture history, and bone mineral density at the start of treatment. After 18 months of treatment, there was a 43% reduction in nonvertebral fracture risk compared to the 28% decrease observed with teriparatide.[49,52] Vertebral fracture risk was decreased by 86% and 80%, respectively. A black box warning for an increased risk of osteosarcoma in rats translates to understanding that this agent is not recommended for those with Paget disease of the bone, elevated alkaline phosphatase, bone metastases, or skeletal malignancies. As with teriparatide, therapy is not recommended to exceed a total of 2 years in a patient's lifetime.[53]

STRUCTURE-ACTIVITY RELATIONSHIP. Abaloparatide is a 34–amino acid synthetic analog of parathyroid hormone-related hormone protein [PTHrP (1-34)]. It retains 76% sequence homology with human PTHrP(1-34) and 41% homology with PTH (1-34).

MECHANISM OF ACTION. Parathyroid hormone receptor type 1 (PTHR1) interacts with two endogenous ligands, PTH and parathyroid hormone-related protein (PTHrP) and can adopt two conformations, R° and RG.[54] As a PTHR1 agonist, abaloparatide has greater selectivity for the RG PTHR1 conformation. Whereas activation of the RG conformation of PTH1R leads to receptor signaling that is short lived, activation of the R° conformation yields a more long-lived response. Given that intermittent PTH receptor activation generally is associated with a bone-forming response, it is no surprise that abaloparatide promotes bone formation with less bone resorption and hypercalcemia than found with PTH (1-34).[54]

PHARMACOKINETICS. Abaloparatide is administered as a once daily subcutaneous injection. Supplementation with calcium and vitamin D is recommended should dietary intake be compromised. It has a mean half-life of 1.7 hours, which allows nearly complete clearance prior to the next injection (hence being considered intermittent vs. continuous dosing).[52,53] It is 36% bioavailable and is largely renally eliminated as peptide fragments. Dosage adjustment is not required in patients with severe renal impairment. It has not been shown to inhibit or induce CYP450 enzymes and is 70% bound by plasma proteins.[52] Adverse effects include hypercalciuria, dizziness, nausea, upper respiratory tract infection, and headache.[52] Patients are also at risk for developing hypercalcemia and therefore should not be administered to those diagnosed with primary hyperparathyroidism or other hypercalcemic conditions. Anti-drug antibodies were present in 49% of patients taking abaloparatide.

Monoclonal Antibody–Based Therapies

RANKL Inhibitor

DENOSUMAB (PROLIA, XGEVA)

Mechanism of Action. Denosumab is approved for the treatment of postmenopausal women with osteoporosis at high risk for fracture. Denosumab is a fully human IgG2 monoclonal antibody to RANKL, where it functions as a RANKL inhibitor (Fig. 23.4). The RANKL receptor is expressed on the surface of osteoclasts and osteoclast precursors. When bound to its receptor, RANKL promotes the formation and activation of osteoclasts. To balance the effects of RANKL, osteoblasts produce osteoprotegerin, which binds to RANKL and prevents it from binding to and activating its receptor, modulating the production and activation of osteoclasts.[30] When an individual develops osteoporosis, this balance is "disrupted," and RANKL overwhelms osteoprotegerin activity, causing significant bone loss. Denosumab was designed to mimic the biochemical effects of osteoprotegerin. Studies show that denosumab is more effective in improving BMD (4%-7%) than weekly administration of alendronate (5%).[30] Denosumab is reported to reduce the risk of vertebral fraction (68%), hip fracture (40%), and nonvertebral facture (20%).[55] This agent has been associated with adverse events including hypocalcemia and osteonecrosis of the jaw.[56]

Pharmacokinetics. Denosumab is administered once every 4 weeks as a subcutaneous injection. It has a bioavailability of 62%.[56] The mean elimination half-life is 28 days, and clearance and volume of distribution are proportional to body weight. Renal impairment has no effect on its pharmacokinetics.

Inorganic Salts

CALCIUM SALTS. Appropriate intake of calcium during childhood, adolescence, and early adulthood increases peak BMD and may reduce the overall risk of developing osteoporosis. For those who are at low risk of developing osteoporosis and have adequate BMD, consumption of the recommended amounts of calcium (1,300 mg/d of elemental calcium for teenagers, 1,000 mg/d for premenopausal women and men, and 1,200 mg/d for postmenopausal women) typically is sufficient to prevent bone loss.[57] This often can be accomplished by eating a well-balanced diet. For patients with established osteoporosis or areas of poorly mineralized bone, calcium supplementation alone is not sufficient to reverse the bone loss or to significantly improve mineralization of the bone.[30]

It should be noted that a study conducted by Bolland et al.[58] reported that calcium supplementation in postmenopausal women may be correlated with significant increases in the rates of vascular events.

The actual amount of elemental calcium that is present in the available calcium salts varies considerably; however, no one particular salt has been identified as an exceptional source of elemental calcium (Table 23.8). Absorption of calcium from the gastrointestinal tract (25%-40%) improves under acidic conditions; therefore, those medications that change the acidic environment of the stomach (e.g., H_2 antagonists, proton pump inhibitors) have an adverse effect on calcium absorption. Total daily doses of elemental calcium that exceed 500 mg should be spaced out over the day to improve absorption.[5] The more water soluble and, therefore, more easily absorbed salts (e.g., citrate, lactate, gluconate) are less dependent on the acidic environment for appropriate absorption[14] and would be appropriate alternatives for patients who produce low levels of acid. Calcium carbonate is a poorly soluble form of calcium, but it is inexpensive and only requires the patient to take a few tablets per day with acidic food or beverages like citrus juice.

DRUG THERAPIES USED TO TREAT HYPERPARATHYROIDISM

Increased levels of PTH lead to moderately to severely elevated serum calcium concentrations and alterations in phosphorous metabolism.[2] To modulate the levels of PTH released from the parathyroid gland chief cells, regulation of calcium-sensing receptor (CaSR) sensitivity is required. An agonist at this receptor, a calcimimetic, serves to activate the receptor, whereas an antagonist at this receptor is classified as a calcilytic. There are two types of calcimimetic agents: agonists that activate the CaSR directly (type I) (e.g., calcium, other divalent cations), and those that are positive allosteric modulators (type II).[59] The type II calcimimetics sensitize the CaSR to calcium. When calcium binds and activates the extracellular portion of the CaSR, the resulting cascade of intracellular signaling suppresses the secretion of PTH, causing a decrease in serum calcium levels.

Cinacalcet Hydrochloride (Sensipar)

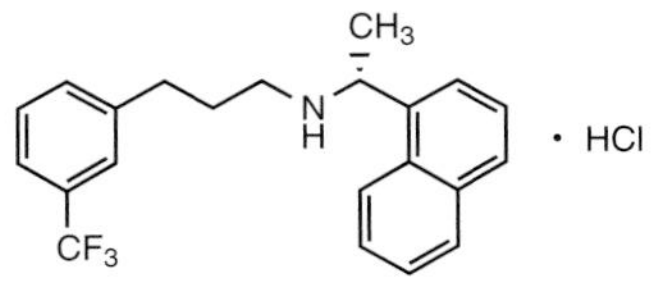

CH_3 N H · HCl CF_3

Cinacalcet hydrochloride (Sensipar)

Mechanism of Action

Cinacalcet hydrochloride is a second-generation calcimimetic approved for the treatment of secondary hyperparathyroidism in patients with chronic kidney disease on dialysis and for the treatment of hypercalcemia in patients with parathyroid cancer. Cinacalcet binds to the transmembrane region of CaSR and induces a conformational change in the receptor such that it is now more sensitive to calcium.[23,59,60] Upon receptor activation phospholipase C is activated, and the secretion of PTH is inhibited. In the presence of cinacalcet, not only is a decrease in PTH levels observed, but a decrease in serum calcium and phosphorous levels is also observed. This represents a significant therapeutic advantage over vitamin D–based treatments for secondary hyperparathyroidism.[23] It can be used alone, with vitamin D and/or with a phosphate binder.[61]

Pharmacokinetics

Administered orally once daily, cinacalcet has an initial half-life of 6 hours and a terminal half-life of 30-40 hours. It is 93%-97% bound to plasma proteins and absorption is enhanced when taken with a high-fat meal. Cinacalcet is metabolized primarily by CYP3A4, less so by CYP2D6 and CYP1A2.[59,60] It is a strong inhibitor of CYP2D6. Caution is advised for coadministration with an inhibitor of either CPY 3A4 and with drugs that are primarily metabolized by CYP2D6. While no dosage adjustment is required for renal impairment, patients with moderate to severe hepatic impairment should be monitored.[61] Common adverse effects include nausea and vomiting.

Etelcalcetide (Parsabiv)

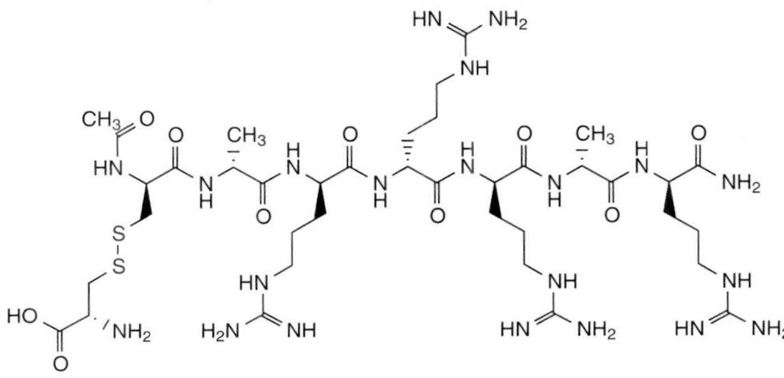

HN NH$_2$ NH CH_3 O O CH_3 H O H O CH_3 H O HN N N N N N NH$_2$ H O H O H O S S HN NH NH HO NH$_2$ H$_2$N NH HN NH$_2$ HN NH$_2$ O

Etelcalcetide

Mechanism of Action

Etelcalcetide is a second generation type II calcimimetic approved for the treatment of secondary hyperparathyroidism in patients with chronic kidney disease who receive dialysis. This agent is a long-acting 8–amino acid peptide CaSR agonist that is associated with receptor activation on the parathyroid gland chief cells. Activation occurs once a disulfide bridge forms between the amino terminal D-cysteine present in etelcalcetide and Cys482 of the CaSR.[62] Unlike cinacalcet, there is slight direct CaSR activation by etelcalcetide under low-calcium conditions. This indicates that etelcalcetide can act as both a direct agonist (minor mechanism) and as an allosteric modulator of CaSR (major mechanism). PTH levels decreased 50% more than what was observed when cinacalcet was administered.[63-65]

PHARMACOKINETICS. Etelcalcetide is administered intravenously three times weekly via the venous line of the hemodialysis blood circuit at the conclusion of hemodialysis.[66] In the plasma a covalent albumin peptide conjugate forms between the D-cysteine in the drug molecule and Cys34 found within serum albumin. Etelcalcetide is not metabolized by CYP450 enzymes.[67] Renal elimination is significant and the terminal elimination half-life is 18.4 hours.[65] The primary adverse effect was an asymptomatic reduction in plasma calcium levels, muscle spasms, diarrhea, nausea, and symptomatic hypocalcemia.[64]

Drug Therapies Used to Treat Hypercalcemia of Malignancy

Zoledronic Acid (Zometa)

Mechanism of Action

Zoledronic acid, a bisphosphonate, is approved for the treatment of hypercalcemia of malignancy, a metabolic complication that can be life-threatening (Fig. 23.8). The primary indication is for adjunct use in patients with multiple myeloma and those with bone metastases from solid tumors.[68] Hypercalcemia of malignancy can occur in up to 50% of patients diagnosed with multiple myeloma, leukemia, and non-Hodgkins lymphoma.[69] This condition arises when chemical moieties produced by the tumor cause overstimulation of osteoclasts. When there is an increase in bone degradation, there is a concomitant release of calcium into the plasma. When serum concentrations of calcium rapidly elevate, the kidneys are unable to handle the overload, and hypercalcemia results. This can lead to dehydration, nausea, vomiting, fatigue, and confusion. Zoledronic acid effectively decreases plasma calcium concentrations via inhibition of bone resorption (inhibition of osteoclastic activity and induction of osteoclast apoptosis).[68] It also prevents the increase in osteoclastic activity caused by tumor-based stimulatory factors.

Cancer treatment–induced bone loss is a major adverse effect associated with endocrine-based cancer therapies. These therapies may depress ovarian function (e.g., goserelin acetate), decrease ER activation (e.g., ER antagonist), and/or inhibit estrogen biosynthesis (e.g., aromatase inhibition) all of which will lead to significant bone loss. Zoledronic acid has demonstrated efficacy in reducing or delaying these complications.

PHARMACOKINETICS. Zoledronic acid is a white, crystalline powder that is available in vials for reconstitution for IV infusion over at least 15 minutes. It does not undergo metabolic transformation and does not inhibit CYP450 enzymes.[68] Clearance of this agent is dependent on the patient's creatinine clearance, not on dose. Serum creatinine levels should be evaluated prior to every treatment. Zoledronic acid is contraindicated in patients with severe renal impairment.

Zoledronic acid should not be mixed with infusion solutions that contain calcium (e.g., lactated Ringer solution) and should be administered via IV infusion in its own line. Because of the possibility of a serious deterioration in renal function, the manufacturer requires strict adherence to the infusion duration being no less than 15 minutes.[68]

Pamidronate Disodium (Aredia)

Pamidronate disodium, a second-generation bisphosphonate, is 100-fold more potent than etidronate disodium for the treatment of hypercalcemia of malignancy (Fig. 23.8).[5] It has also been approved for the treatment of Paget disease of the bone and for osteolytic bone metastases of breast cancer and osteolytic lesions of multiple myeloma.[70] When used to treat bone metastases, pamidronate disodium decreases osteoclast recruitment, decreases osteoclast activity, and increases osteoclast apoptosis.[71] Administered by IV infusion, a single dose is typically sufficient for the treatment of hypercalcemia and Paget disease of the bone. In the treatment of osteolytic lesions of multiple myeloma, monthly administration is indicated.

PHARMACOKINETICS. Pamidronate disodium is cleared renally and therefore is contraindicated in patients with impaired renal function. As with other bisphosphonates, there is a risk of osteonecrosis of the jaw and patients are advised against invasive dental procedures.[70]

Drug Therapy Used in the Treatment of Hypoparathyroidism

Parathyroid Hormone [rhPTH 1-84] (Natpara)

Mechanism of Action

Natpara has an orphan drug designation to treat (along with calcium and Vitamin D) the hypocalcemia associated with hypoparathyroidism (Fig. 23.2). Structurally identical to endogenous PTH, the recombinant human PTH is administered once daily as an SC injection. Although Natpara shares a common mechanism of action with teriparatide it has been suggested that the C-terminal region may possess valuable biologic activity mediated by a novel receptor that specifically interacts with this portion of the peptide hormone.

Representative examples of the common side effects include tingling or burning sensation (paresthesia), hypocalcemia, headache, and nausea.[72] Due to the increase in the reported incidence of osteosarcoma in male and female rats, Natpara is only available through a restricted program (NATPARA REMS—Risk Evaluation and Mitigation Strategy).

Pharmacokinetics

Administered subcutaneously, Natpara has an absolute bioavailability of 53%. Degradation by hepatic cathepsins yields fragments that are renally eliminated. Dosage adjustment is not required in patients with mild to moderate liver or kidney impairment.

Natpara will negate the effects of alendronate and therefore they should not be used in combination.[72] The effectiveness of digoxin is reduced if administered in patients diagnosed with hypocalcemia. Patients should be monitored for calcium levels and digoxin toxicity when taking Natpara.

Structure Challenge

Vitamin D activation is a two-step process (see below) regardless of whether vitamin D_2 (from plants) is consumed or D_3 (from animals and skin biosynthesis) is consumed or produced. Select the correct organ and enzyme for each of the activation steps A and B. Place your answers on the lines provided.

Organs	Liver, Intestine, Kidney, Plasma
Enzymes	Vitamin D 25 hydroxylase; Vitamin D 1α hydroxylase; Vitamin D 24 hydroxylase

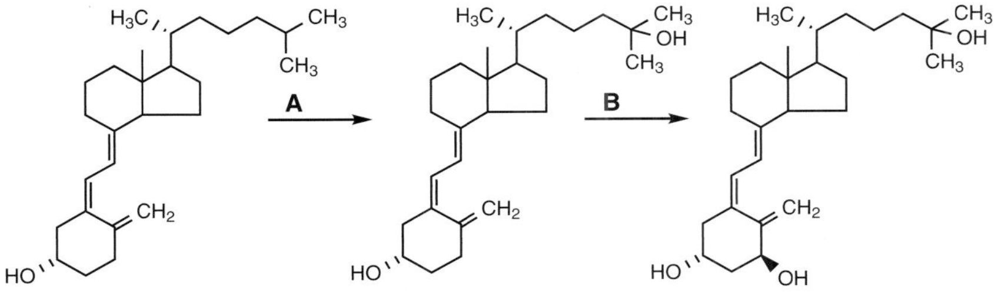

H3C, CH3, CH3 — A → — H3C, CH3, OH, CH3 — B → — H3C, CH3, OH, CH3

CH2, HO — CH2, HO — CH2, HO, OH

A. Organ __________________

Enzyme __________________

B. Organ __________________

Enzyme __________________

An individual must have kidney and liver function in order to activate vitamin D. As we age, both renal and hepatic impairment must be considered when recommending vitamin D supplementation. Based on your knowledge of how vitamin D is activated, determine which patient populations would benefit from the following two vitamin D analogs.

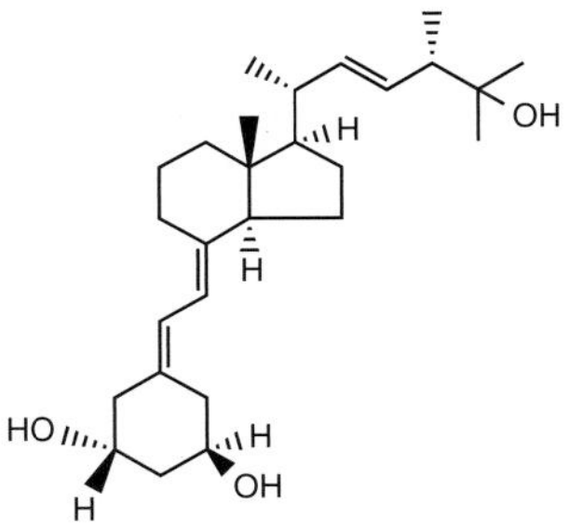

Paricalcitol (Zemplar)

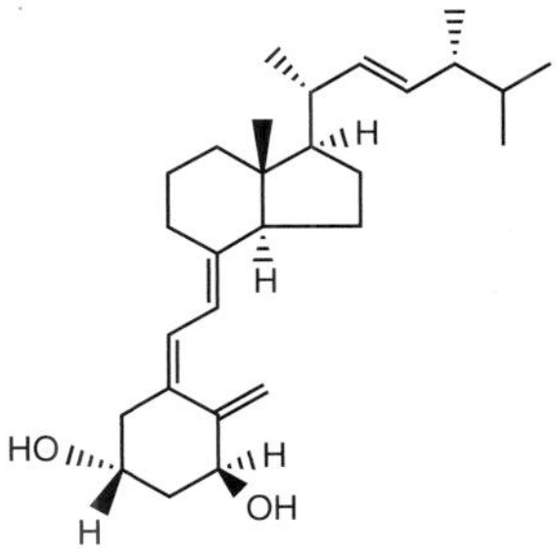

Doxercalciferol (Hectorol)

Structure Challenge answers found immediately after References.

REFERENCES

1. Copp DH. Calcitonin: discovery, development, and clinical application. *Clin Invest Med*. 1994;17:268-277.
2. Bouillon R, Carmeliet G, Boonen S. Aging and calcium metabolism. *Bailliere's Clin Endocrinol Metab*. 1997;11:341-365.
3. Haines ST, Caceres B, Yancey L. Alternatives to estrogen replacement therapy for preventing osteoporosis. *J Am Pharm Assoc*. 1996;NS36:707-715.
4. Christenson RH. Biochemical markers of bone metabolism: an overview. *Clin Biochem*. 1997;30:573-593.
5. Cosman F, de Beur SJ, LeBoff MS, et al. Clinican's guide to prevention and treatment of osteoporosis. *Osteoporos Int*. 2014;25:2359-2381.
6. Khosla S, Riggs BL. Pathophysiology of age-related bone loss and osteoporosis. *Endocrinol Metab Clin North Am*. 2005;34:1015-1030.
7. Slovik DM, Armstrong EJ. Pharmacology of bone mineral homeostasis. In: Golan DE, Armstrong EJ, Armstrong AW, eds. *Principles of Pharmacology: The Pathophysiologic Basis of Drug Therapy*. 4th ed. Philadelphia: Wolters Kluwer Health; 2017.
8. Brown EM, Gamba G, Riccardi D, et al. Cloning and characterization of an extracellular Ca^{2+}-sensing receptor from bovine parathyroid. *Nature*. 1993;366:575-580.
9. Nair R, Maseeh A. Vitamin D: the "sunshine" vitamin. *J Pharmacol Pharmacother*. 2012;3:118-119.
10. Rosen CJ. The epidemiology and pathogenesis of osteoporosis. In: DeGroot LJ, Chrousos G, Dungan K, et al, eds. *Endotext*. South Dartmouth, MA; MDText.com, Inc. 2000–2018. Updated February 21, 2017. Accessed March 23, 2018.
11. Hansen LB, Vondracek SF. Prevention and treatment of nonpostmenopausal osteoporosis. *Am J Health Syst Pharm*. 2004;61:2637-2656.
12. Watts NB, Bilezikian JP, Camacho PM, et al. American Association of Clinical Endocrinologists medical guidelines for clinical practice for the diagnosis and treatment of postmenopausal osteoporosis. *Endocr Pract*. 2010;16:1-37.
13. O'Connell MB, Borgelt LM, Bowles SK, et al. Drug-induced osteoporosis in the older adult. *Aging Health*. 2010;6:501-518.
14. Sözen T, Özişik L, Başaran NC. An overview and management of osteoporosis. *Eur J Rheumatol*. 2017;4:46-56.
15. Diem SJ, Blackwell TL, Stone KL, et al. Use of antidepressants and rates of hip bone loss in older women. *Arch Intern Med*. 2007;167:1240-1245.
16. Gray SL, LaCroix AZ, Larson J, et al. Proton pump inhibitor use, hip fracture and change in bone mineral density in postmenopausal women. *Arch Intern Med*. 2010;170:765-771.
17. Riche DM, King ST. Bone loss and fracture risk associated with thiazolidinedione therapy. *Pharmacotherapy*. 2010;30:716-727.
18. van Brussel MS, Bultink IE, Lems WF. Prevention of glucocorticoid-induced osteoporosis. *Exp Opin Pharmacother*. 2009;10:997-1005.
19. National Osteoporosis Foundation Releases: Updated Data Detailing the Prevalence of Osteoporosis and Low Bone Mass in the U.S. https://www.nof.org/news/54-million-americans-affected-by-osteoporosis-and-low-bone-mass/. Updated June 2, 2014. Accessed March 23, 2018.
20. Wright NC, Looker AC, Saag KG, et al. The recent prevalence of osteoporosis and low bone mass in the United States based on bone mineral density at the femoral neck or lumbar spine. *J Bone Miner Res*. 2014;29;2520-2526.
21. United States National Library of Medicine. Genetics Home Reference Your Guide to Understanding Genetic Conditions. Osteopetrosis https://ghr.nlm.nih.gov/condition/osteopetrosis#-genes. Reviewed September 2010. Published March 27, 2018. Accessed March 28, 2018.
22. Fong J. Hypocalcemia. *Can Fam Physician*. 2012;58:158-162.
23. Block GA, Martin KJ, De Franciso AL. Cinacalcet for secondary hyperparathyroidism in patients receiving hemodialysis. *N Engl J Med*. 2004;350:1516-1525.
24. Creo AL, Tom D, Thacher JM, et al. Nutritional rickets around the world: an update. *Paediatr Int Child Health*. 2017;37:84-98.
25. Abelson A. A review of Paget's disease of bone with a focus on the efficacy and safety of zoledronic acid 5 mg. *Curr Med Res Opin*. 2008;24:695-705.
26. De Silva Jardine P, Thompson D. Antiosteoporosis agents. *Ann Rpts Med Chem*. 1996;31:211-220.
27. Honig SH. Osteoporosis new treatments and updates. *Bull NYU Hosp Jt Dis*. 2010;68:166-170.
28. Rossouw JE, Anderson GL, Prentice RL. et al. Risks and benefits of estrogen plus progestin in healthy postmenopausal women. Principal results from the Women's Health Initiative randomized controlled trial. *JAMA*. 2002;288:321-333.
29. Gizzo S, Saccardi C, Patrelli TS, et al. Update on raloxifene: mechanism of action, clinical efficacy, adverse effects, and contraindications. *Obstet Gynecol Surv*. 2013;68:467-481.
30. Black DM, Rosen CJ. Postmenopausal osteoporosis. *N Engl J Med*. 2016;374:254-262.
31. *Evista® (Raloxifene Hydrochloride) [package insert]*. Indianapolis, IN: Eli Lilly; 2007. Available at https://www.accessdata.fda.gov/drugsatfda_docs/label/2007/020815s018lbl.pdf. Accessed March 28, 2018.
32. Grese TA, Sluka JP, Bryant HU, et al. Benzopyran selective estrogen receptor modulators (SERMs): pharmacological effects and structural correlation with raloxifene. *Bioorg Med Chem Lett*. 1996;6:903-908.
33. Bryant HU, Glasebrook AL, Yang NN, et al. A pharmacologic review of raloxifene. *J Bone Miner Metab*. 1996;14:1-9.
34. Komm BS, Chines AA. Bazedoxifene: the evolving role of third-generation selective estrogen-receptor modulators in the management of postmenopausal osteoporosis. *Ther Adv Musculoskelet Dis*. 2012;4:21-34.
35. Goldberg T, Fidler B. Conjugated estrogens/bazedoxifene (Duavee). *P T*. 2015;40:178-182.
36. Rogers MJ, Crockett JC, Coxon FP, et al. Biochemical and molecular mechanisms of action of bisphosphonates. *Bone*. 2011;49:34-41.
37. Dunford JE, Thompson K, Coxon FP, et al. Structure-activity relationships for inhibition of farnesyl diphosphate synthase in vitro and inhibition of bone resorption in vivo by nitrogen containing bisphosphonates. *J Pharmacol Exp Ther*. 2001;296:235-242.
38. Russell RG. Bisphosphonates: mode of action and pharmacology. *Pediatrics*. 2007;119:S150-S162.
39. Cremers S, Papapoulas S. Pharmacology of bisphosphonates. *Bone*. 2011;49:42-49.
40. Eastell R, Walsh JS, Watts NB, et al. Bisphosphonates for postmenopausal osteoporosis. *Bone*. 2011;49:82-88.
41. Reid IR, Hosking DJ. Bisphosphonates in Paget's disease. *Bone*. 2011;49:89-94.
42. Russell RGG, Bisphosphonates the first 40 years, *Bone*. 2011;49:2-19.
43. *Boniva® (Ibandronate Sodium) [package insert]*. South San Francisco, CA: Genentech; 2015. Available at https://www.accessdata.fda.gov/drugsatfda_docs/label/2015/021455s019lbl.pdf. Accessed March 28, 2018.
44. King AE, Umland EM. Osteonecrosis of the jaw in patients receiving intravenous or oral bisphosphonates. *Pharmacotherapy*. 2008;28:667-677.
45. FDA Drug Safety Communication: Safety Update for Osteoporosis Drugs, Bisphosphonates, and Atypical Fractures. Available at https://www.fda.gov/Drugs/DrugSafety/ucm229009.htm. Updated February 6, 2017. Accessed March 24, 2018.
46. Schmidt GA, Horner KE, McDanel DL, et al. Risks and benefits of long-term bisphosphonate therapy. *Am J Health Syst Pharm*. 2010;67:994-1001.
47. *Miacalcin® (Calcitonin) [package insert]*. East Hanover, NJ: Novartis Pharmaceuticals; 2014. Available at https://www.accessdata.fda.gov/drugsatfda_docs/label/2014/017808s035lbl.pdf. Accessed March 24, 2018.
48. Freeman TR. Teriparatide: a novel agent that builds new bone. *J Am Pharm Assoc*. 2003;43:535-537.

49. McClung MR. Emerging therapies for osteoporosis. *Endocrin Metab.* 2015;30:429-435.
50. Silva BC, Costa AG, Cusano NE, et al. Catabolic and anabolic actions of parathyroid hormone on the skeleton. *J Endocrinol Invest.* 2011;34:801-810.
51. Neer RM, Arnaud CD, Zanchetta JR, et al. Effect of parathyroid hormone (1-34) on fractures and bone mineral density in postmenopausal women with osteoporosis. *N Engl J Med.* 2001;344:1434-1341.
52. Shirley M. Abaloparatide: first global approval. *Drugs.* 2017;77:1363-1368.
53. *Tymlos™ (Abaloparatide) [package insert].* Waltham, MA: Radius; 2017. https://www.accessdata.fda.gov/drugsatfda_docs/label/2017/208743lbl.pdf. Accessed March 18, 2018.
54. Hattersley G, Dean T, Corbon BA, Bahar H, Gardella TJ. Binding selectivity of abaloparatide for PTH-type-1-receptor conformations and effects on downstream signaling. *Endocrinology.* 2016;157:141-149.
55. Cummings SR, San Martin J, McClung MR, et al. Denosumab for prevention of fractures in postmenopausal women with osteoporosis. *N Engl J Med.* 2009;361:756-765.
56. *Xgeva® (Denosumab) [package insert].* Thousand Oaks, CA: Amgen; 2013. Available at https://www.accessdata.fda.gov/drugsatfda_docs/label/2013/125320s094lbl.pdf. Accessed March 24, 2018.
57. Institute of Medicine (US) Committee to Review Dietary Reference Intakes for Vitamin D and Calcium ; Ross CA, Taylor CL, Yaktine AL, eds. *Dietary Reference Intakes for Calcium and Vitamin D.* Washington, DC: National Academies Press (US); 2011. Available at https://www.ncbi.nlm.nih.gov/books/NBK56050/#summary.s5. Accessed March 24, 2018.
58. Bolland MJ, Barber PA, Doughty RN, et al. Vascular events in healthy older women receiving calcium supplementation: randomized controlled trial. *BMJ.* 2008;336:262-266.
59. Pereira L, Meng C, Marques D, et al. Old and new calcimimetics for treatment of secondary hyperparathyroidism: impact on biochemical and relevant clinical outcomes. *Clin Kidney J.* 2018;11:80-88.
60. Poon G. Cinacalcet hydrochloride (Sensipar). *Proc (Bayl Univ Med Cent).* 2015:18(2);181-184.
61. *Sensipar™ (Cinacalcet) [package insert].* Thousand Oaks, CA: Amgen; 2017. https://pi.amgen.com/~/media/amgen/repositorysites/pi-amgen-com/sensipar/sensipar_pi_hcp_english.pdf. Accessed March 18, 2018.
62. Alexander ST, Hunter T, Walter S, et al. Critical cysteine residues in both the calcium-sensing receptor and the allosteric activator AMG 416 underlie the mechanism of action. *Mol Pharmacol.* 2015;88:853-865.
63. Subramanian R, Zhu X, Kerr SJ, et al. Nonclinical pharmacokinetics, disposition, and drug-drug interaction potential of a novel d-amino acid peptide agonist of the calcium-sensing receptor AMG 416 (etelcalcetide). *Drug Metab Dispos.* 2016;44:1319-1331.
64. Cozzolino M, Galassi A, Conte F, et al. Treatment of secondary hyperparathyroidism: the clinical utility of etelcalcetide. *Ther Clin Risk Manag.* 2017;13:679-689.
65. Hamano N, Komaba H, Fukagawa M. Etelcalcetide for the treatment of secondary hyperparathyroidism. *Expert Opin Pharmacother.* 2017;18:529-534.
66. Edson KZ, Wu BM, Iyer A, et al. Determination of etelcalcetide biotransformation and hemodialysis kinetics to guide the timing of its dosing. *Kidney Int Rep.* 2016;1;24-33.
67. *Parsabiv™ (Etelcalcetide) [package insert].* Thousand Oaks, CA: Amgen; 2017. https://www.accessdata.fda.gov/drugsatfda_docs/label/2017/208325Orig1s000Lbledt.pdf. Accessed March 28, 2018.
68. *Zometa® (Zoledronic Acid) [package insert].* East Hanover, NJ: Novartis Pharma Stein AG; 2014. Available at https://www.accessdata.fda.gov/drugsatfda_docs/label/2014/021223s028lbl.pdf. Accessed March 28, 2018.
69. Sternlicht H, Glezerman IG. Hypercalcemia of malignancy and new treatment options. *Ther Clin Risk Manag.* 2015;11:1779-1788.
70. *Pamidronate Disodium [package insert].* Bedford, OH: Ben Venue Laboratories; 2009. Available at https://www.accessdata.fda.gov/drugsatfda_docs/label/2009/021113s008lbl.pdf. Accessed March 28, 2018.
71. Van Poznak CH. The use of bisphosphonates in patients with breast cancer. *Cancer Control.* 2002;9:480-489.
72. *Natpara® (Parathyroid Hormone). [Draft package insert].* Bedminster, NJ: NPS Pharmaceuticals; 2015. Available at https://www.accessdata.fda.gov/drugsatfda_docs/label/2015/125511s000lbl.pdf. Accessed March 28, 2018.

Structure Challenge Answers

A. Liver

Vitamin D25 hydroxylase

B. Kidney

Vitamin D 1α hydroxylase

Patients with renal impairment may be inefficient and/or unable to complete the second step of vitamin D activation. Doxercalciferol, a 1-hydroxy vitamin D analog (normally generated by renal vitamin D activation), would be an appropriate choice for this patient population. This analog would only require hepatic activation to the active 1,25-dihydroxy vitamin D product.

Patients with liver dysfunction will not biosynthesize the 25-hydroxy vitamin D intermediate but will complete the second step of vitamin D activation. Paricalcitol, a fully activated vitamin D analog would be appropriate for this patient population, as it would not require either renal or hepatic activation.

CHAPTER 24

Drugs Used to Advance Men's and Women's Health

Jennifer L. Whetstone, Michael L. Mohler, Ramesh Narayanan, and James T. Dalton

Drugs covered in this chapter:

ESTROGENS
- *Steroidal estrogens*
  - 17β-Estradiol
  - Conjugated estrogens
  - Ethinyl estradiol
  - Estradiol cypionate
  - Estradiol valerate
  - Mestranol
- *Nonsteroidal estrogen*
  - Diethylstilbestrol

PROGESTINS
- Progesterone
- Megestrol acetate
- Medroxyprogesterone
- Synthetic progestins
  - *First generation*
    - Norethindrone
    - Norethindrone acetate
    - Norethynodrel
    - Ethynodiol diacetate
    - Medroxyprogesterone acetate
    - Lynestrenol
  - *Second generation*
    - Norgestrel/levonorgestrel
  - *Third generation*
    - Norgestimate
    - Norelgestromin
    - Desogestrel
    - Etonogestrel
  - *Fourth generation*
    - Dienogest
    - Drospirenone

EMERGENCY CONTRACEPTIVES AND ABORTIFACIENTS
- Mifepristone
- Ulipristal acetate
- Misoprostol
- Carboprost
- Dinoprostone

INFERTILITY DRUGS
- Clomiphene citrate

ANDROGENS
- Testosterone (oral, transdermal, buccal)
- Testosterone esters
- Fluoxymesterone
- Methyltestosterone

ANABOLIC AGENTS
- Nandrolone
- Oxandrolone
- Oxymetholone
- Stanozolol

TREATMENT OF MENOPAUSE

ESTROGENS
- 17β-Estradiol
- Conjugated estrogens
- Esterified estrogens
- Estropipate

PROGESTINS
- Medroxyprogesterone acetate
- Micronized progesterone

SELECTIVE ESTROGEN RECEPTOR MODULATORS (SERMS)
- Bazedoxifene
- Ospemifene

MISCELLANEOUS DRUG
- Prasterone

TREATMENT OF ERECTILE DYSFUNCTION

PHOSPHODIESTERASE-5 INHIBITORS
- Sildenafil
- Tadalafil
- Vardenafil
- Avanafil

MISCELLANEOUS DRUG
- Prostaglandin E_1

TREATMENT OF BENIGN PROSTATIC HYPERPLASIA

α_1-ADRENERGIC ANTAGONISTS
- Alfuzosin
- Terazosin
- Doxazosin
- Tamsulosin
- Silodosin

5α-REDUCTASE INHIBITORS
- Finasteride
- Dutasteride

TREATMENT OF BREAST CANCER

SERMS
- Tamoxifen
- Toremifene

ANTIESTROGENS
- Fulvestrant

AROMATASE INHIBITORS
- Letrozole
- Anastrozole
- Exemestane

TREATMENT OF PROSTATE CANCER

GONADOTROPIN RELEASING HORMONE (GNRH AGONISTS)
- Leuprolide
- Goserelin
- Triptorelin

GNRH ANTAGONIST
- Degarelix

CYP17A1 INHIBITOR
- Abiraterone

ANTIANDROGENS
- Enzalutamide
- Apalutamide
- Bicalutamide
- Flutamide
- Nilutamide

Abbreviations

4-OH TAM 4-hydroxytamoxifen
4-OH-NDM TAM 4-hydroxy-N-desmethyl tamoxifen
4-OH-NDM TOR 4-hydroxy-N-desmethyl toremifene
5AR 5α-reductase
$5AR_1$ 5α-reductase type 1
$5AR_2$ 5α-reductase type 2
$5AR_3$ 5α-reductase type 3
5ARI 5α-reductase inhibitor
3β-HSD 5-ene-3β-hydroxysteroid dehydrogenase/3-oxo-steroid-4,5-isomerase
17β-HSD 17β-hydroxysteroid dehydrogenase
17βHSD3 17β-hydroxysteroid dehydrogenase type 3
17βHSD5 17β-hydroxysteroid dehydrogenase type 5
AC-T anthracycline and cyclophosphamide then taxane
ADME absorption, distribution, metabolism, and excretion
ADT androgen deprivation therapy
AF-1 activation function-1
AF-2 activation function-2
AI aromatase inhibitors
AKR1C3 aldoketoreductase type 1C3
AR androgen receptor
ATAC Arimidex, tamoxifen, alone or in combination
AUA-SI/I-PSS American Urological Association Symptom Index/International Prostate Symptom Score
AUC area under the curve
BIG Breast International Group
BMD bone mineral density
BPH benign prostatic hyperplasia
BRCA breast cancer susceptibility gene
cAMP cyclic adenosine monophosphate
CDK4/6 cyclin-dependent kinase 4/6
CEE conjugated equine estrogens
cGMP cyclic guanosine monophosphate
C_{max} peak serum concentration
COC combined oral contraceptive
CRPC castration-resistant prostate cancer
CSPC castration-sensitive prostate cancer
CYP11A1 cytochrome P-450 side-chain cleavage enzyme
CYP11B2 11β-hydroxylase
CYP17A1 17α-hydroxylase/17,20-lyase
CYP19A1 aromatase
CYP21 21-hydroxylase
DCIS ductal carcinoma in situ
DES diethylstilbestrol
DHEA dehydroepiandrosterone
DHT 5α-dihydrotestosterone
DVT deep vein thrombosis
E1 estrone
E2 17β-estradiol
E3 estriol
ED erectile dysfunction
EE ethinyl estradiol
EGFR epidermal growth factor receptor
ER estrogen receptor
ERα estrogen receptor alpha
ERβ estrogen receptor beta
ERE estrogen response element
FDA U.S. Food and Drug Administration
FSH follicle-stimulating hormone
GABA gamma aminobutyric acid
$GABA_A$ gamma aminobutyric acid receptor subtype A
GI gastrointestinal
GnRH gonadotropin-releasing hormone
GnRH-R gonadotropin-releasing hormone receptor
H12 helix 12
HBA hydrogen bond acceptor
HBD hydrogen bond donor
hCG human chorionic gonadotropin
HER2 human epidermal growth factor receptor type II
HPG hypothalamus pituitary gonadal
HRE hormone response element
IM intramuscular
IUD intrauterine device
LBD ligand binding domain
LH luteinizing hormone
LHRH luteinizing hormone–releasing hormone
LUTS lower urinary tract symptoms
mCRPC metastatic castration-resistant prostate cancer
MFS metastasis-free survival
MPA medroxyprogesterone acetate
mTOR mechanistic target of rapamycin
NAMS North American Menopause Society
NCCN National Comprehensive Cancer Network
NCI National Cancer Institute
NDM TAM N-desmethyl tamoxifen
NDM TOR N-desmethyl toremifene
nmCRPC nonmetastatic castration-resistant prostate cancer
NO nitric oxide
OC oral contraceptive
OTC over the counter
PAP prostatic acid phosphatase
PARP poly(ADP-ribose) polymerase
PDE5 phosphodiesterase type 5
PDE5Is phosphodiesterase 5 inhibitors
PD-L1 programmed death-ligand 1
PMDD postmenopausal dysphoric disorder
POP progestin-only oral contraceptive pills
PR progesterone receptor
PRE progesterone response element
PSA prostate-specific antigen
REMS risk evaluation and mitigation strategy
SARM selective androgen receptor modulator
SCC side-chain cleavage
SERD selective estrogen receptor degrader
SERM selective estrogen receptor modulator
SGRM selective glucocorticoid receptor modulator
SHBG sex hormone–binding globulin
TC taxotere and cyclophosphamide
TNBC triple-negative breast cancer
TOR toremifene
TRT testosterone replacement therapy
UGT UDP-glucuronyl transferase
U.S. United States
VTE venous thromboembolism
WHI Women's Health Initiative

CLINICAL SIGNIFICANCE

Medications that activate or block a sex hormone receptor such as the androgen receptor, estrogen receptor, and progesterone receptor are used regularly to treat a multitude of disorders and diseases. Androgen receptor agonist therapies include testosterone replacement therapy and synthetic steroids for the treatment of disorders requiring anabolic activity. A wide range of parenteral testosterone therapies, as well as many, orally active synthetic androgens, are available, allowing the clinician to tailor the prescribed product to patient needs. The negative aspects of agonist therapies include the inability of approved agents to adequately separate anabolic from androgenic effects mediated through the androgen receptor, causing concern for exacerbation of prostatic disease in men and virilization in females. Nonsteroidal androgen receptor antagonists (and a steroidal inhibitor of androgen synthesis) are used orally in the treatment of advanced prostate cancers to delay metastasis and/or extend survival.

Estrogen receptor and progesterone receptor agonist therapies are commonly used together as oral contraceptives in fertile women or as hormone replacement therapy for women with menopausal symptoms. Oral contraceptives are synthetic steroid combinations or progestin-only formulations available as oral or parenteral drug products, again allowing the clinician to tailor product to patient needs. The negative aspects of agonist therapies include the untoward effects of estrogen receptor and/or progesterone receptor agonism including liability for the development of breast cancer, as well as off-target effects such as antiandrogenism for some agents. Estrogen receptor antagonists (and estrogen biosynthesis inhibitors) are employed in the treatment of hormone-receptor positive breast cancer, alone or as combinations with kinase inhibitors, to increase the time to relapse or progression. Progesterone receptor antagonists are used orally as emergency contraceptives.

A wide variety of sex hormone agonists and antagonists exist in most of the classes above and they are available in an extensive array of formulations and/or combinations. To best serve the diverse populations of patients using these agents, prescribers and pharmacists alike must understand the risks and benefits of individual drugs within each class and combination products and be familiar with how untoward effects of specific agents can be used advantageously in certain patient populations. With a greater understanding of the properties of these medications, pharmacists and physicians can work together to make the best informed decisions regarding the best active ingredient and most appropriate route for their patients while causing the least amount of adverse effects.

INTRODUCTION

This chapter focuses on the physiology, pharmacology, metabolism, and structure-activity relationships of therapeutic and emerging classes of drugs that are indicated for use in men or women based on their sex. Differences in circulating hormones and in the anatomy and physiology of reproductive systems differentiate between males and females and provide the basis for numerous endocrine-based therapies that are exclusive for men or women. Although there are numerous endocrine diseases that are common in both men and women, many of which are associated with adrenocorticoids (see Chapter 21), there are also diseases and medical needs that demonstrate sexual dimorphism and require treatment that is exclusive to men or women (Fig. 24.1). Male and female fertility, sexual function, secondary sex characteristics (e.g., hair growth and muscle mass), and most endocrine cancers (at least in their early stages) rely on the sex hormones. Female hormonal contraceptives are used widely and represent some the earliest endocrine therapies employed, while treatments for benign prostatic hyperplasia (BPH) and erectile dysfunction (ED) in men extend well into the latter decades of the lifespan. The majority of these disorders and their treatments are associated with the male (i.e., androgens) or female (i.e., estrogens and progestins) sex hormones, their pharmacologic targets (i.e., the androgen receptor [AR], estrogen receptors [ERs], and progesterone receptor [PR], respectively), and the tissues that rely on the androgens and estrogens.

THE SEX HORMONES

The sex steroid hormones are steroid molecules that are necessary for reproduction in females and males and that affect the development of secondary sex characteristics in both sexes. The sex steroids comprise three classes: estrogens, progestins, and androgens (Fig. 24.2; carbon numbering system is indicated; see Chapter 21 for more detailed discussion of steroid nomenclature and structure). The two principal classes of female sex steroid hormones are estrogens and progestins, and the principal male sex hormone class is androgens. Chemically, the naturally occurring estrogens are C-18 steroids and they have in common an aromatic A ring with a 3-phenolic group that

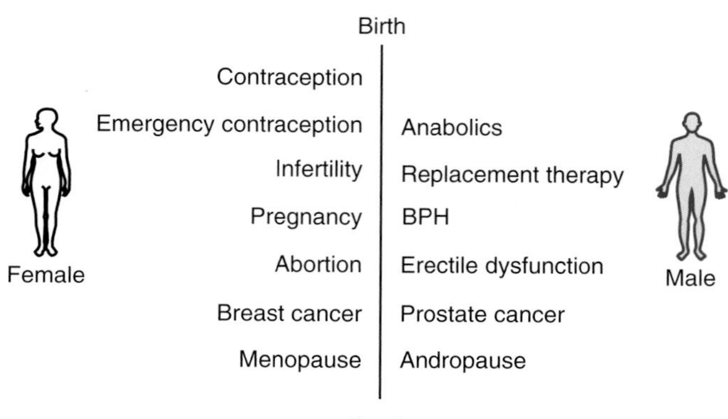

Figure 24.1 Disorders associated with men's and women's health.

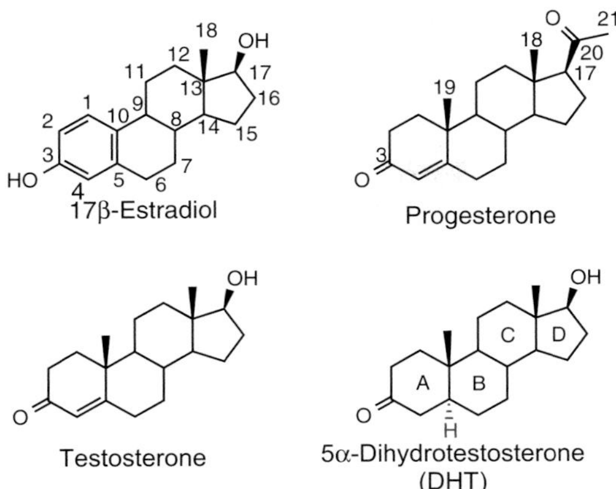

Figure 24.2 Steroidal sex hormones.

distinguishes them from the other sex steroid hormones. The most potent endogenous estrogen is 17β-estradiol (Fig. 24.2). The naturally occurring progestins are C-21 steroids and they have in common an unsaturated 3-keto-4-ene structure in the A ring and a ketone at the C-20 position. The most potent endogenous progestin is progesterone (Fig. 24.2). The naturally occurring androgens are C-19 steroids and they have in common oxygen atoms (as either hydroxyl or ketone groups) at both the C-3 and C-17 positions. Testosterone is a potent androgen that is found in the blood at higher concentrations than other androgens, whereas 5α-dihydrotestosterone (DHT) (Fig. 24.2; note *trans* A/B ring fusion) is a more potent metabolite of testosterone that is formed in certain androgen target tissues including the prostate and scalp. All three classes of endogenous steroids are present in both males and females. The production and circulating plasma levels of estrogens and progestins are higher in females, and the production and circulating plasma levels of androgens are higher in males. Although estrogens are regarded as female hormones, their circulating levels are only a fraction of serum androgen levels. While serum 17β-estradiol in premenopausal women is in the picogram/milliliter range, serum androgen levels are in the nanogram/milliliter range. This discrepancy between the level and activity reflects that the estrogens rely more on local synthesis from androgens by aromatization. In endocrine tissues, cholesterol is the steroid that is stored and converted to estrogen, progesterone, or androgen when the tissue is stimulated by a gonadotropic hormone.

Sexual Hormone Biosynthesis and Metabolism

Biosynthesis

The major pathways for the biosynthesis of the sex steroid hormones are summarized in Figure 24.3, and the synthesis of adrenocorticoids is discussed later (see also Chapter 21 and Fig. 21.8). Briefly, cholesterol is stored in endocrine tissues and is converted to androgen, estrogen, or progesterone when the tissue is stimulated by a gonadotropic hormone. Androgens (male sex hormones) primarily are synthesized from cholesterol in the testes, whereas estrogens are biosynthesized chiefly in the ovary in premenopausal and mature women, and adipose tissue in men and postmenopausal women.[1] Androgens are intermediates in the biosynthesis of estrogens. In the liver, androgens are formed from C-21 steroids. During pregnancy, the placenta is the main source of estrogen biosynthesis and pathways for production change.[2,3] Small amounts of these hormones are also synthesized by the adrenal cortex, the hypothalamus, and the anterior pituitary in both sexes.

Luteinizing hormone (LH), a gonadotropic hormone produced and secreted by the anterior pituitary gland, binds to its receptor on the surface of the Leydig cells of the testis, or theca cells in the ovary, to initiate testosterone, progesterone, and estrogen biosynthesis, respectively. As in other endocrine cells, the binding of gonadotropin (i.e., LH) activates the G_S signal transduction pathway, increasing intracellular cyclic adenosine monophosphate (cAMP) levels via activation of adenylyl cyclase. One of the processes influenced by elevated cAMP levels is the activation of cholesterol esterase, which cleaves cholesterol esters and liberates free cholesterol. The free cholesterol is then converted in mitochondria to pregnenolone via the cholesterol side-chain cleavage (SCC) reaction (step a of Fig. 24.3). Pregnenolone is converted by 17α-hydroxylase to 17α-hydroxypregnenolone (step b) in the endoplasmic reticulum and then to dehydroepiandrosterone (DHEA; a C-19 steroid) via 17,20-lyase (step j), which involves cleavage of the C-17 to C-20 carbon–carbon bond and loss of the 17β-acetyl side chain.[4] Steps b and J are catalyzed by the same bifunctional enzyme CYP17A1. Progesterone can be formed from pregnenolone via the action of another bifunctional enzyme 3b-HSD which catalyzes the 5-ene-3β-hydroxysteroid dehydrogenase and 3-oxosteroid-4,5-isomerase reactions (step c). This same enzyme is responsible for the conversion of DHEA to the 17-ketosteroidal androgen, androstenedione (step c).

Testosterone is formed in the testes by the reduction of the 17-ketone of androstenedione by 17β-hydroxysteroid dehydrogenases, but the reaction is reversible (step g in Fig. 24.3); i.e., testosterone and androstenedione are metabolically interconvertible. 17β-Hydroxysteroid dehydrogenase type 3 is largely responsible for conversion of androstenedione to testosterone in the testes, while type 5 (also known as aldoketoreductase 1C3) is thought to predominate in peripheral (e.g., adipose tissue and prostate) conversion of androstenedione to testosterone. Loss of the C-19 angular methyl group and aromatization of the A ring of testosterone or androstenedione is catalyzed by the microsomal cytochrome P450 enzyme complex, called aromatase, and results in the C-18 steroids—namely, 17β-estradiol or estrone, respectively (step h). 17β-Estradiol and estrone are also metabolically interconvertible and catalyzed by 17β-hydroxysteroid dehydrogenases (step g) but involving different isozymes of 17β-hydroxysteroid dehydrogenase than those responsible for the conversion of androstenedione to testosterone and androstanedione to DHT.

The most potent endogenous androgen is the 5α-reduced steroid, DHT, which is biosynthesized by two

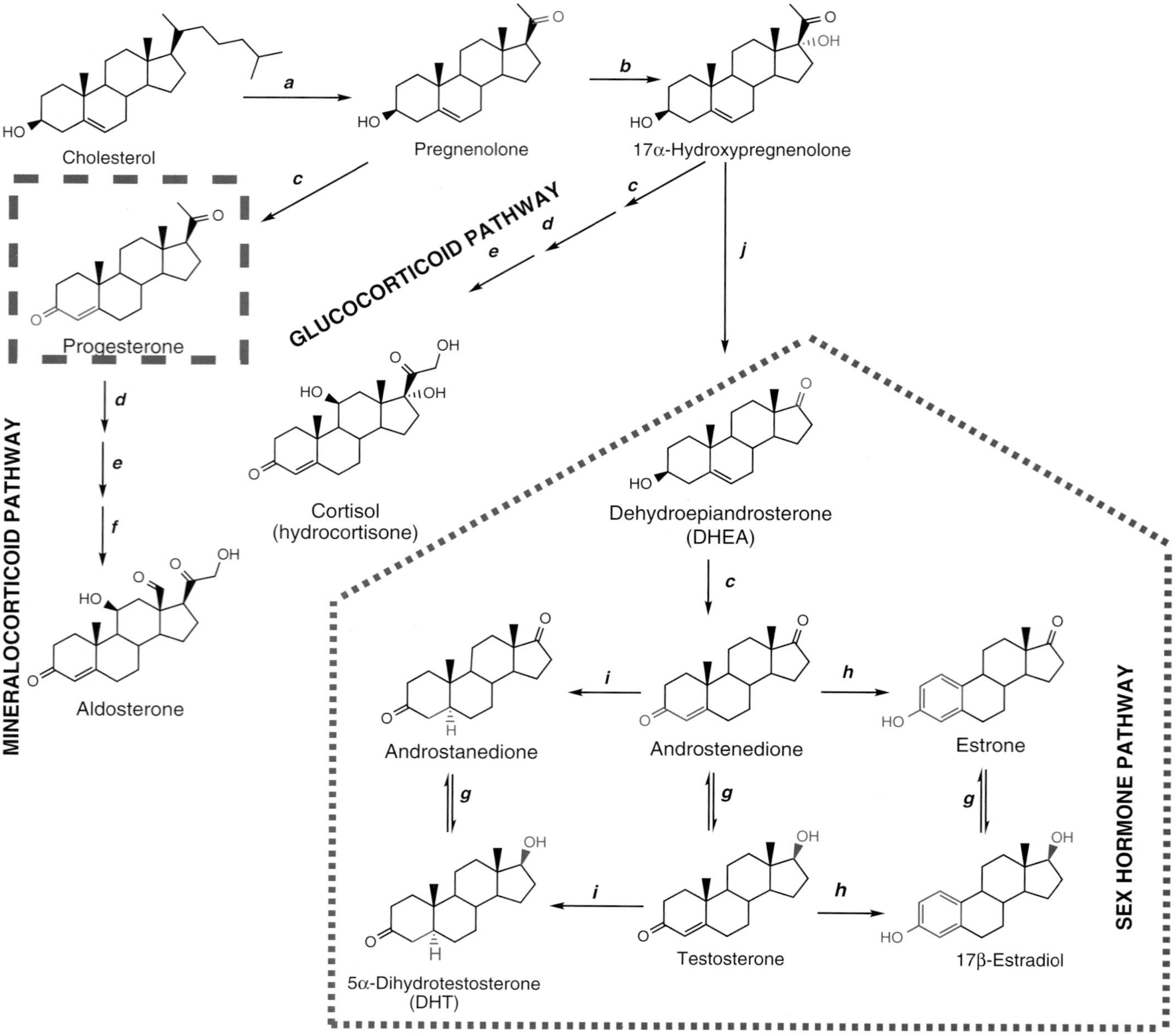

Figure 24.3 Biosynthesis of the adrenocorticoids and sex hormones from cholesterol. The enzymes involved in these biosynthetic pathways are (a) cytochrome P-450 (CYP) cholesterol side-chain cleavage (SCC) enzyme (CYP11A1), (b) 17α-hydroxylase (CYP17A1), (c) 5-ene-3β-hydroxysteroid dehydrogenase/3-oxosteroid-4,5-isomerase (3β-HSD), (d) 21-hydroxylase (CYP21), (e) 11β-hydroxylase (CYP11B2), (f) 18-hydroxyase, (g) 17β-hydroxysteroid dehydrogenases (17β-HSD), (h) aromatase (CYP19A1), (i) 5α-reductase (5AR), and (j) 17,20-lyase (CYP17A1).

5α-reductase (5AR) isoforms, type 1 and type 2. Type 1 5AR is expressed predominantly in sebaceous glands of the skin, scalp, and liver and is responsible for approximately one-third of the circulating DHT (Fig. 24.3). Type 2 5AR is found primarily in the prostate, seminal vesicles, epididymides, genital skin (scrotum), hair follicles, and liver, and it is responsible for two-thirds of the circulating DHT. Approximately 6%-8% of testosterone is converted to DHT. Conversion to DHT amplifies the action of testosterone by three to five times because of the greater binding affinity of DHT as compared to testosterone for the AR.[5]

Progesterone is biosynthesized and secreted by the corpus luteum of the ovary during the luteal phase of the reproductive cycle. LH binds to the LH receptor on the surface of the ovarian cells to initiate progesterone biosynthesis. As in other endocrine cells such as adrenal cortical cells, the binding of LH results in an increase in intracellular cAMP levels via activation of a G-protein and adenylyl cyclase. One of the processes influenced by elevated cAMP levels is the activation of cholesterol esterase, which cleaves cholesterol esters and liberates free cholesterol. The free cholesterol is then converted in mitochondria to pregnenolone via the cholesterol reaction (step a of Fig. 24.3), and progesterone is formed from pregnenolone by the action of 5-ene-3β-hydroxysteroid dehydrogenase/3-oxosteroid-4,5-isomerase (3β-HSD), as discussed previously for 17β-estradiol (and adrenocorticoids) (step c).

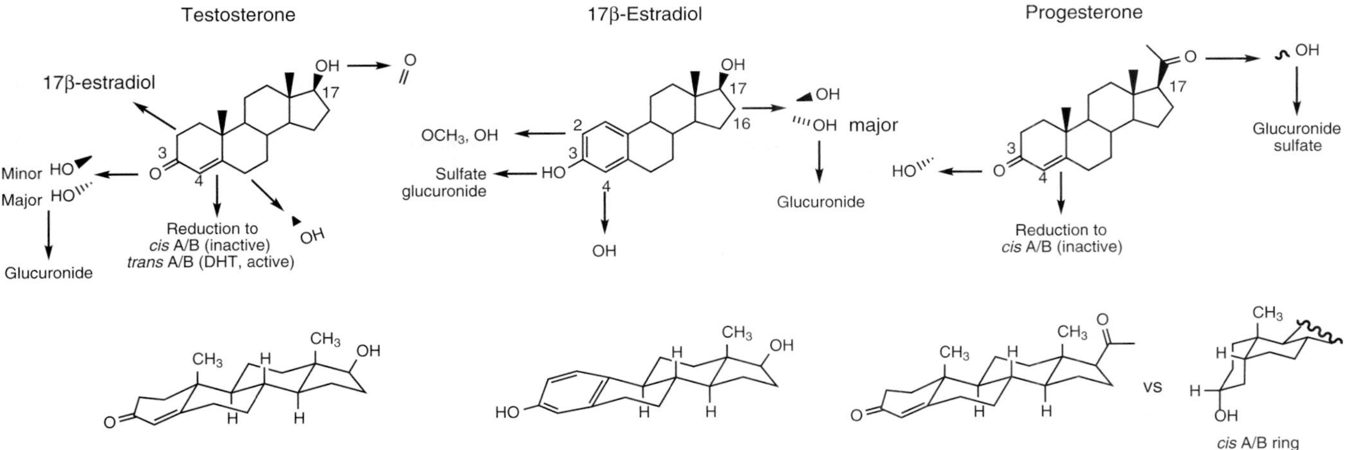

Figure 24.4 General metabolic pathways for androgens, estrogens, and progestins.

Metabolism

The metabolic transformations of androgens, estrogens, and progesterone are similar in many ways (Fig. 24.4). In most cases, metabolic transformations occur predominantly on the A or D rings through phase I hydroxylations followed by phase 2 conjugation reactions (sulfonation or glucuronidation being most common). The stereochemistry of the A/B ring junction upon reduction plays a key three-dimensional conformational role in how these hormones can bind to their respective receptors (Fig. 24.4). By adding a 17α-ethinyl group onto 17β-estradiol, oxidation via first-pass metabolism is prevented allowing for an orally active compound to be used in oral contraceptives. Understanding metabolic transformations is pivotal to understanding why medicinal chemists have added substituents at key positions to prevent their occurrence.

ANDROGEN METABOLISM. Testosterone can be metabolized in either its target tissues or the liver,[6–8] as shown in Figure 24.3. In androgen target tissues, testosterone can be converted to physiologically active metabolites. In the prostate gland, skin, and liver,[9] testosterone is reduced to DHT by 5AR (types 1 and 2).[10] On the other hand, a small amount of testosterone (0.3%) also can be converted to 17β-estradiol by aromatase through cleavage of the C-19 methyl group and aromatization of ring A, which mainly occurs in adipose tissue. This process also occurs in the ovaries of women. In men, approximately 80% of the circulating estrogen arises from aromatization of testosterone in the adipose tissue,[11] with the other 20% being secreted by the Leydig cells in the testes.[12] Both 5α-reduction and aromatization are irreversible processes.

In addition to these pathways to active metabolites, testosterone can also be inactivated in the liver through (1) 6β-oxidation to an inactive hydroxyl metabolite, or (2) 5β-reduction to an inactive cholic acid metabolite then possibly 3α-reduction (Panel B of Fig. 21.9 in Chapter 21 on Adrenocorticoids). Hydroxylated testosterone metabolites are glucuronidated and renally eliminated. Further, testosterone can be metabolized to androstenedione through oxidation of the 17β-OH group which can be further converted to another inactive cholic acid metabolite, etiocholanolone, through 5β- and 3-keto reduction (Fig. 24.4). The 5β reduction of testosterone to its *cis* A/B ring juncture conformation (e.g., 5β-DHT and etiocholanolone) explains its complete loss of activity, because the *cis* A/B ring no longer has affinity for the AR. Most of the other metabolites mentioned earlier undergo extensive glucuronidation as well (e.g., of the 3α- and/or 17β-OH groups) either in the target tissues or in the liver[13] and are excreted in the urine.

After the administration of radiolabeled testosterone, approximately 90% of the radioactivity is found in the urine, and 6% is recovered in the feces through enterohepatic circulation.[14] Major urinary metabolites include androsterone and its 5β-diastereoisomer etiocholanolone, both of which are inactive metabolites. They are excreted mainly as glucuronide conjugates or, to a lesser extent, as sulfate conjugates.[13] Following oral administration, extensive first-pass hepatic metabolism (90% of oral dose) severely limits oral bioavailability and produces a plasma half-life of less than 30 minutes. However, testosterone is commonly delivered by many parenteral dosage forms, and there are ongoing efforts to develop oral dosage forms of testosterone that better circumvent first-pass hepatic metabolism.

Androsterone   5β-Androsterone (etiocholanolone)

ESTROGEN METABOLISM. The endogenous estrogens, estrone and 17β-estradiol, are biochemically interconvertible via the actions of opposing 17β-hydroxysteroid dehydrogenase isozymes, one of which is alternatively referred to as estradiol dehydrogenase, and yield the same metabolic

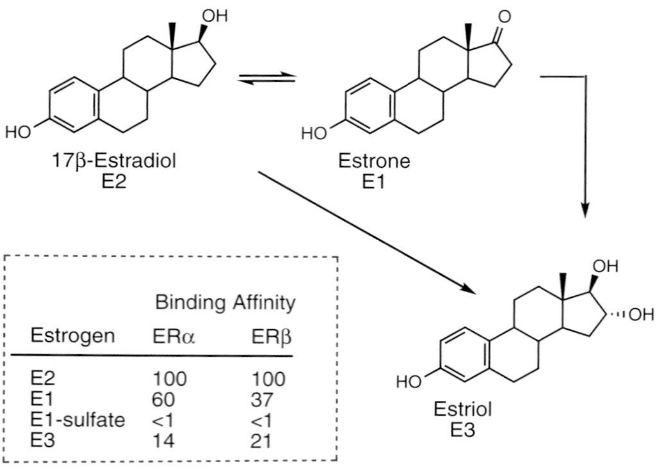

Estrogen	Binding Affinity ERα	ERβ
E2	100	100
E1	60	37
E1-sulfate	<1	<1
E3	14	21

Figure 24.5 Estrogens and their relative binding affinity to ERα and ERβ.

products (Fig. 24.5).[15–17] These hormones are metabolized mainly in the liver and largely excreted as water-soluble glucuronide and sulfate conjugates. Other tissues such as the kidneys and intestines are also involved.

Many metabolites have been isolated from urine, but to date no one has been able to account for all the radioactivity of an administered dose of ^{14}C-labeled 17β-estradiol. The major metabolites are shown in Figure 24.4. Both 17β-estradiol and estrone are converted by CYP3A4 to yield estriol (estra-1,3,5[10]-triene-3,16α,17β-triol). Estriol (Fig. 24.5) is found in the urine as the glucuronide conjugate. Estrogens are also oxidized by CYP3A4 at positions *ortho* to the 3-phenolic group to provide catechol estrogens, 2-hydroxyestrogens and 4-hydroxyestrogens. These metabolites are unstable in vivo, rapidly converted to 2-methoxyestrogen and 4-methoxyestrogen metabolites, and further to glucuronide, sulfate, and glutathione conjugates (Fig. 24.4). These compounds are also found in comparatively large amounts in the urine.[15–17] The catechol estrogens will bind to ERs and produce weak to moderate estrogenic effects. These catechol steroids have also been shown to be produced in certain CNS tissues such as those in the pituitary and hypothalamus, suggesting possible neuroendocrine functions. The formation, metabolism, and biologic effects of catechol estrogens have been reviewed.[18]

PROGESTERONE METABOLISM. Progesterone, the female sex hormone synthesized by the corpus luteum, is metabolized in part by routes similar to those for the adrenocorticoids. Progesterone is mainly excreted as conjugates of 5β-pregnane-3α,20-diol. Reduction of the 20-ketone to an alcohol, reduction of the 4,5-double bond resulting in 5β (i.e., *cis*) ring fusion geometry, and reduction of the 3-ketone to the 3α configuration characterize the production of 5β-pregnane-3α,20-diol from progesterone (Fig. 24.4). Minor pathways of metabolism in the liver can occur, with the side chain at position 17 removed and pathways similar to those for the metabolism of androgens observed.

Understanding Hormone Pharmacotherapy Based Upon the Hypothalamus-Pituitary-Endocrine Axis

The male and female reproductive cycle is regulated by the endocrine and central nervous systems via the hypothalamus-pituitary-endocrine (HPG) axis (Fig. 24.6). Gonadotropin-releasing hormone (GnRH), also known as luteinizing hormone–releasing hormone (LHRH), is a decapeptide that is synthesized by the hypothalamus, secreted, and acts on the GnRH receptor on the anterior pituitary gland. The anterior pituitary gland releases follicle-stimulating hormone (FSH) and LH, glycoproteins of approximately 29,000 molecular weight that are each made of an identical α-subunit (92 amino acids) with differences in the β-subunits that will bind respectively to their receptors (FSH or LH) on the testes/ovary. In the male, the role of FSH is to stimulate spermatogenesis

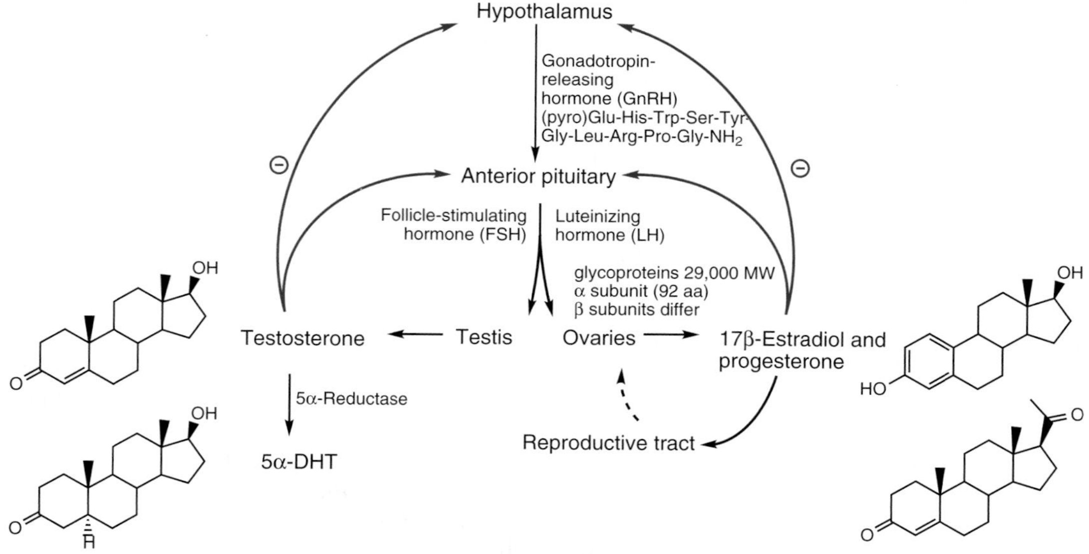

Figure 24.6 Negative feedback role on hypothalamus, pituitary testes/ovary axis, and reproductive tract interrelationships.

in Sertoli cells of testes in addition to testes development, while the role of LH is to stimulate testosterone production from cholesterol in the Leydig cells. In the female, FSH stimulates the growth of follicles, while LH induces luteinization of the ruptured follicle leading to corpus luteum formation. In granulosa cells of the ovary, FSH can regulate expression of aromatase which converts androgens into estrogens, while LH acts on the theca cells to stimulate the synthesis of androstenedione. The production and release of androgens and estrogens from the ovaries/testes allow these hormones to have tissue-specific effects by binding to their respective hormone receptors and resulting in transcription and translation of proteins that can result in altered cell function. These hormones also exhibit negative feedback regulation which allows their precise control of hormone levels.

Knowledge of this axis and the role of hormonal negative feedback can be used to understand how various therapeutic agents work. Disorders of the HPG axis can arise due to changes in concentrations of the sex steroids, as either hyper- or hypogonadism. Changes in concentrations of sex steroids or their effects can lead to infertility, precocious puberty, or delayed puberty. A woman's cycle can be modulated to prevent pregnancy by using estrogen and progestin agonists in oral contraceptive agents. GnRH agonists can help treat central precocious puberty when given in a pulsatile fashion mimicking the normal decapeptide. High concentrations of GnRH given in a continuous fashion help to downregulate the GnRH receptor, thus decreasing androgen and estrogen levels and thus can be used in the treatment of hormone-dependent prostate and breast cancer. Exogenous supply of FSH and LH can allow an endocrinologist to control hormone production and ovaries resulting in hyperstimulation for egg retrieval for in vitro fertilization during infertility problems. Tracking of the LH surge can be used by women in over-the-counter (OTC) ovulation kits to estimate timing of ovulation to increase chances of achieving pregnancy. Progesterone is known as the hormone of pregnancy, and progesterone antagonists can be used to terminate pregnancy. Higher concentrations of progestin antagonists can be used in emergency contraception when taken within 72 hours of unprotected intercourse to prevent pregnancy. During menopause, estrogen and progesterone levels fall giving rise to menopausal side effects that can be alleviated by exogenous administration of agonists of these hormones. Inhibition of the conversion of testosterone to the more potent androgen DHT reduces the size of the male prostate to decrease symptoms of BPH in the aging male. Use of antagonists can be useful in the treatment of hormone-dependent breast and prostate cancers.

This chapter discusses hormonal pharmacotherapy approaches used to modulate a women's fertility (contraceptive agents, infertility, emergency contraception), to improve quality of life in men and women's health (male hypogonadism, andropause, menopause, ED, BPH), and to treat hormone-dependent cancers (breast, prostate).

DRUGS USED IN MODULATING WOMEN'S FERTILITY

Estrogens

Discovery of Estrogens

Allen and Doisy[19] showed in 1923 that an extract of ovaries can produce estrus. Soon thereafter, it was found that a good source of estrogens is the urine of pregnant women. Estrone [3-hydroxyestra-1,3,5(10)-trien-17-one] was the first crystalline estrogen to be isolated from a natural source. Two other C-18 estrogen steroids, 17β-estradiol and estriol, were later isolated and characterized to round out what are considered to be the three classic estrogens (Fig. 24.5).[20,21]

Estrogen Physiology

FEMALE SEX HORMONES AND THE REPRODUCTIVE CYCLE. The ovarian cycle, the preparation of endocrine tissues and release of oocytes, and the menstrual cycle, the preparation and maintenance of the uterine lining, occur concurrently and govern the female reproductive process.[22,23] During the follicular phase of the ovarian cycle, GnRH secreted by the hypothalamus stimulates the release of LH and FSH from the anterior pituitary, which in turn act on the ovaries to regulate the expression of sex hormones (mainly 17β-estradiol) and two protein complexes (activin and inhibin) that govern the reproductive cycle. As the name implies, FSH promotes the initial development of the immature Graafian follicle in the ovary. FSH cannot induce ovulation but must work in conjunction with LH. The combined effect is to promote follicle growth and increase secretion of 17β-estradiol. Growing follicles begin to produce high levels of 17β-estradiol, which acts in concert with activin and inhibin in a negative feedback system to inhibit production of FSH and stimulate output of LH. The level of LH rises to a sharp peak at midpoint, signaling the end of the follicular phase and causing rupture of the follicle and release of its mature oöcyte (ovulation). In contrast, FSH reaches its highest level during menses, falls to a low level during and after ovulation, and then increases again toward the onset of menses.

Once ovulation has taken place, LH induces luteinization of the ruptured follicle, which leads to corpus luteum formation. After luteinization has been initiated, there is an increase in progesterone level from the developing corpus luteum, which in turn suppresses production of LH. Once the corpus luteum is complete, it begins to degenerate toward menses, and the levels of progesterone and 17β-estradiol decline. LH levels remain low during menses. The major events are summarized in Figure 24.7.

The endometrium, the mucous membrane lining of the uterus, passes through different phases which depend on the steroid hormones secreted by the ovary. During the follicular phase, which lasts approximately 12-14 days, the endometrium undergoes proliferation owing to estrogenic stimulation. The luteal phase follows ovulation, lasts

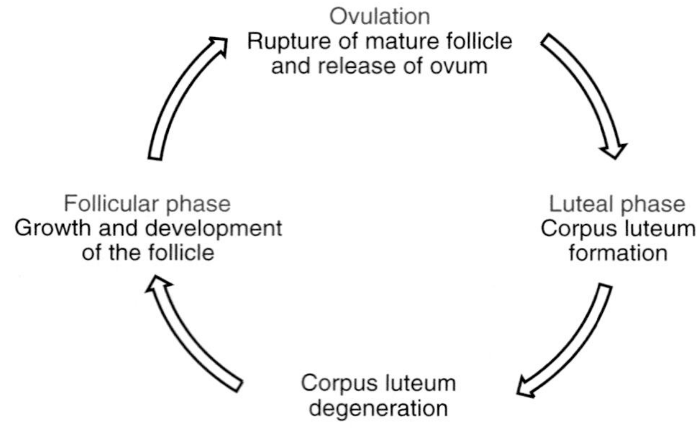

Figure 24.7 Ovarian cycle.

about 14-16 days, and ends at menses. During the luteal phase, the endometrium shows secretory activity, and cell proliferation declines.

In the absence of pregnancy, the levels of 17β-estradiol and progesterone decline; this leads to sloughing of the endometrium. This, together with the flow of interstitial blood through the vagina, is called menses and lasts for 4-6 days. Because the 17β-estradiol and progesterone levels are now low, the hypothalamus releases more GnRH, and the cycle begins again. The reproductive cycle in the female extends from the onset of menses to the next period of menses, with a regular interval varying from 20 to 35 days; the average length is 28 days.

If pregnancy occurs, the menstrual cycle is interrupted because of the release of a fourth gonadotropin. In human pregnancy, the gonadotropin produced by the placenta is referred to as human chorionic gonadotropin (hCG). hCG maintains and prolongs the life of the corpus luteum. The hCG level in the urine rises to the point where it can be detected after 14 days and reaches a maximum around the seventh week of pregnancy. After this peak, the hCG concentration falls to a constant level, which is maintained throughout pregnancy.

The corpus luteum, because of hCG stimulation, provides an adequate level of the steroidal hormones to maintain pregnancy during the first nine weeks. After this period, the placenta can secrete the required level of estrogens and progestational hormones to maintain pregnancy. The levels of estrogen and progesterone increase during pregnancy and finally reach their maximal concentrations a few days before parturition. Because the level of hCG in the urine rises rapidly after conception, it has served as the basis for many pregnancy tests.

Sexual maturation, or the period in which cyclic menstrual bleeding begins to occur, is reached between the ages of 10 and 17; the average age is 13. The period of irregular menstrual cycles before the cessation of menses (usually between the ages of 40 and 50) is commonly known as menopause.

MENOPAUSE. Menopause is defined as the last menstrual cycle due to loss of ovarian function, which results in negligible levels of 17β-estradiol and progesterone. The average age of menopause is 51 years and 90% of women are menopausal by 55 years of age. The period of irregular menstrual cycles before the cessation of menses (menopause) (usually between the ages of 45-55) is commonly known as perimenopause. By 2020, the US population entering perimenopause (45-54) and menopause (55-64) is projected to be 20.6 and 22.1 million, respectively.[24] It typically begins 3-5 years before menopause but can last up to 10 years. It is due to the sporadic failure of ovarian follicles (follicular atresia) and a decrease in estrogen levels, and without a corpus luteum the progesterone levels also decrease. FSH levels will be high during this time and total androgens decrease. Unopposed estrogen and lack of progesterone causes endometrial buildup, resulting in heavier flow in early perimenopause. The length of the cycle is irregular, shorter or longer, and eventually with skipped periods.

Menopausal symptoms are due to negligible levels of 17β-estradiol as the ovaries are no longer functional. The predominant estrogen produced in this stage of a women's life is estrone. It is produced in largest amounts in adipose tissue but also from muscle and the adrenal gland. In these tissues, androstenedione is converted to the weaker estrogen estrone by the action of aromatase. Due to the decline of estrogens, menopausal symptoms can be treated by exogenous administration of estrogen alone (for women without a uterus) or in combination with a progestin (for women with an intact uterus) to help improve quality of life, but recommendations depend on age in relationship to menopause onset. If the exogenous administration of estrogen is too high in the women, side effects such as nausea/vomiting, breast tenderness, weight gain, and vaginal bleeding will develop. Progesterone is known as the hormone of pregnancy in premenopausal women and can have negative symptoms in menopausal women. Unopposed estrogen usage in women with an intact uterus has been shown to cause endometrial hyperplasia and increases the risk of endometrial cancer. Thus, progestin protects the uterus and is included in hormone replacement therapy when women have an intact uterus.

Mechanisms of Estrogen Action

MOLECULAR INTERACTIONS. Steroidal estrogens were first isolated in the 1920s, but the presence of their cognate receptor was not reported until 1962.[25,26] The earliest searches for a biochemical mechanism of action of 17β-estradiol focused on the female reproductive tissues, since estrogens localize and produce dramatic and selective responses in these female tissues. Using labeled 17β-estradiol, Jensen and Jacobson[26] showed that uptake of 17β-estradiol is rapid and that 17β-estradiol is retained to a high degree in the uterus and vagina.

The biochemical mechanism of estrogen action is the regulation of gene expression and subsequent induction of protein biosynthesis via specific, high-affinity ERs, as described in Chapter 7 (Intracellular Cytoplasmic/Nuclear Receptors).[27] ER subtype α (ERα) was successfully cloned in 1986 and was considered to be the sole ER until 1996 when a homologous but novel ER, ERβ, was cloned from rat prostate.[28] This receptor demonstrated sub-nanomolar affinity for 17β-estradiol and offered plausible explanation for the residual ER activity detected in existing ERα knockout mouse models.[29–31] Disparate tissue expression combined with further development of ER knockout models elucidated overlapping but distinct biological roles for these sister receptors.[32–34] Receptor binding sites for 17β-estradiol are located in the cytoplasm and nucleus of target cells[35–38] and exhibit both high affinity ($K_D = 10^{-11}$-10^{-10} M) and low capacity. Binding to the ERs is specific. The uptake of [2,4,6,7-^{3}H]-17β-estradiol by the receptors can be inhibited by pretreatment with unlabeled 17β-estradiol or diethylstilbestrol (DES). Pretreatment with testosterone, cortisol, or progesterone does not inhibit binding of radiolabeled 17β-estradiol. The binding is stereospecific because 17α-estradiol, which differs from 17β-estradiol in the configuration of the hydroxyl group at carbon 17, does not prevent the binding of 17β-estradiol to the ERs.[39]

The two ERs differ in size, with ERα having 595 amino acids and ERβ having 485 amino acids. 17β-Estradiol and other endogenous estrogens have similar affinities for both ERα and ERβ (Fig. 24.5, Table 24.1), whereas nonsteroidal estrogenic compounds and antiestrogens have differing affinities between ERα and ERβ[40] and subtype selectivity is possible to attain via anti-periplanar substitution of the linking element between the hydroxyl groups.

As discussed in Chapter 7 for steroid hormone receptors, when 17β-estradiol binds to the ER, a conformational change of the 17β-estradiol-receptor complex occurs and results in interactions of this complex with particular hormone response element (HRE) regions of the cellular DNA, referred to as estrogen response elements (EREs). Binding of the complex to ERE results in the initiation of transcription of the DNA sequence to produce mRNA. Finally, the elevated levels of mRNA lead to an increase in protein synthesis in the endoplasmic reticulum. For example, levels of PRs increase in uterine tissue, thus preparing the tissue for the actions of progesterone on the uterus during the later half of the reproductive cycle.[41,42]

In addition to the conventional ER actions as mentioned above, a third ER was identified in 2005. This ER, a G-protein–coupled receptor, is localized in the cell membrane and is called GPR30.[43] GPR30 promotes rapid actions of estrogens and has been identified to be responsible for various physiological and pharmacological actions of estrogens. In addition to GPR30, ER is also activated by various posttranslational mechanisms induced by growth factors and kinases. This rapid activation of ER by posttranslational mechanisms and by growth factors is called nongenomic activation or ligand-independent activation. This nongenomic or ligand-independent action of ER has been found to be common in the nuclear receptor family.

Although the two forms of ER are synthesized by two different genes, the PR isoforms, PR-B and PR-A, are synthesized by the same gene as a result of alternate splicing. PR-A lacks the first 164 amino acids of PR-B with the rest of the receptor being completely identical. Despite the sequence homology, PR-A and PR-B have distinct functions; with PR-A under several conditions functioning as a dominant suppressor of PR-B.

Table 24.1 Relative Binding Affinities of Endogenous and Exogenous Estrogens

Estrogen	ERα Binding Affinity	ERβ Binding Affinity
17β-Estradiol (E2)	100	100
Estrone (E1)	60	37
Estrone sulfate	<1	<1
Estriol (E3)	14	21
4-Hydroxy-estradiol	13	7
2-Hydroxy-estradiol	7	11
Coumestrol	94	185
Genistein	5	36
Tamoxifen	7	6
4-Hydroxytamoxifen	178	339
Clomiphene	25	12
Diethylstilbestrol	468	295

Based on Kuiper GG, Carlsson B, Grandien K, et al. Comparison of the ligand binding specificity and transcript tissue distribution of estrogen receptors alpha and beta. *Endocrinology.* 1997;138:863-870.
ER, estrogen receptor.

PHYSIOLOGIC EFFECTS. Estrogens act on many tissues, such as those of the reproductive tract, breast, bone, and CNS. ERα is expressed at high levels in several normal tissues classically associated with estrogenic activity including uterus, ovary (theca cells), bone, and breast. ERα is also expressed at high levels in prostate (stroma) and brain. ERβ is found at its highest levels in normal colon, prostate (epithelium), ovary (granulosa cells), bone marrow, and brain, with smaller amounts reported in uterus, bladder, lung, and testis.[44,45] ERα appears to mediate the ability of 17β-estradiol to provide negative feedback in the brain and to slow bone resorption and maintain bone mineral density (BMD).

The primary physiological action of estrogens is to stimulate the development of secondary sex characteristics, including growth of hair, softening of skin, growth of breasts, widening of the hips, and distribution of fat in the thighs, hips, and buttocks. Estrogens also stimulate the growth and development of the female reproductive tract, including the uterine oviduct, cervix, and vagina. The proliferative changes that occur in the endometrium and myometrium upon administration of exogenous estrogens resemble those that take place naturally. Bleeding often follows withdrawal of the estrogens. The growth and development of tissues in the reproductive tract of animals, in terms of actual weight gained, are not seen for as long as 16 hours after administration of the estrogen, although some biochemical processes in the cell are affected immediately. The growth response produced in the uterus by estrogens is temporary, and the maintenance of such growth requires the hormone to be available almost continuously. The initial growth induced by the estrogen is therefore of limited duration, and atrophy of the uterus occurs if the hormone is withdrawn.

Another physiologic effect of estrogens, observed 1 hour after their administration, is edema in the uterus.

During this period, vasodilation of the uterine pre- and postcapillary arterioles occurs, and there is an increase in permeability to plasma proteins. These effects appear to occur predominantly in the endometrium and not to any great extent in the myometrium.[46] Correspondingly, endometriosis can result from prolonged exposure to estrogens or hormone imbalances among the sex hormones.

Another target of estrogens is breast tissue. Estrogens stimulate the proliferation of breast cells and promote the growth of hormone-dependent mammary carcinoma. Because the breast is the primary site for cancer in women, considerable research has been focused on understanding breast cancer and the factors that influence its growth. 17β-Estradiol will stimulate gene expression and the production of several proteins in breast cancer cells via the ER mechanism. These proteins include both intracellular proteins important for breast cell function and growth, and secreted proteins that can influence tumor growth and metastasis. Intracellular proteins include enzymes needed for DNA synthesis, such as DNA polymerase, thymidine kinase, thymidylate synthetase, and dihydrofolate reductase.[47,48] PRs are induced in breast cells by estrogens,[49] and the content of both ERs and PRs is utilized clinically as markers for hormone responsiveness of the breast cancer in determining hormonal therapy.[50]

PHARMACOLOGY, SIDE EFFECTS, AND CLINICAL APPLICATIONS. Estrogens are used in a wide variety of menstrual disturbances, such as amenorrhea, dysmenorrhea, and oligomenorrhea. They are also effective in failure of ovarian development, acne, and senile vaginitis. For example, a nonsteroidal estrogen is now used in dyspareunia, as will be discussed. After childbirth, estrogens have been used to suppress lactation. One of the most widespread uses of estrogens is in birth control. Hormone replacement therapy and selective estrogen receptor modulators (SERMs) have been used in osteoporosis because it is thought that an estrogen deficiency in postmenopausal women can lead to this serious disorder of the bone. One of the primary therapeutic uses is in the treatment of menopausal symptoms such as hot flashes, chilly sensations, dizziness, fatigue, irritability, and sweating. For many women, menopause does not cause much discomfort; in some, however, both physical and mental discomfort may occur and can usually be prevented through estrogen therapy. Because of feminizing effects, estrogen therapy in males is limited.

Nausea appears to be the main side effect of estrogen therapy; other adverse effects include vomiting, anorexia, and diarrhea. If small doses are used to initiate therapy, and the dose is gradually increased, most of the side effects can be avoided. Excessive doses of estrogens inhibit the development of bones in young patients by accelerating epiphyseal closure.

When estrogens are given in large doses over long periods of time, they can inhibit ovulation because of their feedback action; inhibition of the release of FSH from the adenohypophysis (i.e., anterior pituitary) results in inhibition of ovulation. Administration of these drugs may promote sodium chloride retention; the result is retention of water and subsequent edema. This effect, however, is less pronounced than with glucocorticoids. More detailed information on the pharmacology and toxicology of estrogens can be found in published reviews.[51–54]

CLOMIPHENE, AN ANTIESTROGEN USED FOR INFERTILITY

Clomiphene citrate (first approved in 1982) is an effective first-line treatment used to induce ovulation in anovulatory women. Clomiphene is a nonsteroidal triphenylethylene derivative like tamoxifen. It is administered as a mixture of stereoisomers, in approximately a 3:2 ratio of the *trans*-clomiphene (enclomiphene) and *cis*-clomiphene (zuclomiphene) enantiomers, each with unique pharmacology. The more potent *trans*-isomer is responsible for the ovulation-inducing actions.

In the early follicular phase, plasma estrogen serves as a negative feedback inhibitor to the hypothalamus and anterior pituitary. Clomiphene (oral, 50 mg) is taken by women for 5 days starting on the second to fifth day after the onset of menses. 52% of women ovulate in response to 50 mg treatment of clomiphene; however, a titration may be necessary to determine the lowest effective dose for an individual woman as doses can range daily from 50 to 250 mg.[56] Higher doses may be necessary in women with greater body mass index. By binding to and antagonizing the ER, clomiphene prevents 17β-estradiol from exerting its negative feedback in the hypothalamus. Compensatory mechanisms by the hypothalamus result in increased pulsatile secretions of GnRH secretions and increases of LH and FSH secretion from the pituitary, which in turn increase ovarian follicular activity.[56] The LH surge occurs 5-12 days after the last dose of clomiphene.

Enclomiphene (*trans/E*) + Zuclomiphene (*cis/Z*)

CYP2D6 (Enclomiphene → (*E*)-4-hydroxy-clomiphene)

CYP3A4 ((*E*)-4-hydroxy-clomiphene → (*E*)-4-hydroxy-*N*-desethyl-clomiphene)

(*E*)-4-hydroxy-clomiphene (IC_{50} = 2.5 nM)

(*E*)-4-hydroxy-*N*-desethyl-clomiphene (IC_{50} = 1.4 nM)

Major metabolites of *trans*
100x more potent at ER

Clomiphene has been shown to exhibit both estrogen agonist and antagonist properties.[55] In humans, it is usually considered to be an antiestrogen (competitive estrogen receptor antagonist), and in rats and other species it is considered to be a mixed agonist/antagonist.[55] The estrogenic properties of clomiphene are generally seen only when endogenous estrogen levels are extremely low. By using a cell-based transcription assay, clomiphene has been shown to act as an agonist or antagonist via ERα depending on 17β-estradiol concentration. Serum concentrations of clomiphene in women taking a therapeutic dose are reported to be 10^{-9}-10^{-7} M. Clomiphene acted as a complete antagonist (at 10^{-8} M) of ERα in the presence of lower concentrations of 17β-estradiol (10^{-12} M) but not at 10^{-10} M.[57] Clomiphene exhibits a more pronounced antagonist effect at ERβ as it eliminated the estrogenic activity of 17β-estradiol even at the higher concentrations of 10^{-10} M.

Clomiphene is readily absorbed, reaches peak concentrations in ~6 hours, metabolized predominately by liver via CYP2D6 and 3A4,[58] undergoes enterohepatic recycling, and elimination via feces (42%) and urine (8%). It has a half-life of approximately 5 days. It has been shown that the (*Z*)-4-hydroxylated metabolites produced via CYP2D6 followed by CYP3A4 afford (*Z*)-4-hydroxy-clomiphene and (*Z*)-4-hydroxy-N-desethylclomiphene. These major metabolites are at least 100 times more potent at the ER than their parent compounds. (IC_{50} values for inhibition of 17β-estradiol for ER were reported as 2.5 nM for (*E*)-4-hydroxy-clomiphene and 1.4 nM for (*E*)-4-hydroxy-N-desethylclomiphene.)[59] These results demonstrate that clomiphene is a prodrug with similar metabolic pathways as tamoxifen and toremifene (see information later in this chapter).

The most common side effects of treatment with clomiphene are irritability and mood swings,[60] ovarian enlargement (14%), hot flashes (10%), bloating (≤6%), and visual disturbances (2%, reversible upon discontinuation).[61] Relatively common with clomiphene usage is the 8% increased risk of multiple gestation for anovulatory women due to development of multiple follicles. Although rare, women should be cautioned about ovarian hyperstimulation syndrome that may begin within 24 hours of treatment but may be most severe 7-10 days after therapy.

A women who fails to conceive after three to four successful clomiphene-induced ovulation cycles should be further evaluated for other infertility causes, especially if over the age of 35. Clomiphene can be given in combination with metformin, glucocorticoids, and exogenous gonadotropins when clomiphene only treatment proves unsuccessful for ovulation.

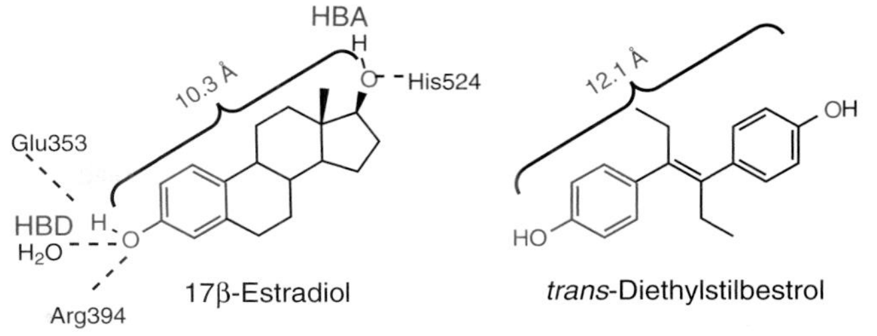

Pharmacophore	Estrogen	Binding Affinity ERα	ERβ
1. Phenol as HBD	E2	100	100
2. Flat, hydrophobic spacer	DES	468	295
3. HBA			

Figure 24.8 Estrogen pharmacophore with important binding interactions to ER shown. The phenol of 17β-estradiol acts as a hydrogen bond donator (HBD) to the amino acids shown and the 17β-OH acts as a hydrogen bond acceptor (HBA) from the amino acid shown. The amino acid numbering shown reflects binding to ERα. Relative binding affinity to ERα and ERβ are given.

Structure-Activity Relationships

Analyses of the biological activities of both steroidal and nonsteroidal estrogens, in vitro investigations with subcellular fractions containing ERs, and X-ray crystallography studies on the ligand binding domain (LBD) of the ERs have resulted in an extensive knowledge of the structure-activity relationships for estrogens.[53,62–64] These studies demonstrated the high affinity and specificity of the most potent endogenous estrogen, 17β-estradiol. There are two polar interactions between 17β-estradiol and ERs which are essential for all estrogens to bind ERα or ERβ: (1) the phenoxy substituent at C-3 (or other hydrogen bond donor if nonsteroidal) of the steroid nucleus (or other hydrophobic, often rigid and/or planar linking element) interacts with ER amino acids Glu353, Arg394, and a conserved/structural water molecule, and (2) the 17β-hydroxyl (or other hydrogen bond acceptor) interacts with His524 (see Fig. 24.8). Importantly, the distance between the two polar groups of the estrogen ligand must be approximately the same as 17β-estradiol and connected by an often rigid and/or planar hydrophobic connecting group, as illustrated with *trans*-DES.

For optimal estrogenic activity, the distance between the oxygen atoms of the two hydroxyl groups ranges from 10.3 to 12.1 Å. The region of the ER that binds the D-ring is flexible and can conform to ligands with different distances (e.g., 10.3 Å for 17β-estradiol and 12.1 Å for DES). Many other potent steroidal and nonsteroidal estrogens conform to the above requirements, but there seems to be few restrictions on the types of linking groups that can be employed. Further, these requirements apply to both ER subtypes as the illustrated amino acids are the same. However, ERβ selectivity can be attained by anti-periplanar substitution of the linking element which would extend toward amino acids that vary between ERα and ERβ.[40] Although many preclinical ERβ agonists exist, none have been U.S. Food and Drug Administration (FDA) approved.

Substituents on the estrogen nucleus significantly modify estrogenic activity. On the A-ring, any functionality at the C-1 position greatly reduces activity, and only small groups can be accommodated at the 2 and 4 positions. Insertion of hydroxyl groups at positions 6, 7, and 11 reduces activity. Removal of the oxygen function from position 3 or 17 or epimerization of the 17-hydroxyl group of estradiol to the α-configuration results in a less active

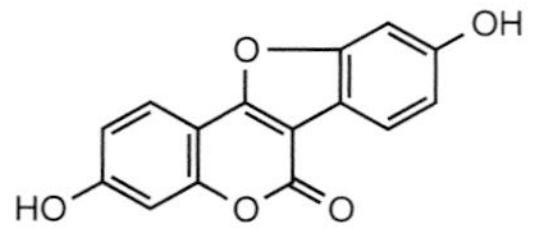

Coumestrol
(legumes)

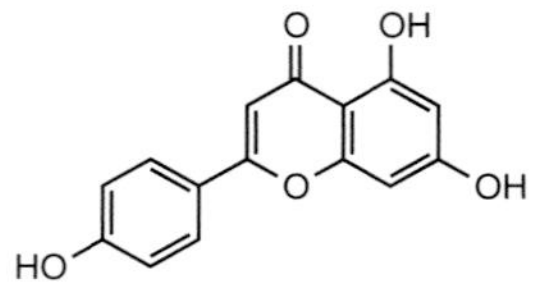

Apigenin
(a flavone from parsley, celery)

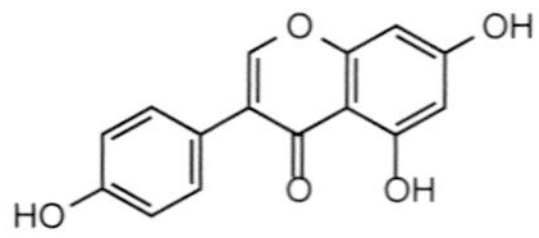

Genistein
(an isoflavone from soy)

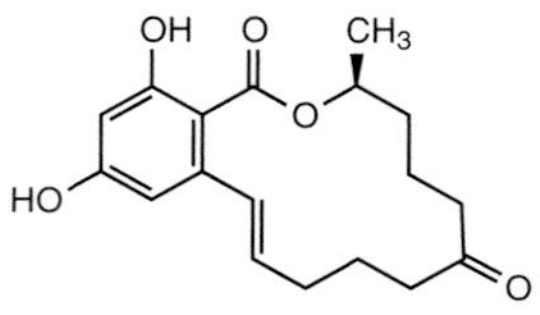

Zearalenone
(fungal metabolite)

Estrogen	Binding Affinity ERα	ERβ
E2	100	100
Coumestrol	94	185
Genistein	5	36

Figure 24.9 Xenoestrogens and their relative binding affinity to ERα and ERβ.

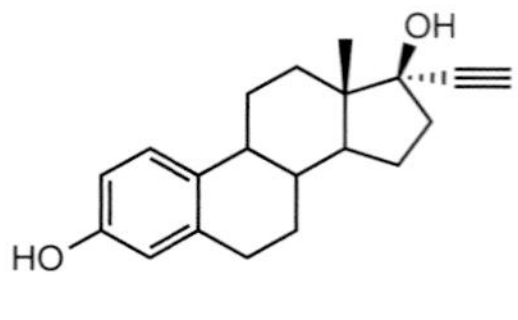

estrogenic substance.[65] Introduction of unsaturation into the B ring similarly reduces potency. Substituents at the 11β position can be well tolerated; for example, 11β-methoxy or 11β-ethyl have significantly greater affinity for ER compared to 17β-estradiol. Modifications at the 17α and 16 positions can lead to enhanced activity. Ethinyl or vinyl groups provide the greatest activity, while highly polar groups are poorly tolerated. At the 16 position, moderate size and polarity are tolerated.

Many compounds of natural origin have estrogenic activity including nonsteroidal xenobiotics consumed as food by humans and livestock (Fig. 24.9).[66] Naturally occurring estrogens are found in a number of plants such as legumes (coumestrol), parsley/celery (apigenin), soy (genistein), or corn/oats (zearalenone).[67] Since these are natural products, they are sold over the counter in products such as Estroven which contains soy isoflavones. Generally, phytoestrogens are weak nonselective estrogens believed to provide some relief for postmenopausal women, but there is controversy about their safety and efficacy relative to hormone replacement therapies using purified and potent estrogens. Although not well studied, it is advisable for those with a history of breast cancer to avoid large amounts of phytoestrogens in foods and supplements.

Steroidal Estrogens

17β-Estradiol is the most potent endogenous estrogen, exhibiting high affinity for the ER and potency when administered parenterally. The naturally occurring estrogens are only weakly active when administered orally. They are thought to be rapidly absorbed from the intestine but can be degraded by microorganisms in the gastrointestinal (GI) tract.[68] The endogenous estrogens are promptly metabolized by the liver to a great extent, resulting in the

Ethinyl estradiol
(EE)

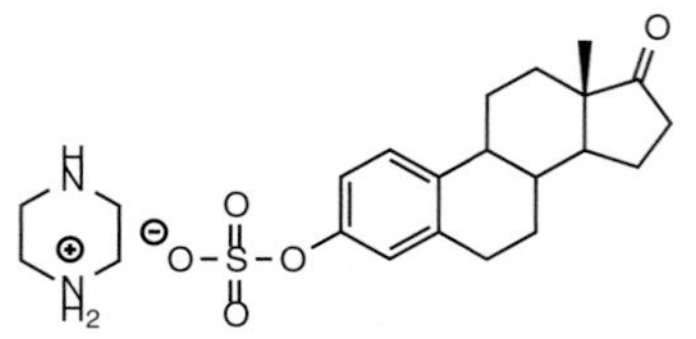

Estropipate
Piperazine estrone sulfate
(prodrug)

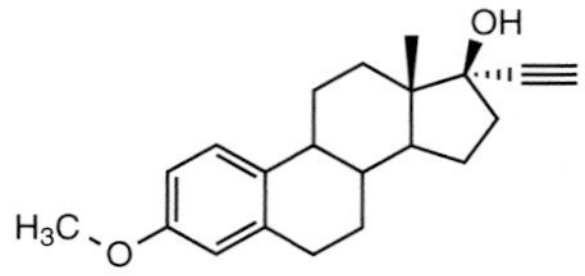

Mestranol
(prodrug)

Figure 24.10 Orally active steroidal estrogens.

observed low therapeutic effectiveness when administered orally. Comparative ER potencies for endogenous estrogens (17β-estradiol, estrone, and estriol) are shown in Figure 24.5. The observed in vivo biologic activity varies with the mode of administration of the estrogens. The order of activity of the three naturally occurring steroids when administered subcutaneously is 17β-estradiol > estrone > estriol. The order changes to estriol > 17β-estradiol > estrone, however, when the drugs are administered orally.[69] Also, metabolic conjugation may produce estrogens that retain some of their activity; it has been reported that estrone sulfate (used as the piperazine salt estropipate; Fig. 24.10) is actually more active than the original hormone when administered orally to rats. The modified drug also retains some activity in humans but is considered a prodrug that will undergo cleavage to estrone.[70,71]

Owing to limited oral bioavailability, 17β-estradiol is administered via once- or twice-weekly transdermal patches (e.g., Alora, Minivelle, Vivelle-Dot, Menostar, and Climara), gels (e.g., Divigel, Estrogel, Elestrin), creams (e.g., EC-RX Estradiol), and a spray (e.g., Evamist) for the prevention of postmenopausal osteoporosis, treatment of moderate to severe vasomotor symptoms associated with menopause (e.g., hot flashes), and treatment of moderate to severe symptoms of vulvar and vaginal atrophy associated with menopause. Transdermal patches are preferably placed on the lower abdomen or buttocks but should not be applied to the breast. Systemic levels of 17β-estradiol concentrations vary by product and the route of administration, and remain generally low (ranging from ~10 to 100 pg/mL) because of rapid hepatic metabolism of the hormone once it enters the circulatory system.[72,73] 17β-Estradiol is also available as a micronized tablet (Estrace) for the same therapeutic applications.

Chemical modifications have led to better orally effective estrogens. One successful method of overcoming this rapid inactivation of 17β-estradiol by the liver has been to stabilize the alcoholic function at C-17 with an appropriate substituent. Ethinyl estradiol (EE) [17α-ethynyl-1,3,5(10)-estratriene-3,17β-diol] (Fig. 24.10) is an estrogenic substance that is very potent when taken orally.[74] EE was synthesized in 1939, is a highly effective oral estrogen due to improved hepatic and intestinal pharmacokinetics, and is the predominantly used estrogen in oral contraceptives. Mestranol, a 3-methoxy ether and orally active prodrug of EE, is also found in some oral contraceptives.[75] EE or mestranol combined with synthetic progestins produce a synergistic suppression of the hypothalamus and pituitary production of FSH and LH, preventing follicular development, ovulation, and implantation.

EE and mestranol are rapidly and nearly completely absorbed in the stomach. Peak serum concentration (C_{max}) values of EE and mestranol are achieved in 1 and 4 hours, respectively. In both cases, EE accumulates in endometrium and ovary compared to plasma. EE is also found in fat and bound to plasma proteins which produces a large volume of distribution. EE is largely converted to various glucuronide and sulfate conjugates of its ethynylated (2-methoxy, unchanged, 16β-hydroxy, 2-hydroxy, and 6α-hydroxy) and de-ethynylated (estrone [E1], 17β-estradiol [E2], estriol [E3], and 2-methoxy) metabolites.[76] Thirty nine percent of radioactivity of EE appears in urine and 53% in feces over a 7-10-day period.[76] The high fecal radioactivity is largely due to biliary excretion of sulfate and glucuronide metabolites. Enterohepatic recirculation occurs as the biliary metabolites are excreted into the intestines, hydrolyzed by microorganisms back to EE, and then reabsorbed and returned to liver (Fig. 24.11). The oral activity of EE results because it is much less susceptible than 17β-estradiol to hepatic first pass metabolism and microbial degradation.

Ester derivatives (i.e., 17β-valerate and 17β-cypionate) of the naturally occurring and synthetic estrogens have been used to prolong estrogenic action (Fig. 24.12). In contrast to the ethynyl derivatives that are administered orally, the ester derivatives of estrogens are given intramuscularly in an oil vehicle that may produce durable estrogenic effects for up to 4 weeks as the ester is slowly hydrolyzed in vivo at the site of injection to release the free hormone. The 17β-valerate (Delestrogen) and the 17β-cyclopentylpropionate (cypionate, Depo-Estradiol) esters of 17β-estradiol are the most commonly used products. A 3-benzoate ester of 17β-estradiol is no longer used therapeutically. However, a 3-acetate ester is available for therapeutic use as a cured silicone elastomer vaginal ring (e.g., Femring) that is inserted into the vagina for

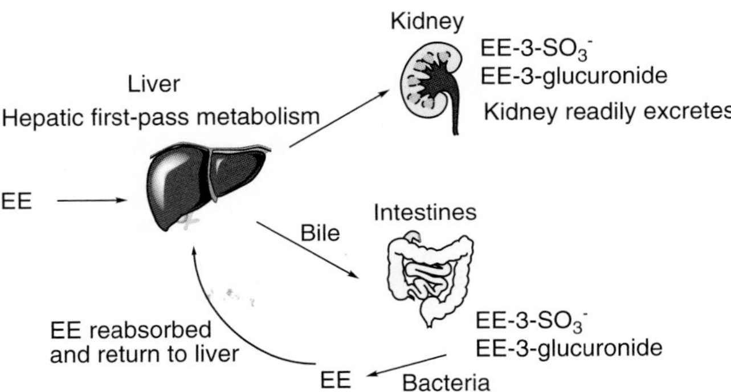

Figure 24.11 Enterohepatic recycling of estrogens using ethinyl estradiol (EE) as an exemplary estrogen.

OR'
RO
Esterases
HO
OH

17β-Esters of estradiol (prodrug) → 17β-Estradiol

Generic name (trade name)	R	R'
Estradiol benzoate	benzoyl	H
Estradiol acetate (Femring)	H_3C–C(=O)–	H
Estradiol cypionate (Depo-estradiol)	H	cyclopentylpropionyl
Estradiol valerate (Delestrogen)	H	valeryl

Figure 24.12 Esterified synthetic estrogens used for long-term estrogen therapy.

the treatment of moderate to severe vasomotor symptoms or vulvar and vaginal atrophy due to menopause. The exact position of the ring is not critical to its function. The elastomeric ring surrounds a central core designed to release 0.10 mg of 17β-estradiol per day for 3 months until removal.

Conjugated, water-soluble forms of naturally occurring estrogens obtained from the urine of pregnant mares, such as Premarin and Menest, are utilized therapeutically, mainly to treat postmenopausal symptoms. Horses produce two unique estrogenic compounds, equilin [3-hydroxyestra-1,3,5(10),7-tetraen-17-one] and equilenin [estra-1,3,5(10),6,8-pentaen-3-ol-17-one], and secrete them in the urine as sodium sulfate conjugates (Fig. 24.13). Estrone and other estrogen metabolites are secreted into the urine as well. Premarin contains six estrogen metabolites as active ingredients, including ~50%-65% sodium estrone sulfate,

Sodium estrone sulfate (prodrug)

Sodium equilin sulfate (prodrug)

Sodium equilenin sulfate (prodrug)

Figure 24.13 Conjugated estrogens.

~20%-35% sodium equilin sulfate, and four other conjugated estrogens in lesser amounts. Cenestin and Enjuvia, both discontinued in 2016, contained nine and ten active compounds, respectively. Enjuvia contained sodium Δ8,9-dehydroestrone sulfate, a plant derived conjugated estrogen. Menest is composed of not less than 90% of two conjugated estrogens derived synthetically, sodium estrone sulfate (75%-85%) and sodium equilin sulfate (6%-15%), in addition to 17α-estradiol.[77] Another sulfate conjugate that is orally effective is estropipate (i.e., piperazine salt of estrone sulfate; Fig. 24.10). This derivative has the same actions and uses as the conjugated naturally occurring estrogens. In an in vivo assay comparing the induction of estrogen-dependent genes following oral administration to postmenopausal women, EE is about 100 times more potent than conjugated estrogen preparations, 500 times more potent than 17β-estradiol and estrone sulfate, and 650 times more potent than 17β-estradiol valerate.[78]

NONSTEROIDAL ESTROGEN: DIETHYLSTILBESTROL

When estrogens were first obtained, the scarcity of the natural hormones led chemists to prepare synthetic materials that could be used as substitutes. *trans*-Diethylstilbestrol (DES; Fig. 24.8) was first prepared in 1939 and was soon thereafter (1941) approved by the FDA as a treatment for menopausal symptoms. The *trans* isomer of DES has 10 times the estrogenic potency of the *cis* isomer because it resembles more closely the natural estrogen, 17β-estradiol.[79] Although many stilbene derivatives have been prepared since, the *trans* isomer of DES remains one of the most active nonsteroidal estrogens known.[80,81] The synthetic estrogens have the same spectrum of effects as the natural steroidal estrogens.

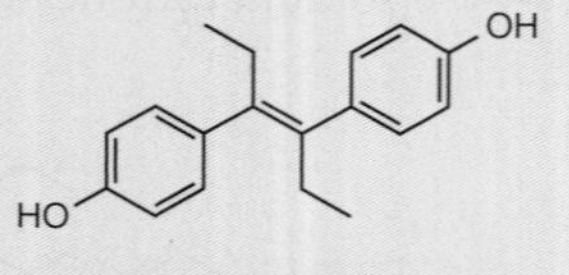

trans-Diethylstilbestrol 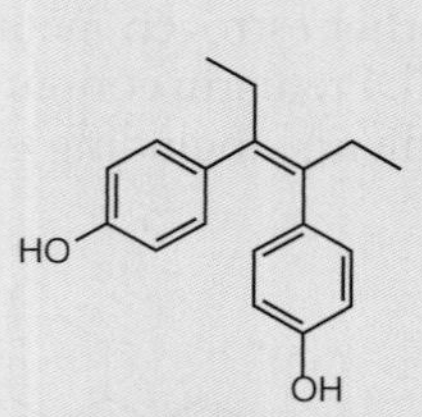 *cis*-Diethylstilbestrol

The therapeutic use of DES expanded greatly in the 1940s, 1950s, and 1960s, being prescribed to pregnant women to prevent miscarriage, premature labor, and related complications of pregnancy. In 1971, a landmark study linking clear cell adenocarcinoma, a type of cancer of the cervix and vagina, in women exposed to DES prior to birth (i.e., prenatally) led FDA to urge doctors to stop prescribing the drug to pregnant women. Surprisingly, FDA did not ban or discontinue DES at that time. Although its use dropped precipitously, an estimated 5-10 million pregnant women and their children born of these pregnancies had already been exposed to DES and similar drugs between 1941 and 1971.[82,83] The consequences of this prenatal exposure were widespread as the daughters of women who used DES during pregnancy, commonly called DES daughters, have ~40 times the risk of developing clear cell adenocarcinoma, and ~1 in every 1,000 of them actually developed the disease. DES daughters also appeared to have a higher incidence of breast cancer, fertility problems, and early menopause.[84,85] There appeared to be few if any effects on the sons of women who used DES during pregnancy. DES, along with the thalidomide tragedy in Europe, remains a somber reminder of the importance and need for harmonized global regulations regarding studies required to characterize the safety and efficacy of new drugs.

Progestins

Discovery of Progestins

Once ovulation has taken place, the tissue remaining from the ruptured follicle forms the corpus luteum, which has the important function of preparing for and maintaining pregnancy if it occurs. Fraenkel[86] first observed in 1903 that removal of the corpus luteum shortly after conception results in termination of the pregnancy. In 1914, Pearl and Surface[87] showed that the corpus luteum can prevent ovulation in animals. In 1929, Corner and Allen[88] developed a method of assay for progestational activity. By 1934, the progestational hormone progesterone (Fig. 24.14) had been isolated by several research groups, and by 1937 it had been shown that pure progesterone alone can maintain pregnancy in animals.[69,89]

The most abundant pregnane steroid found in the urine during pregnancy is 5β-pregnane-3α,20-diol (Fig. 24.14), present as its glucuronide, which is also the main excretory product of exogenous progesterone. Note the *cis* A/B ring junction which makes this metabolite devoid of progestational activity.[90] This conjugated substance can serve as an index of the corpus luteum placental activity, and a premature drop in its level in the urine may be a warning of possible miscarriage.

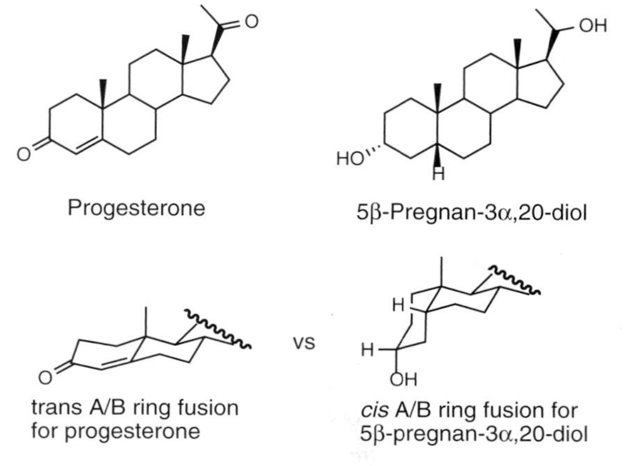

Progesterone 5β-Pregnan-3α,20-diol

trans A/B ring fusion for progesterone vs *cis* A/B ring fusion for 5β-pregnan-3α,20-diol

Figure 24.14 The conformation of progesterone and its predominant metabolite.

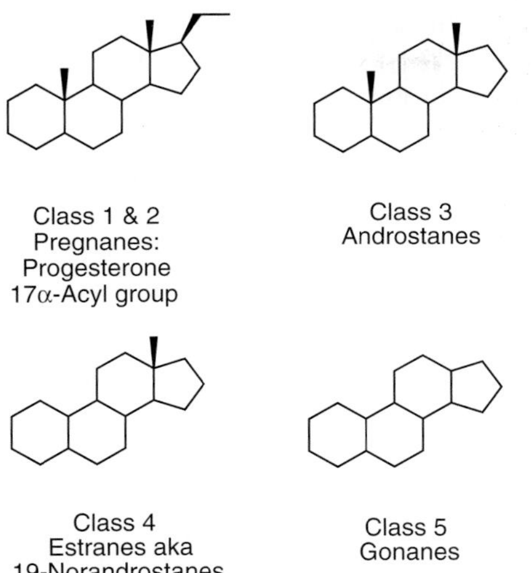

Figure 24.15 Steroidal ring systems present in the five structural classes of synthetic progestins.

Synthetic Progestins

The five structural classes of synthetic progestins are shown in Figure 24.15 and include derivatives of: (1) progesterone (pregnane), (2) 17α-hydroxyprogesterone (pregnane), (3) testosterone (androstane), (4) 19-nortestosterone (estrane), and (5) gonane and miscellaneous agents.

PREGNANES (CLASSES 1 AND 2). Progesterone (class 1), being an important hormone for maintaining pregnancy and normal menstrual bleeding, is used to treat disorders in these areas. Owing to its ability to prevent ovulation during pregnancy and thicken the cervical mucus (thus acting as a sperm barrier), it is considered a natural contraceptive.[91] Early efforts focused on identifying a good source of progesterone. Sequences were devised for the synthesis of progesterone from naturally occurring steroids, including diosgenin, ergosterol, and bile acids. The natural hormone, however, has many drawbacks, including a relatively low potency when orally administered due to poor absorption and almost complete first pass metabolism in the liver. Progesterone is available today as capsules (Prometrium), vaginal gels (Crinone), vaginal suppositories (First-Progesterone VCS), creams for transdermal delivery (9EC-RX Progesterone), and an intramuscular injection in oil (various suppliers) for the treatment of secondary amenorrhea and the prevention of endometrial hyperplasia in postmenopausal women who are also taking conjugated estrogens. Adding progesterone to conjugated estrogen therapy has been shown to reduce the risk of endometrial cancer in women using unopposed estrogens.[92] Progesterone is predominantly administered parenterally for therapeutic effects, and even the injection must be repeatedly administered over relatively short periods for best results.

A variety of orally active, 17α-acyl derivatives of progesterone that maintain the 3-keto-4-ene and the 20-keto pharmacophoric elements were developed (Fig. 24.16). Although many of the early structural modifications of progesterone led to weakly active or inactive progestational agents, it was eventually shown that derivatives of 17α-hydroxyprogesterone (class 2) such as 17α-acetoxyprogesterone had some activity when administered orally even though the parent compound, 17α-hydroxyprogesterone, was inactive.[93] A second derivative of 17α-hydroxyprogesterone, the 17α-caproate ester (Fig. 24.16), is available for therapeutic use via intramuscular or subcutaneous injection (Makena) to reduce the risk of preterm birth or to treat women with uterine adenocarcinoma or amenorrhea. The 17α-acyl groups are not prodrugs of progesterone but rather slow the metabolism of the 20-one to increase their duration of action compared to progesterone. Because of its long duration of action, the drug is administered parenterally for problems related to deficiency of natural progesterone.[94]

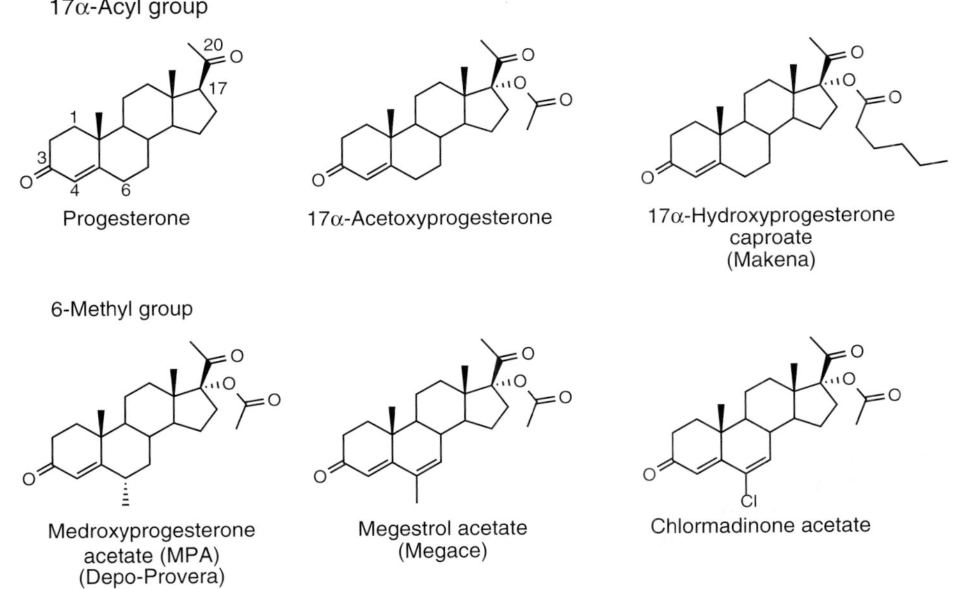

Figure 24.16 Progestins based upon the pregnane nucleus (Class 2) which are 17α-acyl derivatives.

Further structural modifications of 17α-acetoxyprogesterone enhanced its oral contraceptive action. In most instances, these modifications are carried out at the sixth carbon position. Substituents in this position hinder metabolism and increase their lipid solubility, resulting in an enhanced biologic effect.[95] Among the first of these interesting analogs of 17α-acetoxyprogesterone to be used in progestational therapy was medroxyprogesterone acetate (MPA; 6α-methyl-17β-hydroxy-4-pregnene-3,20-dione 17-acetate) (Fig. 24.16), the active pharmaceutical ingredient in Depo-Provera (subcutaneous or intramuscular injection) and Provera (oral tablets).[96] MPA binds the PR with similar affinity to progesterone.[97]

Progestational activity is further enhanced with 6-substituted 17α-acetoxyprogesterones when a double bond is introduced between positions 6 and 7. Megestrol acetate (6-methyl-17α-hydroxy-4,6-pregnadiene-3,20-dione 17-acetate; Megace) is a typical example of a clinically useful progestin. Chlormadinone (6-chloro-17α-hydroxy-4,6-pregnadiene-3,20-dione 17-acetate) is available in Europe (Luteran, Luteral), Japan and South Korea (Prostal) as single-agent treatment for gynecologic indications and in Europe in combination with EE (Belara) for birth control, but is not available in the United States.

ANDROSTANES (CLASS 3). The first synthetic progestin to be used to any extent was synthesized from male sex hormones (androstanes). Ethisterone (17α-ethynyl-17β-hydroxyandrost-4-en-3-one; prepared in 1937), 17α-ethynyl testosterone, proved to be an effective oral progestin and weak androgen, and became useful in the treatment of menstrual dysfunctions (Fig. 24.17).[98,99] 17α-Methyltestosterone also demonstrates some weak progestin activity. Similar to what was seen for the estrogens, 17α-substituents block metabolism to the 17-one, thereby allowing oral activity. Several molecular modifications of ethisterone led to enhanced progestational activity. For example, introduction of a methyl group in the 6α position, as in dimethisterone, provided an active analog (Fig. 24.17).[21] Ethisterone, therefore, paved the way for the synthesis of other progestins that did not have a typical progesterone-type C-17 side chain.

19-NORANDROSTANES OR ESTRANES (CLASS 4). A second breakthrough was made in 1944 when Ehrenstein[100] discovered that the C-19 methyl group on steroids is not necessary for progestational activity. In fact, his work showed that loss of the C-19 methyl (from a compound he thought was progesterone) produced 19-nor-14β,17α-pregn-4-ene-3,20-dione, an estrane with activity equal to or greater than that of parenterally administered progesterone.

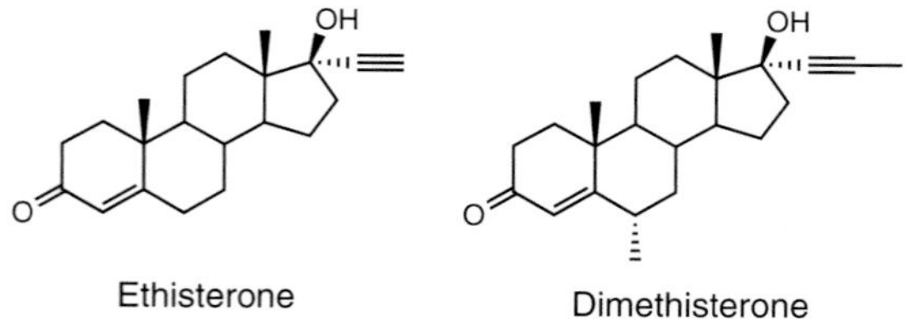

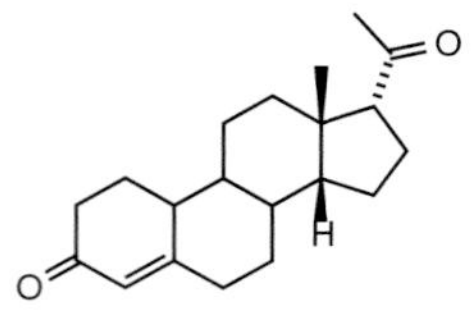

O H O

19-Nor-14β,17α-preg-4-ene-3,20-dione

OH O Ethisterone

OH O Dimethisterone

Figure 24.17 Progestins based upon the androstane nucleus (Class 3) which are 17α-substituted testosterone derivatives.

This work led to intensive attempts to prepare orally active progestins that were devoid of estrogenic and androgenic activities. In 1953, 19-norprogesterone was synthesized[101] and differed from the natural hormone only in replacement of the C-19 angular methyl group by hydrogen. This analog was eight times as active as progesterone when administered parenterally (the Clauberg test) and was the most potent progestin known. Addition of the 17α-ethynyl group to the 19-norsteroids (i.e., estranes) resulted in two potent and orally active progestins, namely norethindrone (17-ethynyl-17β-hydroxyestr-4-en-3-one) and norethynodrel (17-ethynyl-17β-hydroxyestr-5(10)-en-3-one) (Fig. 24.18).[23] The progestational activity of norethynodrel is about one-tenth that of norethindrone, and both compounds appear to have weak estrogenic activity (Fig. 24.18). These two substances were among the first 19-nor-steroids (nor is synonymous for missing 19-methyl) to be used clinically for progestin-related hormonal disorders. Importantly, they also afforded a method, when used with estrogens such as mestranol, for control of conception and ultimately led to the development and widespread introduction of oral contraceptives. The first oral contraceptive, Enovid, was a combination of mestranol and norethynodrel and was introduced in 1960.

The usefulness of norethynodrel and norethindrone for therapy of irregular menses and as oral contraceptive agents provided the impetus to continue research in the area of 19-nor-steroids. Another 19-nor-steroid reported to be effective and exhibit few side effects is ethynodiol diacetate (17-ethynylestr-4-ene-3,17β-diol 3,17-diacetate) (Fig. 24.18). This drug has been used as an oral progestin.[102]

Since the discovery of the first generation of 19-nortestosterone dervatives (estranes), referred to as Class 4 herein, multiple new generations of norsteroids have been discovered. For example, replacement of the 18-methyl group of norethindrone with an ethyl group resulted in a second generation of progestins, represented by norgestrel (a racemic mixture of the dextronorgestrel and levonorgestrel; rac-13-ethyl-17α-ethynyl-19-nortestosterone). The dextro- stereoisomer of norgestrel is inactive, while levonorgestrel is biologically active and one of most widely used progestins in oral contraceptives. Third-generation progestins are analogs of levonorgestrel, including the active progestins norelgestromin (metabolized to levonorgestrel) and etonorgestrel, respectively, and their prodrugs norgestimate and desogestrel. Fourth-generation

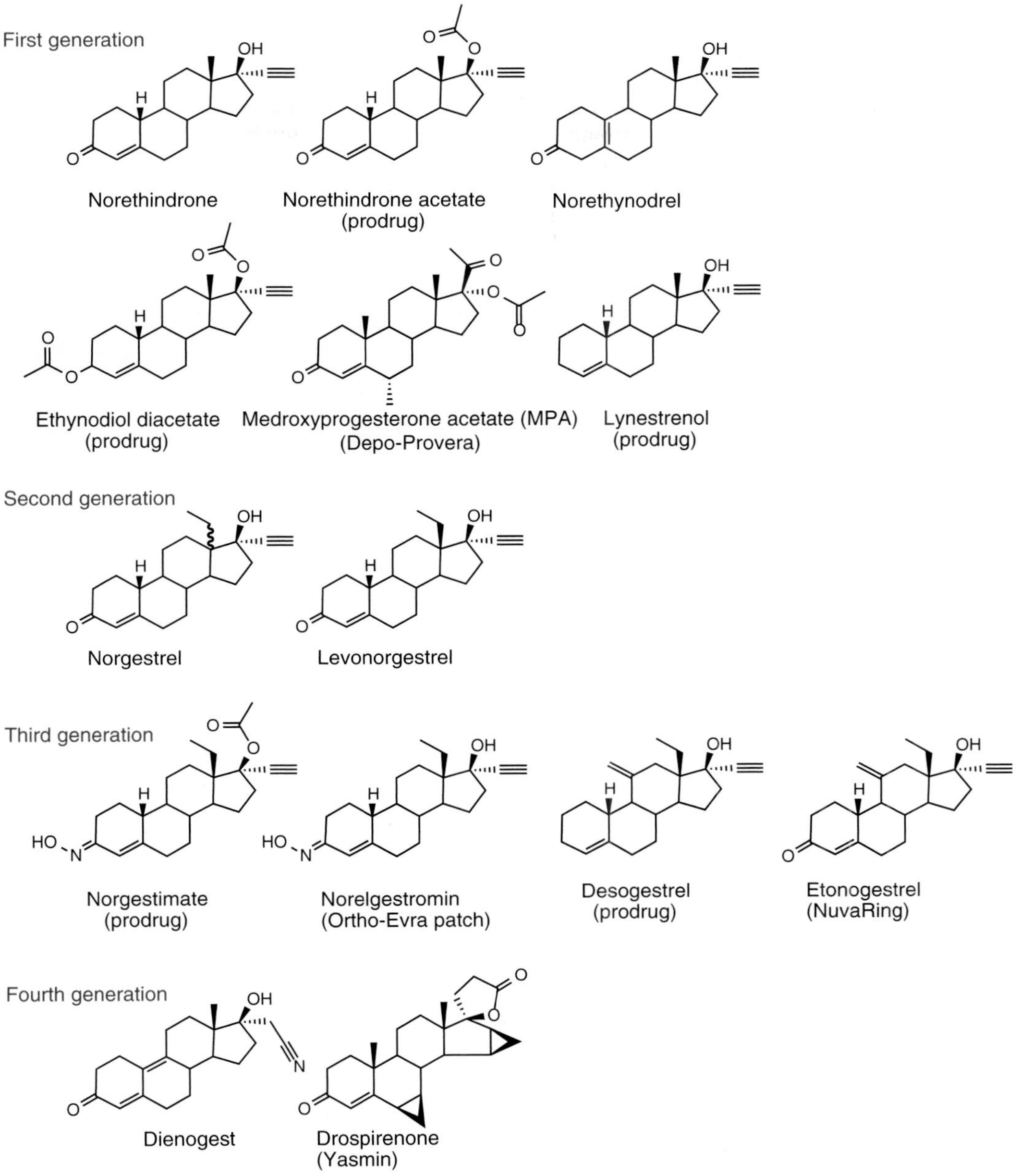

First generation

Norethindrone

Norethindrone acetate (prodrug)

Norethynodrel

Ethynodiol diacetate (prodrug)

Medroxyprogesterone acetate (MPA) (Depo-Provera)

Lynestrenol (prodrug)

Second generation

Norgestrel

Levonorgestrel

Third generation

Norgestimate (prodrug)

Norelgestromin (Ortho-Evra patch)

Desogestrel (prodrug)

Etonogestrel (NuvaRing)

Fourth generation

Dienogest

Drospirenone (Yasmin)

Figure 24.18 Progestins based upon the androstane (Class 3) or estrane (Class 4) nucleus ordered by generation.

progestins include dienogest and drospirenone, the latter of which was first introduced for therapeutic use in combination with an estrogen as an oral contraceptive in 2000.

Structure-Activity Relationships

Currently available progestins are restricted to molecules with a steroid nucleus. Klimstra has pointed out that it is difficult to compare progestins on the basis of studies reported in the literature because there are many ways to do so.[99] Two of the most common methods of measuring uterine glandular development are Clauberg's and McGinty's tests. Other biologic evaluations of the progestins include their effect on uterine carbonic anhydrase, inhibition of gonadotropin hormones, and delay of parturition, and their ability to maintain pregnancy in a spayed female animal. Substances should be evaluated in the same laboratory as the resulting data are more informative.

Ethisterone (Fig. 21.17), the first androgenic compound found to be effective, has about one-third the activity of progesterone in women when taken subcutaneously but is 15 times as active when taken orally. Because this analog is closely related to testosterone, it has androgenic activity. Removal of the methyl group at position 19 leads to norethindrone (norethisterone), which has 5-10 times more progestational activity. The activity of norethindrone may be increased further by substituting a chlorine atom at position 21 (not shown) or by adding a methyl group at carbon 18 (norgestrel). Ethynodiol diacetate is an extremely potent oral progestin; it is more active orally than parenterally and is effective as an oral contraceptive when combined with an estrogen.

Further unsaturation of the B or C ring of 19-androstane derivatives usually enhances progestational activity. Introduction of halogen or methyl substituents in the

6α or 7α position generally increases hormonal activity. Acetylation of the 17β-OH of norethindrone results in a longer duration of action. Removal of the keto function of norethindrone at carbon 3 gives lynestrenol (17-ethynyl-estr-4-en-17β-ol; never marketed in the United States), which retains potent progestational activity and is free of androgenic effects. This hormone is used in combination with an estrogen as a contraceptive agent.

Activity of 17α-hydroxyprogesterones is enhanced by unsaturation at positions 6 and 7 and substitution of a methyl group or a halogen at position 6. This activity may be further increased by introducing a CH_3 group at position 11. These substitutions on the progesterone molecule probably prevent metabolic reduction of the two carbonyl groups and metabolic oxidation at position 6. Substitution of a fluoro group at position 21 apparently prevents hydroxylation at this point and enhances the oral effectiveness. Some of the potent orally administered progestins belong to this series of compounds. A progestin with a prolonged duration of action is 16α,17α-dihydroxyprogesterone acetophenide (also known as algestone; marketed solely in Latin America and Italy). When given parenterally, this agent appears to be devoid of both androgenic and estrogenic activities.

Inversion of the configuration at positions 9 and 10 in progesterone leads to retroprogesterone, which is more active parenterally and orally than progesterone but was never marketed. Further unsaturation at positions 6 and 7 of retroprogesterone gives dydrogesterone (9β,10α-4,6-pregnadiene-3,20-dione), another progestin available alone or in combination with an estrogen outside the United States. The adrenocortical hormone 21-hydroxyprogesterone and the precursor of progesterone, pregnenolone, have minimal or no progestational activity.[103]

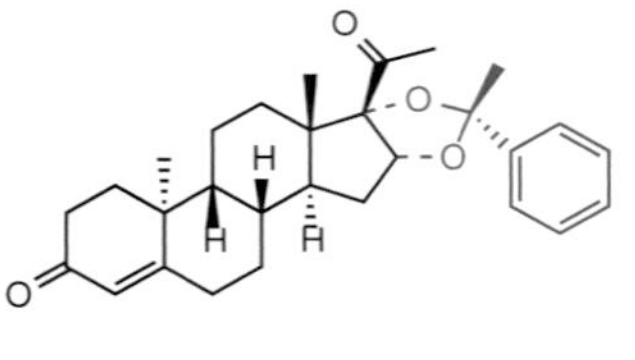

Algestone acetophenide (16α,17α-dihydroxyprogesterone acetophenide)

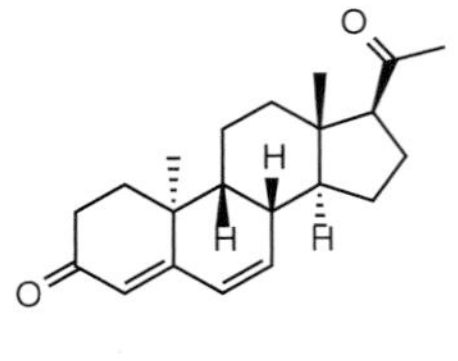

Retroprogesterone

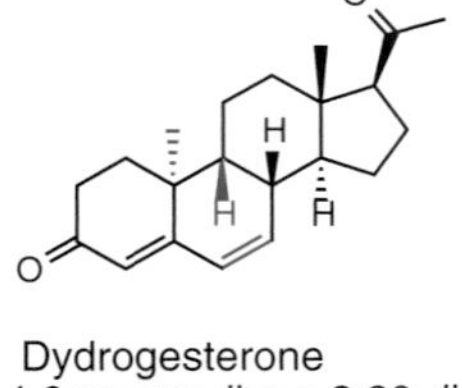

Dydrogesterone (9β,10α-4,6-pregnadiene-3,20-dione)

Because the progestins share the same steroid backbone as adrenocorticoids, androgens, and estrogens, cross-reactivity with other members of the nuclear hormone receptor is common for the progestins.[103]

Progestin Antagonists

The use of an antiprogestin (i.e., competitive PR antagonist) as an abortifacient agent for interfering with the early phases of pregnancy has been approved in the U.S. since 2000. The first antiprogestin, mifepristone[104] contains an 11β-(4-dimethylaminophenyl) side chain believed to destabilize the PR agonist conformation. However, mifepristone also demonstrates potent antiglucocorticoid activity.[105] Additional antiprogestin analogs, such as ulipristal (see Emergency Contraception and Abortifacients), have been developed that exhibit lowered antiglucocorticoid activity[106] and have been approved as emergency contraceptives.

EMERGENCY CONTRACEPTION AND ABORTIFACIENTS

The first approved abortifacient to end an early pregnancy was mifepristone (2000), a progestin antagonist, given in combination with a prostaglandin, misoprostol. In 2016, the use of Mifeprex was revised by the FDA to be approved to end a pregnancy through 70 days of gestation using 200 mg of mifepristone on day 1 of therapy, then 24-48 hours later 800 μg of misoprostol taken buccally, with healthcare provider follow-up 7-14 days later (Fig. 24.19). To ensure safe use, this form of postconception and implantation contraception can only be prescribed and dispensed by or under the supervision of a healthcare provider participating in a risk evaluation and mitigation strategy (REMS) program. The mifepristone acts as an antiprogestin preventing implantation or dislodging implanted fetuses. During pregnancy, the compound sensitizes the myometrium of the uterus to the contraction-inducing activity of prostaglandins. Many women (44.1%) in the U.S. trials expelled the products of conception within 4 hours after taking misoprostol and 62.8% experienced expulsion within 24 hours after the misoprostol administration.[107,108] Mifeprex has a black box warning for very rare but serious and sometimes fatal infections and bleeding. The new approval was intended to address the safety concerns for the mother.

In 2010, ulipristal acetate (Ella, Fig. 24.19) was approved as an emergency contraceptive that can cut the chances of becoming pregnant by about two-thirds (from 5.6% expected to 1.9% observed with a 30 mg dose of ulipristal acetate) for at least 120 hours after a contraceptive failure or unprotected sex. Ulipristal acetate is not intended for routine use as a contraceptive and is not indicated for termination of an existing pregnancy. It works as an antiprogestin by delaying ovulation or preventing implantation of a fertilized egg. A rapid return to fertility is likely following treatment with ulipristal acetate which may interfere pharmacologically with the progestin component of oral contraceptives, requiring barrier methods of contraception for subsequent acts of intercourse that occur in that same menstrual cycle. Oral contraceptive agents with progestins may impair the ability of ulipristal acetate to delay ovulation, and women should start or resume oral contraceptives no sooner than 5 days after taking ulipristal acetate. Ulipristal acetate is metabolized to mono-demethyl-ulipristal acetate and di-demethyl-ulipristal acetate by CYP3A4. Correspondingly, CYP3A4 inducers significantly decreased ulipristal area under the plasma concentration-time curve (AUC) by 93% following 600 mg of rifampin.

Ulipristal is also extremely sensitive to CYP3A4 inhibitors with 400 mg ketoconazoles daily for 7 days increasing ulipristal acetate AUC by 5.9-fold.

A high-dose progestin "morning-after pill" containing only levonorgestrel was approved in 1982 based on its ability to reduce pregnancy rates from the expected 8% with no contraceptive use to approximately 1%[109] if taken less than 72 hours after intercourse, and better efficacy if taken sooner. Clinical studies showed that 84% of expected pregnancies were prevented with a single 1.5 mg dose of levonorgestrel, as compared to only 79% when levonorgestrel was administered as two doses of 0.75 mg administered 12 hours apart. All of the available formulations (Plan B One Step, My Way, Aftera, and others) now provide 1.5 mg of levonorgestrel as an emergency contraceptive indicated for prevention of pregnancy following unprotected intercourse or contraceptive failure. These should be taken as one 1.5 mg tablet taken orally as soon as possible within 72 hours after unprotected intercourse. If vomiting occurs within 2 hours of taking, consider redosing. In 2009, it became available over-the-counter to women over the age of 17 and, after legal challenge, became available over-the counter to all women of reproductive potential in 2013. Approximately 31% of women experience heavier menstrual bleeding after ingesting the 1.5 mg dose.

In recent years, two prostaglandins, PGE_2 (dinoprostone) and carboprost, an analog of $PGF_{2\alpha}$, have been used as abortifacients (Fig. 24.19). The $PGF_{2\alpha}$ analog is injected into the amniotic sac, whereas PGE_2 is given by vaginal suppository to induce abortion.

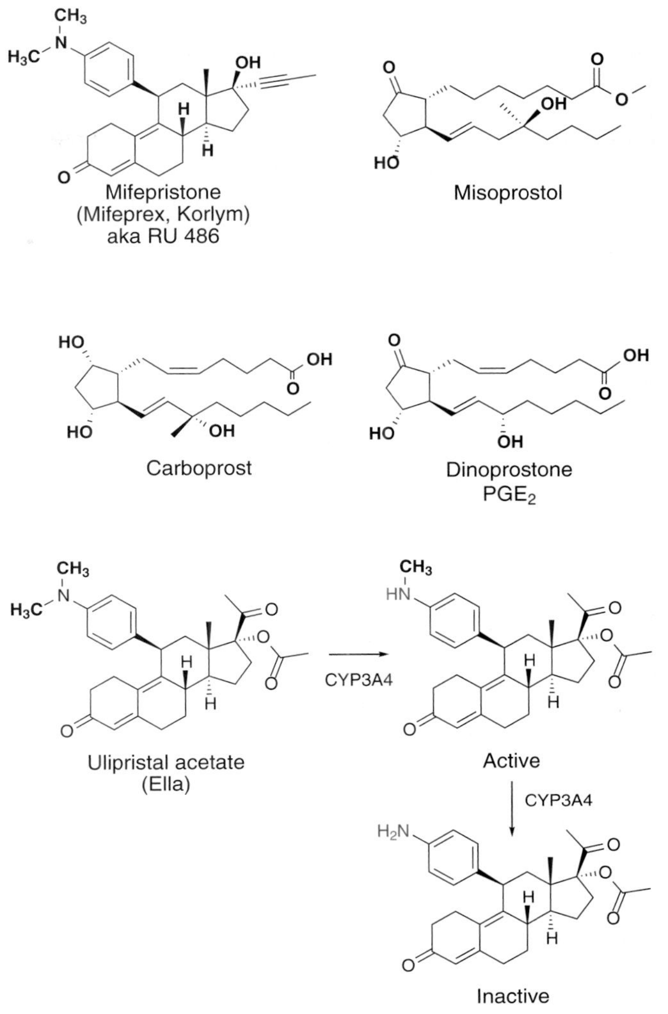

Figure 24.19 Emergency contraceptives and abortifacients.

Mechanism of Progestin Action

MOLECULAR INTERACTIONS. The uterus is the primary site of progesterone action in the female. Once the endometrium proliferates and becomes dense under the influence of estrogens, the levels of progesterone rise. This hormone inhibits the proliferation of the endometrium and initiates a secretory phase of the reproductive cycle. During this stage, the endometrium becomes edematous and glycogen increases in the epithelium of the endometrium.

In an attempt to understand the cellular transformations induced by progesterone that involve gene expression, O'Malley, Schrader, and colleagues studied the effects of progesterone on the chick oviduct, a particularly useful biologic system for the examination of the mechanism of action of progesterone.[110] These studies on PRs extend into mammalian systems as well.[111] The PR consists of two hormone binding proteins, receptors A and B.[112,113] Biologically active PRs are present in the nucleus of target cells, whereas inactive receptors have been found in the cytosol as a complex with HSP90,[114] similar to inactive glucocorticoid complexes. The nuclear PR heterodimer binds progesterone with high affinity, resulting in a conformational change in the complex. The steroid-receptor complex interacts with particular HRE regions of the cellular DNA, referred to as progesterone response element, and initiates transcription of the DNA sequence to produce mRNA. Finally, the elevated levels of mRNA lead to an increase in protein synthesis in the endoplasmic reticulum. Administration of progesterone to estrogen-stimulated chicks resulted in the synthesis of the specific oviduct protein, avidin. In mammals, uteroglobin (a small secretory protein of the uterus) and the enzyme estradiol dehydrogenase have been identified as proteins induced by progesterone.

PHYSIOLOGIC EFFECTS. Progesterone has many biologic functions. The primary site of the physiological action of progesterone is the uterus. The hormone acts on both the endometrium (inner mucous lining) and the myometrium (muscle mass) of the uterus. It acts on the endometrium, which has been primed by the estrogens, to induce the secretory phase, during which the endometrial glands grow and secrete large amounts of carbohydrates that will possibly be used by the fertilized ovum as a source of energy.

The primary function of progesterone with respect to the myometrium is to stop the spontaneous rhythmic contractions of the uterus. The effects of progesterone on the uterus are to prepare the endometrium for reception, implantation, and maintenance of the fertilized ovum and to suppress the myometrial contractions so that the embryo is not dislodged from the uterus.

The corpus luteum is the primary source of progesterone for the first third of pregnancy; subsequently, the developing placenta is the major source of progesterone and estrogens. Both hormones are secreted continually in large amounts until parturition. The high levels of progesterone produced by the corpus luteum and placenta during pregnancy act upon the hypothalamus through the negative feedback system to prevent the formation of new ova. Additionally, this steroid hormone is important for maintenance of pregnancy. Thus, progesterone is often referred to as the "hormone of pregnancy."

Extragenital effects of progesterone, except when secreted in large amounts, are slight. Progesterone is natriuretic, probably because of antagonism of aldosterone. Subsequently, increased sodium excretion stimulates secretion of aldosterone, which affects sodium retention. Progesterone is also catabolic because it increases the total nitrogen excretion brought about by catabolism of amino acids.[115]

The main feedback effects of progesterone in the central nervous system are thought to occur in the hypothalamus; this causes inhibition of pituitary secretion.[22] PRs have been identified in the hypothalamus and are involved in this feedback inhibition. Prior administration of estrogens or progestins does not appear to inhibit ovulation induced by exogenous gonadotropins. Progesterone appears to have a biphasic feedback effect on ovulation. During the first few hours after administration of this hormone, ovulation is produced and the effects are inhibited. It appears that the effects of progesterone are reversed as time passes.

Development of the alveolar sacs in the mammary gland during pregnancy is stimulated by progesterone and estrogens, but lactation does not occur until after the levels of these hormones fall at parturition. Progesterone also increases the basal temperature and decreases the motility of the fallopian tubes. In large doses, progesterone can produce weak analgesia and general anesthesia.

Additional actions of progesterone and progesterone metabolites in the central nervous system have been identified. The identification of various C-21 and C-19 steroids and enzymatic processes for their production in brain tissues led investigators to suggest that these steroids have a possible function in the CNS.[116] Two 5α-reduced metabolites of progesterone, pregnanolone (3α-hydroxy-5α-pregnan-20-one) and its hydroxy derivative (3α,21-dihydroxy-5α-pregnan-20-one), have been shown to bind to the gamma aminobutyric acid (GABA) receptor subtype A ($GABA_A$) complex at 10^{-8} M concentrations and potentiate GABA responses.[117,118] Another C-21 metabolite found in CNS tissues is pregnenolone sulfate, which demonstrates an inhibitory activity on the $GABA_A$ receptor complex.[119] The physiologic relevance of these progestin metabolites in CNS function remains to be determined.

It has been suggested that the temperature-raising effect of progesterone may be due to increased body heat resulting from reduced sweating. This effect is not unique to progesterone; other steroids in the pregnane and androstane series can also produce it.[120]

PHARMACOLOGY, SIDE EFFECTS, AND CLINICAL APPLICATIONS. The mechanism controlling ovarian secretion of progesterone involves the release of LH from the anterior pituitary during ovulation. The LH induces progesterone secretion from the corpus luteum during the second half of the menstrual cycle. As stated earlier, the high levels of progesterone produced by the corpus luteum and placenta during pregnancy act upon the hypothalamus through the negative feedback system to prevent the formation of new ova (Figs. 24.6 and 24.7). This information led to studies involving progesterone and its analogs as contraceptives.[51,121] If conception does not occur, the corpus luteum regresses and progesterone production decreases. This finally leads to sloughing of part of the endometrium during menstruation.

Progesterone, and more recently its synthetic analogs, have been used to treat dysmenorrhea, endometriosis, functional uterine bleeding, and amenorrhea. Progesterone and its derivatives have been used to treat habitual or recurrent abortions, although not always successfully.[122] This seems to be a reasonable use because progesterone is considered a pregnancy-supporting hormone. Because abortion is not always due to a hormonal deficiency, however, progestin treatment has not been as successful as predicted.

Historically, early pregnancy could be diagnosed by giving the combination of an estrogen and a progestin for several days and then withdrawing it. If bleeding occurs in a few days, the patient is not pregnant. Progesterone has also been used in the treatment of carcinoma of the endometrium. The major use of progestins is in combination with estrogens as a contraceptive.

Among the side effects seen with progestins are nausea and vomiting, drowsiness, spotting, and irregular bleeding; these may occur when these drugs are taken for a short time. With prolonged therapy, a greater incidence of side effects may be seen, including edema and weight gain, breast discomfort, breakthrough bleeding, decreased libido, and masculinization of the female fetus.

Female Hormonal Contraceptives

Pincus and his colleagues initiated the use of steroidal hormones in oral contraception (OC) in the early 1950s.[123] Early findings in animals were extended to human subjects in Haiti and Puerto Rico, and such investigations showed that a combination of an estrogen and a progestin prevents conception.[124] Oral contraceptives were approved in 1960s that contained nonselective progestins and much higher (mg) doses of estrogen than are used today (μg); thus the side effects of OCs have been reduced over time. Although early forms of OCs explored estrogen only and estrogen then progestin used sequentially, all current OCs are combination (i.e., estrogen plus progestin) OC (COC) or progestin only contraceptives (discussed below as progestin-only pill [POP]) formulations. A plethora of oral contraceptives (Table 24.2) combining a progestin and estrogen are now available for therapeutic use worldwide. Their pharmacokinetic properties are summarized in Table 24.3.

Table 24.2 Combination Oral Contraceptives: Estimated Relative Progestin/Estrogen/Androgen Activity

		Estrogen		Progestin				
Type of Oral Contraceptive	Trade Name	Estrogen	Dose (µg)	Progestin	Dose (mg)	Estrogen Activity	Progestin Activity	Androgen Activity
Monophasic (one hormone dose over a cycle)	Apri, Desogen, Emoquette, Enskyce, OrthoCept, Reclipsen, Solia	EE	30	Desogestrel	0.15	Intermediate	High	Low
	Beyaz,[a] Gianvi, Loryna, Nikki, Vestura, Yaz	EE	20	Drospirenone	3	Intermediate	High	None
	Ocella, Safyral,[a] Syeda, Yasmin, Zarah	EE	30	Drospirenone	3	Intermediate	High	None
	Kelnor, Zovia	EE	35	Ethynodiol diacetate	1	Low	High	Low
	Zovia	EE	50	Ethynodiol diacetate	1	Intermediate	High	Low
	Aubra, Aviane, Delyla, FaLessa,[a] Falmina, Lessina, Lutera, Orsythia, Sronyx	EE	20	Levonorgestrel		Low	Low	Low
	Altavera, Chateal, Kurvelo, Levora, Marlissa, Portia	EE	30 (28 d)	Levonorgestrel	0.15	Intermediate	Intermediate	Intermediate
	Introvale, Jolessa, Quasense	EE	30 (91 d)	Levonorgestrel	0.15	Low	Intermediate/high	Intermediate/high
	Amethyst, Lybrel	EE	20	Levonorgestrel	0.09	Low	Intermediate/high	Intermediate/high
	Balziva, Briellyn, Femcon-FE, Gildagia, Ovcon, Philith, Vyfemla, Wymzya FE, Zenchent, Zenchent FE	EE	35	Norethindrone	0.4	Intermediate	Low	Low
	Brevicon, Modicon, Necon, Nortrel, Wera	EE	35	Norethindrone	0.5	Low	Low	Low
	Generess FE, Layolis FE	EE	25	Norethindrone	0.8	Intermediate	Low	Low
	Alyacen, Cyclafem, Dasetta, Necon, Norinyl, Nortrel, Ortho-Novum, Pirmella	EE	35	Norethindrone	1	Intermediate	Intermediate	Intermediate
	Necon, Norinyl	Mestranol	50	Norethindrone	1	Intermediate	Intermediate	Intermediate

	Gildess, Gildess FE, Junel, Junel FE, Larin, Larin FE, Loestrin, Loestrin FE, Lomedia FE, Microgestin, Microgestin FE, Minastrin FE, Tarina FE	EE	20	Norethindrone acetate	1	Low	Intermediate/ high	Intermediate/ high
	Gildess, Gildess FE, Junel, Junel FE, Larin, Larin FE, Loestrin, Loestrin FE, Microgestin, Microgestin FE	EE	30	Norethindrone acetate	1.5	Low	Intermediate/ high	Intermediate/ high
	Estarylla, Mono-Linyah, MonoNessa, Ortho-Cyclen, Previfem, Sprintec	EE	35	Norgestimate	0.25	Intermediate	Low	Low
	Cryselle, Elinest, Low-Ogestrel	EE	30	Norgestrel	0.3	Intermediate	Intermediate	Intermediate
	Ogestrel	EE	50	Norgestrel	0.5	High	High	High
Biphasic (two hormone doses over a cycle)	Azurette, Kariva, Kimidess, Pimtrea, Mircette, Viorele	EE	20/10	Desogestrel	0.15	Intermediate		Low
	Amethia Lo, Camrese Lo, LoSeasonique	EE	20/10	Levonorgestrel	0.1	Low	Intermediate/ high	Intermediate/ high
	Amethia, Ashlyna, Camrese, Daysee, Seasonique	EE	30/10	Levonorgestrel	0.15	Low	Intermediate/ high	Intermediate/ high
	Necon	EE	35/35	Norethindrone	0.5/1	Intermediate	Intermediate	Low
	Lo Loestrin FE, Lo Minastrin FE	EE	10/10	Norethindrone	1	Low	Intermediate/ high	Intermediate/ high
Triphasic (three hormone doses over a cycle)	Ortho Tri-Cyclen Lo	EE	25	Norgestimate	0.18/0.215/0.25	Intermediate	Low	Low
	Enpresse, Levonest, Myzilra, Trivora	EE	30/40/30	Levonorgestrel	0.05/0.075/0.125	Intermediate	Low	Low
	Ortho Tri-Cyclen, Tri-Estarylla, Tri-Previfem, TriNessa, Tri-Linyah, Tri-Sprintec	EE	35	Norgestimate	0.18/0.215/0.25	Intermediate	Low	Low
	Aranelle, Leena, Tri-Norinyl	EE	35	Norethindrone	0.5/1/0.5	Low	Low	Low
	Alyacen, Cycalfem, Dasetta, Necon, Nortel, Ortho-Novum, Pirmella	EE	35	Norethindrone	0.5/0.75/1	Intermediate	Intermediate	Low
	Estrostep FE, Tilia FE, Tri-Legest FE	EE	20/30/35	Norethindrone acetate	1	Low	Intermediate/ high	Intermediate/ high
	Caziant, Cesia, Cyclessa, Velivet	EE	25	Desogestrel	0.1/0.125/0.15	Intermediate	Intermediate	Low
Quadriphasic (four hormone doses over a cycle)	Natazia	Estradiol valerate	3/2/2/1	Dienogest	0/2/3/0	Intermediate	High	Low
	Quartette	EE	20/25/30/10	Levonorgestrel	0.15/0.15/0.15/0	Low	Intermediate/ high	Intermediate/ high

Based on Facts and Comparisons. *Oral Contraceptives Monograph*. Available at: http://fco.factsandcomparisons.com/lco/action/doc/retrieve/docid/fc_dfc/5546102.
[a]Also contains levomefolate.
EE, ethinyl estradiol; FE, contains iron; µg, micrograms.

Table 24.3 Pharmacokinetic Properties for Some Estrogenic and Progestational Agents

Drug	Protein[a] Binding	Oral Bioavailability	Biotransformation	Elimination Half-life (hrs)	Time to Peak Conc. (hr)	Peak Serum Conc. (ng/mL)	Elimination (%) Renal[b]	Elimination (%) Fecal
17β-Estradiol	50%-80%	Poor	Hepatic[d]	20 min		0.1-0.2	90	
Ethinyl estradiol (EE)	98%	40%	Hepatic	26 (6-20)	1-2	33		
Progesterone Oral 200 mg micronized IM 45 mg IM 90 mg Vaginal gel 45 mg	>90%	<10%	Hepatic	<5 min 10 wk 19.6 34.8	2-4 28 9.2 6.8	24.3 39.1 53.8 14.9	50-60 10	
Medroxyprogesterone acetate: Oral 10 mg IM 150 mg/mL every 3 mo	>90%	High	Hepatic IM no hepatic	30 50 d	2-4 3 wk	19-35 1-7	15-22	45-80
Megestrol acetate Oral 160 mg Oral 600 mg	>90		Hepatic	38 (13-104)	2-3 2-3	200 753	66	20
Norgestrel	>90%	60%	Hepatic	20	24		45	32
Levonorgestrel 3/12/60 mo implants 216 mg loading dose[c]	>90	60	No hepatic	16 (8-30)	24	1,6 first week, then 0.26-0.4	45	32
Desogestrel (Desogen) (as 3-keto-desogestrel)	>90	76	Hepatic to active 3-ketodesogestrel	12-58	1-2	2-6	43	50
Norethindrone	>80	65	Hepatic	8 (5-14)	0.5-4.0	5-10	50	20-40
Norethindrone acetate	>80	65	Hepatic	8 (5-14)	0.5-4.0	5-10	50	20-40
Norgestimate as (desacetylnorgestimate)	>50-60 >90	60	Hepatic to desacetyl-norgestimate	37	1-2	0.5-0.7	47	37

From USP Drug Information 2000.

[a]Sex hormone–binding globulin (SHBG) synthesis is stimulated by estrogens and inhibited by androgens: levels are twice as high in women as in men. Progesterone binds strongly to cortisol binding globulin (CBG; 17.7%) and SHBG (0.6%) and weakly to albumin (79.3%). Absorption is the rate-limiting step for the elimination half-life. Levonorgestrel: free, 1.1%-1.7%; SHBG, 92%-62%; and albumin, 37.56%; but suppresses SHBG by 33%. Norethindrone: free, 3.5%; SHBG, 35.5%; and albumin, 61%. Medroxyprogesterone does not bind SHBG. 3-Keto-desgestrel, 64%; albumin, 32%. Norgestimate >90% protein bound; not SHBG.

[b]Renal metabolites are primarily conjugates.

[c]A mean dose of 35 μg levonorgestrel is released daily.

[d]Hepatic indicates hepatic first pass metabolism.

Combination Oral Contraceptives

COC regimens are fixed daily doses of an estrogen and a progestin coadministered in a single tablet for 20 or 21 days followed by hormone-free pills (possibly containing iron or folic acid [e.g., levomefolate] supplements) for typically 7 or 8 days to complete a 28-day regimen. The 28-day cyclic regimens are continued for as long as contraception is desired. The hormone-free period allows for a 5-day menstrual period. The predominant estrogen in COCs is EE with mestranol and estradiol valerate also available. Typical doses of EE are 30 or 35 μg, but some products contain low (i.e., 20 μg or below) or high (i.e., around 50 μg) EE doses based on patient needs to either limit estrogenic side effects or ensure adequate contraceptive efficacy. The progestin component of COCs is the major differentiating factor among COC products. The steroid hormone receptor selectivity, pharmacology (e.g., agonist vs. antagonist), and relative potencies vary greatly across the progestins employed in COCs. Some progestins (e.g., norgestrel, levonorgestrel, MPA) possess androgen side effects such as acne, oily skin/scalp, weight gain, increased libido, hirsutism, etc. In some cases, known off-target effects such as antiandrogen (norethindrone; norgestimate) or antimineralocorticoid (drospirenone) activities can be therapeutic in patients with acne or postmenopausal dysphoric disorder (PMDD), respectively. In other cases, COC intolerance can be addressed by changing the progestin component (Table 24.4).

The progestin dose is also variable but in the low to sub-milligram (mg) range. Estrogen and progestin dose is another differentiating factor between COCs with low- and high-dose estrogen products mentioned above. Further, the dose of estrogen or progestin can be static or vary multiple times during the 28-day regimen. The original COCs employed static doses of estrogen and progestin (i.e., estrogen to progestin dose and ratio was fixed throughout each cycle), which are now termed as monophasic regimens. Efforts to more closely simulate the normal menstrual cycle and/or limit the side effects of COC have led to the development of biphasic, triphasic, or quadraphasic formulations where the estrogen and/or progestin doses change two to four times during the 28-day regimen. Consistent with reproductive physiology, often the progestin dose is lower in the initial follicular phase but increases during the luteal phases, whereas the EE dose optionally stays the same or decreases as the menstrual period is approached (Table 24.2). The length of the active hormone pill period is another COC differentiating factor. Extended cycle products that provide 24 days of hormone therapy (e.g., Loestrin-24 FE and Yaz) with only a 4-day hormone-free period and continuous cycle (i.e., no hormone-free period) (e.g., Lybrel) formulations reduce or eliminate menstrual bleeding and may be beneficial when patients present with a history of dysmenorrhea or menstrual (i.e., estrogen withdrawal) migraine headaches.[125] Moreover, Yaz 24/4 is FDA approved for PMDD purportedly due to the strong antimineralocorticoid effects of the progestin drospirenone.[125] An enormous assortment of COC products is engendered by the combination of variables reviewed above, affording the practitioner the opportunity to rationally select an intial COC for a patient or optimize the COC to patient preferences and/or needs. Although extremely popular, in some cases, a COC is not the optimal hormonal contraception for a particular patient and other options are described below.

Table 24.4 Achieving Proper Hormonal Balance in Oral Contraceptive Agents[a]

Estrogen		Progestin		Androgen[a]
Excess	**Deficiency**	**Excess**	**Deficiency**	**Excess**
• Nausea • Bloating • Cervical mucorrhea • Polyposis Melasma • Hypertension • Migraine headache • Increase in breast size • Breast fullness or tenderness • Edema • Urinary tract infection • Uterine enlargement • Uterine fibroid growth	• Early or midcycle breakthrough bleeding • Increased spotting • Hypomenorrhea • Nervousness • Vaginitis atrophic • Vasomotor symptoms	• Increased appetite • Depression • Fatigue • Hypertension • Hypoglycemia symptoms • Hypomenorrhea • Libido decrease • Vaginal yeast infections • Breast regression	• Late breakthrough bleeding • Amenorrhea • Dysmenorrhea • Hypermenorrhea	• Acne • Cholestatic jaundice • Edema • Hirsutism • Libido increase • Oily skin and scalp • Rash and pruritus

From Facts and Comparisons. *Oral Contraceptives Monograph*. Available at: http://fco.factsandcomparisons.com/lco/action/doc/retrieve/docid/fc_dfc/5546102.
[a]Result of androgenic activity of progestins.

Progestin Only Pills

POPs employ a small daily dose of the progestin with all current products using 0.35 mg of norethindrone (0.35 mg) daily (e.g., Micro-Nor or Nor-QD and bioequivalents thereof). POPs are continuous hormone OCs (i.e., there is no hormone-free period during the 28-day regimen and no break between regimens). Further, no estrogen is given at any time which reduces some of the risks associated with the use of estrogens. The time of day of dosing must be consistent as efficacy is compromised in POPs if the dose is delayed by more than 3 hours from normal. In such cases, barrier contraception (e.g., condom) is recommended for 48 hours. POPs may be recommended for breastfeeding patients or patients intolerant of or contraindicated to estrogens. Another major disadvantage is that irregular bleeding is common, especially during the first 18 months of therapy. The major advantage is the absence of estrogen excess side effects reported with the combination methods including serious thromboembolic episodes such as cerebrovascular accidents or other estrogenic side effects such as large, tender, and/or cystic breasts, hypermenorrhea, spider veins, irritability, edema, bloating, nausea, etc. Other serious conditions predisposed by estrogens are increased risk of myocardial infarction, hepatic adenomas, hypertension, severe congenital hyperlipidemia, gallbladder disease, breast cancer, and altered carbohydrate metabolism. A history of any of the above or heavy smoker >35 years old or current pregnancy would each be contraindications to COC, possibly suggesting POP or progestin-only parenteral methods to avoid these estrogenic effects.

Parenteral Hormonal Contraceptives

A variety of parenteral hormonal contraceptives are now available to deliver hormones via transdermal patch, vaginal ring, intramuscular or subcutaneous depot injection, subcutaneous implant, or progesterone-impregnated intrauterine device (IUD). Although similar or identical estrogens and progestins are employed, parenteral administration alters drug exposure. For example, the systemic area under the curve (AUC) of EE from COC (30 μg) is 21.9 versus 35.8 ng-hr/mL and 10.6 ng-hr/mL for patch (20 μg) and ring (15 μg) which suggests relatively high EE levels from patch (possibly due to avoidance of first-pass effects) and low EE levels from ring, qualifying the latter as a low estrogen–dose contraceptive method when compared to COC.[126] A few specific parenteral products are discussed below.

PATCH. Daily transdermal delivery of 20 μg EE and 150 μg of norelgestromin (metabolized to levonorgestrel in liver) is achieved by Xulane patches which are applied weekly for 3 weeks and then no patch for 1 week. Patches typically adhere well to trunk, arm, etc. (do not apply to breasts) despite water/soap exposure. If the patch falls off, patients should replace it within 24 hours. Efficacy is 99% but lower in women >90 kg in body weight. As mentioned above, higher levels of EE suggest the possibility of increased risk of thromboembolism.

VAGINAL RING. Transvaginal delivery of 15 μg/d of EE and continuous release of etonogestrel (0.12 mg/ring) is achieved by NuvaRing, a clear and colorless flexible polymer ring. One ring remains in position for 3 weeks and then no ring for 1 week; if ring falls out, it can be replaced within 3 hours. The ring formulation provides comparable efficacy to other methods despite the low levels of hormones in the product, which is probably attributable to rapid absorption and no first pass effect. NuvaRing produces continuous and relatively low steady-state drug levels, suggesting that this product may be side effect sparing.

INTRAMUSCULAR AND SUBCUTANEOUS INJECTIONS. Depot injections are intermediate-term contraceptive products which use MPA (150 mg IM as Depo-Provera or 104 mg subcutaneous as depo-subQ provera) every 3 months (every 11-13 wk). Advantages include progestin only side effects, amenorrhea, and prevention of endometrial cancer. Disadvantages include weight gain, irregular bleeding, and risk of prolonged infertility and/or side effects due to the 3-month duration. They also require a healthcare provider visit every 3 months.

SUBCUTANEOUS IMPLANTS. Long-term (up to 3 yr) contraception is achieved by Nexplanon which involves implantation of a single EVA (ethylene vinylacetate) rod (4 cm × 2 mm; which is removable) that delivers 67 μg daily of etonogestrel. Advantages include comparable efficacy in obese patients unlike COCs and patches and ensured patient adherence. Further, ease of implantation and removal is much improved compared to Norplant (discontinued; Norplant was relatively large and more difficult to implant/remove). Disadvantages include the possibility of progestin excess side effects including weight gain, depression, fatigue, decreased libido and breast size, as well as bleeding irregularities.

INTRAUTERINE DEVICES. Several brand names of levonorgestrel-impregnated IUDs (Mirena, Liletta, Skyla) release 13.5-20 μg of levonorgestrel daily which is not systemically absorbed. Nonetheless, local progestin thickens cervical mucus and inhibits sperm motility. The IUD may remain for up to 3-7 years, depending on which product is used, with no delay in fertility upon discontinuation. Limitations include that it must be administrated by a healthcare professional and is recommended after having at least one child.

HOW TO TAILOR CONTRACEPTIVE REGIMEN TO A PATIENT NEEDS

Approximately 10 million women use hormonal contraceptives at any given time with the duration of therapy varying from short term (1 or 2 cycles) to up to 30 years. Hormonal contraceptives is highly effective when consistently and correctly used leading to only 5% of unintended pregnancies, whereas 95% of unintended pregnancies result from lack of or inconsistent contraceptive use. Unintended pregnancies in the first year with perfect use of COC are only 0.3% versus 8% for typical use, which takes into account human error. Depo-Provera and progestational IUD/implant methods have comparable perfect use statistics (0.3% and 0.6%) but improved typical use failures (3% and 0.8%, respectively) compared to 0.1% failure with sterilization procedures. Nonhormonal contraception methods such as withdrawal, rhythm, symptothermal, etc. vary in typical use failure rates from 29% (spermicide) to 15% (condom), demonstrating the superiority of hormonal methods at preventing pregnancies.

Like any pharmacotherapy, hormonal contraceptives have a variety of immediate side effects and drug-drug interactions, and should be avoided in certain patient populations with risk factors. Side effects of hormonal contraceptives can be classified according to symptoms of hormonal imbalance as summarized in Table 24.4. Choice of hormonal contraceptive should take into account any symptoms of estrogen, progestin, or androgen excess or deficiency as revealed by the patient on interview or medical history review. For example, acne is an androgen excess symptom and if present could be treated by antiandrogenic progestin containing COC such as Estrostep (norethindrone acetate), Ortho Tri-Cyclen (norgestimate), or Yaz (drospirenone) which are FDA approved for acne. Similarly, estrogen excess or deficiency symptoms can be corrected by employing low or high EE formulations, respectively.

Selection of hormonal contraception should also be made in view of lifestyle (age, level of sexual activity, plans to get pregnant and when, unique characteristics/goals of patient) and risk factors revealed by family history or social history. For example, age in excess of 35 years, family or personal history of cardiovascular problems and coagulopathies, and/or personal history of smoking may predispose patients to estrogenic thromboembolic events, elevating the need to consider progestin-only hormonal contraception methods. Selection of hormonal contraception should further be in view of concurrent medications to avoid drug-drug interactions. OCs are known to interact with multiple anticonvulsants such as carbamazepine, phenytoin, phenobarbital, felbamate, topiramate which are CYP3A4 inducers (but not others, valproic acid, zonisamide, etc. which do not induce) possibly due to induction of first pass effects lowering EE (or progestin levels) to subtherapeutic levels. Although high-dose estrogen COC may be an option, a parenteral hormonal contraceptive may be optimal. Similarly, CYP3A4 inducing antibiotics such as rifampin and griseofulvin may interact with COCs. Broad-spectrum antibiotics such as tetracyclines, metronidazole, and quinolones may cause worrisome breakthrough bleeding with COCs as a consequence of perturbed microbial EE metabolism which returns EE to bloodstream via enterohepatic recycling. It may be prudent to advise use of a backup contraception method for duration of antibiotic course and rest of cycle. Moreover, avoid low-dose COCs if drug-drug interactions are present.

Further patient-specific criteria, including weight (>90 kg start with 35 μg EE or more; avoid patch; consider implant), very young age (start with 20 μg EE), predisposition to therapeutic nonadherence (consider parenterals), and not planning a near term pregnancy within 1-3 years (consider long-acting parenterals) should also be weighed when selecting the appropriate COC. Patients experiencing breakthrough (i.e., midcycle) or dysfunctional bleeding, or with a history of ovarian cyst or endometriosis, and/or a drug-drug interaction may consider a high-dose EE.

Drugs Used in Hormone Replacement Therapy for Menopause

After menopause, the ovaries have atrophied and therefore 17β-estradiol and progesterone are no longer produced, and thus physiologic changes occur including vasomotor symptoms (hot flashes, night sweats, flushing, palpitations, and anxiety), psychological changes (depression, mood swings, memory or concentration changes, fatigue, and irritability), vaginal atrophy and decreased vaginal elasticity, decreased libido, dyspareunia (painful intercourse), urinary tract changes (atrophy of bladder epithelium, stress urinary incontinence, shortening of urethra), risk of cardiovascular disease, bone loss and osteoporosis, and loss of skin elasticity. These menopausal symptoms can greatly affect a women's quality of life. Menopausal symptoms can be alleviated by pharmacologic therapies such as hormone replacement therapy. Nonpharmacological therapies including lifestyle changes, diet, exercise, and stress reduction can also help to a lesser extent. Due to negative, insufficient, or inconclusive data, the North American Menopause Society (NAMS) does not currently recommend cooling techniques, avoidance of triggers, exercise, yoga, relaxation, or OTC supplements and herbal therapies.[127] NAMS recommends cognitive-behavioral therapy using the selective serotonin reuptake inhibitor paroxetine (Bridselle, 7.5 mg) as an effective nonhormonal prescription therapy to alleviate vasomotor symptoms approved by the FDA.[127] At this time, use of soy isoflavones, weight loss, and mindfulness-based stress reduction may be beneficial but should be recommended with caution.[127]

The presence of an intact uterus is a major factor governing the choice to use estrogens alone or in combination with a progestin as hormone replacement therapy. Therapy with an estrogen alone in women with an intact uterus has been shown to cause endometrial hyperplasia and increase the risk of endometrial cancer. Thus, the addition of progestin protects the uterus and is included in hormone replacement therapy when women have an intact uterus. Conversely, progestins can have negative effects in menopausal women. The decision of whether to use hormone replacement therapy by patients should be done in consultation with their physician and/or pharmacist to take patient-relevant risk factors into account.

Since the findings of the Women's Health Initiative (WHI) were released in 2002, U.S. women have decreased the usage of hormone replacement therapy.[128] The objective of the WHI trial was to determine if long-term use of hormone replacement therapy in postmenopausal women (average age 64 yr) reduces risks of heart disease, breast cancer, colon cancer, and fractures. The results of this trial have been since used inappropriately to make therapeutic decisions for women having symptoms during peri- or menopausal years.[128] Based upon WHI findings, the use of hormone replacement therapy is supported in menopausal women, aged 50-59 years, who are experiencing symptoms and have lower risk of breast cancer or cardiovascular disease. Women who initiate hormone replacement therapy within 10 years of menopause to help alleviate bothersome menopausal symptoms are not at increased risk of cardiovascular disease. Women with an intact uterus are at increased risk of endometrial hyperplasia if inadequately opposed estrogen is used. Using the WHI data, a benefit and risk assessment of two hormone therapy formulations was carried out (conjugated equine estrogens [CEE] alone and CEE + MPA) in women aged 50-59 years.[128] The risks and benefits were expressed as the difference in number of events (number in the hormone-therapy group minus the number in the placebo group) per 1,000 women over 5 years. For women on CEE-alone, a risk existed for deep vein thrombosis (DVT) which had 2.5 more events per 1,000 women than placebo. Benefits were seen in the CEE-alone trial, as seen in Table 24.5, as negative values to show the decreased number of events per 1,000 women compared to placebo. Whether on CEE alone or in combination with MPA, benefits for this group of women were seen with diabetes, death from any cause, all fractures, and cancers including colorectal. Additional benefits on CEE alone included protection from breast cancer, stroke, and coronary heart disease. Increased risks were seen in the CEE with or without MPA group for DVT, but only in the CEE with MPA group were risks seen for coronary heart disease, stroke, and breast cancer. These risks were ≤5 events per 1,000 women above the placebo group. Overall, patients and physicians will need to work together to determine options for managing menopausal symptoms. A free mobile app has been developed by the NAMS called MenoPro to aid patients and physicians with treatment options.[129] Starting hormone replacement therapy more than 10 years after menopause can increase risk of cardiovascular disease and other side effects. It is not recommended to initiate systemic hormone replacement therapy more than 10 years after menopause due to risks of coronary heart disease, stroke, venous thromboembolism (VTE), and dementia.[130] A low-dose vaginal estrogen (non-systemic) is safe to use >10 years after menopause.[130]

Table 24.5 Benefits and Risks of Two Formulations (CEE + MPA; CEE-Alone) in the WHI for Women (Aged 50-59)

	Trial[a,b]	
Disease	**CEE + MPA**	**CEE – Alone**
Deep vein thrombosis	5.0	2.5
Coronary heart disease	2.5	−5.5
Stroke	2.5	−0.5
Breast cancer	3.0	−2.5
Colorectal cancer	−0.5	−1.5
All cancers	−0.5	−4.0
All fractures	−12.0	−8.0
Death from any cause	−5.0	−5.5
Diabetes	−5.5	−13.0

Based on Manson JE, Kaunitz AM. Menopause management–getting clinical care back on track. *N Engl J Med.* 2016;374:803-806.

[a]Difference given is number of events per 1,000 women over 5 yr. Number in the hormone-therapy group minus the number in the placebo group. A positive number illustrates a risk and a negative number illustrates a benefit.

[b]CEE, conjugated equine estrogens; MPA, medroxyprogesterone acetate.

Estrogens Used Alone in Hormone Replacement Therapy

The estrogens used in oral hormone replacement therapy include 17β-estradiol and mixtures of sulfate esters of estrone and its derivatives (collectively known as conjugated estrogens or esterified estrogens) (Table 24.6). The structures of the conjugated estrogens used in estrogen replacement therapy are shown in Figure 24.13 and represent mixtures of water-soluble phase 2 metabolites (sulfate esters) of naturally occurring estrogens obtained from the urine of pregnant mares or prepared synthetically. These metabolites are prodrugs that are unable to bind to the ER. However, when orally administered, the sulfates are hydrolyzed in intestines to the phenols which can weakly bind to the ER. In 1941, Ayerst, McKenna & Harrison introduced Premarin, the name coined from pregnant mare urine with subsequent FDA approval in 1942. Premarin was a top-selling prescription drug, and it has been estimated that more than 30 billion doses have been dispensed with yearly sales reaching over $1 billion. Premarin revenues in the United States have been decreasing due to decreases in prescription volume.[131] The other oral estrogens that are approved estrogen replacement therapy are synthetically derived and include 17β-estradiol, piperazine salt of estrone sulfate, or mixtures of sodium sulfate esters of weak estrogens (estrone, equilin, or derivatives). Doses for oral administration of estrogen are typically 60%-80% lower than used for OC, as the smallest dose needed to relieve symptoms is the goal. Treatment typically will start with a low dose of estrogen (Table 24.7) and increase depending on the needs of the patient to maximize symptom relief while minimizing side effects. Estrogen products are available in many formulations including oral, transdermal (patch, gel, emulsion, spray), and vaginal (insert, tablet, ring, cream) (Table 24.8). The estrogens present in these various formulations include 17β-estradiol, micronized 17β-estradiol, 17β-estradiol acetate, estropipate (piperazine estrone sulfate), CEE, and esterified estrogens. The approximate equivalent estrogen doses for postmenopausal use are given in Table 24.9.[132] Due to first-pass metabolism, orally administered estrogens are transformed into estrone and estriol metabolites.

Table 24.6 Estrogens Used Alone in Hormone Replacement Therapy

Product	Generic	Trade Name	Components
Estrogen (oral)	Estrogens (conjugated/ equine, systemic)	Premarin	Sodium estrone sulfate (~50%-65%) Sodium equilin sulfate (~20%-35%) Sodium 17α-dihydroequilin sulfate Sodium 17α-estradiol sulfate Sodium 17β-dihydroequilin sulfate
	Estrogens (esterified)	Menest	Sodium estrone sulfate (75%-85%) Sodium equilin sulfate (6%-15%) Other estrogen components (~10%)
	Estropipate	Ogen	Piperazine estrone sulfate
	Estadiol (Systemic)	Estrace	17β-Estradiol, micronized

From Facts and Comparisons. *Conjugated Estrogens (Systemic) Monograph; Esterified Estrogens Oral Monograph; Estropipate (Piperazine Estrone Sulfate) Oral Monograph*. Available at http://fco.factsandcomparisons.com/lco/action/doc/retrieve/docid/fc_dfc/5546102. Accessed April 17, 2018.
Femtrace, Enjuva, Estratab, Cenestin all discontinued.

17β-Estradiol acetate and CEE are prodrugs and will be active upon hydrolysis of the acetate or sulfate esters at the phenol of A-ring.

Estrogen and Progestin Combinations Used in Hormone Replacement Therapy

Estrogens are given in combination with progestins for women with an intact uterus. The lowest-dose progestin should be administered that prevents endometrial hyperplasia. If the dose is too low, breakthrough bleeding will result. The progestins used in hormone replacement therapy include micronized progesterone, MPA, norethindrone acetate (first generation), levonorgestrel (second generation), norgestimate (third generation), and drospirenone (fourth generation) (Table 24.8). Adverse effects of progestins in hormone replacement therapy include premenopausal symptoms of irritability and depression, headaches, bloating, weight gain, and irregular bleeding. Newer progestins are better tolerated than MPA which has shown more adverse reactions (increased DVT and cardiovascular risk and worsening lipid profile). Nonoral routes of administration of estrogens (transdermal and vaginal) offer the advantage of bypassing first-pass metabolism. In addition, nonoral routes of therapy are recommended for women at increased risk for VTE.[133,134] Many combinations of estrogen and progestins exist and can be found in Table 24.8. Femring is a vaginal ring made of a central core of the prodrug 17β-estradiol acetate which delivers a high enough dose for relief of systemic symptoms even though vaginal delivery. Vaginal atrophy can be treated with vaginal delivery of estrogens which can relieve local or systemic side effects depending on the dose.

Table 24.7 Daily Dose Treatment Options of Estrogen for Postmenopausal Use

	Treatment		
Estrogen	Standard Dose	Low Dose	Ultra-Low Dose
17β-Estradiol, micronized	1 mg	0.5 mg	0.25 mg
Conjugated equine estrogens (CEE)	0.625 mg	0.45 mg	0.3 mg
17β-Estradiol, transdermal	0.1 mg	0.05 mg	0.014 mg
Ethinyl estradiol (EE)		0.005 mg	

Various progestins are given in combination with estrogens in hormone replacement therapy (Fig. 24.18). Progesterone has low oral bioavailability due to poor absorption and almost complete first-pass metabolism in the liver. It is also light sensitive. Micronized progesterone increases oral absorption. MPA is a 6α-methyl-17α-acetyl derivative of progesterone given in combination with CEE (Premopro, Premphase). Both of these structural changes prevent metabolism: 17α-acetyl slows metabolic reduction of 20-ketone to the alcohol and 6α-methyl slows metabolism of the 3-keto-4-ene system. Norethindrone acetate is a first-generation 19-nortestosterone derivative based upon the estrane nucleus and is given in combination with either 17β-estradiol (Activella, CombiPatch) or EE (Femhrt). It is a prodrug and rapidly deacetylated to norethindrone after oral administration. The presence of the 17α-alkynyl group blocks metabolism to 17-ketone, increases progestational activity, and decreases androgenic activity. The absence of the 19β-methyl group increases progestational activity. 19-Nortestosterone derivatives have their primary activity as progestins but do possess some androgenic activity. Levonorgestrel is a

Table 24.8 Hormone Replacement Therapy Products[132]

Category	Trade Name	Components	Dosage Form	Frequency of Dosing
Estrogen (oral)	Estrace	17β-Estradiol (micronized)	Tablet	Once daily
	Menest	Esterified estrogens	Tablet	Once daily
	Ogen	Estropipate	Tablet	Once daily
	Premarin	CEE	Tablet	Once daily
Estrogen (transdermal)	Alora	17β-Estradiol	Patch (matrix)	Twice weekly
	Climara	17β-Estradiol	Patch (matrix)	Once weekly
	Divigel, Elestrin	17β-Estradiol	Gel (topical)	Once daily
	Estraderm	17β-Estradiol	Patch (reservoir)	Twice weekly
	EstroGel	17β-Estradiol	Gel (topical)	1 pump once daily
	Evamist	17β-Estradiol	Spray (topical)	Initially 1 spray daily; may increase to 2-3 sprays if needed
	Menostar	17β-Estradiol	Patch (matrix)	Once daily for osteoporosis
	Vivelle, Vivelle-Dot	17β-Estradiol	Patch (matrix)	Twice weekly
Estrogen (vaginal)	Imvexxy	17β-Estradiol	Vaginal inserts for manual placement	Once daily for 2 wk, then twice weekly
	Vagifem	17β-Estradiol	Vaginal tablets placed by applicator	Once daily for 2 wk, then twice weekly
	Estring	17β-Estradiol	Ring	Once every 90 d
	Femring	Estradiol acetate	Ring	Once every 3 mo (systemic)
	Premarin	CEE	Cream	Daily
Progestin (oral)	Aygestin	Norethindrone acetate	Tablet	Once daily
	Prometrium	Progesterone (micronized)	Capsule	Once daily
	Provera	MPA	Tablet	Once daily
Estrogen + progestin (oral)	Activella	17β-Estradiol/norethindrone acetate	Tablet	Once daily
	Angeliq	17β-Estradiol/drospirenone	Tablet	Once daily
	Femhrt	Ethinyl estradiol/norethindrone acetate	Tablet	Once daily, continuously
	Prefest	17β-Estradiol/norgestimate	Tablet	Once daily, sequentially
	Premphase	CEE/MPA	Tablet	Once daily, sequentially, cyclic
Estrogen + SERM (oral)	Duavee	CEE/bazedoxifene	Tablet	Once daily
Estrogen + progestin (transdermal)	Climara Pro	17β-Estradiol/levonorgestrel	Patch (marix)	Once weekly
	Combipatch	17β-Estradiol/norethindrone acetate	Patch (matrix)	Twice weekly

Based on Facts and Comparisons. *Conjugated Estrogens (Systemic) Monograph; Esterified Estrogens Oral Monograph; Estropipate (Piperazine Estrone Sulfate) Oral Monograph.* Available at http://fco.factsandcomparisons.com/lco/action/doc/retrieve/docid/fc_dfc/5546102. Accessed April 17, 2018 and also based on Straight Healthcare. *Female Hormone Medications.* Available at http://www.straighthealthcare.com/female-hormone-medications.html. Accessed April, 2018.

CEE is conjugated equine estrogens; MPA is medroxyprogesterone acetate; SERM is selective estrogen receptor modulator.

Table 24.9 Approximate Equivalent Doses of Estrogen for Postmenopausal Use

Route	Estrogen	Dose
Oral	17β-Estradiol	1.0 mg
	Conjugated equine estrogens (CEE)	0.625 mg
	Esterified estrogens	0.625 mg
	Estropipate	0.625 mg
	Ethinyl estradiol (EE)	0.005-0.015 mg
Transdermal	17β-Estradiol patch	0.05 mg
	17β-Estradiol gel	1.5 mg/2 metered doses

Based on *Menopause Practice, a Clinician's Guide. 5th ed. Mayfield Heights, OH: North American Menopause Society; 2014.*

second-generation 19-nortestosterone derivative that possesses an 18β-ethyl instead of methyl group. It is given in combination with 17β-estradiol as a transdermal patch (Climara Pro). The 18β-ethyl group decreases androgenic activity while increasing progestational activity; however, second-generation progestins have the most androgenic activity as compared to other generations. In efforts to decrease androgenic activity, an isosteric replacement of an oxime for the 3-keto group of levonorgestrel resulted in the third-generation progestin known as norgestimate. Norgestimate is a prodrug that undergoes cleavage of 17β-ester to the active 17β-hydroxyl group in the intestine and liver. The oxime is active and able to bind to the PR for progestational activity, but it is also metabolized into the 3-keto group in the liver. Norgestimate is given in combination with 17β-estradiol (Prefest). Drospirenone is a fourth-generation progestin and is given in combination with 17β-estradiol (Angeliq) and does not possess androgenic activity.

SERMs Used in Hormone Replacement Therapy

SERMs are nonsteroidal molecules that possess a unique pharmacology in which they behave as an ER agonist in some tissues and as an ER antagonist in other tissues, earning their classification as SERMs. The first SERMs discovered were the ER antagonists tamoxifen and toremifene that are used exclusively for the treatment of breast cancer (discussed later). However, the search for the optimal SERM continued into the early 21st century and resulted in the discovery and development of two SERMs, bazedoxifene and ospemifene, which are used in hormone replacement therapy.

Bazedoxifene, a third-generation SERM, is combined with CEE in an oral product (Duavee). It was approved in 2013 for treatment of menopausal vasomotor symptoms in addition to prevention of postmenopausal osteoporosis in women with a uterus (Fig. 24.20).[135] It is the first nonprogestin drug for use in menopausal women with an intact uterus, as usually they need to take a progestin with the estrogen. Bazedoxifene is a mixed ER agonist/antagonist that acts as an ER agonist in bone and cardiovascular system and relieves menopausal symptoms but acts as an antagonist in breast and uterus, thus reducing risk of endometrial hyperplasia that can occur with CEE.[135,136] Use of bazedoxifene in combination with CEE for up to 2 years has not indicated an increase risk of breast cancer.[137]

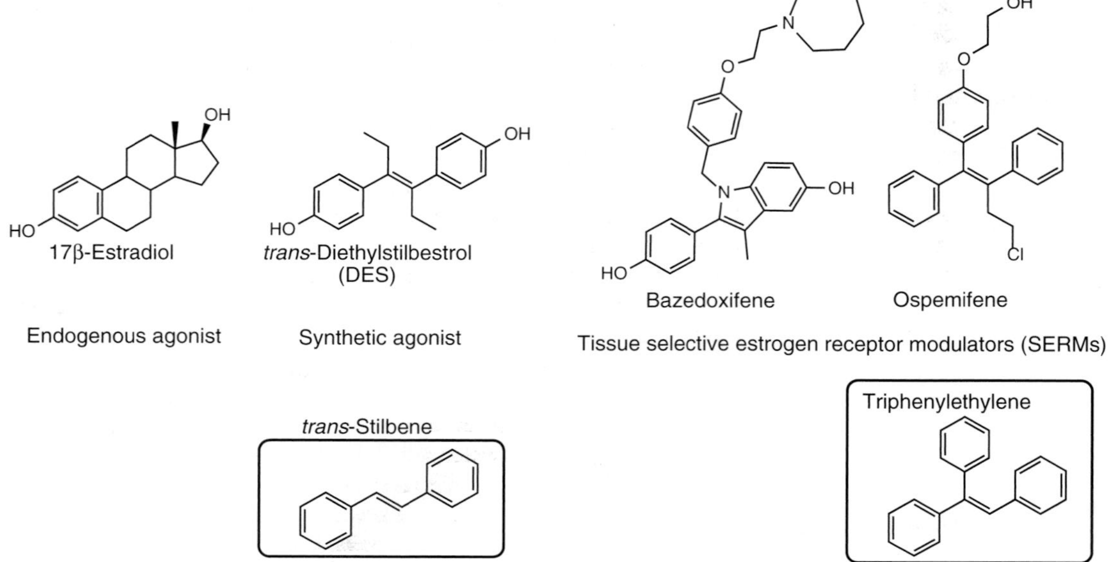

Figure 24.20 17β-Estradiol, non-steroidal agonist DES, and two SERMs used in hormone replacement therapy.

Bazedoxifene is an indole derivative of the benzthiophene raloxifene (see section on SERMs below) and can be envisioned to bind similarly to ERα (compare Figs. 24.8 and 24.20). Bazedoxifene undergoes extensive gluronidation on the indole alcohol to form 5-bazedoxifene glucuronide with little to no CYP-mediated metabolism detected in plasma.[138] The concentration of the glucuronide is 10-fold higher than unchanged drug in plasma. Because it undergoes glucuronidation by the UDP-glucuronyl transferase (UGT) enzyme in the intestinal tract and liver, metabolism of bazedoxifene may be increased by UGT inducers (rifampin, phenobarbital, carbamazepine, phenytoin). Relief of hot flashes of both severity and frequency were seen after 4 weeks of therapy.[139] Bazedoxifene has poor bioavailability (~6%), has elimination half-life of 33 hours for unchanged drug, is excreted primarily in feces (~85%), has time to peak concentration of ~2.5 hours, and is a P-gp substrate.[136,138] It is extensively protein bound (98%-99%) in vitro but not to sex hormone–binding globulin (SHBG). Bazedoxifene is expected to undergo enterohepatic recycling from the gut back to systemic circulation; therefore a decrease in its systemic exposure can be postulated if given in combination with drugs that interfere with the recycling process.[138]

In postmenopausal women, estrogen deficiency causes not only physical changes in the vagina but also thinning of vaginal secretions and vaginal tissue, reduced blood flow, and decreased elasticity and therefore can result in impaired sexual function due to difficult or painful sexual intercourse (dyspareunia). The symptoms of vulvar and vaginal atrophy can affect quality of life, and treatment options can include estrogen replacement therapy, hormone replacement therapy, vaginal moisturizers and lubricants, or SERMs.

Ospemifene (Osphena, approved 2013) is a SERM recommended for postmenopausal women suffering from moderate to severe dyspareunia with vaginal atrophy except if a history of breast cancer exists.[140] Ospemifene is a triphenylethylene and a metabolite of toremifene (see later in this chapter). By binding to the ER, it is an agonist in vaginal epithelia tissue and stimulates endometrial tissue to relieve symptoms of dyspareunia. As it has estrogenic agonist effects in endometrium, there is an increased risk of endometrial hyperplasia and endometrial cancer in women with a uterus who use unopposed estrogens. This can be decreased when a progestin is added to estrogen therapy. Ospemifene has antagonist activity in breast and uterus. It undergoes hepatic metabolism by CYP3A4 (major), 2C9 (major), and 2C19 (minor) to form 4-hydroxyospemifene and is excreted predominantly in feces (75%) and to a lesser extent in the urine (7%; <0.2% as unchanged drug). It has increased bioavailability when taken with food by two- to threefold, and its peak concentration in serum is ~2 hours. Ospemifene binds extensively to plasma proteins (>99%) and half-life is ~26 hours. Fluconazole increases serum concentrations of ospemifene. After 12 weeks of therapy, a significant decrease in vaginal dryness and dyspareunia is seen.[141]

PRASTERONE (INTRAROSA)

Metabolism

Dehydroepiandrosterone (DHEA)
Prasterone (Intrarosa)

Testosterone

Metabolism

17β-Estradiol

Prasterone (dehydroepiandrosterone, DHEA) was approved in 2016 for the treatment of severe pain during sexual intercourse in women (dyspareunia) due to vulvar and vaginal atrophy associated with menopause. It is administered as an intravaginal insert (6.5 mg) once daily at bedtime. While the mechanism of action of prasterone (DHEA) is unknown, it is known that DHEA is metabolized to testosterone and 17β-estradiol. Serum concentrations of DHEA, testosterone, and 17β-estradiol were observed to increase following vaginal administration of the drug demonstrating 100%, 10% and 50% higher AUC values after 7 days of daily prasterone. The role of each of these metabolites is yet to be determined in the relief of dyspareunia. Postmenopausal women with a history of breast cancer should be cautioned when using prasterone as estrogen is a metabolite.

Drugs Used in the Treatment of Androgen Insufficiencies

Androgens

Discovery of Androgens

One of the earliest and most unusual experiments with testicular extracts was carried out in 1889 by the French physiologist Charles Brown-Séquard. He administered such an extract to himself and reported that he felt an increased vigor and capacity for work.[142] In 1911, Pézard showed that extracts of testicular tissue increase comb growth in capons.[143] Early attempts to isolate pure male hormones from the testes failed because only small amounts are present in this tissue.

The earliest report of an isolated androgen was presented by Butenandt[144] in 1931. He isolated 15 mg of crystalline androsterone (see Androgen Metabolism section above for structure) from 15,000 L of human male urine. A second crystalline compound, DHEA (see Prasterone (Intrarosa) box above for structure), which has weak androgenic activity, was isolated by Butenandt and Dannenberg[145] in 1934.

During the following year, testosterone was isolated from bull testes by David et al.[146] This hormone was shown to be 6- to 10-times more active than androsterone.

Shortly after testosterone was isolated, Butenandt and Hanisch[147] reported its synthesis. In that same year, extracts of urine from males were shown to cause nitrogen retention (a measure of protein anabolism) as well as the expected androgenic effects.[148] Many steroids with androgenic activity have subsequently been synthesized. Steroid hormones may have many potent effects on various tissues, and slight chemical alterations of androgenic steroids may increase some of these effects without altering others.

Testosterone was the first androgen to be used clinically for its anabolic activity. Because of its androgenic action, testosterone is limited in its use in humans, especially females, as an anabolic steroid. Many steroids were synthesized in an attempt to separate the androgenic and the anabolic actions. Because testosterone had to be given parenterally, it also was desirable to find orally active agents.

In the U.S., most of the androgens and anabolic steroid products are subject to control by the U.S. Federal Control Substances Act as amended by the Anabolic Steroid Control Act of 1990 as Schedule III drugs.

Androgen Physiology

The overall physiologic effects of endogenous androgens are contributed by testosterone and its active metabolites, DHT and 17β-estradiol. Testosterone and DHT execute their actions predominantly through the AR, which belongs to the nuclear receptor superfamily and functions as a ligand-dependent transcription factor. Circulating testosterone is essential for the differentiation and growth of male accessory reproductive organs (e.g., prostate and seminal vesicles), control of male sexual behavior, and the development and maintenance of male secondary characteristics that involve muscle, bone, larynx, and hair. Healthy young adult men produce approximately 3-10 mg of testosterone per day, with circulating plasma levels ranging from approximately 500-1,000 ng/dL in eugonadal (normal) men. Circulating testosterone and 17β-estradiol participate in the feedback regulation of androgen production by the HPG axis, as shown in Figure 24.21. Testosterone, LH, and GnRH (also known as LHRH) constitute the elements of a negative feedback control mechanism, whereby testosterone controls its own release. Low circulating testosterone levels increase the hypothalamic secretion of GnRH, which leads to increased production of LH and, consequently, increased testosterone production by the Leydig cells. More than 95% of circulating testosterone is synthesized and secreted by the Leydig cells in the testes. GnRH is released from the hypothalamus in short, intermittent pulses every 2 hours and at greater magnitude in the morning, which in turn stimulates the pulsatile secretion of LH and FSH from the pituitary. Thus, testosterone secretion likewise is pulsatile and diurnal, with the highest concentration occurring at approximately 8:00 AM and the lowest at approximately 8:00 PM. In the testis, FSH directly interacts with FSH receptors expressed in Sertoli cells and stimulates spermatogenesis, whereas LH indirectly stimulates spermatogenesis through testosterone synthesized by Leydig cells.

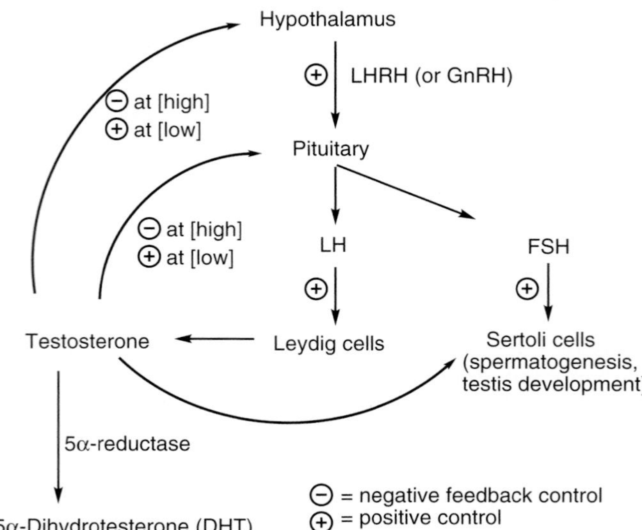

Figure 24.21 Hypothalamic-pituitary-testicular axis.

Testosterone and its aromatized metabolite (17β-estradiol) negatively regulate circulating levels of testosterone in the hypothalamus and pituitary. Activin and inhibin produced by Sertoli cells stimulate or inhibit, respectively, the secretion of FSH from the pituitary.[149] High concentrations of intratesticular testosterone are essential for the initiation and maintenance of spermatogenesis, as evidenced by the infertility of hypogonadal men. Results from both animal models and humans, however, support the idea that both FSH and testosterone are required to achieve quantitative and qualitative spermatogenesis.

In older men, especially those older than 60 years of age, testosterone levels often remain relatively constant, without the morning pulses observed in young adult men. Average plasma testosterone concentrations in older men peak in the morning, with daily ranges of approximately 300-550 ng/dL by 70 years of age. The diurnal cycling is blunted as men age.[150] In women, testosterone levels range from 15 to 100 ng/dL. Starting at approximately 40 years of age, testosterone levels drop by approximately 10% every decade in men. In the normal functioning of the male hormonal system, 97%-98% of plasma testosterone is bound to SHBG, essentially making it unavailable to the body's tissues due to the high binding affinity of testosterone for SHBG. The remaining 2%-3% is known as "bioavailable" or free testosterone. Serum concentrations of SHBG increase with age in men, resulting in a corresponding decrease in free testosterone as men age. Free testosterone levels in serum are positively correlated with muscle strength and BMD in elderly men, but negatively correlated with fat mass.[151]

Androgens also are needed for the development of secondary sex characteristics. The male voice deepens because of thickening of the laryngeal mucosa and lengthening of the vocal cords. In both men and women, they play a role first in stimulating the growth of hair on the face, arms, legs, and pubic areas and later in the recession of the male hairline. The fructose content of human semen and both the size and the secretory capacity of the sebaceous glands also depend on the levels of testosterone.

Testosterone causes nitrogen retention by increasing the rate of protein synthesis and muscle mass while decreasing the rate of protein catabolism. The positive nitrogen balance therefore results from both decreased catabolism and increased anabolism of proteins that are used in male sex accessory apparatus and muscle. The actions of androgen in the reproductive tissues, including prostate, seminal vesicle, testis, and accessory structures, are known as the androgenic effects, whereas the nitrogen-retaining effects of androgen in muscle and bone are known as the anabolic effects. Although the precise mechanism of androgen action on muscle remains unknown, the common hypothesis is that androgens promote muscle protein synthesis. Evidence supports the idea that testosterone supplementation increases muscle protein synthesis in elderly men[152] and young hypogonadal men.[153] Also, androgen-induced increases in muscle mass appear to arise from muscle fiber hypertrophy rather than hyperplasia (i.e., cellular enlargement rather than cellular proliferation).[154]

The thickness and linear growth of bones are stimulated and, later, limited by testosterone because of closure of the epiphyses. Androgens affect BMD by changing overall osteoblast (bone-forming cell) activity and osteoclast (bone-resorbing cell) activity, resulting from changes in the total number of each cell type and individual cell functional capacity.[155,156] Androgens seem to have the ability to decelerate the bone remodeling cycle and tilt the focal balance of that cycle toward bone formation. The loss of androgens is thought to increase the rate of bone remodeling by removing the restraining effects on osteoblastogenesis and osteoclastogenesis.

Mechanisms of Androgen Action

Testosterone, DHT, and other androgens execute their actions predominantly through the AR. The AR is mainly expressed in androgen target tissues, such as the prostate, skeletal muscle, liver, and central nervous system, with the highest expression level being observed in the prostate, adrenal gland, and epididymis.[157] Testosterone is thought to be largely responsible for initiation of AR action in muscle, bone, brain, and bone marrow, whereas DHT plays a major role in genitalia, prostate, skin, and hair follicles due to the higher expression of 5AR enzymes. The mechanism of action of the AR is similar to that of the other nuclear receptors and has been described in detail in Chapter 7.

Besides the genomic pathway, the nongenomic pathway of AR also has been reported in oocytes,[158] skeletal muscle cells,[159] osteoblasts,[160,161] and prostate cancer cells.[162,163] As compared to the genomic pathway, the nongenomic actions of steroid receptors are characterized by the rapidity of the action, which varies from seconds to an hour or so, and by interaction with plasma membrane–associated signaling pathways.[164] Nevertheless, the structural basis for nongenomic action is direct interactions between AR and cytosolic proteins from different signaling pathways, which could be closely related to the ligand-induced conformational change of the LBD or, indirectly, the N-terminal domain. Functionally, the nongenomic action of androgen involves either rapid activation of kinase-signaling cascades or modulation of intracellular calcium levels, which could be related to stimulation of gap junction communication, neuronal plasticity, and aortic relaxation.[165] Separation of the genomic and nongenomic functions of steroid receptors using specific ligands also was proposed as a strategy to achieve tissue selectivity.[164,166]

Male Hypogonadism

Male hypogonadism (testosterone deficiency) is the inability of the testes to produce sufficient testosterone to maintain sexual function, muscle strength, BMD, and fertility (spermatogenesis). Primary hypogonadism refers to a disorder of the testes, wherein LH and/or FSH are elevated and the testes fail to produce sufficient testosterone. LH and FSH levels are generally normal or low in men classified as having secondary hypogonadism, indicating that the problem resides in the brain (i.e., hypothalamic-pituitary failure to stimulate testicles to produce testosterone). Klinefelter syndrome (a chromosomal abnormality resulting in testicular dysfunction), cryptorchidism (failure of the testes to descend), and/or physical damage (e.g., torsion) are disorders associated with very low or absent serum testosterone levels.

Aging-related androgen insufficiency is a physiologic condition characterized by the inability of the testes to produce sufficient testosterone as men age, resulting in deficits in sexual function, muscle strength, BMD, and fertility (spermatogenesis). One in five men older than 50 years will exhibit symptoms of this condition. In men, there is a gradual decline of approximately 1% per year in the production of testosterone beginning around 40 years of age. For most men, testosterone levels naturally decline with advancing age but still remain within the physiologic range throughout their lifetimes, causing no significant problems. Approximately 20% of men older than age 60 years and 30%-40% of men older than 80 years have plasma testosterone levels indicative of hypogonadism (<280-300 ng/dL). Symptoms of aging-related androgen insufficiency may include lethargy or decreased energy, decreased libido or interest in sex, ED (loss of erections), muscle weakness and aches, inability to sleep, hot flashes, night sweats, depression, infertility, thinning of bones or bone loss, and cardiovascular disease. Studies show that a decline in testosterone actually can put men at risk for other health problems, such as heart disease, metabolic syndrome, and weak bones. Psychological stress, alcohol abuse, injuries or surgery, medications, obesity and infections, tobacco, and drugs, such as decongestants, antihypertensives, tranquilizers, statins, or antiseizure agents, can contribute to the onset of these conditions. There is no way of predicting who will experience the symptoms of androgen insufficiency that are of sufficient severity to seek medical help; neither is it predictable at what age the symptoms of aging-related androgen insufficiency will occur in a particular individual. Each man's symptoms also may be different. Because all this happens at a time of life when many men begin to question their values, accomplishments, and direction in life, it often is difficult to realize that the changes occurring are related to more than just external conditions. Now that men are living longer, there is heightened interest in aging-related androgen insufficiency, its risks for other health problems, and its treatment.

Testosterone and structurally related steroidal androgens have been used for decades to treat male hypogonadism, Klinefelter syndrome, anemia secondary to chronic renal failure, aplastic anemia, protein wasting diseases associated with cancer, burns, traumas, AIDS, short stature, breast cancer (as an antiestrogen), and hereditary angioedema. However, these agents have been demoted to the therapy of final resort for anemia and cancer because of serious hepatotoxicity and the recent development of more effective therapies (e.g., erythropoietin, aromatase inhibitors [AIs], and taxanes). Although severe hypogonadism is uncommon, aging-related androgen insufficiency is much more frequent. Low endogenous testosterone concentrations are associated with sarcopenia and frailty arising from decreased fat-free mass, lessened muscle strength, and reduced BMD (osteoporosis). Low testosterone concentrations also are associated with decreased sexual libido and ED. More than 30 million men older than 40 years in the U.S. are estimated to suffer from ED. Although androgens are not essential for erection,[167] transdermal and IM testosterone replacement therapy (TRT) often is employed in hypogonadal men with ED.[168] Furthermore, selective phosphodiesterase type 5 (PDE5) inhibitors that increase penile blood flow are considered to be the treatment of choice for men with ED. Hormone replacement therapy with testosterone in aging men also improves body composition, bone and cartilage metabolism, and memory and cognition, and it even decreases cardiovascular risk.[169]

Testosterone Replacement Therapy

The acceptance of TRT has been hampered by the lack of orally active preparations with good efficacy and, particularly, a safe profile.[170] Progress has been limited over the last three decades in developing synthetic molecules that could separate the desirable physiologic functions normally regulated by endogenous androgens from the undesirable or dose-limiting side effects. The abuse of synthetic anabolic steroids by athletes and body builders has contributed to the general perception of certain undesirable side effects, such as aggressive behavior, liver toxicity, acne, or impotency.

Current formulations for TRT largely are restricted to injectable formulations of testosterone esters, transdermal delivery formulations (scrotal or nonscrotal patches, gels, and pellet implants), or buccal testosterone. Marketed injectable forms of testosterone esters (e.g., testosterone enanthate, cypionate and undecanoate) can produce undesirable fluctuations in testosterone blood levels, with supraphysiologic concentrations early and subphysiologic levels toward the end of the period before the next injection. These fluctuations provide an unsatisfactory benefits profile and, in some cases, undesired side effects. Skin patches provide a better blood level profile of testosterone, but skin irritation and daily application limit the usefulness and acceptability of this form of therapy. Topical gels are widely used for TRT, but must be cautiously used in homes with children due to the risk of virilization. Oral preparations such as fluoxymesterone and 17α-methyltestosterone (see below for structures) are only sparingly used because of concerns about liver toxicity linked to the 17α-alkyl group and because of somewhat lower efficacy.[170] Thus, these oral androgens are generally considered to be obsolete and do not represent a viable form of therapy.

Benefits and Risks of Testosterone Replacement Therapy

Multiple large-scale and long-term clinical trials of TRT have been conducted in aging men to evaluate the risk–benefit ratio of TRT, but no agreement exists regarding the benefits and risks of TRT (Table 24.10) (for review, see Hijazi and Cunningham[171] and Rhoden and Morgentaler[170]). The potential benefits of TRT include increase in BMD and improvement in muscle mass and strength, cognitive function, mood, and sexual function. The potential risks of TRT, however, including those in the cardiovascular system, blood (e.g., hematocrit and hemoglobin levels), and prostate, are routinely experienced. Because the long-term effects of TRT in otherwise healthy men remain unclear, guidelines published by the Endocrine Society recommend a general policy that TRT not be offered to older men with low serum testosterone levels and that TRT only be used in men with clinically significant symptoms of androgen deficiency and serum total testosterone concentrations approaching 200 ng/dL.[172]

Clearly, TRT is beneficial for hypogonadal men with androgen insufficiency to restore sexual function and muscle strength, to prevent bone loss, and to protect against heart disease (atherosclerosis).[170] Increasing testosterone levels with TRT, however, may pose problems by stimulating the growth of the prostate. Long-term TRT could cause prostate gland enlargement, which might exacerbate BPH or fuel the growth of prostate cancer that is already present and could cause breast enlargement in men (gynecomastia). This is especially worrisome because of the high prevalence of BPH in older men and the possibility that many men may have prostate cancer that is undiagnosed. In fact, men with a palpable prostate nodule, a prostate-specific antigen (PSA) level greater than 4 ng/mL, or severe lower urinary tract symptoms (LUTSs) associated with BPH are usually advised to avoid TRT.

In elderly men, testosterone effects on muscle mass and strength have not been consistent or impressive, possibly because of the low dosages used in clinical trials. The high correlation between the dose (and plasma concentration) and the anabolic actions of androgen in muscle suggests that androgen administration of higher doses in elderly men may significantly increase muscle mass and strength, but high doses might increase the adverse effects and the aromatization of testosterone to estrogen.[173]

Types of Testosterone Replacement Therapy

Several types of TRT exist. Choosing a specific therapy depends on the patient's preference of a particular delivery system, the side effects, and the cost. Types include injection, transdermal, buccal mucosal, and oral (Table 24.11).

Table 24.10 Testosterone Replacement Therapy

Benefits	Risks
Improved sexual performance and desire	Stimulated growth of preexisting prostate cancer
More energy and improved quality of life	Greater chance for benign prostatic hyperplasia
More energy and sense of well-being	Increased hemoglobin levels to above the physiologic range
Increased bone mineral density	Problems with voiding; symptoms include poor urine flow and hesitancy before urinating
Improved muscle mass and strength	
Improved (lower) low-density lipoprotein profile	Increased potential for liver damage from oral preparations Sleep apnea (stopping of breathing during sleep)
Decreased irritability and depression	Breast tenderness and swelling (gynecomastia)
Improved cognitive function	Testicular shrinkage (testicular atrophy)
Increased hemoglobin levels to the physiologic range	Infertility (decreased spermatogenesis) Skin reaction from patches or gel
Thickened body hair and skin	Pain, soreness, or bruising from injection Increased fluid retention Increased skin problems (acne, oily skin) Increased body hair

INJECTION. Orally administered testosterone is ineffective in the treatment of male androgen insufficiency syndromes due to extensive presystemic first-pass metabolism. IM injections bypass the problems of first-pass metabolism. IM injections are depot formulations of testosterone esters that undergo differing rates of in vivo ester hydrolysis to release free testosterone over an extended period of time. Typically, the depot esters are administered IM into a large muscle once every 2-4 weeks depending on the depot ester used (Table 24.11). They are safe, effective, and the least expensive androgen preparations available. The major disadvantage with the IM route for the depot esters is that testosterone plasma concentrations exhibit a saw-toothed pattern, with supraphysiologic levels within 2-4 days following the IM injection and subphysiologic levels before the next injection. A more satisfactory physiologic replacement therapy without the fluctuations in free testosterone plasma levels would be to administer a lower IM dose (i.e., 100 mg) on a weekly or biweekly schedule. IM injection of testosterone or its esters causes local irritation. The rate of absorption for IM products may be erratic.

Esters of testosterone prepared for IM administration include the 17β-propionate, 17β-enanthate, and the cypionate (17β-cyclopentylpropionate) (Fig. 24.22). Testosterone enanthate (not currently available) and cypionate demonstrate comparable pharmacokinetics. Testosterone enanthate is formed by esterification of the 17β-hydroxy group of testosterone with heptanoic acid, while testosterone cypionate is formed with cyclopentanepropionic acid. Sterile solutions of these esters are available in a suitable vegetable oil, such as cottonseed oil. Unlike oral testosterone, with a half-life of 10-100 minutes, IM testosterone administration avoids first-pass metabolism and exhibits a longer duration due to the slow hydrolysis and release of testosterone from the depot injection site. Generally, the concentration of SHBG in plasma determines the distribution of testosterone between free and bound forms. The bulky cypionate and enanthate esters of testosterone have durations of action of up to 2-4 weeks, whereas the shorter propionate ester (not currently available) has a shorter duration of action of 1-2 weeks. Doses may be adjusted by aiming for midphysiologic (400-600 ng/dL) testosterone values after 1 week or at the low end (300-400 ng/dL) just before the next injection is due.

IMPLANT. Subcutaneous implantation of testosterone pellets (Testopel) is much less flexible for dose adjustment as compared to transdermal, oral, or IM injection. Fat-soluble pellets containing 75 mg of testosterone can be implanted subcutaneously on the anterior abdominal wall or buttocks to deliver testosterone over a 3- to 4-month period. Recommended doses range from 150 to 450 mg implanted subcutaneously every 3-6 months. The longer duration of action of the pellets is accompanied by a larger dose requirement as compared to weekly or biweekly IM injections. Approximately one-third of the material from the pellet is absorbed in the first month, one-fourth in the second month, and one-sixth in the third month. Adequate effects from the pellets can occasionally continue for as long as 6 months.

TRANSDERMAL. Transdermal TRT systems are, perhaps, the most commonly used systems for delivering testosterone to bypass the rapid first-pass metabolism associated with oral testosterone. Clinical studies have shown that these formulations are effective forms of testosterone replacement, with peak response within 3-6 months. Use of the transdermal formulation should be discontinued

Table 24.11 Testosterone Products and Properties[a]

Product	Trade Name	Onset of Peak Response	Duration of Action	Time to Peak Conc.	Time to Steady-State Conc.	Dose (mg)	Frequency of Dosing	Oral Bioavailability (%)	Elimination Half-life
Methyltestosterone	Android Testred Virilon Oreton Methyl	—	24 hr	2 hr	—	10-50	Daily	70	3 hr
Fluoxymesterone	Androxy	—	24 hr	—	—	5-40	Daily	80	9 hr
Testosterone undecanoate	Aveed	6 hr	10 hr	~6 hr	—	40-120	Daily	<10	3 hr
Testosterone cypionate	Depo-Testosterone	6-24 hr	2-4 wk	24 hr	—	50-400	2-4 wk	—	8 d
Testosterone enanthate	Andro-LA Andryl Delatestryl Delatest Everone Testamon	6-24 hr	2-4 wk	24 hr	—	50-400	2-4 wk	—	8 d
Testosterone pellets	Testopel	1-2 mo	3-6 mo	1 mo	1-2 wk	150-450	3-6 mo	—	—
Trandermal patches	Androderm	3-6 mo	24 hr	2-4 hr	2-3 d	2-5	24 hr	—	10-100 min
Transdermal gels	AndroGel Testim Vogelxo	3-6 mo	5 d	4 (2-6) hours	2-3 d	50-100	24 hr	—	10-100 min
Buccal mucosal	Striant	—	24 hr	5 (0.5-12) hours	2-3 d	30	Every 12 hr	—	6 hr

[a]Thompson Healthcare, Inc. Micromedex Healthcare Series. Available at http://www.Thompsonhc.com.

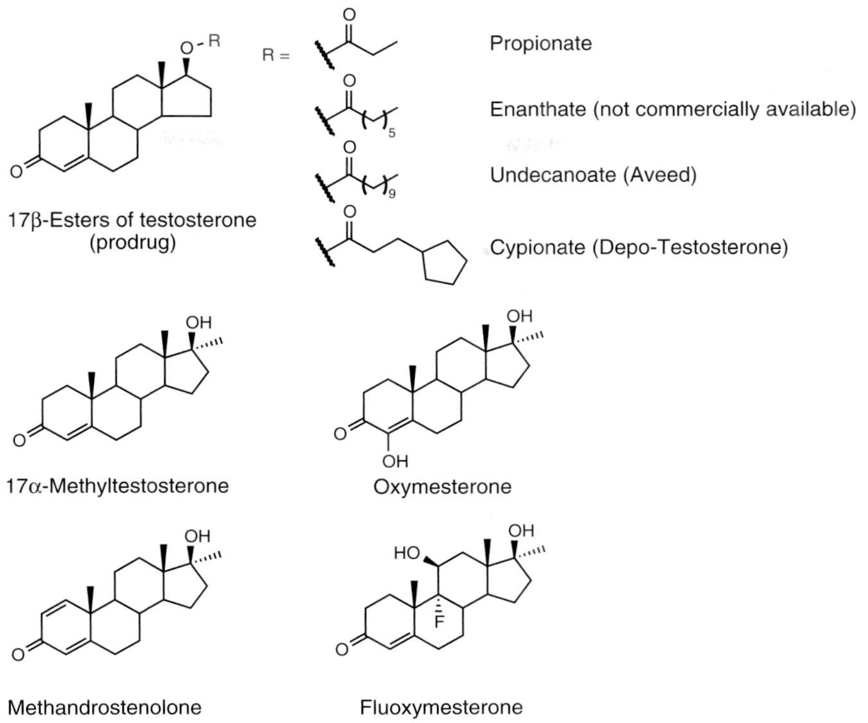

Figure 24.22 Androgenic derivatives of testosterone.

if the desired response is not reached within this time period. Skin irritation is more common with the transdermal formulations, with more than 50% experiencing some form of skin irritation at some point during the treatment. Pretreatment with corticosteroid creams (not with the ointment) has been shown to reduce the severity and incidence of skin irritation without significantly affecting testosterone absorption from the formulation. With the transdermal formulations, testosterone levels are maintained within physiologic values, and a beneficial effect on general mood and sexual functioning is generally observed. A plasma concentration in the midphysiologic range (400-600 ng/dL) is the goal.

Matrix-Type Transdermal Systems. This type of patch (scrotal patch; Testoderm) must be applied to dry, clean (shaven) scrotal skin, which is 5- to 30-times more permeable to testosterone than other skin sites, every 24 hours to produce an adequate testosterone plasma concentration. The matrix system is described as a "drug-in-adhesive film," in which the drug is located on the adhesive layer of the film; thus, it is thinner and less bulky than the reservoir system. The advantage of the matrix system is that it produces supraphysiologic levels of DHT because of the high 5AR enzyme activity of the scrotal tissue. The patches have an occlusive backing that prevents sex partners from coming in contact with the active drug. A matrix transdermal system will not produce adequate plasma testosterone concentrations if applied to nonscrotal skin. Plasma testosterone concentrations are reached in approximately 2-4 hours. Although testosterone is absorbed throughout a 24-hour period, concentrations do not simulate the circadian rhythm of endogenous testosterone in normal (eugonadal) males. Within 24 hours after application of the matrix system, plasma testosterone concentration gradually falls to 60%-80% of the peak plasma concentration, and when the system is removed, testosterone plasma concentration declines to baseline within 2 hours. Inadequate scrotal size and adherence problems are limitations. Skin irritation does occur in those with sensitive scrotal skins.

Reservoir-Type Transdermal Systems. The reservoir-type patch (nonscrotal patch; Androderm, Testoderm TTS) is not applied to scrotal skin but, rather, to the abdomen, back, thighs, or upper arms every 24 hours (see Table 24.11 for dosage strength). This type of patch is membrane-controlled for the drug to diffuse continuously over 24 hours from the reservoir into the skin. Thus, this type of patch is thicker than the matrix (scrotal) patch. The patches have an occlusive backing that prevents sex partners from coming in contact with the active drug. The site of the application is rotated at 7-day intervals between applications to lessen skin reactions at the same application site. The advantage of the reservoir transdermal system is that it achieves normal testosterone circadian rhythm as seen in younger men, peaking in the morning and decreasing throughout the rest of the day. The reservoir-type patch, when applied to nonscrotal skin, produced physiologic DHT and 17β-estradiol plasma concentrations. Steady-state plasma concentrations of testosterone, which are approximately 10-times baseline values, are reached in about 6 hours (range, 4-10 hr depending on application patch location), which then fall to 60%-80% of the peak plasma concentration within 24 hours after application of the transdermal system. Thus, physiologic plasma testosterone concentrations are maintained over 24 hours with this type of patch. Drug accumulation does not occur with repeated applications. When the system is removed, testosterone plasma concentrations decline to baseline within 2 hours. A usual dose for the reservoir-type transdermal results in the systemic absorption of 2-10 mg daily in hypogonadal men.

Gels. Testosterone gel (AndroGel, Testim) is a 1% testosterone hydroalcoholic gel that provides continuous transdermal delivery of testosterone for 24 hours once the gel is rubbed into the skin on the lower abdomen, upper arm, or shoulder. It should not be applied to scrotal tissue (Table 24.11). Because there is a continuous release of testosterone over 24 hours, the normal circadian rhythm is not observed. As the gel dries, approximately 10% of the testosterone is absorbed through the skin. Gel application of TRT appears to cause fewer skin reactions than those that occur with the patches. Men should avoid showering or bathing for several hours after an application to ensure adequate absorption. A potential side effect of the gel is the possibility of transferring the medication to a partner; skin-to-skin contact should be avoided either until the gel is completely dry or by covering the area after an application. Skin-to-skin contact with children is of particular concern and is included as a "black box" warning for these products. Following the application of 5 g of gel, which will deliver 50 mg of testosterone, the mean peak testosterone concentrations are reached in approximately 2 hours, which are about two to three times baseline values. For optimum results, the gel is best applied in the evening to allow maximum concentration to occur early in the morning hours. Doses of the gel may be adjusted by aiming for midphysiologic (400-600 ng/dL) testosterone values after 1 week. When the gel treatment is discontinued, plasma testosterone levels remain in the physiologic range for 24-48 hours, then return to their pretreatment levels within 5 days following the last application. An increase in plasma testosterone can be observed within 30 minutes of application. Plasma concentrations approximate the steady-state level by the end of the first 24 hours and are at steady-state by the second or third day of dosing.

BUCCAL MUCOSAL. Striant is a gel-like drug product that adheres to the gumline, which softens to deliver physiologic amounts of testosterone to the systemic circulation, thereby producing circulating testosterone concentrations in hypogonadal males that approximate physiologic levels seen in healthy young men (400-700 ng/dL). One buccal system (30 mg) is applied to the gum region twice daily, morning and evening, approximately 12 hours apart. Because there is a continuous release of testosterone over 24 hours, the normal circadian rhythm is not observed. Peak plasma testosterone concentrations are reached within 10-12 hours and are stable within a few days of the buccal preparation. The buccal preparation is difficult for patients to get used to, because the side effects may include gum irritation or pain, bitter taste, and headache. A study found that this form of TRT delivers a steadier dose of testosterone throughout the day without significant adverse effects, comparable to the gel.

ORAL. Orally administered testosterone is ineffective in the treatment of male androgen deficiency syndromes because of extensive presystemic first-pass metabolism, primarily to inactive 17-ketosteroids, etiocholanolone and androsterone, and androstenediol (not shown) metabolites in the GI mucosa during absorption and in the liver (Fig. 24.23). Oral administration is generally thought to result in supraphysiologic elevations and undesirable variability in serum testosterone and DHT concentrations. The plasma half-life of testosterone is less than 30 minutes. Generally, the amount of SHBG in plasma determines the distribution of testosterone between free and bound forms. Approximately 90% of a dose of testosterone is metabolized, and its metabolites are

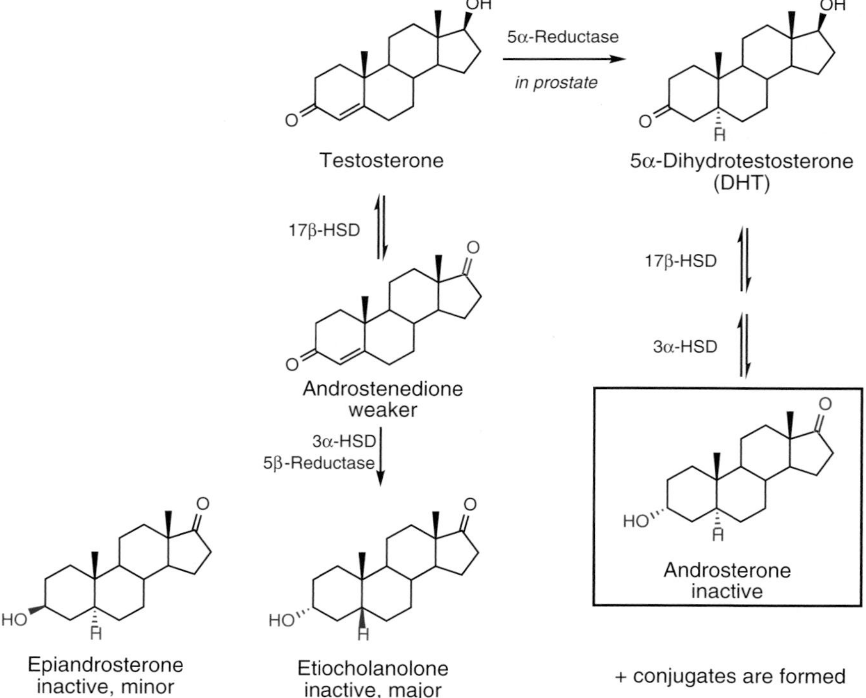

Figure 24.23 Testosterone metabolism. HSD, hydroxysteroid dehydrogenase.

excreted in the urine primarily as glucuronide conjugates, with approximately 6% of a dose being excreted in the feces as unmetabolized testosterone. Comparative dosage ranges for testosterone and its synthetic preparations are shown in Table 24.11. Taking testosterone orally (Android, Testred), in the form of methyltestosterone, is not recommended for long-term replacement. Oral testosterone may cause an unfavorable cholesterol profile and increase the risk of blood clots and heart and liver problems.

The androgenic activity of lipophilic long-chain ester testosterone 17β-undecanoate (Aveed) (Fig. 24.22) has been attributed to formation of testosterone via systemic ester hydrolysis of lymphatically transported testosterone undecanoate.[174] Its oral bioavailability was approximately 3%. Lymphatically transported testosterone undecanoate accounted for between 90% and 100% of the systemically available ester, and 83%-85% of the systemically available testosterone resulted from systemic hydrolysis of lymphatically transported testosterone undecanoate. These data demonstrate that intestinal lymphatic transport of testosterone undecanoate produces increased systemic exposure of testosterone by avoiding the extensive first-pass hepatic metabolism responsible for the inactivation of testosterone after oral administration. New oral formulations in which testosterone undecanoate is formulated in a lipid matrix to enhance oral bioavailability via uptake into the lymphatic system are in late-stage clinical trials and may present an opportunity for oral delivery of testosterone.

SYNTHETIC DERIVATIVES OF TESTOSTERONE. Some of the early studies with androgens included structural modifications of the naturally occurring hormones to avoid first-pass metabolism. Blocking the metabolism of the 17β-hydroxy group with substituents in the 17α-position resulted in androgens with an increased bioavailability and duration of action when given orally. The synthetic androgens include methyltestosterone and fluoxymesterone (Fig. 24.22). The long-term use of these oral androgens has been associated with liver cancer.

17α-METHYLTESTOSTERONE. The synthesis of 17α-methyltestosterone made available a compound that was orally active[175] in daily doses between 10 and 50 mg (Android, Testred), which is equivalent to a 400-mg oral dose of testosterone. The presence of a 17α alkyl group reduces susceptibility to hepatic oxidative metabolism, thereby increasing oral bioavailability (~70%) by slowing metabolism. Following oral administration, methyltestosterone is well absorbed from the GI tract, with a half-life of approximately 3 hours. This drug has the androgenic and anabolic activities of testosterone. Although orally active, it is more effective when administered sublingually. The alkylated oral androgens are seldom used due to their potential hepatotoxicity.

FLUOXYMESTERONE. By substituting a 9α-fluoro group onto an analog of 17α-methyltestosterone, fluoxymesterone has 20 times the anabolic and 10 times the androgenic activity of 17α-methyltestosterone (Fig. 24.22).[175] It has an oral bioavailability of approximately 80% and a mean half-life of 9 hours, and less than 5% of the drug is excreted unchanged. Daily doses of 5-20 mg (Androxy) are generally used for TRT, but, like methyltestosterone, concerns related to the potential hepatotoxicity of alkylated androgens have limited the clinical use of this drug, and there are currently no marketed formulations. Fluoxymesterone is also associated with sodium and water retention, which could lead to edema.

Structure-Activity Relationships of Steroidal Androgens

Until the discovery of nonsteroidal androgens (discussed later), it was believed that a substance must contain a steroid skeleton to have androgenic activity.[176] Oxygen functional groups normally occurring at positions 3 and 17 of the steroid ring system are not essential, because the basic nucleus, 5α-androstane, has androgenic activity. This appears to be the minimal structural requirement for hormonal activity of steroids. For derivatives of etiocholane, in which the hydrogen is in the 5β-position, thereby affording a *cis* A/B ring juncture, no active androgens and anabolic agents are known.[176] Generally, ring expansion (to form homo derivatives by inserting a methylene group into one of the rings in the steroid nucleus) or ring contraction (by removing a methylene group) significantly reduces or destroys the androgenic and anabolic activities.

Introduction of a 3-ketone function or a 3α-OH group enhances androgenic activity. A hydroxyl group in the 17α-position of androstane contributes no androgenic or anabolic activity; no known substituent can approach the effectiveness of a 17β-OH group. Evidence indicates that the longer-acting esters of the 17β-OH compounds are hydrolyzed in vivo to the free alcohol, which is the active species. The 17β-oxygen atom is important for attachment to the receptor site, while 17α-alkyl groups are important for preventing metabolic changes at this position.[175] Such 17α-substituents render the compounds orally active.

Increasing the length of the alkyl side chain at the 17α-position, however, resulted in decreased activity, and the incorporation of other substituents, such as the 17α-ethynyl group, produced compounds with useful progestational activity (progestins), such as ethisterone (Fig. 24.17). Attaching an isoxazole ring to ethisterone produced danazol (Danatrol, Danocrine), which exhibited potent antigonadotropic properties, weak androgen and anabolic properties, and no estrogen or progestin activity.

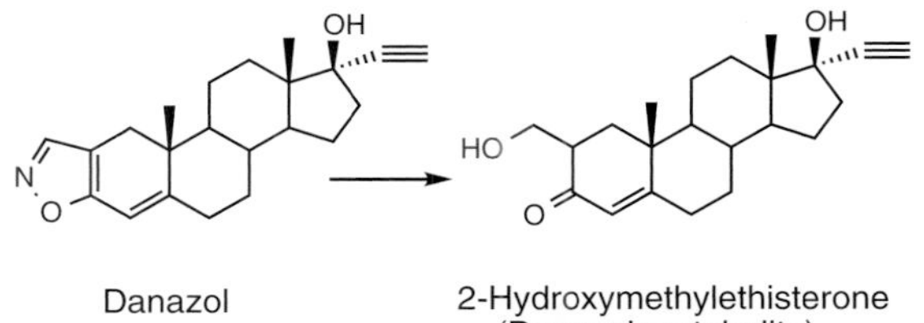

OH N O HO O OH

Danazol

2-Hydroxymethylethisterone (Danazol metabolite)

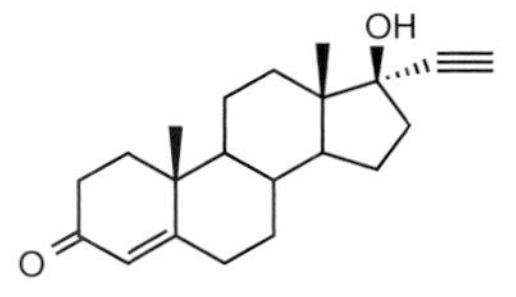

OH O

Ethisterone

As a gonadotropin inhibitor, danazol suppresses the surge of LH and FSH from the pituitary, thus suppressing ovarian steroidogenesis. For this reason, it is used in the treatment of endometriosis. Previous treatment of endometriosis had been surgical or medical, with progestins or a combination of estrogen and progestin. Danazol is metabolized by CYP3A4 to its inactive metabolite, 2-hydroxymethylethisterone.

Several modifications of 17α-methyltestosterone lead to potent, orally active anabolic agents. Two hydroxylated analogs include oxymesterone (Fig. 24.22) and oxymetholone (Fig. 24.24). These drugs have at least three times the anabolic and half the androgenic activity of testosterone.[175]

Halogen substitution produces compounds with decreased activity except when inserted into positions 4 or 9 (e.g., fluoxymesterone). Replacement of a carbon atom in position 2 by oxygen has produced the only clinically successful heterocyclic steroid (oxandrolone) among a number of azasteroids and oxasteroids. Some of the 2-oxasteroids are potent anabolic agents.

Introduction of a sp2-hybridized carbon atom into the A ring (methenolone and testolactone; Fig. 24.24) renders the ring more planar, and in turn, this may be responsible for greater anabolic activity. The 19-norsteroids (nandrolone) are of interest, because these agents seem to produce a more favorable ratio of anabolic to androgenic activity. Vida[175] has extensively reviewed the replacement of various hydrogens on the androgen steroid skeleton by other functional groups. It appears that certain substitutions at positions 1, 2, 7, 17, and 18 may result in compounds with favorable activities that could be of clinical importance.

Adverse Effects

TRT can have undesirable side effects depending on the type of delivery system used. The adverse effects from oral testosterone include stomach upset, headache, acne, increased hair growth on the face or body, jaundice (liver toxicity), anxiety, change in sex drive, sleeplessness, increased urination, depression, enlargement of breasts, and increased frequency and duration of erections.[170,172,173] Breast enlargement can develop because the exogenous testosterone may lead to increased conversion to 17β-estradiol via aromatase. Other adverse effects include water retention, liver toxicity, cardiovascular disease, sleep apnea, and prostate enlargement. These risks are relatively uncommon when the dosage is closely monitored to maintain physiologic plasma testosterone concentrations. TRT is contraindicated in men with carcinoma of the breast or with known or suspected BPH or carcinoma of the prostate. Therefore, pretreatment screening for any prostate dysfunction is mandatory before starting TRT.

Anabolic Agents

Because complete dissociation of anabolic and androgenic effects is not possible, many of the actions of anabolic steroids are similar to those of androgens. Comparative dosage ranges for the anabolic steroids are shown in Table 24.11.

Selenium dioxide dehydrogenation of 17α-methyltestosterone yields the 1,4-diene analog, methandrostenolone (Fig. 24.22), which has severalfold the anabolic activity of the starting material. It has low androgenic activity but, apparently, can produce mammogenic effects in men. These effects are thought to result from estrogenic metabolites.

The 17α-alkylated anabolic steroids (Fig. 24.24) in clinical use are oxandrolone (Oxandrin), oxymetholone (Anadrol-50), and nandrolone decanoate (Deca-Durabolin). Anabolic steroids that are now discontinued are stanozolol (Winstrol) and nandrolone phenpropionate (Durabolin).

A 2-oxasteroid analog of 17α-methyltestosterone is oxandrolone, which contains a lactone in the A ring (oxygen bioisostere of ring A) and, therefore, is susceptible to in vivo hydrolysis. It has three times the anabolic activity

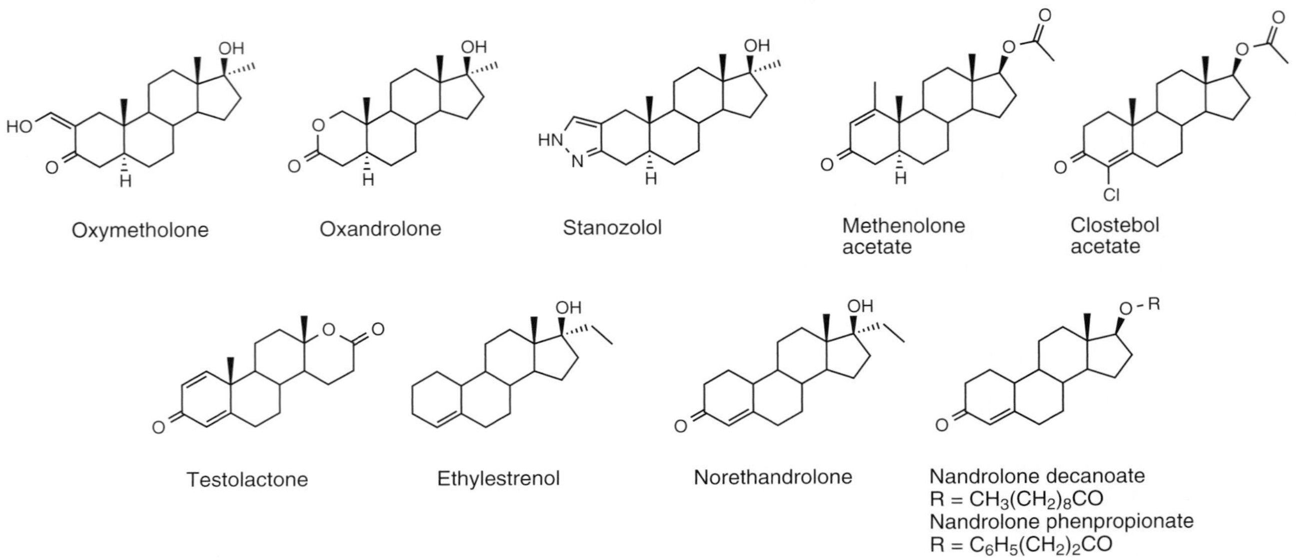

Oxymetholone

Oxandrolone

Stanozolol

Methenolone acetate

Clostebol acetate

Testolactone

Ethylestrenol

Norethandrolone

Nandrolone decanoate
R = $CH_3(CH_2)_8CO$
Nandrolone phenpropionate
R = $C_6H_5(CH_2)_2CO$

Figure 24.24 Anabolic steroids.

of 17α-methyltestosterone but exhibits slight androgenic activity.[177] A pyrazole heterocyclic compound used for its anabolic effects was stanozolol.[177]

The anabolic steroid oxymetholone (Anadrol) was used primarily to stimulate production of erythropoietin in the treatment of anemias resulting from bone marrow failure before the advent of erythropoietin, but is seldom used today due to its association with hepatitis and liver tumors.

Testolactone (Teslac), an 18-oxasteroid, is a D-homo-oxoandrostandienedione analog, with ring D being a six-membered lactone ring. Although testolactone possesses some anabolic activity with weak androgenic effects, before its discontinuation it was used primarily in the treatment of breast cancer as a noncompetitive irreversible inhibitor of aromatase to suppress the formation of estrogens that would stimulate the growth of breast tissue.[178] It is primarily excreted in the urine unchanged, but it is metabolized in the liver by partial reduction of the 4-ene double bond in ring A to the 5β-metabolite (*cis* A/B ring juncture). Testolactone was discontinued in 2008 and is no longer available for clinical use.

Alkylation in the 1, 2, 7, and 18 positions of the androstane molecule generally increases anabolic activity.[175] One of these derivatives, methenolone acetate, is an example of a potent anabolic agent that does not have an alkyl substituent at the 17α-position. It is no longer available for use. A halogenated anabolic agent used in about the same dosage is clostebol acetate (Fig. 24.24; not available in the United States).

Androgens, having no methyl group in position 10 of the steroid nucleus, are an important class of anabolic agents often referred to as the 19-norandrogens, as shown in Figure 24.24. The removal of the 19-CH_3 group of the androgen results in reduction of its androgenic properties but retention of its anabolic, tissue-building properties. These steroids can be synthesized by the Birch reduction of the aromatic A ring of a 3-methoxy estrogen to a 2,5(10)-estradiene. Cleavage of the enol ether with HCl results in the 19-nortestosterone derivative. In animal assays, 19-nortestosterone has about the same anabolic activity as the propionate ester of testosterone, but its androgenic activity is much lower. Because 19-nortestosterone showed some separation of anabolic and androgenic activities, related analogs were synthesized and biologically investigated. Two of the more potent members of the series are norethandrolone and ethylestrenol and are shown in Figure 24.24. Norethandrolone has a better ratio of anabolic to androgenic activity than either 19-nortestosterone (nandrolone) or 17[α]-methyl-19-nortestosterone (not shown).[179] Both androgenic and progestational side effects have been observed with this agent. Ethylestrenol is more potent than norethandrolone as an anabolic agent and before discontinuation was used in a dosage of 4 mg per day orally.

Nandrolone phenpropionate and nandrolone decanoate are esters of 19-nortestosterone, as shown in Figure 24.24. When administered IM, slow in vivo hydrolysis of the ester occurs, releasing free 19-nortestosterone over a prolonged period. Nandrolone decanoate is the longer-acting ester intended for deep IM injection, preferably into the gluteal muscle, in the treatment of anemia associated with renal insufficiency. Nandrolone phenpropionate has a shorter duration of action than the decanoate and is used in the treatment of metastatic breast cancer in women.

Abuse of Steroidal Anabolic Agents to Enhance Athletic Performance

Performance-enhancing substances are now a point of major interest for athletes, government, and news media. These substances are having a major impact on sports and the public in general. It appears that we are headed for much greater antidoping efforts in sports. A great deal of interest has recently been shown in "designer" anabolic steroids for their high-muscle-building effects, as shown in Figure 24.25. Tetrahydrogestrinone and desoxymethyltestosterone brought a great deal of interest to the performance-enhancing area, because their use was very difficult to detect.[180,181] Tetrahydrogestrinone is thought to have been derived from gestrinone, a substance that has been used for the treatment of a variety of gynecologic disorders. Tetrahydrogestrinone also is related to trenbolone, which has been used by body builders and by ranchers to build up cattle before marketing. Before tetrahydrogestrinone, both gestrinone and trenbolone had been on the banned anabolic steroid list of the International Olympic Committee. Tetrahydrogestrinone was very difficult to trace, however, because it was unstable under the normal conditions of testing for anabolic steroids. Once a suitable assay was developed, it was possible to go back and test samples of athletes around the world, and several were found to have taken tetrahydrogestrinone.

Nonsteroidal Androgens

Selective Androgen Receptor Modulators

The successful marketing and clinical application of SERMs raised the possibility of developing selective ligands for other members of the nuclear receptor superfamily. The concept of selective androgen receptor modulator (SARMs)[182–184] emerged more recently; namely, a compound that is an antagonist or weak agonist in the prostate but agonist in the bone and muscle and is orally

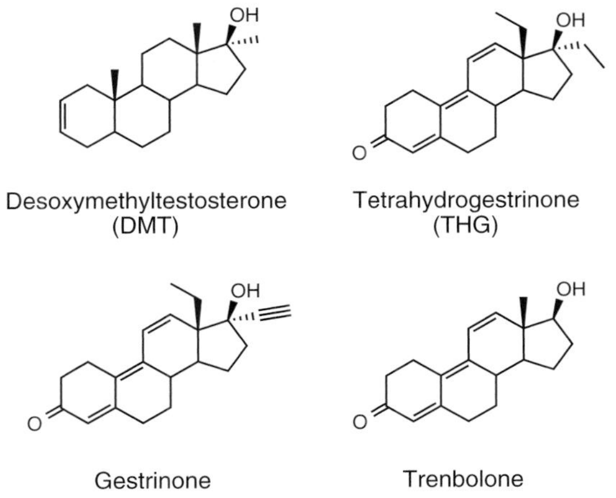

Desoxymethyltestosterone (DMT)

Tetrahydrogestrinone (THG)

Gestrinone

Trenbolone

Figure 24.25 Illegal anabolic agents.

available with low hepatotoxicity. For an ideal SARM, the antagonist or weak agonist activity in the prostate will reduce concern for the potential to stimulate nascent or undetected prostate cancer, whereas the strong agonist activity in the muscle and bone can be used to treat muscle-wasting conditions, hypogonadism, and/or aging-related frailty. SARMs have reached clinical development, but are still looking for a therapeutic indication.

SARM pharmacophores include N-arylpropionamide,[184] bicyclic hydantoin,[185] tricyclic quinolines,[186] and tetrahydroquinoline[187] analogs, as shown in Figure 24.26. These nonsteroidal AR ligands are not substrates for aromatase or 5AR but exhibit affinity as full AR agonists in anabolic organs (e.g., muscle and bone) or as partial AR agonists in androgenic tissues (e.g., prostate and seminal vesicles).

STRUCTURE-ACTIVITY RELATIONSHIPS FOR THE N-ARYLPROPIONAMIDES. The majority of published preclinical research has focused on a series of N-arylpropionamide analogs as AR agonists or partial agonists, using the key structural elements of bicalutamide, an androgen antagonist.[184,188]

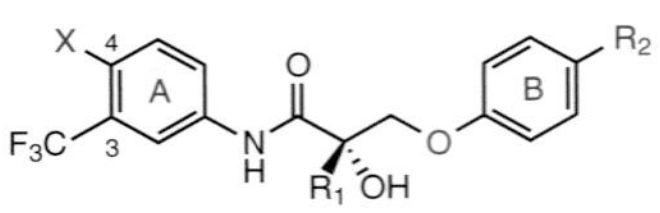

N-Arylpropanamides (ether analogs)

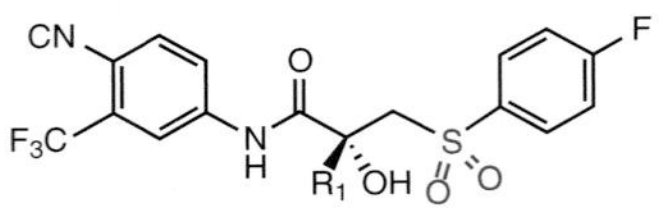

R-Bicalutamide ($R_1 = CH_3$)

SARM Comparison

A series of chiral ether analogs of bicalutamide, which bear electron-withdrawing groups (see variable X of the N-Arylpropanamides structure shown above) in the A-ring and fluoro or acetylamino substituent at the *para* position in ring B (R_2) demonstrated high in vitro AR binding affinity and reduced in vivo androgenicity but full anabolic activity in castrated male rats.[189,190] The sulfide analogs (replacement of ether oxygen with sulfur) exhibited greater AR binding affinity, except that hepatic oxidation of the sulfur to sulfoxides (not shown) or sulfones (like bicalutamide) led to rapid in vivo inactivation and reduced efficacy.

For ether analogs, replacing the aromatic ring A with a heterocyclic ring derivative failed to retain AR binding affinity, which probably arose from steric hinderance on binding with the AR; however, a heterocyclic B ring retained AR binding affinity. Small size electron-withdrawing moieties at R_2, such as fluoro, chloro, nitro, or cyano groups, are optimum. Because aromatic nitro groups are associated with hepatotoxicity, the nitro groups were replaced with a nonreducible electron-withdrawing group (i.e., a cyano group). The dicyano (X and R_2) gave the most potent and efficacious N-arylpropanamide SARM with favorable pharmacokinetic properties. As evidenced from structure–activity relationship studies, minor differences in ligand structure can lead to either agonist or antagonist activity. Full or partial agonist binding to AR is influenced by stereoisomeric conformation as well as by steric and electronic effects of the substituents. Molecular modeling of N-arylpropionamide AR ligands was used in conjunction with pharmacology, pharmacodynamics, pharmacokinetics, and metabolism to examine and optimize structural properties.

Results from in vitro and in vivo animal studies suggest that the therapeutic promise of SARMs as treatment for muscle wasting, osteoporosis, hormonal male contraception, BPH, or other conditions associated with aging or androgen deficiency—without unwanted side effects associated with testosterone—may be realized.[193] The AR specificity and lack of side effects intrinsic to the steroidal backbone such as steroid receptor cross-reactivity, metabolic activation by 5α-reductase and/or aromatase, and hepatotoxicity clearly distinguish these drugs from their steroidal predecessors and open the door for expanded clinical use of androgens. As the molecular mechanisms of action of SARMs on target tissues become more fully understood, the discovery of novel SARMs and expansion into broader therapeutic applications will be more feasible. Currently, research concerning SARMs is in preclinical discovery and the early phase of clinical development with the expectations that SARMs, with the beneficial pharmacologic activity of androgens without the unwanted side effects, will provide individual patients who have various androgen-dependent disorders with a significantly improved quality of life.

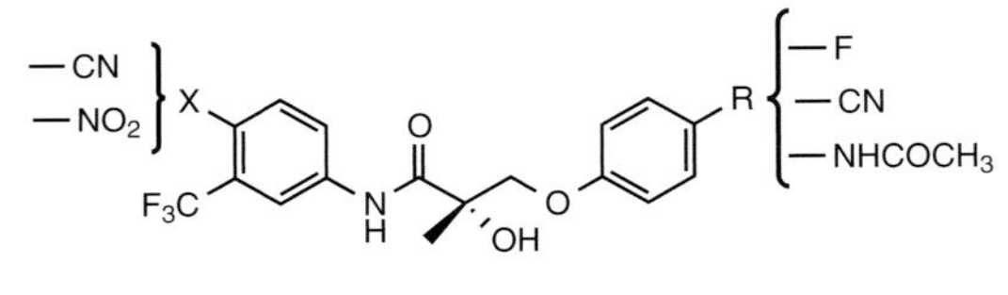

Aryl propionamide

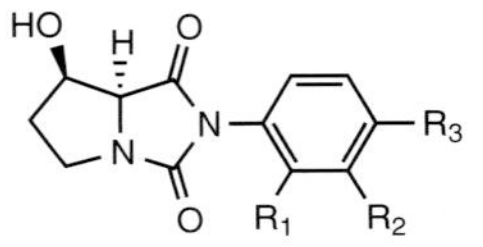

Bicyclic hydantoin

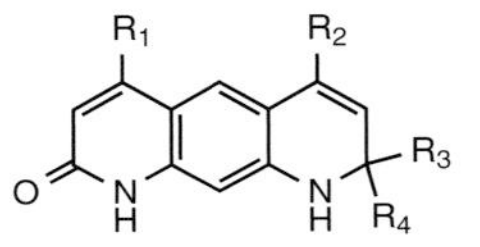

Tricyclic quinoline

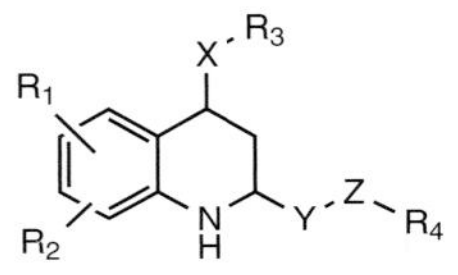

Tetrahydroquinoline

Figure 24.26 Selective androgen receptor modulators (SARMs).

DRUGS USED FOR THE TREATMENT OF ERECTILE DYSFUNCTION

The National Institutes of Health Consensus Development Panel on Impotence defined ED as the inability to achieve or maintain an erection sufficient for satisfactory sexual performance that may substantially influence quality of life. It is estimated that 10-30 million men in the U.S., and more than 100 million men worldwide, experience some form of ED.[191] This condition is strongly associated with age, and according to the community-based Massachusetts Male Aging Study, the prevalence of ED in men between 40 and 70 years of age is 52%.[362] The general classification of ED includes psychogenic ED (e.g., depression, psychological stress, relationship problems, and performance anxiety), organic ED (e.g., diabetes, hypertension, spinal cord injuries, and some medications), and mixed psychogenic and organic ED.

Treatment options for men with ED have changed significantly over the past three decades and have progressed from psychosexual therapy and penile prostheses (1970s) through revascularization, vacuum constriction devices, and intracavernosal injection therapy (1980s) to transurethral and oral drug delivery (1990s). The first line of treatment for ED is PDE5 inhibition because these drugs can be given orally and have a fast onset of action. If the PDE5 inhibitors are not effective, then the cause may be low libido, and men should have their testosterone blood levels checked (in some instances, TRT may help to resolve ED). Other alternative drugs currently available for the treatment of ED include prostaglandin E1, which is given by injection at the base of the penis or by suppository into the tip of the penis, as well as the α1-adrenergic blocker and the nonselective PDE inhibitor papaverine. Apomorphine is a dopamine agonist that can be used for treating ED but, in humans, has the undesirable emetic side effect. Some selective dopamine D4 agents are now being investigated for treatment of ED. Vacuum devices and penile implants are also available.

Phosphodiesterase Inhibitors

The currently available first- and second-generation oral phosphodiesterase 5 inhibitors (PDE5Is), sildenafil, tadalafil, vardenafil, and avanafil have emerged as the first-line treatment for ED because of patient convenience, safety, and clinical efficacy and have markedly improved the quality of life in men with ED of various etiologies. The introduction of the first PDE5I, sildenafil citrate (Viagra), in 1998 revolutionized the treatment of men with ED of a broad-spectrum of etiologies and acknowledged the need for pharmacologic agents in the treatment of ED.[194] With the recognition of the prevalence of ED by the public and the effectiveness of agents like sildenafil, there was an increased effort in the search for new agents with fewer side effects that led to the development of the second-generation PDE5Is, vardenafil (2003), tadalafil (2003), and avanafil (2012) which have since been introduced into the world market at differing potencies and pharmacokinetics (Fig. 24.27).

Sildenafil (Viagra)

In 1998, sildenafil was the first selective PDE inhibitor to be approved and found to be effective in treating ED.[194] Sildenafil has approximately one-sixteenth the selectivity for PDE5 as for PDE6, which is found in the photoreceptors of the human retina. In vitro metabolism studies for sildenafil have shown that the primary metabolite, N-desmethylsildenafil, and the minor metabolite, oxidative opening of the piperazine ring, are mediated by CYP3A4, CYP2C9, CYP2C19, and CYP2D6 (Fig. 24.27). The estimated relative contributions to clearance were 79% for CYP3A4, 20% for CYP2C9, and less than 2% for CYP2C19 and CYP2D6. These results demonstrate that CYP3A4 is the primary cytochrome mediating N-demethylation and that drugs inhibiting CYP3A4 likely impair sildenafil biotransformation and clearance. The pharmacokinetics of radiolabeled sildenafil were consistent with rapid absorption, first-pass metabolism, and

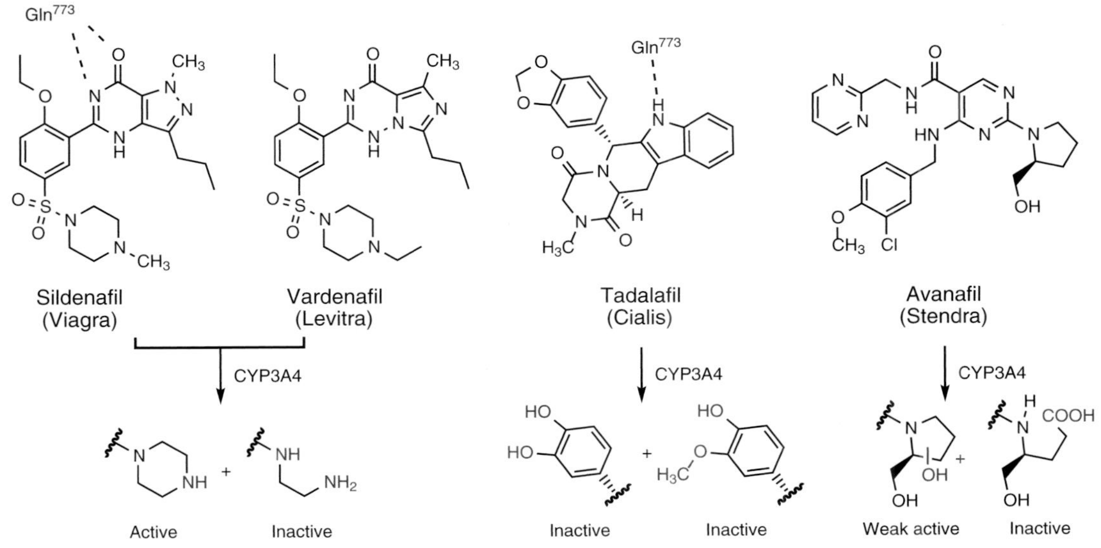

Figure 24.27 Phosphodiesterase 5 inhibitors and primary metabolites.

primarily fecal elimination of N-demethylated metabolites. The absorption of sildenafil following oral administration was rapid (~92%), whereas the oral bioavailability was approximately 38% as a result of first-pass metabolism. Starting doses of 50 mg of sildenafil should be taken approximately 1 hour before sexual activity, however, it may be taken anywhere from 30 minutes to 4 hours before sexual activity. Dosage may be decreased (25 mg) or increased (100 mg) based upon efficacy and tolerability with maximum once per day frequency. If taken after a high fat meal, sildenafil may take longer to start working.

Vardenafil (Levitra)

Vardenafil was the second agent to be marketed and had the advantage that its onset time was not reduced by taking the medication on a full stomach (Table 24.12).[195,196] It is ~20 times more potent as an inhibitor of PDE5 (mean IC_{50} = 0.084 nM) than sildenafil and 48 times more potent than tadalafil, with a greater selectivity (>14,000-times) for human PDE5 than for human PDE2, PDE3, and PDE4 and moderate selectivity (>1000-times) for PDE1 (Table 24.13).[197,198,200] Starting doses of 10 mg of vardenafil should be taken approximately 1 hour before sexual activity. Dosage may be decreased (5 mg) or increased (20 mg) based upon efficacy and tolerability. It may be taken with or without food, but affects are reduced following a fatty meal. Vardenafil is also available as a 10 mg disintegrating oral tablet (Staxyn) which is more rapidly absorbed than oral tablets (Levitra) and provides higher systemic exposure than Levitra. Maximum dosage is 10 mg/d (Staxyn) or 20 mg/d (Levitra).

Tadalafil (Cialis)

Tadalafil was the third agent to be released and can be taken on a full stomach without slowing the onset (Table 24.12).[195] It has a much longer duration of action, lasting up to 48 hours, compared with sildenafil and vardenafil, which last for approximately 4 hours. The longer half-life of tadalafil results in a lengthened period of responsiveness as compared to sildenafil and vardenafil. This longer therapeutic window requires fewer time constraints for the effectiveness of tadalafil and has been interpreted as being advantageous through providing the option for more spontaneous sexual activity. Because of its long half-life, however, tadalafil has been detected in plasma even 5 days after oral administration. This suggests the possibility of accumulation if taken regularly and in short intervals, which may result in an increased risk of side effects with the excessive use of this PDE5I. The 3,4-methylenedioxy

Table 24.12 Some Properties and Pharmacokinetics of the PDE5Is

Drugs	Sildenafil	Vardenafil	Tadalafil	Avanafil
Trade Name	**Viagra**	**Levitra**	**Cialis**	**Stendra**
cLog P[a]	2.3 ± 0.7	3.0 ± 0.7	1.4 ± 0.8	2.42
log D (pH 7)	2.2	3.0	1.4	
Oral bioavailability (%)	38-40	15 (8-25)	~36	
Onset of action (hr)	<0.5	<1	0.5-1	0.25
Duration of action (hr)	<4	<1	<36	
Protein binding (%)	96	94	94	99
Time to peak concentration (hr)	0.5-2	0.5-3	0.5-6	0.5-0.75 (fasting) 1.12-1.25 (high fat meal)
Volume of distribution (L/kg)	105	208	63	
Peak plasma concentration (nmol/L)	1-2	0.03	0.84	
Elimination half-life (hr)	3-5	4-5	18	5
Metabolism	3A4 (major)	3A4 (major)	3A4 (primary)	3A4 (major)
	2C9 (minor)	2C9 (minor)		2C9 (minor)
Active metabolites	N-desmethyl	N-desethyl	None	M4
Excretion (%) Fecal Renal	 ~80 ~13	 >90 <10	 ~60 ~35	 ~62 ~21
PDE5 IC_{50} (nM)[200]	1.6	0.084	4	5.2

[a]Chemical Abstracts, American Chemical Society, calculated using Advanced Chemistry Development (ACD/Labs) Software V8.14 for Solaris (1994-2006 ACD/Labs) or www.drugbank.ca.

IC_{50}, median inhibitory concentration; met, metabolite; PDE, phosphodiesterase.

substitution on the phenyl ring was significant for increasing its potency as a PDE5I. Optimization of the chain on the piperazinedione ring resulted in no significant change in IC_{50}. Tadalafil is a highly potent PDE5 inhibitor (IC_{50} = 4 nM), with high selectivity for PDE5 versus PDE1 through PDE4.[199,200] The PDE6/PDE5 selectivity ratio is 550 (Table 24.13).

Avanafil (Stendra)

Avanafil is a pyrimidine derivative and is the latest PDE5 inhibitor to be approved and exhibits higher potency for PDE5 than other phosphodiesterases (>100-fold for PDE6; >1,000-fold for PDE4, PDE8, and PDE10; >5,000-fold for PDE2 and PDE7; >10,000-fold for PDE1, PDE3, PDE9, and PDE11) (Table 24.13).[200] It is a competitive inhibitor of cGMP binding to PDE5 (K_I of 4.3 nM).[200] Avanafil was found to show potent PDE5 inhibitory activity (IC_{50} = 5 nM) with the (*S*)-enantiomer of the 2-hydroxymethyl group on the pyrrolidine ring being sevenfold more potent than its (*R*)-enantiomer (IC_{50} = 36 nM).[201] Avanafil showed higher selectivity against PDE6 than sildenafil and vardenafil (121-fold vs. 15- to 21-fold) but less than tadalafil (550-fold). The onset of action appears to be shorter (15 min)[202] which can add to its convenience and offers a major advantage during sexual activity. Avanafil is extensively metabolized in the liver predominantly by CYP3A4 and to a minor extent by CYP2C isoforms to produce an active metabolite called M4 (PDE5 inhibitory activity 10% of avanafil) and is responsible for about 4% of pharmacologic activity. The M16 metabolite is inactive and represents about 29% of the parent.[203] Its terminal half-life is 5 hours with the majority excreted in the feces. Dosage adjustments are not necessary based upon hepatic or renal function, age, or gender.[204]

Structure-Activity Relationships

PDE5Is are nonhydrolyzable competitive inhibitors of cGMP. The modified purine ring of sildenafil and vardenafil are thought to mimic the guanine ring systems of cGMP, with the other substituents acting as the ribose and phosphate of cGMP when binding to the PDE. The chemical similarities and distinct differences between PDE5Is regarding their selectivity for inhibition of PDE5 in preference to the 11 other PDE isoforms give rise to pharmacokinetic differences that affect the efficacy profile of these compounds. The obvious difference for the three drugs is the heterocyclic ring systems used to mimic the purine ring of cGMP. Although the heterocyclic ring systems and the N-substituent (ethyl vs. methyl) attached to the piperazine side chain (Fig. 24.27) are the only two structural differences between sildenafil and vardenafil, these differences do not explain why vardenafil has a more than 20 times greater potency than sildenafil for inhibiting PDE5. A structure-activity relationship analysis for the difference in potency between sildenafil and vardenafil revealed that the methyl/ethyl group on the piperazine moiety plays very little role in the potency difference for inhibiting PDE5, whereas the differences in the heterocyclic ring systems play a critical role in higher potency for vardenafil.[197,198]

A comparison of the in vitro inhibition values (IC_{50}) reveals that each drug inhibits PDE5 in the nanomolar range with vardenafil exhibiting higher potency (vardenafil > tadalafil > sildenafil > avanafil) (Table 24.13).[197,200] Selectivity of each drug for PDEs has been determined.[200] The low PDE5/PDE6 selectivity ratio suggests that at therapeutic doses, sildenafil is only approximately 16-fold more selective for PDE5 as for PDE6, which is a retinal enzyme found in the photoreceptors of the human retina. PDE5 and PDE6 are more similar in terms of amino acid sequences and pharmacological properties as compared

Table 24.13 Selectivity of PDE5Is for PDE1-11 Isozymes

	PDE vs. PDE5 Selectivity (Fold Difference)			
PDE	**Sildenafil**	**Vardenafil**	**Tadalafil**	**Avanafil**
1	375	1,012	10,500	10,192
2	39,375	273,810	>25,000	9,808
3	16,250	26,190	>25,000	>19,231
4	3,125	14,296	14,750	1,096
5	1	1	1	1
6	16	21	550	121
7	13,750	17,857	>25,000	5,192
8	>62,500	1,000,000	>25,000	2,308
9	2,250	16,667	>25,000	>19,231
10	3,375	17,857	8,750	1,192
11	4,875	5,952	25	>19,231

Based on Kotera J, Mochida H, Inoue H, et al. Avanafil, a potent and highly selective phosphodiesterase-5 inhibitor for erectile dysfunction. *J Urol.* 2012;188:668-674.

to other PDEs. This lower PDE5/PDE6 selectivity ratio toward PDE6 for sildenafil indicates it is more likely to inhibit PDE6, which is presumed to be the cause for transient color vision abnormalities observed with high doses or plasma levels of sildenafil. A 3D homology model of PDE5 with tadalafil suggests reasons why sildenafil causes visual disorders because of its poor selectivity but tadalafil does not. It suggests that sildenafil binds to PDE6 and PDE5 in a similar pattern and thus may account for its similar inhibitor potencies toward PDE5 and PDE6. The high selectivity of tadalafil for PDE5 versus PDE6 may result from two key amino acid residues in the catalytic sites that vary (Val782 and Leu804 in PDE5 and their corresponding Val738 and Met760 in PDE6).[205] Tadalafil binds PDE6 in a different pattern from sildenafil. Sildenafil forms two hydrogen bonds from the N1 and O6 of the imidazaotriazinone to Gln773 in PDE6 while only the N1 of the indole ring of tadalafil can have a single hydrogen bond to Gln773 giving rise to its lower affinity for PDE6 (Fig. 24.27).[205]

Mechanism of Action

The physiologic mechanism to achieve penile erection is mediated via a nitric oxide (NO)/cyclic guanosine monophosphate (cGMP) pathway (Fig. 24.28). Sexual stimulation is required for a response to treatment with PDE5Is. During sexual stimulation, parasympathetic neurons and vascular endothelial cells release NO, which activates soluble guanylyl cyclase, thereby increasing the level of cGMP in the corpus cavernosum and relaxation (vasodilation) of vascular smooth muscle. PDE5 is a cGMP-specific hydrolyzing enzyme and is present at high concentrations in the smooth muscle of the penile corpus cavernosum.[206,207] One of the more effective methods for elevating cGMP levels in this tissue is to use PDE5Is. Other PDE isoenzymes also found in the human cavernous smooth muscle include PDE3 (cGMP-inhibited PDE) and PDE4 (cAMP-specific PDE). Thus, inhibitors of PDE, especially PDE5, have been shown to be an effective means for treating ED by enhancing and maintaining erections during sexual stimulation through sustaining sufficient cellular levels of cGMP in both the corpus cavernosum and the blood vessels supplying it. The increased vasodilation of the corporeal sinusoids allows more blood flow into the penis, thereby enhancing an erection.

Pharmacokinetics

PDE5Is have only limited oral bioavailability because of extensive presystemic metabolism in the intestine and hepatic first-pass metabolism via the CYP3A isoform family (Table 24.12).[195] They are rapidly absorbed after oral administration and reach peak plasma concentrations within 15-60 minutes. Avanafil has the fastest onset of action, which allows the patient to take the drug 15 minutes prior to sexual activity and offers a major advantage. Rapid absorption and lipophilicity are considered to be a prerequisite for their rapid onset of efficacy and sexual satisfaction. Sildenafil, vardenafil, and tadalafil are rapidly absorbed, but with a significant difference in their mean bioavailability of approximately 15% for vardenafil and ~40% for sildenafil and tadalafil. The administration of a high-fat meal had no significant effect on the rate and extent of absorption of tadalafil but did decrease the rate of absorption for the other three, which is consistent with their calculated lipophilicity (Table 24.12). It remains unclear whether food has any effect on their absorption and therapeutic efficacy. They are all highly protein bound (≥94%), with free plasma concentration fractions of only 4%-6%. The elimination half-life and duration of action for PDE5Is are similar (~5 hr) with exception of tadalafil which has a long duration of action (<36 hr) and half-life of 18 hours suggesting that it is predominately metabolized by hepatic CYP3A4 to catechol metabolites, with minimal presystemic metabolism.

The major route of elimination for the PDE5Is is hepatic metabolism, with renal excretion of unmetabolized drug accounting for 1% or less of the elimination pathways (Fig. 24.27).[195] CYP3A4 is the major drug-metabolizing enzyme for the four PDE5Is. CYP2C9, CYP2C19, and CYP2D6, however, also contribute to the metabolism of sildenafil, and CYP2C9 contributes to the metabolism of vardenafil. Both sildenafil and vardenafil have active metabolites that reach plasma concentrations high enough to contribute to the overall efficacy and safety profile of their parent-drug molecules.

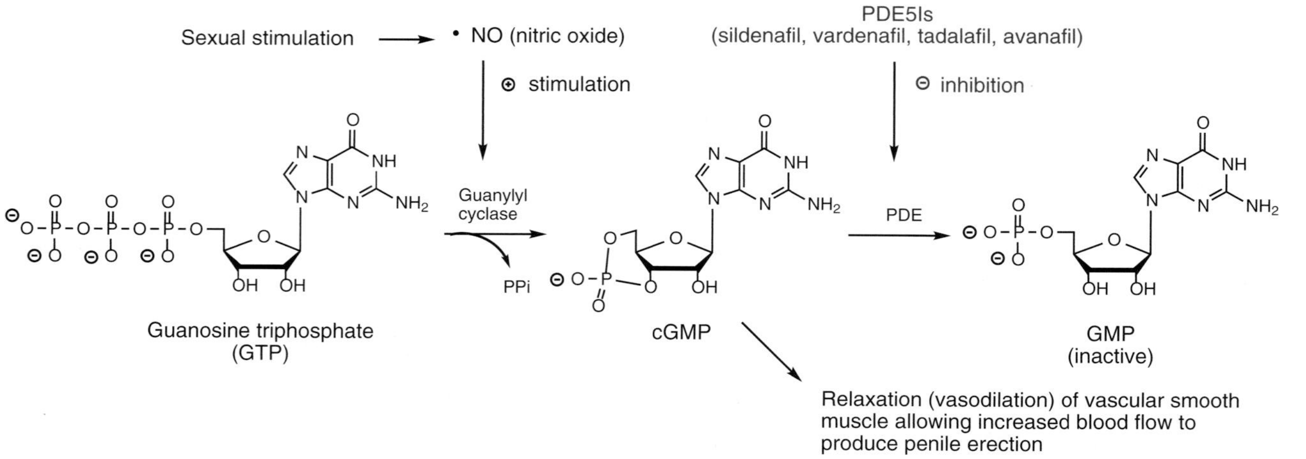

Figure 24.28 Mechanism of action of PDE5 inhibitors.

The larger differences in their volumes of distribution, together with the substantial differences in their systemic clearance, result in distinct differences in their elimination half-lives: 3-5 hours for sildenafil, vardenafil, and avanafil, compared with approximately 18 hours for tadalafil.

Hepatic CYP3A and CYP2C activity has been described as being age-dependent, with reduced activity being exhibited in elderly compared to young individuals. This decrease in metabolic activity is reflected by a corresponding increase in plasma concentrations of PDE5Is, warranting dose reductions for sildenafil and vardenafil in elderly patients. Similarly, ethnicity-dependent differences in the pharmacokinetics of PDE5Is may be expected based on known ethnic differences in CYP3A4/5 activity. Gender differences in pharmacokinetics have not been described for any of the PDE5Is. Severe renal impairment resulted in an increase in plasma concentrations for sildenafil, vardenafil, and tadalafil, and this warrants dose reductions for sildenafil and tadalafil in the affected patient population. Avanafil has not been studied in patients with severe renal disease or on renal dialysis. However, clinical studies of avanafil showed that only minimal changes in avanafil exposure occurred in patients with mild to moderate renal impairment.

Drug-Drug Interactions

PDE5Is have not been identified as CYP inhibitors, including CYP3A or CYP2C substrates. Because metabolism via CYP3A is the major elimination pathway for PDE5Is, all inducers and inhibitors of CYP3A activity have the potential to interfere with the elimination of these drugs. This interaction potential has been verified clinically for inducers of CYP3A activity only for rifampicin and tadalafil.[195] The strong inhibitors of CYP3A4 (ritonavir, indinavir, saquinavir, erythromycin, and ketoconazole) increased the plasma levels for sildenafil, vardenafil, tadalafil, and avanafil. Grapefruit juice, a selective inhibitor of CYP3A intestinal metabolism, also increased the plasma concentrations of sildenafil and vardenafil but not of tadalafil. Grapefruit juice is likely to increase avanafil exposure; however, specific interactions have not been determined. Ritonavir, a strong CYP3A4 and CYP2C9 inhibitor, resulted in increases in vardenafil's AUC (49-fold), C_{max} (13-fold), and half-life (26 hr) and avanafil's AUC (2- and 13-fold) and half-life (9 hr). This is most likely a consequence of the simultaneous inhibition of both CYP3A4 and CYP2C9, the major metabolism pathways for both. The effect of ritonavir on sildenafil was much less pronounced than vardenafil (11 times), because other compensatory CYP-mediated metabolism pathways were still available. Ritonavir increased the plasma levels for tadalafil (CYP3A4) by approximately three times.

Adverse Effects

PDE5Is are generally safe, effective, and well tolerated in patients. The most commonly reported side effects include headaches, flushing, dizziness, visual disturbance (sildenafil), and nasal congestion. There are no significant differences in the efficacy of sildenafil, vardenafil, and avanafil when the recommended maximal doses are used.[208] It is suggested that some of these side effects result from the inhibition of other PDEs, including the isoform PDE6.[195,209] The search is on for even more selective ED agents to see if additional side effects can be eliminated. If one is taking α-adrenergic blockers for high blood pressure, one should consult a physician before using the agents together.[195] Other vasodilators associated with regulating the intracellular levels of cGMP, such as nitroglycerin, should not be used in combination with the PDE5 inhibitors.

Prostaglandin E_1

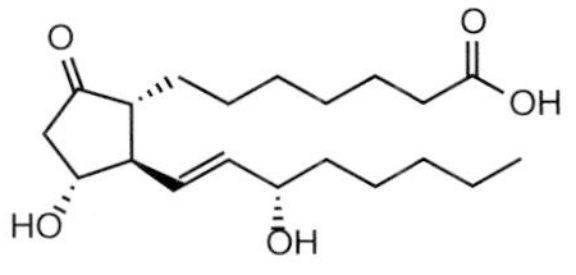

Alprostadil
PGE_1

Prostaglandin E_1 (PGE_1; Alprostadil) is approved for the intracavernosal (Caverject, Edex) or intraurethral suppository (Muse) treatment of ED. A three-drug combination of PGE_1, papaverine, and phentolamine sometimes is used as an intracavernosal injection to achieve a synergistic action. ED that is medication-induced or caused by endocrine problems, such as hypogonadism or hyper- or hypothyroidism, should be evaluated and appropriately treated before PGE_1 treatment is considered. PGE_1 is produced endogenously to relax vascular smooth muscle and cause vasodilation by activating the adenylyl cyclase/cAMP pathway. Recent studies show that cAMP is important in the PGE_1 relaxation of penile erectile tissue and vasodilation of penile resistance arteries.[210] Moreover, agents that stimulate the release of cAMP also cross-activate the NO/cGMP cascade.

When administered by intracavernosal injection or as an intraurethral suppository, PGE_1 acts locally to relax the smooth muscle of the corpora cavernosa and the cavernosal arteries. Swelling, elongation, and rigidity of the penis result when arterial blood rapidly flows into the corpus cavernosum to expand the lacunar spaces. The entrapped blood reduces the venous blood outflow as sinusoids compress against the tunica albuginea. Adding papaverine and phentolamine to the PGE_1 regimen synergistically increases arterial blood flow via separate mechanisms. Papaverine relaxes the sinusoid and the smooth muscle of the helicine arteries, whereas phentolamine relaxes arterial smooth muscle and blocks both of the α-adrenergic receptors that inhibit an erection. PGE_1 is rapidly metabolized within the urethra, prostate, and corpus cavernosum to 7α-hydroxy-5,11-diketotetranorprosta-1,16-dioic acid and 5α,7α-dihydroxy-11-ketotetranor-prostane-1,16-dioic acid.[211] The major route of excretion of PGE_1 metabolites is via the kidney. Its elimination half-life is 5-10 minutes. If any alprostadil is systemically absorbed, it is metabolized by a single pass through the lungs. The onset of action is within 10 minutes, and the time to peak effect is less than 20 minutes. The duration of action is 1-3 hours for the intracavernosal injection and 30-60 minutes for the intraurethral suppository.

MALE OSTEOPOROSIS

Osteoporosis is a common condition in men that usually develops after the age of 70 years and affects approximately 2 million men in the U.S.[212] Osteoporosis occurs less frequently in men because of greater skeletal bone mass during growth (i.e., greater bone size). Approximately 20%-25% of all hip fractures occur in men, however, and the age-adjusted prevalence of vertebral deformities appears to be similar in men and in women. Currently, bisphosphonates (alendronate and risedronate) are the therapy of choice for increasing bone mineral density to decrease the risk of fracture in the treatment of male osteoporosis, and a short course of parathyroid hormone (1-34; teriparatide) may be indicated for men with very low bone mineral density or for those in whom bisphosphonate therapy is unsuccessful. Medical castration (e.g., GnRH agonists and antagonists discussed in this chapter) and antiandrogen therapy for the treatment of prostate cancer, hypogonadism, and diabetes are some of the risk factors for osteoporosis and fracture. Vitamin D and calcium have been shown to help improve bone mineral density. Testosterone replacement therapy is controversial except in men who clearly have hypogonadism and low levels of testosterone; in those men, treatment with testosterone appears to increase bone density.

DRUGS USED FOR BENIGN PROSTATIC HYPERPLASIA

Prostate problems are common in older men, particularly those aged 50 years and older. A man may have prostate problems for a number of reasons, including an infection of the prostate (prostatitis), a noncancerous enlargement of the prostate (BPH), or prostate cancer, the second most common cancer in men. BPH is the most common disease of the prostate, occurring in 50%-60% of men in their 60s and up to 80%-90% of men over the age of 70 years.[213] GlobalData estimated that the 2014 sales for therapeutics to treat BPH at approximately $2 billion and increasing to $4.5 billion by 2024 in the seven major markets (United States, Germany, France, Italy, Spain, United Kingdom, & Japan) with the United States representing 65% of the market share.[214] Prostate problems often are discovered by men themselves. The signs of prostate problems include a frequent urge to urinate, blood in the urine, painful or burning urination, difficulty urinating, or inability to urinate.

BPH is the noncancerous asymmetric proliferation of the prostate gland which can restrict the urethra as it passes through the prostate. Thus, the major problem associated with BPH is LUTSs. The symptoms of BPH stem from obstruction of the urethra by an enlarged prostate and the gradual loss of bladder function, which results in incomplete emptying of the bladder. The two categories of symptoms of BPH include obstructive and irritative. Obstructive symptoms result from factors that reduce bladder emptying (e.g., hesitancy, straining, weak urine stream, dribbling, and urinary retention). Irritative symptoms typically occur late in the disease course and result from long-term obstruction of bladder (e.g., urinary frequency, urgency, incontinence, dysuria, hematuria, and nocturia). The quality of life can be significantly compromised when BPH symptoms wake up the patient every 1-2 hours at night to void (nocturia). The enlarging prostate increases the adrenergic tone of the prostate in patients with BPH, which results in further tightening of the urethra. The consequence to this obstruction can include urinary retention (and can in some cases lead to emergency catheterization), stagnant urine retention leading to urinary infections, and even hydronephrosis.

Short questionnaires exist (American Urological Association Symptom Index/International Prostate Symptom Score [AUA-SI/I-PSS]) that allow practitioners to assess the severity of symptoms regarding urine storage, voiding, and quality of life and make treatment recommendations.[215,216] Management of BPH depends on severity of symptoms and can range from active surveillance, pharmacotherapy (α_1-adrenergic antagonists, 5α-reductase inhibitors [5ARIs], or combination), and surgical/laser reduction of prostate. When partial obstruction is present, urinary retention also can be brought on by alcohol, cold temperatures, a long period of immobility, or the ingestion of over-the-counter cold or allergy medicines that contain a sympathomimetic decongestant drug or anticholinergic. It is important to ask patients if they suffer from BPH when on OTC cold or allergy medications as they may experience acute, severe urinary retention that requires catheterization. First-generation antihistamines can cause urinary retention due to their anticholinergic effects while the decongestant pseudoephedrine, an α_1 agonist, promotes further tightening on urethra.

Although the cause of BPH is not well understood, it occurs mainly in older men and it does not develop in men whose testes were removed before puberty. Before and during adulthood, DHT plays a critical role in determining prostate size, and multiple lines of evidence suggest the importance of DHT in the development of BPH.[217,218] Men who do not produce DHT do not develop BPH.[219] For instance, BPH does not develop in males with certain 5α-reductase type 2 ($5AR_2$) mutations or in males with very low levels of androgen because of prepubertal castration or hypopituitarism-related hypogonadism. Moreover, clinical treatment of BPH either by chemical or surgical castration or by inhibition of $5AR_2$ (e.g., finasteride or dutasteride) induces apoptosis of epithelial cells, which in turn significantly decreases the volume of the prostate.[218] The role of age-dependent changes in the intraprostatic hormonal environment in the development of BPH was evaluated.[220] Despite the aging-related decrease in testosterone and intraprostatic DHT production, an increased 17β-estradiol/DHT ratio was observed in the aging human prostate, which can be relevant to the development of BPH. As men age, the concentration of free testosterone in the blood decreases due to increases in SHBG, while the concentrations of 17β-estradiol increase due to aromatization in adipose tissue. Animal studies have suggested that BPH may result from the increased concentration of 17β-estradiol or 5α-DHT within the gland, which promotes cell growth.[221] Furthermore, 17β-estradiol is capable of inducing precancerous lesions and prostate cancer in aging dogs.[222] Therefore, TRT in older men raises concern regarding acceleration of BPH and/or prostate cancer.

Surgical procedures often are used to reduce a large prostate mass, but there are early pharmacologic treatments for BPH including α_1-adrenergic antagonists and 5ARIs.

α_1-Adrenergic Antagonists

Often the first-line treatment for LUTS and BPH, the α_1-adrenergic antagonists treat the increased adrenergic tone of the sympathetic nervous system by relaxing the muscles at the neck of the bladder and in the prostate, thereby reducing the pressure on the urethra and increasing the flow of urine.[223] They do not cure BPH but, rather, help to alleviate some of the symptoms. For moderate symptoms of BPH, α_1-adrenergic antagonists are often used due to their faster onset of symptom relief as compared with 5ARIs. They can also be used in combination with 5ARIs when prostate volume is large (>40 g) as α_1-adrenergic antagonists do not decrease prostate volume. Approximately 60% of men find that symptoms improve significantly within the first 2-3 weeks of treatment with an α_1-antagonist. Alfuzosin, tamsulosin, and silodosin are used exclusively as first-line α_1-adrenergic antagonists for the treatment of BPH, while doxazosin and terazosin have also been used to treat high blood pressure. Prazosin, another α_1-antagonist, is not indicated for the treatment of BPH. Tamsulosin, alfuzosin, and silodosin are uroselective α_1-adrenergic antagonists developed specifically to treat BPH. When BPH and ED are present, α_1-adrenergic antagonists are used in combination with a phosphodiesterase inhibitor.

Classes of α_1-Adrenergic Antagonists

QUINAZOLINES. Alfuzosin (2003), terazosin (1987), and doxazosin (1990) are nonselective α_1-adrenergic antagonists each bearing a 4-amino-6,7-dimethoxyquinazoline ring system (Fig. 24.29). They differ at the 2-position of the quinazoline ring, having either a piperazine ring (terazosin and doxazosin) or open-chain analog (alfuzosin). The first selective quinazoline α_1-blocker discovered in the late 1960s was prazosin, a commonly used antihypertensive agent that is not recommended for BPH due to multiple doses per day and significant cardiovascular adverse effects. Prazosin is a derivative of terazosin and differs only with respect to a furan ring in place of the hydrofuran of terazosin. Other structural differences exist between the approved quinazolines including the different acyl groups attached to the nitrogen of either the piperazine ring or the open-chain analog. The differences in these groups afford dramatic differences in some of the pharmacokinetic properties for these agents (Table 24.14). Perhaps most significant are the long half-lives (10-22 hr) and duration of action (18-48 hr) for these drugs that permit once-a-day dosing and, generally, lead to increased patient compliance.

Alfuzosin, lacking the piperazine ring, is a first-line uroselective drug for the treatment of BPH, but with no utility in treating hypertension, because it has fewer cardiovascular effects than terazosin and doxazosin. It is hepatically metabolized by 7-O-demethylation and N-dealkylation, primarily by CYP3A4, to inactive metabolites. In patients with moderate or severe hepatic insufficiency, a reduction in clearance resulted in a three to four times increase in its plasma concentration, which may require a reduction in dose.

Doxazosin is extensively metabolized by 7-O-demethylation, hydroxylation of the benzodioxan ring, and oxidation of the piperazine ring to active metabolites in the liver catalyzed by CYP3A4. In patients with renal insufficiency, the elimination half-life was not significantly different from healthy volunteers.

Terazosin is similarly metabolized via 7-O-demethylation and N-dealkylation to four metabolites: 6- and 7-O-demethyl terazosin, the piperazine derivative of terazosin, and the diamine metabolite of the piperazine compound. Terazosin and doxazosin require dose titration to minimize orthostatic hypertension and dizziness.

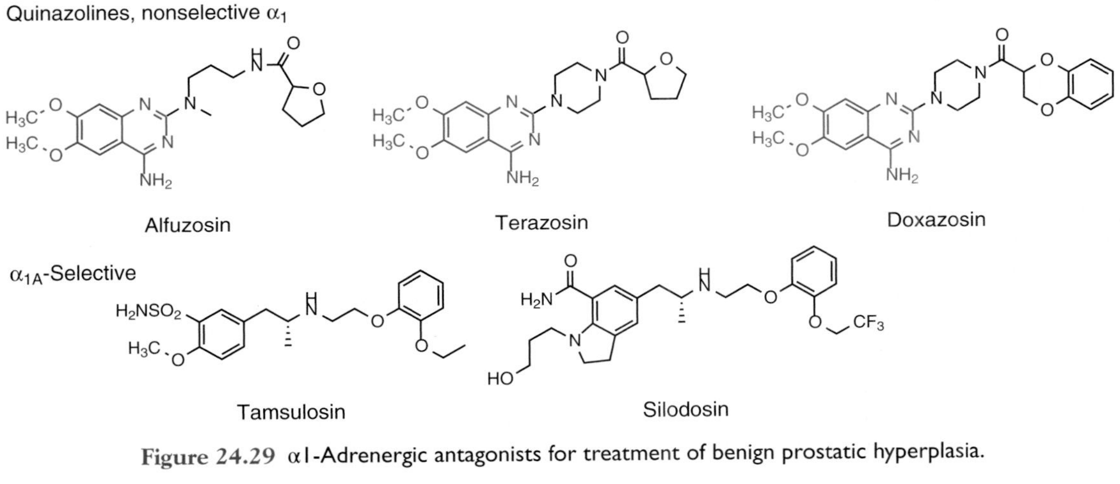

Quinazolines, nonselective α_1

Alfuzosin

Terazosin

Doxazosin

α_{1A}-Selective

Tamsulosin

Silodosin

Figure 24.29 α1-Adrenergic antagonists for treatment of benign prostatic hyperplasia.

CATECHOLAMINE-SULFONAMIDE. Tamsulosin (1997) exhibits uroselectivity for the α_{1A}-adrenergic receptor and is a first-line drug for the treatment of BPH, with no utility for treating hypertension due to lower affinity for vascular α_{1B}-adrenergic receptor. Food decreases oral absorption of tamsulosin; thus it should be taken on empty stomach. Tamsulosin is O-deethylated by CYP3A4 to phenolic metabolites that are conjugated to glucuronide or sulfate before renal excretion and by O-demethylation and 3′-hydroxylation to catechol metabolites that also are conjugated with glucuronide and sulfate. Tamsulosin should be avoided in patients with severe sulfa allergies due to the presence of the aryl sulfonamide.

INDOLE CARBOXAMIDE. Silodosin (2008) is the most uroselective of the α_1-adrenoceptor antagonists, demonstrating 160- and 50-fold higher affinity for binding to α_{1A}- as compared to α_{1B}- and α_{1D}-adrenoceptors, respectively.[224] Silodosin undergoes extensive metabolism through glucuronidation, alcohol and aldehyde dehydrogenase, and CYP3A4. The glucuronide conjugate (formed via direct glucuronidation of the alcohol) of silodosin is active, has a longer half-life (24 hr) than the parent drug, and achieves a plasma exposure (AUC) four times higher than that of silodosin.

Mechanism of Action

α_1-Adrenoceptors are widely distributed in the human body and play important physiologic roles (see Chapter 6). There are three α_1-adrenoceptor subtypes (α_{1A}, α_{1B}, and α_{1D}). Two of these receptors (α_{1A} and α_{1D}) have been shown to mediate smooth muscle contraction. α_{1A}-Adrenoceptors are expressed in prostate and urethral tissue, while α_{1D}-adrenoceptors are expressed mainly in the detrusor muscle of the bladder and the sacral region of the spinal cord. In BPH, α_1-antagonists block adrenergic receptor activation causing relaxation of the prostate smooth muscle and provide relief from the symptoms of LUTS. The vast majority of α-adrenoceptors expressed in the prostate are of the α_{1A} (70%) and α_{1D} subtypes (27%). α_{1B}-Adrenoceptor is known to be important in the regulation of blood pressure.[225] The predominant expression of the α_{1A}-adrenoceptor subtype in the prostatic stromal region and urethral smooth muscle cells led to the design of drugs with uroselectivity for this receptor subtype. Thus, alfuzosin (an aminoquinazoline), tamsulosin (an N-substituted, catecholamine-related sulfonamide), and silodosin (a substituted indole carboxamide) were designed for the treatment of BPH (Fig. 24.29).[218] Doxazosin and terazosin, along with prazosin, originally were used as antihypertensives but also were found to be effective for the treatment of BPH based on their common mechanism of action. Comparisons of the affinities (K_i, nM) of the α_{1A}-adrenoceptor antagonists (Table 24.14) did not show substantial differences for the quinazoline α_{1A}-antagonists (alfuzosin, doxazosin, and terazosin) but some uroselectivity for tamsulosin and silodosin.[223,224,226] In vivo studies showed that those α_{1A}-adrenoceptor antagonists without in vitro adrenoceptor subtype selectivity, such as alfuzosin and doxazosin, showed uroselectivity (terazosin was not uroselective), whereas tamsulosin, which exhibited in vitro selectivity for the α_{1A}-adrenoceptor, did not show the expected in vivo uroselectivity.[227] Silodosin, the most recent addition to this class of drugs, showed both in vitro and in vivo uroselectivity. However, these differences between in vitro and in vivo studies suggest that these drugs modify urethral pressures in a manner that is not directly correlated with their selectivity for the cloned α_{1A}-adrenoceptor subtypes. It is apparent that the existing α_{1A}-adrenoceptor antagonists have different in vivo pharmacologic profiles that are not yet predictable from their receptor based on the current state of knowledge regarding the α_{1A}-adrenoceptor classification.[227]

Thus, tamsulosin, alfuzosin, and silodosin are first-line drugs for the treatment of BPH and have no utility in treating hypertension, because they have fewer cardiovascular effects than terazosin and doxazosin. Some of the basic physicochemical and pharmacokinetic properties of the α_1-antagonists are summarized in Table 24.14. Improvements in urine flow occur 4-8 hours after the first dose and in BPH symptoms within 1 week.

Adverse Reactions

In patients with BPH, the most common adverse effects for α_1-adrenergic antagonists are related to abnormal ejaculation and orthostatic hypotension, with vasodilation, dizziness, headache, and tachycardia also occurring in some patients during the first 2 weeks of treatment.[228] Therefore, a dose titration usually is required, especially in patients taking doxazosin and terazosin or older than 60 years. These cardiovascular side effects are attributed to a nonselective blockade of α_1-adrenoceptors present in vascular smooth muscle in addition to the required blockade of α_1-adrenoceptors in prostate. No first-dose effect and fewer vasodilatory adverse events have been reported with silodosin and the sustained-release formulations of other drugs, which occur more frequently with the immediate-release formulation. At higher doses, orthostatic hypotension occurs more frequently. The first-dose phenomenon of orthostatic hypotension and syncope has been reported occasionally in elderly patients and in those concurrently receiving calcium antagonists, diuretics, and β-blockers. Concomitant use of the α_1-adrenoceptor antagonists with PDE5 inhibitors (used commonly for ED in older men) is associated with a higher risk for dizziness and symptomatic hypotension.

5α-Reductase Inhibitors

The 5ARIs work by suppressing the production of intraprostatic DHT, thereby reducing the size of the prostate.[220] When the prostate volume is large, finasteride and dutasteride are the most commonly used drugs used either alone or in combination with α_1-adrenergic antagonists. Unlike α_1-antagonists, 5ARIs are able to reverse BPH to some extent and so may delay the need for surgery. Several months (6-12 mo) of treatment may be needed before the benefit is noticed by the patient, and thus the patient needs to be encouraged to stay on the medication.

Table 24.14 Some Properties and Pharmacokinetics of the α-Adrenergic Antagonists

Drug	Alfuzosin	Terazosin	Doxazosin	Tamsulosin	Silodosin
Trade Name	Uroxatral	Hytrin	Cardura	Flomax	Rapaflo
cLog P[a]	−1.0 ± 0.4	−1.0 ± 0.4	0.7 ± 0.4	2.2 ± 0.4	2.97
log D[a] (pH 7)	−1.3	−1.0	−0.5	−0.5	0.5
Oral bioavailability (%)	49 fed	90	65 (54-59 XL)	>90 fasted	32
Onset of action (wk)[b]	<2	2	1-2	1	<1
Duration of action (hr)	>48	>18	>24	>24	24
Protein binding (%)	82-90	90-94	98	94-99	97
Time to peak concentration (hr)	8	1	2-3 (8-9 XL)	4-5 fasting/6-7 fed	3
Volume of distribution (L/kg)	3.2	25-30	1.0-3.4	16	49.5
Elimination half-life (hr)	10	12	22 (15-19 XL)	9-15	13
		14 elderly		14-15 elderly	
Cytochrome isoforms	3A4 (inactive metabolites)	—	3A4 (active metabolites)	3A4, 2D6	3A4
Excretion (%)[c] Feces	69/-	60/20 feces	63/5	21/-	55/-
Urine	24/11	40/10	9/4.8	76/<10	34/-
K_i (nM) for α_{1A}	2.4	2.5	2.7	0.5	1.0

XL, extended release tablet formulation.
[a]Chemical Abstracts, American Chemical Society, calculated using Advanced Chemistry Development (ACD/Labs) Software V8.14 for Solaris (1994-2006 ACD/Labs).
[b]Time for improvement in urine flow observed.
[c]% given as metabolites/unchanged

The discovery of the 5ARI finasteride by Merck is an interesting drug discovery story that received inspiration from male pseudohermaphrodites who have an error in the gene that encodes for $5AR_2$.[229,230] This genetic disease was of inspiration to scientists at Merck because the male pseudohermaphrodites had $5AR_2$ deficiency, decreased DHT levels, small prostates throughout life and did not develop BPH, male-pattern baldness, or acne. Except for the associated urogenital defects that were present at birth, no other clinical abnormalities related to 5AR deficiency were observed in these individuals. Thus, scientists hypothesized that DHT was the causative agent. If they could recreate the decreased levels of DHT in men, they hoped they might be able to prevent BPH, acne, and hair loss. In 1992, finasteride was approved for symptomatic treatment of BPH (Proscar, 5 mg) and in 1997 it received approval for androgetic alopecia (Propecia, 1 mg). Dutasteride (Avodart, 0.5 mg) was approved in 2010. 5ARIs may be used to prevent progression of LUTS secondary to BPH only when prostatic enlargement is present and can take 6-12 months for clinical benefit to be felt by patient. Because the clinical efficacy of 5ARIs can be modest at best, 5ARIs can be given in combination with the α_{1A} adrenergic antagonist for additive effects. Dutasteride is available in combination with tamsulosin (Jalyn). 5ARIs may cause decreases in serum PSA concentration in the presence of prostate cancer. 5ARIs are not approved for prostate cancer prevention, but clinical trials have shown they can reduce low-grade prostate cancer by nearly 20%. FDA approval for prostate cancer prevention was prevented as it was also shown there was an increase in high-grade prostate cancer with 5ARIs.[231]

Mechanism of Action

The development of BPH requires a combination of intraprostatic DHT and the aging process. Although not elevated in BPH, levels of DHT in the prostate remain at physiologic levels with aging despite a decrease in plasma testosterone. Inhibitors of DHT biosynthesis can result in a decrease in both circulating and target-tissue (prostate and skin) DHT concentrations, thus blocking its androgenic action in these tissues. The critical enzyme targeted for DHT biosynthesis inhibition is 5AR, which converts testosterone into the more active metabolite DHT (Fig. 24.30). Three different isozymes of 5AR have been reported: 5α-reductase type 1 ($5AR_1$), type 2 ($5AR_2$), and type 3 ($5AR_3$) and their basic biology and role in human diseases reviewed.[232] $5AR_1$ is predominantly expressed in the skin, liver, brain, and prostate, while $5AR_2$ is present in prostate, seminal vesicles, skin, liver, and hair follicles.

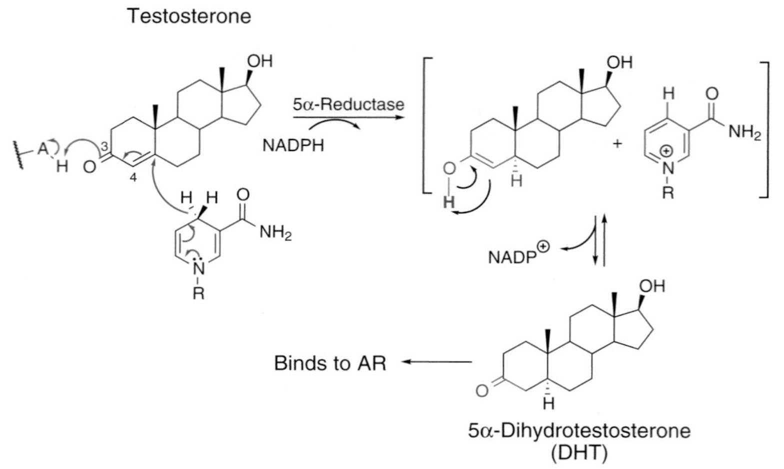

Figure 24.30 Conversion of testosterone into 5α-dihydrotestosterone (DHT) by 5α-reductase.

The mechanism for testosterone reduction to DHT is shown in Figure 24.30 and involves a hydride transfer from the cofactor NADPH to the 5α-position of testosterone, leading to an enol intermediate which can undergo enzyme-mediated tautomerization to form the products of DHT and $NADP^+$.

The first agent to demonstrate 5AR inhibition was a progestin analog, medrogestone (Fig. 24.31).[233] Two azasteroid-17-amide derivatives of medrogestone have been developed as potent competitive inhibitors of 5AR and approved for the treatment of BPH: finasteride, a selective inhibitor of $5AR_2$,[234,235] and dutasteride, a nonselective inhibitor of $5AR_1$ and $5AR_2$ (Fig. 24.31).[236] Thus, the inhibition of $5AR_2$ suppresses the metabolism of testosterone to DHT, resulting in significant decreases in plasma and intraprostatic DHT concentrations.[235–237]

Finasteride and dutasteride are competitive inhibitors of 5AR that also have the ability to work as mechanism-based inhibitors to inactivate 5AR through an apparent irreversible modification of the enzyme.[238,239] They exhibit differing selectivity for 5AR. The inhibition constants (median inhibitory concentrations [IC_{50}]), in Table 24.15, suggest that finasteride is 30 times more selective for $5AR_2$, whereas dutasteride appears to be approximately two times more potent as an inhibitor of $5AR_2$ as compared to $5AR_1$. Finasteride binds to 5AR where testosterone normally binds and accepts a hydride transfer from NADPH to the 1α-position of the A-ring of finasteride forming an enol intermediate (Fig. 24.32). Due to the presence of the 4-aza group, the enol does not tautomerize to the keto group, but rather is postulated to form an enolate that can attack the electrophilic $NADP^+$ still present to form an enzyme-bound, dihydrofinasteride-NADP adduct that slowly releases dihydrofinasteride with a half-life of 1 month.[238] Finasteride and dutasteride are 4-aza steroids with a 1-ene and trans A-B ring junction and are thought to mimic the pathway of testosterone reduction to DHT. It was found that lipophilic groups at the 17β position improve biological activity.[240] The mechanism-based inhibition explains the exceptional potency and specificity of finasteride and dutasteride in the treatment of BPH. This concept of mechanism-based inhibition may have application to the development of other inhibitors of pyridine nucleotide-linked enzymes.

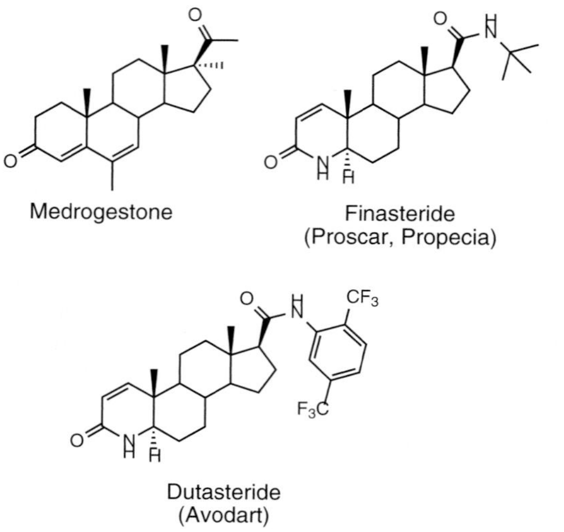

Figure 24.31 5α-Reductase inhibitors.

The 5AR inhibitors are most effective in patients with large prostates (>40 g) and can decrease production of DHT by 50%-70%. A disadvantage of 5AR inhibitors is their slow onset of action as it can take 6-12 months to exert their maximum clinical effect. Common adverse effects of these agents include decreased libido, impotence, and ejaculation disorders which can be bothersome in sexually active patients. 5AR inhibitors can be useful to increase urinary flow rate, decrease prostate volume, prevent acute urinary retention, and avoid surgery in BPH patients. However, if combined with α_1-antagonists, patients get better resolution of their symptoms.

Finasteride (Proscar)

The selective inhibition of the $5AR_2$ isozyme by finasteride produces a rapid reduction in plasma DHT concentration, reaching 65% suppression within 24 hours of administering a 1 mg oral tablet.[241] At steady state, finasteride suppresses DHT levels by approximately 70% in plasma and by as

Table 24.15 Some Properties and Pharmacokinetics of the 5α-Reductases

Drugs	Finasteride	Dutasteride
Tradename	Proscar	Avodart
cLog P[a]	3.2 ± 0.4	5.6 ± 0.6
log D[a](pH 7)	3.2	5.6
Oral bioavailability (%)	65 (26-170)	60 (40-94)
Onset of action (hr)	<24	—
Duration of action (hr)	—	>5 wk
Protein binding (%)	90	99
Time to peak concentration (hr)	—	2-3
Volume of distribution (L/kg)	76 (44-96)	300-500
Elimination half-life (hr)	5-6 (18-60 yr of age)	5 wk
	>8 (60+ years of age)	
Cytochrome isoforms	3A4	3A4
Active metabolites	None	6′-OH
Excretion (%) feces/ urine	57/40 as metabolites	40/5 as metabolites
IC_{50} (nM)	313 (Type I)	3.9 (Type I)
	11 (Type 2)	1.8 (Type 2)

[a]Chemical Abstracts, American Chemical Society, calculated using Advanced Chemistry Development (ACD/Labs) Software V8.14 for Solaris (1994-2006 ACD/Labs).

much as 85%-90% in the prostate. The remaining DHT in the prostate likely is the result of $5AR_1$. The mean circulating levels of testosterone and 17β-estradiol remained within their physiologic concentration range. Long-term therapy with finasteride can reduce clinically significant endpoints of BPH, such as acute urinary retention or surgery. Finasteride is most effective in men with large prostates (>40 g). Finasteride has no affinity for the AR and no androgenic, antiandrogenic, estrogenic, antiestrogenic, or progestational effects.

PHARMACOKINETICS. The mean oral bioavailability of finasteride is 65%, as shown in Table 24.15, and is not affected by food.[241] Approximately 90% of circulating finasteride is bound to plasma proteins.[242] Finasteride has been found to cross the blood brain barrier, but levels in semen were undetectable (<0.2 ng/mL). Finasteride is extensively metabolized in the liver, primarily via CYP3A4, to two major metabolites: monohydroxylation of the *t*-butyl side chain, which is further metabolized via an aldehyde intermediate to the second metabolite, a monocarboxylic acid (Fig. 24.33). The metabolites show approximately 20% the inhibition of finasteride for 5AR.[242] The mean terminal half-life is approximately 5-6 hours in men between 18 and 60 years of age and 8 hours in men older than 70 years of age. Following an oral dose of finasteride, approximately 40% of the dose was excreted in the urine as metabolites and approximately 57% in the feces. Even though the elimination rate of finasteride is decreased in the elderly, no dosage adjustment is necessary. No dosage adjustment is necessary in patients with renal insufficiency. A decrease in the urinary excretion of metabolites was observed in patients with renal impairment, but this was compensated for by an increase in fecal excretion of metabolites. Caution should be used during administration to patients with liver function abnormalities, because finasteride is metabolized extensively in the liver. Finasteride can be absorbed through the skin. As such, tablets, especially broken ones, should not be handled by women who are pregnant or could become pregnant due to a risk of fetal exposure.

Dutasteride (Avodart)

Similar to finasteride, dutasteride is a competitive and mechanism-based inhibitor not only of $5AR_2$ but also of $5AR_1$ isoenzyme, with which stable enzyme-NADP adduct complexes are formed, inhibiting the conversion of testosterone to DHT.[239] The suppression of both $5AR_1$ and $5AR_2$ isoforms results in greater and more consistent reduction of plasma DHT than that observed for finasteride.[243–245] The more effective dual inhibition of $5AR_1$ and $5AR_2$ isoforms lowers circulating DHT to a greater extent than with finasteride and shows advantages in treating BPH and other disease states (e.g., prostate cancer) that are DHT-dependent.

The maximum effect of 0.5 mg daily doses of dutasteride on the suppression of DHT is dose-dependent and is observed within 1-2 weeks. After 2 weeks of 0.5 mg daily dosing, median plasma DHT concentrations were reduced by 90%, and after 1 year, the median decrease in plasma DHT was 94%.[244,245] The median increase in plasma testosterone was 19% but remained within the physiologic range. The drug also reduced serum PSA by approximately 50% at 6 months and total prostate volume by 25% at 2 years. Dutasteride produced improvements in quality of life and peak urinary flow rate and reduction of acute urinary retention without the need for surgery. The main side effects are ED,[246] decreased libido, gynecomastia, and ejaculation disorders. Long-term use (>4 yr), however, did not reveal increased onset of sexual side effects. A combination product (Jalyn) containing dutasteride (0.5 mg) and tamsulosin (0.4 mg) was approved by the U.S. Food and Drug Administration (2010) based on clinical studies showing that the combination was more effective than either monotherapy as assessed by prostate symptom score and maximal urine flow rates. The decreased adrenergic tone associated

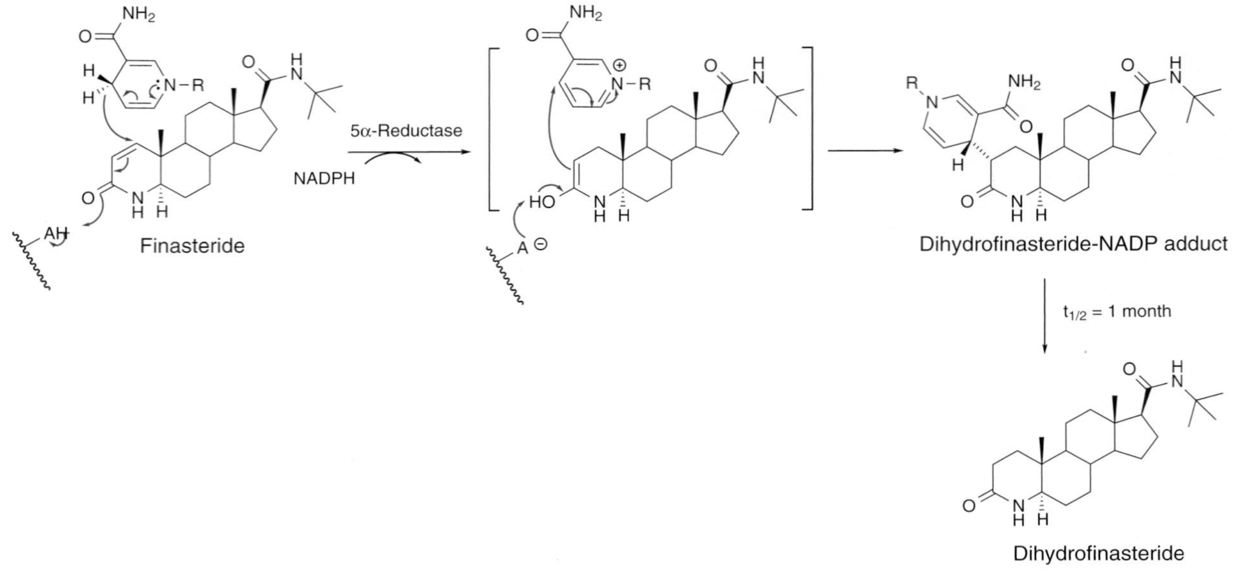

Figure 24.32 Mechanism-based inactivation of 5AR by finasteride.

with tamsulosin and long-term reduction in prostate size (obstruction) associated with dutasteride provide rapid and sustained symptomatic relief for men with BPH.

PHARMACOKINETICS. Following oral administration, peak plasma concentrations of dutasteride occur in approximately 2-3 hours, with a bioavailability of approximately 60% (Table 24.15), and no meaningful reduction in absorption occurs with food.[241,243,247] Dutasteride is highly bound to plasma proteins 99%. The concentrations of dutasteride in semen averaged approximately 3 ng/mL, with no significant effects on DHT plasma levels of sex partners. Dutasteride is extensively metabolized in humans by CYP3A4 to three major metabolites: 4′-hydroxydutasteride and 1,2-dihydrodutasteride, which are less potent than parent drug, and 6′-hydroxydutasteride, which is comparable to the parent drug as an inhibitor of both $5AR_1$ and $5AR_2$ (Fig. 24.33). Dutasteride and its metabolites are excreted mainly (40%) in feces as dutasteride-related metabolites. The terminal elimination half-life of dutasteride is approximately 5 weeks. Because of its long half-life, plasma concentrations remain detectable for up to 4-6 months after discontinuation of treatment. No dose adjustment is necessary in elderly patients, even though its half-life increased with age from approximately 170 hours in men between age 20 and 49 years to 300 hours in men older than age 70 years.[241,248] No adjustment in dosage is necessary for patients with renal impairment. Like finasteride, dutasteride can be absorbed through the skin. As such, dutasteride capsules should not be handled by women who are pregnant or who could become pregnant.

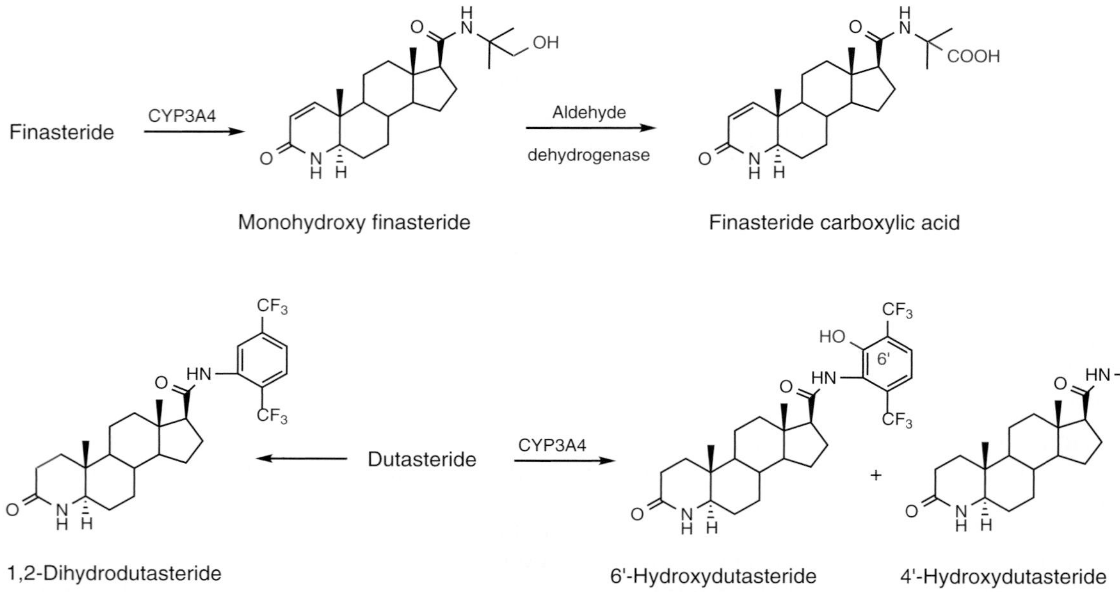

Figure 24.33 Metabolites of finasteride and dutasteride.

Drug-Drug Interactions

Because finasteride and dutasteride are metabolized primarily by CYP3A4, the CYP3A4 inhibitors, such as ritonavir, ketoconazole, verapamil, diltiazem, cimetidine, and ciprofloxacin, may increase these drugs' blood levels and, possibly, cause drug-drug interactions. Clinical drug interaction studies have shown no pharmacokinetic or pharmacodynamic interactions between dutasteride and tamsulosin or terazosin, warfarin, digoxin, and cholestyramine.

Phytotherapy

A number of plant extracts are popularly used to alleviate BPH, although formal evidence that they are effective is often scanty.[248,249] Current guidelines from the American Urological Association do not recommend dietary supplements or combination phytotherapeutic agents for the management of LUTS secondary to BPH.[216] However, extracts of the saw palmetto berry (*Serenoa repens*) are widely used for the treatment of BPH, often as an alternative to pharmaceutical agents. It has been thought that 160 mg twice-daily dose of saw palmetto extract was approximately as effective as 5ARIs over time. However, increasing doses of a saw palmetto fruit extract did not reduce LUTS more than placebo in clinical trials.[249] Other Western herbs that have been investigated for the treatment of BPH include pumpkin seeds (*Cucurbita pepo*), nettle root (*Urtica dioica* or *Urtica urens*), bee pollen (particularly that from the rye plant), African potato (tubers of *Hypoxis rooperi*), and the African tree *Pygeum africanum*, also known as *Prunus africanum*. A detailed discussion of phytotherapy can be found in Chapter 40 of the seventh edition of this book.

TREATMENT OF PROSTATITIS

Prostatitis is a broad term used to identify inflammation of the prostate gland associated with lower urinary tract symptoms in men.[250] Prostatitis rarely occurs in males younger than 30 years; however, it is a common problem in older males, being described as acute bacterial prostatitis, chronic bacterial prostatitis, or nonbacterial prostatitis. Because antimicrobial drug penetration generally is poor into the prostate gland, with poor efficacy of the antimicrobial agents and long duration of treatment, a 30%-40% failure rate occurs with common treatment modalities. Three major factors determine the diffusion and concentration of antimicrobial agents in prostatic fluid and tissue: the lipid solubility of the antimicrobial agent, its dissociation constant (pK_a), and the percentage of plasma protein binding. The physiologic pH of human prostatic fluid is 6.5-6.7, but it increases in chronic prostatitis, ranging from 7.0 to 8.3.[251] A greater concentration of antimicrobial agents in the prostatic fluid occurs in the presence of a pH gradient across the membrane separating plasma from prostatic fluid. Of the available antimicrobial agents, β-lactam drugs have a low pK_a and poor lipid solubility and, thus, penetrate poorly into prostatic fluid, except for some cephalosporins. Good to excellent penetration into prostatic fluid and tissue has been demonstrated with many antimicrobial agents, including tobramycin, tetracyclines, macrolides, fluoroquinolones, sulfonamides, and nitrofurantoin. The diagnosis and therapy of prostatitis remains a challenge. Because prostatitis usually requires prolonged therapy, patients must understand the importance of compliance, and physicians should screen for drug interactions that may decrease compliance and efficacy.

Acute bacterial prostatitis is the least common of the prostate infections and, usually, is accompanied by a urinary tract infection with positive cultures. The symptoms include sudden onset of fever, chills, and low back pain, as well as complaints of urinary obstruction (e.g., dysuria, nocturia, urgency, frequency, and burning) and urinary irritation (e.g., hesitancy, straining, dribbling, weak stream, and incomplete emptying). The most commonly prescribed antimicrobials for acute bacterial prostatitis are trimethoprim-sulfamethoxazole, doxycycline, and the fluoroquinolones, ciprofloxacin, ofloxacin, and norfloxacin (see Chapter 29). The concentrations of these antimicrobial agents in the prostatic fluid are two to three times that in plasma, thus achieving adequate concentrations in prostatic tissues to eradicate the most common causative pathogens. The recommended duration of treatment for acute bacterial prostatitis is 4-6 weeks. A short-course therapy is not recommended because of the risk of relapse or progression to chronic bacterial prostatitis.

Chronic bacterial prostatitis occurs when acute bacterial prostatitis has been inadequately treated because of pathogen resistance, relapse, or short-course therapy or because of blocked drainage of secretions from the prostate. Most men with chronic prostatitis will have had a previous bout of acute prostatitis. The most common clinical feature of chronic prostatitis is recurrent urinary tract infections and the symptoms and complaints of acute bacterial prostatitis. Fluoroquinolones, trimethoprim-sulfamethoxazole, doxycycline, and nitrofurantoin are used in the management of chronic prostatitis. Chronic prostatitis warrants at least 10-12 weeks of therapy. Poor clinical outcomes, however, have been observed because of poor diffusion of antimicrobials into the prostate.

Nonbacterial prostatitis is the most common type of prostatitis. It occurs more frequently than bacterial prostatitis, with the same signs and symptoms as bacterial prostatitis except that prostatic fluid cultures are negative for presence of bacteria. Inflammation is evident on prostate gland examination. Treatment includes minocycline, doxycycline, or erythromycin. Treatment duration is approximately 2-4 weeks.

DRUGS USED FOR THE TREATMENT OF HORMONE-DEPENDENT CANCERS (BREAST, PROSTATE)

As men and women age, hyperproliferation of sexual organs such as the breast and prostate tends to occur under the influence of endogenous estrogens and androgens commonly leading to malignancies derived from these tissues. Breast and prostate cancers are both extremely common cancers having an increased incidence with age which are predominantly dependent on hormones for their growth. Hormone-dependent cancers tend to be slower-growing cancers than other solid malignancies. Whereas surgical hormone-ablation and chemotherapy were once the main treatment options, better understanding of the underlying biology of these cancers has allowed modern treatments to be more personalized, especially for breast cancer. Suppression of the ER- or AR-axis, respectively, has remained the cornerstone of therapy and produced many targeted hormonal therapies to improve the overall survival and quality of life of patients with breast or prostate cancer. Further, earlier intervention to prevent or delay disease recurrence and progression, and rational sequencing of newer agents has become more common, contributing to improved prognosis for these hormone-dependent cancers. Nonetheless, many of the commonly used agents are less than optimal, possessing low potency, intrinsic agonism, dosing-limiting side effects, and/or poor absorption, distribution, metabolism, and excretion (ADME) properties, and the development of resistance to these directed hormonal therapies is common. Consequently, the treatment of hormone-refractory breast and prostate cancers is still a significant unmet medical need, leaving room for improvement of existing therapeutic classes or circumvention of their resistances, as well as extension of the anticancer armamentarium to novel therapeutic classes that are less susceptible to the development of resistance.

Hormone-Dependent Breast Cancer

Personalized Medicine in Breast Cancer

In the U.S., the lifetime risk of developing breast cancer is one in eight, with the greatest incidence in women older than 60 years of age.[252] It is the second leading cause of death from cancer in women (lung cancer is number one). Breast cancer is a diverse collection of diseases that are connected by the formation of tumors in breast tissue. Upon presentation with a breast tumor, in addition to typical staging of the cancer in terms of T (tumor size/aggressiveness/location), N (spread to regional lymph nodes), M (presence of distant metastasis), the prognosis and treatment regimen are largely determined by the types of drug targets that are present in the tumor, as determined by the molecular phenotype of the tumor. The diversity of molecular targets in breast cancer allows for the personalized pharmacotherapy. The majority of breast cancers (~80%) express high levels of the hormone receptors, ER subtype alpha (ERα), and PR, congruent with their origins as hyperproliferative milk duct linings. These cancers depend on the ERα to grow (referred to herein as ER-positive breast cancer) and can be treated with antiestrogen treatments. Typically, ER-positive breast cancer is a better prognosis disease particularly when the PR is also highly expressed and HER2 (human epidermal growth factor receptor [EGFR] type II) is absent. Hormone-dependent breast cancer, i.e., ER-positive breast cancer that is responsive to a variety of hormone therapies, is the main focus of this chapter.

Other Breast Cancers

Approximately 25%-30% of breast cancers[253] are HER2 positive, meaning that they overexpress proteins of the EGFR family. These are more aggressive forms of breast cancer with a poorer prognosis because EGFR activates signaling pathways that promote tumor progression and resistance to treatment.[254] In addition to antiestrogens if ER-positive, the mainstay of directed therapies of HER2-positive tumors is the use of monoclonal antibodies such as trastuzumab (1998), pertuzumab (2013), or ado-trastuzumab emtansine (2013; trastuzumab-directed delivery of chemotherapy to tumor cells) (Chapter 34) that flag the tumor cell for destruction by the body's immune system, i.e., antibody-dependent cellular cytotoxicity. It is also possible to inhibit the kinase function of EGFR using small molecule kinase inhibitors. For example, lapatinib (2007) was approved in breast cancer, and more recently, neratinib (2017) (Chapter 33) was approved in early-stage breast cancer after a woman has completed 1 year of trastuzumab. Unfortunately, resistance can develop to targeted antiestrogen and/or HER2 therapies, and the number of effective pharmacotherapeutic tools starts to diminish, leaving salvage therapies and chemotherapies as the only remaining options.

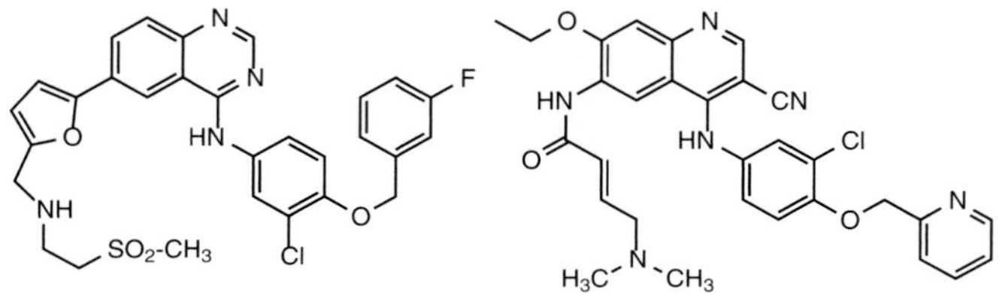

Lapatinib

Neratinib

Unfortunately, approximately 15%-20% of breast cancers upon presentation are triple-negative breast cancers (TNBCs) that do not express any of ERα, PR, or HER2 receptors, leaving no targeted drug therapy options. TNBC is also characterized by more aggressive tumors and poorer prognosis, and TNBC treatment is almost entirely dependent on chemotherapy. Some of the attempts for directed therapies include AR[255]-directed therapies or programmed death-ligand 1(PD-L1)-directed therapies,[256] as TNBC is commonly AR-positive or PD-L1 positive, respectively. However, there are at least six subtypes of TNBC, and responses to these or other targeted therapies are not likely to be univocal[257] across all subtypes. There is also hope that genotyping may be helpful in some TNBC patients.

Genotyping

Genotyping has long been used to screen women who may be genetically predisposed to developing breast cancer. It is another diagnostic or prognostic tool that can be used to determine the availability of therapies. For example, certain women are predisposed to develop breast cancer based on the presence of germline (i.e., inherited) mutations in the breast cancer susceptibility genes (*BRCA*) type 1 (*BRCA1*) or *BRCA2*.[258] A couple of SERMs (discussed in detail below), tamoxifen in 1999 and raloxifene in 2007, were approved for the primary prevention of breast cancer in patient populations that are high risk based on family history and/or genotype considerations.[259,260] However, hysterectomy or prophylactic mastectomy was often considered in these patients as a more definite preventative. In 2018, olaparib (Lynparza), an inhibitor of the enzyme poly(ADP-ribose) polymerase (PARP) (Chapter 33), was approved for metastatic ER-positive and HER2-negative breast cancer patients with certain inherited *BRCA* mutations who have received chemotherapy.[261] Further, there is hope that PARP inhibitors may be helpful in TNBC with inherited *BRCA1* mutations which accounts for ~80% of TNBC.

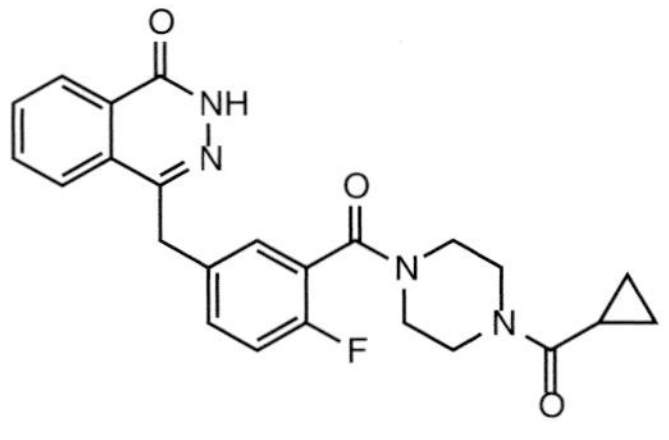

Olaparib

Endocrine Therapy for ER-Positive Breast Cancer

The endogenous female hormone 17β-estradiol is the natural ligand for ER subtype alpha (ERα) and beta (ERβ). ERα's primary role is support of the gender dimorphic female characteristics including primary sexual features such as growth of the mammary glands. Unfortunately, ERα-dependent hyperproliferation of breast tissue (and uterus) is common, affecting ~80% of the one in eight women who develop breast cancer in their lifetime. Suppression of ER signaling is the central feature in the treatment of ER-positive breast cancer and can be accomplished by: (1) direct tissue-selective inhibition of the ER by SERMs (tamoxifen, toremifene, or raloxifene), (2) suppression of endogenous estrogen synthesis, centrally in pre- or perimenopausal women by GnRH agonist (goserelin) which suppresses ovarian production, or peripheral suppression in postmenopausal women by AIs (exemestane, anastrozole, letrozole), or (3) pure antiestrogen activity (discussed below in the Advanced or Metastatic Breast Cancer section) including ER degradation by the selective estrogen receptor degrader (SERD) fulvestrant, the latter of which is reserved for metastatic patients.

While the prognosis of most early stage ER-positive breast cancer patients is relatively good compared to nonhormonal cancers, adjuvant hormone therapy failures do occur resulting in recurrence, including distant metastases (i.e, advanced breast cancer). Metastatic or advanced breast cancer, whether hormone naïve or progressive despite endocrine therapy, is often still ER-positive and still dependent on the ER axis for growth. The treatment of advanced breast cancer is rapidly evolving from the use of an endocrine therapy such as SERM or AI or fulvestrant, to combinations of an endocrine therapy with recently approved kinase inhibitors, including the cyclin-dependent kinase 4/6 (CDK4/6) inhibitors (palbociclib [2015], ribociclib [2017], or abemaciclib [2017]), or mechanistic target of rapamycin (mTOR) inhibitor (everolimus [2012]). These combination therapies delay progression of advanced breast cancer compared to endocrine therapy alone and are supplanting the use of endocrine therapy alone in late breast cancer.

TREATMENT OF EARLY HORMONE RECEPTOR POSITIVE BREAST CANCER. For the sake of clarity, early hormone receptor positive breast cancer is uncomplicated locally invasive breast cancer or noninvasive breast cancer. The initial treatment of hormone receptor positive breast cancer (in the absence of HER2) depends largely on the staging of the tumor. In the absence of distant metastasis, surgical excision (lumpectomy is now favored over radical mastectomy) followed by radiation therapy are common primary treatments. In view of further prognostic criteria such as patient age, tumor lymph node status, tumor size (>1 cm), aggressiveness (e.g., mitotic index, Ki67 staining levels, and the results of gene expression profile[s]), a decision is made with regard to whether adjuvant (refers to treating in the absence of observable active disease) chemotherapy would be beneficial to lower the probability of recurrence. Noninvasive breast cancer (i.e., ductal carcinoma in situ [DCIS]) and the lowest risk invasive carcinoma (e.g., nonaggressive small tumor with no spread to lymph nodes) may not warrant adjuvant chemotherapy. For low- to moderate-risk invasive breast cancers, chemotherapy is typically four cycles of dose-intensive taxotere and cyclophosphamide (TC), whereas good evidence suggests that higher-risk breast cancers should receive six cycles of sequential anthracycline and cyclophosphamide then taxane (AC-T) (Chapter 33)[262] despite the cardiac toxicity of anthracyclines. Unfortunately, chemotherapy only offers a modest benefit in terms of overall survival. A complex array of risk factors, including various biomarkers such as gene expression profiling by OncotypeDx[263] or PAM50,[264] aid in risk assessment and inform decisions regarding whether adjuvant chemotherapy is warranted. National Comprehensive Cancer Network (NCCN) guidelines recommend the use of gene expression profiling in tumors >0.5 cm in node-negative patients, with chemotherapy indicated for intermediate and high recurrence scores; chemotherapy is indicated for all node positive.[265] Neoadjuvant (i.e, before initial treatment with surgery/radiation) chemotherapy is considered in TNBC and HER2-positive patients, but rarely in ER-positive patients.

RISK FACTORS IN EARLY BREAST CANCER

There is little certainty as to which early stage a breast cancer patient is likely to progress. As such, there is little insight as to which patient would benefit from adjuvant chemotherapy. However, the following is a nonexhaustive listing of potential risk factors[266]:

1. ER/PR/HER2 status:
   a. ER or PR positivity are favorable prognostic indicators, but best prognosis is when both are highly expressed. Absence of either is a known risk factor.

b. HER2 is an unfavorable prognostic indicator in ER/PR-positive cancer which suggests more aggressive phenotype which is more likely to develop resistance. In the absence of ER/PR, HER2 provides for targeted therapy albeit still worse prognosis compared to ER/PR-positive and HER2-negative breast cancer.

2. Age at diagnosis: young age at diagnosis is an indicator of poor prognosis.
3. Family history: family history of breast cancer is an indicator of poor prognosis.
4. Initial presentation: Radiologic initial presentation, e.g., on mammogram, is favorable. Clinical initial presentation whereby the cancer progressed until symptomatic issues caused the patient to seek medical care can be considered a risk factor.
5. Nuclear grade: the nuclear grade describes whether the nuclei of cancer cells resemble the nuclei of normal breast cells. In general, the higher the nuclear grade, the more abnormal the nuclei are and the more aggressive the tumor cells tend to be. High nuclear grade is unfavorable and is a part of overall tumor grade.
6. Necrosis: some breast tumors have necrosis apparent upon clinical presentation and this is an unfavorable risk factor.
7. Margins: upon excision of the breast tumor, the pathologist will determine whether or not the surgeon sufficiently removed the tumor. Positive or close margins indicate that residual tumor levels engender an unfavorable risk factor.
8. Number of excisions: a high number of tumors on presentation requiring multiple excisions is a risk factor that suggests an aggressive phenotype.
9. *BRCA* status: inherited *BRCA* mutation positivity suggests that the patient has a genotype predisposed to the development of breast cancer, and it is associated with younger presentation, TNBC molecular phenotype, and more aggressive phenotype.
10. Tumor size: high tumor burden (>1 cm) in breast cancer is also a negative risk factor, indicating inter alia, inability of immune to destroy, increased likelihood of spreading outside the breast, and difficulty in removing the entire tumor.
11. Sentinel node: presence of tumor in the sentinel mode is suggestive of a tumor which is already dedifferentiated to the point that it is viable outside of the breast, and may also suggest that breast cancer is metastatic upon presentation.
12. Obesity: surgeries and chemotherapies limit the patient's ability to maintain an active lifestyle, predisposing to weight gain. Unfortunately, aromatase is highly expressed in adipose tissue and can be a significant source of peripheral estrogen synthesis.

Adjuvant hormonal therapy or endocrine therapy, however, is associated with huge benefits for the vast majority of ER-positive but not ER-negative patients in terms of preventing recurrence (e.g., in the ipsilateral or contralateral breast or distance metastasis) and overall survival. Adjuvant hormonal therapy should only be considered optional in DCIS or small and node-negative invasive carcinoma. All other ER-positive patients will be advised to receive adjuvant hormonal therapy. The main classes of endocrine therapies in the adjuvant setting are SERMs and AIs. Again, many criteria can factor into the selection of which agent to choose, but a few overriding factors include menopausal status and tolerance of side effects. Tamoxifen is preferred for adjuvant therapy of DCIS. Tamoxifen, a SERM, is typically prescribed for pre- and perimenopausal patients as adjuvant therapy of locally invasive carcinoma. Further, premenopausal patients will also receive ovarian suppression using a GnRH agonist with goserelin (Zoladex) being approved for this indication. Perimenopausal patients should be ovarian suppressed and then treated long term with adjuvant AI or SERM. Tamoxifen is typically regarded as having less severe side effects but also inferior ability to prevent recurrence compared to AI. AIs have become favored as adjuvant therapy in postmenopausal locally invasive carcinoma which is the majority of hormone-dependent breast cancer.[267] Usually, patients are treated in the adjuvant setting with a 5-10 year course of SERM (predominantly tamoxifen) or AI (most commonly letrozole or anastrozole), sometimes crossing-over at some point.

Selective Estrogen Receptor Modulators. Since the discovery of the first nonsteroidal estrogen, DES, in 1938 many estrogenic scaffolds have been discovered and explored (Fig. 24.34). The structure of DES belies the simplicity of the pharmacophore for producing ligands of the ER(s). The basic precept is to position two phenol groups approximately the same distance apart as in 17β-estradiol. There seem to be few restraints on the nature of the element linking the phenols, allowing tremendous chemodiversity[40,45]; however, most linking elements are rigidified to orient the phenolic groups in a similar fashion as the steroidal backbone. In the course of structure-activity relationship explorations in the 1960s, it was discovered that addition of steric bulk with a pendant basic amine group to the linking element produced compounds with tissue-selective antagonism in vivo. For example, addition of the N,N-dimethyl(aminoethyl) phenoxy side chain to DES produced tamoxifen which was the first SERM to be FDA approved. Further, addition of a chlorine atom to the ethyl group of tamoxifen produced another FDA-approved SERM toremifene. Historically, these are referred to as antiestrogens due to their use as antagonists of breast tissue growth and utility in treating breast cancer; however, they retain some intrinsic agonist activity as seen in their action in the bone and uterus. The basic pharmacophoric elements of a SERM or antiestrogen are (1) three aromatic groups rigidly held in place by a nonsteroidal linking element; (2) the *trans*-aryl groups must bear either a phenol group or bioisostere, or be metabolized to an active phenolic metabolite; and (3) the *cis*-aryl group must be composed of a phenoxy group linked by a linear alkyl chain (usually ethyl) to a basic tertiary amine. These pharmacophoric features are apparent in the structures of FDA-approved SERMs: tamoxifen, toremifene, raloxifene, and bazedoxifene (see also Chapter 23) (Fig. 24.34).

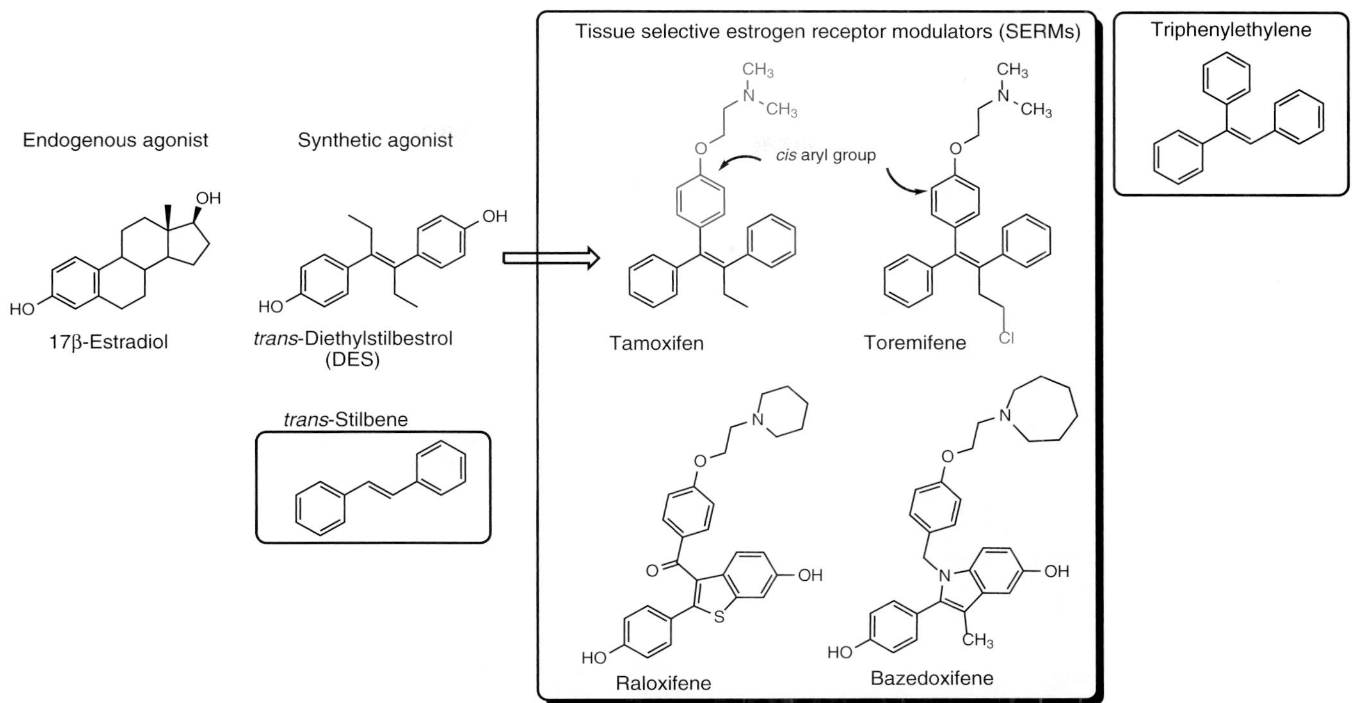

Figure 24.34 17β-Estradiol, nonsteroidal agonist DES, and various SERMs.

SERMs, as a class, possess a unique pharmacology in which they behave as an ER agonist in some favorable estrogenic tissues (e.g., bone and cardiovascular system), and they behave as an ER antagonist in sexual tissues (e.g., the breast and variably and incompletely in the uterus). Triphenylethylene SERMs exhibit a moderately strong and persistent binding to the ER, producing antiestrogen-receptor complexes described below as ERα antagonist conformations. These complexes are believed to translocate into the nucleus of target cells, but normal estrogen transcriptional processes are altered. Hence, antiestrogens interfere with estrogen-dependent tumor growth by competing with estrogens for the receptor site and by turning off the normal processes of the genetic information within the nucleus. Although the full mechanism of action is not completely understood, the molecular basis for tissue-selectivity is apparent from crystallographic studies of the LBD. For example, the DES-ERα LBD co-crystal structure (3ERD.pdb)[64] demonstrated that DES binds analogous to 17β-estradiol (i.e., the ligand is well accommodated by the ERα which completely encloses it within a ligand binding pocket) (Fig. 24.35). Importantly, steroidal agonists and synthetic agonists such as DES promote the formation of, and stabilize, the agonist conformation of ERα in which the C-terminal helix 12 (H12) folds in toward the helical barrel structure of the LBD and encloses the ligand. In the agonist conformation, the activation function-2 (AF-2) located on the exterior of ERα is able to bind to coactivators, recruit the preinitiation complex to ERE sites, and activate transcription of estrogen-driven genes. In contrast, for the antagonist conformations, as seen with 4-hydroxytamoxifen (4-OH-TAM; active metabolite of tamoxifen) (3ERT.pdb),[64] the entire ligand is not accommodated within the interior of the receptor (Fig. 24.35). Instead the basic amine side chain protrudes to the exterior of the ERα helical barrel. The SERM pushes H12 away from the coactivator binding site, preventing coactivator binding and AF-2 function in some tissues; resulting instead in recruitment of corepressors in these tissues (breast and uterus). The antiestrogenic and some of the estrogen-like actions of SERMs can be explained by the different conformations of their ERα complexes which attracts coactivators and/or corepressors that are different depending on the cellular context. In this model, the receptor would be differentially expressed across SERM target tissues.[268] Alternatively, ERα could be modulated by different concentrations of ERβ at different sites. It has been suggested that ERβ could enhance estrogen-like gene activation through a protein-protein interaction at AP-1 (*fos* and *jun*) sites.[269] At present, it is not entirely clear how SERM action is modulated at each target tissue. Indeed, more than one mechanism may occur. This pleiotropic pharmacology can be characterized as the dissociation in vivo of the favorable effects of ERα on bone, heart and brain, from unfavorable growth stimulatory effects of ERα on breast and uterus which is characteristic of SERMs. Similar tissue-selective dissociation of other nuclear hormone receptor effects has been seen with the AR (SARMs)[193] and GR (SGRMs).[270,271] However, there are no approved products yet in those cases. Tissue-selectivity and anticancer effects have also been sought using ERβ agonists which has a distinct tissue distribution and often opposes the growth stimulatory effects of ERα.[40]

Tamoxifen (Nolvadex). Tamoxifen is an example of a compound that was designed for one indication and failed, but was steered toward another indication where

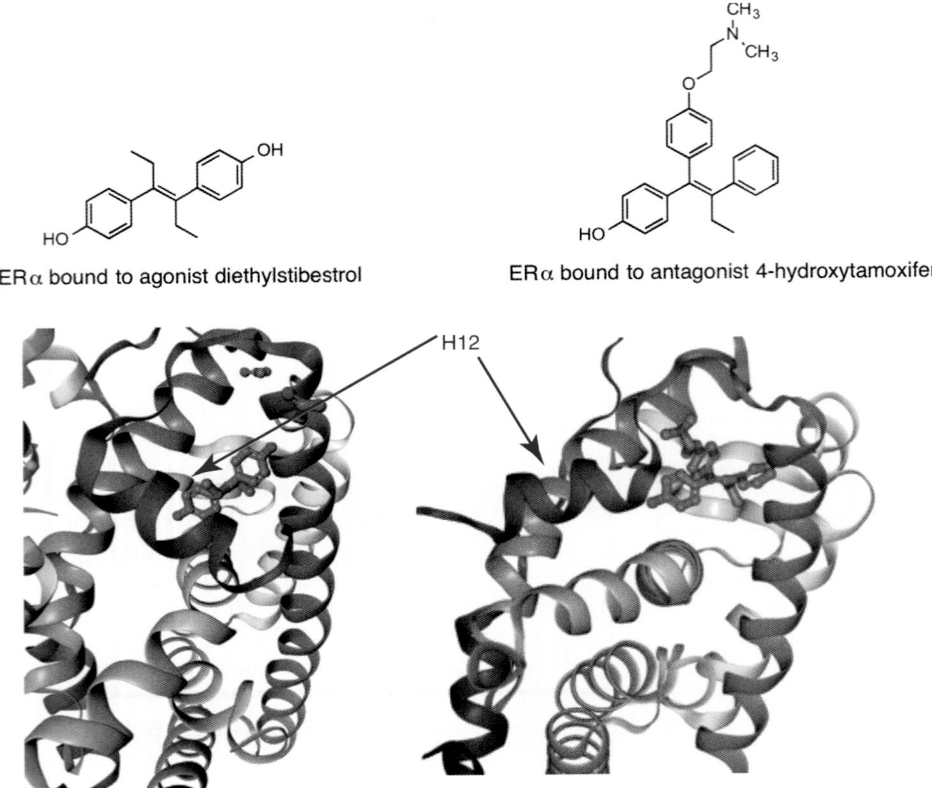

Figure 24.35 Agonist and antagonist conformations of ERα. The left panel demonstrates the agonist conformation of the ERα ligand binding domain when bound to diethylstilbestrol, whereas the right panel demonstrates the antagonist conformation when bound to 4-hydroxytamoxifen. A key difference is the orientation of helix 12 (H12; indicated by red arrows). H12 is a short segment of helix located at the C-terminus of the LBD. In the agonist conformation, H12 folds toward the ligand and completely encloses the ligand within the barrel-shaped binding pocket. Externally, the AF-2 of the agonist conformation forms a coactivator interaction site such that ERα recruits coactivators and activates ERα-dependent transcription. In the antagonist conformation, the basic amino side chain together with the cis aryl group is not accommodated by the receptor. Instead the ligand protrudes toward the exterior of the receptor. H12 is pushed into an alternate orientation which recruits corepressors in breast and uterine tissues, but still acts as an agonist in other tissues such as bone.

it has become the first targeted anticancer therapy and the most prescribed anticancer therapy ever. In the early 1960s, tamoxifen was initially discovered as part of a fertility-control program as a successful postcoital contraceptive in rats and was considered as a possible "morning after pill." However, the reproductive pharmacology of tamoxifen is species specific and in women it induced ovulation (central antagonist) rather than reducing fertility (central agonist). Also in the 1960s, the hormone dependency of breast cancer was further substantiated by the presence of ER (α subtype; ERβ was not discovered until 1996) in breast cancers, prompting Dr. Arthur L. Wadpole to encourage the clinical investigation of tamoxifen in breast cancer patients. In 1977, tamoxifen was FDA approved for the treatment of metastatic breast cancer and since then has been approved for adjuvant hormone therapy of ER-positive breast cancer and chemoprevention in women at high risk for breast cancer.[272] Further, tamoxifen replaced endocrine ablative surgery in both pre- and postmenopausal patients with advanced breast cancer. For decades, tamoxifen was the endocrine treatment of choice for all stages of breast cancer. Over time, AIs have gained favor as a first-line treatment in many settings due to increased efficacy and cost-effectiveness,[273] but tamoxifen remains the treatment of choice for premenopausal and DCIS patients, and a viable first-line option in almost any ER-positive early breast cancer.

Unfortunately, tamoxifen retains some intrinsic agonist activity, and therapy commonly results in tamoxifen resistance and the need to switch to other endocrine therapies, as discussed above. The emergence of tamoxifen resistance seems to be worse in obese patients where, even if gonadal estrogen synthesis is ablated, the fat cells produce estrogens using aromatase. Further, low-adherence patients have shorter time to recurrence, so it is very important to counsel patients to continue taking it on a daily basis throughout their course of therapy. Tamoxifen citrate therapy was associated with serious and life-threatening events including uterine malignancies, stroke, pulmonary embolism, and DVT,[274] with thromboembolic event risk higher when used in combination with cytotoxic agents. Careful risk-benefit evaluation is advised in patients predisposed to thrombotic events. Further, vasomotor and gynecological problems including sexual dysfunction are common with tamoxifen and can be rationalized as symptoms of chemically induced menopause. Fatty liver[275] and occasionally severe liver diseases, myalgias, and eye disorders, e.g., cataracts and retinopathy, have been reported. Fatigue and asthenia have been reported very commonly. Excessive vaginal bleeding or severe pelvic discomfort should be followed up to assess for endometrial cancer versus postmenopausal symptoms.

Tamoxifen citrate is dosed daily as 20-40 mg tablets with the lowest effective dose. In early disease, a 5-year regimen is recommended and should not be taken at the same time as AIs. Tamoxifen is a prodrug that is thought to require metabolic activation by CYP2D6 to produce the 4-hydroxytamoxifen (4-OH TAM) metabolite (Fig. 24.36). Tamoxifen and 4-OH TAM are also metabolized by CYP3A4 to the relatively inactive N-desmethyl tamoxifen (NDM TAM; similar activity as tamoxifen) metabolite and the active 4-hydroxy N-desmethyl tamoxifen (4-OH-NDM TAM; known as endoxifen in the literature) metabolite. These metabolites bind to the ER with up to 30-fold greater affinity than tamoxifen, and this increased potency ER binding translates into enhanced antiestrogen activity.[276,277] Since plasma levels of 4-OH-NDM TAM in patients with functional CYP2D6 frequently exceed the levels of 4-OH TAM, it seems likely that 4-OH-NDM TAM is at least as important as 4-OH TAM to the overall activity of this drug.[277] Consequently, efficacy is lowered by low or null CYP2D6 activity found in patients harboring certain CYP2D6 alleles, e.g., CYP2D6*10/*10.[278] Recent (2018) guidelines suggest consideration of patient genotyping before adjuvant tamoxifen in early breast cancer, and initiating AI (with ovarian suppression if pre- or perimenopausal) if a poor metabolizer genotype is found.[279] Further, coadministration with CYP2D6 inhibitors (e.g., fluoxetine, duloxetine, bupropion, and especially paroxetine) can lead to persistent reduction in the plasma concentrations of the active metabolites. Concurrent chronic use of CYP2D6 inhibitors should be avoided if possible. Although there is still controversy regarding this drug-drug interaction,[280] pragmatism dictates to avoid 2D6 inhibitors in general and prescribe antidepressants that impart lesser 2D6 inhibition (sertraline, citalopram, escitalopram, venlafaxine).[281]

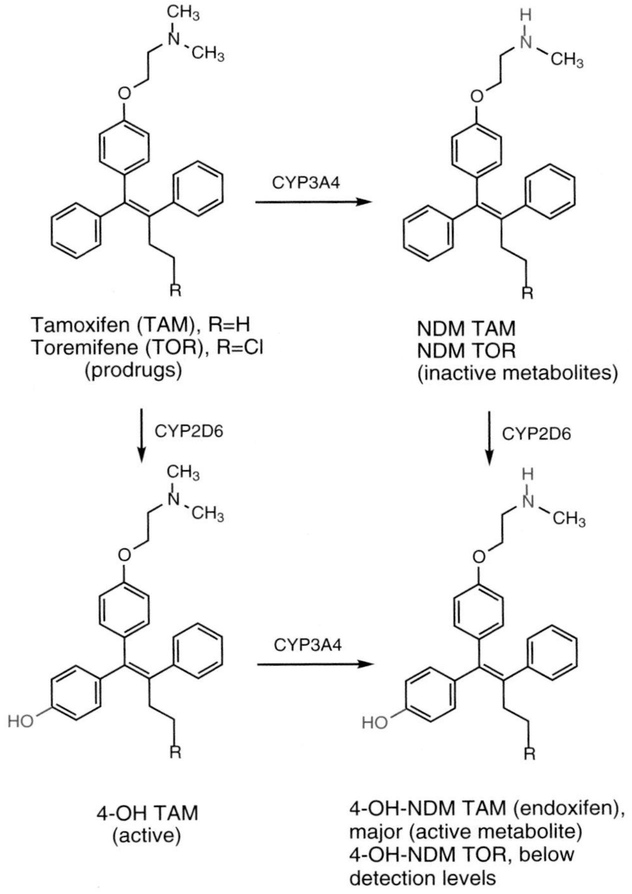

Serum concentrations of tamoxifen vary considerably between patients, possibly due in part to genetic polymorphisms, and these variations can affect efficacy and metabolite levels. Tamoxifen is rapidly and well absorbed (~100%) from the GI tract with C_{max} of 3-7 hours and has a large volume of distribution (20 L/kg) owing to plasma protein binding. High concentrations are found in the uterus and breast tissue. As described above, tamoxifen is metabolized by CYP2D6 and CYP3A4 to active metabolites. Tamoxifen undergoes extensive enterohepatic recycling and is eliminated mostly in the feces (26%-65%) due to bile excretion. The terminal elimination half-life of tamoxifen is 5-7 days with an extremely wide range of 3-21 days.[282] The terminal elimination half-lives of the active metabolites are not provided in the package insert. In female mice, following IV administration of endoxifen as a 1 mg/kg dose, peak plasma concentration, terminal elimination half-life, and plasma clearance values were 0.26 μM, 6.5 hours, and 11.8 L/hr/kg, respectively.[283]

Toremifene (Fareston), approved in 1997, is another triphenylethylene SERM that differs from tamoxifen by the addition of a chlorine atom to the ethyl side chain (Fig. 24.36). The goal of toremifene (TOR) development was to improve the safety profile while retaining the efficacy of tamoxifen, though studies to date suggest similar safety profiles. Toremifene is indicated for the treatment of metastatic breast cancer in postmenopausal women with ER-positive or unknown tumors. Despite a number of clinical trials and over 500,000 patient years of use, many oncologists have limited familiarity with toremifene. Some in vitro evidence suggests that, unlike tamoxifen, toremifene is not a prodrug that requires CYP2D6 metabolism and that the use of TOR in patients with genetically low or null CYP2D6 activity should be investigated.[284,285] The chlorine atom of toremifene was postulated to sterically clash with the CYP2D6 catalytic pocket when the toremifene substrate is oriented for 4-hydroxylation. Further, no 4-hydroxy N-desmethyl toremifene (4-OH-NDM TOR) was detected in the clinical samples evaluated.[284] The endometrial cancer side effect of tamoxifen, which is not as prevalent with toremifene, could be due to the more active 4-hydroxylated tamoxifen metabolites. The pharmacokinetics of toremifene, with the exceptions in the metabolism noted above (i.e., not a substrate for CYP2D6) and below, are comparable to tamoxifen.

Figure 24.36 Metabolism of tamoxifen (TAM) and toremifene (TOR); NDM, N-desmethyl.

Toremifene is rapidly and well-absorbed orally, has a large apparent volume of distribution (580 L) due to extensive albumin binding, is extensively metabolized by CYP3A4 to N-desmethyl toremifene (NDM TOR) (Fig. 24.37), autoinduces its own CYP3A4-mediated metabolism like tamoxifen, and has a terminal elimination half-life of 5 days. Another metabolic divergence from tamoxifen is that toremifene is dealkylated to form deaminohydroxy-toremifene, known as ospemifene (Osphena) which is an FDA-approved SERM for dyspareunia (Fig. 24.37).[286] Notably, a black box warning for QT prolongation exists for toremifene but not tamoxifen, although the two drugs likely have the same effect. Drugs known to prolong the QT interval and strong CYP3A4 inhibitors should be avoided. Efficacy of toremifene for the indicated disease state, advanced breast cancer, seems equivocal when compared to tamoxifen, and the safety profile is at least not worse, suggesting that TOR may serve as a reasonable alternative to tamoxifen when antiestrogens are applicable.[287] Studies in the adjuvant setting (which is off-label for toremifene) also indicated equivocal efficacy.[287]

The search for the optimal SERM continued into the early 21st century with a couple successes, mentioned herein below, but also a few failures.[288] Raloxifene hydrochloride (Evista) is a benzothiophene SERM (Fig. 24.34) that was originally indicated in 1999 for the prevention and treatment of osteoporosis in postmenopausal women. In 2007, raloxifene was FDA approved as a chemopreventive agent to reduce the risk of developing invasive breast cancer in postmenopausal women with osteoporosis and postmenopausal women at high risk for invasive breast cancer. For more information on raloxifene, see Chapter 23. Similarly, bazedoxifene, an indole SERM (Fig. 24.20), was approved in 2007 for prevention and treatment of postmenopausal osteoporosis when administered with conjugated estrogens. Ospemifene was approved in 2013 for postmenopausal women experiencing dyspareunia. These latter SERMs were considered as safer with regard to uterine effects, allowing their use in nononcologic indications, e.g., as antiresorptives in the bone or for climacteric symptoms.

Aromatase Inhibitors. The structures of endogenous estrogens differ most notably from androgens and other endogenous steroids in the A-ring of the steroidal nucleus. The unique requirement of estrogens to have an aromatic A-ring allows the inhibition of estrogen biosynthesis without affecting androgen, progesterone, or adrenocorticoid biosynthesis. All mammalian estrogens (except equine estrogens) are aromatized as their last step in biosynthesis by the action of the enzyme aromatase which converts androstenedione and testosterone to estrone and 17β-estradiol, respectively (Fig. 24.38). In view of the above and the incomplete blockade of estrogen action by tamoxifen, an alternative approach was hypothesized which indirectly blocked the ER axis by decreasing estrogen production.[289]

Aromatization is energetically expensive, and unlike androgen or adrenocorticoid biosynthesis, there is no redundant or salvage metabolic pathways to achieve aromatization of estrogens. Consequently, levels of endogenous estrogens can be very successfully lowered by potent AIs, which indirectly suppress the ER axis in estrogen-dependent breast cancers. Aromatase utilizes three moles of NADPH and O_2 for each mole of estrogen formed, suggesting that aromatization involves three successive hydroxylations (Fig. 24.39, top panel).[290] The first two occur at the 19-methyl group of androgens to produce a C-19 *gem* diol, a hydrated form of the C-19 aldehyde. This is followed by the simultaneous elimination of the 19-methyl group as formate (HCO_2H) and aromatization of the A-ring. Reversible AIs are triazoles that bind tightly with the Fe atom of the heme group to act as competitive inhibitors of aromatase (Fig. 24.39, bottom panel). Two reversible competitive nonsteroidal AIs are available, letrozole and anastrozole, and these are the most commonly used AIs. An irreversible "suicide" inhibitor of aromatase, exemestane, is also approved (Fig. 24.40).

Originally approved for metastatic breast cancer, AIs are now a standard treatment for all postmenopausal patients and are effective as monotherapy in the adjuvant and first-line metastatic settings. It is important not to use AIs in premenopausal patients because the reduction in estrogen levels will induce the expression of ovarian aromatase. The recent favor of AIs over tamoxifen in the postmenopausal setting derives from the adverse partial estrogenic effects of tamoxifen, resulting in incomplete blockage of estrogen action and the development of tamoxifen resistance.[289] It is recommended that postmenopausal women who have completed a 5-year regimen of tamoxifen for the treatment of early-stage, ER–positive breast cancer consider extending their treatment with an AI. It has not yet been definitively established what the optimum duration

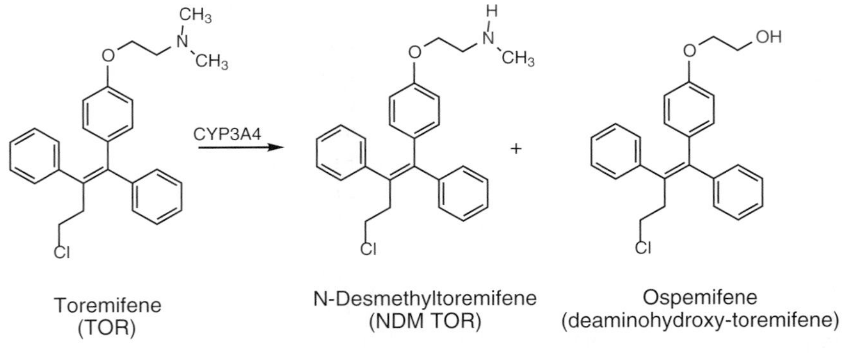

Figure 24.37 Metabolism of toremifene.

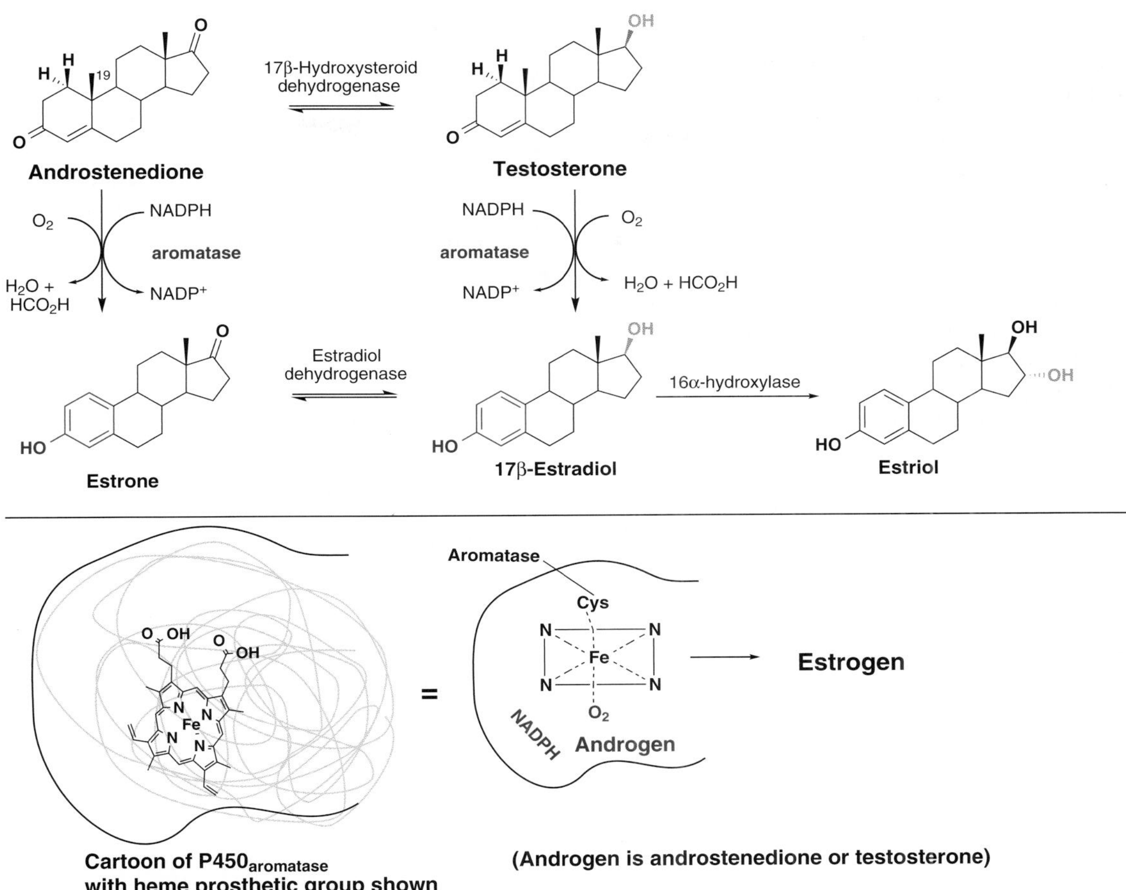

Figure 24.38 Aromatization of androgens to estrogens by aromatase. Top panel: Androstenedione and testosterone are converted by aromatase to the estrogens estrone and 17β-estradiol via an energetically unfavorable reductive dealkylation process, as is shown in red. Biotransformations by other enzymes are shown in gray. Bottom panel: The binding pocket of aromatase contains a heme prosthetic group which is directly involved in the catalytic conversion of androgens to estrogens. Aromatase inhibitors bind strongly to the iron (Fe) atom of the heme group, prevent androgen binding, and inhibit enzyme turnover.

of treatment should be or whether an AI should supplant or be sequenced after tamoxifen therapy. The AIs are associated with a lower risk of endometrial cancer and thromboembolic events but with higher rates of fractures and myalgia as compared to tamoxifen. Unfortunately, resistance to AIs also occurs as a result of pathogenic cross-talk with kinase receptor cell growth pathways,[289] ushering in the recent advent of CDK4/6 inhibitor therapies which are thus far only indicated for advanced breast cancer (discussed below) and are rapidly supplanting AI monotherapy in advanced disease.

Letrozole (Femara). Letrozole was originally approved in 1997 as monotherapy for the treatment of advanced breast cancer in postmenopausal women with disease progression following antiestrogen therapy (Fig. 24.40); however, monotherapy in advanced disease is largely being supplanted by combinations with CDK4/6 inhibitors. In fact, letrozole and ribociclib were approved by FDA for copackaging (Kisqali Femara) in 2017. Letrozole monotherapy is still prevalent and favored in the adjuvant setting where there is a 2%-4% chance each year that the cancer might return or recur. For example, extended adjuvant letrozole monotherapy (switching from tamoxifen to letrozole after 5 years of therapy in the absence of recurrence; approved in 2004) and as initial adjuvant therapy (i.e., to prevent recurrence) in early breast cancer (approved in 2005) can reduce recurrence rates by half. The latter approval was based on a clinical trial (Breast International Group [BIG] 1-98) comparing 5 years of tamoxifen monotherapy to 5 years of letrozole monotherapy. Letrozole had significantly fewer disease-free survival, contralateral breast cancer recurrence, and time-to-distant metastasis events and trended toward an overall survival benefit; however, it was not significant.[291,292] By this and similar trials, it was demonstrated that indirect inhibition of the ER axis by the lowering of endogenous estrogen levels with letrozole was significantly more efficacious than tamoxifen in the neoadjuvant (before any treatment), adjuvant (after treatment but in the absence of evidence of disease), extended adjuvant (switching from tamoxifen to letrozole in absence of disease), and advanced (metastatic or refractory disease) settings,[293] and that such uses were cost effective.[294]

Letrozole is a nonsteroidal reversible (i.e., type I) inhibitor of aromatase that binds via its 1,2,4-triazole ring to the heme group of aromatase (Fig. 24.39, bottom left panel). Letrozole dose-dependently suppresses

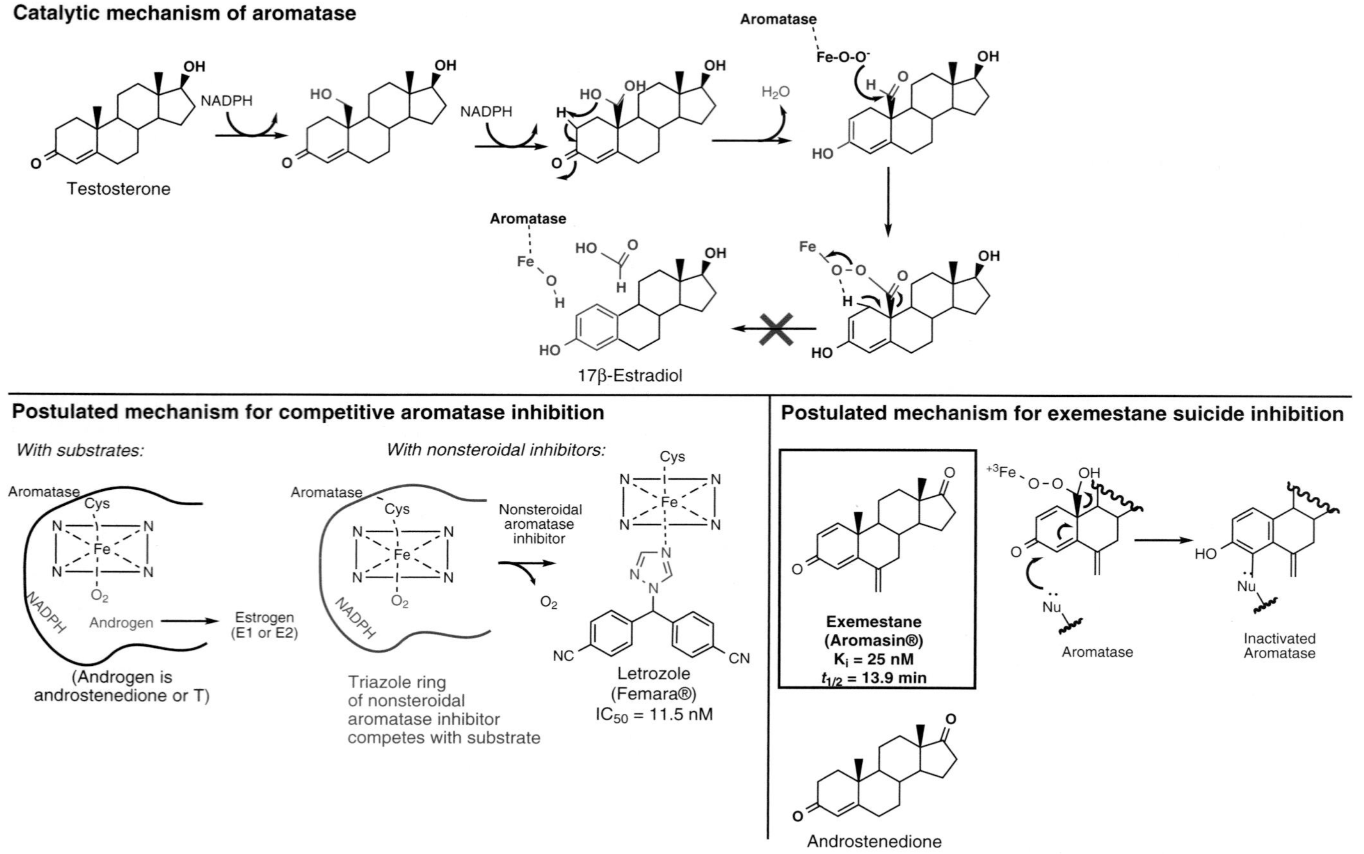

Catalytic mechanism of aromatase

Testosterone → NADPH → NADPH → H_2O → 17β-Estradiol

Postulated mechanism for competitive aromatase inhibition

With substrates: Aromatase, Cys, Fe, O_2, NADPH, Androgen → Estrogen (E1 or E2). (Androgen is androstenedione or T)

With nonsteroidal inhibitors: Aromatase, Cys, Fe, O_2, NADPH, Nonsteroidal aromatase inhibitor. Triazole ring of nonsteroidal aromatase inhibitor competes with substrate. Letrozole (Femara®) IC_{50} = 11.5 nM

Postulated mechanism for exemestane suicide inhibition

Exemestane (Aromasin®) K_i = 25 nM $t_{1/2}$ = 13.9 min; Androstenedione; Aromatase; Inactivated Aromatase

Figure 24.39 Catalytic mechanism of aromatase and postulated mechanisms for its reversible and irreversible inhibition. Top panel: The catalytic mechanism involves two successive NADPH-dependent hydroxylations of the C19 methyl group followed by the 2β hydrogen elimination as H_2O which allows the enolization of the 3-keto group. Aromatization is completed by the attack of the activated oxygen atom of the ferric oxide cofactor on the C19 aldehyde, positioning the other oxygen atom to accept the 1β hydrogen from the steroid and simultaneously eliminate the C19 group as formate. Bottom left panel: Reversible agents bind tightly and competitively with androgen substrate to the iron atom of the heme. Bottom right panel: Exemestane resembles androstenedione allowing the enzyme to form the gem-diol intermediate; however, the 3-keto-$\Delta^{1,4}$ A-ring is aromatized as it captures a nucleophile from the enzyme; thus irreversibly inactivating the enzyme.

the plasma concentration of estrone, estrone sulfate, and 17β-estradiol by 75%-95% with maximal suppression achieved in 2-3 days. This is achieved without accumulation of adrenal androgen substrates and without effects on adrenal steroidogenesis. Letrozole inhibits aromatase which is expressed in, e.g., the gonads, brain, adipose tissue, and the tumor itself. Letrozole reduces uterine weight and regresses estrogen-dependent tumors as effectively as ovariectomy.

Letrozole is administered orally (2.5 mg daily) and is completely and rapidly absorbed from the GI tract, and

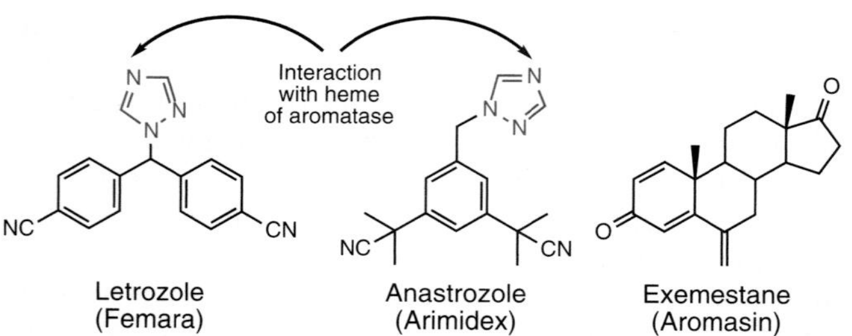

Figure 24.40 Nonsteroidal and steroidal aromatase inhibitors.

absorption is not affected by food. However, when taken with palbociclib it should be taken with a fatty meal to increase the CDK4/6 inhibitor absorption. Steady state is reached in 2-6 weeks. Steady-state plasma concentrations are 1.5 to 2 times higher than predicted from concentrations following single dosing, suggesting a slight nonlinearity of daily dosing of 2.5 mg; however, accumulation does not continue to occur. It is slowly metabolized (CYP3A4 and CYP2A6) to an inactive carbinol metabolite that is subsequently glucuronidated and eliminated renally. Ninety percent of radioactive letrozole is recovered in the urine. Letrozole strongly inhibits CYP2A6 and moderately inhibits CYP2C19. The only notable drug-drug interaction is that coadministration with tamoxifen resulted in 38% reduction in plasma letrozole[295] probably due to CYP3A4 induction by tamoxifen (however, clinical efficacy does not support use of these agents together). Also moderate hepatic impairment increased in letrozole by 37% in normal subjects; thus breast cancer patients with severe impairment are expected to be exposed to higher levels of letrozole. Letrozole increases the risk of osteoporosis and commonly causes hot flashes and night sweats. An increased incidence of hypercholesterolemia also has been documented. Overall, the side effect profile of letrozole compared to tamoxifen is more striking for their similarities than their differences with most adverse events reported at comparable levels. Common adverse events for both included hot flashes (33.7% vs. 38.0% [letrozole vs. tamoxifen]), night sweats (14.1% vs. 16.4%), and weight gain (10.7% vs. 12.9%). Arthralgia (21.1% vs. 13.4%) and bone fractures (5.6% vs. 4.0%) were reported more frequently following treatment with letrozole. Bone loss appears manageable through bisphosphonate therapy[296] and more recently denosumab (Xgeva).

Anastrozole (Arimidex). Anastrozole is FDA approved for a similar set of indications in postmenopausal women as letrozole including initial adjuvant therapy in early breast cancer (2002, see Arimidex, Tamoxifen, Alone or in Combination, ATAC trial),[297] first line in advanced or metastatic breast cancer (2000), and second line in advanced disease with disease progression following tamoxifen therapy (1995). Again, monotherapies in late disease are largely supplanted or augmented by CDK4/6 inhibitor combinations. The registration trial for the initial adjuvant therapy indication, ATAC, tested anastrozole and tamoxifen monotherapy for 5 years and the combination of the two; however, the combination arm was discontinued for lack of efficacy in excess of tamoxifen alone. The two monotherapy arms demonstrated statistically significantly improved disease-free survival for anastrozole at 68 and 120 months, with the latter analysis showing 735 events versus 924 events for the hormone-receptor positive subpopulation. This established the superiority of anastrozole compared to tamoxifen in the adjuvant setting, which is similar to letrozole. In the advanced breast cancer registration trials, anastrozole seemed to produce similar objective tumor rates and time to tumor progression as tamoxifen. Direct head-to-head clinical trials comparing letrozole to anastrozole are not available to our knowledge.[298]

Letrozole is the only AI to demonstrate consistent superiority over tamoxifen in the neoadjuvant and first-line advanced breast cancer settings.[293,299] In direct comparisons with anastrozole, letrozole is significantly more potent in aromatase inhibition in vitro and suppresses estrogen to a greater degree than anastrozole in the serum and breast tumor.[300] Further, it is more efficacious in clinical response in patients as second-line endocrine therapy in advanced metastatic breast cancer.[301] However, a recent trial concluded that letrozole was not significantly superior in efficacy or safety compared with anastrozole in postmenopausal patients with hormone receptor-positive, node-positive early breast cancer.[302]

Anastrozole, a benzyltriazole (Fig. 24.40), is another potent and highly selective, nonsteroidal reversible (type I) AI in which coordination of the triazole ring with the heme iron atom allows potent inhibition of aromatase (Fig. 24.39, bottom left panel).[303,304] Similar to letrozole, anastrozole inhibits aromatase expressed in all tissues and oral 1 mg daily dosing reduced 17β-estradiol by ~70% within 24 hours and by ~80% by 14 days. Anastrozole is rapidly (C_{max} is 2 hr) and well absorbed orally. Food reduces the rate but not overall extent of anastrozole absorption. Linear pharmacokinetics were observed from 1 to 20 mg. Metabolism to inactive metabolites occurs by N-dealkylation to produce triazole as the major circulating metabolite, but hydroxylation and glucuronidation were also observed. Hepatic metabolism accounts for 85% of anastrozole elimination and the terminal elimination half-life is approximately 50 hours.[303] Side effects are similar to letrozole with anastrozole producing adverse changes in hip and lumbar spine BMD and increased fractures (10% vs. 7%), and elevated cholesterol (9% vs. 3.5%) relative to tamoxifen. Unlike letrozole, the anastrozole package insert reported higher incidence of ischemic cardiovascular events than tamoxifen (17% vs. 10%) including angina pectoris (2.3% vs. 1.6%), and risks and benefits should be considered before initiating anastrozole in preexisting ischemic heart disease. However, more recent meta-analysis disputes this conclusion.[298] Otherwise anastrozole and tamoxifen had similar incidence of adverse events, similar to letrozole. Based on clinical and pharmacokinetic results from the ATAC trial, tamoxifen should not be administered with anastrozole (similarly with letrozole).

Exemestane (Aromasin). Exemestane is a steroid-based, irreversible (type II) AI (Fig. 24.40). It is approved as monotherapy for adjuvant therapy after 2-3 years of tamoxifen to complete 5 consecutive years of adjuvant therapy in hormone receptor positive early breast cancer (2005). In this role, exemestane reduced initial disease recurrence events by 9.06% compared to 12.94% for tamoxifen at 34.5 months following exemestane initiation; however, overall survival was equivocal at 119 months. Unlike letrozole and anastrozole, exemestane is not approved as first-line adjuvant therapy. Also unique to exemestane, it is indicated in advanced breast cancer in combination with everolimus (2012; mTOR inhibitor). It is also indicated as monotherapy in advanced breast cancer following tamoxifen failure (1999) like other AIs.

Exemestane resembles androstenedione in structure, acting as a false substrate and thereby binding irreversibly to aromatase as a suicide inhibitor (Fig. 24.39, bottom right panel). Because this agent has high binding affinity and specificity for aromatase, it is able to suppress the activity of this enzyme by 97.7% (anastrozole, 92%-96%; letrozole, 98%).[305] Exemestane is administered orally (25 mg daily) after a meal. Only 42% of radiolabeled exemestane was absorbed from the GI tract with a terminal half-life of about 24 hours. Absorption of exemestane was improved when taken following a high-fat meal, with increases in AUC and C_{max} of 59% and 39%, respectively. Approximately 90% of a dose is bound to plasma proteins including albumin and α_1-acid glycoprotein. Exemestane undergoes extensive metabolism by CYP3A4, and to a minor extent by aldoketoreductases. Dosage adjustments may be necessary if given concomitantly with a CYP3A4 inducer.[305] For example, 600 mg rifampicin for 14 days decreased C_{max} and AUC by 41% and 54% in healthy postmenopausal volunteers; however, the CYP3A4 inhibitor ketoconazole had no effect. The initial steps in metabolism are oxidation of the methelene group at position 6 and reduction of the 17-keto which are inactive or reduced potency metabolites. Radioactive exemestane is excreted equally in the urine and feces (42% each). Adverse reactions reported in patients with early breast cancer include hot flashes (21.2% vs. 19.9% for tamoxifen), arthralgia (14.6% vs. 8.6% for tamoxifen), and fatigue (16.1% vs. 14.7% for tamoxifen), which is similar to other AIs. Also, BMD is lower by exemestane and patients should be evaluated for calcium or vitamin D deficiencies.

Bone Health in Hormone-dependent Cancers. Breast cancer patients in general have a high prevalence of vitamin D deficiency, resulting in bone loss which can be exacerbated by the use of chemotherapy, AIs, and/or pure antiestrogens (i.e., fulvestrant) which further lower BMD, whereas tamoxifen and other SERMs increase BMD compared to placebo. Bone health is extremely important in breast cancer not just to prevent fractures but also to prevent metastasis to the bone. The most common site of metastasis is the bones of the hip and vertebral column where the metastases form lytic lesions and cause compression fractures of vertebrae. Breast cancer patients should be encouraged to take calcium and vitamin D supplements and should consider the use of antiresorptive agents such as denosumab, which is largely supplanting the use of bisphosphonates in breast and prostate cancers.

ADVANCED OR METASTATIC BREAST CANCER. Unfortunately, even though uncomplicated early breast cancer can be thought of as very treatable and curable, Kaplan-Meier curves of ER-positive breast cancers undergoing adjuvant therapy have a steep drop-off for the initial 2 years following surgery and/or initial adjuvant chemotherapy. After this initial higher mortality phase, there is about a 2%-4% recurrence rate per year despite adjuvant therapies. Despite extensive prognostic testing, there is still little insight as to why some patients relapse almost immediately whereas others do well for decades. Further, a certain percentage of ER-positive breast cancers present as advanced or distantly metastatic cancers which is associated with poorer prognosis. Breast cancer most commonly spreads to the bones, liver, lungs, or brain. At this point it is considered stage 4 breast cancer.

Treatment of metastatic breast cancer is less personalized than early breast cancer where multiple therapeutic targets (ER/PR/HER2) are defined as well as a recently approved genotype-guided therapy. The previous notwithstanding, the 21st century has seen an ongoing renaissance in the treatment of advanced breast cancer. Originally, tamoxifen and toremifene were used in advanced breast cancer, as well as salvage therapies such as the progestogens megestrol acetate or medroxyprogesterone or androgens such as oxandrolone. However, responses were short-lived and clinicians resorted to chemotherapy. In the early 21st century, AIs were commonly given as first-line or following recurrence on tamoxifen. Likewise, fulvestrant was approved in 2002 for advanced breast cancer following disease progression on antiestrogen therapy.

Case Study I

CASE

HP is a 45-year-old obese female patient whose menopausal status is unknown and who presents with a large 2.5 cm tumor with a high mitotic index in the left breast near the chest wall close to her heart, making radiation therapy difficult. Molecular phenotyping demonstrates 99% ER staining, 75% PR staining, and HER2 negative status. Genotyping does not reveal known pathogenic mutations in the *BRCA1/2* genes. OncoType Dx suggests a high recurrence score. The sentinel lymph nodes are reported as negative and no further efforts are put into detecting metastatic lesions, but the patient complains of hip pain. Radical double mastectomy with reconstruction is elected as surgery leaving no breast tissue to irradiate. Following a 4-cycle adjuvant TC chemotherapy regimen of docetaxel (taxotere) and cyclophosphamide, the patient is initiated on tamoxifen 20 mg daily.

A. Rationalize whether this patient should have been consider for the 6-cycle adjuvant chemotherapy regimen of TC followed by anthracyclines.
B. Rationalize possible reasons why the patient should or should not receive tamoxifen as adjuvant endocrine therapy? What further information would be needed to decide? What other therapies should be considered for this patient and why?
C. 18 months after initiating tamoxifen therapy, the patient complains of severe hip pain, and musculoskeletal pain in the torso that does not seem to heal. An ultrasound at the gynecologist did not reveal any metastases in the viscera but a strikingly low platelet count.

What is likely to be happening to the patient?

Case Solution found immediately after References.

CDK4/6 inhibitors:

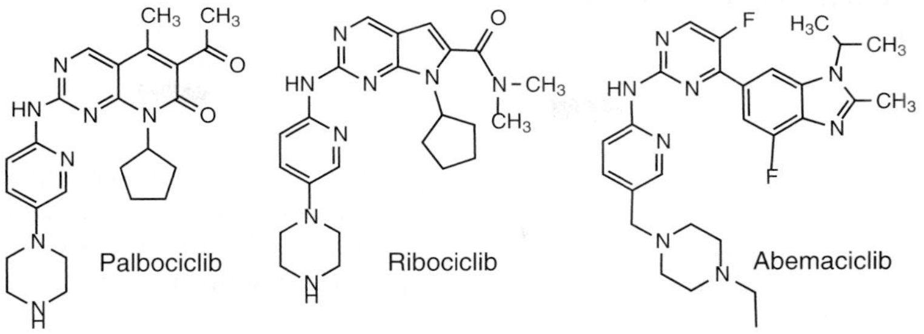

Palbociclib Ribociclib Abemaciclib

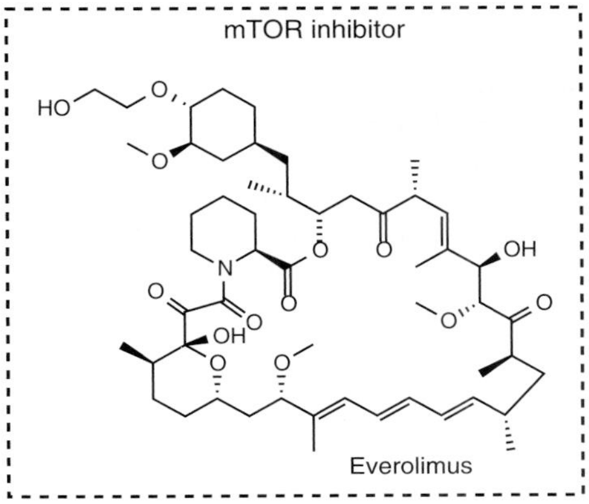

mTOR inhibitor

Everolimus

Since 2012, four kinase inhibitors (everolimus, an mTOR inhibitor) and palbociclib, ribociclib and abemaciclib (which are CDK4/6 inhibitors) have been approved for advanced hormone receptor positive breast cancer and HER2 negative breast cancer; mostly as specific combinations with the endocrine therapies discussed above (see also fulvestrant below), but also as monotherapy. The kinase inhibitor therapies have improved upon the efficacy of AIs and fulvestrant (discussed below) in advanced breast cancer. These combination therapies take advantage of the improved understanding of the interactions between hormone signaling pathways and other important growth factors. Kinase inhibitors modulate hormone signaling and interfere with resistance mechanisms that are yet to be fully understood. CDK4/6 inhibitors consistently improve objective response and progression-free survival.[306] However, they suffer from a lack of biomarkers to aid in patient selection or therapeutic monitoring.[307] As of 2018, the indications for CDK4/6 inhibitors for advanced breast cancer are summarized below. Palbociblib is indicated in advanced disease with letrozole (2015) or fulvestrant (2016) for endocrine therapy failures, or as first line in combination with AIs (2017). Ribociclib is indicated in combination with AIs as initial endocrine-based therapy in advanced or metastatic breast cancer (2017). Abemaciclib is indicated in combination with fulvestrant for endocrine therapy failures (2017). Abemaciclib is also the first CDK4/6 inhibitor approved as monotherapy (2017) in hormone receptor-positive, HER2-negative metastatic disease who previously received endocrine therapy and chemotherapy. For more information on these classes of kinase inhibitors, see Chapter 33.

Pure Antiestrogens. Despite the fact that 30%-40% of patients with advanced breast cancer respond to tamoxifen therapy, this response only lasts for 12-18 months. Tamoxifen resistance is caused, in part, by its intrinsic agonist activity at the ER. In addition, tamoxifen only inhibits the AF-2 activation pathway but does not affect transcription promoted by activation function 1 (AF-1). Pure antiestrogens do not possess any intrinsic estrogenic activity in any target tissue or cellular context and, therefore, offer an additional avenue of treatment when resistance to tamoxifen occurs. In addition, because they are devoid of estrogenic action, these agents cannot be classified as SERMs.

Fulvestrant (Faslodex)

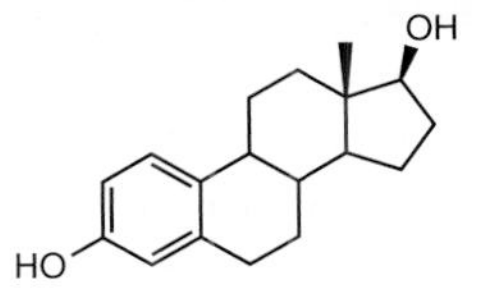

17β-Estradiol

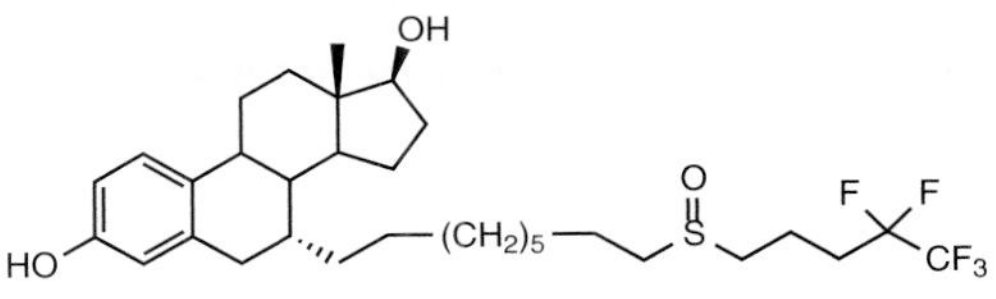

Fulvestrant

Fulvestrant is a pure antiestrogen devoid of ER agonist activity and has high ER binding affinity comparable to 17β-estradiol. It has multiple effects on ER signaling such as blocking dimerization and nuclear localization of the ER, and reducing cellular levels of ER (i.e., acts as a SERD),[308] although the significance of this latter mechanism has been disputed.[309] Despite SERD activity, fulvestrant resistance develops due to activated ERα-independent compensatory growth factor signaling, stimulated downstream kinases, etc., which are at least partially addressed by CDK4/6 inhibition. The search for an orally active SERD that is more effective than AIs in second-line advanced breast cancer is ongoing.[309]

Fulvestrant is effective in preventing the growth of tamoxifen-resistant breast cancers both in the laboratory[310] and in clinical trials.[311] It is indicated for postmenopausal women as monotherapy in the treatment hormone naïve advanced breast cancer (2017) or following antiestrogen therapy for the treatment of ER-positive metastatic breast cancer that has continued to progress (2002).[312] It is indicated in combination with CDK4/6 inhibitors palbociclib (2016) and abemaciclib (2017) in the advanced or metastatic setting following disease progression after endocrine failure. Pre and perimenopausal women treated with these combinations should be treated with GnRH agonists as well.

Fulvestrant is a 17β-estradiol analog with a hydrophobic side chain in the 7α position. Fulvestrant has poor oral bioavailability owing to very poor solubility, despite metabolic protection on the end of the hydrophobic side chain. As a result, it is administered as a 500 mg intramuscular injection once a month. Fulvestrant is 99% plasma protein bound with lipoproteins and SHBG contributing. Metabolism of fulvestrant follows biotransformation pathways similar to endogenous steroids producing both active and less active metabolites. Metabolites include aromatic hydroxylation followed by glucuronic acid and sulfate conjugates at the 2, 3, and 17 positions, and oxidation of the sulfoxide in the side chain.[313] Side effects appear to be minimal and include several arthralgias, GI symptoms, headache, and hot flashes. There is no clinical evidence of uterine stimulation or laboratory evidence of stimulation of endometrial carcinoma models.[314] Fulvestrant should not be administered to women who are pregnant, who are taking anticoagulants, or who have thrombocytopenia.

Treatment of Prostate Cancer

Prostate cancer is the most common noncutaneous cancer and remains the second leading cause of cancer death and the most commonly diagnosed cancer in American men with ~165,000 estimated new cases and ~29,000 estimated deaths in 2018.[315] The growth and maintenance of the prostate is dependent on the endogenous androgens testosterone and 5α-DHT. As men age, the growth of the prostate can become pathogenic due to either BPH or prostate cancer which is typically an adenocarcinoma. Prostate cancer incidence on biopsy is approximately the same as a man's age (i.e., a 50 yr old has ~50% chance of latent prostate cancer and at 90 yr has a 90% chance of having latent prostate cancer). However, men castrated before puberty (eunuchs) or men with inherited deficiency of type II 5AR (i.e., testosterone cannot be converted into DHT) do not develop prostate cancer. Correspondingly, prostate cancer pharmacotherapies primarily block the AR axis. Because prostate cancer typically grows slowly and causes no symptoms, digital rectal examination and the serum PSA test are most often used to screen for prostate cancer. Recently, PSA screening has fallen out of favor.[316] However, PSA is still closely monitored in active disease as a marker of treatment response and/or disease progression. Moreover, PSA is not specific to prostate cancer and can be used to evaluate and manage other prostate problems, most notably BPH.

Treatment of prostate cancer is guided by three initial analyses: (1) staging of the tumor(s) by Gleason score; (2) staging of the cancer following typical tumor/node/metastasis analysis, and (3) PSA biomarker levels and their changes over time. After initial workup, about 40% of prostate cancers present with low grade, low tumor volume, and slow PSA doubling time. These patients are considered to have a good prognosis. For these low-risk patients, therapeutic intervention is trending toward active surveillance because of a popular belief that this population is overtreated with in excess of 1,410 patients treated to prevent 1 death.[317] Moreover, bothersome side effects caused by surgical and X-ray therapies used in early prostate cancer include urinary incontinence

Case Study 2

Four months later, HP, the same patient as from the previous example, presents to the oncologist in extreme and debilitating pain, and using a walking aid. CAT scans show large lytic lesions in the painful hip, and lytic lesions in multiple vertebrae most prominently at T7 and T12, where the spinal canal has been encroached due to multiple pathologic fractures collapsing the spinal column. Radiation therapy of the vertebra is successful at shrinking the tumor and HP's functional status improves. Despite reported adherence with adjuvant tamoxifen, bone biopsy reveals metastatic breast cancer which is still ER and PR positive and HER2 negative. Serum estrogen levels are reported as well above menopausal levels.

A. In addition to therapies for advanced breast cancer, what other issues does HP have that require immediate therapy and what should be the agents chosen?
B. What classes of targeted therapies are available to HP for the advanced breast cancer? Select a targeted treatment and rationalize your choice?
C. Should chemotherapy be considered?

Case Solution found immediately after References.

and impotence. Another 20% of prostate cancers present with high-grade, high-volume tumor and fast PSA doubling times. The prognosis for these patients is relatively poor and pharmacotherapy is clearly indicated in these high-risk patients. Another 40% have a mixture of favorable and unfavorable prognostic indicators, making the decision whether to treat these patients less clear and discussion of risks and benefits with the patient necessary. Further, as PSA screening is also falling out of favor,[316] it is likely that more patients will present with advanced disease. Morbidity and mortality rates may rise, although this may be offset to some extent by the recent advances in the pharmacotherapy.

Traditional treatments for localized prostate cancer include active surveillance, surgery (radical prostatectomy), and external-beam radiation, whereas advanced prostate cancer (i.e., locally advanced or metastasized disease) treatments also include pharmacologic approaches. Chemical or surgical castration has been the cornerstone for advanced prostate cancer since their discovery by Huggins and Hodges in 1941.[318] Initial pharmacotherapy for advanced prostate cancer remains androgen deprivation therapy (ADT) such as GnRH superagonists (1980s) or antagonist (2012), but this approach may evolve soon. Advanced disease is initially controlled by suppression of gonadal androgens, but eventually relapse occurs despite castration levels of testosterone, a condition referred to as castration-resistant prostate cancer (CRPC). Secondary hormonal therapies (discussed under CRPC section) concurrent with ADT were shown to extend survival in nonmetastatic castration-resistant prostate cancer (nmCRPC in 2018; see apalutamide section) and metastatic CRPC (mCRPC in 2011 and 2012; see abiraterone and enzalutamide sections), and even castration-sensitive prostate cancer (CSPC in 2018; see Abiraterone section below). Secondary hormonal therapies can directly and competitively bind and antagonize the AR (e.g., enzalutamide and apalutamide used to suppress the AR axis that is reactivated in CRPC). Alternatively, suppression of androgen biosynthesis (e.g., the lyase inhibitors abiraterone or ketoconazole) can also suppress the reactivated AR axis.

With increased therapeutic options in CRPC, the pharmacotherapy in advanced CSPC is changing to include these agents. Preliminarily it is suggested that younger and healthier patients who have a greater chance of dying from prostate cancer rather than other causes should be considered as candidates for ADT plus docetaxel and/or ADT plus secondary hormonal therapies, whereas older and unhealthy patients may still be candidates for ADT only. For example, the addition of chemotherapy with docetaxel (6 cycles) upon initiation of standard of care has been shown to increase overall survival and reportedly should become standard of care in M1 (metastatic) disease.[319] Recent data with secondary hormonal therapies in the pre-CRPC setting will be discussed below. How these agents will be integrated into advanced prostate cancer therapy is still yet to be seen.

Unfortunately, prostate cancer progresses while taking ADT in virtually all patients who have metastatic disease and in many patients with nonmetastatic disease.[319] CRPC (i.e., prostate cancer that progresses despite testosterone levels less than 50 ng/dL, the level considered as castration by FDA) is induced by ADT. Disease progression can be observed as increasing PSA while taking ADT (biochemical recurrence)[320] or progressive disease on imaging. CRPC can be symptomatic or asymptomatic and metastatic (mCRPC) or nonmetastatic (nmCRPC), affecting the suggested pharmacotherapies. In general, CPRC is treated with ongoing ADT plus secondary hormonal therapies. However, resistance to secondary hormonal therapies is also inevitable with cross-resistance being prevalent. Once CRPC no longer responds to secondary hormonal therapy, then chemotherapy with docetaxel should be considered, followed by cabazitaxel if unresponsive. Moreover, immunotherapy (sipuleucel T) improves survival in asymptomatic CRPC, and radium-223 improves overall survival in men with mCPRC that has spread to the bones. Many of the recently (e.g., since 2010) approved agents for CPRC improve overall survival but only by about 4 months as monotherapy. This indicates that comprehensive studies on proper sequencing or rational combinations of these therapies is needed to maximize pharmacotherapeutic benefits. The modest survival benefits also emphasize the need for the discovery and exploration of novel pharmacotherapies for CRPC with less susceptibility to the development of resistance.

Treatment of Advanced or Metastatic Castration-Sensitive Prostate Cancer

GONADOTROPIN-RELEASING HORMONE THERAPY. Huggins and Hodges won the 1966 Nobel Prize for describing the relationship between testosterone and prostate cancer, having shown in 1941 that marked reductions in serum testosterone by castration or estrogen treatment caused metastatic prostate cancer to regress.[318] ADT has remained an important component in the treatment of prostate cancer since then. Testicular surgery (bilateral orchiectomy) to prevent testosterone production was once the most common treatment for advanced prostate cancer and is still used by some today, but is associated with physical and psychological discomforts. Although this surgery is not a cure, it delays the advance of the disease. Chemical castration to achieve ADT is now the cornerstone of therapy with the goal of reducing serum testosterone to below 50 ng/dL, although some suggest that this threshold should be even lower, e.g., <20 ng/dL. Historically, ADT pharmacotherapy was commonly achieved with DES (seldom used now; used in the 1940s until the advent of GnRH therapies),[321] an estrogen that suppressed testicular testosterone synthesis via a feedback mechanism involving ERs in the brain. Modern ADT was introduced in the 1980s and involves the use of analogs of GnRH which possess greater potency than the natural GnRH hormone. These superagonists bind to GnRH receptors

(GnRH-R) in the pituitary and cause an initial increase in LH and FSH, and, subsequently, increased testosterone[322] synthesis in testes. The initial androgen surge occurs within the first 3-7 days and can be associated with a clinical flare, e.g., increases in prostate volume, bone pain, and spinal cord compression.[323] (Combined androgen blockade through concomitant antiandrogen, e.g., flutamide, to block flare symptoms was common practice, but is now disfavored.) Continuous overstimulation of GnRH-Rs desensitizes the gonadotroph cells and downregulates GnRH-R expression, resulting in decreased LH synthesis and nearly abrogating testicular steroidogenesis. More succinctly, gonadal androgen synthesis is suppressed via feedback inhibition of the HPG axis (see Fig. 24.6). Castration levels of testosterone (i.e., <50 ng/dL) are attained within 2-4 weeks after initiation and maintained long-term. The GnRH agonists (Fig. 24.41), commonly referred to as GnRH superagonists or LHRH agonists, are administered in a continuous, nonpulsatile manner, which is in contrast to the pulsatile release of the endogenous hormone GnRH. Further, they bind with higher affinity to GnRH-R in the pituitary than does the endogenous hormone, cumulatively causing a durable effect in the majority of patients upon constant or intermittent dosing.[324] A wide variety of GnRH agonists have been approved, not just for ADT in prostate cancer but also for use in other indications such as ovarian suppression in breast cancer (nonpulsatile) or dosed in a pulsatile fashion for central precocious puberty as will be reviewed separately. Unfortunately, up to 12% of patients fail to achieve castration levels of testosterone and up to 37% fail to achieve levels <20 ng/dL. Also, breakthrough testosterone levels that increase into the range of 20-50 ng/dL were reported in 32% of patients receiving a GnRH agonist[325] and shortened time to progression to CRPC.[326]

GnRH Agonists. GnRH agonists approved for use in prostate cancer include leuprolide (Lupron), goserelin (Zoladex), and triptorelin (Trelstar). For prostate cancer, these are given via high-dose and constant (nonpulsatile) release formulations. GnRH agonists are peptidic agents that mimic the natural hormone GnRH and consist of an approximately 10-amino-acid segment of GnRH modified to stabilize the N- and C-terminus. Further, modifications at the 6 and 10 positions of the decapeptide block enzyme cleavage sites and increase agonist activity (Fig. 24.41). For example, the first site can be blocked by replacing glycine 6 (Gly6) with a hydrophobic D-amino acid such as D-leucine in leuprolide, D-serine modified with a *t*-Bu group in goserelin, or D-tryptophan in triptorelin. Another enzyme cleavage site can be blocked by eliminating Gly10, as is seen in both leuprolide and goserelin. Changes in GnRH structure at other amino acid positions decrease activity. A variety of depot formulations for subcutaneous or intramuscular administration of leuprolide, goserelin, or triptorelin are available, with durations of action ranging from 1 to 6 months.

Leuprolide (Lupron). Leuprolide acetate (Lupron) is the synthetic nonapeptide: 5-oxo-L-prolyl-L-histidyl-L-tryptophyl-L-seryl-L-tyrosyl-D-leucyl-L-leucyl-L-arginyl-N-ethyl-L-prolinamide acetate (salt) that is inactive orally but can be administered subcutaneously or more often as

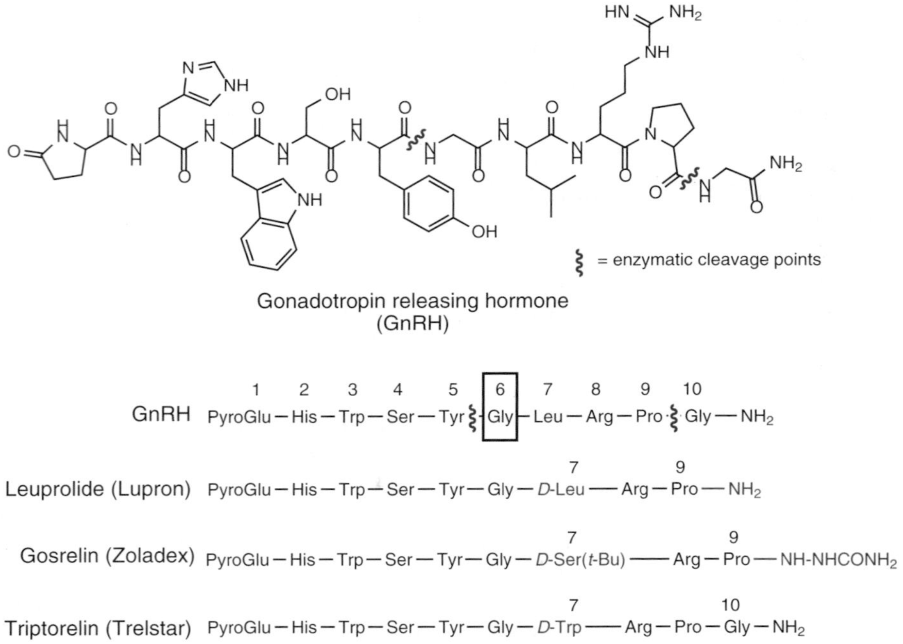

Gonadotropin releasing hormone (GnRH)

= enzymatic cleavage points

GnRH PyroGlu—His—Trp—Ser—Tyr—Gly—Leu—Arg—Pro—Gly—NH2

Leuprolide (Lupron) PyroGlu—His—Trp—Ser—Tyr—Gly—*D*-Leu—Arg—Pro—NH2

Gosrelin (Zoladex) PyroGlu—His—Trp—Ser—Tyr—Gly—*D*-Ser(*t*-Bu)—Arg—Pro—NH-NHCONH2

Triptorelin (Trelstar) PyroGlu—His—Trp—Ser—Tyr—Gly—*D*-Trp—Arg—Pro—Gly—NH2

Figure 24.41 GnRH agonists used for the treatment of prostate cancer. The molecular graph of GnRH decapeptide is shown at the top of the figure with amino acid notation underneath the molecular graph. Enzymatic cleavage sites within GnRH are indicated therein. Amino acid notation of the structures of the GnRH superagonists leuprolide, goserelin, and triptorelin are below the GnRH structure. Modifications at positions 6 and 10 are highlighted in red.

a monthly intramuscular depot injection that allows constant slow release. The 3.75 mg depot formulation is rapidly absorbed producing a C_{max} of 4.6-10.2 ng/mL at 4 hours. Two days after dosing, plasma concentrations were stably maintained at about 0.3 ng/mL for about 4 to 5 weeks. Once released into the plasma, the steady-state volume of distribution was about 27 L with a terminal elimination half-life of about 3 hours. Metabolism is to smaller inactive peptides with only 5% of the intact peptide eliminated in the urine.

Goserlin (Zoladex). Goserlin acetate (Zoladex) is also a synthetic nonapeptide: pyro-Glu-His-Trp-SerTyr-D-Ser(But)-Leu-Arg-Pro-Azgly-NH_2 acetate. It is available as a subcutaneous injectable implant every 28 days (3.6 mg [breast cancer or prostate cancer]) or 12 weeks (10.8 mg [prostate cancer]). The implant is a biodegradable polymer (D,L-lactic and glycolic acids copolymer) that provides rapid initial absorption and constant release over the indicated time periods. For example, for the 3.6 mg depot, mean concentrations gradually rise to reach a peak of about 3 ng/mL at around 15 days after administration and then decline to approximately 0.5 ng/mL by the end of the treatment period. For the 10.8 mg depot, mean concentrations increase to reach a peak of about 8 ng/mL within the first 24 hours and then decline rapidly up to day 4. Thereafter, mean concentrations remain relatively stable in the range of about 0.3-1 ng/mL up to the end of the treatment period. After release into the plasma, goserelin has a large volume of distribution (44 L) and is eliminated similarly to leuprolide as inactive peptides in the urine with only 20% as unchanged peptide.

Triptorelin (Trelstar). Triptorelin pamoate (Trelstar), a synthetic decapeptide: 5-oxo-L-prolyl-L-histidyl-L-tryptophyl-L-seryl-L-tyrosyl-D-tryptophyl-L-leucyl-L-arginyl-L-prolylglycine amide is available as a single intramuscular depot injection in either buttock delivering 3.75, 11.25, or 22.5 mg every 4, 12, or 24 weeks. It is 100-fold more active than native GnRH in vitro. Like leuprolide depot, subcutaneous triptorelin concentrations peak rapidly within 1-3 hours after injection with any of the mentioned doses with a volume of distribution of 30-33 L. Elimination is via a three-compartment model; however, metabolic pathways are unknown as no metabolites of triptorelin have been identified, presumably due to complete degradation. It is eliminated by both liver and kidneys with 42% excreted in the urine as intact peptide, which increased to 62.3% in patients with liver disease.

GnRH Antagonist

Degarelix (Firmagon). Degarelix acetate (Firmagon), approved in 2012, is the only GnRH antagonist for use in the treatment of advanced prostate cancer. (Abarelix was a predecessor which was voluntarily withdrawn from the market in 2005 due unfavorable efficacy compared to agonists.) It competes reversibly with the endogenous GnRH for GnRH-R binding on the pituitary gonadotroph cells and directly suppresses LH and consequently testosterone production, producing chemical castration.

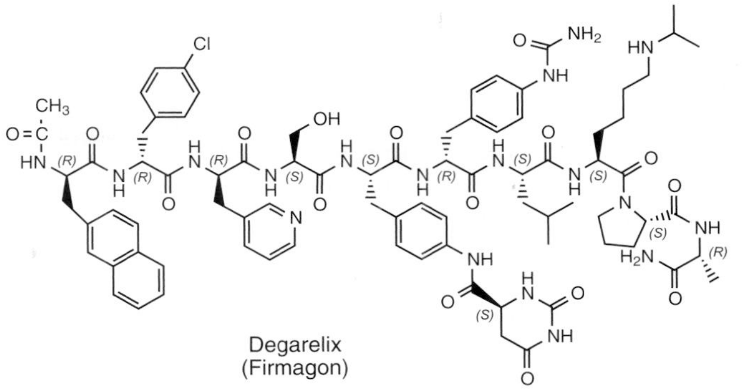

Degarelix
(Firmagon)

Because degarelix acts as an antagonist, there is no surge in pituitary LH or testicular androgen production as is observed with the GnRH agonists, so no clinical flare is manifested. As such, approximately 96% (vs. 0% for leuprolide 7.5 mg) of men achieve castration levels of serum testosterone within 3 days and 99% at 14 days (vs. 18% for leuprolide) of receiving their first (loading) dose of 240 mg of degarelix (administered as two subcutaneous injections of 120 mg). Lower maintenance doses of degarelix (80 mg) are administered every 28 days thereafter to maintain castration. Medical castration rates from days 28-364 were comparable to leuprolide 7.5 mg depot in advanced prostate cancer patients with each achieving >95% efficacy. Subcutaneous administration forms a depot from which degarelix is released to the circulation. After the 240 mg subcutaneous dose (with 40 mg/mL concentration product) the C_{max} occurred within 2 days. (Pharmacokinetic behavior is strongly influenced by its concentration in the injection solution; however, only the 40 mg/mL concentration is approved.) Degarelix is widely distributed throughout the total body water and in vitro plasma protein binding is estimated to be >90% (distribution volume of >1000 L). Degarelix is subject to peptide hydrolysis during passage of the hepatobiliary system and is mainly excreted as peptide fragments in the feces. Terminal elimination half-life of the subcutaneous depot injection is 53 days due to very slow release from the depot. Approximately 20%-30% was renally excreted, whereas 70%-80% was excreted via hepatobiliary excretion. The most common adverse effect was injection site reactions (28% pain and 17% erythema vs. <1% for leuprolide). Most other adverse effects were similar to leuprolide.

ADT with GnRH agonists or the antagonist significantly reduces serum testosterone levels, thereby depriving prostate cancer cells of their primary signal for growth (i.e., testosterone and DHT) and alleviating or easing the symptoms associated with advanced prostate cancer. However, GnRH agonists and the antagonist are not cures for prostate cancer. They are considered as palliative care. Periodic monitoring of PSA and plasma testosterone levels is recommended. Failure of one mode of ADT cannot be compensated for by changing to another mode of ADT; but rather, once castration resistance develops, another class of agents must be added to again suppress the AR axis.

The testosterone deficiency associated with ADT produces a variety of untoward and adverse effects which increase the morbidity of and affect the quality of life of ADT patients. Increased risk morbidities are due to bone and cardiometabolic complications such as osteoporosis and fractures, cardiovascular disease including strokes and acute myocardial infarctions, weight gain, insulin resistance, hyperlipidemia and diabetes, etc. Adverse quality of life issues include genital atrophy, ED, decreased mood and mentation, hot flashes, gynecomastia, etc.[327–329] After induction of castration, some low-risk patients can be considered for intermitent ADT (i.e. patient is not continuously taking ADT) to limit iatrogenic morbidity and cost with comparable overall survival rates.[330] Candidates include those with a robust PSA response and/or if the prostate cancer is asymptomatic.

Castration-Resistant Prostate Cancer

Nearly one-third of patients with prostate cancer develop metastatic disease, and about 80%-90% of those metastatic patients will have good initial responses to treatments such as surgery, radiation or other local therapy, and ADT. However, most advanced prostate cancer patients will go on to develop progressive disease,[331] where they present with increasing PSA or progression observed on imaging despite ongoing ADT (possibly combined with chemotherapy or secondary hormonal therapies). Once castration resistance is verified through testosterone level testing (i.e, levels should be <50 ng/dL or preferably <20 ng/dL), then pharmacotherapy depends on whether the disease is asymptomatic or symptomatic and nonmetastatic (nmCRPC) or metastatic (mCRPC), and pharmacotherapeutic history.

Recently, the CRPC therapeutic landscape has been rapidly expanding. For example, until 2010, the only pharmacotherapy for CRPC was docetaxel (approved for CPRC in 2004); however, six new agents have been approved in the last decade to include sipuleucel-T (2010), cabazitaxel (2010), abiraterone (2011), enzalutamide (2012), Ra-223 (2013), and apalutamide (2018). Most of these were approved in a CRPC setting, e.g., following progression on doxetaxel, but some have subsequently gained approvals or are exploring survival and/or quality-of-life benefits for earlier stage disease, as discussed below for each agent. Although there are a variety of agents, improvements in CRPC survival are typically by only ~4 months, suggesting the need for exploration of optimal sequencing and/or earlier intervention in order to improve outcomes for advanced and castration-resistant prostate cancer patients using existing agents. Novel therapies that are less susceptible to the development of resistance are also needed.

IMMUNOTHERAPY. Sipuleucel-T (Provenge), originally termed a therapeutic cancer vaccine but now referred to as an immunotherapy (e.g., similar to programmed death ligand agents), was approved for the treatment of asymptomatic or minimally symptomatic mCRPC in 2010. Sipuleucel-T was the first immunotherapy and utilizes an autologous cellular immunotherapy. Peripheral blood mononuclear cells, a type of white blood cell which includes antigen-presenting cells, are removed from the patient's blood through leukaphoresis at a treatment center. These cells are then activated ex vivo (i.e., at a separate laboratory) with a recombinant fusion protein (PA2024) so that the cells recognize and target prostate cancer cells. Next, the modified cells are reinfused into the patient. The modified cells, together with the immune system of the patient, find and destroy prostate cancer cells. Although the precise mechanism of action is unknown, sipuleucel-T is designed to induce an immune response targeted against prostatic acid phosphatase (PAP), an antigen expressed in most prostate cancers. Since PAP is only found on prostatic cells, this leads to a localized treatment.[332] However, there is no PSA response or other biomarker to monitor therapy. The treatment course comprises infusions at weeks 0, 2, and 4 that each deliver a minimum of 50 million autologous $CD54^+$ cells activated with PAP-granulocyte-macrophage colony-stimulating factor. Infusions are associated with a high prevalence (~70%) of acute infusion reactions that can be managed via premedication with oral acetaminophen and an antihistamine, such as diphenhydramine, approximately 30 minutes prior to administration. Clinical trials with sipuleucel-T demonstrated a 4-month improvement in survival as compared to placebo[333] in asymptomatic mCRPC. It has been suggested that patients whose cancer is less advanced generally have a more "active" immune system and may benefit the most from this treatment. However, thus far, the expense, narrow indication, and the inconvenience of the workflow (leukaphoresis at specialty clinic, ex vivo cell activation, and reinfusion) have hampered exploration of other indications with little clinical data to suggest indication expansion.[334] Nonetheless, information on its optimal use in combination and/or sequenced with other approved agents is awaited.[332]

SECONDARY HORMONAL THERAPIES AND CHEMOTHERAPY. Last century, disease that progressed despite ongoing ADT was termed androgen-independent prostate cancer suggesting that AR was no longer operant in the growth mechanisms of the prostate cancer. Early in the 21st century (2004), a discovery in recurrent prostate cancer revealed that AR was expressed at levels that were comparable to androgen-stimulated benign prostate.[335] Further, endogenous testosterone levels were also at normal levels in the recurrent prostate cancer tissue with ongoing AR axis activation observable as high expression of AR target genes such as PSA in recurrent cancer. The conclusion was that the AR axis was reactivated despite castration levels of serum testosterone.[335] Importantly, the recurrent prostate cancer, retermed as CRPC, should be sensitive to suppression of the AR axis if more potent agents could be discovered. Many novel AR signaling inhibitor therapies for CRPC were designed and trialed.[336] This stimulated a renaissance in the exploration of secondary hormonal therapies that resulted in the discovery and approval of several new agents such as abiraterone (Zytiga; 2011), enzalutamide (Xtandi; 2012), and most recently apalutamide (Erleada; 2018).

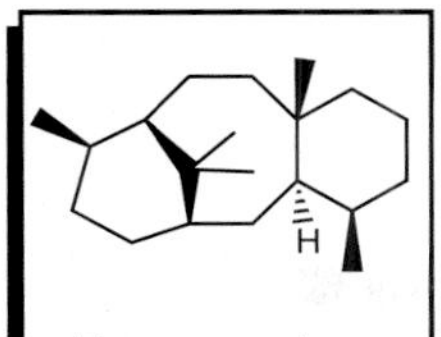

Taxane nucleus

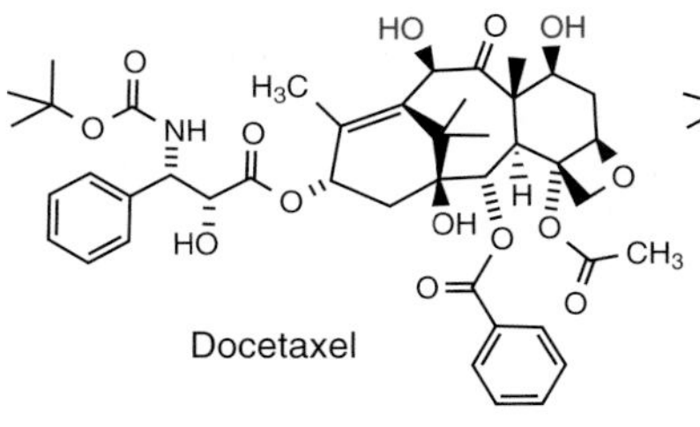

Docetaxel

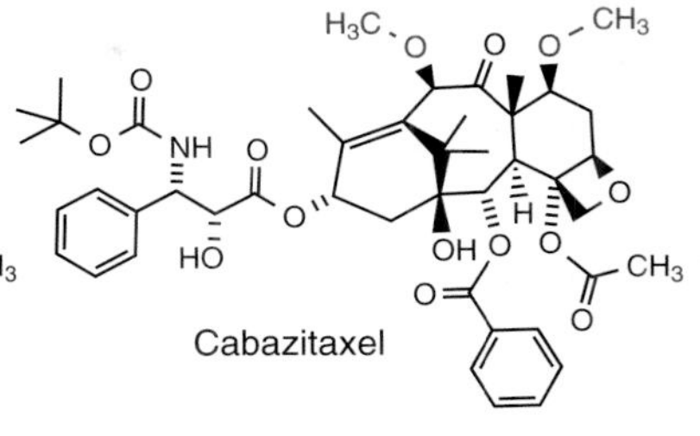

Cabazitaxel

Contemporaneously, advances were being made in chemotherapy for "androgen-independent" prostate cancer. The only FDA-approved chemotherapy for advanced prostate cancer was mitoxantrone (Novantrone) which was approved because it improved pain in approximately one-third of symptomatic patients. However, there was no evidence for a survival advantage. In 2004, docetaxel (Taxotere; Chapter 33) in combination with prednisone became the first chemotherapeutic agent to show increased survival to 18.9 months, or approximately 2 months longer as compared to treatment with mitoxantrone and prednisone.[337] Infusions of 75 mg/m^2 of docetaxel over 1 hour once every 3 weeks in combination with 5 mg of prednisone twice daily for 10 cycles became the standard of care once metastatic patients were demonstrated hormone refractory (i.e., ADT and older generation antiandrogens were ineffective). Today these patients would be classified as mCRPC. In 2011, a cabazitaxel (Jevtana; Chapter 33) dose of 25 mg/m^2 every 3 weeks in combination with 5 mg oral prednisone twice daily was approved as second line after docetaxel exposure or failure in mCRPC.[338] In this population, median survival was 15.1 months for cabazitaxel versus 12.7 months for mitoxantrone, demonstrating a second survival benefit after docetaxel. Recently (2017) a lowered dose of 20 mg/m^2 every 3 weeks with prednisone was approved.[339] A recent study suggested that the lowered dose may not be appropriate if used in combination with enzalutamide due to the possibility of subtherapeutic cabazitaxel exposure.[340]

Inhibitors of Androgen Biosynthesis. Although the antiandrogens bicalutamide (Casodex; 1995), nilutamide (Nilandron; 1996), and flutamide (Eulexin; 1989) were approved for advanced prostate cancer, these agents were weak AR antagonists that had a limited ability to suppress the AR axis. Consequently in 2010, there was still a large unmet need to provide highly potent AR signaling inhibitors to serve as secondary hormonal suppression in CRPC where androgens were demonstrated to be elevated intratumorally despite the castrate environment (<50 ng/dL testosterone in plasma)[335] produced by GnRH agonist or antagonist or orchiectomy. Subsequently, the source of these extragonadal androgens was discovered to be intratumoral and adrenal biosynthetic pathways (among other minor sources) that contributed sufficient endogenous androgens to reactivate the AR axis and sustain prostate tumor growth as CRPC despite ongoing ADT. This left open the possibility of suppressing the AR axis by blocking endogenous biosynthesis. Unlike estrogen biosynthesis, androgen biosynthesis can occur via redundant biosynthetic pathways (see Figs. 24.3 and 24.42). Further, mutant ARs in CRPC cells are promiscuously activated by weak adrenal androgens and glucocorticoids, not just testosterone and DHT. Consequently, simply blocking the last step, as was possible for estrogens (see Aromatase Inhibitors), was not available as an effective treatment modality. Instead, androgen biosynthesis must be blocked at an early and common step to these redundant pathways as will be discussed for the lyase inhibitors below.

Inhibitors of a variety of other enzymes within the redundant biosynthesis pathways have been evaluated to reduce androgen biosynthesis. For example, inhibitors of 17β-hydroxysteroid dehydrogenase (17β-HSD) type 3 (17βHSD3 is gonadal; enzyme **g** in Fig. 24.3)[341] or type 5 (17βHSD5 is peripheral; labeled as AKR1C3 (aldoketoreductase type 1C3)[342] exist, but there is no clinical evidence to support their use. Further, the 5α-ARIs (approved for BPH) were examined for chemoprevention of prostate cancer but were officially advised against by FDA due to more aggressive phenotype cancers in those where chemoprevention failed.

CYP17A1 Inhibitors. 17α-Hydroxylase/17,20-lyase (CYP17A1 or CYP17; sometimes just called lyase) is a bifunctional enzyme which converts pregnenolone into 17α-hydroxyprogesterone (hydroxylase) and subsequently cleaves the 17β side chain (lyase) of this C21 steroid to produce the C19 sex steroid precursor DHEA. These steps are marked with red X's in Figure 24.42. Inhibition of CYP17A1 blocks the synthesis in both the

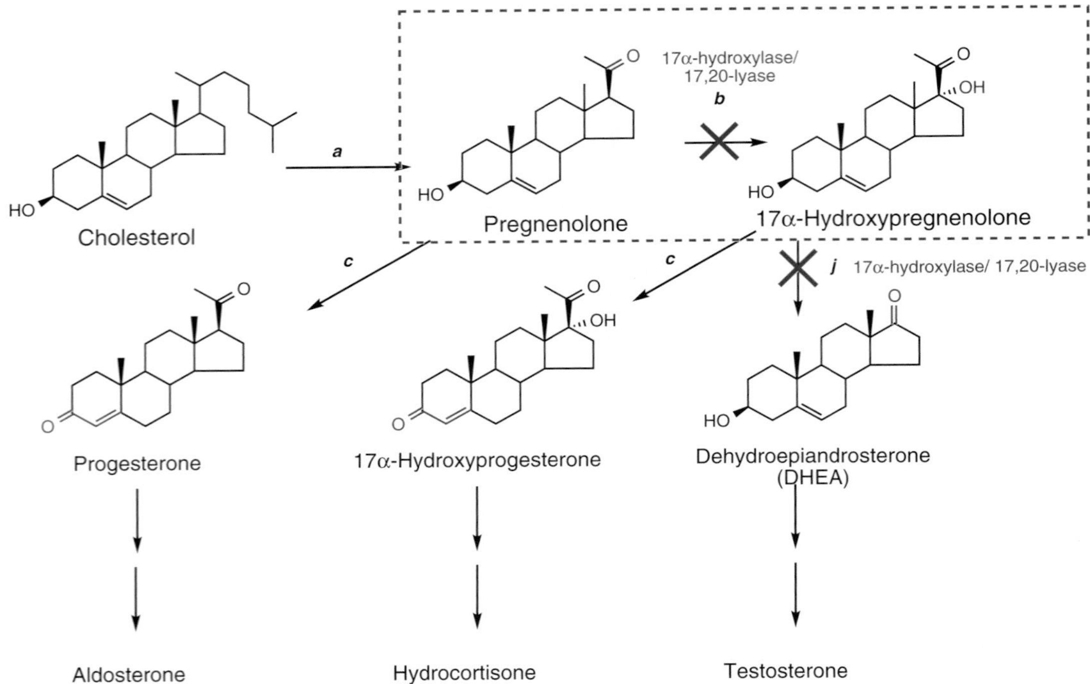

Figure 24.42 Inhibition of androgen synthesis by CYP17A1 inhibitors. Lyase inhibitors block conversion of cholesterol to the precursor of glucocorticoids and androgens through their actions to prevent formation of 17α-hydroxypregnenolone (step b above) and DHEA (step j above). (a) cholesterol side-chain cleavage (SCC)(CYP11A1), (b) 17α-hydroxylase (CYP17A1), (c) 5-ene-3β-hydroxysteroid dehydrogenase/3-oxosteroid-4,5-isomerase (3β-HSD), and (j) 17,20-lyase (CYP17A1).

glucocorticoid and sex hormone pathways due to the common intermediate, 17α-hydroxypregnenolone, and increases the synthesis in the mineralocorticoid pathway. The result is inhibition of androgen biosynthesis in the adrenals, prostatic tumor tissues, or testes leading to decreased levels of weak intermediate androgens, testosterone, and DHT (and 17β-estradiol), but also decreased hydrocortisone levels requiring supplementation of glucocorticoids. Further, the mineralocorticoid excess produces side effects including hypertension, potassium secretion, and fluid retention, which must be monitored.

Ketoconazole
(*racemate)

An early CYP17A1 inhibitor (17α-hydroxylase IC_{50} = 76 nM) that was used in metastatic prostate cancer patients[343] was the antifungal agent ketoconazole. Ketoconazole's role in prostate cancer was supplanted by the approval of abiraterone acetate (Zytiga) plus prednisone in 2011 for mCRPC patients previously treated with docetaxel. Whereas ADT abrogates only gonadal testosterone production, abiraterone (active metabolite of abiraterone acetate) potently inhibits both the hydroxylase and lyase enzymatic actions of CYP17A1 blocking adrenal and tumoral androgen production. Consequently, abiraterone acetate, added to ongoing ADT, was able to effectively suppress the reactivated AR axis in CRPC. Abiraterone acetate (1,000 mg; four 250 mg tablets of Zytiga daily) plus prednisone (5 mg twice daily) resulted in increased overall survival for docetaxel pretreated patients with a median survival benefit of about 4 months (14.8 vs. 10.9 months for placebo). In 2012, the indication was expanded to mCRPC in general (i.e., not requiring previous chemotherapy), based on median radiographic progression-free survival (16.5 vs. 8.3 months with prednisone alone) and a trend toward improved overall survival.[344]

In 2018, the FDA expanded the indication for abiraterone acetate (1,000 mg; Zytiga) in combination with prednisone (5 mg bid) plus ongoing ADT to include metastatic high-risk CSPC based on benefits on overall survival (median overall survival not estimable vs. 34.7 months for placebo) and time to initiation of chemotherapy (median time not reached vs. 38.9 months for placebo).[345]

Abiraterone acetate (Fig. 24.43) is a steroidal prodrug which is rapidly and completely cleaved by unspecified esterases into the active 3β-hydroxy metabolite abiraterone. An oral dose of 1,000 mg daily of abiraterone acetate without food is recommended (combined with 5 mg prednisone twice daily). Following oral

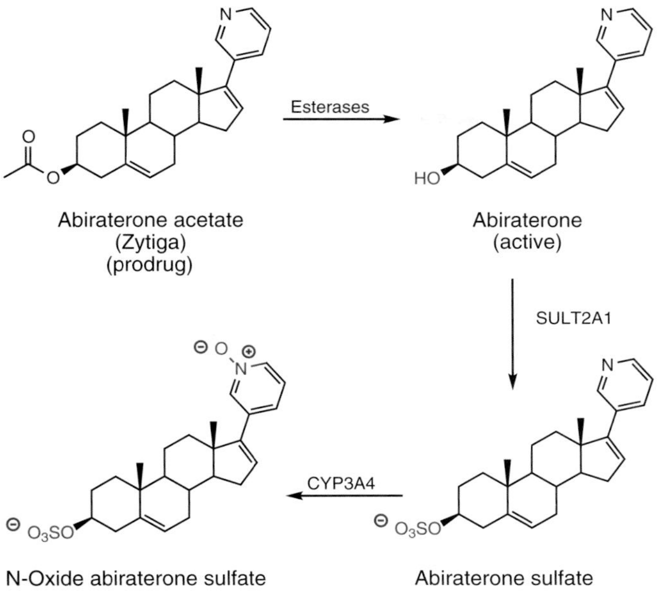

Abiraterone acetate (Zytiga) (prodrug)

Esterases

Abiraterone (active)

SULT2A1

Abiraterone sulfate

CYP3A4

N-Oxide abiraterone sulfate

Figure 24.43 Structure of the CYP17A1 inhibitor abiraterone, its activation, and metabolism.

administration of the inactive prodrug, abiraterone acetate, maximum plasma concentrations of abiraterone were reached in 2 hours. Due to poor solubility, there is a dramatic and inconsistent food effect on absorption with 5- to 7-fold increases with a low-fat (7% fat, 300 calories) meal versus 10- to 17-fold increases with a high-fat (57%, 825 calories) meal. Due to unreliable efficacy and intolerable untoward effects from such wide variations, food is to be avoided for at least 1 hour before and 2 hours after dosing. Abiraterone is highly protein bound (>99%) to the plasma protein albumin and alpha-1 acid glycoprotein, producing an apparent volume of distribution of 19,669 L. The two main circulating metabolites of abiraterone are abiraterone sulfate and N-oxide abiraterone sulfate which are products of SULT2A1 and CYP3A4. The terminal elimination half-life of abiraterone is 12 hours with 88% of the radioactive dose recovered in feces. The major compounds present in feces are unchanged abiraterone acetate and abiraterone (55% and 22%).

The side effect and drug-drug interaction profiles for abiraterone are substantial. In subjects with mild or moderate hepatic impairment, abiraterone systemic exposures were significantly increased and terminal elimination half-life prolonged to 18 hours. For patients with baseline moderate hepatic impairment, dose reduction to 250 mg is recommended. Further, all patients must be monitored for development of hepatotoxicity. Abiraterone is an inhibitor of CYP2D6 and coadministration with narrow therapeutic index CYP2D6 substrates should be avoided. Due to the expected mineralocorticoid excess, prescribers are warned to control hypertension and correct hypokalemia before treatment, and monitor for symptoms of mineralocorticoid excess such as fluid retention or increased blood pressure. Risk benefit analysis should be performed in cardiovascular disease, and safety in patients with Class III or IV heart failure has not been established. Due to the expected adrenocortical insufficiency, daily abiraterone acetate must be taken together with oral prednisone 5 mg twice daily. Further, the prednisone dose may be increased before, during, and after stressful events.

In 2018, a new microparticle formulation of abiraterone acetate, Yonsa, was approved for mCRPC patients in combination with methylprednisolone (4 mg twice daily) and concurrent ADT. Compared to Zytiga, Yonsa had improved abiraterone acetate dissolution rates and oral bioavailability while decreasing the effects of food on efficacy. For example, 500 mg (4 tablets at 125 mg each) of Yonsa had similar absorption as 1,000 mg (4 tablets at 250 mg each) Zytiga and therapeutic bioequivalence based on PSA and testosterone suppressions. Other than dosing and food effects (taken with or without food), the drug profiles for Yonsa and Zytiga are essentially identical.

Antiandrogens (Competitive AR Antagonists). Secondary hormonal therapy to suppress the reactivated AR axis in CRPC patients can also be achieved by antiandrogens that compete with endogenous androgens for binding and antagonize the AR. Early nonsteroidal antiandrogens such as bicalutamide, flutamide, and nilutamide were approved for advanced prostate cancer as combined androgen blockade with ADT (Fig. 24.44). However, these first-generation antiandrogens suffered from low-potency activities and intrinsic agonism, particularly of mutant ARs present in many CRPCs. Although termed, pure antagonists, these first-generation agents were later demonstrated to have less favorable antiandrogen activity profiles than more recently approved antiandrogens, as discussed below, and have been largely supplanted. For example, advances in the understanding of AR biology in CRPC allowed the development of the second-generation antiandrogens, including enzalutamide and apalutamide, that are more potent in vitro (e.g., AR binding and antagonism) and in vivo (e.g., inhibit LNCaP-AR or other CRPC xenograft growth), and possessed novel antiandrogenic properties such as inhibition of AR nuclear translocation, as will be discussed (Fig. 24.44). Importantly, enzalutamide extended overall survival in the mCRPC setting and apalutamide extended the metastasis-free survival in nmCRPC. Both were demonstrated as preclinically and clinically superior compared to bicalutamide, the most efficacious of first generation antiandrogen.

Clinical Use of Second-Generation Antiandrogens

Enzalutamide (Xtandi) and Apalutamide (Erleada). Abiraterone acetate was approved in 2011 for mCRPC following docetaxel, but it only extended survival by ~4 months. Enzalutamide in combination with ADT was approved for the same indication in 2012 and was expanded to include chemotherapy naïve mCRPC in 2014. Enzalutamide (plus ADT) demonstrated the ability to improve the overall survival of docetaxel pretreated (same indication as abiraterone) (18.4 vs. 13.6 months for placebo) or chemotherapy naïve patients (35.3 vs.

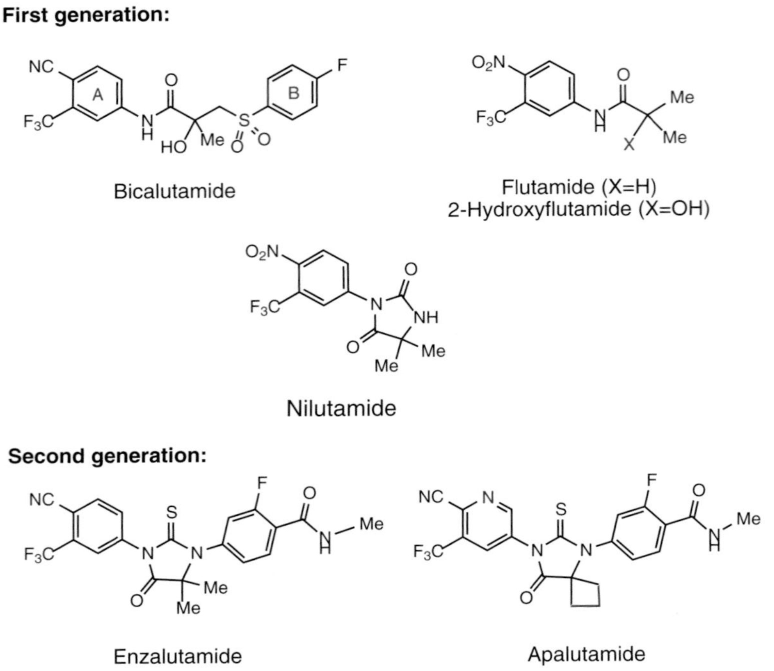

Figure 24.44 First and second generation nonsteroidal antiandrogens.

31.3 months for placebo). Further, this combination demonstrated superiority over bicalutamide in radiographic progression free survival (i.e., the time from randomization to the first objective evidence of radiographic progression) in chemotherapy naïve patients (19.5 vs. 13.4 months for bicalutamide). Although the overall survival benefits of enzalutamide and abiraterone (and other newer agents used in prostate cancer) may seem seem short, the benefit to quality of life should not be overlooked.

In 2018, apalutamide was approved for nonmetastatic CRPC (nmCRPC, also called M0 CRPC), demonstrating improved metastasis-free survival (MFS, the time from randomization until first evidence of distant recurrence) in patients with CRPC who were confirmed nonmetastatic and had a PSA doubling time of <10 months. Concomitant ADT and apalutamide in this population provided dramatically improved MFS of 40.51 months compared to 16.2 months for placebo plus ADT. However, no overall survival benefit has yet been reported.[346] Similarly in the nmCRPC setting, the enzalutamide (Xtandi) and ADT combination extended MFS to 36.6 versus 14.7 months with ADT alone and trended toward overall survival benefit.[347] A supplemental new drug application for enzalutamide in nmCRPC has been filed at the time of writing. As can be seen, use of these agents earlier in the nature history of prostate cancer greatly delays the onset of metastasis (i.e., by almost 2 yr), improving the prognosis of men with nmCRPC. The recent (2018) approval of abiraterone acetate in high-risk CSPC provides further hope that secondary hormonal therapy can dramatically delay progression of disease if used earlier.

Structural Elements of a Nonsteroidal Antiandrogen. Nonsteroidal AR ligands generally contain an electron deficient aniline A-ring that is most often *m*-CF_3 and *p*-CN or NO_2 substituted. All approved nonsteroidal antiandrogens also contain a propanamide segment, which is attached to the aniline N-atom of the A-ring, and can be cyclicized into a hydantoin (nilutamide) or thiohydantoin (enzalutamide and apalutamide). In some cases the propanamide is a linking segment which also attaches to a substituted aromatic B-ring, e.g., in bicalutamide, enzalutamide and apalutamide (Fig. 24.44). All antiandrogens bind to the same binding site on the LBD of AR with a similar predicted binding mode. Although the antagonist conformation of wild-type AR has never been crystallized, the agonist conformation of AR LBD escape mutants bound to first-generation antagonists can be used to rationalize the binding contacts of the conserved structural elements of antiandrogens. For example, the conserved A-ring has polar interactions with Gln711 and Arg752 via the *para* substituent of the A-ring. Similarly, the NH and carbinol OH of bicalutamide (bound to AR mutant Trp741Leu LBD in 1z95.pdb)[192] and hydroxflutamide (active metabolite of flutamide; bound to AR mutant Thr877Ala in 2ax6.pdb)[192] bind to the Leu704 and Asn705, respectively. This latter aspect of the binding mode is not available to enzalutamide and apalutamide, and docking attempts into the cited escape mutants fails (personal experience), suggesting the second-generation antiandrogens cannot be accommodated by the known AR agonist conformations of the first-generation antiandrogens. The divergent antiandrogenicity profile of the thiohydantoins may be explained, in part, by the induction of different AR conformations. Unfortunately, cross-resistant escape mutants for the secondary hormonal therapies (enzalutamide, apalutamide, and abiraterone) are also known, as discussed below.

Pharmacodynamics and Pharmacokinetics of Second-Generation Antiandrogens. Enzalutamide and apalutamide are thiohydantoin antiandrogens, differing only slightly in structure and possessing largely parallel pharmacokinetics and pharmacodynamics. These agents were discovered while screening for antiandrogens that displayed full and pure antagonism in AR overexpressing models of CRPC, unlike bicalutamide. Enzalutamide and apalutamide bind tightly and competitively with ^{18}F-16βF-DHT to AR with 21.4 and 16.0 nM affinities compared to 11.5 nM for ^{18}F-16βF-DHT and 160 nM for bicalutamide (7- to 10-fold weaker) in a whole-cell binding assay. The thiohydantoins are pure antagonists of wild-type AR (wtAR) that produced no agonism of AR-dependent genes such as PSA, even in wtAR-overexpressing models of CRPC[348] (e.g., LNCaP/AR cells). However, the weaker binding antagonist bicalutamide acted as an agonist in prostate cancer cells overexpressing wtAR and could not effectively antagonize R1881, a steroidal agonist commonly used in preclinical research. Bicalutamide acted similarly in VCaP prostate cancer cells (another cell line that overexpresses full-length AR and also expresses an AR-V7 truncated mutant[349]), stimulating cellular proliferation and only partially antagonizing R1881-induced cellular proliferation. The thiohydantoins (including RD 162 [not shown])[350] had no intrinsic stimulatory properties and were also full antagonists in VCaP cells. Further, thiohydantoins inhibit the nuclear translocation of AR, producing nuclear to cytoplasmic ratios of 3.0 (enzalutamide) and 2.5 (apalutamide) versus 29 and 14 for R1881 and bicalutamide, and 0.7 for vehicle, helping to rationalize the relatively high intrinsic agonism of bicalutamide in cells that overexpress the AR as compared to thiohydantoins. Importantly, both enzalutamide and apalutamide are able to shrink (regress) CRPC xenografts in vivo, whereas bicalutamide activity was limited to growth inhibition (only 1 of 10 tumors regressed >50% vs. 8 of 10 for apalutamide) despite threefold lower plasma levels.

Apalutamide appears to be more potent than enzalutamide in vivo. It was more potent preclinically in regressing LNCaP/AR xenografts, requiring a 30 mg/kg dose to achieve tumor volume reduction of >50% in 13 of 20 tumors as compared to a dose of 100 mg/kg of enzalutamide to achieve similar efficacy (>50% reduction of 12 of 20 tumors). Apalutamide also demonstrated slightly better MFS in nmCRPC humans (as discussed above). Increased seizure activity was observed clinically for both drugs. The incidence of seizures was 2.2% for enzalutamide in patients with predisposing risk factors such as use of seizure threshold lowering agents, history of head/brain injury, or cerebrovascular accident or transient ischemic attack in early clinical trials. The incidence of seizures was lower (0.5% and 0.2% for enzalutamide and apalutamide, respectively) in later clinical trials that excluded predisposed patients. Patients experiencing new onset seizures on drug are permanently discontinued.

Enzalutamide and apalutamide have N-desmethyl active metabolites (equipotent and 1/3 as potent as parent) which contribute to the efficacy of the drugs. Following daily oral administration with or without food of enzalutamide (160 mg as four 40 mg tablets) or apalutamide (240 mg as four 60 mg tablets), the thiohydantoins are rapidly (1 and 2 hr, respectively) and completely orally absorbed. Steady state is achieved in 4 weeks with minimal daily fluctuactions (1.25 and 1.63 peak-to-trough ratios) and significant accumulation ratios relative to single dosing (8.3- and 5-fold). Both are highly plasma protein bound. Enzalutamide and apalutamide are metabolized by CYP2C8 and CYP3A4 to N-desmethyl active metabolites with 30% and 40% of total steady state AUC being parent and 49% and 37% being active metabolite. Apalutamide is reported to autoinduce its metabolism via CYP3A4. The terminal elimination half-lives are long at 5.8 and 3 days. Excretion of radioactivity following single oral administration of enzalutamide or apalutamide is slow with 85% and 65% recovered by 77 and 70 days, largely in the urine at 71% and 65% versus 14% and 24% in feces, mostly as inactive metabolites. Single doses of gemfibrozil, a CYP2C8 inhibitor, increased thiohydantoin levels by 220% (AUC of enzalutamide plus metabolite) and 68% (AUC of apalutamide). Both thiohydantoins significantly reduced levels of CYP3A4 (midazolam), CYP2C9 (S-warfarin), and CYP2C19 (omeprazole) substrates suggesting the avoidance of coadministration of narrow therapeutic index substrates of these enzymes. Shared untoward effects compared to placebo include falls and fractures, hot flash, and hypertension, with apalutamide generally having increased prevalence commensurate with increased AR potency.

Resistance to Secondary Hormonal Therapies. Already resistance mechanisms to thiohydantoin therapy have evolved including cross-resistance to apalutamide and enzalutamide, and possibly abiraterone acetate, as conferred by F876L point mutant or F876L_T877A double mutant.[351] Similar to escape mutants of the first-generation antiandrogens (e.g., T877A for flutamide and W741L or W741C for bicalutamide, among other LBD mutations), these mutants operate as agonist switch mutations in which the antiandrogen acts as an agonist when binding to their escape mutant at high concentration. Consequently, antiandrogen withdrawal syndrome is observed clinically and is defined as tumor regression or symptomatic relief on cessation of antiandrogen therapy. Although there is cross-resistance between the different modes of secondary hormonal therapy and there have been no FDA approvals of their sequential use, there is some limited evidence for sequential use (i.e., in mCRPC, apalutamide suppressed PSA >50% for 6 mo in 80% of abiraterone acetate-naïve and 43% of post-abiraterone acetate plus prednisone patients).[352] Various sequential and combinatorial approaches are being explored clinically.[353] At least one LBD-directed antiandrogen, darolutamide (phase 3 trials ongoing [2018]), is in development which is designed to overcome enzalutamide resistance via pan-antagonism of escape mutations in vitro, and in vivo inhibition of xenograft growth and suppression of intratumoral PSA levels in enzaluamide-resistant M49F LNCaP cells which harbor the F876L_T877A double mutant.[354] Darolutamide can be thought of as a diaryl propanamide like bicalutamide (Fig. 24.44) in which the amide is replaced with a pyrazine ring. It also competitively binds the same site of the LBD of AR as other antiandrogens; so darolutamide escape mutants are also likely to evolve. Given the cross-resistance with abiraterone acetate, secondary hormonal therapy resistant CRPC remains an unmet clinical need.

Darolutamide

First-Generation Antiandrogens

Bicalutamide (Casodex). Bicalutamide is a biaryl propanamide (Fig. 24.44) given at a dosage of 50 mg once daily in combination with a GnRH analog or surgical castration for the treatment of advanced prostate cancer in the United States. Bicalutamide is a racemate, and its antiandrogenic activity resides almost exclusively in the (*R*)-enantiomer, which has an approximately fourfold higher affinity for the prostate AR than hydroxyflutamide. The (*S*)-enantiomer has no antiandrogenic activity. (*R*)-Bicalutamide is slowly absorbed, but absorption is unaffected by food.[355] It has a terminal elimination half-life of 1 week and accumulates approximately 10-fold in plasma during daily administration (Table 24.16). (*S*)-Bicalutamide is much more rapidly absorbed and cleared from plasma. At steady state, the plasma levels of (*R*)-bicalutamide are 100 times higher than those of (*S*)-bicalutamide. Although mild to moderate hepatic impairment does not affect its pharmacokinetics, evidence suggests slower elimination of (*R*)-bicalutamide in subjects with severe hepatic impairment.[355] Bicalutamide metabolites are excreted almost equally in urine and feces, with little or no unchanged drug excreted in urine. Unmetabolized drug predominates in the plasma. (*R*)-Bicalutamide is cleared almost exclusively by CYP3A4-mediated metabolism, but glucuronidation is the predominant metabolic route for (*S*)-bicalutamide.

Flutamide (Eulexin). Flutamide is a propanamide lacking the B-ring of bicalutamide (Fig. 24.44). After oral administration (usual dose is 250 mg every 8 hr), flutamide is completely absorbed from the GI tract and

Table 24.16 Some Properties and Pharmacokinetics of the First Generation Antiandrogens

Drugs	Bicalutamide	Flutamide	Nilutamide	Enzalutamide	Apalutamide
Trade Name	Casodex	Eulexin	Nilandron	Xtandi	Erleada
cLog P[a]	4.9 ± 0.7	3.7 ± 0.4	3.3 ± 0.6	3.75	3.05
log D (pH 7)	4.9	3.7	3.3		
Oral bioavailability (%)	80-90	—	—	—	100
Onset of action (wk)[b]	8-12	2-4	1-2		
Duration of action	8 d	3 mo to 2.5 yr	1-3 mo		
Protein binding (%)	96	94-96	80-84	97-98	96
Time to peak concentration (hr)	31	2-3	1-4	0.5-3	2
Elimination half-life	~6 d	8 hr (10 hr for active metabolite)	40-60 hr	5.8 d (7.8-8.6 for active metabolite)	~3 d
Cytochrome isoforms	3A4	1A2	Flavin monooxygenase, CYP2C	2C8	2C8, 3A4
Active metabolites	None	2-hydroxy	Yes	N-desmethyl	N-desmethyl
Excretion: Feces (%) Urine (%)	43 34 (glucuronide)	<10 28	<10% 62	14% 71	24 65

[a]Chemical Abstracts, American Chemical Society, calculated using Advanced Chemistry Development (ACD/Labs) Software V8.14 for Solaris (1994-2006 ACD/Labs) or www.drugbank.ca.

[b]Time for significant improvement in prostate-specific antigen (PSA) or other biomarkers.

undergoes extensive first-pass metabolism by CYP1A2 to its major metabolite, 2-hydroxyflutamide, and its hydrolysis product, 3-trifluoromethyl-4-nitroaniline.[356] 2-Hydroxyflutamide is a more powerful antiandrogen in vivo, with higher affinity for the receptor than that of flutamide.[357] 2-Hydroxyflutamide has a terminal elimination half-life of approximately 10 hours (Table 24.16). These studies show the principal role of CYP1A2 in the metabolism of flutamide to 2-hydroxyflutamide, with minor contribution from CYP3A4. 2-Hydroxyflutamide inhibits the metabolism of flutamide and both 2- and 4-hydroxylation of 17β-estradiol. Flutamide is a pure antagonist, whereas 2-hydroxyflutamide is a more potent AR antagonist but also can activate AR escape mutants at higher concentrations.[357] These findings raise the possibility that increased conversion of flutamide to 2-hydroxyflutamide or accumulation of 2-hydroxyflutamide in cells may contribute to the anomalous responses to flutamide that are observed in some advanced prostate cancers. Rare reports of liver failure have been associated with flutamide, mandating regular monitoring of liver function tests in men taking flutamide therapy.

Nilutamide (Nilandron). Nilutamide is a hydantoin analog of flutamide, as shown in Figure 24.44, that is completely absorbed after oral administration, with a mean terminal elimination half-life of approximately 50 hours (Table 24.16).[358] Daily oral doses of nilutamide range from 150 to 300 mg per day. One of the methyl groups attached to the hydantoin ring is stereoselectively hydroxylated to a chiral metabolite, which subsequently is oxidized to its carboxylic acid metabolite. Less than 2% of nilutamide is excreted unchanged in the urine. In vitro, the nitro group of nilutamide was reduced to the amine and hydroxylamine moieties by nitric oxide (NO) synthases, a flavin monooxygenase system.[359] This reduction proceeds via formation of a nitro anion free radical or via its reduction to its hydroxylamino derivative, which could explain some of the poorly investigated toxic effects of this drug[360] which overshadow the therapeutic effects of nilutamide.

TESTICULAR CANCER

Testicular cancer develops in the testicles and, according to the National Cancer Institute (NCI), accounts only for approximately 1% of all cancers in men with an estimated 9,000 new cases in 2018.[315] Compared with prostate cancer, testicular cancer is relatively rare. It is most common among males between 15 and 40 years of age and is approximately fourfold more common in white men than in black men.

Nearly all testicular tumors originate from germ cells, the specialized sperm-forming cells within the testicles. These tumors fall into one of two types, seminomas or nonseminomas.[361] Seminomas account for approximately 40% of all testicular cancer and are made up of immature germ cells. Seminomas are slow-growing and tend to stay localized in the testicle for long periods. Nonseminomas arise from more mature, specialized germ cells and tend to be more aggressive than seminomas. According to the American Cancer Society, 60%-70% of patients with nonseminomas have cancer that has spread to the lymph nodes. α-Fetoprotein is a tumor-associated marker in blood for testicular cancer. Its measurement can help to show how well the chemotherapeutic drugs are working. Because seminomas are slow-growing, they tend to stay localized and usually are diagnosed at stage I (confined to testicle) or stage II (spread to lymph nodes). Treatment might be a combination of testicle removal, radiation, or chemotherapy. Most nonseminomas are not diagnosed at stage I. Advanced testicular cancer (stage III, metastasized to other tissues) seminomas, as well as stage II and stage III nonseminomas, usually are treated with multidrug chemotherapy. The majority of cases are stage I when first identified; stage III cases are relatively rare.

Chemotherapy is the standard treatment, with or without radiation, when the cancer has spread to other parts of the body. The drugs approved to treat testicular cancer include ifosfamide, etoposide, vinblastine, bleomycin, and cisplatin (Chapter 33). Cisplatin usually is given in combination with bleomycin and etoposide or other chemotherapy drugs following surgery or radiation therapy. Testicular cancer has one of the highest cure rates of all cancers, essentially 100% at stage I. Approximately 90% of men with advanced testicular cancer can be cured, according to the NCI. Because testicular cancer is curable when detected early, the NCI recommends regular monthly testicular self-examination after a hot shower, when the scrotum is looser, feeling for lumps or enlargement.

ACKNOWLEDGMENTS

The authors wish to acknowledge the work of Duane D. Miller, PhD and Dr. Robert W. Brueggemeier, PhD who authored content used within this chapter in a previous edition of this text.

Structure Challenge

The structures of 15 drugs discussed in this chapter are provided. Use your knowledge of medicinal chemistry to identify the indicated hormone or select the appropriate drug as described below.

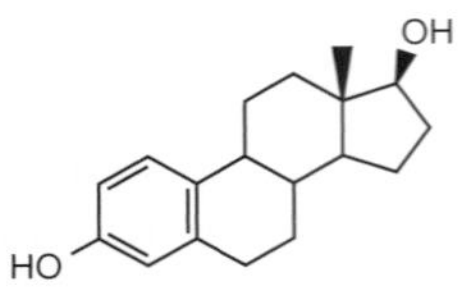

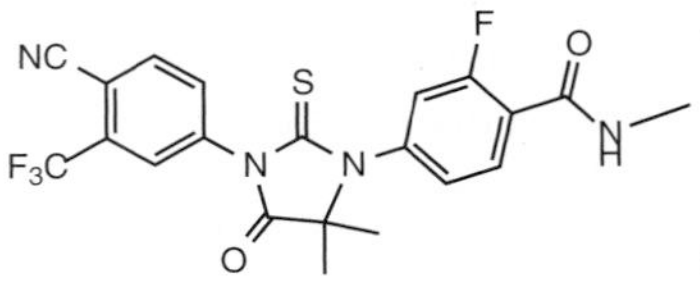

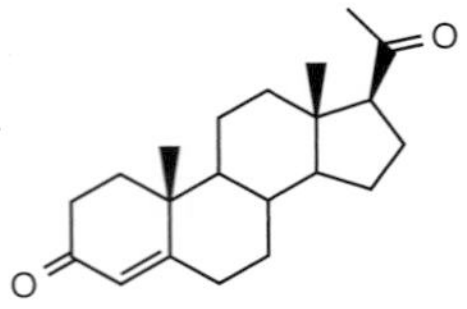

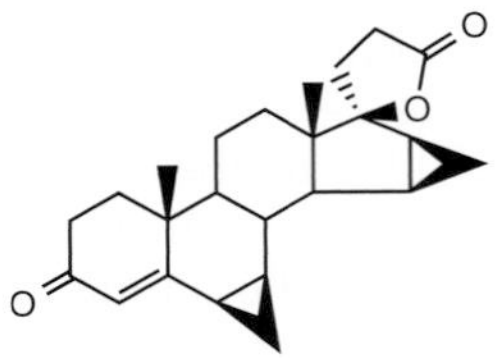

A. The most potent endogenous estrogen. # __
B. A potent endogenous androgen which is also delivered parenterally for hypogonadism. # ___
C. The most potent endogenous progestin. # ___
D. A phosphodiesterase inhibitor used in erectile dysfunction. # ___
E. An orally bioavailable estrogen commonly used in hormone replacement therapies or combination oral contraceptives. # ___
F. A steroidal PR antagonist used in emergency contraception. # __
G. An anabolic AR agonist. # __
H. A selective estrogen receptor modulator used in the treatment of breast cancer. # __
I. A 5α-reductase inhibitor used for benign prostatic hyperplasia. # __
J. A nonsteroidal aromatase inhibitor used in the treatment of breast cancer. # __
K. A second-generation steroidal progestin commonly used in oral contraceptives. # __
L. An α-adrenergic antagonist used for benign prostatic hyperplasia. # __
M. A fourth-generation steroidal progestin commonly used in oral contraceptives. # __
N. A nonsteroidal AR antagonist used in prostate cancer. # __
O. A steroidal ER antagonist used in breast cancer. # __

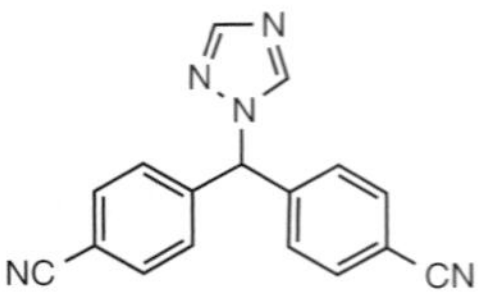

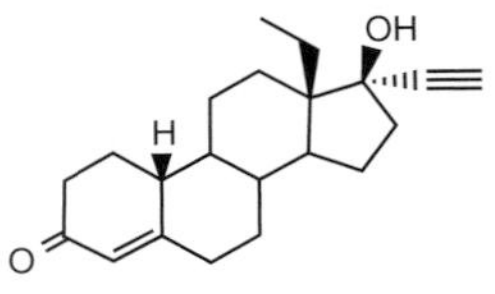

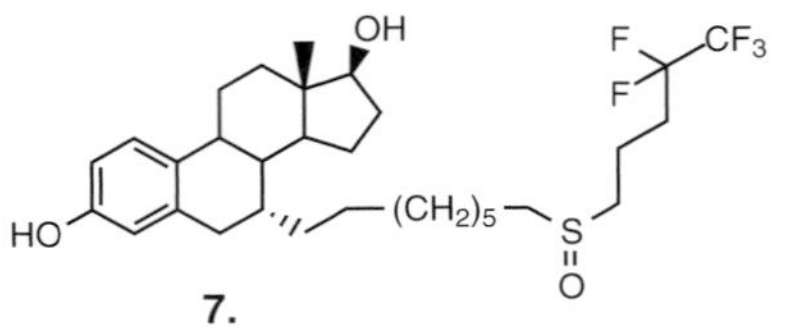

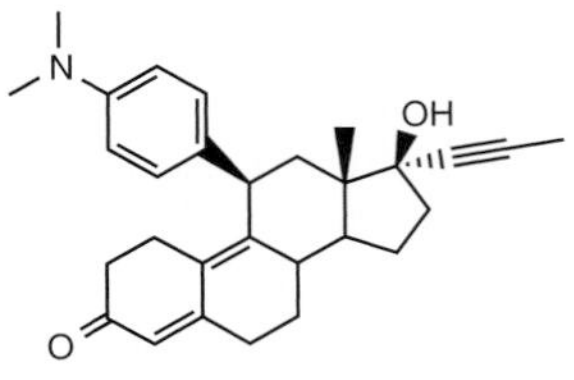

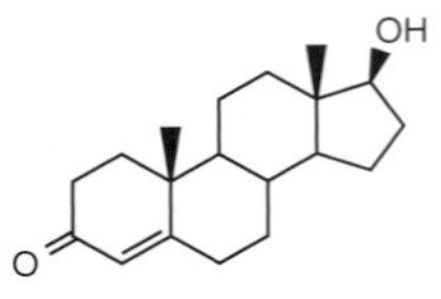

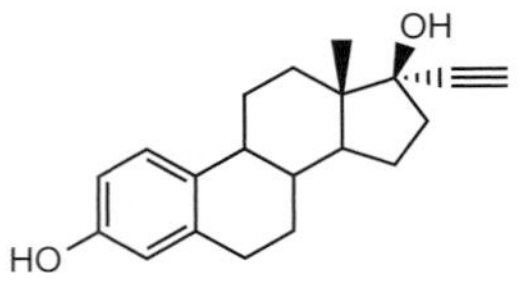

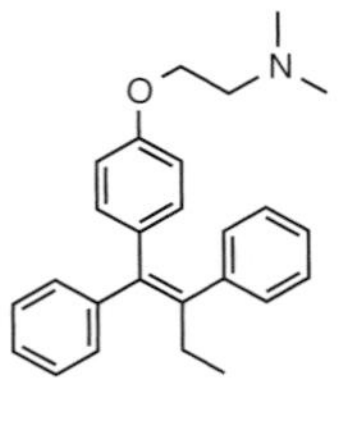

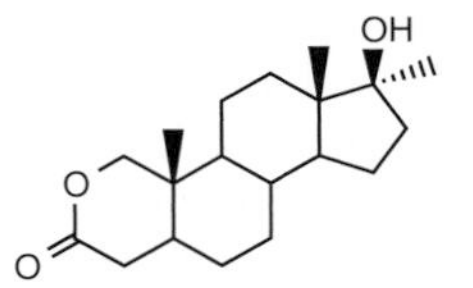

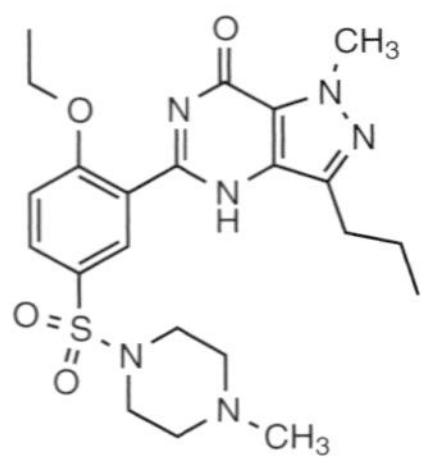

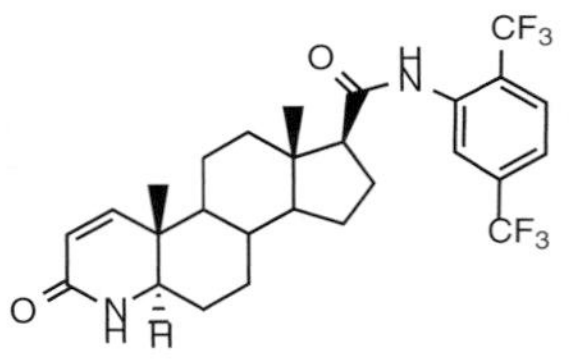

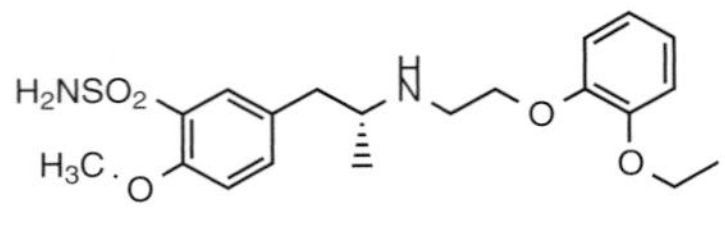

Structure Challenge answers found immediately after References.

REFERENCES

1. Simpson ER, Merrill JC, Hollub AJ, Graham-Lorence S, Mendelson CR. Regulation of estrogen biosynthesis by human adipose cells. *Endocr Rev*. 1989;10:136.
2. Fishman J, Brown JB, Hellman L, Zumoff B, Gallagher TF. Estrogen metabolism in normal and pregnant women. *J Biol Chem*. 1962;237:1489-1494.
3. Gurpide E, Angers M, Vande Wiele RL, Lieberman S. Determination of secretory rates of estrogens in pregnant and non-pregnant women from the specific activities of urinary metabolites. *J Clin Endocrinol Metab*. 1962;22:935-945.
4. Nakajin S, Hall PF. Microsomal cytochrome P-450 from neonatal pig testis. Purification and properties of A C21 steroid side-chain cleavage system (17 alpha-hydroxylase-C17,20 lyase). *J Biol Chem*. 1981;256:3871.
5. Liao S, Liang T, Fang S, Castaneda E, Shao TC. Steroid structure and androgenic activity. Specificities involved in the receptor binding and nuclear retention of various androgens. *J Biol Chem*. 1973;248:6154-6162.
6. Brueggemeier RW. Male sex hormones, analogues, and antagonists. In: Burger A, Abraham DJ, eds. *Burger's Medicinal Chemistry and Drug Discovery*. 6th ed. Hoboken, N.J.: Wiley; 2003.
7. Dorfman RI, Ungar F. *Metabolism of Steroid Hormones*. New York: Academic Press; 1965.
8. Thigpen AE, Silver RI, Guileyardo JM, Casey ML, McConnell JD, Russell DW. Tissue distribution and ontogeny of steroid 5 alpha-reductase isozyme expression. *J Clin Invest*. 1993;92:903-910.
9. Russell DW, Berman DM, Bryant JT, et al. The molecular genetics of steroid 5 alpha-reductases. *Recent Prog Horm Res*. 1994;49:275-284.
10. Johansen KL. Testosterone metabolism and replacement therapy in patients with end-stage renal disease. *Semin Dial*. 2004;17:202-208.
11. Vermeulen A, Kaufman JM, Goemaere S, van Pottelberg I. Estradiol in elderly men. *Aging Male*. 2002;5:98-102.
12. Fotherby K, James F, Atkinson L, Dumasia M. Studies in the aromatization of a synthetic progestin. *J Endocrinol*. 1972;52:v-vi.
13. Dorfman RI, Hamilton JB. Urinary excretion of androgenic substances after intramuscular and oral administration of testosterone propionate to humans. *J Clin Invest*. 1939;18:67-71.
14. Taylor W, Scratcherd T. Steroid metabolism in the rabbit. Biliary and urinary excretion of metabolites of [4-14-C]testosterone. *Biochem J*. 1967;104:250-253.
15. Brown JB. The determination and significance of the natural estrogens. *Adv Clin Chem*. 1960;3:157-233.
16. Diczfalusy E, Lauritzen C. *Oestrogene Beim Menschen*. Berlin: Springer; 1961.
17. Breuer H. Metabolism of the natural estrogens. *Vitam Horm*. 1962;20:285.
18. Merriam GR, Lipsett MB, John E; Fogarty International Center for Advanced Study in the Health Sciences. *Catechol Estrogens*. New York: Raven Press; 1983.
19. Allen E, Doisy EA. Landmark article Sept 8, 1923. An ovarian hormone. Preliminary report on its localization, extraction and partial purification, and action in test animals. By Edgar Allen and Edward A. Doisy. *JAMA*. 1983;250:2681-2683.
20. Williams C, Stancel GM. Chapter 57. In: Goodman LS, Gilman A, Hardman JG, Gilman AG, Limbird LE, eds. *Goodman & Gilman's the Pharmacological Basis of Therapeutics*. 9th ed. New York: McGraw-Hill, Health Professions Division; 1996:1411-1440.
21. Ruentiz PC. Chapter 47. In: Burger A, Wolff ME, eds. *Burger's Medicinal Chemistry and Drug Discovery*. Vol 4. 5th ed. New York: Wiley; 1995:553-558.
22. Harris GW, Naftolin F. The hypothalamus and control of ovulation. *Br Med Bull*. 1970;26:3-9.
23. Jaffe RB, et al. Chapter 1. In: Lednicer D, ed. *Contraception: The Chemical Control of Fertility*. New York: M. Dekker; 1969:xiv, 269 p.
24. U.S. Census Bureau. Population Division. Projections by Age and Sex Composition of the Population (Table 2: Projected 5-Year Age Groups and Sex Composition: Main Projections Series for the United States, 2017-2060). Available at https://census.gov/data/tables/2017/demo/popproj/2017-summary-tables.html. Accessed April 10, 2018.
25. MacGregor JI, Jordan VC. Basic guide to the mechanisms of antiestrogen action. *Pharmacol Rev*. 1998;50:151-196.
26. Jensen EV, Jacobson HI. Basic guides to the mechanism of estrogen action. *Recent Prog Horm Res*. 1962;18:387-414.
27. Greene GL, Gilna P, Waterfield M, Baker A, Hort Y, Shine J. Sequence and expression of human estrogen receptor complementary DNA. *Science*. 1986;231:1150-1154.
28. Green S, Walter P, Kumar V, et al. Human oestrogen receptor cDNA: sequence, expression and homology to v-erb-A. *Nature*. 1986;320:134-139.
29. Couse JF, Curtis SW, Washburn TF, et al. Analysis of transcription and estrogen insensitivity in the female mouse after targeted disruption of the estrogen receptor gene. *Mol Endocrinol*. 1995;9:1441-1454.
30. Kuiper GG, Enmark E, Pelto-Huikko M, Nilsson S, Gustafsson JA. Cloning of a novel receptor expressed in rat prostate and ovary. *Proc Natl Acad Sci USA*. 1996;93:5925-5930.
31. Lubahn DB, Moyer JS, Golding TS, Couse JF, Korach KS, Smithies O. Alteration of reproductive function but not prenatal sexual development after insertional disruption of the mouse estrogen receptor gene. *Proc Natl Acad Sci USA*. 1993;90:11162-11166.
32. Couse JF, Korach KS. Estrogen receptor null mice: what have we learned and where will they lead us? *Endocr Rev*. 1999;20:358-417.
33. Curtis Hewitt S, Couse JF, Korach KS. Estrogen receptor transcription and transactivation: estrogen receptor knockout mice: what their phenotypes reveal about mechanisms of estrogen action. *Breast Cancer Res*. 2000;2:345-352.
34. Deroo BJ, Korach KS. Estrogen receptors and human disease. *J Clin Invest*. 2006;116:561-570.
35. Gorski J, Welshons WV, Sakai D, et al. Evolution of a model of estrogen action. *Recent Prog Horm Res*. 1986;42:297.
36. Chan L, O'Malley BW. Mechanism of action of the sex steroid hormones (third of three parts). *N Engl J Med*. 1976;294:1430.
37. Chan L, O'Malley BW. Mechanism of action of the sex steroid hormones (second of three parts). *N Engl J Med*. 1976;294:1372.
38. Chan L, O'Malley BW. Mechanism of action of the sex steroid hormones (first of three parts). *N Engl J Med*. 1976;294:1322.
39. Noteboom WD, Gorski J. Stereospecific binding of estrogens in the rat uterus. *Arch Biochem Biophys*. 1965;111:559.
40. Mohler ML, Narayanan R, Coss CC, et al. Estrogen receptor beta selective nonsteroidal estrogens: seeking clinical indications. *Expert Opin Ther Pat*. 2010;20:507-534.
41. Ing NH, Tornesi MB. Estradiol up-regulates estrogen receptor and progesterone receptor gene expression in specific ovine uterine cells. *Biol Reprod*. 1997;56:1205-1215.
42. Rasmussen KR, Whelly SM, Barker KL. Estradiol regulation of the synthesis of uterine proteins with clusters of proline- and glycine-rich peptide sequences. *Biochim Biophys Acta*. 1988;970:177-186.
43. Revankar CM, Cimino DF, Sklar LA, Arterburn JB, Prossnitz ER. A transmembrane intracellular estrogen receptor mediates rapid cell signaling. *Science*. 2005;307:1625-1630.
44. Shughrue PJ, Lane MV, Scrimo PJ, Merchenthaler I. Comparative distribution of estrogen receptor-alpha (ER-alpha) and beta (ER-beta) mRNA in the rat pituitary, gonad, and reproductive tract. *Steroids*. 1998;63:498-504.
45. Veeneman GH. Non-steroidal subtype selective estrogens. *Curr Med Chem*. 2005;12:1077-1136.
46. Hechter O, Halkerston IDK. *The Hormones*. Vol 5. New York: Academic Press; 1964.

47. Aitken SC, Lippman ME. Hormonal regulation of de novo pyrimidine synthesis and utilization in human breast cancer cells in tissue culture. *Cancer Res*. 1983;43:4681-4690.
48. Aitken SC, Lippman ME. Effect of estrogens and antiestrogens on growth-regulatory enzymes in human breast cancer cells in tissue culture. *Cancer Res*. 1985;45:1611-1620.
49. Horwitz KB, McGuire WL. Estrogen control of progesterone receptor in human breast cancer. Correlation with nuclear processing of estrogen receptor. *J Biol Chem*. 1978;253:2223.
50. Lippman ME. *Williams Textbook of Endocrinology*. In: Williams RH, Wilson JD, eds. 9th ed. Philadelphia: Saunders; 1998:1675-1692.
51. Murad F, Kuret JA. Chapter 58. In: Goodman LS, Gilman A, eds. *Goodman and Gilman's the Pharmacological Basis of Therapeutics*. New York: Pergamon Press; 1990:1384-1412.
52. Deghenghi R, Givner ML. Chapter 29. In: Wolff ME, ed. *Burger's Medicinal Chemistry*. Vol 2. 6th ed. New York: Wiley; 1979.
53. Bentley PJ. *Endocrine Pharmacology: Physiological Basis and Therapeutic Applications*. New York: Cambridge University Press; 1980.
54. Gruber CJ, Tschugguel W, Schneeberger C, Huber JC. Production and actions of estrogens. *N Engl J Med*. 2002;346:340-352.
55. Clark JH, Guthrie SC. Agonistic and antagonistic effects of clomiphene citrate and its isomers. *Biol Reprod*. 1981;25:667-672.
56. Practice Committee of the American Society for Reproductive M. Use of clomiphene citrate in infertile women: a committee opinion. *Fertil Steril*. 2013;100:341-348.
57. Kurosawa T, Hiroi H, Momoeda M, Inoue S, Taketani Y. Clomiphene citrate elicits estrogen agonistic/antagonistic effects differentially via estrogen receptors alpha and beta. *Endocr J*. 2010;57:517-521.
58. Kim MJ, Byeon JY, Kim YH, et al. Effect of the CYP2D6*10 allele on the pharmacokinetics of clomiphene and its active metabolites. *Arch Pharm Res*. 2018;41:347-353.
59. Murdter TE, Kerb R, Turpeinen M, et al. Genetic polymorphism of cytochrome P450 2D6 determines oestrogen receptor activity of the major infertility drug clomiphene via its active metabolites. *Hum Mol Genet*. 2012;21:1145-1154.
60. Choi SH, Shapiro H, Robinson GE, et al. Psychological side-effects of clomiphene citrate and human menopausal gonadotrophin. *J Psychosom Obstet Gynaecol*. 2005;26:93-100.
61. *Clomid (Clomiphene) [prescribing information]*. Bridgewater, NJ: Sanofi-Aventis US LLC; July 2017.
62. Anstead GM, Carlson KE, Katzenellenbogen JA. The estradiol pharmacophore: ligand structure-estrogen receptor binding affinity relationships and a model for the receptor binding site. *Steroids*. 1997;62:268-303.
63. Brzozowski AM, Pike AC, Dauter Z, et al. Molecular basis of agonism and antagonism in the oestrogen receptor. *Nature*. 1997;389:753-758.
64. Shiau AK, Barstad D, Loria PM, et al. The structural basis of estrogen receptor/coactivator recognition and the antagonism of this interaction by tamoxifen. *Cell*. 1998;95:927-937.
65. Baran JS. A synthesis of 11-beta-hydroxyestrone and related 16- and 17-hydroxyestratrienes. *J Med Chem*. 1967;10:1188-1190.
66. Murkies AL, Wilcox G, Davis SR. Clinical review 92: phytoestrogens. *J Clin Endocrinol Metab*. 1998;83:297-303.
67. Heftmann E. *Steroid Biochemistry*. New York: Academic Press; 1970.
68. Baker JM, Al-Nakkash L, Herbst-Kralovetz MM. Estrogen-gut microbiome axis: physiological and clinical implications. *Maturitas*. 2017;103:45-53.
69. Fieser LF, Feiser M. *Steroids*. New York: Reinhold Pub. Corp.; 1959.
70. Kupperman HS, Blatt MH, Wiesbader H, Filler W. Comparative clinical evaluation of estrogenic preparations by the menopausal and amenorrheal indices. *J Clin Endocrinol Metab*. 1953;13:688-703.
71. Grant GA, Beall D. *Recent Prog Horm Res*. 1950;5:307.
72. Chetkowski RJ, Meldrum DR, Steingold KA, et al. Biologic effects of transdermal estradiol. *N Engl J Med*. 1986;314:1615.
73. Judd H. Efficacy of transdermal estradiol. *Am J Obstet Gynecol*. 1987;156:1326.
74. Inhoffen HH, Hohlweg W. New per os-effective female hipofisis gland hormone derivatives: 17-aethinyl-oesteridol and pregnen-in-on-3-ol-17. *Naturwissenschaften*. 1938;26:96-96.
75. Colton FB, Nysted LN, Riegel B, Raymond AL. 17-Alkyl-19-Nortestosterones. *J Am Chem Soc*. 1957;79:1123-1127.
76. Helton ED, Goldzieher JW. The pharmacokinetics of ethynyl estrogens. A review. *Contraception*. 1977;15:255-284.
77. *Menest (Estrogens, Esterified) [prescribing information]*. Bristol, TN: Monarch Pharmaceuticals; 2011.
78. Helgason S, Damber MG, von Schoultz B, Stigbrand T. Estrogenic potency of oral replacement therapy estimated by the induction of pregnancy zone protein. *Acta Obstet Gynecol Scand*. 1982;61:75-79.
79. Solmssen UV. Synthetic estrogens and the relation between their structure and their activity. *Chem Rev*. 1945;37:481-598.
80. Rubin M, Wishinsky H. Functional variants of diethylstilbestrol. *J Am Chem Soc*. 1944;66:1948-1950.
81. Dodds EC, Golberg L, Lawson W, Robinson R. Estrogenic activity of alkylated stiloestrols. *Nature*. 1938;142:34.
82. Exposure in utero to diethylstilbestrol and related synthetic hormones. Association with vaginal and cervical cancers and other abnormalities. *JAMA*. 1976;236:1107-1109.
83. Giusti RM, Iwamoto K, Hatch EE. Diethylstilbestrol revisited: a review of the long-term health effects. *Ann Intern Med*. 1995;122:778-788.
84. Hoover RN, Hyer M, Pfeiffer RM, et al. Adverse health outcomes in women exposed in utero to diethylstilbestrol. *N Engl J Med*. 2011;365:1304-1314.
85. Palmer JR, Wise LA, Hatch EE, et al. Prenatal diethylstilbestrol exposure and risk of breast cancer. *Cancer Epidemiol Biomarkers Prev*. 2006;15:1509-1514.
86. Fraenkel S. *Arch f Gynaek*. 1903;68:438.
87. Pearl R, Surface FM. *J Biol Chem*. 1914;19:263.
88. Corner GW, Allen WM. Physiology of the corpus luteum II. Production of a special uterine reaction (progestational proliferation) by extracts of the corpus luteum. *Am J Physiol*. 1929;88:326-339.
89. Makepeace AW, Weinstein GL, Friedman MH. The effect of progestin and progesterone on ovulation in the rabbit. *Am J Physiol*. 1937;119:512-516.
90. Heftmann E, Mosettig E. *Biochemistry of Steroids*. New York: Reinhold Pub. Co.; 1960.
91. Djerassi C. Steroid oral contraceptives. *Science*. 1966;151:1055.
92. Greenblatt RB, Gambrell RD Jr, Stoddard LD. The protective role of progesterone in the prevention of endometrial cancer. *Pathol Res Pract*. 1982;174:297-318.
93. Davis ME, Wied GL. 17-Alpha-hydroxyprogesterone-caproate: A new substance with prolonged progestational activity. A comparison iwth chemically pure progesterone. *J Clin Endocrinol Metab*. 1955;15:923-930.
94. Siegel I. Conception control by long-acting progestogens: preliminary report. *Obstet Gynecol*. 1963;21:666-668.
95. Klopper A. Developments in steroidal hormonal contraception. *Br Med Bull*. 1970;26:39-44.
96. Babcock JC, Gutsell ES, Herr ME, et al. 6-Alpha-methyl-17-alpha-hydroxyprogesterone 17-acylates – a new class of potent progestins. *J Am Chem Soc*. 1958;80:2904-2905.
97. Dong Y, Roberge JY, Wang Z, et al. Characterization of a new class of selective nonsteroidal progesterone receptor agonists. *Steroids*. 2004;69:201-217.
98. Ruzicka L, Hofmann K. Se hormones XXIV. On the disposition of acetylene in the 17-constant keto group of trans-androsterone and delta(5)-trans-dehydro-androsterone. *Helv Chim Acta*. 1937;20:1280-1282.

99. Klimstra PD. Progestational agents. *Am J Pharm Educ*. 1970;34:630.
100. Ehrenstein M. Investigations on steroids VIII lower homologs of hormones of the pregnane series 10-nor-11-desoxycorticosterone acetate and 10-norprogesterone. *J Org Chem*. 1944;9:435-456.
101. Djerassi C, Miramontes L, Rosenkranz G. Steroids. XLVIII.1 19-Norprogesterone, a potent progestational hormone. *J Am Chem Soc*. 1953;75:4440-4442.
102. Pincus G, Garcia CR, Paniagua M, Shepard J. Ethynodiol diacetate as a new, highly potent oral inhibitor of ovulation. *Science*. 1962;138:439-440.
103. Africander DJ, Storbeck KH, Hapgood JP. A comparative study of the androgenic properties of progesterone and the progestins, medroxyprogesterone acetate (MPA) and norethisterone acetate (NET-A). *J Steroid Biochem Mol Biol*. 2014;143:404-415.
104. Philibert D, Deraedt R, Teutsch G, Tournemine C, Sakiz E. RU38486 a new lead for steroidal antihormones. Abstract No. 668. 64th Annual Meeting of The Endocrine Society. San Francisco; June 1982.
105. Agarwal MK, Hainque B, Moustaid N, Lazer G. Glucocorticoid antagonists. *FEBS Lett*. 1987;217:221.
106. Melis GB, Piras B, Marotto MF, et al. Pharmacokinetic evaluation of ulipristal acetate for uterine leiomyoma treatment. *Expert Opin Drug Metab Toxicol*. 2012;8:901-908.
107. *Mifeprex (Mifepristone) [prescribing information]*. New York, NY: Danco Laboratories; March 2016.
108. *Cytotec (Misoprostol) [prescribing information]*. New York, NY: Pfizer; January 2017.
109. *Plan B (Levonorgestrel) [prescribing information]*. North Wales, PA: Teva Pharmaceuticals USA Inc.; 2017.
110. O'Malley BW, McGuire WL, Kohler PO, Korenman SG. Studies on the mechanism of steroid hormone regulation of synthesis of specific proteins. *Recent Prog Horm Res*. 1969;25:105.
111. Carson-Jurica MA, Schrader WT, O'Malley BW. Steroid receptor family: structure and functions. *Endocr Rev*. 1990;11:201.
112. Gronemeyer H, Turcotte B, Quirin-Stricker C, et al. The chicken progesterone receptor: sequence, expression and functional analysis. *EMBO J*. 1987;6:3985.
113. Misrahi M, Atger M, d'Auriol L, et al. Complete amino acid sequence of the human progesterone receptor deduced from cloned cDNA. *Biochem Biophys Res Commun*. 1987;143:740.
114. Carson-Jurica MA, Lee AT, Dobson AW, Conneely OM, Schrader WT, O'Malley BW. Interaction of the chicken progesterone receptor with heat shock protein (HSP) 90. *J Steroid Biochem*. 1989;34:1.
115. Fotherby K. The biochemistry of progesterone. *Vitam Horm*. 1964;22:153-204.
116. Baulieu EE. *Steroid Hormone Regulation of the Brain: Proceedings of an International Symposium Held at the Wenner-Gren Center, Stockholm 27-28 October*. Oxford, New York: Pergamon Press; 1981.
117. Majewska MD, Harrison NL, Schwartz RD, Barker JL, Paul SM. Steroid hormone metabolites are barbiturate-like modulators of the GABA receptor. *Science*. 1986;232:1004.
118. Morrow AL, Suzdak PD, Paul SM. Steroid hormone metabolites potentiate GABA receptor-mediated chloride ion flux with nanomolar potency. *Eur J Pharmacol*. 1987;142:483.
119. Baulieu EE, Robel P. Neurosteroids: a new brain function? *J Steroid Biochem Mol Biol*. 1990;37:395.
120. Rothchild I. *Metabolic Effects of Gonadal Hormones and Contraceptive Steroids*. In: Salhanick HA, Kipnis DM, Vande Wiele RL, eds. New York: Plenum Press; 1969:668.
121. Drill VA. *Oral Contraceptives*. New York: McGraw-Hill; 1966.
122. Lewis JJ, Crossland J. *Lewis's Pharmacology*. 4th ed. Baltimore: Williams and Wilkins; 1970.
123. Pincus G. Control of conception by hormonal steroids. *Science*. 1966;153:493.
124. Pincus G, Garcia CR, Rock J, et al. Effectiveness of an oral contraceptive; effects of a progestin-estrogen combination upon fertility, menstrual phenomena, and health. *Science*. 1959;130:81-83.
125. Schindler AE. Non-contraceptive benefits of oral hormonal contraceptives. *Int J Endocrinol Metab*. 2013;11:41-47.
126. van den Heuvel MW, van Bragt AJ, Alnabawy AK, Kaptein MC. Comparison of ethinylestradiol pharmacokinetics in three hormonal contraceptive formulations: the vaginal ring, the transdermal patch and an oral contraceptive. *Contraception*. 2005;72:168-174.
127. Nonhormonal management of menopause-associated vasomotor symptoms: 2015 position statement of The North American Menopause Society. *Menopause*. 2015;22:1155-1172; quiz 1173-1154.
128. Manson JE, Kaunitz AM. Menopause management–getting clinical care back on track. *N Engl J Med*. 2016;374:803-806.
129. Manson JE, Ames JM, Shapiro M, et al. Algorithm and mobile app for menopausal symptom management and hormonal/non-hormonal therapy decision making: a clinical decision-support tool from The North American Menopause Society. *Menopause*. 2015;22:247-253.
130. The Nams Hormone Therapy Position Statement Advisory Panel. The 2017 hormone therapy position statement of The North American Menopause Society. *Menopause*. 2017;24:728-753.
131. Pfizer Inc. 2017 Pfizer Financial Report to Shareholders. Available at https://investors.pfizer.com/financials/annual-reports/default.aspx. Accessed April 11, 2018.
132. *Menopause Practice, a Clinician's Guide*. 5th ed. Mayfield Heights, OH: North American Menopause Society; 2014.
133. Stuenkel CA, Davis SR, Gompel A, et al. Treatment of symptoms of the menopause: an Endocrine Society Clinical Practice Guideline. *J Clin Endocrinol Metab*. 2015;100:3975-4011.
134. Tremollieres F, Brincat M, Erel CT, et al. EMAS position statement: managing menopausal women with a personal or family history of VTE. *Maturitas*. 2011;69:195-198.
135. Pickar JH, Yeh IT, Bachmann G, Speroff L. Endometrial effects of a tissue selective estrogen complex containing bazedoxifene/conjugated estrogens as a menopausal therapy. *Fertil Steril*. 2009;92:1018-1024.
136. *Duavee (Conjugated Estrogens and Bazedoxifene Acetate) [prescribing information]*. New York, NY: Pfizer Inc; 2017.
137. Pickar JH, Komm BS. Selective estrogen receptor modulators and the combination therapy conjugated estrogens/bazedoxifene: A review of effects on the breast. *Post Reprod Health*. 2015;21:112-121.
138. Shen L, Ahmad S, Park S, et al. In vitro metabolism, permeability, and efflux of bazedoxifene in humans. *Drug Metab Dispos*. 2010;38:1471-1479.
139. Pinkerton JV, Utian WH, Constantine GD, Olivier S, Pickar JH. Relief of vasomotor symptoms with the tissue-selective estrogen complex containing bazedoxifene/conjugated estrogens: a randomized, controlled trial. *Menopause*. 2009;16:1116-1124.
140. Stuenkel CA, Santen RJ. An introduction to the Endocrine Society Clinical Practice Guideline on treatment of symptoms of the menopause. *Post Reprod Health*. 2016;22:6-8.
141. Bachmann GA, Komi JO; Ospemifene Study G. Ospemifene effectively treats vulvovaginal atrophy in postmenopausal women: results from a pivotal phase 3 study. *Menopause*. 2010;17:480-486.
142. Brown-Sequard CE. Des effects produits chez Phomme par des injections sous cutanées d'un liquide retire des testicules frais de cobaye et de chien. *CR Seanc Soc Biol*. 1889;1:420-430.
143. Pezard A. Sur la determination des caractéres sexuels secondaire chez les gallinacés. *C R H Acad Sci*. 1911;153:1027-1043.
144. Butenandt A. Chemical investigation of the sex hormones. *Angew Chem*. 1931;44:905-908.
145. Butenandt AH, Dannenberg H. Androsterone, a crystalline male sex hormone. III. Isolation of a new physiologically inert sterol derivative from male urine, its relationship to dehydroandrosterone and androsterone. *Z Physiol Chem*. 1934;229:192-208.
146. David K, Dingemanse E, Freud J, et al. Crystalline male hormone from testes (testosterone), more active than androsterone prepared from urine or cholesterol. *Z Physiol Chem*. 1935:281-282.
147. Butenandt A, Hanisch G. Testosterone. Transformation of dehydroandrosterone into androstenediol and testosterone; a way to the preparation of testosterone from cholestrol. *Chem Ber*. 1935;68B:1859-1862.

148. Kochakian CD, Murlin JR. Effect of male hormone on the protein and energy metabolism of castrate dogs. *J Nutr Biochem*. 1935;10:437-459.
149. Vale W, Wiater E, Gray P, Harrison C, Bilezikjian L, Choe SY. Activins and inhibins and their signaling. *Ann NY Acad Sci*. 2004;1038:142-147.
150. Bremner WJ, Vitiello MV, Prinz PN. Loss of circadian rhythmicity in blood testosterone levels with aging in normal men. *J Clin Endocrinol Metab*. 1983;56:1278-1281.
151. van den Beld AW, de Jong FH, Grobbee DE, Pols HA, Lamberts SW. Measures of bioavailable serum testosterone and estradiol and their relationships with muscle strength, bone density, and body composition in elderly men. *J Clin Endocrinol Metab*. 2000;85:3276-3282.
152. Ferrando AA, Sheffield-Moore M, Yeckel CW, et al. Testosterone administration to older men improves muscle function: molecular and physiological mechanisms. *Am J Physiol Endocrinol Metab*. 2002;282:E601-E607.
153. Brodsky IG, Balagopal P, Nair KS. Effects of testosterone replacement on muscle mass and muscle protein synthesis in hypogonadal men–a clinical research center study. *J Clin Endocrinol Metab*. 1996;81:3469-3475.
154. Bhasin S. Testosterone supplementation for aging-associated sarcopenia. *J Gerontol A Biol Sci Med Sci*. 2003;58:1002-1008.
155. Manolagas SC, Kousteni S, Jilka RL. Sex steroids and bone. *Recent Prog Horm Res*. 2002;57:385-409.
156. Wiren KM. Androgens and bone growth: it's location, location, location. *Curr Opin Pharmacol*. 2005;5:626-632.
157. Gao W, Bohl CE, Dalton JT. Chemistry and structural biology of androgen receptor. *Chem Rev*. 2005;105:3352-3370.
158. Lutz LB, Jamnongjit M, Yang WH, Jahani D, Gill A, Hammes SR. Selective modulation of genomic and nongenomic androgen responses by androgen receptor ligands. *Mol Endocrinol*. 2003;17:1106-1116.
159. Estrada M, Espinosa A, Muller M, Jaimovich E. Testosterone stimulates intracellular calcium release and mitogen-activated protein kinases via a G protein-coupled receptor in skeletal muscle cells. *Endocrinology*. 2003;144:3586-3597.
160. Kousteni S, Bellido T, Plotkin LI, et al. Nongenotropic, sex-nonspecific signaling through the estrogen or androgen receptors: Dissociation from transcriptional activity. *Cell*. 2001;104:719-730.
161. Zagar Y, Chaumaz G, Lieberherr M. Signaling cross-talk from G beta(4) subunit to Elk-1 in the rapid action of androgens. *J Biol Chem*. 2004;279:2403-2413.
162. Kampa M, Papakonstanti EA, Hatzoglou A, Stathopoulos EN, Stournaras C, Castanas E. The human prostate cancer cell line LNCaP bears functional membrane testosterone receptors that increase PSA secretion and modify actin cytoskeleton. *FASEB J*. 2002;16:1429-1431.
163. Unni E, Sun S, Nan B, et al. Changes in androgen receptor nongenotropic signaling correlate with transition of LNCaP cells to androgen independence. *Cancer Res*. 2004;64:7156-7168.
164. Norman AW, Mizwicki MT, Norman DP. Steroid-hormone rapid actions, membrane receptors and a conformational ensemble model. *Nat Rev Drug Discov*. 2004;3:27-41.
165. Simoncini T, Genazzani AR. Non-genomic actions of sex steroid hormones. *Eur J Endocrinol*. 2003;148:281-292.
166. Kousteni S, Chen JR, Bellido T, et al. Reversal of bone loss in mice by nongenotropic signaling of sex steroids. *Science*. 2002;298:843-846.
167. Bancroft J, Wu FC. Changes in erectile responsiveness during androgen replacement therapy. *Arch Sex Behav*. 1983;12:59-66.
168. Arver S, Dobs AS, Meikle AW, Allen RP, Sanders SW, Mazer NA. Improvement of sexual function in testosterone deficient men treated for 1 year with a permeation enhanced testosterone transdermal system. *J Urol*. 1996;155:1604-1608.
169. Oettel M. Testosterone metabolism, dose-response relationships and receptor polymorphisms: selected pharmacological/toxicological considerations on benefits versus risks of testosterone therapy in men. *Aging Male*. 2003;6:230-256.
170. Rhoden EL, Morgentaler A. Risks of testosterone-replacement therapy and recommendations for monitoring. *N Engl J Med*. 2004;350:482-492.
171. Hijazi RA, Cunningham GR. Andropause: is androgen replacement therapy indicated for the aging male? *Annu Rev Med*. 2005;56:117-137.
172. Bhasin S, Cunningham GR, Hayes FJ, et al. Testosterone therapy in men with androgen deficiency syndromes: an Endocrine Society clinical practice guideline. *J Clin Endocrinol Metab*. 2010;95:2536-2559.
173. Basaria S, Coviello AD, Travison TG, et al. Adverse events associated with testosterone administration. *N Engl J Med*. 2010;363:109-122.
174. Shackleford DM, Faassen WA, Houwing N, et al. Contribution of lymphatically transported testosterone undecanoate to the systemic exposure of testosterone after oral administration of two andriol formulations in conscious lymph duct-cannulated dogs. *J Pharmacol Exp Ther*. 2003;306:925-933.
175. Vida JA. *Androgens and Anabolic Agents: Chemistry and Pharmacology*. New York: Academic Press; 1969.
176. Segaloff A, Gabbard RB. 5 Alpha-androstane–an androgenic hydrocarbon. *Endocrinology*. 1960;67:887-889.
177. Arnold A, Potts GO, Beyler AL. The ratio of anabolic to androgenic activity of 7:17-dimethyltestosterone, oxymesterone, mestanolone and fluoxymesterone. *J Endocrinol*. 1963;28:87-92.
178. Cocconi G. First generation aromatase inhibitors–aminoglutethimide and testololactone. *Breast Cancer Res Treat*. 1994;30:57-80.
179. Kicman AT. Pharmacology of anabolic steroids. *Br J Pharmacol*. 2008;154:502-521.
180. Catlin DH, Sekera MH, Ahrens BD, Starcevic B, Chang YC, Hatton CK. Tetrahydrogestrinone: discovery, synthesis, and detection in urine. *Rapid Commun Mass Spectrom*. 2004;18:1245-1049.
181. Jasuja R, Catlin DH, Miller A, et al. Tetrahydrogestrinone is an androgenic steroid that stimulates androgen receptor-mediated, myogenic differentiation in C3H10T1/2 multipotent mesenchymal cells and promotes muscle accretion in orchidectomized male rats. *Endocrinology*. 2005;146:4472-4478.
182. Zhi L, Martinborough E. Chapter 17. Selective androgen receptor modulators (SARMs). *Annu Rep Med Chem*. 2001;36:169-180.
183. Negro-Vilar A. Selective androgen receptor modulators (SARMs): A novel approach to androgen therapy for the new millennium. *J Clin Endocr Metab*. 1999;84:3459-3462.
184. Dalton JT, Mukherjee A, Zhu ZX, Kirkovsky L, Miller DD. Discovery of nonsteroidal androgens. *Biochem Biophys Res Commun*. 1998;244:1-4.
185. Balog A, Salvati ME, Shan WF, et al. The synthesis and evaluation of [2.2.1]-bicycloazahydantoins as androgen receptor antagonists. *Bioorg Med Chem Lett*. 2004;14:6107-6111.
186. Higuchi RI, Edwards JP, Caferro TR, et al. 4-Alkyl- and 3,4-dialkyl-1,2,3,4-tetrahydro-8-pyridono[5,6-g]quinolines: potent, nonsteroidal androgen receptor agonists. *Bioorg Med Chem Lett*. 1999;9:1335-1340.
187. Zhi L, Tegley CM, Marschke KB, Jones TK. Switching androgen receptor antagonists to agonists by modifying C-ring substituents on piperidino[3,2-g]quinolinone. *Bioorg Med Chem Lett*. 1999;9:1009-1012.
188. Tucker H, Crook JW, Chesterson GJ. Nonsteroidal antiandrogens. Synthesis and structure-activity relationships of 3-substituted derivatives of 2-hydroxypropionanilides. *J Med Chem*. 1988;31:954-959.
189. Yin D, He Y, Perera MA, et al. Key structural features of nonsteroidal ligands for binding and activation of the androgen receptor. *Mol Pharmacol*. 2003;63:211-223.
190. He Y, Yin D, Perera M, et al. Novel nonsteroidal ligands with high binding affinity and potent functional activity for the androgen receptor. *Eur J Med Chem*. 2002;37:619-634.
191. Albersen M, Orabi H, Lue TF. Evaluation and treatment of erectile dysfunction in the aging male: a mini-review. *Gerontology*. 2012;58(1):3-14.

192. Bohl CE, Gao W, Miller DD, Bell CE, Dalton JT. Structural basis for antagonism and resistance of bicalutamide in prostate cancer. *Proc Natl Acad Sci USA*. 2005;102:6201-6206.
193. Mohler ML, Bohl CE, Jones A, et al. Nonsteroidal selective androgen receptor modulators (SARMs): dissociating the anabolic and androgenic activities of the androgen receptor for therapeutic benefit. *J Med Chem*. 2009;52:3597-3617.
194. Boolell M, Allen MJ, Ballard SA, et al. Sildenafil: an orally active type 5 cyclic GMP-specific phosphodiesterase inhibitor for the treatment of penile erectile dysfunction. *Int J Impot Res*. 1996;8:47-52.
195. Gupta M, Kovar A, Meibohm B. The clinical pharmacokinetics of phosphodiesterase-5 inhibitors for erectile dysfunction. *J Clin Pharmacol*. 2005;45:987-1003.
196. Porst H, Rosen R, Padma-Nathan H, et al. The efficacy and tolerability of vardenafil, a new, oral, selective phosphodiesterase type 5 inhibitor, in patients with erectile dysfunction: the first at-home clinical trial. *Int J Impot Res*. 2001;13:192-199.
197. Saenz de Tejada I, Angulo J, Cuevas P, et al. The phosphodiesterase inhibitory selectivity and the in vitro and in vivo potency of the new PDE5 inhibitor vardenafil. *Int J Impot Res*. 2001;13:282-290.
198. Corbin JD, Beasley A, Blount MA, Francis SH. Vardenafil: structural basis for higher potency over sildenafil in inhibiting cGMP-specific phosphodiesterase-5 (PDE5). *Neurochem Int*. 2004;45:859-863.
199. Kuan J, Brock G. Selective phosphodiesterase type 5 inhibition using tadalafil for the treatment of erectile dysfunction. *Expert Opin Inv Drug*. 2002;11:1605-1613.
200. Kotera J, Mochida H, Inoue H, et al. Avanafil, a potent and highly selective phosphodiesterase-5 inhibitor for erectile dysfunction. *J Urol*. 2012;188:668-674.
201. Sakamoto T, Koga Y, Hikota M, et al. The discovery of avanafil for the treatment of erectile dysfunction: a novel pyrimidine-5-carboxamide derivative as a potent and highly selective phosphodiesterase 5 inhibitor. *Bioorg Med Chem Lett*. 2014;24:5460-5465.
202. Goldstein I, McCullough AR, Jones LA, et al. A randomized, double-blind, placebo-controlled evaluation of the safety and efficacy of avanafil in subjects with erectile dysfunction. *J Sex Med*. 2012;9:1122-1133.
203. *Stendra (Avanafil) [package insert]*. Cranford, NJ: Mist Pharmaceuticals, LLC; 2017.
204. Kyle JA, Brown DA, Hill JK. Avanafil for erectile dysfunction. *Ann Pharmacother*. 2013;47:1312-1320.
205. Huang YY, Li Z, Cai YH, et al. The molecular basis for the selectivity of tadalafil toward phosphodiesterase 5 and 6: a modeling study. *J Chem Inf Model*. 2013;53:3044-3053.
206. Setter SM, Iltz JL, Fincham JE, Campbell RK, Baker DE. Phosphodiesterase 5 inhibitors for erectile dysfunction. *Ann Pharmacother*. 2005;39:1286-1295.
207. Pissarnitski D. Phosphodiesterase 5 (PDE 5) inhibitors for the treatment of male erectile disorder: attaining selectivity versus PDE6. *Med Res Rev*. 2006;26:369-395.
208. Corona G, Rastrelli G, Burri A, Jannini EA, Maggi M. The safety and efficacy of Avanafil, a new 2(nd) generation PDE5i: comprehensive review and meta-analysis. *Expert Opin Drug Saf*. 2016;15:237-247.
209. Kloner RA. Cardiovascular effects of the 3 phosphodiesterase-5 inhibitors approved for the treatment of erectile dysfunction. *Circulation*. 2004;110:3149-3155.
210. Beckman TJ, Abu-Lebdeh HS, Mynderse LA. Evaluation and medical management of erectile dysfunction. *Mayo Clin Proc*. 2006;81:385-390.
211. Mcdonaldgibson WJ, Mcdonald R, Greaves MW. Prostaglandin-E1 metabolism by human plasma. *Prostaglandins*. 1972;2:251.
212. Kamel HK. Male osteoporosis – new trends in diagnosis and therapy. *Drug Aging*. 2005;22:741-748.
213. Bushman W. Etiology, epidemiology, and natural history of benign prostatic hyperplasia. *Urol Clin North Am*. 2009;36:403-415, v.
214. GlobalData. OpportunityAnalyzer: Benign Prostatic Hyperplasia – Opportunity Analysis and Forecast to 2024. Available at https://www.globaldata.com/store/report/gdhc040poa–opportunityanalyzer-benign-prostatic-hyperplasia-opportunity-analysis-and-forecast-to-2024/#.Vflg0ZddUQ0?utm_source=email&utm_medium=pr&utm_campaign=gdphpr1509&utm_nooveride=1. Accessed April 7, 2018.
215. Barry MJ, Fowler FJ Jr, O'Leary MP, et al. The American Urological Association Symptom Index for Benign Prostatic Hyperplasia. *J Urol*. 2017;197:S189-S197.
216. American Urological Association. Management of Benign Prostatic Hyperplasia (BPH). Available at http://www.auanet.org/guidelines/benign-prostatic-hyperplasia-(2010-reviewed-and-validity-confirmed-2014)#x2513. Accessed April 7, 2018.
217. Tan SY, Antonipillai I, Murphy BE. Inhibition of testosterone metabolism in the human prostate. *J Clin Endocrinol Metab*. 1974;39:936-941.
218. Andriole G, Bruchovsky N, Chung LWK, et al. Dihydrotestosterone and the prostate: the scientific rationale for 5 alpha-reductase inhibitors in the treatment of benign prostatic hyperplasia. *J Urol*. 2004;172:1399-1403.
219. Lee M, Sharifi R. Benign prostatic hyperplasia: diagnosis and treatment guideline. *Ann Pharmacother*. 1997;31:481-486.
220. Tarter TH, Vaughan ED. Inhibitors of 5 alpha-reductase in the treatment of benign prostatic hyperplasia. *Curr Pharm Design*. 2006;12:775-783.
221. Shibata Y, Ito K, Suzuki K, et al. Changes in the endocrine environment of the human prostate transition zone with aging: simultaneous quantitative analysis of prostatic sex steroids and comparison with human prostatic histological composition. *Prostate*. 2000;42:45-55.
222. Liang T, Cascieri MA, Cheung AH, Reynolds GF, Rasmusson GH. Species differences in prostatic steroid 5 alpha-reductases of rat, dog, and human. *Endocrinology*. 1985;117:571.
223. Martin DJ. Preclinical pharmacology of alpha(1)-adrenoceptor antagonists. *Eur Urol*. 1999;36:35-41.
224. Tatemichi S, Tomiyama Y, Maruyama I, et al. Uroselectivity in male dogs of silodosin (KMD-3213), a novel drug for the obstructive component of benign prostatic hyperplasia. *Neurourol Urodyn*. 2006;25:792-799; discussion 800-791.
225. Cavalli A, Lattion AL, Hummler E, et al. Decreased blood pressure response in mice deficient of the alpha(1b)-adrenergic receptor. *Proc Natl Acad Sci USA*. 1997;94:11589-11594.
226. Amadesi S, Varani K, Spisani L, et al. Comparison of prazosin, terazosin and tamsulosin: functional and binding studies in isolated prostatic and vascular human tissues. *Prostate*. 2001;47:231-238.
227. Foglar R, Shibata K, Horie K, Hirasawa A, Tsujimoto G. Use of recombinant alpha(1)-adrenoceptors to characterize subtype selectivity of drugs for the treatment of prostatic hypertrophy. *Eur J Pharmacol*. 1995;288:201-207.
228. Michel MC. The forefront for novel therapeutic agents based on the pathophysiology of lower urinary tract dysfunction: alpha-blockers in the treatment of male voiding dysfunction – how do they work and why do they differ in tolerability? *J Pharmacol Sci*. 2010;112:151-157.
229. Cordes EH. *Hallelujah Moments: Tales of Drug Discovery*. Oxford: Oxford University Press; 2014.
230. Stoner E. The clinical development of a 5 alpha-reductase inhibitor, finasteride. *J Steroid Biochem Mol Biol*. 1990;37:375-378.
231. Liss MA, Thompson IM. Prostate cancer prevention with 5-alpha reductase inhibitors: concepts and controversies. *Curr Opin Urol*. 2018;28:42-45.
232. Azzouni F, Godoy A, Li Y, Mohler J. The 5 alpha-reductase isozyme family: a review of basic biology and their role in human diseases. *Adv Urol*. 2012;2012:530121.
233. Peterson CM. Progestogens, progesterone antagonists, progesterone, androgens – synthesis, classification, and uses. *Clin Obstet Gynecol*. 1995;38:813-820.
234. Rasmusson GH, Reynolds GF, Steinberg NG, et al. Azasteroids: structure-activity relationships for inhibition of 5 alpha- reductase and of androgen receptor binding. *J Med Chem*. 1986;29:2298.

235. McConnell JD, Wilson JD, George FW, Geller J, Pappas F, Stoner E. Finasteride, an inhibitor of 5 alpha-reductase, suppresses prostatic dihydrotestosterone in men with benign prostatic hyperplasia. *J Clin Endocrinol Metab.* 1992;74:505.
236. Djavan B, Milani S, Fong YK. Dutasteride: a novel dual inhibitor of 5 alpha-reductase for benign prostatic hyperplasia. *Expert Opin Pharmaco.* 2005;6:311-317.
237. Vermeulen A, Giagulli VA, De Schepper P, Buntinx A, Stoner E. Hormonal effects of an orally active 4-azasteroid inhibitor of 5 alpha- reductase in humans. *Prostate.* 1989;14:45.
238. Bull HG, GarciaCalvo M, Andersson S, et al. Mechanism-based inhibition of human steroid 5 alpha-reductase by finasteride: enzyme-catalyzed formation of NADP-dihydrofinasteride, a potent bisubstrate analog inhibitor. *J Am Chem Soc.* 1996;118:2359-2365.
239. Stuart JD, Lee FW, Noel DS, et al. Pharmacokinetic parameters and mechanisms of inhibition of rat type 1 and 2 steroid 5 alpha-reductases: determinants for different in vivo activities of GI198745 and finasteride in the rat. *Biochem Pharmacol.* 2001;62:933-942.
240. Bakshi RK, Rasmusson GH, Patel GF, et al. 4-Aza-3-oxo-5 alpha-androst-1-ene-17 beta-N-aryl-carboxamides as dual inhibitors of human type 1 and type 2 steroid 5 alpha-reductases. Dramatic effect of N-aryl substituents on type 1 and type 2 5 alpha-reductase inhibitory potency. *J Med Chem.* 1995;38:3189-3192.
241. Steiner JF. Clinical pharmacokinetics and pharmacodynamics of finasteride. *Clin Pharmacokinet.* 1996;30:16-27.
242. *Proscar (Finasteride) [package insert].* Whitehouse Station, NJ: Merck Sharp & Dohme Corp.; 2013.
243. Frye SV. Discovery and clinical development of dutasteride, a potent dual 5 alpha-reductase inhibitor. *Curr Top Med Chem.* 2006;6:405-421.
244. Dolder CR. Dutasteride: a dual 5-alpha reductase inhibitor for the treatment of symptomatic benign prostatic hyperplasia. *Ann Pharmacother.* 2006;40:658-665.
245. Roehrborn CG, Boyle P, Nickel JC, et al. Efficacy and safety of a dual inhibitor of 5-alpha-reductase types 1 and 2 (dutasteride) in men with benign prostatic hyperplasia. *Urology.* 2002;60:434-441.
246. Corona G, Tirabassi G, Santi D, et al. Sexual dysfunction in subjects treated with inhibitors of 5alpha-reductase for benign prostatic hyperplasia: a comprehensive review and meta-analysis. *Andrology.* 2017;5:671-678.
247. *Avodart (Dutasteride) [package insert].* Research Triangle Park, NC: GlaxoSmithKline; 2014.
248. Buck AC. Is there a scientific basis for the therapeutic effects of serenoa repens in benign prostatic hyperplasia? Mechanisms of action. *J Urol.* 2004;172:1792-1799.
249. Barry MJ, Meleth S, Lee JY, et al. Effect of increasing doses of saw palmetto extract on lower urinary tract symptoms: a randomized trial. *JAMA.* 2011;306:1344-1351.
250. Stevermer JJ, Easley SK. Treatment of prostatitis. *Am Fam Physician.* 2000;61:3015-3022, 3025-3016.
251. Charalabopoulos K, Karachalios G, Baltogiannis D, Charalabopoulos A, Giannakopoulos X, Sofikitis N. Penetration of antimicrobial agents into the prostate. *Chemotherapy.* 2003;49:269-279.
252. Swanson GM. Breast-cancer risk-estimation – a translational statistic for communication to the public. *J Natl Cancer Inst.* 1993;85:848-849.
253. Slamon DJ, Godolphin W, Jones LA, et al. Studies of the HER-2/neu proto-oncogene in human breast and ovarian cancer. *Science.* 1989;244:707-712.
254. Segovia-Mendoza M, Gonzalez-Gonzalez ME, Barrera D, Diaz L, Garcia-Becerra R. Efficacy and mechanism of action of the tyrosine kinase inhibitors gefitinib, lapatinib and neratinib in the treatment of HER2-positive breast cancer: preclinical and clinical evidence. *Am J Cancer Res.* 2015;5:2531-2561.
255. Anestis A, Karamouzis MV, Dalagiorgou G, Papavassiliou AG. Is androgen receptor targeting an emerging treatment strategy for triple negative breast cancer? *Cancer Treat Rev.* 2015;41:547-553.
256. Hartkopf AD, Taran FA, Wallwiener M, et al. PD-1 and PD-L1 immune checkpoint blockade to treat breast cancer. *Breast Care (Basel).* 2016;11:385-390.
257. Abramson VG, Lehmann BD, Ballinger TJ, Pietenpol JA. Subtyping of triple-negative breast cancer: implications for therapy. *Cancer.* 2015;121:8-16.
258. Welcsh PL, King MC. BRCA1 and BRCA2 and the genetics of breast and ovarian cancer. *Hum Mol Genet.* 2001;10:705-713.
259. Grann VR, Jacobson JS, Whang W, et al. Prevention with tamoxifen or other hormones versus prophylactic surgery in BRCA1/2-positive women: a decision analysis. *Cancer J Sci Am.* 2000;6:13-20.
260. King MC, Wieand S, Hale K, et al. Tamoxifen and breast cancer incidence among women with inherited mutations in BRCA1 and BRCA2: National Surgical Adjuvant Breast and Bowel Project (NSABP-P1) Breast Cancer Prevention Trial. *JAMA.* 2001;286:2251-2256.
261. First PARP inhibitor Ok'd for breast cancer. *Cancer Discov.* 2018;8:256-257.
262. Swain SM, Jeong JH, Geyer CE Jr, et al. Longer therapy, iatrogenic amenorrhea, and survival in early breast cancer. *N Engl J Med.* 2010;362:2053-2065.
263. Albain KS, Barlow WE, Shak S, et al. Prognostic and predictive value of the 21-gene recurrence score assay in postmenopausal women with node-positive, oestrogen-receptor-positive breast cancer on chemotherapy: a retrospective analysis of a randomised trial. *Lancet Oncol.* 2010;11:55-65.
264. Ohnstad HO, Borgen E, Falk RS, et al. Prognostic value of PAM50 and risk of recurrence score in patients with early-stage breast cancer with long-term follow-up. *Breast Cancer Res.* 2017;19:120.
265. National Comprehensive Cancer Network. Available at https://www.nccn.org/. Accessed April 2, 2018.
266. Rudloff U, Jacks LM, Goldberg JI, et al. Nomogram for predicting the risk of local recurrence after breast-conserving surgery for ductal carcinoma in situ. *J Clin Oncol.* 2010;28:3762-3769.
267. Breast International Group 1-98 Collaborative G; Thurlimann B, Keshaviah A, et al. A comparison of letrozole and tamoxifen in postmenopausal women with early breast cancer. *N Engl J Med.* 2005;353:2747-2757.
268. Wijayaratne AL, Nagel SC, Paige LA, et al. Comparative analyses of mechanistic differences among antiestrogens. *Endocrinology.* 1999;140:5828-5840.
269. Paech K, Webb P, Kuiper GG, et al. Differential ligand activation of estrogen receptors ERalpha and ERbeta at AP1 sites. *Science.* 1997;277:1508-1510.
270. Schacke H, Berger M, Rehwinkel H, Asadullah K. Selective glucocorticoid receptor agonists (SEGRAs): novel ligands with an improved therapeutic index. *Mol Cell Endocrinol.* 2007;275:109-117.
271. Mohler ML, He Y, Wu Z, Hong SS, Miller DD. Dissociated non-steroidal glucocorticoids: tuning out untoward effects. *Expert Opin Ther Pat.* 2007;17:37-58.
272. Fisher B, Costantino JP, Wickerham DL, et al. Tamoxifen for prevention of breast cancer: report of the National Surgical Adjuvant Breast and Bowel Project P-1 Study. *J Natl Cancer Inst.* 1998;90:1371-1388.
273. Okubo I, Kondo M, Toi M, Ochiai T, Miki S. Cost-effectiveness of letrozole versus tamoxifen as first-line hormonal therapy in treating postmenopausal women with advanced breast cancer in Japan. *Gan To Kagaku Ryoho.* 2005;32:351-363.
274. Day R, Ganz PA, Costantino JP, Cronin WM, Wickerham DL, Fisher B. Health-related quality of life and tamoxifen in breast cancer prevention: a report from the National Surgical Adjuvant Breast and Bowel Project P-1 Study. *J Clin Oncol.* 1999;17:2659-2669.
275. Wickramage I, Tennekoon KH, Ariyaratne MA, Hewage AS, Sundralingam T. CYP2D6 polymorphisms may predict occurrence of adverse effects to tamoxifen: a preliminary retrospective study. *Breast Cancer (Dove Med Press).* 2017;9:111-120.
276. Borgna JL, Rochefort H. Hydroxylated metabolites of tamoxifen are formed in vivo and bound to estrogen receptor in target tissues. *J Biol Chem.* 1981;256:859-868.

277. Johnson MD, Zuo H, Lee KH, et al. Pharmacological characterization of 4-hydroxy-N-desmethyl tamoxifen, a novel active metabolite of tamoxifen. *Breast Cancer Res Treat.* 2004;85:151-159.
278. Sirachainan E, Jaruhathai S, Trachu N, et al. CYP2D6 polymorphisms influence the efficacy of adjuvant tamoxifen in Thai breast cancer patients. *Pharmgenomics Pers Med.* 2012;5:149-153.
279. Goetz MP, Sangkuhl K, Guchelaar HJ, et al. Clinical pharmacogenetics implementation consortium (CPIC) guideline for CYP2D6 and tamoxifen therapy. *Clin Pharmacol Ther.* 2018;103(5):770-777.
280. Donneyong MM, Bykov K, Bosco-Levy P, Dong YH, Levin R, Gagne JJ. Risk of mortality with concomitant use of tamoxifen and selective serotonin reuptake inhibitors: multi-database cohort study. *BMJ.* 2016;354:i5014.
281. Juurlink D. Revisiting the drug interaction between tamoxifen and SSRI antidepressants. *BMJ.* 2016;354:i5309.
282. *Tamoxifen Citrate [package insert].* Corona, CA: Watson Laboratories; 2011.
283. Reid JM, Goetz MP, Buhrow SA, et al. Pharmacokinetics of endoxifen and tamoxifen in female mice: implications for comparative in vivo activity studies. *Cancer Chemother Pharmacol.* 2014;74:1271-1278.
284. Kim J, Coss CC, Barrett CM, et al. Role and pharmacologic significance of cytochrome P-450 2D6 in oxidative metabolism of toremifene and tamoxifen. *Int J Cancer.* 2013;132:1475-1485.
285. Vogel CL, Johnston MA, Capers C, Braccia D. Toremifene for breast cancer: a review of 20 years of data. *Clin Breast Cancer.* 2014;14:1-9.
286. Palacios S, Cancelo MJ. Clinical update on the use of ospemifene in the treatment of severe symptomatic vulvar and vaginal atrophy. *Int J Womens Health.* 2016;8:617-626.
287. Mao C, Yang ZY, He BF, et al. Toremifene versus tamoxifen for advanced breast cancer. *Cochrane Database Syst Rev.* 2012:CD008926.
288. Vogelvang TE, van der Mooren MJ, Mijatovic V, Kenemans P. Emerging selective estrogen receptor modulators: special focus on effects on coronary heart disease in postmenopausal women. *Drugs.* 2006;66:191-221.
289. Chumsri S, Howes T, Bao T, Sabnis G, Brodie A. Aromatase, aromatase inhibitors, and breast cancer. *J Steroid Biochem Mol Biol.* 2011;125:13-22.
290. Fishman J, Raju MS. Mechanism of estrogen biosynthesis. Stereochemistry of C-1 hydrogen elimination in the aromatization of 2 beta-hydroxy-19-oxoandrostenedione. *J Biol Chem.* 1981;256:4472-4477.
291. *Femara (Letrozole) [prescribing information].* East Hanover, NJ: Novartis; 2017.
292. Cohen MH, Johnson JR, Justice R, Pazdur R. Approval summary: letrozole (Femara® tablets) for adjuvant and extended adjuvant postmenopausal breast cancer treatment: conversion of accelerated to full approval. *Oncologist.* 2011;16:1762-1770.
293. Simpson D, Curran MP, Perry CM. Letrozole: a review of its use in postmenopausal women with breast cancer. *Drugs.* 2004;64:1213-1230.
294. Dunn C, Keam SJ. Letrozole: a pharmacoeconomic review of its use in postmenopausal women with breast cancer. *Pharmacoeconomics.* 2006;24:495-517.
295. Morello KC, Wurz GT, DeGregorio MW. Pharmacokinetics of selective estrogen receptor modulators. *Clin Pharmacokinet.* 2003;42:361-372.
296. Monnier A. Adjuvant trials: aromatase inhibitors in early breast cancer–are they alike? *Cancer Treat Rev.* 2006;32:532-540.
297. Howell A, Cuzick J, Baum M, et al. Results of the ATAC (Arimidex, Tamoxifen, Alone or in Combination) trial after completion of 5 years' adjuvant treatment for breast cancer. *Lancet.* 2005;365:60-62.
298. Zhao X, Liu L, Li K, Li W, Zhao L, Zou H. Comparative study on individual aromatase inhibitors on cardiovascular safety profile: a network meta-analysis. *Onco Targets Ther.* 2015;8:2721-2730.
299. Berry J. Are all aromatase inhibitors the same? A review of controlled clinical trials in breast cancer. *Clin Ther.* 2005;27:1671-1684.
300. Dixon JM, Renshaw L, Langridge C, et al. Anastrozole and letrozole: an investigation and comparison of quality of life and tolerability. *Breast Cancer Res Treat.* 2011;125:741-749.
301. Rose C, Vtoraya O, Pluzanska A, et al. An open randomised trial of second-line endocrine therapy in advanced breast cancer. Comparison of the aromatase inhibitors letrozole and anastrozole. *Eur J Cancer.* 2003;39:2318-2327.
302. Smith I, Yardley D, Burris H, et al. Comparative efficacy and safety of adjuvant letrozole versus anastrozole in postmenopausal patients with hormone receptor-positive, node-positive early breast cancer: final results of the randomized phase III Femara versus Anastrozole Clinical Evaluation (FACE) Trial. *J Clin Oncol.* 2017;35:1041-1048.
303. Higa GM, alKhouri N. Anastrozole: a selective aromatase inhibitor for the treatment of breast cancer. *Am J Health Syst Pharm.* 1998;55:445-452.
304. Higa GM. Altering the estrogenic milieu of breast cancer with a focus on the new aromatase inhibitors. *Pharmacotherapy.* 2000;20:280-291.
305. Higa GM. Exemestane: treatment of breast cancer with selective inactivation of aromatase. *Am J Health Syst Pharm.* 2002;59:2194-2201; quiz 2202-2194.
306. Hu X, Huang W, Fan M. Emerging therapies for breast cancer. *J Hematol Oncol.* 2017;10:98.
307. Reinert T, Barrios CH. Optimal management of hormone receptor positive metastatic breast cancer in 2016. *Ther Adv Med Oncol.* 2015;7:304-320.
308. Howell A. Pure oestrogen antagonists for the treatment of advanced breast cancer. *Endocr Relat Cancer.* 2006;13:689-706.
309. Wardell SE, Marks JR, McDonnell DP. The turnover of estrogen receptor alpha by the selective estrogen receptor degrader (SERD) fulvestrant is a saturable process that is not required for antagonist efficacy. *Biochem Pharmacol.* 2011;82:122-130.
310. Brunner N, Frandsen TL, Holst-Hansen C, et al. MCF7/LCC2: a 4-hydroxytamoxifen resistant human breast cancer variant that retains sensitivity to the steroidal antiestrogen ICI 182,780. *Cancer Res.* 1993;53:3229-3232.
311. Howell A, DeFriend DJ, Robertson JF, et al. Pharmacokinetics, pharmacological and anti-tumour effects of the specific anti-oestrogen ICI 182780 in women with advanced breast cancer. *Br J Cancer.* 1996;74:300-308.
312. Bross PF, Cohen MH, Williams GA, Pazdur R. FDA drug approval summaries: fulvestrant. *Oncologist.* 2002;7:477-480.
313. *Faslodex (Fulvestrant) [prescribing information].* Wilmington, DE: AstraZeneca; 2017.
314. O'Regan RM, Cisneros A, England GM, et al. Effects of the antiestrogens tamoxifen, toremifene, and ICI 182,780 on endometrial cancer growth. *J Natl Cancer Inst.* 1998;90:1552-1558.
315. *Cancer Facts and Figures 2018.* In: Society AC, ed. Atlanta: American Cancer Society; 2018.
316. Andriole GL, Crawford ED, Grubb RL 3rd, et al. Mortality results from a randomized prostate-cancer screening trial. *N Engl J Med.* 2009;360:1310-1319.
317. Schroder FH, Hugosson J, Roobol MJ, et al. Screening and prostate-cancer mortality in a randomized European study. *N Engl J Med.* 2009;360:1320-1328.
318. Huggins C, Hodges CV. Studies on prostatic cancer – I The effect of castration, of estrogen and of androgen injection on serum phosphatases in metastatic carcinoma of the prostate. *Cancer Res.* 1941;1:293-297.
319. Vale CL, Burdett S, Rydzewska LHM, et al. Addition of docetaxel or bisphosphonates to standard of care in men with localised or metastatic, hormone-sensitive prostate cancer: a systematic review and meta-analyses of aggregate data. *Lancet Oncol.* 2016;17:243-256.
320. Roberts WB, Han M. Clinical significance and treatment of biochemical recurrence after definitive therapy for localized prostate cancer. *Surg Oncol.* 2009;18:268-274.

321. Wattenberg CA. Carcinoma of the prostate gland, and benefits of diethylstilbestrol or orchiectomy. *Mo Med.* 1945;42:482-485.
322. Tolkach Y, Joniau S, Van Poppel H. Luteinizing hormone-releasing hormone (LHRH) receptor agonists vs antagonists: a matter of the receptors? *BJU Int.* 2013;111:1021-1030.
323. Schroder F, Crawford ED, Axcrona K, Payne H, Keane TE. Androgen deprivation therapy: past, present and future. *BJU Int.* 2012;109(suppl 6):1-12.
324. Oesterling JE. LHRH agonists – a nonsurgical treatment for benign prostatic hyperplasia. *J Androl.* 1991;12:381-388.
325. Morote J, Planas J, Salvador C, Raventos CX, Catalan R, Reventos J. Individual variations of serum testosterone in patients with prostate cancer receiving androgen deprivation therapy. *BJU Int.* 2009;103:332-335; discussion 335.
326. Morote J, Orsola A, Planas J, et al. Redefining clinically significant castration levels in patients with prostate cancer receiving continuous androgen deprivation therapy. *J Urol.* 2007;178:1290-1295.
327. Lepor H, Shore ND. LHRH agonists for the treatment of prostate cancer: 2012. *Rev Urol.* 2012;14:1-12.
328. Allan CA, Collins VR, Frydenberg M, McLachlan RI, Matthiesson KL. Androgen deprivation therapy complications. *Endocr Relat Cancer.* 2014;21:T119-T129.
329. Trost LW, Serefoglu E, Gokce A, Linder BJ, Sartor AO, Hellstrom WJ. Androgen deprivation therapy impact on quality of life and cardiovascular health, monitoring therapeutic replacement. *J Sex Med.* 2013;10(suppl 1):84-101.
330. Schulman C, Cornel E, Matveev V, et al. Intermittent versus continuous androgen deprivation therapy in patients with relapsing or locally advanced prostate cancer: a phase 3b randomised study (ICELAND). *Eur Urol.* 2016;69:720-727.
331. Zhang TY, Agarwal N, Sonpavde G, DiLorenzo G, Bellmunt J, Vogelzang NJ. Management of castrate resistant prostate cancer-recent advances and optimal sequence of treatments. *Curr Urol Rep.* 2013;14:174-183.
332. Mulders PF, De Santis M, Powles T, Fizazi K. Targeted treatment of metastatic castration-resistant prostate cancer with sipuleucel-T immunotherapy. *Cancer Immunol Immunother.* 2015;64:655-663.
333. Kantoff PW, Higano CS, Shore ND, et al. Sipuleucel-T immunotherapy for castration-resistant prostate cancer. *N Engl J Med.* 2010;363:411-422.
334. Hu R, George DJ, Zhang T. What is the role of sipuleucel-T in the treatment of patients with advanced prostate cancer? An update on the evidence. *Ther Adv Urol.* 2016;8:272-278.
335. Mohler JL, Gregory CW, Ford OH 3rd, et al. The androgen axis in recurrent prostate cancer. *Clin Cancer Res.* 2004;10:440-448.
336. Mohler ML, Coss CC, Duke CB III, Patil SA, Miller DD, Dalton JT. Androgen receptor antagonists: a patent review (2008-2011). *Expert Opin Ther Pat.* 2012;22:541-565.
337. Tannock IF, de Wit R, Berry WR, et al. Docetaxel plus prednisone or mitoxantrone plus prednisone for advanced prostate cancer. *New Engl J Med.* 2004;351:1502-1512.
338. de Bono JS, Oudard S, Ozguroglu M, et al. Prednisone plus cabazitaxel or mitoxantrone for metastatic castration-resistant prostate cancer progressing after docetaxel treatment: a randomised open-label trial. *Lancet.* 2010;376:1147-1154.
339. *Jevtana (Cabazitaxel) [prescribing information].* Bridgewater, NJ: Sanofi-Aventis; 2018.
340. Belderbos BPS, Bins S, van Leeuwen RWF, et al. Influence of enzalutamide on cabazitaxel pharmacokinetics: a drug-drug interaction study in metastatic castration-resistant prostate cancer (mCRPC) patients. *Clin Cancer Res.* 2018;24:541-546.
341. Ning X, Yang Y, Deng H, et al. Development of 17beta-hydroxysteroid dehydrogenase type 3 as a target in hormone-dependent prostate cancer therapy. *Steroids.* 2017;121:10-16.
342. Penning TM, Tamae D. Current advances in intratumoral androgen metabolism in castration-resistant prostate cancer. *Curr Opin Endocrinol Diabetes Obes.* 2016;23:264-270.
343. Barrie SE, Potter GA, Goddard PM, Haynes BP, Dowsett M, Jarman M. Pharmacology of novel steroidal inhibitors of cytochrome P450(17-alpha) (17-alpha-hydroxylase C17-20 lyase). *J Steroid Biochem.* 1994;50:267-273.
344. Ryan CJ, Smith MR, de Bono JS, et al. Abiraterone in metastatic prostate cancer without previous chemotherapy. *N Engl J Med.* 2013;368:138-148.
345. Fizazi K, Tran N, Fein L, et al. Abiraterone plus prednisone in metastatic, castration-sensitive prostate cancer. *N Engl J Med.* 2017;377:352-360.
346. Smith MR, Saad F, Chowdhury S, et al. Apalutamide treatment and metastasis-free survival in prostate cancer. *N Engl J Med.* 2018;378(15):1408-1418.
347. Hussain M, Fizazi K, Saad F, et al. PROSPER: a phase 3, randomized, double-blind, placebo (PBO)-controlled study of enzalutamide (ENZA) in men with nonmetastatic castration-resistant prostate cancer (M0 CRPC). *J Clin Oncol.* 2018;36:3-3.
348. Clegg NJ, Wongvipat J, Joseph JD, et al. ARN-509: a novel antiandrogen for prostate cancer treatment. *Cancer Res.* 2012;72:1494-1503.
349. Krause WC, Shafi AA, Nakka M, Weigel NL. Androgen receptor and its splice variant, AR-V7, differentially regulate FOXA1 sensitive genes in LNCaP prostate cancer cells. *Int J Biochem Cell Biol.* 2014;54:49-59.
350. Makkonen H, Kauhanen M, Jaaskelainen T, Palvimo JJ. Androgen receptor amplification is reflected in the transcriptional responses of vertebral-cancer of the prostate cells. *Mol Cell Endocrinol.* 2011;331:57-65.
351. Joseph JD, Lu N, Qian J, et al. A clinically relevant androgen receptor mutation confers resistance to second-generation antiandrogens enzalutamide and ARN-509. *Cancer Discov.* 2013;3:1020-1029.
352. Rathkopf DE, Antonarakis ES, Shore ND, et al. Safety and antitumor activity of apalutamide (ARN-509) in metastatic castration-resistant prostate cancer with and without prior abiraterone acetate and prednisone. *Clin Cancer Res.* 2017;23:3544-3551.
353. Galletti G, Leach BI, Lam L, Tagawa ST. Mechanisms of resistance to systemic therapy in metastatic castration-resistant prostate cancer. *Cancer Treat Rev.* 2017;57:16-27.
354. Borgmann H, Lallous N, Ozistanbullu D, et al. Moving towards precision urologic oncology: targeting enzalutamide-resistant prostate cancer and mutated forms of the androgen receptor using the novel inhibitor darolutamide (ODM-201). *Eur Urol.* 2018;73:4-8.
355. Cockshott ID. Bicalutamide: clinical pharmacokinetics and metabolism. *Clin Pharmacokinet.* 2004;43:855-878.
356. Shet MS, McPhaul M, Fisher CW, Stallings NR, Estabrook RW. Metabolism of the antiandrogenic drug (Flutamide) by human CYP1A2. *Drug Metab Dispos.* 1997;25:1298-1303.
357. Marugo M, Bernasconi D, Miglietta L, et al. Effects of dihydrotestosterone and hydroxyflutamide on androgen receptors in cultured human breast cancer cells (EVSA-T). *J Steroid Biochem Mol Biol.* 1992;42:547-554.
358. Creaven PJ, Pendyala L, Tremblay D. Pharmacokinetics and metabolism of nilutamide. *Urology.* 1991;37:13-19.
359. Ask K, Decologne N, Ginies C, et al. Metabolism of nilutamide in rat lung. *Biochem Pharmacol.* 2006;71:377-385.
360. Ask K, Dijols S, Giroud C, et al. Reduction of nilutamide by NO synthases: implications for the adverse effects of this nitroaromatic antiandrogen drug. *Chem Res Toxicol.* 2003;16:1547-1554.
361. McGlynn KA, Devesa SS, Sigurdson AJ, Brown LM, Tsao L, Tarone RE. Trends in the incidence of testicular germ cell tumors in the United States. *Cancer.* 2003;97:63-70.
362. Feldman HA, Goldstein I, Hatzichristou DG, Krane RJ, McKinlay JB. Impotence and its medical and psychosocial correlates: results of the Massachusetts male aging study. *J Urol.* 1994;151:54-61.

Case Solution 1

A. HP has several risk factors for early recurrence and poor prognosis including large tumor size (2.5 cm), unfavorable Oncotype score, obesity (high aromatase production), and high mitotic index. HP should probably be presented with the option of the 6-cycles of chemotherapy consisting of AC-T, anthracycline, and cyclophosphamide then taxane with clear explanation of the risks and benefits.

B. Tamoxifen is a valid selection for HP, but AIs tend to have better prevention of recurrence in postmenopausal patients. From the initial workup, the menopausal status of the patient is not certain, so endogenous 17β-estradiol levels should be followed from diagnosis through surgery and adjuvant chemo. Ovarian suppression should be considered if estrogen levels are not menopausal. Following ovarian suppression, tamoxifen is generally considered standard of care for premenopausal patients, but AIs are favored in postmenopausal.

C. The most common site of metastasis is the bone and commonly the hip (and spine), which was painful on initial presentation but not evaluated. (Although not the best diagnostic test, ultrasound suggests no visceral metastatis.) Breast cancer tumors grow in the bone marrow and particularly in weak bone, and the low platelet count suggests the possibility of metastasis to the bone. HP should be referred to her oncologist immediately.

Case Solution 2

A. 1. Bone protective agents are needed to prevent further pathologic fractures. In addition to calcium and vitamin D supplements, bisphosphonates have been used historically. However, denosumab has largely supplanted bisphosphonate use in breast and prostate cancer.
   2. Encourage HP to do physical therapy to strengthen bones.
   3. Stabilizing the spinal column to prevent further disability, e.g., kyphoplasty might be considered.

B. Tamoxifen resistance is common and many AIs have been approved for endocrine failures. Letrozole or anastrozole are approved as monotherapies in tamoxifen-resistant patients. However, outcomes are improved by the addition of a CDK4/6 inhibitor to the AI. For example, palbociclib and abemaciclib are approved for endocrine therapy failures in combination with an AI. Letrozole may have the most clinical data to support its use, but anastrozole could also be considered. Fulvestrant is also indicated for endocrine failures as monotherapy or combined with palbociclib or abemaciclib, which also improve outcomes over monotherapy.

C. No. The cancer is still estrogen-receptor positive. So endocrine therapies should be considered first.

Structure Challenge Answers

A-1, B-9, C-3, D-13, E-10, F-8, G-12, H-11, I-14, J-5, K-6, L-15, M-4, N-2, O-7.

SECTION 5

Drugs Impacting Immune, Gastrointestinal and Genitourinary Systems

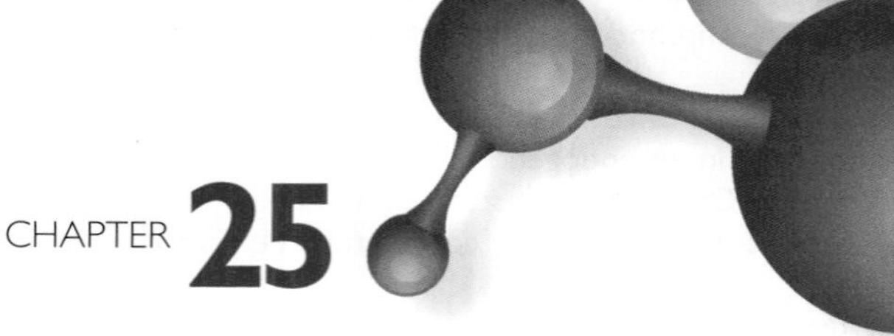

CHAPTER 25

Drugs Used to Treat Allergic Disorders

E. Kim Fifer

Drugs covered in this chapter:

HISTAMINE ANTAGONISTS
- Acrivastine
- Alcaftadine
- Antazoline
- Astemizole
- Azatadine
- Azelastine
- Bepotastine
- Bromodiphenhydramine
- Brompheniramine (dexbrompheniramine)
- Buclizine
- Carbinoxamine
- Cetirizine (levocetirizine)
- Chlorcyclizine
- Chlorpheniramine (dexchlorpheniramine)
- Clemastine
- Cyproheptadine
- Desloratadine
- Dimethindene
- Diphenhydramine (dimenhydrinate)
- Doxylamine
- Emedastine
- Epinastine
- Fexofenadine
- Hydroxyzine
- Ketotifen
- Levocabastine
- Loratadine
- Meclizine
- Methdilazine
- Olopatadine
- Phenindamine
- Piperoxan
- Promethazine
- Pyrrobutamine
- Terfenadine
- Tripelennamine
- Trimeprazine
- Triprolidine

MAST CELL STABILIZERS
- Cromolyn
- Nedocromil
- Lodoxamide
- Pemirolast

Abbreviations

ALDH aldehyde dehydrogenase
AO aldehyde oxidase
cAMP cyclic adenosine monophosphate
CYP cytochrome P450
DAG diacylglycerol
DAO diamine oxidase
ECL enterochromaffin-like cells
Fc fragment crystallizable
GPCRs G protein–coupled receptors
hERG human ether-à-go-go-related gene
hHDC human histidine decarboxylase
HMT histamine N-methyltransferase
5-HT 5-hydroxytryptamine (serotonin)
IgE immunoglobulin E
I_{Kr} inward-rectifying cardiac potassium channel
IL_6 interleukin 6
IP_3 inositol-1,4,5-trisphosphate
MAO-B monoamine oxidase B
OTC over-the-counter
PIP_2 phosphatidylinositol-4,5-bisphosphate
TNF-α tumor necrosis factor alpha
XO xanthine oxidase

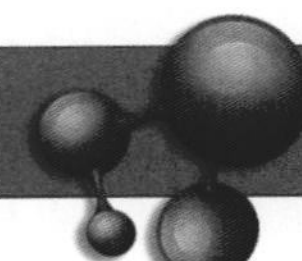

CLINICAL SIGNIFICANCE

Rachel Stafford, PharmD

Antihistamines have several uses and indications for the treatment of various conditions. While they are often simply categorized into two groups (first- vs. second-generation antihistamines), knowing the chemical structure and properties of these compounds and their subclasses can allow for more customized and selective use in clinical practice. Small changes to the structure can increase or decrease antihistaminic, anticholinegic, or sedative activity, which allows for therapy optimization based on the desired effect and clinical use. In some cases, increased anticholinergic activity may be preferred (e.g., rhinorrhea), and in others, limiting anticholinergic activity may be ideal (e.g., use in elderly patients). For example, chlorpheniramine (a *p*-halo–substituted pheniramine) may be beneficial in patients who desire some anticholinergic activity but wish to decrease sedation while maintaining moderate to high antihistaminic effects. In combination with an understanding of a patient's needs and desires, a detailed knowledge of the chemistry of these medications can be very beneficial in clinical care.

THERAPEUTIC CONTEXT

Allergic rhinitis may be considered the second leading cause of chronic disease in the United States.[1] It affects 30-60 million people annually and includes 10%-30% of the nation's adults and up to 40% of the children.[2] The cost associated with treating allergic rhinitis is substantial and increases with disease severity and comorbidity. In 2005 the direct medical cost of treating allergic rhinitis was estimated at $3.4 billion (prescription costs and outpatient visits).[3] In addition to these costs, there are indirect costs associated absenteeism (days off from work) and presenteeism (loss of productivity while at work), as well as with medical costs associated with comorbidities. Allergic rhinitis can have adverse effects on social life and academic performance, especially when treated with an antihistamine that produces sedation. Addressing this condition early can have significant clinical benefits toward improving the patient's quality-of-life while decreasing comorbid disorders such as asthma, rhinosinusitis, allergic conjunctivitis, and sleep apnea.[1]

When John Bostock first described "hay fever," also known as allergic rhinitis or seasonal rhinitis, in 1819, it was a rarely seen condition. Today, the incidence of allergies has reached epidemic proportions in developed nations, with one in two individuals exhibiting some sort of allergic disorder.[4]

Allergic rhinitis is characterized by inflammation of the nasal mucous membranes. When an allergen contacts mucous membranes in sensitized individuals, it binds to immunoglobulin E (IgE) that is bound to mast cells and basophils and triggers release of mediators such as histamine, chemotactic factors, and proteases (Fig. 25.1). This initiates synthesis of prostaglandins, leukotrienes, platelet activating factor, and cytokines, ultimately leading to the characteristic sneezing, watery rhinorrhea, and itching of the nose, eyes, and ears. Seasonal allergic rhinitis occurs in response to allergens such as pollen from trees, grasses, and weeds, while persistent allergic rhinitis lasts year-round and results from exposure to mold, dust mites, and animal dander. Often, patients have a combination of seasonal and persistent rhinitis.

There are four classes of medication used to treat the underlying inflammation associated with allergic rhinitis:

1. antihistamines (inverse agonists at histamine H_1 receptors);
2. intranasal steroids;
3. leukotriene receptor antagonists; and
4. mast cell degranulation inhibitors (histamine release inhibitors).

Treatment with antihistamines and/or intranasal steroids appears to show better clinical outcomes.[1] This chapter will focus on use of antihistamines and degranulation inhibitors. The reader should refer to Chapter 21 for information dealing with use of glucocorticoids and Chapter 28 for leukotriene antagonists.

HISTAMINE

Histamine [2-(imidazole-4-yl)ethylamine] was first synthesized in 1907 by Windaus and Vogt[5] because it possessed structural similarities to the natural alkaloid pilocarpine and the amino acid histidine. In 1910 histamine was discovered to be produced by ergot[6] and as a product of bacterial decarboxylation of histidine.[7] That same year, the pharmacological actions of histamine were reported by Dale and Laidlaw.[8] They observed that it produced smooth muscle contractions, decreased blood pressure, and in some species, produced effects similar to anaphylactic shock. It was not until 1927 that in vivo histamine release due to skin damage and its involvement in immune reactions were reported.[9,10]

NH_2

H-N N

Histamine

Histamine is biosynthesized in many tissues. These include (1) mast cells, basophils, and lymphocytes, where it is involved in allergic and inflammatory responses; (2) gastric enterochromaffin-like (ECL) cells, where it stimulates gastric HCl secretion; and (3) some histaminergic neurons in the CNS, where it functions as a neurotransmitter. In

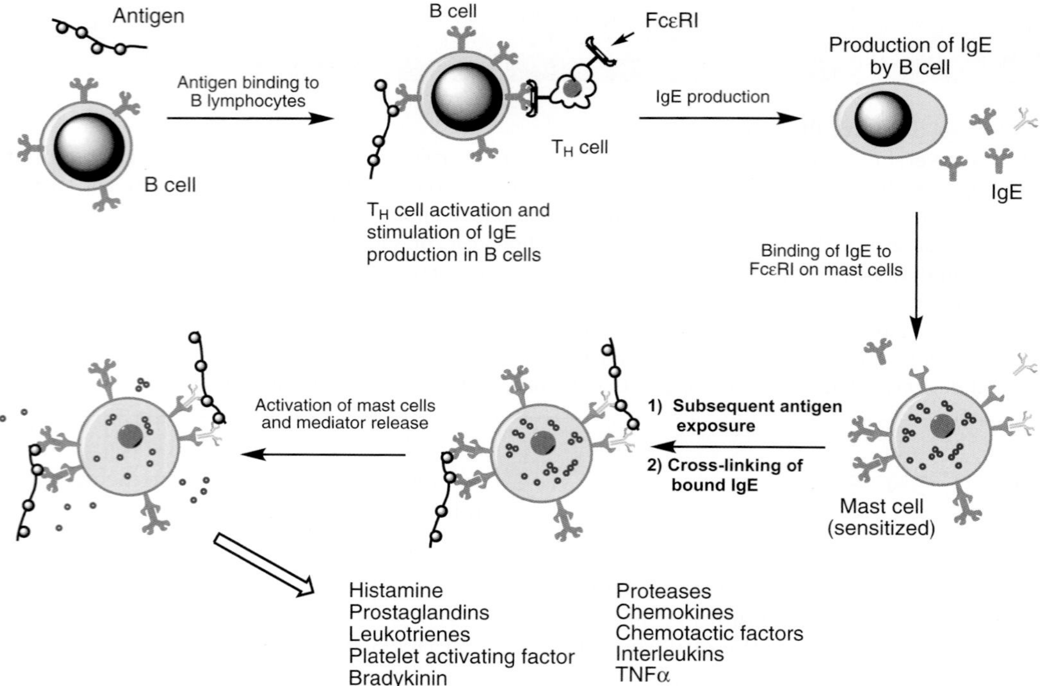

Figure 25.1 IgE-mediated hypersensitivity reaction. Events leading to type I (immediate) hypersensitivity reactions. Upon initial exposure to an antigen, B cells begin to synthesize IgE specific to that antigen. The secreted IgE binds to high-affinity Fcε receptors (FcεRI) on mast cells or basophils. Subsequent exposure to the antigen with cross-linking of the IgE triggers immediate degranulation with histamine release and an inflammatory response.

many tissues histamine acts as an autacoid (local hormone), a molecule that is secreted locally to modulate the activity of nearby cells.

The pharmacologic effects of histamine show marked species differences.[11] In Guinea pigs, a subcutaneous injection of histamine will produce a massive bronchospasm along with effects on smooth muscle and the vasculature that resemble an anaphylactic reaction. These effects are not seen in humans. Its actions in different tissues are mediated through four distinct receptors designated as H_1–H_4. These receptors have been cloned, and they belong to the superfamily of G protein–coupled receptors (GPCRs) (Table 25.1). See Chapter 6 for more detailed information about GPCRs and their signal transduction. Histamine H_1 receptors appear to be closely related to muscarinic receptors, while the H_2 receptors resemble 5-HT_1 receptors. The former may explain the anticholinergic effects of some of the first-generation H_1 antagonists described below. H_3 and H_4 receptors are not closely related to either H_1 or H_2 receptors. For years, H_1 antihistamines were considered traditional receptor antagonists. With the recognition that all of the histamine receptors have some constitutive activity, it is now recognized that the first- and second-generation "H_1 antagonists" are functioning as inverse agonists.

Histamine Chemistry

Histamine is composed of a basic imidazole ring ($pK_a = 5.80$ [HB^+]) connected to a primary aliphatic amino group ($pK_a = 9.40$ [HB^+]) by an ethylene bridge. Although histamine can exist as a mixture of charged and uncharged species at various pH levels, three forms can exist at pH 7.4 (Fig. 25.2), i.e., unionized (1%), monocation (96%), and dication (3%).[12] At lower pH (e.g., the pH of acidic lipids), a much larger proportion of the dication will exist. While the mono- and dication forms are often considered the biologically active species, it is the unprotonated free base form that is believed to penetrate biological membranes. In aqueous solution, the N^{τ}-H/N^{π}-H tautomer ratio of the monocation is 4.2, thus ~80% exits as N^{τ}-H and 20% as N^{π}-H.[12] Studies using the Hammett equation suggest that the tautomeric preference is influenced by the electron withdrawing nature of the side chain.[13] The N^{τ}-H tautomer is also preferred for the free base in aqueous solution. Interestingly, while the monocationic hydrobromide salt crystallizes as the N^{τ}-H tautomer, the free base crystallizes as the N^{π}-H tautomer.[14] The crystalline forms are conformationally "frozen" and can not be related to their tautomeric stability under equilibrating conditions. These solid state findings for the monocation and unionized (free base) form are supported by molecular orbital calculations on isolated molecules.[14] The tautomeric ratios differ with different 4-substituted histamine analogues. As the N^{τ}-H/N^{π}-H tautomer ratio decreases on going from 4-methylhistamine (70%) to 4-chloro-histamine (12%), a similar decrease is observed for the agonist potency. One interpretation of this is that the N^{τ}-H tautomer might be important for agonist interaction with histamine receptors. Structure-activity analysis suggests that the active form of histamine at both the H_1 and H_2 receptor is the N^{τ}-H tautomer of the monocation.

Table 25.1 Histamine Receptors – Signaling and Responses

Receptor	Signaling Mechanism	Tissue	Effect	Clinical Response
H_1	$G_{q/11}$, ⇒ activate phospholipase C, ↑ IP_3 & DAG	Vascular Smooth Muscle	Dilation - Terminal arterioles - Postcapillary venules - Venoconstriction	Erythema
		Vascular endothelium	Contraction and separation of endothelial cells	Edema (wheal response)
		Lungs	Bronchoconstriction	Asthma-like symptoms
		Peripheral nerves	Afferent sensitization	Itch, Pain
H_2	G_s ⇒ stimulate adenylate cyclase, ↑ cAMP	Stomach (parietal cells)	↑ HCl secretion	Heartburn, peptic ulcer disease
		Heart	Small ↑ in rate and contractility	Minor
H_3	$G_{i/o}$ ⇒ inhibit adenylate cyclase, ↓ cAMP	Presynaptic auto- and heteroreceptors: CNS, some peripheral nerves	Neurotransmitter	Cognitive processes, circadian rhythms, wakefulness
H_4	$G_{i/o}$ ⇒ ↓ cAMP, ↑ intracellular Ca^{2+}	Neutrophils, eosinophils, CD4,T cells	Chemotaxis / Inflammation	

cAMP, cyclic adenosine monophosphate; DAG, diacylglycerol; IP_3, inositol 1,4,5- triphosphate

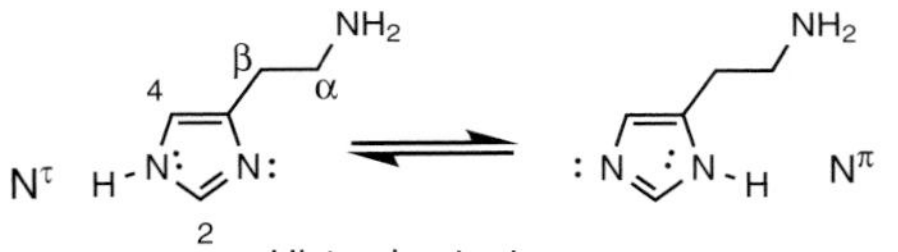

Histamine tautomers
(numbering according to Black and Ganellin[15])

Both *anti (transoid)* and *gauche* conformations of histamine can exist in solution (Fig. 25.3).[16] It has been suggested that the *trans* conformation is preferred at H_1- and H_2-receptors since both α- and β-methylhistamine, which exist predominately in the *gauche*-conformation due to steric hindrance, exhibit greatly reduced agonist activity at both H_1 and H_2 receptors. α-Methylhistamine and other conformationally restricted histamine analogues that predominately exist in the *gauche* conformation have been shown to be active H_3-agonists.

While 2-methylhistamine and 4-methylhistamine are selective H_1 and H_2 agonists, respectively, methyl substitution at the N^{τ} or N^{π} position of the imidazole produces compounds that are nearly inactive. Methylation of the aliphatic amine nitrogen also results in decreased activity (decreasing activity: $-NH_2 > -NHMe > -NMe_2 > -N^+Me_3$ [quaternary ammonium salt]) at H_1 and H_2 receptors.[14]

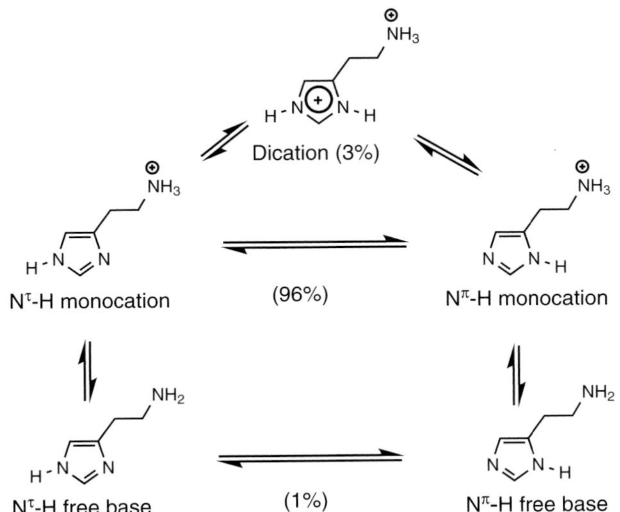

Figure 25.2 Ionization states and tautomerizaton of histamine. pK_a 5.0 (imidazole: HB^+), 9.4 (aliphatic amine: HB^+).

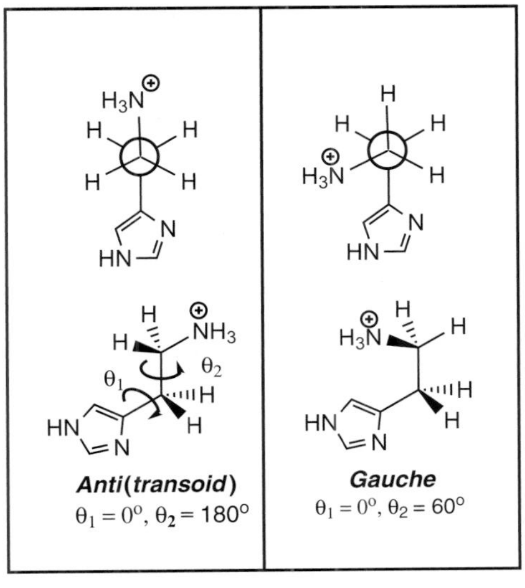

Anti(transoid) $\theta_1 = 0°, \theta_2 = 180°$

Gauche $\theta_1 = 0°, \theta_2 = 60°$

Figure 25.3 Conformers of histamine.

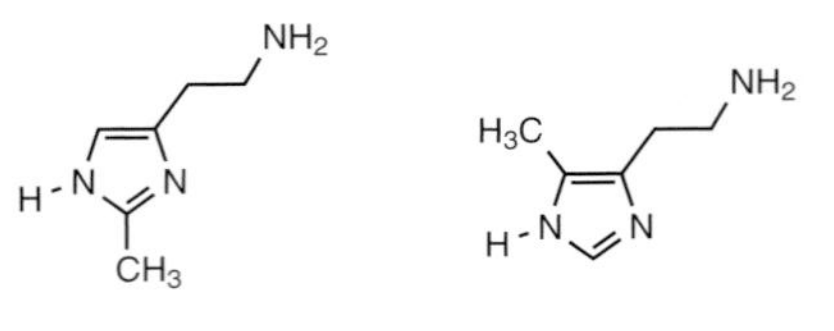

2-Methylhistamine 4-Methylhistamine

For histamine binding at H_1 receptors, there is a strict requirement for the following: (1) a protonated, cationic side chain amine, (2) a nitrogen atom with a lone pair of electrons in the position adjacent to the protonated aminoethyl side chain, which is fulfilled by the N^{τ}-H tautomer, and (3) a freely rotating imidazole ring that can achieve coplanarity with the side chain.[14] SAR studies also suggest that the following are required of histamine at the H_2 receptor: (1) a protonated, cationic side chain amine, (2) a N^{τ}-H tautomer/amidine system, and (3) imidazole N^{τ}-H tautomer involvement in a static hydrogen bonding or a dynamic proton transfer. The proton transfer via tautomerization has been suggested to be necessary for histamine to activate the H_2 receptor.[14] Quantum chemical studies have been used to explain the agonistic activities of nontautomeric H_2 agonists.[17]

Histamine Physiology

Histamine Biosynthesis and Metabolism

Histamine is biosynthesized by mammals in the Golgi apparatus of basophils and mast cells via decarboxylation of the amino acid L-histidine. The reaction is catalyzed by the dimeric enzyme, L-histidine decarboxylase (HDC), a pyridoxal phosphate (PLP)-dependent enzyme.[18] The mechanism (Fig. 25.4) is similar to that seen for other α-amino acids and involves the "internal aldimine" (hHDC-PLP), a Schiff base, formed between Lys305 on HDC and its coenzyme, PLP.[19] In a transaldimination, the substrate, His, displaces Lys305 of HDC to produce an "external aldamine" (His-PLP). Subsequent to decarboxylation, a second transaldimination involving Lys305 of HDC occurs to release histamine, the product, and regenerate original HDC-PLP "internal aldamine". α-Fluoromethylhistidine, a mechanism-based inhibitor, can decrease the rate of histamine synthesis and thus, deplete cells of histamine.[20] Theoretically, inhibition of histamine biosynthesis might be of use in the treatment of allergic inflammatory disorders, peptic ulcers, or motion sickness, but it has not found clinical utility.

Once released, histamine is rapidly metabolized via both phase 1 and phase 2 metabolic reactions (Fig. 25.5). One pathway involves histamine N-methyltransferase (HMT) catalyzed N-methylation of the N^{τ} position of the imidazole ring. The methyl group is transferred from the coenzyme, S-adenosylmethionine, to give the inactive 3-methylhistamine. This undergoes oxidative deamination by either diamine oxidase (DAO) or monoamine oxidase B (MAO-B) to produce the corresponding aldehyde, which is quickly oxidized by aldehyde dehydrogenase (ALDH), aldehyde oxidase (AO), or xanthine oxidase (XO) to give 3-methylimidazole acetic acid. Similarly, histamine can undergo oxidative deamination and aldehyde oxidation to afford imidazole acetic acid. This undergoes conjugation to afford the corresponding ribonucleoside.

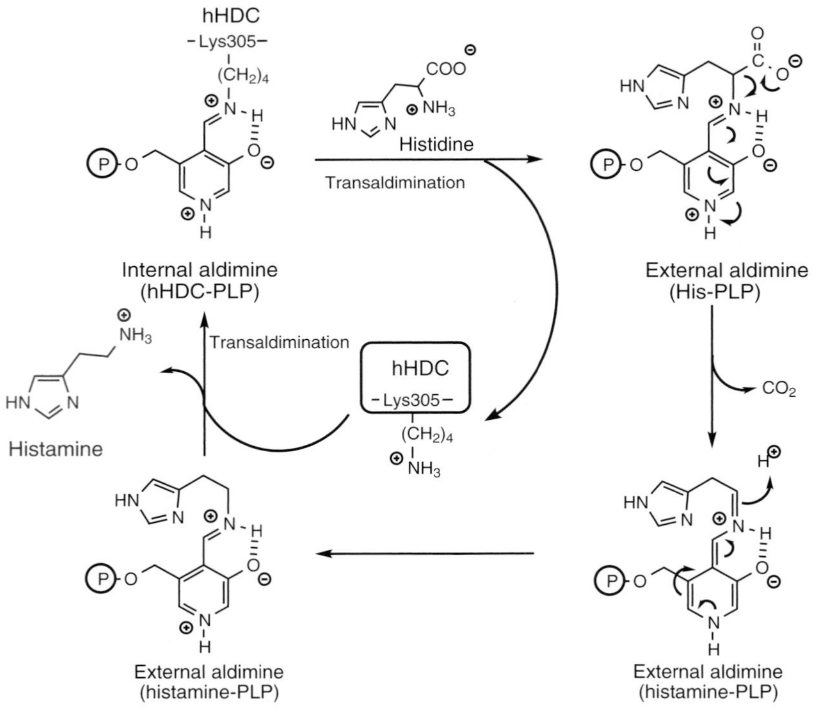

Figure 25.4 Histidine decarboxylase–catalyzed formation of histamine.[19] *hHDC*, human histidine decarboxylase; *His*, histidine; *PLP*, pyridoxal phosphate.

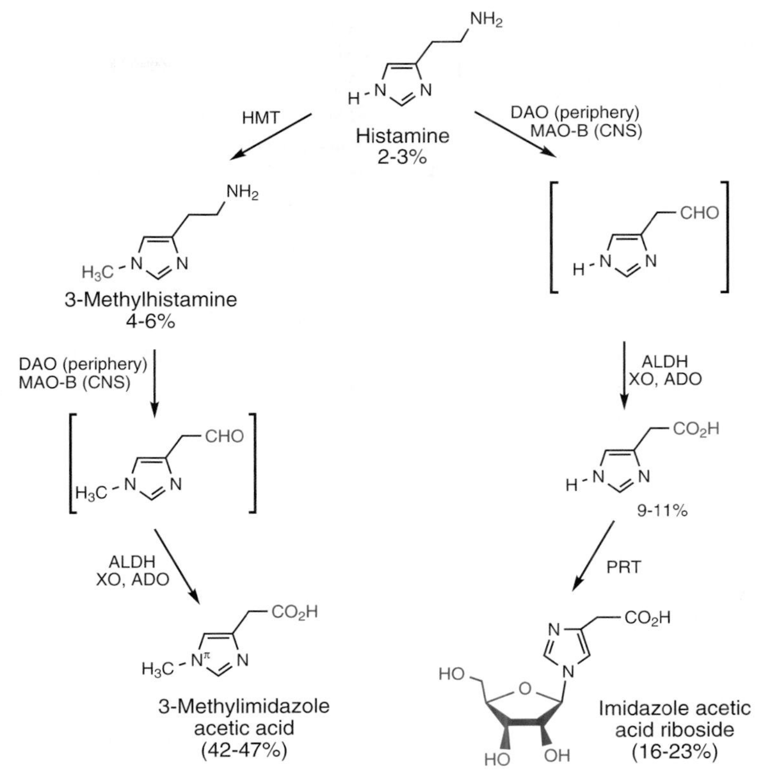

Figure 25.5 Histamine metabolism. Metabolites are found in urine over a 12-hour period after an intradermal histamine injection.[21] *ADO*, aldehyde oxidase; *ALDH*, aldehyde dehydrogenase; *DAO*, diamine oxidase; *HMT*, histamine N-methyltransferase; *MAO-B*, monoamine oxidase B; *PRT*, phosphoribosyl transferase; *XO*, xanthine oxidase.

Histamine Storage and Release

Histamine is found in many tissues throughout the body, but most is stored in secretory granules of tissue-bound mast cells and circulating basophils. In mast cells it is stored as a complex with the acidic residues of heparin, while in basophils it is complexed with chondroitin sulfate.[22,23] Histamine is also found in some non–mast cell sites, e.g., the CNS, where it functions as a neurotransmitter, and enterochromaffin-like cells of the stomach fundus, where it functions as a secretagogue to stimulate parietal cells to release HCl. Degranulation (i.e., release of histamine) may be triggered by allergic reactions, anaphylaxis, cellular trauma, cold, etc. The tissue-bound form of histamine is not biologically active. Drugs such as tubocurarine and morphine are known to cause itching and other reactions due to their displacement of histamine from its binding sites. This process is energy independent and not associated with mast cell injury or degranulation. Chemical and mechanical injury to mast cells can also lead to degranulation and release.[24]

As a mediator of immune and inflammatory reactions, histamine plays a prominent role in allergic responses (i.e., immunoglobulin E [IgE]-mediated type I hypersensitivity reaction).[25] These reactions are also referred to as immediate hypersensitivity reactions because they occur within an hour of initial exposure. In this type of reaction, the antigen (allergen) must penetrate an epithelial surface (e.g., skin or nasal mucosa), or it could be delivered systemically, as seen with penicillin allergy. With the aid of T-helper cells, the antigen comes in contact with B lymphocytes and stimulates production of IgE antibodies (Fig. 25.1). These antibodies are specific for a particular antigen. "Sensitization" occurs upon binding of the specific IgE antibodies to Fc receptors on mast cells or basophils. Once sensitized with IgE antibodies, immune cells are able to recognize and quickly respond to the next exposure to the antigen. Upon subsequent exposure, antigen binds and cross-links the IgE/Fc receptor complexes leading to degranulation and release of histamine and other inflammatory mediators.

Released histamine activates H_1 receptors on vascular smooth muscle and endothelial cells, leading to the initial stage of the inflammatory response, i.e., increased local blood flow and vascular permeability. Other immune cells are required for prolonged inflammation. Histamine-induced local vasodilation provides other immune cells with greater access to the injured area, and vasodilation aids movement of the immune cells into the tissue.[25] An immune response is not always required for mast cell degranulation. Physical disruption of mast cells by trauma or chemicals can lead to degranulation. Released histamine facilitates access of macrophages and other immune cells to the damaged area, which initiates the repair process.

Histamine Receptors

All histamine receptors, H_1–H_4, are GPCRs (see Chapter 6) and are widely distributed throughout the body (Table 25.1). This chapter will consider the H_1 receptor. They are found on nerve cells, airway and vascular smooth muscle, hepatocytes, chondrocytes, endothelial cells, eosinophils, monocytes, macrophages, dendritic cells, and T and B lymphocytes. H_1 receptor stimulation results in vasodilation, edema, bronchoconstriction, itching, and pain. Stimulation also affects maturation of cells of the immune system, altering their activation, chemotactic, and effector functions.[26,27] The human H_1 receptor gene encodes for a 487-amino acid G coupled-protein composed of seven transmembrane domains, N-terminal glycosylation sites, phosphorylation sites for protein kinase A and C, and a large intracellular loop with multiple Ser and Thr residues.[28,29] Results from site-directed mutagenesis studies suggest that Asp107 in transmembrane domain three (TM3) coordinates with the protonated amine group of the aminoethyl side chain of histamine, while the N^{τ}-nitrogen and the N^{π}-nitrogen of histamine interact with Arg207 and Lys200 of TM5, respectively.[29,30] There is about 40% homology between the human H_1 receptor and muscarinic M_1 and M_2 receptors.

H_1 receptor signal transduction involves $G_{q/11}$-coupled activation of phospholipase C and its subsequent hydrolysis of phosphatidylinositol-4,5-bisphosphate (PIP_2) to afford the second messengers inositol-1,4,5-trisphosphate (IP_3) and 1,2-diacylglycerol (DAG). IP_3 is an intracellular messenger that opens ligand-gated calcium channels on the endoplasmic reticulum, leading to intracellular calcium release, while DAG remains in the membrane and activates protein kinase C (Table 25.1).

INHIBITORS OF RELEASED HISTAMINE

Background (Inverse Agonists)

From a historical context, H_1 antihistamines have been considered "neutral" H_1 receptor antagonists. As such, they were believed to have no intrinsic activity in the absence of either an agonist or inverse agonist. This belief was supported by the parallel shift in concentration-response relationships in tracheal smooth muscle. However, advances in histamine pharmacology have demonstrated that they are not antagonists. They are actually inverse agonists. In the absence of histamine or another ligand, such as an antihistamine, H_1 receptors exist in equilibrium between two conformational states, active and inactive. With no ligand bound, the receptor exhibits constitutive activity. Bound histamine acts as an agonist, and the receptor equilibrium is shifted toward the active state. However, when an antihistamine is bound, the receptor equilibrium shifts toward the inactive state, and activity is reduced. The term inverse agonists is used because these structures preferentially bind to the inactive conformation of the H_1 receptor and reduce its constitutive activity, even in the absence of histamine.

Forneau and Bovet were the first to report a compound, piperoxan, that would protect guinea pigs against the bronchospasm produced by histamine.[31] The dramatic response observed in the guinea pig toward histamine was originally believed to be a good model for asthma. It should be noted that not all species respond to the same extent as guinea pigs. Piperoxan also exhibits antagonistic properties at α-adrenergic receptors, a characteristic seen with many of the older, first-generation H_1 antihistamines. These antihistamines have been shown to be useful for treatment of allergic and inflammatory disorders, but they do not antagonize the effects of histamine on the stomach (increased gastric acid secretion) or the heart (positive chronotropic and inotropic effects). These observations led to speculation that there was more than one histamine receptor and ultimately to discovery of H_2 receptors and development of selective H_2 antagonists. Subsequently, H_3 receptors have been reported. They function as presynaptic autoreceptors and heteroreceptors. As autoreceptors in the CNS, they presynaptically control the biosynthesis and release of histamine, whereas, as heteroreceptors, they control release of other neurotransmitters. H_3 receptors affect cognitive processes, circadian rhythms, and wakefulness. The recently discovered H_4 receptors are primarily found on eosinophils and mast cells where they are involved in inflammatory responses.

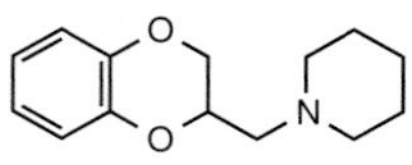

Piperoxan

This discussion will refer to antihistamines as either first- or second-generation. The first-generation antihistamines may be divided into five chemical groups: (1) ethylenediamines, (2) ethanolamine ethers (aminoalkyl ethers), (3) piperazines (cyclizines), (4) alkylamines (propylamines or pheniramines), and (5) tricyclic antihistamine (phenothiazines and other tricyclics). They have variable efficacy in the treatment of allergic disorders and also exhibit numerous side effects through interaction with cholinergic, adrenergic, dopaminergic, and serotonergic receptors. Adverse CNS effects vary according to the class and include drowsiness, sedation, decreased cognitive function, and somnolence. CNS depression is so pronounced with some agents that they are marketed as over-the-counter sleep aids, rather than for treatment of allergic disorders. Peripheral anticholinergic effects include blurred vision, dry mouth and eyes, urinary retention, and constipation. Other undesirable effects include muscle spasm, anxiety, confusion, irritability, tremor, appetite stimulation, and tachycardia. Because of the potential for significant anticholinergic and CNS depressant effects, the first-generation antihistamines are considered potentially inappropriate for use in older adults according to the AGS Beers Criteria.[32] Development of the second-generation antihistamines proved to be a great step forward in the treatment of allergic rhinitis and similar conditions. These agents exhibit separation of the peripheral H_1 antihistamine activity from the CNS depressant and anticholinergic side effects and have improved the quality-of-life of allergy sufferers worldwide.

The numerous side effects associated with first-generation H_1 antihistamines, developed in the 1940s and 1950s, often limit their clinical use. It was originally thought that the sedative properties were unrelated to the H_1 blockade, but it is now known that the sedation is actually due to H_1 receptor blockade in the CNS, and that these H_1 receptors are identical to those in the periphery. Early attempts to develop nonsedating antihistamines were aimed at designing compounds that were more polar than first-generation compounds so that they would not cross the blood-brain barrier. Although these efforts were unsuccessful, the goal of a nonsedating antihistamine was ultimately achieved with development of peripherally selective terfenadine. This was

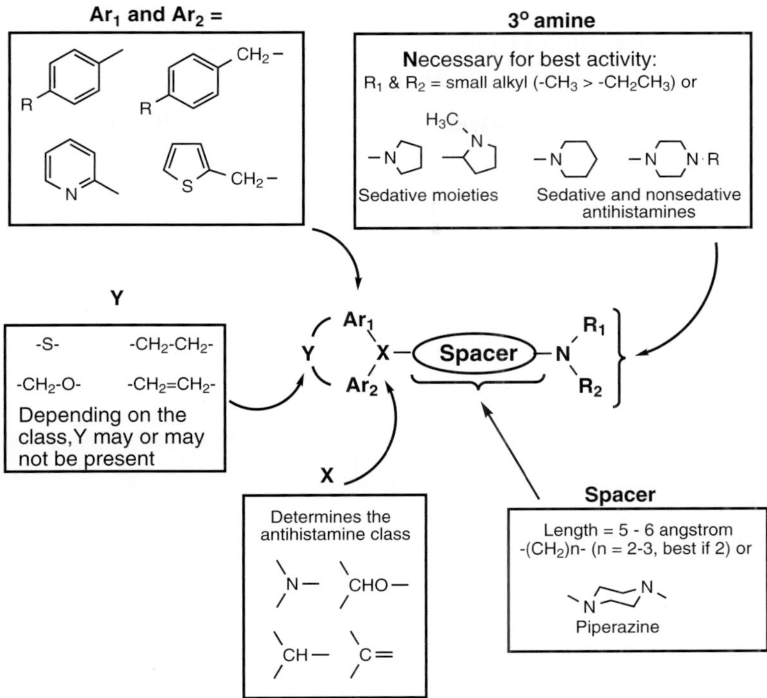

Figure 25.6 General structure of first-generation antihistamines.

the first example of what is now considered a second-generation H_1 antihistamine. It was later found that the lack of sedation exhibited by second-generation (nonsedating) antihistamines was the result of their being substrates for the permeability glycoprotein (P-gp) transporter system.

First-Generation Antihistamines

General SAR

A general structure for various chemical classes of first-generation antihistamines may be represented by two aromatic rings linked to a tertiary amine via a short spacer chain (Fig. 25.6), usually two or three carbons or a heterocycle such as piperazine as seen in the piperazines (cyclizines) class. One of the aromatic groups (AR_1) is often a phenyl, substituted phenyl, or a heteroaromatic such as 2-pyridyl. A 2-pyridyl group in place of a phenyl often increases antihistaminic activity while reducing anticholinergic and sedative properties. The second group (AR_2) may be aryl or arylmethyl group, but only one arylmethyl group is permitted in this part of the structure, and it is restricted to the ring that will orient in a *cis* fashion relative to the cationic amine when the drug binds to the H_1 receptor. This diaryl substitution is required for good H_1-receptor affinity and may be seen in both first- and second-generation antihistamines. The two aryl groups in Ar_1-X-Ar_2 must be noncoplanar or able to become noncoplanar in order to exhibit receptor affinity.[33] Substituents on the aryl rings should not be hydrophilic. When substituted in the *p*-position of the Ar moiety that orients in a *cis* fashion relative to the cationic amine, an increase both in antihistaminic and anticholinergic activity is generally observed, while *o*-substitution decreases H_1-receptor affinity and favors anticholinergic activity. Substitution is not allowed on the Ar moiety that orients *trans* relative to the cationic amine, as the receptor is sterically restricted in this binding area. Replacing a phenyl ring with a 2-pyridyl increases antihistaminic activity and decreases both anticholinergic and sedative properties. Benzyl-like groups (Ar-CH_2-) are seen in the ethylenediamine class but, again, are only allowed for one Ar moiety. Methapyrilene, an early example containing the 2-thienylmethyl group as a bioisosteric replacement for a benzyl group, proved to be carcinogenic and is no longer used. The two aromatic rings may or may not be linked via a bridge, Y. This connection is seen in the tricyclic antihistamines, e.g., phenothiazines (Y = -S-), dibenzoheptanes (Y = -CH_2-CH_2-), or dibenzoheptenes (Y = -CH = CH-).

The aryl substituents are connected to a group, X, that determines the subclass of the first-generation antihistamine classes. Group X is a nitrogen atom in the ethylenediamines, an ether in the ethanolamine ethers, or a sp^3 or sp^2 carbon in the alkylamine series.

The terminal nitrogen must be basic and is most often a tertiary dimethyl substituted amine. Antihistaminic activity is best when the substitution is with small alkyl groups to minimize steric hindrance to ion-ion anchoring at the H_1 receptor Asp107. Methyl substitution is better than ethyl, but sterically constrained five to six member nonaromatic heterocycles (pyrrolidine, piperidine, and imidazoline) have been used. The pK_a of these groups usually ranges from 8.5 to 10.3; thus, they will be significantly cationic at physiological pH.

Ethylenediamines

The ethylenediamine antihistamines were the earliest to find clinical use. With the exception of antazoline, which contains an amidine as part of an imidazoline ring, compounds in this series possess two nitrogen atoms separated by a two-carbon spacer. Examples of bioisosteric aromatic ring replacements (e.g., pyridine, pyrimidine, furan, thiazole) can be seen in this class, although no such antihistamines are currently marketed in the United States. As noted above, the thiophene-containing congener, known as methapyrilene, was removed from the market after it was shown to induce cancer in rats.[34] As a class, ethylenediamines exhibit low antihistaminic and anticholinergic effects and moderate sedative effects. Although tripelennamine is still available, the ethylenediamines find little clinical use today.

Tripelennamine
Salt form = citrate
pK_a 9.04
log P 2.78
$t_{1/2}$ = 2.9-5.3 hr

There are limited data on the pharmacokinetics and metabolism of the ethylenediamines and the first-generation antihistamines in general. As a representative example, tripelennamine undergoes, N-demethylation, aryl hydroxylation, N-oxide formation, glucuronic acid conjugation.[35]

DISCONTINUED OR *LESS COMMONLY USED DRUGS OF STRUCTURAL INTEREST

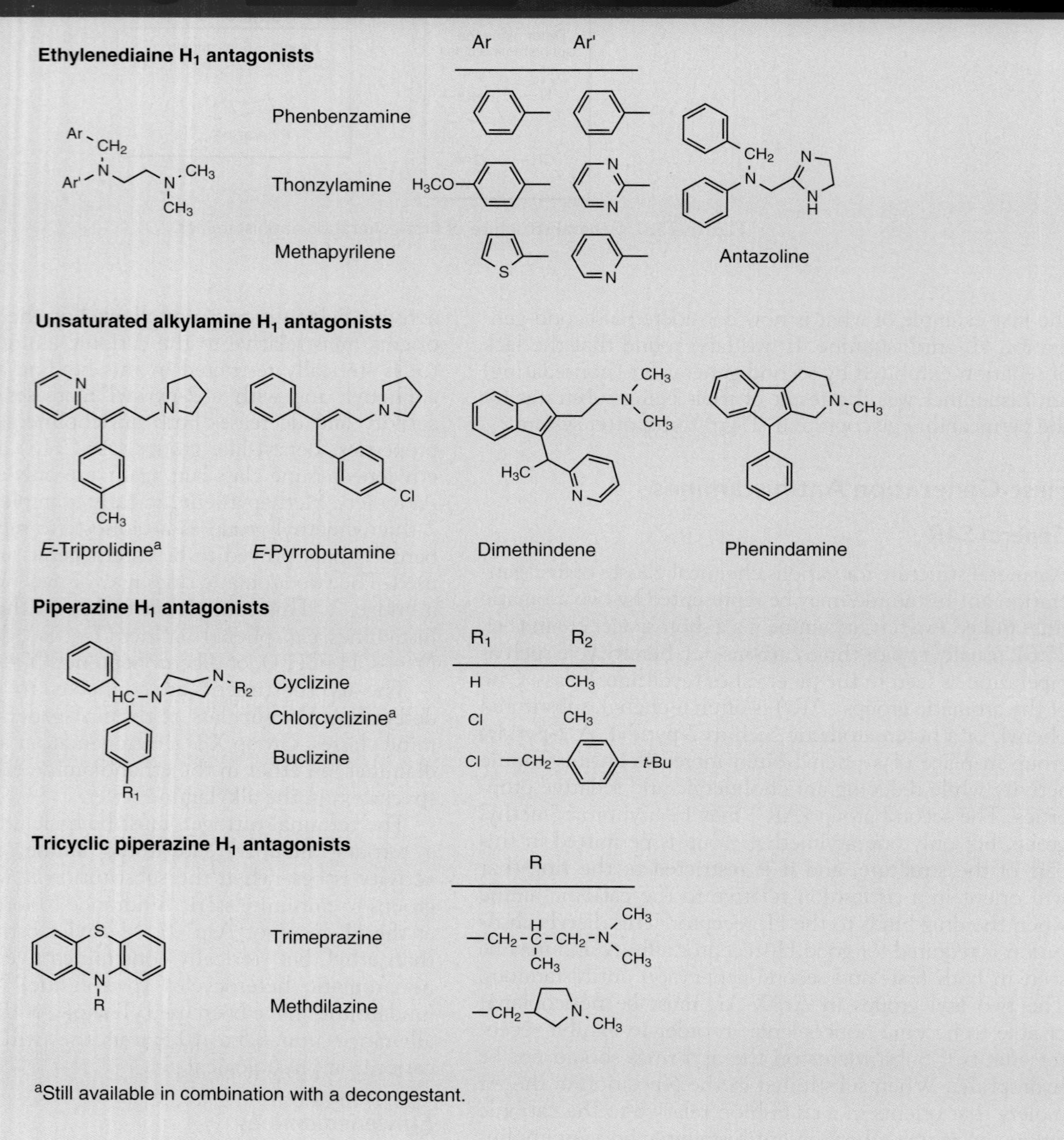

aStill available in combination with a decongestant.

Table 25.2 Ethanolamine Ether Antihistamines

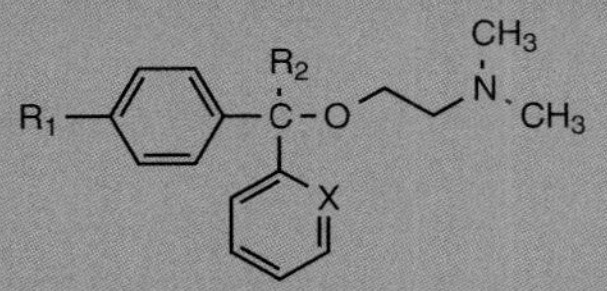

Drug	Salt	R_1	R_2	X	pK_a[a]	cLog P[a]	$t_{1/2}$[b]
Diphenhydramine (Benadryl) Dimenhydrinate (Dramamine)	HCl, citrate, tannate (8-Chlorotheophyllinate)	H	H	CH	8.76	2.99	4-8
Bromodiphenhydramine (Ambodryl)	HCl	Br	H	CH	8.71	4.03	–
Carbinoxamine (Clistin)	Maleate	Cl	H	N	8.65	2.69	10-20
Doxylamine (Unisom)	Succinate	H	CH_3	N	4.4 (pyr HB^+) 9.2 (HB^+)	2.34	7-13
Clemastine (Tavist)	Fumarate	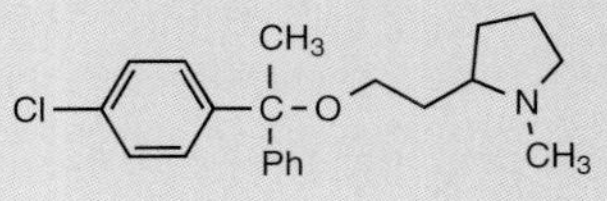			10.23	5.30	21

[a]pK_a and cLog P (calculated Log P) from Advanced Chemistry Development Software V11.02.
[b]From Baselt RC. *Disposition of Toxic Drugs and Chemicals in Man.* 11th ed. Seal Beach: Biomedical Publications; 2017 (monographs and references therein) or Micromedex.

Ethanolamine Ethers (Aminoalkyl Ethers)

Diphenhydramine, a benzhydryl (diphenylmethyl) ether (Table 25.2), is considered the prototype of the ethanolamine ether antihistamine class and continues to be widely used today. Several *p*-substituted phenyl ring analogues of diphenhydramine have been developed (CH_3, OCH_3, Cl, Br), as have 2-pyridyl aromatic ring bioisosteres.

Although the antihistaminic effect of the ethanolamine ethers is considered to be low to moderate, the antimuscarinic (anticholinergic or atropine-like) effects are generally considered to be high. As noted previously, these effects include tachycardia, dry mouth and mucous membranes, blurred vision, urinary retention, and constipation. The central anticholinergic effects of the ethanolamine ethers and other structurally related antihistamines have allowed some to find use in the treatment of Parkinson's disease, where they bring the central dopamine:acetylcholine ratio into better balance. Because they also produce a moderate to high degree of sedation, have relatively short half-lives, and enjoy a wide safety margin, some are used as OTC sleep aids. Their sedative properties require that they be used with caution in the elderly, when taking other sedative agents or consuming alcohol, and when engaging in activities that require alertness (e.g., operating dangerous machinery). They exhibit good antiemetic effects, and the 8-chlorotheophyllinate salt of diphenhydramine, marketed as dimenhydrinate, is used for prophylaxis and treatment of motion sickness.

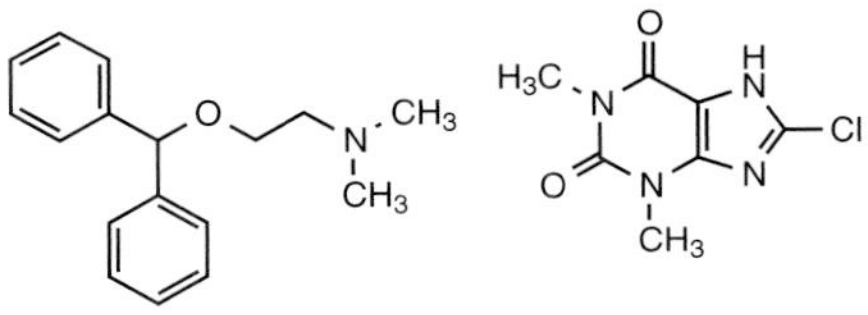

Dimenhydrinate
(diphenhydramine 8-chlorotheophyllinate)

Both the *p*-Cl-Ph and the 2-pyridyl ring found in carbinoxamine contribute to increased antihistaminic activity. Removal of the *p*-Cl and substitution of a methyl on the benzylic carbon, α to the ether oxygen affords doxylamine. It has good hypnotic activity when compared to secobarbital.[36] Clemastine has an additional carbon between the ether oxygen and the basic nitrogen, and the nitrogen is incorporated into a pyrrolidine ring. Because the ring is incorporated into the connecting chain, clemastine can exist as two enantiomeric pairs (I & II) and (III & IV) and thus, four diastereomeric pairs (I & III), (I & IV), (II & III), and (II & IV) (Table 25.3). The *R*,*R*-stereoisomer (I) is the form marketed. Like observations with similar compounds, the stereochemistry at the benzhydryl carbon has a greater influence on potency than the chiral center in the pyrrolidine ring.

ANTIHISTAMINIC VERSUS ANTICHOLINERGIC ACTIVITY. Selectivity for the histamine H_1 receptor over the muscarinic receptor may be affected by ortho versus para-substitution of one of the aromatic rings (the one that orients *cis* with respect to the cationic amine). With o-alkyl–substituted analogues, rotation of the two aromatic rings

Table 25.3 Stereoisomers of clemastine

Compound	Stereoisomer	ED_{50} (mg/kg)[a]	pA_2[b]
I Clemastine	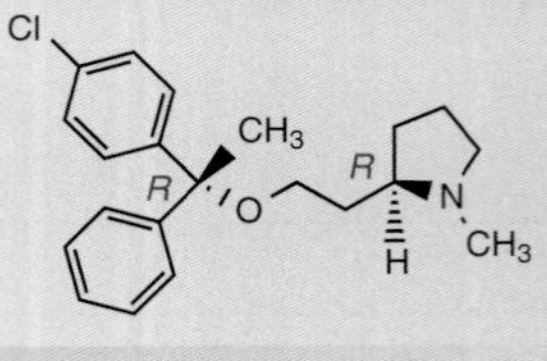 (R,R)	0.04	9.45
II	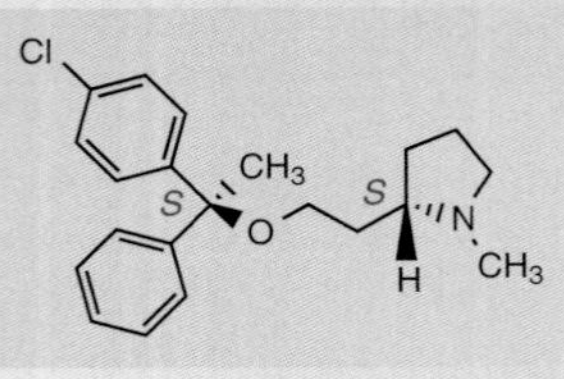 (S,S)	5.0	7.99
III	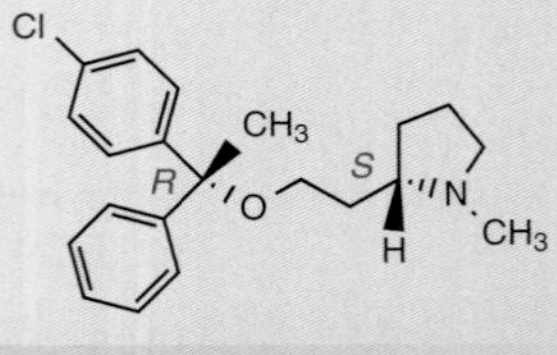 (R,S)	0.28	9.44
IV	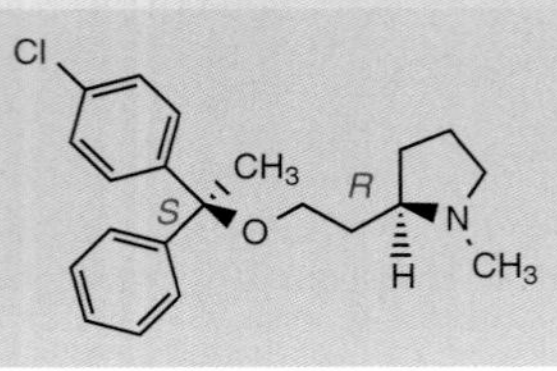 (S,R)	11.0	8.57

[a] ED_{50} for a lethal dose of histamine in guinea pigs.[37]

[b] The negative log of the molar concentration of an antagonist that requires doubling the concentration of an agonist in order to elicit the original submaximal response obtained in the absence of the antagonist.

Enantiomeric pairs: (I & II); (III & IV)

Diastereomeric pairs: (I & III); (I & IV); (II & III); (II & IV)

is restricted, and decreased antihistaminic and increased anticholinergic activity is observed as the size of the alkyl group increases.[37] *p*-Substitution results in decreased anticholinergic activity along with a small increase in antihistaminic activity. Both *o*- and *p*-substitution introduce chirality into the molecule, and enantiomeric differences in activity and receptor affinity are observed.

METABOLISM. There is limited information on metabolism of ethanolamine ether antihistamines. As one would predict, they commonly undergo sequential oxidative N-dealkylation to form the less active secondary and primary amines. This may be followed by inactivating oxidative deamination and oxidation to the corresponding carboxylic acid, which may be conjugated. O-Dealkylation has been reported for some members of this class.[35]

SPECIFIC DRUGS (TABLE 25.2)

Diphenhydramine. Diphenhydramine was introduced in the mid-1940s. The hydrochloride salt is available in tablet, capsule, oral solution, topical gel, and injectable forms. In addition to its use for allergic rhinitis, other approved uses include as an adjunct in anaphylaxis and in treatment of dermal pruritus, insomnia, motion sickness, Parkinsonism, and the common cold. Its use in Parkinsonism is associated with its central anticholinergic effects, and it can suppress the extrapyramidal effects of some antipsychotic drugs. As noted above, diphenhydramine is also marketed as the 8-chlorotheophyllinate salt under the generic name dimenhydrinate for treatment and prophylaxis of motion sickness.

The pK_a of diphenhydramine hydrochloride is 8.76. Therefore, it is predominately ionized at physiologic pH and exhibits high water solubility (1 g/mL). Diphenhydramine undergoes extensive oxidative N-dealkylation to the secondary and primary amines, followed by deamination and oxidation to form the diphenylmethoxyacetic acid (Fig. 25.7). The primary amine metabolite undergoes conjugation to form the N-glucuronide, while the carboxylic acid metabolite is likely excreted as a glycine or glutamine conjugate.[35]

Only about 1% of an oral dose of diphenhydramine is excreted unchanged, with about 64% excreted as metabolites in the urine.[38] Its elimination half-life is 4-8 hours in young adults but shows a significant increase (13.5 hr) in the elderly. The onset of action after an oral dose of diphenhydramine is 15-60 minutes with a duration of action of 4-6 hours for allergic reactions. Its bioavailability is about 65%. Protein binding varies from 76% to 85%. The volume of distribution varies from 480 to 292 L/70 kg.[39]

Adverse effects associated with diphenhydramine are typical for all first-generation antihistamines and include dry mouth, blurred vision, and sedation (see above). These effects may be exaggerated in the elderly due their slower rate of elimination in this often hepatically and renally

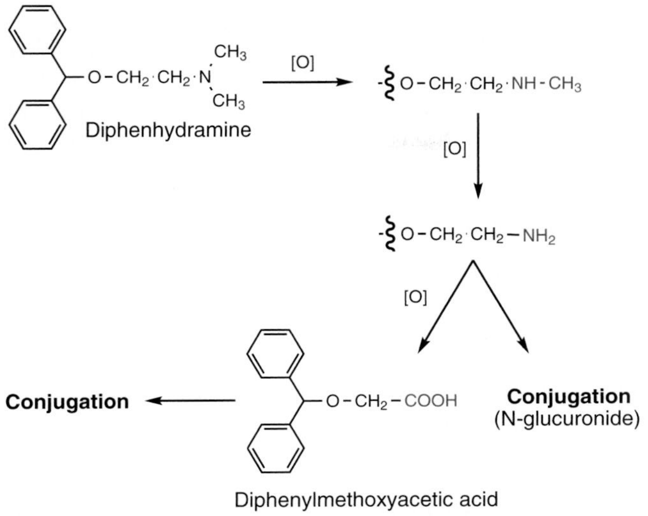

Figure 25.7 Diphenhydramine metabolism.

compromised population. Concurrent use with drugs that produce CNS depression may increase the risk of CNS and respiratory depression. Thus, patients should avoid use while driving, while operating dangerous machinery, or whenever it is essential to remain alert. Use along with other anticholinergic agents may increase the risk for paralytic ileus. Interestingly, diphenhydramine has been shown to inhibit the metabolism of CYP2D6 substrates. One such interaction is its inhibition of metoprolol metabolism in extensive metabolizers. In this population, the negative chronotropic and inotropic effects are prolonged, resulting in excessive drops in heart rate and blood pressure.[40]

Bromodiphenhydramine. Bromodiphenhydramine hydrochloride is used in combination products for relief of symptoms associated with allergies and the common cold. It is more lipophilic than diphenhydramine and has similar side effects and contraindications as diphenhydramine and other members of the ethanolamine ether class. In humans, it primarily undergoes mono and didemethylation to form the corresponding amines, as well as oxidation to the N-oxide. *p*-Bromobenzhydrol and *p*-bromobenzophenone, the reductive and oxidative products of O-dealkylation, respectively, as well as the phenol, *p*-hydroxybenzophenone, have been identified. Glucuronide conjugates are formed with the primary amine, alcohol, and phenol metabolites.[41]

Carbinoxamine. Carbinoxamine is a potent antihistaminic agent that is marketed as the racemate of the maleate salt. The (*S*)-enantiomer is the more potent isomer. Carbinoxamine is more lipophilic than diphenhydramine by virtue of its *p*-Cl substituent, and it is generally the more potent and longer lasting of two antihistamines. It is extensively metabolized, and its side effects and drug interactions are similar to other ethanolamine antihistamines. Carbinoxamine appears to undergo extensive metabolic transformation since no parent drug is found in the urine after therapeutic doses.[35]

Doxylamine. Doxylamine has two basic nitrogen atoms with pK_a values of 4.4 (pyridine HB^+) and 9.2 (aliphatic amine HB^+), and it is marketed as the succinate salt of the more basic aliphatic amine. It was introduced in 1948 and is primarily used as a sleep-inducing agent, as the α-methyl group enhances antimuscarinic action and sedative potential. It is also indicated for allergic rhinitis and for symptom control in the common cold. It is comparable to diphenhydramine in potency as an antihistamine, and its hypnotic potential is comparable to secobarbital and pentobarbital. Doxylamine is well absorbed orally, and its absorption is unaffected by food. Its Log P is 2.34 and, despite the addition of the α-methyl, it is less lipophilic than diphenhydramine, due to the bioisosteric replacement of phenyl ring of diphenhydramine with the more polar 2-pyridyl ring. Its onset and duration for treatment of insomnia are 30 minutes and 3-6 hours, respectively, with a mean elimination half-life of 13.11 hours.[42] The half-life is increased in geriatric and pediatric patients.

There are few studies examining the metabolism of doxylamine in man, but it is known to be excreted in the urine as unchanged doxylamine, the desmethyl and didesmethylated metabolites, and the N-acetyl conjugates.[43]

Clemastine. Clemastine fumerate has some unique features compared to other clinically available ethanolamine ethers. While it has a *p*-chlorophenyl ring similar to carbinoxamine and a quaternary, methyl substituted benzhydryl carbon similar to doxylamine, it is also a homologue with one extra carbon between the ether oxygen and the tertiary amine. The additional carbon atom in the spacer chain is accepted because the molecule is flexible enough to "bend" to ensure the appropriate 5-6 angstrom distance between anchoring cationic amine and the receptor-binding aromatic moieties. In addition, the carbon α to the amine is chiral because it is tied to one of the N-substituents via a pyrrolidine ring. Because clemastine possess two chiral centers, it exists as four stereoisomers, two enantiomeric pairs, and four diastereomeric pairs (Table 25.3). The (*R*,*R*) enantiomer is in clinical use and is the most potent of the four possible isomers. The chiral center at the benzhydryl carbon appears to influence receptor selectivity to a greater extent than the one in the pyrrolidine ring.[44]

Clemastine is well absorbed on oral administration and has an onset of 2 hours. It is primarily excreted via the kidneys with an elimination half-life of 21 hours. Its duration of action with multiple dosing is 10-12 hours. Clemastine undergoes extensive metabolism. The major urinary metabolite (M3) is the product of oxidative O-dealkylation (Fig. 25.8). A number of oxidative metabolites and dehydration products are also formed.[45] Its side effects and drug interactions are similar to others in this class and primarily involve its anticholinergic effects and sedation. Thus, like the others, it should be used with caution in the elderly, when operating machinery, or taking other anticholinergic drugs or CNS depressants.

Alkylamines (Propylamines)

A carbon atom replaces the heteroatom spacer (X) in the general structure of the alkylamine antihistamines (Fig. 25.6 and Table 25.4). This atom can be either sp^3 to afford a propylamine (Table 25.4) or sp^2 to give an olefinic propene analogue (see "DISCONTINUED OR LESS COMMONLY USED DRUGS OF STRUCTURAL INTEREST") with the *E*-isomer being more potent than the *Z*-isomer. The more active *E* isomer places the bulkier of the two aromatic rings *cis* to the protonated amine, allowing the unsubstituted *trans* ring to reach the sterically restricted binding site on the H_1 receptor. In the case of phenindamine, both aromatic rings

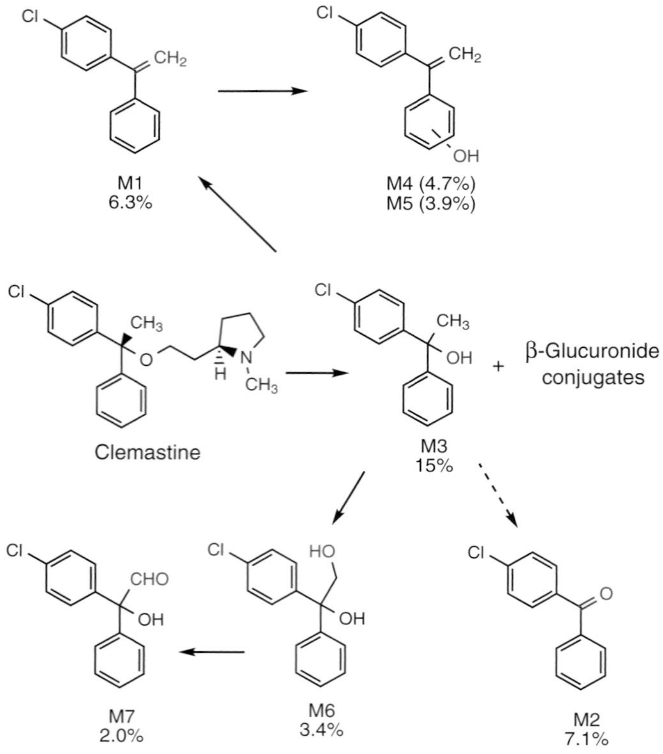

Figure 25.8 Phase I metabolites of clemastine in man.

are unsubstituted and would be accepted at either site. The saturated propylamines are often referred to as pheniramines. Three of these, pheniramine (*p*-H), chlorpheniramine (*p*-Cl), and brompheniramine (*p*-Br), are currently in clinical use. The halogen-substituted analogues exhibit much greater potency, likely due to an increase in lipophilicity. They have good antihistaminic properties and a long duration of action, and thus, have been widely used for the OTC treatment of allergic rhinitis, often in combination with decongestants, expectorants, antitussives, and analgesics.

The *p*-halo–substituted pheniramines generally produce less sedation than the ethylenediamines and ethanolamine ethers. In addition, they exhibit only moderate anticholinergic effects in comparison to the ethanolamine ethers. Those in clinical use have a 2-substituted pyridine ring, making them chiral. Racemic chlorpheniramine and brompheniramine were the most widely used antihistamines until the "nonsedating" second-generation antihistamines were introduced.

STRUCTURAL AND STEREOCHEMICAL EFFECTS. As mentioned above, in tissue-based assays, the *E*-isomers of the olefinic analogues exhibit a much greater potency than the corresponding *Z*-isomers. The *E*-isomers of pyrrobutamine and triprolidine are 165- and 1,000-fold more potent, respectively, than their *Z*-isomers.[16] Studies with compounds with varying degrees of conformational restriction, e.g., dimethindene and phenindamine, suggested that the receptor requires a 5-6 angstrom distance between the binding site for the cationic tertiary aliphatic amine and one of the aromatic rings,[46,47] and that the binding sites for the two aromatic moieties differ in their degree of steric restriction.

Potency differences between the enantiomers of the pheniramine derivatives have also been observed. In radioligand displacement and tissue-based assays the (+)-*S*-enantiomer of chlorpheniramine (Ar = Cl-Ph, 2-pyridyl) exhibits 200- to 1,000-fold greater affinity for H_1 receptors than its (−)-*R*-enantiomer. The (+)-*S*-enantiomer also shows greater selectivity for H_1 receptors relative to muscarinic and adrenergic receptors, and it is also more potent.

Both chlorpheniramine and brompheniramine, and to a lesser extent their *dextro*-isomers, have been used as the maleate or tannate salts in over-the-counter and prescription products. They are sometimes formulated with decongestants, expectorants, antitussives, and analgesics.

SPECIFIC DRUGS

Chlorpheniramine. Chlorpheniramine is used for treatment of allergic rhinitis and symptoms associated with the common cold in adults and children over the age of six.

Table 25.4 Alkylamine Antihistamines

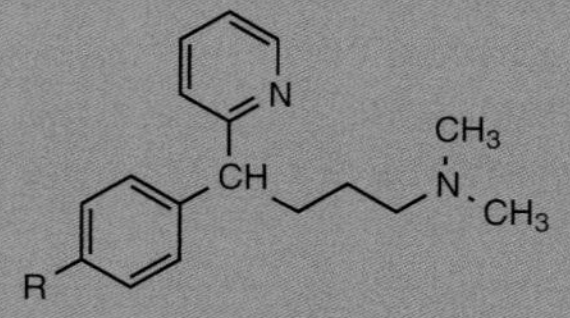

Drug	Salt	R	pK_a[a]	cLog P[a]	$t_{1/2}$ (hr)[b]
Pheniramine	Maleate	H	9.36	2.20	16-19
Chlorpheniramine (Chlor-Trimeton) (Dexchlorpheniramine)	Maleate	Cl	9.33	2.97	20
Brompheniramine (Dimetapp) (Dexbrompheniramine) (D-isomer)	Maleate, tannate (Maleate)	Br	9.33	3.24	25

[a] pK_a and cLog P (calculated Log P) from Advanced Chemistry Development Software V11.02.
[b] From Baselt RC. *Disposition of Toxic Drugs and Chemicals in Man.* 11th ed. Seal Beach: Biomedical Publications; 2017 (monographs and references therein) or Micromedex.

Off-label uses include atopic dermatitis, urticaria, psoriasis, and mastocytosis. Like others in this class, it exhibits low sedative effects, moderate anticholinergic effects, and moderate to high antihistaminic effects. While its average half-life is about 20 hours, it can vary from 12 to 43 hours depending on the individual and urine pH. The lipophilicity contributed by the chloro- group contributes to the longer half-life. Chlorpheniramine undergoes oxidative N-dealkylation to form the mono- and didemethylated amines as well as other oxidized products.[48] On chronic administration of 4 mg, urinary metabolites have been reported to include unchanged drug (13%), monodemethylated (13%) and didemethylated (6%) over a 24-hour period.[49] Deamination has not been reported for chlorpheniramine.

Chlorpheniramine maleate is primarily marketed as a racemic mixture, often in combination with a decongestant. Although not as widely used, the (+)-enantiomer, dexchlorpheniramine maleate, is also available. The dose of the (+)-isomer is half that of the racemic mixture. It is available as oral, single, and extended release tablets and as an oral solution. It is sometimes formulated with decongestants, expectorants, antitussives, and analgesics.

Brompheniramine. Brompheniramine is indicated for treatment of allergic rhinitis, as an adjunct to epinephrine for anaphylaxis, urticaria, urticarial transfusion reaction, and vasomotor rhinitis. Because a bromo group imparts greater lipophilicity than a chloro group, brompheniramine is more lipophilic than chlorpheniramine. This likely contributes to its greater potency and longer half-life than chlorpheniramine; 20 and 25 hours for chlorpheniramine and brompheniramine, respectively. Brompheniramine undergoes mono- and di-N-demethylation. It also undergoes deamination, followed by oxidation to the diarylpropionic acid and conjugation with glycine.[50]

Pheniramine. Pheniramine is not available in the United States as a single-ingredient product. It is marketed for ophthalmic use in combination with naphazoline for treatment of ocular inflammatory conditions. A nasal spray containing phenylephrine is also available. It is found in several oral extended release tablet or capsule formulations and oral liquids for treatment of nasal and sinus congestion. Other ingredients in these oral products may include phenylephrine, phenylpropanolamine, guaifenesin, sodium salicylate, dextromethorphan, codeine, or hydrocodone. Like its halogen-substituted analogues, pheniramine undergoes oxidative N-dealkylation to the mono- and didealkylated amines.[51,52]

Piperazines

Examination of the structure of the piperazine class of H_1 antagonists (Table 25.5) reveals direct similarities with the ethylenediamines and bioisosteric similarities with the ethanolamine ethers. The two nitrogen atoms found in the ethylenediamines are incorporated into a piperazine ring in this class, thus providing a two-carbon separation between the nitrogen atoms as seen in the ethylendiamines. The diaryl-substituted methylene or benzhydryl group is attached to one of the nitrogen atoms of the piperazine ring. The other, a basic aliphatic amine, is attached to an alkyl or aralkyl group.

Members of this class include meclizine, hydroxyzine, and its metabolite, cetirizine (discussed with the second-generation antihistamines below). The piperazines are moderately potent as antihistamines, and they exhibit significant anticholinergic side effects. Because of their ability to penetrate the CNS, they also cause sedation and psychomotor and cognitive dysfunction. They are among the more effective antihistamine-based antiemetics and can be used to treat motion sickness. Their anticholinergic actions likely contribute to this therapeutic action. While teratogenic effects have been observed in rodents, this has not been studied in humans. Nevertheless, these agents should be used with caution in pregnant women and children.

SPECIFIC DRUGS

Hydroxyzine. Hydroxyzine is marketed as the hydrochloride (intramuscular and oral) and pamoate (oral) salt forms. While it is rarely used as an antihistamine because of

Table 25.5 Piperazine Antihistamines

HC–N (piperazine) N–R; Cl

Drug	Salt	R_1	R_2	pK_a[a]	cLog P[a]	$t_{1/2}$ (hr)[b]
Meclizine (Antivert)	HCl, diHCl	Cl	$-CH_2$–(3-methylphenyl) (CH_3)	3.1, 6.2	5.28	5-6
Hydroxyzine (Atarax, Vistaril)	HCl, pamoate	Cl	$-CH_2CH_2OCH_2CH_2OH$	2.1, 7.1	2.32	13-27

[a]pK_a and cLog P (calculated Log P) from Advanced Chemistry Development Software V11.02.
[b]From Baselt RC. *Disposition of Toxic Drugs and Chemicals in Man.* 11th ed. Seal Beach: Biomedical Publications; 2017 (monographs and references therein) or Micromedex.

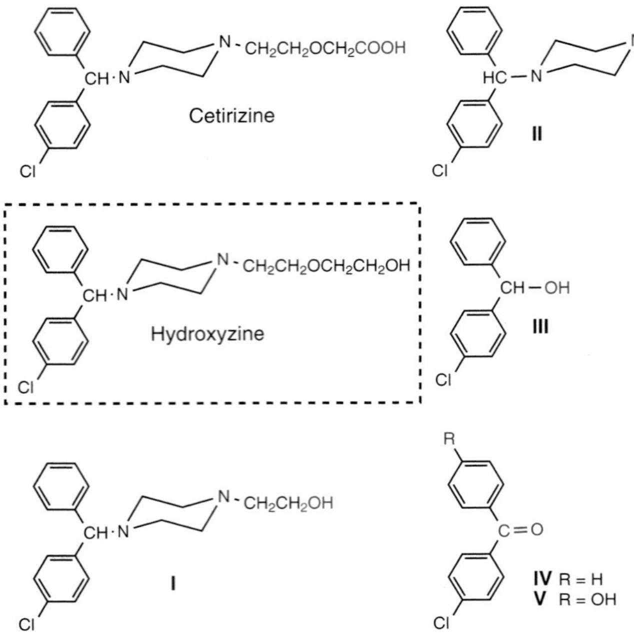

Figure 25.9 Phase I metabolites of hydroxyzine.

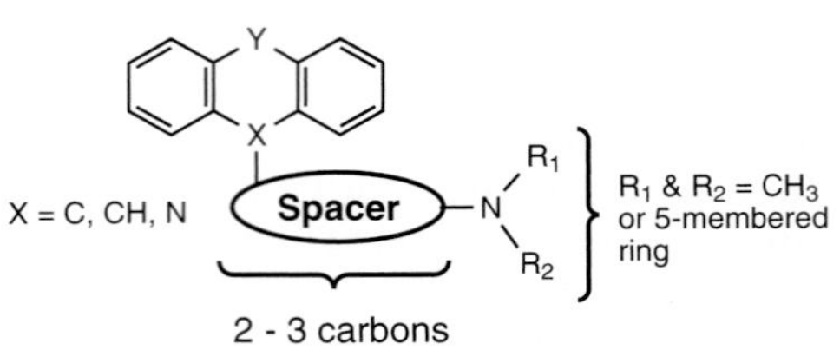

Figure 25.10 General structure of tricyclic antihistamines.

its sedative properties, it is used pre- and post-op for nausea, anxiety, pruritus, and allergic rhinitis, as well as a sedative. Phase 1 metabolites of hydroxyzine are illustrated in Figure 25.9. The terminal hydroxymethyl group of hydroxyzine undergoes sequential oxidation by cytosolic alcohol dehydrogenase and aldehyde dehydrogenase to provide the active carboxylic acid metabolite, cetirizine. Oxidative O-dealkylation and N-dealkylation of the ether side chain gives the ethanolamine (I) and norhydroxyzine (II) analogues, respectively. N-Dealkylation at the benzhydryl carbon affords *p*-chlorobenzophenone (IV). Reductions of IV gives III. *p*-Hydroxylation (aromatic oxidation) of the phenyl ring of IV also occurs to yield the phenol (V). Similar metabolic patterns occur for others in this class.

Meclizine. Meclizine is an analogue of hydroxyzine in which the hydroxy ether side chain has been replaced with a 3-methylbenzyl group. The 3-methylbenzyl significantly increases lipophilicity relative to hydroxyzine. It is marketed as both the hydrochloride and the dihydrochloride salt. It is metabolized via N-dealkylation similar to hydroxyzine to afford normeclizine, which is the same structure as norhydroxyzine and has only minimal pharmacologic activity.[35]

Tricyclic H_1 Antihistamines

Connection of the two aromatic rings found in some classes of first-generation antihistamines can afford active H_1 antagonists known as tricyclic antihistamines. The two rings may be connected via a heteroatom such as sulfur or oxygen or with a one- or two-carbon chain (Fig. 25.10 and Table 25.6). Compounds with a phenothiazine ring system (Y = S, X = N) were the earliest tricyclic antihistamines (e.g., promethazine, Table 25.6). The aromatic rings on antihistaminic phenothiazines are unsubstituted and have a branched two- or three-carbon aliphatic amine side chain attached to the nonbasic diarylamine.

Antipsychotic phenothiazines differ in that they have an electron-withdrawing substituent on an aromatic ring and possess a three-carbon, unbranched aliphatic amine side chain.

Tricyclic antihistamines are typically used to treat nausea and vomiting associated with anesthesia and motion sickness and for their antipruritic effect in the treatment of urticaria.

CONFORMATIONAL AND STEREOCHEMICAL EFFECTS. Connection of the two aromatic rings results in steric restrictions. At first glance, one might think these rings are flat or in the same plane, when in fact they are slightly puckered or noncoplaner. These possible conformations may rapidly

Table 25.6 Tricyclic First-Generation Antihistamines

Drug	Salt	pK_a[a]	cLog P[a]	$t_{1/2}$ (hr)[b]
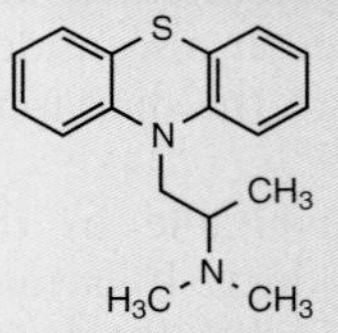 Promethazine (Phenergan)	HCl	8.89	4.89	10-20
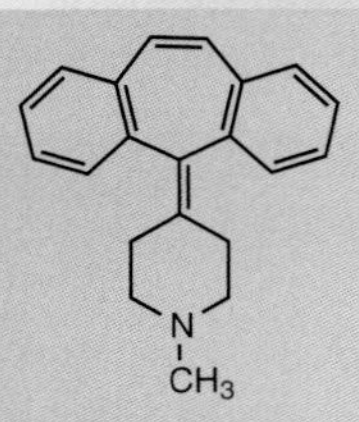 Cyproheptadine (Periactin)	HCl	8.95	5.82	20-70
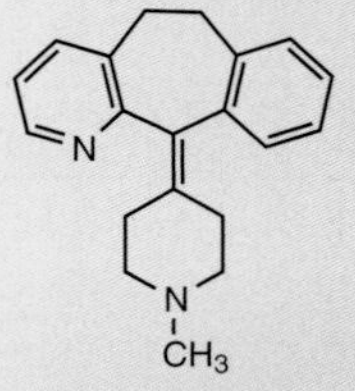 Azatadine	maleate	8.74	2.69	9

[a]pK_a and cLog P (calculated Log P) from Advanced Chemistry Development Software V11.02.

[b]From Baselt RC. *Disposition of Toxic Drugs and Chemicals in Man*. 11th ed. Seal Beach: Biomedical Publications; 2017 (monographs and references therein) or Micromedex.

interconvert, but in some related systems, where the interconversion is slow, conformational enantiomers (i.e., atropoisomers) may exist.[53,54] These have been studied with cyproheptadine, doxepin, and hydroxylated metabolites of loratadine (discussed below).[55] The pharmacological potency is significantly different (9- to 60-fold) for the conformational enantiomers of 3-methoxycyproheptadine as antihistamine, antiserotonin, and anticholinergic agents. The (−)-isomer retained the antihistaminic, antiserotonin, and appetite-stimulant effects, while the (+)-isomer showed greater anticholinergic potency.

Replacement of the sulfur atom of the phenothiazine ring system with a two-carbon unsaturated or saturated bridge connecting the two aromatic rings produced related compounds such as cyproheptadine and azatadine. Replacement with $-CH_2$-O- affords doxepin.

SPECIFIC DRUGS

Promethazine. Promethazine is considered to be a good antiemetic, and it has high antihistaminic and anticholinergic effects. While it is used for its antihistaminic effects to treat allergic rhinitis, it is used more often as a sedative, an antiemetic in the prevention of motion sickness, and pre- and postoperatively to prevent and treat nausea and vomiting associated with surgical procedures. It is sometimes used to potentiate the pain-relieving effects of analgesics. Promethazine metabolism has not been extensively studied in man, but the metabolites norpromethazine (N-demethylation) and the sulfoxide have been reported.[35]

Cyproheptadine. Cyproheptadine could be considered an analogue of a phenothiazine in which the sulfur is replaced with an unsaturated ethylene (vinyl) bridge. Similarities may also be seen to the olefinic alkylamines, where the two aromatic rings are connected through an unsaturated ethylene bridge. In addition to its antihistaminic activity, cyproheptadine exhibits moderate anticholinergic and low sedative effects. It also acts as a serotonin antagonist, which explains its ability to stimulate appetite. While appetite stimulation and weight gain are not approved uses, it is used "off-label" to promote weight gain in conditions where this is needed, such as cancer. FDA-approved uses include allergic conjunctivitis and rhinitis, dermatologic urticaria, hypersensitivity to blood or plasma, urticaria due to cold, and vasomotor rhinitis.

Cyproheptadine is eliminated as unchanged drug (1%), the quaternary ammonium glucuronide (10%), and the remainder as metabolites resulting from N-demethylation, aromatic hydroxylation, heterocyclic ring oxidation, and conjugation.[35]

Azatadine. Azatadine is an analogue of cyproheptadine. It has a saturated ethylene bridge between the two aromatic rings, one of which is a fused pyridine rather than a fused benzene ring. It is a potent antihistamine and has been shown to be more potent than chlorpheniramine and cyproheptadine in protecting guinea pigs from histamine challenge.[56] It is approved for used in allergic rhinitis, Eustachian tube obstruction, and urticaria. Like cyproheptadine, azatadine exhibits anticholinergic and antiserotonin activity. It has also been shown to inhibit mediator release from human mast cells.[57]

Second-Generation (Nonsedating) H_1 Antihistamines

Selectivity and Lack of CNS Effects

Introduction of the second-generation, nonsedating H_1 antihistamines in the 1980s improved the quality of life of patients suffering from allergic conditions. Agents in this class may be found in Table 25.7 and Figure 25.11. In contrast to first-generation antihistamines, these new antihistamines have greater selectivity for peripheral H_1 receptors and are relatively free from adverse CNS effects, as well as anticholinergic, antiserotonergic, and antiadrenergic effects.[58] Their lack of sedative properties is likely due to a greatly reduced ability to penetrate the blood-brain barrier. This is the result of their being substrates for the drug efflux P-gp transporter[59] or the organic anion transporter, or because of poor partitioning characteristics resulting from their being amphoteric and existing as zwitterions at physiologic pH.[58] While the first-generation antihistamines are lipophilic amines that readily penetrate the blood-brain-barrier, causing sedation as a side-effect, some of the second-generation antihistamines possess both the basic amine required for activity, as well as a carboxylic acid group. These latter agents exist as zwitterions at physiologic pH and are more polar than those agents containing only the basic amine. For example, at pH 7.4, the log D of the first-generation antihistamine hydroxyzine is 3.1, while cetirizine, its zwitterionic carboxylic acid metabolite, has a log D of 1.5, making it much less lipophilic. The decrease in lipophilicity exhibited by cetirizine would be even greater were it not for the ability of the carboxylate anion to fold around and form an intramolecular ionic bond with the protonated amine. As a result, these zwitterionic molecules exhibit lower CNS penetration and an improved side effect profile. The CNS activity of the second-generation agents varies from 0% (fexofenadine) to 30% (cetirizine).

The carboxylic acid group also contributes to enhanced H_1 receptor affinity. It can form an ionic bond with Lys191 of the receptor.[60] This contributes to the slow receptor dissociation kinetics seen with these agents.

There is a large variation in structure in the second-generation antihistamines. For some, structural similarities with first-generation agents are readily apparent, while for others, they are not obvious. The large N-substituents found on these agents when compared to the first-generation antihistamines may contribute to their lack of affinity for cholinergic, α-adrenergic, or serotonergic receptors.

Extensive clinical use of astemizole and terfenadine revealed that concurrent use with drugs that are inhibitors of, or cosubstrates for, CYP3A4 is associated with dangerous cardiac arrhythmias.[61] This combination could lead to prolongation of the QT interval and torsades de points, a life-threatening ventricular arrhythmia. These effects are associated with blockade of the hERG gene product, a subunit of an inward-rectifying cardiac potassium channel (I_{Kr}).[62,63] The arrhythmias are observed at high concentrations of these lipophilic amines, such as when they are concurrently used with inhibitors of CYP3A4 or with competing CYP3A4 substrates, such as ketoconazole or macrolide antibiotics like erythromycin. This is not a class effect and is only associated with astemizole and terfenadine. Both are no longer marketed in the United States.

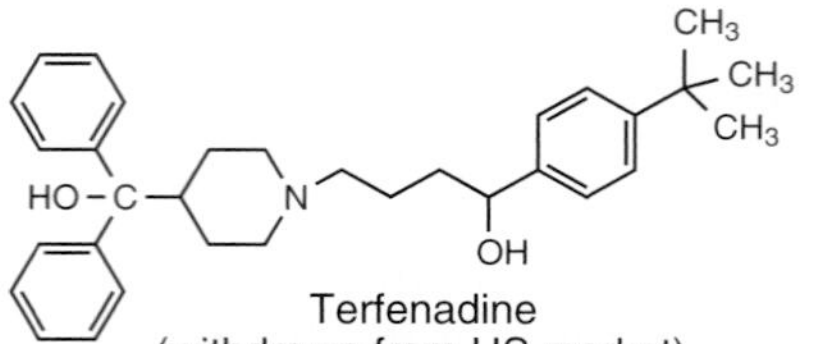

Terfenadine
(withdrawn from US market)

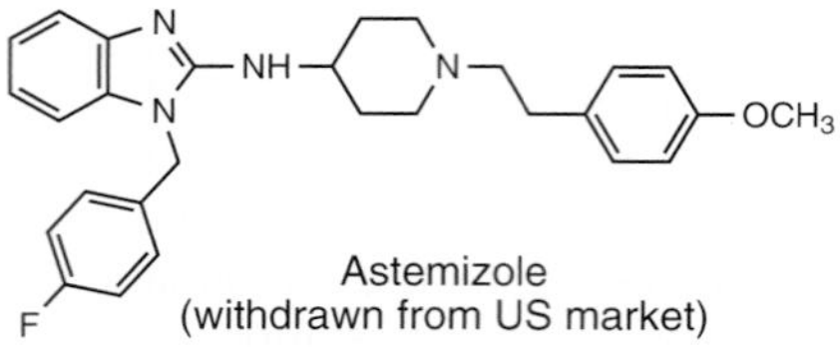

Astemizole
(withdrawn from US market)

THE RISE, FALL, AND RESURRECTION OF TERFENADINE

Terfenadine (Seldane) was the first nonsedative antihistamine to be marketed in the United States and, as such, it was a blockbuster. It was known to be highly cardiotoxic, but in most individuals it was readily converted via CYP3A4 and cytosolic enzymes to noncardiotoxic metabolites. These metabolites not only retained the nonsedative properties of terfenadine, the carboxylic acid metabolite exhibited antihistaminic action up to four times that of the parent drug. However, the risk of potentially fatal arrhythmia, including torsades de pointes and cardiac arrest, when given to vulnerable patients, those with hepatic disease and/or when coadministered drugs or foods that inhibit CYP3A4 (e.g., conazole antifungal agents, erythromycin, grapefruit juice), resulted in a "Black Box Warning."

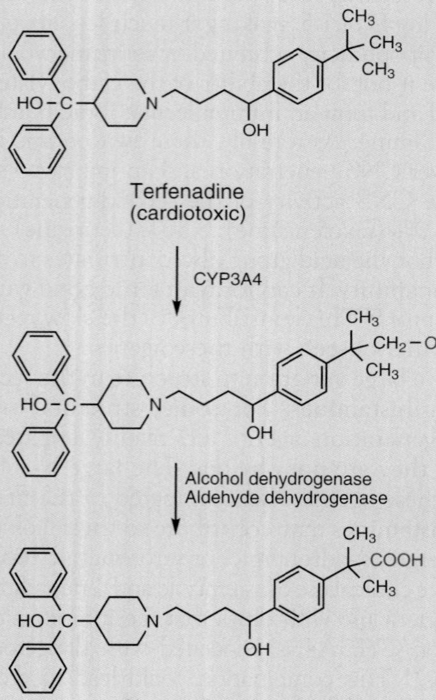

Terfenadine
(cardiotoxic)

CYP3A4

Alcohol dehydrogenase
Aldehyde dehydrogenase

Noncardiotoxic carboxylic acid

In 1996, the Pharmacy profession was collectively reminded of their critical role in protecting the public health when approximately one-third of practitioners in selected Washington D.C. area pharmacies dispensed terfenadine along with erythromycin without comment or warning when presented with simultaneous prescriptions in a study conducted by Georgetown University researchers. The study received much attention in the professional literature and lay press, and within 3 years, terfenadine was withdrawn from the US market.

However, the manufactures of terfenadine took clinical and economic advantage of their understanding of terfenadine metabolism to bring the noncardiotoxic carboxylic acid metabolite to the market as fexofenadine (Allegra, the Italian word for "happy"). Allegra has enjoyed significant success and has been joined by other second-generation antihistamines that owe their nonsedating properties to their zwitterionic character, which drives a folded conformation that prevents their accumulation in the CNS.

SPECIFIC DRUGS USED SYSTEMICALLY IN ALLERGIC RHINITIS (FIG. 25.11, TABLE 25.7)

Fexofenadine. Fexofenadine is the carboxylic acid metabolite produced by rapid CYP3A4-catalyzed oxidation of one of the methyl groups on the t-butyl group of terfenadine. Fexofenadine is believed responsible for the antihistaminic properties seen with terfenadine, but it has none of terfenadine's life-threatening arrhythmic actions. It is a long-acting (>12 hr), lipophilic, selective H_1 antagonist that shows little affinity for the cholinergic, adrenergic, or serotonergic receptors. The N-phenylbutanol group is believed to be, at least in part, responsible for the high H_1 receptor selectivity. The enantiomers of terfenadine have been shown to have approximately equal activity,[64] but there are little data on the activity of the enantiomers of fexofenadine. However, the drug efflux transporter P-glycoprotein and organic anion transporter proteins may show some stereoselectivity, since higher plasma concentrations are seen for the *R*-enantiomer. The N-phenylbutanol group is linked to affinity for the P-glycoprotein efflux pump and thus, reduced CNS accumulation. Fexofenadine is primarily eliminated unchanged with 80% appearing in the feces and 11% in the urine.[35]

Loratadine and Desloratadine. Loratadine and its metabolite desloratadine are both peripherally selective, nonsedating, antihistamines used for treatment of idiopathic urticarial and chronic and seasonal allergic rhinitis. They have structural similarities with tricyclic first-generation antihistamines and tricyclic antidepressants. Desloratadine is the descarboethoxy metabolite of loratadine, and it has a longer half-life than the parent drug. Thus, with chronic administration, its plasma concentration will exceed that of loratadine. The potency of desloratadine is greater than that of loratadine as both an H_1 antagonist and as an inhibitor of histamine release. Because of its longer half-life, greater potency, and essentially complete generation from loratadine on first pass, desloratadine likely contributes

Table 25.7 Second-Generation Antihistamines

Drug	Salt	pK_a[a]	cLog P[a]	$t_{1/2}$ (hr)[b]
Systemic Agents				
Acrivastine	–	1.99	2.41	1.5-1.9
Cetirizine (Levocetirizine)	Hydrochloride (dihydrochloride)	2.7 (HA), 8 (HB^+)	1.61	6.5-10
Desloratadine	–	4.2 (HA), 9.7 (HB^+)	3.5	17-27
Fexofenadine	Hydrochloride	4.3 (HA), 9.5 (HB^+)	3.73	6-20
Loratadine	–	5.0 (HB^+)	3.9	3-20
Ophthalmic Agents				
Alcaftadine	–	8.76	2.66	1.7-3.5
Azelastine[c]	Hydrochloride	9.16 (HB^+)	3.47	22
Bepotastine	Besilate	4.4 (HA)	3.01	3-7
Emedastine	Difumarate	4.5 (HA), 8.5 (HB^+)	2.78	3-8
Epinastine	Hydrochloride	11.98 (HB^+)	3.5	12
Ketotifen	Fumarate	8.4	2.19	7-27
Olopatadine[a]	Hydrochloride	4.2 (HA), 9.8 (HB^+)	2.96	9-10

[a]pK_a and cLog P (calculated Log P) from Advanced Chemistry Development Software V11.02.
[b]From Baselt RC. *Disposition of Toxic Drugs and Chemicals in Man.* 11th ed. Seal Beach: Biomedical Publications; 2017 (monographs and references therein) or Micromedex.
[c]Opthalmic drops and nasal spray.

significantly to the overall activity of loratadine. When compared to first-generation antihistamines, desloratadine has a 100-fold slower receptor dissociation rate.[65]

The metabolic removal of the carbamate group of loratadine to afford the descarboethoxy analogue, desloratadine, is not via direct hydrolysis as one might first expect. Rather, it involves oxidation by CYP2D6 and CYP3A4 at the methylene group of the carbamate (Fig. 25.12).[66] This unstable hydroxylated intermediate readily undergoes O-deethylation and decarboxylation to give the secondary amine, desloratadine. When orally administered, loratadine is extensively converted to desloratadine on first pass through the liver. Thus, little, if any, loratadine parent drug reaches the general circulation or H_1 receptors. Concurrent use with CYP3A4 inhibitors or competitive substrates does not lead to significant drug-drug interactions, and they both lack effects on hERG K^+ ion channels in the heart. Desloratadine also undergoes oxidation to 3-hydroxydesloratadine, the principle hydroxylated metabolite. Other hydroxylated aliphatic and aromatic metabolites have been identified, with many appearing as products of O-glucuronidation.[67,68]

Desloratadine does not penetrate the CNS in significant concentration and has a long half-life, 17-27 hours in humans, with about 41% of an administered dose being excreted in the urine and a 47% in the feces over a 10-day period.[35,67,68]

Cetirizine and Levocetirizine. Cetirizine is the carboxylic acid metabolite formed upon oxidation of the primary alcohol of the first-generation antihistamine, hydroxyzine.[69] It has a long duration of action and no cardiotoxicity. Although many consider cetirizine to have decreased sedative effects, they are not absent. As described above, the "decreased sedation" is likely the result of its amphoteric nature.

The *R*-enantiomer is now marketed as levocetirizine, and its affinity for the H_1 receptor is more than 30-fold greater than that of the *S*-enantiomer, and its receptor dissociation rate is more than 20-fold slower.[70] Thus, most antihistaminic properties observed with cetirizine are likely due to the *R*-enantiomer. Levocetirizine is largely excreted unchanged (77%) in the urine with eight minor products of oxidation and glucuronide conjugation.[71]

Acrivastine. Acrivastine is a second-generation, acrylic acid–substituted analogue of the first-generation antihistamine triprolidine. Its CNS penetration is limited and it is less sedating than triprolidine. It is used in combination with the decongestant pseudoephedrine in seasonal rhinitis. Urinary excretion products include unchanged drug, the product of reduction of the double bond in the acrylic acid side chain, and some unidentified products. The reduction product is pharmacologically active but probably contributes little to overall activity because it is a minor product compared to the parent.

Second-Generation Topical (Ophthalmic and Nasal) H_1 Antihistamines

THERAPEUTIC APPLICATIONS. Several H_1 antihistamines have been formulated for topical application in the eye to relieve itching, congestion of the conjunctiva,

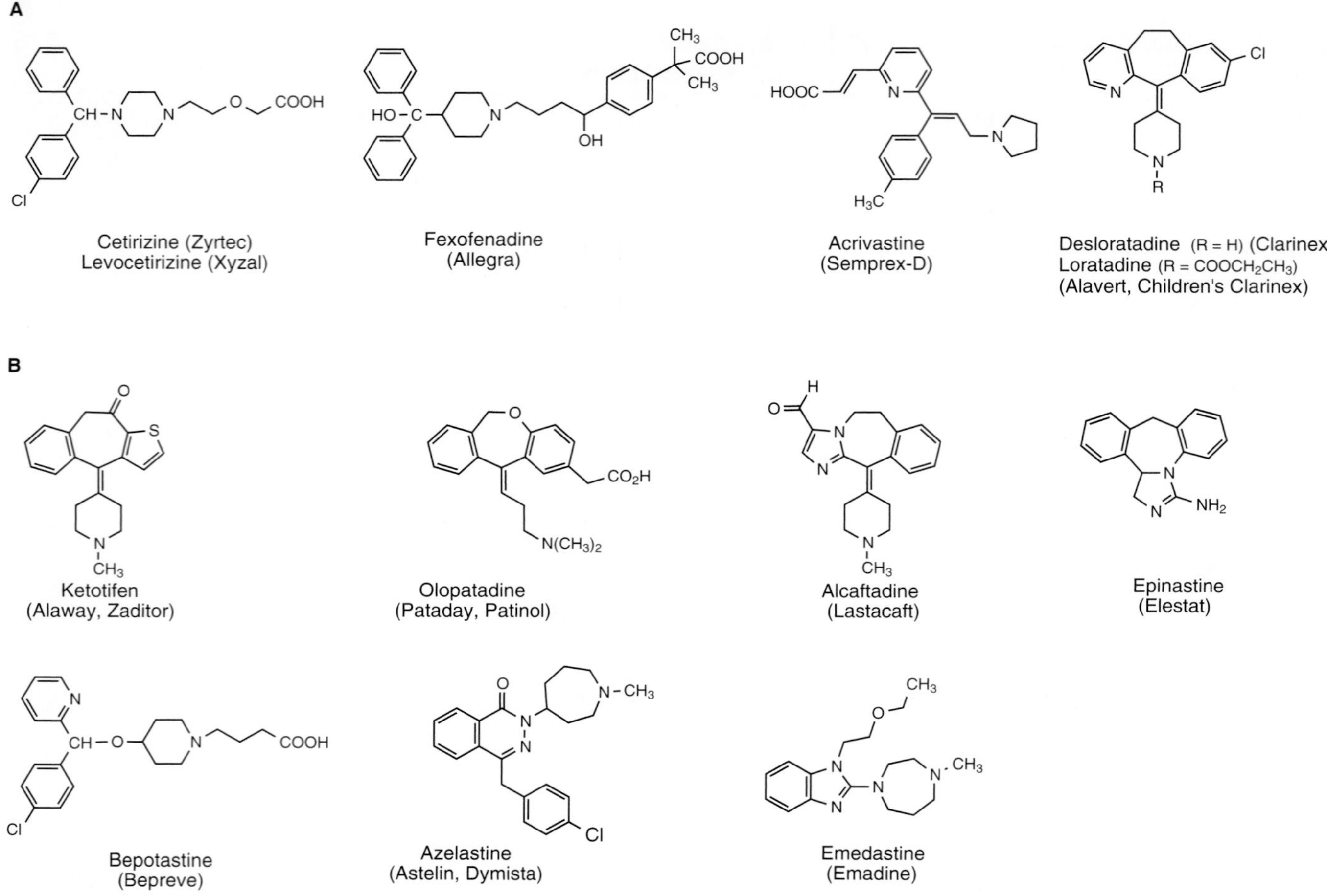

Figure 25.11 Second-generation antihistamines. A, Second-generation antihistamines used for their systemic action. B, Second-generation antihistamines for topical use (ophthalmic and nasal).

and erythema (Fig. 25.11 and Table 25.7; also see Chapter 27).[27,72] Ocular allergic reactions are common in seasonal allergy sufferers since the density of mast cells in the conjunctiva is high, and there is a significant concentration of histamine in the tear film. Only about 1%-5% of an antihistamine penetrates the cornea when topically applied. More of the drug is systemically absorbed via the conjunctiva and nasal mucosa, as well as from being swallowed from tear duct and nasal drainage. The first topical ocular antihistamines were the antazoline and pheniramine, first-generation agents in the ethylenediamine and alkylamine class, respectively. They are used in combination with sympathomimetic vasoconstrictors.

The more recently developed ocular antihistamines exhibit slow receptor dissociation kinetics and a long systemic duration of action. Those antihistamines with a log D near 1.0 ± 0.5 at pH 7.4 are the most efficacious, and their water-soluble salts exhibit a low incidence of ocular irritation. Log D takes into consideration the lipid/water distribution of both ionized and unionized forms at a given pH. The relationship between partitioning characteristics of an antihistamine and receptor affinity (moderate at the least) suggests that a particular range of lipophilicity is best for topical ocular antihistamines with minimum ocular irritation.[73]

SPECIFIC DRUGS (FIG. 25.11, TABLE 25.7)

Ketotifen. Ketotifen is a tricyclic antihistamine with structural similarities to cyproheptadine. It differs from cyproheptadine in that it has a bioisosteric thiophene ring in place of the benzene ring, and the bridge between the two aromatic rings is saturated and oxidized to a ketone at the benzylic position. It is a potent, selective dual action H_1 antihistamine that, in addition to its antihistamine actions, also stabilizes mast cells and prevents degranulation of eosinophils. It is used in the United States in OTC ophthalmic drops for treatment and prevention of itching associated with allergic conjunctivitis, and it is used systemically in other countries for seasonal allergic rhinitis, hay fever, and asthma. Ketotifen undergoes metabolic N-dealkylation to give norketotifen and N-oxidation to the N-oxide. Reduction of the exocyclic double bond produces dihydroketotifen. Glucuronic acid conjugation at the tertiary amine gives the quaternary N-glucuronide.[35,74]

Olopatadine. Olopatadine is a substituted dibenzoxepine that shows obvious structural similarities to the tricyclic antihistamines. It is formulated for topical use in the eye to treat allergic conjunctivitis and as a nasal spray for nasal symptoms of allergic rhinitis. It is a "dual-action" antihistamine because, in addition to its antihistaminic

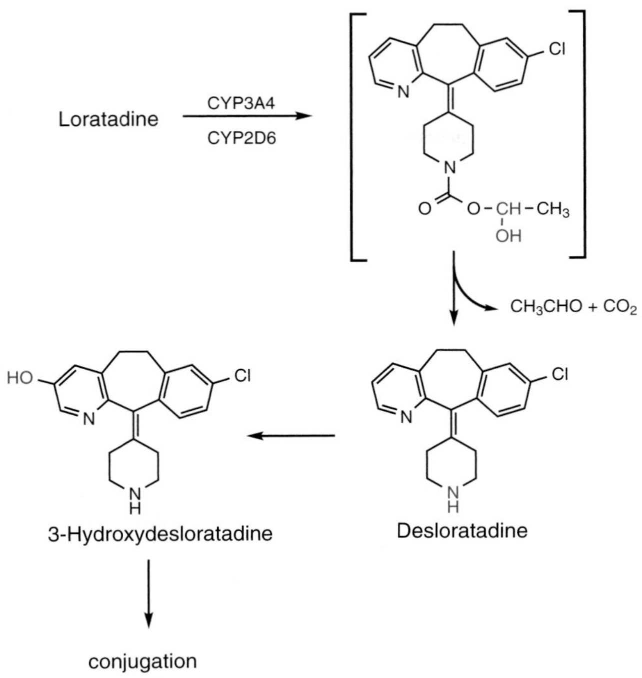

Loratadine → (CYP3A4, CYP2D6) → [intermediate] → ($CH_3CHO + CO_2$) Desloratadine → 3-Hydroxydesloratadine → conjugation

Figure 25.12 Metabolism of loratadine.

properties, it also exhibits mast cell–stabilizing properties, i.e., it inhibits release of other inflammatory mediators from mast cells (see below). Olopatadine is highly specific for H_1 receptors over H_2, H_3, α-adrenergic, dopaminergic, serotonergic, and muscarinic receptors. It has a rapid onset and long duration of action, indicative of high receptor affinity and slow dissociation kinetics. The carboxylic acid containing aromatic substituent is likely responsible for its lack of muscarinic effects. At pH 7.4, olopatadine would exist as a zwitterion, and the carboxylate group of the Z-isomer could form an ionic bond with protonated amine side chain. This likely contributes in some part to its limited CNS penetration. When binding to the receptor, the carboxylic acid extends out of the binding pocket and interacts with Lys191 and Tyr108 without displacing a phosphate ion that is also interacting with these residues.[60]

Olopatadine is only metabolized to a minor extent. In a 48-hour, single-dose study using labeled olopatadine in healthy adults, urine collection afforded parent drug (63%-72%), norolopatadine (1%), and olopatadine-N-oxide (3%).[75]

Alcaftadine. Alcaftadine is an aldehyde-substituted imidazobenzazpine H_1 antagonist that can be related to the other tricyclic H_1 antagonists. It is indicated for treatment of allergic conjunctivitis. It also inhibits histamine release from mast cells and inhibits eosinophil activation. The aldehyde group on the imidazole ring is metabolically oxidized to the carboxylic acid and excreted in the urine.

Epinastine. Epinastine is a dibenzazepine that is fused to a dihydroimidazolamine. Embedded within the structure is a basic guanidine moiety that is more basic than the typical aliphatic amine (Table 25.7). It is indicated for treatment of allergic conjunctivitis. Epinastine is selective for the H_1 receptor but also has some affinity for histamine H_2 receptors, adrenergic α_1 and α_2 receptors, and 5-HT_2 receptors. In humans it is eliminated largely unchanged in the urine (25%) and feces (70%).[35]

Emedastine. Emedastine is a relatively selective H_1 antagonist that is structurally related to the benzimidazoles (e.g., astemizole) and is formulated for ophthalmic administration for treatment of allergic conjunctivitis. It is relatively selective for H_1 receptors and has been shown to stabilize mast cells. Emedastine is metabolized to the phenols, 5- and 6-hydroxyemedastine, via aromatic oxidation, emedastine-N-oxide, and conjugates of the phenols.[76]

Azelastine. Azelastine is a substituted phthalazine-1(2H)-one that has some structural similarities to the benzimidazole emedastine. It is a dual-action antihistamine. Thus, like olopatadine, it also stabilizes mast cells and prevents release of histamine, leukotrienes, PGD_2, etc. It is used as a nasal spray and as eye drops in the United States for seasonal and perennial allergic rhinitis, allergic conjunctivitis, and vasomotor rhinitis. In Europe, it is available for systemic treatment of seasonal allergies and asthma. Azelastine undergoes oxidative N-dealkylation to give the active metabolite, N-desmethylazelastine which has a half-life twice that of the parent.[35]

Bepotastine. Bepotastine is substituted piperidine structurally related to the aminoalkyl ethers. Similarities to cetirizine and fexofenadine are also readily apparent. It is formulated as an ophthalmic solution for treatment of allergic conjunctivitis. In addition to its antihistaminic properties, it also inhibits release of histamine from mast cells. In a 24-hour study following a single oral dose in Japanese men, the parent drug was eliminated (76%-88%) in the urine along with an unidentified metabolite (1%).[77]

Histamine Release Inhibitors (Mast Cell Stabilizers)

Background

Khellin, a chromone found in the fruit of *Ammi visnaga*, also known as toothpick weed, possess bronchodilatory activity and has been used as a spasmolytic in the Mediterranean region as far back as ancient Egypt. Its use stimulated the search for related compounds with similar pharmacologic activity.[78] Cromolyn sodium, the first in this class, was developed while studying a large number of bischromones. Other agents in this class include nedocromil, pemirolast, and lodoxamide (Table 25.8). They are classified as mast cell stabilizers because they prevent release of histamine and other mediators from mast cells and other inflammatory cells associated with allergy and asthma. While they will prevent bronchospasm, they do not reverse antigen-induced bronchoconstriction. They exhibit no intrinsic bronchodilator, antihistaminic, anticholinergic, glucocorticoid, vasoconstrictor, or other systemic activity.

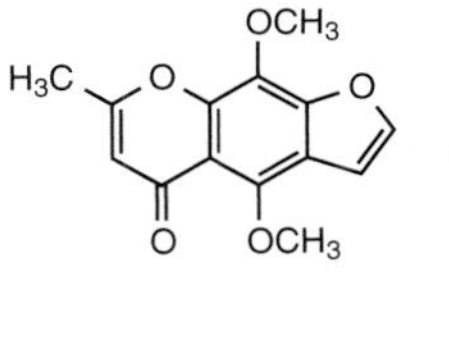

Khellin
cLog P = 1.73

Mechanism of Action

The mechanism by which cromolyn and nedocromil prevent degranulation of mast cells has been studied.[79] They stimulate protein kinase C–catalyzed phosphorylation of Ser residues of moesin, a protein involved in the bridging of actin cytoskeleton and cell membranes. This induces a conformational change in moesin that promotes its association with actin and other proteins of the secretory granules, leading to immobilization of the granules and inhibition of their exocytosis.[7] Another proposed mechanism involves inhibition of antigen-induced calcium ion influx into mast cells. This stabilizes the cells and prevents release of histamine, leukotrienes, and other inflammatory mediators that are involved in allergic reactions.

Cromolyn and the other mast cell stabilizers also inhibit activation and mediator release from eosinophils, macrophages, neutrophils, monocytes, and platelets.

Specific Drugs (Table 25.8)

CROMOLYN. Cromolyn is a bischromone carboxylic acid complex that is marketed as the sodium salt.

It is used prophylactically by inhalation via a nebulizer or a metered dose inhaler for prevention of asthma and exercise-induced bronchospasm, and as a nasal spray for prevention of seasonal and perennial allergic rhinitis. It is formulated for topical use as eye drops to prevent allergic conjunctivitis and keratitis. An oral dosage form is available for the treatment of mastocytosis, an uncommon disorder that involves abnormal elevation of mast cell density in the skin, bone marrow, and/or internal organs. On oral administration, its bioavailability is low due to poor absorption, and less than 10% reaches systemic circulation on inhalation. To be effective, cromolyn must be administered at least 30 minutes prior to antigen exposure. Overuse can lead to development of tolerance.

NEDOCROMIL. Nedocromil is a pyranoquinolone dicarboxylic acid derivative related to cromoloyn. Its sodium salt is formulated as an ophthalmic solution for prevention of seasonal and perennial allergic conjunctivitis. Aerosols have previously been used for prophylaxis of asthma, but they are not currently available due to difficulties finding a qualified manufacturer for the chlorofluorocarbon propellant inhaler. Its mechanism is like that of cromolyn.

LODOXAMIDE. Lodoxamide is a dicarboxylic acid, with some structural similarities to both cromolyn and nedocromil. It is marketed as the tromethamine (1,1,1-tris(hydroxymethyl)aminomethane salt. Its molecular mechanism(s) of action is (are) not completely understood, but are believed to be similar to that of cromolyn and others in this class. It is used as an ophthalmic solution for treatment of vernal conjunctivitis and vernal keratitis.

PEMIROLAST. Pemirolast potassium is unique among the clinically used mast cell stabilizers because it has a bioisosteric tetrazole (pK_a = 4) in place of the carboxylic acid seen in the others. The acidic proton on the tetrazole ring

Table 25.8 Mast Cell Stabilizers (Degranulation Inhibitors)

Drug	pK_a[a]	cLog P[a]	$t_{1/2}$ (hr)[b]
Cromolyn (Intal)	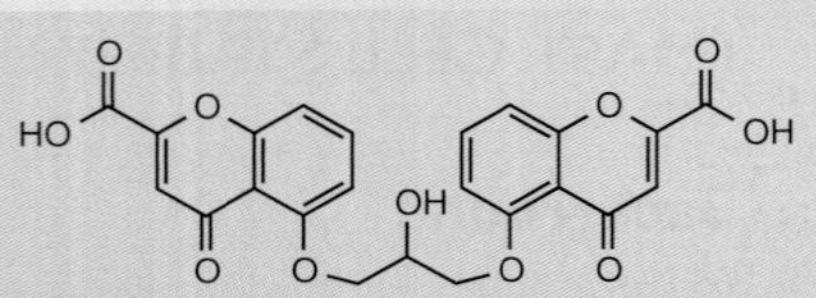 4.00	2.0	1.5-2.0
Nedocromil (Alocril)	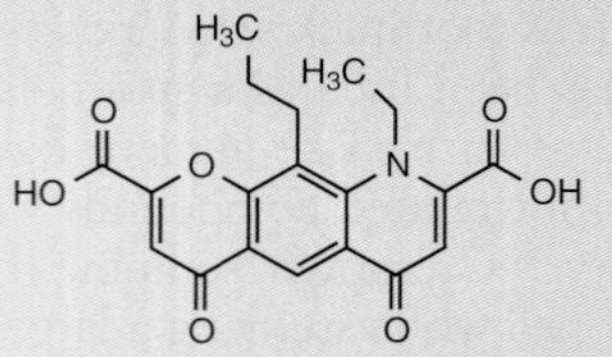 2.19	1.30	1-3
Lodoxamide (Alomide)	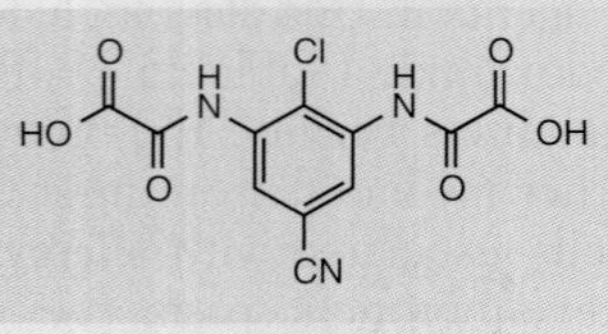 2.07	−0.40	8.5
Pemirolast (Alamast)	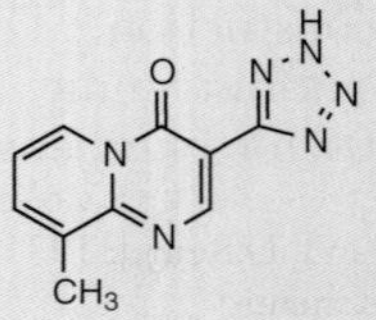 4.00	0.22	4-5

[a]pK_a and cLog P (calculated Log P) from Advanced Chemistry Development Software V11.02.

[b]From Baselt RC. *Disposition of Toxic Drugs and Chemicals in Man.* 11th ed. Seal Beach: Biomedical Publications; 2017 (monographs and references therein) or Micromedex.

is the site of salt formation. This group is attached to a pyrido[1,2α]pyrimidin-4-one ring system. It is used as an ophthalmic solution for prophylaxis of itching associated with allergic conjunctivitis. Like cromolyn it inhibits release of histamine and other inflammatory mediators from mast cells.

ACKNOWLEDGMENT

The author wishes to acknowledge the work of Wendel L. Nelson, PhD, who authored content used within this chapter in a previous edition of this text.

Structure Challenge

The structures of five antihistamines are provided below. Use your understanding of antihistaminic SAR to identify the appropriate agent for each of the following descriptors.

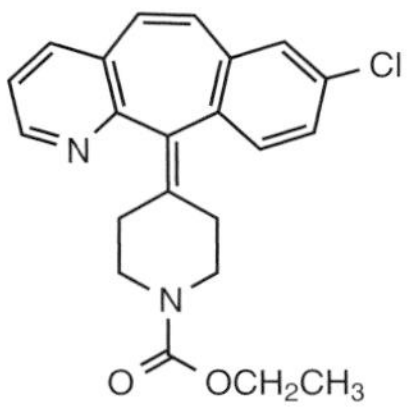

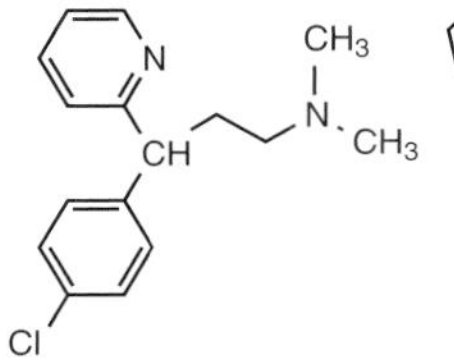

a. Which could be used as an OTC sleep aid?
b. Which should not be used in a man who has benign prostatic hypertrophy (BPH)?
c. Which is sometimes used to stimulate appetite to produce weight gain?
d. Which is metabolized via CYP-catalyzed O-dealkylation and subsequent decarboxylation to form a metabolite that is likely responsible for most of the antihistamine activity of the parent?
e. Which owes its nonsedative properties to its ability to exist as a zwitterion at physiologic pH?
f. What effect would replacing the 2-pyridyl ring of compound II with a phenyl ring have on its antihistaminic activity?

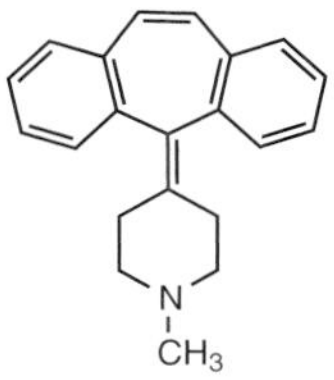

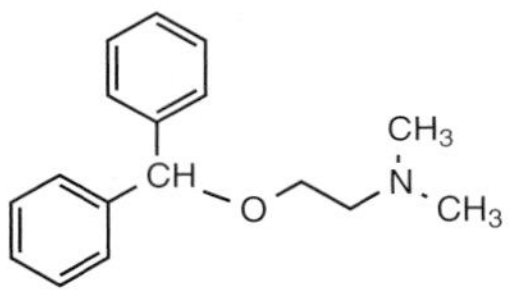

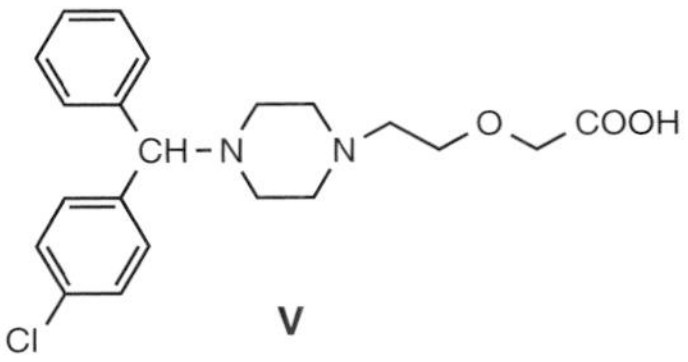

Structure Challenge answers found immediately after References.

REFERENCES

1. Benninger M, Farrar JR, Blaiss M, et al. Evaluataing approved medications to treat rhinitis in the United States: an evidence-based review of efficacy for nasal symptoms by class. *Ann Allergy Asthma Immunol*. 2010;104:13-29.
2. Meltzer EO, Bukstein DA. The economic impact of allergic rhinitis and current guidelines for treatment. *Ann Allergy Asthma Immunol*. 2011;106:S12-S16.
3. Stempel DA, Woolf R. The cost of treating allergic rhinitis. *Curr Allergy Asthma Rep*. 2007;28:223-230.
4. Ramachandran M, Aronson JK. John Bostock's first description of hayfever. *J R Soc Med*. 2011;104:237-240.
5. Windaus A, Vogt W. Synthesis of iminazolylethylethylamine. *Chem Ber*. 1907;40:3691-3698.
6. Barger G, Dale HH. 4β-Aminoethylglycoxaline (β-Iminazolylethylamine) and the other active principles of ergot. *J Chem Soc Trans*. 1910;97:2592-2595.
7. Ackermann D. Uber den bacteriellen Abbau des Histadine. *Hopp-Seylers Z Physiol Chem*. 1911;65:504-510.
8. Dale HH, Laidlaw PP. The physiological action of β-imidazolylethylamine. *J Physiol (London)*. 1910;41:318-344.
9. Lewis T. *The Blood Vessels of the Human Skin and Their Responses*. London: Shaw and Sons, Ltd; 1927.
10. Dale HH. Some chemical factors in the control of the circulation. *Lancet*. 1929;1:1233-1237.
11. Zhang MQ, Leurs R, Timmerman H. Histamine H_1-receptor antagonists. In: Wolff ME, ed. *Burger's Medicinal Chemistry and Drug Discovery*. 5th ed. New York: John Wiley & Sons; 1997:495-559.
12. Ganellen CR. The tautomer ratio of histamine. *J Pharm Pharmacol*. 1973;25:787-792.
13. Ganellin CR. Imidazole tautomerism of histamine derivatives. In: Bergmann ED, Pullman B, eds. *Molecular and Quantum Pharmacology*. Dordrecht-Holland: D Reidel; 1974:43-44.
14. Ganellin CR. Chemistry and structure-activity relationships of drugs acting at histamine receptors. In: Ganellin CR, Parsons ME, eds. *Pharmacology of Histamine Receptors*. Bristol: Wright PSG; 1982:10-102.
15. Black JW, Ganellin CR. Naming of substituted histamines. *Experientia*. 1974;30:111-113.

16. Cooper DG, Young RC, Durant GJ, et al. Histamine receptors. In: Emmett JC, ed. *Comprehensive Medicinal Chemistry: The Rational Design, Mechanistic Study, and Therapeutic Application of Chemical Compounds. Vol. 3: Membranes and Receptors*. Oxford UK: Pergamon Press; 1990:343-421.
17. Eriks JC, Van Der Goot H, Timmerman H. New activation model for the histamine H2 receptor, explaining the activity of the different classes of histamine H2 receptor agonists. *Mol Pharm*. 1993;44:884-894.
18. Moya-Garcia AA, Pino-Angeles A, Gil-Redondo R, et al. Structural features of mammalian histidine decarboxylase reveal the basis for specific inhibition. *Br J Pharmacol*. 2009;157:4-13.
19. Wu F, Yu J, Gehring H. Inhibitory and structural studies of novel coenzyme-substrate analogs of human histidine decarboxylase. *FASEB J*. 2008;22:890-897.
20. Watanabe T, Yamatodani A, Maeyama K, et al. Pharmacology of α-fluoromethylhistidine, a specific inhibitor of histidine decarboxylase. *Trends Pharmacol Sci*. 1990;11:363-367.
21. Schayer RC, Cooper JAD, Smiley RL, et al. Metabolism of ^{14}C histamine in man. *J Appl Physiol*. 1956;9:481-483.
22. Marone G, Genovese A, Granata F, et al. Pharmacological modulation of human mast cells and basophils. *Clin Exp Allergy*. 2002;32:1682-1689.
23. Oliver JM, Kepley CL, Ortega E, et al. Immunologically mediated signaling in basophils and mast cells: finding therapeutic targets for allergic diseases in the human FceR1 signaling pathway. *Immunopharmacology*. 2000;48:269-281.
24. Katzung BG. Histamine, serotonin & the ergot alkaloids. In: Katzung BG, ed. *Basic & Clinical Pharmacology*. New York: McGraw Hill; 2018:277-299.
25. Chambers C, Kvedar JC, Armstrong AW. Histamine pharmacology. In: Golan DE, Tashjian AH, Armstrong EJ, Armstrong AW, eds. *Principles of Pharmacology: The Pathophysiologic Basis of Drug Therapy*. 3rd ed. Philadelphia: Wolters Kluwer; 2018:765-775.
26. Jutel M, Akdis M, Akdis CA. Histamine, histamine receptors and their role in immune pathology. *Clin Exp Allergy*. 2009;39:1786-1800.
27. Simons FER, Akdis CA. Histamine and H_1-antihistamines. In: Adkinson NF, Bochner BS, Busse WW, eds. *Middleton's Allergy: Principles and Practice*. 7th ed. Philadelphia: Mosby; 2009:1517-1547.
28. Bakker RA, Timmerman H, Leurs R. Histamine receptors: specific ligands, receptor biochemistry, and signal transduction. In: Simons FER, ed. *Histamine and H_1-Antihistamines in Allergic Disease*. 2nd ed. New York: Marcel Dekker; 2002:27-64.
29. Leurs R, Vollinga RC, Timmerman H. The medicinal chemistry and therapeutic potentials of ligands of the histamine H_3 receptor. *Prog Drug Res*. 1995;45:107-165.
30. Luers R, Smit MJ, Tensen CP, et al. Site-directed mutagenesis of the histamine H1-receptor reveals a selective interaction of asparagine 207 with subclasses of H1-receptor agonists. *Biochem Biophys Res Commun*. 1994;201:295-301.
31. Forneau E, Bovet D. Recherches sur l'action sypmathicolytique d'un nouveau derive du dioxane. *Arch Int Pharmacodyn*. 1933;46:178-191.
32. A Pocket Guide to the AGS 2015 Beers Criteria, American Geriatrics Society.
33. Ahlquist RP. A study of the adrenotropic receptors. *Am J Physiol*. 1948;153:586-600.
34. Lijinsky W, Rueber MD, Blackwell BN. Liver tumors induced in rats by oral administration of the antihistaminic methapyrilene hydrochloride. *Science*. 1980;209:817-819.
35. Baselt RC. *Disposition of Toxic Drugs and Chemicals in Man*. 11th ed. Seal Beach: Biomedical Publications; 2017 (monographs and references therein).
36. Sjoqvist F, Lasagna L. The hypnotic efficacy of doxylamine. *Clin Pharmacol Ther*. 1967;8:48-54.
37. Ariens EJ. Stereoselectivity of bioactive agents: general aspects. In: Ariens EJ, Soudijn W, Timmermans PBM, eds. *Stereochemistry and Biological Activity*. Oxford, UK: Blackwell Scientific Publications; 1983:11-32.
38. Glazko AJ, Dill WA, Young RM, et al. Metabolic disposition of diphenhydramine. *Clin Pharmacol Ther*. 1974;16:1066-1076.
39. Spector R, Choudhury AK, Chiang CK, et al. Diphenhydramine in orientals and caucasians. *Clin Pharmacol Ther*. 1980;28:229-234.
40. Hamelin BA, Bouayad A, Méthot J, et al. Significant interaction between the nonprescription antihistamine diphenhydramine and the CYP2D6 substrate metoprolol in healthy men with high or low CYP2D6 activity. *Clin Pharmacol Ther*. 2000;67:466-477.
41. Goenechea S, Eckhardt G, Fahr W. Isolation and identification of some metabolites of bromazine from human urine. *Arzneimittel-Forschung*. 1980;30:1580-1584.
42. Videla S1, Lahjou M, Guibord P, et al. Food effects on the pharmacokinetics of doxylamine hydrogen succinate 25 mg film-coated tablets: a single-dose, randomized, two-period crossover study in healthy volunteers. *Drugs R D*. 2012;12:217-225.
43. Ganes DA, Midha KK. Identification in in vivo acetylation pathway for N-dealkylated metabolites of doxylamine in humans. *Xenobiotica*. 1987;17:993-999.
44. Ebnöther A, Weber HP. Synthesis and absolute konfiguration von clemastine und seiner isomern. *Helv Chim Acta*. 1976;59:2462-2468.
45. Choi MH, Jung BH, Chung BC. Identification of urinary metabolites of clemastine after oral administration to man. *J Pharmacy Pharmacol*. 1999;51:53-59.
46. Towart R, Sautel M, Moret E, et al. Investigation of the antihistaminic action of dimethindene maleate (Fenistil) and its optical isomers. In: Timmerman H, van der Goot H, eds. *Agents Actions Supplements*. Vol. 33: New Perspectives in Histamine Research. 1991:403-408.
47. Hanna PE, Ahmed AE. Conformationally restricted analogs of histamine H1 receptor antagonists: trans- and cis-1,5-diphenyl-3-dimethylaminopyrrolidine. *J Med Chem*. 1973;16:963-968.
48. Peets EA, Jackson M, Symchowicz S. Metabolism of chlorpheniramine maleate in man. *J Pharmacol Exp Ther*. 1972;180:464-474.
49. Kabasakalian P, Taggart M, Townley E. Urinary excretion of chlorpheniramine and its N-demethylated metabolites in man. *J Pharm Sci*. 1968;57:856-858.
50. Bruce RB, Turnbull LB, Newman JH, et al. Metabolism of brompheniramine. *J Med Chem*. 1968;11:1031-1034.
51. Witte PU, Irmisch R, Hajdu P. Pharmacokinetics of pheniramine (Avil®) and metabolites in healthy subjects after oral and intravenous administration. *Int J Clin Pharmacol Ther Toxicol*. 1985;23:59-62.
52. Kabasakalian P, Taggart M, Townley E. Urinary excretion of pheniramine and its N-demethylated metabolites in man – comparison with chlorpheniramine and brompheniramine data. *J Pharm Sci*. 1968;57:621-623.
53. Piwinski JJ, Wong JK, Chan TM, et al. Hydroxylated metabolites of loratadine: an example of conformational diastereomers due to atropisomerism. *J Org Chem*. 1990;55:3341-3350.
54. Otsuki I, Ishiko J, Sakai M, et al. Pharmacological activities of doxepin hydrochloride in relation to its geometrical isomers. *Oyo Yakuri*. 1972;6:973-984.
55. Remy DC, Rittle KE, Hunt CA, et al. (+)- and (−)-3-Methoxycyproheptadine. A comparative evaluation of the antiserotonin, antihistaminic, anticholinergic, and orexigenic properties with cyproheptadine. *J Med Chem*. 1977;20:1681-1684.
56. Tozzi S, Roth FE, Tabachnick II A. The pharmacology of azatadine, a potential antiallergy drug. *Agents Actions*. 1974;4:264-270.
57. Togias AG, Naclerio RM, Warner J. Demonstration of inhibition of mediator release from human mast cells by azatadine base. *J Am Med Assoc*. 1986;255:225-229.
58. Simons FE, Simons KJ. Histamine and H1-antihistamines: celebrating a century of progress. *J Allergy Clin Immunol*. 2011;128:1139-1150.
59. Chen C, Hanson E, Watson JW, et al. P-Glycoprotein limits the brain penetration of nonsedatinig but not sedating H1-antagonists. *Drug Metabol Dispo*. 2003;31:312-318.
60. Shimamura T, Shiroishi M, Weyland S, et al. Structure of the human histamine H1 receptor complex with doxepin. *Nature*. 2011;475(7354):65-70.
61. Soldovieri MV, Miceli F, Taglialatela M. Cardiotoxic effects of antihistamines: from basics to clinics (...and back). *Chem Res Toxicol*. 2008;21:997-1004.

62. Aronov AM. Predictive in silico modeling for hERG channel blockers. *Drug Discov Today*. 2005;10:149-155.
63. Pearlstein R, Vaz R, Rampe D. Understanding the structure-activity relationship of the human ether-a-go-go-related gene cardiac K^+ channel. A model for bad behavior. *J Med Chem*. 2003;46:2017-2022.
64. Zhang MQ, Caldirola P, Timmerman H. Chiral manipulation of drug selectivity: studies on a series of terfenadine-derived dual antagonists of H1-receptors and calcium channels. *Agents Actions*. 1994;41:C140-C142.
65. DuBuske LM. Pharmacology of desloratadine: special characteristics. *Clin Drug Investigation*. 2002;22(suppl 2):1-11.
66. Yumibe N, Huie K, Chen KJ, et al. Identification of human liver cytochrome P450 enzymes that metabolize the nonsedating antihistamine loratadine. Formation of descarboethoxyloratadine by CYP3A4 and CYP2D6. *Biochem Pharmacol*. 1996;51:165-172.
67. Ramanathan R, Reyderman L, Kulmatycki K, et al. Disposition of loratadine in healthy volunteers. *Xenobiotica*. 2007;37:753-769.
68. Ramanathan R, Reyderman L, Su AD, et al. Disposition of desloratadine in healthy volunteers. *Xenobiotica*. 2007;37:770-787.
69. Curran MP, Scott LJ, Perry CM. Cetirizine: a review of its use in allergic disorders. *Drugs*. 2004;64:523-561.
70. Gillard M, Van Der Perren C, Moguilevsky N, et al. Binding characteristics of cetirizine and levocetirizine to human H1 histamine receptors: contribution of Lys191 and Thr194. *Mol Pharmacol*. 2002;61:391-399.
71. Benedetti MS, Plisnier M, Kaise J, et al. Absorption, distribution, metabolism and excretion of [^{14}C]levocetirizine, the R enantiomer of cetirizine, in healthy volunteers. *Eur J Clin Pharmacol*. 2001;57:571-582.
72. Bielory L, Lien KW, Bigelsen S. Efficacy and tolerability of newer antihistamines in the treatment of allergic conjunctivitis. *Drugs*. 2005;65:215-228.
73. Sharif NA, Hellberg MR, Yanni JM. Antihistamines, topical ocular. In: Wolff ME, ed. *Burger's Medicinal Chemistry and Drug Discovery*. 5th ed. New York: John Wiley & Sons, Inc.; 1997:255-279.
74. Mey U, Wachmuth H, Breyer-Pfaff U. Conjugation of enantiomers of ketitofen to four isomeric quaternary ammonium glucuronides in humans in vivo and in liver microsomes. *Drug Metab Disp*. 1999;27:1281-1292.
75. Tsunoo M, Momomura S, Masuo M, et al. Phase 1 clinical study on KW-4679, an antiallergic drug: safety and pharmacokinetics in the single and repeated administration study to healthy subjects. *Kiso To Rinsho*. 1995;29:4129-4147.
76. Brunner M, Kletter K, Assandi A. Pharmacokinetic and mass balance study of unlabeled and ^{14}C-labeled emedastine difumarate in healthy volunteers. *Xenobiotica*. 2002;32:761-770.
77. Yokota H, Mizuuchi H, Maki T, et al. Phase I study of TAU-284 – single oral dose administration in healthy male volunteers. *J Clin Ther Med*. 1997;4:1137-1153.
78. Edwards AM, Holgate ST. The chromones: cromolyn sodium and neodocromil sodium. In: Adkinson NF, Bochner BS, Busse WW, et al, eds. *Middleton's Allergy: Principles and Practice*. 7th ed. Philadelphia: Mosby; 2009:1591-1601.
79. Cook EB, Stahl JL, Barney NP, et al. Mechanisms of antihistamines and mast cell stabilizers in ocular allergic inflammation. *Med Chem Rev*. 2004;1:333-347.

Structure Challenge Answers

a. Compound IV: It is a first-generation antihistamine (diphenhydramine) in the ethanolamine class. This class of antihistamine is very lipid soluble and easily crosses the blood-brain barrier to produce a high degree of sedation when compared with the other classes.
b. Compound IV: The ethanolamine class of antihistamines produces a high degree of anticholinergic effects. Compare compound IV to the anticholinergic structures shown in Chapters 10 and 26.
c. Compound III: Cyproheptadine exhibits antiserotonin properties and stimulates increased appetite and weight gain.
d. Compound I: Loratadine is rapidly converted to the secondary amine, desloratadine, on first pass through the liver. Desloratadine has higher receptor affinity than the parent.
e. Compound V: At pH 7.4, cetirizine would be zwitterionic. The carboxylic acid would be anionic and the piperazine nitrogen attached acetoxyethyl side chain would be protonated.
f. Replacing the 2-pyridyl ring of compound II (diphenhydramine) with a phenyl ring would decrease antihistaminic activity and increase anticholinergic and sedative effects.

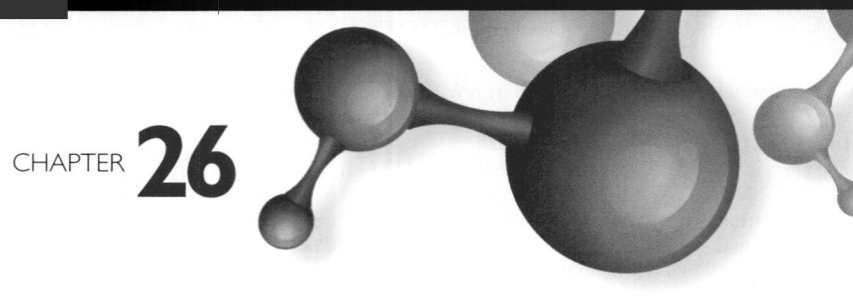

CHAPTER **26**

Drugs Used to Treat Gastrointestinal and Genitourinary Disorders

Sabesan Yoganathan

Drugs covered in this chapter:

H_2 RECEPTOR ANTAGONISTS
- Cimetidine
- Famotidine
- Nizatidine
- Ranitidine

PROTON PUMP INHIBITORS (PPIs)
- Dexlansoprazole
- Esomeprazole
- Lansoprazole
- Omeprazole
- Pantoprazole sodium
- Rabeprazole sodium
- Tenatoprazole

OTHER ANTIULCER AGENTS
- Bismuth subsalicylate
- Dexpanthenol
- Metoclopramide
- Misoprostol
- Prostaglandin E1
- Sucralfate

ANTI-EMETICS AND IBS DRUGS
- Alosetron
- Dolasetron
- Granisetron
- Linaclotide
- Ondansetron
- Palonosetron
- Plecanatide
- Prochlorperazine
- Promethazine
- Tropisetron
- Tegaserod

MONOCLONAL ANTIBODY FOR INFLAMMATORY GI DISEASES
- Adalimumab
- Certolizumab
- Golimumab
- Infliximab
- Vedolizumab

MUSCARINIC ANTAGONISTS
- Atropine
- Darifenacin
- Fesoterodine
- Mirabegron
- Oxybutynin
- Scopolamine
- Solifenacin
- Tolterodine
- Trospium chloride

Abbreviations

ACh acetylcholine
AChE acetylcholinesterase
AChEI acetylcholinesterase inhibitor
ATP adenosine triphosphate
AUC area under the plasma concentration curve
cAMP cyclic adenosine monophosphate
CNS central nervous system
CTZ chemoreceptor trigger zone
CYP cytochrome P450
CoA coenzyme A
COPD chronic obstructive pulmonary disease
COX cyclooxygenase
CTZ chemoreceptor trigger zone
ECL enterochromaffin-like cells
EM extensive metabolizer
ENS enteric nervous system
FDA U.S. Food and Drug Administration
GABA γ-aminobutyric acid
GLP glucagon-like peptide
GI gastrointestinal
GU genitourinary
GPCR G protein–coupled receptor
GERD gastroesophageal reflux disease
5-HT 5-hydroxytryptamine (serotonin)
IBD inflammatory bowel disease
IBS irritable bowel syndrome
IL interleukin
IM intermediate metabolizer
mAChR muscarinic acetylcholine receptor
nAChR nicotinic acetylcholine receptor

Abbreviations—Continued

NSAIDs nonsteroidal anti-inflammatory drugs
OAB overactive bladder
MOA monoamine oxidase
NSAID nonsteroidal anti-inflammatory drug
OTC over the counter
PEG polyethylene glycol
PLP pyridoxal phosphate
PG prostaglandin
P-gp P-glycoprotein
PM poor metabolizer
PPI proton pump inhibitor
SAR structure-activity relationships
SERT serotonin transporter
TNF-α tumor necrosis factor alpha

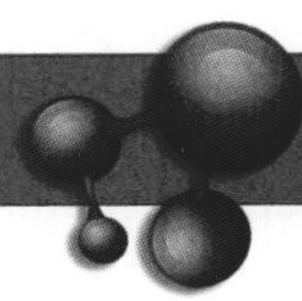

CLINICAL SIGNIFICANCE

Emily M. Ambizas, PharmD

Pharmacists will commonly encounter patients with gastrointestinal and urologic conditions regardless of their practice site. There are a multitude of medications utilized to treat these conditions, some of which are available over the counter (OTC). Many of these agents can be used to treat a different number of disease states. Although commonly used for the management of allergies, antihistamines can also be utilized in the management of motion sickness, gastroesophageal acid reflux disease, and ulcers. Alpha-1 antagonists can be used to treat benign hypertrophic prostate disease as well as hypertension. Cholinergic agents are used in impaired or excessive gastric motility disorders as well as urinary incontinence. Having a thorough understanding of the structural relationship of these various compounds helps the pharmacist determine the how and why of drug therapy. A first-generation antihistamine, such as meclizine, should be recommended for motion sickness, as the second-generation agents only act peripherally and possess no antiemetic effect. A patient who has been on omeprazole but is experiencing no relief of symptoms may be a rapid CYP2C19 metabolizer; this patient may benefit from the *S*-isomer, esomeprazole, which is biotransformed by CYP2C19 at about one-third the rate of omeprazole. This understanding has led to agents that have increased efficacy and selectivity for receptors, while minimizing unwanted or harmful effects. With this knowledge, pharmacists are best equipped to select the most appropriate drug regimen for their patients.

INTRODUCTION

Gastrointestinal Disorders

Gastrointestinal (GI) disorders are broadly characterized by illnesses associated with upper GI tract (esophagus, stomach, and duodenum) and lower GI tract (small and large intestine) and/or diseases associated with liver, gallbladder, and pancreas. In general, GI disorders are (1) structural, (2) malabsorptive, (3) inflammatory, and/or (4) neoplastic in nature. The most common GI diseases include acid reflux, peptic ulcer, inflammation-associated diseases, constipation, infection, diarrhea, celiac disease, and cancer. These diseases substantially diminish the quality of life and are a huge economic burden in terms of health care costs. GI diseases affect close to 70 million people in the United States annually, and over 200,000 deaths are related to GI diseases. Moreover, the direct and indirect cost of managing GI diseases in the United States has been estimated to be $142 billion per year.[1,2] This chapter focuses on drugs that are clinically used for the treatment of acid reflux, peptic ulcer, irritable bowel syndrome (IBS), inflammatory bowel disease (IBD), as well as nausea and vomiting. Many other drug classes covered elsewhere in this text are also used for the treatment of other GI disorders, including infections and cancer.

Gastroesophageal reflux disease (GERD) is one of the most common GI disorders and affects a significant number of people in the United States and worldwide.[3,4] GERD is typically associated with the esophageal mucosa being continuously exposed to gastric secretions. This often occurs when the lower esophageal sphincter relaxes and the duration of esophageal acid exposure is considerably prolonged. Typically, when gastric secretions enter the esophagus, innate clearing mechanisms limit the duration of exposure by rapidly pushing the refluxed content into the stomach. Additionally, bicarbonate-rich secretions by esophageal glands help neutralize the residual acid trapped within the mucosa. Since GERD is associated with gastric acid reflux and associated symptoms, most treatment options are directed toward reducing the acidic nature of the refluxate. An effective therapeutic option should heal esophageal damage while providing symptomatic relief. Current therapy for acid reflux–related GI diseases focuses on inhibiting biological pathways that directly or indirectly play a role in stomach acid secretion. Two such pathways involve inhibition of the histamine H_2 receptor and inhibition of the proton pump (H^+/K^+-ATPase) in the stomach. Selective muscarinic receptor antagonists and prokinetic agents can also be used for the treatment of GERD.[5,6]

Other common GI disorders include IBS and IBD. Ulcerative colitis (UC) and Crohn's diseases (CD) are two examples of IBD, which are chronic diseases of the GI tract caused by inflammation in the gut mucosal tissue.[7] The pathogenesis of IBD is linked to multiple inflammatory cell types, including neutrophils, macrophages, and lymphocytes. In most cases, modulation of inflammation in the GI tract is a viable approach that provides symptomatic treatment of IBDs.[8] Additionally, serotonergic agents and anti-inflammatory monoclonal antibodies have also been considered as useful therapeutic options for the treatment of IBDs.

Genitourinary Disorders

The genitourinary (GU) system consists of the genital or reproductive organs and urinary system. Some of the primary functions of the GU system include (1) excretion of cellular waste products, (2) regulation of blood volume via conservation or excretion of fluids, (3) regulation of electrolytes, (4) balancing pH via regulation of H^+ and HCO_3^- ions reabsorbed or excreted, (5) arterial blood pressure control via regulation of sodium excretion and renin secretion, and (6) erythropoietin secretion. Taken together, the GU system plays an important role in maintaining homeostasis. Several pathological conditions are associated with the GU tract, ranging from infections, inflammation, dysuria, nocturia, and kidney-related diseases. The focus of this chapter is on managing urination frequency from an overactive bladder with the use of antimuscarinic agents. Other chapters within this text provide more detailed discussions on therapeutic agents used as diuretics and for the treatment of GU tract infections and inflammation.

Overactive bladder (OAB) is characterized as symptoms of urgency to urinate, with or without urge urinary incontinence. This happens because the detrusor muscle is overactive and inconsistently contracts. The smooth muscle in bladder is controlled by the parasympathetic nervous system and, more specifically, by the action of acetylcholine (ACh) on the muscarinic acetylcholine receptor (mAChR). There are several subtypes of the mAChR (see Chapter 6), and the M_2 and M_3 subtypes are mainly present in urinary bladder. Although the M_2 subtype is the predominant mAChR in bladder, the M_3 subtype appears to play a more important role in directly mediating detrusor contraction.[9] Inhibition of these receptors in the urinary bladder results in decreased bladder contraction, providing relief from OAB. Several antimuscarinic agents have been developed from the structure-activity relationships (SARs) of atropine, a natural alkaloid and antimuscarinic agent. The detailed structure, function, and SAR of this class of medicinal agents are discussed later in this chapter.

Histamine and Histamine Receptors

Histamine plays an important role in mediating biochemical responses through different signaling pathways. Its action on endothelial cells and vascular smooth muscle cells results in the symptoms of allergic reactions, and it also acts on parietal cells to stimulate gastric acid secretion.[10,11] Inhibition of the histamine-based signaling pathway in specific tissues has been proven to be an effective approach to treat allergic reactions or GI disorders.

Histamine is a basic compound with an imidazole ring and a primary amine motif. The imidazole has a pK_a of 5.80 and the aliphatic amine has a pK_a of 9.40. Due to its basic nature, histamine protonates to form cations at physiological pH, including a monocation (major) and a dication (minor). Both species are considered biologically active. When the imidazole ring of histamine is protonated, it tautomerizes, forming a mixture of the N^{τ}-H tautomer and N^{π}-H tautomer with a ratio of 4:1, respectively. Chemical modifications of the imidazole ring change the rate of formation of one or the other tautomer.[12,13] More specifically, the electronic nature of the substituent at the 4-position (e.g., CH_3 vs. Cl) changes the proportion existing as the N^{τ}-H tautomer. The electron-withdrawing chlorine substitution provides 12% of the N^{τ}-H tautomer versus 70% for the electron donating 4-methylhistamine. Additionally, this change in composition decreases agonist potency, indicating that tautomeric composition is important in the agonist-receptor interaction.[13]

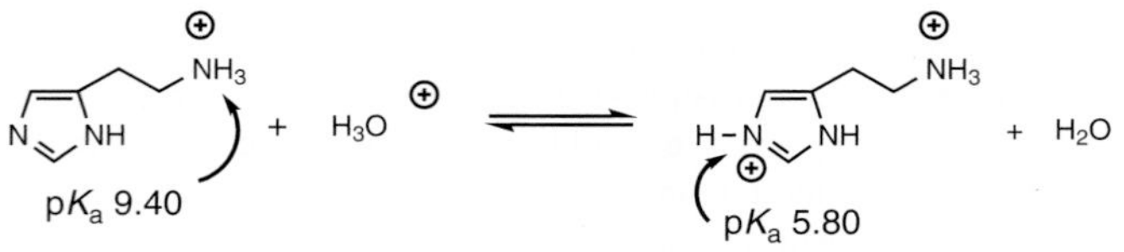

pK_a 9.40 + H_3O^+ ⇌ pK_a 5.80 + H_2O

pK_a of histamine

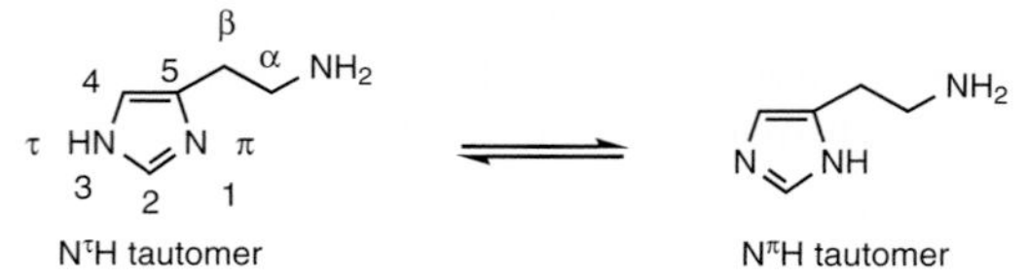

$N^{\tau}H$ tautomer ⇌ $N^{\pi}H$ tautomer

Tautomers of histamine

Histamine exists as both *trans* and *gauche* conformations in solution (Fig. 26.1),[13] and studies have shown that the conformational isomerism impacts selectivity toward the different histamine receptors (H_1, H_2, H_3, and H_4).[13] Although histamine has no chiral centers, the selectivity toward the receptor binding arises from its ability to form the *trans/gauche* conformational isomers. Based on experimental studies done using conformationally restricted analogues of histamine, it is evident that *trans* conformer selectively binds to H_1 and H_2 receptors, while the *gauche* conformer binds to the H_3 receptor. Synthesis and evaluation of histamine analogues have yielded some important information about the SAR of histamine. Introduction of alkyl groups typically produces compounds with reduced activity toward H_1 and H_2 receptors. Introduction of a methyl group at the 2- or 4-position produces selective compounds toward the H_1 receptor and H_2 receptor, respectively. However, imidazole N-substitution produces inactive compounds. Additionally, modification of the aliphatic amine through substitution decreases histamine's activity ($R\text{-}NH_2 > R\text{-}NHMe > R\text{-}NMe_2 > R\text{-}N^+Me_3$) at both H_1 and H_2 receptors.[13,14]

Histamine is synthesized in various tissues, including mast cells, parietal cells of the gastric mucosa, and neurons in the CNS and periphery. The biosynthesis of histamine occurs in the Golgi apparatus of these cells via an enzymatic decarboxylation of histidine. A decarboxylase

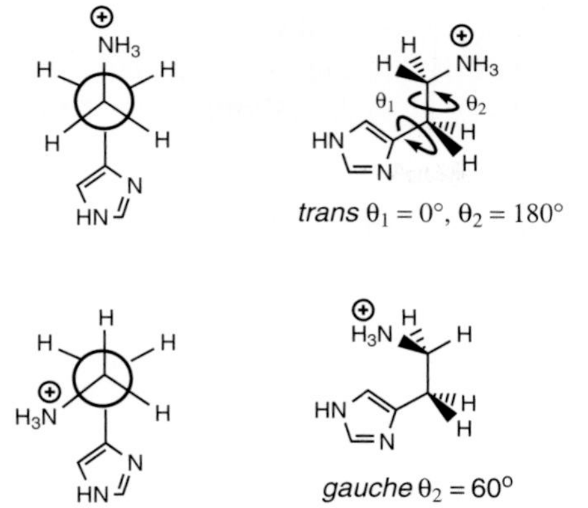

Figure 26.1 Conformers of histamine.

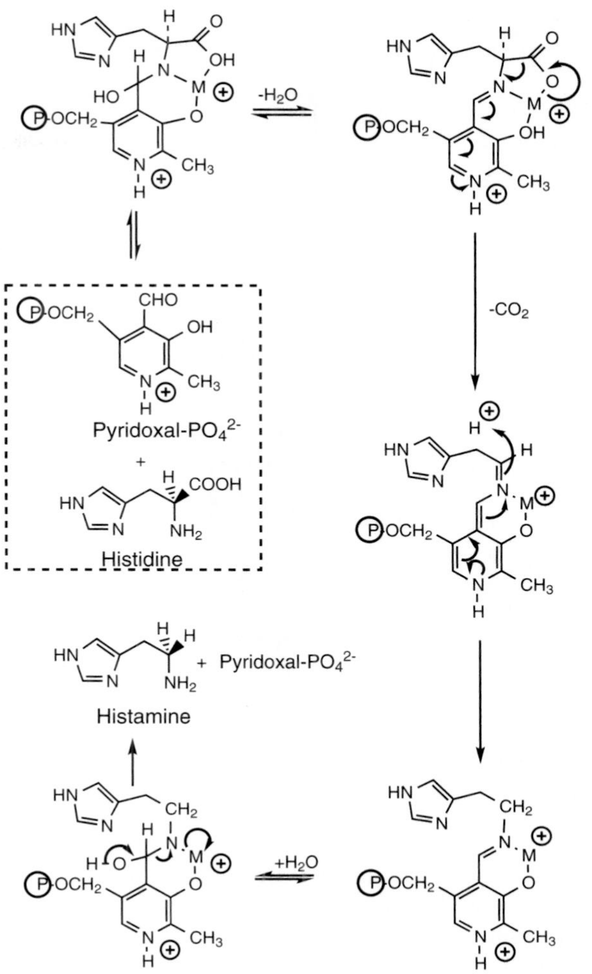

Figure 26.2 Biosynthesis of histamine.

enzyme utilizes pyridoxal phosphate (PLP) as a cofactor to convert L-histidine into histamine (Fig. 26.2). The reaction mechanism for this process involves condensation of histidine with PLP, which forms an imine intermediate. Subsequently, loss of the carboxylate group in the form of carbon dioxide generates the histamine-PLP adduct. Finally, histamine is released from PLP via hydrolysis of the intermediate. This type of PLP-dependent decarboxylation of amino acids is a common catalytic transformation known to generate amino acid–derived endogenous small molecules. Based on the mechanism of histamine biosynthesis, α-fluoromethylhistidine was identified as an inhibitor of histidine decarboxylase.[15] Although this small molecule was a useful tool to inhibit histamine biosynthesis, such an approach has not yielded any successful drug leads for the treatment of histamine-induced disorders, including peptic ulcer or motion sickness.

Once histamine is released from mast cells or parietal cells, its physiological effect is mediated by binding to the various histamine receptors. The histamine receptors belong to the G protein–coupled receptor (GPCR) family, which are a diverse family of transmembrane proteins (see Chapter 6).[16] Histamine plays a central role in immune responses and regulates physiological function in the gut as well as in the CNS. Due to its important role in various physiological functions that relates to several diseases, histamine receptors have been targeted for the treatment of many disorders. In fact, scientist Daniel Bovet was awarded the 1957 Nobel Prize for Physiology or Medicine for his work on substances that inhibit the action of histamine, called "antihistamines." Histamine's role in allergy and inflammation is extensively discussed in Chapter 25. Drugs for the treatment of allergy and inflammatory disorders target the H_1 receptor, whereas drugs that target the H_2 receptor inhibit acid secretion in the stomach. As noted previously, this chapter focuses on the H_2 receptor and its role in GI disorders.[17]

In addition to H_2 receptors, the proton pump found in the canaliculus of parietal cells of the gastric mucosa is also commonly targeted for the treatment of GI disorders. Activation of H_2 histamine, M_3, and gastrin receptors initiates a stimulatory signaling pathway for acid secretion. The H_2 receptor acts through the cyclic adenosine monophosphate (cAMP) dependent pathway, while M_3 and gastrin receptors act via the Ca^{2+} dependent pathway to activate the proton pump. Once activated and facilitated by a trio of anionic residues (Asp824, Glu820, and Glu795), the proton pump exchanges cytoplasmic H^+ and extracytoplasmic K^+ ions across the gastric membrane to maintain an acidic pH in the stomach (Fig. 26.3).[17-19] The proton pump is Cys-rich, containing a total of 28 of these nucleophilic residues, and at least two will be critical to the action of the inhibitors used in the treatment of gastric ulcers (discussed below).

Drugs Used for the Treatment of GI Disorders, Including Ulcer and GERD

As noted above, gastric acid secretion occurs at the level of parietal cells in the gastric mucosa. Remarkably, these cells can secrete up to 3 L of gastric juice daily, where the hydrochloric acid can drop the pH to ~1. The parietal cells contain receptors for ACh, histamine, and gastrin,

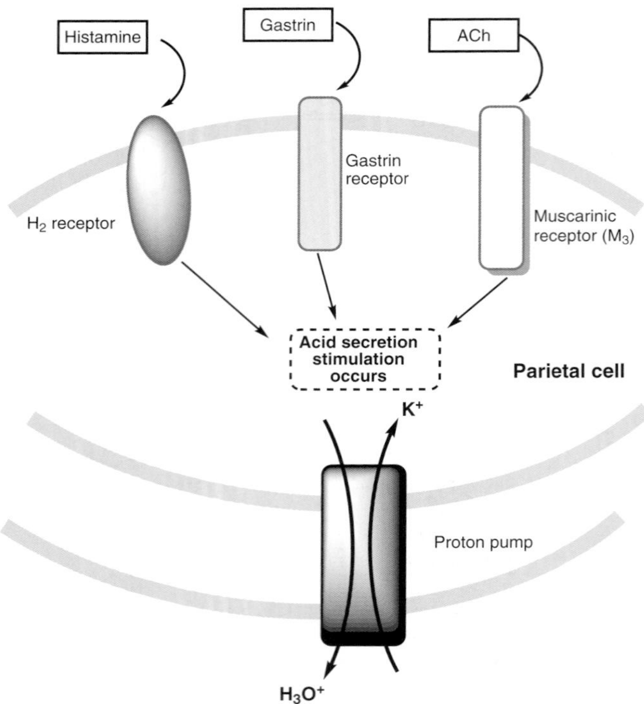

Figure 26.3 Physiological mechanism of gastric acid secretion in parietal cells.

which are signal molecules that stimulate acid production. ACh binds to the muscarinic receptor (M_3 subtype), and histamine binds to the H_2 receptor on parietal cells to stimulate acid secretion. It is proposed that gastrin also mediates acid secretion indirectly via the release of histamine from ECL cells. Although the receptor stimulation and gastric acid secretion steps are highly regulated, in many cases *Helicobacter pylori* infection has been associated with hypersecretion of gastric acid.[20] Such an event is likely to contribute to gastric mucosal deterioration and can lead to gastric ulceration.

Antacids

Patients suffering from mild dyspepsia and/or gastric acid–induced disorders typically find relief with the use of nonprescription antacids. These have been used for centuries, at least until the advent of H_2 antihistamines and proton pump inhibitors (PPIs). However, common antacids continue to be used by patients as readily available remedies for intermittent heartburn. Antacids are weak inorganic bases that neutralize stomach acid to generate water and a metal-containing chloride salt. Some of the common antacids are pharmaceutical formulations containing sodium bicarbonate, calcium carbonate, magnesium hydroxide, and aluminum hydroxide (Table 26.1). Both sodium bicarbonate and calcium carbonate may cause belching or metabolic alkalosis due to the production of carbon dioxide (CO_2). Additionally, excessive intake of calcium carbonate with calcium-rich dairy products can lead to hypercalcemia and potential renal insufficiency. Magnesium- and aluminum-based antacids may impact bowel function. Since both magnesium and aluminum are absorbed and excreted by the kidneys, intake of these antacids must be limited in patients with renal insufficiency.

Table 26.1 Composition of Selected Antacids

Product	Composition (mg)[a]
Tablets	
Rolaids—regular strength	$CaCO_3$—550 $Mg(OH)_2$—110
Rolaids—advanced	$CaCO_3$—1,000 $Mg(OH)_2$—200 Simethicone—40
Tums—regular strength	$CaCO_3$—500
Tums—extra strength	$CaCO_3$—750
Maalox	$CaCO_3$—600
Gelusil	$Mg(OH)_2$—200 $Al(OH)_3$—200 Simethicone—25
Liquids	
Milk of magnesia	$Mg(OH)_2$—400
Mylanta—maximum strength	$Mg(OH)_2$—400 $Al(OH)_3$—400 Simethicone—40
Maalox—therapeutic concentrate	$Mg(OH)_2$—300 $Al(OH)_3$—600

[a] mg per tablet or 5 mL liquid

H_2 Antihistamines

The role of H_2 receptors in GI disorders directly relates to their role in the stimulation and secretion of stomach acid. Histamine binds to H_2 receptors on parietal cells, which results in activation of adenylyl cyclase. Activation of this enzyme increases intracellular cAMP, which in turn activates kinases that stimulate the proton pump. Cimetidine, ranitidine, famotidine, and nizatidine are the four H_2 antihistamines currently in clinical use (Fig. 26.4).[21] These agents are available OTC and used for the treatment of gastric ulcers, GERD, and upper GI bleeding. H_2 antihistamines are considered inverse agonists that block the basal level activity of H_2 receptors by promoting a shift from an active to an inactive conformation.[22]

Structural Features and Mechanism of Action of H_2 Antihistamines

The H_2 antihistamines were designed based on extensive medicinal chemistry research on the partial agonists that are structurally similar to histamine. Cimetidine was the first drug developed for clinical use in the treatment of heartburn and peptic ulcers.[23] Cimetidine has an imidazole ring that mimics the structural feature of histamine.

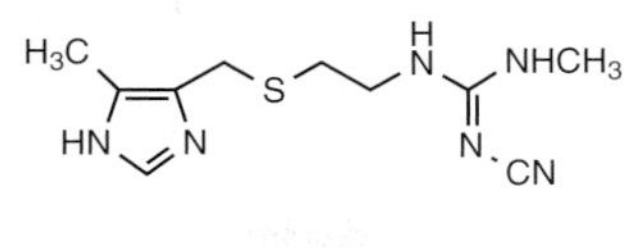

Cimetidine (Tagamet)

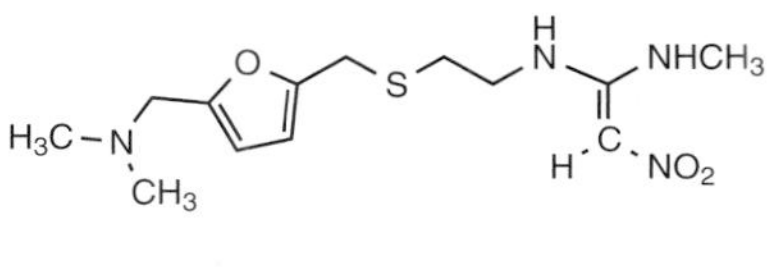

Ranitidine (Zantac)

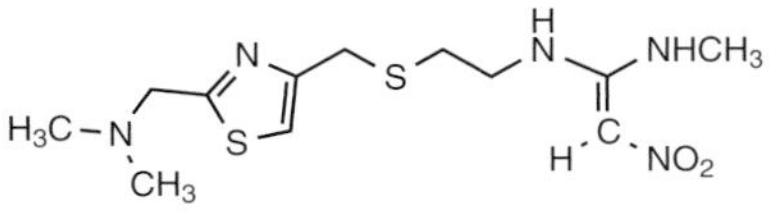

Nizatidine (Axid)

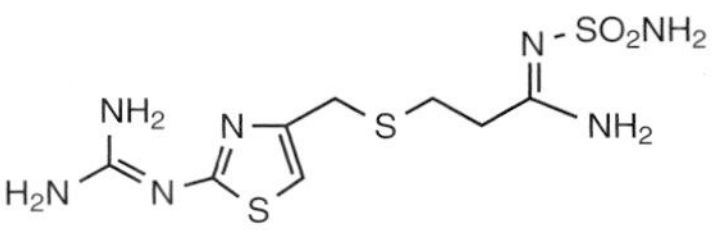

Famotidine (Pepcid)

Figure 26.4 H_2 receptor antihistamines.

Introduction of a C-4 methyl group afforded selectivity toward the H_2 receptor by stabilizing the N^{τ}-H tautomer required for receptor recognition.

All four clinically used H_2 antihistamines have a thioether-containing four-atom side chain, a heterocyclic structure with a basic functional group, and a guanidine group with different substituents. The sulfur atom in the side chain increases potency compared to carbon or oxygen analogues. The guanidine moiety is substituted with an electron-withdrawing group (i.e., cyano, nitro, sulfonamido) that significantly decreases the basicity of the guanidine; thus the guanidine group is not protonated under physiological conditions. Initial structure-based research that led to the discovery of cimetidine showed that protonation of the guanidine group abolishes H_2 antagonist activity. Based on the binding model of ranitidine with the H_2 receptor, it has been shown that the basic amino group attached to (or, in the case of cimetidine, a component of) the heterocycle interacts with Asp98 via an ionic interaction, and the guanidine NH forms a hydrogen bond with Asp186 within the binding pocket.[24] Through these interactions, these drugs prevent histamine binding, and thus, inhibit the action of H_2 receptors. Cimetidine has an imidazole ring; however, other heterocyclic motifs (i.e. furan, thiazole) are utilized to generate ranitidine, famotidine, and nizatidine. These newer structures have a basic amine or guanidine motif attached to these heterocycles because a basic group is necessary for binding.

Metabolism and Drug Interactions of H_2 Antihistamines

Cimetidine, ranitidine, and famotidine undergo first-pass metabolism, and their oral bioavailability is 40%-60% in patients with GI issues (Fig. 26.5). On the other hand, nizatidine has a high oral bioavailability (90%). The half-lives of these four H_2 antihistamines are between 1 and 4 hours, and they are generally excreted unaltered in urine. The primary metabolic pathways can involve oxidation of the sulfur atom, the nitrogen atom of the amine functional group, and C-H oxidation (Fig. 26.5). Cimetidine undergoes both thioether oxidation to the sulfoxide and oxidation at the C-4 methyl group to yield a hydroxylated metabolite. Ranitidine undergoes minor metabolic modifications via N-demethylation, N-oxidation, and S-oxidation. Nizatidine undergoes minor modification via similar reactions as ranitidine. Famotidine undergoes S-oxidation. Except for nizatidine, metabolites of H_2 antihistamines do not contribute to the therapeutic properties of the parent drug. The N-monodesmethyl metabolite of nizatidine exhibits about 61% of the H_2 antihistaminic activity of the parent drug.[25]

Metabolites of cimetidine:

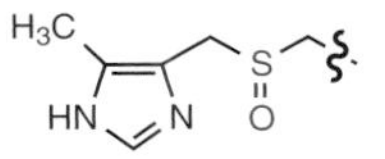

Cimetidine sulfoxide

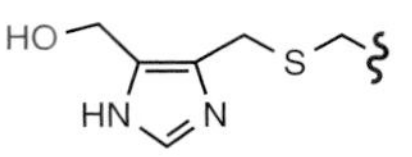

4-Hydroxymethyl cimetidine

Metabolites of ranitidine:

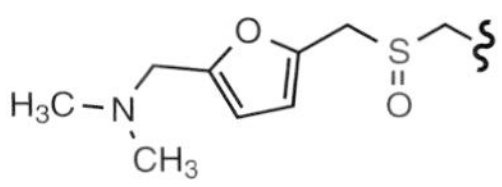

Ranitidine sulfoxide

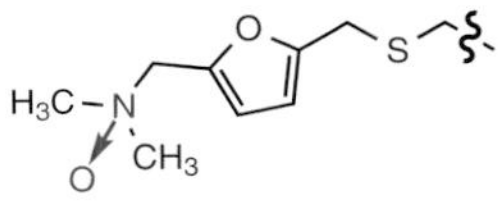

Ranitidine N-oxide

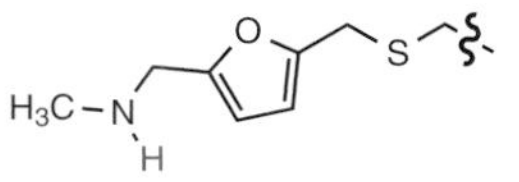

Monodesmethyl ranitidine

Metabolites of nizatidine:

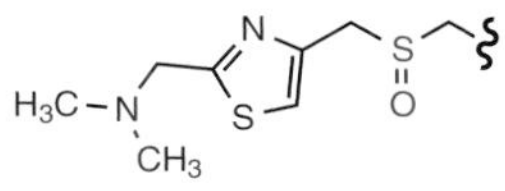

Nizatidine sulfoxide

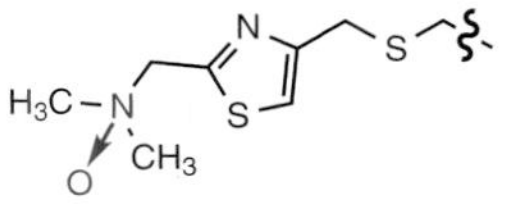

Nizatidine N-oxide

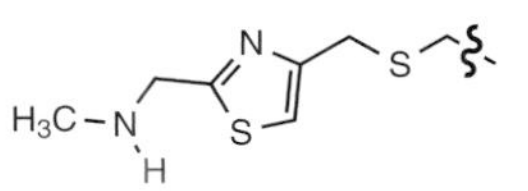

Monodesmethyl nizatidine

Metabolite of famotidine:

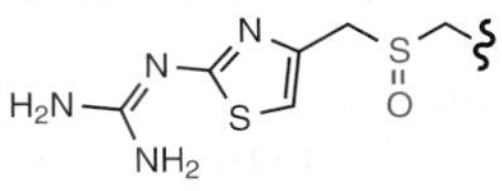

Famotidine sulfoxide

Figure 26.5 Major metabolites of H_2 antihistamines.

Drug interactions of H_2 antihistamines are certainly a concern, especially with cimetidine.[26] Cimetidine's imidazole ring inhibits CYP450-dependent oxidation of drugs, causing an increased duration of action of several agents. Based on this observation, other members of this class of drugs were specifically developed with different heterocyclic motifs to prevent their ability to inhibit CYP450. Cimetidine is also a known inhibitor of renal tubular secretion of some drugs (i.e., procainamide), where other members of the class show little or no effect.

Specific Drugs

Famotidine and ranitidine are viewed as the most commonly utilized OTC H_2 antihistamines for relief of GI distress, and they are described in more detail below, along with the historically relevant agent cimetidine. The fourth H_2 antagonist, nizatidine is a "patchwork" of structural features found in other antagonists, incorporating the thiazole ring of famotidine, the basic dimethylaminomethyl and neutral diaminonitroethene moiety of ranitidine, and the methylthioethyl connecting chain found in all marketed H_2 antagonists.

CIMETIDINE. As previously mentioned, cimetidine was the first H_2 antagonist developed and is an OTC drug available for the treatment of acid reflux and related GI disorders. It is available in tablet form (200, 300, 400, 600, or 800 mg). An injection formulation (cimetidine hydrochloride injection, 300 mg/2 mL) is also available by prescription for administration by providers in a clinic setting. The 4-methylimidazole ring mimics the imidazole motif found in histamine, and due to conformational preference driven by the stabilization of the N^{τ}-H tautomer, it is more selective toward the H_2 receptor. Additionally, the nonionizable cyanoguanidine motif is key to high H_2 receptor affinity and antagonistic activity, and it is held at the proper distance from the anchoring cationic nitrogen of the imidazole ring by the methylthioethyl connecting chain. The electron-withdrawing sulfur atom in this chain also helps stabilize the N^{τ}-H tautomer required for receptor recognition. Cimetidine has an oral bioavailability of 60%-70%, and about 20% is bound to plasma protein. The estimated elimination half-life is about 2 hours and about 40%-80% of drug is excreted in the urine in unaltered form.[27]

Cimetidine undergoes hepatic metabolic transformation, providing the sulfoxide and 4-hydroxymethyl metabolites shown in Figure 26.5. One of the major clinical limitations is the reversible inhibition of CYP enzymes, which occurs through competition for heme iron (Fe^{2+}) binding between cimetidine's imidazole ring and the identical ring of a His residue on the CYP protein.[28] This leads to many drug-drug interactions (some of them serious), particularly in elderly patients who commonly take many CYP vulnerable drugs. It inhibits the hepatic metabolism of warfarin, phenytoin, propranolol, lidocaine, and diazepam, to name a few, leading to increased plasma level of these drugs and the risk of serious or potentially fatal toxicity.[29]

Following administration, cimetidine is widely distributed in various tissues; thus it exhibits some adverse effects, including dizziness, headache, drowsiness, and nausea. The later generation H_2 antagonists to some extent address some of these adverse effects, primarily by the replacement of the CYP-inhibiting imidazole ring with aromatic isosteres less capable (but not incapable) of competing with the CYP His residue for heme Fe^{2+}.

RANITIDINE. Ranitidine is a commonly recommended H_2 antagonist that is available OTC and by prescription. It is available in tablet form (150 or 300 mg) and as ranitidine injection (25 mg/mL). Ranitidine has a furan ring, a heterocyclic motif that mimics the aromaticity of the imidazole ring, a dimethyl amino group that serves as the cationic center for ion-ion anchoring to Asp98, and a modified guanidine moiety with a nitro group (diaminonitroethene) attached to eliminate basicity. Based on cimetidine's binding interactions, the guanidine moiety and the dimethyl ammonium motif are envisioned to form a hydrogen bond and an ionic interaction, respectively, with the H_2 receptor.[24] Ranitidine is about four to nine times more potent than cimetidine.

Absorption of ranitidine is rapid, and peak plasma concentrations are observed within 3 hours. Although bioavailability is only 50%-60%, it is more effective and exhibits reduced adverse effects compared to cimetidine. Renal excretion is the principal mode of elimination of this drug, and it has an elimination half-life of 2-3 hours. Ranitidine is metabolized by CYP to ranitidine sulfoxide, ranitidine N-oxide, and monodesmethylranitidine, which are all minor metabolites (1%-4%) (Fig. 26.5). Unlike cimetidine, ranitidine is not a known CYP enzyme inhibitor at the therapeutic level and does not affect the action of drugs that depend on CYP enzyme activity for clearance (e.g., phenytoin, diazepam, lidocaine, and propranolol). CYP inhibition is possible at higher doses, but the clinical impact is significantly less than observed with cimetidine. Since ranitidine alters the gastric pH, absorption of certain drugs that depend on a highly acid gastric environment can be affected. Based on pH variability, the absorption of triazolam and midazolam can increase, and the absorption of ketoconazole, atazanavir, and gefitnib can decrease.[30] Although adverse effects are rare, if signs of hepatotoxicity are observed, ranitidine should be discontinued.

FAMOTIDINE. Famotidine is another H_2 antagonist that is used for the treatment of GERD, duodenal ulcers, and stomach ulcers. It is available in a tablet form, as well as for injection. In the United States, 10 and 20 mg tablets are available OTC. A prescription is required for higher doses and the injectable formulation. Famotidine has a 2-guanidothiazole ring in place of the imidazole ring found in cimetidine, and this basic guanidine provides the cation needed for anchoring to the H_2 receptor Asp98. The second guanidine moiety attached to the ethylthiomethyl connecting chain is modified via the addition of an electron-withdrawing sulfonamide group, which lowers the basicity of this guanidine moiety and improves potency by ensuring a lack of positive charge at physiologic pH. Famotidine is about 7.5 times more potent than famotidine and about 20 times more potent than cimetidine.[31]

Famotidine is not completely absorbed, providing a bioavailability of about 40%-45% when orally administered. About 15%-20% of the drug is bound to plasma protein.

Famotidine has an elimination half-life of 4.5 hours, and a large portion (65%-70%) is eliminated via renal excretion. Famotidine is metabolized by CYP enzymes, and the only metabolite identified is the famotidine sulfoxide (Fig. 26.5). Unlike cimetidine, this drug does not exhibit significant inhibitory effect on CYP enzyme activity, indicating minimal drug-drug interactions.

Proton Pump Inhibitors

A second class of drugs that are commonly and more frequently used in the treatment of peptic ulcer is PPIs.[32] This class of drugs covalently inhibits the gastric H^+/K^+-ATPase that is responsible for secretion of stomach acid in parietal cells of the gastric mucosa.[33,34] The gastric proton pump is very similar to Na^+/K^+-ATPase,[19] and also similar in structure and function to the H^+/K^+-ATPase found in osteoclasts, which play an important role in bone resorption. PPIs enable healing of peptic ulcer, erosive esophagitis, GERD, GERD-related laryngitis, Barrett's esophagus, and Zollinger-Ellison syndrome, as well as the infection caused by *H. pylori*, the latter in combination with antibiotics.[33,34]

Since the H^+/K^+-ATPase–mediated process is the final step in gastric acid secretion, inhibiting this enzyme is considered the most effective approach to acid suppression. PPI discovery began with the early investigation of timoprazole. This compound is a pyridylmethylsulfinylbenzimidazole, which is the conserved pharmacophore for subsequently developed PPIs. Based on its acid-dependent activity, it was identified as an acid-activated prodrug. Omeprazole was later synthesized and, in 1989, became the first drug of this class available for clinical use.[35] Other clinically available PPIs include lansoprazole, dexlansoprazole, esomeprazole, pantoprazole sodium, and rabeprazole sodium (Fig. 26.6). Dexlansoprazole and esomeprazole are enantiomerically pure forms of lansoprazole and omeprazole, respectively. Omeprazole and lansoprazole are both also marketed as racemic mixtures.

Structural Features and Mechanism of Action of PPIs

The 2-pyridylmethylsulfinylbenzimidazole motif is conserved in all members of the PPI family, as it is necessary for bioactivity through acid-catalyzed decomposition to the reactive sulfenic acid and sulfenamide structures. Typically, the structural modifications are done on the pyridine ring or at the benzo component of the benzimidazole to generate drugs with differing levels of acid stability, which impacts duration of proton pump inhibiting action. The investigational drug, tenatoprazole is slightly different in that it has an imidazopyridine isostere, instead of the traditional benzimidazole scaffold.

PPIs are weak bases with a pyridine pK_a between 3.8 and 4.9, which enables them to selectively accumulate through ion trapping in the stimulated parietal cell (pH~1.0). This acidic environment-selective accumulation of PPIs is an important property that contributes to their selectivity and activity. As mentioned, PPIs are prodrugs, and acid-catalyzed activation generates the active form of the drug. The active form has electrophilic sulfenic acid and sulfenamide sulfur atoms capable of reacting with the thiol group of a Cys residue of the ATPase, forming a covalent adduct.[36] Covalent inhibition of the proton pump results in inactivation of the catalytic function of this enzyme.[19]

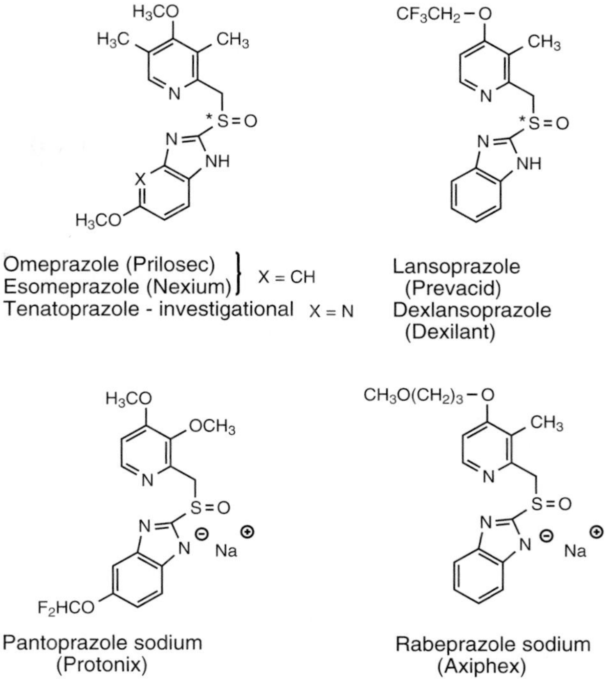

Omeprazole (Prilosec) / Esomeprazole (Nexium) X = CH; Tenatoprazole - investigational X = N

Lansoprazole (Prevacid); Dexlansoprazole (Dexilant)

Pantoprazole sodium (Protonix)

Rabeprazole sodium (Axiphex)

Figure 26.6 Proton pump inhibitors.

The chemical mechanism of activation of omeprazole and subsequent covalent interaction is described in Figure 26.7.[33] All PPIs follow a similar mechanism of action. The imidazole ring N3, an exceptionally weak base with a pK_a <0.8, is first protonated under the very low pH of the parietal cell through proton transfer from pyridine N1. Nucleophilic attack by the unionized pyridine nitrogen at benzimidazole C2 (made electron deficient by cationic N3) generates a highly electrophilic and unstable electrophilic spiro intermediate, which rearranges to generate the sulfenic acid intermediate that preferentially forms the inactivating disulfide bond with the proton pump Cys (Fig. 26.7). The following step involves loss of water and the formation of a reactive sulfenamide intermediate, which can also covalently modify the Cys thiol of the proton pump.[36]

Within the proton pump, several different Cys residues are potential sites for covalent modification. The different substituents on the pyridine or benzimidazole ring of PPIs determine which Cys residue the drug preferentially reacts with, which subsequently determines the permanency of the covalent attachment, as discussed below. Electron-donating groups on the C5-position of benzimidazole enhance reactivity by increasing the extent of benzimidazole N3 protonation and the strength of the δ^+ charge on the carbon at the C2 position of benzimidazole moiety. Electron-donating groups at the C4 position of the pyridine ring increase the nucleophilicity of pyridine nitrogen, enhancing the rate at which N1 attacks electrophilic benzimidazole C2. Conversely, electron-withdrawing groups at either site have been shown to decrease reactivity.[37]

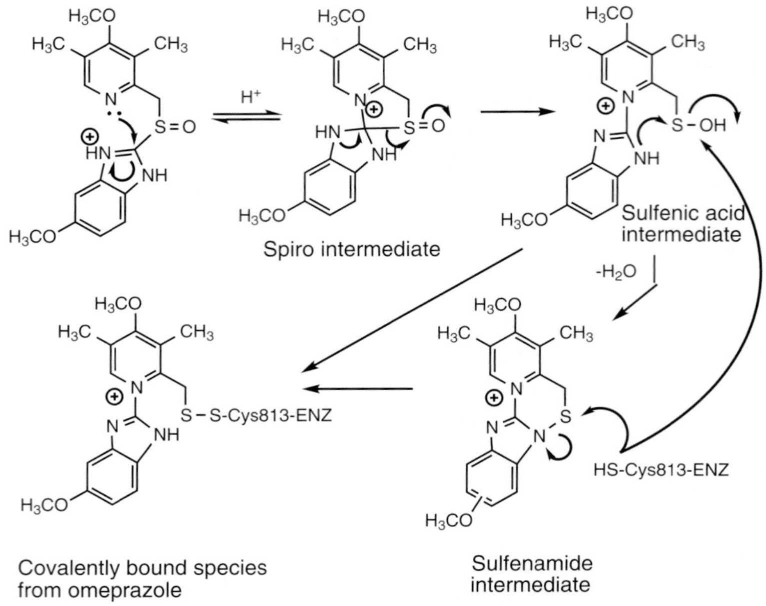

Figure 26.7 Acid-catalyzed activation of omeprazole to reactive sulfenic acid and sulfenamide.

All PPIs can react with the readily accessible Cys813 of the ATPase. It has been observed that activated molecules of omeprazole can bind to either Cys813 or Cys892 of the proton pump.[37,38] Similarly, lansoprazole is known to covalently modify Cys813 or Cys321. Pantoprazole, the most sluggish-reacting of the PPIs, can react with either Cys813 or the more deeply recessed and less accessible Cys822. Although PPIs are covalently bound to the proton pump, the interaction with accessible Cys residues can be reversed by reduced glutathione (GSH). The disulfide bond formed between the drug and receptor can be cleaved by this endogenous reducing agent, regenerating the essential Cys thiol of the pump and prompting the excretion of the drug fragment as a glutathione conjugate. Due to low concentration of GSH in the body, regeneration of proton pumps inhibited through Cys813 is incomplete. Pantoprazole binding is found to be less susceptible to GSH-mediated removal. These observations suggest that modification of Cys813 is more easily reversed, providing a fast phase of recovery, while modification of Cys822 is difficult to reverse, as GSH may not easily reach this site.[37]

Since the activation and rearrangement of PPIs take place at a strongly acidic pH, all of the oral formulations of PPIs have been developed to be acid-stable. This allows for better dissolution and absorption of PPIs (typically enteric-coated formulations) from the intestines. Both lansoprazole (enteric-coated) and omeprazole (either enteric coated or formulated with $NaHCO_3$) are available in granular form. This allows for the drug to be absorbed readily with minimal drug destruction in the stomach. Rearrangement selectively occurs in the acidic environment of the canaliculus within parietal cells after the drug is absorbed from the intestine and delivered to that target site. Typically, the half-life of PPIs is relatively short (~1 hr); however, the duration of action is long (~20-48 hr) because of their ability to irreversibly inhibit the proton pump.

Benzimidazole N1 is typically nonionizable at physiological pH and considered neutral in nature. However, as noted in Figure 26.6, benzimidazole N1 within PPIs is slightly acidic due to the electron-withdrawing property of the attached sulfinyl moiety. Due to this change in acidity, PPIs can be made into salt forms when benzimidazole N1 ionizes (loses proton) through treatment with strong base and becomes paired with the resultant metal cation (e.g., Na^+ or Mg^{2+}). Due to this property, some of the PPIs are marketed in the salt form, which provides improved aqueous solubility.

Metabolism and Drug Interactions

CYP enzymes in the liver extensively metabolize all PPIs, with CYP2C19 and CYP3A4 isoforms catalyzing most of the oxidations. The investigational drug tenatoprazole is an exception, in that it is less readily metabolized, yielding a longer plasma half-life of 7-9 hours. Excretion of PPI metabolites is predominantly renal. The CYP2C19 metabolizer phenotype determines the extent of metabolic transformation of PPIs. The three common phenotypes include extensive metabolizers (EM, "normal," *1 allele), ultrafast metabolizers (UM, *17 allele), and poor metabolizers (PM, *2 and *3 alleles).[39] About 3% of Caucasians and 15%-20% of Asians are considered PMs.[37,39] Omeprazole is found to exhibit significant inhibition of CYP2C19, and it may increases the plasma concentration of other drugs that are substrates for this isoform (i.e., diazepam) when administered at the same time. Lansoprazole is also found to inhibit CYP2C19 at therapeutically relevant concentration and exhibits drug-drug interactions.

Omeprazole undergoes three possible metabolic transformations: (1) CYP2C19-catalyzed hydroxylation of the 5′-methyl group on the pyridine ring, (2) CYP3A4-catalyzed sulfone formation, and (3) CYP2C19-catalyzed 5-O-demethylation (Fig. 26.8). Pantoprazole is metabolized into the O-desmethyl metabolite, pantoprazole sulfone, and pantoprazole thioether (a minor metabolite).

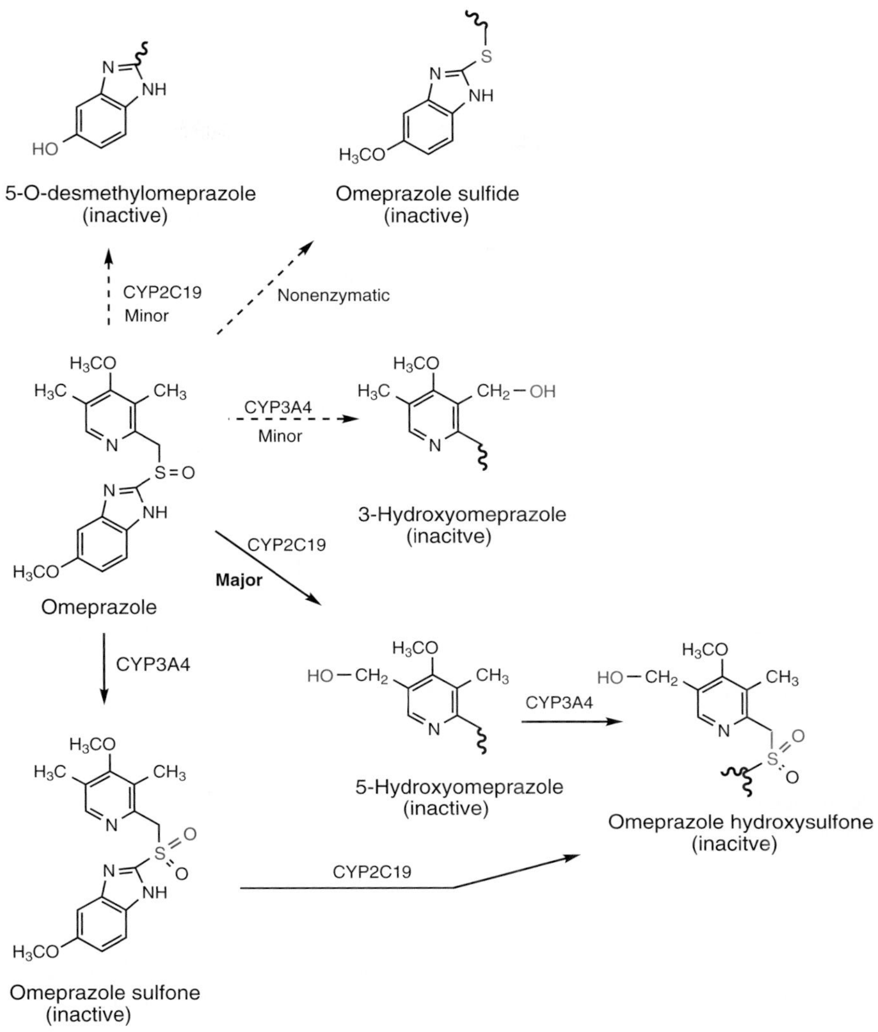

Figure 26.8 Omeprazole metabolism. Reprinted from Roche VF. The chemically elegant proton pump inhibitors. *Am J Pharm Educ.* 2006; 70(5): article 101, with permission.

The 4-desmethylpantoprazole is further modified via phase 2 metabolic transformation into 4-desmethylpantoprazole sulfate (Fig. 26.9). Lansoprazole also undergoes sulfone and thioether formation similar to pantoprazole. Additionally, a major pathway involves 5-hydroxylation of the benzimidazole motif (Fig. 26.10). Finally, rabeprazole is metabolized to generate sulfone, thioether, and demethylated derivatives. The desmethylrabeprazole thioether further undergoes oxidation to yield the carboxylic acid derivative as well (Fig. 26.11).[33,40,41]

The thioether metabolite of rabeprazole has been shown to undergo oxidation by microsomal enzymes (CYP2C19 and CYP3A4) under experimental conditions to generate the parent drug with the regenerated sulfoxide moiety. Rabeprazole is found to exhibit significantly fewer drug interactions compared to other PPIs; however, its thioether metabolite, which is formed via a nonenzymatic pathway, does inhibit CYP2C19, CYP2C9, CYP2D6, and CYP3A4.[42,43] Although the pyridyl-5-methyl group readily oxidized by CYP2C19 is not present in rabeprazole, lansoprazole, and pantoprazole, other sites in each of these drugs are modified by the same enzyme.

Similar to clinically available PPIs, investigational tenatoprazole also undergoes hepatic metabolism. The *S*-isomer of tenatoprazole is predominantly metabolized by CYP3A4 and the *R*-isomer is metabolized by CYP2C19.[44]

The structure of all PPIs contains a sulfoxide (also called sulfinyl) group where the sulfur atom is chiral. The stereochemistry of this functional group plays an important role in the pharmacological activity and metabolic profile. The *R*-enantiomer of omeprazole is metabolized more rapidly by CYP2C19 than the *S*-enantiomer. Thus, the single enantiomer, esomeprazole, provides improved bioavailability in those individuals who are EM or UM CYP2C19 metabolizers. Systemic drug exposure (AUC) is greater for esomeprazole compared to racemic omeprazole in EM and UM patients. Therefore, duration of drug exposure is extended and the gastric pH achieved from therapy is >4. All these correlate with improved healing rates.

Lansoprazole is metabolized by CYP2C19 and CYP3A4 in the liver. The CYP2C19 genotype has been shown to influence the metabolism of *S*-lansoprazole to a greater extent than the *R*-enantiomer. Since the potency of both

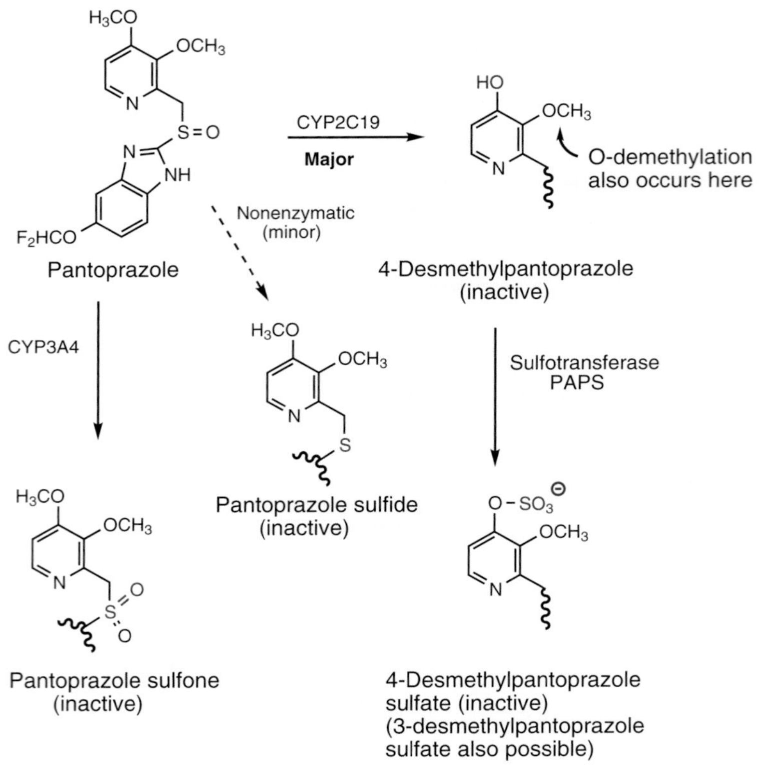

H_3CO
OCH_3
S=O
NH
F_2HCO
Pantoprazole
CYP2C19
Major
Nonenzymatic (minor)
CYP3A4
HO
OCH_3
O-demethylation also occurs here
4-Desmethylpantoprazole (inactive)
Sulfotransferase PAPS
Pantoprazole sulfide (inactive)
Pantoprazole sulfone (inactive)
$O-SO_3^{\ominus}$
4-Desmethylpantoprazole sulfate (inactive) (3-desmethylpantoprazole sulfate also possible)

Figure 26.9 Pantoprazole metabolism. Reprinted from Roche VF. The chemically elegant proton pump inhibitors. *Am J Pharm Educ.* 2006; 70(5): article 101, with permission.

enantiomers is equal, the use of *R*-lansoprazole would be more desirable, as it has less interpatient variability. Pantoprazole is metabolized by CYP2C19, and via a subsequent sulfonation pathway. It is less susceptible to CYP3A4-catalyzed metabolism. The enantiomers of pantoprazole are also differentially affected by CYP2C19 genotype.[44] Rabeprazole on the other hand is less sensitive to CYP-catalyzed metabolism.

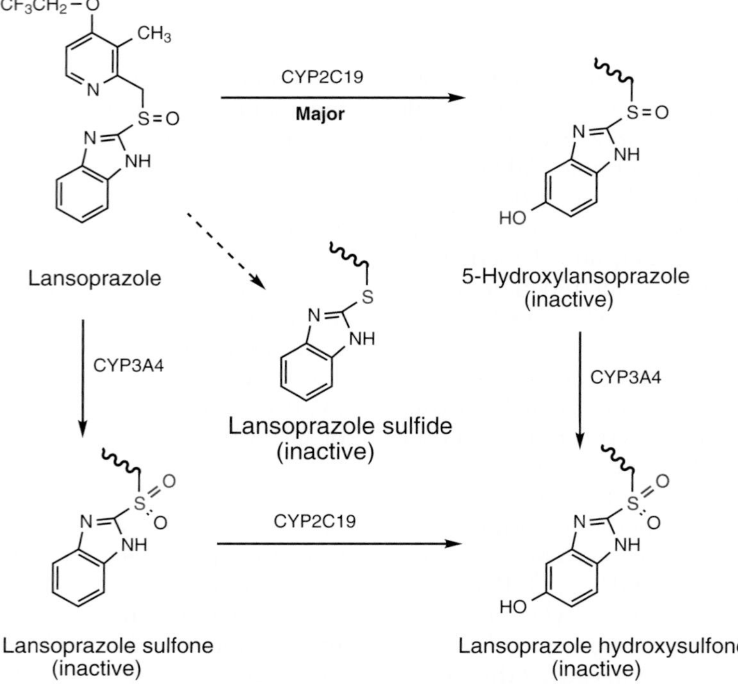

Figure 26.10 Lansoprazole metabolism. Reprinted from Roche VF. The chemically elegant proton pump inhibitors. *Am J Pharm Educ.* 2006; 70(5): article 101, with permission.

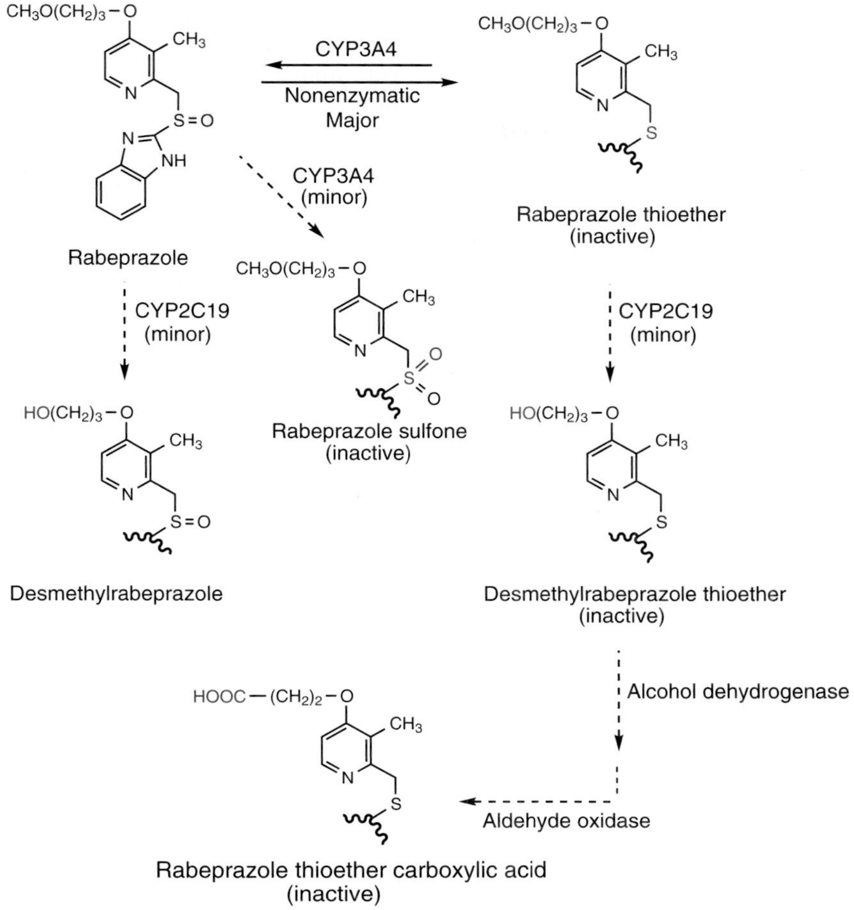

Figure 26.11 Rabeprazole metabolism. Reprinted from Roche VF. The chemically elegant proton pump inhibitors. *Am J Pharm Educ.* 2006; 70(5): article 101, with permission.

Omeprazole and esomeprazole are both substrates and strong inhibitors of the CYP2C19 isoform, and they compete with drugs that depend on this isoform for metabolic activation or clearance while limiting the availability of the isoform. For example, clopidogrel is an antiplatelet prodrug that is activated by CYP2C19 and is commonly prescribed to patients who have suffered a stroke or have a high risk of ischemia.[45] These patients may also be prescribed a PPI due to higher risk of GI ulceration from clopidogrel therapy. In this case, omeprazole and esomeprazole should be avoided because inhibition of CYP2C19 will inhibit clopidogrel activation and put patients at a risk for a potentially fatal cardiovascular event.[46] Lansoprazole has been a suitable option for patients when a PPI and clopidogrel need to be coadministered but pantoprazole, the weakest CYP2C19 inhibitor of the PPIs, is now considered the preferred agent.[32] In addition, due to the possibility of PPIs interfering with bone remodeling, prolonged usage of PPIs (more than 1 yr) is likely to increase the risk of bone fracture. Additionally, recent studies have indicated that PPI use is linked to chronic kidney disease. Since the use of PPIs is frequently extended beyond recommended durations, the risk of renal toxicity may be higher than normally anticipated.[47,48] The exact mechanism of damage is unclear at this stage.

The reason for the discovery and development of enantiomers of omeprazole and lansoprazole relates to their different metabolic profile and efficacy. The interest in developing single enantiomers as drugs has been at the forefront of medicinal chemistry and drug discovery. The single bioactive enantiomer of a drug, if it exists, provides more specificity and generally less toxicity than a racemic mixture. The development of improved chemical methods to synthesize pure enantiomers and the ability to investigate each enantiomer against a specific disease model have facilitated the development of enantiomerically pure drugs. During such investigations, "isomeric ballast" is used as an informal term to describe the enantiomer that is less active or inactive (also called the distomer). On the other hand, the eutomer is the pharmacologically active enantiomer.

In the case of PPIs, both enantiomers are biologically active because the activated form has no chiral center (the chiral sulfoxide is converted into achiral structures upon activation). The difference is related to their metabolic conversion by CYP2C19 and CYP3A4. In the case of omeprazole (racemic mixture), the AUC of the *S*-enantiomer exhibits an activity difference of 3-fold between EM and PM patients, where the *R*-enantiomer shows about a 7.5-fold difference. This indicates that omeprazole (*R*-isomer) exhibits more significant variability between patients and potentially improved therapeutic outcomes in PMs.[49,50] Dexlansoprazole is the *R*-enantiomer of lansoprazole, and it has a higher plasma concentration than the *S*-enantiomer due to less rapid inactivating metabolism. *S*-pantoprazole has been shown to be more potent than the *R*-enantiomer, and its pharmacokinetic profile is less dependent on CYP2C19 genotype. Therefore, although pantoprazole is marketed as a racemic mixture, the *S*-enantiomer is considered to have pharmacokinetic and pharmacodynamic advantages for clinical use. In the case of racemic rabeprazole, the *R*-enantiomer is more potent than the *S*-enantiomer, providing a superior pharmacokinetic profile.

Another major GI issue where PPIs can have therapeutic value relates to infection by *H. pylori*, which is likened to peptic ulcer in a majority of patients.[51] *H. pylori* infects the gastric mucosa and produces ammonia and CO_2 in order to withstand the acidic pH. The process involves hydrolysis of urea by the bacterial enzyme urease. Once a diagnosis has been made to show that *H. pylori* infection is the cause, eradication regimens involve a combination of PPI and antibiotics. Typically, PPIs with amoxicillin and clarithromycin or metronidazole are recommended. More details on bacterial infections and available antibiotics to treat them are discussed in Chapter 29.

Specific Drugs (Fig. 26.6)

The chemistry, reactivity, and metabolism of the clinically available PPIs have been discussed above, but three of the more commonly used and/or kinetically unique drugs are summarized in greater depth below.

OMEPRAZOLE. The pyridine substituents of omeprazole (and esomeprazole) promote the nucleophilicity of N1 through electron release via π (methoxy) and σ (methyl) bonds. Protonation of benzimidazole N3 (with subsequent enhancement of the electrophilic character of adjacent C2) is augmented by the electron-releasing property of the C5-methoxy, resulting in a readily activated drug that inactivates the proton pump predominantly through covalent interaction with Cys813. Recovery through reduced GSH and *de novo* protein synthesis yields a duration of approximately 20 hours, although it can range up to 72 hours.

Absorption of the enteric-coated oral dosage form is rapid and bioavailability ranges from 30% to 40%. Activity often begins within 1 hour. Omeprazole is 96% protein bound, and a magnesium salt formulation is available.[32,52] The combination product with sodium bicarbonate (Zegerid) does not require that omeprazole be enteric coated because the bicarbonate increases gastric pH from the normal (close to 1) to 4.2-5.2. At this elevated pH, benzimidazole N3 will not protonate and the nucleophilic attack by pyridine N1 cannot occur. Thus, the drug is safe from premature activation in the stomach. In addition, without an enteric coating, once the drug reaches the intestine, absorption can proceed immediately.

PANTOPRAZOLE SODIUM. Pantoprazole sodium is marketed as a racemic mixture of *R*- and *S*-enantiomers. It is a prescription drug and available for oral administration (20, 40 mg) and IV administration. Pantoprazole has two electron-releasing methoxy groups conjugated with the pyridine ring. While the σ electron–withdrawing effect of the C3 methoxy group can impact pyridine N1, the nitrogen is still reasonably and sufficiently nucleophilic for the drug to be activated at the acidic canalicular pH. However, the strongly electron-withdrawing difluoromethyl substitution at benzimidazole C5 is instrumental in lowering the pK_a of benzimidazole N3, which decreases the extent of protonation and detracts from the δ^+ character of benzimidazole C2. This significantly slows nucleophilic attack by the pyridine N1 nucleophile, which is a requirement for drug activation. Pantoprazole is the most sluggishly activated PPI of those currently marketed, and this is directly related to its long duration. Despite a short half-life of approximately 1-2 hours,[32] pantoprazole in its active form has time to reach and bind to a deeply recessed and less accessible Cys822 within the proton pump. Since the inactivated pump cannot be rescued by reduced GSH, the therapeutic effect lasts for a longer period of time (47 hr) than other PPIs (approximately 20 hr).[37]

Since PPIs are sensitive to stomach acid, pantoprazole sodium is available as an enteric-coated tablet, where the drug release begins only after the tablet leaves the stomach. Bioavailability of pantoprazole is about 77% and it takes about 2-3 hours to reach maximum plasma level. A significant percentage (98%) of this drug is bound to plasma protein. Pantoprazole undergoes hepatic metabolic clearance by the action of CYP2C19 and CYP3A4 (Fig. 26.9). Studies have shown that there are no significant drug interactions observed with pantoprazole in combination with other common drugs metabolized by CYP2C19, 3A4, 2D6, or 1A2.

DEXLANSOPRAZOLE. Dexlansoprazole is the newest PPI introduced for the treatment of gastric acid–related GI diseases. It is the *R*-enantiomer of lansoprazole, marketed as a dual delayed release pharmaceutical formulation. The variation in CYP2C19 genotype influences the metabolism of *S*-lansoprazole to a greater extent than the *R*-enantiomer. Thus, dexlansoprazole is more desirable, as it has less interpatient variability. It is available as a 30 or 60 mg capsules for use. The recommended regimen for nonerosive GERD in adult is 30 mg twice daily for 4 weeks. A 60 mg twice-daily regimen is recommended for healing of erosive esophagitis for about 8 weeks.

As noted, dexlansoprazole is formulated with a dual delayed release formulation using two different copolymer-coated granules. These are pH-sensitive granules, and about 25% of the drug is released within 2 hours and the other 75% is released at 4-5 hours from the distal intestine.[53] While the resulting duration does not quite mimic that of twice-daily dosing and distress from nocturnal acid rebound can still occur, there is more likely to be "round the clock" coverage than from simple enteric-coated formulations like racemic lansoprazole or omeprazole. By 6.5 hours postadministration, the canaliculus "residence time" of isomerically pure dexlansoprazole is approximately twice that of the racemic mixture, Like other PPIs, since dexlansoprazole lowers the pH of stomach contents, absorption of drugs that depend on low gastric pH can be negatively affected, including ampicillin esters, digoxin, and ketoconazole.

Prokinetic Agents

Gastrointestinal hypomotility is linked to various GI disorders, including GERD, gastroparesis IBS, and colonic pseudo-obstruction. One approach to managing these pathological events is administration of prokinetic

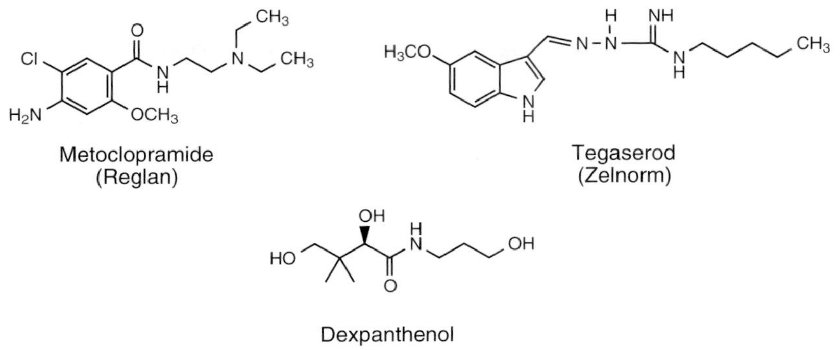

Figure 26.12 Examples of prokinetic agents.

agents.[54,55] This class of drugs stimulates and facilitates GI motility. Increased gastric emptying takes place via drug-induced peristalsis, which improves the symptoms of the above-mentioned GI disorders. Traditionally, prokinetic agents are classified into three categories: (1) agents that target cholinergic or 5-HT_4 receptors, (2) agents that target dopamine or opioid receptors, and (3) agents with agonistic activity on GI hormone receptors (motilin receptor agonists or somatostatin agonists). This section only focuses on selected prokinetic agents, namely metoclopramide, dexpanthenol, and tegaserod (Fig. 26.12). The reader is directed toward specific sections within this chapter for more detail on how cholinergic and serotonin (5-HT) receptors are targeted for the treatment of various GI disorders.

Metoclopramide

Metoclopramide is a procainamide derivative which does not exhibit antiarrhythmic or topical anesthetic activity, and which was initially developed as an antiemetic agent. Later, its ability to stimulate upper GI tract motility was realized, and it was used as a drug for improving gastric emptying. Metoclopramide is either orally administered or injected to alleviate GERD, diabetic gastropharesis, and chemotherapy-induced nausea and vomiting. Metoclopramide exhibits an agonistic effect at 5-HT_4 receptors and an antagonistic effect at dopamine D_2 and 5-HT_3 receptors. Inhibition of dopamine secretion by metoclopramide increases the release of acetylcholine (ACh) in the myenteric plexus in the GI tract and increases GI motility.[54] However, some of the adverse effects caused by this agent are also related to D_2 antagonistic effects, particularly in the CNS, where patients may develop irreversible tardive dyskinesia. To prevent potential complications, metoclopramide treatment is often restricted to less than 3 months and discontinued at the first observation of involuntary muscle movement. Metoclopramide should not be given to patients who take monoamine oxidase inhibitors, tricyclic antidepressants, or phenothiazines due to the risk for serious drug-drug interactions.

CYP and phase 2 conjugating enzymes metabolize metoclopramide to a significant extent. Some of the commonly observed metabolites include the N-deethylated derivative (CYP2D6), N-oxidation (CYP2D6), and glucuronide and sulfate conjugates of the aryl amine (Fig. 26.13).[56]

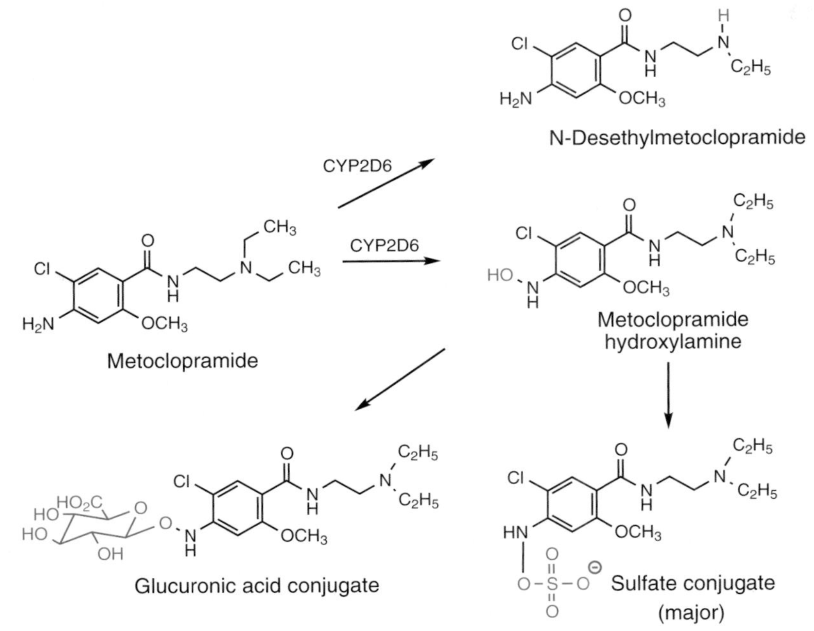

Figure 26.13 Metabolism of metoclopramide.

Other Prokinetic Agents

Several other prokinetic agents structurally similar to metoclopramide are available outside of the United States and/or are in clinical trials. Some of these include prucalopride, mosapride, and itopride. These are used for either chronic constipation or gastritis.[57-59] Prucalopride and mosapride are 5-HT_4 receptor agonists while itopride is an acetylcholinesterase (AChE) inhibitor and D_2 receptor antagonist. Centrally active dopamine antagonists provide an anti-emetic property, while peripherally these antagonists stimulate GI tract motility.[60,61]

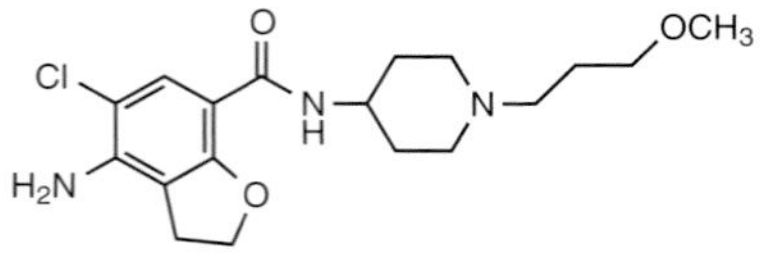

Prucalopride

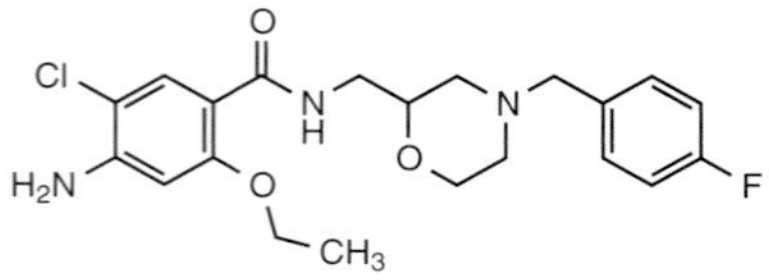

Mosapride

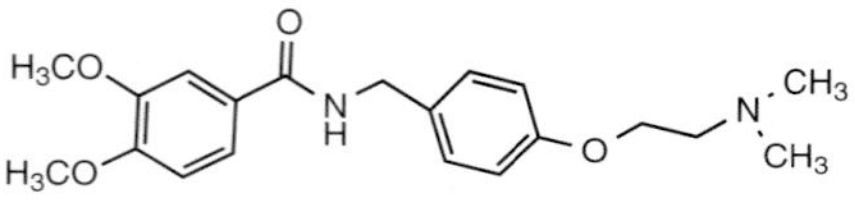

Itopride

Dexpanthenol is used for paralytic ileus and intestinal atonia. The administration is IM for these conditions. Dexpanthenol is the alcohol analogue of endogenous pantothenic acid, a precursor of coenzyme A (CoA). The biosynthesis of ACh requires CoA and, as previously emphasized, ACh plays an important role in controlling GI muscle movement.

Tegaserod is also a selective 5-HT_4 partial agonist and has been shown to be an effective prokinetic agent. It is clinically used for the treatment of IBS.[62] A more detail discussion on IBS is given in a later section of this chapter.

Prostaglandins

Prostaglandins exhibit antisecretory effects by inhibiting adenylyl cyclase activity in parietal cells. This in turn results in inhibition of gastric acid secretion. Additionally, prostaglandins stimulate secretion of mucus and bicarbonate to prevent acid-related erosion in the GI tract.[63] Endogenous prostaglandin E1 and a more stable synthetic derivative, misoprostol, exhibit cytoprotective effects. The active form of this class of molecules has a terminal carboxylic acid, so misoprostol, a methyl ester, is a prodrug with the advantage of oral bioavailability. The ester is hydrolyzed to the corresponding bioactive carboxylic acid in the bloodstream. Other structural differences are at C15 and C16. Prostaglandin E1 has a secondary alcohol at the C15 position, where misoprostol has no hydroxyl group at C15 and an alcohol at C16. The hydroxyl at C16 is a tertiary alcohol which is stable to oxidation compared to the allylic secondary alcohol at C15 of prostaglandin E1. Combined with the need for hydrolytic activation, this prolongs duration of action.

Misoprostol reduces the basal levels of gastric acid secretion, resulting in GI mucosal protection.[64] In terms of GI disorders, misoprostol has been recommended for the treatment of duodenal ulcers that are unresponsive to traditional H_2 antagonists. Due to its ability to induce smooth muscle contraction, misoprostol's adverse effects relate to diarrhea and abdominal pain. It is contraindicated in pregnant women due to its ability to stimulate uterine contraction. In the United States, misoprostol can be administered in combination with nonsteroidal anti-inflammatory drugs (NSAIDs) because it reduces the risk of gastric ulceration associated with extended use of NSAIDs.[63]

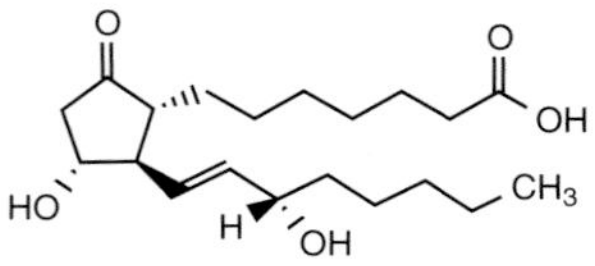

Prostaglandin E1

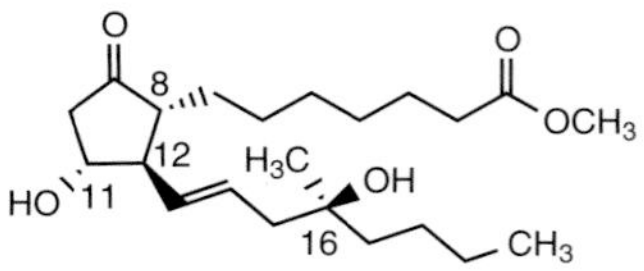

Misoprostol

GI Mucosal Protectants

Sucralfate

Sucralfate is a poly-sulfuric acid ester of sucrose complexed with aluminum hydroxide and is used in gastric ulcer disease.[65,66] These poorly dissociated complexes are insoluble in stomach. The physical complex sits in the crater of the ulcerated area and serves as a physical and chemical barrier to protect the ulcer from erosion by enzymes and bile salts in the stomach. The chemical barrier is the result of the basic metal hydroxide neutralization of gastric acid. It is also observed that sucralfate stimulates prostaglandin synthesis and bicarbonate release, which may be beneficial in peptic ulcers. Systemic absorption of sucralfate is negligible but it reduces the absorption of other drugs, such as H_2 antihistamines, quinolone antibiotics, phenytoin, and warfarin.[67] As aluminum is part of this complex, there is a risk of aluminum accumulation from absorbed material in patients with renal impairment.

Bismuth Subsalicylate

Bismuth-based preparations, such as bismuth subsalicylate, exhibit a similar protective effect as sucralfate and by a similar mechanism. A combination therapy involving an H_2 antihistamine, antibiotic (metronidazole, tetracycline), and potassium bismuth subsalicylate is used as a second-line option for *H. pylori* eradication and treatment of associated ulcers.

ANTIEMETIC AGENTS

Serotonergics

Serotonin is one of the prominent neurotransmitters that has generated remarkable interest in drug development.[68] Although its physiological importance was underappreciated in the early days, later it became an important focus of scientific and clinical investigation. Serotonin has been associated with many disorders, including anxiety, depression, drug abuse, cardiovascular disorders, sexual behavior, appetite control, gastric motility, nausea, and irritable bowel disorders.[69] This section discusses the role of serotonin and its receptors in nausea and IBD.

Serotonin (5-hydroxytryptamine, 5-HT) was discovered independently in the United States and in Italy. In addition to various homeostatic physiological actions, 5-HT is also associated with certain mental/behavioral disorders. This was realized due to the structural similarity of 5-HT to a hallucinogenic agent, (+)-lysergic acid diethylamide (LSD). This drug was shown to be a potent 5-HT receptor agonist at certain receptor subtypes and an antagonist at others. With the development of sophisticated biochemical methods, substantial research has been undertaken to understand the structure and function of 5-HT receptors and the physiological roles of 5-HT.[70,71]

To date, seven distinct families or subtypes of 5-HT receptors have been discovered, which are designated as 5-HT_1 to 5-HT_7. Within each subtype, several subpopulations of receptors are also known.[72] All 5-HT receptors are G protein–coupled receptors except for 5-HT_4, which belongs to the Cys-loop–containing ligand-gated ion channels (see Chapter 6).[16,73] This chapter specifically focuses on drugs developed to target 5-HT_3 and 5-HT_4 receptors closely associated with GI disorders.[74-77]

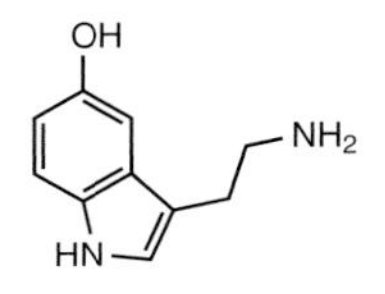

Serotonin

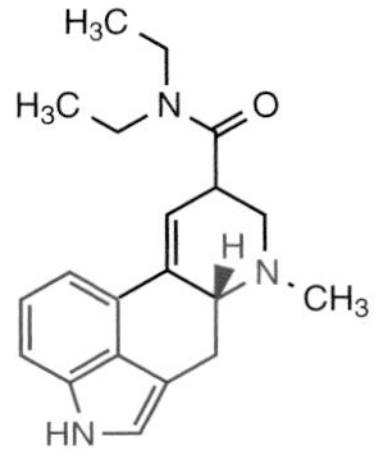

(+)-Lysergic acid diethylamide

The biosynthesis of 5-HT begins with the hydroxylation of dietary tryptophan by tryptophan hydroxylase, which generates 5-hydroxytryptophan (5-HTP). Subsequently, a nonselective amino acid decarboxylase called 5-HTP decarboxylase converts 5-HTP into 5-HT. The major metabolic pathway involves oxidative deamination by monoamine oxidase (MAO) to the corresponding aldehyde, which further undergoes oxidation to the carboxylic acid or reduction to the primary alcohol (Fig. 26.14). In addition, acylation of 5-HT by N-acetyltransferase occurs to yield N-acetylserotonin. It is interesting to note that O-methylation of acetylated 5-HT generates melatonin, the endogenous hormone associated with circadian rhythms and sleep. From a drug discovery standpoint, it is important to realize that each step in 5-HT biosynthesis and metabolism, along with the understanding of the nature of important receptor interactions, is a potential target for drug development.

5-HT_3 Antagonists

A large proportion of 5-HT is found in the GI tract, where it regulates physiological functions and changes.[78] 5-HT is found in the mucosal enterochromaffin cells, which release 5-HT to activate 5-HT_3 and 5-HT_4 receptors. Stimulation of 5-HT_3 receptors inhibits gastric secretions and stimulates ion migrating motor complexes in the gut.[74] This enhances the intestinal secretions to facilitate bowel movements. Activation of intestinal 5-HT_3 receptors also stimulates antral contractions and vagal afferent nerves which induce nausea. It is understood that chemotherapy agents induce nausea, at least in part, through the release of large amount of 5-HT in the enterochromaffin cells, which stimulates vagal afferent nerves and initiates the vomiting reflex. Several 5-HT_3 receptor antagonists have been developed as anti-emetics to inhibit this process (Fig. 26.15).

Structural Features and Mechanism of Action

Ondansetron, palonosetron, granisetron, alosetron, dolasetron, and tropisetron are the clinically available 5-HT_3 receptor antagonists (Fig. 26.15). The first-generation agents can be categorized into three major structural classes: (1) carbazole derivatives, (2) indazole derivatives, and (3) indole derivatives. Palonosetron is a second-generation agent that is highly selective toward the 5-HT_3 receptor.

The first selective 5-HT_3 antagonist (bemesetron) was developed based on the structure of cocaine, which was previously shown to weakly inhibit the 5-HT_3 receptor and exhibit an antiemetic property.[76] The tropane core from cocaine is an important structural feature and retained in many of the early 5-HT_3 antagonists, including tropisetron. This nitrogen-containing heterocycle was slightly modified to introduce similar looking bicyclic cores to generate newer members of this class of agents, including granisetron, dolasetron, and palonosetron. Both ondansetron and alosetron have an imidazole or similar amine-containing heterocyclic structure.

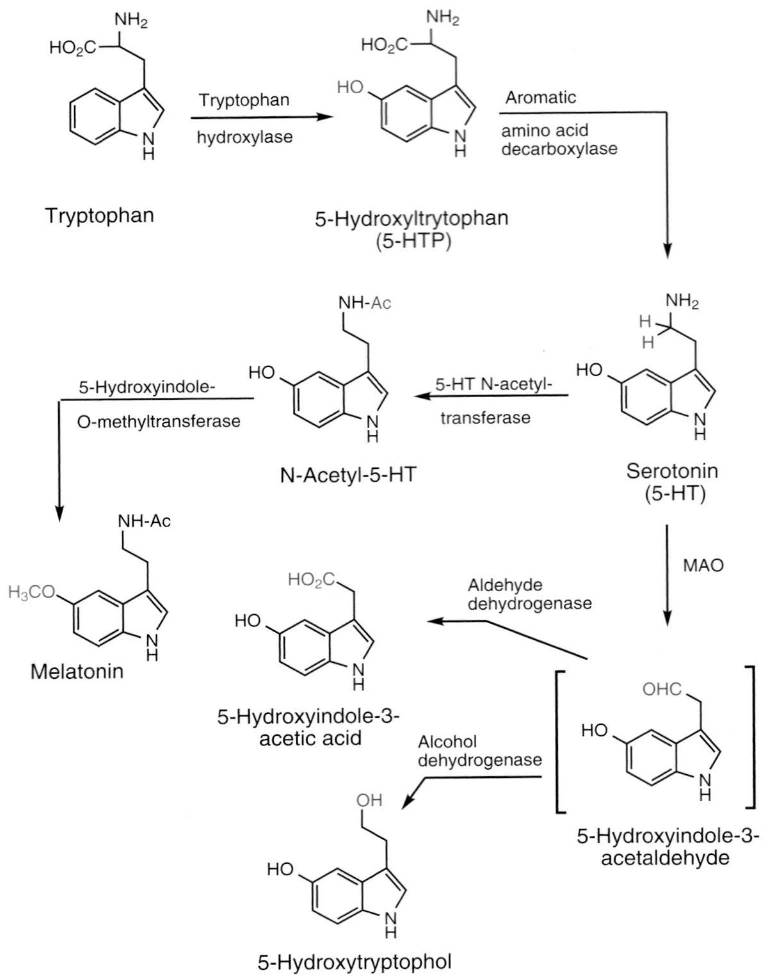

Figure 26.14 Biosynthesis and catabolism of serotonin (5-HT).

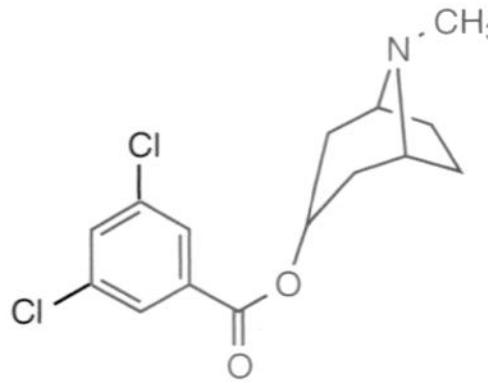

Bemesetron (cocaine core is highlighted in red)

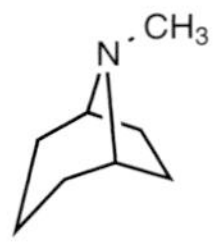

Tropane core

Based on the SAR of 5-HT_3 antagonists, a number of structural features have been identified as important motifs for receptor binding.[76,79,80] A proposed pharmacophore model is provided in Figure 26.16. It has been speculated that ring A may not be required for binding but, rather, acts as a spacer between ring B and the carbonyl oxygen atom. Ring B may be more important for binding and associated hydrophobic binding regions have been proposed. An aromatic centroid (A)-to-oxygen distance of 3.3-3.5 Å is thought to be optimal. Distances calculated from the terminal amine to the oxygen atom, and from the terminal amine to centroid A, are 5.1-5.2 Å and 6.7-7.2 Å, respectively.

As mentioned previously, the cocaine scaffold was an inspiration for the design of early 5-HT_3 antagonists. The tropane or amine-containing bicyclic motifs are linked to the aromatic component via an ester or amide bond. The aromatic component has a fused benzene ring and nitrogen heterocycle as part of the indole, indazole, or carbazole core. The distance between the aromatic ring segment and the terminal basic amine is optimal at 6.7 Å. The nitrogen heterocycle of the aromatic ring moiety is important to provide the needed electron density for the observed cation-π interaction with Arg92 of the 5-HT_3 receptor. Based on proposed pharmacophoric models, the aromatic ring segment is also involved in hydrophobic interactions. Additionally, the carbonyl oxygen of the amide bond forms a water-mediated hydrogen bond, and the amine-containing ring (in protonated form) forms a cation-π interaction with Trp183 and Tyr193 (Fig. 26.17).[81]

Palonosetron (Fig. 26.15), a more recent 5-HT_3 antagonist, also contains a similar pharmacophore, yet it has a longer half-life (40 hours) and greater receptor binding affinity compared to first-generation agents. The stronger binding affinity can be attributed to the following drug-receptor interactions: (1) a hydrogen bond between Tyr153

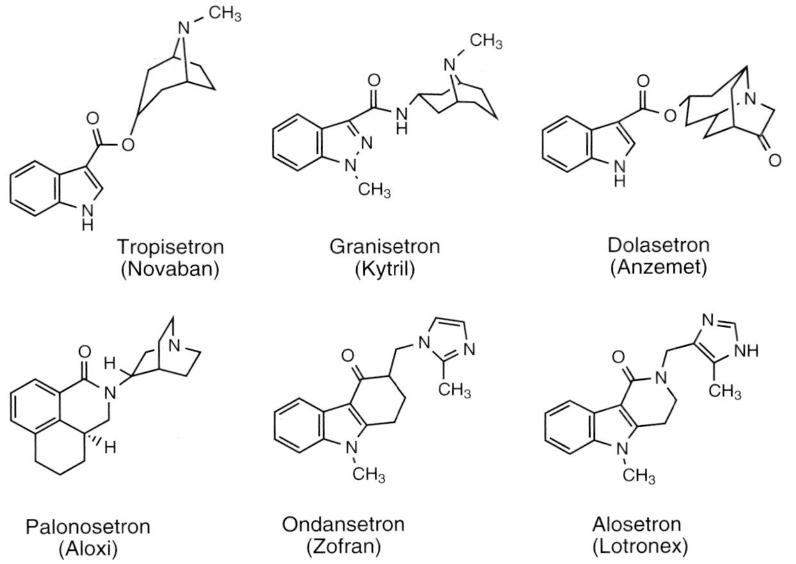

Tropisetron (Novaban) Granisetron (Kytril) Dolasetron (Anzemet)

Palonosetron (Aloxi) Ondansetron (Zofran) Alosetron (Lotronex)

Figure 26.15 5-HT_3 receptor antagonists.

and the carbonyl oxygen of the amide group of palonosetron, which is consistent with the role of this residue interacting with 5-HT, and (2) a cation-π interaction of the quinuclidine nitrogen (in its protonated form) with Tyr153 and Trp183. The precision of the angle and distance of these functional groups within palonosetron is proposed to be crucial for its high binding affinity.[82]

Currently available 5-HT_3 receptor antagonists are important in the treatment of chemotherapy- and radiation-induced nausea and vomiting. These are unavoidable and often dose-limiting adverse effects for patients undergoing such treatments. Many of the 5-HT_3 antagonists exhibit comparable efficacy and safety, yet their pharmacological and pharmacokinetic properties are different.[83-86] The half-lives of these drugs vary widely. The selection of a specific agent relates, in part, to the emetogenic potential and properties of the chemotherapeutic regimen, the patient's ability to tolerate adverse effects, and patient history. The metabolic profile of the drug also plays a role in selecting the most suitable drug for a specific population of patients.

Ondansetron is a competitive, reversible antagonist of 5-HT_3 receptor, whereas granisetron, tropisetron, and palonosetron produce an insurmountable antagonism.[86] Ondansetron has an alkylimidazole moiety as the nitrogen-containing heterocycle, and a ketone moiety between the aromatic segment and the nitrogen-containing heterocycle (Fig. 26.15). The other members of this class have a tertiary alkyl amine–containing heterocycle (a stronger base) and an amide or ester moiety (a better hydrogen bond acceptor). Based on these structural features, it is highly likely that granisetron, tropisetron, and palonosetron can make stronger cation-π and hydrogen bond interactions, which are key interactions for tighter receptor binding.

Ondansetron also has some affinity for the 5-HT_1 (B and C subtypes), α-adrenergic, and opioid receptors, while dolasetron is considered a very selective 5-HT_3 receptor antagonist. Dolasetron readily undergoes a reduction by carbonyl reductase to generate hydrodolasetron, which is an active metabolite with a half-life of 4-8 hours. The

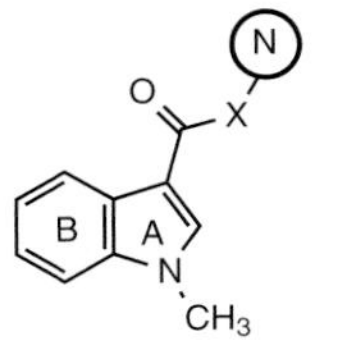

Figure 26.16 A general pharmacophore model for 5-HT_3 antagonists.

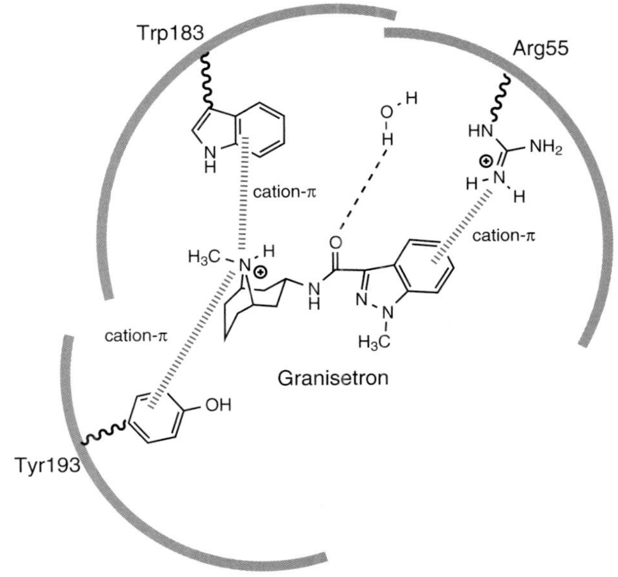

Figure 26.17 Proposed binding interactions of granisetron with the 5-HT_3 receptor.

bioavailability of orally administered dolasetron is high and makes it a therapeutically useful option for those who can tolerate oral medications. Although IV administration was available in earlier times, the FDA suspended this mode of administration in 2010 due to the risk of hemodynamically unstable tachyarrhythmia. The mechanism of this adverse effect is related to slowing or delaying of cardiac depolarization by sodium or potassium channel blockade.[87]

Selected pharmacokinetic properties of common 5-HT_3 antagonists are summarized in Table 26.2.

Hydrodolasetron

Metabolism

Although all 5-HT_3 receptor antagonists exhibit a similar mechanism of action, their structural differences alter their binding affinities and pharmacokinetic profiles. Dolasetron undergoes reduction of the carbonyl group by carbonyl reductase and aryl hydroxylation and N-oxidation catalyzed by CYP2D6 and CYP3A4. As indicated previously, hydrodolasetron is an active metabolite that exhibits about 20-60 times greater 5-HT_3 receptor affinity than dolasetron.[88,89] Granisetron is primarily metabolized by CYP3A4 to the N-demethylated metabolite and by CYP1A1 to the 7-hydroxy derivative.[90] Chemical inhibitors of CYP3A4, such as ketoconazole, affect the metabolism of granisetron. Palonosetron typically undergoes an N-oxidation and 6S-hydroxylation. Well-known genetic variations in CYP2D6 are known to produce patients who are intermediate metabolizers (IMs), PMs, or UMs related to this isoform, and this affects the metabolic profile of 5-HT_3 antagonists, leading to inconsistent therapeutic response and risk of adverse effects. In addition to the phase 1 metabolic transformations, most of the 5-HT_3 receptor antagonists also undergo phase 2 transformations, including glucuronidation and sulfate conjugation. The phase 2 metabolites are excreted in the urine, in addition to 10%-60% of the unmodified parent drug.

Specific Drugs

The 5-HT_3 antagonists described below are the two most commonly prescribed antiemetics in this class.

ONDANSETRON. Ondansetron is a carbazole-based 5-HT_3 antagonist indicated for the prevention of chemotherapy-induced nausea/vomiting in adults and children 4 years and older. It is available for oral and IV administration. Based on a proposed receptor binding model, the carbazole interacts with the 5-HT_3 receptor via hydrophobic and cation-π interactions. The weakly basic methylimidazole moiety, in a protonated state, can form a cation-π interaction with conserved active site Tyr and Trp residues.[81] Ondansetron is a reversible antagonist and exhibits relatively weaker binding compared to other members, perhaps due to reduced basicity of the imidazole nitrogen.

Ondansetron is primarily metabolized by CYP3A4 and follows a secondary metabolic pathway catalyzed by CYP1A2, CYP2D6, and CYP2E1. Significant drug-drug interactions based on this metabolic profile are known. Major metabolic reactions include aryl hydroxylation at positions 6, 7, or 8, and demethylation of the carbazole nitrogen.[91] There has not been any reported major adverse effect linked to ondansetron besides headache.

PALONOSETRON. Palonosetron is the most recent 5-HT_3 antagonist approved for therapeutic use. Despite having an aryl ring, an amide bond, and a nitrogen heterocycle like all members of this therapeutic class, it is structurally slightly different than other classical 5-HT_3 antagonists. It has a tricyclic aryl amide linked to a quinuclidine ring via the amide nitrogen. Based on the binding models with the receptor, the stronger cation-π interaction introduced by the highly basic quinuclidine (in its protonated form) and the conformation achieved by the rigid tricyclic core within this molecule may help explain its strong binding affinity. Palonosetron is available as capsules (0.5 mg) and for IV injection (0.25 mg/5 mL). It is currently used for the prevention of cancer chemotherapy-induced nausea and vomiting in adult and geriatric patients. It has the longest half-life of about 40 hours among clinically used 5-HT_3 antagonists. Palonosetron is well distributed in tissues and exhibits moderate plasma protein binding.[92] Its metabolism is primarily hepatic, and CYP2C9, CYP3A4, and CYP1A2 are the common isoforms responsible for its biotransformation.[93] Drug-drug interactions based on CYP3A4 vulnerability are less common than with ondansetron, and it can be a viable alternative when serious or otherwise significant interactions rule out ondansetron use.

Other Anti-Emetic Agents

Although several 5-HT_3 antagonists are available as antiemetic agents for the treatment of nausea and vomiting, promethazine and prochlorperazine are two other agents with non-5-HT_3 mechanisms that are commonly used as well.

Promethazine

Promethazine is a phenothiazine derivative and falls in the category of a tricyclic H_1-antihistamine (see Chapter 25). Phenothiazine antihistamines have a short, branched carbon chain between the nonbasic phenothiazine nitrogen and the basic aliphatic amine. The branched side chain is an important structural difference between promethazine and antipsychotic phenothiazines, which have a straight chain connection between nitrogen atoms. In addition to being used to reverse the symptoms of allergic reaction (a common H_1 antihistamine indication), promethazine is widely used for the treatment of nausea and vomiting associated with anesthesia, and for the treatment of motion

Table 26.2 Pharmacokinetic Properties of 5-HT_3 Antagonists

Parameters	Ondansetron (Zofran)	Dolasetron (Anzemet)	Granisetron (Kytril)	Alosetron (Lotronex)	Palonosetron (Aloxi)	Tropisetron (Navoban)
cLog P (calc)[a]	2.1 ± 0.5	2.8 ± 0.5	1.5 ± 0.5	0.88 ± 0.8	2.6 ± 0.5	3.6 ± 0.3
Log D (pH 7) (calc)[a]	1.5	2.8	1.5	0.4	0.01	0.8
Bioavailability (%)	56-70[d]	Hydrodolasetron: 60-80	60[d]	50-60[b,c]	NA (administered IV)	60 (60-100)
Protein binding (%)	70-76	Hydrodolasetron: 70-80	65	82	62	71
Volume of distribution (L/kg)	PO: 2.2-2.5	Hydrodolasetron: PO: 5.8-10	PO: 3.9	PO: 70 (65-95)	IV: 6.8-12.5	IV: 500
		PO: 6-7				
Elimination half-life (hr)	PO: 3-6	PO: <10 min	IV: 4-5	PO: 1.5-2.0	PO: 30-40	EM: PO: 6-8
	Elderly: PO: 11	Hydrodolasetron: PO: 4-9	PO: ~6			PM: PO: 30
Metabolism	Hydroxylation	Reduction of carbonyl	N-Demethylation	6-Hydroxylation	N-oxidation	Hydrolysis
	Glucuronidation	Hydroxylation	Hepatic	N-Demethylation	6S-Hydroxylation	Glucuronidation
	Hepatic	N-Demethylation			Hepatic: 50%	
Metabolizing enzyme	CYP3A4	Carbonyl reductase	CYP3A4	CYP2C9: 30%	CYP2D6	CYP2D6
	CYP2D6	CYP2D6		CYP3A4: 20	CYP3A4	
		CYP3A4 (N-oxide)		CYP1A2: 10%	CYP1A2	
Time to peak plasma concentration (hr)	PO: 1-2	Hydrodolasetron IV: <0.5	PO: 2-3	PO: 0.5-2	IV: injected over 30 sec	EM: PO: 3
		Hydrodolasetron PO: <1				PM: PO: 4
Excretion (%)	Urine metabolites (40-60)	Urine metabolites (45)	Urine metabolites (48)	Urine metabolites (70)	Urine metabolites (80)	Urine metabolites (~70)
	Feces metabolites (25)	Feces metabolites (30)	Feces metabolites (38)	Feces metabolites (25)		Feces metabolites (~15)
	Unchanged (<10)	Unchanged hydrodolasetron (60)	Unchanged (<10)	Unchanged (<10)	Unchanged (40)	Unchanged (<10)
Duration (hr)	–	–	8-24	1-10	>24	–

[a] Chemical Abstracts, American Chemical Society, calculated using Advanced Chemistry Development (ACD/Labs) Software V8.14 for Solaris (1994-2006 ACD/Labs).
[b] First-pass metabolism.
[c] Food delays absorption and peak plasma concentrations.
[d] Food increases extent of absorption.
IM, intramuscular; IV, intravenous; PO, oral.

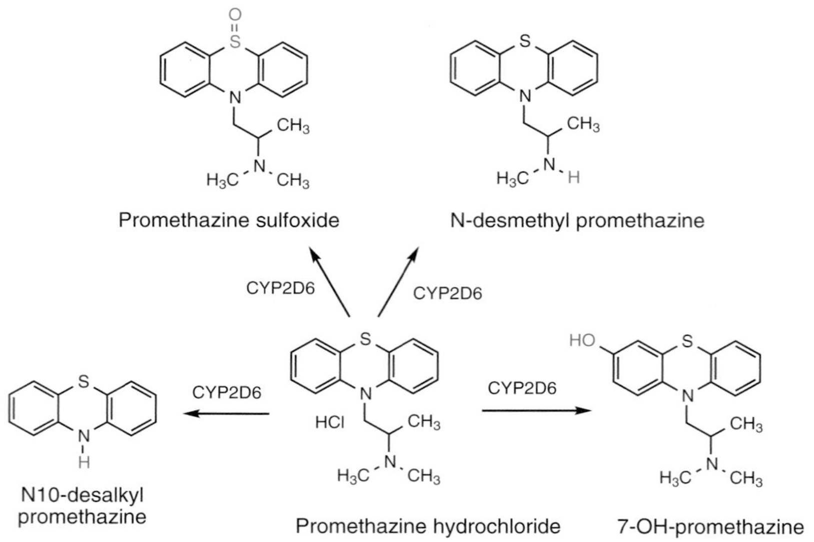

Figure 26.18 Metabolism of promethazine.

sickness. The sedative properties of H_1 antihistamines have been instrumental in treating nausea caused by analgesic drugs and/or chemotherapeutics.

For patients at high risk of postoperative nausea and vomiting, combination therapy including granisetron and promethazine has been shown to be more effective than promethazine alone. Promethazine is also an antagonist at muscarinic (M_1) and dopamine (D_2) receptors, and these actions contribute to its anti-emetic action. However, these nonspecific actions cause several adverse effects, including dystonic reactions and neuroleptic malignant syndrome. A high percentage of absorbed promethazine undergoes first-pass hepatic N-glucuronidation and sulfoxidation, leading to relatively low absolute bioavailability. Additionally, promethazine undergoes CYP2D6-catalyzed aryl-oxidation and dealkylation, where the methyl group or the entire aminoalkyl chain is lost from the tricyclic structure (Fig. 26.18).[94]

Prochlorperazine

Prochlorperazine is a D_2-antagonist and belongs to the phenothiazine class of compounds. It also exhibits mild H_1 antihistaminic activity, although that activity is kept low by the aromatic Cl atom. Inhibition of D_2-receptors in the chemoreceptor trigger zone (CTZ) is the primary mechanism leading to the observed anti-emetic property of this agent.

Structurally, prochlorperazine has a chlorinated tricyclic phenothiazine core, and the aliphatic amino group is a three-carbon chain attached to an N-methylpiperazine motif. Prochlorperazine is closely related to the first antipsychotic agent, chlorpromazine, which has a dimethyl amine motif at the alkyl side chain. It is known to exhibit lower sedative and anticholinergic effects than other D_2 antagonists, activities attributed to the phenothiazine component of the structure. Similar to promethazine, prochlorperazine also undergoes significant first-pass metabolism, including aryl-oxidation, sulfoxidation, and N-dealkylation (Fig. 26.19).[95]

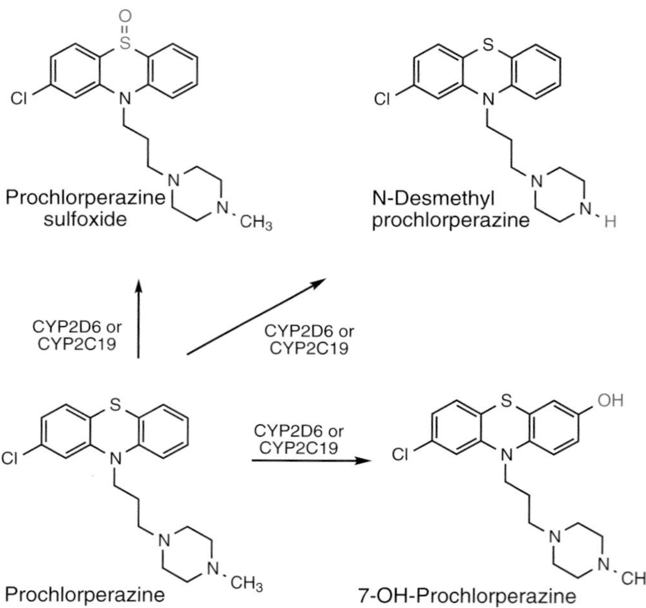

Figure 26.19 Metabolism of prochlorperazine.

Irritable Bowel Syndrome and Treatment Options

IBS is often a debilitating GI disorder that affects a significant proportion of population in the United States and worldwide.[96] The difficulty in managing IBS with limited therapeutic interventions affects the quality of life of millions of people.[97] It has been estimated that about 1.4 million people in the United States are affected by IBS, and the economic impact associated with diagnosis and care is substantial.[98]

IBS is described as a disorder of the brain-GI tract connection, where GI motility is affected and the sensitivity of the gut is heightened. The symptoms include cramping, abdominal pain, bloating, and diarrhea or constipation.[55,97,99] Based on the symptoms, IBS can be designated as diarrhea predominant (IBS-D), constipation predominant (IBS-C), or a third category where patients experience diarrhea alternating with constipation (IBS-A).[100] The management of IBS has been guided by a better understanding of the pathology of the disorder, collaborative physician-patient relationships, and judicious use of treatment options based on symptoms. In general, only those patients suffering from severe symptoms are treated with medications.

Serotonin Receptor Antagonists and Agonists

Until recently, available treatment options for IBS were limited by poor efficacy or adverse effects. Typically, laxatives, antispasmodics and smooth muscle relaxants, and tricyclic antidepressants are used, but with limited patient satisfaction. However, important drug targets that have emerged for the treatment of IBS are $5HT_3$ and $5\text{-}HT_4$ receptors.

Alosetron

$5\text{-}HT_3$ receptor stimulation causes increased motility, secretion, and excitation in the gut. Thus, $5\text{-}HT_3$ antagonists can reduce colonic transit and improve fluid absorption. Alosetron (Fig. 26.15), a $5\text{-}HT_3$ antagonist, is one of the agents used for IBS treatment. Since $5\text{-}HT_3$ antagonists can inhibit the action of $5\text{-}HT_3$ receptors on extrinsic afferent neurons, they can decrease the visceral pain associated with IBS as well.[55,98,100-102]

Tegaserod

On the other hand, $5\text{-}HT_4$ receptors mediate the initiation of peristalsis through a coupled process with $5\text{-}HT_{1p}$ receptors. Tegaserod (Fig. 26.12), a prokinetic agent discussed earlier, is a partial agonist of presynaptic $5\text{-}HT_4$ receptors which entered clinical use for the treatment of IBS in 2002.[103] It is an aminoguanidine indole derivative of 5-HT. Tegaserod accelerates small bowel and colonic transit in IBS patients. It is absorbed readily, and peak plasma concentrations are reached in approximately 1 hour. It is significantly bound to plasma proteins (98%), more specifically to α1-acid glycoprotein. In terms of metabolism, tegaserod undergoes acid-catalyzed hydrolysis in the stomach to lose the indole component in the form of an aldehyde. Hepatic oxidation further converts the aldehyde metabolite into the inactive 4-methoxyindole-3-carboxylic acid. Tegaserod is also modified by phase 2 metabolism to yield the three isomeric N-glucuronides.[104,105]

Although tegaserod is an efficacious drug for the treatment of IBS, it was removed from the US market due to increased risk of myocardial infractions or stroke. In the past, it was only available through a restricted distribution program for life-threatening circumstances. However, as of 2019, tegaserod has been reintroduced for the treatment of IBS-C in women younger than 65 years who have no history of cardiovascular ischemic diseases and those who have no more than one risk factor for cardiovascular diseases.

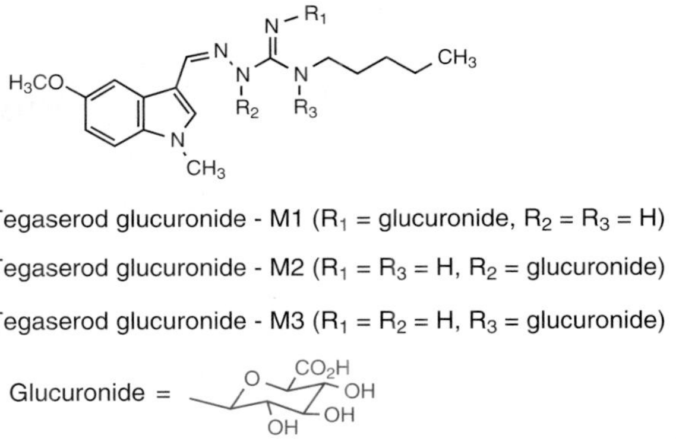

Tegaserod glucuronide - M1 (R_1 = glucuronide, $R_2 = R_3$ = H)

Tegaserod glucuronide - M2 ($R_1 = R_3$ = H, R_2 = glucuronide)

Tegaserod glucuronide - M3 ($R_1 = R_2$ = H, R_3 = glucuronide)

Glucuronide =

Renzapride

Renzapride is another example of a $5\text{-}HT_4$ agonist that is useful as gastroprokinetic and anti-emetic agent. It is currently an investigational drug and has the potential to be useful for the treatment for IBS. It stimulates GI tract motility and has been shown to be potentially effective for IBS-C and IBS-A. Renzapride is a benzamide derivative and structurally similar to metoclopramide. The structure retains the biologically important tertiary amine in the form of a bulky bicyclic amine. Renzapride is predominantly metabolized by CYP enzymes to the N-oxide, which exhibits reduced binding affinity to $5\text{-}HT_4$ receptors.[106]

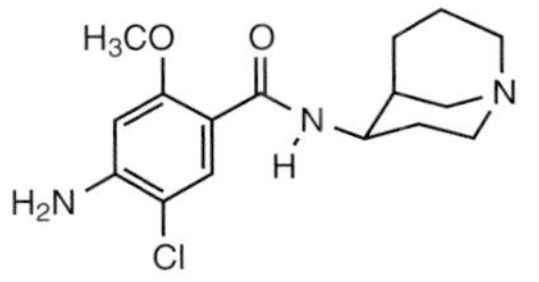

Renzapride

Guanylyl Cyclase-C Agonists

Agonists of guanylyl cyclase-C have been useful therapeutic options for IBS-C and chronic idiopathic constipation. Plecanatide and linaclotide are two peptide-derived agonists of this enzyme approved for therapeutic use.[107] Guanylyl cyclase-C is expressed mainly in the GI neurons, and binding of endogenous guanylin and uroguanylin regulates water and electrolyte transport in the gut. Guanylin is a 15 amino acid peptide with defined secondary structure. It is secreted in the colon, and binding to its receptor induces chloride secretion and decreases intestinal fluid absorption, which causes diarrhea. This process is similar to the binding of enterotoxins in the gut, which leads to diarrhea.[108] Uroguanylin is a 16 amino acid oligopeptide that is secreted in the duodenum and proximal small intestine. This peptide ligand functions in a similar fashion to guanylin.[109] Based on the structure and biological role of these endogenous ligands, both plecanatide and linaclotide have been developed into therapeutic agents.[110]

Plecanatide is a structural analogue of uroguanylin that is 16 amino acids long. The structural change involves modification of the third residue of uroguanylin into glutamic acid. All Cys residues within the structure are preserved, as they all are involved in the formation of disulfide bonds to generate the secondary structure. Linaclotide is a peptide mimic of endogenous guanylin and uroguanylin that is a 14 amino acid synthetic peptide.

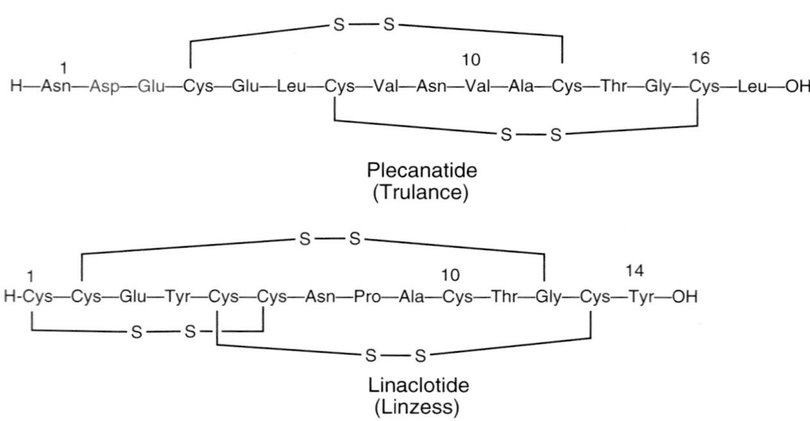

Systemic absorption of these agents after oral administration is minimal; however, since these agents act on receptors present on the apical side of the endothelium of GI tract, there is no need for them to be systemically absorbed. The acidic residues (Asp2 and Glu3) of plecanatide are important for binding to the receptor, and optimal binding is observed at pH 5. One of the limitations of peptide agents is metabolic instability in the GI tract and, as one can expect, plecanatide and linaclotide are degraded by intestinal proteases. Linaclotide is an effective drug; however, it has a boxed warning against use in children less than 6 years old and it is not recommended for patients who are 6-18 years old due to a high risk of dehydration.

Humanized Monoclonal Antibodies for IBD

IBDs are characterized by chronic inflammation of GI tract, which is related to an immunological imbalance of the intestinal mucosa.[7,8,111] The cells of the adaptive immune system are observed to respond against self-antigens that lead to inflammatory conditions. It is also associated with an imbalance in the gut microflora. Crohn's disease (CD) and ulcerative colitis (UC) are the most common types of IBD and have a very high prevalence in the world population.[112-114] The pathophysiological mechanism of IBD is not well understood; however, substantial efforts have been dedicated to discover drugs to target inflammatory pathways.

Given the role of tumor necrosis factor-alpha (TNF-α) as a proinflammatory cytokine and its ability to promote production of other proinflammatory cytokines, chemokines, and adhesion molecules (e.g., α4β7-integrin), this pathway is a highly investigated target for IBD drug development. To date, various monoclonal antibodies (MAbs) have been developed against the offending proinflammatory molecules named above as treatment options. Given the pleiotropic effect of TNF-α, therapeutic agents targeting TNF-α are being developed for the treatment of IBD.

An antibody is a large Y-shaped protein that is used by immune system to neutralize pathogens (see Chapters 5 and 34). A MAb is a monovalent antibody and it binds to an epitope on an antigen. MAbs are one of the fastest growing classes of therapeutics agents, and about 30 are currently in clinical use (see Chapter 34). In recent years, several MAbs have been developed for the treatment of IBS by targeting some of the key proinflammatory molecules, as well as integrins, a specific type of cell surface adhesion protein.[115-117]

Adalimumab, certolizumab, infliximab, and golimumab are the four clinically available anti-TNF-α MAbs that are prescribed to achieve clinical remission from moderate to severe CD, and in adults to induce and sustain remission from UC (Table 26.3). All carry a boxed warning relative to the risk of developing serious or life-threatening infection and/or malignancies.[118] Vedolizumab is a MAb that targets the adhesion protein integrin a4b7, rather than TNF-α. Due to its unique mechanism of action, it has been shown to exhibit gut-selective anti-inflammatory activity. Vedolizumab is approved for the treatment of moderate to severe UC or CD, and as an alternative option for patients who do not respond to MAb treatments that target TNF-α.[119] Although it carries no boxed warning, there is a risk of infection, leukoencephalopathy, and hepatotoxicity associated with its use.

MAbs target inflammatory pathways to treat diseases linked to autoimmune response. In this regard, they are also useful therapies for other inflammatory diseases, including rheumatoid arthritis, psoriatic arthritis, and ankylosing spondylitis. As noted above, one of the concerning adverse effects is the risk of serious infections, including tuberculosis. Since anti-inflammatory MAbs compromise immune function, a patient's ability to fight infections becomes difficult.

Although MAbs have been developed to target various diseases, developing novel, safe, and efficacious drugs of this type is very challenging. Some of the challenges

Table 26.3 Monoclonal Antibodies for the Management of Ulcerative Colitis and Crohn's Disease

Name	Antibody Type	Mechanism of Action	Indication
Adalimumab (Humira)	Recombinant	Anti-TNF-α	Crohn's disease and ulcerative colitis
Certolizumab (Cimzia)	Humanized (pegylated)	Anti-TNF-α	Crohn's disease
Infliximab (Remicade)	Chimeric	Anti-TNF-α	Crohn's disease and ulcerative colitis
Golimumab (Simponi)	Human	Anti-TNF-α	Ulcerative colitis
Vedolizumab (Entyvio)	Humanized	Anti-α4β7 integrin	Crohn's disease and ulcerative colitis

include (1) the use of inefficient biological models for generating human antibodies, (2) a lack of efficacy for targeted diseases, and (3) the cost-effectiveness associated with MAb-based treatment. Current efforts are focused on addressing one or more these limitations. It seems that, with new technologies and expanding knowledge, future MAb treatment options can be more efficacious and much more personalized to address the need of individual patients.[120]

AGENTS THAT IMPACT GASTROINTESTINAL AND GENITOURINARY SMOOTH MUSCLE AND GLANDS

Cholinergic Nervous System

ACh is released by cholinergic neurons in the autonomic nervous system and somatic nervous system and by some neurons in the CNS.[121,122] Cholinergic receptors are classified as either muscarinic (mAChR) or nicotinic (nAChR) based on their affinity for the naturally occurring alkaloids muscarine and nicotine, respectively (Fig. 26.20).[123] The mAChR is the receptor of relevance for cholinergic drugs targeting the GI and GU systems.

Parasympathetic nerve activities stimulate GI and urinary tract muscle contraction and relaxation of vascular smooth muscle and lower heart contractility. Direct-acting cholinergic agonists bind directly to receptors, whereas inhibitors of AChE indirectly stimulate cholinergic receptors by increasing the concentration of the ACh neurotransmitter in the synapse. AChE is responsible for hydrolyzing ACh into choline and acetate, that latter of which can supplement pools needed to generate cofactors like acetyl coenzyme A. Cholinergic antagonists have affinity for cholinergic receptors; however, they cannot stimulate them. ACh-mediated activation of cholinergic receptors in parasympathetic nervous system is a therapeutically important process, and the pathway has been extensively investigated for drug discovery.[124]

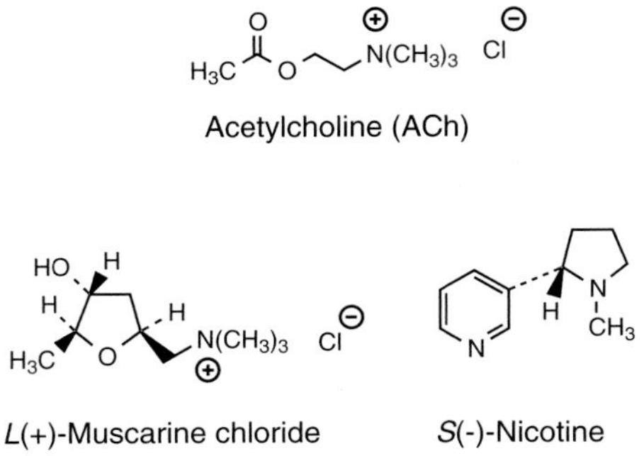

Acetylcholine (ACh)

L(+)-Muscarine chloride

S(-)-Nicotine

Figure 26.20 Structures of naturally occurring cholinergic agonists.

Acetylcholine Biosynthesis Metabolism and Stereochemistry

ACh biosynthesis, storage, release, and metabolism are illustrated in Figure 26.21.[124] The biosynthesis of this important neurotransmitter begins in the cholinergic neuron, where the transfer of an acetyl group from acetyl-CoA to choline is catalyzed by choline acetyltransferase. When ACh is hydrolyzed by AChE in the synaptic space, the generated choline is transported into the neurons to be used for ACh biosynthesis. Most newly synthesized ACh is kept in cytosolic storage vesicles in presynaptic nerve endings. The release of ACh into the synapse is triggered by an action potential that opens voltage-gated calcium channels, allowing influx of calcium ion and exocytotic release of ACh. Once released, ACh in the synapse binds with cholinergic receptors and produces a response.

Although ACh is an achiral molecule, the stereochemical impact resides in conformational isomerism. Four of the most commonly studied conformations of ACh are shown in Figure 26.22. Based on the activity of ACh analogues, it is likely that the less-favored anticlinal conformation binds to the mAChR.[125]

Muscarinic Cholinergic Receptors

As noted earlier, multiple mAChR subtypes exist and are designated as M_1 through M_5.[123,126] All are GPCRs (Chapter 6).[16] Activation of M_3 receptors found in smooth muscle stimulates contraction, and activation in glands stimulates secretion. Understanding their effect on smooth muscle of the bladder has led to the development of M_3 receptor antagonists as therapeutic agents for OAB (discussed below). Although M_3 receptors are also found in the CNS, their concentration is much lower than other receptor subtypes in that tissue. When these receptor subtypes are activated in smooth muscle and secretary glands, it leads to inhibition of potassium and calcium channels.

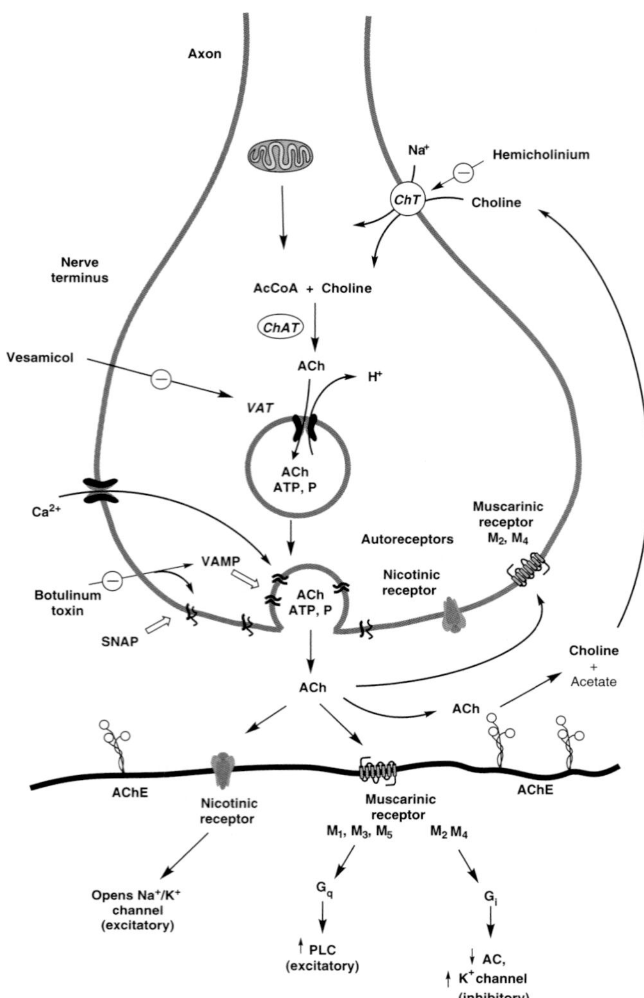

Figure 26.21 Cholinergic neuron site of biosynthesis, storage, release, and receptor activation.

SAR of Acetylcholine and Its Analogues

The synthetic design for many cholinergic agonists and antagonists comes from the SAR of ACh analogues. The structure of ACh can be divided into three segments to explain the SAR: (1) the acyloxy group or acetyl group, (2) the ethylene group that connects the acyloxy and quaternary ammonium motif, and (3) the quaternary ammonium group.[127] Briefly, a cationic amine is important for muscarinic agonist activity.[127] Replacement of a single methyl group of ACh with a longer alkyl group (i.e. ethyl, propyl) lowers the muscarinic activity, as does sequential replacement of each methyl group with hydrogen to generate tertiary, secondary, or primary amine analogues.[128] The "Rule of Five" by Ing[127] states that there should be no more than five atoms between the cationic nitrogen and the terminal hydrogen atom (e.g., on the acetyl group of ACh) for optimal mAChR binding and stimulation. Methyl substituents on the ethylene chain are permitted, and methacholine (the β-methyl analogue of ACh) exhibits muscarinic activity that is equal to ACh and has improved selectivity toward the mAChR over the nAChR. The *S*-isomer of chiral methacholine is 20 times more active at the mAChR than the *R*-enantiomer and is also much more slowly hydrolyzed by AChE due to both steric hindrance and a less electrophilic carbonyl carbon. Modification of the terminal acyloxy group (e.g., extending the length to propionyl or butanoyl) provides less effective agonists, as expected based on Ing's Rule of Five.[127] However, conversion of the acetate ester to a carbamate retains high mAChR affinity, as discussed below.

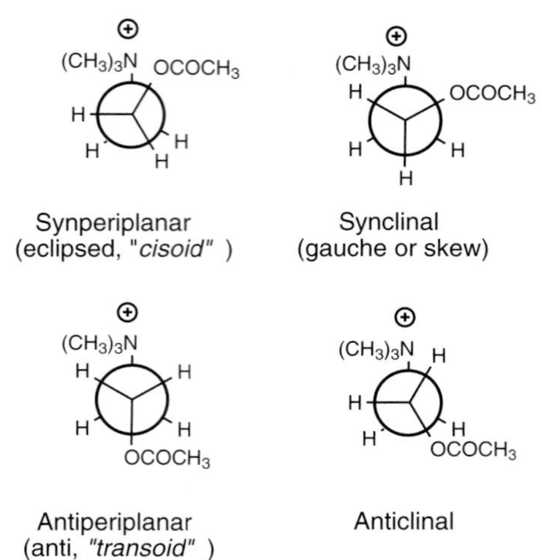

Figure 26.22 Conformational isomers of acetylcholine.

As noted previously, ACh is rapidly degraded by AChE and ubiquitous plasma esterases via the hydrolysis of acetyl group. To improve the stability of ACh in the synapse, analogues have been developed by replacing the ester functionality with a hydrolytically more stable isostere. Carbamates are esters derived from carbamic acid (and therefore are hybrids of an ester and an amide) and are much more stable to hydrolysis compared to simple esters. Using this bioisosteric replacement strategy, carbachol and bethanechol have been developed, which are the carbamate derivatives of ACh and methacholine, respectively. The conversion of a terminal acetate to a carbamate is tolerated at the mAChR, and so these are both potent direct-acting cholinergic agonists with improved stability to AChE and other esterases. Once they do hydrolyze, they reversibly inactivate AChE by carbamylating the catalytic Ser residue responsible for its hydrolyzing action, allowing ACh to enjoy a longer duration in cholinergic synapses.

The SARs for mAChR agonists are developed based on the binding interactions of ACh with its receptor. The oxygen atoms of the acetate ester moiety form a hydrogen bond with an active site Asn residue, while the quaternary ammonium nitrogen forms an ionic interaction with active site Asp residue. The methyl groups occupy the hydrophobic pockets within the receptor. Considering the importance of these interactions, the SARs of mAChR agonists can be summarized as follows: (1) they contain a quaternary ammonium functional group with a permanent positive charge,[127,128] (2) improved binding and agonist potency is achieved when the onium nitrogen is substituted with small alkyl groups, with methyl group being optimal,[128] (3) an ester-like oxygen atom that can be a hydrogen bond

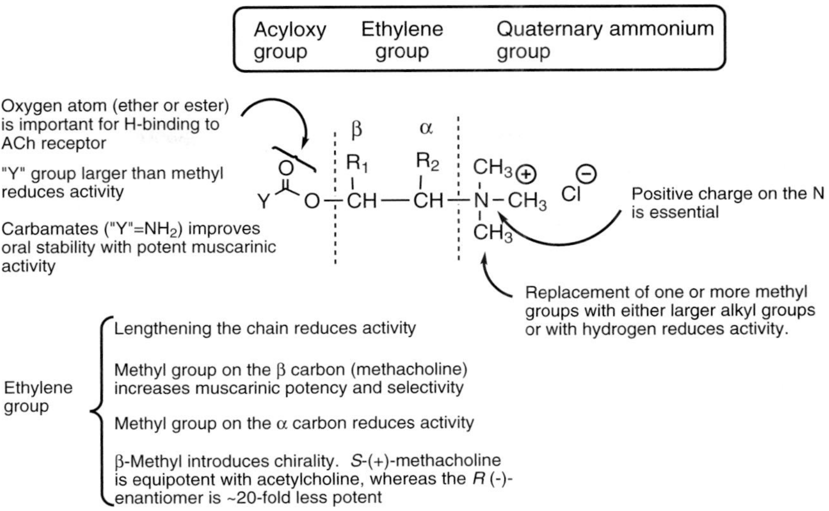

Figure 26.23 SAR summary for muscarinic agonists.

acceptor at the mAChR is required, and (4) the quaternary ammonium nitrogen and the oxygen atom should be connected by a two-carbon bridge (Fig. 26.23).[129]

Muscarinic Receptor Agonists

Since mAChRs play a crucial role in regulating GI and urinary tract functions, agonists can be used to reestablish smooth muscle tone of the GI and urinary tract following surgical procedures. These agents can relieve abdominal distention and urinary retention and stimulate glandular secretions. To be therapeutically useful in treating GI and GU disorders, they must have a sufficiently long duration of action, and the close structural analogues of ACh, methacholine, and carbachol do not qualify. However, bethanechol can be used in the treatment of postsurgical and postpartum urinary retention, and two mAChR analogues that are structurally distinct from ACh have some therapeutic utility in treating dry mouth (a GI disorder) (Fig. 26.24).

Specific Drugs

BETHANECHOL CHLORIDE. Bethanechol chloride is the carbamate analogue of methacholine and a selective agonist at the mAChR. Its localized action (ammonium head), direct action selectivity (β-methyl), and prolonged duration (carbamate and β-methyl) make it useful for the treatment of postsurgical and postpartum urinary retention and abdominal distension. Similar to carbachol, the carbamate functional group makes this drug hydrolytically stable and, when it does hydrolyze, it reversibly inhibits AChE through Ser carbamylation. It is an orally administered drug and, due to concern about more system-wide cholinergic effects, it is not given by IV or IM injection. Some of the more serious adverse effects associated with this drug relate to cardiovascular events and bronchoconstriction. Because it is administered orally and retained locally, adverse events are uncommon.

PILOCARPINE. Pilocarpine is a natural alkaloid isolated from *Pilocarpus jaborandi* that exhibits potent muscarinic agonistic activity. It was discovered in 1876, and the N-methylimidazole-containing lactone structure was determined in 1901. The naturally occurring compound is 3*S*,4*R*-(+)-pilocarpine, and the specific stereochemistry is important for bioactivity. Pilocarpine exhibits affinity for the M_3 receptor subtype.

Pilocarpine is available as tablets, ophthalmic solution, and gel. It is a useful drug for the treatment of dry mouth caused by radiation therapy based on the activity of cholinergic agents as sialagogues (salivation inducers). Due to its lactone motif, the α-stereocenter (C3 position) is sensitive

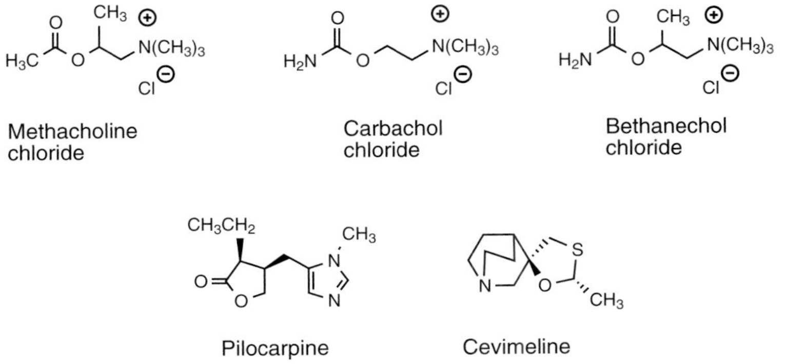

Methacholine chloride
Carbachol chloride
Bethanechol chloride
Pilocarpine
Cevimeline

Figure 26.24 Muscarinic agonists.

to epimerization when stored in solution. The epimerized product is called isopilocarpine. The lactone functionality is also susceptible to hydrolysis, yielding pilocarpic acid as the inactive product. Epimerization is expected to be a problem only if the drug is improperly stored. One approach to enhancing in vitro stability is conversion of the lactone into a carbamate, which increases the lactone moiety's hydrolytic stability and minimizes the extent of epimerization.

CEVIMELINE. Cevimeline is a nonclassical agonist of the mAChR. It is derived from a cyclic amine called quinuclidine. Cevimeline exhibits affinity for M_1 receptors in the central nervous system (CNS) and M_3 receptors in epithelial tissue of lacrimal and salivary glands. It is administered orally for the treatment of dry mouth and acts in the same manner as pilocarpine. Some of the important contraindications to the use of these mAChR agonists include asthma, GU or GI tract obstructions, and peptic acid–related illnesses. The metabolic profile of cevimeline includes CYP2D6-, CYP3A3-, and CYP3A4-catalyzed oxidations. The thioether is oxidized to the sulfoxide, and the amine is converted to the N-oxide. It is also metabolized by phase 2 glucuronidation.

Muscarinic Receptor Antagonists

Muscarinic antagonists competitively and reversibly bind to mAChR and prevent the binding of ACh. It is proposed that binding of muscarinic antagonists induces a conformational change in the receptor that is different from the conformation induced by agonists and uncouples the receptor from its G protein. By blocking ACh access to the mAChR, antimuscarinic agents decrease the contraction of smooth muscle of the GI and urinary tracts and reduce gastric, mucociliary, and salivary secretions. Due to their relaxant effect, they are useful therapeutic agents for the treatment of smooth muscle spasm and OAB. Since they also reduce gastric secretions, they were at one time useful therapeutic agents for the management of peptic ulcers. However, these drugs lost their place in clinical practice due to the introduction of more effective H_2 antagonists and proton pump inhibitors (as previously discussed).

A recent study has illuminated the mode of binding of antimuscarinics with the M_2 receptor. It is proposed that binding of sterically bulky molecules (i.e., muscarinic antagonists) blocks the activation-related contraction of the binding pocket, which locks the M_2 receptor in an inactive conformation (Fig. 26.25).[130] This leads to the observed antagonistic activity.

Antimuscarinic agents exhibit several predictable adverse effects based on their inhibition of ACh-induced actions, including blurred vision, photophobia, dry mouth, and difficulty in urination. Antimuscarinics that act centrally are sedative, which can be viewed as either an adverse effect or, when needed to avoid motion sickness, a therapeutic benefit (e.g., scopolamine, discussed below). Taken together, the effect of antimuscarinic agents has been very useful in treating various GI and GU disorders,[124] and selected agents are available as both prescription-based and OTC drugs.

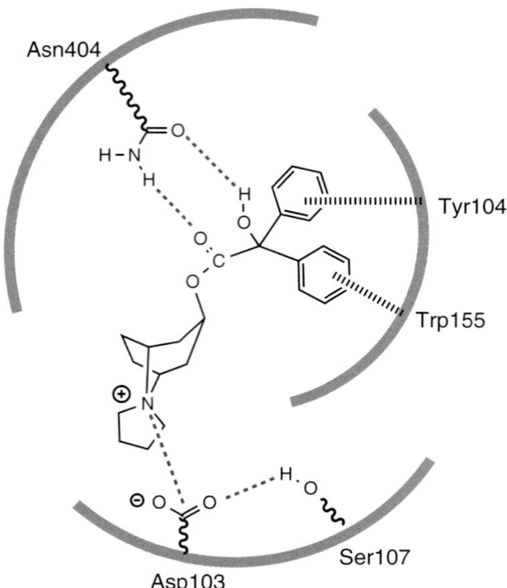

Figure 26.25 Proposed binding interactions of a model anticholinergic drug (3-quinuclidinyl benzilate) with the M_2 receptor.

Alkaloids From Solanaceae Family—Atropine and Scopolamine

Atropine and scopolamine are two natural products from the plant family *Solanaceae* and the earliest known anticholinergic agents. They are competitive mAChR antagonists and prevent the action of ACh and other direct- and indirect-acting muscarinic agonists. While they are not used in the treatment of GI or GU disorders, they served as the template for the design of new antimuscarinics that are structurally similar, and their chemistry is briefly summarized below.

Atropine is a tropine ester of tropic acid (Fig. 26.26). The tertiary amine functionality within this molecule makes it a basic drug, and it is clinically available as the sulfate salt. The naturally occurring (−)-hyoscyamine undergoes racemization during isolation and yields the racemic mixture of (+) and (−)-isomers known as atropine. The tropic acid component has the stereogenic center that undergoes racemization. The bicyclic tropane-scaffold is the other preserved component of these natural products. Atropine has been used as a preoperative agent to reduce secretions prior to a surgery. Following administration of atropine sulfate, approximately half is excreted in the urine in its parent form, while the remainder is excreted as the N-demethylated noratropine metabolite, the N-oxide, and hydrolysis products.

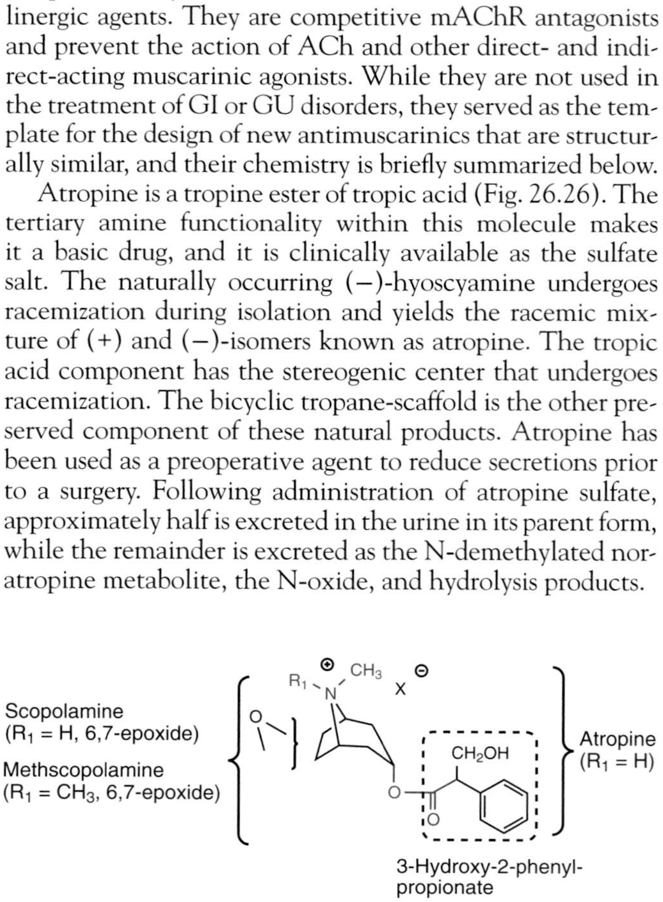

Scopolamine (R_1 = H, 6,7-epoxide)
Methscopolamine (R_1 = CH_3, 6,7-epoxide)
Atropine (R_1 = H)
3-Hydroxy-2-phenylpropionate

Figure 26.26 Solanaceous alkaloid-based antimuscarinics with key structural features of ACh highlighted in red.

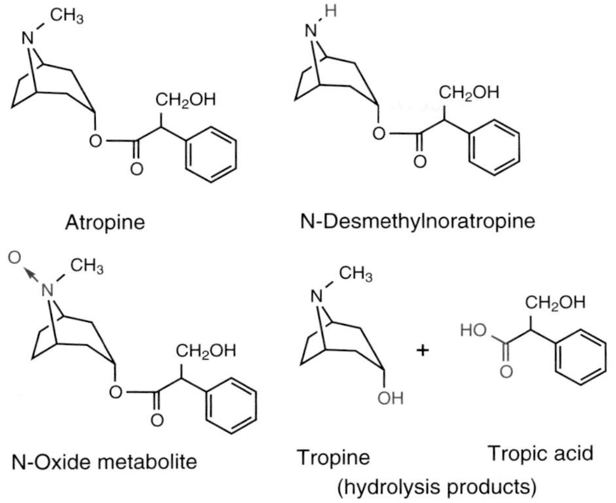

The other natural alkaloid, scopolamine ((−)-hyoscine) is structurally very similar to atropine. It is also a tropane ester of tropic acid, but the tropane core in scopolamine has a 6,7-epoxide functionality (Fig. 26.26). Scopolamine is available as the hydrobromide salt for clinical use. The interesting pharmacological difference between atropine and scopolamine is that atropine is a CNS stimulant and scopolamine is a CNS depressant. Scopolamine is clinically used for the treatment of iritis, uveitis, and Parkinsonism. Scopolamine is extensively metabolized by hepatic enzymes via phase 1 reactions that are similar to atropine metabolism and through glucuronide conjugation of the hydroxyl group.[131]

Structural Features and SAR

The SAR of atropine has provided the structural information needed for designing synthetic antimuscarinic agents. As discussed previously, the ester- and the nitrogen-containing functional groups of the endogenous mAChR ligand ACh are important for binding. Similarly, the ester and tertiary amine group found in atropine and scopolamine are important structural features. Antimuscarinics bind to the mAChR in a similar fashion to ACh, where the ester group forms a hydrogen bond with a conserved active site Asn residue, and the quaternary ammonium nitrogen forms an ionic interaction with conserved active site Asp residue. Additionally, several aromatic residues within the active site, such as Phe, Trp, and Tyr, provide additional hydrophobic regions for stronger binding affinity of antimuscarinics.[130] Although the ester and amine groups within atropine are separated by more than two carbons (unlike in ACh), the conformation assumed by the tropane ring places these two functional groups close to each other, with a distance similar to that found in ACh. The key structural difference between ACh and atropine is the size of the acyl portion. Based on the proposal that sterically larger molecules tend to block mAChR and behave as antagonists, several analogues of atropine have been designed and synthesized as potential antimuscarinic agents. Based on the structural modifications and bioactivity profile, it was evident that most potent mAChR antagonists contain two lipophilic ring substitutions on the acyl group (α to the carbonyl group of the ester). Antimuscarinic SAR that describes the impact of substituents on the antimuscarinic pharmacophore is briefly summarized below.[124,132]

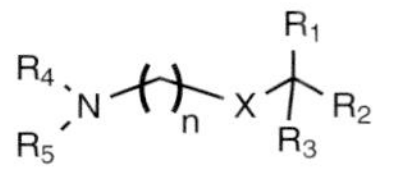

- R_1 and R_2 should be carbocyclic or heterocyclic rings and bind to the mAChR through hydrophobic and/or π stacking interactions with active site Tyr, Phe, and Trp residues that lie outside of the ACh binding pocket (Fig. 26.25).[132] Optimal potency is observed when one ring is aromatic and the other is saturated. Typically, five- or six-membered ring substituents are optimal. Analogues containing larger ring structures, such as naphthalene, tend to be inactive, perhaps due to increased steric bulk.
- The R_3 substituent is variable, with hydrogen, hydroxy, hydroxymethyl, or carboxamide all acceptable. H-bonding hydroxy or hydroxymethyl substituents are optimal and can be a substituent on the R_1 or R_2 ring system. These groups interact with a conserved Asn residue within the mAChR active site through two hydrogen bonding interactions.
- The connecting functional group "X" in most analogues is an ester, mimicking ACh. However, ether and carbon X moieties also produce active compounds. The nature of the connecting group allows antimuscarinic agents to be chemically classified as aminoalkyl esters, aminoalkyl ethers, or aminoalcohols. The nitrogen is typically a quaternary ammonium species (most potent) or a tertiary amine. The tertiary amine will be extensively protonated at physiological pH to generate the cationic species needed for ionic interaction with the conserved active site Asp residue.
- R_4 and R_5 are typically small alkyl groups such methyl, ethyl, propyl, or isopropyl. Some compounds contain a cyclic motif to yield the quaternary nitrogen.
- Due to molecular flexibility, the distance between the nitrogen atom of the tertiary or quaternary amine and the ring-substituted carbon seems to be less critical for activity. Normally, the linking chain is two (optimal) to four carbons.

Synthetic Muscarinic Antagonists

As discussed above, the atropine scaffold has been used as the structural model for developing antimuscarinic SAR that led to synthetic antimuscarinic agents. Because the outer regions of the mAChR are largely hydrophobic in nature, they bind more strongly than ACh and in a competitive manner. The most common synthetic antimuscarinic agents used to treat OAB are given in Figure 26.27. There are representatives from the aminoalkyl ester class (solifenacin, oxybutynin, trospium chloride) and modified aminoalcohols (X = carbon) where the OH has been replaced by an aromatic ether substituent (tolterodine,

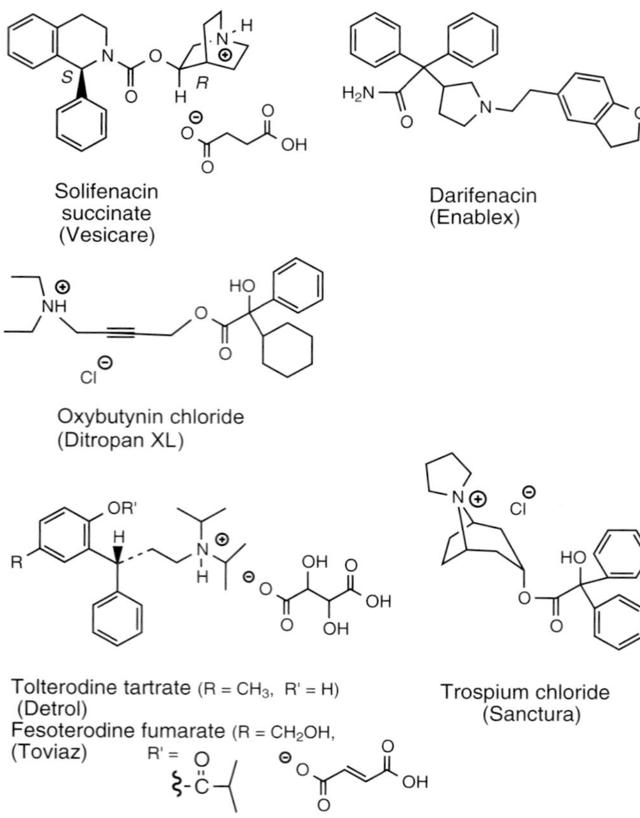

Figure 26.27 Antimuscarinics used in overactive bladder.

fesoterodine) or an amide (darifenacin). These agents all follow the classical SAR, where a tertiary amine or quaternary ammonium motif and a bulky hydrophobic structure are present.[133,134]

Therapeutic Use in Overactive Bladder

OAB is associated with urinary frequency or nocturia. It is a common health disorder that affects the quality of life for many and can be successfully treated with antimuscarinics.[135] As discussed above, antimuscarinics decrease smooth muscle contraction in bladder by acting on M_2 or M_3 subtypes.[136,137] The common mAChR antagonists used for the treatment of OAB are oxybutynin, trospium chloride, tolterodine, fesoterodine, darifenacin, and solifenacin (Fig. 26.27).[138] These agents are also able to control GI motility and secretions by inhibiting the effects of parasympathetic activity in the gut. Antimuscarinics reduce gastric and salivary gland secretions by acting on the M_1 subtype; however, they produce pronounced adverse effects due to their nonselective binding to other muscarinic receptor subtypes. While they were once widely used to manage peptic ulcer, their utility in that disease state has significantly declined.

Chemically, trospium chloride contains a quaternary ammonium motif that is permanently cationic, so it is generally not well absorbed from the GI tract. The remainder of the antimuscarinics used in OAB possess a basic tertiary amine motif (and, therefore, exist in both cationic and unionized conjugate forms in the gut), are better absorbed relative to the quaternary ammonium salt, and are better distributed systemically via all routes of administration. The tertiary amine-containing drugs also cross the blood-brain barrier very well, leading to central adverse effects.

Although these are all effective antimuscarinic agents, their nonspecific binding to mAChR subtypes causes several predictable adverse effects, including xerostomia (dry mouth), blurred vision, constipation, and dyspepsia. Binding of antimuscarinics to receptors in CNS causes drowsiness, dizziness, and confusion. Oxybutynin is the oldest mAChR antagonist clinically used for the treatment of OAB, and it is often associated with an increased incidence of adverse effects, including xerostomia. Improved formulations and delivery methods (i.e., transdermal delivery, extended-release formulations) have been developed to minimize these unwanted actions. Solifenacin and darifenacin show selectivity toward M_3 receptors, giving a desirable ratio of efficacy to adverse effects.[139]

The pharmacological properties and receptor-subtype selectivity of the synthetic antimuscarinics used in OAB are given in Table 26.4.

Metabolism

The synthetic anticholinergic agents discussed here are all extensively metabolized by hepatic enzymes and, if they contain an ester linkage, undergo both enzymatic (plasma esterase) and nonenzymatic (acidic or basic pH) hydrolysis. One of the most common hepatic oxidation reactions of antimuscarinic agents is N-oxidation. Since many of these compounds possess a tertiary amine group, CYP enzyme–catalyzed oxidation leads to an inactive N-oxide metabolite. Another common reaction is oxidative N-dealkylation. A summary of common metabolic reactions for selected anticholinergic agents is given in Table 26.4 and Figure 26.28. To illustrate the metabolic reactions in this class of agents, some common metabolic transformations are summarized here. Several of the phase 1 metabolites undergo conjugation via phase 2 metabolite transformations.[134]

- Trospium is predominantly metabolized via hydrolysis.
- Darifenacin is oxidized by CYP2D6 and CYP3A4 to generate a benzylic alcohol and a ring-opened carboxylic acid metabolite (Fig. 26.28). An N-dealkylated metabolite is generated via the action of CYP3A4.[140]
- Tolterodine (active) and fesoterodine (a tolterodine prodrug) undergo CYP2D6-mediated oxidation and esterase-mediated hydrolysis, respectively, to a common active benzylic alcohol metabolite that is further oxidized by CYP3A4 and 2D6 to an inactive carboxylic acid. The N-dealkylated metabolite of tolterodine and fesoterodine is inactive.
- Solifenacin is converted into the inactive N-oxide by the action of CYP3A4. A benzylic oxidation of solifenacin yields the corresponding hydroxy metabolite, which is active. The hydroxy metabolite subsequently forms a glucuronide conjugate and is excreted.
- Oxybutynin is metabolized by CYP3A4 to the corresponding dealkylated metabolite, which retains biological activity. The carboxylic acid metabolite generated via hydrolysis is pharmacologically inactive.

Table 26.4 Antimuscarinic Agents Used in Overactive Bladder

Name	Calculated[a] Log P and Log D (pH 7)	Half-Life (hr)	Metabolism	Comments
Trospium chloride (Sanctura)	–	20	Hydrolysis; conjugation	High affinity for M_1 and M_3 receptors; lesser affinity for M_2
Oxybutynin (oral: Ditropan and Ditropan XL; transdermal: Oxytrol)	5.19 (Log P) 3.93 (Log D)	2-5	CYP3A4; hydrolysis; N-dealkylation	Nonselective muscarinic antagonist
Solifenacin (Vesicare)	3.70 (Log P) 1.70 (Log D)	55	4-(*R*)-Hydroxy (active); N-glucuronide; N-oxide; 4*R*-hydroxy-N-oxide	Selective M_3 antagonist
Tolterodine (Detrol)	5.77(Log P) 2.79 (Log D)	2-4 (extensive metabolizers); 9.6 (poor metabolizers)	Primary pathway: CYP2D6 (primary); 7% of Caucasians and 2% of African Americans lack CYP2D6; CYP3A4 is the primary pathway in the latter. Metabolites: 5-hydroxymethyl (active), 5-carboxylic acid, N-dealkylated-5-carboxylic acid	Nonselective muscarinic antagonist
Fesoterodine fumarate (Toviaz)	5.08 (Log P) 2.09 (Log D)	7	Hydrolysis to 5-hydroxymethyl tolterodine, followed by CYP2D6 and CYP3A4 to give carboxy, carboxy-N-desisopropy, N-desisopropyl metabolites	Prodrug of 5-hydroxymethyl tolterodine, a nonselective muscarinic agonist
Darifenacin (Enablex)	4.50 (Log P) 2.25 (Log D)	–	CYP2D6 (primary; see tolterodine above); hydroxylation of the dihydrobenzofuran; ring opening (dihydrobenzofuran); N-dealkylation	Selective M_3 antagonist

[a]Values calculated using ACD Lab Solarius, Chemical Abstracts Service, 2006, Columbus, OH (values for quaternary compounds are not listed).

Specific Drugs

OXYBUTYNIN. Oxybutynin is one of the oldest mAChR antagonists used in OAB. It relaxes bladder urothelium, calms overactive detrusor smooth muscle contractions, and interferes with cholinergic neurotransmission in bladder afferent pathways, resulting in a decrease in urinary urgency and frequency.[138] While the M_2 mAChR subtype is most prevalent in human bladder, M_3 is viewed as the critical receptor mediating the therapeutic utility of antimuscarinics in OAB.[138]

The dealkylated desethyl metabolite (DEO, Fig. 26.28) noted above is generated in both gut and liver and binds with high affinity to salivary mAChRs (M_1 and M_3 subtypes[141,142]), resulting in a high incidence of dry mouth which can limit patient acceptability.[138,141] While the parent drug has low affinity for the M_2 subtype,[143] the DEO metabolite is deemed responsible for the potential induction of cardiac arrhythmias (an M_2 effect[141]) that negatively impacts adherence.[143] In fact, it has been estimated that between 43% and 83% of women patients stop antimuscarinic therapy (including oxybutynin, which carries the highest risk of adverse effects) within a month of initiation.[144]

Oxybutynin is marketed as the racemic mixture, but its antimuscarinic action is isolated to the *R*-isomer.[142] It is over 99% protein bound. In addition to tablet and syrup formulations, extended-release tablets and transdermal gel and patch dosage forms that limit DEO formation (and, therefore, adverse effects) are clinically available.[138,144] With regard to therapeutic efficacy, oxybutynin immediate- and extended-release formulations are comparable and statistically equivalent to tolterodine and darifenacin (see below).[138,142] Combination therapy that includes oxybutynin (e.g., in combination with solifenacin or tolterodine) has been shown to provide symptom relief superior to the partner product alone.[144] The transdermal gel and patch formulations have demonstrated efficacy compared to placebo, and patients may experience mild-moderate application site pruritis from their use.[138]

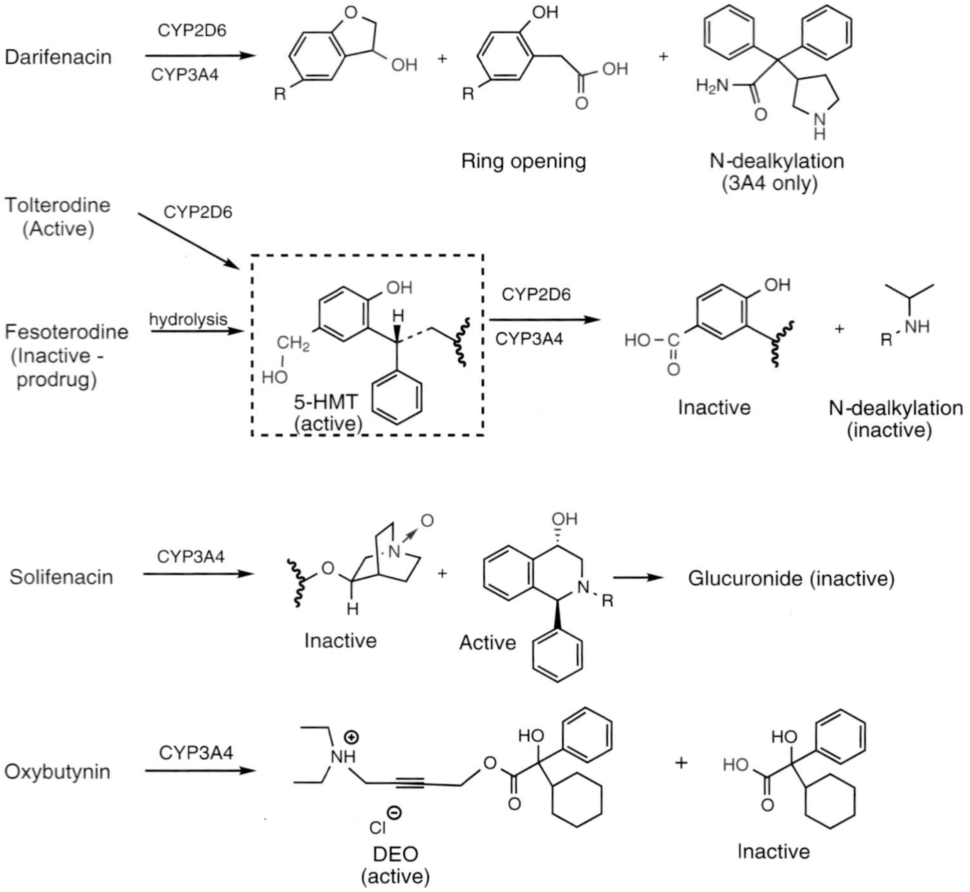

Figure 26.28 Metabolism of selected antimuscarinics.

OAB incidence rises as patients age[138] and caution must be used when treating elderly patients, particularly frail elderly, as antimuscarinic agents can negatively impact gait stability and cognition.[141,144] Oxybutynin in particular has been associated with serious decreases in attention and cognitive function due to central M_1 receptor antagonism, and the benefits of its use in vulnerable patients should clearly outweigh the risks. Safer choices include the quaternary trospium chloride (which does not penetrate the blood-brain barrier) and the M_3-selective antagonist darifenacin, which also has a low level of CNS accumulation due to active efflux from the brain via P-glycoprotein (P-gp) (Fig. 26.27).[144]

Oxybutynin, and all antimuscarinic OAB agents, should be used with extreme caution or avoided altogether in patients with urinary obstructions, compromised GI motility, or uncontrolled narrow angle glaucoma. This agent can exacerbate gastroesophageal reflux, which can be a use-limiting adverse effect in patients already suffering from GERD.

DARIFENACIN. Darifenacin is an M_3 selective antimuscarinic that acts quickly to improve OAB symptoms, often within the first week of therapy. It is available in extended-release tablets and costs more per dose than any of the other orally available OAB options.[142] Dry mouth and constipation are its most commonly observed adverse effects, but they are normally not severe enough to prompt discontinuation.[138,142] As alluded to above, cognition impairment with darifenacin use is not significantly different from placebo,[138,144] and its safety and tolerability in patients over the age of 65 years has been documented.[145]

Darifenacin is metabolized by both CYP3A4 and 2D6 (Fig. 26.28). Manufacturer dosing guidelines recommend a downward adjustment when darifenacin is coadministered with strong CYP3A4 inhibitors, but the caution does not apply to coadministered CYP2D6 inhibitors.[142] It is highly protein bound and the inactive metabolites are excreted in both urine and feces.

TOLTERODINE/FESOTERODINE. Tolterodine and fesoterodine are structurally related nonselective aminoalkyl antimuscarinics (Fig. 26.27). While the former contains a phenolic OH essential to pharmacological action, the latter is an inactive isobutyrate ester of that phenol and must hydrolyze to provide therapeutic utility. The hydrolyzing enzymes are nonspecific esterases. As shown in Figure 26.28, tolterodine undergoes CYP2D6-mediated benzylic hydroxylation to provide the identical active metabolite, 5-hydroxymethyltolterodine (5-HMT), and the elimination half-life in 2D6 PMs rise from 2 to 10 hours (immediate-release tablet) and from 7 to 18 hours (extended-release capsule). As shown in Figure 26.28, the active 5-HMT metabolite is inactivated by both CYP3A4 and 2D6. Excretion of both drugs and their metabolites is predominantly renal, and the presence of 5-HMT in the urinary bladder has been proposed to potentially play a role in their therapeutic action.[143]

Tolterodine binds to mAChRs in the bladder and submaxillary gland with approximately equal affinity, although the binding to bladder receptors is more prolonged. The 5-HMT metabolite preferentially binds to the M_3 receptor in bladder.[138] As noted earlier, tolterodine has OAB efficacy comparable to oxybutynin with a much lower risk of adverse effects, although the incidence of dry mouth is significantly higher than placebo.[138] Once-daily administration of the extended-release capsule formulation is claimed to be slightly more effective in attenuating urinary urge incontinence than twice-daily administration of the immediate-release tablets and may result in less dry mouth.[142] Tolterodine (but not fesoterodine) can prolong the QT interval at therapeutic doses and must be used with care in patients vulnerable to arrhythmia.[142] While tolterodine is over 96% protein bound, 5-HMT is only modestly sequestered by albumin (36%-54%).[143]

Fesoterodine's pharmacokinetics is less complex than tolterodine's, given its lack of dependence on the highly polymorphic CYP2D6 for the generation of the active 5-HMT metabolite. Hydrolysis to this active metabolite is rapid and complete, and the elimination half-life of the extended-release tablet (the only formulation marketed) is 7 hours. A head-to-head comparison of the OAB therapeutic efficacy of 8 mg fesoterodine vs. 4 mg extended-release tolterodine showed fesoterodine to be superior in decreasing urinary urge incontinence episodes, increasing the ability of the bladder to hold urine and providing patients with a perceived enhanced physical and emotional quality of life.[146] Neither fesoterodine nor 5-HMT concentrates in the CNS due to limited blood-brain barrier penetration and active efflux from central sites by P-gp.[138] In contrast, tolterodine is not a P-gp substrate and the risk of cognitive impairment would conceivably be higher.[145] However, the safety of tolterodine in the elderly is generally viewed as comparable with younger patient populations.[147]

SOLIFENACIN. Solifenacin enjoys a high M_3 receptor selectivity and, thus, is less problematic for OAB patients as far as M_1- and M_2-mediated adverse reactions are concerned.[138] Its primary mechanism of action is inhibition of detrusor smooth muscle contraction, and it is marketed as the pure 1*S*, 3*R*-isomer (Fig. 26.27). Efficacy studies have given it the edge over tolterodine in terms of urinary urgency, frequency, and urinary urge incontinence episodes. The OAB efficacy is viewed as comparable to fesoterodine.[138] In addition to decreasing daytime urinary frequency and urge incontinence, solifenacin provides therapeutic benefit to patients experiencing nocturia.[142]

Solifenacin has a decreased incidence of dry mouth when compared to tolterodine. The drug is not a P-gp substrate, but no worsening of cognition impairment in mildly impaired elders has been observed, likely due to its high M_3 selectivity.[138,144] However, the AUC can increase between 20% and 25% in elderly patients[148] which may put them at risk for other adverse effects. Like tolterodine, prolongation of the QT interval is possible.[142] Patient adherence to the prescribed regimen of solifenacin has been found to be higher than for other antimuscarinic agents.[144]

Solifenacin is available as immediate-release tablets and has a prolonged elimination half-life of 45-68 hours. Like most OAB antimuscarinics, solifenacin is strongly protein bound (>98%).[148] CYP3A4 is the principal isoform involved in its metabolism and, like darifenacin, the manufacturer recommends decreasing the dose if strong CYP3A4 inhibitors must be coadministered.[142] The most abundant metabolite, 4*R*-hydroxysolifenacin (Fig. 26.28) is comparatively active with the parent structure but is unlikely to contribute to therapeutic efficacy due to its low concentration.[149] The N-oxides of the 4*R*-hydroxymetabolite (generated by CYP3A4) and the parent drug (generated by multiple CYP isoforms) are inactive.

TROSPIUM CHLORIDE. While not used clinically to the extent of the other drugs described in this section, trospium chloride bears mentioning because it is the only quaternary amine antimuscarinic available for OAB. It has the highest affinity for all mAChR subtypes and is a powerful inhibitor of bladder and detrusor smooth muscle contractions.[138] Immediate-release tablets and extended-release capsules are marketed, and dry mouth and constipation are the major adverse effects. The extended-release dosage form has an elimination half-life of 35 hours (approximately 15 hours longer than the immediate-release formulation) and maintains efficacy over 24 hours.[138,150] Trospium is effective in patients experiencing nocturia.

As a quaternary amine, trospium chloride's ability to penetrate membranes is poor. Oral absorption is <10%,[150] and it does not cross the blood-brain barrier. While ester hydrolysis can occur, the majority of a dose is excreted unchanged in feces.

Beta Adrenergic Agonists

Mirabegron

Mirabegron
(Myrbetriq)

Mirabegron is a recently approved orally active agent for the treatment of OAB. It is a potent β_3-adrenoreceptor agonist that activates receptors in bladder tissue and causes dose-dependent detrusor relaxation. Once administered, it is rapidly absorbed and well distributed. A large percentage (71%) is bound to plasma proteins. The fat content of the food affects the bioavailability of mirabegron. Several metabolic pathways have been identified through which mirabegron is metabolized, including dealkylation, oxidation, hydrolysis, and glucuronidation. The oxidative biotransformations are linked to the activity of CYP3A4, CYP2D6, and alcohol dehydrogenase. Due to its dependence on CYP2D6, polymorphism of CYP2D6 causes pharmacokinetic differences among PM, EM, and UM phenotypes.[151,152]

CLINICAL SCENARIO

Clinical Scenario

Sum Lam, PharmD

SCENARIO

Mrs. A. M., a 68 year-old woman (height 5′ 4″, weight 80 kg), sought assistance in selecting an OTC medication for heartburn frequently experienced within an hour of eating. The burning feeling in her abdomen was sometimes accompanied by acid reflux or regurgitation, particularly after eating spicy or fatty food. Gastroesophageal reflux disease had been diagnosed 6 months ago. She tried OTC famotidine (10 mg twice daily) with good symptom relief. However, after 2 months of treatment, she decided to take famotidine once daily for convenience.

OUTCOME

The pharmacist reviewed lifestyle modifications, including weight loss and avoiding aggravating food (alcohol, fats, spicy foods, orange juice, and coffee), and then recommended one of the nonprescription proton pump inhibitors, omeprazole or lansoprazole, to be swallowed whole once daily before breakfast. Mrs. A. M. was advised to seek medical attention if symptoms were not relieved within 2 weeks. Since PPIs provide long-lasting relief from gastric acid–induced GI conditions, it is a better choice compared to OTC H_2 antihistamines. In addition, taking recommended PPI once daily may be more convenient for the patient. Mrs. A. M. was asked to follow up with her physician to discuss the improvement of symptoms after taking the recommended PPI for 4 days.

Chemical Analysis found immediately after References.

ACKNOWLEDGMENTS

The author wishes to acknowledge the work of E. Kim Fifer, PhD, Richard A. Glennon, PhD, and Wendel L. Nelson, PhD, who authored content used within this chapter in a previous edition of this text. The author also acknowledges Victoria F. Roche, PhD, for contributing a subsection of text to the chapter.

REFERENCES

1. Everhart JE, Ruhl CE. Burden of digestive diseases in the United States part I: overall and upper gastrointestinal diseases. *Gastroenterology*. 2009;136:376-386.
2. Everhart JE, Ruhl CE. Burden of digestive diseases in the United States part II: lower gastrointestinal diseases. *Gastroenterology*. 2009;136:741-754.
3. Katz PO, Gerson LB, Vela MF. Guidelines for the diagnosis and management of gastroesophageal reflux disease. *Am J Gastroenterol*. 2013;108:308-328.
4. Sobieraj DM, Coleman SM, Coleman CI. US prevalence of upper gastrointestinal symptoms: a systematic literature review. *Am J Manag Care*. 2011;17:e449-e458.
5. Vakil N. New pharmacological agents for the treatment of gastroesophageal reflux disease. *Rev Gastroenterol Disord*. 2008;8:117-122.
6. Sharkey KA, MacNaughton WK. Pharmacotherapy for gastric acicity, peptic ulcer, and gastroesophageal reflux disease. In: Brunton LL, Hilal-Dandan R, Knollmann BC, eds. *Goodman & Gilman's the Pharmacological Basis of Therapeutics*. 13th ed. New York: McGraw-Hill Medical; 2018:909-920.
7. Kaser A, Zeissig S, Blumberg RS. Inflammatory bowel disease. *Annu Rev Immunol*. 2010;28:573-621.
8. D'Haens GR, Sartor RB, Silverberg MS, et al. Future directions in inflammatory bowel disease management. *J Crohns Colitis*. 2014;8:726-734.
9. Chapple CR, Yamanishi T, Chess-Williams R. Muscarinic receptor subtypes and management of the overactive bladder. *Urology*. 2002;60:82-88; discussion 88-89.
10. Parsons ME, Ganellin CR. Histamine and its receptors. *Br J Pharmacol*. 2006;147(suppl 1):S127-S135.
11. Pino-Angeles A, Reyes-Palomares A, Melgarejo E, et al. Histamine: an undercover agent in multiple rare diseases? *J Cell Mol Med*. 2012;16:1947-1960.
12. Zhang M-Q, Leurs R, Timmerman H. Histamine H1-receptor antagonists. In: Wolff ME, ed. *Burger's Medicinal Chemisry and Drug Discovery*. 5th ed. New York: John Wiley & Sons; 1997:495-559.
13. Cooper DG, Young RC, Durant GJ, et al. Histamine receptors. In: Emmett JC, ed. *Comprehensive Medicinal Chemistry: The Rational Design, Mechanistic Study and Therapeutic Application of Chemical Compounds*. Vol 3. Oxford, UK: Pergamon Press; 1990:343-421.
14. Watanabe T, Yamatodani A, Maeyama K, et al. Pharmacology of a-fluoromethylhistidine, a specific inhibitor of histidine decarboxylase. *Trends Pharmacol Sci*. 1990;11:363-367.
15. Moya-Garcia AA, Pino-Angeles A, Gil-Redondo R, et al. Structural features of mammalian histidine decarboxylase reveal the basis for specific inhibition. *Br J Pharmacol*. 2009;157:4-13.
16. Katritch V, Cherezov V, Stevens RC. Structure-function of the G protein-coupled receptor superfamily. *Annu Rev Pharmacol Toxicol*. 2013;53:531-556.
17. Nelson WL. Antihistamines and related antiallergic and antiulcer agents. In: Lemke TL, Williams DA, Roche VF, Zito SW, eds. *Foye's Principles of Medicinal Chemistry*. 7th ed. Philadelphia: Lippincott Williams & Wilkins; 2012:1045-1072.
18. Hoogerwerf WA, Pasricha PJ. Pharmacotherapy of gastric acidity, peptic ulcers, and gastroesophageal reflux disease. In: Hardman JG, Limbird LE, Mollinoff PB, et al. eds. *Goodman and Gilman's the Pharmacological Basis of Therapeutics*. 11th ed. New York: McGraw-Hill; 2005:968.
19. Shin JM, Munson K, Vagin O, et al. The gastric HK-ATPase: structure, function, and inhibition. *Pflugers Arch*. 2009;457:609-622.
20. Pace F, Porro GB. Gastroesophageal reflux and Helicobacter pylori: a review. *World J Gastroenterol*. 2000;6:311-314.
21. Jones AW. Perspectives in drug development and clinical pharmacology: the discovery of histamine H1 and H2 antagonists. *Clin Pharmacol Drug Dev*. 2016;5:5-12.

22. Roberts S, McDonald IM. Inhibitors of gastric acid secretion. In: Abraham DJ, ed. *Burger's Medicinal Chemistry and Drug Discovery*. 6th ed. Hoboken, NJ: Wiley-Interscience; 2003:85-127.
23. Ganellin CR. Discovery of cimetidine. In: Roberts SM, Price AH, eds. *Medicinal Chemistry: The Role of Organic Chemistry in Drug Research*. London: Academic Press; 1985:93-118.
24. Gantz I, DelValle J, Wang LD, et al. Molecular basis for the interaction of histamine with the histamine H2 receptor. *J Biol Chem*. 1992;267:20840-20843.
25. Price AH, Brogden RN. Nizatidine – a preliminary review of its pharmacodynamic and pharmacokinetic properties, and its therapeutic use in peptic-ulcer disease. *Drugs*. 1988;36:521-539.
26. Penston J, Wormsley KG. Adverse reactions and interactions with H2-receptor antagonists. *Med Toxicol*. 1986;1:192-216.
27. Lin JH. Pharmacokinetic and pharmacodynamic properties of histamine H2-receptor antagonists. Relationship between intrinsic potency and effective plasma concentrations. *Clinical Pharmacokinetics*. 1991;20:218-236.
28. Stadel R, Yang J, Nalwalk JW, et al. High-affinity binding of [3H] cimetidine to a heme-containing protein in rat brain. *Drug Metab Dispos*. 2008;36:614-621.
29. Sedman AJ. Cimetidine-drug interactions. *Am J Med*. 1984;76:109-114.
30. Klotz U, Kroemer HK. The drug interaction potential of ranitidine: an update. *Pharmacol Ther*. 1991;50:233-244.
31. Berardi RR, Tankanow RM, Nostrant TT. Comparison of famotidine with cimetidine and ranitidine. *Clin Pharm*. 1988;7:271-284.
32. Strand DS, Kim D, Peura DA. 25 Years of proton pump inhibitors: a comprehensive review. *Gut Liver*. 2017;11:27-37.
33. Roche VF. The chemically elegant proton pump inhibitors. *Am J Pharm Educ*. 2006;70:101.
34. Robinson M. Proton pump inhibitors: update on their role in acid-related gastrointestinal diseases. *Int J Clin Pract*. 2005;59:709-715.
35. Lindberg P, Brandstrom A, Wallmark B, et al. Omeprazole: the first proton pump inhibitor. *Med Res Rev*. 1990;10:1-54.
36. Jana K, Bandyopadhyay T, Ganguly B. Revealing the mechanistic pathway of acid activation of proton pump inhibitors to inhibit the gastric proton pump: a DFT study. *J Phys Chem B*. 2016;120:13031-13038.
37. Shin JM, Sachs G. Pharmacology of proton pump inhibitors. *Curr Gastroenterol Rep*. 2008;10:528-534.
38. Shin JM, Cho YM, Sachs G. Chemistry of covalent inhibition of the gastric (H^+, K^+)-ATPase by proton pump inhibitors. *J Am Chem Soc*. 2004;126:7800-7811.
39. Scott SA, Sangkuhl K, Shuldiner AR, et al. PharmGKB summary: very important pharmacogene information for cytochrome P450, family 2, subfamily C, polypeptide 19. *Pharmacogenet Genomics*. 2012;22:159-165.
40. Andersson T. Pharmacokinetics, metabolism and interactions of acid pump inhibitors – focus on omeprazole, lansoprazole and pantoprazole. *Clin Pharmacokinet*. 1996;31:9-28.
41. Andersson T. Single-isomer drugs – true therapeutic advances. *Clin Pharmacokinet*. 2004;43:279-285.
42. Ishizaki T, Horai Y. Review article: cytochrome P450 and the metabolism of proton pump inhibitors–emphasis on rabeprazole. *Aliment Pharmacol Ther*. 1999;13(suppl 3):27-36.
43. Shin JM, Kim N. Pharmacokinetics and pharmacodynamics of the proton pump inhibitors. *J Neurogastroenterol Motil*. 2013;19:25-35.
44. Zhou Q, Yan XF, Pan WS, et al. Is the required therapeutic effect always achieved by racemic switch of proton-pump inhibitors? *World J Gastroenterol*. 2008;14:2617-2619.
45. Huang B, Huang Y, Li Y, et al. Adverse cardiovascular effects of concomitant use of proton pump inhibitors and clopidogrel in patients with coronary artery disease: a systematic review and meta-analysis. *Arch Med Res*. 2012;43:212-224.
46. Drepper MD, Spahr L, Frossard JL. Clopidogrel and proton pump inhibitors–where do we stand in 2012? *World J Gastroenterol*. 2012;18:2161-2171.
47. Hung SC, Liao KF, Hung HC, et al. Using proton pump inhibitors correlates with an increased risk of chronic kidney disease: a nationwide database-derived case-controlled study. *Fam Pract*. 2018;35:166-171.
48. Lazarus B, Chen Y, Wilson FP, et al. Proton pump inhibitor use and the risk of chronic kidney disease. *JAMA Intern Med*. 2016;176:238-246.
49. Lind T, Rydberg L, Kyleback A, et al. Esomeprazole provides improved acid control vs. omeprazole in patients with symptoms of gastro-oesophageal reflux disease. *Aliment Pharmacol Ther*. 2000;14:861-867.
50. Andersson T, Weidolf L. Stereoselective disposition of proton pump inhibitors. *Clin Drug Investig*. 2008;28:263-279.
51. Souza RC, Lima JH. Helicobacter pylori and gastroesophageal reflux disease: a review of this intriguing relationship. *Dis Esophagus*. 2009;22:256-263.
52. *Omeprazole. Drug Facts and Comparisons. Facts & Comparisons eAnswers [database online]*. St. Louis, MO: Wolters Kluwer Health, Inc; March 2005. Accessed November 07, 2018.
53. Metz DC, Vakily M, Dixit T, et al. Review article: dual delayed release formulation of dexlansoprazole MR, a novel approach to overcome the limitations of conventional single release proton pump inhibitor therapy. *Aliment Pharmacol Ther*. 2009;29:928-937.
54. Acosta A, Camilleri M. Prokinetics in gastroparesis. *Gastroenterol Clin North Am*. 2015;44:97-111.
55. Gershon MD. Review article: serotonin receptors and transporters – roles in normal and abnormal gastrointestinal motility. *Aliment Pharmacol Ther*. 2004;20(suppl 7):3-14.
56. Livezey MR, Briggs ED, Bolles AK, et al. Metoclopramide is metabolized by CYP2D6 and is a reversible inhibitor, but not inactivator, of CYP2D6. *Xenobiotica*. 2014;44:309-319.
57. Curran MP, Robinson DM. Mosapride in gastrointestinal disorders. *Drugs*. 2008;68:981-991.
58. Frampton JE. Prucalopride. *Drugs*. 2009;69:2463-2476.
59. Holtmann G, Talley NJ, Liebregts T, et al. A placebo-controlled trial of itopride in functional dyspepsia. *N Engl J Med*. 2006;354:832-840.
60. Quigley EM. Prokinetics in the management of functional gastrointestinal disorders. *J Neurogastroenterol Motil*. 2015;21:330-336.
61. Quigley EMM. Prokinetics in the management of functional gastrointestinal disorders. *Curr Gastroenterol Rep*. 2017;19:53.
62. Patel S, Berrada D, Lembo A. Review of tegaserod in the treatment of irritable bowel syndrome. *Expert Opin Pharmacother*. 2004;5:2369-2379.
63. Wallace JL. Prostaglandins, NSAIDs, and gastric mucosal protection: why doesn't the stomach digest itself? *Physiol Rev*. 2008;88:1547-1565.
64. Collins PW. Misoprostol: discovery, development, and clinical applications. *Med Res Rev*. 1990;10:149-172.
65. Nagashima R, Yoshida N. Sucralfate, a basic aluminum salt of sucrose sulfate. I. Behaviors in gastroduodenal pH. *Arzneimittelforschung*. 1979;29:1668-1676.
66. Nagashima R, Yoshida N, Terao N. Sucralfate, a basic aluminum salt of sucrose sulfate. II. Inhibition of peptic hydrolysis as it results from sucrose sulfate interaction with protein substrate, serum albumins. *Arzneimittelforschung*. 1980;30:73-76.
67. Marks IN. Sucralfate: worldwide experience in recurrence therapy. *J Clin Gastroenterol*. 1987;9(suppl 1):18-22.
68. Frazer A, Hensler JG. Serotonin. In: Siegel GJ, Agranoff BW, Albers RW, et al, eds. *Basic Neurochemistry*. New York: Raven Press; 1993:283-308.
69. Langlois M, Fischmeister R. 5-HT4 receptor ligands: applications and new prospects. *J Med Chem*. 2003;46:319-344.
70. Glennon RA, Dukat M. Serotonin receptors and drugs affecting serotonergic neurotransmission. In: Lemke TL, Williams DA, Roche VF, et al, eds. *Foye's Principles of Medicinal Chemistry*. 6th ed. Philadelphia: Lippincott Williams & Wilkins; 2008:415-443.
71. Nichols DE, Nichols CD. Serotonin receptors. *Chem Rev*. 2008;108:1614-1641.

72. Hoyer D, Clarke DE, Fozard JR, et al. International union of pharmacology classification of receptors for 5-hydroxytryptamine (serotonin). *Pharmacol Rev*. 1994;46:157-203.
73. Lameh J, Cone RI, Maeda S, et al. Structure and function of G-protein coupled receptors. *Pharm Res*. 1990;7:1213-1221.
74. Barnes NM, Hales TG, Lummis SCR, et al. The 5-HT3 receptor – the relationship between structure and function. *Neuropharmacology*. 2009;56:273-284.
75. Bockaert J, Claeysen S, Compan V, et al. 5-HT4 receptors. *Curr Drug Targets CNS Neurol Disord*. 2004;3:39-51.
76. Gaster LM, King FD. Serotonin 5-HT3 and 5-HT4 receptor antagonists. *Med Res Rev*. 1997;17:163-214.
77. Glennon RA, Dukat M. Serotonin receptors and drugs affecting adrenergic neurotransmission. In: Lemke TL, Williams DA, Roche VF, Zito SW, eds. *Foye's Principles of Medicinal Chemistry*. 7th ed. Philadelphia: Lippincott Williams & Wilkins; 2012:365-396.
78. Gershon MD. 5-Hydroxytryptamine (serotonin) in the gastrointestinal tract. *Curr Opin Endocrinol Diabetes Obes*. 2013;20:14-21.
79. Gozlan H. 5-HT3 receptors. In: Olivier B, van Wijngaarden I, Soudin W, eds. *Serotonin Receptors and Their Ligands*. Amsterdam: Elsevier; 1997:221-258.
80. Heidempergher F, Pillan A, Pinciroli V, et al. Phenylimidazolidin-2-one derivatives as selective 5-HT3 receptor antagonists and refinement of the pharmacophore model for 5-HT3 receptor binding. *J Med Chem*. 1997;40:3369-3380.
81. Kesters D, Thompson AJ, Brams M, et al. Structural basis of ligand recognition in 5-HT3 receptors. *EMBO Rep*. 2013;14:49-56.
82. Price KL, Lillestol RK, Ulens C, et al. Palonosetron-5-HT3 receptor interactions as shown by a binding protein cocrystal structure. *ACS Chem Neurosci*. 2016;7:1641-1646.
83. Aapro M, Blower P. 5-Hydroxytryptamine type-3 receptor antagonists for chemotherapy-induced and radiotherapy-induced nausea and emesis – can we safely reduce the dose of administered agents? *Cancer*. 2005;104:1-13.
84. de Wit R, Aapro M, Blower PR. Is there a pharmacological basis for differences in 5-HT3-receptor antagonist efficacy in refractory patients? *Cancer Chemother Pharmacol*. 2005;56:231-238.
85. Jordan K, Kasper C, Schmoll HJ. Chemotherapy-induced nausea and vomiting: current and new standards in the antiemetic prophylaxis and treatment. *Eur J Cancer*. 2005;41:199-205.
86. Aapro M. Optimising antiemetic therapy: what are the problems and how can they be overcome? *Curr Med Res Opin*. 2005;21:885-897.
87. Roberts SM, Bezinover DS, Janicki PK. Reappraisal of the role of dolasetron in prevention and treatment of nausea and vomiting associated with surgery or chemotherapy. *Cancer Manag Res*. 2012;4:67-73.
88. Obach RS. Pharmacologically active drug metabolites: impact on drug discovery and pharmacotherapy. *Pharmacol Rev*. 2013;65:578-640.
89. Reith MK, Sproles GD, Cheng LK. Human metabolism of dolasetron mesylate, a 5-HT3 receptor antagonist. *Drug Metab Dispos*. 1995;23:806-812.
90. Nakamura H, Ariyoshi N, Okada K, et al. CYP1A1 is a major enzyme responsible for the metabolism of granisetron in human liver microsomes. *Curr Drug Metab*. 2005;6:469-480.
91. Pritchard JF. Ondansetron metabolism and pharmacokinetics. *Semin Oncol*. 1992;19:9-15.
92. Navari RM. Palonosetron for the treatment of chemotherapy-induced nausea and vomiting. *Expert Opin Pharmacother*. 2014;15:2599-2608.
93. Stoltz R, Parisi S, Shah A, et al. Pharmacokinetics, metabolism and excretion of intravenous [l4C]-palonosetron in healthy human volunteers. *Biopharm Drug Dispos*. 2004;25:329-337.
94. Huang M, Gao JY, Zhai ZG, et al. An HPLC-ESI-MS method for simultaneous determination of fourteen metabolites of promethazine and caffeine and its application to pharmacokinetic study of the combination therapy against motion sickness. *J Pharm Biomed Anal*. 2012;62:119-128.
95. Finn A, Collins J, Voyksner R, et al. Bioavailability and metabolism of prochlorperazine administered via the buccal and oral delivery route. *J Clin Pharmacol*. 2005;45:1383-1390.
96. Khan S, Chang L. Diagnosis and management of IBS. *Nat Rev Gastroenterol Hepatol*. 2010;7:565-581.
97. Camilleri M. Pharmacology of the new treatments for lower gastrointestinal motility disorders and irritable bowel syndrome. *Clin Pharmacol Ther*. 2012;91:44-59.
98. Fayyaz M, Lackner JM. Serotonin receptor modulators in the treatment of irritable bowel syndrome. *Ther Clin Risk Manag*. 2008;4:41-48.
99. Dinning PG, Smith TK, Scott SM. Pathophysiology of colonic causes of chronic constipation. *Neurogastroenterol Motil*. 2009;21(suppl 2):20-30.
100. Camilleri M. Current and future pharmacological treatments for diarrhea-predominant irritable bowel syndrome. *Expert Opin Pharmacother*. 2013;14:1151-1160.
101. Gershon MD, Tack J. The serotonin signaling system: from basic understanding to drug development for functional GI disorders. *Gastroenterology*. 2007;132:397-414.
102. Hornby PJ. Drug discovery approaches to irritable bowel syndrome. *Expert Opin Drug Discov*. 2015;10:809-824.
103. Layer P, Keller J, Loeffler H, et al. Tegaserod in the treatment of irritable bowel syndrome (IBS) with constipation as the prime symptom. *Ther Clin Risk Manag*. 2007;3:107-118.
104. Vickers AE, Zollinger M, Dannecker R, et al. In vitro metabolism of tegaserod in human liver and intestine: assessment of drug interactions. *Drug Metab Dispos*. 2001;29:1269-1276.
105. Chiu SH, Huskey SW. Species differences in N-glucuronidation. *Drug Metab Dispos*. 1998;26:838-847.
106. Meyers NL, Hickling RI. Pharmacology and metabolism of renzapride: a novel therapeutic agent for the potential treatment of irritable bowel syndrome. *Drugs R D*. 2008;9: 37-63.
107. Love BL, Johnson A, Smith LS. Linaclotide: a novel agent for chronic constipation and irritable bowel syndrome. *Am J Health Syst Pharm*. 2014;71:1081-1091.
108. Currie MG, Fok KF, Kato J, et al. Guanylin: an endogenous activator of intestinal guanylate cyclase. *Proc Natl Acad Sci USA*. 1992;89:947-951.
109. Hamra FK, Forte LR, Eber SL, et al. Uroguanylin: structure and activity of a second endogenous peptide that stimulates intestinal guanylate cyclase. *Proc Natl Acad Sci USA*. 1993;90:10464-10468.
110. Corsetti M, Tack J. Linaclotide: a new drug for the treatment of chronic constipation and irritable bowel syndrome with constipation. *United European Gastroenterol J*. 2013;1:7-20.
111. de Mattos BR, Garcia MP, Nogueira JB, et al. Inflammatory bowel disease: an overview of immune mechanisms and biological treatments. *Mediators Inflamm*. 2015;2015:1-11.
112. Ordas I, Eckmann L, Talamini M, et al. Ulcerative colitis. *Lancet*. 2012;380:1606-1619.
113. Sandborn WJ, Feagan BG, Lichtenstein GR. Medical management of mild to moderate Crohn's disease: evidence-based treatment algorithms for induction and maintenance of remission. *Aliment Pharmacol Ther*. 2007;26:987-1003.
114. Sartor RB. Mechanisms of disease: pathogenesis of Crohn's disease and ulcerative colitis. *Nat Clin Pract Gastroenterol Hepatol*. 2006;3:390-407.
115. Jovani M, Danese S. Vedolizumab for the treatment of IBD: a selective therapeutic approach targeting pathogenic a4b7 cells. *Curr Drug Targets*. 2013;14:1433-1443.
116. Khanna R, Preiss JC, MacDonald JK, et al. Anti-IL-12/23p40 antibodies for induction of remission in Crohn's disease. *Cochrane Database Syst Rev*. 2015:CD007572.
117. Shah B, Mayer L. Current status of monoclonal antibody therapy for the treatment of inflammatory bowel disease. *Expert Rev Clin Immunol*. 2010;6:607-620.
118. Sofia MA, Rubin DT. The impact of therapeutic antibodies on the management of digestive diseases: history, current practice, and future directions. *Dig Dis Sci*. 2017;62:833-842.

119. Soler D, Chapman T, Yang LL, et al. The binding specificity and selective antagonism of vedolizumab, an anti-alpha4beta7 integrin therapeutic antibody in development for inflammatory bowel diseases. *J Pharmacol Exp Ther*. 2009;330:864-875.
120. Liu JK. The history of monoclonal antibody development – progress, remaining challenges and future innovations. *Ann Med Surg (Lond)*. 2014;3:113-116.
121. Katzung BG. Introduction to autonomic pharmacology. In: Katzung BG, ed. *Basic and Clinical Pharmacology*. 11th ed. New York: McGraw-Hill; 2009:77-94.
122. Changeux JP, Devillers-Thiery A, Chemouilli P. Acetylcholine receptor: an allosteric protein. *Science*. 1984;225:1335-1345.
123. Lukas RJ, Bencherif M. Heterogeneity and regulation of nicotinic acetylcholine receptors. *Int Rev Neurobiol*. 1992;34:25-131.
124. Fifer EK. Drugs affecting cholinergic neurotransmission. In: Lemke TL, Williams DA, Roche VF, Zito SW, eds. *Foye's Principles of Medicinal Chemistry*. 7th ed. Philadelphia: Lippincott Williams & Wilkins; 2012:309-339.
125. Armstrong PD, Cannon JG, Long JP. Conformationally rigid analogues of acetylcholine. *Nature*. 1968;220:65-66.
126. Caulfield MP, Birdsall NJ. International Union of Pharmacology. XVII. Classification of muscarinic acetylcholine receptors. *Pharmacol Rev*. 1998;50:279-290.
127. Ing HR. The structure-action relationships to the choline group. *Science*. 1949;109:264-266.
128. Ing HR, Kordik P, Williams DP. Studies on the structure-action relationships of the choline group. *Br J Pharmacol Chemother*. 1952;7:103-116.
129. Holton P, Ing HR. The specificity of the trimethylammonium group in acetylcholine. *Br J Pharmacol Chemother*. 1949;4:190-196.
130. Haga K, Kruse AC, Asada H, et al. Structure of the human M2 muscarinic acetylcholine receptor bound to an antagonist. *Nature*. 2012;482:547-551.
131. Renner UD, Oertel R, Kirch W. Pharmacokinetics and pharmacodynamics in clinical use of scopolamine. *Ther Drug Monit*. 2005;27:655-665.
132. Ariens EJ. Receptor theory and structure activity relationships. *Adv Drug Res*. 1966;3:235-285.
133. Tzefos M, Dolder C, Olin JL. Fesoterodine for the treatment of overactive bladder. *Ann Pharmacother*. 2009;43:1992-2000.
134. Malhotra B, Gandelman K, Sachse R, et al. The design and development of fesoterodine as a prodrug of 5-hydroxymethyl tolterodine (5-HMT), the active metabolite of tolterodine. *Curr Med Chem*. 2009;16:4481-4489.
135. Jayarajan J, Radomski SB. Pharmacotherapy of overactive bladder in adults: a review of efficacy, tolerability, and quality of life. *Res Rep Urol*. 2013;6:1-16.
136. Chapple C, Khullar V, Gabriel Z, et al. The effects of antimuscarinic treatments in overactive bladder: a systematic review and meta-analysis. *Eur Urol*. 2005;48:5-26.
137. Chapple CR, Khullar V, Gabriel Z, et al. The effects of antimuscarinic treatments in overactive bladder: an update of a systematic review and meta-analysis. *Eur Urol*. 2008;54:543-562.
138. Yamada S, Ito Y, Nishijima S, et al. Basic and clinical aspects of antimuscarinic agents used to treat overactive bladder. *Pharmacol Ther*. 2018;189:130-148.
139. Chapple CR, Rechberger T, Al-Shukri S, et al. Randomized, double-blind placebo- and tolterodine-controlled trial of the once-daily antimuscarinic agent solifenacin in patients with symptomatic overactive bladder. *BJU Int*. 2004;93:303-310.
140. Skerjanec A. The clinical pharmacokinetics of darifenacin. *Clin Pharmacokinet*. 2006;45:325-350.
141. Fonseca AM, Meinberg MF, Monteiro MV, et al. The effectiveness of anticholinergic therapy for overactive bladders: systematic review and meta-analysis. *Rev Bras Ginecol Obstet*. 2018;38. doi:10.1055/s-0036-1594289.
142. Hesch K. Agents for treatment of overactive bladder: a therapeutic class review. *Proc (Bayl Univ Med Cent)*. 2007;20:307-314.
143. Mansfield KJ. Role of fesoterodine in the treatment of overactive bladder. *Open Access J Urol*. 2009;2:1-9.
144. Marcelissen T, Rashid T, Antunes Lopes T, et al. Oral pharmacologic management of overactive bladder syndrome: where do we stand? *Eur Urol Focus*. 2018. doi:10.4172/2167-4065X.1000156.
145. McFerren SC, Gomelsky A. Treatment of overactive bladder in the elderly female: the case for trospium, oxybutynin, fesoterodine and darifenacin. *Drugs Aging*. 2015;32:809-819.
146. Herschorn S, Swift S, Guan Z, et al. Comparison of fesoterodine and tolterodine extended release for the treatment of overactive bladder: a head-to-head placebo-controlled trial. *BJU Int*. 2010;105:58-66.
147. *Tolterodine. Drug Facts and Comparisons. Facts & Comparisons eAnswers [database online]*. St. Louis, MO: Wolters Kluwer Health, Inc; March 2005. Accessed November 07, 2018.
148. *Solifenacin. Drug Facts and Comparisons. Facts & Comparisons eAnswers [database online]*. St. Louis, MO: Wolters Kluwer Health, Inc; March 2005. Accessed November 07, 2018.
149. Doroshyenko O, Fuhr U. Clinical pharmacokinetics and pharmacodynamics of solifenacin. *Clin Pharmacokinet*. 2009;48:281-302.
150. *Trospium chloride. Drug Facts and Comparisons. Facts & Comparisons eAnswers [database online]*. St. Louis, MO: Wolters Kluwer Health, Inc; March 2005. Accessed November 07, 2018.
151. Sacco E, Bientinesi R. Mirabegron: a review of recent data and its prospects in the management of overactive bladder. *Ther Adv Urol*. 2012;4:315-324.
152. Sacco E, Bientinesi R, Tienforti D, et al. Discovery history and clinical development of mirabegron for the treatment of overactive bladder and urinary incontinence. *Expert Opin Drug Discov*. 2014;9:433-448.

Clinical Scenario

Sabesan Yoganathan, PhD

CHEMICAL ANALYSIS

Omeprazole and lansoprazole are two of the commonly recommended proton pump inhibitors for GERD or related GI disorders. These drugs target the H^+, K^+-ATPase (proton pump) that is in the parietal cells, where acid secretion occurs. Proton pump inhibitors (PPIs) are irreversible inhibitors and they stop the secretion of stomach acid. Omeprazole and lansoprazole belong to 2-pyridylmethylsulfinylbenzimidazole class of compounds. The sulfinyl group is a chiral center, where omeprazole and lansoprazole exist as a racemate (*R* and *S* isomers). PPIs are weak bases with the highest pK_a being between 3.8 and 4.9, which enables them to selectively reach the canaliculus. These drugs are considered prodrugs because they are activated in the acidic parietal cell environment, yielding the active drug.

(Continued)

Clinical Scenario—*Continued*

The mechanism involves protonation of the benzimidazole nitrogen that initiates the conversion of the sulfoxide motif into a sulfenic acid intermediate. Subsequently, a reactive sulfenamide intermediate is formed. The activated forms covalently interact with a cysteine thiol of the proton pump (Cys813) to inhibit stomach acid secretion. The covalently bound drug can be released from the proton pump by the action of reduced form of glutathione (GSH). However, limited physiological concentration of GSH and its ability to reach the pocket containing the bound proton pump makes this process difficult.

This chemical mechanism of action of PPIs allows one to take a recommended PPI once daily, as compared to a H_2 antagonist which exhibits reversible action and a short half-life, thus must be taken multiple times a day. From a patient's perspective, the multiple daily-dose regimen could be an inconvenience and could result in nonadherence to the therapeutic regimen.

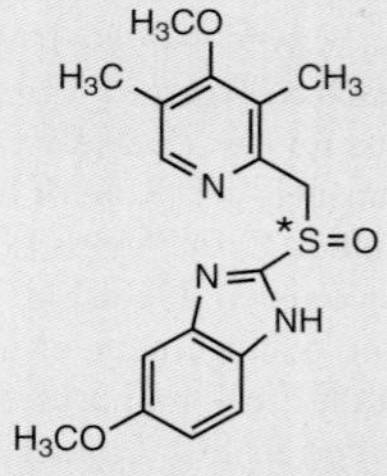

H_3CO, H_3C, CH_3, N, *S=O, N, NH, H_3CO

Omeprazole (Prilosec)

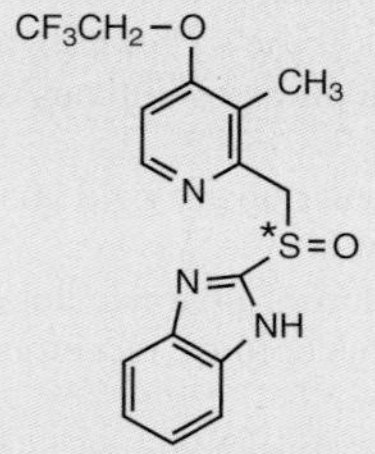

CF_3CH_2-O, CH_3, N, *S=O, N, NH

Lansoprazole (Prevacid)

Due to the chiral nature of the sulfoxide motif, the different isomers (*R* and *S*) have different metabolic profiles, which impacts bioavailability and plasma clearance. Omeprazole and lansoprazole are both metabolized by CYP2C19 and CYP3A4 to inactive metabolites.

If the patient experiences insufficient relief of symptoms with omeprazole or lansoprazole, she may be a rapid (ultrafast) CYP2C19 metabolizer. In that case, the *S*-isomer of omeprazole, esomeprazole, which is biotransformed to a lesser extent by CYP2C19, may be the better option.

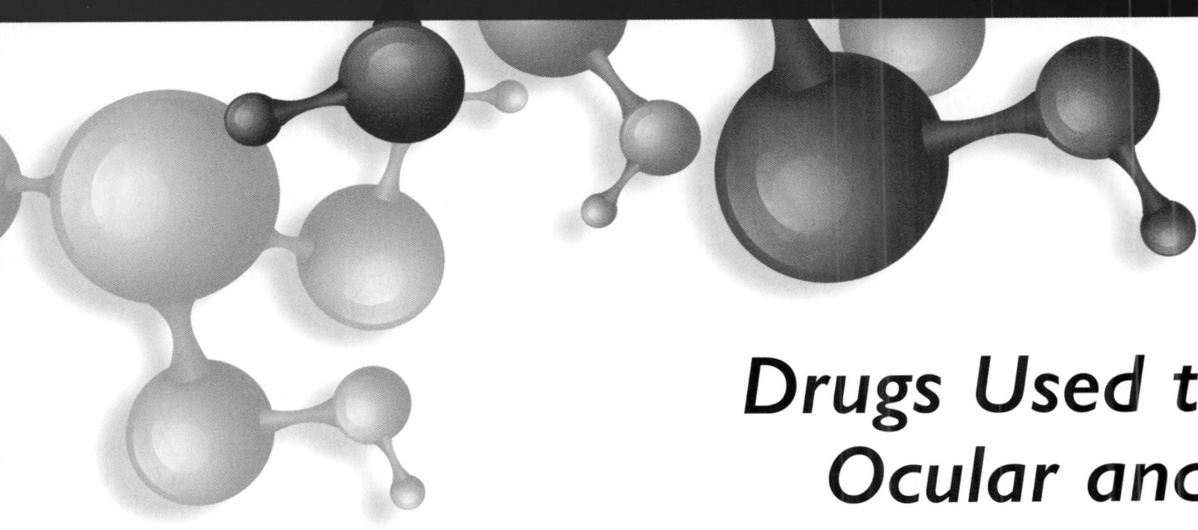

CHAPTER 27

Drugs Used to Treat Ocular and Nasal Congestion Disorders

Srikanth Kolluru

Drugs covered in this chapter:

ACETYLCHOLINESTERASE INHIBITORS (ANTICHOLINESTERASES)
- Echothiophate iodide

α_1-ADRENERGIC AGONISTS
- Naphazoline
- Oxymetazoline
- Phenylephrine
- Tetrahydrozoline
- Xylometazoline

α_2-ADRENERGIC AGONISTS
- Apraclonidine
- Brimonidine

β-ADRENERGIC RECEPTOR BLOCKERS
- Betaxolol
- Carteolol
- Levobunolol
- Metipranolol
- Timolol

CARBONIC ANHYDRASE INHIBITORS
- Acetazolamide
- Methazolamide
- Dorzolamide
- Brinzolamide

MIXED-ACTING SYMPATHOMIMETICS

PHENYLPROPANOLAMINES
- (−)-Ephedrine
- (+)-Pseudoephedrine
- (+)-Phenylpropanolamine

PHENYLISOPROPYLAMINES
- Amphetamine
- Methamphetamine

MUSCARINIC AGONISTS
- Acetylcholine
- Carbachol chloride
- Pilocarpine

PROSTAGLANDINS
- Bimatoprost
- Latanoprost
- Tafluprost
- Travoprost

RHO KINASE INHIBITORS
- Netarsudil

TOPICAL OPHTHALMIC NONSTEROIDAL ANTI-INFLAMMATORY DRUGS
- Bromfenac
- Flurbiprofen
- Ketorolac tromethamine
- Nepafenac

TOPICAL OPHTHALMIC STEROIDS
- Dexamethasone
- Difluprednate
- Fluorometholone
- Loteprednol etabonate
- Prednisolone acetate
- Prednisolone sodium phosphate

TOPICAL OPHTHALMIC ANTIHISTAMINES
- Alcaftadine
- Azelastine
- Bepotastine
- Cetirizine
- Emedastine
- Epinastine
- Ketotifen
- Olopatadine

Abbreviations

AChE acetylcholinesterase
AChEI acetylcholinesterase inhibitor
BBB blood-brain barrier
CA carbonic anhydrase
CAI carbonic anhydrase inhibitor
cAMP cyclic adenosine monophosphate
CNS central nervous system
COMT catechol-O-methyltransferase
COPD chronic obstructive pulmonary disorder
COX cyclooxygenase
DAG 1,2-diacylglycerol
DOPGAL 3,4-dihydroxyphenylglycolaldehyde
EPI epinephrine
GDP guanosine diphosphate
GPCR G protein–coupled receptor
GTP guanosine triphosphate
IOP intraocular pressure
IP_3 inositol-1,4,5-triphosphate
L-DOPA L-dihydroxyphenylalanine
mAChR muscarinic acetylcholinergic receptor
MAO monoamine oxidase
MAOI monoamine oxidase inhibitor
nAChR nicotinic acetylcholinergic receptor
NE norepinephrine
NET norepinephrine reuptake transporter
NSAID nonsteroidal anti-inflammatory drug
OTC over-the-counter
PLC phospholipase-C
ROCK rho kinase
SAR structure-activity relationship
TMD transmembrane domain

INTRODUCTION

Congestion is an abnormal accumulation of fluids in tissues leading to swollen membranes, dilated blood vessels, and blockade of passages. Vasodilation widens gaps between cells lining blood vessels allowing fluids to escape to the surrounding tissue causing itching, sneezing, runny nose, and watery eyes. If congestion is untreated, it may facilitate infections via the movement of mucus from the nose to throat causing throat infection, accumulation of fluids in the sinus cavities causing sinus infections. Congestion can be responsible for anywhere from mild discomfort to a life-threatening situation. Nasal congestion may also lead to headaches, sleep apnea, snoring and interfere with hearing and speech. Risk factors for nasal congestion include allergic rhinitis, influenza, gastroesophageal reflux disorder,[1] sinus infection, deviated septum, drug addiction, enlarged adenoids, hormonal changes, nasal polyps, nonallergic rhinitis, occupational asthma, respiratory syncytial virus, stress, thyroid disorders, hay fever, and common cold to mention a few.[2] Allergic rhinitis is the most common cause for nasal congestion and affects about 60 million people each year in the United States.[3,4] In 2016, there were about 16 million adult and 5.5 million childhood hay fever cases reported in the United States.[5] Nasal congestion may also occur due to structural abnormalities of nose and nasal septum, enlargement of adenoids, and nasal tumors.

Ocular congestion is associated with burning, pain, itchy, swollen, and watery eyes. Common causes for ocular congestion include allergic conjunctivitis, infection, glaucoma, migraine, sinus infection, and influenza. Seasonal allergic rhinoconjunctivitis affects about 16% of the US population annually.[6] Nasal or ocular decongestants help relieve discomfort caused by congestion, but the root cause may need treatment with other medications. Common symptoms associated with congestion are inflammation and vasodilation. Pathophysiology of nasal congestion involves inflammation, increased venous engorgement, increased nasal secretions, and edema. It may also alter sensory perception and physical structure of nasal passage.[7]

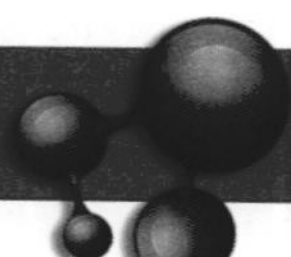

CLINICAL SIGNIFICANCE

Michelle M. Hughes, PharmD, BCPS, BCACP

This chapter focuses on medications used to treat common conditions such as nasal and ocular congestion. The chemical structures of these medications are derived from endogenous catecholamines, epinephrine and norepinephrine. The structure plays an important role in determining whether the medication will be nonselective or selective for the α_1 receptor, which is the main therapeutic target for congestion. One example is phenylephrine which is a common medication used to treat congestion. Its chemical structure contains a phenyl ring with a hydroxyl group substituted at the 3′ position, which confers selectivity for the α_1 receptor. This targeted action results in vasodilation and has minimal effect on other adrenergic receptors such as the β_1 receptors in the heart. Phenylephrine is available as both oral and topical formulations. Topical delivery has the advantage of a more localized effect at the site of action, which minimizes the risk for systemic adverse effects.

Another disease state reviewed in this chapter is glaucoma. The complex anatomy of the eye poses a significant barrier for effective drug delivery to the anterior segment of the eye where glaucoma medications exert their pharmacologic action. In general, ocular drug formulations have amphipathic properties, which allow the drug to overcome the hydrophilic nature of the tear film as well as permeate through lipophilic layers of the cornea. One example is latanoprost, which is an ester prodrug of prostaglandin $F_{2\alpha}$. The presence of an ester group functions to enhance corneal permeability. Latanoprost is then bioactivated by esterases and exerts its pharmacologic action to increase aqueous humor outflow and reduce intraocular pressure (IOP). Prostaglandin analogues are considered first-line agents owing to their efficacy for reducing IOP and favorable risk-benefit profile. They have the advantage of reducing IOP for up to 24 hours which allows for once daily dosing. They are also minimally absorbed into the systemic circulation which reduces the risk for side effects.

Therapeutic Classes of Drugs Used to Treat Nasal and Ocular Congestion

Treating the two common symptoms, vasodilation and inflammation, is critical to help relieve nasal and ocular congestion. Smooth muscle tone of vasculature is maintained through a balance between the sympathetic and the parasympathetic nervous systems with opposing functions. Sympathetic activation causes vasoconstriction and parasympathetic activation inhibits vasoconstriction. Vasodilation is due to the shift of balance to the parasympathetic nervous system over the sympathetic nervous system. Congestion can be treated by constricting the dilated vasculature, which brings cells together and reduces fluid leakage. Thus, drugs that are agonists at adrenergic receptors or antagonists at cholinergic receptors can be implicated in the treatment of congestion disorders. Due to several systemic adverse effects and availability of safer alternatives, cholinergic antagonists are no longer used for treating congestion disorders.

A second symptom of congestion disorders is inflammation, due to the release of inflammatory substances such as inflammatory prostaglandins, interleukins, histamine, leukotrienes, and various other hormones. Antihistamines play a big role and are used widely in treating nasal congestion. Antihistamines are discussed in detail in a dedicated Chapter 25. Drugs discussed in this chapter target adrenergic receptors, cholinergic receptors, or pathways responsible for the synthesis or release of inflammatory autacoids.

α_1-Adrenergic Agonists

Why do agonists at α_1-receptors help relieve congestion? What is the tissue distribution of α_1-receptors in the body? What are the endogenous substrates for these receptors? What structural features are important for these drugs to exhibit α_1-receptor selectivity? What are the preferred routes of administration for these drugs? To address these questions, a general understanding of adrenergic receptors, their tissue distribution, and the receptor binding of the endogenous substrates norepinephrine (NE) and epinephrine (EPI) is necessary.

Vascular smooth muscles of the nasal pathway and the eye are rich in adrenergic α_1-receptors. Activation of α_1-receptors causes vasoconstriction and smooth muscle contraction that is needed for treating congestion. Detailed information about various adrenergic receptors in the body is discussed in Chapters 16 and 17. Tissue distribution and physiological functions of α_1-receptor activation are listed in Table 27.1. Except in the vasculature of skeletal muscles, α_1-receptors are widely distributed in arterioles and veins throughout the body.

As indicated above, vasodilation widens the gap between endothelial cells lining blood vessels allowing fluids to escape to the surrounding tissue causing congestion. Therefore, agonists at adrenergic α_1-receptors can constrict

Table 27.1 Tissue Distribution and Physiological Effects of the Activation of Adrenergic α_1-Receptors

Organ	Physiological Effects of α_1-Receptors
Eye	
Iris radial muscle contraction	Dilation—mydriasis
Arterioles except for muscle	Contraction—increases blood pressure
Veins	Contraction—increases blood pressure
Stomach and Intestine	
Sphincters	Contraction—closes sphincters
Glandular Secretions	
Lacrimal glands	Increases
Salivary glands	Increases
Bronchial	Decreases
Pancreatic gland	Decreases
Mucosal	Decreases
Sweat	Increases
Bladder sphincter	Contraction – closes
Sex organs—male (seminal track)	Ejaculation
Uterus	Contraction—premature labor

blood vessels thereby reducing the amount of fluid release. However, adrenergic receptors are widely distributed in various tissues and organs as well as on the neurons of both the peripheral and central nervous system (CNS). Because of their wider distribution, the patients taking oral or other systemic adrenergic agonists may experience systemic adverse effects such as hypertension. Caution must be exercised while administering oral adrenergic agonists to treat congestion disorders in hypertensive patients. Since the target site is vascular smooth muscles in the nose and eye, the topical route is the most preferred route of drug delivery for both nasal and ocular decongestants.

Endogenous Substrates Norepinephrine (NE) and Epinephrine (EPI)

OH
HO NHR
HO

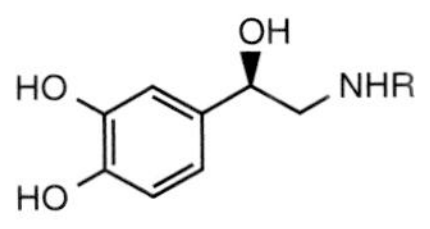

Norepinephrine, R = H
Epinephrine, R = CH_3

NE and EPI are members of a class of pharmacologically active substances known as catecholamines. The catecholamine structure has an ethanolamine and an *ortho* dihydroxy phenyl moiety. Most adrenergic drugs are catecholamine derivatives.

BIOSYNTHESIS AND METABOLISM NOREPINEPHRINE. Biosynthesis of NE takes place within the adrenergic neurons whereas EPI's biosynthesis occurs within the chromaffin cells of adrenal medulla. The general biosynthetic pathway[8] is illustrated in Figure 27.1. Starting with L-tyrosine, the enzyme tyrosine hydroxylase catalyzes the hydroxylation at the *meta* position of tyrosine to form a catechol, L-dihydroxyphenylalanine (L-DOPA). This is the rate-limiting step in NE biosynthesis. The activity of tyrosine hydroxylase is inhibited by the negative feedback mechanism upon excessive synthesis of NE.[9]

Decarboxylation of L-DOPA by L-DOPA decarboxylase, also known as aromatic L-amino acid decarboxylase, leads to the synthesis of dopamine. Dopamine is further hydroxylated on the β-carbon by dopamine β-hydroxylase giving rise to NE. NE is converted to EPI by N-methylation catalyzed by phenylethanolamine N-methyltransferase. Two major enzymes, monoamine oxidase (MAO) and catechol O-methyltransferase (COMT), metabolize NE. MAO converts a primary amine into an aldehyde through oxidative deamination. COMT metabolizes via selective transfer of a methyl group on to the *meta* hydroxyl function of the catechol moiety. Drugs that are resistant to both MAO and COMT metabolism are expected to have a longer duration of action. Since both metabolizing enzymes are present in abundance in the body, drugs inhibiting any one of the two enzymes may not improve their duration of action. General metabolic pathways for NE are given in Figure 27.2. Refer to Chapters 16, 17, or 28 for a detailed discussion.

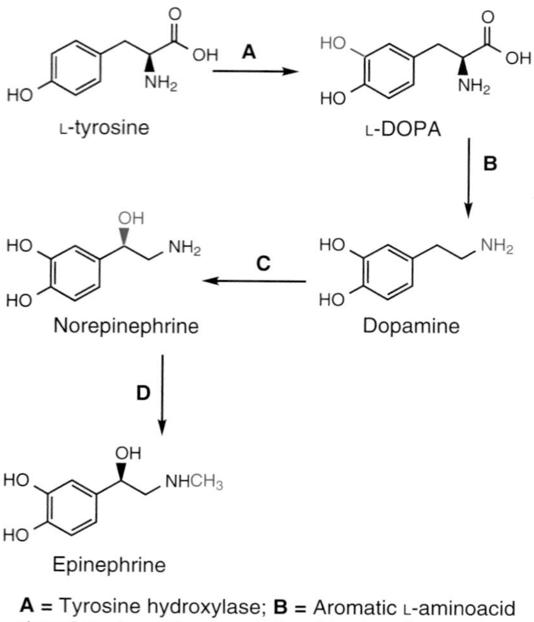

L-tyrosine → (A) → L-DOPA → (B) → Dopamine → (C) → Norepinephrine → (D) → Epinephrine

A = Tyrosine hydroxylase; B = Aromatic L-aminoacid decarboxylase; C = Dopamine β-hydroxylase; D = Phenylethanolamine N-methyl transferase.

Figure 27.1 Biosynthesis of norepinephrine and epinephrine.

Adrenergic Receptors

Adrenergic receptors are classified into α- and β-adrenoreceptors. α-Receptors are further classified into the α_1 and α_2 subtypes, and β-adrenoceptors are classified into β_1, β_2, and β_3 subtypes. Currently, three types of α_1-adrenoceptors, α_{1A}, α_{1B}, and α_{1D}, and three subtypes of α_2 receptors α_{2A}, α_{2B}, and α_{2C}, have been identified.[10] α_1-Receptors are predominantly postsynaptic, G_q-coupled receptors and are found in the vascular smooth muscles and the CNS. α_1-Receptor stimulation activates phospholipase C, which increases cellular levels of inositol 1,4,5-triphosphate (IP_3) and diacylglycerol (DAG). Released IP_3 induces the opening of the voltage-gated calcium channels allowing the influx of calcium. This leads to the activation of myosin light chain kinase (MLCK), which in turn phosphorylates myosin filaments of smooth muscles causing muscle contraction. DAG also contributes to smooth muscle contraction by activating cytosolic protein kinase C. Thus, the agonists at adrenergic α_1-receptors cause vasoconstriction thereby having utility in treating shock and nasal congestion. Nasal decongestants are most commonly administered topically to avoid systemic adverse effects such as hypertension. α_2-Receptors are presynaptic and G-inhibitory (G_i) coupled. α_2-Receptors stimulation inhibits adenylyl cyclase, which decreases intracellular cyclic adenosine monophosphate (cAMP). This action inhibits the release of NE from presynaptic terminals leading to reduced blood pressure as well as reduced intraocular pressure. α_2-Adrenergic agonists therefore have the therapeutic utility in treating hypertension and glaucoma. Stimulation of α_2-receptors found in the ciliary epithelium of the eye reduces aqueous humor production thereby reducing intraocular pressure (IOP). β_1- and β_2-receptors are predominantly postsynaptic and G-stimulatory (G_s) coupled. Stimulation activates adenylyl cyclase, which increases intracellular cAMP. β_1-Receptors are primarily present in the myocardium of the heart. Stimulation results in increased chronotropic (heart rate) and inotropic (force of contraction) effects. β_2-Receptors are found in the lungs, uterus, vascular smooth muscle, and skeletal muscle. β_2-Receptors are also present in the ciliary muscle and ciliary epithelium of the eye. Activation leads to ciliary muscle relaxation, dilation of the pupil (mydriasis) and increased aqueous humor production thereby increasing IOP (Fig. 27.3). Thus, β-blockers have found utility in the treatment of ocular hypertension. Nonselective β-blockers

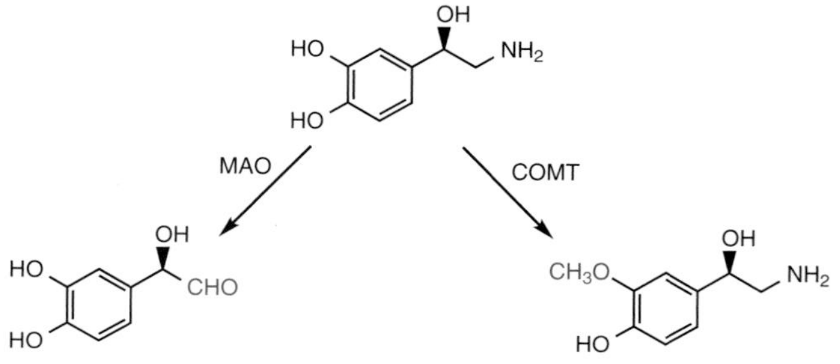

MAO / COMT

COMT= catechol-O-methyltransferase; MAO = monoamine oxidase

Figure 27.2 General metabolism of norepinephrine.

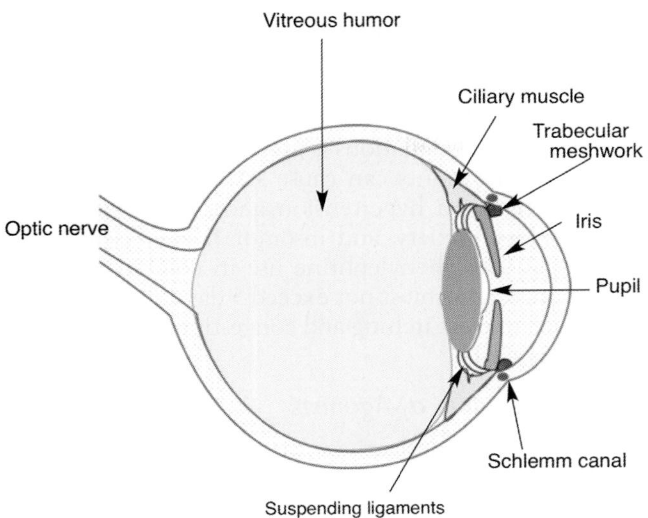

Figure 27.3 Diagram of the eyeball and key components of the eye.

such as timolol, carteolol, levobunolol, and selective β_1-blocker betaxolol are currently used in the treatment of glaucoma. Only adrenergic agonists that target α-receptors are used in treating nasal and ocular congestion.

Adrenergic Receptor Ligand Interactions

All adrenergic receptors are G protein–coupled receptors (GPCRs). In all of the adrenoceptors, the agonist/antagonist recognition site is located within the membrane-bound portion of the receptor. This binding site is within a pocket formed by the membrane-spanning regions of the peptide. The adrenergic receptor site was identified based on the mutational studies and the crystal structure of the β_2 adrenoceptor with isoproterenol. These studies identified the key amino acid residues and their interactions with the ligand functional groups at the adrenergic receptor site. Figure 27.4 illustrates binding sites for isoproterenol bound to the human β_2-receptor. Isoproterenol shows interactions with amino acid residues from transmembrane domains (TMD) 3, 5, 6, and 7.

Asp113 in transmembrane domain 3 (TMD3) of the β_2-receptor exhibits ionic or a salt bridge binding with the positively charged amine functional group of adrenergic agonists. This is a common interaction among all adrenergic receptors. Serine amino acid residues at 204 and 207 positions of TMD5 show hydrogen bonds with the catechol hydroxyl groups.[11,12] Ser204 interacts with the *meta*-hydroxyl group of the ligand, whereas Ser207 interacts specifically with the *para*-hydroxyl group of the catechol. Phenylalanine and tryptophan residues of TMD6 show van der Waals interactions with the catechol ring. Phe289, His296 of TMD6, and Asn312 of TMD7 show hydrophobic interactions with the isopropyl group of isoproterenol. In the case of α-receptors TMD7 does not have any involvement in the agonist interactions due to a smaller hydrophobic pocket in the region of the isopropyl group. This is a significant difference between α- and β-receptors. Therefore, drugs having smaller substituents on the nitrogen such as hydrogen or methyl groups bind to both α- and β-receptors, whereas nitrogen substituents larger than the methyl group shifts their selectivity to β-receptors.

When the N-alkyl group is isopropyl or larger, the agonist completely loses α-activity leaving behind only β-activity. Other critical binding sites within the α-receptors are similar to those seen in β-receptors.

Mechanism of Action of Adrenergic Agonists

There are three categories of adrenergic agonists based on their mechanism of action: direct-acting, indirect-acting, and mixed-acting adrenergic agonists. As the name itself indicates, direct-acting agonists bind directly to the adrenergic receptors and elicit intrinsic activity similar to NE. They can be selective to adrenergic receptor subtypes.

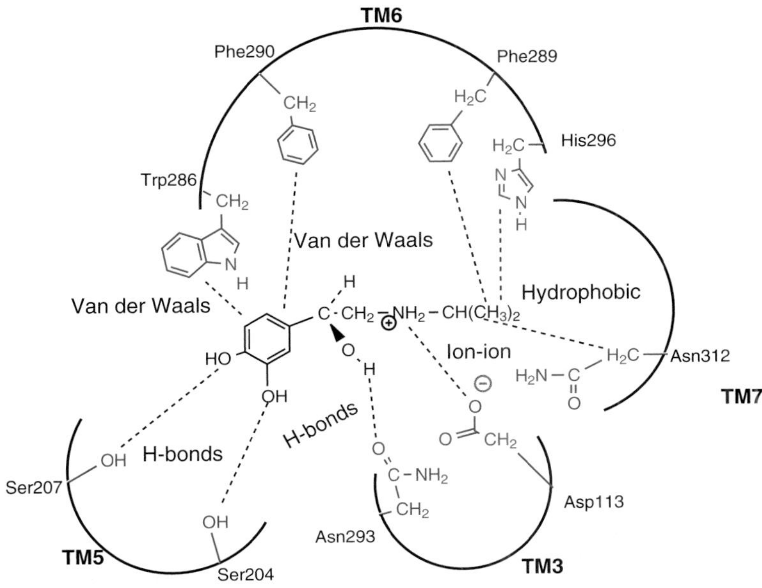

Figure 27.4 Isoproterenol-human β_2-adrenergic receptor binding interactions.

Indirect-acting adrenergic agonists act by indirect mechanisms such as inhibiting metabolism of NE, inhibiting reuptake of NE from the synapse or increasing the release of NE from synaptic vesicles. All these mechanisms increase the amount of NE at the synaptic cleft and its time spent at the receptor site. Therefore, indirect-acting agonists are nonselective to receptor subtypes as NE activates all adrenergic receptors. Mixed-acting adrenergic agonists act by the combination of both direct and indirect mechanisms.

Specific Adrenergic Receptor Agonists Used in the Treatment of Congestion Disorders

Epinephrine

EPI is an endogenous adrenergic agonist synthesized in the adrenal medulla. It binds and activates all adrenergic receptors eliciting responses similar to NE. It has a poor oral bioavailability due to extensive metabolism by MAO and COMT. It is used as a nasal decongestant due to its agonistic activity at α-adrenergic receptors. Activation of α_1-adrenergic receptors in the dilated blood vessels of the mucous membranes causes vasoconstriction and reduces nasal congestion. EPI has a limited clinical utility for treating congestion disorders due to rebound congestion. Its onset of action is about 5 minutes with less than 1-hour duration of action. Since it has a catechol functional group, it rapidly undergoes oxidation to produce a potentially toxic *o*-quinone metabolite in aqueous conditions or when exposed to light or oxygen. Therefore, it is formulated in combination with antioxidants and must be stored away from light. It must be used with caution in patients with cardiovascular disease or diabetes, as it may cause hypertension upon systemic absorption.

Phenylephrine

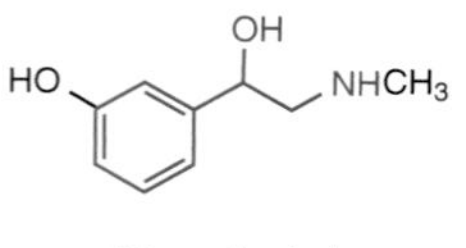

HO OH NHCH$_3$

Phenylephrine

Phenylephrine has a phenylethanolamine pharmacophore. The presence of the 3′-phenolic hydroxyl moiety improves α_1-receptor selectivity while decreasing β-receptor binding. As a result, phenylephrine has minimal cardiac stimulatory properties. Phenylephrine is very frequently found in over-the-counter decongestant in cold medications. It is not a substrate for COMT unlike EPI and hence, the duration of action is longer than EPI. Its oral bioavailability is less than 10% because of its hydrophilic properties and intestinal metabolism by MAO and 3′-O-glucuronidation/sulfate conjugation. Phenylephrine as an oral formulation is used to treat nasal and sinus congestion as well as to relieve symptoms such as sneezing, lacrimation, and itchy eyes. It is given very commonly in combination with other drugs such as anti-inflammatory drugs and antihistamines. Phenylephrine preparations applied topically to the eye to constrict the dilated blood vessels of bloodshot eyes. During surgery, a higher dose phenylephrine formulations is used to dilate pupil.

Oral decongestants can cause systemic adverse effects such as tachycardia, hypertension, and CNS adverse effects (e.g., tremors, anxiety, and insomnia). Hence, in hypertensive patients phenylephrine use in combination with oral decongestants must not exceed 5 days. Phenylephrine is also used to treat itching and congestion caused by allergic conjunctivitis.

2-Arylimidazoline α_1-Agonists

The imidazoline derivatives shown in Figure 27.5 are selective α_1-agonists with vasoconstrictor/vasopressor activity.[13] Arylimidazoline analogues are structurally very different from traditional adrenergic agonists and NE/EPI. The α-adrenoceptors can accommodate a very diverse assortment of ligand structures.

STRUCTURE-ACTIVITY RELATIONSHIPS. The imidazolines contain a one-carbon bridge between the C-2 of the imidazoline ring (pK_a range, 10-11) and a phenyl substituent. The phenylethylamine pharmacophore exists within the heterocyclic arylimidazoline structures as indicated in Figure 27.5.

Lipophilic substitution (e.g., methyl) on the phenyl ring *ortho* to the methylene bridge appears to be required for agonist activity at α_1- and α_2-receptors.[14] Presumably, the bulky lipophilic groups attached to the phenyl ring at the *para* positions provide selectivity for the α_1-receptor by diminishing affinity for α_2-receptors. The arylimidazolines do not have a chiral center unlike most adrenergic agonists. Quaternization of the imidazoline nitrogen or replacement of nitrogen with another heteroatom (e.g., oxygen) significantly reduces activity.

Imidazoline derivatives bind differently at the adrenergic α_1-receptor active site compared to the phenylethanolamines. The arylimidazolines bind more like antagonists through van der Waals interactions with Phe308 and Phe312 in the transmembrane domain 7 (TMD-7) (Fig. 27.6A). This could be the reason for their partial agonistic properties. Mutations at either Phe308 or Phe312 significantly reduces imidazoline's agonist affinity compared to

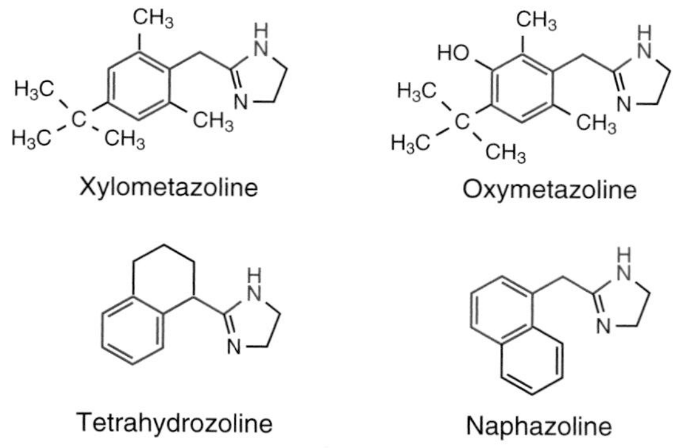

Xylometazoline

Oxymetazoline

Tetrahydrozoline

Naphazoline

Figure 27.5 Imidazoline α_1-adrenergic agonists.

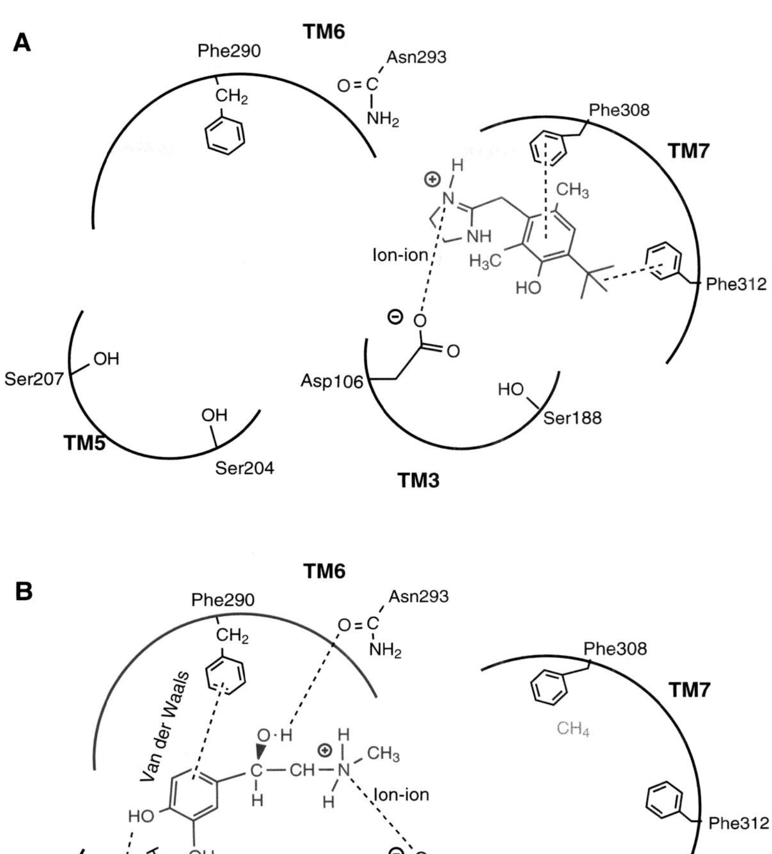

Figure 27.6 Representation of oxymetazoline and epinephrine (EPI) binding to the α_1-adrenergic receptor pocket. A, Oxymetazoline, α_2-arylimidazoline α_1-adrenergic agonist binding to the receptor pocket, as compared to (B), EPI binding to the same receptor pocket.

phenylethanolamines or EPI at the adrenergic α_1-receptors.[15] The lipophilic functional groups on the aryl ring of imidazolines show essential van der waals interactions with Phe308 and Phe312 in the TM-7. These groups are also responsible for their selectivity for α_1-receptors. The orientation of arylimidazolines at the α_1-receptor is in sharp contrast to epinephrine binding where the phenyl ring is oriented toward TM-5 (Fig. 27.6B). Nitrogen on the imidazole ring undergoes protonation under physiological pH and shows required hydrogen bonding with Asp106 on TM3. A general overview of structure-activity relationship (SAR) studies for arylimidazolines is given in Figure 27.7.

PHARMACOKINETICS. Arylimidazoline adrenergic agonists are highly ionic in nature. They are widely used in topical preparations as nasal decongestants and eye drops for conditions associated with the common cold, influenza, sinusitis, allergic and nonallergic rhinitis, and upper respiratory track infections (Table 27.2). Due to potent vasoconstrictor activity they are not used systemically.

Upon topical administration, oxymetazoline gets minimally absorbed into the systemic circulation. The absorbed drug is metabolized by CYP2C19 resulting in hydroxylation of the *t*-butyl group to produce a monohydroxy derivative. The resultant phenolic hydroxyl group is conjugated via UGT-mediated glucoronidation. An imidazole metabolite produced through CYP2C19 catalyzed oxidative dehydrogenation of imidazoline ring has been reported as shown in Figure 27.8. Additionally, oxymetazoline can undergo bioactivation to produce a reactive toxic intermediate, which is converted in to glutathione conjugation in the liver.[16,17] Xylometazoline is rapidly absorbed in to the nasal mucosa with rapid onset of action.

Clinical Application

The duration of action of topical α_1-adrenergic agonists used in nasal and ocular decongestants differ significantly. Phenylephrine has a short duration of action of less than 4 hours; naphazoline and tetrahydrozoline have intermediate duration of action of approximately 4-6 hours; and oxymetazoline and xylometazoline have a longer duration of action of nearly 12 hours. Prolonged use of these medications will lead to rebound congestion which may

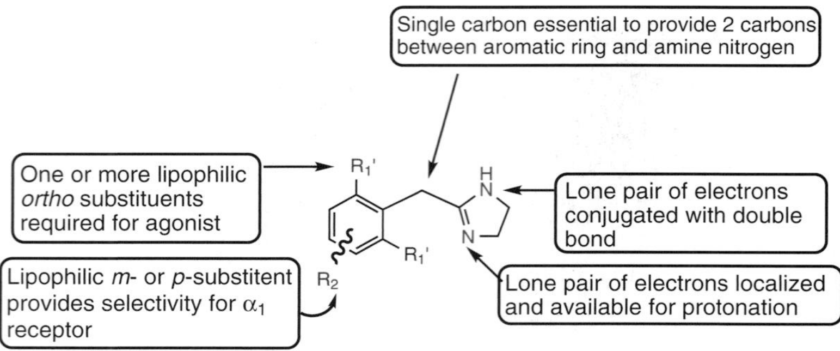

Figure 27.7 Structure-activity relationship (SAR) of arylimidazoline agonists.

be severe.[13] Their use should be restricted to less than 5 days, and patient counseling on rebound congestion upon prolonged usage should occur. Caution must be exercised while using in an elderly population or patients with cardiovascular disease, glaucoma, and diabetes.[18] It should be noted that these products are often found in combination with an antihistamine (i.e., pheniramine).

Mixed-Acting Sympathomimetics

Mixed-acting sympathomimetics are common ingredients in many cold medications with oral decongestant formulations. These are commonly given in combination with antihistamines. The systemic sympathomimetic products generally have a slower onset but longer duration of action compared to topical decongestants and do not cause irritation to the nasal membranes or rebound congestion after completion of the therapy as is seen with topical decongestants.

PHENYLPROPANOLAMINES

Mechanism of Action. The mixed-acting sympathomimetics with the phenylpropanolamine pharmacophore have no substituents on the phenyl ring (Fig. 27.9). This makes them both direct- and indirect-acting agonists. Their direct action comes from binding to both α- and β-adrenoceptors and Indirect action results from displacing NE from the synaptic vesicles or reuptake inhibition thereby increasing NE concentration at the adrenergic receptors. Because NE stimulates both α- and β-adrenoceptors, indirect activity cannot be selective. These drugs are more frequently used as oral decongestants. The stereochemistry of the various substituents can also play a role in determining the extent of direct/indirect activity. For example, ephedrine and pseudoephedrine have the same substitution pattern (Fig. 27.9), but substitution at both chiral carbons produces four stereoisomers.

Racemic (±)-ephedrine is a mixture of the *erythro* enantiomers 1*R*,2*S* and 1*S*,2*R*, whereas the *threo* pair of enantiomers, 1*R*,2*R* and 1*S*,2*S*, are found in racemic pseudoephedrine (ψ-ephedrine). (−)-Ephedrine is the naturally occurring stereoisomer and has the 1*R*,2*S* absolute configuration with a mixed activity on both α- and β-receptors and some indirect activity. Its 1*S*,2*R*-(+)-enantiomer exhibits primarily indirect activity. 1*S*,2*S*-(+)-Pseudoephedrine has virtually no direct receptor activity but with indirect activity.

Specific Drugs

(-)-Ephedrine. Ephedrine (Fig. 27.9) is a natural product isolated from several species of ephedra plants, used for centuries in Chinese folk medicine. Its occurrence in ephedra represents approximately 80%-90% of the alkaloid content. Other alkaloids also found include (+)-pseudoephedrine (10%-15%) and N-methylephedrine (2%-5%). Ephedrine's sympathomimetic activity was not recognized until 1917, and the pure drug was used clinically even before epinephrine and norepinephrine were isolated and characterized. Ephedrine does not have any phenolic substituents, making it a mixed-acting adrenergic agonist. It has good oral bioavailability because it lacks a catechol function and therefore is not a substrate for COMT. Additionally, ephedrine is not metabolized by MAO due to the presence of an α-methyl group which

Table 27.2 Imidazoline α_1-Agonists in Over-the-Counter Vasoconstrictors

Generic Name	Nasal Decongestant: Trade Names	Dosage Form	Duration of Action	Eye Drops: Trade Names	Dosage Form
Xylometazoline	Otrivin, Inspire	Drop/spray	12 hr	—	
Oxymetazoline	Afrin, Duration, Neo-Synephrine, Vicks Sinex	Spray	12 hr	Visine L.R.	Drops/solution
Tetrahydrozoline	Tyzine	Spray/solution	4-6 hr	Murine, Visine, Soothe	Drops
Naphazoline	4-Way Fast Acting, Privine	Spray	4-6 hr	Naphcon, Clear Eyes	Drops/solution

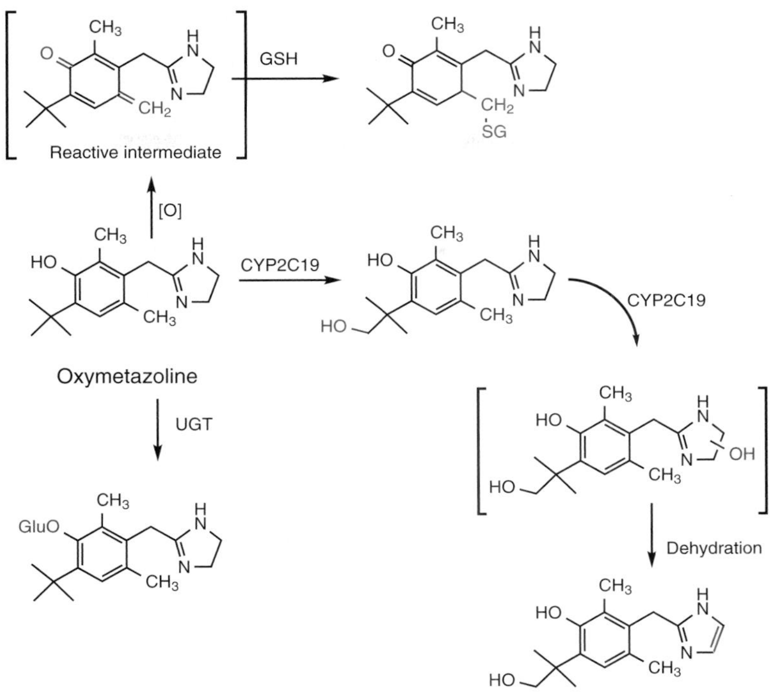

Figure 27.8 Metabolism of oxymetazoline.

sterically hinders metabolism by MAO. Lacking hydrogen-bonding phenolic substituents, ephedrine is more lipophilic and crosses the blood-brain barrier (BBB) far better than the catechol containing agonists, thus causing CNS adverse effects. Because of its ability to penetrate the BBB, ephedrine has also been used as a CNS stimulant. Ephedrine is widely used for many of the same indications as EPI, including use as a bronchodilator, vasopressor, cardiac stimulant, and nasal decongestant.

(+)-Pseudoephedrine. Pseudoephedrine (Fig. 27.9), as previously discussed, is the *threo* (*S*,*S*) diastereomer of ephedrine, with virtually no direct activity and fewer CNS adverse effects than ephedrine. (+)-Pseudoephedrine is widely used as a nasal decongestant. The most common adverse effects of pseudoephedrine include restlessness, nausea, vomiting, weakness, and headache. Currently its sales is restricted because it can be used in the illicit manufacture of the widely abused drug methamphetamine. Pseudoephedrine is sold from behind the counter to control its availability. Pseudoephedrine is available in both sustained as well as controlled release formulations. Due to vasoconstriction effects of pseudoephedrine, it is used with caution in hypertensive patients. It might antagonize the actions of antihypertensive drugs such methyldopa, carvedilol, and labetalol. It is contraindicated in combination with MAOIs, as it can lead to life threatening hypertension.

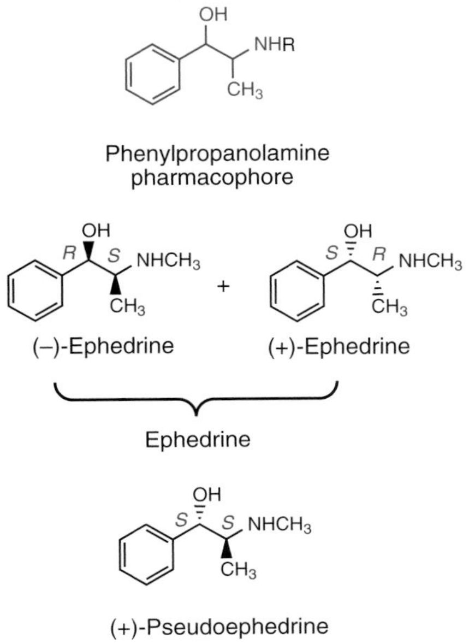

Figure 27.9 Ephedrine and pseudoephedrine

Intranasal Corticosteroids

Sneezing, nasal congestions, and rhinorrhea are the common symptoms of allergic rhinitis and occur in response to the release of histamine, prostaglandins, and leukotrienes following exposure to external allergens. The nasal steroids have proven effective in reducing inflammation arising from the exposure to allergens as well as relieve the symptoms of congestion and mucus production.

MECHANISM OF ACTION. Steroids work through a multitude of mechanisms including inhibition of immunoglobulin E (IgE)–dependent release of histamine and inhibition of the synthesis and release of cytokines and chemokines from T-lymphocytes, epithelial cells, eosinophils, and mast cells.[19] The exact mechanism of action of the intranasal corticosteroids remains unclear.

STRUCTURE-ACTIVITY RELATIONSHIP STUDIES. The steroid basic structure has the cyclopentanoperhydrophenanthrene nucleus with specific functional groups essential for both glucocorticoid and mineralocorticoid activity. These include the unsaturation and a ketone in ring A, free hydroxyl groups at C-11 in ring B, and a ketol and hydroxyl groups at the C-17 side chain. By esterifying at the C-21 hydroxyl a prodrug can be produced (see metabolism below).

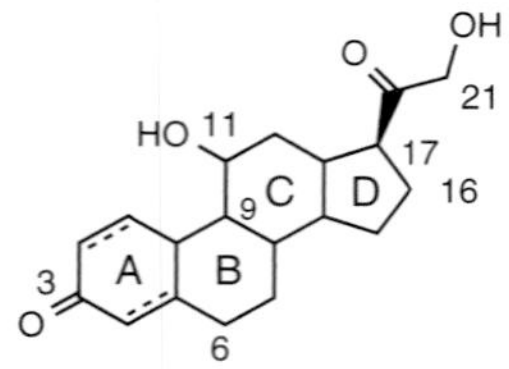

Basic nucleus required for gluco- and mineralocorticoid activity

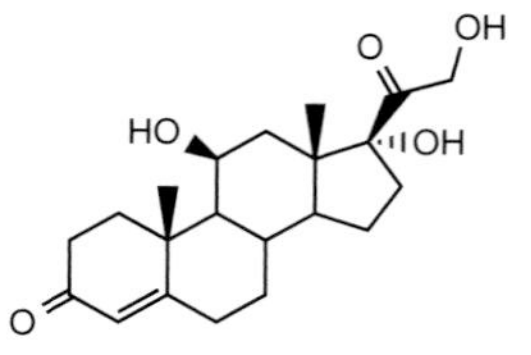

Hydrocortisone

Additionally this position is commonly used to adjust the lipophilicity of the drug thereby the duration of action. Substituents at other locations also affect lipophilicity and activity such as a methyl substitution at C-6 position and substitution at C-16. Both of these substitutions abolishes mineralocorticoid activity leaving behind only glucocorticoid activity. Lipophilic halogen substitutions at C-9 increases both glucocorticoid and mineralocorticoid activity whereas halogen substitution at C-6 increases only glucocorticoid activity without altering mineralocorticoid activity.[20] Hydrocortisone represents the prototype corticosteroid.

The commonly used nasal corticosteroids include beclomethosone dipropionate and beclomethosone dipropionate monohydrate, budesonide, ciclesonide, fluticasone furoate, fluticasone propionate, mometasone furoate monohydrate, and triamconolone acetonide (Fig. 27.10).

PHARMACOKINETICS. Intranasal corticosteroids are generally available as nasal sprays, as their action is on the tissue of the nasal passage. While the benefit of the intranasal corticosteroids for treatment of allergic rhinitis is local, varying amounts of the administered drug is swallowed and absorbed from the intestinal track. As a result, plasma levels of the administered drug can be measured and systemic drug metabolism does occur to some extent. Additionally, several corticosteroids are prodrugs (i.e., beclomethasone dipropionate and ciclesonide). The C-21 ester group must be metabolized to a free alcohol, which is the active form, and as a result, awareness of the active form of the drug and the metabolism of the corticosteroids is important (Fig. 27.11).[21-23] An exception to this is that both fluticasone and mometasone are active as such even without a free –OH group at C-21 position.

As indicated in Figure 27.10 the intranasal corticosteroids are available as prescription products as well as over-the-counter (OTC) products. Local adverse effects include nasal irritation, burning, stinging, sore throat, and, in rare cases, bleeding. The benefits of nasal steroids are seen only after 2-3 weeks. Detailed steroidal drugs mechanism, SAR, and metabolism are discussed in Chapters 21 and 28.

Drugs Used for Treating Glaucoma

Glaucoma is the major leading cause for irreversible vision loss due to damage to the optic nerve head. There are two types of glaucoma, open-angle glaucoma and angle-closure glaucoma. Open-angle glaucoma is most commonly seen in the United States. The pathophysiology of glaucoma is not clearly understood but the optic neuropathy is associated with the increase in the intraocular pressure (IOP). Therefore, the drugs that help reduce IOP can prevent or delay optic nerve damage leading to blindness. It is estimated about 70 million people worldwide are affected by glaucoma with nearly 10% being classified as bilaterally

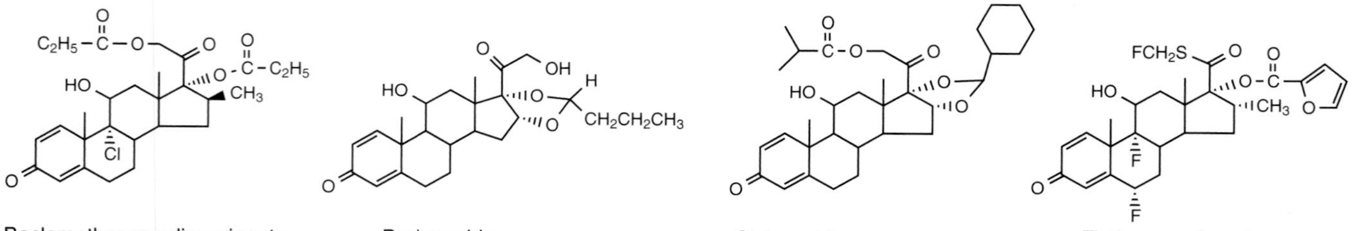

Beclomethasone dipropionate (Beconase AQ, Qnasl)

Budesonide (Rhinocort Allergy**)

Ciclesonide (Omnaris)

Fluticasone furoate (Flonase Sensimist Allergy Relief**)

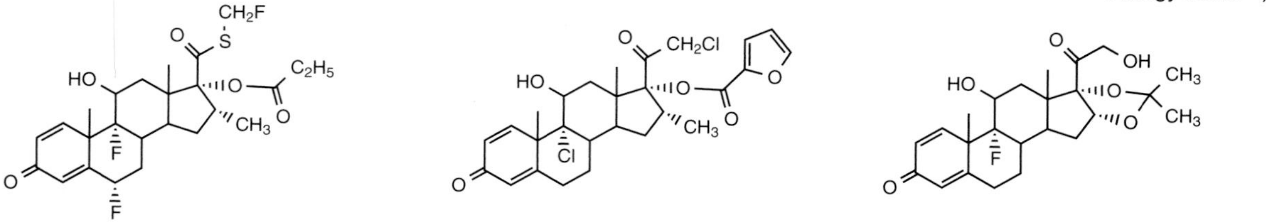

Fluticasone propionate (Flonase Allergy Relief**)

Mometasone furoate (Nasonex)

Triamcinolone acetonide (Nasacort Allergy 24 hr**)

**Indicates products that are available over-the-counter.

Figure 27.10 Intranasal corticosteroids.

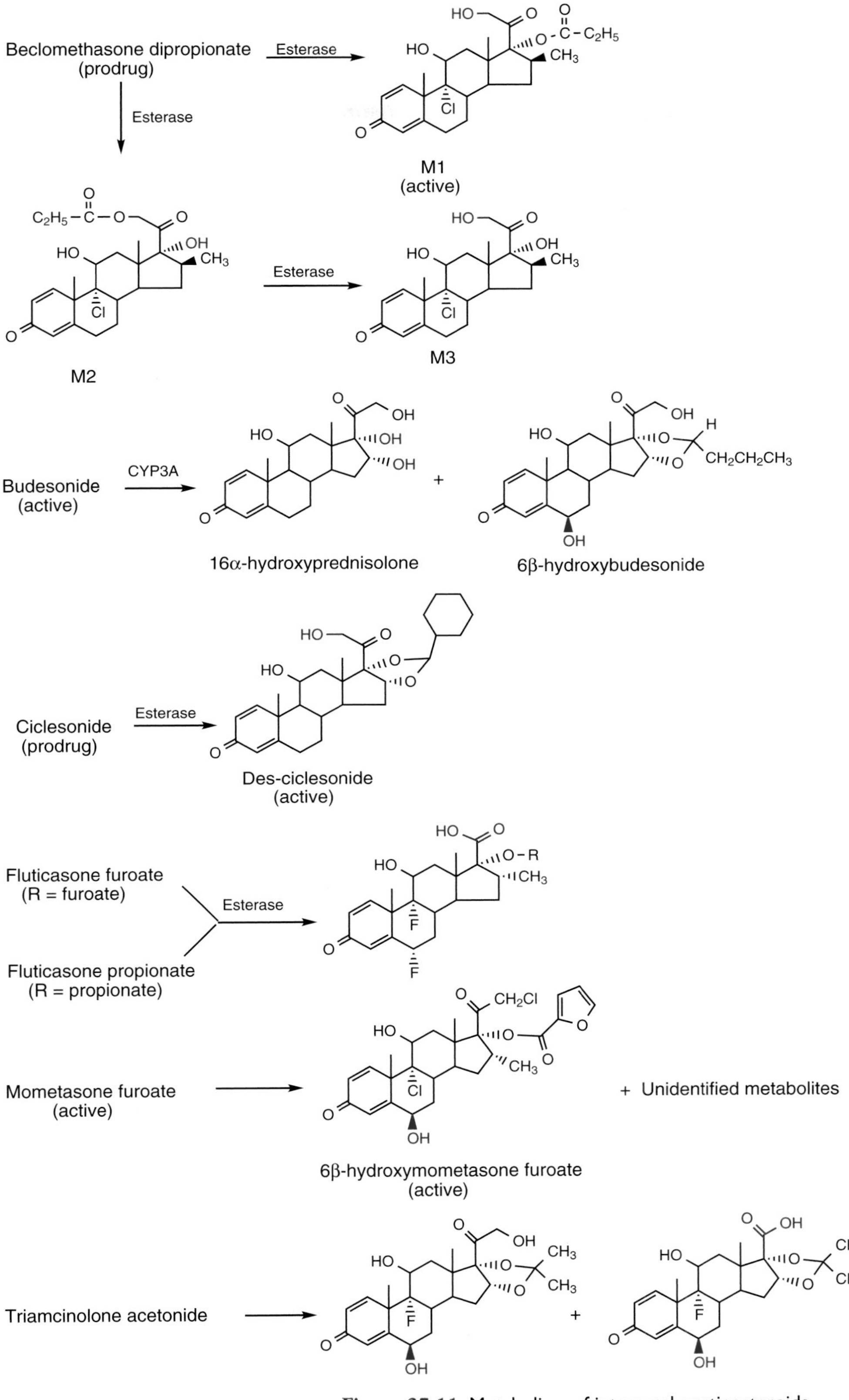

Figure 27.11 Metabolism of intranasal corticosteroids.

blind.[24] An estimated six million people worldwide may go blind by 2020 if untreated. In a majority of cases glaucoma is asymptomatic until which time the diagnosis and treatment become quite difficult. Major risk factors include high IOP, old age, hypertension, diabetes, and thin central cornea.[25]

In normal conditions, aqueous humor from the eye flows out through trabecular network. In open-angle glaucoma, the trabecular network is blocked internally, whereas in angle-closure glaucoma, it is blocked by the iris (see Fig. 27.3). When the trabecular network is blocked,

IOP increases leading to damage to the optic nerve head, interfering with the transmission of optical images to the brain. Increased pressure in the eye is manifested via eye pain, headache, and blurred vision. Genetic defects may also lead to glaucoma. There are about 15 genes identified that contribute to the development of glaucoma. The major treatment goal for glaucoma is to reduce the IOP, which has shown to delay or prevent the disease onset and progression. Prostaglandin analogues are used as first-line agents to treat glaucoma. Apart from that muscarinic agonists, β-blockers, adrenergic α-agonists, and carbonic anhydrase inhibitors are also used.[26] In most cases, the ophthalmic drugs are administered topically. Absorption and duration of action for topical ophthalmic formulations can be adjusted by varying the formulation or vehicle used. Topical medications work either by increasing the outflow of aqueous humor (prostaglandin analogues, adrenergic and cholinergic agonists) or by reducing aqueous humor production (α-adrenergic agonists, β-blockers, and carbonic anhydrase inhibitors). The various classes of drugs used are discussed below.

α_2-Adrenergic Agonists—Their Role in Treatment of Glaucoma

The agonist action at α_2-receptors in the eye reduces IOP by decreasing the aqueous humor production and increasing its outflow thus reducing the IOP. The α_2-receptors are presynaptic receptors present on the outer membrane of the nerve terminus. The α_2-receptor serves as a sensor and modulator of the quantity of neurotransmitter present in the synapse at any given moment. Thus, during periods of rapid nerve firing and neurotransmitter release, the α_2-receptor is stimulated and causes an inhibition of further release of neurotransmitter. This is a well-characterized mechanism for modulation of neurotransmission. But not all α_2-receptors are presynaptic, and the physiologic significance of postsynaptic α_2-receptors is less well understood.[27] The α_2-receptor can use more than one effector system depending on the location of the receptor. The best-understood effector system of the α_2-receptor appears to be similar to that of the β-receptors, except that linkage via a G protein (G_i) leads to inhibition of adenylyl cyclase instead of activation.

α_2-Adrenoceptors are of three subtypes α_{2A}, α_{2B}, and α_{2C}, and agonists at these sites find clinical utility as antiglaucoma drugs, antihypertensives, and analgesics. Clonidine, was introduced as an antihypertensive drug, an effect attributed to its action on central α_{2A}-adrenoceptors.[28] The imidazolines, which include clonidine, are effective in the treatment of glaucoma through their α_2-adrenergic agonist activity are shown in Figure 27.12.

IMIDAZOLINE α_2-RECEPTOR AGONISTS. Structural modification of the previously reported nasal decongestant arylimidazolines in which the aryl and imidazoline are connected by a CH_2 group (X = CH_2; Fig. 27.12) is replaced with an -NH- group gave rise to the arylaminoimidazolines class (X = NH; Fig. 27.12). Unlike the nasal decongestant arylimidazolines which possess α_1-agonist activity (Fig. 27.5) the newly discovered drugs exhibit α_2-receptors agonist activity.

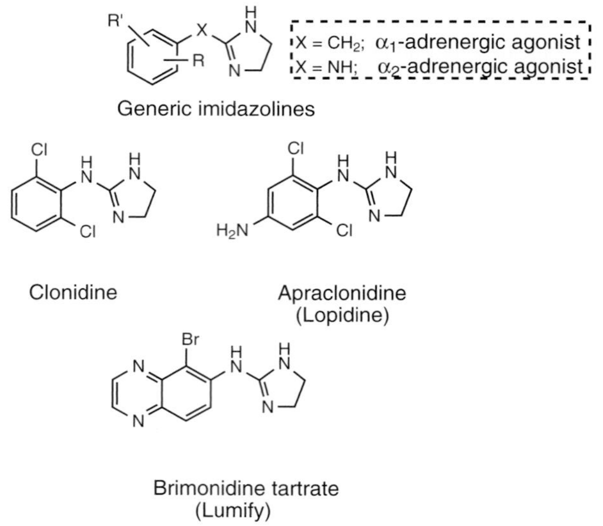

X = CH_2; α_1-adrenergic agonist
X = NH; α_2-adrenergic agonist

Generic imidazolines

Clonidine

Apraclonidine (Lopidine)

Brimonidine tartrate (Lumify)

Figure 27.12 Imidazoline α_2-adrenergic agonists.

Clonidine is the prototype α_2-agonist. By replacing the CH_2 with a NH gives rise to a guanidine functional group. Clonidine in the uncharged form exists as a pair of tautomers with the physiochemical properties of pK_a of 8.3 and a log $D_{pH\ 7.4}$ = 1.03.

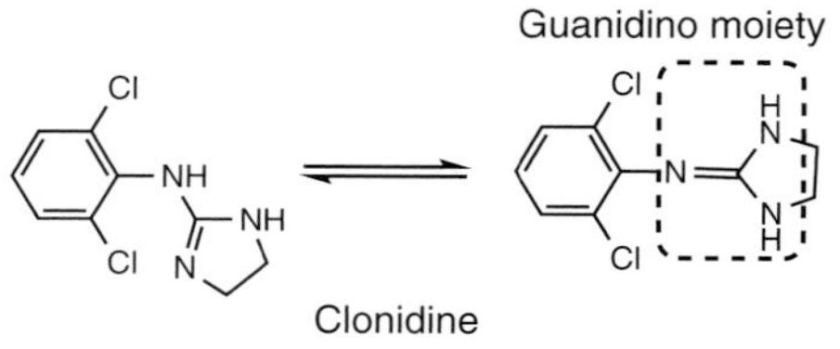

Guanidino moiety

Clonidine

The pK_a value indicates an approximately 80% ionization at physiological pH, and the log D is the result of the lipophilic *ortho*-dichloro substituents on the phenyl ring.

While developed as a potential nasal decongestant, clonidine was found to possess hypotensive activity along with potential therapeutic benefit of reducing high IOP in glaucoma. Because of the high lipophilicity, the drug has the ability to cross the blood-brain barrier, causing significant CNS effects which has limited its utility for treating glaucoma. This led to the development of its close analogues apraclonidine and brimonidine (Fig. 27.12).

Apraclonidine and Brimonidine. Apraclonidine (pK_a = 9.22; log $D_{pH\ 7.4}$ = 0.01) is highly ionized at physiological pH and is much more polar, and as a result, it does not cross the blood-brain barrier as readily making a good candidate for treating glaucoma with fewer CNS adverse effects. Brimonidine (pK_a = 7.4; log $D_{pH\ 7.4}$ = 0.49) is lipophilic enough to cross BBB causing fatigue and/or drowsiness in some patients.

Both drugs through stimulation of α_2-receptors in the eye reduces production of aqueous humor and enhances its outflow, thus reducing intraocular pressure. They also have a neuroprotective effect apparently through α_{2A}-receptors located in the retina.[29,30] Apraclonidine's primary mechanism of action is due to a reduction of aqueous humor formation, whereas brimonidine lowers intraocular pressure by reducing aqueous humor production and increasing uveoscleral outflow. Brimonidine is approximately 1,000-fold more selective for α_2-receptors than are clonidine or apraclonidine. It exhibits minimal cardio stimulatory effects. Although both are applied topically to the eye, measurable quantities of these drugs are detectable in plasma, so caution must be employed when cardiovascular agents are coadministered. Plasma brimonidine levels peaked within 1-4 hours and declined with a systemic half-life of approximately 3 hours. Apraclonidine and briminidine, have a duration of action of 4 and 8 hours, respectively, requiring twice or thrice a day dosing. That is why they are considered second line agents for treating glaucoma after the introduction of prostaglandin analogues. Both drugs are contraindicated in patients receiving MAOI therapy. Tricyclic antidepressants have been shown to reduce the therapeutic effects of apraclonidine. Major adverse effects of apraclonidine include discomfort, hyperemia, and pruritis in the eye. Major adverse effects of brimonidine include allergic conjunctivitis, conjunctival hyperemia, and eye pruritus.

β-Adrenergic Receptor Blockers

MECHANISM OF ACTION. As previously discussed, intraocular pressure can be reduced by decreasing the production of aqueous humor from the ciliary body or increasing the outflow from the anterior chamber through the trabecular network. β-Adrenergic receptor blockers decrease the aqueous humor production by blocking β-adrenergic receptors on the ciliary body. Adrenergic β-receptors are of three subtypes, β_1, β_2, and β_3. Apart from the eye, these receptors are distributed in other organs such as β_1-receptors in cardiac smooth muscle, β_2-receptors in bronchioles, and β_3-receptors in adipose tissue. β-blockers that are currently used in the treatment of glaucoma include betaxolol, carteolol, levobunolol, metipranolol, and timolol. All of these are nonselective β-blockers except for betaxolol, which is selective β_1-blocker.

STRUCTURE-ACTIVITY RELATIONSHIPS. All β-blockers used in the treatment of glaucoma have an aryloxypropanolamine pharmacophore. These agents are more potent β-blockers than the corresponding arylethanolamines. In addition to the use of β-blockers for the treatment of glaucoma these drugs have found wide spread use in treating hypertension (see Chapter 17).

OH H
O N-R1
R2

Aryloxypropanolamine pharmacophore

For maximum effectiveness in receptor binding, the hydroxy group in aryloxypropanolamines must occupy the same region in space as it does for the phenylethanolamine agonists in the *R* absolute configuration. Because of the insertion of an oxygen atom in the side chain of the aryloxypropanolamines, the Cahn-Ingold-Prelog priority of the substituents around the asymmetric carbon changes, and the isomer with the required special arrangement now has the *S* absolute configuration. General overview of SAR is given in Figure 27.13.

Substitution at the 4 position of the aryl group results in selectivity as β_1-blockers (Fig. 27.14). Metipranolol is an exception to this rule in that although it has substitution at the 4-position it is a non-selective β-blocker.

PHARMACOKINETICS. In general the aryloxypropanolamine β-blockers have a rapid onset (1-2 hr) and duration of action (verses other β-blockers) ranging from 12-24 hours and are normally administered one or two times daily.[31] While some systemic absorption is possible this is usually minimal and as a result little is reported concerning metabolism or excretion.

ADVERSE EFFECTS. Dose-dependent follicular conjunctivitis is a common adverse effect.[26] Systemic absorption of β-blockers used in treating glaucoma may present adverse effects associated with their binding elsewhere in the body such as bradycardia (β_1), bronchospasms (β_2) as well as other adverse effects including depression, fatigue and ocular dryness. Some of these adverse effects can be lowered or avoided by closing the eyelid for at least 1 minute after administering the topical formulation that prevents

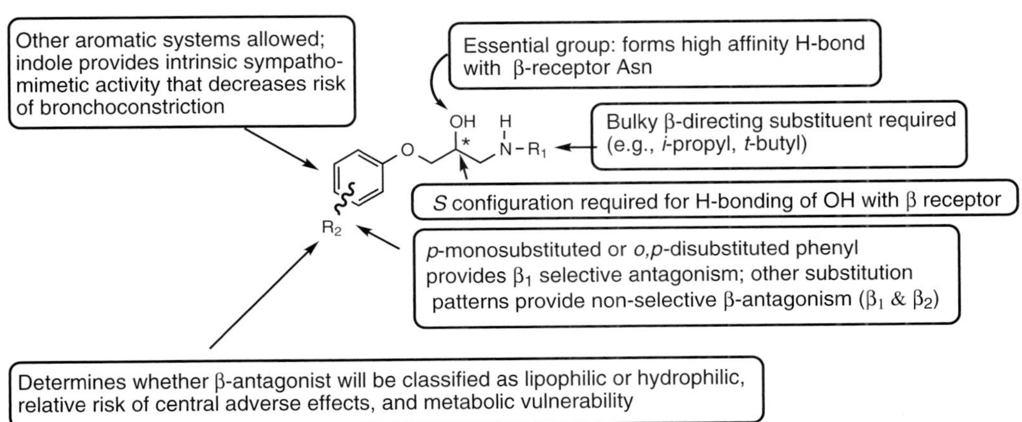

Figure 27.13 Aryloxypropanolamine β-adrenergic antagonist structure-activity relationship (SAR).

Nonselective:

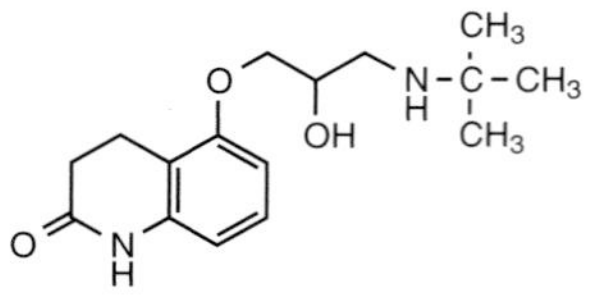

Carteolol
(generic)

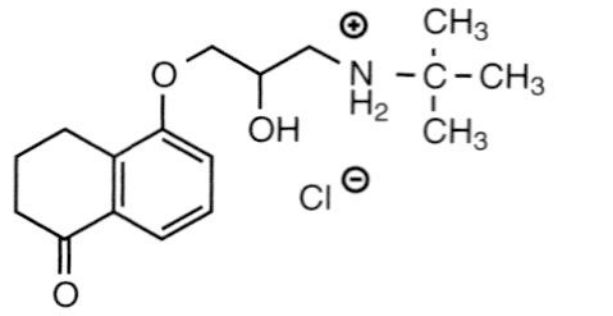

Levobunolol HCl
(Akbet, Betagan)

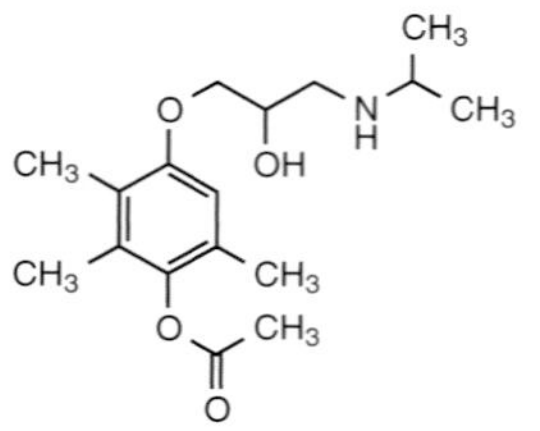

Metipranolol
(Optipranolol)

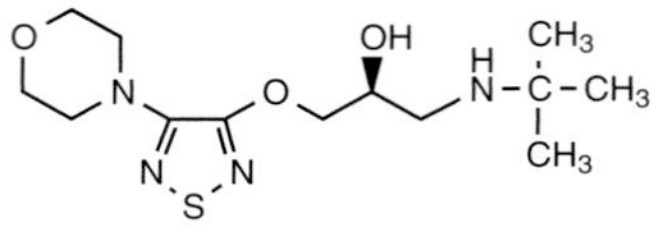

Timolol
(Betimol, Istalol, Timoptic)

β_1-selective:

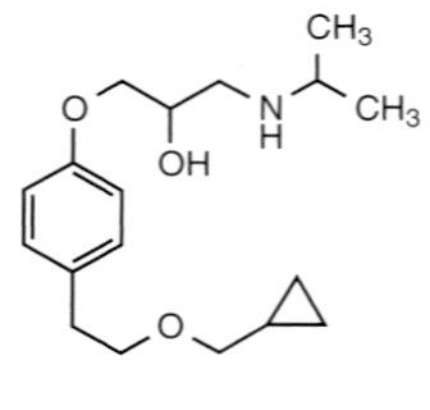

Betaxolol HCl
(Betoptic)

Figure 27.14 β-Blockers used in the treatment of glaucoma.

systemic absorption through nasolacrimal duct. Betaxolol being a selective β_1-blocker presents fewer respiratory adverse effects.[32] In general β-blockers are contraindicated in patients with bronchial asthma, COPD, sinus bradycardia, or cardiac failure. Coadministration of oral β-blockers may lead to additive effects. β-blockers were previously considered first-line therapy for glaucoma until the advent of prostaglandin analogue therapy.

Prostaglandin Analogues

Prostaglandin analogues are the first-line therapy for glaucoma. Bimatoprost, latanoprost, tafluprost, and travoprost (Fig. 27.15) are currently indicated for treating glaucoma or ocular hypertension.

MECHANISM OF ACTION. As previously indicated an increase in the ocular pressure is one of the major causes of optic nerve damage in primary open-angle glaucoma patients. This is due to the increase in the production and/or decrease in the out flow of aqueous humor in the eye. In the normal eye, outflow of aqueous humor occurs mostly through the trabecular meshwork while the uveoscleral pathway (also referred to as the unconventional outflow pathway) is a minor pathway. The prostaglandin derivatives increase the aqueous humor outflow from the anterior chamber of the eye thereby reducing IOP, but the exact mechanism is presently unknown. The action of these drugs include agonistic binding at the prostaglandin F (FP) receptor an action similar to that of the natural ($PGF_{2\alpha}$), but there is mounting evidence that these drugs may act through a mimicking action on the uveoscleral pathway. The relative affinity of prostaglandins for

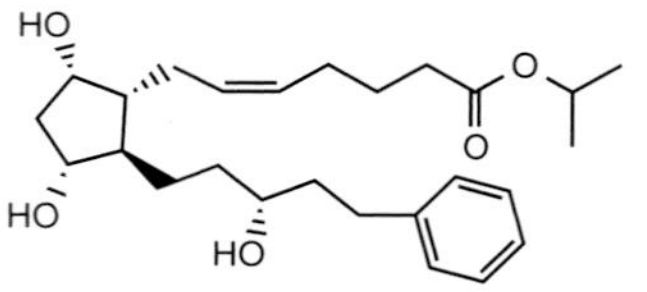

Latanoprost
(Vyzulta, Xalatan, Xelpros)

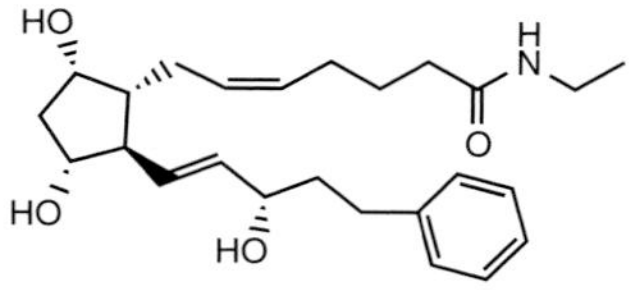

Bimatoprost
(Latisse, Lumigan)

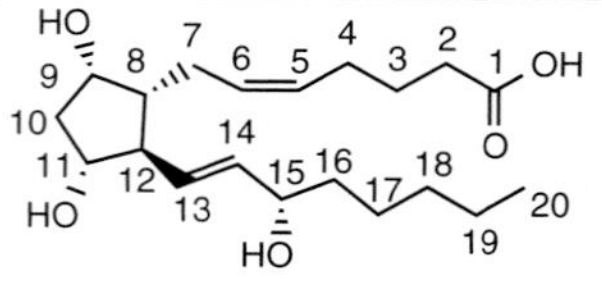

Prostaglandin $F_{2\alpha}$

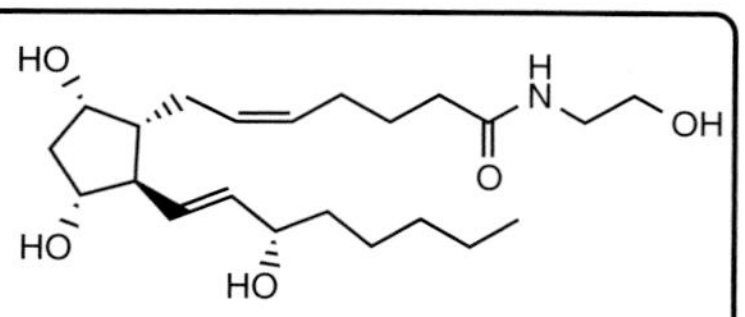

Prostamide $F_{2\alpha}$

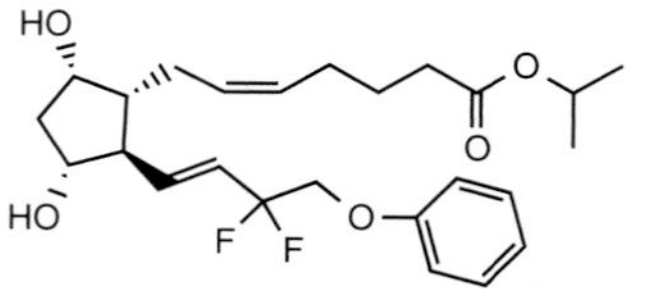

Tafluprost
(Zioptan)

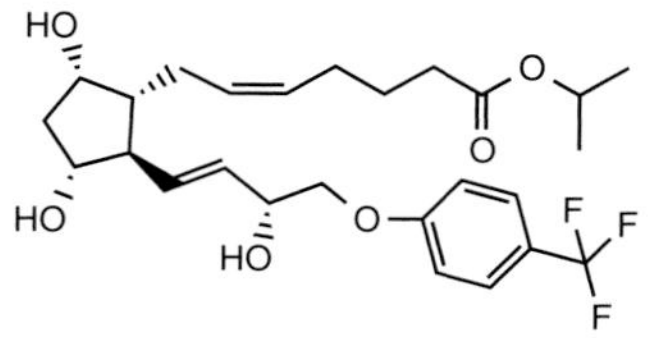

Travoprost
(Travatan Z)

Figure 27.15 Prostaglandin analogues.

FP receptor are $PGF_{2\alpha}$ > PGD_2 > PGE_2 > PGI_2 = TXA_2. The FP receptor is a G protein–coupled receptor (GPCR) and is a G_q type. Upon activation, this receptor couples to G-protein Rho via G_q independent mechanisms resulting in the activation of phospholipase C which causes muscle contraction.[33] FP receptors are found in the ciliary muscle and trabecular meshwork cells of the eye and upon their activation leads to a widening and drainage of the channels (uveoscleral pathway), increasing the outflow of aqueous humor from the anterior chamber through the Schlemm canal. Prostaglandin analogues reduce IOP by 25%-30%.

SPECIFIC DRUGS

Latanoprost. Latanoprost is a $PGF_{2\alpha}$ analogue, which is formulated as a sterile, isotonic, buffered aqueous solution. Latanoprost is a prodrug, which is rapidly metabolized in the cornea by esterase to produce the active metabolite latanoprost acid (Fig. 27.16). Further metabolism of latanoprost acid occurs in the liver via successive β-oxidations the first of which results in removal of two carbons (dinor) and then two additional carbons (tetranor) to give an acid, which can exist as a lactone (these same metabolic reactions occur with all four of the prostaglandin derivatives [Fig. 27.15]). The only metabolites found in the urine are oxidative products.[34] The plasma half-life of latanoprost is ~17 minutes. Reduction of IOP starts within 3-4 hours and peaks after 8-12 hours. The drug is indicated to treat elevated intraocular pressure in patients with open-angle glaucoma or ocular hypertension.

BIMATOPROST. Bimatoprost is also a prostaglandin $F_{2\alpha}$ analogue (Fig. 27.15), indicated for treating ocular hypertension. Unlike latanoprost, tafluprost, and travoprost the amide nature of this drug results in a significantly more stable product, which is active in its own right.[35,36] It has been suggested that bimatoprost may be active by virtue of its ability to interfere with the biosynthesis of prostamide $F_{2\alpha}$ at a yet to be defined FP receptor. An agonist at this receptor might be expected to increase the aqueous humor outflow via the uveoscleral pathway without effecting production of aqueous humor. In addition to its stability the amide helps improve the lipophilicity, which facilitate absorption through the corneal membrane. There is no indication that bimatoprost is hydrolyzed in the eye nor has the activity due to bimatoprost acid formation unlike the action of latanoprost acid or travoprost acid.[37] Bimatoprost is well absorbed through the cornea reaching peak plasma concentration within 10 minutes. It is highly bound to plasma protein (88%) and is eliminated within 90 minutes of administration. Bimatoprost is metabolized by oxidation, N-deethylation, and glucuronidation. It is a substrate of CYP3A4. Bimatoprost is available as 0.01% and 0.03% solutions. Common adverse effects associated with bimatoprost include eye irritation, hyperpigmentation of the iris, periorbital tissue and eyelashes, eyelash growth, and conjunctival hyperemia. One of the significant side effects of bimatoprost is increasing length and thickness of eyelashes. In 2008, it was approved by the FDA for cosmetic use of lengthening and darkening of eyelashes under the brand name Latisse.

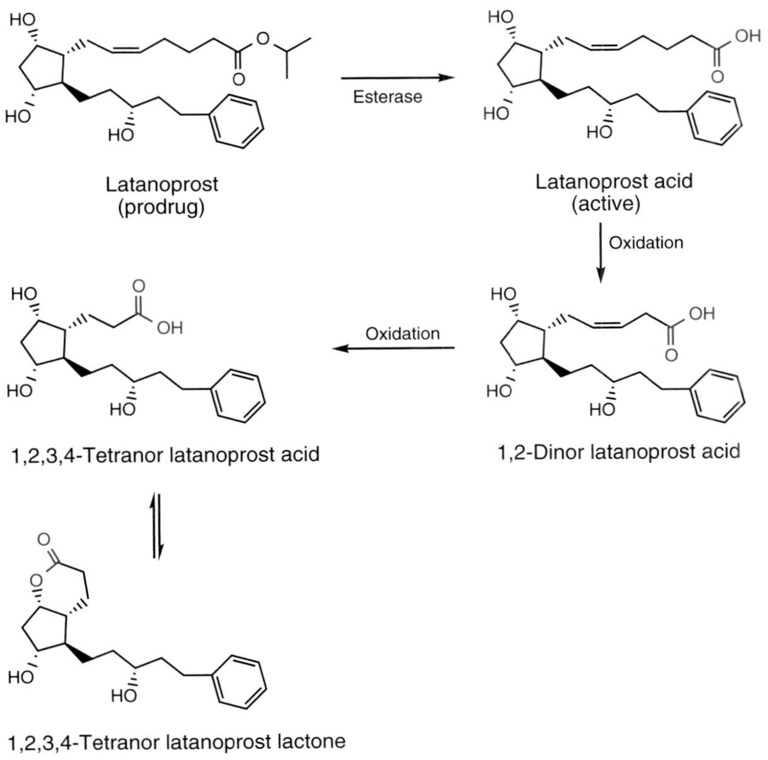

Latanoprost (prodrug) → Esterase → Latanoprost acid (active)

Latanoprost acid (active) → Oxidation → 1,2-Dinor latanoprost acid

1,2-Dinor latanoprost acid → Oxidation → 1,2,3,4-Tetranor latanoprost acid

1,2,3,4-Tetranor latanoprost acid ⇌ 1,2,3,4-Tetranor latanoprost lactone

Figure 27.16 Metabolism of latanoprost.

TRAVOPROST. Travoprost is an isopropyl ester prodrug, which is converted to active acid metabolite by esterases in the eye. It follows similar metabolism and elimination profile as latanoprost (Fig. 27.16). Travoprost metabolism includes β-oxidation to give 1,2-dinor travoprost acid and 1,2,3,4-tetranor travoprost acid. Further, oxidation of the15-OH group as well as reduction of 13, 14 double bond have also been reported.[38]

TAFLUPROST. The design of tafluprost was based upon the replacement of both the 15-hydroxy and hydrogen with two fluorides with the intent of decreasing the potential for 15-hydroxydehydrogenase catalyzed oxidation. In addition, this replacement results in increased lipophilicity to improve corneal absorption. As with latanoprost and travopost, tafluprost is a prodrug which is rapidly hydrolyzed to the active tafluprost acid. As indicated in Figure 27.16, β-oxidation leads to the 1,2-dinor and then 1,2,3,4-tetranor tafluprost.[39,40]

Tafluprost is the only preservative-free prostaglandin analogue; thus, it is packaged in unit dose, to be discarded after single use. It is a lipophilic ester, which readily crosses the cornea (~75% absorption in rats). Its onset of action is 2-4 hours with maximal effect reaching after 12 hours. The drug is administered once daily. No CYP enzymes are involved in its metabolism.

CLINICAL APPLICATION. Once daily dosing and fewer systemic adverse effects make prostaglandin analogues first-line agents. Maximum therapeutic effect is reached in 2 weeks. FP receptors are also highly expressed in dermal papillae, which increases the eyelash growth, one of the major adverse effects reported for prostaglandin analogues.[41] However, this side effect is temporary and will be relieved after discontinuation of the therapy. Other common adverse effects include pigmentation on the iris and eyelashes, redness, stinging, hyperemia, ocular inflammation, and ocular pruritus. These medications should be avoided in patients with active intraocular inflammation. Due to instability, prostaglandin analogues should be stored away from light below room temperature.[42] Patients should be advised to discard any unused medication after 4-6 weeks.

Rho Kinase Inhibitors

Rho kinases are serine/threonine kinases that act as effectors for Rho proteins. There are two types of Rho kinases, ROCK1 and ROCK2. ROCK1 is an important downstream effector for Rho-GTP protein. Rho proteins (RhoA, RhoB, RhoC) are small G-proteins bound to guanosine diphosphate (GDP) in their inactive state. Upon external stimuli, GDP is converted into GTP. Rho proteins are active when bound to GTP. The active Rho-GTP protein binds to Rho kinase at the Rho binding pocket. Rho kinase phosphorylates a number of downstream proteins including myosin light chain. All these actions result in a contractile state of the cells increasing their stiffness and smooth muscle contraction. Due to the increase in contractile nature of cells in the trabecular meshwork, changes in the extracellular matrix composition and/or a decrease in the conductance of the inner wall endothelial cells of Schlemm canal in the eye leads to clogging and buildup of IOP. Rho kinase inhibitors can help relax these muscles by reducing cell contraction, stiffness and decreasing the concentration of fibrosis related proteins, thereby increasing aqueous humor outflow through the trabecular meshwork.[43]

Aqueous humor outflow occurs in two ways, conventional trabecular outflow and unconventional uveoscleral pathway. Of the aqueous humor outflow, 90% happens through trabecular meshwork. Traditional glaucoma drugs work by increasing the aqueous humor outflow through unconventional uveoscleral pathway without having much effect on the clogged trabecular meshwork. Contrary to this, a Rho kinase inhibitor would work to unclog trabecular meshwork, increasing its outflow. Due to this unique mechanism of action, a Rho kinase inhibitor can be used in combination with other classes of glaucoma drugs. It has also been suggested that ROCK inhibitors could have a dual mechanisms of action.[44]

A second mechanism reported involves inhibition of norepinephrine reuptake transporter (NET) in ciliary body synapses causing vasoconstriction of arteries that supply blood to ciliary body, which in turn reduces aqueous humor production.

Rho kinase inhibitors have found number of clinical uses including the treatment of glaucoma and cerebral vasospasm among several others. These are the newest class of drugs used for treating high IOP associated with glaucoma or ocular hypertension. Netarsudil is the first Rho kinase inhibitor to enter the US market. Several other Rho kinase inhibitors are currently under development.

NETARSUDIL

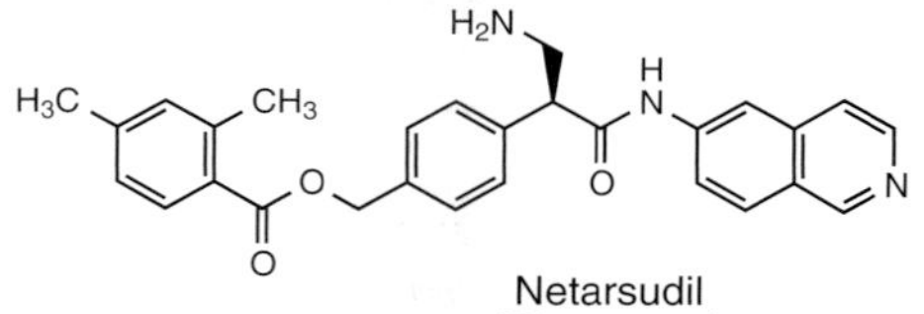

Netarsudil
(Rhopressa)

Mechanism of Action. Netarsudil is approved for treating elevated intraocular pressure in open-angle glaucoma and ocular hypertension.[45] Similar to the use of prostaglandin esters to improve corneal drug absorption, it is administered as a prodrug, which undergoes hydrolysis by esterases present in the eye to produce the active metabolite M1 (Fig. 27.17). Netarsudil-M1 is an active inhibitor of ROCK 1 and ROCK 2. In vitro studies have shown that netarsudil-M1 is approximately fivefold more active than netarsudil. It does not appear that M1 possess NET inhibition activity in humans but studies are continuing.[46]

Conjunctival hyperemia is a common adverse effect seen. Less common adverse effects include corneal verticillata, instillation site pain, and conjunctival hemorrhage. Netarsudil is administered once daily.

The FDA has recently approved the fixed combination of netarsudil and latanoprost (Rocklatan) for the treatment of open-angle glaucoma or ocular hypertension as a once-daily product. Both netarsudil and latanoprost have previously been approved as single agents.

Carbonic Anhydrase Inhibitors

Carbonic anhydrase (CA) is a very important enzyme in our body, which regulates secretions and fluid transport.

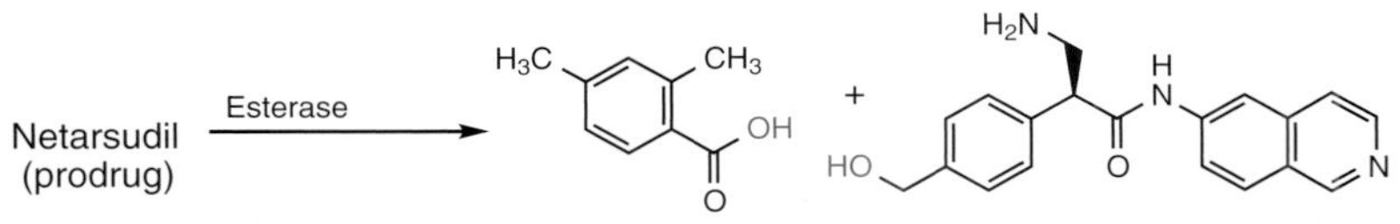

Netarsudil (prodrug) Esterase → + Netarsudil-M1 (Active)

Figure 27.17 Metabolism of netarsudil.

There are several different families of carbonic anhydrases (i.e., α-CA, β-CA) that have been identified of which α-CA is found in humans. CAs have minimal sequence similarity among themselves. Over 10 different isoforms of α-CA have been identified. They are present throughout the body and with various functions based on tissue location. Carbonic anhydrase II (CA-II) which belongs to α-CA family is highly expressed in the ciliary body of the eye, where its role is to regulate aqueous humor production through pH changes. CA rapidly interconverts carbon dioxide and water into dissociated carbonic acid, bicarbonate and a hydrogen ion, and thus regulates fluid pH. Due to its wide array of functions in the body, systemic use of carbonic anhydrase inhibitors are expected to cause numerous biological effects.

$$CO_2 + H_2O \underset{\text{anhydrase}}{\overset{\text{Carbonic}}{\rightleftharpoons}} HCHO_3^{\ominus} + H^{\oplus}$$

For their role in treatment of glaucoma, it would be desirable to develop topical carbonic anhydrase inhibitors to reduce potential for systemic effects. Unfortunately, topical application of carbonic anhydrase inhibitors is less effective compared to oral formulations. Of the drugs available, the first-generation inhibitors, acetazolamide and methazolamide, are used as systemic drugs while the second-generation drugs, dorzolamide and brinzolamide, are available in topical dosage forms (Fig. 27.18).

MECHANISM OF ACTION. Carbonic anhydrase as previously discussed converts water and carbon dioxide to carbonic acid and bicarbonate. CA is a zinc- metalloenzyme, which has zinc (Zn) in its catalytic site. The Zn prosthetic ion is coordinated to three histidine residues as well as a water molecule (Fig. 27.19A).[47]

Glutamine (Gln) and threonine (Thr) are key catalytic amino acids, which are bound to carbon dioxide and facilitate the reaction process to generate carbonic acid. The resulting dissociated carbonic acid brings about a change in pH and the movement of sodium ions that eventually promotes fluid secretion.[47] Carbonic anhydrase inhibitors (CAIs) interfere with interactions of water molecule with zinc ion as well as prevent carbon dioxide from entering the active site through their interactions with the threonine amino acid. Binding interactions of the carbonic anhydrase inhibitor dorzolamide in the carbonic anhydrase active site is shown in Figure 27.19B. All carbonic anhydrase inhibitors used in the treatment of glaucoma are sulfonamide derivatives. As seen in Figure 27.18, the sulfonamide functional group exhibits key hydrogen bonding interaction with Thr199 amino acid as well as chelation to the zinc metal. The alicyclic sulfone oxygen also shows hydrogen bonding interaction with the Gln92.[47]

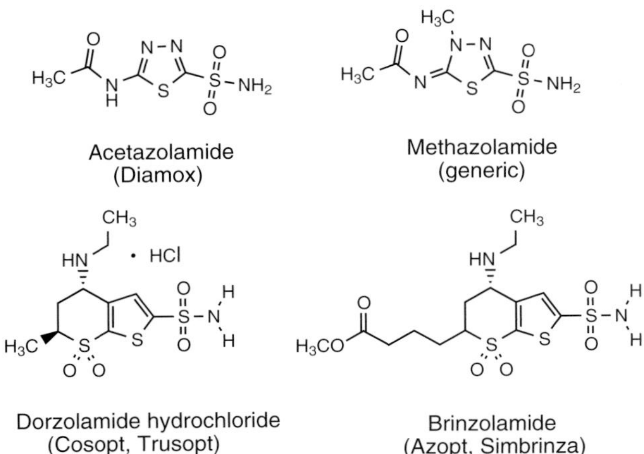

Figure 27.18 Carbonic anhydrase inhibitors.

SPECIFIC DRUGS

Acetazolamide and Methazolamide. Acetazolamide and methazolamide are potent first-generation CAIs, which are administered orally. They effectively inhibit most of the CA isoforms (Fig. 27.18). They decrease the aqueous humor production reducing IOP by 25%-30%. Because of their poor solubility, they are unable to pass through the cornea to reach the ciliary body, which limits their use to oral administration. Most of the acetazolamide is excreted unchanged while methazolamide undergoes N-dealkylation to produce an active metabolite. Both drugs are indicated for the treatment of refractory glaucoma that does not respond to adrenergic antagonists or prostaglandin analogues. In general, due to systemic adverse effects, they have been replaced with topical agents.

Dorzolamide and Brinzolamide. Dorzolamide and brinzolamide are second-generation CAIs, developed as topical formulations (Fig. 27.18). They selectively inhibit CA-II. Their pharmacokinetic profiles suggest a more favorable ability to cross the cornea and reach the ciliary body, the location of CA enzymes. Both of these drugs have a good hydrophilic/lipophilic balance. Upon topical application, more than 50% of the drug is absorbed with significant amounts reaching systemic circulation where the drug is absorbed by red blood cells. It should be noted that 90% of body's CA is stored in red blood cells. Both drugs are extremely effective in inhibiting CA in ciliary bodies (~100% inhibition). Dorzolamide

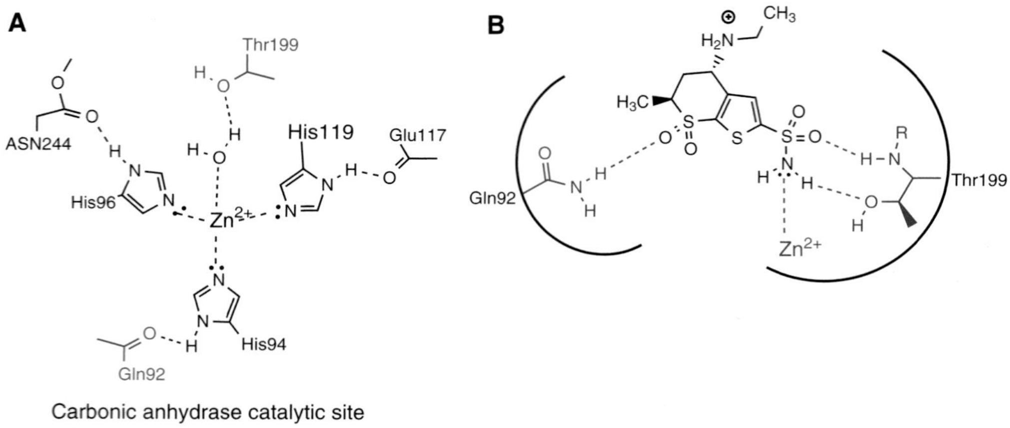

Figure 27.19 A, Carbonic anhydrase catalytic site. B, The binding interactions of dorzolamide at the carbonic anhydrase catalytic site.

and brinzolamide undergoes N-deethylation catalyzed by CYP2B1/2, CYP2E2, and CYP3A to produce the corresponding desethyl active metabolites (Fig. 27.20). These drugs and their metabolites are eliminated through the kidneys.[48]

The second-generation CAIs are devoid of most systemic adverse effects unlike first-generation drugs. Common adverse effects include stinging, burning of the eye, blurred vision, pruritus, and bitter taste. Brinzolamide produces less stinging/burning adverse effects but more blurred vision in comparison to dorzolamide. Additional adverse effects associated with dorzolamide include contact allergy, nephrolithiasis, anorexia, depression, dementia, and irreversible corneal decompensation in patients with established corneal problems.

Muscarinic Agonists

Several muscarinic agonists continue to be used in the treatment of ocular conditions.

MECHANISM OF ACTION. Interaction of cholinergic agonists with muscarinic acetylcholinergic receptors (mAChRs) leads to well-defined pharmacologic responses depending on the tissue or organ in which the receptor is located. These responses include contractions of smooth muscle, vasodilation, increased secretion from exocrine glands, miosis, and decreased heart rate and force of contraction. Muscarinic receptors are G protein–coupled receptors (GPCRs) of five types M_1 through M_5, of which M_3 muscarinic receptors are highly populated in the ciliary body and iris sphincter of the eye.[49] Signal transduction at the stimulatory M_3 mAChR occurs via coupling with a $G_{q/11}$ protein that is involved with mobilization of intracellular calcium. Agonist

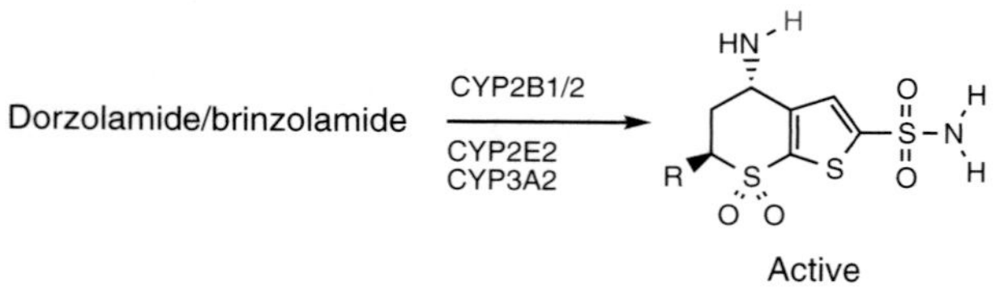

Figure 27.20 Metabolism of dorzolamide and brinzolamide.

binding to this receptor results in activation of phospholipase C, with subsequent production of the second messengers, diacylglycerol and inositol-1,4,5-triphosphate (IP_3). Stimulation of IP_3 ion channel receptors leads to release of intracellular calcium from the endoplasmic reticulum. The diacylglycerol produced, along with calcium, activates protein kinase C, which phosphorylates proteins to afford ciliary muscle contraction in the eye causing miosis. This opens up the trabecular meshwork allowing the aqueous humor to flow out, thus lowering IOP. Topical muscarinic agonists are used for reducing the intraocular pressure in treating glaucoma and ocular hypertension. They also find utility in inducing miosis during surgery.

ACETYLCHOLINE. Acetylcholine is the prototypical muscarinic and nicotinic agonist because it is the physiologic chemical neurotransmitter for the cholinergic nervous system. However, it is a poor therapeutic agent due to its lack of specificity for both nicotinic acetylcholinergic receptors (nAChRs) and mAChRs. In addition, the chemical properties associated with the ester and the quaternary ammonium functional group create potential problems. Although very stable in the solid crystalline form, ACh undergoes rapid hydrolysis in aqueous solution. This hydrolysis is accelerated in the presence of catalytic amounts of either acid or base. For this reason, acetylcholine cannot be administered orally due to rapid hydrolysis in the gastrointestinal tract. Even when administered parenterally, its pharmacologic action is fleeting as a result of hydrolysis by butyrylcholinesterase (also known as pseudocholinesterase or plasma cholinesterase) in serum. The quaternary ammonium functional group of acetylcholine imparts excellent water solubility, but quaternary ammonium salts are poorly absorbed across lipid membranes due to their high hydrophilic and ionic character. Thus, even if acetylcholine were stable enough to be administered orally, it would be poorly absorbed. When used during ocular surgery to produce complete miosis, acetylcholine must be directly instilled into the anterior chamber. It cannot be administered topically because it is not lipophilic enough to penetrate the cornea, and it must be reconstituted immediately before instillation into the eye due to its hydrolytic liability. It is therefore not used in the treating glaucoma.

STRUCTURE-ACTIVITY RELATIONSHIP. The classic SAR for muscarinic agonist activity is summarized in Figure 27.21. Key SAR points are listed below:

- The molecule must possess a nitrogen atom capable of bearing a positive charge, preferably a quaternary ammonium salt.
- For maximum potency, the size of the alkyl groups substituted on the nitrogen should not exceed the size of a methyl group.
- The molecule should have an oxygen atom, preferably an ester-like oxygen, capable of participating in a hydrogen bond.
- There should be a two-carbon unit between the oxygen atom and the nitrogen atom.

SPECIFIC DRUGS

Carbachol Chloride (Miostat)

Carbachol
(Miostat)

Carbachol, the carbamate analogue of acetylcholine, exhibits affinity for both mAChRs and nAChRs. Because it is a carbamate, carbachol is more resistant toward acid-, base-, or enzyme (AChE)–catalyzed hydrolysis than acetylcholine. It is also reported to exhibit weak anticholinesterase activity. Both of these actions work to prolong the duration of action of carbachol. Carbachol is used for the treatment of glaucoma and for the induction of miosis in ocular surgery. Carbachol is available as an intraocular solution and an ophthalmic solution.

Pilocarpine Hydrochloride (Isopto Carpine)

3*S*,4*R*-pilocarpine hydrochloride
(Isopto Carpine)

Pilocarpine hydrochloride, the salt of an alkaloid obtained from *Pilocarpus jaborandi*, is a selective M_3 mAChR agonist that does not adhere to the traditional SAR of muscarinic agonists. It possesses two chiral centers at C-3 and C-4. Thus, four optical isomers (two enantiomeric pairs) are possible, and of these, the naturally occurring alkaloid is 3*S*,4*R*-(+)-pilocarpine, with a pK_a of 6.8 and a log D at pH 7.4 of 1.03.

Pilocarpine is marketed as tablets (for treatment of dry mouth) and an ophthalmic solution. It penetrates the eye well and is the miotic of choice for open-angle glaucoma and to terminate acute angle-closure attacks. Because pilocarpine is a lactone, its solutions are subject to (1) hydrolysis to afford the pharmacologically inactive pilocarpic acid and (2) base-catalyzed epimerization at C-3 in the lactone to give isopilocarpine, an inactive stereoisomer of pilocarpine (Fig. 27.22).

Epimerization is not believed to be a serious problem if the drug is properly stored. Its solutions can be stored at room temperature. Pilocarpine is metabolized by esterases as well as CYP2A6. It is also an inhibitor of CYP2A6. Given the low amounts of pilocarpine, systemic absorption upon topical administration is minimal and is not expected to show significant drug-drug interactions. Pilocarpine is approved for treating elevated ocular pressure in patients with ocular hypertension or open-angle glaucoma, the management of acute angle-closure glaucoma, the prevention of postoperative elevated IOP associated with laser surgery, and induction of miosis.[50]

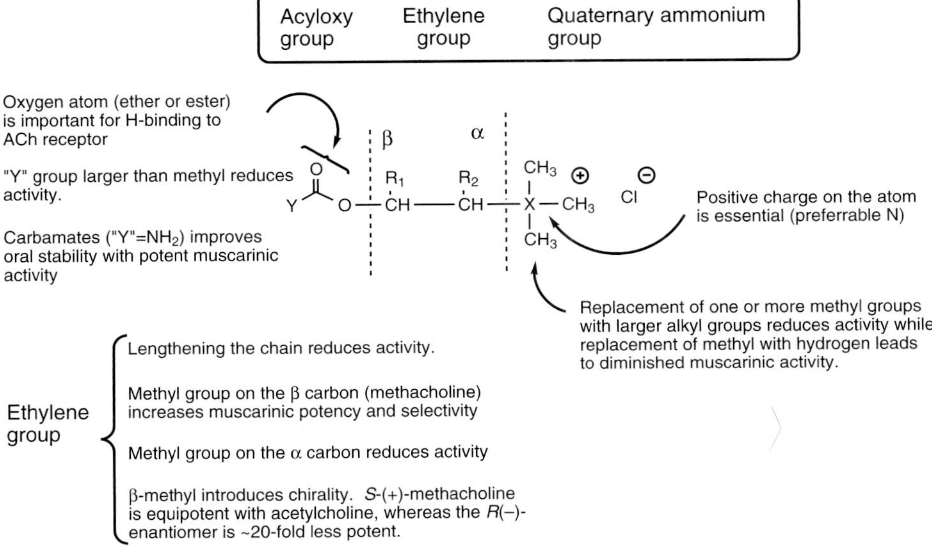

Figure 27.21 Summary of muscarinic agonists structure-activity relationship (SAR).

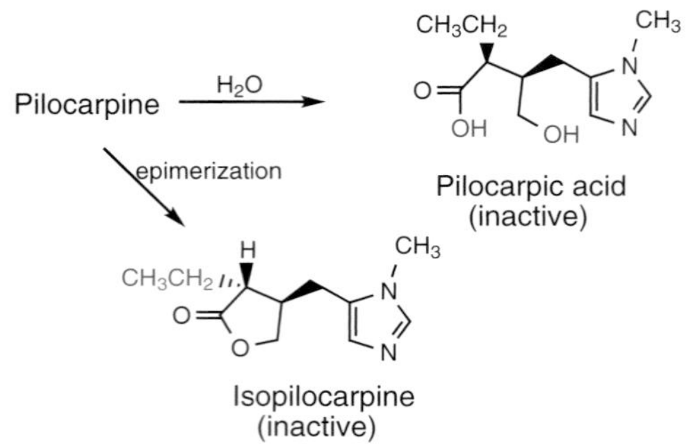

Pilocarpine $\xrightarrow{H_2O}$ Pilocarpic acid (inactive)

Pilocarpine → epimerization → Isopilocarpine (inactive)

Figure 27.22 Chemical instabilities of pilocarpine.

Acetylcholinesterase Inhibitors

Acetylcholine esterase inhibitors inhibit the metabolism of acetylcholine by acetylcholine esterase (AChE) enzyme. Thus, inhibition of hydrolysis by AChE increases the concentration of acetylcholine in the synapse and results in potentiation and/or prolonged activation of both muscarinic and nicotinic effects.

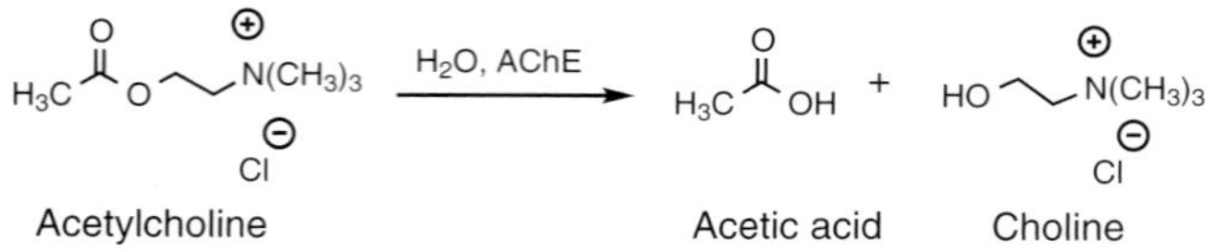

Acetylcholine $\xrightarrow{H_2O,\ AChE}$ Acetic acid + Choline

Acetylcholinesterase inhibitors (AChEIs), sometimes referred to as anticholinesterases, are classified as indirect cholinomimetics because their principle mechanism of action does not involve binding to cholinergic receptors but indirectly increasing the synaptic concentration of acetylcholine. AChEIs are used in open-angle glaucoma to decrease intraocular pressure by stimulating contraction of the ciliary muscle and sphincter of the iris. This facilitates outflow of aqueous humor via the canal of Schlemm.

Mechanism of Acetylcholinesterase-Catalyzed Hydrolysis of Acetylcholine

The active site of AChE consists of the ester binding site at which hydrolysis of the ester occurs and an "anionic binding site" where the cationic amine of acetylcholine binds (Fig. 27.23).

Instead of regular ionic bond, the quaternary nitrogen binds to the π-electrons of a tryptophan residue forming a cation-π bonding interaction.[51] Like other serine hydrolases, the functional catalytic unit of AChE is composed of a catalytic triad of glutamate, histidine, and serine at the ester binding site.[52,53] During hydrolysis the serine amino acid is acetylated. The acylated enzyme then undergoes rapid hydrolysis to regenerate the active form of AChE and a molecule of acetic acid.

Hydrolysis of the acylated enzyme (deacylation) is important in the development of AChEIs. If the enzyme becomes acylated by a functional group (i.e., carbamyl or phosphate) that is more stable toward hydrolysis than a carboxylate ester, the enzyme remains inactive for a longer period of time. Application of this chemical principle regarding rates of hydrolysis led to discovery and design of two classes of AChEIs, the reversible inhibitors and the irreversible inhibitors.

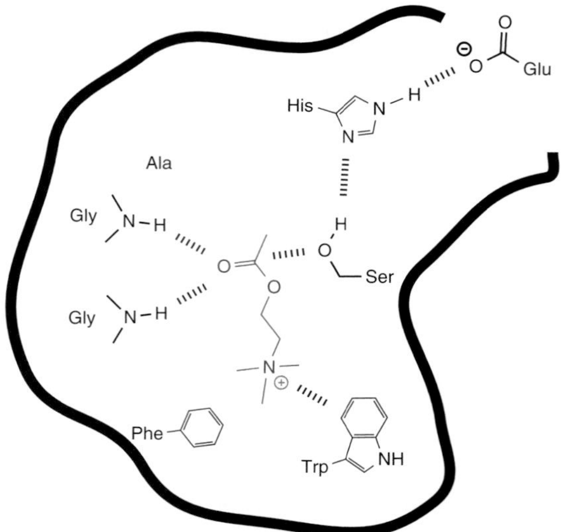

Figure 27.23 Binding of acetylcholine to catalytic site of acetylcholinesterase; role of serine and histidine residues is illustrated.

Reversible Inhibitors of Acetylcholinesterase

PHYSOSTIGMINE

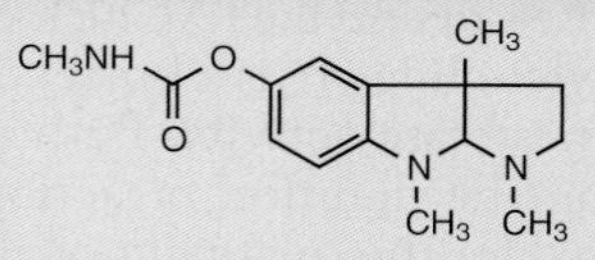

Physostigmine

For many years, physostigmine was a marketed drug available for the treatment of glaucoma. Physostigmine has exceptionally high affinity ($K_i \sim 10^{-9}$ M) for the catalytic site of AChE where it acted as a reversible AChEI. The carbamylated AChE was regenerated very slowly. Because physostigmine is lipophilic, it was able to diffuse across lipophilic membranes including the blood-brain barrier. Physostigmine is no longer marketed in the United States, although there has been some interest in its potential use in the treatment of Alzheimer disease.

Irreversible Inhibitors of Acetylcholinesterase

MECHANISM OF ACTION. The chemical logic involved in the development of AChEIs was to synthesize compounds that would be substrates for AChE and result in an acylated enzyme more stable to hydrolysis than a carboxylate ester. Phosphate esters are very stable to hydrolysis even more so than many amides. Application of this chemical property to the design of AChEIs led to derivatives of phosphoric, pyrophosphoric, and phosphonic acids that are effective inhibitors of AChE. These act as inhibitors by the same mechanism as the previously available carbamate inhibitor physostigmine, except that they form phosphate esters with the enzyme. The rate of hydrolysis of the phosphorylated enzyme is very slow with its rate being measured in hours (e.g., the half-lives for diethyl phosphates are ~8 hr). Because of their exceptionally longer duration of action, these compounds, are referred to as irreversible inhibitors of AChE. Knowledge of the chemical mechanisms associated with irreversible inhibition of AChE has led to the development of a series of phosphoester insecticides (i.e., malathion, parathion, chlorpyrifos, etc.,) as well as the development of deadly phosphorus-derived chemical warfare "nerve agents," one of which is sarin.

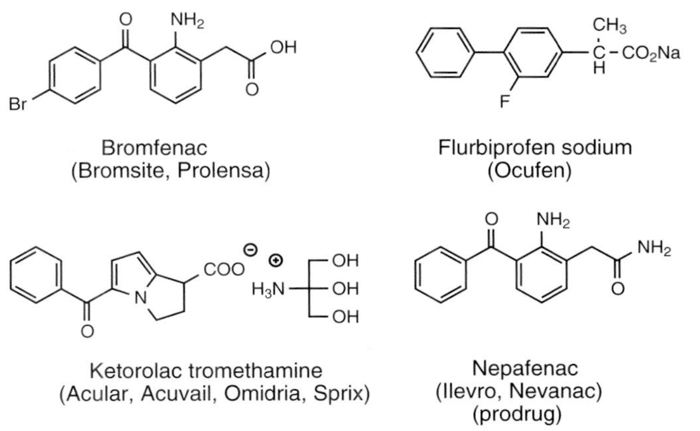

ECHOTHIOPHATE IODIDE (PHOSPHOLINE IODIDE)

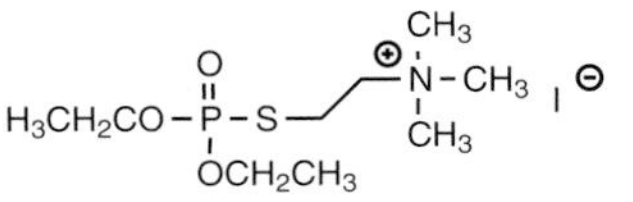

Echothiophate iodide
(Phospholine iodide)

Echothiophate iodide has found therapeutic application for the treatment of glaucoma and strabismus. Echothiophate is applied topically as a solution and is the only irreversible AChEI for the treatment of glaucoma. The decrease in intraocular pressure observed which can last up to 4 weeks. Phosphoester AChEIs exhibit cataractogenic properties; thus, their use should be reserved for patients who are refractory to other forms of treatment (i.e., short-acting miotics, β-blockers, epinephrine, and, possibly, carbonic anhydrase inhibitors). Because of its toxicity, echothiophate is not used for its systemic action. Adverse effects include stinging, burning, lacrimation, eyelid muscle twitching, reddening, and blurred vision.

Topical Ophthalmic Nonsteroidal Anti-Inflammatory Drugs (NSAIDs)

There has been considerable interest in the safety and effectiveness of topical ophthalmic NSAIDs for treatment of inflammation of the anterior segment of the eye (the cornea, iris, ciliary body, and lens) as a result of corneal damage from diclofenac ophthalmic solution.[54] Since 1999, several replacement ophthalmic NSAID products have been introduced including flurbiprofen ophthalmic solution, ketorolac tromethamine ophthalmic solution, bromfenac ophthalmic solution, and nepafenac ophthalmic suspension for postoperative pain and inflammation after cataract extraction or from corneal refractive surgery (Fig. 27.24). Chemistry and pharmacology of diclofenac, flurbiprofen, and ketorolac are discussed in Chapter 15. Systemic toxicity from topical NSAIDs are rare due to minimal absorption, but there are some reports of asthma exacerbations with the use of ophthalmic NSAIDs.[52] Thus, their use should be avoided in patients allergic to NSAIDs. Most common ocular toxicities include burning, irritation, and conjunctival hyperemia. Prolonged use may result in corneal thinning, ulcerations, and corneal perforations in susceptible individuals.[55]

Bromfenac
(Bromsite, Prolensa)

Flurbiprofen sodium
(Ocufen)

Ketorolac tromethamine
(Acular, Acuvail, Omidria, Sprix)

Nepafenac
(Ilevro, Nevanac)
(prodrug)

Figure 27.24 Topical nonsteroid anti-inflammatory drugs (NSAIDs).

MECHANISM OF ACTION. Nonsteroidal anti-inflammatory drugs (NSAIDs) are competitive and reversible inhibitors of two closely related cyclooxygenase enzymes, COX-1 and COX-2. These are the rate-limiting enzymes in the synthesis of the inflammatory prostaglandins PGE_2 and $PGF_{2\alpha}$ and the vasoactive prostanoids thromboxane A_2 (TXA_2) and prostacyclin (PGI_2) (Fig. 27.25).

COX-1 is constitutive and continually expressed. Conversely, COX-2 is inducible and actively expressed during inflammatory episodes. COX-2 is the ideal target for NSAIDs, as it is the enzyme expressed and active in pathological states; however, most anti-inflammatory NSAIDs in clinical use are nonselective in their action. The optimal structural features for all nonselective NSAIDs that promote high affinity binding at the COX active site include (1) an acidic functional group with pKa between 3 and 6 (i.e., anionic at pH 7.4) and (2) one or two aromatic rings that can achieve a noncoplanar orientation with respect to one another. Functional groups that add lipophilicity to the compounds (thus enhancing distribution through membranes) or which block degradative metabolism will increase potency and duration of action.

SPECIFIC DRUGS

Nepafenac. Nepafenac (Fig. 27.24) is unique among ophthalmic NSAIDs. It is an amide prodrug that requires intraocular hydrolysis to the more active amfenac, a potent nonselective COX inhibitor (Fig. 27.26). An important factor in the design of NSAIDs as topical ophthalmic drugs is the degree of penetration through the corneal epithelium. Corneal absorption of an NSAID into the anterior segment depends on its lipid solubility and degree of ionization (pH range of normal tears 6.5-7.6). Due to the inherent water solubility and the degree of ionization of phenylalkanoic acid NSAIDs (~pK_4), it would be predicted that these agents would have limited ability to penetrate corneal epithelium. However, nepafenac as an unionized amide prodrug would be expected to readily

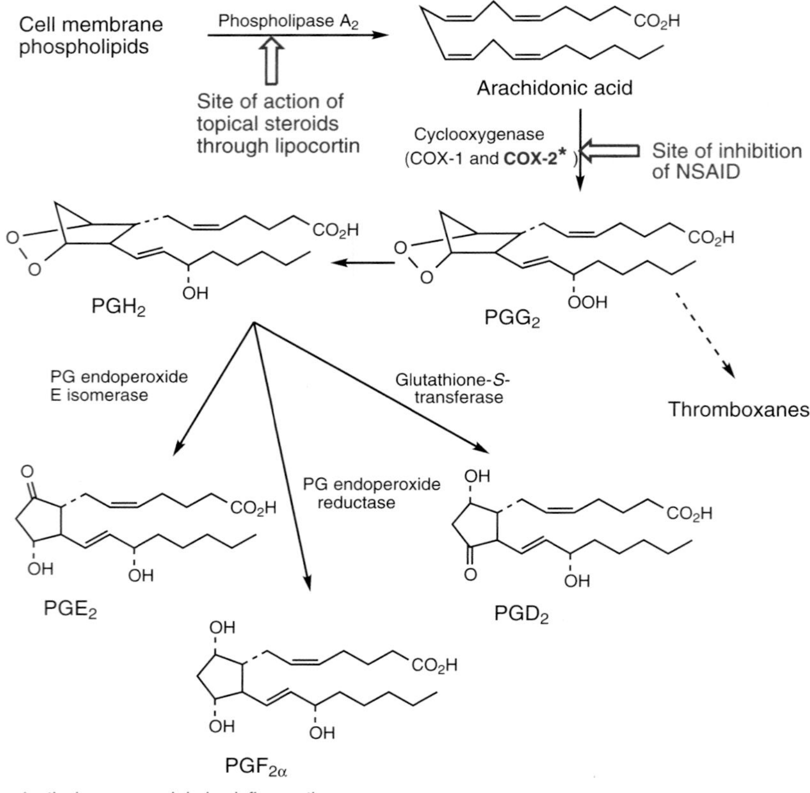

Figure 27.25 Biosynthesis of prostaglandins from arachidonic acid.

penetrate the corneal epithelium and enter into all ocular tissues including aqueous humor, iris, ciliary body, and retina.[56] In a rabbit model, corneal permeability of nepafenac was approximately 19- and 28-fold greater than bromfenac and ketorolac, respectively.[57] Another important factor for nepafenac is that the drug has no inherent COX inhibition activity before absorption.

Mechanism of Action. Nepafenac exhibits weak COX inhibition. However, its active metabolite, amfenac inhibits both COX-1 and COX-2 prostaglandin synthesis for up to 6 hours, with greater selectivity for COX-2 than does ketorolac. The COX-2/COX-1 ratio was approximately ninefold that of ketorolac, which suggests greater COX-2 anti-inflammatory activity for nepafenac than with ketorolac ophthalmic suspensions.[56] Nepafenac exhibited a longer duration of action than ketorolac.

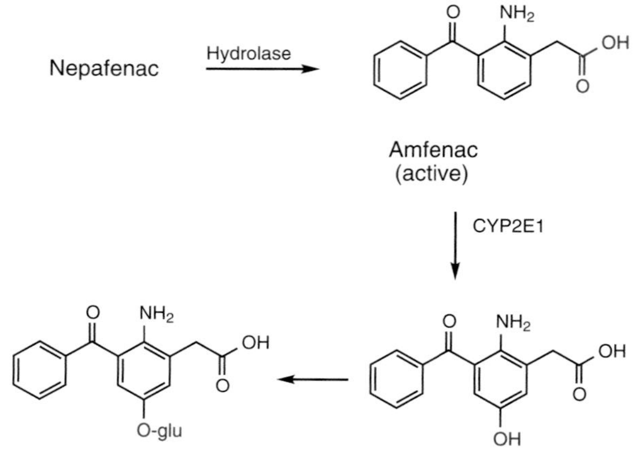

Figure 27.26 Metabolic activation and metabolism of nepafenac.

Pharmacokinetics. Nepafenac is rapidly absorbed when administered topically as a 0.1% ophthalmic suspension. Amfenac has high affinity (~95%) for serum albumin proteins. Following topical application, the onset of napafenac is ~15 minutes and the duration of action is greater than 8 hours. Small quantifiable plasma concentrations of nepafenace and amfenac have been observed in subjects in 2-3 hours after topical application. In rabbits, nepafenac conversion to active metabolite is seen mostly in the retina, the iris and ciliary body and minimal conversion in the cornea.[57] Bioactivation of nepafenac in aqueous humor appears to be negligible; however, it is possible that nepafenac could undergo water hydrolysis once reaching the aqueous humor.[58] Amfenac undergoes CYP2E1-catalyzed oxidation followed by conjugation to its glucuronide (Fig. 27.26). The major route of elimination is via the urine.

BROMFENAC. Bromfenac is a nonselective COX inhibitor approved for the treatment of postoperative inflammation and reduction of ocular pain in patients who had undergone cataract surgery (Fig. 27.24).[59] It is available as 0.07% ophthalmic solution with once daily dosing starting one day before and continuing until 14 days after the surgery. It has a minimal systemic absorption.

Most common adverse effects include anterior chamber inflammation, foreign body sensation, eye pain, photophobia, and blurred vision.

THERAPEUTIC USE. The ophthalmic dosage forms of these drugs are used to treat postoperative pain and inflammation associated with cataract surgery. Additionally, they might have value to reduce swelling and stinging sensations following cataract surgery or corneal refractory surgery.

Topical ophthalmic nepafenac is also approved for use as a preoperative agent. The dosage is one drop two to four times a day for 2 weeks following the surgery. The topical application is preferred over systemic dosing due to the higher ocular drug concentration that can be gained as well as a reduction in adverse effects. In general, there are minimal adverse effects and few if any drug-drug interactions.

Topical Ophthalmic Steroids

Topical ophthalmic steroids are commonly used for the management of inflammation due to external injury, allergies, ocular surgeries, and infections. Topical steroidal drugs that are currently used for treating ocular inflammation are dexamethasone, difluprednate, fluorometholone, loteprednol etabonate, prednisolone acetate, and prednisolone sodium phosphate (Fig. 27.27).

MECHANISM OF ACTION. During ocular injury or infection, the body releases prostaglandins causing inflammation, vasodilation, miosis, and increased aqueous humor production. The mechanism of action of the topical ophthalmic steroids is not totally understood. They are believed to act by inhibiting phospholipase A_2, an enzyme that catalyzes the first step in the biosynthesis of prostaglandins. (Fig. 27.25). Furthermore, it is suggested that glucocorticoids induce the production of lipocortin and related proteins by increasing gene expression through activation of the glucocorticoid receptor (GR). The inhibition of phospholipase A_2 blocks the release of arachidonic acid leading to reduction in the inflammatory prostaglandins and thromboxanes. Through the action of lipocortin other inflammatory responses can be reduced such as cellular infiltration and capillary permeability, which adds to the inflammatory condition. For more details concerning the steroidal mechanism of action, the reader is referred to Chapter 21.

PHARMACOKINETICS. The most unique of the topical ophthalmic steroids is loteprednol, which was developed with the goal of being an effective agent for treatment of various ocular inflammatory conditions (i.e., giant papillary conjunctivitis, seasonal allergic conjunctivitis, uveitis, inflammation, and pain following cataract surgery) with minimal adverse effects. Common to topical ophthalmic steroids is the development of cataracts and IOP elevation upon long-term use. Loterednol is a lipophilic drug that penetrates the cornea and exhibit strong affinity for the GR. However, the drug is rapidly metabolized to an inactive metabolite without the adverse effects reported for other ophthalmic steroids. Loterednol has met these goals and is rapidly metabolized as shown in Figure 27.28.[60]

Dexamethasone ophthalmic, is available in combination with various antibiotics, but has limited availability as a single agent (suspension).

Difluprednate is a lipophilic prodrug indicated for the treatment of inflammation and pain associated with ocular surgery. The drug is rapidly deacetylated to an active drug. Fluorometholone is available as such or as its acetate ester. The ester prodrug is more lipophilic that help facilitate corneal transport.

THERAPEUTIC APPLICATION. The topical ophthalmic steroids are used for the management of inflammation due to external injury, allergies, ocular surgeries, and infections. The therapy is usually started immediately after the refractive surgeries and tapered off over a few days

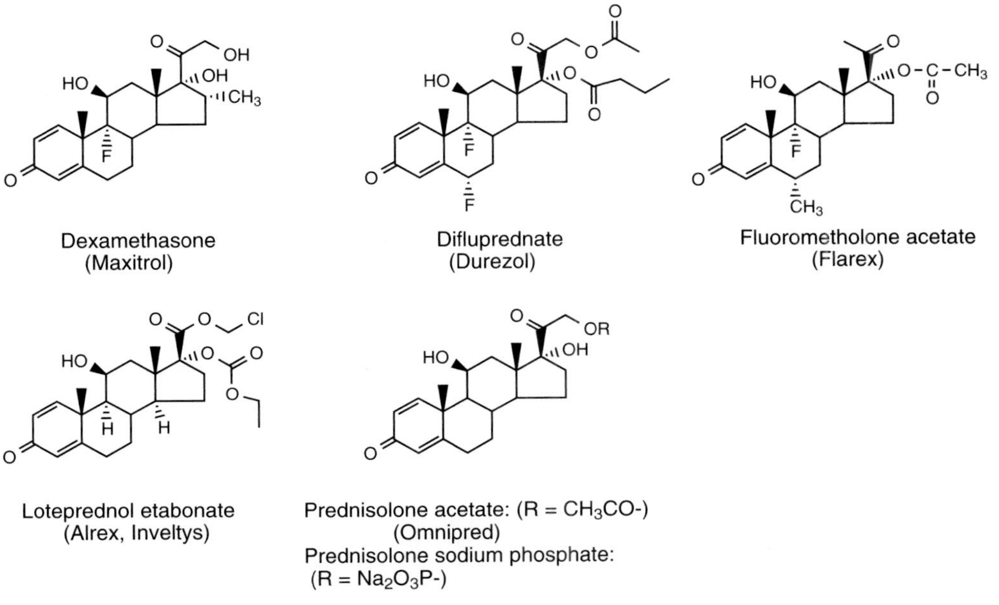

Dexamethasone (Maxitrol)

Difluprednate (Durezol)

Fluorometholone acetate (Flarex)

Loteprednol etabonate (Alrex, Inveltys)

Prednisolone acetate: (R = CH_3CO-) (Omnipred)
Prednisolone sodium phosphate: (R = Na_2O_3P-)

Figure 27.27 Ophthalmic topical steroids.

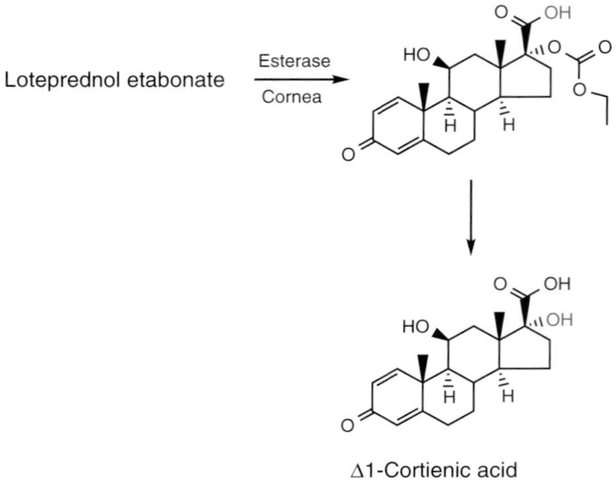

Loteprednol etabonate
Esterase
Cornea

Δ1-Cortienic acid

Figure 27.28 Metabolism of loteprednol.

to weeks and sometimes months. They may have better anti-inflammatory effects when combined with NSAIDs than as a monotherapy in treating cystoid macular edema. The biggest concern results from prolonged usage, which may result in glaucoma with damage to the optic nerve. Prolong usage may also suppress the immune response increasing the possibility of a secondary ocular infection. These drugs are contraindicated in viral infections of cornea and conjunctiva, varicella and mycobacterial as well as fungal infections of eye.

Topical Antihistamines

The topical antihistamines are formulated with the intent of being used directly in the eye for treatment of allergic conjunctivitis. They play an important role in providing quick symptomatic relief. The ophthalmic antihistamines most commonly used are shown in Figure 27.29.

MECHANISM OF ACTION. Topical antihistamines used in the treatment of allergic conjunctivitis are all potent H_1 inverse agonists. They also have a certain degree of inhibition of H_2 and H_4 receptors. The eyelids and conjunctiva are rich of mast cells, which upon exposure to allergens produce immunoglobulin E (IgE) leading to mast cells degranulation releasing inflammatory mediators including histamine. The activation of histamine receptors present in the conjunctival epithelium and goblet cells of the upper eyelid leads to redness, tearing, eyelid swelling, and associated symptoms (often referred to as early phase symptoms). Antihistamines, such as emedastine, pheniramine, bepotastine, and cetirizine, act by antagonizing histamine action at H_1 receptors thereby alleviating early phase symptoms of allergic conjunctivitis. These early phase symptoms can also be inhibited by preventing IgE-mediated mast cell degranulation. Several dual-acting drugs are available such as azelestine, epinastine, alcaftadine, ketotifen, and olopatadine, which act by both blocking H_1 receptors as well as stabilizing mast cells from degranulation. This dual-acting therapy has improved patient compliance

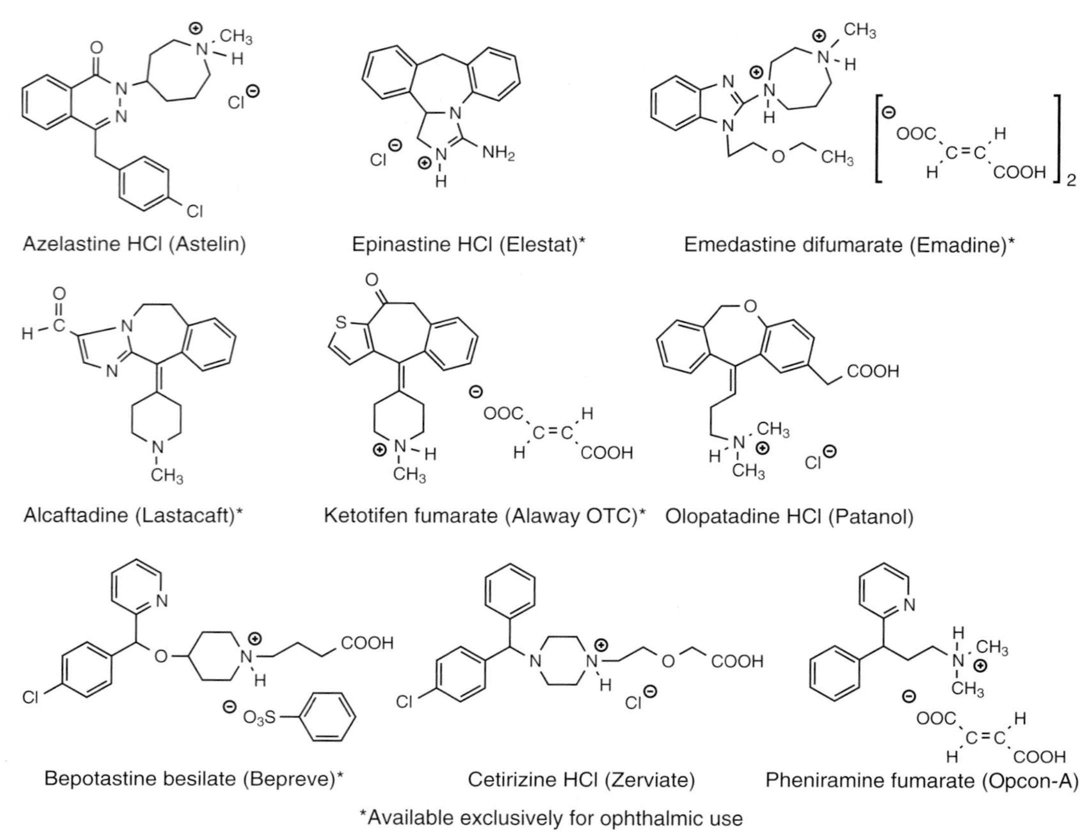

Figure 27.29 Topical antihistamines.

and management of allergic conjunctivitis.[61] One of the newer drugs, alcaftadine also works as an inverse agonist at H_4 receptors resulting in inhibiting the recruitment of immune cells and release of inflammatory chemokines and cytokines.[62] Burning is a very commonly seen adverse effect with dual-acting drugs.[58] Topical antihistamine pheniramine is available in combination with adrenergic α_1 agonist naphazoline. Most common side effects seen with ophthalmic antihistamines include burning, stinging, and headache.

PHARMACOKINETICS. Less than 10% of the topically administered antihistamines crosses corneal membrane and enters into the aqueous humor and ocular structures. A large amount of drug escapes into the systemic circulation via conjunctiva and scleral routes. Higher corneal absorption is observed for drugs having higher lipophilicity. However, systemic side effects are very rarely observed with ophthalmic antihistamines due to the low doses. Minor systemic side effects observed include dry mouth, nausea, headache, and dizziness. Onset of action for ophthalmic antihistamines is much faster compared to oral antihistamines, ranging from 3-15 minutes with a duration of action ranging from 8-12 hours. Due to high lipophilic nature, H_1 antihistamines dissociate very slowly from the receptor site providing longer duration of action. Metabolites of various topical antihistamines are shown in Figure 27.30.

THERAPEUTIC APPLICATION. Topical antihistamines are commonly used to treat mild to moderate symptoms associated with seasonal and perineal allergic conjunctivitis. They are used alone or in combination with mast cell stabilizers or adrenergic α_1 agonists (vasoconstrictors). Topical antihistamines are contraindicated in closed-angle glaucoma patients, as they may increase intraocular pressure through pupillary dilation. Prophylactic treatment of ocular antihistamines also proved beneficial. Dosing parameters are shown in Table 27.3.

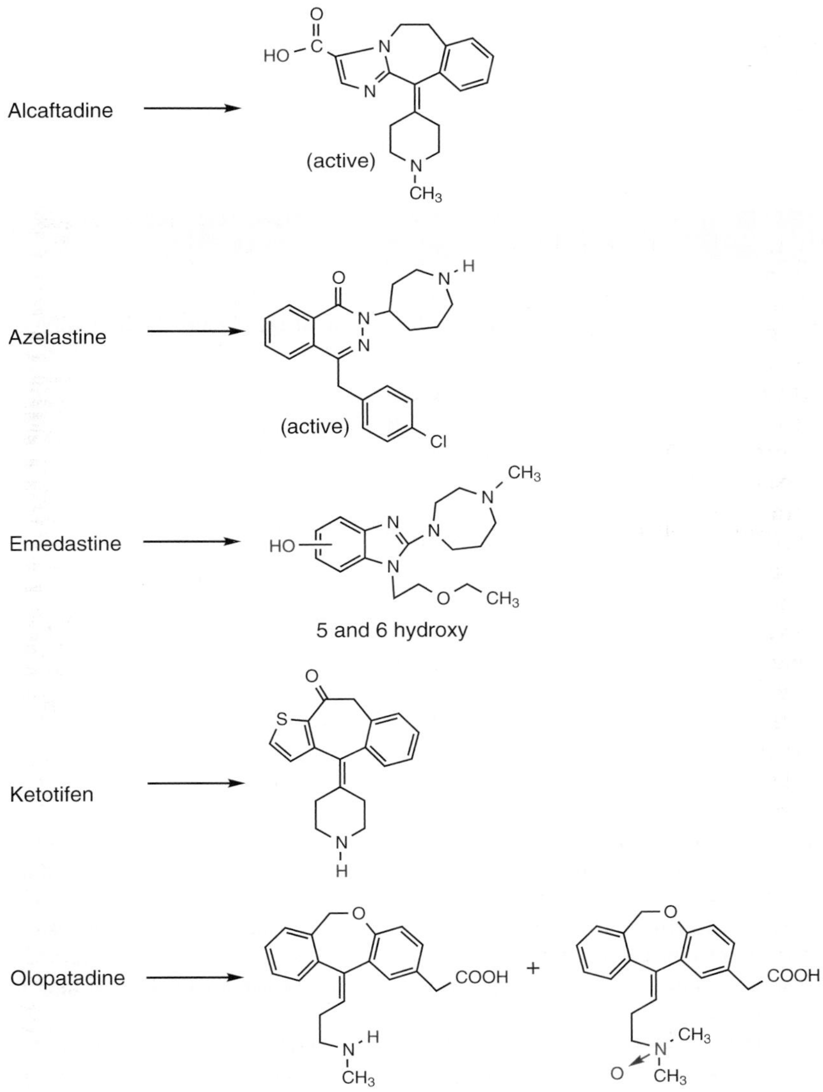

Alcaftadine → (active)

Azelastine → (active)

Emedastine → 5 and 6 hydroxy

Ketotifen →

Olopatadine →

Figure 27.30 Metabolism of topical antihistamines.

Table 27.3 Dosing Parameters for Topical Antihistamines

Topical Antihistamine	Ophthalmic Solution Strengths	Ophthalmic Dosing (Drops Each Eye)	Nasal Solution Strengths	Nasal Dosing (Each Nostril)
Alcaftadine	0.25%	1/daily	NA	NA
Azelastine	0.05%	1/twice daily	137 μg/spray 15%	1-2 sprays twice daily
Bepotastine	1.5%	1/twice daily	NA	NA
Cetirizine	0.24%	1/twice daily	NA	NA
Emedastine	0.05%	1/up to four times daily	NA	NA
Epinastine	0.05%	1/twice daily	NA	NA
Pheniramine	0.135%	1-2/four times daily		
Ketotifen	0.025%	1/twice daily	NA	NA
Olopatadine	0.1%, 0.2%	1/daily (0.2%) 1/twice daily (0.1%)	0.6%	2 sprays twice daily

NA, not available.

ACKNOWLEDGMENTS

The author wishes to acknowledge the work of E. Kim Fifer, PhD, and Robert K. Griffith, PhD, who authored content used within this chapter in a previous edition of this text.

Structure Challenge

Several drug structures that are agonists (direct or indirect) and antagonists at adrenergic receptors are given below. Based on the information learned from the SAR studies and properties of each of those drugs, identify the best choice for the questions below.

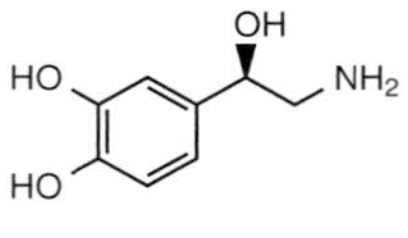

A 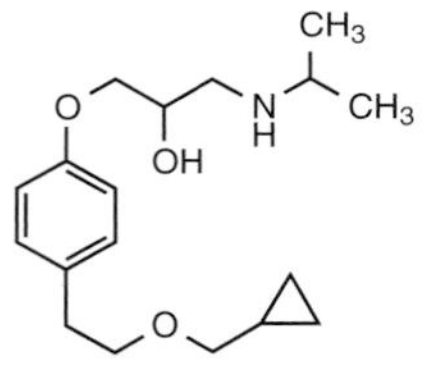 B 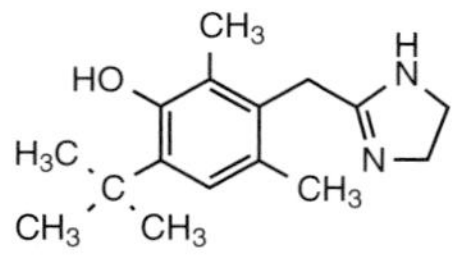 C 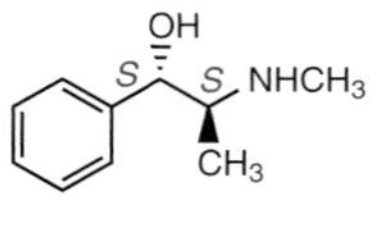 D 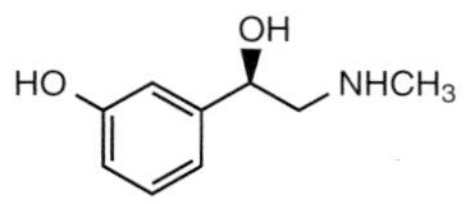 E

1. Which drug readily undergoes oxidation when exposed to air or light producing toxic metabolite? Therefore, it has to be stored away from light in air tight amber color bottles. Draw the toxic metabolite, and if ingested show how body handles toxicity.
2. Identify the drug that is selective to α_1-receptors and is commonly used in oral decongestant medications. Identify the functional group that is responsible for this selectivity.
3. Which nasal decongestant binds at the adrenergic α_1-receptor more like an antagonist? Identify the functional group in this drug that is responsible for this α_1-receptor selectivity.
4. Which drug is an indirect adrenergic agonist? Explains reasons why, from the SAR analysis.
5. Identify the antiglaucoma drug from the list. Which adrenergic receptor does it target and the functional group that is responsible for its selectivity?

Structure Challenge answers found immediately after References.

REFERENCES

1. Pacheco-Galvan A, Hart SP, Morice AH. Relationship between gastro-oesophageal reflux and airway diseases: the airway reflux paradigm. *Arch Bronconeumol*. 2011;47:195-203.
2. Mayo Clinic Staff. Nasal Congestion: Causes. Mayo Clinic. Available at https://www.mayoclinic.org/symptoms/nasal-congestion/basics/causes/sym-20050644. Accessed July 19, 2018.
3. Bush RK. Etiopathogenesis and management of perennial allergic rhinitis: a state-of-the-art review. *Treat Respir Med*. 2004;3:45-57.
4. Meltzer EO, Blaiss MS, Derebery MJ, et al. Burden of allergic rhinitis: results from the pediatric allergies in America survey. *J Allergy Clin Immunol*. 2009;124:S43-S70.
5. Center for Disease Control. *Summary Health Statistics Tables for U.S. Children: National Health Interview Survey*. National Center for Health Statistics; March 30, 2017. Available at https://www.cdc.gov/nchs/fastats/allergies.htm. Accessed July 18, 2018.
6. Meltzer EO, Farrar JR, Sennett C. Findings from an online survey assessing the burden and management of seasonal allergic rhinoconjunctivitis in US patients. *J Allergy Clin Immunol Pract*. 2017;5:779-789, e776.
7. Naclerio RM, Bachert C, Baraniuk JN. Pathophysiology of nasal congestion. *Int J Gen Med*. 2010;3:47-57.
8. Von Euler US. Synthesis, uptake, and storage of catecholamines in adrenergic nerves: the effect of drugs. In: Blaschko H, Marshall E, eds. *Catecholamines*. New York: Springer; 1972:186-230.
9. Kaufman S, Nelson TJ. Studies on the regulation of tyrosine hydroxylase activity by phosphorylation and dephosphorylation. In: Dahlstrom A, Belmaker RH, Sandler M, eds. *Progress in Catecholamine Research. Part A: Basic Aspects and Peripheral Mechanisms*. New York: Alan R Liss; 1988:57-60.
10. Harrison JK, Pearson WR, Lynch KR. Molecular characterization of alpha 1- and alpha 2-adrenoceptors. *Trends Pharmacol Sci*. 1991;12:62-67.
11. Strader CD, Candelore MR, Hill WS, et al. Identification of two serine residues involved in agonist activation of the beta-adrenergic receptor. *J Biol Chem*. 1989;264:13572-13578.
12. Strader CD, Sigal IS, Register RB, et al. Identification of residues required for ligand binding to the beta-adrenergic receptor. *Proc Natl Acad Sci USA*. 1987;84:4384-4388.
13. Melvin TA, Patel AA. Pharmacotherapy for allergic rhinitis. *Otolaryngol Clin North Am*. 2011;44:727-739.
14. Nichols AJ, Ruffolo RRJ. Structure–activity relationships for α-adrenoceptor agonists and antagonists. *α-Adrenoceptors: Molecular Biology, Biochemistry, and Pharmacology*. Karger; 1991:75-114.
15. Waugh DJ, Gaivin RJ, Zuscik MJ, et al. Phe-308 and Phe-312 in transmembrane domain 7 are major sites of alpha 1-adrenergic receptor antagonist binding. Imidazoline agonists bind like antagonists. *J Biol Chem*. 2001;276:25366-25371.
16. Mahajan MK, Uttamsingh V, Daniels JS, et al. In vitro metabolism of oxymetazoline: evidence for bioactivation to a reactive metabolite. *Drug Metab Dispos*. 2011;39:693-702.
17. Mahajan MK, Uttamsingh V, Gan LS, et al. Identification and characterization of oxymetazoline glucuronidation in human liver microsomes: evidence for the involvement of UGT1A9. *J Pharm Sci*. 2011;100:784-793.
18. Kushnir NM. The role of decongestants, cromolyn, guafenesin, saline washes, capsaicin, leukotriene antagonists, and other treatments on rhinitis. *Immunol Allergy Clin North Am*. 2011;31:601-617.
19. Nelson HS. Mechanisms of intranasal steroids in the management of upper respiratory allergic diseases. *J Allergy Clin Immunol*. 1999;104:S138-S143.
20. Bush IE. Chemical and biological factors in the activity of adrenocortical steroids. *Pharmacol Rev*. 1962;14:317-445.
21. Teng XW, Cutler DJ, Davies NM. Mometasone furoate degradation and metabolism in human biological fluids and tissues. *Biopharm Drug Dispos*. 2003;24:321-333.
22. Sahasranaman S, Issar M, Hochhaus G. Metabolism of mometasone furoate and biological activity of the metabolites. *Drug Metab Dispos*. 2006;34:225-233.
23. Roberts JK, Moore CD, Ward RM, et al. Metabolism of beclomethasone dipropionate by cytochrome P450 3A enzymes. *J Pharmacol Exp Ther*. 2013;345:308-316.
24. Weinreb RN, Aung T, Medeiros FA. The pathophysiology and treatment of glaucoma: a review. *JAMA*. 2014;311:1901-1911.
25. Quigley HA, Broman AT. The number of people with glaucoma worldwide in 2010 and 2020. *Br J Ophthalmol*. 2006;90:262-267.
26. Weinreb RN, Leung CK, Crowston JG, et al. Primary open-angle glaucoma. *Nat Rev Dis Primers*. 2016;2:16067.
27. Timmermans PB, van Zwieten PA. Alpha 2 adrenoceptors: classification, localization, mechanisms, and targets for drugs. *J Med Chem*. 1982;25:1389-1401.
28. Kanagy NL. Alpha(2)-adrenergic receptor signalling in hypertension. *Clin Sci (Lond)*. 2005;109:431-437.
29. Wheeler LA, Woldemussie E. Alpha-2 adrenergic receptor agonists are neuroprotective in experimental models of glaucoma. *Eur J Ophthalmol*. 2001;11(suppl 2):S30-S35.
30. Wheeler LA, Gil DW, WoldeMussie E. Role of alpha-2 adrenergic receptors in neuroprotection and glaucoma. *Surv Ophthalmol*. 2001;45(suppl 3):S290-S294; discussion S295–296.
31. Frishman WH, Fuksbrumer MS, Tannenbaum M. Topical ophthalmic beta-adrenergic blockade for the treatment of glaucoma and ocular hypertension. *J Clin Pharmacol*. 1994;34:795-803.
32. Gupta D, Chen PP. Glaucoma. *Am Fam Physician*. 2016;93:668-674.
33. Ricciotti E, FitzGerald GA. Prostaglandins and inflammation. *Arterioscler Thromb Vasc Biol*. 2011;31:986-1000.
34. Sjoquist B, Stjernschantz J. Ocular and systemic pharmacokinetics of latanoprost in humans. *Surv Ophthalmol*. 2002;47(suppl 1):S6-S12.
35. Woodward DF, Krauss AH, Chen J, et al. The pharmacology of bimatoprost (Lumigan). *Surv Ophthalmol*. 2001;45(suppl 4):S337-S345.
36. Brubaker RF. Mechanism of action of bimatoprost (Lumigan). *Surv Ophthalmol*. 2001;45(suppl 4):S347-S351.
37. Shafiee A, Bowman LM, Hou E, et al. Ocular pharmacokinetics of bimatoprost formulated in DuraSite compared to bimatoprost 0.03% ophthalmic solution in pigmented rabbit eyes. *Clin Ophthalmol*. 2013;7:1549-1556.
38. CORP NP. FDA Label. Available at https://www.accessdata.fda.gov/scripts/cder/daf/index.cfm?event=overview.process&ApplNo=021994. Accessed October 20, 2018.
39. Liu Y, Mao W. Tafluprost once daily for treatment of elevated intraocular pressure in patients with open-angle glaucoma. *Clin Ophthalmol*. 2013;7:7-14.
40. Fukano Y, Kawazu K. Disposition and metabolism of a novel prostanoid antiglaucoma medication, tafluprost, following ocular administration to rats. *Drug Metab Dispos*. 2009;37:1622-1634.
41. Woodward DF, Jones RL, Narumiya S. International Union of Basic and Clinical Pharmacology. LXXXIII: classification of prostanoid receptors, updating 15 years of progress. *Pharmacol Rev*. 2011;63:471-538.
42. Johnson TV, Gupta PK, Vudathala DK, et al. Thermal stability of bimatoprost, latanoprost, and travoprost under simulated daily use. *J Ocul Pharmacol Ther*. 2011;27:51-59.
43. Tanna AP, Johnson M. Rho kinase inhibitors as a novel treatment for glaucoma and ocular hypertension. *Ophthalmology*. 2018. 125(11):1741-1756.
44. Ren R, Li G, Le TD, et al. Netarsudil increases outflow facility in human eyes through multiple mechanisms. *Investig Ophthalmol Vis Sci*. 2016;57:6197-6209.
45. Sturdivant JM, Royalty SM, Lin CW, et al. Discovery of the ROCK inhibitor netarsudil for the treatment of open-angle glaucoma. *Bioorg Med Chem Lett*. 2016;26:2475-2480.
46. Wang RF, Williamson JE, Kopczynski C, et al. Effect of 0.04% AR-13324, a ROCK, and norepinephrine transporter inhibitor, on aqueous humor dynamics in normotensive monkey eyes. *J Glaucoma*. 2015;24:51-54.
47. Smith GM, Alexander RS, Christianson DW, et al. Positions of His-64 and a bound water in human carbonic anhydrase II upon binding three structurally related inhibitors. *Protein Sci*. 1994;3:118-125.

48. Martens-Lobenhoffer J, Banditt P. Clinical pharmacokinetics of dorzolamide. *Clin Pharmacokinet*. 2002;41:197-205.
49. Gil DW, Krauss HA, Bogardus AM, et al. Muscarinic receptor subtypes in human iris-ciliary body measured by immunoprecipitation. *Investig Ophthalmol Vis Sci*. 1997;38:1434-1442.
50. Administration FAD. Isopto Carpine Ophthalmic Solution. FDA. Available at https://www.accessdata.fda.gov/drugsatfda_docs/nda/2010/200890_carpine_toc.cfm. Accessed September 24, 2018.
51. Ordentlich A, Barak D, Kronman C, et al. Dissection of the human acetylcholinesterase active center determinants of substrate specificity. Identification of residues constituting the anionic site, the hydrophobic site, and the acyl pocket. *J Biol Chem*. 1993;268:17083-17095.
52. Shafferman A, Kronman C, Flashner Y, et al. Mutagenesis of human acetylcholinesterase. Identification of residues involved in catalytic activity and in polypeptide folding. *J Biol Chem*. 1992;267:17640-17648.
53. Zhang Y, Kua J, McCammon JA. Role of the catalytic triad and oxyanion hole in acetylcholinesterase catalysis: an ab initio QM/MM study. *J Am Chem Soc*. 2002;124:10572-10577.
54. Gaynes BI, Onyekwuluje A. Topical ophthalmic NSAIDs: a discussion with focus on nepafenac ophthalmic suspension. *Clin Ophthalmol*. 2008;2:355-368.
55. Aragona P, Tripodi G, Spinella R, et al. The effects of the topical administration of non-steroidal anti-inflammatory drugs on corneal epithelium and corneal sensitivity in normal subjects. *Eye (Lond)*. 2000;14(pt 2):206-210.
56. Gamache DA, Graff G, Brady MT, et al. Nepafenac, a unique nonsteroidal prodrug with potential utility in the treatment of trauma-induced ocular inflammation: I. Assessment of anti-inflammatory efficacy. *Inflammation*. 2000;24:357-370.
57. Ke TL, Graff G, Spellman JM, et al. Nepafenac, a unique nonsteroidal prodrug with potential utility in the treatment of trauma-induced ocular inflammation: II. In vitro bioactivation and permeation of external ocular barriers. *Inflammation*. 2000;24:371-384.
58. Walters T, Raizman M, Ernest P, et al. In vivo pharmacokinetics and in vitro pharmacodynamics of nepafenac, amfenac, ketorolac, and bromfenac. *J Cataract Refract Surg*. 2007;33:1539-1545.
59. FDA. FDA Label. Available at https://www.accessdata.fda.gov/scripts/cder/daf/index.cfm?event=overview.process&ApplNo=203168. Accessed September 26, 2018.
60. Comstock TL, Paterno MR, Bateman KM, et al. Safety and tolerability of loteprednol etabonate 0.5% and tobramycin 0.3% ophthalmic suspension in pediatric subjects. *Paediatr Drugs*. 2012;14:119-130.
61. del Cuvillo A, Sastre J, Montoro J, et al. Allergic conjunctivitis and H1 antihistamines. *J Investig Allergol Clin Immunol*. 2009;19(suppl 1):11-18.
62. Gong H, Blaiss MS. Topical corticosteroids and antihistamines-mast cell stabilizers for the treatment of allergic conjuctivitis. *US Ophthalmic Review*. 2013;6:78-85.

Structure Challenge Answers

1. A: The catechol functional group readily undergoes oxidation when exposed to air or light to a toxic *o*-quinone metabolite. Small amount of this metabolite produced in the body is neutralized by the glutathione reserves in the liver via conjugation.
2. E: This drug contains phenylethanolamine pharmacophore. The *m*-hydroxyl group on the phenyl ring brings its selectivity for α_1-receptors. If –OH group is present on the *para* position, it will make the drug selective to β-receptors.
3. C: The lipophilic *ortho* and *para* substituents show van der Waals interactions with Phe 308 and 312 present on the transmembrane domain 7 (TM-7) which is different from all catecholamine derivatives which bind at the receptor site.
4. D: This drug does not have a required phenolic hydroxyl group to show H-bonding interactions with the serine amino acid residues at the adrenergic receptors. However, the rest of the structure is similar to that of NE; thus, it displaces more of NE from the synaptic vesicles and inhibits NE reuptake thereby increasing its release and prolongs its duration of action.
5. B: Beta blockers have an aryloxypropanolamine pharmacophore. When this aryl group has a substituent at the *para* position that is capable of showing H-bonding interaction, selectivity for β_1-receptors is seen. β_2-Receptors do not have this space to accommodate *para* substituents. These drugs are a good choice for treating glaucoma in patients with respiratory problems.

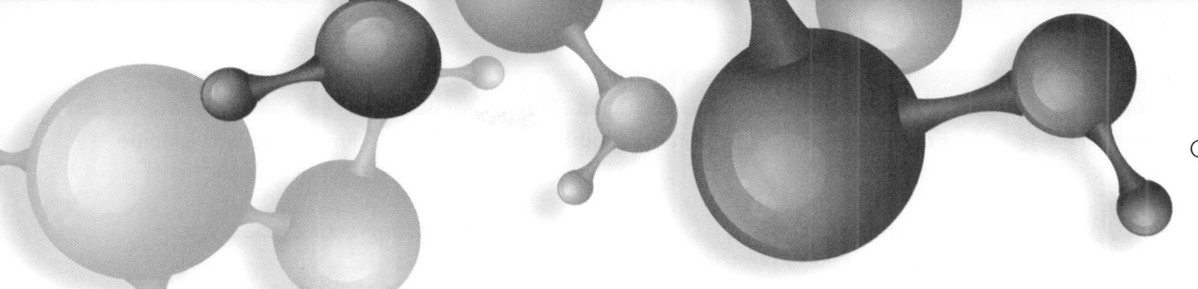

CHAPTER **28**

Drugs Used to Treat Pulmonary Disorders

S. William Zito and Srikanth Kolluru

Drugs covered in this chapter:

DRUGS USED FOR TREATING ASTHMA AND COPD

ADRENOCORTICOIDS
- Beclomethasone dipropionate
- Budesonide
- Ciclesonide
- Flunisolide
- Fluticasone propionate
- Hydrocortisone
- Methylprednisolone
- Mometasone furoate
- Prednisolone
- Triamcinolone acetonide

β_2-ADRENERGIC AGONISTS
- Albuterol sulfate
- Bitolterol mesylate
- Epinephrine (adrenalin)
- Formoterol fumarate (arformoterol)
- Indacaterol maleate
- Metaproterenol sulfate
- Olodaterol hydrochloride
- Salmeterol xinafoate
- Terbutaline sulfate
- Vilanterol trifenatate

ANTIMUSCARINICS
- Aclidinium bromide
- Glycopyrrolate bromide
- Ipratropium hydrobromide
- Tiotropium bromide
- Umeclidinium bromide

LEUKOTRIENE MODIFIERS
- Montelukast
- Zafirlukast
- Zileuton

MAST CELL DEGRANULATION INHIBITORS
- Cromolyn sodium (sodium cromoglycate)
- Nedocromil sodium

METHYLXANTHINES
- Dyphylline
- Theophylline

MONOCLONAL ANTI-IGE ANTIBODIES
- Benralizumab
- Mepolizumab
- Omalizumab
- Reslizumab

PHOSPHODIESTERASE INHIBITORS
- Roflumilast

SMOKING CESSATION MEDICATIONS
- Bupropion
- Varenicline

DRUGS USED TO TREAT CYSTIC FIBROSIS

CFTR CORRECTORS
- Lumacaftor
- Tezacaftor

CFTR POTENTIATORS
- Ivacaftor

DRUGS USED TO TREAT IDIOPATHIC PULMONARY FIBROSIS
- Nintedanib
- Pirfenidone

DRUGS USED TO TREAT PULMONARY ARTERIAL HYPERTENSION

PROSTACYCLIN RECEPTOR AGONISTS
- Epoprostenol
- Iloprost
- Treprostinil
- Selexipag

ENDOTHELIN RECEPTOR ANTAGONISTS
- Ambrisentan
- Bosentan
- Macitentan

PDE-5 INHIBITORS
- Sildenafil
- Tadalafil

SOLUBLE GUANYL CYCLASE STIMULATORS
- Riociguat

Abbreviations

AEC alveolar epithethial cells
AMP adenosine monophosphate
ATT α_1-antitrypsin
cAMP cyclic adenosine monophosphate
cGMP cyclic guanosine monophosphate
CF cystic fibrosis
CFTR cystic fibrosis transmembrane conductance regulator
CLRD chronic lower respiratory disease
CDC Centers for Disease Control and Prevention
COMT catechol O-methyl transferase
COPD chronic obstructive pulmonary disease
CRF corticotrophin-releasing factor
cysLT cysteinyl leukotriene
EPI epinephrine
FcεRI high-affinity Fc immunoglobulin E receptor
FDA U.S. Food and Drug Administration
FEV$_1$ forced expiratory volume in 1 second
FLAP 5-lipoxygenase–activating protein
FVC forced vital capacity
GI gastrointestinal
GOLD Global Initiative for Chronic Lung Disease
GR glucocorticoid receptor
HDAC2 histone deacetylase 2
HPA hypothalamus-pituitary-adrenal
HRE hormone response element
Ig immunoglobulin
IL interleukin
ICS inhaled corticosteroid
IPF idiopathic pulmonary fibrosis
IV intravenous
L-DOPA L-dihydroxyphenylalanine
LAMA long-acting muscarinic antagonist
LABA long-acting β2-adrenergic agonist
MAbs monoclonal antibodies
MAO monoamine oxidase
MSD1 membrane spanning domain 1
NE norepinephrine
NIH National Institutes of Health
NBD1 nucleotide-binding domain 1
PAH pulmonary arterial hypertension
PDE phosphodiesterase
PEF peak expiratory flow
SABA short-acting β_2-adrenergic agonist
SAMA short-acting muscarinic antagonist
SRS-A slow-reacting substance of anaphylaxis
TSLP thymic stromal lymphopoietin

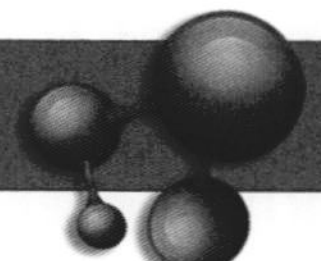

CLINICAL SIGNIFICANCE

Joseph V. Etzel, PharmD

The therapeutic approach to the pharmacologic management of both asthma and chronic obstructive pulmonary disease (COPD) have evolved over several decades, as we have gained new insights into the underlying pathophysiology of these conditions. Although both conditions are characterized by chronic inflammation and pulmonary obstruction, the nature of such abnormalities and their clinical presentations differ. Treatment guidelines have changed over the years based on a better understanding of the pathophysiology of these disease states, as well as the role of mediators such as cytokines and inflammatory cells. In addition, the application of structure-activity relationship (SAR) principles has led to the development of newer, more effective agents in the management of these conditions.

The current approach to managing these disease states is twofold: the use of rapidly acting drugs to relieve acute symptoms, as well as maintenance medications to minimize pulmonary inflammation and prevent disease exacerbations. Rapidly acting β_2-adrenergic agonists are the agents most commonly used to manage acute disease exacerbations. Older agents such as epinephrine and isoproterenol were effective in relieving symptoms but were limited because of their poor pharmacokinetic profiles and lack of pulmonary selectivity. Modification of the chemical structure of these agents has resulted in the availability of newer agents with significant clinical advantages in terms of duration of action, pulmonary specificity, and tolerability. Likewise, modification of the chemical structure of antimuscarinic agents such as atropine has resulted in the development of inhaled anticholinergic agents with superior tolerability because of minimal systemic absorption.

Multiple classes of agents are employed as maintenance therapies to prevent clinical exacerbations and minimize disease progression of both asthma and COPD. The application of SAR principles in the development of corticosteroids, long-acting adrenergic agonists, leukotriene antagonists, mast cell stabilizers, phosphodiesterase-4 inhibitors, and monoclonal antibodies have resulted in the availability of superior long-term controlling agents in terms of enhanced efficacy, greater potency, and better tolerated adverse effect profiles.

Numerous agents are approved for use in both the acute and chronic management of patients with asthma and COPD. Current treatment guidelines often provide the clinician with several pharmacologic options to employ based upon patient symptomatology and disease severity. Clinicians should be mindful of the SAR principles of these agents and use these principles to guide them in the selection of the most appropriate drug therapy based on patient-specific needs and desired clinical outcomes. As research continues, it is likely that newer and more clinically appropriate drugs will become available for clinicians to utilize in managing patients with these chronic conditions.

INTRODUCTION

The respiratory system consists of the mouth, nose, lungs, trachea, bronchi, bronchioles, and diaphragm that are collectively concerned with the exchange of oxygen and carbon dioxide. Every cell in the body requires oxygen. Anything that affects lung function has a direct impact on the quality of life. Smoking, radon, air pollution, and infections are considered major causes for most respiratory disorders.

Pulmonary diseases are disorders that affect lung function, causing breathing problems. They are classified into four categories: (1) airway diseases that include asthma and chronic obstructive pulmonary disease (COPD); (2) interstitial lung diseases, which cause scarring and inflammation, leading to reduced elasticity that make it difficult for the lungs to expand fully, such as cystic fibrosis/pulmonary fibrosis and sarcoidosis; (3) pulmonary circulation diseases affecting blood pressure in the pulmonary arteries due to scarring, inflammation, or vasoconstriction of blood vessels, leading to reduced gaseous exchange, such as pulmonary hypertension and pulmonary embolism; and (4) lung disorders due to infection, causing severe and potentially fatal inflammation of the lungs, such as influenza and pneumonia.[1]

Respiratory disorders are the third leading cause of mortality in the United States after cardiovascular diseases and cancer. Of all lung diseases, asthma, COPD, and lung cancer account for substantial morbidity in the United States. This chapter focuses on asthma, COPD, cystic fibrosis, idiopathic pulmonary fibrosis, and pulmonary arterial hypertension. Drugs that are used for respiratory disorders due to infections, such as pneumonia and influenza, are covered in Chapter 29 (antibacterial agents) and Chapter 30 (antiviral agents).

ASTHMA

Epidemiology

Asthma has been known since antiquity. The earliest reference to asthma can be found in Homer's *Iliad*, where it is a noun used to denote breathlessness or panting. The earliest use of the term as a medical condition dates back to ancient Greece, in Hippocrates' *Corpus Hippocraticum*, and the best clinical description of asthma from antiquity was offered by the physician Aretaeus of Cappadocia who practiced in the first century AD.[2]

Asthma prevalence was on the rise in the United States until 1999 but, since then, has plateaued. In addition, asthma-related mortality and hospitalizations have decreased, which may be an indication of improved disease state management.[3,4] According to US population data gathered by the national and state surveillance systems administered by the Centers for Disease Control and Prevention (CDC), asthma prevalence as of 2016 is 26.5 million. The current percentage for asthma prevalence for both children younger than 18 years and adults over age 18 years is the same at 8.3%. Boys have a higher incidence of asthma than girls (9.2% vs. 7.4%); however, this reverses in adulthood, where females show a higher prevalence compared to males (9.7% vs. 6.9%).[5] In a 2008 study, over a 1-year period (2004-2005), 15% of all children in the study population (>4 million) younger than 17 years were dispensed an asthma-related medication.[6] Race/ethnicity plays a significant role in the prevalence of asthma. Blacks have the highest prevalence, followed by whites and Hispanics (11.6% vs. 8.3% vs. 6.6%, respectively).[5] If asthma is not controlled, it can result in death. According to 2016 data, 3,518 asthma-related deaths were recorded, of which 3,309 occurred in persons older than 18 years.[5] These prevalence, morbidity, and mortality data demonstrate the significant public health burden of asthma in the United States and why the CDC has established an asthma public health approach, which includes the collection of standardized comprehensive surveillance data.[4]

A study analyzing data collected from 2008 to 2013 revealed that the economic burden of asthma in the United States was $3,266 dollars annually per person. Of this total, prescription drugs represented $1,830; office visits, $640; hospitalizations, $529; out-patient hospital visits, $176; and emergency room visits, $105 dollars. Overall, asthma cost the US economy $3 billion dollars due to missed work and school days, $53 billion in medical costs, and $29 billion due to asthma-related mortality. It is obvious that asthma poses not only a significant health burden but also an economic burden in the United States.[7]

Etiology, Signs, and Symptoms

Asthma is a common chronic, complex airway disorder that is characterized by airflow obstruction, bronchial hyperresponsiveness, and an underlying inflammation that leads to variable degrees of symptoms, such as difficulty breathing (paroxysmal dyspnea), wheezing, and cough.[8] The National Institutes of Health (NIH) Expert Panel Report 3, "Guidelines for the Diagnosis and Management of Asthma," simply defines asthma as a chronic inflammatory response of the airways.[8,9]

The most common form of asthma is allergic asthma (atopic or extrinsic asthma), and it is associated with environmental allergens, such as plant pollens, house dust mites (*Dermatophagoides farinae*), domestic pet dander, molds, and foods. The less common form, intrinsic asthma (i.e., nonallergic), has no known allergic cause and usually occurs in adults older than 35 years. Intrinsic asthma may result from an autonomic dysfunction characterized by excess cholinergic and/or tachykinin activity, but this hypothesis has never been proven.[10] Aside from environmental allergens, an asthmatic attack may be precipitated by respiratory infection, strenuous physical exercise, polyps, drugs (e.g., aspirin and β-adrenergic antagonists), and environmental pollutants, primarily cigarette smoke. Strong emotional stress and breathing cold dry air can also precipitate an asthmatic onset.[11]

Why has there been a marked increase in asthma in affluent industrialized countries? To answer this question, recent thought has focused on the "hygiene hypothesis," which implicates an imbalance of TH1 and TH2 lymphocytes as a major cause of the increased prevalence of asthma.[12] The TH1 lymphocytes are the type of CD4+ T lymphocyte associated with defense against bacterial infection, whereas the TH2 type predominates in allergic inflammation. The hypothesis claims that because bacterial infections have significantly decreased in industrialized nations, there is an imbalance in susceptible children in favor of the TH2-type lymphocytes, and this imbalance therefore favors allergic asthma.[13,14] However, it is an oversimplification to claim that asthma inflammation is simply an overproduction of TH2-type lymphocytes. Recent studies have discovered that a number of other T-helper cell subtypes are also involved in allergic inflammation, including TH9, TH17, TH25, and TH3 cells, and that regulatory T cells also contribute to asthma pathogenesis.[15]

Asthma phenotyping has been particularly difficult due to the lack of specific cellular biomarkers. The NIH sponsored Severe Asthma Research Program (SARP) reported that a few groups in Europe and the United Kingdom had initiated statistically based asthma phenotyping using different variables such as age, onset of disease, severity of the disease, etc. Based on their analysis, the following asthma phenotypes were identified.

Early-onset asthma: This type commonly starts in childhood with mild to moderate allergies. It represents about 50% of the patient population. These patients show high allergen-specific immunoglobulin E (IgE) antibodies and TH2 cytokines and respond well to corticosteroid therapy.

Late-onset asthma: This type starts later in life, usually after 35 years of age. It is often severe and nonallergic. Women are more susceptible than men; they show higher IL-5 levels and are refractory to corticosteroid therapy. Patients may respond better to IL-5 antibody and cysteinyl leukotriene modifiers.

Exercise-induced asthma: This type is usually mild and occurs during exercise. Asthma symptoms are mainly due to mast cell activation and elevation of TH2 cytokines and cysteinyl leukotrienes. These patients are expected to respond better to cysteinyl leukotriene modifiers, β-agonists, and Il-9 antibody.

Obesity-related asthma: This type affects mostly women, primarily at a later age in life. Weight loss is the best treatment available, but antioxidants and hormonal therapy might also help.

Asthma frequently occurs in families, and studies have shown that this results, at least in part, from mutually shared genes.[16,17] Asthma is a complex disorder and lacks a Mendelian genetic pattern, so it is difficult to study. To date, genetic research indicates that what is inherited is the susceptibility to develop the disease. It is clear that genes alone are not the whole development story because environmental factors also play a major role. Numerous genes on various chromosomes have been linked to asthma, and Table 28.1 shows several gene products that may influence disease development.[16–21] In reality, however, there is little correlation between gene expression and clinical symptoms.

Table 28.1 Putative Asthma-Associated Gene Products

Gene Products
β_2-adrenergic receptor
Interleukin-4, -5, -9, and -13
Interleukin-4 receptor α (Il-4Rα)
β chain of the high-affinity immunoglobulin E receptor (FcεRIβ)
Tumor necrosis factor α (TNFα)
Major histochemical complex (MHC)
T-cell receptor a/δ complex
ADAM33 (a disintegrin and metalloproteinase)
Dipeptidyl peptidase 10
PHD finer protein 11
Prostanoid DP1 receptor
Macrophage migration inhibitory factor (MIF)

Pathogenesis of Asthma

For a long time, asthmatic symptoms were thought to be the result of episodic bronchoconstriction–related airway smooth muscle abnormalities. Today, however, it is clear that the constriction of bronchial smooth muscle is only one of many effects of chronic airway inflammation. Evidence of inflammation appears very soon after the onset of symptoms; therefore, treatment algorithms for asthma now emphasize quick relief of the bronchoconstriction and the amelioration of the underlying inflammation.[22]

Inflammation in asthma is characterized by mucous plugging, epithelial shedding, basement membrane thickening, inflammatory cell infiltration, and smooth muscle hypertrophy, and hyperplasia. An acute extrinsic asthmatic attack begins when allergens interact with lung epithelia, which causes the release of cytokines (thymic stromal lymphopoietin [TSLP] and interleukin [IL], primarily IL-33 and IL-25). TSLP mediates migration and maturation of dendritic cells and production of IL-4 from competent T-helper cells (TFH). This leads to the activation of B cells to produce immunoglobulin IgE antibody, which in turn binds to high-affinity Fc IgE receptors (FCεRI) on the mast cells. Activation of mast cells occurs when an antigen cross-links with IgEs on their surface. This IgE complex triggers mast cell degranulation, leading to the rapid release of inflammatory mediators, such as histamine, prostaglandins, leukotrienes, and cytokines (including tumor necrosis factor-α and ILs). The initial attack generally resolves within an hour; however, a second phase begins 4-6 hours after exposure and can last up to 24 hours. This late phase is the result of recruitment of additional inflammatory cells, primarily eosinophils, by the release of cytokines (IL-4, IL-13, IL-5, IL-9, and IL-3) from macrophages and TH_2-type lymphocytes in the lower lung (Fig. 28.1).[23,24]

Clinical Evaluation

Most patients with asthma are asymptomatic between acute exacerbations. The onset of symptoms can be sudden or gradual and frequently occurs during the night or early in the morning. Acute symptoms include shortness of breath, wheezing or whistling at the end of exhalation, cough, and chest tightness. Patients with chronic and poorly controlled asthma develop barrel chest and diminished diaphragm movement, both of which are evidence of chronic pulmonary hyperinflation.

Acute asthmatic attacks may be mild, moderate, or severe depending on the degree of airway obstruction. The determination of the degree of airflow obstruction is accomplished by pulmonary function testing. The most common pulmonary function test uses spirometry, which measures the rate at which the lung changes volume during forced breathing maneuvers. The most important spirometric measure is the forced vital capacity (FVC). This requires the patient to exhale as rapidly and as completely as possible after a maximal inhalation. Normal lungs generally can empty their volume in 6 seconds or less. When airflow is obstructed, however, the expiratory time may increase by as much as fivefold. In practice, the forced expiratory volume in 1 second (FEV_1) is measured and compared to the FVC and then recorded as the ratio of FEV_1 to FVC (FEV_1/FVC) (Fig. 28.2) (measurement is done by means of a spirometer). Healthy persons normally can expel at least 75% of their FVC in the first second. Decreases in the FEV_1/FVC ratio indicate obstruction, and a decrease below 40% indicates severe asthma.[22]

A more convenient way to measure airway obstruction is to determine the peak expiratory flow (PEF) rate. The PEF rate correlates well with the FEV_1, can be determined using inexpensive, handheld, peak flow meters, and is easily and simply measured at home. The PEF rate is the maximal rate of flow that is produced through forced expiration. Peak flow meters come with a chart that lists predicted PEF rates based on the patient's age, gender, and height. The patient or clinician can then compare the determined PEF rate with the predicted PEF rate and make an evaluation regarding the severity of an asthmatic attack. The PEF rate or the FEV_1/FVC ratio, along with the frequency of daytime and nighttime symptoms, forms the basis for the classification of the severity of an asthmatic attack. Table 28.2 shows the severity classification of asthma established by the NIH Expert Panel Report 3, "Guidelines for the Diagnosis and Management of Asthma."[8]

Alternatively, it has become common to estimate asthma severity based upon the treatment necessary to control symptoms after the patient has been on a regular controller treatment for several months. Mild asthma is defined when the patient is well controlled with reliever medication alone or with a low-dose controller medication such as an inhaled corticosteroid (ICS), leukotriene receptor antagonist, or a chromone. Moderate asthma is asthma

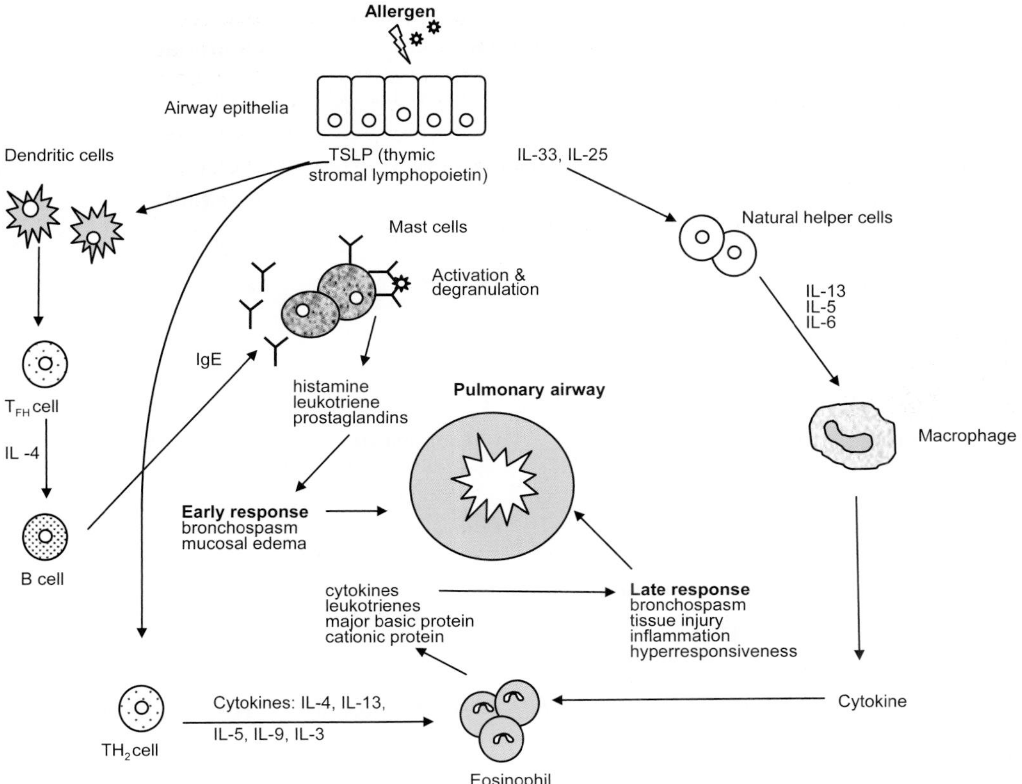

Figure 28.1 Pictorial summary of asthma pathogenesis. *IL*, interleukin.

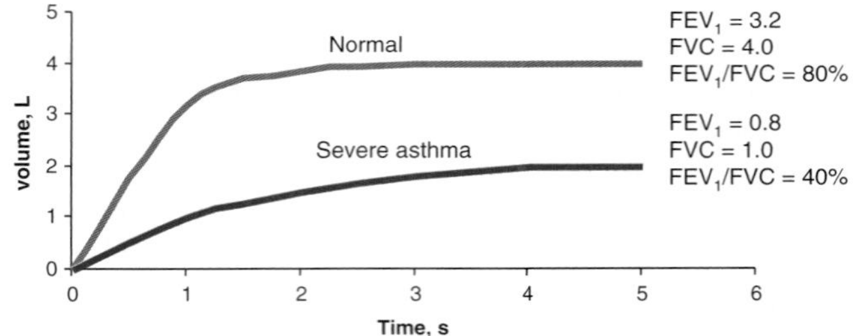

Figure 28.2 Spirometric comparison of normal and severe asthma. FEV_1, forced expiratory volume in 1 second; FVC, forced vital capacity.

that is well controlled with low-dose ICS in combination with a long-acting β agonist (LABA). Severe asthma is asthma that needs to be prevented from becoming uncontrolled in spite of treatment with high-dose ICS/LABA.[25,26]

Patients with uncontrolled (refractory) asthma may benefit from biomarker identification of their particular asthma phenotype. There are three major asthma phenotypes: (1) trigger-induced asthma (allergen, nonallergenic, aspirin, exercise, infection); (2) clinical presentation of asthma (multitrigger wheezing, exacerbation-prone asthma, irreversible airflow limitation), and (3) inflammatory markers of asthma (eosinophilic and neutrophilic asthma).[27]

Biological markers can aid in the understanding of phenotypes and might help identify other treatments for patients who respond poorly to first-line pharmacotherapy. IgE is allergen specific and stimulated early in the asthma episode by the release of IL-4, IL-5, and IL-13 through activated TH2 cells. IgE binds to FcεRI expressed on mast cells, basophils, eosinophils, and B lymphocytes, releasing proinflammatory mediators (tryptase, histamine, prostaglandins, leukotrienes). Eosinophils are recruited into areas of inflammation, usually late in the onset, and are associated with modulation of the immune response. They promote airway hyperresponsiveness and remodeling under the influence of IL-4 and IL-13. IL-5 is necessary for the maturation, activation, and survival of eosinophils. High levels of IgE and eosinophils (among other markers) are related to severe refractory asthma. Neutrophils are found in high numbers in sputum and are associated with severe asthma and in patients experiencing exacerbations. IL-8 activates neutrophils to secrete enzymes and other factors that contribute to eosinophil activity. In addition to the IgE, eosinophils, and neutrophils, many cytokines mediate asthma inflammation, including ILs-4, 5, 9, 11, 13, 17, 25, and 33. Monoclonal antibodies (MAbs) developed to target components of the inflammatory cascade have added to the management of severe refractory asthma.[24]

Table 28.2 Classification of Asthma Severity[8]

Components of Severity		Intermittent Step 1	Persistent: Mild Step 2	Persistent: Moderate Step 3	Persistent: Severe Step 4 or 5
	Symptoms	≤2 d/wk	>2 d/wk but not daily	Daily	Throughout the day
Impairment	Nighttime awakenings	≤2×/month	3-4×/mo	>1×/wk but not nightly	Often 7×/wk
Normal FEV_1/FVC:	Rescue inhaler use	≤2 d/wk	>2 d/wk but not daily and not >1× on any day	Daily	Several times per day
8-19 yr 85%					
20-39 yr 80%					
40-59 yr 75%	Interference with normal activity	None	Minor limitation	Some limitation	Extremely limited
60-80 yr 70%					
	Lung function	Normal FEV_1 between exacerbation			
		FEV_1 >80% predicted	FEV_1 >80% predicted	FEV_1 >60% but <80% predicted	FEV_1 <60% predicted
		FEV_1/FVC normal	FEV_1/FVC normal	FEV_1/FVC reduced 5%	FEV_1/FVC reduced >5%

FEV1, forced expiratory volume in 1 s; FVC, forced vital capacity.

General Therapeutic Approaches to the Treatment and Management of Asthma

Asthma symptoms are caused by bronchoconstriction and inflammation, and approaches to treatment are directed at both of these physiologic problems. Therefore, drugs that affect adrenergic/cholinergic bronchial smooth muscle tone and drugs that inhibit the inflammatory process are used to treat and control asthma symptoms. In the normal lung, bronchiole smooth muscle tone results from the balance between the bronchoconstrictive effects of the cholinergic system and the bronchodilating effects of the adrenergic system on the smooth muscles of the bronchioles. Pharmacologic treatment of asthmatic bronchoconstriction consists of either increasing adrenergic tone with an adrenergic agonist or inhibiting cholinergic tone with an anticholinergic agent.

The inflammatory effects seen in asthma are the result of the release of physiologically active chemicals from a variety of inflammatory cells. Pharmacologic treatment, therefore, uses anti-inflammatory drugs (corticosteroids), mast cell stabilizers, leukotriene modifiers, and IgE monoclonal antibodies. Figure 28.3 depicts the overall approach to the pharmacologic treatment of asthma.

Therapeutic management of asthma requires the use of quick-acting drugs to relieve an acute attack, as well as drugs that control symptoms over the long term. The current approach to asthma management uses a stepwise approach.[8] The quick-reliever (rescue) medication is almost always an inhaled short-acting β_2-adrenergic agonist (SABA), whereas controller drugs are inhaled corticosteroids, LABAs, leukotriene modifiers, cromolyn sodium, and/or methylxanthines. The dose, route of administration, and number of controller drugs depend on the severity of the patient's disease. The U.S. Food and Drug Administration (FDA), in 2011, required a boxed warning on LABAs, stating they should never be used alone or in combination in the treatment of asthma in children or adults based on analyses of studies showing an increased risk of severe worsening of asthma symptoms, leading to hospitalizations and even death in some patients. However in 2017, after several trials, the FDA removed the boxed warning on LABA combinations with ICs, but it still remains on LABA use alone.[28] Table 28.3 shows the stepwise approach to asthma management based on disease severity.

Bronchial smooth muscle tone

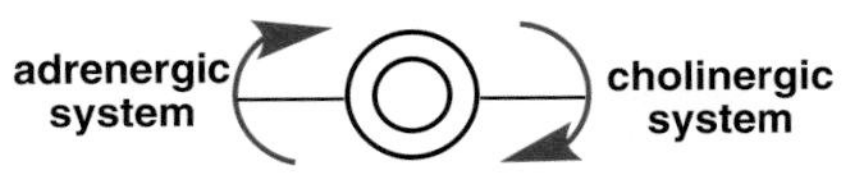

bronchodilation **bronchoconstriction**

Treatment

Increase bronchodilation by using an adrenergic agonist
Decrease bronchoconstriction by using an anticholinergic

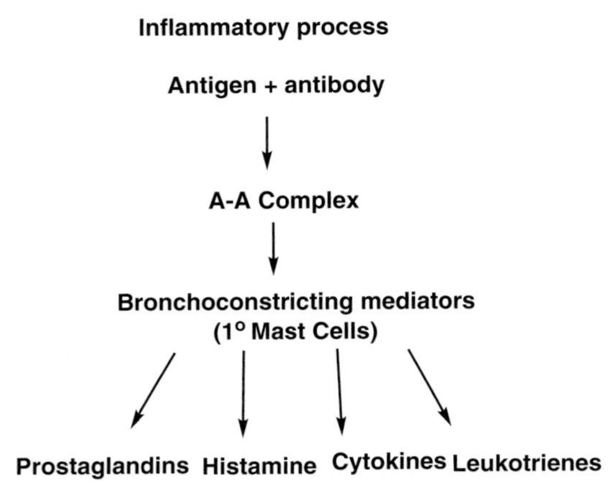

Treatment

Corticosteroids; mast cell stabilizers; leukotriene modifiers; and monoclonal anti-IGE antibodies

Figure 28.3 Overview of pharmacologic treatment for asthma.

Therapeutic Classes of Drugs Used to Treat Asthma and Chronic Obstructive Pulmonary Disease

β_2-Adrenergic Agonists

What structural features make a drug an adrenergic agonist? What features make it a selective β_2-agonist? The answers to these questions lie in the structural relationship of a drug to that of norepinephrine (NE), the physiologic neurotransmitter of the sympathetic branch of the autonomic nervous system. Drugs that act on postsynaptic sympathetic receptors in the same way as NE are called sympathomimetics or, more commonly, adrenergic agonists. The related natural agonist epinephrine (EPI; adrenalin, a neurohormone) is the predominant adrenergic hormone produced in the chromaffin cells of the adrenal medulla. EPI interacts just like NE at all adrenergic receptors, only with slightly higher affinity due to hydrophobic bonding of the N-CH_3 group.

Chemistry and Biochemistry of Norepinephrine and Epinephrine

Chemically, NE is classified as a catecholamine. A catechol is a 1,2-dihydroxybenzene, and NE is a β-hydroxyethylamino-3,4-dihydroxybenzene. EPI is the N-methyl derivative of NE, and they both have acidic and basic functional groups. Physiologically, however, they behave as bases, being more than 90% protonated at pH 7.4 (amine $pK_a = 9.6$) and functioning as an ionized acid. The acidic phenols have pH values of approximately 9 and remain significantly unionized at physiologic pH.

HO, HO, OH, NHR

Norepinephrine R = H
Epinephrine R = CH_3

Table 28.3 Stepwise Medication Management of Asthma

All Asthma Patients: Short-Acting Inhaled β_2-Agonist (SABA) as Needed for Acute Exacerbations

Severity Classification	Long-Term Control
Step 1: Intermittent asthma	*Preferred:* SABA PRN
Persistent Asthma	
Step 2: Mild	*Preferred:* Low-dose inhaled corticosteroid (ICS)
	Alternative: Cromolyn, nedocromil, leukotriene receptor antagonist (LTRA) or theophylline
Step 3: Moderate	*Preferred:* Low-dose ICS + long-acting $\beta_2$agonist (LABA) or medium-dose ICS
	Alternative: Low-dose ICS + either LTRA, theophylline, or zileuton
Step 4: Severe	*Preferred:* Medium-dose ICS + LABA
	Alternative: Medium-dose ICS + either LTRA, theophylline, or zileuton
Step 5: Severe	*Preferred:* High-dose ICS + LABA
	Consider: Omalizumab for patients who have allergies *Consider:* Mepolizumab, reslizumab, benralizumab for patients with eosinophilic asthma
Step 6: Severe	*Preferred:* High-dose ICS + LABA + oral corticosteroid
	Consider: Omalizumab for patients who have allergies

NE is biosynthesized in the neurons of both the central nervous system and the autonomic nervous system, whereas EPI is formed in and secreted from the chromaffin cells of the adrenal medulla. Both NE and EPI are derived from L-tyrosine by a series of enzyme-catalyzed reactions (Fig. 28.4 depicts the overall pathway). L-tyrosine hydroxylase hydroxylates the *m*-position of L-tyrosine, producing L-dihydroxyphenylalanine (L-DOPA), and is the rate-limiting step. The L-DOPA is then decarboxylated by L-aromatic amino acid decarboxylase to form dopamine, which is converted to NE by the action of dopamine β-hydroxylase. Dopamine β-hydroxylase is found in storage vesicles of the nerve ending, and the NE formed is stored there until it is released into the synaptic cleft upon nerve depolarization. In the chromaffin cells, the formed NE is converted to EPI by N-methylation catalyzed by phenylethanolamine N-methyltransferase.

Termination of Neurotransmission

Stimulated adrenergic neurons release NE into the synaptic cleft, which then binds reversibly with receptors to produce a characteristic adrenergic response. Termination of the adrenergic response occurs primarily by reuptake (uptake-1) into the presynaptic neuron; however, diffusion away from the receptors and extracellular metabolism also occur to a limited extent. The NE that is taken back up into the presynaptic neuron is either used again as a neurotransmitter or is metabolized by mitochondrial monoamine oxidase (MAO). The extraneuronal NE that diffuses away from the neurons is either metabolized by catechol O-methyl transferase (COMT) in situ or reaches the circulatory system and is metabolized by COMT and MAO in various tissues, most importantly the liver, gastrointestinal (GI) tract, and the lungs. Figure 28.5 depicts the possible metabolic pathways for both NE and EPI. It is important to note that agonists that are resistant to MAO and/or COMT have greater oral availability and a longer duration of action.

Adrenergic Receptors

The adrenergic receptors have long been pharmacologically classified as α or β based on their interaction with NE, EPI, and the β adrenergic agonist prototype, isoproterenol.[29] NE and EPI are nonselective and interact with all adrenergic receptors, but isoproterenol selectively interacts only with the β-receptors.

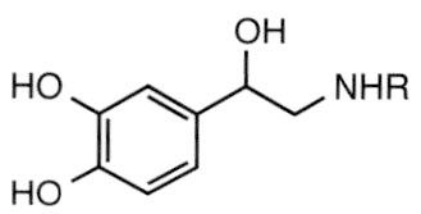

HO, HO, OH, NHR

Norepinephrine (NE) R = H

Epinephrine (EPI) R = CH_3

Isoproterenol (ISO) R = $HC(CH_3)_2$

The adrenergic receptors have been further divided into three groups, α_1, α_2, and β, each of which has been further divided into three receptor subtypes based on their organ distribution and physiologic activities.[29] Therefore, there are now a total of nine adrenergic receptor subtypes, but the most important in relation to the treatment of asthma and chronic obstructive pulmonary disease (COPD) are the β_1 and β_2 subtypes that are found primarily in the heart and the lung, respectively. As may be deduced from Table 28.4, adrenergic agonists that are selective for the β_2 subtype will cause bronchial dilation and might be expected to relieve the bronchospasm of an asthmatic attack. Nonselective β-agonists, however, will have stimulatory cardiac effects and, therefore, would have limited use in cardiac patients with asthma.

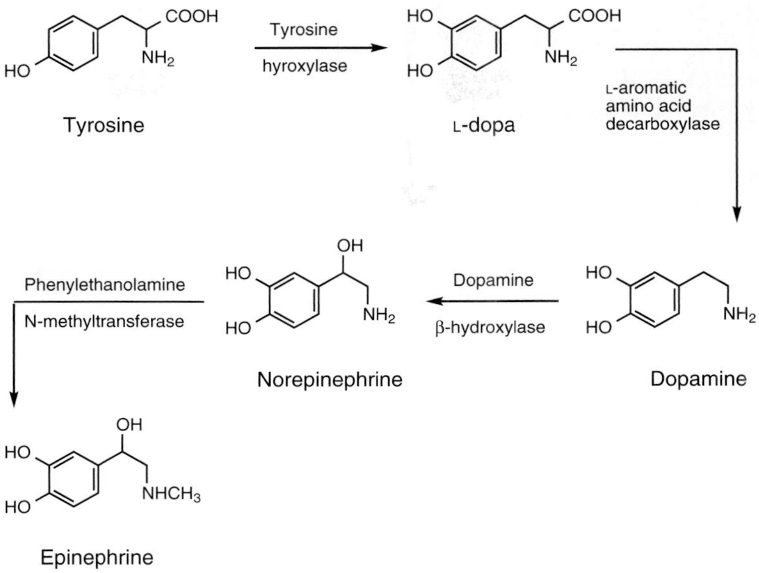

COOH
NH2
HO
Tyrosine
Tyrosine hyroxylase
HO
HO
COOH
NH2
L-dopa
L-aromatic amino acid decarboxylase
HO
HO
NH2
Dopamine
Dopamine β-hydroxylase
OH
HO
HO
NH2
Norepinephrine
Phenylethanolamine N-methyltransferase
OH
HO
HO
NHCH3
Epinephrine

Figure 28.4 The biosynthesis of norepinephrine and epinephrine from tyrosine.

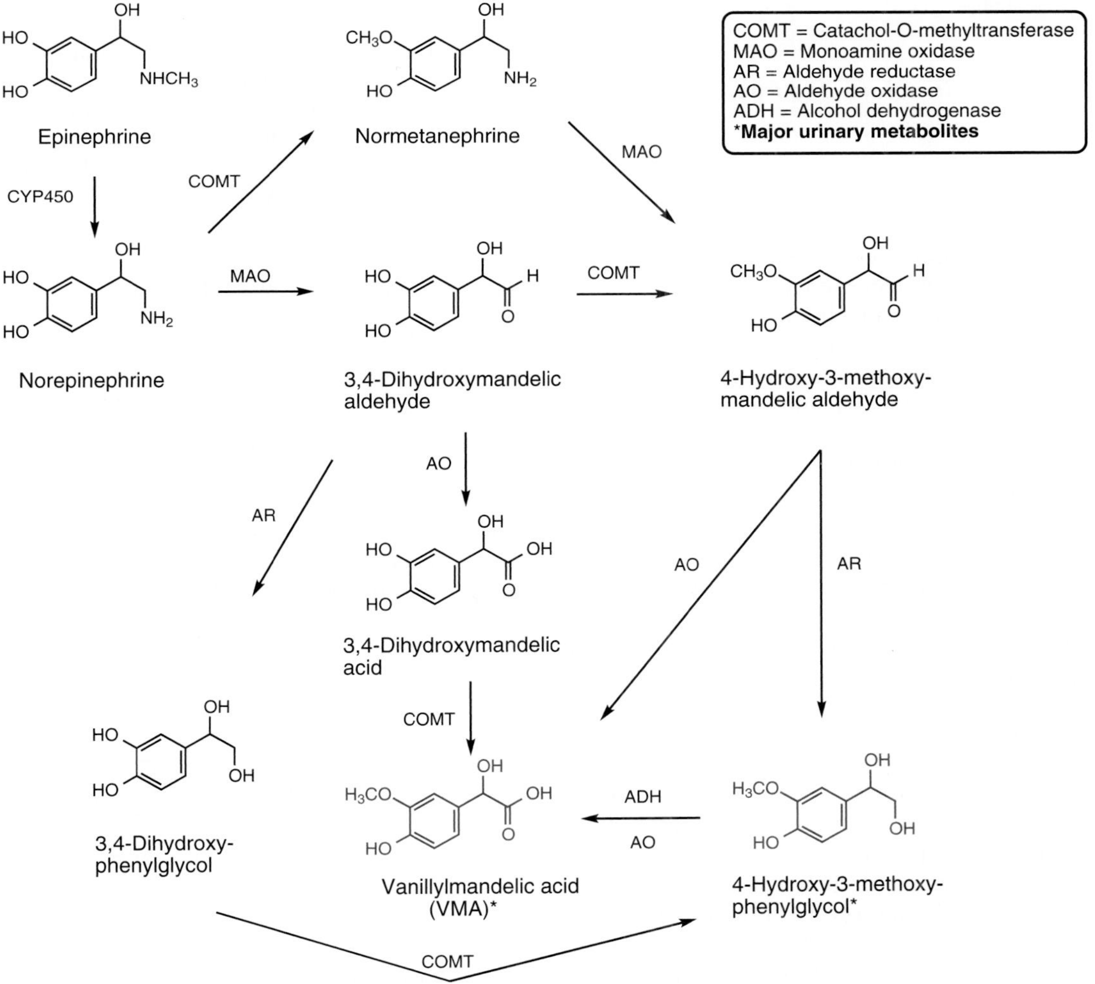

Figure 28.5 Metabolic pathways for norepinephrine and epinephrine.

Table 28.4 Physiologic Response in Relationship to β-Receptor Subtype and Organ Site

Receptor Subtype	Organ Location	Response
β_1	Heart	Increased rate and force
		Increased conduction velocity
β_2	Bronchiole smooth muscle	Dilation
	Intestine	Decreased motility
	Liver	Increased gluconeogenesis
		Increased glycogenolysis
	Uterus	Contraction
	Lungs	Bronchial dilation

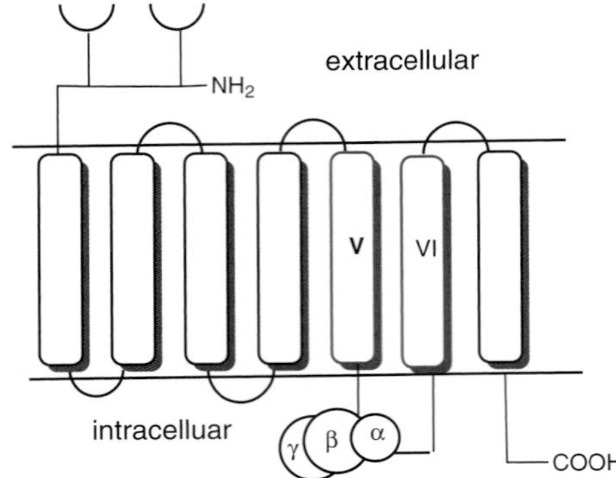

Figure 28.6 Representations of the G protein–coupled receptor.

Adrenergic Receptor Structure and Agonist Interactions

The adrenergic receptors are members of the guanine nucleotide-binding regulatory protein–coupled receptor family more commonly referred to as G protein–coupled receptors (GPCRs, see Chapter 8). They affect biologic activity by releasing second messenger molecules inside the cell after they bind an extracellular agonist. This process is usually referred to as signal transduction and is common to hormone and neurotransmitter receptors found in the muscarinic, serotonergic, dopaminergic, and adrenergic systems. All GPCRs are structurally similar, being comprised of seven transmembrane α-helix bundles. The helices are connected by short stretches of hydrophilic residues, which form multiple loops in the intracellular and extracellular domains. The G proteins generally are bound to the third intracellular loop and imbedded in the inner membrane (Fig. 28.6).

All β-adrenergic receptors are coupled to adenylyl cyclase via specific stimulatory G proteins (Gs). When agonist binds to the β-adrenergic receptors, the α-subunit migrates through the membrane and stimulates adenylyl cyclase to form cyclic adenosine monophosphate (cAMP) from adenosine triphosphate (ATP). Once formed in the cell, cAMP activates protein kinase A, which catalyzes the phosphorylation of numerous proteins, thereby regulating their activity and leading to characteristic cellular responses. The intracellular enzyme phosphodiesterase (PDE) hydrolyzes cAMP to form adenosine monophosphate (AMP) and terminates its action (Fig. 28.7).

A great deal of research has been done to identify the binding residues of the adrenergic receptors. Molecular modeling methods have been used to construct three-dimensional models for agonist complexes with the β_2-adrenergic receptor. The picture that has emerged is that NE binds ionically via its protonated amine to Asp113 in helix 3 and hydrogen bonds to both hydroxyls of the catechol ring with Ser204 and Ser207 in helix 5. That binding limits its configurational and rotational freedoms, which allows reinforcing van der Waals interactions between the aromatic ring with residues Phe290 in helix 6 and Val114 in helix 3. The N-alkyl substituents are believed to fit into a pocket formed between aliphatic residues in helix 6 and helix 7. Stereochemistry also plays an important role in receptor binding. The β-carbon in NE/EPI is chiral and can be either R or S in configuration. Endogenous NE/EPI exists in the R configuration so that the β-hydroxy is oriented toward the receptor Asn293[30–33] (Fig. 28.8). This bond is deemed essential at β-receptors, and every direct-acting β agonist (including the β_2-selective agonists used in asthma) will have a β–OH group in the R configuration.

Adrenergic Agonist Structure-Activity Relationships

The fundamental pharmacophore for all adrenergic agonists is a substituted β-phenylethylamine (as in EPI and NE). The nature and number of substituents on the pharmacophore influences whether an analogue will be direct acting, indirect acting, or have a mixture of direct and indirect action. In addition, the nature and number of substituents also influences the specificity for the β-receptor subtypes. Direct-acting adrenergic agonists

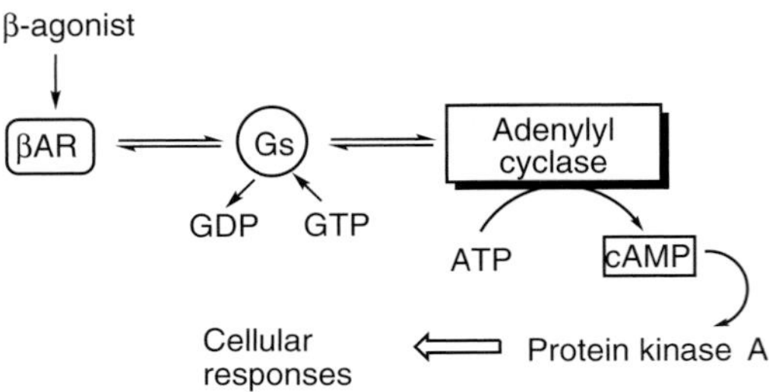

Figure 28.7 β-adrenergic receptor (β-AR) G protein coupling to adenylyl cyclase. ATP, adenosine triphosphate; cAMP, cyclic adenosine monophosphate; GDP, guanosine diphosphate; Gs, G proteins; GTP, guanosine triphosphate.

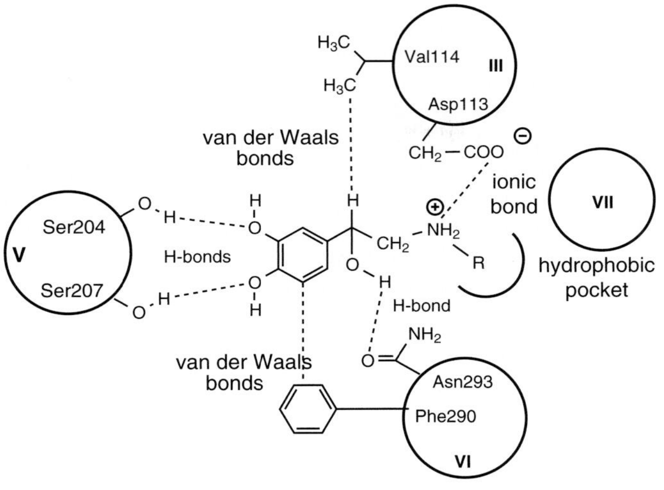

Figure 28.8 Ligand binding to key residues in the adrenergic receptor.

bind the β-adrenergic receptors just like NE/EPI, producing a sympathetic response. Indirect-acting agonists cause their effect by a number of mechanisms. They can stimulate the release of NE from the presynaptic terminal, inhibit the reuptake of released NE, or inhibit the metabolic degradation of NE by neuronal MAO (i.e., MAO inhibitors). Mixed-acting agonists work as their name implies (i.e., they have both direct and indirect abilities).

Relationship of Structure to α- or β-Receptor Selectivity

The substituents on the amino group determine α- or β-receptor selectivity. As was noted earlier, when the N-substituent is changed from hydrogen (NE) to methyl (EPI) to isopropyl (isoproterenol), the receptor affinity transitions from nonselective (NE/EPI) to β-selective. Therefore, one can say that bulk greater than CH_3 on the amino N confers selectivity for the β-receptor. As a matter of fact, if R_1 is *t*-butyl, there is not only a complete loss of α-receptor affinity, but also the β affinity shows preference for the β_2-receptor. It must be said that receptor selectivity is dose related, and when the dose is high enough, all selectivity can be lost.

Substituents on the α-carbon (R_2) other than hydrogen will show an increased duration of action, because they make the compound resistant to metabolism by MAO. In addition, if the substituent is ethyl, there is selectivity for the β_2-receptor, which is enhanced by a bulky N-substituent. Interestingly, α-methyl substitution shows a slight β-receptor enhancement and only for the *S*-configuration. The β-receptor is clearly more tolerant of steric bulk than the α-receptor.

For an adrenergic agonist to demonstrate significant β_2-receptor selectivity, there needs to be, in addition to the bulky N-substituent, an appropriately substituted phenyl ring. The currently marketed adrenergic agonists contain either a resorcinol ring, a salicyl alcohol moiety, a *m*-formamide group, or a quinoline-based 6-hydroxybenzoxazine-3-one or 8-hydroxybenzquinolin-2-one group (Fig. 28.9). In addition, these ring configurations are resistant to COMT metabolism and will increase the duration of action.

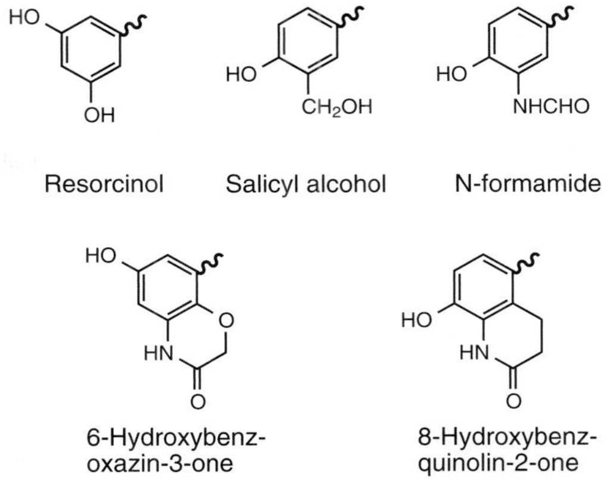

Figure 28.9 Ring configurations that contribute to β_2-receptor selectivity.

Specific Adrenergic Drugs Used to Treat Asthma

Epinephrine (Adrenalin)

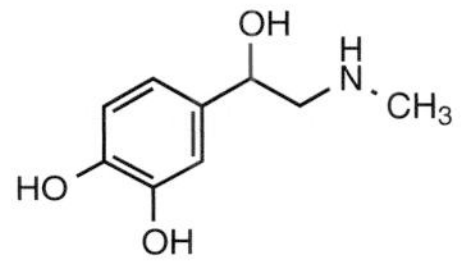

Epinephrine

The combination of the catechol nucleus, the β-hydroxy group, and the N-methyl gives EPI direct action and high affinity for all adrenergic receptors. Epinephrine and all other catechols are chemically susceptible to oxygen and other oxidizing agents, especially in the presence of base and/or light, quickly decomposing to inactive quinones. Therefore, all catechol-containing drugs are stabilized with antioxidants and dispensed in air-tight amber containers.

Epinephrine is ultimately metabolized by COMT and MAO to 3-methoxy-4-hydroxymandelic acid (vanillylmandelic acid), which is excreted as the sulfate or glucuronide conjugate in the urine (Fig. 28.5). Only a very small amount is excreted unchanged.

Epinephrine usually is administered slowly by intravenous (IV) injection to relieve acute asthmatic attacks not controlled by other treatments. IV injection produces an immediate response. Use of EPI with drugs that enhance cardiac arrhythmias (digitalis or quinidine) is not recommended. Tricyclic antidepressants and MAO inhibitors will potentiate the effects of EPI on the heart. Epinephrine should be used with caution in individuals suffering from hyperthyroidism, cardiovascular disease, hypertension, or diabetes. Adverse effects include palpitations, tachycardia, sweating, nausea and vomiting, respiratory difficulty, dizziness, tremor, apprehension, and anxiety.

Metaproterenol Sulfate

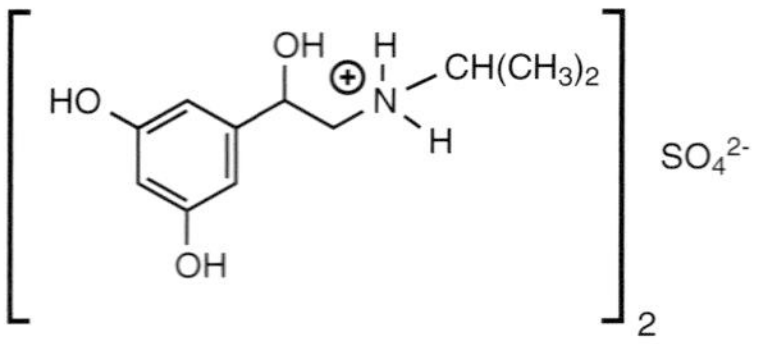

Metaproterenol sulfate
(Alupent, Metaprel)

Metaproterenol is a direct-acting resorcinol analogue of isoproterenol. The N-isopropyl is β-directing, and the combination with the resorcinol ring system enhances the selectivity for β_2-receptors. It is the least potent of the β_2-selective agonists.

Metaproterenol has good oral bioavailability, as it is resistant to COMT and only slowly metabolized by MAO. As a phenol, it is subject to sulfonation in the gut (the preferred phase 2 reaction of SABAs); however, the dose administered ensures a sufficient amount is absorbed for therapeutically relevant action. When administered orally, it has an onset of approximately 30 minutes with a 4-hour duration. Inhaled metaproterenol can have an onset as rapid as 5 minutes; however, it can be as long as 30 minutes in some individuals. Metaproterenol is available in tablet, syrup, and inhalation dosage forms and is recommended for bronchial asthma attacks and treatment of acute asthmatic attacks in children 6 years of age and older (5% solution for inhalation only). Metaproterenol has the same adverse effect profile as other β-adrenergic agonists but with a decreased incidence of arrhythmias.

Terbutaline Sulfate

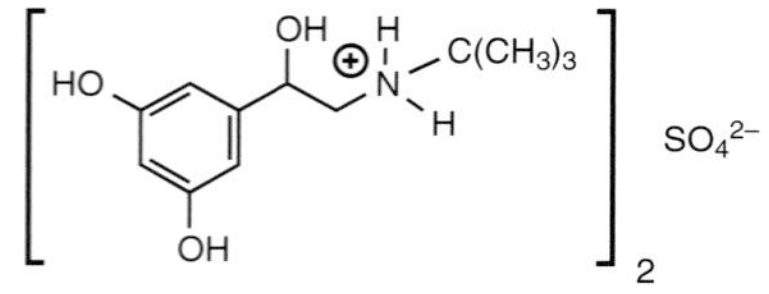

Terbutaline sulfate
(Brethine, Brethaire)

Terbutaline is the N-*t*-butyl analogue of metaproterenol and, as such, would be expected to have a more potent β_2-selectivity. When compared to metaproterenol, terbutaline has a threefold greater potency at the β_2-receptor. Like metaproterenol, it is resistant to COMT (although vulnerable to intestinal and hepatic sulfonation) and slowly metabolized by MAO and thus has good oral bioavailability, with similar onset and duration. Terbutaline is available as tablets and solutions for injection and inhalation. Adverse effects are similar to other direct-acting β_2-selective agonists but with a greater incidence of palpitations.

Bitolterol Mesylate

Although bitolterol mesylate has been withdrawn from the market, it is presented here as an excellent example of a prodrug designed for enhanced duration of action via lipophilic ester formation.[34] Upon inhalation, it sequesters in lipophilic bronchial membranes and slowly releases colterol on activation by hydrolytic esterases in the lung (Fig. 28.10). Colterol is a direct-acting agonist, and the N-*t*-butyl group makes it β_2-selective with a binding potency equivalent to that of terbutaline. The ester also provides resistance to COMT, which adds to its increased duration of action. Onset begins 2-4 minutes after administration, and the effect can last as long as 8 hours. It has an adverse effect profile similar to that of other β_2-selective agonists, with less drowsiness and restlessness compared to other direct-acting β_2 agonists.

Albuterol

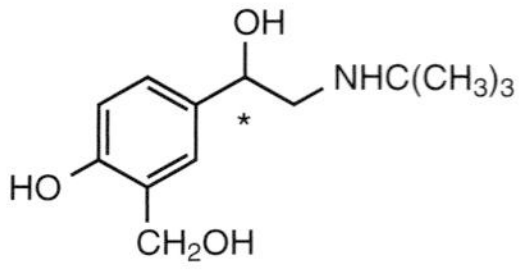

dl-Albuterol (Proventil, Ventolin)
Levalbuterol (Xopenex)

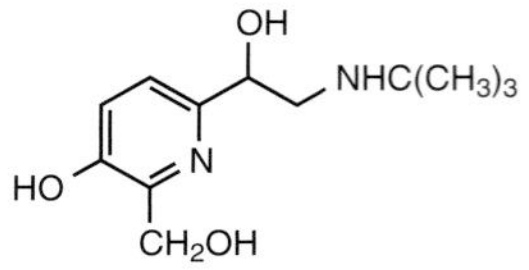

Pirbuterol (Maxair)

Albuterol has the N-*t*-butyl and a salicyl alcohol phenyl ring, which gives it optimal β_2-selectivity. It is resistant to COMT (although vulnerable to sulfonation) and slowly metabolized by MAO, thus having good oral bioavailability. Its onset by inhalation is within 5 minutes and has a duration of action between 4 and 8 hours. It currently is the drug of choice for relief of the acute bronchospasm of an asthmatic attack.

Levalbuterol is the *R*-(−)-isomer of albuterol and is available only in solution to be administered via nebulizer of albuterol. Studies with the *R*/*S* enantiomers of albuterol have shown that the *S*-enantiomer can be proinflammatory, exacerbating airway reactivity to a variety of

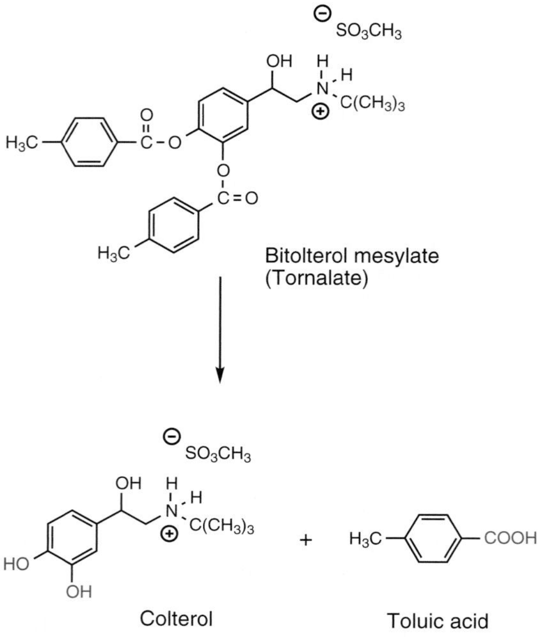

Bitolterol mesylate
(Tornalate)

Colterol

Toluic acid

Figure 28.10 Esterase hydrolysis of bitolterol.

spasmogens and, thereby, enhancing bronhiolar smooth muscle contraction. This opposes the bronchodilation effects of the *R*-enantiomer levoalbuterol. Moreover, racemic albuterol exhibits enantioselective presystemic metabolism. Levalbuterol undergoes more rapid metabolism (sulfation) than the *S*-(+)-isomer, resulting in a lower oral bioavailability and rapid elimination. Because of its slower metabolism, *S*-albuterol has a higher and more prolonged tissue concentration than levalbuterol, increasing airway reactivity. These adverse effects of *S*-albuterol are completely avoided by using the *R*-enantiomer, levalbuterol (Xopenex). Thus, the removal of *S*-albuterol from racemic albuterol increases the clinical potency of levalbuterol, such that bronchodilator efficacy is achieved at one-fourth the dose of racemic albuterol along with a marked reduction in side effects. Racemic albuterol is still a primary drug of choice for occasional users, as *S*-enantiomer also will be eliminated before administering the next dose. Levalbuterol is recommended for chronic use to avoid the proinflammatory effects caused by the accumulation of inactive *S*-isomer.

Pirbuterol is the pyridine isostere of albuterol. It exhibits pharmacokinetic properties similar to albuterol but is half as potent at the β_2-receptor. Pirbuterol is only available as an inhaler, whereas albuterol comes in tablet, syrup, solution, and aerosol formulations. Adverse effects of pirbuterol are nervousness, tremor, and headache, which are less extensive than the profile for albuterol, which adds nausea, vomiting, dizziness, hypertension, insomnia, tachycardia, and palpitations. The difference in adverse effects may be due to pirbuterol being 9 times more selective for pulmonary tissue than albuterol.[35]

Salmeterol Xinafoate

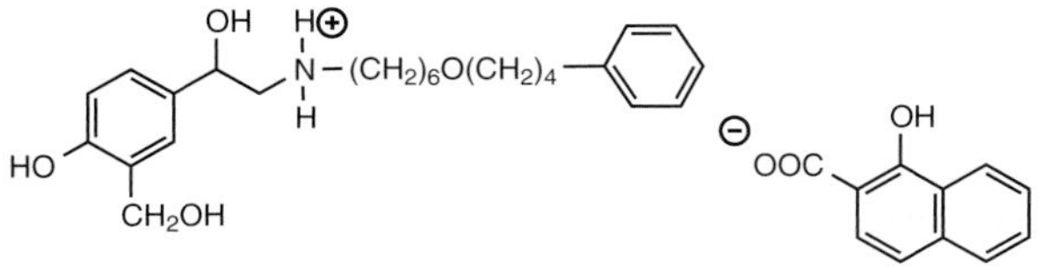

Salmeterol xinafoate
(Serevent diskus)

Salmeterol, a partial β_2 receptor agonist, has an N-phenylbutoxyhexyl substituent in combination with a β-hydroxy group and a salicyl alcohol phenyl ring for optimal direct-acting β_2-receptor selectivity and potency. It is resistant to both MAO and COMT, and that, together with its increased lipophilicity, gives salmeterol a long duration of action. It has been postulated that the phenylbutoxyhexyl N-substituent binds outside of the receptor site and keeps the active pharmacophore moiety in position for prolonged receptor stimulation. While this may be true, there is now evidence that its long duration of action may also be due to its lipid solubility (log $D_{pH\ 7.4}$ >2.5) and ability to form a depot in lung tissue membranes.[36] It is available only as a powder for inhalation, with a 20-minute onset of action and a 12-hour duration. It is used as a controller for the long-term treatment of asthma and is not recommended for quick relief of an acute attack. It also is available in combination with the steroid fluticasone propionate (Advair Diskus).

There was a small but significant increase in asthma-related deaths among patients receiving salmeterol during a large clinical trial, and as a result, the FDA has recommended that it not be used as monotherapy for asthma in either children or adults. Subgroup analyses suggested that the risk may be greater in black patients compared with Caucasian patients.[28,37] Salmeterol is metabolized extensively by CYP3A4 in the liver through benzylic hydroxylation. Caution must be exercised while using salmeterol in combination with strong CYP3A4 inhibitors such as ketoconazole.[38]

Formoterol Fumarate

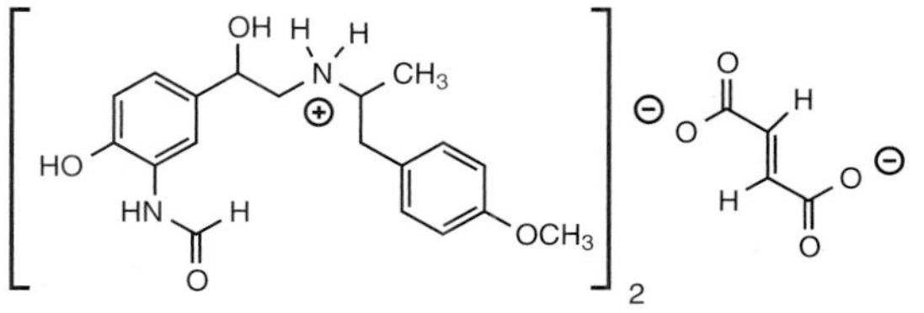

Formoterol fumarate (Foradil aerosolizer)
Arformoterol (*R,R*-Formoterol [Brovana])

Formoterol has a β-directing N-isopropyl-p-methoxyphenyl group and a unique *m*-formamide and *p*-methoxyphenyl ring, which provides selectivity for β_2-receptors. It is resistant to MAO and COMT, making it a long-acting agonist. The most prominent metabolic pathway involves direct glucuronidation at the phenolic hydroxy group.[39] O-demethylation followed by conjugation at the phenolic 2′-hydroxy group also occurs and the phase 1 oxidation appears to involve four cytochrome P450 isozymes (CYP2D6, CYP2C19, CYP2C9, and CYP2A6).

Formoterol has a more rapid onset as compared to salmeterol while maintaining the same long duration of action. The quicker onset is believed to result from formoterol's greater water solubility, allowing it to get to receptor sites faster, while its moderate lipophilicity still allows it to stay localized in the lungs. Its long duration of action is not primarily due to membrane sequestration, as seen with salmeterol but, rather, to a highly stable formoterol-β2 receptor complex.[36] It is indicated for the long-term maintenance treatment of asthma and for patients with symptoms of nocturnal asthma who require regular treatment with inhaled short-acting β_2-agonists. It is not indicated for patients whose asthma can be managed by occasional use of inhaled short-acting β_2-agonists. Formoterol is available only as a powder in a capsule for administration via an aerosolizer. Patients should be cautioned not to take the capsules orally and to keep them in a safe place to avoid accidental oral administration.

Formoterol has two asymmetric centers and, therefore, can exist in four possible enantiomers. The *R,R*-enantiomer is active and reported to be 1,000 times more active than the *S,S*-enantiomer and twice as potent as racemic formoterol. It is available under the name arformoterol (Brovana), undergoes the same metabolism, and is only indicated for the treatment of COPD.

Olodaterol

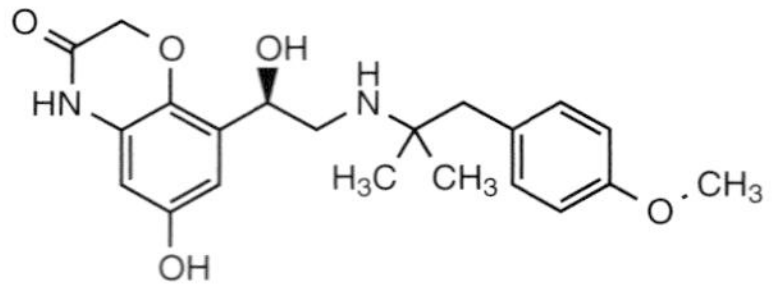

Olodaterol

Olodaterol has a β_2-directing N-isobutyl joined to a p-methoxyphenyl ring (aralkyl substituent) and a unique 6-hydroxybenzoxazine-3-one ring that provides selectivity for the β_2-receptors. The *m*-orientation of the phenolic OH group relative to the ethanolamine moiety of the pharmacophore is believed to contribute to the observed selectivity. It is resistant to both COMT and MAO making it a long-acting agonist. It is metabolized to an O-demethylated product by CYP2C9 and 2C8 as well as glucuronidated via UGT to inactive conjugates. Both olodaterol and its O-demethylated metabolite form glucuronides. Concurrent administration of potent CYP2C8 and 2C9 inhibitors such as ketoconazole increase plasma concentrations of olodaterol by 70%, but no dosage adjustments are recommended.

Olodaterol's long duration of action is enhanced by its fast and high affinity association with the β_2-receptor and its slow dissociation half-life of 17 hours. Olodaterol binds to the β_2-receptor through segments 5, 6, and 7 of the transmembrane G protein in addition to an exosite on the β_2 receptor. The β-hydroxy, carbonyl oxygen, the amino functions, and the p-methoxy group are also involved in receptor binding.[40] Olodaterol provides a lasting bronchodilation (24 hr), allowing for once daily dosing. It is administered via an aerosol inhaler and is approved for the treatment of COPD.[41,42] Most common adverse reactions include nasopharyngitis, upper respiratory tract infection, bronchitis, cough, rash, dizziness, diarrhea, and arthralgia.

Indacaterol

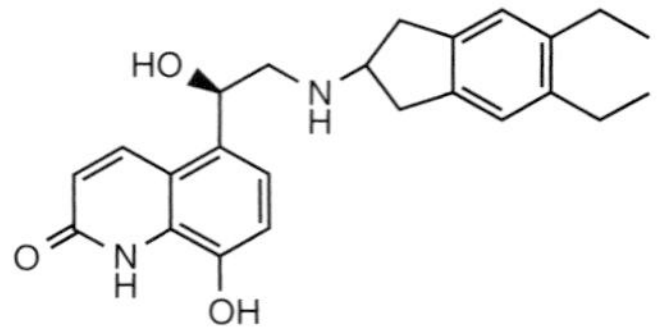

Indacaterol

Indacaterol is a selective β_2-receptor agonist. It has an N-diethyldihydroindane aralkyl group and that, coupled with the 8-hydroxyquinolinone aromatic ring system, is responsible for its receptor selectivity. It is resistant to metabolism by COMT and MAO and is excreted primarily in feces as unchanged indacaterol. CYP3A4-catalyzed benzylic hydroxylation of one ethyl moiety occurs, and UGT1A1-catalyzed glucuronic acid conjugation can take place at either the CYP-generated or the phenolic OH group. In addition, N-dealkylation also occurs to a limited extent. All are urinary metabolites, none of which amount to greater than 0.3% of the administered dose.[43]

Drug interactions are similar to other CYP3A4-vulnerable LABAs. Indacaterol showed a significantly reduced rate of exacerbations when combined with glycopyrronium. Indacaterol is recommended for the treatment of COPD including chronic bronchitis and emphysema via inhalation once every 24 hours. Peak serum levels occur after 15 minutes, and the absolute bioavailability is 45%.[44]

Vilanterol

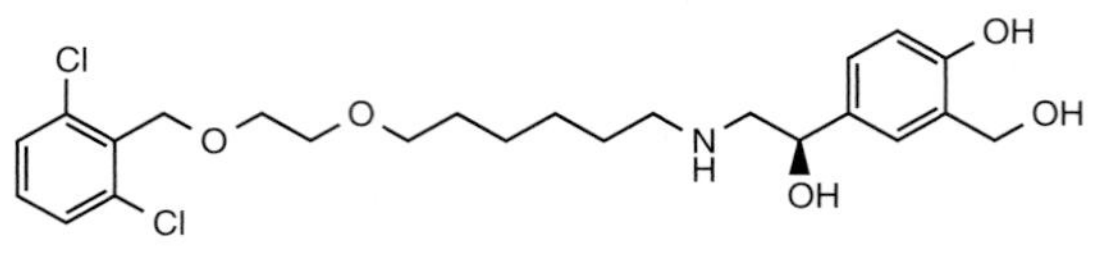

Vilanterol

Vilanterol is an LABA similar in structure to salmeterol, having the salicyl alcohol ring system and essential β-hydroxy group in common. However the N-hexyloxy moiety of salmeterol is extended with a dichlorobenzyloxyethyl group instead of a phenylbutyl group. This combination confers a greater intrinsic activity and optimal direct-acting β_2-receptor selectivity than salmeterol. Its long duration of action suggests that vilanterol has strong binding to the β_2-receptor. Docking experiments demonstrated strong H-bonding in transmembrane helix 5 between Ser207 and its phenolic hydroxy group, as well as between Asn293 and the benzylic hydroxy, interactions common to all β_2 agonists. Asp113 in transmembrane 5 also shows the anticipated ionic interaction with the cationic amine. In addition, the central ether oxygen H-bonds to Asn318 of transmembrane 7 and the benzylic ether can H-bond with the Ser in transmembrane 3 and an Asn of transmembrane 7, enhancing vilanterol's receptor affinity. Vilanterol has a rapid onset and long duration of action. It undergoes extensive first-pass metabolism primarily via CYP3A4-mediated O-demethylation to a primary alcohol and 2,6-dichlorobenzoic acid. The alcohol metabolite retains only a very small β_2-receptor agonist activity. Vilanterol serum drug concentration is increased by 70% when administered concurrently with potent CYP3A4 inhibitors. Vilanterol, in combination with fluticasone, is approved for the treatment of long-term chronic COPD that can include bronchitis and/or emphysema. The combination is a once daily medication for airflow maintenance treatment.[33,45,46]

Antimuscarinics

Acetylcholine is the endogenous neurotransmitter of the parasympathetic nervous system. The parasympathetic nerve fibers are found in both the autonomic and central nervous systems. These fibers are classified into those that are stimulated by muscarine and those that are stimulated by nicotine. Nicotine, an alkaloid from *Nicotiana tabacum*, stimulates preganglionic fibers in both the parasympathetic and sympathetic systems, as well as the somatic

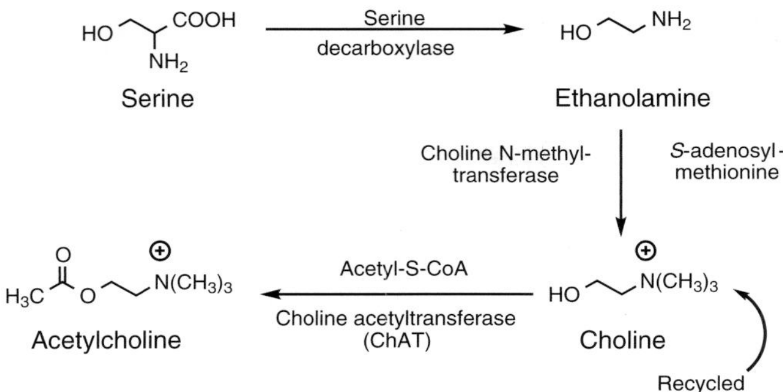

Figure 28.11 Biosynthesis of acetylcholine.

motor fibers of the skeletal system. Muscarine, an alkaloid from the poisonous mushroom *Amanita muscaria*, stimulates postganglionic parasympathetic fibers with receptors found on autonomic effector cells. The central nervous system has fibers that contain both nicotinic and muscarinic receptors. In this chapter, we are most interested in the drugs that block the muscarinic fibers (antimuscarinics) because blockade results in cardiovascular, mydriatic, antispasmodic, antisecretory, and bronchodilatory effects.

Biochemistry and Metabolism of Acetylcholine

Acetylcholine is the ester formed between acetylcoenzyme A and choline by the action of choline acetyltransferase in the presynaptic cholinergic neurons. Most of the choline used to biosynthesize acetylcholine comes via uptake from the synaptic space, where it is produced from the hydrolysis of acetylcholine by acetylcholinesterase, a membrane-bound serine hydroxylase. Additionally, some choline is biosynthesized in the presynaptic neurons from serine (Fig. 28.11). Once formed, acetylcholine is stored in vesicles from which it is released on stimulation.

The duration of action of acetylcholine is very short because it is rapidly hydrolyzed by the acetylcholinesterase present on postsynaptic terminals in the synaptic space. This hydrolysis is a straightforward splitting of the acetylcholine into acetic acid and choline; however, the way this happens is very interesting and begins by the proper binding of acetylcholine in the catalytic pocket. Binding of the cationic N-end to Tyr, Glu, and Trp via a combination of π-cation and electrostatic forces places the acyl head of acetylcholine in the correct position for attack by the Ser hydroxy group (Fig. 28.12).

Once properly bound, the hydrolysis actually involves two hydrolytic steps. The first step is the hydrolysis of acetylcholine by nucleophilic attack at the carbonyl carbon by the Ser hydroxy group, which liberates choline and leaves the enzyme acetylated. A triad formed between Glu, His, and the Ser at the catalytic site activates the Ser for the nucleophilic attack. The second step is the hydrolysis of the acetylated enzyme by water to regenerate the free enzyme. The water is activated by hydrogen-bonding to the His residue, which increases the nucleophilic character of the oxygen of water. The activated water attacks the electrophilic carbonyl carbon of the acetyl group to generate acetate and regenerate the free hydroxy group of Ser (Fig. 28.13).[47]

Muscarinic Receptor Structure and Agonist/Antagonist Interactions

The muscarinic receptors are members of the superfamily of G protein–coupled receptors (see Chapter 8). They consist of seven transmembrane helices and are linked to their G protein through interaction with the second and third intracellular loops.[48] There are five receptor subtypes, designated M_{1-5}, and the odd-numbered receptors (M_1, M_3, and M_5) are coupled to the G_q/G_{11} class. This class of receptors activates intracellular phospholipase C to hydrolyze phosphatidylinositol 4,5-diphosphate (PIP_2) to diacylglycerol (DAG) and inositol triphosphate (IP_3) as membrane-bound and intracellular second messengers, respectively. The even-numbered receptors (M_2 and M_4) are coupled to the G_i/G_o class, which mediates the inhibition of adenylyl cyclase (Fig. 28.14).

Table 28.5 lists the physiologic action of the M_3 receptors. Because the M_3 receptors cause bronchoconstriction, they counterbalance the bronchodilation mediated by the β_2-adrenergic receptors in the lung, resulting in maintenance of bronchiole tone. This forms the basis for the therapeutic use of inhaled antimuscarinics, as they block cholinergic bronchiole constriction and allow adrenergic bronchodilation to help overcome the pulmonary constriction associated with an asthmatic attack.

Affinity labeling and mutagenic studies have established that acetylcholine binds to its receptor in a narrow region of the circular arrangement of the seven transmembrane helices approximately 10-15 Å away from the membrane surface. The permanently cationic nitrogen of acetylcholine binds to the anionic carboxylate of an Asp located in helix 3.[49] As depicted in Figure 28.15, the ionic interaction is stabilized

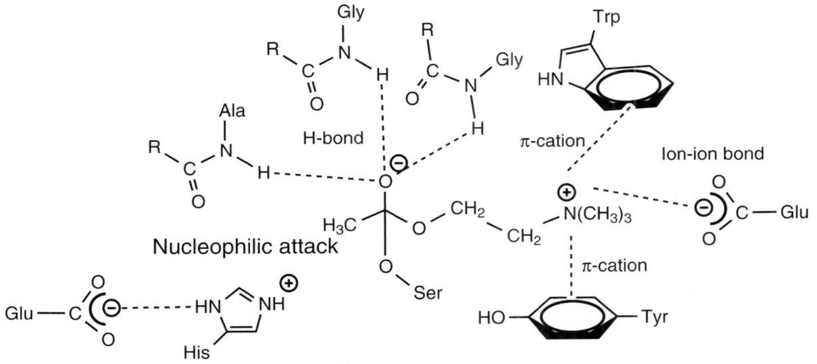

Figure 28.12 Binding of acetylcholine in the catalytic site of acetylcholinesterase.

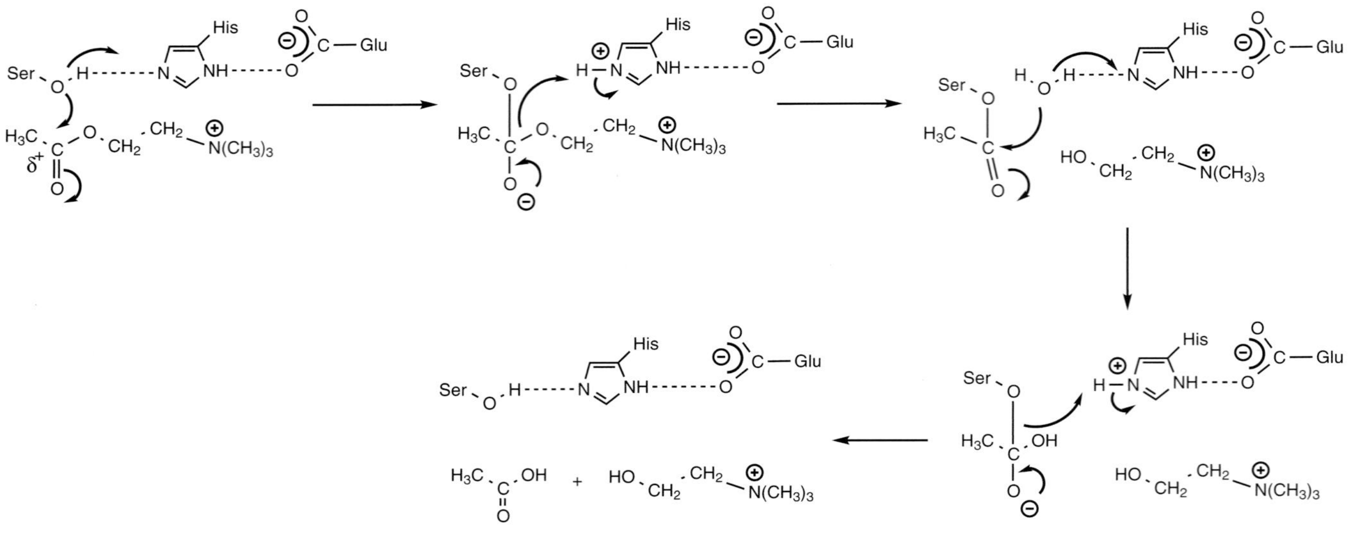

Figure 28.13 The role of the triad formed between glutamine, histidine, and serine in the hydrolysis of acetylcholine by acetylcholinesterase.

by hydrogen bonding with a Tyr in helix 5 and a Thr in helix 5. It is postulated that muscarinic antagonists bind to the Asp and contain hydrophobic substituents that bind within a hydrophobic pocket in the receptor, which does not allow the change in conformation needed to transfer the agonist signal to the coupled G protein[50] (see Structure-Activity Relationships of Antimuscarinic Agents below).

Structure-Activity Relationships of Antimuscarinic Agents

The structural pharmacophore for all antimuscarinic drugs is an acetylcholine analogue in which the acetyl methyl group is substituted with at least one phenyl ring. This pharmacophore is generally classified as an aminoalcohol ester. The ester function can be replaced with different moieties to produce different classes of antimuscarinic drugs. When the ester function is replaced by an ether function, the aminoalcohol ether class is produced. When the ester function is replaced by a saturated carbon, the aminoalcohols are obtained when R_1 is a hydroxy group, and the amino amides are obtained when R_1 is an amido group (Fig. 28.16). Antimuscarinic action in all classes is greatly enhanced if R_2 is a second aromatic or five- to six-membered alicyclic ring with the higher activity achieved with the alicyclic substitution.

The classic chemical prototype for the antimuscarinics is atropine, an alkaloid from *Atropa belladonna*. Buried within its structure is the aminoalcohol ester pharmacophore, where R_1 is a hydroxymethyl group, R_2 is hydrogen, and the nitrogen

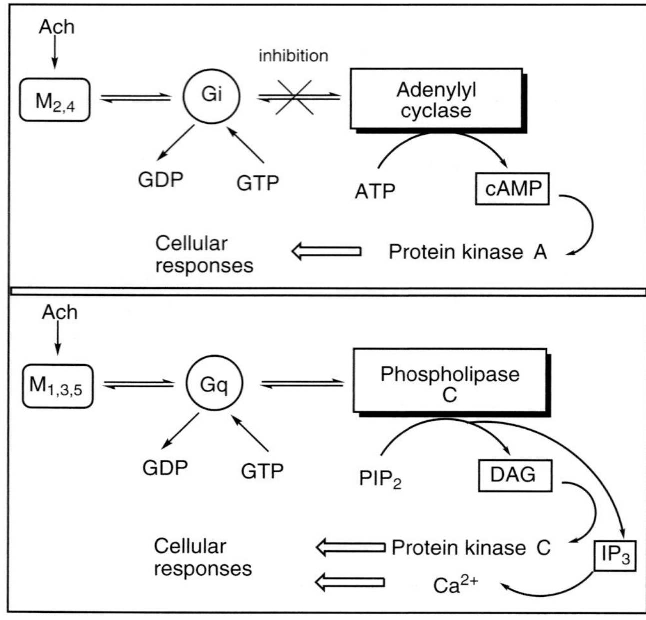

Figure 28.14 Comparison of the role of G protein in odd- and even-numbered muscarinic receptors. ATP, adenosine triphosphate; cAMP, cyclic adenosine monophosphate; DAG, diacylglycerol; GDP, guanosine diphosphate; GTP, guanosine triphosphate; IP_3, inositol triphosphate; PIP_2, phosphatidylinositol biphosphate.

Table 28.5 Physiologic Action Associated With the M_3 Muscarinic Receptors

Organ	M_3-Receptor Effect
Eye	
Iris circular muscle	Contracts
Ciliary muscle	Contracts
Heart	
Sinoatrial node	Decelerates
Atrial contractility	Decelerates
Bronchiole smooth muscle	Contracts
Gastrointestinal tract	
Smooth muscle	Contracts
Secretions	Increases
Sphincters	Relaxes

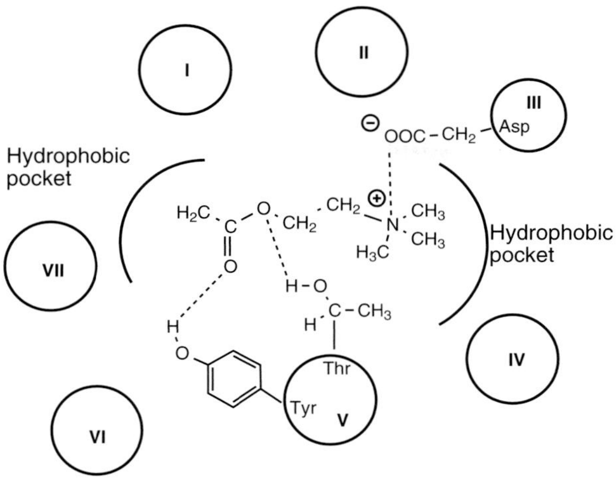

Figure 28.15 Acetylcholine binding to residues in the muscarinic receptor.

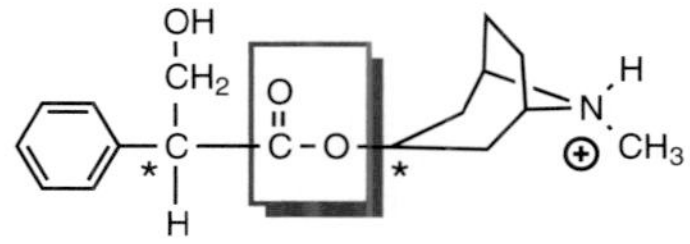

Figure 28.17 Atropine, an aminoalcohol ester antimuscarinic (*designates chirality).

is part of a bicyclic ring system called tropine. To form atropine, tropine is esterified with tropic acid; a common chemical name for atropine is tropine tropate (Fig. 28.17).

Although atropine does not have a quaternary nitrogen, the tertiary amine is protonated at physiologic pH; therefore, it can bind to the anionic Asp residue in the muscarinic receptor. The nitrogen can be substituted with alkyl groups (tertiary and quaternary amines are the most active), and methyl is the optimal size to minimize steric hindrance to ion-ion anchoring. When the nitrogen is made quaternary, the molecule loses its oral availability but leads to compounds that can be administered effectively by inhalation. When chirality exists in the aminoalcohol moiety (e.g., tropine), there is little difference between the activities of the *R*- and *S*-configurations. When chirality is found in the acid moiety (e.g., tropic acid), however, the *R* configuration is approximately 100-fold more active than the *S*-isomer. This indicates the importance of the binding role for the phenyl ring in causing the uncoupling from the G protein, which leads to receptor inhibition.

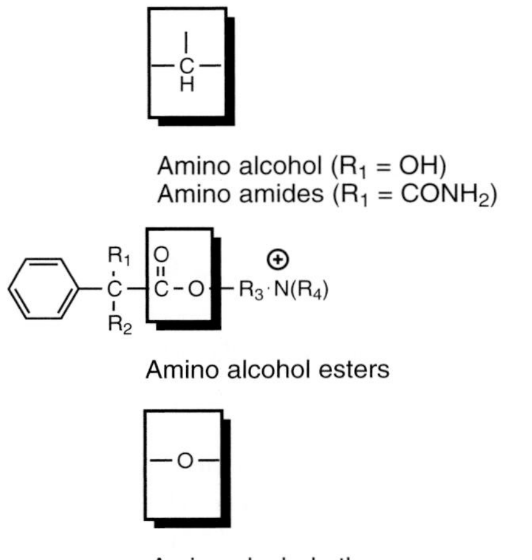

Figure 28.16 The pharmacophore for all classes of antimuscarinic agents.

Specific Antimuscarinic Drugs Used to Treat Asthma and COPD

Ipratropium Hydrobromide

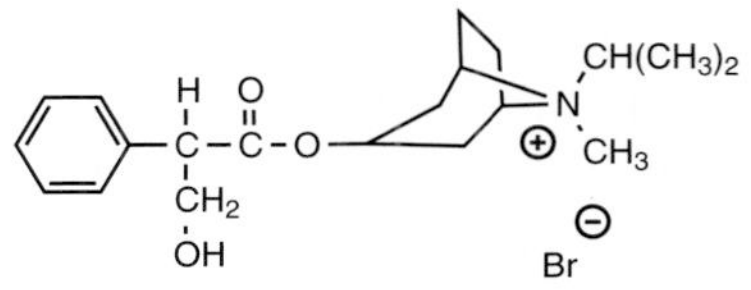

Ipratropium hydrobromide
(Atrovent)

Ipratropium is the N-isopropyl analogue of atropine. Its quaternary cationic nature makes it highly hydrophilic and poorly absorbed from the lungs after inhalation via solution or aerosol; therefore, the bronchodilation effect can be considered to be a local, site-specific effect. Much of an inhaled dose is swallowed and excreted without significant absorption. Ipratropium is indicated primarily for the relief of bronchospasms associated with COPD and has seen little application for the treatment of asthma. It also is administered by nasal spray for the relief of rhinorrhea associated with the common cold and perennial rhinitis. Inhaled ipratropium has a 15-minute onset of action and a rather short duration of action (<4 hr); therefore, it is dosed four times a day. Other drugs, including adrenergic agonists, methylxanthines, steroids, and cromolyn sodium can be coadministered with ipratropium in COPD without adverse drug-drug interactions. The little ipatropium that reaches the circulation is minimally protein bound and is partially metabolized by esterase to inactive products. Most adverse effects from ipratropium are common to antimuscarinics and include blurred vision, dry mouth, tachycardia, urinary difficulty, and headache. Patients should be careful not to spray ipratropium into their eyes because its dilation effects can precipitate or exacerbate narrow-angle glaucoma.[51]

Tiotropium Bromide

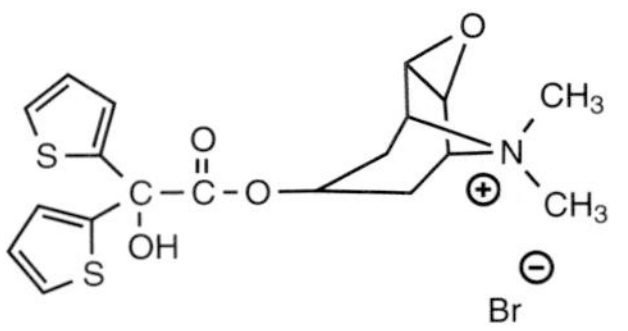

Tiotropium bromide
(Spiriva)

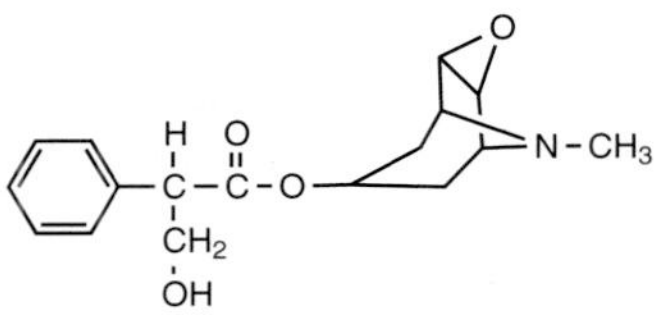

Scopolamine

Tiotropium is the α,α-dithienyl derivative of N-methyl scopolamine, a quaternary analogue of naturally occurring scopolamine in *Atropa belladonna*. Scopolamine differs from atropine only in the insertion of an ether oxygen between tropine carbons 2 and 3. Tiotropium is indicated primarily for the relief of bronchospasms associated with COPD and, when inhaled, can be considered a site-specific, local medication to the lung. Tiotropium is administered as a dry powder via inhalation using a HandiHaler, in which the drug capsule is placed. As with formoterol inhalation capsules, patients should be cautioned not to take the medication orally. Systemic distribution following oral inhalation is minimal, essentially because of its hydrophilic character. If swallowed, only approximately 14% of the dose is eliminated in the urine, with the remainder being found in the feces. Inhaled tiotropium has a 30-minute onset but a much longer duration than ipratropium (24 hr vs. <4 hr, respectively). Tiotropium is metabolized by both CYP3A4 and CYP2D6, followed by glutathione conjugation to a variety of metabolites. Only a very small amount is nonenzymatically hydrolyzed to inactive products N-methylscopine and dithienylglycolic acid. Tiotropium has an adverse reaction profile similar to that of ipratropium, with dry mouth being the most common adverse effect; however, blurred vision, tachycardia, urinary difficulty, headache precipitation, and exacerbation of narrow-angle glaucoma have been reported.[51]

Aclidinium Bromide

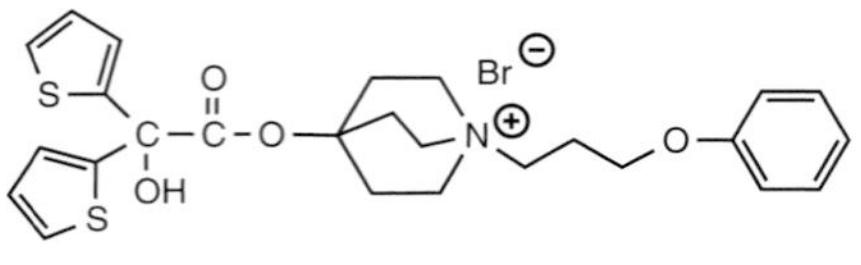

Aclidinium bromide
(Tudorza)

Aclidinium bromide was approved in 2012 for the inhalation treatment of COPD. It is structurally related to tiotropium in that it is an α,α-dithienyl substituted quaternary amine where the N-methyl scopolamine moiety is replaced by an N-phenoxypropyl-1-azabicyclo[2,2,2]octane ring system. Aclidinium has a kinetic selectivity for the M_3 versus the M_2 muscarinic receptors. Aclidinium is a long-acting bronchodilator with a quick onset of action. It undergoes rapid hydrolysis of its ester in plasma to inactive acid and alcohol components with a half-life of 2.4 minutes. In comparison, more than 70% of tiotropium remains intact in plasma after 1 hour. The short half-life, combined with the lack of antimuscarinic activity of its hydrolysis products, suggest that aclidinium may have reduced antimuscarinic side effects. In addition to hydrolysis, aclidinium also undergoes CYP metabolism yielding a monooxygenated phenyl ring and the loss of one of the thienyl rings, mediated by 3A4 and 2D6 CYP isoforms. In a clinical trial with patients with mild to severe COPD, aclidinium demonstrated significant elevation of FEV1 from baseline, producing sustained bronchodilation over 24 hours with no side effects related to the treatment protocol.[52,53]

Umeclidinium Bromide

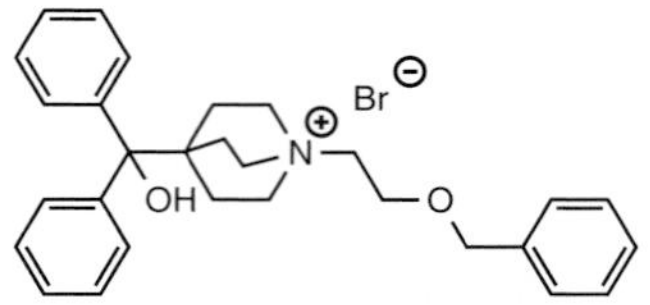

Umeclidinium bromide
(Incruse Ellipta)

Umeclidinium was approved by the FDA in 2014 for the long-term maintenance treatment of airflow obstruction in patients with COPD. It is structurally related to aclidinium in that it has the same azabicyclic ring system, but the thienyl rings have been replaced with phenyl and the oxygen atom of the N-aralkylether has shifted its position within the carbon chain. It is inhaled using the Ellipta inhaler. Umeclidinium is a competitive, reversible antagonist selective for the M_3 muscarinic receptor; however, it does show some affinity for all muscarinic receptors.

Upon inhalation, umeclidinium stays localized in the lung and plasma levels are insignificant. Following IV administration the drug is highly bound to plasma protein (89%). Umeclidinium is a substrate for P-glycoprotein as well as CYP2D6, with O-dealkylated, hydroxylated and glucuronidated metabolites being formed. Elimination occurs primarily in the feces (58%) with a lesser amount eliminated in urine (22%). Less than 10% of the drug is absorbed following oral administration, so no oral dosage forms are marketed. Umeclidinium may worsen acute narrow-angle glaucoma as well as urinary retention, especially in patients with prostate hyperplasia or bladder-neck obstruction. Umeclidinium is used singly or in fixed-combination with vilanterol trifenatate. It is a long-acting bronchodilator used in once-a-day dosing regimens.[54,55]

Glycopyrrolate Bromide

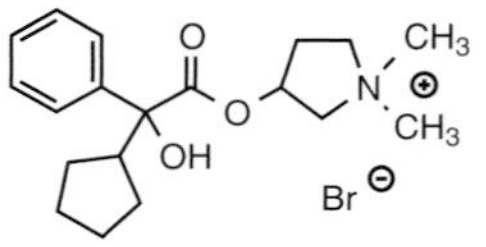

Glycopyrrolate bromide
(Seebri)

Glycopyyrolate is an aminoalcohol ester anticholinergic. The acetyl methyl carbon is optimally substituted with one aromatic (phenyl) and one alicyclic (cyclohexane) ring, and the amino group is quaternized within a pyrrolidine ring. Glycopyrolate is a bronchodilator recommended for the inhalation-based treatment of COPD in a dose of 15.6 mcg twice daily. Glycopyrrolate competitively and reversibly inhibits the action of acetylcholine at the three muscarinic receptors with greater affinity for the M_1 and M_3 subtypes. Its T_{max} occurs in 5 minutes with a volume of distribution at steady state of 83L following IV administration. It undergoes minimal ester hydrolysis in the liver and is excreted in both the urine and bile. Only a slight increase in total systemic exposure is seen in patients with moderate renal impairment. Glycopyrrolate, just as with all anticholinergics, should be used with caution in patients with glaucoma, BPH (benign prostatic hyperplasia), diabetes and myasthenia gravis. Glycopyrrolate adverse effects include abdominal pain, diarrhea, nausea, arthralgia, back pain, dyspnea, nasopharyngitis and induction of bronchospasms.[56] It also is used in combination with formoterol fumarate (Brevespi).

Methylxanthines

The methylxanthines naturally occur in coffee (*Coffea arabica*), cacao (*Theobroma cacao*), and tea (*Camellia sinensis*).[57] The major methylxanthines are caffeine, theophylline, and theobromine, and they differ in the position and number of methyl groups on their xanthine ring system (Fig. 28.18).

The most common source of these xanthines is in the beverages coffee, tea, and cocoa, which are universally consumed, often for their stimulant properties. A cup of coffee or tea contains between 60 and 85 mg of caffeine, and a cup of cocoa can have as much as 250 mg of theobromine. Caffeine frequently is added to cola drinks and to over-the-counter analgesics and stimulants. Theophylline is used for its bronchodilating effects in the treatment of asthma. Its importance has declined greatly since the development of the inhaled β_2-adrenergic agonists and inhaled corticosteroids and because it has a narrow therapeutic window, which requires close patient monitoring and periodic blood level determination to avoid serious side effects.

Theophylline Mechanism of Action and Metabolism

Despite a great deal of investigation, just how theophylline causes bronchodilation is not clearly understood. Inhibition of the enzyme PDE, which is responsible for the hydrolysis of cAMP and cyclic guanosine monophosphate (cGMP), generally is put forth as the mechanism of action; however, theophylline also is an adenosine antagonist and has been implicated in the stimulation of the release of NE and EPI. It has been clearly shown that theophylline does inhibit PDEs in vitro, and x-ray crystallographic studies have identified the binding residues that interact with the methylxanthines (Fig. 28.19).

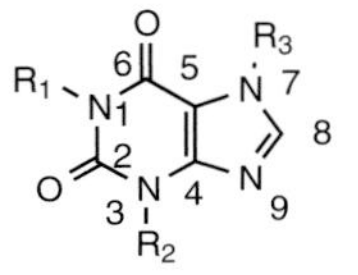

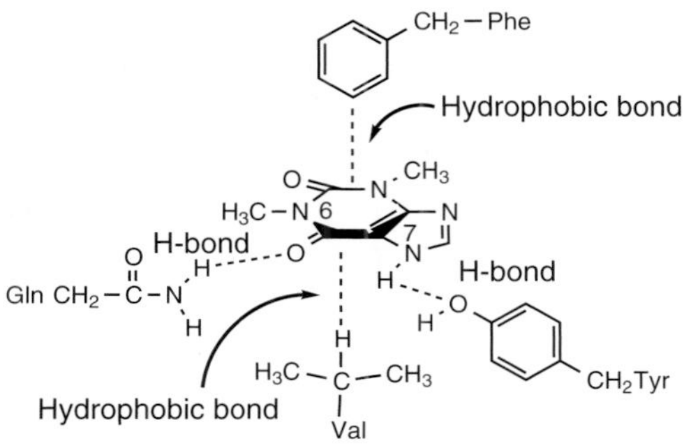

Figure 28.19 Methylxanthine binding interactions in the catalytic pocket of phosphodiesterase.

Theophylline binds to a subpocket of the active site and appears to be sandwiched between a Phe and a Val by forming hydrophobic bonds with both. Its binding affinity is reinforced by hydrogen-bonding between a Tyr and the N7 and a Glu and the O6 of the xanthine ring system. There are more than 11 families of PDEs, and studies have shown that theophylline binds in a similar manner to both the PDE4 and PDE5 family isoforms.[58]

Chemically, theophylline is 1,3-dimethylxanthine and contains both an acidic and a basic nitrogen (N7 and N9, respectively; see Fig. 28.18). Physiologically, it behaves as an acid (pK_a = 8.6), and its poor aqueous solubility can be enhanced by salt formation with organic bases. Theophylline is metabolized by a combination of C-8 oxidation by xanthine oxidase and N-demethylation by CYP to yield methyluric acid metabolites (Fig. 28.20). The major urinary metabolite is 1,3-dimethyl uric acid, which is the product of the action of xanthine oxidase alone. Because none of the metabolites is uric acid itself, theophylline can be safely given to patients who suffer from gout.

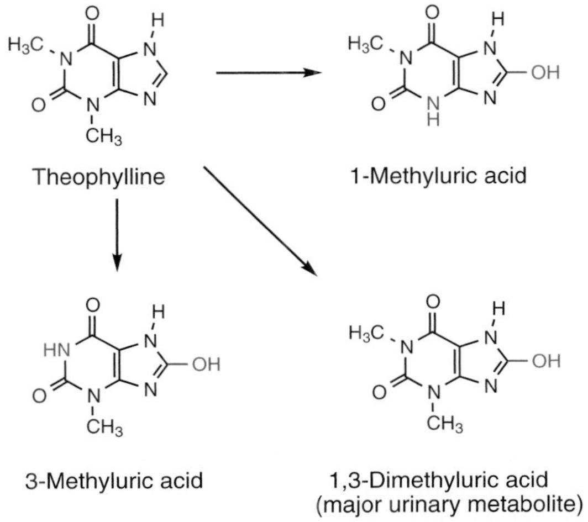

	R_1	R_2	R_3
Caffeine	CH_3	CH_3	CH_3
Theophylline	CH_3	CH_3	H
Theobromine	H	CH_3	CH_3

Figure 28.18 Structural differences between the methylxanthines.

Figure 28.20 Metabolism of theophylline.

Methylxanthine Drugs Used to Treat Asthma

Theophylline

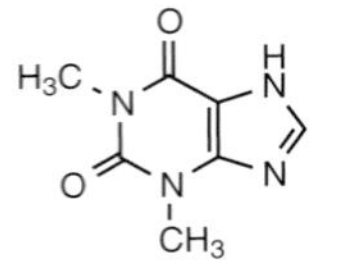

Theophylline
(Elixophylline, Bronkodyl, various others)

The primary indication for theophylline is as a controller medication for the treatment of bronchospasm of asthma and COPD. In addition to bronchodilation effects, theophylline dilates pulmonary blood vessels, acts centrally to stimulate respiration, acts as a diuretic, increases gastric acid secretion, and inhibits uterine contractions. Dosing requires the determination of plasma levels, with 10-20 μg/mL associated with the lowest incidence of side effects. Theophylline overdose can result in a quick onset of ventricular arrhythmias, convulsions, or even death without any warning. Many drugs increase the plasma concentration of theophylline, including quinolone and macrolide antibiotics, nonselective β-blockers, ephedrine, calcium channel blockers, cimetidine, and oral contraceptives. Theophylline is available in tablet, capsule, liquid, and parenteral dosage preparations. There also are combination products with guaifenesin and ephedrine available as tablet and liquid dosage forms. There are two products that are theophylline salts. Aminophylline is theophylline ethylenediamine, which contains 70% theophylline and is available in tablets, liquid, parenteral, and suppository dosage forms. Oxytriphylline is the choline salt of theophylline, and it contains 64% theophylline in tablets and liquid dosage forms. Care must be taken to correctly calculate the equivalent dose when switching a patient from theophylline to one of its salts.

Dyphylline (Dihydroxypropyl Theophylline)

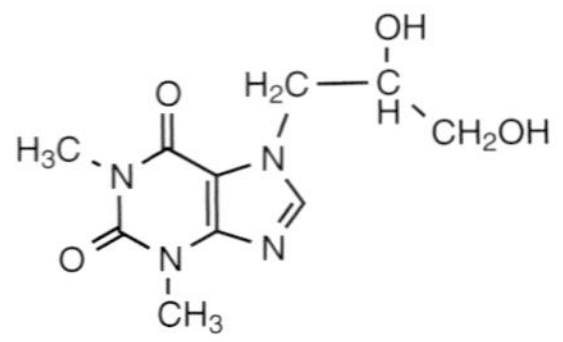

Dyphylline
(Dilor, Lufyllin)

Dyphylline is the N7 2,3-dihydroxypropyl derivative of theophylline and is not a theophylline salt. Dyphylline is not metabolized to theophylline in vivo, and even though it contains 70% theophylline by molecular weight ratio, the equivalent amount to theophylline is not known. Dosing must be determined independently by monitoring dyphylline blood levels. Dyphylline has a diminished bronchodilator effect compared to theophylline, but it may have lower and less serious side effects. Dosage forms available are an elixir and tablets.

Adrenocorticoids Used to Treat Asthma and COPD

Steroids are a class of tetracyclic terpene compounds that are widely distributed in plants and animals. Many synthetic analogues have been made to take advantages of their various pharmacologic activities. There are four major classes of steroids: the adrenocorticoids, the sex hormones, the bile acids, and the vitamins. The adrenocorticoids are formed in the adrenal cortex and are subdivided into the glucocorticoids and mineralocorticoids. The glucocorticoids are so named because they affect glucose homeostasis, but they also have significant anti-inflammatory activity. The mineralocorticoids affect sodium and water retention. The reproductive organs in both the male and female produce steroid hormones, which are responsible for the differentiation of the sex characteristics and the development of muscle and hair. The bile acids are derived from cholesterol and are an essential aid to the action of lipase in the digestion of fats, and vitamin D and its derivatives are associated with calcium homeostasis. We will limit our discussion to the glucocorticoids because their anti-inflammatory activity makes them useful for the treatment of asthma and COPD.

Of note, because the major role of the glucocorticoids is to provide the body with levels of glucose that are compatible with life, they should be used with caution in patients with diabetes. Similarly, because the major role of the mineralocorticoids is to maintain blood volume and regulate electrolyte balance, their use in patients with hypertension should be monitored carefully.

Steroid Nomenclature

The basic structure of a steroid is a tetracyclic cyclopentanoperhydrophenanthrene, referred to as the steroid nucleus, as depicted in Figure 28.21. The addition of methyl groups at C10 and C13 and of an ethyl group at C17 to the steroid nucleus gives a 21-carbon base structure

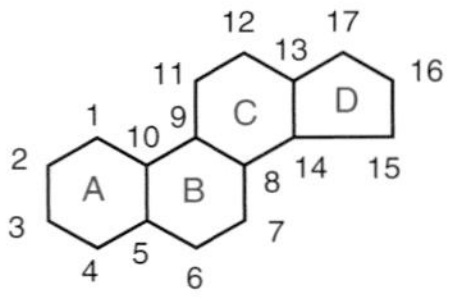

Cyclopentanoperhydrophenanthrene

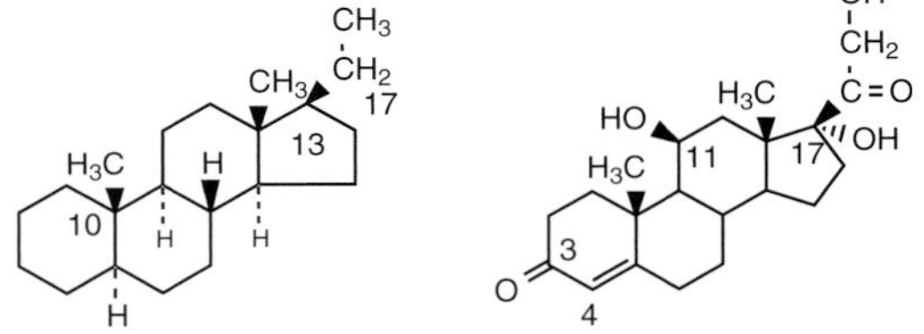

5α-Pregnane

Δ4-11β,17α,21-Trihydroxy-3,20-pregenedione
(Hydrocortisone)

Figure 28.21 Basic skeletons for steroid structures, numbering, and nomenclature.

called pregnane. All glucocorticoids are substituted pregnanes (see Chapter 21). Rings A, B, and C are in the chair conformation, and all ring junctions are *trans*, giving the glucocorticoids a rigid, flat backbone with α and β faces. The glucocorticoids bind to their receptor via the β face. All glucocorticoids have at least one double bond in ring A and hydroxy groups at C11, C17, and C21 as well as 3- and 20-keto groups. For example, hydrocortisone is Δ^4-11β,17α,21-trihydroxy-3,20-pregnenedione (Fig. 28.21). A more complete discussion of steroid nomenclature and stereochemistry has been published elsewhere.[59]

Steroid Biosynthesis and Secretion

Steroids are biosynthesized from cholesterol. Cholesterol is obtained through diet (~0.3 g/d), but the majority is biosynthesized from acetate in the liver (~1 g/d). The complete pathway is provided in Figure 28.22. Of note is the central branching role played by pregnenolone, leading to both classes of the adrenocorticoids.

Once formed, the adrenocorticoids are secreted into the circulatory system and circulating levels are maintained via a feedback mechanism (Fig. 28.23). When circulating levels are low, the hypothalamus secretes

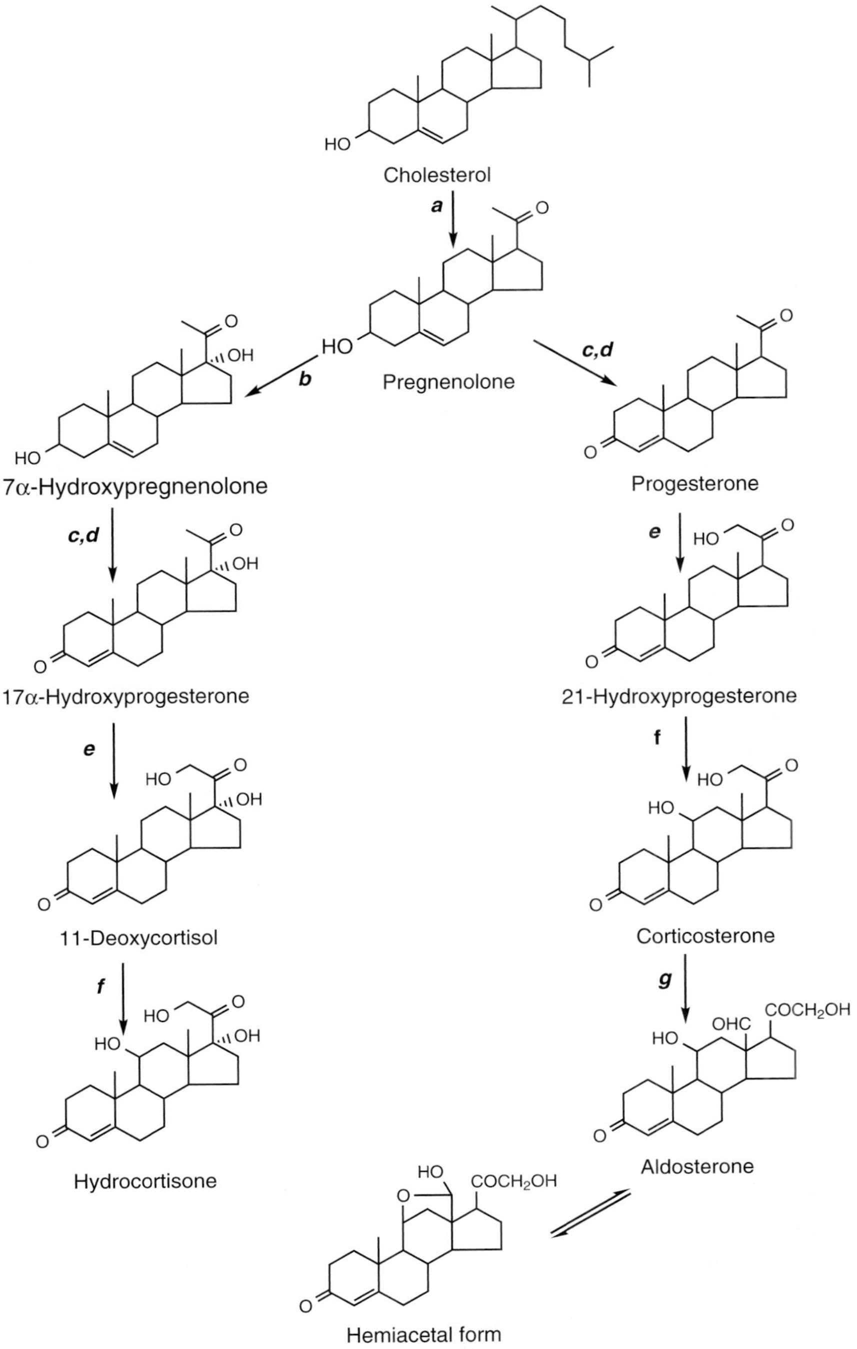

Cholesterol

a

Pregnenolone

b

c,d

17α-Hydroxypregnenolone

Progesterone

c,d

e

17α-Hydroxyprogesterone

21-Hydroxyprogesterone

e

f

11-Deoxycortisol

Corticosterone

f

g

Hydrocortisone

Aldosterone

Hemiacetal form

Figure 28.22 Biosynthesis of the adrenocorticoids from cholesterol. The enzymes involved are (*a*) side chain cleavage, (*b*) 17α-hydroxylase, (*c*) 5-ene-3β-hydroxy-steroid dehydrogenase, (*d*) 3-oxosteroid-4,5-isomerase, (*e*) 21-hydroxylase, (*f*) 11β-hydroxylase, and (*g*) 18-hydroxylate.

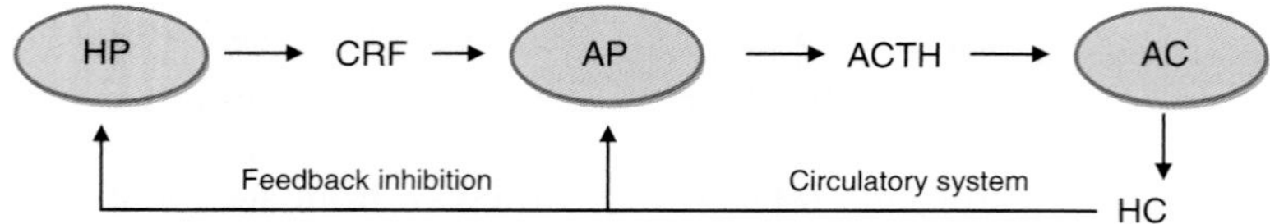

Figure 28.23 Mechanism of adrenocorticoid secretion and control. AC, adrenal cortex; ACTH, adrenocorticotrophic hormone; AP, anterior pituitary; CRF, corticotrophin-releasing factor; HC, hydrocortisone; HP, hypothalamus.

corticotrophin-releasing factor (CRF). In turn, CRF stimulates the anterior pituitary to secrete adrenocorticotrophic hormone, which stimulates the adrenal cortex to synthesize and secrete the adrenocorticoids (mainly hydrocortisone and aldosterone). When circulating levels of the adrenocorticoids are sufficiently high, they induce a feedback inhibition of CRF secretion from the hypothalamus and adrenocorticotrophic hormone release from the anterior pituitary gland. It should be noted that chronic use of steroids inhibits the adrenal cortex from producing glucocorticoids. This is known as hypothalamus-pituitary-adrenal (HPA) axis suppression. If steroid therapy is stopped abruptly, the lack of endogenous glucocorticoids can be life-threatening. A slow and gradual withdrawal from exogenous steroid therapy is always warranted to allow the HPA axis to recover.

Steroid Pharmacologic Action (See Chapter 21)

The major pharmacologic activities of the glucocorticoids are anti-inflammation realized through three distinct mechanisms. The most well-recognized mechanism of glucocorticoid-induced anti-inflammatory activity is derived from their ability to affect protein synthesis. Specifically, they stimulate the synthesis of lipocortin, a protein that inhibits phospholipase A_2, which is an enzyme that catalyzes the breakdown of membranes to release arachidonic acid, the first step in the arachidonic acid cascade that results in the production of inflammatory prostaglandins and leukotrienes (Figs. 28.24 and 28.25). Therefore, inhibition of phospholipase A_2 ultimately results in the reduction of the inflammatory prostaglandins and leukotrienes.

A second anti-inflammatory mechanism of glucocorticoids involves inhibition of IL-1. IL-1 stimulates the proliferation of T and B lymphocytes that are responsible for the production of the cytokines and antibodies, which in turn are important in the inflammatory and immune responses to antigens. The glucocorticoids, by their ability to inhibit IL-1, cause a decrease in T and B lymphocytes, leading to immunosuppression, and therefore must be used with caution in patients with infection. A third action of glucocorticoids is inhibition of the synthesis and release

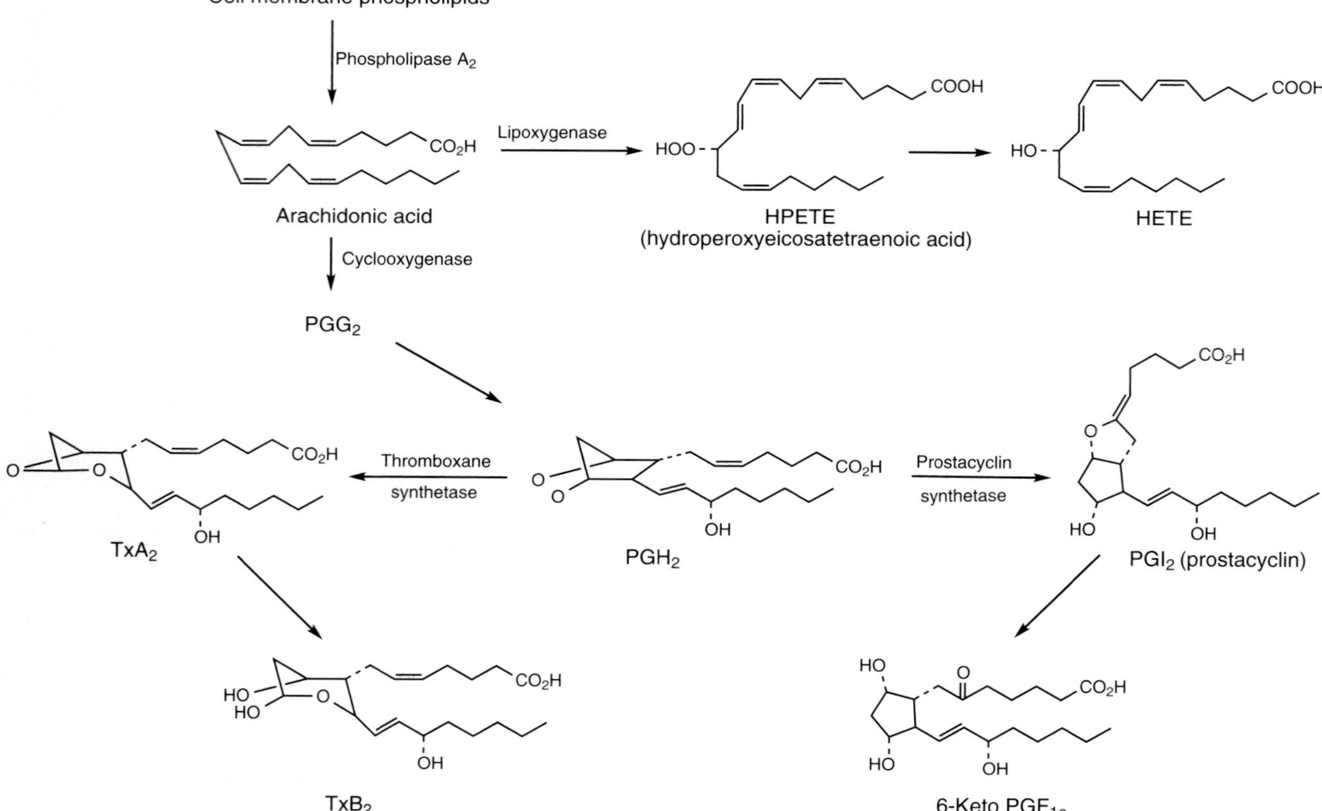

Figure 28.24 Biosynthesis of thromboxanes (TxA_2 and TxB_2), prostacyclin (PGI_2), and prostaglandins (PGG_2, PGF_2, and PGH_2). HETE, hydroxyeicosatetraenoic acid.

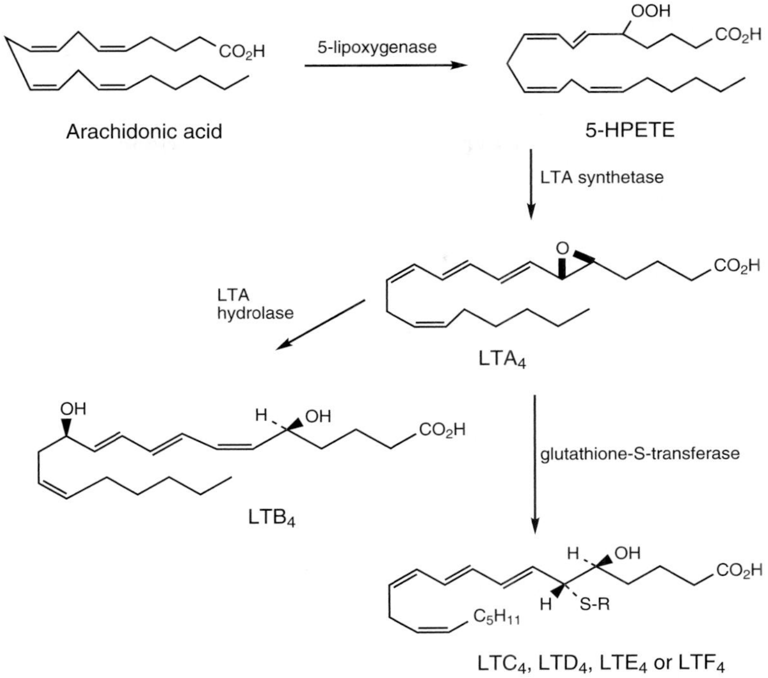

Arachidonic acid → 5-lipoxygenase → 5-HPETE (OOH, CO_2H)

5-HPETE → LTA synthetase → LTA_4 (O, CO_2H)

LTA_4 → LTA hydrolase → LTB_4 (OH, H, OH, CO_2H)

LTA_4 → glutathione-S-transferase → LTC_4, LTD_4, LTE_4 or LTF_4 (H, OH, CO_2H, H, S-R, C_5H_{11})

Figure 28.25 Biosynthesis of leukotrienes. HPETE, hydroperoxyeicosatetraenoic acid; LT, leukotriene.

of histamine and other autocoids from mast cells. These pharmacologic activities make the glucocorticoids especially useful for treating the inflammatory processes associated with asthma and COPD.

Steroid Mechanism of Action

How do glucocorticoids and other adrenocorticoids affect the levels of proteins and other biologically important compounds? The short answer is that these steroids bind to their receptor in the cytoplasm and that the glucocorticoid-receptor complex travels into the nucleus, where it binds to DNA and affects gene transcription. This increases, and sometimes decreases, the production of important biologically active compounds. How the glucocorticoids accomplish this is quite interesting and is depicted in Figure 28.26.

Circulating glucocorticoids enter the target cell by simple diffusion because they are relatively lipophilic (e.g., Log P hydrocortisone = 2.86). The glucocorticoid receptor resides inside the cell in combination with a

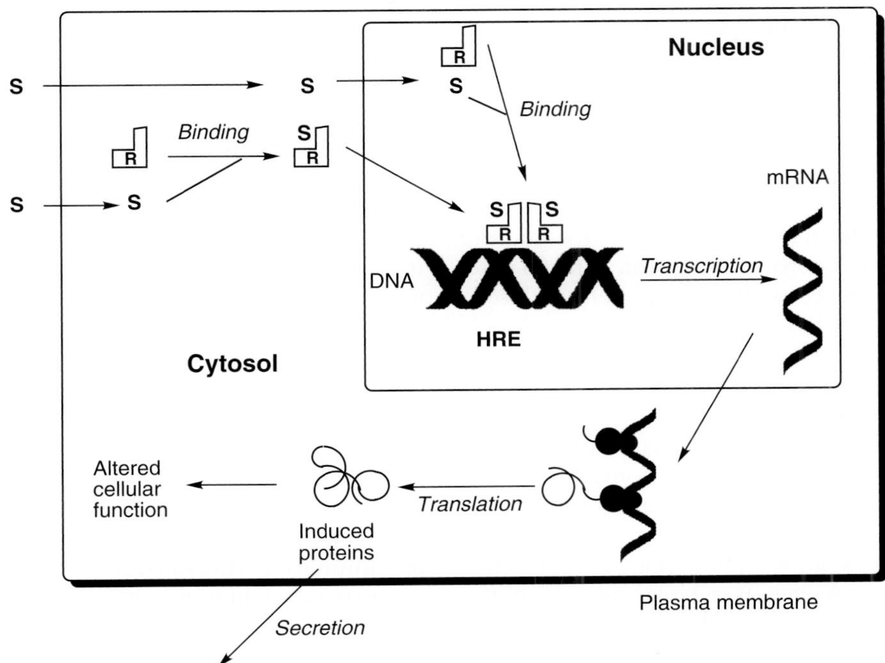

Figure 28.26 Mechanism of steroid hormone action. HRE, hormone response element; R, receptor; S, steroid.

heat shock protein. The glucocorticoid receptor has three distinct regions: the amino terminus for trans-activating functions (e.g., nuclear translocation, phosphorylation and other protein interactions), a middle region for binding to DNA, and the carboxy terminus, where the glucocorticoids bind. When the glucocorticoid binds to its receptor, the heat shock protein is released, resulting in a conformational change in the steroid-receptor complex. The glucocorticoid-receptor complex then translocates into the nucleus of the cell, where it binds to specific sequences of DNA called hormone response elements (HREs) which are located in the promoter areas of hormone-responsive genes. The DNA-binding region of the glucocorticoid receptor contains eight Cys amino acid residues that coordinate two zinc ions that form peptide loops called zinc fingers. When the zinc finger domains bind to the HRE of DNA, it dimerizes the glucocorticoid-receptor complex, placing each subunit in adjacent binding grooves.

In most cases, binding causes gene transcription and protein synthesis; however, in some instances, binding will block transcription.[60] A more precise understanding of just how the glucocorticoids inhibit the expression of inflammatory proteins has only recently become understood. In the inflammatory cells, such as macrophages, inflammatory protein genes are activated by the acetylation of core histones, which are entwined in DNA. This acetylation opens the chromatin structure allowing gene transcription and synthesis of inflammatory proteins. Glucocorticoids recruit histone deacetylase 2 (HDAC2) to actively transcribe genes, which reverses this process and switches off inflammatory gene transcription.[61]

Receptor Structure and Glucocorticoid Binding

The glucocorticoid receptor is a member of the nuclear receptor superfamily, which includes the receptors for the steroid hormones, retinoids, peroxisomal activators, vitamin D, and thyroid hormones (see Chapter 7). The steroid receptor is a soluble protein found in the cytosol of the cell. The binding domain of all the steroid receptors consists of 11 α-helices and 4 β-strands. X-ray crystallographic structural analysis, however, has revealed a unique binding pocket for the glucocorticoid receptor, which makes it distinct from the estrogen receptor, androgen receptor, and mineralocorticoid receptor. When a glucocorticoid binds to its receptor, it is completely enclosed within a pocket formed by helices 3, 4, 5, 6, 7, and 10 and β-strands 1 and 2.

The strong binding affinity for the glucocorticoids is a result of the hydrophobic and hydrophilic interactions with amino acid residues in the ligand binding domain. Nearly every atom of the glucocorticoid contacts one or more amino acid residues. The most significant contacts are the hydrogen-bonding between every hydrophilic group on the glucocorticoid structure (Fig. 28.27). The carbonyl group on ring A acts as a H-acceptor to both Arg611 and the amide of Gln570. The hydroxys at C-11 and C-21 are H-donors to the side chain carbonyl oxygen of Asn564. The C-17 hydroxy group hydrogen bonds with Gln642, and the C-20 carbonyl oxygen bonds with Thr739. Glucocorticoid binding to the ligand binding domain releases the heat shock protein and stabilizes the receptor in an active form capable of dimerization subsequent to HRE site binding.[62,63]

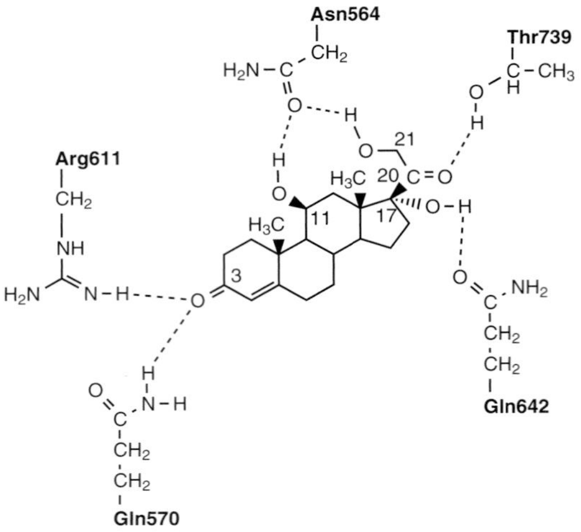

Figure 28.27 Important glucocorticoid receptor-ligand binding residues.

Glucocorticoid Structure-Activity Relationships

There are essential structural features that are necessary for glucocorticoid activity. The natural glucocorticoids also interact with the mineralocorticoid receptor and, therefore, will have salt-retaining properties. A large number of synthetic analogues have been prepared to decrease the mineralocorticoid effects in favor of increasing the relative glucocorticoid (anti-inflammatory) action of the steroids. In addition, many derivatives are prepared to enhance pharmacokinetic parameters, most notably the synthesis of lipophilic and hydrophilic esters.

Functional groups that are essential for both mineralocorticoid and glucocorticoid activity include the pregnane skeleton with an all-*trans* backbone, the A-ring enone system (Δ^4-3-one), and the 17β-ketol side chain (C-20-keto-C-21-hydroxy). The C-21 hydroxy group must be free for both mineralocorticoid and glucocorticoid activity. Exceptions to this rule are the C-21-chloro and C-20-fluoromethylthio ester ($-SCH_2F$) derivatives that retain anti-inflammatory activity when applied topically or by inhalation. Glucocorticoids that are used for their anti-inflammatory effects and that have both glucocorticoid and mineralocorticoid activities are hydrocortisone, cortisone, prednisone, and prednisolone.

Many derivatives of the fundamental glucocorticoid skeleton have been synthesized with the intention of enhancing anti-inflammatory activity and decreasing or eliminating the salt-retaining properties of the glucocorticoids when administered in therapeutic doses. Figure 28.28 depicts those positions where substituents will affect anti-inflammatory and/or mineralocorticoid

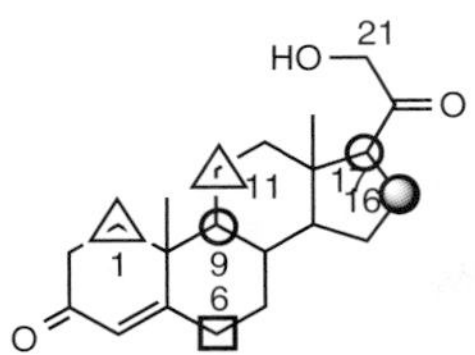

Both anti-inflammatory and mineralcorticoid activity increased (open circle)	Anti-inflammatory activity increased (triangle and square)	Mineralocorticoid activity decreased (closed circle and square)
17α-OH	1-dehydro	6α-CH_3
9α-F	6α-F	16α-& 16β-CH_3
9α-Cl	11β-OH	16α,17α-acetonide
21-OH		16α-OH

Figure 28.28 Glucocorticoid structure-activity relationship.

activity. The triangles indicate those positions where substitutions will increase the anti-inflammatory activity, the open circles indicate those positions where substituents will increase both anti-inflammatory and mineralocorticoid properties, the closed circle is the position where substituents will decrease the mineralocorticoid activity, and the open box is where specific substituents can either increase anti-inflammatory activity or decrease mineralocorticoid properties depending on the specific substituent. Therefore, the anti-inflammatory activity will be greatly increased by flattening ring A by adding a double bond at C-1 (Δ^1) and also by adding a hydroxy group at C-11β. A 17α-hydroxy increases both activities, as does 9α-fluoro or 9α-chloro. Mineralocorticoid activity is substantially eliminated by 16α- or 16β-methyl groups, a 16α-hydroxy group, or a 16α,17α-acetonide. A C6α-methyl group only slightly enhances the anti-inflammatory activity, whereas a C6-α-fluoro has twice as much anti-inflammatory effect. Both substituents, in combination with a C-16 substituent, will greatly decrease the mineralocorticoid effects.

Therefore, synthetic compounds can be prepared with marked glucocorticoid activity and little if any significant mineralocorticoid activity. These include triamcinolone, methylprednisolone, fluticasone, beclomethasone, budesonide, mometasone, and ciclesonide.

Glucocorticoid Metabolism

If one or more of the essential functional groups on the glucocorticoid skeleton are modified by metabolism, glucocorticoid activity will be lost. There are three major metabolic reactions that will eliminate glucocorticoid activity. They are ring A reductions, C-17 oxidation, and C-11 keto-enol isomerization. Reduction of the ring A 3-keto to a 3α-hydroxy by 3α-hydroxysteroid dehydrogenase and the reduction of the 4,5-double bond by 5β-reductase to produce the A/B *cis*-fused ring give rise to inactive metabolites (Fig. 28.29). Oxidation of the C-17 side chain to produce a 17-keto steroid requires both the C-17 hydroxy group and a free C-21 hydroxy group. Esterification of one or both will inhibit this metabolism and prolong the duration of action. The rapid in vivo equilibrium that exists between cortisone (11-keto) and hydrocortisone (11β-hydroxy) is catalyzed by 11β-hydroxysteroid dehydrogenase and produces the keto form that is inactive but also regenerates the hydroxy form that is highly glucocorticoid enhancing and found on all glucocorticoids. Figure 28.29 summarizes the metabolism of hydrocortisone.

Synthetic Steroid Esters

The glucocorticoids are lipophilic despite having at least three hydroxy groups. The hydroxy groups can be esterified with an appropriate acid that will either enhance or decrease that lipophilicity. The C-21 hydroxy group is the most accessible and, therefore, is the easiest to esterify. The C-17 hydroxy group also is easily esterified, but because it is slightly hindered by the C-17 side chain, it will react more slowly. The C-11 hydroxy group is highly hindered by the C-10 and C-13 methyl groups and will not react with acids to form esters. In addition, esterification has an effect on both receptor affinity and glucocorticoid metabolism. Because the C-21 hydroxy must be free to hydrogen bond to the Arg564 in the glucocorticoid receptor, C-21 esters are prodrugs requiring hydrolysis to become active. Also, the C-17 hydroxy group needs to be free to be metabolically oxidized; therefore, esterification of the C-17 hydroxy group inhibits oxidation to the C-17 keto group and prolongs duration of action. Duration also is prolonged because the lipophilic glucocorticoid esters do not concentrate in the urine (i.e., they undergo tubular reabsorption after glomerular filtration).

The lipophilicity of a glucocorticoid can be enhanced by esterification with lipophilic acids. Doing so results in a number of effects, including an increased log P which provides local activity with less systemic absorption and decreased side effects. The fact that C-21 lipophilic esters are prodrugs means that they have longer durations of action. They also have a slower onset because the lipophilic esters generally are bulky and retard hydrolytic enzymes.

Hydrocortisone

Cortisone

Metabolizing enzymes: 1 = 11β-hydroxysteroid dehydrogenase
2 = 3α-hydroxysteroid dehydrogenase
3 = 5β-reductase
4 = C-17 oxidase

Figure 28.29 Metabolic pathways for hydrocortisone.

These lipophilic prodrugs can be administered orally to treat a variety of conditions, by inhalation to treat asthma and COPD, and topically to treat various types of dermatitis. When administered orally, their longer duration of action means that they can be given less frequently, which often results in better patient adherence. When administered topically, C-21 lipophilic ester prodrugs are activated by hydrolysis by skin esterases,[63,64] which slows their systemic absorption. Systemically absorbed glucocorticoids are further metabolized in the liver as depicted in Figure 28.29. Figure 28.30 shows the structures of the most common C-21 lipophilic esters found on commercially available glucocorticoids.

Diesters and ketals provide a further enhancement of log P (i.e., increased lipophilicity) and an increased duration of action because they are slow to metabolize. It should be noted that diesters and hexacetonides (Fig. 28.31) are prodrugs, whereas simple ketals are not (i.e., they already have a free C-21 hydroxy group). Diesters are formed at C-21 and at either the C-17α or, if present, the C-16α hydroxyl groups, although 16α is a more sterically constrained position compared to 17α. The diesters are prodrugs due to esterification of the C-21-OH; however, esters at C-17α or C-16α are active intact. The most common diesters are the diacetate and dipropionate.

A ketal is a cyclic derivative formed between hydroxy groups on adjacent carbons and a carbonyl carbon of a ketone. The most common ketal found in glucocorticoids is called an acetonide and is the condensation product formed between the C-16α and C-17α hydroxy groups and the carbonyl carbon of acetone (CH_3COCH_3) (Fig. 28.31). If the acetonide is found along with a C-21-t-butylacetate ester, it is named a hexacetonide; the "hex" refers to the total number of carbons found in the butylacetate group. The hexacetonides are prodrugs and must hydrolyze at C-21to become active. The buteprate (i.e., probutate) is a diester consisting of a propionate at C-21 and a butyrate at C-17α (Fig. 28.31). It also is a prodrug, and the C-21 ester must be hydrolyzed to yield the active form.

Esterification also can be used to increase the hydrophilicity of the glucocorticoids, making them water-soluble prodrugs. The synthetic approach here is to use either a dicarboxylic acid or phosphoric acid to condense with the C-21 hydroxy group (Fig. 28.31). This places an ionizable group (a carboxylate or phosphate) on the prodrug, yielding water-soluble esters. These derivatives are used to prepare aqueous injectable products that can be administered intramuscularly or IV.

Hydrophilic glucocorticoid prodrugs have a rapid onset because they are readily hydrolyzed by plasma esterases. In contrast to the lipophilic prodrugs, their water solubility allows them to be easily excreted through the kidney,

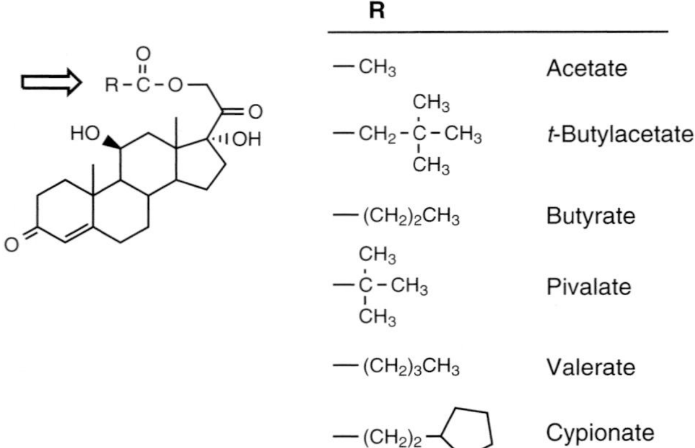

R	
$-CH_3$	Acetate
$-CH_2-C(CH_3)_2-CH_3$	*t*-Butylacetate
$-(CH_2)_2CH_3$	Butyrate
$-C(CH_3)_2-CH_3$	Pivalate
$-(CH_2)_3CH_3$	Valerate
$-(CH_2)_2$-cyclopentyl	Cypionate

Figure 28.30 Common lipophilic esters of glucocorticoids.

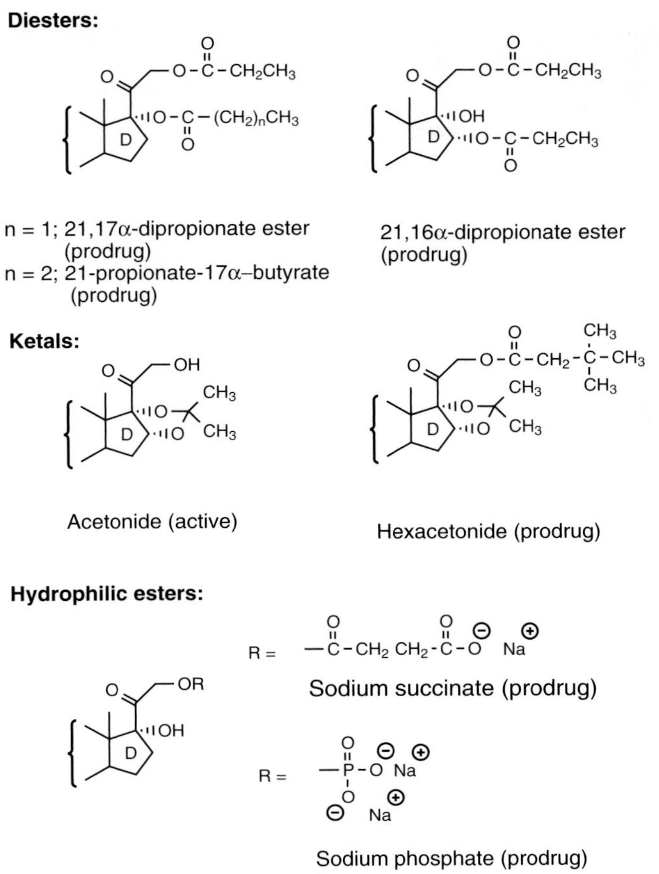

Diesters:

n = 1; 21,17α-dipropionate ester (prodrug)
n = 2; 21-propionate-17α–butyrate (prodrug)

21,16α-dipropionate ester (prodrug)

Ketals:

Acetonide (active)

Hexacetonide (prodrug)

Hydrophilic esters:

Sodium succinate (prodrug)

Sodium phosphate (prodrug)

Figure 28.31 Examples of glucocorticoid lipophilic diesters and ketals and hydrophilic esters.

resulting in a shorter duration of action. Hydrophilic prodrugs have more systemic side effects because of the wide distribution that comes from their high solubility in the blood. Along with their ability to be injected IV, this property makes them useful in asthmatic emergencies (i.e., status asthmaticus) during which the patient is unable to take oral medication. Table 28.6 summarizes glucocorticoid prodrug derivatives.

Glucocorticoid Drugs Used to Treat Asthma

Systemic Glucocorticoids

HYDROCORTISONE[65]

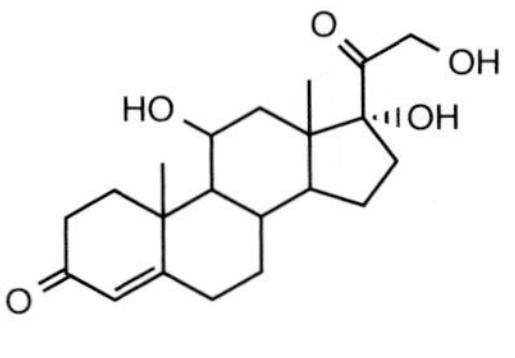

Hydrocortisone (Cortisol)

Δ^4-11β,17α,21-Trihydroxy-3,20-pregnenedione

Hydrocortisone is endogenous, and it has both glucocorticoid and mineralocorticoid activity. It is the fundamental structure by which the glucocorticoid and mineralocorticoid activities of all other corticosteroids are judged. Functional groups that are essential for both mineralocorticoid and glucocorticoid activity include the pregnane skeleton with an all-*trans* backbone, the A ring Δ^4-3-one system, and the 17β-ketol side chain. The glucocorticoid activity is enhanced by the C-11β and C-17α hydroxy groups. Hydrocortisone can be used to treat severe asthmatic attacks that do not respond to conventional treatment. It is available as various ester forms (Table 28.6). Due to its mineralocorticoid activity, it is not recommended for patients with hypertension.

Prednisolone[66]

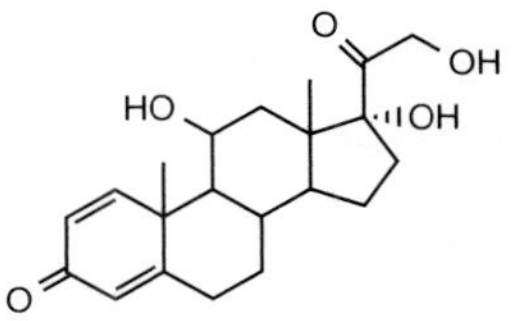

Prednisolone (Delta-Cortef)

$\Delta^{1,4}$-11β,17α,21-trihydroxy-pregnadiene-3,20-dione

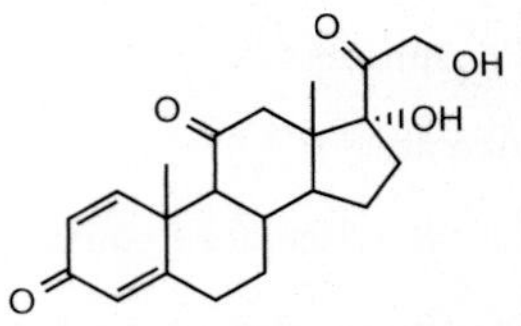

Prednisone (Deltasone, Meticortin)

$\Delta^{1,4}$-17α,21-dihydroxy-pregnadiene-3,11,20-trione

Prednisolone is hydrocortisone with an additional Δ^1 double bond. This forms an A ring that is conjugated from C-1 to C-5, and the trigonal coplanar sp^2 hybridized carbons flatten the ring increase glucocorticoid action at the expense of mineralocorticoid activity. Prednisolone has fourfold the glucocorticoid activity of hydrocortisone while having approximately half its mineralocorticoid activity. In addition, prednisolone has an increased duration of action compared to hydrocortisone because the extra double bond in ring A retards metabolic reduction.

Prednisolone can be used to treat severe asthmatic attacks that do not respond to conventional treatment, and it is available as the free alcohol for oral administration. The C-21 sodium phosphate ester (Hydeltrasol) is available for parenteral use. Various ester prodrugs are available, as listed in Table 28.6. A nonester prodrug of prednisolone is prednisone. It is the 11-keto analogue of prednisolone and must be converted in vivo to the active 11β-hydroxy metabolite, which is necessary to serve as an H-donor in a hydrogen bond to Asn564 in the glucocorticoid receptor. Prednisone should not be used in patients with hepatic dysfunction, because their ability to reduce the 11-keto group with 11β-hydroxysteroid dehydrogenase to the active metabolite may be impaired.

When orally administered, prednisone and prednisolone are almost completely absorbed, with a bioavailability greater than 80%. Prednisolone is metabolized into a number of hydrophilic and less active metabolites.

Table 28.6 Glucocorticoid Prodrug Ester Derivatives

Drug	Trade Name	Site of Ester	Route of Administration
Hydrocortisone Derivatives			
Phosphate		C-21	IM, IV, SC
Sodium succinate	A-Hydrocort Solu-Cortef	C-21	IM, IV
Cypionate	Cortef	C-21	PO
Acetate	Cortaid	C-21	Topical
Butyrate	Locoid	C-21	Topical
Buteprate	Pandel	C-21	Topical
Valerate	Westcort	C-21	Topical
Prednisolone Derivatives			
Phosphate	Hydeltrasol	C-21	IV, IM
Acetate	Key-Pred	C-21	Topical
Di-*t*-butylacetate (tebutate)	Prednisol TBA	C-17, 21	Topical
Methylprednisolone Derivatives			
Sodium succinate	Solu-Medrol	C-21	IV, IM
	A-Methapred		
Acetate	Depo-Medrol		
	Depoject	C-21	IM

IM, intramuscular; IV, intravenous; PO, oral; SC, subcutaneous.

The major metabolites (6β- and 16β-hydroxy analogues) are primarily excreted as glucuronide conjugates in the urine.

Methylprednisolone[67]

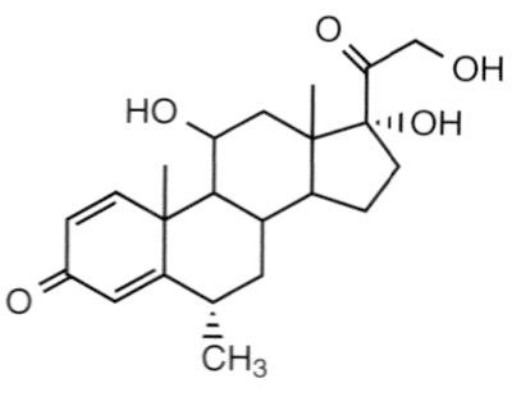

6-Methylprednisolone
(Medrol)

$\Delta^{1,4}$-6α-methyl-11β,17α,21-trihydroxy-pregnadiene-3,20-dione

Adding a 6α-methyl group to prednisolone increases the glucocorticoid activity and effectively abolishes mineralocorticoid action. It has fivefold the glucocorticoid activity of hydrocortisone (25% more than prednisolone) and none of its mineralocorticoid properties. It is used almost exclusively as a systemic agent and is available as the free alcohol for oral administration and in ester prodrug form for parenteral use (Table 28.6). For example, methylprednisolone is administered IV as its water-soluble sodium salt of the 21-succinate ester. The succinate ester is slowly and incompletely hydrolyzed, and peak plasma levels attained in approximately 30-60 minutes. Approximately 10% of an IV dose is recovered unchanged in urine.[68]

Methylprednisolone is extensively metabolized, with approximately 10% recovered unchanged in urine. The metabolic pathways include reduction of the C-20 ketone, oxidation of 17β-ketol group to both the C-21-COOH and C-20-COOH metabolites, and 6β-hydroxylation (CYP3A4). CYP3A4 inhibitors such as the antifungals, ketoconazole, and itraconazole can potentiate the effects of prednisolone.

Side Effects

Systemic administration of glucocorticoids can result in a large number of adverse effects on prolonged use. As previously stated, there is the serious risk of HPA axis suppression, requiring the slow tapering of the dose. In addition, glucocorticoids can affect the following systems:

- cardiovascular (thromboembolism, hypertension, and arrhythmias)
- central nervous system (convulsions and steroid psychosis)
- dermatologic (impaired wound healing and hair growth)

- endocrine (amenorrhea, postmenstrual bleeding, and suppression of growth in children)
- GI (pancreatitis, increased appetite, and peptic ulcer)
- musculoskeletal (muscle weakness, steroid myopathy, and osteoporosis)
- ophthalmic (cataracts, increased intraocular pressure, and glaucoma)
- electrolyte disturbances (sodium and fluid retention, hypertension, and metabolic alkalosis)

Glucocorticoids for Inhalation

Beclomethasone Dipropionate[69,70]

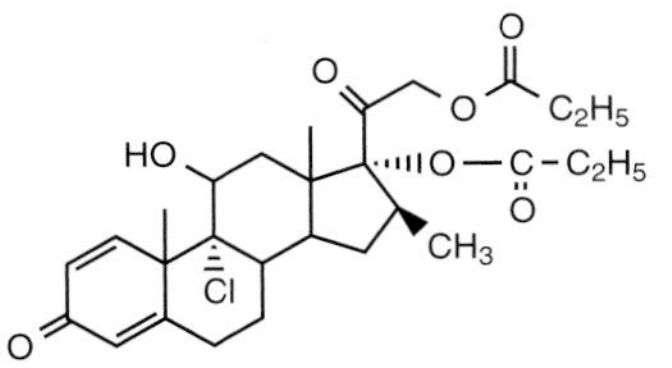

Beclomethasone dipropionate
(QVAR, Vanceril)

9α-Chloro-16β-methyl-11β,17α,21-trihydroxypregna-1,4-diene-3,20-dione 17,21-dipropionate

Beclomethasone dipropionate is a lipophilic prodrug that, when inhaled, shows a systemic bioavailability of approximately 20%. While the 9α-chloro substituent normally increases both glucocorticoid and mineralocorticoid activity, the 16β-methyl group essentially abolishes mineralocorticoid action, resulting in potent anti-inflammatory activity with little or no salt-retaining effects. The main adverse effects are headache, sinusitis, and sinus pain. Beclomethasone dipropionate is hydrolyzed to the active 17α-monopropionate derivative during absorption from the lungs and then further metabolized to the free 17α alcohol in the liver. Less commonly, the dipropionate can also metabolized to the inactive C-21-monopropionate in the liver. Beclomethasone dipropionate and its metabolites are mainly excreted in the feces, with less than 10% excreted in the urine.

Budesonide[71]

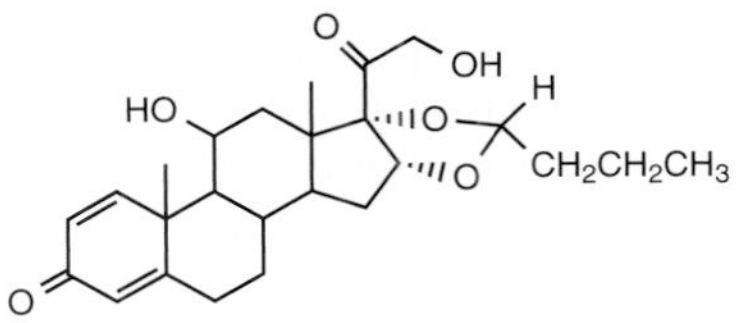

Budesonide
(Pulmacort tubuhaler, Respules)

16α,17-[(*R,S*-butylidenebis(oxy))]-11β,21-dihydroxypregna-1,4-diene-3,20-dione

Budesonide is an acetal formed between the 16α,17α-dihydroxy groups and butanal. It is a nonhalogenated glucocorticoid with decreased mineralocorticoid activity due to the presence of a 16α oxygen. In receptor affinity studies, the acetal *R*-epimer was twofold more active than the S. Because the C-21 hydroxy is free, budesonide is not a prodrug and is active as administered.

Only 34% of the metered dose of inhaled budesonide reaches the lung. Systemically absorbed budesonide is highly protein bound and metabolized by CYP3A4 to 16α-hydroxyprednisolone and 6β-hydroxybudesonide in the liver. Both metabolites have less than 1% of the glucocorticoid activity of the parent compound. It is known that the polar 16α-OH decreases glucocorticoid affinity (the complimentary receptor residues are lipophilic), and activity can be retained only if augmented by other glucocorticoid-enhancing groups (e.g., 9α-F as found in triamcinolone, discussed below). Inhaled budesonide is excreted mainly as metabolites via both feces (15%) and urine (32%). Following inhalation, approximately 70%-80% is reversibly esterified by free fatty acids in the airway tissue. These inactive esters behave like an intracellular depot drug by slowly regenerating free budesonide. Thus, this reversible esterification prolongs the local anti-inflammatory action of budesonide in the airways and may contribute to high efficacy and safety in the treatment of mild asthma when inhaled once daily.[72,73] Budesonide is available as a powder delivered as an aerosol or as a suspension for inhalation.

Ciclesonide[74]

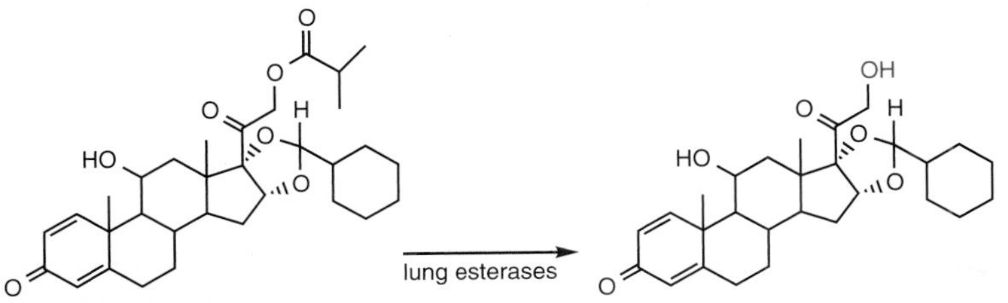

lung esterases

Ciclesonide (Alvesco, Omnaris)

16α,17-[(*R*-cyclohexylmethene]bis(oxy)]-11β-hydroxy-21-(2-methyl-1-oxopropoxy)-pregna-1,4-diene-3,20-dione]

Desisobutyrylciclesonide
(active metabolite)

Ciclesonide is a glucocorticoid with an acetal formed at positions C16α and C17α with cyclohexylcarboxaldehyde. A 16α–oxygen atom, including the one found in glucocorticoid acetals, decreases mineralocorticoid activity. In addition, ciclesonide has a Δ^1 that retards ring A reduction, promoting a longer duration of action, and increasing glucocorticoid action at the expense of mineralocorticoid activity through conformational influences, as previously described. Ciclesonide is a prodrug that is converted to the active desisobutyrylciclesonide via esterases in the lung. It is reported to have a relative potency equivalent to budesonide and beclomethasone dipropionate, as well as fluticasone and mometasone (discussed below). Lung deposition on inhalation is 52%, and the oral bioavailability is less than 1%, presumably due to low GI absorption and high first-pass metabolism. Desisobutyrylciclesonide is metabolized in the liver to polar metabolites mainly dihydroxylated desisobutyrylciclesonide.

Ciclesonide is available in a hydrofluoroalkane propellant metered-dose formulation for inhalation. Ciclesonide is also available in a nasal spray (Omnaris) for the treatment of hay fever.

Flunisolide[75,76]

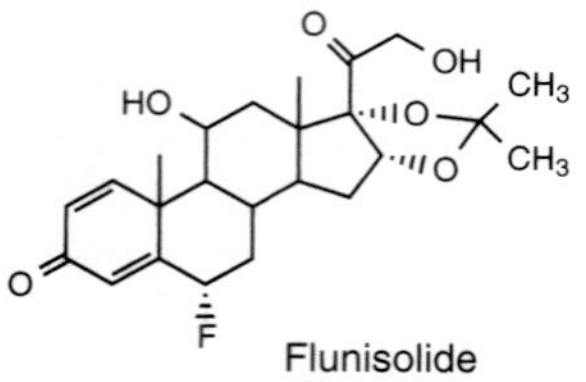

Flunisolide (Aerobid)

6α–Fluoro-11β,21-dihydroxy-16α,17-[(1-methylethylidene)bis(oxy)]pregna-1,4-diene-3,20-dione

Flunisolide is an active acetone ketal (acetonide) with a 6α-fluoro group and a free C-21 hydroxyl group. As with other acetonides, the 16α-oxygen decreases mineralocorticoid activity and the 6α-fluoro group increases glucocorticoid activity. Flunisolide has approximately 20% of the receptor affinity as budesonide, and approximately 40% of the inhaled dose is systemically bioavailable. Flunisolide is quickly metabolized by CYP3A4 to the 6β-hydroxy metabolite, which has less than 1% of the activity of the parent compound. This, along with the rapid elimination of both flunisolide and its hydroxy metabolite as glucuronides, greatly limits any systemic adverse effects. Flunisolide is available as a microcrystalline powder aerosol.

Fluticasone Propionate[77,78]

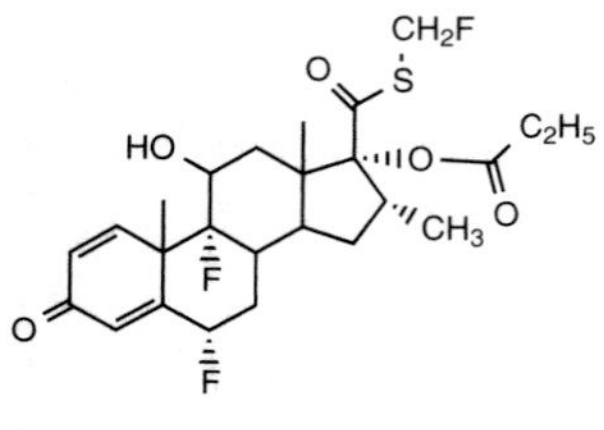

Fluticasone propionate (Flovent, Flonase)

6α,9α-Difluoro-S-fluoromethyl-11β-hydroxy-16α-methyl-3-oxo-17α-propionyloxyandrosta-1, 4-diene-17α-carbothioate

Fluticasone propionate has a unique C-20 thiofluoromethyl group, and that, in combination with the 17α-propionate ester, gives it 36-fold the glucocorticoid receptor affinity compared to beclomethasone dipropionate and twofold the affinity compared to budesonide. The 9α-fluoro group increases both glucocorticoid and mineralocorticoid activities, and the 6α-fluoro group enhances only the glucocorticoid action. Studies have determined that the effectiveness of inhaled fluticasone propionate results from a local, rather than a systemic, effect. Interestingly, less than 1% of the swallowed dose is bioavailable, in contrast to the systemic bioavailability of a majority of the inhaled dose. Once in plasma it is highly protein bound.

Despite the unusual substitution pattern at C-20, fluticasone propionate is not a prodrug. It is extensively metabolized by the liver, with the only detectable metabolite being the 17β-carboxylic acid derived from CYP3A4 oxidation of the thioester. This metabolite has a 2,000-fold lower affinity for the glucocorticoid receptor than the parent drug. Elimination is through both the feces and the urine, with the relative amounts determined by the route of administration. Fluticasone propionate is available in aerosol and powder inhalation formulations.

Mometasone Furoate[79,80]

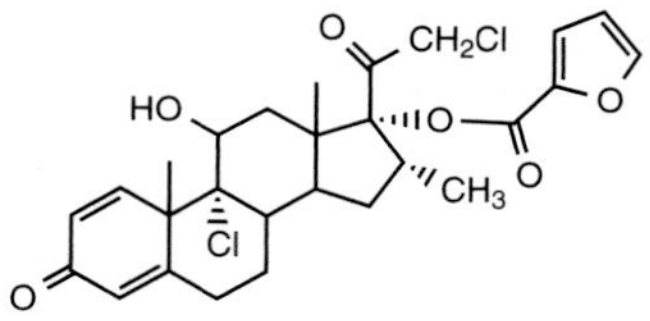

Mometasone furoate (Asmanex Twisthaler)

9α,21-dichloro-17α–[(2-furanylcarbonyl)oxy]-11β-hydroxy-16α-methylpregna-1,4-diene-3,20-dione

Mometasone furoate has a number of unique functional groups that confer enhanced glucocorticoid activity, as well as pharmacokinetic advantages. The combination of the C-21 chloro substituent and the furoic acid ester at C-17α results in the highest glucocorticoid receptor affinity of any topical corticosteroid. As with beclomethasone, while the 9α-chloro group is known to increase both glucocorticoid and mineralocorticoid activity, the 16α-methyl eliminates mineralocorticoid action in the same way beclomethasone's 16β-methyl does. Inhaled mometasone furoate acts locally as an anti-inflammatory treatment for asthma and has the lowest systemic bioavailability of all the inhaled glucocorticoids (<1%). It is extensively metabolized, with 6β-hydroxymometasone and C-21-hydroxymometasone being found among the metabolites. Inhaled mometasone furoate is mainly excreted in the feces (~74%) as metabolites and only minimally excreted in the urine (~8%). It has a relatively long half-life in the lung and is administered once daily, usually in the evening.

Triamcinolone Acetonide[81]

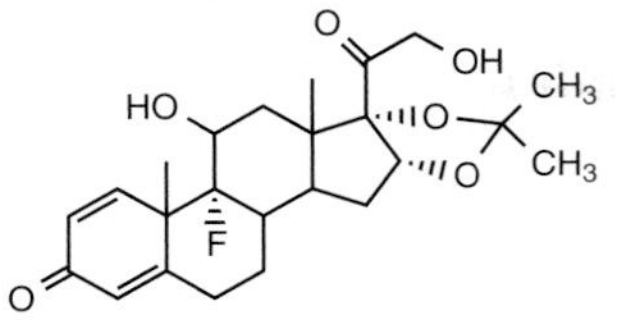

Triamcinolone acetonide (Azmacort)

9α–Fluoro-11β,17α,21-trihydroxypregna-1,4-diene-3,20-dione-16α,17-acetonide

Triamcinolone acetonide has the essentially abolished mineralocorticoid activity of all acetonides. The 9α-fluoro group, known to increase both the glucocorticoid and the mineralocorticoid activities, essentially promotes only glucocorticoid action in drugs with mineralo-abolishing functional groups. Triamcinolone acetonide has a gluco receptor affinity that is 10-fold that of beclomethasone dipropionate but 6-fold less than that of mometasone furoate. After oral inhalation, as much as 25% of triamcinolone acetonide can be detected systemically; a good proportion of that is assumed to be secondary to absorption from the GI tract after swallowing. It is metabolized in the liver to a number of metabolites, including 6β-hydroxytriamcinolone acetonide and the C-21 carboxy-6β-hydroxytriamcinolone acetonide, both of which are readily excreted via the kidneys. The acetonide remains intact during metabolic transformation and, therefore, is highly resistant to hydrolytic cleavage. Triamcinolone acetonide is excreted mainly as metabolites in the urine (40%) and feces (60%), with less than 1% being excreted unchanged.

Mast Cell Degranulation Inhibitors

The discovery that a Middle Eastern herb, *Ammi visnaga* (Khella, Bishop's weed), had mild bronchodilation effects led to the isolation of a benzopyrone (a chromone), khellin. Khellin had only weak bronchodilator effects, so synthetic analogues were prepared in an attempt to enhance the bronchodilation. All analogues were less active; however, it was noted by Dr. Roger Altounyans, who was experimenting on himself with these analogues, that one of them, if inhaled before an asthmatic attack, gave excellent protection against the attack's severity.[82] The active compound was identified as a bischromone and named cromolyn sodium in the United States and sodium cromoglycate in Europe (Fig. 28.32).

This class of mast cell degranulation inhibitors prevents the release of histamine, leukotrienes, prostaglandins, and other inflammatory autocoids by interaction with the sensitized mast cell before antigenic challenge and does not inhibit the binding of IgE to the mast cell or the antigen to IgE. The exact mechanism of action is still not completely understood; however, it is clear that inhibition of the role of calcium in the degranulation process is involved. A number of membrane and cellular proteins that bind cromolyn sodium are known to regulate intracellular calcium levels, including basophilic membrane protein, nucleoside diphosphate kinase, calgranulins B and C, and annexins I through V.[83,84] Mast cell degranulation inhibitors also are used topically in the eye to treat allergic reactions.

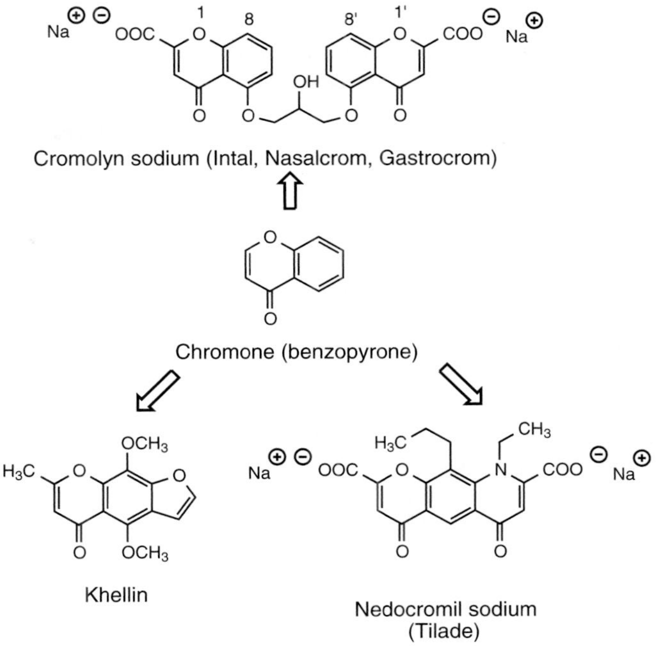

Cromolyn sodium (Intal, Nasalcrom, Gastrocrom)

Chromone (benzopyrone)

Khellin

Nedocromil sodium (Tilade)

Figure 28.32 Structures of several chromone mast cell stabilizers.

Mast Cell Stabilizers Used to Treat Asthma

Cromolyn Sodium

Cromolyn sodium is a bischromone that contains the fundamental benzopyrone moiety of khellin (Fig. 28.32). The two chromone rings are necessary for activity and must be coplanar, with a linking chain of no longer than six carbons. If one changes the linking chain to positions 8 and 8′, coplanarity cannot be maintained, and the compound loses all activity. Cromolyn sodium is poorly absorbed from the lungs (~8%), insignificantly from the eye (~0.07%), and approximately 1% from the GI tract. What little that finds its way into systemic circulation is eliminated intact in the urine and the bile. For the treatment of asthma, cromolyn sodium is available as a solution for both intranasal and inhalation administration. There also is an oral concentrate (100 mg/5 mL) which is administered as a 200-mg dose given four times a day.[85]

Nedocromil Sodium

Nedocromil sodium was developed by changing the dihydropyranone ring of khellin to a dihydropyridinone ring (Fig. 28.32). In vitro, nedocromil sodium inhibits the release of inflammatory response mediators from a variety of cells, including neutrophils, mast cells, macrophages, and platelets. Inhaled nedocromil sodium is poorly absorbed into the systemic circulation, with approximately 3% of an inhaled dose excreted in the urine during the first 6 hours after administration. Only 2% of orally dosed nedocromil sodium is bioavailable, 89% of which is protein bound. When administered IV, nedocromil sodium is not metabolized and is excreted unchanged in the bile and the urine. Nedocromil sodium is available in aerosol canisters for oral inhalation via a mouthpiece.[85,86]

Leukotriene Modifiers

It has been known for more than 40 years that a substance called SRS-A (slow-reacting substance of anaphylaxis) produced a slowly developing, long-lasting contraction of isolated guinea pig ileum, and that this same substance was associated with the pathophysiology of asthma. Subsequently, it was determined that SRS-A was actually a mixture of triene-containing lipids, designated as Cys-leukotrienes: LTC_4, LTD_4, and LTE_4. Determination of the chemical structure of these biologically active compounds led to the development of inhibitors of their biosynthesis, as well as receptor antagonists that are useful in the treatment of asthma.[87]

Biosynthesis of Leukotrienes

The leukotrienes occur in a variety of inflammatory cells that are abundant in asthma, including eosinophils, mast cells, and macrophages. They are derived from arachidonic acid via a branch of the common pathway to the prostacyclins and thromboxanes. Arachidonic acid itself is produced by the action of phospholipase A_2 on cell membranes. Unlike the prostacyclins and thromboxanes, excess arachidonic acid does not activate the leukotriene pathway. Instead, the first step in the conversion of arachidonic acid to leukotrienes is controlled by an activating protein, 5-lipoxygenase–activating protein (FLAP), which regulates the interaction of 5-lipoxygenase with its substrate. Figure 28.33 depicts the biosynthetic pathway and shows that 5-lipoxygenase oxidizes arachidonic acid to the unstable peroxide intermediate, 5-hydroperoxyeicosatetraenoic acid, which is quickly dehydrated to LTA_4, which in turn is further metabolized by (1) LTA_4 hydrolase to LTB_4 and (2) LTA_4 synthase to the glutathione adduct, LTC_4. Cleavage of γ-glutamic acid by γ-glutamyl transpeptidase converts LTC_4 to LTD_4, which in turn is converted to LTE_4 by the removal of Gly under the action of dipeptidase. Of the four leukotrienes produced from LTA_4, all but LTB_4 have strong bronchoconstrictive activity: LTD_4 is the most potent bronchoconstrictor with the fastest onset of action. While LTB_4 has no bronchoconstrictive activity, it is a potent neutrophil chemotactic agent.[87]

Leukotriene Receptors

The cysteinyl leukotriene (cysLT) receptors are of the rhodopsin family of the GPCRs. As such, they consist of seven transmembrane-spanning helices that activate intracellular signaling pathways in response to their endogenous ligands (LTC_4, LTD_4, and LTE_4). Studies have identified two distinct cysLT receptors, and molecular biologists have cloned the human genes for both $cysLT_1$ and $cysLT_2$.[88] Studies have distinguished between the two cysLT receptors by evaluating their interaction with known antagonists, showing that the $cysLT_1$ receptor was competitively inhibited from binding LTD_4, whereas the $cysLT_2$ receptor was not. In addition, there is a slight difference in ligand-binding affinities between the two

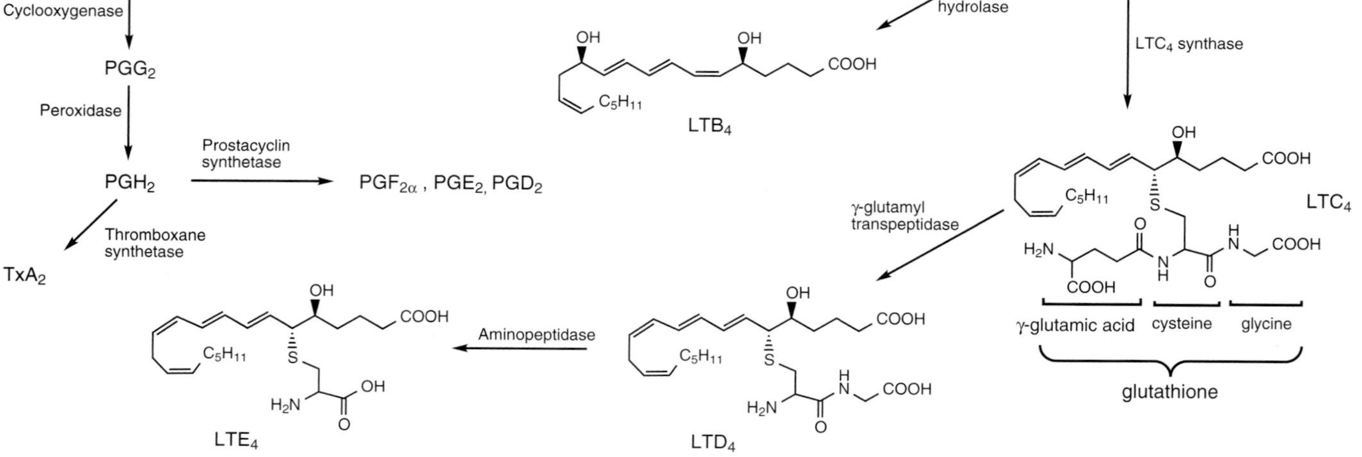

Figure 28.33 Biochemical pathways leading to the leukotrienes. FLAP, 5-lipoxygenase–activating protein; LT, leukotriene; PG, prostaglandin.

receptors. The cysLT$_1$ receptors have an affinity profile of LTD$_4$ > LTC$_4$ = LTE$_4$, whereas the cysLT$_2$ receptors show an affinity profile of LTC$_4$ = LTD$_4$ > LTE$_4$. Both receptor types occur in the lungs and spleen. The cysLT$_1$ receptor is also found in the placenta and small intestines, whereas the cysLT$_2$ receptor occurs in the heart, lymph nodes, and brain. The incomplete overlap of tissue distribution, along with distinct ligand-binding properties, suggests cysLT$_1$ and cysLT$_2$ receptors might serve different functions in vivo.[89] Because the cysLT$_1$ receptors are inhibited by selective antagonists, they have importance in the treatment of leukotriene-related bronchoconstriction in asthma.

There are two leukotriene receptors for LTB$_4$, designated as BLT$_1$ and BLT$_2$. They are also GPCRs and are expressed in mast cells. There is growing evidence supporting the involvement of BLT$_1$ and BLT$_2$ receptor activation in the pathophysiology of asthma. BLT$_1$ receptors are also expressed in bronchial fibroblasts, neutrophils and macrophages, and glucocorticoids upregulate BLT$_1$ receptors in steroid-resistant inflammatory cells potentially involved in causing inflammation.[90]Therefore, developing therapies to antagonize LTB$_4$/BLT$_1$ interaction could provide a promising treatment for steroid-resistant asthma. A possible role of BLT$_2$ in asthma pathogenesis is also being explored.[91]

Leukotriene Modifier Drugs

Two approaches to the development of leukotriene modifiers have been taken. The first approach was to block their biosynthesis by designing compounds that inhibit one or more of the enzymes involved in their biochemical pathway. The second approach was to identify antagonists with selective affinity for the cysLT$_1$ receptor.

Leukotriene Biosynthesis Inhibitors

The search for orally active 5-lipoxygenase inhibitors has resulted in only a few classes of investigational compounds that are effective in animals and humans, with the N-hydroxyureas yielding a useful product.[92] The 5-lipoxygenase inhibitors block the production of LTB$_4$, as well as LTC$_4$, LTD$_4$, and LTE$_4$, thereby decreasing both the bronchoconstrictive and chemotactic effects of the leukotrienes.

ZILEUTON

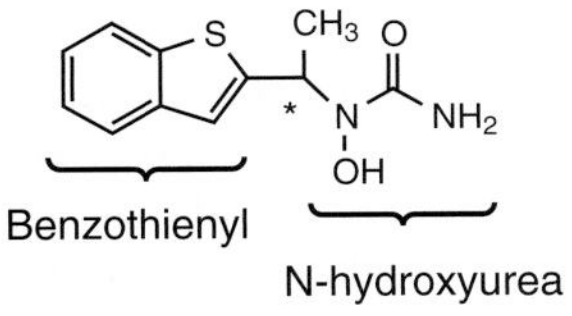

Benzothienyl

N-hydroxyurea

Zileuton (Zyflo)

Zileuton is the first N-hydroxyurea 5-lipoxygenase inhibitor to be marketed. It is the benzothienylethyl derivative of N-hydroxyurea and is marketed as the racemic mixture, as both isomers are pharmacologically active. The N-hydroxy group is essential for inhibitory activity, with the benzothienyl group contributing to its overall lipophilicity. Zileuton is rapidly absorbed after oral administration and is 93% protein bound. Metabolism occurs in the liver, with the inactive O-glucuronide being the major metabolite, along with less than 0.5% inactive N-dehydroxylated and unchanged zileuton. Glucuronidation is stereoselective, with the S-isomer being metabolized and eliminated more quickly.[93] Greater than 90% of an oral dose is bioavailable, and 95% is excreted as metabolites in the urine. The short 2.5 hour half-life requires four-times-a-day dosing.

Zileuton increases the plasma levels of propranolol, theophylline, and warfarin, and dosing of these drugs should be reduced and the serum levels monitored carefully in patients taking one or more in combination with zileuton. The most serious side effect of zileuton is elevation of liver enzymes; if symptoms of liver dysfunction (e.g., nausea, fatigue, pruritus, jaundice, or flu-like symptoms) occur, the drug should be discontinued.[94] Zileuton is used as an alternative to LABAs, and in addition to ICSs, for the treatment of moderate persistent asthma.

Leukotriene Receptor Antagonists

The search for leukotriene receptor antagonists began without the aid of ligand-receptor binding data and took three distinct approaches: (1) design of leukotriene structural analogues, (2) exploration of quinoline analogues, and (3) random screening from compound libraries. The combination of these efforts led to a simple structure-activity relationship: (1) the lipophilic tetraene tail of LTD$_4$ can be mimicked by a variety of more stable aromatic rings, (2) the thioether of the glycinylcysteinyl dipeptide can be replaced by an alkyl carboxylic acid, and (3) the C1 carboxylate of LTD$_4$ is essential and must be retained. Additional research focusing on the three-dimensional requirements for antagonist binding to the cysLT receptors further clarified that the pharmacophore needs to consist of an acidic functional group that can generate an anion at physiologic pH, a hydrogen bond H-acceptor function, and three hydrophobic regions.[95] Based on this background, synthetic efforts resulted in the development of montelukast and zafirlukast as cysLT$_1$ receptor antagonists. Figure 28.34 demonstrates how both these antagonists fit the pharmacophore model. Leukotriene receptor antagonists, just as with zileuton, are used as an alternative to LABAs, and in addition to ICSs, for the treatment of moderate persistent asthma.

MONTELUKAST SODIUM

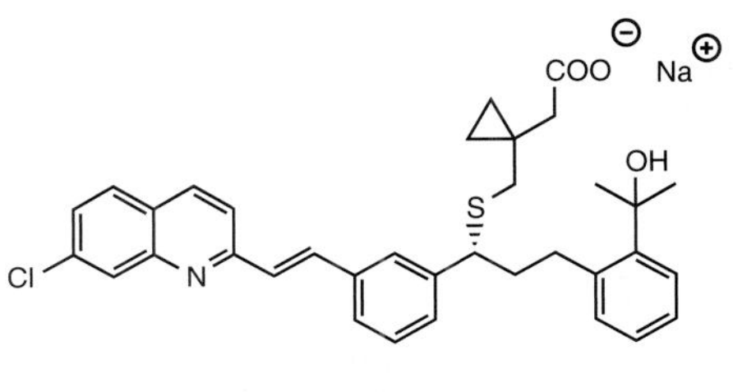

Montelukast (Singulair)

Montelukast sodium is a high-affinity, selective antagonist of the cysLT$_1$ receptor that was developed from other weakly antagonistic quinoline derivatives. A number of

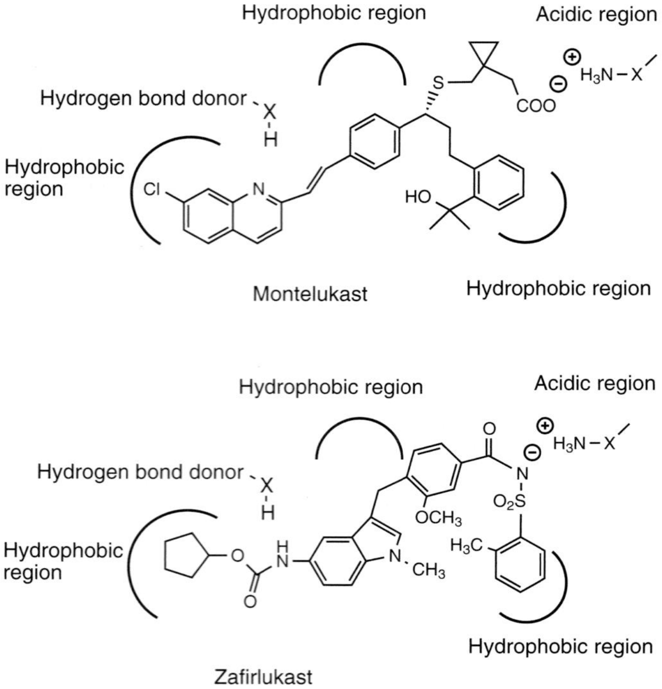

Figure 28.34 Interaction of montelukast and zafirlukast with cysteinyl leukotriene (cysLT) receptor model.

changes can be made to the structure without the loss of activity. These include changing the double bond between the two aromatic rings to an ether linkage, reducing the quinoline ring, changing the chlorine to fluorine, and/or exchanging the sulfur for an amide group. It is rapidly absorbed orally, with a bioavailability of 64%. Montelukast is 99% bound to plasma proteins and is metabolized extensively in the liver by CYP3A4 and CYP2C9 to oxidized products. As shown in Figure 28.35, CYP3A4 oxidizes the sulfur and the C21 benzylic carbon, whereas CYP2C9 is selectively responsible for methyl hydroxylation. Figure 28.35 shows the primary metabolic pathway for montelukast in humans.[96] More than 86% of an oral dose is eliminated as metabolites through the bile. Montelukast did not demonstrate any significant adverse effects greater than placebo in clinical trials; however, because CYP450 enzymes metabolize it, its plasma levels should be monitored when coadministered with CYP450-inducing drugs, such as phenobarbital, rifampin, and phenytoin. Montelukast is also an inhibitor of CYP2C8. Montelukast is available in tablet, chewable tablet, and granules for administration mixed with food.[97]

Zafirlukast

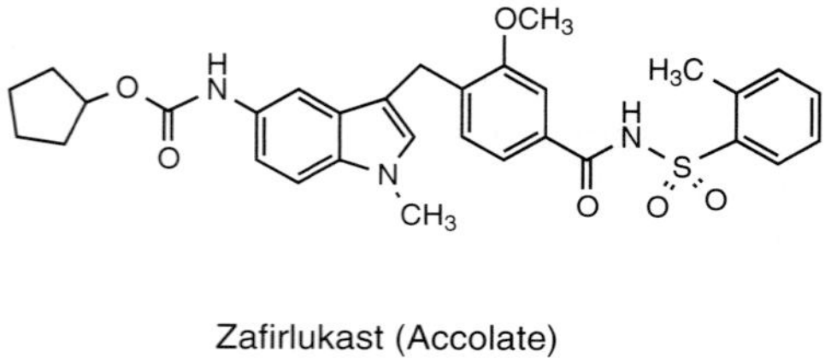

Zafirlukast (Accolate)

Zafirlukast is an indole derivative with a sulfonamide group that fulfills the need for an anion-generating moiety on the pharmacophore. A large number of analogues have been prepared; however, they all resulted in a decrease in antagonist activity. Zafirlukast, like montelukast, is a selective antagonist for the cysLT$_1$ receptor and antagonizes the bronchoconstrictive effects of all leukotrienes (LTC$_4$, LTD$_4$, and LTE$_4$). It is well absorbed orally; however, food will decrease its absorption by as much as 40%. Zafirlukast is primarily metabolized in the liver by CYP2C9 and CYP3A4 to hydroxylated metabolites[98] and has also been shown to undergo carbamate hydrolysis followed by N-acetylation. Additionally, zafirlukast is known to produce an idiosyncratic hepatotoxicity in susceptible patients. This appears to result from the formation of an electrophilic α,β-unsaturated iminium intermediate evidenced by the formation of a glutathione adduct on the methylene carbon bridging the indole ring to the methoxyphenyl moiety of the molecule.[99]

Figure 28.36 summarizes the metabolism of zafirlukast. More than 90% of its metabolites are excreted in the feces, with the remainder found in the urine. Zafirlukast inhibits CYP3A4 and CYP2C9 in concentrations equivalent to clinical plasma levels and, therefore, inhibits its own metabolism. It should be used with caution in patients taking other drugs metabolized by these enzymes. Specifically, coadministration with warfarin results in a significant increase in prothrombin time. Other drugs with a narrow therapeutic index that are metabolized by CYP2C9 include phenytoin and carbamazepine. CYP3A4-metabolized drugs of concern are cyclosporine and the dihydropyridine class of calcium channel blockers. Of particular interest is the fact that aspirin and theophylline respectively increase and decrease the plasma levels of zafirlukast. Care should be taken when coadministering with erythromycin because this decreases the bioavailability of zafirlukast. Zafirlukast is only available in tablet formulations.[100]

Monoclonal Antibodies (MAbs)

The pathophysiology of allergic asthma, as already discussed, ultimately results in the production of allergen-specific IgE by activated B lymphocytes. The IgE binds to high-affinity FcεRI receptors on mast cells. The site where IgE binds to the receptor is located on the Fc fragment area of the C-ε-3 region, hence the acronym FcεRI (Fig. 28.37A). Subsequent allergen exposure causes cross-linking of bound IgE molecules, which triggers degranulation of these cells and results in the release of asthma mediators. Monoclonal anti-IgE antibody development is designed to moderate the role of IgE in activating mast cells, thereby decreasing the severity of allergic asthmatic attacks, and may also have beneficial effects in treating seasonal allergic rhinitis.

The success of IgE antibodies that moderate the role of mast cells has stimulated the development of antibodies to cytokines involved in the asthmatic inflammatory processes. There are now MAbs to IL-5, the major cytokine responsible for the growth and differentiation, recruitment, activation, and survival of eosinophils. The naming

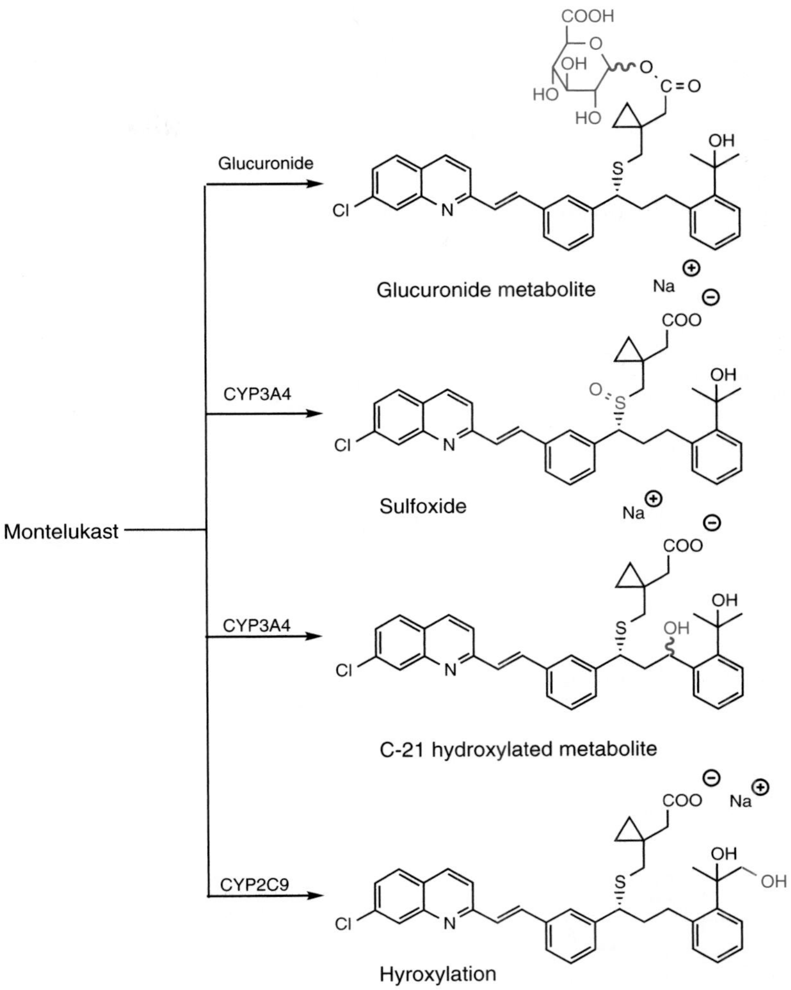

Figure 28.35 Metabolism of montelukast.

of MAbs provides clues to their target, source and potential immunogenicity. MAb nomenclature is based on a specific structure developed by the International Nonproprietary Names Working Group under the direction of the World Health Organization. The naming structure consists of a Prefix, Substem A, Substem B, and a Suffix. The Prefix does not follow any specific criteria and only serves to distinguish MAbs from one another. The Suffix will always be MAb, noting the drug is a monoclonal antibody. The Substem A denotes the target of the antibody and Substem B specifies the source (organism) from which the antibody is derived, providing insight into possible immunogenicity. For example, OMALIZUMAB has a Prefix OMA with Substem A as –LI meaning its target is the immune system. Substem B is –ZU meaning it is humanized and therefore will have diminished immunogenicity compared to murine derived antibodies.[101]

Omalizumab

Omalizumab is a MAb developed through somatic cell hybridization techniques and was identified as a murine anti–human IgE antibody originally called MAE11.[102] It is designed to interact with the IgE site that binds to FcεRI on mast cells. Additional amino acid sequences have been incorporated into the antibody so that a humanized product resulted that only contains 5% nonhuman amino acid residues.

In vitro, omalizumab has been shown to complex with free IgE, forming trimers consisting of a 2:1 and 1:2 complexes of IgE:omalizumab. In addition, larger complexes also are formed consisting of a 3:3 ratio of each (Fig. 28.37B). Omalizumab does not bind to IgE already bound to mast cells and, therefore, does not prevent the degranulation that might be expected from such interaction. Thus, omalizumab effectively neutralizes free IgE and, aside from the obvious decrease of available IgE, also causes the down-regulation of FcεRI receptors on the mast cell surface, resulting in a decrease of IgE bound to the mast cell.

The clinical role for omalizumab is in the treatment of allergic asthma. It is approved for the treatment of adults and adolescents 12 years of age and older whose symptoms are not controlled with inhaled glucocorticoids and who have a positive skin test for airborne allergens. The bioavailability after subcutaneous administration is 62%, with slow absorption resulting in peak serum levels from a single dose in 7-8 days. Steady-state plasma concentration is reached in 14-29 days with multiple dosing regimens.

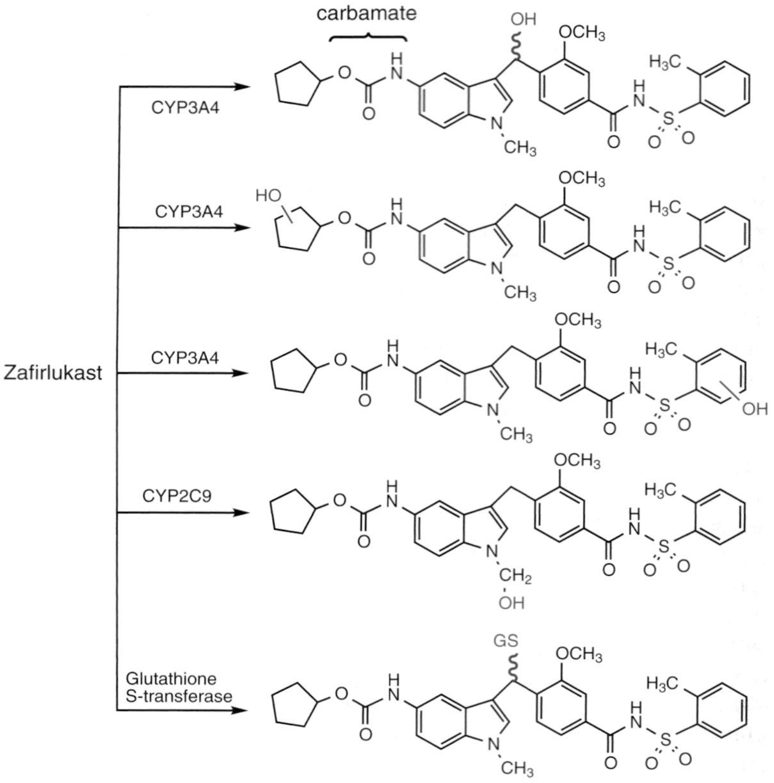

Figure 28.36 Metabolism of zafirlukast to oxidative products and a glutathione adduct.

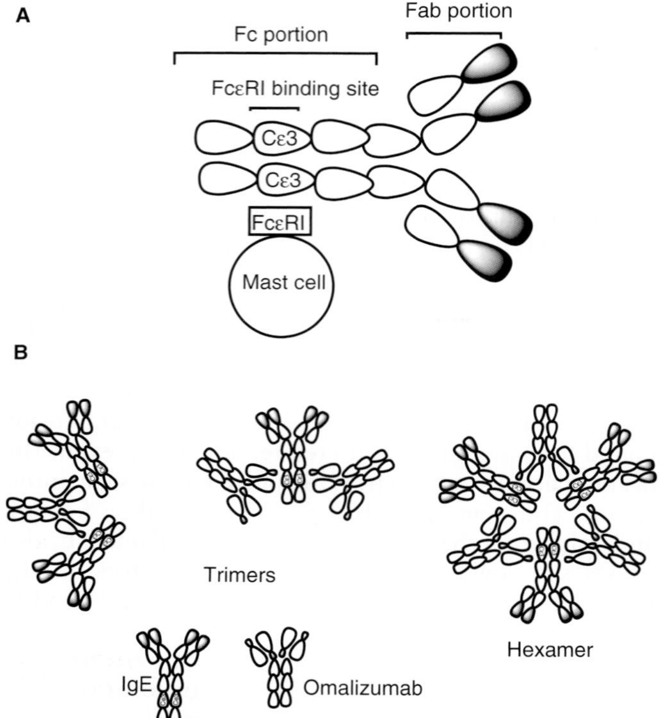

Figure 28.37 (A) Graphic representation of IgE binding to the high-affinity Fc immunoglobulin E receptor (FcεRI) on a mast cell. (B) Graphic representation of immune complexes formed between omalizumab. Hexamers predominate when components are in a 1:1 ratio, and the trimers predominate when one of the components is in excess.

The elimination of omalizumab is not clearly understood; however, studies have determined that intact IgE is excreted via the bile and that omalizumab:IgE complexes are cleared faster than uncomplexed omalizumab and more slowly than free IgE. This means that, over time, total IgE concentrations (free and complexed) increase because the complex is cleared more slowly. The metabolism of omalizumab is not known, and the clearance of the complex is similar to the hepatic elimination of another immunoglobulin, IgG. The reticuloendothelial system degrades IgG, and it is believed that the same process occurs for the omalizumab:IgE complex. Omalizumab is available as a lyophilized powder for injection in single-use, 5-mL vials.[103,104]

Benralizumab

Benralizumab is an IL-5 receptor antagonist. The IL-5 receptor, a GPCR, is highly expressed in eosinophils, basophils, and mast cells and contains monomeric α and dimeric β subunits. IL-5 binds to the α subunit of the IL-5 receptor on the cell surface, initiating hetero-oligomerization of the α and β subunits. The β subunit is responsible for signal transduction leading to cell differentiation. Benralizumab binding inhibits oligodimerization and signal transduction, resulting in inhibition of IL-5 receptor expressed cells.[105] IL-5 is the major cytokine responsible for the maturation and survival of eosinophils, and high levels of eosinophils are implicated in severe treatment-resistant asthma. Therefore, benralizumab attenuation of eosinophil viability can ameliorate the symptoms of asthma.

As the name indicates benralizumab targets the immune system (substem A –li) and is humanized (substem B –zu). It is an add-on medication for the treatment of severe asthma in adults and children ≥12 years of age with an eosinophilic phenotype.[27] It is administered subcutaneously in a 30 mg dose every 4 weeks for the first three doses and then once every 8 weeks. It has ~58% bioavailability with an elimination half-life of 15 days (nonrenal). It undergoes proteolytic degradation throughout the body. Adverse reactions include immunological development of antibodies, headache, pharyngitis, and fever. It is available as a 30 mg/mL solution in prefilled syringes.[106,107]

Mepolizumab

Mepolizumab, another IL-5 receptor antagonist, has the same therapeutic indication as benralizumab. It acts by binding to IL-5 and inhibits its binding to the IL-5 receptor complex expressed on the eosinophil cell surface. This results in reduction in eosinophil production and survival. However, the exact mechanism of action is not clearly established. It also has the same nomenclature with the –li and –zu substems indicating its immune system targeting and humanized structure.

Mepolizumab is administered SC in a dose of 100 mg every 4 weeks. It is 80% bioavailable with a 3.6 L volume of distribution. Like benralizumab, it is metabolized by proteases and not renally excreted. It has a terminal half-life of 16-22 days. The most significant adverse reactions are headache and injection site irritation. Other adverse effects include fatigue, pruritus, eczema, and infections (influenza and urinary tract infections). For subcutaneous administration, meprolizumab the lyophilized powder is diluted to 100 mg/mL concentration using sterile water for injection.[108]

Reslizumab

Reslizumab is yet another IL-5 antagonist similar to benralizumab and mepolizumab with the same therapeutic indication. It has the same nomenclature with the –li and –zu substems indicating its immune system targeting and humanized structure. It is only administered by IV infusion at a 3 mg/kg dose every 4 weeks, and is metabolized by proteases. It has a 5 L volume of distribution and a terminal half-life of approximately 24 days. Reslizumab has fewer adverse effects compared to both benralizumab and mepolizumab, with the major toxicities being antigenicity, myalgia, and oropharyngeal pain.[109,110]

CHRONIC OBSTRUCTIVE PULMONARY DISEASE

Definition and Epidemiology

COPD is characterized by persistent breathing difficulty that is not completely reversible and is progressive over time. It usually is the result of an abnormal inflammatory response to airborne toxic chemicals. Thus, COPD is a general term and most commonly refers to chronic bronchitis and emphysema. Asthma is considered to be a disease entity unto itself and is not included in the definition of COPD. Both COPD and asthma are considered inflammatory diseases; however, the nature of the inflammation is different. Asthma is associated with the release of inflammatory mediators from mast cells and eosinophils, whereas chronic bronchitis is primarily associated with neutrophils and emphysema with alveoli damage. In addition, asthma is more often than not allergenic, whereas chronic bronchitis and emphysema have no allergic component. Finally, it is uncommon for asthma to be associated with smoking, whereas there is a very high incidence of both chronic bronchitis and emphysema in smokers.[111]

Patients with COPD display a variety of symptoms, ranging from chronic productive cough to severe dyspnea requiring hospitalization. Other chronic illnesses, including cardiac, endocrine, and renal disease, often occur along with COPD in many patients. In the United States, COPD is the third leading cause of death, being responsible for more than 150,000 deaths per year.[112] According to the National Ambulatory Medical Care Survey, in 2015 there were 7.3 million visits to emergency departments and the number of respiratory disease deaths (including from asthma) totaled 155,041 which equates to 48 deaths per 100,00 population. The number of adults with diagnosed chronic bronchitis in the year 2016 was 8.9 million. Rates of COPD-related death among women have tripled over the last 30 years, and this is being attributed to an increase in smoking. COPD is recognized as a global health problem, and in 2017, the NIH and the World Health Organization developed the Global Initiative for Chronic Lung Disease (GOLD) guidelines, which present only evidence-based recommendations for the treatment of COPD.[113,114]

Pathogenesis

The single most important risk factor for the development of COPD is smoking. It is estimated that 85% of COPD cases are attributable to cigarette smoking. Not all people who smoke, however, develop the disease, which means other factors are involved. It seems that genetics, environmental pollutants, and infection, along with bronchial hyperreactivity, all play an important role.

Cigarette smoke attracts inflammatory cells into the lungs and stimulates the release of the proteolytic enzyme elastase. Elastase breaks down elastin, which is a required structural component of lung tissue. Normally, the lung is protected from elastase by an inhibitor, α_1-antitrypsin (ATT). Cigarette smoke, however, causes an abnormal amount of elastase to be produced, more than ATT can counter, leading to lung damage. Smokers with an inherited deficiency of ATT have a greatly increased risk of developing emphysema, especially at an early age. Patients with COPD show an accelerated decline in lung function (50-90 mL FEV_1/yr) as compared to nonsmokers (20-30 mL/yr) (see earlier discussion of FEV_1 under General Therapeutic Approaches to the Treatment and Management of Asthma). Patients with COPD who stop smoking slow the progression of the disease. Unfortunately, however, they do not improve because the symptoms are an indication of irreparable lung tissue damage.

The role of other risk factors for developing COPD is not clear. Air pollution and occupational exposure to gases and particulates from the incomplete combustion of coal, diesel, and gasoline are related to the development of cough and sputum, but development of COPD seems to occur only in susceptible individuals. Passive cigarette smoke comes from the burning end of the cigarette and actually is higher in toxic substances compared with exhaled smoke. It has been established that respiratory infections, as well as cough and sputum production, are more common in children who live in households where one or both parents smoke. Chinese and Afro-Caribbean races have a reduced incidence of COPD, whereas COPD in American blacks is on the rise.[115]

COPD is a disease of the small airways and their adjacent aveoli. Permanent destructive enlargement of the air spaces distal to the terminal bronchioles without obvious fibrosis is the pathologic characteristic of emphysema. Inflammation and alveolar wall destruction lead to loss of lung elastic recoil. On the other hand, chronic bronchitis is characterized by hypersecretion of mucus, most of which is produced by the trachea and first branches of the bronchi. The smaller bronchi and terminal bronchioles are the site of the increased airway resistance, primarily due to narrowing from persistent inflammatory irritation. In the early stages of chronic bronchitis, the mucus and inflammation contribute to "smoker's cough," with little effect on airway obstruction. As inflammation continues, cell membrane edema and the production of large amounts of mucus contribute to airway narrowing and the difficulty in breathing associated with COPD. Even though bronchospasm may seem to be involved in COPD, there is little related pathogenesis.

Both emphysema and chronic bronchitis often occur together, with one predominating over the other. An important distinguishing clinical manifestation is that there is significant hypoxia and carbon dioxide retention with chronic bronchitis that does not happen with emphysema. Because of this, emphysema patients are referred to as "pink puffers," whereas patients with chronic bronchitis are called "blue bloaters."[116]

Pharmacotherapy

All the medications used to treat COPD have already been covered in the previous section on asthma. The 2018 GOLD guidelines no longer use only airflow limitation based on FEV_1 for the determination of pharmacotherapy for COPD. Instead the guidelines use protocols that also take into consideration the patient's exacerbation history.

Pharmacotherapy is divided into four classes denoted as A, B, C, and D. Using FEV_1, patients are first divided into four airflow limitation groups (GOLD 1-4). In the GOLD 1 group the patient has minor airway limitation (i.e., FEV_1 ≥80%). Patients in GOLD 2 group demonstrate an FEV_1 between 50% and 79% and are considered to be in moderate airway limitation. Patients with FEV_1 between 30% and 49 are in severe airway limitation and are in the GOLD 3 group, and those with FEV_1 <30% are the most severe cases and are placed in the GOLD 4 grouping. Patients are then evaluated for their exacerbation history and placed into two categories: those that experienced 0 or 1 exacerbations in the past year not leading to hospitalization and those who had 2 or more exacerbations in the past year or one or more that led to hospitalization admission. Based on these criteria patients are placed into one of pharmacotherapy classes A, B, C, or D. This allows treatment to distinguish patients who have the same GOLD number but more exacerbations so all can receive appropriate pharmacotherapy as described below.

Patients who fall into class A have mild to moderate COPD and 0-1 exacerbations a year and are started on a bronchodilator, either an SABA or LABA. These patients are labeled GOLD class A. Patients who are labeled GOLD class B have had >2 exacerbations in the past year and should be initiated on a long-acting bronchodilator, either an LABA or a muscarinic antagonist (LAMA) as needed. For patients in this class with persistent breathlessness it is recommended to use two bronchodilators (LABA + LAMA). Patients who fall into GOLD class C, experiencing >2 exacerbations but reporting breathlessness only when hurrying on level ground or upon strenuous exercise, should be started on an LAMA (not an LABA). Patients in this group who continue to have further exacerbations may benefit from the addition of either an LABA (LAMA + LABA) or an inhaled corticosteroid (LABA + ICS). Patients in GOLD class D suffer the most severe breathlessness, having to stop walking after about 300 feet or even when they are getting dressed. It is recommended starting these patients on an LABA + LAMA or an LABA + ICS. In patients who are still uncontrolled on the combination therapy, it is recommended to add in an ICS (LABA + LAMA + ICS). If triple therapy still does not control breathlessness, it is recommended to add a fourth medication, usually roflumilast (discussed below).[113,114,117]

Phosphodiesterase Inhibitors (PDE)

A number of important therapeutic agents owe their pharmacologic action to their ability to inhibit the enzyme PDE. In the treatment of asthma, theophylline, at least in part, relaxes bronchospasm by relaxing bronchiole smooth muscles; amrinone and milrinone are ionotropic agents that relax vasculature, causing vasodilation that results in a compensatory increase in heart rate; sildenafil and vardenafil relax smooth muscle of the vasculature in the penis; dipyramidole inhibits platelet aggregation; and the alkaloid papaverine relieves smooth and cardiac muscle spasms through its ability to inhibit PDE. These pharmacologic effects are the result of inhibiting the ability of PDE to break down cAMP and cGMP, prolonging their action as second messengers within a variety of cell and tissue types throughout the body. The PDE inhibitors also are implicated in an anti-inflammatory role by increasing cAMP and cGMP levels in cell types associated with the release of inflammatory chemicals from T and B cells, monocytes, neutrophils, and eosinophils. This last discovery was the impetus to develop PDE inhibitors to treat asthma (eosinophils) and COPD (neutrophils).

DEVELOPMENT OF PHOSPHODIESTERASE INHIBITORS. Progress in the development of PDE inhibitors to treat COPD and asthma awaited the basic pharmacologic research that identified the specific PDE isoforms associated with inflammatory cells so that selective inhibitors could be designed and synthesized.[118] There are 11 families of PDEs, with PDE4 being associated with inflammatory processes. Specifically, three PDE4 subtypes (PDE4A, PDE4B, and PDE4D) are found in inflammatory cells, with PDE4B being predominant. Therefore, efforts in this area have been directed toward the development and synthesis of selective PDE4 inhibitors. Progress in the development of PDE4 inhibitors has been slow because of a lack of clinical efficacy and dose-limiting side effects (nausea, diarrhea, and headache). The primary problem is the low therapeutic ratio of these compounds because the tolerated dose is either subtherapeutic or at the very bottom of the effective dose-response curve.[119,120] To date only one PDE4 inhibitor, roflumilast, has made it to the market.

ROFLUMILAST

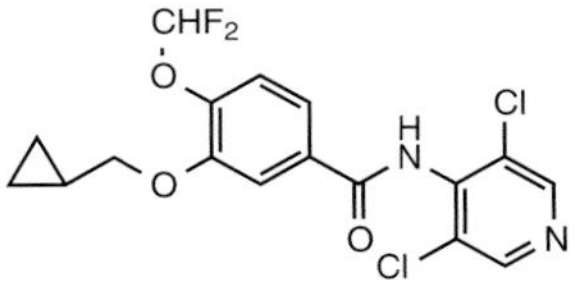

Roflumilast
(Daliresp)

The PDE4 enzyme has a compact α-helical structure with three domains. The active site forms a pocket at the junction of these three domains. The active site is composed of three subpockets; a metal binding pocket (Mg^{2+} and Zn^{2+}) with hydrophobic and polar residues to coordinate the metal ions (M-pocket), a solvent pocket filled with water molecules (S-pocket), and a pocket containing a purine-selective Gln and a pair of residues that form a hydrophobic clamp (Q-pocket). The ether oxygens of roflumilast hydrogen bond to the γ-carboxamide group of Gln deep inside the Q-pocket. The difluoromethoxy group and the cyclopropyl group contribute hydrophobic bonds in the Q-pocket as well. The dichloropyridyl group of roflumilast forms one hydrogen bond with the water molecule coordinated to the Mg^{2+} within the M-pocket.[121,122] Roflumilast is well absorbed on oral administration and has a half-life of 10 hours. It is metabolized in the liver by CYP3A4 and 1A2 to its N-oxide derivative, which also is a PDE4 inhibitor with a plasma half-life of 20 hours (Fig 28.38). Roflumilast's preclinical pharmacology continues to evolve, but it is known to be an effective oral treatment for COPD with an acceptable tolerability profile.[123] Roflumilast was approved for treatment of COPD associated with chronic bronchitis in the European Union in 2010 and in the United States in 2011.

SMOKING CESSATION

It has already been stated that COPD is most often associated with smoking.[111] In a recent population-based survey of adult smokers, it was found that prolonged smoking was associated with an increase in the likelihood of developing COPD, frequent productive cough, and frequent shortness of breath. In contrast, former smokers who had quit smoking for more than 10 years had a significantly lower incidence of COPD. At all levels of smoking duration, the prevalence of COPD was higher in women than in men.[124] It follows that it is most important for smokers to

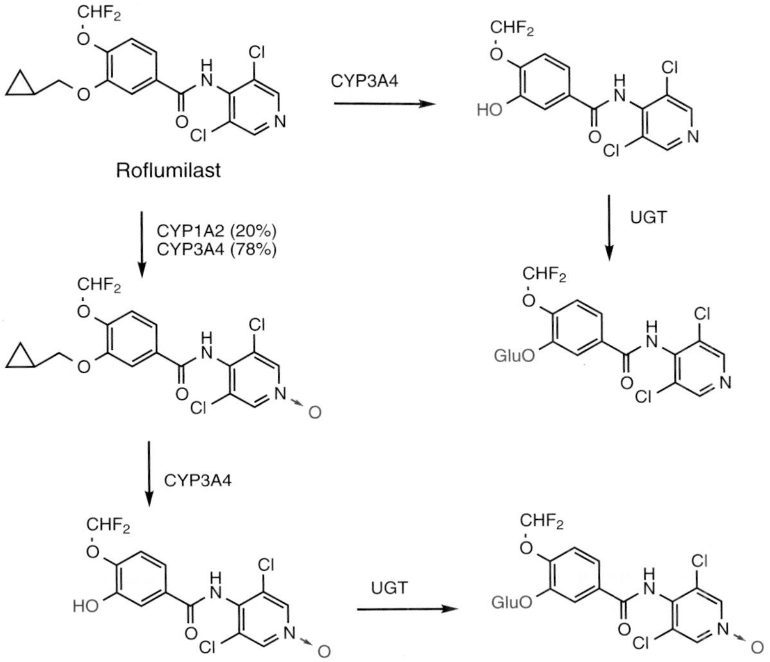

Roflumilast

CYP3A4

UGT

CYP1A2 (20%)
CYP3A4 (78%)

CYP3A4

UGT

Figure 28.38 Roflumilast metabolism.

stop smoking before they develop COPD. Unfortunately, the highly addicting nature of nicotine in tobacco makes it difficult for many to stop smoking, and only about 6% of smokers who attempt to quit actually succeed.[125]

Nicotine

Nicotine   Acetylcholine

Nicotine's addicting properties stem from its binding to the nicotinic acetylcholine receptor (nAChR). The nAChRs are actually named from their ability to bind nicotine, a nonendogenous molecule. The nAChRs are found at the neuromuscular junction, adrenal medulla, and autonomic ganglia and are chemically and mechanistically distinct from the muscarinic acetylcholine receptors (mAChRs) found mainly at postganglionic fibers in the parasympathetic system. The mAChRs are GPCR whereas the nAChRs are ligand gated ion channels (see Chapter 8). Figure 28.39 is a stylized drawing of the nAChR. The receptor consists of five transmembrane proteins made up of subunits designated as α, β, δ, and γ with the α subunit occurring twice. There are various types of nAChRs depending upon their tissue distribution made of different α (α1–α6) and β (β2–β4) subunits. Each of the five transmembrane subunits is composed of four hydrophobic membrane spanning segments (M1-M4). The acetylcholine binding sites are found on the α subunits located at the αγ and αδ junctions.

Nicotine binding to the nAChRs opens the ion channel (mainly for Na^+ or K^+) which stimulates a large number of physiological systems, including the skeletal, cardiovascular, gastrointestinal, and the central nervous system, as well as exocrine glands. Nicotine's action is biphasic, i.e., binding initially stimulates the neuromuscular system however prolonged application causes persistent blockage of transmission.[126] Nicotine dependence is primarily attributed to its binding to the $\alpha_4\beta_2$ nicotinic receptor subtype, which produces pleasurable feelings by releasing dopamine from central dopaminergic neurons.[127]

Approaches to Smoking Cessation

Quitting smoking is difficult because it involves withdrawal of nicotine, which causes anxiety, irritability, depression, and stress. Like the treatment for most addicting substances, smoking cessation should involve the slow removal of nicotine over a period of time so that nicotinic receptors will normalize in the brain to avoid withdrawal symptoms. Approaches to smoking cessation include nicotine replacement therapy (NRT) and prescription cessation medications such as varenicline and bupropion. Counseling along with medication has been shown to have good quit rates within the first 3 months (~60%) but half relapse, giving an overall quit rate of ~30% after 12 months.[128]

Nicotine Replacement Therapy (NRT)

NRT in combination with behavioral and/or pharmacotherapy has the best cessation results.[128] Nicotine replacement products include nicotine patches, gum, lozenges, and prescription nasal spray. Nicotine gum and lozenges come in 2 and 4 mg doses. Heavy smokers (>40 cigarettes/d) should chew or suck the 4 mg dose q1-2hr prn to a maximum of 20 doses per day. The NRT patch comes in 7 and 21 mg patches. They are applied in doses from 7-42 mg for light (<10 cigarettes/d) to heavy smokers, respectively.[129] The FDA approved the nicotine nasal spray in 1996. The spray requires a prescription and delivers 0.5 mg of nicotine per activation. The recommended dose is 1 mg (2 sprays) in each nostril as needed, with up to 5 doses/hr or 40 doses per day permitted. Approximately 53% of the dose enters the systemic circulation with an absorption half-life of 3 minutes. This dose approximates the same level reached from smoking one cigarette.[130] Absorbed nicotine is metabolized (Fig. 28.40) primarily by CYP2A6. The major metabolites are cotinine and nicotine-N1′-oxide. Nicotine and its metabolites are rapidly excreted via the kidney with $T_{1/2}$ of 2 hours.[131]

Bupropion

Bupropion (Zyban)   Methamphetamine

Bupropion is an antidepressant that acts as a weak dopamine and norepinephrine reuptake inhibitor (DNRI) at

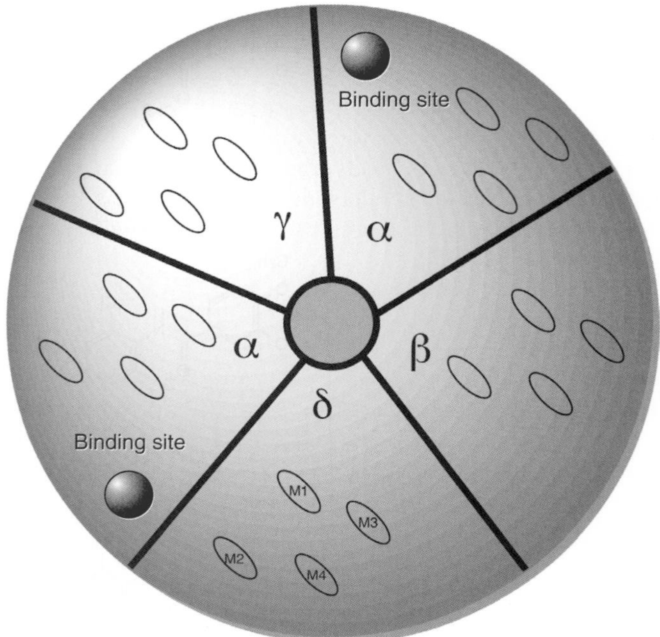

Figure 28.39 Stylized drawing of the nicotinic acetylcholine receptor (nAChR).

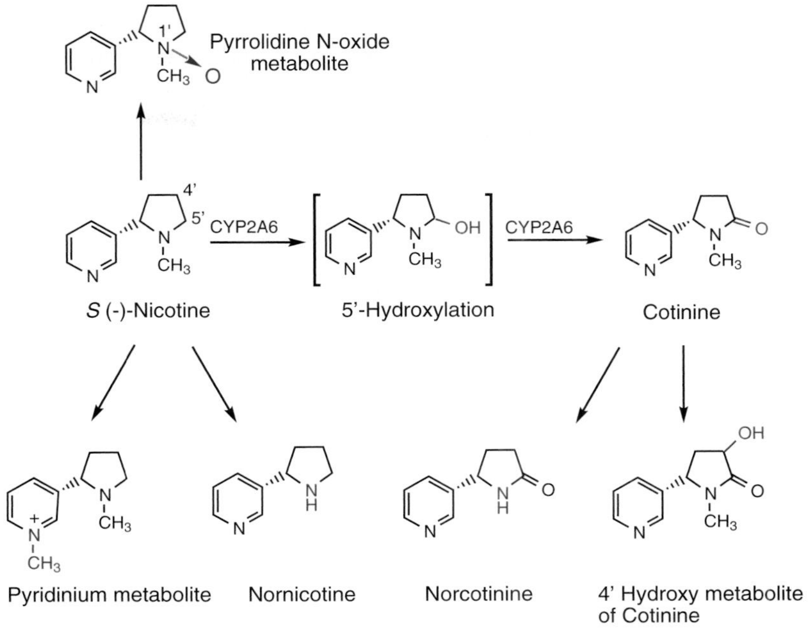

Pyrrolidine N-oxide metabolite

S (-)-Nicotine → CYP2A6 → [5'-Hydroxylation] → CYP2A6 → Cotinine

Pyridinium metabolite   Nornicotine   Norcotinine   4' Hydroxy metabolite of Cotinine

Figure 28.40 Nicotine metabolism.

the presynaptic neuronal membrane. In addition, bupropion also inhibits the nAChR, giving it antinicotinic activity and utility as a medication for smoking cessation. Structurally, bupropion is related to methamphetamine, where the benzyl carbon has been oxidized to a ketone and the N-methyl changed to a *t*-butyl group.

Bupropion has a half-life of 21 hours and is metabolized by CYP2B6 in the liver. The primary metabolite is hydroxybupropion, which is half as active as bupropion and cyclizes to an inactive phenylmorpholinol structure (Fig. 28.41). Racemic threohydrobupropion and erythrohydrobupropion also form and are each 20% as active as the parent drug. In addition, bupropion inhibits CYP2D6 and may reduce clearance of drugs metabolized by this isoform.

Bupropion is available in a 150 mg sustained release tablet, usually taken twice a day with therapy beginning 1-2 weeks prior to anticipated quitting date.[132] The drug demonstrates a number of adverse reactions and side effects, including headache, dizziness, decreased libido, hallucinations, unusual thoughts and behaviors, and seizures.

Varenicline

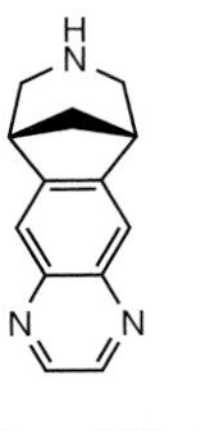

Varenicline

Varenicline is a partial agonist at $\alpha 4\beta 2$ and a full agonist at $\alpha 7$ nAChRs. Varenicline was developed from structural studies of the substructures of both morphine and cytisine (Fig. 28.42). Cyticine is a naturally occurring $\alpha 4\beta 2$ nAChR antagonist from *Laburnum* species (*Laburnam alpinum*; golden rain tree).[133]

Varenicline was approved by the FDA in 2006 as an aid to smoking cessation. However, in response to reports of suicidal ideation and erratic behaviors, the FDA in 2009 required varenicline to carry a boxed warning that the drug should be stopped if any of these symptoms manifest. Subsequently, in 2016, the FDA removed the boxed warning after reviewing a number of systematic reviews that found no evidence of increased risks for suicide or neuropsychiatric side effects. Patients are still advised to stop the medication if they notice any side effects related to altered mood, behavior, or thinking.[134]

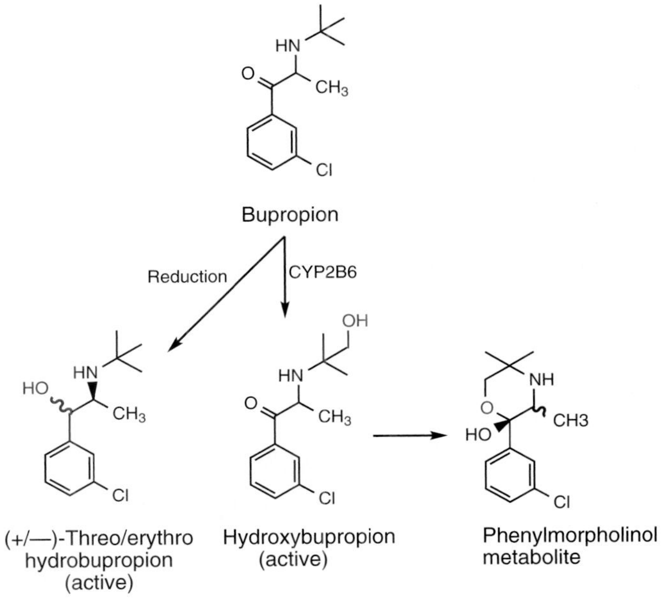

Bupropion

Reduction   CYP2B6

(+/—)-Threo/erythro hydrobupropion (active)   Hydroxybupropion (active)   Phenylmorpholinol metabolite

Figure 28.41 Bupropion metabolism.

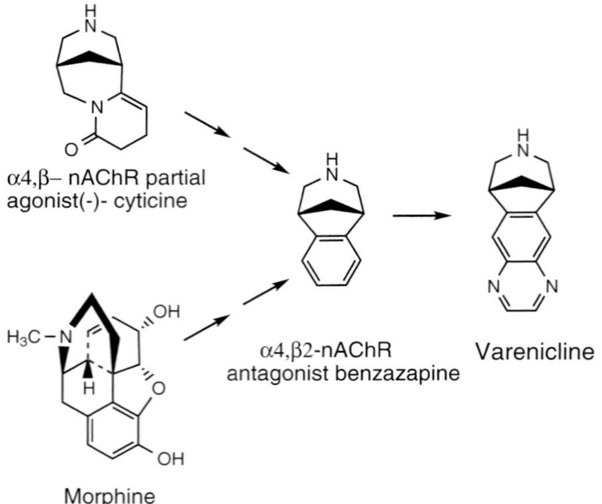

Figure 28.42 Structure activity studies of cyticine and morphine substructures ultimately led to varenicline.

Varenicline does not undergo significant metabolism and is almost exclusively excreted unchanged in the urine, mostly by glomerular filtration with some active tubular secretion via the organic cation transporter-2 (OCT-2). It is well absorbed (~90%), and oral bioavailability is unaffected by food. Maximum plasma levels occur within 3-4 hours, and protein binding is ~20%. There are no significant drug-drug interactions, and varenicline demonstrates linear pharmacokinetics.[135]

Patients should begin taking varenicline for smoking cessation 1 week before their quit date and follow a prescribed dosing regimen: days 1-2 take 0.5 mg daily; days 4-7 take 0.5 mg bid; and weeks 2-12 take 1 mg bid. Quitting success rate is greatly enhanced when taken along with NRT.[136]

CYSTIC FIBROSIS

Cystic fibrosis (CF) is an inherited life-threatening genetic disorder that damages the lungs, pancreas, liver, and other organs and afflicts about 30 thousand Americans. It affects cells that produce mucous, sweat, and digestive juices. People with CF have sticky mucous build up in their lungs, making them susceptible to bacterial infections. Mucous clogging in the airways also leads to inflammation and injury to the lung tissue.

There are several drugs that are approved for treating CF patients, which can be classified into two major classes: drugs that are used to treat symptoms such as inflammation, infection, and congestion due to thickened mucous and drugs that modulate the effect of gene mutation in certain patients. Congestion is treated with dornase alfa and hypertonic saline both of which are used as mucous thinners. Dornase alfa breaks up mucous by cutting DNA strands in white blood cells. Hypertonic saline thins mucous by increasing sodium levels in the airways, making it easier to cough. Inflammation is treated with ibuprofen, which is the only nonsteroidal anti-inflammatory drug (NSAID) approved for treating inflammation associated with CF. Several antibiotics and antiviral drugs are being evaluated for their effectiveness in treating infections caused by CF. Tobramycin, aztreonam, and azithromycin are the approved antibiotics to treat patients with CF infected with *Pseudomonas aeruginosa*.

The second class of drugs include those that modulate the effect of mutated genes responsible for the symptoms of CF. This chapter emphasizes the development of gene modulators. Patients who developed CF inherit two faulty cystic fibrosis transmembrane conductance regulator (*CFTR*) genes, one from each parent. CFTR regulator protein produced from the CFTR gene works as an ATP-gated chloride ion channel (Fig. 28.43). Its normal function is to allow chloride ions and water to maintain the correct fluid balance in the cells surrounding the airways, keeping the airway surface moist. Several mutations are reported to affect translation, folding or the functioning of the CFTR protein, causing reduced chloride and water release resulting in mucous thickening. Mucous thickening makes the lungs susceptible to infections and tissue damage characteristic of CF. The mutations that are known to affect the CFTR protein are as follows:

- G542X, W1282X, and R553X mutations leads to the production of nonsense proteins due to miscoding. These mutations are seen in 22% of CF patients.
- F508del, N1303K, and I507del mutations causes improper folding of the CFTR protein in the cytoplasm which prevents it from moving to the cell surface. These are the most common mutations and found in 88% of patients with CF.
- G551D and S549N mutations affect 6% of the population, producing a CFTR protein ion channel that does not open.
- D115H, R347P, or R117H mutations affect approximately 6% of CF patients and which produces faulty CFTR proteins.
- 3,849 + 10kbc → T, 2,789 + 5G → A and A455E mutations produce a decreased amount of CFTR proteins.

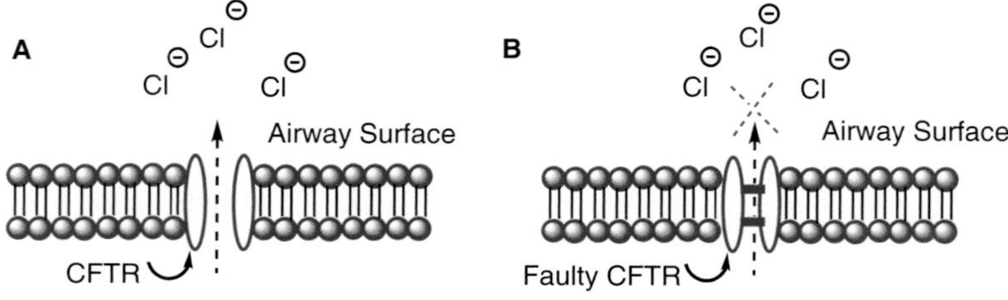

Figure 28.43 Cystic fibrosis transmembrane conductance regulator (CFTR) normal function and mutations (A) Normal CFTR protein on the cell surface working as a chloride ion channel allowing for salt and water balance in airways. (B) Defective CFRT protein resulting from genetic mutations, e.g., D1152H, R347P, R117H, etc.

Several drugs are under development to address the mutations that affect various stages of CFTR biosynthesis or function.[137]

CFTR Modulators

CFTR modulators are divided into three classes based on their function as either CFTR potentiators, correctors, or amplifiers.[138]

CFTR Potentiators

Depending on the type, mutations may induce the synthesis of nonfunctioning or faulty functioning CFTR or produce a decrease in CFTR protein levels. CFTR potentiators help open the CFTR channels and enhance the residual function of faulty, as well as normal, CFTR channels, thereby increasing chloride ion transport.

IVACAFTOR

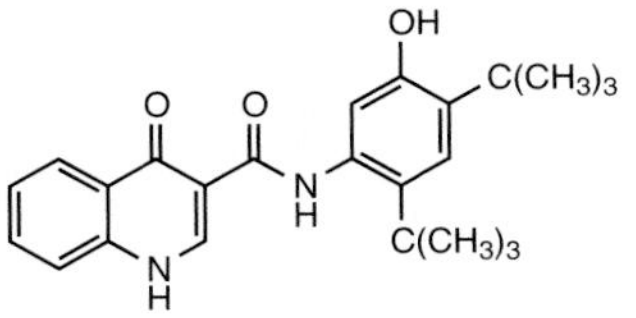

Ivacaftor (Kalydeco)

Ivacaftor was the first CFTR modulator approved for the treatment of CF. The FDA has recently expanded the approval of the drug for treatment of any of the 33 CFTR gene mutations. Ivacaftor is thought to increase CFTR function by increasing the secretion of chloride ions through the activated CFTR channel, possibly through activation of cAMP/protein kinase A (PKA) signaling.[139] It is orally effective, highly bound to plasma proteins (99%), and exhibits a biological half-life of ~12 hours. It is metabolized by CYP3A4 to metabolites M1 and M6 (Fig. 28.44); M1 is an active metabolite that retains about 15%-20% of parent drug's activity. Drugs that affect CYP3A4 may cause drug-drug interactions with ivacaftor. For example, concurrent administration with ketoconazole, a potent CYP3A4 inhibitor, doubles ivacaftor's plasma levels. It is recommended to halve the dose when coadministering with ketoconazole. Similar dosing adjustments should be considered with other strong 3A4 inhibitors. The majority of the ivacaftor dose is eliminated through feces.

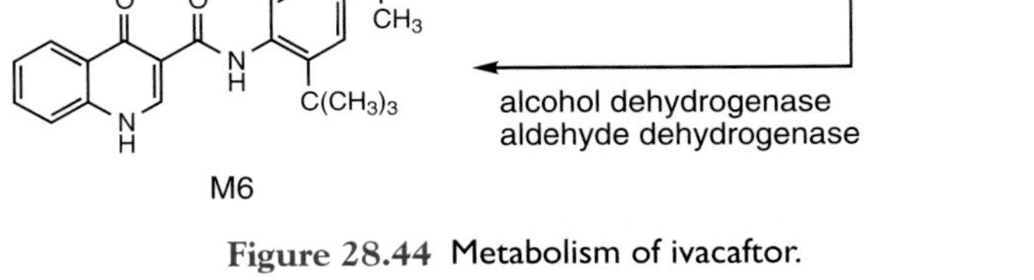

Ivacaftor → (CYP3A4) → M1 → (alcohol dehydrogenase, aldehyde dehydrogenase) → M6

Figure 28.44 Metabolism of ivacaftor.

The most common adverse effects include headache, upper respiratory infections, stomach pain, and diarrhea. The drug may also result in increased levels of transminases in the liver and cataracts in children.

CFTR Correctors

More than 50% of CF patients have the F508del mutation, resulting in the deletion of a Phe at position 508 (ΔF508) which causes the misfolding of the CFTR protein in the cytoplasm and prevents it from moving onto the cell surface. As noted previously, this is the most common mutation responsible for CF. CFTR correctors help defective CFTR fold correctly and translocate to the cell surface.

LUMACAFTOR

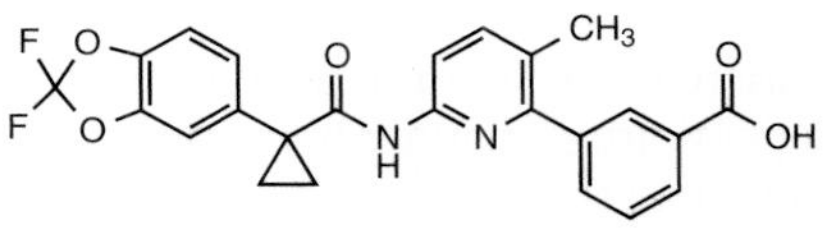

Lumacaftor (VX-809)

Lumacaftor is indicated in combination with ivacaftor to treat CF in patients 2 years and older who are homozygous for the CFTR F508del mutation. An FDA-cleared CF mutation test should be used in patients with unknown F508del mutation status. Lumacaftor is reported to act by increasing the amount of ΔF508-CFTR protein delivered to the cell surface through suppression of misfolding. This leads to a partial restoration of chloride ion transport. If ΔF508-CFTR protein does not misfold, then proteolytic degrading enzymes will not recognize it. It is thought that lumacaftor binds to MSD1 in a region near the interphase with NBD1 of the CFTR protein, altering and stabilizing its conformation.[140,141] By positively impacting CFTR protein conformational stability, lumacaftor increases mature protein transport to the cell surface, where the coadministered ivacaftor subsequently potentiates the opening and function of the chloride ion channel.

Lumacaftor undergoes minimal metabolism and is excreted primarily unchanged in the feces. The drug is reported to be a strong inducer of CYP3A4. As a result, when administered in combination with ivacaftor, lumacaftor greatly decreases the serum concentration of ivacaftor (Fig. 28.44). Both lumacaftor and ivacaftor exhibit significantly increased absorption when administered with fatty foods (lumacaftor 2X and ivacaftor 3X). Like ivacaftor, lumacaftor is both 99% bound to plasma proteins, and the most common adverse effects involve the GI (nausea, diarrhea, flatulence) and respiratory tract (upper respiratory tract infection, rhinorrhea, influenza). Elevations in blood phosphokinase bilirubin-transaminases are also noted.

TEZACAFTOR

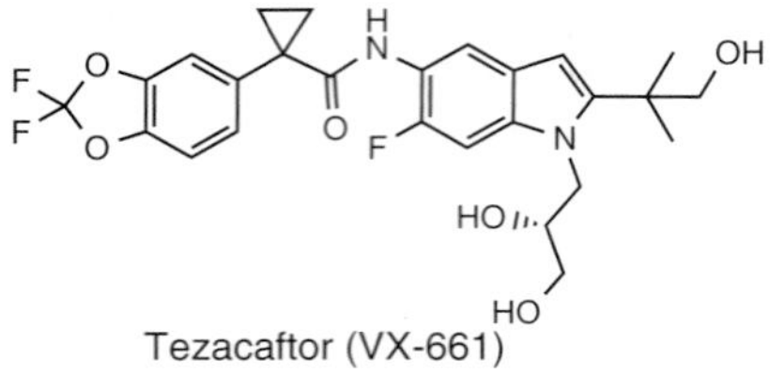

Tezacaftor (VX-661)

Tezacaftor is a CFTR corrector drug approved in February 2018 for use in combination with ivacaftor in CF patients with the F508del mutation.[142] Its mechanism of action is similar to that of lumacaftor. Like the CFTR modifiers discussed thus far, tezacaftor is approximately 99% bound to plasma proteins, and it is metabolized extensively by CYP3A4/5. M1, M2, and M5 are three major tezacaftor metabolites. M1 is an active metabolite with a similar potency to the parent drug (Fig. 28.45). Dosage adjustments are needed when coadministered with CYP3A4 inducers or inhibitors.

CFTR Amplifiers

Amplifiers increase the amount CFTR protein made. There are several drugs that are being developed, but none have yet made it to the clinic.

IDIOPATHIC PULMONARY FIBROSIS

Idiopathic pulmonary fibrosis (IPF) is a slow, progressive, irreversible disease of unknown cause that leads to scarring of the interstitial tissue of the lungs. Over time, the body cannot get enough oxygen, and it becomes harder to breathe. Typical IPF symptoms include shortness of breath, dry cough, and nail clubbing (disfiguration of fingertips). The etiology of the disease is unknown, but smoking is thought to be the most common risk factor. Other risk factors include environmental and occupational exposure to noxious chemicals, gastroesophageal reflux disorder (GERD), and genetic predisposition.[143] The pathogenesis of IPF is believed to be due to aberrant repair processes of the damaged alveolar epithelial cells (AEC). There are two types of AECs, Type I and Type II. Type I AECs line the majority of the alveolar surface on the basement membrane. Under normal conditions, when Type I AECs are damaged, Type II AECs undergo hyperproliferation to cover the exposed basement membrane. When repair mechanisms regenerate Type I AECs, Type II AECs undergo regulated apoptosis. In pathological conditions, fibroblasts accumulate at the damaged sites and differentiate into α-smooth muscle actin–expressing myofibroblasts that secrete collagen and extracellular matrix (ECM) proteins. These released substances interfere with normal repair mechanisms, causing scaring and eventual alveolar collapse.[144]

The destructive effects of IPF are associated with proliferation and migration of lung fibroblasts and myofibroblasts that require growth factors such as fibroblastic growth factor (FGF) and platelet derived growth factor (PDGF). These growth factors require tyrosine kinases for signal transduction. While a number of medications were investigated for use in IPF, currently only two drugs are available for treatment. Typical therapy consists of oxygen supplementation, pulmonary rehabilitation, and lung transplant, along with treating comorbidities such as GERD.

IPF tends to occur in people older than 50 years and is most commonly seen in males. Median survival time is less than 5 years after diagnosis. There is no cure for IPF but, as noted, symptoms may be treated to enhance quality of life.

Nintedanib

VEGFR kinase inhibitor

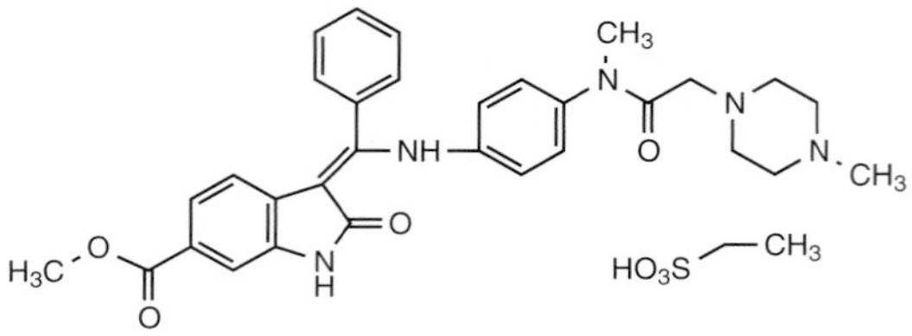

Nintedanib esylate
(Ofev)

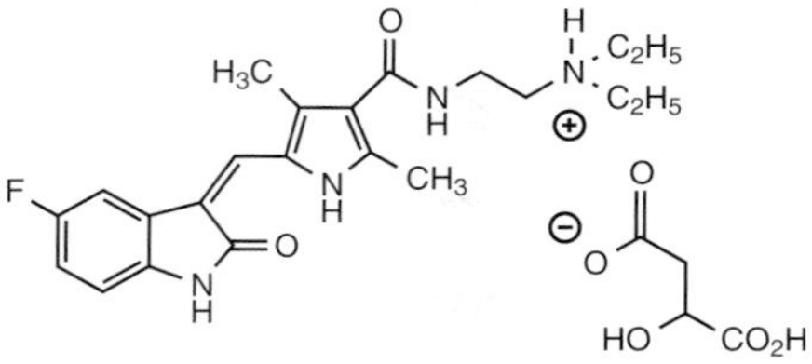

Sunitinib malate
(Sutent)

Nintedanib is a tyrosine kinase inhibitor which targets vascular endothelial growth factor receptors (VEGFR), fibroblastic growth factor receptors (FGFR), and platelet-derived growth factor receptors (PDGFR). A chemical similarity is suggested between nintedanib and the VEGFR kinase inhibitor sunitinib (discussed in Chapter 33). It should be noted that nintedanib exhibits activity against non–small cell lung cancer as well as IPF (sunitinib is an anticancer agent used in renal cell carcinoma). It is reported that nintedanib is a competitive inhibitor that binds to the ATP-binding site (hinge region) of the tyrosine kinase receptor, inhibiting cell proliferation and migration. The indolinone moiety may be capable of hydrogen bonding to specific amino acids in the hinge region of the ATP-site.[145,146] Sunitinib also has an indolinone ring known to be involved in kinase binding (see Chapter 33).

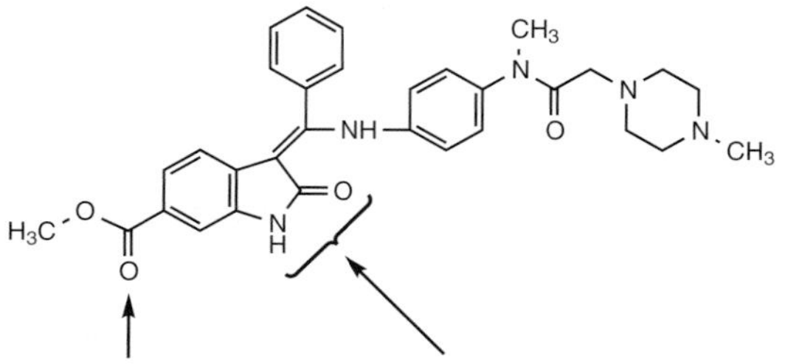

Nintedanib critical sites involved in binding to amino acids in the ATP site of FGFR

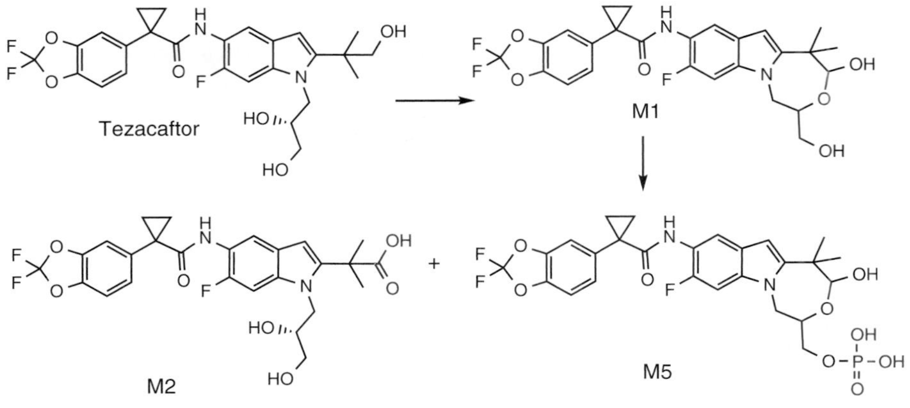

Figure 28.45 Metabolism of tezacaftor.

Nintedanib is reported to exhibit a low bioavailability (~5%) with a majority of the drug/metabolites being excreted in the feces. The major metabolic reactions of nintedanib include acetate ester hydrolysis followed by glucuronidation of the resulting aromatic carboxylic acid. Neither of these metabolites is active. Common adverse effects following oral administration are gastrointestinal (diarrhea, nausea, abdominal pain, vomiting). Additionally, an increase in liver transaminases was reported. Major cardiovascular events were also reported in a small number of patients.

Pirfenidone

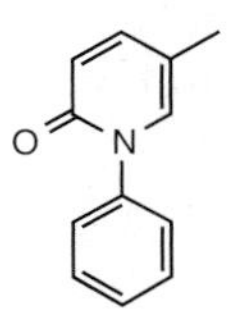

Pirfenidone (Esbriet)

Pirfenidone has been approved for the treatment of IPF and joins nintedanib as the only drugs approved for this indication. Pirfenidone exhibits antifibrotic effects that are thought to be associated with inhibitory action on collagen type I expression but may also involve inhibition of heat shock protein (HSP) 47 expression in lung fibroblasts.[147] Studies in mice suggest that pirfenidone is rapidly absorbed, completely metabolized as shown in Figure 28.46, and readily excreted in the urine following oral administration (terminal half-life in mice following IV administration is 8.6 min). The drug is rapidly distributed to the heart, lung, and kidney tissue. Metabolism consists of benzylic hydroxylation followed by cytosolic oxidation to the carboxylic acid.[148]

Pulmonary Arterial Hypertension

Pulmonary arterial hypertension (PAH) is elevation of blood pressure in the pulmonary arteries due to increased vascular resistance. This results in reduced blood flow and a reduced oxygen supply. It affects 50 out of every one million Americans. Median survival time of untreated PAH patients is about 3 years, whereas treated patients survive about 9 years. The etiology of PAH is poorly understood.

Pulmonary vasodilation is mediated by cGMP and cAMP, cyclic nucleotides that are released via multiple physiological triggers, some of which are illustrated in Figure 28.47. PGI_2 (prostacyclin) is a vasoactive prostaglandin highly expressed in pulmonary vascular endothelial cells. Binding to the prostanoid IP receptor activates the adenylyl cyclase enzyme which converts AMP to cAMP. cAMP increases protein kinase activity, leading to several physiologic events including vasodilation. Reduced levels of prostacyclin synthase (and, therefore, PGI_2) are observed in PAH patients. The IP receptor offers an excellent drug target for treating PAH.

cGMP mediated vasodilation is initiated by nitric oxide (NO). PGI_2 and NO both have antiproliferative and anticoagulant properties which inhibit pulmonary vascular thickening and clot formation. Endothelin-1 (ET-1) is an endogenous vasoconstrictor produced in the pulmonary vascular smooth muscles that facilitates smooth muscle proliferation. ET-1 binds to two subtype receptors, ET_A and ET_B receptors. Binding at ET_A receptors leads to vasoconstriction and smooth muscle proliferation whereas ET_B binding leads to vasodilation via activating NO-cGMP pathway catalyzed by the guanylyl cyclase enzyme. ET_A receptors are overexpressed in vascular smooth muscles of PAH patients, and antagonists at ET_A receptors could help alleviate PAH symptoms. Direct activators of the soluble guanylyl cyclase (sGC) enzyme are also clinically available to treat PAH.

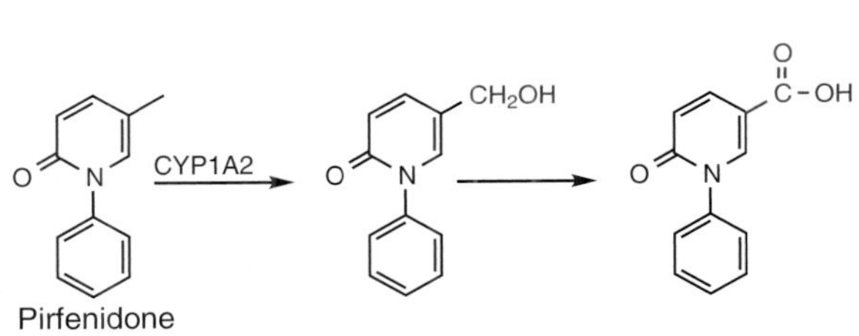

Figure 28.46 Metabolism of pirfenidone.

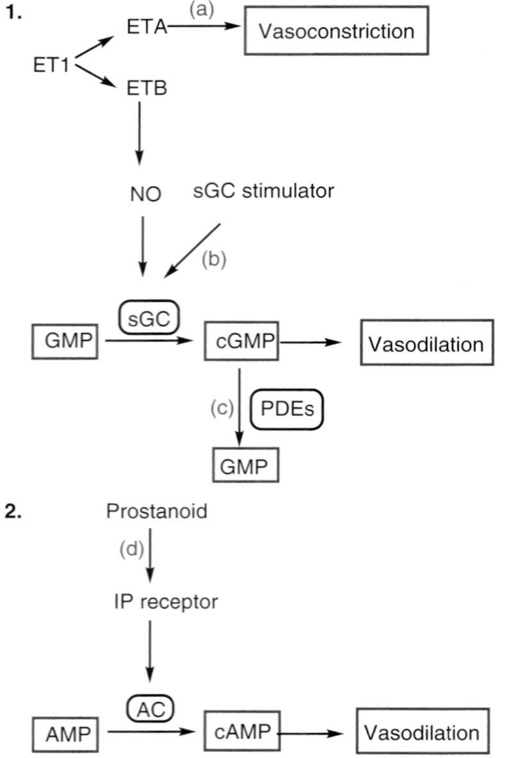

Figure 28.47 Various pathways of vasodilation in pulmonary arteries along with drug targets for the currently available drugs. (1) cGMP-mediated vasodilation pathway; (2) cAMP-mediated vasodilation pathway; (a) endothelic receptor antagonist; (b) sGC stimulator; (c) phosphodiesterase-5 inhibitors; (d) prostacyclin receptor agonists. AC, adenylyl cyclase; AMP, adenosine monophosphate; ET1, endothelin-1; ET_A, endothelin receptor A; ET_B, endothelin receptor B; GMP, guanosine monophosphate; NO, nitric oxide; sGC, soluble guanylyl cyclase; PDE, phosphodiesterase.

cGMP and cAMP are eventually metabolized by phosphodiesterase enzymes to GMP and AMP respectively. Phosphodiesterase-5 (PDE5) is highly expressed in lungs and, hence, PDE5 inhibitors provide therapeutic benefit in PAH patients.[149]

Therapeutic Classes of Drugs Used for Treating Pulmonary Arterial Hypertension

Prostacyclin Receptor Agonists

PGI_2 is an endogenous prostaglandins that activates IP receptors resulting in vasodilation along with antiproliferative and anticoagulant effects. Prostacyclin synthase is downregulated in PAH patients, leading to decreased levels of PGI_2. Hence, agonists at IP receptors help alleviate symptoms in patients by compensating for the loss of endogenous PGI_2.

PGI_2 ANALOGUES. Epoprostenol sodium, iloprost, and treprostinil are synthetic PGI_2 analogues indicated to improve exercise capacity in PAH.

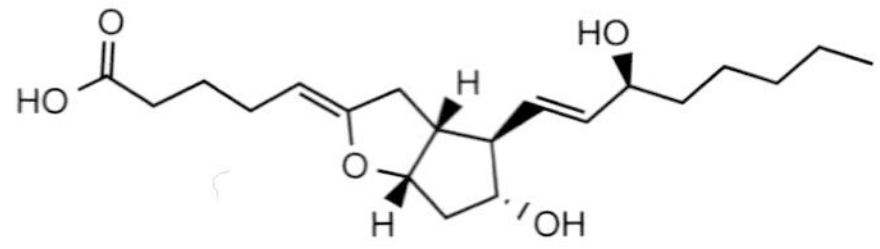

Epoprostenol

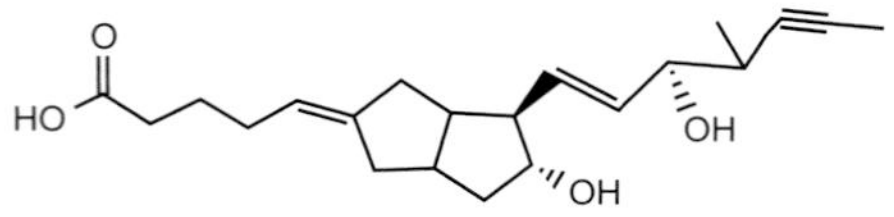

Iloprost

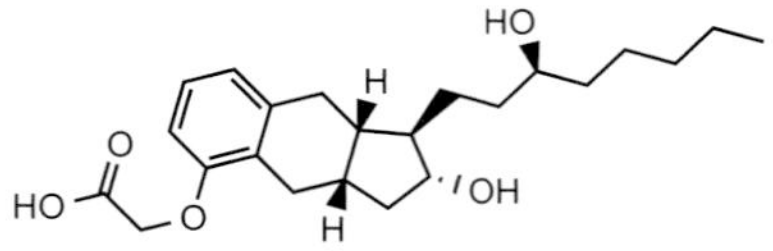

Treprostinil

Epoprostenol is highly unstable with a half-life of less than 5 minutes. Iloprost is the carbocyclic analogue of PGI_2 with a half-life of 20-30 minutes and better stability than epoprostenol. Treprostinil has an even longer half-life of 4 hours and improved stability compared to epoprostenol. Epoprostenol undergoes metabolism to inactive 6-keto-$PGF_{1\alpha}$ (nonenzymatic) and 6,15-diketo-13,14-dihydro-$PGF_{1\alpha}$ (Fig. 28.48). Treprostinil undergoes extensive first-pass metabolism by CYP2C8 and to lesser extend by 2C9 (Fig. 28.49).

PGI_2 is a powerful proaggregatory prostaglandin so, apart from vasodilation, these agonists also possess a strong anticoagulant effect. Hence, caution must be observed in patients with bleeding risk. The most common adverse reactions are dizziness, jaw pain, headache,

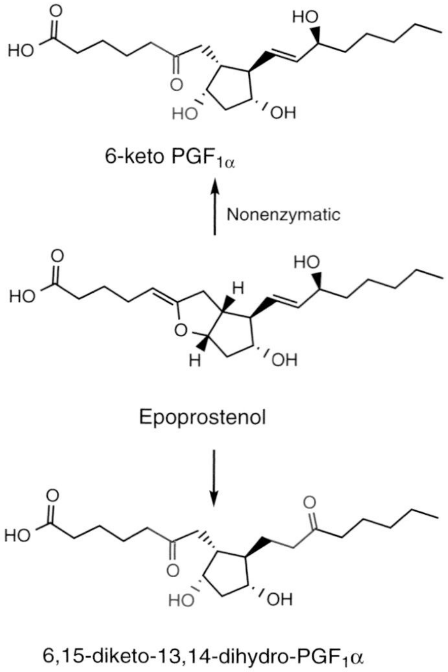

6-keto $PGF_{1\alpha}$

Nonenzymatic

Epoprostenol

6,15-diketo-13,14-dihydro-$PGF_{1\alpha}$

Figure 28.48 Metabolism of epoprostenol.

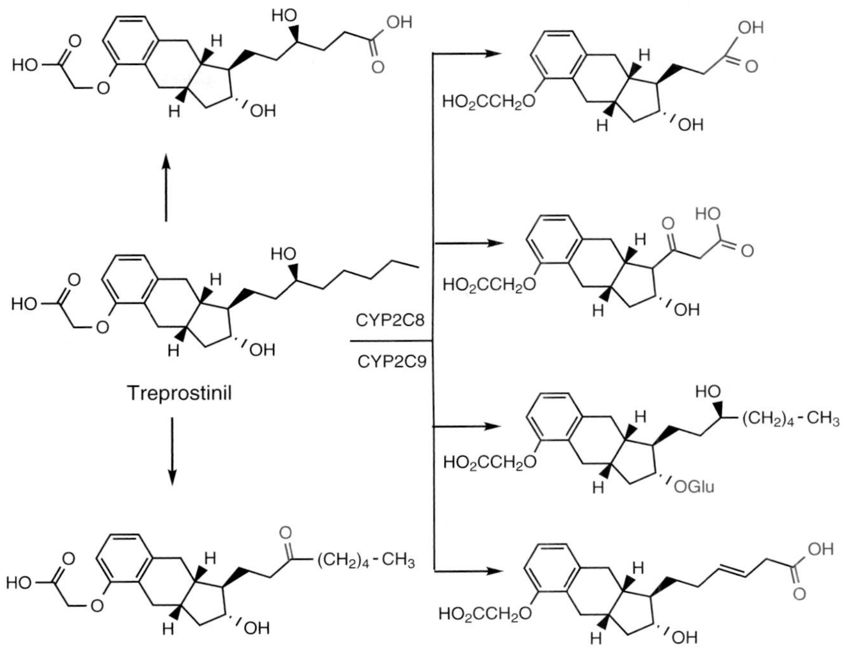

Figure 28.49 Metabolism of treprostinil.

musculoskeletal pain, and nausea/vomiting, and all are generally associated with vasodilation. Therapy should not be abruptly stopped or patients run the risk of rebound PAH.

SELEXIPAG

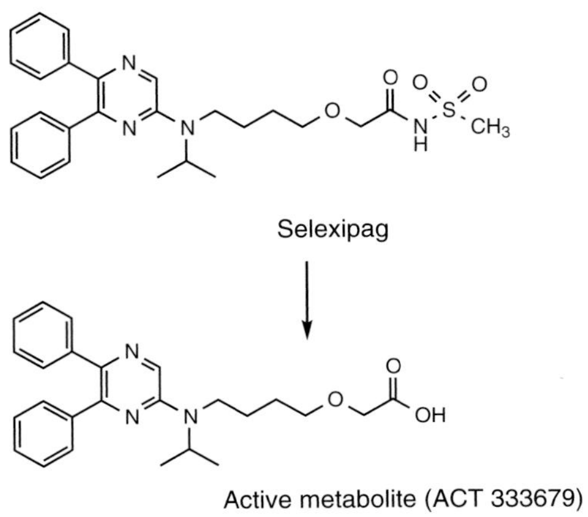

Selexipag has been approved for the treatment of PAH. It is reported that patients suffering from PAH have a deficiency of prostacyclin synthase, leading to increases in pulmonary vascular resistance and pulmonary artery pressure which, in turn, leads to right-sided heart failure. Selexipag is reported to act as an IP prostacyclin receptor agonist, resulting in the relaxation of muscles in the walls of blood vessels, vasodilation of vessels leading to the lungs, and reduction of blood pressure. The prostacyclin receptors (IP_1 and IP_2) are GPCRs, which respond to prostacyclin formed from cyclooxygenase-catalyzed oxidation of arachidonic acid. A prostacyclin agonist working via reaction with the IP receptor changes the conformation of the receptor such that protein kinase A activity is promoted, providing the therapeutic vasodilation.

Selexipag is rapidly absorbed following oral administration and rapidly hydrolyzed to the carboxylic acid, which is a major contributor to the biological activity of the drug (ratio of metabolite to selexipag reported as 4:1). Maximum plasma concentrations of selexipag and its metabolite are reached within 3 hours, and the terminal half-life for both is 9.4-12.6 hours. When administered with food, absorption is reduced, as is the blood level of the metabolite, but adverse effects are also significantly reduced. Very little selexipag or its metabolite are recovered in the urine, suggesting that the major route of elimination is hepatobiliary excretion. The common adverse effects reported for selexipag consist of dizziness and vomiting.

Endothelin Receptor Antagonists

MACITENTAN, AMBRISENTAN, AND BOSENTAN

Macitentan

Bosentan

Ambrisentan

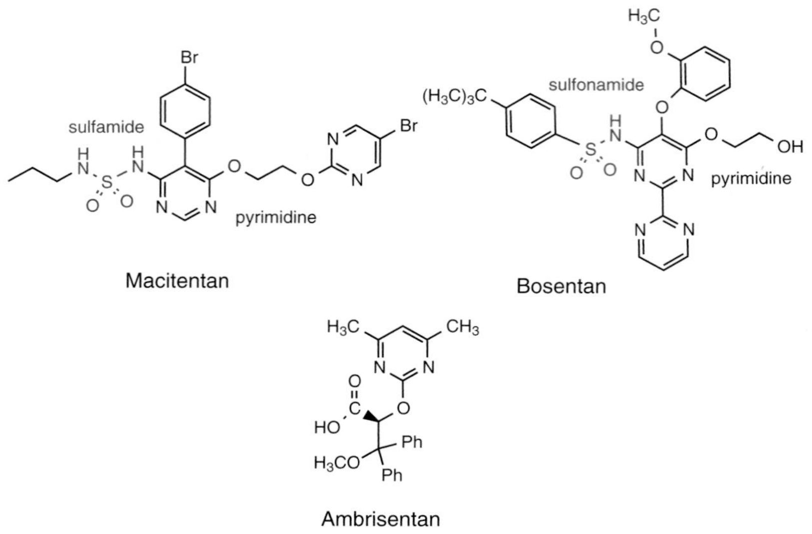

Macitentan has been approved for the treatment of PAH[150] and joins ambrisentan and bosentan which have similar mechanisms of action. They act as endothelin receptor antagonists (ERAs), blocking the action of the protein endothelin (specifically ET-1 the most common endothelin) at this GPCR. The action of macitentan and bosentan are on both the ERA subtypes ET_A and ET_B receptors,[151] but macitentan exhibits a 50-fold increased selectivity for ET_A receptors. Because macitentan has a high receptor occupancy half-life ($t_{1/2}$ 17 min) compared to bosenten ($t_{1/2}$ 70 sec) and ambrisentan ($t_{1/2}$ 40 sec), macitentan is considered a noncompetitive antagonist. Like macitentan, ambrisentan is also a selective ET_A receptor antagonist. Macitentan is a substituted pyrimidine with structural similarity to bosentan and some similarity to ambrisentan, but unlike bosentan, macitentan is a sulfamide rather than a sulfonamide (ambrisentan has no sulfur-containing functional group).

Macitentan is administered once daily in tablet form, and it has a terminal elimination $t_{1/2}$ of ~16 hours. The drug undergoes CYP3A4 metabolism to an active and several inactive metabolites (Fig. 28.50), and drug-drug interactions may be expected if coadministered with CYP CYP3A4 inhibitors or inducers.[152] For example, rifampicin (a 3A4 inducer) is reported to decrease the area under the plasma concentration curve (AUC) of macitentan by 79% while ketoconazole (a 3A4 inhibitor) may double AUC. Macitentan is primarily excreted via the urine (~50%) and to a lesser extent in feces

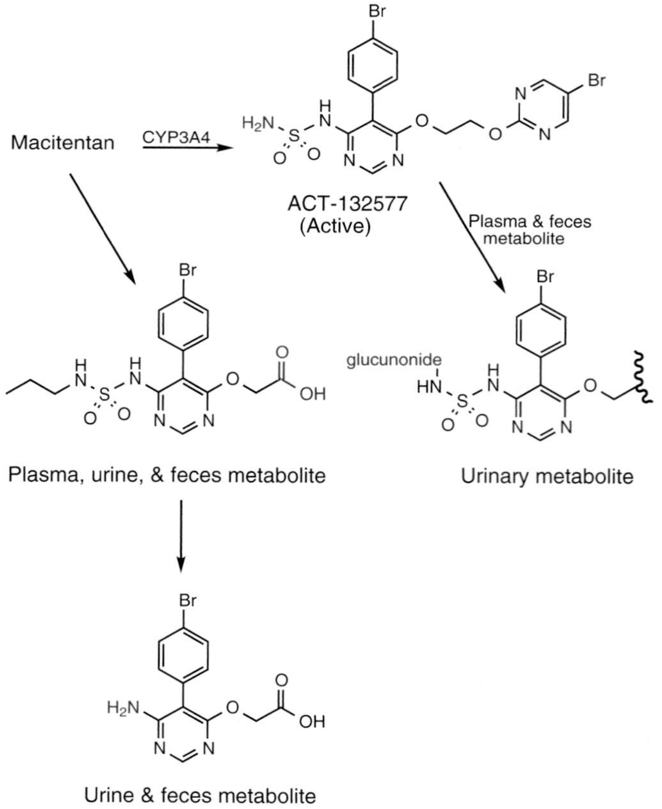

Macitentan → CYP3A4 → ACT-132577 (Active)

Plasma & feces metabolite → Urinary metabolite

Plasma, urine, & feces metabolite

Urine & feces metabolite

Figure 28.50 Metabolism of macitentan.

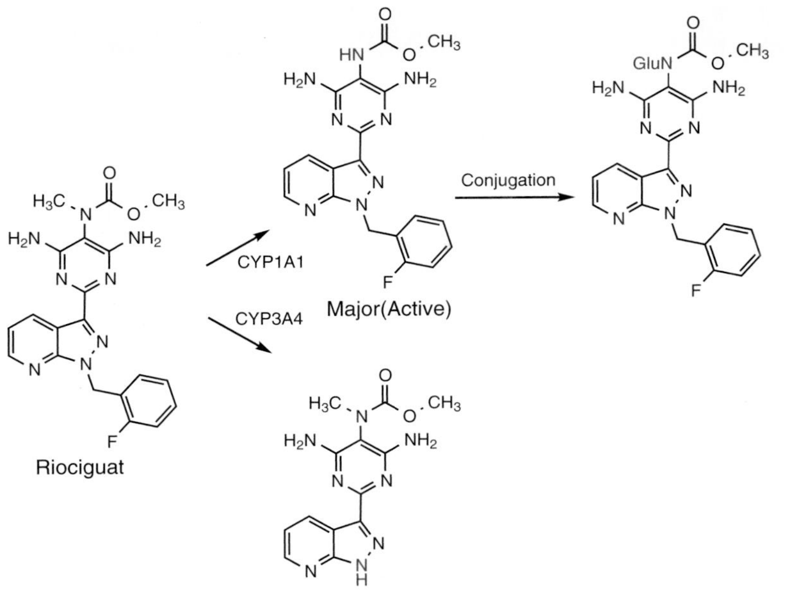

Figure 28.51 Metabolism of riociguat.

(~23%). While macitentan was identified in the plasma, the active metabolite ACT-13257 was the major plasma component. AT-13257 has a much longer half-life than macitentan.[152]

The most common adverse effects of ERAs consist of headache, nausea, and vomiting, but an important warning is associated with macitentan: the drug can cause serious birth defects, and therefore it should not be taken during pregnancy. Females are advised to have a negative pregnancy test prior to starting on macitentan. Previously approved endothelin receptor antagonists have been reported to cause hepatotoxicity as indicated by elevated liver aminotransferases. It has been suggested that this adverse effect may be associated with inhibition of the bile salt export pump (BSEP) leading to reduced secretion of the bile salts across the canalicular plasma membrane of the hepatocyte. At present, there is no evidence of this toxicity with macitentan.

Phosphodiestase-5 Inhibitors

Phosphodiesterases metabolize cGMP and cAMP, important mediators for vasodilation. PDE-5 is highly expressed in pulmonary vascular smooth muscle cells of PAH patients. Inhibiting PDE5 extends the duration of cGMP and cAMP and promotes vasodilation. Sildenafil and tadalafil are the two PDE5 inhibitors approved for treating PAH patients. It is important to note that tadalafil has a longer half-life allowing one daily dosing rather than the three times daily dosing for sildenafil. Detailed mechanism and metabolism information for this class of drugs can be found in Chapter 24.

Soluble Guanylyl Cyclase Stimulators

RIOCIGUAT

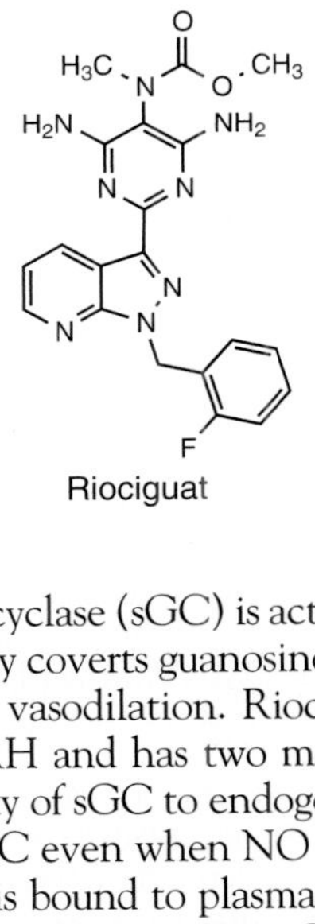

Riociguat

Soluble guanylyl cyclase (sGC) is activated by endogenous NO and subsequently coverts guanosine triphosphate (GTP) to cGMP, initiating vasodilation. Riociguat is indicated for the treatment of PAH and has two mechanisms of actions; it increases sensitivity of sGC to endogenous NO, and it also directly activates sGC even when NO is absent. Ninety-five percent of the drug is bound to plasma proteins. It is metabolized by CYP1A1 (major), CYP3A, CYP2C8, and CYP2J2 with one active metabolite (1A1), as shown in Figure 28.51. It is also a substrate of P-glycoprotein/ABCB1. CYP1A1 is induced by cigarette smoke, making riociguat subtherapeutic in chronic smokers. Its elimination half-life is about 7 hours and is excreted almost equally via feces and urine. Common side effects seen are headache, dizziness, dyspepsia, nausea, diarrhea, and anemia.

Structure Challenge

Using your knowledge of the structures of the drugs presented in this chapter, identify the compound that would be the best to use in each patient scenario described below.

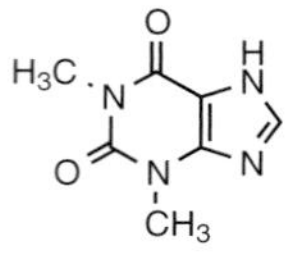

A

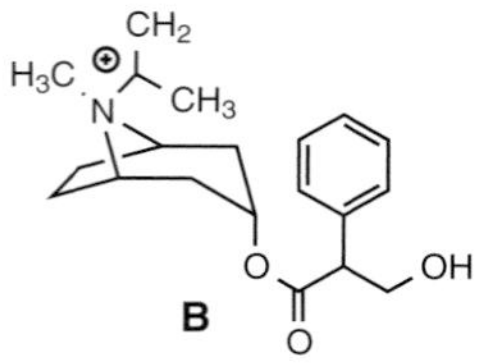

B

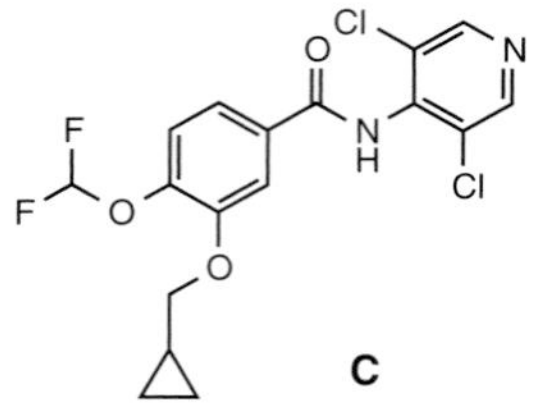

C

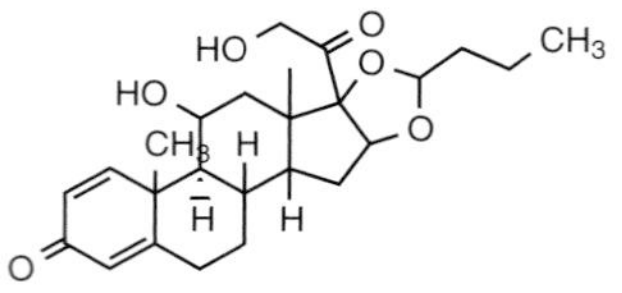

D

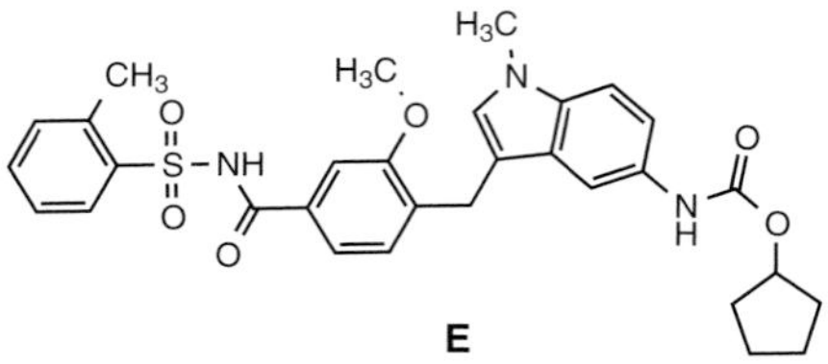

E

1. A COPD patient whose breathlessness is uncontrolled by the combination of an LABA, LAMA, or ICS.
2. An asthma patient unable to tolerate an LABA/ICS combination may be switched to which compound?
3. In addition to a rescue inhaler, which of the structures drawn is the first-line treatment for treating asthma?
4. An asthma patient who does not receive adequate relief for moderate symptoms or cannot tolerate other bronchodilator medications might be put on this compound, even though it has a narrow therapeutic window.
5. Which of the given options is primary treatment for the treatment of mild COPD?

Structure Challenge Answers found immediately after References.

REFERENCES

1. Shoopman J. Disorders of ventilation and gas exchange. In: Porch CM, Gaspard KJ, eds. *Essentials of Pathophysilogy Concepts of Altered Health States*. Lippincott Williams and Wilkins; 2014. http://pharmacy.lwwhealthlibrary.com.ccl.idm.oclc.org/content.aspx?sectionid=55478681&bookid=1008.
2. Marketos SG, Ballas CN. Bronchial asthma in the medical literature of Greek antiquity. *J Asthma Off J Assoc Care Asthma*. 1982;19:263-269.
3. Mannino DM, Homa DM, Akinbami LJ, et al. Surveillance for asthma–United States, 1980-1999. *Morb Mortal Wkly Rep Surveill Summ Wash DC 2002*. 2002;51:1-13.
4. Moorman JE, Rudd RA, Johnson CA, et al. National surveillance for asthma–United States, 1980-2004. *Morb Mortal Wkly Rep Surveill Summ Wash DC 2002*. 2007;56:1-54.
5. CDC – Asthma – Most Recent Asthma Data; 2018. https://www.cdc.gov/asthma/most_recent_data.htm. Accessed 26 June 2018.
6. Korelitz JJ, Zito JM, Gavin NI, et al. Asthma-related medication use among children in the United States. *Ann Allergy Asthma Immunol Off Publ Am Coll Allergy Asthma Immunol*. 2008;100:222-229.
7. Nurmagambetov T, Kuwahara R, Garbe P. The economic burden of asthma in the United States, 2008-2013. *Ann Am Thorac Soc*. 2018;15:348-356.
8. Busse WW. Expert panel report 3 (EPR-3): guidelines for the diagnosis and management of asthma-summary report 2007. *J Allergy Clin Immunol*. 2007;120:S94-S138.
9. Guidelines for the Diagnosis and Management of Asthma (EPR-3) | National Heart, Lung, and Blood Institute (NHLBI). https://www.nhlbi.nih.gov/health-topics/guidelines-for-diagnosis-management-of-asthma. Accessed 29 June 2018.
10. Elias JA, Lee CG, Zheng T, et al. New insights into the pathogenesis of asthma. *J Clin Invest*. 2003;111:291-297.
11. CDC - Asthma - Common Asthma Triggers; 2018. https://www.cdc.gov/asthma/triggers.html. Accessed 30 June 2018.
12. Weiss ST. Eat dirt–the hygiene hypothesis and allergic diseases. *N Engl J Med Boston*. 2002;347:930-931.
13. Bach J-F. The effect of infections on susceptibility to autoimmune and allergic diseases. *N Engl J Med Boston*. 2002;347:911-920.
14. Kuo C-H, Kuo H-F, Huang C-H, et al. Early life exposure to antibiotics and the risk of childhood allergic diseases: an update from the perspective of the hygiene hypothesis. *J Microbiol Immunol Infect*. 2013;46:320-329.
15. Vock C, Hauber H-P, Wegmann M. The other T helper cells in asthma pathogenesis. *J Allergy*. 2010;2010:519298.
16. Cookson W. The alliance of genes and environment in asthma and allergy. *Nature*. 1999;402:B5-B11.
17. Ober C. Perspectives on the past decade of asthma genetics. *J Allergy Clin Immunol*. 2005;116:274-278.
18. Sandford AJ, Paré PD. The genetics of asthma. The important questions. *Am J Respir Crit Care Med*. 2000;161:S202-S206.
19. Tattersfield AE, Knox AJ, Britton JR, et al. Asthma. *Lancet Lond Engl*. 2002;360:1313-1322.
20. Bochner BS, Busse WW. Allergy and asthma. *J Allergy Clin Immunol*. 2005;115:953-959.
21. Lilly CM. Diversity of asthma: evolving concepts of pathophysiology and lessons from genetics. *J Allergy Clin Immunol*. 2005;115:S526-S531.
22. Sorkness C, Blake K. Asthma. In: DiPiro JT, Talbert RL, Yee GC, et al, eds. *Pharmacotherapy: A Pathophysiological Approach*. New York, NY: McGraw-Hill Education; 2018. http://accesspharmacy.mhmedical.com/content.aspx?aid=1148572282.

23. Locksley RM. Asthma and allergic inflammation. *Cell.* 2010;140:777-783.
24. Kim H, Ellis AK, Fischer D, et al. Asthma biomarkers in the age of biologics. *Allergy Asthma Clin Immunol Off J Can Soc Allergy Clin Immunol.* 2017;13. doi:10.1186/s13223-017-0219-4. Epub ahead of print.
25. Carr TF, Kraft M. Management of severe asthma before referral to the severe asthma specialist. *J Allergy Clin Immunol Pract.* 2017;5:877-886.
26. Bateman ED, Hurd SS, Barnes PJ, et al. Global strategy for asthma management and prevention: GINA executive summary. *Eur Respir J.* 2008;31:143-178.
27. Kiley J, Smith R, Noel P. Asthma phenotypes. *Curr Opin Pulm Med.* 2007;13:19-23.
28. Drug Safety and Availability – FDA Drug Safety Communication: FDA review finds no significant increase in risk of serious asthma outcomes with long-acting beta agonists (LABAs) used in combination with inhaled corticosteroids (ICS). https://www.fda.gov/Drugs/DrugSafety/ucm589587.htm. Accessed 2 July 2018.
29. Ahlquist RP. A study of the adrenotropic receptors. *Am J Physiol.* 1948;153:586-600.
30. Bikker JA, Trumpp-Kallmeyer S, Humblet C. G-Protein coupled receptors: models, mutagenesis, and drug design. *J Med Chem.* 1998;41:2911-2927.
31. Furse KE, Lybrand TP. Three-dimensional models for beta-adrenergic receptor complexes with agonists and antagonists. *J Med Chem.* 2003;46:4450-4462.
32. Goodsell DS. Adrenergic receptors. *RCSB Protein Data Bank.* 2008. doi:10.2210/rcsb_pdb/mom_2008_4. Epub ahead of print.
33. Rasmussen SGF, Choi H-J, Rosenbaum DM, et al. Crystal structure of the human β2 adrenergic G-protein-coupled receptor. *Nature.* 2007;450:383-387.
34. Walker SB, Kradjan WA, Bierman CW. Bitolterol mesylate: a beta-adrenergic agent. Chemistry, pharmacokinetics, pharmacodynamics, adverse effects and clinical efficacy in asthma. *Pharmacotherapy.* 1985;5:127-137.
35. Pirbuterol – An Overview | ScienceDirect Topics, https://www.sciencedirect.com/topics/immunology-and-microbiology/pirbuterol. Accessed 17 October 2018.
36. Casarosa P, Kollak I, Kiechle T, et al. Functional and biochemical rationales for the 24-hour-long duration of action of olodaterol. *J Pharmacol Exp Ther.* 2011;337:600-609.
37. Nelson HS, Weiss ST, Bleecker ER, et al. The Salmeterol Multicenter Asthma Research Trial: a comparison of usual pharmacotherapy for asthma or usual pharmacotherapy plus salmeterol. *Chest.* 2006;129:15-26.
38. The Food & Drug Administration. Salmeterol Label; 2017. https://www.accessdata.fda.gov/drugsatfda_docs/label/2017/021077s056s057lbl.pdf. Accessed 8 July 2018.
39. Zhang M, Fawcett JP, Kennedy JM, et al. Stereoselective glucuronidation of formoterol by human liver microsomes. *Br J Clin Pharmacol.* 2000;49:152-157.
40. Rasmussen SGF, Choi H-J, Fung JJ, et al. Structure of a nanobody-stabilized active state of the β(2) adrenoceptor. *Nature.* 2011;469:175-180.
41. Ramadan WH, Kabbara WK, Abilmona RM. Olodaterol for the treatment of chronic obstructive pulmonary disease. *Am J Health-Syst Pharm AJHP Off J Am Soc Health-Syst Pharm.* 2016;73:1135-1143.
42. Deeks ED. Olodaterol: a review of its use in chronic obstructive pulmonary disease. *Drugs.* 2015;75:665-673.
43. Kagan M, Dain J, Peng L, et al. Metabolism and pharmacokinetics of indacaterol in humans. *Drug Metab Dispos Biol Fate Chem.* 2012;40:1712-1722.
44. Indacaterol.pdf. https://www.accessdata.fda.gov/drugsatfda_docs/label/2011/022383s000lbl.pdf. Accessed 6 July 2018.
45. Harrell AW, Siederer SK, Bal J, et al. Metabolism and disposition of vilanterol, a long-acting β(2)-adrenoceptor agonist for inhalation use in humans. *Drug Metab Dispos Biol Fate Chem.* 2013;41:89-100.
46. Biggadike K, Bledsoe RK, Hassell AM, et al. X-ray crystal structure of the novel enhanced-affinity glucocorticoid agonist fluticasone furoate in the glucocorticoid receptor-ligand binding domain. *J Med Chem.* 2008;51:3349-3352.
47. Kua J, Zhang Y, Eslami AC, et al. Studying the roles of W86, E202, and Y337 in binding of acetylcholine to acetylcholinesterase using a combined molecular dynamics and multiple docking approach. *Protein Sci Publ Protein Soc.* 2003;12:2675-2684.
48. Kostenis E, Zeng FY, Wess J. Structure-function analysis of muscarinic acetylcholine receptors. *J Physiol Paris.* 1998;92:265-268.
49. Katzung BG. Introduction to autonomic pharmacology. In: Katzung BG, ed. *Basic & Clinical Pharmacology.* New York, NY: McGraw-Hill Education; 2017. https://accessmedicine.mhmedical.com/content.aspx?aid=1148433176. Accessed 7 July 2018.
50. Wess J, Blin N, Mutschler E, et al. Muscarinic acetylcholine receptors: structural basis of ligand binding and G protein coupling. *Life Sci.* 1995;56:915-922.
51. Cheyne L, Irvin-Sellers MJ, White J. Tiotropium versus ipratropium bromide for chronic obstructive pulmonary disease. *Cochrane Database Syst Rev.* 2015;16:CD009552.
52. Albertí JJ, Sentellas S, Salvà M. In vitro liver metabolism of aclidinium bromide in preclinical animal species and humans: identification of the human enzymes involved in its oxidative metabolism. *Biochem Pharmacol.* 2011;81:761-776.
53. Reid DJ, Carlson AA. Clinical use of aclidinium in patients with COPD. *Int J Chron Obstruct Pulmon Dis.* 2014;9:369-379.
54. Segreti A, Calzetta L, Rogliani P, et al. Umeclidinium for the treatment of chronic obstructive pulmonary disease. *Expert Rev Respir Med.* 2014;8:665-671.
55. Spyratos D, Sichletidis L. Umeclidinium bromide/vilanterol combination in the treatment of chronic obstructive pulmonary disease: a review. *Ther Clin Risk Manag.* 2015;11:481-487.
56. Glycopyyrolate Facts & Comparisons eAnswers. https://fco-factsandcomparisons-com.jerome.stjohns.edu/lco/action/doc/retrieve/docid/fc_dfc/5940257. Accessed 11 July 2018.
57. Ashihara H, Kato M, Crozier A. Distribution, biosynthesis and catabolism of methylxanthines in plants. *Handb Exp Pharmacol.* 2011;(200):11-31.
58. Huai Q, Liu Y, Francis SH, et al. Crystal structures of phosphodiesterases 4 and 5 in complex with inhibitor 3-isobutyl-1-methylxanthine suggest a conformation determinant of inhibitor selectivity. *J Biol Chem.* 2004;279:13095-13101.
59. IUPAC-IUB Joint Commission on Biochemical Nomenclature (JCBN). The nomenclature of steroids. Recommendations 1989. *Eur J Biochem.* 1989;186:429-458.
60. Luisi BF, Xu WX, Otwinowski Z, et al. Crystallographic analysis of the interaction of the glucocorticoid receptor with DNA. *Nature.* 1991;352:497-505.
61. Bhavsar P, Ahmad T, Adcock IM. The role of histone deacetylases in asthma and allergic diseases. *J Allergy Clin Immunol.* 2008;121:580-584.
62. Bledsoe RK, Montana VG, Stanley TB, et al. Crystal structure of the glucocorticoid receptor ligand binding domain reveals a novel mode of receptor dimerization and coactivator recognition. *Cell.* 2002;110:93-105.
63. Hammer S, Spika I, Sippl W, et al. Glucocorticoid receptor interactions with glucocorticoids: evaluation by molecular modeling and functional analysis of glucocorticoid receptor mutants. *Steroids.* 2003;68:329-339.
64. Jewell C, Prusakiewicz JJ, Ackermann C, et al. The distribution of esterases in the skin of the minipig. *Toxicol Lett.* 2007;173:118-123.
65. Gupta P, Bhatia V. Corticosteroid physiology and principles of therapy. *Indian J Pediatr.* 2008;75:1039-1044.
66. Zhai Y, Zhang H, Sun T, et al. Comparative efficacies of inhaled corticosteroids and systemic corticosteroids in treatment of chronic obstructive pulmonary disease exacerbations: a systematic review and meta-analysis. *J Aerosol Med Pulm Drug Deliv.* 2017;30:289-298.
67. Methylprednisolone Facts & Comparisons eAnswers. https://fco-factsandcomparisons-com.jerome.stjohns.edu/lco/action/doc/retrieve/docid/martindale_f/1353663. Accessed 8 July 2018.

68. Rohatagi S, Barth J, Mollmann H, et al. Pharmacokinetics of methylprednisolone and prednisolone after single and multiple oral administration. *J Clin Pharmacol.* 1997;37:916-925.
69. Beclomethasone Dipropionate Facts & Comparisons eAnswers. https://fco-factsandcomparisons-com.jerome.stjohns.edu/lco/action/search?q=Beclomethasone%20Dipropionate%20Inhalation&t=name&va=Beclomethasone%20Dipropionate. Accessed 8 July 2018.
70. Jentzsch NS, Camargos P, Sarinho ESC, et al. Adherence rate to beclomethasone dipropionate and the level of asthma control. *Respir Med.* 2012;106:338-343.
71. Pelaia G, Vatrella A, Busceti MT, et al. Molecular and cellular mechanisms underlying the therapeutic effects of budesonide in asthma. *Pulm Pharmacol Ther.* 2016;40:15-21.
72. Miller-Larsson A, Jansson P, Runstrom A, et al. Prolonged airway activity and improved selectivity of budesonide possibly due to esterification. *Am J Respir Crit Care Med.* 2000;162:1455-1461.
73. Miller-Larsson A, Mattsson H, Hjertberg E, et al. Reversible fatty acid conjugation of budesonide. Novel mechanism for prolonged retention of topically applied steroid in airway tissue. *Drug Metab Dispos.* 1998;26:623-630.
74. Ciclesonide Inhalation (Drug Facts and Comparisons) Facts & Comparisons eAnswers. https://fco-factsandcomparisons-com.jerome.stjohns.edu/lco/action/doc/retrieve/docid/fc_dfc/5549025. Accessed 8 July 2018.
75. Dickens GR, Wermeling DP, Matheny CJ, et al. Pharmacokinetics of flunisolide administered via metered dose inhaler with and without a spacer device and following oral administration. *Ann Allergy Asthma Immunol.* 2000;84:528-532.
76. Corren J, Tashkin DP. Evaluation of efficacy and safety of flunisolide hydrofluoroalkane for the treatment of asthma. *Clin Ther.* 2003;25:776-798.
77. Kuo L-Y, Hung C-H, Tseng H-I, et al. Effects of budesonide and fluticasone propionate in pediatric asthma patients. *Pediatr Neonatol.* 2010;51:31-36.
78. Biggadike K. Fluticasone furoate/fluticasone propionate – different drugs with different properties: letter to the editor. *Clin Respir J.* 2011;5:183-184.
79. Crim C, Pierre LN, Daley-Yates PT. A review of the pharmacology and pharmacokinetics of inhaled fluticasone propionate and mometasone furoate. *Clin Ther.* 2001;23:1339-1354.
80. Mometasone Facts & Comparisons eAnswers. https://fco-factsandcomparisons-com.jerome.stjohns.edu/lco/action/search?q=Mometasone%20Furoate%20Oral%20Inhalation&t=name&va=mometasone. Accessed 8 July 2018.
81. Heffler E, Madeira LNG, Ferrando M, et al. Inhaled corticosteroids safety and adverse effects in patients with asthma. *J Allergy Clin Immunol Pract.* 2018;6:776-781.
82. Howell J. Roger Altounyan and the discovery of cromolyn (sodium cromoglycate). *J Allergy Clin Immunol.* 2005;115:882-885.
83. Hemmerich S, Yarden Y, Pecht I. A cromoglycate binding protein from rat mast cells of a leukemia line is a nucleoside diphosphate kinase. *Biochemistry.* 1992;31:4574-4579.
84. Oyama Y, Shishibori T, Yamashita K, et al. Two distinct anti-allergic drugs, amlexanox and cromolyn, bind to the same kinds of calcium binding proteins, except calmodulin, in bovine lung extract. *Biochem Biophys Res Commun.* 1997;240:341-347.
85. Zhang T, Finn DF, Barlow JW, et al. Mast cell stabilisers. *Eur J Pharmacol.* 2016;778:158-168.
86. Nedocromil Facts & Comparisons eAnswers. https://fco-factsandcomparisons-com.jerome.stjohns.edu/lco/action/doc/retrieve/docid/martindale_f/1352900. Accessed 8 July 2018.
87. Samuelsson B, Dahlén SE, Lindgren JA, et al. Leukotrienes and lipoxins: structures, biosynthesis, and biological effects. *Science.* 1987;237:1171-1176.
88. Capra V. Molecular and functional aspects of human cysteinyl leukotriene receptors. *Pharmacol Res.* 2004;50:1-11.
89. Kanaoka Y, Boyce JA. Cysteinyl leukotrienes and their receptors: cellular distribution and function in immune and inflammatory responses. *J Immunol Baltim Md 1950.* 2004;173:1503-1510.
90. Montuschi P, Peters-Golden ML. Leukotriene modifiers for asthma treatment. *Clin Exp Allergy.* 2010;40:1732-1741.
91. Cho KJ, Seo JM, Shin Y, et al. Blockade of airway inflammation and hyperresponsiveness by inhibition of BLT2, a low-affinity leukotriene B4 receptor. *Am J Respir Cell Mol Biol.* 2010;42:294-303.
92. Brooks CD, Summers JB. Modulators of leukotriene biosynthesis and receptor activation. *J Med Chem.* 1996;39:2629-2654.
93. Sweeny DJ, Nellans HN. Stereoselective glucuronidation of zileuton isomers by human hepatic microsomes. *Drug Metab Dispos Biol Fate Chem.* 1995;23:149-153.
94. Zileutin Facts & Comparisons eAnswers. https://fco-factsandcomparisons-com.jerome.stjohns.edu/lco/action/search?q=Zileuton%20Oral&t=name&va=zil. Accessed 9 July 2018.
95. Palomer A, Pascual J, Cabré F, et al. Derivation of pharmacophore and CoMFA models for leukotriene D(4) receptor antagonists of the quinolinyl(bridged)aryl series. *J Med Chem.* 2000;43:392-400.
96. Chiba M, Xu X, Nishime JA, et al. Hepatic microsomal metabolism of montelukast, a potent leukotriene D4 receptor antagonist, in humans. *Drug Metab Dispos Biol Fate Chem.* 1997;25:1022-1031.
97. Montelukast Facts & Comparisons eAnswers. https://fco-factsandcomparisons-com.jerome.stjohns.edu/lco/action/doc/retrieve/docid/fc_atoz2/3763754. Accessed 9 July 2018.
98. Savidge RD, Bui KH, Birmingham BK, et al. Metabolism and excretion of zafirlukast in dogs, rats, and mice. *Drug Metab Dispos Biol Fate Chem.* 1998;26:1069-1076.
99. Kassahun K, Skordos K, McIntosh I, et al. Zafirlukast metabolism by cytochrome P450 3A4 produces an electrophilic alpha,beta-unsaturated iminium species that results in the selective mechanism-based inactivation of the enzyme. *Chem Res Toxicol.* 2005;18:1427-1437.
100. Zafirlukast Facts & Comparisons eAnswers. https://fco-factsandcomparisons-com.jerome.stjohns.edu/lco/action/search?q=Zafirlukast%20Oral&t=name&va=zaf. Accessed 9 July 2018.
101. General Policies for Monoclonal Antibodies; 2009. http://www.who.int/medicines/services/inn/Generalpoliciesformonoclonalantibodies2009.pdf. Accessed 12 July 2018.
102. Buhl R. Anti-IgE antibodies for the treatment of asthma. *Curr Opin Pulm Med.* 2005;11:27-34.
103. Jensen RK, Plum M, Tjerrild L, et al. Structure of the omalizumab Fab. *Acta Crystallogr Sect F Struct Biol Commun.* 2015;71:419-426.
104. Normansell R, Walker S, Milan SJ, et al. Omalizumab for asthma in adults and children. *Cochrane Database Syst Rev.* 2014;13:CD003559.
105. Ghazi A, Trikha A, Calhoun WJ. Benralizumab – a humanized mAb to IL-5Rα with enhanced antibody-dependent cell-mediated cytotoxicity – a novel approach for the treatment of asthma. *Expert Opin Biol Ther.* 2012;12:113-118.
106. Laviolette M, Gossage DL, Gauvreau G, et al. Effects of benralizumab on airway eosinophils in asthmatic patients with sputum eosinophilia. *J Allergy Clin Immunol.* 2013;132:1086-1096, e5.
107. Bleecker ER, FitzGerald JM, Chanez P, et al. Efficacy and safety of benralizumab for patients with severe asthma uncontrolled with high-dosage inhaled corticosteroids and long-acting β2-agonists (SIROCCO): a randomised, multicentre, placebo-controlled phase 3 trial. *Lancet Lond Engl.* 2016;388:2115-2127.
108. Ortega HG, Liu MC, Pavord ID, et al. Mepolizumab treatment in patients with severe eosinophilic asthma. *N Engl J Med.* 2014;371:1198-1207.
109. Maselli DJ, Velez MI, Rogers L. Reslizumab in the management of poorly controlled asthma: the data so far. *J Asthma Allergy.* 2016;9:155-162.
110. Lim HF, Nair P. Efficacy and safety of reslizumab in patients with moderate to severe eosinophilic asthma. *Expert Rev Respir Med.* 2015;9:135-142.
111. Ferguson GT, Cherniack RM. Management of chronic obstructive pulmonary disease. *N Engl J Med.* 1993;328:1017-1022.
112. CDC – Data and Statistics – Chronic Obstructive Pulmonary Disease (COPD); 2017. https://www.cdc.gov/copd/data.html. Accessed 26 June 2018.

113. GOLD 2017 Global Strategy for the Diagnosis, Management and Prevention of COPD. Global Initiative for Chronic Obstructive Lung Disease – GOLD. https://goldcopd.org/gold-2017-global-strategy-diagnosis-management-prevention-copd/. Accessed 12 July 2018.
114. GOLD-2017-Pocket-Guide.pdf. https://goldcopd.org/wp-content/uploads/2016/12/wms-GOLD-2017-Pocket-Guide.pdf. Accessed 12 July 2018.
115. Raherison C, Girodet P-O. Epidemiology of COPD. *Eur Respir Rev*. 2009;18:213-221.
116. Chapter 16. Chronic Obstructive Pulmonary Disease | Pharmacotherapy: A Pathophysiologic Approach, 9e | AccessPharmacy | McGraw-Hill Medical. https://accesspharmacy.mhmedical.com/content.aspx?bookid=689&Sectionid=48811464.
117. GOLD-2018-v6.0-FINAL-revised-20-Nov_WMS.pdf. https://goldcopd.org/wp-content/uploads/2017/11/GOLD-2018-v6.0-FINAL-revised-20-Nov_WMS.pdf. Accessed 15 July 2018.
118. Lipworth BJ. Phosphodiesterase-4 inhibitors for asthma and chronic obstructive pulmonary disease. *Lancet Lond Engl*. 2005;365:167-175.
119. Spina D. PDE4 inhibitors: current status. *Br J Pharmacol*. 2008;155:308-315.
120. Giembycz MA. Can the anti-inflammatory potential of PDE4 inhibitors be realized: guarded optimism or wishful thinking? *Br J Pharmacol*. 2008;155:288-290.
121. Moussa BA, El-Zaher AA, El-Ashrey MK, et al. Synthesis and molecular docking of new roflumilast analogues as preferential-selective potent PDE-4B inhibitors with improved pharmacokinetic profile. *Eur J Med Chem*. 2018;148:477-486.
122. Card GL, England BP, Suzuki Y, et al. Structural basis for the activity of drugs that inhibit phosphodiesterases. *Struct Lond Engl 1993*. 2004;12:2233-2247.
123. Hatzelmann A, Morcillo EJ, Lungarella G, et al. The preclinical pharmacology of roflumilast–a selective, oral phosphodiesterase 4 inhibitor in development for chronic obstructive pulmonary disease. *Pulm Pharmacol Ther*. 2010;23:235-256.
124. Liu Y, Pleasants RA, Croft JB, et al. Smoking duration, respiratory symptoms, and COPD in adults aged ≥45 years with a smoking history. *Int J Chron Obstruct Pulmon Dis*. 2015;10:1409-1416.
125. Is nicotine addictive?. https://www.drugabuse.gov/publications/research-reports/tobacco-nicotine-e-cigarettes/nicotine-addictive. Accessed 7 August 2018.
126. Leonard S, Bertrand D. Neuronal nicotinic receptors: from structure to function. *Nicotine Tob Res Off J Soc Res Nicotine Tob*. 2001;3:203-223.
127. Benowitz NL. Nicotine addiction. *N Engl J Med*. 2010;362:2295-2303.
128. Tønnesen P. Smoking cessation and COPD. *Eur Respir Rev Off J Eur Respir Soc*. 2013;22:37-43.
129. Stead LF, Perera R, Bullen C, et al. Nicotine replacement therapy for smoking cessation. *Cochrane Database Syst Rev*. 2012;11:CD000146.
130. Nicotine Replacement Therapy for Quitting Tobacco. https://www.cancer.org/healthy/stay-away-from-tobacco/guide-quitting-smoking/nicotine-replacement-therapy.html. Accessed 8 August 2018).
131. Sobkowiak R, Lesicki A. Absorption, metabolism and excretion of nicotine in humans. *Postepy Biochem*. 2013;59:33-44.
132. Jefferson JW, Pradko JF, Muir KT. Bupropion for major depressive disorder: pharmacokinetic and formulation considerations. *Clin Ther*. 2005;27:1685-1695.
133. Rollema H, Coe JW, Chambers LK, et al. Rationale, pharmacology and clinical efficacy of partial agonists of alpha4beta2 nACh receptors for smoking cessation. *Trends Pharmacol Sci*. 2007;28:316-325.
134. Research C for DE and. Drug Safety and Availability - FDA Drug Safety Communication: FDA revises description of mental health side effects of the stop-smoking medicines Chantix (varenicline) and Zyban (bupropion) to reflect clinical trial findings. https://www.fda.gov/Drugs/DrugSafety/ucm532221.htm. Accessed 13 August 2018.
135. Faessel HM, Obach RS, Rollema H, et al. A review of the clinical pharmacokinetics and pharmacodynamics of varenicline for smoking cessation. *Clin Pharmacokinet*. 2010;49:799-816.
136. Chang P-H, Chiang C-H, Ho W-C, et al. Combination therapy of varenicline with nicotine replacement therapy is better than varenicline alone: a systematic review and meta-analysis of randomized controlled trials. *BMC Public Health*. 2015;15:689.
137. Prickett M, Jain M. Gene therapy in cystic fibrosis. *Transl Res J Lab Clin Med*. 2013;161:255-264.
138. Bethesda CFF 4550 MAS 1100 N, Md 20814301-951-4422 800-344-4823. CFTR Modulator Therapies. http://www.cff.org/Life-With-CF/Treatments-And-Therapies/Medications/CFTR-Modulator-Therapies/. Accessed 14 September 2018.
139. Van Goor F, Hadida S, Grootenhuis PD, et al. Rescue of CF airway epithelial cell function in vitro by a CFTR potentiator, VX-770. *Proc Natl Acad Sci USA*. 2009;106:18825-18830.
140. Ren HY, Grove DE, De La Rosa O, et al. VX-809 corrects folding defects in cystic fibrosis transmembrane conductance regulator protein through action on membrane-spanning domain 1. *Mol Biol Cell*. 2013;24:3016-3024.
141. Eckford PD, Li C, Ramjeesingh M, et al. Cystic fibrosis transmembrane conductance regulator (CFTR) potentiator VX-770 (ivacaftor) opens the defective channel gate of mutant CFTR in a phosphorylation-dependent but ATP-independent manner. *J Biol Chem*. 2012;287:36639-36649.
142. Kirby T. Tezacaftor-ivacaftor is safe and efficacious in patients with cystic fibrosis with Phe508del mutations. *Lancet Respir Med*. 2018;6:13-14.
143. Garcia-Sancho C, Buendia-Roldan I, Fernandez-Plata MR, et al. Familial pulmonary fibrosis is the strongest risk factor for idiopathic pulmonary fibrosis. *Respir Med*. 2011;105:1902-1907.
144. Loomis-King H, Flaherty KR, Moore BB. Pathogenesis, current treatments and future directions for idiopathic pulmonary fibrosis. *Curr Opin Pharmacol*. 2013;13:377-385.
145. Roth GJ, Binder R, Colbatzky F, et al. Nintedanib: from discovery to the clinic. *J Med Chem*. 2015;58:1053-1063.
146. Wollin L, Wex E, Pautsch A, et al. Mode of action of nintedanib in the treatment of idiopathic pulmonary fibrosis. *Eur Respir J*. 2015;45:1434-1445.
147. Nakayama S, Mukae H, Sakamoto N, et al. Pirfenidone inhibits the expression of HSP47 in TGF-beta1-stimulated human lung fibroblasts. *Life Sci*. 2008;82:210-217.
148. Giri SN, Wang Q, Xie Y, et al. Pharmacokinetics and metabolism of a novel antifibrotic drug pirfenidone, in mice following intravenous administration. *Biopharm Drug Dispos*. 2002;23:203-211.
149. Humbert M, Ghofrani HA. The molecular targets of approved treatments for pulmonary arterial hypertension. *Thorax*. 2016;71:73-83.
150. Sidharta PN, van Giersbergen PL, Halabi A, et al. Macitentan: entry-into-humans study with a new endothelin receptor antagonist. *Eur J Clin Pharmacol*. 2011;67:977-984.
151. Bolli MH, Boss C, Binkert C, et al. The discovery of N-[5-(4-bromophenyl)-6-[2-[(5-bromo-2-pyrimidinyl)oxy]ethoxy]-4-pyrimidinyl]-N'-p ropylsulfamide (Macitentan), an orally active, potent dual endothelin receptor antagonist. *J Med Chem*. 2012;55:7849-7861.
152. Bruderer S, Hopfgartner G, Seiberling M, et al. Absorption, distribution, metabolism, and excretion of macitentan, a dual endothelin receptor antagonist, in humans. *Xenobiotica*. 2012;42:901-910.

Structure Challenge Answers

1-C, 2-E, 3-D, 4-A, 5-B.

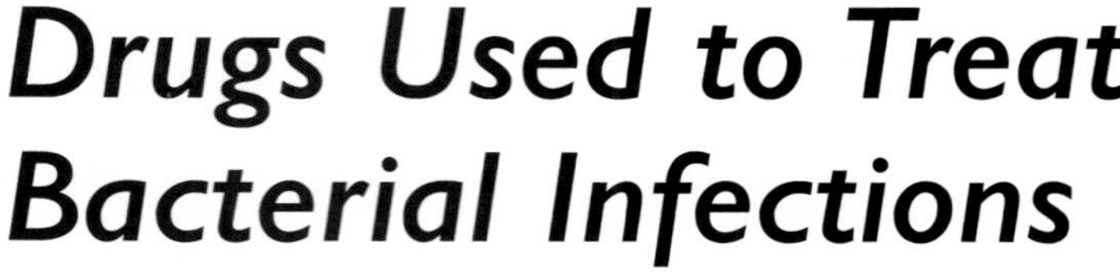

CHAPTER 29

Drugs Used to Treat Bacterial Infections

Elmer J. Gentry, E. Jeffrey North, and Robin M. Zavod

Drugs covered in this chapter[a]:

ANTIBACTERIALS

Sulfonamide class
- Silver sulfadiazine
- Sulfacetamide
- Sulfamethoxazole
- Sulfisoxazole
- Trimethoprim

Nitroheteroaromatic compounds
- Nitrofurantoin
- Metronidazole
- Tinidazole
- Secnidazole
- Fosfomycin

Quinolone class
- Besifloxacin
- Ciprofloxacin
- Delafloxacin
- Finafloxacin
- Gatifloxacin
- Gemifloxacin
- Levofloxacin, ofloxacin
- Moxifloxacin
- *Norfloxacin*

ANTIBIOTICS

Penicillin class
- Amoxicillin
- Ampicillin
- Benzylpenicillin
- Dicloxacillin
- Nafcillin
- Oxacillin
- Phenoxymethylpenicillin
- Piperacillin
- Ticarcillin

β-lactamase inhibitors
- Clavulanic acid
- Sulbactam
- Tazobactam
- Avibactam
- Vaborbactam

Cephalosporin class
- Cefaclor
- Cefadroxil
- Cefazolin
- Cefdinir
- Cefditoren pivoxil
- Cefepime
- Cefixime
- Cefotaxime
- Cefotetan
- Cefoxitin
- Cefpodoxime proxetil
- Cefprozil
- Ceftaroline fosamil
- Ceftazidime
- Ceftibuten
- Ceftizoxime
- Ceftolozane
- Ceftriaxone
- Cefuroxime
- Cephalexin

Carbapenems
- Doripenem
- Ertapenem
- Imipenem/cilastatin
- Meropenem

Monobactams
- Aztreonam

Aminoglycosides
- Amikacin
- Gentamicin
- Neomycin
- Plazomicin
- Streptomycin
- Tobramycin

Macrolides and ketolides
- Azithromycin
- Clarithromycin
- Erythromycin ethylsuccinate
- Erythromycin stearate
- Fidaxomicin
- Telithromycin

Lincosamides
- Clindamycin
- Lincomycin

Tetracyclines and glycylcyclines
- Demeclocycline
- Doxycycline
- Minocycline
- Tetracycline
- Tigecycline

Drugs covered in this chapter—Continued

Special purpose antibiotics
- Bacitracin
- Chloramphenicol
- Dalbavancin
- Daptomycin
- Linezolid
- Mupirocin
- Oritavancin
- Polymyxin B
- Quinupristin/dalfopristin
- Retapamulin
- Tedizolid phosphate
- Telavancin
- Vancomycin

Antitubercular drugs
- Capreomycin
- Cycloserine
- Ethambutol
- Ethionamide
- Isoniazid
- Kanamycin
- *Para*-aminobenzoic acid
- Pyrazinamide
- Rifabutin
- Rifampin
- Rifapentine
- Streptomycin

Nontuberculous mycobacteria therapeutics
- Clofazimine
- Dapsone
- Thalidomide

[a]Drugs listed include those available inside and outside of the United States; drugs available outside of the United States are shown in italics.

Abbreviations

AAC aminoglycoside acetylase
AG arabinogalactan
ANT aminoglycoside nucleotide transferase
6-APA 6-aminopenicillanic acid
APH aminoglycoside phosphorylase
ATP adenosine triphosphate
CDC Centers for Disease Control and Prevention
CNS central nervous system
DDRP DNA-dependent RNA polymerase
DOTS direct observed treatment, short-course
EMB ethambutol
ENL erythema nodosum leprosum
FDA U.S. Food and Drug Administration
G6PD glucose-6-phosphate dehydrogenase
GABA γ-aminobutyric acid
GI gastrointestinal
HABA L-hydroxyaminobutyryl amide
INH isoniazid
LAM lipoarabinomannan
MAC *Mycobacterium avium–intracellulare* complex
MBC minimum bacteriocidal concentration
MDR-TB multidrug-resistant tuberculosis
MIC minimum inhibitory concentration
MRSA methicillin-resistant *Staphylococcus aureus*
MTT methylthiotetrazole
PABA *p*-aminobenzoic acid
PAS *p*-aminosalicylic acid
PBP penicillin-binding protein
RIF rifampin
SAR structure-activity relationship
STM streptomycin
TB tuberculosis
XTR-TB extensively drug-resistant tuberculosis

INTRODUCTION

Antibiotics are microbial metabolites or synthetic analogues that, in small doses, inhibit the growth and survival of microorganisms without serious toxicity to the host. Selective toxicity is the key concept. Antibiotics are among the most frequently prescribed medications today, although microbial resistance due to evolutionary pressures and misuse threatens their continued efficacy. In many cases, the utility of natural antibiotics has been improved through medicinal chemical manipulation of the original structure, leading to broader antimicrobial spectrum, greater potency, lesser toxicity, more convenient administration, and additional pharmacokinetic advantages. Synthetic substances that are unrelated to natural products but still inhibit or kill microorganisms are referred to as antimicrobial agents.

All of the parts of our bodies that are in contact with the environment support microbial life. It is estimated that our body contains approximately 10 times more bacterial cells than human cells. These organisms are generally harmless to the host and actually provide a number of benefits.

However, all of our internal fluids, organs, and body structures are sterile under normal circumstances, and the presence of bacteria, fungi, viruses, or other organisms in these places is diagnostic evidence of infection. When mild microbial disease occurs, an otherwise healthy patient will often recover without requiring treatment because their immune system is called upon to kill invasive microorganisms. When this is insufficient to protect us, appropriate therapeutic intervention is indicated.

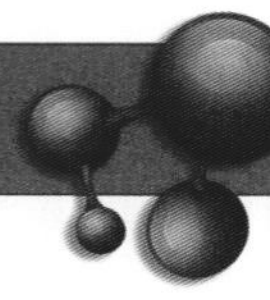

CLINICAL SIGNIFICANCE

Sean Avedissian, PharmD

Sheila Wang, PharmD BCPS-AQID

Clinicians are responsible for the selection of appropriate antimicrobials that are both safe and effective. This process of selection has become complicated by antimicrobial resistance often leaving very few susceptible treatment options to choose from. The rise and significance of antimicrobial resistance has led to global action plans to not only encourage appropriate use of antimicrobials but to advance research in developing new agents to effectively combat multidrug-resistant (MDR) pathogens. However, we have entered a dormant phase of novel antimicrobial development. The capacity for new drug discovery targeted toward specific bacteria and their resistant mechanisms continues to lag the rate of emerging bacterial resistance. Analogues of existing antibiotics and newer generation β-lactam and β-lactamase inhibitor combinations have been recently marketed with activity against MDR pathogens but with wavering clinical outcomes. As a result, clinicians have availed old-generation antibiotics and considered unique combinations of existing agents to improve therapeutic efficacy. With these alternative approaches, it is imperative that clinicians understand the properties of existing antimicrobials, such as mechanism of action and resistance, spectrum of activity, dose effects, pharmacokinetic and pharmacodynamics influences, and adverse drug outcomes. Knowledge of the drug effects and limitations assists the clinician in choosing antimicrobials that are not only optimal for MDR pathogens but also patient specific to minimize untoward adverse effects. With the few antimicrobial options available today for MDR pathogens, understanding the basic principles of medicinal chemistry will be key in assessing and selecting the most appropriate treatment options.

HISTORY

Humankind has been subject to infection by microorganisms since before recorded history. One presumes that mankind has been searching for suitable therapy for nearly as long. This was a desperately difficult enterprise given the acute nature of most infections and the nearly total lack of understanding of their origins until the 19th century. Although one can find indications in ancient medical writings of folkloric use of plant and animal preparations, these factors were inefficiently applied, and they often failed. Until the discovery of bacteria by van Leeuwenhoek in 1676 and subsequent understanding of their role in infection about 150 years later, there was no hope for rational therapy.

In the 19th century, Robert Koch showed that specific microorganisms could always be isolated from the excreta and tissues of people with particular infectious diseases and that these same microorganisms were usually absent in healthy individuals. They could then be grown on culture media and be administered to healthy individuals so as to reproduce in healthy individuals all of the classic symptoms of the same disease. Finally, the identical microorganism could then be isolated from this deliberately infected person. Following these rules, at long last, a chain of evidence connecting cause and effect was forged between certain microorganisms and specific infectious diseases. This work laid the foundation for rational prevention and therapy of infectious diseases.

Louis Pasteur reported in 1877 that when what he termed "common bacteria" were introduced into a pure culture of anthrax bacilli, the bacilli died, and that an injection of deadly anthrax bacillus into a laboratory animal was harmless if "common bacteria" were injected along with it. This did not always work but led to the appreciation of antibiosis, wherein two or more microorganisms competed with one another for survival.[1] However, it was more than a half century later that the underlying mechanisms began to be appreciated and applied to achieve successful therapy.

The modern anti-infective era opened with the discovery of the sulfonamides in France and Germany in 1936 as an offshoot of Paul Ehrlich's earlier achievements in treating infections with organometallics and his theories of vital staining.[2] The well-known observation of a clear zone of inhibition (lysis) in a bacterial colony surrounding a colony of contaminating airborne *Penicillium* mold by Alexander Fleming in England in 1929 and the subsequent purification of penicillin from it in the late 1930s and early 1940s by Florey, Chain, Abraham, and Heatley provided important additional impetus.[3,4] With the first successful clinical trial of crude penicillin in 1941 and the requirements of war times, an explosion of successful activity ensued that continues into the 21st century. In rapid succession, deliberate searches of the metabolic products of a wide variety of soil microbes led to discovery of tyrothricin (1939), streptomycin (1943), chloramphenicol (1947), chlortetracycline (1948), neomycin (1949), and erythromycin (1952). These discoveries ushered in the age of the so-called miracle drugs. The discovery of antibiotics is widely considered to be one of the top five discoveries/inventions of the 20th century.

Microbes of soil origin remain to this day one of the more fruitful sources of antibiotics, although the specific means employed for their discovery are more sophisticated today than those employed 70 years ago. Initially, extracts of fermentations were screened simply for their ability to kill pathogenic microorganisms in vitro. Those that did were pushed along through ever more complex pharmacologic and toxicologic tests in attempts to discover clinically useful agents. Today, many thousands of such extracts of increasingly unusual microbes are tested each year, and the tests now include sophisticated assays for agents operating through particular biochemical mechanisms or possessing particular properties.

Combinatorial chemical synthesis coupled with high-throughput screening today make it possible to screen hundreds of thousands of compounds in a short time for antimicrobial activity. This is coupled with dramatic advances in all of the relevant sciences. One would logically suppose that this would lead to the emergence of a large number of new antimicrobial agents.

That this is yet to happen is a measure of the complexity of the task. The impact of genomics and proteomics is predicted to have a larger effect on this effort. The genome of *Haemophilus influenzae* was determined in 1995, and currently more than 1,000 microbial genomes have been deciphered and are publicly available.[5,6] Of the more than 1,700 genes of *H. influenzae*, it is thought that 642 are essential and thus are potential targets for antimicrobial drug development.[7]

These exciting new possibilities have yet to yield many practical results due to the inherent complexity of the task.

This picture has an increasingly dark side, however, because of the increasing impact of bacterial resistance. Intrinsic resistance to antimicrobial agents (resistance present before exposure to antibiotics) was recognized from the beginning. Some bacteria are immune to treatment from the outset because they do not take up the antibiotic or lack a susceptible target. Starting in the 1940s, however, and encountered with increasing frequency to this day, bacteria that were previously expected to respond were found to be resistant, many bacteria became resistant during the course of chemotherapy, and others were simultaneously resistant to several different antibiotics. The organisms were found to be capable of passing this trait on to other bacteria, even to those belonging to different genera. The spread of this phenomenon is aided by microorganisms' short generation time (sometimes measured in fractions of an hour) and genetic versatility, as well as by poor antibiotic prescribing and utilization practices. Some authorities predict an impending return to the defenseless days of the preantibiotic era. An understanding of these phenomena and the devising of appropriate practical response measures are important contemporary priorities.

GENERAL THERAPEUTIC APPROACH

Drug Nomenclature

The names given to antimicrobials and antibiotics are highly varied yet some helpful unifying conventions are followed. For example, the penicillins are derived from fungi and have names ending in the suffix -cillin, as in the term ampicillin. The cephalosporins are likewise fungal products, although their names mostly begin with the prefix cef- (or sometimes, following the English practice, spelled ceph-). The synthetic fluoroquinolones mostly end in the suffix -floxacin. Although helpful in many respects, this nomenclature does result in many related substances possessing quite similar names. This can make remembering them difficult. Most of the remaining antibiotics are produced by fermentation of soil microorganisms belonging to various *Streptomyces* species. By convention, these have names ending in the suffix -mycin, as in streptomycin. Some prominent antibiotics are produced by fermentation of various soil microbes known as *Micromonospora* sp. These antibiotics have names ending in -micin (e.g., gentamicin).

In earlier times, the terms "broad spectrum" and "narrow spectrum" had specific clinical meaning. The widespread emergence of microbes resistant to single agents and multiple agents has made these terms less meaningful. It is, nonetheless, still valuable to remember that some antimicrobial families have the potential of inhibiting a wide range of bacterial genera belonging to both gram-positive and gram-negative cultures and so are called broad spectrum (such as the tetracyclines). Others inhibit only a few bacterial genera and are termed narrow spectrum (such as the glycopeptides, typified by vancomycin, which are used almost exclusively for a few gram-positive and anaerobic microorganisms).

The Importance of Identification of the Pathogen

Empiric-Based Therapy

Fundamental to appropriate antimicrobial therapy is an appreciation that individual species of bacteria are associated with particular infective diseases and that specific antibiotics are more likely to be useful than others for killing them. Sometimes this can be used as the basis for successful empiric therapy. For example, first-course community-acquired urinary tract infections in otherwise healthy individuals are commonly caused by gram-negative *Escherichia coli*. Even just knowing this much can give the physician several convenient choices for useful therapy. Likewise, skin infections, such as boils, are commonly the result of hair-follicle infection with gram-positive *Staphylococcus aureus*. In most other cases, the cause of the disease is less obvious and so likewise is the agent that might be useful against it. It is important to determine the specific disease one is dealing with in these cases and what susceptibility patterns are exhibited by the causative microorganism. Knowing these factors enables the clinician to narrow the range of therapeutic choices. The only certainty, however, is that inability of a given antibiotic to kill or inhibit a given pathogen in vitro is a virtual guarantee that the drug will fail in vivo.

Unfortunately, activity in vitro often also results in failure to cure in vivo, but in these cases, at least, there is a significant possibility of success. Before the emergence of widespread bacterial resistance, identification of the causative microorganism often was sufficient for selecting a useful antibiotic. Now this is only a useful first step, and much more detailed laboratory studies are needed in order to make a successful choice.

GRAM STAIN

Hans C.J. Gram, a Danish microbiologist, developed the Gram staining method for staining bacteria so that they were more readily visible under the microscope. The term has proven to be particularly useful in describing antibiotics as well because antibiotics are conveniently classified by their activity against microorganisms depending on their reaction to this method. Gram-positive microorganisms are stained purple by contact with a methyl violet-iodine process. This is largely a consequence of their lack of an outer membrane and the nature of the thick cell wall surrounding them. Gram-negative microorganisms do not retain the methyl violet-iodine stain when washed with alcohol but rather are colored pink when subsequently treated with the red dye safranin. The lipopolysaccharides on their outer membrane apparently are responsible for the staining behavior of gram-negative cells.

Since Gram stain is dependent on the outer layers of bacterial cells and this also strongly influences the ability of antimicrobial agents to reach their cellular targets, knowing the Gram staining behavior of infectious bacteria helps one decide which antimicrobial might be effective in therapy.

Not all bacteria can be stained by the Gram procedure. These often require special staining processes for visualization. Among the more prominent of these for our purposes are the mycobacteria (the causative agents of tuberculosis, for example). These very waxy cells are called acid-fast and are stained by a carbol fuchsin mixture.

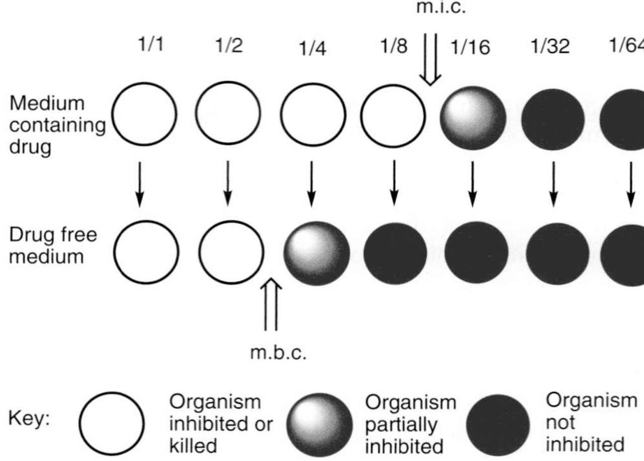

Figure 29.1 In the top tubes (viewed from the top), a serially decreasing amount of antimicrobial agent is added to a suitable growth medium innoculated with a microorganism. Following incubation, microbial growth is detected by turbidity. The last concentration that produces no visible growth is scored as the minimum inhibitory concentration (m.i.c.) (1/8). Next a loopful is taken from each tube and placed in fresh medium (bottom row). In tubes where the organisms were killed by the drug there is no resumption of growth. Where the organisms were inhibited but not killed, removal of drug allows for resumption of growth. The last concentration that produces no visible growth under these conditions is scored as the minimum bactericidal concentration (m.b.c.) (1/2).

Experimentally Based Therapy

The modern clinical application of Koch's discoveries to the selection of an appropriate antibiotic involves sampling infectious material from a patient before instituting anti-infective chemotherapy, culturing the microorganism on suitable growth media, and identifying its genus and species. The bacterium in question is then grown in the presence of a variety of antibiotics to see which of them will inhibit its growth or survival and what concentrations will be needed to achieve this result. This is expressed in minimum inhibitory concentration (MIC) units. The term MIC refers to the concentration that will inhibit 99% or more of the microbe in question and represents the minimum quantity that must reach the site of the infection in order to be useful.

These concepts are illustrated in Figure 29.1. To "cure" the infection, it is usually desirable to have several multiples of the MIC at the site of infection. This requires not only an understanding of the MIC, but also an understanding of pharmacokinetic and pharmacodynamic considerations as well as the results of accumulated clinical experience. The choice of anti-infective agent is made from among those that are active. One of the most convenient experimental procedures is that of Kirby and Bauer. With this technique, sterile filter paper disks impregnated with fixed doses of commercially available antibiotics are placed on the seeded Petri dish. The dish is then incubated for a period of time. If the antibiotic is active against the particular strain of bacterium isolated from the patient, a clear zone of inhibition will be seen around the disk. If a given antimicrobial agent is ineffective, the bacterium may even grow right up to the edge of the disk. The diameter of the inhibition zone is directly proportional to the degree of sensitivity of the bacterial strain and the concentration of the antibiotic in question.

Currently, a given zone size in millimeters is dictated above which the bacterium is sensitive and below which it is resistant. When the zone size obtained is near this break point (the break point represents the maximum clinically achievable concentration of an anti-infective agent), the drug is regarded as intermediate in sensitivity, and clinical failure can occur. This powerful methodology gives the clinician a choice of possible antibiotics to use. This method is illustrated in Figure 29.2. The widespread occurrence of resistance of certain strains of bacteria to given antibiotics reinforces the need to perform susceptibility testing. Other laboratory methods can be employed for similar purposes. Of particular note is the Epsilometer test (E-test), which uses the same idea but employs a gradient of drug concentrations on a filter paper strip. This high level of scientific medicine requires significant expertise and equipment and thus is practiced mainly in medical centers. In outpatient practice, the choice of antimicrobial agents is more commonly made empirically.

Bactericidal Versus Bacteriostatic

Almost all antibiotics have the capacity to be bactericidal in vitro; that is, they will kill bacteria if the concentration

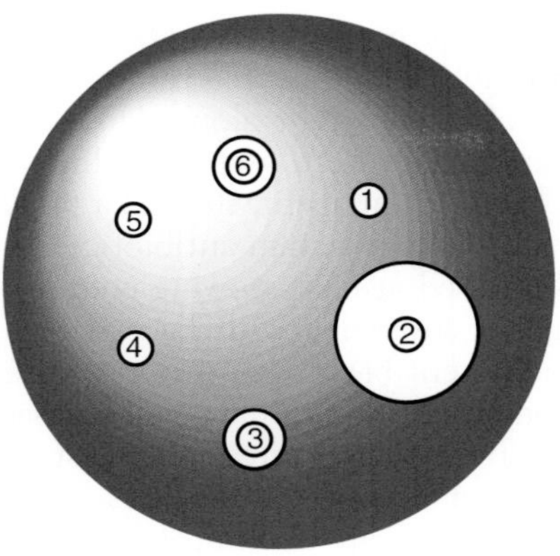

Figure 29.2 Looking down upon a Petri dish containing solidified nutrient agar to which had been added a suspension of a bacterial species. Next, six filter paper discs containing six different antimicrobials were added followed by overnight incubation. The antimicrobials in discs 1, 4, and 5 were inactive. Of the active agents in discs 2, 3, and 6, antibiotic 2 was much more active, as the microorganism was not able to grow as near this impregnated disc.

or dose is sufficiently high. In the laboratory, it is almost always possible to use such doses. Subsequent inoculation of fresh, antibiotic-free media with a culture that has been so treated will not produce growth of the culture because the cells are dead. When such doses are achievable in live patients, such drugs are clinically bactericidal. At somewhat lower concentrations, bacterial multiplication is prevented even though the microorganism remains viable (bacteriostatic action).

The smallest concentration that will kill a bacterial colony is the minimum bactericidal concentration. The difference between a minimum bactericidal dose and a bacteriostatic dose is characteristic of given families of antibiotics. With gentamicin, for example, doubling or quadrupling the dose changes the effect on bacteria from bacteriostatic to bactericidal. Such doses are usually achievable in the clinic, so gentamicin is termed bactericidal. However, the difference between bactericidal and bacteriostatic doses with tetracycline is approximately 40-fold, and it is not possible to achieve such doses safely in patients, so tetracycline is referred to as bacteriostatic. If a bacteriostatic antibiotic is withdrawn prematurely from a patient, the microorganism can resume growth, and the infection can reestablish itself because the organism is still viable. When a patient is immunocompetent or the infection is not severe, a bacteriostatic concentration will break the fulminating stage of the infection (when bacterial cell numbers are increasing at a logarithmic rate). With *E. coli*, for example, the number of cells doubles approximately every 2 hours. A bacteriostatic agent will interrupt this rapid growth and give the immune system a chance to deal with the disease. Cure usually follows if the numbers of live bacteria are not excessive at this time. Obviously, in immunocompromised patients who are unable to contribute natural defenses to fight their own disease, having the drug kill the bacteria is more important for recovery. Thus, although it is preferred that an antibiotic be bactericidal, bacteriostatic antibiotics are widely used and are usually satisfactory.

Microbial Susceptibility

Resistance

Resistance is the failure of microorganisms to be killed or inhibited by antimicrobial treatment. Resistance can either be intrinsic (be present before exposure to drug) or acquired (develop subsequent to exposure to a drug). Resistance of bacteria to the toxic effects of antimicrobial agents and to antibiotics develops fairly easily both in the laboratory and in the clinic and is an ever-increasing public health hazard. Challenging a culture in the laboratory with sublethal quantities of an antibiotic kills the most intrinsically sensitive percentage of the strains in the colony. Those not killed or seriously inhibited continue to grow and have access to the remainder of the nutrients. A mutation to lower sensitivity also enables individual bacteria to survive against the selecting pressure of the antimicrobial agent. If the culture is treated several times in succession with sublethal doses in this manner, the concentration of antibiotic required to prevent growth becomes ever higher. When the origin of this form of resistance is explored, it is almost always found to be due to an alteration in the biochemistry of the colony so that the molecular target of the antibiotic has become less sensitive, or it can be due to decreased uptake of antibiotic into the cells. This is genomically preserved and passes to the next generation. The altered progeny may be weaker than the wild strain so that they die out if the antibiotic is not present to give them a competitive advantage. In some cases, additional compensatory mutations can occur that restore the vigor of the resistant organisms. Resistance of this type is usually expressed toward other antibiotics with the same mode of action and thus is a familial characteristic; most tetracyclines, for example, show extensive cross-resistance with other agents in the tetracycline family. This is very enlightening with respect to discovery of the molecular mode of action but is not very relevant to the clinical situation.

In the clinic, resistance more commonly takes place by resistance (R) factor mechanisms. In this case, enzymes are elaborated that attack the antibiotic and inactivate it. Mutations leading to resistance occur by many mechanisms. They can result from point mutations, insertions, deletions, inversions, duplications, and transpositions of segments of genes or by acquisition of foreign DNA from plasmids, bacteriophages, and transposable genetic elements. The genetic material coding for this form of resistance is often carried on extrachromosomal elements consisting of small circular DNA molecules known as plasmids. A bacterial cell may have many plasmids or none. The plasmid may carry DNA for several different enzymes capable of destroying structurally dissimilar antibiotics. Such plasmid DNA may migrate within the cell from plasmid to plasmid or from plasmid to chromosome by a process known as transposition. Such plasmids may migrate from cell to cell by conjugation (passage through a sexual pilus), transduction (carriage by a virus vector), or transformation (uptake of exogenous DNA from the environment). These mechanisms can convert an antibiotic-sensitive cell to an antibiotic-resistant cell. This can take place many times in a bacterium's already short generation time. The positive selecting pressure of inadequate levels of an antibiotic favors explosive spread of R-factor resistance. This provides a rationale for conservative but aggressive application of appropriate antimicrobial chemotherapy. Bacterial resistance is generally mediated through one of three mechanisms: failure of the drug to penetrate into or stay in the cell, destruction of the drug by defensive enzymes, or alterations in the cellular target of the drug. It is rarely an all-or-nothing effect. In many cases, a resistant microorganism can still be controlled by achievable, although higher, doses than are required to control sensitive populations.

Persistence

Sensitive bacteria may not all be killed. Survivors are thought to have been resting (not metabolizing) during the drug treatment time and are still viable. These bacteria are still sensitive to the drug even though they survived an otherwise toxic dose. Some bacteria also can aggregate in films. A poorly penetrating antibiotic may not reach the cells lying deep within such a film.

Such cells, although intrinsically sensitive, may survive antibiotic treatment. Bacteria living in host cells, living in cysts, or existing as an abscess are also harder to reach by drugs and thus are more difficult to control.

Combination Therapy

It could be assumed that use of combinations of antibiotics would be superior to the use of individual antibiotics because this would broaden the antimicrobial spectrum and make less critical the accurate identification of the pathogen. It has been found, however, that many times, such combinations are antagonistic. A useful generalization, but one that is not always correct, is that one can often successfully combine two bactericidal antibiotics, particularly if their molecular mode of action is different. A common example is the use of a β-lactam antibiotic and an aminoglycoside for empiric therapy of overwhelming sepsis of unknown etiology. Therapy must be instituted as soon as a specimen is obtained, or the patient may die. This often does not allow the microbiologic laboratory sufficient time to identify the offending microorganism or to determine its antibiotic susceptibility. Both of the antibiotic families applied in this example are bactericidal in readily achievable parenteral doses. As will be detailed later in this chapter, the β-lactams inhibit bacterial cell wall formation, and the aminoglycosides interfere with protein biosynthesis and membrane function. Their modes of action are supplementary. Because of toxicity considerations and the potential for adverse effects, this empiric therapy is replaced by suitable specific monotherapy at the first opportunity after the sensitivity of the bacterium is experimentally established.

One may also often successfully combine two bacteriostatic antibiotics for special purposes, for example, a macrolide and a sulfonamide. This combination is occasionally used for the treatment of an upper respiratory tract infection caused by *Haemophilus influenzae* because the combination of a protein biosynthesis inhibitor and an inhibitor of DNA biosynthesis results in fewer relapses than the use of either agent alone. However, the use of a bacteriostatic agent, such as tetracycline, in combination with a bactericidal agent, such as a β-lactam, is usually discouraged. The β-lactam antibiotics are much more effective when used against growing cultures, and a bacteriostatic agent interferes with bacterial growth, often giving an indifferent or antagonistic response when such agents are combined. Additional possible disadvantages of combination chemotherapy are higher cost, greater likelihood of adverse effects, and difficulties in demonstrating synergism. The rising rate of clinical failure due to antibiotic resistance is overcoming these reservations, and combination therapy is becoming more common.

Serum Protein Binding

The influence of serum protein binding on antibiotic effectiveness is fairly straightforward. It is considered in most instances that the percentage of antibiotic that is protein bound is not available at that moment for the treatment of infections so must be subtracted from the total blood level in order to get the effective blood level. The tightness of the binding is also a consideration. Thus, a heavily and firmly serum protein-bound antibiotic would not generally be a good choice for the treatment of septicemias or infections in deep tissue, even though the microorganism involved is susceptible in in vitro tests. If the antibiotic is rapidly released from the protein, however, this factor decreases in importance, and the binding becomes a depot source. Distinguishing between these two types of protein binding is accomplished by comparing the percentages of binding to the excretion half-life. A highly bound but readily released antibiotic will have a comparatively short half-life and work well for systemic infections. An antibiotic that is not significantly protein bound will normally be rapidly excreted and have a short half-life. Thus, some protein binding of poorly water-soluble agents is normally regarded as helpful.

Preferred Means of Dosing

Under ideal circumstances, it is desirable for an antibiotic to be available in both parenteral and oral forms. Although there is no question that the convenience of oral medication makes this ideal for outpatient and community use, very ill patients often require parenteral therapy. It would be consistent with today's practice of discharging patients sooner to send them home from the hospital with an efficacious oral version of the same antibiotic that led to the possibility of discharge in the first place. In this way, the patient would not have to come back to the hospital at intervals for drug administration and would not have to risk treatment failure by starting therapy with a new drug.

Cost

Antibiotics are often expensive, but so is morbidity and mortality. For many patients, however, cost is a significant consideration. The pharmacist is in an ideal position to guide the physician and the patient on the question of possible alternative equivalent treatments that might be more affordable. The most frequent comparisons are based on the cost of the usual dose of a given agent for a single course of therapy (usually the wholesale cost to the pharmacist for 10 d worth of drug).

Agricultural Use of Antibiotics

It is estimated that more than half of the antibiotics of commerce are used for agricultural purposes. Their use for treatment of infections of plants and animals is not to be discouraged so long as drug residues from the treatment do not contaminate foods. In contamination, problems such as penicillin allergy or subsequent infection higher up the food chain by drug-resistant microbes can occur. Animals demonstrably grow more rapidly to marketable size when antibiotics are added to their feed even though the animals have no apparent infection. This is believed to be due in large part to suppression of subclinical infections that would consequently divert protein biosynthesis from muscle and tissue growth into proteins needed to combat the infection. Under appropriate conditions, antibiotic feed supplementation is partly responsible for the comparative wholesomeness and cheapness of our food supplies. This practice has the potential, however, to contaminate the food we consume or to provide reservoirs of drug-resistant enteric microorganisms, so it is imperative that antibiotics used for agriculture be utilized appropriately.

THERAPEUTIC CLASSES

Synthetic Antimicrobial Agents

Synthetic antimicrobial agents have not been modeled after any natural product, so they may not properly be called "antibiotics." Some synthetics are extremely effective for treatment of infections and are widely used. Very few antibiotics are known to work in precisely the same way as these agents in antibacterial action.

Sulfonamides

The antibacterial properties of the sulfonamides were discovered in the mid-1930s after an incorrect hypothesis, but after observing the results carefully and drawing correct conclusions. Prontosil rubrum, a red dye, was one of a series of dyes examined by Gerhard Domagk of Bayer of Germany in the belief that it might be taken up selectively by certain pathogenic bacteria and not by human cells, in a manner analogous to the way that the Gram stain works, and thus serve as a selective poison to kill these cells.[2] The dye, indeed, proved active in vivo against streptococcal infections in mice. Curiously, it was not active in vitro. Trefouel and others soon showed that the urine of prontosil rubrum–treated animals was bioactive in vitro.[8] Fractionation led to identification of the active substance as *p*-aminobenzenesulfonic acid amide (sulfanilamide), a colorless cleavage product formed by reductive liver metabolism of the administered dye. Today, we would call prontosil rubrum a prodrug.

NH$_2$ N=N SO$_2$NH$_2$ H$_2$N —Liver [H]→ H$_2$N SO$_2$NH$_2$

Prontosil rubrum Sulfanilamide

The discovery of sulfanilamide's in vivo antibacterial properties ushered in the modern anti-infective era, and Domagk was awarded a Nobel Prize for Medicine in 1939.

Once mainstays of antimicrobial chemotherapy, the sulfonamides have decreased enormously in popularity and are now comparatively minor drugs. The relative inexpensiveness of the sulfonamides is one of their most attractive features and accounts for much of their persistence on the market.

MECHANISM OF ACTION. The sulfonamides are bacteriostatic when administered to humans in achievable doses. They inhibit the enzyme dihydropteroate synthase, an important enzyme needed for the biosynthesis of folic acid derivatives and, ultimately, the thymidine required for DNA.[9] They do this by competing at the active site with *p*-aminobenzoic acid (PABA), a normal structural component of folic acid derivatives. PABA is otherwise incorporated into the developing tetrahydrofolic acid molecule by enzyme-catalyzed condensation with 6-hydroxymethyl-7,8-dihydropterin-pyrophosphate to form 7,8-dihydropteroate and pyrophosphate. Thus, sulfonamides may also be classified as antimetabolites (Fig. 29.3). Indeed, the antimicrobial efficacy of sulfonamides can be reversed by adding significant quantities of PABA into the diet (in some multivitamin preparations and as metabolites of certain local anesthetics) or into the culture medium. Most susceptible bacteria are unable to take up preformed folic acid from their environment and convert it to a tetrahydrofolic acid but, instead, synthesize their own folates de novo. Folates are essential intermediates for the biosynthesis of thymidine without which bacteria cannot multiply. Thus, inhibition of the dihydropteroate synthase is bacteriostatic. Humans are unable to synthesize folates from component parts, lacking the necessary enzymes (including dihydropteroate synthase), and folic acid is supplied to humans in our diet. Sulfonamides consequently have no similarly lethal effect on human cell growth, and the basis for the selective toxicity of sulfonamides is clear.

In a few strains of bacteria, however, the picture is somewhat more complex. Here, sulfonamides are attached to the dihydropteroate diphosphate in place of the normal PABA. The resulting unnatural product, however, is not capable of undergoing the next necessary reaction, condensation with glutamic acid. This false metabolite is also an enzyme inhibitor, and the net result is inability of the bacteria to multiply when the folic acid in their cells is used up, and further nucleic acid biosynthesis becomes impossible. The net result is the same, but the molecular basis of

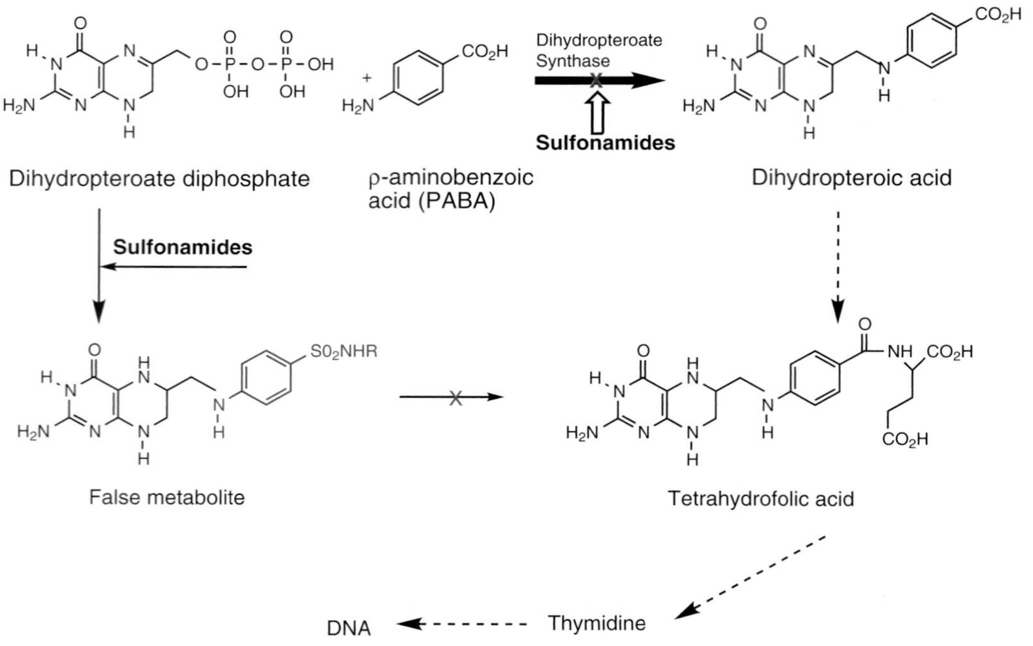

Figure 29.3 Microbial biosynthetic pathway leading to tetrahydrofolic acid synthesis and major site of action (⇧) of sulfonamides as well as site of action seen in some bacteria (←), resulting in incorporation of sulfanamide as a false metabolite.

the effect is somewhat different in these strains (Fig. 29.3). Bacteria that are able to take up preformed folic acid into their cells are intrinsically resistant to sulfonamides.

STRUCTURE-ACTIVITY RELATIONSHIPS. The basis of the structural resemblance of sulfonamides to PABA is clear. The functional group that differs in the two molecules is the carboxyl of PABA and the sulfonamide moiety of sulfanilamide. The strongly electron-withdrawing character of the aromatic SO_2 group makes the nitrogen atom to which it is directly attached partially electropositive. This, in turn, increases the acidity of the hydrogen atoms attached to the nitrogen so that this functional group is slightly acidic (pK_a = 10.4). The pKa of the carboxyl group of PABA is approximately 4.9. It was soon found that replacement of one of the NH_2 hydrogens by an electron-withdrawing heteroaromatic ring enhanced the acidity of the remaining hydrogen and dramatically enhanced potency. With suitable groups in place, the pK_a is reduced to the same range as that of PABA itself. Not only did this markedly increase the antibacterial potency of the product, but it also dramatically increased the water solubility under physiologic conditions. The pK_a of sulfisoxazole, one of the sulfonamides in present use, is approximately 5.0. The poor water solubility of the earliest sulfonamides led to occasional crystallization in the urine (crystalluria) and resulted in kidney damage because the molecules were un-ionized at urine pH values. It is still recommended to drink increased quantities of water to avoid crystalluria when taking certain sulfonamides, but this form of toxicity is now comparatively uncommon with the more important agents used today because they form sodium salts that are at least partly ionized and hence reasonably water soluble at urinary pH values. They are poorly tolerated on injection, however, because these salts are corrosive to tissues.

Structural variation among the clinically useful sulfonamides is restricted primarily to installation of various heterocyclic aromatic substituents on the sulfonamide nitrogen.

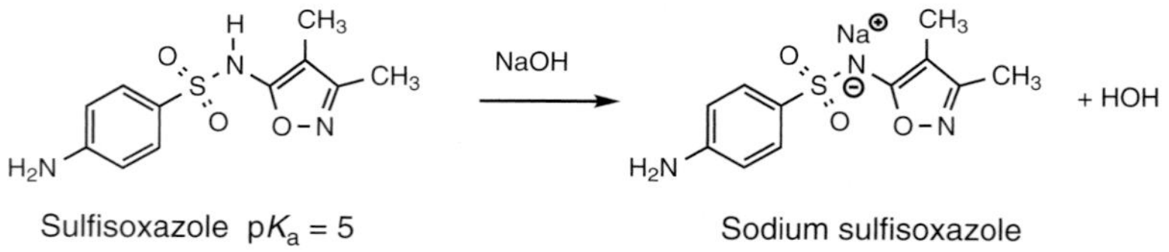

Pharmacokinetics

The orally administered sulfonamides are well absorbed from the gastrointestinal (GI) tract, distributed fairly widely, and excreted by the kidney. The drugs are bound to plasma protein (sulfisoxazole 30%-70%, sulfamethoxazole 70%) and, as such, may displace other protein-bound drugs as well as bilirubin. The latter phenomenon disqualifies them for use in late-term pregnancy because they can cause neonatal jaundice. Sulfonamides are partly deactivated by acetylation at N-4 and glucuronidation of the anilino nitrogen in the liver.[10]

Plasmid-mediated resistance development is common, particularly among gram-negative microorganisms and usually takes the form of decreased sensitivity of dihydropteroate synthase or increased production of PABA.[11]

Therapeutic Applications

Of the thousands of sulfonamides that have been evaluated, only a few are still available and are often used in combination with other agents. The surviving sulfonamides (Table 29.1) include sulfisoxazole, which is used in combination with erythromycin. It has a comparatively broad antimicrobial spectrum in vitro, especially against gram-negative organisms, but clinical use is generally restricted due to the development of bacterial resistance. Susceptible organisms may include enterobacteriaceae (*E. coli*, *Klebsiella*, and *Proteus*) and *Streptococcus pyogenes*, *Streptococcus pneumoniae*, and *Haemophilus*.[12] Sulfamethoxazole in combination with trimethoprim is more commonly seen and is further described in the discussion of trimethoprim.

The remaining sulfonamides are not used systemically. Sulfadiazine in the form of its silver salt is used topically for treatment of burns and is effective against a range of bacteria and fungus, whereas sulfacetamide is used ophthalmically for treatment of eye infections caused by susceptible organisms and is used as a topical lotion in the treatment of acne vulgaris.

Adverse Effects

Allergic reactions are the most common and take the form of rash, photosensitivity, and drug fever. Less common problems are kidney and liver damage, hemolytic anemia, and other blood problems. The most serious adverse effect is the Stevens-Johnson syndrome characterized by sometimes fatal erythema multiforme and ulceration of mucous membranes of the eye, mouth, and urethra.[10] Fortunately, these effects are comparatively rare.

Trimethoprim

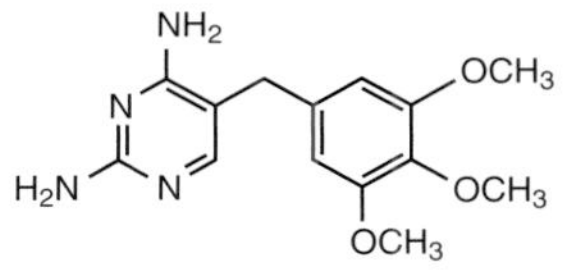

NH_2 OCH_3 N H_2N N OCH_3 OCH_3

Trimethoprim

MECHANISM OF ACTION. A further step in the pathway leading from the pteroates to folic acid and on to DNA bases requires the enzyme dihydrofolate reductase. Exogenous folic acid must be reduced stepwise to dihydrofolic acid and then to tetrahydrofolic acid, an important cofactor essential for supplying a one-carbon unit in thymidine biosynthesis and ultimately for DNA synthesis (Fig. 29.4). The same enzyme must also reduce endogenously produced dihydrofolate. Inhibition of this key enzyme had been widely studied in attempts to find anticancer agents by starving rapidly dividing cancer cells of needed DNA precursors. Antifolates such as methotrexate arose from

Table 29.1 Clinically Relevent Sulfonamides

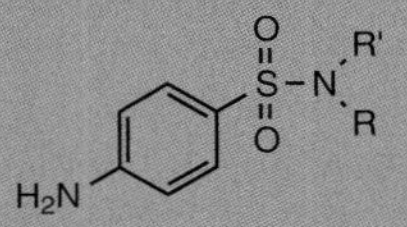

General structure: $H_2N-C_6H_4-SO_2-N(R)(R')$

Drug: Generic Name	Product	R	R′	pK_a
Sulfisoxazole acetyl (prodrug)	In combination with erythromycin ethylsuccinate	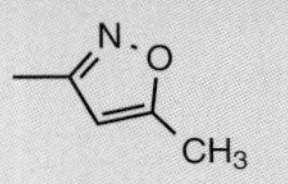 N, O, CH_3 (isoxazolyl)	$-C(=O)-CH_3$	5.6 after hydrolysis
Sulfamethoxazole	In combination with trimethoprim	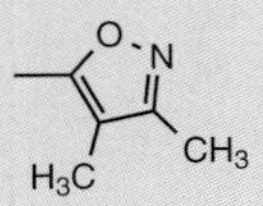 O, N, CH_3, H_3C (isoxazolyl)	—H	5.0
Sulfadiazine	Oral dosage form	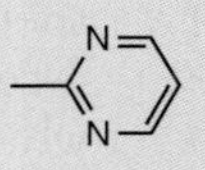 N, N (pyrimidinyl)	—H	6.52
Silver sulfadiazine	Topical dosage form	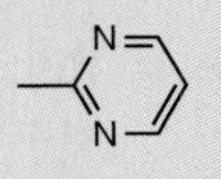 N, N (pyrimidinyl)	⊖ Ag ⊕	
Sulfacetamide sodium	Opthalmic dosage form	$-C(=O)-CH_3$	⊖ Na ⊕	5.4 free acid
Sulfasalazine	Gastrointestinal oral dosage form	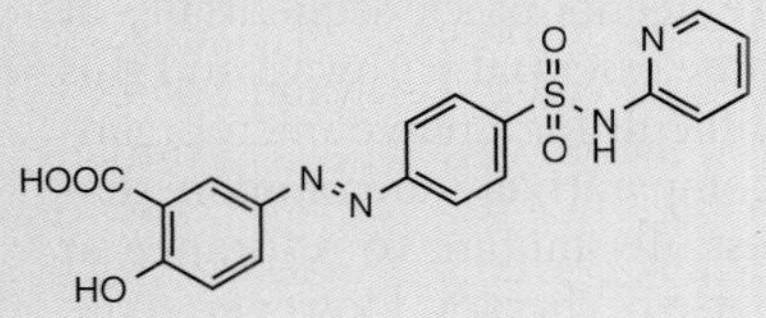 HOOC, HO, N=N, SO_2, N-H, N (structure)		

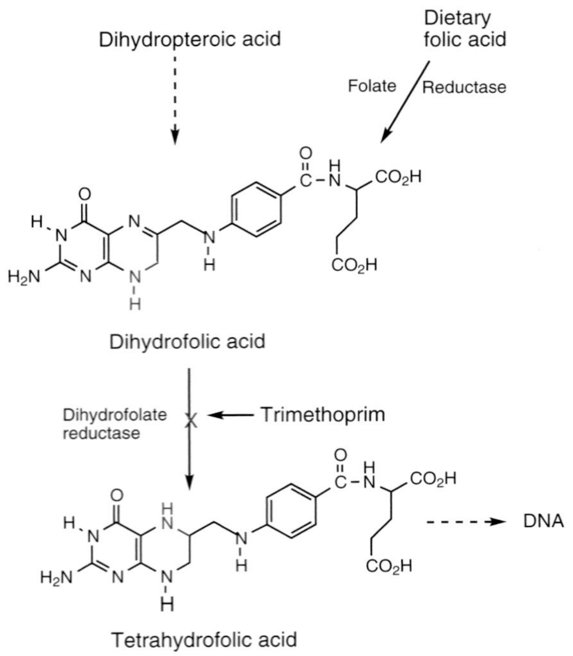

Figure 29.4 Site of action of trimethoprim.

such studies. Methotrexate, however, is much too toxic to be used as an antibiotic. Subsequently, however, trimethoprim was developed in 1969 by George Hitchings and Gertrude Elion (who shared a Nobel Prize for this and other contributions to chemotherapy in 1988). This inhibitor prevents tetrahydrofolic acid biosynthesis and results in bacteriostasis. Trimethoprim selectivity between bacterial and mammalian dihydrofolate reductases results from the subtle but significant architectural differences between these enzyme systems. Whereas the bacterial enzyme and the mammalian enzyme both efficiently catalyze the conversion of dihydrofolic acid to tetrahydrofolic acid, the bacterial enzyme is sensitive to inhibition by trimethoprim by up to 100,000 times lower concentrations than is vertebrate enzyme.[13] This difference explains the useful selective toxicity of trimethoprim.

THERAPEUTIC APPLICATION. Trimethoprim can be used as a single agent clinically for the oral treatment of uncomplicated urinary tract infections caused by susceptible bacteria (predominantly community-acquired *E. coli* and other gram-negative rods).[14] It is, however, most commonly used in a 1:5 fixed concentration ratio with the sulfonamide sulfamethoxazole (Bactrim, Septra). This combination is not only synergistic in vitro but is less likely to induce bacterial resistance than either agent alone. It is rationalized that microorganisms not completely inhibited by sulfamethoxazole at the pteroate condensation step will not likely be able to push the lessened amount of substrates that leak through past a subsequent blockade of dihydrofolate reductase. Thus these agents block sequentially at two different steps in the same essential pathway, and this combination is extremely difficult for a naive microorganism to survive. It is also comparatively uncommon that a microorganism will successfully mutate to resistance at both enzymes during the course of therapy. However, if the organism is already resistant to either drug at the outset of therapy, much of the advantage of the combination is lost.

Pairing these two particular antibacterial agents was based on pharmacokinetic factors. For such a combination to be useful in vivo, the two agents must arrive at the necessary tissue compartment where the infection is at the correct time and in the right ratio. In this context, the optimum ratio of these two agents in vitro is 1:20. Administration of the 1:5 combination of the two drugs orally produces the desired 1:20 ratio in the body once steady state is reached.[10] The combination is used for oral treatment of urinary tract infections, shigellosis, otitis media, traveler's diarrhea, community-acquired methicillin-resistant *Staphylococcus aureus* (MRSA), acute exacerbations of chronic bronchitis, and pneumocystis pneumonia.[10] The pneumonia-causing fungus *Pneumocystis jiroveci* (previously classified as *Pneumocystis carinii*) is an opportunistic pathogen for immunocompromised individuals.

The most frequent side effects of trimethoprim-sulfamethoxazole are rash, nausea, and vomiting. Blood dyscrasias are less common, as is pseudomembranous colitis (caused by non–antibiotic-sensitive opportunistic gut anaerobes, often *Clostridium difficile*).[10] Despite a significant effort, no structurally related analogue has emerged to compete with trimethoprim.

RESISTANCE. Bacterial resistance to trimethoprim is increasingly common. In pneumococcal infections, it can result from a single amino acid mutation (Ile100 to Leu100) in the dihydrofolate reductase enzyme. Overexpression of dihydrofolate reductase by *Staphylococcus aureus* has also been reported in resistant strains.[11]

Quinolones

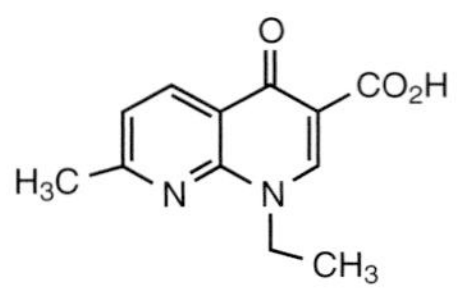

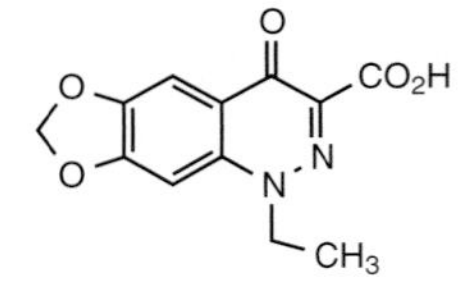

The quinolone antimicrobials comprise a group of synthetic substances possessing in common an N-1-alkylated 3-carboxypyrid-4-one ring fused to another aromatic ring, which itself carries other substituents. The first quinolone to be marketed was nalidixic acid, which has since been discontinued. Nalidixic acid was classified as a first-generation quinolone based on its spectrum of activity and pharmacokinetic properties. The spectrum of activity was limited to a small number of gram-negative organisms. Thus, the quinolones were of little clinical significance until the discovery that the addition of a fluoro group to the 6 position of the basic nucleus greatly increased the biologic activity.[15,16] Agents that contain the 6-fluoro substitution are referred to as fluoroquinolones and represent an important therapeutic class of antimicrobials. Norfloxacin was approved for use in 1986 and represents the first of the second-generation quinolones; it is considered to be broad spectrum and equivalent in potency to many of the fermentation-derived antibiotics.[15] Following its introduction, intense research ensued, and over a thousand analogues have now been made. Ciprofloxacin, gemifloxacin, ofloxacin, levofloxacin, moxifloxacin, and delafloxacin are currently marketed for systemic use in the United States. In addition, ciprofloxacin, levofloxacin, moxifloxacin, and ofloxacin along with besifloxacin and gatifloxacin are available for ophthalmic use. Finafloxacin joins ofloxacin and ciprofloxacin for topical otic administration (Fig. 29.5).

Mechanism of Action. The quinolones are rapidly bactericidal, largely as a consequence of inhibition of DNA gyrase and topoisomerase IV, key bacterial enzymes that dictate the conformation of DNA.[16,17] Using the energy generated by adenosine triphosphate (ATP) hydrolysis, DNA is progressively wound about itself in a positive supercoil. In the absence of ATP, the process is reversed, relaxing the molecule. It must also be partially unwound so that the cell has access to the genetic information it contains. This requires reversible conformational changes so that it can be stored properly, unwound, replicated, repaired, and transcribed on demand. DNA gyrase alters the conformation of DNA by catalyzing transient double-strand cuts, passing the uncut portion of the molecule through the gap, and resealing the molecule back together (Fig. 29.6).[16] In this way, DNA gyrase alters the degree of twisting of DNA by introducing negative DNA supercoils releasing tensional stress in the molecule. DNA topoisomerase IV, on the other hand, decatenates (unties) enchained daughter DNA molecules produced through replication of circular DNA.[16] Inhibition of DNA gyrase and topoisomerase IV makes a cell's DNA inaccessible and leads to cell death, particularly if the cell must deal with other toxic effects at the same time. Different quinolones inhibit these essential enzymes to different extents, which explains some of the differences in the spectrum of activity of the fluoroquinolones. Topoisomerase IV seems more important to some gram-positive organisms, and DNA gyrase seems more important to some gram-negative organisms.

Humans shape their DNA with a topoisomerase II, an analogous enzyme to DNA gyrase that, however, does not bind quinolones at normally achievable doses, so the quinolones of commerce do not kill host cells.

Structure-Activity Relationship. The structural features of the quinolones strongly influence the antimicrobial and pharmacokinetic properties of this class of drugs.[18,19] The essential pharmacophore for activity is the carboxy-4-pyridone nucleus (Fig. 29.7). Apparently, the carboxylic acid and the ketone are involved in binding to the DNA/DNA-gyrase enzyme system. Reduction of the 2,3-double bond or the 4-keto group inactivates the molecule, and substitution at C-2 interferes with enzyme-substrate complexation. Fluoro substitution at

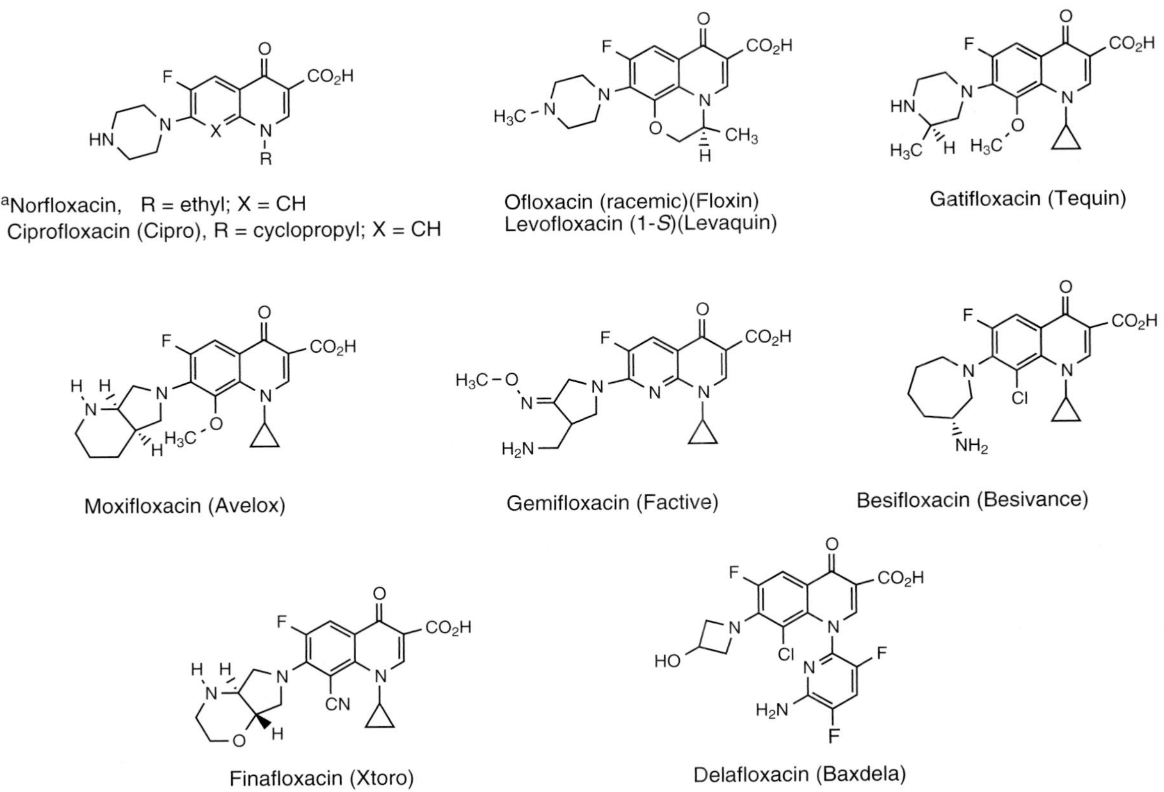

Figure 29.5 Second-, third-, and fourth-generation quinolones.

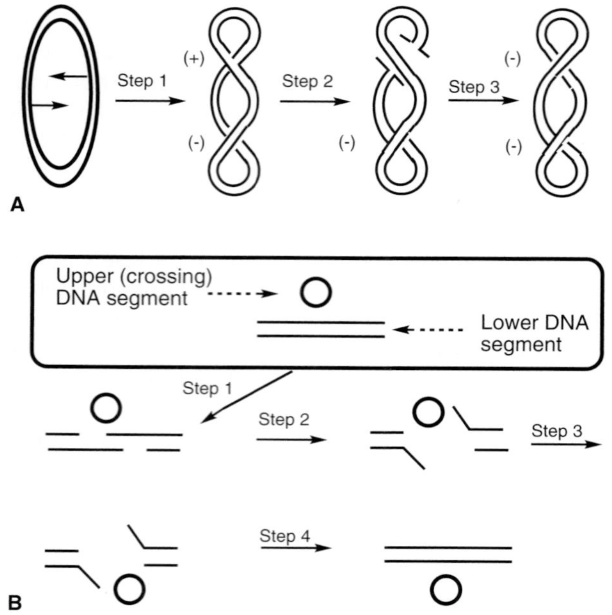

Figure 29.6 Schematic depicting supercoiling of circular DNA catalyzed by DNA gyrase. A, View from the top: Step 1, stabilize positive node. Step 2, break both strands of the back segment. Step 3, pass unbroken segment through the break and reseal on the front side. B, View from the side: Step 1, staggered cuts in each strand. Step 2, gate opens. Step 3, transverse segment passed through the break. Step 4, reseal cut segment.

the C-6 position greatly improves antimicrobial activity by increasing the lipophilicity of the molecule, which in turn improves the drug's penetration through the bacterial cell wall. C-6 fluoro also increases the DNA gyrase/topoisomerase IV inhibitory action. An additional fluoro group at C-8 further improves drug absorption and half-life, but also increases drug-induced photosensitivity. Substitution of a methoxy group at C-8 reduces the photosensitivity (moxifloxacin and gatifloxacin). Heterocyclic substitution at C-7 improves the spectrum of activity especially against gram-negative organisms. The piperazinyl (ciprofloxacin) and pyrrolidinyl (moxifloxacin) represent the most significant antimicrobial improvement. Unfortunately, the piperazinyl group at C-7 also increases binding to central nervous system (CNS) γ-aminobutyric acid (GABA) receptors, which accounts for CNS side effects. Alkyl substitution on the piperazine nitrogen (ofloxacin and levofloxacin) is reported to decrease binding to GABA. The cyclopropyl substitution at N-1 appears to broaden activity of the

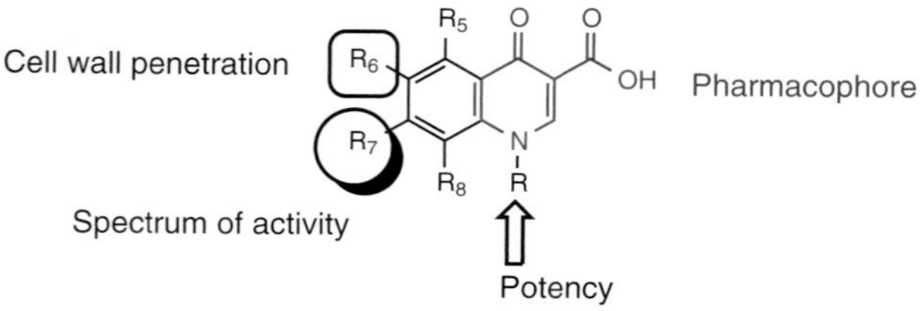

Figure 29.7 Major structure-activity relationship (SAR) features of 4-quinolones.

quinolones to include activity against atypical bacteria including *Mycoplasma*, *Chlamydia*, and *Legionella* species. Substitution of a 2,4-difluorophenyl at N-1 also improves antimicrobial potency, but agents with this substitution (trovafloxacin and temafloxacin) have been withdrawn from the market due to serious adverse effects.

The introduction of a third ring to the nucleus of the quinolones gives rise to ofloxacin. Additionally, ofloxacin has an asymmetric carbon at the C-3′ position. The S-(-)-isomer (levofloxacin) is twice as active as ofloxacin and 8-128 times more potent than the *R*-(+)-isomer resulting from increased binding to the DNA gyrase. Finally, a chemical incompatibility common to all of the quinolones involves the ability of these drugs to chelate polyvalent metal ions (Ca^{2+}, Mg^{2+}, Zn^{2+}, Fe^{2+}, Al^{3+}), resulting in decreased solubility and reduced drug absorption. Chelation occurs between the metal and the 3-carboxylic acid and 4-keto groups. Agents containing polyvalent metals should be administered separately from the quinolones.

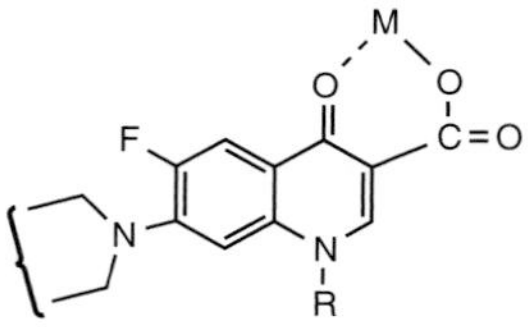

PHARMACOKINETICS. The fluoroquinolones are well absorbed following oral administration, with excellent bioavailability. The maximum plasma concentration is usually reached within a few hours, and the drugs are moderately bound to plasma protein, leading to comparatively long half-lives (Table 29.2). Earlier, quinolones were rapidly excreted into the urine, which limited their therapeutic application to urinary tract infections, whereas the newer drugs are distributed to alveolar macrophages, bronchial mucosa, epithelial lining fluid, and saliva, improving the use in various systemic infections.

THERAPEUTIC APPLICATIONS. The quinolones therapeutically fall into one of four classifications (Table 29.3). The specific drugs within each classification include nalidixic acid and cinoxacin as first-generation agents both of which have been discontinued in the United States. The second-generation quinolones include norfloxacin and ciprofloxacin. Ciprofloxacin has a broader spectrum of activity and is used for urinary tract infections (*Enterobacter*, *Enterococcus*, or *Pseudomonas aeruginosa*), prostatitis, gonorrhea, upper respiratory tract infections, bone infections, septicemia, staphylococcal and pseudomonal endocarditis, meningitis, and anthrax infections.[20,21] The third-generation quinolones include levofloxacin, gatifloxacin, and gemifloxacin. These agents find use in the treatment of bacterial exacerbation of chronic bronchitis and community-acquired pneumonia.[22,23] Levofloxacin is also used to treat respiratory infections caused by *Legionella*, *Chlamydia*, and *Mycoplasma* as well as other nosocomial pneumonias.

Table 29.2 Pharmacokinetic Properties for Select Quinolones

Drug	Bioavailability (%)	Protein Binding (%)	Half-Life (hr)
Ciprofloxacin	70	30	3.5
Norfloxacin	30-40	10-15	3-4
Enoxacin	90	40	3-6
Levofloxacin	99	31	6.9
Gatifloxacin	96	20	8.0
Gemifloxacin	71	60-70	8.0
Delafloxacin	59	84	8.0
Ofloxacin	98	32	9
Moxifloxacin	86	47	12.1

Additional indications for levofloxacin include skin and skin structure infections and acute sinusitis caused by *Streptococcus pneumoniae*, *Haemophilus influenzae*, and *Moraxella catarrhalis*.[23] The fourth-generation quinolones include moxifloxacin and have a spectrum of activity that includes *Bacteroides fragilis*.[24] Moxifloxacin and levofloxacin are also recommended as second-line agents for tuberculosis as an off-label use.[23,24]

RESISTANCE. Resistance to the quinolones is becoming more frequent and is associated with spontaneous mutations in genes (*gyrA* and *gyrB*) that encode for the quinolone target protein, DNA gyrase, and genes (*parC* and *parE*) that encode for topoisomerase IV.[25] A single mutation can lead to low-level resistance, whereas mutations in more than one gene lead to high-level resistance. This mechanism of resistance would be expected to produce differing levels of cross-resistance within the class of quinolones. In addition, there are suggestions that resistance may be associated with an increase in drug efflux or a decrease in outer membrane permeability affecting drug influx.

Such a mechanism of resistance would be expected to be more common in gram-negative organisms with a more complex cell wall than in gram-positive organisms with their cell envelope.

Table 29.3 Therapeutic Classification of Quinolones

Generation	Characteristics
First generation	Poor serum and tissue concentration Not valuable for systemic infections Lack activity against *Pseudomonas aeruginosa*, gram-positive organisms, and anaerobes
Second generation	Adequate serum and tissue concentration Good for systemic infections Active against gram-negative organisms including *P. aeruginosa*; weak activity against *Streptococcus pneumoniae*; and no activity against anaerobes
Third generation	Once-daily dosing Active against *S. pneumoniae* and atypical bacteria; less active against *P. aeruginosa*
Fourth generation	Active against anaerobes and aerobic gram-positive and gram-negative organisms

ADVERSE EFFECTS. The quinolone class is associated with more side effects than the β-lactam and macrolide classes but nonetheless see widespread medicinal use. All of the fluoroquinolones have a black box warning for possible tendonitis and tendon rupture. They are also not for use in myasthenia gravis patients. Another side effect associated with quinolones is a proconvulsant action, especially when coadministered with nonsteroidal anti-inflammatory drugs. Other CNS problems include hallucinations, insomnia, and visual disturbances. Some patients also experience diarrhea, vomiting, abdominal pain, and anorexia. The quinolones are associated with erosion of the load-bearing joints of young animals. As a precaution, these drugs are not used casually in children less than 18 years of age or in sexually active females of childbearing age. They are also potentially damaging in the first trimester of pregnancy because of a risk of severe metabolic acidosis and of hemolytic anemia. Some of the quinolones may potentiate the action of theophylline and should be monitored closely. They also have been linked to QT prolongation and may increase the risk of torsades de pointes when used with other QT-prolonging agents such as some antiarrhythmic agents.[21-26]

SEVERE TOXICITIES. Certain members of the fluoroquinolone family were marketed for a while but were subsequently severely limited in use or withdrawn because of the unacceptable toxicities experienced by some patients. These agents, because of their breadth of spectrum and potency against resistant microorganisms, were introduced with great hope. Temafloxacin, for example, was removed from the market because of hemolysis, renal failure, and thrombocytopenia (the hemolytic uremic syndrome). These effects only became apparent when large numbers of patients received the drug. Severe liver toxicity led to the removal from the market of trovafloxacin. Grepafloxacin was introduced on the market in late 1997 as a broad-spectrum fluoroquinolone and withdrawn from the market in 1999 because of cardiovascular toxicity. Analogues with a C-8 chloro substituent, such as clinafloxacin and sitafloxacin, were also very potent but have been withdrawn due to excessive phototoxicity.

Miscellaneous Agents

NITROHETEROAROMATIC COMPOUNDS

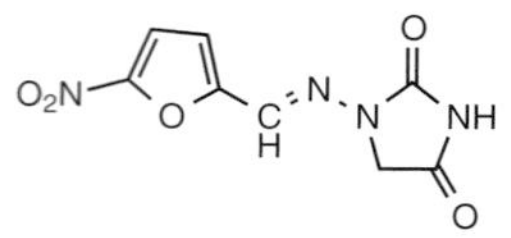

Nitrofurantoin (Furadantin, Macrodantin)

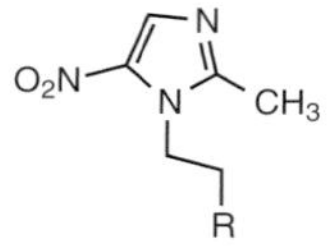

Metronidazole, R = OH (Flagyl)
Tinidazole R = $SO_2C_2H_5$(Fasigyn)

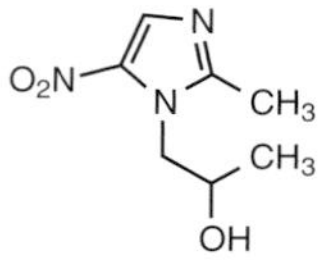

Secnidazole (Solosec)

Nitrofurantoin, a widely used oral antibacterial nitrofuran, has been available since World War II. It is used for prophylaxis or treatment of acute urinary tract infections when kidney function is not impaired, and it inhibits kidney stone growth. Nausea and vomiting are common side effects. This is avoided in part by slowing the rate of absorption of the drug through use of wax-coated large particles (Macrodantin). Nitrofurantoin inhibits DNA and RNA functions through mechanisms that are not well understood, although bioreductive activation is suspected to be an important component of this. There is little acquired resistance to this agent. Severe side effects can be experienced when using this drug (acute pulmonary reactions, peripheral neuropathy, hemolytic anemia, liver toxicity, and fertility impairment).[27]

Metronidazole was initially introduced for the treatment of vaginal infections caused by amoeba. This nitroimidazole is also useful orally for the treatment of trichomoniasis, giardiasis, and *Gardnerella vaginalis* infections. It has found increasing use of late in the parenteral treatment of anaerobic infections and for treatment of pseudomembranous colitis due to *Clostridium difficile*. *C. difficile* is an opportunistic pathogen that occasionally flourishes as a consequence of broad-spectrum antibiotic therapy, and infections can be life-threatening. The drug is believed to be metabolically activated by reduction of its nitro group to produce metabolites that interfere with DNA and RNA function. Metronidazole is also a component of a multidrug cocktail used to treat *Helicobacter pylori* infections associated with gastric ulcers.[28] Tinidazole, another nitroimidazole, has been introduced primarily as an antiprotozoal agent.[29] Because of the similarities in structure and action, tinidazole is believed to have a similar spectrum and mechanism to metronidazole. Both drugs can cause disulfiram-like adverse reactions when alcohol is consumed. Metronidazole use is associated with allergic rashes and CNS disturbances, including convulsions, in some patients. It is carcinogenic in rodents.[28] Secnidazole is a recently introduced agent for bacterial vaginosis. It is administered orally as granules that are swallowed whole in applesauce or pudding. It is believed to work by the same mechanism as other nitroimidazoles but does not appear to cause a disulfuram-like reaction with alcohol.[30]

FOSFOMYCIN

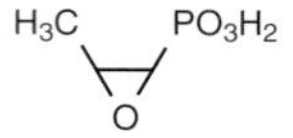

Phosphomycin (Monurol)

Fosfomycin (also known as phosphomycin) inhibits enolpyruvial transferase, an enzyme catalyzing an early step in bacterial cell wall biosynthesis. Inhibition results in reduced synthesis of peptidoglycan, an important component in the bacterial cell wall. Fosfomycin is bactericidal against *Escherichia coli* and *Enterobacter faecalis* infections. It is used for treatment of uncomplicated urinary tract infections by susceptible organisms.

Antibiotics: Inhibitors of Bacterial Cell Wall Biosynthesis

THE BACTERIAL CELL WALL. Bacterial cells are enclosed within a complex and largely rigid cell wall. This differs dramatically from mammalian cells that are surrounded by a flexible membrane whose chemical composition is dramatically different. This provides a number of potentially attractive targets for selective chemotherapy of bacterial infections. For one thing, enzymes that have no direct counterpart in mammalian cells construct the bacterial cell wall. Three of the main functions of the bacterial cell wall are (1) to provide a semipermeable barrier interfacing with the environment through which only desirable substances may pass; (2) to provide a sufficiently strong barrier so that the bacterial cell is protected from changes in the osmotic pressure of its environment; and (3) to prevent digestion by host enzymes. The initial units of the cell wall are constructed within the cell, but soon the growing and increasingly complex structure must be extruded; final assembly takes place outside of the inner membrane. This circumstance makes the enzymes involved in late steps more vulnerable to inhibition because they are at or near

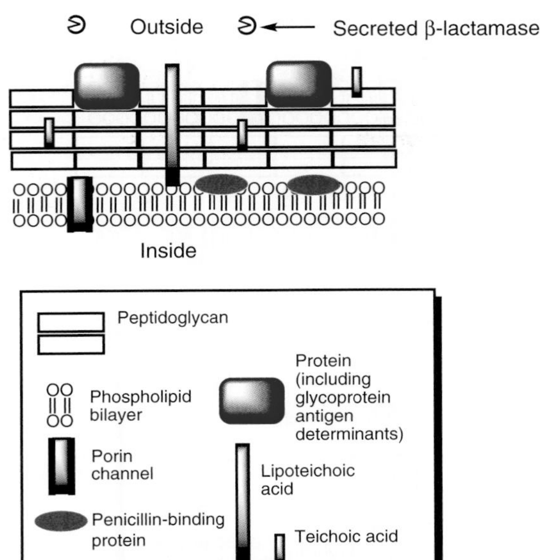

Figure 29.8 Schematic of some features of the gram-positive bacterial cell wall.

the cell surface. Whereas individual bacterial species differ in specific details, the following generalized picture of the process is sufficiently accurate to illustrate the process.

Gram-Positive Bacteria. The cell wall of gram-positive bacteria, although complex enough, is simpler than that of gram-negative organisms. A schematic representation is shown in Figure 29.8. On the very outside of the cell is a set of characteristic carbohydrates and proteins that together make up the antigenic determinants that differ from species to species and that also cause adherence to particular target cells. There may also be a lipid-rich capsule surrounding the cell (not shown in the diagram). The next barrier that the wall presents is the peptidoglycan layer. This is a spongy, gel-forming layer consisting of a series of alternating sugars (N-acetylglucosamine and N-acetylmuramic acid) linked (1,4)-β in a long chain (Fig. 29.9). To the lactic acid carboxyl moieties of the N-acetylmuramic acid units is attached, through an amide linkage, a series of amino acids of which L-alanyl-D-glutamyl-L-lysyl-D-alanine is typical of *Staphylococcus aureus*. One notes the D-stereochemistry of the glutamate and the terminal alanine. This feature is presumably important in protecting the peptidoglycan from hydrolysis by host peptidases, particularly in the GI tract.

The early steps in the biosynthesis of the peptidoglycan unit result in formation of a complex polymeric sheet. This is then cross-linked to form a thickened wall. This bonds the terminal D-alanyl unit to the lysyl unit of an adjacent tetrapeptide strand through a pentaglycyl unit. This last step is an enzyme-catalyzed transamidation by which the terminal amino moiety on the last glycine unit of the A strand displaces the terminal D-ala unit on the nearby B strand. The cell wall transamidase, one of the penicillin-binding proteins (PBPs), forms a transient covalent bond during the synthesis phase with a particular serine hydroxyl on the enzyme. Completion of the catalytic cycle involves displacement of the enzyme by a glycine residue, which regenerates the enzyme. This process gives the wall additional rigidity. This strong barrier protects against osmotic

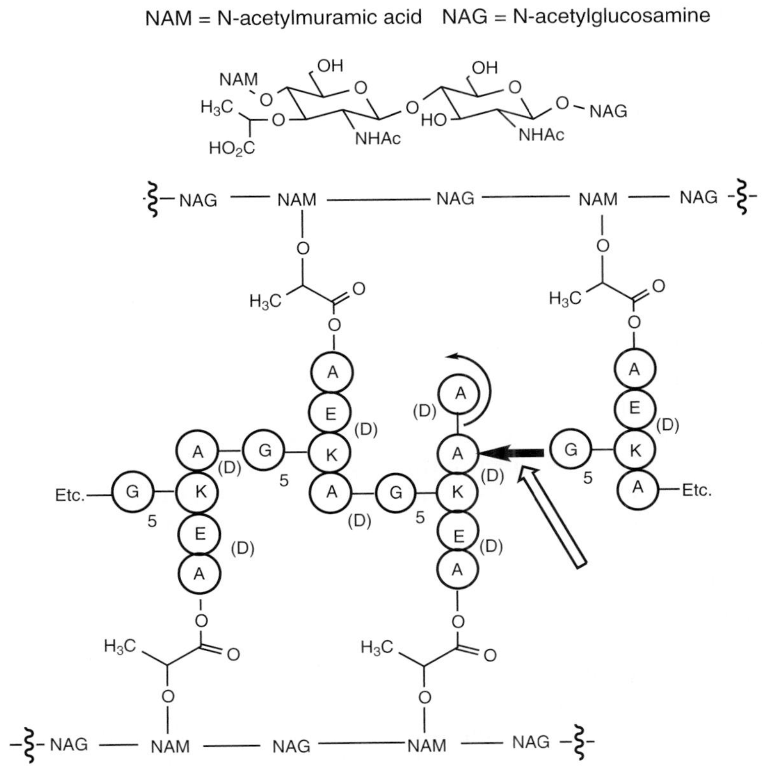

NAM = N-acetylmuramic acid NAG = N-acetylglucosamine

Figure 29.9 Schematic of cell wall cross-linking. Pentaglycyl group replaces terminal D-alanine.

stress and accounts for the retention of characteristic morphologic shape of gram-positive bacteria (globes and rods, for example). This step is highly sensitive to inhibition of β-lactam antibiotics. It is also the target of the glycopeptide antibiotics (such as vancomycin), as will be discussed later.

The peptidoglycan layer is traversed by complex glycophospholipids called teichoic and teichuronic acids. These are largely responsible for the acid mantle of gram-positive bacteria. Beneath the peptidoglycan layer is the lipoidal cytoplasmic cell membrane in which a number of important protein molecules float in a lipid bilayer. Among these proteins are the β-lactam targets, the PBPs.[31] These are enzymes that are important in cell wall formation and remodeling. In gram-positive bacteria, the outer layers are relatively ineffective in keeping antibiotics out.

The inner membrane and its protein components provide the principal barrier to uptake of antibiotics. There are a number of different types of PBPs (PBP-1a, PBP-1b, PBP-2, PBP2a, PBP-3, etc.), and their function is dependent on the species of bacteria and has been more fully reviewed elsewhere.[32] The functions of all of the PBPs are not entirely understood, but they are important in construction and repair of the cell wall. β-Lactam antibiotics bind to these proteins and kill bacteria by preventing the biosynthesis of a functional cell wall. Various β-lactam antibiotics display different patterns of binding to the PBPs. These proteins must alternate in a controlled and systematic way between their active and inert states so that bacterial cells can grow and multiply in an orderly manner. Selective interference by β-lactam antibiotics with their functioning prevents normal growth and repair and creates serious problems for bacteria, particularly young cells needing to grow and mature cells needing to repair damage or to divide.

Gram-Negative Bacteria. With the gram-negative bacteria, the cell wall is more complex and more lipoidal (Fig. 29.10). These cells usually contain an additional outer lipid membrane that differs considerably from the inner membrane. The outer layer contains complex lipopolysaccharides that encode antigenic responses, cause septic shock, provide the serotype, and influence morphology. This exterior layer also contains a number of enzymes and exclusionary proteins. Important among these are the porins. These are transmembranal supermolecules made up of two or three monomeric proteins. The center of this array is a transmembranal pore of various dimensions. Some allow many kinds of small molecules to pass, and others contain specific receptors that allow only certain molecules to come in. The size, shape, and lipophilicity of drugs are important considerations controlling porin passage. Antibiotics have greater difficulty in penetrating into gram-negative bacterial cells as a consequence. Next comes a periplasmic space containing a somewhat less impressive and thinner, as compared to gram-positive organisms, layer of peptidoglycan. Also present is a phospholipid-rich cytoplasmic membrane in which floats a series of characteristic proteins with various functions. The β-lactam targets (PBPs) are found here.

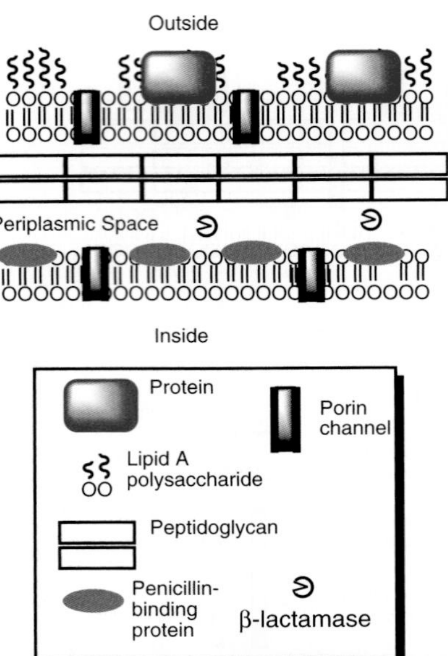

Figure 29.10 Schematic of some features of the gram-negative bacterial cell wall.

Other inner membrane proteins are involved in transport, energy, and biosynthesis. In many such cells, there are proteins that actively pump out antibiotics and other substances at the expense of energy and that may require the simultaneous entrance of oppositely charged materials to maintain an electrostatic balance.

β-LACTAM ANTIBIOTICS

α β

O N H

β-lactam
azetidinone

The name lactam is given to cyclic amides and is analogous to the name lactone given to cyclic esters. In an older nomenclature, the second carbon in an aliphatic carboxylic acid was designated alpha, the third beta, and so on. Thus a β-lactam is a cyclic amide with four atoms in its ring. The contemporary name for this ring system is azetidinone. This structural feature was very rare when it was found to be a feature of the structure of the penicillins, so the name β-lactam came to be a generic descriptor for the whole family. Ultimately, this ring proved to be the main component of the pharmacophore, so the term possesses medicinal as well as chemical significance. The penicillin subclass of β-lactam antibiotics is characterized by the presence of a substituted five-membered thiazolidine ring fused to the β-lactam ring. This fusion and the chirality of the β-lactam ring result in the molecule roughly possessing a "V" shape. This drastically interferes with the planarity of the lactam bond and inhibits resonance of the lactam nitrogen with its carbonyl group. Consequently, the β-lactam ring is much more reactive and thus more sensitive to nucleophilic attack when compared with normal planar amides.

History. The general story of the discovery of the penicillins was previously discussed. The earliest penicillins were produced by fungi from media constituents. The bicyclic heterocyclic nucleus of 6-aminopenicillanic acid is constructed by a process catalyzed by enzymes. The side chain was added essentially intact from media constituents. It was discovered that certain arylacetic acids, when added to the medium, were used to form the side chain amide moiety and that this was very important for stability and breadth of spectrum.[33] It was later discovered that exclusion of such materials from the medium allowed the production of 6-aminopenicillanic acid without a side chain.[34] Chemists could then add a wider variety of side chains without being limited by the specific requirements of the fungal enzymes. With this breakthrough, the penicillin field expanded to include orally active, broad-spectrum, and enzymatically stable penicillins. The cephalosporins were discovered as secondary metabolites of a different fungal species.[35] Because it was stable to many activity-destroying β-lactamases, its core nucleus, 7-aminocephalosporanic acid was substituted with a wide variety of unnatural side chains, and three generations of clinically useful analogues have resulted. Later work produced the carbapenems, monobactams, and β-lactamase inhibitors.[36-38] Many thousands of these compounds have been prepared by partial or total chemical synthesis, and a significant number of these remain on the market many years after their discovery.

Penicillins. The medicinal classifications, chemical structures, and generic names of the penicillins currently available are provided in Table 29.4.

Preparation of Penicillins. The original fermentation-derived penicillins were produced by growth of the fungus *Penicillium chrysogenum* on complex solid media with the result that they were mixtures differing from one another in the identity of the side chain moiety. When a sufficient supply of phenylacetic acid is present in liquid media, this is preferentially incorporated into the molecule to produce mainly benzylpenicillin (penicillin G in the old nomenclature). Use of phenoxyacetic acid instead leads to phenoxymethylpenicillin (penicillin V). More than two dozen different penicillins have been made in this way, but these two are the only ones that remain in clinical use. The complete exclusion of side chain precursor acids from the medium produces the fundamental penicillin nucleus, 6-aminopenicillanic acid (6-APA), but in poor yield. By itself, 6-APA has only very weak antibiotic activity, but when substituted on its primary amino group with a suitable acid to give amide side chains, its potency and antibacterial spectrum are profoundly enhanced. With this key precursor isolated, limitations caused by enzyme specificities in biosynthesis could be overcome by use of partial chemical synthesis.

The sodium and potassium salts of penicillins are crystalline, hydroscopic, and water soluble. They can be employed orally or parentally. When dry, they are stable for long periods, but they hydrolyze rapidly when in solution. Their best stability is noted at pH values between 5.5 and 8, especially at pH 6.0-7.2. The procaine and benzathine salts of benzylpenicillin, on the other hand, are water insoluble. Because they dissolve slowly, they are used for repository purposes following injection when long-term blood levels are required.

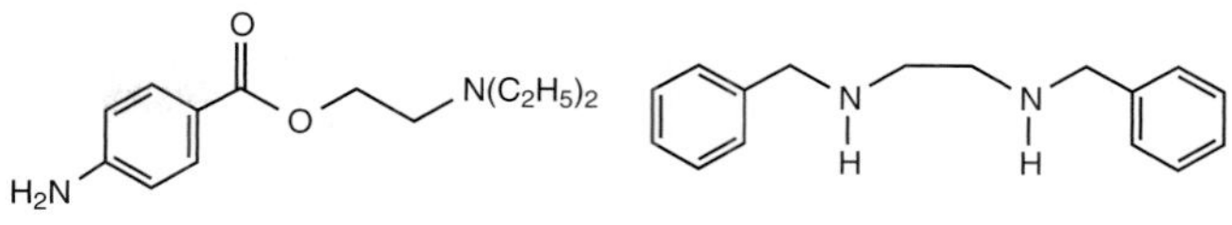

O
H_2N
O
$N(C_2H_5)_2$
N
H
N
H

Procaine   Benzathine

Nomenclature. The nomenclature of the penicillins, as with most antibiotics, is complex. The Chemical Abstracts system is definitive and unambiguous but too complex for ordinary use (Fig. 29.11). For example, the chemical name for benzylpenicillin sodium is monosodium (2*S*,5*R*,6*R*)-3,3-dimethyl-7-oxo)-6-(2-phenylacetamido)-4-thia-l-azabicyclo[3.2.0]heptane-2-carboxylate. A simpler system has stood the test of time and involves taking the repeating unit, carbonyl-6-APA, and adding to this the chemical trivial name for the added radical that completes the structure. The use of the names benzylpenicillin and phenoxymethylpenicillin makes practical sense. There are three asymmetric centers in the benzylpenicillin molecule as indicated by the asterisk in Table 29.4. This absolute stereochemistry must be preserved for useful antibiotic activity.

Clinically Relevant Chemical Instabilities. The most unstable bond in the penicillin molecule is the highly strained and reactive β-lactam amide bond. This bond cleaves moderately slowly in water unless heated, but breaks down much more rapidly in alkaline solutions to produce penicilloic acid, which readily decarboxylates to produce penilloic acid (Fig. 29.12). Penicilloic acid has a negligible tendency to reclose to the corresponding penicillin, so this reaction is essentially irreversible under physiologic conditions. Because the β-lactam ring is an essential portion of the pharmacophore, its hydrolysis deactivates the antibiotic. A fairly significant degree of hydrolysis also takes place in the liver. The bacterial enzyme, β-lactamase, catalyzes this reaction also and is a principal cause of bacterial resistance in the clinic. Alcohols and amines bring about the same cleavage reaction, but the products are the corresponding esters and amides. These products are inactive. A reaction with a specific primary amino group of aminoglycoside antibiotics is of clinical relevance as it inactivates penicillins and cephalosporins and will be discussed later in the chapter. When proteins serve as the nucleophiles in this reaction, the antigenic conjugates that cause many penicillin allergies are produced. Small molecules that are not inherently antigenic but react with proteins to produce antigens in this manner are called haptens. Commercially available penicillin salts may be contaminated with small amounts of these antigenic penicilloyl proteins derived from reaction with proteins encountered in their fermentative production or by high-molecular-weight self-condensation–derived polymers resulting when penicillins are concentrated and react with themselves. Both of these classes of impurities are antigenic and may sensitize some patients.

In acidic solutions, the hydrolysis of penicillins is complex. Hydrolysis of the β-lactam bond can be shown

Table 29.4 Commercially Significant Penicillins and Related Molecules

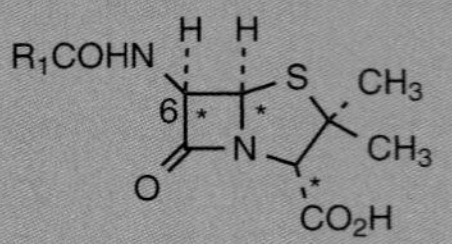

(Core structure: R_1COHN–6-position penicillin nucleus with S, CH_3, CH_3, CO_2H)

Generic Name	Trade Name	R_1
Fermentation-Derived Penicillins		
6-Aminopenicillanic acid		H
Benzylpenicillin (Penicillin G)	Generic	C_6H_5-CH_2–
Phenoxymethylpenicillin (Penicillin V)	Generic	C_6H_5-OCH_2–
Semisynthetic Penicillinase-Resistant Parenteral Penicillins		
Nafcillin	Nallpen, Unipen	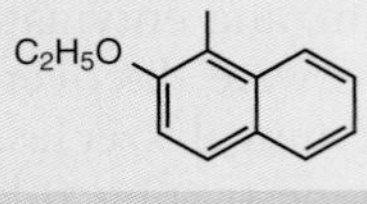 C_2H_5O (naphthyl structure)
Semisynthetic Penicillinase-Resistant Oral Penicillins		
Oxacillin (X = Y = H)	Generic	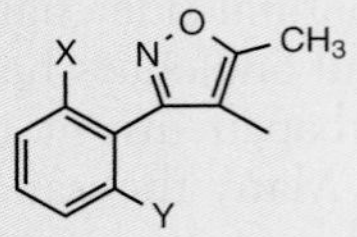 X, Y, CH_3 (isoxazolyl structure)
Dicloxacillin (X = Y = Cl)	Generic	
Semisynthetic Penicillinase-Sensitive, Broad Spectrum, Parenteral Penicillins		
Ticarcillin (in combination with clavulanic acid)	Timentin	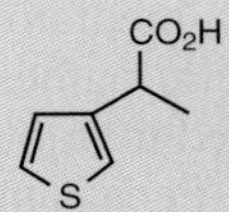 CO_2H, S (thienyl structure)
Piperacillin (in combination with tazobactam)	Zosyn	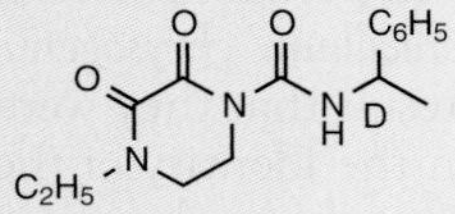 C_6H_5, D, C_2H_5 (piperazinedione structure)
Semisynthetic Penicillinase-Sensitive, Broad-Spectrum, Oral Penicillins		
Ampicillin (X = H)	Generic	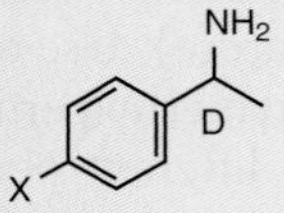 NH_2, D, X (phenylglycyl structure)
Amoxicillin (X = OH)	Amoxil, Trimox	

through kinetic analysis to involve participation of the side chain amide oxygen because the rate of this reaction differs widely depending on the nature of the *R* group. The main end products of the acidic degradation are penicillamine, penilloic acid, and penilloaldehyde (Fig. 29.13). The intermediate penicillenic acid is highly unstable and undergoes subsequent hydrolysis to the corresponding penicilloic acid. An alternate pathway involves sulfur ejection to a product that in turn fragments to liberate penicilloic acid also. Penicilloic acid readily decarboxylates to penilloic acid. The latter hydrolyzes to produce penilloaldehyde and penicillamine (itself used clinically as a chelating agent). Several related fragmentations to a variety of other products take place. None of these products has antibacterial activity. At gastric pH (~2.0) and a temperature of 37°C, benzylpenicillin has a half-life measured in minutes. The less water-soluble amine salts are more stable.

Structure-Activity Relationship. The chemical substituents attached to the penicillin nucleus can greatly influence the stability of the penicillins as well as the spectrum of activity. It is important to recognize whether the structural changes affect drug stability on the shelf or in the GI tract (in vivo), improve stability toward bacterial metabolism, or enlarge the spectrum of activity.

The substitution of a side chain R group on the primary amine of 6-APA with an electron-withdrawing group decreases the electron density on the side chain carbonyl and protects these penicillins in part from acid degradation.

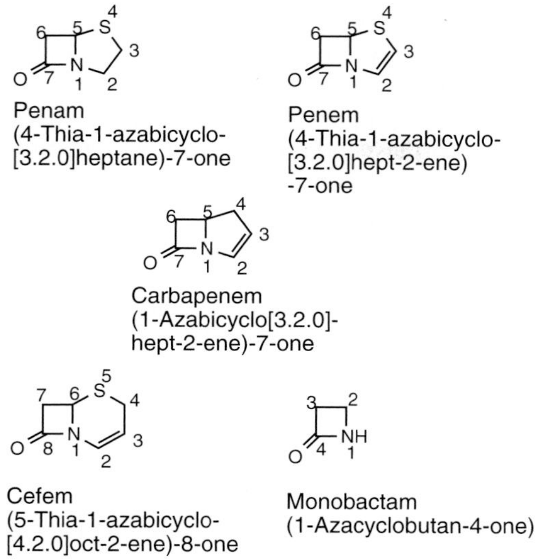

Penam
(4-Thia-1-azabicyclo-[3.2.0]heptane)-7-one

Penem
(4-Thia-1-azabicyclo-[3.2.0]hept-2-ene)-7-one

Carbapenem
(1-Azabicyclo[3.2.0]-hept-2-ene)-7-one

Cefem
(5-Thia-1-azabicyclo-[4.2.0]oct-2-ene)-8-one

Monobactam
(1-Azacyclobutan-4-one)

Figure 29.11 Ring and numbering systems of clinically available β-lactam antibiotic types.

This property has clinical implications because these compounds survive passage through the stomach better and many can be given orally for systemic purposes. The survival of passage and degree of absorption under fasting conditions are shown in Table 29.5.

In addition, in vitro degradation reactions of penicillins can be retarded by keeping the pH of solutions between 6.0 and 6.8 and by refrigerating them. Metal ions such as mercury, zinc, and copper catalyze the degradation of penicillins so they should be kept from contact with penicillin solutions. The lids of containers used today are commonly made from inert materials in part to minimize such problems.

The more lipophilic the side chain of a penicillin, the more serum protein bound the antibiotic (Table 29.6).

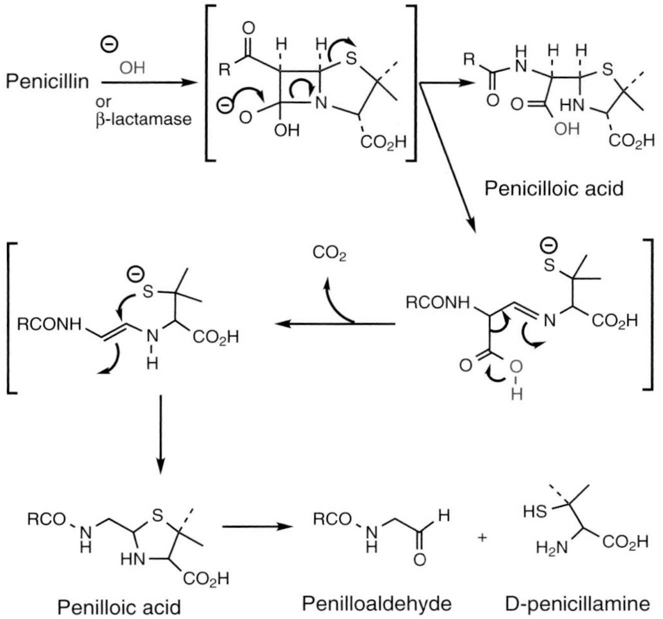

Penicillin —(OH⁻ or β-lactamase)→ ... Penicilloic acid → ... (CO_2) → Penilloic acid → Penilloaldehyde + D-penicillamine

Figure 29.12 Instability of β-lactams to nucleophiles.

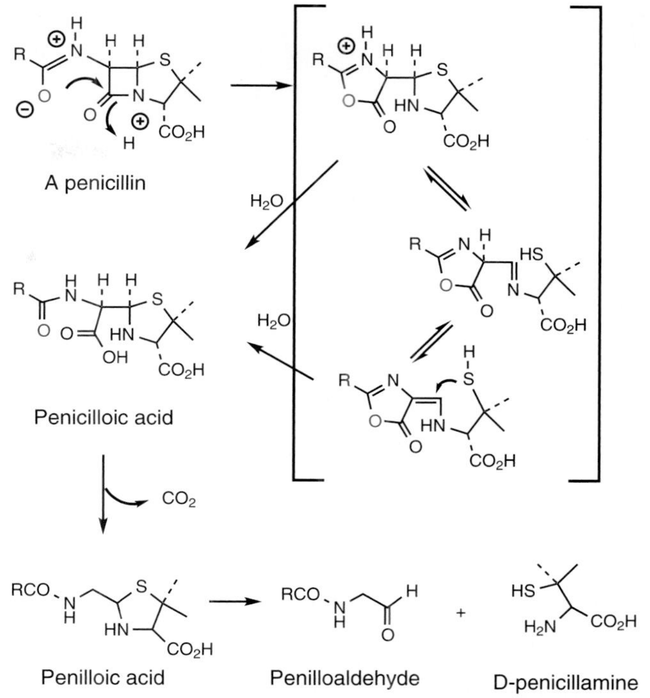

A penicillin → ... (H_2O) → Penicilloic acid; → (CO_2) → Penilloic acid → Penilloaldehyde + D-penicillamine

Figure 29.13 Instability of penicillins in acid. Hydrolysis involves the C-6 side chain.

Although this has some advantages in terms of protection from degradation, it does reduce measurably the effective bactericidal concentration of the drug in whole blood. The degree of serum protein binding of the penicillins has comparatively little influence on their half-lives. The penicillins are actively excreted into the urine via an active

Table 29.5 Improved Acid Stability and Absorption of Substituted Penicillins

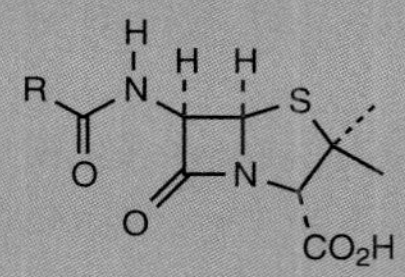

Drug	R	% Absorption Intact Drug
Benzylpenicillin	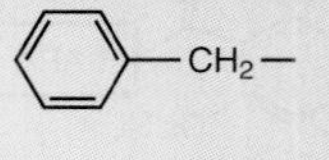 C_6H_5—CH_2—	15-30
Penicillin V	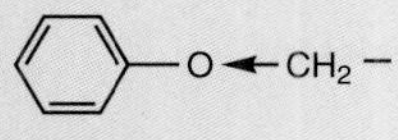 C_6H_5—O—CH_2—	60-73
Ampicillin	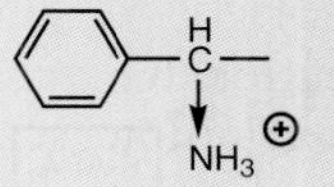 C_6H_5—CH(NH_3^+)—	30-50
Amoxicillin	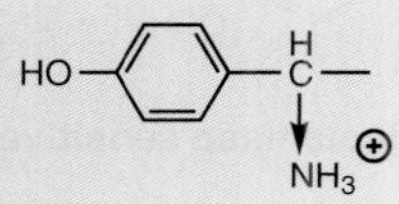 HO—C_6H_4—CH(NH_3^+)—	75-90

Table 29.6 Protein Binding of Penicillins

Penicillin	Protein Binding (%)
Benzyl penicillin	45-68
Phenoxymethyl penicillin	75-89
Methicillin	35-80
Ampicillin	25-30
Amoxicillin	25-30
Carbenicillin	~50
Oxacillin	>90
Cloxacillin	>90

transport system for weak acids, and the rate of release from their protein-bound form is sufficiently rapid that the controlling rate is the kidney secretion rate. The serum half-life of penicillin G is about 0.4-0.9 hours, and that of phenoxymethylpenicillin is about 0.5 hours. Both are excreted into the urine by tubular excretion. Probenecid, when present, competes effectively for excretion and thus prolongs the half-life.

Stability of the penicillins toward β-lactamase is influenced by the bulk in the acyl group attached to the primary amine. β-Lactamases are much less tolerant to the presence of steric hindrance near the side chain amide bond than are the PBPs. The stability of methicillin (discontinued in the United States) to β-lactamases is an example of this. When the aromatic ring is attached directly to the side chain carbonyl and both ortho positions are substituted by methoxy groups, β-lactamase stability results (Fig. 29.14). Movement of one of the methoxy groups to the para position or replacing one of them with a hydrogen results in an analogue sensitive to β-lactamases. Putting in a methylene between the aromatic ring and 6-APA likewise produces a β-lactamase–sensitive agent (Fig. 29.14). These findings provide strong support for the hypothesis that its resistance to enzyme degradation is based on differential steric hindrance. Prime examples of this effect are seen in nafcillin and dicloxacillin (Table 29.4).

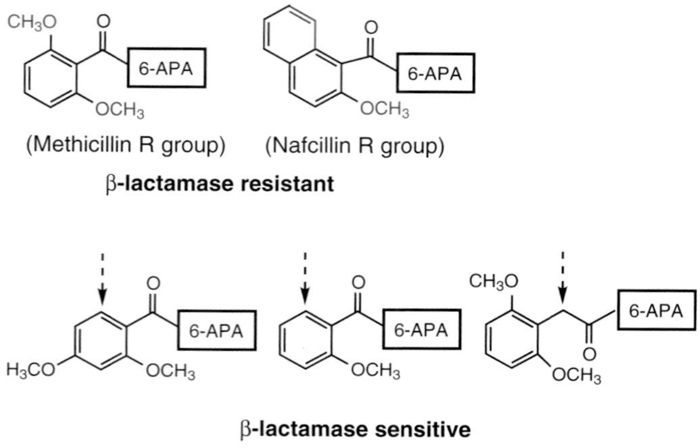

Figure 29.14 β-lactamase–resistant/–sensitive structural features.

Mechanism of Action. The molecular mode of action of the β-lactam antibiotics is a selective and irreversible inhibition of the enzymes processing the developing peptidoglycan layer (Fig. 29.15). Just before cross-linking occurs, the peptide pendant from the lactate carboxyl of a muramic acid unit terminates in a D-alanyl-D-alanine unit. The terminal D-alanine unit is exchanged for a glycine unit on an adjacent strand in a reaction catalyzed by a cell wall transamidase. This enzyme is one of the PBPs (carboxypeptidases, endopeptidases, and transpeptidases) that normally reside in the bacterial inner membrane and perform construction, repair, and housekeeping functions, maintaining cell wall integrity and playing a vital role in cell growth and division. They differ significantly between species and even individual strains, and this fact is used to rationalize different potency and morphologic outcomes following β-lactam attack on the different bacteria. The cell wall transamidase uses a serine hydroxyl group to attack the penultimate D-alanyl unit forming a covalent ester bond, and the terminal D-alanine, which is released by this action, diffuses away. The enzyme-peptidoglycan ester bond is attacked by the free amino end of a pentaglycyl unit of an adjacent strand, regenerating the transpeptidase's active site for further catalytic action and producing a new amide bond, which connects two adjacent strands together.

The three-dimensional geometry of the active site of the enzyme perfectly accommodates to the shape and separation of the amino acids of its substrate. Because the substrate has unnatural stereochemistry at the critical residues, this enzyme is not expected to attack host peptides or even other bacterial peptides composed of natural amino acids.

The penicillins and the other β-lactam antibiotics have a structure that closely resembles that of acylated D-alanyl-D-alanine. The enzyme mistakenly accepts the penicillin as though it were its normal substrate. The highly strained β-lactam ring is much more reactive than a normal amide moiety, particularly when fused into the appropriate bicyclic system. The intermediate acyl-enzyme complex, however, is rather different structurally from the normal intermediate in that the hydrolysis does not break penicillin into two pieces as it does with its normal substrate. In the penicillins, a heterocyclic residue is still covalently bonded and cannot diffuse away as the natural terminal D-alanine unit does. This presents a steric barrier to approach by the nearby pentaglycyl unit and thus keeps the enzyme's active site from being regenerated and the cell wall precursors from being cross-linked. The result is a defective cell wall and an inactivated enzyme. The relief of strain that is obtained on enzymatic β-lactam bond cleavage is so pronounced that there is virtually no tendency for the reaction to reverse. Water is also an insufficiently effective nucleophile and cannot hydrolyze the complex either. Thus, the cell wall transamidase is stoichiometrically inactivated. The gaps in the cell wall produced by this covalent interruption are not filled in because the enzyme is now inactivated. The resulting cell wall is structurally weak and subject to osmotic stress. Cell lysis can result, and the cell rapidly dies assisted by another class of bacterial enzymes, the autolysins.[39]

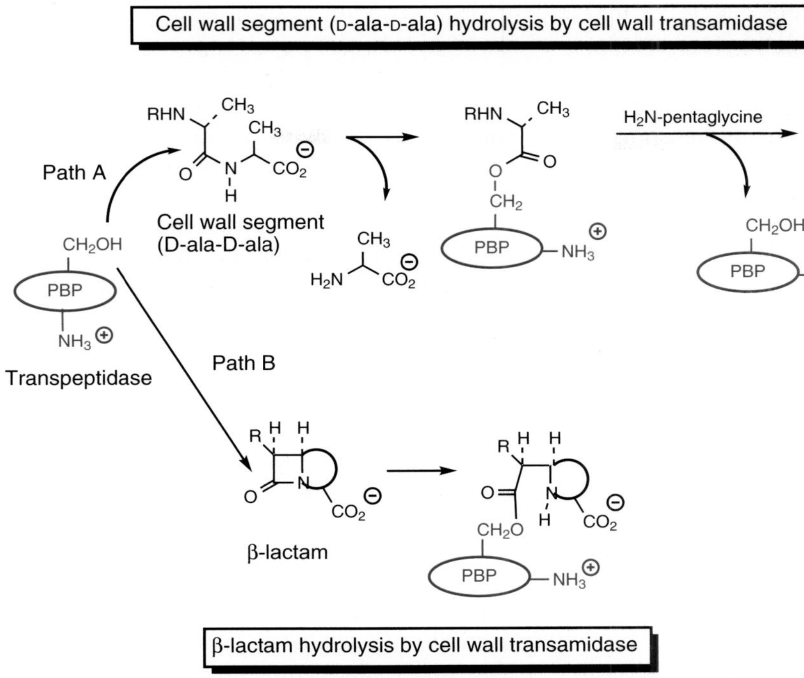

Figure 29.15 Cell wall cross-linking and mechanism of action of β-lactams. Path A represents the normal cross-linking mechanism. Path B illustrates the reaction of β-lactam antibiotics with the penicillin-binding protein (PBP).

Resistance. The first literature reports of a penicillinase were published in 1940.[40] This phenomenon was rare at the time and caused no particular alarm. Resistance to β-lactam antibiotics is unfortunately increasingly common and is rather alarming. It can be intrinsic and involve decreased cellular uptake of drug, or involve lower binding affinity to the PBPs. This is particularly the case with MRSA. MRSA produces a mutated PBP-2 (PBP-2a) that does not efficiently bind methicillin any longer. More common, however, is the production of β-lactamases. β-Lactamases are enzymes (usually serine proteases) elaborated by microorganisms that catalyze hydrolysis of the β-lactam bond and inactivate β-lactam antibiotics to penicilloic acids before they can reach the PBPs (Fig. 29.16). They somewhat resemble the cell wall transamidase, which is the usual target. Hydrolytic regeneration of the active site is dramatically more facile with β-lactamases than is the case with cell wall transamidase, so that the enzyme can turn over many times and a comparatively small amount of enzyme can destroy a large amount of drug. With gram-positive bacteria, such as staphylococci, the β-lactamases are usually shed continuously into the medium and meet the drug outside the cell wall (see Fig. 29.8). They are biosynthesized in significant quantities. With gram-negative bacteria, a more conservative course is followed. Here the β-lactamases are secreted into the periplasmic space between the inner and outer membrane so, while still distal to the PBPs, they do not readily escape into the medium and need not be resynthesized as often (see Fig. 29.10). Numerous β-lactamases with various antibiotic substrate specificities are now known. Various classification systems are used for β-lactamases and have been extensively reviewed.[32] The clinical relevance of β-lactamases is becoming increasingly important as more destructive examples known as ESBL's (extended spectrum β-lactamases) become more commonly encountered. These β-lactamases are capable of inactivation of many previously stable β-lactams. This is an intensive area of research and is frequently updated as new information is discovered.[41] Elaboration of β-lactamases is often R-factor mediated and, in some cases, is even induced by the presence of β-lactam antibiotics.

Allergenicity. It is estimated that 2%-8% of the US population is allergic to β-lactam antibiotics. The actual number is very difficult to determine due to overreporting. Most commonly, the allergy is expressed as a mild drug rash or itching and is of delayed onset. Occasionally, the reaction is immediate and profound. It may include cardiovascular collapse and shock and can result in death. Sometimes penicillin allergy can be anticipated by taking a medication history, and often, patients likely to be allergic are those with a history of hypersensitivity to a wide variety of allergens (e.g.,

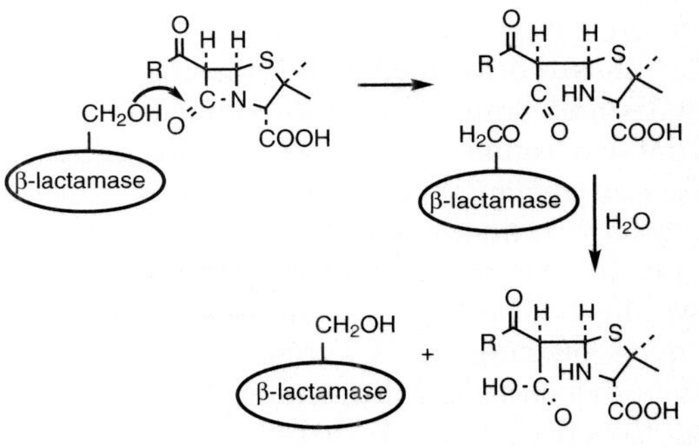

Figure 29.16 β-lactamase–catalyzed hydrolysis of penicillins.

foods and pollens). A prior history of allergy to penicillins is a contraindicating factor to their use. Skin tests are available when there is doubt. When an allergic reaction develops, the drug must be discontinued and, because cross-sensitivity is relatively common, other β-lactam families should be used carefully. Considering all therapeutic categories, penicillins are probably the drugs most associated with allergy. Erythromycin and clindamycin are useful alternate choices for therapy in many cases of penicillin allergy.

In some cases, the patient may have become sensitized without knowing it due to prior passive exposure through contaminated foodstuffs or cross-contaminated medications. Generally, penicillins are manufactured in facilities separate from those used to prepare other drugs in order to prevent cross contamination and possible sensitization. Animals treated with penicillins are required to be drug free for a significant time before products prepared from them can be consumed. Because the origin of the allergy is a haptenic reaction with host proteins and the responsible bond in the drug is the β-lactam moiety, this side effect is caused by the pharmacophore of the drug and is unlikely to be overcome by molecular manipulation.

Individual Penicillins. The penicillins are usually discussed under various groups based on spectrum of activity and sensitivity or resistance toward β-lactamase. One of the earliest and still most commonly used penicillins is benzylpenicillin.

Benzylpenicillin Group

Benzylpenicillin (Penicillin G, Table 29.4). With the exception of *Neisseria gonorrhoeae* and *Haemophilus influenzae*, and a few bacteria encountered less frequently, the useful antimicrobial spectrum of benzylpenicillin is primarily against gram-positive cocci. Because of its cheapness, efficacy, and lack of toxicity (except for acutely allergic patients), benzylpenicillin remains a remarkably useful agent for treatment of diseases caused by susceptible microorganisms. As with most antibiotics, susceptibility tests must be performed because many formerly highly sensitive microorganisms are now comparatively resistant. Infections of the upper and lower respiratory tract and the genitourinary tract are the particular province of benzylpenicillin. Infections caused by group A β-hemolytic streptococci (pharyngitis, scarlet fever, cellulitis, pelvic infections, and septicemia) are commonly responsive. Group B hemolytic streptococci infections, especially of neonates (acute respiratory distress, pneumonia, meningitis, septic shock, and septicemia), also may respond.

Pneumococcal pneumonia, *H. influenzae* pneumonia of children, *Streptococcus pneumoniae*– and *Streptococcus pyogenes*–caused otitis media and sinusitis, meningococcal meningitis and brain abscess, meningococcal and pneumococcal septicemia, streptococcal endocarditis (often by *Streptococcus viridans*), pelvic inflammatory disease (often by *Neisseria gonorrhoeae* and *S. pyogenes*), uncomplicated gonorrhea (*N. gonorrhoeae*), meningitis (*Neisseria meningitidis*), syphilis (*Treponema pallidum*), Lyme disease (*Borrelia burgdorferi*), gas gangrene (*Clostridium perfringens*), and tetanus (*Clostridium tetani*) are among the diseases that may respond to benzylpenicillin therapy, either alone or sometimes with other drugs used in combination.

Non–penicillinase-producing *Staphylococcus aureus* and *Staphylococcus epidermidis* are quite sensitive but are very rare today. Other, less common, bacterial diseases also respond, such as those caused by *Bacillus anthracis* (anthrax) and *Corynebacterium diphtheriae* (diphtheria).

Because of its low cost, mild infections with susceptible microorganisms can be treated with comparatively large oral doses, although the most effective route of administration is parenteral because five times the blood level can be regularly achieved in this manner. As previously discussed (see previous section Clinically Relevant Chemical Instabilities), penicillin G is unstable under the acidic conditions of the stomach.

Very water-insoluble penicillin salts form with procaine and with N,N′-bibenzyl ethylenediamine. These find therapeutic application for intramuscular injections. This produces lower but prolonged levels of penicillin as the drug slowly diffuses from the injection site.

The need to improve defects in benzylpenicillin stimulated an intense research effort that persists to this day. Overcoming such negative features as comparative instability (particularly to acid), comparatively poor oral absorption, allergenicity, sensitivity to β-lactamases, and relatively narrow antimicrobial spectrum has been an objective of this work.

Phenoxymethylpenicillin (Penicillin V, Table 29.4). Penicillin V is produced by fermentation where the medium is enriched in phenoxyacetic acid. It can also be prepared by semisynthesis. It is considerably more acid stable than benzylpenicillin as indicated by oral absorption (Table 29.5). This is rationalized as being due to the electronegative oxygen atom in the C-7 amide side chain inhibiting participation in β-lactam bond hydrolysis. In any case, penicillin V was the first of the so-called oral penicillins giving higher and more prolonged blood levels than penicillin G itself. Its antimicrobial and clinical spectrum is roughly the same as that of benzylpenicillin, although it is somewhat less potent and is not used for acutely serious infections. Penicillin V has approximately the same sensitivity to β-lactamases and allergenicity as penicillin G.

HISTORICALLY SIGNIFICANT PENICILLINS

Methicillin is now archaic but was the first penicillinase-resistant agent to reach the clinic.[42] This compound was developed in response to the production of β-lactamases by gram-positive organisms against early penicillins. Although it has a narrow spectrum, it represented an effective therapy against these organisms.

Penicillinase-Resistant Penicillins

Nafcillin (Table 29.4). Nafcillin has a 2-ethoxynaphthyl side chain. This bulky group serves to inhibit destruction by β-lactamases analogous to methicillin. As discussed previously, increased steric bulk in the side chain leads to a β-lactamase–resistant drug. Nafcillin has a narrow antimicrobial spectrum so is used clinically for parenteral use in infections due to β-lactamase–producing *S. aureus* and a few other gram-positive organisms. An increasing number of infections are caused by MRSA. In these organisms, an altered PBP (PBP2A) is formed which has very low affinity for any of the β-lactams except for ceftaroline, a cephalosporin that was designed to target this altered PBP.

Dicloxacillin. Using a substituted isoxazolyl ring as a bioisosteric replacement for the benzene ring of penicillin G produces the isoxazolyl penicillins (oxacillin and dicloxacillin). These drugs are generally less potent than benzylpenicillin against gram-positive microorganisms (generally staphylococci and streptococci) that do not produce a β-lactamase but retain their potency against those that do. An added bonus exists in that they are somewhat more acid stable; thus they may be taken orally. Because they are highly serum protein bound (Table 29.6), they are not good choices for treatment of septicemia. Like nafcillin, the isoxazolyl group of penicillins is primarily used against penicillinase-producing *S. aureus*.[43,44]

Penicillinase-Sensitive, Broad-Spectrum, Oral Penicillins

Ampicillin. The first member of this group, ampicillin, is a benzylpenicillin analogue in which one of the hydrogen atoms of the side chain methylene has been replaced with a primary amino group to produce an *R*-phenylglycine moiety (Table 29.4). In addition to significant acid stability enhancing its successful oral use, the antimicrobial spectrum is shifted so that many common gram-negative pathogens are sensitive to ampicillin. This is believed to be due to greater penetration of ampicillin into gram-negative bacteria. The acid stability is generally believed to be caused by the electron-withdrawing character of the protonated primary amine group reducing the side chain carbonyl participation in hydrolysis of the β-lactam bond as well as to the comparative difficulty of bringing another positively charged species (H_3O^+) into the vicinity of the protonated amino group. The oral activity is also enhanced, in part, to active uptake by the dipeptide transporters.[45] It unfortunately lacks stability toward β-lactamases, and resistance is increasingly common. To assist with this, several β-lactamase inhibitors for coadministration (discussed below) have been developed that restore many penicillinase-producing strains to the clinical spectrum of the aminopenicillins. Ampicillin is essentially equivalent to benzylpenicillin for pneumococcal, streptococcal, and meningococcal infections, and many strains of gram-negative *Salmonella*, *Shigella*, *P. mirabilis*, and *E. coli*, as well as many strains of *H. influenzae* and *N. gonorrhoeae* respond well to oral treatment with ampicillin.

Amoxicillin (Table 29.4). Amoxicillin is a close analogue of ampicillin in which a para-phenolic hydroxyl group has been introduced into the side chain phenyl moiety. This adjusts the isoelectric point of the drug to a more acidic value and is believed to be partially responsible, along with the intestine dipeptide transporter, for the enhanced blood levels obtained with amoxicillin compared with ampicillin itself (Table 29.5). Better oral absorption leads to less disturbance of the normal GI flora and, therefore, less drug-induced diarrhea. The antimicrobial spectrum and clinical uses of amoxicillin are approximately the same as those of ampicillin.

The addition of clavulanic acid (below) to amoxicillin gives a combination (Augmentin) in which the clavulanic acid serves to protect amoxicillin to a considerable extent against β-lactamases. This expands the spectrum of activity to include organisms and strains that produce β-lactamases.

Clavulanic Acid

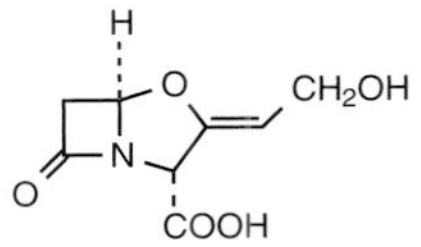

H O CH_2OH N O COOH

Clavulanic acid

Clavulanic acid is a mold product that has only weak intrinsic antibacterial activity but is an excellent irreversible inhibitor of most β-lactamases. It is believed to acylate the active site serine by mimicking the normal substrate. While hydrolysis occurs with some β-lactamases, in many cases, subsequent reactions occur that inhibit the enzyme irreversibly. This leads to its classification as a mechanism-based inhibitor (or so-called suicide substrate). The precise chemistry is not well understood (Fig. 29.17), but when clavulanic acid is added to amoxicillin and ticarcillin preparations, the potency against β-lactamase–producing strains is markedly enhanced.

Sulbactam

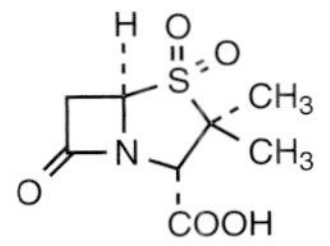

H O S O CH_3 CH_3 N O COOH

Sulbactam

Another β-lactamase inhibitor is sulbactam. Sulbactam is prepared by partial chemical synthesis from penicillins. The oxidation of the sulfur atom to a sulfone greatly enhances the potency of sulbactam. The combination of sulbactam and ampicillin (Unasyn) is also clinically popular. Not all β-lactamases are sensitive to the presence of clavulanic acid or sulbactam.

Penicillinase-Sensitive, Broad-Spectrum, Parenteral Penicillins

Ticarcillin. Ticarcillin is a sulfur-based bioisostere of benzylpenicillin in which one of the methylene hydrogens of the side chain has been substituted with a carboxylic acid moiety (Table 29.4). Ticarcillin is classified as a carboxy penicillin. The addition of this functional group increases the water solubility of the drug and significantly enhances the potency against gram-negative organisms by increasing penetration through hydrophilic porins in these organisms. The drug is susceptible to β-lactamases and is acid unstable and thus must be given by injection.

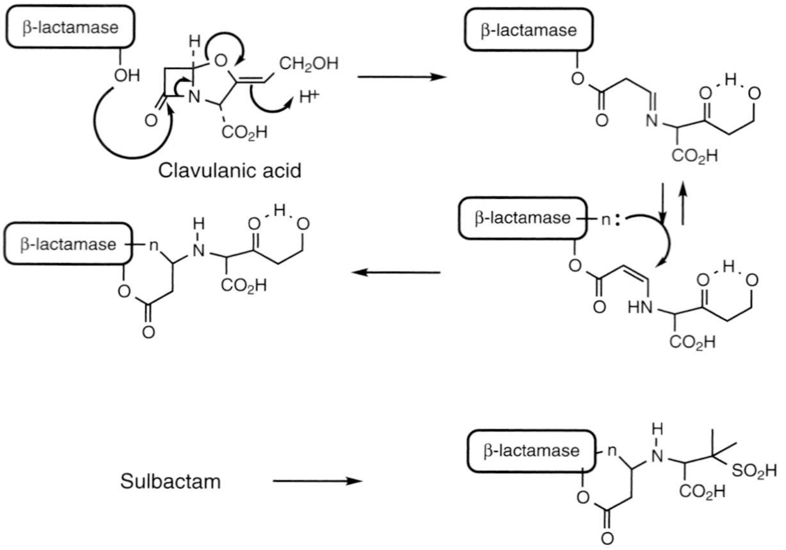

Figure 29.17 Speculative mechanism for irreversible inactivation of β-lactamase by clavulanic acid and sulbactam.

When potassium clavulanate is added to ticarcillin (Timentin), the combination has enhanced spectrum due to its enhanced stability to lactamases.

Piperacillin. Piperacillin is an ampicillin derivative in which the D-side chain amino group has been converted by chemical processes to a substituted urea analogue (Table 29.4). This ampicillin analogue is referred to as an acylureidopenicillin and preserve the useful anti–gram-positive activity of ampicillin but has a higher anti–gram-negative potency. Some strains of *P. aeruginosa* are sensitive to this agent. It is speculated that the added side chain moiety mimics a longer segment of the peptidoglycan chain than ampicillin does. This cell wall fragment is usually a tetrapeptide, so there is expected to be room for an extension in this direction. This would give more possible points of attachment to the penicillin-binding proteins, and perhaps these features are responsible for the enhanced antibacterial properties. This agent is used parenterally with particular emphasis on gram-negative bacteria, especially *K. pneumoniae* and the anaerobe, *B. fragilis*.[46] Resistance due to β-lactamases is a prominent feature of its use, so antimicrobial susceptibility testing and incorporation of additional agents (such as an aminoglycoside) for the treatment of severe infections are advisable.

Piperacillin and Tazobactam Combination (Zosyn)

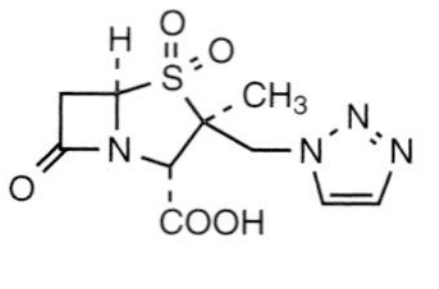

Tazobactam

Tazobactam is often coadministered with piperacillin because of tazobactam's ability to inhibit β-lactamases. Tazobactam, like other β-lactamase inhibitors, has little or no antibacterial activity.

This effect is analogous to that of clavulanic acid and sulbactam discussed earlier. This combination is the broadest spectrum penicillin currently available.[46]

Summary. The penicillins ushered in the era of powerful antibiotics, and their use transformed the practice of antimicrobial chemotherapy. A significant percentage of the population that is alive today owes their longevity and relative freedom from morbidity to the use of these agents. The pace of discovery has fallen off dramatically, and no new penicillin has been introduced into the market for many years. Instead, although retaining their important place in contemporary medicine, research has turned elsewhere for novel agents.

Cephalosporins

History. In contrast to the discovery of the penicillins, in which the first agent had such outstanding biologic antibiotic properties that it entered clinical use with comparatively little modification, the cephalosporins are remarkable for the level of persistence required before their initial discovery yielded economic returns. Abraham and Newton described the structure of the first cephalosporin, cephalosporin C.[35] The compound was interesting because, although it was not very potent, it had activity against some penicillin-resistant cultures due to its stability to β-lactamases. Cephalosporin C is not potent enough to be a useful antibiotic, but removal, through chemical means, of the natural side chain produced 7-aminocephalosporanic acid, which, analogous to 6-APA, could be fitted with unnatural side chains (Fig. 29.18). Many of the compounds produced in this way are remarkably useful antibiotics. They differ from one another in antimicrobial spectrum, β-lactamase stability, absorption from the GI tract, metabolism, stability, and side effects as detailed below.

Chemical Properties. The cephalosporins have their β-lactam ring annealed to a six-membered dihydrothiazine ring, in contrast to the penicillins where the β-lactam ring is fused to a five-membered thiazolidine ring.

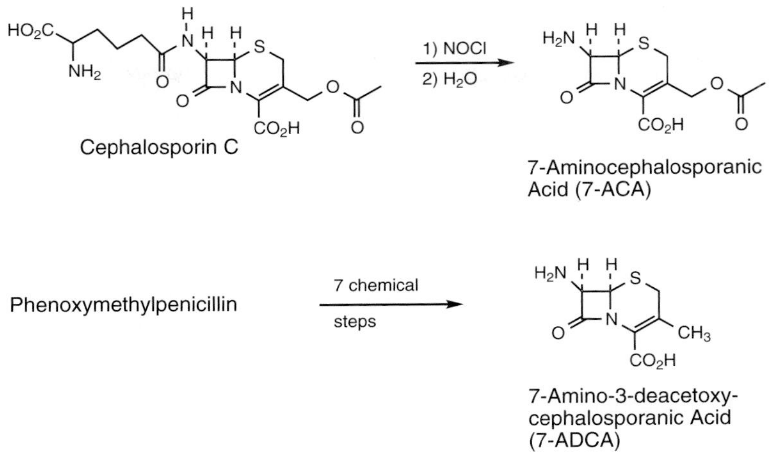

Figure 29.18 Chemical preparation of 7-ACA and 7-ADCA.

As a consequence of the bigger ring, the cephalosporins should be less strained and less reactive/potent. However, much of the reactivity loss is made up by possession of an olefinic linkage at C-2,3 and a methyleneacetoxy or other leaving group at C-3. When the β-lactam ring is opened by hydrolysis, the leaving group can be ejected, carrying away the developing negative charge. This greatly reduces the energy required for the process. Thus the facility with which the β-lactam bond of the cephalosporins is broken is modulated both by the nature of the C-7 substituent (analogous to the penicillins) as well as the nature of the C-3 substituent and its ability to serve as a leaving group. Considerable support for this hypothesis comes from the finding that isomerization of the olefinic linkage to C-3,4 leads to great losses in antibiotic activity. In practice, most cephalosporins are comparatively unstable in aqueous solutions, and the pharmacist is often directed to keep injectable preparations frozen before use. Being carboxylic acids, they form water-soluble sodium salts, whereas the free acids are comparatively water insoluble.

Clinically Relevant Chemical Instabilities. The principal chemical instability of the cephalosporins is associated with β-lactam bond hydrolysis. The role of the C-7 and C-3 side chains in these reactions was discussed previously. Ejection of the C-3 substituent following β-lactam–bond cleavage is usually drawn for convenience as though this is an unbroken (concerted) process, although ejection of the side chain may at certain times and with specific cephalosporins involve a discrete intermediate with the β-lactam bond broken, but the C-3 substituent not yet eliminated, while other cephalosporins have nonejectable C-3 substituents. The methylthiotetrazole (MTT) group, found in a number of cephalosporins, is capable of elimination. When this happens, this moiety is believed to be responsible in part for clotting difficulties and acute alcohol intolerance in certain patients. The role of the C-7 side chain in all of these processes is clearly important, but active participation of the amide moiety in a manner analogous to the penicillins is rarely specifically involed. The same considerations that modulate the chemical stability of cephalosporins are also involved in dictating β-lactamase sensitivity, potency, and allergenicity.

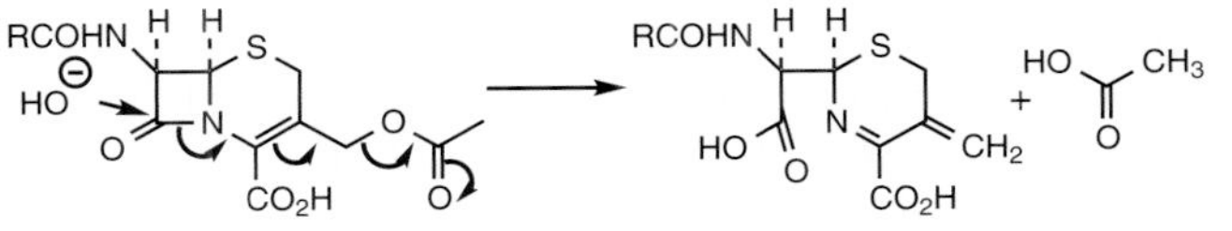

Metabolism. Those cephalosporins that have an acetyl group in the side chain are subject to enzymatic hydrolysis in the body. This results in a molecule with a hydroxymethyl moiety at C-3. A hydroxy moiety is a poor leaving group, so this change is considerably deactivating with respect to breakage of the β-lactam bond. In addition, the particular geometry of this part of the molecule leads to facile lactonization with the carboxyl group attached to C-2 (Fig. 29.19). In principle, this should result in formation of a different but reasonable leaving group. The result is, instead, inactivation of the drugs involved. The PBPs have an absolute requirement for a free carboxyl group to mimic that of the terminal carboxyl of the D-alanyl-D-alanine moiety in their normal substrate. Lactonization masks this docking functional group and, as a result, blocks affinity of the inhibitor for the enzyme.

Structure-Activity Relationship

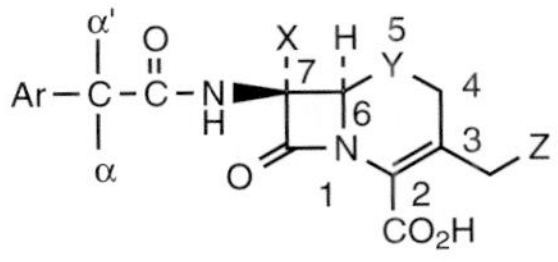

As with the penicillins, various molecular changes in the cephalosporin can improve in vitro stability, antibacterial activity, and stability toward β-lactamases.[47] The addition of an amino and a hydrogen to the α and α′ positions, respectively, results in a basic compound that is protonated under the acidic conditions of the stomach. The ammonium ion improves the stability of the β-lactam of the cephalosporin, leading to orally active drugs.

The 7β amino group is essential for antimicrobial activity (X = H), whereas replacement of the hydrogen at C-7 (X = H) with an alkoxy (X = OR) results in improvement of the antibacterial activity of the cephalosporin.

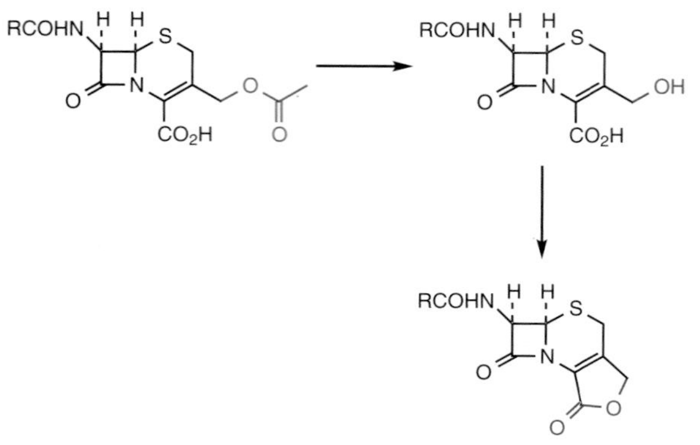

Figure 29.19 Metabolism of C-3-acetyl–substituted cephalosporins.

Within specific cephalosporin derivatives, the addition of a 7α methoxy also improves the drugs stability toward β-lactamase. The derivatives where Y = S exhibit greater antibacterial activity than if Y = O, but the reverse is true when stability toward β-lactamase is considered. The 6α hydrogen is essential for biologic activity. And finally, antibacterial activity is improved when Z is a five-membered heterocycle versus a six-membered heterocycle.

In a study examining stability of cephalosporins toward β-lactamase, it was noted that the following changes improved β-lactamase resistance: (1) the L-isomer of an α amino α′ hydrogen derivative of a cephalosporin was 30-40 times more stable than the D-isomer; (2) the addition of a methoxyoxime to the α and α′ positions increased stability nearly 100-fold; and (3) the Z-oxime was as much as 20,000-fold more stable than the *E*-oxime (Fig. 29.20).[47] These changes have been incorporated into a number of marketed and experimental cephalosporins (e.g., cefuroxime, ceftizoxime, ceftazidime, cefixime).

Mechanism of Action. The cephalosporins are believed to act in a manner analogous to that of the penicillins by binding to the penicillin-binding proteins followed by cell lysis (Fig. 29.15). Cephalosporins are bactericidal in clinical terms.

Resistance. Analogous to the penicillins, susceptible cephalosporins can be hydrolyzed by β-lactamases before they reach the penicillin-binding proteins. Certain β-lactamases are constitutive (chromosomally encoded) in certain strains of gram-negative bacteria (*Citrobacter*, *Enterobacter*, *Pseudomonas*, and *Serratia*) and are normally repressed. These can be induced by certain β-lactam antibiotics (e.g., imipenem, cefotetan, and cefoxitin). As with the penicillins, specific examples will be seen below wherein resistance to β-lactamase hydrolysis is conveyed by strategic steric bulk near the side chain amide linkage. Penetration barriers to the cephalosporins are also known.

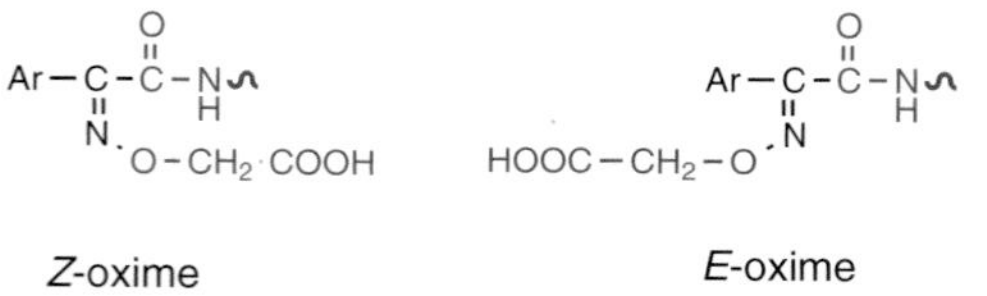

Z-oxime

E-oxime

Figure 29.20 Z and E oxime configuation.

Allergenicity. Allergenicity is less commonly experienced and is less severe with cephalosporins than with penicillins. Cephalosporins are frequently administered to patients who have had a mild or delayed penicillin reaction; however, cross allergenicity is possible, and this should be done with caution for patients with a history of allergies. Patients who have had a rapid and severe reaction to penicillins should not be treated with cephalosporins.

Nomenclature and Classification. Most cephalosporins have generic names beginning with cef- or ceph-. This is convenient for classification but makes discriminating between individual members a true memory test. The cephalosporins are classified by a trivial nomenclature system loosely derived from the chronology of their introduction but more closely related to their antimicrobial spectrum. The first-generation cephalosporins are primarily active in vitro against gram-positive cocci (penicillinase-positive and -negative *S. aureus* and *S. epidermis*), group A β-hemolytic streptococci (*S. pyogenes*), group B streptococci (*S. agalactiae*), and *S. pneumoniae*. They are not effective against MRSA. They are not significantly active against gram-negative bacteria, although some strains of *E. coli*, *K. pneumoniae*, *P. mirabilis*, and *Shigella* sp. may be sensitive.[48] The second-generation cephalosporins generally retain the anti–gram-positive activity of the first-generation agents but include *H. influenzae* as well and add to this better anti–gram-negative activity, so that some strains of *Acinetobacter*, *Citrobacter*, *Enterobacter*, *E. coli*, *Klebsiella*, *Neisseria*, *Proteus*, *Providencia*, and *Serratia* are also sensitive.[49] Cefotetan and cefoxitin also have anti-anaerobic activity as well.[50] The third-generation cephalosporins are less active against staphylococci than the first-generation agents but are much more active against gram-negative bacteria than either the first- or the second-generation drugs.[51] They are frequently particularly useful against nosocomial multidrug-resistant hospital-acquired strains. *Morganella* sp. and *P. aeruginosa* can also be added to the list of species that are often sensitive. Newer third-generation agents have been combined with β-lactamase inhibitors to further improve the spectrum against β-lactamase–producing strains. The fourth-generation cephalosporins have an antibacterial spectrum like the third-generation drugs but add some enterobacteria that are resistant to the third-generation cephalosporins. They are also more active against some gram-positive organisms.[52]

Therapeutic Application. The incidence of cephalosporin resistance is such that it is usually preferable to do sensitivity testing before instituting therapy. Infections of the upper and lower respiratory tract, skin and related soft tissue, urinary tract, bones, and joints, as well as septicemias, endocarditis, intra-abdominal, and bile tract infections caused by susceptible gram-positive organisms are usually responsive to cephalosporins. When gram-positive bacteria are involved, a first-generation agent is preferable. When the pathogen is gram-negative and the infection is serious, parenteral use of a third-generation agent is recommended.

Adverse Effects. Aside from mild or severe allergic reaction, the most commonly experienced cephalosporin toxicities are mild and temporary nausea, vomiting, and diarrhea associated with disturbance of the normal flora. Rarely, a life-threatening pseudomembranous colitis diarrhea associated with the opportunistic and toxin-producing anaerobic pathogen, *C. difficile*, can be experienced. Rare blood dyscrasias, which can even include aplastic anemia, can also be seen. Cephalosporins containing a methylthiotetrazole side chain (MTT) are associated with prolonged bleeding times and a disulfiram-like acute alcohol intolerance. Most of these agents are no longer widely used.

First-Generation Cephalosporins (Table 29.7)

Cefazolin. Cefazolin has the natural acetyl side chain at C-3 replaced by a thio-linked thiadiazole ring. Although this group is an activating leaving group, the moiety is not subject to the inactivating host hydrolysis reaction. At C-7, it possesses a tetrazoylmethylene unit. Its dosing should be reduced in the presence of renal impairment. It is comparatively unstable and should be protected from heat and light.

Cephalexin. Use of the ampicillin-type side chain conveys oral activity to cephalexin. Whereas it no longer has an activating side chain at C-3, and as a consequence is somewhat less potent, it does not undergo metabolic deactivation and thus maintains potency. It is rapidly and completely absorbed from the GI tract and has become quite popular. Somewhat puzzling is the fact that the use of the ampicillin side chain in the cephalosporins does not result in a comparable shift in antimicrobial spectrum. Cephalexin, like the other first-generation cephalosporins is active against many gram-positive aerobic cocci but is limited against gram-negative bacteria. It is a widely used drug, particularly against gram-negative bacteria causing urinary tract infections, gram-positive infections (*S. aureus*, *S. pneumoniae*, and *S. pyogenes*) of soft tissues, pharyngitis, and minor wounds.[48]

Cefadroxil. Cefadroxil has an amoxicillin-like side chain at C-7 and is orally active. The prolonged biologic half-life of cefadroxil allows for once-a-day dosage.

Second-Generation Cephalosporins (Table 29.8)

One of the second-generation cephalosporins contains an N-methyl-5-thiotetrazole (commonly referred to by the acronym, MTT) at the C-3 position.

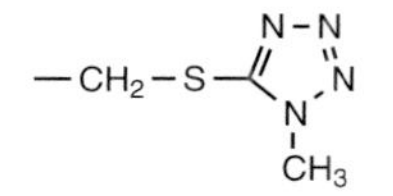

—CH_2—S—(N-methyltetrazolyl, CH_3)

MTT

Loss of the MTT group is associated with prothrombin deficiency and bleeding problems, as well as with a disulfiram-like acute alcohol intolerance.[53] However, this grouping enhances potency and prevents metabolism by deacetylation.

Cefuroxime. Cefuroxime has a Z-oriented methoxyimino moiety as part of its C-7 side chain (Fig. 29.20). This conveys considerable resistance to attack by many β-lactamases but not by all. This is believed to result from the steric demands of this group. Resistance by *P. aeruginosa*, on the other hand, is attributed to lack of penetration of the drug rather than to enzymatic hydrolysis. The carbamoyl moiety at C-3 is intermediate in metabolic stability between the classic acetyl moieties and the thiotetrazoles.

In the form of its axetil ester (1-[acetyloxy]ethyl ester) prodrug, cefuroxime axetil, a more lipophilic drug is produced that results in satisfactory blood levels on oral administration. The ester bond is cleaved metabolically, and the resulting intermediate form loses acetaldehyde spontaneously to produce cefuroxime itself. The axetil is officially labeled for treatment of Lyme disease (although doxycycline is often the first choice).[49]

Table 29.7 First-Generation Cephalosporins

(Core structure: RCOHN–cephem nucleus with S, N, CH_2X at C-3, CO_2H)

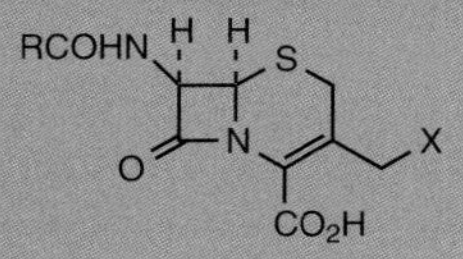

Generic Names	Trade Names	R	X	Salt
Parenteral Agents				
Cefazolin	Ancef, Kefzol, Zolicef	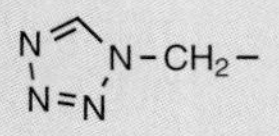 tetrazol-1-yl–CH_2–	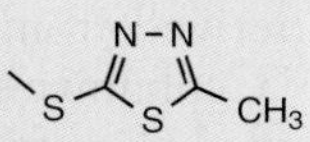 –S–(5-methyl-1,3,4-thiadiazol-2-yl), CH_3	Na
Oral Agents				
Cephalexin	Keflex, Biocef Keftab	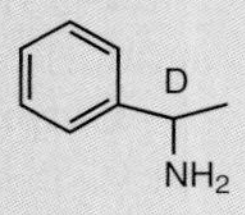 phenyl–CH(D)–NH_2	H	HCl
Cefadroxil	Duricef	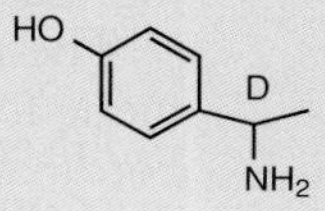 HO–phenyl–CH(D)–NH_2	H	-

Table 29.8 Second-Generation Cephalosporins

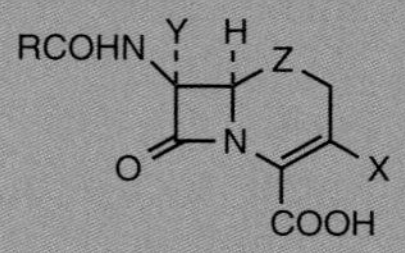

Generic Name	Trade Name	R	X	Y	Z	Salt
Parenteral Agents						
Cefuroxime	Ceftin Kefurox Zinacef	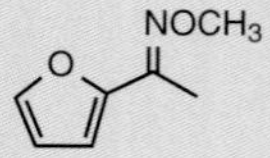 NOCH$_3$	$-CH_2OCONH_2$	H	S	Na
Cefoxitin	Mefoxin	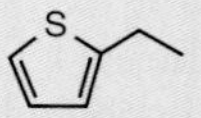 S	$-CH_2OCONH_2$	OCH_3	S	Na
Cefotetan	Cefotan	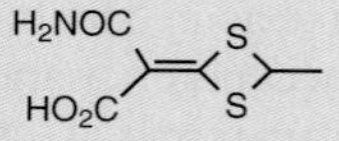 H_2NOC, S, S, HO_2C	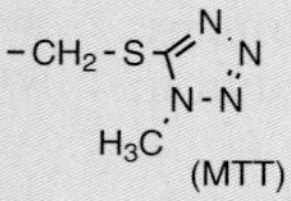 $-CH_2-S$, N, N, N-N, H_3C (MTT)	OCH_3	S	diNa
Oral Agents						
Cefaclor	Ceclor	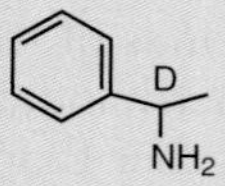 D, NH_2	Cl	H	S	-
Cefprozil	Cefzil	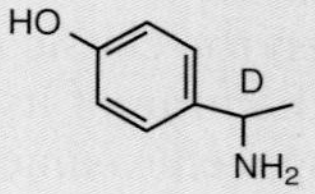 HO, D, NH_2	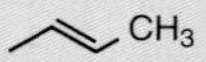 CH_3	H	S	-

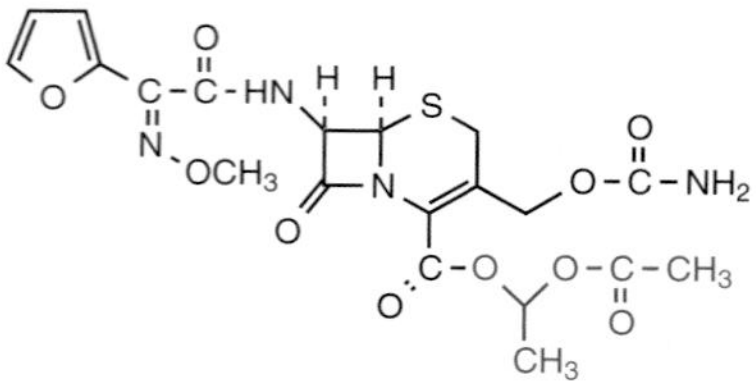

Cefuroxime axetil

Cefoxitin. The most novel chemical feature of cefoxitin is the possession of an α-oriented methoxyl group in place of the normal H-atom at C-7. This increased steric bulk conveys very significant stability against β-lactamases. The inspiration for these functional groups was provided by the discovery of the naturally occurring antibiotic cephamycin C derived from fermentation of *Streptomyces lactamdurans*.[54] Cephamycin C itself has not seen clinical use but provided the structural clue that led to useful agents such as cefoxitin. Agents that contain this 7α methoxy group are commonly referred to as cephamycins.

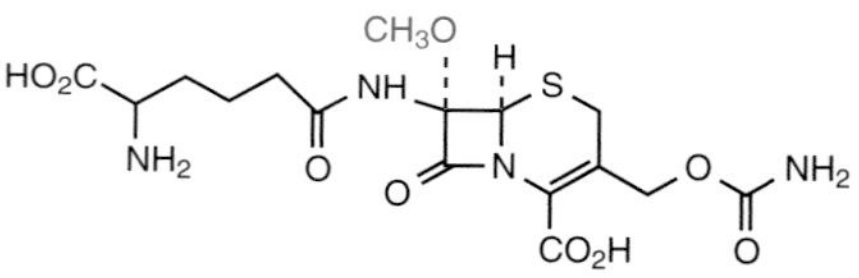

Cephamycin C

Cefoxitin has useful activity against gonorrhea and against some anaerobic infections (including *B. fragilis*) as compared with its second-generation relatives. On the negative side, cefoxitin has the capacity to induce certain broad-spectrum β-lactamases.

Cefotetan. Cefotetan is also a cephamycin but has a rather unusual sulfur-containing C-7 side chain amide. Possession of two carboxyl groups leads to its marketing as a disodium salt. The C-3 MTT side chain suggests caution in monitoring bleeding as well as care in ingesting alcohol when using this agent. Like cefoxitin, cefotetan has better activity against anaerobes than the rest of this group. Like cefoxitin, it is stable to a wide range of β-lactamases but is also an inducer in some bacteria.

Cefaclor. Cefaclor differs from cephalexin primarily in the bioisosteric replacement of methyl by chlorine at C-3 and is quite acid stable, allowing for oral administration. It is also quite stable to metabolism. It is less active against gram-negative bacteria than the other second-generation cephalosporins but is more active against gram-negative bacteria than the first-generation drugs.

Cefprozil. Cefprozil has an amoxicillin-like side chain at C-7, but at C-3, there is now an l-propenyl group conjugated with the double bond in the six-membered ring.

The double bond is present in its two geometric isomeric forms, both of which exhibit antibacterial activity. Fortunately, the predominant trans form (illustrated in Table 29.8) is much more active against gram-negative organisms. Cefprozil most closely resembles cefaclor in its properties but is a little more potent.

Third-Generation Cephalosporins (Table 29.9)

Cefotaxime. Cefotaxime, like cefuroxime, has a Z-methoxyimino moiety at C-7 that conveys significant β-lactamase resistance. The oxime moiety of cefotaxime is connected to an aminothiazole ring. Like other third-generation cephalosporins, it has excellent anti–gram-negative activity. It has a metabolically vulnerable acetoxy group attached to C-3 and loses about 90% of its activity when this is hydrolyzed. This metabolic feature also complicates the pharmacokinetic data because both structures are present and have different properties. Cefotaxime should be protected from heat and light and may color slightly without significant loss of potency. Like other third-generation cephalosporins, cefotaxime has less activity against staphylococci but has greater activity against gram-negative organisms.[55]

Ceftizoxime. In ceftizoxime, the whole C-3 side chain has been omitted to prevent deactivation by hydrolysis. It rather resembles cefotaxime in its properties; however, not being subject to metabolism, its pharmacokinetic properties are much less complex.

Ceftriaxone. Ceftriaxone has the same C-7 side chain moiety as cefotaxime and ceftizoxime, but the C-3 side chain consists of a metabolically stable and activating thiotriazinedione in place of the normal acetyl group. The C-3 side chain is sufficiently acidic that at normal pH, it forms an enolic sodium salt, and thus the commercial product is a disodium salt. It is useful for many severe infections and notably in the treatment of some meningitis infections caused by gram-negative bacteria. It is quite stable to many β-lactamases but is sensitive to some inducible chromosomal β-lactamases.[51]

Ceftazidime With Avibactam. In ceftazidime, the oxime moiety is more complex, containing two methyl groups and a carboxylic acid. This assemblage conveys even more pronounced β-lactamase stability, greater *P. aeruginosa* activity, and increased activity against gram-positive organisms. The C-3 side chain has been replaced by a charged pyridinium moiety. The latter considerably enhances water solubility and also highly activates the β-lactam bond toward cleavage. It is not stable under some conditions, such as in the presence of aminoglycosides and vancomycin. It is also attacked readily in sodium bicarbonate solutions. Resistance is mediated by chromosomally

Table 29.9 Third-Generation Cephalosporins

RCOHN, H, H, S, O, N, X, COOH

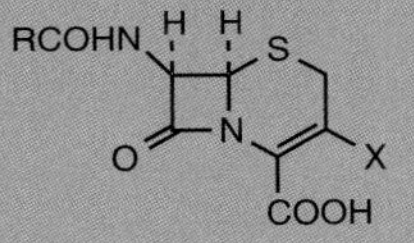

Generic Name	Trade Name	R	X	Salt
Parenteral Agents				
Cefotaxime	Claforan	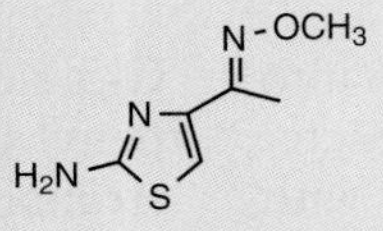 N-OCH$_3$; N; H$_2$N; S	CH_2OAc	Na
Ceftizoxime	Cefizox	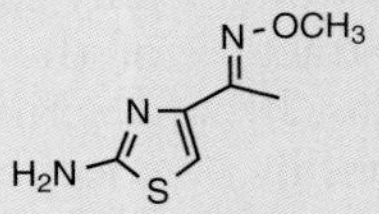 N-OCH$_3$; N; H$_2$N; S	H	Na
Ceftriaxone	Rocephin	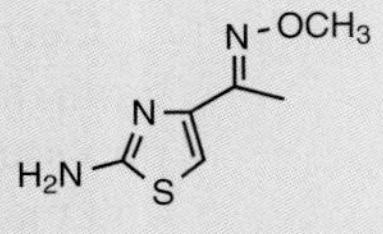 N-OCH$_3$; N; H$_2$N; S	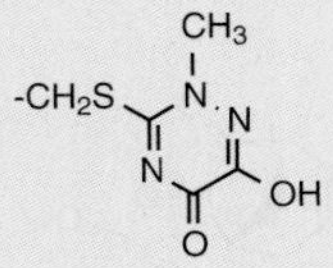 CH$_3$; -CH$_2$S; N; N; N; OH; O	diNa
Ceftazidime w/ avibactam	Avycaz	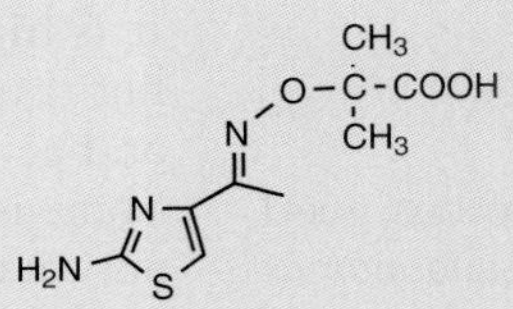 CH$_3$; O-C-COOH; N; CH$_3$; N; H$_2$N; S	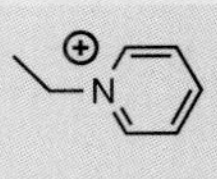 ⊕; N	H or Na
Ceftolozane w/ tazobactam	Zerbaxa	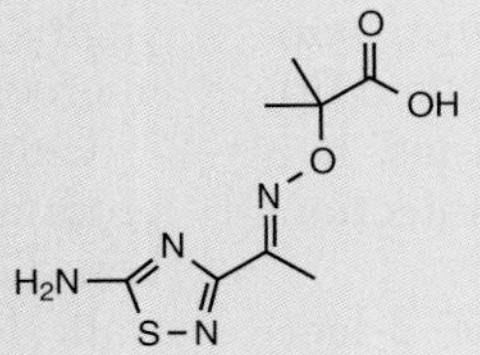 O; OH; O; N; N; H$_2$N; S-N	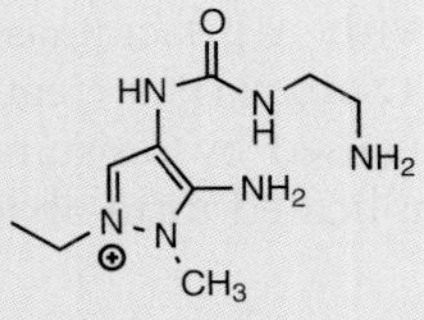 O; HN; N; H; NH$_2$; NH$_2$; N; N; ⊕; N; CH$_3$	

(continued)

Table 29.9 Third-Generation Cephalosporins (Continued)

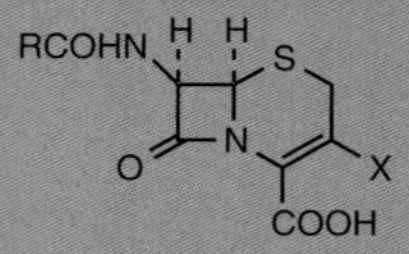

(Core structure: RCOHN–cephem nucleus with X at C-3 and COOH)

Generic Name	Trade Name	R	X	Salt
Oral Agents				
Cefixime	Suprax	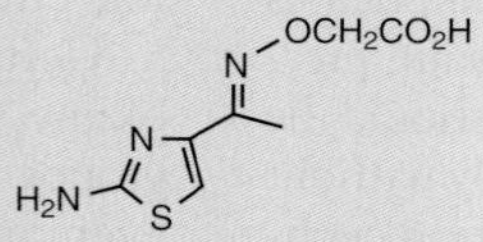 2-aminothiazolyl–C(=N–OCH_2CO_2H)–	$-CH=CH_2$	-
Ceftibuten	Cedax	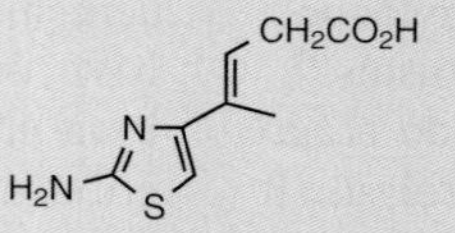 2-aminothiazolyl–C(=CH–CH_2CO_2H)–	H	-
Cefpodoxime proxetil (2-carboxyester 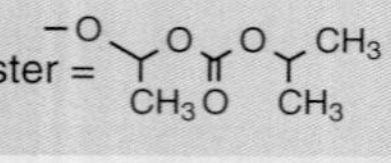 = –O–CH(CH_3)–O–C(=O)–O–CH(CH_3)–CH_3)	Vantin	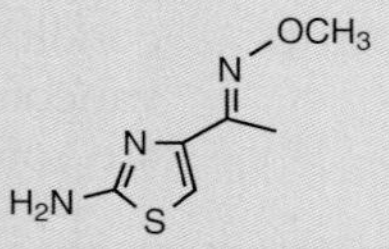 2-aminothiazolyl–C(=N–OCH_3)–	$-CH_2OCH_3$	-
Cefdinir	Omnicef	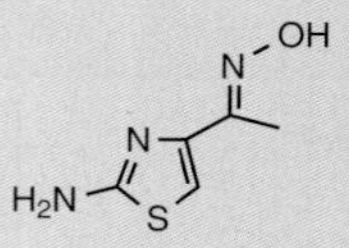 2-aminothiazolyl–C(=N–OH)–	$-CH=CH_2$	-
Cefditoren pivoxil (2-carboxyester 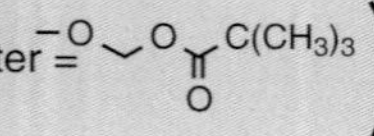 = –O–CH_2–O–C(=O)–$C(CH_3)_3$)	Spectracef	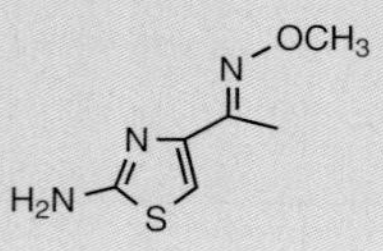 2-aminothiazolyl–C(=N–OCH_3)–	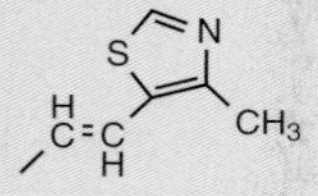 –CH=CH–(4-methylthiazol-5-yl)	-

mediated β-lactamases and also by lack of penetration into target bacteria. Otherwise, it has a very broad antibacterial spectrum. It has more recently been combined with avibactam, a novel, broad-spectrum β-lactamase inhibitor, in a product (Avycaz) to treat complicated urinary tract infections caused by β-lactamase–producing organisms. It is also used for complicated intra-abdominal infections in combination with metronidazole.[56]

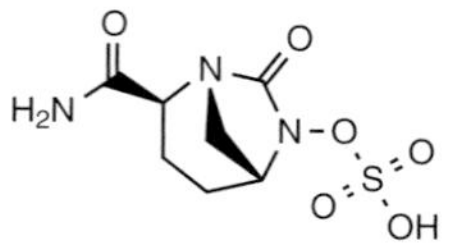

Avibactam

Ceftolozane With Tazobactam. Ceftolozane has good gram-negative activity especially against *Pseudomonas aeruginosa* and good stability to many β-lactamases. It has been combined with a β-lactamase inhibitor, tazobactam, in a product (Zerbaxa) to treat complicated urinary tract infections caused by resistant organisms. It is also approved for complicated intra-abdominal infections (with metronidazole).[57]

Cefixime. In cefixime, in addition to the β-lactamase stabilizing Z-oximino acidic ether at C-7, the C-3 side chain is a vinyl group analogous to the propenyl group of cefprozil. This is believed to contribute strongly to the oral activity of the drug. Cefixime has anti–gram-negative activity intermediate between that of the second-generation and third-generation agents described previously. It is poorly active against staphylococci because it does not bind satisfactorily to a specific PBP (PBP-2).

Ceftibuten. Ceftibuten has a Z-ethylidinecarboxyl group at C-7 instead of the Z-oximino ether linkages seen previously. This conveys enhanced β-lactamase stability and may contribute to oral activity as well. Ceftibuten has no C-3 side chain and thus is not measurably metabolized. It is highly (75%-90%) absorbed on oral administration, but this is decreased significantly by food. Being lipophilic and acidic, it is significantly serum protein bound (65%). Some isomerization of the geometry of the olefinic linkage appears to take place in vivo before excretion. It is mainly used for respiratory tract infections, otitis media, and pharyngitis, as well as urinary tract infections by susceptible microorganisms.[58]

Cefpodoxime Proxetil. Cefpodoxime proxetil is a prodrug. It is cleaved enzymically to isopropanol, carbon dioxide, acetaldehyde, and cefpodoxime in the gut wall. It has better anti–*Staphylococcus aureus* activity than cefixime and is used to treat pharyngitis, urinary tract infections, upper and lower respiratory tract infections, otitis media, skin and soft tissue infections, and gonorrhea.

Cefdinir. Cefdinir has an unsubstituted Z-oxime in its C-7 side chain, the consequence of which is attributed to its somewhat enhanced anti–gram-positive activity—its main distinguishing feature. It has a vinyl moiety attached to C-3 that is associated with its oral activity. It has reasonable resistance to β-lactamases.

Cefditoren Pivoxil. Cefditoren pivoxil is an orally active prodrug. Similar to cefpodoxime proxetil, the pivoxil ester is hydrolyzed following intestinal absorption to release the active drug, cefditoren, along with formaldehyde and pivalic acid. Cefditoren pivoxil should not be administered with drugs that reduce stomach acidity because this may result in decreased absorption. The bioavailability of cefditoren pivoxil is increased if taken with food. Cefditoren pivoxil is indicated for mild to moderate infections in adults and adolescents with chronic bronchitis, pharyngitis/tonsillitis, and uncomplicated skin infections associated with gram-negative bacteria.[59]

Fourth-Generation Cephalosporins

Cefepime

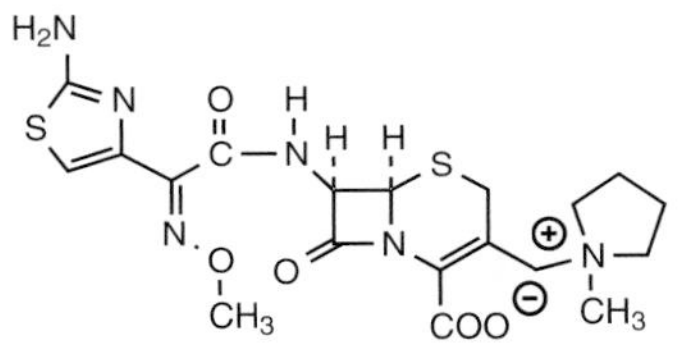

Cefepime (Maxipime)

Cefepime is a semisynthetic agent containing a Z-methoxyimine moiety and an aminothiazolyl group at C-7, broadening its spectrum, increasing its β-lactamase stability, and increasing its antistaphylococcal activity. The quaternary N-methylpyrrolidine group at C-3 seems to help penetration into gram-negative bacteria. The fourth-generation cephalosporins are characterized by enhanced antistaphylococcal activity and broader anti–gram-negative activity than the third-generation group. Cefepime is used intramuscularly and intravenously against urinary tract infections, skin and skin structure infections, pneumonia, and intra-abdominal infections.[52]

Special Use Cephalosporins

Ceftaroline Fosamil

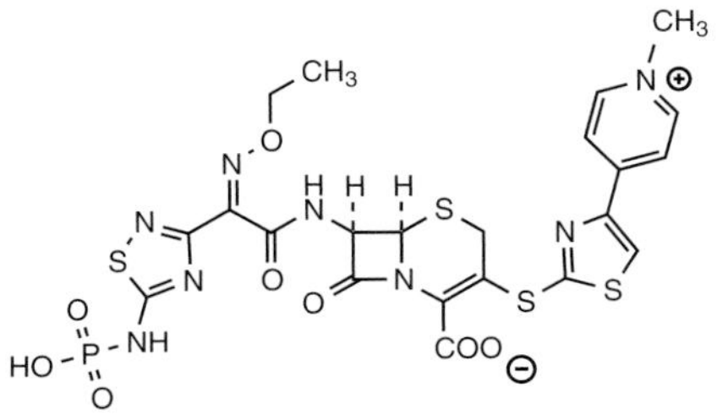

Ceftaroline fosamil (Teflaro)
(prodrug of ceftaroline)

Ceftaroline fosamil is currently unique among the marketed β-lactams because of its affinity for "abnormal" PBPs, in addition to having affinity for normal PBPs. It is bactericidal against MRSA due to its affinity for PBP-2a and against *S. pneumoniae* due to its affinity for PBP-2x. It can be used to treat MRSA infections of skin and soft tissues. It is administered as a water-soluble prodrug that is readily hydrolyzed to the active ceftaroline (loss of the phosphate ester).

The most common adverse effects are nausea, diarrhea, and rash.[60]

Summary. With their broader spectrum including many very dangerous bacteria, the cephalosporins have come to dominate β-lactam chemotherapy, despite often lacking oral activity. Because the cephalosporin field is still being very actively pursued, additional introduction of new agents in the future is expected.

Carbapenems

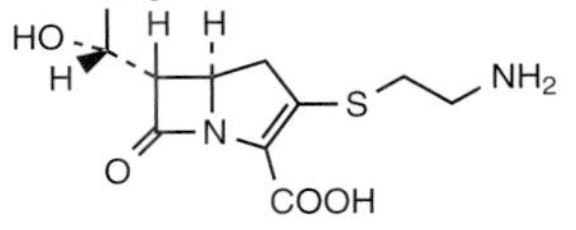

Thienamycin

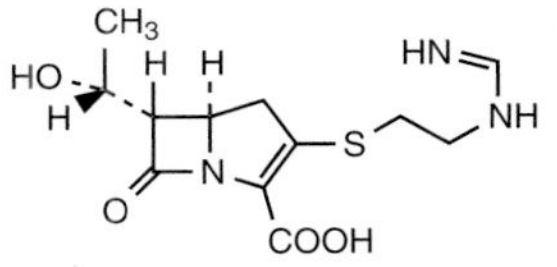

Imipenem

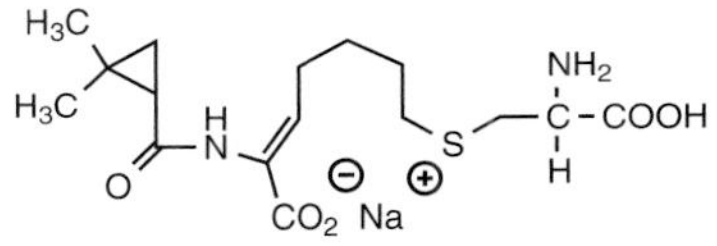

Cilastatin sodium

Thienamycin, the first of the carbapenems, was isolated from *Streptomyces cattleya*.[61] It differs structurally from the penicillins and cephalosporins. The sulfur atom is not part of the five-membered ring but rather has been replaced by a methylene moiety at that position.

Consequently, the carbapenem ring system is highly strained and very susceptible to reactions cleaving the β-lactam bond (including reaction between two molecules resulting in inactivation) (Fig. 29.21). At C-6, there is a 2-hydroxyethyl group attached with α-stereochemistry. Thus, the absolute stereochemistry of the molecule is 5*R*,6*S*,8*S*. With these differences from the penicillins and cephalosporins, it is not surprising that carbapenems bind differently to the penicillin-binding proteins (especially strongly to PBP-2), but the result is very potent broad-spectrum activity.[62] However, none of the current carbapenems have activity against MRSA.

Imipenem. Imipenem (Fig. 29.22), like thienamycin, penetrates very well through porins and is very stable, even inhibitory, to many β-lactamases. Imipenem is not orally active. Renal dehydropeptidase-l metabolizes imipenem through hydrolysis of the β-lactam and deactivates it. An inhibitor for this enzyme, cilastatin, is coadministered with imipenem to protect it.[62] Inhibition of human dehydropeptidase does not seem to have deleterious consequences to the patient, making this combination highly efficacious.

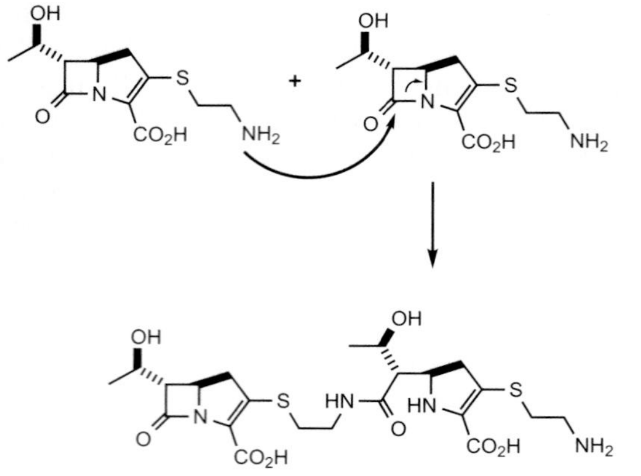

Figure 29.21 Inactivation of thienamycin via intermolecular reaction.

The combination of imipenem and cilastatin (Primaxin) is about 25% serum protein bound. On injection, it penetrates well into most tissues, but not cerebrospinal fluid, and it is subsequently excreted in the urine. This very potent combination is especially useful for treatment of serious infections by aerobic gram-negative bacilli, anaerobes, and *S. aureus*. It is used clinically for a number of significant infections. The more common adverse effects are irritation at the infusion site, nausea, vomiting, diarrhea, and pruritus. Of greater concern is the ability of imipenem to induce seizures. The risk factors for seizure development include impaired renal function, preexisting CNS disease or infection, and use of large doses.[63]

Meropenem. Meropenem (Fig. 29.22) is a synthetic carbapenem possessing a complex side chain at C-3. It also has a chiral methyl group at C-4. This methyl group conveys intrinsic resistance to hydrolysis by dehydropeptidase-1.[64] As a consequence, it can be administered as a single agent for the treatment of severe bacterial infections. While the common adverse effects are similar to imipenem/cilastatin, the risk of seizures is significantly less.[65] Meropenem in combination with a novel non–β-lactam, β-lactamase inhibitor vaborbactam (Fig. 29.22) (Vabomere) was recently approved for use against complicated urinary tract infections (cUTI) and pyelonephritis.[66,67] The adverse effects for the combination product are similar to meropenem.

Doripenem. Doripenem (Fig. 29.22) also contains the 4-β-methyl group, which confers stability toward dehydropeptidase-1, so it is given as a single agent. It is similar in spectrum to imipenem and meropenem but is considered more potent against *Pseudomonas* species.[68]

Ertapenem. Ertapenem (Fig. 29.22) is another synthetic carbapenem with a rather complex side chain at C-3. As with meropenem and doripenem, the 4-β-methyl group confers stability toward dehydropeptidase-1. It is not active against *Pseudomonas* or *Acinetobacter* and thus should not be substituted for other carbapenems for these organisms.[68] This class of antimicrobial agents is under intensive investigation, and several analogues are currently in various phases of preclinical investigation, including tebipenem, an oral prodrug carbapenem that is currently available in Japan.[69]

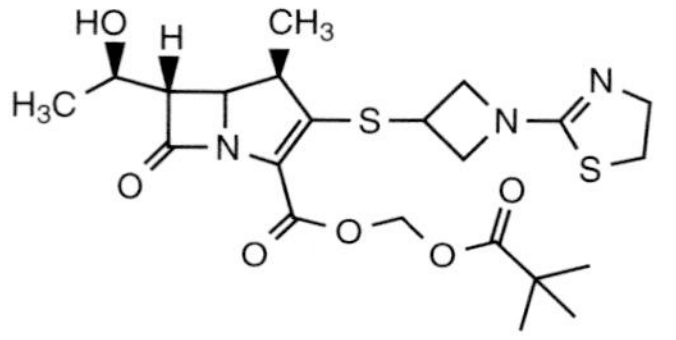

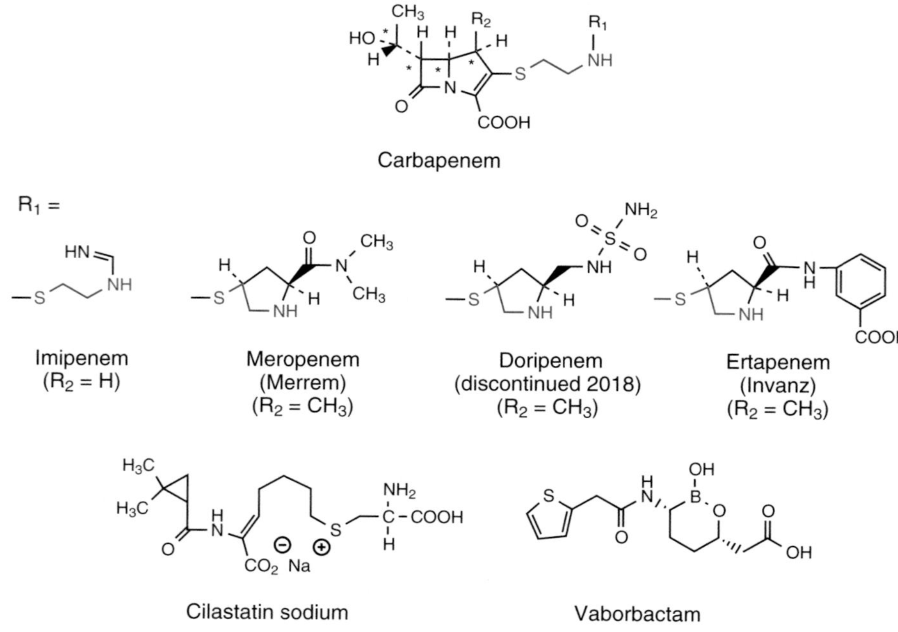

Figure 29.22 Carbapenem antibiotics and coadministered compounds.

Monobactams

Aztreonam

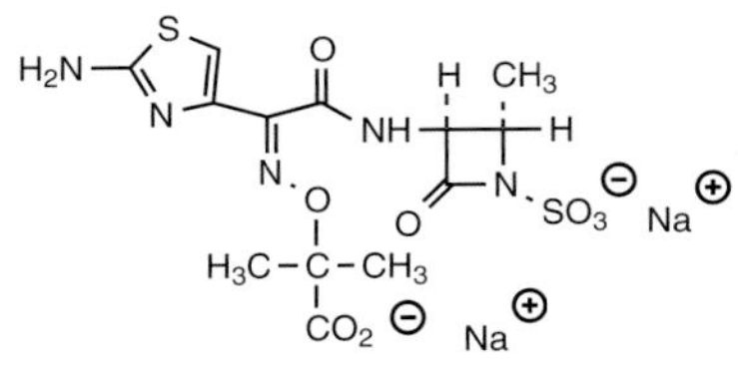

Aztreonam disodium (Azactam)

Fermentation of unusual microorganisms led to the discovery of a class of monocyclic β-lactam antibiotics, named monobactams.[37,38] None of these natural molecules have proven to be important, but the group served as the inspiration for the synthesis of aztreonam. Aztreonam is a totally synthetic parenteral antibiotic whose antimicrobial spectrum is devoted almost exclusively to gram-negative microorganisms, and it is capable of inactivating some β-lactamases. Its molecular mode of action is closely similar to that of the penicillins, cephalosporins, and carbapenems, the action being characterized by strong affinity for PBP-3, producing filamentous cells as a consequence. Whereas the principal side chain closely resembles that of ceftazidime, the sulfamic acid moiety attached to the β-lactam ring was unprecedented. Remembering the comparatively large size of sulfur atoms, this assembly may sufficiently spatially resemble the corresponding C-2 carboxyl group of the precedent β-lactam antibiotics to confuse the PBPs. The strongly electron-withdrawing character of the sulfamic acid group probably also makes the β-lactam bond more vulnerable to hydrolysis. In any case, the monobactams demonstrate that a fused ring is not essential for antibiotic activity. The α-oriented methyl group at C-2 is associated with the stability of aztreonam toward β-lactamases. The protein binding is moderate (~50%), and the drug is nearly unchanged by metabolism. Aztreonam is given by injection and is primarily excreted in the urine. The primary clinical use of aztreonam is against severe infections caused by gram-negative microorganisms, especially those acquired in the hospital. These are mainly urinary tract, upper respiratory tract, bone, cartilage, abdominal, obstetric, and gynecologic infections and septicemias. The drug is well tolerated, and adverse effects are infrequent.[70] Interestingly, allergy would not be unexpected, but cross-allergenicity with penicillins and cephalosporins has not often been reported.[70]

ANTIBIOTICS: INHIBITORS OF PROTEIN BIOSYNTHESIS

Basis for Selectivity. Once the bacterial cell wall is traversed, complex cellular machinery deeper within the cell becomes available to antibiotics. Some of the most successful antibiotic families exert their lethal effects on bacteria by inhibiting ribosomally mediated protein biosynthesis. At first glimpse, this may seem problematic because eukaryotic organisms also construct their essential proteins on ribosomal organelles and the sequence of biochemical steps is closely analogous to that in prokaryotic microorganisms. At a molecular level, however, the apparent anomaly resolves itself because the detailed architecture of prokaryotic ribosomes is rather different. In *E. coli*, for example, the 70S ribosomal particle is composed not only of three RNA molecules, but also of 55 different structural and functional proteins arranged in a nonsymmetrical manner. The small (30S) subunit has a 16S rRNA molecule and about 20 different proteins. The large subunit has a 23S and a 5S rRNA and over 30 proteins. The x-ray crystal structure of the components of the bacterial ribosome has been determined.[71,72] This was a landmark achievement given the size and complexity of this organelle. The picture is still not complete but allows one to unravel the molecular details not only of how proteins are biosynthesized but also where important antibiotics bind when they interrupt this process. The functioning parts of the ribosome organize and catalyze some portions of the biosynthetic cycle. The tRNA molecules bind roughly at the interface where the 50S and 30S subparticles come together. The codon-anticodon interaction with mRNA takes place in the 30S subunit, and the incoming amino acid and the growing peptide chain being made lie in the 50S subunit. Upsetting the view held for decades that the antibiotics bind to ribosomal proteins, it is now known that they bind to the rRNA instead. Aside from this important fact, most of the other key beliefs are still valid. Of key importance is the repeated movement of the tRNA bases, which mostly take place near interfaces between the individual rRNA molecules where this would be easiest. In agreement with this theory, it has been found that this region is comparatively disordered, which is consistent with that movement (Fig. 29.23).

At normal doses, antibiotics do not bind to or interfere with the function of eukaryotic 80S ribosomal particles. The basis for the selective toxicity of these antibiotics is apparent.

Interference with bacterial protein biosynthesis prevents repair, cellular growth, and reproduction and can be clinically bacteriostatic or bactericidal.

AMINOGLYCOSIDES AND AMINOCYCLITOLS. The aminoglycoside/aminocyclitol class of antibiotics contains the pharmacophore 1,3-diaminoinositol moiety consisting either of streptamine, 2-deoxystreptamine, or spectinamine (Fig. 29.24). Several of the alcoholic functions of the 1,3-diaminoinositol are substituted through glycosidic bonds with characteristic amino sugars to form pseudooligosaccharides. The chemistry, spectrum, potency, toxicity, and pharmacokinetics of these agents are a function of the specific identity of the diaminoinositol unit and the arrangement and identity of the attachments. The various aminoglycoside antibiotics are freely water soluble across the pH scale, are basic and form acid salts, are not absorbed in significant amounts from the GI tract, and are excreted in high concentrations in the urine following injection as the active form. When the kidneys are not functioning efficiently, the dose must be reduced to prevent accumulation to toxic levels. When given orally, their action is confined to the GI tract. Aminoglycosides are used topically as solutions or ointments for ophthalmic infections. They can be given intramuscularly but are more commonly

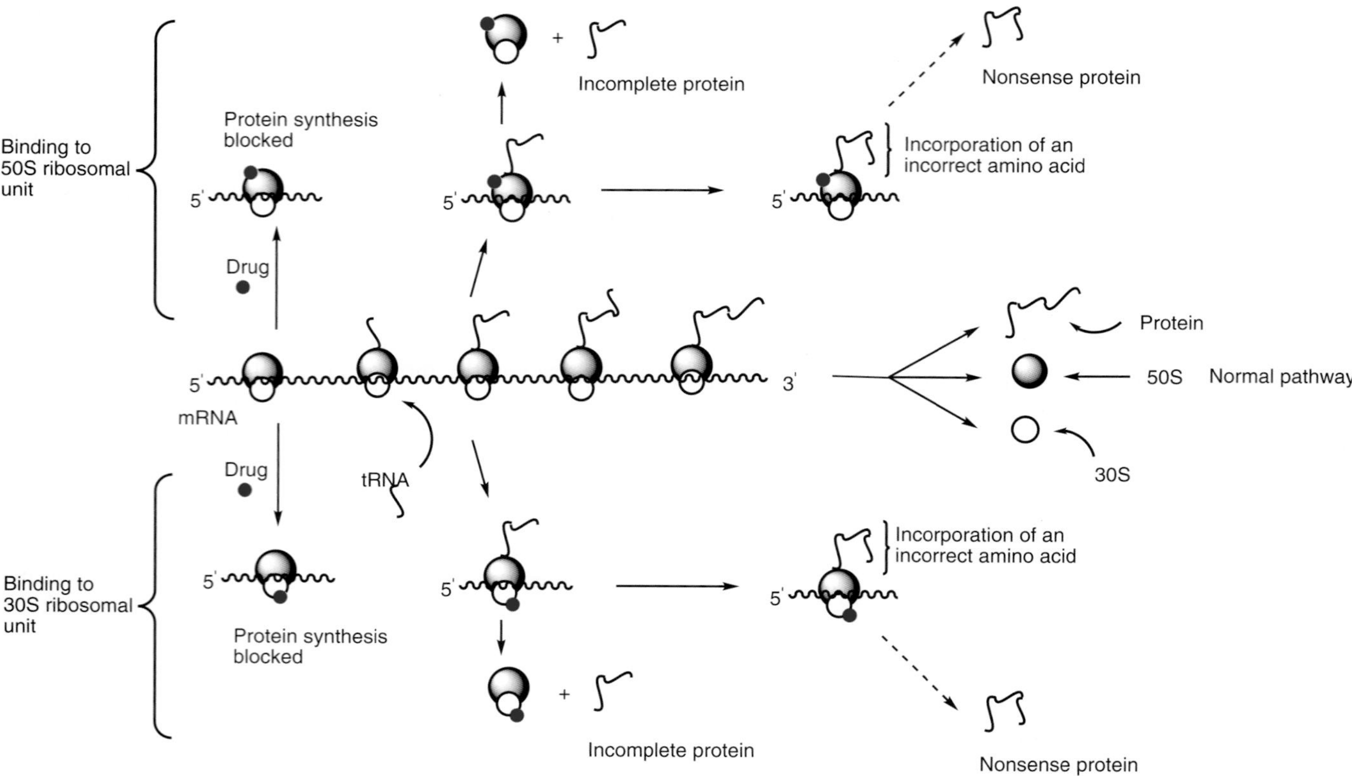

Figure 29.23 General mechanism of action of drugs that block protein synthesis by binding to ribosomal units.

delivered by intravenous infusion. In addition, tobramycin is available for inhalation to treat *P. aeruginosa* infections in cystic fibrosis patients and has led to improved pediatric treatment and improved patient compliance.[73,74] Currently, liposomal amikacin for inhalation is under phase 2 clinical trials for the treatment of *Mycobacterium abscessus* infections in cystic fibrosis patients.[75] Inhalation route of administration results in significantly reduced toxicity to the patient. These agents have intrinsically broad antimicrobial spectra, but their toxicity potential limits their clinical use to infections by gram-negative bacteria. The aminoglycoside antibiotics are widely distributed (mainly in extracellular fluids) and have low levels of protein binding.

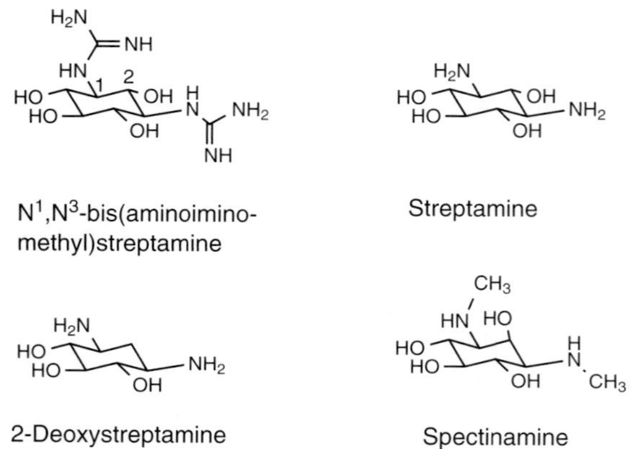

Figure 29.24 1,3-Diaminoinositol moieties present in aminoglycosides.

Mechanism of Action. The aminoglycosides are bactericidal due to a combination of toxic effects. At less than toxic doses, they bind to the 16S ribosomal DNA portion of the 30S ribosomal subunit, impairing the proofreading function of the ribosome. A conformational change occurs in the peptidyl A site of the ribosome upon aminoglycoside binding. This leads to mistranslation of RNA templates and the selection of wrong amino acids and formation of so-called nonsense proteins (Fig. 29.23).

The most relevant of these unnatural proteins are involved in upsetting bacterial membrane function. Their presence destroys the semipermeability of the membrane, and this damage cannot be repaired without de novo programmed protein biosynthesis. Among the substances that are admitted by the damaged membrane are large additional quantities of aminoglycoside. At these increased concentrations, protein biosynthesis ceases altogether. These combined effects are devastating to the target bacterial cells. Aminoglycosides are highly polar drugs, and cellular permeability through diffusion is expected to be low. However, they bind to external lipopolysaccharides, and this complex is thought to diffuse across the bacterial cell membrane. The uptake process is inhibited by Ca^{2+} and Mg^{2+} ions. These ions are, then, partially incompatible therapeutically. Passage through the cytoplasmic membrane is dependent on electron transport and energy generation. At high concentrations, eukaryotic protein biosynthesis can also be inhibited by aminoglycoside/aminocyclitol antibiotics.[76,77]

Bacterial Resistance. Bacterial resistance to aminoglycoside antibiotics in the clinic is most commonly due to bacterial elaboration of R-factor–mediated enzymes that N-acetylate (aminoglycoside acetylase [AAC]), O-phosphorylate (aminoglycoside phosphorylase [APH]), and O-adenylate (aminoglycoside nucleotide transferase [ANT]) specific functional groups, preventing subsequent ribosomal binding (Fig. 29.25). In some cases, chemical deletion of the functional groups transformed by these enzymes leaves a molecule that is still antibiotic but no longer a substrate; thus, semisynthetic agents with intrinsically broader spectrum are a viable option with this in mind. In other cases, novel functional groups can be attached to remote functionality, which converts these antibiotics to poorer substrates for these R-factor–mediated enzymes, and this expands their spectra. It is important to note that resistance mediated in this way is not necessarily class-wide; therefore, susceptibility testing with multiple aminoglycosides should be used. Resistance can also involve point mutations of the ribosomal A site. These involve single nucleotide residues at specific position.[77] The substituent at position 6′ of the aminoglycoside, the number of protonated amino groups, and the linkage between the sugar rings and the central deoxystreptamine moiety are particularly important in the interactions with rRNA.

Therapeutic Application. Intrinsically, aminoglycosides have broad antibiotic spectra against aerobic gram-positive and gram-negative bacteria but are reserved for use in serious infections caused by gram-negative organisms because of serious toxicities that are often delayed in onset. They are active against gram-negative aerobes such as *Acinetobacter* sp., *Citrobacter* sp., *Enterobacter* sp., *Escherichia coli*, *Klebsiella* sp., *Proteus vulgaris*, *Providencia* sp., *Pseudomonas aeruginosa*, *Salmonella* sp., *Serratia marcesans*, *Shigella* sp., and gram-positive aerobes such as *Staphylococcus epidermidis*.[77]

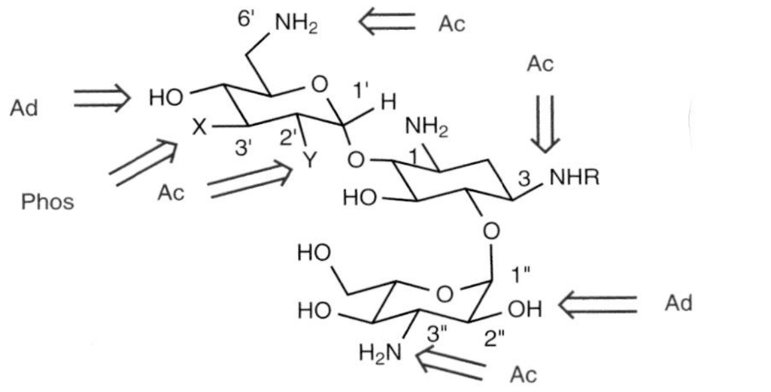

Streptomycin and spectinomycin differ from the others in their useful antimicrobial spectra. Streptomycin is most commonly used for the treatment of tuberculosis and spectinomycin for treatment of gonorrhea, although spectinomycin is no longer marketed in the United States. Some aminoglycoside antibiotics in present clinical use are illustrated in Figure 29.25, along with some of their sites of enzymatic inactivation.

Adverse Effects. The toxicities associated with the aminoglycosides involve toxicity to functions mediated by the eighth cranial nerve, such as hearing loss and vertigo. Their use can also lead to kidney tubular necrosis, leading to decreases in glomerular function. These toxic effects are related to blood levels and are apparently mediated by the special affinity of these aminoglycosides to kidney cells and to the sensory cells of the inner ear.[78] The effects may have a delayed onset, making them all the more dangerous because the patient can be injured significantly before symptoms appear. Less commonly, curare-like neuromuscular blockade can exaggerate the muscle weakness of myasthenia gravis and patients with Parkinson's disease.[79] In current practice, all of these toxic phenomena are well known; therefore, creatinine clearance should be determined and the dose adjusted downward accordingly so that these adverse effects are less common and less severe.

Specific Agents

Amikacin (Amikin). Amikacin is a semisynthetic form of the natural product kanamycin A (Fig. 29.25). Interestingly, the L-hydroxyaminobutyryl amide (HABA) moiety attached to N-3 inhibits adenylation and phosphorylation in the distant amino sugar ring (at C-2′ and C-3′) even though the HABA substituent is not where the enzymatic reaction takes place. This effect is attributed to decreased binding to the R-factor–mediated enzymes. With this change, potency and spectrum are strongly enhanced, and amikacin is used for the treatment of sensitive strains of M. *tuberculosis*, *Yersinia tularensis*, and severe *P. aeruginosa* infections resistant to other agents.

Tobramycin (Nebcin). Tobramycin is one component of a mixture produced by fermentation of *Streptomyces tenebrarius* (Fig. 29.25). Lacking the C-3′ hydroxyl group, it is not a substrate for APH(3′)-I and–II, and thus has an intrinsically broader spectrum than kanamycin. It is a substrate, however, for adenylation at C-2′ by ANT(2′) and acetylation at C-3 by AAC(3)-I and –II and at C-2′ by AAC(2′) (Fig. 29.25). It is used parenterally for difficult infections, especially those by gentamicin-resistant *P. aeruginosa*. Tobramycin is also available as ophthalmic drops to treat superficial eye infections.

Gentamicin (Garamycin). Gentamicin is a mixture of several antibiotic components produced by fermentation of *Micromonospora purpurea* and other related soil microorganisms (hence its name is spelled with an

Tobramycin (X=H, Y= NH_2, R =H)

Kanamycin A (X=OH, Y = OH, R =H)

Amikacin (X=Y=OH, R=$COCHOHCH_2CH_2NH_2$)

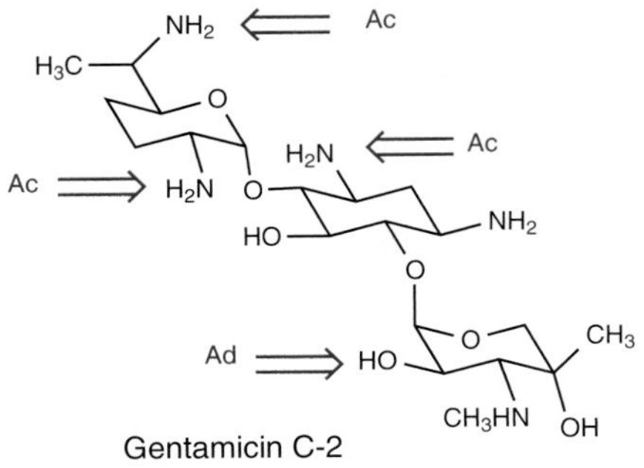

Gentamicin C-2

Figure 29.25 Commercially important 2-desylstreptamine–containing aminoglycosides. Some points of inactivating attack by specific R-factor–mediated enzymes are indicated by the following: Ac, acetylation; Ad, adenylation; Phos, phosphorylation. APH(3′)-I, for example, is an acronym for an enzyme that phosphorylates aminoglycosides at the 3′-OH position.

"i" instead of a "y"). Gentamicins C-1, C-2, and C-1a are most prominent (gentamicin C-2 is shown in Fig. 29.25). Gentamicin was one of the first antibiotics to have significant activity against *P. aeruginosa* infections. This water-loving opportunistic pathogen is frequently encountered in burns, pneumonias, and urinary tract infections. It is highly virulent. As noted earlier, some of the functional groups that serve as targets for R-factor–mediated enzymes are missing in the structure of gentamicins, so their antibacterial spectrum is enhanced. They are, however, inactivated through C-2′ adenylation by enzyme ANT(2′) and acetylation at C-6′ by AAC(6′), at C-1 by AAC(1)-I and -II, and at C-2′ by AAC(2′). Gentamicin is often combined with other anti-infective agents, and an interesting incompatibility has been uncovered. With certain β-lactam antibiotics, the two drugs react with each other so that N-acylation on C-1 of gentamicin by the β-lactam antibiotic takes place, thus inactivating both antibiotics (Fig. 29.26). The two agents should not, therefore, be mixed in the same solution and should ideally be administered into different tissue compartments to prevent this. This incompatibility is likely to be associated with other aminoglycoside antibiotics as well. Gentamicin is used for urinary tract infections, burns, some pneumonias, and bone and joint infections caused by susceptible gram-negative bacteria.

Streptomycin

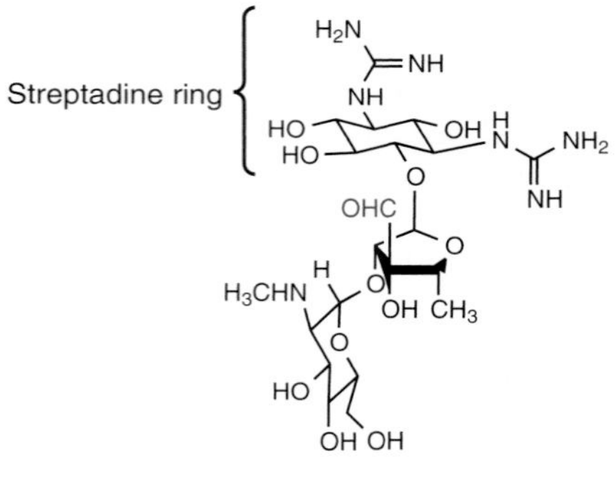

Streptadine ring

Streptomycin

Streptomycin is produced by fermentation of *S. griseus* and several related soil microorganisms. It was introduced in 1943 primarily for the treatment of tuberculosis. It was the first antibiotic effective for this devastating disease, and Selmon Waksman, the discoverer of streptomycin, received a Nobel Prize in 1952.[80] Streptomycin differs from the typical aminoglycosides with a modified pharmacophore in that the diaminoinositol unit is streptamine, and streptomycin has an axial hydroxyl group at C-2 and two highly basic guanido groups at C-1 and C-3 in place of the primary amine moieties of 2-deoxystreptamine. It is possible that the unusual pharmacophore of streptomycin accounts in large measure for its unusual antibacterial spectrum. Another molecular feature, the α-hydroxyaldehyde moiety, is a center of instability such that streptomycin cannot be sterilized by autoclaving, so streptomycin sulfate solutions that need sterilization are made by ultrafiltration. Streptomycin is rarely used today as a single agent. Resistance to streptomycin takes the familiar course of N-acetylation, O-phosphorylation, and O-adenylation of specific functional groups.

Gentamicin C-2a (active) + β-lactam antibiotic (active)

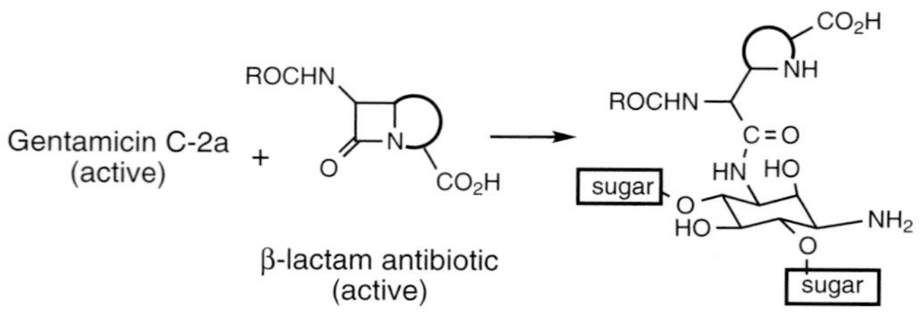

Figure 29.26 A chemical drug-drug incompatibility between gentamicin C-2a and β-lactams.

Orally Used Aminoglycosides. Neomycin, as part of a combination of agents, finds some oral use for the suppression of gut flora in preparation for bowel surgery. Paromomycin (Humatin) is also used for the oral treatment of amoebic dysentery. Amoebas are persistent pathogens causing chronic diarrhea and are acquired most frequently by travelers who consume food supplies contaminated with human waste.

Neomycin

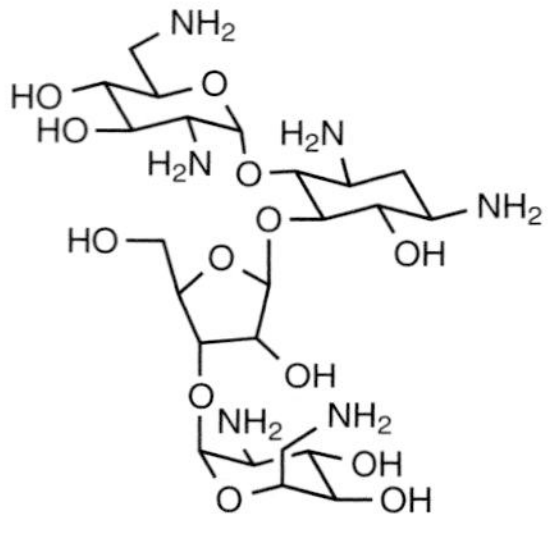

Neomycin B

Neomycin is a mixture of three compounds produced by fermentation of *Streptomyces fradiae*, with neomycin B predominating. Although it is not normally considered to have systemic absorption when administered orally, neomycin now has a black box warning related to systemic toxicities due to absorption in ulcerated or denuded areas of the GI tract.[81] It is also found in nonprescription ointments and used topically for treatment of bacterial skin infections. When applied to intact skin, the drug is not absorbed, but if applied to large denuded areas, systemic absorption occurs with the potential to cause toxic side effects.

Newer Aminoglycosides

Plazomicin

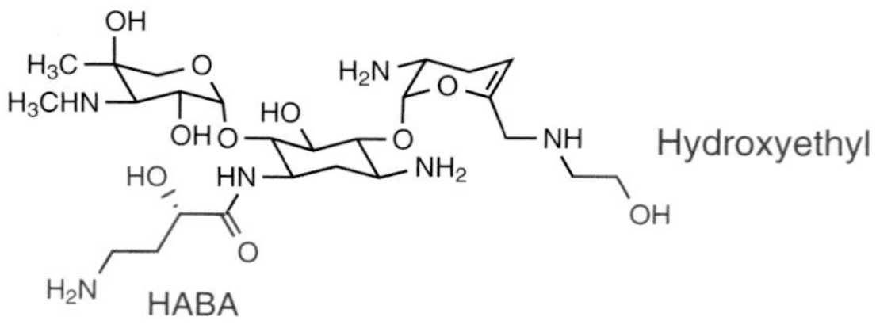

Hydroxyethyl

HABA

Plazomicin

Plazomicin (Zemdri) is considered a next generation aminoglycoside that is resistant to many aminoglycoside-modifying enzymes and was recently approved for treatment of complicated urinary tract infections in adults. It has been demonstrated to be effective in infections associated with *E. coli*, *K. pneumoniae*, *P. mirabilis*, and *E. cloacae*.[82] Plazomicin is a semi-synthetic derivative of the archaic aminoglycoside sisomicin which is isolated from *Micromonospora*. A hydroxyaminobutyrylamide (HABA) group and a hydroxyethyl group have been added to the sisomicin structure to produce plazomicin.[83]

Macrolide Antibiotics. The term macrolide is derived from the characteristic large lactone (cyclic ester) ring found in these antibiotics. The clinically important members of this antibiotic family (Fig. 29.27) have two or more characteristic sugars (usually cladinose and desosamine) attached to the 14-membered ring. One of these sugars usually carries a substituted amino group, so their overall chemical character is weakly basic (pK_a ~8). They are not very water soluble as free bases, but salt formation with certain acids (lactobionic acids in Fig. 29.27) increases water solubility, whereas other salts decrease solubility (stearic). Macrolide antibiotics with 16-membered rings are popular outside the United States, but one example, tylosin, finds extensive agricultural use in the United States. The 14-membered ring macrolides are biosynthesized from propionic acid units so that every second carbon of erythromycin, for example, bears a methyl group and the rest of the carbons, with one exception, are oxygen bearing. Two carbons bear so-called "extra" oxygen atoms introduced later in the biosynthesis (not present in a propionic acid unit), and two hydroxyls are glycosylated (Fig. 29.28).[84]

Chemical Properties. The early macrolides of the erythromycin class are chemically unstable due to rapid acid-catalyzed internal cyclic ketal formation, leading to inactivity (Fig. 29.29). This reaction, which occurs in the GI tract, is clinically important. Most acid-susceptible macrolides are administered in coated tablets to minimize this. Analogues have been prepared semisynthetically that are structurally incapable of undergoing this reaction and have become very popular in the clinic.[85]

Many macrolides have an unpleasant taste, which is partially overcome with water-insoluble dosage forms that also reduce acid instability and the gut cramps. Enteric coatings are also beneficial in reducing these adverse effects.

Mechanism of Action. The macrolides inhibit bacteria by interfering with programmed ribosomal protein biosynthesis by binding to the 23S rRNA in the polypeptide exit tunnel adjacent to the peptidyl transferase center in the 50S ribosomal subunit (Fig. 29.23). This prevents the growing peptide from becoming longer than a few residues, resulting in the dissociation of peptidyl tRNA molecules. Clindamycin, lincomycin, and chloramphenicol bind in the same vicinity, leading to extensive cross-resistance between them.

Resistance. Developed bacterial resistance is primarily caused by bacteria possessing R-factor enzymes that methylate a specific guanine residue on their own ribosomal RNA making them somewhat less efficient at protein biosynthesis but comparatively poor binders of macrolides.[86] The erythromycin-producing soil organism uses the same ribosomal methylation technique to protect itself against the toxic effects of its own metabolite.[86] This leads to the speculation that the origin of some antibiotic resistance genes may lie in the producing organism itself and that this genetic material is acquired by bacteria from this source. A second mechanism of resistance is associated with the

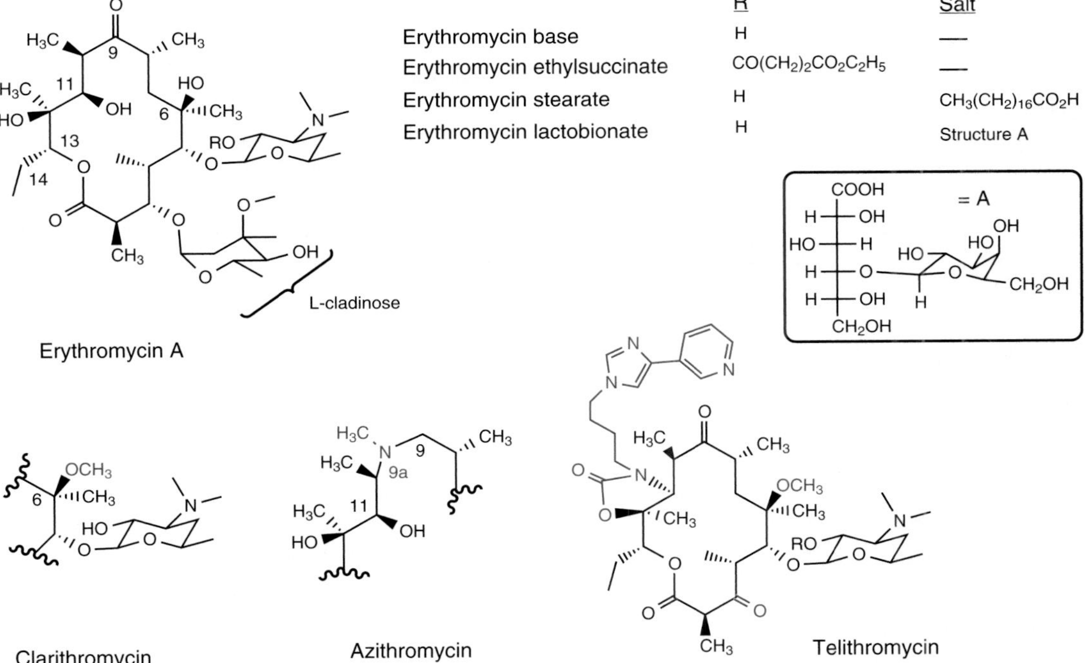

Figure 29.27 Clinically important macrolide antibiotics.

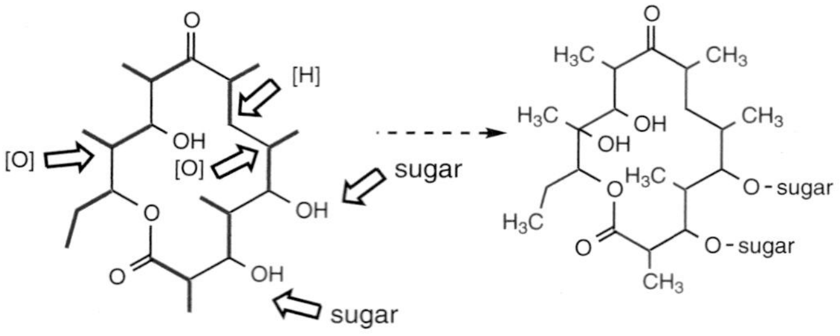

Figure 29.28 Biosynthetic pathway to erythromycins from propionic acid units. ⇧ refers to modifications to the basic ring skeleton.

mutation of adenine to guanine that occurs in domain V at A2058. This change results in a 10,000-fold reduction of binding capacity of erythromycin and clarithromycin to the 23S rRNA.[86] Some bacterial strains, however, appear to be resistant to macrolides due to the operation of an active efflux process in which the drug is expelled from the cell at the cost of energy.[86] Intrinsic resistance of gram-negative bacteria is primarily caused by lack of penetration as the isolated ribosomes from these organisms are often susceptible.

Drug Interactions. Drug-drug interactions with macrolides are comparatively common and usually involve inhibition of CYP3A4 of the cytochrome P450 oxidase family.[87] There is also evidence suggesting that these interactions are intensified by the inhibition of P-glycoprotein.[88] These interactions can have severely negative consequences for the patient. The result of this interaction is a longer half-life and enhanced potential toxicity by increasing the effective dose over time. The main product of liver metabolism of erythromycin is the N-demethylated analogue.

Therapeutic Application. The macrolides are among the safest of the antibiotics in common use and are often used for the treatment of upper and lower respiratory tract and soft tissue infections primarily caused by gram-positive microorganisms like *S. pyogenes* and *S. pneumoniae*, Legionnaires' disease, prophylaxis of bacterial endocarditis by *S. viridans*, otitis media caused by *H. influenzae* (with a sulfonamide added), mycoplasmal pneumonia, and *Mycobacterium avium* complex infections in AIDS patients (in combination with rifabutin). They are also used for certain sexually transmitted diseases, such as gonorrhea and pelvic inflammatory disease, caused by mixed infections involving cell wall–free organisms such as *C. trachomatis*. Clarithromycin is also used to treat gastric ulcers due to *H. pylori* infection as a component of multidrug cocktails. The macrolides have a comparatively narrow antimicrobial spectrum, reminiscent of the medium-spectrum penicillins, but the organisms involved include many of the more commonly encountered community-acquired microorganisms. The utility of the macrolides against upper respiratory tract infections is enhanced by their particular affinity for these tissues. Tissue levels in the upper respiratory tract are often several times those seen in the blood. They are considered bacteriostatic against most organisms in achievable concentrations.

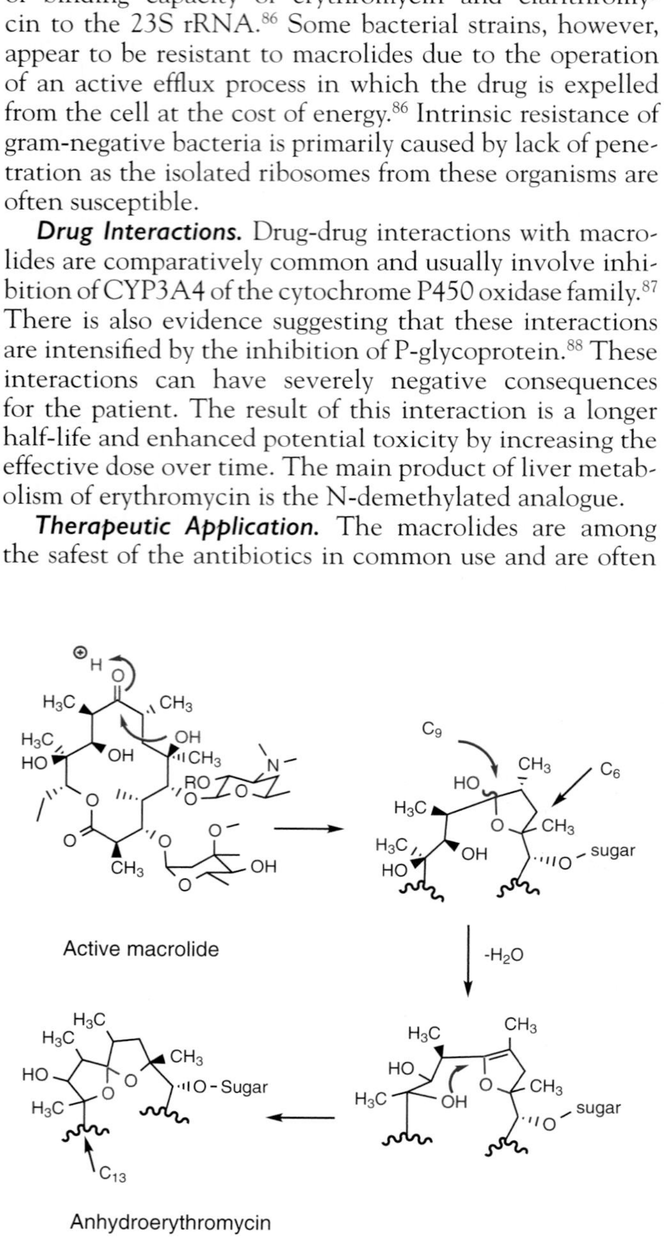

Figure 29.29 Acid-catalyzed intramolecular ketal formation with erythromycin.

Specific Agents

Erythromycin Esters and Salts

Ethylsuccinate (EryPed, EES). Erythromycin ethyl succinate is a mixed double-ester prodrug in which one carboxyl of succinic acid esterifies the C-2′ hydroxyl of erythromycin and the other ethanol (Fig. 29.27). This prodrug is frequently used in an oral suspension for pediatric use largely to mask the bitter taste of the drug. Film-coated tablets are also used to deal with this. Some cholestatic jaundice is associated with the use of erythromycin ethyl succinate.[89]

Stearate. Erythromycin stearate is a very insoluble salt form of erythromycin. The water insolubility helps mask the taste of the drug and enhances its stability in the stomach.

Lactobionate. Erythromycin lactobionate is a salt with enhanced water solubility that is used for injections.

Clarithromycin (Biaxin). Clarithromycin differs from erythromycin in that the C-6 hydroxy group has been converted semisynthetically to a methyl ether (Fig. 29.27). The C-6 hydroxy group is involved in the process, initiated by protons, leading to internal cyclic ketal formation in erythromycin that results in drug inactivation (Fig. 29.29). This ketal, or one of the products of its subsequent degradation, is also associated with GI cramping. Conversion of the molecule to its more lipophilic methyl ether prevents internal ketal formation, which not only gives better blood levels through chemical stabilization, but also results in less gastric upset. An extensive saturable first-pass liver metabolism of clarithromycin leads to formation of its C-14 hydroxy analogue, which has even greater antimicrobial potency, especially against *Haemophilus influenzae*.[90] The enhanced lipophilicity of clarithromycin also allows for lower and less frequent dosage for mild infections. Recently, the FDA issued a safety communication recommending alternative antibiotics in patients with heart disease.[91]

Azithromycin (Zithromax, Zmax). Azithromycin, called an "azalide," has been formed by semisynthetic conversion of erythromycin to a ring-expanded analogue in which an N-methyl group has been inserted between carbons 9 and 10 and the carbonyl moiety is thus absent (Fig. 29.27). Azithromycin has a 15-membered lactone ring. This new functionality does not form a cyclic internal ketal. Not only is azithromycin more stable to acid degradation than erythromycin, but it also has a considerably longer half-life, attributed to greater and longer tissue penetration, allowing once-a-day dosage.[92] A popular treatment schedule with azithromycin is to take two tablets on the first day and one a day for the following 5 days and then to discontinue treatment. This is convenient for patients who comply poorly. The drug should be taken on an empty stomach. Azithromycin tends to be broader spectrum than either erythromycin or clarithromycin. Azithromycin has a significant postantibiotic effect against a number of pathogens.[92] Azithromycin is now commonly the first choice for treatment of infections that require a macrolide.

Fidaxomicin (Dificid)

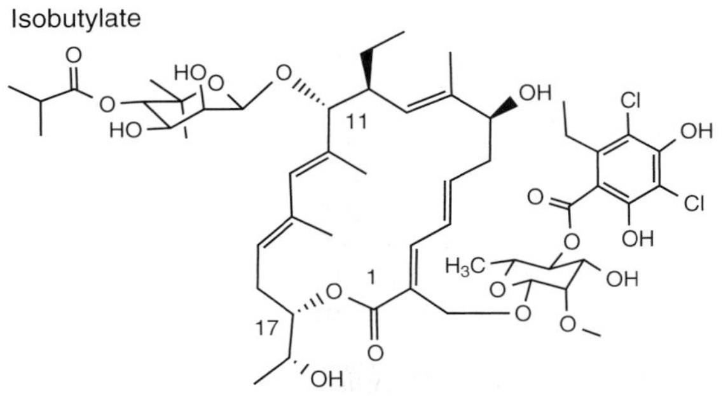

Isobutylate

Fidaxomicin (Dificid)

Fidaxomicin is a unique 18-membered macrolide that is poorly absorbed upon oral administration. It is specifically used to treat gastrointestinal infections caused by *C. difficile*. The narrow spectrum of activity against this organism leads to minimal disruption of normal intestinal flora. The mechanism of action is distinct from other macrolides, in that it is bactericidal and inhibits RNA synthesis by inhibiting RNA polymerases. The lack of oral absorption leads to minimal adverse effects. Hydrolysis of the isobutyl ester on the C-11 sugar by intestinal enzymes produces a compound which retains significant activity.[93]

Ketolides; research activity in the macrolide antibiotic class has been intense recently in attempts to reduce side effects and to broaden their antimicrobial spectra. The ketolides are a group of agents that are characterized by oxidation of the 3 position from an alcohol to a ketone. They are active against a significant number of erythromycin-resistant microorganisms.

Telithromycin (Fig. 29.27) was approved for oral treatment of community-acquired pneumonia, acute bacterial exacerbations of chronic bronchitis, and acute sinusitis in 2004. Significant controversy about the safety of this agent arose after approval by the U.S. Food and Drug Administration and ultimately led to removal of two indications, additional warning information about liver toxicity and a black box warning regarding use in myasthenia gravis patients. The drug was withdrawn from the US market shortly after the decision by the FDA. The toxicity reported for telithromycin appears to be associated with the pyridine portion of the molecule and the antagonist action of the drug on cholinergic receptors.

Lincosamides

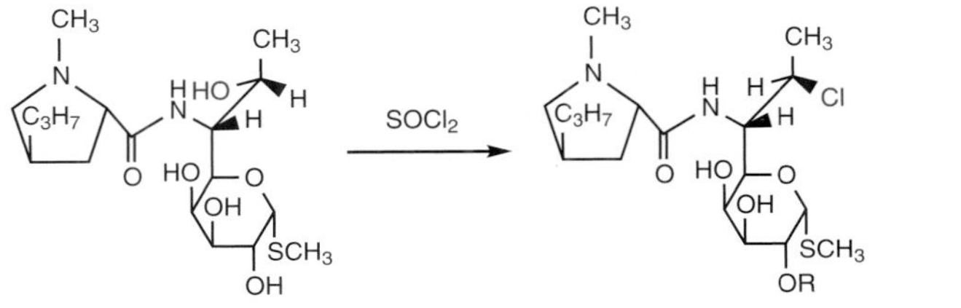

Lincomycin

$SOCl_2$

Clindamycin, R = H (Cleocin)
Clindamycin phosphate, R = PO_3H

The lincosamides contain an unusual 8-carbon sugar, a thiomethyl amino-octoside (O-thio-lincosamide), linked by an amide bond to an *n*-propyl–substituted N-methylpyrrolidylcarboxylic acid (N-methyl-*n*-propyl-*trans*-hygric acid). Lincosamides are weakly basic and form clinically useful hydrochloric acid salts. They are chemically distinct from the macrolide antibiotics but possess many pharmacologic similarities to them. The lincosamides bind to 50S ribosomal subparticles at a site partly overlapping with the macrolide site and are mutually cross-resistant with macrolides and work through essentially the same molecular mechanism of action (Fig. 29.23). The lincosamides undergo extensive liver metabolism resulting primarily in N-demethylation. The N-desmethyl analogue retains biologic activity.

Specific Agents

Lincomycin (Lincocin). Lincomycin is a natural product isolated from fermentations of *Streptomyces lincolnensis*. It is active against gram-positive organisms including some anaerobes. It is indicated for treatment of serious infections caused by sensitive strains of streptococci, pneumococci, and staphylococci. It is generally reserved for penicillin-allergic patients due to the increased risk of pseudomembranous colitis (described below). It also serves as the starting material for the synthesis of clindamycin (by an S_N2 reaction that inverts the *R*-stereochemistry of the C-7 hydroxyl to a C-7 *S*-chloride).

Clindamycin (Cleocin). The substitution of the chloride for the hydroxy group consequently makes clindamycin more bioactive and lipophilic than lincomycin, and thus, it is better absorbed following oral administration. It is about 90% absorbed when taken orally. Clindamycin has a clinical spectrum rather like the macrolides, although it distributes better into bones. Clindamycin works well for gram-positive coccal infections, especially in patients allergic to β-lactams, and also has generally better activity against anaerobes. However, as with lincomycin, it is associated with GI complaints (nausea, vomiting, cramps, and drug-related diarrheas).[94] The most severe of these (black box warning) is pseudomembranous colitis caused *C. difficile*, an opportunistic anaerobe. Its overgrowth results from suppression of the normal flora whose presence otherwise preserves a healthier ecologic balance. The popularity of clindamycin in the clinic has decreased even though pseudomembranous colitis is comparatively rare and is also associated with several other broad-spectrum antibiotics. A less common side effect is exudative erythema multiform (Stevens-Johnson syndrome). Clindamycin has excellent activity against *Propionibacterium* acnes when applied topically.[94] A very water-insoluble palmitate hydrochloride prodrug of clindamycin is also available (lacks bitter taste).

Tetracyclines and Glycylcyclines. The tetracycline family is widely but not intensively used in office practice. Of the agents in this family, minocycline and doxycycline are still frequently prescribed in the United States. This family of antibiotics is characterized by a highly functionalized, partially reduced naphthacene (four linearly fused six-membered rings) ring system from which both the family name and numbering system are derived.

Naphthacene

Tetracycline

(1,2,3,4,4a,5,5a,6,11,11a ,12,12a-dodecahydronaphthacene)

They possess a number of adverse effects, although most of them are annoying rather than dangerous. Because their antimicrobial spectrum is broad enough to include many of the pathogens encountered in a community setting, they were once very widely used. The advent of other choices and the high incidence of resistance that has developed have greatly decreased their medicinal prominence in recent years. Presently, they are recommended primarily for use against *Rickettsia*, *Chlamydia*, *Mycoplasma*, anthrax, plague, and *Helicobacter*.

Chemical Properties. The tetracyclines are amphoteric substances with three pK_a values revealed by titration (2.8-3.4, 7.2-7.8, and 9.1-9.7) and have an isoelectric point at about pH 5. The basic function is the C-4-α-dimethylamino moiety. Commercially available tetracyclines (Table 29.10) are generally administered as comparatively water-soluble hydrochloride salts. The conjugated phenolic enone system extending from C-10 to C-12 is associated with the pK_a at about 7.5, whereas the conjugated trione system extending from C-1 to C-3 in ring A is nearly as acidic as acetic acid (pK_a ~3).[95] These resonating systems can be drawn in a number of essentially equivalent ways with the double bonds in alternate positions. The formulae normally shown are those settled upon by popular convention.

Chelation. Chelation is an important feature of the chemical and clinical properties of the tetracyclines. The acidic functions of the tetracyclines are capable of forming salts through chelation with metal ions. The salts of polyvalent metal ions, such as Fe^{2+}, Ca^{2+}, Mg^{2+}, and Al^{3+}, are all quite insoluble at neutral pHs (Fig. 29.30). This insolubility is not only inconvenient for the preparation of solutions, but also interferes with blood levels on oral administration

Consequently, the tetracyclines are incompatible with coadministered multivalent ion-rich antacids, and concomitant consumption of daily products rich in calcium ion is also contraindicated.[95] When concomitant oral therapy with tetracyclines and incompatible metal ions must be done, the ions should be given 1 hour before or 2 hours after the tetracyclines. Further, the bones, of which the teeth are the most visible, are calcium-rich structures at

Table 29.10 Commercially Available Tetracyclines

Generic Name	Trade Name	X	Y	R_1	R_2	R_3
Tetracycline	Generic	H	H	OH	CH_3	H
Demeclocycline	Declomycin	Cl	H	OH	H	H
Minocycline	Minocin	$N(CH_3)_2$	H	H	H	H
Doxycycline	Vibramycin	H	H	H	CH_3	OH
Tigecycline	Tygacil	$N(CH_3)_2$	NH–C(=O)–CH₂–NH–t-Bu	H	H	H

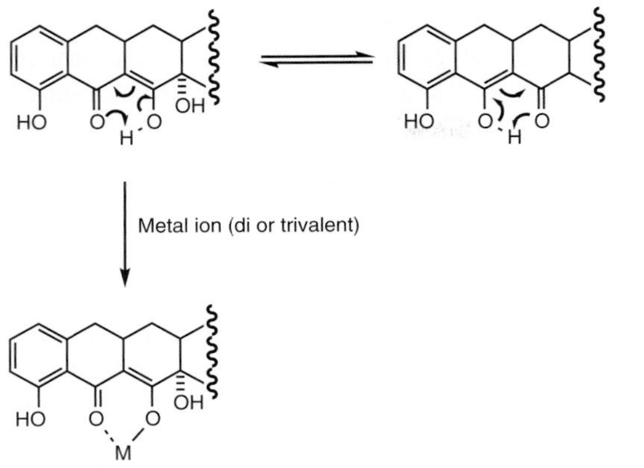

Metal ion (di or trivalent)

Figure 29.30 Metal chelation with the tetracyclines.

Tetracycline (active)

Anhydrotetracycline (inactive)

4-Epitetracycline (inactive)

4-Epianhydrotetracycline (inactive)

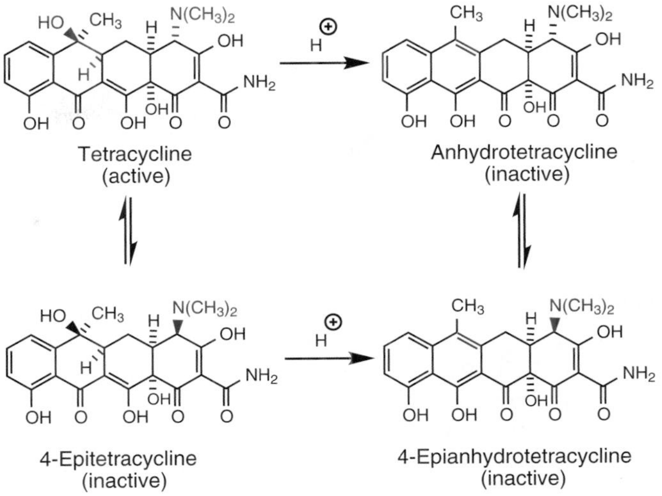

Figure 29.32 Acid-catalyzed instability of tetracyclines.

nearly neutral pHs and so accumulate tetracyclines in proportion to the amount and duration of therapy when bones and teeth are being formed. Because the tetracyclines are yellow, this leads to a progressive and essentially permanent discoloration in which, in advanced cases, the teeth are even brown. The intensification of discoloration with time is thought to be a photochemical process. This is cosmetically unattractive but does not seem to be deleterious except in extreme cases where so much antibiotic is taken up that the structure of bone is mechanically weakened. To avoid this, tetracyclines are not normally given to children.[95]

Epimerization. The α-stereo orientation of the C-4 dimethylamino moiety of the tetracyclines is essential for their bioactivity. The presence of the tricarbonyl system of ring A allows enolization involving loss of the C-4 hydrogen (Fig. 29.31). Reprotonation can take place from either the top or bottom of the molecule. Reprotonation from the top of the enol regenerates tetracycline. Reprotonation from the bottom, however, produces inactive 4-epitetracycline. At equilibrium, the mixture consists of nearly equal amounts of the two diastereomers.

Dehydration. Most of the natural tetracyclines have a tertiary and benzylic hydroxyl group at C-6. This function has the ideal geometry for acid-catalyzed dehydration involving the C-5a α-oriented hydrogen (antiperiplanar *trans*). The resulting product is a naphthalene derivative, so there are energetic reasons for the reaction proceeding in that direction (Fig. 29.32). C-5a,6-anhydrotetracycline is much deeper in color than tetracycline and is biologically inactive.

Not only can inactive 4-epitetracyclines dehydrate to produce 4-epianhydrotetracyclines, but also anhydrotetracycline can epimerize to produce the same product. This degradation product is toxic to the kidneys and produces a Fanconi-like syndrome that, in extreme cases, has been fatal.[96] Tetracyclines that have no C-6-hydroxyl groups, such as minocycline and doxycycline, cannot undergo dehydration and thus are completely free of this toxicity.

Cleavage in Base. Another untoward degradation reaction involving a C-6-hydroxyl group is cleavage of the C-ring in alkaline solutions at or above pH 8.5 (Fig. 29.33). The lactonic product, an isotetracycline, is inactive. The clinical impact of this degradation under normal conditions is uncertain.

Phototoxicity. Certain tetracyclines, most notably those with a C-7-chlorine, absorb light in the visible region, leading to free radical generation and potentially causing severe erythema to sensitive patients on exposure to strong sunlight. Patients should be advised to be cautious about such exposure for at least their first few doses to avoid potentially severe sunburn. This effect is comparatively rare with most currently popular tetracyclines.[96]

Mechanism of Action. The tetracyclines of clinical importance interfere with protein biosynthesis at the ribosomal level, leading to bacteriostasis. Tetracyclines bind to rRNA in the 30S subparticle with the possible cooperation of a 50S site by a process that remains imprecisely understood despite intensive study (Fig. 29.23). There is more than one binding site, but only one is believed to be critical for its action. The points of contact with the rRNA are those associated with antibiosis, with the puzzling exception of the dimethylamino function (Fig. 29.34). This latter is known to be essential for activity but does not appear to bind in the X-ray structures that are available.[97-99] Once the tetracycline binds, it inhibits subsequent binding of

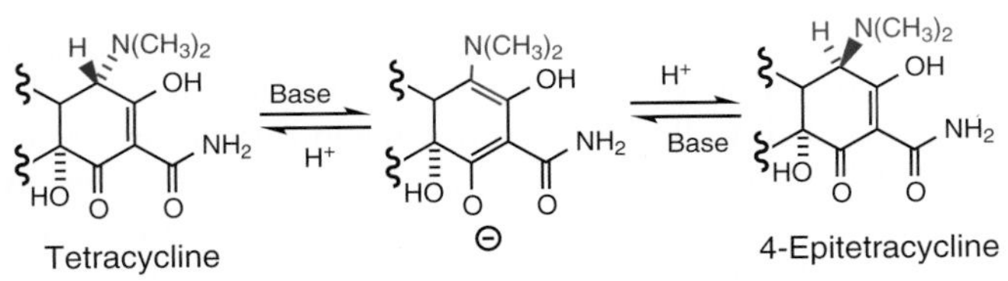

Base H+ H+ Base

Tetracycline 4-Epitetracycline

Figure 29.31 Epimerization of tetracyclines.

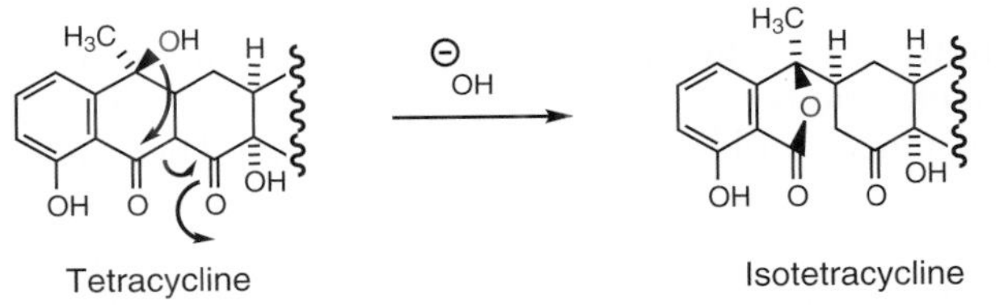

Tetracycline Isotetracycline

Figure 29.33 Base-catalyzed instability of tetracyclines.

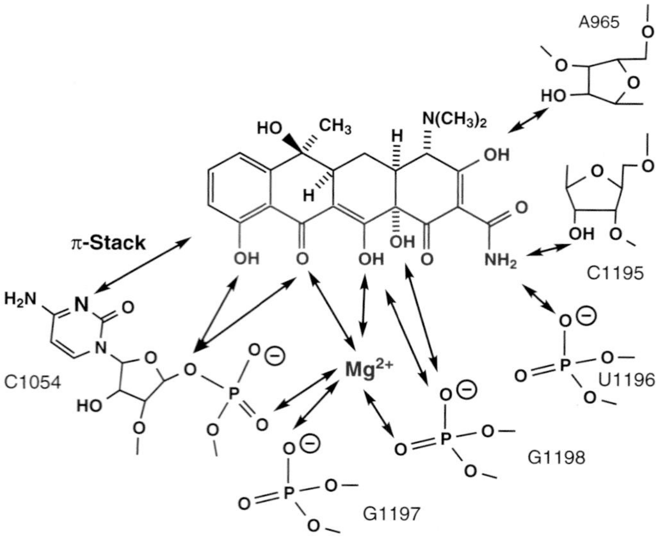

Figure 29.34 Schematic representation of the primary binding site for a tetracycline and the sugar phosphate groups of 16S rRNA which also involves a magnesium ion and the critical functional groups on the "southern" and "eastern" face of the tetracycline. Redrawn and modified from Brodersen, et al. *Cell.* 2000;103:1143-1154.

aminoacyltransfer-RNA to the ribosomes, resulting in termination of peptide chain growth. The more lipophilic tetracyclines, typified by minocycline, are also capable of disrupting cytoplasmic membrane function, causing leakage of nucleotides and other essential cellular components from the cell, and have bactericidal properties.

Resistance. Resistance to tetracyclines results in part from an unusual ribosomal protection process involving elaboration of bacterial proteins. These proteins associate with the ribosome, thus allowing protein biosynthesis to proceed even in the presence of bound tetracycline, although exactly how this works is not well understood. Another important resistance mechanism involves R-factor–mediated, energy-requiring, active efflux of tetracyclines from the bacterial cells.[100] Some of the efflux proteins have activity that is limited to older tetracyclines, whereas others confer resistance to the entire family with the exception of glycylcyclines. Certain other microbes, such as *Mycoplasma* and *Neisseria*, seem to have modified membranes that either accumulate fewer tetracyclines or have porins through which tetracyclines have difficulty passing. Because resistance is now widespread, these once extremely popular antibiotics are falling into comparative disuse

Therapeutic Application. The tetracyclines possess very wide bacteriostatic antibacterial activity. Because of the resistance phenomenon and the comparative frequency of troublesome side effects, they are rarely the drugs of first choice. The differences between the antimicrobial spectra of various tetracyclines are not large, although greater resistance to older agents limits their use. They are used for low-dose oral and topical therapy for acne, first-course community-acquired urinary tract infections (largely due to *E. coli*), brucellosis, borreliosis, sexually transmitted diseases (especially chlamydia), rickettsial infections, mycoplasmal pneumonia, prophylaxis of malaria, prevention of traveler's diarrhea, cholera, *Enterobacter* infections, as part of *Helicobacter* cocktails, Lyme disease, Rocky Mountain spotted fever, anthrax, and many other less common problems.[95] The tetracyclines are also widely used for agricultural purposes.

Adverse Effects. In addition to the adverse effects mentioned earlier (tooth staining, phototoxicity, and potential kidney damage with outdated drug), the tetracyclines are associated with nausea, vomiting, diarrhea, and some CNS effects (dizziness and vertigo). Rapid administration or prolonged intravenous use can lead to thrombophlebitis, so tetracyclines are generally administered orally because they are well absorbed. They also distinguish imperfectly between the bacterial 70S ribosomes and the mammalian 80S ribosomes, so in high doses or special situations (i.e., intravenous use during pregnancy), these drugs also demonstrate a significant antianabolic effect. In cases of significant renal impairment, higher serum levels of tetracyclines can lead to azotemia. Additionally, inducers of CYP450 metabolism (i.e., rifampin, barbiturates, carbamazepine) increase metabolism of tetracyclines (especially doxycycline), so the dose of the tetracycline may require adjustment.[96]

Specific Agents (Table 29.10)

Tetracycline. Tetracycline is produced by fermentation of *Streptomyces aureofaciens* and related species or by catalytic reduction of chlortetracycline. The blood levels achieved on oral administration are often irregular. Food and milk lower absorption by about 50%.[95]

Demeclocycline. Demeclocycline lacks the C-6-methyl of tetracycline and is produced by a genetically altered strain of *S. aureofaciens*. Because it is a secondary alcohol, it is more chemically stable than tetracycline against dehydration. Food and milk co-consumption decreases absorption by half, although it is 60%-80% absorbed by fasting adults. It is the tetracycline most highly associated with phototoxicity and also has been shown to produce dose-dependent, reversible diabetes insipidus with extended use. Demeclocycline is commonly used off label for treatment of inappropriate secretion of antidiuretic hormone.

Minocycline (Minocin and Others). An important antibiotic produced by semisynthesis from demeclocycline is minocycline. It is much more lipophilic than its precursors, gives excellent blood levels following oral administration (90%-100% available), and can be given once a day. Its absorption is lowered by about 20% when taken with food or milk. It is less dependent on active uptake mechanisms and has a somewhat broader antimicrobial spectrum. It has vestibular toxicities (e.g., vertigo, ataxia, and nausea) not generally shared by other tetracyclines.[101]

Doxycycline (Vibramycin and Others). It is produced by semisynthesis from other tetracycline molecules and is the most widely used of the tetracycline family. Doxycycline is well absorbed on oral administration (90%-100% when fasting; reduced by 20% by co-consumption with food or milk), has a half-life permitting once-a-day dosing for mild infections, and is excreted partly in the feces and partly in the urine.

Tigecycline (Tygacil). The increased incidence of resistance to the tetracyclines led to a renewed research effort to find novel agents within this class. This effort led to the discovery of a new class of antibiotics, the glycylcyclines, that are closely structurally related to the tetracyclines but lack many of the clinical resistance issues.[102,103] They are characterized by having an additional glyclamido substitution at the 9 position. Tigecycline is the first of these agents to be marketed. Although it has limited indications, treatment of complicated skin/skin structure and complicated intra-abdominal infections, this agent is a broad-spectrum antibiotic based on the in vitro data. It is administered intravenously and, like the tetracyclines, can cause injection site pain and thrombophlebitis. It has other adverse effects similar to the tetracyclines.

Special Purpose Antibiotics. This group of antibiotics consists of a miscellaneous collection of structural types whose toxicities or narrow range of applicability give them a more specialized place in antimicrobial chemotherapy than those covered to this point. They are generally reserved for special purposes.

Chloramphenicol (Chloromycetin)

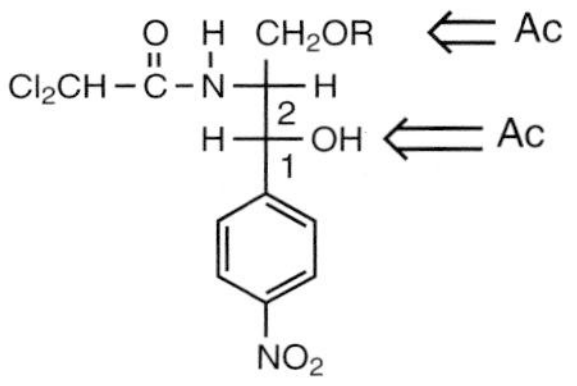

Chloramphenicol hemisuccinate R = $COCH_2CH_2CO_2H$

Chloramphenicol was originally produced by fermentation of *Streptomyces venezuelae*, but its comparatively simple chemical structure soon resulted in several efficient total chemical syntheses. With two asymmetric centers, it is one of four diastereomers, only one of which (1*R*,2*R*) is significantly active. Because total synthesis produces a mixture of all four, the unwanted isomers must be removed before use. Chloramphenicol is a neutral substance only moderately soluble in water because both nitrogen atoms are nonbasic under physiologic conditions (one is an amide and the other a nitro moiety). It was the first broad-spectrum oral antibiotic used in the United States (1947) and was once very popular. Severe potential blood dyscrasia has greatly decreased its use in North America, although its cheapness and efficacy make it still very popular in many places in the world where it can often be purchased over the counter without a prescription.

Mechanism of Action. Chloramphenicol is bacteriostatic by virtue of inhibition of protein biosynthesis in both bacterial and, to a lesser extent, the host ribosomes. Chloramphenicol binds to the 50S subparticle in a region near where the macrolides and lincosamides bind (Fig. 29.23).

Resistance is mediated by several R-factor enzymes that catalyze acetylation of the secondary and, to some extent, the primary hydroxyl groups in the aliphatic side chain.[104] These products no longer bind to the ribosomes and thus are inactivated.

Metabolism. When given orally, chloramphenicol is rapidly and completely absorbed but has a fairly short half-life. It is mainly excreted in the urine in the form of its metabolites, which are C-3 and C-1 glucuronides, and, to a lesser extent, its deamidation product and the product of dehalogenation and reduction. These metabolites are all inactive. The aromatic nitro group is also reduced metabolically, and this product can undergo amide hydrolysis. The reduction of the nitro group, however, does not take place efficiently in humans but primarily occurs in the gut by the action of the normal flora.[105] Chloramphenicol potentiates the activity of some other drugs by inducing liver metabolism. Such agents include anticoagulant coumarins, sulfonamides, oral hypoglycemics, and phenytoin.[105]

Prodrug Forms. Two prodrug forms of chloramphenicol are available (only the injectable form is available in the United States). The drug is intensively bitter. This can be masked for use as a pediatric oral suspension by use of the C-3 palmitate, which is cleaved in the duodenum to liberate the drug.

Chloramphenicol's poor water solubility is largely overcome by conversion to the C-3 hemisuccinoyl ester, which forms a water-soluble sodium salt. This is cleaved in the body by lung, liver, kidney, and blood esterases to produce active chloramphenicol. Because cleavage in muscles is slow, this prodrug is used intravenously rather than intramuscularly.

Therapeutic Applications. Despite potentially serious limitations, chloramphenicol is an effective drug when used carefully. Its special value is in typhoid fever, *Haemophilus* infections (especially epiglottitis and meningitis, when given along with ampicillin), and rickettsial infections and in cases where susceptible organisms have proven resistant to other therapies. Safer antibiotics should be used whenever possible. It is about 60% serum protein bound and diffuses well into tissues, especially into inflamed cerebrospinal fluid, and is, therefore, of value for meningitis. It also penetrates well into lymph and mesenteric ganglions, rationalizing its particular value in typhoid fever.

Adverse Effects. Toxicities prevent chloramphenicol from being more widely used. Blood dyscrasias are seen in patients predisposed to them.[105] The more serious form is a pancytopenia of the blood that is fatal in about 70% of cases and is believed to be caused by one of the reduction products of the aromatic nitro group. This side effect is known as aplastic anemia and has even occurred following use of the drug as an ophthalmic ointment. There seems to be a genetic predisposition toward this in a very small percentage of the population. Less severe, but much more common, is a reversible inhibition of hematopoiesis, seen in older patients or in those with renal insufficiency. If cell counts are taken, this can be controlled because it is dose related and marrow function will recover if the drug is withdrawn.

The so-called "gray" or "gray baby" syndrome, a form of cardiovascular collapse, is encountered when chloramphenicol is given to young infants (especially premature infants) when liver glucuronidation is underdeveloped, and successive doses will lead to rapid accumulation of the drug due to impaired excretion. A dose-related profound anemia accompanied by an ashen gray pallor is seen, as are vomiting, loss of appetite, and cyanosis. Deaths have resulted, often involving cardiovascular collapse.

Glycopeptides. A variety of cyclic peptides are utilized for their antibiotic properties. The usual physiologically significant peptides are linear. Several bacterial species, however, produce antibiotic mixtures of cyclic peptides, some with uncommon amino acids and some with common amino acids but with the D absolute stereochemistry. These cyclic substances often have a pendant fatty acid chain as well. One of the consequences of this unusual architecture is that these glycopeptide agents are not readily metabolized. These drugs are usually water soluble and are highly lethal to susceptible bacteria because they attach themselves to the bacterial membranes and interfere with their semipermeability so that essential metabolites leak out and undesirable substances pass in. Unfortunately, they are also highly toxic in humans, so their use is reserved for serious situations where there are few alternatives or to topical uses. Bacteria are rarely able to develop significant resistance to this group of antibiotics. They are generally unstable, so solutions should be protected from heat, light, and extremes of pH.

Vancomycin (Vancocin, Generic). Vancomycin (Table 29.11) is produced by fermentation of *Amycolatopsis orientalis* (formerly called *Nocardia orientalis*). It has been available for about 40 years, but its popularity has increased significantly with the emergence of MRSA in the early 1980s. Chemically, vancomycin has a glycosylated hexapeptide chain rich in unusual amino acids, many of which contain aromatic rings cross-linked by aryl ether bonds into a rigid molecular framework.

Mechanism of Action. Vancomycin is a bacterial cell wall biosynthesis inhibitor. There is evidence that the active species is a homodimer of two vancomycin units. The binding site for its target is a peptide-lined cleft having high affinity for acetyl-D-alanyl-D-alanine and related peptides through five hydrogen bonds (Fig. 29.35).[106] It inhibits both transglycosylases (inhibiting the linking between muramic acid and acetyl glucosamine units) and transpeptidase (inhibiting peptide cross-linking) activities in cell wall biosynthesis (Fig. 29.9). Thus, vancomycin functions like a peptide receptor and interrupts bacterial cell wall biosynthesis at the same step as does the β-lactams but by a different mechanism. By covering the substrate for cell wall transamidase, it prevents cross-linking, resulting in osmotically defective cell walls.

Resistance. Only recently, despite decades of intensive use, have some vancomycin-resistant bacteria emerged (vancomycin-resistant *Enterococcus* and vancomycin-resistant *S. aureus*).[107] The mechanism of resistance appears to be alteration of the target D-alanyl-D-alanine units on the peptidoglycan cell wall precursors to D-alanyl-D-lactate. This results in lowered affinity for vancomycin. It is feared that this form of resistance will become more common in the bacteria for which vancomycin presently is used for successful chemotherapy.

Therapeutic Applications. Although a number of adverse effects can result from intravenous infusion (see below), vancomycin has negligible oral activity. It can be used orally for action in the GI tract, especially in cases of *C. difficile* overgrowth. The useful spectrum is restricted to gram-positive pathogens with particular utility against multiply resistant coagulase-negative staphylococci and MRSA, which causes septicemias, endocarditis, skin and soft tissue infections, and infections associated with venous catheters.[108]

Adverse Effects. Vancomycin is highly associated with adverse infusion-related events. These are especially prevalent with higher doses and a rapid infusion rate. Rapid infusion rate has been shown to cause anaphylactoid reactions, including hypotension, wheezing, dyspnea, urticaria, and pruritus. A significant drug rash (the so-called red man syndrome) can also occur. These events are much less frequent with a slower infusion rate.

In addition to the danger of infusion-related events, higher doses of vancomycin can cause nephrotoxicity and auditory nerve damage. The risk of these effects is increased with elevated, prolonged concentrations, so vancomycin use should be monitored, especially in patients with decreased renal function. The ototoxicity may be transient or permanent and more commonly occurs in patients on high doses, those who have underlying hearing loss, and those treated concomitantly with other ototoxic agents (i.e., aminoglycosides).[108]

Telavancin (Vibativ), Dalbavancin (Dalvance), and Oritavancin (Orbactiv). Telavancin, dalbavancin, and oritavancin (Table 29.11) are semisynthetic derivatives of vancomycin that have been altered at the R7 substituent.[109-111] This change has an effect on the half-life of the derivatives that allows for less frequent dosing of the drugs. Telavancin is dosed once per day; dalbavancin and oritavancin can be given as single dose therapy. Although they inhibit cell wall biosynthesis in the same manner as vancomycin, it appears that the structural change also causes disruption of cell membrane integrity (similar to a detergent) as part of their mechanism. Oritavancin also binds to the pentaglycyl bridging structure to further inhibit peptidoglycan crosslinking.[111] These additional mechanisms likely account for retention of antibacterial activity against some vancomycin-resistant organisms. They are indicated for treatment of skin and skin structure infections by gram-positive organisms including MRSA. Telavancin is also indicated for hospital- or

Table 29.11 Structures of the Glycopeptide Antibiotics

Glycopeptide nucleus

	X	R_1	R_2	R_3	R_4	R_5	R_6	R_7
Dalbavancin (Dalvance)		H				H	H	
Telavancin (Vibativ)	OH0		H			OH	Cl	
Vancomycin (Vancocin)	OH	H	H			OH	Cl	
Oritavancin (Orbactiv)	OH	H	H			OH	Cl	

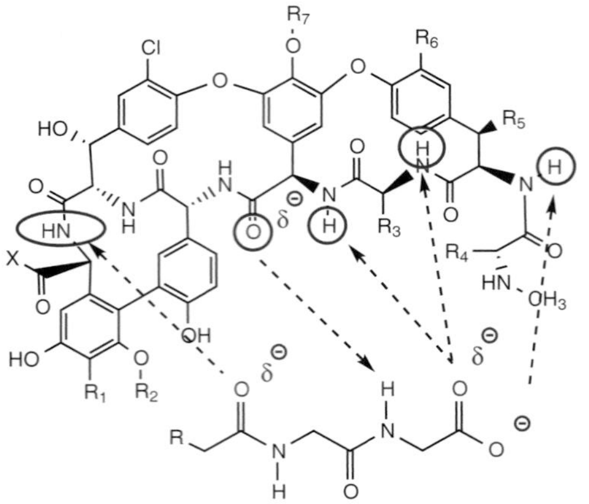

Figure 29.35 Binding of glycopeptide antibiotics to bacterial cell wall D-alanine-D-alanine moiety.

ventilator-acquired bacterial pneumonia when alternative treatments are not suitable. They should not be used in pregnancy, and like vancomycin, telavancin and dalbavancin require dose adjustment with renal impairment. Oritavancin does not require adjusted doses for mild or moderate renal impairment. They also produce infusion-related toxicities, so slow infusion is recommended to reduce the toxicities.

Daptomycin (Cubicin)

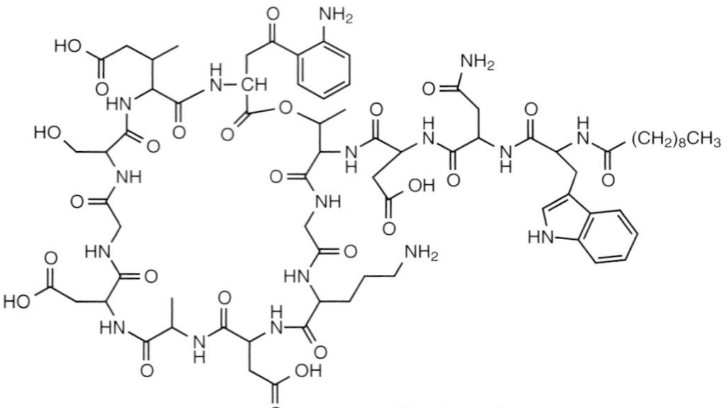

Daptomycin

Daptomycin is a fermentation product having a cyclic lipopeptide structure.[112] It is primarily active against gram-positive infections, especially skin and skin structure infections. It is given intravenously but must be administered over a period of 30 minutes or more. It binds to cell membranes and causes depolarization, which interrupts protein, DNA, and RNA synthesis.

Daptomycin is bactericidal. Although resistance can be achieved in vitro, resistance has been slow to emerge in the clinic. Patients should be monitored for muscle pain or weakness because some incidence of elevated serum creatinine phosphokinase is associated with its use. Daptomycin is eliminated primarily by the kidney, so dose adjustment may be necessary in cases of renal insufficiency.[113]

Quinupristin/Dalfopristin (Synercid)

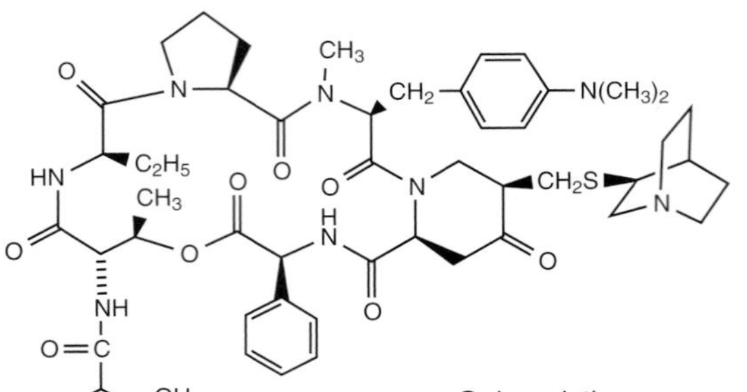

Quinupristin (Streptogramin B)

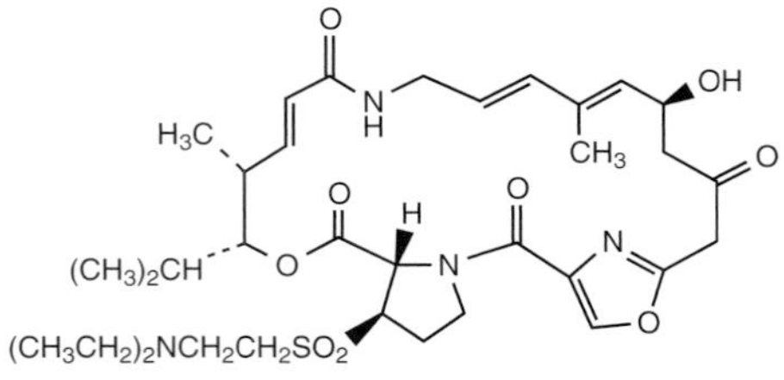

Dalfopristin (Streptogramin A)

A combination of the streptogramins quinupristin and dalfopristin is approved for intravenous use in the treatment of infections caused by vancomycin-resistant *E. faecium* bacteremia as well as skin and skin structure infections caused by methicillin-sensitive *S. aureus* and *S. pyogenes*. Certain strains of *E. faecium* are resistant to essentially all other antibiotics, including vancomycin. Dalfopristin binds to the 23S portion of the 50S ribosomal subunit and causes a conformational change that enhances quinupristin binding to the 50S subunit by 100X.[114] The two drugs are bacteriostatic when administered individually but are found to act synergistically when combined (quinupristin:dalfopristin [30:70 w/w]) to produce a bactericidal effect. It appears that dalfopristin binding creates a high-affinity binding site for quinupristin, accounting for the synergy. The combination is found to inhibit protein synthesis by binding to the 70S ribosome that is thought to account for the mechanism of action. Synercid is a strong inhibitor of the CYP3A4 isozyme, and a number of drug interactions are to be expected. Although the combination does not appear to prolong the QTc interval, it inhibits the metabolism of a number of agents that have been shown to have this effect, so concomitant administration should be avoided. Synercid also can produce a number of other adverse effects including infusion site reactions (pain, edema, and inflammation), arthralgia and myalgia, and hyperbilirubinemia.[115]

Polymyxin B

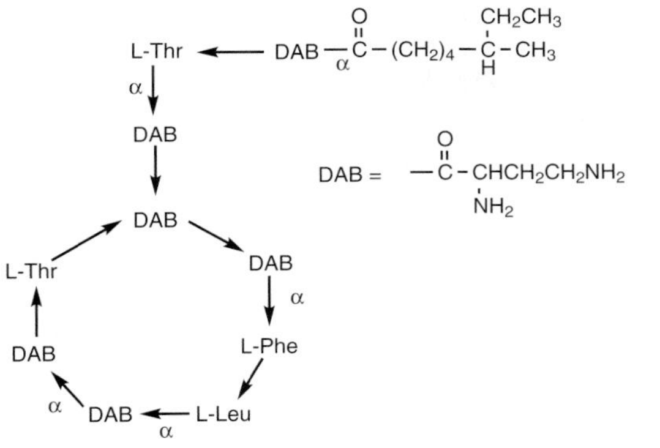

L-Thr ← DAB —α— C(=O) – $(CH_2)_4$ – CH(CH_2CH_3) – CH_3

DAB = –C(=O)–CH(NH_2)$CH_2CH_2NH_2$

Polymyxin B

Polymyxin B is produced by fermentation of *Bacillus polymyxa*. It is separated from a mixture of related cyclic peptides and is primarily active against gram-negative microorganisms. It apparently binds to phosphate groups in bacterial cytoplasmic membranes and disrupts their integrity. It is used intramuscularly or intravenously as a sulfate salt to treat serious urinary tract infections, meningitis, and septicemia primarily caused by *P. aeruginosa*, but some other gram-negative bacteria will also respond. It is also used orally to treat enteropathogenic *E. coli* and *Shigella* sp. diarrheas. Irrigation of the urinary bladder with solutions of polymyxin B sulfate is also employed by some to reduce the incidence of infections subsequent to installation of indwelling catheters. When given parenterally, the drug is neuro- and nephrotoxic and thus is used only after other drugs have failed.

Bacitracin

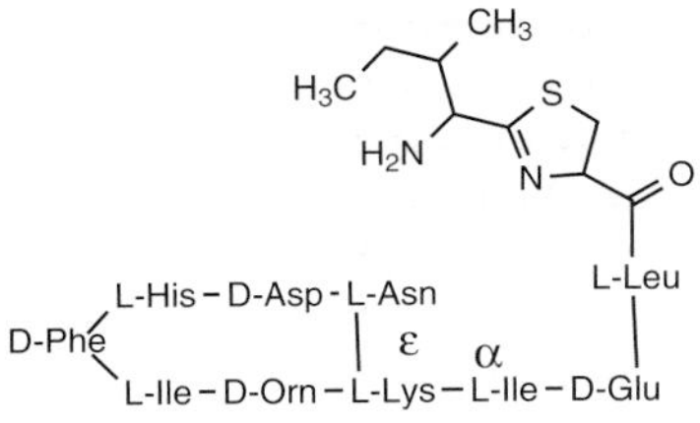

Bacitracin A

Bacitracin is a mixture of similar peptides produced by fermentation of the bacterium *Bacillus subtilis*. The A component predominates. Its mode of action is to inhibit both peptidoglycan biosynthesis at a late stage (probably at the dephosphorylation of the phospholipid carrier step) and disruptions of plasma membrane function. It is predominantly active against gram-positive microorganisms, and parenteral use is limited to intramuscular injection for infants with pneumonia and empyema caused by staphylococci resistant to other agents. It is rather neuro- and nephrotoxic and thus is used in this manner with caution. Bacitracin is also widely used topically to prevent infection in minor cuts, scrapes, and burns.

Oxazolidinones

Linezolid (Zyvox) and Tedizolid Phosphate (Sivextro)

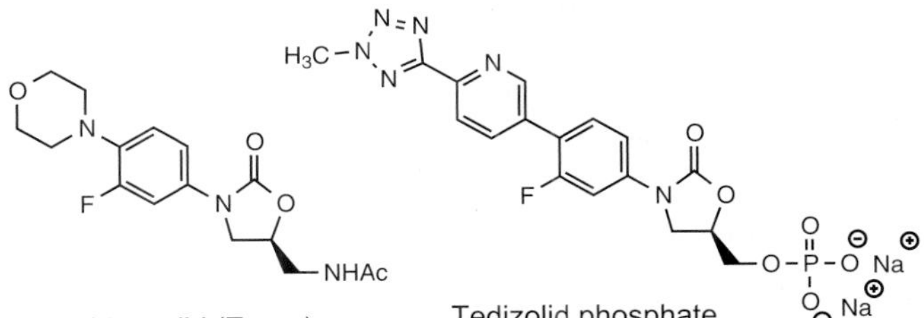

Linezolid (Zyvox)

Tedizolid phosphate disodium (Sivextro)

The oxazolidinones are bacteriostatic (bactericidal against some bacteria) antibacterial agents that are effective against primarily gram-positive bacteria. They are available in injectable and tablet forms. Linezolid is also available as an oral suspension dosage forms. Linezolid is effective against MRSA and are used to treat nosocomial pneumonia, community-acquired pneumonia, complicated and uncomplicated skin and skin structure infections, and vancomycin-resistant *E. faecium* infections.[116] Tedizolid phosphate is a prodrug of tedizolid and has a similar microbial spectrum but is specifically approved for treatment of acute skin and skin structure infections.[117]

The mechanism of action of oxazolidinones is associated with inhibition of protein synthesis but at a stage different from that of other protein synthesis inhibitors. The oxazolidinones inhibit the initiation of protein synthesis by binding to the 50S subparticle, preventing the formation of a functional initiation complex including N-formylmethionyl-tRNA ($tRNA^{fMet}$), the 30S subunit, mRNA, and initiation factors. It is believed that the drug distorts the binding site for the initiator-tRNA, which overlaps both 30S and 50S ribosomal subunits.[118] The result of this is that translation of the mRNA is prevented. The other prominent ribosomal protein biosynthesis inhibitors inhibit after a functional initiation complex forms. In those cases, mRNA translation begins, but elongation of the growing peptide chain is blocked.

Resistance to oxazolidinones is encountered in the clinic due to a mutation in the 23S rRNA associated with the 50S ribosomal subunit.[119] This is believed to distort the binding site. Gram-negative microorganisms are intrinsically resistant to oxazolidinones due to the presence of endogenous efflux pumps that keep them from accumulating in the cells.

Linezolid is well absorbed orally and is generally well to moderately tolerated; however, some severe cases of reversible blood dyscrasias have been noted, resulting in a package insert warning that complete blood counts should be monitored weekly, especially in patients with poorly draining infections and who are receiving prolonged therapy with the drug.[116] Both agents are inhibitors of monoamine oxidase, so patients should be cautious about eating tyramine-containing foods. Coadministration with adrenergic and serotonergic agents is also unadvisable. Significant oxidative metabolism occurs for linezolid by oxidation of the morpholine ring, and the antimicrobially inactive metabolites are excreted primarily in the urine.[115]

Tedizolid is not significantly metabolized by phase I pathways and is primarily excreted as a sulfate conjugate of the primary alcohol.[117]

Mupirocin (Bactroban)

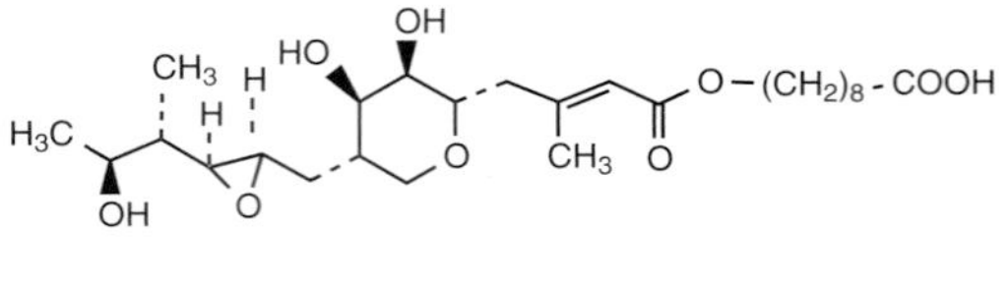

Mupirocin

Mupirocin is a member of a group of lipid acids produced by fermentation of *Pseudomonas fluorescens*. It can only be used topically because of hydrolysis in vivo that inactivates the drug. It is intrinsically broad spectrum, but its primary indication is topically against staphylococcal and streptococcal skin infections. Mupirocin binds to bacterial isoleucyl tRNA synthase, preventing incorporation of isoleucine into bacterial proteins. Resistance is due to alterations of the synthase target such that the enzyme still functions but does not bind mupirocin.

Retapamulin (Altabax)

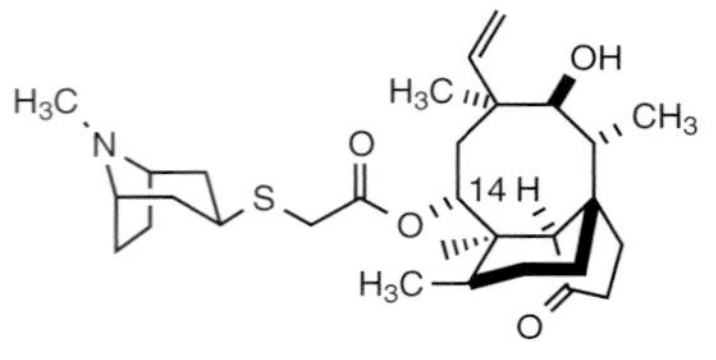

Retapamulin

Retapamulin is approved for use in adults and children over the age of 9 months for the treatment of impetigo caused by methicillin-susceptible *S. aureus* and *S. pyogenes*. Impetigo is a highly contagious infection found most commonly in children involving the upper layers of the skin and spread through close contact. Retapamulin is a semisynthetic diterpene derivative of the naturally occurring pleuromutilins, a group of chemicals produced by the fungus *Pleurotus mutilus* (also referred to as *Clitopilus scyphoides*).[120]

Retapamulin is a bacteriostatic topically used drug that inhibits protein synthesis by binding to the 50S ribosomal subunit. It is a semisynthetic derivative of the natural product mutilin (alcohol at C-14) and pleuromutilin (C-14 hydroxyacetate). The drug is selective for inhibiting translational bacterial protein syntheses and is inactive in eukaryotic translation. Retapamulin is active at a site distinct from that occupied by macrolide antibiotics, both of which inhibit protein synthesis at the 50S ribosomal subunit. It inhibits ribosomal peptidyl transferase, thus preventing peptide bond formation. The C-14 sulfamylacetate moiety appears important for binding to the peptidyl transferase center in the 50S ribosomal subunit of the susceptible bacteria. By occupying this site, the pleuromutilins block peptide bond formation, thus inhibiting bacterial protein synthesis. The pleuromutilins interact with the 23S RNA domain V. There are indications because of the unique binding of retapamulin to the 50S ribosomal subunit that bacterial resistance will be low. Additionally, it has been reported that retapamulin inhibits the biosynthesis of the 50S ribosomal subunit itself in susceptible gram-positive bacteria, leading to the suggestion of a dual antibacterial action.[121-123]

Retapamulin is well tolerated, with minimal adverse events. The most common adverse effects are pruritus, diarrhea, and nasopharyngitis. The drug does not appear to be absorbed to any great degree when applied topically, although it is a substrate for CYP3A4.[120]

ANTIMYCOBACTERIAL AGENTS

Introduction

Mycobacteria are a genus of acid-fast bacilli belonging to the mycobacteriaceae, which include the organisms responsible for tuberculosis and leprosy as well as a number of other, less common diseases. Mycobacteria tend to be slow-growing and difficult to stain pathogens and, when they are stained with basic dye, can resist decolorization with acid alcohol. The staining characteristics relate to the abnormally high lipid content of the cell wall. In fact, the cell wall or cell envelope of the mycobacterium holds the secret to many of the characteristics of this genus of organisms. The cell envelope is unique in both structure and complexity. It has been suggested that the cell envelope is responsible for mycobacterium pathogenicity or virulence, multiple drug resistance, cell permeability, immunoreactivity, and inhibition of antigen responsiveness, as well as disease persistence and recrudescence. In addition, several of the successful chemotherapeutic agents are known to inhibit the cell envelope synthesis as their mechanism of action. It is no wonder that significant effort has been put forth to define the chemical structure of the mycobacterial cell envelope.

The mycobacterial cell envelope contains, on the interior surface, a plasma membrane similar to that found in most bacteria (Fig. 29.36). A conventional peptidoglycan layer affording the organism rigidity appears next. This layer is composed of alternating N-acetyl-D-glucosamines (Glu) linked to N-glycoyl-D-muramic acids (Mur) through 1-4 linkages that, in turn, is attached to the peptido chain of D-alanine (A), D-glutamine (G), meso-diaminopimelic acid (DP), and L-alanine (A). A novel disaccharide phosphodiester linker made up of N-acetyl-D-glucosamine and rhamnose connects the muramic acid to a polygalactan and polyarabinose chain. The latter polysaccharides are referred to as the arabinogalactan (AG) portion of the cell envelope. The manner in which the arabinosyl and galactosyl residues are arranged is still under investigation. It is known that the arabinosyl chains terminate in mycolic acid residues. Noncovalently bound to the mycolates are a number of free nonpolar and polar lipids (the phthiocerol lipids and the glycopeptidolipids, respectively). Finally, spanning from the interior, embedded in the plasma membrane, to the exterior is the lipoarabinomannan (LAM)

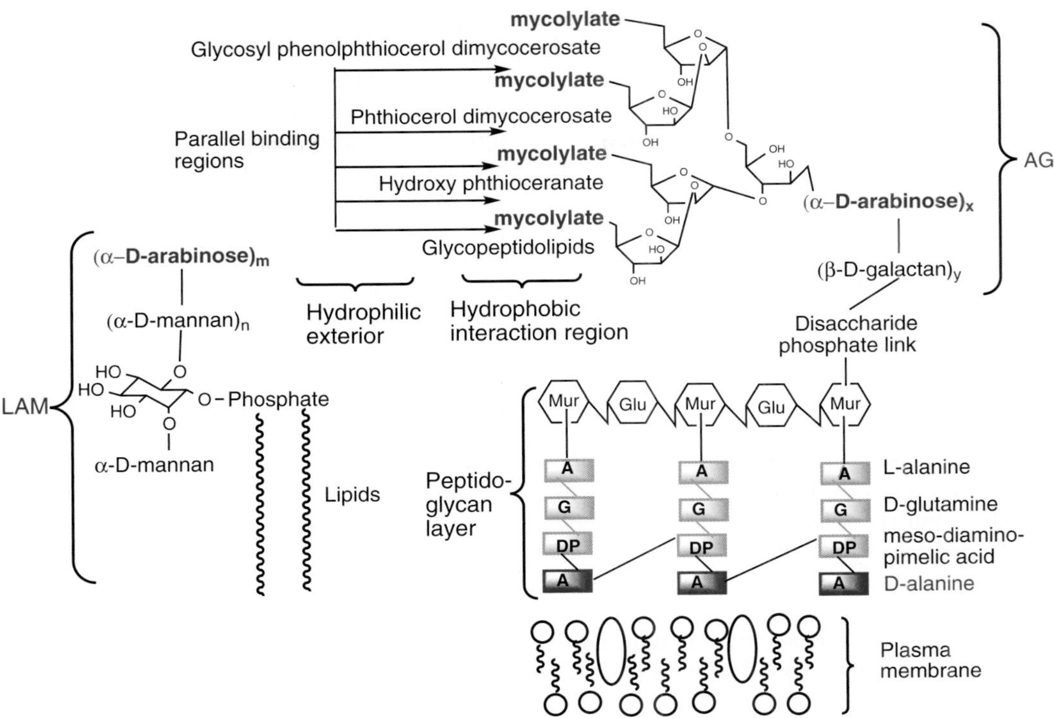

Figure 29.36 Diagrammatic representation of the cell wall/cell envelope of mycobacterium with drug sites of action highlighted in red. AG, arabinogalactan; LAM, lipoarabinomannan.

polymer. As indicated, this unit is composed of polyarabinose, polymannan, and various lipids attached through a phosphatidylinositol moiety.[124,125]

Specific Diseases

Tuberculosis

Tuberculosis (TB) is a disease that has been known from the earliest recorded history and is a current global epidemic. TB is a chronic bacterial infection caused by *Mycobacterium tuberculosis*, an acid-fast, aerobic bacillus with the previously discussed, unusual cell wall. The cell wall has a high lipid content, resulting in a high degree of hydrophobicity and resistance to alcohol, acids, alkali, and some disinfectants. After staining with a dye, the *M. tuberculosis* cell wall cannot subsequently be decolorized with acid wash, thus the characteristic of being an acid-fast bacillus. According to the World Health Organization's (WHO) Global Tuberculosis Report 2017, 1.7 million people died from TB and it is one of the top ten causes of death worldwide.[126] Before 1984, only 10% of the organisms isolated from patients with TB were resistant to any drug. In 1984, 52% of the organisms were resistant to at least one drug, and 32% were resistant to more than one drug. Multidrug-resistant TB is associated with resistance to the two most potent first-line anti-TB drugs (i.e., isoniazid and rifampicin). More patients are being diagnosed with extensively drug-resistant TB (XTR-TB), a condition in which the organism is resistant to either isoniazid or rifampicin, any fluoroquinolone, and at least one of the three second-line injectable drugs (i.e., capreomycin, kanamycin, and amikacin). As a result of MDR-TB and XTR-TB, isolates of *M. tuberculosis* should be tested for antimicrobial susceptibility. In fact, drug resistance is encountered in patients who have never been treated with any of the TB drugs.

Nontuberculous Mycobacterial Infections

LEPROSY (HANSEN DISEASE). Leprosy (Hansen disease) is recognized as a chronic granulomatous infection caused by *Mycobacterium leprae*. The disease can consist of lepromatous leprosy, tuberculoid leprosy, or a condition with characteristics between these two poles and referred to as borderline leprosy. The disease is more common in tropical countries but is not limited to warm climate regions. It is thought to afflict some 10-20 million individuals. Children appear to be the most susceptible population, but the signs and symptoms do not usually occur until much later in life. The incubation period is usually 3-5 years. The disease is contagious, but the infectiousness is quite low. Person-to-person contact appears to be the means by which the disease is spread, with entrance into the body occurring through the skin or the mucosa of the upper respiratory tract. Skin and peripheral nerves are the regions most susceptible to attack. The first signs of the disease consist of hypopigmented or hyperpigmented macules. Anesthetic or paresthetic patches can be additionally experienced by the patient. Neural involvement in the extremities leads ultimately to muscle atrophy, resorption of small bones, and spontaneous amputation. When facial nerves are involved, corneal ulceration and blindness can occur. The identification of *M. leprae* in skin or blood samples is not always possible, but the detection of the antibody to the organism is an effective diagnostic test, especially for the lepromatous form of the disease.

***Mycobacterium avium-intracellulare* AND *Mycobacterium abscessus*.** Complexes *Mycobacterium avium* and *Mycobacterium intracellulare* are atypical acid-fast bacilli that are ubiquitous in the environment and considered usually to be nonpathogenic in healthy individuals. Unfortunately, in immunocompromised individuals, these and possibly other, unidentified mycobacteria cause severe, life-threatening infections. Disseminated *Mycobacterium avium-intracellulare* complex (MAC) is the most common bacterial opportunistic infection seen in patients with AIDS and the third most common opportunistic infection behind candidal esophagitis and primary *Pneumocystis jirovecii* pneumonia (PCP) reported in patients with AIDS. Between 1981 and 1987 and before the availability of effective antiretroviral medication, the incidence of MAC was reported as 5%. Today, approximately half of all patients with AIDS develop an infection caused by MAC. The lungs are the organs most commonly involved in patients without AIDS, but the infection can involve bone marrow, lymph nodes, liver, and blood in patients with AIDS. The CD4 T-lymphocyte count is used as a predictor for risk of disseminated MAC; a count of less than 50 cells/mm^3 in an HIV-infected person (adult or adolescent) is an indication of a potential infection and a recommendation for chemoprophylaxis. Of concern is the increasing prevalence of *M. abscessus* infections among patients with structural lung diseases such as chronic obstructive lung disease (COPD) and cystic fibrosis.[127,128] The MAC and MABSC organisms grow within macrophages; therefore, the drug must be capable of penetration of the macrophage. Treatment of MAC and MABSC, both prophylactically and for diagnosed infections, requires the use of multidrug therapy, and for disseminated MAC, this treatment is for the life of the patient.

General Approaches to Drug Therapy

The mycobacteria have a number of characteristics in common, but it is important to recognize that the species vary widely in their susceptibility to the different drugs and that, in turn, this can relate to significant differences in the organisms. Some species, such as *M. tuberculosis*, are very slow-growing, with a doubling time of approximately 24 hours, whereas others, such as *M. smegmatis*, double in 2-3 hours. The pathogenic mycobacterial organism can be divided into organisms that are actively metabolizing and rapidly growing; semidormant bacilli, which exhibit spurts of metabolism; bacilli that exist at low pH and exhibit low metabolic activity; and dormant or persisters. The latter characteristic is the most problematic and responsible for treatment failures. Most current TB drugs are those that are effective against actively metabolizing and rapidly growing bacilli. Thus, successful chemotherapy calls for drugs with bactericidal action against all stages of the organisms—but especially against the persisters. The use of combination therapy over an extended period of time is one answer to successful treatment.

Drug Therapy for Tuberculosis

Drug therapy for the treatment of TB has been greatly hampered by the development of MDR-TB (and more recently XDR-TB) and the lack of new classes of drugs. In fact, no new drugs have been developed for drug susceptible TB in the last 60 years. The only change in the treatment of TB has been the strategy of using direct observed treatment, short-course (DOTS), with an emphasis on patient-centered care.[129] Currently, the short course treatment consists of a four-drug cocktail comprised of isoniazid, rifampicin, pyrazinamide, and ethambutol or streptomycin for a two-month "intensive phase" followed by a four-month "continuation phase" with the two most powerful TB chemotherapeutics, isoniazid and rifampicin.[130] Additionally, patient compliance continues to be a serious problem, which in turn can be associated with the development of bacterial resistance.

First-Line Antitubercular Agents

ISONIAZID

O C N–NH_2 H N

Isoniazid

Isoniazid (INH) is a synthetic antibacterial agent with bactericidal action against *M. tuberculosis*. The drug was discovered in the 1950s as a beneficial agent effective against intracellular and extracellular bacilli, and it is generally considered to be the primary drug for treatment of *M. tuberculosis*. Its action is bactericidal against replicating organisms, but it appears to be only bacteriostatic at best against semidormant and dormant populations. After treatment with INH, *M. tuberculosis* loses its acid fastness, which can be interpreted as indicating that the drug interferes with cell wall development.

Mechanism of Action. INH is a prodrug that is activated through an oxidation reaction catalyzed by an endogenous enzyme.[131] This enzyme, katG, which exhibits catalase-peroxidase activity, converts INH to a reactive species capable of acylation of an enzyme system found exclusively in *M. tuberculosis*. Evidence in support of the activation of INH reveals that INH-resistant isolates have decreased catalase activity and that the loss of catalase activity is associated with the deletion of the catalase gene, katG. Furthermore, reintroduction of the gene into resistant organisms results in restored sensitivity of the organism to the drug. Reaction of INH with catalase-peroxidase results in formation of isonicotinaldehyde, isonicotinic acid, and isonicotinamide, which can be accounted for through the reactive intermediate isonicotinoyl radical or isonicotinic peroxide (Fig. 29.37).[132]

Mycolic acids (Fig. 29.38) are the primary lipid component of the mycobacterial cell wall in that they provide a permeability barrier to hydrophilic solutes as well as virulence.[133,134] The enzyme inhA, produced under the control of the inhA gene, is an NADH-dependent, enoyl reductase protein thought to be involved in double-bond reduction during fatty acid elongation (Fig. 29.39). Isoniazid specifically inhibits long-chain fatty acid synthesis (>26 carbon atoms). It should be noted that the mycolic acids are α-alkylated β-hydroxylated lipids having a "short" α-chain of 20-26 carbons and a "long" meromycolyl chain of 40-60 carbons. It has been proposed that INH is activated to an electrophilic

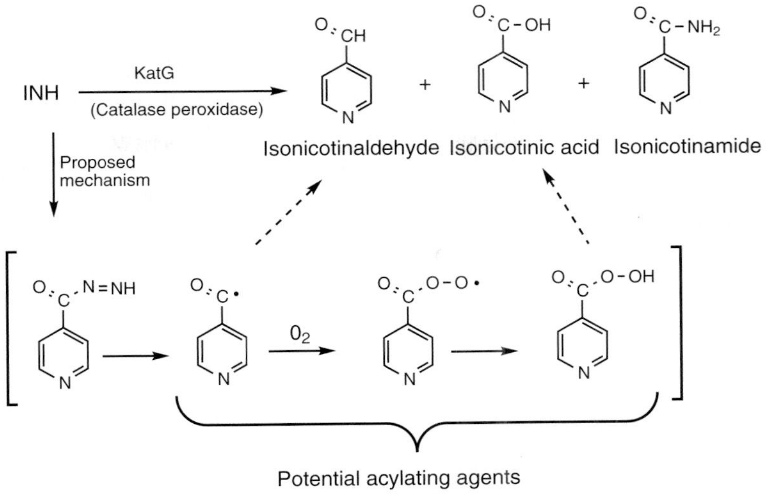

Figure 29.37 Reaction products formed from catalase-peroxidase reaction with isoniazid (INH).

species that acylates the 4 position of the NADH (Fig. 29.40). The acylated NADH is no longer capable of catalyzing the reduction of unsaturated fatty acids, which are essential for the synthesis of the mycolic acids.[135-137]

The mechanism of resistance to INH appears to be a very complicated process, possibly involving mutations in multiple genes including katG and inhA. It is possible that different mutations result in different degrees of resistance. This seems to be especially true in MDR-TB. A high level of resistance is reported to occur through katG mutation, which leads to a Ser315 to Thr315 in KatG catalase-peroxidase and prevents INH activation.[138]

Structure-Activity Relationship. An extensive series of derivatives of nicotinaldehyde, isonicotinaldehyde, and substituted isonicotinic acid hydrazides have been prepared and investigated for their tuberculostatic activity. Isoniazid hydrazones were found to possess activity, but these compounds were shown to be unstable in the gastrointestinal (GI) tract, releasing the active isonicotinic acid hydrazide (i.e., INH). Thus, it would appear that their activity resulted from INH and not from the derivatives.[139,140] Substitution of the hydrazine portion of INH with alkyl and aralkyl substituents resulted in a series of active and inactive derivatives. Substitution on the N-2 position resulted in active compounds (R1 and/or R2 = alkyl; R3 = H), whereas any substitution of the N-1 hydrogen with alkyl groups destroyed the activity (R1 and R2 = H; R3 = alkyl). None of these changes produced compounds with activity superior to that of INH.

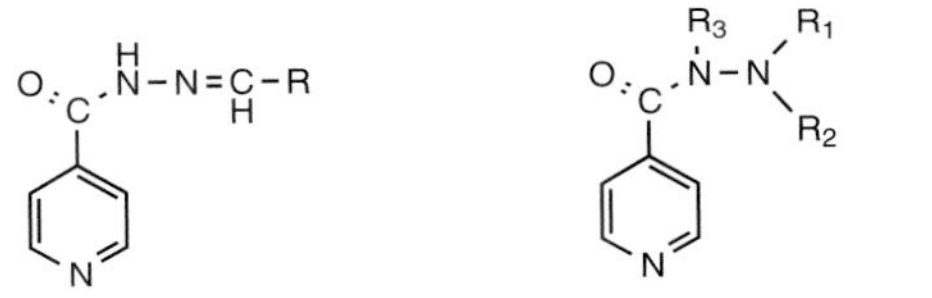

Metabolism. Isoniazid is extensively metabolized to inactive metabolites (Fig. 29.41).[141,142] The major metabolite is N-acetylisoniazid. The enzyme responsible for acetylation, cytosolic N-acetyltransferase, is produced under genetic control in an inherited autosomal fashion. Individuals who possess high concentrations of the enzyme are referred to as

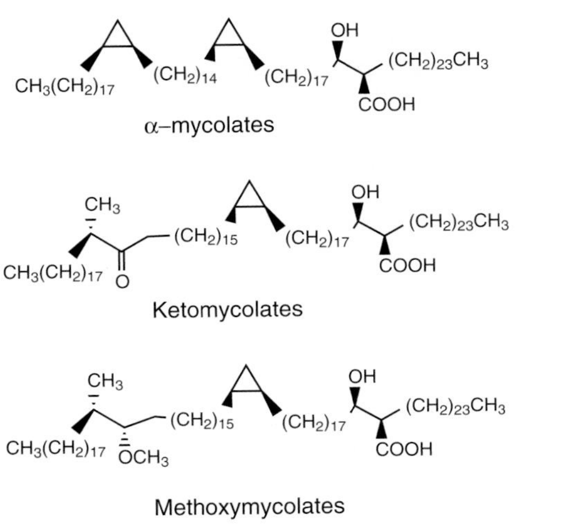

Figure 29.38 Representative structures of mycolic acids.

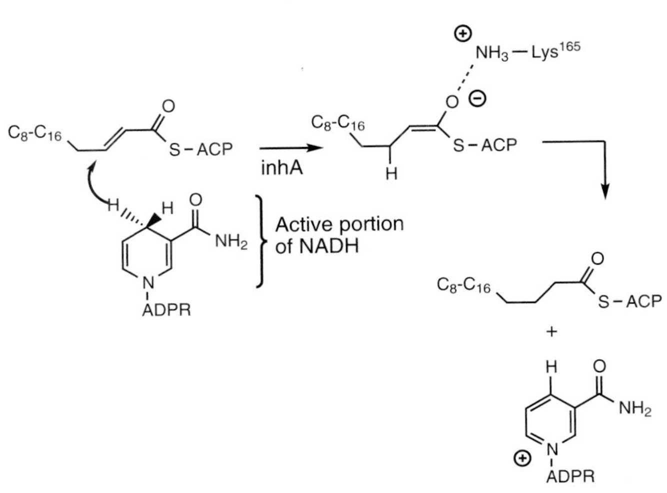

Figure 29.39 Enoylthioester (ACP, acyl carrier protein) reduction catalyzed by NADH (reduced nicotinamide adenine dinucleotide) and InhA (enoyl-acyl carrier protein reductase)

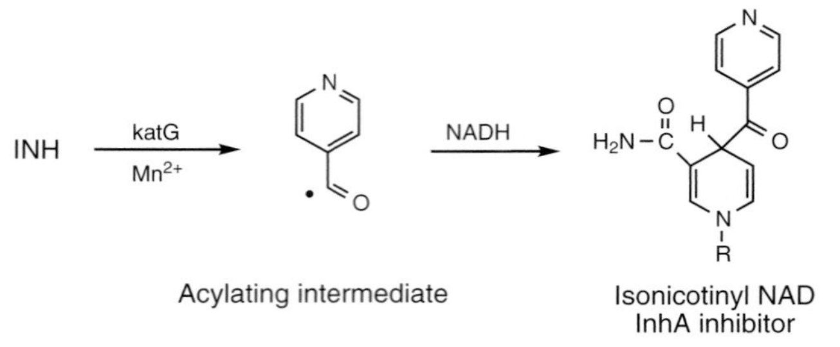

Figure 29.40 Acylation of NADH of NADH-dependent enoylacyl protein (InhA).

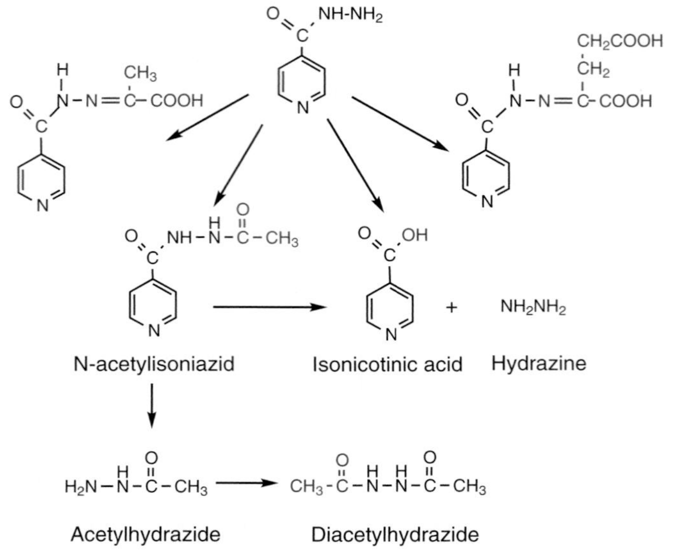

Figure 29.41 Metabolism of isoniazid.

rapid acetylators, whereas those with low concentrations are slow acetylators. This can result in a need to adjust the dosage for fast acetylators. The N-acetyltransferase is located primarily in the liver and small intestine. Other metabolites include isonicotinic acid, which is found in the urine as a glycine conjugate, and hydrazine. Isonicotinic acid can also result from hydrolysis of N-acetylisoniazid, but in this case, the second product of hydrolysis is acetylhydrazine. Mono-N-acetylhydrazine is acetylated by N-acetyltransferase to the inactive N-diacetyl product. This reaction occurs more rapidly in rapid acetylators. The formation of N-acetylhydrazine is significant in that this compound has been associated with hepatotoxicity, which can occur during INH therapy. N-acetylhydrazine has been postulated to serve as a substrate for microsomal P450, resulting in the formation of a reactive intermediate that is capable of acetylating liver proteins, in turn resulting in liver necrosis.[143] It has been suggested that an N-hydroxylamine intermediate is formed that results in a reactive acetylating agent (Fig. 29.42). The acetyl radical/cation acylates liver protein.

Pharmacokinetics. Isoniazid is readily absorbed following oral administration. Food and various antacids, especially aluminum-containing antacids, can interfere with or delay the absorption; therefore, it is recommended that the drug be taken on an empty stomach. The drug is well distributed to body tissues, including infected tissue. A long-standing concern about the use of INH during preventive therapy for latent TB has been the high incidence of hepatotoxicity. Recent studies have concluded that, excluding patients over 35 years of age, if relevant clinical monitoring is employed, the rate of hepatotoxicity is quite low.[144] The risk of hepatotoxicity is associated with increasing age and, for unknown reasons, appears to be higher in women than in men.

RIFAMYCIN ANTIBIOTICS. The rifamycins are members of the ansamycin class of natural products produced by *Streptomyces mediterranei*. This chemical class is characterized as molecules with an aliphatic chain forming a bridge between two nonadjacent positions of an aromatic moiety.

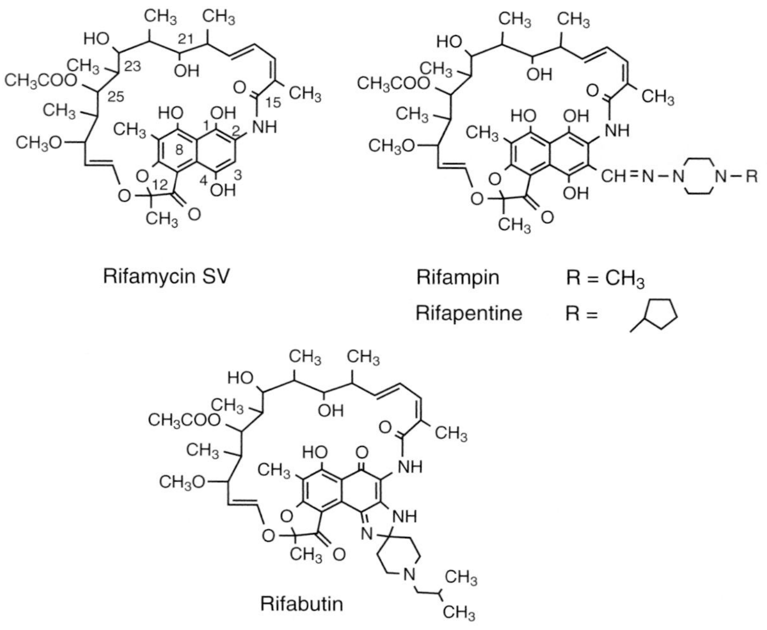

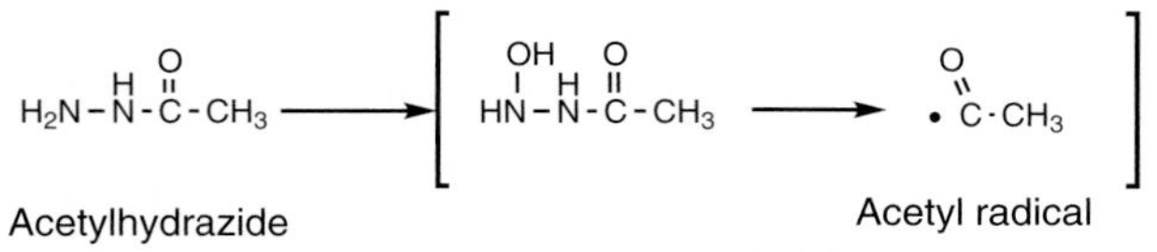

$H_2N-NH-C(=O)-CH_3 \longrightarrow [\, HN(OH)-NH-C(=O)-CH_3 \longrightarrow \cdot C(=O)-CH_3 \,]$

Acetylhydrazide — Acetyl radical

Figure 29.42 Acylating metabolite of isoniazid.

While investigating the biologic activity of the naturally occurring rifamycins (B, O, and S), a spontaneous reaction gave the biologically active rifamycin SV, which was later isolated from natural sources. Rifamycin SV was the original rifamycin antibiotic chosen for clinical development. Semisynthetic derivatives are prepared via conversion of the natural rifamycins to 3-formylrifamycin, which is derivatized with various hydrazines to give products such as rifampin (RIF) and rifapentine. RIF and rifapentine have significant benefit over previously investigated rifamycins in that they are orally active, are highly effective against a variety of both gram-positive and gram-negative organisms, and have high clinical efficacy in the treatment of TB. The rifamycin antibiotics are active against both growing and slow-metabolizing, nongrowing bacilli.

Mechanism of Action. The rifamycins inhibit bacterial DNA-dependent RNA polymerase (DDRP) by binding to the β-subunit of the enzyme and are highly active against rapidly dividing intracellular and extracellular bacilli. RIF is active against DDRP from both gram-positive and gram-negative bacteria, but because of poor penetration of the cell wall of gram-negative organisms by RIF, the drug has less value in infections caused by such organisms. Inhibition of DDRP leads to blocking the initiation of chain formation in RNA synthesis. It has been suggested that the naphthalene ring of the rifamycins π-π bonds to an aromatic amino acid ring in the DDRP protein (Fig. 29.43).[145] The DDRP is a metalloenzyme that contains two zinc atoms. It is further postulated that the oxygens at C-1 and C-8 of a rifamycin can chelate to a zinc atom, which increases the binding to DDRP, and finally, the oxygens at C-21 and C-23 form strong hydrogen bonds to the DDRP. The binding of the rifamycins to DDRP results in the inhibition of the RNA synthesis. Specifically, RIF has been shown to inhibit the elongation of full-length transcripts, but it has no effect on transcription initiation.[146] Resistance develops when a mutation occurs in the gene responsible for the β-subunit of the RNA polymerase (rpoB gene), resulting in an inability of the antibiotic to readily bind to the RNA polymerase.[147]

Structure-Activity Relationship. A large number of derivatives of the naturally occurring rifamycins have been prepared.[148] From these compounds, the following generalizations can be made concerning the structure-activity relationship (SAR): (1) Free –OH groups are required at C-1, C-8, C-21, and C-23; (2) these groups appear to lie in a plane and to be important binding groups for attachment to DDRP, as previously indicated; (3) acetylation of C-21 and/or C-23 produces inactive compounds; (4) reduction of the double bonds in the macro ring results in a progressive decrease in activity; and (5) opening of the macro ring also gives inactive compounds. These latter two changes greatly affect the conformational structure of the rifamycins, which in turn decreases binding to DDRP. Substitution at C-3 or C-4 results in compounds with varying degrees of antibacterial activity. The substitution at these positions appears to affect transport across the bacterial cell wall. In vitro studies have shown rapid tissue sterilization and encouraging results concerning combination therapy for TB and, possibly, MAC.

Metabolism. RIF and rifapentine are readily absorbed from the intestine, although food in the tract can affect absorption. RIF's absorption can be reduced by food in the intestine; therefore, the drug should be taken on an empty stomach.[142] Intestinal absorption of rifapentine has been reported to be enhanced when taken after a meal.[149] Neither drug appears to interfere with the absorption of other antitubercular agents, but there are conflicting reports on whether INH affects absorption of RIF. The major metabolism of RIF and rifapentine is deacetylation, which occurs at the C-25 acetate (Fig. 29.44). The resulting products, desacetylrifampin and desacetylrifapentine, are still active antibacterial agents. The majority of both desacetyl products are found in the feces, but desacetylrifampin glucuronide can be found in the urine as well. 3-Formylrifamycin SV has been reported as a second metabolite after administration of both RIF and rifapentine. This product is thought to arise in the gut from an acid-catalyzed hydrolysis reaction. Formylrifamycin is reported to possess a broad spectrum of antibacterial activity.[150]

Physicochemical Properties. RIF and rifapentine are red-orange, crystalline compounds with zwitterionic

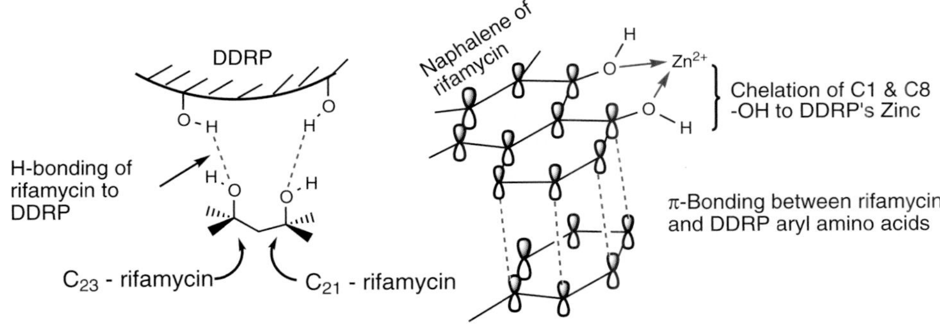

Figure 29.43 Binding of rifamycin to DNA-dependent RNA polymerase (DDRP).

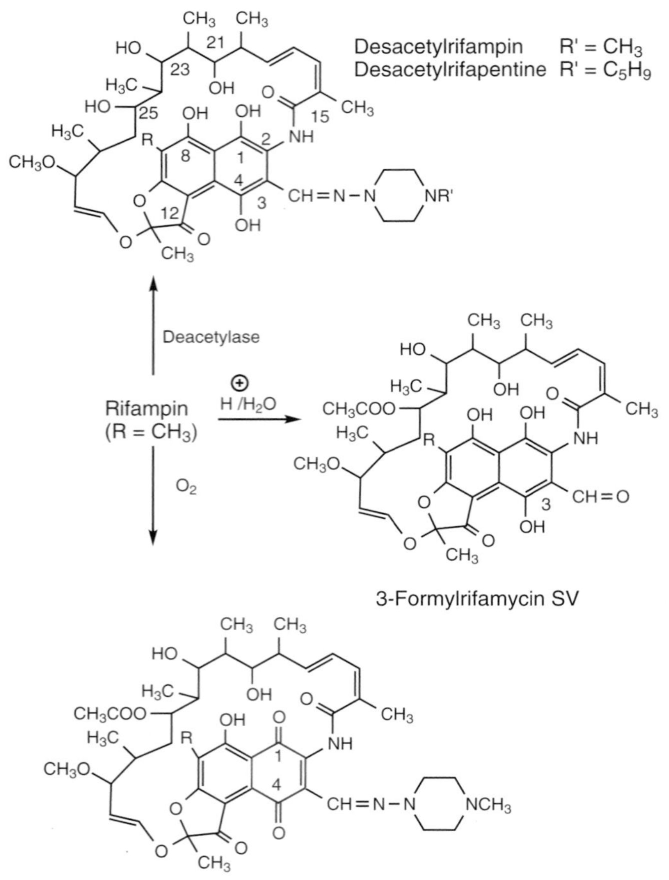

Desacetylrifampin R' = CH_3
Desacetylrifapentine R' = C_5H_9

Deacetylase

Rifampin (R = CH_3)

H^+/H_2O

O_2

3-Formylrifamycin SV

Figure 29.44 Metabolism and in vitro reactions of rifampin.

properties. The presence of the phenolic groups results in acidic properties (pK_a ~1.7), whereas the piperazine moiety gives basic properties (pK_a ~7.9). These compounds are prone to acid hydrolysis, giving rise to 3-formylrifamycin SV, as indicated earlier. RIF and presumably rifapentine are prone to air oxidation of the *p*-phenolic groups in the naphthalene ring to give the *p*-quinone (C-1,4 quinone) (Fig. 29.44). RIF, rifapentine, and their metabolites are excreted in the urine, feces (biliary excretion), saliva, sweat, and tears. Because these agents have dye characteristics, one can note discoloration of the body fluids containing the drug. Notably, the tears can be discolored, and permanent staining of contact lenses can occur.

Therapeutic Application

Rifampin (Rifadin, Rimactane). With the introduction of RIF in 1967, the duration of combination therapy for the treatment of TB was significantly reduced (from 18 to 9 mo). RIF is nearly always used in combination with one or more other antitubercular agents. The drug is potentially hepatotoxic and can produce GI disturbances, rash, and thrombocytopenic purpura. RIF is known to be a potent inducer of the hepatic CYP3A4 and can decrease the effectiveness of oral contraceptives, corticosteroids, warfarin, quinidine, methadone, zidovudine, clarithromycin, and the azole antifungal agents. In addition, the rifamycins appear to increase the expression of P-glycoproteins, which increase the efflux of various drugs.

Because of the decreased effectiveness of protease inhibitors and nonnucleoside reverse transcriptase inhibitors used in the treatment of HIV, the CDC has recommended avoidance of RIF in treatment of HIV-infected patients presently on these HIV therapies.

Rifapentine (Priftin). Rifapentine is a relatively new agent introduced for the treatment of pulmonary TB, approved in the last 25 years. The drug's major advantage over RIF is the fact that when used in combination therapy, rifapentine can be administered twice weekly during the "intense" phase of therapy, followed by once-a-week administration during the "continuous" phase. In contrast, RIF normally is administered daily during the "intense" phase, followed by twice-a-week dosing during the "continuous" phase. Because relapse and the emergence of resistant strains of bacteria are associated with poor patient compliance, reduced dosing is expected to increase compliance. Initial clinical studies actually showed that the relapse rates in patients treated with rifapentine (10%) were higher than those in patients treated with RIF (5%). It was found that poor compliance with the nonrifamycin antituberculin agents was responsible for the increased relapse.[149] Rifapentine is readily absorbed following oral administration and is highly bound to plasma protein (97.7% vs. 80% for RIF). Related to the higher plasma binding, rifapentine has a longer mean elimination half-life (13.2 hr in healthy male volunteers) in comparison with the half-life reported for RIF (~2-5 hr). Greater than 70% of either drug is excreted in the feces. Rifapentine is generally considered to be more active than RIF and can be used in patients with varying degrees of hepatic dysfunction without the need for dose adjustment.[151] This drug, similar to what is seen with RIF, induces hepatic microsomal enzymes (CYP3A4 and CYP2C8/9) but appears to have less of an inducing effect on cytochrome P450 than RIF. Rifapentine has been reported to be teratogenic in rats and rabbits.[149]

Rifabutin (Mycobutin). Rifabutin was approved for the treatment of both M. *tuberculosis* and MAC infections in 1992. Rifabutin can be used in first-line treatment for TB in lieu of RIF; however, this is not commonly practiced due to its higher cost. Where rifabutin is more commonly used, is with patients co-infected with both M. *tuberculosis* and HIV, where RIF is commonly not tolerated by common antiretroviral therapy.[152] There are less drug-drug interactions among HIV antiretroviral therapy and rifabutin than RIF.[152]

PYRAZINAMIDE

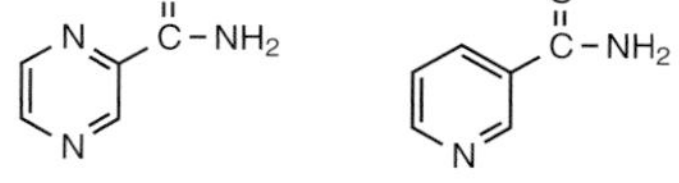

Pyrazinamide Nicotinamide

Pyrazinamide (pyrazinecarboxamide) was discovered while investigating analogues of nicotinamide. Pyrazinamide is a bioisostere of nicotinamide and possesses bactericidal action against M. *tuberculosis*. Pyrazinamide has become one of the more popular antituberculin agents despite the fact that resistance develops quickly. Combination therapy, however, has proven to be an effective means of reducing the rate of resistant strain development. The activity of pyrazinamide is pH dependent with good in vivo activity at pH 5.5, but the compound is nearly inactive at neutral pH.

Mechanism of Action. The mechanism of action of pyrazinamide is unknown, but recent findings suggest that pyrazinamide can be active either totally or in part as a prodrug. Susceptible organisms produce pyrazinamidase, which is responsible for conversion of pyrazinamide to pyrazinoic acid intracellularly.[146] Mutation in the pyrazinamidase gene (pncA) results in resistant strains of *M. tuberculosis*.[153] Pyrazinoic acid has been shown to possess biologic activity at a pH 5.4 or lower, in contrast in vitro tests that show pyrazinoic acid is 8- to 16-fold less active than pyrazinamide.[154] Pyrazinoic acid can lower the pH in the immediate surroundings of the *M. tuberculosis* to such an extent that the organism is unable to grow, but this physicochemical property appears to account for only some of the activity. The protonated pyrazinoic acid can also permeate the mycobacterial membrane to lower the pH of the cytoplasm. Recent evidence suggests that pyrazinoic acid decreases membrane potential in older, nonreplicating bacilli, thus decreasing membrane transport, and interferes with the energetics of the membrane.[155]

Structure-Activity Relationship. Previous structural modification of pyrazinamide has proven to be ineffective in developing analogues with increased biologic activity. Substitution on the pyrazine ring or use of alternate heterocyclic aromatic rings has given compounds with reduced activity.[156] Using quantitative SAR, a series of analogues have been prepared with improved biologic activity. The requirements for successful analogues include (1) provision for hydrophilicity to allow sufficient plasma concentrations such that the drug can be delivered to the site of infection, (2) lipophilicity to allow penetration into the mycobacterial cell, and (3) susceptibility to hydrolysis such that the prodrug is unaffected by the "extracellular" enzymes but is readily hydrolyzed at the site of action. Two compounds have been found that meet these criteria: *tert*-butyl 5-chloropyrazinamide and 2′-(2′-methyldecyl) 5-chloropyrazinamide.[157]

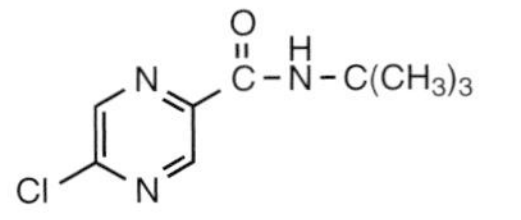

tert-Butyl 5-chloropyrazinoate

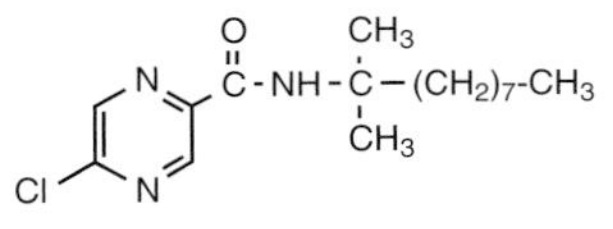

2'-(2'-Methyldecyl) 5-chloropyrazinoate

Metabolism. Pyrazinamide is readily absorbed after oral administration, but little of the intact molecule is excreted unchanged (Fig. 29.45). The major metabolic route consists of hydrolysis by hepatic microsomal pyrazinamidase to pyrazinoic acid, which can then be oxidized by xanthine oxidase to 5-hydroxypyrazinoic acid. The latter compound can appear in the urine either free or as a conjugate with glycine.[141]

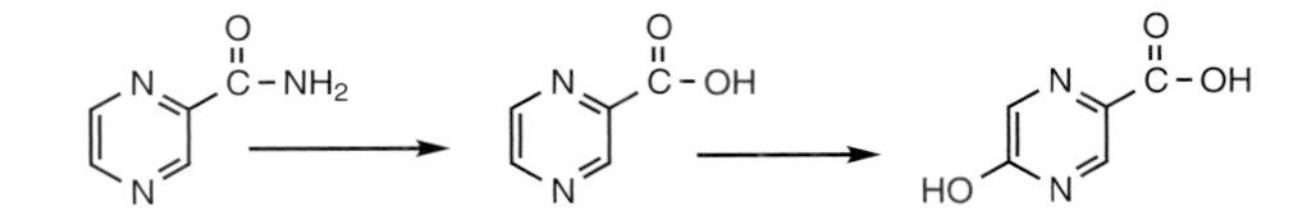

Pyrazinamide → Pyrazinoic acid → 5-Hydroxypyrazinoic acid

Figure 29.45 Metabolism of pyrazinamide.

Therapeutic Application. Pyrazinamide has gained acceptance as an essential component in combination therapy for the treatment of TB (component of Rifater with INH and RIF). The drug is especially beneficial in that it is active against semidormant intracellular tubercle bacilli that are not affected by other drugs.[129,151] Evidence suggests that pyrazinamide is active against nonreplicating persister bacilli. The introduction of pyrazinamide combinations has reduced treatment regimens to 6 months from the previous 9-month therapy. The major serious side effect of pyrazinamide is the potential for hepatotoxicity. This effect is associated with dose and length of treatment.

Pyrazinamide is not affected by the presence of food in the GI tract or by the use of aluminum-magnesium antacids.[158]

ETHAMBUTOL (MYAMBUTOL)

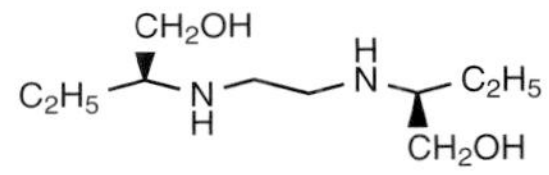

Ethambutol

Ethambutol (EMB), an ethylenediiminobutanol, is administered as its (+)-enantiomer, which is 200- to 500-fold more active than its (−)-enantiomer. The difference in activity between the two isomers suggests a specific receptor for its site of action. EMB is a water-soluble, bacteriostatic agent that is readily absorbed (75%-80%) after oral administration.

Mechanism of Action. The mechanism of action of EMB remains unknown, although mounting evidence suggests a specific site of action for EMB. It has been known for some time that EMB affects mycobacterial cell wall synthesis; however, the complicated nature of the mycobacterial cell wall has made pinpointing the site of action difficult. In addition to the peptidoglycan portion of the cell wall, the mycobacterium have a unique outer envelope consisting of arabinofuranose and galactose (AG), which is covalently attached to the peptidoglycan and an intercalated framework of LAM. The AG portion of the cell wall is highly branched and contains distinct segments of galactan and distinct segments of arabinan. At various locations within the arabinan segments (terminal and penultimate), the mycolic acids are attached to the C-5′ position of arabinan.[159,160] Initially, Takayama and colleagues reported that EMB inhibited the synthesis β-D-arabinofuranosyl-1-monphosphoryldecaprenol

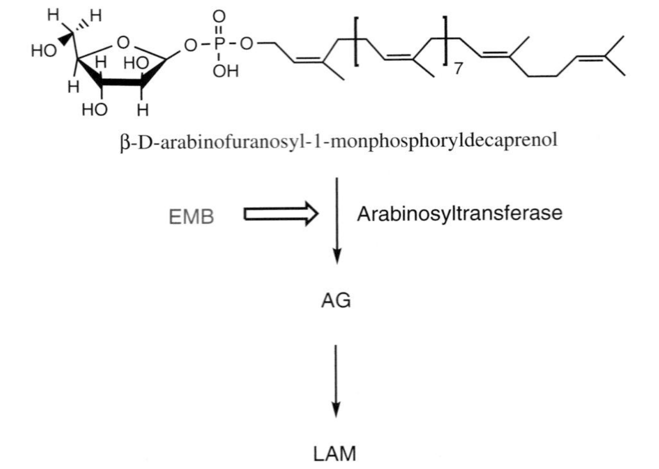

EMB ⟹ Arabinosyltransferase

AG

LAM

Figure 29.46 Site of action of ethambutol (EMB) in cell wall synthesis. AG, arabinogalactan; LAM, lipoarabinomannan.

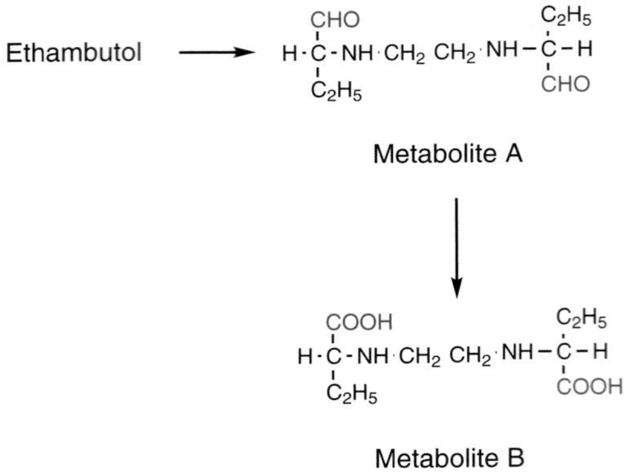

Ethambutol ⟶ Metabolite A ⟶ Metabolite B

Figure 29.47 Metabolism of ethambutol.

of the AG portion of the cell wall.[161] It has also been reported that EMB inhibits the enzyme arabinosyl transferase. One action of arabinosyl transferase is to catalyze the polymerization of D-arabinofuranose, leading to AG (Fig. 29.46).[162,163] EMB mimics arabinan, resulting in a buildup of the arabinan precursor β-D-arabinofuranosyl-L-monophosphoryldecaprenol and, as a result, a block of the synthesis of both AG and LAM (Fig. 29.36).[164] The mechanism of resistance to EMB involves a gene overexpression of arabinosyl transferase, which is controlled by the embAB gene.[165]

This mechanism of action also accounts for the synergism seen between EMB and intracellular drugs, such as RIF. Damage to the cell wall created by EMB improves the cell penetration of the intracellular drugs, resulting in increased biologic activity.

Structure-Activity Relationship. An extensive number of analogues of EMB have been prepared, but none has proven to be superior to EMB itself. Extension of the ethylenediamine chain, replacement of either nitrogen, increasing the size of the nitrogen substituents, and moving the location of the alcohol groups are all changes that drastically reduce or destroy biologic activity.

Metabolism. The majority of the administered EMB is excreted unchanged (73%), with no more than 15% appearing in the urine as either metabolite A or metabolite B (Fig. 29.47). Both metabolites are devoid of biologic activity.

STREPTOMYCIN

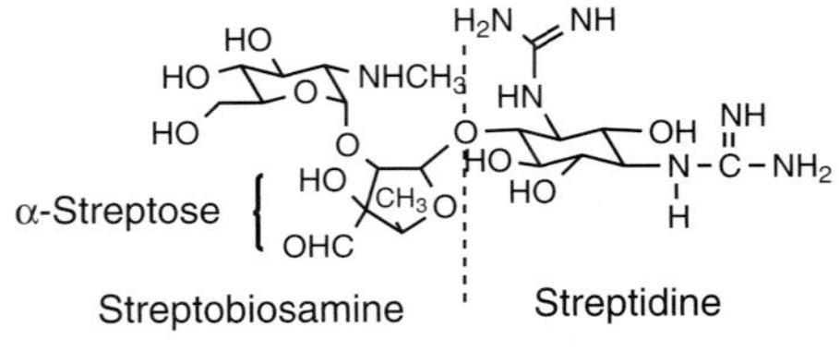

α-Streptose

Streptobiosamine

Streptidine

Streptomycin

Streptomycin (STM) was first isolated by Waksman and coworkers in 1944 and represented the first biologically active aminoglycoside. The material was isolated from a manure-containing soil sample and, ultimately, was shown to be produced by *S. griseus*. The structure was proposed and later confirmed by Kuehl and colleagues in 1948.[166] STM is water soluble, with basic properties. The compound is usually available as the trihydrochloride or sesquisulfate salt, both of which are quite soluble in water. The hydrophilic nature of STM results in very poor absorption from the GI tract. Orally administered STM is recovered intact from the feces, indicating that the lack of biologic activity results from poor absorption and not chemical degradation.

Mechanism of Action. The mechanism of action of STM and the aminoglycosides in general has not been fully elucidated. It is known that the STM inhibits protein synthesis, but additional effects on misreading of an mRNA template and membrane damage can contribute to the bactericidal action of STM. STM is able to diffuse across the outer membrane of *M. tuberculosis* and, ultimately, to penetrate the cytoplasmic membrane through an electron-dependent process. Through studies regarding the mechanism of drug resistance, it has been proposed that STM induces a misreading of the genetic code and, thus, inhibits translational initiation. In STM-resistant organisms, two changes have been discovered: first, S12 protein undergoes a change in which the lysine present at amino acids 43 and 88 in ribosomal protein S12 is replaced with arginine or threonine; second, the pseudoknot conformation of 16S rRNA, which results from intramolecular base pairing between GCC bases in regions 524-526 of the rRNA to CGG bases in regions 505-507, is perturbed.[167] It is thought that S12 protein stabilizes the pseudoknot, which is essential for 16S rRNA function. By some yet-to-be-defined mechanism, STM interferes with one or both of the normal actions of the 16S protein and 16S rRNA.

Structure-Activity Relationship. All of the aminoglycosides have very similar pharmacologic, pharmacodynamic, and toxic properties, but only STM and, to a lesser extent, kanamycin and possibly amikacin are used to treat TB. This is an indication for the narrow band of structurally allowed modifications giving rise to active analogues. Modification of the α-streptose portion of STM has been extensively studied. Reduction of the aldehyde to the alcohol results in a compound, dihydrostreptomycin, that has activity similar to STM but with a greater potential for producing delayed, severe deafness. Oxidation of the aldehyde to a carboxyl group or conversion to Schiff base derivatives (oxime, semicarbazone, or phenylhydrazone) results in inactive analogues. Oxidation of the methyl group in α-streptose to a methylene hydroxy gives an active analogue that has no advantage over STM. Modification of the aminomethyl group in the glucosamine portion of the molecule by demethylation or by replacement with larger alkyl groups reduces activity; removal or modification of either guanidine in the streptidine nucleus also decreases activity.

Metabolism. No human metabolites of STM have been isolated in the urine of patients who have been administered the drug, with approximately 50%-60% of the dose being recovered unchanged in the urine.[142] Metabolism appears to be insignificant on a large scale, but it is implicated as a major mechanism of resistance. One problem with STM that was recognized early was the development of resistant strains of *M. tuberculosis*. Combination drug therapy was partially successful in reducing this problem, but over time, resistance has greatly reduced the value of STM as a chemotherapeutic agent for treatment of TB. Various mechanisms can lead to the resistance seen in *M. tuberculosis*. Permeability barriers can result in STM not being transported through the cytoplasmic membrane, but the evidence appears to suggest that enzymatic inactivation of STM represents the major problem. The enzymes responsible for inactivation are adenyltransferase, which catalyzes adenylation of the C-3 hydroxyl group in the N-methylglucosamine moiety to give the O-3-adenylated metabolite, and phosphotransferase, which phosphorylates the same C-3 hydroxyl to give the O-3-phosphorylate metabolite (Fig. 29.48). This latter reaction appears to be the most significant clinically. The result of these chemical modifications is that the metabolites produced will not bind to ribosomes.

Second-Line Antitubercular Agents

A number of drugs, including ethionamide, *p*-aminosalicylic acid, cycloserine, bedaquline, capreomycin, kanamycin, and amikacin are considered to be second-line agents (it should be noted that some authorities classify STM as a second-line agent). These agents are active antibacterial agents, but they are usually less well tolerated or have a higher incidence of adverse effects. These agents are used in cases of resistance (MDR-TB), retreatment, or intolerance to the first-line drugs.

ETHIONAMIDE (TRECATOR-SC)

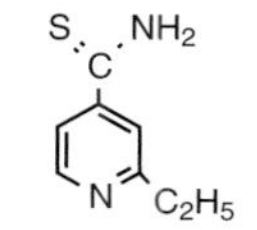

Ethionamide

The synthesis of analogues of isonicotinamide resulted in the discovery of ethionamide and a homolog in which the ethyl group is replaced with a propyl (prothionamide). Both compounds have proven to be bactericidal against *M. tuberculosis* and *Mycobacterium leprae*.

Mechanism of Action. Evidence has been presented suggesting that the mechanism of action of ethionamide is similar to that of INH (see Mechanism of Action under Isoniazid).[136,168] Similar to INH, ethionamide is considered to be a prodrug that is converted via oxidation by catalase-peroxidase to an active acylating agent, ethionamide sulfoxide, which in turn inactivates the inhA enoyl reductase enzyme (Fig. 29.49). In the case of ethionamide, it has been proposed that the ethionamide sulfoxide acylates Cys243 in InhA protein.

Metabolism. Ethionamide is orally active but is not well tolerated in a single large dose (>500 mg). The GI irritation can be reduced by administration with meals. Additional side effects can include central nervous system (CNS) effects, hepatitis, and hypersensitivities. Less than 1% of the drug is excreted in the free form, with the remainder of the drug appearing as one of six metabolites. Among the metabolites are ethionamide sulfoxide, 2-ethylisonicotinamide, and the N-methylated-6-oxodihydropyridines (compounds A, B, and C in Fig. 29.50).[169]

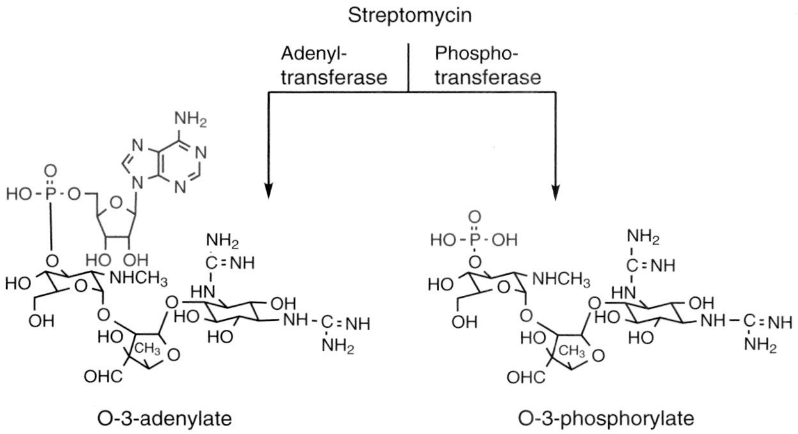

Streptomycin

Adenyltransferase | Phosphotransferase

O-3-adenylate

O-3-phosphorylate

Figure 29.48 Metabolism of streptomycin (STM) as a mechanism of resistance.

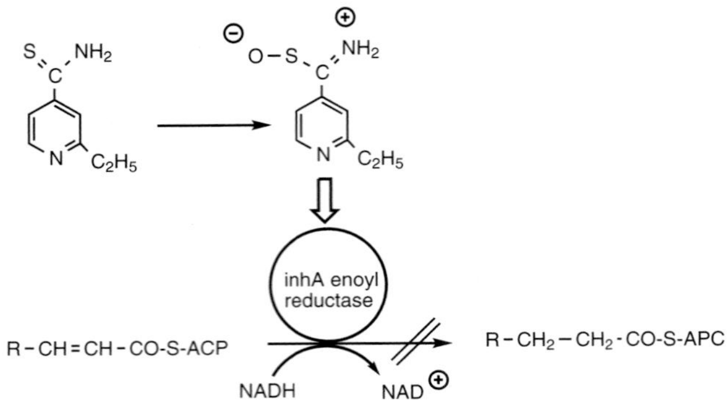

Figure 29.49 Mechanism of action of ethionamide.

p-AMINOSALICYLIC ACID

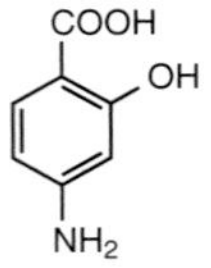

Para-aminosalicylic acid

Once a very popular component in TB therapy, p-aminosalicylic acid (PAS) is used as a second-line agent today. A combination of bacterial resistance and severe side effects has greatly reduced its value. As a bacteriostatic agent, PAS is used at a dose of up to 12 g/d, which causes considerable GI irritation. In addition, hypersensitivity reactions occur in 5%-10% of the patients, with some of these reactions being life-threatening.

Mechanism of Action. PAS is thought to act as an antimetabolite interfering with the incorporation of p-aminobenzoic acid into folic acid. When coadministered with INH, PAS is found to reduce the acetylation of INH, itself being the substrate for acetylation, thus increasing the plasma levels of INH. This action can be especially valuable in patients who are rapid acetylators.

Metabolism. PAS is extensively metabolized by acetylation of the amino group and by conjugation with glucuronic acid and glycine at the carboxyl group. It is used primarily in cases of resistance, retreatment, and intolerance of other agents and is available from the CDC.

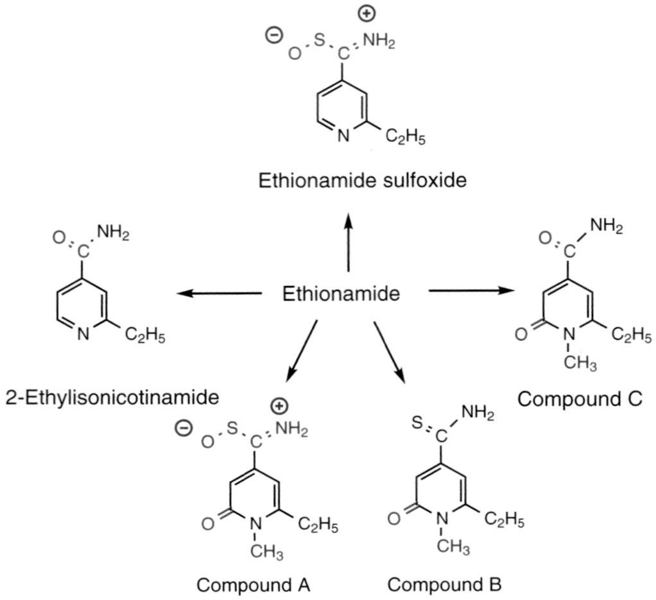

Figure 29.50 Metabolism of ethionamide.

CYCLOSERINE (SEROMYCIN)

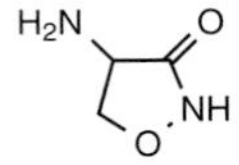

Cycloserine

Cycloserine is a natural product isolated from *Streptomyces orchidaceus* as the D-(+)-enantiomer.

Mechanism of Action. D-cycloserine is considered to be the active form of the drug, having its action associated with the ability to inhibit two key enzymes, D-alanine racemase and D-alanine ligase. D-Alanine is an important component of the peptidoglycan portion of the mycobacterial cell wall. Mycobacteria are capable of using naturally occurring L-alanine and converting the L-alanine to D-alanine via the enzyme D-alanine racemase. The resulting D-alanine is coupled with itself to form a D-alanine-D-alanine complex under the influence of D-alanine ligase, and this complex is incorporated into the peptidoglycan of the mycobacterial cell wall (Fig. 29.51). D-Cycloserine is a rigid analogue of D-alanine; therefore, it competitively inhibits the binding of D-alanine to both of these enzymes and its incorporation into the peptidoglycan (Fig. 29.51).[170] Resistance is associated with an overexpression of D-alanine racemase.

Adverse Effects. Cycloserine is readily absorbed after oral administration and is widely distributed, including the CNS. Unfortunately, D-cycloserine binds to neuronal N-methylasparate receptors and, in addition, affects synthesis and metabolism of γ-aminobutyric acid, leading to a complex series of CNS effects. As a second-line agent, cycloserine should only be used when retreatment is

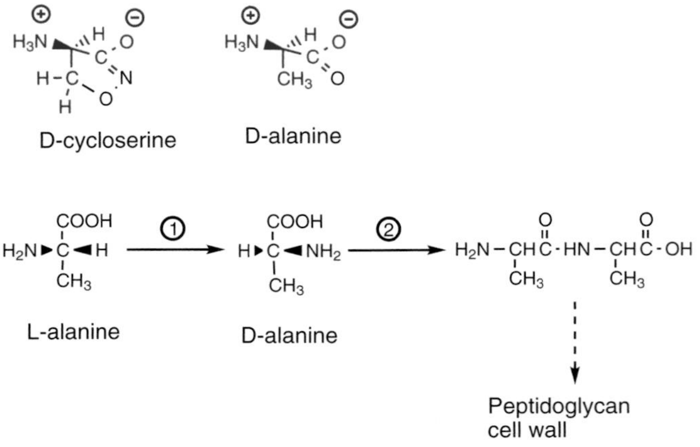

Figure 29.51 Sites of action of D-cycloserine: 1, D-alanine racemase and 2, D-alanine ligase.

necessary or when the organism is resistant to other drugs. Cycloserine should not be used as a single drug; it must be used in combination.

BEDAQUILINE FUMARATE (SIRTURO)

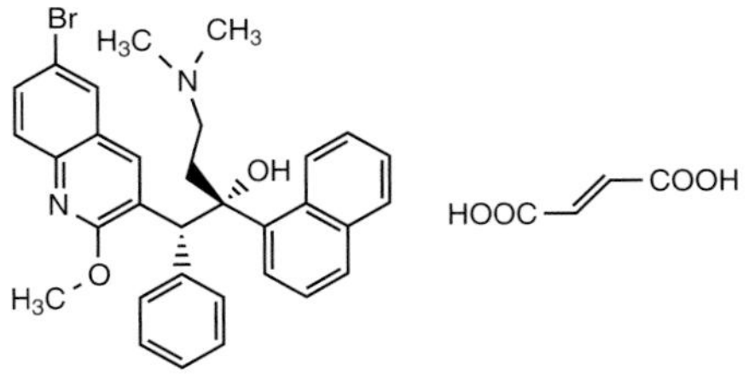

Bedaqules fumarate

Bedaquiline is a diarylquinoline and is one of the newest approved drugs for treatment of MDR-TB.[171-173] It has been shown to have activity against NTM strains including *M. abscessus*, *M. avium*, *M. fortuitum*, and *M. kansasii*; however, bedaquline is not approved for clinical use in patients diagnosed with these infections. Bedaquiline is marketed in a 100 mg oral tablet and should be used in combination with at least three other antitubercular drugs. Maximum plasma concentrations are observed five hours after dosing and is >99% bound to plasma proteins.[174] Food increases the bioavailability of bedaquline by approximately 2x, and thus it is recommended to be taken with meals.

Mechanism of Action. Bedaquline is a time-dependent mycobacterial growth inhibitor acting through the C-ring of mycobacterial ATP synthase, blocking the electrochemical gradient energy source (Fig. 29.52).[174-177] This is a unique mechanism of action compared to the other antitubercular drugs; thus, cross-resistance is low, and it is the reason why bedaquiline is used against the drug-resistant strains.

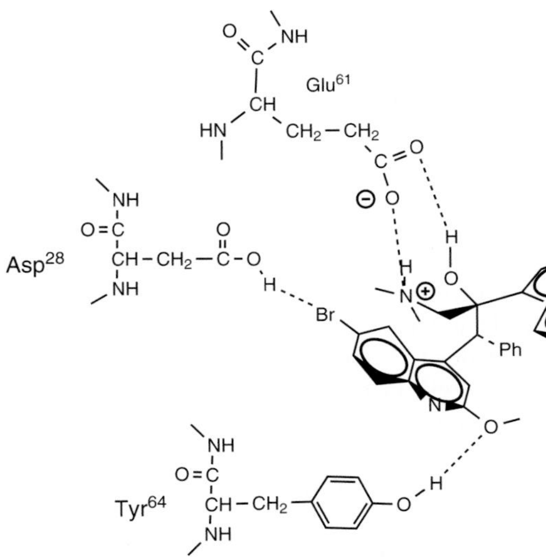

Figure 29.52 Binding of bedaquiline and amino acids in ATP (adenosine triphosphate) synthase C-subunit of *Mycobacterium tuberculosis*.

Metabolism. Bedaquiline is primarily metabolized through CYP3A4 N-dealkylation to the N-monodesmethyl metabolite. This metabolite is approximately 4-6 times less potent against whole cell *M. tuberculosis*; however, the impact on clinical efficacy is not significant. Elimination occurs primarily through the feces with very little (≤0.001%) excreted unchanged in the urine.

CAPREOMYCIN (CAPASTAT)

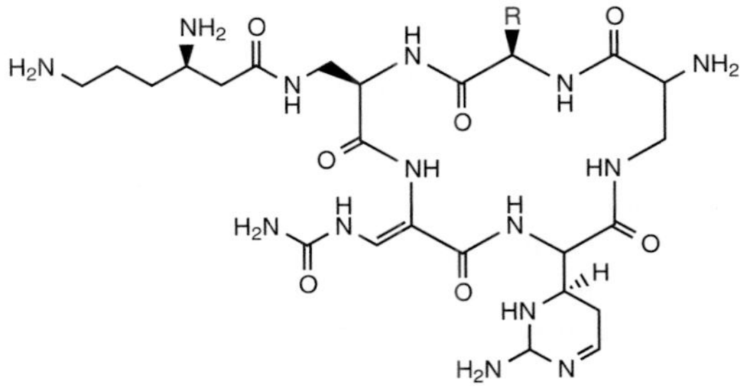

Capreomycin

Capreomycin is a mixture of four cyclic polypeptides, of which capreomycin Ia (R = OH) and Ib (R = H) make up 90% of the mixture. Capreomycin is produced by *Streptomyces capreolus* and is quite similar to the antibiotic viomycin. Little is known about its mechanism of action, but if the chemical and pharmacologic similarity to viomycin carries over to the mechanism of action, then one might expect something similar. Viomycin is a potent inhibitor of protein synthesis, particularly that which depends on mRNA at the 70S ribosome.[178] Viomycin blocks chain elongation by binding to either or both the 50S and 30S ribosomal subunits. As a polypeptide, capreomycin must be administered parenterally, with the preferred route of administration being intramuscular. As a second-line bacteriostatic antituberculin drug, it is reserved for "resistant" infections and cases of treatment failure. The drug should not be given as a single agent; rather, it should be used in combination with EMB or INH. Reported toxicity of capreomycin includes renal and hepatic damage, hearing loss, and allergic reactions.

AMIKACIN. A member of the aminoglycoside class, amikacin is a second-line agent commonly used in the treatment of MDR-TB (Fig. 29.25). Amikacin is an analogue of kanamycin, which is a mixture of at least three components (A, B, and C, with A predominating; Fig. 29.25), isolated from *S. kanamyceticus*. The drug is used to treat drug-resistant *M. tuberculosis* pathogens and should be used in combination with other effective agents. In addition, amikacin is also used to treat other mycobacterium infections, including *M. avium*, *M. abcessus*, *M. chelonae*, and *M. fortuitum*.

The parenteral form of the drug is used because, as an aminoglycoside, the drug is poorly absorbed via the oral route. Of note, the narrow range of effectiveness and the severe toxicity of kanamycin, especially if the drug is administered over a long period of time, have limited its usefulness and thus has been discontinued in the United States.

FLUOROQUINOLONES

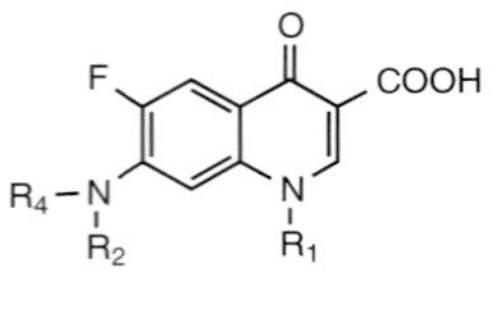

6-Fluoro-4-quinolones

The fluoroquinolones are a broad-spectrum class of antibacterials that have been demonstrated to have activity against a wide range of gram-negative and gram-positive pathogens, including M. *tuberculosis*, M. *kansasii*, M. *xenopi*, M. *fortuitum*, MAC, and M. *leprae*. The quinolones are attractive in that they are active at low concentrations, concentrate within macrophages, and have a low frequency of side effects.

Mechanism of Action. The mechanism of action of the fluoroquinolones involves binding to DNA gyrase-DNA complex (GyrA and GyrB), inhibiting bacterial DNA replication and transcription. As a result, these drugs exhibit bactericidal activity (see earlier discussion as an antibacterial for more detail).

Structure-Activity Relationship. The structural requirements for activity against mycobacterium and, specifically, for activity against the MAC have been explored.[179,180] It is known that nonfluorinated quinolones are inactive against mycobacteria. In addition, it has been reported that certain fragments or substructures within the quinolones improve activity toward the MAC (biophores), whereas other fragments deactivate the quinolones (biophobes). The important structural features acting as biophores include (1) a cyclopropyl ring at the N-1 position, (2) fluorine atoms at positions C-6 and C-8, and (3) a C-7 heterocyclic substituent. Excessive lipophilicity at N-1 can decrease activity (i.e., 2,4-difluorobenzene). The C-7 substituents with greatest activity against mycobacteria include the substituted piperazines and pyrrolidines (Fig. 29.53).

Several C-8 methoxy–substituted fluoroquinolones have been reported with superior activity over earlier quinolones (Fig. 29.54).[181,182] Moxifloxacin is reported to be active against M. *tuberculosis* when combined with INH.

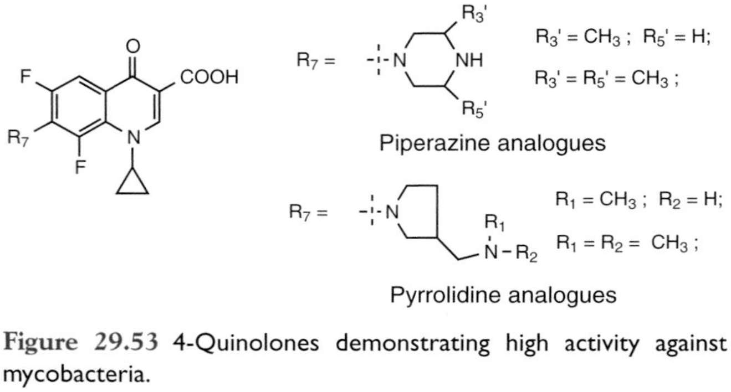

R_7 = Piperazine: $R_3' = CH_3$; $R_5' = H$; $R_3' = R_5' = CH_3$;

Piperazine analogues

R_7 = Pyrrolidine: $R_1 = CH_3$; $R_2 = H$; $R_1 = R_2 = CH_3$;

Pyrrolidine analogues

Figure 29.53 4-Quinolones demonstrating high activity against mycobacteria.

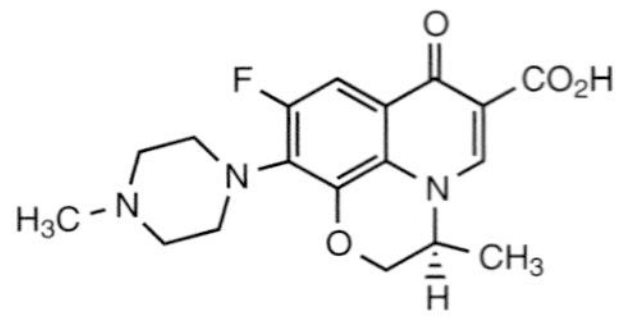

Ofloxacin (racemic)(Floxin)
Levofloxacin (1-*S*)(Levaquin)

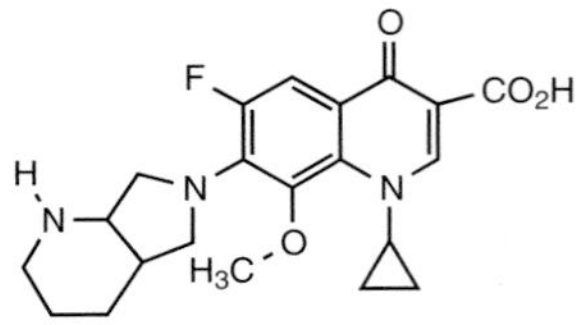

Moxifloxacin (Avelox)

Figure 29.54 Fluoroquinolones active against *Mycobacterium tuberculosis*.

Therapeutic Considerations for Treatment of Tuberculosis

Various stages of infectious organisms have been identified that can require special consideration for chemotherapy. The organism can be in a dormant stage, which is usually not affected by drugs. The continuously growing stage of the organism can find the bacteria either in an extracellular or an intracellular location. A stage of the organism, which is classified as the very slowly metabolizing bacteria, exists also in a relatively acidic environment. Finally, the organism can exhibit a stage in which it is dormant, followed by spurts of growth. As noted in the discussion of specific drugs, one stage or another can be more or less susceptible to a particular drug based on the above characteristics. It is also recognized that organisms from some geographic regions can show a low incidence of drug resistance, whereas those from other regions have a high incidence of drug resistance.

For patients with TB likely to be infected with organisms suspected of showing low rates of drug resistance, the American Thoracic Society currently recommends a minimum 26-week treatment period, consisting of an initial 2-month (8-week) phase, followed by a continuation phase of either 4 or 7 months. Four basic regimens are recommended for treatment of susceptible M. *tuberculosis* infections in adults. During the initial phase, three of the four regimens use a combination of INH, RIF, pyrazinamide, and EMB, given either 7, 5, or 3 days per week. The fourth regimen uses INH, RIF, and EMB given 7 or 5 days per week (when drugs are administered DOTS, the drugs can be given less often). The four-drug regimen is administered based on the assumption that a proportion of the organisms are resistant to INH. For treatment of children when visual acuity cannot be tested, EMB is usually not recommended. Several options for drug treatment exist for the continuation phase of treatment.[183] In a majority of cases, the continuation phase will last 4 months. Here again, if DOTS is used, the patient might only need to be treated two or three times weekly; without DOTS, the treatment is daily. The drug combination of INH and RIF is used during the continuation phase. Typical daily doses are 300 mg of INH, 600 mg of RIF, 2 g of pyrazinamide, and 1 g of EMB. The addition of pyrazinamide to the drug regimen results in a reduction of treatment time from

9 to 6 months. Individuals on any of these regimens are considered to be noninfectious after the first 2 weeks. This same group of drugs is recommended for patients with both TB and AIDS. The "cardinal rules" for all TB regimens are as follows: (1) get drug susceptibility information as soon as possible; (2) always begin therapy with at least three drugs; (3) at all costs, avoid a regimen using only one effective drug; and (4) always add at least two drugs to a failing regimen.[184] In addition, it is recommended that consideration be given to treating all patients with DOTS.

The only proven treatment for prophylaxis of TB (patients with a positive skin test or a high-risk factor) is INH used for 6 or 12 months. High-risk persons are considered to be adults and children with HIV infection, close contacts of infectious cases, and those with fibrotic lesions on chest radiographs. Adverse effects when using INH over a long treatment period can be a serious problem. Isoniazid can cause severe liver damage, and the drug should be removed if serum aminotransferase activity increases to three- to fivefold the normal level, or the patient develops symptoms of hepatitis. Peripheral neuropathy can be seen with INH therapy. This condition can be prevented by coadministration of pyridoxine. Persons who are presumed to be infected with INH-resistant organisms should be treated with RIF rather than INH. Hepatitis, thrombocytopenia, and nephrotoxicity can be seen with RIF therapy. RIF is thought to potentiate the hepatitis caused by INH. GI upset and staining effects caused by RIF are of minor importance. Although drug-susceptible TB has been successfully treated, the long period of treatment and low patient adherence have in part led to the development of drug-resistant TB, both MDR-TB and XDR-TB. In such situations, a new treatment paradigm has become necessary. For treatment of MDR-TB a five- to six-drug regimen is commonly used (Table 29.12).[185,186] The particular regimen should be based on drug susceptibility testing or previous treatment history. With dual mycobacterium resistance to INH and RIF, a combination of an aminoglycoside from group III drugs, a fluoroquinolone from group II drugs, along with EMB and pyrazinamide and ethionamide or prothionamide from groups I and IV, respectively, can be used at the doses indicated. If resistance to all group I drugs occurs, then *p*-aminosalicylic acid and cycloserine are added to the previously indicated drug list of an aminoglycoside, a fluoroquinolone, and ethionamide or prothionamide. The treatment should continue for up to 18 months after smear conversion to negativity as recommended by the WHO.

Table 29.12 Grouping of Drugs Used to Treat MDR-TB and XDR-TB

Drug Group	Drugs	Doses
I. First-line oral TB drugs	Isoniazid	5 mg/kg
	Rifampicin	10 mg/kg
	Ethambutol	15-25 mg/kg
	Pyrazinamide	30 mg/kg
II. Fluoroquinolones	Ofloxacin	15 mg/kg
	Levofloxacin	15 mg/kg
	Moxifloxacin	7.5-10 mg/kg
III. Injectable TB drugs	Streptomycin	15 mg/kg
	Kanamycin	15 mg/kg
	Amikacin	15 mg/kg
	Capreomycin	15 mg/kg
IV. Second-line TB drugs	Ethionamide/prothionamide	15 mg/kg
	Cycloserine/terizidone	15 mg/kg
	p-Aminosalicylic acid	150 mg/kg
	Bedaquiline	400 mg daily for 2 wk followed by 200 mg thrice weekly
V. Less effective drugs (efficacy uncertain)	Clofazimine	100 mg
	Amoxicillin/clavulanate	875/125 mg every 12 hr
	Linezolid	600 mg
	Imipenem	500-1,000 mg every 6 hr
	Clarithromycin	500 mg every 12 hr
	Thioacetazone	150 mg

MDR-TB, multidrug-resistant tuberculosis; XDR-TB, extensively drug-resistant tuberculosis.

Drug Therapy for Nontuberculous Mycobacterial Infections

Drug Therapy for Leprosy

SULFONES. The diaryl sulfones represent the major class of agents used to treat leprosy. The initial discovery of the sulfones came about as a result of studies directed at exploring the SAR of sulfonamides (Fig. 29.55). A variety of additional chemical modifications have produced several other active agents, but none has proved to be more beneficial than the original lead, 4,4′-diaminodiphenylsulfone. Dapsone was first introduced into the treatment of leprosy in 1943.

Sulfone

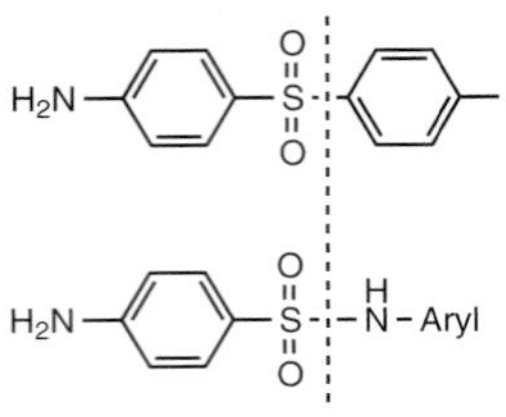

Sulfonamide

Figure 29.55 Structural comparison of sulfones versus sulfonamide.

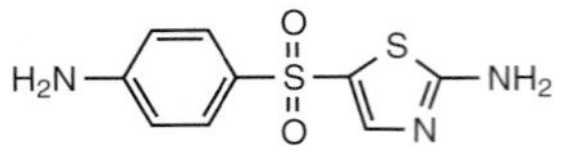

Thiazolsulfone

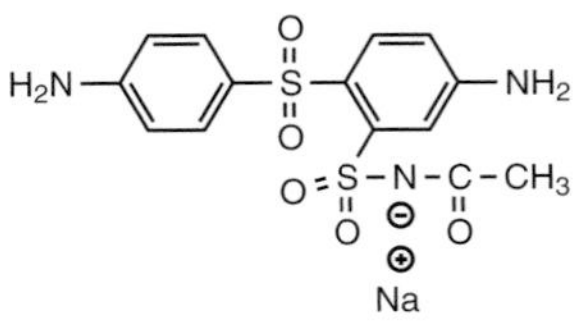

Acetosulfone

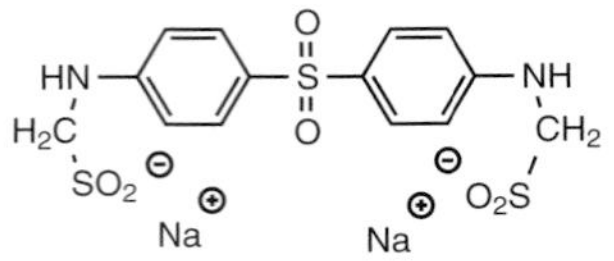

Sulfoxone sodium

DAPSONE

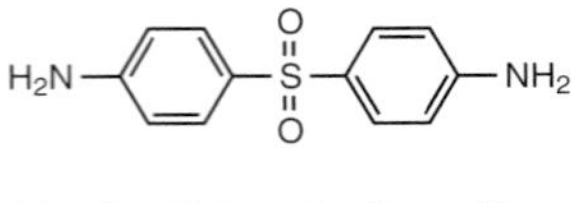

4,4'-Diaminodiphenylsulfone (Dapsone)

Dapsone, a diaminodiphenylsulfone, is a nearly water-insoluble agent that is very weakly basic (pK_a ~1.0). The lack of solubility can account, in part, for the occurrence of GI irritation.

Despite the lack of solubility, the drug is efficiently absorbed from the GI tract. Although dapsone is bound to plasma protein (~70%), it is distributed throughout the body.

Mechanism of Action. Dapsone, a bacteriostatic agent, is thought to act in a manner similar to that of the sulfonamides—namely, through competitive inhibition of *p*-aminobenzoic acid incorporation into folic acid. Bacteria synthesize folic acid, but host cells do not. As a result, coadministration of dapsone and *p*-aminobenzoic acid will inactivate dapsone. Both dapsone and clofazimine have significant anti-inflammatory actions, which may or may not play a role in the antimicrobial action. The anti-inflammatory action can also be a beneficial side effect, offsetting the complication of erythema nodosum leprosum seen in some patients. The anti-inflammatory action can come about by inhibition of myeloperoxidase-catalyzed reactions.[187]

Structure-Activity Relationship. Several derivatives of dapsone have been prepared in an attempt to increase the activity. Isosteric replacement of one benzene ring resulted in the formation of thiazolsulfone. Although still active, it is less effective than dapsone. Substitution on the aromatic ring, to produce acetosulfone, reduced activity while increasing water solubility and decreasing GI irritation. A successful substitution consists of adding methanesulfinate to dapsone to give sulfoxone sodium. This water-soluble form of dapsone is hydrolyzed in vivo to produce dapsone. Sulfoxone sodium is used in individuals who are unable to tolerate dapsone because of GI irritation, but it must be used in a dose threefold that of dapsone because of inefficient metabolism to dapsone. The chemical modification of dapsone derivatives continues to be pursued with the intent of finding newer agents useful for the treatment of resistant strains of M. *leprae*.[188]

Metabolism. The major metabolic product of dapsone results from N-acetylation in the liver by N-acetyltransferase. Dapsone is also N-hydroxylated to the hydroxylamine derivative. These metabolic reactions are catalyzed by CYP3A4 isoforms. Neither of these compounds possesses significant leprostatic activity, although N-acetyldiaminodiphenylsulfone can be deacetylated back to dapsone. Products found in the urine consist of small amounts of dapsone, the metabolites N-acetyldiaminodiphenylsulfone and N-hydroxydiaminodiphenylsulfone, and glucuronide and sulfates of each of these substances (Fig. 29.56).

CLOFAZIMINE (LAMPRENE)

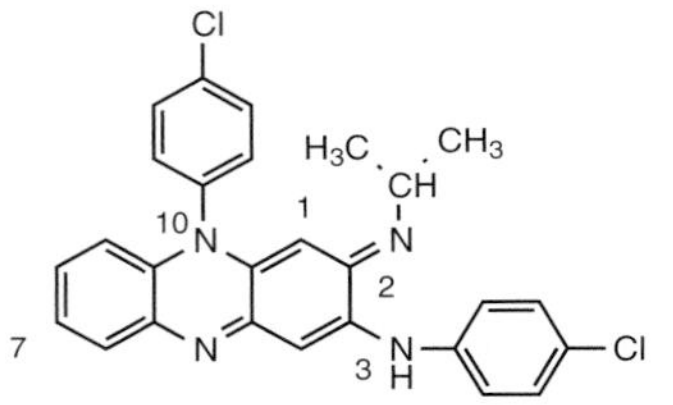

Clofazimine

Although classified as a secondary drug for the treatment of leprosy and commonly used as a component of multidrug therapy, clofazimine appears to be increasing in use for nontuberculous mycobacterial infections. Clofazimine was first used to treat advanced leprosy unresponsive to dapsone or STM in 1966. Currently, clofazimine is not commercially available in the United States; however, there are two mechanisms by which physicians

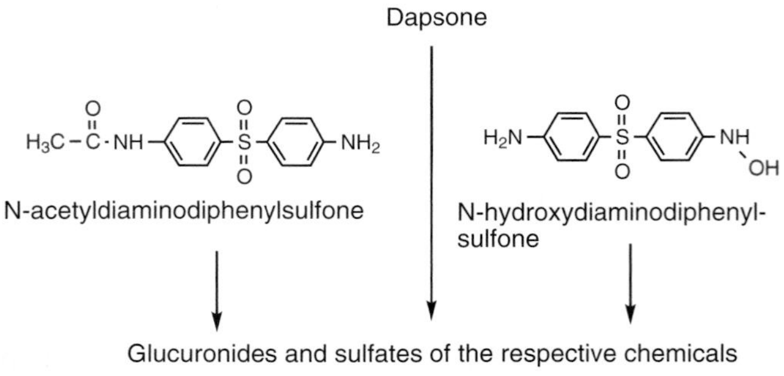

Dapsone

N-acetyldiaminodiphenylsulfone

N-hydroxydiaminodiphenyl-sulfone

Glucuronides and sulfates of the respective chemicals

Figure 29.56 Metabolites of dapsone.

can acquire this drug. The first mechanism is through Novartis Pharmaceuticals Corporation, which currently produces clofazimine sold as Lamprene (generic name for clofazimine), for patients not currently being treated under an existing single patient investigational new drug (IND). The second mechanism is for the health care provider to go through the patient's hospital's Independent Review Board (IRB) and submit an individual IND to the FDA. Clofazimine is a phenazine-based compound and is a water-insoluble dye (dark-red crystals) that leads to pigmentation of the skin. In addition, discoloration (pink, red, or brownish-black) of the feces, eyelid lining, sputum, sweat, tears, and urine is seen.

Mechanism of Action. The mechanism of action remains unclear at the present time; however, many studies have shown that clofazimine has at least two putative mechanisms of action—(1) microbial intracellular redox cycling and (2) membrane disruption.[189] The molecule possesses direct antimycobacterial and immunosuppressive properties. It has been shown that clofazimine increases prostaglandin synthesis and the generation of antimicrobial reactive oxidants from neutrophils, which can play a role in the antileprosy effects. The host cell defense can be stimulated by clofazimine, resulting in the generation of oxidants, such as the superoxide anion, which in turn could have a lethal effect on the organism.[190,191]

Structure-Activity Relationship. Several investigators have reported studies directed toward an understanding of the SAR of clofazimine.[192-194] Substituents on the imino group at position 2, *p*-chloro substitution on the phenyls at C-3 and N-10, and substituents at position 7 have been investigated. The imino group at C-2 appears to be essential, with activity increased when the imino group is substituted with alkyl and cycloalkyl groups. Halogen substitution on the para position of the two phenyls at C-3 and N-10 enhance activity but are not essential to activity. The following order of activity has been reported: Br > Cl > CH_3 > EtO > H or F. In the analogues studied, the increased activity correlates well with pro-oxidative activities of the molecule (e.g., ability to generate superoxide anion) as well as increased lipophilicity.

Metabolism. Various metabolites of clofazimine have been identified, but these account for less than 1% of the administered dose. The lack of higher concentrations of the metabolites can, in part, result from the very slow elimination of clofazimine from the body, which has an estimated half-life of 8.8-69 days. The lipophilic nature of clofazimine results in distribution and storage of the drug in fat tissue. There appears to be some discrepancy as to the structures of the metabolites.[194] The most recent studies suggest the presence of two conjugates, with the possibility of intermediates (Fig. 29.57). Clofazimine is thought to undergo hydroxylic dehalogenation on the 3-chloroaniline, followed by sulfate conjugation and 4-hydroxylation, followed by glucuronic acid conjugation.[195]

RIFAMPIN (RIFADIN, RIMACTANE). RIF, an antituberculin drug, has already been discussed. Its actions against *M. leprae* parallel those effects reported for *M. tuberculosis*. Today, RIF is considered to be an effective antileprosy agent when used in combination with the sulfones.

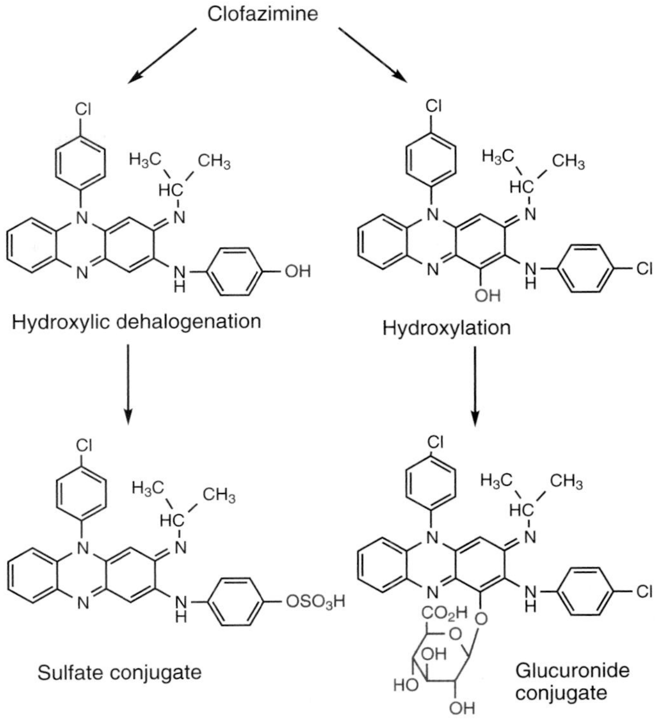

Figure 29.57 Human metabolic products of clofazimine.

THALIDOMIDE (THALOMID)

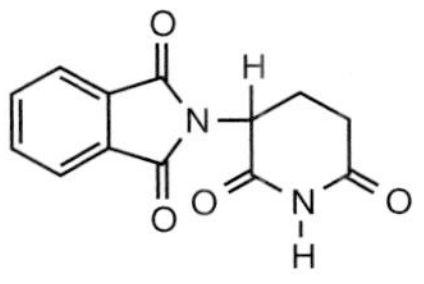

The development of painful, tender, inflamed, subcutaneous nodules that can last a week or two but can reappear and last for long periods is seen in a number of diseases. In the case of leprosy, the condition is referred to as erythema nodosum leprosum (ENL). The condition appears to be a hypersensitivity reaction, and although it can appear in nontreated patients, it commonly is seen as a complication of the chemotherapy of leprosy. In addition to painful nodules, the patient can experience fever, malaise, wasting, vasculitis, and peripheral neuritis. This condition has been successfully treated with thalidomide. Thalidomide has been approved by the FDA for treatment of ENL and is considered to be the drug of choice.[196] The mechanism whereby thalidomide produces relief is thought to be associated with the drug's ability to control inflammatory cytokines. Specifically, thalidomide inhibits the synthesis and release of tumor necrosis factor-α, which is synthesized and released by blood mononuclear cells and appears in the serum during ENL; concentrations drop when the patient is treated with thalidomide. In addition to the treatment of ENL, thalidomide has been reported to exhibit beneficial effects in the treatment of aphthous ulcers in HIV-positive patients, Behcet disease, chronic graft-versus-host disease, rash caused by systemic or cutaneous lupus erythematosus, pyoderma gangrenosum, and multiple myeloma. Thalidomide is a very potent teratogenic agent, with a history of an estimated 10,000 deformed infants born to mothers who used the drug during pregnancy. It can be used safely in postmenopausal women, but strict controls are required for women of childbearing age. Although no evidence suggests that men can transmit the drug during sex, the use of condoms by male patients will be required.

Therapeutic Considerations for Leprosy. Since its introduction into the chemotherapy of leprosy in 1947, dapsone has proved to be the single most effective agent. This drug was used as a monotherapeutic agent despite the recognition that resistant strains were beginning to emerge. Since 1977, monotherapy with dapsone is no longer recognized as an acceptable method for the treatment of leprosy. Today, combination chemotherapy is the method of choice. The combination consists of RIF (600 mg monthly), dapsone (100 mg daily), and clofazimine (300 mg monthly, with 50 mg daily added for patients with multibacillary leprosy, which is defined as five or more skin lesions). Therapy is usually continued for at least 2 years or as long as skin smears are positive. The patient is kept under supervision for 5 years following completion of chemotherapy. A similar treatment regimen is recommended for treatment of paucibacillary leprosy (defined as five or fewer skin lesions) except that treatment is continued for 6 months and the patient is kept under observation for an additional 2 years.[197,198] It should be noted that the patient is noninfectious within 72 hours of starting treatment. Other combinations that have been reported include RIF plus ofloxacin and minocycline or ofloxacin plus minocycline. The new regimens allow a shortened treatment period and a reduced rate of relapse. An important aspect of therapy for leprosy involves the treatment of peripheral nerve damage. This nerve damage can be treated with steroids, such as prednisolone. For severe cases, however, thalidomide is used.

Drug Therapy for MAC

Drug therapy for the treatment of MAC is complicated. It underwent significant changes in the early 1990s, but little has changed during the last 30 years. Recommendations for treatment are presently based on small and, in some cases, incomplete studies; more changes can be expected in the future. The 1997 guidelines for prophylaxis of MAC advise that all adults and adolescents with HIV infection and a CD4 lymphocyte count of less than 50 cells/mL receive clarithromycin 500 mg twice a day or azithromycin 1,200 mg once a week. This recommendation is considered to be a standard of care.[199-201] For treatment of MAC, it is recommended that a combination therapy be used that includes either clarithromycin or azithromycin plus EMB and either RIF or rifabutin.[202] Fluoroquinolones and amikacin can be added to the combination. It should be noted that INH and pyrazinamide are ineffective in the treatment of disseminated MAC.

MACROLIDES. Both clarithromycin and azithromycin (Fig. 29.27) are considered to be first-line agents for the prevention and treatment of MAC and have replaced rifabutin. Both macrolides are concentrated in macrophages (clarithromycin concentration is 17.3-fold higher in macrophage cells than in extracellular fluid) and appear to be equally effective, although clarithromycin has a lower minimum inhibitory concentration. Azithromycin has an intra-alveolar macrophage half-life of 195 hours, compared to a 4-hour half-life for clarithromycin. For prevention, the macrolides can be used as single agents, although there is a risk of resistant organisms forming and of a cross-resistance between clarithromycin and azithromycin. In one study, the combination of azithromycin and rifabutin proved to be more effective than either drug used alone. For the treatment of MAC, combination therapy is recommended.

Mechanism of Action. The macrolide antibiotics are bacteriostatic agents that inhibit protein synthesis by binding to the 50S ribosomal units as previously discussed in the chapter.

Metabolism. Clarithromycin is metabolized in the liver to an active metabolite, 14-hydroxyclarithromycin, which is less active than the parent molecule. In addition, the drug is an inhibitor of CYP3A4, which could lead to increased concentrations of some drugs, such as rifabutin (see below). Azithromycin is primarily excreted unchanged in the gut, and at present, there is no evidence of CYP3A4 induction or inhibition.

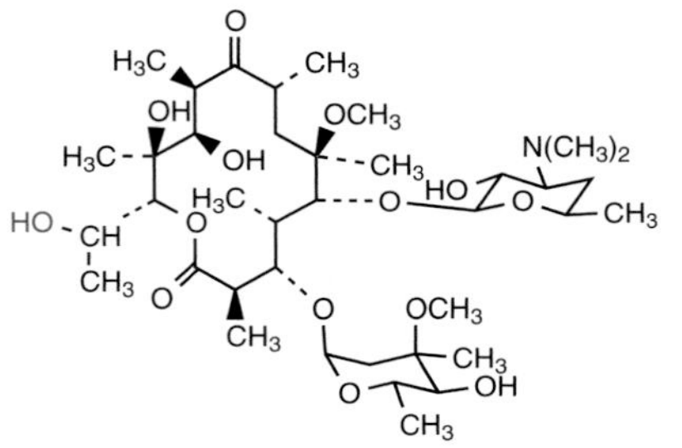

14-Hydroxyclarithromycin

RIFAMYCINS. Various rifamycin derivatives have been investigated or are under investigation for use in the prevention and treatment of MAC. Up until 1997, rifabutin (Mycobutin) was considered to be the drug of choice for prophylaxis of MAC-infected patients. Studies since 1995, however, have suggested that the macrolides are more effective (survival rates), present fewer side effects, and cause less drug interactions than rifabutin. Early treatment of MAC bacteremia consists of multidrug regimens, usually involving four or five drugs. Drug interactions and, in some studies, exceptionally high drug doses have given confusing results. It is generally agreed that rifabutin should be used in treatment when macrolides have failed or can be combined with azithromycin for prophylaxis or treatment when clarithromycin is unsuccessful.

Drug Interactions. The most significant drug interaction identified with rifabutin is associated with the fact that the drugs in this class are inducers of CYP3A4 and the CYP2C family. As a result, certain drugs that are substrates for these isoforms will show reduced activity.

Rifabutin has been shown to reduce the area under the curve and the maximum concentration of clarithromycin and most HIV protease inhibitors. This action could lead to inactivity or resistance to these agents. In addition, because the HIV protease inhibitors are inhibitors of CYP3A4, a combination of rifabutin plus an HIV protease inhibitor is expected to increase the rifabutin area under the curve and maximum concentration, thus increasing the risk of rifabutin side effects. The most serious side effect of rifabutin is uveitis (inflammation of the iris). Under these conditions, appropriate changes in dosing are required. If combination therapy is desirable for the treatment of MAC, the combination of azithromycin and rifabutin is recommended because no significant change in mean serum drug concentration is reported to occur with either agent when used in combination.

Drug Metabolism. The hepatic metabolism of rifabutin is complex, with as many as 20 metabolites having been reported. The structure of most of the metabolites remains unknown, but several have been identified, including 25-desacetylrifabutin, 25-desacetylrifabutin-N-oxide, 31-hydroxyrifabutin, 32-hydroxyrifabutin, and 32-hydroxy-25-desacetylrifabutin. The metabolites appear in the urine (50%) and in the feces (30%). Based on the activity of other rifamycins, it might be expected that one or more of the metabolites possess antimycobacterial activity.

Structure Challenge

Choose which of the following β-lactam antibiotic structures is appropriate for the listed class and infection.

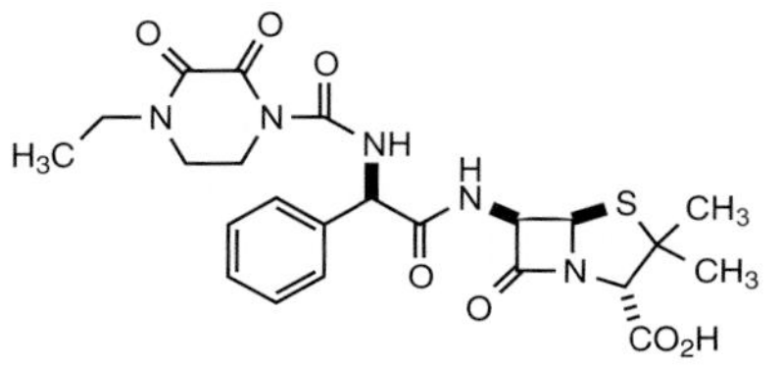

Sructure A

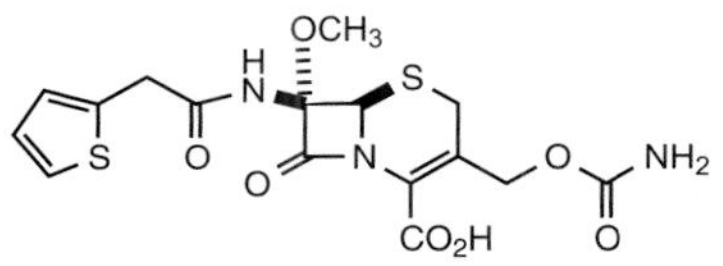

Structure B

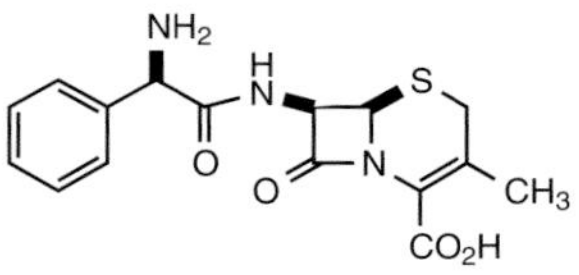

Structure C

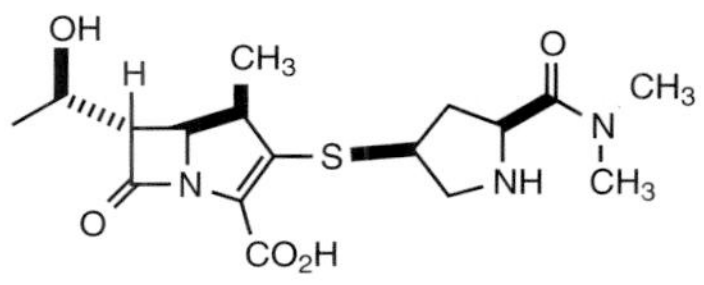

Structure D

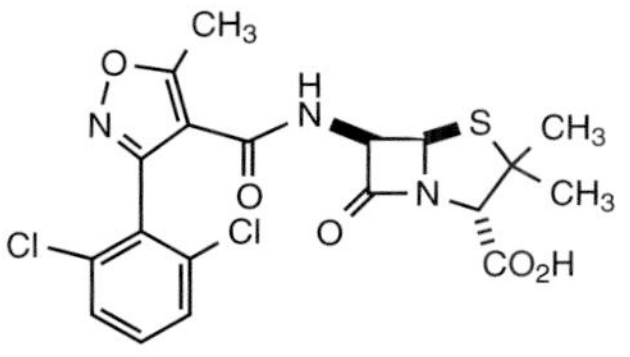

Structure E

1. Cephalosporin antibiotic to treat *S. aureus* infection
2. Carbapenem antibiotic to treat *P. aeruginosa* infection
3. Penicillin antibiotic to treat penicillinase-producing *S. aureus* infection
4. Cephalosporin antibiotic to treat *B. fragilis* infection
5. Penicillin antibiotic to treat *P. aeruginosa* infection

Evaluate the antimycobacterial structures drawn below, and identify which would be the most appropriate for each numbered description below.

(continued)

Structure Challenge—Continued

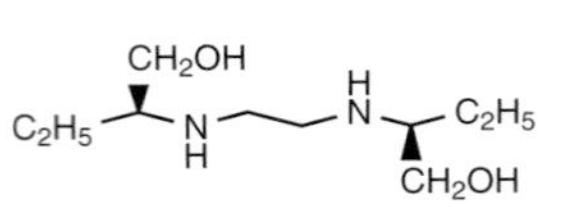

Structure A

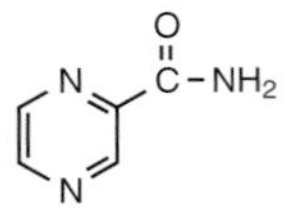

Structure B

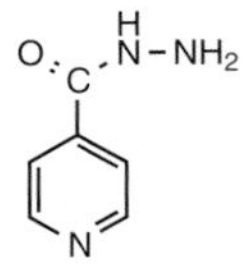

Structure C

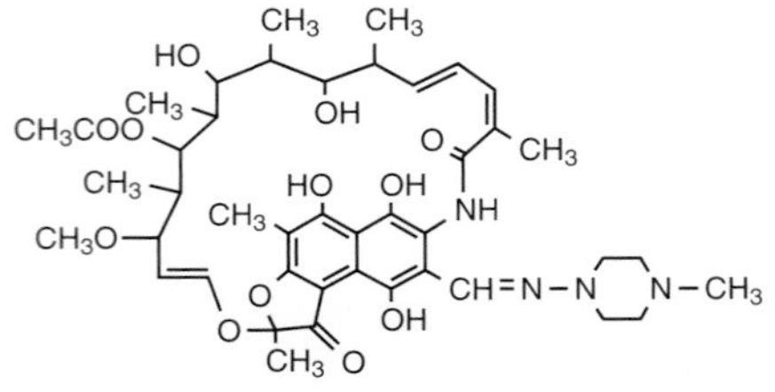

Structure D

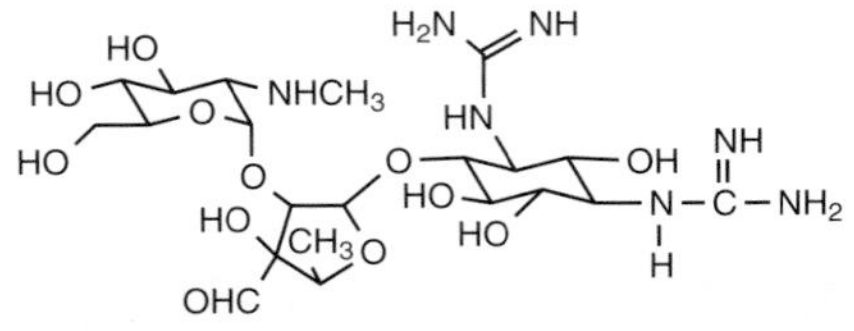

Structure E

6. What is the mechanism of action of each drug?
7. Combination therapy is used to treat *Mycobacterium tuberculosis* infections to reduce the emergence of drug resistance. Based on your answer to the previous question, pick four drugs that would be effective to be used in combination to treat a patient infected with *Mycobacterium tuberculosis*. Why did you think the four drugs you chose would reduce drug resistance?
8. Which of these agents is/are a prodrug?
9. Which of these drugs inhibit mycobacterial cell wall biosynthesis? Why are these compounds **not** cross-resistant with each other?
10. Which of these have activity against the dormant phase of *Mycobacterium tuberculosis*?

Structure Challenge answers found immediately after References.

REFERENCES

1. Pasteur L, Joubert J. Charbon et septicemia. *CR Acad Sci Paris*. 1877;85:101-115.
2. Domagk GJ. Ein Beitrag zur chemotherapie der bakteriellen infektionen. *Dtsch Med Wochenschr*. 1935;61:250-253.
3. Fleming A. On the antibacterial action of cultures of a penicillum, with special reference to their use in the isolation of *B. influenza*. *Br J Exp Pathol*. 1929;10:226-236.
4. Abraham EP, Chain E, Fletcher CM, et al. Further observations on penicillin. *Eur J Clin Pharmacol*. 1941;42:3-9.
5. Fleischmann RD, Adams MD, White O, et al. Whole-genome random sequencing and assembly of *Haemophilus influenzae* Rd. *Science*. 1995;269:496-512.
6. National Institutes of Health. Complete Microbial Genomes. Available at http://www.ncbi.nlm.nih.gov/genomes/lproks.cgi?view=1. Accessed May 2018.
7. Tianjin University. Database of Essential Genes. Available at http://tubic.tju.edu.cn/deg/. Accessed May 2018.
8. Tréfouël JT, Nitti F, Bovet D. Activité du *p*-aminophénylsulfamide sur l'infection streptococcique expérimentale de la souris et du lapin. *CR Soc Biol*. 1935;120:756.
9. Anand N. Sulfonamides: structure-activity relationships and mechanism of action. In: Hitchings GH, ed. *Inhibition of Folate Metabolism in Chemotherapy. Handbook of Experimental Pharmacology (Continuation of Handbuch der experimentellen Pharmakologie)*. Vol 64. Berlin, Heidelberg: Springer; 1983.
10. *Bactrim Tablets and Double Strength Tablets [package insert]*. Philadelphia, PA: AR Scientific. Revised June 2013. Accessed May 2018.
11. Sköld O. Sulfonamides and trimethoprim. *Expert Rev Anti Infect Ther*. 2010;8(1):1-6.
12. *Erythromycin Ethylsuccinate and Sulfisoxazole Acetyl for Oral Suspension [package insert]*. Pomona, NY: Duramed; 2007. Revised November 2009/Physicians Total Care, Inc.
13. Roberts VA, Dauber-Osguthorpe P, Osguthorpe DJ, et al. A comparison of the binding of the ligand trimethoprim to bacterial and vertebrate dihydrofolate reductases. *Israel J Chem*. 1986;27(2):198-210.
14. Trimethoprim 100 mg Tablets [package insert]. Medically reviewed November 2017. Available at https://www.drugs.com/pro/trimethoprim.html. Accessed May 2018.
15. Andriole VT, The quinolones: past, present, and future. *Clin Infect Dis*. 2005;41(suppl 2):S113-S119.
16. Drlica K, Zhao X. DNA gyrase, topoisomerase IV and the 4-quinolones. *Microbiol Mol Biol Rev*. 1997;61:377-392.
17. Cheng G, Hao H, Dai M, Liu Z, Yuan Z. Antibacterial action of quinolones: from target to network. *Eur J Med Chem*. 2013;66:555-562.
18. Domagala JM. Structure-activity and structure-side effect relationships for the quinolone antibacterials. *J Antimicrob Chemother*. 1994;33:685-706.
19. Blondeau JM. Fluoroquinolones: mechanism of action, classification, and development of resistance. *Surv Ophthalmol*. 2004;49(suppl 2).

20. *Noroxin [package insert].* Whitehouse Station, NJ: Merck & Co.; 2013.
21. *Cipro [package insert].* Wayne, NJ: Bayer HealthCare Pharmaceuticals, Inc.; 2009.
22. *Factive [package insert].* Waltham, MA: Oscient Pharmaceuticals; 2007.
23. *Levaquin [package insert].* Raritan, NJ: Ortho-McNeil-Janssen Pharmaceuticals; 2008.
24. *Avelox [package insert].* Kenilworth, NJ: Schering-Plough Corp.; 2010.
25. Hooper DC, Jacoby GA. Mechanisms of drug resistance: quinolone resistance. *Ann NY Acad Sci.* 2015;1354:12-31.
26. Kang J, Wang L, Chen X, et al. Interactions of a series of fluoroquinolone antibacterial drugs with the human cardiac K^+ channel HERG. *Mol Pharmacol.* 2001;59:122-126.
27. *Macrodantin (Nitrofurantoin Macrocrystals) [package insert].* Cincinnati, OH: Procter & Gamble Pharmaceuticals; 2009.
28. *Flagyl [package insert].* New York: Pfizer; 2018.
29. *Tindamax [package insert].* San Antonio, TX: Mission Pharmacal Company; 2007.
30. *Solosec [package insert].* Baltimore, MD: Lupin Pharmaceuticals Inc.; 2017.
31. Wise EM, Park JT. Penicillin: its basic site of action as an inhibitor of a peptide cross-linking reaction in cell wall mucopeptide synthesis. *Proc Natl Acad Sci USA.* 1965;54:75-81.
32. Kong KF, Schneper L, Mathee K. Beta-lactam antibiotics: from antibiosis to resistance and bacteriology. *APMIS.* 2010;118:1-36.
33. Behrens OK, Corse JW, Jones RG, et al. Process and culture media for producing new penicillins. U.S. Patent 2479297. 1949.
34. Peter DF, Charles NJH, Newbolt RG. Recovery of solid 6-aminopenicillanic acid. U.S. Patent 2941995. 1960.
35. Abraham EP, Newton GGF. The structure of cephalosporin-C. *Biochem J.* 1961;79:377-393.
36. Nagarajan R, Boeck LD, Gorman M, et al. Beta-lactam antibiotics from Streptomyces. *J Am Chem Soc.* 1971;93:2308-2310.
37. Imada A, Kitano K, Kintaka K, et al. Sulfazecin and isosulfazecin, novel beta-lactam antibiotics of bacterial origin. *Nature.* 1981;289:590-591.
38. Sykes RB, Cimarusti CM, Bonner DP, et al. Monocyclic beta-lactam antibiotics produced by bacteria. *Nature.* 1981;291:489-491.
39. Tomasz A, Waks S. Mechanism of action of penicillin: triggering of the pneumococcal autolytic enzyme by inhibitors of cell wall synthesis. *Proc Natl Acad Sci USA.* 1975;72:4162-4166.
40. Abraham EP, Chain E. An enzyme from bacteria able to destroy penicillin. *Nature.* 1940;146:837-838.
41. UpToDate. Extended-Spectrum Beta-Lactamases. Available at https://www.uptodate.com/contents/extended-spectrum-beta-lactamases#!. Accessed May 2018.
42. Fairbrother RW, Taylor G. Sodium methicillin in routine therapy. *Lancet.* 1961;1:473-476.
43. Nafcillin [package insert]. Medically reviewed September 2017. Available at https://www.drugs.com/pro/nafcillin.html. Accessed May 2018.
44. Dicloxacillin [package insert]. Medically reviewed June 2018. Available at https://www.drugs.com/pro/dicloxacillin.html. Accessed May 2018.
45. Ganapathy ME, Brandsch M, Prasad PD, et al. Differential recognition of β-lactam antibiotics by intestinal and real peptide transporters, PEPT 1 and PEPT 2. *J Biol Chem.* 1995;270:25672-25677.
46. *Zosyn [package insert].* Philadelphia, PA: Wyeth Pharmaceuticals; 2012.
47. Dunn GL. Ceftizoxime and other third generation cephalosporins: structure-activity relationships. *J Antimicrob Chemother.* 1982;10(suppl C):1-10.
48. Cephalexin [package insert]. Medically reviewed December 2017. Available at https://www.drugs.com/pro/cephalexin.html. Accessed May 2018.
49. *Ceftin [package insert].* Research Triangle Park, NC: GlaxoSmithKline; 2017.
50. Cuchural GJ, Tally FP, Jacobus NV, et al. Comparative activities of newer β-lactam agents against members of the *Bacteroides fragilis* group. *Antimicrob Agents Chemother.* 1990;3:479-480.
51. Ceftriaxone [package insert]. Medically reviewed December 2017. Available at https://www.drugs.com/pro/ceftriaxone.html. Accessed May 2018.
52. *Maxipime [package insert].* Lake Forest, IL: Hospira; 2012.
53. Lipsky JJ. Mechanism of the inhibition of γ-carboxylation of glutamic acid by *N*-methylthiotetrazole antibiotics. *Proc Natl Acad Sci USA.* 1984;81:2893-2897.
54. Wildman GT, Datta R. Isolation of antibiotic cephamycin C. U.S. Patent 4137405. 1979.
55. Claforan [package insert]. Medically reviewed April 2018. Available at https://www.drugs.com/pro/claforan.html. Accessed May 2018.
56. Sharma R, Park TE, Moy S. Ceftazidime-avibactam: a novel cephalosporin/β-lactamase inhibitor combination for the treatment of resistant gram-negative organisms. *Clin Ther.* 2016;38(3):431-444.
57. Zhanel GG, Chung P, Adam H, et al. Ceftolozane/tazobactam: a novel cephalosporin/B lactamase inhibitor combination with activity against multidrug-resistant gram-negative bacilli. *Drugs.* 2014;74(1):31-51.
58. Cedax [package insert]. Medically reviewed August 2017. Available at https://www.drugs.com/pro/cedax.html. Accessed May 2018.
59. Cefditoren Pivoxil [package insert]. Medically reviewed March 2018. Available at https://www.drugs.com/pro/cefditoren-pivoxil.html. Accessed May 2018.
60. *Teflaro [package insert].* St. Louis, MO: Forest Pharmaceuticals; 2016.
61. Kahan JS, Kahan FM, Goegelman R, et al. Thienamycin, a new beta-lactam antibiotic I. Discovery, taxonomy, isolation, and physical properties. *J Antibiot.* 1979;32:1-12.
62. Birnbaum J, Kahan FM, Kropp H, et al. Carbapenems, a new class of beta-lactam antibiotics. Discovery and development of ipenem/cilastatin. *Am J Med.* 1985;78(6A):3-21.
63. *Primaxin [package insert].* Whitehouse Station, NJ: Merck, Sharp & Dohme; 2017.
64. Tsuji M, Ishii Y, Ohno A, et al. In vitro and in vivo antibacterial activities of S-4661, a new carbapenem. *Antimicrob Agents Chemother.* 1998;42:94-99.
65. Norrby SR. Neurotoxicity of carbapenem antibiotics: consequences for their use in bacterial meningitis. *J Antimicrob Chemother.* 2000;45:5-7.
66. Hecker SJ, Reddy KR, Totrov M, et al. Discovery of a cyclic boronic acid β-lactamase inhibitor (RPX7009) with utility vs class A serine carbapenemases. *J Med Chem.* 2015;58:3682-3692.
67. *Vabomere [package insert].* Lincolnshire, IL: Melinta Therapeutics Inc.; 2018.
68. Zhanel GC, Wiebe R, Dialy L, et al. Comparative review of the carbapenems. *Drugs.* 2007;67:1027-1052.
69. Kobayashi R, Komoni M, Hasegawa K, et al. In vitro activity of tebipenem, a new oral carbapenem antibiotic, against penicillin-nonsusceptible Streptococcus pneumoniae. *Antimicrob Agents Chemother.* 2005;49:889-994.
70. *Azactam [package insert].* Princeton, NJ: Bristol-Myers Squibb Company; 2013.
71. Schuwirth BS, Borovinskava MA, Hau CW, et al. Structures of the bacterial ribosome at 3.5A resolution. *Science.* 2005;310:827-834.
72. Selmer M, Dunham CM, Murphy FV 4th, et al. Structure of the 70S ribosome complexed with mRNA and tRNA. *Science.* 2006;313:1935-1942.
73. Ratjen F, Moeller A, McKinney ML, et al. Eradication of early P. aeruginosa infection in children <7 years of age with cystic fibrosis: the early study. *J Cyst Fibros.* 2019;18(1):78-85.
74. Blasi F, Carnovale V, Cimino G, et al. Treatment compliance in cystic fibrosis patients with chronic Pseudomonas aeruginosa infection treated with tobramycin inhalation powder: the FREE study. *Respir Med.* 2018;138:88-94.
75. *Liposomal Amikacin for Inhalation (LAI) in the Treatment of Mycobacterium abscessus Lung Disease.* Bethesda (MD): ClinicalTrials.gov; 2018. Identifier NCT03038178. Available at https://clinicaltrials.gov/ct2/show/NCT03038178?cond=amikacin&rank=4. Accessed June 13, 2018.

76. Jana S, Deb JK. Molecular understanding of aminoglycoside action and resistance. *App Microbiol Biotech*. 2006;70:140-150.
77. Magnet S, Blanchard JS. Molecular insights into aminoglycoside action and resistance. *Chem Rev*. 2005;105:477-498.
78. Kahlmeter G, Dahlager JI. Aminoglycoside toxicity – a review of clinical studies published between 1975 and 1982. *J Antimicrob Chemother*. 1984;13(suppl A):9-22.
79. Warner WA, Sanders E. Neuromuscular blockade associated with gentamicin therapy. *JAMA*. 1971;215:1153-1154.
80. Schatz A, Bugie E, Waksman SA. Streptomycin, a substance exhibiting antibiotic activity against gram-positive and gram-negative bacteria. 1944. *Clin Ortho Rel Res*. 2005;(437):3-6.
81. Masur H, Whelton PK, Whelton A. Neomycin toxicity revisited. *Arch Surg (Chicago, Ill: 1960)*. 1976;111:822-825.
82. Walkty A, Adam H, Baxter M, et al. In vitro activity of plazomicin against 5,015 gram-negative and gram-positive clinical isolates obtained from patients in Canadian hospitals as part of the CANWARD study, 2011-2012. *Antimicrob Agents Chemother*. 2014;58:2554-2563.
83. Aggen JB, Armstrong ES, Goldblum AA, et al. Synthesis and spectrum of the neoglycoside ACHN-490. *Antimicrob Agents Chemother*. 2010;54:4636-4642.
84. Stauton J, Wilkinson B. Biosynthesis of erythromycin and rapamycin. *Chem Rev*. 1997;97:2611-2629.
85. Fiese EF, Steffen SH. Comparison of the acid stability of azithromycin and erythromycin A. *J Antimicrob Chemother*. 1990;25(suppl A):39-47.
86. Roberts MC, Sutcliffe J, Courvalin P, et al. Nomenclature for macrolide and macrolide- lincosamide-streptogramin B resistance determinants. *Antimicrob Agents Chemother*. 1999;43:2823-2830.
87. Westphal JF. Macrolide-induced clinically relevant drug interactions with cytochrome P- 450A (CYP) 3A4: an update focused on clarithromycin, azithromycin, and dirythromycin. *Br J Clin Pharmacol*. 2000;50:285-295.
88. Yasuda K, Lan L, Sanglard D, et al. Interaction of cytochrome P450 3A inhibitors with P- glycoprotein. *J Pharmacol Exp Ther*. 2002;303:323-332.
89. *Ery-Ped [package insert]*. Atlanta, GA: Arbor Pharmaceuticals; 2012.
90. Ferrero JL, Bopp BA, Marsh KC, et al. Metabolism and disposition of clarithromycin in man. *Drug Metab Dispos*. 1990;18:441-446.
91. Safety Alerts for Human Medical Products – Clarithromycin (Biaxin): Drug Safety Communication – Potential Increased Risk of Heart Problems or Death in Patients with Heart Disease. FDA. Retrieved June 12, 2018. Accessed May 2018.
92. *Zithromax [package insert]*. New York: Pfizer Labs; 2017.
93. *Dificid [package insert]*. Whitehouse Station, NJ: Merck, Sharpe & Dohme; 2015.
94. *Cleocin [package insert]*. New York: Pharmacia & Upjohn; 2018.
95. Chopra I, Roberts M. Tetracycline antibiotics: mode of action, applications, molecular biology, and epidemiology of bacterial resistance. *Microb Mol Biol Rev*. 2001;65:232-260.
96. *Tetracycline Hydrochloride Capsules [package insert]*. Corona, CA: Watson Pharma; 2010.
97. Broderson DE, Clemons WM Jr, Carter AP, et al. The structural basis for the action of the antibiotics tetracycline, pactamycin, and hygromycin B on the 30S ribosomal subunit. *Cell*. 2000;103:1143-1154.
98. Pioletti M, Schlunzen F, Harms J, et al. Crystal structures of complexes of the small ribosomal subunit with tetracycline, edeine, and IF3. *EMBO J*. 2001;20:1829-1839.
99. Anokhina MM, Barta A, Nierhaus KH, et al. Mapping of the second tetracycline binding site on the ribosomal small subunit of *E. coli*. *Nucl Acids Res*. 2004;92:2594-2597.
100. Speer BS, Shoemaker NB, Salyers AA. Bacterial resistance to tetracycline: mechanisms, transfer, and clinical significance. *Clin Microbiol Rev*. 1992;5:387-399.
101. Minocin [package insert]. Medically reviewed April 2017. Available at https://www.drugs.com/pro/minocin.html. Accessed May 2018.
102. Goldstein FW, Kitzis MD, Acar JF. *N,N*-Dimethylglycyl-amido derivative of minocycline and 6-demethyl-6-desoxytetracycline, two new glycylcyclines highly effective against tetracycline-resistant Gram-positive cocci. *Antimicrob Agents Chemother*. 1994;38:2218-2220.
103. Sum PE, Peterson P. Synthesis and structure-activity relationship of novel glycylcycline derivative leading to the discovery of GAR-936. *Bioorg Med Chem Lett*. 1999;9:1459-1462.
104. Shaw WV, Packman LC, Burleigh BD, et al. Primary structure of a chloramphenicol acetyltransferase specified by R plasmids. *Nature*. 1979;282: 870-872.
105. Chloramphenicol Sodium Succinate [package insert]. Medically Reviewed August 2017. Available at https://www.drugs.com/pro/chloramphenicol-sodium-succinate.html. Accessed May 2018.
106. Barna JCJ, Williams DH. The structure and mode of action of glycopeptide antibiotics of the vancomycin group. *Ann Rev Microbiol*. 1984;38:339-357.
107. Arthur M, Courvalin P. Genetics and mechanisms of glycopeptide resistance in enterococci. *Antimicrob Agents Chemother*. 1993;37:1563-1571.
108. *Vancomycin Hydrochloride [package insert]*. New York: Pfizer Labs; 2010.
109. Higgins DL, Chang R, Debabov DV, et al. Telavancin, a multifunctional lipoglycopeptide, disrupts both cell wall synthesis and membrane integrity in methicillin-resistant *Staphylococcus aureus*. *Antimicrob Agents Chemother*. 2005;49:1127-1134.
110. *Dalvance [package insert]*. Parsippany, NJ: Durata Therapeutics; 2016.
111. *Orbactiv [package insert]*. Lincolnshire, IL: Melinta Therapeutics; 2018.
112. Tally FP, DeBruin MF. Development of daptomycin for gram positive infections. *J Antimicrob Chemother*. 2000;46:523-526.
113. *Cubicin [package insert]*. Whitehouse, NJ: Merck, Sharp & Dohme; 2018.
114. Vasquez D. The streptogramin family of antibiotics. In: Gottlieb D, Shaw PD, eds. *Antibiotics*. New York: Springer-Verlag; 1967:387-403.
115. *Synercid [package insert]*. New York: Pfizer Inc.; 2017.
116. *Zyvox [package insert]*. New York: Pharmacia and Upjohn; 2018.
117. *Sivextro [package insert]*. Whitehouse, NJ: Merck, Sharp & Dohme; 2017.
118. Colca JR, McDonald WG, Waldon DJ, et al. Cross-linking in the living cell locates the site of action of oxazolidinone antibiotics. *J Biol Chem*. 2003;278:21972-21979.
119. Lincopan N, de Almeida LM, Elmor de Araújo MR, et al. Linezolid resistance in *Staphylococcus epidermidis* associated with a G2603T mutation in the 23S rRNA gene. *Int J Antimicrob Agents*. 2009;34:281-282.
120. *Altabax [package insert]*. Extron, PA: Aqua Pharmaceuticals; 2015.
121. Yan K, Madden L, Choudhry AE, et al. Biochemical characterization of the interactions of the novel pleuromutilin derivative retapamulin with bacterial ribosomes. *Antimicrob Agents Chemother*. 2006;50:3875-3881.
122. Davidovich C, Bashan A, Auerbach-Nevo T, et al. Induced-fit tightens pleuromutilins binding to ribosomes and remote interactions enable their selectivity. *Proc Nat Acad Sci USA*. 2007;104:4291-4296.
123. Champney WS, Rodgers WK. Retapamulin inhibition of translation and 50S ribosomal subunit formation in *Staphylococcus aureus* cells. *Antimicrob Agents Chemother*. 2007;51:3385-3387.
124. McNeil MR, Brennan PJ. Structure, function and biogenesis of the cell envelope of mycobacteria in relation to bacterial physiology, pathogenesis and drug resistance; some thoughts and possibilities arising from recent structural information. *Res Microbiol*. 1991;142:451-463.
125. Jackson M. The mycobacterial cell envelope—lipids. *Cold Spring Harb Perspect Med*. 2014;4:a021105.
126. WHO. *Global Tuberculosis Report*; 2017.
127. Prevots DR, Shaw PA, Strickland D, et al. Nontuberculous mycobacterial lung disease prevalence at four integrated health care delivery systems. *Am J Respir Crit Care Med*. 2010;182:970-976.

128. Park IK, Olivier KN. Nontuberculous mycobacteria in cystic fibrosis and non-cystic fibrosis bronchiectasis. *Semin Respir Crit Care Med.* 2015;36:217-224.
129. Zhang Y. The magic bullets and tuberculosis drug targets. *Annu Rev Pharmacol Toxicol.* 2005;45:529-564.
130. WHO. *Treatment of Tuberculosis: Guidelines for National Programmes.* 4th ed. Geneva, Switzerland: World Health Organization; 2010.
131. Zhang Y, Heym B, Allen B, et al. The catalase-peroxidase gene and isoniazid resistance of Mycobacterium tuberculosis. *Nature.* 1992;358:591-593.
132. Johnsson K, Schultz PG. Mechanistic studies of the oxidation of isoniazid by the catalase peroxidase from *Mycobacterium tuberculosis. J Am Chem Soc.* 1994;116:7425-7426.
133. Dubnau E, Chan J, Raynaud C, et al. Oxygenated mycolic acids are necessary for virulence of *Mycobacterium tuberculosis* in mice. *Mol Microbiol.* 2000;36:630-637.
134. Glickman MS, Cox JS, Jacobs WR Jr. A novel mycolic acid cyclopropane synthetase is required for cording, persistence, and virulence of Mycobacterium tuberculosis. *Mol Cell.* 2000;5:717-727.
135. Quemard A, Sacchettini JC, Dessen A, et al. Enzymatic characterization of the target for isoniazid in *Mycobacterium tuberculosis. Biochemistry.* 1995;34:8235-8241.
136. Johnsson K, King DS, Schultz PG. Studies on the mechanism of action of isoniazid and ethionamide in the chemotherapy of tuberculosis. *J Am Chem Soc.* 1995;117:5009-5010.
137. Rozwarski DA, Grant GA, Barton DH, et al. Modification of the NADH of the isoniazid target (InhA) from *Mycobacterium tuberculosis. Science (New York NY).* 1998;279:98-102.
138. van Soolingen D, de Haas PE, van Doorn HR, et al. Mutations at amino acid position 315 of the katG gene are associated with high-level resistance to isoniazid, other drug resistance, and successful transmission of *Mycobacterium tuberculosis* in The Netherlands. *J Infect Dis.* 2000;182:1788-1790.
139. Bavin EM, James B, Kay E, et al. Further observations on the antibacterial activity to *Mycobacterium tuberculosis* of a derivative of isoniazid, omicron-hydroxybenzal isonicotinylhydrazone (nupasal-213). *J Pharm Pharmacol.* 1955;7:1032-1038.
140. Bavin EM, Drain DJ, Seiler M, et al. Some further studies on tuberculostatic compounds. *J Pharm Pharmacol.* 1952;4:844-855.
141. Weber WW, Hein DW. Clinical pharmacokinetics of isoniazid. *Clin Pharmacokinet.* 1979;4:401-422.
142. Holdiness MR. Clinical pharmacokinetics of the antituberculosis drugs. *Clin Pharmacokinet.* 1984;9:511-544.
143. Timbrell JA, Mitchell JR, Snodgrass WR, et al. Isoniazid hepatoxicity: the relationship between covalent binding and metabolism in vivo. *J Pharmacol Exp Ther.* 1980;213:364-369.
144. Nolan CM, Goldberg SV, Buskin SE. Hepatotoxicity associated with isoniazid preventive therapy: a 7-year survey from a public health tuberculosis clinic. *JAMA.* 1999;281:1014-1018.
145. Arora SK. Correlation of structure and activity in ansamycins: structure, conformation, and interactions of antibiotic rifamycin S. *J Med Chem.* 1985;28:1099-1102.
146. Blanchard JS. Molecular mechanisms of drug resistance in *Mycobacterium tuberculosis. Annu Rev Biochem.* 1996;65:215-239.
147. Levin ME, Hatfull GF. Mycobacterium smegmatis RNA polymerase: DNA supercoiling, action of rifampicin and mechanism of rifampicin resistance. *Mol Microbiol.* 1993;8:277-285.
148. Lancini G, Zanchelli W. Structure–activity relationship in rifamycins. In: Perlman D, ed. *Structure–Activity Relationship Among the Semisynthetic Antibiotics.* New York: Academic Press; 1977.
149. Jarvis B, Lamb HM. Rifapentine. *Drugs.* 1998;56:607-616.
150. Reith K, Keung A, Toren PC, et al. Disposition and metabolism of ^{14}C-rifapentine in healthy volunteers. *Drug Metab Dispos.* 1998;26:732-738.
151. Keung AC, Eller MG, Weir SJ. Pharmacokinetics of rifapentine in patients with varying degrees of hepatic dysfunction. *J Clin Pharmacol.* 1998;38:517-524.
152. Crabol Y, Catherinot E, Veziris N, et al. Rifabutin: where do we stand in 2016? *J Antimicrob Chemother.* 2016;71:1759-1771.
153. Scorpio A, Zhang Y. Mutations in pncA, a gene encoding pyrazinamidase/nicotinamidase, cause resistance to the antituberculous drug pyrazinamide in tubercle bacillus. *Nat Med.* 1996;2:662-667.
154. Heifets LB, Flory MA, Lindholm-Levy PJ. Does pyrazinoic acid as an active moiety of pyrazinamide have specific activity against *Mycobacterium tuberculosis? Antimicrob Agents Chemother.* 1989;33:1252-1254.
155. Zhang Y, Wade MM, Scorpio A, et al. Mode of action of pyrazinamide: disruption of Mycobacterium tuberculosis membrane transport and energetics by pyrazinoic acid. *J Antimicrob Chemother.* 2003;52:790-795.
156. Kushner S, Dalalian H, Sanjurjo JL, et al. Experimental chemotherapy of tuberculosis. II. The synthesis of pyrazinamides and related Compounds1. *J Am Chem Soc.* 1952;74:3617-3621.
157. Bergmann KE, Cynamon MH, Welch JT. Quantitative structure-activity relationships for the in vitro antimycobacterial activity of pyrazinoic acid esters. *J Med Chem.* 1996;39:3394-3400.
158. Peloquin CA, Bulpitt AE, Jaresko GS, et al. Pharmacokinetics of pyrazinamide under fasting conditions, with food, and with antacids. *Pharmacotherapy.* 1998;18:1205-1211.
159. Daffe M, Brennan PJ, McNeil M. Predominant structural features of the cell wall arabinogalactan of *Mycobacterium tuberculosis* as revealed through characterization of oligoglycosyl alditol fragments by gas chromatography/mass spectrometry and by 1H and 13C NMR analyses. *J Biol Chem.* 1990;265:6734-6743.
160. Wolucka BA, McNeil MR, de Hoffmann E, et al. Recognition of the lipid intermediate for arabinogalactan/arabinomannan biosynthesis and its relation to the mode of action of ethambutol on mycobacteria. *J Biol Chem.* 1994;269:23328-23335.
161. Takayama K, Kilburn JO. Inhibition of synthesis of arabinogalactan by ethambutol in *Mycobacterium smegmatis. Antimicrob Agents Chemother.* 1989;33:1493-1499.
162. Mikusová K, Slayden RA, Besra GS, et al. Biogenesis of the mycobacterial cell wall and the site of action of ethambutol. *Antimicrob Agents Chemother.* 1995;39:2484-2489.
163. Lee RE, Mikusova K, Brennan PJ, et al. Synthesis of the Arabinose Donor .beta.-D-arabinofuranosyl-1-monophosphoryldecaprenol, development of a basic arabinosyl-transferase assay, and identification of ethambutol as an arabinosyl transferase inhibitor. *J Am Chem Soc.* 1995;117:11829-11832.
164. Khoo KH, Douglas E, Azadi P, et al. Truncated structural variants of lipoarabinomannan in ethambutol drug-resistant strains of *Mycobacterium smegmatis.* Inhibition of arabinan biosynthesis by ethambutol. *J Biol Chem.* 1996;271:28682-28690.
165. Belanger AE, Besra GS, Ford ME, et al. The embAB genes of *Mycobacterium avium* encode an arabinosyl transferase involved in cell wall arabinan biosynthesis that is the target for the antimycobacterial drug ethambutol. *Proc Nat Acad Sci USA.* 1996;93:11919-11924.
166. Kuehl FA, Peck RL, Hoffhine CE, et al. Streptomyces antibiotics. XVIII. Structure of streptomycin. *J Am Chem Soc.* 1948;70:2325-2330.
167. Finken M, Kirschner P, Meier A, et al. Molecular basis of streptomycin resistance in Mycobacterium tuberculosis: alterations of the ribosomal protein S12 gene and point mutations within a functional 16S ribosomal RNA pseudoknot. *Mol Microbiol.* 1993;9:1239-1246.
168. Banerjee A, Dubnau E, Quemard A, et al. inhA, a gene encoding a target for isoniazid and ethionamide in *Mycobacterium tuberculosis. Science (New York, NY).* 1994;263:227-230.
169. Auclair B, Nix DE, Adam RD, et al. Pharmacokinetics of ethionamide administered under fasting conditions or with orange juice, food, or antacids. *Antimicrob Agents Chemother.* 2001;45:810-814.
170. Caceres NE, Harris NB, Wellehan JF, et al. Overexpression of the D-alanine racemase gene confers resistance to D-cycloserine in *Mycobacterium smegmatis. J Bacteriol.* 1997;179:5046-5055.
171. Wong EB, Cohen KA, Bishai WR. Rising to the challenge: new therapies for tuberculosis. *Trends Microbiol.* 2013;21:493-501.
172. Hoffmann H, Kohl TA, Hofmann-Thiel S, et al. Delamanid and bedaquiline resistance in *Mycobacterium tuberculosis* ancestral Beijing genotype causing extensively drug- resistant tuberculosis in a Tibetan refugee. *Am J Respir Crit Care Med.* 2016;193:337-340.

173. Bonnet M, Bastard M, du Cros P, et al. Identification of patients who could benefit from bedaquiline or delamanid: a multisite MDR-TB cohort study. *Int J Tuberc Lung Dis*. 2016;20:177-186.
174. Andries K, Verhasselt P, Guillemont J, et al. A diarylquinoline drug active on the ATP synthase of *Mycobacterium tuberculosis*. *Science (New York, NY)*. 2005;307:223-227.
175. Koul A, Dendouga N, Vergauwen K, et al. Diarylquinolines target subunit c of mycobacterial ATP synthase. *Nat Chem Biol*. 2007;3:323-324.
176. Cole ST, Alzari PM. Microbiology. TB–a new target, a new drug. *Science (New York, NY)*. 2005;307:214-215.
177. Segala E, Sougakoff W, Nevejans-Chauffour A, et al. New mutations in the mycobacterial ATP synthase: new insights into the binding of the diarylquinoline TMC207 to the ATP synthase C-ring structure. *Antimicrob Agents Chemother*. 2012;56:2326-2334.
178. Gale EF, Cundliffe E, Reynolds PE, et al. *The Molecular Basis of Antibiotic Action*. 2nd ed. London: Wiley & Sons; 1981.
179. Jacobs MR. Activity of quinolones against mycobacteria. *Drugs*. 1999;58(suppl 2):19-22.
180. Renau TE, Sanchez JP, Gage JW, et al. Structure-activity relationships of the quinolone antibacterials against mycobacteria: effect of structural changes at N-1 and C-7. *J Med Chem*. 1996;39:729-735.
181. Miyazaki E, Miyazaki M, Chen JM, et al. Moxifloxacin (BAY12-8039), a new 8-methoxyquinolone, is active in a mouse model of tuberculosis. *Antimicrob Agents Chemother*. 1999;43:85-89.
182. Zhao BY, Pine R, Domagala J, et al. Fluoroquinolone action against clinical isolates of Mycobacterium tuberculosis: effects of a C-8 methoxyl group on survival in liquid media and in human macrophages. *Antimicrob Agents Chemother*. 1999;43:661-666.
183. Blumberg HM, Burman WJ, Chaisson RE, et al. American Thoracic Society/Centers for Disease Control and Prevention/Infectious Diseases Society of America: treatment of tuberculosis. *Am J Respir Crit Care Med*. 2003;167:603-662.
184. Taylor HG. The tuberculosis epidemic and the pharmacist's role. *Am Pharm*. 1992;Ns32:41-44.
185. Nuermberger EL, Spigelman MK, Yew WW. Current development and future prospects in chemotherapy of tuberculosis. *Respirology*. 2010;15:764-778.
186. Caminero JA, Sotgiu G, Zumla A, et al. Best drug treatment for multidrug-resistant and extensively drug-resistant tuberculosis. *Lancet Infect Dis*. 2010;10:621-629.
187. van Zyl JM, Basson K, Kriegler A, et al. Mechanisms by which clofazimine and dapsone inhibit the myeloperoxidase system. A possible correlation with their anti-inflammatory properties. *Biochem Pharmacol*. 1991;42:599-608.
188. Dhople AM. In vitro and in vivo activity of K-130, a dihydrofolate reductase inhibitor, against *Mycobacterium leprae*. *Arzneimittelforschung*. 1999;49:267-271.
189. Cholo MC, Mothiba MT, Fourie B, Anderson R. Mechanisms of action and therapeutic efficacies of the lipophilic antimycobacterial agents clofazimine and bedaquiline. *J Antimicrob Chemother*. 2017;72:338-353.
190. Savage JE, O'Sullivan JF, Zeis BM, et al. Investigation of the structural properties of dihydrophenazines which contribute to their pro-oxidative interactions with human phagocytes. *J Antimicrob Chemother*. 1989;23:691-700.
191. Franzblau SG, White KE, O'Sullivan JF. Structure-activity relationships of tetramethylpiperidine-substituted phenazines against *Mycobacterium leprae* in vitro. *Antimicrob Agents Chemother*. 1989;33:2004-2005.
192. Arutla S, Arra GS, Prabhakar CM, et al. Pro- and anti-oxidant effects of some antileprotic drugs in vitro and their influence on super oxide dismutase activity. *Arzneimittelforschung*. 1998;48:1024-1027.
193. Liu B, Liu K, Lu Y, et al. Systematic evaluation of structure-activity relationships of the riminophenazine class and discovery of a C2 pyridylamino series for the treatment of multidrug-resistant tuberculosis. *Molecules*. 2012;17:4545-4559.
194. O'Sullivan JF, Conalty ML, Morrison NE. Clofazimine analogues active against a clofazimine-resistant organism. *J Med Chem*. 1988;31:567-572.
195. Krishna DR, Mamidi RN, Hofmann U, et al. Characterization of clofazimine metabolites in humans by HPLC-electrospray mass spectrometry. *Arzneimittelforschung*. 1997;47:303-306.
196. Stirling D, Sherman M, Strauss S. Thalidomide. A surprising recovery. *J Am Pharm Assoc*. 1997;Ns37:306-313.
197. Lockwood DNJ, Kumar B. Treatment of leprosy. *BMJ*. 2004;328:1447.
198. Finch R, Greenwood D, Whitley R, et al. *Antibiotic and Chemotherapy*. 9th ed. Saunders; 2010.
199. Amsden GW, Peloquin CA, Berning SE. The role of advanced generation macrolides in the prophylaxis and treatment of Mycobacterium avium complex (MAC) infections. *Drugs*. 1997;54:69-80.
200. Faris MA, Raasch RH, Hopfer RL, et al. Treatment and prophylaxis of disseminated *Mycobacterium avium* complex in HIV-infected individuals. *Ann Pharmacother*. 1998;32:564-573.
201. Wright J. Current strategies for the prevention and treatment of disseminated *Mycobacterium avium* complex infection in patients with AIDS. *Pharmacotherapy*. 1998;18:738-747.
202. Ryu YJ, Koh WJ, Daley CL. Diagnosis and treatment of nontuberculous mycobacterial lung disease: clinicians' perspectives. *Tuberc Respir Dis (Seoul)*. 2016;79:74-84.

Structure Challenge Answers

1. C
2. D
3. E
4. B
5. A
6. D
7. A, B, C, D or B, C, D, E. Each of the chosen drugs have unique mechanisms of action, which helps to prevent the emergence of resistance.
8. B and C
9. A and C. Structure C (Isoniazid) inhibits InhA, an enzyme involved in the biosynthesis of mycolic acids. Structure A (Ethambutol) is inhibits cell wall biosynthesis downstream from C (isoniazid), thus, A and C inhibit two unique steps of the mycobacterial cell wall biosynthesis.
10. B, C, and D

CHAPTER **30**

Drugs Used to Treat Viral Infections

Patrick M. Woster

Drugs covered in this chapter:

INHIBITORS OF VIRAL ATTACHMENT, PENETRATION OR EARLY REPLICATION
- Amantadine
- Amphotericin B methyl
- Ester
- Interferon/PEG-IFN
- Rimantadine
- Tecovirimat

NEURAMINIDASE INHIBITORS
- Oseltamivir
- Peramivir
- Zanamivir
- Baloxavir marboxil

FUSION INHIBITORS
- Enfuvirtide
- Maraviroc

ACYCLIC NUCLEOLSIDE ANALOGUES
- Acyclovir
- Adefovir dipivoxil
- Cidofovir
- Famciclovir
- Ganciclovir
- Penciclovir
- Valacyclovir

CONVENTIONAL NUCLEOSIDE ANALOGUES
- Ribavirin

NONNUCLEOSIDE ANALOGUES
- Foscarnet
- Letermovir

ANTIRETROVIRAL AGENTS—NUCLEOSIDE REVERSE TRANSCRIPTASE INHIBITORS
- Abacavir
- Didanosine
- Emtricitabine
- Lamivudine
- Stavudine
- Tenofovir disoproxil
- Zidovudine

ANTIRETROVIRAL AGENTS—NONNUCLEOSIDE REVERSE TRANSCRIPTASE INHIBITORS
- Delavirdine
- Doravirine
- Efavirenz
- Etravirine
- Nevirapine
- Rilpivirine

HIV PROTEASE INHIBITORS
- Atazanavir
- Darunavir
- Fosamprenavir
- Indinavir
- Lopinavir
- Nelfinavir
- Ritonavir
- Saquinavir
- Tipranavir

INHIBITORS OF HCV PROTEASE NS3/NS4A
- Glecaprevir
- Grazoprevir
- Paritaprevir
- Voxilaprevir

INHIBITORS OF HCV PROTEASE NS5A AND NS5B
- Daclatasvir
- Dasabuvir
- Elbasvir
- Ledipasvir
- Ombitasvir
- Pibrentasvir
- Sofosbuvir
- Velpatasvir

DRUG COMBINATIONS FOR HCV INFECTION
- Epclusa
- Harvoni
- Mavyret
- Technivie
- Viekira Pak/Viekira XR
- Zepatier

HIV INTEGRASE INHIBITORS
- Dolutegravir
- Elvitegravir
- Raltegravir
- Bictegravir

Abbreviations

AIDS acquired immune deficiency syndrome
ARC AIDS-related complex
CMV cytomegalovirus
CNS central nervous system
D4T stavudine
ddI didanosine
EBV Epstein-Barr virus
FDA United States Food and Drug Administration
HA hemagglutinin
HAART highly active antiretroviral therapy
HAV hepatitis A virus
HBV hepatitis B virus
HCC hepatocellular carcinoma
HCMV human cytomegalovirus
HCV hepatitis C virus;
HEV hepatitis E virus
HHV-8 human herpesvirus 8
HPV human papillomavirus
HTLV human adult T-cell leukemia virus
HIV human immunodeficiency virus
HSV herpes simplex virus
MHC major histocompatibility complex
NA neuraminidase
NS nonstructural protein
NRTI nucleoside reverse transcriptase inhibitors
RT reverse transcriptase
3TC lamivudine
ZDV zidovudine

INTRODUCTION

Viruses are the smallest of the human infectious agents and range in size from about 20 nm to about 300 nm in diameter.[1,2] They contain one kind of nucleic acid, either RNA or DNA, as their entire genome, which codes for a variety of enzymes and other proteins used in replication and transmission of the organism. It can be argued that a virus does not qualify as a true life form, as it is nothing more than a nucleic acid strand with associated proteins, and it cannot move on its own power. However, when it attaches itself to a host cell, it internalizes itself and forces the host to make additional copies of the virus, demonstrating a clear reproductive plan. During replication, it utilizes host cellular biochemicals and processes and thus, in a sense, takes in "nutrients" in order to survive and multiply. In some cases, viruses respond to external conditions and escape the immune response by integrating into the host DNA, demonstrating the ability to respond to external stimuli. Although viruses are simple organisms, they are a significant causative agent for numerous human diseases and as such represent one of the major challenges in the area of drug discovery. Agents that are used clinically for a variety of viral diseases act by targeting processes that are specific to the virus, such as a unique viral enzyme or a necessary process such as transcription. However, to date, no drug has been discovered that is truly curative for viral infection. In addition, because viruses have the ability to undergo mutations, resistance to existing therapies can develop. The discovery of new antiviral agents is thus an important ongoing effort in medicinal chemistry.

CLINICAL SIGNIFICANCE

Christopher Destache, PharmD

When viral isolates infect the human host, it can result in signs and symptoms that can range from a nuisance to life-threatening shock. Hepatitis B and C infections are manageable with identification of plasma antigens. Acute respiratory viral infections (e.g., influenza, respiratory syncytial virus [RSV]) can be life-threatening for both immunocompromised and normal patients. HIV has undergone a significant medical transition from a life-threatening infection to one that is chronic and manageable thanks to a growing understanding of molecular biology and the structural elements of therapeutic entities that are essential to targeting and eradicating this virus.

Antiviral agent mechanisms are different from most other drugs, as they involve inhibition different viral enzymes in contrast to human receptor modulation. The recommendation of an appropriate antiviral agent is based on identification of the viral isolate causing the disease. Diagnostic testing, therefore, becomes critical to isolate and identify the infecting viral pathogen. Once the virus has been identified, selection of appropriate antiviral drug therapy is based on overall efficacy, toxicity, patient adherence, and cost. Understanding the impact of drug structure on all of these parameters is critical to the therapeutic decision-making process because structure (1) dictates the molecular targets available to the drug, (2) restricts where that drug can go within the body, and (3) determines length of drug action.

Development of resistance has occurred with a number of antiviral drugs. Viruses maintain a balancing act between viral fitness and circumventing a drug's destructive mechanism. The concept of a "barrier to resistance" has been proposed. Drugs with "high barrier to resistance" will be used significantly more than drugs with a "low barrier to resistance". High barrier drugs will reduce or eliminate the probability of virus developing resistance during therapy. As a general rule, viruses will eventually find a way to evade antiviral agents. Thus, new agents with new mechanisms are always needed to counter drug resistant isolates. Finally, when a new virus (or new viral strain) infects humans, a major treatment strategy is vaccine development (e.g., Ebola). For all of the aforementioned reasons, an understanding of how drug structure impacts mechanism, pharmacologic action, and ultimate therapeutic utility is essential to rational drug discovery and development, including biotechnologically-derived therapeutic agents and vaccines.

VIRUS STRUCTURE AND CLASSIFICATION[1,2]

Numerous species of virus that infect bacteria, plants, and animals have been identified, and they exhibit a remarkable range of diversity. All viruses exist as obligate cellular parasites, and as such they do not need possess the complex biochemical machinery that is characteristic of higher organisms. However, they do have a defined macromolecular structure that is designed to protect them from the environment and facilitate their entry into cells. The basic subunit of a virus is its genome, which can be made up of either DNA or RNA. The nucleic acid portion of a virus can be single or double stranded and may be present in linear or circular form. Viral genomic DNA or RNA is often associated with basic nucleoproteins and may be surrounded by a symmetrical protein known as a capsid. The capsid is made up of repeating structural units known as protomers, which themselves are made up of nonidentical protein subunits. The combination of the nucleic acid core and the capsid is termed the nucleocapsid, and in some cases, this comprises the entire virus. In other cases, the nucleocapsid structure is surrounded by a lipid-containing membrane that is derived during viral maturation, when the virus undergoes budding through the host cell membrane. The complete virus particle, with or without an envelope, is termed the virion. Viral architecture can be grouped into three types based on the arrangement of morphologic subunits, and each virus exhibits cubic (icosahedral) symmetry or helical symmetry or has a complex structure. Icosahedral virions are symmetrical structures that contain 20 surfaces, each of which is an equilateral triangle. A sufficient number of capsid structural units must be employed in the icosahedron to make a capsid large enough to encapsulate the viral genome. Morphologic units called capsomeres are seen on the surface of icosahedral virus particles. These structures are clusters of polypeptides, but they do not necessarily correspond to the chemically defined structural units. Some viruses arrange their structural subunits into a standard helical formation. In viruses with helical symmetry, protein subunits systematically bind to the viral nucleic acid, ultimately forming a nucleocapsid helix. The filamentous nucleocapsid is then coiled inside a lipid-containing envelope. Unlike icosahedral virions, regular, periodic interaction between capsid protein and viral nucleic acid prevents the formation of "empty" helical particles. Finally, some virus particles, such as the large and complex poxviruses, do not exhibit cubic or helical symmetry, but instead form more complicated structures that can be spherical, brick-shaped, or ovoid. A subset of complex viruses are termed pleomorphic, in that they assume multiple complex morphologies. Advances in the visualization of viral capsid structure suggest that the assembly and processing of viral proteins could serve as a new target for antiviral drug development.[3]

Viral taxonomy is complex, and viruses are classified according to a number of factors, including morphology, properties of the genome (i.e., DNA vs. RNA, single strand vs. double strand, linear or circular, sense or antisense), physicochemical properties, structure of associated proteins, replication strategy, and so on. Viruses are separated into major groups called families, with names that end in the suffix –viridae, and then into genera that end in –virus. Thus poxviruses are in the family Poxviridae, and in the genus poxvirus. A comparison of the genetic and structural features of viral families with members that can infect humans appears in Table 30.1.

VIRAL REPLICATION, CELLULAR EFFECTS, AND PATHOGENESIS[2,4]

As was mentioned above, all viruses exist as obligate intracellular parasites, and as such, they rely on the cellular machinery of the host for their growth, development, and replication. In order to synthesize the proteins needed for viral replication, the organism must be capable of producing usable mRNA in sufficient quantities to compete with host mRNA for protein synthesis. During viral replication, all of the macromolecules required by the virus are synthesized in a highly organized sequence. The replication cycle (Fig. 30.1) begins when the intact virion binds to a host cell through electrostatic adsorption to a specific "receptor" site.

This process is known as the attachment phase. Attachment is most likely a fortuitous event resulting from structural complementarity between the exterior structure of the virion and a normal cell surface structure on the host cell. For example, human immunodeficiency virus binds to the CD4 receptor on cells of the immune system, rhinoviruses bind ICAM-1, and *Epstein-Barr virus* recognizes the CD21 receptor on B cells. Recent studies suggest that some mammalian cells can develop proteins that restrict the binding of viral capsid structures,[5] thus preventing entry into noninfected cells. When attachment has been achieved, the virion enters the penetration phase, the process by which it gains entry into the host cell. Penetration may occur by receptor-mediated endocytosis, fusion of the viral envelope with the cell membrane, or in some cases by direct penetration of the membrane. Following penetration of the cell, viruses must be uncoated, resulting either in the naked nucleic acid or in the nucleocapsid form, which usually contains polymerase enzymes. After they have been uncoated, viruses are no longer infectious.

Once the virus has penetrated the cell and uncoated, it enters a segment of its life cycle known as the eclipse period, the length of which varies with the type of virus. It is during this time that the virus utilizes host resources to replicate and produce necessary viral proteins. Cells that can support viral reproduction are termed permissive, and as a result, the infection is known as productive, as it results in new viral particles. When new infectious viral particles are produced, host cellular metabolism may be completely directed to the production of viral products, resulting in destruction of the cell. In other cases, host cell metabolism is not dramatically altered, and the infected cell can survive. During viral reproduction, up to 100,000 new virions can be produced, and the replication cycle can vary from a few hours to more than 3 days. Some cells types,

Table 30.1 Characteristics of Virus Families Containing Members That Infect Humans

Family	Examples	Genome	Capsid Symmetry	Size (nm^{-1})	Envelope	Diseases
Parvoviridae	Parvovirus B19	ss DNA sense or anti-sense	Icosahedral	18-26	No	Erythema infectiosum (fifth disease); poly-arthralgia arthritis; aplastic crisis, anemia
Papillomaviridae	Human papilloma (wart) virus; poly-oma virus; SV 40	ds, cir-cular DNA	Icosahedral	55	No	Warts; salivary gland infection; multifocal leukoencephalop-athy; tumors (i.e., cervical)
Adenoviridae	Multiple types (40 adenoviruses, mastadenovirus)	ds DNA	Icosahedral	70-90	No	Infections of the eye and respiratory tract; tumors
Hepadnaviridae	Hepadnavirus, hepatitis B virus	ds DNA, circular, one ss region	Icosahedral	40-48	Yes	Hepatitis B; tumors
Herpesviridae	Herpes simplex I and II; varicella zoster; herpes zoster; cytomegalovirus; Epstein-Barr virus	ds DNA	Icosahedral	150-200	Yes	Eye, skin, and genital infection; chick-enpox; shingles; mononucleosis; tumors
Poxviridae	Variola; vaccinia	ds DNA	Complex	230 × 400	Complex	Smallpox; cowpox; chickenpox; tumors
Picornaviridae	Hepatitis A virus; polio-virus; enterovirus; rhinovirus, coxsackie virus A and B	ss RNA, sense	Icosahedral	28-30	No	Respiratory diseases; gastrointestinal dis-eases; polio; aseptic meningitis
Astroviridae	Astrovirus	ss RNA, sense	Icosahedral	28-30	No	Diarrhea in infants and immune-com-promised patients
Caliciviridae	Norwalk virus	ss RNA, sense	Icosahedral	27-40	No	Epidemic gastroenteritis
Togaviridae	Rubella virus; alphavi-rus, arbovirus	ss RNA, sense	Icosahedral	50-70	Yes	Measles (rubella)
Flaviviridae	Hepatitis C virus; arbovirus; yellow fever virus; dengue virus; West Nile virus	ss RNA, sense	Complex	40-60	Yes	Hepatitis C; yellow fever; dengue fever; encephalitis; tumors
Coronaviridae	Coronavirus	ss RNA, sense	Complex	120-160	Yes	Colds; gastroenteritis in infants; SARS
Retroviridae	HIV I and II; Lentivirus; human T-cell lym-photropic viruses	ss RNA as dimer	Complex	80-100	Yes	AIDS; AIDS-related complex; breast cancer; human T-cell leukemia; nasopha-ryngeal carcinoma
Arenaviridae	Arenavirus	ss RNA, anti-sense	Complex	50-300	Yes	Lassa fever; hem-orrhagic fever; choriomeningitis

Table 30.1 Characteristics of Virus Families Containing Members That Infect Humans (Continued)

Family	Examples	Genome	Capsid Symmetry	Size (nm^{-1})	Envelope	Diseases
Orthomyxoviridae	Influenza virus A, B, C	ss RNA, anti-sense	Helical	80-120	Yes	Influenza
Bunyaviridae	Hantavirus	ss RNA, anti-sense	Helical	80-120	Yes	Hemorrhagic fever
Rhabdoviridae	Rhabdovirus; rabies virus; encephalitis virus	ss RNA, anti-sense	Helical	75 × 180	Yes	Rabies; encephalitis
Paramyxoviridae	Syncytial virus; parainfluenze virus	ss RNA, anti-sense	Helical	150-300	Yes	Mumps; measles (rubeola)
Filoviridae	Marburg virus; Ebola virus	ss RNA, anti-sense	Helical	80 × 800	Yes	Marburg viral fever; Ebola hemorrhagic fever
Reoviridae	Rheovirus; rotavirus; orbivirus	ds RNA in 10-12 pieces	Icosahedral	60-80	No	Mild respiratory and gastrointestinal infection; Colorado tick fever
Prion	Prion proteinaceous material	None	NA	NA	No	Bovine spongiform encephalopathy; Cruetzfeldt-Jakob disease

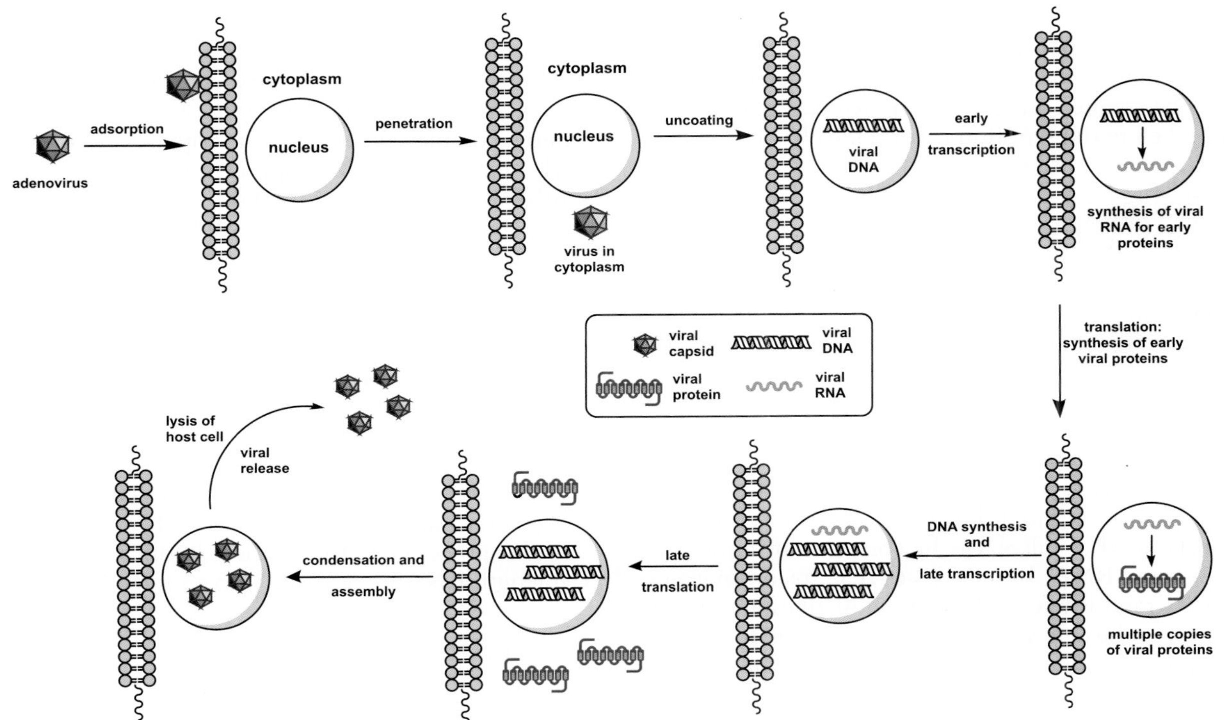

Figure 30.1 Steps involved in the viral life cycle.

called nonpermissive, are unable to support the reproduction of an infective virion, resulting in an abortive infection. Abortive infections also occur when the virus itself is defective. Either situation can lead to a latent infection, where the viral genome may persist in a surviving host cell. As will be described below, such an infection can lead to the transformation of a cell from normal to malignant.

DNA Viruses

The strategies used by various viruses to replicate vary widely, but all are characterized by the need to transcribe mRNA that is suitable for translation of viral proteins. There are several pathways leading to the required mRNA, after which the host enzymes and raw materials are used to make viral proteins. Early viral proteins used in replication are synthesized immediately after infection, while late proteins used to produce the complete virion structure are synthesized after viral nucleic acid synthesis. Most DNA viruses contain double-stranded DNA as their genome and thus can replicate using host cell machinery to produce mRNA directly. Papillomavirus, adenovirus, and herpesvirus are replicated in the host nucleus and thus use transcriptional enzymes of the host (i.e., DNA-dependent RNA polymerase) to synthesize mRNA. This mRNA is then translated to form proteins needed by the virus, including enzymes (e.g., DNA-dependent DNA polymerase) used to produce progeny DNA copies. These progeny DNA strands are infectious. By contrast, poxviruses replicate in the cytoplasm using a mechanism that is not well understood, wherein the genome is initially transcribed by a viral enzyme in the virion core. Parvoviruses contain a single-stranded DNA genome and must synthesize double-stranded DNA in the host nucleus prior to synthesis of mRNA and translation of proteins. This process may or may not require a helper virus such as herpes simplex. The hepatitis B viral genome, comprised of double-stranded DNA, contains numerous gaps that must be repaired using a DNA polymerase packaged in the virion before transcription to form mRNA.

RNA Viruses

Compared to DNA viruses, those viruses with RNA-based genomes have evolved a wide variety of reproductive strategies. The single-stranded RNA viruses may be divided into three groups that differ in the method by which the RNA genome is utilized. In all three groups, the RNA genome must serve two functions: to be translated to form protein and to be replicated to form progeny RNA strands. The first group is comprised of viruses such as picornaviruses, flaviviruses, and togaviruses that have an RNA genome that can be used directly as mRNA. Viral RNA that can be used as mRNA is by convention termed (+) or sense-strand RNA. In most cases (e.g., picornoviruses) this sense-strand RNA binds to the host ribosome shortly after entering the cell, where it is read and used to produce a single polypeptide called the polyprotein. The polyprotein is then processed by autocatalysis and various proteolytic enzymes to produce the required viral proteins. In some cases (e.g., togaviruses), only a portion of the RNA genome is available to be translated by the host ribosome. Following the initial translation of the sense strand, it serves a second function, namely to serve as a template for the synthesis of a (−) or antisense strand via an RNA-dependent RNA polymerase. This antisense strand then can be used to produce additional sense strand RNAs that are infectious and can also serve as mRNA. These progeny sense RNA strands are then packaged into an intact virion prior to transmission to another host cell.

The second group of single-stranded RNA viruses, including orthomyxoviruses, bunyaviruses, arenaviruses, paramyxoviruses, filoviruses, and rhabdoviruses, all contain an antisense RNA genome that can only be used for transcription of new RNA. All antisense RNA viruses contain an RNA transcriptase as part of their virion because the host cell does not have this type of RNA-dependent RNA polymerase. In the first round of genome expression, a series of short sense strand RNAs are made, and then translated to form the required viral enzymes for replication. Ultimately, these enzymes are used to produce a full-length sense RNA strand, which is then used to make multiple copies of the antisense viral genome. The progeny antisense DNA strands by themselves are not infectious, because they have not yet been packaged with the required RNA transcriptase. When the progeny antisense RNA has been synthesized, it is packaged into an intact virion, in which form it becomes infectious prior to transmission to another cell.

The third group of RNA viruses are the retroviruses, in which single-stranded RNA exists as a dimer of a sense- and antisense strand. The genomic RNA strands can be base-paired, although the structure of this complex is not well understood, or the strands can be hydrogen bonded to other macromolecules in the virion. Retroviral genomic RNA serves a single function, namely, to act as a template for the formation of double-stranded viral DNA. Host cells do not contain an enzyme which can form DNA from viral RNA, and thus the virion of a retrovirus must contain a reverse transcriptase (RT) enzyme, as well as various host tRNA molecules. Transcription of the genome begins when a complex of reverse transcriptase and tRNA binds to the viral genome. A complimentary DNA strand is then synthesized using one of the host tRNAs as a primer, and the original RNA strand is digested by RNAse H and viral ribonuclease packaged in the virion. A complimentary DNA strand is then synthesized, and the resulting double-stranded DNA is translocated to the nucleus, where viral enzymes incorporate genome-length viral DNA into the host genome. In some cases, the viral portion of the genome can remain dormant for long periods, or it may be immediately used to make progeny viral RNA, a process that is catalyzed by host RNA polymerase II. Transcription produces both shortened segments that are used to make polyproteins and full length progeny RNA. The polyproteins are processed to form various viral proteins, while the full length RNA is packaged into an infectious virion.

Viral Proteins

In addition to replication of the viral genome, a number of other structures associated with the complete virion can also be made. A number of viral proteins may be synthesized that have important functions in the structure, transmission and survival of the virus. These proteins can protect the genetic material in the virus from destruction by nucleases, participate in the attachment process and provide structure and symmetry to the virion. In addition, in certain cases where the virus requires an enzymatic process for which there is no host enzyme, a virion may include enzymes such as RNA polymerases or a reverse transcriptase. Some viruses require a lipid envelope that contains transmembrane proteins specifically coded for by the virus and which envelopes the genetic material during viral budding. Viral envelopes contain glycoproteins that are involved in cell recognition during attachment to the host cell. These glycoproteins often reflect the composition of glycoproteins in the host cell. They are a determinant of the antigenic nature of viruses and thus facilitate recognition by the immune system of the host. However, depending on their composition, they can also help the virus elude neutralization by the immune system.

Viral Egress From the Host Cell

Viruses use one of two strategies for exiting infected cells. Nonenveloped viruses (picornoviruses, rheoviruses, etc.) complete their maturation by assembling into their corresponding virion within the cell nucleus or the cytoplasm. For example, picornoviruses assemble by clustering 60 copies of each of three viral proteins, called VP0, VP1, and VP3, into a structure called a procapsid. Viral RNA is then packaged into the procapsid, and proteolytic cleavage of VP0 produces two new viral proteins called VP2 and VP4. The resulting conformational change produces a stable and symmetrical structure that shields the genome from degradation by host nucleases. In most cases, destruction of the host cell is required when the virion exits. Enveloped viruses (all antisense RNA viruses, togaviruses, flaviviruses, coronaviruses, hepadnaviruses, herpesviruses, and retroviruses) contain proteins that carry signal sequences and markers that cause them to be inserted into the inner and outer surface of the host cell cytoplasmic membrane. Viral proteins on the outer surface are glycosylated using host enzymes, and then displace host cell surface proteins and collect into patches. Viral nucleocapsids recognize proteins on the inner surface of the membrane, where they bind and are engulfed by the patch area of the membrane. The completed virion exits the cell by budding and release into the extracellular space. Viral egress can have a variety of effects on the host cell, ranging from destruction of the cell to minimal noncytolytic effects. Herpesviruses differ from other enveloped viruses in the manner in which they form their envelope. The nucleocapsid is formed in the nucleus, and final maturation of the virion occurs only on the inner surface of the host cell membrane, forming vesicles that are stored in between the inner and outer aspect of the cell membrane. Egress of the herpesvirus vesicle always occurs through destruction of the host cell.

Viral Pathogenesis

A complete discussion of viral pathogenesis is beyond the scope of this chapter. However, in general, it may be considered that the symptoms of a viral infection arise from the response to viral replication and cell injury in the host. These responses range from asymptomatic or subclinical to severe clinical manifestations and may be either local or systemic. Understanding the biochemical events that produce viral diseases can aid in the design of effective and specific therapies. Not surprisingly, viral pathogenesis occurs in distinct steps: (1) viral entry into the host and primary viral replication; (2) viral spread; (3) cellular injury and host immune response; (4) viral clearance or establishment of persistent infection; and (5) viral shedding. Most viruses enter the host through the respiratory or gastrointestinal tract but may also penetrate the skin, urogenital tract, or conjunctiva. In a few cases, virus particles can enter through direct injection (e.g., HIV and hepatitis) or through insect bites (arboviruses). When a local infection occurs, the virus replicates near the site of entry, and the underlying tissue is not affected. However, some viruses are able to migrate to other sites, usually through the bloodstream or lymphatic system, to produce systemic infections. When infection occurs at a remote site, most viruses demonstrate tissue or organ preference (e.g., herpesvirus localizes in nerve ganglia, and the rabies virus migrates to the central nervous system [CNS]). Localization of a virus in a particular tissue can be the result of cell receptor specificity or can arise because a virus may be activated by proteolytic enzymes in a specific cell type.

Clinical disease develops through a complex series of events when virus-infected cells are destroyed or their function is impaired, and some symptoms such as malaise and anorexia can result from host responses such as cytokine release. Disease-mediated damage may become chronic when cell types that do not regenerate (e.g., brain tissue) are involved. Ultimately, the host either succumbs to the infection, develops a chronic, latent or subclinical infection, or completely recovers. In chronic infections, the virus can be continuously detected, at low levels, and either mild or no clinical symptoms may present. By contrast, latent infections are those in which the virus persists for extended periods of time in an inactive form or a location not exposed to the immune response. Intermittent flare-ups of clinical disease can occur, during which time infectious virus can be detected. Subclinical infections are those that give no overt sign of their presence. Humoral and cell-mediated immunity, interferon and other cytokines, and other host defense factors, depending on the type of virus, are common mediators of recovery and begin to develop very soon after infection. Infiltration with mononuclear cells and lymphocytes is responsible for the inflammatory reaction in uncomplicated viral lesions. Virus-infected cells can be lysed by T lymphocytes through recognition of viral polypeptides on the cell surface, and humoral immunity protects the host against reinfection by the same virus. Neutralizing antibodies that are directed against capsid proteins can prevent viral infection by disrupting viral attachment or uncoating. Interestingly, viruses have evolved a variety of survival tactics that serve to suppress or evade the host immune response. Because viruses are obligate intracellular parasites, a method of transmission from one host to another is required for survival of the species. Thus, during an active infection, shedding of the infectious virion into the environment is a required step in the life cycle of the virus and ensures transmission of the virus to new hosts. Shedding usually occurs at the same site where the infection was initiated and can occur at various stages of the disease course.

VIRAL DISEASES[6,7]

Human Immunodeficiency Virus

The human immunodeficiency virus (HIV-1) was first identified in 1979 and was found to be the cause of acquired immune deficiency syndrome (AIDS) in 1981.[8] Since that time, AIDS had become a serious worldwide epidemic that continues to expand. The Joint United Nations Program on HIV/AIDS estimated that by the end of 2005, a total of 40.3 million people worldwide were living with HIV/AIDS, the majority having been infected by heterosexual contact. In the four decades since AIDS was first described, a total of 77.3 million people have been infected, and the disease has claimed more than 35 million lives worldwide. At the end of 2017, there were 36.9 million people living with AIDS worldwide, 1.8 million of whom were newly diagnosed cases.[9] Also during 2017, 940,000 people died from HIV-related causes, including over 110,000 children.[9] While these statistics appear to be bleak, the rate of new infections and the rate of AIDS-related deaths have both declined sharply.[10] Annual deaths around the world due to AIDS-related complications have declined from a peak of 1.9 million in 2004 to 940,000 in 2017. The incidence of the disease varies by location, with eastern and southern Africa having the highest incidence of the disease (53% of all infected individuals). In the Third World, HIV infection is often comorbid with neglected tropical diseases (trypnosomiasis, leishmania), malaria and tuberculosis, causing a higher level of mortality.[11] In 2017, 1 in 3 HIV-related deaths was due to tuberculosis. Because it is sexually transmitted, a high percentage of infected individuals are young adult workers, and as such, the disease has a significant economic impact in some regions. In addition, infected mother-to-fetus transmission occurs between 13% and 40% of the time. Although a variety of drugs have been developed for treating AIDS patients, none have proven successful in curing the disease. The basic difficulty experienced with this viral infection is the ability of virus to mutate leading to rapid drug resistance.

The HIV-1 genome consists of two identical 9.2 kb single-stranded RNA molecules within the virion, each of which contains information for only 9 genes. Following infection of the host cell, the persistent form of the HIV-1 genome is proviral double-stranded DNA. Mature HIV virions are spherical and consist of a lipid bilayer membrane surrounding a nucleocapsid that contains genomic RNA, a viral protease, reverse transcriptase, an integrase, and some other cellular factors. The HIV life cycle is depicted in Figure 30.2 and begins when the viral extracellular protein gp120 attaches to the CD4 receptor on T-lymphocytes. Following attachment, the viral envelope and host cell membrane are fused, and the nucleocapsid is released into the cytoplasm. The nucleocapsid is uncoated,

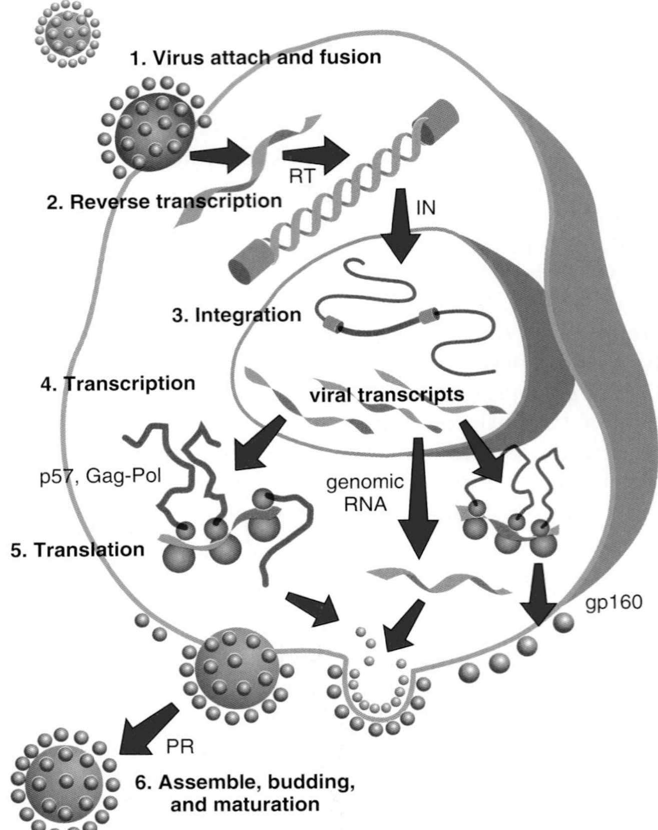

Figure 30.2 Replicative cycle of human immunodeficiency virus (HIV). (1) The virus gp120 protein binds to CD4 resulting in fusion of the viral envelope and the cellular membrane and the release of viral nucleocapsid into the cytoplasm. (2) The nucleocapsid is uncoated and viral RNA is reverse transcribed by reverse transcriptase (RT). (3) The resulting double-stranded proviral DNA migrates into the cell nucleus and is integrated into the cellular DNA by integrase (IN). (4) Proviral DNA is transcribed by the cellular RNA polymerase II. (5) The mRNAs are translated by the cellular polysomes. (6) Viral proteins and genomic RNA are transported to the cellular membrane and assemble. Immature virions are released. Polypeptide precursors are processed by the viral protease (PR) to produce mature viral particles. Used with permission from Tyler KL, Fields BN. *Fields Virology*. 2nd ed. New York: Raven Press; 1990:191-239.

and the resulting RNA serves as a substrate for reverse transcriptase, producing a proviral double-stranded DNA that migrates to the nucleus and is incorporated into host DNA by integrase. This DNA is not expressed in resting T-lymphocytes, but when the cell is activated, proviral DNA is transcribed by host RNA polymerase II. The viral RNA and proteins are transported to the cell membrane, where they assemble, form a viral bud and are released from the lymphocyte membrane. This produces an immature virion, and processing of the viral surface proteins by HIV protease then affords the mature, infectious virus. About 50% of HIV infections are asymptomatic, while the other 50% produce flu-like symptoms within 4 weeks. During this initial phase, viral titers are very high, and decline as specific antibodies are formed. The latent period is mediated by factors that are not well understood and can last several years.

During this time, viral replication continues, and the level of CD4-positive T-lymphocytes steadily declines. Eventually, the patient immune system becomes compromised, resulting in a variety of opportunistic infections. Reverse transcriptase sometimes makes mistakes reading the viral RNA sequence, leading to mutations in the virus, and changes in the structure of the surface proteins. Thus vaccines, which induce the production of antibodies that recognize and binding to very specific viral surface molecules, are unlikely to be effective in HIV therapy. As will be discussed below, other viral processes, such as reverse transcription and proteolytic processing, are viable targets for small molecule therapy.

Kaposi's sarcoma is a common complication of AIDS and has been shown to arise from a complex interaction between HIV and the human herpes virus 8 (HHV-8). This disease presents as a reddish or purple lesion on various areas of the skin and, in advanced state, may involve the lungs or gastrointestinal tract. HHV-8 does not work alone but rather in combination with a patient's altered response to cytokines and the HIV-1 transactivating protein Tat which promotes the growth of endothelial cells. HHV-8 can then encode interleukin 6 viral proteins, specific cytokines that stimulate cell growth in the skin. HHV-8 destroys the immune system further by directing a cell to remove the major histocompatibility complex (MHC-1) proteins that protect it from invasion. These proteins are then transferred to the interior of the cell and are destroyed, leaving the cell unguarded and vulnerable to pathogens that would normally be cleared by the immune system. It has recently been discovered that xCT, the 12-transmembrane light chain of the human cystine/glutamate exchange transporter system, serves as a receptor for internalization of HHV-8.[12]

Herpesvirus[2]

The herpesvirus family contains several of the most important human pathogens and is responsible for causing a spectrum of common diseases. A common and significant feature of the herpesviruses is their ability to establish lifelong persistent infections in their hosts and to undergo periodic reactivation. Herpesviruses possess a large number of genes, and some of the resulting proteins are targets for antiviral chemotherapy. The herpesviruses that commonly infect humans include herpes simplex virus (HSV) types 1 and 2, varicella-zoster virus, cytomegalovirus, Epstein-Barr virus, human herpesviruses 6 and 7, and Kaposi's sarcoma–associated herpesvirus HHV-8 (also known as KSHV). Herpesviruses are large viruses that have identical morphology, and consist of a core of linear, double-stranded DNA surrounded by a protein coat that exhibits icosahedral symmetry and has 162 capsomeres. The genome is large and encodes at least 100 different proteins, including polypeptides involved in viral structure, the viral envelope and enzymes involved in nucleic acid metabolism, DNA synthesis, and protein regulation. Oral cold sores and genital herpes infections are caused by herpes simplex viruses HSV1 and HSV2, respectively. These viruses can establish a latent infection in the ganglia of nerves that supply the site of the primary infection, and the latent disease is reactivated by a number of stress factors. It is estimated that virtually 100% of adult humans are infected with HSV1, although many infections are subclinical and asymptomatic. The varicella virus is the cause of chickenpox, and the herpes zoster virus is responsible for shingles. Human cytomegalovirus (HCMV) rarely causes disease in healthy people, but when infection occurs in adulthood it may cause an infectious mononucleosis-like illness. Primary infection with the Epstein-Barr virus is the cause of infectious mononucleosis, and this virus is thought to be a factor in the development of Burkitt's lymphoma and other malignancies. Human herpesvirus 6 (HHV-6) is thought to cause roseola and mononucleosis, while HHV-7 is probably not involved in any human diseases. The role of HHV-8 in the pathogenesis of Kaposi's sarcoma has been discussed above.

Hepatitis[2]

Viral hepatitis is a systemic disease but primarily involves the liver. Hepatitis A virus (HAV) is responsible for infectious hepatitis, hepatitis B virus (HBV) is associated with serum hepatitis, and hepatitis C virus (HCV) is a common cause of posttransfusion hepatitis. Another viral agent, hepatitis E virus (HEV) causes an enterically transmitted form of hepatitis. On occasion, disease can arise from hepatic infection with yellow fever virus, cytomegalovirus, Epstein-Barr virus, herpes simplex virus, rubella virus, and the enteroviruses. Viral hepatitis usually involves acute inflammation of the liver, fever, nausea, vomiting, and jaundice, and all forms of hepatitis produce identical histopathologic lesions in the liver during acute disease. HAV is a member of the picornavirus family and carries a single-stranded RNA genome, and only one strain of the virus exists. The onset of HAV hepatitis occurs within 24 hours, in contrast to the slower onset of clinical symptoms with HBV and HCV infection. Complete recovery occurs in most hepatitis A cases, and chronic infection never occurs. HBV is classified as a hepadnavirus with a double-stranded circular DNA genome. The outcome of HBV infection ranges from complete recovery to progression to chronic hepatitis and, rarely, death. HBV establishes chronic infections, especially in infants; 80%-95% of infants and young children infected with HBV become chronic carriers and are at high risk of developing hepatocellular carcinoma. In adults, 65%-80% of infections are asymptomatic, and 90%-95% of all patients recover completely. HCV is a positive-stranded RNA flavivirus and exists in at least six major genotypes. Most cases of posttransfusion hepatitis are caused by HCV, and these infections are usually subclinical with minor elevation of liver enzymes and a low incidence of jaundice. However, 70%-90% of HCV patients develop chronic hepatitis, and many are at risk of progressing to chronic active hepatitis and cirrhosis decades later. HEV is transmitted enterically and occurs in epidemic form in developing countries, where water supplies are sometimes contaminated with feces. The disease is more severe in adults than in children, who are usually asymptomatic.

Hepatitis C and Hepatocellular Carcinoma

It is estimated that 80 million people worldwide have a chronic infection with HCV. HCV is the cause of hepatitis C, as indicated above, and some cancers such as liver cancer (hepatocellular carcinoma, abbreviated HCC) and lymphomas in humans. HCC is the most common primary malignant tumor of the liver, and it ranks fifth in overall frequency relative to all cancers. An estimated 372,000 new cases of HCC are diagnosed each year, constituting 4.6% of all new human cancers (6.3% in men; 2.7% in women). While many factors can contribute to the development of HCC, such as liver cirrhosis, HCV infection, and alcohol abuse, the cellular event leading to the initiation of HCC appears to be inactivation of the p53 tumor suppressor protein.[13] HCC has the fourth highest mortality rate of cancers worldwide and is responsible for an estimated one million deaths annually.[14,15] The overall survival rate for HCC is poor. Surgical resection and orthotopic liver transplantation are the only curative treatment options but are suitable for few patients. The disease often has a fulminant course (i.e., occurring suddenly, with great severity), and screening of even at-risk populations has been insufficient, so in most cases HCCs are diagnosed only at an advanced stage when surgical therapy is not possible. There is no standard treatment for patients with unresectable HCC, and when untreated, patients with inoperable HCC have a median survival of three months. Furthermore, following resection and liver transplantation, there is a high recurrence rate of HCC. However, although HCC has historically had a dismal prognosis, it is now being detected earlier as a result of improved radiological imaging and surveillance. Such screening offers the best hope for early detection, eligibility for treatment, and improved survival.

The Hepatitis C Genome

HCV belongs to the *Hepacivirinae* genus within the Flaviviridae family.[16] The HCV particle measures 30-60 nm in diameter and consists of a core of single-stranded RNA encased in an icosahedral protective shell that is surrounded by a lipid envelope derived from the host cell. Two viral envelope glycoproteins, E1 and E2, are embedded in the lipid envelope. The HCV genome features a 5′-noncoding region with an internal ribosome entry site, a long open-reading frame that is translated to produce a single polyprotein of about 3,010 amino acids, and a 3′-noncoding region (Fig. 30.3). The ribosomal entry site serves as a promoter for the expression of the open reading frame, forming a polyprotein precursor that is cleaved to form structural and nonstructural proteins. This polyprotein is co- and posttranslationally cleaved into at least ten polypeptides, including three structural proteins (C, E1 and E2) at the N-terminal end and multiple nonstructural proteins (NS2 to NS5). The C protein is a nonglycosylated, basic, 19-22 kDa nucleocapsid protein also known as p22. Its amino acid sequence is highly conserved among different isolates of HCV. The other structural proteins formed by cleavage at the N-terminal end are E1 (aka gp35) and E2 (gp70), which are surface proteins in the viral envelope. The NS1 protein appears to act as a viroporin, a small protein of 100-120 amino acid residues that facilitates the release of mature viral particles from the cell. The NS proteins NS2–5 include enzymes necessary for protein processing (proteases) and viral replication (RNA polymerase). The NS2 region consists of 217 amino acid residues and is extremely hydrophobic. It appears to exist at least in part as a transmembrane protein that is necessary for viral assembly. The NS2/NS3 polyprotein contains

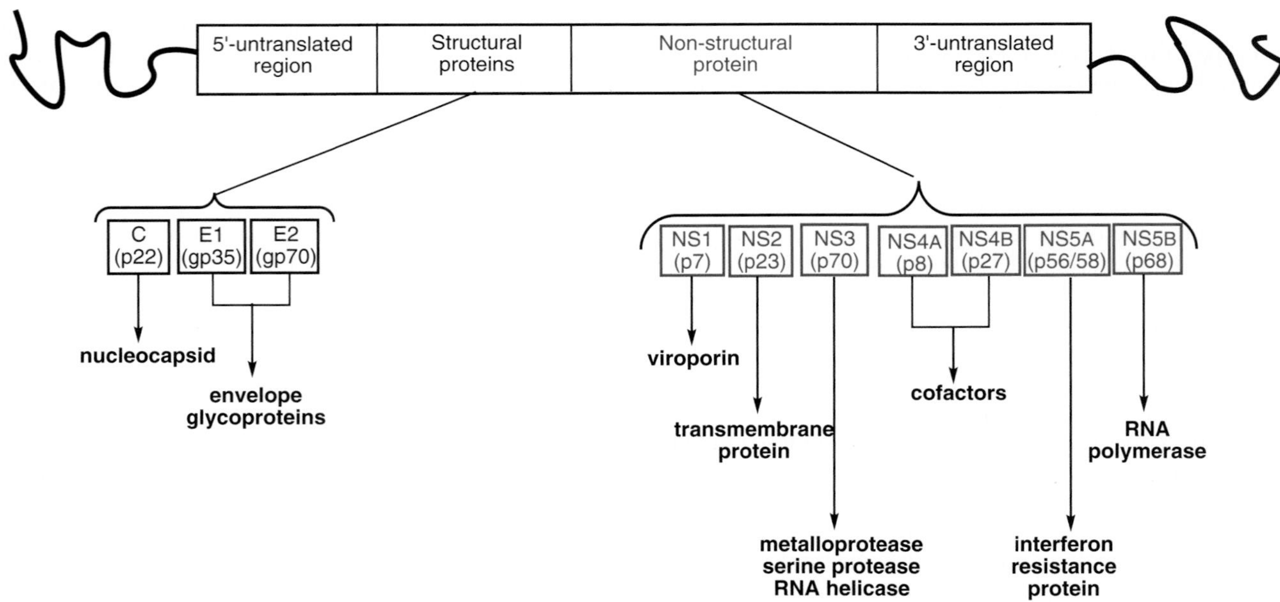

Figure 30.3 Proteins encoded by the hepatitis C virus (HCV) genome. The genome carries a long open-reading frame (ORF) encoding a polyprotein precursor of 3,010 amino acids. The HCV polyprotein is cleaved co- and posttranslationally by cellular and viral proteases into ten different products, with the structural proteins (core [C], E1 and E2) located in the N-terminal third and the nonstructural (NS2–5) replicative proteins in the remainder. Putative functions of the cleavage products are shown.

an autocatalyzing metalloprotease activity that cleaves the polypeptide at the NS2/NS3 junction. The NS3 region encodes a 70 kDa protein that contains two functional domains: a viral protease involved in cleavage of the nonstructural region of the polyprotein and a helicase enzyme that is probably involved in unwinding the RNA genome for replication. The NS4 region is also extremely hydrophobic and shows 50% sequence homology among the different HCV types, but its function is unknown. The NS5B region encodes a 116 kDa RNA polymerase that replicates the RNA genome and contains the Gly-Asp-Asp motif common to viral RNA-dependent RNA polymerases. No function has yet been attributed to NS5A. However, it has been reported to be a cytoplasmic, zinc-binding, and proline-rich hydrophilic phosphoprotein that plays a key role in HCV viral assembly, replication and secretion.

Influenza[2]

Respiratory illnesses commonly known as colds and flu account for more than half of all acute illnesses in the United States each year. Influenza viruses belong to the orthomyxoviridae family, and are a major source of morbidity and mortality caused by respiratory disease. Outbreaks of infection can occur in worldwide epidemics that have resulted in millions of deaths. Genetic mutations often cause antigenic changes in the structure of viral surface glycoproteins, making influenza viruses extremely difficult to control. Three immunologic types of influenza viruses are known and are termed influenza A, B, and C. Antigenic changes are very common in type A group of influenza viruses, which are responsible for the majority of influenza epidemics. Influenza type B undergoes more infrequent antigenic changes and is less often the cause of an influenza epidemic, while influenza type C is antigenically stable and causes only mild illness in immunocompetent individuals. The viruses carry a single-stranded, negative-sense RNA genome that has eight segments in influenza A and B. Influenza C viruses contain only seven segments of RNA and lack a neuraminidase gene (see below). The complete virion in each type contains nine different structural proteins. A nucleoprotein associates with viral RNA to form a ribonucleoprotein structure that makes up the viral nucleocapsid. Three other large proteins are bound to the viral ribonuclear protein and are responsible for RNA transcription and replication. A matrix protein is also included in the virion that forms a shell underneath the viral lipid envelope, and comprises about 40% of all viral protein.

The influenza virion structure also includes a lipid envelope derived from the host cell. This envelope contains two viral surface glycoproteins called hemagglutinin (HA) and neuraminidase (NA). Mutations cause antigenic changes in the structure of these two surface glycoproteins, and thus they are the main determinants of antigenicity and host immunity. The ability of the virus to change the structure of HA on the virus surface is primarily responsible for the continual evolution of new strains, sometimes leading to subsequent influenza epidemics. NA is an enzyme that removes sialic acid from surface glycoproteins during viral maturation and is required to produce infectious particles and lower the viscosity of the mucin layer of the respiratory tract. Influenza virus spreads through airborne droplets or contact with contaminated hands or surfaces and has an incubation period that varies from 1 to 4 days. However, transmission of the virus begins to occur 24 hours prior to the onset of symptoms. Interferon is detectable in respiratory secretions at the onset of symptoms, and the host response to interferon response contributes to recovery. Antibodies and other cell-mediated responses are seen 1-2 weeks after infection. It is well established that secondary infections from other viruses or bacteria can occur, and Reye's syndrome, an acute encephalopathy occurring in children and adolescents, is a rare complication of influenza B, influenza A, and herpesvirus varicella-zoster infections. The chances of contracting Reye's syndrome are increased when salicylates are used in children suffering from influenza and related respiratory diseases.

Tumor Viruses[2,17-21]

Viruses are etiologic factors in the development of several types of human tumors, most notably cervical cancer and liver cancer. At least 15% of all human tumors worldwide have a viral cause. Tumor viruses can be found in both the RNA and DNA virus kingdoms.[22] The list of human viruses presently known to be involved in tumor development includes four DNA viruses, Epstein-Barr virus (EBV), certain papillomaviruses, hepatitis B virus (HBV), and the Kaposi's sarcoma herpesvirus (HHV-8), and two RNA viruses, human adult T-cell leukemia virus (HTLV-1) and the hepatitis virus (HCV). Nearly every case of cervical cancer is known to be caused by human papillomavirus (HPV), a fact that spurred the development of the HPV vaccines Gardasil and Cervarix.[23] Tumor viruses alter cellular behavior through the use of a small amount of genetic information, using two general strategies. The tumor virus either introduces a new "transforming gene" into the cell (direct-acting), or the virus alters the expression of a preexisting cellular gene or genes (indirect-acting). In both cases, normal regulation of cellular growth processes is lost. Viruses alone cannot act as carcinogens, and other events are necessary to disable regulatory pathways and checkpoints in order to produce transformed, malignant cells. The processes used in the transformation of host cells by human tumor viruses are very diverse.

Cellular transformation may be defined as a stable, heritable change in the growth control of cells that results in tumor formation. Transformation from a normal to a neoplastic cell generally requires the retention of viral genes in the host cell. In the majority of cases, this is accomplished by the integration of certain viral genes into the host cell genome. Retroviruses incorporate their proviral DNA, formed through the action of reverse transcriptase, into host cell DNA. By contrast, DNA tumor viruses integrate a portion of the DNA of the viral genome into the host cell chromosome.

All RNA tumor viruses are members of the retrovirus family and belong to one of two classes.[18,19,21] Class I RNA viruses are direct transforming and carry an oncogene obtained through accidental incorporation from the host cell. No class I RNA viruses are known to produce tumors in humans. Class II or chronic RNA tumor viruses are weakly transforming and do not carry host cell–derived oncogenes. The two known cancer-causing retroviruses in humans act indirectly. They often act by inserting their proviral DNA into the immediate neighborhood of a host cellular oncogene. HTLV-1 acts in this manner, thus increasing the number of preneoplastic cells and facilitating secondary cellular changes leading to transformation.

DNA tumor virus strains exist among the papilloma-, polyoma-, adeno-, herpes-, hepadna-, and poxvirus groups.[20] DNA tumor viruses encode viral oncoproteins that not only are important for viral replication but also affect cellular growth control pathways. For example, inactivation of the Rb and the p53 pathway by viral transforming proteins is a common strategy used by papillomaviruses and adenoviruses. As was mentioned above, all DNA tumor viruses kill their host cell when the infectious virion is released to infect other cells. Thus, transformation and tumorigenicity are entirely dependent on a host cell interaction with the virus that do not involve viral spread to other cells, and cells transformed by DNA tumor viruses depend on the continued expression of the virally encoded oncogene.

Recent studies have revealed that the human tumor viruses EBV, HHV-8, HPV, HBV, HCV, and HTLV-1 express proteins that are targeted to the mitochondria.[17] Because the mitochondria play a critical role in energy production, cell death, calcium homeostasis, and redox balance, these proteins have profound effects on host cell physiology. Further study of these proteins and their interactions with mitochondria will aid in the understanding of the mechanisms of viral replication and tumorigenesis and could reveal important new targets for antitumor therapy.

Prion Diseases[24-26]

Although they are not viruses, the infective proteins known as prions have sufficient similarities to viruses to warrant their discussion in this chapter. Prions are small proteins that have been shown to cause a variety of transmissible spongiform encephalopathies (TSEs), which are rare neurodegenerative disorders typified by symptoms in the CNS such as spongiform changes, neuronal loss, glial activation, and the accumulation of amyloid aggregates of an abnormally folded host protein. Human prion diseases include Kuru, Creutzfeldt-Jakob disease (variant, sporadic, familial and iatrogenic), Gerstmann-Sträussler-Scheinker syndrome, and fatal familial insomnia. The disease in cattle known as bovine spongiform encephalopathy and the related disease scrapie in sheep exhibit similar pathologic features. Following exposure, prions accumulate in lymphoid tissue such as the spleen, lymph nodes, tonsils, and in Peyer's patches (specialized lymphoid follicles located in the submucosa of the small intestine). This accumulation of the infectious agent is necessary for invasion of the CNS. In humans, the incubation period of the disease can vary between 18 months and 40 years. Prions appear to be variant, improperly folded versions of a normal cellular protein called PrP^c, a 30-35 kDa protein with two sites for N-glycosylation that is anchored in the neuronal cell membrane. PrP^c proteins contain three α-helices, a short β-pleated sheet region, and a long, unstructured portion that comprises half of the molecule. The variant, infectious form of the protein is known as PrP^{sc} and is produced autocatalytically from PrP^c. Prion diseases are always fatal, with no known cases of remission or recovery. The host shows no inflammatory response or immune response, as there is no production of interferon, and there is no effect on host B cell or T cell function. At the present time, there are no effective agents to treat prion diseases.

VIRAL CHEMOTHERAPY—GENERAL APPROACHES[27,28]

The principles involved in the design of antiviral agents are similar to those used in the design of all chemotherapeutic agents. Drugs in this category are targeted to some process in the virus that is not present in the host cell. The earliest examples of antiviral agents did not achieve this goal, and these drugs were toxic at therapeutic levels or had a limited spectrum of activity. A variety of factors make the design of effective antiviral agents difficult, including their ability to undergo antigenic changes, the latent period during which there are no symptoms, and their reliance on host enzymes and other processes. This problem is compounded by the fact that host immunity is not well understood and that symptoms of viral infection may not appear until replication is complete and the viral genome has been incorporated into infected cells. None the less, the continuing identification of new targets for antiviral agents provides new avenues for the discovery of small molecule therapies. The following section includes information on currently marketed antiviral compounds that have been designed in eight general areas:

1. Agents that disrupt virus attachment to host cell receptors, penetration, or uncoating.
2. Agents that inhibit virus-associated enzymes such as DNA polymerases and others.
3. Agents that inhibit viral transcription.
4. Agents that inhibit viral translation.
5. Agents that interfere with viral regulatory proteins.
6. Agents that interfere with glycosylation, phosphorylation, sulfation etc.
7. Agents that interfere with the assembly of viral proteins.
8. Agents that prohibit the release of viruses from cell surface membranes.

The remainder of this chapter deals primarily with small molecule antiviral agents that have been approved by the United States Food and Drug Administration (FDA) and are clinically effective in the treatment of viral infection. Immunizing biological agents such as vaccines, as well as antineoplastic agents with antiviral activity, are not covered. Some compounds used primarily in the treatment of bacterial infections, such as rifampicin, bleomycin, adriamycin, and actinomycin, also inhibit viral replication. However, these antibiotics do not affect the transcription or translation of viral mRNA, and are only effective in high concentrations. Therefore, such antibiotics are not commonly used for viral infections. There is a continuing need for new antiviral agents, primarily because viral infections are not curable after the virus invades the host cell and begins to replicate. Vaccines are effective, but they are only able to prevent an infection, and only in cases where specific virus strains are involved. For example, immunization against influenza, which is a yearly routine in many parts of the world, can only provide immunity against specific strains that are represented in that preparation. New virulent strains may arise from nonhuman sources, such as the so-called swine flu or avian flu viruses, and currently available vaccines would have no effect against these new strains. With regard to small molecule antiviral agents, the ideal drug would have broad-spectrum antiviral activity, completely inhibit viral replication, maintain efficacy against mutant viral strains, and reach the target organ without interfering with normal cellular processes or the immune system of the host.

Amantadine · HCl

Rimantadine · HCl

Amphotericin B methyl ester

Tecovirimat (Tpoxx)

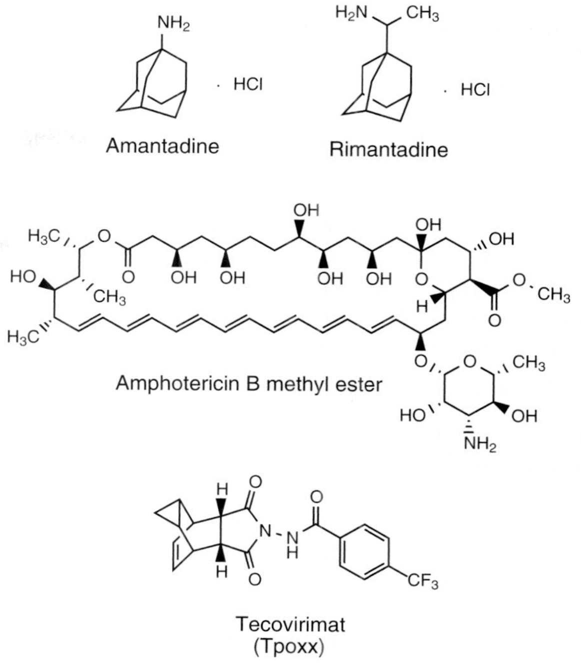

Figure 30.4 Agents that inhibit virus attachment, penetration, and early viral replication.

ANTIVIRAL AGENTS[27,28]

Agents Inhibiting Virus Attachment, Penetration, and Early Viral Replication

Amantadine and Rimantadine

Amantadine hydrochloride (1-adamantanamine hydrochloride) (Fig. 30.4) is a symmetric tricyclic primary amine that inhibits penetration of RNA virus particles into the host cell.[29] It also inhibits the early stages of viral replication by blocking the uncoating of the viral genome and the transferring of nucleic acid into the host cell. Amantadine is clinically effective in preventing and treating all A strains of influenza, particularly A2 strains of Asian influenza virus, and, to a lesser extent, German measles (rubella) or togavirus. It also shows in vitro activity against influenza B, parainfluenza (paramyxovirus), RSV, and some RNA viruses (murine, Rous, and Esh sarcoma viruses). Many prototype influenza A viruses of different human subtypes (H1N1, Fort Dix, H2N2, Asian type and H3N2, Hongkong type) are also inhibited by amantadine hydrochloride in vitro and in animal model systems. If given within the first 48 hours of onset of symptoms, amantadine hydrochloride is effective in respiratory tract illness resulting from influenza A but not influenza B virus infection, adenoviruses, and RSV.

PHARMACOKINETICS. Amantadine (Fig. 30.4) is well absorbed orally, and the usual dosage for oral administration is 100 mg twice daily. A 100 mg oral dose produces blood serum levels of 0.3 mg/mL within 1-8 hours. Maximum tissue concentration is reached in 48 hours when a 100 mg dose is given every 12 hours. In healthy adults receiving 25, 100, or 150 mg dose of the drug twice daily, steady-state trough plasma concentrations were 110, 302, or 588 mg/mL, respectively. Usually, no neurotoxicity is observed if the plasma level of amantadine is no more than 1.00 mg/mL. Amantadine crosses the blood-brain barrier and is distributed in saliva, nasal secretions, and breast milk.[30] Approximately 90% of the drug is excreted unchanged by the kidney, primarily through glomerular filtration and tubular secretion, and there are no reports of metabolic products. Acidification of urine increases the rate of amantadine excretion. The half-life of the drug is 15-20 hours in patients with normal renal function.

ADVERSE EFFECTS. Generally, the drug has low toxicity at therapeutic levels but may cause severe central nervous system (CNS) symptoms such as nervousness, confusion, headache, drowsiness, insomnia, depression, and hallucinations. GI side effects include nausea, diarrhea, constipation, and anorexia. Convulsions and coma occur with high doses and in patients with cerebral arteriosclerosis and convulsive disorders. Chronic toxicity with amantadine is unexpected, as few side effects have been experienced when the drug has been used for long-term therapy for Parkinson's disease. Some serious reactions, however, include depression, orthostatic hypotension, psychosis, urinary retention, and congestive heart failure. Amantadine hydrochloride should be used with caution in patients who have a history of epilepsy, severe arteriosclerosis, liver diseases, and eczematoid dermatitis. Because amantadine does not appear to interfere with the immunogenicity of inactivated influenza A virus vaccine, patients may continue the use of amantadine for 1 week after influenza A vaccination. A virus resistant to amantadine has been obtained in cell culture and from animals, but these reports are not confirmed in humans.

Rimantidine

Rimantadine hydrochloride (α-methyl-1-adamantanemethylamine hydrochloride) (Fig. 30.4) is a synthetic adamantane derivative, which is structurally and pharmacologically related to amantadine.[31,32] It appears to be more effective than amantadine hydrochloride against influenza A virus with fewer CNS side effects. Rimantadine hydrochloride is thought to interfere with virus uncoating by inhibiting the release of specific proteins. It may act by inhibiting RT or the synthesis of virus-specific RNA but does not inhibit virus adsorption or penetration and has activity against most strains of influenza A including H1N1, H2N2, and H3N2 but has no activity against influenza B virus. Rimantidine is approved for use in the United States but is not commonly prescribed.

Amphotericin B Methyl Ester

Amphotericin B is a well-known polyene macrolide antifungal agent that is used for serious fungal infections and also for leishmaniasis. It was first isolated from *Streptomyces nodosus*, an aerobic, Gram-positive filamentous soil bacteria, in 1955. The methyl ester form of amphotericin B (Fig. 30.4) retains antifungal activity, is water soluble, and is less toxic than the parent molecule. It was first shown in 1978 that the methyl ester of amphotericin B had dose-dependent activity against vesicular stomatitis virus, herpes simplex types 1 and 2, Sindbis virus, and vaccinia in a plate reduction assay.[33] It was postulated that amphotericin B methyl ester could bind to sterol components of the host membrane that would be incorporated into the viral envelope, thus reducing their virulence. It also potently inhibits viral replication in a panel of HIV-1 isolates due to profoundly impaired virulence and a defect in viral particle production. It is thought that amphotericin B methyl ester binds preferentially to the HIV envelope due to its high cholesterol content and prevents viral fusion. It has also been suggested that the drug produces a mutation in the G41 viral glycoperotein.[34] More recently, amphotericin B methyl ester was shown to arrest the replication of enterovirus 71 and 68 by impairing the attachment and internalization of enterovirus 71.[35]

Interferon[36,37]

Isaacs and Lindenmann discovered interferon in 1957. When they infected cells with viruses, interference with the cellular effects of viral infection was observed. Interferon was subsequently isolated and found to protect the cells from further infection. When interferon was administered to other cells or animals, it displayed biological properties such as inhibition of viral growth, cell multiplication, and immunomodulatory activities. The results led to the speculation that interferon may be a natural antiviral factor, possibly formed before antibody production, and may be involved in the normal mechanism of resistance displayed against viral infection. Some investigators relate interferon to the polypeptide hormones and suggest that interferon functions in cell-to-cell communication by transmitting specific messages. Recently, antitumor and anticancer properties of interferon have evoked worldwide interest in the possible use of this agent in therapy for viral diseases, cancer, and immunodeficiency disorders. Host cells in response to various inducers synthesize interferons.

Interferon consists of a mixture of small proteins with molecular weights ranging from 20 to 160 kDa. They are glycoproteins that exhibit species-specific antiviral activity. Human interferons are classified into three types[38]: alpha (α), beta (β), and gamma (γ). The α-type is secreted by human leukocytes (white blood cells, non-T-lymphocytes) and the β-type secreted by human fibroblasts. Lymphoid cells (T lymphocytes), which either have been exposed to a presensitized antigen or have been stimulated to divide by mitogens, secrete α-interferon. γ-interferon is also called "immune" interferon. Interferons are active in extremely low concentrations.

Interferon has been tested for use in chronic hepatitis B virus infection, herpetic keratitis, herpes genitalis, herpes zoster, varicella-zoster, chronic hepatitis, influenza, and common cold infections. Other uses of interferon are in the treatment of cancers, such as breast cancer, lung carcinoma, and multiple myeloma. Interferon has had some success when used as a prophylactic agent for HCMV infection in renal transplant recipients. The scarcity of interferon and the difficulty in purifying it have limited clinical trials. Supplies have been augmented by recombinant DNA technology, which allows cloning of the interferon gene,[39] although the high cost still hinders clinical application. The FDA has approved recombinant interferon α-2a, α-2b, and γ-interferon for the treatment of hairy cell leukemia (a rare form of cancer), AIDS-related Kaposi's sarcoma, and genital warts (condyloma acuminatum). Subcutaneous injection of recombinant interferon α-2b has been approved for the treatment of chronic hepatitis C. Some foreign countries have approved α-interferon for the treatment of cancers such as multiple myeloma (cancer of plasma cells), malignant melanoma (skin cancer), and Kaposi's sarcoma (cancer associated with AIDS). Both β- and γ-interferons and interleukin-2 may be commercial drugs of the future for the treatment of cancers and viral infections, including genital warts and the common cold.

MECHANISM OF ACTION. Although, interferons are mediators of immune response, different mechanisms for the antiviral action of interferon have been proposed. α-interferon possesses broad-spectrum antiviral activity and acts on virus-infected cells by binding to specific cell surface receptors. It inhibits the transcription and translation of mRNA into viral nucleic acid and protein. Studies in cell free systems have shown that the addition of adenosine triphosphate and double-stranded RNA to extracts of interferon-treated cells activates cellular RNA proteins and a cellular endonuclease. This activation causes the formation of translation inhibitory protein, which terminates production of viral enzyme, nucleic acid, and structural proteins.[40] Interferon may also act by blocking synthesis of a cleaving enzyme required for viral release.

PHARMACOKINETICS. The pharmacokinetics of interferon is not well understood. Maximum levels in blood after intramuscular injection were obtained in 5-8 hours. Interferon does not penetrate well into cerebrospinal fluid (CSF). Oral administration of interferon does not indicate a detectable serum level, and as such, oral administration is clinically ineffective. After intramuscular or subcutaneous injection, drug concentration in plasma is dose related. Clinical use of interferon is limited to topical administration (nasal sprays) for prophylaxis and treatment of rhinovirus infections. Adverse reactions and toxicity include influenza-like syndrome of fever, chills, headache, myalgias, nausea, vomiting, diarrhea, bone marrow suppression, mental confusion, and behavioral changes. Intranasal administration produces mucosal friability, ulceration, and dryness.

Because viruses were found to induce the release of interferon, efforts were made to induce the production or release of interferon in humans by the administration of chemical "inducers."[41] Various small molecules (substituted propanediamine) and large polymers (double-stranded polynucleotides) were used to induce interferons. Statolon, a natural double-stranded RNA produced in *Penicillium stoloniferum* culture, and a double-stranded complex of polyriboinosinic acid and polyribocytidylic acid (poly I:C) have been used as nonviral inducers for releasing preformed interferons. A modification of poly I:C stabilized with poly-L-lysine and carboxymethylcellulose (poly ICLC) has been used experimentally in humans. Clinically, it prevented coryza when used locally in the nose and conjunctival sacs. This substance was found to be a better interferon inducer than poly I:C. Another interferon inducer is ampligen, a polynucleotide derivative of poly I:C with spaced uridines. It has anti-HIV activity in vitro and is an immunomodulator. Other chemical inducers, such as pyran copolymers, tilorone, diethylaminoethyl dextran, and heparin, have also been used.

Tecovirimat

Tecovirimat (Fig. 30.4), also known as ST-246, was approved by the FDA on July 13, 2018 for the treatment of variola, the virus that causes smallpox. It is the only approved treatment for pox virus and is effective against vaccinia, monkeypox, and cowpox as well as variola.[42] Tecovirimat is highly specific for orthopoxviruses and targets the viral p37 protein, a highly conserved protein that has no homologs outside the *Orthopoxvirus* genus. The drug disrupts the cellular localization of p37 and prevents its association with cellular protein involved in membrane trafficking.[43] In this way, tecovirimat inhibits the ability of the virus to form a viral envelope.

PHARMACOKINETICS. Following oral administration, tecovirimat is absorbed rapidly, achieves C_{max} within 6 hours, and has an elimination half-life of 20 hours.[44] Tecovirimat is metabolized by hydrolysis of the amide bond and is conjugated as the glucuronide. Approximately 95% of the dose is recovered in urine and feces (~73/23% respectively), indicating that the urinary pathway is the major route of excretion. The urinary excretion of parent compound is minimal, accounting for less than 0.02%. The majority of excreted drug in urine is in a glucuronidated form.

Neuraminidase Inhibitors[45]

Role of NA in Viral Infections

The role played by the surface glycoproteins hemagglutinin (HA), an enzyme important for viral binding to host cell receptors via a terminal sialic acid residue, and NA, an enzyme involved in various aspects of activation of influenza viruses, was discussed above. Freshly shed virus particles are coated with sialic acid residues. NA is found in both influenza A and B viruses and is thought to be involved in catalytically cleaving glycosidic bonds between terminal sialic acid residues and adjacent sugars on HA. The cleavage of sialic acid bonds facilitates the spread of viruses by enhancing adsorption to cell surface receptors and thus increases the infective level of the virus. In the absence of sialic acid cleavage from HA, viral aggregation or inappropriate binding to hemagglutinin will occur, interfering with the spread of the infection. NA also appears to play a role in preventing viral inactivation by respiratory mucus.

As NA plays such an important role in the activation of newly formed viruses, it is not surprising that the development of NA inhibitors has become an important potential means of inhibiting the spread of viral infections. X-ray crystallography of NA has shown that while the amino acid sequence of NA from various viruses is considerably different, the sialic acid binding site is quite similar for type A and B influenza viruses. In addition, it is believed that the hydrolysis of sialic acid proceeds through an oxonium cation–stabilized carbonium ion as shown in Figure 30.5. Mimicking the transition state with novel carbocyclic derivatives of sialic acid has led to the development of transition-state–based inhibitors.[46] The first of these compounds, 2-deoxy-2,3-dehydro-N-acetylneuraminic acid (DANA, Fig. 30.6), was found to be an active neuraminidase inhibitor but lacked specificity for viral neuraminidase. Upon determination of the crystal structure of neuraminidase, more sophisticated measurements of the binding site for sialic acid lead to the development of zanamivir and later oseltamivir, peramivir, and baloxavir (Fig. 30.6).

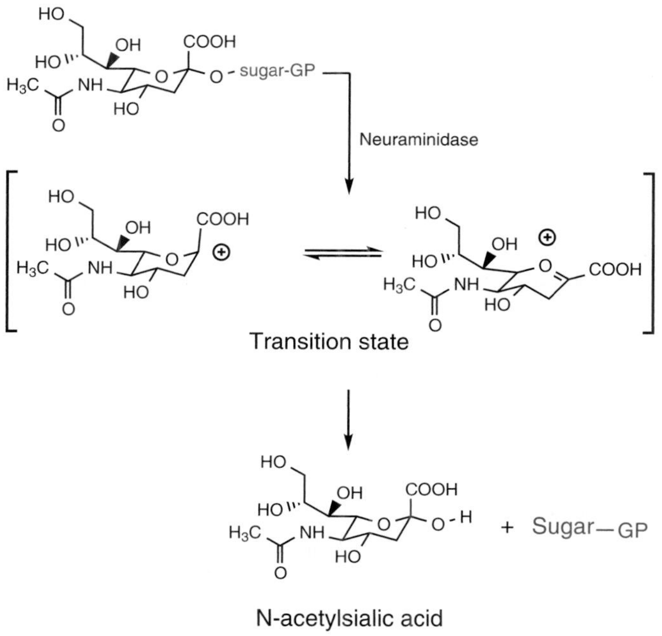

Figure 30.5 Neuraminidase-catalyzed removal of a sialic acid residue from a glycoprotein chain. *NA*, neuraminidase; *GP*, glycoprotein.

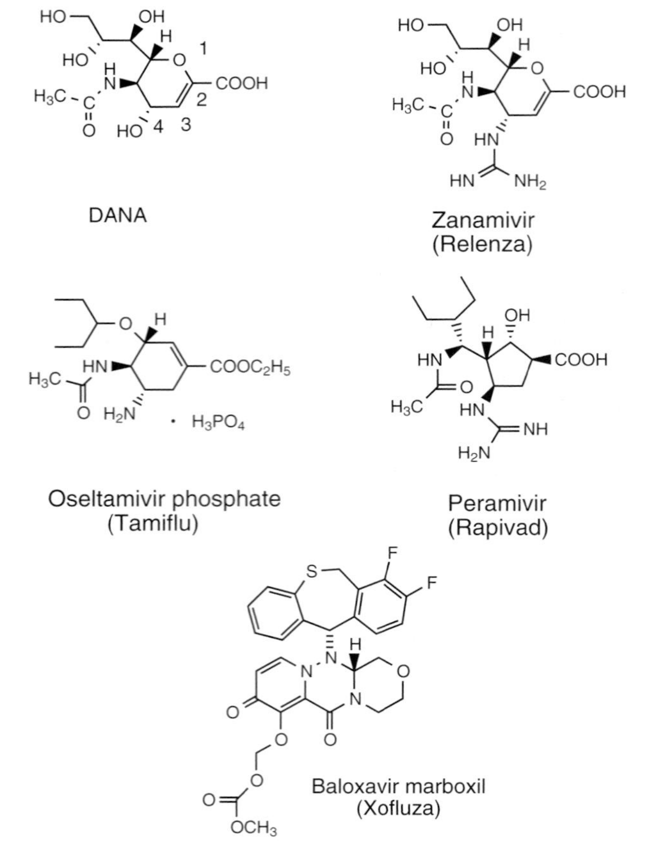

Figure 30.6 Sialic acid derivatives DANA (2-deoxy-2,3-dehydro-N-acetylneuraminic acid), zanamivir, oseltamivir phosphate, peramivir, and baloxavir that act as inhibitors of neuraminidase.

Zanamivir

MECHANISM OF ACTION. Crystallographic studies of DANA (Fig. 30.6) bound to NA defined the receptor site to which the sialic acid portion of the virus binds. These studies suggested that substitution of the 4-hydroxy with an amino group or the larger guanidino group should increase binding of the inhibitor to NA. The 4-amino derivative was found to bind to a glutamic acid (Glu 119) in the receptor through a salt bridge while the 4-guanidino derivative (zanamivir) was able to form both a salt bridge to Glu 119 and a charge-charge interaction with a glutamic acid at position 227. The result of these substitutions was a dramatic increase in binding capacity of the 4-amino and 4-guanidino derivatives to NA leading to effective competitive inhibition of the enzyme. The result has been the development of the 4-guanidino analogue zanamivir (Fig. 30.6), which has become an effective agent against influenza A and B virus.

PHARMACOKINETICS. Zanamivir (Fig. 30.6) is effective when administered via the nasal, intraperitoneal, and intravenous routes but is inactive when given orally (Table 30.2). Animal studies have shown 68% recovery of the drug in the urine following intraperitoneal administration, 43% urinary recovery following nasal administration, and only 3% urinary recovery following oral administration. Human data gave similar results to those obtained in animal models. Human efficacy studies with nasal drops or sprays demonstrated that the drug was effective when administered before exposure and after exposure to influenza A or B virus. When given before viral inoculation,

Table 30.2 Antiviral Agents Interfering With Cellular Penetration and Early Replication

Generic Name	Spectrum of Activity	Dosage Form (mg/unit)
Amantadine	Influenza A	Cap (100), Syrup (50 mg/5 mL)
Rimantadine	Influenza A	Cap (100)
Interferon α-2a	Chronic hepatitis, HCMV, HSV, papillomavirus, rhinovirus, and others	Injectable (3, 5, 10, 18, 25, and 50 million units/mL)
Interferon α-2b	Chronic hepatitis B and C, many other viruses	Injectable (3, 5, 10, 18, 25, and 50 million units/mL)
γ-interferon	Chronic hepatitis B and C, many other viruses	Injectable (100 mcg/0.5 mL)
Amphotericin B methyl ester	Vesicular stomatitis virus, herpes simplex types 1 and 2, Sindbis virus, vaccinia, HIV	Injectable (5/kg over 3 hr)
Baloxavir	Influenza A and B	Tab (40 mg—patient wt. 40-79 kg; 80 mg—patient wt. >80 kg)
Enfuvirtide	HIV	SQ injectable (Adult: 90/BID) Child SQ (Age 6-16 yr: 2/kg BID)
Maraviroc	HIV	Tab (300/BID)
Oseltamivir	Influenza A and B	Cap (75)
Peramivir	H1N1	IV (600 single dose) (200/20 mL sterile injection)
Tecovirimat	Variola virus (smallpox)	Cap (600) BID for 14 d
Zanamivir	Influenza A and B	Inhaled powder (5/inhalation)

HCMV, human cytomegalovirus; *HIV*, human immunodeficiency virus; *HSV*, herpes simplex virus; *IV*, intravenous; *SQ*, subcutaneous.

the drug reduced viral shedding, infection, and symptoms. When administered beginning at either 26 or 32 hours after inoculation, there was a reduction in shedding, viral titer, and fever. Presently the drug is available as a dry powder for oral inhalation by adults and adolescents who have been symptomatic for no more than 2 days. Zanamivir is able to more rapidly resolve influenza symptoms and improve recovery (from 7 d with placebo to 4 d with treatment). Additional studies have suggested the prophylactic benefit of zanamivir when administered to family members after one member of the family developed flu-like symptoms. As a result, the manufacturer has submitted an application for the use of the drug for the prevention of influenza A and B.

Oseltamivir Phosphate

X-ray crystallographic studies further demonstrated that additional binding sites exist between NA and substrate involving the C-5 acetamido carbonyl and an arginine (Arg 152), the C-2 carboxyl and arginines as 118, 292, and 371, and the potential for hydrophobic binding to substituents at C-6 (with glutamic acid, alanine, arginine, and isoleucine). Structure-activity relationship studies showed that maximum binding occurred to NA when C-6 was substituted with the 3-pentyloxy side chain such as the one found in oseltamivir. In addition, esterification with ethanol gave rise to a compound that is orally effective.

PHARMACOKINETICS. Oseltamivir phosphate (Fig. 30.6) was approved as the first orally administered NA inhibitor used against influenza A and B (Table 30.2). The drug is indicated for the treatment of uncomplicated acute illness due to influenza infection. Recently, the manufacturer has submitted a request for approval of the drug for prevention of influenza A and B for use in adults, adolescents, and children one year of age and older. The drug is effective in treating influenza if administered within 2 days after onset of symptoms. The recommended dose is 75 mg twice daily for 5 days. The prophylactic dose is 75 mg taken once daily for 7 days. Oseltamivir is readily absorbed from the GI tract following oral administration. It is a prodrug which is extensively metabolized in the liver undergoing ester hydrolysis to the active carboxylic acid (Fig. 30.7A). Two oxidative metabolites have also been isolated with the major oxidation product being the ω-carboxylic acid shown in Figure 30.7.[47] Side effects with oseltamivir are minor, consisting of nausea and vomiting that occur primarily in the first 2 days of therapy.

Peramivir

More recently, the experimental neuraminidase inhibitor peramivir (Fig. 30.6; Table 30.2) has received emergency approval for use in severe H1N1 influenza cases where other antiviral agents (including neuraminidase inhibitors) have failed.[48] The recommended dose of peramivir in adult and adolescent patients 13 years of age or older with acute uncomplicated influenza is a single 600 mg dose administered via intravenous infusion for 15-30 minutes. In patients 2-12 years of age, the recommended dose for acute uncomplicated influenza is a single 12 mg/kg dose (up to a maximum dose of 600 mg) administered via intravenous infusion for 15-30 minutes.

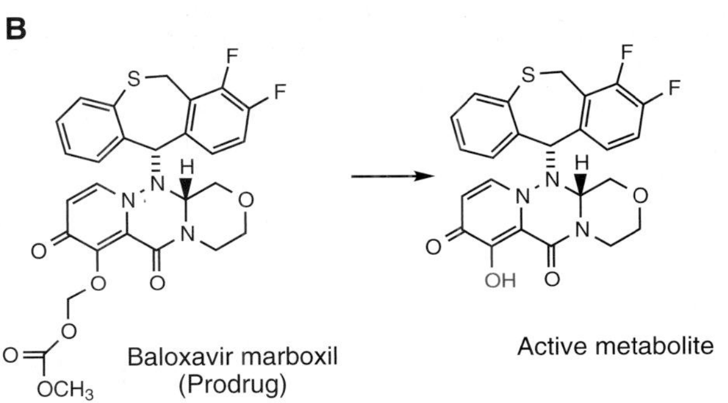

Figure 30.7 A, Metabolism of oseltamivir by deethylation and ω-oxidation. B, Metabolic activation of baloxavir marboxil.

Baloxavir Marboxil

Baloxavir marboxil (Fig. 30.6) was approved in the United States in late 2018 for the treatment of uncomplicated influenza. Like oseltamivir, it is also administered as a prodrug form that requires metabolic activation (Fig. 30.7B). The influenza RNA polymerase is a heterotrimeric protein that consists of 3 subunits termed PA, PB1, and PB2. The transcription of viral mRNA proceeds through a unique "cap snatching" mechanism. As the RNA transcripts are formed, PB2 binds to the nascent strand, after which an oligonucleotide of approximately 12 bases is cleaved from the 5′-end of the chain by cap-dependent endonuclease (CEN). The resulting oligonucleotides are then used as primers for subsequent mRNA synthesis. CEN is a metalloenzyme that requires divalent cations for activity, and it is a critical step in the influenza viral life cycle. Baloxavir marboxil enters the infected cell and is metabolically activated (Fig. 30.7B) to form a phenolic residue.[49] In this form, baloxavir is a potent metal chelator and deprives CEN of the required metal cations, thus disrupting viral replication.

PHARMACOKINETICS. Baloxavir marboxil is orally active and, when given as a single dose, is well tolerated with a favorable safety profile.[50] It is dosed according to body weight (Table 30.2). The drug has a long half-life (79 hr) and is approximately 93% protein bound in plasma. It is primarily metabolized by conjugation mediated by the UDP-glucuronosyltransferase UGT1A3 and is also a substrate for CYP3A4. Baloxavir is excreted in the feces (80.1%).

Entry (Fusion) Inhibitors

Enfuvirtide[51,52]

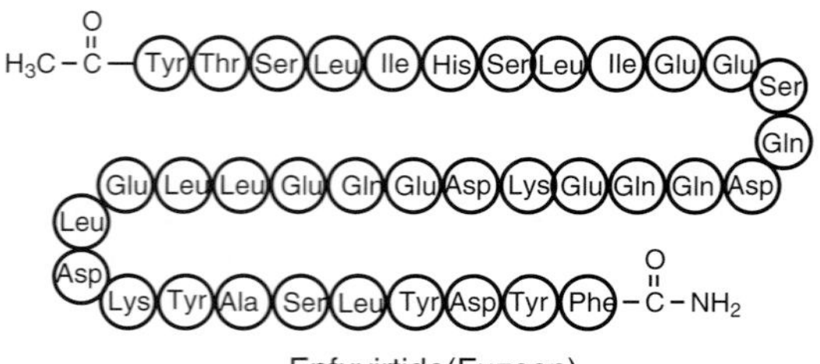

Enfuvirtide(Fuzeon)

MECHANISM OF ACTION. Entry inhibitors, also known as fusion inhibitors, are a new class of drugs for the treatment of HIV infection, and enfuvirtide is the first compound of this family to be approved for clinical use. Enfuvirtide is an oligopeptide consisting of 36 amino acids. It is a synthetic peptide that mimics an HR2 fragment of gp41, blocking the formation of a six-helix bundle structure which is critical in the fusion of the HIV-1 virion to a CD4-positive T-lymphocyte. Specifically, it binds to the tryptophan-rich region of the gp41 protein.

CLINICAL APPLICATION. Enfuvirtide is used in combination with other antiretrovirals and works against a variety of HIV-1 variants, but it is not active against HIV-2. Resistance to enfuvirtide can develop when the virus produces changes in a 10-amino acid domain between residues 36-45 in the gp41 HIV surface glycoprotein. The drug is administered twice daily as a subcutaneous injection and has a complex absorption pattern (Table 30.2). Enfuvirtide is highly bound to plasma protein (~92%) and is prone to proteolytic metabolism. Adverse reactions are common at the site of injection (pain, erythema, pruritus) and insomnia.

Maraviroc

Maraviroc (Selzentry)

Maraviroc metabolite

MECHANISM OF ACTION. The binding of HIV-1 cell surface gp41 and gp120 to CD4 cells in host T-cells is assisted in some individuals by CCR5 protein (Fig. 30.2). The CCR5 protein is a chemokine found on the host cell, which functions as a coreceptor for HIV fusion and penetration of the HIV virion. A second coreceptor associated with HIV-1 penetration into host cells is the CXCR4 chemokine protein, which may be present on some T-cells.

Maraviroc selectively binds to CCR5 inhibiting the binding of HIV-1 to the CCR5~gp120/gp41 complex. As a result of this inhibition, HIV-1 binding to the host cell prevents fusion and penetration into the host cells. Individuals with a genetic mutation in the *CCR5* gene (*CCR5*-δ32) may be unresponsive to maraviroc. Maraviroc is not effective on cells exhibiting CXCR4 coreceptors; therefore, a viral tropism assay is required, and the drug is not recommended for patients with dual/mixed or CXCR4-topic HIV-1 infections.

PHARMACOKINETICS. Maraviroc is orally administered and effectively absorbed. The drug exhibits poor bioavailability (~23%) which is possibly due to P-glycoprotein transport for which it is a substrate. Maraviroc is highly bound to plasma protein (~76%). As shown above, maraviroc is metabolized by CYP3A4, giving rise to the inactive N-dealkylated product. The potential for drug-drug interactions with other drugs metabolized by CYP3A4 should be considered (as an example care should be taken with atazanair, saquinavir, and ritonavir, which are CYP3A4 inhibitors).

CLINICAL APPLICATION. Maraviroc should be used in combination with other antiretroviral therapy regimens when treating HIV-1 patients. Combination therapy should include at least three different drugs from at least two different classes: nucleoside reverse transcriptase inhibitors, nonnucleoside reverse transcriptase inhibitors, protease inhibitors, and the entry inhibitor enfuvirtide. Allergic reactions and potential liver diseases are associated with the use of maraviroc.

Agents Interfering With Viral Nucleic Acid Replication—Acyclic Nucleoside Analogues

Acyclovir

MECHANISM OF ACTION. Acyclovir (Fig. 30.8) is a synthetic analogue of deoxyguanosine in which the carbohydrate moiety is acyclic.[53] Because of this difference in structure as compared to other antiviral compounds (idoxuridine, vidarabine, and trifluridine, see below), acyclovir possesses a unique mechanism of antiviral activity. The mode of action of acyclovir consists of three consecutive mechanisms.[54] The first of these mechanisms involves conversion of the drug to active acyclovir monophosphate within cells by viral thymidine kinase, as shown in Figure 30.9. This phosphorylation reaction occurs faster within cells infected by herpesvirus than in normal cells because acyclovir is a poor substrate for the normal cell thymidine kinase. Acyclovir is further converted to di- and triphosphates by a normal cellular enzyme called guanosine monophosphate kinase. The viral DNA polymerase

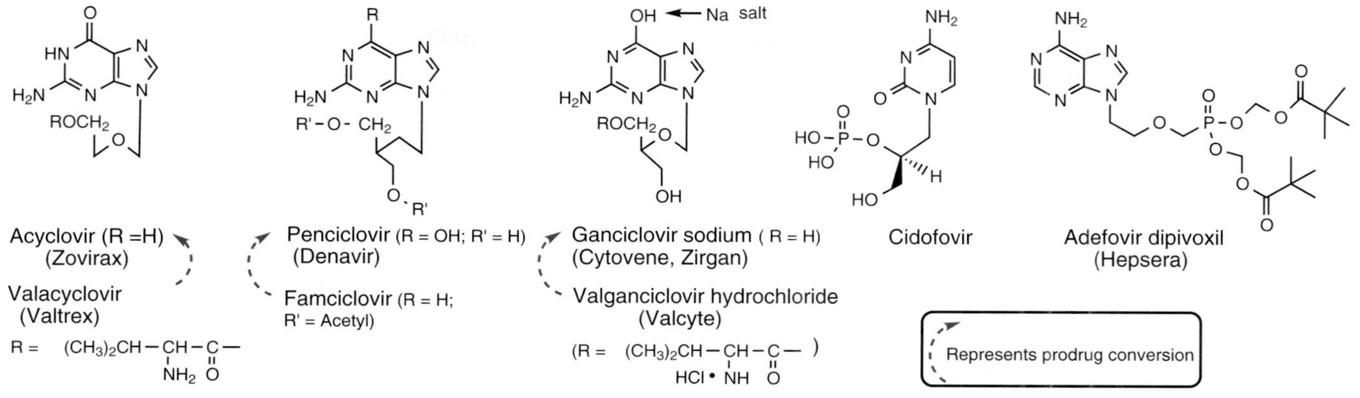

Acyclovir (R =H) (Zovirax)
Valacyclovir (Valtrex)
R = $(CH_3)_2CH-CH(NH_2)-C(=O)-$
Penciclovir (R = OH; R' = H) (Denavir)
Famciclovir (R = H; R' = Acetyl)
Ganciclovir sodium (R = H) (Cytovene, Zirgan)
Valganciclovir hydrochloride (Valcyte)
(R = $(CH_3)_2CH-CH(NH \cdot HCl)-C(=O)-$)
Cidofovir
Adefovir dipivoxil (Hepsera)
Represents prodrug conversion

Figure 30.8 Agents that interfere with viral nucleic acid replication: acyclic nucleosides.

is competitively inhibited by acyclovir triphosphate with a lower IC_{50} concentration than that for cellular DNA polymerase.

In the second mechanism, acyclovir triphosphate is incorporated into the viral DNA chain during DNA synthesis. Because acyclovir triphosphate lacks the 3′-hydroxyl group of a cyclic sugar, it terminates further elongation of the DNA chain. The third mechanism depends on preferential uptake of acyclovir by herpes-infected cells as compared to uninfected cells, resulting in a higher concentration of acyclovir triphosphate and leading to a high therapeutic index between herpes-infected cells to normal cells. Acyclovir is active against certain herpes virus infections. These viruses induce virus-specific thymidine kinase and DNA polymerase, which are inhibited by acyclovir. Thus, acyclovir significantly reduces DNA synthesis in virus-infected cells without significantly disturbing the active replication of uninfected cells.

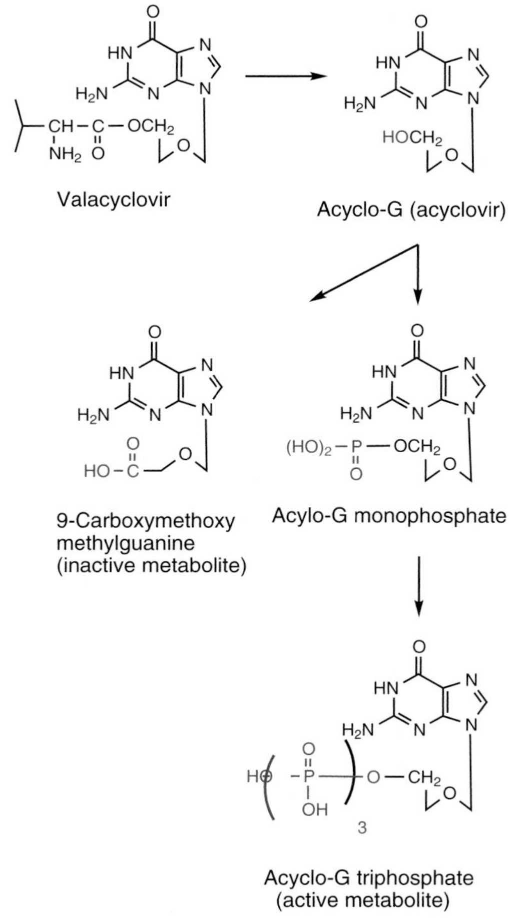

Valacyclovir
Acyclo-G (acyclovir)
9-Carboxymethoxy methylguanine (inactive metabolite)
Acylo-G monophosphate
Acyclo-G triphosphate (active metabolite)

Figure 30.9 Metabolic reactions of acyclovir and valacyclovir.

PHARMACOKINETICS. Pharmacokinetic studies show that IV dose administration of 2.5 mg/kg, acyclovir results in peak plasma concentrations of 3.4-6.8 mg/mL.[55,56] The bioavailability of acyclovir is 15%-30%, and it is metabolized to 9-carboxymethoxymethylguanine, which is inactive (Fig. 30.9). Plasma protein binding averages 15%, and approximately 70% of acyclovir is excreted unchanged in the urine by both glomerular filtration and tubular secretion. The half-life of the drug is approximately 3 hours in patients with normal renal function. In an individual with renal diseases, the half-life of the drug is prolonged. Therefore, acyclovir dosage adjustment is necessary for patients with renal impairment. Acyclovir easily penetrates the lung, brain, muscle, spleen, uterus, vaginal mucosa, intestine, liver, and kidney.

Valacyclovir Hydrochloride

Valacyclovir hydrochloride (Fig. 30.8) is an amino acid ester prodrug of acyclovir, which exhibits antiviral activity only after metabolism in the intestine or liver to acyclovir followed by conversion to the triphosphate as shown in Figure 30.9.[57] Structurally, it differs from acyclovir by the presence of the amino acid valine attached to the 5′-hydroxyl group of the nucleoside. Valacyclovir's benefit comes from an increased GI absorption resulting in higher plasma concentrations of acyclovir, which is normally poorly absorbed from the GI tract. The binding of valacyclovir to human plasma proteins ranged between 13.5% and 17.9%. The plasma elimination half-life of acyclovir is 2.5-3.3 hours. The bioavailability of valacyclovir hydrochloride is 54% compared to approximately 20% for oral acyclovir.

CLINICAL APPLICATIONS OF ACYCLOVIR AND VALACYCLOVIR. Both acyclovir and valacyclovir have potent activity against several DNA viruses including

HSV-1, the common cause of labial herpes (cold sore), and HSV-2, common cause of genital herpes.[58] Varicella zoster virus (VZV) and some isolates of Epstein-Barr virus (EBV) are affected to a lesser extent by acyclovir. On the other hand, cytomegalovirus (HCMV) is less sensitive to acyclovir, which has no activity against vaccinia virus, adenovirus, and parainfluenza infections. An ointment containing 5% acyclovir has been used in a regimen of five times a day for up to 14 days for the treatment of herpetic keratitis and primary and recurrent infections of herpes genitalis. Mild pain, transient burning, stinging, pruritus, rash, and vulvitis have been noted. The FDA has approved topical and intravenous (IV) acyclovir preparations for initial herpes genitalis and HSV-1 and HSV-2 infections in immunocompromised patients.[59] In these individuals, early use of acyclovir shortens the duration of viral shedding and lesion pain. Oral valacyclovir is used for the treatment of acute, localized herpes zoster (shingles) in immunocompetent patients and may be given without meals. It is also used for the initial and recurrent episodes of genital herpes infections. Oral doses of 200 mg of acyclovir, taken five times a day for 5-10 days, have not proven successful because of the low bioavailability of current preparations. Oral doses of 800 mg of the drug given five times daily for 7-10 days have been approved by the FDA for treatment of herpes zoster infection. This treatment shortens the duration of viral shedding in chickenpox and shingles. The IV injection of acylovir (given 10 mg/kg three times daily for 10-12 d) has been approved for the treatment of herpes simplex encephalitis.[60] Excessive and high doses of acyclovir have, however, caused viruses to develop resistance to the drug. This resistance results from reduction of virus-encoded thymidine kinase, which does not effectively activate the drug. Both drugs are effective in decreasing the duration of pain associated with posttherapeutic neuralgia and episodes of genital lesion healing. Similar adverse effects are seen with both acyclovir and valacylovir, which include nausea, headache, vomiting, constipation, and anorexia.

Cidofovir

MECHANISM OF ACTION. Cidofovir (1-[(*S*)-3-hydroxy-2-(phosphonomethoxy)propyl]cytosine) is a synthetic acyclic purine nucleotide analogue of cytosine (Fig. 30.8).[61] It is a phosphorylated nucleotide that is additionally phosphorylated by host cell enzymes to its active intracellular metabolite, cidofovir diphosphate. This reaction occurs without initial virus-dependent phosphorylation by viral nucleoside kinases. It produces antiviral effects through interfering with DNA synthesis and inhibiting viral replication. More specifically, the diphosphate competitively inhibits incorporation of deoxycytodine triphosphate into viral DNA via inhibition of DNA polymerase.

CLINICAL APPLICATIONS. Cidofovir is active against herpesviruses including, HSV-1 and HSV-2, VZV, HCMV, and EBV. It is effective against acyclovir-resistant strains of HSV and ganciclovir-resistant strains of HCMV. Cidofovir is a long-acting drug for the treatment of HCMV retinitis in AIDS patients given as IV infusion or intravitreal injection. It is not a curative drug, and its benefit over foscarnet or ganciclovir is yet to be determined. The major adverse effect is nephrotoxicity, which appears to result in renal tubular damage. Concomitant administration of cidofovir with probenecid is contraindicated because of increased risk of nephrotoxicity. Topical cidofovir (0.2%) is as effective as trifluridine (1%) in reducing HSV-1 shedding and healing time in rabbits with dendritic keratitis. Cidofovir is administered IV, topically, and by ocular implant (Table 30.3). Peak plasma concentration of 3.1-23.6 mg/mL is achieved with doses of 1.0-10.0 mg/kg, respectively. The terminal plasma half-life is 2.6 hours, and 90% drug is excreted in the urine. It has a variable bioavailability (2%-26%).

Famciclovir

Famciclovir is a synthetic purine nucleoside analogue related to guanine (Fig. 30.8).[62,63] It is the diacetyl 6-deoxy ester of penciclovir (PCV) which is structurally related to ganciclovir. Its pharmacologic and microbiologic activities are similar to acyclovir. Famciclovir is a prodrug of penciclovir (Fig. 30.8), which is formed in vivo by hydrolysis of the acetyl groups and oxidation at the 6-position by cytochrome P450 enzymes. Penciclovir and its metabolite penciclovir triphosphate possess antiviral activity resulting from inhibition of viral DNA polymerase. Famciclovir is active against recurrent HSV (genital herpes and cold sores), VZV, and EBV but less active against HCMV (Table 30.3). It is used in the treatment of recurrent localized herpes zoster and genital herpes in immunocompetent adults and is also promising for the treatment of chronic hepatitis B virus (HBV) reinfection after liver transplantation.

Famciclovir can be given with or without food. The most common adverse effects are headache and GI disturbances. Concomitant use of famciclovir with probenecid results in increased plasma concentrations of penciclovir. The recommended dose of famciclovir is 500 mg every 8 hours for 7 days. The absolute bioavailability of famciclovir is 77%, and area under plasma-concentration-time curve (AUC) is 86 mcg/mL. Famciclovir with digoxin increased plasma concentration of digoxin to 19% as compared to digoxin given alone.

Ganciclovir Sodium and Valganciclovir

The relationship of valganciclovir to ganciclovir (Fig. 30.8) is similar to that found with valacyclovir and acyclovir in which valganciclovir is a prodrug of ganciclovir which in turn is phosphorylated to the active ganciclovir triphosphate. Ganciclovir an acyclic deoxyguanosine analogue of acyclovir.[64] Ganciclovir triphosphate is an inhibitor of viral rather than cellular DNA polymerase. The phosphorylation of ganciclovir does not require a virus-specific thymidine kinase for its activity against HCMV. The mechanism of action is similar to that of acyclovir; however, ganciclovir is more toxic to human cells than is acyclovir. Ganciclovir has greater activity than acyclovir against HCMV and EBV infection in immunocompromised patients. It is also active against HSV infection and,

Table 30.3 Antiviral Agents Interfering With Viral Nucleic Acid Replication

Generic Name	Common Name	Spectrum of Activity	Dosage Form (mg/unit)
Acyclic Nucleoside Analogues (Fig. 30.8)			
Acyclovir	Acyclo-G	HSV-1; HSV-2; VZV; EBV	5% Oint, Inj (5/mL), Cap (200), Tab (400, 800), Susp (200/5 mL)
Adefovir dipivoxil		Hepatitis B	Tab (10)
Cidofovir	HPMPC	HCMV; HSV-1; HSV-2; VZV; EBV	Inj (75 mg/mL)
Famciclovir	FCV	HSV; VZV; EB; Chronic HBV	Tab (125, 250, 500)
Ganciclovir	DHPG	HCMV retinitis	Inj (50/mL), Cap (250,500) Insert (4.5/insert)
Valacyclovir		HSV-1; VZV; HCMV	Tab (500)
Valganciclovir		HCMV retinitis	Tab (450) Powder (oral use)
Conventional Nucleoside Analogues (Fig. 30.11)			
Ribavirin		RSV; Influenza A and B; HIV-1; Parainfluenza	Aerosol (20/mL)
Nonnucleoside Analogues (Fig. 30.12)			
Foscarnet	PFA	HCMV retinitis; HSV	Inj (24/mL)
Letermovir	AIC 246	HCMV	Tab (240, 480); Inj (20/mL)

EBV, Epstein-Barr virus; *HBV*, hepatitis B virus; *HCMV*, human cytomegalovirus; *HSV*, herpes simplex virus; *RSV*, respiratory syncytial virus; *VZV*, varicella zoster virus.

in some mutants, resistant to acyclovir. In AIDS patients, ganciclovir stopped progressive hemorragic retinitis and symptomatic pneumonitis related to HCMV infection.

Ganciclovir is absorbed and phosphorylated by infection-induced kinases of HSV and VZV infections. Ganciclovir is available only as an IV infusion because oral bioavailability is poor (Table 30.3). It is given in doses of 5 mg/kg twice daily for 14-21 days. The maintenance dose of ganciclovir is 900 mg taken once daily. Additionally, ganciclovir exhibits superior oral bioavailability (~60%). When ganciclovir is given by IV administration, concentrations of the drug in the CSF and the brain vary from 25% to 70% of the plasma concentration. After minimal metabolism, ganciclovir is excreted in the urine. In adults with normal renal function, the serum half-life of the drug is approximately 3 hours. Ganciclovir has been approved by the FDA for the treatment of HCMV retinitis in immunocompromised and AIDS patients.

Common side effects are leukopenia, neutropenia, and thrombocytopenia. Ganciclovir with ZDV causes severe hematologic toxicity.

Adefovir Dipivoxil[65]

Adefovir dipivoxil (Fig. 30.8) is an orally active prodrug indicated for the treatment of chronic hepatitis B. The drug is hydrolyzed by extracellular esterases to produce adefovir, which in turn is phosphorylated by adenylate kinase to adefovir diphosphate, which inhibits hepatitis B virus (HBV) DNA polymerase (Fig. 30.10). Incorporation of adefovir into viral DNA also leads to DNA chain termination.

PHARMACOKINETICS. Adefovir is poorly absorbed orally, but the bioavailability of adefovir dipivoxil reaches approximately 59%. The drug is absorbed to an equal extent with or without the presence of food, and it is excreted unchanged by the kidney. Adefovir dipivoxil

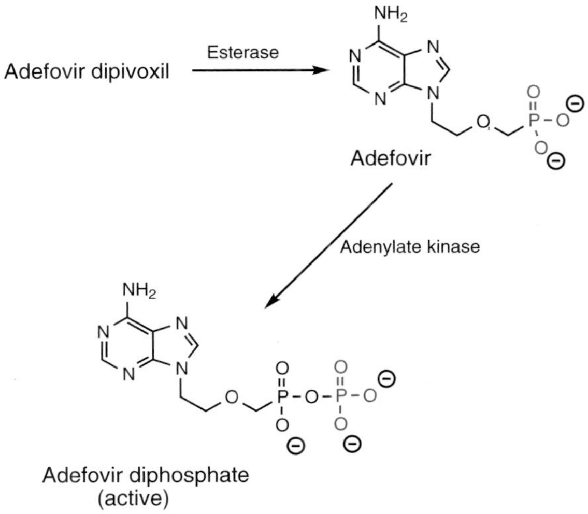

Figure 30.10 Activation of the prodrug adefovir dipivoxyl by esterase and adenylate kinase.

joins interferon and lamivudine in the treatment of chronic HBV. It can be used singly or in combination with lamivudine. Early clinical studies indicate benefit of the use of adefovir dipivoxil to treat lamivudine-resistant HBV with a low level of resistant virus developing to monotherapy with adefovir dipivoxil.

Agent Interfering With Viral Nucleic Acid Replication—Conventional Nucleoside Part I

Historically a number of important drugs appeared under this classification (idoxuridine, trifluorothymidine, vidarabine, and cytarabine), but over time these drugs have been replaced with more effective antiviral agents. Several these drugs are listed in the FDA-Approved Drug Products as discontinued or have such limited benefits that they no longer warrant extensive coverage. They are presented in the accompanying side box under the title Agents Interfering with Viral Nucleic Acid Replication—Conventional Nucleoside Part II.

Ribavirin

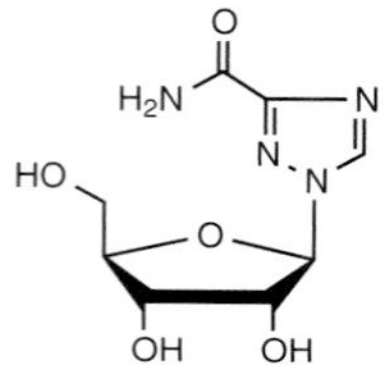

Ribavirin
(Virazole)

MECHANISM OF ACTION. Ribavirin is a guanosine analogue that has broad-spectrum antiviral activity against both DNA and RNA viruses.[66,67] It is a prodrug which requires activation through phosphorylation by adenosine kinase to the triphosphate (Fig. 30.11). The resulting derivative inhibits viral-specific RNA polymerase, disrupting messenger RNA and nucleic acid synthesis.

PHARMACOKINETICS. Oral or IV forms of ribavirin are useful in the prevention and treatment of Lassa fever. The oral bioavailability is approximately 45% and serum half-life is 9 hours. Peak plasma level after one hour is 1-3 mg/mL. IV administration of the drug has higher peak plasma levels. Aerosol preparation delivery of drug (0.8 mg/kg/hr)

Ribavirin —Adenosine kinase→ Active

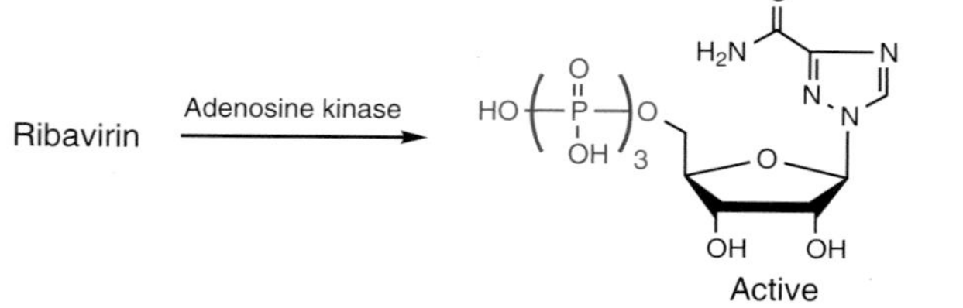

Figure 30.11 Agents that interfere with viral nucleic acid replication: conventional nucleosides.

produced drug levels in respiratory secretions of 50-200 mg/mL (Table 30.3). The clinical benefits of this agent are yet to be confirmed. Its few side effects are generally limited to GI disturbances, such as nausea, vomiting, and diarrhea. The drug is contraindicated in asthma patients because of deterioration of pulmonary function. Viral strains susceptible to ribavirin have not been found to develop drug resistance.

CLINICAL APPLICATION. Ribavirin is highly active against influenza A and B and the parainfluenza group of viruses, genital herpes, herpes zoster, measles, and acute hepatitis types A, B, and C. Aerosolized ribavirin has been approved by the FDA for the treatment of lower respiratory tract infections (bronchiolitis and pneumonia) and serious respiratory syncytial virus (RSV) infections, but it can cause cardiopulmonary and immunologic disorders in children. Ribavirin inhibits in vitro replication of HIV-1; clinically, ribavirin was shown to delay the onset of full-blown AIDS in patients with early symptoms of HIV infection. Some viruses are less susceptible, for example, poliovirus and herpesviruses excluding varicella, vaccinia, mumps, reovirus, and rotavirus. A randomized double-blind study of aerosolized ribavirin treatment of infants with RSV infections indicated significant improvement in the severity of infection with a decrease in viral shedding.[68]

Agents Interfering With Viral Nucleic Acid Replication—Nonnucleoside Analogues

AGENTS INTERFERING WITH VIRAL NUCLEIC ACID REPLICATION—CONVENTIONAL NUCLEOSIDE PART II

Early drug development often consisted of the replacement of an atom or a group of atoms within a natural metabolite with another atom or group of atoms with the intent that the newly formed substance would produce an effective drug (bioisosterism) and thus the development of nucleoside analogues of thymidine such as idoxuridine and trifluorothymidine.[61]

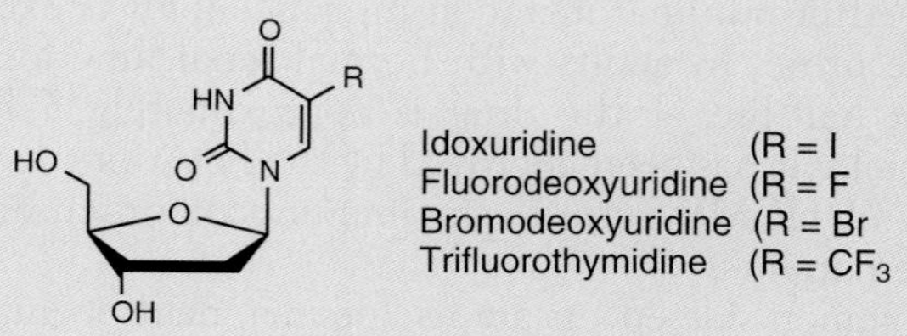

Idoxuridine (R = I
Fluorodeoxyuridine (R = F
Bromodeoxyuridine (R = Br
Trifluorothymidine (R = CF_3

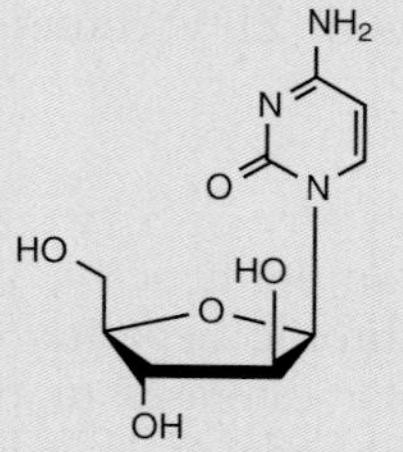

Cytarabine

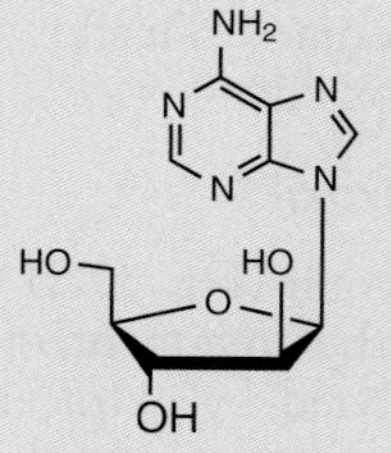

Vidarabine (ara-A)

As with ribavirin, idoxuridine is a prodrug which requires phosphorylation to the active triphosphate form (Fig. 30.11). The phosphorylated drug inhibits cellular DNA polymerase. This triphosphate is also incorporated into viral nucleic acid through a false pairing system that replaces thymidine. When transcription occurs, faulty viral proteins are formed, resulting in defective viral particles.[69] In a similar manner, trifluorothymidine is converted to its triphosphate derivative which is then incorporated into viral DNA in place of thymidine to stop the formation of late virus mRNA and subsequent synthesis of the virion proteins. Both drugs were often used for topical HSV infections. Fluorodeoxyuridine was also investigated and was shown to have in vitro antiviral activity as was bromodeoxyuridine but neither drugs were used in clinical practice.

Cytarabine and vidarabine, both prodrugs, consist of a pyrimidine and purine base attached to unnatural arabinofuranosyl sugar, respectively. As with the previous drugs both of these agents are activated via phosphorylation to the triphosphates which interfere with DNA synthesis. Cytarabine while exhibiting antiviral activity actually found considerable use in the treatment of Burkett's lymphoma. As an antiviral, cytarabine has been used topically for herpes infections. Vidarabine utility among other uses has been used to treat HSV infections.

Foscarnet Sodium

Foscarnet sodium (Fig. 30.12) is a trisodium phosphoformate hexahydrate that inhibits DNA polymerase of herpesviruses including HCMV and retroviral RT.[70] It is not phosphorylated into an active form by viral host cell enzymes. Therefore, it has the advantage of not requiring an activation step before attacking the target viral enzyme. Foscarnet sodium was approved by the FDA for the treatment of HCMV retinitis in AIDS patients. In combination with ganciclovir, the results have been promising, even in progressive disease with ganciclovir-resistant strains. Foscarnet sodium is also effective in the treatment of mucocutaneous diseases caused by acyclovir-resistant strains of HSV and VZV in AIDS patients. The drug is administered intravenously (60 mg/kg) three times a day for initial therapy and 90-120 mg/kg daily for maintenance therapy (Table 30.3). The plasma-half life is 3-6 hours.

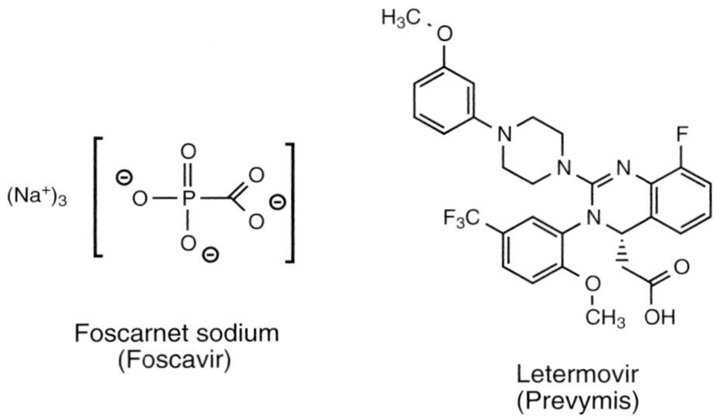

Foscarnet sodium
(Foscavir)

Letermovir
(Prevymis)

Figure 30.12 Nonnucleoside inhibitors of viral replication.

Foscarnet sodium penetrates into the CSF and the eye. The drug is neurotoxic, and common adverse effects include phlebitis, anemia, nausea, vomiting, and seizures. Foscarnet sodium carries risk of severe hypocalcemia, especially with concurrent use of IV pentamidine. Foscarnet sodium used with zidovudine (ZDV) has an additive effect against HCMV and acts synergistically against HIV.

Letermovir

Letermovir (Fig. 30.12) has been approved by the FDA for the prevention of HCMV infections in patients exposed to common virus while receiving allogeneic hematopoietic stem cell transplant (HSCT) also known as bone marrow transplant. HCMV is a leading cause of birth defects and life-threatening disease in immunocompromised patients and treatment with commonly used drugs are associated with potential toxicities including teratogenic, mutagenic, and carcinogenic actions.

Mechanism of Action. The majority of drugs available for treatment of HCMV target DNA polymerase pUL54. However, letermovir has been shown to act at a completely different site. Studies suggest that letermovir targets the viral terminase subunit pUL56.[71,72] This enzyme is involved in viral DNA cleavage and packaging. The drug may block viral DNA concatemer cleavage to monomeric genomes that are required for procapsid formation.

Pharmacokinetics. Letermovir is administered once daily and appears to be well absorbed following oral administration.[73] The drug is also available in an IV solution. It has been reported that the drug is excreted mainly unchanged via the biliary route. No known drug-drug interactions have been reported, but adverse effects including nausea, diarrhea, vomiting, swelling in the arms and legs, cough, and headache have been reported.

Antiretroviral (Anti-HIV) Agents[74,75]

While there can be no permanent cure of AIDS without prevention or elimination of HIV infection, AIDS patients can prolong their life if the disease is diagnosed early, and treatment is promptly initiated. Initial HIV treatment requires specific drugs that inhibit RT and HIV protease. In advanced HIV infection, AIDS is complicated by other organisms that proliferate in immunocompromised hosts, known as opportunistic infections. Such patients are treated symptomatically with a variety of drugs depending upon the opportunistic infections.[76-78] Anti-HIV agents have side effects, but patients can be managed by a careful monitoring of the drugs. Opportunistic diseases include infections by parasites, bacteria, fungi, and viruses. Neoplasms including Kaposi's sarcoma and Burkitt's lymphoma also commonly occur.

Anti-HIV agents are classified according to the mode of action. The drugs inhibiting RT interfere with replication of HIV and stop synthesis of infective viral particles. They are further classified into nucleoside and nonnucleoside RT inhibitors. The drugs inhibiting HIV protease inactivate RT activity and block release of viral particles from the infected cells. The chemistry, pharmacokinetics, side effects, toxicity, and drug interactions of RT inhibitors and PIs are discussed below.

Antiretroviral (Anti-HIV) Agents—Nucleoside Reverse Transcriptase Inhibitors (NRTI)[79,80]

The synthesis of viral DNA under the direction of reverse transcriptase (RT) (Table 30.4) requires availability of purines and pyrimidine nucleosides and nucleotides. Therefore, it is not surprising that a variety of chemical modifications of natural nucleosides have been investigated. Two such modifications have resulted in active drugs. Removal of the ribosyl 3′-hydroxyl group of the deoxynucleosides has given rise to dideoxy*adenosine* (didanosine is the prodrug for this derivative),[81,82] dideoxy*cytidine*,[83-85] and didehydrodideoxy*thymidine*.[86] Replacement of the 3′-deoxy with an azido group has given 3′-azido*thymidine*[87-90] and 3′-azido*uridine* (no longer used as a drug).[91] All of these drugs have similar mechanisms of action in that their incorporation into the viral DNA will ultimately lead to chain terminating blockade due to the lack of a 3′-hydroxyl needed for the DNA propagation.

Zidovudine

MECHANISM OF ACTION. Zidovudine (Fig. 30.13) is an analogue of thymidine in which the azido group is substituted at the 3-carbon atom of the dideoxyribose moiety. It is active against RNA tumor viruses (retroviruses) that are the causative agents of AIDS and T cell leukemia. Retroviruses, by virtue of RT, direct the synthesis of a provirus (DNA copy of a viral RNA genome). Proviral DNA integrates into the normal cell DNA, leading to the HIV infection.

Table 30.4 HIV Reverse Transcriptase (RT) and Integrase Inhibitors

Generic Name	Common Name	Dosage Form (mg/unit)
Nucleoside Reverse Transcriptase Inhibitors (NRTIs)		
Abacavir	ABC	Tab (300), Sol (20/mL) Trizivir (300), abacavir, 150 mg of lamivudine and 300 mg of zidovudine
Didanosine	ddI	Tab (25, 50, 100, 150, 200)
Emtricitabine		Cap (200)
Lamivudine	3TC	Epivir-HPV: Tab (150), Sol (10/mL); Tab (100), Sol (5, 10/mL)
Stavudine	D4T	Cap (15, 20, 30, 40); Powder for oral soln. (1/mL)
Tenofovir disoproxil		Tab (300)
Zidovudine	AZT, ZDV	Tab (300), Cap (100), Syrup (50/5 mL), Inj (10/mL)
Nonnucleoside Reverse Transcriptase Inhibitors (NNRTIs)		
Delavirdine		Tab (100, 200)
Doravirine		Pifeltro: Tab (100) Delstrigo: Tab doravirine (100), lamivudine (300), tenofir disproxil (300)
Efavirenz	EFV	Cap (50, 100, 200)
Etravirine		Tab (25, 100, 200)
Nevirapine		Tab (200)
Rilpivirine		Edurant: Tab (25); Odefsey: Tab emtricitabine (200), pilpirivine (25) and tenofovir alafenemide (25); Juluca: Tab rilpivirine (25) and dolutegravir (50)
Integrase Strand Transfer Inhibitors (INSTIs)		
Bictegravir		Biktarvy: Tab bictegravir (50), emtricitabine (200), tenofovir alafenamide (25)
Dolutegravir		Tivicay: Tab (5, 10 and 20) Triumeq: Tab abacavir (600), dolutegravir (50), lamivudine (300);
Elvitegravir		Genvoya: Tab elvitegravir (150), cobicistat (150), emtricitabine (200) and tenofivir alafenamide (10); Stribild: Tab elvitegravir (150), cobicistat (150), emtricitabine (200) and tenofovir disproxil (300)
Raltegravir		Tab (400, 600), Chewable (25, 100) and Powder (100)

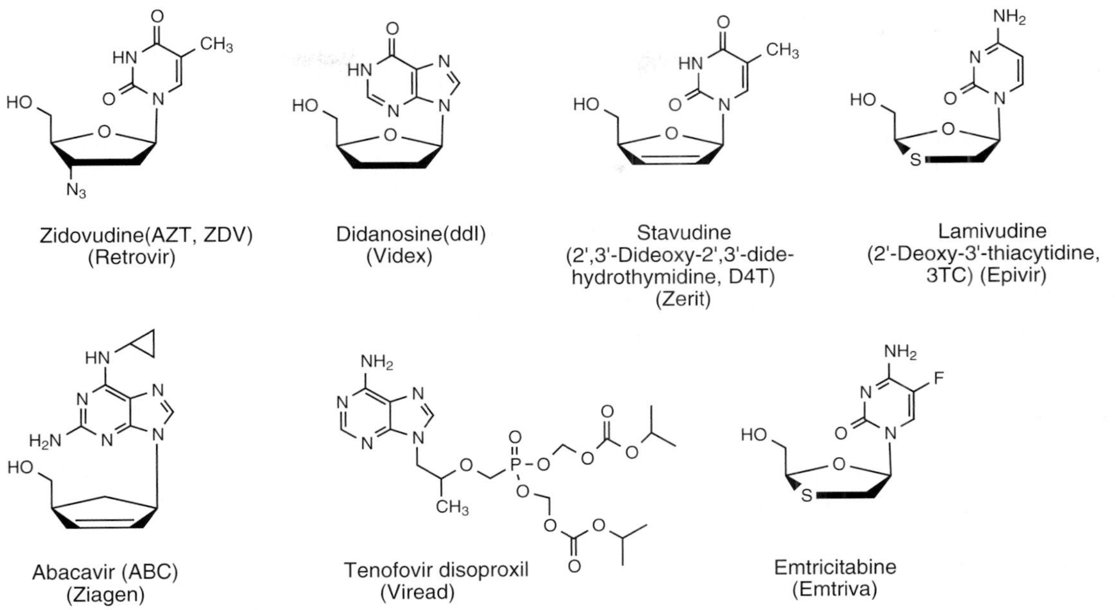

Figure 30.13 Nucleoside reverse transcriptase inhibitors (NRTIs).

ZDV is converted to 5′-mono-, di-, and triphosphates by the cellular thymidine kinase. The triphosphates are then incorporated into proviral DNA since RT uses ZDV triphosphate as a substrate. This process prevents normal 5′,3′-phosphodiester bonding, resulting in termination of DNA chain elongation owing to the presence of an azido group in ZDV. The multiplication of HIV is halted by selective inhibition of reverse transcriptase, and thus viral DNA polymerase by ZDV-triphosphate at the required dose concentration. ZDV is a potent inhibitor of HIV-1 but also inhibits HIV-2 and EBV.

PHARMACOKINETICS. ZDV is available in various dosage forms (Table 30.4). For asymptomatic adults, the initial recommended dosage is 1,200 mg daily (200 mg every 4 hr) reducing to 600 mg daily (100 mg every 4 hr) for patients with advanced disease. The maintenance dose is 600 mg daily in symptomatic patients. ZDV is sensitive to heat and light because of its azide group and should be stored in colored bottles at 15-25°C. ZDV is well absorbed through the GI tract. It concentrates in the body tissues and fluids, including CSF. The bioavailability of the drug was found to be approximately 65%. Its half-life is approximately 1 hour. IV doses of 2.5 mg/kg or oral doses of 5 mg/kg yielded peak plasma concentrations of 5 mg mol/L. Plasma protein binding was approximately 30%. Most of the drug is converted to its inactive glucuronide metabolite (GZDV) and is excreted as such in the urine. ZDV also crosses the blood-brain barrier. Pentamidine, dapsone, amphotericin B, flucytosine, and doxorubicin may increase the toxic effects of ZDV. Probenecid prolongs the plasma half-life of the drug.

CLINICAL APPLICATION. ZDV is used in AIDS and AIDS-related complex (ARC) to control opportunistic infections by raising absolute $CD4^+$ lymphocyte counts. ZDV was first synthesized by Horwitz (1964)[92]; its biologic activity was reported by Ostertag (1974); and in 1986, Yarchoan demonstrated application of ZDV in clinical trials of AIDS and related diseases.[93,94] ZDV is recommended in the control of the disease in asymptomatic patients in whom absolute $CD4^+$ lymphocyte counts are less than 200/mm^3. It prolongs the life of patients affected with *Pneumocystis jirovecii* pneumonia (PCP) and improves the condition of patients with advanced ARC by reducing the severity and frequency of opportunistic infections. Substantial benefits are obtained when the drug is given after the $CD4^+$ cell counts fall below 500/mm^3. Therefore, ZDV is used in early and advanced symptomatic treatment of AIDS or ARC patients. ZDV with other RT inhibitors or in combination with PIs are more beneficial when resistance to ZDV occurs.

HIV attacks susceptible cells and interacts mainly with $CD4^+$ cell surface proteins of helper T cells. As was discussed above, the viral glycoprotein gp120 forms a complex with CD4 receptor on host cells and enters the cells by endocytosis. This sequence of events is shown in Figure 30.2. Ultimately, the immune system of the host is altered and AIDS symptoms appear. AIDS patients have symptoms, such as high fever, weight loss, lymphadenopathy, chronic diarrhea, myalgias, fatigue, and night sweats. ZDV is given in such conditions. However, the drug is toxic to the bone marrow and causes macrocytic anemia, neutropenia, and granulocytopenia. Other adverse reactions include headache, insomnia, nausea, vomiting, seizures, myalgias, and confusion.

Didanosine

MECHANISM OF ACTION. Didanosine (Fig. 30.13) is a purine dideoxynucleoside analogue of inosine. Chemically, it is 2′, 3′-dideoxyinosine, and differs from inosine by having hydrogen atoms in place of 2′- and 3′-hydroxyl groups on the ribose ring. Didanosine is a prodrug which is bioactivated by metabolism to dideoxyadenosine triphosphate (ddATP). ddATP is a competitive inhibitor of viral reverse transcriptase and is incorporated into the developing viral DNA in place of deoxyladenosine triphosphate. As such this agent causes chain termination due to the absence of a 3′-hydroxyl group. Didanosine inhibits HIV RT and exerts a virustatic effect on the retroviruses. Combined with ZDV, antiretroviral activity of ddI is increased.

PHARMACOKINETICS. Didanosine has a plasma half-life of 1.5 hours, and it is given in 200-mg dose twice daily. Oral bioavailability of the drug is approximately 25% at doses of 7 mg/kg or less. It significantly decreased p24 antigen levels and increased $CD4^+$ cell counts. In some cases, viral resistance to ddI has been known to occur after treatment for one year. It is given in advanced HIV infection, ZDV intolerance or significant clinical/immunologic deterioration. The major side effects of ddI are painful peripheral neuropathy and pancreatitis. Some of the minor side effects include abdominal pain, nausea, and vomiting. The use of products such as pentamidine, sulfonamides, and cimetidine should be avoided with ddI.

Stavudine

Stavudine (D4T) (Fig. 30.13) is a pyrimidine nucleoside analogue that has significant activity against HIV-1 after intracellular conversion of the drug to a D4T-triphosphate. It differs in structure from thymidine by the replacement of the 3′-hydroxyl group with a hydrogen atom and a double bond in the 2′ and 3′ positions on the deoxyribose ring. It decreased p24 antigen and raised $CD4^+$ cell counts. D4T is beneficial for patients where $CD4^+$ cell counts do not decrease below 300 cells/mm^3 with ZDV and ddI. It was more effective than ZDV treated patients in delaying the progression of HIV infection. It is recommended for patients with advanced HIV infection.

PHARMACOKINETICS. Stavudine is rapidly absorbed and absolute bioavailability in adults is 85% at an oral dose of 4 mg/kg. A peak plasma concentration in dose-dependent manner occurs within an hour. It can be taken with food. The apparent volume distribution after oral dose is 66 L. The plasma half-life of D4T is approximately 1.5 hours and intracellular half-life of D4T-triphosphate is 3.5 hours. It is less toxic to bone marrow but causes peripheral neuropathic toxicity. The side effects include pain, tingling, and numbness in the hands and feet.

Lamivudine

Lamivudine, also known as 3TC (Fig. 30.13), it is formed by replacement of the 3′-methylene hydroxyide group with a sulfur (S) atom in the ribose ring.[95] It exerts virustatic effect against retroviruses by competitively inhibiting HIV RT after intracellular conversion of the drug to its active 5′-3TC-triphosphate form. It is usually given with other antiretroviral agents, such as ZDV or D4T. 3TC in 600 mg/d dose reduced HIV cells by 75%, and in combination with ZDV, the reduction in viral load was 94%.

PHARMACOKINETICS. Lamivudine is rapidly absorbed through the GI tract. Its bioavailability is approximately 86% after oral administration of 2 mg/kg twice daily, and peak serum 3TC concentration was approximately 2 mg/mL. 3TC binding to human plasma were approximately 36%. In vivo, it is converted to transsulfoxide metabolite, and a majority of the drug is eliminated unchanged in urine. The FDA approved 3TC in combination with ZDV for the treatment of disease progression caused by HIV infection (see Table 30.5 and discussion below). The combinations of 3TC with ddI or D4T also are used for advanced HIV infection. Such combinations have the ability to delay resistance to ZDV and restore ZDV sensitivity in AIDS patients. Recently, lamivudine oral therapy in lower doses (Table 30.4) has been approved by the FDA for treatment of chronic hepatitis B (trade name Epivir-HBV). Peripheral neuropathy and GI disturbances are the major side effects of 3TC. The minor side effects are nausea, vomiting, and diarrhea.

Abacavir Sulfate

Abacavir sulfate (Fig. 30.13) was approved in 1998 as an NRTI to be used in combination with other drugs for the treatment of HIV and AIDS. The drug is extensively metabolized via stepwise phosphorylation to 5′-mono-, di-, and triphosphate. Abacavir is well absorb (>75%) and penetrates the CNS. The drug can be taken without regard to meals. The drug does not show any clinically significant drug-drug interactions. The drug has been reported to produce life-threatening hypersensitivity reactions. The major use of abacavir appears to be in combination with other NRTIs. A fixed combination product has recently been approved by the FDA under the trade name of Trizivir (see Table 30.5 and discussion below). This product contains 300 mg of ABC, 150 mg of lamivudine, and 300 mg of ZDV. The combination has been shown to be superior to other combinations in reducing viral load as well as showing improvement in $CD4^+$ cell count. The most common adverse effects reported with abacavir include headache, nausea, vomiting, malaise, and diarrhea.

Tenofovir Disoproxil

Tenofovir disproxil (Fig. 30.13) is a prodrug with good bioavailability (25%), which is improved in the presence of food (35%). The drug is approved for the treatment of HIV infections in adult patients. Tenofovir diphosphate is an HIV reverse transcriptase inhibitor (RTI). The drug is hydrolyzed via plasma esterase to tenofovir, which is then phosphorated to the active tenofovir diphosphate, as shown in Figure 30.14. The diphosphate competes with dATP for incorporation into viral DNA, and when incorporated tenofovir diphosphate results in premature termination of DNA growth and inhibition of DNA polymerase.

Tenofovir disoproxil is indicated for treatment-experienced patients with HIV-1. The drug appears to also be effective in treatment-naive patients, but initial approval is for treatment-experienced patients. The drug is administered as one tablet once daily (300 mg). It is recommended that the drug be combined with other RTIs or HIV protease inhibitors, which results in additive or synergistic activity (see Table 30.5 and discussion below).[96]

Table 30.5 Fixed Combination Antiretroviral Drugs Used in the Treatment of HIV Infections

Fixed Combinations	**Abacavir**	**Bictegravir**	Doravirine	Dolutegravir	Efavirenz	Elvitegravir	**Emtricitabine**	**Lamivudine**	Lopinavir	Rilpivirine	Ritonavir	**Tenofovir diso-proxil fumarate**	**Zidovudine**
Atripla					✓		✓					✓	
Biktarvy		✓					✓					✓	
Combirvir								✓					✓
Complera							✓			✓		✓	
Delstrigo			✓					✓				✓	
Epzicom	✓							✓					
Genvoya						✓	✓					✓	
Juluca				✓						✓			
Kaletra									✓		✓		
Odefsey							✓			✓		✓	
Stribild						✓	✓					✓	
Trizivir	✓							✓					✓
Truvada							✓					✓	

NRTIs shown in **bold**. NNRTIs shown in red.

Emtricitabine

Emtricitabine (Fig. 30.13) is an orally active nucleoside reverse transcriptase inhibitor. It is metabolized in vivo to the 5′-triphosphate, which in turn competes with the normal substrate (deoxycytidine-5′-triphosphate) for incorporation into DNA. In addition, incorporation of emtricitabine into viral DNA inhibits further chain elongation resulting in chain termination. The drug is administered orally once daily. The (−) enantiomer is the most active form of the drug although the (+) isomer is also active. Emtricitabine is not bound to plasma protein, and approximately 86% is excreted unchanged in the urine. The only metabolites identified consist of the 3′-sulfoxide and the 2′-hydroxymethyl-O-glucuronide. Emtricitabine is reported to be more active than lamivudine with a low level of resistance developing when used in combination therapy with efavirenz and didanosine.[97]

Antiretroviral (Anti-HIV) Agents—Nonnucleoside RT Inhibitors (NNRTI) (Table 30.4; Fig. 30.15)

The FDA has recently approved several nonnucleosides that inhibit RT activity. They are used with nucleoside drugs to obtain synergistic activity in decreasing the viral load and increasing CD4$^+$ cell count. These drugs are primarily designed and synthesized by protein structure-based drug design methodologies. Their use as monotherapy may be limited because of rapid onset of resistance and hypersensitivity reactions. However, interaction of nonnucleoside drugs with other protease inhibitors, such as saquinavir, indinavir, and ritonavir, is being investigated. Also, interaction of these drugs with clarithromycin, ketoconazole, rifabutin, and rifampin are under study.

Nevirapine

MECHANISM OF ACTION. Nevirapine (Fig. 30.15) is a dipyridodiazepinone derivative that binds directly to RT. Thus, it blocks RNA- and DNA-dependent polymerase activities by causing a disruption of the RT catalytic site. HIV-2 RT and human DNA polymerases are not inhibited by nevirapine. The 50% inhibitory concentration ranged within 10-100 nM against HIV-1.

PHARMACOKINETICS. Nevirapine is rapidly absorbed after oral administration, and its bioavailability is approximately 95%. Peak plasma nevirapine concentrations of 2 ± 0.4 mg/mL (7.5 mM) are obtained in 4 hours following a single 200 mg dose (Table 30.4). Following multiple doses, nevirapine concentrations appear to increase linearly in the dose range of 200-400 mg/d. Nevirapine is bound to plasma proteins (~60%) in the plasma concentration range of 1-10 mg/mL. It readily crossed the placenta and was found in breast milk. Nevirapine is metabolized via CYP to a number of hydroxylated metabolites, which are excreted in urine (Fig. 30.16).

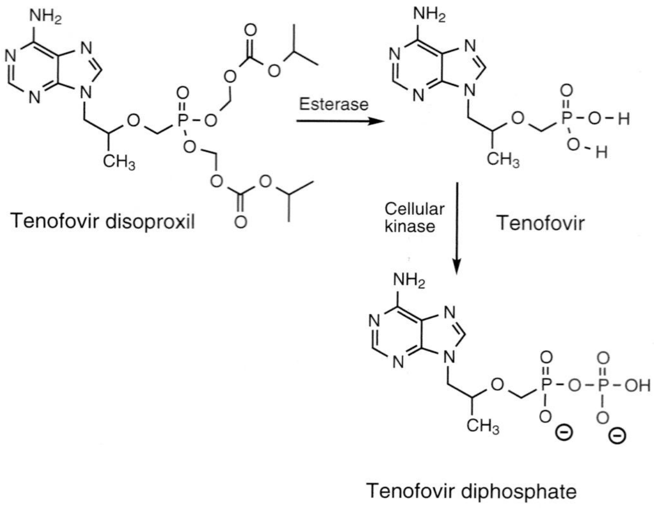

Figure 30.14 Metabolic activation of tenofir disoproxil.

CLINICAL APPLICATION. Nevirapine and its analogues exhibit antiretroviral effects against AZT-resistant HIV strains.[98] Nevirapine in combination with ZDV and ddI produced approximately 18% higher $CD4^+$ cell counts and a decrease in viral load compared with patients who took ZDV and ddI. Nevirapine is recommended with nucleosides for HIV-1 infected patients who have experienced clinical or immunologic deterioration. The significant side effects of nevirapine are liver dysfunction and skin rashes. In vivo, ketoconazole did not produce any significant inhibitory effect on nevirapine metabolism. The plasma concentrations of nevirapine were elevated or reduced in patients receiving cimetidine or rifabutin, respectively.

Delavirdine

Delavirdine (Fig. 30.15), a bisheteroarylpiperazine derivative, is a potent nonnucleoside RT inhibitor with activity specific for HIV-1.[99] In phase I/II study trials, it demonstrated sustained improvements in $CD4^+$ cell counts, p24 antigen levels and RNA viral load. Promising results were obtained when the drug was used in two- or three-drug combination with nucleoside drugs. Administration of delavirdine with ddI, ddC, or ZDV demonstrated additive or synergistic effect. However, delavirdine with ZDV was more beneficial in early HIV infection. Combinations of nevirapine and delavirdine had an antagonistic effect on HIV-1 RT inhibition. Delavirdine directly inhibits RT and DNA-directed DNA polymerase activities of HIV-1 after the formation of the enzyme-substrate complexes thereby causing chain termination effects.

PHARMACOKINETICS. Delavardine is rapidly absorbed by oral administration, and peak plasma concentration is obtained in one hour. The single dose bioavailability of delaviridine tablets relative to oral solution was approximate 85%. The 50% inhibitory concentration for delavirdine against RT activity was 6.0 nM. Delaviridine is extensively bound to plasma protein (about 98%). Delavirdine is metabolized to its N-desisopropyl metabolite in liver, and the pharmacokinetics is nonlinear. Skin rashes are the major side effect of delavirdine therapy. Cross-resistance between delavidine and PIs, such as indinavir, nelfinavir, ritonavir, and saquinavir is unlikely because they act at different target enzymes.

Efavirenz

Efavirenz (Fig. 30.15) is a nonnucleoside RT inhibitor that has been approved by the FDA as a single agent and in several combinations (see Table 30.5) (Table 30.4).[100] It is a potent inhibitor of wild-type as well as resistant mutants HIV-1 that is inhibited up to 95% in efavirenz concentration of 1.5 mM. In combination with indinavir, a mean reduction in HIV-RNA of 1.68 log and an increase in $CD4^+$ cell counts of 96 cells/mm^3 were reported. Coadministration of efavirenz with indinavir reduced indinavir concentration (AUC) by approximately 35%. Efavirenz is administered

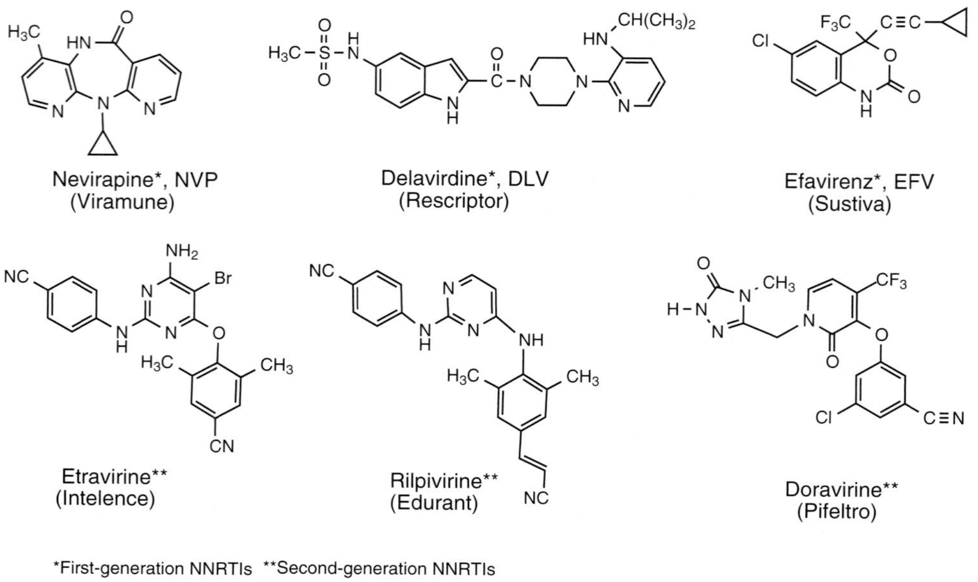

Figure 30.15 Nonnucleoside reverse transcriptase inhibitors (NNRTIs).

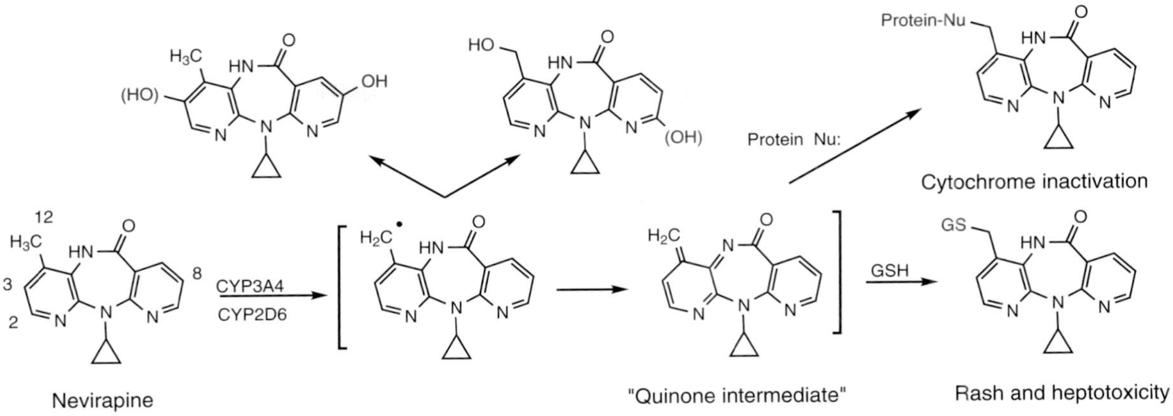

Figure 30.16 Metabolic oxidation of nevirapine by CYP3A4 leading to C2 or C12 hydroxylation or by CYP2D6 leading to C3 or C8 hydroxylation and an explanation for side effects associated with a quinone intermediate.

once a day and can be used as a substitute for indinavir in combination therapy with standard drugs, such as ZDV and 3TC. Since, it is given once a day, it cuts down the number of pills that an AIDS patient has to swallow. In the current cocktail therapy of AIDS patients, efavirenz is a good option for reducing the many side effects of cocktail therapy. It is administered to both adults and children and may be less expensive than indinavir.

The side effects of efavirenz include dizziness, insomnia, impaired concentration, abnormal dreams, and drowsiness. The most common adverse effect is a skin rash. Other side effects are diarrhea, headache, and dizziness. Efavirenz is recommended to be taken at bedtime with or without food. Avoiding driving or operating machinery and intake of high-fat meals are recommended. It should always be taken in combination with at least one other anti-HIV agent. Efavirenz is contraindicated with midazolam, triazolam, or ergot derivatives.

Etravirine

Etravine (Fig. 30.15) is a second-generation NNRTI that was approved for use in treatment-experienced patients in 2008.[101] The drug is highly bound (96%-99%) to plasma proteins, primarily albumin and α-1-acid glycoprotein. Unlike the first-generation NNRTIs nevirapine, efavirenz, and delavirdine, which have a low genetic barrier to resistance, etravirine is less likely to produce resistant strains. Etravirine (as well as rilpivirine and doravirine below) binds at an allosteric site adjacent to the reverse transcriptase catalytic site, resulting in inhibition of both RNA- and DNA-dependent polymerases and the synthesis of the viral cDNA. Etravirine is metabolized by CYP450 (Fig. 30.17) and is a weak inducer of CYP3A4 and a weak inhibitor of CYP2C9, CYP2C19 and P-glycoprotein resulting in potentially altered metabolism of other drugs, when coadministered. Currently, 200 mg twice a day is the recommended dose for clinical use in adult patients.

Rilpivirine

Rilpivirine (Fig. 30.15), previously known as TMC278, is a diarylpyrimidine derivative that acts as a potent oral NNRTI.[102] It was approved by the FDA in 2011, and is now widely used as a first line therapy in antiretroviral naive patients and in individuals on suppressive Highly active antiretroviral therapy (HAART) therapy (see below). Orally, it is available as single drug (25 mg once daily) and as a component of two combination products (Odefsey and Juluca see Table 30.5). Like etravirine, rilpivirine has a high genetic barrier to initiating resistance and exhibits antiretroviral activity against viruses with reduced sensibility to first-generation NNRTIs (nevirapine, efavirenz and delavirdine).

PHARMACOKINETICS. Rilpivirine is primarily metabolized by cytochrome P450 (CYP3A), and drugs that induce or inhibit CYP3A may thus affect the clearance of rilpivirine.

The development of the injectable formulation of rilpivirine in combination with the integrase strand transfer agent cabotegravir is currently in clinical trials, and results are encouraging. This formulation could potentially overcome the patient compliance issues in HIV-infected patients that ultimately lead to the development of resistant viral strains.

Doravirine

Doravirine (Fig. 30.15) is the newest NNRTI and was approved by the FDA in August of 2018.[103] It is available as a single drug and in combination with tenofovir disproxil and lamuvidine (Table 30.5). As a single drug or as a combination, it is only indicated for patients who have had no prior antiretroviral therapy. It appears to have the highest genetic barrier to the development of HIV resistance and a better safety profile. Doravirine is eliminated by oxidative metabolism and conjugation, since it is a substrate for CYP3A4 and P-glycoprotein. Most importantly, it has a favorable pharmacokinetic profile that allows once a day dosing.

Antiretroviral (Anti-HIV) Agents—Integrase Strand Transfer Inhibitors (INSTIs) (Fig. 30.18)

Mechanism of Action

Inhibitors of the HIV-1 integrase (IN) enzyme represent one of the most important advances in HIV care (Fig. 30.2). Integrase is one of three core enzymes encoded by

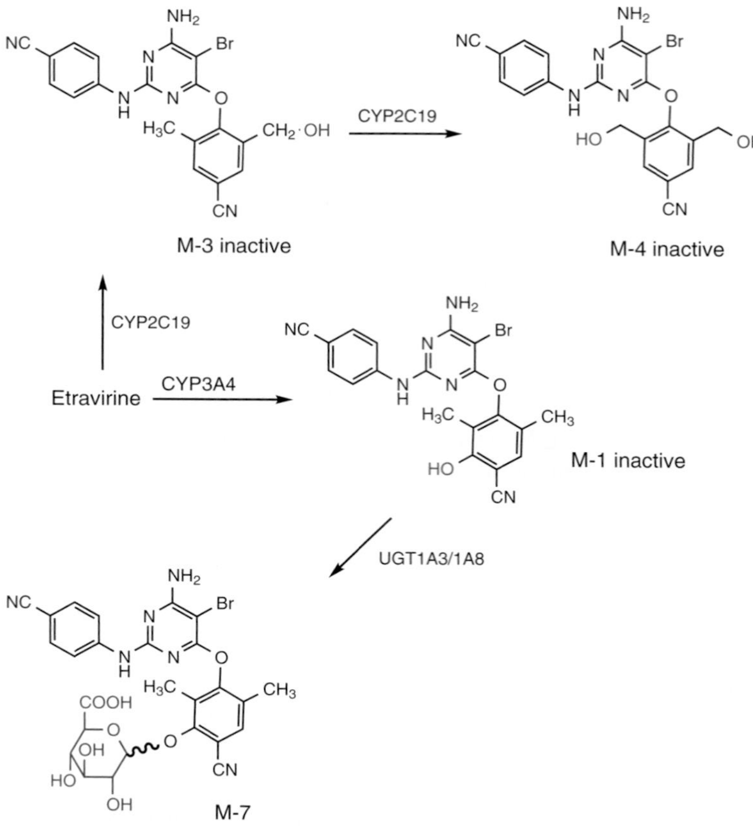

M-3 inactive

M-4 inactive

M-1 inactive

M-7

Figure 30.17 Metabolic inactivation of etravirine.

the HIV genome and is essential for successful integration of viral genetic material into the host genome and successful replication of the virus. Integrase strand transfer inhibitors (INSTIs) are drugs targeted to integrase, a viral enzyme that inserts the viral genome into the DNA of the host cell.[104] Strand integration is a critical step that occurs during retroviral replication, and thus inhibition of integrase prevents replication and prevents spread of the virus. INSTIs exert their effects by binding the integrase-viral DNA complex in the catalytic core domain (CCD), consequently interfering with integration of viral DNA integration into host DNA. It has been proposed that the INSTs bind to key metals that are involved the action of integrase and thus block the viral enzyme (Fig. 30.19). Because INSTIs target a distinct step in retroviral replication, they are often used in combination with antiretroviral drugs that have distinct mechanisms of action, thereby reducing the possibility of viral mutation and development of resistance.

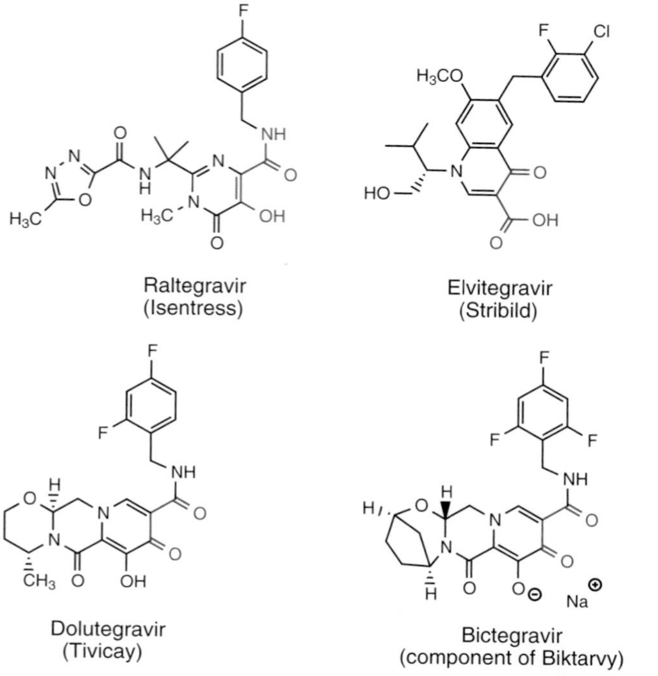

Raltegravir (Isentress)

Elvitegravir (Stribild)

Dolutegravir (Tivicay)

Bictegravir (component of Biktarvy)

Figure 30.18 Integrase strand transfer inhibitors (INSTIs). Red highlight indicates the pharmacophore in INSTIs.

Raltegravir

Raltegravir (Fig. 30.18) was the first FDA-approved treatment for HIV that acts by inhibition of HIV integrase, entering the market on October 12, 2017.[105] It was approved in 2008 for use in individuals whose infection has proven resistant to HAART drugs (see below), and in 2009, the FDA expanded approval for use in all patients. It is taken twice daily, and doses of 400 and 600 mg have been used. Raltegravir is now considered a first-line agent in the US HIV treatment guidelines, and is considered one of the best tolerated antiretroviral medications, due to limited side effects and few long-term safety concerns. It is metabolically stable, and plays an important role in the management of HIV infection. Due to lack of significant

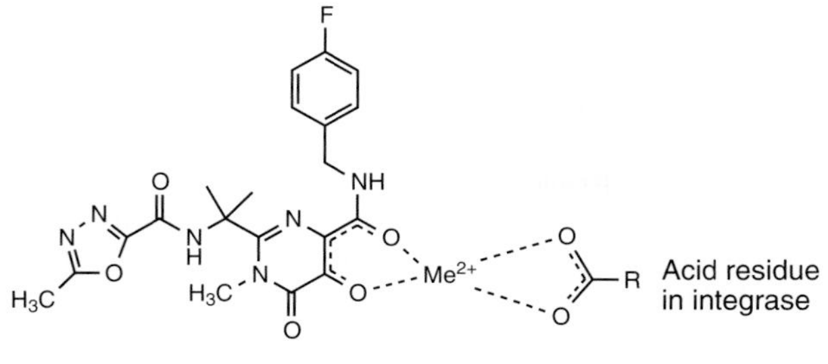

Figure 30.19 Chelation complex between raltegravir and integrase.

drug-drug interactions, raltegravir may be used in the treatment of a number of special patient populations, such as patients with renal disease, malignancy, tuberculosis, and hepatitis coinfection. For example, rategravir is effective and safe for the treatment of patients coinfected with HIV and tuberculosis and is used in combination with rifampicin at the two standard raltegravir doses (400 mg twice a day) instead of 800 mg twice a day.

Elvitegravir

Elvitegravir (Fig. 30.18) is the second INSTI that was approved in the United States for the treatment of HIV in adults who have never received treatment for the disease.[106] As a single drug, it is available in 85 and 150 mg tablets (Vitekta). However, this drug is usually administered in combination with cobicastat, emtricitabine, and tenofivir (see Tables 30.4 and 30.5). Cobicastat is a highly selective and irreversible inhibitor of CYP3A4. Additionally, it is a competitive inhibitor of P-glycoprotein efflux which increases absorption of tenofovir disoproxil fumarate.

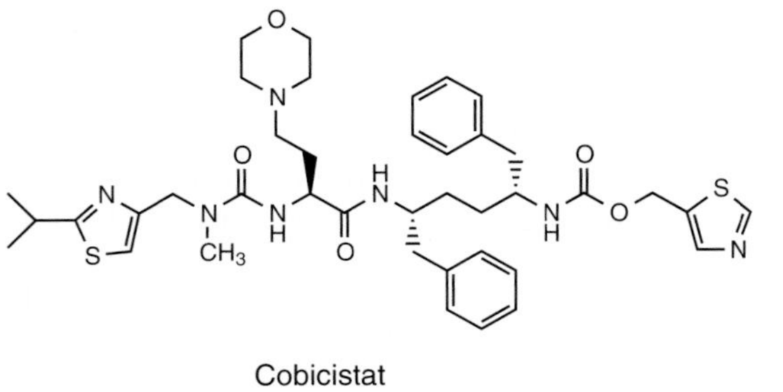

PHARMACOKINETICS. Elvitegravir is nearly entirely bound to plasma proteins, with only 1% of the dose circulating in free form. It is metabolized to inactive metabolites primarily through CYP3A4 oxidation, followed by glucuronidation and excretion. Resistance to elvitegravir can occur, although it is rare, and occurs in only 3% of patients over a 144-week period.

Dolutegravir

Dolutegravir (Fig. 30.18) is the latest INSTI approved for the treatment of HIV-1 in infected adults and adolescent children. It is well tolerated, with little potential for drug-drug interactions, and it has a long serum half-life that allows once-daily dosing in patients who have not become resistant to another INSTI. Twice-daily administration is recommended in patients with known or suspected resistance mutations to first-generation INSTIs. Like other INSTIs, dolutegravir is well tolerated. However, dolutegravir has the lowest incidence of resistance among the currently available INSTIs due to a higher genetic barrier to resistance. It has also been reported to cause very few adverse drug-drug interactions. Dolutegravir is unique in that it does not require "boosting," which is the practice of administering a drug with a cytochrome p450 inhibitor to limit its metabolism (i.e., cobicistat).

Bictegravir

Bictegravir (Fig. 30.18) is a new INSTI that was approved for use in 2018 in the combination product Biktarvy.[107] Biktarvy contains bictegravir, emtricitabine, and tenofovir alafenamide in a single tablet (Table 30.4) and is indicated for patients who have not had previous exposure to antiretroviral therapy. The combination was also studied in "switch studies" where patients were switched to Biktarvy from other combination therapies, and although it was essentially equipotent, there was no meaningful benefit to switching therapies.[108]

PHARMACOKINETICS. In pharmacokinetic studies, bictegravir produced significant reductions in HIV-1 RNA in serum by day 11, with a median T_{max} at 1.0-1.8 hours and a half-life of 15.9-20.0 hours. It is well tolerated, is rapidly absorbed, and does not require boosting with a cytochrome P450 inhibitor.[109] Bictegravir is mainly metabolized through CYP3A4 oxidation and glucuronidation, followed by renal excretion. About 1% of the dose is excreted unchanged.

Combination Drug Therapy[110,111]

When several antiretroviral drugs, typically three or four, are taken in combination for the treatment of HIV, the approach is known as highly active antiretroviral Therapy, or HAART. Multiple approaches to HAART therapy have been undertaken, and the National Institutes of Health recommend that all infected patients should be treated by this method.[105] However, unlike clinical practice in cancer chemotherapy, there are no standard combination therapies for HIV infection. In fact, there is a move toward individualized HIV combination therapy that takes into account the patient's pharmacokinetic profile, mutated forms of the virus, comorbidities, and degree of immune recovery.[112] The synergistic antiviral effects of rimantadine with ribavirin against influenza B virus and DHPG with foscarnet against HSV-1 and 2 are noteworthy. The synergistic action of acyclovir with leukocyte interferon has been used in the topical treatment of human herpetic keratitis. During the past decade, research into combination antiretroviral therapy for AIDS patients has made remarkable progress. ZDV, the first approved drug for HIV-infected patients, produced bone marrow toxicity. To overcome toxic effects, combinations of ZDV with foscarnet or ddI have been used. Such combination therapy indicated improved efficacy and decreased side effects as compared to either drug used alone. The combination of ZDV with α-interferon has been used to treat patients with AIDS-related Kaposi's sarcoma. This combination drug therapy delayed emergence of ZDV-resistant HIV strains.

A combination of granulocyte-macrophage colony-stimulating factor with ZDV and α-interferon has been successful in managing treatment-related cytopenia in HIV-infected patients. The advantages of combination therapy include therapeutic antiviral effect, decreased toxicity, and low incidence of drug-resistant infection. In recent years, emergence of drug resistance has been demonstrated in patients receiving single antiviral agent therapy. Resistance to amantadine, acyclovir, ribavirin, ganciclovir, ZDV, and other antiviral agents is noteworthy.

Combined antiretroviral drug therapy serves different purposes. It prolongs the life of AIDS patients; removes drug resistance and/or reduces toxicity of drugs. With these objectives, successful combinations of ZDV have been reported with, ddI, 3TC or D4T. Recently, combination of nucleosides drugs (ZDV, ddI and 3TC) are used with protease inhibitors (saquinavir, indinavir, ritonavir) for delaying HIV infection. Combined nucleoside drugs are known to delay progression of HIV infection.

Antiretroviral therapy includes nucleosides or nonnucleoside RT inhibitors and protease inhibitors in fixed combinations (Table 30.5). These drugs inhibit HIV replication at different stage of viral infection. Nucleoside and nonnucleoside drugs inhibit RT by preventing RNA formation or viral protein synthesis. Nonnucleoside drugs inhibit RT by inactivating the catalytic site of the enzyme while protease inhibitors act after HIV provirus has integrated into the human genome. These latter drugs inhibit protease, which is an enzyme responsible for cleaving viral precursor polypeptides into effective virions. Thus, protease inhibitors combined with RT inhibitors act by a synergistic mechanism to interrupt HIV replication.

Two-drug combination, such as ZDV plus ddI, 3TC and ZDV, and D4T and ddI, has been successful in raising $CD4^+$ cell counts and decreasing HIV RNA viral load. Triple drug therapy consisting of ZDV, 3TC, and one of protease inhibitors (indinavir, ritonavir, nelfinavir) has been more effective than double drug therapy consisting of two nonnucleoside analogue combinations. Also fewer opportunistic infections were noted when patients took the three-drug combination. ZDV can also be combined with immunomodulators to increase immunologic response in AIDS patients. ZDV has been combined with alpha interferon to obtain synergistic activity of the drug. An ideal approach of combined antiretroviral drug therapy would be drugs acting at different stages of HIV cell replication.

HIV Protease Inhibitors[113]

Mechanism of Action

The HIV genome contains various structural genes, such as the gag and gag-pol genes, that are translated into precursor polyproteins that form immature viral particles. These precursor protein molecules are processed (cleaved) by an essential viral *pol-encoded* aspartic proteinase, HIV protease, to form the desired structural proteins of the mature viral particle that are necessary for virus replication and survival. For example, the structural proteins p7, p9, p17, and p24, which play important roles in infectivity of HIV, are products of the *pol* gene. HIV protease also activates RT and plays an important role in the release of infectious viral particles. Thus, an area of considerable interest has been the development of drugs that act as inhibitors of HIV protease. Such inhibitors act on HIV protease and prevent posttranslational processing and budding of immature viral particles from the infected cells. This group of drugs represents a major breakthrough in treatment of HIV when used in combination with RT inhibitors, and their development is one of the most significant advances in medicinal chemistry.

Functional HIV protease exists as a dimer in which each monomer contains one of two conserved aspartate residues at the active site. There are several HIV protease cleavage sites on the polyprotein precursors, but the enzyme prefers to perform the hydrolysis of the peptide bond on the amino terminal side of a proline.[114] As shown in Figure 30.20A, the amino acid R-groups flanking the scissile bond are designated $\mathbf{P_1}$, $\mathbf{P_2}$, etc., on the amino terminus, and $\mathbf{P_1'}$, $\mathbf{P_2'}$, etc., on the carboxyl terminus of the cleavage site.

The corresponding pockets on the enzyme that are responsible for binding the P groups are termed S_1, S_2, $S_{1'}$, $S_{2'}$, etc. In the active site, a pair of aspartates (the Asp25 on each of the 2 subunits of the protein) work together to complete the reaction (Fig. 30.20B). One coordinates the water that performs the hydrolysis, while the other coordinates the carboxyl group on the $P_{1'}$ amino acid. Rationally designed drugs that inhibit HIV protease are designed as transition-state mimics that align at the active site of HIV-1 protease, as defined by three-dimensional crystallographic analysis of the protein structure. Figure 30.20C shows the aspartic protease inhibitor pepstatin bound in the HIV protease active site. Pepstatin is an inhibitor of all aspartic proteases, but can be used to illustrate the mechanism by which transition state analogues inhibit HIV protease.[115] Pepstatin contains an unnatural amino acid core known as statine (Fig. 30.21), and the hydroxyl-bearing sp3 carbon of this core mimics the tetrahedral transition state that occurs during hydrolysis of the peptide bond.

Other transition state cores have been used in the design of highly potent aspartic protease inhibitors, including the hydroxyethylene and hydroxyethylamine cores (Fig. 30.21). The crystal structure of several HIV protease inhibitors bound to wild type and mutant HIV proteases have been solved by X-ray crystallography. The structure of the HIV protease inhibitor lopinavir bound to wild type HIV protease is depicted in Figure 30.22. Note that the hydroxyl group of the transition state core is hydrogen bonded to the two Asp25 carboxylate moieties at a distance of about 3 angstroms.

A number of oligopeptide-like analogues have been synthesized that differentially inhibit viral and mammalian aspartic proteases, and the most useful of these

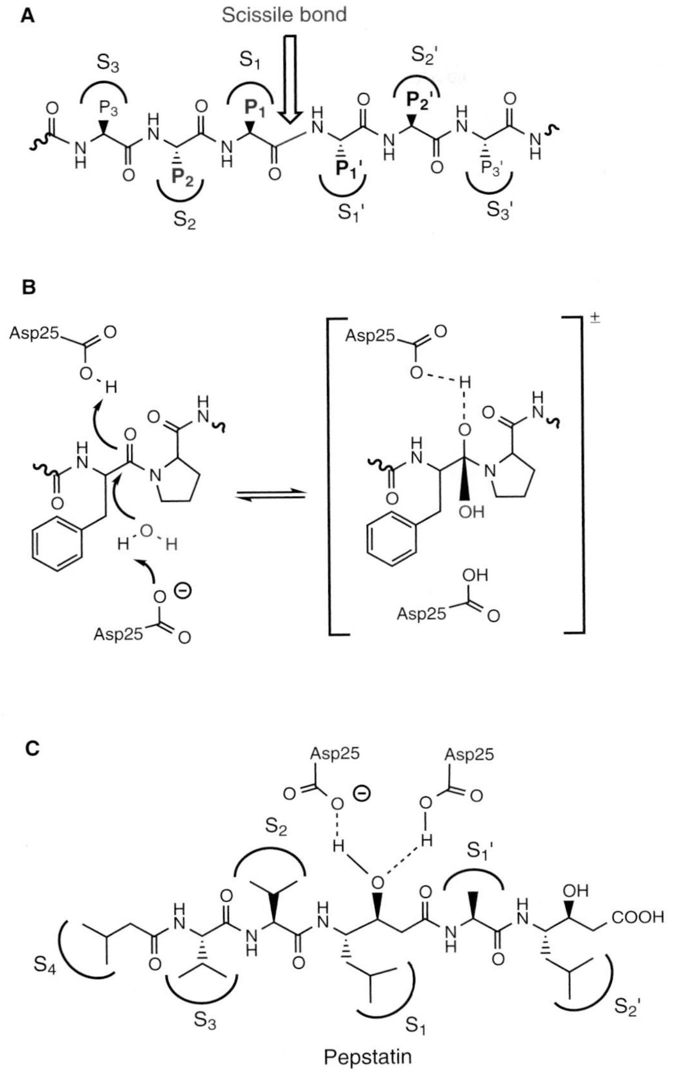

Figure 30.20 Principles of the design of transition state analogue inhibitors of HIV protease. A, Nomenclature of amino acid side chains (P) and binding pockets (S) surrounding a protease cleavage site. B, Role of two Asp25 residues in formation of the hydrolytic transition state. C, Coordination of the Asp25 residues by the transition state analogue pepstatin.

are selective for the viral enzyme HIV-1 protease. Structurally, these agents are either peptidomimetic or nonpeptide compounds. Their effectiveness is related to their ability to inhibit the processing of the gag-pol precursor polyprotein to p24, p55, and p160. Consequently, the infectivity of HIV-1 is diminished. Although some compounds exhibit in vitro and in vivo antiviral activities, optimization of their pharmacokinetic and pharmacodynamic properties have presented major problems. In view of the great demand for successful anti-AIDS drugs, the FDA has approved the protease inhibitors described below using the accelerated approval process. The structures of currently marketed HIV protease inhibitors are shown in Figure 30.23.

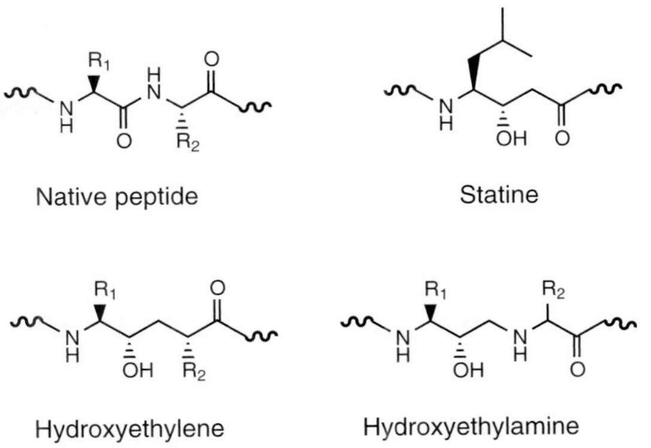

Figure 30.21 Transition state mimics used in the design of HIV protease inhibitors.

Potential Drug Interactions

Protease inhibitors have a high potential for drug interactions, stemming from the fact that they are substrates for and inhibitors of the CYP3A4 enzyme system. As a result, concurrent use of protease inhibitors with other drugs metabolized by CYP3A4 may be contraindicated, and in some cases, the resulting drug interactions can be life-threatening. The most potent CYP450 inhibitor in this class is ritonavir (used to advantage in a fixed combination with lopinavir and other HIV protease inhibitors, Table 30.6), followed by indinavir, nelfinavir (moderate inhibitors), and saquinavir as the least potent inhibitor. Drug interactions have been reported with bepridil, dihydroergotamine, and a number of benzodiazepines. Marked increases in the activity of amiodarone, lidocaine (systemic), quinidine, the tricyclic antidepressants, and warfarin might be expected.[116] Other interactions have been reported to include rifampin, rifabutin, phenobarbital, phenytoin, dexamethasone, or carbazepine. As the protease inhibitors are themselves metabolized by CYP450, their action may be altered by other agents that induce or inhibit this system. In the case of rifabutin, which inhibits CYP3A4 in the gut, relative bioavailability of the protease inhibitors is increased, and the dose of the protease inhibitor may need to be decreased.

Pharmacokinetics

The pharmacokinetics of the HIV protease inhibitors are summarized in Table 30.6. In general, these drugs exhibit poor bioavailability, are highly bound to plasma protein, have a short half-life due to rapid metabolism as indicated above, and are eliminated primarily in the feces. Variable effects are seen if the drugs are taken with or without food. A common metabolic feature of the HIV protease inhibitors is that they are substrates for CYP450. Representative metabolic routes for HIV protease inhibitors are shown in Figure 30.24. Their oxidative metabolism usually results in inactive or less active metabolites with the exception of nelfinavir in which the hydroxylated metabolites exhibit activity. Fosamprenavir undergoes an initial hydrolysis to the active drug amprenavir, but further metabolism leads to inactive metabolites.

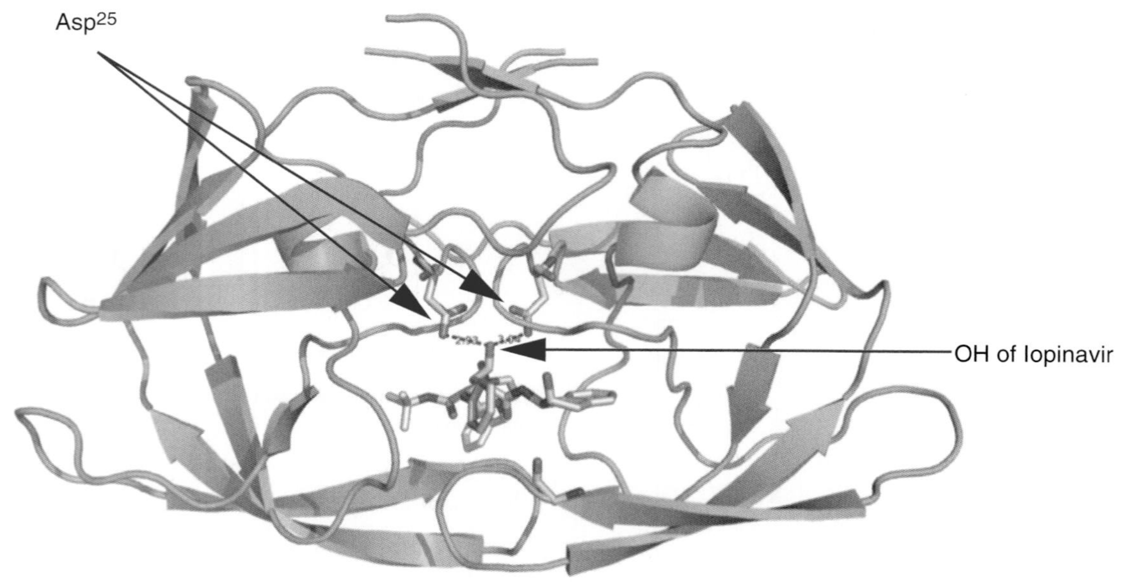

Figure 30.22 Model of the HIV protease inhibitor lopinavir bound to wild type HIV protease.

The rapid inactivation of HIV protease inhibitors oxidative metabolism has been dealt with in two ways. In the case of atazanavir, darunavir, and tipranivir, it is suggested that these drugs be used in combination with ritonavir while lopinavir is marketed as a fix combination of lopinavir and ritonavir. The role of ritonavir is the same in both situations. Ritonavir is not added to the therapy as an antiviral agent, but rather it serves as the preferentially metabolized substrate for CYP3A thus sparing the oxidative metabolism of second drug leading to an improved drug half-life of the HIV protease inhibitor (Table 30.6).[117,118]

HIV Protease Inhibitors That are Used Clinically

Saquinavir

Saquinavir (Fig. 30.23) mesylate was the first protease inhibitor approved by the FDA in December 1995.[119,120] It is a carboxamide derivative used in the treatment of advanced HIV infection in selected patients. Saquinavir is used concomitantly in either ZDV-untreated patients or patients previously treated with prolonged ZDV therapy. Although combined therapy did not slow progression of disease, CD4$^+$ cell counts were increased in patients infected with HIV in the United States and European countries. The resistance of HIV isolates to saquinavir was found to be due to mutations in the HIV protease at amino acid positions 48 (glycine to valine) and 90 (leucine to methionine). Saquinavir is well tolerated in combination with ZDV and has few side effects, but GI disturbances were common adverse effects. Saquinavir has a few mild side effects, such as headache, rhinitis, nausea, and diarrhea.

Ritonavir

Ritonavir (Fig. 30.23) is another HIV protease inhibitor that was approved by the FDA in March 1996.[121] Ritonavir is a peptidomimetic inhibitor of both the HIV-1 and HIV-2 proteases. The drug is often used in combination with other protease inhibitors to prevent their metabolism by cytochrome P450, as ritonavir is partially converted to an active metabolite. Ritonavir is contraindicated with several compounds, such as clarithromycin, desipramine, ethinyl estradiol, rifabutin, sulfamethoxazole, and trimethoprim, because of increased concentrations of these drugs in the plasma due inhibited oxidative metabolism. Ritonavir alone or in combination with 3TC, ZDV, or saquinavir increased CD4$^+$ cell counts and decreased HIV RNA particle levels. Cross-resistance between ritonavir and RT inhibitors is unlikely because of the different mode of action and enzymes involved. Common adverse reactions, such as nausea, diarrhea, vomiting, anorexia, abdominal pain, and neurologic disturbances were reported with the use of ritonavir alone or in combination with other nucleoside analogues. Ritonavir is used for the treatment of advanced HIV infection including opportunistic infections. In combination with nucleoside drugs, ritonavir reduced the risk of mortality and clinical progression.

Indinavir Sulfate

Indinavir (Fig. 30.23), a pentanoic acid amide derivative, was approved by the FDA in March 1996.[122] Because of indinavir's metabolism, a number of drug interactions are possible with rifabutin or ketoconazole leading to increased or decreased indinavir concentration, respectively, in the blood plasma. Administration of drug combinations of indinavir with antiviral nucleoside analogues, cimetidine, quinidine, trimethoprim/sulfamethoxazole, fluconazole,

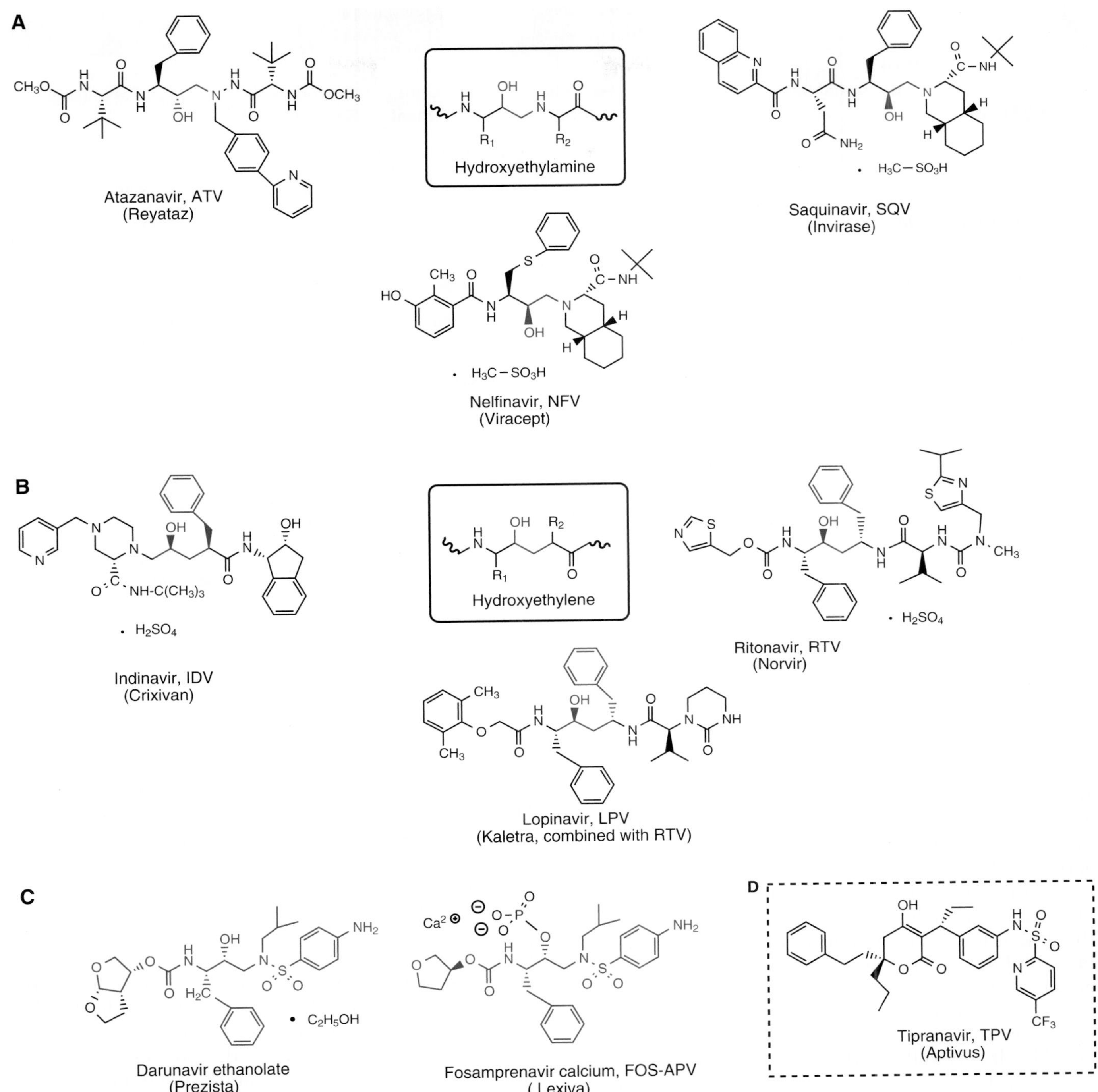

Figure 30.23 Structures of HIV protease inhibitors that are used clinically.

or isoniazid resulted in an increased activity of indinavir. Indinavir is contraindicated in patients taking triazolam or midazolam because of inhibition of metabolism of these drugs may result in prolonged sedation, nephrolithiasis, asymptomatic hyperbilirubinemia, and GI problems (anorexia, constipation, dyspepsia, and gastritis).

Nelfinavir Mesylate

Nefinavir (Fig. 30.23) is a peptidomimetic drug which is effective in HIV-1 and 2 wild type and ZDV-resistant strains, with an ED_{50} concentrations ranging from 9 to 60 nM (95% effective dose was 0.04 mg/mL).[123] After IV administration, the elimination half-life of nelfinavir was about an hour. In combination with D4T, nelfinavir reduced HIV viral load by about 98% after 4 weeks. It is well tolerated when used with azole antifungals (ketoconazole, fluconazole, or itraconazole) or macrolide antibiotics (erythromycin, clarithromycin or azithromycin). However, it causes diarrhea and other side effects common to nonnucleoside drugs.

Table 30.6 Pharmacokinetic Properties of HIV Protease Inhibitors

Drug Name	Oral Bioavailability (%)	Protein Binding (%)	Half-Life (hrs)	Absorption: With Meal	Excretion Route (%)	Dosage Form (mg/unit)
Atazanavir	NA	86	6.5/8.6[a]	Increase		Cap (150, 200)
Darunavir[b]	37-82	95	15[a]	Increase	Feces (80)	Tab (75, 800)
Fosamprenavir	NA	90	~7.7	None	Feces (75) Urine (14)	Tab (700) Susp (50/mL)
Indinavir	~65	60	1.8	Decrease	Urine (20)	Cap (200 mg, 400 mg)
Lopinavir/Ritonavir[c]	NA	>98		Increased	Feces-major	Tab (100 mg, 200 mg) Sol (80 mg/20 mL)
Nelfinavir	20-80	>98	3.5-5	Increase	Feces-major	Tab (250), Powder (50/g)
Ritonavir	~60	~99	3-5	Minimal	Feces (34) Urine (5)	Cap (200)
Saquinavir	13	98	1.8	None	Feces (88) Urine (19)	Cap (200)
Tipranivir[b]	NA	~99	~5[a]	None	Feces-major	Cap (250) Sol (100)

NA, Not available.
[a]half-life when combined with ritonavir.
[b]atazanavir, darunavir and tipranivir should be coadministered with ritonavir to block there metabolism and improve half-life.
[c]combination product in which ritonavir inhibits lopinavir metabolism.

Atazanavir Calcium[124]

Atazanavir (Fig. 30.23) is an antiretroviral agent approved for use in combination with other antiretroviral agents for the treatment of HIV infections. It targets HIV-1 protease and reduces viral replication and thus virulence of HIV-1. Similar to saquinavir, ritonavir, indinavir, nelfinavir, amprenavir, and lopinavir, the drug is used in combination with reverse transcriptase inhibitors to produce excellent efficacy in AIDS patients. Atazanavir is dosed orally once daily, thus reducing "pill burden," and appears to have a minimum impact on lipid parameters but does increase total bilirubin. The drug is well absorbed when administered orally with food (bioavailability ~68%). The drug is highly bound to plasma protein (86%) and is metabolized by CYP3A. Atazanavir is a moderate inhibitor of CYP3A, and potential drug-drug interactions are possible with CYP3A inhibitors and inducers.

Fosamprenavir Calcium[125]

Fosamprenavir (Fig. 30.23) has been approved for the treatment of HIV in adults when used in combination with other anti-HIV drugs. It is a prodrug that, upon hydrolysis by serum phosphatases, gives rise to amprenavir, which is a peptidomimetric transition state inhibitor that targets HIV-1 protease and reduces viral replication and thus, infectiousness of HIV-1. It is commonly administered in combination with reverse transcriptase inhibitors to produce excellent efficacy in AIDS patients. The drug is administered as two 700 mg tablets twice daily or in combination with ritonavir can be given as two 700 mg tablets once daily or one 700 mg tablet twice daily. As a result, formaprenavir lowers the "pill burden" in AIDS patients.

Tipranavir

Tipranavir (Fig. 30.23) was approved in 2005 as a nonpeptidic inhibitor of HIV protease.[126] It is indicated for patients who have developed resistance to other antiretroviral drugs, including other HIV protease inhibitors. Although it is very potent, it also exhibits more severe side effects than other HIV protease inhibitors, including intracranial hemorrhage, hepatitis, and diabetes mellitus. It is dosed at 500 mg twice daily in combination with 200 mg of ritonavir to suppress metabolism by cytochrome P450.[127] There is evidence that tipranavir induces its own metabolism, but using twice-daily coadministration of tipranavir and ritonavir at varying doses, tipranavir levels were 24–70-fold higher than levels achieved with administration of tipranavir alone.

Darunavir

Darunavir (Fig. 30.23) is a second-generation HIV protease inhibitor that can be used in treatment-naive and treatment-experienced adult and pediatric patients.[128]

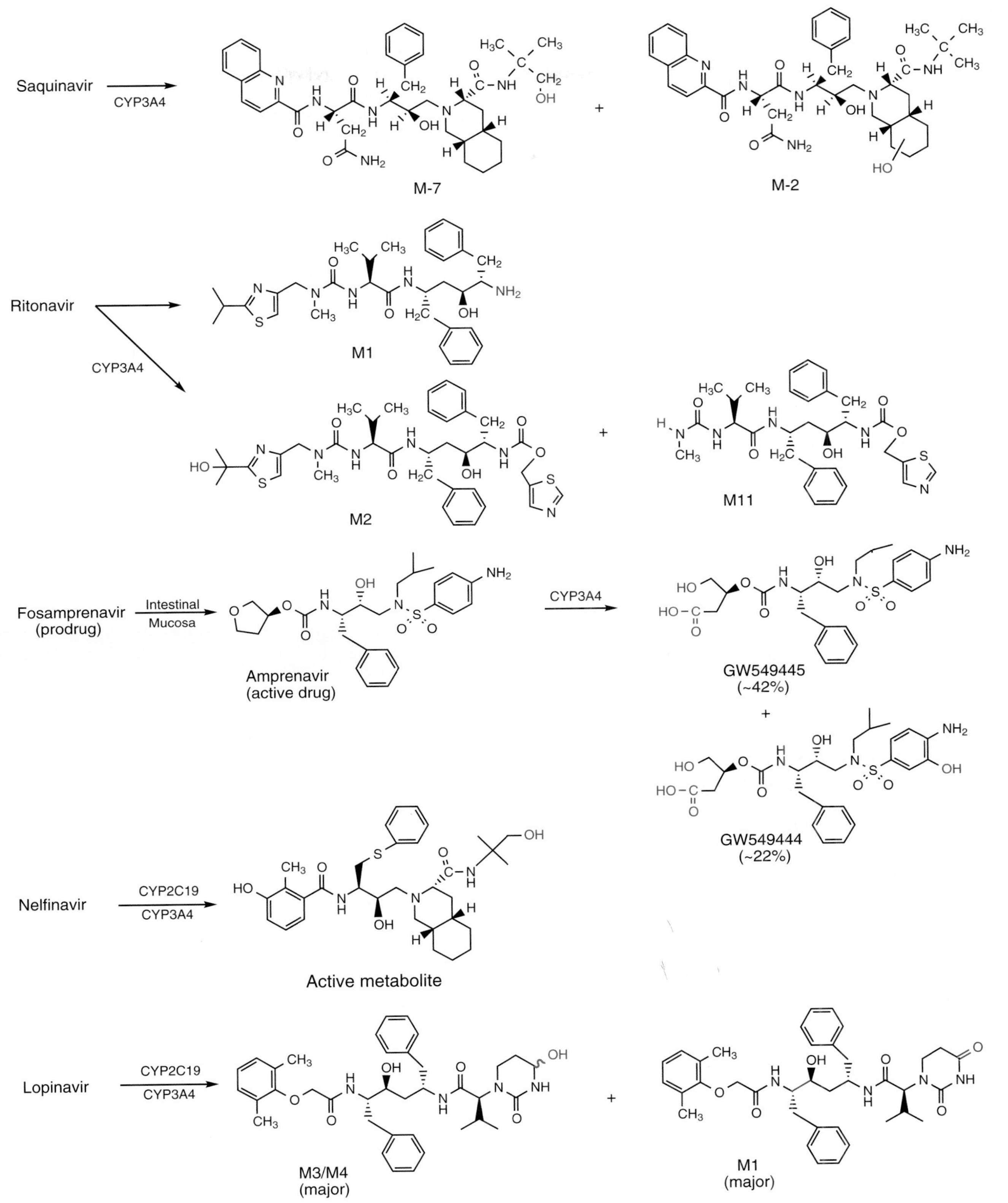

Figure 30.24 Metabolism of HIV protease inhibitors.

It was designed to bind tightly and specifically to HIV protease and thereby overcome the problems associated with first-generation drugs, including toxicity, high dose, expensive manufacture, and susceptibility to resistance.

Like other HIV protease inhibitors, darunavir is metabolized by cytochrome P450, and so the drug is dosed at 800 mg once daily in combination with 100 mg of ritonavir.[129]

Drugs for Hepatitis C Virus (HCV): Inhibitors of Protease NS3/4A

As indicated earlier (see Hepatitis C Genome and Fig. 30.3) the HCV has a number of structural and nonstructural proteins (NS) that arise from a large polyprotein. These NS proteins are found in the endoplasmic reticulum of the infected cell and their roles involve replication of HCV in infected cells via RNA polymerase, mediation of HCV resistance to interferon, inhibition of apoptosis, and possibly promotion of tumorigenesis. The essential HCV enzyme NS3/4A protease is responsible for cleaving this HCV polyprotein at four sites to generate four peptides called NS4A, NS4B, NS5A, and NS5B.

Mechanism of Action of NS3/4A Inhibitors

In general, it is proposed that the NS3/4A inhibitors act to block the processing of the HCV polyprotein and prevents the virus from replicating. These drugs are often referred to as the direct-acting nonnucleoside NS3/4A protease inhibitors and are effective against HCV genotypes 1-6. These drugs bind noncovalently to the NS3/4A HCV protease preventing the cleaving of HCV-encoded polyprotein, which is necessary for development of the HCV.

Specific Drugs

GLECAPREVIR. Glecaprevir[130] (Fig. 30.25, formerly ABT-493) is a potent NS3/4A protease inhibitor with activity against all HCV genotypes 1-6. It is administered in combination with the NS5A protease inhibitor pibrentasvir (Fig. 30.26) and marketed as Mavyret (Table 30.7). When taken together as a fixed dose in a ribavirin-free regimen, the combination produces cures in 98% of patients, due to the synergy of the two agents. The glecaprevir/pibrentasvir combination has a high barrier to resistance. Its excretion is primarily biliary, with negligible excretion by the kidney, and as such it is suitable for patients with renal insufficiency.

GRAZOPREVIR. The HCV NS3/4A inhibitor grazoprevir (Fig. 30.25), like other HCV protease inhibitors, is administered in combination with an NS5A inhibitor, in this case elbasvir (Fig. 30.26).[131] The trade name for the combination product is Zepatier. It is indicated for patients with chronic HCV genotypes 1a, 1b, 4, or 6. Treatment with the combination of grazoprevir/elbasvir at a fixed-dose for 12 or 16 weeks with or without ribavirin resulted in a potent antiviral response at 12 weeks in treatment-naïve and treatment-experienced patients. The combination was also effective in individuals with advanced chronic

Telaprevir (2011), boceprevir (2011), and simeprevir (2013) were early FDA approvals for the treatment HCV infection.[129-131] These drugs were the first of the so-called direct-acting antiviral agents, which effectively inhibited NS3/NS4A protease and revolutionized HCV therapy, producing cures in as many as 98% of patients. Unfortunately all three have been discontinued in 2014, 2015, and 2018, respectively, for what was listed as business reasons and may have involved diminished demand for the product caused by significant competition from newer agents (Fig. 30.25). Also, adverse effects may have entered into the decision. Telaprevir was reported to cause severe skin reactions (Stevens-Johnson syndrome) and boceprevir's adverse effects included anemia and neutropenia.

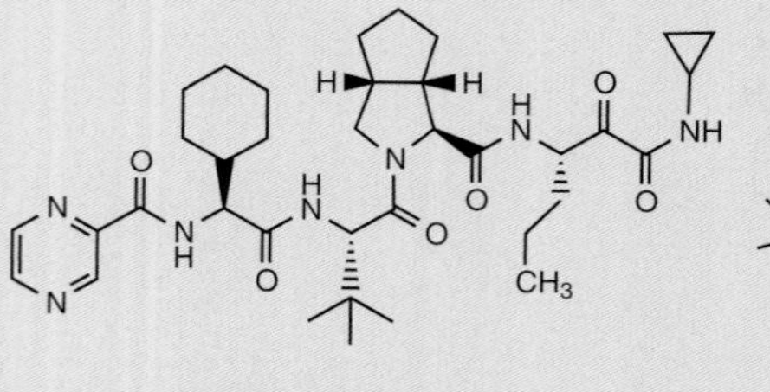

Telaprevir

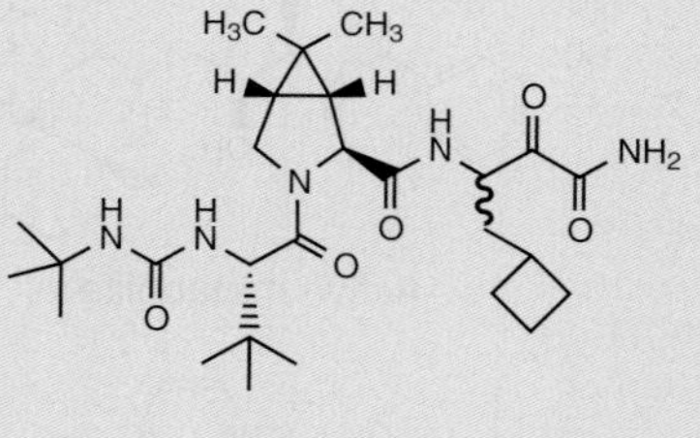

Boceprevir

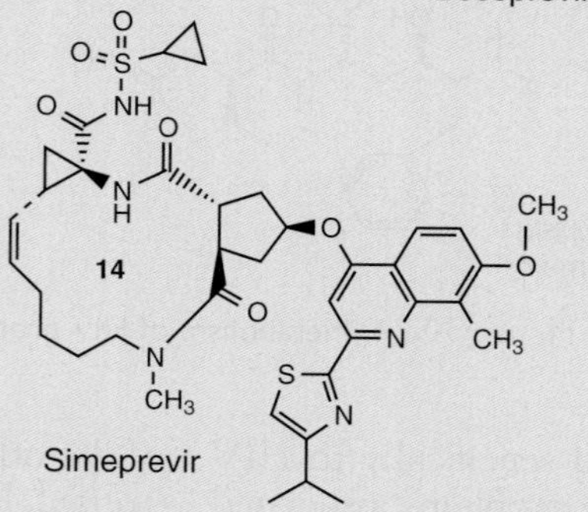

Simeprevir

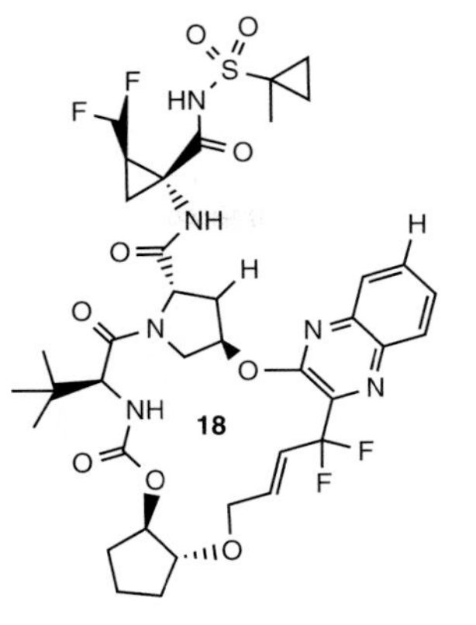

Glecaprevir
(component of Mavyret)

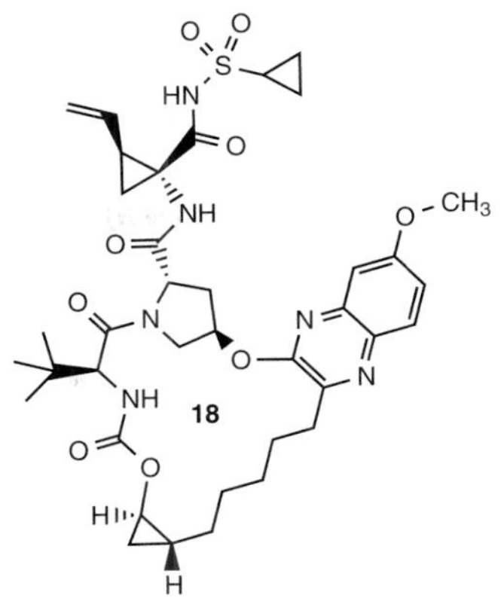

Grazoprevir
(component of Zepatier)

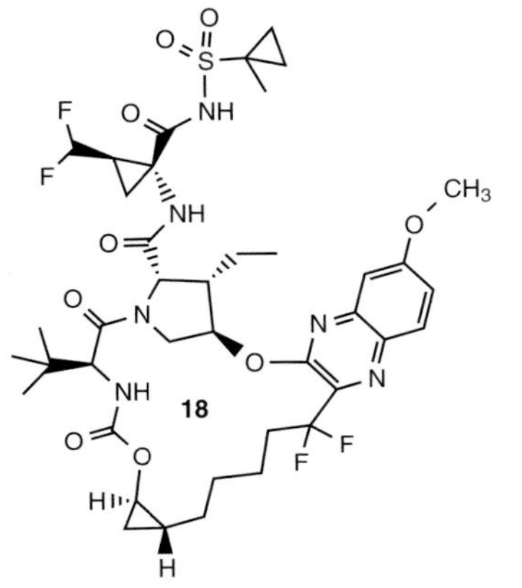

Voxilaprevir
(component of Vosevi)

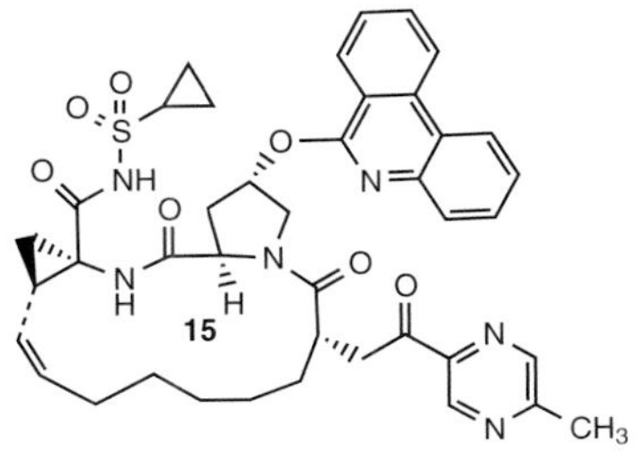

Paritaprevir
(component of Viekira Pak)

Figure 30.25 Inhibitors of HCV protease NS3/4A.

kidney disease, HCV-HIV coinfection, or cirrhosis of the liver. Zepatier is administered once daily as a tablet containing grazoprevir and elbasvir (Table 30.7). Peak plasma concentrations of both drugs are reached in 2-3 hours after oral administration, and steady-state pharmacokinetics are reached within 6 days. Both grazoprevir and elbasvir are highly bound to plasma proteins (98.8% for grazoprevir and 99.9% for elbasvir) and are metabolized by CYP3A and excreted in the feces, with half-lives of 31 and 24 hours, respectively. Zepatier is also effective in patients who have failed therapy with peginterferon alfa.

PARITAPREVIR. Paritaprevir (Fig. 30.25)[132] is marketed as an oral regimen (Viekera Pak) available as a fixed-dose combination of paritaprevir, ritonavir, and ombitasvir in one tablet, which is taken once daily, plus a dasabuvir tablet taken twice daily (Table 30.7). This dosage regimen is continued for 12-24 weeks, with or without ribavirin, depending on the HCV strain involved. Viekera Pak is indicated for HCV genotype 1a and 1b, and can be used in patients with cirrhosis of the liver. Paritaprevir is also sold as Technivie, which is the same preparation as Viekera, except dasabuvir is not included. Technivie is only indicated for HCV genotype 4 in combination with ribavirin. The medications in these combination products act additively, in that they target multiple steps in the HCV life cycle. Paritaprevir is an inhibitor of the HCV NS3/4A protease, and ritonavir is an HIV-1 protease inhibitor that is included as a pharmacokinetic booster for paritaprevir. Ombitasvir is an inhibitor of HCV NS5A and is active against all HCV genotypes with EC_{50} values in the low to mid picomolar range, while dasabuvir is an allosteric inhibitor of NS5B RNA-dependent RNA polymerase that reduces the expression of NS5B, which is essential for viral RNA replication and HCV virion assembly. All four drugs are highly bound to plasma proteins and are metabolized by cytochrome P450, except for dasabuvir, which is metabolized by amide hydrolysis. Viekera Pak and Technivie are safe for use in patients with renal impairment, but because of their reliance on metabolism by cytochrome P450, they are not recommended for patients with moderate hepatic impairment and contraindicated in severe hepatic impairment.

VOXILAPREVIR. The HCV NS3/4A protease inhibitor voxilaprevir (Fig. 30.25)[133] is administered as a single-dose tablet in combination with the NS5B inhibitor, sofosbuvir, and an NS5A inhibitor, velpatasvir. This combination was approved in 2017 (Vosevi, Table 30.7) based on data from the POLARIS-1 study (12 wk of treatment among adults

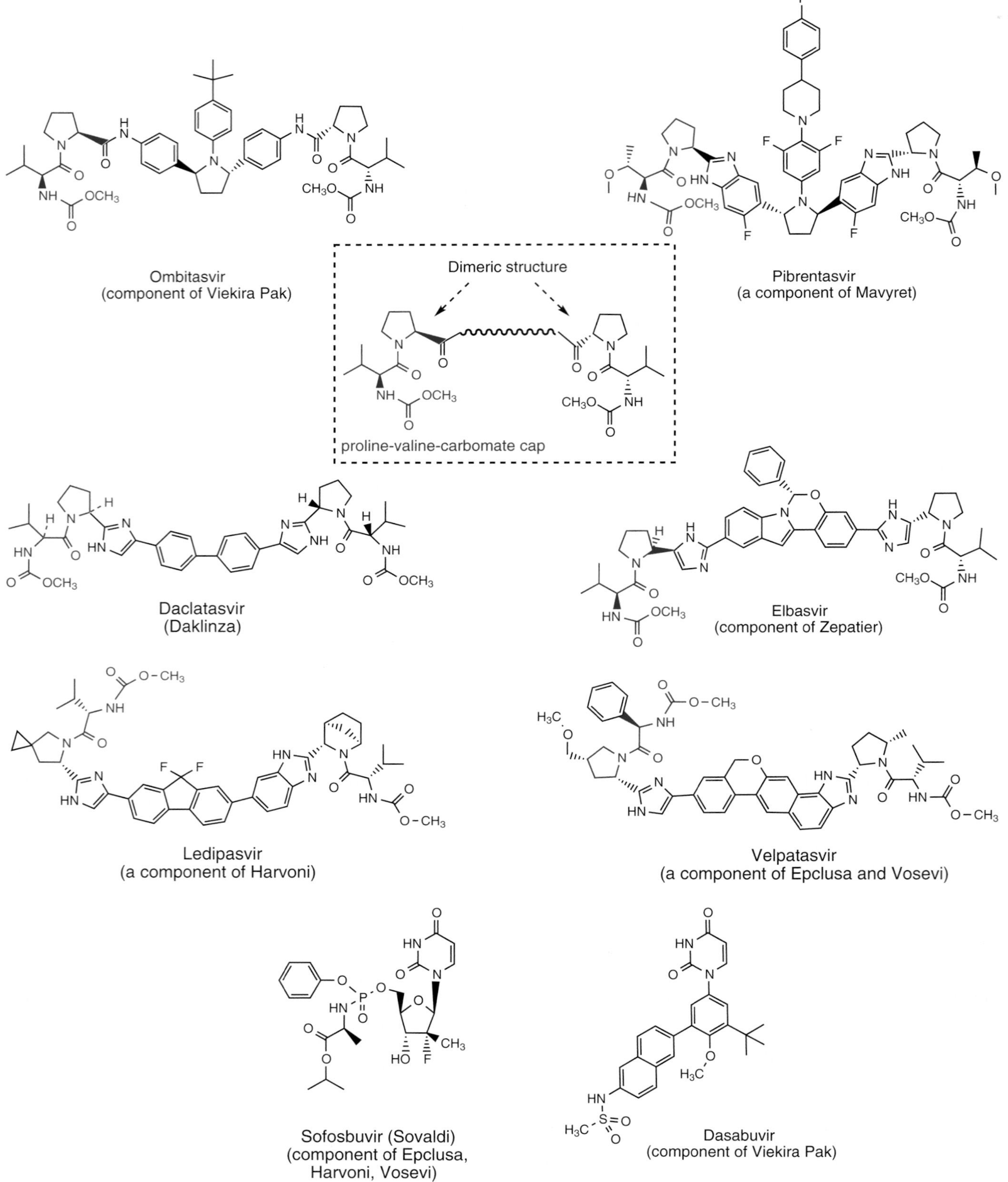

Figure 30.26 Inhibitors of HCV protease NS5A and NS5B.

with any HCV genotype who had failed prior treatment with an NS5A inhibitor-containing regimen) and the POLARIS-4 study (12 wk of treatment among adults with HCV genotypes 1a and 3 who had failed prior treatment with a sofosbuvir-containing regimen that did not include an NS5A inhibitor). Voxilaprevir has potent activity against HCV genotypes 1-6 and features an improved resistance profile compared to other NS3/4A protease

Table 30.7 HCV Protease Inhibitors

Generic Name	Trade Name	Dosage Form (mg/unit)
Inhibitors of HCV Protease NS3/4A		
Glecaprevir	Mavyret (with pibrentasvir)	Tab: glecaprevir (300), pibrentasvir (120). Dosed at 3 tabs daily for 8, 12 or 16 wk, depending on HCV genotype
Grazoprevir	Zepatier	Tab: grazoprevir (100), elbasvir (50)
Paritaprevir	Viekira Pak Technivie	Tab: Ombitasvir (12.5), paritaprevir (75), ritonavir (50), plus Tab: dasabuvir (250) Tab: Ombitasvir (12.5), paritaprevir (75) ritonavir (50)
Voxilaprevir	Vosevi	Tab:Velpatasvir (100), voxilaprevir (100), sofosbuvir (400)
Inhibitors of HCV Protease NS5A and NS5B		
Daclatasvir	Daklinza	Tab: (30, 60, 90)
Dasabuvir	Viekira Pak	Tab: ombitasvir (12.5), paritaprevir (75) ritonavir (50), dasabuvir (250)
Elbasvir	Zepatier	Tab: grazoprevir (100), elbasvir (50)
Ledipasvir	Harvoni	Tab: ledipasvir (90) sofosbuvir (400)
Ombitasvir	Viekira Pak Technivie	Tab: ombitasvir (12.5), paritaprevir (75), ritonavir (50), dasabuvir (250) Tab: ombitasvir (12.5), paritaprevir (75), ritonavir (50)
Pibrentasvir	Mavyret (with glecaprevir)	Tab: glecaprevir (300), pibrentasvir (120). Dosed at 3 tabs daily for 8, 12 or 16 wk, depending on HCV genotype
Sofosbuvir	Sovaldi Harvoni Epclusa	Tab film-coated: (400) Tab: ledipasvir (90) sofosbuvir (400) Tab: velpatasvir (100), sofosbuvir (400)
Velpatasvir	Epclusa Vosevi	Tab: velpatasvir (100), sofosbuvir (400) Tab: velpatasvir (100), voxilaprevir (100), sofosbuvir (400)

inhibitors. Up to 96% cure rates were achieved, despite the difficulty encountered in treating this population. Voxilaprevir is 99% bound to plasma proteins following administration, serves as a substrate for CYP3A4, and 94% of the dose is excreted in the feces.

Drugs for Hepatitis C Virus (HCV): Inhibitors of Protease NS5A and NS5B

General Mechanism of Action

NS5A is one of six nonstructural proteins encoded in the single-stranded envelope of HCV RNA (Fig. 30.3). NS5A consists of a 447–amino acid, zinc-binding phosphoprotein consisting of three domains connected by two linker regions. The NS5A has multiple roles during replication; one is to interact with host cell membranes during virus replication. There are suggestions that NS5A may also play a role in assembly/release of infectious HCV particles. Studies have shown that with ledipasvir and ombitasvir (and presumably ebasvir and pibrentasvir) bind to the NS5A protein to inhibit the development of HCV. The dimeric nature of these drugs is critical as is the proline-valine-carbamate cap found in the NS5A inhibitors (Fig. 30.26).[134]

The two other drugs in Figure 30.26, sofosbuvir and dasabuvir, are potent inhibitors of HCV NS5B and act on the viral RNA-dependent RNA polymerase. This inhibition leads to nonobligate chain termination. Sofosbuvir is a nucleoside prodrug (discussed below) while dasabuvir is a nonnucleoside with high selectivity for HSV genotype 1 polymerase of NS5B.[135]

Specific Drugs

OMBITASVIR. Ombitasvir (Fig. 30.26)[136] is approved in the United States for use in two combination products, both produced by Abbvie: with paritaprevir, ritonavir, and dasabuvir in the product Viekira Pak used for HCV genotype 1, and with paritaprevir and ritonavir in the product Technivie for HCV genotype 4 (Table 30.7). The use of ombitasvir in the combination products Viekira Pak and Technivie is described in the section on the NS3/4A inhibitor paritaprevir above (see also Table 30.7). For pharmacokinetic properties of the NS5A and NS5B protease inhibitors see Table 30.8.

PIBRENTASVIR. Pibrentasvir (Fig. 30.26)[137] is a NS5A inhibitor that has potent activity against HCV genotype 1-6 and a low liability for producing resistance, as compared to previously discovered NS5A inhibitors. Pibrentasvir is approved for use in the United States in combination with the NS3/4A inhibitor glecaprevir (Fig. 30.23; Table 30.7). Glecaprevir is an HCV NS3/NS4A protease inhibitor. Both of these direct-acting antivirals are effective against all six major HCV genotypes with a high barrier to the selection of common variants with resistance-associated

Table 30.8 Pharmacokinetic Properties of HCV Protease NS5A/NS5B Inhibitors

Drug	Bioavailability (%)	Protein Binding (%)	Half-Life (hr)	Elimination
Daclatasvir	~67	>99	12-15	Feces
Dasabuvir	~70	99.5	5-6	Feces
Elbasvir		~99	~24	Feces
Ledipasvir		100		Feces
Ombitasvir	~48	100		Feces
Pibrentasvir	48-53	97-100	~13	Feces
Sofosbuvir		61-65	0.4/17.8 tri-phosphate	Urine
Velpatasvir		>99.5	~15	Feces

substitutions. The use of pibrentasvir in the combination product Mavyret is described in the section on the NS3/4A inhibitor paritaprevir (above). Glecaprevir plus pibrentasvir is well tolerated and achieved excellent sustained virologic response rates in HCV genotypes 1-6 over an 8- or 12-week course of therapy.[138]

DACLATASVIR. Daclatasvir (Fig. 30.26) is an inhibitor of the HCV NS5A, and computer modeling data indicate that daclatasvir interacts with the N-terminus of Domain 1 of NS5A, which causes structural distortions that interfere with NS5A functions. This drug is indicated for use with sofosbuvir, with or without ribavirin, for the treatment of patients with chronic HCV infection of genotype 1 or 3. As such, it represents a newer strategy of including newer direct-acting antivirals in combination therapy to attain sustained virological response, high efficacy, and enhanced patient tolerance. This combination, taken orally with or without food, has an excellent pharmacokinetic and pharmacodynamic profile (Table 30.8). Like all drugs in this class that are metabolized by cytochrome P450, daclatasvir is contraindicated with drugs that induce cytochrome P450.

LEDIPASVIR. Ledipasvir (Fig. 30.26) is an inhibitor of the HCV phosphoprotein NS5A and is combined with ledipasvir/sofosbuvir (Harvoni, Table 30.7) with or without ribavirin for use in the United States for the treatment of chronic hepatitis C in adults and adolescents aged 12-18 years. The introduction of Harvoni and other combination regimens containing direct-acting antivirals has created a paradigm shift in the treatment of HCV. The combination of ledipasvir/sofosbuvir produces high sustained virological response rates 12 weeks post treatment in treatment-naive and treatment-experienced patients with HCV genotype 1 infections, including patients with cirrhosis of the liver or HIV coinfections. Ledipasvir is highly active against HCV genotype 1a and 1b, with moderate activity against genotypes 4a, 4b, 5a, and 6a. Sofosbuvir is a potent antiviral that is active against HCV genotypes 1a, 1b, 2a, 2b, 3a, 4a, 5a, and 6a. The pharmacokinetic properties are presented in Table 30.8.

DASABUVIR. Dasabuvir (Fig. 30.26) is effective as a single agent against HCV genotypes 1a and 1b, but in the United States, it is only approved for use in combination of paritaprevir, ritonavir, and ombitasvir (Viekera Pak), with or without ribavirin. While dasabuvir represents an important medical advance in the treatment of HCV infection, it does suffer from low genotypic coverage. However, it is synergistic when used in combination with other direct-acting antivirals, as in Viekera Pak.[139] For pharmacokinetic properties of dasabuvir see Table 30.7. Dasabuvir is metabolized by cytochrome P450 oxidation, followed by glucuronidation and excretion in the feces (Fig. 30.27).[134]

SOFOSBUVIR. Sofosbuvir (Fig. 30.26) represents a significant advance in the treatment of HCV,[140] in that was the first NS5B RNA-dependent RNA-polymerase inhibitor to be marketed in the United States. As a single agent, sofosbuvir produces low toxicity, a high barrier to the development of resistance, and has excellent compatibility with other direct-acting antiviral agents. It was originally marketed as Sovaldi and was approved in 2013 for use against HCV genotypes 2 and 3 in combination with ribovirin and against genotypes 1 and 4 in

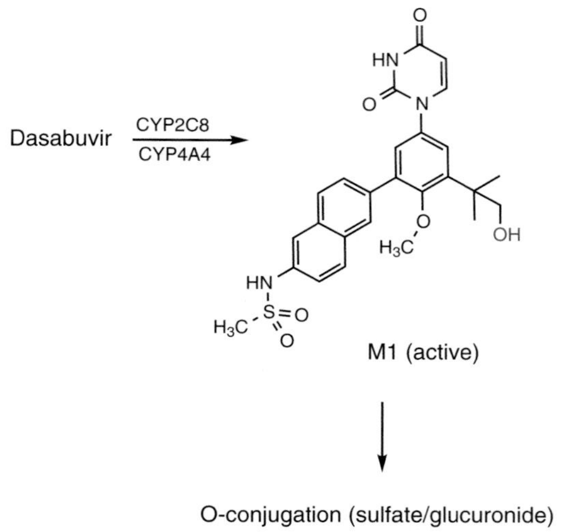

Dasabuvir —CYP2C8 / CYP4A4→ M1 (active) → O-conjugation (sulfate/glucuronide)

Figure 30.27 Metabolism of dasabuvir.

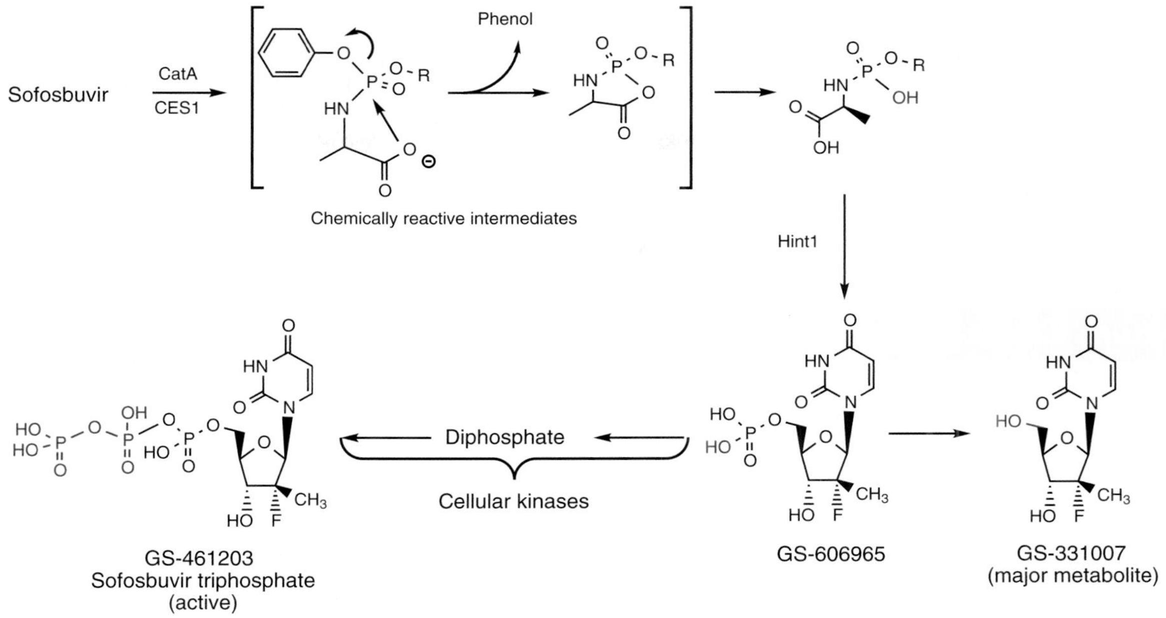

Figure 30.28 Metabolic activation of sofosbuvir to the active triphosphate form. This process is sequentially catalyzed by cathepsin A (CatA), carboxylesterase I (CESI) and histidine triad nucleotide-binding protein (Hint1). The intermediate constituent GS-606965 is inactivated by dephosphorylation, or activated to the triphosphate by celluar kinases.

combination with pegylated alfa-interferon and ribavirin. This approval provided the first interferon-free therapy for chronic viral infection by HCV and requires a shorter course of therapy. Sofosbuvir is a uridine-based nucleoside analogue that is well absorbed orally and rapidly taken up into hepatocytes. There it is metabolized to the monophosphate form GS-606965, and ultimately to the triphosphate active metabolite GS-461203 (Fig. 30.28).[141] The triphosphate is then incorporated into the growing viral RNA chain and acts as a chain terminator, preventing any further elongation of the viral RNA strand. The pharmacokinetic properties of sofosbuvir are presented in Table 30.7. Sofosbuvir triphosphate has a 17.8-hour half-life in hepatocytes, allowing it to be dosed once daily.

Clinically, sofosbuvir in combination with other direct-acting antivirals produces HCV cures in as many as 99% of patients. It is marketed in three forms, Epclusa (velpatasvir and sofosbuvir), Harvoni (ledipasvir and sofosbuvir tablets), and Vosevi (velpatasvir, voxilaprevir, and sofosbuvir tablets) (Table 30.9). Harvoni is taken once daily as a single tablet and produces a 94%

Table 30.9 Fix Combination Antiretroviral Drugs Used in the Treatment of HIV Infections

Fixed Combinations	Dasabuvir	Elbasvir	**Glecaprevir**	**Grazoprevir**	Ledipasvir	Ombitasvir	**Paritaprevir**	Pibrentasvir	Ritonavir	Sofosbuvir	Velpatasvir	**Voxilaprevir**
Epclusa										✓	✓	
Harvoni					✓					✓		
Mavyret			✓					✓				
Technivie						✓	✓		✓			
Viekira Pak	✓					✓	✓		✓			
Vosevi										✓	✓	✓
Zepatier		✓		✓								

NS5A/NS5B inhibitors shown in red; NS3/4A inhibitors shown in **bold.**

cure rate after 8 weeks and a 96%-99% cure rate after 12 weeks. The combination of ledpasvir and sofosbuvir is an effective treatment for HCV infection, and Harvoni currently ranks as the second most profitable drug product in the United States. According to Gilead Sciences, a 12-week course of Harvoni has a total cost of $94,500, boosting sales of the preparation to $13,864 million USD in 2015.

VELPATASVIR. Velpatasvir is an HCV NS5A inhibitor with activity similar to pibrentasvir.[142] It is only approved for use in fixed combination with sofosbuvir (Epclusa) or with sofosbuvir and voxilaprevir (Vosevi) (Table 30.9). All three drugs are pan-inhibitors of the HCV virus, meaning they are all effective against genotyopes 1-6. On oral administration, velpatasvir reaches peak plasma levels in three hours when taken together with sofosbuvir.

Structure Challenge

Zidovudine (AZT)

Lopinavir

Velpatasvir

As our knowledge of the structure and biochemistry of viruses has advanced, new opportunities to design effective antivirals have been created. Consider the structures of the three antiviral agents shown in the figure above. These agents represent antivirals that were created based on knowledge that existed at the time they were synthesized.

1. Describe the antiviral activity of each agent as it relates to a specific biochemical target within the life cycle of a virus.
2. Based on what you have learned in this chapter, postulate the methods that were used to design these three agents. What enzymatic processes have been targeted by these agents, and how was this information used in their design? How has antiviral drug discovery evolved during the time these three agents were created?

SUGGESTED READINGS

Bamford DH, Burnett RM, Stuart DI. Evolution of viral structure. *Theor Popul Biol*. 2002;61:461.

Brooks GF, Butel JS, Morse SA, et al. *Jawetz, Melnick and Adelberg's* Medical Microbiology. 23rd ed. McGraw-Hill Companies; 2004.

De Clercq E. Antiviral drug discovery and development: where chemistry meets with biomedicine. *Antivir Res*. 2005;67:56.

De Clercq E, Field HJ. Antiviral prodrugs–the development of successful prodrug strategies for antiviral chemotherapy. *Br J Pharmacol*. 2006;147:1-11.

Mabbott NA, MacPherson GG. Prions and their lethal journey to the brain. *Nat Rev Micro*. 2006;4:201.

Wong E, Trustman N, Yalong A. HIV pharmacotherapy: a review of integrase inhibitors. *JAAPA*. 2016;29:36-40.

Zhengtong L, Chu Y, Wang Y. HIV protease inhibitors: a review of molecular selectivity and toxicity. *HIV AIDS*. 2015;7:95-104.

de Leuw P, Stephan C. Protease inhibitor therapy for hepatitis C virus-infection. *Expert Opin Pharmacother*. 2018;19:577-587.

Scott LJ. Ledipasvir/sofosbuvir: a review in chronic hepatitis C. *Drugs*. 2018;78:245-256.

Vermehren J, Park JS, Jacobson IM, et al. Challenges and perspectives of direct antivirals for the treatment of hepatitis C virus infection. *J Hepatol*. 2018.

REFERENCES

1. Baron S. *Medical Microbiology*. 3rd ed. New York, NY: Churchill Livingstone; 1991.
2. Brooks GF, Butel JS, Morse SA, et al. *Jawetz, Melnick and Adelberg's Medical Microbiology*. 23rd ed. McGraw-Hill Companies; 2004.
3. Pornillos O, Ganser-Pornillos BK, Yeager M. Atomic-level modelling of the HIV capsid. *Nature*. 2011;469:424-427.
4. Tyler KL, Fields BN. *Fields Virology*. 2nd ed. New York, NY: Raven Press; 1990.

5. Ganser-Pornillos BK, Chandrasekaran V, Pornillos O, et al. Hexagonal assembly of a restricting TRIM5alpha protein. *Proc Natl Acad Sci USA*. 2011;108:534-539.
6. Gallo RC. History of the discoveries of the first human retroviruses: HTLV-1 and HTLV-2. *Oncogene*. 2005;24:5926-5930.
7. Sierra S, Kupfer B, Kaiser R. Basics of the virology of HIV-1 and its replication. *J Clin Virol*. 2005;34:233.
8. Gallo RC, Montagnier L. The discovery of HIV as the cause of AIDS. *N Engl J Med*. 2003;349:2283-2285.
9. World Health Organization (WHO). *HIV: Key Facts*; 2018. http://www.who.int/en/news-room/fact-sheets/detail/hiv-aids.
10. UNAIDS. *UNAIDS Report on the Global AIDS Epidemic 2018*. 2018:1-370.
11. Hotez PJ, Molyneux DH, Fenwick A, et al. Incorporating a rapid-impact package for neglected tropical diseases with programs for HIV/AIDS, tuberculosis, and malaria. *PLoS Med*. 2006;3:e102.
12. Kaleeba JAR, Berger EA. Kaposi's sarcoma-associated herpesvirus fusion-entry receptor: cystine transporter xCT. *Science*. 2006;311:1921-1924.
13. Anzola M, Burgos JJ. Hepatocellular carcinoma: molecular interactions between hepatitis C virus and p53 in hepatocarcinogenesis. *Expert Rev Mol Med*. 2003;5:1-16.
14. Brechot C, Gozuacik D, Murakami Y, et al. Molecular bases for the development of hepatitis B virus (HBV)-related hepatocellular carcinoma (HCC). *Semin Cancer Biol*. 2000;10:211-231.
15. Hussain SA, Ferry DR, El-Gazzaz G, et al. Hepatocellular carcinoma. *Ann Oncol*. 2001;12:161-172.
16. Pawlotsky JM. NS5A inhibitors in the treatment of hepatitis C. *J Hepatol*. 2013;59:375-382.
17. D'Agostino DM, Bernardi P, ChiecoBianchi L, et al. Mitochondria as functional targets of proteins coded by human tumor viruses. *Adv Cancer Res*. 2005:87-142.
18. Grassmann R, Aboud M, Jeang K-T. Molecular mechanisms of cellular transformation by HTLV-1 tax. *Oncogene*. 2005;24:5976.
19. Mikkers H, Berns A. Retroviral insertional mutagenesis: tagging cancer pathways. *Adv Cancer Res*. 2003;88:53-99.
20. O'Shea CC. DNA tumor viruses – the spies who lyse us. *Curr Opin Genet Dev*. 2005;15:18.
21. Robinson HL. Retroviruses and cancer. *Rev Infect Dis*. 1982;4:1015-1025.
22. Klein G. Perspectives in studies of human tumor viruses. *Front Biosci*. 2002;7:d268-d274.
23. Saslow D, Castle PE, Cox JT, et al. American cancer society guideline for human papillomavirus (HPV) vaccine use to prevent cervical cancer and its precursors. *CA Cancer J Clin*. 2007;57:7-28.
24. Johnson RT. Prion diseases. *Lancet Neurol*. 2005;4:635.
25. Mabbott NA, MacPherson GG. Prions and their lethal journey to the brain. *Nat Rev Micro*. 2006;4:201.
26. Weissmann C. Birth of a prion: spontaneous generation revisited. *Cell*. 2005;122:165.
27. Mandell GL. *Principles and Practice of Infectious Diseases*. New York, NY: Churchill Livingstone; 1995.
28. Mills J, Corey L. *Antiviral Chemotherapy: New Directions for Clinical Application and Research*. Englewood Cliffs, NJ: PTR Prentice Hall; 1993.
29. Burlington DB, Meiklejohn G, Mostow SR. Anti-influenza a virus activity of amantadine hydrochloride and rimantadine hydrochloride in ferret tracheal ciliated epithelium. *Antimicrob Agents Chemother*. 1982;21:794-799.
30. Hayden FG. Combinations of antiviral agents for treatment of influenza virus infections. *J Antimicrob Chemother*. 1986;18(suppl B):177-183.
31. Wingfield WL, Pollack D, Grunert RR. Therapeutic efficacy of amantadine HCL and rimantadine HCL in naturally occurring influenza A2 respiratory illness in man. *N Engl J Med*. 1969;281:579-584.
32. Wintermeyer SM, Nahata MC. Rimantadine: a clinical perspective. *Ann Pharmacother*. 1995;29:299-310.
33. Jordan GW, Seet EC. Antiviral effects of amphotericin B methyl ester. *Antimicrob Agents Chemother*. 1978;13:199-204.
34. Hartsel S, Bolard J. Amphotericin B: new life for an old drug. *Trends Pharmacol Sci*. 1996;17:445-449.
35. Xu F, Zhao X, Hu S, et al. Amphotericin B inhibits enterovirus 71 replication by impeding viral entry. *Sci Rep*. 2016;6:33150.
36. Francis ML, Meltzer MS, Gendelman HE. Interferons in the persistence, pathogenesis, and treatment of HIV infection. *AIDS Res Hum Retroviruses*. 1992;8:199-207.
37. Hayden FG. *Clinical Aspects of Interferons*. Boston: Kluwer Academic Publishers; 1988.
38. Streuli M, Nagata S, Weissmann C. At least three human type alpha interferons: structure of alpha 2. *Science*. 1980;209:1343-1347.
39. Taniguchi T, Guarente L, Roberts TM, et al. Expression of the human fibroblast interferon gene in *Escherichia coli*. *Proc Natl Acad Sci USA*. 1980;77:5230-5233.
40. Baglioni C, Maroney PA. Mechanisms of action of human interferons. Induction of 2′5′-oligo(A) polymerase. *J Biol Chem*. 1980;255:8390-8393.
41. Pollard RB. Interferons and interferon inducers: development of clinical usefulness and therapeutic promise. *Drugs*. 1982;23:37-55.
42. Yang G, Pevear DC, Davies MH, et al. An orally bioavailable antipoxvirus compound (ST-246) inhibits extracellular virus formation and protects mice from lethal orthopoxvirus challenge. *J Virol*. 2005;79:13139-13149.
43. Jordan R, Leeds JM, Tyavanagimatt S, et al. Development of ST-246® for treatment of poxvirus infections. *Viruses*. 2010;2:2409-2435.
44. Leeds JM, Fenneteau F, Gosselin NH, et al. Pharmacokinetic and pharmacodynamic modeling to determine the dose of ST-246 to protect against smallpox in humans. *Antimicrob Agents Chemother*. 2013;57:1136-1143.
45. Calfee DP, Hayden FG. New approaches to influenza chemotherapy. Neuraminidase inhibitors. *Drugs*. 1998;56:537-553.
46. Kim CU, Lew W, Williams MA, et al. Influenza neuraminidase inhibitors possessing a novel hydrophobic interaction in the enzyme active site: design, synthesis, and structural analysis of carbocyclic sialic acid analogues with potent anti-influenza activity. *J Am Chem Soc*. 1997;119:681-690.
47. Sweeny DJ, Lynch G, Bidgood AM, et al. Metabolism of the influenza neuraminidase inhibitor prodrug oseltamivir in the rat. *Drug Metab Dispos*. 2000;28:737-741.
48. Mancuso CE, Gabay MP, Steinke LM, et al. Peramivir: an intravenous neuraminidase inhibitor for the treatment of 2009 H1N1 influenza. *Ann Pharmacother*. 2010;44:1240-1249.
49. Noshi T, Kitano M, Taniguchi K, et al. In vitro characterization of baloxavir acid, a first-in-class cap-dependent endonuclease inhibitor of the influenza virus polymerase pa subunit. *Antiviral Res*. 2018;160:109-117.
50. Koshimichi H, Ishibashi T, Kawaguchi N, et al. Safety, tolerability, and pharmacokinetics of the novel anti-influenza agent baloxavir marboxil in healthy adults: phase I study findings. *Clin Drug Investig*. 2018;38(12):1189-1196.
51. Lalezari JP, Henry K, O'Hearn M, et al. Enfuvirtide, an HIV-1 fusion inhibitor, for drug-resistant HIV infection in north and south America. *N Engl J Med*. 2003;348:2175-2185.
52. Poveda E, Briz V, Soriano V. Enfuvirtide, the first fusion inhibitor to treat HIV infection. *AIDS Rev*. 2005;7:139-147.
53. Field HJ. A perspective on resistance to acyclovir in herpes simplex virus. *J Antimicrob Chemother*. 1983;12(suppl B):129-135.
54. Elion GB, Furman PA, Fyfe JA, et al. Selectivity of action of an antiherpetic agent, 9-(2-hydroxyethoxymethyl) guanine. *Proc Natl Acad Sci USA*. 1977;74:5716-5720.
55. Brigden D, Bye A, Fowle AS, et al. Human pharmacokinetics of acyclovir (an antiviral agent) following rapid intravenous injection. *J Antimicrob Chemother*. 1981;7:399-404.
56. de Miranda P, Whitley RJ, Blum MR, et al. Acyclovir kinetics after intravenous infusion. *Clin Pharmacol Ther*. 1979;26:718-728.
57. Perry CM, Faulds D. Valaciclovir. A review of its antiviral activity, pharmacokinetic properties and therapeutic efficacy in herpesvirus infections. *Drugs*. 1996;52:754-772.

58. Whitley RJ, Alford CA. Antiviral agents: clinical status report. *Hosp Pract (Off Ed)*. 1981;16:109-121.
59. Mitchell CD, Bean B, Gentry SR, et al. Acyclovir therapy for mucocutaneous herpes simplex infections in immunocompromised patients. *Lancet*. 1981;1:1389-1392.
60. Whitley RJ, Alford CA, Hirsch MS, et al. Vidarabine versus acyclovir therapy in herpes simplex encephalitis. *N Engl J Med*. 1986;314:144-149.
61. Martinez CM, Luks-Golger DB. Cidofovir use in acyclovir-resistant herpes infection. *Ann Pharmacother*. 1997;31:1519-1521.
62. De Clercq E, Field HJ. Antiviral prodrugs–the development of successful prodrug strategies for antiviral chemotherapy. 2006;147:1-11.
63. Schacker T, Hu HL, Koelle DM, et al. Famciclovir for the suppression of symptomatic and asymptomatic herpes simplex virus reactivation in HIV-infected persons. A double-blind, placebo-controlled trial. *Ann Intern Med*. 1998;128:21-28.
64. Fletcher CV, Balfour HH Jr. Evaluation of ganciclovir for cytomegalovirus disease. *DICP*. 1989;23:5-12.
65. Dando T, Plosker G. Adefovir dipivoxil: a review of its use in chronic hepatitis B. *Drugs*. 2003;63:2215-2234.
66. Hall CB, McBride JT. Vapors, viruses, and views. Ribavirin and respiratory syncytial virus. *Am J Dis Child*. 1986;140:331-332.
67. Sidwell RW, Huffman JH, Khare GP, et al. Broad-spectrum antiviral activity of virazole: 1-beta-D-ribofuranosyl-1,2,4-triazole-3-carboxamide. *Science*. 1972;177:705-706.
68. Fox CF, Robinson WS. *Virus Research*. New York: Academic Press; 1973.
69. Farah A. *Handbook of Experimental Biology*. Berlin: Springer; 1975.
70. Chrisp P, Clissold SP. Foscarnet. A review of its antiviral activity, pharmacokinetic properties and therapeutic use in immunocompromised patients with cytomegalovirus retinitis. *Drugs*. 1991;41:104-129.
71. Goldner T, Hewlett G, Ettischer N, et al. The novel anticytomegalovirus compound AIC246 (letermovir) inhibits human cytomegalovirus replication through a specific antiviral mechanism that involves the viral terminase. *J Virol*. 2011;85:10884-10893.
72. Lischka P, Hewlett G, Wunberg T, et al. In vitro and in vivo activities of the novel anticytomegalovirus compound AIC246. *Antimicrob Agents Chemother*. 2010;54:1290-1297.
73. Kropeit D, Scheuenpflug J, Erb-Zohar K, et al. Pharmacokinetics and safety of letermovir, a novel anti-human cytomegalovirus drug, in patients with renal impairment. *Br J Clin Pharmacol*. 2017;83:1944-1953.
74. Mohan P, Baba M. *Anti-AIDS Drug Development: Challenges, Strategies and Prospects*. Chur: Harwood Academic; 1995.
75. Sethi ML. Current concepts in HIV/AIDS pharmacotherapy. *Consult Pharma*. 1998;13:1224-1245.
76. Berger TG. Treatment of bacterial, fungal, and parasitic infections in the HIV-infected host. *Semin Dermatol*. 1993;12:296-300.
77. Goa KL, Barradell LB. Fluconazole. An update of its pharmacodynamic and pharmacokinetic properties and therapeutic use in major superficial and systemic mycoses in immunocompromised patients. *Drugs*. 1995;50:658-690.
78. Sattler FR, Feinberg J. New developments in the treatment of pneumocystis carinii pneumonia. *Chest*. 1992;101:451-457.
79. Mitsuya H. *Anti-HIV Nucleosides: Past, Present and Future*. New York, NY: Chapman and Hall; 1997.
80. Gorbach SL, Barlett JG, Blacklow NR. *Infectious Diseases*. Philadelphia: W.B. Saunders Company; 1998.
81. MacDonald L, Kazanjian P. Antiretroviral therapy in HIV-infection: an update. *Formulary*. 1996;31:780-804.
82. Faulds D, Brogden RN. Didanosine. A review of its antiviral activity, pharmacokinetic properties and therapeutic potential in human immunodeficiency virus infection. *Drugs*. 1992;44:94-116.
83. Beach JW. Chemotherapeutic agents for human immunodeficiency virus infection: mechanism of action, pharmacokinetics, metabolism, and adverse reactions. *Clin Ther*. 1998;20:2-25; discussion l.
84. Lipsky JJ. Zalcitabine and didanosine. *Lancet*. 1993;341:30-32.
85. Shelton MJ, O'Donnell AM, Morse GD. Zalcitabine. *Ann Pharmacother*. 1993;27:480-489.
86. Neuzil KM. Pharmacologic therapy for human immunodeficiency virus infection: a review. *Am J Med Sci*. 1994;307:368-373.
87. Fischl MA, Richman DD, Grieco MH, et al. The efficacy of azidothymidine (AZT) in the treatment of patients with AIDS and AIDS-related complex. A double-blind, placebo-controlled trial. *N Engl J Med*. 1987;317:185-191.
88. Fischl MA, Richman DD, Hansen N, et al. The safety and efficacy of zidovudine (AZT) in the treatment of subjects with mildly symptomatic human immunodeficiency virus type 1 (HIV) infection. A double-blind, placebo-controlled trial. The AIDS clinical trials group. *Ann Intern Med*. 1990;112:727-737.
89. Nasr M, Litterst C, McGowan J. Computer-assisted structure-activity correlations of dideoxynucleoside analogs as potential anti-HIV drugs. *Antiviral Res*. 1990;14:125-148.
90. Sethi ML. *Zidovudine*. San Diego: Academic Press; 1991.
91. Hoth DF Jr, Myers MW, Stein DS. Current status of HIV therapy: I. Antiretroviral agents. *Hosp Pract (Off Ed)*. 1992;27:145-156.
92. Horwitz JP, Chua J, Noel M, et al. Nucleosides. IV. 1-(2-deoxy-beta-D-lyxofuranosyl)-5-iodouracil. *J Med Chem*. 1964;7:385-386.
93. Ostertag W, Roesler G, Krieg CJ, et al. Induction of endogenous virus and of thymidine kinase by bromodeoxyuridine in cell cultures transformed by friend virus. *Proc Natl Acad Sci USA*. 1974;71:4980-4985.
94. Yarchoan R, Klecker RW, Weinhold KJ, et al. Administration of 3′-azido-3′-deoxythymidine, an inhibitor of HTLV-III/LAV replication, to patients with AIDS or AIDS-related complex. *Lancet*. 1986;1:575-580.
95. Perry CM, Faulds D. Lamivudine. A review of its antiviral activity, pharmacokinetic properties and therapeutic efficacy in the management of HIV infection. *Drugs*. 1997;53:657-680.
96. Barditch-Crovo P, Deeks SG, Collier A, et al. Phase I/II trial of the pharmacokinetics, safety, and antiretroviral activity of tenofovir disoproxil fumarate in human immunodeficiency virus-infected adults. *Antimicrob Agents Chemother*. 2001;45:2733-2739.
97. Bang LM, Scott LJ. Emtricitabine: an antiretroviral agent for HIV infection. *Drugs*. 2003;63:2413-2424; discussion 2425-2416.
98. Tan B, Ratner L. The use of new antiretroviral therapy in combination with chemotherapy. *Curr Opin Oncol*. 1997;9:455-464.
99. Freimuth WW. Delavirdine mesylate, a potent non-nucleoside HIV-1 reverse transcriptase inhibitor. *Adv Exp Med Biol*. 1996;394:279-289.
100. Graul AI, Rabesseda X, Castaner J. Efavirenz. *Drugs Future*. 1998;23:133-141.
101. Schrijvers R. Etravirine for the treatment of HIV/AIDS. *Expert Opin Pharmacother*. 2013;14:1087-1096.
102. Ferretti F, Boffito M. Rilpivirine long-acting for the prevention and treatment of HIV infection. *Curr Opin HIV AIDS*. 2018;13:300-307.
103. Colombier MA, Molina JM. Doravirine: a review. *Curr Opin HIV AIDS*. 2018;13:308-314.
104. Blanco JL, Whitlock G, Milinkovic A, et al. HIV integrase inhibitors: a new era in the treatment of HIV. *Expert Opin Pharmacother*. 2015;16:1313-1324.
105. Al-Mawsawi LQ, Neamati N. Allosteric inhibitor development targeting HIV-1 integrase. *ChemMedChem*. 2011;6:228-241.
106. Unger NR, Worley MV, Kisgen JJ, et al. Elvitegravir for the treatment of HIV. *Expert Opin Pharmacother*. 2016;17:2359-2370.
107. Gallant J, Lazzarin A, Mills A, et al. Bictegravir, emtricitabine, and tenofovir alafenamide versus dolutegravir, abacavir, and lamivudine for initial treatment of HIV-1 infection (GS-US-380-1489): a double-blind, multicentre, phase 3, randomised controlled non-inferiority trial. *Lancet*. 2017;390:2063-2072.
108. Harris M. What did we learn from the bictegravir switch studies? *Lancet HIV*. 2018;5:e336-e337.
109. Gallant JE, Thompson M, DeJesus E, et al. Antiviral activity, safety, and pharmacokinetics of bictegravir as 10-day monotherapy in HIV-1-infected adults. *J Acquir Immune Defic Syndr*. 2017;75:61-66.

110. Fischl MA, Stanley K, Collier AC, et al. Combination and monotherapy with zidovudine and zalcitabine in patients with advanced HIV disease. The niaid AIDS clinical trials group. *Ann Intern Med.* 1995;122:24-32.
111. Havlir DV, Lange JM. New antiretrovirals and new combinations. *AIDS.* 1998;12(suppl A):S165-S174.
112. Mu Y, Kodidela S, Wang Y, et al. The dawn of precision medicine in HIV: state of the art of pharmacotherapy. *Expert Opin Pharmacother.* 2018;19:1581-1595.
113. Deeks SG, Volberding PA. HIV-1 protease inhibitors. *AIDS Clin Rev.* 1997;145-185.
114. Bihani S, Das A, Prashar V, et al. X-ray structure of HIV-1 protease in situ product complex. *Proteins.* 2009;74:594-602.
115. Rich DH, Sun ET. Mechanism of inhibition of pepsin by pepstatin. Effect of inhibitor structure on dissociation constant and time-dependent inhibition. *Biochem Pharmacol.* 1980;29:2205-2212.
116. Josephson F. Drug-drug interactions in the treatment of HIV infection: focus on pharmacokinetic enhancement through CYP3A inhibition. *J Intern Med.* 2010;268:530-539.
117. Kumar GN, Dykstra J, Roberts EM, et al. Potent inhibition of the cytochrome P-450 3A-mediated human liver microsomal metabolism of a novel HIV protease inhibitor by ritonavir: a positive drug-drug interaction. *Drug Metab Dispos.* 1999;27:902-908.
118. Kumar GN, Jayanti V, Lee RD, et al. In vitro metabolism of the HIV-1 protease inhibitor ABT-378: species comparison and metabolite identification. *Drug Metab Dispos.* 1999;27:86-91.
119. Hoetelmans RM, Meenhorst PL, Mulder JW, et al. Clinical pharmacology of HIV protease inhibitors: focus on saquinavir, indinavir, and ritonavir. *Pharm World Sci.* 1997;19:159-175.
120. Perry CM, Noble S. Saquinavir soft-gel capsule formulation. A review of its use in patients with HIV infection. *Drugs.* 1998;55:461-486.
121. Markowitz M, Saag M, Powderly WG, et al. A preliminary study of ritonavir, an inhibitor of HIV-1 protease, to treat HIV-1 infection. *N Engl J Med.* 1995;333:1534-1539.
122. Deeks SG, Smith M, Holodniy M, et al. HIV-1 protease inhibitors. A review for clinicians. *JAMA.* 1997;277:145-153.
123. Perry CM, Benfield P. Nelfinavir. *Drugs.* 1997;54:81-87; discussion 88.
124. Colonno RJ, Thiry A, Limoli K, et al. Activities of atazanavir (BMS-232632) against a large panel of human immunodeficiency virus type 1 clinical isolates resistant to one or more approved protease inhibitors. *Antimicrob Agents Chemother.* 2003;47:1324-1333.
125. Falcoz C, Jenkins JM, Bye C, et al. Pharmacokinetics of GW433908, a prodrug of amprenavir, in healthy male volunteers. *J Clin Pharmacol.* 2002;42:887-898.
126. Courter JD, Teevan CJ, Li MH, et al. Role of tipranavir in treatment of patients with multidrug-resistant HIV. *Ther Clin Risk Manag.* 2010;6:431-441.
127. Hughes CA, Robinson L, Tseng A, et al. New antiretroviral drugs: a review of the efficacy, safety, pharmacokinetics, and resistance profile of tipranavir, darunavir, etravirine, rilpivirine, maraviroc, and raltegravir. *Expert Opin Pharmacother.* 2009;10:2445-2466.
128. Boyd MA, Hill AM. Clinical management of treatment-experienced, HIV/AIDS patients in the combination antiretroviral therapy era. *Pharmacoeconomics.* 2010;28(suppl 1):17-34.
129. McCoy C. Darunavir: a nonpeptidic antiretroviral protease inhibitor. *Clin Ther.* 2007;29:1559-1576.
130. Hubbard H, Lawitz E. Glecaprevir + pibrentasvir (ABT493 + ABT-530) for the treatment of hepatitis C. *Expert Rev Gastroenterol Hepatol.* 2018;12:9-17.
131. Morikawa K, Nakamura A, Shimazaki T, et al. Safety and efficacy of elbasvir/grazoprevir for the treatment of chronic hepatitis C: current evidence. *Drug Des Devel Ther.* 2018;12:2749-2756.
132. Geddawy A, Ibrahim YF, Elbahie NM, et al. Direct acting anti-hepatitis C virus drugs: clinical pharmacology and future direction. *J Transl Int Med.* 2017;5:8-17.
133. Soriano V, Benitez-Gutierrez L, Arias A, et al. Evaluation of sofosbuvir, velpatasvir plus voxilaprevir as fixed-dose co-formulation for treating hepatitis C. *Expert Opin Drug Metab Toxicol.* 2017;13:1015-1022.
134. Kohler JJ, Nettles JH, Amblard F, et al. Approaches to hepatitis C treatment and cure using NS5A inhibitors. *Infect Drug Resist.* 2014;7:41-56.
135. Shen J, Serby M, Reed A, et al. Metabolism and disposition of hepatitis C polymerase inhibitor dasabuvir in humans. *Drug Metab Dispos.* 2016;44:1139-1147.
136. Ahmed H, Abushouk AI, Menshawy A, et al. Safety and efficacy of ombitasvir/paritaprevir/ritonavir and dasabuvir with or without ribavirin for treatment of hepatitis C virus genotype 1: a systematic review and meta-analysis. *Clin Drug Investig.* 2017;37:1009-1023.
137. Wagner R, Randolph JT, Patel SV, et al. Highlights of the structure-activity relationships of benzimidazole linked pyrrolidines leading to the discovery of the hepatitis C virus NS5A inhibitor pibrentasvir (ABT-530). *J Med Chem.* 2018;61:4052-4066.
138. Kwo PY, Poordad F, Asatryan A, et al. Glecaprevir and pibrentasvir yield high response rates in patients with HCV genotype 1-6 without cirrhosis. *J Hepatol.* 2017;67:263-271.
139. El Kassas M, Elbaz T, Hafez E, et al. Discovery and preclinical development of dasabuvir for the treatment of hepatitis C infection. *Expert Opin Drug Discov.* 2017;12:635-642.
140. Kayali Z, Schmidt WN. Finally sofosbuvir: an oral anti-HCV drug with wide performance capability. *Pharmgenomics Pers Med.* 2014;7:387-398.
141. Kirby BJ, Symonds WT, Kearney BP, et al. Pharmacokinetic, pharmacodynamic, and drug-interaction profile of the hepatitis C virus NS5B polymerase inhibitor sofosbuvir. *Clin Pharmacokinet.* 2015;54:677-690.
142. Heo YA, Deeks ED. Sofosbuvir/velpatasvir/voxilaprevir: a review in chronic hepatitis C. *Drugs.* 2018;78:577-587.

CHAPTER **31**

Drugs Used to Treat Fungal Infections

Robert K. Griffith

Drugs covered in this chapter[a]:

POLYENES
- Amphotericin B
- Natamycin
- Nystatin

AZOLES
- Butoconazole
- Clotrimazole
- Econazole
- Efinaconazole
- Fluconazole
- Flutrimazole
- Isavuconazole
- Itraconazole
- Ketoconazole
- Luliconazole
- Miconazole
- Oxiconazole
- Posaconazole
- Sertaconazole
- Sulconazole
- Terconazole
- Tioconazole
- Voriconazole

ALLYL AMINES
- Butenafine
- Naftifine
- Terbinafine

ECHINOCANDINS
- Anidulafungin
- Caspofungin
- Micafungin

MISCELLANEOUS
- *Amorolfine*[a]
- Ciclopirox
- Flucytosine
- Griseofulvin
- Tavaborole
- Tolnaftate
- Undecylenic acid

[a]Not approved for market in the United States, but is approved in Australia and the UK and can readily be purchased online.

Abbreviations

AUC area under the curve
CNS central nervous system
CYP450 cytochrome P450
5-FU 5-fluorouracil
IC_{50} median inhibitory concentration
IV intravenous
spp multiple species

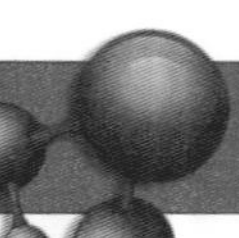

CLINICAL SIGNIFICANCE

Douglas Slain, PharmD, BCPS, FCCP, FASHP

Antifungal agents include diverse compounds with varied actions. A few key examples can highlight the importance of medicinal chemistry to clinical practice. Understanding the molecular structure of polyene antifungal agents such as amphotericin B is essential in understanding how they work. These agents are macrocyclic lactones with distinct hydrophilic and lipophilic regions. One of the putative mechanisms of polyene action involves the formation of pores in the fungal cell membrane. The lipophilic regions of the polyene molecules facilitate the binding to the cell membrane sterols. The hydrophilic portions of the molecule align to create a hydrophilic pore in the sterol-containing cell membrane. As a result, there is membrane depolarization and increased membrane permeability, and eventual fungal cell death. The lipophilic regions of amphotericin B also contribute to its poor solubility in aqueous solutions. The traditional intravenous formulation of amphotericin B includes a dispersing agent, deoxycholate, which facilitates formation of the required micellular dispersion when administered in a 5% dextrose in water solution.

5-Flucytosine (5-FC) is an analogue of the natural pyrimidine cytosine that is converted to 5-fluorouracil (5-FU) in susceptible fungi. Metabolic formation of the 5-FU is essential to the antimycotic effect of 5-FC. 5-FU acts as a pyrimidine antimetabolite and is phosphorylated to the cytotoxic agent 5-fluorodeoxyuridine monophosphate. Readers are probably aware that 5-FU is a chemotherapeutic agent that causes myelosuppression as its major toxicity. Therefore, it should not be surprising that the same side effect can be seen in patients receiving 5-FC.

The triazole antifungals are the most widely used class of antifungal agent used for serious systemic infections. The agents in this class include fluconazole, itraconazole, voriconazole, posaconazole, and the newer isavuconazole (administered as the prodrug isavuconazonium sulfate). With the exception of narrow spectrum fluconazole, the other agents are nonpolar with higher lipophilicity. It is therefore difficult to make intravenous (IV) formulations of these nonpolar agents, which are needed for serious infections. To overcome this difficulty, itraconazole, posaconazole, and voriconazole are administered with a cyclodextrin carrier molecule to facilitate aqueous IV solubility. Cyclodextrins are not advocated for patients with poor renal function due to the possibility of contributing to renal dysfunction. By administering isavuconazole as a water-soluble prodrug, an intravenous formulation can be made without a cyclodextrin. The prodrug undergoes rapid hydrolysis to form the active isavuconazole. Thus an understanding of the metabolic fate of a drug and its conversion to an active drug is critical to understanding the use of this drug.

INTRODUCTION

Because most humans with a normally functioning immune system are able to ward off invading fungal pathogens with little difficulty, the demand for improvements in antifungal therapy had been low until in recent decades a dramatic increase in immunocompromised patients has led to a similarly dramatic increase in potentially lethal invasive fungal infections. The onset of the AIDS epidemic, combined with the increased use of powerful immunosuppressive drugs for organ transplants, cancer chemotherapy, and recent introduction of several monoclonal antibody drugs, has resulted in a greatly increased incidence of life-threatening fungal infections and a corresponding increase in demand for new agents to treat these infections. The number of effective antifungal agents available is quite small compared to that available to treat bacterial infections, but research in this area is quite active. Several new agents have been introduced in the last few years, but more are needed.[1]

FUNGAL DISEASES

The fungal kingdom includes yeasts, molds, rusts, and mushrooms. Most fungi are saprophytic, which means that they live on dead organic matter in the soil or on decaying leaves or wood. Few fungi cause disease in humans (Table 31.1), and those that do can be limited to superficial topical infections, systemic, or both. A few of these fungi can cause opportunistic infections if they are introduced into a human through wounds or by inhalation. Some of these infections can be fatal. There are relatively few obligate animal parasites (i.e., microorganisms that can only live on mammalian hosts) among the fungi, although *Candida albicans* is commonly found as part of the normal flora of the gastrointestinal tract and vagina. The obligatory parasites are limited to dermatophytes that have evolved to live on/in the keratin-containing hair and skin of mammals, where they cause diseases such as ringworm and athletes foot. (Ringworm is not caused by a parasitic worm, but rather is named for the ringlike appearance of this fungal infection of the skin.) A detailed description of fungal infections is beyond the scope of this chapter, but comprehensive treatises are available.[2]

Most fungal infections are caused primarily by various yeasts and molds. Yeasts, such as the opportunistic pathogen *Candida albicans* and the bakers' yeast *Saccharomyces cerevisiae*, typically grow as single oval cells and reproduce by budding. *Candida albicans* and some other pathogenic yeasts also can grow in multicellular chains called hyphae. Infection sites may contain both yeast and hyphal forms of the microorganism. Molds, such as *Trichophyton rubrum*, one of the causative agents of ringworm, grow in clusters of hyphae called a mycelium. All fungi produce spores, which may be transported by direct contact or through the air. Although most topical fungal infections are readily treated, the incidence of life-threatening systemic fungal infections, including those caused by yeasts such as *Candida albicans* and molds such as *Aspergillus fumigatus* are increasing, and mortality is high.[3]

Dermatophytes

Dermatophytes are fungi causing infections of the skin, hair, and nails.[4] The dermatophytes obtain nutrients from attacking the cross-linked structural protein keratin, which other fungi cannot use as a food source. Dermatophytic infections, known as tinea, are caused by various species of three genera (*Trichophyton*, *Microsporum*, and *Epidermophyton*) and are named for the site of infection rather than for the causative organism. Tinea capitis is a fungal infection of the hair and scalp. Tinea pedis refers to infections of the feet, including athlete's foot, tinea manuum to fungal infection of the hands, tinea cruris to infection of the groin (jock itch), tinea unguium to infection of the fingernails or toenails, and tinea corporis to ring-shaped infections of the torso. Tinea corporis is more commonly known as ringworm even though there are no worms involved. Athlete's foot in particular may be an infection involving several different fungi, including yeasts. Tinea unguium, also known as onychomycosis,

Table 31.1 Common Infectious Fungal Organisms

Disease State	Common Organisms	Topical/ Systemic
Dermatomycosis: • Tinea capitis • Tinea pedis (athlete foot) • Tinea cruris (jock itch) • Tinea unguium (nail infection) • Tinea corporis (ringworm)	*Epidermophyton* *Microsporum* *Trichophyton*	Topical
Aspergillosis	*Aspergillus fumigatus, niger, flavus*	Systemic
Blastomycosis	*Blastomyces*	Systemic
Candidiasis	*Candida albicans*	Topical/ systemic
Coccidioidomycosis, valley fever	*Coccidioides immitis*	Systemic
Cryptococcosis	*Cryptococcus neoformans*	Systemic
Histoplasmosis	*Histoplasma capsulatum*	Systemic
Mucormycosis	*Rhizopus, Mucor, Absidia*	Topical/ systemic
Pneumocystosis	*Pneumocystis jirovecii*	Systemic

whether of the fingernails or toenails, can be particularly difficult to treat because the fungi invade the nail itself which is difficult for drugs to penetrate. Appropriate drug therapy prevents the fungus from spreading to the newly formed nail. Penetration of drugs into previously existing nail is problematic, however, and with some drug regimens, the infection is not cured until an entirely new, fungus-free nail has grown in. Because this takes months, patient compliance with a lengthy drug regimen can be a problem.

Yeasts

The most common cause of yeast infections is *Candida albicans*, which is part of the normal flora in a significant portion of the population where it resides in the oropharynx, gastrointestinal tract, vagina, and surrounding skin.[5] It is the principal cause of vaginal yeast infections and oral yeast infections (thrush). These commonly occur in mucosal tissue when the normal population of flora has been disturbed by treatment of a bacterial infection with an antibiotic or when growth conditions are changed by hormonal fluctuations, such as occur in pregnancy. *Candida albicans* can cause infections of the skin and nails, although the latter are not common. In persons with healthy immune systems, *Candida* infections are limited to superficial infections of the skin and mucosa. In persons with impaired immune systems, however, *Candida albicans* also may cause deep-seated systemic infections, which can be fatal. Several other infections with *Candida* species occur, including *C. tropicalis*, *C. krusei*, *C. parapsilosis*, and *C. glabrata* (also known as *Torulopsis glabrata*). These organisms are becoming more common and often do not respond to antifungal therapy as readily as *Candida albicans*.

Cryptococcus neoformans is a yeast commonly found in bird droppings, particularly pigeon droppings.[6] When dust contaminated with spores is inhaled by persons with a competent immune system, the organism causes a minor self-limiting lung infection. Such infections frequently are mistaken for a cold, and medical treatment is not sought. In immunocompromised persons, however, the organism can be carried by the circulatory system from the lungs to many other organs of the body, including the central nervous system (CNS). Infection of the CNS is uniformly fatal unless treated.

Although most yeast infections are caused by various species of *Candida* or *Cryptococcus*, other yeasts also can cause infections in humans, including *Malassezium furfur*, *Trichosporon beigelii*, and *Blastoschizomyces capitatus*.[7] These infections are relatively rare and are difficult to treat.

Molds

Various *Aspergillus* species are found worldwide and are virtually ubiquitous in the environment.[8] The most common organisms causing disease are *A. fumigatus*, *A. niger*, and *A. flavus*. Several other *Aspergillus* species are known to cause infection and some, such as *A. nidulans*, are becoming more common. *Aspergillus* spp. very rarely cause disease in persons with normal immune systems but are very dangerous to persons with suppressed immune systems. Because *Aspergillus* spores are found everywhere, inhalation is the most common route of inoculation, but infection through wounds, burns, and implanted devices (e.g., catheters) is also possible. Nosocomial (hospital-derived) aspergillosis is a major source of infection in persons with leukemia and in those receiving organ or bone marrow transplants. Aspergillosis of the lungs may be contained, but systemic aspergillosis has a high mortality rate.

Zygomycosis (mucormycosis) is a term used to describe infections caused by the genera *Rhizopus*, *Mucor*, and *Absidia* of the fungal order Mucorales.[9] As with several other opportunistic fungal pathogens, these soil microorganisms generally are harmless to those with a competent immune system but can cause rapidly developing, fatal infections in an immunosuppressed patient. These organisms can infect the sinus cavity, from which they spread rapidly to the CNS. Blood vessels also may be attacked and ruptured, and Zygomycoses spread rapidly and are often fatal.

Endemic Mycoses

The group of fungi known as endemic mycoses or thermally dimorphic fungi is saprophytes that grow in one form at room temperature and in a different form in a human host at 37°C.[10] The most common infectious agents are *Blastomyces dermatitidus*, *Paracoccidiodes brasiliensis*, *Coccidioides immitus*, and *Histoplasma capsulatum*, the causative agents of blastomycosis, paracoccidiomycosis, coccidiomycosis (valley fever), and histoplasmosis, respectively. All these organisms live in soil and cause disease through inhalation of contaminated dust. The resulting lung infections are often mild and self-limiting, but they may progress on to a serious lung infection. The circulatory system may transport the organisms to other tissues, where the resulting systemic infection may be fatal. *Blastomyces dermatitidus* is endemic to South Central United States and *P. brasiliensis* to Central and South America, where it is the most common cause of fungal pulmonary infections. *Coccidioides immitus* is endemic to the dry areas of the Southwestern United States and Northern Mexico. It is particularly prevalent in the San Joaquin Valley of California, hence the name valley fever. *Histoplasma capsulatum* is endemic to the Mississippi and Ohio River valleys of the United States, where nearly 90% of the population tests positive for exposure to the organism.

BIOCHEMICAL TARGETS OF ANTIFUNGAL CHEMOTHERAPY

Antifungal chemotherapy depends on biochemical differences between fungi and mammals.[1] Unlike bacteria, which are prokaryotes, both fungi and mammals are eukaryotes, and the biochemical differences between them are not as great as one might expect. At the cellular level, the greatest difference between fungal cells and mammalian cells is that fungal cells have cell walls but that mammalian cells do not. The fungal cell wall is a logical target for a similar class of drugs, which would be expected to be potent antifungals yet have little human toxicity. However, only a few potent inhibitors of fungal cell wall biosynthesis have become available for clinical use.[11,12] Other targets for antifungal agents include inhibitors of DNA biosynthesis, disruption of mitotic spindles, and general interference with intermediary metabolism. The difference between fungal and mammalian cells that is most widely exploited, however, is that the cell membranes of fungi and mammals contain different sterols. Mammalian cell membranes contain cholesterol as the sterol component, whereas fungi contain ergosterol.[13]

Cholesterol

Ergosterol

Although the two sterols are quite similar, the side chains are slightly different, and when three-dimensional models are constructed, the ring system of ergosterol is slightly flatter because of the additional double bonds in the B ring. Nevertheless, with only a few exceptions, this difference in sterol components provides the biochemical basis of selective toxicity for most of the currently available antifungal drugs.

Polyene Membrane Disruptors: Nystatin, Amphotericin B, and Natamycin

Before the mid-1950s, no reliable treatments existed for the few cases of deep-seated, highly lethal, systemic fungal infections that did occur. The discovery of the polyene antifungal agents (Fig. 31.1) provided a breakthrough and the first drug found to be effective against deep-seated fungal infections.[14]

The polyenes are macrocyclic lactones with distinct hydrophilic and lipophilic regions. The hydrophilic region contains several alcohols, a carboxylic acid, and usually, a sugar. The lipophilic region contains, in part, a

Nystatin

Amphotericin B

Natamycin

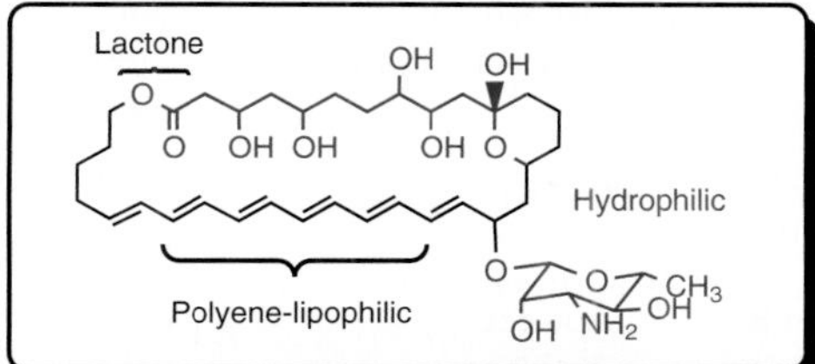

Figure 31.1 Commercially available polyenes. Insert indicates chemical features of this class of antifungal agents.

chromophore of four to seven conjugated double bonds. The number of conjugated double bonds correlates directly with antifungal activity in vitro and inversely with the degree of toxicity to mammalian cells. That is, not only are the compounds with seven conjugated double bonds, such as amphotericin B, approximately 10-fold more fungitoxic, amphotericin B is the only one that may be used systemically (Table 31.2).[15]

Polyene Mechanism of Action

The polyenes have an affinity for sterol-containing membranes, insert into those membranes, and disrupt membrane functions. The lipophilic polyene portion crosses the cell lipid bilayer forming a pore in the cell membrane. The membranes of cells treated with polyenes become leaky, and eventually, the cells die because of the loss of essential cell constituents, such as ions and small organic molecules.[16] Polyenes have a demonstrably higher affinity for membranes containing ergosterol over membranes containing cholesterol.[17] This is the basis for their greater toxicity to fungal cells. Some evidence suggests that the mechanism of insertion differs between the types of cells. Polyene molecules may insert individually into ergosterol-containing membranes but require prior formation of polyene micelles before inserting into cholesterol-containing membranes.

Specific Drugs

NYSTATIN. Nystatin is a conjugated tetraene isolated from cultures of the bacterium *Streptomyces noursei* in 1951.[14] Nystatin is an effective topical antifungal against a wide variety of organisms and is available in a variety of creams and ointments. Nystatin is too toxic to be used systemically, but because very little drug is absorbed following oral administration, it may be administered by mouth to treat fungal infections of the mouth and gastrointestinal tract.[18,19]

AMPHOTERICIN B. Amphotericin B, which as a heptaene, has low enough toxicity to mammalian cells to permit intravenous (IV) administration. Amphotericin B is nevertheless a very toxic drug and must be used with caution.[20] Adverse effects include fever, shaking chills, hypotension, and severe kidney toxicity. Despite its toxicity, amphotericin B is considered to be the drug of choice for many systemic, life-threatening fungal infections. The drug cannot cross the blood-brain barrier and must be administered intrathecally for treatment of fungal infections of the CNS.[21]

The nephrotoxicity of amphotericin B was a serious drawback to the use of this drug upon its introduction. However, the toxicity of the drug has been decreased substantially by changes in formulation (Table 31.2). More recently developed formulations of amphotericin B, such as liposomal encapsulation and lipid complexes, have dramatically decreased the toxicity of the drug which permits higher plasma levels to be employed.[22]

The mechanisms by which the new formulations decrease the toxicity are not entirely clear, but altered distribution is clearly a factor. Because the blood vessels at the site of infection are more permeable than those of normal tissue, the large suspended particles of the lipid formulations can penetrate the site of infection more readily than they can penetrate healthy tissue. The result is selective delivery of drug to the site of infection. Some evidence also indicates that the newer formulations transfer amphotericin B to ergosterol-containing fungal cells more efficiently than to cholesterol-containing mammalian cells.

NATAMYCIN. Natamycin, a tetraene, is available in the United States as a 5% suspension applied topically for the treatment of fungal infections of the eye (Table 31.2).

Table 31.2 Polyene Formulations

Generic Name	Trade Name	Dosage Form
Nystatin	Mycostatin, Nilstat, Nystex	Cream, ointment, powder
Natamycin	Natacyn	Ophthalmic solution
Amphotericin B Injection solution Lipid complex Liposomal	Abelcet AmBisome	Injectables

Ergosterol Biosynthesis Inhibitors

A schematic of fungal ergosterol biosynthesis starting from squalene is shown in Figure 31.2. The biosynthetic pathway has been simplified to emphasize steps important to the action of currently employed antifungal drugs.[1] The last nonsteroidal precursor to both ergosterol and cholesterol is the hydrocarbon squalene. Squalene is converted to squalene epoxide by the enzyme squalene epoxidase. Squalene epoxide is then cyclized to lanosterol, the first steroid in the pathway. The steps involved in converting the side chain of lanosterol to the side chain of ergosterol, and the steps in removal of the geminal dimethyl groups on position 4, are not shown, because none of these reactions is targeted by clinically employed antifungal agents.

A key step in conversion of lanosterol to both cholesterol and ergosterol is removal of the 14α-methyl group. This reaction is carried out by a cytochrome P450 enzyme, sterol-14α-demethylase, also known as cytochrome P450-51 (CYP51).[23] The mechanism of this reaction involves three successive hydroxylations of the 14α-methyl group, converting it from a hydrocarbon through the alcohol, aldehyde, and carboxylic acid oxidation states (Fig. 31.3). The methyl group is eliminated as formic acid to afford a double bond between C-14 and C-15 of the D ring. This enzyme is the primary target of the azole antifungal agents discussed below.

Eventually, either before or after modification of the side chain, the Δ^{14} double bond is reduced by a Δ^{14}-reductase to form a *trans* ring juncture between the C and D rings. Several steps later, the double bond between C-8

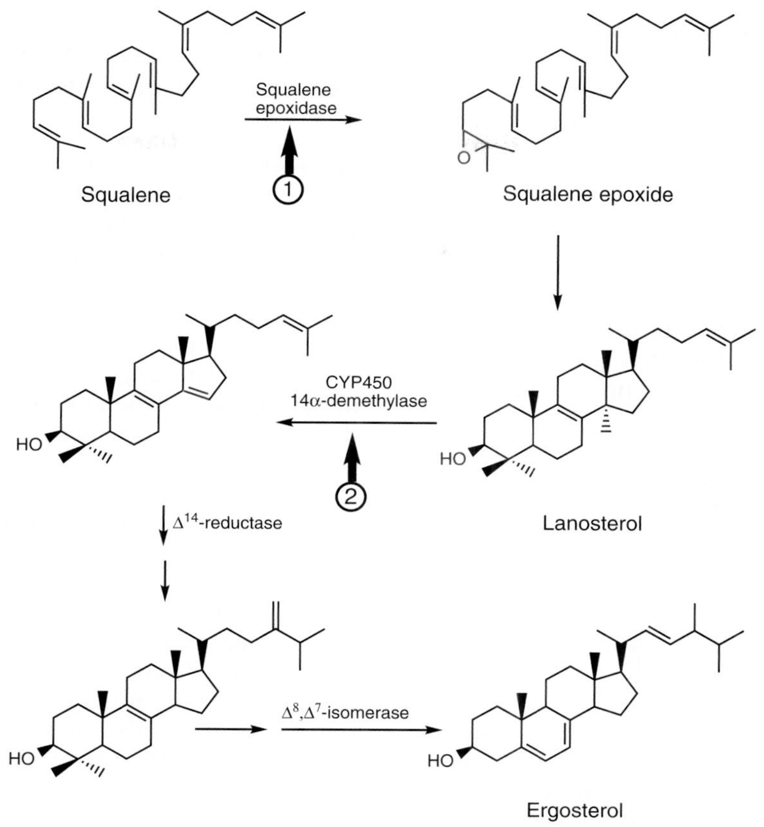

Squalene epoxidase
Squalene
1
Squalene epoxide
CYP450
14α-demethylase
HO
2
HO
Lanosterol
Δ[14]-reductase
Δ[8],Δ[7]-isomerase
HO
HO
Ergosterol

Figure 31.2 Key steps in the biosynthesis of ergosterol by fungi. Enzymatic steps known to be the site of action of currently employed anti-fungal agents are indicated by a heavy black arrow and a number.

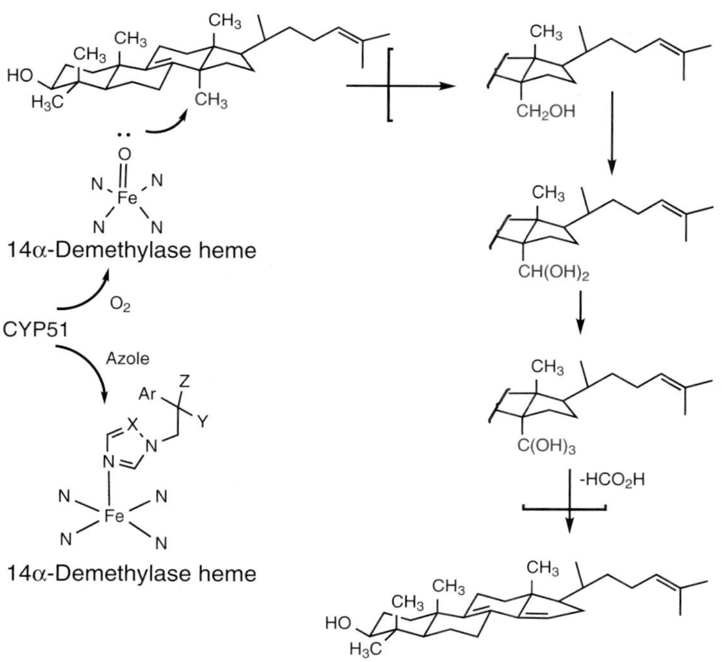

Figure 31.3 Demethylation of the 14α-methyl group from lanosterol via the CYP450 enzyme sterol 14α-demethylase, CYP51. Three successive heme catalyzed insertions of activated oxygen into the three carbon-hydrogen bonds of the 14α-methyl group which raises the oxidation state of the methyl group to a carboxylic acid. The azoles bind to CYP51 through the N3 atom of the azole preventing oxygen transfer.

and C-9 is isomerized to a Δ^7 double bond by the enzyme Δ^8,Δ^7-isomerase. Many of the steps are identical to those involved in mammalian cholesterol biosynthesis, and the basis for selective toxicity to fungal cells will be discussed under the specific agents.

Azoles—Imidazoles and Triazoles

The characteristic chemical feature of azoles from which their name is derived is the presence of a five-membered aromatic ring containing either two or three nitrogen atoms. Imidazole rings have two nitrogens and triazoles have three. In both cases, the azole ring is attached through N-1 to a side chain containing at least one aromatic ring.

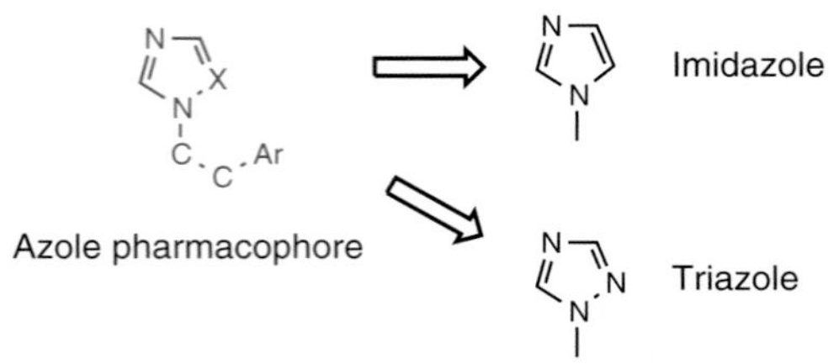

Azole pharmacophore

Imidazole

Triazole

Azole antifungal agents are the largest class of antimycotics available today, with more than 20 drugs on the market in the Unites States or other countries. The antifungal imidazoles (Fig. 31.4) are primarily used topically to treat superficial dermatophytic and yeast infections.

The antifungal triazoles (Fig. 31.5) are administered orally for the treatment of systemic fungal infections, or topically against dermatophytes. The oral bioavailability of some azoles, in contrast to amphotericin B, combined with their generally broad spectrum of activity has led to their widespread use in treating a variety of serious fungal infections.

Mechanism of Action. All antifungal azoles act by inhibiting ergosterol biosynthesis through inhibition of the 14α-demethylase, CYP51, discussed above under ergosterol biosynthesis (Fig. 31.2, Site 2). The basic N3 atom of the azole forms a bond with the heme iron of the CYP450 prosthetic group in the position normally occupied by the activated oxygen (Fig. 31.3). The remainder of the azole antifungal forms bonds with the apoprotein in a manner that determines the relative selectivity of the drug for the fungal demethylase versus other CYP450 enzymes.

Inhibition of the 14α-demethylase results in accumulation in the fungal cell membrane of sterols still bearing a 14α-methyl group. These sterols do not have the exact shape and physical properties of the normal membrane sterol ergosterol. This results in permeability changes, leaky membranes, and malfunction of membrane-imbedded proteins. These effects taken together lead to fungal cell death.[24] Biosynthesis of the mammalian membrane sterol cholesterol also employs a CYP450 14α-demethylase, but 14α-methyl sterols do not accumulate in human cell membranes because of the relative strength of inhibition of the same enzyme from different species. For example, the median inhibitory concentration (IC_{50}) for ketoconazole against the enzyme from *Candida albicans* is approximately 10^{-8} M versus approximately 10^{-6} M for mammalian enzymes.[25] This two orders of magnitude

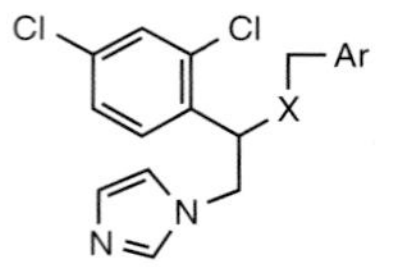

Generic name	Trade Name	X	Ar
Miconazole	Generic, Desenex, Fungoid, Monistat Oravig, Zeasorb	O	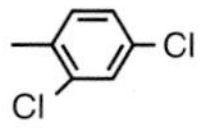
Econazole	Generic	O	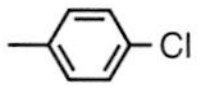
Sulconazole	Exelderm	S	Same
Sertaconazole	Ertaczo	O	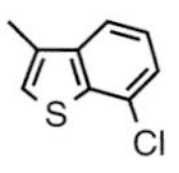
Tioconazole	Vagistat, TZ-3	O	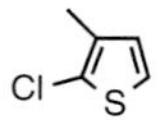

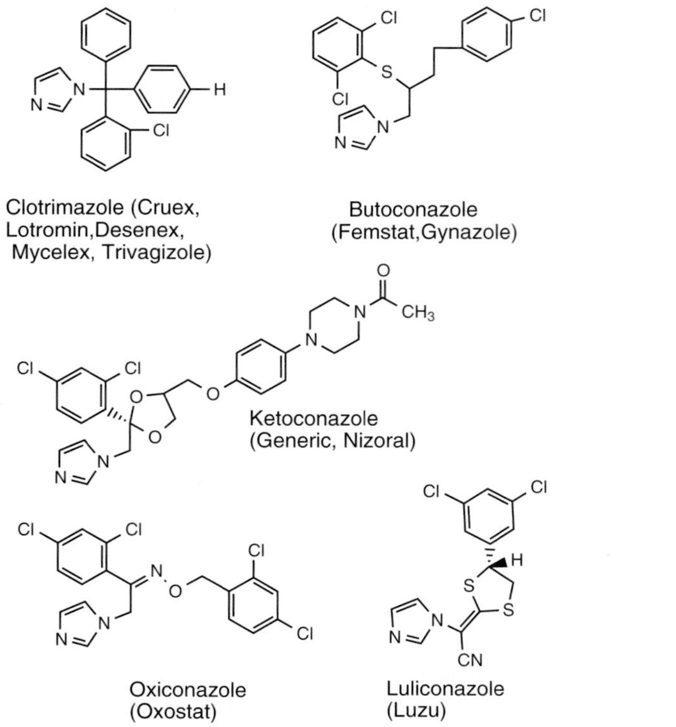

Clotrimazole (Cruex, Lotromin,Desenex, Mycelex, Trivagizole)

Butoconazole (Femstat,Gynazole)

Ketoconazole (Generic, Nizoral)

Oxiconazole (Oxostat)

Luliconazole (Luzu)

Figure 31.4 Imidazole antifungal agents. All imidazoles are used topically with the exception of ketoconazole which is available in both a topical and systemic dosage form.

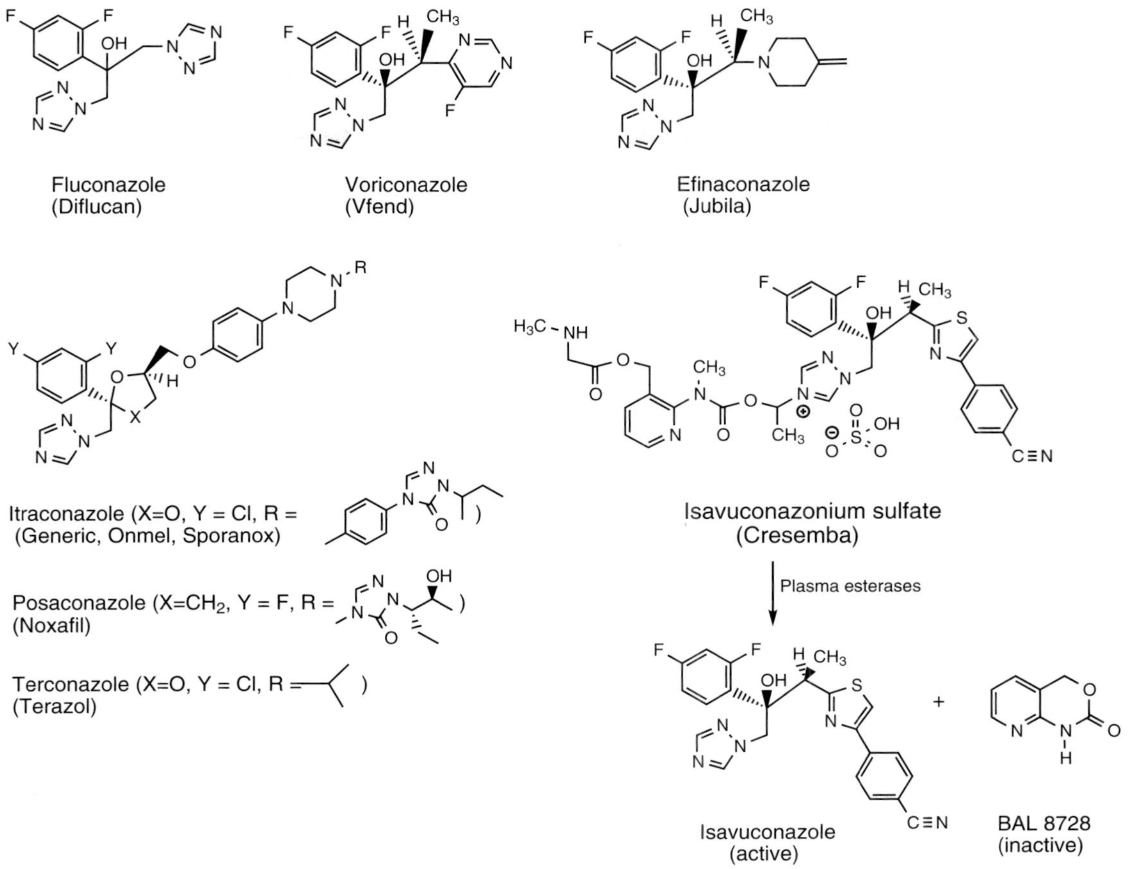

Figure 31.5 Triazole antifungal agents. While efinaconazole, isavuconazole, and terconazole are used topically, the remaining triazoles are used systemically.

difference in strength of inhibition provides the therapeutic index with respect to this particular enzyme. However, many of the azoles used systemically are inhibitors or substrates for other mammalian CYP450 enzymes (Table 31.3).

The early azole antifungal drugs were all either extensively and rapidly degraded by first-pass metabolism, or too toxic for systemic use. As a result, only those drugs with reduced or slow first-pass metabolism (ketoconazole, fluconazole, itraconazole, voriconazole, posaconazole, and isavuconazole) are used systemically.

The other azoles are available in a variety of creams and ointments for topical treatments of dermatophytic infections, and intravaginal use for vaginal yeast infections.

One recently introduced triazole, efinaconazole (Fig. 31.5), is the first azole to be employed in treatment of onychomycosis as a 10% solution applied topically to the infected nail.[26] The antifungal activity resides almost exclusively in the *R*,*R*-diastereomer.[27] The low affinity of efinaconazole for the nail protein keratin is thought to be a significant factor in the drug's effectiveness versus other topical antimycotics.[28]

Table 31.3 Azole as Inhibitors and Substrates for Cytochrome P450 Enzymes

	CYP Inhibitor	Substrate	Drug-Drug Interaction
Ketoconazole	1A2, 2C19, 3A4	3A4	Yes
Fluconazole	2C19, 2C9, 3A4	Low metabolism	Yes
Itraconazole	3A4	3A4	Yes
Voriconazole	2C19, 2C9, 3A4	2C19, 2C9, 3A4	Yes
Posaconazole	3A4	Low metabolism	Lower potential
Isavuconazole	3A4/5, 2C8, 2C19, 2D6, all weak	3A4	Lower potential

Specific Drugs Used Systemically

KETOCONAZOLE. Ketoconazole (Fig. 31.4), an imidazole, was the first orally active antifungal azole to be discovered and has been widely studied and employed for the treatment of systemic fungal infections, primarily candidiasis. Ketoconazole has little effect on *Aspergillus* or *Cryptococcus*. Ketoconazole is highly dependent on low stomach pH for absorption, and antacids or drugs that raise stomach pH will lower the bioavailability of ketoconazole. As with other azoles, it is extensively metabolized by microsomal enzymes (Fig. 31.6).

All the metabolites are inactive. CYP3A4 plays a significant role in metabolism of ketoconazole, and coadministration of CYP3A4 inducers, such as phenytoin, carbamazepine, and rifampin, can cause as much as a 50% reduction in levels of ketoconazole.[29] Ketoconazole also is a powerful inhibitor of human CYP3A4 and, as a consequence, has many serious interactions with other drugs. For example, coadministration of ketoconazole with the hypnotic triazolam results in a 22-fold increase in triazolam's area under the curve (AUC) and a 7-fold increase in half-life. Ketoconazole is also a weak inhibitor of CYP2C9, which is the enzyme responsible for the metabolism of several narrow therapeutic index drugs, such as warfarin and phenytoin. As better systemic agents have become available, ketoconazole's clinical use has generally become limited to topical applications in a variety of dosage forms, including creams, lotions, suppositories, and shampoos.

ITRACONAZOLE. Itraconazole, along with fluconazole, was one of the first triazoles introduced into clinical use (Fig. 31.5).[30] Itraconazole's oral bioavailability is variable and is influenced by food and stomach pH, a strongly acidic pH being required for good absorption. Like ketoconazole, itraconazole is extensively metabolized by CYP3A4 following oral administration (Fig. 31.6), and levels are markedly reduced by coadministration of the CYP3A4 inducers phenytoin, carbamazepine, and rifampin.[29] Additionally, like ketoconazole, itraconazole has been demonstrated to be a strong inhibitor of CYP3A4.[31] This interaction has

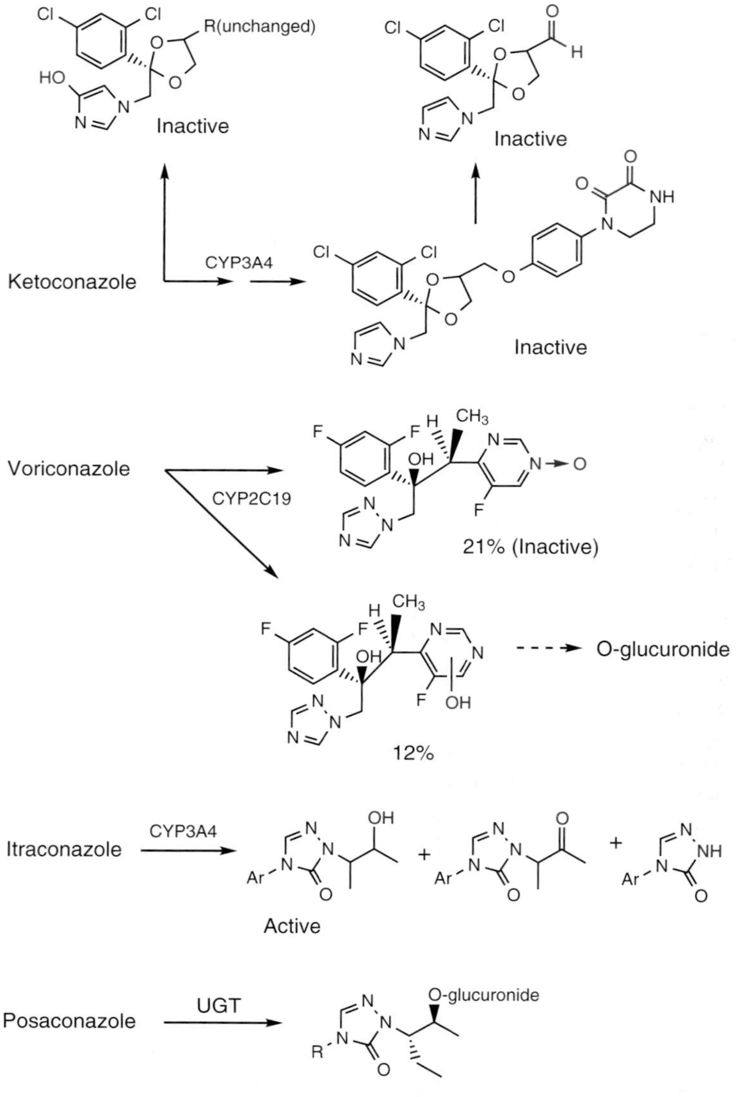

Figure 31.6 Major metabolic products formed from metabolism of systemic azoles.

proven to be of clinical significance because of the risk of developing rhabdomyolysis following lovastatin or simvastatin therapy with coadministration of itraconazole.[32–34] Itraconazole therefore is likely to have serious interactions with any other drug metabolized by CYP3A4. Like ketoconazole, itraconazole appears to have little or no effect on CYP2C9-mediated metabolism of warfarin and phenytoin.

FLUCONAZOLE. Fluconazole (Fig. 31.5), which was introduced at the same time as itraconazole, differs from ketoconazole and itraconazole in that it is equally bioavailable when given orally or IV. Fluconazole is not extensively metabolized and is mostly excreted unchanged.[35] Two major advantages of fluconazole over other antifungal agents are that it can cross the blood-brain barrier and has efficacy against *Cryptococcus neoformans*.[36] Fluconazole also differs in that it is only a weak inhibitor of CYP3A4 but a strong inhibitor of CYP2C9.[37] For instance, fluconazole doubles the AUC of (*S*)-warfarin (the active enantiomer) and greatly prolongs the prothrombin time in patients receiving warfarin anticoagulant therapy.[38] Because warfarin has such a narrow therapeutic index and excessive anticoagulation can be extremely harmful, this interaction is considered to be of major clinical significance. Fluconazole also decreases the metabolism of the CYP2C9 substrate phenytoin, an antiepileptic agent that also has a narrow therapeutic index.[39] Depending on the dose of fluconazole, coadministration with phenytoin can result in a 75% to 150% increase in the phenytoin AUC, and numerous case reports have documented substantial adverse effects following this regimen. Fluconazole also will inhibit CYP3A4, though not to the same degree as ketoconazole and itraconazole. Fluconazole exhibits a dose-dependent inhibition of triazolam metabolism (a CYP3A4 reaction) causing as much as a 4-fold increase in triazolam AUC.

VORICONAZOLE. Voriconazole (Fig. 31.5) is an analogue of fluconazole that was developed to overcome some of the limitations of fluconazole[40] and has a broader spectrum of activity than fluconazole, being active against *Aspergillus* and fluconazole-resistant strains of *Candida* and *Cryptococcus*.[41] Voriconazole is orally absorbed and penetrates the blood-brain barrier. Unfortunately, voriconazole is extensively metabolized CYP450 enzymes (Fig. 31.6) and is an inhibitor of CYP2C19, CYP2C9, and CYP3A4, leading to many drug interactions.[42,43] Voriconazole exhibits nonlinear, saturable kinetics, and because CYP2C19 exhibits genetic polymorphisms, plasma levels can be higher in poor metabolizers versus extensive metabolizers.[44,45]

POSACONAZOLE. Posaconazole (Fig. 31.5) has a number of advantages over previous agents.[46,47] Posaconazole has a wide spectrum of activity compared to other azoles, particularly against *Aspergillus* and other increasingly common nosocomial infections resistant to treatment by other antifungal drugs. *Aspergillus* resistance to azole antifungals has been attributed to the unique presence in *Aspergillus* of two distinct 14α-demethylases CYP51A and CYP51B.[48] *Aspergillus* CYP51B is sensitive to fluconazole and itraconazole, but CYP51A remains functional, allowing the fungus to synthesize needed ergosterol. Posaconazole is active against both *Aspergillus* CYP51 enzymes accounting for its greater activity against the fungus compared to other azoles.[49]

Posaconazole is metabolized primarily by Phase II glucuronide conjugation (Fig. 31.6) and has little interaction with most oxidative CYP450 drug-metabolizing enzymes, but it is an inhibitor of CYP3A4.[50,51] Posaconazole is structurally similar to itraconazole and saperconazole, but it contains a tetrahydrofuran ring in place of the dioxolan ring of those agents, which may account for some of its unique properties.

ISAVUCONAZONIUM SULFATE AND ISAVUCONAZOLE. The prodrug isavuconazonium sulfate and its active metabolite isavuconazole (Fig. 31.5) are the newest triazoles for systemic use.[52,53] The prodrug isavuconazonium is available in both a water-soluble injectable formulation and capsules for oral administration. The prodrug is rapidly converted to the active form, isavuconazole, by plasma esterases. Isavuconazole is slowly but thoroughly further metabolized by CYP3A4 and 3A5 to a variety of inactive oxidized products (not shown) which are conjugated as glucuronides. Isavuconazole is a substrate for CYP3A4/5 and a weak inhibitor of CYP3A4, 2C8, 2C9, 2C19, and 2D6. Because the inhibition is weak, the potential for drug-drug interactions is small. Isavuconazole shows great promise as a systemic antifungal with a broad spectrum of activity.

Azole Antifungals and P-Glycoprotein

In addition to being substrates and inhibitors of various cytochrome P450 enzymes, azole antifungals can also be inhibitors and/or substrates for the multidrug resistance enzyme P-glycoprotein. As discussed in Chapter 3, P-glycoprotein is an ATP-dependent pump that expels some drugs from blood circulation into the lumen of the small intestine and is also a component part of the blood-brain barrier. Therefore P-glycoprotein is an important contributor to drug distribution and plasma levels and can be a major factor in drug-drug interactions. Fluconazole[54] and voriconazole[55] have little or no effect on P-glycoprotein, being neither substrates nor inhibitors. Itraconazole and ketoconazole bind tightly to P-glycoprotein and appear to be substrates for the transporter as well as strong inhibitors of its actions on other drugs.[54] Posaconazole is also both a substrate and inhibitor of P-glycoprotein,[56] whereas the most recently introduced triazole, isavuconazole is a weak inhibitor of P-glycoprotein.[52]

Allyl Amines

The group of agents generally known as allyl amines[57] includes naftifine, terbinafine, and butenafine (Fig. 31.7). One can consider the benzyl group of butenafine to be bioisosteric with the allyl group of naftifine and terbinafine. These drugs have a more limited spectrum of activity than the azoles and are effective only against dermatophytes. Therefore, they are employed in the treatment of fungal infections of the skin and nails.[58]

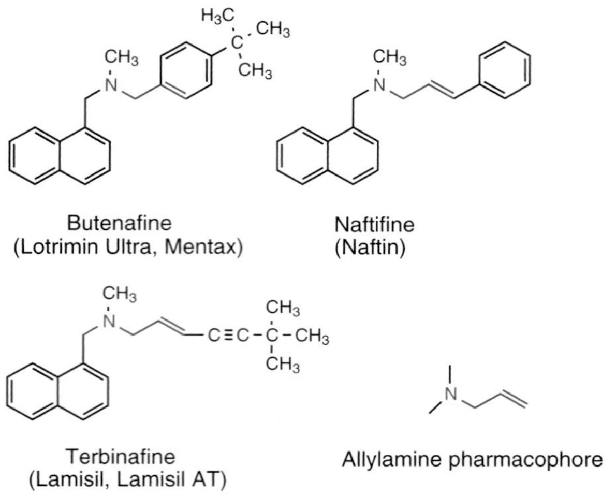

Butenafine
(Lotrimin Ultra, Mentax)

Naftifine
(Naftin)

Terbinafine
(Lamisil, Lamisil AT)

Allylamine pharmacophore

Figure 31.7 Allyl amine squalene epoxidase inhibitors. Butenafine and nafttifine are topical only. Terbinafine may be used topically or systemically.

MECHANISM OF ACTION. All of the drugs in Figure 31.7 act through inhibition of the enzyme squalene epoxidase (Fig. 31.2, Site 1). Inhibition of this enzyme has two effects, both of which appear to be involved in the fungitoxic mechanism of this class.[59] First, inhibition of squalene epoxidase results in a decrease in total sterol content of the fungal cell membrane. This decrease alters the physicochemical properties of the membrane, resulting in malfunctions of membrane-imbedded transport proteins involved in nutrient transport and pH balance. Second, inhibition of squalene epoxidase results in a buildup within the fungal cell of the hydrocarbon squalene, which is itself toxic when present in abnormally high amounts. Mammals also employ the enzyme squalene epoxidase in the biosynthesis of cholesterol, but a desirable therapeutic index arises from the fact that the fungal squalene epoxidase enzyme is far more sensitive to the allyl amines than the corresponding mammalian enzyme. Terbinafine has a K_i of 0.03 μM versus squalene epoxidase from *Candida albicans* but only 77 μM versus the same enzyme from rat liver—a 2,500-fold difference.[60]

Specific Drugs

NAFTIFINE. Naftifine (Fig. 31.7) was the first allyl amine to be discovered and marketed.[57] It is also too subject to extensive first-pass metabolism to be orally active and, consequently, is only available in topical preparations. The widest use of naftifine is against various tinea infections of the skin.

TERBINAFINE. Terbinafine (Fig. 31.7) is available in both topical and oral dosage forms and is effective against a variety of dermatophytic infections when employed topically or systemically.[60] A unique property of terbinafine is its effectiveness in the treatment of onychomycoses (nail infections).[61] Given orally, the highly lipophilic drug redistributes from the plasma into the nail bed and into the nail itself where the infection resides,[62,63] making terbinafine superior to other agents for treating this type of infection. Terbinafine is extensively metabolized by several CYP450 enzymes, including CYP1A2, CYP2C19, CYP2C9, CYP2C8, CYP3A4, and CYP2B6.[64] Because there are so many pathways for terbinafine metabolism, inhibition of any one has very little effect on overall clearance of the drug. Drugs that inhibit several CYP450 enzymes, such as cimetidine, can increase terbinafine plasma levels. Although not a substrate for the enzyme, terbinafine is a strong inhibitor of CYP2D6 and can have significant interactions with drugs that are metabolized by this enzyme, such as codeine and desipramine.[37,65] Terbinafine has also been associated with severe liver toxicity[66] and alcohol consumption should be avoided when taking terbinafine.

BUTENAFINE. Butenafine (Fig. 31.7), like naftifine, is only available in topical preparations for the treatment of dermatophytic infections. Butenafine is active against superficial *Candida albicans* infections[67] but is otherwise considered equivalent to naftifine.

Inhibitors of Cell Wall Biosynthesis—Echinocandins

The most notable difference between fungal and mammalian cells is that fungi have a cell wall and mammals do not, so drugs interfering with cell wall biosynthesis would be expected to be relatively nontoxic to mammals. Such drugs have been the foundation of antibacterial therapy since the discovery of penicillin and the development of dozens of effective penicillins and cephalosporins. However, only a few drugs affecting fungal cell wall biosynthesis have become available. Echinocandins (Fig. 31.8), a group of cyclic peptides with long lipophilic side chains, sometimes called lipopeptides, have been under investigation for a number of years.[68] Echinocandins interfere with cell wall biosynthesis through inhibition of the enzyme β-1,3-glucan synthase. β-Glucan is an important polymer component of many fungal cell walls, and reduction in the glucan content severely weakens the cell wall, leading to rupture of the fungal cell.[69]

Caspofungin, Anidulafungin, and Micafungin

Three semisynthetic echinocandins have been approved for use in treating life-threatening systemic fungal infections, caspofungin, anidulafungin, and micafungin (Fig. 31.8).[11] These are effective against a variety of *Candida* species that have proven to be resistant to other agents as well as effective against azole-resistant *Aspergillus*. Therefore, these drugs are truly life-saving for those afflicted with these previously resistant fungi. Unfortunately these echinocandins are not effective against *Cryptococcus neoformans*. None of these drugs is orally active, and all must be administered by IV infusion. Because of limited hepatic metabolism, drug-drug interactions are not a problem. Caspofungin is metabolized by hydrolysis in two portions of the hexapeptide ring (Fig. 31.9),[70] whereas anidulafungin does not appear to be actively metabolized but rather slowly degrades.[71] Micafungin is metabolized by a sulfotransferase and by catechol-O-methyltransferase (COMT), but no significant drug interactions are known.[72]

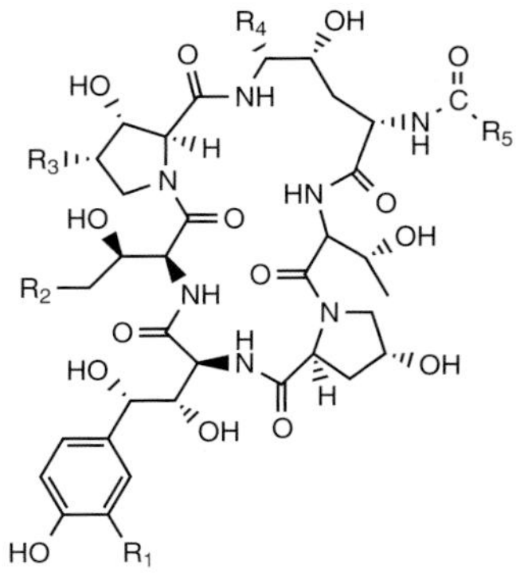

Drug	R_1	R_2	R_3	R_4	R_5
Caspofungin (Cancidas)	H	CH_2NH_2	H	$NHCH_2CH_2NH_2$	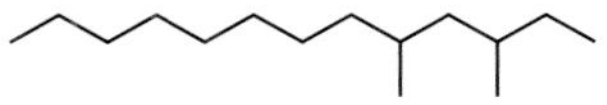
Anidulafungin (Eraxis)	H	H	CH_3	OH	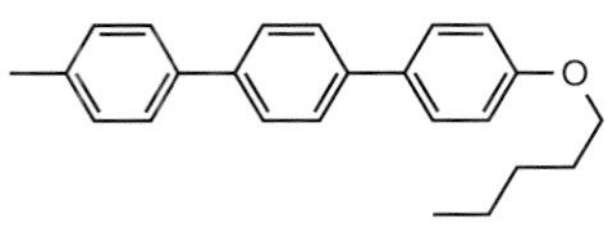
Micafungin (Mycamine)	OSO_3H	$CONH_2$	CH_3	OH	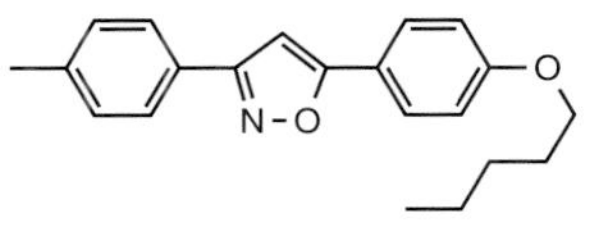

Figure 31.8 Echinocandins.

Miscellaneous Antifungals Acting Through Other Mechanisms

Amorolfine

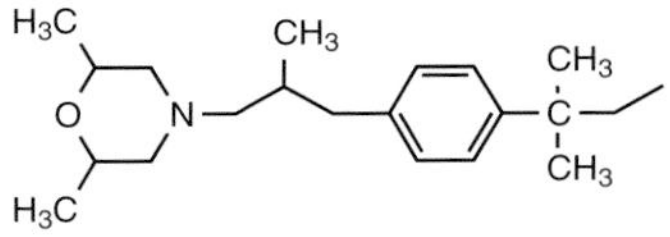

Amorolfine

Amorolfine is not FDA approved in the United States but is approved in the United Kingdom and Australia and can be purchased from a variety of online sources. Amorolfine is used topically to treat nail infections and has good penetration of the nail.[73] Amorolfine acts by inhibiting ergosterol biosynthesis through inhibition of Δ^{14}-reductase and Δ^8,Δ^7-isomerase (Fig. 31.1).[74] Inhibition of these enzymes results in incorporation into fungal cell membranes of sterols retaining a Δ^{14} double bond, a Δ^8 double bond, or both. None of these will have the same overall shape and physicochemical properties as the preferred sterol, ergosterol. As with the antifungals already discussed, this results in membranes with altered properties and malfunctioning of membrane-embedded proteins.

Flucytosine

Flucytosine is a powerful antifungal agent used in the treatment of serious systemic fungal infections, such as *Cryptococcus neoformans* and *Candida* spp. (Table 31.1).

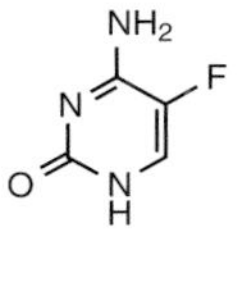

Flucytosine
(Ancobon)

Flucytosine itself is not cytotoxic but is a prodrug that is taken up by fungi and metabolized to 5-fluorouracil (5-FU) by fungal cytidine deaminase (Fig. 31.10).[75] Then 5-FU is converted to 5-fluorodeoxyuridine, a thymidylate synthase inhibitor that interferes with both protein and RNA biosynthesis. 5-Fluorouracil is cytotoxic and is employed in cancer chemotherapy (see Chapter 33). Human cells do not contain cytosine deaminase

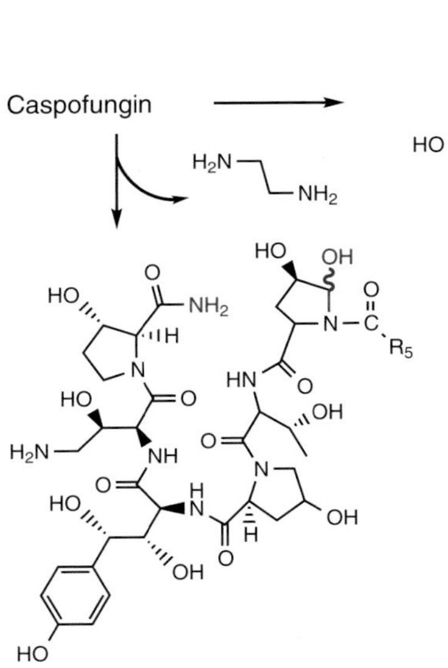

Caspofungin

Figure 31.9 Metabolic products formed from caspofungin.

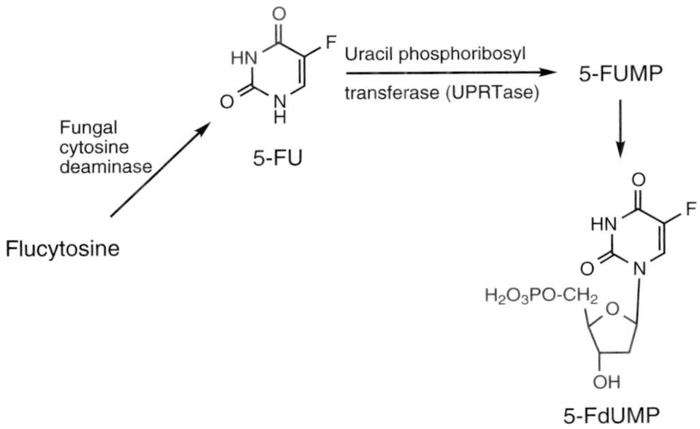

Flucytosine → Fungal cytosine deaminase → 5-FU → Uracil phosphoribosyl transferase (UPRTase) → 5-FUMP → 5-FdUMP

Figure 31.10 Metabolic activation of flucytosine by deamination, conjugated with ribosylphosphate to 5-fluorouracil monophosphate (5-FUMP) and onto 5-fluorodeoxyuridine monophosphate (5-FdUMP).

and therefore do not convert flucytosine to 5-FU. Some intestinal flora, however, do convert the drug to 5-FU, so human toxicity can result from this metabolism.[76] Resistance rapidly develops to flucytosine when used alone, so it is almost always used in conjunction with amphotericin B. Use of flucytosine has declined since the discovery of fluconazole.

Ciclopirox

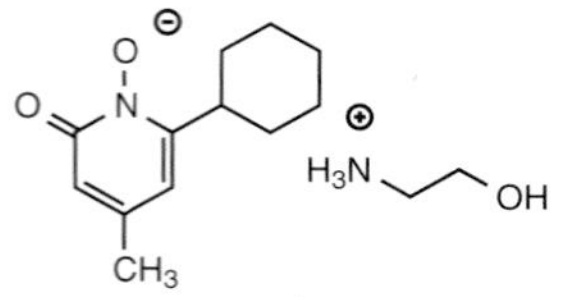

Ciclopirox olamine
(Loprox, Penlac)

Ciclopirox is a hydroxylated pyridinone that is employed for superficial dermatophytic infections, principally onychomycosis. The mechanism of action of ciclopirox is poorly understood but likely involves interference with many biochemical pathways through chelation of polyvalent cations, such as Fe^{3+}, which causes inhibition of a number of metal-dependent enzymes within the fungal cell.[77] Ciclopirox has been available for many years in a variety of topical dosage forms including formulation of an 8% lacquer for treating nail infections.[78]

Tolnaftate

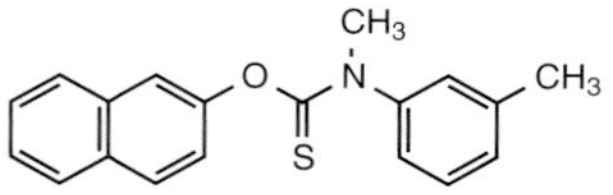

Tolnaftate

Tolnaftate is an old drug which was used topically to treat dermatophytic infections for years before its mechanism was discovered to be the same as the allyl amines, inhibition of squalene epoxidase.[79] Tolnaftate is widely employed in nonprescription antifungal preparations for treating athlete's foot.

Undecylenic Acid

$H_2C{=}CH(CH_2)_8COOH$

Undecylenic acid

Undecylenic acid is widely employed, frequently as the zinc salt, in over-the-counter preparations for topical treatment of infections by dermatophytes.[80] Undecylenic acid is fungistatic and acts through a nonspecific interaction with components in the fungal cell membrane.

Tavaborole

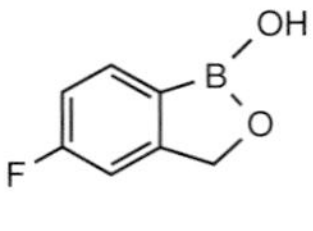

Tavaborole (Kerydin)

Tavaborole is a completely novel antifungal agent recently introduced for the treatment of onychomycosis (nail infections).[81,82] Tavaborole has excellent penetration of human nails when applied topically.[83] The mechanism of action is also unique in that inhibits protein biosynthesis by binding the terminal adenosine of leucine tRNA preventing peptide elongation (Fig. 31.11).[84]

Griseofulvin

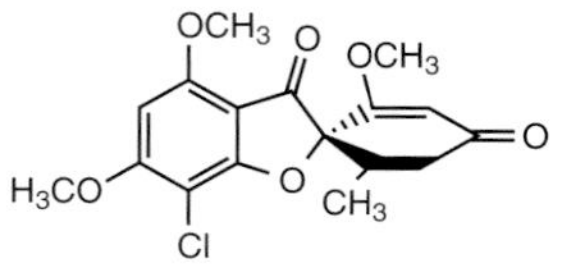

Griseofulvin

Griseofulvin is an antifungal antibiotic produced by an unusual strain of *Penicillium*.[85] It is used orally to treat superficial fungal infections, primarily fingernail and toenail infections, but it does not penetrate skin or nails if used topically. When given orally, however, plasma-borne griseofulvin becomes incorporated into keratin precursor cells and, ultimately, into keratin, which cannot then support fungal growth. The infection is cured when the diseased tissue is replaced by new uninfected tissue, which can take months. The mechanism of action of griseofulvin is binding to the protein tubulin, which interferes with the function of the mitotic spindle and thereby inhibits cell division. Griseofulvin also may interfere directly with DNA replication. Griseofulvin is gradually being replaced by newer agents.[86]

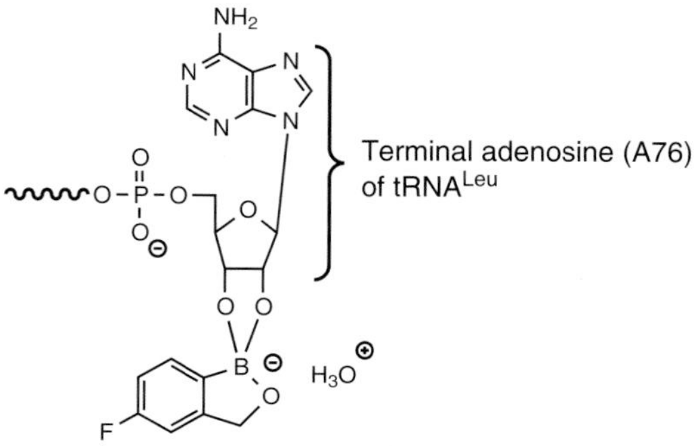

Terminal adenosine (A76) of $tRNA^{Leu}$

Figure 31.11 Binding between tavaborole and tRNA in the editing active site of leucine-tRNA synthetase (LeuRS).

Structure Challenge

The structures of 10 drugs discussed in this chapter are provided. Use your knowledge of drug chemistry to identify the agent or agents that would be the most appropriate answer for each statement below.

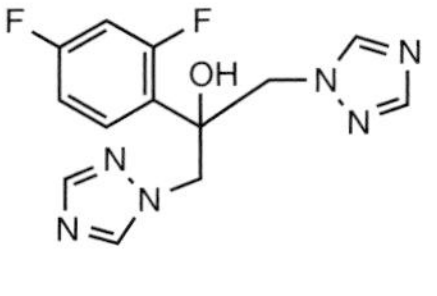

1 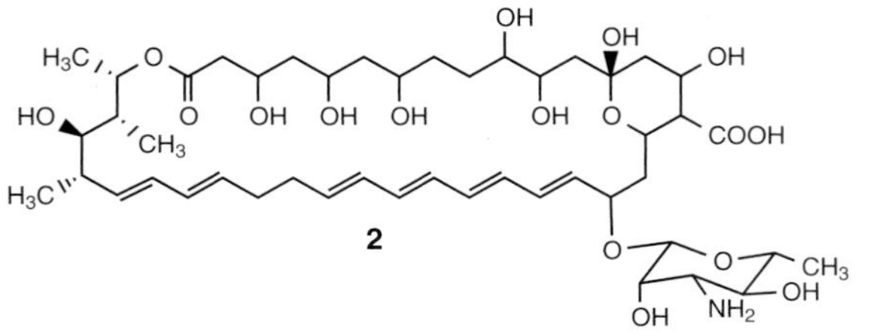 2 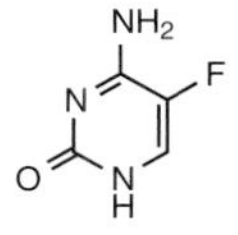 3 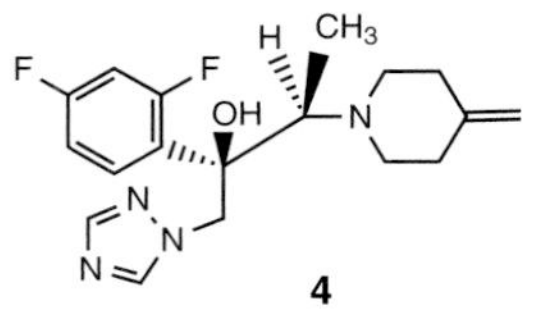 4

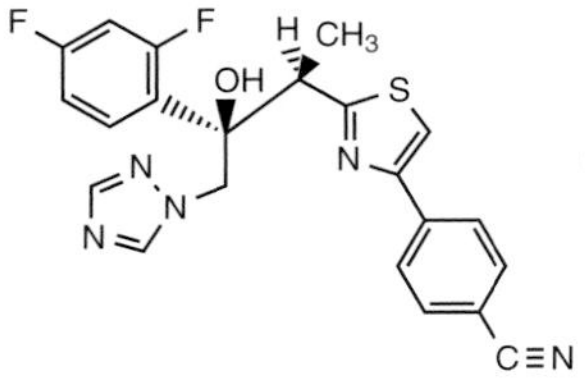

5 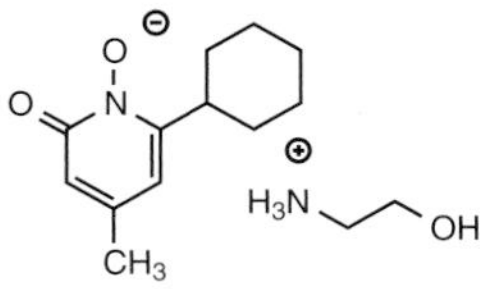 6 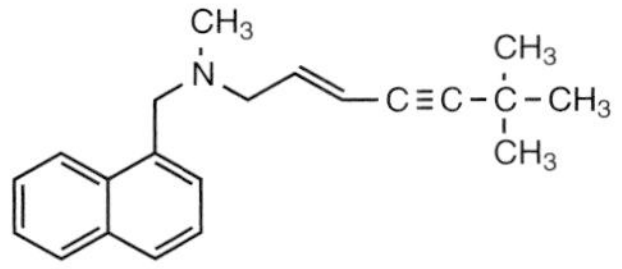 7 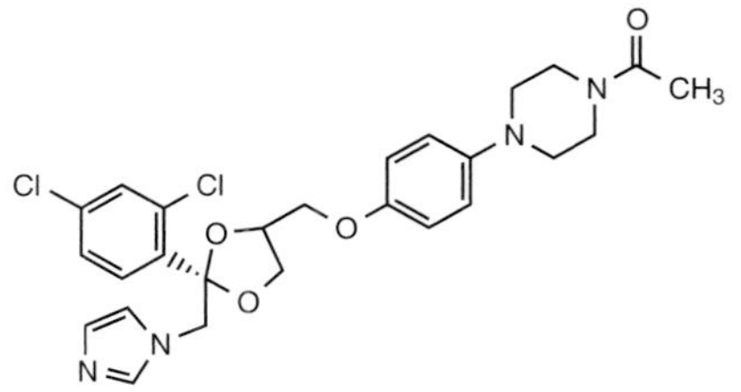 8

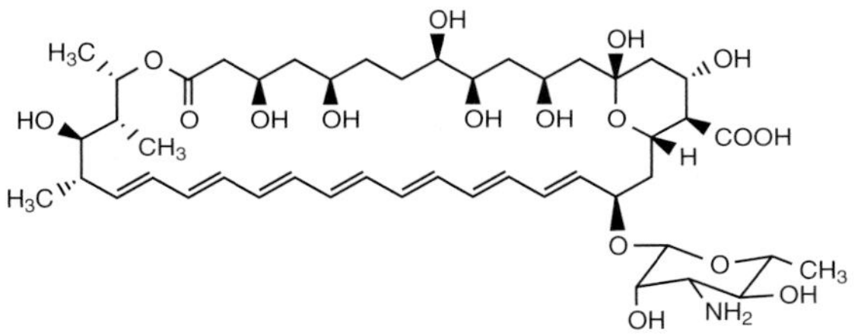

9 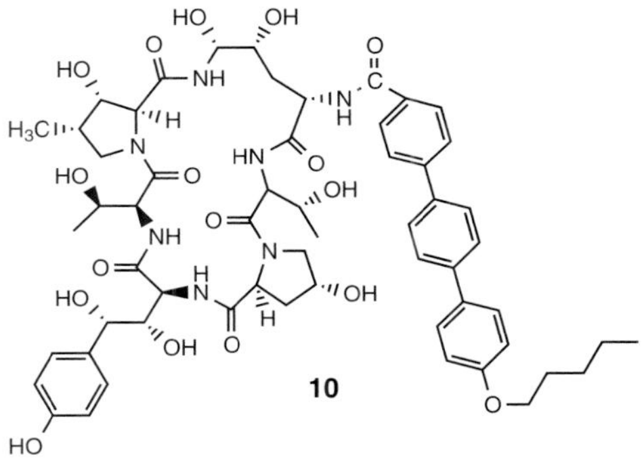 10

A. Acts by inhibiting fungal cell wall biosynthesis. #____
B. Can be given orally for oropharyngeal candidiasis but is too toxic for systemic use. #____
C. Is/are effective orally for treatment of onychomycoses. #____
D. Is a prodrug converted by fungi to the active antifungal agent. #____
E. Antifungal mechanism is inhibition of the enzyme sterol-14α-demethylase. #____
F. Applied topically for treatment of onychomycoses. #____

Structure Challenge answers found immediately after References.

REFERENCES

1. Campoy S, Adrio JL. Antifungals. *Biochem Pharmacol.* 2017;133:86-96.
2. Anaissie EJ, McGinnis MR, Pfaller MA. *Clinical Mycology*. 2nd ed. New York: Elsevier; 2009.
3. Lockhart SR, Diekema DJ, Pfaller MA. The epidemiology of fungal infections. In: Anaissie EJ, McGinnis MR, Pfaller MA, eds. *Clinical Mycology*. 2nd ed. New York: Elsevier; 2009:1-14.
4. Ghannoum MA, Isham NC. Dermatophytes and dermatophytoses. In: Anaissie EJ, McGinnis MR, Pfaller MA, eds. *Clinical Mycology*. 2nd ed. New York: Elsevier; 2009:375-384.
5. Dignani MC, Solomkin JS, Anaissie EJ. Candida. In: Anaissie EJ, McGinnis MR, Pfaller MA, eds. *Clinical Mycology*. 2nd ed. New York: Elsevier; 2009:197-229.
6. Viviani MA, Tortorano AM. Cryptococcus. In: Anaissie EJ, McGinnis MR, Pfaller MA, eds. *Clinical Mycology*. 2nd ed. Elsevier; 2009:231-249.
7. Pfaller MA, Diekema DJ, Merz WG. Infections caused by non-Candida, non-Cryptococcus yeasts. In: Anaissie EJ, McGinnis MR, Pfaller MA, eds. *Clinical Mycology*. 2nd ed. Elsevier; 2009:251-270.
8. Malcolm D, Richardson KB, Hope W. Aspergillus. In: Anaissie EJ, McGinnis MR, Pfaller MA, eds. *Clinical Mycology*. 2nd ed. Elsevier; 2009:271-296.
9. Ostrosky-Zeichner L, Smith M, McGinnis MR. Zygomycosis. In: Anaissie EJ, McGinnis MR, Pfaller MA, eds. *Clinical Mycology*. 2nd ed. Elsevier; 2009:297-307.
10. Anstead GM, Patterson TF. Endemic mycoses. In: Anaissie EJ, McGinnis MR, Pfaller MA, eds. *Clinical Mycology*. 2nd ed. Elsevier; 2009:355-373.

11. Denning DW. Echinocandin antifungal drugs. *Lancet.* 2003;362:1142-1151.
12. Zaas AK, Alexander BD. Echinocandins: role in antifungal therapy, 2005. *Expert Opin Pharmacother.* 2005;6:1657-1668.
13. Koller W. Antifungal agents with target sites in sterol functions and biosynthesis. In: Koller W, ed. *Target Sites of Fungicide Action.* Boca Raton. CRC Press; 1992:119-206.
14. Hamilton-Miller JM. Chemistry and biology of the polyene macrolide antibiotics. *Bacteriol Rev.* 1973;37:166-196.
15. Kotler-Brajtburg J, Medoff G, Kobayashi GS, et al. Classification of polyene antibiotics according to chemical structure and biological effects. *Antimicrob Agents Chemother.* 1979;15:716-722.
16. Bolard J. Interaction of polyene antibiotics with membrane lipids: physicochemical studies of the molecular basis of selectivity. *Drugs Exp Clin Res.* 1986;12:613-618.
17. Cotero BV, Rebolledo-Antunez S, Ortega-Blake I. On the role of sterol in the formation of the amphotericin B channel. *Biochim Biophys Acta.* 1998;1375:43-51.
18. Hellfritzsch M, Pottegard A, Pedersen AJ, et al. Topical antimycotics for oral candidiasis in warfarin users. *Basic Clin Pharmacol Toxicol.* 2017;120:368-372.
19. Russo A, Carriero G, Farcomeni A, Ceccarelli G, Tritapepe L, Venditti M. Role of oral nystatin prophylaxis in cardiac surgery with prolongedextracorporeal circulation. *Mycoses.* 2017; 60:826-829.
20. Laniado-Laborin R, Cabrales-Vargas MN. Amphotericin B: side effects and toxicity. *Rev Iberoam Micol.* 2009;26:223-227.
21. Ho J, Fowler P, Heidari A, Johnson RH. Intrathecal amphotericin B: a 60-year experience in treating coccidioidal meningitis. *Clin Infect Dis.* 2017;64:519-524.
22. Wong-Beringer A, Jacobs RA, Guglielmo BJ. Lipid formulations of amphotericin B: clinical efficacy and toxicities. *Clin Infect Dis.* 1998;27:603-618.
23. Lepesheva GI, Waterman MR. Sterol 14alpha-demethylase cytochrome P450 (CYP51), a P450 in all biological kingdoms. *Biochim Biophys Acta.* 2007;1770:467-477.
24. Prasad R, Shah AH, Rawal MK. Antifungals: mechanism of action and drug resistance. *Adv Exp Med Biol.* 2016;892:327-349.
25. Bossche HV, Janssen PA. Target sites of sterol biosynthesis inhibitors: secondary activities on cytochrome P-450 dependent reactions. In: Koller W, ed. *Target Sites of Fungicide Action.* Boca Raton: CRC Press; 1992:227-254.
26. Patel T, Dhillon S. Efinaconazole: first global approval. *Drugs.* 2013;73:1977-1983.
27. Tatsumi Y, Yokoo M, Arika T, Yamaguchi H. In vitro antifungal activity of KP-103, a novel triazole derivative, and its therapeutic efficacy against experimental plantar tinea pedis and cutaneous candidiasis in Guinea pigs. *Antimicrob Agents Chemother.* 2001;45:1493-1499.
28. Sugiura K, Sugimoto N, Hosaka S, et al. The low keratin affinity of efinaconazole contributes to its nail penetration and fungicidal activity in topical onychomycosis treatment. *Antimicrob Agents Chemother.* 2014;58:3837-3842.
29. Tucker RM, Denning DW, Hanson LH, et al. Interaction of azoles with rifampin, phenytoin, and carbamazepine: in vitro and clinical observations. *Clin Infect Dis.* 1992;14:165-174.
30. Warnock DW. Itraconazole and fluconazole: new drugs for deep fungal infection. *J Antimicrob Chemother.* 1989;24:275-277.
31. Colburn DE, Giles FJ, Oladovich D, Smith JA. In vitro evaluation of cytochrome P450-mediated drug interactions between cytarabine, idarubicin, itraconazole and caspofungin. *Hematology.* 2004;9:217-221.
32. Horn M. Coadministration of itraconazole with hypolipidemic agents may induce rhabdomyolysis in healthy individuals. *Arch Dermatol.* 1996;132:1254.
33. Neuvonen PJ, Jalava KM. Itraconazole drastically increases plasma concentrations of lovastatin and lovastatin acid. *Clin Pharmacol Ther.* 1996;60:54-61.
34. Vlahakos DV, Manginas A, Chilidou D, Zamanika C, Alivizatos PA. Itraconazole-induced rhabdomyolysis and acute renal failure in a heart transplant recipient treated with simvastatin and cyclosporine. *Transplantation.* 2002;73:1962-1964.
35. Brammer KW, Farrow PR, Faulkner JK. Pharmacokinetics and tissue penetration of fluconazole in humans. *Rev Infect Dis.* 1990;12:S318-S326.
36. Bailey EM, Krakovsky DJ, Rybak MJ. The triazole antifungal agents: a review of itraconazole and fluconazole. *Pharmacotherapy.* 1990;10:146-153.
37. Venkatakrishnan K, von Moltke LL, Greenblatt DJ. Effects of the antifungal agents on oxidative drug metabolism: clinical relevance. *Clin Pharmacokinet.* 2000;38:111-180.
38. Kunze KL, Wienkers LC, Thummel KE, Trager WF. Warfarin-fluconazole I. Inhibition of the human cytochrome P450-dependent metabolism of warfarin by fluconazole: in vitro studies. *Drug Metab Dispos.* 1996;24:414-421.
39. Niwa T, Shiraga T, Takagi A. Effect of antifungal drugs on cytochrome P450 (CYP) 2C9, CYP2C19, and CYP3A4 activities in human liver microsomes. *Biol Pharm Bull.* 2005;28:1805-1808.
40. Sabo JA, Abdel-Rahman SM. Voriconazole: a new triazole antifungal. *Ann Pharmacother.* 2000;34:1032-1043.
41. Herbrecht R, Denning DW, Patterson TF, et al. Voriconazole versus amphotericin B for primary therapy of invasive aspergillosis. *N Engl J Med.* 2002;347:408-415.
42. Niwa T, Inoue-Yamamoto S, Shiraga T, Takagi A. Effect of antifungal drugs on cytochrome P450 (CYP) 1A2, CYP2D6, and CYP2E1 activities in human liver microsomes. *Biol Pharm Bull.* 2005;28:1813-1816.
43. Roffey SJ, Cole S, Comby P, et al. The disposition of voriconazole in mouse, rat, rabbit, Guinea pig, dog, and human. *Drug Metab Dispos.* 2003;31:731-741.
44. Cocchi S, Codeluppi M, Guaraldi G, et al. Invasive pulmonary and cerebral aspergillosis in a patient with Weil's disease. *Scand J Infect Dis.* 2005;37:396-398.
45. Ghannoum MA, Kuhn DM. Voriconazole – better chances for patients with invasive mycoses. *Eur J Med Res.* 2002;7:242-256.
46. Barchiesi F, Schimizzi AM, Caselli F, et al. Activity of the new antifungal triazole, posaconazole, against *Cryptococcus neoformans. J Antimicrob Chemother.* 2001;48:769-773.
47. Torres HA, Hachem RY, Chemaly RF, Kontoyiannis DP, Raad II. Posaconazole: a broad-spectrum triazole antifungal. *Lancet Infect Dis.* 2005;5:775-785.
48. Mellado E, Diaz-Guerra TM, Cuenca-Estrella M, Rodriguez-Tudela JL. Identification of two different 14-alpha sterol demethylase-related genes (CYP51A and CYP51B) in *Aspergillus fumigatus* and other *Aspergillus* species. *J Clin Microbiol.* 2001;39:2431-2438.
49. Warrilow AG, Melo N, Martel CM, et al. Expression, purification, and characterization of Aspergillus fumigatus sterol 14-alpha demethylase (CYP51) isoenzymes A and B. *Antimicrob Agents Chemother.* 2010;54:4225-4234.
50. Krieter P, Flannery B, Musick T, Gohdes M, Martinho M, Courtney R. Disposition of posaconazole following single-dose oral administration in healthy subjects. *Antimicrob Agents Chemother.* 2004;48:3543-3551.
51. Wexler D, Courtney R, Richards W, Banfield C, Lim J, Laughlin M. Effect of posaconazole on cytochrome P450 enzymes: a randomized, open-label, two-way crossover study. *Eur J Pharm Sci.* 2004;21:645-653.
52. Pettit NN, Carver PL. Isavuconazole: a new option for the management of invasive fungal infections. *Ann Pharmacother.* 2015;49:825-842.
53. Falci DR, Pasqualotto AC. Profile of isavuconazole and its potential in the treatment of severe invasive fungal infections. *Infect Drug Resist.* 2013;6:163-174.
54. Wang EJ, Lew K, Casciano CN, Clement RP, Johnson WW. Interaction of common azole antifungals with P glycoprotein. *Antimicrob Agents Chemother.* 2002;46:160-165.

55. Leveque D, Nivoix Y, Jehl F, Herbrecht R. Clinical pharmacokinetics of voriconazole. *Int J Antimicrob Agents*. 2006;27:274-284.
56. Sansone-Parsons A, Krishna G, Simon J, et al. Effects of age, gender, and race/ethnicity on the pharmacokinetics of posaconazole in healthy volunteers. *Antimicrob Agents Chemother*. 2007;51:495-502.
57. Petranyi G, Ryder NS, Stutz A. Allylamine derivatives: new class of synthetic antifungal agents inhibiting fungal squalene epoxidase. *Science*. 1984;224:1239-1241.
58. Gupta AK, Sauder DN, Shear NH. Antifungal agents: an overview. Part II. *J Am Acad Dermatol*. 1994;30:911-933; quiz 934-936.
59. Georgopapadakou NH, Bertasso A. Effects of squalene epoxidase inhibitors on *Candida albicans*. *Antimicrob Agents Chemother*. 1992;36:1779-1781.
60. Petranyi G, Stutz A, Ryder NS. Experimental antimycotic activity of naftifine and terbinafine. In: Fromtling RA, ed. *Recent Trends in the Discovery, Development, and Evaluation of Antifungal Agents*. Barcelona: Prous Science; 1987:441-459.
61. Gupta AK, Ryder JE, Chow M, Cooper EA. Dermatophytosis: the management of fungal infections. *Skinmed*. 2005;4:305-310.
62. Zaias N. Management of onychomycosis with oral terbinafine. *J Am Acad Dermatol*. 1990;:810-812.
63. Finlay AY. Pharmacokinetics of terbinafine in the nail. *Br J Dermatol*. 1992;:28-32.
64. Vickers AE, Sinclair JR, Zollinger M, et al. Multiple cytochrome P-450s involved in the metabolism of terbinafine suggest a limited potential for drug-drug interactions. *Drug Metab Dispos*. 1999;27:1029-1038.
65. Abdel-Rahman SM, Marcucci K, Boge T, Gotschall RR, Kearns GL, Leeder JS. Potent inhibition of cytochrome P-450 2D6-mediated dextromethorphan O-demethylation by terbinafine. *Drug Metab Dispos*. 1999;27:770-775.
66. Ajit C, Suvannasankha A, Zaeri N, Munoz SJ. Terbinafine-associated hepatotoxicity. *Am J Med Sci*. 2003;325:292-295.
67. Odom RB. Update on topical therapy for superficial fungal infections: focus on butenafine. *J Am Acad Dermatol*. 1997;36:S1-S2.
68. Debono M, Gordee RS. Antibiotics that inhibit fungal cell wall development. *Annu Rev Microbiol*. 1994;48:471-497.
69. Patil A, Majumdar S. Echinocandins in antifungal pharmacotherapy. *J Pharm Pharmacol*. 2017;69:1635-1660.
70. Balani SK, Xu X, Arison BH, et al. Metabolites of caspofungin acetate, a potent antifungal agent, in human plasma and urine. *Drug Metab Dispos*. 2000;28:1274-1278.
71. Raasch RH. Anidulafungin: review of a new echinocandin antifungal agent. *Expert Rev Anti Infect Ther*. 2004;2:499-508.
72. Hebert MF, Smith HE, Marbury TC, et al. Pharmacokinetics of micafungin in healthy volunteers, volunteers with moderate liver disease, and volunteers with renal dysfunction. *J Clin Pharmacol*. 2005;45:1145-1152.
73. Zaug M, Bergstraesser M. Amorolfine in the treatment of onychomycoses and dermatomycoses (an overview). *Clin Exp Dermatol*. 1992;:61-70.
74. Polak A. Preclinical data and mode of action of amorolfine. *Dermatology*. 1992;:3-7.
75. Gubbins PO, Anaissie EJ. Antifungal therapy. In: Anaissie EJ, McGinnis MR, Pfaller MA, eds. *Clinical Mycology*. 2nd ed. New York: Elsevier; 2009:161-195.
76. Harris BE, Manning BW, Federle TW, Diasio RB. Conversion of 5-fluorocytosine to f-fluorouracil by intestinal microflora. *Antimicrob Agents Chemother*. 1986;29:44-48.
77. Leem SH, Park JE, Kim IS, Chae JY, Sugino A, Sunwoo Y. The possible mechanism of action of ciclopirox olamine in the yeast Saccharomyces cerevisiae. *Mol Cells*. 2003;15:55-61.
78. Gupta AK, Fleckman P, Baran R. Ciclopirox nail lacquer topical solution 8% in the treatment of toenail onychomycosis. *J Am Acad Dermatol*. 2000;43:S70-S80.
79. Barrett-Bee KJ, Lane AC, Turner RW. The mode of antifungal action of tolnaftate. *J Med Vet Mycol*. 1986;24:155-160.
80. Diehl KB. Topical antifungal agents: an update. *Am Fam Physician*. 1996;54:1687-1692.
81. Baker SJ, Zhang YK, Akama T, et al. Discovery of a new boron-containing antifungal agent, 5-fluoro-1,3-dihydro-1-hydroxy-2,1- benzoxaborole (AN2690), for the potential treatment of onychomycosis. *J Med Chem*. 2006;49:4447-4450.
82. Coronado D, Merchant T, Chanda S, Zane LT. In vitro nail penetration and antifungal activity of tavaborole, a boron-based pharmaceutical. *J Drugs Dermatol*. 2015;14:609-614.
83. Hui X, Baker SJ, Wester RC, et al. In vitro penetration of a novel oxaborole antifungal (AN2690) into the human nail plate. *J Pharm Sci*. 2007;96:2622-2631.
84. Ferrer E. Spotlight on targeting aminoacyl-tRNA synthetases for the treatment of fungal infections. *Drug News Perspect*. 2006;19:347-348.
85. Hunter PA, Darby GK, Russell NJ, eds. *Fifty Years of Antimicrobials: Past Perspectives and Future Trends*. Symposia of the Society for General Microbiology. Cambridge: Cambridge University Press; 1995.
86. Cole GW, Stricklin G. A comparison of a new oral antifungal, terbinafine, with griseofulvin as therapy for tinea corporis. *Arch Dermatol*. 1989;125:1537-1539.

Structure Challenge Answers

Answers: A-10; B-2; C-7; D-3; E-1,4,5,8; F-4,6.

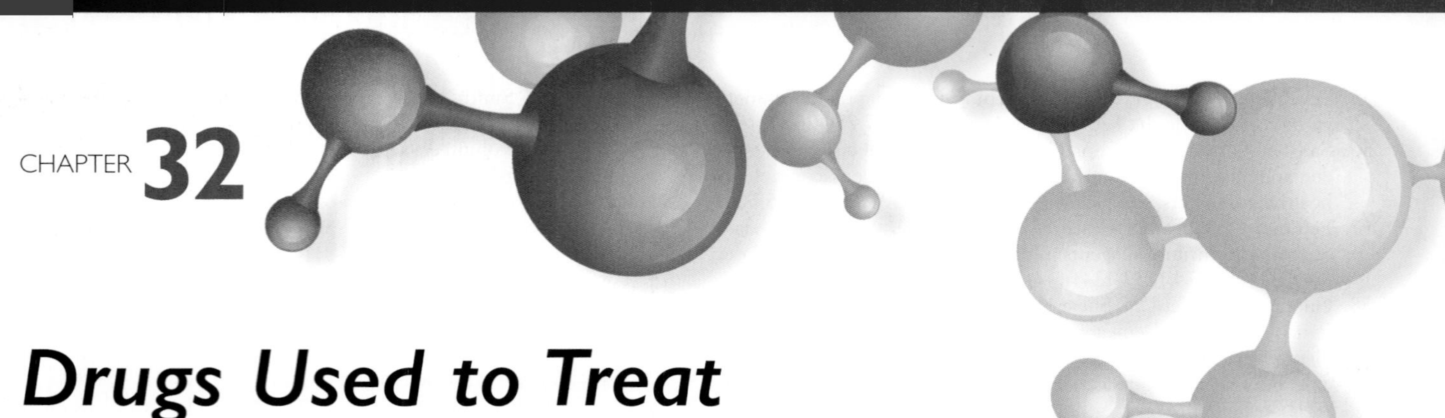

CHAPTER 32

Drugs Used to Treat Parasitic Infections

Thomas L. Lemke

Drugs covered in this chapter:

TREATMENT OF AMEBIASIS, GIARDIASIS, AND TRICHOMONIASIS:
- Metronidazole
- Nitazoxanide
- Tinidazole

TREATMENT OF PNEUMOCYSTIS:
- Atovaquone
- Penamidine isethionate
- Sulfamethoxazole-trimethoprim

TREATMENT OF TRYPANOSOMIASIS:
- Benznidazole
- Eflornithine
- Melarsoprol
- Niturtimox
- Pentamidine isethionate
- Suramin sodium

TREATMENT OF LEISHMANIASIS:
- Sodium stibogluconate
- Miltefosine

TREATMENT OF MALARIA:
- Artemisinins (artemether, artesunate, dihydroartemisinin)
- Atovaquone-proguanil
- Chloroquine
- Lumefantrine
- Mefloquine
- Piperaquine, primaquine, quinine
- Tafenoquine

TREATMENT OF HELMINTH INFECTIONS:
- Albendazole
- Ivermectin
- Mebendazole
- Moxidectin
- Praziquantel
- Pyrantel pamoate

TREATMENT OF SCABIES AND PEDICULOSIS:
- Benzyl alcohol
- Crotamiton
- Lindane
- Permethrin
- Spinosad

Abbreviations

ACT artemisinin-based combination therapy
ATP adenosine 5′-triphosphate
CDC Center for Disease Control
CNS Central nervous system
DDT dichlorodiphenyltrichlorethane
DHFR dihydrofolate reductase
FDA U.S. Food and Drug Administration
GABA gamma aminobenzoic acid
GI gastrointestinal tract
HM 2-hydroxymethylmetronidazole
IV intravenous
IVM ivermectin
NPIs neglected parasitic infections
NTZ nitazoxanide
ODC ornithine decarboxylase
OYE old yellow enzyme (a prostaglandin $F_{2\alpha}$ synthase)
OTC over the counter
PCP *Pneumocystis pneumonia*
PJP *Pneumocystis (jirovecii) pneumonia*
PABA *p*-aminobenzoic acid
PZQ praziquantel
RBC red blood cell
ROS reactive oxygen species
TIZ tizoxanide
WHO World Health Organization

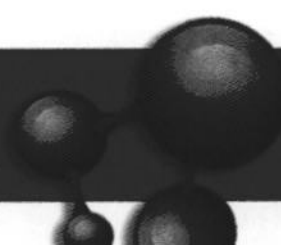

CLINICAL SIGNIFICANCE

Joseph Etzel, PharmD

Parasitic diseases remain the most common cause of serious infections worldwide and are responsible for significant morbidity and mortality. It is estimated that over half of the world's population are infected by parasites and over one million deaths occur annually. The majority of these infections are found in developing countries, but a number of parasites are endemic to developed countries including the United States. Unfortunately, efforts to control these diseases have been moderately effective at best, partly due to the inability to develop effective vaccines, the high cost of drug development, and limited access to proper health care in many of the marginalized populations in which these diseases are endemic.

Because of the limited effectiveness of vaccine development and public health initiatives, drug therapy remains important in the prevention and treatment of these infections. The pharmacologic management of these conditions is often complicated for several reasons. Parasitic infections are caused by a diverse group of organisms with different metabolic processes including protozoa, helminths, and ectoparasites. In addition, many parasites are often only susceptible to chemotherapeutic agents during specific stages of their life cycle. The effective treatment of many of these conditions is also complicated because the availability of medications is often limited in many countries. Lastly, clinicians may often be unfamiliar with proper use and monitoring of these agents because of limited clinical studies and personal experience with their use.

An understanding of the medicinal chemistry of agents used in the management of parasitic infections is essential for the clinician in order to properly utilize these agents and achieve optimal outcomes. For example, the ionic nature of certain agents like suramin prevent the drug from entering the central nervous system (CNS) and therefore limits its use to only the early stages of trypanosomiasis, whereas eflornithine enters the CNS readily and can be used for both early and advanced infection. The physiochemical properties of agents also affect their adverse effect profile and tolerability; inhaled pentamadine has minimal toxicity compared to the intravenous formulation due to its poor absorption from pulmonary tissue. Nitazoxanide is not considered to be mutagentic because it does not fragment DNA in a manner similar to metronidazole and tinidazole. The clinician should use an understanding of a drug's physiochemical principles in order to determine the most appropriate therapy and monitoring plan for their patients.

The pharmacologic management of parasitic infections remains challenging because of the development of resistance to many of the agents currently in use. Unfortunately, many of the more common parasitic infections are considered neglected diseases and research for them has been lacking. The development of newer agents, utilizing knowledge of structure-activity relationship principles, is warranted to provide clinicians with more effective and safer therapies to combat these common and burdensome conditions.

INTRODUCTION

Generally, the antiparasitic agents covered in this chapter include those drugs which are used to treat what the World Health Organization (WHO) calls vector-transmitted infectious diseases. The vectors commonly referred to are mosquitoes, sandflies, ticks, triatomine bugs, tsetse flies, fleas, black flies, aquatic snails, and lice. This chapter will discuss drugs used to treat the following disease producing organisms: protozoa (responsible for amebiasis, giardiasis, trichomoniasis, leishmaniasis, malaria), protozoan/yeast-like organism (responsible for pneumocystis pneumonia), helminthes (responsible for intestinal worm infections and systemic infections such as schistosomiasis and onchocerciasis), and ectoparasites (responsible for scabies, pediculosis, chiggers and bedbugs [Cimicidae family]). It should be noted that the Center for Disease Control (CDC) has targeted for surveillance, prevention, and treatment five neglected parasitic infections (NPIs), which include Chagas disease (transmitted by a blood-sucking triatomine), cysticercosis and toxocariasis (infections associated with helminthes), and toxoplasmosis and trichomoniasis (infections caused by a protozoans).

It is estimated that well over one billion people are infected with parasitic diseases worldwide with a majority of these parasitic infections being found in developing nations. It has been estimated that more than 700,000 deaths occur worldwide by these infections and their complications.

PROTOZOAL DISEASES (TABLE 32.1)

Amebiasis is a disease of the large intestine caused by *Entamoeba histolytica*. The disease occurs mainly in the tropics, but it is also seen in temperate climates. Amebiasis can be carried without significant symptoms, or it can lead to severe, life-threatening dysentery. The organism exists in one of two forms: the motile trophozoite form or the dormant cyst form. The trophozoite form is found in the intestine or in the wall of the colon and can be expelled from the body with the feces. The cyst form is encased by a chitinous wall that protects the organism from the environment, including chlorine used in water purification; thus, the organism can be transmitted through contaminated water and foods.

The cyst form is responsible for transmission of the disease. The cyst is spread by direct person-to-person contact and is commonly associated with living conditions in which poor personal hygiene, poor sanitation, poverty, and ignorance of sound public health practices exist. The hosts can be rendered susceptible to infection by preexisting conditions, such as protein malnutrition, pregnancy, HIV

Table 32.1 Diseases Associated With Protozoal Infections and Their Characteristics

Disease	Organism	Life Stages	Infected Organ/Cells	Transmitter
Amebiasis	*Entamoeba histolytica*	Cyst/trophozoite	Intestine/liver	Contaminated food/ water
Giardiasis	*Giardia lamblia*	Cyst/trophozoite	Intestine/liver	Contaminated water
Trichomoniasis	*Trichomonas vaginalis*	Trophozoite	Vagina/urethra/prostate	Sexual contact
Pneumocyctis pneu- monia (PCP)	*Pnemocystis jirovecii*	Yeastlike	Lung	Airborne
Trypanosomiasis				
Sleeping Sickness	*Trypanosoma brucei*	Trypomasbigotes	CNS	Tsetse fly
Chagas Disease	*Trypanosoma cruzi*	Trypomasbigotes/ amastigote	Heart	Reduviid bug
Leishmaniasis	*Leishmania spp*	Promastigote/amastigote	Skin/systemic	Female sandflies
Malaria	*Plasmodium spp*	Sporozoite/merozoite/ trophozoite/gametes	Liver/red blood cells	*Anopheles* mosquito

infection, or high carbohydrate intake. Under these conditions, the organism is capable of invading body tissue. The protozoal invasion is not well understood, but it does appear to involve the processes indicated in Table 32.1. Symptoms can range from intermittent diarrhea (foul-smelling loose/watery stools) to tenderness and enlargement of the liver (with the extraintestinal form) to acute amebic dysentery. Some patients may experience no symptoms.

Giardiasis (Table 32.1)

Giardiasis is a disease that shows considerable similarity to amebiasis. It is caused by *Giardia lamblia*, an organism that can be found in the duodenum and jejunum. The organism exists in a motile trophozoite form and an infectious cyst form. The cyst form can be deposited in water (lives up to 2 mo), and the contaminated water can then be ingested by the human. The trophozoite, if expelled from the gastrointestinal (GI) tract, normally will not survive. *Giardia lamblia* is the single most common cause of waterborne diarrhea in the United States. Giardiasis is a common disease among campers who drink water from contaminated streams. It also can be spread between family members, children in day care centers, and dogs and their owners. The organism can attach to the mucosal wall via a ventral sucking disk and, similar to amebiasis, the patient can be asymptomatic or develop watery diarrhea, abdominal cramps, distention and flatulence, anorexia, nausea, and vomiting. Usually, the condition is self-limiting in 1-4 weeks.

Trichomoniasis (Table 32.1)

Trichomoniasis is a protozoal infection caused by *Trichomonas vaginalis*, which exists only in a trophozoite form. The organs most commonly involved in the infection include the vagina, urethra, and prostate; thus, the disease is considered to be a venereal infection. The condition is transmitted by sexual contact, and it is estimated that trichomoniasis affects 180 million individuals worldwide. Infections in the male can be asymptomatic, whereas in the female, the symptoms can consist of vaginitis, profuse and foul-smelling discharge, burning and soreness on urination; and vulvar itching. Diagnosis is based on microscopic identification of the organism in fluids from the vagina, prostate, or urethra.

ORGANISMS THAT COMMONLY CAUSE VAGINITIS

Vaginitis also can be caused by *Haemophilus vaginalis* (bacteria) or *Candida albicans* (fungus), which are treated differently from the protozoal infection.

Pneumocystis (Table 32.1)

The disease pneumocystis, commonly referred to as PCP, incorrectly derived its name from what was thought to be the causative organism, *Pneumocystis carinii* and the disease state of *pneumonia*. The organism *Pneumocystis carinii* was originally isolated and reported to grow in both humans and rats. The organism itself was difficult to characterize since it had morphologic characteristics of a protozoan (i.e., lack of ergosterol in its cell membrane), but its rRNA and mitochondrial DNA pattern resembles that of fungi. It was only later recognized that the organism infecting humans and responsible for the disease pneumocystes pneumonia was actually *Pneumocystis jirovecii*, a yeast-like fungus which can only be cultured in humans.

Acute pneumocystis rarely strikes healthy individuals, although the organism is harbored in most humans without any apparent adverse effect. *Pneumocystis jirovecii* becomes active only in those individuals who have a serious impairment of their immune systems. Thus, the organism is considered to be an opportunistic pathogen. More recently, this disease has appeared in patients with HIV/AIDS, 80% of whom ultimately contract *P. jirovecii* pneumonia (Note: the disease PCP is now derived from the *Pneumocystis [jirovecii] pneumonia* and may be referred to as PJP). *P. jirovecii* pneumonia is one of the main causes of death in these patients. The disease also occurs in those receiving immunosuppressive drugs to prevent rejection following organ transplantation or for the treatment of malignant disease. Additionally, pneumocystis is seen in malnourished infants whose immunologic systems are impaired. The disease is thought to be transmitted via an airborne route. PCP is characterized by a severe pneumonia caused by rapid multiplication of the organisms, almost exclusively in lung tissue, with the organism lining the walls of the alveoli and gradually filling the alveolar spaces. Untreated, the acute form of the disease generally is fatal. Even patients who recover from pneumocystosis are at risk of recurrent episodes. Patients with AIDS experience a recurrence rate of approximately 50%.

Extrapulmonary pneumocystosis—that is, pneumocystosis outside of the lungs—is also known to exist and can be more common than presently recognized. This infection can be complicated by the presence of coinfectious organisms. Fortunately, the commonly employed antibacterial and antiprotozoal drug therapy utilized for treatment of the pulmonary infection is beneficial for the extrapulmonary condition, although intravenous (IV) administration of the drugs can be necessary.

Tritryps (Table 32.1)

Three protozoan pathogens that belong to the family Trypanosomatidae, the order Kinetoplastida, and the genus *Trypanosoma* are *Leishmania major*, which is responsible for leishmaniasis; *Trypanosoma brucei*, which is responsible for African trypanosomiasis (African sleeping sickness); and *Trypanosoma cruzi*, which is the responsible organism for Chagas disease. Referred to as the "tritryps," these eukaryotic organisms share characteristic subcellular structures of a kinetoplast (a network of circular DNA) and glycosomes (an organelle containing glycolytic enzymes), are unicellular motile protozoa, are transmitted by various insect vectors, and infect mammalian hosts. The genomes of tritryps have recently been reported.[1-3] Together, they infect hundreds of millions of people annually.

Trypanosomiasis

There are two distinct forms of trypanosomiasis: Chagas disease, and African sleeping sickness.[4]

CHAGAS DISEASE. Chagas disease, also known as American trypanosomiasis, is caused by the parasitic protozoa *Trypanosoma cruzi* and is found only in the Americas, primarily in Brazil but also in the southern United States. The protozoan lives in mammals and is spread by the blood-sucking insect known as the reduviid bug, assassin bug, or kissing bug. The insect becomes infected by drawing blood from an infected mammal and releases the protozoa with discharged feces. The pathogen then enters the new host through breaks in the skin. Inflammatory lesions are seen at the site of entry. The disease also can be spread through transfusion with contaminated blood. Signs of initial infection can include malaise, fever, anorexia, and skin edema at the site where the protozoa entered the host. The disease ultimately can invade the heart, where after decades of infection with chronic Chagas disease, the patient can experience an infection-associated heart attack. It is estimated that 5% of the Salvadorian and Nicaraguan immigrants to the United States can have chronic Chagas disease.

AFRICAN TRYPANOSOMIASIS. African trypanosomiasis, or sleeping sickness, is caused by several subspecies of *Trypanosoma brucei* (*T. brucei rhodesiense* [east African sleeping sickness] and *T. brucei gambiense* [west African sleeping sickness]). In this case, the infected animal is bitten by the blood-sucking tsetse fly. The protozoa, initially present in the gut of the vector, appear in the salivary gland for inoculation during the subsequent biting of a human. It is estimated that some 50 million people are at risk of African sleeping sickness, with 300,000-500,000 cases occurring in sub-Saharan Africa each year.

The infection progresses through two stages. Stage I can present as fever and high temperatures lasting several days; hematologic and immunologic changes occur during this stage. Stage II occurs after the organism enters the central nervous system (CNS) and can involve symptoms suggesting the disease name—daytime somnolence, loss of spontaneity, halting speech, listless gaze, and extrapyramidal signs (e.g., tremors and choreiform movements). A breakdown of neurological function leading to coma and death can occur. Death can occur within weeks if untreated (*T. brucei rhodesiense*) or only after several years (*T. brucei gambiense*).

It should be noted that the sole source of energy for the trypanosomal organism is glycolysis, which in turn can account for the hypoglycemia seen in the host. In addition, the migration of the organism into the CNS can be associated with the organism's search for a rich source of available glucose.

Leishmaniasis

Leishmaniasis is a disease caused by a number of protozoa in the genus *Leishmania*. The protozoa can be harbored in diseased rodents, canines, and various other mammals. Once transmitted from the infected mammal to man by bites from female sandflies of the genus *Phlebotomus*, it then appears in one of four major clinical syndromes: visceral leishmaniasis, cutaneous leishmaniasis, mucocutaneous leishmaniasis, or diffuse cutaneous leishmaniasis. The sandfly, the vector involved in spreading the disease, breeds in warm, humid climates; thus, the disease is more common in the tropics. As many as 12 million individuals, worldwide are infected by this organism with an estimate of 600,000-1,000,000 new cases annually.

The visceral leishmaniasis, also known as kala azar (black fever), is caused by *Leishmania donovani*. This form of the disease is systemic and is characterized in patients by fever (typically nocturnal), diarrhea, cough, and enlarged liver and spleen. The skin of the patient can become darkened. Without treatment, death can occur in 20 months and is commonly associated with diarrhea, superinfections, or GI hemorrhage. Visceral leishmaniasis is most commonly found in India and Sudan.

Both cutaneous and monocutaneous leishmaniasis are characterized by single or multiple localized lesions. These slow-healing and possibly painful ulcers can lead to secondary bacterial infections. The Old World cutaneous leishmaniasis is caused by *Leishmania topica*, which is found most commonly in children and young adults in regions bordering the Mediterranean, the Middle East, Southern Russia, and India. *Leishmania major* is endemic to desert areas in Africa, the Middle East, and Russia, whereas *Leishmania aethiopica* is found in the Kenyan highlands and Ethiopia. The New World disease caused by *Leishmania peruviana*, *Leishmania braziliensis*, and *Leishmania panamensis* is found in South and Central America, whereas *Leishmania mexicana* can be endemic to southcentral Texas. The incubation period for cutaneous leishmaniasis ranges from a few weeks to several months. The slow-healing lesions can be seen on the skin in various regions of the body depending on the specific strain of organism. Usually, these conditions exhibit spontaneous healing, but this also can occur over an extended period of time (1-2 yr).

Malaria (Table 32.1)

Malaria is transmitted by the infected female *Anopheles* mosquito. The specific protozoan organisms causing malaria are from the genus *Plasmodium*. Only four of approximately 100 species cause malaria in humans. The remaining species affect birds, monkeys, livestock, rodents, and reptiles. The four species that affect humans are *Plasmodium falciparum*, *Plasmodium vivax*, *Plasmodium malariae*, and *Plasmodium ovale*. Concurrent infections by more than one of these species are seen in endemically affected regions of the world. Such multiple infections further complicate patient management and the choice of treatment regimens.

It is estimated that two billion individuals are at risk of developing malaria and that the disease affects as many as 500 million humans globally and causes more than two million deaths annually. It is estimated that a third of these fatalities occur in children younger than 5 years. Although this disease is found primarily in the tropics and subtropics, it has been observed far beyond these boundaries. Malaria was virtually eradicated from the United States between 1947 and 1951 through the use of the insecticide DDT (dichlorodiphenyltrichlorethane) which destroyed the insect vector, and in 1955 the World Health Organization (WHO) launched a program titled the Global Malaria Eradication Program. The program intended to irradicate the disease worldwide through the use of DDT and disease treatment with chloroquine, but due to the development of DDT-resistant *Anopheles* mosquitoes, drug-resistant plasmodium, and political resistance, WHO abandoned its program in 1972. Recently, there has been an increased global interest in addressing the disease through the use of preventative measures and development of multidrug treatments, although at present nearly nothing new has reached the market.

While malaria has essentially been eradicated in most temperate-zone countries, more than 1,000 cases were documented recently in US citizens returning from travel abroad. Today, malaria is found in most countries of Africa, Central and South America, and Southeast Asia. It is reported to be on the increase in Afghanistan, Bangladesh, Brazil, Myanmar, Cambodia, Colombia, China, Iran, India, Indonesia, Mexico, the Philippines, Thailand, and Vietnam. Infection from plasmodia can cause anemia, pulmonary edema, renal failure, jaundice, shock, cerebral malaria, and, if not treated in a timely manner, even death.

Types of Malaria

Malarial infections are known according to the species of the parasite involved.

PLASMODIUM FALCIPARUM. Infection with *Plasmodium falciparum* has an incubation period (time from mosquito bite to clinical symptoms) of 1-3 weeks (average, 12 d). The *P. falciparum* life cycle in humans begins with the bite of an infected female mosquito. The parasites in the sporozoite stage enter the circulatory system, through which they can reach the liver in approximately 1 hour. These organisms grow and multiply 30,000- to 40,000-fold by asexual division within liver cells in 5-7 days. Then, as merozoites, they leave the liver to reenter the bloodstream and invade the erythrocytes, or red blood cells (RBCs), where they continue to grow and multiply further for 1-3 days. Specific receptors on the surface of the erythrocytes serve as binding sites for the merozoite. These infected RBCs rupture, releasing merozoites in intervals of approximately 48 hours. Chemicals released by the ruptured cells in turn cause activation and release of additional substances associated with the patient's symptoms. The clinical symptoms include chills, fever, sweating, headaches, fatigue, anorexia, nausea, vomiting, and diarrhea.

Some of the released merozoites are sequestered in vital organs (brain and heart), where they continue to grow. Recurrence of the clinical symptoms on alternate days leads to the terminology of tertian malaria. The *P. falciparum* parasite also can cause RBCs to clump and adhere to the wall of blood vessels. Such a phenomenon has been known to cause partial obstruction and, sometimes, restriction of the blood flow to vital organs like the brain, liver, and kidneys. Reinfection of RBCs can occur, allowing further multiplication and remanifestation of the malaria symptoms. Some merozoites develop into male and female sexual forms, called gametocytes, which can then be acquired by the female mosquito after biting the infected human. Gametocytes mature in the mosquito's stomach to form zygotes. Growth of the zygotes leads to the formation of oocysts (spherical structures located on the outside wall of the stomach). Sporozoites develop from the oocysts, are released into the body cavity of the mosquito, and migrate to the salivary gland of the insect, from which they can be transmitted to another human following a mosquito bite. The life cycle of the malaria parasites is shown in Figure 32.1. The genome of the *P. falciparum*, as well as that of the *Anpheles* mosquito, are now known and are expected to provide potential new avenues for drug development. Genome information is also expected to give insight regarding the mechanisms of resistance and improve drug treatment.

PLASMODIUM VIVAX. *Plasmodium vivax* (benign tertian) is the most prevalent form of malaria. It has an incubation period of 1-4 weeks (average, 2 wk). This form of malaria can cause spleen rupture and anemia. Relapses (renewed manifestations of erythrocytic infection) can occur. This results from the periodic release of dormant parasites (hypnozoites) from the liver cells. The erythrocytic forms generally are considered to be susceptible to treatment.

PLASMODIUM MALARIAE. *Plasmodium malariae* is responsible for quartan malaria. It has an incubation period of 2-4 weeks (average, 3 wk). The asexual cycle occurs every 72 hours. In addition to the usual symptoms, this form also causes nephritis. This is the mildest form of malaria and does not relapse. The RBC infection associated with *P. malariae* can last for many years, and the organism is quite unlikely to become resistant.

PLASMODIUM OVALE. Infection with *Plasmodium ovale* has an incubation period of 9-18 days (average, 14 d). Relapses have been known to occur in individuals infected with this plasmodium. The relapse can be indicative of ovale tertian malaria and is associated with the ability of the organism to lay dormant (hypnozoites) in hepatic tissue for extended periods of time.

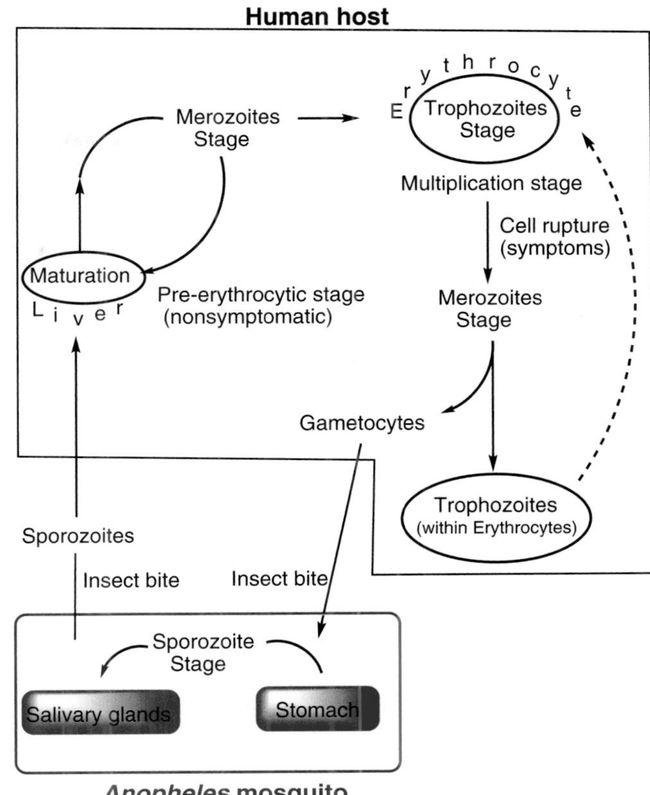

Figure 32.1 Life cycle of malarial protozoa.

General Approaches to Antimalarial Chemotherapy

DRUG CLASSIFICATION

Generally the antimalarial drugs are classified by the life cycle stage (see Fig. 32.1) that the drugs are effective against, although they can be also classified by their structural type. Listed below are the theoretical approaches through which drugs can intervene to destroy the organism. Presently, the majority of drugs act upon the intracellular erythrocyctic form of the disease. It should be noted that some antimalarials can be effective against more than one form of the organism while others may be species specific.

Tissue Schizonticides. These drugs eradicate the exo-erythrocytic liver-tissue stages of the plasmodium parasite, which prevents the parasite's entry into the blood. Drugs of this type are useful for prophylaxis. Some tissue schizonticides can act on the long-lived tissue form (hypnozoites of *P. vivax* and *P. ovale*) and, thus, can prevent relapses.

Blood Schizonticides. These drugs destroy the erythrocytic stages of parasites and can cure cases of falciparum malaria or suppress relapses. This is the easiest phase to treat because drug delivery into the bloodstream can be accomplished rapidly.

Gametocytocides. Agents of this type kill the sexual forms of the plasmodia (gametocytes), which are transmittable to the *Anopheles* mosquito, thereby preventing transmission of the disease.

Sporontocides (Sporozooiticides). These drugs act against sporozoites and are capable of killing these organisms as soon as they enter the bloodstream following a mosquito bite.

Despite the history of malaria, the epidemiology and clinical features of the disease are not that well documented. In many parts of Africa, the diagnosis of the disease is not routinely done, and therefore, the success of prevention efforts and treatment cannot be known. For more details on these difficulties, the reader is directed to an excellent review by Greenwood, et al. (Malaria: progress, perils, and prospects for eradication. *The J Clin Invest.* 2008;118(4):1266-1276).

GENERAL APPROACHES TO PROTOZOAL THERAPY

Amebiasis and Giardiasis

The most appropriate approach for treatment of this type of protozoal infection is through prevention. Because the infection usually occurs by consumption of contaminated drinking water and food, avoidance is the key to prevention. Drinking bottled water, or boiling or disinfecting the water, will reduce the risk. Improvements in personal hygiene and general sanitation are also beneficial.

Trypanosomiasis, Leishmaniasis, and Malaria

For these diseases that are spread by insect vectors, the use of insecticides, protective clothing, and insect repellents can greatly reduce the incidence of the disease. Unfortunately, many of these protozoal infections also can infect other hosts beside humans; thus, even the most successful insect irradiation methods cannot destroy all the reservoirs of the protozoa. The use of insect repellents and protective clothing can be useful for visitors to regions with endemic infections, but these procedures can prove to be ineffective for those living in the area. For such individuals, early detection and drug therapy is the method of treatment.

DRUG THERAPY FOR PROTOZOAL INFECTIONS

Treatment of Amebiasis, Giardiasis, and Trichomoniasis

Metronidazole (Flagyl, Generic Forms)

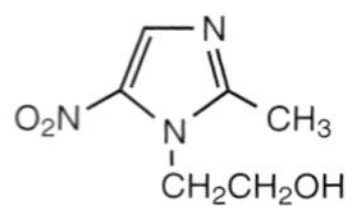

Metronidazole

Metronidazole was initially introduced for the treatment of vaginal infections caused by *Trichomonas vaginalis* but has since been shown to be effective for treatment of amebiasis, giardiasis, and anaerobic bacterial infections, including *Clostridium difficile*.

MECHANISM OF ACTION. Despite the availability of metronidazole since the late 1950s, the mechanism of action of the drug is still unknown. It is generally agreed that metronidazole is a prodrug and that anaerobic organisms reduce the nitro group in metronidazole to a hydroxylamine, as shown in Figure 32.2, during which a reactive derivative or reactive species are produced that cause destructive effects on cell components (i.e., DNA, proteins, and membranes). Specifically, DoCampo[5] has reported that nitroaryl compounds (nitroimidazoles, metronidazole; nitrofurans, nifurtomox) are reduced to nitro radical anions, which in turn react with oxygen to regenerate the nitroaryl and the superoxide radical anion (Fig. 32.3). Further reduction of superoxide radical anion leads to hydrogen peroxide, and

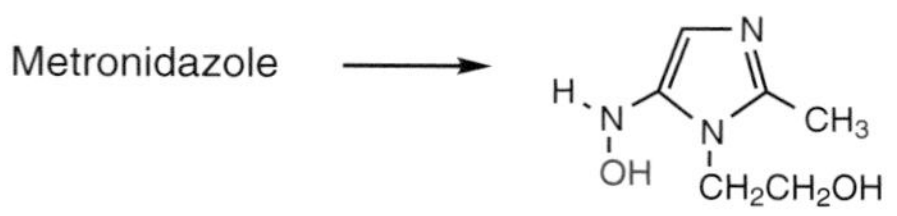

Figure 32.2 Anaerobic metabolic activation of metronidazole.

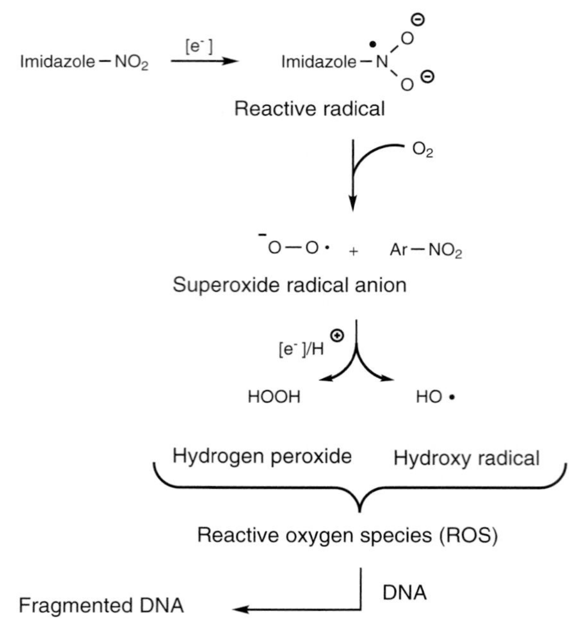

Figure 32.3 Formation of reactive oxygen species (ROS) from nitroimidazole compounds.

homolytic cleavage of the latter leads to hydroxyl radical formation. Superoxide radical anion, hydrogen peroxide, and hydroxyl radicals are referred to as reactive oxygen species (ROS) and are the reactive substances that are implicated in damage to critical cellular components of the parasite.

METABOLISM. Liver metabolism of metronidazole leads to two major metabolites: hydroxylation of the 2-methyl group to 2-hydroxymethylmetronidazole (HM) and its oxidation to metronidazole acetic acid.[6] Both compounds possess biological activity. Additionally, HM is found in the urine as glucuronide and sulfate conjugates. In addition, a small amount of metronidazole is oxidized to acetamide, a known carcinogen in rats but not in humans, and to the oxalate derivative shown in Figure 32.4.[7]

PHARMACOKINETICS[6]
Metronidazole is available in a variety of dosage forms, including IV, oral, topical, rectal, and vaginal suppositories. The bioavailability of metronidazole is nearly 100% when administered orally but is significantly less when administered via the rectal (67%-82%) or the vaginal (19%-56%) routes. The drug is not bound to plasma protein. Distribution of the drug is fairly uniform throughout the body, including mother's milk.

THERAPEUTIC APPLICATION. Metronidazole is considered to be the drug of choice for treatment of the protozoal infections amebiasis (intestinal and extraintestinal), giardiasis, and trichomoniasis.[8] It is the drug of choice for treatment of the Gram-positive bacilli *Clostridium difficile* and in combination is an alternative therapy for *Helicobacter pylori* infections.[9] The common side effects exhibited with metronidazole include abdominal distress, a metallic taste, and a disulfiram-like effect if taken

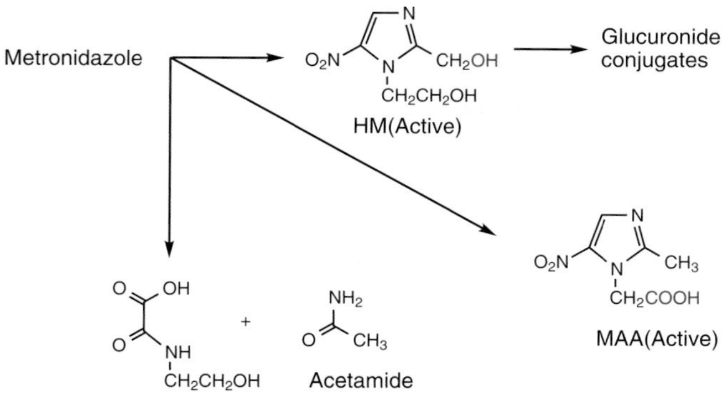

Figure 32.4 Hepatic metabolism of metronidazole. *HM*, 2-hydroxymethylmetronidazole; *MAA*, metronidazole acetic acid.

with alcohol. The drug is reported to be carcinogenic in mice, possibly related to the metabolite acetamide, and as a result should not be used during the first trimester of pregnancy.

Tinidazole (Tindamax)

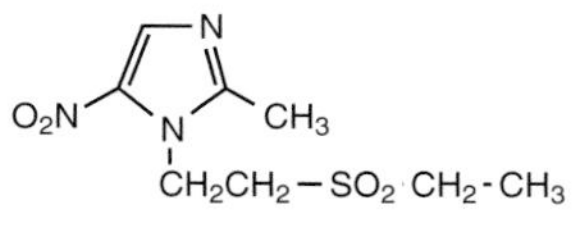

Tinidazole has been approved by the U.S. Food and Drug Administration (FDA) for the treatment of amebiasis, giardiasis, and trichomoniasis. It also appears to be highly effective against *Helicobacter pylori* infections, although it is not approved for this use. The drug is rapidly and completely absorbed following oral administration and can be administered with food to reduce GI disturbance. Tinidazole has a mechanism of action that parallels that of metronidazole, as well as a similar metabolic pathway leading to hydroxylation at the 2-methyl group catalyzed by CYP3A4. Basically, tinidazole appears to mimic the actions of metronidazole, although there are reports that it is effective against some protozoa which are resistant to metronidazole.

Nitazoxanide (Alinia)

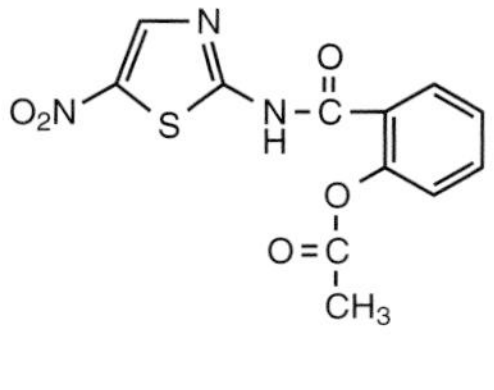

Nitazoxanide (NTZ) was originally approved as an orphan drug for the treatment of diarrhea associated with giardiasis in children 1-11 years of age, but it is also approved for diarrhea caused by crytosporidiosis in patients with AIDS. Crytosporidiosis is a protozoal infection caused by *Cryptosporidium parvum*. The condition is uncommon in healthy individuals but can be life-threatening in immunosuppressed patients, including those with HIV infections.

MECHANISM OF ACTION[10]
Nitazoxanide is a prodrug that is metabolically converted into the deacetylated drug tizoxanide (TIZ) (Fig. 32.5). TIZ then undergoes a four-electron reduction of the 5-nitro group giving various short-lived intermediates, which can include the hydroxylamine derivative. These reduced products represent the active forms of NTZ. Whereas these intermediates would suggest that NTZ has the same mechanism of action as metronidazole, this does not appear to be the case. Nitazoxanide is thought to inhibit the enzyme pyruvate:ferredoxin oxidoreductase in *Trichomonas vaginalis*, *Entamoeba histolytica*, and *Clostridium perfingens*. The result of this inhibition is disruption of the bioenergetics of these organisms. Unlike metronidazole and tinidazole, which fragment DNA and are suspected mutagenic agents, NTZ and TIZ do not cause DNA fragmentation and are not considered to be mutagenic. This might be associated with the higher redox potential of NTZ, a nitrothiazole, in comparison with very low redox potential found for the nitroimidazoles, such as metronidazole and tinidazole. Additional metabolites of TIZ include the glucuronide, which shows some biological activity, and small amounts of an aromatic hydroxylation product (Fig. 32.5). A more recent study suggests that NTZ may act on an ion channel via its action on the *avr-14* gene.[11]

PHARMACOKINETICS. Nitazoxanide is available as a powder that is reconstituted and dispensed as an oral suspension and as a tablet. The drug is well absorbed from the GI tract and rapidly metabolized, with elimination products appearing in the urine and feces. The only identified products in the plasma are TIZ and its glucuronide.[12] The product can be taken with food.

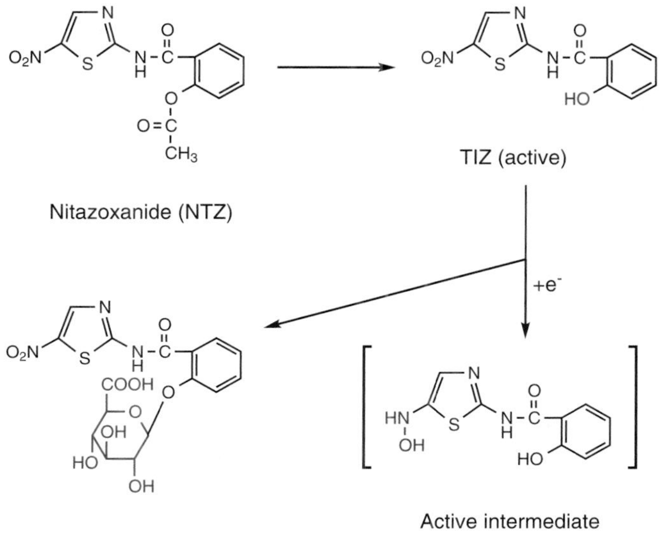

Figure 32.5 Metabolic activation of nitazoxanide. *TIZ*, tizoxanide.

THERAPEUTIC APPLICATION. NTZ was previously approved for treatment of pediatric patients with *Giardia lamblia*, and it is now approved for diarrhea caused by this organism in adults and children over 12 years of age. The drug is also effective for treatment of *Cryptosporidium parvum*, as well as the protozoa *Entamoeba histolytica* and *Trichomonas vaginalis*, the bacteria *Helicobacter pylori* and *Clostridium perfringens*, and various helminths, including *Ascaris lumbricoides*, *Enterobius vermicularis*, *Ancylostoma doudenale*, and *Strongyloides stercoralis*.[13]

Treatment of Pneumocystis[14,15]

Sulfamethoxazole-Trimethoprim; Cotrimoxazole (Bactrim, Septra, Cotrim)

The combination of sulfamethoxazole and trimethoprim has proven to be the most successful method for treatment and prophylaxis of pneumocystis in patients with AIDS. This combination was first reported as being effective against PCP in 1975, and by 1980, it had become the preferred method of treatment, with a response rate of 65%-94%. The combination is effective against both pneumocystic pneumonia and the extrapulmonary disease. *Pneumocystis jirovecii* appears to be especially susceptible to the sequential blocking action of cotrimazole, which inhibits both the incorporation of *p*-aminobenzoic acid (PABA) into folic acid as well as the reduction of dihydrofolic acid to tetrahydrofolic acid by dihydrofolate reductase (DHFR). (A detailed discussion of the mechanism of action and the structure-activity relationship of these drugs can be found in Chapter 29.) Depending on the severity of the infection, the combination is administered in doses of 20 mg/kg/d of trimethoprim and 100 mg/kg/d of sulfamethoxazole in four divided doses over a period of 14-21 days. The incidence of side effects of this combination is high and generally reflects the effects of the sulfa drug component. Side effects can be significant enough to terminate treatment.

Pentamidine Isethionate (Pentam 300, Nebupent)

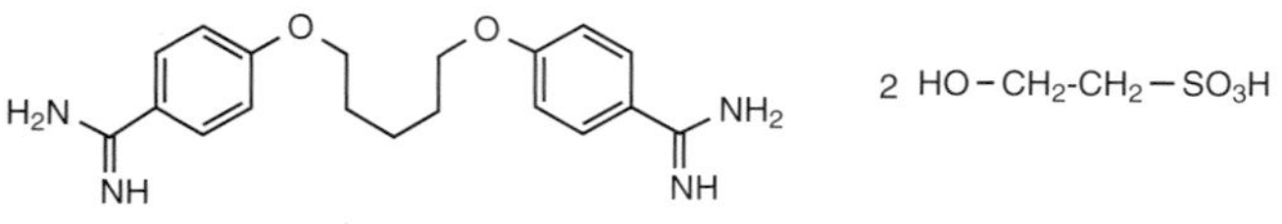

H_2N … NH_2, NH, NH; 2 $HO-CH_2-CH_2-SO_3H$

Pentamidine isethionate

Pentamidine is available as the water-soluble isethionate salt, which is used both IV and as an aerosol. The drug can be used via the intramuscular route, but significant complications have been reported, and therefore, this route of administration is not recommended. The drug has fungicidal and antiprotozoal activity but is used primarily for prevention of PCP.

MECHANISM OF ACTION. The mechanism of action of pentamidine is not known with certainty, but strong evidence supports involvement of a DNA cleavage process. Pentamidine selectively binds to the DNA in the trypanosoma parasite (see below) and has also been shown to inhibit topoisomerase in *Pneumocystis jirovecii*, which leads to double-strand cleavage of DNA in trypanosome.[13-15] It has been suggested that pentamidine's mechanism of action can be different in different organisms and, therefore, that the actions reported for trypanosoma may not carry over to pneumocystis.

PHARMACOKINETICS. Pentamidine must be administered IV and, after multiple injections daily or on alternate days, accumulates in body tissue. The drug is not readily absorbed orally and exhibits binding to plasma protein (~70%). Plasma concentrations are measurable up to 8 months following a single 2-hour IV infusion. The accumulation aids in treatment, as well as in prophylaxis. The drug shows poor penetration of the CNS but is distributed to the lungs.

THERAPEUTIC APPLICATION. Pentamidine is used as a second-line agent either by itself or in combination for the treatment and prophylaxis of PCP. For prophylaxis, the aerosol form of the drug is indicated and has minimum toxicity. The need for IV administration can be associated with the potential for severe toxicity, which includes breathlessness, tachycardia, dizziness, headache, and vomiting. These symptoms can occur in as many as 50% of the patients, representing a serious therapeutic limitation. These effects are thought to be associated with excessively rapid IV administration, resulting in the release of histamine.

Atovaquone (Mepron)

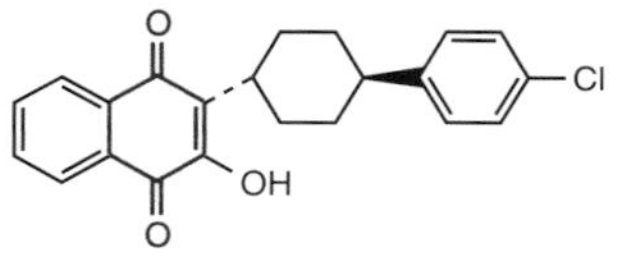

O, O, OH, Cl; CH_3O, CH_3O, O, O, CH_3, CH_3, H, 6-10

Atovaquone 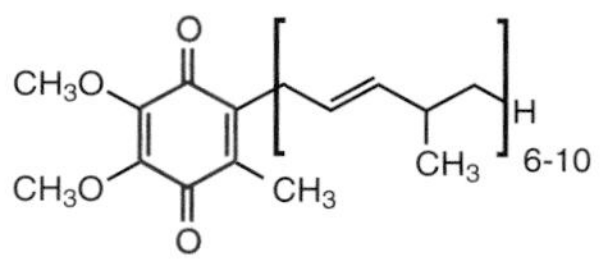 | Ubiquinone

Atovaquone, a chemical with structural similarity to the ubiquinone metabolites, was initially synthesized and investigated as an antimalarial, a use for which it has recently gained acceptance when used in combination with other antimalarial agents. Today, its usefulness is primarily directed toward the treatment of PCP.

MECHANISM OF ACTION. Atovaquone is thought to produce its antiparasitic action by virtue of its ability to inhibit the mitochondrial respiratory chain. More specifically, atovaquone is a ubiquinone reductase inhibitor, inhibiting at the cytochrome bc_1 complex.[16] This action leads to a collapse of the mitochondrial membrane potential. The compound shows stereospecific inhibition, with the *trans* isomer being more active than the *cis* isomer.

PHARMACOKINETICS. Atovaquone is poorly absorbed from the GI tract because of its poor water solubility and high fat solubility, but the absorption can be significantly increased if taken with a fat-rich meal. The drug is highly bound to plasma protein (94%) and, despite its high lipophilicity, does not enter the CNS in significant quantities. It is not significantly metabolized in humans and is exclusively eliminated in feces via the bile.

THERAPEUTIC APPLICATIONS. With as many as 70% of patients with AIDS developing pneumocystis and, of these, with nearly 60% on cotrimoxazole developing serious side effects to this combination, atovaquone is an important alternative drug.[17] Atovaquone also has been reported to be effective for the treatment of toxoplasmosis caused by *Toxoplasma gondii*, although it has not been approved for this use.

Treatment of Trypanosomiasis[18]

Suramin Sodium (Available From the CDC)

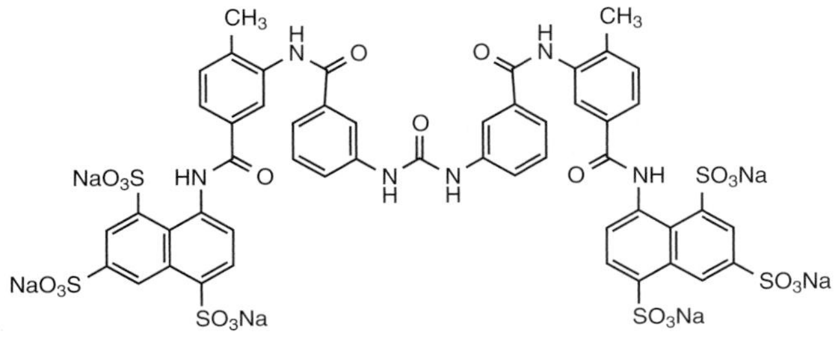

Suramin Sodium

Introduced into therapy for the treatment of first-stage African trypanosomiasis (sleeping sickness) in the 1920s, suramin, a bis-hexasulfonatednaphthylurea, is still considered to be the drug of choice for treatment of non–CNS-associated African trypanosomiasis.

MECHANISM OF ACTION. The mechanism of action of suramin is unproven, but the drug is known to have a high affinity for binding to a number of critical enzymes in the pathogen. Among the enzymes to which suramin has been shown to bind are several dehydrogenases and kinases. As a result of binding, suramin has been shown to be an inhibitor of DHFR (a crucial enzyme in folate metabolism) and thymidine kinase. In addition, suramin is an inhibitor of glycolytic enzymes in *Trypanosoma brucei*, with binding constants much lower than those seen in mammalian cells. Inhibition of glycolysis would be expected to block energy sources of the pathogen, leading to lysis. Whether one or more of these inhibitor actions represent the toxic action of suramin on the pathogen remains unproven.

PHARMACOKINETICS. Suramin sodium is a water-soluble compound that is poorly absorbed via oral administration and must be administered IV in multiple injections. Because of its highly ionic nature, suramin will not cross the blood-brain barrier and, therefore, is ineffective for the treatment of trypanosomal infections that reach the CNS. In addition, suramin is tightly bound to serum albumin (~98%). Despite this binding, the drug is preferentially absorbed by trypanosomes through a receptor-mediated endocytosis of serum protein. Because the drug remains in the bloodstream for an extended period of time ($t_{1/2}$–50 d), suramin has value as a prophylactic drug.

THERAPEUTIC APPLICATION. Seramin sodium is effective against east African trypanosomiasis, but it has limited value against west African trypanosomiasis. As indicated, because the drug will not enter the CNS, it is only useful for treatment of early stages of the disease. The drug exhibits a wide variety of side effects which can be severe in debilitated individuals and includes nausea, vomiting, and fatigue.

Pentamidine Isethionate (Pentam 300, Nebupent)

First introduced as a therapy for trypanosomiasis in 1937, pentamidine is now used in a variety of protozoal and fungal infections and finds use in the treatment of trypanosomiasis, leishmaniasis, and pneumocystis (PCP). The drug is primarily used for treatment of PCP. When used for trypanosomiasis, pentamidine is only effective against *Trypanosoma brucei rhodesiense* (east African sleeping sickness) and, even then, only during the early stage of the disease because the drug does not readily cross the blood-brain barrier.

MECHANISM OF ACTION. As indicated above, several biochemical actions have been reported for pentamidine. The drug has been shown to bind to DNA through hydrogen-bonding of the amidine proton with the adenine-thymine–rich regions of DNA. More specifically, pentamidine binds to the N-3 of adenine, spans four to five base pairs, and binds to a second adenine to form interstrand cross-bonding.[19] In addition to, and possibly separate from, this action, pentamidine appears to be a potent inhibitor of type II topoisomerase of mitochondrial DNA (kinetoplast DNA) of the trypanosoma parasite.[20] The mitochondrial DNA is a cyclic DNA. This inhibition leads to double-stand breaks and linearization of the DNA. The relationship between binding to specific regions of the DNA and inhibition of topoisomerase is unclear.

In the case of *Trypanosoma brucei*, resistant strains are common. It is thought that resistance develops through an inability of the drug to reach the mitochondrial DNA.[21] Transport into the mitochondria is a carrier-mediated process, with the absence of carrier in the resistant strains.

Eflornithine (Available From the CDC)

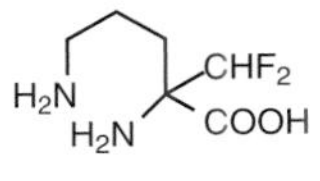

Eflornithine

Metcalf et al.[22] reported the synthesis of eflornithine in 1978. Their interest arose from the desire to prepare ornithine decarboxylase (ODC) inhibitors as tools for studying the role of polyamines as regulators of growth processes. Ornithine decarboxylase catalyzes the conversion of ornithine to putrescine (1,4-diaminobutane), which in turn leads to the formation of the polyamines, spermine, and spermidine. It was not until 1980 that Bacchi et al.[23] demonstrated the potential of eflornithine in the treatment of trypanosomiasis.

MECHANISM OF ACTION. Difluoromethyl ornithine is a suicide inhibitor of ODC, a pyridoxal phosphate–dependent enzyme, as shown in Figure 32.6. Evidence suggests that cysteine-360 in ODC is the site of eflornithine alkylation.[24] Alkylation of ODC blocks the synthesis of putrescine, the rate-determining step in the synthesis of polyamines. Mammalian ODC also can be inhibited, but because the turnover of ODC is so rapid in mammals, eflornithine does not produce serious side effects.

PHARMACOKINETICS. Eflornithine can be administered either IV or orally. IV administration requires large doses and frequent dosing, whereas poor oral absorption and rapid excretion because of the zwitterionic nature of the drug (an amino acid) has limited that route of administration. The drug does not bind to plasma protein and enters the CNS readily, most likely via an amino acid transport system. As a result, the drug can be used for both early and late stages of trypanosomiasis.

THERAPEUTIC APPLICATION. Eflornithine is indicated for the treatment of west African trypanosomiasis caused by *Trypanosoma brucei gambiense* but has proven to be ineffective against east African trypanosomiasis. The cause of this ineffectiveness remains a mystery, although evidence suggests that in the resistant organism, endogenous ornithine plus increased activity of S-adenosylmethionine decarboxylase allow sufficient synthesis of spermidine and spermine to support cell division, thus bypassing the need for organism-synthesized ornithine.[25] Side effects reported for eflornithine consist of anemia, diarrhea, and leukopenia.

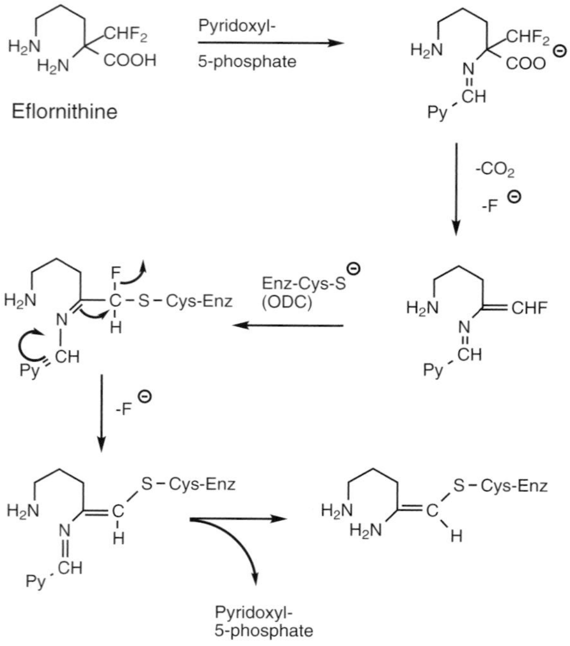

Eflornithine

Pyridoxyl-5-phosphate

$-CO_2$, $-F^{\ominus}$

Enz-Cys-S$^{\ominus}$ (ODC)

$-F^{\ominus}$

Pyridoxyl-5-phosphate

Figure 32.6 Inhibition of ornithine decarboxylase (Enz-Cys-SH) by eflornithine.

Nifurtimox (Available From the CDC)

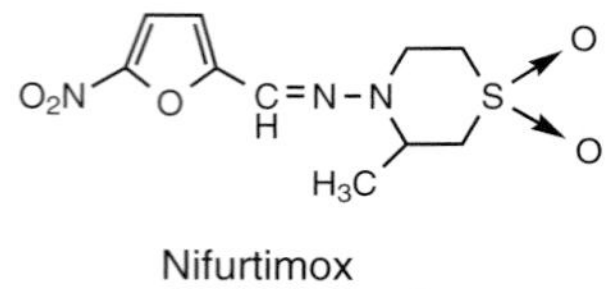

Nifurtimox

Another of the nitroaryl compounds, nifurtimox has proven to be useful as a drug for the treatment of trypanosomiasis. It is one of two drugs approved for use in the treatment of Chagas disease. It has been estimated by the CDC that eight million individuals in the Americas have Chagas disease.

MECHANISM OF ACTION. As discussed for metronidazole, nifurtimox is thought to undergo reduction followed by oxidation and, in the process, generate ROS such as the superoxide radical anion, hydrogen peroxide, and hydroxyl radical (Fig. 32.3).[5] These species are potent oxidants, producing oxidative stress that can induce damage to DNA and lipids that can affect cellular membranes. In addition, Henderson et al.[26] have reported that nifurtimox inhibits trypanothione reductase, which results in the inhibition of trypanothione formation (93% inhibition). Trypanothione is a critical protective enzyme found uniquely in trypanosomal parasites.

THERAPEUTIC APPLICATION. Nifurtimox is the drug of choice for the treatment of acute Chagas disease. The drug is not effective for the chronic stages of the disease. In the acute stage, the drug has an 80% cure rate. Side effects of the drug include hypersensitivity reactions, GI complications (nausea and vomiting), myalgia, and weakness.

Benznidazole (Generic)

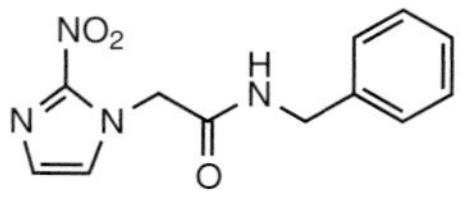

Benznidazole

Benznidazole is the first drug approved for treatment of Chagas disease in the United States. Specifically the drug is approved for treatment of pediatric patients 2-12 years of age. Like nifurtimox, it is effective against the circulating form of *Trypanosoma cruzi* during the acute phase of the disease, but also like nifurtimox, it is ineffective during the chronic stage of the disease.

MECHANISM OF ACTION. The mechanism of action of benznidazole remains under investigation. Studies suggest that benznidazole may partially catalyze the formation of ROS through the action of type I nitroreductase, leading to cell death (Fig. 32.7). Additionally it has been proposed that benznidazole undergoes metabolic activation via a protazoal prostaglandin $F_{2\alpha}$ synthase refered to as old

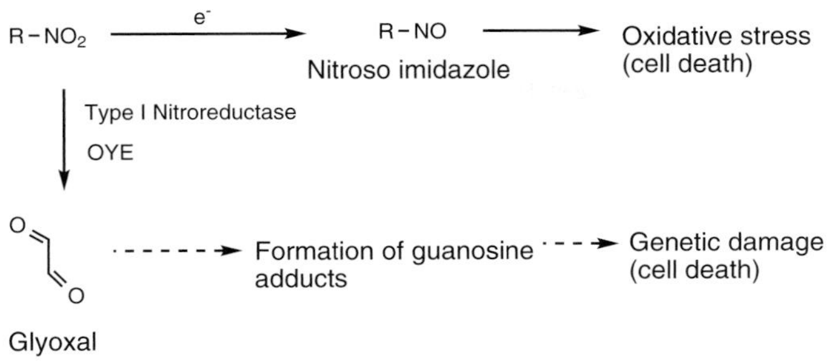

R−NO₂ → (e⁻) R−NO Nitroso imidazole → Oxidative stress (cell death)
Type I Nitroreductase OYE
Glyoxal - - → Formation of guanosine adducts - - → Genetic damage (cell death)

Figure 32.7 Proposed mechanism of action of benznidazole. *OYE*, old yellow enzyme (a prostaglandin $F_{2\alpha}$ synthase).

yellow enzyme (OYE), leading to the formation of glyoxal which, in turn, forms an adduct with the guanosine of DNA that results in genetic damage and cell death.[27]

THERAPEUTIC APPLICATION. Benznidazole, as with nifurtimox, is only of value for the treatment of acute Chagas disease. The drug is not effective for the chronic stages of the disease. Benznidazole has only recently been approved in the United States. It is administered orally in a tablet form.

ADVERSE EFFECTS. A number of serious adverse effects have been reported, including the potential for genotoxicity, carcinogenicity, and mutagenicity. Additionally, hypersentivity skin reactions, manifestations of bone marrow depression, and peripheral neuropathy may occur. The drug should not be administered with disulfiram.

Melarsoprol (Available From the CDC, Arsobal)

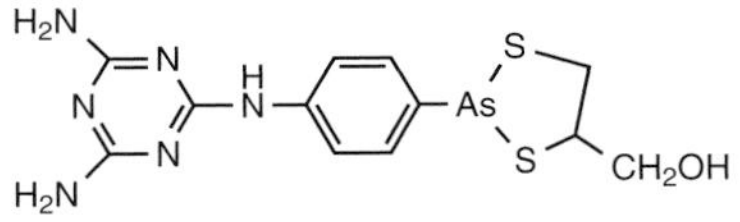

Melarsoprol

Knowingly or unknowingly, arsenic-containing drugs have been used for treatment of parasitic conditions for thousands of years. In the late 1800s and early 1900s, Paul Ehrlich introduced the use of trivalent arsenicals. Melarsoprol, an organoarsenical, came into use in the late 1940s, and it remains the first-choice drug in the treatment of second-stage African trypanosomiasis (sleeping sickness). Until 1990, it also was the only treatment for late-stage sleeping sickness.

MECHANISM OF ACTION. It is known that trivalent arsenic reacts rapidly and reversibly with sulfhydryl-containing proteins, as shown in Figure 32.8. It is generally accepted that the enzyme with which melarsoprol reacts is involved in glycolysis, and as a result, inhibition of pyruvate kinase occurs. It is argued, however, that the inhibition cannot occur at pyruvate kinase but rather at a step before the pyruvate kinase. Blockage of glycolysis would be expected to lead to loss of motility and cell lysis. More recently, Fairlamb et al.[28] have proposed a mechanism of action that results in the inhibition of trypanothione reductase through the

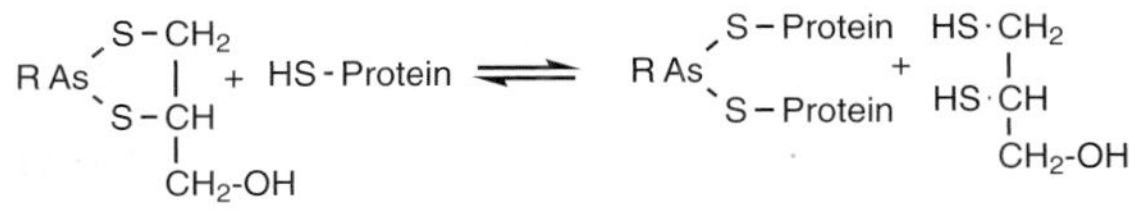

Figure 32.8 Mechanism of action of trivalent arsenic compounds with trypanosoma organism.

formation of a stable complex between melarsoprol and trypanothione. Melarsoprol reacts with the cysteine sulfhydryl of trypanothione to form the stable adduct shown in Figure 32.9. Supportive of this mechanism is the synergistic action of melarsoprol with eflornithine, two drugs that produce sequential blockage of the synthesis of trypanothione.

PHARMACOKINETICS. Melarsoprol is administered IV in multiple doses and multiple sessions. Its major metabolite in humans is the lipophilic melarsen oxide, which can penetrate into the CNS. This metabolite apparently is responsible for the protein-binding characteristic for melarsoprol.

THERAPEUTIC APPLICATION. Melarsoprol is the drug of choice for the treatment of late-stage meningoencephalitic trypanosomiasis caused by the west and east African strains of the disease. Because the drug has the potential for serious nervous system toxicities (e.g., convulsions, acute cerebral edema, and coma), it is usually administered in a hospital setting with supervision. An additional problem with melarsoprol is the development of resistance by the parasite.

Treatment of Leishmaniasis

Sodium Stibogluconate (Pentostam, Available From the CDC)

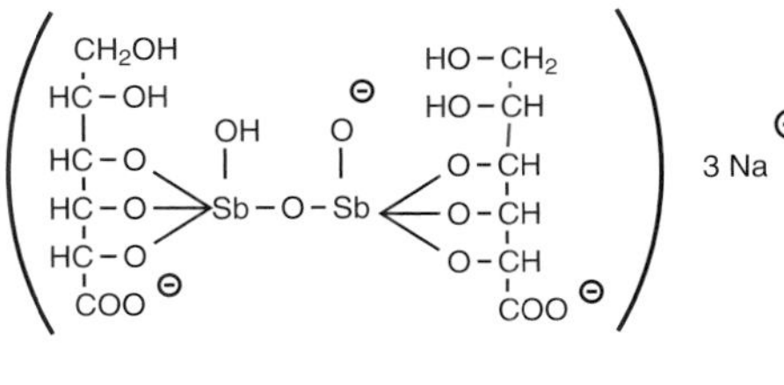

Sodium stibogluconate

Leishmaniasis was first described in the medical literature by Deishman and Donovan in 1903, and shortly after that, the use of antimony-based drugs were introduced as

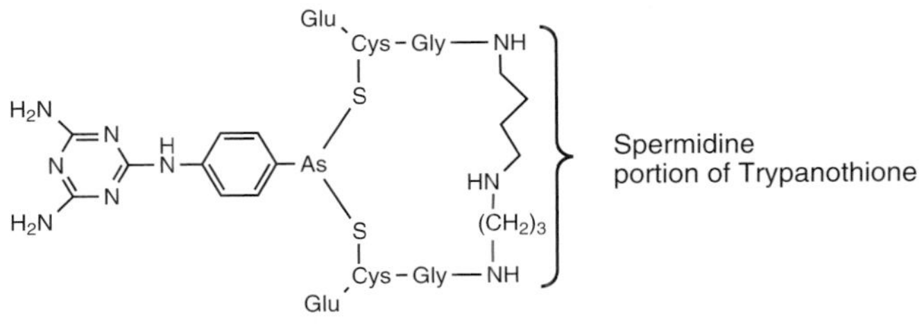

Spermidine portion of Trypanothione

Figure 32.9 Structure of melarsoprol trypanothione complex.

therapeutic agents to treat this disease.[29] Although the structure of sodium stibogluconate is commonly drawn as shown, the actual compound probably is much more complex. The drug is a water-soluble preparation that is administered IM or IV. Pentavalent antimony compounds are thought to inhibit bioenergetic processes in the pathogen, with catabolism of glucose and inhibition of glycolytic enzymes being the primary mechanism of action (glucose catabolism is 86%-94% inhibited). This in turn results in inhibition of adenosine triphosphate (ATP)/guanosine triphosphate formation.

Sodium sibogluconate (or meglumine antimonate, another pentavalent antimony agent) is the drug of choice for the treatment of most forms of leishmaniasis. The recommended dose is 20 mg antimony/kg/d, not to exceed 850 mg antimony/d. A number of other drugs have been reported to be effective in the treatment of leishmaniasis, and these include pentamidine, amphotericin B, paromomycin, alkylphosphocholine analogues, rifampicin, and ketoconazole.[30,31]

Miltefosine (Impavido)

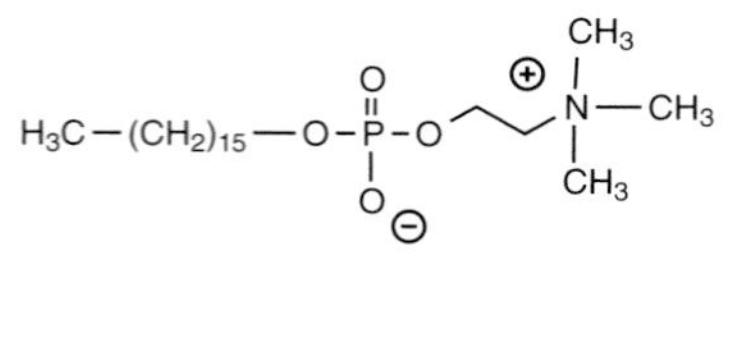

$H_3C-(CH_2)_{15}-O-P(=O)(O^-)-O-CH_2CH_2-N^+(CH_3)_3$

Miltefosine

Miltefosine is an orally active drug, which is effective against mucosal, visceral, and cutaneous leishmaniasis. The drug is approved by the FDA for adults and adolescents ≥12 years of age. This drug is especially important since the only other drug available is sodium stibogluconate which is administered IM or IV, thus limiting its utility, and has a high potential for toxicity associated with the antimony component of the drug. Miltefosine has been reported to exhibit activity in vitro against a broad range of leishmanial strains.

MECHANISM OF ACTION. Although the mechanism of action of miltefosine remains unknown, it has been suggested that the drug acts directly on the promastigote and amastigote stages of the parasite and not through stimulation of the immune system.[32] This distinction is important since patients who are immuno compromised can also suffer from leishmaniasis. It has been suggested that the drug may interact with the organism's lipid by inhibiting cytochrome c oxidase causing the death of the organism. In addition the drug may inhibit phosphatidylcholine synthesis. Recent work has demonstrated that miltefosine can increase accumulation of intracellular Ca^{2+} via opening sphingosine-activated plasma membrane Ca^{2+} channels in the parasite.[33]

PHARMACOKINETICS. The drug is well absorbed via the oral route and well distributed with a half-life of 6-8 days. Miltefosine is highly bound to plasma protein (~98%).

ADVERSE EFFECTS. Miltefosine is contraindicated in pregnant women since it has been reported to cause fetal death and teratogenicity in animals. Reduced fertility and testicular atrophy have been reported in male rats. Other adverse effects reported include decreased appetite and headaches, GI disorders, edema, jaundice and seizures.

Treatment of Malaria

Historical Background

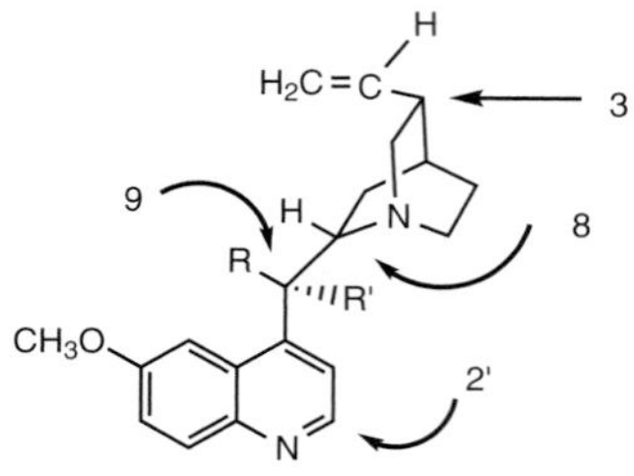

Quinine (R = OH, R' = H)
Quinidine (R = H, R' = OH)

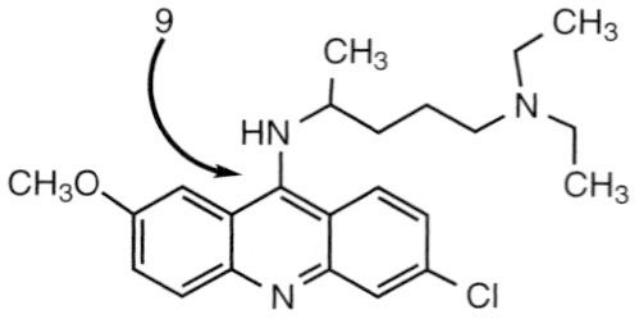

Quinacrine

Quinine was the first known antimalarial. It is a 4-quinolinemethanol derivative bearing a substituted quinuclidine ring. The use of quinine in Europe began in the 17th century, after the Incas of Peru informed the Spanish Jesuits about the antimalarial properties of the bark of an evergreen mountain tree they called quinquina (later called cinchona, after Dona Franciscoa Henriquez de Ribera [1576-1639], Countess of Chinchon and wife of the Peruvian Viceroy). The bark, when made into an aqueous solution, was capable of curing most forms of malaria. It was listed in the London Pharmacopeia of 1677. The alkaloid derived from the bark, quinine, was isolated in the mid-1820s. Quinine, a very bitter substance, has been used by millions of malaria sufferers. Recently, it has been employed successfully to treat chloroquine-resistant strains of *Plasmodium falciparum* and is considered to be the drug of choice for these resistant strains.

Quinidine, the C-9 stereoisomer of quinine, is also an effective antimalarial but suffers from the fact that it is considerably more toxic than quinine. Its use is usually limited to treatment of severe malarial infections. Quinidine is also used as an antiarrthymic agent.

A second class of chemicals that played a role in the development of synthetic antimalarials is the 9-aminoacridines. 9-Aminoacridine was known to exhibit antibacterial activity, whereas a derivative of 9-aminoacridine synthesized in 1934, quinacrine, was found to possess weak antimalarial activity.

With the beginning of World War II and concern about an interruption in the supply of cinchona bark from the East Indies, a massive effort was begun to search for synthetic alternatives to quinine and to develop more effective antimalarial agents than quinacrine. With a basic understanding of the structure-activity relationship of quinine (see Quinine, below) and the chemical

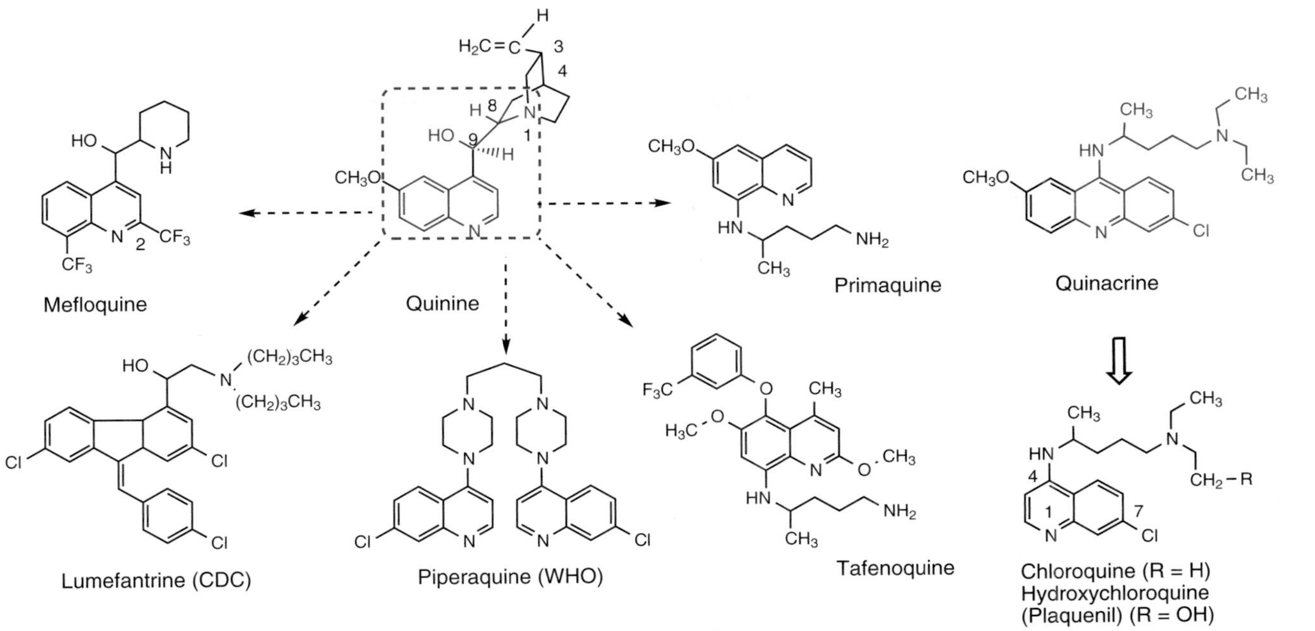

Figure 32.10 Structure similarity between the lead antimalarials (quinine and quinacrine) and the available antimalarials. *CDC*, Center for Disease Control; *WHO*, World Health Organization.

similarities seen with quinacrine, it is easy to visualize the relationship between these agents and the synthetic antimalarials (Fig. 32.10).

A third class of chemicals, which today represents the first-line standard treatment of malaria, is the artemisinins and the semisynthetic derivatives of this natural product. Artemisinin was first isolated over 2000 year ago from the sweet wormwood or annual wormwood plant *qing hao* (*Artemisia annua*). This natural product was used as an herbal medicine through the Chinese culture, and in the late 1500s was used for the treatment of malaria. Major developments in the chemistry of artemisinin were not reported until the 1970s, which lead to the development of semisynthetic analogues. The 2015 Nobel Prize in Physiology and Medicine was awarded to Tu Youyou for her contributions to the development of artemisinin and dihydroartemisinin and their use in treating malaria. Today artemisinin-based combination therapy (ACT) utilizing artemether, artesunate, and dihyroartemisinin serve as the main stay of antimalarial treatments (Fig. 32.11).

4-Substituted Quinolines

Eight compounds can be considered within this class of drugs: quinine, chloroquine and hydroxychloroquine, mefloquine, primaquine, tafenoquine, lumefantrine, and piperaquine. These compounds not only share a structural similarity but are also thought to have similar mechanisms of action, are effective on the same stage of the parasite, and can share similar mechanisms of resistance.

MECHANISM OF ACTION. The mechanism of action of chloroquine has been studied in depth, and the results of these studies have been assumed to be applicable to the other 4-substituted quinolines.[34] Various mechanisms of actions have been offered to explain the action of this class of drugs, including the DNA intercalation mechanism, the weak base hypothesis, and the ferriprotoporphyrin hypothesis. The present understanding about the mechanism of action would appear to utilize various aspects of each of these three mechanisms. It is known that hemoglobin is transported into the food vacuoles of the plasmodium (Figs. 32.12 and 32.13), where digestion of the hemoglobin supplies the organism with a source of amino acids.

One of the products of this digestion is a free heme called hematin. Hematin is toxic to the plasmodium cell, but it has been demonstrated that within the plasmodium vacuole the organism is capable of converting the hematin to nontoxic hemozoin. While it was initially thought that hemozoin was a polymeric form of hematin, it is now thought that the detoxification occurs through biocrystallization.[35,36] The

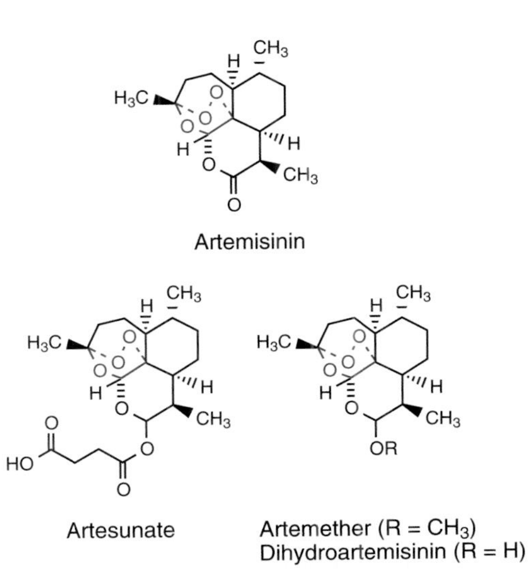

Figure 32.11 Structures of artemisinin and artemisinin derivatives.

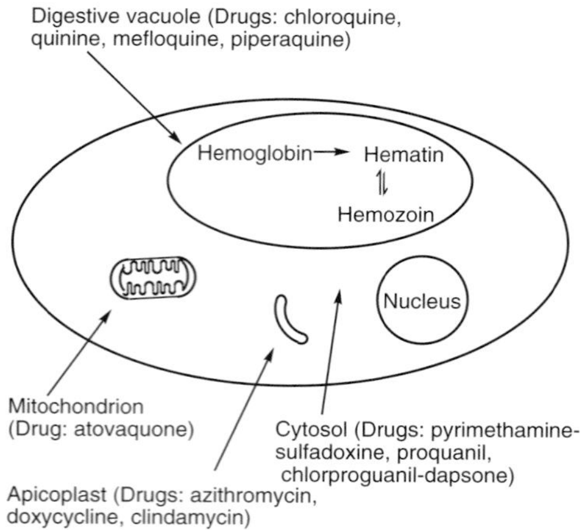

Figure 32.12 *Plasmodium* parasite cell as present within the erythrocyte and sites of drug action.

dimeric hemozoin as a biocrystal is insoluble and chemically inert and, therefore, has no biologic effect on the plasmodium. The quinolines bind to hematin through a drug-heme complex in which the aromatic quinoline ring binds via π-stacking to the porphyrin nucleus.[37] This drug-heme complex blocks further biocrystallization. The result of this complexation is that newly formed, free toxic hematin is now present, which leads to the death of the plasmodium. Additionally, since heme is not a component of plasmodium, it appears unlikely that the organism will be capable of developing a resistance mechanism to this type of activity. The accumulation of the 4-substituted quinolines in the acidic food vacuoles (pH 4.8-5.2) is based on the fact that these drugs are weak bases, as indicated by their pK_a values. The extracellular fluid of the parasite is at pH 7.4, and as a result, the weak base will move toward the more acidic pH of the vacuoles, reaching concentrations hundreds of times those in the plasma. Additionally, the binding of the quinoline to the heme draws additional quantities into the vacuole.

Mechanism of Resistance. A limiting factor for most of the antimalarial drugs is the development of resistant strains of plasmodium. It should be noted that resistance differs from region to region, and in some cases, a resistant strain can develop to a particular drug without that drug ever having been introduced to the region (possible cross-resistance). The development of resistance is thought to be due to a spontaneous gene mutation. Several mechanisms of resistance appear to be operating. One of these mechanisms is based on the *Plasmodium falciparium* chloroquine-resistance transporter (*pfrcrt*) mechanism, which is sufficient and necessary to impart resistance.[38] A gene encodes for a transmembrane transporter protein found in the membrane of the food vacuole. Multiple mutations within a specific region of this gene result in reduced accumulation of chloroquine, resulting from the increased efflux of the drug. Additional transporter proteins also can be involved in resistance.

Rapid metabolism of the antimalarials by resistant strains of plasmodium also might be considered to play a significant role in the development of resistance. It has been shown that cytochrome P450 activity parallels increased resistance to specific drugs.

Pharmacokinetics. In general, the quinolines are well absorbed via the oral route, with the exception of the fat-soluble drugs (e.g., lumefantrine and piperaquine), and have similar pharmacokinetic properties (Table 32.2).

Therapeutic Application. The 4-substituted quinolines are referred to as rapidly acting blood schizonticides, with activity against plasmodium in the erythrocytic stage. Chloroquine is the drug of choice, but unfortunately, the incidence of chloroquine-resistant infections is extremely common today. The spread of chloroquine resistance has reached almost all malarious areas of the world. In addition, multidrug-resistant and cross-resistant strains of plasmodium are now common. The drug of choice for the treatment of malaria caused by *Plasmodium falciparum*, *Plasmodium ovale*, *Plasmodium vivax*, and *Plasmodium malariae* in regions infected by chloroquine-resistant *P. falciparum* is quinine in combination with traditional antibiotics, mefloquine, or various other combinations as alternative treatment agents (Table 32.3). Of interest is the observation that after years of nonuse of chloroquine, a reemergence of chloroquine-sensitive parasites has been found.

The 4-substituted quinolines, depending on the specific drug in question, can also be used for prophylaxis of malaria. Two types of prophylaxis are possible: causal prophylaxis and suppressive prophylaxis. The former prevents the establishment of hepatic forms of the parasite, whereas the latter eradicates the erythrocytic parasites but has no effect on the hepatic forms. Several of the 4-substituted quinolines are effective suppressive prophylactics.

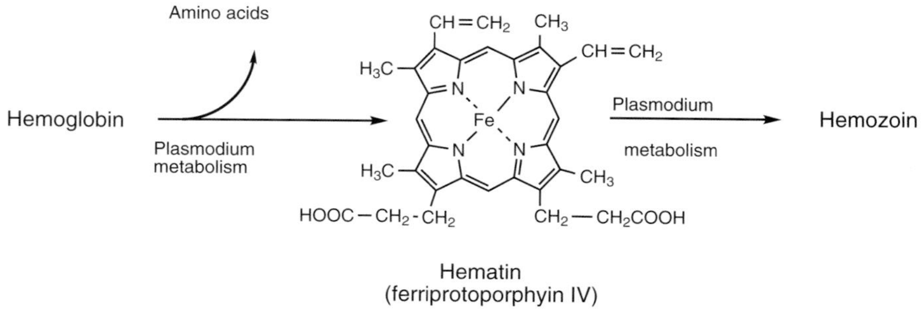

Hemoglobin → (Plasmodium metabolism; Amino acids) → Hematin (ferriprotoporphyin IV) → (Plasmodium metabolism) → Hemozoin

Figure 32.13 Proteolytic degradation of hemoglobin by the plasmodium organism to the potentially toxic hematin and then to the nontoxic dimers hemozoin.

Table 32.2 Pharmacokinetic of Quinoline Antimalarials

Generic Name	Protein Binding	Bioavailability	Half-Life (Days)	Route of Excretion
Quinine	69-92%	~85 %	~0.5	Urine
Chloroquine	~55%	75 %	3-9	Urine/feces
Hydroxychloroquine	30-40%	~74%	~40-50	Urine/feces
Mefloquine	>98%	~85%	20 median	–
Primaquine	NA	75%	~6 hr	Urine
Lumefantrine	99%	Low (5-11%)	3-6	Feces
Piperaquine	~97%	Not reported	20-30	Urine

Specific 4-Substituted Quinolines

Quinine. Quinine is the most prevalent alkaloid present in the bark extracts (~5%) of cinchona. Four stereochemical centers exist in the molecule (at C-3, C-4, C-8, and C-9) (Fig. 32.10). Quinine (absolute configuration of 3*R*:4*S*:8*S*:9*R*), quinidine (absolute configuration of 3*R*:4*S*:8*R*:9*S*), and their enantiomers all have antimalarial activity, whereas their diasteriomeric C-9 epimers (i.e., the epi-series having either 3*R*:4*S*:8*R*:9*R* or 3*R*:4*S*:8*S*:9*S* configurations) are inactive. Modification of the secondary alcohol at C-9, through oxidation, esterification, or similar processes, diminishes activity. The quinuclidine portion is not necessary for activity; however, an alkyl tertiary amine at C-9 is important.

Quinine is metabolized in the liver to the 2′-hydroxy derivative, followed by additional hydroxylation on the quinuclidine ring, with the 2,2′-dihydroxy derivative as the major metabolite. This metabolite has low antimalarial activity and is rapidly excreted. The metabolizing enzyme of quinine is CYP3A4. With the increased use of quinine and its use in combination with other drugs, the potential for drug interactions based on the many known substrates for CYP3A4 (see Chapter 3) is of concern.[39]

A quinine overdose causes tinnitus and visual disturbances; these side effects disappear on discontinuation of the drug. Quinine also can cause premature contractions during the late stages of pregnancy. Although quinine is suitable for parenteral administration, this route is considered to be hazardous because of its ability to cause hemolysis. Quinidine, the (+)-enantiomer of quinine, has been shown to be more effective in combating the disease, but it has undesirable cardiac side effects. When used for severe malaria, quinidine gluconate is administered IV.

Table 32.3 Guidelines for Treatment of Malaria in the United States[a]

Clinical Diagnosis	Sensitivity	Drug Recommendation
Uncomplicated malaria *P. falciparum*	Chloroquine sensitive	Chloroquine phosphate
	Chloroquine resistant or unknown	A. Atovaquone-proguanil (Malarone) B. Artemether-lumefantrine (Coartem) C. Quinine sulfate + one of the following: Doxycycline Tetracycline Clindamycin D. Mefloquine
Uncomplicated malaria *P. malariae, P. knowlesi*	Chloroquine sensitive	A. Chloroquine phosphate B. Hydroxychloroquine
Uncomplicated malaria *P. vivax or P. ovale*	Chloroquine sensitive	Chloroquine phosphate + Primaquine phosphate
Uncomplicated malaria *P. vivax*	Chloroquine resistant	A. Quinine sulfate + Doxycycline or Tetracycline B. Atovaquone-proguanil + Primaquine phosphate C. Mefloquine + Primaquine phosphate
Severe malaria	Chloroquine sensitive/resistant	Quinidine gluconate (parenteral) + one of the following: Doxycycline Tetracycline Clindamycin

[a]Information taken from the CDC Guideline for Treatment of Malaria in the United States. Updated July 1, 2013. For more details including infectious region and dosing go to: www.cdc.gov/malaria/diagnosis_treatment/treatment and then CDC treatment guidelines.pdf.

Chloroquine, Hydroxychloroquine (Fig. 32.10). Chloroquine is the most effective of the hundreds of 4-aminoquinolines synthesized and tested during World War II as potential antimalarials. Structure-activity relationships demonstrated that the chloro at the 8-position increased activity, whereas alkylation at C-3 and C-8 diminished activity. The replacement of one of its N-ethyl groups with a hydroxyethyl produced hydroxychloroquine, a compound with reduced toxicity that is rarely used today except in cases of rheumatoid arthritis.

Chloroquine is commonly administered as the racemic mixture because little is gained by using the individual isomers, which are more costly to produce. The drug is well absorbed from the GI tract and distributed to many tissues, where it is tightly bound and slowly eliminated. The drug is metabolized by N-dealkylation by CYP2D6 and CYP3A4 isoforms. It has been reported that the level of metabolism correlates closely with the degree of resistance. The suggestion has been made to coadminister chloroquine with CYP2D6 and CYP3A4 inhibitors to potentate activity and reduce resistance. Although this can be possible, it is not commonly practiced.

Chloroquine is an excellent suppressive agent for treating acute attacks of malaria caused by *Plasmodium vivax* and *Plasmodium ovale.* The drug is also effective for cure and as a suppressive prophylactic for the treatment of *Plasmodium malariae* and susceptible *Plasmodium falciparum.* Chloroquine is generally a safe drug, with toxicity occurring at high doses of medication, if the drug is administered too rapidly via parenteral routes. With oral administration, the side effects primarily are GI upset, mild headache, visual disturbances, and urticaria.

ADDITIONAL THERAPEUTIC INDICATIONS FOR CHLOROQUINE

Chloroquine is also prescribed for treatment of rheumatoid arthritis, discoid lupus erythematosus, and photosensitivity diseases.

Mefloquine (Fig. 32.10)[40]. Mefloquine, which was synthesized with the intent of blocking the site of metabolism in quinine with the chemically stable CF_3 group, exists as four optical isomers of nearly equal activity. The drug is active against chloroquine-resistant strains of plasmodium, yet cross-resistance is not uncommon. Metabolism is cited as the possible mechanism of resistance. Mefloquine is slowly metabolized through CYP3A4 oxidation to its major inactive metabolite, carboxymefloquine (Fig. 32.14). Most of the parent drug is excreted unchanged into the urine. Its coadministration with CYP3A4 inhibitors (e.g., ketoconazole) has increased the area under the curve for mefloquine by inhibiting its metabolism to carboxymefloquine.

Mefloquine is only available in an oral dosage form, which is well absorbed. The presence of food in the GI tract affects the pharmacokinetic properties of the drug, usually enhancing absorption. The lipophilic nature of the drug accounts for the extensive tissue binding and low clearance of total drug, although the drug does not accumulate after prolonged administration. The drug has a high affinity for erythrocyte membranes.

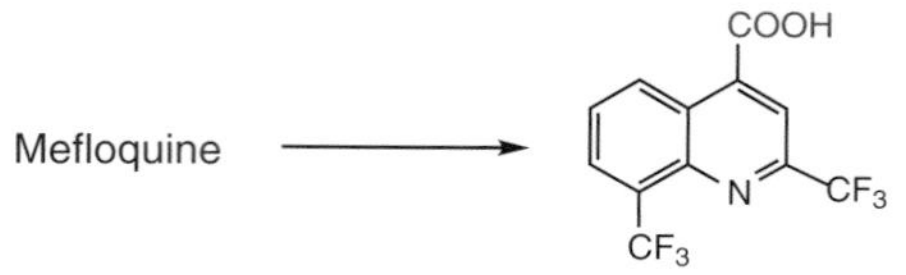

Mefloquine → [quinoline structure with COOH at C-4, CF_3 at C-2 and C-8]

Figure 32.14 *P. falciparumn* metabolism of mefloquine.

Mefloquine is an effective suppressive prophylactic agent against *Plasmodium falciparum*, both in nonimmune populations (travelers coming into regions of malaria) and in resident populations. The drug has also high efficacy against falciparum malaria, with a low incidence of recrudescence. The drug is ineffective against sexual forms of the organism.

The incidence of side effects with mefloquine is considered to be high. The effects are classified as neuropsychiatric, GI, dermatologic, and cardiovascular. The neuropsychiatric effects can be serious (e.g., suicidal tendencies or seizures) or relatively minor (e.g., dizziness, vertigo, ataxia, and headaches). Gastrointestinal side effects included nausea, vomiting, and diarrhea, whereas the dermatologic effects include rash, pruritus, and urticaria. Finally, cardiovascular side effects can include bradycardia, arrhythmias, and extrasystoles.

Lumefantrine (Fig. 32.10). Lumefantrine, an effective erythrocytic schizonticide, has been reported to exhibit antimalarial activity when combined with artemether in the treatment of multidrug-resistant *Plasmodium falciparium.* The drug is only used in combination with artemether (artemisinin-based combination therapies [ACTs]) in which a synergistic effect has been noted (see combinations with artemisinins). Lumefantrine has a relatively long half-life of 3-6 days, which makes it ideal for combination with the short half-life artemisinins. The drug is quite lipophilic, and a diet rich in fat increases the bioavailability of the drug. Unfortunately, many patients suffering from malaria do not tolerate food, and therefore the bioavailability of lumefantrine is not very high. No evidence of cardiotoxicity has been reported with this combination, which can offer promise for successful treatment of resistant organisms.

Piperaquine (Fig. 32.10). Piperaquine has been available since the 1960s but has not found significant use until the 1990s. With the development of chloroquine-resistant strains, piperaquine gained importance especially when used in combination with dihydroartemisinin. As with other quinolines, the drug enters the food vacuole of the plasmodium where it is suggested to have a mechanism of action similar to the other quinolines. Piperaquine has basically replaced chloroquinoline as a first-line agent. The long half-life combined with a shorter acting artemisinin has been useful in combination therapy.[41,42] Metabolism has been reported to involve oxidation to the carboxylic acid (Fig. 32.15).

8-AMINOQUINOLINES

Primaquine (Fig. 32.10). Primaquine is active against latent tissue forms of *Plasmodium vivax* and *Plasmodium ovale*, and it is active against the hepatic stages of

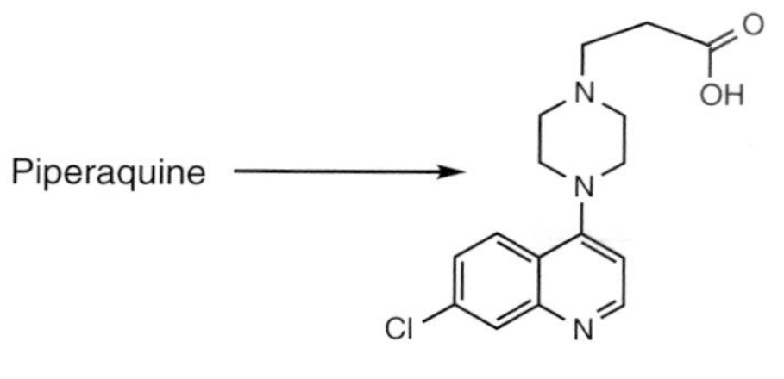

Figure 32.15 Metabolism of piperaquine.

Plasmodium falciparum. The drug is not active against erythrocytic stages of the parasite but does possess gametocidal activity against all strains of plasmodium.

Mechanism of Action. The mechanism of action of the 8-aminoquinolines is unknown, but primaquine can generate ROS via an autoxidation of the 8-amino group. The formation of a radical anion at the 8-amino group has been proposed by Augusto et al.[43] As a result, cell-destructive oxidants, such as hydrogen peroxide, superoxide, and hydroxyl radical can be formed, as shown in Figure 32.3, leading to oxidative damage to critical cellular components of the organism.

Metabolism. Primaquine is almost totally metabolized by CYP3A4 (99%), with the primary metabolite being carboxyprimaquine (Fig. 32.16).[44] Trace amounts of N-acetylprimaquine plus aromatic hydroxylation and conjugation metabolites also have been reported.

Tafenoquine (Krintafel) (Fig. 32.10). An exciting breakthrough in the treatment of relapse *P. vivax* has been reported utilizing tafenoquine, which like primaquine is effective against the latent liver stage (hypnozoites) of this disease. While the 4-aminoquinolines are effective against the blood stage (erythrocytic stage) of the disease (Fig. 32.1), the 8-aminoquinolines are active against the hypnozoites (liver stage).

Mechanism of Action. Tafenoquine has shed additional light on the action of the 8-aminoquinone. Tafenoquine is considered a prodrug, which requires metabolism by CYP2D6 to produce the active tafenoquine 5,6-quinone (Fig. 32.17), a source of reactive oxygen species.[45,46]

Therapeutic Application. Primaquine is classified as the drug of choice for the treatment of relapsing vivax and ovale forms of malaria and will produce a radical cure of the condition. It is recommended that the drug be combined with chloroquine to eradicate the erythrocytic stages of malaria. A major problem with primaquine is its short half-life (Table 32.2) and the fact that it cannot be given for long-term treatment because of potential toxicity and sensitization. The sensitivity appears most commonly in individuals who have glucose-6-phosphate dehydrogenase deficiency (G6PD). In these cases, hemolytic anemia can develop. While tafenoquine should still be limited in G6PD patients, its long half-life ($t_{1/2}$ 14-19 d) allows the drug to be used as a single dose treatment with better compliance.

Tafenoquine's bioavailability can be improved if administered with a high-fat meal, and the drug is reported to exhibit high protein binding (>99.5%). This combined with the slow metabolic activation may account for the long half-life.

PYRIMETHAMINE (DARAPRIM)

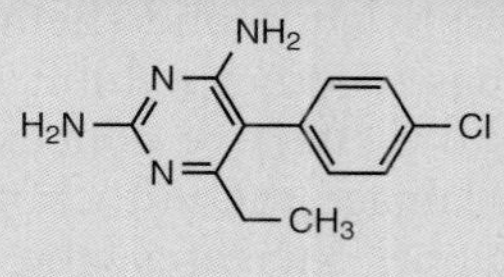

Pyrimethamine

Pyrimethamine was previously available as a fixed-dose combination with a sulfonamide (sulfadoxine, trade name Fansidar) but has been discontinued through the FDA due in part to potential toxicity. A black box warning indicated that fatalities and severe adverse reactions had occurred when the combination was used as an antimalarial. The combination is still listed by WHO for use in treatment of malaria in combination with artesunate. Pyrimethamine is available individually in the United States for treatment of toxoplasmosis a parasitic disease caused by *Toxoplasma gondii*. When used for treatment of this parasite, it is suggested that the drug be used conjointly with a synergic sulfonamide. Pyrimethamine is a potent inhibitor of dihydrofolate reductase.

Atovaquone-Proguanil (Malarone)

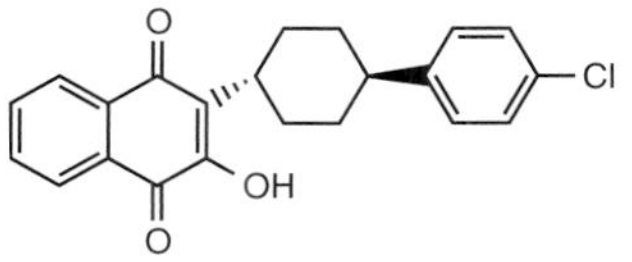

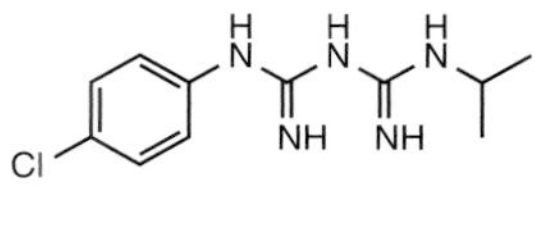

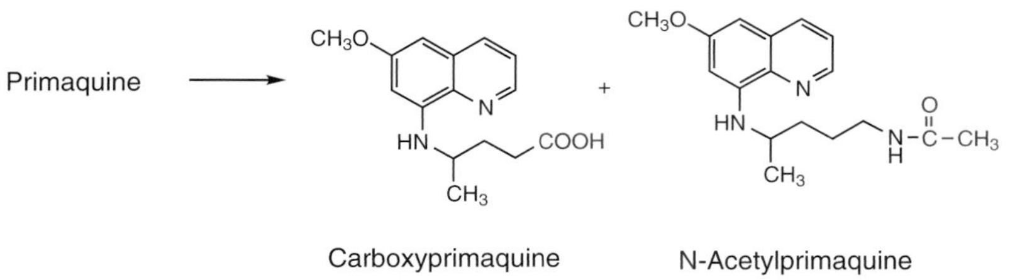

Figure 32.16 Metabolism of primaquine.

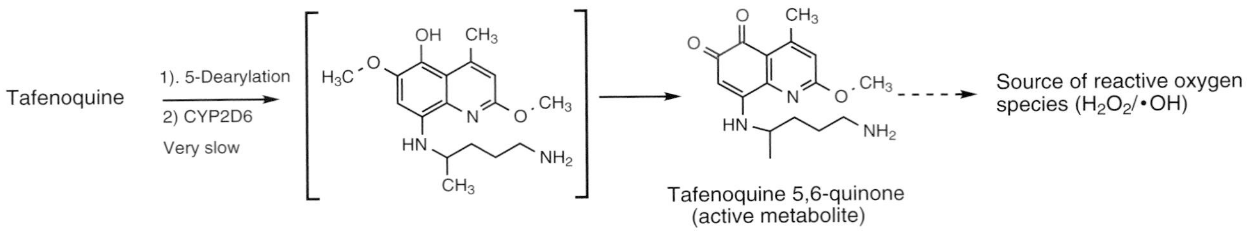

Figure 32.17 Metabolic activation of tafeoquine.

Atovaquone was originally developed as an antimalarial, but because of the high failure rate (~30%), it is not prescribed as a single chemical entity but rather is used to treat pneumocystis (see p. 29). More recently, however, atovaquone has been combined with proguanil as an effective prophylactic and therapeutic antimalarial.[38] The two drugs together exhibit synergy in which proguanil reduces the effective concentration of atovaquone needed to damage the mitochondrial membrane. In turn, atovaquone increases the effectiveness of proguanil but not its active metabolite (for the mechanism of action of atovaquone, see p. XXX). Proguanil was developed decades earlier as a folic acid antagonist and functions as a prodrug. The active form of proguanil is cycloguanil (Fig. 32.18), which acts as a DHFR inhibitor. Later, this discovery led to the development of pyrimethamine. The action of this combination occurs at two different locations. Atovaquone is active within the mitochondrion of the plasmodium while the proguanil acts as an antifolate in the cytosol (Fig. 32.12).

Resistance to atovaquone used as a monotherapy might have been associated with the pharmacokinetics of the drug. Atovaquone is quite lipophilic and has slow uptake resulting in the pathogen experiencing low concentrations of the drug over an extended period of time, both of which encourage the development of resistance. A single point mutation appears to be sufficient for resistance.[47] To date, resistance to the combination has not been reported, but treatment failure to the combination is possible.[48]

ARTEMISININS[49-52]. The most recent additions to the drug therapy for malaria are artemisinin and its derivatives (Fig. 32.11). Isolated from *Artemisia annua* (qinghao, sweetworm wood), this material has been used by Chinese herbalists since 168 BC. Artemisinin and the synthetic and semisynthetic derivatives, artemether, artesunate, and arteflene, are active by virtue of the endoperoxide. The artemisinin derivatives are built upon the 1,2,4-trioxanes or 1,2-dioxane ring systems.

The recommendation for treatment of malaria with artemisinins is that these drugs should not be used individually but rather in combination with at least one other effective medication with a different mechanism of action.

Mechanism of Action. Two mechanisms have been suggested to account for the antimalarial action of the artemisinins. In the first mechanism, the artemisinins appear to kill the parasite by a free radical mechanism—not by the generation of ROS but rather by virtue of a free radical associated with the endoperoxide, possibly involving a carbon radical. It is proposed that the heme in the form of hemazoin within the digestive vacuole is a source of Fe^{2+} which reacts with the peroxide to generate an oxy radical and Fe^{3+}. A carbon radical is formed from the oxy radical, which is then lethal to the plasmodium within the erythrocyte. The second mechanism suggests endoperoxide activation via an iron-dependent mechanism, but the activated artemisinins target sarcoplasmic/endoplasmic reticulum Ca^{2+}-ATPase of the *Plasmodium falciparum* (PfATP6), altering calcium stores.[53,54] The artemisinins actually can form covalent adducts to specific membrane-associated proteins after concentrating in infected erythrocytes.

Pharmacokinetics. The artemisinins are hydrophobic in nature with the exception of artesunate, which is available as a water-soluble hemisuccinate salt, and are partitioned into the membrane of the plasmodium. The artemisinin derivatives are available in various dosage forms, including oral tablets, intramuscular injectables, and rectal suppositories. Artemether and dihydroartemisinin are highly bound to plasma protein (93%-95%) with rapid elimination ($t_{1/2}$ 1-5 h). Artesunate is rapidly metabolized (~2 min via esterases) to dihydroartemisinin as is artemether via CYP3A4 and to a lesser extent by other cytochromes (Fig. 32.19).

Therapeutic Application. The artemisinins have gametocytocidal activity, as well as activity against all asexual stages of the parasites. These agents are short acting with relatively short half-lives. Little or no cross-resistance has been reported, with the drugs rapidly clearing the blood of parasites. The drugs have limited availability in the United States, but they are being utilized elsewhere

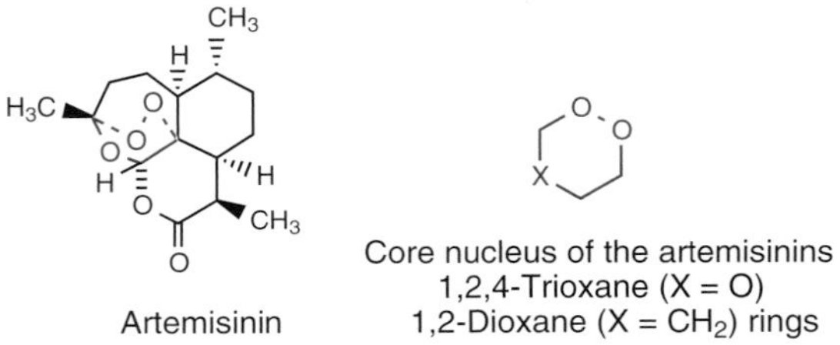

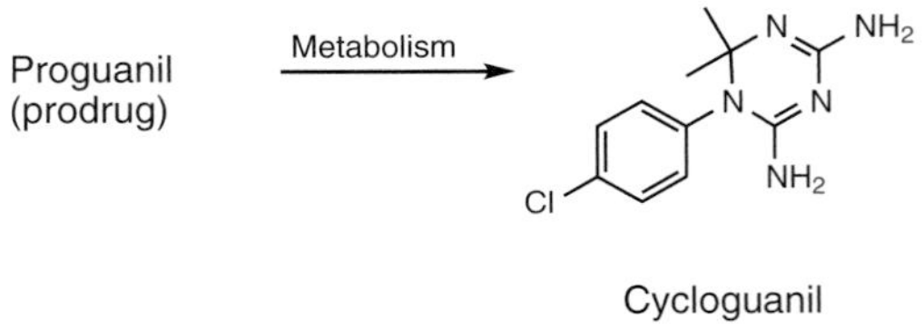

Figure 32.18 Activation of proguanil leading to cycloguanil.

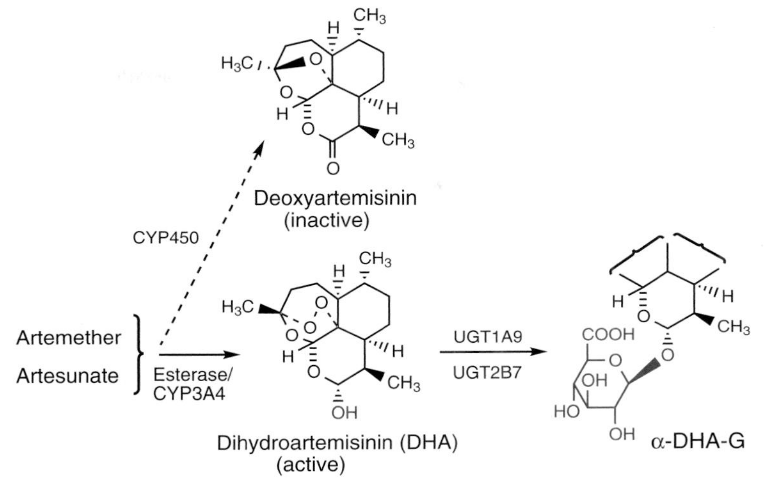

Figure 32.19 Metabolism of artemisinins.

as commercial or experimental agents in combination therapy (Table 32.4). Combination therapy has the goal of reducing resistance with the hope for synergism and, when combined with longer acting drugs, an improved therapy.

The ACTs have been reported to show cure rates of greater than 90%. The fixed-dose combination Coartem has been used in more than 10 million treatments, with significant increases being forecast. Common adverse effects include hypersensitivity reactions, GI disturbance, dizziness, and elevated liver enzymes.

The use of the artemisinins and artemisinin derivatives in other parasitic infections has received recent attention.[54] Specifially, several derivatives of artemisinin exhibited activity as antileishmaniasis agents, in treatment of shistosomiasis, and in treatment of trypanosomiasis. Combinations of artesunate-sulfamethoxypyrazine-pyrimethamine and artemether-lumefantrine are effective against *S. mansoni*, and artemisinin was reported to show activity against *T.b. rhodesiense*, *T. cruzi*, and *L. donovani* in vitro.

Antibiotics

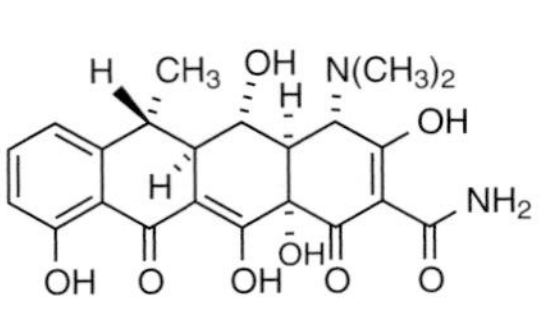

Doxycycline (Vibramycin)

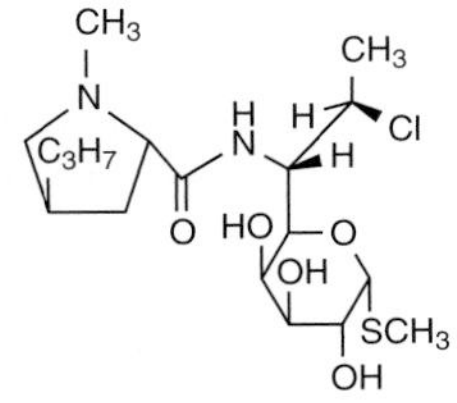

Clindamycin (Cleocin)

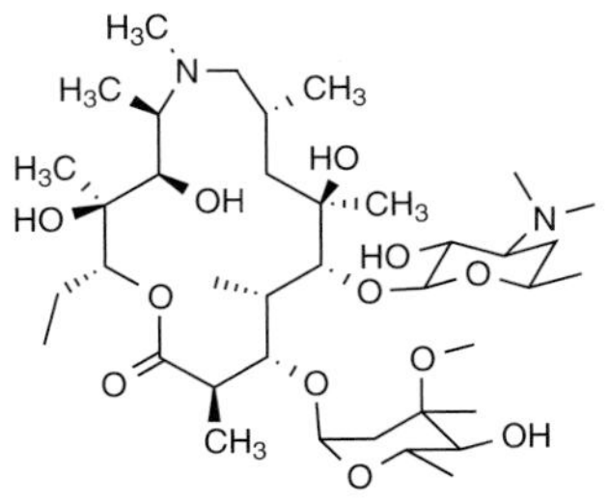

Azithromycin (Zithromax, Zmax)

Various antibiotics have proven useful in the treatment of malaria. They can be used alone as prophylaxis or in combination with quinine or artesunate as treatment measures. The most commonly used antibiotics are doxycycline, clindamycin, and azithromycin.[55] Their mechanisms of action are the same as those seen when treating a bacterial infection and involve interference in protein synthesis. What is unique about the use of the antibiotics in malaria is the site of action. The antibiotics affect protein synthesis within the apicoplast (Fig. 32.12). The apicoplast is an organelle found in most Apicomplexa (a group of eukaryotic microorganisms which include plasmodium). The apicoplast is a nonphotosynthesizing plastid with undefined function, although it does contain tRNAs, rRNAs, RNA polymerases, and ribosomal protein and is essential to the parasite's survival. Interference with protein synthesis blocks replication of the apicoplast organelle and prevents a second replication of the life cycle of the plasmodium and thus the prophylactic action. Limitations on the use of doxycycline include children and pregnant women, two major groups of malarial patients, which explain the use of clindamycin and azithromycin as backup drugs. Azithromycin has proven valuable in prophylaxis against *P. vivax*, although its use has been questioned.[56]

Table 32.4 Artemisinins Used in Artemisinin-Based Combination Therapy(ACT)

Artemisinin	Second Component of ACT	Trade Name/ Alternative Name
Artemether	Lumefantrine	Coartem[a]
Artesunate	Amodiaquine	ASAQWinthrop
Artesunate	Mefloquine	ASMQ
Artesunate	Pyrimethamine/ Sulfadoxine	SPAQ-CO
Dihyroartemisinin	Piperquine	Eurartesim

[a]The only FDA-approved artemisinin in the United States.

Clinical Application of Antimalarials

The treatment of malaria in children and adults as defined by WHO requires an integrated approach involving prompt treatment with effective drugs. Over the years, drug therapy has gone from monotherapy with quinolines to the use of ACT today. The treatment of uncomplicated malaria requires the cure of the infection as rapidly as possible, while the goal for severe malaria is to prevent death. In addition, it is important to use preventive therapy in healthy people. The goal is to eliminate the parasite from the blood, and to do so WHO recommends ACT for uncomplicated *P. falciparum* malaria. The ACT drugs should be active against the erythrocytic form of the disease. Activity against the gamete form of the disease is also important to prevent the spread of the disease. The site and spectrum of activity for the presented drugs are shown in Table 32.5. For a detailed review of the disease and its treatment, the reader is referred to the WHO *Guidelines for the Treatment of Malaria*, third edition, April 2015 (available at http://www.who.int/malaria/publications/atoz/9789241549127/en/).

HELMINTH INFECTIONS

Helminthiasis, or worm infestation, is one of the most prevalent diseases—and one of the most serious public health problems—in the world. Many worms are parasitic in humans and cause serious complications. Hundreds of millions (if not billions) of human infections by helminths exist worldwide, and with increased world travel and immigration from developing countries, one might expect to see this pattern of infection continue. It is estimated that one-fourth of the world population can be infected. It is interesting to note that helminths differ from many other parasites in that these organisms multiply outside of the definitive host and have the unique ability to evade host immune defenses for reasons that are not fully understood. As a result, helminth infections tend to be chronic, possibly lasting for the entire lifetime of the host. Interested readers are directed to a classic review of helminth infections published by Maizels, et al. (Immunological modulation and evasion by helminth parasites in human populations. *Nature* 1993; 365:797–805).

Helminths that infect human hosts are divided into two categories, or phyla: platyhelminths (flatworms) and aschelminths or nematodes (roundworms). The nematode class includes helminths common to the United States: roundworm, hookworm, pinworm, and whipworm. These worms are cylindrical in shape, with significant variations in size, proportion, and structure. The flatworms include the classes cestode (tapeworms) and trematode (flukes or schistosomes). A list of common human helminthes is shown in Table 32.6.

Nematode Infections

Ancylostomiasis or Hookworm Infection

The two most widespread types of hookworm in humans are the American hookworm (*Necator americanus*) and the "Old World" hookworm (*Ancylostoma doudenale*). The life cycles of both are similar. The larvae are found in the soil and are transmitted either by penetrating the skin or being ingested orally. The circulatory system transports the larvae via the respiratory tree to the digestive tract, where they mature and live for 9-15 years if left untreated. These worms feed on intestinal tissue and blood. Infestations cause pulmonary lesions, skin reactions, intestinal ulceration, and anemia. The worms are most prevalent in regions of the world with temperatures of 23-33°C, abundant rainfall, and well-drained, sandy soil.

*Enterobiasis or Pinworm Infection (*Enterobius Vermicularis*)*

These worms are widespread in temperate zones and are a common infestation of households and institutions. The pinworm lives in the lumen of the GI tract, attaching itself by the mouth to the mucosa of the cecum. Mature worms reach 10 mm in size. The female migrates to the

Table 32.5 Site and Spectrum of Action of Antimalarial Drugs

	Site of Action			*Plasmodium sp.*			
Drug/Drug Class	**Liver**	**Erythrocyte**	**Gametocyte**	***falciparum***	***ovale***	***vivax***	***malariae***
Artemisinins		√	√	√	√		√
Chloroquine		√		√	√	√	√
Hydroxychloroquine		√		√	√	√	√
Mefloquine		√		√	√	?	√
Lumefantrine		√		√		√	
Piperaquine		√		√			
Primaquine	√		√			√	
Pyrimethamine		√		√	?	√	?

Table 32.6 Human Infection Helminthes

Common Name	Phylum/Latin Name	Diseases	Location in Host
Roundworms	**Nematode**		
Hookworm	*Nector americanus*	Ancylostomiasis	Digestive tract
Hookworm	*Ancylostoma doudenale*	Ancylostomiasis	Digestive tract
Pinworm	*Enterobius vermicularis*	Enterobiasis	Digestive tract
Roundworm	*Ascaris lumbricoides*	Ascariasis	Small intestine
Whipworm	*Trichuris trichiura*	Trichuriasis	Intestinal wall
	Trichinella spiralis	Trichuriasis	Intestinal wall
Eyeworm	*Mansonella streptocerca*[a]	Filariasis	Subcutaneous layer
River blindness	*Onchocerca volvulus*	Onchoceriasis	Dermis
Timor filariasis	*Wuchereria bancrofti*	Elephantiasis	Lymphatic-dwelling
	Brugia malayi	Elephantiasis	Lymphatic-dwelling
	Brugia timori	Elephantiasis	Lymphatic-dwelling
Flatworms	**Cestode**		
Beef tapeworm	*Taenia saginata*	Taeniasis	Digestive tract
Pork tapeworm	*Taenia solium*	Cysticercosis	Digestive tract
Dwarf tapeworm	*Hymenolepis nana*		Digestive tract
Fish tapeworm	*Diphyllobothrium latum*		Digestive tract
	Trematode		
	Schistosoma hemaetobium	Schistosomiasis	Urinary bladder
	Schistosoma mansoni	Schistosomiasis	Blood vessels of GI tract
	Schistosoma japonicum	Schistosomiasis	Blood vessels of GI tract

[a]*M. streptocerca*, *O. volvulus*, *W. bancrofti*, *B. malayi*, and *B. timori* are commonly referred to as lymphatic-dwelling filariae. An early stage of these parasites is the microfilariae stage.

rectum, usually at night, to deposit her eggs. This event is noted by the symptom of perianal pruritus. The eggs infect fingers and contaminate nightclothes and bed linen, where they remain infective for up to three weeks. Eggs resist drying and can be inhaled with household dust to continue the life cycle. Detection of the worm in the perianal region can be accomplished by means of a cellophane tape swabbed in the perianal region in the evening. The worms can be visible with the naked eye. The eggs can be collected in a similar manner but can only be seen under a microscope.

*Ascariasis or Roundworm Infections (*Ascaris lumbricoides*)*

These roundworms are common in developing countries, with the adult roundworm reaching 25-30 cm in length and lodging in the small intestine. Some infections are without symptoms, but abdominal discomfort and pain are common with heavy infestation. Roundworm eggs are released into the soil, where they incubate and remain viable for up to 6 years. When the egg is ingested, the larvae are released in the small intestine, penetrate the intestinal walls, and are carried via the blood to the lungs. The pulmonary phase of the disease lasts approximately 10 days, with the larvae passing through the bronchioles, bronchi, and trachea before being swallowed and returning to the small intestine. Some patients have reported adult worms exiting the esophagus through the oral cavity, and it is not unusual for live ascaris to be expelled with a bowel movement. Poor or absent sanitary facilities expose the population to infestation through contaminated foods and beverages.

*Trichuriasis or Whipworm Infections (*Trichuris trichiura*)*

Infections by this parasite are caused by swallowing eggs from contaminated foods and beverages. The eggs are passed with the feces from an infected individual. These eggs can live in the soil for many years. The ingested eggs hatch in the small intestine, and the larvae embed in the intestinal wall. The worms then migrate to the large intestine, where they mature. Adult worms, which reach approximately 5 cm in length, thread their bodies into the epithelium of the colon. They feed on tissue fluids and blood. Infections from this worm cause symptoms of irritation and inflammation of the colonic mucosa, abdominal pain, diarrhea, and distention. Infections can last five or more years if not treated. Whipworm infections are commonly seen in individuals returning from visits to the subtropics and are more common in rural areas of the southeastern United States.

*Trichinosis or Trichina Infection (*Trichinella spiralis*)*

Trichinella spiralis produces an infection that can be both intestinal and systemic. The worm is found in muscle meat, where the organism exists as an encysted larva. Traditionally, the worm has been associated with domestic pork that feeds on untreated garbage. More recently, outbreaks have occurred in individuals eating infected game, such as wild boar, bear, or walrus. Trichinosis infections are more likely to occur after consumption of homemade pork or wild game sausages. After ingestion, the larvae are released from the cyst form and then migrate into the intestinal mucosa. After maturation and reproduction, the newly released larvae penetrate the mucosal lining and are distributed throughout the body, where they enter skeletal muscle. During the adult intestinal stage, diarrhea, abdominal pain, and nausea are the most common symptoms, whereas the muscular form of the disease has symptoms that can include muscle pain and tenderness, edema, conjunctivitis, and weakness.

Filariasis

The term "filariasis" denotes infections with any of the Filarioidea, although it is commonly used to refer to lymphatic-dwelling filariae, such as *Wuchereria bancrofti*, *Brugia malayi*, and *Brugia timori*. Other filarial infections include *Loa loa* and *Onchocerca volvulus*. The latter two are known as the eyeworm and the river blindness worm, respectively. Elephantiasis is the most common disease associated with filariasis. These parasites vary in length from 6 cm for *Brugia* to 50 cm for *Onchocerca*. The incubation periods also vary from 2 months for brugian to 12 months for bancroftian filaria. It is estimated that 400 million persons are infected with human filarial parasites. Depending on the specific organism, various intermediate hosts are involved in spreading the infection. Mosquitoes are involved with the spread of *Wuchereria bancrofti*, *Brugia malayi*, and *Brugia timori*, whereas the female blackfly spreads river blindness. The larvae released by the female filaria are referred to as microfilariae and commonly can be found in the lymphatics.

Cestode and Trematode Infections

Cysticercosis or Tapeworm Infection

Helminths of this class that are of concern as potential parasites in humans include the following.

BEEF TAPEWORM (*Taenia saginata*)
This worm is found worldwide and infects people who eat undercooked beef. The worm reaches a length of more than 5 m, and it contains approximately 100 segments/m. Each of these segments contains its own reproductive organs.

PORK TAPEWORM (*Taenia solium*)
Pork tapeworms sometimes are called bladder worms and occasionally are found in uncooked pork. The worm attaches itself to the intestinal wall of the human host. The adult worm reaches 5 m in length and, if untreated, survives in the host for many years.

DWARF TAPEWORM (*Hymenolepis nana*)
This infection is transmitted directly from one human to another without an intermediate host. *Hymenolepis nana* reaches only 3-4 cm in length. It is found in temperate zones, and children are most frequently infected.

FISH TAPEWORM (*Diphyllobothrium latum*)
The fish tapeworm reaches a length of 10 m and contains approximately 400 segments/m. These tapeworms attach themselves to the intestinal wall and rob the host of nutrients. They especially absorb vitamin B_{12} and folic acid. Depletion of these critical nutrients, especially vitamin B_{12}, can lead to pernicious anemia. Tapeworm eggs are passed in the patient's feces, and contamination of food and drink can result in transmission of the infection.

Schistosomiasis or Blood Flukes

Three primary trematode species cause schistosomiasis in humans: *Schistosoma hematobium*, *Schistosoma mansoni*, and *Schistosoma japonicum*. Infections result from the penetration of normal skin by living (free-swimming) cercaria (the name given to the infectious stage of the parasite) with the aid of secreted enzymes. The cercariae develop to preadult forms in the lungs and skin. Then, these parasites travel in pairs via the bloodstream and invade various tissues. The adult worm reaches approximately 2 cm in length. The female deposits her eggs near the capillary beds, where granulomas form. Some of the eggs will move into the lumen of the intestines, bladder, or ureters and are released into the environmental surroundings, where the parasite will seek out the intermediate snail vector. Asexual reproduction occurs in the snail. After a period of time, the cercariae are again released from the snail to continue the cycle.

Patients might experience headache, fatigue, fever, and GI disturbances during the early stages of the disease. Hepatic fibrosis and ascites occur during later stages. Untreated patients can harbor as many as 100 pairs of worms. Untreated worms can live 5-10 years within the host. As many as 200 million persons worldwide are estimated to be infected with schistosomes. Depending on the species of schistosome, the disease is found in parts of South America, the Caribbean Islands, Africa, and the Middle East.

Drug Therapy for Helminth Infections[57]

Helminths represent a biologically diverse group of parasitic organisms differing in size, life cycle, site of infection (local and systemic), and susceptibility to chemotherapy. With such variation in infectious organisms, it is not surprising that the drugs used to control helminth infections also represent a varied group of chemical classes.

Benzimidazoles

The benzimidazoles (Table 32.7) are a broad-spectrum group of drugs discovered in the 1960s with activity against

Table 32.7 Benzimidazole Anthelmintics

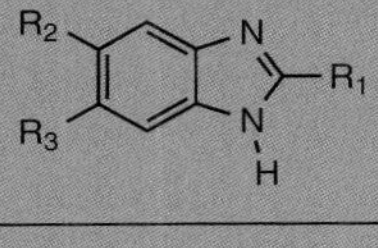

Drugs	Trade Name	R_1	R_2	R_3
Mebendazole	Emverm Vermox	$-NH-C(=O)-OCH_3$	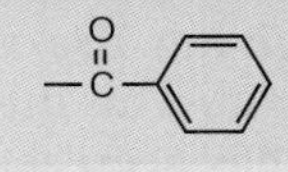 $-C(=O)-C_6H_5$	H
Albendazole	Albenza	$-NH-C(=O)-OCH_3$	$-SCH_2CH_2CH_3$	H
Triclabendazole	Egaten[a] Fasinex[b]	$-S-CH_3$	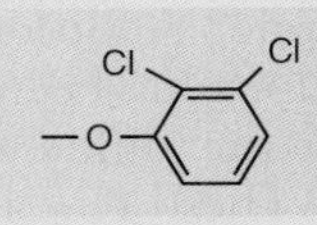 $-O-C_6H_3Cl_2$ (2,3-dichlorophenoxy)	Cl
Fenbendazole	Several brand names[b]	$-NH-C(=O)-OCH_3$	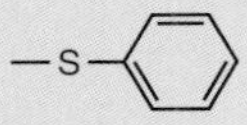 $-S-C_6H_5$	H
Flubendazole	Several brand names[b]	$-NH-C(=O)-OCH_3$	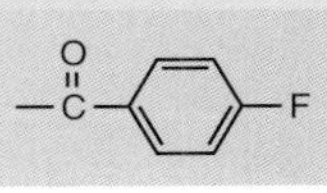 $-C(=O)-C_6H_4-F$	H

[a]Egaten has recently been shown to be useful for treatment of fascioliasis by WHO.
[b]Used in veterinary practice for protection and treatment of parasite and worm infections.

GI helminths. Several thousand benzimidazoles have been synthesized and screened for anthelmintic activity, with albendazole and mebendazole representing the only benzimidazoles marketed in the United States today. The development and chemistry of this class of agents has been reviewed by Townsend and Wise.[58]

MECHANISM OF ACTION. Two mechanisms have been proposed to account for the action of the benzimidazoles. Fumarate reductase is an important enzyme in helminths that appears to be involved in oxidation of NADH to NAD. The benzimidazoles are capable of inhibiting fumarate reductase.[59] Inhibition of fumarate reductase ultimately uncouples oxidative phosphorylation, which is important in ATP production.

A second mechanism, and probably the primary action of the benzimidazoles, is associated with their ability to bind to the protein tubulin and, thus, prevent tubulin polymerization to microtubules.[60,61] Tubulin is a dimeric protein that is in dynamic equilibrium with the polymeric microtubules. Binding to the tubulin prevents the self-association of tubulin subunits and creates a "capping" of the microtubule at the associating or polymerizing end. The microtubule continues to dissociate or erode from the opposite end, with a net loss of microtubule length. What is interesting is the unique selectivity of the benzimidazoles. Benzimidazole can also bind to mammalian tubulin, but when used as anthelmintics, these drugs are destructive to the helminth with minimal toxicity to the host. It has been suggested that the selectivity is associated with differing pharmacokinetics between binding to the two different tubulin proteins.

METABOLISM. The benzimidazoles have limited water solubility and, as a result, are poorly absorbed from the GI tract (a fatty meal will increase absorption). Poor absorption can be beneficial because the drugs are used primarily to treat intestinal helminths. To the extent that the drugs are absorbed, they undergo rapid metabolism in the liver and are excreted in the bile (Fig. 32.20).[62,63] In most cases, the parent compound is rapidly and nearly completely metabolized, with oxidative and hydrolytic processes predominating. The phase 1 oxidative reaction commonly is

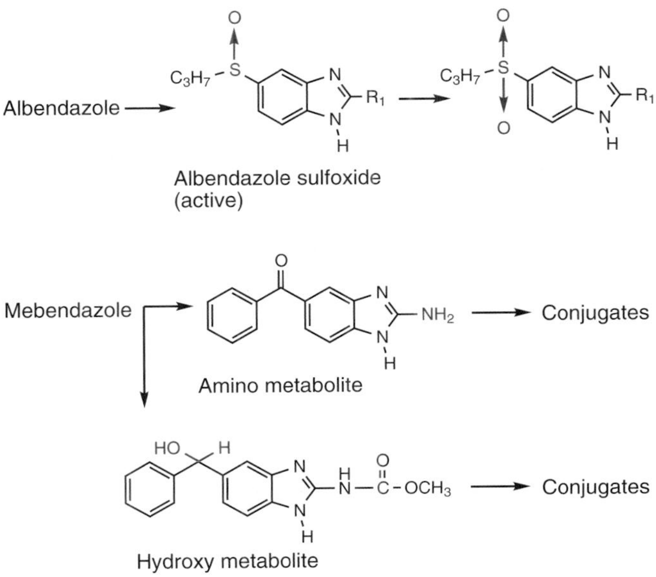

Figure 32.20 Metabolism of benzimidazoles.

a cytochrome P450–catalyzed reaction, which can then be followed by a phase 2 conjugation.

Albendazole is unique in two ways. First, the presence of a thioether substituent at the 5-position increases the likelihood of sulfur oxidation. Second, the initial metabolite, albendazole sulfoxide, is a potent anthelmintic. This initial oxidation is catalyzed principally (70%) by CYP3A4 and CYP1A2 and 30% is metabolized by flavin-containing monooxygenase, giving rise to a compound that is bound to plasma protein. This intermediate has an expanded utility in that it has been shown to be active against the hydatid cyst found in echinococciasis, a tapeworm disease.[64] Further oxidation by cytochrome P450 leads to the inactive sulfone. Additional metabolic biotransformation of the sulfone has been reported, including carbamate hydrolysis to the amine and oxidation of the 5-propyl side chain. These reactions occur only to a minor extent.

Metabolism of mebendazole occurs primarily by reduction of the 5-carbonyl to a secondary alcohol, which greatly increases the water solubility of this compound. An additional phase 1 metabolite resulting from carbamate hydrolysis has been reported as well. Both the secondary alcohol and the amine are readily conjugated (a phase 2 reaction). Evidence would suggest that the anthelmintic activity of mebendazole resides in the parent drug and not in the metabolites.

THERAPEUTIC APPLICATION. As indicated in Table 32.8, mebendazole and albendazole have a wide spectrum of activity against intestinal nematodes. The drugs are useful and effective against mixed infections. The adverse reactions are commonly GI in nature (nausea, vomiting, and diarrhea). Both drugs have been reported to be teratogenic in rats and, therefore, should not be used during the first trimester of pregnancy.

Table 32.8 Therapeutic Application of Anthelmintics for Specific Helminth Infections

	M	A	IVM	PZQ	PP
Nematode infections:					
Necator americanus	✓	✓			
Ancylostoma doudenale	✓	✓			✓
Enterobius vermicularis	✓		✓		✓
Ascaris lumbricoides	✓	✓	✓		✓
Trichuris trichiura	✓	✓	✓		
Trichinella spiralis	✓	✓			
Wuchereria bancrofti			✓		
Brugia malayi			✓		
Brugia timori.					
Loa Loa		✓	✓		
Onchocerca volvulus		✓	✓		
Cestode Infections:					
Taenia saginata	✓	✓		✓	
Taenia solium	✓	✓		✓	
Hymenolepis nana	✓			✓	
Diphyllobothrium latum				✓	
Trematode Infections:					
Schistosoma hematobium				✓	
Schistosoma mansoni				✓	
Schistosoma japonicum				✓	

Benzimidazoles: A, albendazole; IVM, ivermectin; M, mebendazole; PP, prantel pamoate; PZQ, praziquantel.

DIETHYLCARBAMAZINE CITRATE

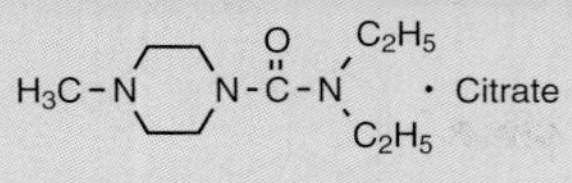

Diethylcarbamazine citrate

Diethylcarbamazine has been discontinued in the United States but is listed in the WHO Model List of Essential Medicines 20th List (March 2017) for treatment of filariasis.

Ivermectin (Stromectol)

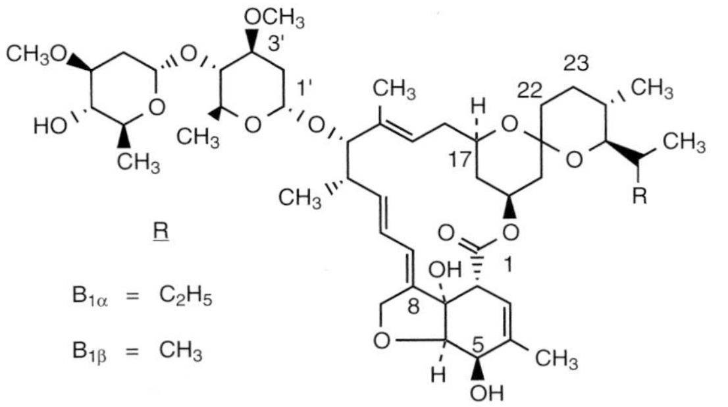

Ivermectin

Extracted from the soil actinomycete *Streptomyces avermitilis*, the natural avermectins are 16-membered macrocyclic lactones which are 80:20 mixtures of avermectin $B_{1\alpha}$ and $B_{1\beta}$, respectively, and used under the generic name abamectin. As such the product is used for the control of various insects, mite pests, fire ants and as a veterinary antihelmintic. Reduction of the $C_{22\text{-}23}$ double bond, gives rise to ivermectin (IVM), which is an 80:20 mixture of dihydroavermectin $B_{1\alpha}$ and $B_{1\beta}$, respectively. The natural avermectins have minimal biological activity, but IVM has proven to be quite beneficial in the treatment of various nematode infections.

MECHANISM OF ACTION. Two mechanisms of action are thought to be involved in the action of IVM.[57,65] The first is an indirect action in which motility of microfalaria is reduced, which in turn allows cytotoxic cells of the host to adhere to the parasite, resulting in elimination from the host. This action can occur by virtue of the ability of IVM to act either as a γ-aminobutyric acid (GABA) agonist or as an inducer of chloride ion influx, leading to hyperpolarization and muscle paralysis. The chloride ion influx appears to be the more plausible mechanism.[66] Recently, it has been shown that IVM binds irreversibly to the glutamate-gated chloride channel of the nematode *Haemonchus contortus*, where the channel is in an open conformation. The binding then remains locked in the open conformation, allowing ions to cross the membrane, leading to the paralytic action of IVM.[67] The result of this action is a rapid decrease in microfilarial concentrations.

A second action of IVM leads to the degeneration of microfilariae in utero. This action would result in fewer microfilariae being released from the female worms, and it occurs over a longer period of time. The presence of degenerated microfilariae in utero prevents further fertilization and production of microfilariae.

MOXIDECTIN

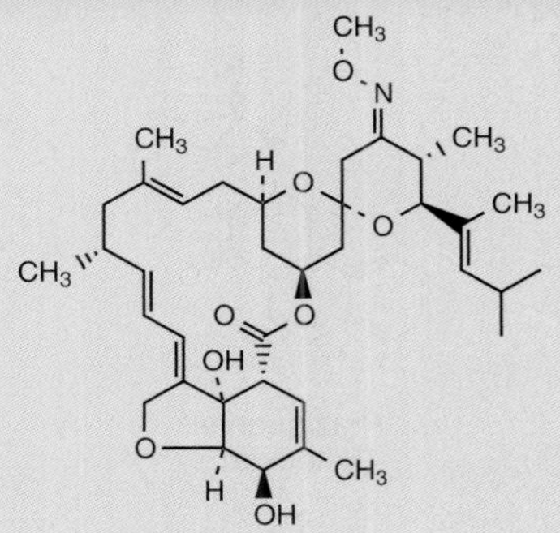

Moxidectin

Moxidectin, an orally administered drug, has recently been approved for treatment of patients aged 12 years or older with onchocerciasis (river blindness) due to *Onchocerca volvulus*. The drug is effective against the microfilaria and not effective against the adult form of the worm. Studies would suggest improved effectiveness verses ivermectin with a similar pattern of adverse effects. As an analog of ivermectin, moxidectin's mechanism of action is reported to be the same. Moxidectin has been available for some time for veterinary use for prevention and treatment of worms in dogs, cats, cattle, sheep, and horses.

METABOLISM. Ivermectin is rapidly absorbed, bound to a great extent to plasma protein, and excreted in the urine or feces either unchanged or as the 3′-O-demethyl-22,23-dihydroavermectin $B_{1\alpha}$ or dihydroavermectin $B_{1\alpha}$ monosaccharide metabolites. The absorption of IVM is significantly affected by the presence of alcohol. Administration of IVM as an alcoholic solution can result in as much as a 100% increase in absorption.

THERAPEUTIC APPLICATION. Although IVM has activity against a variety of microfalaria, including *Wuchereria bancrofti*, *Brugia malayi*, *Loa loa*, and *Mansonella ozzardi*, as well as activity against *Strongyloides stercoralis*, the drug is used primarily in the treatment of onchocerciasis (African river blindness) caused by *Onchocerca volvulus*. It is estimated that 20 million people are affected by this condition and an additional 123 million are at risk of the infection. The drug is effective against both the eyeworm as well as skin infections of *O. volvulus*. Ivermectin has the distinct advantage over the previously available diethylcarbamazine (recently discontinued in the United States) in that IVM can be used as a single dose (150 μg/kg) once a year (although there is support for dosing every 6 mo), has far less likelihood of causing the potentially fatal anaphylactic reaction (Mazzotti reaction), and can be used for mass treatment programs.

It should be noted that two topical dosage forms are available for the treatment of head lice (Sklice) and rosacea lesions (Soolantra).

Praziquantel (Biltricide)

Praziquantel
(Biltricide)

Praziquantel (PZQ) is an isoquinoline derivative with most of the biological activity found in the levo enantiomer. The compound has no activity against nematodes, but it is highly effective against cestodes and trematodes.

MECHANISM OF ACTION. More than one mechanism of action can exist for PZQ, possibly depending on the type of parasite being treated. The mechanism of action appears to involve Ca^{2+} redistribution, either directly or indirectly. In the case of helminths found in the lumen of the host (cestode infection), the drug leads to muscle contraction and paralysis, leading in turn to worm expulsion. Additionally, PZQ has been shown to inhibit phosphoinositide metabolism, which by an undetermined mechanism, leads to the worm paralysis.[68] With intravascular-dwelling schistosomes, PZQ leads to drug-induced damage of the tegument of the worm. As a result, antigens in the helminth are subject to attack by immune antibodies of the host.[69,70] An antigen-antibody immunological reaction leads to the death of the parasite. Finally, PZQ affects glycogen content and energy metabolism.[71,72]

METABOLISM. Praziquantel is rapidly absorbed and undergoes hepatic first-pass metabolism. The metabolites are either less active or inactive and consist of hydroxylated compounds. In the serum, the major metabolite appears to be the monohydroxylated 4-hydroxycyclohexylcarboxylate, whereas in the urine 50%-60% of the initial PZQ exists as dihydroxylated products (Fig. 32.21).[73] These hydroxylation reactions are catalyzed by CYP2B6 and CYP3A4. The metabolites would be expected to exist in the conjugated form in the urine.

THERAPEUTIC APPLICATION. PZQ is the drug of choice for treatment of schistosomiasis and liver flukes (trematode and cestode infections). The drug is stage specific, with activity against the invasive stages. This includes the cercariae and young schistosomula and the mature worms but not the liver stages. Although an approved drug, PZQ is considered to be an investigational drug by the FDA in

Praziquantel (PZQ)

Urinary metabolites

Serum metabolite

Figure 32.21 Metabolism of praziquantel (PZQ).

the treatment of schistosomiasis and liver flukes. The drug has a bitter taste and, therefore, should not be chewed. The side effects usually are not severe and consist of abdominal discomfort (pain and diarrhea). Mounting evidence suggests that resistance can become a significant problem.

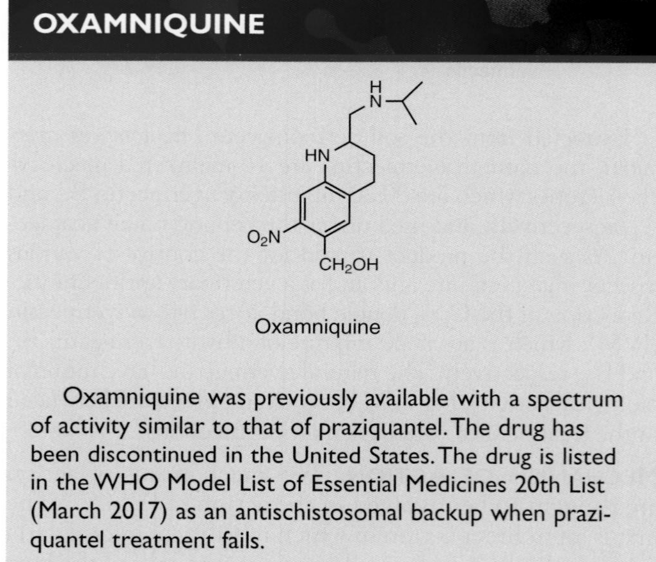

OXAMNIQUINE

Oxamniquine

Oxamniquine was previously available with a spectrum of activity similar to that of praziquantel. The drug has been discontinued in the United States. The drug is listed in the WHO Model List of Essential Medicines 20th List (March 2017) as an antischistosomal backup when praziquantel treatment fails.

Pyrantel Pamoate (Various Over-the-Counter Products)

Pyrantel pamoate

Pyrantel was first reported for its anthelmintic activity in 1966.[74] Although it has activity against most intestinal roundworm infections, it is considered to be the drug of choice in the treatment of pinworms. The drug is used as the pamoate salt, which is quite insoluble and, as a result, is not readily absorbed. This property improves the usefulness of the drug for treatment of intestinal helminths. In addition to its value in treating enterobiasis, the drug is effective for hookworm and roundworm (ascariasis) infections.

MECHANISM OF ACTION. Pyrantel acts as a depolarizing neuromuscular blocking agent that activates nicotinic receptors and inhibits cholinesterase, ultimately leading to worm paralysis.

THERAPEUTIC APPLICATIONS. Pyrantel pamoate is generally effective in the treatment of roundworm infections and is considered the drug of choice for treatment of pinworm infections (*Enterobius vemicularis* as indicated in Table 32.8).

ECTOPARASITIC INFECTIONS

Three parasitic organisms that cause common topical infections are *Sarcoptes scabiei*, which is responsible for scabies, *Pediculus humanus*, which is responsible for lice infections, and *Cimex lectularius* the common bedbug which is an insect living exclusively on the blood of warm-blooded animals. This latter organism has shown a recent reemergence, and while its bite is normally not responsible for a primary or secondary infection, the topical irritation and the social implications can be quite disturbing to the patient. The only treatment is the use of antipruretics and the hiring of a professional exterminator.

Scabies

Scabies, commonly referred to as the "seven-year itch," is a condition caused by *Sarcoptes scabiei*, or the itch mite. The condition is commonly spread by direct, person-to-person contact, although the organism is capable of living for 2-3 days in clothing, bedding, or house dust. Sharing of clothing is a common means whereby the condition spreads. The organism burrows into the epidermis, usually in the folds of the skin of the fingers, the elbows, female breast, penis, scrotum, and buttocks. The female parasite lays eggs in the skin, which then hatch and mature to adults. The itch mite can live for 30-60 days. The infections are most common in children, but they also can be found in adults in institutional settings. The primary symptom of severe itching can foster secondary infections at the site of scratching. Because of the potential for spread to other members of a family, it is common to treat all family members. This will prevent reinfection from a second family member after successful therapy of the first family member.

Lice

Pediculosis (lice associated disease) is caused by any of the parasites *Pediculus humanus capitis*, the head louse; *Pediculus humanus corporis*, the body louse; or *Phthirius pubis*, the crab louse (found in the genital area). Lice are blood-sucking insects that live for 30-40 days on the body of the host. The organisms reproduce, and the female lays her eggs, the nits, which become attached to hair. The nits are white in color and hatch in 8-10 days. For the parasite to live, it must feed on blood, which it sucks through punctures in the skin. A hypersensitivity reaction occurs at these puncture sites, which then leads to pruritus, host scratching, and possible secondary infection. In addition to the scalp and skin, the eyebrows, eyelids, and beard can become sites of infection. The transfer of infection can occur through person-to-person contact and from infected clothing, on which the organism can survive for up to 1 week. The sharing of clothing is a common means for the spread of body lice. Head lice are quite common among children in grade school, whereas crab lice are common among individuals who are sexually active. Treatment of family members is recommended, and clothing and bed linens should be removed and washed in very hot water.

Drug Therapy for Scabies and Pediculosis

Lindane

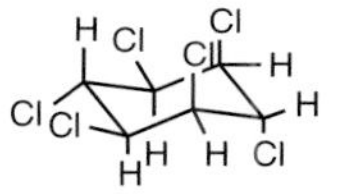

H Cl Cl Cl H Cl Cl H H H H H Cl

γ-Benzene hexachloride
(Lindane)

Chlorination and reduction of benzene leads to a mixture of hexachlorocyclohexanes. The insecticidal activity resides primarily in the γ-isomer of hexachlorocyclohexane (γ-benzene hexachloride). The compound is thought to produce its insecticidal action by virtue of a CNS stimulatory action that occurs by blockage of GABA. The compound is readily absorbed through the chitinous exoskeleton of the parasite. Unfortunately, lindane is also readily absorbed through intact human skin, especially the scalp, and has the potential for systemic neurotoxicity in the host. Infants, children, and possibly the elderly are most prone to the neurotoxic effects of the drug. Because lindane is quite lipophilic and is applied to the scalp as a shampoo, it can be absorbed and readily enter the CNS of the patient producing signs of neurotoxicity (convulsions, dizziness, clumsiness, and unsteadiness).

The drug is available in a lotion and a shampoo and is recommended for the treatment of both pediculosis and scabies. When using the lotion topically, it should be applied to dry skin (covering the entire surface) and left in place for 8 hours. The lindane then should be removed by washing thoroughly. If the shampoo is used for *Pediculosis capitis*, the hair should be cleaned of oil and dried before application of the lindane shampoo. The shampoo is then worked into the hair and scalp, being applied in such a way as to prevent other parts of the body from coming into contact with the drug. After approximately 4 minutes, the drug is removed by rinsing with water, and the hair is dried and then combed with a fine-toothed comb to remove nits.

Pyrethrum and Pyrethroids

The naturally occurring pyrethrums have been used as insecticides since the 1800s. These compounds are extracted from the flowering portion of the *Chrysanthemum* plant. The flowers produced in Kenya have, on average, 1.3% pyrethrins. These pyrethrum extracts have been a major agricultural product for that country.

CHEMISTRY. The *Chrysanthemum* extract is a mixture of alcohols and esters including chrysanthemic and pyrethric acids (Fig. 32.22). The esters are prone to hydrolysis and oxidation and, as a result, should be stored in the cold and protected from light. Because of the high cost, limited availability, and rapid degradation, the natural pyrethrum mixture has limited utility today and is found in only a few over-the-counter (OTC) products. Commonly in products using pyrethrums, piperonyl butoxide, a synergist, is added to reduce insect metabolism. The synthetic pyrethroid derivatives have replaced pyrethrins. The pyrethroids have the same mechanism of action as pyrethrum.

MECHANISM OF ACTION.[75-78] The pyrethrins and pyrethroids are nerve membrane sodium channel toxins that do not affect potassium channels. The compounds bind to specific sodium channel proteins and slow the rate of inactivation of the sodium current elicited by membrane depolarization and, as a result, prolong the open time of the sodium channel. At low concentrations, the pyrethroids produce repetitive action potentials and neuron firing; at high concentrations, the nerve membrane is depolarized completely, and excitation is blocked.

The receptor interaction of the pyrethrums with the sodium channel complex is stereospecific and dependent on the stereochemistry of the carboxylic acid. In the case of the pyrethroids, the most active isomers are the 1*R*,3-*cis*- and 1*R*,3-*trans*-cyclopropanecarboxylates. The 1*S*-*cis*- and -*trans*-isomers are inactive and actually are antagonists to the action of the 1*R*-isomers.

METABOLISM. A property that enhances the usefulness of the pyrethroids is that these compounds are highly toxic to the ectoparasites but relatively nontoxic to mammals if absorbed. The apparent lack of toxicity is associated with the rapid metabolism of these drugs through hydrolysis and/or oxidation.[79,80] The rapid breakdown of these agents also accounts for their low persistence in the environment.

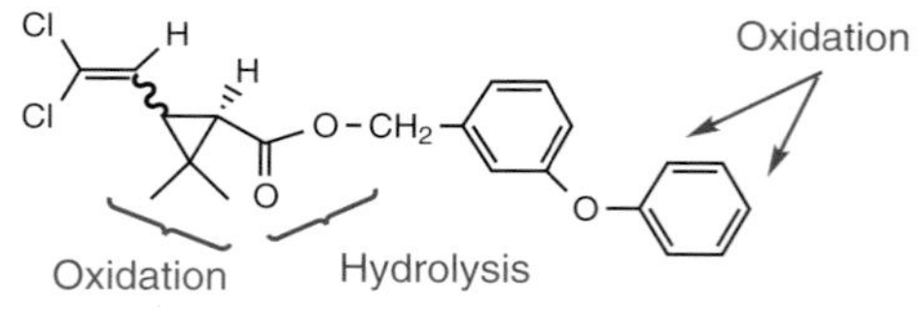

Cl H H O-CH2 O O Cl Oxidation Oxidation Hydrolysis

Permethrin

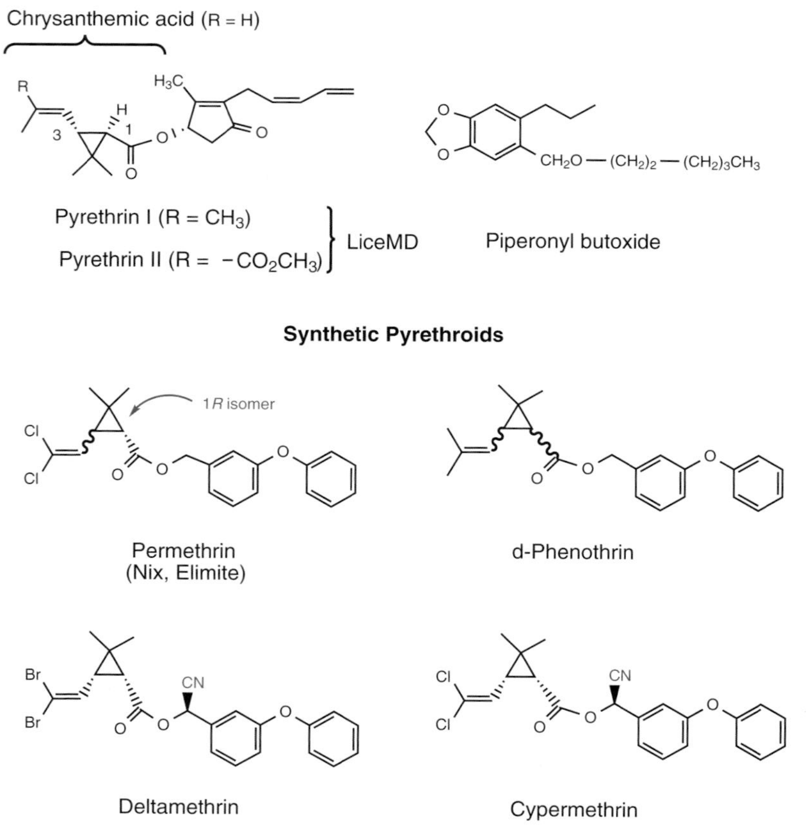

Chrysanthemic acid (R = H)

R H_3C H 3 1 O O O

Pyrethrin I (R = CH_3)
Pyrethrin II (R = $-CO_2CH_3$)
} LiceMD

O O $CH_2O-(CH_2)_2-(CH_2)_3CH_3$

Piperonyl butoxide

Synthetic Pyrethroids

1*R* isomer Cl Cl O O O

Permethrin (Nix, Elimite)

O O O

d-Phenothrin

Br Br CN O O O

Deltamethrin

Cl Cl CN O O O

Cypermethrin

Figure 32.22 Structures of the naturally occuring pyrethrins, the synergist piperonyl butoxide, and the pyrethroid derivatives.

THERAPEUTIC APPLICATION.

Permethrin (Nix-1% Lotion, Elimite-5% Cream). Permethrin, because of its increased stability and its synthetic availability, is not used with a synergist. The compound is used in a 1% lotion for the treatment of pediculosis capitis and in a 5% cream as a scabicide. The 5% product is a prescription product while the 1% solution is available in OTC products. The permethrins are meant to kill the scabies mite and eggs.

The pyrethroids are also commonly found in OTC backyard insecticides and agricultural and veterinary products. These pyrethroids are divided into two classes depending on the absence (type I: permethrin, d-phenothrin) or presence (type II: cypermethrin, deltamethrin) of a cyano group. The type II products are the more potent insecticides.[81]

CROTAMITON (CROTAN, EURAX).

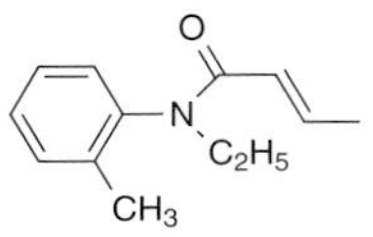

Crotamiton

Crotamiton is available as a 10% cream for the treatment of scabies, although it is less effective than pyrethrins or permethrin.[82,83] Because crotamiton may need to be applied a second time for successful treatment of scabies (permethrin requires a single application), poor patient compliance with crotamiton can reduce its effectiveness. The advantage of crotamiton over lindane comes from the fact that lindane has potential neurotoxicity if absorbed, especially in infants and children, whereas crotamiton has less systemic neurotoxicity. The most common side effect reported for crotamiton is skin irritation.

SPINOSAD (NATROBA).

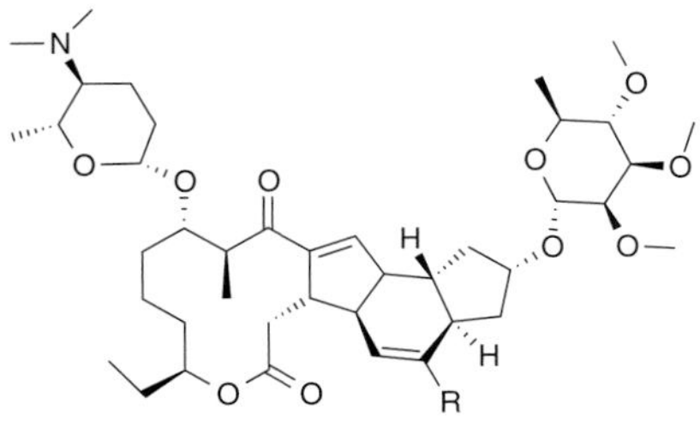

Spinosad (Natroba)

(Spinosyn A: R = H, Spinosyn D: R = CH_3)

Spinosad is a naturally occurring 12-member macrolide which consists of a mixture of spinosyn A and D produced by the bacterium *Saccharopholyspora spinose*, a member of the actinomycete family. The product was a serendipitous discovery isolated from a soil sample found in an abandoned rum distillery on a Caribbean Island by an employee of Eli Lilly. The mixture has a broad spectrum of activity and was approved for agricultural use by the Environmental Protection Agency in 1995.[84]

Mechanism of Action. The mechanism of action has been investigated and found to lead to death of the insect via rapid excitation of the insect's nervous system. Spinosad is an insecticide by virtue of its ability to act as an agonist at the nicotinic acetylcholine receptors (nAChRs) and more specifically at the Da6 subunit.[85,86] Thus, spinosad has a novel mechanism of action compared to other insecticides. The results are that spinosad creates prolonged hyperexcitation of the CNS of the insects and eventually paralysis and death of the organism. It has also been suggested that the drug may function as an antagonist at GABA receptors.

Therapeutic Application. The product is available as a 0.9% topical suspension, which is applied to a dry scalp and hair for a period of 10 minutes and then rinsed with water. Because spinosad has ovicidal activity, nit combing is not required. Studies would suggest that spinosad, which requires a single treatment, is more effective (~80%) than permethrin (~45%) especially after a single treatment. Fewer topical adverse events were noted with spinosad versus permethrin and presently resistance, a growing problem with the permethrin, has not been reported for spinosad.[87]

IVERMECTIN. As indicated earlier (see p. 26 in this chapter) ivermectin in the form of a topical lotion (Sklice) is approved for the treatment of head lice. IVM binds to glutamate and GABA-gated chloride ion channels and, as a result, leads to parasite paralysis and death. The drug can be used without nit combing, and although it does not kill nits, the nits die following hatching since the nymphs are unable to feed due to the paralysis of mouthparts caused by the IVM. Minimal absorption of the drug is found following topical application, and few dermatological adverse effects have been reported.

BENZYL ALCOHOL (ULESFIA).

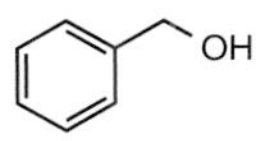

Benzyl alcohol

Benzyl alcohol in a 5% concentration along with mineral oil is reported to be effective in the treatment of head lice in individuals 6 month of age and older. Benzyl alcohol is not insecticidal but acts to prevent the insect from closing their respiratory spiracles (external openings which allow gases to enter the internal respiratory system) which, in turn, allows mineral oil to obstruct the spiracles leading to asphyxiation of the organism.[88]

Clinical Scenario

Kathleen A. Packard, PharmD, BCPS
Thomas L. Lemke, PhD

SCENARIO

A 2-year-old female presented to the clinic in the Dominican Republic campos of Sonador. Her parents reported that she had been experiencing difficulty sleeping secondary to nocturnal perianal pruritus for several weeks. The symptoms were most pronounced in the early evening. She co-sleeps with her 6-year-old sister, who was not having difficulty sleeping. The perianal area was examined and was inflamed with the presence of white, pin-shaped, adult pinworms, approximately 10 mm long. No secondary bacterial infection was observed. The diagnosis of *Enterobius vermicularis* or pinworms was made.

The child was treated with mebendazole 100 mg po (chewable) one time. She was given a second dose to repeat two weeks later. Even though asymptomatic, the 6-year-old sister and both parents were also treated in an effort to prevent reinfection.

OUTCOME

The family was also counseled regarding hand hygiene and encouraged to shower every morning during treatment, if possible. They were also encouraged to keep fingernails trimmed and avoid nail biting and scratching. After the second dose, the 2-year-old's symptoms completely resolved.

Chemical Analysis found immediately after References.

REFERENCES

1. El-Sayed NM, Myler PJ, Blandin G, et al. Comparative genomics of trypanosomatid parasitic protozoa. *Science*. 2005;309:404-409.
2. El-Sayed NM, Myler PJ, Bartholoneu DS, et al. The genome sequence of *Trypanosoma cruzi*, etiologic agent of Chagas' disease. *Science*. 2005;309:409-415.
3. Berriamn M, Ghedin E, Hertz-Fowler C, et al. The genome of the African trypanosome *Trypanosoma brucei*. *Science*. 2005;309:416-422.
4. Barrett MP, Burchmore RJB, Stich A, et al. The trypanosomiases. *Lancet*. 2003;362:1469-1480.
5. DoCampo R. Sensitivity of parasites to free radical damage by antiparasitic drugs. *Chem Biol Interact*. 1990;73:1-27.
6. Lau AH, Lam NP, Piscitelli SC, et al. Clinical pharmacokinetics of metronidazole anti-infectives. *Clin Pharmacokinet*. 1992;23:328-364.
7. Koch R, Beaulieu BB, Chrystal EJT, et al. Metronidazole metabolite in urine and its risk. *Science*. 1981;211:399-400.
8. Drugs for parasitic infections. *Med Lett*. 1998;40:1-12.
9. The choice of antibacterial drugs. *Med Lett*. 1998;40:33-42.
10. Sisson G, Goodwin A, Raudonikiene A, et al. Enzyme associated with reductive activation and action of nitrazoxande, nitrofurans, and metronidazole in *Helicobacter pylori*. *Antimicrob Agents Chemother*. 2002;46:2116-2123.
11. Somvanshi VS, Ellis BL, Hu Y, et al. Nitazoxanide: nematicidal mode of action and drug combination studies. *Mol Biochem Parasitol*. 2014;193:1-8.
12. Stockis A, DeBruyn S, Gengler C, et al. Nitazoxanide pharmacokinetics and tolerability in man during 7 days dosing with 0.5 g and 1 g b.i.d. *Int J Clin Pharmacol Ther*. 2002;40:221-2v27.
13. Nitazoxanide (Alinia)—a new antiprotozoal agent. *Med Lett*. 2003;45:29-31.
14. Vohringer H-F, Arasteh K. Pharmacokinetic optimization in the treatment of *Pneumocystis carinii* pneumonia. *Clin Pharmacokinet*. 1993;24:388-412.
15. Fishman JA. Treatment of infections due to *Pneumocystis carinii*. *Antimicrob Agents Chemother*. 1998;42:1309-1314.
16. Fry M, Pudney M. Site of action of the antimalarial hydroxymaphthoquinoine, 2-[*trans*-4-(4′- chlorophenyl)cyclohexyl]-3-hydroxy-1,4-naphthoquinone (566C80). *Biochem Pharmacol*. 1992;43:1545-1553.
17. Hughes WT, Gray VL, Gutteridge WE, et al. Efficacy of a hydroxynaphthoquinone, 566C80, in experimental *Pneumocystis carinii* pneumonitis. *J Antimicrob Chemother*. 1990;34:225-228.
18. Wang CC. Molecular mechanisms and therapeutic approaches to the treatment of African trypanosomiasis. *Annu Rev Pharmacol Toxicol*. 1995;35:93-127.
19. Edwards KJ, Jenkins T, Neidle S. Crystal structure of a pentamidine–oligonucleotide complex: implications for DNA-binding properties. *Biochemistry*. 1992;31:7104-7109.
20. Shapiro T, Englund PT. Selective cleavage of kinetoplast DNA minicircles promoted by antitrypanosomal drugs. *Proc Natl Acad Sci USA*. 1990;87:950-954.
21. Dykstra CC, Tidwell RR. Inhibition of topoisomerase from *Pneumocystis carinii* by aromatic dicationic molecules. *J Protozool*. 1991;38:78S-81S.
22. Metcalf BW, Bey P, Danzin C, et al. Catalytic irreversible inhibition of mammalian ornithine decarboxylase (E.C. 4.1.1.17) by substrate and product analogues. *J Am Chem Soc*. 1978;100:2551-2553.
23. Bacchi CJ, Nathan HC, Hutner SH, et al. Polyamine metabolism: a potential therapeutic target in trypanosomes. *Science*. 1980;210:332-334.
24. Poulin R, Lu L, Ackermann B, et al. Mechanism of the irreversible inactivation of mouse ornithine decarboxylase by α-difluoromethylornithine. *J Biol Chem*. 1992;267:150-158.
25. Bacchi CJ, Garofalo J, Ciminelli M, et al. Resistance to DL-α-difluoromethylornithine by clinical isolates of Trypanosoma brucei rhodeniense: role of S-adenosylmethionine. *Biochem Pharmacol*. 1993;46:471-481.
26. Henderson GB, Ulrich P, Fairlamb AH, et al. "Subversive" substrates for the enzyme trypanothione disulfide reductase. Alternative approach to chemotherapy of Chagas' disease. *Proc Natl Acad Sci USA*. 1988;85:5374-5378.
27. García-Huertas P, Mejía-Jaramillo AM, Machado CR, et al. Prostaglandin F2α synthase in Trypanosoma cruzi plays critical roles in oxidative stress and susceptibility to benznidazole. *Royal Soc Open Sci*. 2017;4(9):170773. doi:10.1098/rsos.170773. eCollection 2017.
28. Fairlamb AH, Henderson GB, Cerami A. Trypanothione is the primary target for arsenical drugs against African trypanosomes. *Proc Natl Acad Sci USA*. 1989;86:2607-2611.
29. Berman JD. Chemotherapy for leishmaniasis: biochemical mechanisms, clinical efficacy, and future strategies. *Rev Infect Dis*. 1988;10:560-586.
30. Cook GC. Leishmaniasis: some recent developments in chemotherapy. *J Antimicrob Chemother*. 1993;31:327-330.

31. Singh S, Sivakumar R. Challenges and new discoveries in the treatment of leishmaniasis. *J Infect Chemother*. 2004;10:307-331.
32. Griewank K, Gazeau C, Eichhorn A, von Stebut E. Miltefosine efficiently eliminates Leishmania major amastigotes from infected murine dendritic cells without altering their immune functions. *Antimicro Agents Chemo*. 2010;54(2):652-659.
33. Pinto-Martinez AK, Rodriguez-Durán J, Serrano-Martin X, et al. Mechanism of action of miltefosine on Leishmania donovani involves the impairment of acidocalcisomes function and the activation of the sphingosine-dependent plasma membrane Ca^{2+} channel. *Antimicrob Agents Chemother*. 2017:01614-01617. doi:10.1128/AAC.01614-17. pii:AAC.
34. Ward SA. Mechanisms of chloroquine resistance in malarial chemotherapy. *Trends Pharmacol Sci*. 1988;9:241-246.
35. Hempelmann E. Hemozoin biocrystallization in *Plasmodium falciparum* and the antimalarial activity of crystallization inhibitors. *Parasitol Res*. 2007;100:671-676.
36. Kurosawa Y, Dorn A, Kitsuji-Shirane M, Shimada H, et al. Hematin polymerization assay as a high-throughput screen for identification of new antimalarial pharmacophores. *Antimicrob Agents Chemother*. 2000;44(10):2638-2644.
37. Sullivan DJ, Gluzman IY, Russell DG, et al. On the molecular mechanism of chloroquine's antimalarial action. *Proc Natl Acad Sci USA*. 1996;93:11865-11869.
38. Arav-Boger R, Shapiro TA. Molecular mechanisms of resistance in antimalarial chemotherapy: the unmet challenge. *Annu Rev Pharmacol Toxicol*. 2005;45:565-585.
39. Zhao X-J, Ishizaki T. Metabolic interactions of selected antimalarial and nonantimalarial drugs with the major pathway (3-hydroxylation) of quinine in human liver microsomes. *Br J Clin Pharmacol*. 1997;44:505-511.
40. Palmer KJ, Holliday SM, Brogden RN. Mefloquine: a review of its antimalarial activity, pharmacokinetic properties, and therapeutic efficacy. *Drugs*. 1993;45:430-475.
41. Davis TME, Hung T, Sim I, et al. Piperaquine a resurgent antimalarial drug. *Drugs*. 2005;65(1):75-87.
42. Tarning J, Lindegardh N, Sandberg S, et al. Pharmacokinetics and metabolism of the antimalarial piperaquine after intravenous and oral single doses to the rat. *J Pharm Sci*. 2008;97(8):3400-3410.
43. Augusto O, Schrieber J, Mason RP. Direct ESR detection of a free radical intermediate drug in the peroxidase-catalyzed oxidation of the antimalarial drug primaquine. *Biochem Pharmacol*. 1988;37:2791-2797.
44. Mihaly GW, Ward SA, Edwards G, et al. Pharmacokinetics of primaquine in man: identification of the carboxylic acid derivative as a major plasma metabolite. *Br J Clin Pharmacol*. 1984;17:441-446.
45. Ebstie YA, Abay SM, Tadesse WT, et al. Tafenoquine and its potential treatment and relapse prevention of Plasmodium vivax malaria: the evidence to date. *Drug Design, Develop Ther*. 2016;10:2387-2399.
46. Vuong C, Xie LH, Potter BM, et al. Diffenertial cytochrome P450 2D metabolism alters tafenoquine pharmacokinetics. *Antimicrob Agents Chemother*. 2016;59:3864-3869.
47. Olliaro P. Mode of action and mechanisms of resistance for antimalarial drugs. *Pharmacol Ther*. 2001;89:207-219.
48. Cottrell G, Musset L, Hu V, et al. Emergence of resistance to atovaquone-proguanil in malaria parasites: insights from computational modeling and clinical case reports. *Antimicrob Agents Chemother*. 2014;58(8):4504-4514.
49. Cumming JN, Ploypradith P, Posner GH. Antimalarial activity of artemisinin (Qinghaosu) and related trioxanes: mechanism(s) of action. *Adv Pharmacol*. 1997;37:253-297.
50. Meshnick SR, Taylor TE, Kamchonwongpaisan S. Artemisinin and the antimalarial endoperoxides: from herbal remedy to targeted chemotherapy. *Microbiol Rev*. 1996;60:301-315.
51. Posner GH, Cumming JN, Woo S-H, et al. Orally active antimalarial 3-substituted trioxanes: new synthetic methodology and biological evaluation. *J Med Chem*. 1998;41:940-951.
52. Cumming JN, Wang D, Shapiro TA, et al. Design, synthesis, derivatization, and structure–activity relationships of simplified, tetracyclic, 1,2,4-trioxane alcohol analogues of the antimalarial artemisinin. *J Med Chem*. 1998;41:952-964.
53. Eckstein-Ludwig U, Webb RJ, van Goethem ID, et al. Artemisinins target the SERCA of *Plasmodium falciparum*. *Nature*. 2003;424:957-961.
54. Hencken CP, Kalinda AS, D'Angelo JG. The anti-infective and anti-cancer properties of artemisinin and its derivatives. *Ann Rev Med Chem*. 2009;44:359-378.
55. Wiesner J, Ortmann R, Jomaa H, Schlitzer M. New antimalarial drugs. *Angew Chem Int Ed*. 2003;42:5274-5293.
56. Schachterle SE, Mtove G, Levens JP, et al. Short-term malaria reduction by single dose azithromycin during mass drug administration for trachoma, Tanzania. *Emerging Infect Dis*. 2014;20(6):941-949.
57. de Silva N, Guyatt H, Bundy D. Anthelmintics: a comparative review of their clinical pharmacology. *Drugs*. 1997;53:769-786.
58. Townsend LB, Wise DS. The synthesis and chemistry of certain anthelmintic benzimidazoles. *Parasitol Today*. 1990;6:107-112.
59. Prichard RK. Mode of action of the anthelmintic thiabendazole in *Haemonchus contortus*. *Nature*. 1970;228:684-685.
60. Friedman PA, Platzer EG. Interaction of anthelmintic benzimidazoles and benzimidazole derivatives with bovine brain tubulin. *Biochim Biophys Acta*. 1978;544:605-614.
61. Lacey E. Mode of action of benzimidazoles. *Parasitol Today*. 1990;6:112-115.
62. Braithwaite PA, Roberts MS, Allan RJ, et al. Clinical pharmacokinetics of high-dose mebendazole in patients treated for hydatid disease. *Eur J Clin Pharmaco*. 1982;22:161-169.
63. Gottschall DW, Theodorides EJ, Wang R. The metabolism of benzimidazole anthelmintics. *Parasitol Today*. 1990;6:115-124.
64. Marriner SE, Morris DL, Dickson B, et al. Pharmacokinetics of albendazole in man. *Eur J Clin Pharmacol*. 1986;30:705-708.
65. Goa KL, McTavish D, Clissold SP. Ivermectin: a review of its antifilarial activity, pharmacokinetic properties and clinical efficacy in onchocerciasis. *Drugs*. 1991;42:640-658.
66. Ottesen EA, Campbell WC. Ivermectin in human medicine. *J Antimicrob Chemother*. 1994;34:195-203.
67. Forrester SG, Beech RN, Prichard RK. Agonist enhancement of macrocyclic lactone activity at a glutamate-gated chloride channel subunit from *Haemonchus contortus*. *Biochem Pharmacol*. 2004;67:1019-1024.
68. Wiest PM, Li Y, Olds GR, et al. Inhibition of phosphoinositide turnover by praziquantel in *Schistosoma mansoni*. *J Parasitol*. 1992;78:753-755.
69. Xiao S-H, Catto BA, Webster LT. Effects of praziquantel on different developmental stages of *Schistosoma mansoni* in vitro and in vivo. *J Infect Dis*. 1985;151:1130-1137.
70. Fallon PG, Cooper RO, Probert AJ, et al. Immune-dependent chemotherapy of schistosomiasis. *Parasitology*. 1992;105:S41-S48.
71. Utzinger J, Keiser J, Shuhua X, et al. Combination chemotherapy of schistosomiasis in laboratory studies and clinical trials. *Antimicrob Agents Chemother*. 2003;47:1487-1495.
72. Cioli D, Pica-Mattoccia L, Archer S. Antischistosomal drugs: past, present and future? *Pharmacol Ther*. 1995;68:35-85.
73. Buhring KU, Diekmann HW, Muller H, et al. Metabolism of praziquantel in man. *Eur J Drug Metab Pharmacokinet*. 1978;3:179-190.
74. Austin WC, Courtney WC, Danilewicz W, et al. Pyrantal tartrate, a new anthelmintic effective against infections of domestic animals. *Nature*. 1966;212:1273-1274.
75. Narahashi T. Nerve membrane ionic channels as the primary target of pyrethroids. *Neurotoxicology*. 1985;6:3-22.
76. Vijverberg HPM, de Weille JR. The interaction of pyrethroids with voltage-dependent Na channels. *Neurotoxicology*. 1985;6:23-34.
77. Grammon DW, Sanders G. Pyrethroid–receptor interactions: stereospecific binding and effects on sodium channels in mouse brain preparations. *Neurotoxicology*. 1985;6:35-46.
78. Lombet A, Mourre C, Lazdunski M. Interaction of insecticides of the pyrethroid family with specific binding sites on the voltage-dependent sodium channel from mammalian brain. *Brain Res*. 1988;459:44-53.

79. Soderund DM. Metabolic consideration in pyrethroid design. *Xenobiotic*. 1992;22:1185-1194.
80. Ruzo LO, Casida JE. Metabolism and toxicology of pyrethroids with dihalovinyl substituents. *Environ Health Perspect*. 1977;21:285-292.
81. Anand SS, Bruckner JV, Haines WT, et al. Characterization of deltamethrin metabolism by rat plasma and liver microsomes. *Tox Appl Pharmacol*. 2006;212:156-166.
82. Taplin D, Meinkin TL, Joaquin BA, et al. Comparison of critamiton 10% cream (Eurax) and permethrin 5% cream (Elimite) for the treatment of scabies in children. *Pediatr Dermatol*. 1990;7:67-73.
83. Amer M, El-Ghariband I. Permethrin versus crotamiton and lindane in the treatment of scabies. *Int J Dermatol*. 1992;31:357-358.
84. Stough D, Shallenbarger S, Quiring J, et al. Effecicacy and safetly of spiosad and permetring cream rinses for pdeiculosis capitis (head lice). *Pediatrics*. 2009;124:e389-e395
85. Spinosad: a new organically accepted insecticide. Available at: www.jlgardencenter.com/uploads/handouts/Spinosad.pdf. Accessed 13 March 2011.
86. Millar NS, Denholm I. Nicotinic acetylcholine receptors: targets for commercially important insecticides. *Invert Neurosci*. 2007;7(1):53-66.
87. Salgado VL,1 Sheets JJ, Watson GB. Studies on the mode of action of spinosad:the internal effective concentration and the concentration dependence of neural excitationStudies on the mode of action of spinosad:the internal effective concentration and the concentration dependence of neural excitationStudies on the mode of action of spinosad:the internal effective concentration and the concentration dependence of neural excitation. *Pest Biochem Physiol*. 1998;60:103-110.
88. Koch E, Clark JM, Cohn B, et al. Management of head louse infectations in the United States – a literature review. *Ped Derm*. 2016;5:466-472.

Clinical Scenario

Kathleen A. Packard, PharmD, BCPS
Thomas L. Lemke, PhD

CHEMICAL ANALYSIS

Three chemical classes of drugs are commonly utilized for the treatment of *Enterobius vermicularis* (pinworms). They are the benzimidazoles, ivermectin, and pyrantel pamoate. Since pinworms infections are limited to the GI tract, it is important to choose a drug which remains local with little or no systemic absorption. A physiochemical property of the benzimidazoles is that they show limited water solubility and thus are poorly absorbed following oral administration. Additionally, any absorption leads to rapid metabolism and elimination via biliary excretion. Without absorption, the potential for adverse effects is greatly reduced, although stomach and abdominal pain along with vomiting and diarrhea may occur.

Mebendazole, a benzimidazole, is active against adult worm, larva, and eggs. Given that the medication used in the Dominican Republic service mission are donated and clinicians must make the best therapeutic decisions they can with what is at hand, it was fortunate that a drug with the desired physiochemical and therapeutic profile (mebendazole) was available. It was an appropriate therapeutic choice, particularly given that it kills eggs; something no alternative therapy does. This would keep eggs released from the infected child from spreading to her sibling.

Although not available to the clinicians in the DR, pyrantel pamoate could have been an acceptable alternative to mebendazole. The pamoic acid moiety prevents absorption, thus limiting systemic effects. This drug exhibits similar adverse effects to those reported for mebendazole, but it does not kill eggs, which is a significant drawback in this patient care situation.

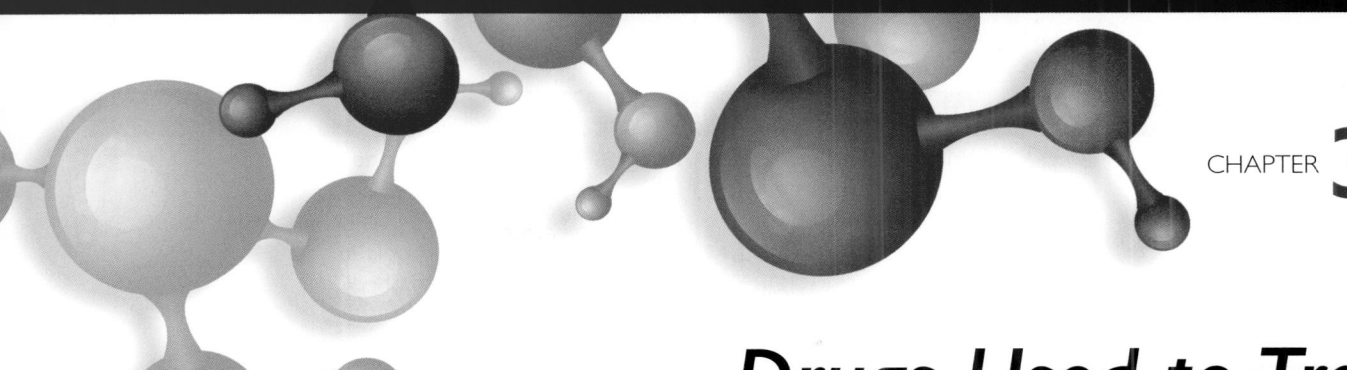

CHAPTER **33**

Drugs Used to Treat Neoplastic Diseases

Victoria F. Roche

Drugs covered or mentioned in this chapter:

TYROSINE KINASE INHIBITORS
- Acalabrutinib
- Afatinib
- Alectinib
- Axitinib
- Bosutinib
- Brigatinib
- Cabozantinib
- Ceritinib
- Crizotinib
- Dasatinib
- Erlotinib
- Gefitinib
- Ibrutinib
- Imatinib
- Lapatinib
- Lenvatinib
- Midostaurin
- Neratinib
- Nilotinib
- Omacetaxine mepesuccinate
- Osimertinib
- Pazopanib
- Ponatinib
- Regorafenib
- Ruxolitinib
- Sorafenib
- Sunitinib
- Vandetanib

SERINE/THREONINE KINASE INHIBITORS

CYCLIN-DEPENDENT KINASE INHIBITORS
- Abemaciclib
- Palbociclib
- Ribociclib

BRAF INHIBITORS
- Dabrafenib
- Vemurafenib

MEK INHIBITORS
- Cobimetinib
- Trametinib

mTOR INHIBITORS
- Everolimus
- Temsirolimus

LIPID KINASE INHIBITORS

PHOSPHATIDYLINOSITOL 3 KINASE INHIBITORS
- Copanlisib
- Idelalisib

IDH1/2 INHIBITORS
- Enasidenib
- Ivosidenib

BCL-2 INHIBITORS
- Venetoclax

PARP INHIBITORS
- Niraparib
- Olaparib
- Rucaparib

PROTEASOME INHIBITORS
- Bortezomib
- Carfilzomib
- Ixazomib

HORMONE-BASED ANTINEOPLASTIC AGENTS (REPRESENTATIVE)

AROMATASE INHIBITORS
- Anastrozole

ANTIESTROGENS
- Tamoxifen

ANTIANDROGENS
- Enzalutamide

GONADOTROPIN-RELEASING HORMONE MODULATORS
- Leuprolide
- Degarelix

IMMUNOMODULATORS
- Lenalidomide
- Pomalidomide
- Thalidomide

HISTONE DEACETYLASE INHIBITORS
- Belinostat
- Panobinostat
- Romidepsin
- Vorinostat

TOPOISOMERASE POISONS

CAMPTOTHECINS
- Irinotecan
- Topotecan

EPIPODOPHYLLOTOXINS
- Etoposide
- Teniposide

ANTHRACYCLINES AND ANTHRACENEDIONES
- Aldoxorubicin
- Daunorubicin
- Doxorubicin
- Epirubicin
- Idarubicin
- Mitoxantrone
- Valrubicin

MITOSIS INHIBITORS
- Cabazitaxel
- Docetaxel
- Eribulin
- Ixabepilone
- Paclitaxel
- Vinblastine
- Vincristine
- Vinorelbine

ANTIMETABOLITES

PURINE ANTAGONISTS
- Mercaptopurine
- Thioguanine

Drugs covered or mentioned in this chapter—Continued

PYRIMIDINE ANTAGONISTS
- Capecitabine
- Floxuridine
- Fluorouracil

ANTIFOLATES
- Methotrexate
- Pemetrexed
- Pralatrexate

DNA POLYMERASE INHIBITORS
- Cladribine
- Clofarabine
- Cytarabine
- Fludarabine
- Gemcitabine
- Trifluridine/tipiracil

DNA METHYLTRANSFERASE INHIBITORS
- Azacitidine
- Decitabine
- Nelarabine

MISCELLANEOUS ANTIMETABOLITES
- Hydroxyurea
- Pentostatin

DNA CROSS-LINKING AGENTS

NITROGEN MUSTARDS
- Bendamustine
- Chlorambucil
- Cyclophosphamide
- Ifosfamide
- Mechlorethamine
- Melphalan
- Thiotepa

TRIAZENES AND PROCARBAZINE
- Dacarbazine
- Procarbazine
- Temozolomide

NITROSOUREAS
- Carmustine
- Lomustine
- Streptozocin

ORGANOPLATINUM COMPLEXES
- Carboplatin
- Cisplatin
- Oxaliplatin

MISCELLANEOUS ANTICANCER AGENTS
- Arsenic trioxide
- Bexarotene
- Bleomycin
- Dactinomycin
- Gemtuzumab ozogamicin conjugate
- Inotuzumab ozogamicin conjugate
- Mitomycin
- Mitotane
- Trabectedin
- Tretinoin

Abbreviations

ABC ATP-binding cassette
ABL Abelson
AIC 5-aminoimidazole-4-carboxamide
AKR aldo-keto reductase
ALK anaplastic lymphoma kinase
ALL acute lymphoblastic leukemia
ALT alanine transaminase
AML acute myeloid leukemia
AMP adenosine monophosphate
APL acute promyelocytic leukemia
ATP adenosine triphosphate
AUC area under the curve
BBB blood-brain barrier
BCL B-cell lymphoma
BCR breakpoint cluster region
B-CR B-cell receptor
BCRP breast cancer resistance protein
BRAF/B-Raf B-rapidly accelerated fibrosarcoma
BTK Bruton tyrosine kinase
CBR carbonyl reductase
CEA carcinoembryonic antigen
CDK cyclin-dependent kinase
CLL chronic lymphocytic leukemia
C_{max} maximum plasma concentration
CML chronic myelogenous leukemia
CNS central nervous system
CNU chloroethyl-containing nitrosourea
CRPC castration-resistant prostate cancer
CSF cerebrospinal fluid
CTR copper transporter
CYP cytochrome P450
DACH diaminocyclohexane
DCIS ductal carcinoma in situ
DDI drug-drug interaction
DHF dihydrofolate
DHFR dihydrofolate reductase
DNMT DNA methyltransferase
DPD dihydropyrimidine dehydrogenase
dTMP deoxythymidine monophosphate
dUMP deoxyuridine monophosphate
EGCG epigallocatechin-3-gallate
EGFR epidermal growth factor receptor
ERK extracellular signal–regulated kinase
FDA U.S. Food and Drug Administration
FPGS folylpolyglutamate synthase
FSH follicle-stimulating hormone
FU fluorouracil
GAR glycinamide ribonucleotide
GI/GIT gastrointestinal/gastrointestinal tract
GIST gastrointestinal stromal tumors
GMP guanosine monophosphate
GnRH gonadotropin-releasing hormone
GSH reduced glutathione
GTP guanosine triphosphate
HAT histone acetyltransferase
HCC hepatocellular carcinoma
HDAC/HDACi histone deacetylase/histone deacetylase inhibitors
HER human epidermal growth factor receptor
HG hydroxyglutarate
HGPRT hypoxanthine guanine phosphoribosyl transferase
HIF hypoxia-inducible factor
HR homologous recombination
hTS human thymidylate synthase
IDH isocitrate dehydrogenase
IM intramuscular
IMP inosine monophosphate
ITD internal tandem duplication
ITPA inositol triphosphate pyrophosphatase
IV intravenous
KI kinase inhibitor
LH/LHRH luteinizing hormone/luteinizing hormone–releasing hormone
MAb monoclonal antibody
MAP microtubule-associated protein
MAPK/MEK mitogen-activated protein kinase
MBC metastatic breast cancer
MCL mantle cell lymphoma
MDR multidrug resistance
MMR mismatch repair
MMR major molecular response
MPN myeloproliferative neoplasms
MTC medullary thyroid cancer

Abbreviations—Continued

MTIC 3-methyl-(triazen-1-yl) imidazole-4-carboxamide
mTOR mammalian target of rapamycin
NCCN National Comprehensive Cancer Network
NER nucleotide excision repair protein
NHL non-Hodgkin lymphoma
NSCLC non–small cell lung cancer
OAT/OATP organic anion transporter/organic anion transporting protein
OCT organic cation transporter
OS overall survival
PARP poly(ADP-ribose) polymerase
PCFT proton-coupled folate transporter
PDGFR platelet-derived growth factor receptor
PD-L1 programmed death ligand 1
PFS progression-free survival
P-gp P-glycoprotein
Ph Philadelphia chromosome
PI3K phosphatidylinositol 3 kinase
PLC phospholipase C
PM poor metabolizer
PSA prostate-specific antigen
RAS rat sarcoma
Rb retinoblastoma
RCC renal cell carcinoma
REMS Risk Evaluation and Mitigation Strategy
RET rearranged during transfection
RFC1 reduced folate carrier 1
ROS reactive oxygen species
SAM S-adenosylmethionine
SAR structure-activity relationships
SC subcutaneous
SERM selective estrogen receptor modulator
SHMT serine hydroxymethyltransferase
SNP single nucleotide polymorphism
SPF sun protection factor
STAT signal transducer and activator of transcription
STEPS System for Thalidomide Education and Prescribing Safety
SYK spleen tyrosine kinase
6TGN 6-thioguanine nucleotide
THF tetrahydrofolate
TK tyrosine kinase
TKI tyrosine kinase inhibitor
T_{max} time to maximum plasma concentration
TNM tumor-node-metastasis
TopI topoisomerase I
TopIIα topoisomerase IIα
TPMT thiopurine methyl transferase
VEGFR vascular endothelial growth factor receptor

CLINICAL SIGNIFICANCE

Kelly K. Nystrom, PharmD, BCOP

The American Cancer Society estimates that over 1.7 million people will be diagnosed with cancer in 2018, and it is estimated that by 2026 there will be more than 20.2 million survivors. While cytotoxic chemotherapy agents are still an ingrained component of the antineoplastic arsenal, newer chemotherapy agents and targeted therapies have dramatically changed the way we treat cancer and the outcomes for patients.

The disadvantage of traditional chemotherapy agents is the inability of the agent to recognize the difference between normal and cancer cells. Understanding chemical mechanisms of action helps us choose multiple chemotherapy agents to include in one regimen that not only approach cell death in different ways, avoiding resistance for as long as possible, but also help us avoid overlapping toxicities that would make the regimen intolerable. An understanding of genetic mutations is also important. Patients with dihydropyrimidine dehydrogenase (DPD) deficiency or UGT1A1 deficiency can see life-threatening toxicities from 5-fluorouracil and irinotecan, respectively. On the other hand, patients with tumors that have epidermal growth factor receptor (EGFR) mutations can benefit from targeted drugs like erlotinib. It is important to understand what implications various mutations have on the efficacy of treatment in different disease states.

Targeted therapies are not without toxicities but are generally better tolerated than traditional chemotherapy. Many targeted therapies are metabolized in the liver and thus have potentially significant drug interactions. One example of this is seen with neratinib, a newer targeted therapy approved for human epidermal growth factor receptor 2 (HER2/neu) positive breast cancer patients. Neratinib is a CYP3A4 substrate and should be avoided with moderate or strong CYP3A4 inhibitors. Normally moderate inhibitors are only recommended to be used with caution, but because strong inhibitors have been shown to increase neratinib levels by 481%, it is recommended to avoid moderate inhibitors as well because of the potential for significant risk of increased exposure of neratinib, leading to increased toxicity. As pharmacists, one of our roles is to understand the significant probability of drug interactions occurring and informing health care professionals and patients so all can monitor for increased toxicity. Pharmacists should understand which interactions can just be monitored and which require action up front.

Unfortunately, resistance is a problem even with targeted therapies. Upregulation of the anexelekto (AXL) pathway is a common pathway for resistance, is seen in multiple disease states, and is associated with a poorer prognosis. An in vitro study adding an investigational AXL-specific inhibitor to targeted therapy for AML showed increased cell death when compared with treatment without the AXL inhibitor. Understanding these various pathways can allow us to treat various cancers more effectively for a longer period of time.

This is an exciting time for cancer treatment, and understanding the mutations and pathways that are being targeted to treat individual cancers is more important than ever. While these agents are better tolerated than traditional chemotherapy, understanding how and what toxicities to monitor are important so they can be managed effectively, ultimately improving not only survival, but quality of life as well.

CANCER

"Cancer does not have a face until it's yours or someone you know" (Anthony Del Monte)

Public Health and Economic Burdens

The link to the American Cancer Society website proclaims that "Cancer Affects Us All." As the second leading cause of death in the United States, it is indeed seemingly difficult to find anyone who has not been touched in some way by this constellation of diseases. In March, 2017 the National Cancer Institute projected the U.S. incidence of cancer at 454.8 per 100,000 population and cancer mortality at 171.2 per 100,000.[1] Siegel et al.[2] estimate that 1,688,780 new cancer diagnoses will be made in the United States in 2017, and 600,920 cancer patients will die in that same year. The projected number of new cancer diagnoses in women edge out those in men by a slim margin (852,630 vs. 836,150), but men appear more likely to succumb to their illness (318,420 vs. 282,500). For males, colorectal, prostate, and respiratory system cancers top both the morbidity and mortality lists. Breast cancer is by far the most commonly diagnosed cancer in females and joins with colorectal and respiratory system cancers to claim the most lives. For both sexes, pulmonary neoplasms are predicted to be the second most commonly diagnosed in 2017 and the most deadly. With melanoma and liver cancer, men have a poorer prognosis when compared to women. Race/ethnicity, poverty, and access to health care resources also impact cancer morbidity and mortality risk.[2-4]

However, survival statistics are encouraging.[1] As of January 1, 2016, there were over 15.5 million U.S. citizens living with a cancer diagnosis, and that number is expected to climb to close to 20.3 million by 2026.[5] From 2000 to 2013, the incidence of the most lethal cancers in men has declined, thanks in part to education and the ready availability of screening procedures such as prostate-specific antigen (PSA) and colonoscopy. During the same time period, colorectal cancer incidence in woman declined, pulmonary-related cancer incidence began declining in 2006, and breast cancer incidence was essentially flat. Liver cancer, melanoma, and thyroid cancer diagnoses, on the rise for some time, appear to show signs of slowing, particularly in younger age-groups.[2] Advances in the understanding of blood- and lymph-related cancers, along with the establishment of targeted therapeutic approaches to treatment, prompted the optimistically titled editorial "The best of times in hematologic malignancies" in a recent issue of *Current Opinion in Hematology*.[6]

Siegel et al[2] document the significant slowing of the U.S. cancer death rate since 1991, with an estimated 2.14 million deaths prevented due to smoking cessation/avoidance and early diagnosis and treatment. Early detection public awareness campaigns designed to improve survival odds have also been championed in the United Kingdom.[7] The intense global cancer research enterprise that has resulted in the development and marketing of many innovative targeted antineoplastic drugs, including kinase inhibitors, immunologic- and monoclonal antibody (MAb)–based therapies, is surely also contributing to the positive prognosis picture, as is the commitment to collaboration among scientific, clinical, and patient-related stakeholders.[8]

Still, the economic burden of the collection of diseases called cancer is staggering. In 2017, the American Cancer Society Cancer Action Network published a report that documented an $87.8 billion dollar price tag on cancer-associated care in the United States in 2014, with approximately $4 billion (4%) being paid out of pocket by patients and families.[9] Of the almost $85 billion remainder, private insurance picked up 44%, Medicare and Medicaid paid 33% and 4%, respectively, and other sources covered the balance. Approximately 12% of expenditures went for prescription medications, with 58% covering provider visits and 27% paying for inpatient services. Regarding medications, insurance coverage for IV-administered chemotherapy may be distinct from coverage for supportive therapy to treat pain, nausea/vomiting, or other adverse effects from the disease or its treatment. The report urges all to keep in mind the significant, but often overlooked, indirect costs related to cancer, including mental health services, childcare, transportation and caregiving expenses, cosmetic support, and lost wages.[9]

Financially, patients can be hit hardest at the beginning of their cancer journey, as they seek to meet the often high deductible required by low-premium insurance plans. Patients lacking insurance coverage are anticipated to incur expenses totaling "tens to possibly hundreds of thousands of dollars," but even with insurance, allowed out-of-pocket costs can reach between $7,000 and 14,000 annually.[9] Costs can escalate if insured patients use out-of-network providers or require procedures not covered by their health plan. To keep cancer care costs down, the American Cancer Society advocates for no-cost prevention and early detection services, continued emphasis on healthy lifestyles, ensuring tobacco-free environments, access to affordable health insurance, and support for palliative care.

Etiology

Healthy cells are under strict biochemical control for growth and differentiation. Cells divide and proliferate under the influence of various growth stimulators and are subject to arrested growth (senescence) and programmed cell death (apoptosis). In cancer, these regulatory processes have gone awry, and cells grow and divide uncontrollably, consuming energy and losing both structure and function due to an inability to adequately differentiate. To add insult to injury, rampant cell division is accompanied by disabled cell death processes, leading first to cellular immortality and, eventually, to genetic instability.[10,11] Cancers can usually be classified as lymphatic, epithelial, nerve, or connective tissue–related, and tumor nomenclature is based on tissue of origin as follows: carcinoma (epithelial origin), sarcoma (muscle or connective tissue origin), leukemia and lymphoma (lymphatic or hematologic origin), and glioma (neural origin). The risk of receiving a cancer diagnosis commonly increases with age.[12]

The causes of cancer are many and varied (e.g., chemical, environmental, viral, and mutagenic), but all ultimately lead to an aberration in the expression of proto-oncogenes and tumor suppressor genes, the products of which control normal cell life.[13] The development of cancer occurs in four discrete steps or phases: initiation, promotion, transformation, and progression. Exposure to a carcinogen **initiates** the neoplastic process (irreversible), which is **promoted** by environmental factors that favor proliferation of precancerous cells (reversible). It is at this promotion phase of carcinogenesis when healthy lifestyle modifications (including diet, exercise, vaccination, and smoking cessation) can have a positive impact on outcome. However, if proto-oncogenes **transform** over time (commonly 5-20 yr) in a sequential multistep process to become oncogenes, cancer results. Oncogenes (e.g., *myc* and *ras*) can either overexpress or underexpress regulatory biochemicals, resulting in preferential and accelerated cellular growth. Concomitantly, tumor suppressor genes (e.g., antioncogenes like *TP53* and *Rb1*) and DNA repair genes (e.g., *PARP1*) can be inhibited.

As the cancer develops, genetic and epigenetic alterations amass and are passed on to subsequent generations of cells. The cancer **progresses** as genetically fueled cellular proliferation leads to augmented invasion of the primary site and migration to new tissues through the metastatic highways of the bloodstream or lymphatic system.[10,11] Many cancers have the ability to generate new blood vessels (angiogenesis) to ensure an ongoing supply of essential nutrients, and to provide an "escape hatch" for meandering cells to travel to distant sites and establish metastatic tumors. Vascular endothelial growth factor (VEGF) and platelet-derived growth factor (PDGF) promote angiogenesis and serve as the molecular targets of some of the newer protein kinase inhibitor antineoplastic agents. Fortunately, there are also many opportunities within the metastatic cascade for the body to mount a successful immunological defense and destroy the would-be invaders.

Environmental carcinogens are all around us (Table 33.1),[14] but individuals can do many things to protect themselves from exposure or from the negative consequences of limited exposure. The chemicals deposited in the lungs from inhaling cigarette smoke are the primary cause of lung cancer in the United States, but smokers who quit decrease their risk of dying from this often-fatal cancer by approximately half after 10 smoke-free years.[15,16] Many other cancers are also causally linked to cigarette smoking and, not surprisingly, the longer and more intense the smoking history, the greater the risk.[17] Nonsmokers can protect themselves from the cancer-promoting effects of secondhand smoke by removing themselves from smoke-filled environments. Smoking combined with alcohol has a synergistic effect in promoting the development of oral cancer. In addition to quitting smoking, abstaining from alcohol or drinking in moderation is a choice that individuals can make in an effort to decrease their overall risk of developing cancer. Other protective measures that patients can take include avoiding damaging ultraviolet rays through the use of high-SPF (sun protection factor) sunscreens, the consumption of foods that are low in fat but rich in carotenoids, vitamins A and C, folate, selenium, and/or fiber, and being vaccinated against human papillomavirus (HPV). DNA and RNA viruses associated with carcinogenesis, including HPV, are provided in Table 33.2.[18]

Table 33.1 Some Environmental Precipitants of Cancer

Environmental Cancer Precipitant	Cancer Type
Tobacco	Lung, oral, bladder, pancreatic, stomach, and renal cancer
Alcohol	Liver, rectal, and breast cancer
Tobacco plus alcohol	Oral cancer
Radon	Lung cancer
Halogenated compounds	Bladder cancer
Immunosuppressive agents	Lymphoma
Herbicides	Lymphoma
Ionizing or ultraviolet radiation	Leukemia and breast, thyroid, lung, and skin cancer

Staging and Clinical Response

Clinicians need to have a common language through which to communicate about disease severity to make the best team-based decisions about the relative risks and benefits of treatment options. In the tumor-node-metastasis (TNM) cancer staging classification system, the severity of solid tumor neoplastic growth is characterized by the size

Table 33.2 RNA and DNA Viruses Associated With Cancer Development[a]

Virus	Cancer
RNA Virus	
Hepatitis C	Hepatocellular carcinoma
Human T-cell leukemia	Adult T-cell leukemia
DNA Virus	
Papilloma	Skin cancer, cervical cancer, anogenital cancer
Hepatitis B	Hepatocellular carcinoma
Epstein-Barr	Burkitt lymphoma, non-Hodgkin lymphoma, nasopharyngeal carcinoma
Kaposi sarcoma herpes	Kaposi sarcoma

[a]Listed within each viral category in decreasing order of cancer induction incidence.

of the tumor mass (T_1 to T_4), the extent of lymph node involvement (N_0 to N_3), and whether distant metastasis has occurred (M_0 or M_1). The larger the subscripted number in each of these parameters, the more advanced and/or disseminated the disease. Taken together, the TNM characteristics of a tumor can be translated into a comprehensive staging scale ranging from I (localized) to IV (metastatic). The intermediate disease severity stages indicate local (stage II) or regional (stage III) tissue invasion.[11] Staging is an essential prerequisite for the prediction of prognosis and the identification of the most appropriate treatment plan and optimal dosing regimen.

Likewise, it is equally beneficial to quantify a patient's clinical response to therapy in a manner that is consistent and universally understood by all health care providers, as well as patients. Five discrete anticancer therapy response categories in solid tumors have been defined, with criteria established for each. Although **cure** is obviously the most noble goal, it is very difficult to achieve in most types of cancer. For cancers deemed "curable" (which excludes breast cancer and melanoma), cure equates to no evidence of disease for a minimum of 5 years. More commonly, the response category viewed as the pinnacle is **complete response**, in which the patient has no evidence of cancer, but where relapses are still possible. A **partial response** is claimed when tumor size has been reduced by 30% or more from baseline and there is no evidence of new lesions at the primary site or elsewhere. The term **clinical benefit** has been used if this level of improvement is not reached, yet the patient has experienced significant attenuation of symptoms and/or enhancement of quality of life. A less optimistic response category is **stable disease**, in which tumor size has increased by less than 20% or decreased by less than 30%. Most dire is **progression**, a category that is characterized by tumor growth at the 20% or higher level relative to the lowest lesion diameter since beginning therapy and/or the formation of new lesions during treatment. In hematologic cancers, clinical response is evaluated based on the extent of malignant cell absence, positive improvement in the levels of tumor or cytogenic markers, and restoration of normal organ function.[11]

Treatment Options

Surgery, radiation, and chemotherapy represent the triad of approaches to the treatment, and ideally eradication, of a diagnosed and potentially life-threatening cancer. Commonly given in combination, the order and timing of the interventions are dictated by many factors, including specific diagnosis, disease stage, and anticipated response based on clinical trials.

When a solid tumor is localized and surgically accessible, surgery may be the first option,[13] with radiation or chemotherapy preceding surgery if needed to shrink large lesions. The use of fluorescent dyes, with or without a conjugated targeting antibody, to guide the removal of as much cancerous tissue as possible, is currently being investigated in colorectal, breast, ovarian, uterine, lung, liver, and brain cancer.[19-21] Radiation may replace surgery as the first intervention in localized disease,[13] but early- and late-stage toxicities, including tissue necrosis and secondary cancers, are possible. Postsurgical or postradiation chemotherapy can be administered to eradicate metastatic cells that are too few in number to be clinically visible (micrometastasis). Known as adjuvant chemotherapy, this chemical "insurance policy" is designed to attenuate the risk of recurrence and extend survival. When the goal is symptom attenuation, rather than disease eradication, chemotherapy is called palliative.[11]

Chemotherapy, with or without radiation, may be the only option in hematological or metastatic disease.[11,13] Chemotherapy administered as primary therapy for hematologic malignancies is termed induction therapy. When used to eliminate subclinical neoplastic cells, it is referred to as consolidation therapy, which may possibly be followed with ongoing maintenance therapy.

Evolution of Cancer Chemotherapy[4,22]

> *Those who have not been trained in chemistry or medicine, which after all is only applied chemistry, may not realize how difficult the problem of [cancer] treatment really is. It is almost, not quite, but almost as hard as finding some agent that will dissolve away the left ear, say, yet leave the right ear unharmed: so slight is the difference between the cancer cell and its normal ancestor.*[23]

Thus wrote noted cancer researcher and physician William H. Woglom in a monograph published by the American Association for the Advancement of Science in 1947. Although somewhat predictive of what we now know to be true regarding the relationship between resident genes and oncogenes, Dr. Woglom's rather gloomy prognosis of our ability to meet cancer on its own ground and beat it was underpinned by centuries of unsuccessful attempts to treat neoplastic disease with toxic metals, including lead, arsenic, silver, zinc, antimony, mercury, and bismuth. However, the era of more promising cytotoxic chemotherapy was just on the horizon even as Woglom penned his words of therapeutic woe.

Among the first nonmetallic therapeutic agents to show benefit in the treatment of cancer were cortisone and, later, prednisone. In the 1940s, these glucocorticoids were shown to induce tumor regression in a murine lymphosarcoma and in acute leukemia. In the same decade, the retrospective recognition that World War I soldiers exposed to sulfur mustard gas, as well as World War II gas exposure victims, suffered from damaged lymphoid tissue and bone marrow led to the development of the cytotoxic nitrogen mustards for the treatment of lymphoma. Chemists used their understanding of mustard reactivity to design agents where nitrogen replaced sulfur and conjugated aromatic rings attenuated lone pair nucleophilicity. These "kinder, gentler" nitrogen mustards were orally active agents and less systemically toxic. More recently, oxazaphosphorine-based prodrug mustards, activated predominantly by CYP2B6 (cyclophosphamide) and CYP3A4 (ifosfamide), have enjoyed widespread clinical use in the treatment of hematologic cancers, and testicular cancer and pediatric solid tumors, respectively.

The discovery in 1940 that *p*-aminobenzenesulfonamide was effective against streptococcal infections ushered in the era of antimetabolite chemotherapy. The development of antifolate antineoplastics, which were shown to be effective in combating childhood leukemias, got its start in the late 1940s. In the mid to late 1950s, on the heels of the success of antifolates, came the development of antimetabolites based on the structures of endogenous purine and pyrimidine bases. Perhaps the most exciting discovery in this regard was the recognition that a very simple analogue of the endogenous pyrimidine uracil (5-fluorouracil) was a potent inhibitor of deoxythymidine monophosphate biosynthesis, and that inhibiting the production of this essential nucleotide produced positive results in patients suffering from colon, stomach, pancreatic, and breast cancers. Antimetabolites that target DNA polymerase (e.g., gemcitabine) were first conceptualized and synthesized in the late 1950s and have found use in a variety of solid tumor and hematological cancers.

The antibiotic antineoplastics came into clinical use when the highly toxic actinomycin (discovered in the 1940s) was found to be effective in the treatment of human testicular cancer and uterine choriocarcinoma. Other natural anticancer antibiotics, such as bleomycin, were subsequently found to be active against various hematologic cancers and solid tumors (1960s), which led in more recent times to the development of semisynthetic analogues with both high potency and wider margins of safety. The antimitotic vinca alkaloids vincristine and vinblastine were shown to have activity against Hodgkin disease and acute lymphoblastic leukemia around the same time that the antibiotic antineoplastics were being developed.

Cancer chemotherapy appears to have come full circle since the "metal-intense Renaissance," with the introduction of organometallic platinum complexes to the antineoplastic arsenal in the early 1970s. The fortuitous discovery of organoplatinum complexes in the treatment of cancer is attributed to Dr. Barnett Rosenberg, who was studying the impact of electromagnetic radiation on bacterial cell growth using platinum electrodes.[24] He followed up on the astute observation that the bacteria exposed to the electrodes experienced profound changes in cellular structure, which ultimately were attributed to the in situ generation of cisplatin, the first organoplatinum complex to be marketed. Subsequent additions to the organoplatinum complex family were designed to either attenuate use-limiting toxicity (carboplatin) and/or overcome cisplatin resistance (oxaliplatin). In addition to organometallics, the efficacy of sex hormones and hormone antagonists in fighting hormone-dependent cancers (e.g., estrogen receptor–positive breast cancer and prostate cancer) and the advent of therapeutic biologic response modifiers with direct antiproliferative effects (e.g., interferons) have added significantly to the therapeutic options available to providers and the cancer patients for whom they care.

The later 1990s saw the introduction of the tyrosine kinase inhibitors (TKIs),[25] which ushered in a new era of targeted cancer chemotherapy (discussed below). The recognition in 1960 that a mutant chromosome known as BCR-ABL (or the Philadelphia [Ph] chromosome) appeared consistently in the cells of patients with chronic myelogenous leukemia (CML) represented the first time a chromosomal aberration had been directly linked to a neoplastic disorder. The product of this abbreviated chromosome, the Bcr-Abl protein, is an unregulated tyrosine kinase that promotes cellular proliferation at the expense of apoptosis. Imatinib, the first rationally designed drug in the TKI class,[26] was made available in 2001 and dramatically changed the treatment and clinical outcome of Ph^+ leukemias. Although imatinib selectively targets the Bcr-Abl protein, other inhibitors with selectivity for epidermal growth factor receptor (EGFR) and vascular endothelial growth factor receptor (VEGFR) kinases soon followed. These growth factor–selective TKIs show efficacy in the treatment of solid tumors of the lung, breast, pancreas, and kidney.

From a biologicals perspective, several MAbs targeted to tumor cell antigens or proteins critical to cellular proliferation (e.g., human EGF, VEGF, tyrosine kinase, and proteasomes) have also found their way to the U.S. market (see Chapter 34). In addition to therapeutic efficacy, the goal of the more target-specific kinase inhibitor and biologic therapies is attenuation of the mechanism-related destruction of healthy cells (particularly those with short half-lives) for which cytotoxic chemotherapy is well known.[13]

It is important to note that many molecules derived from plant or marine animal sources have demonstrated value either as cytotoxic chemotherapeutic agents themselves, or as synthetic springboards to anticancer drugs that can be readily produced in the laboratory.[4] Prime examples of anticancer drugs or precursors found in plants include paclitaxel and its precursor 10-deacetylbaccatin III, vinca alkaloids (e.g., vincristine, vinblastine), podophyllotoxin (precursor to the epipodophyllotoxins etoposide and teniposide) and camptothecin (precursor to topotecan and irinotecan). Sea sponges have added cytarabine and eribulin to the antineoplastic war chest. These discoveries point clearly to the need to be good stewards of Mother Nature's medicine cabinet, which undoubtedly holds many yet-to-be discovered therapies that could literally serve as a patient's lifeline.

Contemporary Directions and Developments in Cancer Chemotherapy

BIOMARKERS. Cancer could be more effectively and safely treated if clinicians could identify clues within the patient's genetic and biochemical machinery to disease vulnerability, presence, and aggressiveness, as well as anticipated responsiveness to therapeutic options and susceptibility to resistance mechanisms. The keen interest in discovering reliable cancer biomarkers and exploiting them for therapeutic benefit is evidenced by the dedication of a 2015 special issue of *Molecular Aspects of Medicine* to this topic.[27]

Biomarkers are most commonly proteins able to be detected by immunohistochemical means, and they can be generally classified as prognostic markers (telling clinicians whom to treat) and predictive markers (informing clinicians on how to treat).[28] By "interrogate(ing) the genomics of cancer cells"[29] neoplasms once thought to be uniform in nature can be distinguished into subtypes based on defining molecular properties. The science was intensively applied to non–small cell lung cancer (NSCLC), which can now be stratified with regard to prognosis, treatment responsiveness, and/or acquired resistance by evaluating mutations in genes expressing epidermal growth factor receptor (EGFR) and anaplastic lymphoma kinase (ALK).[29] For example, patients with *EGFR* exon 19 deletions (ex19del) are more responsive to EGFR kinase inhibitor therapy than those with exon 21 mutations (e.g., L858R), and more than half of patients who express a T790M EGFR mutant after exposure to inhibitor therapy become resistant to that therapy. The National Comprehensive Cancer Network (NCCN)[30] also recommends testing NSCLC patients for ROS1, B-Raf (BRAF), and programmed death ligand 1 (PD-L1). Insights gained from the groundbreaking exploration of biomarker-driven NSCLC therapy[31] are now being applied to other solid tumors, underscoring the ongoing need for genomics-facilitated drug discovery.

TARGETED CHEMOTHERAPY. "Precision oncology"[32] involves the use of prodrug (gene-directed or antibody-directed), kinase inhibitor (that specifically target molecular determinants of selected cancers identified through genetic screening), and MAb-based therapies. As with biomarkers discussed above, this antineoplastic "hot topic" has been the focus of intense research and dedicated issues of cancer-related journals.[33] The goal of targeted chemotherapy is to sidestep the nonspecific toxicity inherent in cytotoxic chemotherapy by directing drugs selectively to the genes or proteins within cancer cells that mediate uncontrolled growth. While feasible, targeted chemotherapy comes with its own set of specific toxicities and adverse effects. Still, the excitement over the therapeutic value of this more neoplasm-specific approach is evidenced by the fact that, from 2000 to 2014, 79.5% of new cancer drugs approved by the FDA have been targeted therapeutic agents.[13]

Prodrugs. Gene-directed (GDEPT) or virus-directed (VDEPT) enzyme prodrug therapy delivers to cancer cells a gene that encodes an unnatural enzyme capable of selectively activating a prodrug toxin that is nontoxic to cells not expressing the activating enzyme. Antibody-directed enzyme prodrug therapy (ADEPT) conjugates the activating enzyme to an MAb specific for tumor cell antigens. As before, the administered prodrug anticancer agent will only be activated in (hence, only toxic to) tumor cells.[34] ADEPT therapy is restricted to use in highly vascularized tumors, and in all cases, the activating enzyme should have a pH activity optimum close to the pH of the tumor cell.

Kinase Inhibitors. An array of orally active small molecule enzyme inhibitors have been developed that target kinases known to drive dysfunctional neoplastic-related processes in selected cancers. BCR-ABL, EGFR, ALK, human epidermal growth factor receptor 2 (HER2), vascular endothelial growth factor receptor (VEGFR), BRAF, and mammalian target of rapamycin (mTOR) are among the protein kinases serving as targets for these highly specific inhibitors.[34-36] Kinase inhibitors have clearly changed the face of cancer chemotherapy in responding neoplasms, but serious challenges with their use demand ongoing research to optimize long-term therapeutic utility. Among these challenges are: (1) acquired resistance secondary to gene mutation, with expression of proteins that no longer bind or respond to drug,[29] and (2) risk of clinically significant drug-drug interactions (DDIs) with CYP and/or P-glycoprotein (P-gp) inhibitors and inducers, as well as with drugs that raise gastric pH (e.g, proton pump inhibitors [PPIs], H_2 antagonists).[36] CYP3A4, which metabolizes the greatest number of clinically relevant drugs (see Chapter 3), is the most problematic isoform involved in serious and/or life-threating DDIs involving kinase inhibitors.[36]

Immunotherapy.[37,38] As noted previously, the body's own immunochemical surveillance and defense mechanisms are called into play when primary or metastatic neoplastic cells threaten. Immunotherapy can bolster this self-preservation response by activating T-lymphocytes designed to destroy invading cancer cells. Called an antineoplastic "game changer" and potentially "the beginning of the end of cancer,"[37] immunotherapy commonly employs MAbs that either target tumor cells by binding to specific antigens expressed on their surface, or home in on immune cells to undo the cancer's inhibitory damage to normal immune response pathways. Successful examples of the former approach include antibodies targeting antigens presented by HER2$^+$ breast cancer, B-cell lymphoma, EGFR-expressing colorectal cancer, and VEGF-expressing NSCLC. The latter approach, termed checkpoint blockade therapy, has thus far focused on inhibiting T-lymphocyte–associated protein 4 (CTLA-4) and programmed cell death 1 protein (PD-1), resulting in the liberation of the suppressed immune response.[37,38] Based on its positive impact on long-term survival of advanced melanoma patients, checkpoint blockade immunotherapy is being actively investigated in other solid tumors, including breast, prostate, kidney, and lung. The search for new targets appropriate to this therapeutic strategy is ongoing. The strategies described below may be effective as monotherapy in some patients, although most will likely be used in combination, either with other immunotherapies or with traditional cytotoxic chemotherapy or radiotherapy.[37]

The concept of conjugating a cell-specific antibody to a cell-killing drug (e.g., doxorubicin, methotrexate), toxin (e.g., ricin A), or radionuclide (e.g, ^{131}I, ^{90}Y) is not new. However, with over 50 antineoplastic drug-antibody conjugates currently in clinical trial,[39] the strategy is experiencing a clinical renaissance in cancer chemotherapy. Conjugation allows the delivery of two synergistic cytotoxic entities (antibody and drug/toxin/nuclide) to the tumor, and the use of humanized and fully human antibodies has attenuated immunogenicity that was a therapeutic deal-breaker with previously employed murine antibodies.[40] In addition to being tumor-specific or -selective, the target antigen should be readily internalized when bound to antibody so as to transport the cytotoxic drug to intracellular sites of action.[41]

The chemical moiety linking drug and antibody is critical to the action of the conjugate, as it must (1) ensure stability in the bloodstream until the target cell is reached, (2) allow penetration of the conjugate into tumor vasculature, and (3) release the toxin in tumor lysosomes or endosomes, either through hydrolysis or reduction (cleavable linkers) or degradation (noncleavable linkers).[39-41] The drugs selected for conjugation must be stable in the acidic environment of the drug-liberating organelle, and potent in sub-nanomolar concentrations since only a few conjugates (1%-2% of the administered dose) actually reach their intended target.[39] The cytotoxic payload should be high enough to ensure maximum drug delivery to the tumor, but not so high as to negatively impact the stability and pharmacokinetic properties of the conjugate. In general, a drug:antibody ratio of approximately 4 has proven effective, with the drug linked through antibody Lys residues.[40] The most common classes of antineoplastic drugs used to generate therapeutic antibody conjugates include mitosis inhibitors (e.g., monomethylauristatin E) and DNA toxins (e.g., the bacterial natural products duocarmycin and calicheamicin).[40]

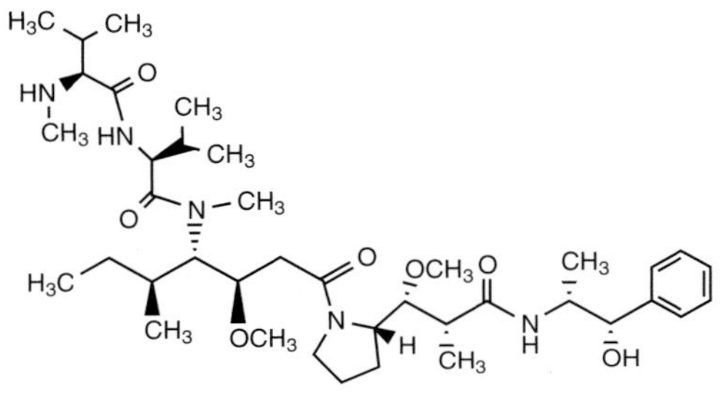

Monomethylauristatin E

The antibody-based cancer chemotherapy drugs currently on the U.S. market are provided in Table 33.3.

A novel nonantibody immunotherapeutic approach that has been used in metastatic melanoma is termed adoptive cell transfer (ACT). ACT involves collecting T-lymphocytes activated to attack neoplastic cells from tissue adjacent to the tumor, and infusing them back into the patient in combination with interleukin-2 (IL-2) to stimulate antigen specific T-cell proliferation. This approach is possible with melanoma because, unlike other cancers, the T-lymphocytes are readily harvested. Administering vaccines that target dendritic cells presenting tumor cell antigen to T-cells is another approach to boost cytotoxic T-lymphocyte action within tumors,[37] and it has been employed in trials with many solid (e.g., breast, prostate, pancreatic) and hematological (lymphoma) cancers. The hope is that antineoplastic vaccines could conceivably provide immunity from the cancer beyond the time of immediate treatment.[38]

NANOCARRIERS.[13] Similar to the antigen-homing antibody component of a drug-antibody conjugate, colloidal nanocarriers are designed to transport high concentrations (payloads) of cytotoxic chemotherapeutic agents selectively to neoplastic cells. While conjugated to or incorporated within the nanocarrier system, the drug is stable from metabolic and chemical degradation and spared elimination, thus increasing its biological half-life. The nanocarrier is designed to exploit the high permeability of the new

Table 33.3 Antibody-Based Chemotherapeutics on the U.S. Market

MAb	Antibody Type	Antigenic Target	Indications
Alemtuzumab	Humanized	CD52	B-cell CLL
Atezolizumab	Humanized	Programmed death ligand 1 (PD-L1)	Metastatic NSCLC, advanced/metastatic urothelial carcinoma
Avelumab	Human	PD-L1	Metastatic Merkel cell carcinoma, advanced/metastatic urothelial carcinoma
Ado-trastuzumab emtansine	Humanized, conjugated with DM1 (maytansine-based mitosis inhibitor)	HER2	$HER2^+$ MBC
Bevacizumab	Humanized	VEGF	Metastatic/recurrent/progressive cervical, colorectal, ovarian, glioblastoma, non-squamous NSCLC, renal cell cancers
Blinatumomab	Mouse	CD19, CD3	Relapsed/refractory ALL
Brentuximab vedotin	Human/mouse chimeric, conjugated with monomethylauristatin E (mitosis inhibitor) and a protease labile dipeptide linker	CD30	Primary or systemic anaplastic large cell lymphoma, relapsed/refractory Hodgkin lymphoma
Cetuximab	Human/mouse chimeric	EGFR	Metastatic/recurrent colorectal, squamous cell head and neck cancers
Daratumumab	Human	CD38	Relapsed/refractory multiple myeloma

(continued)

Table 33.3 Antibody-Based Chemotherapeutics on the U.S. Market (Continued)

MAb	Antibody Type	Antigenic Target	Indications
Dinutuximab	Human/mouse chimeric	GD2	Neuroblastoma
Durvalumab	Human	PD-1	Unresectable NSCLC, advanced/metastatic urothelial carcinoma
Elotuzumab	Humanized	SLAMF7 (also known as CS1)	Relapsed/refractory multiple myeloma
Gemtuzumab ozogamicin	Humanized, conjugated with a calicheamicin analogue	CD33	AML
Ibritumomab tiuxetan	Mouse, chelated with ^{90}Y (β-emitting isotope)	CD20	Relapsed/refractory NHL
Inotuzumab ozogamicin	Humanized, conjugated with a calicheamicin analogue	CD22	Relapsed/refractory ALL
Ipilimumab	Human	CTLA-4	Unresectable/metastatic melanoma
Necitumumab	Human	EGFR	Metastatic squamous NSCLC
Nivolumab	Human	PD-1	Metastatic/recurrent/progressive NSCLC, colorectal, squamous cell head and neck and renal cell cancers, Hodgkin lymphoma, urothelial carcinoma, hepatocellular carcinoma, melanoma
Obinutuzumab	Humanized	CD20	Previously untreated CLL, previously untreated or relapsed/refractory follicular lymphoma
Ofatumumab	Human	CD20	Relapsed, refractory, or previously untreated CLL
Olaratumab	Human	PDGFR-α	Soft tissue sarcoma
Panitumumab	Human	EGFR	Metastatic colorectal cancer
Pertuzumab	Humanized	HER2	Early or metastatic HER2$^+$ breast cancer
Ramucirumab	Human	VEGFR2	Advanced/metastatic NSCLC, colorectal, gastric cancers
Rituximab	Mouse/human chimeric	CD20	CLL, NHL, previously untreated diffuse large B-cell lymphoma (with recombinant human hyaluronidase), follicular lymphoma (with recombinant human hyaluronidase)
Trastuzumab	Humanized	HER2	HER2$^+$ MBC and gastric cancer

ALL, acute lymphoblastic leukemia; AML, acute myeloid leukemia; CLL, chronic lymphocytic leukemia; MBC, metastatic breast cancer; NHL, non-Hodgkin lymphoma; NSCLC, non–small cell lung cancer.

blood vessels generated by tumors through angiogenesis, bypassing the normal barriers the cytotoxic drug molecule would face if "going it alone." Once inside the tumor cell, the cytotoxic drug is released from the carrier to do its cell-killing work.

In order to escape being phagocytized by the reticuloendothelial and mononuclear phagocyte cellular guardian systems, nanocarriers must have a diameter no larger than 400 nm and ideally less than or equal to 200 nm.[13,42] While the nanocarrier surface must be hydrophilic and either charge balanced (i.e., neutral) or slightly anionic to sidestep sequestration by plasma proteins, excessive negative charge must be avoided to minimize the risk of repulsion by the negatively charged surface of tumor blood vessels. Hydrophilic or amphiphilic polymers such as polyethylene glycol (PEG) or polyethylene oxide-propylene oxide copolymers have been successfully employed to provide the desired nanocarrier surface properties.

Nanocarriers are categorized into two major types: polymeric nanocarriers directly conjugate drug while particulate nanocarriers physically trap drug within the carrier.

Polymeric Nanocarriers. An example of a polymeric nanotherapeutic is the albumin bound nanoparticle formulation of paclitaxel (marketed as Abraxane for use in metastatic breast cancer, metastatic pancreatic cancer, and advanced NSCLC). Once internalized into tumor cells by a mechanism facilitated by albumin-activated endocytosis, the drug is cleaved from the carrier by a tumor-secreted protein known as SPARC (secreted protein acidic and rich in cysteine).[43] Abraxane is currently the only polymeric drug-nanocarrier conjugate on the U.S. market, although several are in clinical trials. Many of these investigational polymeric nanoparticles also use albumin as the drug-delivery scaffold.[13]

Targeting antibodies can also be conjugated to the drug-loaded nanocarrier, which has the potential to improve tumor cell selectivity and uptake and dodge multidrug resistance mechanisms. However, these advantages are currently overcome by the potential for premature docking that limits tumor cell penetration, as well as enhanced plasma protein binding and the potential for immunogenicity. Despite the hypothetical promise, the therapeutic efficacy of antibody-conjugated nanocarriers evaluated to date has been no greater (and often lower) than nontargeted carriers.[13]

The downside of polymeric nanoparticles is hepatic and splenic accumulation, tumor cell distribution challenges, and relatively low therapeutic efficacy. If these challenges can be overcome, in addition to more marketed nanocarrier-conjugated drugs, the future may see the use of magnetized nanoparticles as imaging agents in MRI (theragnostics) and/or to generate cytotoxicity-augmenting heat within the tumor after exposure to an externally applied oscillating magnetic field.[13]

Particulate Nanocarriers. Of the various particulate nanocarrier systems, liposomes are perhaps the most familiar. Liposomes are spherical aqueous vesicles, enclosed by a lipid bilayer and into which drugs can be incorporated.[13,42] Cholesterol and biologically safe phospholipids are the common starting materials for liposome production.[42] The anthracycline doxorubicin was the first anticancer drug to be marketed in this formulation (Doxil, FDA-approved in 1995 for use in advanced ovarian cancer, multiple myeloma and AIDS-related Kaposi sarcoma). While only four liposomal anticancer drug products have followed, several formulations of cytotoxic antineoplastics from a wide range of chemical classes, as well as gene-silencing short interfering RNA (siRNA), are currently in clinical trials.[13]

As with polymer therapeutics, the nanocarrier persists in the bloodstream (particularly if conjugated with PEG; so called stealth liposomes), enhances the chemical and metabolic stability of its cytotoxic payload, and facilitates tumor cell vasculature penetration and interstitial space sequestration through a process known as the enhanced permeability and retention (EPR) effect.[13,42] Liposomes are also heat sensitive and can be induced to release their cytotoxic payload if ambient temperature is raised with IR lasers or microwave irradiation.

The downside of liposomes as nanocarriers includes their ability to induce a hypersensitivity reaction after IV administration (despite being otherwise biocompatible), the incorporation preference for water-soluble drugs, and the relatively low number of drug molecules tolerated.[13] Like polymeric nanoparticles, they can accumulate in the liver and spleen, particularly if their diameter is less than 70 nm or greater than 300 nm.[42] Being less highly vascularized, metastatic tumors are inherently less responsive to liposomal drug delivery systems than primary tumors.

Although they are plagued by tumor cell penetration, phagocytic, and immunogenicity challenges, research to optimize the therapeutic value of ligand-targeting (e.g., antibody conjugated) liposomes is ongoing. If successful strategies can be developed to minimize the formation of the protein corona generated around antibody-conjugated liposomes by interacting proteins, the future may hold a ligand targeting cytotoxic liposome of unprecedented selectivity and potency.[42]

BIOSIMILARS. Biosimilars are synthetic macromolecules that are highly similar to, but not identical with, biological therapeutic agents. The first biosimilar was made available to U.S. patients in 2015 with the FDA approval of Zarxio (filgrastim-sndz), a biosimilar of the granulocyte colony-stimulating factor filgastrim.[44,45] To be termed a biosimilar, the therapeutic entity must be equivalent to the reference biologic in terms of safety, purity, and potency, with any structural, in vitro/in vivo property, and clinical activity differences deemed clinically insignificant.

Biosimilars are generated through reverse engineering of the natural product using recombinant DNA technology. Positive data from extensive immunogenicity, pharmacokinetic, and pharmacodynamics studies in humans, along with direct comparative studies with the reference biologic, must be presented to regulatory agencies in order to achieve final marketing approval. Clinical trials should take place with the most "sensitive patient populations" so that response rate outcomes data can be clearly tied to the biosimilar and not confounded by the characteristics of the population under study.[44] The FDA has mandated that approved biosimilars must demonstrate that they "produce the same clinical result as the reference product in any given patient and, if the biological product is administered more than once to an individual, the risk in terms of safety or diminished efficacy of alternating or switching between the use of the biological product and the reference product is not greater than the risk of using the reference product without such alternation or switch."[46] In other words, the biosimilar must "first do no harm."

With patents on current biologic anticancer therapies set to expire in the next several years (e.g., the MAbs rituximab, trastuzumab, and bevacizumab), several biosimilars clinical trials are in the final stages, and the global health care market can logically expect to see more of these drugs made available to clinicians and patients fairly soon. It has been hypothesized that biosimilars could be cost-effective options that would allow more patients worldwide to gain access to therapies that could augment quality (and possibly quantity) of life.[45] This may be particularly significant in the growing geriatric oncology population, where compromised renal, hepatic, and cardiovascular function often complicates the choice of chemotherapy and prohibits enrollment in clinical trials.[45] The decision on whether to use a biosimilar to treat neoplastic disease should involve an analysis of postmarketing surveillance data relative to therapeutic scope, efficacy, and safety in the broader patient population over time. This, of course, demands that clinicians employing biosimilars contribute to the postmarketing safety monitoring systems so that reliable information can be made available to all practitioners.[44]

GENE THERAPY. The first anticancer cell-based gene therapy available in the United States, tisagenlecleucel (Kymriah), was FDA approved in late August, 2017 for refractory or relapsing acute B-cell lymphoblastic leukemia (ALL) in patients up to 25 years of age. Tisagenlecleucel is an example of a chimeric antigen receptor T-cell (CAR-T) therapy, where patient-derived T-cells are genetically manipulated to fuse an antibody that targets the CD19 antigen expressed by that individual leukemia patient's cancer. Upon binding to the target antigen after reinfusion, modified CAR-T proliferation with release of cancer-cell annihilating cytokines occurs.[47] Clinical trials have demonstrated 80% one-year survival statistics and 25% six-month recurrence rates, which currently bests alternative therapies.[47] While only 600 ALL patients per year are estimated to be eligible for treatment, the $470,000 per one-time infused dose price tag makes it a fiscally viable industrial investment. The manufacturer has stated that patients non-responsive by one month post-infusion would not be charged for the drug.[47]

Anticipated toxicities from CAR-T therapies like tisagenlecleucel include cytokine release syndrome (boxed warning), which can induce adverse effects ranging from mild to fatal, neurologic damage, infection, hepatotoxicity, and destruction of healthy cells expressing the target antigen.[47] In one multi-center global phase II tisagenlecleucel clinical trial involving 75 relapsed or refractory ALL patients, serious drug-related toxicity occurred in 73%, with 77% experiencing symptoms of cytokine release syndrome and 40% experiencing neurologic toxicity (e.g., encephalopathy, confusion).[48] Due to the potential for serious or fatal toxicity, tisagenlecleucel can only be administered in certified health centers under a Risk Evaluation and Mitigation Strategy (REMS) program.

CAR-T therapies are not inherently limited to ALL, and research investigating their potential in diffuse large B-cell lymphoma and high-incidence solid tumors is ongoing.[47,49]

EPIGENETIC THERAPY. Epigenetics describes the study of how gene function, independent of DNA sequence changes, leads to significant alterations in gene expression.[50] Important players in epigenetic gene modification include histone proteins that can undergo a wide array of posttranslational modifications and transcription-impacting cytosine methylation processes. It is known that cancer DNA is predominantly hypomethylated, but with site-dependent patches of hypermethylation that can quell tumor suppressor gene function.

Currently marketed anticancer agents that fall under the category of epigenetic therapy include the histone deacetylase inhibitors romidepsin and vorinostat, and the DNA methyl transferase inhibitor 5-azacytidine. However, the lack of tumor cell specificity of these agents cries out for the development of more selective epigenetic modifying drugs. Research uncovering new neoplastic targets, such as histone lysine methylase EZH2 (which is often mutated in diffuse large B-cell lymphoma), holds promise for the future.[50] The Human Epigenome Project[51-53] is expected to reveal additional mechanistic pathways ripe for the rational development of drugs that can right the wayward epigenetic ship and result in the selective destruction of cancer cells.

HYPERTHERMIC CHEMOTHERAPY. While not currently the standard of care because of toxicity, procedure-related and cost concerns, hyperthermic chemotherapy with cytotoxic drugs has been explored as a treatment approach in selected advanced intraperitoneal cancers (e.g., ovarian, appendiceal, colorectal).[54] The drugs employed most commonly include a DNA cross-linking organoplatinum complex (i.e., cisplatin, oxaliplatin, or carboplatin). During the procedure, a heated solution of drug is directly infused and circulated in the abdominal cavity. Heat damages malignant cells to a greater extent than surrounding healthy cells and induces more extensive DNA cross-linking by the organoplatinum complex. Administered at the time of surgical intervention, the chemotherapy can be concentrated at the site where it is most needed and for the amount of time envisioned to provide the highest effect-to-toxicity benefit. Both open abdomen and closed abdomen techniques have been shown to be safe,[54] although advantages and disadvantages of each approach have been identified.[55]

While there is currently no uniformity in procedure, tissue exposure to the antineoplastic drug for 10-60 minutes at temperatures of 42-45°C has been shown to effectively kill cancer cells. In 2017, there were 11 clinical trials of hyperthermic intraoperative intraperitoneal chemotherapy (HIPEC) ongoing across the globe, including in the United States[54] The hope is that these trials will provide the data needed to scientifically evaluate the risk:benefit ratio of HIPEC for use in patients with these advanced and often lethal cancers.

Resistance to Cancer Chemotherapy

Unfortunately, cancer cells do not simply lie down in the face of chemotherapeutic intervention. Rather, these aggressive cells fight back in an attempt to retain their immortality. Some cancer cells acquire resistance to anticancer drugs by downregulating enzymes and carriers essential for drug transport or for the activation of antineoplastic prodrugs, or by upregulating enzymes involved in inactivating biotransformation. Other mechanisms of biochemical retaliation include downregulation of target enzymes or antigens, activation of kinase-associated biochemical pathways, altered drug uptake, inhibition of cellular repair proteins, apoptosis inhibition, and upregulated drug efflux mechanisms.[11,40] Efflux proteins involved in cancer chemotherapy resistance include classic multidrug resistance (MDR; e.g., P-gp) and multidrug resistance–associated (MRP) proteins. Both are classified as adenosine triphosphate (ATP)–binding cassette (ABC) transporters, but MRP (but not MDR) action depends on phase 2 biotransformations such as glucuronidation, sulfonation, and glutathione conjugation.[56]

It has been estimated that up to 90% of cancer-related deaths can be linked in some way to intrinsic (phenotype-related) or acquired resistance to therapy,[56] and the identification and development of compounds that combat acquired resistance is an active area of research. Fortunately, Mother Nature's medicine cabinet is known to house molecules with this desirable property,[56,57] underscoring the need to actively preserve the world's natural resources for generations to come.

THERAPEUTIC CLASSES OF ANTICANCER DRUGS

The remainder of this chapter will focus on anticancer drugs that either enjoy widespread clinical use or are considered first- or second-line therapy in very specific indications with narrowly defined patient populations. Drugs that have fallen out of favor due to the availability of more effective, safer and/or targeted therapies may not be covered. Interested readers are referred to the seventh edition of this textbook for chemical discussions on those less commonly employed antineoplastics.

Kinase Inhibitors

Few classes of anticancer drugs have experienced the explosion of research and new product development more than the small molecule inhibitors of protein kinase enzymes. In 2015, it was reported that (1) from 2001 (the year the first such anticancer agent, imatinib, was approved) to 2010, essentially one new kinase inhibitor (KI) was approved by the FDA each year, (2) 15 of the 28 approved inhibitors at that time had been made available within the past three years, and (3) over 1 million research articles on kinases had been published and over 5,000 kinase crystal structures (some bound to inhibitor) solved.[58] Yet, despite very intense and clinically productive research in this area over the last two decades, the literature assures us that the era of targeted KI drug discovery is just beginning.[59-64]

Mechanisms of Action

Kinases are phosphorylating enzymes that are highly conserved in the three-dimensional structure of the catalytic (ATP-binding) domain. They regulate cell proliferation, differentiation, metabolism, and survival, and when functioning in a deregulated manner, can accelerate cell signaling cascades and cellular growth, induce tumors, and augment antiapoptotic processes. Aberrations in protein phosphorylation by kinases, stimulated by "'mutation hotspots," have been called "drivers" in neoplastic disease, underscoring the potential value of kinase inhibition in cancer chemotherapy. Indeed, the use of these targeted therapeutic molecules in patients carefully screened for genomic markers that would predict susceptibility have shown superior clinical results compared to more generalized chemotherapeutic approaches.[59]

KIs bind to the hydrophobic hinge region (the ATP-binding domain) that connects the N-terminal and C-terminal lobes of the kinase. A minimum of five potential binding pockets surround this site, which may help explain the otherwise surprising degree of selectivity exhibited by many anticancer KIs.[25]

Most marketed inhibitors bind reversibly to their residues, and do so in one of four distinct ways.[58]

- Type I inhibitors compete with ATP and bind to the enzyme in its active form.
- Type II inhibitors bind to the inactive kinase conformer, which differs from the active form in the outward versus inward orientation, respectively, of a critical Asp residue that's part of a DFG residue trio (motif).
- Type III molecules fit into a binding pocket adjacent to the active site (allosteric binding).
- Type IV inhibitors seek out an allosteric binding site that is distant from the ATP-binding site.

SAR (Structure-activity Relationships)

In general, type I inhibitors will contain a heteroaromatic ring that directly competes with ATP for access to the adenine-binding domain of the hinge region. Lipophilic and hydrogen-bonding functional groups attached to the heteroaromatic system insert into allosteric and hydrophobic pockets adjacent to the adenine pocket, enhancing affinity. Many contain polar functional groups that extend into the solvent interface. Type II inhibitors access the same binding areas as type I, so many of the structural elements found on type I inhibitors are retained.

Since type III inhibitors bind in allosteric pockets adjacent to the adenine-binding site and do not compete directly with ATP, hydrophobic, π-stacking, and hydrogen-bonding groups will be important to affinity and potency. In addition, with ATP located "next door," electrostatic interactions between the inhibitor and the anionic terminal phosphate of the bound nucleotide, and/or with charged or polar residues lining the catalytic site, are often possible. Since they bind a distance from the adenine pocket, no such interactions are of importance to type IV inhibitors.[25,65]

Four electrophilic kinase inhibitors contain a Michael alkylating moiety that allows them to act irreversibly through covalent bond formation with a nucleophilic Cys797 residue that flanks the ATP-binding site.

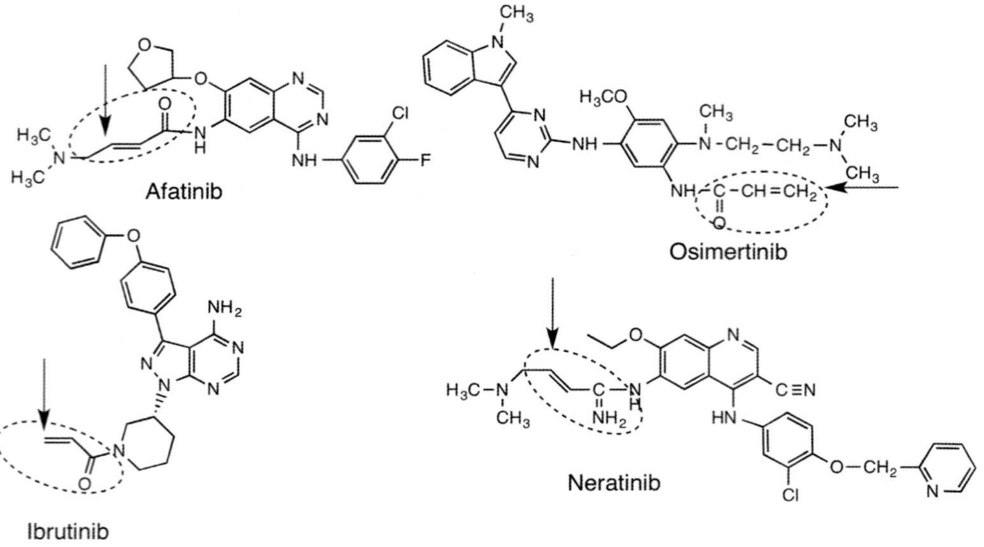

Michael alkylating moieties of irreversibly acting kinase inhibitors (arrow indicates site of Cys attack)

Resistance

Resistance to KIs is also multifaceted, with predominant "on target" resistance pathways mediated through affinity-attenuating mutations or conformational changes in the kinase enzyme. On-target resistance can also involve enhanced kinase affinity for the endogenous ATP ligand. Alternative resistance mechanisms include disruption of destructive processes that follow kinase inhibition ("on-pathway" resistance), upregulation of parallel pathways that accomplish the biochemical goals of the inhibited kinase, epigenetic modification of the tumor cell's phenotype, and negative influences on inhibitor pharmacokinetics or metabolic stability.[59] The ability to screen tumor cells for operational resistance mechanisms is paving the way for the design of more tenacious therapies for use in mutation-nimble neoplasms. The use of combination KI therapy, selected to target-specific or parallel kinase pathways or crucial tumor cell properties, is another approach to delaying or overcoming resistance.[59]

Tyrosine Kinase Inhibitors (TKIs)

Of the 39 currently marketed kinase inhibitors, 28 target one or more tyrosine kinase enzymes (Fig. 33.1). These enzymes are most commonly receptor-associated, but a few are cellular (nonreceptor-associated). Compared to healthy cells, genetically deregulated malignant cells are more highly dependent on glycolytic activity without a concomitant increase in reliance on oxidative phosphorylation (the Warburg effect),[66] and the kinases of greatest neoplastic relevance appear to regulate glycolysis, lipid, and energy (TCA cycle) metabolism. TKIs act by inhibiting the binding of ATP in the catalytic hinge region of the kinase, with a resultant decrease in glucose uptake, disruption of mitochondria metabolism, and a possible decrease in fatty acid metabolism (the understanding of the impact of TKIs on lipid metabolism is still evolving).[66] These inhibitors can be highly selective for one enzyme type, or they can target multiple kinases, but they are usually fairly well tolerated by nonmalignant cells.

TKs that serve as targets for anticancer TKIs commonly include EGFR, VEGFR, human epidermal growth factor receptor (HER1 and HER2), platelet-derived growth factor receptor (PDGFR), anaplastic lymphoma kinase (ALK), Bcr-Abl (a product of the translocated breakpoint cluster [*Bcr*]-Abelson [*Abl*] gene known as the Philadelphia, or Ph, chromosome) and Src. Bcr-Abl and Src are nonreceptor kinases, whereas the remainder are receptor-associated enzymes.

As noted previously, type I inhibitors bind to the active conformation of the kinase, whereas type II TKIs inhibit the enzyme in its inactive conformation. Type II inhibitors share common structural features, including a heterocyclic ring that binds to the hydrophobic adenine pocket, up to three hydrogen-bonding moieties that interact with hinge region residues, and a lipophilic carbo- or heterocyclic aromatic ring that binds within a hydrophobic pocket.[62] Since the inactive conformations of TKs differ in structure to a greater degree than the active conformers, it has been proposed that type II inhibitors may have a better opportunity for selectivity,[25,67] although that presumption has recently been questioned.[58,62] Promiscuous TKIs that inhibit several kinase enzymes are referred to as multikinase inhibitors.

CYP3A4 is a common TKI-metabolizing isoform (Table 33.4), leading to a high risk of drug-drug interactions (DDIs) with 3A4 substrates, inducers and inhibitors, including grapefruit juice.[68-75] Cautions against coadministration of drugs and foods that strongly impact CYP3A4 activity are routine, and dosing adjustments are required if coadministration cannot be avoided. Several TKIs generate active metabolites that contribute to their antineoplastic activity (Fig. 33.2), and many inhibit one or more CYP isoforms and/or are substrates for (and inhibitors of) cellular efflux pumps like P-gp and breast cancer resistance protein (BCRP). All TKIs are excreted predominantly in the feces.

Adverse effects are common to drugs within a given TKI class and between classes. Several TKIs show pH-dependent solubility, with oral absorption and subsequent drug exposure significantly compromised with elevated gastric pH. Coadministration of antacids, H_2 antagonists, and proton pump inhibitors (PPIs) with these TKIs should be separated by at least two hours or avoided altogether.

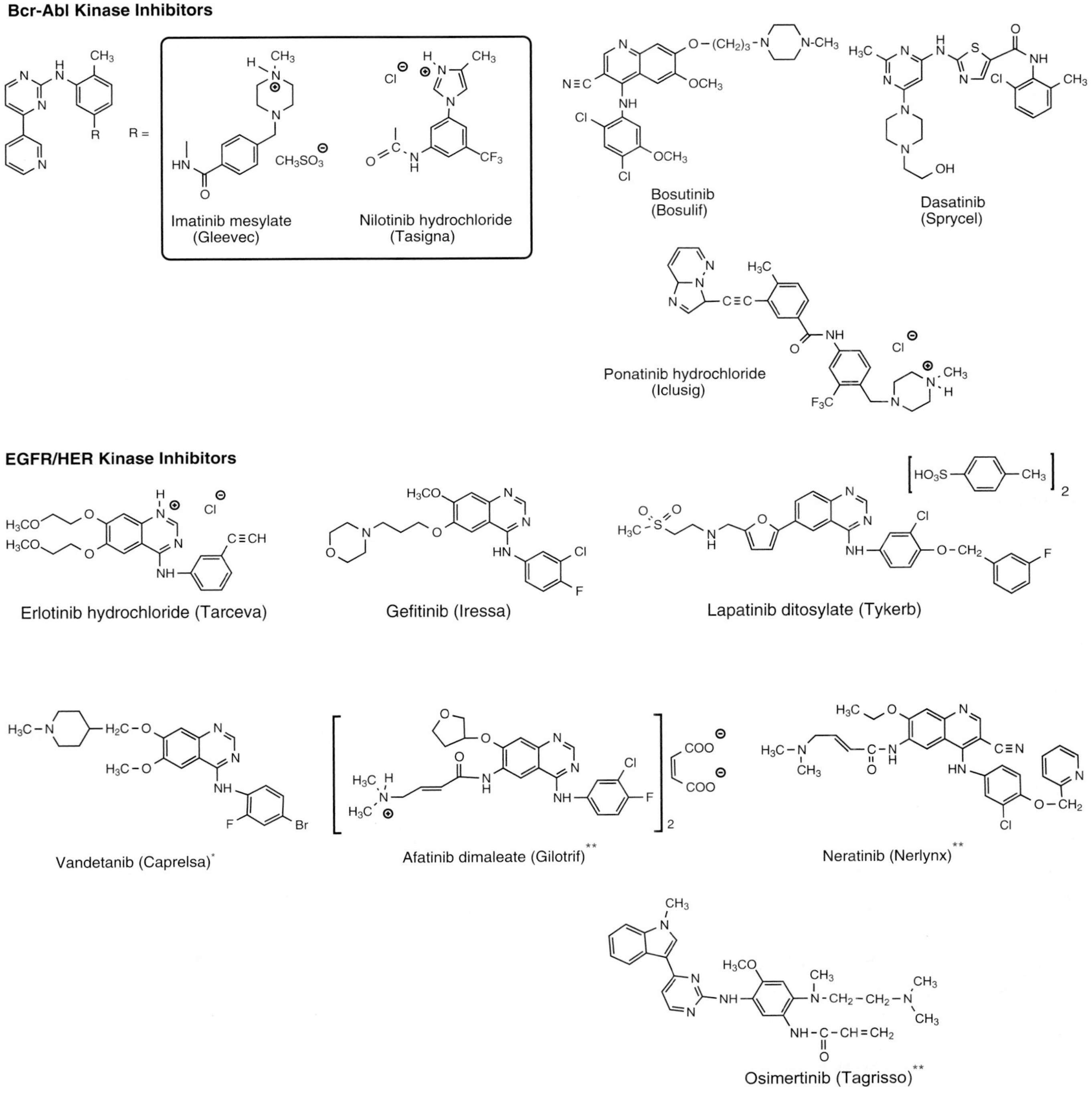

Bcr-Abl Kinase Inhibitors

Imatinib mesylate (Gleevec)

Nilotinib hydrochloride (Tasigna)

Bosutinib (Bosulif)

Dasatinib (Sprycel)

Ponatinib hydrochloride (Iclusig)

EGFR/HER Kinase Inhibitors

Erlotinib hydrochloride (Tarceva)

Gefitinib (Iressa)

Lapatinib ditosylate (Tykerb)

Vandetanib (Caprelsa)*

Afatinib dimaleate (Gilotrif)**

Neratinib (Nerlynx)**

Osimertinib (Tagrisso)**

*Inhibits multiple kinases; **Irreversible kinase inhibitor

Figure 33.1 Tyrosine kinase inhibitors.

VEGFR kinase inhibitors

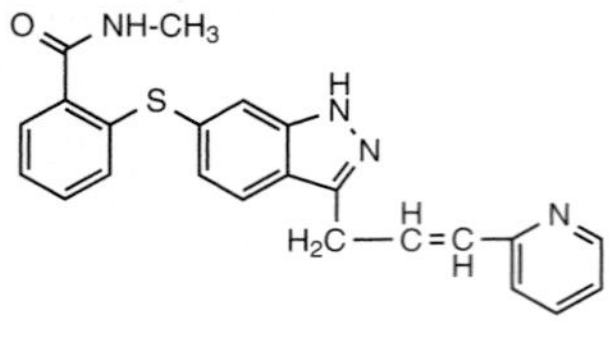

Axitinib (Inlyta)

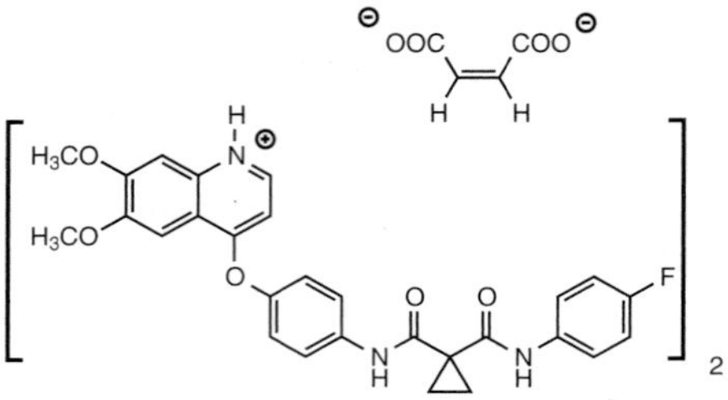

Cabozantinib maleate (Exelixis)*

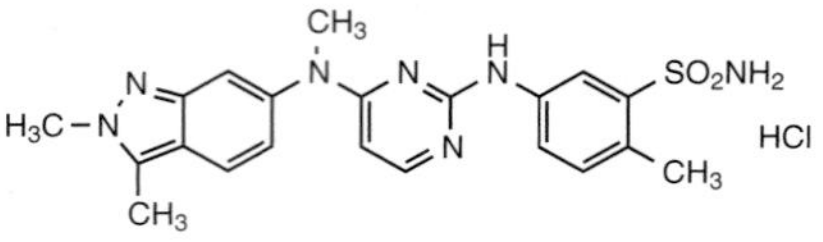

Pazopanib hydrochloride (Votrient)*

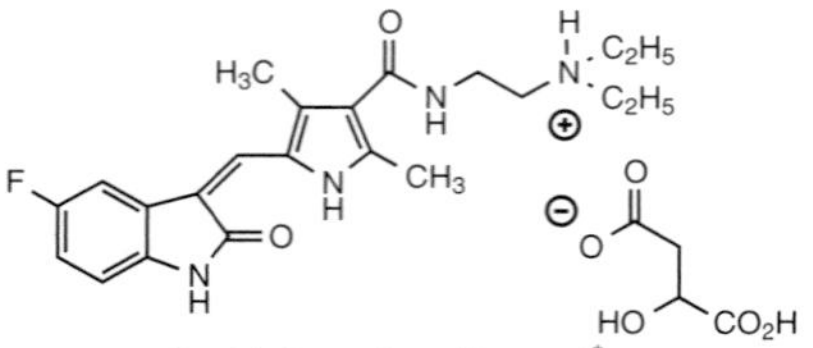

Sunitinib malate (Sutent)*

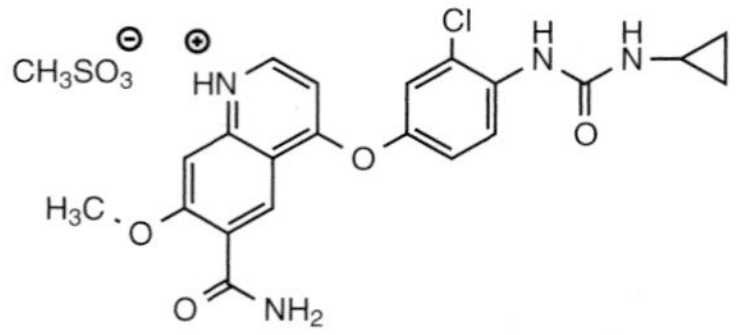

Lenvatinib mesylate (Lenvima)*

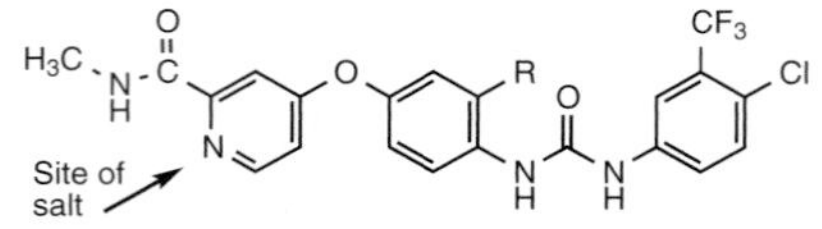

Sorafenib tosylate (R = H, tosylate = $C_7H_7SO_3^-$) (Nexavar)*
Regorafenib (R = F) (Stivarga)*

ALK inhibitors

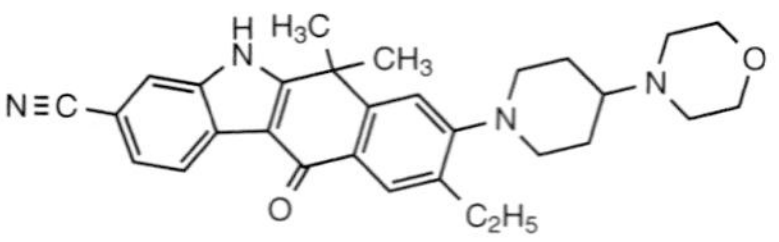

Alectinib (Alecensa)

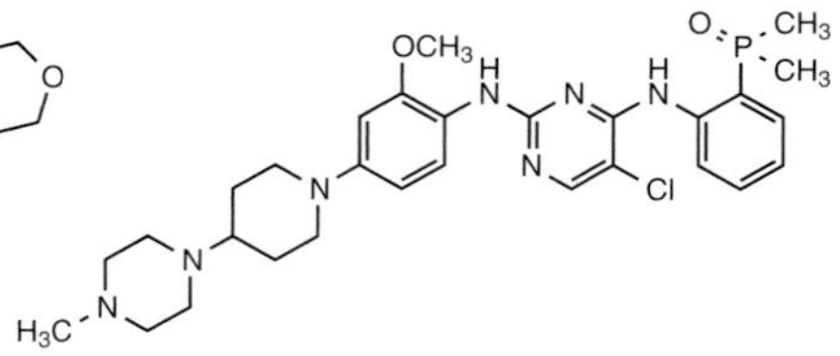

Brigatinib (Alunbrig)*

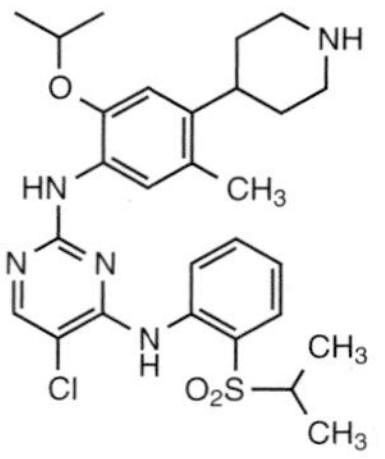

Ceritinib (Zykadia)

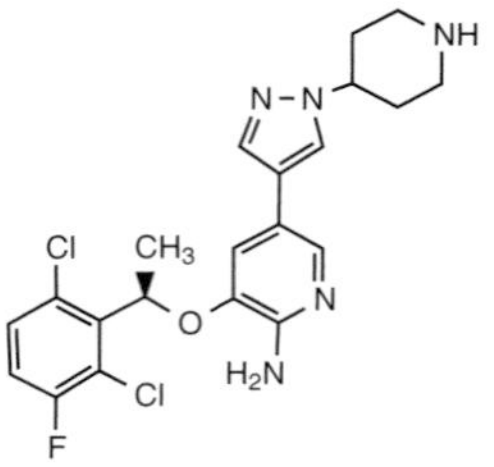

Crizotinib (Xalkori)*

Bruton tyrosine kinase inhibitors

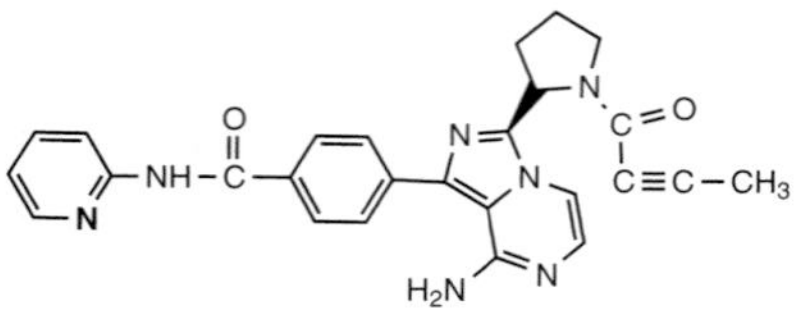

Acalabrutinib (Calquence)**

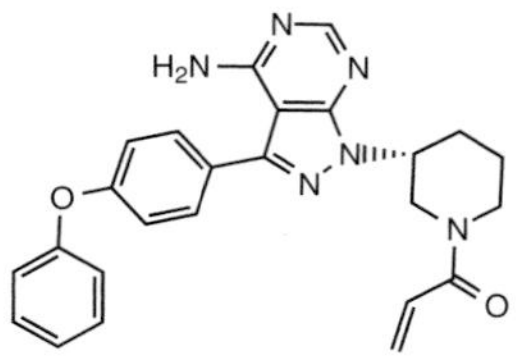

Ibrutinib (Imbruvica)**

FLT3 kinase inhibitor

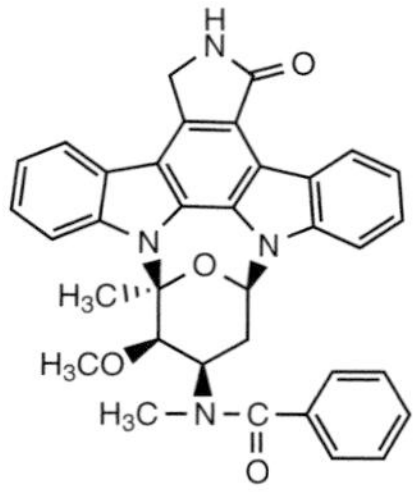

Midostaurin (Rydapt)*

JAK inhibitor

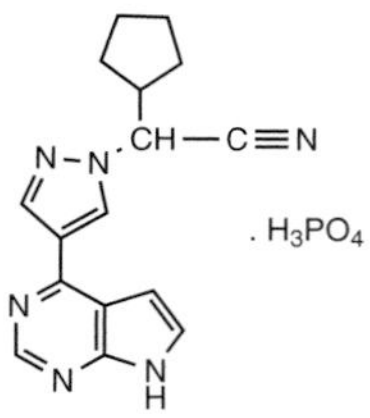

Ruxolitinib phosphate (Jakafi)

*Inhibits multiple kinases; **Irreversible kinase inhibitor

Figure 33.1 Cont'd

Table 33.4 CYP-Mediated Metabolism of Tyrosine Kinase and Multikinase Inhibitors

TKI	Reaction (Site)	Major Metabolizing CYP Isoform	Active CYP Metabolite?
BCR-ABL Kinase Inhibitors			
Imatinib	N-dealkylation (piperazine)	3A4	Yes
Nilotinib	Methyl hydroxylation (imidazole)	3A4	No
Ponatinib	N-dealkylation (piperazine)	3A4	Yes
Dasatinib	Aromatic hydroxylation (phenyl), benzylic hydroxylation (phenyl), N-dealkylation (piperazine), N-oxidation (piperazine N4)	3A4	Questionable significance

Table 33.4 CYP-Mediated Metabolism of Tyrosine Kinase and Multikinase Inhibitors (Continued)

TKI	Reaction (Site)	Major Metabolizing CYP Isoform	Active CYP Metabolite?
Bosutinib	N-dealkylation (piperazine), oxidative dechlorination (chlorinated phenyl)	3A4	No
Omacetaxine mepesuccinate[a]	Minimal non-hydrolytic metabolism	NA	No
EGFR/HER Kinase Inhibitors			
Erlotinib	O-demethylation, aromatic hydroxylation (acetylenated phenyl)	3A4, 1A1, 1A2	Yes (desmethyl metabolite)
Gefitinib	Morpholine oxidation/ring opening (3A4) O-demethylation (2D6)	3A4, 2D6	Yes (phenol)
Lapatinib	Dealkylation (fluorobenzyl)	3A4	No
Vandetanib	N-dealkylation	3A4	Yes
Afatinib	Minimal metabolism	NA	NA
Neratinib	N-oxidation (pyridine), N-dealkylation	3A4	Yes
Osimertinib	N-demethylation (indole, terminal amine)	3A4	Yes
VEGFR Kinase Inhibitors			
Cabozantinib	N-oxidation	3A4	No
Lenvatinib	N-dealkylation (cyclopropyl), O-demethylation, O-dearylation (pyridine), N-oxidation (pyridine)	3A4	No
Axitinib	Sulfoxidation	3A4	No
Pazopanib	Benzylic hydroxylation	3A4	Yes
Sunitinib	N-deethylation to secondary amine	3A4	Yes
Sorafenib	N-oxidation (pyridine)	3A4	Yes
Regorafenib	N-oxidation (pyridine), N-demethylation	3A4	Yes
ALK Inhibitors			
Crizotinib	Oxidation to lactam (piperidine), O-dealkylation	3A4	Yes (lactam)
Ceritinib	O-dealkylation (isopropoxy), monooxygenation	3A4	Questionable significance
Alectinib	Deethylation/ring opening (morpholine)	3A4	Yes
Brigatinib	N-demethylation (piperazine), cysteine conjugation	2C8, 3A4	Yes
Bruton Tyrosine Kinase Inhibitors			
Ibrutinib	Epoxidation to diol (ethylene), aromatic hydroxylation, ring opening (piperidine)	3A4	Yes (diol)
Acalabrutinib	Not reported	3A4	Yes
FLT3 Kinase Inhibitor			
Midostaurin	Hydroxylation (pyrrolidinone), O-dealkylation, N-demethylation	3A4	Yes (7-hydroxypyrrolidinone epimers, hydroxytetrahydropyran metabolite)
Janus-Associated Kinase Inhibitor			
Ruxolitinib	Hydroxylation (cyclopentane)	3A4	Yes

[a]Protein synthesis inhibitor targeting TKI-resistant Bcr-Abl CML.

COMMON ADVERSE EFFECTS OF TYROSINE KINASE INHIBITORS

All TKIs

- Edema
- Fatigue
- Bone marrow suppression
- GI distress with diarrhea or constipation
- Rash and other dermatologic reactions (some severe)
- Headache

Bcr-Abl

- Muscle cramps, arthralgia

EGFR

- Hepatotoxicity

VEGFR

- Hypertension
- Palmar-plantar erythrodysethesia (hand-foot syndrome)

ALK

- Cardiovascular toxicity (bradycardia, hypertension, QT interval prolongation)
- Hepatotoxicity
- Hyperglycemia

Bruton

- Musculoskeletal pain

FLT3

- Urinary, upper respiratory tract, and other infections
- Hyperglycemia
- Musculoskeletal pain
- Hepatotoxicity

JAK

- Dyslipidemia
- Dyspnea
- Muscle spasm

Specific metabolic pathways are shown below for selected TKIs, and other key pharmacokinetic properties of currently marketed inhibitors are provided in Table 33.5. Important therapeutic parameters of these anticancer agents are listed in Table 33.6.[76]

BCR-ABL KINASE INHIBITORS—IMATINIB, NILOTINIB, PONATINIB, DASATINIB, BOSUTINIB. Bcr-Abl inhibitors were the first TKIs to be introduced, and they literally changed the face of CML therapy.[66] The fusion of the Abelson (*Abl*) gene on chromosome 9 with the breakpoint cluster region (*Bcr*) of chromosome 22 results in the *Bcr-Abl* fusion gene known as the Philadelphia (Ph) chromosome. The aberrant Ph chromosome is considered the cause of 95% of adult CML[77] and is also found in approximately 25% of patients with acute ALL. It is a harbinger of a poor prognosis.[78]

The clinical availability of imatinib, discovered serendipitously in a search for new anti-inflammatory agents, allowed CML patients to realistically anticipate a 5-year survival, as opposed to the 2- to 3-year prognosis in untreated disease. The drug is known to revert glucose metabolism in Bcr-Abl positive cells from anaerobic to aerobic in a concentration-dependent manner and to decrease glucose uptake through a 90% downregulation of the GLUT1 transporter.[66] It has its greatest effect in the initial (chronic) phase of CML, when the malignant cells are proliferating fairly slowly. Fortunately, approximately 95% of patients are diagnosed in this treatable phase, since Bcr-Abl kinase inhibitors are significantly less effective in the accelerated or highly fatal blastic phases.

As is the case with so many chemotherapeutic agents, acquired resistance has undermined the positive clinical outcomes imatinib first promised. Resistance mechanisms are often associated with point mutations in the Abl (kinase) domain,[58] in particular a Thr to Ile mutation at position 315 (T315I). Residue 315 is known as the "gatekeeper" to the hydrophobic binding pocket. The more significant bulk of the Ile residue, along with the loss of the polar OH moiety that Thr provided, blocks imatinib's access to this receptor through steric interference with the benzyl moiety and prevents affinity-enhancing H-bonding.[25,79,80] Of all Bcr-Abl mutations 12 % are T315I, and CML patients carrying this mutation have a poor prognosis. Alternate mechanisms of resistance are related to *BRC-ABL* gene amplification, P-gp overexpression, underexpression of an organic cation transporter-1 (OCT1) protein that helps some TKIs (including imatinib) gain access to cells, and activation of Src kinases.

Chemistry (Fig. 33.3)[58,62]

The Bcr-Abl inhibitors imatinib and nilotinib contain a 2-phenylaminopyrimidine pharmacophore. They are relatively large, extended structures that bind to both the ATP-binding hinge region (adenine pocket) and to adjacent hydrophobic subdomains of the Bcr-Abl protein. As type II inhibitors, they bind to the inactive conformation of the kinase known as the "DFG-out state."[67] In this conformation, an enzymatic aspartate (Asp381; D)-Mg^{2+} interaction is broken, and a Phe residue is pushed out toward the aqueous environment, occluding the approach of ATP and generating a new binding area that attracts type II Bcr-Abl inhibitors. This conformation is also stabilized by a non-phosphorylated Tyr393, which orients toward the center of the enzyme and H-bonds with Asn363.[81]

The *o*-methyl substituent found on imatinib and nilotinib confers selectivity for the cytosolic Bcr-Abl protein in its inactive conformation, although the benzamide moiety permits some inhibition of PDGFR kinase. It is the PDGFR-related component of the activity profile that is believed responsible for the fluid retention induced by these two TKIs. These agents also contain a pyridyl substituent at C4 of the pyrimidine ring, which enhances affinity through H-bonding with the amide NH of Met318 within the hinge region (Fig. 33.3).[58] The amide moiety, inverted in nilotinib compared to imatinib, forms H-bonds with Glu286 and Asp381.[58,82,83] Yet another H-bond is formed between gatekeeper Thr315 and the NH group connecting the pyrimidine and phenyl rings.[58] Thus, while nilotinib can show activity in some imatinib-resistant mutants, it cannot overcome the resistance induced by T315I.

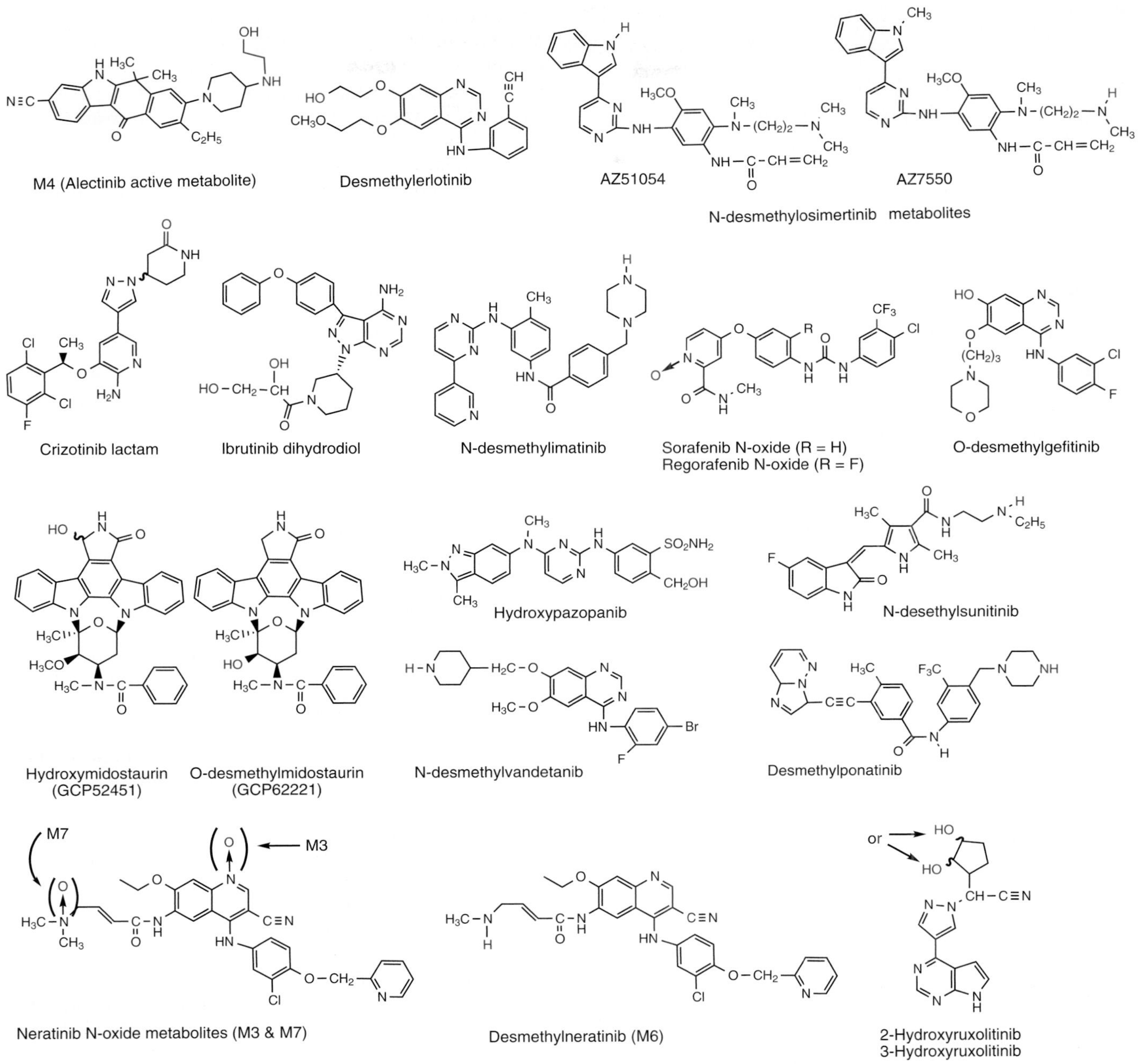

M4 (Alectinib active metabolite) Desmethylerlotinib AZ51054 AZ7550

N-desmethylosimertinib metabolites

Crizotinib lactam Ibrutinib dihydrodiol N-desmethylimatinib Sorafenib N-oxide (R = H) Regorafenib N-oxide (R = F) O-desmethylgefitinib

Hydroxypazopanib N-desethylsunitinib

Hydroxymidostaurin (GCP52451) O-desmethylmidostaurin (GCP62221) N-desmethylvandetanib Desmethylponatinib

Neratinib N-oxide metabolites (M3 & M7) Desmethylneratinib (M6) 2-Hydroxyruxolitinib 3-Hydroxyruxolitinib

Figure 33.2 Active metabolites of tyrosine kinase inhibitors.

The [(piperazinyl)methyl]phenyl moiety of imatinib seeks out an allosteric pocket, where the cationic piperazine nitrogen atom bonds with His361 and Ile360. Nilotinib's trifluoromethylated imidazole-phenyl group allows for tighter binding deeper within this allosteric site.[58] The affinity-enhancing hydrophobic interactions with Leu298, Val299, and Phe359 are, in part, responsible for nilotinib's 10- to 50-fold increase in TK-inhibiting potency compared to imatinib.[77] The methylimidazole moiety also augments affinity through hydrophobic interactions with Leu285, Glu286, and Val289, while leaving the basic nitrogen exposed to the aqueous environment.[25,67,80,81]

Ponatinib, the third type II Bcr-Abl inhibitor, was designed to circumvent resistance due to the T315I mutation that has been the bane of imatinib and nilotinib chemotherapy. The linear alkyne moiety connecting the tolyl and imidazo[1,2-b]pyridazinyl rings can navigate around Ile's bulk, and the trifluromethylphenyl substituent on the benzamide moiety (shared with nilotinib) ensures tight binding deep within the allosteric pocket.[58,78] Binding of the tolyl ring occurs within a hydrophobic pocket, and hydrogen bonding further enhances affinity.[79] The potency of ponatinib is claimed to be 520 times that of imatinib.[78]

Water solubility of these three type II TKIs is conferred by the substituted piperazine (imatinib, ponatinib) and imidazole (nilotinib) rings. The lower pK_a of imidazole compared to piperazine explains why nilotinib is not a substrate for the OCT1 protein that ferries imatinib

Table 33.5 Selected Pharmacokinetic Properties of Tyrosine Kinase Inhibitors

TKI	Dosage Form	T_{max} (hr)	$T_{1/2}$ (hr)	Protein Binding (%)	Oral Bioavailability (%)	Administration
BCR-ABL Kinase Inhibitors						
Imatinib	Tablet	2-4	18	95	98	Administer with food
Nilotinib	Capsule	3	17	98	50	Administer on empty stomach
Ponatinib	Tablet	≤6	12-66	<99	Not available	Food independent
Dasatinib	Tablet	0.5-6	3-5	96	Incomplete	Food independent
Bosutinib	Tablet	6	22-27	94	34	Administer with food
Omacetaxine mepesuccinate[a]	SC injection	0.5	14.6	≤50	NA	Administer q 12 hr.
EGFR/HER Kinase Inhibitors						
Erlotinib	Tablet	4	36	93	60 (fasted) 100 (fed) Smoking ↓AUC (64%)	Administer on empty stomach
Gefitinib	Tablet	3-7	48	90	60	Food independent
Lapatinib	Tablet	4	24	>99	Variable absorption	Administer on empty stomach
Vandetanib	Tablet	4-10	456	90	Not available	Food independent
Afatinib	Tablet	2-5	37	95	92	Administer on empty stomach
Neratinib	Tablet	2-8	7-17	>99	High-fat meal↑C_{max} (1.7X)	Administer with food
Osimertinib	Tablet	3-24	48	95	70 High-fat meal↑AUC (19%)	Food independent
VEGFR Kinase Inhibitors						
Cabozantinib	Tablet, capsule	2-5	55 (capsule); 99 (tablet)	>99	tablet > capsule	Administer on empty stomach
Lenvatinib	Capsule	1-4	28	98-99	Not available	Food independent
Axitinib	Tablet	2.5-4	2.5-6.1	>99	58 High-fat meal ↓bioavailability (19%)	Food independent
Pazopanib	Tablet	2-4	31	>99	Food ↑bioavailability (2X)	Administer on empty stomach
Sunitinib	Capsule	6-12	40-60	95	Not available	Food independent
Sorafenib	Tablet	3	25-48	99.5	38-49 High-fat meal ↓bioavailability (41%)	Administer on empty stomach
Regorafenib	Tablet	4	28	99.5	69 High-fat meal ↑AUC (48%) Low-fat meal ↑AUC (36%)	Administer with food (low fat)

Table 33.5 Selected Pharmacokinetic Properties of Tyrosine Kinase Inhibitors (Continued)

TKI	Dosage Form	T_{max} (hr)	$T_{1/2}$ (hr)	Protein Binding (%)	Oral Bioavailability (%)	Administration
ALK Inhibitors						
Crizotinib	Capsule	4-6	42	91	43 High-fat meal ↓bioavailability (14%)	Food independent
Ceritinib	Capsule	4-6	41 (fasted)	97	High-fat meal ↑C_{max} (41%)	Administer with food
Alectinib	Capsule	4	33	>99	37 High-fat meal ↑drug exposure	Administer with food
Brigatinib	Tablet	1-4	25	66	High-fat meal ↓ C_{max} (13%)	Food independent
Bruton Tyrosine Kinase Inhibitors						
Ibrutinib	Tablet, capsule	1-2 (fasted) 4 (fed)	4-6	97	Food ↑C_{max} (2-4X)	Food independent
Acalabrutinib	Capsule	0.75	0.6-2.8	97.5	25 High-fat meal ↓ C_{max} (73%); ↑T_{max} (1-2 hr)	Food independent
FLT3 Kinase Inhibitor						
Midostaurin	Capsule	1-3 (fasted) 2.5-3 (fed)	21	>99.8	High-fat meal ↑drug exposure (1.6X) ↓C_{max} (27%)	Administer with food
Janus-Associated Kinase Inhibitor						
Ruxolitinib	Tablet	1-2	3	97	>95	Food independent

[a]Protein synthesis inhibitor targeting TKI-resistant Bcr-Abl CML.
AUC, area under the concentration curve; SC, subcutaneous; $T_{1/2}$, elimination half-life; T_{max}, time to peak plasma concentration.

Table 33.6 Selected Therapeutic Parameters of Tyrosine Kinase Inhibitors

TKI	Indications	Usual Adult Dose (mg/d)	Precautions
BCR-ABL Kinase Inhibitors			
Imatinib	Ph⁺ CML, ALL GIST Not effective in T315I mutants	400-600 (CML) 600 (ALL) 400 (GIST)	Heart failure and hepatotoxicity possible Inhibits BCRP, CYP3A4
Nilotinib	Imatinib-resistant Ph⁺ CML Not effective in T315I mutants	600-800 (2 divided doses)	**Boxed warning:** QT interval prolongation leading to sudden death Elevated gastric pH decreases bioavailability Inhibits CYP3A4, 2D6, 2C8/9, UGT1A1
Ponatinib	Imatinib-resistant Ph⁺ CML, ALL Effective in T315I mutants	45	**Boxed warning:** Vascular occlusion, heart failure, hepatotoxicity, venous thromboembolism Inhibits BCRP
Dasatinib	Imatinib-resistant Ph⁺ CML, ALL Not effective in T315I mutants	100-180 (CML) 140-180 (ALL)	QT interval prolongation and hemorrhage possible Elevated gastric pH decreases bioavailability

(continued)

Table 33.6 Selected Therapeutic Parameters of Tyrosine Kinase Inhibitors (Continued)

TKI	Indications	Usual Adult Dose (mg/d)	Precautions
Bosutinib	Imatinib-resistant Ph⁺ CML Not effective in T315I mutants	400-600	Elevated gastric pH decreases bioavailability
Omacetaxine mepesuccinate[a]	TKI-resistant or -intolerant CML	2.50 mg/m^2 (two divided doses)	Significant hyperglycemia possible. Avoid in poorly controlled diabetic patients
EGFR/HER Kinase Inhibitors			
Erlotinib	Exon 19 deletion or L858R⁺ NSCLC Pancreatic cancer	150 (NSCLC) 100 (pancreatic)	Pulmonary toxicity possible 24% increase in clearance in smokers Elevated gastric pH decreases bioavailability May not increase survival when used as maintenance therapy in nonmutated NSCLC Inhibits UGT1A1
Gefitinib	Exon 19 deletion or L858R⁺ NSCLC	250	Pulmonary toxicity possible Elevated gastric pH decreases bioavailability Inhibits BCRP
Lapatinib	HER2⁺ BC	1250-1500	**Boxed warning:** Potentially fatal hepatotoxicity Decreased left ventricular ejection fraction and QT interval prolongation possible Inhibits BCRP, P-gp
Vandetanib	MTC	300	**Boxed warning:** QT interval prolongation leading to torsades de pointes, sudden death Pulmonary toxicity possible Inhibits BCRP, OCT2
Afatinib	NSCLC	40	Patients of Asian heritage at high risk for pulmonary toxicity Inhibits BCRP
Neratinib	HER2⁺ BC	240	Elevated gastric pH decreases bioavailability Inhibits P-gp
Osimertinib	T790M⁺ NSCLC	80	Cardiomyopathy and pulmonary toxicity possible Inhibits BCRP
VEGFR Kinase Inhibitors			
Cabozantinib	Advanced RCC MTC	60-80 (RCC) 140-180 (MTC)	**Boxed warning:** Perforations, fistulas, hemorrhage
Lenvatinib	Advanced RCC Iodine-refractory differentiated TC	18 (RCC) 24 (TC)	Decreased ejection fraction possible Inhibits OATs, OCTs, UGT1A1, UGT1A9
Axitinib	Advanced RCC	10 (2 divided doses)	Hemorrhage and cardiovascular events possible
Pazopanib	Advanced RCC Advanced soft tissue sarcoma	800	**Boxed warning:** Potentially fatal hepatotoxicity QT interval prolongation with torsades de pointes, heart failure and hemorrhage possible Elevated gastric pH decreases bioavailability Inhibits OATP1B1, UGT1A1
Sunitinib	Advanced RCC Advanced pancreatic NET Imatinib-resistant GIST	50 (RCC, GIST) 37.5 (NET)	**Boxed warning:** Potentially fatal hepatotoxicity Cardiomyopathy, including QT interval prolongation, heart failure, and hemorrhage possible Inhibits BCRP

Table 33.6 Selected Therapeutic Parameters of Tyrosine Kinase Inhibitors (Continued)

TKI	Indications	Usual Adult Dose (mg/d)	Precautions
Sorafenib	Advanced RCC TC HCC	800 (2 divided doses)	Cardiac ischemia and hemorrhage possible Inhibits BCRP, UGT1A9
Regorafenib	GIST Metastatic CRC HCC	160	**Boxed warning:** Potentially fatal hepatotoxicity Infection, hemorrhage, and cardiotoxicity possible Inhibits BCRP, UGT1A1, UGT1A9
ALK Inhibitors			
Crizotinib	ALK⁺ NSCLC	500 (2 divided doses)	QT interval prolongation with torsades de pointes, pulmonary toxicity and visual disturbances possible Inhibits CYP3A4, OCT1, OCT2
Ceritinib	ALK⁺ NSCLC	450	QT interval prolongation with torsades de pointes and pulmonary toxicity possible Elevated gastric pH may decrease bioavailability
Alectinib	ALK⁺ NSCLC	1200 (2 divided doses)	Pulmonary toxicity possible
Brigatinib	ALK⁺ NSCLC	90 (7 d) -180 (if 90 mg dose is tolerated)	Pulmonary toxicity and visual disturbances possible
Bruton Tyrosine Kinase Inhibitors			
Ibrutinib	MCL (previously treated), refractory MZL, CLL, SLL	560 (MCL, MZL) 420 (CLL, SLL)	Hemorrhage, infections, hypertension, and cardiac arrhythmias possible
Acalabrutinib	MCL (previously treated)	200 (2 divided doses)	Hemorrhage, infections, and atrial arrhythmias possible
FLT3 Kinase Inhibitor			
Midostaurin	FLT3⁺ AML	100 (2 divided doses)	Pulmonary toxicity possible Inhibits OATP1A1 Induces MRP2
Janus-Associated Kinase Inhibitor			
Ruxolitinib	Myeloproliferative neoplasms (myelofibrosis, polycythemia vera)	10-40 (MF, 2 divided doses) 20-50 (CV, 2 divided doses)	Secondary non-melanoma skin cancers possible Relapse possible upon dose tapering or discontinuation

[a]Protein synthesis inhibitor targeting TKI-resistant Bcr-Abl CML..

ALL, acute lymphoblastic leukemia; AML, acute myeloid leukemia; BC, breast cancer; BCRP, breast cancer resistance protein; CLL, chronic lymphocytic leukemia; CML, chronic myelogenous leukemia; CRC, colorectal cancer; GIST, gastrointestinal stromal tumor; HCC, hepatocellular carcinoma; MCL, mantle cell lymphoma; MRP2, multidrug-resistant protein 2; MTC, medullary thyroid cancer; MZL, marginal zone lymphoma; NET, neuroendocrine tumors; NSCLC, non–small cell lung cancer; OAT, organic anion transporter; OCT, organic cation transporter; RCC, renal cell carcinoma; SLL, small lymphocytic lymphoma; TC, thyroid carcinoma.

(but not ponatinib) into cells and contributes to imatinib resistance.[84] At 98%, the oral bioavailability of imatinib is the highest of the three drugs; the bioavailabilty of nilotinib (50%-82%), and possibly ponatinib (≈65%), may be compromised by coadministered drugs that elevate gastric pH and, subsequently, decrease solubility. A low gastric pH is also required for the effective absorption of dasatinib and bosutinib, discussed below.

Dasatinib and bosutinib are primarily type I Bcr-Abl kinase inhibitors. Although dasatinib contains a pyrimidine ring, this moiety does not bind in the hinge region as the pyrimidine rings of imatinib and nilotinib do. Rather, this binding honor goes to aminothiazole, and it is facilitated by a critical hydrogen bond between the thiazole nitrogen and the amide NH of Met318.[58] Met318's carbonyl oxygen also binds to the hydrogen of the amino group connecting the thiazole and pyrimidine rings. A third hydrogen bond between the drug's amide nitrogen and the hydroxyl of gatekeeper residue Thr315 ensures high affinity for the active (DFG-in) state of the kinase[80] but also causes the drug to fall prey to T315I-induced resistance.[58,85]

The 2-chloro-6-methylbenzamide segment of dasatinib binds deep within the hydrophobic pocket of the kinase in

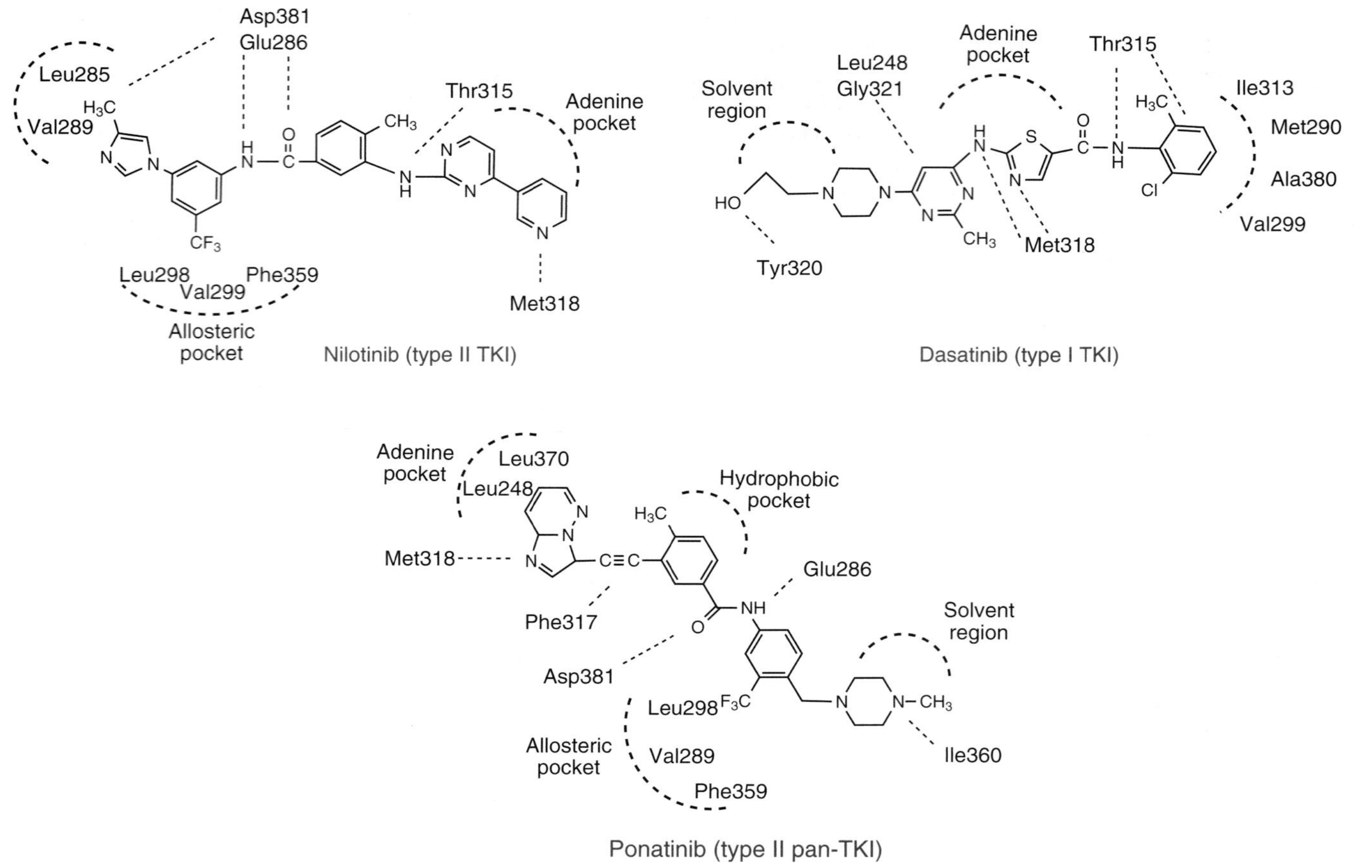

Figure 33.3 Binding interactions between Bcr-Abl tyrosine kinase and representative inhibitors.

an area distinct from the ATP-binding site. Interactions between this aromatic moiety and Thr315, Met290, Val299, Ile313, and Ala380 are known.[86] Hydrophobic interactions with Leu248 and Gly321 also hold the pyrimidine ring to the kinase. As in imatinib, dasatinib's water solubility is assured through the hydroxyethyl-substituted piperazine ring, which is oriented toward the hinge region and is solvent exposed. An H-bond between this moiety and the backbone carbonyl oxygen of Tyr320 is known to occur.

Dasatinib's ability to bind to the active kinase conformation has been attributed to the fact that it does not insert into the hydrophobic pocket containing Phe(F)382, as the substituted benzyl moiety of imatinib does.[25] It can bind to both the active and inactive conformations of Bcr-Abl kinase. Dasatinib retains activity in cells made resistant to imatinib via activation of Src kinases. Most mutations that confer resistance to imatinib occur in the P-loop of the kinase, an area not important to dasatinib binding.[86]

The quinoline nitrogen atom of bosutinib forms the crucial bond with the amide moiety of Met318. The sterically unobtrusive nitrile and the aniline nitrogen atom that bridges the quinoline and chlorinated phenyl rings bind within separate hydrophobic pockets adjacent to Thr315, providing a bound kinase conformation distinct from that formed with dasatinib.[58] Bosutinib has a similar resistance profile to dasatinib and is ineffective in T315I mutants.

Specific Drugs (Figs. 33.1 and 33.2, Tables 33.4-33.6). While the drugs discussed below are classified as Bcr-Abl kinase inhibitors, their spectrum of action is actually broader, commonly also blocking Src, c-Kit, and/or PDGFR. The therapeutic goals in the use of Bcr-Abl kinase inhibitors in CML is attainment of complete cytogenetic response and major molecular response (MMR), which is defined as BCR-ABL RNA <0.1%.[87] All Bcr-Abl inhibitors are associated with significant myelosuppression and fatigue. Coadministration of CYP3A4 inducers or inhibitors should be accompanied by dosage adjustment or avoided altogether.

The reversible protein synthesis inhibitor omacetaxine mepesuccinate is included due to its ability to bind to Bcr-Abl kinase and its therapeutic use in TKI-resistant CML. Its anticancer mechanism is believed to be independent of Bcr-Abl kinase binding.

Imatinib Mesylate. Imatinib was the first kinase inhibitor employed as an antineoplastic agent and the springboard to the multitude of TKIs currently on the U.S. market. Referred to as a "wonder drug" for its impact on patient care and practitioner understanding of molecular mechanisms of cancer, its ability to induce complete hematologic and cytogenic responses in 95% and 74% of CML patients, respectively, has led to significant increases in survival (5-year: 89% vs. 50%)[78] and quality of life.[88] However, less than 35% of patients treated with imatinib achieve MMR within 12 months of initiating therapy, and some become intolerant to the drug.[87] While 6-year event-free survival has been cited at 83%,[77] 4-year resistance, usually around 20% in the chronic phase of the disease, can rise to as high as 70%-90% in advanced (accelerated and/or blastic) CML.[89] The development of second- and third-generation Bcr-Abl kinase inhibitors was driven, in part, to assure efficacy in imatinib-resistant CML, including T315I-mediated resistance.

Imatinib's duration of action is extended due to the 40 hour half-life of its active desmethyl metabolite (Fig. 33.2). Its groundbreaking success in the treatment of adult CML led to its approval for use in pediatric patients and, until recently, it was only TKI approved in this population[90] (dasatinib and nilotinib now share this indication). Imatinib is a P-gp substrate, and the presence or absence of certain single nucleotide polymorphisms in the gene encoding this transporter may predict the likely response to this anticancer drug.[91]

Nilotinib Hydrochloride. Nilotinib is significantly more potent than imatinib and generally well-tolerated. A meta-analysis comparing achievement of MMR by 12 months on three Bcr-Abl kinase inhibitors documented the superiority of nilotinib to either imatinib or dasatinib, with an estimated 28% and 10% increase in patients achieving this efficacy goal, respectively.[87] On the downside, its use is associated with life-threatening toxicities, including QT interval prolongation that can progress to torsades de pointes and sudden death. The risk of potentially fatal myocardial toxicity is elevated if the drug is taken with potent CYP3A4 inhibitors, and the dose should be halved if coadministration with 3A4 inhibitors is required.

Nilotinib is modestly bioavailable, and a high-fat meal can increase drug exposure from 50% to 82%. To attenuate the risk of serious toxicity the drug should be administered in a fasted state.[92] As noted in Table 33.6, solubility is pH-dependent, and elevating gastric pH through the concomitant administration of antacids, H_2 antagonists, or PPIs significantly impairs absorption.[77]

Nilotinib biotransformation is limited, with the major metabolite being an inactive carboxylic acid arising from CYP3A4-mediated hydroxylation of an aromatic methyl group. Sixty-nine percent of a dose is excreted unchanged,[93] and dose reductions are recommended in hepatic impairment.

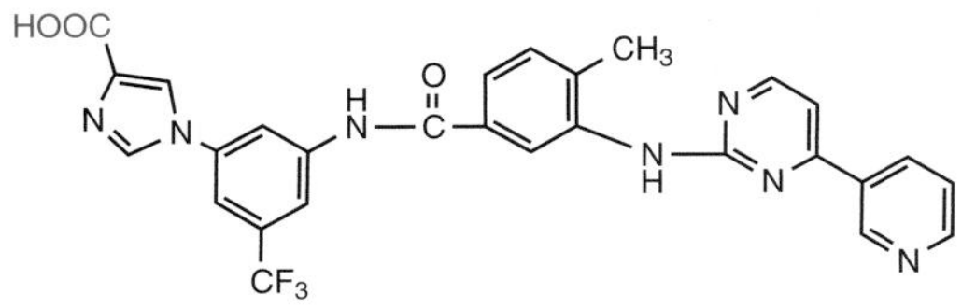

Nilotinib carboxylic acid metabolite (inactive)

Ponatinib Hydrochloride. Ponatinib is a third-generation type II Bcr-Abl TKI. With affinity for the broadest range of TKs of all drugs in its class, it has been referred to as a "pan-tyrosine kinase inhibitor."[78,94] It is also the only Bcr-Abl kinase inhibitor that retains efficacy in T315I mutants, and its use is reserved for mutant-positive CML or ALL patients, those who have failed or progressed on at least two first-line TKIs, or those who have accelerated or blast phase disease. It is among the most toxic of these inhibitors and carries a boxed warning related to life-threatening cardiovascular (infarct, stroke, heart failure, embolism) and hepatotoxity. In fact, the risk of arterial and venous occlusions prompted a temporary suspension of U.S. marketing in 2013 before the drug was reintroduced with a restricted indication and the boxed warning.[95] Hypertension can occur in up to 74% of patients taking this drug.

Like nilotinib and dasatinib, ponatinib absorption requires gastric acidity (pH $\leq$3.7), and the same contraindication against concomitant antacid/PPI use applies.[78] The toxicities that drive dosing modifications include bone marrow suppression, hepatotoxicity, and pancreatitis. Serum lipase levels should be closely monitored during therapy and the drug discontinued if levels rise above 1.5 times the normal upper limit. Attention should also be paid to liver function throughout therapy. The CYP3A4-generated desmethyl metabolite is fourfold less active than the parent drug, and inactivating hydrolysis occurs prior to fecal excretion.[79]

Although all TKI therapies are costly, ponatinib is among the highest. In 2016, a 1-month supply of this drug was over $16.5K.[96]

Dasatinib. Dasatinib is a mixed type I/type II Bcr-Abl inhibitor which lacks affinity for OCT1 and P-gp. It has a potency approximately 325 times that of imatinib in the treatment of CML and is effective against all imatinib-resistant mutants except T315I.[85,89] Oral bioavailability is compromised by poor absorption and rapid first-pass CYP3A4-mediated biotransformation.[85] All phase 1 metabolites retain activity but, since they represent only 5% of the area under the concentration curve, their clinical relevance is questionable (Fig. 33.4). Of potential importance to dasatinib's toxicity profile is the ability of the *p*-hydroxylated metabolite to oxidize to a potentially hepatotoxic quinoneimine,[93] a property this TKI shares with several others that contain an aniline moiety vulnerable to CYP-mediated *p*-hydroxylation.

The clinical choice between dasatinib and another second- or third-generation TKI depends on the specific point mutation expressed by the enzyme (e.g., the F317L mutant is uniquely dasatinib-resistant),[89] patient vulnerability to individual TKI toxicity, and/or patient preference related to differences in drug administration (e.g., once vs. twice daily, fasted vs. fed state). Unlike nilotinib, there is no boxed warning related to QT interval prolongation, but the potential of dasatinib to exacerbate the toxicity of agents that do should not be ruled out.[85]

Bosutinib. Bosutinib has many properties in common with dasatinib. It is a mixed type I/type II Bcr-Abl kinase inhibitor that is effective in non-T315I mutant imatinib-resistant CML; it exhibits pH-dependent solubility and should not be coadministered with drugs that raise gastric pH, and it has little or no effect on the expression or activity of CYP enzymes. Unlike dasatinib, it is a P-gp substrate and has no inhibiting action on c-kit or PDGFR kinases.[97]

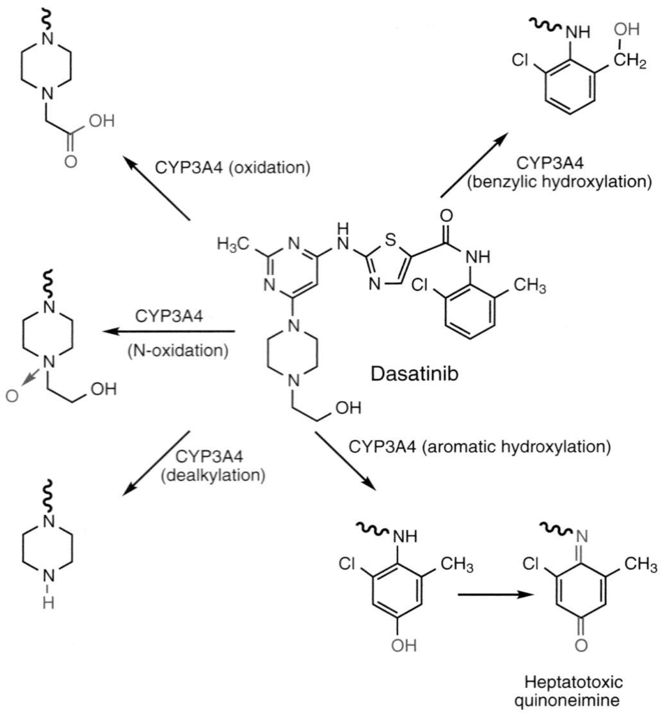

Figure 33.4 Dasatinib metabolism.

It has been reported that patients placed on bosutinib after demonstrating intolerance to imatinib, nilotinib, or dasatinib generally did well, with relatively few patients having to withdraw from therapy due to adverse effects that prompted discontinuation of the original TKI.[97,98] In fact, a major advantage claimed for bosutinib over its "classmates" is an improved safety profile; the risk of edema, cardiovascular toxicity, and electrolyte imbalance that can lead to muscle cramping is comparatively low.[97-99] Another is retention of efficacy in CML that has developed resistance to dasatinib and nilotinib.[97]

Omacetaxine Mepesuccinate (a Protein Synthesis Inhibitor)

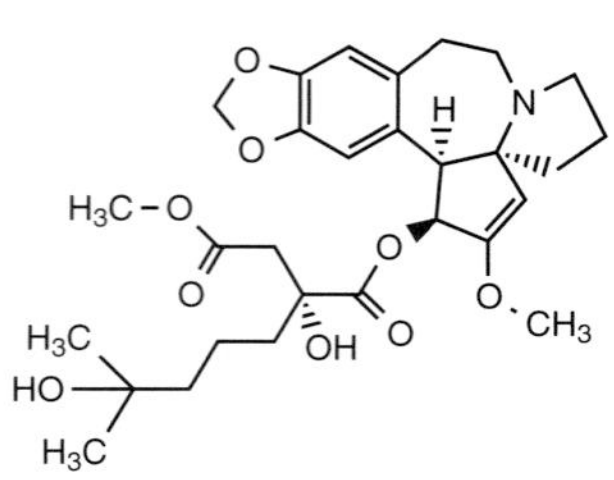

Omacetacine mepesuccinate
(Homoharringtonine)

Omacetaxine mepesuccinate, also known as homoharringtonine, is a natural product, isolated from the Chinese evergreen *Cephalotaxus harringtonia*. Although often mentioned in the same breath with Bcr-Abl kinase inhibitors because of its ability to bind to this enzyme,[78] its antineoplastic mechanism of action is protein synthesis inhibition secondary to binding to the hydrophobic A-site cleft in the peptidyl transferase center of the large ribosome subunit. Affinity for this site is augmented by π-stacking interactions involving the aromatic ring which, along with the fused dioxylane ring, fills this space. Hydrogen bonding of the polar terminal tertiary alcohol and amine moieties to ribosomal residues augments affinity.[100] In the human myeloid leukemia cell line K562, omacetaxine reduced the expression of Bcr-Abl, as well decreased levels of a stabilizing protein (HSP90) which resulted in the degradation of the kinase. Cell death is also promoted by the downregulation of the apoptotic protein Mcl-1.[101]

As with ponatinib, omacetaxine mepesuccinate is reserved for use in CML patients who have failed or progressed on at least two other first-line TKIs. It is not orally active but, rather, is administered by subcutaneous (SC) injection, where it is rapidly absorbed into the bloodstream (bioavailability 70%-90%). The major metabolite is 4-desoxyhomoharringtonine (4-DMHHT), generated by hydrolysis of the methyl ester.[102]

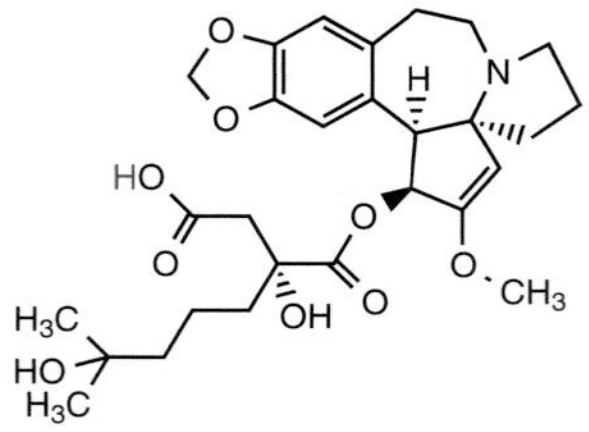

4'-DMHHT

EGFR/HER2 KINASE INHIBITORS. EGFR and HER2 are closely related membrane-bound TKs. EGFR expression in solid tumors of the breast, lung, bladder, esophagus, and oral cavity has been clearly correlated with decreased life expectancy, and it is a consistent presence in almost all epithelial-derived cancers. Likewise, HER2 overexpression is a classic feature of treatment-resistant breast, ovarian, lung, and gastric cancers, and it endows tumors with what's been called an "antiapoptotic shield."[103]

As observed with Bcr-Abl kinase inhibitors, the efficacy of EGFR/HER2 inhibitors can be thwarted by mutations in the "gatekeeper" (Thr790) residue, specifically T790M. This therapeutically challenging genetic transformation is found in approximately 60% of resistant non–small cell lung cancer (NSCLC).[104] The mutant enzyme has enhanced affinity for the endogenous ATP substrate such that only excessively large doses of reversible EGFR inhibitors can compete. One approach to overcoming this resistance is the development of irreversibly acting inhibitors. A unique Cys797 residue is located at the edge of the ATP-binding domain,[58] and electrophilic TKIs capable of irreversibly inactivating the protein through covalent bond formation showed promise in these resistant mutants.[104] Unfortunately, two (afatinib and neratinib) did not produce the anticipated positive impact on T790M positive patient survival, although afatinib is effective in ex19del and L858R mutations (two so-called activating mutations because they provide a distinguishing tumor-based target sensitive to inhibition by the TKIs).[105] However, osimertinib, a structure containing a terminal electrophilic target for the nucleophilic Cys797, is an effective inhibitor of T790M-positive EGFR, and has provided new hope to NSCLC patients.[106] The search for even more clinically promising structures is, of course, ongoing.

While not all EGFR/HER2 inhibitors are marketed in salt form, all contain at least two basic nitrogen atoms capable of in vitro protonation. The pKas range from 9.13 (vandetanib) to 4.59 (erlotinib)

Chemistry (Fig. 33.5)[58,62]

Reversible EGFR/HER Kinase Inhibitors: Erlotinib, Gefitinb, Lapatinib, Vandetanib. The currently marketed reversible EGFR/HER TKIs (along with two irreversibly acting agents) all contain a 4-anilinoquinazoline pharmacophore with an oxygen-containing substituent at C6. Ether-containing moieties of varying size are also permitted at C7. An electron-withdrawing substituent at position 3′ of the aniline phenyl ring provides high selectivity for EGFR kinase as long as the 4′ position remains unsubstituted (erlotinib) or is modified with a very small substituent such as fluorine (gefitinib). Erlotinib and gefitinib are quintessential type I TKIs, with the *m*-substituted phenyl ring of the aniline moiety enhancing affinity through binding with hydrophobic pocket residues of the active (open) enzyme. The H-bonds formed between the quinazoline nitrogen atoms and hinge residues Met793 (N1) and Thr790 (N3) are crucial to activity. The halogenated and acetylene-substituted phenyl rings of gefitinib and erlotinib, respectively, are maintained at a 42-degree angle relative to the quinazoline ring and, in this orientation, bind well in the hydrophobic pocket near Thr790 as long as this gatekeeper residue remains small.[25] As noted previously, a T790M mutation is believed responsible for acquired resistance to these highly selective TKIs.[58,107] Unlike the acquired Bcr-Abl kinase resistance, which was predominantly steric in nature, an unfavorable TKI/ATP binding affinity ratio in the T790M mutant has been proposed to explain acquired resistance to EGFR TKIs.[25]

Increasing the size of the 4′ substituent with groups like *m*-fluorobenzyloxy (lapatinib) restricts access to only the inactive conformation of EGFR[25] and broadens TK specificity to include HER2. The entire substituted aniline structural component of lapatinib binds within a lipophilic pocket of the HER2 kinase in its inactive (closed) conformation. The quinazoline ring of EGFR/HER2 inhibitors again affiliates with residues in the hinge region of the ATP-binding domain (adenine pocket). Selectivity for the inactive conformation of its target kinases (which requires a conformational change to dislodge the inhibitor) may contribute to the very slow (300 min) enzyme dissociation half-life compared to erlotinib and gefitinib (30 min).[25]

Lapatinib's 2-furanyl substituent can be further substituted at position 5 with long, unbranched chains that extend out into the aqueous environment. The addition of a methylsulfone moiety to the chain terminus enhances water solubility. The ionizable morpholine ring of gefitinib serves a similar purpose, as should the strongly basic moieties of vandetanib (piperidine), afatinib, and neratinib (dimethylamine). The water solubility of erlotinib is predictably low given the relative lack of polar functional groups in this area of the molecule.

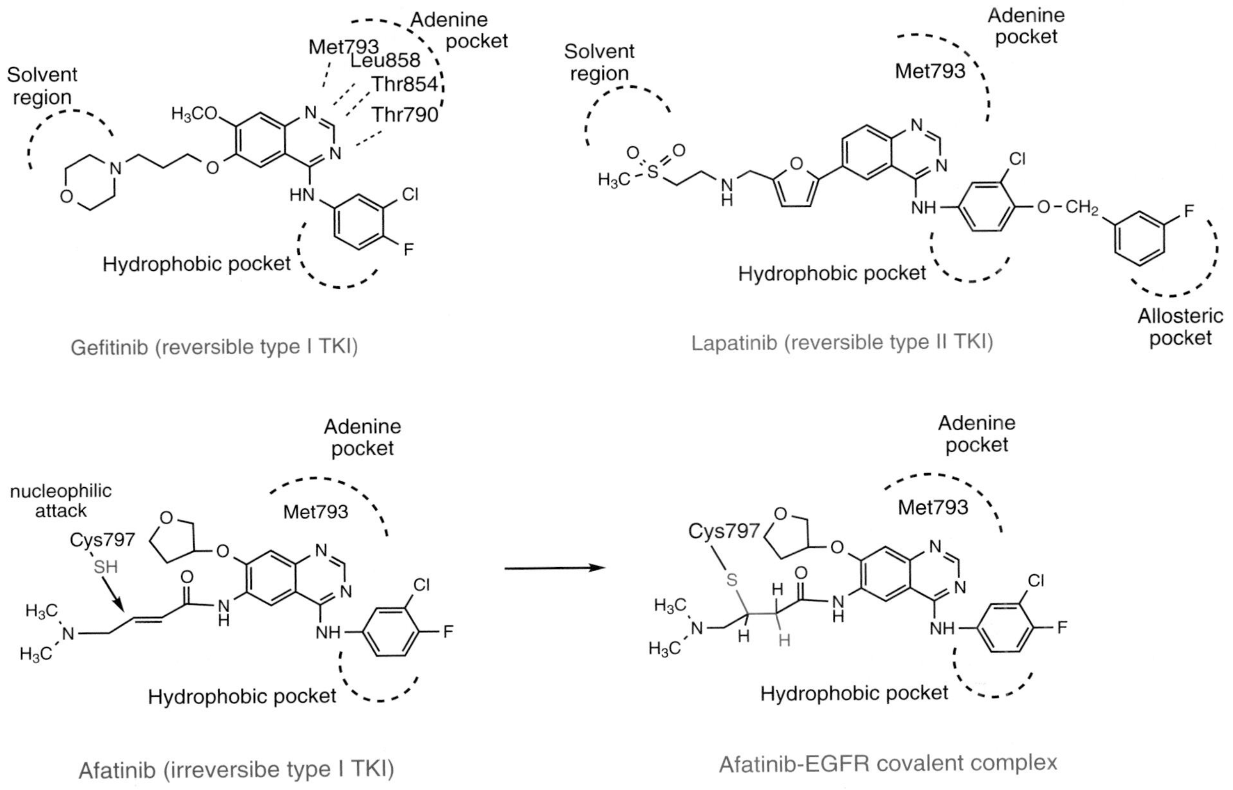

Figure 33.5 Binding interactions between EGFR/HER2 tyrosine kinase and representative inhibitors.

A vandetanib-EGFR complex has not yet been crystallized, but a cocrystal with the molecule bound to RET showed similarities to erlotinib- and gefitinib-kinase interactions.[108]

Irreversible EGFR/HER Kinase Inhibitors: Afatinib, Neratinib, Osimertinib. As noted above, a unique Cys797 residue is located within the ATP-binding domain of EFGR and HER2, and three electrophilic TKIs capable of forming a covalent complex through this residue are marketed.[58] As shown in Figure 33.5 with afatinib as the model Michael alkylating inhibitor, the SH group of Cys797 is positioned to conduct a nucleophilic attack at the electrophilic terminal carbon of the acrylamide, forming the irreversibly bound adduct. Osimertinib and neratinib also contain this electrophilic moiety within their structures, and it serves the same permanently enzyme-inactivating purpose.

Metabolism to Hepatotoxic Quinoneimines. As with other TKIs, EGFR/HER2 inhibitors are generally vulnerable to CYP3A4-catalyzed biotransformation (Table 33.4), and several are capable of generating a hepatotoxic quinoneimine in the manner described for dasatinib (Fig. 33.4). In structures with an unsubstituted aniline moiety (e.g., erlotinib), direct CYP-mediated hydroxylation generates a *p*-hydroxyaniline group that is vulnerable to further CYP-catalyzed oxidation to the electrophilic quinoneimine.[93] Structures where the *p*-position is blocked by halogen can undergo oxidative dehalogenation followed by hydroxylation to the labile *p*-hydroxyaniline (e.g., gefitinib).[109] The *o*-Cl group increases the electrophilic character of the ring, making it more vulnerable to attack by reduced glutathione (GSH), and after stores of that scavenger are exhausted, cell nucleophiles (e.g., Cys residues). While it appears vulnerable to this same series of reactions, afatinib is resistant to CYP-mediated metabolism,[73] and the *p*-bromo group of vandetanib is stable in vivo.[110]

Lapatinib forms the *p*-hydroxyaniline precursor to the toxic quinoneimine through O-dealkylation of the *m*-fluorobenzyl group.[93] While osimertinib undergoes modest rates of N-dealkylation at both the indole (8%) and terminal amine (6%), O-dealkylation of the methoxy ether to provide a *p*-hydroxyaniline structure does not occur.[70] As an electrophilic irreversible TKI, osimertinib binds to protein nucleophiles and can be excreted as drug-protein conjugates.[70] Afatinib[73] and neratinib[111] also conjugate with biologic proteins and could conceivably find their way to the feces in conjugated form.

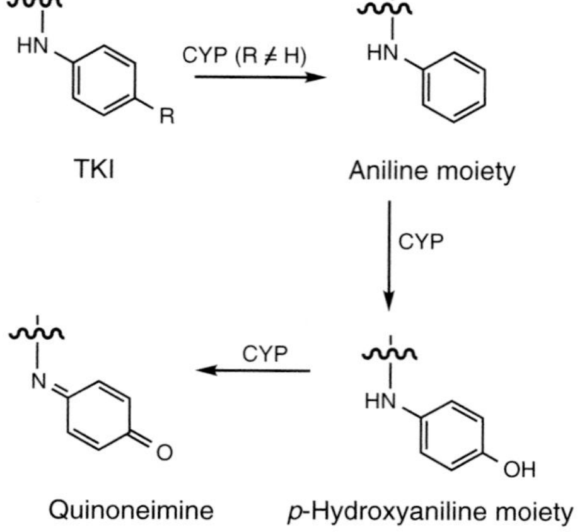

Specific Drugs (Figs. 33.1-33.2, Tables 33.4-33.6)

Erlotinib Hydrochloride. Erlotinib is used in the treatment of NSCLC cancer in patients whose disease has either stabilized after four rounds of organoplatinum therapy or progressed after completion of a non–TKI-based chemotherapeutic regimen. It is also used in combination with the DNA polymerase inhibitor gemcitabine as first-line therapy in advanced or metastatic pancreatic cancer. It is more effective in tumors expressing activating ex19del or exon 21 L858R mutations compared to wild type (normal) kinase, and it has been shown to be essentially equally effective with gefitinib and afatinib when used as first-line therapy in NSCLC.[112] Median progression-free survival (PFS) with all of these agents is in the range of 9-14 months, but resistance to therapy invariably arises. Over half the time, resistance is due to the development of the "gatekeeper" T790M mutation.[113]

Extensive CYP3A4-mediated O-dealkylation of the terminal methoxy of the C6 side chain occurs, and some molecules of the primary alcohol are further oxidized by cytosolic enzymes to the carboxylic acid (Fig. 33.6). CYP1A1 and CYP1A2 can also catalyze the O-dealkylation reaction, resulting in a 24% increase in erlotinib clearance in smokers. Both half-life and AUC decrease, and increased doses are warranted.[93]

The maculopapular rash induced by erlotinib has been positively correlated with therapeutic efficacy and worsens when exposed to sunlight. Hepatotoxicity risk might be due, in part, to the formation of an electrophilic quinoneimine from a CYP3A4- and CYP1A1-generated phenolic metabolite[93] and may be more severe in hepatocompromised patients (Fig. 33.6).

Gefitinib. Gefitinib is used in the treatment of NSCLC that presents with ex19del or L858R mutation. EGFR is often robustly expressed in this neoplastic disease.

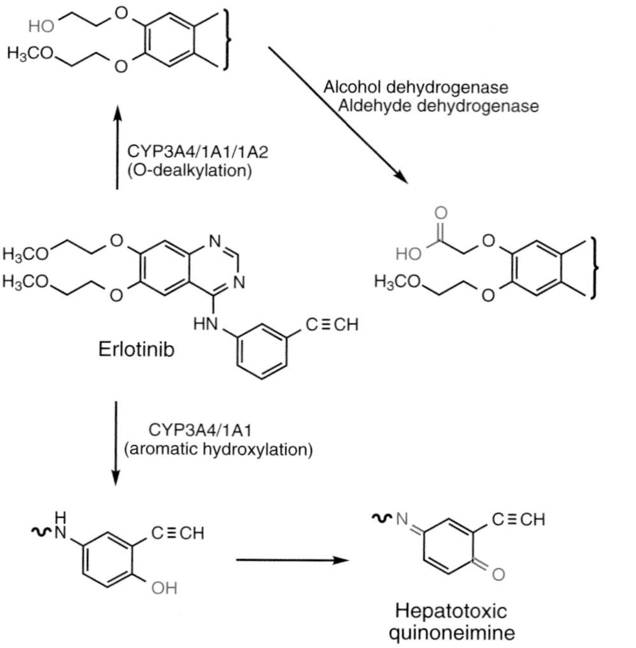

Figure 33.6 Erlotinib metabolism.

Resistance generally develops at 10 months, commonly due to the development of the T790M mutation.[114]

The active demethylated metabolite is generated primarily by CYP2D6, although its clinical relevance has been questioned due to polarity-induced difficulties in tumor cell penetration.[92] Interestingly, poor 2D6 metabolizers are at increased risk for the characteristic EGFR kinase inhibitor-induced rash.[115] As with erlotinib, CYP1A1 oxidation of the *p*-phenol (generated after oxidative defluorination by CYP3A4/5 in the liver and 1A1 in the lung) to a reactive quinoneimine can occur[109] (Fig. 33.7). Cigarette smoking, which induces 1A1, speeds metabolic inactivation of gefitinib, resulting in a poor response and an increased risk of quinoneimine-induced interstitial lung disease and hepatotoxicity. Smokers can generate up to 12 times more reactive quinoneimine metabolite than nonsmokers.[93,109,114] The drug induces aberrant eyelash growth which can induce eye pain.

Gefitinib is a P-gp substrate, and this transporter is believed to play a role in resistance and the drug's dermal adverse effects. In contrast, OCT1 is not involved in gefitinib uptake.[114]

Lapatinib Ditosylate. Lapatinib is a dual kinase inhibitor with affinity for both EGFR and HER2. It is used in combination with the pyrimidine antagonist capecitabine or the aromatase inhibitor letrozole in HER2+ breast cancer patients (approximately 25%-30% of cases)[116] who have failed on first-line therapies, including the MAb trastuzumab that targets HER2. HER2 overexpression in breast cancer is associated with poor prognosis and limited survival, and lapatinib is one of only two TKIs available to treat it. The drug is very expensive (approximately $1,500 per month), and the fact that the area under the curve can be increased threefold by taking the drug with a high-fat meal has caused some to question whether this pharmacokinetic profile could be safely harnessed to lower costs without compromising clinical outcomes.[93] Lapatinib inhibits P-gp and BCRP. As noted above, CYP3A4-catalyzed dealkylation of the *m*-fluorobenzyl moiety sets the metabolic stage for oxidation to the hepatotoxic quinoneimine.[93]

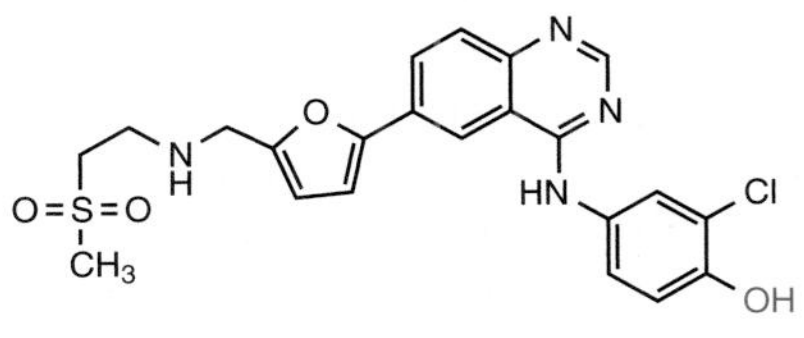

Lapatinib dealkylated metabolite

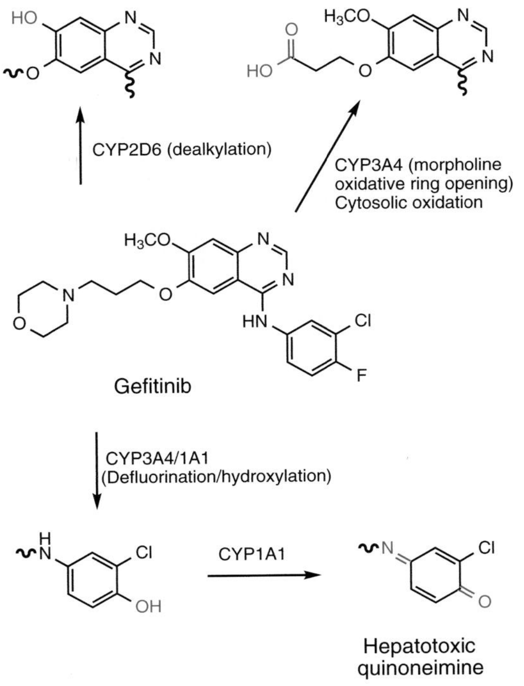

As with other drugs in this class, resistance sabotages therapeutic efficacy. Resistance mechanisms are multifaceted and may include activation of compensatory pathways, HER2 mutation, and amplification of the gene expressing this protein.[116] It has been estimated that 78% of patients will be nonresponders (intrinsic resistance), and those who do respond will develop resistance within one year (acquired resistance).[117] With approximately 300,000 new cases of breast cancer diagnosed annually and over 40,000 deaths per year from the disease,[118] investigations into the complex mechanisms driving lapatinib resistance are urgently underway. The goal is the development of resistance-countering therapies and the optimization of patient selection to ensure the best possible therapeutic outcomes.[116,117]

Vandetanib. With a mean survival of 8.6 years, unresectable locally advanced or metastatic medullary thyroid cancer (MTC; 3%-12% of cases) has a challenging prognosis.[119,120] Vandetanib is one of only a few targeted therapies available to attenuate cell proliferation, halt angiogenesis, and slow tumor growth in this aggressive disease. It does so via the inhibition of several targets in addition to EGFR, including VEGFR, rearranged during transfection (RET) proto-oncogene, and SRC. As a VEGFR inhibitor, vandetanib stems angiogenesis that would otherwise feed the tumor, an action deemed very important to its mechanism of antineoplastic action. Its inhibitory action on RET halts cell signaling in an attempt to check uncontrolled tumor cell proliferation.[120] The drug has a positive impact on PFS (11.2 mo compared to placebo), although not on overall survival (OS).[119] Tumors expressing the M918T RET mutation generally have a poor prognosis, but vandetanib can still promote a better quality of life for these patients.[119]

Due to the risk of life-threatening adverse effects, including sudden cardiac death, vandetanib is only available to trained providers through the Risk Evaluation and Mitigation Strategy (REMS) program. Resistance arises, likely involving RET expression/function (e.g., mutation) and activation of downstream signaling pathways.[120]

In addition to the active N-demethylated metabolite (Fig. 33.2), vandetanib undergoes inactivating FMO-catalyzed N-oxidation.[110,119]

Figure 33.7 Gefitinib metabolism.

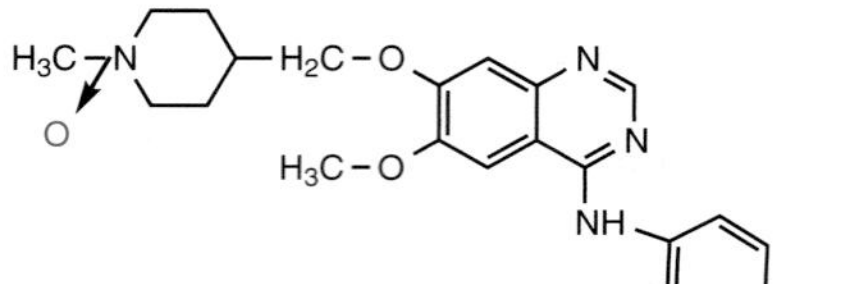

Vandetanib N-oxide

Afatinib Dimaleate. Afatinib is a second-generation EGFR kinase inhibitor approved as first-line therapy for treatment of NSCLC that has developed non-resistant mutations which can render first-generation agents erlotinib and gefitinib ineffective within a year's time.[121] As described above, this electrophilic agent forms a covalent bond with Cys797 on EGFR (and with Cys805 and Cys803 of HER2 and HER4, respectively) to irreversibly inactivate the kinase. While CYP-resistant, plasma protein conjugates circulate in the bloodstream and decompose to release free or potentially conjugated drug before fecal excretion. Activity is generally independent of patient-specific characteristics, although compromised renal function, female sex, and/or lean body mass may increase exposure.[73]

Afatinib has been shown to increase OS in squamous NSCLC compared to erlotinib.[73,121] It is effective in ex19del and L858R mutants, promotes OS in patients with ex19del mutations, and may delay manifestation of the drug-resistant T790M mutation.[122] Janus-activated kinase-1 (JAK1) may play a role in acquired resistance, and combination therapy with JAK1 inhibitors has been suggested.[123] Afatinib is a substrate and mild inhibitor of P-gp and BCRP.[123]

Neratinib. While neratinib's therapeutic indication is similar to lapatinib (HER2$^+$ breast cancer in patients previously administered trastuzumab), the electrophilic acrylamide within its structure assures that its antineoplastic mechanism mirrors that of afatinib, namely irreversible kinase inhibition through covalent bond formation with a Cys residue; Cys805 in HER2.[124]

Even when provided with the current standard of care (presurgical chemotherapy, surgery, trastuzumab), it is estimated that 25%-30% of breast cancer patients will experience disease recurrence within 10 years,[125] which underscores the need for effective long-term therapy to extend both PFS and OS. While there is much to be learned from ongoing clinical trials, neratinib has shown promise when used either pre- or postsurgery. Because it binds to a different HER2 domain than trastuzumab (intracellular vs. extracellular, respectively), there is no cross resistance with the MAb and coadministration can be beneficial.[126] There is also evidence that combination therapy with a mitosis inhibitor (e.g., paclitaxel) in metastatic breast cancer can be synergistic.[127] Investigations to better define neratinib resistance mechanisms are ongoing, but in vitro studies have suggested the potential involvement of the insulin-like growth factor 1 pathway.[124]

Neratinib is metabolized by CYP3A4[128] and, to a lesser extent, by FMO. Three active metabolites are known[129] and have been identified as the N-oxides of the pyridine (M3) and dimethylamine (M7) moieties, and the monodesmethyl secondary amine (M6).[130] M7 is the metabolite generated by FMO.

Osimertinib. The goal of therapeutic efficacy in T790M positive NSCLC was finally achieved with the design and clinical development of osimertinib, an acrylamide-containing third-generation irreversible TKI. Osimertinib promotes PFS in T790M positive patients compared to alternative therapies (e.g., organoplatinum-antifolate), significantly decreases the risk of death, and can elicit clinical responses in patients with commonly encountered central metastases due to its ability to penetrate the blood-brain barrier (BBB).[131-133] Unlike other irreversible inhibitors, osimertinib shows selectivity for the T790M mutant over the wild type kinase, with a potency ratio of 184 in recombinant enzyme assays.[113] As a result, the adverse effect profile, while qualitatively similar to other drugs in this class, is of lower frequency and severity.[113] The NCCN currently recommends the drug as second-line therapy for T790M positive metastatic NSCLC that has progressed after treatment with a first- or second-generation TKI.[131]

Underscoring the seemingly inexhaustible ability of tumors to fight back, a C797S mutation was identified in 22% of an NSCLC patient population involved in an osimertinib clinical trial (AURA) at the time of disease progression.[113] The loss of the highly nucleophilic Cys residue at the critical gatekeeper 797 position renders the drug's alkylating acrylamide moiety useless in irreversibly inactivating the kinase.[134] Importantly, if the C797S mutation occurs on a different allele than the T790M mutation, sensitivity to combination therapy with osimertinib and a first-generation TKI is retained; if the mutations are present on the same allele, the cell will be completely TKI resistant.[113,134] Alterations in downstream signaling pathways (e.g., MET, BRAF) are also believed to play a role in acquired osimertinib resistance, which can develop after approximately 10 months of therapy.[133] The ever-present reality of resistance makes clear that logically sequenced combination therapy will continue to be the state-of-the-art in treating constantly "morphing" tumor cells for some time to come.

CYP3A4 catalyzes osimertinib N-dealkylation at the indole and terminal amine moieties, generating two active metabolites known as AZ5104 and AZ7550, respectively[70] (Fig. 33.2). AZ7550 retains both the potency and the desired selectivity of the parent drug. While AZ5014 is eight times more potent than osimertinib in inhibiting T790M and ex19del positive kinases, it lacks selectivity, as its wild type kinase inhibiting potency is effectively twice that value (15 fold more potent).[131] Osimertinib is a substrate of P-gp, but not OCT1.[105] It inhibits CYP3A4 and BCRP.[131]

VEGFR Kinase Inhibitors. Along with Bcr-Abl and EGFR kinases, VEGFR has been the focus of significant investigation related to targeted cancer chemotherapy. Three VEGFR isoforms bind the angiogenesis-promoting VEGF protein, resulting in the development of new blood vessels that supply oxygen and nutrients to growing neoplasms. The rationale behind inhibiting VEGFR is clear; starve malignant cells and block the production of metastatic highways. The buildup of cellular waste no longer able to be readily discharged into the vasculature also contributes to the cell-killing action of VEGFR-targeting TKIs. Augmenting the cytotoxic effect is the fact that VEGF inhibition decreases the permeability of tumor cell vasculature and eases intracellular delivery of chemotherapeutic agents.[135]

Chemistry. The type II binding of sorafenib and its fluorinated analogue regorafenib to VEGFR is believed to be similar to its interaction with its originally recognized kinase target B-RAF, a component of the RAS signal transduction network. The pyridine nitrogen in its unionized form and the adjacent methylamide NH moiety H-bond with the amide group of Cys919 in the ATP-binding hinge region (NH and carbonyl oxygen, respectively). The indolinone and indazole ring systems of sunitinib and axitinib, respectively, occupy this same space, as do pazopanib's pyrimidine-2-amino group and lenvatinib's quinoline ring system. By analogy, the quinoline ring of cabozantinib would be anticipated to bind within the adenine pocket. In addition to Cys919, Glu917 is also an important hinge region H-bonding residue.

The hydrophobic pocket adjacent to the ATP-binding region interacts with the phenyl rings of sorafenib, regorafenib, axitinib, lenvatinib, and (presumably) cabozantinib, and captures a component of sunitinib's fluorinated indolinone ring. The allosteric pocket is poised to receive sorafenib/regorafenib's trifluoromethylphenyl moiety, axitinib's benzamide group, pazopanib's indazole ring, (presumably) the cyclopropyl substituent on lenvantinib's urea moiety, and the fluorinated phenyl ring of cabozantinib. Sunitinib is not believed to bind within this pocket. As in the hinge region, hydrogen bonding within the allosteric site is important. Binding residues include Asp1046 and Phe1047 of the DFG trio, as well as Glu885 (Fig. 33.8).[25,58] Sunitinib and lenvatinib can inhibit VEGFR in both its active and inactive conformations.[58]

The VEGFR inhibitors are solvated to differing degrees when bound to the enzyme. Soratinib and regorafenib bind deep within the allosteric pocket and are not solvated, while axitinib's pyridylvinyl moiety reaches the edge solvent front. The comparatively long diethylaminoethyl group of sunitinib extends further out from the pocket and is more extensively solvated.

Geometric isomerism is important to the TKI activity of sunitinib, with the lower energy *Z* isomer being over 100 times as potent as the higher energy *E* isomer. The drug is marketed in its pure eutomeric (*Z*) form. Exposure to light will prompt a *Z* to *E* isomeric inversion, with a return to the lower energy *Z* state over time in the dark.[93] Axitinib also contains an olefinic linkage, and computational and molecular docking studies confirmed that the *E* isomer binds with highest affinity to the modeled VEGFR-2 protein due to the ability to form a greater number of intermolecular hydrogen bonds.[136] Only the *E* isomer of axitinib is marketed.

The selectivity of VEGFR kinase inhibitors is low since the ATP binding domain is replicated in many closely related enzymes, such as PDGFRα and c-kit that

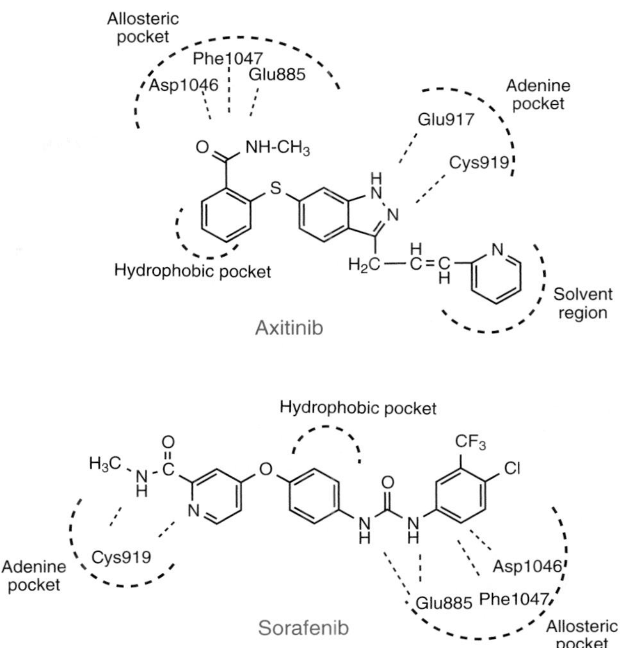

Figure 33.8 Binding interactions between VEGFR tyrosine kinase and representative inhibitors.

are associated with GI stromal tumors (GISTs). Sorafenib and regorafenib in particular are categorized in some drug information references as "multikinase inhibitors."[76]

Specific Drugs (Figs. 33.1-33.2, Tables 33.4-33.6). With the exception of regorafenib, all VEGFR inhibitors are indicated for use in advanced renal cell carcinoma (RCC), the most common kidney-related cancer which claimed 14,240 U.S. lives in 2016 and has a 5 year survival of 12%.[137,138]

Sorafenib Tosylate. In 2017, it was estimated that close to 64,000 new cases of kidney and renal cancer would be diagnosed and approximately 14,400 people would die from this neoplastic disease.[2] Sorafenib was the first TKI approved to treat metastatic RCC, and its affinity for multiple kinases (including RAF, RET, c-kit and FLT3, in addition to VEGFR) is important to its activity. Its ability to extend PFS by a few months when compared to placebo in patients previously treated with cytokines appeared promising, but this benefit was not observed in chemotherapy naïve RCC patients. A meta-analysis of over 3,000 RCC patients found sorafenib to be most valuable in patients with an intermediate prognosis who has progressed on a different antineoplastic.[139] However, perhaps because it had a similar impact on OS and, in some cases, a milder adverse effect profile when compared to other targeted agents, its use is not restricted to second-line therapy.[140,141]

Sorafenib was also the first TKI approved for the treatment of radioactive iodine refractory advanced differentiated thyroid cancer, a type of thyroid cancer with a poor prognosis (3-5 yr median survival). Clinical trials documented disease stabilization with a 5-month gain in PFS compared to placebo, although OS benefits were not observed.[142] It is also the first systemic drug approved to treat hepatocellular carcinoma, a disease caused by hepatitis C and B viral infections. Data from both clinical trials and "real-world" studies support its use in this cancer, with survival outcomes in the latter performance evaluation environment often besting the former.[143] Its fluorinated analogue, regorafenib, shares this indication, although it comes with a potentially fatal hepatotoxicity risk.

CYP3A4 oxidizes sorafenib to a similarly active N-oxide metabolite (Fig. 33.2), and the glucuronide conjugate that forms as a result of UGT1A9 catalysis can be cleaved in the gut, resulting in the recycling of active drug. CYP3A4 inducers and inhibitors should not be coadministered if at all possible. Resistance to sorafenib ultimately develops within 1-2 years through multifacted, complex, and incompletely understood mechanisms.[142,143]

Sorafenib distribution is restricted and prescriptions must be filled at specialty pharmacies. Only patients enrolled in the Resources for Expert Assistance and Care Helpline (REACH) program can receive this drug.

Lenvatinib Mesylate. Lenvatinib, a positive alternative to sorafenib in patients with differentiated thyroid cancer,[144] inhibits tumor growth through its antiangiogenic action. In clinical trials, its impact on PFS compared to placebo was three times that of sorafenib, and it retains efficacy in patients previously treated with a VEGFR inhibitor. Although a known substrate of CYP3A4 (Table 33.4) and P-gp, lenvatinib is claimed to have a low drug-drug interaction liability and does not require dosing adjustments in patients coadministered inhibitors or inducers of these proteins.[145] No metabolites are active (Fig. 33.9). The drug is a BCRP substrate but does not bind to OCT1.

When used in the treatment of advanced RCC, lenvatinib is coadministered with the mTOR inhibitor everolimus to patients who failed on prior antiangiogenic TKI monotherapy.[146] Phase II trials with this synergistic combination demonstrated increases in median PFS, with a lower toxicity incidence compared to lenvatinib (but not everolimus) alone.[147,148]

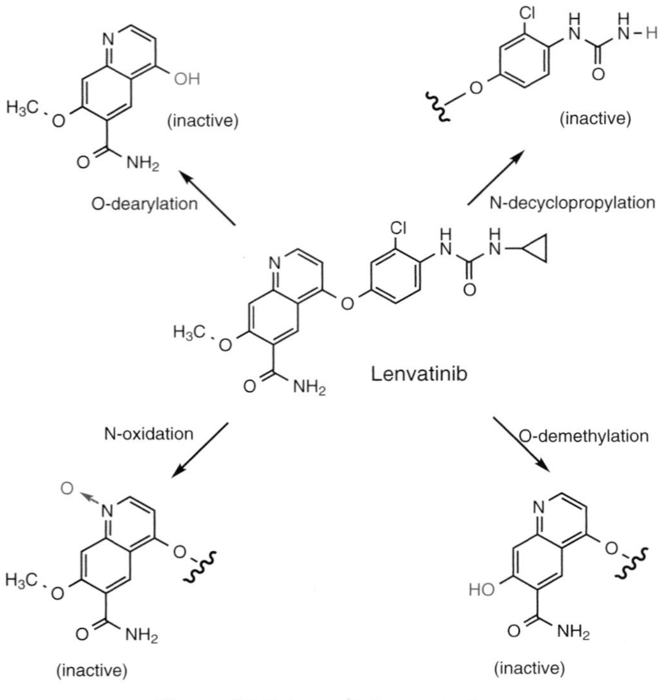

Figure 33.9 Lenvatinib metabolism.

Cabozantinib Maleate. Cabozantinib is the third VEGFR inhibitor used in the treatment of thyroid cancer; in this case, metastatic medullary disease (MTC). MTC can be sporadic (80%) or inherited, and as noted above under the vandetanib discussion, it often arises from a genetic mutation in the *RET* proto-oncogene (e.g., M918T). In advanced disease, when surgical resection with or without radiation is not curative, targeted chemotherapy with cabozantinib gives patients the best chance for an increase in PFS,[149] including those with the M918T mutation and those previously treated with vandetanib (a EGFR TKI). This indicates that, like lenvatinib, the therapeutic effect of cabozantinib is likely related to inhibition of VEGFR, as opposed to RET (a TK for which it also has affinity).[150] Cabozantinib therapy also attenuates serum levels of the MTC biomarkers calcitonin and carcinoembryonic antigen (CEA).[149]

Clinical trials indirectly comparing cabozantinib and vandetanib in MTC must be interpreted with caution, but there is evidence that cabozantinib might provide greater benefit.[150] It would clearly be the drug of choice in patients with cardiac dysfunction due to vandetanib's propensity to prolong the QT interval.

With regard to RCC therapy, cabozantinib has been called "the most efficacious TKI" in both previously treated and treatment naïve patients.[151] It has demonstrated efficacy in advancing both PFS and OS in previously TKI-treated RCC patients, providing median increases of 3.6 months and 4.9 months, respectively, when compared to the mTOR inhibitor everolimus. When compared to sunitinib (discussed below), clinical trials showed a 34% lower rate of disease progression or death.[137] Of significance, this multikinase inhibitor blocks AXL and MET signaling, both of which are believed to be involved in the development of secondary resistance to VEGFR inhibition.[151] AXL overexpression in particular is associated with poor prognoses in a variety of neoplastic diseases and resistance to several targeted therapies. Medicinal chemists are actively investigating the design of selective inhibitors of this protein as one strategy to improve patient care outcomes.[152]

Adverse effects with cabozantinib can be severe, prompting dose reduction and/or discontinuation. As noted in Table 33.6, the drug carries a boxed warning relative to GI perforations (3%) and fistulas (1%), as well as the potential for severe/fatal hemorrhage (3%).[76] Clinical trials have shown that serious adverse effects occur in close to 80% of patients[150] but, unlike vandetanib, prescribers do not require REMS certification.

All cabozantinib metabolites are inactive. The major circulating metabolite is the product of amide cleavage, O-dealkylation, and sulfate conjugation. This metabolite and the parent drug are inhibitors of CYP2C8, and cabozantinib also inhibits CYPs 2B6, 2C19 3A4, and P-gp.[153] Coadministration of 3A4 inhibitors or inducers should be avoided. As cabozantinib solubility drops with increasing pH, concomitant administration of PPIs may result in compromised oral absorption.[149]

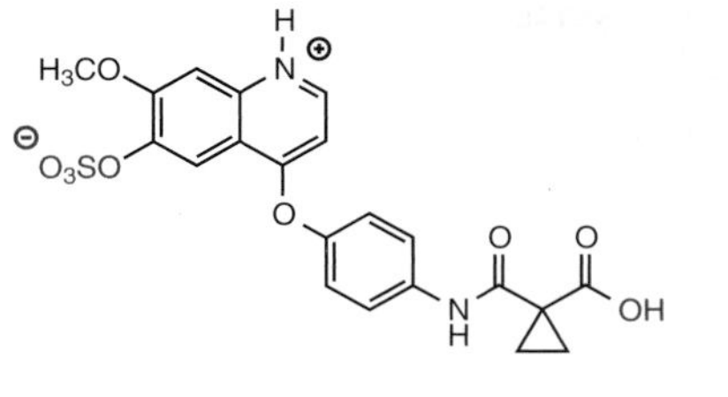

6-Desmethyl amide cleavage product sulfate cabozantinib metabolite

Axitinib. Axitinib is a potent VEGFR inhibitor with approximately 10 times the affinity of other TKIs for this kinase. With close to a 10-fold lower activity against other kinases such as c-kit or PDGFR, it is also highly selective. It is considered second-line therapy in RCC patients who have failed on at least one systemic antineoplastic regimen. With the introduction of cabozantinib and the check point inhibitor nivolumab to the RCC therapeutic arsenal, some believe the future of axitinib in the treatment of this cancer may be uncertain.[137] Clinical trials have shown little difference in OS between these two TKIs. Similar results were obtained when axitinib was compared against sorafenib, although axitinib may provide a PFS advantage particularly in previously treated patients.[154-156] Trials that pair axitinib with an immunotherapeutic agent or a different angiogenesis inhibitor are ongoing.

Unlike many VEGFR inhibitors, axitinib does not inhibit CYP enzymes; however, it is a substrate for P-gp, BCRP, and organic anion transporting protein 1B1 (OATP1B1). It is inactivated primarily by CYP3A4-catalyzed sulfoxidation and phase 2 N-glucuronidation,[157] and doses should be halved if coadministration with strong 3A4 inhibitors cannot be avoided. Solubility is pH dependent, but the AUC is not significantly impacted by coadministration of antacids or PPIs.[137] The hypertension that is commonly associated with VEGFR inhibitor therapy is viewed as a potential predictor of a positive therapeutic effect.[154]

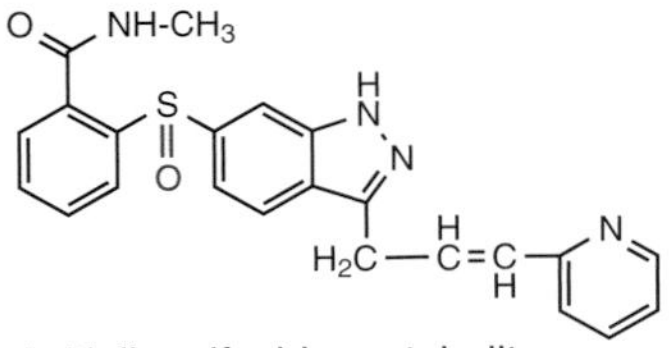

Axitinib sulfoxide metabolite

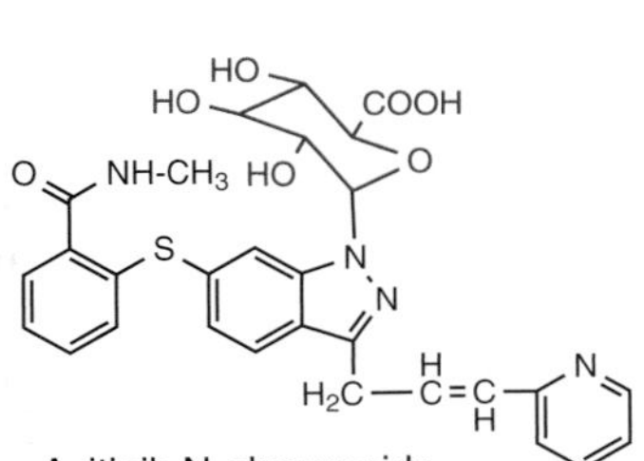

Axitinib N-glucuronide

Sunitinib Malate. Sunitinib is used as postsurgical therapy in RCC patients, in metastatic/advanced pancreatic neuroendocrine tumors, and in the treatment of imatinib-resistant GIST. Its introduction in 2006 more than doubled the rate of positive therapeutic outcomes previously achieved with interferon-α or interleukin-2 in RCC patients (40% vs. 2%-20% response rates).[93] Its relative efficacy in promoting PFS compared to other VEGFR inhibitors has been previously noted.

Sunitinib's use in highly VEGFR-dependent pancreatic neuroendocrine tumors has been shown to double PFS compared to placebo (12.6 vs. 5.8 mo), and there is evidence (albeit not statistically significant) that median 5-year OS increases as well (38.6 vs. 29.1 mo).[158] The phase III trial that generated these data noted a higher rate of serious adverse effects and death in the placebo group, prompting the shift of 69% of the placebo-treated patients to sunitinib that likely impacted the evaluation of OS.

GIST is another highly vascularized neoplasm where sunitinib has shown clinical benefit. In patients resistant to imatinib (the "gold standard" therapy), sunitinib enhances PSF, particularly in patients harboring exon 9 *KIT* mutations.[159]

As with many TKIs, the potential therapeutic value of sunitinib is undercut by the development of resistance. While there is still much to understand, tumor hypoxia appears to be a major player in resistance mechanisms. Starving the tumor of oxygen results in upregulation of several proangiogenic molecules via the action of hypoxia inducible factor 1 (HIF1) and an increased aggressiveness of surviving tumor cells. Attempts to overcome resistance with combination therapies (e.g., the mTOR inhibitor everolimus) come with excessive toxicity, although cabozantinib (which inhibits tumor invasiveness-advancing cMET and resistance-promoting AXL) may be a viable approach in sunitinib-resistant RCC. The fact that some resistant patients respond anew after a sunitinib "holiday" indicates that resistance may be temporary.[160]

An interesting study by Carlisle et al. investigated the patient burden associated with the clinical development of sunitinib.[161] After evaluating literature reporting on over 9,000 patients who received sunitinib monotherapy for 32 distinct malignancies, they found 15.7% achieved objective tumor response, 13.7% suffered from serious drug-related adverse effects, and 1% died from drug-related toxicity. After the first positive clinical responses were identified, the risk/benefit in subsequent trials continually worsened as investigators attempted to identify new therapeutic uses for sunitinib. The negative impact on patient well-being of this "indication hunt" prompted a call for a more holistic review of research findings to minimize unnecessary patient risk during the drug development process.

CYP3A4 deethylates sunitinib to an equally active secondary amine metabolite (Fig. 33.2) whose serum levels are approximately one-third of the parent drug. Appropriate precautions related to coadministration of strong CYP3A4 inhibitors or inducers should be taken.[93] The highly conjugated structure imparts a yellow color to the drug and its metabolites, which can be transferred to skin and body fluids.

Pazopanib Hydrochloride. Pazopanib is first-line therapy in the treatment of RCC. It inhibits multiple kinases, including PDGFR and c-kit, but it has the highest affinity for VEGFR. Related to PFS and OS, clinical trials have shown it to be superior to placebo[138] and "noninferior" to sunitinib with a better margin of safety (not including hepatotoxicity risk) and tolerability.[138,162,163] Real-world experience with pazopanib has confirmed these findings, with health-related quality of life assessments related to fatigue, hand/foot and mouth discomfort increased compared to sunitinib.[138] The use of targeted therapy, including pazopanib, has effectively replaced toxic high-dose cytokine therapy (e.g., IL-2, interferon-α) in this most common of kidney-related neoplasms.[162]

Soft tissue sarcoma is a rare and commonly fatal cancer traditionally treated with anthracycline-based chemotherapy regimens. Pazopanib now offers an oral and safer alternative to patients who have failed on, or are unable to tolerate, these more toxic agents. It has shown positive results relative to disease stabilization and PFS, and it can be used in patients undergoing radiation therapy with limited additional toxicity. While the search for reliable biomarkers to predict pazopanib response are ongoing, some are advocating for the earlier use of this TKI, at least in patients with less aggressive tumors and limited prior exposure to cytotoxic chemotherapy.[163,164]

Of the seven known metabolites, only hydroxypazopanib is active (Fig. 33.2), and the drug is predominantly excreted unchanged. It is a P-gp and BCRP substrate, a weak inhibitor of several CYP isoforms, and moderately induces CYP3A4 and 2B6. The boxed warning of severe hepatotoxicity is shared with sunitinib and regorafenib, and coadministration with the lipophilic antihyperlipidemic agent simvastatin significantly elevates the hepatotoxicity marker alanine transaminase (ALT).[162]

Regorafenib. Regorafenib and its nonfluorinated analogue sorafenib share only one indication; hepatocellular carcinoma (HCC). Until the mid-2017 approval of this multikinase inhibitor for this indication, there were essentially no alternatives for advanced HCC patients who progressed on sorafenib.[165] It is now second-line therapy for these patients and has been shown to increase OS (10.6 vs. 7.8 mo for placebo) as well as PFS. Although highly structurally similar, regorafenib's fluorine atom provides a broader kinase inhibiting profile than sorafenib and higher affinities for the kinase targets they share.[166]

Regorafenib is also second-line therapy in imatinib-resistant GIST that has progressed on sunitinib, the only other VEGFR kinase inhibitor with this indication. Its ability to inhibit c-Kit and TIE-2 kinase (an angiopoietin-binding protein) is believed to play a major role in its PFS-promoting efficacy (4.8 vs. 0.9 mo). Although it carries a boxed warning for potentially fatal hepatotoxicity (Table 33.6), regorafenib appears to be well-tolerated by most patients. Its multiple targets gives rise to hope that resistance might be minimized, prompting some to suggest earlier use in GIST.[159] Treatment strategies for regorafenib nonresponders have focused on PI3 kinase inhibition (e.g., mTOR inhibitors), combination TKI therapy with attention to dose scheduling, and immunotherapies. A thorough, pharmacist-targeted review of regorafenib use in GIST has been published.[167]

The use of regorafenib in colorectal cancer is reserved for patients who have not responded to a variety of first- and second-line therapies. A meta-analysis of 24 phase III clinical trials showed significant increases in survival benefit (1.4-2.5 mo) compared to placebo.[168]

Regorafenib is a CYP3A4 substrate. While the pyridine N-oxide shown in Figure 33.2 is the most predominant active metabolite after a single dose of drug, the N-demethylated N-oxide also has activity comparable to the parent drug. Exposure to the desmethyl metabolite is effectively equal to the secondary amide at steady state, but neither is believed to contribute extensively to regorafenib's therapeutic effect. An inactive N-glucuronide is generated through the action of UGT1A9, but it undergoes enterohepatic cycling and is cleaved back to the parent drug by gut flora. The N-oxide is also believed to be reduced to regorafenib in the gut upon recycling.[169]

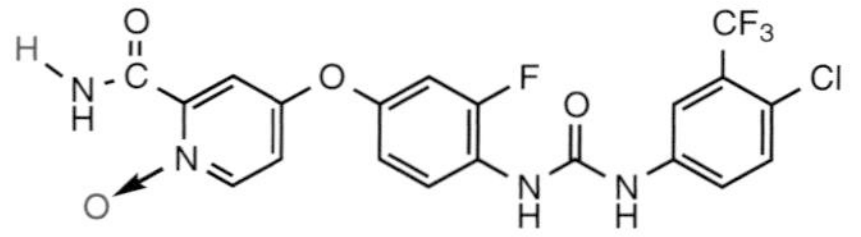

Desmethylregorafenib-N-oxide metabolite

ALK INHIBITORS. Anaplastic lymphoma kinase (ALK) belongs to the insulin receptor superfamily.[170] While ALK expression is essentially absent in the adult population,[171] the fusion of ALK with proteins such as nucleophosmin (NPM) or echinoderm microtubule-associated protein-like 4 (EML4) results in kinase activation and subsequent deregulation of homeostatic cell signaling processes. This, in turn, leads to an increase in the aggressiveness of tumors expressing these ALK fusion proteins or carrying other *ALK* gene mutations. By targeting these hyperactive kinases, ALK inhibitors derail their tumor-accelerating mission and, until resistance develops, promote disease stability or regression and PFS. While currently indicated for ALK$^+$ NSCLC (approximately 3%-5% of cases),[171] preclinical studies hold promise that ALK inhibitors will be effective in all ALK-expressing neoplastic diseases.[172] Interestingly, the EML4-ALK fusion protein is found more frequently in NSCLC patients who are light or "never" smokers, compared to heavy smokers.[173]

Chemistry (Fig. 33.10)

Like the TKIs before them, type I ALK inhibitors seek out hinge region residues in the ATP binding pocket and insert lipophilic moieties into adjacent hydrophobic pockets (Fig. 33.10). Cocrystal structures of the first two FDA-approved ALK inhibitors, crizotinib and ceritinib, with ALK are known. The isopropylsulfonylphenyl moiety of ceritinib is known to embed deeper into the hydrophobic pocket than the methyl group of crizotinib, and crizotinib's relatively meager engagement with residues within the adenine pocket is one explanation for its relative lack of ALK selectivity. Potentially cationic nitrogen atoms of

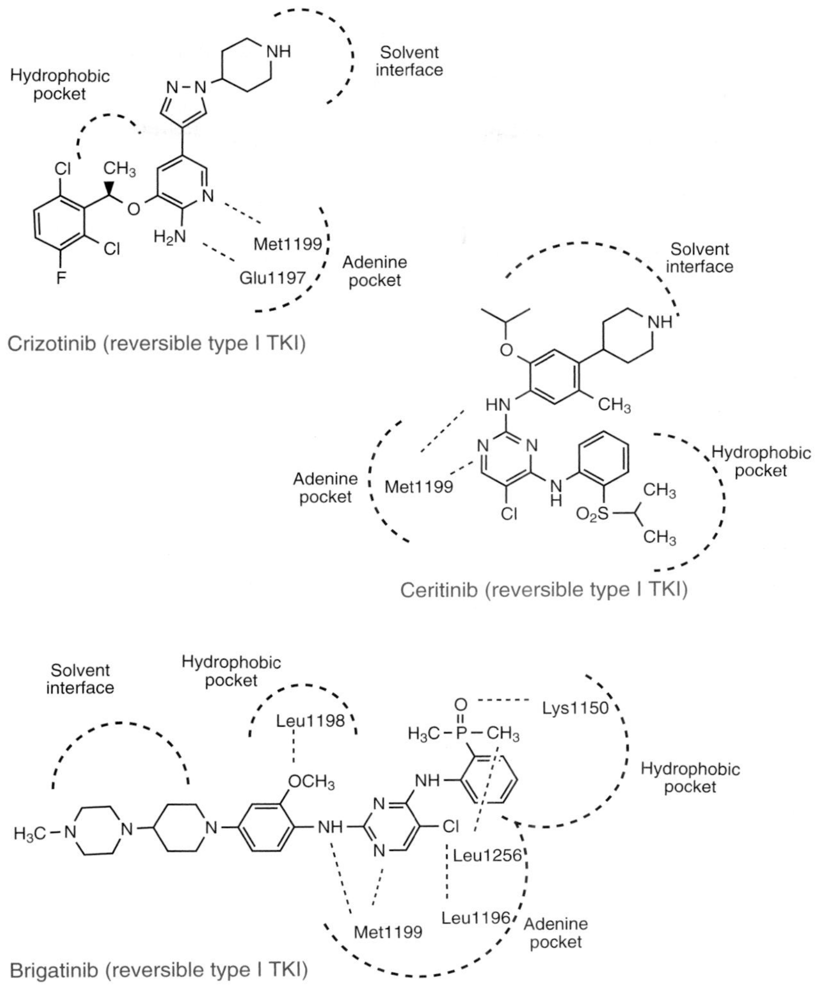

Crizotinib (reversible type I TKI)

Ceritinib (reversible type I TKI)

Brigatinib (reversible type I TKI)

Figure 33.10 Binding interactions between ALK and representative inhibitors.

ALK inhibitors are stabilized by association with solvent at its interface with the adenine pocket.[58] The newest ALK inhibitor, brigatinib, has many structural features in common with ceritinib (chlorinated 2,4-diaminopyrimidine, phenyl moiety substituted with a dimethylated oxygen-containing polar group, ionizable nitrogen heterocycle) and binds at ALK via similar modes. An X-ray crystal structure of ALK bound to brigatinib has allowed for the identification of key intermolecular interactions.[174] A stabilizing intramolecular hydrogen bond between the phosphine oxide and anilino NH group assures the proper U-shaped conformation important to high affinity binding.[174]

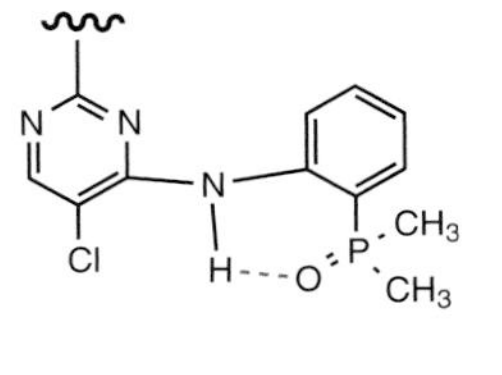

Brigatinib intramolecular H-bond

Not surprisingly, resistance to ALK inhibitors is a multifaceted biochemical phenomenon that is incompletely understood. In addition to gene amplification/mutation and activation of alternative signaling pathways in response to TKI exposure[171] (a common mechanism of acquired resistance), it has been suggested that the presence of cancer stem cells might play a role in intrinsic resistance.[171,172]

ALK^+ NSCLC contains the oncogenic *EML4-ALK* fusion gene. L1196M is considered the "gatekeeper mutation" (viewed as comparable to T790M and T315I in EGFR and Bcr-Abl kinases, respectively), and second-generation ALK inhibitors are capable of eliciting positive therapeutic outcomes in cancers expressing this mutant. The G1202R mutation is a therapeutic deal-breaker for all ALK inhibitors except brigatinib, although E1210K combined with S1206C or D1203N can halt clinical benefit from this fairly "resistance-resistant" TKI. Clearly, sequencing ALK inhibitors to be most effective in "rolling resistance" is a wise therapeutic strategy, albeit one challenging to discern.[171,175] Amplification of *cKIT*, *MET*, Scr, and stem cell factor is also believed to be involved in ALK inhibitor resistance.

Specific Drugs (Fig. 33.1). All currently marketed ALK inhibitors are used in the treatment of ALK^+ NSCLC, and all are metabolized by CYP3A4 to at least one active metabolite (Fig. 33.2).

Crizotinib. Crizotinib, FDA-approved in mid-2011, was the first ALK inhibitor on the U.S. market. This TKI also demonstrates high affinity for MET and ROS1, the latter of which has a strong structural similarity to ALK in the ATP-binding domain of the catalytic site.[171] Therefore, unlike other ALK inhibitors, its indication also includes ROS1⁺ NSCLC. In clinical trials in previously untreated and organoplatinum-resistant patients, crizotinib documented a median PFS of 10.9 and 7.7 months, respectively. The positive outcomes were supported by real-world studies in which crizotinib therapy produced estimated median PFS statistics of 9.6 (first-line) and 9.0 (second-line) months, respectively, a 1-year survival probability of 82%, and an overall objective response rate of 66%.[176]

As noted earlier, resistance undermines therapeutic efficacy and generally manifests within 8-15 months.[176,177] The L1196M mutation, along with the C1156Y mutation, alter the structure of the adenine pocket such that crizotinib can no longer bind effectively.[170] The G1269A mutant also interferes with crizotinib efficacy. Crizotinib does not effectively distribute into the central nervous system (CNS) and is also actively effluxed by P-gp; therefore, it is not effective in brain metastases that occur in approximately 60% of crizotinib-treated NSCLC patients.[170,171] Unlike other ALK inhibitors, visual disturbances are a common adverse effect (60%-71%) but do not generally result in drug discontinuation.[177]

Slightly over half of the crizotinib dose is excreted unchanged in feces, potentially representing unabsorbed drug. Diasteriometic lactams generated by CYP3A4 are the major metabolites (Fig. 33.2). They are between 2.5 and 7.7 times less active than crizotinib as ALK inhibitors and exhibit stereoselectivity with regard to inhibitory action and pharmacokinetic parameters. O-dealkylation of the pyridine ring of the parent drug and lactam metabolites to inactive aromatic alcohols, followed by conjugation with glucuronic acid or sulfate, also occurs, but to a lesser extent. The inactivity of the O-dealkylated metabolites is not surprising given the role the lost methyl group plays in binding the inhibitor to the ALK hydrophobic site.[173]

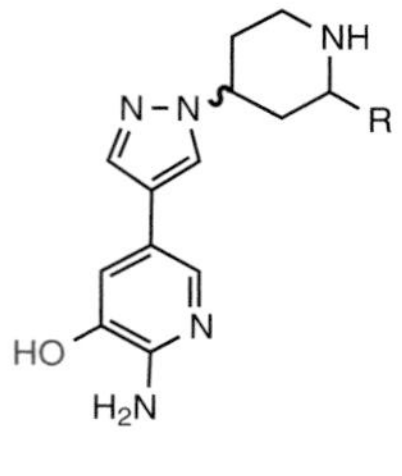

Inactive O-dealkylated crizotinib metabolites (R = H, =O)

Although present in urine in only trace amounts, Cys conjugates generated from GSH attack of a quinoneimine lactam metabolite are of chemical interest (Fig. 33.11).[173]

Ceritinib. Ceritinib, a 20-fold more potent, highly ALK-selective TKI, was FDA-approved approximately 3 years

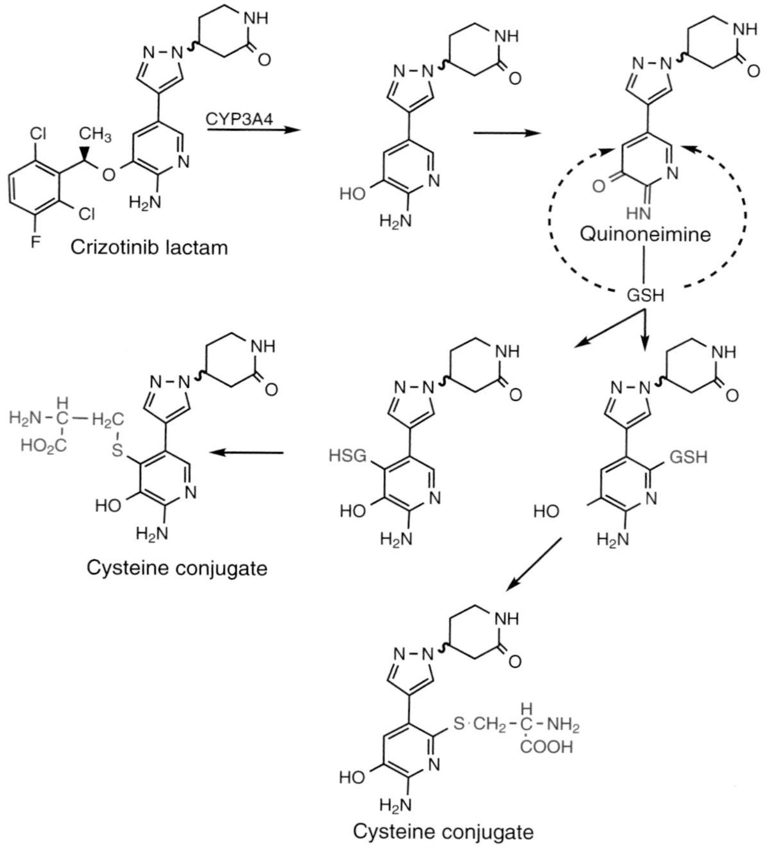

Figure 33.11 Formation of cysteine metabolites of crizotinib lactam.

after crizotinib and has shown value in crizotinib-resistant NSCLC. It retains efficacy in L1196M and G1269A mutants, although not in C1156Y transformed cells.[170] Clinical trials have shown overall response rates of 56.4% in patients previously treated with crizotinib, as well as median PFS and OS gains of 6.9 and 16.7 months, respectively.[170,175] Of significance is that treatment outcomes were similar regardless of the presence or absence of crizotinib resistance-promoting mutations in the ALK protein. In a continuation study, complete/partial remission or disease stability statistics ranged from 38% to 39%. When compared against platinum-based chemotherapy, ceritinib showed a 16.6 month improvement in median PFS with stronger OS predictions.[170] Importantly, ceritinib (and alectinib, discussed below) show higher activity against brain metastases compared to crizotinib or cytotoxic chemotherapy due to an enhanced ability to penetrate the BBB, although is a substrate for P-gp and can therefore be effluxed from the CNS.[170,178]

Ceritinib is primarily excreted unchanged (68%) in feces and, like crizotinib, some is eliminated prior to absorption. Ceritinib phase 1 biotransformation is CYP3A4 catalyzed (Table 33.4) with some phase 2 glucuronide and sulfate conjugation following.[179] The parent drug is the primary species found in plasma, and the low level of circulating metabolites (each <2.3% of the AUC) calls into question the clinical relevance of the O-dealkylated or monooxygenated structures.[180]

Although solubility is inversely related to gastric pH, coadministration of PPIs is not contraindicated since drug exposure in the presence of these achlorhydria-inducing agents was not seriously impacted.[170] However, coadministration of strong CYP3A4 inhibitors or inducers should be avoided if at all possible. A primer on ceritinib targeted to pharmacy practitioners has been published.[181]

Alectinib. This second-generation ALK inhibitor has much in common with ceritinib, including high ALK selectivity, efficacy in crizotinib-resistant ALK⁺ NSCLC, and the ability to treat brain metastases. Unlike ceritinib, it is a poor substrate for P-gp and, thus, able to concentrate in the cerebrospinal fluid.[175,178] Also unlike ceritinib, it is effective in cells expressing the C1156Y mutation, but does succumb to other ALK genetic transformations, including G1202R.

As second-line therapy in crizotinib-resistant ALK⁺ NSCLC, a clinical trial conducted in Japan documented an overall alectinib response rate of 92% (vs. 79% for crizotinib) and a median PFS greater than crizotinib's 10.2 months.[182] A real-world retrospective chart review of alectinib outcomes in 207 crizotinib-resistant patients cared for by 95 U.S. oncologists documented an objective response rate of 67.1% and a disease control rate of 89.9%, both higher than observed in clinical trials.[178] The response rate was highest in patients of Asian ancestry, of relatively good functional status, and/or who were former or "never" smokers (compared to current smokers). While overall response rates between patients with and without a history of chemotherapy were comparable, chemotherapy-naïve patients exhibited a higher rate of stable disease than those with previous chemotherapy exposure (25.8% vs. 11.4%). Tolerance to alectinib's adverse effects was generally good,[178] although it should be noted that alectinib-induced bradycardia is responsible for essentially all major drug-drug interactions (DDIs) identified for this TKI.[76]

In TKI-naïve ALK⁺ NSCLC patients, another Japanese trial evaluating alectinib as first-line therapy showed an overall response rate of 93.5%, a PSF of greater than 29 months, and a 4-year OS of 70%.[171,182] A worldwide clinical trial in treatment-naïve patients confirmed alectinib's superiority to crizotinib in terms of median PFS, overall response rate, and effectiveness in treating brain metastases.[182] NCCN guidelines now accept alectinib as a first-line "standard of care" in ALK⁺ NSCLC.

The major alectinib metabolite is the CYP3A4-generated morpholine ring-opened structure shown as M4 in Figure 33.2. Although present in plasma at concentrations less than the parent drug (5.8% vs. 84%, respectively) it retains activity comparable to the parent and contributes to the therapeutic response elicited by alectinib.[183] A pharmacologically inactive carboxylate metabolite (M1b) also forms (~7% of the dose), and a small amount of M4 will lose the hydroxyethyl moiety to yield the unsubstituted 4-aminopiperine metabolite, M6 (0.2% of the dose).[68,183]

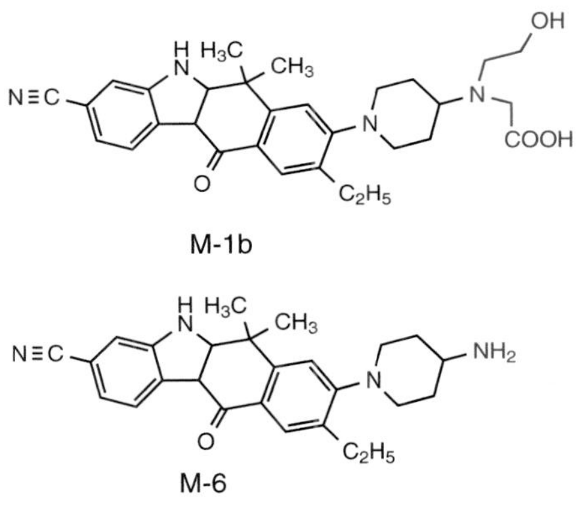

M-1b

M-6

Inactive alectinib metabolites

Brigatinib. Brigatinib, FDA approved in mid-2017, is active against several ALK mutants that confer resistance to other ALK inhibitors. Used in crizotinib-resistant NSCLC, this third-generation agent is claimed to retain efficacy in the face of L1196M, C1156Y, and G1202R mutations,[74,184,185] although some G1202R mutants have been identified in brigatinib-resistant NSCLC.[170,171] Like crizotinib, it has affinity for related kinases (albeit with 11-35 fold higher IC_{50} values), including ROS1, FLT-3, and the EGFR T790M mutant. The unique phosphine oxide moiety's ability to engage in strong inter- and intramolecular hydrogen bonding is believed responsible for the high ALK selectivity, as well as brigatinib's beneficial pharmacokinetic profile. For example, the higher polarity of the dimethylphosphine oxide moiety, compared to the isopropylsulfone group of certinib, results in significantly lower binding to serum proteins (Table 33.5).[184]

Clinical trials in crizotinib-resistant patients administered 180 mg brigatinib once daily after a week at 90 mg/d showed a 55% objective response rate and a median PFS of 15.6 months after a median 18.6 month follow-up. Median OS was 27.6 months. The drug also shows promise in eliciting response and promoting PFS in crizotinib-resistant patients with brain metastases. In another study, 100% of crizotinib-naïve patients responded to brigatinib, although the numbers were small.[184] Several clinical trials are ongoing in the United States and around the world to evaluate its use as first-line therapy, in addition to second-line therapy in crizotinib resistant NSCLC.[74,184,185]

CYP3A4 and 2C8-catalyzed N-demethylation and Cys conjugation represent the two major brigatinib metabolic routes. Unchanged brigatinib and the unidentified 3-fold less active primary metabolite account for 92% and 3.5% of the circulating drug, respectively. In addition to being biotransformed by CYP3A4, brigatinib can induce this isoform.[74] Given the risk of serious adverse effects when blood levels rise (including pulmonary toxicity, hypertension and visual disturbances), coadministration with strong CYP3A4 inhibitors should be avoided.[74,171]

Bruton Tyrosine Kinase (BTK) Inhibitors. BTK, a nonreceptor kinase essential to proper B-lymphocyte development and B-cell receptor (B-CR) signaling, is expressed by a gene associated with the X chromosome. It was named for a U.S. Navy pediatrician Ogden Bruton, who first described an X-linked immunodeficiency syndrome (XLA) caused by mutations in the *BTK* gene.[186] Under normal circumstances, the kinase phosphorylates phospholipase C-γ2 (PLCγ2), mobilizing Ca^{2+} and activating pathways critical to B-cell homeostasis. Aberrations in the function of BTK are associated with B-cell-related hematological cancers, and inhibiting this kinase results in a complex series of biochemical events that terminates in apoptosis. Importantly, BTK inhibition spares T-cells since the protein is not found there, thus also sparing patient immune function.[187] Myelosuppression with these antineoplastic agents is claimed to be rare,[188] although thrombocytopenia and neutropenia can occur in up to half (or more) of ibrutinib-treated patients.[76]

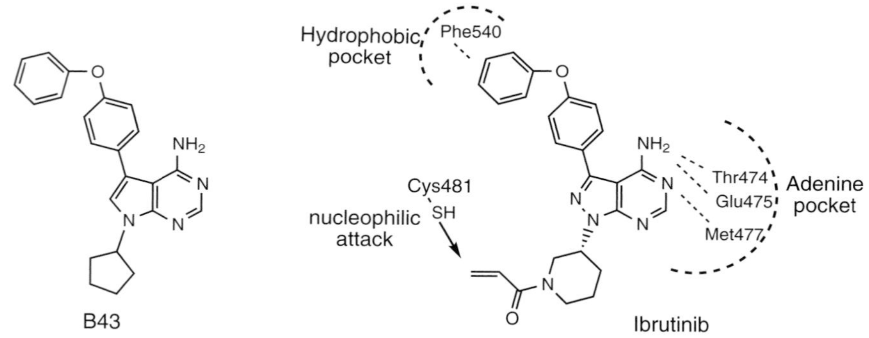

Chemistry. The binding of the first marketed BTK inhibitor (ibrutinib) to the kinase was originally modeled after a cocrystal of bound reversible analogue B43, and subsequently confirmed through crystal structure evaluation.[58,189,190] Like the TKIs afatinib, neratinib and osimertinib, ibrutinib has an electrophilic acrylamide moiety that undergoes attack by a nucleophilic Cys residue in the catalytic domain, irreversibly alkylating the protein[188] (see Fig. 33.5, afatinib interaction with EGFR). The *R* enantiomer is the active enzyme-alkylating isomer.

Acalabrutinib, the only other currently marketed BTK inhibitor, has an electrophilic butynamide group that serves the same covalent bond-generating purpose as ibrutinib's acrylamide. In this case, it's the *S* isomer that properly positions the butynamide for Cys attack.[191] Modeling of acalabrutinib bound to BTK shows interactions with the same adenine pocket residues that hold ibrutinib to the catalytic site, as well as interactions of the butynamide carbonyl and pyridine nitrogen with Ser538 and Asp539, respectively. This likely contributes to acalabrutinib's higher BTK inhibiting potency.[191]

A combination of high affinity for BTK with a short half-life of unbound drug (Table 33.5) promotes selectivity of these agents.[186,188] This appears particularly true for acalabrutinib, as the butynamide confers an attenuated reactivity that decreases alkylation of "off-target" kinases, such as EGFR. The fact that it is capable of alkylating Cys481 is attributed to the close proximity of the electron withdrawing (and, therefore, activating) imidazopyrazine ring system.

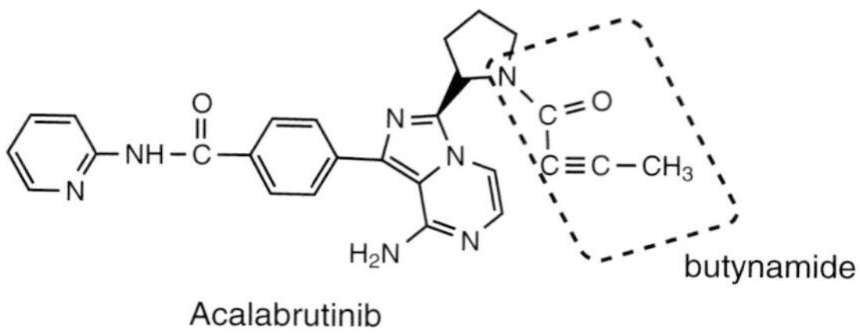

Resistance to irreversible BTK inhibitors occurs primarily through a C481S mutation, which destroys the ability of the enzyme to attack the electrophilic acrylamide or butynamide moiety. A similar mutation (C797S) was previously described for the irreversibly acting EGFR/HER inhibitor osimertinib. T316A mutations, as well as R665W PLCγ2 mutants, are also known to result in ibrutinib-resistant cells.[192-195] In one clinical study, the median time to drug discontinuation due to ibrutinib resistance was 13 months, which had a negative impact on survival.[196]

Specific Drugs (Fig. 33.1)

Ibrutinib. Ibrutinib is used in a number of B-cell lymphomas and leukemias. Chronic lymphocytic leukemia (CLL) is the most common leukemia the United States, and ibrutinib has shown a positive impact on overall response rate (67%) and PFS (75% at two years) in patients with previously treated relapsing or refractory disease. A phase III trial comparing ibrutinib to the MAb ofatumumab in previously treated patients showed superior outcomes for the BTK inhibitor related to PFS and risk of death. The 30-month PFS rate for treatment naïve CLL patients given ibrutinib was 96%.[193]

In marginal zone lymphoma, a cancer without a defined standard of treatment, ibrutinib therapy in patients previously treated with an anti-CD20 MAb resulted in a 48% overall response rate and a median PFS of 14.2 months upon evaluation at 19.4 months. Little outcomes variance was observed between clinically defined subgroups.[197] Positive outcomes were also obtained in a phase II trial evaluating ibrutinib in bortezomib-treated and -naïve patients with relapsed/refractory mantle cell lymphoma (MCL; median PFS of almost 14 mo when evaluated at 15.3 mo).[187]

As noted in Table 33.4, ibrutinib is a CYP3A4 substrate, and three oxidation products predominate.[69] The dihydrodiol metabolite (Fig. 33.2) is about 15-fold less active as a BTK inhibitor, and the remaining two metabolites result from aromatic hydroxylation and piperidine ring opening with subsequent reduction or oxidation to the primary alcohol (M34) and carboxylic acid (M25), respectively. In addition to GI distress, rash, headache and other adverse effects common to all kinase inhibitors, urinary tract, upper respiratory, and other infections, hemorrhage, hypertension, as well as dry eye syndrome, can manifest in patients taking ibrutinib, but drug discontinuation is rare.

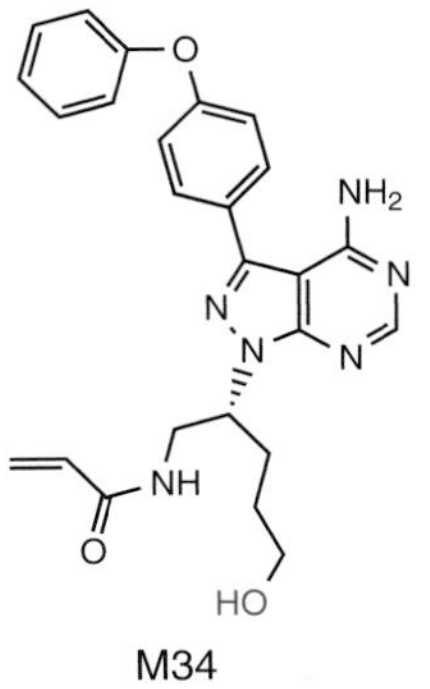

M34 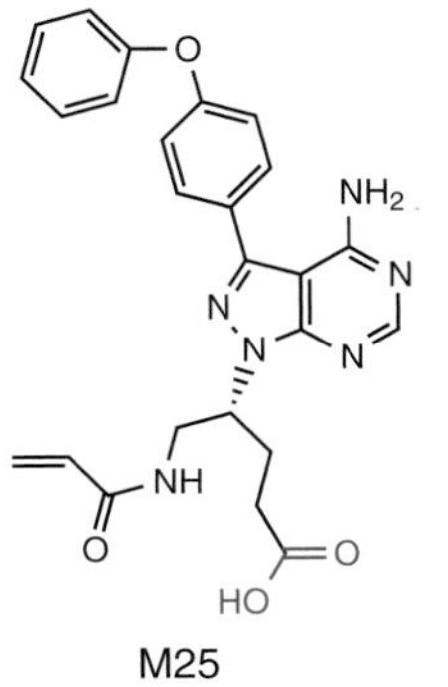 M25

Acalabrutinib. Acalabrutinib's only current indication is previously treated MCL, although clinical trials are underway to assess its potential value in CLL and solid tumors.[198] Ibrutinib resistance in MCL is believed to be mediated by activation of the P13K-AKT pathway, rather than by a loss of BTK inhibition efficacy.[195] As a more selective BTK inhibitor, acalabrutinib has shown promise as second-line therapy in this disease and may be better tolerated (e.g., lower risk of infection, hemorrhage) with fewer drug-drug interactions. In a recent phase II global clinical trial with 124 refractory/relapsed MCL patients who had failed on one to five previous therapies (only four patients had ibrutinib exposure), the overall response rate was 80%, which was evenly divided between complete and partial response. At one year, investigators estimated that 67% of the study population achieved PFS, and the estimated 1-year survival was 87%. Headache was the most common adverse effect.[199]

Acalabrutinib is metabolized predominantly by CYP3A and to a minor extent by glutathione conjugation and amide hydrolysis. Strong CYP3A inducers and inhibitors can be expected to significantly affect the maximum plasma concentration (C_{max}) of the drug. The metabolite known as ACP-5862 has approximately half the activity of the parent, but its structure has not yet been reported.

FLT3 Kinase Inhibitor

Midostaurin (Fig. 33.1). Midostaurin is the N-benzoyl derivative of staurosporin, an alkaloid produced by *Streptomyces staurosporeus*. A reversible type I TKI, it is indicated for the treatment of acute myeloid leukemia (AML) in the ~30% of patients who carry a genetic mutation in *FLT3* that puts them at risk for poor disease remission and survival outcomes.[200] *FLT3*'s primary function is hematopoietic homeostasis, but internal tandem duplications (ITDs) and point mutations in the TK domain result in dysregulated signaling systems. The TK point mutations of highest relevance to AML involve replacement of an Asp835 residue with Tyr, Val, His, Glu, Ala, or Asn.[200]

Midosaurin's inhibition of mutation-positive Fms-like tyrosine kinase-3 ($FLT3^+$) and spleen tyrosine kinase (SYK, a "signaling partner" of FLT3) is responsible for its myeloid cell antiproliferative effect.[201] SYK is an essential element for the transformation and advancement of AML and a biochemical driver for several leukemias and lymphomas. Unrestrained SYK activity can induce resistance in AML drugs that selectively target FLT3 kinase. Inhibition of both kinases is a key to therapeutic success.[201] Midostaurin is used in combination with cytotoxic induction (cytarabine, daunorubicin) and consolidation (cytarabine) chemotherapy in patients who test positive for a FLT3 mutation. CDx FLT3 Mutation Assay (LeukoStrat), a companion diagnostic which detects ITD and TK domain point mutations, was simultaneously approved with midostaurin.

In a phase III clinical trial with 717 $FLT3^+$ patients undergoing standard induction and consolidation chemotherapy, midostaurin essentially tripled the OS rate compared to placebo (74.7 vs. 26.0 mo, respectively). Positive outcomes related to complete remission rate in newly diagnosed $FLT3^+$ AML patients undergoing chemotherapy was also achieved in earlier phase II trials.[200]

Midostaurin is also an inhibitor of many other kinases, including protein kinase C (PKC), VEGFR, PDGFR, c-kit and cyclin-dependent kinase I (cdsk1). Its broad spectrum has resulted in its classification as a multikinase inhibitor in drug information resources.[76] The potential role of these other targets in midostaurin's antileukemic action has been described.[200]

Once absorbed from the gastrointestinal tract (GIT), midostaurin is transported in plasma bound to α-1 acidic glycoprotein and extensively metabolized via CYP3A4. Two active FLT3 kinase and SYK-inhibiting metabolites are produced; the epimeric mixture of the 7-hydroxy derivative (CGP52421) and the O-demethylation product (CGP62221) (Fig. 33.2). CGP62221 is equipotent with the parent as an inhibitor of FLT3-ITD-dependent cell proliferation, while CGP52421 is approximately 10-fold less active.[71] CGP52421 has a long terminal elimination half-life (~36 d)[202] likely associated with protein binding. Clinically relevant drug-drug interactions are anticipated if midostaurin is coadministered with moderate-strong CYP3A4 inhibitor or inducers.

As with many other TKIs, there is a risk of pulmonary toxicity (specifically interstitial lung disease) with midostaurin use. It has been proposed that the drug's ability to inhibit VEGFR may, in some cases, play a role in this potentially fatal event. Toxicity appears to be dose-dependent. Sequential, rather than concurrent, administration of cytotoxic chemotherapy has been shown to enhance tolerance of midostaurin which, in turn, should decrease the risk of drug discontinuation.[200]

JANUS-ASSOCIATED KINASE INHIBITORS. The Janus-associated kinases (JAKs) are a family of cytoplasmic tyrosine kinases (JAK1, JAK2, JAK3, and nonreceptor tyrosine kinase 2 [TYK2]). They associate with the cytoplasmic end of cytokine receptors and mediate signals that impact hematopoiesis and immune function. Integral to the action of JAK are the *s*ignal *t*ransducer and *a*ctivator of *t*ranscription (STAT) proteins. JAK enzymes phosphorylate STAT, which then translocate from the cytosol to the nucleus where they activate gene transcription processes leading to angiogenesis and immunosuppression.

While JAK activity is essential for proper immune function, dysregulation has been associated with the initiation and progression of blood-based cancers. Point mutations, specifically JAK2 V617F that results in a "supercharged" kinase, have been linked to myeloproliferative neoplasms (MPN) such as polycythemia vera and myelofibrosis. Mutations leading to ALL and various lymphomas have also been identified, which underscore the rationale behind the use of JAK inhibitors in the treatment of vulnerable hematologic malignancies.[203] The JAK2 V617F mutation is the primary TK contributing to MPN pathology and results from a guanine to thymine nucleotide shift at position 1849 in the *JAK2* gene (G1849T).[204] JAK2 phosphorylates STAT3 and STAT5, and inhibiting this kinase in MPN results in dose- and time-dependent decreases in STAT3 activation.

Ruxolitinib Phosphate (Fig. 33.1). Ruxolitinib has been approved for the treatment of myelofibrosis and polycythemia vera, conditions that fall under the "umbrella" neoplastic category of MPN. As noted above, the JAK2 V617F is the primary TK contributing to MPN pathology, and ruxolitinib competes with ATP for access to the adenosine site of the enzyme. Hinge residues Leu932 and Glu930 are thought to be important to drug-kinase binding, and are hypothesized to H-bond with N1 (pyrimidine) and N7 (pyrrole) of ruxolitinib.[58]

The clinical signs of MPN include progressive myelofibrosis, anemia and splenomegaly, which results in weight loss, fatigue, and bone pain. Approximately 1-2 in 10 patients will develop AML within 10 years of initial diagnosis, and post-diagnosis survival is commonly between 5 and 6 years. Ruxolitinib therapy has been shown to attenuate spleen enlargement, decrease levels of inflammatory cytokines, and induce apoptosis in JAK V617F positive cells, leading to an improved quality and a potentially increased duration of life.[203]

Phase III trials in intermediate-high risk myelofibrosis patients comparing ruxolitinib to either placebo (COMFORT-I) or first-line hydroxyurea therapy (COMFORT-II) documented statistically significant positive therapeutic outcomes, including OS, with generally manageable adverse effects (e.g., myelosuppression, diarrhea). However, slightly over one-third (38%) of patients in the COMFORT-II trial had discontinued therapy within the 48 weeks due to drug-related toxicity or disease exacerbation.[205] A phase III trial in polycythemia vera patients who had progressed on hydroxyurea demonstrated similar benefits related to spleen size reduction, as well as blood cell profile and hematocrit control at 32 weeks. Patients who achieved hematocrit control at 32 weeks had an 89% chance of a persistent response at 80 weeks.[206]

The dose of ruxolitinib in myelofibrosis increases with elevated platelet count, ranging from 5 mg twice daily (platelet count 50-100 × 10^3/mm^3) to 20 mg twice daily (platelet count >200 × 10^3/mm^3). The initial dose of 10 mg twice daily in polycythemia vera should be adjusted based on platelet count and hemoglobin levels, but the dose in both disease states should not exceed 50 mg/d.

Ruxolitinib is rapidly and almost completely absorbed after oral administration. The half-life is short (3 hr) due to oxidative metabolism primarily catalyzed by CYP3A4 and, to a lesser extent, by CYP2C9. Ruxolitinib represents the major component (~50%) in the plasma, and active isomeric metabolites contributing 18% to the therapeutic action result from cyclopentane hydroxylation at positions 2 or 3 (17% and 8.3% of the $AUC_{0\text{-}24}$, respectively).[207,208] Oxidation of the 3-hydroxy metabolite to the ketone is known to occur. Coadministration of ruxolitinib with CYP3A4 inhibitors or inducers should be undertaken only with careful monitoring, and strong CYP3A4 inhibitor cotherapy should be avoided. The drug is eliminated via renal (~70%) and biliary (~22%) routes, with <1% excreted unchanged.

Ser/Thr Kinase Inhibitors

CYCLIN-DEPENDENT KINASE INHIBITORS (FIG. 33.12)

COMMON ADVERSE EFFECTS OF SER/THR KINASE INHIBITORS

All Ser/Thr kinase inhibitors

- Myelosuppression
- Fatigue
- GI distress
- Hair loss/thinning
- Rash/cutaneous reactions

CDK
- Neutropenia

BRAF
- Hyperglycemia
- Joint/muscle pain

MEK
- Hypertension
- Edema
- Hypoalbuminemia
- Hepatotoxicity

mTOR
- Hyperglycemia
- Hyperlipidemia
- Pulmonary toxicity

PI3K
- Infection
- Hyperglycemia
- Pulmonary toxicity

Abberant cyclin-dependent kinase (CDK) activity, particularly CDK2, CDK4, and CDK6 is associated with carcinogenic transformations in gene transcription and cellular regulatory mechanisms. The 20 known CDKs exist in active and inactive conformations, with action demanding complexation with a cyclin subunit and subsequent ATP-catalyzed phosphorylation of (most commonly) Thr.[209] CDKs 4 and 6, which contain the regulatory cyclin D1 and three subunits, respectively,[210] have structural variances from the 18 other enzymes, which has proven valuable in the design of targeted inhibitors for use in therapy for advanced or metastatic hormone receptor positive (HR^+)/HER2 negative breast cancer (the common indication of the three marketed CDK inhibitors). Importantly, CDK4/6 has been shown to be intimately involved in breast cancer initiation and invasive progression, and it induces attenuation of retinoblastoma gene (Rb) phosphorylation and cell cycle arrest at G1.[210] Patients who respond to these drugs must be Rb^+.[210]

Research continues to identify potent type I inhibitors less likely to induce the dose-limiting myelosuppression common to the currently available compounds, as well as inhibitors that target the more structurally diverse inactive conformations (type II), or allosteric binding pockets (type III and IV) of the enzymes.[211]

Chemistry and SAR. Like all kinases, CDK proteins have N-and C-terminal lobes connected through a hinge region that serves as the ATP-binding catalytic site. Planar (aromatic) structures that mimic adenine, along with H-bonding moieties are critical to holding inhibitors to the catalytic site. The catalytic pocket is large and contains a Phe gatekeeper residue (Phe98 for CDK6) that can be targeted for inactivating interaction in the active conformation to which type I KIs bind. Other key residues believed involved in inhibitor binding to CDK6 include Thr107 (Thr99 or Thr102 in CDK4),[209,211] Asp104 and Asn150. A cationic Lys residue found on other CDKs decreases affinity for therapeutic inhibitors and promotes selectivity for CDK4/6.[209] A crystal structure of active CDK4/6-cyclin D bound to inhibitor is yet to be solved, so a more definitive description of inhibitor interaction with these kinase proteins awaits this important scientific advancement.

SAR studies on selective CDK4/6 inhibitors demonstrated the importance of incorporating a cationic moiety (e.g., piperazine) positioned to form an affinity-enhancing ion-dipole bond with the CDK4/6 Thr residue while repelling the cationic Lys reside found on other CDKs (e.g., CDK1/2). The 2-aminopyrimidine group binds to the hinge region adenine site, as it has in many other KIs. Using palbociclib (Fig. 33.12) as an example, N1 of the pyridopyrimidine nucleus may promote affinity through interaction with a unique His residue in the hinge region of CDK4 (His92) and CDK6 (His100). The affinity-enhancing piperazine terminus and pyridopyrimidine N8-cyclopentyl ring were declared important to potency, while the C5-CH_3 and C6-acetyl moieties promoted CDK4 selectivity. As noted earlier, the cationic piperazine should also enhance selectivity by repelling the cationic Lys residue found in other CDKs. While SAR data on ribociclib and abemaciclib are scarce, the structural similarities with palbociclib are obvious, particularly for ribociclib (Fig. 33.12).[211]

Resistance to CDK4/6 inhibitors has been linked to Rb deficiency and the associated high levels of tumor suppressor protein $p16^{INK4A}$ and the deletion or inactivation of the *CDKN2A* gene.[212]

Specific Drugs (Fig. 33.12). As noted above, all currently marketed CDK4/6 inhibitors are used in the treatment of $HR^+/HER2^-$ metastatic breast cancer (MBC), and given in combination with the aromatase inhibitor letrozole (see Chapter 24). Two agents, palbociclib and abemaciclib, have found value in combination with the estrogen receptor antagonist fluvestrant (see Chapter 24) in MBC that has progressed on endocrine therapy alone. Myelosuppression (potentially leading to infection), fatigue, and GI distress, rash, and hair loss/thinning are common adverse effects.

All three CKD4/6 inhibitors are vulnerable to CYP3A4-catalyzed metabolism, and ribociclib and abemaciclib have clinically relevant active metabolites (Table 33.7). Fecal elimination predominates. The CYP-mediated metabolic properties of the marketed CDKs are provided in Table 33.7 and selected pharmacokinetic and therapeutic properties appear in Table 33.8.

Palbociclib. The MBC 5-year OS statistic of 25% is grim, but patients have been given the gift of time and better life quality with the introduction of palbociclib. The PALOMA clinical trials series documented significant benefits of palbociclib plus letrozole in promoting PFS and clinical benefit compared to letrozole alone. While the specifics varied between trials, median PFS of up to 2 years (vs. approximately 1 yr) was achieved for combination therapy and, in some cases, overall response rate significantly increased. Overall response and clinical benefit outcomes also favored fulvstrant plus palbociclib over fulvestrant plus placebo in endocrine therapy-resistant disease, and some speculate that the CKD inhibitor

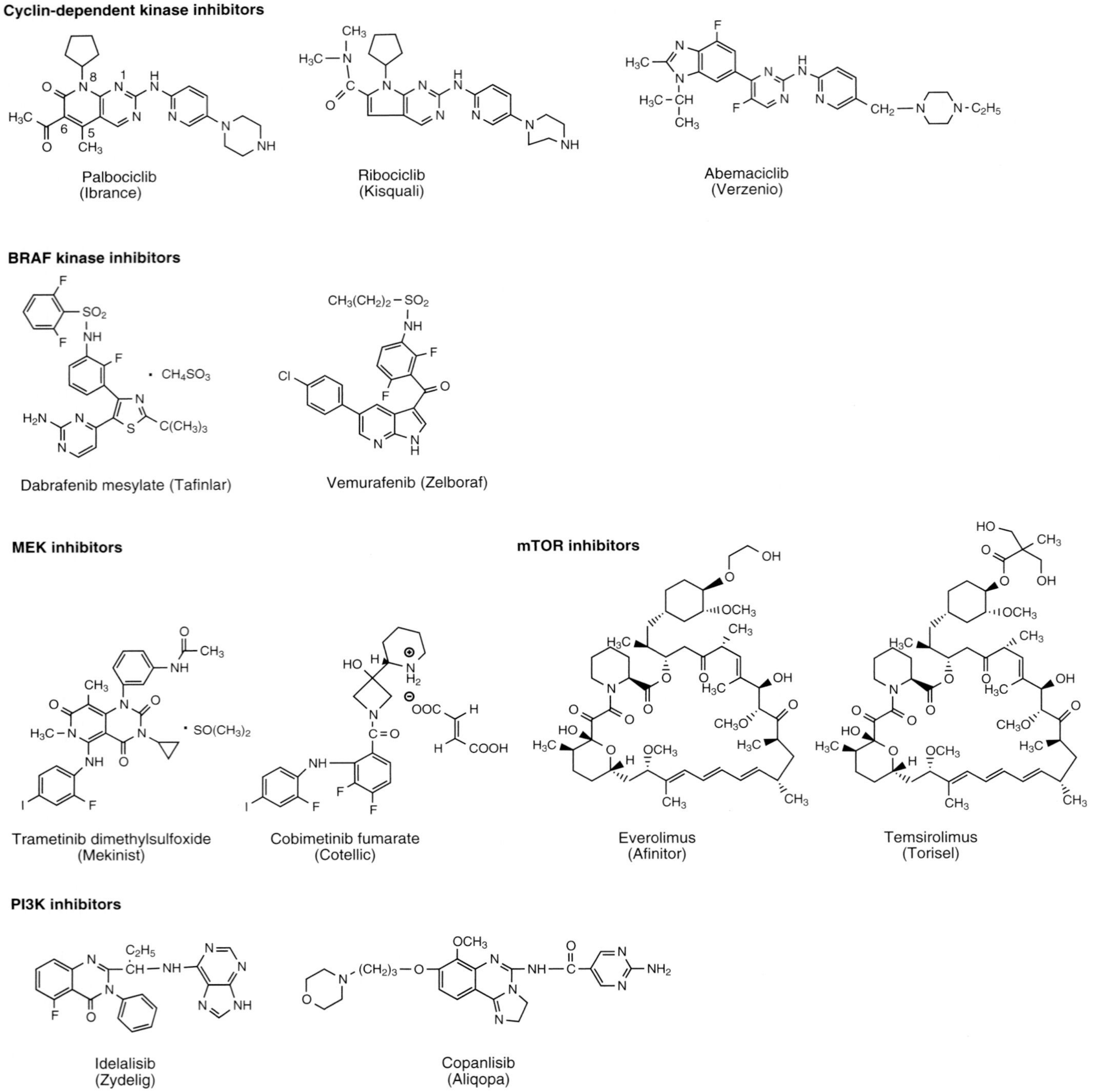

Cyclin-dependent kinase inhibitors

Palbociclib (Ibrance)

Ribociclib (Kisquali)

Abemaciclib (Verzenio)

BRAF kinase inhibitors

Dabrafenib mesylate (Tafinlar)

Vemurafenib (Zelboraf)

MEK inhibitors

Trametinib dimethylsulfoxide (Mekinist)

Cobimetinib fumarate (Cotellic)

mTOR inhibitors

Everolimus (Afinitor)

Temsirolimus (Torisel)

PI3K inhibitors

Idelalisib (Zydelig)

Copanlisib (Aliqopa)

Figure 33.12 Serine/threonine kinase inhibitors.

may reverse endocrine resistance. In preoperative studies, two weeks of palbociclib therapy significantly halted disease progression compared to placebo (58% vs. 10%).[210] The potential role of palbociclib in HR^+/$HER2^+$ MBC is currently being investigated.[213]

Palbociclib undergoes CYP3A4-mediated oxidation and phase 2 sulfonation to inactive metabolites. The sulfate conjugate is the major metabolite found in feces (26% of the administered dose). Coadministration of strong CYP3A4 inhibitors and inducers can alter AUC up to 87% (increase) and 85% (decrease), respectively, and, therefore, is not advised. Palbociclib is also a time-dependent 3A4 inhibitor.[214] Glucuronidation is a minor metabolic pathway but produces the major circulating metabolite, although fecal concentrations account for only 1.5% of the dose.

Ribociclib. In a phase III placebo-controlled clinical trial with HR^+/$HER2^-$ MBC patients, evaluation at 1.5 years documented that ribociclib in combination with letrozole provided significant increases in PFS (63% vs. 42.2%) and overall response (52.7% vs. 37.1%). There may be a synergistic action when mTOR inhibitors (discussed later in this chapter) are added to the ribociclib/aromatase inhibitor regimen.[210,212,215]

Table 33.7 CYP-Mediated Metabolism of Ser/Thr Kinase Inhibitors

Kinase Inhibitor	Reaction (Site)	Major Metabolizing CYP Isoform	Active CYP Metabolite?
Cyclin-Dependent Kinase Inhibitors			
Abemaciclib	N-dealkylation, hydroxylation	3A4	Yes (desethyl, hydroxylated, desethyl-hydroxylated)
Palbociclib	Not reported	3A4	No
Ribociclib	Not reported	3A4	Yes (LEQ803)
BRAF Kinase Inhibitors			
Dabrafenib	Hydroxylation, dealkylation (*t*-butyl)	3A4, 2C8	Yes (hydroxy- and desmethyl dabrafenib)
Vemurafenib	Aromatic hydroxylation (various), aliphatic hydroxylation (propyl)	3A4	Not investigated
MEK Inhibitors			
Cobimetinib	Aromatic, alicyclic hydroxylation, N-oxidation	3A4	No
Trametinib	No CYP metabolism	No CYP metabolism	NA
mTOR Inhibitors			
Everolimus	O-dealkylation, aliphatic/alicyclic hydroxylation (multiple sites)	3A4	No
Temsirolimus	O-dealkylation, aliphatic/alicyclic hydroxylation (multiple sites)	3A4	No
PI3K Inhibitors			
Idelalisib	Hydroxylation	3A4	No
Copanlisib	Oxidation (morpholine), ring opening (morpholine), O-dealkylation (C_8)	3A4, 1A1	Questionable significance clinical

Plasma concentrations of the main CYP3A4-generated active metabolite, known as LEQ803, represent approximately 10% of the dose, so the majority of the drug's activity is attributed to the parent structure. As with palbociclib, coadministration of strong CYP3A4 inhibitors or inducers should be avoided if at all possible. Minor metabolites are generated through oxidation and desaturation (M9) and oxygenation (M13) and, unlike palbociclib, there is no evidence of phase 2 sulfoconjugation. The drug inhibits CYP3A4 and possibly 1A2.[213,215]

Abemaciclib. Abemaciclib, the most recently approved of the three inhibitors, shows a preference for CDK4.[210] It has shown positive disease control results in several phase II and III clinical trials (most currently ongoing) when coadministered with aromatase inhibitors letrozol or anastrozole, or the antiestrogen tamoxifen. As noted earlier, abemaciclib may have benefit in treating patients who have advanced on previous endocrine therapy, particularly in combination with fluvestrant.[210]

CYP3A4 catalyzes the conversion of abemaciclib to N-desethyl (M2; 13%), hydroxylated (M18; 5%) and N-desethyl-hydroxylated (M20; 26%) metabolites that are all equally active with the parent drug.[216] Abemaciclib induces less neutropenia compared to palbociclib and ribociclib, potentially due to its preference for CDK4 (cyclin D1) versus CDK5 (cyclin D3). However, the risk of diarrhea is significantly higher (90% vs. 25%-35%), particularly with ongoing therapy and likely due to a lower level of drug absorption from the GIT.

Desethylabemaciclib (M2—major metabolite—active)

BRAF KINASE INHIBITORS. B-rapidly accelerated fibrosarcoma (BRAF) kinase is one component of a complex cell signaling system that also includes rat sarcoma (RAS), mitogen activated protein kinase (MEK or MAPK/ERK), and extracellular signal-regulated kinase (ERK), along with ARAF and CRAF. When activated through homo- or heterodimerization (e.g., BRAF-BRAF or BRAF-CRAF,

Table 33.8 Selected Pharmacokinetic and Therapeutic Properties of Ser/Thr Kinase Inhibitors

Kinase Inhibitor	Indication	Usual Adult Dose (mg/d)	T_{max} (hr)	$T_{1/2}$ (hr)	Oral Bioavailability (%)	Protein Binding (%)	Precautions
Cyclin-Dependent Kinase Inhibitors							
Abemaciclib	HR$^+$/HER2$^-$ MBC	300-400 (2 divided doses)	8	18.3	45	96	
Palbociclib	HR$^+$/HER2$^-$ MBC	125	6-12	29	46	85	
Ribociclib	HR$^+$/HER2$^-$ MBC	600	1-4	30-55		70	QT interval prolongation
BRAF Kinase Inhibitors							
Dabrafenib	Melanoma NSCLC TC	300 (2 divided doses	2	8 (parent)	95 High-fat meal ↓ T_{max}	>99	Dermatologic toxicities and malignancies possible Inhibits BCRP, OATP1B1 Induces CYP3A4
Vemurafenib	Melanoma	1920 (2 divided doses)	3	57		>99	Dermatologic toxicities and malignancies possible Inhibits CYP1A2, P-gp, BCRP
MEK Inhibitors							
Cobimetinib	Melanoma	60	2.4	44	95	46	Dermatologic malignancies, hemorrhage, cardiomyopathy and ocular toxicity possible
Trametinib	Melanoma NSCLC TC	2	1.5	4-5 d	72	97	Cardiac, pulmonary, and ocular toxicity possible
mTOR Inhibitors							
Everolimus	Advanced RCC HR$^+$/HER2$^-$ Advanced BC Neuroendocrine tumors	10	1-2	30	30 High-fat meal ↓ AUC (16%-22%)	74	Pulmonary toxicity, nephotoxicity, and mucositis possible
Temsirolimus	Advanced RCC	25 weekly (IV)	End of infusion	17	NA		Hyperglycemia, hyperlipidemia and pulmonary toxicity possible H_1 antagonist premedication required to minimize risk of hypersensitivity

Table 33.8 Selected Pharmacokinetic and Therapeutic Properties of Ser/Thr Kinase Inhibitors (Continued)

Kinase Inhibitor	Indication	Usual Adult Dose (mg/d)	T_{max} (hr)	$T_{1/2}$ (hr)	Oral Bioavailability (%)	Protein Binding (%)	Precautions
PI3K Inhibitors							
Idelalisib	CLL Small lymphocytic lymphoma Follicular B-cell non-Hodgkin lymphoma	300 (2 divided doses)	1.5	8.2	High-fat meal ↑AUC (40%)	≥84	**Boxed warning:** Potentially fatal hepatotoxicity, diarrhea, pneumonitis, infection and intestinal perforation Inhibits CYP3A4, P-gp, OATP1B1/1B3
Copanlisib	Relapsed follicular lymphoma	60	End of infusion	39.1	NA	84.2	Infection, hypertension and hyperglycemia possible

BC, breast cancer; CLL, chronic lymphocytic leukemia; HR, hormone receptor; IV, intravenous; MBC, metastatic breast cancer; NSCLC, non-small cell lung cancer; RCC, renal cell carcinoma; TC, thyroid cancer

respectively), BRAF phosphorylates MEK, which then phosphorylates ERK. The end result is regulation of cellular functions that support viability and controlled growth.[217,218]

Oncogenic BRAF mutants are present in several human malignancies, including approximately 50% of melanomas, 24%-45% of thyroid cancers, and some lung cancers. The V600E mutant that represents approximately 90% of the oncogenic transformations allows the kinase to function in both dimeric and monomeric forms, as well as to ignore feedback inhibition prompts from phosphorylated ERK. The result is a loss of control of homeostatic signaling in the malignant cells and, in turn, tumor proliferation. In cultured melanocytes, the V600E mutation is known to "addictively" activate the MAPK pathway, and promote malignant transformation both in vitro and in vivo.[219]

Chemistry. The currently available BRAF kinase inhibitors vemurafenib and dabrafenib are type I1/2. They bind to the active conformation of the enzyme as it relates to the DFG motif (DFG-in), but the conformation of a structural component called the αC-helix is "out," rather than "in" (as it is in classical type I inhibitors). Once the inhibitor binds to one of the enzymes in the dimer and induces the αC-out conformation, the αC-helix of the second enzyme shifts to the "in" conformation, which inhibits additional drug binding.[217] Interestingly, while BRAF kinase inhibitors block the action of the V600E mutant, they activate wild type BRAF and, in turn, ERK cellular action. Thus, cancer patients prescribed these agents must express the mutant kinase, and the drugs should be avoided in patients who do not.

The structures of the two BRAF kinase inhibitors currently marketed show distinct structural similarities (Fig. 33.12). The heteroaromatic pyrrolopyridine (vemurafenib) or aminopyrimidine (dabrafenib) ring accesses the hinge region adenosine site where ATP normally binds, placing the difluorinated (vemurafenib) or monofluorinated (dabrafenib) ring in the adjacent hydrophobic pocket. The sulfonamide moiety with its attached fluorinated phenyl ring inserts into another site known as the type I pocket, which contains the regulatory Phe595 of the DFG motif. The thiazole ring of dabrafenib binds within the domain that normally accommodates the ribose of the nucleotide substrate, and the *p*-chlorophenyl moiety of vemurafenib is solvent exposed.[217] A graphic illustrating dabrafenib binding to the kinase is provided in Figure 33.13.

Intrinsic resistance to BRAF kinase inhibition runs at approximately 20%. Acquired resistance to BRAF inhibitors that target the V600E mutation normally

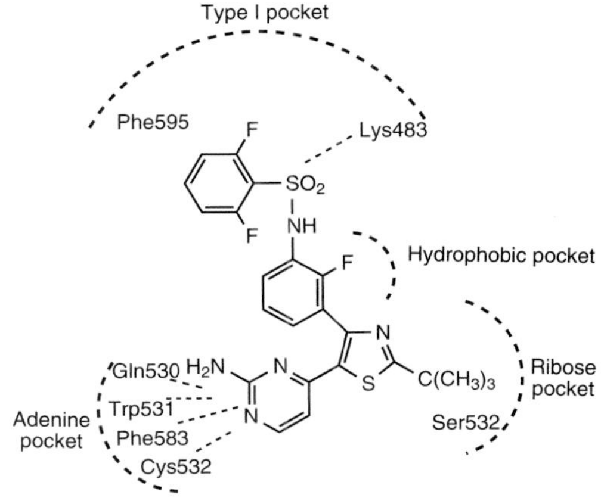

Figure 33.13 Binding interactions between BRAF kinase and dabrafenib.

develops within a year's time, with altered homo- or heterodimeric signaling, re-activation of the MAPK signaling pathway, and/or splice variants of the mutant believed responsible.[217-219] Approaches to providing a more sustained therapeutic response from BRAF kinase inhibitors include combination therapy with MEK inhibitors (e.g., trametinib, discussed later in this chapter) and/or checkpoint inhibitor antibodies targeting CTLA-4 (ipilimumab) or PD-1(nivolumab) (Table 13.3). Promising outcomes in preclinical studies and clinical trials are hoped to translate into positive survival benefits for patients.

Specific Drugs

Vemurafenib and Dabrafenib Mesylate (Fig. 33.12). Both of these BRAF kinase inhibitors have shown clinical benefit compared to cytotoxic chemotherapy (dacarbazine) in the treatment of advanced, unresectable melanoma that carries the BRAF V500E mutation.[220] Melanoma is an aggressive disease that is responsible for approximately 75% of skin cancer deaths.[221] Phase III trials have documented response rates of 48%-50% compared to 5%-6% for dacarbazine, along with a decreased risk of death and tumor progression and an increase in PFS.

Dabrafenib is also employed in thyroid carcinoma and NSCLC that is BRAF V6003 positive and, regardless of indication, is always given in combination with the MEK inhibitor trametinib. In a small phase II clinical trial in patients with advanced or metastatic anaplastic thyroid cancer, dabrafenib plus trametinib provided an overall response rate of 69%, and the 1-year estimates of median duration of response, PFS and OS were 90%, 79% and 80%, respectively.[222] The documented value of dabrafenib plus trametinib in the treatment of NSCLC has been recently reviewed.[223]

Both drugs are vulnerable to CYP3A4-mediated metabolism, and CYP2C8 also plays a role in dabrafenib biotransformation. Vemurafenib is minimally metabolized, but does undergo hydroxylation at various positions on the aromatic rings and on the propyl chain adjacent to the sulfonamide, with subsequent glucuronidation.[224]

Dabrafenib's metabolic pathway yields three primary metabolites, hydroxydabrafenib (short lived), carboxydabrafenib (most abundant in plasma with time) and desmethyldabrafenib. Conversion of carboxydabrafenib to the desmethyl metabolite is proposed to proceed via non-enzymatic, pH-dependent decarboxylation facilitated by the adjacent thiazole nitrogen atom (Fig. 33.14).[225] The hydroxy and desmethyl metabolites, while less potent than the parent drug, are believed to contribute to the therapeutic action of dabrafenib.[225] While the dabrafenib parent has a half-life of 8 hours, the active desmethyl metabolite's half-life extends to 21-22 hours.[76]

Dabrafenib is a moderate inducer of CYP3A4 and a weak inducer of CYP2C9; appropriate precautions should be taken when considering drug coadministration. Vemurafenib only weakly inhibits CYP3A4, but caution is still indicated if strong 3A4 inducers or inhibitors must be coadministered. Both drugs are P-gp substrates and BCRP inhibitors.

An adverse effect of note when these BRAF inhibitors are used in the treatment of melanoma is their ability to

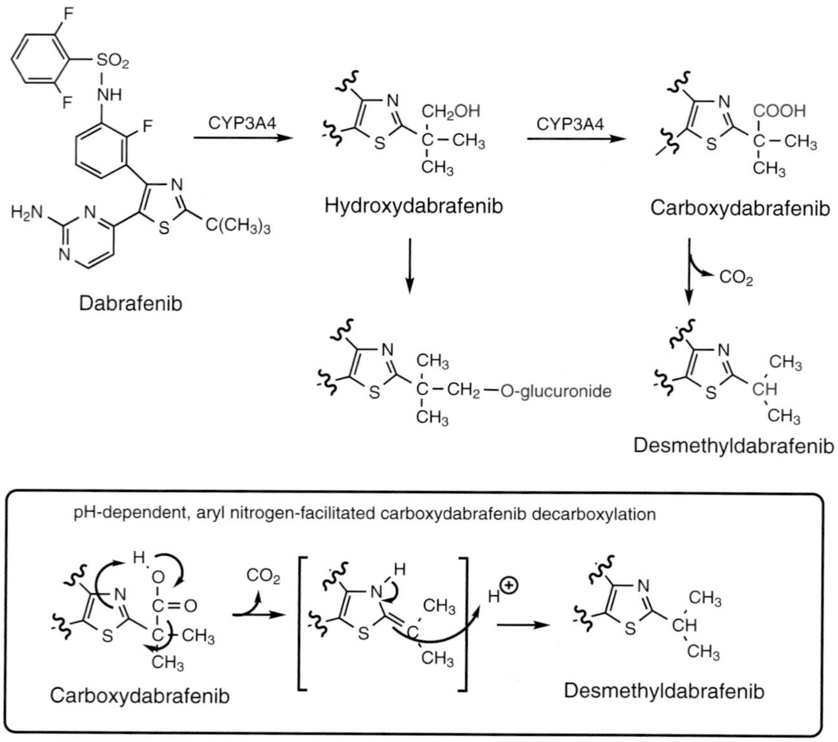

Dabrafenib — CYP3A4 → Hydroxydabrafenib — CYP3A4 → Carboxydabrafenib

Hydroxydabrafenib → $C-CH_2-O$-glucuronide

Carboxydabrafenib → (CO_2) → Desmethyldabrafenib

pH-dependent, aryl nitrogen-facilitated carboxydabrafenib decarboxylation

Carboxydabrafenib → (CO_2) → [intermediate] → ($H^{\oplus}$) → Desmethyldabrafenib

Figure 33.14 Dabrafenib metabolism.

induce dermatologic malignancies, including squamous cell carcinoma and keratoacanthoma. The cause of this serious toxic effect is the "paradoxical activation" of CRAF in established keratinocytic lesions with wild type BRAF. These secondary malignancies usually appear within the first 2-3 mo of therapy. Surgical intervention may be required, and the risk:benefit of drug discontinuation should be considered.[217,219]

MEK INHIBITORS (FIG. 33.12). The pivotal role of the MAPK/ERK (MEK) in the complex RAS-initiated signaling cascade has been described above, as has the value of MEK inhibition in extending the therapeutic life of BRAF kinase inhibitors (see BRAF Kinase Inhibitors section).

Chemistry. The currently marketed MEK inhibitors target MEK1 and MEK2 (MEK1/2) and are type III enzyme antagonists. That is, they bind within an allosteric site adjacent to the adenine site and do not directly compete with ATP. An X-ray crystal structure of cobimetinib bound to activated (ATP-bound) MEK1 is known, and was used to develop a model of trametinib-MEK1 binding. Models of cobimetinib and trametinib binding to MEK2 have been published.[226]

Models of trametinib binding to MEK1[58,221] predict positioning of the pyridopyrimidinedione within the allosteric pocket where the pyridine carbonyl oxygen can H-bond with Val211 and Ser212 (Fig. 33.15). Lys97 binds with a pyrimidinedione carbonyl oxygen, and the fluorinated/iodinated phenyl ring inserts into a hydrophobic pocket within the allosteric site. The acetamide carbonyl oxygen interacts with cationic Arg189. Hydrophobic and van der Waals bonding with several aliphatic and aromatic residues within the αC-helix and C-lobe activation segment of the kinase (where two Ser residues are phosphorylated during kinase activation) occurs.[221]

Cobimetinib lacks the heteroaromatic pyridopyrimidinedione ring system of trametinib, and important interactions include H-bonding between an aromatic fluorine with Ser212 and the carbonyl oxygen with Lys97 in the allosteric site[226] (Fig. 33.15). Asp190 and a γ-phosphate oxygen from ATP interact with the piperidine N-H and also form stabilizing bonds with the OH on the azetidine ring.[221,227] Asn195 from the catalytic loop also bonds to the azetidine-OH, reinforcing the importance of this moiety to pharmacologic activity.[221] Hydrophobic and van der Waals interactions within the αC-helix and activation segment are known to occur and served as the prediction model for the interactions with trametinib.[221] While not shown in the figure, it may be that cobimetinib's unrestrained fluorinated/iodinated phenyl ring accesses the hydrophobic pocket of the allosteric site in the manner predicted for trametinib's identical ring, as the affinity of cobimetinib for activated MEK1 is high (IC_{50} = 0.9 nM).[228] The *S* isomer has approximately 10 times the activity of the *R* enantiomer.[227]

Intrinsic and acquired resistance to MEK inhibitors may be linked to phosphatidylinositol 3-kinase/protein

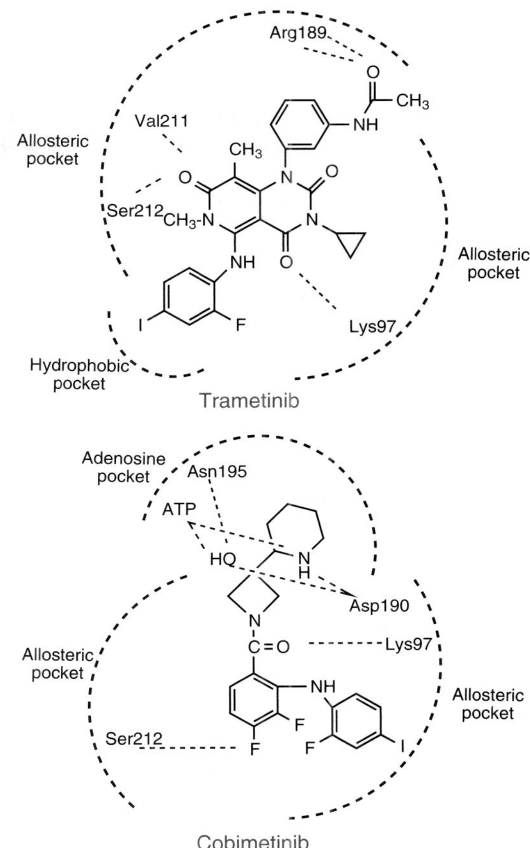

Figure 33.15 Binding interactions between MEK1 and inhibitors trametinib and cobimetinib.

kinase B (PI3K/AKT) activation, as well as to the previously discussed reactivation of the MAPK signaling pathway.[229,230]

Specific Drugs

Trametinib Dimethylsulfoxide and Cobimetanib fumarate. While documented to be effective when used alone in the treatment of BRAF V600E mutated melanoma, trametinib is most commonly coadministered with the BRAF kinase inhibitor dabrafenib to metastatic melanoma, NSCLC, and thyroid cancer patients whose tumors express this mutant (see section on dabrafenib, above). Clinical trials have shown significantly positive clinical outcomes, including survival, for the combination therapy compared to BRAF kinase inhibitor monotherapy. For example, in a multicentered study of patients with stage IV NSCLC, the overall response to combination therapy increased from 27% (dabrafenib alone) to 60%, and median PFS rose from 5.5 to over 9 months.[228]

Cobimetinib is indicated only in unresectable or metastatic melanoma with BRAF V600E mutation and is coadministered with the BRAF kinase inhibitor vermuafenib. Like trametinib, it has shown positive results in extending PFS and can stimulate renewed clinical response in BRAF kinase–resistant cancer.[221,228,230] Both of these agents are in clinical trials to evaluate efficacy in a wide range of solid tumor and hematologic malignancies,[221] and several new structurally related MEK inhibitors are currently in active development.[228]

The major trametinib biotransformation reaction is conversion to the desacetylated metabolite, M1. M1 is approximately equipotent with the parent, although it may not contribute significantly to therapeutic action. Some molecules of this metabolite will be hydroxylated in a CYP-independent fashion (M3), and fewer will form the N-glucuronide (M2). The parent drug is the predominant entity in plasma and feces. Trametinib is retained in "deep compartments" and eliminated slowly over the course of several days.[231] Although cobimetinib also undergoes significant amide cleavage (followed, in this case, by glycine conjugation), the molecule and its hydrolyzed metabolite are extensively biotransformed by CYP3A4 to multiple hydroxylated or N-oxidized metabolites, none of which are significantly active.[232]

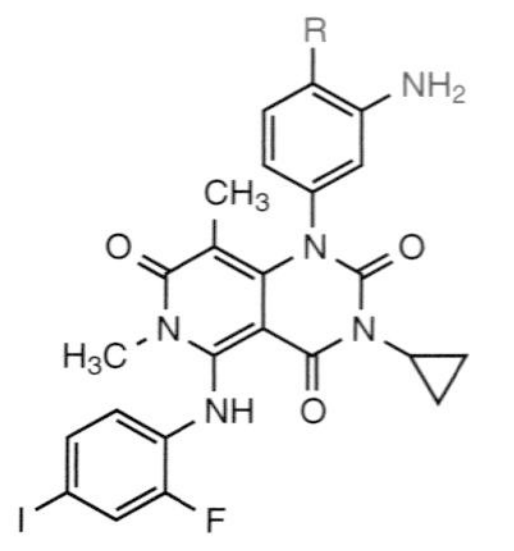

Trametinib deacetylated metabolites (M1; R = H: M3; R = OH)

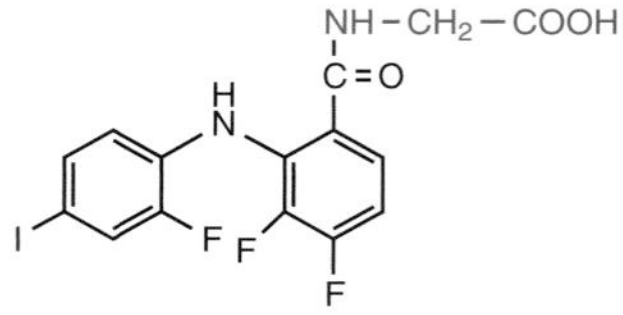

Glycine conjugate of hydrolyzed cobimetinib

While trametinib and cobimetinib are claimed to be fairly well tolerated, adverse effects of rash, GI distress, dermatologic reactions, and elevated blood pressure can commonly occur.

mTOR INHIBITORS (FIG. 33.12). Mammalian target of rapamycin (mTOR) is a component of the PI3K/AKT/mTOR signaling pathway, and like the pathways discussed previously, it is intimately involved in regulating cellular homeostasis. When activated, mTOR phosphorylates kinases that ultimately result in the de novo synthesis of proteins (including VEGF) that stimulate angiogenesis and promote cellular growth. When system control is lost, commonly through the dysfunction of a genetic inhibitor of the PI3K pathway (*PTEN*), cellular proliferation is unchecked and differentiation is lost; i.e., cancer results.

The systems and tissues most commonly impacted by PI3K/AKT/mTOR dysregulation are neuroendocrine, kidney, and breast.[233] Blocking key enzymatic elements of this malignancy-promoting supercharged signaling pathway (e.g., inhibiting mTOR and PI3K) have proven valuable in the treatment of cancers driven by this dysregulated system. The two marketed mTOR inhibitors, everolimus and temsirolimus, are O13 analogues of rapamycin (also known as sirolimus), an antibiotic isolated from soil. In addition to being antiproliferative, this macrolide is also immunosuppressive, a property shared by the structurally related mTOR inhibitors.[234]

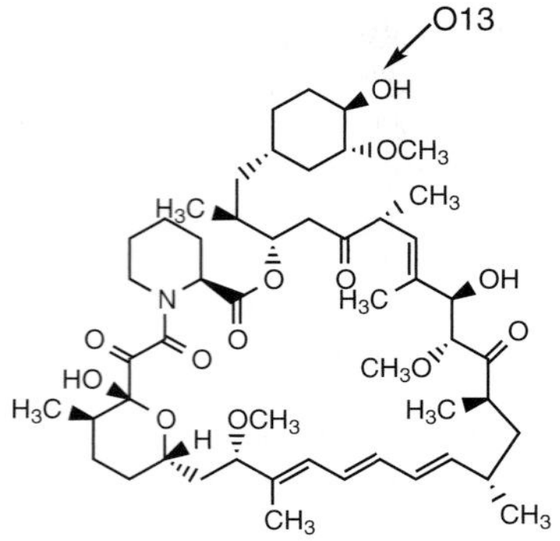

Rapamycin (Sirolimus)

CHEMISTRY. The kinase domain of the 289-kd mTOR protein resides in the C-terminal area, with the 100-residue macrolide-binding domain (known as FKBP12-FRB) located just to its N-terminal side. The ATP-binding hinge region common to all kinases joins the C- and N-terminal lobes. mTOR forms two complexes (mTORC1 and mTORC2) that serve distinct functions; regulating cell growth and promoting cell survival, respectively.[234]

Rapamycin binds tightly to FKBP12-FRB and, by burrowing into a deep "gap" between these proteins, promotes an interaction that is not observed in the absence of the macrolide. This inhibits the ability of the kinase to function. Van der Waals interactions with a number of Tyr, Phe, and Trp residues in the FKBP12 domain, along with H-bonds with Asp and Tyr side chains promotes high-affinity binding between inhibitor and enzyme. Hydrophobic interactions between the carbon-rich macrolide and the kinase are known to occur and are the only interactions believed to form with the FRB domain.[25] Rapamycin is 92% buried when bound to these two mTOR domains, and only O13 (the site of modification in the commercially available rapamycin-based inhibitors), C40, and C41 (of the cyclohexane ring) contact the surrounding environment. The polar nature of the O13 ester and alcoholic substituents of temsirolimus and everolimus would promote solubility in these aqueous fluids.

mTOR inhibitors bind to the allosteric FKBP12-FRB domain of mTORC1, which is adjacent to the catalytic ATP-binding domain. Hence, they fit the definition of type III kinase inhibitors. Once bound, they prevent a regulatory protein (called regulatory-associated protein of mTOR, or "raptor") from binding to the complex. Cell growth is arrested at the G1 phase, and inhibition of hypoxia-inducible factors (HIF) resulting from mTOR blockade halts angiogenesis by attenuating levels of VEGF and PDGF.[233,234] While selective for mTORC1 at therapeutic doses, in high concentrations, the inhibitors may inhibit both complexes via a process that does not involve FKBP12.[234]

The *MTOR* gene is vulnerable to mutation, leading to changes in the kinase structure that induce mTOR inhibitor resistance. Alterations in the rate of phosphorylation of the S6K1 protein, which happens after normal mTOR activation, is another harbinger of resistance, as it indicates tumor-driven "work arounds" of normal signaling pathways. A multitude of other resistance mechanisms, including "survival-promoting signaling feedback loops," have been identified.[234]

Specific Drugs

Everolimus. Everolimus is indicated in solid tumors that have progressed on first-line therapy. In advanced renal cell carcinoma no longer responsive to VEGFR kinase inhibitors sunitinib and sorafenib, everolimus has been shown to increase PFS by 2 months compared to placebo. A "head-to-head" comparison of everolimus and sunitinib as first-line therapy confirmed the appropriateness of the current use of everolimus post sunitinib (or sorafenib) failure. In $HR^+/HER2^-$ breast cancer resistant to the aromatase inhibitors letrozole and anastrozole, everolimus plus exemestane (another aromatase inhibitor) increased median PFS by 4.1-6.9 months compared to exemestane plus placebo. Everolimus has demonstrated a similar PFS benefit in patients with advanced neuroendocrine tumors and is used in aggressive tumors of the pancreas, GIT, and lung.[233] A meta-analysis of the outcome of 32 clinical trials of mTOR inhibitor use in other solid tumor malignancies (either alone or in combination with other agents) showed disappointing results.[235]

Metabolically, everolimus is hydroxylated and O-dealkylated by CYP3A4 at several positions around the macrolide, and coadministration of strong 3A4 inducers or inhibitors should be avoided.[233] Cleavage of lactone functional groups can also occur, and a novel phosphocholine ester metabolite has been identified.[236] As noted previously, in addition to other commonly observed kinase inhibitor adverse effects (e.g., fatigue, rash, GI distress), everolimus is immunosuppressive, explaining its use in renal transplantation for rejection prophylaxis. It is orally active and available in tablet and soluble tablet forms.

Temsirolimus. In contrast to orally active and poly-indicated everolimus, temsirolimus is used IV in the treatment of just one malignancy, advanced RCC. Clinical trials comparing temsirolimus alone, interferon alone, and combination therapy showed the highest survival benefit from the mTOR inhibitor as a single agent, particularly in patients with at least three conditions that normally predict a poor prognosis.[233] IV administration allows doses to be kept low enough to attenuate immunosuppression risk.[237] The drug has no ionizable functional groups and must be solubilized for IV administration with polysorbate 80 (Tween). This solubilizer can induce a hypersensitivity reaction that can manifest as hypotension and breathing difficulties, so patients must be pretreated with an H_1 antagonist (e.g., diphenhydramine) before each administration. Drug discontinuation and supportive therapy are required in the event of a hypersensitivity reaction.

Temsirolimus is hydrolyzed to sirolimus (rapamycin), which retains the activity of the parent and has a significantly longer elimination half-life (55 vs. 17 hr).[237] Additional CYP3A4-catalyzed hydroxylation, dealkylation, and N-oxidation reactions occur (along with lactone cleavage), but none of the metabolites retain therapeutically relevant activity. Only six of the 15 CYP-generated metabolites are considered major,[238] and the same precautions noted for everolimus regarding coadministration of strong CYP3A4 inhibitors and inducers apply. Patients on temsirolimus can experience hyperglycemia and serum cholesterol and triglyceride elevations.

Lipid Kinase Inhibitors

PHOSPHATIDYLINOSITOL 3 KINASE INHIBITORS (FIG. 33.12). The rationale for the use of inhibitors of PI3K was laid out in the mTOR inhibitor discussion above. PI3K is a lipid kinase family composed of three classes and several subtypes, and they are the most frequently mutated kinase enzymes in neoplastic disease. The class I_A kinases that are the targets of currently marketed inhibitors are heterodimers with a catalytic subunit known as p110 (α, β, or δ) and a regulatory p85 subunit.

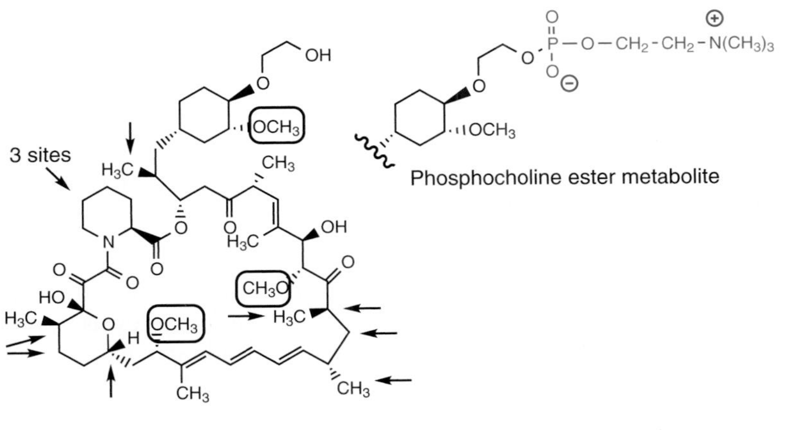

3 sites

Phosphocholine ester metabolite

Sites of everolimus 3A4-catalyzed hydroxylation (arrows) and dealkylation (boxes)

They phosphorylate phosphatidylinositol bisphosphate (IP_2) to generate the second messenger inositol triphosphate (IP_3) which, in turn, phosphorylates AKT and mTOR. PI3K inhibitors are of the type II variety. Those which interact selectively with p110δ (PI3Kδ inhibitors such as idelalisib) adopt a "propeller conformation", where the two aromatic moieties are oriented at right angles to one another.[239]

Idelalisib (propeller conformation)

Chemistry. PIK3 inhibitors are commonly built around a quinazoline or related heteroaromatic scaffold. The proposed binding of idelalisib with PI3Kδ is shown in Figure 33.16.[58,239] Val828 and Glu826 are important H-bonding residues in the hinge region and interact with the purine ring that seeks out the ATP-binding site (adenine pocket). The fluorinated quinazolinone aromatic system induces an allosteric "specificity pocket" that is hydrophobic in nature and fits tightly within it. The phenyl substituent seeks out its own hydrophobic pocket near the solvent region.

As noted above, the three Class I_A PI3K subtypes are α, β, and δ. PI3Kδ is found predominantly in blood cells, and inhibition leads to serious immunosuppression and infection risk. PI3Kα is involved in glucose metabolism and associated with neoplastic cells. PI3Kβ is associated with platelet activation and more likely to be found in cancer cells deficient in the tumor suppressor PTEN (the product of the *PTEN* gene).[240]

Unlike the PI3Kδ-specific inhibitor idelalisib, the second molecule in the class to be marketed, copanlisib, is a "pan PI3K" inhibitor, although it has the highest affinity for the α and δ subtypes.[240,241] Copanlisib was rationally designed to exhibit strong binding to the catalytic site, as well as within all allosteric pockets.[240] Key SAR findings, along with binding interactions with PI3Kγ, are shown in Figure 33.17.

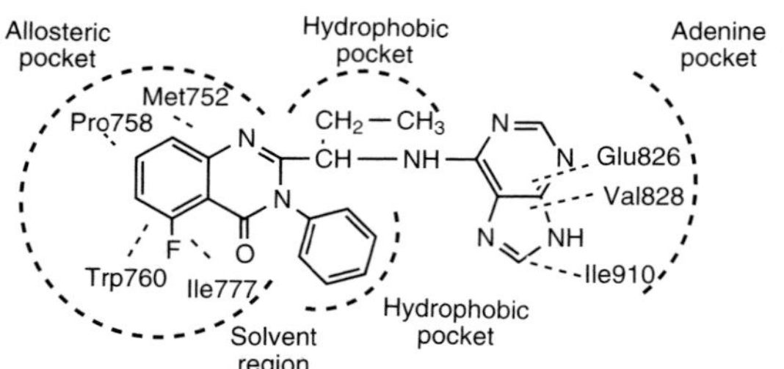

Idelalisib (type II inhibitor)

Figure 33.16 Binding interactions between PI3Kδ and idelalisib.

The resistance story now familiar with all kinase inhibitors can be told of the PI3K inhibitor structures. Neither agent is approved for first-line therapy due to indirect (feedback) activation of alternative signaling pathways and mechanism-dependent and -independent toxicities. Idelalisib and copanlisib are CYP3A4 and P-gp substrates, and idelalisib is a strong inhibitor of both (the former through its inactive metabolite).[242]

Specific Drugs

Idelalisib. Idelalisib is a PI3Kδ selective inhibitor with a 30-fold higher affinity for this protein compared to other class I_A subtypes.[241] The δ subtype is a key player in B-lymphocyte signaling and extensively expressed in cancers of B-cell origin. It is used orally in various relapsed or refractory leukemias and lymphomas, sometimes in combination with immunotherapy.

In relapsed CLL, idelalisib is coadministered with rituximab, and the combination has demonstrated partial response rates of up to 81% and an overall 1-year survival of 91%, compared with 13% and 80%, respectively for rituximab alone. Median PFS at 1 year was 66% (combination) vs. 13% (MAb alone), and idelalisib retained efficacy in the face of genetic mutations.[242] The drug is used alone in refractory small lymphocytoic and follicular B-cell NHL. An international phase II trial in refractory B-cell lymphomas documented an overall response rate of 57%, and a median PFS and OS at 9.7 months of 11 and 20.3 months, respectively, as well as a median 12.5 month duration of response.[243]

Aldehyde oxidase is the primary metabolizing enzyme of idelalisib, generating the inactive circulating imidazolinone metabolite GS-563117. CYP3A4 plays a relatively minor role in idelalisib metabolism (19%), as does phase 2 glucuronidation (7%).[244] None of these minor metabolites is found plasma.[245]

GS-563117 (Idelalisib inactive metabolite)

Idelalisib is both a substrate and an inhibitor of CYP3A4, and coadministration of other 3A4 inhibitors can increase serum levels by almost 2-fold (79% increase in AUC), leading to excess toxicity of a drug that already carries a boxed warning for several potentially fatal adverse effects. Conversely, the drug's AUC can drop by 75% in the presence of CYP3A4 inducers, leading to a loss of therapeutic efficacy. Appropriate precautions are warranted.[242,246] Prescribers of idelalisib must be REMS certified.

Copanlisib. Like the mTOR inhibitor temsirolimus, copanlisib is administered IV and is indicated in a single neoplastic disease; relapsed follicular lymphoma that has failed on at least two other regimens. As noted earlier,

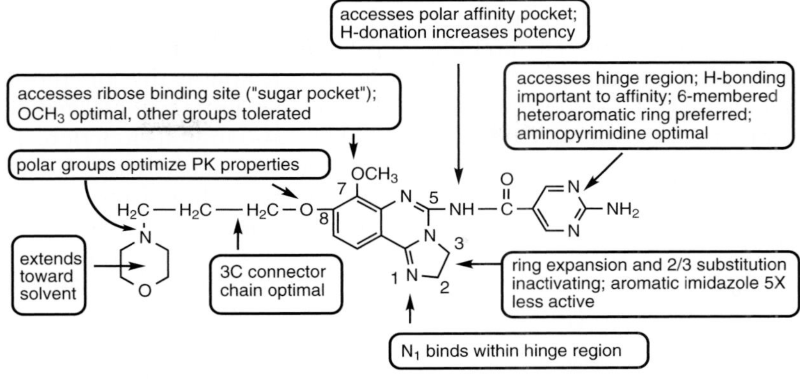

Copanlisib SAR

Solvent channel · Ribose pocket · Polar affinity pocket · Trp812 · Solvent region · Val882 · Lys833 · Asp836 · Asp841 · Asp964 · Adenine pocket

Copanlisib-PI3Kγ interactions

Figure 33.17 Copanlisib SAR and binding to PI3Kγ.

this PI3K inhibitor has its highest affinity for the δ and α subtypes; the former being the subtype targeted by idelalisib and the latter potentially being upregulated in idelalisib-resistant lymphoma.[247] Unlike idelalisib, copanlisib carries no boxed warnings and has a lower risk of serious adverse effects, although hypertension occurs in about a third of patients receiving the drug.

A multisite international phase II clinical trial of copanlisib in relapsed B-cell lymphoma patients who have failed on rituximab and cytotoxic chemotherapy (DNA alkylating agent), 47% achieved a partial response while 12% documented a complete response to therapy. In patients with follicular lymphoma, the partial and complete response rates were 44% and 14%, respectively, and the median duration of response was 12.2 months with a median PFS of 11.2 months.[247]

Copanlisib is vulnerable to CYP3A4-mediated metabolism, generating a number of oxidized, dealkylated and morpholine ring-opened metabolites in fairly small amounts (1%-12% of the dose). Therapy should be closely monitored if the coadministration of drugs impacting CYP3A4 expression/activity cannot be avoided. The only circulating metabolite is the morpholine lactam (M1). Although equipotent to the parent, it represents only 5% of drug exposure and is, therefore, of questionable clinical relevance. Unchanged copanlisib is the compound found in highest concentration in excretia.[248]

M1 (Copanlisib active, but clinically irrelevant, metabolite)

Nonkinase-Targeted Enzyme/Protein Inhibitors

IDH1/2 Inhibitors

Isocitrate dehydrogenase 2 (IDH2), an $NADP^+$-dependent enzyme active in the tricarboxylic acid (TCA) cycle, converts isocitrate to α-ketoglutarate and generates NADPH and, in so doing, promotes mitochondrial oxidative respiration. Mutations in mitochondrial IDH2 or its cytosolic isozyme IDH1 (collectively referred to as IDH1/2) are found in approximately 20% of patients diagnosed with AML and drive the neoplastic process.[249,250]

CHEMISTRY. Oncogenic IDH1 mutations occur at the highly conserved Arg132 (e.g., R132H)[251] while, at IDH2, positions 172 and 140 are involved (R172K, R140Q).[252] The guanidinium moiety of the Arg residues in the wild-type enzymes stabilizes β-carboxyl addition in the interconversion of isocitrate and α-ketoglutarate, and loss of this critical residue shifts the product formed by the aberrant enzymes to β-hydroxyglutarate (2-HG). IDH mutants are unable to convert isocitrate to α-ketoglutarate.[250,252]

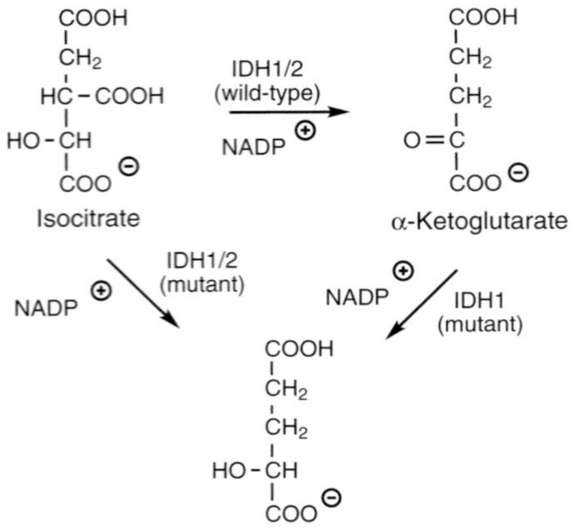

Isocitrate

α-Ketoglutarate

2-Hydroxyglutarate

IDH enzymes normally exist as homodimers, and mutant IDH enzymes retain the ability to dimerize with wild-type proteins which, in the case of IDH1 mutants, has been proposed to facilitate reduction of α-ketoglutarate to 2-HG. The ability of IDH2 mutants to catalyze this reaction is unknown.[252] Regardless of how it forms, 2-HG accumulates in the cancer cell at concentrations over 100 times normal and serves as an oncometabolite by hypermethylating DNA and histones, inhibiting cellular differentiation, and dysregulating homeostatic biochemical pathways.[252] The "epigenetic signature" of IDH1/2 mutants in AML involves cytosine 5-methylation throughout the genome.[251,253]

Inhibiting mutant IDH with targeted chemotherapy has revolutionalized the treatment of AML in patients harboring IDH mutations, and spared those eligible for therapy from the often intolerable adverse effects associated with cytotoxic chemotherapy. That was their only option until the arrival of the IDH2 inhibitor enasidenib to the U.S. market in 2017, followed by the IDH1 inhibitor ivosidenib in 2018. Now, quality of life and, at least for some, OS statistics have improved.

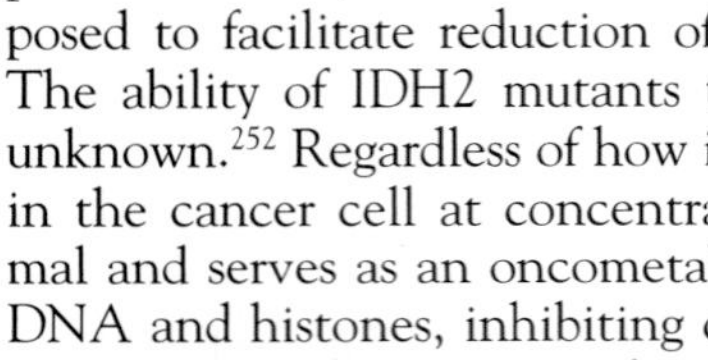

Enasidenib (Idhifa)

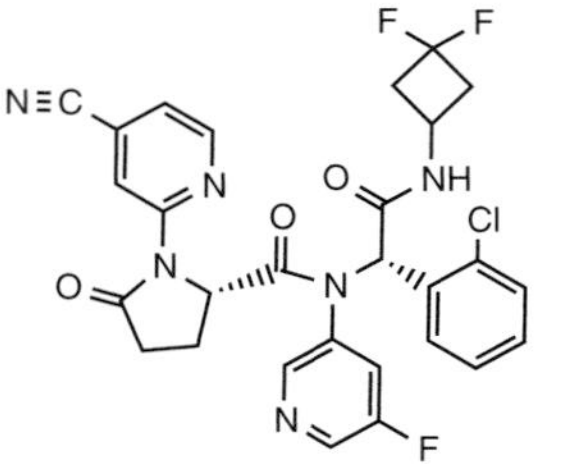

Ivosidenib (Tibsovo)

Enasidenib. IDH2 mutants are more commonly encountered in AML than IDH1 mutants (8%-19% vs. 7%-14%, respectively).[250] Enasidenib, a weakly basic and selective IDH2 inhibitor, binds to the divalent cation binding region at the juncture of the IDH2 dimer, forcing an open protein conformation which lowers affinity for $NADP^+$ and inhibits function. The affinity for the mutant enzyme is 40 times that of the wild-type, promoting tumor selectivity.[249] Phase I trials have demonstrated the drug's ability to inhibit 2-HG formation by as much as 90.6% and restore cellular differentiation.

While results of phase III trials are pending, in a phase II trial of 239 AML patients on 100 mg enasidenib once daily, 19.3% with relapsed/refractory disease achieved complete remission for a median of 8.8 months. The median OS for this cohort was 9.3 months (19.7 mo for those who achieved complete remission) and 1 year survival was estimated at 39%. One-year overall AML survival statistics prior to the introduction of enasidenib ranged from 10% to 50%. While enasidenib intervention produced positive outcomes in patients with very few viable options, the relatively low remission rate clearly communicates that there is much research left to be done to optimize its therapeutic value.[250]

Hyperbilirubinemia and nausea were among the most common adverse effects experienced by patients on enasidenib, although some experienced tumor lysis syndrome (characterized by altered levels of serum electrolytes and nitrogenous compounds released by destroyed cells). IDH differentiation syndrome (characterized by fluid redistribution leading to edema and effusions) was also experienced by 11.7% of the patients in the aforementioned phase II study and is responsible for a boxed warning for this drug. While potentially fatal, IDH differentiation syndrome generally responds to glucocorticoids (e.g., dexamethasone) and hemodynamic monitoring.

Enasidenib (100 mg daily) has a T_{max} of 4 hours, a half-life of around 5.7 days, and an absolute oral bioavailability of 57%.[250] N-dealkylation by a wide variety of CYP isoforms generates an active metabolite (AGI-16903) which accounts for 10% of the circulating drug concentration. Both the parent drug and metabolite are highly protein bound. Several glucuronidating isoforms are involved in phase 2 metabolism, and biliary excretion predominates over renal (89% vs. 11%). Unchanged drug accounts for 34% and 1% of the dose eliminated in feces and urine, respectively.[76,250] No significant drug-drug interactions have been reported.

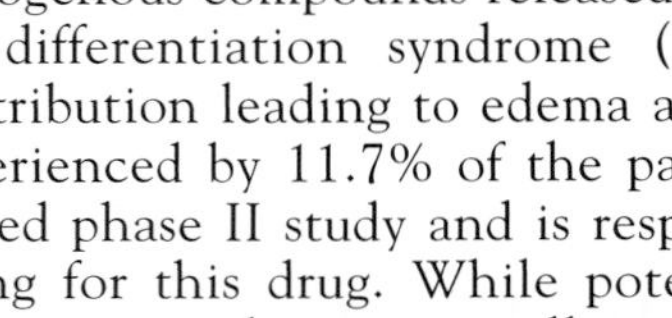

AGI-16903

Ivosidenib. Ivosidenib, an IDH1 inhibitor FDA-approved in July 2018, is used orally in the treatment of relapsed/refractory AML in patients expressing mutated

IDH1. It is a strong inhibitor of 2-HG synthesis and promotes differentiation and maturation of malignant cells.[254] It was the first such inhibitor to be shown effective in clinical trials and was specifically designed for enhanced metabolic stability compared to precursor leads. Specifically, stable *o*-Cl and difluorocyclobutyl moieties replaced oxidatively vulnerable *o*-CH_3 and cyclohexyl groups, respectively, and a 1-(4-cyano-2-pyridyl)pyrrolidine-2-one ring system was employed in lieu of metabolically labile 2-methylimidazole.[255]

The standard dose of ivosidenib is 500 mg (two 250 mg tablets) once daily for a minimum of 6 months. Clinical trials have documented sustained remission in patients with advanced *IHD1*-mutated AML with a low risk of serious adverse effects. In a pivotal trial, complete remissions were obtained in 21.6% of the study population with a median duration of approximately 9 months.[254]

Ivosidenib is rapidly absorbed and has a prolonged half-life of 3-6 days.[254] While CYP3A4 is known to play a metabolic role, the parent drug is the major entity found in plasma and is excreted predominantly unchanged in feces. The most serious toxicity is IDH differentiation syndrome (boxed warning, similar to enasidenib and similarly managed). QT interval prolongation, leukocytosis, fatigue, rash, GI distress, and respiratory events (e.g., dyspnea, cough) are the most commonly encountered adverse effects.

BCL-2 Inhibitors

B-cell lymphoma-2 (BCL-2) is an antiapoptotic protein associated with cell survival, and dysregulation of its normal biochemical pathway to augment expression is common in hematological malignancies, including CLL. High levels of BCL-2 in CLL cells block the action of apoptosis mediator proteins BAX and BAK, leading to mitochondrial membrane stabilization and cellular immortality. BCL-2 arrests cells in the G_0 phase, which also contributes to its oncogenic potential.

BH3-only proteins, a BCL-2 subfamily, are BCL-2 inhibitors and BAX/BAK facilitators and are induced under cellular stress. They are also vigorously expressed in CLL cells but sequestered by BCL-2. BCL-2 inhibitors, by binding to the protein as BH3 mimetics, displace apoptotic BAX and BAK proteins, allowing them to realize their cell-killing purpose.[256] Some have hypothesized that BH3 profiling may help identify CLL patients most likely to respond to BCL-2 inhibitor therapy.[249,257]

The mutant IDH enzymes discussed previously promote a BCL-2 dependent state within AML cells. While the one BCL-2 inhibitor currently on the market (venetoclax) is indicated only in CLL patients with a chromosome17p deletion in the tumor suppressor gene *TP53*, clinical trials are ongoing to evaluate its potential use in IDH2-mutated AML and other hematologic cancers.[249,258,259] Interestingly, despite the indication, one study found the therapeutic action of venetoclax in CLL was independent of 17p deletion and tumor suppressor gene *TP53* mutation and TP53 function.[257]

VENETOCLAX

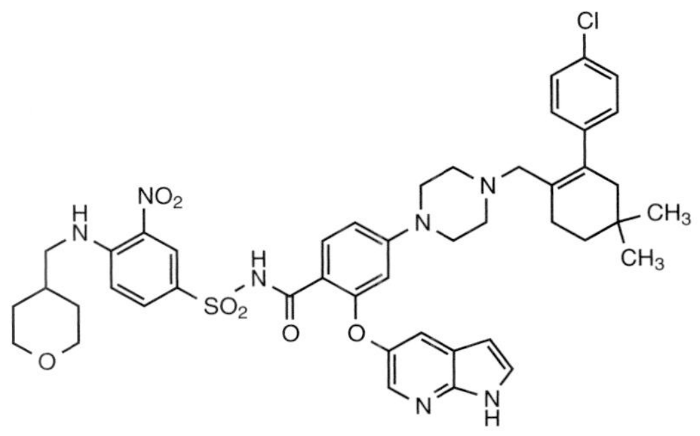

Venetoclax (Venclexta)

As noted above, venetoclax binds directly to the BCL-2 protein in the manner of BH3 and liberates the apoptotic BAX and BAK proteins that restore cancer cell mortality.[256] Binding interactions of importance include hydrophobic tethering through the *p*-chlorophenyl and dimethylcyclohexene rings, as well as an electrostatic interaction between an anionic center on venetoclax (potentially the sulfonylbenzamide moiety) and cationic Arg103 of the protein.[258]

Clinical trials have shown that ventoclax works quickly to restore apoptotic processes in CLL patients, and is associated with high response rates whether used alone or in combination with the MAb rituximab.[257,258] A phase II trial with 107 CLL patients with relapsed/refractory disease and who carried the *TP53* 17p chromosome deletion (a poor prognosis predictor) found overall and complete response rates of 79% and 8%, respectively. The median time to complete response was 8.2 months.[260]

Venetoclax's lack of affinity for a related antiapoptotic protein (BCL-X_L) decreases the potential for thrombocytopenia which plagued a precursor BCL-2 inhibitor, navitoclax. Adverse effects observed most frequently include diarrhea, neutropenia, fatigue, upper respiratory tract infections and cough. The risk of potentially fatal tumor lysis syndrome can be lessened by incrementally increasing the daily dose from 20 mg (initial) to 400 mg (maintenance) over 5 weeks in accordance with a recommended schedule.[258]

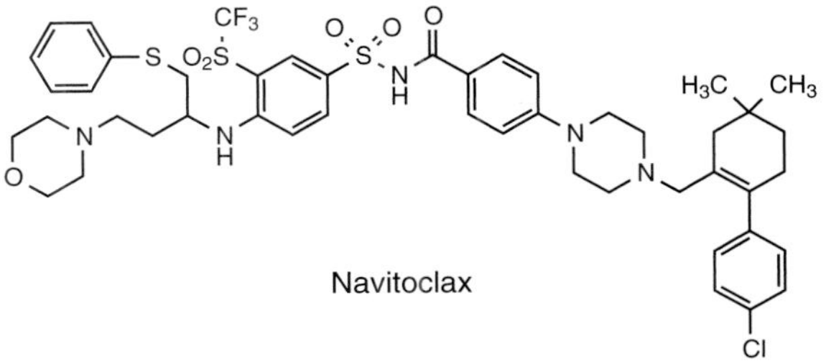

Navitoclax

The half-life of venetoclax runs between 19 and 26 hours and the T_{max} is 6-8 hours.[259] It is strongly protein bound. CYP3A4 hydroxylation at position 6 of the cyclohexene ring followed by cyclization generates a significantly less active metabolite (M27) that represents 30% of total drug concentration at the 400 mg maintenance dose.[261] The route of elimination is almost exclusively biliary, with 21% of the drug being excreted unchanged in feces. Venetoclax is also a P-gp substrate, and the coadministration of CYP3A4 inducers or inhibitors, as well as P-gp inhibitors, should be avoided.

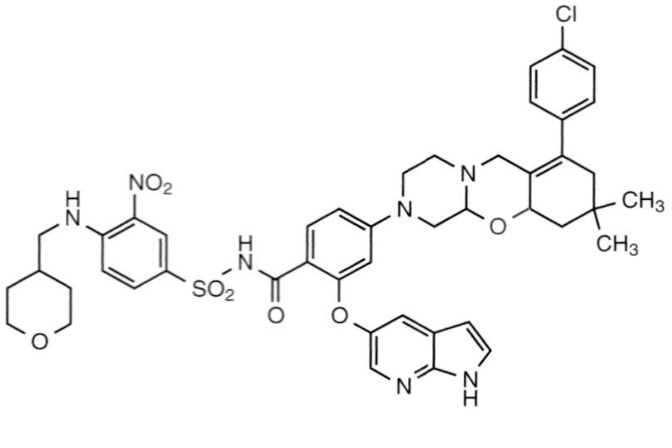

M27 (Venetoclax active metabolite)

While not officially listed by the National Institute for Occupational Safety and Health as a hazardous drug, venetoclax may be teratogenic and damaging to reproductive organs. It should be handled with extreme care, and gloves should be worn during drug administration. Tablets should be swallowed whole (never crushed or chewed) and taken with food and water at approximately the same time each day.[76]

PARP Inhibitors (Fig. 33.18)

Poly(ADP-ribose) polymerase isozymes PARP1 and PARP2 are active in the repair of DNA that has suffered single-strand breaks or base excision. Damaged DNA recruits these enzymes, which bind via a zinc finger moiety and cleave NAD^+ into nicotinamide and ADP-ribose, which is then extensively polymerized. At some point, a conformational change in PARP allows its disengagement, leaving the final repair process to other biochemical entities that have been summoned to the scene by the polymerized ADP-ribose.[262,263]

If PARP activity is inhibited, single-strand breaks progress to double-strand breaks, which will kill the cell if not repaired by a process called homologous recombination (HR). Tumors harboring homozygous mutated *BRCA1* and *BRCA2* genes have deficient HR repair capabilities and are incapable of righting the damaged DNA ship. Thus, PARP inhibitors have found value in treating cancers characterized by these genetic mutations (e.g., ovarian and breast cancers). This is an example of "synthetic lethality," in which two independently nonlethal entities (PARP inhibitors and mutated *BRAC*) become lethal in combination.[262] Importantly, mutated *BRAC* found in healthy cells is generally heterogyzous with the wild-type enzyme, which allows DNA repair to proceed in the presence of PARP inhibition. This promotes tumor cell selectivity and attenuates the risk of use-limiting adverse effects.[262]

Acquired resistance to PARP inhibitors undermines long-term therapeutic benefits and shortens survival. Resistance mechanisms are multifaceted and the focus of intense research. Restoration of HR DNA repair capability via secondary reversion mutations in *BRAC1/2* is believed to be the most common path to resistance, and excessive activation of an alternative repair process (nonhomologous end-joining) also plays a role. Two other strategies that cancer cells employ to thwart PARP inhibitor–induced apoptosis involve the upregulation of P-gp that expels the inhibitors and RAD51, an essential HR-associated protein.[262,264]

CHEMISTRY. The currently marketed PARP inhibitors mimic the nicotinamide component of the NAD^+ substrate. The benzamide moiety binds to the nicotinamide binding domain on PARP, and the optimal *s-trans* conformation is promoted through incorporation into a ring (olaparib, rucaparib) or via an intramolecular H-bond (niraparib). The aromatic sidechain seeks out the adenosine-ribose binding pocket, with *m*- and *p*-substituents showing favorable binding compared to *o*-substituents. A variety of substituents are tolerated. Insertion of a fluorine atom at the *m*-position of the side chain phenyl (olaparib), as well as *m* to the carboxamide (rucaparib), promotes

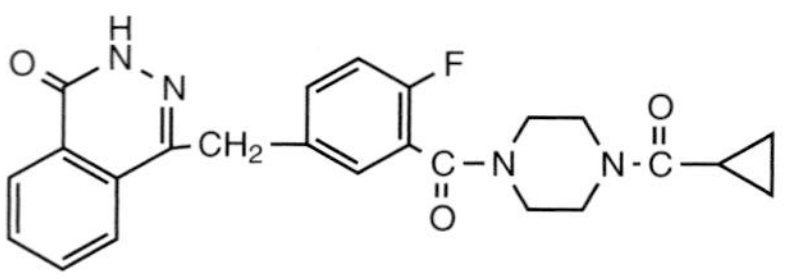

Olaparib (Lynparza)

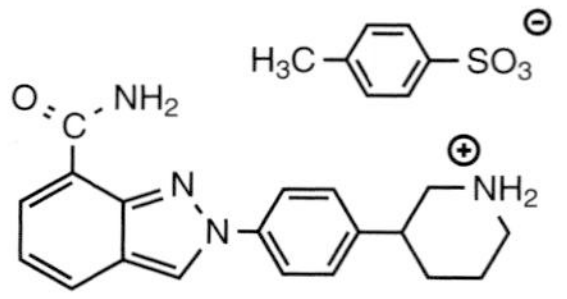

Niraparib tosylate (Zejula)

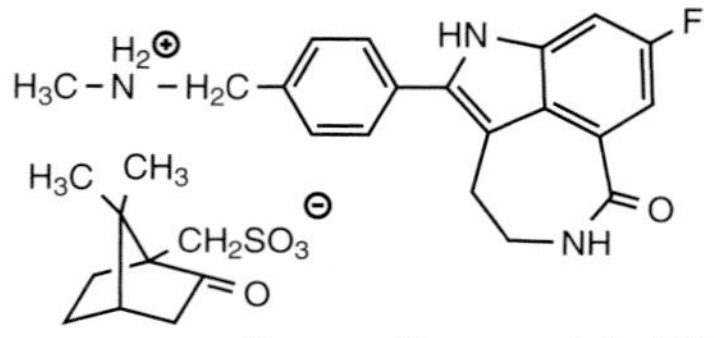

Rucaparib camsylate (Rubraca)

Figure 33.18 PARP inhibitors.

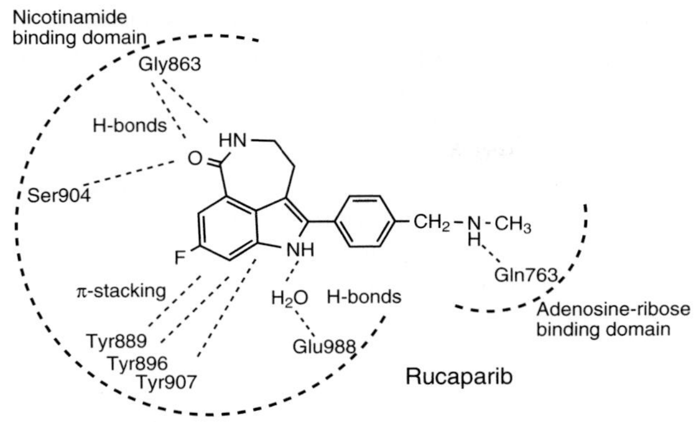

Figure 33.19 PARP1-rucaparib binding interactions.

activity.[265] A cocrystal of PARP1 bound to rucaparib has been solved, and specific binding interactions identified (Fig. 33.19)[263]

SPECIFIC DRUGS (FIG. 33.18). Ovarian cancer claimed over 14,000 U.S. lives in 2017, and almost 22.5 thousand women received this diagnosis that year.[266] Since this malignancy is usually well advanced when discovered, survival statistics are dismal. Platinum-based chemotherapy is considered first-line treatment, but PARP inhibitors are now available for use in patients who have failed on that therapy and/or as maintenance therapy in patients who have completely or partially responded. The results of clinical trials of the three marketed PARP inhibitors, administered as mono- or combination therapy, have been recently reviewed.[267] These drugs are potential teratogens and reproductive system toxins and must be handled with significant care. Selected pharmacokinetic properties of the PARP inhibitors are provided in Table 33.9.

Olaparib. In addition to epithelial and germline ovarian cancers with mutated *BRAC1/2*, olaparib can be used in HER$^+$ MBC that carries these mutations. The tablet formulation is used in breast cancer patients and ovarian cancer patients on maintenance therapy (300 mg twice daily), while capsules or tablets are used in advanced ovarian disease (400 mg and 300 mg, respectively, both twice daily).

The clinical trial that prompted FDA approval of olaparib included 193 patients with advanced ovarian cancer. These patients achieved a median PFS of 7 months, a median OS of 16.6 months, and a tumor response rate of 31%. GI distress and fatigue were the most common adverse effects.[267] Myelosuppression, peripheral edema, and rash are also possible with this agent.

Olaparib is extensively biotransformed by CYP3A4 into a number of oxidized metabolites of unknown activity. The metabolites are readily excreted, often as glucuronide or sulfate conjugates, leaving the unchanged drug as the primary circulating entity. Coadministration of drugs or foods known to be moderate-strong inducers or inhibitors of CYP3A4 can impact serum levels of active drug and should be avoided.[268] In addition to grapefruit juice, consumption of Seville oranges and juice (which contain naringin, one of the intestinal CYP3A4-inhibiting compounds in grapefruit) is contraindicated. Olaparib is also a P-gp substrate.

Rucaparib. Rucaparib has the same ovarian cancer indications as olaparib, and the tablet formulation is dosed on a 600 mg twice daily basis. The pivotal clinical trials in patients with advanced ovarian cancer who progressed on at least two prior chemotherapy regimens (and which prompted FDA-approval) demonstrated an 80%-86% response rate, with adverse effects qualitatively similar to olaparib.[269,270]

Unlike olaparib, CYP3A4 plays a minor role in rucaparib metabolism. Phase 1 biotransformation is catalyzed primarily by CYP2D6, although hepatic turnover of the parent drug is low.[271] Likely for that reason, 2D6 phenotype does not impact steady state plasma concentrations.[270]

Table 33.9 Selected Pharmacokinetic Properties of PARP Inhibitors

PARP Inhibitor	T_{max} (hr)	$T_{1/2}$ (hr)	Bioavailability (%)	Protein Binding (%)	Excretion (%)
Niraparib	≤3	36	73	83	Renal (48) Fecal (39)
Olaparib	1.5 (tablet) 1-3 (capsule)	14.9 (tablet) 11.9 (capsule)	Tablet > capsule High-fat meal delays absorption	82	Renal (44) Fecal (42)
Rucaparib	1.9	17-19	36 High-fat meal ↑ AUC, delays T_{max}	70	Fecal (≥79)

Niraparib. Naraparib, the third PARP inhibitor to be approved by the FDA, is indicated for maintenance treatment of recurrent epithelial ovarian cancer patients who have responded to platinum-based chemotherapy.[272] Clinical trials have demonstrated its ability to prolong median PFS and decrease progression risk.[273] Unlike the other two agents, its use is independent of *BRAC* mutation status. It is available as capsules and administered in 300 mg daily doses. The dose can be reduced in 100 mg daily increments if unacceptable toxicity occurs. In addition to the adverse effects mentioned above, approximately 20% of patients will experience drug-induced hypertension.

Niraparib is not a CYP substrate. It is metabolized by carboxyesterase to the inactive carboxylic acid, which is excreted as the glucuronide conjugate.[273]

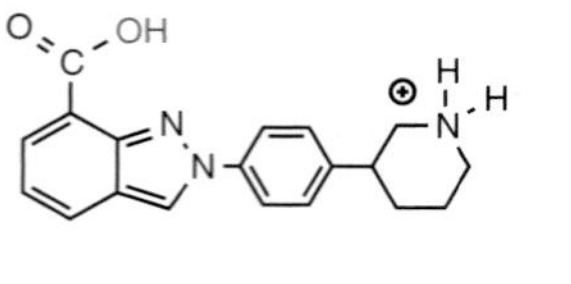

Niraparib carboxylic acid metabolite (inactive)

Proteasome Inhibitors (Fig. 33.20)

Facilitated by ubiquitin tagging, proteasomes selectively clear cells of cytoplasmic regulatory proteins by cleaving them into short peptides. The 26S proteasome serves as the recognition site for doomed ubiquitinated proteins. Through the action of an ATP-dependent 19S regulatory unit, they are transferred to the 20S "core particle" proteolytic domain (a chamber from which there is no escape) for destruction. The β-OH group of the N-terminal threonine residue (Thr1) serves as the proteolytic nucleophile responsible for peptide bond cleavage.[274]

Inhibition of this homeostatic process through the blockade of the 20S proteasome induces apoptosis via a build-up of aged or conformationally altered proteins.[275] It was originally proposed that suppression of nuclear factor-κB was involved in the apoptotic mechanism, but that hypothesis is now under scrutiny.[276,277] Two dipeptide proteasome inhibitors (bortezomib and ixazomib) are reversibly acting boronic acid derivatives, and the third (carfilzomib, an epoxyketone) was designed for irreversible 20S proteasome inhibition.

CHEMISTRY. The crystal structure of the bortezomib-20S proteasome complex from yeast has been reported and specific drug-proteasome interactions with the chymotrypsin-like site (also known as the β5 subunit) identified (Fig. 33.21).[278] The phenylmethyl moiety of the Phe component of the dipeptide inserts into a proteasome pocket but does not interact with the protein, so its loss in ixazomib is tolerated. Ixazomib has chlorine atoms in the same relative position as bortezomib's pyrazine nitrogen atoms. Since Asp114 is proposed to interact in free acid form with one unionized bortezomib pyrazine nitrogen, an electron-rich chlorine can serve the same binding function. The boronic acid moiety is essential to the proteasome-specific action of the reversible inhibitors, as CYP-mediated deboronation of bortezomib yields an inactive metabolite.

More recently, the human 20S proteasome bound to the irreversible proteasome inhibitor carfilzomib has been crystallized (Fig. 33.21).[274] Unlike bortezomib and ixazomib, this inhibitor shows high selectivity for the chymotrypsin-like (β5) site (vs. the trypsin- (β2) and caspase-like (β1) sites) of constitutive proteasomes. The nucleophilic β-OH of Thr1 attacks the electrophilic epoxyketone at the carbonyl carbon and the electron-deficient oxirane carbon alkylates the terminal NH_2, forming an adduct where drug and enzyme are covalently joined through a newly

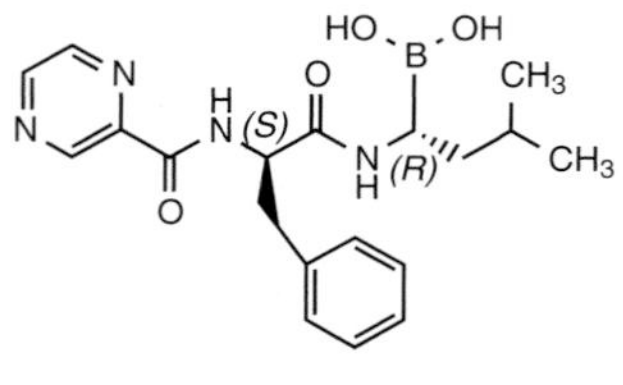

Bortezomib (Velcade)

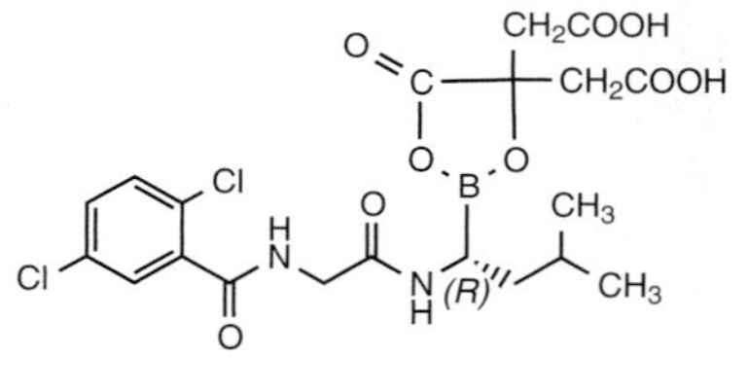

Ixazomib citrate (Ninlaro)

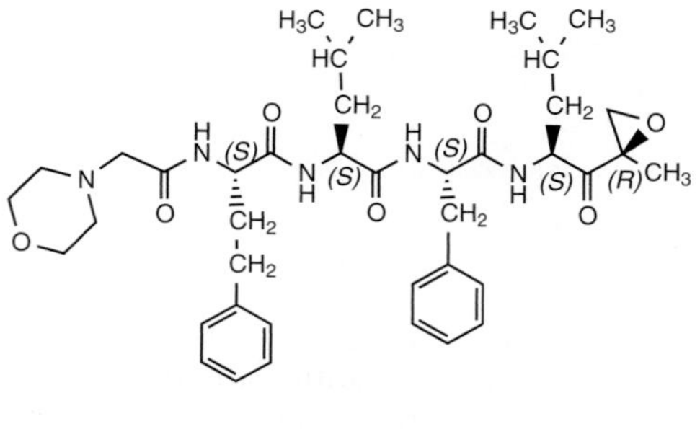

Carfilzomib (Kyprolis)

Figure 33.20 Proteasome inhibitors.

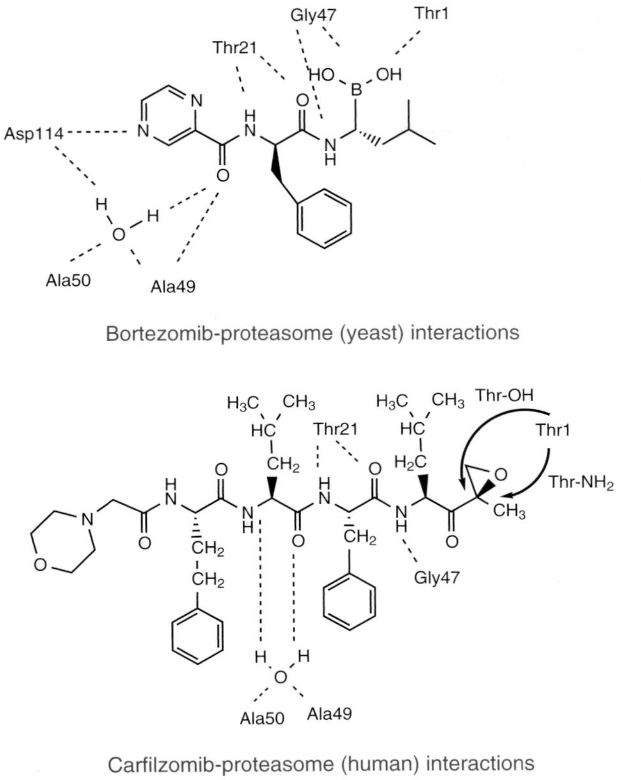

Bortezomib-proteasome (yeast) interactions

Carfilzomib-proteasome (human) interactions

Figure 33.21 Proteasome-inhibitor interactions.

generated morpholine ring. Like the phenylmethyl of bortezomib, the morpholine ring on the N-terminal end of the parent drug does not bind to any proteasome residues.

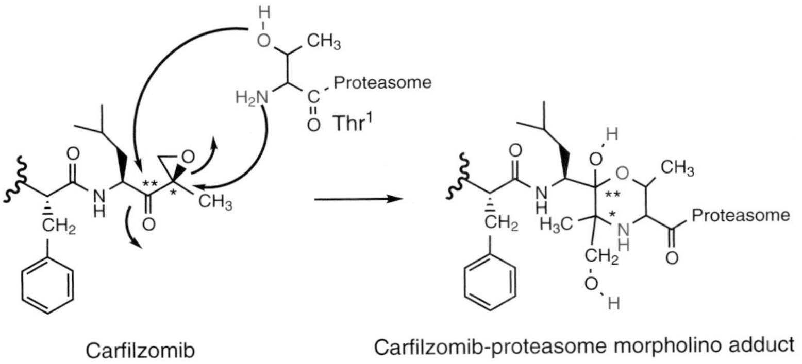

β5 subunit gene (e.g., A40T, A50V), altered expression of β5 ubiquitin-proteasome pathway proteins, induction of homeostatic heat shock (cell repair) proteins, and P-gp upregulation have all been implicated.

Bortezomib. Bortezomib is used IV (1 mg/mL concentration) or SC (2.5 mg/mL concentration) in the treatment of multiple myeloma and MCL. Because it can be fatal if delivered intrathecally, it should not be given at the same time as drugs administered by this route. While the initial dose of 1.3 mg/m^3 applies to both IV and SC administration, providers should take care that dosing calculations are based on the appropriate concentration for the prescribed route.[279] The drug is administered either twice weekly for the first two weeks of a 3-week regimen, or once weekly in a 4-week regimen. Bortezomib as first-line therapy in MCL is administered IV, but either the IV or SC route is acceptable in relapsed disease.

Phase III trials have documented superior PFS and OS statistics with bortezomib versus dexamethasone in refractory multiple myeloma. Similar survival benefits to the above were observed when bortezomib was added to melphalan/prednisone in newly diagnosed patients,[279] and it also prolongs life when used with the immunomodulatory lenalidomide and dexamethasone in this population.[280] Based on these trials, bortezomib combination therapy is considered the "standard of care" for newly diagnosed multiple myeloma patients.[280]

Following inactivating deboronization, bortezomib is hydroxylated at various positions prior to excretion. The CYP isoforms involved in the biotransformation include primarily CYP3A4 and CYP2C19, although the 1A2 and 2D6 are also involved to a minor extent. Like many other

Carfilzomib

Carfilzomib-proteasome morpholino adduct

SPECIFIC DRUGS. The marketed proteasome inhibitors are all used in multiple myeloma, an incurable hematologic cancer that is most common in older individuals who are least likely to tolerate cytotoxic chemotherapy. By inhibiting the 20S proteasome, these drugs impair homeostatic clearance of cellular proteins whose time has come, and they induce fatal endoplasmic reticular stress by rendering the malignant cells incapable of managing the high amounts of mis-folded immunoglobulin produced. Apoptosis results.[276] As with many targeted therapies, resistance can manifest. Bortezomib resistance has been the most intensely studied, and point mutations in the

anticancer agents, the drug suppresses bone marrow leading to neutropenia and thrombocytopenia and can induce serious sensory (and less commonly motor) peripheral neuropathy. Use-limiting neuropathy is less common with the SC route of administration[279] and can often be managed with dose reduction, although drug discontinuation is required with grade 4 dysfunction. In addition to GI distress, cardiac and pulmonary complications have also been reported, including left ventricular ejection fraction dysfunction, arrhythmia, and acute respiratory distress syndrome.

Ixazomib Citrate. Ixazomib is an orally active analogue of bortezomib used in combination with lenalidomide and dexamethasone in multiple myeloma patients who have progressed on at least one prior therapy. It is available in capsule form and initially dosed at 4 mg once per week for the first three weeks of a 4-week cycle. The extended 9.5 day half-life permits the once-weekly dosage regimen. Doses should be reduced sequentially to 3 mg or, if needed, 2.3 mg if adverse drug reactions occur. The oral bioavailability is 58% and peak plasma concentrations are achieved in approximately 1 hour. Administration with a high-fat meal can decrease AUC and C_{max} by 28% and 69%, respectively so the drug should be taken no later than 1 hour before, or no earlier than 2 hours after, eating.

Ixazomib's affinity for the chymotrypsin-like (β5) site of the 20S proteasome is higher than for the β1 and β2 sites, and it dissociates from this site significantly faster than bortezomib (half-life of 18 vs. 110 min.), leading to better tissue penetration properties. Compared to bortezomib, the maximum plasma concentration is 19 times greater, the AUC slightly more than two times higher, and protein binding more extensive (99% vs. 83%).[277,281]

Ninlaro capsules contain ixazomib citrate, a prodrug that rapidly provides the active boronic acid when exposed to an aqueous environment.[277,281] It acts synergistically with dexamethasone and retains efficacy in bortezomib-resistant disease.[279] The clinical trial resulting in FDA approval demonstrated the superior survival outcomes when ixazomib was added to a lenalidomide/dexamethasone regimen in patients with relapsed/refractory multiple myeloma. The positive survival benefits impacted all subgroups, including elders, previously treated, advanced disease, and/or genetically high-risk patients. As with bortezomib, GI distress was the most common adverse effect. Myelosuppression also occurred but peripheral neuropathy was less problematic, likely due to ixazomib's higher selectivity for the β5 site.[277]

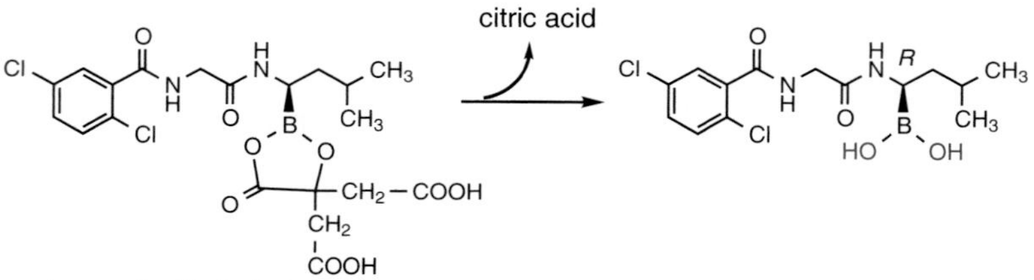

Carfilzomib. Carfilzomib is administered IV and dosed in accordance with the patient's body surface area and the prescribed regimen. It is used in refractory/relapsed disease either as monotherapy or in combination with lenalidomide and/or dexamethasone, and has demonstrated positive response and survival outcomes in patients unresponsive or intolerant to bortezomib and lenalidomide.[279] Clinical trials have documented superiority to bortezomib in terms of efficacy and adverse effect profile; for example, one trial documented a 50% increase in PFS, increased OS, and less use-limiting peripheral neuropathy with carfilzomib (vs. bortezomib) in combination with dexamethasone.[279] The complete response rates in newly diagnosed patients administered lenalidomide/dexamethasone/carfilzomib therapy has been described as "unprecedented."[281] Although there is a lower incidence of serious peripheral neuropathy, myelosuppression, fatigue and GI distress, along with serious cardiovascular and pulmonary toxicity, can occur.[281]

From a pharmacokinetic standpoint, carfilzomib has a short plasma half-life due to covalent bonding to the β5 site of the 20S proteasome. The C_{max} is over 37 times that of bortezomib and it is 97% protein bound. Carfilzomib is not metabolized to any appreciable extent by CYP enzymes but is extensively transformed by peptidase-catalyzed cleavage and epoxide hydrolysis prior to excretion.[76]

An orally active carfilzomib analogue, oprozomib, has shown promise in clinical trials. As an epoxyketone, it is an irreversible 20S proteasome inhibitor, but additional studies in larger patient populations are needed to determine what place it will have in the treatment of multiple myeloma. In addition, a structurally unrelated proteasome inhibitor that crosses into the CNS (marizomib) is under clinical investigation for multiple myeloma and may show value in other hematological and solid tumor malignancies.[283]

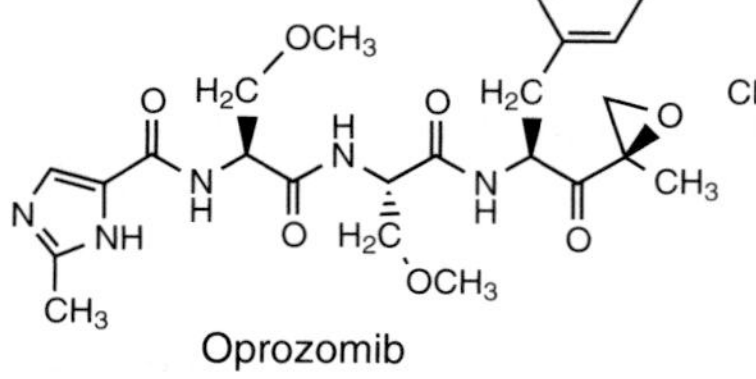

citric acid

Ixazomib citrate (prodrug)

Ixazomib (active)

Ixazomib is metabolized by a wide variety of CYP and non-CYP enzymes, and the oxidatively deboronated hemiaminal (M1) is the major metabolite. The parent drug is the most predominant entity in plasma, and excretion of the metabolites is both renal (62%) and biliary (22%). Less than 3.5% of the dose is excreted as unchanged drug in urine.[282]

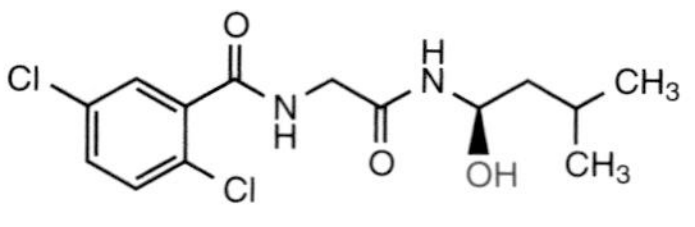

Ixazomib hemiaminal metabolite (M1)

Oprozomib

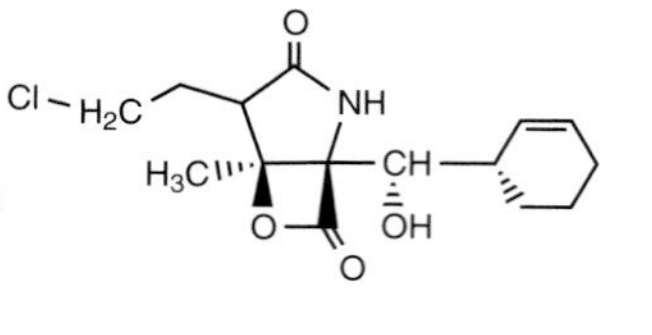

Marizomib

Hormone-Based Antineoplastic Agents (Representative)

Structures that modulate the activity of estrogen and androgen receptors or influence levels of circulating hormones that can impact steroid-dependent tumors are available as antineoplastic agents. These therapeutic entities are discussed in detail in Chapter 24, but one representative molecule from each pharmacological class is highlighted below (Fig. 33.22).

Aromatase Inhibitors

Aromatase inhibitors are used in the treatment of postmenopausal ER^+ breast cancer, as adjuvant (early), first-line (locally advanced or metastatic) and/or alternate (disease that has progressed on estrogen antagonists) therapy. In postmenopausal women, estrogen is biosynthesized in breast via the oxidation of androstenedione. The catalyzing enzyme is CYP19A1 (aromatase), and the estrogen generated in situ fuels the progression of HR^+ breast cancers. Of the three currently marketed agents in this class, one is steroidal (exemestane, an irreversible inhibitor by virtue of a 1,2-double bond that traps the enzyme upon nucleophilic attack at C4), and two are non-steroidal reversible inhibitors of the aromatase enzyme (anastrozole, letrozole).

ANASTROZOLE[76,284] **(FIG. 33.22).** Anastrozole binds competitively and selectively to the heme moiety of the aromatase enzyme, interfering with its oxidizing potential. As a result, cellular levels of estrone (the product of androstenedione oxidation) fall up to 85%. This leads to a significant decrease in its metabolite, the most potent receptor estrogen estradiol, which is generated reversibly from estrone by 17β-hydroxysteroid dehydrogenase (17β-HSD).

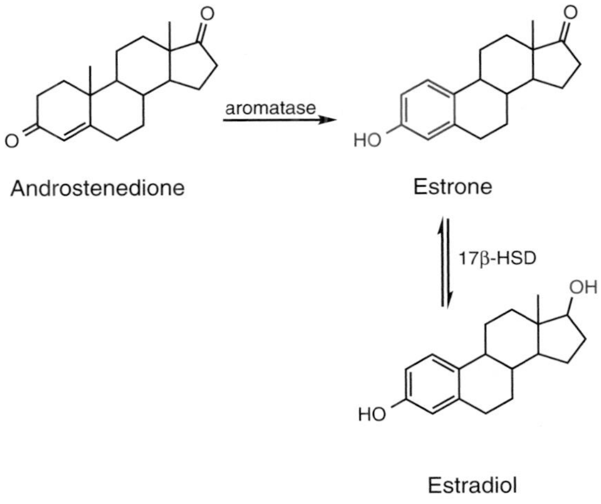

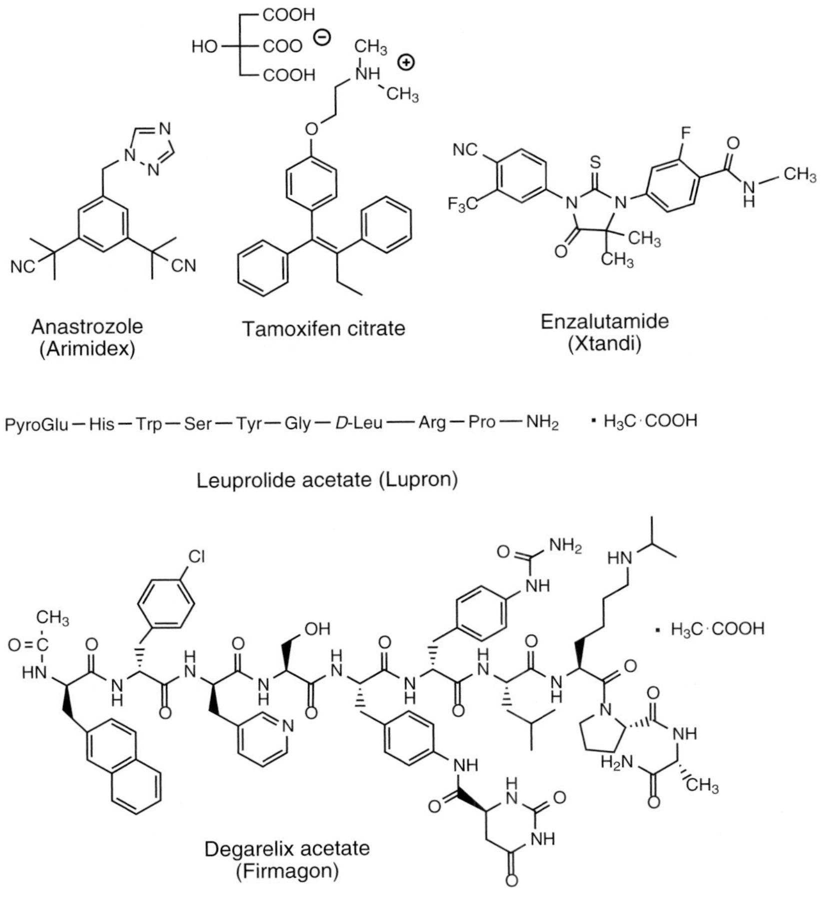

Androstenedione —aromatase→ Estrone ⇌ (17β-HSD) Estradiol

Anastrozole (Arimidex)

Tamoxifen citrate

Enzalutamide (Xtandi)

PyroGlu—His—Trp—Ser—Tyr—Gly—*D*-Leu—Arg—Pro—NH_2 · $H_3C{\cdot}COOH$

Leuprolide acetate (Lupron)

Degarelix acetate (Firmagon)

Figure 33.22 Representative hormone-based antineoplastic agents.

Anastrozole has demonstrated efficacy in all of the aforementioned clinical situations, and one 1 mg tablet is administered once daily. While it can be administered without regard to food, absorption is faster on an empty stomach. A 70% reduction in estrogen levels is achieved within 1 day, with an additional 10% reduction after two weeks on therapy. The drug undergoes aromatic hydroxylation at C4, methyl hydroxylation at the cyanopropyl moiety, and N-dealkylation to release the primary inactive metabolite, triazole.[285] Glucuronide conjugates are excreted primarily in urine.

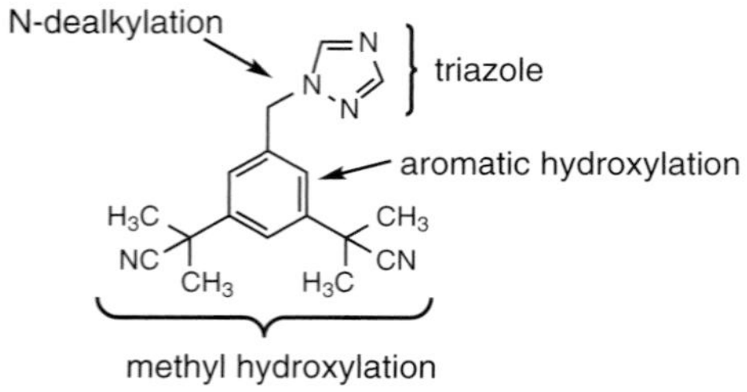

Anastrozole phase 1 metabolism

Antiestrogens

The antiestrogens used in the treatment of breast cancer often exhibit tissue-specific action at estrogen receptors, blocking hormone binding in breast and reproductive organs while displaying agonist actions in other tissues (e.g., uterus, bone). These dual-acting agents are more accurately referred to as selective estrogen receptor modulators, or SERMs. The three-fold structural requirements for estrogen receptor blockade by SERMs include: (1) three aromatic (phenyl) rings with a strictly maintained 3-dimensional structure, (2) a *cis* ring that bears a potentially cationic amine moiety linked through an alkylether group, and (3) a phenol-bearing *trans* ring, where the OH (or isostere) is either a component of the parent drug or generated via metabolism. The binding of SERMs to the estrogen receptor has been well-characterized (see Chapter 24). One anticancer agent in this pharmacologic class, fulvestrant, is a pure antiestrogen and decreases cellular levels of the receptor protein through degradation.

TAMOXIFEN CITRATE[76,286] **(FIG. 33.22).** It is hard to overestimate the positive therapeutic benefit of the relatively simple molecule tamoxifen. It has been termed "ground-breaking" and "pioneering" in that it introduced the SERM pharmacologic concept and ushered in the era of targeted breast cancer treatment and prevention therapy. This drug has saved countless lives with few use-limiting adverse effects. Unlike many targeted cancer therapies, it is inexpensive (generally <\$2 US/d) and, therefore, accessible to essentially all patients worldwide. Its indications range from disease prevention in high-risk patients to early-advanced breast cancer to ductal carcinoma in situ (DCIS). A boxed warning on potentially fatal uterine malignancies (adenocarcinoma and sarcoma) and cardiovascular events, including stroke and pulmonary embolism, applies to high risk breast cancer patients and those with DCIS.

Therapeutic action is realized through two major metabolites of isomerically pure Z (*trans*) tamoxifen, both of which have the essential phenolic OH generated through CYP2D6 metabolism. The CYP3A4-generated desmethyl metabolite is only active if 2D6-catalyzed *p*-hydroxylation has occurred. Patients who are 2D6 intermediate or poor metabolizers may see little or no clinical benefit from tamoxifen, and the concomitant use of drugs that inhibit this isoform should be avoided.

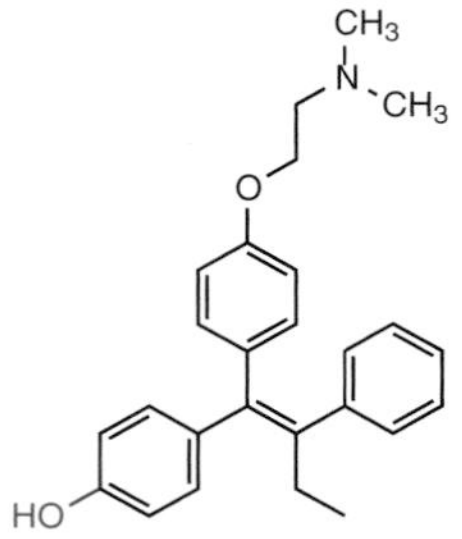

4-hydroxytamoxifen (active)

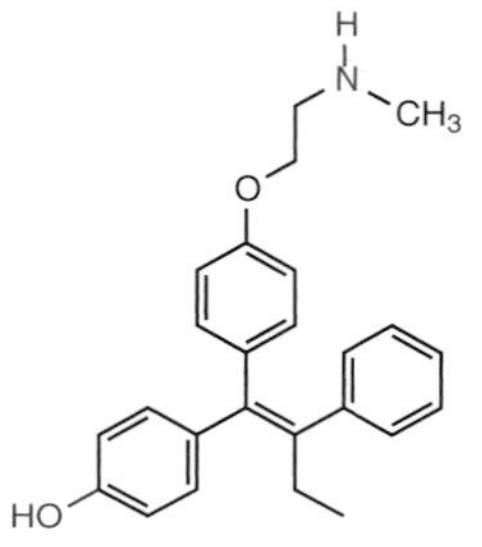

N-desmethyl-4-hydroxytamoxifen (active)

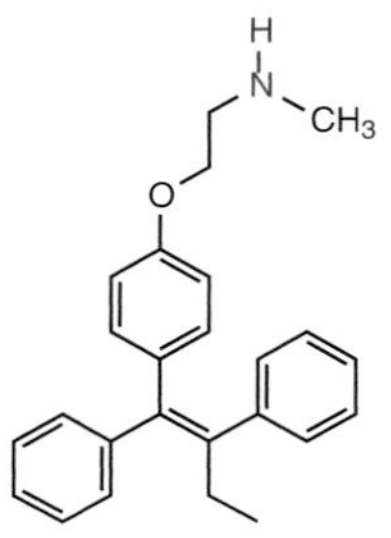

N-desmethyltamoxifen (inactive)

The usual dosage regimen of tamoxifen is 20-40 mg/d for 5 years, with the higher doses being used in metastatic disease. The drug is administered in tablet form, and concentrates in the breast (antiestrogen action) and uterus/endometrium (estrogen agonist action). It is highly protein bound, and the half-life of the parent drug and desmethyl metabolite ranges from 1 to 2 weeks, respectively. Excretion is predominantly, but not exclusively, fecal. The significant risk of metabolic and other DDIs warrants vigilant monitoring by the pharmacist.

Antiandrogens (Fig. 33.22)

Compounds that antagonize or otherwise disrupt the function of androgen receptors have value in castration-resistant prostate cancer (CRPC), a disease characterized by dysregulated androgen receptor signaling with subsequent loss of the homeostatic balance between cellular proliferation and apoptosis. Antiandrogens are used when disease progression is realized or anticipated despite androgen deprivation therapy (see GnRH Modulators discussion below) or testicular removal (orchidectomy). While the prognosis for CRPC is poor, early use of selected agents (i.e., with androgen deprivation or surgical castration) may delay progression and/or metastasis.

Structural requirements for high affinity androgen receptor binding of these antagonists include an aniline ring substituted with an electron withdrawing group at the *m*- and *p*-positions, and a propanamide moiety (often cyclic) that may serve as a bridge between the aniline core and a second aromatic ring. The common interactions of antiandrogens with key ligand binding domain residues have been identified (see Chapter 24).

ENZALUTAMIDE.[76,287] Enzalutamide, a second-generation pure antiandrogen, meets the structural requirements for an androgen receptor antagonist. In addition to blocking testosterone/dihydrotestosterone binding to the cytoplasmic receptor, it also inhibits translocation of the occupied receptor dimer to the nucleus (where it would normally regulate DNA transcription) and interferes with the binding of any nuclear receptor dimers with the androgen response elements of DNA. These latter actions are important, as CRPC is often characterized by androgen receptor overexpression secondary to gene amplification, which provides greater opportunity for androgen receptor signaling that can drive tumor growth.

Enzalutamide is marketed as 40 mg capsules, and the usual dose is 4 capsules (160 mg) taken at once at a consistent time of day. Absorption is rapid and food-independent, and peak plasma levels are achieved within 3 hours (most commonly by 1 hour). An active N-desmethyl metabolite is generated by CYP2C8, and the parent drug and metabolite have half-lives of 5.8 and 7.8-8.6 days, respectively. Urinary excretion predominates.

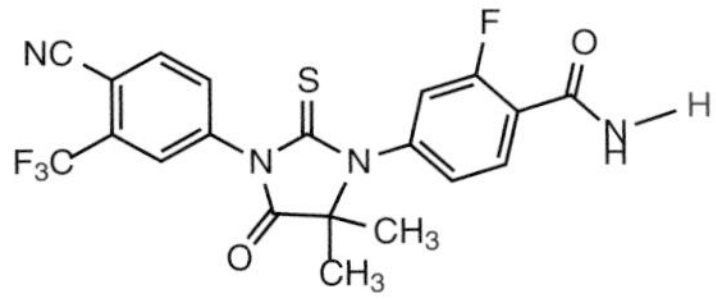

NC F O S F_3C N N N H H CH_3 O CH_3

Desmethylenzalutamide (active metabolite)

Resistance to enzalutamide has been linked to tumor cell expression of androgen splice variant AR-V7. Drug-associated seizures requiring enzalutamide discontinuation have been noted in patients with predisposing risk factors.

Gonadotropin Releasing Hormone (GnRH) Modulators

LEUPROLIDE ACETATE.[76,288] Leuprolide is a potent GnRH (also called luteinizing hormone releasing hormone or LHRH) agonist administered by depot injection to provide constantly elevated plasma levels of drug. While it initially stimulates the release of LH and follicle stimulating hormone (FSH) from the anterior pituitary (which promotes steroidogenesis), the unrelenting agonism of the GnRH receptor induces a profound desensitization due to the negative feedback inhibition of the hypothalamus by the high serum concentrations of sex steroids. Testicular biosynthesis of androgens is essentially halted, and testosterone levels drop to below castrate level, usually within 4 weeks. As noted previously, androgen deprivation therapy, or chemical castration, has significant therapeutic benefit in advanced prostate cancer.

Leuprolide acetate has been used to induce androgen deficiency in prostate cancer for over two decades. The drug is commonly administered intramuscularly (IM), where the delivery system (microsphere or biodegradable polymer) generates a depot that provides continuous release of the high affinity and metabolically stable GnRH-mimetic leuprolide. Concentrations are available to deliver drug anywhere from 1 to 6 months, but formulations should not be used in combination nor fractionated. During the initial steroidogenesis stage, patients can experience tumor exacerbation, bone pain, hematuria, and neuropathy, but these adverse effects usually subside as testosterone biosynthesis attenuates. Once testosterone levels drop, gynecomastia, breast pain and hot flashes can be problematic. Leuprolide prolongs the QT interval and can lead to life-threatening arrhythmia if other drugs with this effect are coadministered. Seizures have also been noted with leuprolide use, and depressive symptoms can worsen.

The major leuprolide metabolite is an inactive pentapeptide (M1) generated by peptidase enzymes.

DEGARELIX ACETATE.[76,289,290] Another approach to androgen deprivation therapy in the treatment of advanced prostate cancer is the direct inhibition of the GnRH receptor in the anterior pituitary; essentially the opposite of the GnRH "superagonism" approach exemplified by leuprolide and other GnRH agonists, but with the same biochemical outcome. One important goal of this therapy is to suppress the LH and FSH-mediated surge in steroidogenesis and potentially delay the seemingly inevitable progression to CRPC.

Degarelix is delivered in a mannitol solution and forms a gel-like depot on SC administration. An initial dose of two 120 mg injections is followed in 28 days by an 80 mg maintenance dose that is repeated every 28 days. Drug release from the SC depot is initially rapid, but then slows to give a maintenance dose elimination half-life of 31 days. Patients normally respond within 3 days (testosterone levels ≤50 ng/dL, although <20 ng/dL is now proposed to be the more appropriate target).[288] Studies have shown that degarelix works more quickly than GnRH agonists to lower testosterone to castrate levels, although both therapies are able to maintain target levels of this androgen over the long term (1 yr). There was no statistically significant difference in the degree of attenuation of PSA (a key prostate cancer marker) from baseline, but degarelix provided a significantly higher PSA progression-free survival compared to GnRH agonists.[289] Potentially contributing to the positive outcome is the fact that tumor growth promoting FSH is also suppressed by degarelix.[290]

As with leuprolide, inactivating metabolism is via peptidase cleavage and QT prolongation leading to potentially life-threatening DDIs occurs. Bone demineralization can put patients at increased risk for fractures.

Immunomodulators

Three closely related immunomodulatory drugs are used as maintenance therapy (lenalidomide) or in active treatment of newly diagnosed (thalidomide) or relapsed/

refractory (pomalidomide) multiple myeloma, the latter two indications in combination with dexamethasone. All are dioxopiperadin-3-yl (glutarimide) substituted isoindolinones; thalidomide and pomalidomide have the isoindoline-1,3-dione (phthalimide) structure, and lenalidomide and pomalidomide are aniline derivatives.

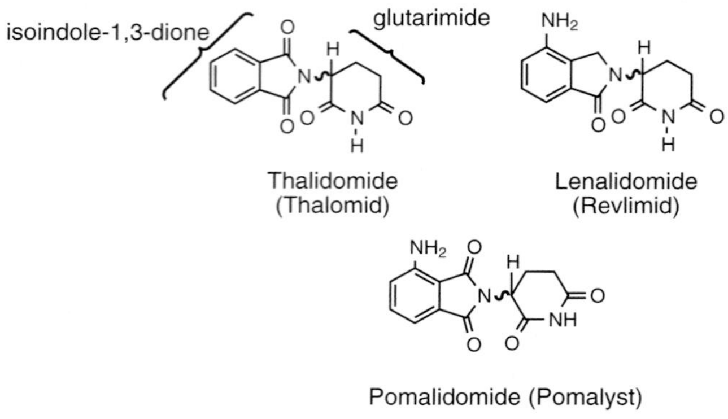

isoindole-1,3-dione glutarimide

Thalidomide (Thalomid)

Lenalidomide (Revlimid)

Pomalidomide (Pomalyst)

Immunomodulatory agents used in multiple myeloma

Anyone of the "baby boomer" or World War II generation will recognize the name of the drug thalidomide because it induced perhaps the most well-known incident of drug-associated birth defects in recent history.[291] Used in the late 1950s and early 1960s as an antiemetic and sedative in pregnant women, more than 10,000 European children were born with flipper-like arms and legs, a condition called phocomelia or "seal limb." Although it is known that the teratogenic and sedative actions of chiral thalidomide are mediated by different stereoisomers,[292] the in vivo inversion of the therapeutic *R*-isomer to its cytotoxic *S*-enantiomer prohibited the use of this drug in women who were or could become pregnant. Although not licensed in the United States during those years, the drug was banned by the FDA until 1997.

Thalidomide's antiproliferative and proapoptotic actions allowed its very cautious use in multiple myeloma.[279,293] In addition to arresting uncontrolled cell growth, thalidomide and its analogues deny multiple myeloma cells access to bone marrow stromal cells and various growth factors needed for tumor cell survival and augment circulating levels of natural killer cells, interleukin-2, and interferon-γ.[292] Lenalidomide and pomalidomide, as more potent and less toxic immunomodulatory analogues, have effectively taken thalidomide's therapeutic place, but all of these agents are contraindicated in pregnancy. Boxed warnings mandate that female patients capable of becoming pregnant document they are not pregnant for two months prior to beginning therapy, and either use two contraceptive methods or opt for total abstinence from heterosexual intercourse during, and for one month following, therapy. During and for one month following therapy, male patients must use condoms during intercourse with childbearing-capable women. These drugs are only available through the appropriate restricted distribution (REMS) program.

Specific Drugs

LENALIDOMIDE. Lenalidomide exerts its antitumor activity through interaction with, and regulation of, an E3 ubiquitin ligase complex protein called cereblon,[294] and its ability to stem angiogenesis has made it valuable in multiple myeloma maintenance therapy. It is used in doses approximately 1/10 that of thalidomide (25 vs. 200 mg. once daily on specific days of a 28 day cycle), and has been shown to augment PFS and OS compared to placebo, and PFS and quality of life when added as combination and maintenance therapy to a melphalan/prednisolone regimen. The drug is also used in MCL at the same dose and for the same 21 (out of 28) day regimen. Low frequency dexamethasone (40 mg once weekly in a 28 day cycle) appears safer and more efficacious than high frequency (40 mg on 12 days of a 28 day cycle). As noted previously, addition of a proteasome inhibitor (e.g., bortezomib) to lenalidomide/dexamethasone therapy has advanced therapeutic outcomes in relapsed/refractory multiple myeloma.[279]

Lenalidomide is marketed as the racemic mixture, and chiral inversion converts 5% of the *R* isomer to *S* within an hour after administration. Slow non-enzymatic hydrolysis of the glutarimide ring occurs, but CYP2C19-catalyzed oxidation (5-hydroxylation) and phase 2 N-acetylation (at the primary aromatic NH_2) is minimal, as is the risk of kinetics-related DDIs. Approximately 82% of a dose is excreted unchanged in urine. Kidney function impacts drug exposure more than any other factor, and the dose should be tailored in the face of renal impairment (creatinine clearance <60 mL/min) and when dialysis is required.[294]

Lenalidomide oral bioavailablity is high (>90%) and the drug is only about 30% bound to serum proteins. Doses should be administered at the same time of day and, while high-fat foods decreases the AUC and C_{max} by 20% and 50%, respectively, patients can take the medication without regard to meals. Lenalidomide's adverse effect profile is milder than thalidomide's, but because the drug is coadministered with dexamethasone, significant venous thromboembolic events can still occur. Neutropenia and thrombocytopenia can also be dose-limiting, and GI distress and drug-induced rash may be problematic. Secondary malignancies have occurred, but are generally less life-threatening than the primary neoplastic disease being treated.[279,294]

POMALIDOMIDE. Pomalidomide is the most potent immunomodulator of the three substituted isoindolinones and is considered the "standard of care" in patients who have progressed on lenalidomide/bortezomib and at least one other therapy. Until the introduction of pomalidomide, these patients had a survival expectancy of less than one year, but a pivotal phase III trial has shown the drug in combination with low dose dexamethasone can increase PFS (2 mo benefit), OS (5 mo benefit), and overall response (21% increased benefit) compared to high dose dexamethasone alone. The reported overall response is thought to be underestimated, since patients in the dexamethasone-only arm were allowed to cross over to the pomalidomide arm of the study. Like lenalidomide, pomalidomide has an absolute dependence on cereblon for its immunodulatory activity, and the protein has been suggested as a biomarker for sensitivity to these agents.[295,296]

Pomalidomide is formulated as capsules, and the 4 mg dose is administered once daily on days 1-21 of a 28 day cycle, along with 40 mg dexamethasone once per week. Studies evaluating the benefit of adding pomalidomide to other anti-multiple therapies, including the DNA alkylator cyclophosphamide and immunotherapeutic MAbs, are onoing.[296]

Pomalidomide has oral bioavailability, protein binding characteristics, and an adverse effect profile qualitatively similar to lenalidomide. Hematologic toxicities predominate and infections (including pneumonia) can be a source of concern in a heavily pre-treated population already at risk. Unlike lenalidomide, pomalidomide can prolong the QT interval.[279,295,296]

While in vivo isomeric inversion and glutarimide hydrolysis occur, pomalidomide is vulnerable to CYP-catalyzed oxidation (principally 3A4 and 1A2, and possibly 2C19), with hydroxylation occurring predominantly on the aniline side of the isoindolinedione ring. Only about 10% of a dose is excreted unchanged, and glucuronidation of the 5-phenol, as well as N-acetylation of the aromatic NH_2 group, can precede mostly urinary elimination. None of the metabolites contributes to therapeutic activity.[297,298]

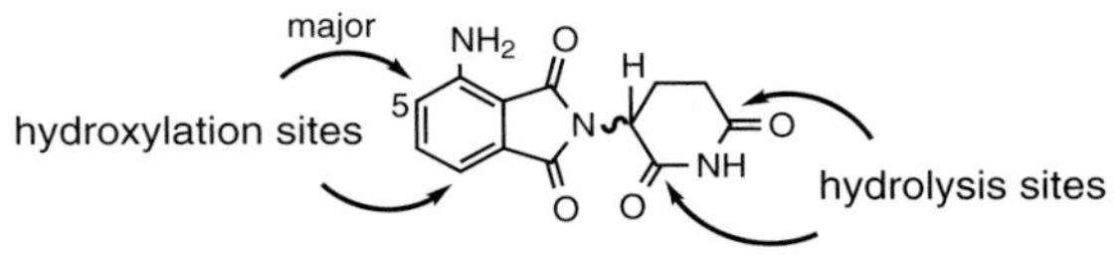

major NH_2 O H 5 N O NH O O hydroxylation sites hydrolysis sites

Sites of pomalidomide metabolism

Histone Deacetylase Inhibitors (HDACi)

Histones are highly basic, Lys-rich proteins that process DNA into nucleosomes required for chromatin formation, and they are substrates for specific histone acetyltransferase (HAT) and deacetylase (HDAC) enzymes. Destruction of the basicity of Lys' terminal amine (and thus, its ability to become cationic) through HAT-catalyzed acetylation provides a more open chromatin conformation, allowing transcription factors to readily access DNA and initiate RNA synthesis. Halting the HDAC-catalyzed loss of the neutralizing acetyl moiety by administering HDACi keeps the chromatin in its relaxed conformation and blocks transcriptional repression and tumor suppression silencing that results from the more structurally tight (closed) chromatin conformation favored by cationic histones.[299,300]

While excessive histone acetylation can be associated with aggressive neoplastic disease, reduction in the extent of Lys acetylation of selected histones (particularly Lys16 on H4) is also a common finding in many human cancers. Several structural prototypes can selectively inhibit enzymatic histone deacetylation and positively impact gene transcription regulation by these proteins. Three of the four classes of HDAC enzymes require Zn^{2+} as a cofactor, including Class I members HDAC1 and HDAC2 that are overexpressed in lymphoma. These enzymes are the targets of several clinically available HDACi.

Many other non-histone proteins acetylated through post-translational modification are impacted by the administration of HDACi, including nuclear factor κB, transcription repressor protein Yin Yang 1, and oncoprotein-stabilizing Hsp90. Through a variety of complex mechanisms, exposure to these therapeutic inhibitors is associated with: (1) an increase in *p21* antioncogenes, (2) inhibition of cyclin/CDK, (3) induction of cell cycle arrest, (4) angiogenesis suppression, (5) DNA damage initiation and repair inhibition, and (6) tumor cell apoptosis. Fortunately, non-cancerous cells are fairly resistant to the lethal actions of these antineoplastic agents.[300]

Three of the four clinically available HDACi are used in the treatment of cutaneous and/or peripheral T-cell lymphoma (romidepsin, vorinostat, belinostat), while the newest drug (panobinostat) is indicated in relapsed/refractory multiple myeloma. Romidepsin, the first drug in this class, is a macrolide prodrug. The remaining agents are active hydroxamic acids that contain a terminal aromatic moiety (phenyl or indole) and a long lipophilic connecting chain that may (or may not) incorporate a second aromatic ring (Fig. 33.23). Vorinostat and panobinostat are oral medications while romidepsin and belinostat are administered by IV infusion.

A thorough review of HDACi chemistry, SAR, rational drug design, and therapeutic utility has recently been published.[301]

Specific Drugs (Fig. 33.23)

ROMIDEPSIN. Romidepsin, the original HDACi, is an inactive depsipeptide macrolide that, once activated through glutathione-catalyzed reduction to the thiol, sequesters the Zn^{2+} cofactor associated with Class I HDAC1 andHDAC2 enzymes that regulate cellular proliferation. Only one free sulfhydryl moiety of the reduced active metabolite interacts with the Zn^{2+}. Romidepsin induces a caspase-dependent apoptosis and retains efficacy in cutaneous and peripheral T-cell lymphoma cells overexpressing the prosurvival protein Bcl-2 (an advantage over the other marketed HDACi agents).[299] It is used by IV infusion in refractory forms of the disease that have progressed after at least one previous therapeutic intervention. The standard adult dose is 14 mg/m^2 administered over 4 hours once weekly for three weeks of a 4-week cycle. Overall response rates in clinical trials have ranged from 25% to 35%.

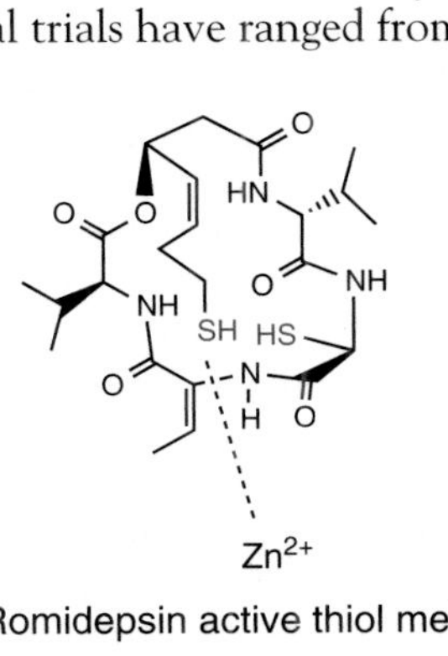

O HN O O O NH NH SH HS O N H O Zn^{2+}

Romidepsin active thiol metabolite

Romidepsin is a moderate emetogen, and pretreatment with an anti-nauseant is advised. Myelosuppression with

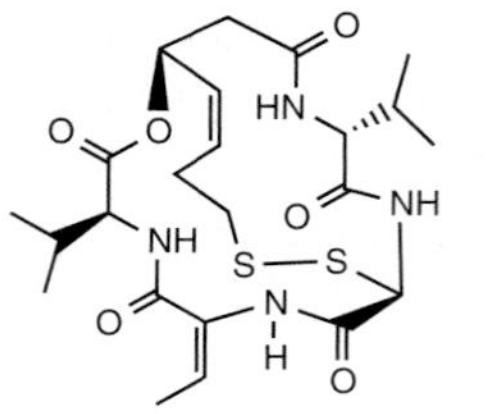

Romidepsin (Istodax)

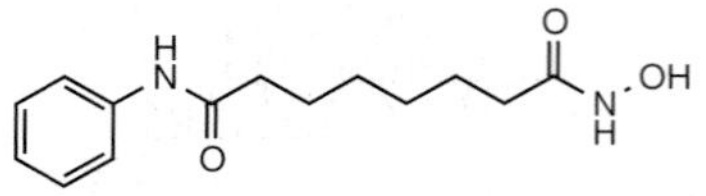

Vorinostat (Zolinza)

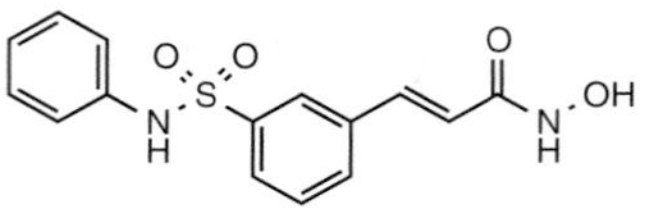

Belinostat (Beleodaq)

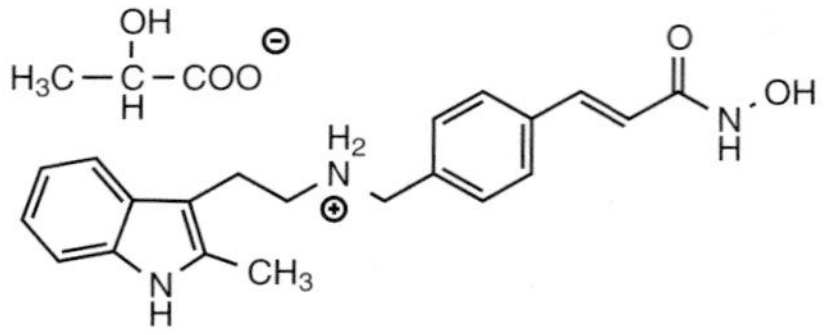

Panobinostat lactate (Farydak)

Figure 33.23 Histone deacetylase inhibitors (HDACi).

fatigue and infection are among the more likely adverse effects. Cardiac toxicities with all HDACi antineoplatics are possible, and romidepsin use has been linked to QT prolongation (potentially via HERG K^+ interaction or changes in HERG expression) and other electrocardiogram abnormalities. While rare, sudden cardiac death has been observed.[300]

Romidepsin is strongly protein bound (92%-94%) and has a $t_{1/2}$ of approximately 3 hours. After activation, it is extensively metabolized primarily by CYP3A4, generating up to 30 metabolites of minor significance. The drug is also a P-gp substrate, and appropriate precautions should be taken with coadministered inhibitors or inducers of these proteins, as well as with drugs that could augment cardiotoxicity risk.

VORINOSTAT AND BELINOSTAT. Vorinostat and belinostat are hydroxyamic acid derivatives used in relapsed/refractory cutaneous and peripheral T-cell lymphoma, respectively. Like romidepsin, these agents block Class I HDACs by chemically sequestering the critical Zn^{2+} cofactor of their target enzymes, but do so via a different mechanism. In this case, the hydroxamic acid anion serves as the Zn-chelating entity, and the long, slender hydrocarbon chain allows these drugs to dangle their cation magnet into the tube-like "fishing hole" that shelters the metal ion. The aromatic moiety at the opposite end of the structure caps the entrance to the tubular pocket, ensuring effective inhibition of the cofactor.[302] Clinical trials have documented the value of both drugs in terms of overall response, but they are not effective in lymphoma cells made HDACi-resistant through Bcl-2 overexpression.[299,303]

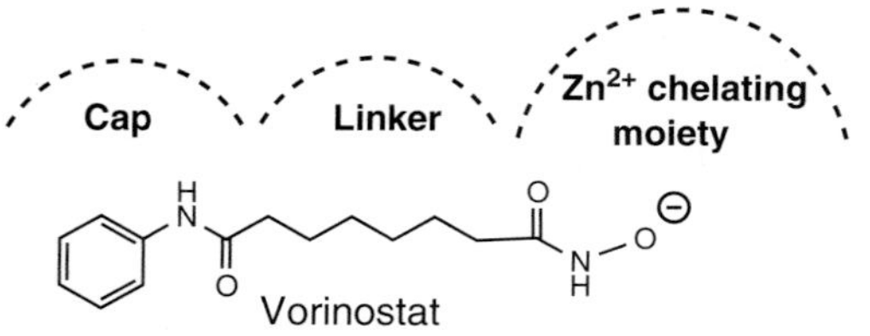

Cap Linker Zn^{2+} chelating moiety

Vorinostat

Selected therapeutic and pharmacokinetic properties of vorinostat and belinostat are provided in Table 33.10. CYP is not important to the metabolism of either inhibitor. Both are directly glucuronidated, and vorinostat also undergoes hydrolysis and β-oxidation to 4-anilino-oxobutanoic acid.

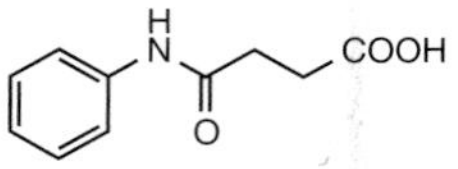

4-Anilino-4-oxobutanoic acid

PANOBINOSTAT LACTATE. Panobinostat is the only HDACi used in multiple myeloma, and the most potent drug in this therapeutic category (10 times vorinostat).[302] It is an orally active hydroxamic acid-based pan-inhibitor that blocks several Class I, II and IV isozymes (all Zn^{2+} dependent), and 20 mg is administered daily in a complex regimen.[300] Clinical studies evaluating its use as monotherapy were disappointing, and it is given in combination with bortezomib and dexamethasone. This combination produced an overall response rate of 73% in a phase I clinical trial. In a multicenter phase III trial in relapsed/refractory multiple myeloma patients being treated with bortezomib and dexamethasone with and without panobinostat, the median PFS increased by almost 4 months and a significantly higher percentage of patients achieved a complete/near complete response with the HDACi in the regimen.[302] The adverse effects most commonly observed are myelosuppression and GI distress (nausea, diarrhea). The oral dosage form induces much less QT interval prolongation than the IV formulation, which is the primary reason the latter is not marketed. The drug carries a boxed warning related to severe diarrhea and potentially fatal cardiovascular events (including ischemia and arrhythmia), and it is administered through a REMS program to ensure appropriate patient education and safety.

Table 33.10 Selected Therapeutic and Pharmacokinetic Properties of Vorinostat and Belinostat

	Vorinostat	Belinostat
Indication	Refractory cutaneous T-cell lymphoma	Refractory peripheral T-cell lymphoma
Formulation	Capsules (taken with food)	IV solution
Usual adult dose	400 mg once daily	1000 mg/m² daily on days 1-5 of a 21 d regimen
$T_{1/2}$ (hrs)	2	1.1
Protein binding (%)	71	93-96
Metabolism	Hydrolysis, β-oxidation, glucuronidation	Glucuronidation, CYP-catalyzed oxidation (minor)
Excretion	Primarily renal	Primarily renal
Adverse effects	Diarrhea, fatigue, nausea, anorexia	Anemia, thrombocytopenia, QTc prolongation, nausea

Panobinostat is most effectively absorbed in the absence of food but can be administered without regard to meals. It is 90% protein bound and extensively biotransformed, with approximately 40 out of at least 77 metabolites circulating in plasma. Reduction and hydrolysis of the hydroxamic acid moiety, along with α- and β-oxidation and aromatic and benzylic hydroxylation, generate the most prevalent phase 1 metabolites, none of which are active (Fig. 33.24). While CYP metabolism is less important than alternate pathways, 3A4 accounts for approximately 40% of the clearance. The acyl glucuronide of the β-oxidation product is the most abundant metabolite, and excretion of parent drug (<7%) and metabolites is both renal and biliary.[304]

Topoisomerase Poisons

Topoisomerases are enzymes that control the degree of DNA supercoiling and, in so doing, maintain proper DNA structure during replication and transcription to RNA. Topoisomerase IIα (topIIα) cleaves double-stranded DNA during the replication phase via a transesterification reaction involving a topoisomerase Tyr residue and a terminal 5′ phosphate but, through a reverse transesterification, repairs its own damage after replication is complete.[305] Topoisomerase I (topI) functions in essentially the same way, but cuts and religates a single DNA strand. Antineoplastic agents that function as topoisomerase poisons stimulate the DNA cleavage

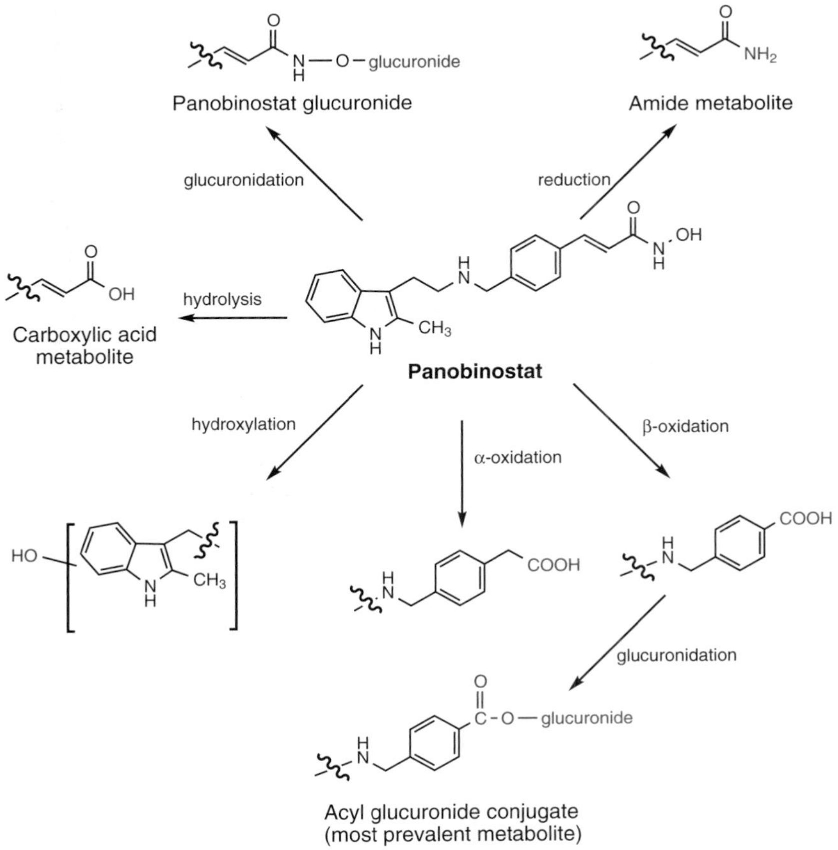

Figure 33.24 Panobinostat metabolism.

reaction but inhibit the DNA resealing activity of the enzymes, leaving the DNA irreversibly damaged and unable to replicate.

Three chemically distinct classes of anticancer agents can be classified as topoisomerase poisons: camptothecins, epipodophyllotoxins, and anthracyclines and related anthracenediones.

Camptothecins

MECHANISM OF ACTION. Camptothecins are chiral, extensively conjugated pentacyclic lactones (Fig. 33.25). The biologic target of camptothecins is topI, rather than the topIIα enzyme that serves as the target for the epipodophyllotoxins and anthracyclines. However, the mechanism of antineoplastic action of both enzyme inhibitors is stabilization of a cleavable ternary (drug-enzyme-DNA) complex that does not permit the resealing of nicked DNA. Although the fragmented DNA is capable of resealing in the absence of drug, when DNA replication forks encounter the fragmented DNA, shear stress induces a double-stranded DNA break, killing the cell.[306] Camptothecins are most toxic to cells undergoing active DNA replication and cell division (e.g., they are S-G2 phase specific).[306]

The binding of camptothecins occurs in such a way as to stabilize a covalent DNA–topoisomerase bond at the point of single-strand breakage (Tyr723 on the human enzyme) but sterically keep a topI Lys532 residue from catalyzing the DNA religation reaction.[307,308] The binding pocket, located within the DNA strand, is revealed only after the normal DNA nicking has occurred, explaining why these poisons preferentially bind to the enzyme–DNA complex rather than to unoccupied DNA or enzyme. The flat camptothecin ring system intercalates DNA at the site of cleavage, mimicking a DNA base pair.[308] The crystal structures of human ternary complexes involving the parent alkaloid (the water insoluble natural product camptothecin), and the semisynthetic analogue, topotecan have been solved, and important drug-protein interacting entities are noted in Table 33.11.[307-309] The C7, C9, and/or C10 substituents of the marketed compounds, which project into the major groove of DNA, do not hinder binding, and may actually enhance it through hydrophobic and/or H-bonding interactions.[310] Position 7 is viewed as the most ripe for activity-enhancing modifications, as the topI region accommodating substituents at this position is spacious.[311]

Proposed camptothecin resistance mechanisms are similar to those operational in many other classes of cytotoxic antineoplastic drugs, including downregulation or mutation of the target enzyme and cellular efflux. BCRP and MDR-associated proteins MAP-2 and MAP-3 (rather than P-gp) have been suggested as resistance mediators, but a recent publication claims proteasomal destruction of topI may hold the key to resistance. TopI degradation in diseased cells is distinct from enzyme processing in healthy cells, and the extent of topI-Ser10 phosphorylation in tumors appears directly related to the rate of ubiquitin tagging, proteasome destruction and camptothecin resistance.[312]

CHEMISTRY. The parent camptothecin alkaloid, isolated from the bark of *Camptotheca acuminata* (the Chinese xi shu or "happy tree"),[306,313] has antitumor activity, but its limited water solubility necessitated delivery as the sodium salt of the significantly less active hydrolyzed lactone. Lactonization of the hydroxy acid in acidic urine is significant, and elevated levels of active intact alkaloid in the kidney accounted for the hemorrhagic cystitis induced by this compound. For these reasons, development of this natural product as a chemotherapeutic agent was abandoned in the 1970s.[306] It would take another two decades before the currently available agents irinotecan and topotecan received FDA approval.

While camptothecin's quinoline ring system is primarily unsubstituted, the currently marketed analogues have a basic side chain incorporated at either C9 (topotecan)

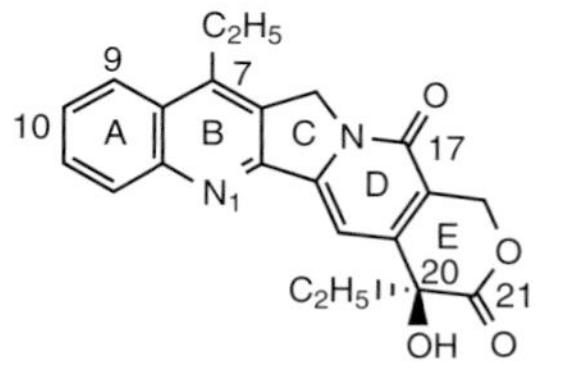

Camptothecin
(water-insoluble natural product)

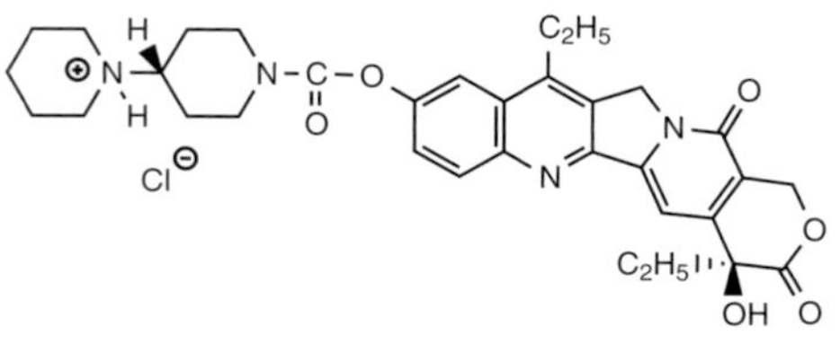

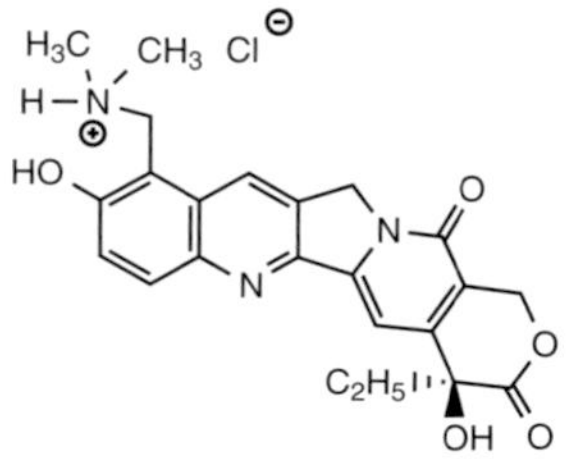

Irinotecan hydrochloride
(Camptosar, Oinvyde)

Topotecan hydrochloride
(Hycamtin)

Figure 33.25 Camptothecin topoisomerase I (TopI) poisons.

Table 33.11 Topotecan Topisomerase I Interactions

Topotecan Functional Group	Topoisomerase I Residue
Pyridine N_1	Arg364
C_{10}-OH	Enzyme-associated water (H-bond)
C_{17}-pyridone carbonyl	Asn722
C_{20}-OH	Asp533 (H-bond)
C_{21}-lactone carbonyl	Tyr723-phosphate, Lys532

or C10 (irinotecan), allowing the formation of water-soluble salts of the intact semisynthetic alkaloid. At pH 7.4, the active lactone exists in equilibrium with the hydroxy acid hydrolysis product, with the direction dictated by the extent of binding to serum albumin. The preferential protein binding of the lactone, which occurs with irinotecan, shifts the equilibrium to favor the production of the more active lactone, thus enhancing potency.

While the love affair between the scientific community and camptothecins has been an "on again-off again" thing, there is currently renewed interest in mining this structural prototype for novel agents of therapeutic value. A quantitative study on camptothecin structure-property relationships has been published,[314] as have reviews summarizing current literature on the chemical and pharmacological activities of both well-known and new entities.[306,310]

SPECIFIC DRUGS. Despite significant camptothecin-related drug discovery research, the two originally marketed analogues irinotecan and topotecan remain the only clinically available drugs in this class in the United States. It has been suggested that the likelihood of finding topI-inhibiting camptothecins with greater potency and/or margins of safety than these two "war horses" is slim.[306]

Irinotecan Hydrochloride

Conventional Formulation. In combination with fluorouracil (5-FU) and leucovorin, this prodrug camptothecin is considered first-line therapy in the treatment of metastatic colorectal cancer, and can be used as second-line therapy in 5-FU resistant patients. With a 22% increase in 1-year survival in 5-FU refractory disease (monotherapy), and an OS beyond 30 months when combined with 5-FU/leucovorin/oxaliplatin/bevacizumab in clinical trials, irinotecan is a major player in colorectal cancer chemotherapy.[315] Fortunately, no significant DDIs with commonly coadministered chemotherapeutic agents have been noted.[316]

Given IV at a usual initial dose of 125 mg/m^2, conventional irinotecan is slowly bioactivated in the liver through hydrolysis of the C10-carbamate ester. The metabolite, known as SN-38, is 100-1000 times more active than the parent (Fig. 33.26). OATP1B1 facilitates hepatic uptake of irinotecan, and the primary activating enzyme is the saturable carboxylesterase CES2. Butyrylcholinesterase can also activate irinotecan in plasma.[316] Levels of SN-38 are

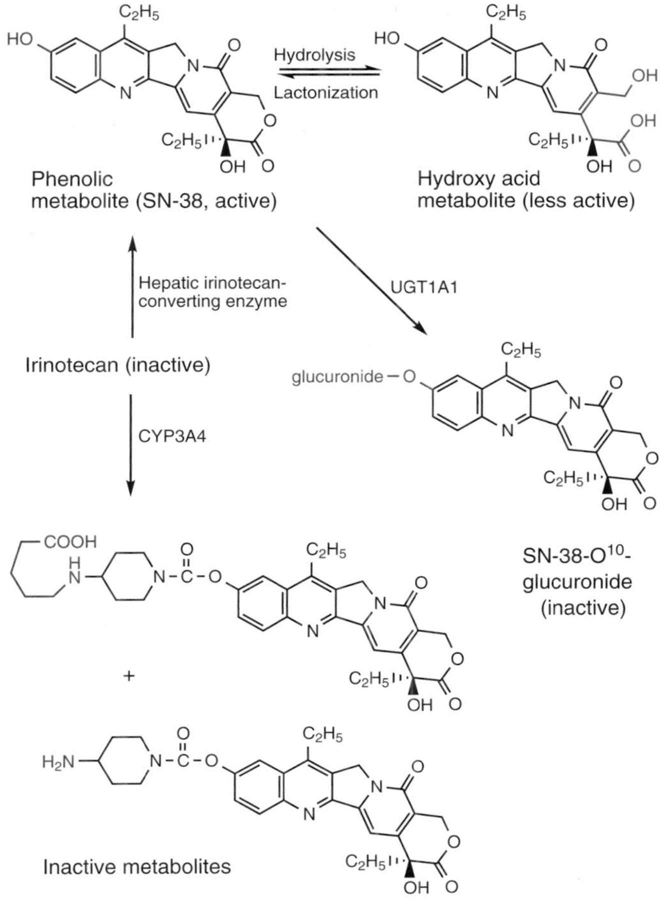

Figure 33.26 Irinotecan metabolism.

50-100 times lower than the parent drug, but preferential protein binding of the lactone (95%) permits significant plasma levels of SN-38 compared to the less active hydroxy acid metabolite. There is significant individual variability in kinetics and clearance for irinotecan (30%) and SN-38 (80%), and a SN-38 terminal half-life of between 6 and 32 hours has been reported (compared to 5-18 hr for the prodrug parent).[315,316] CYP3A4 cleaves the terminal piperidine ring through oxidation at the α-carbons, which is followed by hydrolysis of the resultant amides to inactive metabolites. Drug-induced toxicity can be exacerbated if strong CYP3A4 inhibitors are coadministered. Prior to elimination, irinotecan is glucuronidated by UGT1A1 or sulfonated at the C10 phenol. Elimination of the parent drug and all metabolites except SN-38 glucuronide is predominantly fecal (66%), and biliary excretion is facilitated by ATP-binding cassette (ABC) transporting proteins.[315,316]

Diarrhea is a hallmark irinotecan adverse effect, potentially exacerbated by coadministered 5-FU. Acute episodes that can begin during drug administration are attributed to acetylcholinesterase inhibition. Pretreatment with an anticholinergic agent (e.g., atropine) can effectively address this toxicity and help patients avoid "cholinergic syndrome," a collection of effects that include abdominal pain, sweating, blurred vision, and less commonly, bradycardia. The delayed diarrhea that occurs approximately

7-10 days post-administration is attributed to drug-induced mucosal damage. It is dose-limiting and potentially fatal, and the primary impetus behind a boxed warning. Vigorous loperamide therapy should be instituted at the first sign of symptoms, and fluid, electrolytes and antibiotics administered as needed. Camptothecins are also myelosuppressive, and neutropenia (also potentially worsened by 5-FU) can be severe, particularly in females or patients with elevated bilirubin levels or prolonged systemic exposure to SN-38.[316] Extensive biotransformation also demands cautious use of irinotecan in patients with hepatic dysfunction. Prophylactic antiemetic therapy should be given at least 30 minutes before the administration of irinotecan to minimize the nausea and vomiting associated with this anticancer agent.

It is now recognized that some patients may be pharmacogenetically predisposed to serious camptothecin-induced toxicity. Variations in expression of genes involved in the inactivating glucuronidation of irinotecan, specifically overexpression of the low activity *UGT1A1*6* and *UGT1A1*28* alleles more common in Asian and Caucasian populations, respectively, are deemed responsible. Doses must be decreased in patients homogyzous (e.g., *UGT1A1*28/*28*) or double heterozygous (e.g, *UGT1A1*6/*28*) for these poor metabolizer alleles to circumvent life-threatening neutropenia and diarrhea. While precise dose reduction guidelines are lacking, a minimum 20%-25% starting dose reduction in *UGT1A1*28/*28* carriers has been recommended.[76,316] While not yet standard procedure, genotyping prior to initiating therapy can more safely and effectively individualize therapy in at-risk individuals.[315-317]

Liposomal Formulation. A pegylated liposomal formulation of irinotecan is marketed as Onivyde for use in combination with 5-FU/leucovorin in metastatic pancreatic adenocarcinoma patients who have relapsed after gemcitabine (DNA polymerase inhibitor) therapy.[318] The usual starting dose of 70 mg/m^2 should be reduced to 50 mg/m^2 in *UGT1A1*28/*28* carriers, and slowly increased as tolerated. As with most liposomal formulations, the drug is stable in the circulation, and is preferentially taken up and retained for a longer period of time in the tumor cell. This results in a more potent therapeutic effect with fewer adverse reactions, although the boxed warning for life-threatening neutropenia and diarrhea noted for the conventional formulation still applies. The elimination $t_{1/2}$ of liposomal irinotecan and SN-38 is approximately 26 and 68 hours, respectively, significantly longer than the most commonly cited half-lives of these entities after conventional IV administration.[76] Binding to serum proteins is blocked by the polyethylene glycol attached to the liposomal surface.

Clinical trials have documented the value of liposomal irinotecan in promoting median OS, PFS and objective response rate in metastatic pancreatic adenocarcinoma compared to 5-FU/leucovorin alone.[318] As with conventional IV irinotecan, pre-treatment with antiemetic and anticholinergic medications prior to infusion is advised.

Topotecan[76,319]**.** This active camptothecin analogue is used by the IV route in the treatment of ovarian, cervical and small cell lung cancer that has either not responded to or relapsed after first-line therapy. An oral dosage form is available for use in relapsed small cell lung cancer. The drug carries a boxed warning for myelosuppression, particularly neutropenia, which precludes combination therapy with other bone marrow-suppressing drugs. Thrombocytopenia and anemia occur in approximately one-third of treated patients.

When administered IV, topotecan is commonly infused in doses of 1.5 mg/m^2 for 5 consecutive days of a 21 day cycle in ovarian and small cell lung cancer, and at 0.75 mg/m^2 on days 1-3 of a 21 day cycle in recurrent/resistant cervical cancer. Schedules that call for 5 consecutive day administration can result in serious mucositis and diarrhea. For the oral formulation, the appropriate number of 1 and 0.25 mg capsules is administered to provide a final dose of 2.3 mg/m^2 (rounded to the nearest 0.25 mg). Oral absorption is rapid, and bioavailability approaches 40%.

Topotecan elimination is biphasic with a terminal $t_{1/2}$ of 2-3 hours after IV administration. Plasma clearance is approximately 24% higher in males, but pharmacokinetic behavior after oral administration appears gender-independent. Lactone hydrolysis is rapid, reversible, and pH dependent, and binding to serum proteins is limited to approximately 35%. CYP3A4-mediated N-dealkylation to mono- and di-dealkylated metabolites occurs to a limited extent, and the O-glucuronides that form at multiple points along the metabolic path are excreted via the kidney (Fig. 33.27). Extensive renal clearance demands dosage adjustment in patients with kidney disease.

Because both topotecan and irinotecan are metabolized by CYP3A4, coadministration of strong CYP3A4 inducers and inhibitors should be avoided. It has been reported that Asian patients have greater topotecan exposure than Caucasian patients with similar renal function, and the possibility of a genetic difference in the ABCG2 transporter (specifically, the potential for a Q141K mutant in Asians that can increase oral bioavailability) was proposed.[320] The total topotecan exposure difference in patients with normal renal function is 30%, and rises to 60%-70% in moderate-severe impairment. At the time of this writing, there have been no published reports correlating topotecan toxicity to UGT1A1 polymorphism.

There is no topotecan liposomal formulation currently marketed, in part because of difficulties with low encapsulation efficiency and rapid plasma clearance, although explorations to address these challenges are ongoing.[321-323] Nanotechnology approaches to topotecan delivery are also being actively investigated.[324]

Epipodophyllotoxins

The epipodophyllotoxins (Fig. 33.28) are semisynthetic glycosidic derivatives of podophyllotoxin, the major component of the resinous podophyllin isolated from the dried roots of the American mandrake or mayapple plant (*Podophyllum peltatum*). Although these compounds are capable of binding to tubulin and inhibiting mitosis, their primary mechanism of antineoplastic action is topIIα poisoning, a mechanism that they share with anthracyclines (see below). TopIIα has two distinct DNA-independent binding sites for the epipodophyllotoxins, one within the catalytic domain and a second within the N-terminal ATP-binding domain.[325] Once bound, the toxins stabilize the cleavable ternary complex, stimulating DNA ligation

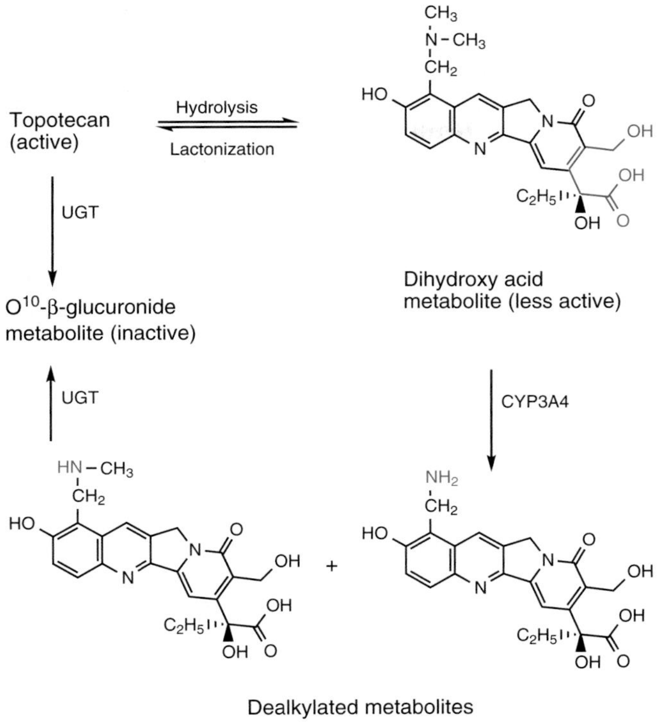

Topotecan (active) — Hydrolysis / Lactonization — Dihydroxy acid metabolite (less active)

UGT → O^{10}-β-glucuronide metabolite (inactive)

CYP3A4 → Dealkylated metabolites

Figure 33.27 Topotecan metabolism.

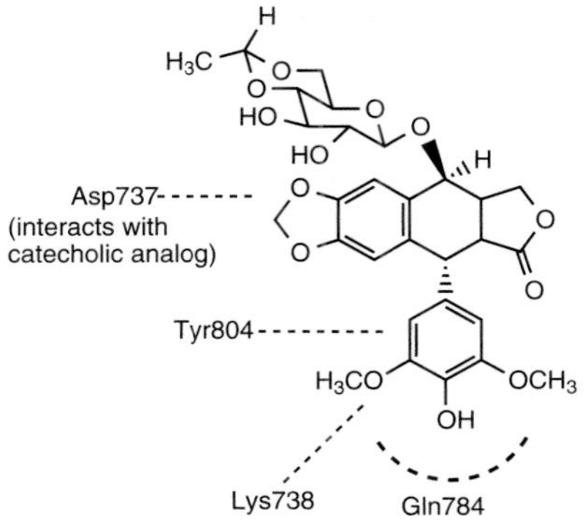

but inhibiting resealing. The DNA-topoisomerase fragments accumulate in the cell, ultimately resulting in apoptosis. The RNA transcription processes are also disrupted by the interaction of epipodophyllotoxins with topIIα.

The epipodophyllotoxin binding site has been probed with a carbene-generating diazirine photoaffinity label,[326] and a virtual library of 143 epipodophyllotoxin derivatives has been docked to a three-dimensional human topIIα receptor model in order to identify key drug-enzyme interactions (Fig. 33.29).[327] More recently, an X-ray crystal of two etoposide molecules bound in a ternary complex with cleaved DNA and topIIβ (an isoform found in myocardium) has been solved, documenting that the area that binds the glycoside moiety of epipodophyllotoxins is unhindered.[328]

Etoposide (VePesid)

Etoposide phosphate (Etopophos)

Teniposide hydrochlorde (Vumon)

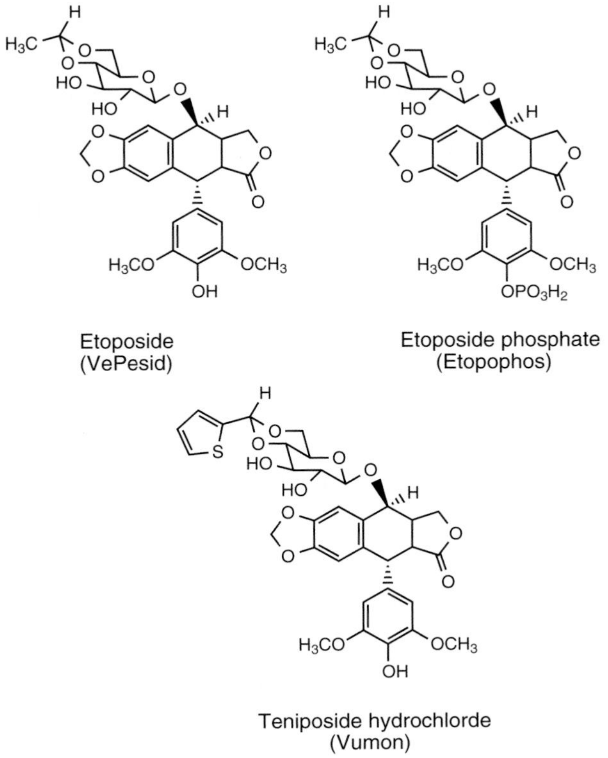

Figure 33.28 Epipodophyllotoxin topoisomerase IIα (TopIIα) poisons.

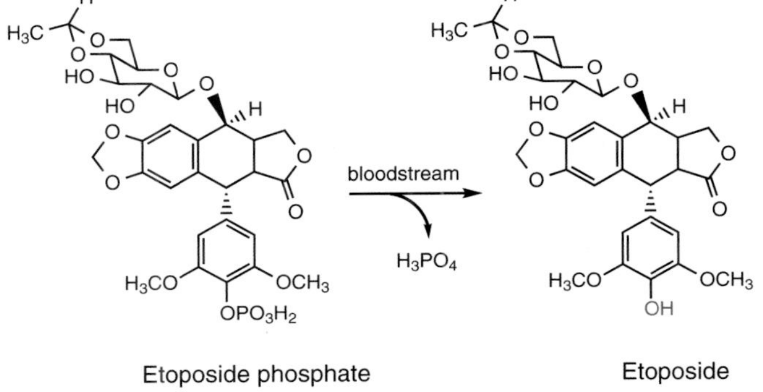

Asp737 (interacts with catecholic analog)

Tyr804

Lys738

Gln784

Figure 33.29 Proposed etoposide-TopIIα binding interactions.

Epipodophyllotoxins are cell cycle specific and have their most devastating impact on cells in the S or early G_2 phase. For this reason, doses are divided and administered over several days. Resistance is multifaceted and involves downregulation of topIIα, attenuation of enzymatic activity levels, development of novel DNA repair mechanisms, and P-gp–mediated cellular efflux.

CHEMISTRY. Structurally, the two marketed epipodophyllotoxins, etoposide and teniposide, differ only in the nature of one β-D-glucopyranosyl substituent (methyl or thienyl, respectively). Both are highly water insoluble, but teniposide's higher lipophilicity facilitates cellular uptake and results in a 10-fold enhancement of potency. The need for solubility enhancers, such as polysorbate 80 (Tween, etoposide) or polyoxyethylated castor oil (Kolliphor EL, teniposide), in intravenous formulations puts patients at risk for hypersensitivity reactions that can manifest as hypotension and thrombophlebitis. Antihistamines and corticosteroids are often coadministered to minimize this toxic liability. A water-soluble phosphate ester analogue of etoposide can be administered in standard aqueous vehicles, permitting higher doses than the oil-modified formulations would allow. The phosphate ester is rapidly cleaved to the free alcohol in the bloodstream.

Etoposide phosphate — bloodstream (H_3PO_4) → Etoposide

METABOLISM. Epipodophyllotoxins are subject to metabolic transformation before renal and biliary elimination (Fig. 33.30). Etoposide is stable enough for oral administration, although a dose approximately twice that of the IV formulation must be administered. Teniposide is more extensively metabolized, presumably due to its enhanced ability to penetrate into hepatocytes, and no oral dosage form is marketed. Both drugs undergo lactone hydrolysis to generate the inactive hydroxy acid as the major metabolite, but the parent drugs can also be transformed by CYP3A4-catalyzed O-demethylation and phase 2 glucuronide or sulfate conjugation. Phase 2 metabolism accounts for between 5% and 22% of the dose. Clinically significant interactions between epipodophyllotoxins and CYP3A4 inducers have been documented, and coadministration can enhance antineoplastic drug clearance by as much as 77%. Conversely, CYP3A4 inhibitors can decrease clearance, leading to unwanted toxicity.

Both etoposide and teniposide carry a boxed warning for severe myelosuppression that can result in infection (leukopenia) or hemorrhage (thrombocytopenia). Teniposide's warning extends to hypersensitivity due to the need for the more problematic solubilizer, Kolliphor EL (also known as Cremophor EL). The catechol metabolite can oxidize to a reactive orthoquinone, and both have been proposed to promote topoisomerase-mediated DNA cleavage, potentially enhancing the risk of the translocations that result in therapy-induced AML in children treated with these drugs. While the orthoquinone can be detoxified with reduced glutathione,[329] endogenous supplies of this electrophile scavenger are limited. Epipodophyllotoxin-induced leukemia occurs in 2% to 12% of patients and is believed to result from translocation of the *MLL* gene at chromosome band 11q23. The mean latency period of 2 years is shorter than the 5- to 7-year latency for leukemia induced by DNA alkylators, and the drug-induced cancer is often resistant to standard treatment, including bone marrow transplantation.[330] Another serious adverse effect is dose-limiting mucositis. Alopecia is common, and nausea and vomiting, most noticeable with the oral dosage form, are generally mild.

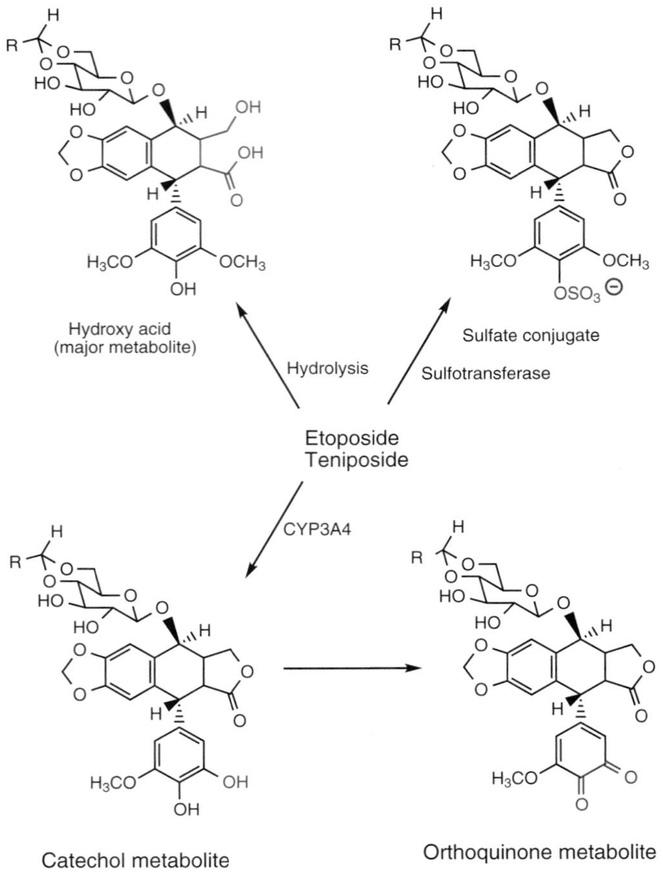

Figure 33.30 Epipodophyllotoxin metabolism.

SPECIFIC DRUGS

Etoposide. Etoposide and etoposide phosphate ester are used IV in combination with an organoplatinum agent (cisplatin, carboplatin) in the treatment of small cell lung cancer, and in combination with other agents in refractory testicular cancer. The dose of both runs from 35 to 50 mg/m^2 depending on whether a 5 or 4 day administration per cycle regimen is prescribed. Despite the fact that the phosphate ester prodrug does not require an oil-based solubilizer, etoposide is the more commonly employed agent, likely because polysorbate 80-induced hypersensitivity can usually be thwarted with corticosteroid/antihistamine pretreatment, coupled with the significantly higher cost of the prodrug. The phosphate ester would be a viable choice in patients who do exhibit hypersensitivity to etoposide despite pretreatment. The oral formulation is reserved for lung cancer patients. Oral bioavailability is concentration-dependent and runs approximately 50% for the 50 mg capsule. Doses twice the IV dose (rounded to the nearest 50 mg) are administered.

Etoposide is approximately 97% protein bound, undergoes biphasic elimination, and has a terminal half-life of 4 to 11 hours. Approximately 56% of a dose is eliminated via the kidneys the remainder is excreted in feces. The drug should be used with caution in patients with renal impairment or liver disease that impacts protein binding sites (e.g., hyperbilirubinemia). Specifically, doses should be decreased in patients with creatinine clearance ≤50 mL/min or bilirubin levels >1.5 mg/dL. Organoplatinum anticancer agents decrease etoposide clearance, especially in children. If used in combination, administration must be separated by at least 2 days. The list of drugs interacting with etoposide via metabolic or other mechanisms is extensive.

Teniposide. Teniposide is used in combination with other agents for the treatment of refractory childhood ALL. The common dose is 165 mg/m^2 twice weekly. Compared to etoposide, it is more highly protein bound (>99%), more extensively metabolized, more slowly cleared (terminal half-life of 5-40 hr), and less dependent on renal elimination (10%-21%). The lack of oral bioavailability precludes the marketing of an oral dosage form, and no phosphate ester prodrug formulations are available. The hypersensitivity risk from Kolliphor EL is significant and, although normally controlled with pretreatment, patients should be closely observed throughout the infusion. The infusion is given over the course of 0.5-1 hour to avoid a drop in blood pressure.[76]

Exposure to heparin can cause teniposide to precipitate, so lines must be thoroughly flushed before and after teniposide administration. The drug can also spontaneously precipitate, particularly if solutions are over-agitated, and patients receiving prolonged infusions should be monitored for blockage of access catheters.

Anthracyclines and Anthracenediones

Anthracycline antineoplastics are very closely related to the tetracycline antibacterials. Structurally, they are glycosides and contain a sugar portion (L-daunosamine) and a nonsugar (aglycone) organic portion. The aglycone moiety of anthracyclines is referred to as the anthracyclinone or anthroquinone.

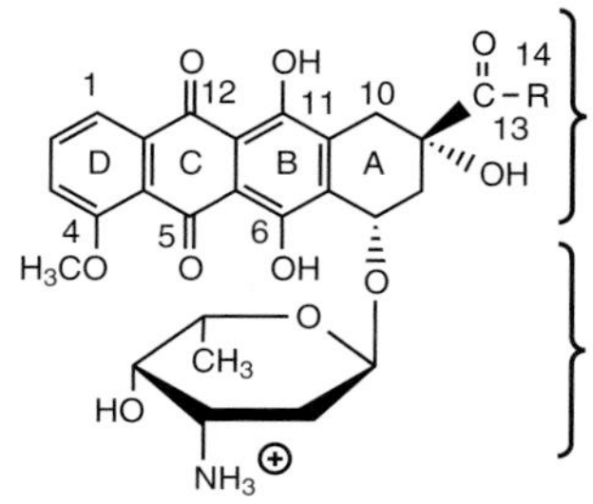

Anthracyclinone aglycone

Protonated L-daunosamine

MECHANISM OF ACTION. TopIIα, the topII isoform that predominates in rapidly dividing cells, is the molecular target for anthracycline anticancer agents. Like the poisons discussed earlier, they stabilize the cleavable ternary drug-enzyme-DNA complex, allowing DNA to be cut and covalently linked to the conserved Tyr residue. However, by inhibiting proper alignment of the cleaved DNA segments, they inhibit the resealing reaction. The aromatic portion of the anthracyclinone and the daunosamine sugar bind to DNA, with the anthracyclinone A ring bridging the gap between DNA and enzyme.[331] The site of DNA cleavage contains an essential thymine-adenine (T-A) dinucleotide, and a small number of anthracycline-induced DNA breaks here results in a high level of cell death.[332]

CHEMISTRY. DNA intercalation by rings B, C and D of the anthracyclinone initiates antineoplastic action.[305] The cyclic structure orients perpendicular to the long axis of DNA and the complex is stabilized through π-stacking and other affinity-enhancing interactions. A study which docked doxorubicin in a modeled DNA "postcleavage" intercalation site proposed highly efficacious H-bonds between topIIα Ser740 and the C5 quinone oxygen (ring C), Thr744 and the C4-OCH_3 (ring D), and a DNA thymine base and the C9-OH (ring A).[305] If present, a C14-OH should H-bond with the carbonyl oxygen of a DNA thymine base (Fig. 33.31). Although the C4-OCH_3 helps hold drug to enzyme, its removal increases planarity, facilitates intercalation, and directs daunosamine binding to better stabilize the ternary cleavable complex, thus increasing antineoplastic potency.[333]

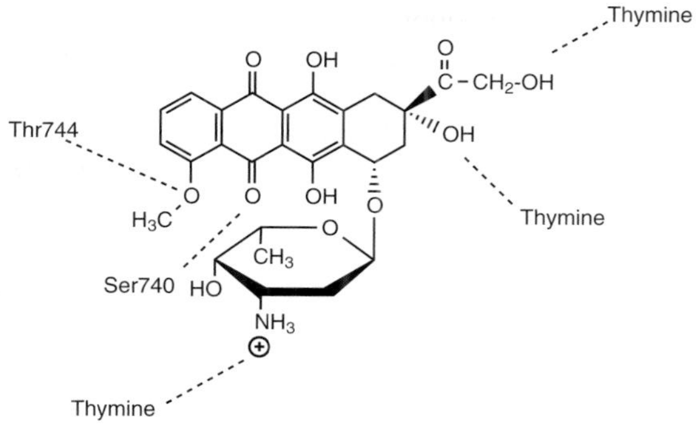

Figure 33.31 Proposed interaction between doxorubicin, DNA, and topoisomerase IIα.

Daunosamine binds in the DNA minor groove at the interface with topIIα and orchestrates DNA intercalation and the overall poisoning process.[333] The aforementioned molecular modeling study suggested that the cationic daunosamine 3′-amino binds with high affinity to the carbonyl oxygen of a DNA thymine base when in the naturally occurring α configuration. In the epimerized β configuration, the distance between these two moieties increases and unfavorable steric interactions with other DNA residues occur, yet cytotoxic potency increases. Antitumor activity of anthracyclines is thought to be related more to the proper positioning and stabilization of the drug within the cleavable ternary complex than to the actual drug affinity for DNA.[333] The daunosamine 3′-amino group is in the natural α configuration in all marketed anthracycline antineoplastics.

Resistance to anthracycline chemotherapy can be intrinsic or acquired. Major resistance mechanisms include: (1) compromised drug transport across cell membranes, (2) active efflux via P-gp and MDR transporters, (3) changes in tumor cell responsiveness to apoptotic triggers, (4) alterations in topIIα expression and activity, and (5) augmented biochemical defenses against anthracycline-induced oxidative stress.[334] Recently, upregulation of the reductase enzymes that convert anthracyclines to their less active or inactive secondary alcohol (rubicinol) metabolites has been proposed as a potential mechanism of acquired resistance.[335] The reason for the drop in cytotoxic activity is three-fold: in addition to having a lower DNA binding potential, rubicinols can be retained in lysosomes and are more vigorously effluxed from tumor cells by P-gp. As noted below, rubicinols concentrate in myocardial tissue and mediate the chronic cardiac toxicity that is the major use-limiting adverse effect of these drugs. Therefore, inhibiting these enzymes could conceivably help prevent/reverse resistance and could potentially protect against myocardial damage.[335]

Interestingly, the polyphenol epigallocatechin-3-gallate (EGCG, found in green tea) has been shown to inhibit cellular efflux of the anthracycline doxorubicin[57,336] and to sensitize doxorubicin-treated/resistant human colon carcinoma cells.[337] In addition to the scientific evidence supporting the positive doxorubicin–EGCG interaction, Sadzuka and colleagues holistically state, "We think that the intake of a favorite beverage favors a positive mental attitude of the patient and increases the efficacy of the chemotherapeutic index, and that this efficacy is useful for improving the quality of life on cancer chemotherapy."[57]

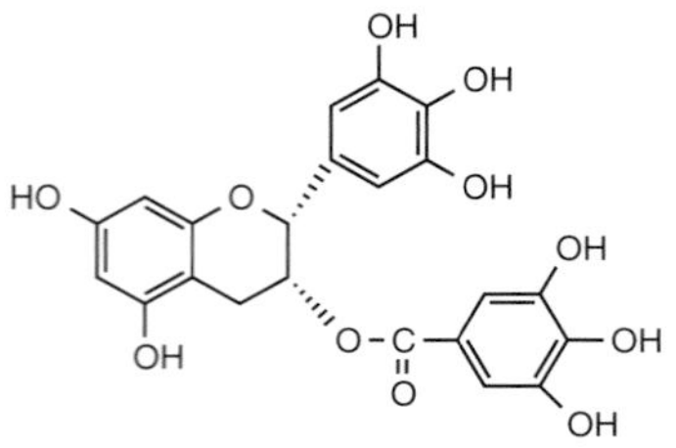

Epigallocatechin 3-gallate
(EGCG from Green tea)

Chemical Mechanism of Cardiotoxicity

Acute Toxicity. Approximately 11% of patients treated with anthracyclines will develop acute, reversible cardiac toxicity, and about 1.7% will suffer from chronic, delayed and potentially life-threatening damage.[335] Some estimate the percentage experiencing drug-induced cardiomyopathy as high as 20%, with 9% exhibiting delayed left ventricular systolic pathology within 1-year post therapy.[338,339]

The traditional and potentially still relevant mechanism, particularly in the acute phase, is the formation of reactive oxygen species (ROS). Of particular importance is the generation of superoxide radical anion and hydroxyl radical (·OH), both of which are formed via a one-electron reduction of the anthracyclinone quinone (ring C) to hydroquinone via a free radical semiquinone intermediate by NADPH/CYP450 reductase (Fig. 33.32). Superoxide radical anions generate hydrogen peroxide (H_2O_2) in a Cu^{2+}-dependent process that requires superoxide dismutase and proton.

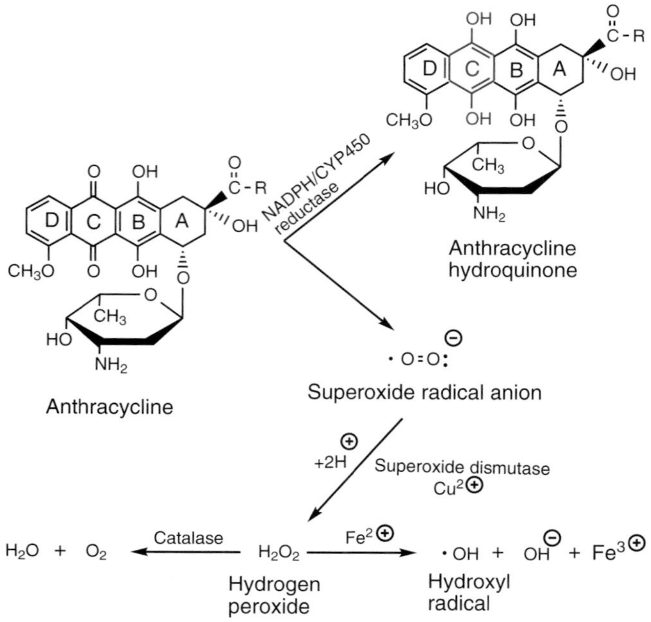

Anthracycline

Anthracycline hydroquinone

Superoxide radical anion

Hydrogen peroxide

Hydroxyl radical

Figure 33.32 Anthracycline-mediated free radical formation.

The fate of H_2O_2 dictates the degree of acute myotoxicity observed from the anthracycline. In the presence of catalase, H_2O_2 is rapidly converted to water and oxygen. However, in the absence of catalase and in the presence of ferrous ion (Fe^{2+}), the highly damaging hydroxyl radical is generated via the Fenton reaction (Fig. 33.32). Anthracyclines chelate strongly with di- and trivalent cations, including intracellular Fe^{3+}, which can be reduced to Fe^{2+} enzymatically or via auto-reduction if the C13 substituent is CH_2OH.[340-342] Therefore, the ready availability of the iron needed to generate hydroxyl radicals from H_2O_2 is essentially guaranteed.

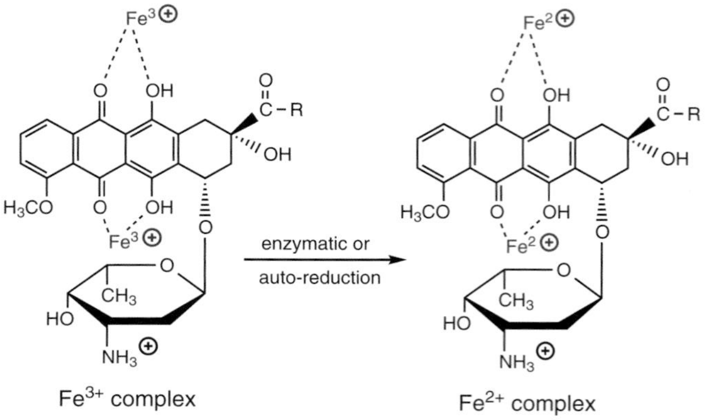

Fe^{3+} complex

Fe^{2+} complex

Hydroxyl radicals promote single-strand breaks in DNA and could conceivably augment the cytotoxic action of anthracyclines; however, this is uncommon in tumor cells at standard antineoplastic doses.[332] In contrast, hydroxyl radicals are readily generated in the myocardium because cardiac tissue does not contain significant amounts of catalase and other relevant cytoprotective enzymes.[343] When H_2O_2 forms in the myocardium, it has no choice but to go down the Fenton pathway.

Cardiac toxicity is the major use-limiting side effect of anthracyclines, but coadministration of dexrazoxane (an antioxidant and iron chelator) has been shown to lower its incidence when used with the C13-CH_2OH substituted anthracyclines doxorubicin and epirubicin.[344,345] As discussed below, dexrazoxane's mechanism of cardioprotective action likely lies outside of its iron-chelating ability.

Chronic (Delayed) Cardiotoxicity. Rubicinol metabolites are believed responsible for the more life-threatening chronic cardiotoxicity that some patients experience. The C13-carbonyl is reduced via a two-electron mechanism to a usually less active[346,347] or inactive[342] rubicinol via cytosolic aldo-keto reductase (AKR1C3) and carbonyl reductase (CBR1) enzymes[335] (Fig. 33.33). Before excretion, anthracyclines can be further metabolized via hydrolytic or reductive deglycosidation to their 7-hydroxy or 7-deoxy aglycones, respectively, followed by O-dealkylation of the C4 methoxy ether (if present) and conjugation with either glucuronic acid or sulfate. The aglycones may also have cardiotoxic properties.[339,342]

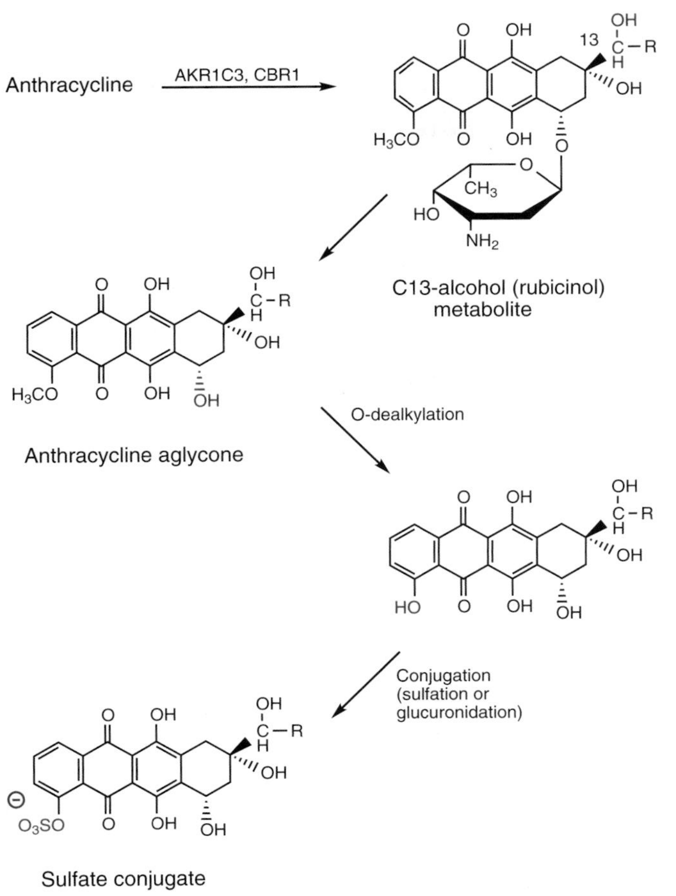

Figure 33.33 Anthracycline metabolism (AKR, aldo-keto reductase; CBR, carbonyl reductase).

The larger the C13-substituent the slower the AKR/CBR-catalyzed reduction reaction, and the longer the duration of cytotoxic activity. C13-substituents found on most marketed anthracyclines include CH_3 (daunorubicin and idarubicin) and CH_2OH (doxorubicin and epirubicin).

Rubicinol metabolites concentrate in cardiomyocytes and induce profound increases in intracellular calcium concentrations through a variety of mechanisms, which can include: (1) prolonged inhibition of calcium loading, (2) inhibition of Ca^{2+}, Mg^{2+}-ATPase and simulation of vesicular calcium release in the sarcoplasmic reticulum, and (3) inhibition of Na^+, K^+-ATPase in the sarcolemma.[335] The synthesis of sarcomeric proteins essential to cardiomyocyte integrity is also impaired.[339,348] As a result, myocardial contractility is compromised, and the myopathy presents as severe congestive heart failure involving systolic and diastolic dysfunction.

TopIIβ, the predominant topII isoform in quiescent cells, is the only isoform found in the myocardium, and a critical role for this protein in anthracycline-induced cardiotoxicity has been proposed.[349] Anthracycline binding to myocardial topIIβ disrupts mitochondrial function, initiates DNA double-strand breaks, stimulates p53-induced apoptosis in cardiomyocytes, and may facilitate formation of ROS.[350] Studies in mice genetically engineered to be topIIβ deficient were resistant to anthracycline-induced cardiac toxicity, and a small isolated study found patients sensitive to anthracycline-induced cardiac effects had significantly higher peripheral blood leukocyte levels of topIIβ than resistant patients.[350] TopIIβ is currently viewed as a highly significant (and likely a primary) mediator of anthracycline-related cardiotoxicity.

Although the acute and chronic phases of anthracycline-induced cardiomyopathy appear metabolically distinct, a unifying hypothesis suggests that induction of ROS-mediated oxidative stress may upregulate AKR, thereby facilitating the development of rubicinol-induced chronic cardiotoxicity.[342] It is also thought that rubicinol metabolites can generate ROS, and that acute toxicity (e.g., left ventricular systolic dysfunction) from "real time" drug exposure can predispose patients to worsening myopathy over time, as described below.[339]

Clinical Aspects. Fortunately, acute anthracycline-induced cardiotoxicity is generally self-limiting. It commonly manifests during or a few weeks after therapy, and often presents as disturbances in EEG, cardiac rhythm, and ventricular function. Symptoms commonly resolve within 1 week, although the caution about early damage predisposing to chronic pathology must be noted.[339,351]

In contrast, rubicinols form long-lived reservoirs of cardiotoxic drug within the myocardium,[339] and chronic anthracycline-induced heart failure can manifest without warning years (even decades) after therapy concludes. It is often unresponsive to therapeutic intervention, and more than half of the patients so diagnosed die within 2 years.[342,351] Elevated risk occurs with high cumulative doses, age extremes, genetic polymorphisms impacting ROS production, rubicinol formation and/or anthracycline transport, coadministration of other cardiotoxic drugs, and underlying cardiovascular disease.[338,339] Females and Blacks are at risk for increased incidence or severity of drug-induced cardiomyopathy.[350,352] Because toxicity is dose-dependent,[350] dosage adjustments must be made in patients with liver dysfunction who cannot adequately metabolize and clear anthracyclines to avoid life-threatening toxicity.

Dexrazoxane. As noted above, coadministration of dexrazoxane, an antioxidant and prodrug iron chelating agent, can attenuate anthracycline-induced cardiotoxicity (including chronic, delayed heart failure) from the 13-CH_2OH substituted anthracyclines doxorubicin and epirubicin in both adults and children. The level of protection has been estimated at 80%.[338,339] Dexrazoxane readily enters cells and is hydrolyzed to the active Fe^{2+} and Fe^{3+} chelating form ADR-925. It is administered IV 30 minutes prior to the anthracycline to allow distribution to cells where it will be needed. Although the affinity of ADR-925 for iron surpasses that of doxorubicin, chelation-independent mechanisms for cardioprotection by dexrazoxane have been proposed, including altering topIIβ configuration in a way that inhibits anthracycline binding and inducing transient topIIβ depletion.[338,342,350,353] The fact that: (1) other iron chelators and free radical scavengers are ineffective in providing cardioprotection, (2) inhibition of dexrazoxane hydrolysis does not abolish its cardioprotective effect, and (3) direct application of ADR-925 to cardiomyocytes does not protect against anthracycline-induced damage lends strong support to these alternative mechanisms of action, and to the dexrazoxane parent structure as the active entity.[338]

Whether dexrazoxane should be administered early or later in the anthracycline regimen has been subject to debate. On one hand, early administration initiates cardioprotection before the first dose of anthracycline hits the heart.[349] However, it has been proposed that dexrazoxane can deplete the topIIβ (as well as topIIα) that's expressed in over 90% of breast cancers, resulting in reduced early tumor shrinkage. Although studies have not shown any significant impact of dexrazoxane therapy on PFS, OS and tumor response rate in advanced breast cancer, the concern remains because tumor shrinkage is positively associated with tumor response.[338] The latter argument is winning out, as current therapeutic guidelines for dexrazoxane administration call for it to be given after patients have received a cumulative doxorubicin dose of 300 mg/m^2 (i.e., later in the regimen).

Dexrazoxane can also be used to attenuate serious tissue injury following accidental anthracycline extravasation.[354] For this indication, it is administered IV once daily for three days, beginning within 6 hours of the extravasation incident.

Dexrazoxane ADR-925

In addition to dexrazoxane administration, other suggested strategies for attenuating anthracycline-induced cardiomyopathy include limiting the cumulative (lifetime) dose, administering the anthracycline by continuous infusion and in divided doses (vs. bolus administration), and electing liposomal formulations when appropriate.[350]

OTHER TOXICITIES. In addition to cardiac toxicity, all anthracycline antineoplastics can cause severe myelosuppression (especially leukocytopenia) as well as moderate to severe nausea and vomiting, mucositis leading to hemorrhage and potentially fatal infection, and alopecia. Boxed warnings for these life-threatening adverse effects are in effect for all anthracyclines. Side effects are dose-dependent.

Most of the anthracyclines are orally inactive and must be given by intravenous injection. They are highly necrotic to skin and, if extravasation occurs, can cause such severe blistering and ulceration that skin excision, followed by plastic surgery, may be indicated. The anthracyclines contain photosensitive phenolic groups that must be protected from light and air. The highly conjugated structure imparts a reddish-orange color to these compounds (implied in the name "rubicin"), which is maintained when these compounds are excreted in the urine.

SPECIFIC DRUGS. The structures of the currently marketed anthracycline anticancer agents, and a related anthracenedione, are provided in Figure 33.34.

Doxorubicin Hydrochloride. Doxorubicin is used either alone or in combination therapy to treat a wide range of neoplastic disorders, including hematologic cancers and solid tumors in breast, ovary, stomach, bladder, and thyroid gland. In addition to cardiomyopathy and myelosuppression, the boxed warning advises on the dangers of extravasation and the risk of secondary AML.[76]

The C13 substituent of doxorubicin is hydroxymethyl, which retards the action of cytosolic reductase and slows conversion to the less active and chronically cardiotoxic doxorubicinol. This contributes to the longer duration of action compared to analogues that have CH_3 at this position (e.g., daunorubicin). It is given IV in starting doses that range from 25 to 75 mg/m^2, and cumulative doses above 550 mg/m^2 are associated with an elevated risk of cardiac toxicity. As previously noted, doses are decreased in hepatic impairment, and the cardioprotectant dexrazoxane should be coadministered when cumulative doses reach 300 mg/m^2.

Doxorubicin is highly lipophilic and concentrates in the liver, lymph nodes, muscle, bone marrow, fat, and skin. Elimination is triphasic, and the drug has a terminal half-life of 30-40 hours. It is 75% protein bound. The majority of an administered dose is excreted in the feces, approximately half of it unchanged.[342]

A liposomal formulation of doxorubicin, marketed as Doxil, is used in the treatment of AIDS-related Kaposi sarcoma, refractory multiple myeloma (in combination with bortezomib), and organoplatinum-resistant ovarian cancer.[350] Liposomes are taken up selectively into tumor cells, presumably due to their persistence in the bloodstream and enhanced permeability of tumor vascular membranes. In liposomal form, the drug is protected against enzymes that generate cardiotoxic metabolites and is less likely to concentrate in the heart.[355] However, because this form of the drug can still induce potentially fatal congestive heart failure (i.e., the boxed warning for conventional doxorubicin applies) all precautions outlined for the use of doxorubicin should be taken.

The half-life of Doxil is extended to approximately 55 hours, and it is administered in doses ranging from 20 to 50 mg/m^2 every 3-4 weeks. The AUC of the liposomal formulation is approximately three-times that of the free drug formulation. It is cleared more slowly than conventional doxorubicin and generates very little of the doxorubicinol metabolite. Significant adverse effects have occurred when the liposomal formulation is erroneously dispensed, so pharmacists must be vigilant when interpreting therapeutic orders.

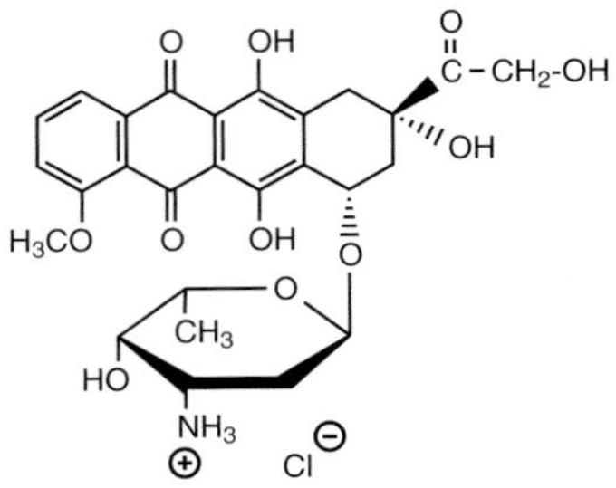

Doxorubicin hydrochloride (Adriamycin)

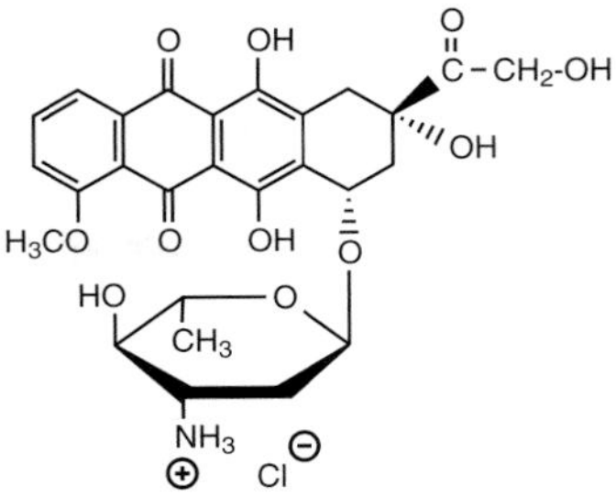

Epirubicin hydrochloride (Ellence)

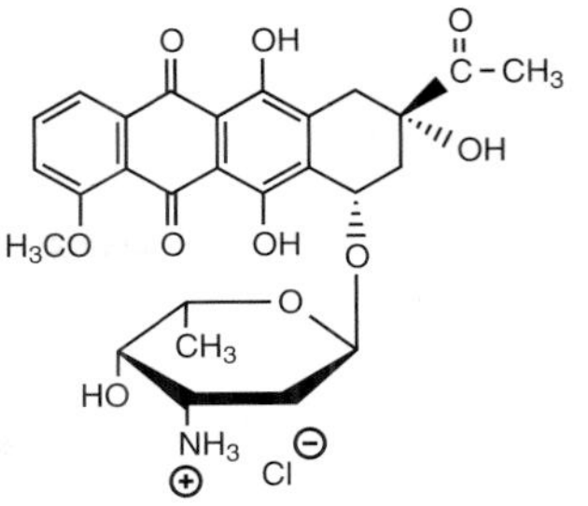

Daunorubicin hydrochloride (Cerubidine)

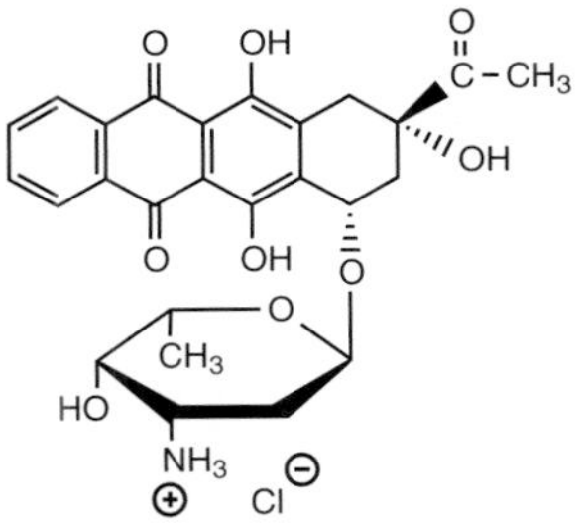

Idarubicin hydrochloride (Idamycin PFS)

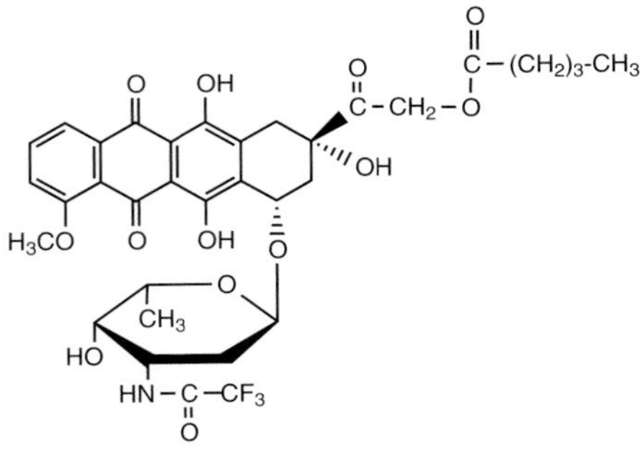

Valrubicin (Valstar)

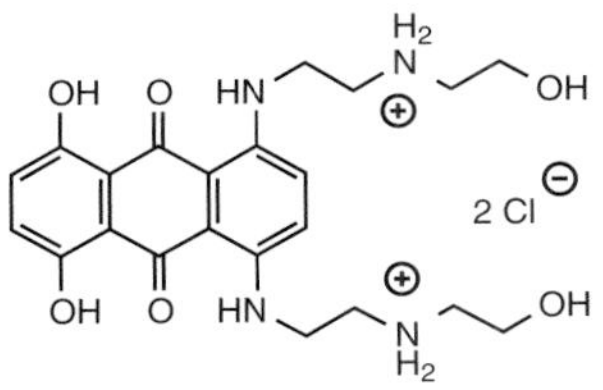

Mitoxantrone hydrochloride (Novantrone)

Figure 33.34 Anthracycline and related anticancer agents.

A maleimide-containing hydrazone prodrug of doxorubicin, aldoxorubicin, is in clinical trials for the treatment of advanced, relapsed/refractory soft tissue sarcoma. First-line therapy for this aggressive cancer is currently doxorubicin in combination with the DNA alkylating agent ifosfamide, but dose-limiting doxorubicin-induced cardiotoxicity can limit treatment options. Aldoxorubicin is delivered to tumor cells covalently bound to albumin and selectively released in situ, providing targeted therapy with minimal risk of doxorubicin's hallmark toxicities.[356-359]

ALDOXORUBICIN

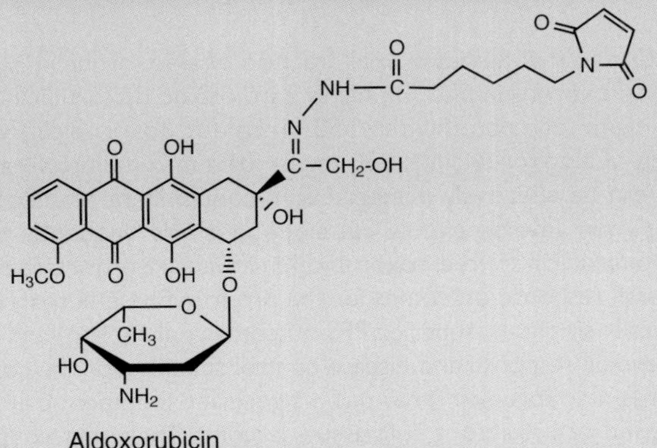

Aldoxorubicin

Aldoxorubicin is a doxorubicin prodrug that takes full chemical advantage of (1) an accessible Cys34 residue on serum albumin, (2) the propensity of tumors to accumulate macromolecules, and (3) the acidic pH of the hypoxic tumor cell. Equipped with a sterically unhindered Michael-alkylating maleimido moiety that specifically reacts with sulfhydryl (thiol) groups at physiologic pH, aldoxorubicin is attacked by Cys34 within minutes of IV administration. The covalent complex is transported throughout the bloodstream and drawn into the highly permeable tumor cells, where the acidic environment catalyzes the hydrolysis of the hydrazone linker and achieves targeted delivery of doxorubicin exactly where it is needed.[359]

SH
Cys34-Albumin
Aldoxorubicin
Aldoxorubicin covalently bound to albumin
H^+ Acid-catalyzed hydrolysis
S-Cys34-Albumin
H^+
Doxorubicin

Pharmacokinetic studies have confirmed that all but a small fraction of aldoxorubicin is securely tethered to circulating albumin, and serum concentrations of free doxorubicin and the highly cardiotoxic doxorubicinol metabolite are minimal. This allows for higher cumulative dosing (>2000 mg/m^2 compared with <550 mg/m^2 for doxorubicin) with essentially no serious cardiotoxicity risk. The standard dosing regimen of aldoxorubicin is 350 mg/m^2 (the maximum tolerated dose) every three weeks. The neutropenia induced by this prodrug can be effectively managed with concomitant granulocyte colony-stimulating factor (GCSF) therapy. Fatigue and mucositis are common adverse effects, but alopecia is less frequently observed than with doxorubicin.[356-358]

Phase II clinical trials comparing aldoxorubicin to free doxorubicin in advanced or metastatic soft tissue sarcoma patients documented superior median PFS and overall response outcomes for the prodrug. Phase III trials comparing aldoxorubicin to oncologists' choice of therapy showed statistically significant superior PFS outcomes only in lipo- and leiomyosarcoma patients (L-sarcomas), but improved PFS at 4 and 6 months, overall response and disease control statistics for the complete study cohort.[356-358]

The prevailing clinical opinion is that aldoxorubicin provides a significant therapeutic and safety advantage over doxorubicin as first-line therapy in advanced, relapsed or refractory soft tissue sarcoma. Trials that couple aldoxorubicin with the PDGF-α MAb olaratumab (which improves outcomes when paired with doxorubicin) and/or explores efficacy in other doxorubicin-sensitive cancers are eagerly awaited.

Epirubicin Hydrochloride. This stereoisomer of doxorubicin has the 4′-hydroxy group of the daunosamine sugar oriented in the unnatural β-position. However, this relatively modest structural change has a major impact on pharmacodynamics and pharmacokinetic properties. The higher starting dose of 100-120 mg/m^2 for epirubicin in breast cancer (its only indication) compared to doxorubicin's single agent dose of 60-75 mg/m^2 indicates a less potent topIIα-inhibiting action. Although excretion is primarily biliary, dose reduction in severe renal impairment, as well as in hepatic dysfunction, is warranted.

Epirubicin is reduced to the C13 alcohol (epirubicinol) to a much lower (60%) extent than doxorubicin, preferentially generating the reduced aglycone doxorubicinolone that is more easily eliminated. The rate of C4-glucuronidation of the O-dealkylated phenol is faster than that of doxorubicin, and the terminal half-life of 33 hours is shorter. Because it is readily trapped in lysosomes and other acidic organelles, it is not highly susceptible to ROS-generating one-electron oxidation. The overall cardiotoxicity has been estimated at 30% lower than doxorubicin. However, the margin of safety is mitigated by epirubicin's greater propensity to accumulate in myocardiocytes.[339,342,360] Other adverse effects and precautions are as outlined for doxorubicin.

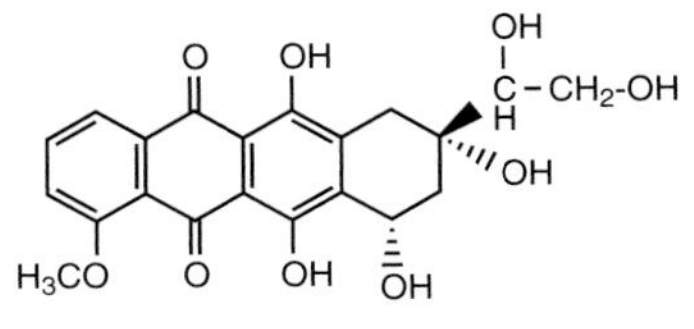

Doxorubicinolone

Daunorubicin Hydrochloride. The absence of the OH group at C14 in daunorubicin results in a faster conversion to the less active and chronically cardiotoxic daunorubicinol compared to CH_2OH-substituted anthracyclines like doxorubicin. The 18.5-hour terminal half-life is approximately half that of doxorubicin, and the terminal half-life of the daunorubicinol metabolite is 27 hours. Excretion is approximately 40% biliary and 25% urinary. Daunorubicin is administered IV at a dose of 45 mg/m^2 for the treatment of lymphocytic leukemia and AML. The toxicity and side effect profile of this anthracycline is similar to that of doxorubicin, and all previously identified precautions apply.[76]

The citrate salt of daunorubicin is marketed as a liposomal formulation, which promotes the use of this agent in solid tumors. Like Doxil (the liposomal formulation of doxorubicin), DaunoXome is indicated for use in AIDS-related Kaposi sarcoma and is administered IV at a dose of 40 mg/m^2 every 2 weeks. The pharmacokinetic profiles of Doxil and DaunoXome are similar.[76]

Idarubicin Hydrochloride. Idarubicin is the 4-desmethoxy analogue of daunorubicin, which facilitates intercalation between DNA base pairs. In turn, this orients the daunosamine sugar in the minor groove in a way that better stabilizes the ternary complex for the DNA cleavage reaction.[333] The loss of the 4-methoxy moiety also makes this compound more lipophilic than other anthracyclines, resulting in better penetration into tumor cells.

Idarubicin is reduced to idarubicinol which, unlike other rubicinols, is as active an antitumor agent as the parent drug.[335,347] Importantly, idarubicin has limited affinity for P-gp (a major anthracycline resistance mechanism), although the idarubicinol metabolite is still actively effluxed from tumor cells.[335] The elimination half-lives of idarubicin and idarubicinol are 22 and 45 hours, respectively.

Idarubicin's primary indication is AML, and it is administered in combination with other cytotoxic agents at a dose of 10-12 mg/m^2 (much lower than other anthracyclines). Its higher potency can be attributed to its four previously highlighted pharmacodynamics and pharmacokinetic distinctions: (1) better DNA intercalation, (2) more effective tumor cell penetration, (3) resistance to P-gp efflux, and (4) an equally cytotoxic idarubicinol metabolite. In addition, the lack of the C4-methoxy means no O-dealkylation and no phenolic conjugation with glucuronic acid. The major metabolite is idarubicinol and, like other anthracyclines, excretion is predominantly fecal with a lesser dependence on renal elimination.

Some authors have shown that idarubicin is transported into cardiac tissue via a saturable transporter and that coadministration of methylxanthines (e.g., caffeine) can increase both myocardial drug concentrations and the risk of idarubicin-induced cardiotoxicity.[361]

Valrubicin. Chemically, valrubicin differs from doxorubicin by the addition of a carbon-rich C14-valerate ester and a nonionizable 3′-trifluoroacetamide moiety. After solubilizing with Kolliphor EL, the drug is instilled intervesically in the treatment of bacille Calmette-Guérin (BCG)-refractory carcinoma in situ of the bladder.[362] Its high lipophilicity effectively traps it at the site of action, so therapy can be considered local.

Valrubicin is not a doxorubicin prodrug; the trifluroacetamide and valerate ester remain intact within the bladder. The drug should not be given to patients with compromised bladder wall integrity, as it can reach the bloodstream and hydrolyze to doxorubicin, initiating serious toxicity that would not otherwise manifest. Its primary mechanism is cell chromosomal damage and cell cycle arrest through the inhibition of DNA synthesis.[363] The patient population is small, sustained positive outcomes are rare,[364] and this drug is not in common use.

Mitoxantrone Hydrochloride. Chemically, mitoxantrone is classified as an anthracenedione. The cationic sidechain amines bind to the anionic phosphate residue of the DNA backbone in the same fashion that the anthracycline cationic amino group is believed to do. The anthracenedione ring system intercalates DNA to initiate topIIα inhibition, but the enhanced stability of the quinone ring (possibly through an increased potential for intramolecular hydrogen bonding) results in an 8-fold lower ability to chelate Fe^{3+}.[341] This limits the formation of highly toxic ROS. In addition, there is no rubicinol to induce chronic toxicity.

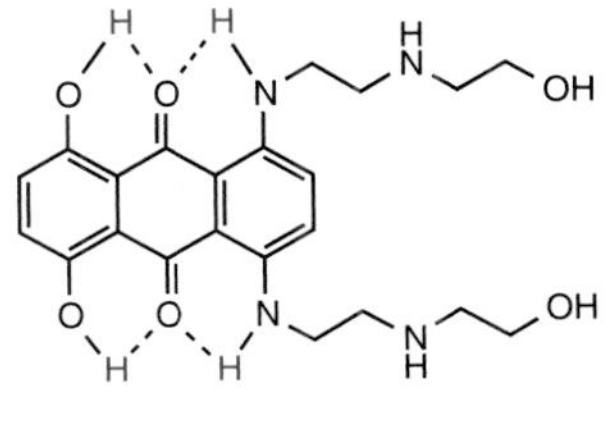

Mitoxantrone

The chance of cardiac toxicity from mitoxantrone is significantly decreased compared to true anthracyclines, although patients, particularly those who have previously received anthracycline therapy, are still at risk. While the symptoms mimic anthracycline-induced toxicity, the mechanism is unknown and cardioprotection therapy is not available. The drug carries a maximum lifetime cumulative dose of 140 mg/m^2.[365] It is also myelosuppressive, but non-hematological toxicities are less serious than observed with anthracyclines.

The major mitoxantrone metabolites are mono- and dicarboxylic acid products of N-dealkylation and CYP oxidation, and they are inactive and excreted as glucuronide conjugates in urine (along with 65% unchanged drug). However, a naphthoquinoxaline metabolite also forms that retains cytotoxic action and has been found to be less cardiotoxic than mitoxantrone in isolated differentiated H9c2 cells. Consideration of the development of this metabolite as a potential anticancer drug has been encouraged.[365]

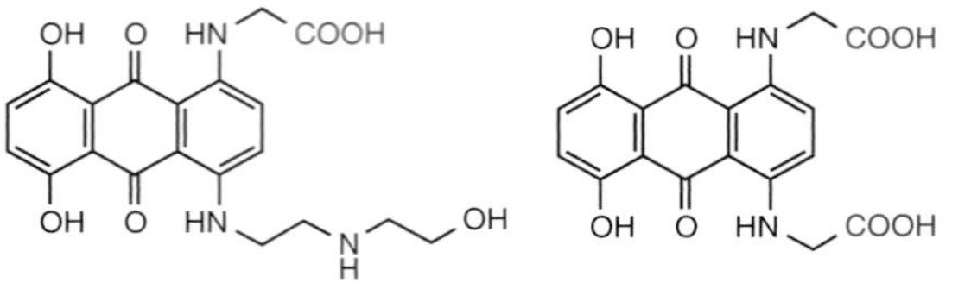

Mitoxantrone mono- and dicarboxylic acid metabolites (inactive)

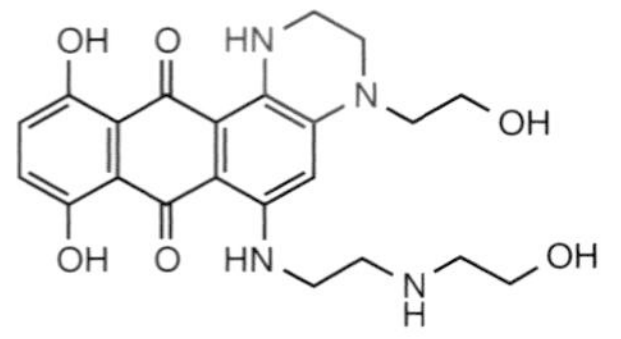

Naphthoquinoxaline metabolite (active)

Mitoxantrone is used in combination with other agents during the initial treatment of acute nonlymphocytic leukemia and CRPC. In contrast to the "fire engine red" color of the anthracyclines, the conjugated anthracenedione is a vibrant blue, a color that can be apparent in urine and the whites of the eyes.

Mitosis Inhibitors

The mitotic process depends on the structural and functional viability of microtubules, which are polymeric heterodimers consisting of isotypes of α- and β-tubulin. These distinct but nearly identical 50-kd proteins lie adjacent to one another and roll up to form an open, pipe-like cylinder akin to a hollow peppermint candy stick. A γ-tubulin protein is found at the organizational center of the microtubule. The tubulin isotypes found in the microtubule are conserved throughout specific tissues within a given species and will impact the cell's sensitivity to mitosis inhibitors.

During cell division, tubulin undergoes alternating periods of structural growth and erosion known as "dynamic instability." The proteins alternatively polymerize and depolymerize through guanosine triphosphate (GTP)- and Ca^{2+}-dependent processes, respectively. Polymerization involves the addition of tubulin dimers to either end of the tubule, although the faster-growing (+) end is more commonly involved. Polymerization results in tubular elongation, whereas depolymerization results in structural shortening. The frenetic alteration in structure, facilitated by microtubule-associated proteins (MAPs), ultimately allows for the formation of the mitotic spindle and the attachment of chromosomes that are prerequisites to cell division. Inhibiting the essential hyperdynamic changes in microtubular structure results in mitotic arrest and apoptosis.

Two general chemical classes of mitosis inhibitors have historically been marketed for the treatment of cancer: taxanes, and vinca alkaloids. The epothilone ixabepilone (Fig. 33.35) is also available, although it does not yet enjoy the widespread clinical use of taxane and vinca-derived therapies. Estramustine, an estrogen-based nitrogen mustard-like carbamate originally thought to act via DNA alkylation, is no longer recommended for use in metastatic CRPC (its only original indication) due to a lack of clinical benefit.[76] Only 20 papers with "estramustine" in the title were published between January, 2014 and July, 2018, and most confirmed an increased risk of adverse effects with no counterbalancing positive impact on OS.[366-368]

Taxanes

MECHANISM OF ACTION. Antineoplastic taxanes were originally isolated from the bark of the Pacific yew (*Taxus brevifolia*) but are now produced semisynthetically from an inactive natural precursor (10-deactetylbaccatin III) found in the leaves of the European yew (*Taxus baccata*), a renewable resource. Taxanes bind to polymerized β-tubulin at a specific hydrophobic receptor site comprised of the 31 N-terminal residues located deep within the tubular lumen.[369] At standard therapeutic doses, binding promotes a stable tubulin conformation similar to that of the GTP-bound protein, rendering the microtubules prone to further polymerization and resistant to erosion. Dynamic instability is disrupted, the mitotic spindle does not form, and microtubules collapse into dense aberrant structures known as asters. In other words, mitosis stops and the cell dies.

In contrast to taxanes, vinca-based mitosis inhibitors promote microtubule erosion over polymerization. Patients expressing a mutant variety of the *p53* oncogene that causes MAP4 overexpression, and subsequently promotes microtubular polymerization/elongation, show enhanced sensitivity to taxane chemotherapy and resistance to vinca alkaloids.[370] Cellular efflux by P-gp is a major mechanism of taxane resistance, as is β-tubulin mutation and overexpression of another isotype, βIII-tubulin.[371,372]

CHEMISTRY. Diterpenoid taxanes consist of a 15-membered tricyclic taxane ring system (tricyclo[9.3.1.0]pentadecane) fused to an oxetane (D) ring, and contain an esterified β-phenylisoserine side chain at C13. As shown in Figure 33.35, the three marketed taxane antineoplastics differ in substitution pattern at C13 (benzamido or *t*-butoxycarboxamido), C10 (secondary alcohol, acetate ester, or methoxy ether), and/or C7 (secondary alcohol or methoxy ether). The taxane ring system is conceptualized as having "northern" and "southern" halves. The southern

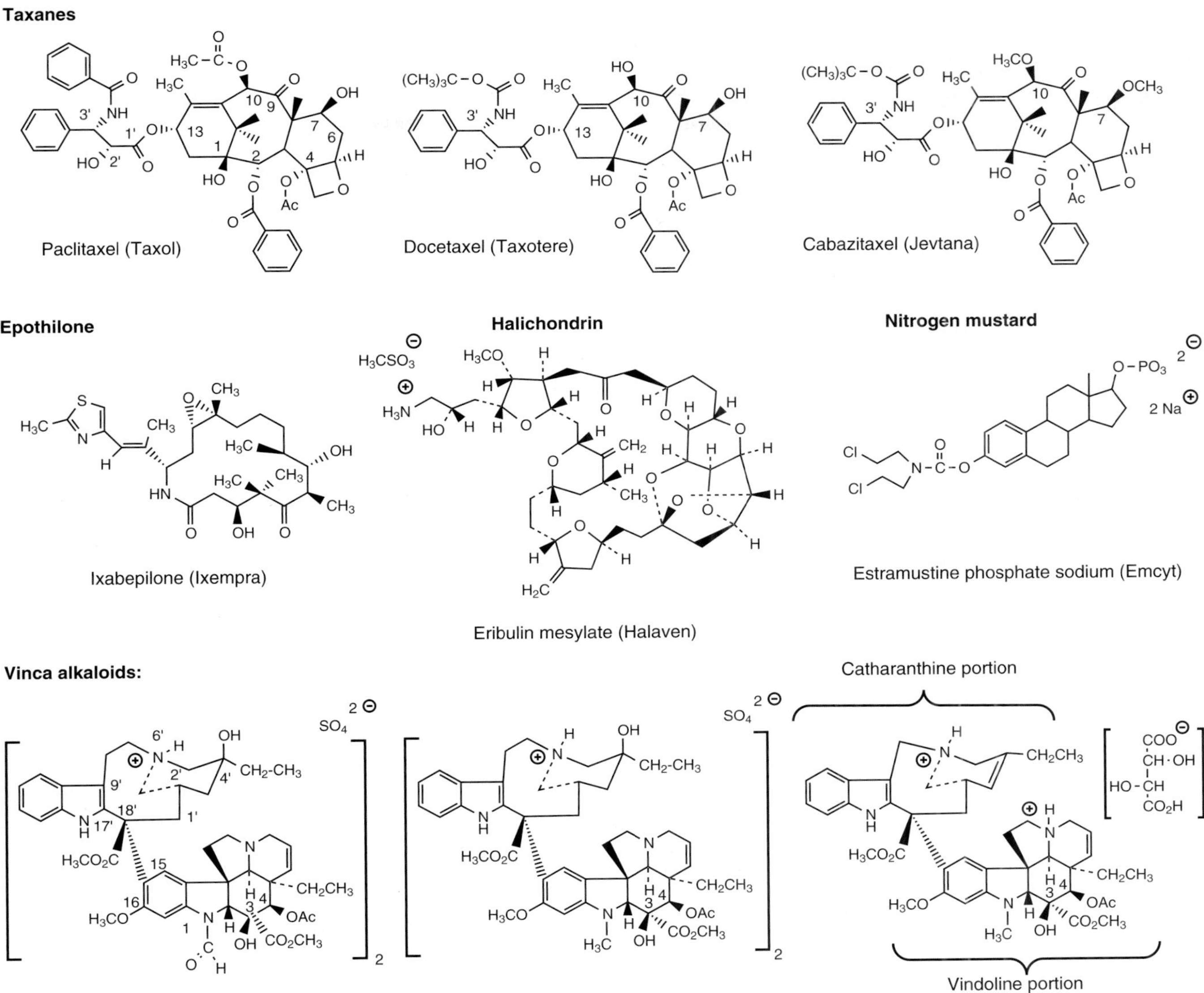

Figure 33.35 Mitosis inhibitors.

segment is critical to receptor binding, while the northern section ensures the proper conformation of critical functional groups, including the C13-isoserine side chain [with its C1′-carbonyl, free C2'-(*R*)-OH and C3'-(*S*)-benzamido or *t*-butoxycarboxamido groups], the benzoyloxy and acetoxy groups at C2 and C4, respectively, and the intact oxetane ring. The free C2′ hydroxyl in particular is essential to taxane antimitotic action.[373,374]

The key taxane-tubulin binding interactions are identified in Table 33.12 using paclitaxel as ligand.[375,376] Paclitaxel interacts in a folded ("T" or "butterfly") conformation that places the C2-benzoyloxy and C3′-benzamido groups in close proximity.[374,376,377] Their independent intermolecular engagement with a critical β-tubulin His residue perfectly positioned between them keeps them from interacting with one another. The oxetane ring, although capable of hydrogen bonding with receptor residues, is believed to serve a more critical role in properly orienting the C4-acetoxy moiety for interaction within its hydrophobic binding pocket.[375,378] The C1-OH also promotes conformational stability through intramolecular interaction with the carbonyl oxygen of the C2 benzoyloxy moiety.[374] The areas of the paclitaxel structure where steric influences are most critical to receptor binding have been identified.[373]

METABOLISM. The taxanes are metabolized to significantly less cytotoxic metabolites by CYP enzymes (Fig. 33.36). In humans, CYP2C8 converts paclitaxel to 6α-hydroxypaclitaxel, the major metabolite, which is 30-fold less active than the parent structure.[379] CYP3A4 mediates the formation of additional minor *p*-hydroxylated metabolites of the benzamido and benzoyloxy moieties at C3′ and C2 respectively, and the 10-desacetyl metabolite has been documented in urine and plasma.

Docetaxel is oxidized exclusively by CYP3A4/5, with CYP3A4 having a 10-fold higher affinity for the drug

Table 33.12 Paclitaxel-β-Tubulin Binding Interactions

Paclitaxel Functional Group	β-Tubulin Binding Residues	Interaction
C_2-benzoyloxy phenyl	Leu217, Leu219, His229, Leu230	Hydrophobic
C_2-benzoyloxy carbonyl	Arg278	Hydrogen bond
$C_{3'}$-benzamido NH	Asp26	Hydrogen bond
$C_{3'}$-benzamido carbonyl	His229	Hydrogen bond
$C_{3'}$-phenyl	Ala233, Ser236, Phe272	Hydrophobic
C_4-acetoxy	Leu217, Leu230, Phe272, Leu275	Hydrophobic
C_7-OH	Thr276 Ser277, Arg278	Hydrogen bond
C_{12}-CH_3	Leu217, Leu230, Phe272, Leu275	Hydrophobic
$C_{2'}$-OH	Arg369, Gly370 (NH)	Hydrogen bond
$C_{1'}$-carbonyl	Gly370 (NH)	Hydrogen bond
Oxetane oxygen	Thr276 (NH)	Hydrogen bond

From Yue Q, Liu X, Guo D. Microtubule-binding natural products for cancer therapy. *Planta Med.* 2010;76:1037-1043; Maccari L, Manetti F, Corelli F, et al. 3D QSAR studies for the β-tubulin binding site of microtubule-stabilizing anticancer agents (MSAAs). A pseudoreceptor model for taxanes based on the experimental structure of tubulin. *Il Farmaco.* 2003;58:659-668; Gueritte F. General and recent aspects of the chemistry and structure-activity relationships of taxoids. *Curr Pharm Des.* 2001;7:1229-1249.

than CYP3A5. The major metabolite, known as hydroxydocetaxel, is the hydroxymethyl derivative of the 3′-*t*-butoxycarboxamide side chain.[379] Hydroxydocetaxel can be further oxidized and cyclized to oxazolidinedione and diasteriomeric hydroxyoxazolidinone metabolites prior to excretion. The oxazolidinedione has been linked to the edema and weight gain that are problematic adverse effects of docetaxel.[380]

Cabazitaxel is metabolized predominantly (80%-90%) by CYP3A4/5, with CYP2C8 taking on a minor biotransformation role. Three active metabolites (including docetaxel) result from O-demethylation at C7 and/or C10. The elimination of taxanes is predominantly biliary.

The C13 side chain is believed to guide the positioning of taxanes within the catalytic site of CYP enzymes. Specifically, the 3′-phenyl of paclitaxel has been proposed to properly orient C6 for hydroxylation through π-stacking interactions with CYP2C8 active site residues while decreasing affinity for CYP3A4 binding groups. The hydrophobic character of the 10-acetoxy group, found in paclitaxel, enhances CYP-mediated hydroxylation 2-5 fold by facilitating substrate binding and/or augmenting catalytic capability. Both isoforms are impacted by the presence of this ester, often to the same extent.[379]

Epothilones

CHEMISTRY. Low water solubility is a significant drawback to the therapeutic utility of the taxanes. This is particularly true of paclitaxel, which has a more lipophilic acetate moiety at C10 compared to docetaxel's polar hydroxyl group. Paclitaxel is administered in a vehicle of 50% alcohol/50% Kolliphor EL, which can lead to an enhanced risk of hypersensitivity reactions (dyspnea, hypotension, angioedema, and urticaria) in patients not pretreated with H_1 and H_2 antagonists and dexamethasone. As noted previously, high P-gp-mediated cellular efflux of paclitaxel and docetaxel can result in drug resistance.

To overcome these problems, epothilones, 16-membered macrolides structurally unrelated to the taxanes but with functional groups properly positioned to mimic critical tubulin-binding groups, have been investigated for use in a variety of solid tumor and hematologic cancers (Fig. 33.37). Epothilone B binds with high affinity to the taxane binding site on polymerized β-tubulin, and acts through the same cytotoxic mechanism (microtubule polymerization and stabilization).[381] In addition to enhanced water solubility and a lack of P-gp affinity, epothilone B is more efficiently produced through fermentation with the myxobacterium *Sorangium cellulosum* and has a higher antineoplastic potency.[376,382,383] The lactam analogue ixabepilone has a comparable anticancer activity with an even higher water solubility and better in vivo and in vitro stability[381] (Fig. 33.38). The story of the discovery and subsequent development of this lactam as the lead compound in the search for a paclitaxel alternative makes for interesting reading.[384]

Epothilones and taxanes bind to a shared tubulin binding site in distinct ways.[372,385,386] A comparison of the crystal structures of tubulin-bound epothilone A (the 12-desmethyl derivative of epothilone B) and paclitaxel documented that the smaller macrolide fills only about half the binding site volume of the larger taxane ligand. The binding site is plastic, and residues adjust their side-chain conformations to accommodate either drug. Despite being surrounded by identical tubulin residues, the only common binding interaction is a hydrogen bond between Arg282 and the 7-OH group of taxanes and epothilones,[385] although the relevance of this interaction to epothilone affinity has been questioned.[386]

Although epothilone B is nearly identical in structure to epothiolone A, it binds to β-tubulin via a distinct mode. Molecular dynamics simulations with the native protein complexed with epothilone B have identified key binding interactions (Fig. 33.39), while studies with selected mutant proteins revealed mechanisms of epothilone resistance. Specifically, T274I, R282Q and Q292E mutations alter the protein's M-loop conformation, disrupting important polar interactions with the ligand that decrease β-tubulin affinity. Gln292 does not bind directly to epothiolone B, but it does assure favorable interactions between tubulin dimers important to microtubule formation. Mutation of Gln292 to anionic

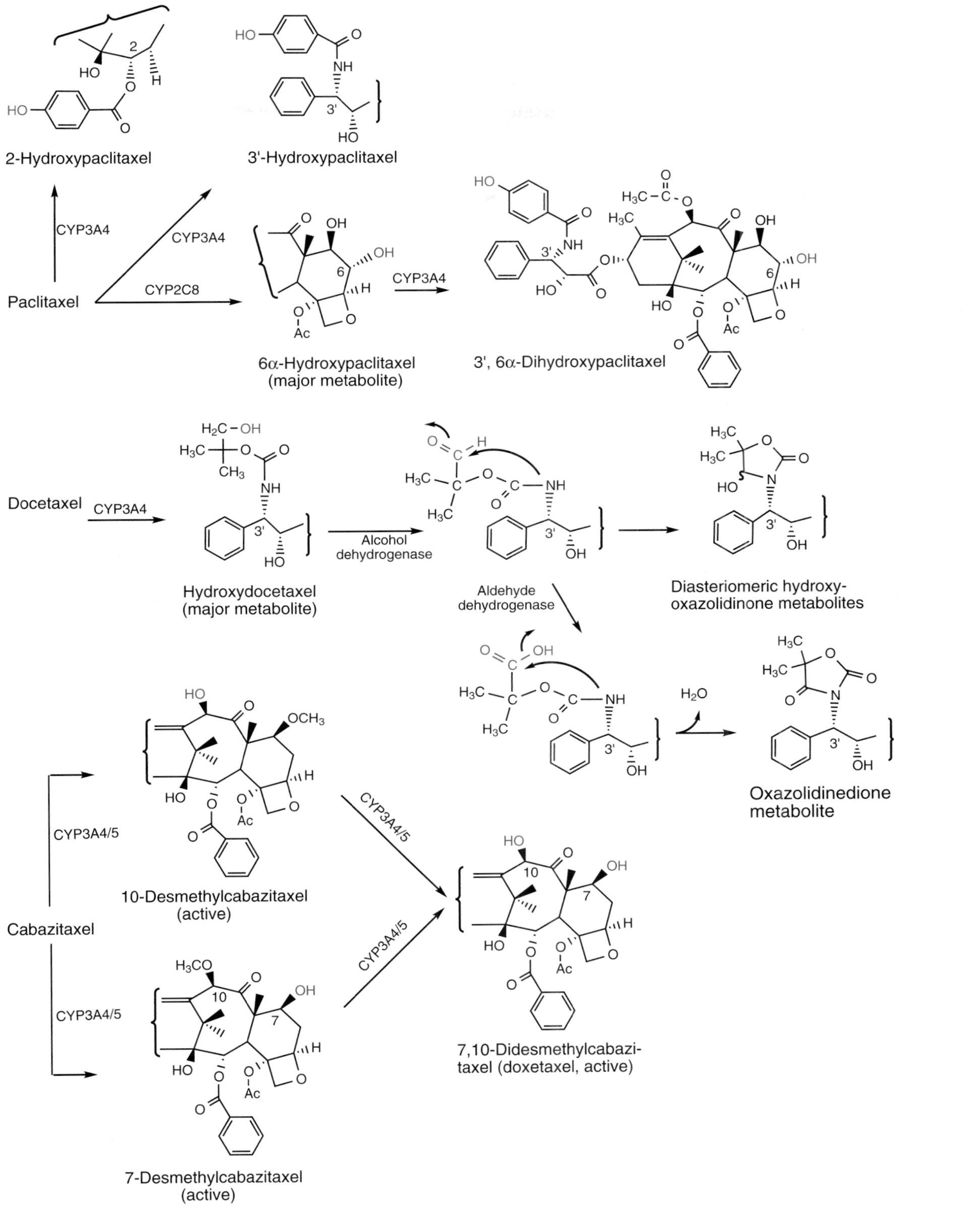

Figure 33.36 Taxane metabolism.

Glu produces the most profound resistance of any of the mutants studied. Phe270 engages in a critical interaction with the epoxide oxygen of epothilone B. While mutation to Val (F270V) also significantly decreases ligand affinity, the impact on resistance was the lowest of the four mutants.[386]

Specific Drugs

PACLITAXEL. Paclitaxel is claimed to be "one of the most successful drugs ever used in cancer chemotherapy",[387] and also the "best-selling".[374] It is available in conventional injection (Taxol) and albumin bound nanoparticle (Abraxane) formulations.

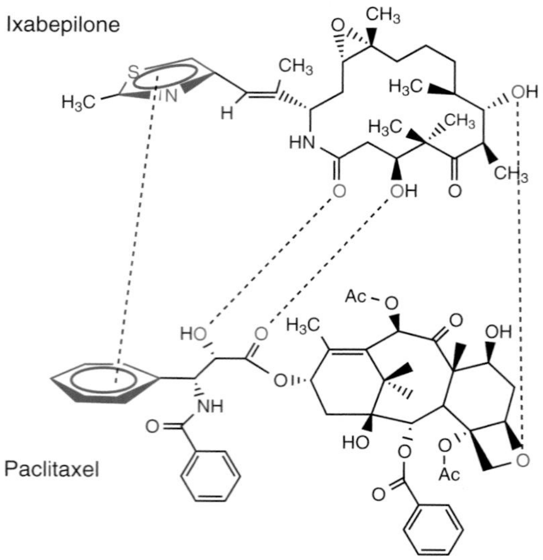

Figure 33.37 Complementary ixabepilone and paclitaxel functional groups.

Conventional Injection. Paclitaxel conventional injection is indicated for IV use in combination with cisplatin as first-line therapy for advanced ovarian and NSCLC. It is also used alone or in combination with the fluorouracil prodrug capecitabine in anthracycline-resistant MBC. Paxclitaxel's ability to upregulate thymidine phosphorylase, one of capecitabine's activating enzymes, is the rationale behind the combination therapy.[388]

The Kolliphor EL-solubilized drug is infused in doses of 135-175 mg/m^2, most commonly over 3 hours, and can be passed through an in-line, 0.22-μm filter to reduce vehicle-related cloudiness. In addition to hypersensitivity reactions (generally kept at bay by antihistamine/corticosteroid pretreatment), the major use-limiting adverse effect of paclitaxel is dose-dependent myelosuppression, particularly neutropenia, and first doses might need to be decreased in patients with hepatic dysfunction. Subsequent dose reductions, if any, should be tailored to individual

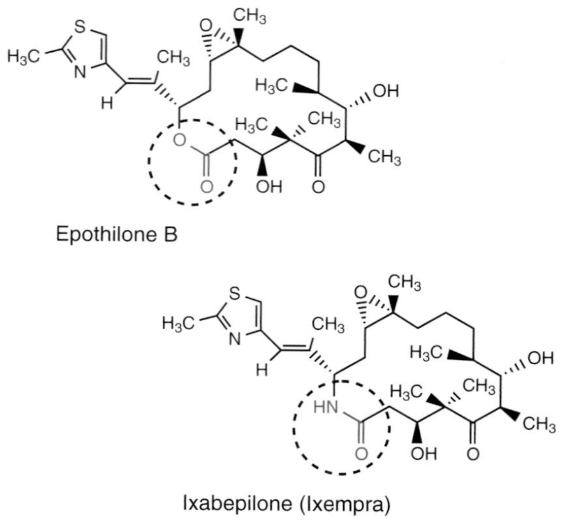

Epothilone B

Ixabepilone (Ixempra)

Figure 33.38 Epothilones.

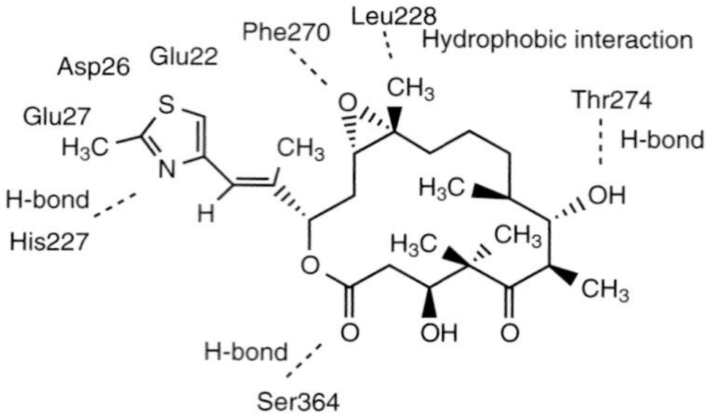

Figure 33.39 Epothilone B-β-tubulin interactions.

response. The drug should not be given to patients who have baseline neutrophil counts below 1,500 cells/mm^3. The drug carries a boxed warning for both of these serious toxicity risks.[76]

Peripheral sensory neuropathy is a frequently observed adverse effect. This toxicity is cumulative and, while usually reversible, it can progress to become painful and permanent. Kolliphor El is known to potentiate the myelosuppressive and neurotoxic adverse effects of this agent.[389] GI disturbances are common and alopecia is essentially a given. The drug can severely irritate skin, and hyaluronidase should be administered IV or SC if extravasation occurs. Paclitaxel is a Category D teratogen and carries a high risk of fetal intrauterine mortality. Both male and female patients are advised not to attempt conception while on this drug. Due caution should be observed when coadministering paclitaxel with drugs that inhibit or compete for metabolizing enzymes, particularly CYP2C8 (e.g., 17α-ethinylestradiol and diazepam).

As noted previously, paclitaxel resistance is mediated primarily through P-gp and βIII-tubulin overexpression. Regarding the latter, it is proposed that the exchange of Ala for Ser at position 277 in βIII-tubulin disrupts the critical H-bond with the C7-OH, resulting in a loss of affinity.[372]

Albumin-Bound. Albumin-bound paclitaxel nanoparticles (sometimes referred to as nab-paclitaxel) are administered IV in the same disease states as the conventional injection, although pancreatic carcinoma replaces advanced ovarian cancer as an indication. The boxed warning accompanying this formulation relates to the severe myelosuppression (primarily neutropenia) and a caution against interchanging with the conventional injection. The colloidal suspension of paclitaxel nanoparticles contains 3%-4% albumin, which surrounds and solubilizes the drug, eliminating the need for Kolliphor EL. Infusion times drop to 30 minutes, and disease-specific doses of 100-260 mg/m^2 are employed.

In addition to the naturally high permeability and impaired lymphatic drainage of neovascularlized tumors, targeted delivery to malignant cells is facilitated by active transport of the nanoparticles secondary to albumin binding to gp60 receptors found on the surface of tumor vascular endothelial cells. Binding activates a membrane protein called caveolin-1, which stimulates the formation of vesicles (or caveolae) that fill up with drug-bound albumin and traverse the endothelial cell, ultimately depositing in the interstitial space. In their hunger for albumin-bound nutrients, some tumor cells (including NSCLC, pancreatic and ovarian cancer cells) overexpress an albumin-binding glycoprotein known as SPARC (secreted protein acidic and rich in cysteine). As the SPARC-bound albumin approaches the lipophilic cell membrane, fatty acids initiate the jettison of any water insoluble compounds bound to the albumin. In the case of nab-paclitaxel, that water insoluble molecule is free paclitaxel, which readily penetrates the tumor cell membrane and makes its way to the nucleus (its site of action). Albumin-bound drug can also penetrate the membrane.[389,390] Either way, the tumor cell has effectively signed its own death warrant.

The literature is replete with reports of Abraxane trials in various cancers, often in combination with other drugs. In NSCLC, a multinational phase III trial in patients with advanced disease showed nab-paclitaxel to provide PFS and OS outcomes statistically equivalent to conventional paclitaxel, while providing a statistically significant increase in overall response rate, particularly among patients with squamous cell pathology.[389] A lower frequency of neuropathy was noted in the nab-paclitaxel arm of the study, possibly due to the absence of Kolliphor EL. Still, it has been reported that the overall response rate elicited by Abraxane is 21%, which has fueled the ongoing quest for novel paclitaxel delivery systems that retain all of nab-paclitaxel's clinical advantages and improves upon its therapeutic efficacy.[387]

DOCETAXEL. The indications for docetaxel include cancers of the breast, prostate and head/neck, as well as NSCLC and gastric adenocarcinoma. It has greater water solubility than paclitaxel due to the unesterified C10-OH group, and it is formulated with polysorbate 80 (Tween) rather than with Kolliphor EL. Hypersensitivity reactions, while less likely, are still possible, and all patients should receive antihistamine/corticosteroid premedication. In addition to neutropenia and teratogenicity, this taxane can induce significant fluid retention, and 2-kg weight gains are not uncommon. As noted previously, fluid retention has been associated with the cyclized oxazolidinedione metabolite (Fig. 33.36). A boxed warning advises about hypersensitivity, edema, myelosuppression, and use in patients with significant liver impairment. While uncommon, treatment-related deaths from sepsis have also been reported.

DDIs have been noted when docetaxel is coadministered with drugs that inhibit or compete for CYP3A4 enzymes.[391] Like paclitaxel, docetaxel is a P-gp substrate, and strict attention must be paid when drugs that bind to or inhibit this efflux protein are a part of the patient's therapeutic regimen.

CABAZITAXEL. Although currently less widely used than paclitaxel or docetaxel, cabazitaxel has some unique activities and advantages that deserve mention.

The 7,10-dimethoxy ether moieties of cabazitaxel dramatically lower affinity for P-gp, resulting in sustained retention in tumor cells (twice that of docetaxel) and efficacy in docetaxel-resistant cell lines where resistance is due to P-gp overexpression.[371,392] It is currently approved for use only in metastatic CRPC that has progressed despite docetaxel therapy. A recent meta analysis comparing the efficacy of cabazitaxel against other CRPC therapies (including docetaxel, both in combination with prednisolone) identified cabazitaxel as the most suitable agent in this disease due to equitable or superior efficacy as evaluated by PFS, OS and PSA attenuation.[367] In addition, cabazitaxel was viewed as having a better overall margin of safety. Other studies comparing these two taxanes have reported similar findings, and claim that their different adverse effect profiles may help practitioners optimize safety and quality of life for individual patients.[393]

Neutropenia is the most problematic dose-limiting reaction of cabazitaxel, although its incidence and severity are no worse than observed with other taxanes. It does not promote the fluid retention commonly observed with docetaxel. Peripheral neuropathy can be persistent, although some studies have claimed the incidence of this adverse effect is low.[394] The relatively high incidence of diarrhea (up to 47%) may be explained by the accumulation of the drug in enterocytes, cells that constitutively express P-gp and, therefore, actively evict other taxanes. The use of the recommended starting dose of 20 mg/m^2 has been associated with fewer adverse effects than the upper limit dose of 25 mg/m^2. Importantly, the lower dose demonstrated non-inferiority in terms of efficacy.[394] Administration is via a 1-hour IV infusion once every 3 weeks.

Despite the conversion of the two secondary alcohols to more lipophilic ethers, cabazitaxel's aqueous solubility is on a par with docetaxel's. Like docetaxel, it is formulated with polysorbate 80 rather than the more hypersensitivity-inducing Kolliphor EL. It is administered by IV infusion in doses of 25 mg/m^2 every 3 weeks, and a boxed warning cautions against both hypersensitivity and neutropenia.[76]

IXABEPILONE. The epothilone ixabepilone is used in combination with the thymidylate synthesis inhibitor capecitabine in anthracycline- and/or taxane-resistant advanced breast cancer or MBC, or when these alternative drugs are contraindicated. Like cabazitaxel, it retains activity in tumors overexpressing P-gp, although the literature differs on the issue of efficacy in βIII-tubulin expressing cells.[372,381] The lactam moiety provides stability to carboxyesterase-catalyzed hydrolysis, but the drug is extensively metabolized by CYP3A4 to over 30 inactive metabolites prior to predominately fecal excretion.[381] DDIs with CYP3A4 substrates, inducers, or inhibitors have been reported, and dosage adjustments may be warranted if coadministration cannot be avoided. Dose reductions are also required in patients with compromised hepatic function. A boxed warning cautions against administration to patients with elevated liver enzymes and/or bilirubin due to an increased risk of neutropenia-associated fatalities.[76]

Some phase II clinical trials have shown overall response rates to this agent as high as 57% in previously untreated breast cancer patients and up to 30% in patients who had been heavily pretreated.[395] Ixabepilone-capecitabine combination therapy provides superior outcomes compared to capecitabine monotherapy, but with a higher risk of adverse cardiac events, including ischemia and ventricular dysfunction. Ixabepilone is less effective than paclitaxel in advancing PFS and OS, but essentially equivalent in efficacy and safety to eribulin, a synthetic analogue of a marine-derived natural product (halichondrin B) also used in the treatment of MBC (see below).[396]

Like cabazitaxel, ixabepilone's serious use-limiting adverse effects include peripheral neuropathy and neutropenia. Diarrhea can occur, likely due to retention of drug in enterocytes, but the incidence with monotherapy (22%) is less than half that of cabazitaxel. Like paclitaxel, it uses Kolliphor EL for solubilization, so prophylactic premedication to protect against hypersensitivity reactions is required. The most common IV dosage regimen is 40 mg/m^2 administered over 3 hours every third week. This regimen increases overall response rate compared to once-weekly dosing, but with an elevated incidence of peripheral neuropathy. The once-weekly regimen may be valuable in patients in whom neutropenia risk must be minimized. Diarrhea incidence between the two regimens is similar.[396]

Vinca Alkaloids

MECHANISM OF ACTION. Several alkaloids found naturally in *Catharanthus roseus* (periwinkle) have potent antimitotic activity. In contrast to taxanes and epothilones, vinca alkaloids halt cell division by inhibiting polymerization. They bind to a single high-affinity β-tubulin site at the interface of two heterodimers within the tubular lumen near the GTP binding site on the (+) end of the tubules. Once bound, these alkaloids attenuate the uptake of the GTP essential to tubule elongation.[397] Simultaneous binding to α- and β-tubulin results in protein cross-linking, which promotes a stabilized protofilament structure.[398] Inhibition of microtubule elongation occurs at substoichiometric concentrations, at which alkaloid occupation of only 1%-2% of the total number of high-affinity sites can result in up to a 50% inhibition of microtubule assembly.[399,400] At high concentrations, when alkaloid binding to high-affinity sites becomes stoichiometric and lower-affinity binding sites on the tubule wall are also occupied, microtubular depolymerization is stimulated, leading to the exposure of additional alkaloidal binding sites and resulting in dramatic changes in microtubular conformation. Spiral aggregates, protofilaments, and highly structured crystals form, and the mitotic spindle ultimately disintegrates.[388] The loss of the directing mitotic spindle promotes chromosome "clumping" in unnatural shapes (balls and stars), leading to cell death. Other nonmitotic toxicities related to the microtubule-disrupting action of vinca alkaloids include inhibition of axonal transport and secretory processes, and disturbances in platelet structure and function.[399]

As noted earlier, the mutant *p53* oncogene is associated with resistance to vinca alkaloid-induced cytotoxicity due to its augmentation of MAP4-mediated microtubulin polymerization, which counteracts the depolymerizing mechanism of the alkaloids. In addition, the mutant oncogene gives a degree of immortality to stathmin, a cytosolic protein that must be inactivated for mitosis to begin. Finally, *p53* upregulates the MRP-1 efflux protein that ejects vinca alkaloids from cells. It has been suggested that *p53* phenotype could be harnessed to better predict a patient's anticipated susceptibility to various mitosis inhibitor antineoplastic therapy options.[370]

CHEMISTRY. The vinca alkaloids are complex structures composed of two polycyclic segments, catharanthine and vindoline (Fig. 33.35), both of which are essential for high-affinity tubulin binding. Of the three marketed vinca-based mitosis inhibitors, two are natural products (vincristine and vinblastine) and one is a semisynthetic alkaloid derivative (vinorelbine), but all will be included under the general "vinca alkaloids" descriptor. Vincristine and vinblastine have the highest and lowest tubulin affinity, respectively.[400]

Molecular simulation and docking studies with crystal structures of tubulin and vinblastine have allowed for the identification of potential tubulin binding modes and suggested specific drug-tubulin interactions.[401,402] Chi et al.[401] have proposed a "double faces sticking mechanism", where the polar functional groups of the catharanthine and vindoline moieties (the two "faces") seek out identical polar/charged residues on the dimerized tubulin, including residues within the 178-226 range on β-tubulin and 326-336 on α-tubulin. The point of difference in the binding options is the replacement of an α-tubulin Lys352 in the catharanthine mode by a β-tubulin Lys176 in the vindoline approach.

The three available vinca structures differ in the length of the alkyl chain bridging positions 6′ and 9′ of the catharanthine moiety (methylene or ethylene), in the substituents at position 4′ (olefin or tertiary alcohol), and in the vindoline indole nitrogen substituent (methyl or formyl). Although subtle, these structural changes lead to significant differences in clinical spectrum, potency, and toxicity. For example, vincristine's relative lack of bone marrow toxicity at standard therapeutic doses makes it popular in combination therapy with more myelosuppressive anticancer agents, whereas vinblastine's relative lack of neurotoxicity permits its coadministration with cisplatin. It is known that acetylation of either hydroxyl group destroys antineoplastic action and reduction of the vindoline olefinic linkage greatly attenuates activity. The C18′-methoxycarbonyl and the stereochemistry at positions 18′ and 2′ are believed to be critical to activity, as is the dihedral angle involving carbons 17′, 18′, 15 and 16 that connects the catharanthine and vindoline moieties of the alkaloids.[402,403]

Because vinca alkaloids enter cells by passive diffusion, unbound vinorelbine and vinblastine (being more lipophilic than vincristine) may be more extensively taken up into tissues. Vincristine, however, is cleared more slowly from the system and has the longest terminal half-life of the three agents, resulting in a more prolonged tumor cell exposure. Like paclitaxel and docetaxel, resistance is mediated, in part, through P-gp.

Vinca alkaloids undergo O4-deacetylation to yield metabolites that are equipotent to or more active than the parent drug. They are also subject to extensive CYP3A4/5-mediated metabolism before biliary excretion.[404-409] Vincristine alone is selectively metabolized by the 3A5 isoform.[406] A representative hydrolyzed metabolite of vinblastine and the major CYP3A-generated metabolites of the other vinca alkaloids are shown in Figure 33.40. As CYP metabolism is inactivating and CYP3A overexpression has been noted in human tumors, it has been proposed that CYP3A enzymes could contribute to vinca resistance.[408]

SPECIFIC DRUGS. Vinca alkaloids contain two ionizable nitrogen atoms and are marketed as water soluble salts. No oil-based solubilizers are required for IV administration.

Vincristine Sulfate. Vincristine is employed in many hematologic malignancies, and is a common choice in pediatric (as well as adult) ALL. It is also given in Wilms tumor (an almost exclusively pediatric cancer), rhabdomyosarcoma and neuroblastoma. The drug is given by IV infusion over 5-10 minutes using a minibag, via a 1 minute IV push or, less commonly, infused over 24 hours. Continuous infusion may result in more pronounced toxicity, and the drug is fatal if administered by the intrathecal route. A liposomal formulation, marketed as Marqibo, is available to treat relapsed ALL. As with the liposomal anticancer agents discussed previously, this formulation is not interchangeable with the conventional IV dosage form. The urinary elimination half-life of liposomal vincristine is approximately 45 hours.

Elimination of conventional vincristine is triphasic, with the first phase (5 min) representing rapid uptake into tissues and the terminal phase (85 hr) representing release back to the plasma from tubulin-containing cells. Since the drug is extensively metabolized by O4-deacetylation and selective CYP3A5-catalyzed oxidation in the liver, patients with hepatic dysfunction are at an increased risk for toxicity, and dosage reductions should be considered.

The most significant dose-limiting adverse effect is peripheral neuropathy, which initially manifests as numbness and painful paresthesias in the extremities and progresses to muscular pain, severe weakness, and loss of coordination. Caucasian children receiving vincristine experience a higher level of drug-induced neurotoxicity compared to African American pediatric patients, and the significantly higher incidence of the *CYP3A5*1* allele that translates to a rapid 3A5 metabolizing phenotype in the latter population (75% vs. 19%) may explain the toxicity difference.[406] Patients can also experience constipation secondary to intestinal neurotoxicity, which may require treatment with cathartics. Myelosuppression is not particularly problematic because it occurs at doses higher than those that can be tolerated.

All vinca alkaloids are severe vesicants that can induce necrosis, cellulitis, and/or thrombophlebitis. Proper needle placement before administration should be assured to eliminate the risk of extravasation. Unlike the tissue damage caused by the vesicant action of nitrogen mustards (discussed below) and anthracyclines, cold exacerbates tissue destruction. If extravasation occurs, apply heat for 1 hour 4 times a day for 3-5 days, coupled with local hyaluronidase injections.

Vincristine and vinblastine carry boxed warnings for extravasation risk and appropriate administration route.

Vinblastine Sulfate. Vinblastine is used as palliative therapy in hematologic malignancies and has found utility in the treatment of advanced testicular carcinoma (often in combination with bleomycin), advanced mycosis fungoides, and Kaposi sarcoma. Leukopenia is the dose-limiting adverse effect, and the dose should be cut in half for patients with serum bilirubin levels between 3 and 5 mg/dL. Patients with serum bilirubin above 5 mg/dL should not

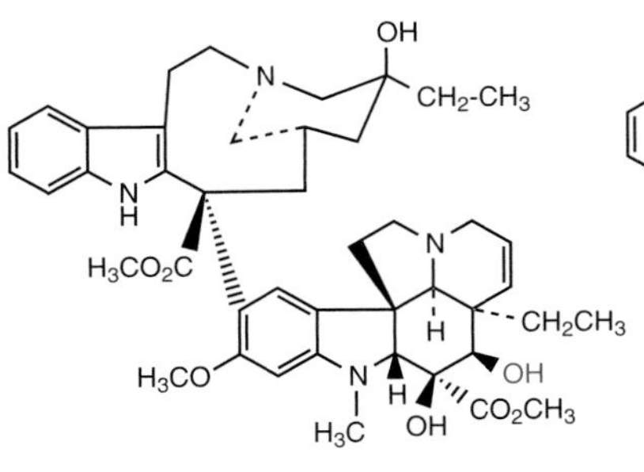

Desacetylvinblastine (active)

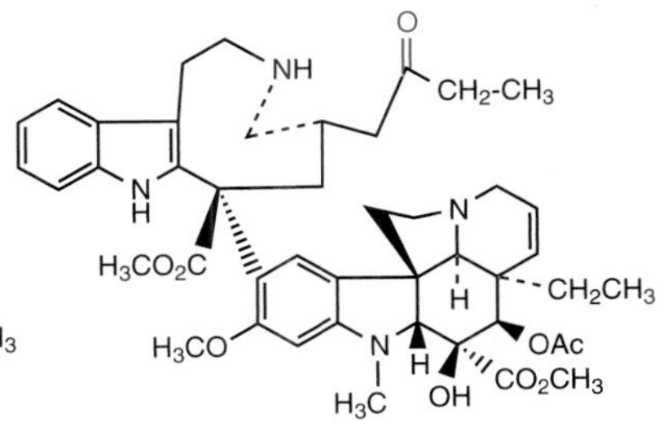

Vincristine M1 metabolite (inactive)

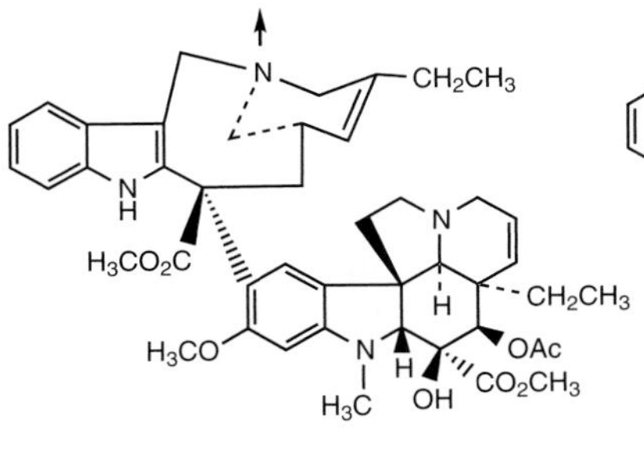

Vinorelbine N-oxide metabolite (inactive)

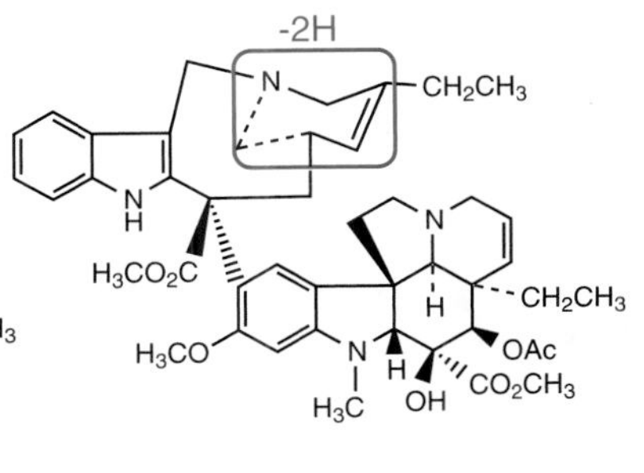

Vinorelbine didehydro metabolite (inactive)

Figure 33.40 Major metabolites of vinca alkaloids.

receive vinblastine. The drug-related impact on erythrocyte and thrombocyte levels is usually insignificant.

Short IV infusions through a minibag are the preferred administration route, but 1 minute infusions into a free flowing IV line are allowed. Prolonged infusion (more than 0.5-1 hr) increases the risk of extravasation. The initial elimination half-life of 3.7 minutes is similar to vincristine, but the 25-hour terminal half-life is significantly shorter. Since CYP3A metabolism is not specific for the 3A5 isoform, pharmacogenetic-related variability in efficacy and safety is of no concern.

Vinorelbine Tartrate. Vinorelbine is used alone or in combination with cisplatin for first-line treatment of NSCLC. It is administered by IV push or rapid bolus over 6-10 minutes. Administration over a longer time period can result in phlebitis and injection pain. As with the other drugs in this class, intrathecal administration is fatal.

Vinorelbine's initial phase elimination half-life is on a par with that of vincristine and vinblastine, and the terminal half-life is between 28 and 44 hours. Although dose-limiting granulocytopenia is the major adverse effect (and myelosuppression the reason behind its boxed warning), potentially fatal interstitial pulmonary changes have been noted. Patients with symptoms of respiratory distress should be promptly evaluated. As with all vinca alkaloids, elimination is primarily biliary, and dosage reduction should be considered in patients with liver dysfunction. CYP3A4 and 3A5 are both involved in inactivating metabolism, so there is no pharmacogenetic-based impact on tumor response or rate/severity of adverse effects.

Halichondrins

Halichondrin B is a chemical found in *Halichondria okadai*, a rare Japanese sea sponge. This structure, and its therapeutically active macrolide component known as eribulin, destabilize microtubules by interfering with the elongation phase of dynamic instability, inhibiting polymerization without any direct impact on erosion.[410] The interaction of these two large molecules with β-tubulin have been modeled.[411] Their binding site is within the vinca alkaloid domain on the ends of β-tubulin, approximately 16 Å from vinblastine's binding site, and they serve as competitive inhibitors of vinblastine binding. Eribulin's affinity for this binding site is three times higher than that of halichondrin B. Five hydrogen bonds involving O3, O7, O11 and N1 are particularly crucial to eribulin-tubulin binding.

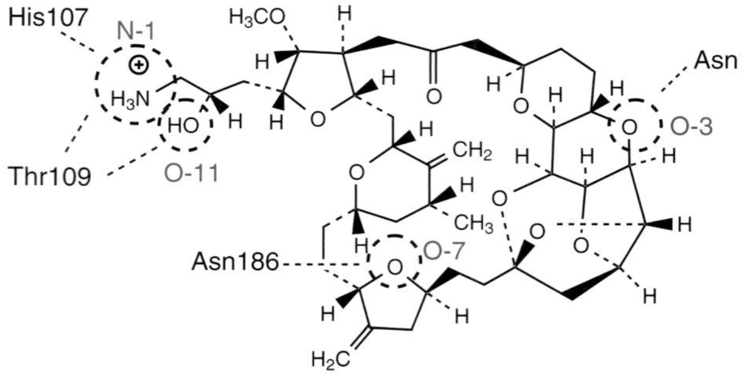

Eribulin-tubulin interactions

Eribulin Mesylate. Eribulin mesylate is indicated in MBC patients who have received as least two prior regimens that included a taxane and an anthracycline. Phase III trials comparing eribulin to physician's choice of alternative chemotherapy have documented significant improvement in median OS and objective response rate; PFS was also augmented.[412] As noted above, one clinical trial found eribulin's efficacy to be equivalent to ixabepilone.[396]

Eribulin is administered by IV infusion over 2-5 minutes, and patients seem to do better when the drug is given on days 1 and 8 of a 21 day cycle than on days 1, 8 and 15 of a 28 day cycle.[413] Serious side effects include myelosuppression (specifically neutropenia and anemia) constipation and peripheral neuropathy (the most common cause of drug discontinuation). Many patients experience fatigue. QT interval prolongation can sometimes occur on day 8 (but not on day 1) of eribulin therapy. The effect can be additive with other drugs that also prolong the QT interval.[76]

Eribulin is not significantly metabolized. Four very minor CYP3A4-generated metabolites form, but the risk of DDIs with CYP substrates, inhibitors or inducers is insignificant.[410] Fecal excretion of unchanged drug predominates.

Like vinca alkaloids, eribulin contains a basic amino nitrogen that readily protonates at physiologic pH. The water soluble mesylate salt can be administered directly or diluted with normal saline.

Antimetabolites

Many antimetabolites stop de novo DNA biosynthesis by inhibiting the formation of the nucleotides that make up these life-sustaining polymers. The rate-limiting enzymes of nucleotide biosynthesis are the primary targets for the antimetabolites, since inhibition of these key enzymes is the most efficient way to shut down any biochemical reaction sequence. Other enzymes required in DNA biosynthesis can be inhibited, or chain elongation can be arrested through the incorporation of false nucleotides into the growing DNA strand.

The antimetabolites serve as false substrates for critical nucleotide biosynthesis or polymerizing enzymes. These enzyme inhibitors are structurally designed to look like a super attractive version of the normal (endogenous) substrate. Speaking anthropomorphically, through a form of chemical entrapment, they entice the enzymes to choose them over the endogenous substrate and, once they do, the antimetabolites bind them irreversibly or pseudoirreversibly. If the building block nucleotides cannot be synthesized or DNA polymerization is blocked, then DNA synthesis (and tumor growth) is stopped dead in its tracks.

Many antimetabolite antineoplastics are categorized by the class of nucleotide they inhibit. Purine antagonists inhibit the synthesis of adenosine monophosphate (AMP) and guanosine monophosphate (GMP), while pyrimidine antagonists stop the production of deoxythymidine monophosphate (dTMP). Antifolates shut down purine and pyrimidine biosynthesis pathways since folate cofactors are essential to both. DNA polymerase inhibitors are false nucleotides which, when added to a growing DNA chain, put the chemical kibosh on further chain elongation. The structures of the anticancer antimetabolites are provided in Figure 33.41.

Purine Antagonists

AMP AND GMP BIOSYNTHESIS. Purine antagonists that inhibit the de novo biosynthesis of AMP and GMP target the rate-limiting enzyme amidophosphoribosyltransferase (also known as glutamine-5-phosphoribosylpyrophosphate amidotransferase (Fig. 33.42)). The rate-limiting step is the first of the pathway; if that step is inhibited no other step can proceed. Since the rate-limiting transferase enzyme works on a phosphorylated ribose substrate, no enzyme in the sequence will function without its presence. The formylation reaction catalyzed by GAR formyltransferase requires the methyl-donating 10-formyltetrahydrofolate and can be inhibited by the antifolates methotrexate and pemetrexed (discussed below).

CHEMISTRY. The two currently marketed purine antagonists are 6-thiol analogues of the endogenous purine bases guanine and purine, the latter also known as inosine (Fig. 33.41). They are prodrugs and must be converted to

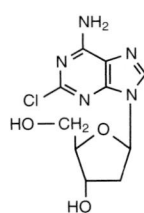

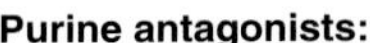

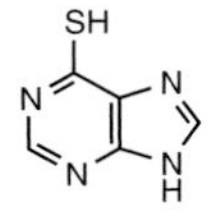

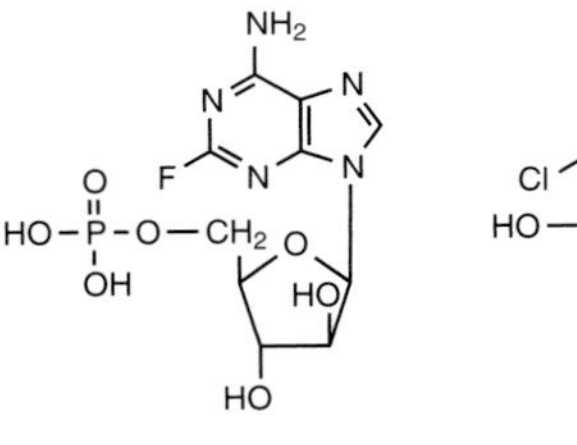

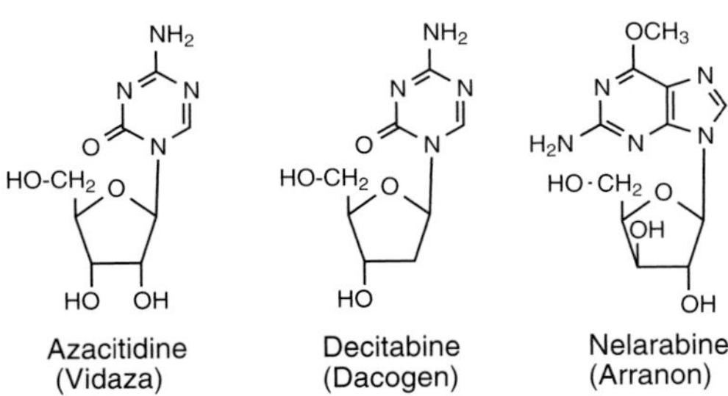

Figure 33.41 Antimetabolites.

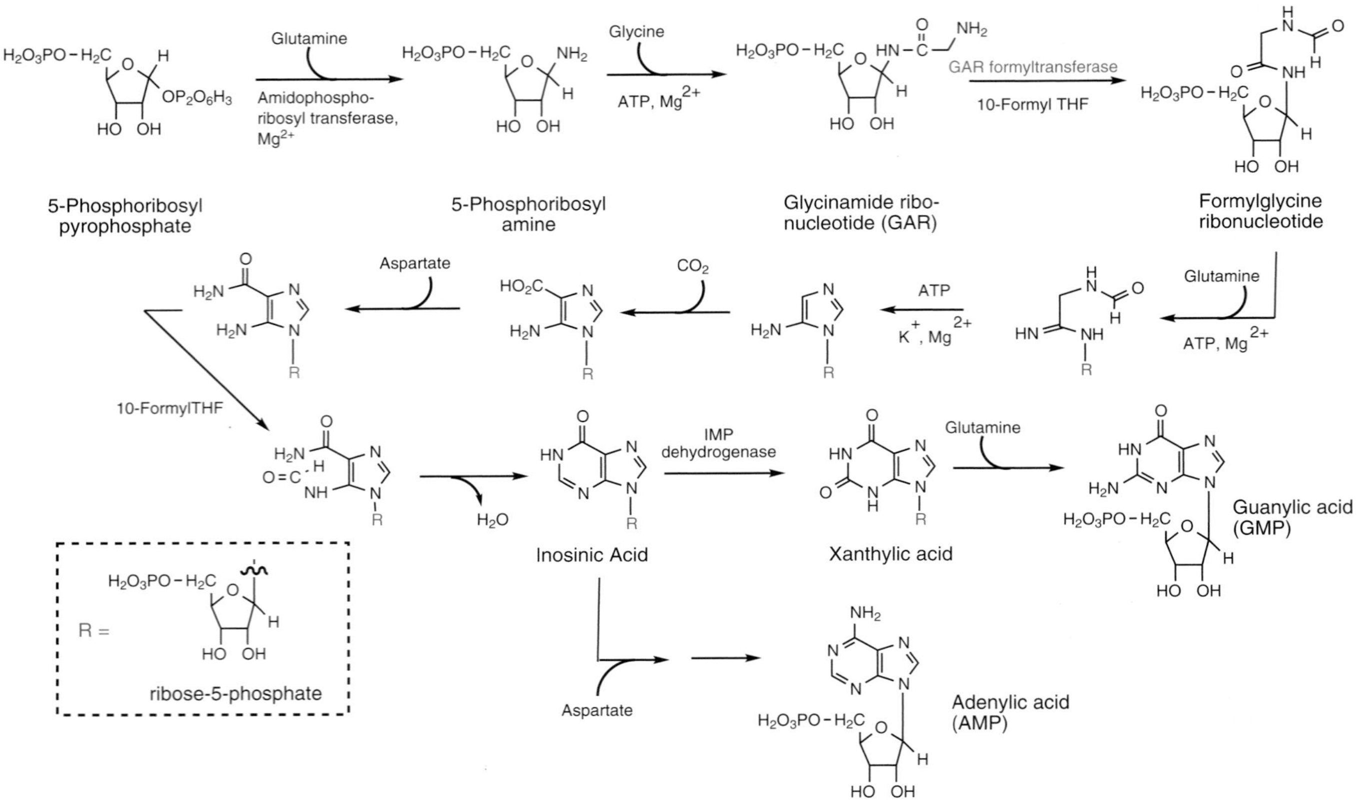

Figure 33.42 Biosynthesis of purine nucleotides.

ribonucleotides by hypoxanthine guanine phosphoribosyltransferase (HGPRT) before they can exert their cytotoxic actions (Fig. 33.43). Mercaptopurine and its S-methylated ribonucleotide metabolite inhibit the target amidophosphoribosyltransferase and the inosine monophosphate (IMP) dehydrogenase enzyme that generates xanthylic acid from inosinic acid later in the pathway; AMP and GMP biosynthesis are halted. A second mechanism, believed to be the more therapeutically important one for both thiopurines, involves the incorporation of thioguanine di- and triphosphate deoxyribo- and ribonucleotides (generally referred to as 6-thioguanine nucleotides, or 6TGNs) generated within the tumor cell into DNA and RNA, respectively.[414,415] This illicit substitution inhibits further strand elongation and results in cleavage, cell-cycle arrest and apoptosis.[415]

As alluded to above, thiopurines are metabolized by S-methylation via the polymorphic enzyme thiopurine methyl transferase (TPMT) with S-adenosylmethionine (SAM) serving as cofactor. The 6-methylthioinosinic acid ribonucleotide metabolite is a potent inhibitor of the amidophosphoribosyltransferase enzyme and can contribute to the cytotoxic action of the parent nucleotide (Fig. 33.43). However, since the primary therapeutic mechanism of thiopurines is cell-cycle arrest and apoptosis secondary to the incorporation of 6TGNs into DNA, methylation is viewed as detracting from therapeutic efficacy.[415,416] In contrast to 6-methylthioinosinic acid, little or no 6-methylthioguanylic acid is produced inside the cell.[417,418] The thiopurine bases can also be methylated by TPMT, but these metabolites do not react with HGPRT and remain permanently inactive, a fact drug manufacturers take into account when establishing dosing regimens.

TPMT is polymorphic, and the *3, *3A, *3B and *3C alleles are associated with 80%-95% of poor metabolizing phenotypes.[415] Patients who are poor TPMT metabolizers (approximately 10% of Caucasians, but also evident in other races) will not experience inactivating methylation of the prodrug structure and will generate more active 6-thioinosinic acid per dose than patients with normal or excessive levels of the enzyme. The TPMT genotype of patients should be assessed before initiating thiopurine therapy because poor metabolizers are at a high risk of life-threatening myelosuppression and serious infection from elevated levels of 6TGNs, even when standard doses are administered.[415-417] In addition, the accumulation of mutagenic thiopurine-based ribonucleotides puts these patients at higher risk for secondary malignancies.[416,418] Thiopurines can still be used in poor TPMT metabolizers, but the dose should be significantly decreased in accordance with published guidelines[76] and white blood cell counts monitored vigilantly. Mercaptopurine appears to be more significantly impacted by TPMT genotype than thioguanine.[419]

On the flipside, extensive TPMT metabolizers, who represent up to 90% of patients on thiopurine therapy, will form lower amounts of apoptotic 6TGNs. In the case of mercaptopurine, the molecules of ribonucleotide generated will be methylated very rapidly to 6-methylthioinosinic acid, and this can predispose to drug-induced

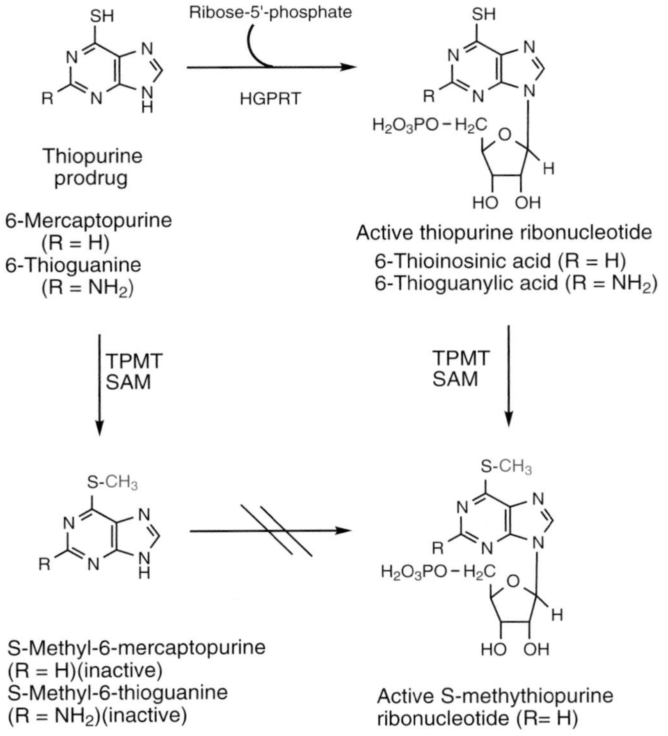

Figure 33.43 Thiopurine metabolism leading to activation and inactivation.

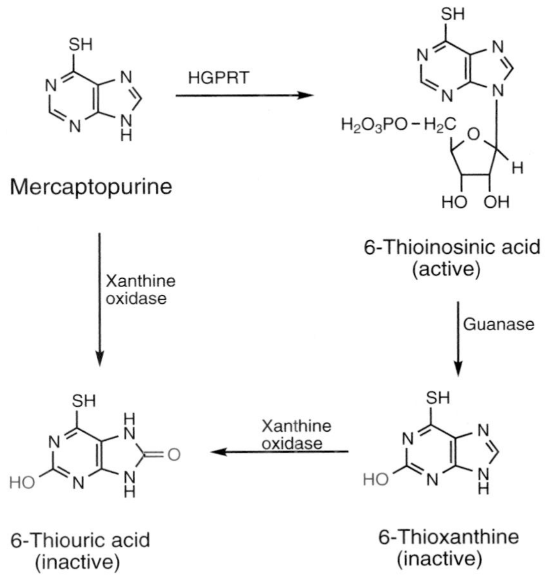

Figure 33.44 Xanthine oxidase inactivation of mercaptopurine and 6-thioinosinic acid.

hepatotoxicity and treatment failure.[415-417] Higher doses of mercaptopurine are required in these patients.[420] In contrast, extensive TPMT metabolizers show a decreased sensitivity to thioguanine because there is no compensatory increase in the formation of methylated ribonucleotide to offset the decreased production of 6-thioguanylic acid.[418]

It is claimed that approximately 70% of patients who experience adverse effects from thiopurines have normal TPMT levels, so TPMT genetic testing (as important as it is) is not a panacea.[415] Genes that encode for inositol triphosphate pyrophosphatase (ITPA) are also known to impact the metabolic and toxicity profiles of mercaptopurines. ITPA normally converts ITP to the monophosphate and, in so doing, advances AMP and GMP biosynthesis. However it also hydrolyzes 6-mercaptopurine triphosphate to the monophosphate.[416] Carriers of the rs41329251 ITPA allele appear to be at significantly higher risk for the development of mercaptopurine-induced febrile neutropenia even after TPMT genotype-based dosage adjustment.[421,422] Other potential pharmacogenetic-based influences on thiopurine drug disposition in children have been proposed.[416]

Xanthine oxidase competes with TPMT for mercaptopurine (but not thioguanine) and converts it to inactive 6-thiouric acid, which is excreted in the urine (Fig. 33.44).[423] 6-Thioinosinic acid is also subject to metabolism via the xanthine oxidase pathway, ultimately forming the same inactive metabolite. Allopurinol, which inhibits xanthine oxidase and increases levels of active 6-thioinosinic acid, can be coadministered with mercaptopurine to increase duration of action and antineoplastic potency. However, the mercaptopurine dose must be cut to 25%-33% of the standard dose to avoid serious toxicity.[76,414] There are literature reports of children with ALL who experienced use-limiting hepato- or pancreatic toxicity on standard mercaptopurine doses, but who were able to continue treatment on a much lower dose (commonly 33% of normal) when this combination therapy strategy was employed.[420,424] Importantly, coadministration of allopurinol decreases the formation of methylated mercaptopurine metabolites, shifting the metabolic balance to the more therapeutically relevant 6TGNs. The mechanism by which this occurs is not well understood.[420] In contrast to mercaptopurine, allopurinol cotherapy is not warranted with thioguanine since the impact of xanthine oxidase on its metabolic degradation is minor.

SPECIFIC DRUGS (FIG. 33.41)

Mercaptopurine. Mercaptopurine is used in the treatment of ALL, and its role in maintenance therapy is believed to have contributed to the 90% OS rate in children with this malignancy.[424] It is available in an oral dosage form, but absorption can be erratic and is reduced by the presence of food. The usual daily dose is 1.5-2.5 mg/kg (50-75 mg/m^2) in adults and children, with appropriate adjustment if excessive leukopenia, thrombocytopenia and/or anemia is noted. Dosage adjustments should be considered in the face of renal or hepatic impairment. In addition to myelosuppression, immunosuppression and GI distress are common. High levels of methylated metabolites can induce potentially fatal hepatotoxicity requiring drug discontinuation. As noted previously, coadministration of allopurinol can significantly decrease the effective dose of mercaptopurine, potentially permitting continuation of therapy after recovery from drug-induced toxicity.

Resistance to mercaptopurine (and thioguanine) therapy involves deficiency in the activating HGPRT enzyme, increases in alkaline phosphatase, TPMT high metabolizer phenotype, and attenuated active uptake via nucleoside transporters.[425,426]

Thioguanine. Thioguanine is administered orally at a daily dose of 2 mg/kg in the acute treatment of AML. It's value when added to other antineoplastic agents has been questioned,[414] and it is not recommended for maintenance therapy due to a high risk of hepatotoxicity.[76] Like mercaptopurine, absorption is incomplete and variable, and the toxicities are qualitatively similar. The risk of secondary malignancies may be greater since 6-thioguanylate is not an effective inhibitor of the amidotransferase enzyme, and acts almost exclusively through the DNA/RNA incorporation of false guanine nucleotides.

Pyrimidine Antagonists

DTMP BIOSYNTHESIS. Looked at simply, dTMP is produced via C5-methylation of deoxyuridine monophosphate (dUMP). The rate-limiting enzyme of the dTMP synthetic pathway is the sulfhydryl-containing thymidylate synthase, with 5,10-methylenetetrahydrofolate (5,10-methylene-THF) serving as the methyl-donating cofactor. All dTMP synthesis inhibitors will inhibit thymidylate synthase either directly or indirectly, and this will result in a "thymineless death" in actively dividing cells. Without dTMP and its deoxythymidine triphosphate metabolite, DNA will fragment and the cell will die.

To understand how an antimetabolite inhibits a biochemical pathway, we must first understand completely how the pathway normally functions. A quick look at the dTMP synthesis pathway (Fig. 33.45) will confirm that our "simple methylation reaction" is comprised of several important steps, each of which is analyzed in turn below.

The thymidylate synthase enzyme is very large, and the active site binding motifs for both substrate and cofactor are highly conserved regardless of source.[427] The human enzyme (hTS) has been crystallized, and key binding residues for substrate and cofactor have been identified (Fig. 33.46).[428-430] Many of the residues identified in Figure 33.46 have been confirmed in a binding study with mutant (R163K) human thymidylate synthase and dUMP, as well as the high affinity false substrate 5-F-dUMP.[431]

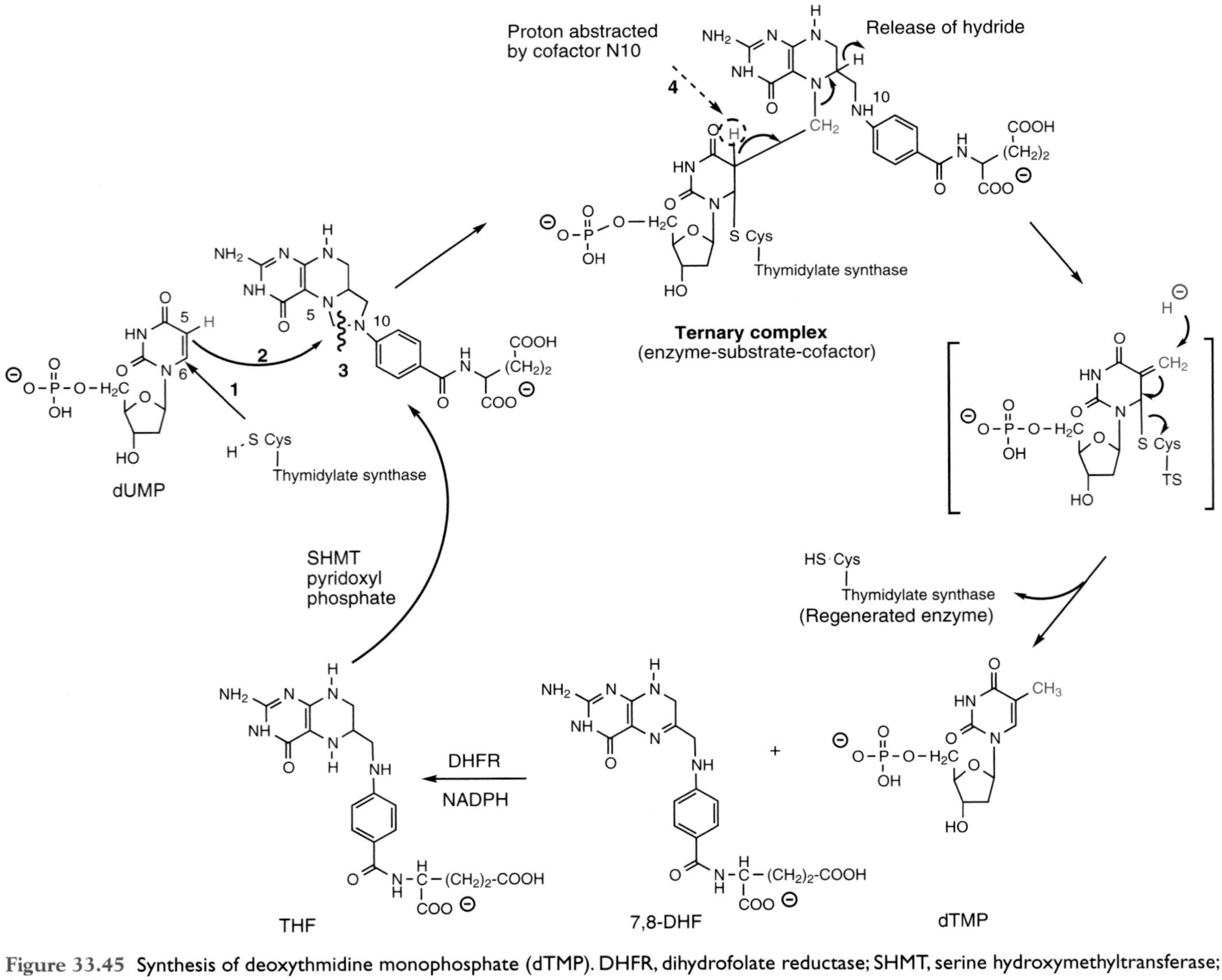

Figure 33.45 Synthesis of deoxythmidine monophosphate (dTMP). DHFR, dihydrofolate reductase; SHMT, serine hydroxymethyltransferase; TS, thymidylate synthase.

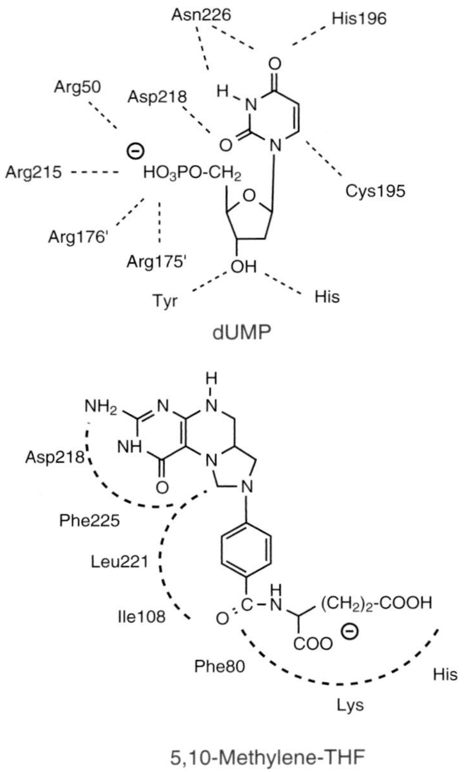

Figure 33.46 dUMP and 5,10-methylene-THF binding to thymidylate synthase.

The non-covalent binding of both substrate and cofactor promotes a conformational change in the synthase, causing the N-terminal portion of the enzyme to shift. The conformational change positions the pteridine ring of the folate cofactor "face to face" with the dUMP substrate, permitting the ring stacking that properly orients all key functional groups for the reaction to come.[428]

CHEMISTRY. With substrate and cofactor properly positioned, the nucleophilic sulfhydryl moiety of synthase Cys195 launches an intermolecular nucleophilic attack on the highly electrophilic C6 of dUMP, forming a new (albeit transient) covalent bond (step 1). The bond that breaks as a result is the 5,6-double bond of dUMP, and the released electrons are accepted by the perfectly positioned δ^+ methylene group of the cofactor (step 2). When substrate C5 covalently joins with the cofactor methylene carbon, the imidazolidine ring breaks (step 3), releasing steric constraints on N10. Taken together, steps 1-3 generate a ternary complex of enzyme, substrate, and cofactor (Fig. 33.45).[431] Liberated N10 then abstracts the C5-H of the cofactor (step 4) which, through a series of electronic rearrangements, releases the cofactor C6-hydrogen as hydride (H^-). H^- attacks the δ^+ methylene moiety of the substrate, which restores the essential 5,6-pyrimidine double bond of the product (dTMP) and regenerates thymidylate synthase. To complete the biochemical cycle, the released 7,8-DHF byproduct must be reduced to tetrahydrofolate (THF) via dihydrofolate reductase (DHFR) using NADPH. Finally, THF is converted to 5,10-methylene-THF through the action of serine hydroxymethyltransferase (SHMT) and vitamin B_6.

With the enzyme and cofactor both regenerated, the cell is ready to synthesize another molecule of dTMP utilizing stored dUMP. This happens at a normal pace in healthy cells and at an uncontrolled rate in tumor cells.

SPECIFIC DRUGS: PYRIMIDINE ANALOGUES (FIG. 33.41)

Fluorouracil. This fluorinated pyrimidine prodrug must be converted to its deoxyribonucleotide before it will be recognized by thymidylate synthase (Fig. 33.47). The active form differs from the endogenous substrate only by the presence of the 5-F group, which holds the key to the DNA biosynthesis inhibiting action of this drug. The C6 position of the false substrate is significantly more δ^+ than normal due to the strong electron-withdrawing effect of the adjacent C5 fluorine. This greatly increases the rate of attack by Cys195, resulting in a very fast formation of a fluorinated ternary complex (Fig. 33.48). The small size of the fluorine atom assures no steric hindrance to the formation of this false complex.

The next step in the pathway requires the abstraction of the C5-H (as proton) by the lone pair of electrons on N10 of the cofactor (kept primarily in unionized form by

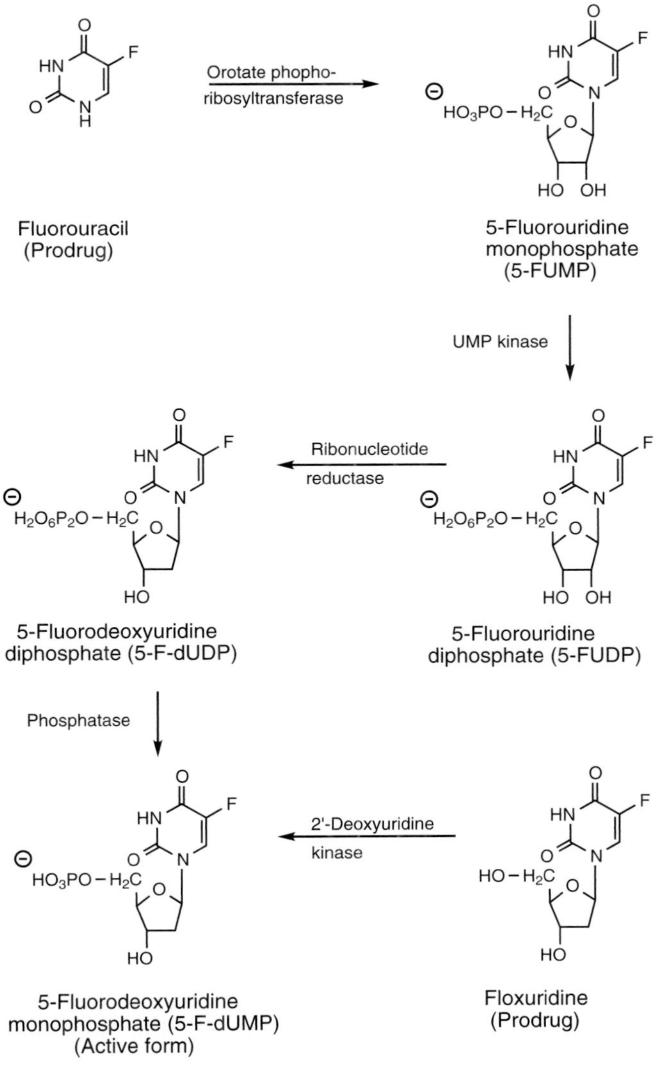

Figure 33.47 Activation of fluorouracil and floxuridine.

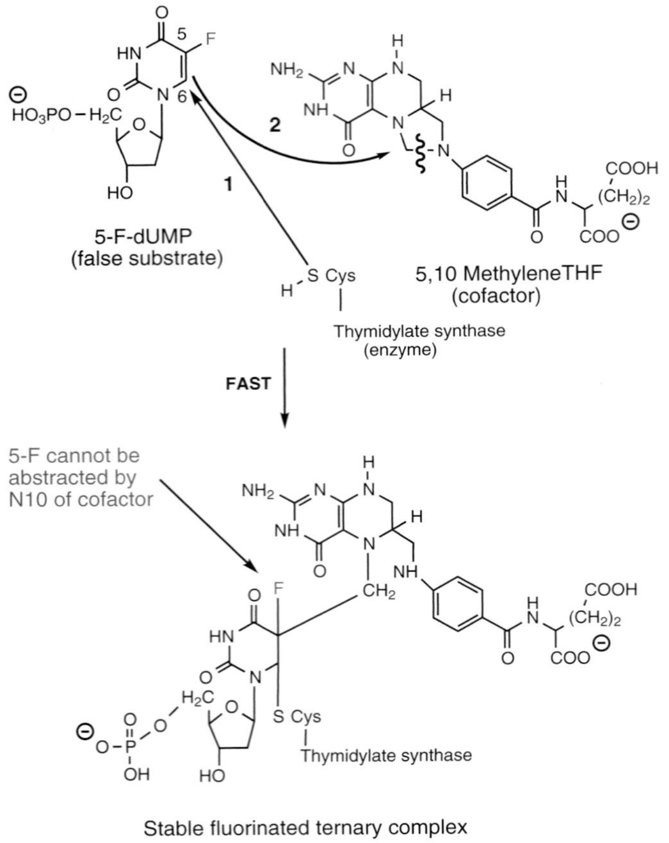

Figure 33.48 Mechanism of action of fluorouracil.

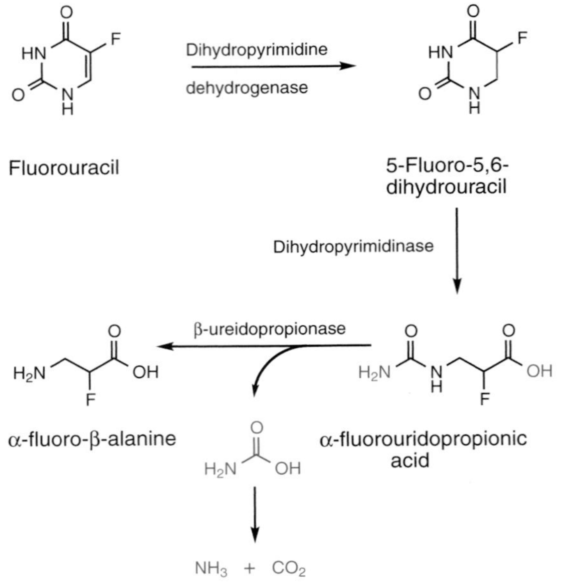

Figure 33.49 Fluorouracil metabolism.

a resonance-facilitated low pK_a), but this is no longer possible. Not only is the C5-fluorine bond stable to cleavage, the δ^- fluorine atom and unionized N10 would repel one another because they are both electron rich. The false ternary complex cannot break down, no thymidine-based product is formed, no folate cofactor is released, and most importantly, the rate-limiting thymidylate synthase enzyme is not regenerated. With thymidylate synthase directly and irreversibly inhibited, dTMP can no longer be synthesized, DNA will be irreversibly damaged, and the cell will die.

Importantly, a secondary mechanism of therapeutic fluorouracil toxicity is the incorporation of the false triphosphorylated ribonucleotide (5-F-UTP) into RNA, a chemical deal breaker for RNA viability.[432] Therefore, fluorinated uracil antimetabolites inhibit the biosynthesis of both DNA and RNA.

Fluorouracil is administered IV in the palliative treatment of colorectal, breast, stomach, and pancreatic cancers, with disease state-dependent doses and regimens. It is rapidly cleared from the bloodstream, and although up to 20% of a dose is excreted unchanged in the urine, most undergoes hepatic catabolism via a series of enzymes that includes the polymorphic dihydropyrimidine dehydrogenase (DPD) (Fig. 33.49). The approximately 5% of the population genetically deficient in this enzyme will experience a more pronounced effect from this drug, and are at significant risk for use-limiting or life-threatening toxicity unless doses are appropriately adjusted.[433] Neutropenia, neurotoxicity, diarrhea, mucositis and cardiotoxicity most commonly manifest, and no dosage reduction rubric currently exists to guide practitioners.

It has been estimated that between 40% and 60% of patients who experience severe toxicity from fluorouracil are DPD-deficient.[434] The incidence of DPD deficiency in African Americans is 3-fold higher than in Caucasians, and Black women have a 3-fold higher incidence of DPD deficiency than Black men.[434] A simple "bedside" mechanism of determining DPD phenotype based on the serum dihydrouracil:uracil ratio has been reported (ratio <4 indicating a poor metabolizer (PM) phenotype).[435] Fluorouracil dose in PM patients being treated for digestive tract cancers was decreased by an average of 35%, which retained therapeutic efficacy while significantly decreasing the incidence of serious toxicity.

A recent publication documents the efficacy of uridine triacetate (Vistogard, a uridine prodrug) as an antidote for fluorouracil or capecitabine (discussed below) toxicity due to overdose or DPD deficiency. Regardless of the toxicity mechanism, the uridine generated by Vistogard hydrolysis competes with fluorouracil for access to target enzymes and prevents cellular damage and destruction.[432] In animal studies designed to mimic clinical toxicity, the greatest protection benefit was observed when uridine triacetate was administered within 24 hours of the last dose of antimetabolite.[436]

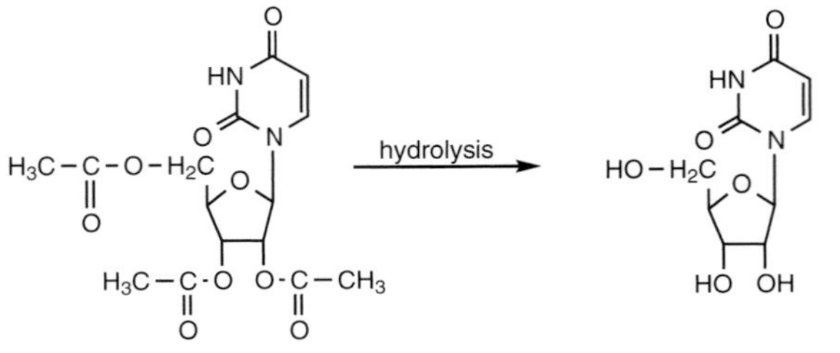

In patients with normal DPD activity, dosage adjustments are usually not required in hepatic or renal dysfunction. Major toxicities are related to bone marrow depression, stomatitis/esophagopharyngitis, and potential GI ulceration. Nausea and vomiting are common.

Solutions of fluorouracil are light sensitive, but discolored products that have been properly stored and protected from light are still safe to use.

Floxuridine. This deoxyribonucleoside prodrug is bioconverted via 2′-deoxyuridine kinase-mediated phosphorylation to the same active 5-fluoro-dUMP structure generated in the multistep biotransformation of fluorouracil (Fig. 33.47). It is given by intra-arterial infusion for the palliative treatment of GI adenocarcinoma that has metastasized to the liver and that cannot be managed surgically. Because floxuridine does not generate fluorouracil, its kinetic profile is not impacted by DPD pharmacogenetic status.

Capecitabine. Although capecitabine is a carbamylated analogue of cytidine, the drug actually is another 5-fluoro-dUMP prodrug (Fig. 33.50). Given orally, it is extensively metabolized to fluorouracil, which is then converted to the active fluorinated deoxyribonucleotide as previously described. Thymidine phosphorylase, an enzyme involved in this biotransformation, is much more active in tumors than in normal tissue, which improves the tumor-selective generation of fluorouracil. Levels of active drug in the tumor can be up to 3.5-fold higher than in surrounding tissue, leading to a lower incidence of adverse effects compared to fluorouracil therapy.[437] Because capecitabine is biotransformed to fluorouracil, it follows the same catabolic and elimination pathways reported for fluorouracil (Figs. 33.47 and 33.49). Doses should be decreased by 25% in moderate renal impairment, and the caution relative to the augmented risk of toxicity in patients with DPD deficiency applies.

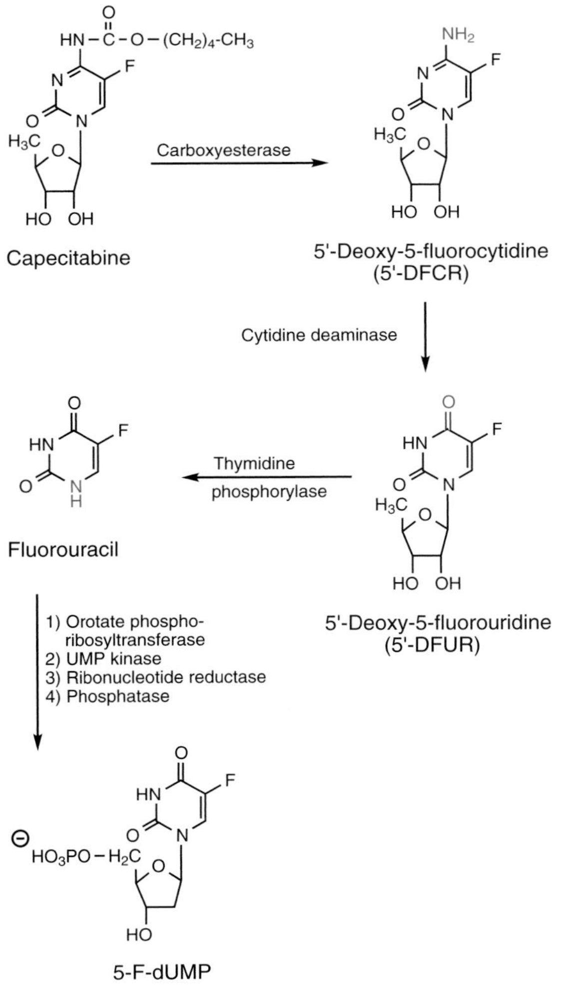

Figure 33.50 Capecitabine activation.

Capecitabine is currently indicated for use as first-line therapy in patients with colorectal cancer. It is also used alone or in combination with docetaxel in patients with MBC cancer who have experienced disease progression or recurrence after anthracycline therapy. However, it is being investigated for use in several other malignancies in combination with kinase inhibitors, DNA crosslinking antineoplastics, mitosis inhibitors and MAbs. Given twice daily in tablet form, the total daily dose is calculated based on patient body surface area and is taken 30 minutes after eating to avoid food-induced decreases in absorption. In addition to bone marrow suppression, nausea and vomiting, the drug can induce severe diarrhea and a potentially disabling disorder termed "hand-and-foot syndrome" (palmar-plantar erythrodysesthesia). As noted above, since capecitabine acts through the generation of 5-fluorouracil, uridine triacetate can be used to reduce toxicity in overdose or in DPD PMs.

Capecitabine inhibits CYP2C9 and, along with competition for serum protein binding sites, results in clinically significant DDIs with both warfarin and phenytoin. The interaction with warfarin carries a boxed warning, as it can result in potentially fatal bleeding episodes that appear within days of combination therapy or can be delayed up to 1 month after discontinuation of capecitabine therapy.

SPECIFIC DRUGS: ANTIFOLATES (FIG. 33.41)

Methotrexate. Methotrexate is a folic acid antagonist structurally designed to compete successfully with 7,8-DHF for the DHFR enzyme. The direct inhibition of DHFR causes cellular levels of 7,8-DHF to rise, which in turn results in feedback (indirect) inhibition of thymidylate synthase. Methotrexate also inhibits glycinamide ribonucleotide (GAR) formyltransferase, a key enzyme in the synthesis of purine nucleotides (Fig. 33.42).

Methotrexate's C4-NH_2 substituent and the fully aromatic pteridine ring system hold the key to its DHFR-inhibiting action. It has been proposed that the N5 position of endogenous DHF is protonated by Glu30 of DHFR[438] and, in cationic form, binds to DHFR Asp27 (Fig. 33.51). N5 is the strongest base in the DHF structure, in part due to the attenuating impact of the C4 carbonyl on N1 electron density. Additional affinity-enhancing interactions between enzyme and substrate have also been identified.[439-441] Once bound, the substrate's 5,6-double bond is positioned close to the NADPH cofactor so that the transfer of hydride can proceed.

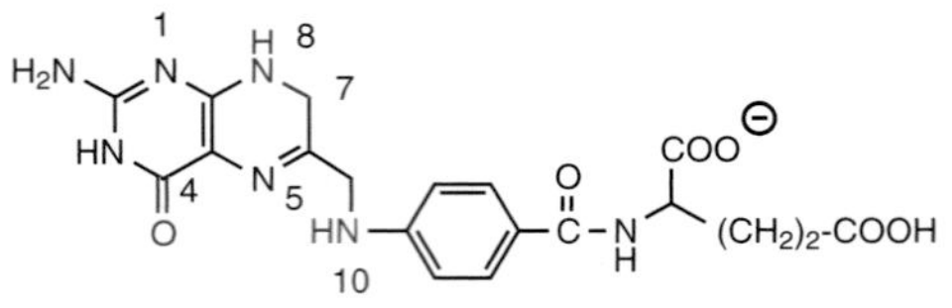

7,8-Dihydrofolate

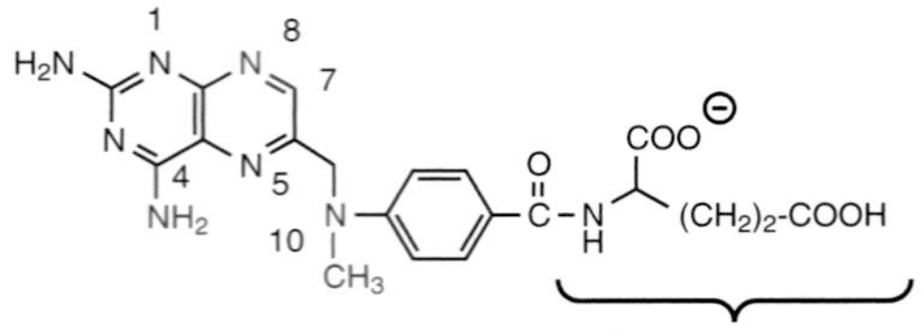

Methotrexate

Glutamate tail

In contrast, the C4-NH_2 substituent of methotrexate enriches electron density at N1 through π-electron donation, increasing its basic character between 10- and 1,000-fold and promoting protonation by Glu30 at the expense of N5. Because N1 and N5 are across the pteridine ring from one another, the interaction of N1 with the DHFR Asp27 will effectively stand the false substrate "on its head" relative to the orientation of 7,8-DHF (Fig. 33.51).[439,441,442] With the 5,6-double bond of methotrexate 180° away from the bound NADPH cofactor, and stabilized by the fully aromatic pteridine ring, the possibility for reduction is eliminated.[439] The DHFR enzyme will be pseudoirreversibly bound to a molecule it cannot reduce, which ties up the DHFR enzyme and prevents the conversion of DHF to THF. In turn, this halts the synthesis of the 5,10-methylene-THF cofactor required for dTMP biosynthesis and causes feedback inhibition of the thymidylate synthase enzyme. The cell will die a "thymineless death."

Methotrexate is given orally in the treatment of breast, head and neck, and various lung cancers as well as in non-Hodgkin lymphoma (NHL). The sodium salt form is also marketed for IV, IM, intra-arterial, or intrathecal injection. Oral absorption is dose-dependent and peaks at 80 mg/m^2 due to site saturation.

7,8-Dihydrofolate (properly oriented)

Methotrexate (misoriented)

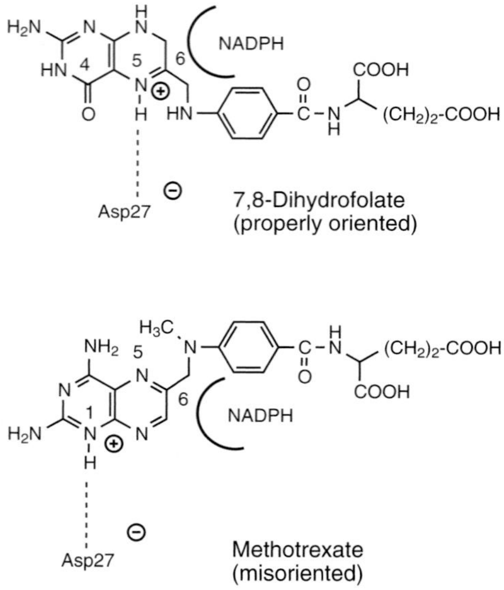

Figure 33.51 Misorientation of methotrexate at DHFR.

The monoglutamate tail of methotrexate permits active transport into cells via a reduced folate carrier (RFC1, a transporter extensively expressed on tumor cell membranes), where it subsequently undergoes intracellular folylpolyglutamate synthase (FPGS)-catalyzed polyglutamation. This process adds several anionic carboxylate groups to the molecule and traps the drug at the site of action.[443] Polyglutamation is more efficient in tumor cells than in healthy cells, which promotes the selective toxicity of this drug.[444] The polyglutamated drug will be hydrolyzed back to the parent structure by γ-glutamyl hydrolase before renal elimination. Up to 90% of an administered dose is excreted unchanged in the urine within 24 hours.

Several boxed warnings have been issued for methotrexate use.[76] Toxicity occurs if drug is allowed to accumulate in ascites and pleural effusions and/or when renal excretion is impaired by kidney disease. Methotrexate-induced lung disease is a particularly critical problem because it arises at any time and at any dose, and can be fatal. Severe GI adverse effects, including ulcerative stomatitis and hemorrhagic enteritis leading to intestinal perforation, can also occur. Potentially fatal skin reactions are a risk as well. Methotrexate and its aldehyde oxidase-generated 7-hydroxy metabolite (which has a 3-5 fold lower water solubility) can precipitate in the renal tubule, causing damaging crystal nephropathy (crystalluria). The drug should not be given to patients unless urinary pH is at or above 7.5, and parenterally and/or enterally-administered urinary alkalinizing agents should be given (along with vigorous hydration) if high doses (≥1000 mg/m^2) are to be used.[445,446] As a Category X teratogen, this drug should not be given to women who are pregnant or planning to become pregnant.

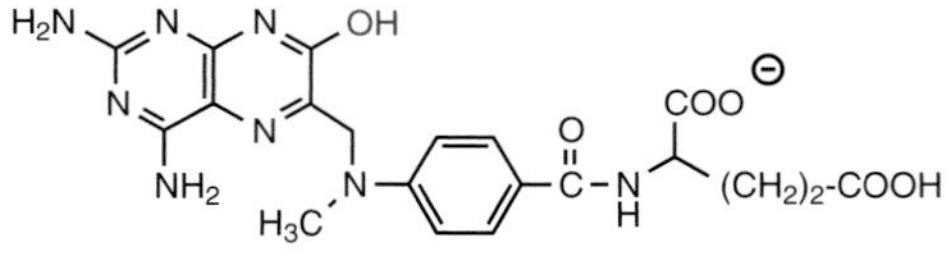

7-hydroxymethotrexate

If severe methotrexate toxicity occurs, reduced folate replacement therapy with 5-formyltetrahydrofolate (leucovorin) must be initiated as soon as possible. Leucovorin generates the folate cofactors needed by DHFR and GAR formyltransferase to ensure the continued synthesis of pyrimidine and purine nucleotides in healthy cells. "Leucovorin rescue" is often given prophylactically after high-dose methotrexate therapy.[446,447]

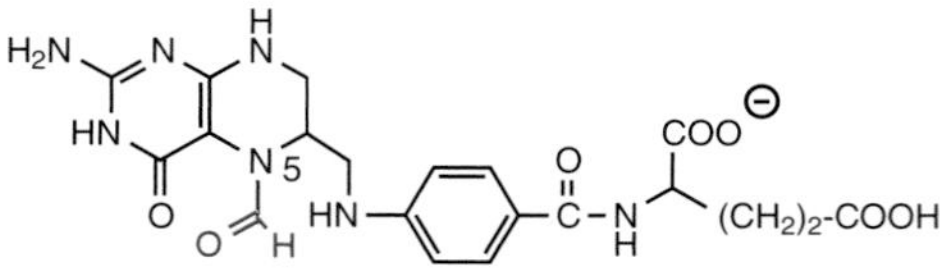

5-Formyltetrahydrofolate (Leucovorin)

Cancer cells can become resistant to methotrexate over time. Acquired resistance mechanisms include increased of expression of DHFR and other enzyme targets, impaired RFC1-mediated transport, active cellular efflux by P-gp, and/or attenuated intracellular polyglutamation.[443]

Pemetrexed Disodium. Pemetrexed is a multitarget antifolate administered by IV in combination with an organoplatinum agent for the treatment of advanced or metastatic nonsquamous NSCLC[448] and malignant pleural mesothelioma. Pemetrexed/carboplatin therapy has demonstrated a more positive impact on PFS and OS in NSCLC patients than paclitaxel/carboplatin, but at a significantly higher economic cost (approximately $20,000 in 2013).[449] A recent systematic review of the literature related to pemetrexed use in nonsquamous NSCLC patients with EGFR mutations who failed on TKI therapy concluded favorable survival outcomes compared to regimens without this antifolate, although patient numbers were relatively small and no formal statistical comparisons could be made.[450]

Pemetrexed's affinity for RFC1 is approximately twice that of methotrexate.[451] While methotrexate transport reaches a plateau after a relatively short drug exposure time, pemetrexed uptake continues to increase for a prolonged period, resulting in significantly more drug being ferried into the tumor cell over time.[451] If RFC1 transport is impaired, a second carrier protein (proton-coupled folate transporter or PCFT) takes over pemetrexed intracellular transport. PCFT is found in a majority of solid tumor cell lines, and the affinity of pemetrexed for this carrier is approximately 20 times that of methotrexate.[451]

The K_m of pemetrexed for FPGS is 100-fold lower than methotrexate, and this higher affinity results in more polyglutamated drug being rapidly generated (and trapped) inside the cancer cell.[451] Tetra- and pentaglutamates predominate. Both mono- and polyglutamated forms of pemetrexed are capable of inhibiting DHFR, and they do so with comparable activity.[452,453] Unlike methotrexate, pemetrexed does not distribute centrally to any significant extent.[453] It is minimally metabolized and up to 90% is excreted unchanged in urine.

In addition to DHFR, polyglutamated pemetrexed (but not the monoglutamated parent) binds tightly to thymidylate synthase and, to a lesser extent, GAR formyltransferase.[451,452,454,455] Since intracellular polyglutamation of pemetrexed is so efficient, this drug realizes a significant portion of its potent anticancer activity through the inhibition of these two enzymes. In fact, thymidylate synthase is considered its primary target, and a lack of overexpression of this enzyme (which can lead to tumor cell viability despite therapy) may predict positive outcomes in terms of PFS and OS.[448,456] Fortunately, the affinities of the polyglutamated forms of pemetrexed for this enzyme are higher than that of the monoglutamate parent, so efficacy is not sacrificed for enhanced localization at the site of action. As noted above, pemetrexed is used in combination with an organometallic, most commonly cisplatin.[452] A synergistic effect with gemcitabine (a DNA polymerase inhibitor) in the treatment of lung cancer patients has also been noted as long as gemcitabine is administered immediately prior to the antifolate.[453]

Patients on pemetrexed must take folic acid (commonly 400 μg daily) and vitamin B_{12} (1 mg IM on an established schedule) to reduce the risk of bone marrow suppression (neutropenia, thrombocytopenia, and anemia) and use-limiting GI adverse effects like mucositis and stomatitis. A 3-day course of corticosteroid therapy beginning the day before pemetrexed can reduce the risk of drug-induced skin rash.[76] Antiemetic therapy to proactively combat drug-induced nausea and vomiting is also warranted.[453] Pemetrexed has a half-life of 3.5 hours and is excreted primarily unchanged via the kidneys.

Resistance to pemetrexed is mediated predominantly through a decrease in FPGS activity, enhanced hydrolysis of pemetrexed polyglutamates via γ-glutamyl hydrolase, and upregulation of the thymidylate synthase target.[452,456] In contrast to methotrexate, downregulation of RFC1 is not involved in acquired resistance to pemetrexed as long as PCFT is functioning.[451] Likewise, upregulation of DHFR is not a pemetrexed resistance mechanism since DHFR is not a primary target of this antifolate.

In addition to the level of thymidylate synthase expression, differences in ATP-binding cassette (ABC) C11 transporters may be an important predictor of sensitivity to pemetrexed chemotherapy.[457] In the ABCC11 SNP 538G>A, the A/A variant (unlike the G/G or G/A) does not promote pemetrexed efflux from the cancer cell. ABCC11 genotype also impacts the nature of earwax, and it has been noted that East Asians (80%-95% of whom express the A/A variant and have dry earwax) are particularly responsive to pemetrexed–cisplatin chemotherapy. Patients expressing the other ABCC11 variants would be at risk for pemetrexed resistance due to excessive drug efflux.

Pralatrexate. Pralatrexate is a 10-deaza analogue of methotrexate where the chiral carbon atom replacing N10 has been substituted with a propargyl moiety. This structural alteration results in a significantly enhanced tumor cell uptake via RFC1.[458] The rate of active transport of pralatrexate by RFC1 has been measured at approximately 10-14 times that of methotrexate. In addition, pralatrexate is polyglutamated by FPGS at a rate that is comparable to pemetrexed and 10-fold higher than methotrexate.[459,460] This translates to more active drug inside the tumor cell for a longer period of time.

Unlike pemetrexed, which is also more extensively polyglutamated than methotrexate, pralatrexate's primary antineoplastic enzymatic target is DHFR. Although it interacts with and inhibits the isolated DHFR enzyme 2-3 fold less vigorously than methotrexate (K_i apparent = 26 and 45 nmol/L, respectively), the RFC1 cellular influx and FPGS polyglutamation first-order rate constants (V_{max}/K_m) are 12- and 10-fold greater, respectively.[461] Higher concentrations of active polyglutamated drug trapped within the cell provide a more potent DHFR inhibitory effect compared to methotrexate and a greater antitumor response than either methotrexate or pemetrexed.[458,461]

Like pemetrexed, pralatrexate is not significantly metabolized and is excreted in both urine and feces. The marketed product is a racemic mixture, and the two isomers have differing volumes of distribution (37 vs. 105 L for the *R* and *S* isomers, respectively).

Pralatrexate is currently used exclusively in peripheral T-cell lymphoma,[462] although it might eventually find use in other cancers (e.g., NSCLC, NHL). Some T-cell lymphoma patients treated with pralatrexate have achieved complete remission.[460] Dosing is based on body surface area in order to standardize exposure to active drug. When used in combination with gemcitabine, the synergistic apoptotic effect is maximized when the antifolate is administered before the polymerase inhibitor.[461] Pralatrexate is not effective against B-cell lymphoma.[459] Unlike methotrexate, acquired resistance is believed to be more highly dependent on reduced RFC1 expression than on an increased expression of DHFR.[463]

As with other antifolates, patients on pralatrexate should receive daily folic acid supplementation and vitamin B_{12} to reduce the risk of mucositis/stomatitis and bone marrow suppression. Whereas the latter adverse effect is viewed as a minor risk,[461] mucositis has been termed the major dose-limiting adverse reaction. Folic acid/vitamin B_{12} normalizes levels of methylmalonic acid, which decreases mucositis risk without compromising antineoplastic activity.[464] Mucositis generally occurs early in therapy (e.g., in the first cycle) so gradual dose escalation can potentially minimize risk, as can concomitant oral leucovorin prophylaxis (15 mg daily other than the day before, after and of pralatrexate therapy). Unlike methotrexate, pralatrexate's efficacy is not negatively impacted by leucovorin, an advantage likely due to pralatrexate's very rapid and extensive intracellular transport via RCF1.[465]

O O HO OH CH_3

Methylmalonic acid

A review of pralatrexate pharmacologic and therapeutic actions after 8 years of clinical use has been published and has reinforced the mechanistic understandings described above.[465] These authors also noted pralatrexate's low affinity for PCFT, confirming the primary importance of RFC1 for intracellular transport, as well as the synergistic efficacy of pralatrexate/romidepsin combination therapy. They also interestingly reveal that pralatrexate's remarkable utility in refractory peripheral T-cell lymphoma was serendipitously discovered when a single individual with this disorder in a group of B-cell lymphoma patients (all of whom had failed completely on pralatrexate) exhibited a complete response after a single dose. When three additional highly refractory T-cell lymphoma patients responded in the same "miraculous" way, pralatrexate's place in the antineoplastic armamentarium was assured.

DNA Polymerase/DNA Chain Elongation Inhibitors

MECHANISM OF ACTION. Six halogenated and/or ribose-modified DNA nucleoside analogues (including one nucleotide) are marketed for the treatment of a wide variety of hematologic cancers and solid tumors (Fig. 33.41). These agents have complex and multifaceted mechanisms, but all include inhibition of DNA polymerase and/or DNA chain elongation among their actions. The nucleosides are actively transported into tumor cells where they are converted to triphosphorylated nucleotides by specific kinases and subsequently incorporated into the growing DNA chain, thus arresting further elongation. Tumors deficient in the nucleoside transporter will be resistant to these anticancer agents. In mono- and diphosphorylated forms, these drugs may also inhibit the biosynthesis of essential deoxyribonucleotides, but this is viewed as a secondary mechanism of toxicity.[466]

Gemcitabine's structure provides one example of how DNA halogenated polymerase inhibitors work (Fig. 33.52). When incorporating the false nucleotide into the growing DNA chain, DNA polymerase activity is not impacted by the substitution at 2′ (no larger than hydrogen) because the enzyme is working at the phosphate end of the structure, attaching it to the 3′-OH of the last nucleotide in the chain. One more nucleotide can be added to the incorporated gemcitabine. However, when it's time to add the next nucleotide, the highly electronegative 2′-fluorine atoms inhibit the polymerase enzyme and chain elongation stops. While DNA polymerase has "proofreading" capabilities and can correct the mis-incorporation of a "wrong" nucleotide, the false nucleotide looks so much like the expected dCTP that it is not recognized by this "seek and repair" enzyme machinery.[467]

With the exception of trifluridine, all drugs in this pharmacologic class are administered IV. They are excreted predominantly via the kidneys and induce myelosuppression as their major use-limiting adverse effect. Resistance can involve aberrations in the expression of metabolizing enzymes as well as of transporting and efflux proteins. Some in vitro evidence points to the loss of functional nucleoside transporter proteins (specifically hENT1/SLC29A1) and deoxycytidine kinase enzymes as the primary causes of acquired resistance to DNA polymerase inhibitors.[468]

SPECIFIC DRUGS (FIG. 33.41)

Fludarabine, Cladribine, and Clofarabine. These 3-halogenated adenosine-based nucleosides undergo conversion to the active triphosphate nucleotides after facilitated transport into tumor cells. All are initially phosphorylated by deoxycytidine kinase, and cells with high levels of this enzyme should respond well to these agents. Mono- and diphosphate kinases complete the metabolic conversion to the active form. The C2-halogen renders the molecules relatively resistant to the degradative action of adenosine deaminase, and a significant fraction of the dose is eliminated unchanged in urine. Fludarabine, an arabinoside, is marketed as the monophosphate nucleotide to enhance water solubility for intravenous administration, but this group is cleaved rapidly in the bloodstream, allowing the free nucleoside to take advantage of the nucleoside-specific transporting proteins.

Cladribine is indicated in the treatment of hairy cell leukemia, whereas fludarabine phosphate is used in refractory/progressive CLL. In addition to myelosuppression, fludarabine can induce hemolytic anemia, along with

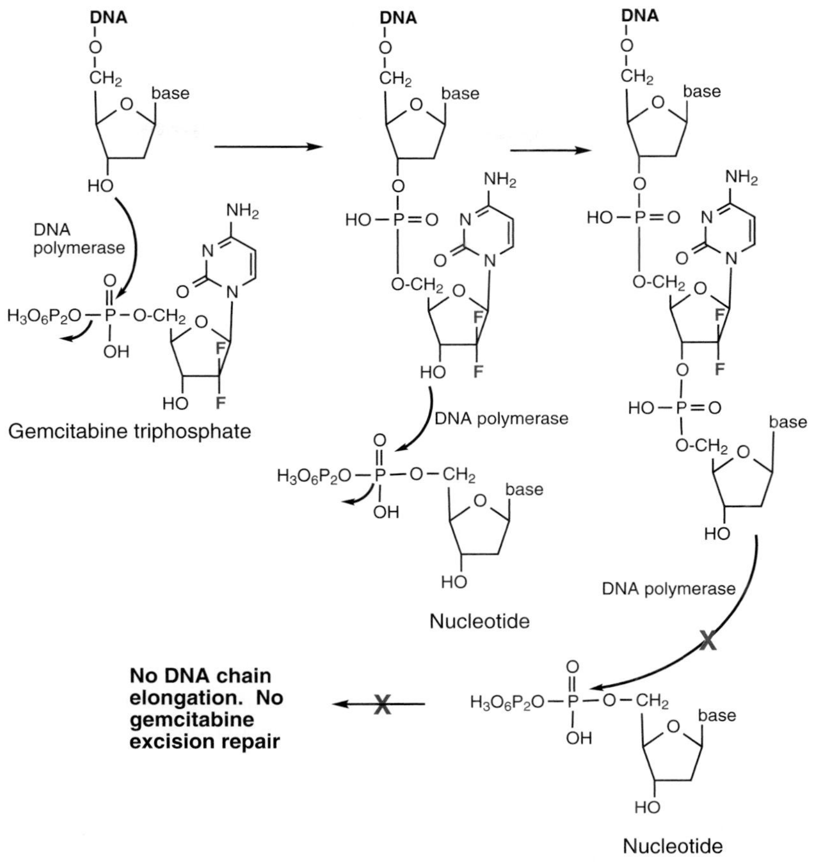

Figure 33.52 Gemcitabine triphosphate inhibition of DNA polymerase.

severe CNS toxicity when used in high doses, and this has resulted in a boxed warning. The warning also cautions on the high incidence of fatal pulmonary toxicity when fludarabine phosphate is used in combination with pentostatin. The boxed warning for cladribine is focused on myelosuppression, neurotoxicity, and nephrotoxicity.

Clofarabine is used in relapsed/refractory ALL patients 21 years or younger who have failed on at least two previous regimens. In addition to inhibiting DNA chain elongation, this drug also inhibits ribonucleotide reductase (required for the conversion of ribonucleotides to deoxyribonucleotides) and facilitates the release of proapoptotic proteins from mitochondria. The rapid attenuation of leukemia cells after administration of this agent can result in a condition known as tumor lysis syndrome, and respiratory and cardiac toxicities can occur secondary to cytokine release. Toxicity can progress to potentially fatal capillary leak syndrome and organ failure, and patients should receive IV fluids for the entire 5-day course of therapy to minimize risk of serious adverse events. Despite these serious toxicities, this DNA polymerase inhibitor carries no boxed warning.

Cytarabine, Gemcitabine and Trifluridine. All of these pyrimidine-based anticancer agents undergo initial phosphorylation by deoxycytidine kinase (cytarabine, gemcitabine) or thymidine kinase (trifluridine) to the monophosphate with subsequent phosphorylation catalyzed by pyrimidine monophosphate and diphosphate kinases. Cytarabine, an arabinoside, is catabolized by cytidine and deoxycytidylate (deoxycytidine monophosphate or dCMP) deaminases to inactive uracil analogues (Fig. 33.53). The significantly longer half-life of gemcitabine (19 hr) compared to conventional cytarabine (3.6 hr) is due to the inhibitory action of the difluorodeoxycytidine triphosphate metabolite on the dCMP deaminase enzyme.[437] Gemcitabine elimination is gender-dependent, with women having the greater risk for toxicity due to lower renal clearance.

Gemcitabine is indicated in the treatment of breast, pancreatic, and non-small cell lung cancers. Cytarabine, which can be administered SC and intrathecally as well as IV, is used in the treatment of various leukemias. A liposomal formulation of cytarabine is available for the treatment of lymphomatous meningitis.

Trifluridine, the only orally administered DNA polymerase inhibitor, is highly vulnerable to the inactivating enzyme thymidine phosphorylase, which cleaves the deoxyribose moiety from the trifluorothymidine base. Although this reaction occurs rapidly and extensively via pre-hepatic (gut) and first pass metabolism, therapeutic utility is assured because the marketed product also contains the thymidine phosphorylase inhibitor tipiracil hydrochloride in a 2:1 molar ratio (trifluridine/tipiracil). When administered orally in combination with tipiracil, trifluridine's

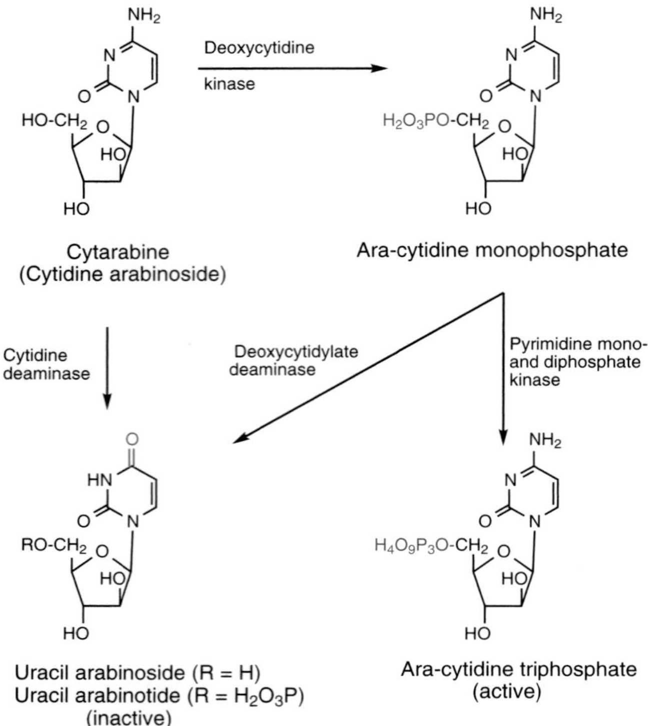

Figure 33.53 Cytarabine metabolism.

AUC increases by 100-fold and the C_{max} is over 70-fold higher compared to trifluridine alone. Tipiracil itself is not extensively absorbed from the GIT.[469]

Tipiricil hydrochloride

Trifluridine is used in metastatic colon cancer refractory to first-line cytotoxic and targeted chemotherapies from several chemical/pharmacologic classes. In addition to DNA polymerase inhibition by trifluridine triphosphate, the monophosphorylated nucleotide inhibits thymidylate synthase, binding directly to Tyr146 within the active site.[466] Trifluridine is claimed to be tumoristatic, rather than tumoricidal with modest PFS and OS benefits, supporting the ongoing search for response enhancing cotherapies and predictive biomarkers.[469,470] Neutropenia, leukopenia, anemia, thrombocytopenia and GI distress are the major adverse effects, with myelosuppression being dose limiting. Neutropenia of grade 3 or higher during any cycle of trifluridine therapy has been associated with better survival outcomes.[470,471] The drug is administered twice daily within 1 hour after morning and evening meals to enhance tolerability.[472]

DNA Methyltransferase Inhibitors

MECHANISM OF ACTION. Three nucleic acid-based chemotherapeutic agents, azacitidine, decitabine, and nelarabine (Fig. 33.41), block abnormal cellular proliferation by inhibiting DNA alkylation (specifically methylation) on genes responsible for differentiation and growth. Aberrant epigenetic DNA methylation in cancer most commonly occurs at C5 of cytidine nucleotides that precede guanylate residues (CpG dinucleotides or "islands"), and results in tumor-suppressor-, apoptosis- and DNA repair-related gene silencing and overall genomic instability.[473-476] SAM serves as the methyl donor. The hypomethylation effect of these agents, mediated through the inhibition of DNA methyltransferase (DNMT) subtype 1, can sometimes restore normal gene function while selectively killing cells that have stopped responding to the body's cellular proliferation control processes. A recent review of decitabine's impact on gene expression proposes a multifaceted mechanism involving activation of genes beyond those influencing DNA methylation.[476]

All of the marketed DNMT inhibitors are nucleosides that, once actively transported and converted to triphosphate nucleotides inside the cell, are mistakenly incorporated into DNA in lieu of their cytidine or guanine nucleotide counterparts. Interaction of the false nucleotide with DNMT1 results in covalent bond formation that irreversibly inhibits the enzyme, which is followed by destruction via proteasomal cleavage.[475,477] The therapeutic effect manifests slowly over several drug administration cycles, and only between 30% and 40% of eligible patients respond.[475] Research in this area has branched out into non-nucleoside small molecules that mimic SAM and oligonucleotides that mimic DNA and RNA, but more work is needed to identify novel DNMT inhibitors with both high therapeutic efficacy and selectivity.[474]

CHEMISTRY. The nucleoside-based DNMT inhibitors hydrolyze in aqueous solution and must be administered soon after the dose is constituted. Their vulnerability to deaminase enzymes explains their short elimination half-lives of less than or equal to 4 hours.[475] Nelarabine will be O-demethylated to ara-G by adenosine deaminase prior to phosphorylation and DNA incorporation,[478] and can be further metabolized to guanine, xanthine, and uric acid. Anemia, neutropenia, and thrombocytopenia are among the most common side effects of this class of drugs, and low grade GI disturbances are frequent.

Ara-G

SPECIFIC DRUGS (FIG. 33.41)

Azacitidine and Decitabine. Decitabine is the deoxyribonucleoside analogue of azacitidine. Decitabine is phosphorylated by deoxycytidine kinase and, in triphosphorylated nucleotide form, incorporated exclusively into DNA.[479] In contrast, azacitidine is phosphorylated by uridine-cytidine kinase. At the diphosphate stage of azacitidine activation, up to 20% will be converted to decitabine diphosphate via ribonucleotide reductase and, after conversion to the triphosphate, will inhibit DNMT1 as described above. The remainder of the azacitidine diphosphate metabolite will add a final phosphate residue and be incorporated into RNA, where it interferes with the synthesis of mRNA and proteins (Fig. 33.54).[473,475,477,479] Given the significant difference in pharmacodynamics, it may not be surprising that in vitro studies have demonstrated no cross-resistance between the two structurally related agents.[479]

Azacitidine and decitabine are given IV (and, in the case of azacitidine, SC) for the treatment of myelodysplastic syndrome, a disorder of blood-forming stem cells known to express a hypermethylated *p5(INK4B)* gene, and which can progress to AML.[473] The absolute bioavailablity of SC-administered azacitidine is approximately 89%, and administration by this route results in twice the half-life achieved after IV administration.[475,479] Doses of azacitidine (either route) and decitabine are 75 and 15 mg/m^2, respectively, and the number and duration of the cycles are drug-specific. Both drugs have off-label indications in AML.

Azacitidine has demonstrated significant survival value in phase III trials that compared it to three "standard of care" therapies that ranged from supportive to strong chemotherapy. Additional trials pairing it with a variety of chemotherapeutic agents (including targeted therapies) are ongoing. This drug is also being studied as first-line and salvage therapy in AML patients deemed unfit for standard therapy (e.g., frail elderly), and an oral dosage form is in development.[473,479] The low oral bioavailability of decitabine precludes administration via this route unless a cytidine deaminase inhibitor is coadministered.[475] While preclinical studies favor decitabine as an antileukemic agent, there have not been randomized "head-to-head" trials of these two DNMT inhibitors in AML.[475]

Both azacitidine and decitabine are resistant to CYP and phase 2 conjugating enzymes, but are inactivated via cytidine deaminase and/or non-enzymatic hydrolysis.[76,479] Unchanged azacitidine and its metabolites are excreted in urine, but the excretion profile of decitabine is currently unknown.

Patients on either azacitidine or decitabine should be monitored for hematologic and renal toxicities. Both drugs are known to cause fetal harm, and patients should be actively counseled to take appropriate reproductive precautions.[76] Resistance related to genetic adaptations and instability is, unfortunately, commonly encountered.[473] As with so many other anticancer drugs, the search is on for predictive biomarkers to facilitate identification of patients most likely to respond favorably to these agents.[473,479]

Nelarabine. Nelarabine is considered third-line treatment for T-cell acute lymphoblastic leukemia or lymphoma. It is rapidly and efficiently converted to ara-G in the bloodstream, and then selectively accumulates in malignant T-cells for phosphorylation and DNA

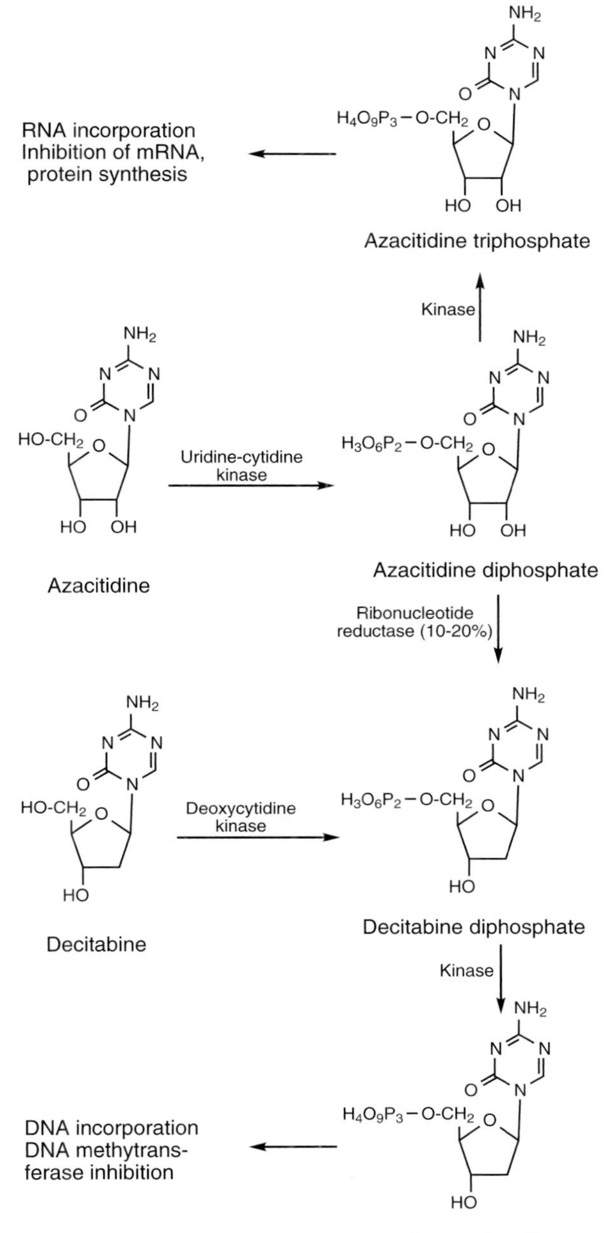

Figure 33.54 Azacitidine and decitabine metabolism and mechanism.

incorporation.[478] It is administered by IV infusion over 1 or 2 hours in pediatric and adult patients, respectively. The drug can induce severe and potentially irreversible neurologic symptoms including convulsions, severe central depression, and peripheral neuropathy that can mimic Guillain-Barré syndrome, and carries a boxed warning as a result. These adverse effects are dose-limiting, but there is early evidence that administration via 24 hour continuous infusion might attenuate these serious toxicities.[478] As noted earlier, nelarabine can be metabolized to uric acid. Along with hydration and urine basification, the xanthine oxidase inhibitor allopurinol can be given prophylactically to minimize risk of nelarabine-induced hyperuricemia.

Miscellaneous Antimetabolites

The antimetabolites described below are less widely used than those discussed above.

SPECIFIC DRUGS

Pentostatin. Pentostatin is a ring-expanded purine ribonucleoside that inhibits adenosine deaminase and is primarily used in the treatment of hairy cell leukemia. The elevated levels of dATP that result from inhibition of this degradative enzyme inhibit the action of ribonucleotide reductase (the enzyme that converts ribose diphosphate to deoxyribose diphosphate), thus halting DNA synthesis within the tumor cell. When used in CLL, some authors claim pentostatin offers a therapeutic efficacy comparable to fludarabine, but with a lower risk of toxicity.[480,481] The combination of pentostatin and fludarabine in this disease state has resulted in fatal pulmonary toxicity, which prompted the issuance of a boxed warning.[76]

Several phase II clinical trials conducted in a total of 288 patients with progressive, treatment naïve CLL that employed pentostatin-based chemoimmunotherapy documented overall response rates >90%, a complete remission rate of 41%, an approximately 10-year median OS, and a median treatment-free survival of almost 4 years.[481]

Hydroxyurea. Hydroxyurea, a drug with a 100-plus year history, blocks the synthesis of DNA by trapping a tyrosyl free radical species at the catalytic site of ribonucleotide reductase, thereby inhibiting the enzyme that converts ribonucleotide diphosphates into their corresponding deoxyribonucleotides. It is used orally for the treatment of resistant CML and as an adjunct to radiation in the treatment of squamous cell head and neck cancer. Hydroxyurea increases the effectiveness of radiation therapy through its selective toxicity to cells in the radiation-resistant S phase and by stalling the cell cycle in the G_1 stage, in which radiation therapy does the greatest damage. It addition, hydroxyurea thwarts the normal damage repair mechanisms of surviving cells. A review of its chemical, pharmacologic, metabolic, and therapeutic properties has been published.[482]

Hydroxyurea has excellent oral bioavailability (80%-100%), and serum levels peak within 2 hours of administration. If a positive response is noted within 6 weeks, toxicities are mostly mild enough to permit long-term or indefinite therapy on either a daily or every-3-day basis. Mucositis risk is augmented with high dose therapy (≥75 mg/kg/d).[483] Leukopenia and, less commonly, thrombocytopenia and/or anemia are the most serious adverse effects, and the drug carries a boxed warning for severe myelosuppression and the induction of secondary malignancies. Excretion of the unchanged drug and the urea metabolite is via the kidneys. The carbon dioxide produced as a by-product of hydroxyurea metabolism is excreted in the expired air.

DNA Alkylating and Crosslinking Agents

The primary target of DNA alkylating and cross-linking agents is the actively dividing DNA molecule. The DNA cross-linkers are extremely reactive electrophilic structures. The nucleophilic groups on various DNA bases (particularly, but not exclusively, the N7 of guanine) readily attack the electrophilic drug, resulting in irreversible alkylation or complexation of the DNA base.

Some DNA alkylating agents, such as the nitrogen mustards and nitrosoureas, are bifunctional, meaning that one molecule of the drug can bind two distinct DNA bases. Most commonly, the alkylated bases are on different DNA molecules, and interstrand DNA cross-linking through two guanine N7 atoms results. Cell cycle arrest and apoptosis follow as the cell tries unsuccessfully to repair the chemical insult. The DNA alkylating antineoplastics are not cell cycle specific, but they are more toxic to cells in the late G_1 or S phases of the cycle. This is the time when DNA is unwinding and exposing its nucleotides, increasing the chance that vulnerable DNA functional groups will encounter the electrophilic antineoplastic drug and launch the nucleophilic attack that leads to its own destruction. The DNA alkylators have a great capacity for inducing both mutagenesis and carcinogenesis.

Organoplatinum complexes also cross-link DNA, and many do so by binding to adjacent guanine nucleotides (called diguanosine dinucleotides) on a single strand of DNA. This leads to intrastrand DNA cross-linking. The anionic phosphate group on a second strand of DNA stabilizes the drug-DNA complex and makes the damage to DNA replication irreversible. Some organoplatinum agents also damage DNA through interstrand cross-linking.

The DNA alkylating and crosslinking antineoplastics are shown in Figure 33.55. Those that enjoy the most widespread clinical use will be described in some detail under the **Specific Drugs** sections below. Interested readers are referred to the 7th Edition of this text for descriptions of agents less commonly used in contemporary patient care (e.g., thiotepa, streptozocin, busulfan, altretamine).

Nitrogen Mustards and Aziridine-Mediated Alkylators

Nitrogen mustards are bis(β-haloalkyl)amines. The term "bis" means two, and the "halo" (short for halogen) in the nomenclature is invariably chlorine. The two chlorine atoms dramatically decrease the basic strength of the amino nitrogen through a strong negative inductive effect. As a result, the unionized conjugate of these drugs predominates at physiologic pH. This is intentional because it is the lone pair of electrons on the unionized amine that allows for the formation of the highly electrophilic aziridinium ion, which is the reactive DNA-destroying intermediate generated by all true mustards.

$$\mathrm{Cl-\overset{\beta}{C}H_2-\overset{\alpha}{C}H_2-\overset{R}{N}-\overset{\alpha}{C}H_2-\overset{\beta}{C}H_2-Cl}$$

Bis-β-haloalkylamine

MECHANISM OF ACTION. The mechanism of action of the nitrogen mustards is depicted in Figure 33.56.[484,485] In step 1, the lone pair of electrons on the unionized amine conducts an intramolecular nucleophilic attack at the

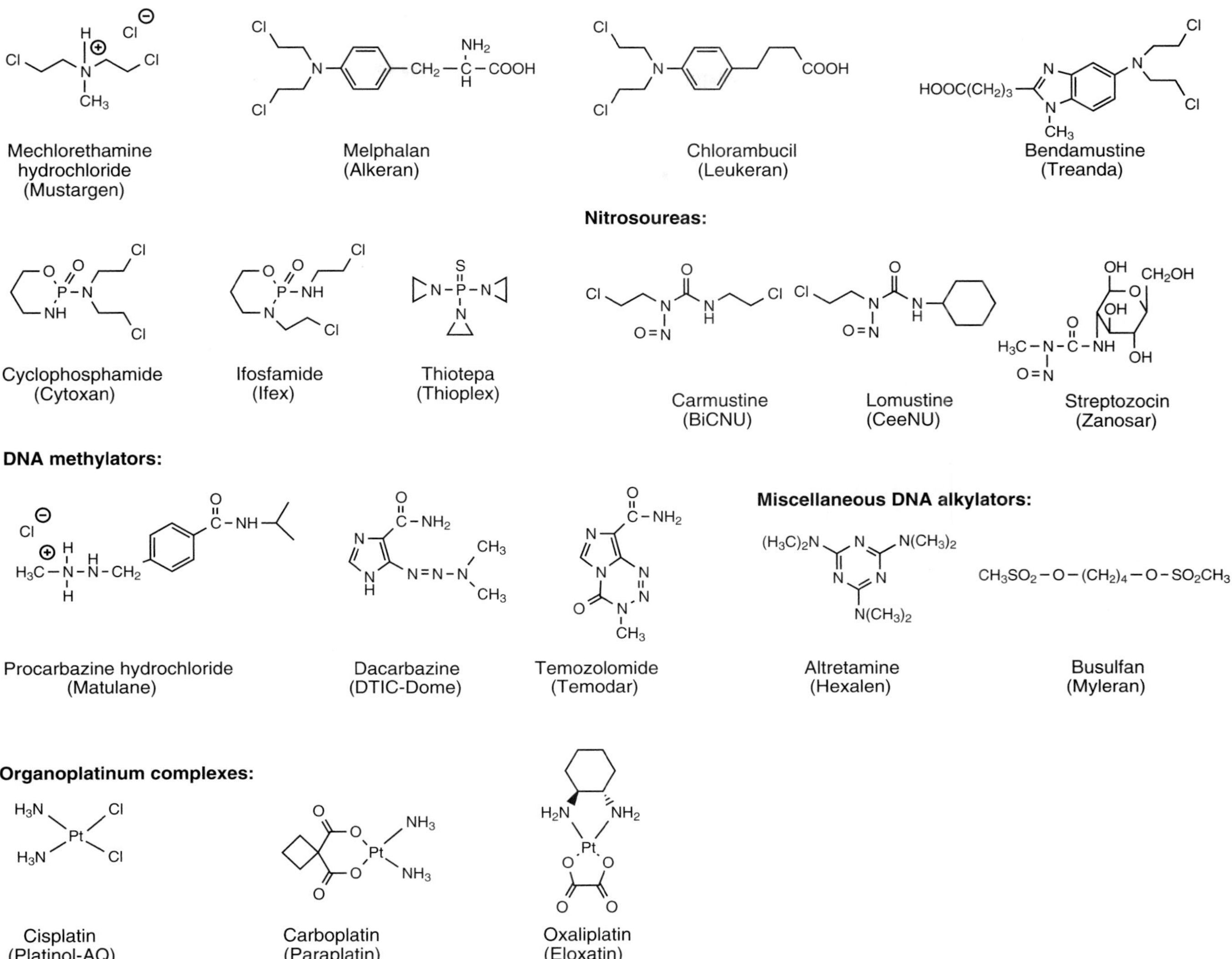

Figure 33.55 DNA alkylating and cross-linking agents.

β-carbon of the mustard, displacing chloride anion and forming the highly electrophilic aziridinium ion intermediate. The carbon atoms of this strained quaternary amine are highly electrophilic due to the strong negative inductive effect of the cationic nitrogen.

In step 2, a DNA nucleophile conducts an intermolecular nucleophilic attack, which breaks the aziridine ring and alkylates DNA. Although guanine is the preferred nucleic acid base involved, the less nucleophilic adenine is also known to react.[485] Of critical importance is the fact that the lone pair of electrons on the mustard nitrogen is regenerated when the aziridine ring cleaves.

Steps 3 and 4 are simply repetitions of steps 1 and 2, respectively, involving the second arm of the mustard and a second molecule of DNA. Ultimately, two molecules of DNA will be cross-linked through the carbon atoms of what was once the nitrogen mustard. Tethered together, the DNA strands cannot separate nor replicate, so transcription of DNA to RNA is halted. In an attempt to liberate the DNA from the mustard's covalent stranglehold, hydrolytic depurination (step 5) cleaves the bound guanine residues from the DNA strand. However, the DNA released from this mustard trap is damaged and unable to replicate, and cell death is the inevitable result. If this is happening in a tumor cell, the therapeutic goal has been accomplished. If it is happening in a healthy cell, particularly one with a short half-life, the patient may experience adverse effects that can be use-limiting.

CHEMISTRY. The structure of nitrogen mustards differs only in the nature of the third group (R) attached to the amino nitrogen. This group, which can be either aliphatic or aromatic, is the prime determinant of chemical reactivity, oral bioavailability, and the nature and extent of advese effects.

An aliphatic nitrogen substituent (e.g., CH_3) will release electrons to the amine through σ bonds. This electronic enrichment enhances the nucleophilic character of the lone pair of electrons and increases the speed at which

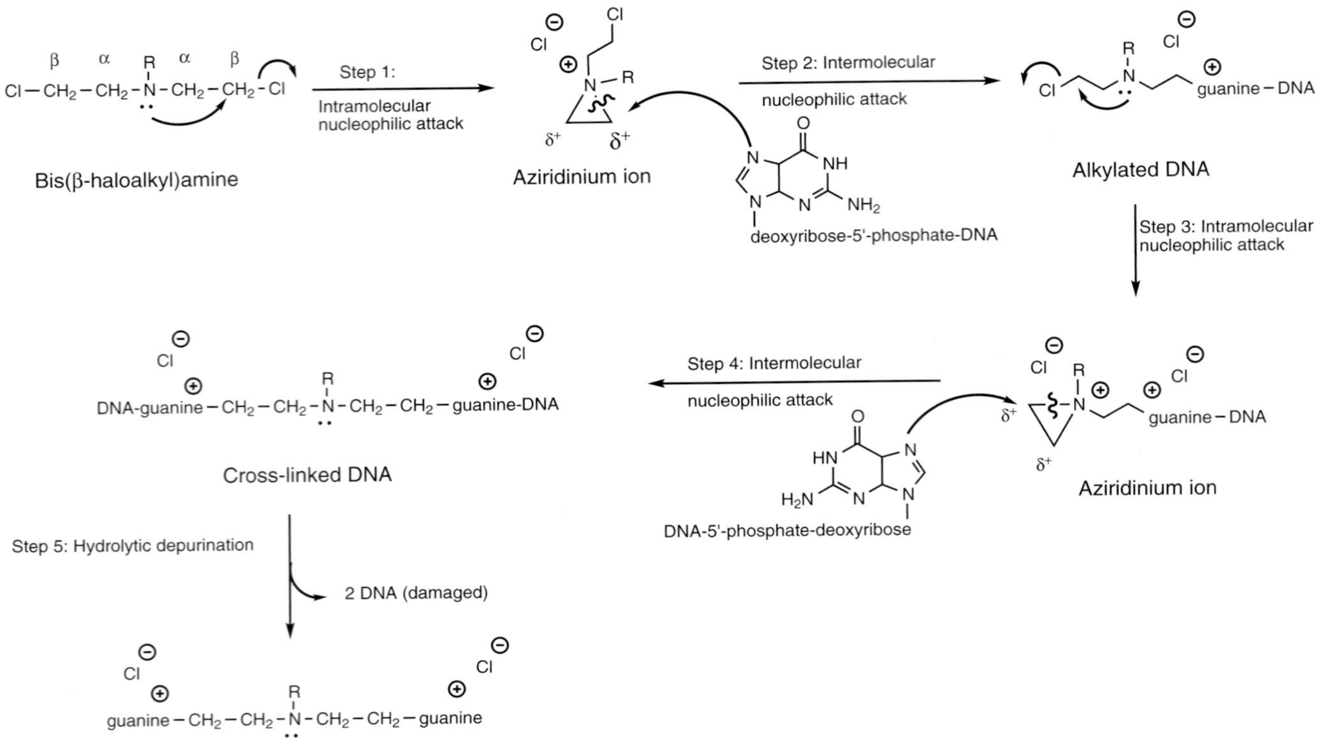

Figure 33.56 DNA destruction through nitrogen mustard-mediated alkylation.

the δ⁺ β-carbon of the mustard will be attacked. Whether in a tumor cell or a healthy cell, as soon as the aziridinium ion forms, it will react with unpaired DNA and/or other cell nucleophiles, such as electron-rich SH, OH and NH groups of amino acids on enzymes or membrane-bound receptors.[485] The body's water can also react with (and inactivate) the aziridinium ion. The intra- and intermolecular reactions designated as steps 1 through 4 in Figure 33.56 happen rapidly, so little opportunity exists for tissue or cell specificity. This means a greatly increased risk of serious adverse effects and use-limiting toxicity.

Conversely, an aromatic nitrogen substituent (e.g., phenyl) conjugated with the mustard nitrogen will stabilize the lone pair of electrons through resonance. Resonance delocalization significantly slows the rate of intramolecular nucleophilic attack, aziridinium ion formation, and DNA alkylation. Aromatic mustards have a reactivity sufficiently controlled to permit oral administration and attenuate the severity of adverse effects. The higher stability also provides the chance for enhanced tissue selectivity by giving the intact mustard time to reach malignant cells before generating the cytotoxic aziridinium ion.

Nitrogen mustards can decompose in aqueous media through formation of the inactive dehalogenated diol shown in Figure 33.57. Both the mustard nitrogen (pathway a) and the oxygen of water (pathway b) can act as nucleophiles to advance this degradative process. The decomposition reactions can be inhibited if the nucleophilic character of these atoms is eliminated through protonation, so buffering solutions to an acidic pH (e.g., 3-5) helps to enhance stability in aqueous solution.

SPECIFIC DRUGS (FIG. 33.55)

Mechlorethamine Hydrochloride. While mechlorethamine's high toxicity relegates it to use in combination therapy in primarily hematological malignancies where the potential benefits outweigh the risks, it bears mentioning because it is the only aliphatic nitrogen mustard currently on the U.S. market. Its extremely high reactivity leads to

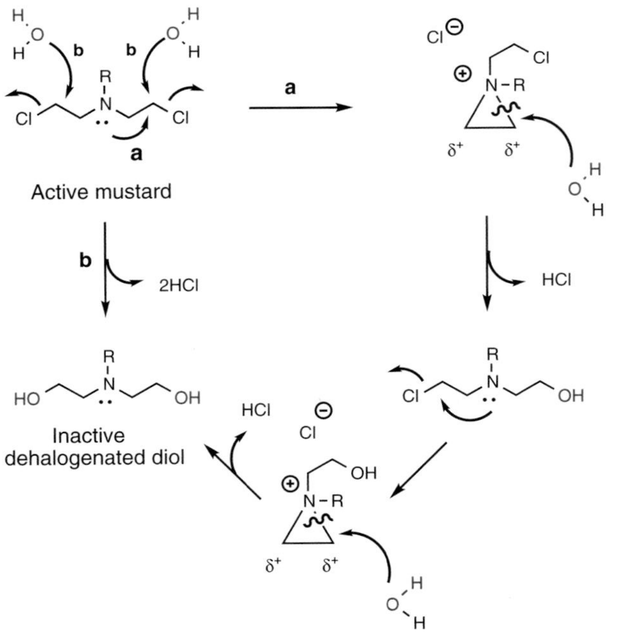

Figure 33.57 Aqueous decomposition of nitrogen mustards.

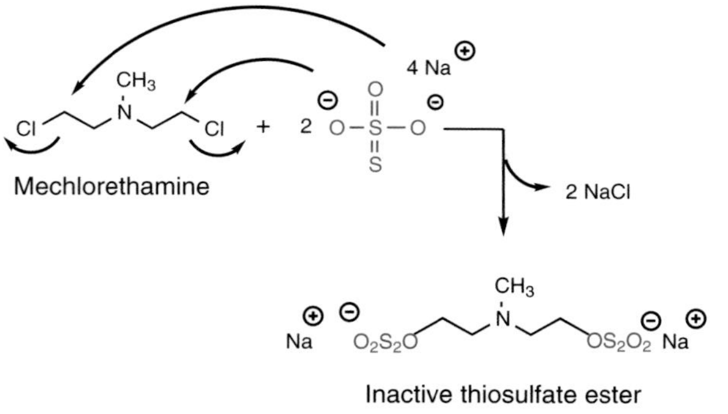

Mechlorethamine

2 NaCl

Inactive thiosulfate ester

Figure 33.58 Mechlorethamine inactivation by sodium thiosulfate.

rapid and nonspecific alkylation of cell nucleophiles. It is a severe vesicant, and if skin contact occurs, the drug must be inactivated with 2% sodium thiosulfate ($Na_2S_2O_3$) solution.[76] This reagent reacts with the mustard to create an inactive, highly ionized, and water-soluble thiosulfate ester that can be washed away (Fig. 33.58). The affected tissue should also be treated with an ice compress for 6-12 hours.

Mechlorethamine is marketed in hydrochloride salt form to provide water solubility for IV or intracavitary administration. In addition to severe nausea and vomiting, myelosuppression (lymphocytopenia and granulocytopenia) and alopecia, it can cause myelogenous leukemia with extended use due to its mutagenic/carcinogenic effects on bone marrow stem cells.

Chlorambucil. Chlorambucil is one of three aromatic nitrogen mustards with a resonance-stabilized amine that results in oral activity and fewer adverse effects than aliphatic mechlorethamine. The drug is active intact and also undergoes β-oxidation to provide an active phenylacetic acid mustard metabolite which is responsible for some of the observed antineoplastic activity. There is a reduced incidence of nausea and vomiting, but patients still experience myelosuppression which is severe enough to carry a boxed warning. It is also mutagenic, teratogenic and carcinogenic; it can induce nonlymphocytic leukemia, although secondary malignancies are considered rare events.[486] It is administered in tablet form in doses ranging from 0.1 to 0.2 mg/kg/d for the management of CLL, NHL and Hodgkin lymphoma. Patients with Hodgkin disease generally require doses on the high end of this range. Absorption is over 70% and, although decreased by the presence of food, regimens do not demand an empty stomach. C_{max} is achieved within an hour and the drug is extensively bound to serum protein. Elimination of inactive mono- and dihydroxy spontaneous hydrolysis products[487] of both the parent drug and phenylacetic acid metabolite is primarily via the urine.[76]

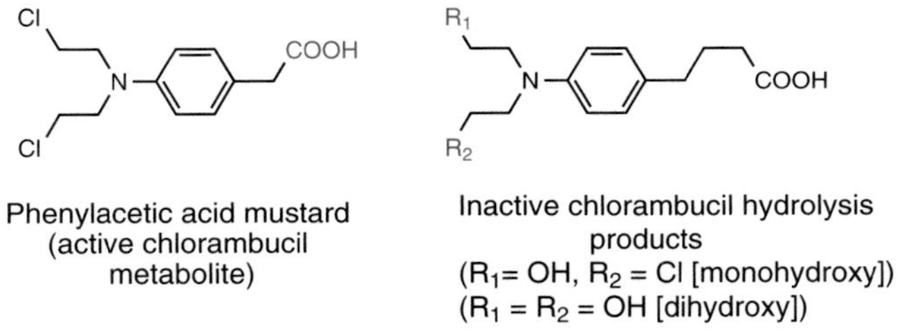

Phenylacetic acid mustard (active chlorambucil metabolite)

Inactive chlorambucil hydrolysis products (R_1= OH, R_2 = Cl [monohydroxy]) (R_1 = R_2 = OH [dihydroxy])

Recent meta-analyses of chlorambucil use in B-cell malignancies such as CLL have found no disadvantage relative to OS when compared with more commonly employed regimens. Authors have advocated for its use in combination with ibrutinib or obinutuzumab (an anti-CD20 MAb) in patients unfit for more aggressive chemotherapy with fludarabine, cyclophosphamide and rituximab.[486,488]

A structurally similar aromatic mustard, melphalan (Fig. 33.55), is used primarily in the treatment of multiple myeloma. L-Phe was purposefully incorporated into this antineoplastic to promote active transport into tumor cells, however studies indicate that melphalan enters cells through facilitated diffusion rather than by active transport.[489]

Bendamustine Hydrochloride. Bendamustine, an antineoplastic "old timer" first synthesized in 1963, is the N-methylbenzimidazole analogue of chlorambucil. The incorporation of this purine-like aromatic ring was purposefully done to promote an antimetabolite mechanism in addition to DNA alkylation. DNA damage is more extensive and less repairable than that induced by other aromatic alkylating agents,[490] and the drug is unique in its ability to stimulate *p21* and *p53*-induced apoptosis, S-phase cell cycle arrest, and "mitotic catastrophe".[491] The risk of acquired resistance and cross-resistance via the upregulation of alkylguanyl transferase appears lower than with other DNA alkylators.[490,492]

Unlike chlorambucil, bendamustine is given only IV on days 1 and 2 of a 21-day (NHL) or 28-day (CLL) cycle. The dose in these disease states is commonly 100 and 120 mg/m^2, respectively, and it can be given alone or in combination with other antineoplastic agents (e.g., the anti-CD20 MAbs rituximab or obinutuzumab). It has a rapid attenuating effect on lymphocyte count and lymphadenopathy and may be valuable as a debulking agent prior to treatment with targeted therapies.[490]

Compared to chlorambucil, bendamustine therapy in CLL results in higher response rates but at the cost of an increased risk of infection.[486] Myelosuppression, hypersensitivity/anaphylaxis, and skin reactions have also been noted with its use, along with fatigue, anticholinergic actions and delayed nausea. Despite this, the long-term safety of bendamustine in both CLL and NHL is generally viewed as acceptable.[493] Pretreatment with antihistamines and corticosteroids can help minimize infusion reactions, a major cause of drug discontinuation. Like chlorambucil, it is viewed as a viable alternative in elderly and/or frail patients unable to withstand more aggressive chemotherapy regimens.[490]

Bendamustine undergoes minor CYP1A2-catalyzed N-demethylation and γ-hydroxylation.[490] While active, these metabolites are clinically insignificant and the drug is eliminated almost exclusively (90%) in feces. There is currently no evidence of serious metabolism-based interactions or toxicities associated with bendamustine.

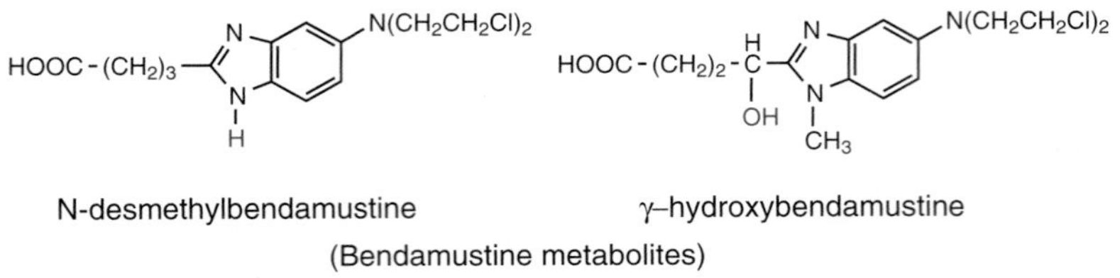

(Bendamustine metabolites)

Cyclophosphamide. Cyclophosphamide is a chiral prodrug antineoplastic agent requiring activation by metabolic and nonenzymatic processes (Fig. 33.59).[494] The initial metabolic step is mediated primarily by CYP2B6 (and, to a lesser extent, by CYP3A4 and CYP2C isoforms) and involves regioselective hydroxylation at C4 of the oxazaphosphorine ring to generate a carbinolamine.[494,495] This hydroxylation reaction must occur before the molecule will be transported into cells, and approximately 90% of an administered dose will be appropriately converted.[494] CYP3A4 and CYP2B6 stereospecifically catalyze an inactivating N-dechloroethylation reaction on the *R* and *S* isomers, respectively, which yields highly nephrotoxic and neurotoxic chloroacetaldehyde.[494,495] Chloroacetaldehyde toxicity is accompanied by GSH depletion, indicating that (as expected) this electrophilic byproduct alkylates Cys residues of critical cell proteins.[496] Alkylation of Lys, adenosine, and cytidine residues is also possible.

The CYP-generated carbinolamine undergoes nonenzymatic, reversible cleavage to provide the aldophosphamide tautomer, either in the bloodstream or inside cells.[497] Acrolein, a highly reactive α,β-unsaturated aldehyde, is cleaved from aldophosphamide via intracellular spontaneous β-elimination, generating phosphoramide mustard. With a pK_a of 4.75, the mustard will be persistently anionic at intracellular pH and trapped inside the cell.

The fate of phosphoramide mustard is varied. Most cyclizes to the quaternary aziridinium ion, which alkylates DNA in the manner of all mustards. Some decomposes, losing phosphoric acid and ammonia. This leaves the secondary bis(β-chloroethyl)amine mustard, which cyclizes to form a tertiary aziridine (rather than a quaternary aziridinium) species. The free tertiary aziridine will protonate at intracellular pH to provide the cationic conjugate acid, and the carbon atoms of both conjugates are still sufficiently δ^+ to attract DNA nucleophiles, albeit less vigorously than the permanently cationic quaternary amine. The net result is DNA alkylation and cell death. Oxidation of oxazaphosphorine intermediates along the metabolic pathway by cytosolic alcohol or aldehyde dehydrogenase is inactivating.[494,497]

The need for metabolic activation in the liver means lowered GI toxicity and less nonspecific toxicity for cyclophosphamide compared with other DNA alkylating agents, but cyclophosphamide is not without its toxic effects. Acrolein, generated during the decomposition of aldophosphamide, is a very electrophilic and highly reactive species, and it causes extensive damage to cells of the kidney and bladder. While acrolein can be produced in kidney via CYP3A4-mediated metabolism, it is predominantly generated in liver, where it readily conjugates with GSH (Fig. 33.60).[498,499] However, when the acrolein-GSH or mercapturic acid (N-acetylcysteine) conjugate is delivered to the bladder for excretion, the conjugate can cause direct toxicity or cleave to release electrophilic acrolein to the cells.[498] Without additional GSH to re-scavenge liberated toxin, the acrolein will be attacked at its δ^+ terminus by the nucleophilic SH of bladder cell Cys residues (Fig. 33.60). More complex

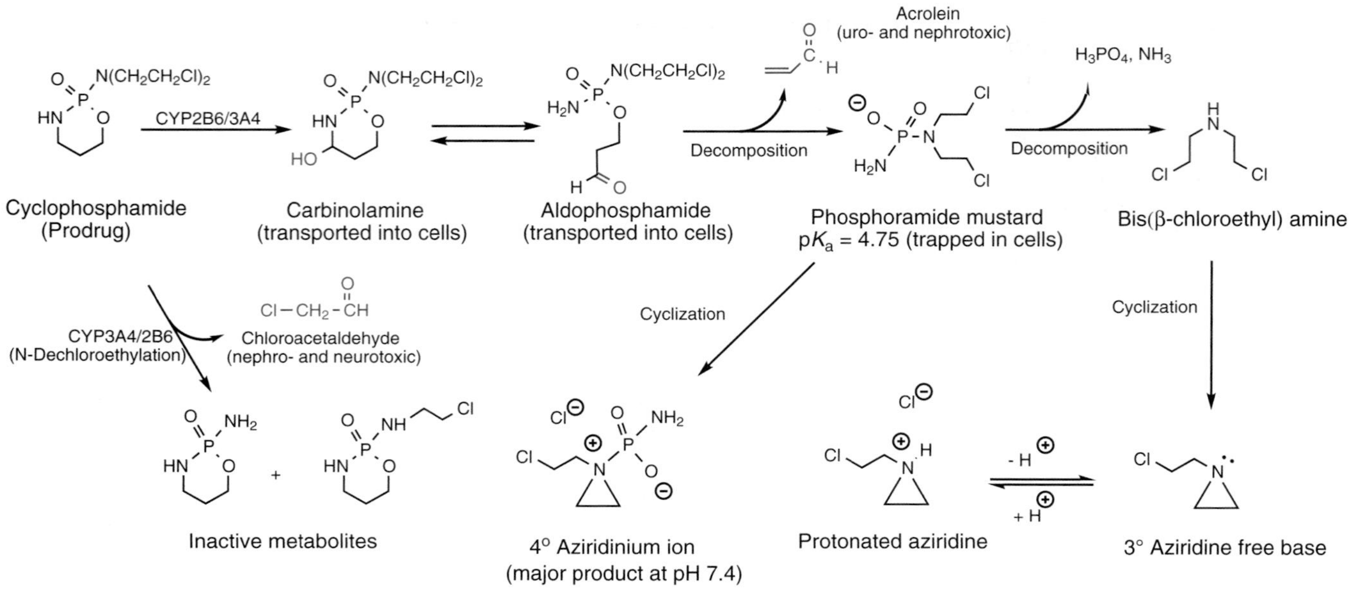

Figure 33.59 Cyclophosphamide metabolism.

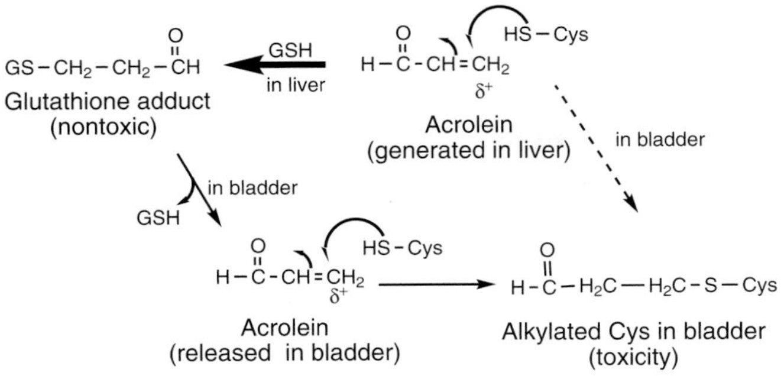

Figure 33.60 GSH conjugation with acrolein.

biochemical cascades involving the generation of ROS, increased levels of preoxynitrite and subsequent lipid peroxidation also contribute to the observed urotoxicity.[494,500] Physiologic results can include severe hemorrhage that can progress to sclerosis and fibrosis. Secondary bladder cancer that can develop years after treatment completion is a dose-dependent liability, and ovarian cancer patients administered cyclophosphamide have a 4-fold increased risk for this diagnosis.[501] Acrolein also damages the nephron, particularly when used in high doses, in children, in patients with only one kidney, or when coadministered with other nephrotoxic agents (e.g., cisplatin).

To minimize the risk of acrolein-induced hemorrhagic cystitis (a known risk factor for delayed secondary malignancies), administer the drug during daylight hours, force fluids to prompt frequent voiding, and consider bladder irrigation. Mesna (Mesnex) is available as adjuvant therapy in case of overt toxicity or as a prophylactic protectant. A sulfhydryl reagent, mesna is transported in the bloodstream as the inactive disulfide (dimesna) and reduced by glutathione dehydrogenase to the reactive sulfhydryl in the proximal tubules.[500] After delivery to the bladder, the SH group competes with Cys residues for the alkylating acrolein, as shown in Figure 33.61. Many investigators have sought alternatives to mesna as prophylaxis against hemorrhagic cystitis, but most potential substitutes had fatal flaws and none provided superior protection.[500]

Mesna concentrates in the bladder and will prevent damage to those cells. It does not concentrate to any appreciable extent in the nephron and, therefore, is not good protection against acrolein-induced nephrotoxicity. It also does little to spare the kidney and nerve cells from chloroacetaldehyde, the other toxic by-product of cyclophosphamide metabolism.[502] Fortunately, only about 10% of a standard dose of cyclophosphamide undergoes the dechloroethylation reaction, and most of the chloroacetaldehyde generated can be scavenged by GSH. Since the competing hydroxylation reaction is saturable, this percentage can rise if higher doses are used.[495]

Cyclophosphamide is most commonly used in combination with other antineoplastic agents to treat a wide range of neoplasms, including leukemias, lymphomas, multiple myeloma, ovarian adenocarcinoma, and breast cancer. In 2016 the American Cancer Society estimated that over 400,000 new cancer diagnoses per year could be treated with this powerful antineoplastic.[500] It is metabolized in the liver and eliminated via the kidney, with approximately 10%-20% of a given dose being excreted unchanged. While the parent drug is only 20% protein bound, some metabolites show up to 3-times the affinity for serum protein.

When given IV, initial divided doses of 40-50 mg/kg administered over 2-5 days are usual. Doses should be reduced by one-third to one-half in myelosuppressed (leukopenic) patients, and a 25% reduction considered if creatinine clearance falls below 10 mL/min or serum bilirubin is between 3.1 and 5 mg/dL.[76] The drug is also administered in capsule form in some hematologic malignancies (1-5 mg/kg/d). When used in these lower doses (1-3 mg/kg), a significant component of the anticancer activity has been proposed to be mediated by regulatory T-cell depletion and concomitant effector T-cell activation.[497] Significant stereochemistry-based variation in the metabolic, enzyme inhibition, excretion, and toxicity profiles of cyclophosphamide and related oxazaphosphorine antineoplastic agents have been described in the literature.[494]

Ifosfamide. Ifosfamide, a cyclophosphamide analogue, has the two arms of the mustard on different nitrogen atoms. It also requires metabolic activation (Fig. 33.62), but this time, it is the CYP3A4 isoform that converts the majority of the dose to the carbinolamine, with CYP2B6 taking on a minor supporting role.[503] Because ifosfamide has a lower affinity for the hydroxylating CYP3A4 and CYP2B6 enzymes, presumably as a result of steric

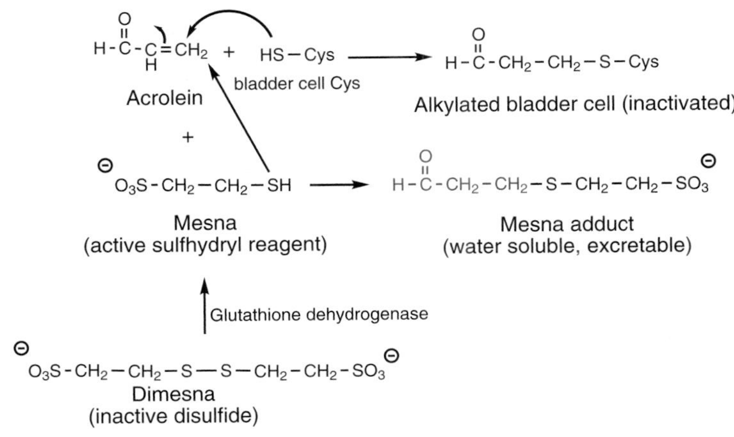

Figure 33.61 Acrolein detoxification by mesna.

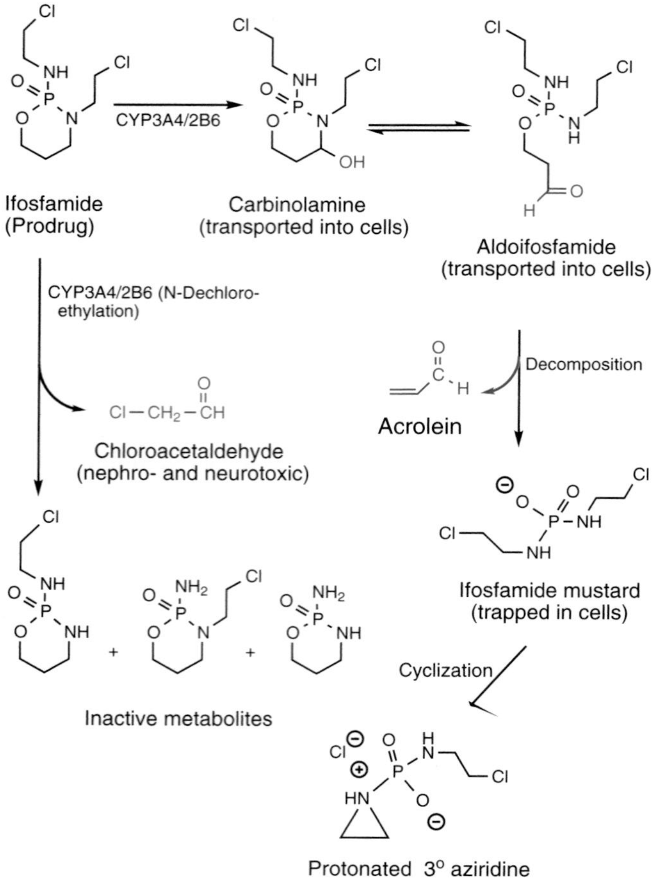

Figure 33.62 Ifosfamide metabolism.

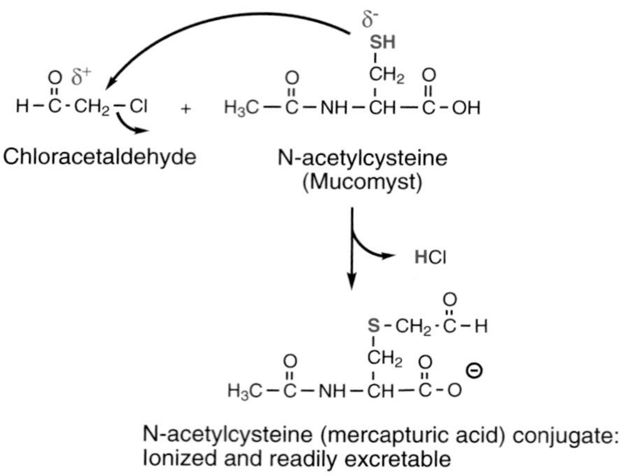

Figure 33.63 Chloroacetaldehyde detoxification by N-acetylcysteine.

hindrance, bioactivation proceeds at a slower rate.[504] Doses 3-4 fold higher than cyclophosphamide are required to achieve the same antineoplastic result.

Unlike cyclophosphamide, dechloroethylation is a significant metabolic pathway for ifosfamide, and up to 60% of a standard dose will undergo this toxicity-inducing biotransformation.[494,505] CYP3A4/3A5 catalyzes approximately 70% of ifosfamide dechloroethylation, with CYP2B6 taking care of the remainder.[495] Ultimately, both chloroalkyl groups are lost before the compound is excreted. So much chloroacetaldehyde is generated that endogenous GSH (available in limited quantities) is overwhelmed. The fact that this reaction can occur in the renal tubule, generating chloroacetaldehyde right in the nephron, contributes to a significantly higher nephrotoxicity that can result in glomerular and renal tubular failure.[504] Neurotoxicity is most commonly central in origin (e.g., mental status dysfunction, seizures) and, in severe forms, can progress to coma and death.

Because acrolein is generated during the bioactivation of ifosfamide, the same precautions against hemorrhagic cystitis that were outlined for cyclophosphamide must be taken: hydrate well, irrigate thoroughly, and administer mesna prophylactically. Ifosfamide is more water soluble than cyclophosphamide and will concentrate in the renal system. In addition, since higher doses must be administered to achieve the same degree of antineoplastic action, more molecules of nephro- and urotoxic acrolein will be produced. It is claimed that some urothelial and mucosal damage will occur even with standard prophylactic doses of mesna.[500]

As previously stated, mesna will not prevent chloroacetaldehyde-induced nephro- and neurotoxicity. However, strategies for successfully treating pediatric patients at risk for ifosfamide-induced nephrotoxicity with N-acetylcysteine (Mucomyst) have been published,[506] and the approach has been supported by the work of others[507] (Fig. 33.63). While N-acetylcysteine is not yet a standard of care in pediatric patients receiving ifosfamide, it is certainly possible that it may at some point be included in the treatment protocol, and it could also be a legitimate therapeutic approach to adult patients at risk for serious nephrotoxicity secondary to ifosfamide therapy. Because N-acetylcysteine does not penetrate the BBB, it would be of little value in central neurotoxicity prophylaxis.[494]

Ifosfamide is currently used in combination with other antineoplastics as third-line therapy in testicular cancer, although it has also shown activity in a number of other solid tumors and hematologic malignancies. For its primary indication, 1.2 g/m^2 is administered IV for 5 consecutive days and, if tolerated, repeated every 3 weeks. In addition to the acrolein- and chloroacetaldehyde-related toxicities discussed above, the drug carries a boxed warning for severe myelosuppression leading to potential fatal infections. It does not bind to serum protein, and as much as 18% (low dose) and 61% (high dose) can be excreted unchanged in urine.[76]

DNA Methylators: Triazenes and Procarbazine

The triazenes (temozolomide and dacarbazine) and procarbazine act by different mechanisms, but they both exert an antineoplastic effect through the O6-methylation of guanine nucleotides. O6-Methylguanine pairs preferentially with thymine, and these "mispairings" prompt point mutations during subsequent DNA replication cycles and trigger cell destruction through the activation of the normal postreplication mismatch repair system. Patients who are able to repair this damage through the action of O6-alkylguanine-DNA-alkyltransferase, which transfers the offending CH_3 group to Cys145 on the alkyltransferase protein, will exhibit resistance to these agents, whereas those who underexpress this protein should respond well.[508]

Since the alkyltransferase is irreversibly inactivated in the DNA rescue process, enzyme depletion with subsequent loss of DNA repair capability is a significant risk.

The triazenes methylate DNA guanine via diazomethane and/or methyl carbocation generated in situ. Although temozolomide is converted to the diazomethane precursor 3-methyl-(triazen-l-yl)imidazole-4-carboxamide (MTIC) through nonenzymatic mechanisms, the conversion of dacarbazine to MTIC depends on the action of CYP1A1 and CYP1A2 enzymes, with a smaller contribution by CYP2E1 (Fig. 33.64)[508-510] The O6 and N7 positions of guanine are the most vulnerable to triazene methylation.

In contrast, procarbazine metabolism involves CYP1A and CYP2B enzymes,[509] and DNA alkylation operates through a free radical mechanism (Fig. 33.65). The major degradation pathway involves benzylic oxidation of azo-procarbazine, producing methylhydrazine that generates a methyl radical through an unstable diazene intermediate.[511,512] In addition to O6, the reactive methyl radical formed can alkylate the C8 and N7 positions of guanine.

SPECIFIC DRUGS (FIG. 33.55)

Temozolomide. This imidazolotetrazine derivative is the most widely used agent within the DNA methylator class of antineoplastics. It is administered IV or in capsule form for the treatment of glioblastoma multiforme, a brain cancer with a dire prognosis, and in patients with anaplastic astrocytoma who have not responded to procarbazine or nitrosoureas (see below). The dosing for both routes is identical and based on body surface area. Oral absorption is rapid and complete, although decreased by food. Administration on an empty stomach also attenuates drug-induced nausea and vomiting. The literature also documents efficacy in aggressive pituitary cancers, so the approved indications for this agent may ultimately expand.[508]

While CYP enzymes are not extensively involved in temozolomide metabolism, less than 6% of the drug is excreted unchanged in the urine. Women clear the drug less effectively than men and have a higher incidence of severe neutropenia and thrombocytopenia in the initial therapy cycle. Myelosuppression is the most significant adverse effect.

Resistance to temozolomide primarily involves drug-induced damage reversal by overexpressed O6-methylguanine-DNA methyltransferase.[513] Disappointingly, inhibitors of this DNA repair enzyme, while effective in augmenting temozolomide activity in tumor cells that overexpress the methyltransferase, have shown unacceptably high myelotoxicity in clinical trials.[514] Other potential mechanisms of resistance are currently being explored, including overexpression of the base excision repair protein methylpurine-N-glycosylase, EGFR upregulation, and drug-induced genetic alterations (e.g., *p53*) that favor tumor cell survival. Challenges to the development of therapeutically viable resistance inhibitors include assurance of efficacy in multifaceted resistance systems and the ability to cross the BBB.[508,514] Inhibition of specific mRNA through a strategy termed RNA interference (RNAi) may hold promise in keeping glioblastoma cells responsive to the lethal effects of temozolomide.[515]

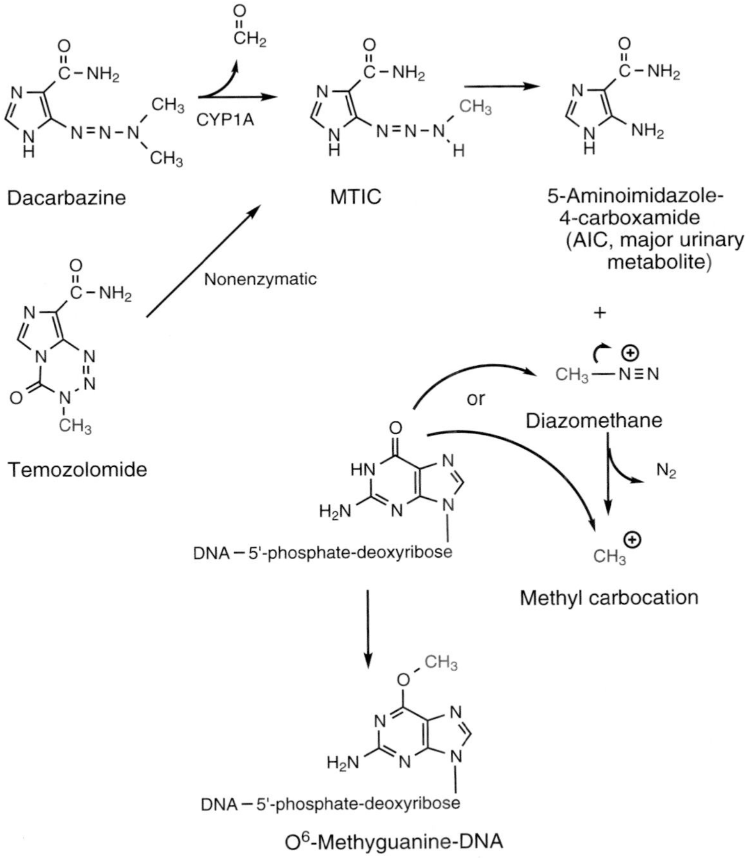

Dacarbazine
CYP1A
MTIC
5-Aminoimidazole-4-carboxamide (AIC, major urinary metabolite)
Temozolomide
Nonenzymatic
Diazomethane
or
N_2
Methyl carbocation
DNA – 5'-phosphate-deoxyribose
O^6-Methyguanine-DNA

Figure 33.64 Metabolic activation of triazenes.

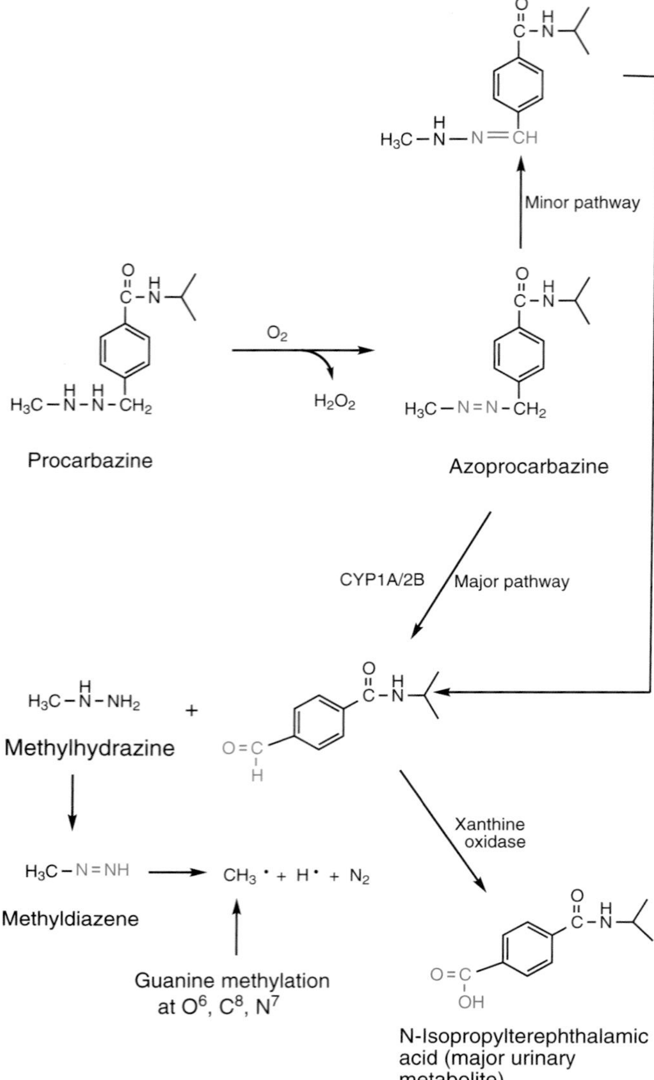

Figure 33.65 Procarbazine metabolism and mechanism of action.

Dacarbazine. This DNA methylating agent is administered IV as a single agent in the treatment of metastatic malignant melanoma and in combination with other agents in the treatment of Hodgkin lymphoma. Approximately 40% of the drug is excreted unchanged, but both the 5-aminoimidazole-4-carboxamide (AIC, formed through the action of CYP1A enzymes) and the carboxylic acid (AIC hydrolysis product) are major urinary metabolites (Fig. 33.64). Leukopenia and thrombocytopenia are the most common adverse effects and can be fatal. Patients are also at risk for hepatotoxicity, including hepatocellular necrosis, and the drug carries a boxed warning for all of these serious potential toxicities.

The advent of effective and less toxic targeted and immunotherapies for the first- and second-line treatment of dacarbazine's primary indications have diminished this agent's importance in contemporary chemotherapy.[516]

Procarbazine. This methyl radical generator is used primarily in the treatment of Hodgkin disease. It is administered as part of a multidrug regimen that also includes a nitrogen mustard (mechlorethamine, cyclophosphamide), a mitosis inhibitor (vincristine), and prednisone. It is administered as capsules and is well absorbed after oral administration. Procarbazine is extensively metabolized in the liver, and 70% of an administered dose is excreted in the urine as N-isopropylterephthalamic acid (Fig. 33.65). In addition to methylating DNA guanine residues, it is proposed to inhibit the de novo synthesis of proteins and nucleic acids.

Procarbazine inhibits monoamine oxidase, leading to several significant and potentially fatal DDIs and drug-food interactions. Facial flushing and other disulfiram-like symptoms are noted when alcohol is concomitantly consumed because the drug also inhibits enzymes involved in ethanol metabolism.

Nitrosoureas

The chloroethyl-containing nitrosoureas (CNUs) are unstable structures that decompose readily in the aqueous environment of the cell to generate electrophilic chloroethyl- and hydroxyethyl carbocations that target both the N7 and O6 positions of guanine (Figs. 33.66 and 33.67). Guanine N7 is the most commonly alkylated atom, although all DNA bases are vulnerable. The N7-hydroxyethyl analogue could be envisioned to form directly from the chloroethylated guanine, but hydrolysis is known to be sluggish. Rather, direct N7-hydroxyethylation has been proposed, as has "progressive alkylation," where rearrangements transfer the chloroethyl or hydroxyethyl group to various positions on the DNA base.[517] Pyrimidine bases are consistently alkylated at N3. DNA alkylation by CNUs results in apoptosis and necrosis in the impacted cell.[518]

While less commonly generated, O6-chloroethylguanine is particularly unstable, and spontaneously cyclizes to form N1-O6-ethanoguanine that covalently links via the purine's N1 position to a complementary cytosine residue through the pyrimidine's N3 position (Fig. 33.67).[517-519] In contrast, the stable O6-hydroxyethyl analogue does not cyclize, but is presumed to mismatch during DNA replication and transcription, stimulating mutagenesis.[517] While base alkylation with or without subsequent cyclization is toxic, the more interstrand crosslinks generated the more lethal the cellular response. Twenty-forty links normally result in cell death if repair mechanisms are absent or ineffective.[518]

Resistance to CNU chemotherapy is known to involve O6-alkylguanine-DNA alkyltransferase, the same enzyme that thwarts the cytotoxic action of triazenes and procarbazine. Transfer of the aberrant alkyl moiety to Cys145 is the common mechanism.[517,518] Interstrand crosslinks can also be reversed by nucleotide excision repair (NER) proteins, and Fanconi-associated nuclease 1 (FAN1) has also been proposed to play a DNA restorative role.[518] Drug sequestration by neuroprotective metallothionein proteins may also be involved in CNU resistance.[520]

$(C_2H_5)_2N-C(=S)-S-S-C(=S)-N(C_2H_5)_2$

Disulfiram

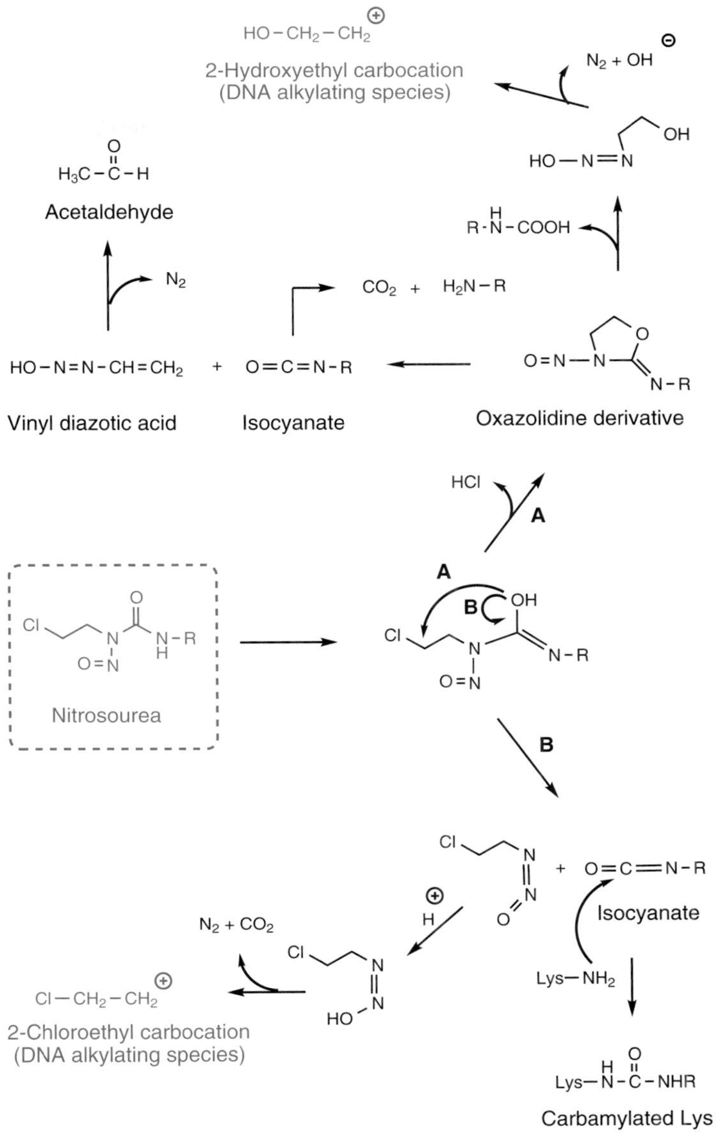

Figure 33.66 Nitrosourea decomposition to cytotoxic electrophiles.

SPECIFIC DRUGS

Carmustine and Lomustine. Carmustine and lomustine are both highly lipophilic CNUs marketed for use in brain tumors and Hodgkin disease.[518] Carmustine has also shown value in the treatment of NHL and multiple myeloma, and it is given IV or incorporated into biodegradable wafers that are implanted directly into the CNS after tumor resection. The high lipophilicity of carmustine precludes a totally aqueous IV formulation, and the drug is administered in 10% ethanol. Although carmustine degrades within 15 minutes of IV administration, lomustine is stable enough for oral use and is marketed in capsule form. Excretion of both drugs is predominantly via the urine, although any CO_2 generated from decomposition will be exhaled. Carmustine can decompose in vitro if exposed to temperatures around 90°F. Pure carmustine is a low-melting solid, but the decomposed product is an oil and, therefore, readily detected. Vials of carmustine that appear oily should be discarded.

Combination therapy with dacarbazine pretreatment has been proposed to deplete O6-guanine-DNA alkyltransferase, thus enhancing sensitivity to CNUs in tumors overexpressing the resistance-promoting enzyme. Dacarbazine and lomustine coadministration in glioblastoma multiforme has resulted in greater disease stability compared to dacarbazine alone. Small molecule inhibitors of the alkyltransferase, including the thiol scavenger disulfiram, are also being investigated as possible adjuncts to CNU chemotherapy.[518]

Both carmustine and lomustine can induce thrombocytopenia and leukopenia, leading to hemorrhage and massive infection, and the drugs carry boxed warnings for these toxicities. Acute and delayed pulmonary toxicity is also a risk with carmustine (boxed warning). Pulmonary toxicity is dose-related, and individuals who received the drug in childhood or early adolescence are at higher risk for the potentially fatal delayed reaction. The grand mal seizures that are possible with the wafer formulation of carmustine appear to result from the wafer itself, rather than from the nitrosourea.

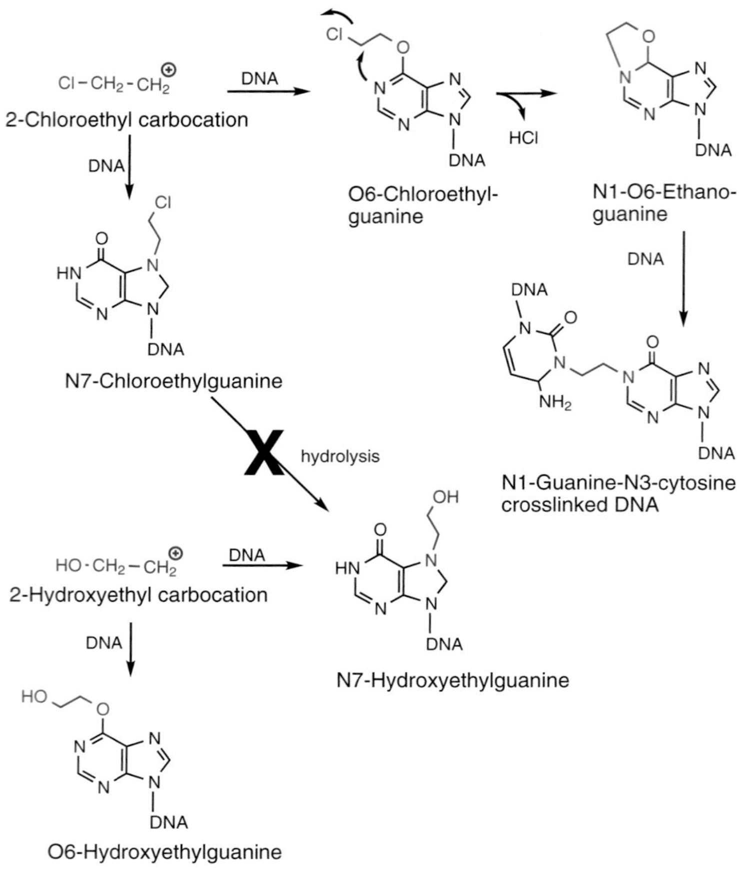

Figure 33.67 DNA cross-linking by 2-chloroethyl carbocation.

Organoplatinum Complexes

MECHANISM OF ACTION. Organoplatinum antineoplastic agents contain an electron-deficient metal atom that acts as a magnet for electron-rich DNA nucleophiles. Like nitrogen mustards, organoplatinum complexes are bifunctional and can accept electrons from two DNA nucleophiles. Intrastrand cross-links most frequently occur between adjacent guanine residues referred to as diguanosine dinucleotides (60%-65%) or adjacent guanine and adenine residues (25%-30%).[521] Interstrand cross-linking, which occurs much less frequently (1%-3%), usually involves guanine and adenine bases.[522]

CHEMISTRY. All currently marketed organoplatinum anticancer agents are Pt(II) complexes with square planar geometry. Platinum is inherently electron deficient, but the net charge on the organometallic complex is zero due to the contribution of electrons by two of the four ligands bound to the parent structure. Most commonly, the electron-donating ligand is chloride. Before reacting with DNA, the electron-donating ligands are displaced through nucleophilic attack by cellular water. When the displaced ligands are chloride anions (e.g., cisplatin), the chloride-poor environment of the tumor cell facilitates the process, driving the generation of the active, cytotoxic hydrated forms (Fig. 33.68). Since the original ligands leave the metal with their electrons, the hydrated organoplatinum molecule has a net positive charge.

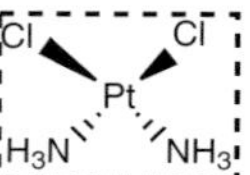

Cisplatin (square planar geometry)

The hydrated Pt analogues are readily attacked by DNA nucleophiles (e.g., the N7 of adjacent guanine residues) due to the net positive charge that has been regained on the Pt atom (Fig. 33.68). The DNA bases coordinate with the Pt, and in the *cis* configuration, DNA repair mechanisms are unable to permanently correct the damage. The net result is a major change in DNA conformation such that base pairs that normally engage in hydrogen bond formation are not permitted to interact. The two ammine ligands of the complex are bound irreversibly to the Pt atom through very strong coordinate covalent bonds. They cannot be displaced by DNA nucleophiles, but they do stabilize the cross-linked DNA-Pt complex by forming strong ion-dipole bonds with the anionic phosphate residues on DNA. The DNA distortion prompts a futile cycle of damage recognition and repair before succumbing to cell cycle arrest and apoptosis.

SPECIFIC DRUGS (FIG. 33.55)

Cisplatin. The simplest of the organometallic antineoplastic agents, cisplatin is used IV in the treatment of metastatic testicular and ovarian cancer and advanced bladder

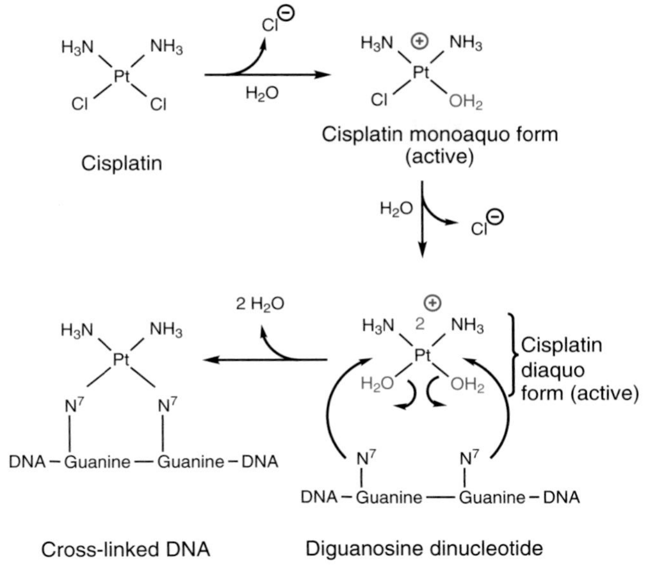

Cisplatin
Cisplatin monoaquo form (active)
Cisplatin diaquo form (active)
Cross-linked DNA
Diguanosine dinucleotide

Figure 33.68 Cisplatin activation and DNA cross-linking.

cancer. It is rapidly hydrated, resulting in a short plasma half-life of less than 30 minutes. It is eliminated predominantly via the kidney, but approximately 10% of a given dose undergoes biliary excretion. It is highly nephrotoxic and can cause significant damage to the renal tubules, especially in patients with preexisting kidney disease or who are concurrently receiving other nephrotoxic drugs (e.g., cyclophosphamide or ifosfamide). Dosages should be reduced in any of these situations. Clearance decreases with chronic therapy, and toxicities can manifest at a later date.

To proactively protect against kidney damage, patients should be aggressively hydrated with chloride-containing solutions and magnesium supplementation should be initiated. Mannitol diuretics can be administered to promote continuous excretion of the drug and its hydrated analogues.[523,524] Sodium thiosulfate, which accumulates in the renal tubules, has also been used to neutralize active drug in the kidneys in an effort to avoid nephrotoxicity (Fig. 33.69). The potential inactivation of cisplatin in the bloodstream is not of concern since the drug does not concentrate there, and what is there is very strongly bound to serum proteins. The very strong protein binding explains why dialysis, even when prolonged, cannot rescue patients from cisplatin toxicity.

Cisplatin carries a boxed warning for many serious toxicities. In addition to cumulative nephrotoxicity, myelosuppression is common. Cisplatin is also a very severe emetogen, and vomiting almost always occurs unless antiemetic therapy is coadministered. Hypersensitivity reactions can occur within minutes of administration, and can result in a respiratory and/or cardiovascular emergency; epinephrine, corticosteroids and/or antihistamines should be at hand for immediate administration in the event of anaphylaxis. Ototoxicity that can lead to irreversible hearing loss can also occur with cisplatin use. The ototoxicity is related to a high cochlear uptake of cisplatin with subsequent destruction of sensory hair cells by ROS that can be generated by this drug.[525] High frequency hearing is the first to be impacted.[526]

Amifostine, a thiol-generating prodrug, has been evaluated as a means to decrease risk of serious hearing loss secondary to cisplatin therapy. It is activated by alkaline phosphatase, an enzyme with higher activity in normal tissue compared to tumor cells.[527] It is proposed that activated amifostine interacts with cisplatin to reduce the number of drug-DNA adducts,[527,528] perhaps via the mechanism shown in Figure 33.70. Unfortunately, clinical trials assessing the protective value of amifostine cotherapy have produced inconsistent results. On the positive side, one study demonstrated that, in young patients 3-21 year old with average risk (for a poor prognosis) medulloblastoma, bolus administration of amifostine immediately before and during cisplatin infusion significantly decreased ototoxicity and the need for a hearing aid post therapy.[529] A later study confirmed the potential value of amifostine cotherapy in preventing hearing loss in average risk (but not high risk) pediatric medulloblastoma patients.[526] However, while one research group noted an apparent benefit of cotherapy in adults,[530] a meta-analysis of four nonblinded, randomized and controlled amifostine otoprotection trials found only a strong trend toward efficacy that did not achieve statistical significance.[531] Other studies have produced negative results.[532] It is possible that these inconsistent outcomes could be due to amifostine being concentrated near cochlear capillaries that are distant from the sensory hair cells that are the target of cisplatin destruction.[527] Clearly more controlled clinical trials in large adult and pediatric patient populations are needed to determine if there is therapeutic benefit of amifostine cotherapy in protecting patients from cisplatin-induced hearing loss. The same can be said for amifostine protection against drug-induced nephrotoxicity.[533,534]

Resistance to cisplatin therapy can be intrinsic in colorectal, prostate, and lung cancer, or acquired after multiple courses of therapy (e.g., in ovarian cancer).[535] Resistance is mediated through several distinct mechanisms, including: (1) compromised carrier-mediated cellular transport via the copper transporting protein CTR1; (2) enhanced intracellular inactivation through drug trapping in vesicles; (3) drug inactivation through conjugation to Cys and/or Met-containing GSH and metallothionein proteins; (4) uncontrolled expression of noncoding RNA (lncRNA), (5) cellular efflux by P-type ATP 7A/7B, MDR, and (possibly) P-gp proteins, and (6) increased DNA repair and/or tolerance to cisplatin-induced DNA damage.[535,536] Regarding the latter mechanism, cisplatin damage can be successfully repaired by NER proteins, which

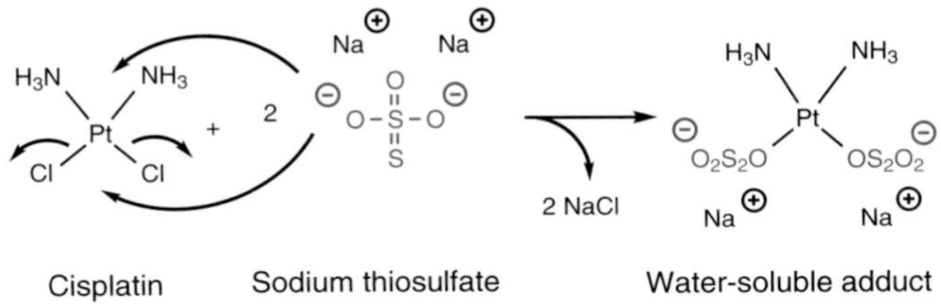

Cisplatin
Sodium thiosulfate
Water-soluble adduct

Figure 33.69 Cisplatin inactivation by sodium thiosulfate.

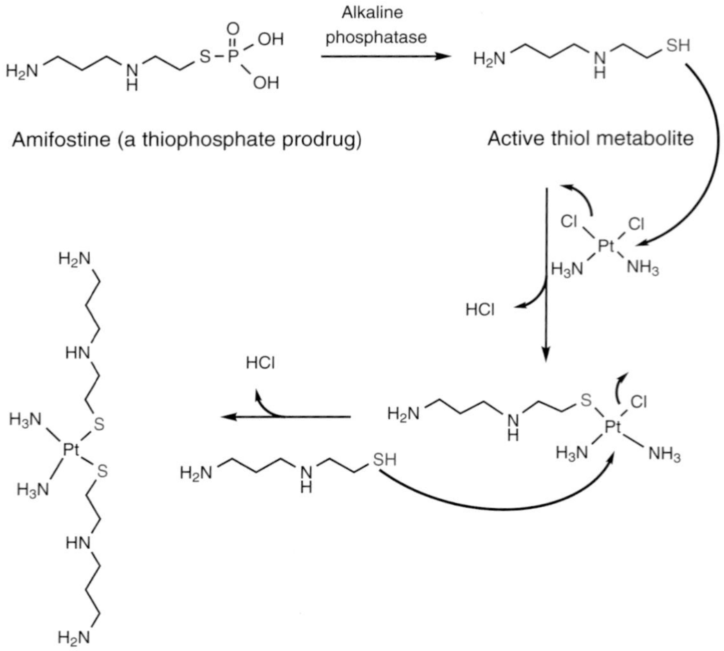

Figure 33.70 Amifostine activation and reaction with cisplatin.

remove platinum-damaged segments from the DNA, and these proteins are often upregulated in cisplatin-resistant tumors. Cisplatin-DNA (and carboplatin-DNA, discussed below) adducts are also recognized by mismatch repair (MMR) proteins. The downregulation of MMR in cisplatin and carboplatin-treated cancer cells induces resistance through the loss of an apoptotic response that normally follows several ill-fated attempts to repair organoplatinum-induced damage.[535] Testicular tumors are particularly responsive to cisplatin due to their inherent deficiency in DNA repair processes.

Cisplatin is administered IV in accordance with disease-specific regimens. It is a vesicant in high doses and can blister skin. Extravasation should be managed with IV and SC sodium thiosulfate (Fig. 33.69) and the affected limb elevated. Cisplatin and the other organoplatinum anticancer agents react with aluminum and cannot be administered through aluminum-containing needles. The drug is photosensitive, is packaged in amber bottles, and must be protected from light.[76]

A comprehensive review of the historical development, chemistry, molecular mechanisms, and toxicity of cisplatin and oxaliplatin (discussed below) has recently been published.[537]

Carboplatin. Carboplatin forms the same cytotoxic hydrated intermediate as cisplatin but does so at a 10-fold slower rate, making it a 20- to 40-fold less potent chemotherapeutic agent.[536] The ultimate damage done to cells as a result of carboplatin use approaches that of cisplatin, but the adverse effect profile is significantly milder. Suppression of platelets and white blood cells is the most significant toxic reaction, and nonhematologic toxicities (e.g., emesis, nephrotoxicity, and ototoxicity) are rare. The plasma half-life of carboplatin is 3 hours, and the drug is less extensively bound to serum proteins than cisplatin. Excretion is still predominantly renal, however, and doses must be reduced in patients with kidney disease.

Carboplatin is only approved for use in the treatment of advanced ovarian cancer, although clinical trials have shown that it may have a future in the treatment of hormone-refractory prostate cancer. Carboplatin can be used in combination with docetaxel (often considered the standard of care for prostate cancer) and estramustine (a less commonly used mitosis inhibitor). This drug has provided therapeutic benefit as a single agent in patients whose cancer has progressed after docetaxel therapy. Unlabeled uses for carboplatin include combination therapy in myriad solid and hematological malignancies (including NSCLC, head and neck cancer, and GI and reproductive tract cancers), in which it has been shown to be a reasonable and often less toxic alternative to cisplatin.[538,539]

Oxaliplatin. This Pt(II) complex loses oxalate dianion ($^-$OOC-COO$^-$) in vivo to form the mono- and dihydrated diaminocyclohexane (DACH) platinum analogues shown in Figure 33.71. The *trans*-(*R*,*R*)-DACH structure serves as the carrier for the cytotoxic hydrated platinum and extends into the major groove of DNA when the DNA-Pt complex forms.[540] Hydrophobic DNA intrusion is believed to contribute to the cytotoxicity of this organometallic. Oxaliplatin engages primarily in intrastrand cross-linking with diguanosine dinucleotides, adjacent A-G nucleotides, and guanines that are separated by one nucleotide (G-X-G). Interstrand cross-linking, although less common, also occurs.

The adduct formed between oxaliplatin and DNA diguanosine dinucleotides is conformationally distinct from the adduct formed with cisplatin or carboplatin. Specifically, whereas the cisplatin diguanosine dinucleotide adduct bends the DNA by 60-80° and presents a relatively wide minor groove, the oxaliplatin adduct produces a 31-degree

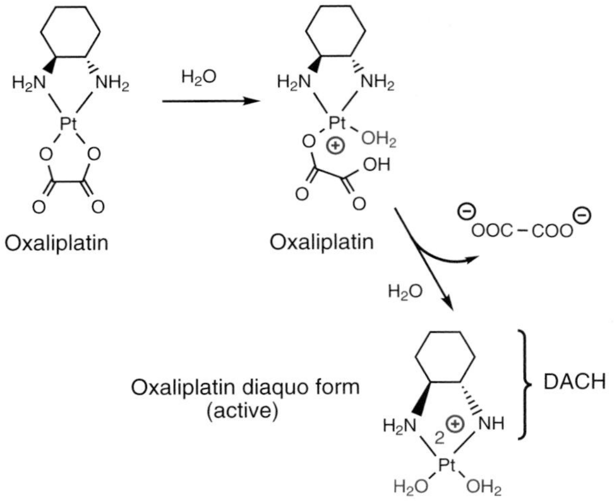

Figure 33.71 Activation of oxaliplatin.

bend with a comparatively narrow minor groove.[541] This distinct oxaliplatin conformation is believed to result from the steric impact of the (*R*,*R*)-DACH carrier, which permits the *cis*-NH_3 moieties to hydrogen bond with a guanine-O6, a bond that the inactive (*S*,*S*)-isomer cannot make.[542] The conformation of the oxaliplatin-DNA adduct is much less likely to be recognized by MMR proteins, and the effectiveness of oxaliplatin in MMR-deficient cells is, at least in part, responsible for the lack of resistance that has plagued cisplatin and carboplatin.[543,544] Oxaliplatin is also less dependent on CRT1 for intracellular access and often retains activity in patients who are no longer responding to the first-generation organoplatinum agents. It is significantly less mutagenic, nephrotoxic, hematotoxic, and ototoxic than cisplatin. Excretion is via the kidney. Oxaliplatin decomposes in alkaline media and should not be coadministered with drugs that will increase the pH of the IV solution.

Oxaliplatin is used in the treatment of metastatic colon or rectal cancer in combination with fluorouracil/leucovorin (FOLFOX regimen). The usual adult dose is 85 mg/m^2 infused over two hours to minimize hypersensitivity risk (the reason for oxaliplatin's boxed warning), repeating every two weeks. Literature suggests that faster infusion rates of 1 mg/m^2/min can be used to expedite drug delivery without increasing the hypersensitivity reaction risk.[545] Pulmonary fibrosis and anaphylaxis can be life-threatening, and dose- and/or use-liming peripheral sensory neuropathy that can become permanent and painful significantly impacts patient quality of life. The acute neuropathy that occurs in up to 98% of oxaliplatin-treated patients is reversible. Chronic neuropathy (often with negative functional consequences) will manifest in approximately 15% of patients who receive cumulative doses of 780-850 mg/m^2.[546] Neuropathy has been attributed to the chelation of intracellular Ca^{2+} by the oxalate dianion that is displaced from the parent drug by water, which disrupts the function of calcium-gated ion channels in sensory nerve cells.[547]

The concurrent IV administration of calcium gluconate and magnesium sulfate (known as CaMg) was first reported to significantly attenuate the risk of sensory neuropathy in patients receiving oxaliplatin in a 2004 retrospective study,[548] and the practice was subsequently adopted by approximately half of oncologists worldwide.[549] Various reports, including meta analyses, supported these findings.[546,550-552] However, a randomized, placebo-controlled, double-blind study in 343 colon cancer patients failed to document a statistically significant neuroprotective effect of CaMg coadministration with oxaliplatin.[549] A very interesting summary of this therapeutic controversy and its explicit and rapid impact on oncology practice patterns was subsequently published.[553] The most recent review of the evidence from randomized controlled trials involving nearly 700 patients was negative relative to the value of CaMg as a neurotoxicity protectant,[554] and the practice is no longer routinely recommended. Patients at risk are more commonly given oxaliplatin at a slower infusion rate, and those with persistent neuropathy are given a holiday from oxaliplatin, with therapy resuming when benefits outweigh risks. All patients should avoid exposure to cold, which exacerbates neuropathic pain. Investigations on the possible neuroprotectant effect of 5-HT/NE reuptake inhibitors are ongoing, and one retrospective study suggests that calcium channel blockers may attenuate acute neuropathy.[555] Of interest in this age of culturally informed care, a meta-analysis of therapeutic outcomes when traditional plant-based medicines were administered to colorectal cancer patients on oxaliplatin showed positive total response rate benefits.[556] Studies exploring the impact of pharmacogenetics on patient response to therapy that includes oxaliplatin are being reported, and exploitation of genetic differences in the expression of various repair proteins, growth factors, and metabolizing enzymes may ultimately allow the tailoring of oxaliplatin therapy based on an individual's pharmacogenetic profile.[543]

Miscellaneous Antineoplastic Agents

The anticancer agents included in Table 33.13 are "one of a kind" structures that do not fit neatly into other antineoplastic drug classes. Those in more common clinical use are described below.

SPECIFIC DRUGS

Arsenic Trioxide. The toxic effects of arsenic, a name derived from the Greek word for "potent," have been recognized for millennia.[557,558] Arsenic trioxide (As_2O_3, the "King of Poisons")[559] is an odorless and tasteless toxin well known in ancient Chinese medicine. It was originally introduced into Western medicine in the late 19th century for the treatment of leukemia, subsequently falling out of favor as newer chemotherapeutic and radiation-based approaches to care became available. The drug experienced a pharmacotherapeutic renaissance in the late 20th century, and it is currently used IV to induce remission in patients with acute promyelocytic leukemia (APL).[558,559] APL is characterized by the reciprocal translocation of chromosomes 15 and 17, resulting in the abnormal joining of the promyelocytic gene and retinoic acid receptor α (RARα) gene which produces a PML-RARα fusion protein.[560] This, in turn, results in the generation of immature leukemia cells, differentiation

Table 33.13 Selected Therapeutic Properties of Miscellaneous Anticancer Agents

Anticancer Agent	Mechanism	Indication	Administration Route	Metabolism/ Metabolizing Enzymes	Boxed Warning
As_2O_3 Arsenic trioxide (Trisenox)	PLM-RARα fusion protein–induced toxicity	Acute PML	IV	NA	Differentiation syndrome, QT prolongation
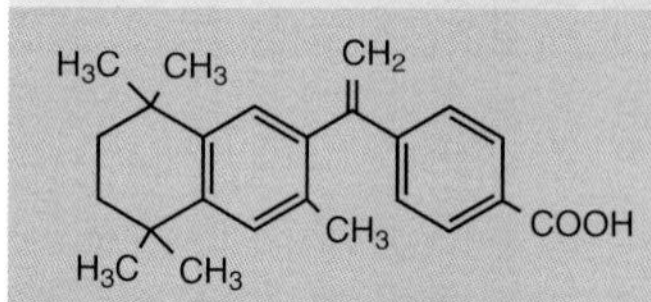 Bexarotene (Targretin)	Retinoid X receptor agonist	Cutaneous T-cell lymphoma	p.o., topical	3A4, glucuronidation	Teratogenic
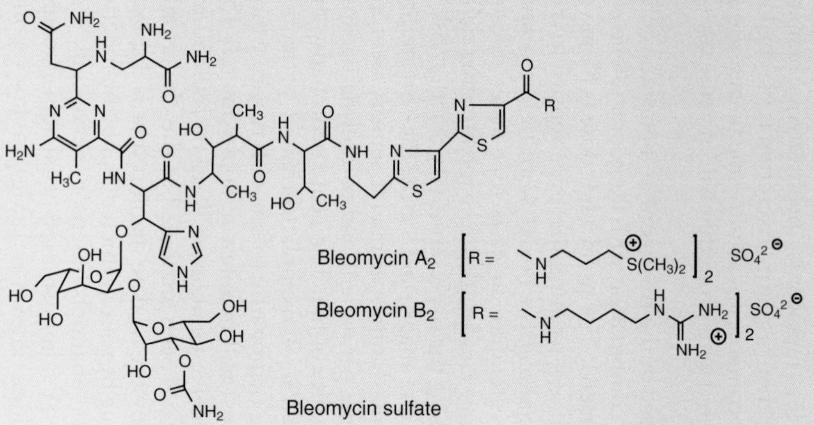 Bleomycin sulfate (Bleomycin A_2 [R = $-NH(CH_2)_3S^{\oplus}(CH_3)_2$]$_2$ $SO_4^{2\ominus}$; Bleomycin B_2 [R = $-NH(CH_2)_4NHC(=NH_2^{\oplus})NH_2$]$_2$ $SO_4^{2\ominus}$)	Free radical-induced DNA cleavage	Head and neck cancer, testicular cancer, Hodgkin lymphoma, malignant pleural effusion	IV, intrapleural injection	Bleomycin hydrolase	Pulmonary fibrosis, idiosyncratic reaction

Dactinomycin (Cosmegen)	DNA intercalation	Ewing sarcoma, Wilms tumor, childhood rhabdosarcoma, testicular cancer	IV	Negligible metabolism	Teratotogenic, mutagenic, carcinogenic, corrosive
Inotuzumab ozogamicin (Besponsa)	DNA cleavage	AML	IV	Non-enzymatic reduction	Hepatotoxic, post-HSCT mortality
Mitomycin (Mutamycin)	DNA alkylation	Gastric cancer, pancreatic cancer	IV	NQO1 reductase, NADPH/CYP450 reductase	Myelotoxicity, hemolytic uremic syndrome

(continued)

Table 33.13 Selected Therapeutic Properties of Miscellaneous Anticancer Agents (Continued)

Anticancer Agent	Mechanism	Indication	Administration Route	Metabolism/ Metabolizing Enzymes	Boxed Warning
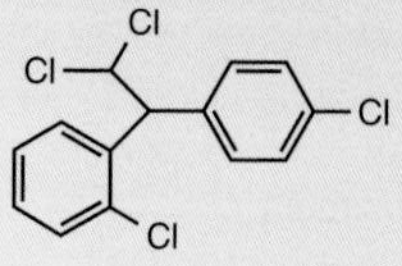 Mitotane (Lysodren)	Adrenolytic	Adenocortical carcinoma	p.o.	Unknown	Adrenal crisis
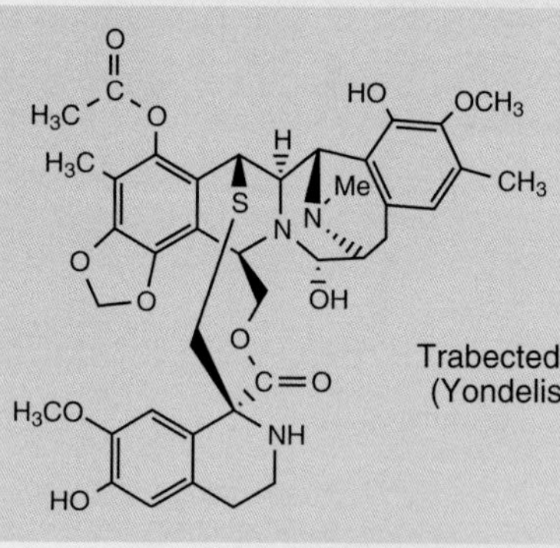 Trabectedin (Yondelis)	DNA alkylation	Soft tissue sarcoma	IV	CYP3A4	None
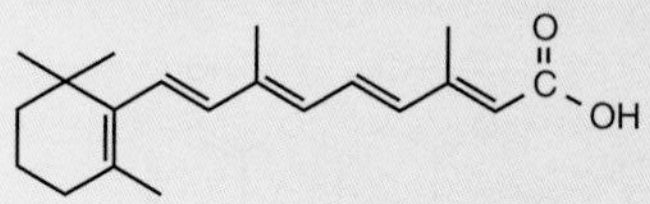 Tretinoin (*trans*-retinoic acid)	APL proliferation inhibitor and differentiation inducer	Remission induction	p.o.	CYP	Teratogenic, leukocytosis, retinoic acid-APL syndrome

APL, acute promyelocytic leukemia; HSCT, hematopoietic stem cell therapy; IV, intravenous; PML, promyelocytic leukemia; p.o., oral; RAR, retinoic acid receptor.

arrest, and the induction of serious/fatal hemorrhagic and other coagulation-related disorders. As_2O_3 induces remission in APL patients through the destruction of the offending fusion protein, promotion of promyelocyte differentiation, and stimulation of apoptosis in malignant cells. One documented chemical apoptotic mechanism is inhibition of intracellular catalase and glutathione peroxidase, with the resultant accumulation of the free radical precursor H_2O_2. Another is the downregulation of the antiapoptotic protein Bcl-2.[557]

As_2O_3 can be used as initial therapy in combination with tretinoin (all *trans*-retinoic acid, Table 33.13) in patients with low-risk disease, as well as alone in those who have relapsed after tretinoin/anthracycline chemotherapy. Clinical trials have shown first-line therapy with As_2O_3 in newly diagnosed patients lowers relapse rate, and complete remission and 3-year OS rates of up to 86% have been achieved.[558] Superior relapse-free survival outcomes have been documented with As_2O_3 and tretinoin maintenance therapy (compared to tretinoin plus mercaptopurine and methotrexate) in patients who have achieved complete remission after consolidation therapy.[561] An interesting historical sidebar to APL treatment is the 1988 clinical trial in which tretinoin monotherapy in 24 patients (8 of whom had received previous chemotherapy) resulted in complete remission in 23 (96%), dispelling the notion that cancer is invariably progressive. As_2O_3 acts synergistically with tretinoin to destroy the PML-RARα fusion protein, justifying the cotherapy approach.[558]

The pentavalent As(V) in the parent drug is rapidly reduced to the active trivalent As(III) by arsenate reductase. Along with oncogenic, antiangiogenesis, and cytokine signaling pathway mechanisms yet to be fully elucidated, As(III) is known to generate ROS in mitochondria that damage DNA and stimulate apoptosis.[558] Prior to urinary excretion, As(III) is methylated to mono- and dimethylarsonic acid. Although As_2O_3 is usually well tolerated, the possibility of QT interval prolongation, torsades de pointes, and complete atrioventricular block demands an assessment of serum electrolytes (particularly magnesium and potassium) prior to the initiation of therapy. APL differentiation syndrome (also known as retinoic acid syndrome and characterized by pleural/pericardial/pulmonary infiltrates or effusions, dyspnea, weight gain, and fatigue) responds to corticosteroid intervention. Reversible hepatotoxicity has also been noted, and the strong emetogenic potential of As_2O_3 warrants coadministration of drugs to control nausea and vomiting.

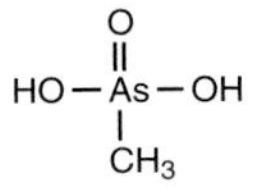

$HO-As(=O)(CH_3)-OH$ — Monomethylarsonic acid

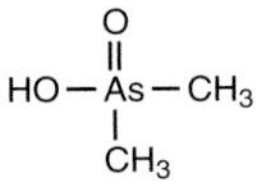

$HO-As(=O)(CH_3)-CH_3$ — Dimethylarsonic acid

The rapid clearance of As(III) and its methylated metabolites from the blood precludes As_2O_3 use in solid tumors, although studies in multiple solid tumor cell lines document efficacy. Strategies to harness the power of this ancient toxin in treating solid malignancies without increasing the dose to intolerable levels have included combination therapy with GSH depleting agents and encapsulation in nanoparticles, liposomes and polymersomes.[558,559] Clinical trials are ongoing, and preliminary findings are encouraging.

A timely review of the evolution of arsenic as the agent of choice for medieval "professional poisoners" during the Renaissance to a valued antineoplastic used to prolong life is well worth the read for pharmacy professionals and history enthusiasts alike.[558]

Bleomycin Sulfate. The commercially available bleomycin drug product is a mixture of naturally occurring glycopeptides, predominantly bleomycin A_2. Through DNA intercalation in guanine-rich regions, the aromatic bithiazole ring system (in partnership with the pyrimidine ring on the opposite side of the structure) positions bleomycin for DNA destruction via cytotoxic free radicals.[562] The disaccharide, polyamine, imidazole, and pyrimidine structures are very electron rich and readily chelate intracellular Fe^{2+}. Once chelated, Fe^{2+} is oxidized to Fe^{3+} with a concomitant reduction of bound oxygen and the release of the highly reactive and cytotoxic hydroxyl radical. The ferric hydroperoxide bleomycin complex is considered the cytotoxic form responsible for both single- and double-stranded DNA breaks.[563] Through the direct abstraction of a hydrogen atom from 4′ of a deoxyribose, a free radical is generated that subsequently decomposes to a DNA-destroying 4′-hydroperoxide. A highly electrophilic pyrimidine base propenal that inactivates essential cellular proteins via Cys alkylation is also produced (Fig. 33.72). Reduced GSH is proposed to serve a protective role by acting as propenal scavenger and, until depleted, saves cellular proteins from alkylation.[562,564] A review of the multifaceted mechanisms of bleomycin-induced DNA/chromosomal damage and damage repair has been recently published.[565]

Bleomycin is a natural product isolated from *Streptomyces verticillus*. It is naturally chelated with Cu^{2+}, which must be removed via catalytic reduction before marketing. This increases the cost of the drug, but is essential to the liberation of critical bleomycin functional groups for chelation with intracellular Fe^{2+}.

The action of bleomycin is terminated through the action of bleomycin hydrolase, a cytosolic aminopeptidase that cleaves the terminal amide moiety to form the inactive carboxylate metabolite (Fig. 33.73). The metabolic conversion of the electron-withdrawing amide to an electron-donating carboxylate increases the pK_a of the α-amino group, which normally interacts with DNA in the unionized conjugate form. After hydrolysis, the ratio of ionized to unionized amine increases approximately 126-fold, destroying DNA affinity and leading to the loss of therapeutic action. Drug destruction via the bleomycin hydrolase pathway is rapid, and tumors will be resistant to bleomycin if they contain high concentrations of the enzyme. Conversely, tumors that are poor in bleomycin hydrolase (e.g., squamous cell carcinoma) respond well to this agent.

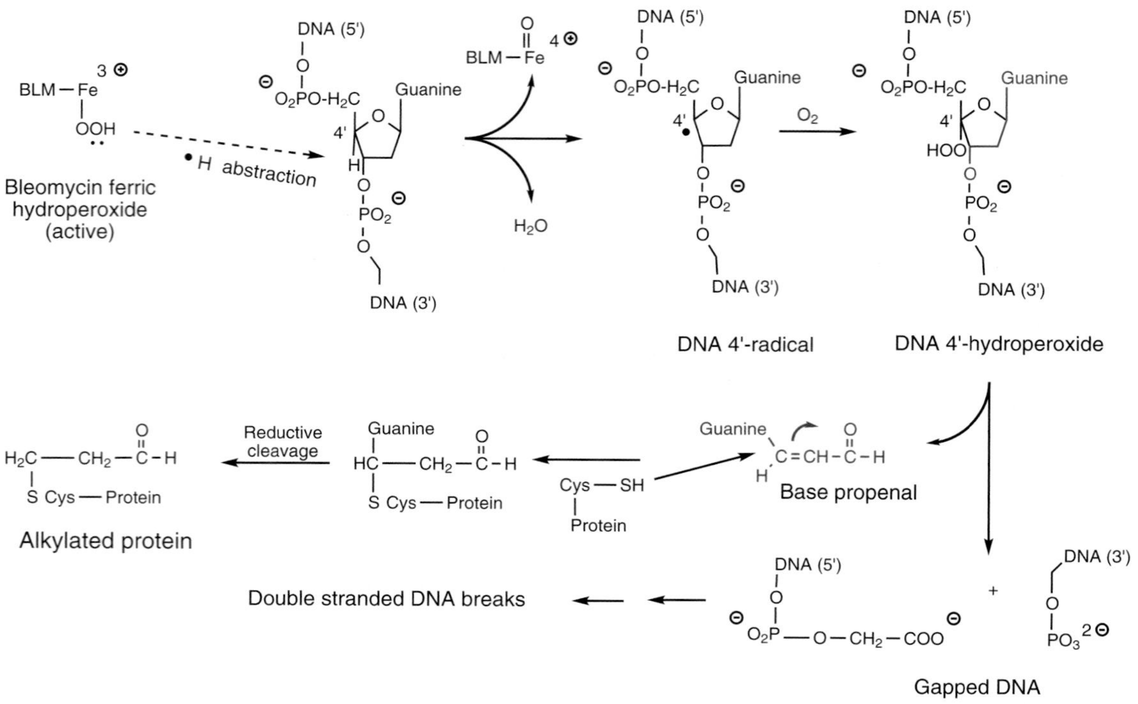

Figure 33.72 Mechanism of bleomycin-induced damage of DNA and proteins.

Bleomycin hydrolase is found in all tissues except skin and lung. Approximately 10% of patients who are administered bleomycin will experience potentially fatal pulmonary fibrosis, which can occur during therapy or several months following termination of therapy, often without warning. The copper-complexing agent tetrathiomolybdate may reduce the risk of bleomycin-induced fibrosis by inhibiting the action of copper-dependent inflammatory cytokines.[566] A recent report also supports the protective effect of inhibitors of the N-terminal catalytic site of angiotensin-converting enzyme (e.g., N-acetyl-Ser-Asp-Lys-Pro or AcSDKP).[567] Erythema and hypertrophic modifications in skin are also common adverse effects that manifest after 2-3 weeks of bleomycin therapy.

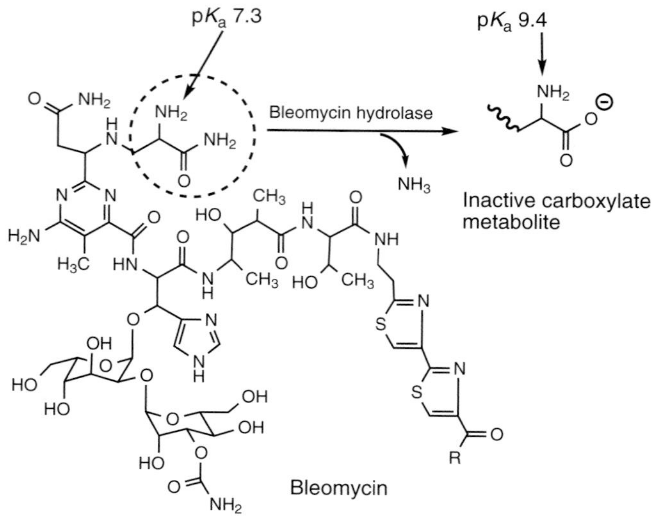

Figure 33.73 Bleomycin hydrolase–mediated inactivation of bleomycin.

Bleomycin is used IV in the palliative treatment of squamous cell head and neck cancers, testicular and other genital carcinomas, and Hodgkin lymphoma. It is excreted via the kidneys, and serum concentrations of active drug are increased in patients with renal disease. The elimination half-life can rise from 2 to 4 hours to more than 20 hours in renal failure, resulting in significant toxicity, especially pulmonary toxicity. Dosage adjustments are warranted. Unlike many antineoplastic agents, bleomycin does not suppress the bone marrow[565] and it is often given in combination with compounds that do so that the dose of all drugs can be optimized. Nausea and vomiting are also relatively mild, but approximately 1% of lymphoma patients who are treated with bleomycin will experience an immediate or delayed severe idiosyncratic reaction that mimics anaphylaxis.

Inotuzumab Ozogamicin Conjugate. Inotuzumab ozogamicin, a targeted chemotherapeutic agent, was approved in mid-2017 for use in adults with relapsed or refractory B-cell precursor ALL. The drug contains 6 molecules of a cytotoxic N-acetylated hydrazine derivative of γ-calicheamicin conjugated with a Chinese hamster ovary (CHO)-derived human MAb. It was preceded on the U.S. market by another calicheamicin-MAb conjugate, gemtuzumab ozogamicin, which is used in newly diagnosed and/or refractory AML. Both antibodies bind specifically to antigenic markers expressed on the surface of B-cell (CD22) and myeloid cell (CD33) malignancies, respectively, allowing internalization of the conjugate where it is needed. Hydrolysis of the acid-labile hydrazone linker at the low pH of lysosomes (~6) releases N-acetyl-γ-calicheamicin dimethylhydrazide, which undergoes further hydrolysis to generate calicheamicin, the active enediyne which binds within the minor grove of DNA. The enediyne moiety of the DNA-bound calicheamicin is vulnerable to SH-dependent conformational changes that generate di-radicals, leading to H-abstraction from the DNA phosphodiester group and subsequent double-strand breaks in the DNA.[568,569]

CD22 is known to be a very readily endocytic B-cell antigen that is not released into the extracellular fluids, thus being retained as the cellular gateway for the inotuzumab ozogamicin conjugate into malignant B-cells. The cellular uptake of the conjugate is superior to that of calicheamicin alone, as the antibody has subnanomolar affinity for the antigen. The MAb minus calicheamicin is nontoxic to malignant B-cells.[568] Clinical trials have demonstrated significantly higher rates of complete remission, PFS, and 2-year survival probability in ALL patients compared to standard chemotherapy.[570] It is currently being investigated in combination with the MAb rituximab for use in relapsed/refractory CD22$^+$ B-cell NHL.[571]

Trabectedin. Trabectedin, a tri-tetrahydroisoquinoline–containing alkaloid derived from the marine tunicate *Ecteinascidia turbinate*, is indicated in unresectable, metastatic, refractory soft tissue sarcoma (liposarcoma and leiomyosarcoma; the "L-sarcomas"). Treatment of this rare cancer is challenged by the more than 50-60 histological subtypes that exist, and prognosis after first-line chemotherapy with doxorubicin (alone or with ifosfamide) is dismal.[572,573] The availability in 2015 of this naturally occurring chemotherapy, which has demonstrated value in anthracycline- and nitrogen mustard-resistant tumors, provided a new option to patients who previously had very few. It is proposed to act by several mechanisms, including alkylation of guanine N2 within a CGG-rich region of the minor groove. This binding leads to DNA double strand cleavage and, through simultaneous interaction with nearby proteins, RNA polymerase II degradation and transcription inhibition via a NER-dependent process. The cell cycle is arrested in the G2-M phase and apoptosis results. Trabectedin also interferes with oncogenic transcription factor FUS-CHOP function in liposarcomas, which promotes normalizing adipocyte differentiation. Of prime importance to its mechanism is attenuation of inflammation and angiogenesis through selective interference with monocytes and macrophages within the tumor microenvironment.[572-574]

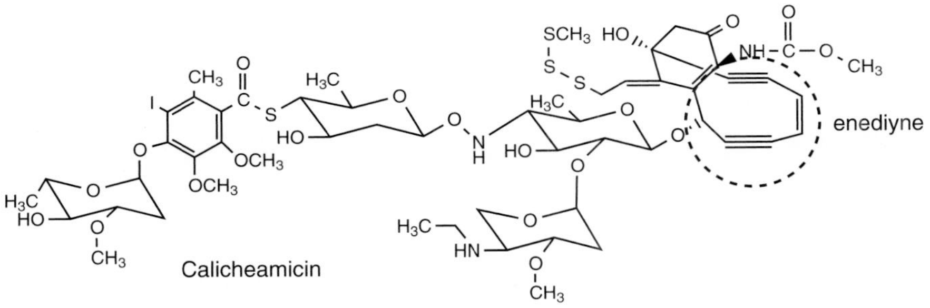

Calicheamicin

enediyne

Inotuzumab ozogamicin is administered IV in doses of either 0.5 or 0.8 mg/m^2 for a maximum of six 21- or 28-day cycles. The maximum tolerated dose has been reported at 1.8 mg/m^2.[569] The drug is highly bound to plasma protein (~97%) with a terminal half-life of 12.3 days. The N-acetyl-γ-calicheamicin dimethylhydrazide is a substrate for P-gp, which negates the therapeutic value of the conjugate in P-gp positive malignant cells.[569] While the targeted nature of conjugate delivery spares cells that do not express CD22 from calicheamicin toxicity, the drug is myelosuppressive (which increases infection risk) and carries a boxed warning for potentially severe hepatotoxicity and an increased risk of posthematopoietic stem cell therapy mortality unrelated to relapse. As research into the place of this antineoplastic conjugate in ALL therapy continues, emphasis will be needed on optimal dosing and how (or if) to integrate it with cytotoxic chemotherapy without narrowing its therapeutic index.[569]

Trabectedin is administered via 24-hour continuous IV infusion through a central venous catheter in a usual dose of 1.5 mg/m^2. While efficacy is slightly superior in patients with L-sarcoma versus unselected disease, use in all soft tissue sarcoma subtypes is feasible, particularly if tumor burden is manageable and disease stabilization with a positive quality of life is the objective.[574] Combination therapy with doxorubicin may provide a response advantage and is being explored.[573]

Trabectedin is 94%-98% protein bound, rapidly converted to many metabolites (Fig. 33.74) and eliminated in feces.[575] The terminal half-life is long at approximately 7.5 days. As multiple CYP isoforms (including 3A4) are presumed involved in the complex metabolic pathway of trabectedin, coadministration with CYP inhibitors or enhancers should be undertaken with caution.[575] The most commonly observed adverse effects are myelosuppression (neutropenia, thrombocytopenia), GI distress, and hepatic enzyme elevation.[573]

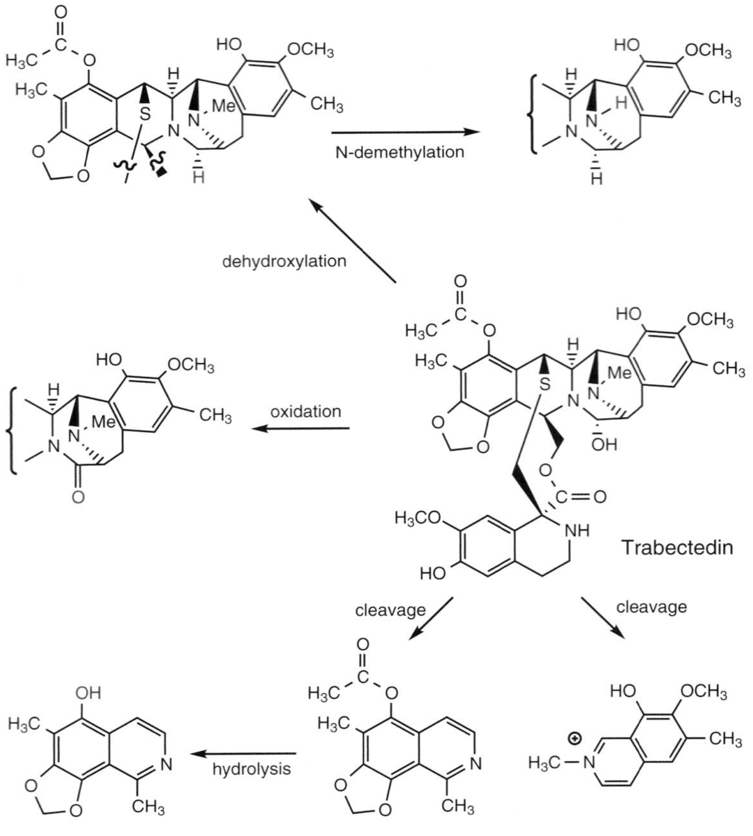

Figure 33.74 Proposed trabectedin metabolism.

Clinical Scenario

Kelly K. Nystrom, PharmD, BCOP

MF is a 67-year-old female who was recently diagnosed with extensive stage small cell lung cancer. She has a performance status of 1 and presents to the clinic for her first cycle of cisplatin and etoposide. Chemotherapy orders were received, but it was noted that the physician ordered hydration with D5W before and after the cisplatin. The oncologist was contacted, and it was recommended to change the D5W hydration to normal saline with 20 mEq of magnesium sulfate per liter to run over 3 hours prior to cisplatin.

OUTCOME

The oncologist agreed with the pharmacist's recommendation, and MF's renal function remained stable.

Chemical Analysis found immediately after References.

REFERENCES

1. Cancer Statistics. National Cancer Institute. Available at https://www.cancer.gov/about-cancer/understanding/statistics. Accessed September 29, 2018.
2. Siegel R, Miller K, Jemal A. Cancer statistics, 2017. *CA Cancer J Clin*. 2017;67:7-30.
3. Morris P. Pushing back against the long shadow of cancer. *N C Med J*. 2014;75:247.
4. Masood I, Kiani M, Ahmad M, et al. Major contributions towards finding a cure for cancer: a historical perspective. *Tumori*. 2016;102:6-17.
5. Cancer Treatment and Survivorship Facts and Figures 2016-2017. American Cancer Society. Available at https://www.cancer.org/content/dam/cancer-org/research/cancer-facts-and-statistics/cancer-treatment-and-survivorship-facts-and-figures/cancer-treatment-and-survivorship-facts-and-figures-2016-2017.pdf. Accessed April 6, 2018.
6. Tallman M. The best of times in hematologic malignancies. *Curr Opin Hematol*. 2015;22:75-76.
7. Hiom S. Diagnosing cancer earlier: reviewing the evidence for improving cancer survival. *Br J Cancer*. 2015;112:S1-S5.
8. Hudson M, Meyer W, Pui C-H. Progress born from a legacy of collaboration. *J Clin Oncol*. 2015;33:2935-2937.

9. Singleterry J. The Cost of Cancer: Addressing Patient Costs. American Chemical Society Cancer Action Network. Available at https://www.acscan.org/sites/default/files/Costs%20of%20Cancer%20-%20Final%20Web.pdf. Accessed April 5, 2018.
10. Liu ET. Oncogenes and suppressor genes: genetic control of cancer. In: Goldman L, Ausiello D, eds. *Cecil Textbook of Medicine*. Philadelphia: W.B. Saunders; 2004:1108-1116.
11. Shord S, Cordes L. Cancer treatment and chemotherapy. In: DiPiro J, Talbert R, Yee G, et al, eds. *Pharmacotherapy: A Pathophysiologic Approach*. 10th ed. USA: McGraw-Hill; 2017.
12. *Preventing One of the Nation's Leading Causes of Death at a Glance*. U.S. Department of Health and Human Services; 2016. Available at https://www.cdc.gov/chronicdisease/resources/publications/aag/dcpc.htm. Accessed March 6, 2018.
13. Perez-Herrero E, Fernandez-Medarde A. Advanced targeted therapies in cancer: drug nanocarriers, the future of chemotherapy. *Eur J Pharm Biopharm*. 2015;93:52-79.
14. Blot W. Epidemiology of cancer. In: Goldman L, Ausiello D, eds. *Cecil Textbook of Medicine*. 22nd ed. Philadelphia, PA: W.B. Saunders; 2004:1116-1120.
15. Benefits of Quitting Smoking Over Time. American Cancer Society. Available at https://www.cancer.org/healthy/stay-away-from-tobacco/benefits-of-quitting-smoking-over-time.html. Accessed September 28 2018.
16. *Tobacco Control: Reversal of Risks After Quitting Smoking*. Lyon, France: International Agency for Research on Cancer; 2007.
17. O'Connor R. Etiology of cancer. In: DeVita V, Lawrence T, Rosenberg S, eds. *DeVita, Hellmen and Rosenberg's Cancer: Principles and Practices of Oncology*. 10th ed. Philadelphia, PA: Wolters Kluwer Health; 2011.
18. Buck C, Ratner L. Oncogenic viruses. In: DeVita V, Lawrence T, Rosenberg S, eds. *DeVita, Hellman and Rosenberg's Cancer: Principles and Practices of Oncology*. 10th ed. Philadelpha, PA: Wolters Kluwer Health; 2011.
19. Buda A, Papadia A, Di Martino G, et al. Real-time fluorescent sentinel lymph node mapping with indocyanine green in women with previous conization undergoing laparoscopic surgery for early invasive cervical cancer: comparison with radiotracer ± blue dye. *J Minim Invasive Gynecol*. 2018;25:455-460.
20. Gutowski M, Framery B, Boonstra M, et al. SGM-101: an innovative near-infrared dye-antibody conjugate that targets CEA for fluorescence-guided surgery. *Surg Oncol*. 2017;26:153-162.
21. Lv P-C, Roy J, Putt K, et al. Evaluation of a carbonic anhydrase IX-targeted near infrared dye for fluroescent-guided surgery of hypoxic tumors. *Mol Pharm*. 2016;13:1618-1625.
22. Burchenal J. The historical development of cancer chemotherapy. *Semin Oncol*. 1977;4:135-146.
23. Woglom W. General review of cancer therapy. In: Moulton F, ed. *Approaches to Tumor Chemotherapy*. Vol 1. Washington, DC: AAAS; 1947.
24. Rosenberg B, VanCamp L, Krigas T. Inhibition of cell division in *Escherichia coli* by electrolysis products from a platinum electrode. *Nature*. 1965;205:698-699.
25. Johnson L. Protein kinase inhibitors: contributions from structure to clinical compounds. *Q Rev Biophys*. 2009;42:1-40.
26. Drucker B, Talpaz M, Resta D, et al. Efficacy and safety of a specific inhibitor of the BRC-ABL tyrosine kinase in chronic myeloid leukemia. *N Engl J Med*. 2001;344:1031-1037.
27. Kucuk O, McBride M, Rida PCG, et al. Cancer biomarkers. *Mol Aspects Med: Special Issue*. 2015;45:1-102.
28. Bosman F, True L. Prognostic biomarkers: an introduction. *Virchows Arch*. 2014;464:253-256.
29. Kumar M, Ernani V, Owonikoko T. Biomarkers and targeted systemic therapeies in advanced non-small cell lung cancer. *Mol Aspects Med*. 2015;45:55-66.
30. National Comprehensive Cancer Network. Available at https://www.nccn.org/. Accessed March 20, 2018.
31. Steuer C, Ramalingam S. Targeting EGFR in lung cancer: lessons learned and future perspectives. *Mol Aspects Med*. 2015;45:67-73.
32. Bao J, Qiao L. New developments on targeted cancer chemotherapy: multi-faceted issues in targeted cancer therapy. *Cancer Lett*. 2017;387:1-2.
33. Abdelmoez A, Coraca-Huber DC, Thurner GC, et al. New developments on targeted cancer chemotherapy. *Cancer Lett: Special Issue*. 2017;387:1-126.
34. Padma V. An overview of targeted cancer chemotherapy. *BioMed*. 2015;5:1-6.
35. Baudino T. Targeted cancer therapy: the next generation of cancer treatment. *Curr Drug Discov Technol*. 2015;12:3-20.
36. Conde-Estevez D. Targeted cancer therapy: interactions with other medicines. *Clin Transl Oncol*. 2017;19:21-30.
37. Farkona S, Diamandis E, Blasutig I. Cancer immunotherapy: the beginning of the end of cancer? *BMC Med*. 2016;14:73. doi:10.1186/s12916-016-0623-5.
38. Meiliana A, Dewi N, Wijaya A. Cancer immunotherapy: a review. *Indones Biomed J*. 2016;8:1-20.
39. Nasiri H, Valedkarimi Z, Aghebati-Maleki L, et al. Antibody-drug conjugates: promising and efficient tools for targeted cancer therapy. *J Cell Physiol*. 2018;233(9):6441-6457.
40. Diamantis N, Banerji Y. Antibody-drug conjugates – an emerging class of cancer treatment. *Br J Cancer*. 2016;114:362-367.
41. Smaglo B, Aldeghaither D, Weiner L. The development of immunoconjugates for targeted cancer therapy. *Nat Rev Clin Oncol*. 2014;11:637-648.
42. Fathi S, Oyelere A. Liposomal drug delivery systems for targeted cancer therapy: is active targeting the best choice? *Future Med Chem*. 2016;8:2091-2112.
43. Iglesias J. nab-Paclitaxel (Abraxane): an albumin-bound cytotoxic exploiting natural delivery mechanisms into tumors. *Breast Cancer Res*. 2009;11(suppl 1):S21.
44. Rugo H, Linton K, Cervi P, et al. A clinician's guide to biosimilars in oncology. *Cancer Treat Rev*. 2016;46:73-79.
45. Lichtman S, Reske T, Jacobs I. Biosimilars and cancer treatment of older patients. *J Geriatr Oncol*. 2016;7:S1-S8.
46. *Biosimilars: Questions and Answers Regarding Implementation of the Biologics Price Competition and Innovation Act of 2009/Guidance for Industry*. Silver Spring, MD: U.S. Food and Drug Administration; Center for Drug Evaluation and Research; 2015.
47. Bach P, Giralt S, Saltz L. FDA approval of tisagenlecleucel: promise and complexities of a $470,000 cancer drug. *J Amer Med Assoc*. 2017;318:1861-1862.
48. Maude S, Laetsch T, Rives S, et al. Tisagenlecleucel in children and young adults with B-cell lymphoblastic leukemia. *New Engl J Med*. 2018;378:439-448.
49. Schuster S, Svoboda J, Chong E, et al. Chimeric antigen receptor T cells in refractory B-cell lymphomas. *New Engl J Med*. 2017;377:2545-2554.
50. Walton E. On the road to epigenetic therapy. *Biomed J*. 2016;39:161-165.
51. Bradbury J. Human epigenome project – up and running. *PLoS Biol*. 2003;1(3):e82. doi:10.1371/journal.pbio.0000082.
52. Esteller M. The necessity of a human epigenome project. *Carcinogenesis*. 2006;27:1121-1125.
53. Jones P, Archer T, Baylin S. Moving AHEAD with an international human epigenome project. *Nature*. 2008;454:711-715.
54. Cowan R, O'Cearbhaill R, Zivanovic O, et al. Current status and future prospects of hyperthermic intraoperative intraperitoneal chemotherapy (HIPEC) clinical trials in ovarian cancer. *Int J Hyperthermia*. 2017;33:548-553.
55. Gonzalez-Moreno S, Gonzalez-Bayon L, Ortega-Perez G. Hyperthermic intraperitoneal chemotherapy: rationale and technique. *World J Gastrointest Oncol*. 2010;2:68-75.
56. Yuan R, Hou Y, Sun W, et al. Natural products to prevent drug resistance in cancer chemotherapy: a review. *Ann NY Acad Sci*. 2017;1401:19-27.
57. Sadzuka Y, Sugiyama T, Sonobe T. Efficacies of tea components on doxorubicin induced antitumor activity and reversal of multidrug resistance. *Toxicol Lett*. 2000;114:155-162.

58. Wu P, Nielsen T, Clausen M. FDA-approved small-molecule kinase inhibitors. *Trends Pharm Sci*. 2015;36:422-439.
59. Gross S, Rami R, Stransky N, et al. Targeting cancer with kinase inhibitors. *J Clin Invest*. 2018;125:1780-1789.
60. Ma X, Lv X, Zhang J. Exploiting polypharmacology for improving therapeutic outcome of kinase inhibitors (KIs): an update of recent medicinal chemistry efforts. *Eur J Med Chem*. 2018;143:449-463.
61. Wang Y, Sun Y, Cao R, et al. In silico identification of a novel hinge-binding scaffold for kinase inhibitor discovery. *J Med Chem*. 2017;60:8552-8564.
62. Zhao Z, Wu H, Wang L, et al. Exploration of type II binding mode: a privileged approach for kinase inhibitor focused drug discovery? *ACS Chem Biol*. 2014;9:1230-1241.
63. Furtmann N, Hu Y, Bajorath J. Comprehensive analysis of three-dimensional activity cliffs formed by kinase inhibitors with different binding modes and cliff mapping of structural analogs. *J Med Chem*. 2015;58:252-264.
64. Ferguson F, Gray N. Kinase inhibitors: the road ahead. *Nat Rev Drug Discov*. 2018;17(5):353-377. doi:10.1038/nrd.2018.21.
65. McInnes C, Fisher P. Strategies for the design of potent and selective kinase inhibitors. *Curr Pharm Des*. 2005;11:1845-1863.
66. Poliakova M, Aebersold D, Zimmer Y, et al. The relevance of tyrosine kinase inhibitors for global metabolic pathways in cancer. *Mol Cancer*. 2018;17(1):27. doi:10.1186/s12943-018-0798-9.
67. Morphy R. Selectively nonselective kinase inhibition: striking the right balance. *J Med Chem*. 2010;53:1413-1437.
68. Morcos P, Yu L, Bogman Y, et al. Absorption, distribution, metabolism and excretion (ADME) of the ALK inhibitor alectinib: results from an absolute bioavailability and mass balance study in healthy subjects. *Xenobiotica*. 2017;47:217-229.
69. Scheers E, Leclercq L, deJong J, et al. Absorption, metabolism, and excretion of oral 14C radiolabeled ibrutinib: an open-label, phase I, single-dose study in healthy men. *Drug Metab Dispos*. 2015;43:289-297.
70. Dickinson P, Cantarini M, Collier J, et al. Metabolic disposition of osimertinib in rats, dogs, and humans: insights into a drug designed to bind covalently to a cysteine residue of epidermal growth factor receptor. *Drug Metab Dispos*. 2016;44:1201-1212.
71. He H, Tran P, Gu H, et al. Midostaurin, a novel protein kinase inhibitor for the treatment of acute myelogenous leukemia: insights from human absorption, metabolism, and excretion studies of a BDDCS II drug. *Drug Metab Dispos*. 2017;45:540-555.
72. Dubbelman A-C, Rosing H, Nijenhuis C, et al. Pharmacokinetics and excretion of 14C-lenvatinib in patients with advanced solid tumors of lymphomas. *Invest New Drugs*. 2015;33:233-240.
73. Wind S, Schnell D, Ebner T, et al. Clinical pharmacokinetics and pharmacodynamics of afatinib. *Clin Pharmacokinet*. 2017;56:235-250.
74. Markham A. Brigatinib: first global approval. *Drugs*. 2017;77:1131-1135.
75. Abbas R, Hsyu P. Clinical pharmacokinetics and pharmacodynamics of bosutinib. *Clin Pharmacokinet*. 2016;55:1191-1204.
76. *Facts & Comparisons* [database online]. St. Louis, MO: Wolters Kluwer Health, Inc.; March 2005.
77. Emole J, Talabi T, Pinilla-Ibarz J. Update on the management of Philadelphia chromosome positive chronic myelogenous leukemia: role of nilotinib. *Biologics*. 2016;10:23-31.
78. Shamroe C, Comeau J. Ponatinib: a new tyrosine kinase inhibitor for the treatment of chromic myeloid leukemia and Philadelphia chromosome-positive acute lymphoblastic leukemia. *Ann Pharmacol*. 2013;47:1540-1546.
79. Massaro F, Molica M, Breccia M. Ponatinib: a review of efficacy and safety. *Curr Cancer Drug Targets*. 2017;17:1-10.
80. Muller B. Imatinib and its successors: how modern chemistry has changed drug development. *Curr Pharm Des*. 2009;15:120-133.
81. Deininger M, Druker B. Specific targeted therapy of chronic myelogenous leukemia with imatinib. *Pharmacol Rev*. 2003;55:401-422.
82. Schenone S, Bruno O, Radi M, et al. New insights into small-molecule inhibitors of Bcr-Abl. *Med Res Rev*. 2009;31:1-41.
83. Weisberg E, Manley P, Breitenstein W, et al. Characterization of AMN107, a selective inhibitor of native and mutant Bcr-Abl. *Cancer Cell*. 2005;7:129-141.
84. Jarkowski AI, Sweeny R. Nilotinib: a new tyrosine kinase inhibitor for the treatment of chronic myelogenous leukemia. *Pharmacotherapy*. 2008;28:1374-1382.
85. Keskin D, Sadri S, Eskazan A. Dasatinib for the treatment of chronic myeloid leukemia: patient selection and special considerations. *Drug Des Devel Ther*. 2016;10:3355-3361.
86. Tokarski J, Newitt J, Chang C, et al. The structure of dasatinib (BMS-354825) bound to activated Abl kinase domain elucidates its inhibitory activity against imatinib-resistant Abl mutants. *Cancer Res*. 2006;66:5790-5797.
87. Signorovitch J, Ayyagari R, Reichmann W, et al. Major molecular response during the first year of dasatinib, imatinib or nilotinib treatment for newly diagnosed chronic myeloid leukemia; a network meta-analysis. *Cancer Treat Rev*. 2014;40:285-292.
88. Iqbal N, Iqbal N. Imatinib: a breakthrough of targeted therapy in cancer. *Chemother Res Pract*. 2014;2014:e357027.
89. Chen R, Chen B. The role of dasatinib in the management of chronic myeloid leukemia. *Drug Des Devel Ther*. 2015;9:773-779.
90. Suttorp M, Bornhauser M, Metzler M, et al. Pharmacology and pharmacokinetics of imatinib in pediatric patients. *Clin Pharmacol*. 2018;11:219-231.
91. Zheng Q, Wu P, Yu Q, et al. ABCB1 polymorphisms predict imatinib response in chronic myeloid leukemia patients: a systematic review and meta-analysis. *Pharmacogenomics J*. 2015;15:127-134.
92. Van Erp N, Gelderblom H, Guchelaar H-J. Clinical pharmacokinetics of tyrosine kinase inhibitors. *Cancer Treat Rev*. 2009;35:692-706.
93. Duckett D, Cameron M. Metabolism considerations for kinase inhibitors in cancer treatment. *Expert Opin*. 2010;6:1775-1793.
94. Huang W-S, Metcalf C, Sundaramoorthi R, et al. Discovery of 3-[2-(Imidazo[1,2-b]pyridazin-3-yl)ethynyl]-4-methyl-N-{4-[(4-methylpiperazin-1-yl)-methyl]-3-(trifluoromethyl)phenyl} benzamide (AP24534), a potent, orally active pan-inhibitor of breakpoint cluster region-abelson (BCR-ABL) kinase including the T315I gatekeeper mutant. *J Med Chem*. 2010;53:4701-4719.
95. Gainor J, Chabner B. Ponatinib: accelerated disapproval. *Oncologist*. 2015;20:847-848.
96. Hagen T. *Ponatinib (CML) Pricing Gets a Blast From Congress*. OncLive; 2016. Available at https://www.onclive.com/web-exclusives/ponatinib-cml-pricing-gets-a-blast-from-congress. Accessed April 23, 2018.
97. Breccia M, Binotto G. Bosutinib for chromic myeloid leukemia. *Rare Cancers Ther*. 2015;3:35-46.
98. Ault P, Rose J, Nodzon L, et al. Bosutinib therapy in patients with chromic myeloid leukemia: practical considerations for management of side effects. *J Adv Pract Oncol*. 2016;7:160-175.
99. Kong G, Kim A, Hill B, et al. The safety of bosutinib for the treatment of chronic myeloid leukemia. *Expert Opin Drug Saf*. 2017;16:1203-1209.
100. Gurel G, Blaha G, Moore P, et al. U2504 determines the species specificity of the A-site cleft antibiotics: the structures of tiamulin, homoharringtonine and bruceantin bound to the ribosome. *J Mol Biol*. 2009;389:146-156.
101. Chen Y, Hu Y, Michaels S, et al. Inhibitory effects of omacetaxine on leukemic stem cells and BCR-ABL-induced chronic myeloid leukemia and acute lymphoblastic leukemia in mice. *Leukemia*. 2009;23:1446-1454.
102. Nemunaitis J, Mita A, Stephenson J, et al. Pharmacokinetic study of omacetaxine mepesuccinate administered subcutaneously to patients with advanced solid and hematologic tumors. *Cancer Chemother Pharmacol*. 2013;71:35-41.
103. Levitzki A. Protein tyrosine kinase inhibitors as novel therapeutic agents. *Pharmacol Ther*. 1999;82:231-239.
104. Sjin R, Lee K, Walter A, et al. In vitro and in vivo characterization of irreversible mutant-selective EGFR inhibitors that are wild-type sparing. *Mol Cancer Ther*. 2014;13(6):1468-1479.

105. Ricciuti B, Baglivo S, Paglialunga L, et al. Osimertinib in patients with advanced epidermal growth factor receptor T790M mutation-positive non-small cell lung cancer: rationale, evidence and place in therapy. *Ther Adv Med Oncol.* 2017;9:387-403.
106. Cross D, Ashton S, Ghiorghiu S, et al. AZD9291, an irreversible EGFR TKI, overcomes T790M-mediated resistance to EGFR inhibitors in lung cancer. *Cancer Discov.* 2014;4:1046-1061.
107. Kettle J, Ward R. Toward the comprehensive systematic enumeration and synthesis of novel kinase inhibitors based on a 4-anilinoquinazoline binding mode. *J Chem Inf Model.* 2010;50:525-533.
108. Knowles P, Murray-Rust J, Kjaer S, et al. Structure and chemical inhibition of the RET tyrosine kinase domain. *J Biol Chem.* 2006;281:33577-33587.
109. Li X, Kamenecka T, Cameron M. Bioactivation of the epidermal-growth factor receptor inhibitor gefitinib: implications for pulmonary and hepatic toxicities. *Chem Res Toxicol.* 2009;22:1736-1742.
110. Martin P, Oliver S, Kennedy S-J, et al. Pharmacokinetics of vandetanib: three phase I studies in healthy subjects. *Clin Ther.* 2012;34:221-237.
111. Tailor A, Waddington J, Meng X, et al. Mass spectrometric and functional aspects of drug–protein conjugation. *Chem Res Toxicol.* 2016;29:1912-1935.
112. Yang Z, Hackshaw A, Feng Q, et al. Comparison of gefitinib, erlotinib and afatinib in non-small cell lung cancer: a meta-analysis. *Int J Cancer.* 2017;140:2805-2819.
113. Skoulidis F, Papadimitrakopoulou V. Targeting the gatekeeper: osimertinib in EGFR T790M mutation-positive non-small cell lung cancer. *Clin Cancer Res.* 2017;23:618-622.
114. Zhao C, Han S-Y, Li P-P. Pharmacokinetics of gefitinib: roles of drug metabolizing enzymes and transporters. *Curr Drug Deliv.* 2017;14:282-288.
115. Suzumura T, Kimura T, Kudoh S, et al. Reduced CYP2D6 function is associated with gefitinib-induced rash in patients with non-small cell lung cancer. *BMC Cancer.* 2012;12. doi:10.1186/471-2407-12-568.
116. D'Amato V, Raimondo L, Formisano L, et al. Mechanisms of lapatinib resistance in HER2-driven breast cancer. *Cancer Treat Rev.* 2015;41:377-388.
117. Shi H, Zhang W, Zhi Q, et al. Lapatinib resistance in HER2+ cancers: latest findings and new concepts on molecular mechanisms. *Tumor Biol.* 2016;37:15411-15431.
118. Breast Cancer Facts and Figures 2015–2016. American Cancer Society. Available at https://www.cancer.org/content/dam/cancer-org/research/cancer-facts-and-statistics/breast-cancer-facts-and-figures/breast-cancer-facts-and-figures-2015-2016.pdf. Accessed April 25, 2018.
119. Cooper M, Yi S, Alghamdi W, et al. Vandetanib for the treatment of medullary thyroid carcinoma. *Ann Pharmacother.* 2014;48:387-394.
120. Deshpande H, Marler V, Sosa J. Clinical utility of vandetanib in the treament of patients with advanced medullary thyroid cancer. *Onco Targets Ther.* 2011;4:209-215.
121. Hirsh V. Next-generation covalent irreversible kinase inhibitors in NSCLC: focus on afatinib. *BioDrugs.* 2015;29:167-183.
122. Kim Y, Ko J, Cui Z-Y. The EGFR T790M mutation in acquired resistance to an irreversible second-generation EGFR inhibitor. *Mol Cancer Ther.* 2012;11:784-791.
123. Keating G. Afatinib: a review of its use in the treatment of advanced non-small cell lung cancer. *Drugs.* 2014;74:207-221.
124. Feldinger K, Kong A. Profile of neratinib and its potential in the treatment of breast cancer. *Breast Cancer.* 2015;7:147-162.
125. Kourie H, El Rassy E, Clatot F, et al. Emerging treatments for HER2-positive early stage breast cancer: focus on neratinib. *Onco Targets Ther.* 2017;10:3363-3372.
126. Tiwari S, Mishra P, Abraham J. Neratinib, a novel HER2-targeted tyrosine kinase inhibitor. *Clin Breast Cancer.* 2016;5:344-348.
127. Burstein H, Sun Y, Dirix L, et al. Neratinib, an irreversible ErbB receptor tyrosine kinase inhibitor, in patients with advanced ErbB2-positive breast cancer. *J Clin Oncol.* 2010;28:1301-1307.
128. Kourie H, Chaix M, Gombos A, et al. Pharmacodynamics, pharmacokinetics and clinical efficacy of neratinib in HER2-positive breast cancer and breast cancer with HER2 mutations. *Expert Opin Drug Metab Toxicol.* 2016;12:947-957.
129. Nerlynx (Neratinib) Puma Biotechnology. Available at https://www.accessdata.fda.gov/drugsatfda_docs/label/2017/208051s000lbl.pdf. Accessed April 25, 2018.
130. *Multi-discipline Review: Nerlynx (Neratinib Maleate 33ts).* Silver Spring, MD: U.S. Food and Drug Administration; Center for Drug Evaluation and Research; 2017.
131. Lamb Y, Scott L. Osimertinib: a review in T790M-positive advanced non-small cell lung cancer. *Targ Oncol.* 2017;12: 555-562.
132. Santarpia M, Liguori A, Karachaliou N, et al. Osimertinib in the treatment of non-small cell lung cancer: design, development and place in therapy. *Lung Cancer.* 2017;8:109-125.
133. Rossi A, Muscarella L, Di Micco C, et al. Pharmacokinetic drug evaluation of osimertinib for the treatment of non-small cell lung cancer. *Expert Opin Drug Metab Toxicol.* 2017;13:1281-1288.
134. Tang Z-H, Lu J-J. Osimertinib resistance in non-small cell lung cancer: mechanisms and therapeutic strategies. *Cancer Lett.* 2018;420:242-246.
135. Erman M. Molecular mechanisms of signal transduction: epidermal growth factor receptor family, vascular endothelial growth factor family, kit, platelet-derived growth factor receptor, ras. *J BUON.* 2007;12(suppl 1):S83-S94.
136. Mirzaei M, Taherpour A. Tautomeric preferences of the *cis* and *trans* isomers of axitinib. *Chem Phys.* 2018;507:10-18.
137. Bellesoeur A, Carton E, Alexandre J, et al. Axitinib in the treatment of renal cell carcinoma: design, development, and place in therapy. *Drug Des Devel Ther.* 2017;11:2801-2811.
138. Cella D, Beaumont J. Pazopanib in the treatment of advanced renal cell carcinoma. *Ther Adv Urol.* 2016;8:61-69.
139. Iacovelli R, Verri E, Rocca M, et al. Is there still a role for sorafenib in metastatic renal carcinoma? A systematic review and meta-analysis of the effectiveness of sorafenib over other targeted agents. *Crit Rev Oncol Hematol.* 2016;99:324-331.
140. Hutson T, Al-Shukri S, Stus V, et al. Axitinib versus sorafenib in first-line metastatic renal cell carcinoma: overall survival from a randomized Phase III trial. *Clin Genitourin Cancer.* 2017;15:72-76.
141. Qin F, Yu H, Bai J. Safety and toxicity of axitinib and sorafenib monotherapy for patients with renal cell carcinoma: a meta-analysis. *J Biomed Res.* 2017;31. doi:10.7555/JBR.31.20170080.
142. Pitoia F, Jerkovich F. Selective use of sorafenib in the treatment of thyroid cancer. *Drugs Des Devel Therp.* 2016;10:1119-1131.
143. Keating G. Sorafenib: a review in hepatocellular carcinoma. *Targ Oncol.* 2017;12:243-253.
144. Kawalec P, Malinowska-Lipien I, Brzostek T, et al. Lenvatinib for the treatment of radioactive-refractory differentiated thyroid carcinoma: a systematic review and indirect comparison with sorafenib. *Expert Rev Anticancer Ther.* 2016;16:1303-1309.
145. Frampton J. Lenvatinib: a review in refractory thyroid cancer. *Targ Oncol.* 2016;11:115-122.
146. Grande E, Glen H, Aller J, et al. Recommendations on managing lenvatinib and everolimus in patients with advanced or metastatic renal cell carcinoma. *Expert Opin Drug Saf.* 2017;16: 1413-1426.
147. Leonetti A, Leonardi F, Bersanelli M, et al. Clinical use of lenvatinib in combination with everolimus for the treatment of advanced renal cell carcinoma. *Ther Clin Risk Manag.* 2017;13:799-806.
148. De Lisi D, De Giorgi U, Lolli C, et al. Lenvatinib in the management of metastatic renal cell carcinoma: a promising combination therapy? *Expert Opin Drug Metab Toxicol.* 2018;14:461-467.
149. Hoy S. Cabozantinib: a review of its use in patients with medullary thyroid cancer. *Drugs.* 2014;74:1435-1444.
150. Colombo J, Wein R. Cabozantinib for progressive metastatinc medullary thyroid cancer: a review. *Ther Clin Risk Manag.* 2014;10:395-404.

151. Bersanelli M, Buti S. Cabozantinib in metastatic renal cell carcinoma: latest findings and clinical potential. *Ther Adv Med Oncol.* 2017;9:627-636.
152. Myers S, Brunton V, Unciti-Broceta A. AXL Inhibitors in cancer: a medicinal chemistry perspective. *J Med Chem.* 2016;59:3593-3608.
153. Lacy S, Hsu B, Miles D, et al. Metabolism and disposition of cabozantinib in healthy male volunteers and pharmacologic characterization of its major metabolites. *Drug Metab Dispos.* 2015;43:1190-1207.
154. Narayan V, Haas N. Axitinib in the treatment of renal cell carcinoma: patient selection and perspectives. *Int J Nephrol Renovasc Dis.* 2016;9:65-72.
155. Keating G. Axitinib: a review in advanced renal cell carcioma. *Drugs.* 2015;75:1903-1913.
156. Wang H, Man L, Li G, et al. Comparative efficacy and safety of axitinib versus sorafenib in metastatic renal cell carcinoma: a systematic review and meta-analysis. *Onco Targets Ther.* 2016;9:3423-3432.
157. Verzoni E, Grassi P, Testa I, et al. Targeted treatments in advanced renal cell carcinoma: focus on axitinib. *Pharmgenomics Pers Med.* 2014;7:107-116.
158. Faivre S, Noccoli P, Castellano D, et al. Sunitinib in pancreatic neuroendocrine tumors: updated progression-free survival and final overall survival from a phase III randominzed study. *Ann Oncol.* 2017;28:339-343.
159. Schroeder B, Li Z, Cranmer L, et al. Targeting gastrointestinal stromal tumors: the role of regorafenib. *Onco Targets Ther.* 2016;9:3009-3016.
160. Joosten S, Hamming L, Soetekouw P, et al. Resistance to sunitinib in renal cell carcinoma: from molecular mechanisms to predictive markers and future perspectives. *Biochem Biophys Acta.* 2015;1885:1-16.
161. Carlisle B, Demko N, Freeman G, et al. Benefit, risk and outcomes in drug development: aasystematic review of sunitinib. *J Natl Cancer Inst.* 2016;108. doi:10.1093/jnci/djv292.
162. McCormack P. Panzopanib: a review of its use in the management of advanced renal cell carcinoma. *Drugs.* 2014;74:1111-1125.
163. Miyamoto S, Katutani S, Sato Y, et al. Drug review: pazopanib. *Jpn J Clin Oncol.* 2018. doi:10.1093/jjco/hyy053.
164. Alavi S, Florou V, Tinoco G, et al. A precision medicine approach in sarcoma: identification of patients who may benefit from early use of pazopanib. *Discov Med.* 2018;25:131-144.
165. Thillai K, Srikandarajah K, Ross P. Regorafenib as treatment for patients with advanced haptocellular cancer. *Future Oncol.* 2017;13:2223-2232.
166. Tovoli F, Granito A, De Lorenzo S, et al. Regorafenib for the treatment of hepatocellular carcinoma. *Drugs Today.* 2018;54:5-13.
167. Rey J-B, Launay-Vacher V, Tournigand C. Regorafenib as a single-agent in the treatment of patients with gastrointestinal tumors: an overview for pharmacists. *Targ Oncol.* 2015;10:199-213.
168. Skarderud M, Polk A, Kjeldgaard K, et al. Efficacy and safety of regoafenib in the treatment of metastatic colorectal cancer: a systemic review. *Cancer Treat Rev.* 2018;62:61-73.
169. Gerish M, Hafner F-T, Lang D, et al. Mass balance, metabolic disposition, and pharmacokinetics of a single oral dose of regorafenib in healthy human subjects. *Cancer Chemother Pharmacol.* 2018;81:195-206.
170. De Pas T, Pala L, Catania C, et al. Molecular and clinical features of second-generation anaplastic lymphoma kinase inhibitors ceritinib. *Future Oncol.* 2017;13:2629-2644.
171. Katayama R. Drug resistance in anaplastic lymphoma kinase-rearranged lung cancer. *Cancer Sci.* 2017;109:572-580.
172. Alshareef A. Novel molecular challenges in targeting anaplastic lymphoma kinase in ALK-expressing human cancers. *Cancers.* 2017;9. doi:10.3390/cancers9110148.
173. Johnson T, Tan W, Goulet L, et al. Metabolism, excretion and pharmacokinetics of [^{14}C]crizotinib following oral administration to healthy subjects. *Xenobiotica.* 2015;45:45-59.
174. Huang W-S, Liu S, Zou D, et al. Discovery of brigatinib (AP26113), a phosphine oxide-containing potent, orally active inhibitor of anaplastic lymphoma kinase. *J Med Chem.* 2016;59:4948-4964.
175. Katayama R. Therapeutic strategies and mechanisms of drug resistance in anaplastic lymphoma kinase (ALK)-rearranged lung cancer. *Pharmacol Ther.* 2017;177:1-8.
176. Davis K, Kaye J, Masters E, et al. Real-world outcomes in patients with ALK-positive non-small cell lung cancer treated with crizotinib. *Curr Oncol.* 2018;25:e40-9.
177. Arbour K, Riely G. Diagnosis and treament of anaplastic lymphoma kinase-positive non-small cell lung cancer. *Hematol Oncol Clin N Am.* 2017;31:101-111.
178. DiBonaventura M, Wong W, Shah-Manek B, et al. Real world usage and clinical outcomes of alectinib among post-crizotinib progression anaplasatic lymphoma kinase positive non-small cell lung cancer patients in the USA. *Onco Targets Ther.* 2018;11:75-82.
179. Hong Y, Passos V, Huang P-H, et al. Population pharmacokinetics of ceritinib in adult patients with tumors characterized by genetic abnormalities in anaplastic lymphoma kinase. *J Clin Pharmacol.* 2017;57:652-662.
180. *Zykadia: Ceritinib Capsules.* Dorval, Quebec: Norvartis Pharmaceuticals; 2015:1-48.
181. Au T, Cavalieri C, Stenehjem D. Ceritinib: a primer for pharmacists. *J Oncol Pharm Pract.* 2017;23:602-614.
182. Gadgeel S. The use of alectinib in the first-line treatment of anaplastic lymphoma kinase-positive non-small-cell lung cancer. *Future Oncol.* 2018. doi:10.2217/fon-018–0027.
183. Sato-Nakai M, Kawashima K, Nakagawa T, et al. Metabolites of alectinib in human: their identification and pharmacological activity. *Heliyon.* 2017;3. doi:10.1016/j.heliyon. 2017. e00354.
184. Mezquita L, Planchard D. The role of brigatinib in crizotinib-resistant non-small cell lung cancer. *Cancer Manag Res.* 2018;10:123-130.
185. Jain R, Chen H. Spotlight on brigatinib and its potential in the treatment of patients with metastatic ALK-positive non-small cell lung cancer who are resistant or intolerant to crizotinib. *Lung Cancer Targ Ther.* 2017;8:169-177.
186. Buggy J, Elias L. Bruton tyrosine kinase (BTK) and its role in B-cell malignancy. *Int Rev Immunol.* 2012;31:119-132.
187. Aalipour A, Advani R. Bruton tyrosine kinase inhibitors: a promising novel targeted treatment for B cell lymphoma. *Br J Haematol.* 2013;163:436-443.
188. Burger J, Buggy J. Bruton tyrosine kinase inhibitor ibrutinib (PCI-32765). *Leuk Lymphoma.* 2013;54:2385-2391.
189. Zheng N, Pan J, Hao Q, et al. Design, synthesis and biological evaluation of novel 3-substituted pyrazolopyrimidine derivatives as potent Bruton's tyrosine kinase (BTK) inhibitors. *Bioorg Med Chem.* 2018;26:2165-2172.
190. Bender A, Gardberg A, Pereira A, et al. Ability of Bruton's tyrosine kinase inhibitors to sequester Y551 and prevent phosphorylation determines potency for inhibition of Fc receptor but not B-cell receptor signaling. *Mol Pharmacol.* 2017;91:208-219.
191. Barf T, Covey T, Izumi R, et al. Acalabrutinib (ACP-196): a covalent Bruton tyrosine kinase inhibitor with a differentiated selectivity and in vivo potency profile. *J Pharmacol Exp Ther.* 2017;363:240-252.
192. Sharma S, Galanina N, Guo A, et al. Identification of a structurally novel BTK mutation that drives ibrutinib resistance in CLL. *Oncotarget.* 2016;7:68833-68841.
193. Foluso O, Glick A, Stender M, et al. Ibrutinib as a Bruton kinase inhibitor in the management of chronic lymphocytic leukemia: a new agent with great promise. *Clin Lymphoma Myeloma Leuk.* 2016;16:63-69.
194. Wu J, Zhang M, Delong L. Bruton tyrosine kinase inhibitor ONO/GS-4056: from bench to bedside. *Oncotarget.* 2017;8:7201-7207.
195. Wu J, Liu C, Tsui S, et al. Second generation inhibitors of Bruton tyrosine kinase. *J Hematol Oncol.* 2016;9. doi:10.1186/s13045-016-0313-y.

196. Jain P, Keating M, Wierda W, et al. Outcomes of patients with chronic lymphocytic leukemia after discontinuing ibrutinib. *Blood*. 2015;125:2062-2067.
197. Noy A, de Vos S, Thieblemont C, et al. Targeting Bruton tyrosine kinse with ibrutinib in relapsed/refractory marginal zone lymphoma. *Blood*. 2018;20:2224-2232.
198. Wu J, Zhang M, Liu D. Acalabrutinib (ACP-196): a selective second-generation BTK inhibitor. *J Hematol Oncol*. 2016;9. doi:10.1186/s13045-016-2050-9.
199. Wang M, Rule S, Zinzani P, et al. Acalabrutinib in relapsed or refractory mantle cell lymphoma (ACE-LY-004): a single-arm, multicentre, phase 2 trial. *Expert Rev Hematol*. 2018;391:659-667.
200. Weisberg E, Sattler M, Manley P, et al. Spotlight on midostaurin in the treatment of FLT3-mutated acute myeloid leukemia and systemic mastocytosis: design, development and potential place in therapy. *Onco Targets Ther*. 2018;11:175-182.
201. Weisberg E, Puissant A, Stone R, et al. Characterization of midostaurin as a dual inhibitor of FLT3 and SKY and potentiation of FLT3 inhibition against FLT3-ITD-driven leukemia harboring activated SKY kinase. *Oncotarget*. 2017;8:52026-52044.
202. Monnerat C, Henriksson R, Le Chevalier T, et al. Phase I study of PKC412 (N-benzyl-staurosporine), a novel oral protein kinase C inhibitor, combined with gemcitabine and cisplatin in patients with non-small-cell lung cancer. *Ann Oncol*. 2004;15:316-323.
203. Senkevitch E, Durum S. The promise of janus kinase inhibitors in the treatment of hematological malignancies. *Cytokine*. 2017;98:33-41.
204. Delhommeau F, Dupont S, Tonetti C, et al. Evidence that the JAK2 G1849T (V617F) mutation occurs in a lymphomyeloid progenitor in polycythemia vera and idopathic myelofibrosis. *Blood*. 2007;109:71-77.
205. Wade R, Hodgson R, Biswas M, et al. A review of ruxolitinib for the treatment of myelofibrosis: a critique of the evidence. *Pharmacoeconomics*. 2017;35:203-213.
206. McKeage K. Ruxolitinib: a review in polycythaemia vera. *Drugs*. 2015;75:1773-1781.
207. Shilling A, Nedza F, Emm T, et al. Metabolism, excretion and pharmacokinetics of [^{14}C]INCB018424, a selective Janus tyrosine kinase 1/2 inhibitor in humans. *Drug Metab Dispos*. 2010;38:2023-2031.
208. Summary of Product Characteristics (Ruxolitinib). European Medicines Agency. Available at http://www.ema.europa.eu/docs/en_GB/document_library/EPAR_-_Product_Information/human/002464/WC500133223.pdf. Accessed June 28, 2018.
209. Martin M, Endicott J, Noble M. Structure-based discovery of cyclin-dependent protein kinase inhibitors. *Essays Biochem*. 2017;61:439-452.
210. Bilgin B, Sendur M, Sdede D, et al. A current and comprehensive review of cyclin-dependent kinase inhibitors for the treatment of metastatic breast cancer. *Curr Med Res Opin*. 2017;33:1559-1569.
211. Li T, Tianwei W, Zuo M, et al. Recent progress of cyclin-dependent kinase inhibitors as potential anticancer agents. *Future Med Chem*. 2016;8:2047-2076.
212. Xu H, Yu S, Liu Q, et al. Recent advances of highly selective CDK4/6 inhibitors in breast cancer. *J Hematol Oncol*. 2017;10. doi:10.1186/s13045-017-0467-2.
213. Kwapisz D. Cyclin-dependent kinase 4/6 inhibitors in breast cancer: palbociclib, ribocicilb, and abemaciclib. *Breast Cancer Res*. 2017;166:41-54.
214. Yu Y, Loi C-M, Hoffman J, et al. Physiologically based pharmacokinetic modeling of palbociclib. *J Clin Pharmacol*. 2017;57:173-184.
215. Curigliano G, Criscitiello C, Esposito A, et al. Phamacokinetic drug evaluation of ribociclib for the treatment of metastatic hormone-positive breast cancer. *Expert Opin Drug Metab Toxicol*. 2017;13:575-581.
216. Burke T, Torres R, McNulty A, et al. The major human metabolites of abemaciclib are inhibitors of CDK4 and CDK6. *Cancer Res*. 2016;76 (14 suppl). doi:10.1158/538-7445.AM2016-830.
217. Agianian B, Gavathiotis E. Current insights of BRAF inhibitors in cancer. *J Med Chem*. 2018;61. doi:10.1021/acs.jmedchem.7b01306.
218. Griffin M, Scotto D, Josephs D, et al. BRAF inhibitors: resistance and the promise of combination treatments for melanoma. *Oncotarget*. 2017;8:78174-78192.
219. Arozarena I, Wellbrock C. Overcoming resistance to BRAF inhibitors. *Ann Transl Med*. 2017;5. doi:10.21037/atm.2017.06.09.
220. Cabanillas M, Patel A, Danysh B, et al. BRAF inhibitors: experience in thyroid cancer and general review of toxicity. *Horm Canc*. 2015;6:21-36.
221. Roskoski R Jr. Allosteric MEK1/2 inhibitors including cobimetanib and trametinib in the treament of cutaneous melanomas. *Pharmacol Res*. 2017;117:20-31.
222. Subbiah V, Kreitman R, Wainberg Z, et al. Dabrafenib and trametinib treatment in patients with locally advanced or metastatic BRAF V600E-mutant anaplastic thryoid cancer. *J Clin Oncol*. 2018;36:7-13.
223. Weart T, Miller K, Simone C II. Spotlight on dabrafenib/trametinib in the treatment on non-small cell lung cancer: place in therapy. *Cancer Manag Res*. 2018;10:647-652.
224. Goldinger S, Rinderknecht J, Dummer R, et al. A single-dose mass balance and metabolite-profiling study of vemurafenib in patients with metastatic melanoma. *Pharmacol Res Perspect*. 2015;3. doi:10.1002/prp2.113.
225. Bershas D, Ouellet D, Mamaril-Fishman D, et al. Metabolism and disposition of oral dabrafenib in cancer patients: proposed participation of aryl nitrogen in carbon-carbon bond cleavage via decarboxylation following enzymatic oxidation. *Drug Metab Dispos*. 2013;41:2215-2224.
226. Hatzivassiliou G, Haling J, Chen H, et al. Mechanism of MEK inhibition determines efficacy in mutant KRAS-versus BRAF-driven cancers. *Nature*. 2013;501:232-236.
227. Rice K, Aay N, Anand N, et al. Novel carboxamide-based allosteric MEK inhibitors: discovery and optimization efforts towards XL518 (GDC-0973). *Med Chem Lett*. 2012;3:416-421.
228. Cheng Y, Tian H. Current development status of MEK inhibitors. *Molecules*. 2017;22. doi:10.3390.
229. Park K-S, Oh B, Lee M-H, et al. The HSP90 inhibitor, NVP-AUY922, sensitizes KRAS-mutant non-small cell lung cancer with intrinsic resistance to MEK inhibitor trametinib. *Cancer Lett*. 2016;372:75-81.
230. Wahid M, Jawed A, Mandal R, et al. Recent developments and obstacles in the treatment of melanoma with BRAF and MET inhibitors. *Crit Rev Oncol Hematol*. 2018;125:84-88.
231. Ho M, Morris M, Pirhalla J, et al. Trametinib, a first-in-class oral MEK inhibitor mass balance study with limited enrollment of two male subjects with advanced cancers. *Xenobiotica*. 2014;44:352-368.
232. Takahashi R, Choo E, Ma S, et al. Absorption, metabolism, excretion and the contribution of intestinal metabolism to the oral disposition of [^{14}C] cobimetinib, a MEK inhibitor, in humans. *Drug Metab Dispos*. 2015;44:28-39.
233. Lin T, Leung C, Nguyen K, et al. Mammalian target of rapamycin (mTOR) inhibitors in solid tumors. *Clin Pharmacist*. 2016;8. doi:10.1211/CP.2016.20200813.
234. Saran U, Foti M, Dufour J-F. Cellular and molecular effects of the mTOR inhibitor everolimus. *Clin Sci*. 2015;129:895-914.
235. Huang Z, Wu Y, Zhou X, et al. Clinical efficacy of mTOR inhibitors in solid tumors: a systematic review. *Future Oncol*. 2015;11:1687-1699.
236. Zollinger M, Sayer C, Dannecker R, et al. The macrolide everolimus forms an unusual metabolite in animals and humans: identification of a phosphocholine ester. *Drug Metab Dispos*. 2008;36:1457-1460.
237. Boni J, Hug B, Leister C, et al. Intravenous temsirolimus in cancer patients: clinical pharmacology and dosing considerations. *Sem Oncol*. 2007;36:S18-S25.
238. Cai P, Tsao R, Ruppen M. In vitro metabolic study of temsirolimus: preparation, isolation and identification of the metabolites. *Drug Metab Dispos*. 2007;35:1554-1563.

239. Berndt A, Miller S, Williams O, et al. The p110d crystal structure uncovers mechanisms for selectivity and potency of novel PI3K inhibitors. *Nat Chem Biol.* 2010;6:117-124.
240. Scott W, Hentemann M, Rowley R, et al. Discovery and SAR of novel 2,3-dihydroimidazo[1,2-c]-quinazoline PI3K inhibitors: identification of copanlisib (BAY 80-6946). *Chem Med Chem.* 2016;11:1517-1530.
241. Zhao W, Qiu Y, Kong D. Class I phosphatidylinositol 3-kinase inhibitors for cancer therapy. *Acta Pharm Sin B.* 2017;7:27-37.
242. Shah A, Mangaonkar A. Idelalisib: a novel PI3Kd inhibitor for chronic lymphocytic leukemia. *Ann Pharmacother.* 2015;49:1162-1170.
243. Cheah C, Fowler N. Idelalisib in the management of lymphoma. *Blood.* 2016;128:331-336.
244. Clinical Pharmacology and Biopharmaceutics Reviews. Available at https://www.accessdata.fda.gov/drugsatfda_docs/nda/2014/206545 Orig1s000ClinPharmR.pdf. Accessed June 3, 2018.
245. Jin F, Robeson M, Zhou H, et al. Pharmacokinetics, metabolism and excretion of idelalisib. *Blood.* 2013;122:5570.
246. Ramanathan S, Jin F, Sharma S, et al. Clinical pharmacokinetic and pharmacodynamic profile of idelalisib. *Clin Pharmacokinet.* 2016;55:33-45.
247. Dreyling M, Santoro A, Mollica L, et al. Phosphatidylinositol 3-kinase inhibition by copanlisib in relapsed or refractor indolent lymphoma. *J Clin Oncol.* 2017;35:3898-3905.
248. Gerish M, Schwarz T, Lang D, et al. Pharmacokinetics of intravenous pan-class I phosphatidylinositol 3-kinase (PI3K) inhibitor [^{14}C]copanlisib (BAY 80-6946) in a mass balance study in healthy male volunteers. *Cancer Chemother Pharmacol.* 2017;80:535-544.
249. Buege M, DiPippo A, DiNardo C. Evolving treatment strategies for elderly leukemia patients with IDH mutations. *Cancers.* 2018;10. doi:10.3390/cancers10060187.
250. Dugan J, Pollyea D. Enasidenib for the treatment of acute myeloid leukemia. *Expert Rev Clin Pharmacol.* 2018. doi:10.1080/17512433 .2018.1477585.
251. Figueroa M, Abdel-Wahab O, Lu C, et al. Leukemic IDH1 and IDH2 mutations result in a hypermethylation phenotype, disrupt TET2 function, and impair hematopoietic differentiation. *Cancer Cell.* 2010;18:553-567.
252. Ward P, Patel J, Wise D, et al. The common feature of leukemia-associated IDH1 and IDH2 mutations is a neomorphic enzyme activiting converting a-ketoglutarate to 2-hydroxyglutarate. *Cancer Cell.* 2010;17:225-234.
253. Xu W, Yang H, Liu Y, et al. Oncometabolite 2-hydroxyglutarate is a competitive inhibitor of a-ketoglutarate-dependent dioxygenases. *Cancer Cell.* 2011;19:17-30.
254. DiNardo CD, Stein EM, deBotton S, et al. Durable remissions with ivosidenib in IDH1-mutated relapsed or refractory AML. *New Engl J Med.* 2018;378:2386-2398.
255. Popovici-Muller J, Lemieux RM, Artin E, et al. Discovery of AG-120 (Ivosidenib): a first-in-class mutant IDH1 inhibitor for the treatment of IDH1 mutant cancers. *Med Chem Lett.* 2018;9:300-305.
256. Pullarkat V, Newman E. BCL2 inhibition by venetoclax: targeting the Achilles' heel of the acute myeloid leukemia stem cell? *Cancer Discov.* 2016;6:1082-1083.
257. Anderson M, Deng J, Seymour J, et al. The BCL2 selective inhibitor venetoclax induces rapid onset apoptosis of CLL cells in patients via a TP43-independent mechanism. *Blood.* 2016;127:3215-3224.
258. Cang S, Iragavarapu C, Savooji J, et al. ABT-199 (venetoclax) and BCL-2 inhibitors in clinical development. *J Hematol Oncol.* 2015;8. doi:10.1186/s13045-015-0224-3.
259. King A, Peterson T, Horvat T, et al. Venetoclax: a first-in-class oral BCL-2 inhibitor for the management of lymphoid malignancies. *Ann Pharmacother.* 2017;51:410-416.
260. Stilgenbauer S, Eichhorst B, Schetelig J, et al. Venetoclax in relapsed or refractory chronic lymphocytic leukaemia with 17p deletion: a mutlicentre, open-label, phase 2 study. *Lancet Oncol.* 2016;17:768-778.
261. *Pharmacological Reviews (Venetoclax).* Silver Spring, MD: U.S. Food and Drug Administration; Center for Drug Evaluation and Research; 2016.
262. Dziadkowiec K, Gasiorowska E, Nowak-Markwitz E, et al. PARP inhibitors: review of mechanisms of action and BRCA1/2 mutation. *Menopause Rev.* 2016;15:215-219.
263. Canan S, Maegley K, Curtin N. Strategies employed for the development of PARP inhibitors. In: Tulin AV, ed. *Poly(ADP-Ribose) Polymerase: Methods and Protocols.* Vol 1608. Humana Press; 2017:271-297.
264. Bitler B, Watson Z, Wheeler L, et al. PARP inhibitors: clinical utility and possibilities of overcoming resistance. *Gynecol Oncol.* 2017;147:695-704.
265. Scarpelli R, Boueres J, Cerratani M, et al. Synthesis and biological evaluation of substituted 2-phenyl-2H-indazole-7-carboxamides as potent poly(ADP-ribose)polymerase (PARP) inhibitors. *Bioorg Med Chem Lett.* 2010;20:488-492.
266. Chen Y, Du H. The promising PARP inhibitors in ovarian cancer therapy: from olaparib to others. *Biomed Pharmacother.* 2018;99:552-560.
267. Walsh C. Targeted therapy for ovarian cancer: the rapidly evolving landscape of PARP inhibitor use. *Minera Ginecol.* 2018;70:150-170.
268. Munroe M, Kolesar J. Olaparib for the treatment of BRAC-mutated advanced ovarian cancer. *Am J Health-Syst Pharm.* 2016;73:1037-1041.
269. Musella A, Bardhi E, Marchetti C. Rucaparib: an emerging parp inhibitor for treatment of recurrent ovarian cancer. *Cancer Treat Rev.* 2018;66:7-14.
270. Dockery L, Gunderson C, Moore K. Rucaparib: the past, present and future of a newly approved PARP inhibitor for ovarian cancer. *Onco Targets Ther.* 2017;10:3029-3037.
271. Rucaparib Prescribing Information. Clovis Oncology. Available at https://www.accessdata.fda.gov/drugsatfda_docs/label/2016/ 209115s000lbl.pdf. Accessed July 2, 2018.
272. Ethier J-L, Lheureux S, Oza A. The role of niraparib for the treatment of ovarian cancer. *Future Oncol.* 2018. doi:10:2217/fon-018–0101.
273. Scott L. Niraparib: first global approval. *Drugs.* 2017;77:1029-1034.
274. Harshbarger W, Miller C, Diedrich C, et al. Crystal structure of the human 20S proteasome in complex with carfilzomib. *Structure.* 2015;23:418-424.
275. Myung J, Kim K, Crews C. The ubiquitin-proteasome pathway and proteasome inhibitors. *Med Res Rev.* 2001;21:245-273.
276. Wallington-Beddoe C, Sobieraj-Teague M, Kuss B, et al. Resistance to proteasome inhibitors and other targeted therapies in myeloma. *Br J Haematol.* 2018;182:11-28.
277. Offidani M, Corvatta L, Caraffa P, et al. An evidence-based review of ixazomib citrate and its potential in the treatment of newly diagnosed multiple myeloma. *Onco Targets Ther.* 2014;7:1793-1800.
278. Groll M, Berkers C, Ploegh H, et al. Crystal structure of the boronic acid-based proteasome inhibitor bortezomib in complex with the yeast 20S proteasome. *Structure.* 2006;14:451-456.
279. Noonan K, Colson K. Immunomodulatory agents and proteasome inhibitors in the treatment of multiple myeloma. *Sem Oncol.* 2017;33:279-291.
280. Vandross A. Proteasome inhibitor-based therapy for treatment of newly diagnosed multiple myeloma. *Sem Oncol.* 2017;44:381-384.
281. Brayer J, Baz R. The potential of ixazomib, a second-generation proteasome inhibitor, in the treatment of multiple myeloma. *Ther Adv Hematol.* 2017;8:209-220.
282. *Assessment Report: Ninlaro (Ixazomib).* London: European Medicines Agency; 2016.
283. Scalzulli E, Grammatico S, Vozella F, et al. Proteasome inhibitors for the treatment of multiple myeloma. *Expert Opin Pharmacother.* 2018;19:375-386.
284. Barros-Oliveira M, Costa-Silva D, De Andrade D, et al. Use of anastrozole in the chemoprevention and treatment of breast cancer: a literature review. *Rev Assoc Med Bras.* 2017;63:371-378.
285. Kamdem L, Liu Y, Stearms V, et al. In vitro and in vivo oxidative metabolism and glucuronidation of anastrozole. *Br J Clin Pharmacol.* 2010;70:854-869.
286. Shagufta I. Tamoxifen a pioneering drug: an update on the therapeutic potential of tamoxifen derivatives. *Eur J Med Chem.* 2018;143:515-531.

287. Schalken J, Fitzpatrick J. Enzalutamide: targeting the androgen signalling pathway in metastatic castration-resistant prostate cancer. *BJU Int*. 2016;117:215-225.
288. Hoda M, Kramer M, Merseburger A, et al. Androgen deprivation therapy with leuprolide acetate for treatment of advanced prostate cancer. *Expert Opin Pharmacother*. 2017;18:105-113.
289. Sciarra A, Fasulo A, Ciardi A, et al. A meta-analysis and systematic review of randomized controlled trials with degarelix versus gonadotropin-releasing hormone agonists for advanced prostate cancer. *Medicine* 2016;95. doi:10.1097/MD.0000000000003845.
290. Clinton T, Woldu S, Raj G. Degarelix versus luteinizing hormone-releasing hormone agonists for the treatment of prostate cancer. *Expert Opin Pharmacother*. 2017;18:825-832.
291. Lecutier M. Phocomelia and internal defects due to thalidomide. *Br Med J*. 1962;2:1147-1148.
292. Copur M, Rose M, Gettinger S. Miscellaneous chemotherapeutic agents. In: DeVita VJ, Lawrence T, Rosenberg S, eds. *Cancer: Principles and Practice of Oncology*. 8 ed. Baltimore: Lippincott Williams & Wilkins; 2008:490-495.
293. Cavello F, Boccadoro M, Palumbo A. Review of thalidomide in the treatment of newly diagnosed multiple myeloma. *Ther Clin Risk Manag*. 2007;3:543-552.
294. Chen N, Zhou S, Palmisano M. Clinical pharmacokinetics and pharmacodynamics of lenalidomide. *Clin Pharmcokinet*. 2017;56:139-152.
295. Hanaizi Z, Flores B, Hemmings R, et al. The European medicines agency review of pomalidomide in combination with low-dose dexamethasone for the treatment of adult patients with multiple myeloma: summary of the scientific assessment of the committee for medicinal products for human use. *Oncologist*. 2015;20:329-334.
296. Touzeau C, Moreau P. Pomalidomide in the management of relapsed multiple myeloma. *Future Oncol*. 2016;12:1975-1983.
297. Hoffman M, Kasserra C, Reyes J, et al. Absorption, metabolism and excretion of [^{14}C]pomalidomide in humans following oral administration. *Cancer Chemother Pharmacol*. 2013;71:489-501.
298. Chowdhury G, Shibata N, Yamakazi H, et al. Human cytochrome P450 oxidation of 5-hydroxythalidomide and pomalidomide, an amino analogue of thalidomide. *Chem Res Toxicol*. 2014;27:147-156.
299. McGraw A. Romidepsin for the treatment of T-cell lymphomas. *Am J Health-Syst Pharm*. 2013;70:1115-1122.
300. Chun P. Histone deacetylase inhibitors in hematological malignancies and solid tumors. *Arch Pharm Res*. 2015;38:933-949.
301. Sultana F, Manasa K, Shaik S, et al. Zinc dependent histone deacetylase inhibitors in cancer chemotherapy: recent update. *Curr Med Chem*. 2018;25:1-66.
302. Cheng T, Grasse L, Shah J, et al. Panobinostat, a pan-histone deacetylase inhibitor: rationale for and application to treatment of multiple myeloma. *Drugs Today*. 2015;51:491-504.
303. Newbold A, Lindemann R, Cluse L, et al. Characterisation of the novel apoptotic and therapeutic activities of the histone deacetylase inhibitor romidepsin. *Mol Cancer Ther*. 2008;7:1066-1079.
304. Clive S, Woo M, Nydam T, et al. Characterizing the disposition, metabolism, and excretion of an orally active pan-deacetylase inhibitor, panobinostat, via trace radiolabeled ^{14}C material in advanced cancer patients. *Cancer Chemother Pharmacol*. 2012;70:513-522.
305. Dal Ben D, Palumbo M, Zagotto G, et al. DNA topoisomerase II structures and anthracycline activity: insights into ternary complex formation. *Curr Pharm Des*. 2007;13:2766-2780.
306. Li F, Jiang T, Li Q, et al. Camptothecin (CPT) and its derivatives and known to target topoisomerase I (Top1) as their mechanism of action: did we miss something in CPT analogue moleular targets for treating human disease such as cancer? *Am J Cancer Res*. 2017;7:2350-2394.
307. Giordano M, D'Annessa I, Coletta A, et al. Structural and dynamical effects induced by the anticancer drug topotecan on the human topoisomerase I-DNA complex. *PLoS One*. 2010;5. doi:10.1371/journal.pone.0010934.
308. Staker B, Hjerrild K, Feese M, et al. The mechanism of topoisomerase I poisoning by a camptothecin analog. *Proc Natl Acad Sci*. 2002;99:15387-15392.
309. Staker B, Feese M, Cushman M, et al. Structures of three classes of anticancer agents bound to the human topoisomerase I-DNA covalent complex. *J Med Chem*. 2005;48:2336-2345.
310. Liu Y-Q, Li W-Q, Morris-Natschke S, et al. Perspectives on biologically active camptothecin derivatives. *Med Res Rev*. 2015;35:753-789.
311. Liu W, Zhu L, Guo W, et al. Synthesis and biological evaluation of novel 7-acyl homocamptothecins as topoisomerase I inhibitors. *Eur J Med Chem*. 2011;46:2408-2414.
312. Ando K, Shah A, Sachdev V, et al. Camptothecin resistance is determined by the regulation of topoisomerase I degradation mediated by ubiquitin proteasome pathway. *Oncotarget*. 2017;8:43733-43751.
313. Kirschbaum M. A comeback for camptothecins? *Leuk Lymphoma*. 2009;50:1914-1915.
314. Xu C, Barchet T, Mager D. Quantitative structure-property relationships of camptothecins in humans. *Cancer Chemother Pharmacol*. 2009;65:325-333.
315. Fujita K, Kubota Y, Ishida H, et al. Irinotecan, a key chemotherapy drug for metastatic colorectal cancer. *World J Gastroenterol*. 2015;21:12234-12248.
316. de Man F, Goey A, van Schaik R. Individualization of irinotecan treatment: a review of pharmacokinetics, pharmacodynamics and pharmacogenetics. *Clin Pharmacokinet*. 2018. doi:10.1007/s40262-018-0644-7.
317. Takano M, Sugiyama T. UGT1A1 polymorphisms in cancer: impact on irinotecan treatment. *Pharmacogenomics Pers Med*. 2017;10:61-68.
318. Lamb Y, Scott L. Liposomal irinotecan: a review in metastatic pancreatic adenocarcinoma. *Drugs*. 2017;77:785-792.
319. *Hycamtin (Topotecan) for Injection*. East Hanover, NY: Novartis Pharmaceuticals; 2015:1-16.
320. Devriese L, Witteveen P, Mergui-Roelvink M, et al. Pharmacodynamics and pharmacokinetics of oral topotecan in patients with advanced solid tumors and impaired renal function. *Br J Clin Pharmacol*. 2015;80:253-266.
321. Saraf S, Jain A, Hurkat P, et al. Topotecan liposomes: a visit from a molecular to a therapeutic platform. *Crit Rev Ther Drug Carrier Syst*. 2016;33:401-432.
322. Gilabert-Oriol R, Chernov L, Anantha M, et al. In vitro assay for measuring real time topotecan release from liposomes: release kinetics and cellular internalization. *Drug Deliv Transl Res*. 2017;7:544-557.
323. Jain A, Jain S. Multipronged, strategic delivery of paclitaxel-topotecan using engineered liposomes to ovarian cancer. *Drug Dev Ind Pharm*. 2016;42:136-149.
324. Padhi S, Kapoor R, Verma D, et al. Formulation and optimization of topotecan nanoparticles: in vitro characterization, cytotoxicity, cellular update and pharmacokinetic outcomes. *J Photochem Photobiol B*. 2018;183:222-232.
325. Vilain N, Tsai-Pflugfelder M, Benoit A, et al. Modulation of drug sensitivity in yeast cells by the ATP-binding domain of human DNA topoisomerase IIalpha. *Nucleic Acids Res*. 2003;31:5714-5722.
326. Chee G, Yalowich J, Bodner A, et al. A diazirine-based photoaffinity etoposide probe for labeling topoisomerase II. *Bioorg Med Chem*. 2010;18:830-838.
327. Naik P, Dubey A, Soni K, et al. The binding modes and binding affinities of epipodophyllotoxin derivatives with human topoisomerase IIα. *J Molec Graph Model*. 2010;29:546-564.
328. Yadav A, Chee G-L, Wu X, et al. Structure-based design, synthesis, and biological testing of piperazine-linked bis-epipodophyllotoxin etoposide analogs. *Bioorg Med Chem*. 2015;23:3542-3551.
329. Mans D, Lafleur M, Westmijze I, et al. Reactions of glutathione with the catechol, the ortho quinone, and the semi-quinone free radical of etoposide. Consequences for DNA inactivation. *Biochem Pharmacol*. 1992;43:1761-1768.

330. Felix C. Secondary leukemias induced by topoisomerase-targeted drugs. *Biochim Biophys Acta*. 1998;1400:233-255.
331. Pommier Y, Leo E, Zhang H, et al. DNA topoisomerases and their poisoning by anticancer and antibacterial drugs. *Chem Biol Rev*. 2010;17:421-433.
332. Gerwirtz D. A critical evaluation of the mechanisms of action proposed for the antitumor effects of the anthracycline antibiotics adriamycin and daunorubicin. *Biochem Pharmacol*. 1999;57:727-741.
333. Zunino F, Pratesi G, Perego P. Role of the sugar moiety in the pharmacological activity of anthracyclines: development of a novel series of disaccharide analogs. *Biochem Pharmacol*. 2001;61:933-938.
334. Chien A, Moasser M. Cellular mechanisms of resistance against taxanes and anthracyclines in cancer: intrinsic and acquired. *Semin Oncol*. 2008;35(suppl 2):S1-S14.
335. Piska K, Koczurkiewicz P, Bucki A, et al. Metabolic carbonyl reduction of anthracyclines – role in cardiotoxicity and cancer resistance. Reducing enzymes as putative targets for novel cardioprotective and chemosensitizing agents. *Invest New Drugs*. 2017;35(35).
336. Mei Y, Qian F, Wei M, et al. Reversal of cancer by green tea polyphenols. *J Pharm Pharmacol*. 2004;56:1307-1314.
337. Stammler G, Volm M. Green tea catechins (EGCG and EGC) have modulating effects on the activity of doxorubicin in drug resistant cell lines. *Anticancer Drugs*. 1997;8:265-268.
338. Deng S, Yan T, Jendrny C, et al. Dexrazoxane may prevent doxorubicin-induced DNA damage via depleting both topoisomerase II isoforms. *BMC Cancer*. 2014;14. doi:10.1186/471-2407-14-842.
339. Mele D, Nardozza M, Spallarossa P, et al. Current views on anthracycline cardiotoxicity. *Heart Fail Rev*. 2016;21:621-634.
340. Malisza K, Hasinhoff B. Production of hydroxyl radical by iron(III) – anthraquinone complexes through self-reduction and through reductive activation by the xanthine oxidase/hypoxanthine systen. *Arch Biochem Biophys*. 1995;1:51-60.
341. Hasinhoff B, Wu X, Patel D, et al. Mechanisms of action and reduced cardiotoxicity of pixantrone: a topisomerase II targeting agents with cellular selectivity for the topoisomerase IIa isoform. *J Pharmacol Exp Ther*. 2016;356:397-409.
342. Mordente A, Meucci E, Silvestrini G, et al. New developments in anthracycline-induced cardiotoxicity. *Curr Med Chem*. 2009;16:1656-1672.
343. Lothstein L, Israel M, Sweatman T. Anthracycline drug targeting: cytoplasmic versus nuclear-a fork in the road. *Drug Res Updat*. 2001;4:169-177.
344. Swain S, Vici P. The current and future role of dexrazoxane as a cardioprotectant in anthracycline treatment: expert panel review. *J Cancer Res Clin Oncol*. 2004;130:1-7.
345. Malisza K, Hasinhoff B. Inhibition of anthracycline semiquinone formation by ICRF-187 (dexrazoxane) in cells. *Free Radic Biol Med*. 1996;20:905-914.
346. Kassner N, Huse K, Martin H, et al. Carbonyl reductase 1 is a predominant doxorubicin reductase in human liver. *Drug Metab Dispos*. 2008;36:2113-2120.
347. Yamashita T, Fukushima T, Ueda T. Pharmacokinetic self-potentiation of idarubicin by induction of anthracycline carbonyl reducing enzymes. *Leuk Lymphoma*. 2008;49:809-814.
348. Giesberg C, Sawyer D. Mechanisms of anthracycline cardiotoxicity and strategies to decrease cardiac damage. *Curr Hypertens Rep*. 2010:12.
349. Vejpongsa P, Yeh E. Topisomerase 2b; a promising molecular target for primary prevention of anthracycline-induced cardiotoxicity. *Clin Pharmacol Ther*. 2014;95:45-52.
350. Vejpongsa P, Yeh E. Prevention of anthracycline-induced cardiotoxicity. *J Am Coll Cardiol*. 2014;64:938-945.
351. Tahover E, Patil Y, Gabizon A. Emerging delivery systems to reduce doxorubicin cardiotoxicity and improve therapeutic index: focus on liposomes. *Anticancer Drugs*. 2014;26:241-258.
352. Hasan S, Dinh K, Lombardo F, et al. Doxorubicin cardiotoxicity in African Americans. *J Natl Med Assoc*. 2004;96:196-199.
353. Lyu Y, Kerrigan J, Lin C, et al. Topoisomerase IIbeta mediated DNA double-strand breaks: implications in doxorubicin cariotoxicity and prevention by dexrazoxane. *Cancer Res*. 2007;67:8839-8846.
354. Hasinoff B. The use of dexrazoxane for the prevention of anthracycline extravasation injury. *Expert Opin Invest Drugs*. 2008;17:217-223.
355. Waterhouse D, Tardi P, Mayer L, et al. A comparison of liposomal formulations of doxorubicin with drug administered in free form: changing toxicity profiles. *Drug Saf*. 2001;24:903-920.
356. Gong J, Yan J, Forscher C, et al. Aldoxrubicin: a tumor-targeted doxorubicin conjugate for relapsed or refractory soft tissue sarcomas. *Drug Des Devel Ther*. 2018;12:777-786.
357. Sachdev E, Sachdev D, Mita M. Aldoxorubicin for the treament of soft tissue sarcoma. *Expert Opin Invest Drugs*. 2017;26:1175-1179.
358. Seetharam M, Kolla K, Ganjoo K. Aldoxorubicin therapy for the treatment of patients with advanced soft tissue sarcoma. *Future Oncol*. 2018.
359. Kratz F, Warnecke A, Scheuermann K, et al. Probing the cysteine-34 position of endogenous serum albumin with thiol-binding doxorubicin derivatives. Improved efficacy of an acid-sensitive doxorubicin derivative with specific albumin-binding properties compared to that of the parent compound. *J Med Chem*. 2002;45:5523-5533.
360. Salvatorelli E, Menna P, Lusini M, et al. Doxorubicinolone formation and efflux: a salvage pathway against epirubicin accumulation in human heart. *J Pharmacol Exp Ther*. 2009;329:175-184.
361. Kang W, Weiss M. Caffeine enhances the myocardial uptake of idarubicin but reverses its negative inotropic effect. *Naunyn Schmiedelbergs Arch Pharmacol*. 2003;367:151-155.
362. Sharma P, Zarger-Shoshtari K, Sexton W, et al. Valrubicin in refractory non-muscle invasive bladder cancer. *Expert Rev Anticancer Ther*. 2015;15:1379-1389.
363. Grossman H, O'Donnell M, Cookson M, et al. Bacillus Calmette-Guerin failures and beyond: contemporary management of non-muscle invasive bladder cancer. *Rev Urol*. 2008;10:281-289.
364. Expert to Discuss Treatment of BCG Refractory Carcinoma In situ. American Urological Association. Available at http://www.auadailynews.org/expert-to-discuss-treatment-of-bcg-refractory-carcinoma-in-situ/. Accessed July 19, 2018.
365. Reis-Mendes A, Gomes A, Carvalho R, et al. Naphthoquinoxaline metabolite of mitoxantrone is less cardiotoxic than the parent compound and it can be a more cardiosafe drug in anticancer therapy. *Arch Toxicol*. 2017;91:1871-1890.
366. Qin Z, Li X, Zhang J, et al. Chemotherapy with or without estramustine for treatment of castration-resistant prostate cancer: a systematic review and meta-analysis. *Medicine*. 2016;95:e4801.
367. Song P, Huang C, Wang Y. The efficacy and safety comparison of docetaxel, cabazitaxel, estraumustine, and mitoxantrone for castration-resistant prostate cancer: a network meta-analysis. *Int J Surg*. 2018;56:133-140.
368. Zhang C, Jing T, Wang F, et al. Chemotherapy plus estramustine for management of castration-resistant prostate cancer: meta-analysis of randomized controlled trials. *Actas Urol Esp*. 2014;38:184-191.
369. Yue Q, Liu X, Guo D. Microtubule-binding natural products for cancer therapy. *Planta Med*. 2010;76:1037-1043.
370. Hait W, Yang J-M. The individualization of cancer therapy: the unexpected role of p53. *Transact Am Clin Climatol Assoc*. 2006;117:85-101.
371. Duran G, Derdau V, Weitz D, et al. Cabazetaxil is more active than first generation taxanes in ABCB1(+) cell lines due to its reduced affinity for P-glycoprotein. *Cancer Chemother Pharmacol*. 2018;81:1095-1103.
372. Lopus M, Smiyun G, Miller H, et al. Mechanism of action of ixabepilone and its interaction with the bIII-tubulin isotype. *Cancer Chemother Pharmacol*. 2015;76:1013-1024.
373. Islam M, Song Y, Iskander M. Investigation of structural requirements of anticancer activity at the paclitaxel/tubulin binding site using CoMFA and CoMSIA. *J Mol Graph Model*. 2003;21:263-272.

374. Maccari L, Manetti F, Corelli F, et al. 3D QSAR studies for the β-tubulin binding site of microtubule-stabilizing anticancer agents (MSAAs). A pseudoreceptor model for taxanes based on the experimental structure of tubulin. *Il Farmaco*. 2003;58:659-668.
375. Manetti F, Forli S, Maccari L, et al. 3D QSAR studies of the interaction between β-tubulin and microtubule stabilizing antimitotic agents (MSAA): a combined pharmacophore generation and pseudoreceptor modeling approach applied to taxanes and epothilones. *Il Farmaco*. 2003;58:357-361.
376. Manetti F, Maccari L, Corelli F, et al. 3D QSAR models of interactions between β-tubulin and microtubule stabilizing antimitotic agents (MSAA): a survey on taxanes and epothilones. *Curr Topics Med Chem*. 2004;4:203-217.
377. Yang Y, Alcaraz A, Snyder J. The tubulin-bound conformation of paclitaxel: T-taxol vs. "PTX-NY." *J Natl Prod*. 2009;72:422-429.
378. Gueritte F. General and recent aspects of the chemistry and structure-activity relationships of taxoids. *Curr Pharm Des*. 2001;7:1229-1249.
379. Cresteil T, Monsarrat B, DuBois J, et al. Regioselective metabolism of taxoids by human CYP3A4 and 2C8: structure-activity relationship. *Drug Metab Dispos*. 2002;39:438-445.
380. Omran M, Badary O, Helal A, et al. A prospective phamacokinetic study of docetaxel in breast cancer patients in relation to CYP3A4 activity. *Clin Pharmacol Biopharm*. 2016;5. doi:10.4172/2167–065X.1000156.
381. De Luca A, D'Alessio A, Maiello M, et al. Evaluation of the pharmacokinetics of ixabepilone for the treatment of breast cancer. *Expert Opin Drug Metab Toxicol*. 2015;11:1177-1185.
382. Altmann K-H. Epothilone B and its analogs: a new family of anticancer agents. *Mini Rev Med Chem*. 2003;3:149-158.
383. Buey R, Diaz J, Andreu J, et al. Interation of epothilone analogs with the paclitaxel binding site: relationship between binding affinity, microtubule stabilization, and cytotoxicity. *Chem Biol Rev*. 2004;11:225-236.
384. Hunt J. Discovery of ixabepilone. *Mol Cancer Ther*. 2009;8:275-281.
385. Heinz D, Schubert W-D, Hofle G. Much anticipated–the bioactive conformation of epothilone and its binding to tubulin. *Angew Chem Int Ed*. 2005;44:1298-1301.
386. Navarrete K, Alderete J, Jimenez V. Structural basis for drug resistance conferred by b tubulin mutations: a molecular modeling study on native and mutated tubulin complexes with epothilone B. *J Biomol Struct Dyn*. 2015;33:2530-2540.
387. Wang F, Porter M, Konstantopoulos A, et al. Preclinical development of drug delivery systems for paclitaxel-based cancer chemotherapy. *J Control Release*. 2017;267:100-118.
388. Hait W, Rubin E, Goodin S. Tubulin-targeting agents. In: Giaconne G, Schilsky R, Sondel P, eds. *Cancer Chemotherapy and Biological Response Modifiers*. New York: Elsevier B.V.; 2003:41-67.
389. Gupta N, Hatoum H, Dy G. First line treatment of advanced non-small cell lung cancer – specific focus on albumin bound paclitaxel. *Int J Nanomedicine*. 2014;9:209-221.
390. Mechanism of Action for Abraxane (Nab-Paclitaxel, Paclitaxel albumin). *Européenne de Formation pour les Pharmaciens*. Available at https://www.youtube.com/watch?v=BsLLZxXLSfA. Accessed July 30, 2018.
391. Engles F, Ten-Tije A, Baker S, et al. Effect of cytochrome P450 3A4 inhibition on the pharmacokinetics of docetaxel. *Clin Pharmacol Ther*. 2004;75:448-454.
392. Mita A, Denis L, Rowinsky E, et al. Phase I and pharmacokinetic study of XRP6258 (RPR 116258A), a novel taxane, administered as a 1-hour infusion every 3 weeks in patients with advanced solid tumors. *Clin Cancer Res*. 2009;15:723-730.
393. Oudard S, Kizazi K, Sengelov L, et al. Cabazitaxel vs. docetaxel as first-line therapy for patients with metastatic castration-resistant prostate cancer: a randomized phase III trial-FIRSTANA. *J Clin Oncol*. 2017;35:3189-3197.
394. Eisenberger M, Hardy-Bessard A, Kim C, et al. Phase III study comparing a reduced dose of cabazitaxel (20 mg/m^2) and the currently approved dose (25 mg/m^2) in postdocetaxel patients with metastatic castration-resistant prostate cancer-PROSELICA. *J Clin Oncol*. 2017;35:3198-3206.
395. Donovan D, Vahdat L. Epothilones: clinical update and future directions. *Oncology*. 2008;22:408-416.
396. Li J, Ren J, Sun W. Systematic review of ixabepilone for treating metastatic breast cancer. *Breast Cancer*. 2017;24:171-179.
397. Pellegrini F, Budman D. Review: tubulin function, actions of antitubulin drugs, and new drug development. *Cancer Invest*. 2005;23:264-273.
398. Gigant B, Wang C, Ravelli R, et al. Structual basis for the regulation of tubulin by vinblastine. *Nature*. 2005;435:519-522.
399. Beck W, Cass C, Houghton P. Microtubule-targeting anticancer drugs derived from plants and microbes: vinca alkaloids, taxanes and epothiolones. In: Bast RJ, Kufe D, Pollock R, et al, eds. *Cancer Medicine*. Vol 5. New York: BC Decker Inc.; 2003:680-698.
400. Islam M, Iskander M. Microtubulin binding sites as target for developing anticancer agents. *Mini Rev Med Chem*. 2004;4:1077-1104.
401. Chi S, Xie W, Zhang J, et al. Theoretical insight into the structural mechanism for the binding of vinblastine with tubulin. *J Biomol Struct Dyn*. 2015;33:2234-2254.
402. Kelly E, Tuszynski J, Klobukowski M. QM and QM/MD simulations of the vinca alkaloids docked to tubulin. *J Mol Graph Model*. 2011;30:50-66.
403. Chabner B, Ryan D, Paz-Ares L, et al. Antineoplastic agents. In: Hardman J, Limbird L, eds. *Goodman & Gilman's the Pharmacological Basis of Therapeutics*. 10 ed. New York: McGraw Hill; 2001:1389–1459.
404. Beulz-Riche D, Grude P, Puozzo C, et al. Characterization of human cytochrome P450 isoenzymes involved in the metabolism of vinorelbine. *Fundam Clin Pharmacol*. 2005;19:545-553.
405. Egbelakin A, Ferguson M, MacGill E. Increased risk of vincristine neurotoxicity associated with low CYP3A5 expression genotype in children with acute lymphoblastic leukemia. *Pediatr Blood Cancer*. 2011;56:361-367.
406. Dennison J, Mohutsky M, Barbuch R, et al. Apparent high CYP3A5 expression is required for significant metabolism of vincristine by human cryopreserved hepatocytes. *J Pharmacol Exp Ther*. 2008;327:248-257.
407. Topletz A, Dennison J, Barbuch R, et al. The relative contributions of CYP3A4 and CYP3A5 to the metabolism of vinorelbine. *Drug Metab Dispos*. 2013;41:1651-1661.
408. Yao D, Ding S, Burchell B, et al. Detoxication of vinca alkaloids by human P450 CYP3A4-mediated metabolism: implications for the develoment of drug resistance. *J Pharmacol Exp Ther*. 2000;294:387-395.
409. KSangkuhl. Vinca Alkaloid Pathway, Pharmacokinetics. PharmGKB. Available at https://www.pharmgkb.org/pathway/PA150981002. Accessed August 1, 2018.
410. Preston J, Trivedi M. Eribulin: a novel cytotoxic chemotherapy agent. *Ann Pharmacother*. 2012;46:802-810.
411. Bai R, Nguyen T, Burnett J, et al. Interactions of halichondrin B and eribulin with tubulin. *J Chem Inf Model*. 2011;51:1393-1404.
412. Jain S, Cigler T. Eribulin mesylate in the treatment of metastatic breast cancer. *Biologics*. 2012;6:21-29.
413. Vahdat L, Pruitt B, Fabian C, et al. Phase II study of eribulin mesylate, a Halichondrin B analog, in patients with mestastatic breast cancer previously treated with an anthracycline and a taxane. *J Clin Oncol*. 2009;27:2954-2961.
414. Gerson S, Caimi P, William B, et al. Pharmacology and molecular mechanisms of antineoplastic agents for hematologic malignancies. In: Hoffman R, Benz E, Silberstein L, et al, eds. *Hematology: Basic Principles and Practice*. 7th ed. Philadelphia: Elsevier; 2018:895.
415. Asadov C, Aliyeva G, Mustafayeva K. Thiopurine S-methyltransferase as a pharmacogenetic biomarker: significance of testing and reivew of major methods. *Cardiovasc Hematol Agents Med Chem*. 2017;15:23-30.

416. de Beaumais T, Jacqz-Aigrain E. Pharmacogenetic determinants of mercaptopurine disposition in children with acute lymphoblastic leukemia. *Eur J Clin Pharmacol.* 2012;68:1233-1242.
417. Cara C, Pena A, Sans M, et al. Reviewing the mechanism of action of thiopurine drugs: towards a new paradigm in clinical practice. *Med Sci Mont.* 2004;10:247-254.
418. Coulthard S, Hogarth L, Little M, et al. The effect of thiopurine methyltransferase expression on sensitivity to thiopurine drugs. *Mol Pharmacol.* 2002;62:102-109.
419. Hartford C, Vasquez E, Schwab M, et al. Differential effects of targeted disruption of thiopurine methyltransferase on mercaptopurine and thioguanine pharmacodynamics. *Cancer Res.* 2007;67:4965-4972.
420. Giamanco N, Cunningham B, Klein L, et al. Allopurinol use during maintenance therapy for acute lymphoblastic leukemia avoids mercaptopurine-related hepatoxicity. *J Pediatr Hematol Oncol.* 2016;38:147-151.
421. Marsh S, Booven D. The increasing complexity of mercaptopurine pharmacogenomics. *Clin Pharmacol Ther.* 2009;85:139-141.
422. Stocco G, Cheok M, Crews K, et al. Genetic polymorphism of inositol triphosphate pyrophosphatase is a determinant of mercaptopurine metabolism and toxicity during treatment for lymphoblastic leukemia. *Clin Pharmacol Ther.* 2009;85:164-172.
423. Coulthard S, Hogarth L. The thiopurines: an update. *Invest New Drugs.* 2005;23:523-532.
424. Zerra P, Bergsagel J, Keller F, et al. Maintenance treatment with low-dose mercaptopurine in combination with allopurinol in children with acute lymphoblastic leukemia and mercaptopurine-induced pancreatitis. *Pediatr Blood Cancer.* 2016;63:712-715.
425. Fotoohi A, Lindqvist M, Peterson C, et al. Impaired transport as a mechanism of resistance to thiopurines in human T-lymphoblastic leukemia cells. *Nucleosides Nucleotides Nucleic Acids.* 2006;25:1039-1044.
426. Saif M, Chu E. Antimetabolites. In: DeVita V, Lawrence T, Rosenberg S, eds. *DeVita, Hellman and Rosenberg's Cancer: Principles & Practice of Oncology.* 10th ed. Philadelphia: Wolters Kluwer; 2015.
427. Guliana S, Polkinghorne I, Smith GA, et al. Macropodid herpesvirus 1 encodes genes for both thymidylate synthase and ICP34.5. *Virus Genes.* 2002;24:207-213.
428. Jarmula A, Fraczyk T, Cieplak P, et al. Mechanism of influence of phosphorylation on serine 124 on a decrease of catalytic activity of human thymidylate synthase. *Bioorg Med Chem.* 2010;18:3361-3370.
429. Schiffer C, Clifton I, Davisson V, et al. Crystal structure of human thymidylate synthase: a structural mechanism for guiding substrates into the active site. *Biochemistry.* 1995;34:16279-16287.
430. Kamb A, Finer-Moore J, Calvert A, et al. Structural basis for recognition of polyglutamyl folates by thymidylate synthase. *Biochemistry.* 1992;31:9883-9890.
431. Gibson L, Celeste L, Lovelace L, et al. Structures of human thymidylate synthase R163K with dUMP, FdUMP and glutathione show asymmetric ligand binding. *Acta Crystallogr D Biol Crystallogr.* 2011;67(pt 1):60-66.
432. Ma W, Saif M, El-Rayes B, et al. Emergency use of uridine triacetate for the prevention and treatment of life-threatening 5-fluro-uracil and capecitabine toxicity. *Cancer.* 2017;123:345-356.
433. Lee A, Ezzeldin H, Fourie J, et al. Dihydropyrimidine dehydrogenase deficiency: impact of pharmacogenetics on 5-fluorouracil therapy. *Virchows Arch.* 2004;2:527-532.
434. Mattison L, Fourie J, Desmond R, et al. Increased prevalence of dihydropyrimidine dehydrogenase deficiency in African-Americans compared to Caucasians. *Cancer Ther Clin.* 2006;12:5491-5495.
435. Launay M, Dahan L, Duval M, et al. Beating the odds: efficacy and toxicity of dihydropyrimidine dehydrogenase-driven adaptive dosing of 5-FU in patients with digestive cancer. *Br J Clin Pharmacol.* 2016;81:124-130.
436. Garcia R, Saydoff J, Bamat M, et al. Prompt treatment with uridine triacetate improves survival and reduces toxicity due to fluorouracil and capecitabine overdose or dihydropyrimidine dehydrogenase deficiency. *Toxicol Appl Pharmacol.* 2018;353:67-73.
437. Kummar S, Noronha V, Chu E. Antimetabolites. In: DeVita VJ, Hellman S, Rosenberg S, eds. *Cancer: Principles and Practice of Oncology.* 7th ed. Baltimore, MD: Lippincott Williams & Wilkins; 2005:365-374.
438. Dummins P, Gready J. Energetically most likely substrate and active-site protonation sites and pathways in the catalytic mechanism of dihydrofolate reductase. *J Am Chem Soc.* 2001;123:3418-3428.
439. Cannon W, Garrison B, Benkovic S. Consideration of the pH-dependent inhibition of dihydrofolate reductase by methotrexate. *J Mol Biol.* 1997;271:656-668.
440. Cody V, Luft J, Ciszak E, et al. Crystal structure determination at 2.3 angstrom of recombinant human dihydrofolate reductase ternary complex with NADPH and methotrexate-γ-tetrazole. *Anticancer Drug Des.* 1992;7:483-491.
441. Klon A, Heroux A, Ross L, et al. Atomic structures of human dihydrofolate reductase complexed with NADPH and two lipophilic antifolates at 1.09 angstrom and 1.05 angstrom resolution. *J Mol Biol.* 2002;320:677-693.
442. Meiering E, Li H, Delcamp T, et al. Contributions of tryptophan 24 and glutamate 30 to binding long-lived water molecules in the ternary complex of human dihydrofolate reductase with methotrexate and NADPH studies by site directed mutagenesis and nuclear magnetic resonance spectroscopy. *J Mol Biol.* 1995;241:309-325.
443. Wojtuszkiewicz A, Peters G, van Woerden N, et al. Methotrexate resistance in relation to treatment outcome in childhood acute lymphoblastic leukemia. *J Hematol Oncol.* 2015;8. doi:10.1186/s13045-015-0158-9.
444. Visentin M, Unal E, Zhao R, et al. The membrane transport and polyglutamation of pralatrexate: a new generation dihydrofolate reducatase inhibitor. *Cancer Chemother Pharmacol.* 2013;72:597-606.
445. Rouch J, Burton B, Dabb A, et al. Comparison of enteral and parenteral methods of urine alkalinization in patients receiving high-dose methotrexate. *J Oncol Pharm Pract.* 2017;23:3-9.
446. Zelcer S, Kellick M, Wexler L, et al. The Memorial Sloan Kettering Cancer Center experience with outpatient administration of high dose methotrexate with leucovorin rescue. *Pediatr Blood Cancer.* 2008;50:1176-1180.
447. Flombaum C, Meyers P. High dose leucovorin as sole therapy for methotrexate toxicity. *J Clin Oncol.* 1999;17:1589-1594.
448. Perez-Moreno M, Galvan-Banqueri M, Flores-Moreno S, et al. Systematic review of efficacy and safety of pemetrexed in non-small-cell-lung cancer. *Int J Clin Pharm.* 2014;36:476-487.
449. Shah M, Winfree K, Peterson P, et al. Cost effectiveness of first-line pemetrexed plus platinum compared with other regimens in the treatment of patients with nonsquamous non-small cell lung cancer in the US outpatient setting. *Lung Cancer.* 2013;82:121-127.
450. Han B, Yang L, Wang X, et al. Efficacy of pemetrexed-based regimens in advanced non-small cell lung cancer patients with activating epidermal growth factor receptor mutations after tyrosine kinase inhibitor failure: a systematic review. *Onco Targets Ther.* 2018;11:2121-2129.
451. Chattopadhyay S, Moran R, Goldman D. Pemetrexed: biochemical and cellular pharmacology, mechanisms, and clinical applications. *Mol Cancer Ther.* 2007;6:404-417.
452. Joerger M, Omlin A, Cerny T, et al. The role of pemetrexed in advanced non small-cell lung cancer: special focus on pharmacology and mechanism of action. *Curr Drug Topics.* 2010;11:37-47.
453. Villela L, Stanford B, Shah S. Pemetrexed, a novel antifolate therapeutic alternative for cancer chemotherapy. *Pharmacotherapy.* 2006;26:641-654.
454. Mendelsohn L, Shih C, Chen V, et al. Enzyme inhibition, polyglutamation and the effect of LY231514 (MTA) on purine biosynthesis. *Semin Oncol.* 1999;26(suppl 6):42-47.
455. Sayre P, Finer-Moore J, Fritz T, et al. Multi-targeted antifolates aimed at avoiding drug resistance form covalent closed inhibitory complexes with human and *Escherichia coli* thymidylate synthases. *J Mol Biol.* 2001;313:813-829.

456. Liu Y, Yin T-J, Zhou R, et al. Expression of thymidylate synthase predicts clinical outcomes of pemetrexed-containing chemotherapy for non-small-cell lung cancer: a systematic review and meta-analysis. *Cancer Chemother Pharmacol*. 2013;72:1125-1132.
457. Uemura T, Oguri T, Ozasa H, et al. ABCC11/MRP8 confers pemetrexed resistance in lung cancer. *Cancer Sci*. 2010;101:2404-2410.
458. Izbicka E, Diaz A, Streeper R, et al. Distinct mechanistic activity profile of pralatrexate in comparison to other antifolates in in vitro and in vivo models of human cancers. *Cancer Chemother Pharmacol*. 2009;64:993-999.
459. O'Connor O. Pralatreate: an emerging new agent with activity in T-cell lymphoma. *Curr Opin Oncol*. 2006;18:591-597.
460. O'Connor O, Hamlin P, Portlock C, et al. Pralatrexate, a novel class of antifol with high affinity for the reduced folate carrier-type 1, produces marked complete and durable remissions in a diversity of chemotherapy refractor cases of T-cell lymphoma. *Br J Haematol*. 2007;139:425-428.
461. Molina J. Pralatrexate, a dihydrofolate reductase inhibitor for the potential treatment of several malignancies. *IDrugs*. 2008;11:508-521.
462. Rueda A, Casanova M, Quero C, et al. Pralatrexate, a new hope for aggressive T-cell lymphoma? *Clin Transl Oncol*. 2009;11:215-220.
463. Serova M, Bieche I, Sablin M, et al. Single agent and combination studies of pralatexate and molecular correlates of sensitivity. *Br J Cancer*. 2011;104:272-280.
464. Mould D, Sweeney K, Duffull S, et al. A population pharmacokinetic and pharmacodynamic evaluation of pralatrexate in patients with relapsed or refractory non-Hodgkin's or Hodgkin's lymphoma. *Clin Pharmacol Ther*. 2008;86:190-196.
465. O'Connor O, Amengual J, Colbourn D, et al. Pralatrexate: a comprehensive update on pharmacology, clinical activity and strategies to optimize use. *Leuk Lymphoma*. 2017;58:2548-2557.
466. Weinberg B, Marshall J, Salem M. Trifluridine/tipiracil and regorafenib: new weapons in the war against metastatic colorectal cancer. *Clin Adv Hematol Oncol*. 2016;14:630-639.
467. Plunkett W, Huang P, Xu Y, et al. Gemcitabine: metabolism, mechanism of action, and self-potentiation. *Semin Oncol*. 1995;22:3-10.
468. Cai J, Damaraju V, Grouix N, et al. Two distinct molecular mechanisms underlying cytarabine resistance in human leukemic cells. *Cancer Res*. 2008;68:2349-2357.
469. van der Velden D, Opdam F, Voest E. TAS-102 for treatment of advanced colorectal cancers that are no longer responding to other therapies. *Clin Cancer Res*. 2016;22:2835-2839.
470. Puthiamadathil J, Weinberg B. Emerging combination therapies for metastatic colorectal cancer-impact of trifluridine/tipiracil. *Cancer Manag Res*. 2017;9:461-469.
471. Lee J, Chu E. Adherence, dosing, and managing toxicites with trifluridine/tipiracil (TAS-102). *Clin Colorectal Cancer*. 2017;16:85-92.
472. White T, Larson H, Minnella A, et al. Metastatic colorectal cancer. *Clin J Oncol Nurs*. 2017;21:E30-E7.
473. Fakih R, Komrokji R, Shaheen M, et al. Azacitidine use for myeloid neoplasms. *Clin Lymphoma Myeloma Leuk*. 2018;18:e147-e155.
474. Xu P, Hu G, Luo C, et al. DNA methyltransferase inhibitors: an updated patent review (2012-2015). *Expert Opin Ther Pat*. 2016;26:1017-1030.
475. Bohl S, Bullinger L, Rucker F. Epigenetic therapy: azacytidine and decitabine in acute myeloid leukemia. *Expert Rev Hematol*. 2018;11:361-371.
476. Seelan R, Mukhopadhyay P, Piasano M, et al. Effects of 5-aza-2'-deoxycytidine (decitabine) on gene expression. *Drug Metab Rev*. 2018;50:193-207.
477. Anders N, Liu J, Wanjiku T, et al. Simultaneous quantitative determination of 5-aza-2'-deoxycytidine genomic incorporation and DNA methylation by liquid chromatography tandem mass spectrometry as exposure-response measures of nucleoside analog DNA methyltransferase inhibitors. *J Chromatogr B Analyt Technol Biomed Life Sci*. 2016;1022:38-45.
478. Kadia T, Gandhi V. Nelarabine in the treatment of pediatric and adult patients with T-cell acute lymphoblastic leukemia and lymphoma. *Expert Rev Hematol*. 2017;10:1-8.
479. Scott L. Azacitidine: a review in myelodyspastic syndromes and acute myeloid leukaemia. *Drugs*. 2016;76:889-900.
480. Lamanna N, Kay N. Pentostatin treatment combinations in chronic lymphocytic leukemia. *Clin Adv Hematol Oncol*. 2009;7:386-392.
481. Kay N, LaPlant B, Pettinger A, et al. Cumulative experience and long term follow-up of pentostatin-based chemoimmunotherapy trials for patients with chronic lymphocytic leukemia. *Expert Rev Hematol*. 2018;11:337-349.
482. Kovacic P. Hydroxyurea (therapeutics and mechanism): metabolism, carbamoyl nitroso, nitroxyl, radicals, cell signaling and clinical applications. *Med Hypotheses*. 2011;76:24-31.
483. Trepte M, Auten J, Clark S, et al. Dose related mucositic with hydroxyurea for cytoreduction in acute myeloid leukemia. *J Oncol Pharm Pract*. 2018. doi:10.1177/1078155218758499.
484. Ludeman S. The chemistry of the metabolites of cyclophosphamide. *Curr Pharm Des*. 1999;5:627-643.
485. Larranaga O, de Cozar A, Cossio F. Mono- and di-alkylation process of DNA bases by nitrogen mustard mechlorethamine. *Chem Phys Chem*. 2017;18:3390-3401.
486. Vidal L, Gurion R, Ram R, et al. Chlorambucil for the treatment of patients with chronic lymphocytic leukemia (CLL) – a systematic review and meta-analysis of randomized trials. *Leuk Lymphoma*. 2016;57:2047-2057.
487. Dulik D, Colvin O, Fenselau C. Characterizaton of glutathione conjugates of chlorambucil by fast atom bombardment and thermospray liquid chromatography/mass spectrometry. *Biomed Environ Mass Spectrom*. 1990;19:248-252.
488. Lepretre S, Dartigeas C, Feugier P, et al. Systematic review of the recent evidence for the efficacy and safety of chlorambucil in the treatment of B-cell malignancies. *Leuk Lymphoma*. 2016;57:852-865.
489. Goldenberg G, Lee M, Lam H, et al. Evidence for carrier-mediated transport of melphalan by L5178Y lymphoblasts in vitro. *Cancer Res*. 1977;37:755-760.
490. Al-Sawaf O, Cramer P, Goede V, et al. Bendamustine and its role in the treatment of unfit patients with chronic lymphocytic leukemia: a perspective review. *Ther Adv Hematol*. 2017;8:197-205.
491. Tageja N, Nagi J. Bendamustine: something old, something new. *Cancer Chemother Pharmacol*. 2010;66:413-423.
492. Montillo M, Ricci F, Tedeschi A, et al. Bendamustine: new perspective for an old drug in lymphoproliferative disorders. *Expert Rev Hematol*. 2010;3:131-148.
493. Martin P, Barr P, James L, et al. Long-term safety experience with bendamustine for injection in a real-world setting. *Expert Opin Drug Saf*. 2017;16:647-650.
494. Giraud B, Herbert G, Deroussent A, et al. Oxazaphosphorines: new therapeutic strategies for an old class of drugs. *Expert Opin Drug Metab Toxicol*. 2010;6:919-938.
495. Huang A, Roy P, Waxman D. Role of human liver microsomal CYP3A4 and CYP2B6 in catalyzing N-dechloroethylation of cyclophosphamide and ifosfamide. *Biochem Pharmacol*. 2000;59:961-972.
496. Lind M, McGown A, Hadfield J, et al. The effect of ifosfamide and its metabolites on intracellular glutathione levels in vitro and in vivo. *Biochem Pharmacol*. 1989;38:1835-1840.
497. Madondo M, Quinn M, Plebanski M. Low dose cyclophosphamide: mechanisms of T cell modulation. *Cancer Treat Rev*. 2016;42:3-9.
498. Ramu K, Fraiser L, Mamiya B, et al. Acrolein mercapturates: synthesis, characterization and assessment of their role in the bladder toxicity of cyclophosphamide. *Chem Res Toxicol*. 1995;8:515-524.
499. Ramu K, Perry C, Ahmed T, et al. Studies on the basis for the toxicity of acrolein mercapturates. *Toxicol Appl Pharmacol*. 1996;140:487-498.
500. Matz E, Hsieh M. Review of advances in uroprotective agents for cyclophosphamide-and ifosfanide-induced hemorrhagic cystitis. *Urolology*. 2017;100:16-19.
501. Sannu A, Radha R, Mathews A, et al. Ifosfamide-induced malignancy of ureter and bladder. *Cureus*. 2017;9:e1594.
502. Springate J. Ifosfamide metabolite chloroacetaldehyde causes renal dysfunction in vivo. *J Appl Toxicol*. 1997;17:75-79.

503. Roy P, Yu L, Crespi C, et al. Development of a substrate-activity based approach to identify the major human liver P-450 catalysts of cyclophosphamide and ifosfamide activation based on cDNA-expressed activities and liver microsomal P-450 profiles. *Drug Metab Dispos*. 1999;27:655-666.
504. Woodland D, Ito S, Granvil C, et al. Evidence of renal metabolism of ifosfamide to nephrotoxic metabolites. *Life Sci*. 2000;68:109-117.
505. Storme T, Deroussent A, Mercier L, et al. New ifosfamide analogs designed for lower associated neurotoxicity and nephrotoxicity with modified alkylating kinetics leading to enhanced in vitro anticancer activity. *J Pharmacol Exp Ther*. 2009;328:598-609.
506. Hanly L, Chen N, Aleksa K, et al. N-acetylcysteine as a novel prophylactic treatment for ifosfamide-induced nephrotoxicity in children: translational pharmacokinetics. *J Clin Pharmacol*. 2012;52:55-64.
507. El-Din A, El-Sisi E, El-Syaad M, et al. Protective effects of alpha lipoic acid versus N-acetylcysteine on ifosfamide-induced nephrotoxicity. *Toxicol Ind Health*. 2015;31:97-107.
508. Syro L, Rotondo F, Camargo M, et al. Temozolomide and pituitary tumors: current understanding, unresolved issues, and future directions. *Front Endocrinol*. 2018;9:318.
509. Patterson L, Murray G. Tumour cytochrome P450 and drug activation. *Curr Pharm Des*. 2002;8:1335-1347.
510. Yamagata S, Ohmori S, Suzuki N, et al. Metabolism of dacarbazine by rat liver microsomes: contribution of CYP1A enzymes to dacarbazine N-demethylation. *Drug Metab Dispos*. 1998;26:379-382.
511. Moloney S, Prough R. Studies on the pathway of methane formation from procarbazine, a 2-methylbenzylhydrazine derivative, by rat liver microsomes. *Arch Biochem Biophys*. 1983;221:577-584.
512. Moloney S, Wiebkin P, Cummings S, et al. Metabolic activation of the terminal N-methyl group of N-isopropyl-alpha-(2-methylhydrazino)-p-toluamide hydrochloride (procarbazine). *Carcinogenesis*. 1985;6:397-401.
513. Jiang G, Jiang A-J, Xin Y, et al. Progression of O^6-methylguanine-DNA methyltransferase and temozolomide resistance in cancer research. *Mol Biol Rep*. 2014;41:6659-6665.
514. Messaoudi K, Clavreul A, Lagarce F. Toward an effective strategy in glioblastoma treatment. Part I: resistance mechanisms and strategies to overcome resistance of glioblastoma to temozolomide. *Drug Discov Today*. 2015;20:899-905.
515. Messaoudi K, Clavreul A, Lagarce F. Toward an effective strategy in glioblastoma treatment. Part II: RNA interference as a promising way to sensitize glioblastomas to temozolomide. *Drug Discov Today*. 2015;20:772-779.
516. Quinn C, Ma Q, Kudlac A, et al. Relative efficacy of granulocyte-macrophage colony-stimulating factor, dacarbazine, and glycoprotein 100 in metastatic melanoma: an indirect treatment comparison. *Adv Ther*. 2017;34:495-512.
517. Ludlum D. DNA alkylation by the haloethylnitrosoureas: nature of modifications produced and their enzymatic repair or removal. *Mut Res*. 1990;233:117-126.
518. Nikolova T, Roos W, Kramer O, et al. Chloroethylating nitrosoureas in cancer therapy: DNA damage, repair and cell death signaling. *Biochim Biophys Acta*. 2017;1868:29-39.
519. Eisenbrand G, Muller N, Denkel E, et al. DNA adducts and DNA damage by antineoplastic and carcinogenic N-nitrosocompounds. *J Cancer Res Clin Oncol*. 1986;112:196-204.
520. Bacolod M, Fehdrau R, Johnson S, et al. BCNU sequestration by metallothioneines may contribute to resistance in a medulloblastoma cell line. *Cancer Chemother Pharmacol*. 2009;63:753-758.
521. Teicher B. Newer cytotoxic agents: attacking cancer broadly. *Clin Cancer Res*. 2008;24:1610-1617.
522. Chaney S, Campbell S, Bassett E, et al. Recognition and processing of cisplatin- and oxaliplatin-DNA adducts. *Crit Rev Oncol Hematol*. 2005;53:3-11.
523. Duffy E, Fitzgerald W, Boyle K, et al. Nephrotoxicity: evidence in patients receiving cisplatin therapy. *Clin J Oncol Nurs*. 2018;22:175-183.
524. Crona D, Faso A, Nishijima T, et al. A systematic review of strategies to prevent cisplatin-induced nephrotoxicity. *Oncologist*. 2017;22:609-619.
525. Sheth S, Mukherjea D, Rybak L, et al. Mechanisms of cisplatin-induced ototoxicity and otoprotection. *Front Cell Neurosci*. 2017;11:338.
526. Gurney J, Bass J, Onar-Thomas A, et al. Evaluation of amifostine for protection against cisplatin-induced serious hearing loss in children treated for average-risk or high-risk medulloblastoma. *Neuro-Oncol*. 2014;16:848-855.
527. Ekborn A, Hansson J, Ehrsson H, et al. High-dose cisplatin with amifostine: ototoxicity and pharmacokinetics. *Laryngoscope*. 2004;114:1660-1667.
528. Johnsson A, Wennerberg J. Amifostine as a protector against cisplatin-induced toxicity in nude mice. *Acta Oncol*. 1999;38:247-253.
529. Fouladi M, Chintagumpala M, Ashley D, et al. Amifostine protects against cisplatin-induced ototoxicity in children with average-risk medulloblastoma. *J Clin Oncol*. 2008;26:3749-3755.
530. Fisher M, Lange B, Needle M, et al. Amifostine for children with medulloblastoma treated with cisplatin-based chemotherapy. *Pediatr Blood Cancer*. 2004;43:780-784.
531. Duval M, Daniel S. Meta-analysis of the efficacy of amifostine in the prevention of cisplatin ototoxicity. *Otolaryngol Head Neck Surg*. 2012;41:309-315.
532. Marina N, Chang K, Malogolowkin M, et al. Amifostine does not protect against the ototoxicity of high dose cisplatin combined with etoposide and bleomycin in pediatric germ-cell tumors: a Children's Oncology Group study. *Cancer*. 2005;104:841-847.
533. Asna N, Lewy H, Ashkenazi I, et al. Time dependent protection of amifostine from renal and hematopoietic cisplatin induced toxicity. *Life Sci*. 2005;76:1825-1834.
534. Gallegos-Castorena S, Martinez-Avalos A, Mohar-Betancourt A, et al. Toxcity prevention with amifostine in pediatric osteosarcoma patients treated with cisplatin and doxorubicin. *Pediatr Hematol Oncol*. 2007;24:403-408.
535. Hu Y, Zhu Q, Deng J, et al. Emerging role of non-coding RNAs in cisplatin resistance. *Onco Targets Ther*. 2018;11:3185-3194.
536. Kelland L. The resurgence of platinum-based cancer chemotherapy. *Nat Rev Clin Oncol*. 2007;7:573-584.
537. Riddell I. Cisplatin and oxaliplatin: our current understanding of their actions. *Met Ions Life Sci*. 2018;18. doi:10.1515/9783110470734–007.
538. Aguiar PJ, Tadokoro H, daSilva G, et al. Definitive chemoradiotherapy for squamous head and neck cancer: cisplatin vs. carboplatin? A meta-analysis. *Future Oncol*. 2016;12:2755-2764.
539. Ho G, Woodward N, Coward J. Cisplatin versus carboplatin: comparative review of therapeutic management in solid maligancies. *Crit Rev Oncol Hematol*. 2016;102:37-46.
540. Mishima M, Samimi G, Kondo A, et al. The cellular pharmacology of oxaliplatin resistance. *Eur J Cancer*. 2002;38:1405-1412.
541. Chaney S, Campbell S, Temple B, et al. Protein interactions with platinum-DNA adducts: from structure to function. *J Inorg Biochem*. 2004;98:1551-1559.
542. Barnes K, Lippard S. Cisplatin and related anticancer drugs: recent advances and insights. *Met Ions Biol Syst*. 2004;42:143-177.
543. Kweekel D, Gelderblom H, Guchelaar H-J. Pharmacology of oxaliplatin and the use of pharmacogenomics to individualize therapy. *Cancer Treat Rev*. 2005;31:90-105.
544. McKeage M. New-generation platinum drugs in the treatment of cisplatin-resistant cancers. *Expert Opin Invest Drugs*. 2005;14:1033-1046.
545. Cercek A, Park V, Yaeger R, et al. Faster FOLFOX: oxaliplatin can be safely infused at a rate of 1 mg/m2/min. *J Oncol Pract*. 2016;12:e548-53.
546. Wen F, Zhou Y, Wang W, et al. Ca/Mg infusions for the prevention of oxaliplatin-related neuropathy in patients with colorectal cancer: a meta analysis. *Ann Oncol*. 2013;24:171-178.

547. Grolleau F, Gamelin L, Boisdron-Celle M, et al. A possible explanation for a neurotoxic effect of the anticancer agent oxaliplatin on neuronal voltage-gated sodium channels. *J Neurophysiol.* 2001;85:2293-2297.
548. Gamelin L, Boisdron-Celle M, Delva R, et al. Prevention of oxaliplatin-related neurotoxicity by calcium and magnesium infusions: a retrospective study of 161 patients receiving oxaliplatin combined with 5-fluorouracil and leucovorin for advanced colorectal cancer. *Clin Cancer Res.* 2004;10:4055-4061.
549. Loprinzi C, Qin R, Dakhil S, et al. Phase III randomized, placebo-controlled, double-blind study of intravenous calcium and magnesium to prevent oxaliplatin-induced sensory neurotoxicity (N08CB/Alliance). *J Clin Oncol.* 2014;32:997-1005.
550. Grothy A, Nikcevich D, Sloan J, et al. Intervenous calicum and magnesium for oxaliplatin-induced sensory neurotoxicity in adjuvant colon cancer: NCCTG N04C7. *J Clin Oncol.* 2011;29:421-427.
551. Chaves J, Patel K, Abdelghany O, et al. Outcome of intravenious calcium and magnesium (Ca/Mg) in oxaliplatin-containing regimens compared with no Ca/Mg. *J Clin Oncol.* 2011;29(suppl):e19861.
552. Knijn N, Tol J, Koopman M, et al. The effect of prophylactic calcium and magnesium infusions on the incidence of neurotoxicity and clinical outcome of oxaliplatin-based system treatment in advanced colorectal cancer patients. *Eur J Cancer.* 2011;47:369-374.
553. Pachman D, Ruddy K, Sangaralingham L, et al. Calcium and magnesium use for oxaliplatin-induced neuropathy: a case study to assess how quickly evidence translates into practice. *J Natl Compr Canc Netw.* 2015;13:1097-1101.
554. Jordan B, Jahn F, Beckmann J, et al. Calcium and magnesium infusions for the prevention of oxaliplatin-induced peripheral neurotoxicity: a systematic review. *Oncology.* 2016;90:299-306.
555. Tatsushima Y, Egashira N, Narishige Y, et al. Calcium channel blockers reduce oxaliplatin-induced acute neuropathy: a retrospective study of 69 male patients receiving modified FOLFOX6 therapy. *Biomed Pharmacother.* 2013;67:39-42.
556. Chen M, May B, Zhou I, et al. Meta-analysis of oxaliplatin-based chemotherapy combined with traditional medicines for colorectal cancer: contributions of specific plants to tumor response. *Integr Cancer Ther.* 2016;15:40-59.
557. Bairey O, Vanichkin A, Shpilberg O. Arsenic-trioxide-induced apoptosis of chronic lymphocytic leukemia cells. *Int J Lab Hematol.* 2010;32:e77-85.
558. Hoonjan M, Jadhav V, Bhatt P, et al. Arsenic trioxide: insights into its evolution as an anticancer agent. *J Biol Inorg Chem.* 2018;23:313-329.
559. Akhtar A, Wang XS, Ghali L, et al. Recent advances in arsenic trioxide encapsulated nanoparticles as drug delivery agents to solid cancers. *J Biomed Res.* 2017;31:177-188.
560. Leu L, Mohassel L. Arsenic trioxide as first line treatment for acute promyelocytic leukemia. *Am J Health Syst Pharm.* 2009;66:1913-1918.
561. Liang B, Zheng Z, Shi Y, et al. Maintenance therapy with all-trans retinoic acid and arsenic trioxide improves relapse-free survival in adults with low- to intermediate-risk acute promyelocytic leukemia who have achieved complete remission after consolidation therapy. *Onco Targ Ther.* 2017;10:2305-2313.
562. Chen J, Stubbe J. Bleomycins: towards better therapeutics. *Nat Rev Cancer.* 2005;5:102-112.
563. Chow MS, Liu LV, Soloman EI. Further insights into the mechanism of the reaction of activated bleomycin with DNA. *Proc Natl Acad Sci.* 2008;105:13241-13245.
564. Grollman AP, Takeshita M, Pillai KMR, et al. Origin and cytotoxic properties of base propenals derived from DNA. *Cancer Res.* 1985;45:1127-1131.
565. Bolzan AD, Bianchi MS. DNA and chromosome damage induced by bleomycin in mammalian cells: an update. *Mutat Res Rev Mutat Res.* 2018;775:51-62.
566. Brewer GJ, Dick R, Ullenbruch MR, et al. Inhibition of key cytokines by tetrathiomolybdate in the bleomycin model of pulmonary fibrosis. *J Inorg Biochem.* 2004;98:2160-2167.
567. Li P, Xiao HD, Xu J, et al. Angiotensin converting enzyme N-terminal inactivation alleviates bleomycin-induced lung injury. *Am J Pathol.* 2010;177:1113-1121.
568. DiJoseph JF, Armellino DC, Bofhaert ER, et al. Antibody-targeted chemotherapy with CMC-544, a CD22-targeted immunoconjugate of calicheamicin for the treatment of B-lymphoid malignancies. *Blood.* 2004;103:1807-1814.
569. Ricart AD. Antibody-drug conjugates of calicheamicin derivative: gemtuzumab ozogamicin and inotuzumab ozogamicin. *Clin Cancer Res.* 2011;17:6417-6427.
570. Al-Salama ZT. Inotuzumab ozogamicin: a review in relaped/refractory B-cell acute lymphoblastic leukemia. *Target Oncol.* 2018;13:525-532.
571. Dang NH, Ogura M, Castaigne S, et al. Randomized, phase 3 trial of inotuzumab ozogamicin plus rituximab versus chemotherapy plus rituximab for relapsed/refractory aggressive B-cell non-Hodgkin lymphoma. *Br J Haematol.* 2018;182:583-586.
572. Petek BJ, Loggers ET, Pollack SM, et al. Trabectedin in soft tissue sarcomas. *Mar Drugs.* 2015;13:974-983.
573. Desar IME, Constantinidou A, Kaal S, et al. Advanced soft-tissue sarcoma and treatment options: critical appraisal of trabectedin. *Cancer Manag Res.* 2016;8:95-104.
574. DeSanctis R, Marrari A, Santoro A. Trabectedin for the treatment of soft tissue sarcomas. *Exp Opin Pharmacother.* 2016;17:1569-1577.
575. Beumer JH, Rademaker-Lakhai JM, Rosing H, et al. Metabolism of trabectedin (ET-43, YondelisTM) in patients with advanced cancer. *Cancer Chemother Pharmacol.* 2007;59:825-837.

Clinical Scenario

Victoria F. Roche, PhD

CHEMICAL ANALYSIS

This was a very sound recommendation to protect MF from drug-induced renal toxicity. Cisplatin is activated through the displacement of Cl^- by cellular water, generating the monoaquo and diaquo species capable of complexing with and cross-linking DNA, respectively. By increasing the concentration of chloride anions in the glomerular filtrate, the stability of the inactive cisplatin parent drug in the kidney is increased. It is much less likely that additional chloride anions will be displaced to add to an already enriched Cl^- aqueous environment, so drug activation will be minimized and renal function will be maintained.

(continued)

Clinical Scenario—Continued

Activation inhibited when $Cl^{\ominus}$ concentration is high

$$cis\text{-}[Pt(NH_3)_2Cl_2] \xrightarrow[H_2O]{-Cl^{\ominus}} [Pt(NH_3)_2Cl(OH_2)]^{\oplus} \xrightarrow[H_2O]{-Cl^{\ominus}} [Pt(NH_3)_2(OH_2)_2]^{2\oplus}$$

Cisplatin (inactive) — Cisplatin monoaquo form (active) — Cisplatin diaquo form (active)

In addition, magnesium deficiency has been linked to acute renal toxicity from cisplatin through increased platinum accumulation in the kidney and induction of drug-induced oxidative stress. Magnesium replacement/augmentation can reduce these risks and/or reverse these effects, attenuating acute kidney injury (AKI) risk without negatively impacting therapeutic action in tumor cells.

SECTION 8

Therapeutic Biologics

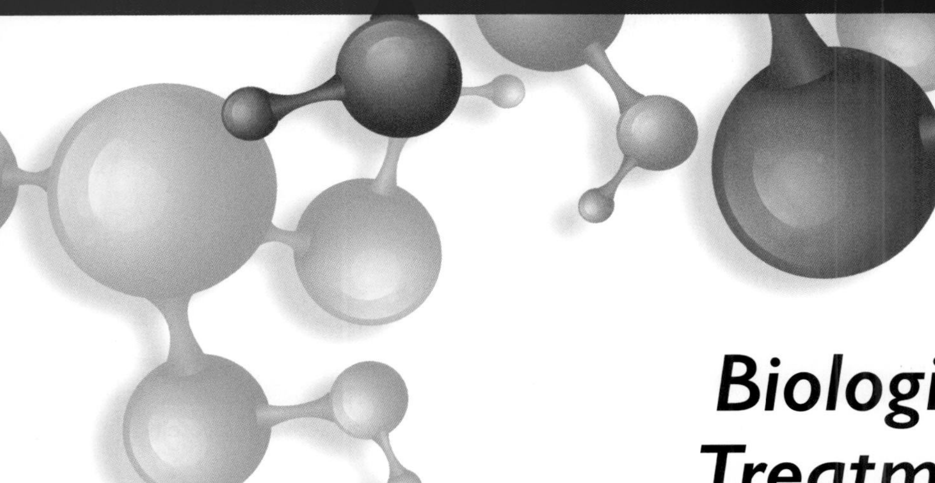

CHAPTER 34

Biologics Used in the Treatment of Disease

Vijaya L. Korlipara and Tanaji T. Talele

Drugs covered in this chapter:

ADRENOCORTICOTROPIC HORMONES
- Adrenocorticotropic hormone
- Cosyntropin

ANTIBODY-DRUG CONJUGATES
- Ado-trastuzumab emtansine
- Brentuximab vedotin
- Gemtuzumab ozogamicin
- Inotuzumab ozogamicin

ANTISENSE OLIGONUCLEOTIDES
- Nusinersen

CORTICOTROPIN-RELEASING FACTOR
- Corticorelin ovine triflutate

CYTOKINES
- Anakinra
- Consensus interferon
- Denileukin diftitox
- Interferon α
- Interferon β
- Interferon γ
- Interleukin-1
- Interleukin-2/aldesleukin
- Interleukin-2 fusion protein
- Interleukin-11/oprelvekin
- Rilonacept

ENZYMES
- Tissue plasminogen activators
- Alteplase
- Dornase α
- Reteplase
- Tenecteplase

ENZYME REPLACEMENT THERAPY
- Alglucosidase α
- Idursulfase
- Imiglucerase

GONADOTROPINS
- Follitropin α
- Follitropin β
- Lutropin α
- Menotropins
- Urofollitropin

GONADOTROPIN-RELEASING HORMONE AGONISTS AND ANTAGONISTS
- Cetrorelix acetate
- Degarelix acetate
- Ganirelix acetate
- Goserelin acetate
- Histrelin acetate
- Leuprolide acetate
- Nafarelin acetate
- Triptorelin pamoate

GROWTH HORMONES
- Pegvisomant
- Somatropin

HEMATOPOIETIC GROWTH FACTORS
- Erythropoietin (epoetin α)
- Filgrastim
- Sargramostim

MISCELLANEOUS PEPTIDIC DRUGS
- Larazotide
- Linaclotide
- Plecanatide
- Teduglutide
- Uroguanylin

MONOCLONAL ANTIBODIES
- Alemtuzumab
- Basiliximab
- Belimumab
- Bevacizumab
- Blinatumomab
- Canakinumab
- Catumaxomab
- Certolizumab pegol
- Cetuximab
- Denosumab
- Eculizumab
- Golimumab
- Ibritumomab tiuxetan
- Ipilimumab
- Ofatumumab
- Olaratumab
- Panitumumab
- Ranibizumab
- Tositumomab
- Trastuzumab
- Ustekinumab

PANCREATIC HORMONES
- Amylin
- Glucagon
- Insulin
- Pramlintide acetate

Drugs covered in this chapter—Continued

PARATHYROID HORMONES
- Teriparatide

PITUITARY HORMONES
- Desmopressin acetate
- Oxytocin
- Vasopressin

PLACENTAL HORMONES
- Choriogonadotropin α
- Human chorionic gonadotropin

SOMATOSTATINS
- Indium pentetreotide
- Octreotide acetate

THYROTROPIN

THYROID HORMONES
- Calcitonin salmon

TUMOR NECROSIS FACTORS
- Abatacept
- Etanercept

OTHER GROWTH FACTORS
- Clotting factor VIII, factor IX, and anticoagulants

Abbreviations

ACTH adrenocorticotropic hormone
ADC antibody-drug conjugate
a-GVHD acute graft-versus-host disease
ALCL anaplastic large cell leukemia
ALL acute lymphoblastic leukemia
AML acute myeloid leukemia
ART assisted reproductive therapy
ASCT autologous stem cell transplant
ASO antisense oligonucleotide
BAFF B cell–activating factor
cDNA complementary DNA
CF cystic fibrosis
CFTR cystic fibrosis transmembrane conductance regulator
cGMP cyclic guanosine monophosphate
CHO Chinese hamster ovary
CIC chronic idiopathic constipation
CLL chronic lymphocytic leukemia
CMV cytomegalovirus
CRF corticotropin-releasing factor
CSF colony-stimulating factor
CT calcitonin
CTCL cutaneous T cell lymphoma
CTLA-4 cytotoxic T-lymphocyte–associated antigen-4
DDAVP desamino-D-arginine vasopressin
DM diabetes mellitus
DMARD disease-modifying antirheumatic drug
DMD Duchenne muscular dystrophy
DPP-IV dipeptidyl peptidase IV
DTPA diethylenetriaminepentaacetic acid
EGF epidermal growth factor
EGFR epidermal growth factor receptor
EpCAM epithelial cell adhesion molecule
EPO erythropoietin
ERT enzyme replacement therapy
Fab functional human antibody
FDA U.S. Food and Drug Administration
FSH follicle-stimulating hormone
GAG glycosaminoglycan
GC-C guanylyl cyclase C
G-CSF granulocyte colony-stimulating factor
GH growth hormone
GLP-2 glucagon-like peptide-2
GM-CSF granulocyte-macrophage colony-stimulating factor
GnRH gonadotropin-releasing hormone
HAART high-activity antiretroviral therapy
HAMA human anti-mouse antibody
hCG human chorionic gonadotropin
HER2 human epidermal growth factor receptor 2
hGH human growth hormone
IBS-C irritable bowel syndrome accompanied by constipation
IL interleukin
IFN interferon
IgG immunoglobulin G
111In indium-111
IRR infusion-related reaction
IVF in vitro fertilization
LH luteinizing hormone
MAb monoclonal antibody
MAPK mitogen-activated protein kinase
M-CSF macrophage colony-stimulating factor
MMAE monomethyl auristatin E
MPS mucopolysaccharidosis
mRNA messenger RNA
MS multiple sclerosis
MTX methotrexate
MW molecular weight
NHL non-Hodgkin lymphoma
oCRF sheep corticotropin-releasing factor
PDC peptide-drug conjugate
PDGF platelet-derived growth factor
PEG polyethylene glycol
PI3K phosphatidylinositol 3-kinase
PTH parathyroid hormone
RA rheumatoid arthritis
RANK receptor activator of nuclear factor-κB
RANKL receptor activator of nuclear factor-κB ligand
rDNA recombinant DNA
SC subcutaneous
SBS short bowel disease
SMA spinal muscular atrophy
SMN survival motor neuron
STS soft tissue sarcoma
TNF tumor necrosis factor
TPN total parenteral nutrition
t-PA tissue-type plasminogen activator
VEGF vascular endothelial growth factor
VEGFR vascular endothelial growth factor receptor
VIP vasoactive intestinal peptide

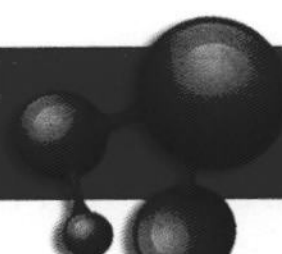

CLINICAL SIGNIFICANCE

Tina Kanmaz, PharmD, AAHIVE, BCMAS

Since the late 1980s, biotechnology has helped identify compounds with new mechanisms of action to treat serious and chronic diseases, including rheumatoid arthritis, cancers, and diabetes. The top 10 biologics in the United States as of June 2018 were adalimumab, rituximab, etanercept, trastuzumab, bevacizumab, infliximab, insulin glargine, pegfilgrastim, interferon β-1a, and ranibizumab.

Development of trastuzumab, a monoclonal antibody that binds to the extracellular domain of human epidermal growth factor receptor 2 protein (HER2) and mediates proliferation of cells that overexpress HER2, has improved disease-free progression and overall survival in patients with HER2+ breast cancer. The advent of small molecule-antibody conjugates has the potential to further impact the personalized treatment of diseases with enhanced therapeutic index. This class of drug molecules involves synthetic medicinal chemistry principles combined with biotechnology tools. For example, the design and development of ado-trastuzumab emtansine involved conjugating the highly cytotoxic small molecule emtansine to HER-2–targeted trastuzumab. Ado-trastuzumab emtansine is indicated in patients with HER2-positive metastatic breast cancer that relapses within 6 months of completing adjuvant trastuzumab therapy. Ado-trastuzumab alone has also resulted in significant pathologic complete response rates in early HER2-positive, hormone receptor–positive breast cancer, saving patients from experiencing the toxic effects of chemotherapy.

INTRODUCTION

Banting and Best demonstrated nearly a century ago that pancreatic extract markedly reduces blood sugar, even to normal levels, with relatively low toxicity in human diabetes mellitus.[1] The internal secretion of pancreas that was responsible for this miraculous achievement was the 51–amino acid peptide hormone insulin. Animal-derived insulin became the first commercially available peptide drug in 1923, and with the introduction of human insulin in 1982, it achieved the distinction of being the first recombinant drug. The introduction of a number of other peptide hormones followed in the first half of the 20th century. The perception that the disadvantages of peptide drugs far outweigh their advantages led to their loss of prominence in clinical development. Rapid biotechnological advances toward the end of 20th century resulted in a renaissance of peptidic drugs in the last two decades. An estimated 60 peptides are currently approved for human use worldwide. In addition, more than 140 peptidic drugs are in various stages of therapeutic development.[2,3]

Recombinant therapeutic proteins provide interventions for some of the most intractable diseases and, in addition, find applications as diagnostic tools. More than 100 protein therapeutic agents are approved, and several others are currently being evaluated in different phases of clinical trials. Protein therapeutics include antibody-drug conjugates, peptide-drug conjugates, monoclonal antibodies (MAbs), vaccines, enzymes, natural/recombinant cytokines, and interferons.

Peptide and protein therapeutics elicit a high degree of specificity toward molecular targets and are attractive because of their low toxicity. More than 200 peptide and protein therapeutics have been approved for the treatment of neoplastic and infectious diseases, as well as a range of disorders which include metabolic, hematologic, immunologic, genetic, bone, cardiac, eye, neurologic, respiratory, malabsorption, and hormonal disorders.[4]

THERAPEUTIC PEPTIDE AND PROTEIN DRUGS

The following sections introduce a variety of peptide and protein hormones, both natural and synthetic, and their recombinant analogues that are commercially available for the treatment of various diseases. The peptide hormones are obtained synthetically, from natural sources or via genetic engineering. They are categorized, for the most part, according to their endocrine organ of origin. Table 34.1 summarizes some of the interesting peptides and proteins used in medicine.

Recombinant DNA (rDNA) technology provides a powerful tool for new pharmaceutical product development and production. Biotechnology-produced medicinal agents discussed in this chapter include hormones, enzymes, cytokines, hematopoietic growth factors, other growth factors, blood clotting factors and anticoagulants, vaccines, MAbs, antibody-drug conjugates, and peptide-drug conjugates. Some MAb-based in-home test kits are summarized in Chapter 5 (Table 5.3), and FDA-approved MAb therapeutic agents are discussed later in this chapter.

Peptide and Protein Hormones and Analogues

Hormones of Hypothalamic Origin

The hypothalamus, a relatively small organ located in the brain and responsible for thermoregulation and other functions, is the secretory source for a number of peptide hormones that are transported to the pituitary gland situated immediately below it. These hormones regulate the synthesis of other peptide hormones produced by the anterior pituitary (adenohypophysis) and are thus called releasing hormones, releasing factors, or inhibitory factors. The

Table 34.1 Peptides and Proteins of Biologic Interest

Generic Name	Trade Name	Indication
Exenatide	Byetta	Type 2 diabetes mellitus
Liraglutide	Victoza	Type 2 diabetes mellitus
Insulin-like growth factor-I (human)		Treatment of major burns requiring hospitalization
Secretin, synthetic human	ChiRhoStim	Diagnostic agent for gastrinoma (Zollinger-Ellison syndrome)
Thymopentin	Timunox	Immunomodulator
Thyrotropin α	Thyrogen	Diagnostic agent for serum thyroglobulin testing
Carfilzomib		Multiple myeloma
Nesiritide	Natrecor	Acute decompensated congestive heart failure
Enfuvirtide	Fuzeon	HIV-1 infection
Ziconotide	Prialt	Chronic pain
Lanreotide	Somatuline	Acromegaly
Romiplostim	Nplate	Chronic idiopathic thrombocytopenic purpura
Degarelix	Firmagon	Advanced prostate cancer
Botulinum toxin A	Dysport	Excessive efferent activity in motor nerves
Ecallantide	Kalbitor	Acute attacks of hereditary angioedema
Tesamorelin acetate	Egrifta	HIV-associated lipodystrophy

release of these hypothalamic hormones is regulated via cholinergic and dopaminergic stimuli from higher brain centers, and their synthesis and release are controlled by feedback mechanisms from their target organs.

GONADOTROPIN-RELEASING HORMONE. Gonadotropin-releasing hormone (GnRH) is a decapeptide (Fig. 34.1) that causes the release of the gonadotropins luteinizing hormone (LH) and follicle-stimulating hormone (FSH) from the anterior pituitary gland but not in equal amounts. Therefore, GnRH is closely involved in the control of both male and female reproduction. Medicinal chemists have capitalized on the relatively simple decapeptide structure of GnRH by preparing several analogues as potential fertility and antifertility agents, some of which are commercially available. It is known that GnRH can be degraded by enzymatic cleavage between Tyr5-Gly6 and Pro9-Gly10. Structure-activity relationship studies of GnRH analogues have shown that when Gly6 is replaced with certain hydrophobic D-amino acids, as well as with changes in the peptide C-terminus, they generally are less susceptible to proteolytic enzymes, resulting in a longer duration of action. For that reason, they are referred to as superagonists.

In physiologic doses, GnRH agonists are able to induce ovulation and spermatogenesis by increasing LH and FSH levels and the resulting sex steroid levels, as does the normal hormone. In larger pharmacologic (therapeutic) doses, GnRH agonists, especially the superagonists, block implantation of the fertilized egg, cause luteolysis of the corpus luteum, and can act as postcoital contraceptive agents (although they are not approved for this latter use). This "paradoxical" antifertility effect seen with the superagonists has been attributed to the fact that GnRH must be administered in a low-dose, pulsatile manner that mimics natural hypothalamic GnRH release for it to be therapeutically effective as a fertility agent. When GnRH or a superagonist is administered in pharmacologic doses each day, LH and FSH levels will initially rise but then begin to fall after a few days because of target tissue desensitization/downregulation of pituitary GnRH receptors. The continued use of these agents in a nonpulsatile manner will result in a drastic drop of the gonadal steroid levels to near castrate levels in both males and females, thereby giving rise to their use in such conditions as precocious puberty, endometriosis, and advanced metastatic breast and prostate carcinoma. Typically, the GnRH superagonists take approximately 2 weeks to finally desensitize the GnRH receptors. During this time, there is a transient rise in LH and FSH levels, which often results in an initial "flare-up" of the original symptoms.

The following discussion is focused on the medicinal chemistry and medical use of the commercially available GnRH analogues.[5-7]

Specific Drugs

Leuprolide Acetate (Lupron). Leuprolide acetate, a synthetic nonapeptide analogue of GnRH that possesses greater potency than the natural hormone, is a commercially available superagonist. Leuprolide acetate contains substitutions that hinder enzymatic degradation, D-Leu and NH-Et in place of Gly6 and Gly10-NH_2, respectively (Fig. 34.1). Leuprolide acetate exhibits 15-fold higher potency than natural GnRH. When given continuously and in therapeutic doses, leuprolide acetate inhibits LH and FSH secretion by desensitizing/downregulating the GnRH receptors, as discussed previously. After an initial stimulation, chronic administration of leuprolide acetate results in suppression of ovarian and testicular steroidogenesis. In premenopausal females, estrogens are reduced to postmenopausal levels; in males, testosterone is reduced to castrate levels.[8]

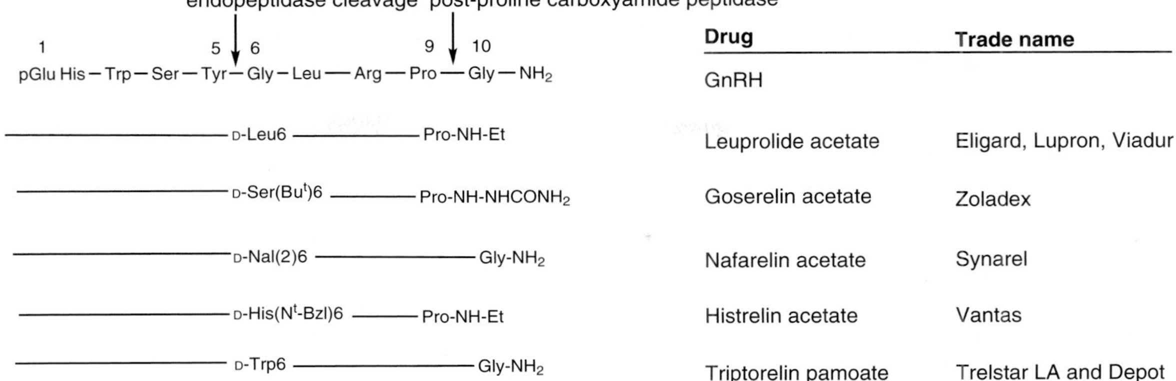

Figure 34.1 GnRH-based drugs that are commercially available. Note that leuprolide, goserelin, nafarelin, histrelin, and triptorelin are all superagonists and contain a D-amino acid in place of Gly6 and that three of the five are missing the C-terminal Gly (the line indicates an identical sequence of amino acids). Note: pGlu = pryoglutamic acid = Bu^t = t-butyl; D-Nal(2) = D-3-(2-naphthyl)alanine; N^t-Bzl = 1-benzyl-D-histamine.

Leuprolide acetate is administered by daily injections or as depot injections that can be given once every 1-6 months as a palliative treatment in advanced prostatic carcinoma (as an alternative to orchiectomy, see Chapter 33). An implant version (Viadur) also is available for long-term palliative therapy; after implantation of the device into the upper arm, leuprolide acetate is continuously released over a 12-month period. Because dihydrotestosterone, a metabolite of testosterone, is able to stimulate the growth of prostate cancer, the ability of leuprolide acetate to bring testosterone to near castrate levels is responsible for its use as a palliative in advanced disease. The addition of a nonpeptidic antiandrogen, such as flutamide or bicalutamide, to the leuprolide acetate regimen inhibits adrenal and testicular synthesized androgens from binding to, or being taken up by, target prostate cancer tissue. This combination therapy helps to control the initial flare-up by blocking all sources of androgen and is referred to as maximal androgen blockade.

Leuprolide acetate, in monthly and every 3-month depot formulations, is useful in treating women diagnosed with endometriosis, but not for longer than 6 months because of the chance of developing osteoporosis. Because estrogens stimulate the growth of endometrial tissue, the ability of this drug to drastically reduce estrogen levels suggests its beneficial effect in treating endometriosis.

Central precocious puberty that is idiopathic or gonadotropin dependent can cause the development of secondary sexual characteristics in girls before the age of 8 years and in boys before the age of 9 years. In addition to the psychological and physiologic changes that occur because of entering puberty too early, there is the risk of the child failing to reach his or her full adult height. Therefore, leuprolide acetate's ability to suppress LH and sex steroid levels (testosterone and estradiol) to prepubertal levels is the reason that leuprolide acetate is approved for treating children with this disease. Use of this drug in a child with precocious puberty will slow or stop that child's secondary sexual development, slow linear growth and skeletal maturation, and, in girls, bring about the cessation of menstruation.

Uterine leiomyomas (fibroids), which are benign neoplasms derived from smooth muscle, can cause excessive vaginal bleeding that may progress to anemia. Leuprolide acetate, concomitant with iron therapy, is used in treating the anemia that arises from uterine leiomyoma. The decrease in the formation of the steroid sex hormones reduces fibroid and uterine volume, produces relief in the clinical symptoms (pelvic pain), and stops the excessive vaginal bleeding, thus correcting the anemia.

Goserelin Acetate (Zoladex). Goserelin acetate, like leuprolide acetate, is a synthetic superagonist nonapeptide analogue of GnRH that demonstrates greater potency than the natural hormone. It contains D-Ser (t-butyl) and NH-NHCONH$_2$ in place of Gly6 and Gly10-NH$_2$, respectively (Fig. 34.1). That is, the C-terminal modification simply has an NH substituting for the CH$_2$ of glycine, and like the C-terminal change in leuprolide acetate, this inhibits enzymatic degradation of the peptide by the post-proline carboxyamide peptidase.

Goserelin acetate is available in the form of a small solid pellet that is administered as a subcutaneous (SC) implant for the palliative treatment of advanced metastatic breast cancer in pre- and perimenopausal women or, similarly, as a palliative in advanced prostatic cancer. The rationale for this superagonist's use is its ability to bring the levels of estradiol or testosterone to near castrate levels, thus slowing the progression of breast or prostate carcinoma, respectively. Additionally, goserelin acetate is approved for the treatment of endometriosis for up to 6 months.

Goserelin acetate also is used in combination with the antiandrogen flutamide for shrinking prostate carcinoma before radiation therapy. This maximal androgen blockade combination is used when the prostate carcinoma has been staged as locally confined to the prostate gland, with one or both lobes, as well as the seminal vesicles, involved. The treatment should start 8 weeks before radiation treatment begins and be continued throughout the radiation therapy.

Furthermore, women who are to undergo hysterectomy for menorrhagia (heavy menstrual bleeding) can benefit from pretreatment with goserelin acetate because it is able to induce endometrial thinning. This thinning of the endometrium improves the operating environment by causing less intrauterine bleeding, increases postoperative amenorrhea, and decreases dysmenorrhea following surgery.

Nafarelin Acetate (Synarel). Nafarelin acetate, another synthetic superagonist decapeptide analogue of GnRH, contains D-Nal(2) 6 [Nal = 3-(2-naphthyl)-Ala] in place of Gly6, but the C-terminal Gly10-NH_2 is identical with natural GnRH (Fig. 34.1). Nafarelin acetate is available as a 0.2% nasal spray for the relief of endometriosis. Estrogen is needed for the growth of endometrial tissue; thus, decreased estrogen leads to shrinkage of errant endometrial tissue. The observed adverse effects of nafarelin acetate are related to falling estrogen levels and include decreased libido, amenorrhea, hot flashes, and vaginal dryness. When used consistently, nafarelin acetate will inhibit ovulation and stop menstruation.

Nafarelin acetate also is used in male and female children for the treatment of central precocious puberty. By suppressing the release of LH, the estradiol or testosterone levels fall to prepubertal levels; early secondary sexual development is arrested; linear growth and skeletal maturation are slowed; and in girls, menstruation stops.

Histrelin Acetate (Supprelin, Vantas). Histrelin acetate, a superagonist analogue of GnRH, contains D-His (N1-Bzl) 6 in place of Gly6, and the C-terminus is identical to leuprolide acetate namely, NH-Et in place of Gly10-NH_2 (Fig. 34.1). This GnRH analogue is commercially available in the form of an implantable device (SC in the upper arm) that slowly releases the drug over a 12-month period, resulting in decreased testicular steroidogenesis. It is used for the palliative treatment of advanced prostate cancer.

Triptorelin Pamoate (Trelstar). Triptorelin pamoate is another superagonist analogue of GnRH which, like nafarelin acetate, contains only a single amino acid substitution (D-Trp6 for Gly6) when compared to the natural hormone (Fig. 34.1). As described above, the treatment of advanced prostate cancer involves reduction of serum testosterone to very low levels, which can be achieved surgically by orchiectomy. When this surgical method is unacceptable to the patient, an alternative approach is "chemical castration," which can be achieved by use of estrogen therapy, leuprolide, goserelin or histrelin acetates, or triptorelin pamoate. This product is available for intramuscular depot injection (monthly or every 3 mo), and treatment drops serum testosterone concentrations to a level generally seen in surgically castrated men.

Ganirelix Acetate (Antagon). Ganirelix acetate is an analogue of GnRH with substitutions at residues 1, 2, 3, 6, 8, and 10 (Fig. 34.2).[9] It is not a superagonist but, rather, is a synthetic decapeptide with high antagonist activity and the first GnRH antagonist to be marketed. It is approved for the suppression of LH surges in women who are undergoing ovarian hyperstimulation fertility treatment; LH surges normally promote ovulation. The therapeutic goal of this drug is to significantly reduce the number of medication days necessary to suppress the LH surge, thereby maintaining eggs in the ovaries. In vitro fertilization (IVF) treatment cycles were historically initiated by the administration of leuprolide acetate to suppress the premature release of LH. This inhibits ovulation so that the eggs remain available for retrieval by a fertility specialist. For this purpose, leuprolide acetate usually is injected for as many as 26 days. Clinical studies have shown that ganirelix acetate can shut down the LH surge with only 5 days of treatment, that the suppression of LH is more pronounced than that induced by FSH, and that the shorter treatment time minimizes unpleasant side effects, such as hot flashes and headaches.

Cetrorelix Acetate (Cetrotide). Cetrorelix acetate[10] is an analogue of GnRH with amino acid substitutions at residues 1, 2, 3, 6, and 10 and differing from ganirelix at amino acids 1, 6, and 8 (Fig. 34.2). These substitutions are synthetic, non–DNA-directed amino acids and, like ganirelix acetate, impart GnRH antagonist activity to cetrorelix acetate. This drug is also marketed for use in women undergoing assisted reproductive therapy (ART) procedures, in which it is necessary to control their LH surge. This allows the follicles to develop to a size, as determined by ultrasound, which increases the success of timed insemination and oocyte retrieval for IVF. Like ganirelix acetate, cetrorelix acetate has an advantage over GnRH agonists such as leuprolide acetate because it reduces the fertility therapy cycle to days rather than weeks.

Degarelix acetate (Firmagon). Degarelix acetate is an analogue of GnRH with amino acid substitutions at residues 1, 2, 3, 5, 6, 8, and 10 (Fig. 34.2). These substitutions are synthetic, non–DNA-directed amino acids and, like ganirelix acetate, impart competitive and reversible GnRH

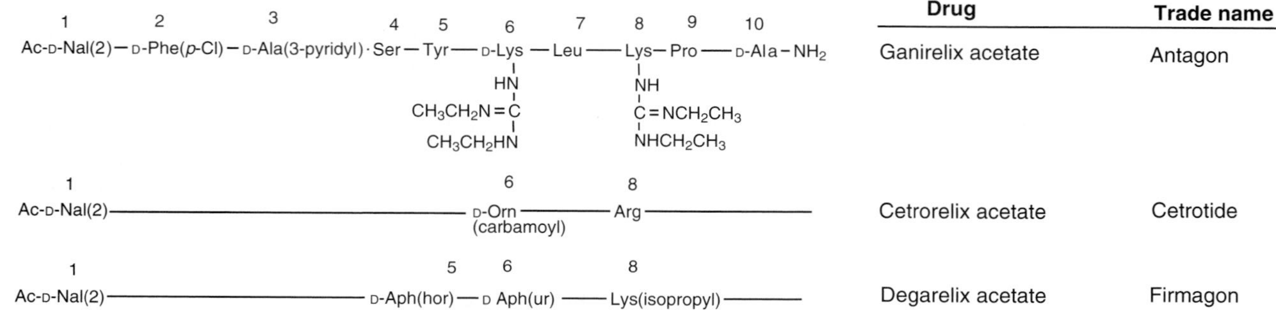

Figure 34.2 GnRH receptor antagonists. Note: Ac-D-Nal(2) = N-acetyl-D-2-naphthylalanine; D-Orn(carbamoyl) = D-ornithine; D-Aph(hor) = 4-dihydroorotoylamino-D-phenylalanine; D-Aph(ur) = 4-ureido-D-phenylalanine.

antagonist activity leading to suppression of LH release from the pituitary gland. Degarelix acetate is indicated for treatment of patients with advanced prostate cancer (see Chapter 33).[11] Like the superagonists, degarelix affords a drop in testosterone to castrate levels. Degarelix does not, however, produce the initial rise in testosterone levels and the resulting flare-up of symptoms often seen with the superagonists. Relative to its predecessors, degarelix has increased aqueous solubility due to the presence of unnatural amino acids at positions 5 and 6 with polar dihydropyrimidinedione carboxamide and urea moieties that have extensive hydrogen bonding capabilities. Replacement of Arg8 by (Nε-isopropyl)Lys minimizes the histamine-releasing properties, an unwanted side effect with other GnRH antagonists.

SOMATOSTATINS. Somatostatin is a cyclic 14–amino acid peptide that was first isolated by Guillemin in 1973 and is probably the most thoroughly investigated and most important of the inhibitory factors produced by the hypothalamus (Fig. 34.3).[12] The principal activity of somatostatin is inhibition of the release of growth hormone (GH) from the anterior pituitary. Too much GH, as in pituitary tumors, causes acromegaly, a form of gigantism. Conversely, too little GH leads to dwarfism. Somatostatin has also been found in the pancreas and the gastrointestinal tract, where it inhibits the secretion of both insulin and glucagon from the pancreas, as well as the secretion of a variety of intestinal peptides (e.g., gastrin, secretin, pepsin, and renin). The short half-life of somatostatin, which is less than 3 minutes, has precluded its use as a therapeutic agent. Consequently, many derivatives of somatostatin were developed to increase duration of action and/or to enhance the selectivity profile. The culmination of these structure-activity relationship studies was the development of octreotide acetate.

Specific Drugs

Octreotide Acetate (Sandostatin). Octreotide acetate, a long-acting octapeptide analogue of somatostatin, has a half-life of approximately 100 minutes. A comparison of the primary structures of octreotide and somatostatin suggests little similarity, but studies have shown that the essential fragment for its activity was the tetrapeptide Phe7-Trp8-Lys9-Thr10 (Fig. 34.3). These studies helped in the design of the potent drug now known as octreotide acetate, which incorporates D-Trp in the essential tetrapeptide segment.[13] This drug suppresses the secretion of gastroenteropancreatic peptides, such as gastrin, vasoactive intestinal peptide (VIP), insulin, and glucagon, as well as pituitary GH. Furthermore, it is more potent than natural somatostatin in inhibiting the release of glucagon, insulin, and GH.

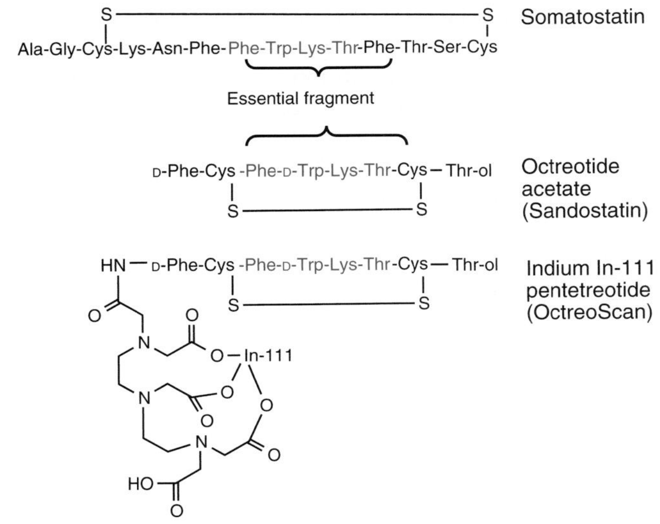

Octreotide acetate is used by SC injection in the palliative treatment of metastatic carcinoid tumors, which are tumors of the endocrine system, gastrointestinal tract, and lung. It is also used in the palliative management of VIP-secreting tumors (VIPomas, usually pancreatic tumors). Patients with VIPomas suffer a profuse, watery diarrhea syndrome, and octreotide acetate is able to help by decreasing the release of damaging intestinal tumor cell secretions. Octreotide also helps to reduce hypokalemia by correcting electrolyte imbalances.

Octreotide acetate is able to decrease the secretion of GH from the pituitary and is used in patients with acromegaly who are unresponsive to pituitary radiation therapy or surgery. It is used in the treatment of acromegaly because it reduces the blood levels of both GH and insulin-like growth factor-1. The long-acting repository form of octreotide acetate is administered as monthly depot injections for all of the above indications.

Octreotide for intravenous (IV) injection is used for the treatment of acute bleeding from esophageal varices. Variceal bleeding occurs in about half the patients with cirrhosis of the liver and is responsible for about one-third of deaths in these patients. Octreotide is a potent vasoconstrictor that reduces portal and collateral blood flow by constricting visceral vessels, which leads to reduced portal blood pressure and decreased bleeding.

Indium-111 Pentetreotide (OctreoScan). Somatostatin receptors have a broad distribution in normal tissue, as well as in a variety of human malignancies (e.g., small-cell lung, brain, breast, pituitary, and endocrine pancreatic cancers). For this reason, octreotide, which binds to somatostatin receptors, was converted to a radionuclide-containing peptide by reacting the amino terminus with an active ester of diethylenetriaminepentaacetic acid (DTPA) to give DTPA-octreotide and then chelated to the radionuclide indium-111 (111In) (Fig. 34.3). This radiopharmaceutical, marketed as OctreoScan, is used as a diagnostic agent for the early detection and localization of small tumors and their metastases, especially tumors that originate from neuroendocrine cells.[14] Administration of this diagnostic agent in total parenteral nutrition (TPN) admixtures or injection into TPN IV administration lines may lead to the formation of a complex glycosyl octreotide conjugate and is contraindicated.

CORTICOTROPIN-RELEASING FACTOR. The primary function of corticotropin-releasing factor (CRF), a hypothalamic 41–amino acid peptide, is the regulation of the

Ala-Gly-Cys-Lys-Asn-Phe-Phe-Trp-Lys-Thr-Phe-Thr-Ser-Cys — Somatostatin

Essential fragment

D-Phe-Cys-Phe-D-Trp-Lys-Thr-Cys—Thr-ol — Octreotide acetate (Sandostatin)

HN—D-Phe-Cys-Phe-D-Trp-Lys-Thr-Cys—Thr-ol — Indium In-111 pentetreotide (OctreoScan)

Figure 34.3 Somatostatin and its analogues.

release of adrenocorticotropic hormone (ACTH) from the anterior pituitary gland, which subsequently stimulates the release of hydrocortisone from the adrenal gland. Human CRF, which was previously commercially available, has been replaced by the sheep CRF (oCRF).

Corticorelin Ovine Triflutate (Acthrel). The ovine form of the human CRF hormone (oCRF), which shares 83% homology with the human form, has a longer half-life and greater potency.[15] ACTH deficiency in humans is usually associated with a pituitary disorder, rather than with a deficiency of CRF, and oCRF can be used to distinguish between pituitary hypersecretion of ACTH (Cushing syndrome) and ectopic ACTH secretion, both of which are conditions that cause a hypersecretion of hydrocortisone. In the case of ectopic ACTH secretion, the administration of oCRF will elicit little to no response in the production of ACTH and hydrocortisone. Therefore, synthetic oCRF trifluoroacetate salt is marketed as a diagnostic agent for patients with ACTH-dependent Cushing syndrome.

Hormones Originating in the Anterior Lobe of the Pituitary Gland

The pituitary, located just below the hypothalamus, is a small gland that can be divided into an anterior and a posterior lobe. This gland is responsible for the secretion of several important peptide hormones, two of which are released by the posterior lobe (oxytocin and vasopressin). The remaining anterior pituitary peptide hormones control important functions such as growth, reproduction, metabolic and ion balance, as well as a number of other functions.

GROWTH HORMONE. Human GH, a 191–amino acid protein with a molecular weight (MW) of 22 kDa, is roughly spherical with a hydrophobic interior. GH is secreted by the anterior pituitary in response to the liberation of GH-releasing factor from the hypothalamus. This contrasts with somatostatin, which inhibits the release of GH. The primary function of GH is to promote skeletal growth. When GH is absent during childhood, or if there is an inadequate supply, dwarfism results. Before 1985, children of short stature were sometimes treated with human GH (hGH) of pituitary origin, which was obtained from cadavers, but hGH of natural origin was discontinued by the U.S. Food and Drug Administration (FDA) when several young adults who had received hGH died. Their deaths were attributed to contaminated hGH, and the contaminant was later found to be an infective agent, known as a prion, that causes Creutzfeldt-Jakob disease, a rare and fatal neurodegenerative disease.[16] Naturally occurring hGH has been replaced by the product that is derived from rDNA methodology.

Specific Drugs

Somatropin (Genotropin, Nutropin, Saizen). Somatropin, which is an hGH prepared by rDNA procedures, contains the identical sequence of 191 amino acids as the natural hormone. Several of these products are indicated for the long-term treatment of children who fail to grow because of inadequate secretion of endogenous GH and for growth problems associated with chronic renal failure.[17] Even adults who are diagnosed with GH deficiency, which can arise as a result of pituitary or hypothalamic disease, surgery, radiation therapy, or other reasons, can benefit from hGH replacement therapy. Turner syndrome, a genetic disease in which there is a complete or partial absence of one of the two X chromosomes in females, causes short stature as one of its many symptoms. Girls suffering from Turner syndrome can benefit from the use of Humatrope, Norditropin, or Nutropin during their growth years. A long-acting dosage form of somatotropin is approved for use in children with Prader-Willi syndrome, a rare genetic disorder that causes short stature, an involuntary, continuous urge to eat that is life-long and may be life-threatening, low muscle tone, and cognitive disorders. The formulation was designed to reduce the frequency of injections to once or twice a month by encapsulating the agent in biodegradable microspheres.

The anabolic properties of hGH are the basis for the orphan drug uses of several of these recombinant products. hGH is used in AIDS-associated catabolism or weight loss, in cachexia resulting from AIDS, and as an anabolic agent in patients with severe burns. In addition, the anabolic property of recombinant hGH is the reason for the use of Zorbtive, along with specialized nutritional support, in the treatment of short bowel syndrome.

Pegvisomant (Somavert). This recombinant product contains 191 amino acid residues, the same number as in GH, but there are substitutions at residues 18, 21, 120, 167, 168, 171, 172, 174, and 179. This product is covalently linked to several polyethylene glycol (PEG) molecules, and the PEGylated protein becomes a GH receptor antagonist. As such, pegvisomant binds to the GH receptor and blocks endogenous GH from binding. The result is a blocking of the GH-stimulated overproduction of insulin-like growth factor-1 that contributes to the disabling symptoms and long-term health problems associated with acromegaly.[18]

GONADOTROPINS. The gonadotropins FSH and LH are large glycoproteins released by the anterior pituitary upon stimulation by GnRH produced in the hypothalamus. Both FSH and LH consist of two noncovalently associated α and β subunits. The α subunits contain 92 amino acids and are identical in both hormones, whereas the β subunit consists of 121 amino acids in LH and 111 amino acids in FSH. As the β subunit structures are dissimilar,[19] they are responsible for each hormone's bioactivity and rate of degradation (biological half-life of LH is 20 min which is shorter than that of FSH's 3-4 hr).

Both LH and FSH are referred to as gonadotropins because they act on the male and female gonads, which results in the production of the sex steroids testosterone and estradiol, respectively. FSH is a 34 kDa glycoprotein (~14% carbohydrate), and LH is a 26 kDa glycoprotein. In the female, FSH and LH act in concert in regulating ovarian function; egg maturation and estradiol secretion are stimulated by FSH while ovulation, transformation of the ruptured follicle into the corpus luteum, and progesterone secretion are LH-mediated actions. In males, spermatogenesis is dependent on these two hormones. FSH stimulates the maturation of sperm in the testes while LH enables the testicular secretion of testosterone.

Male infertility is generally caused by the quality and/or quantity of the sperm produced. Female infertility, however, may be caused by several factors, such as the inability to produce an egg, to ovulate, to achieve fertilization, and for implantation of the fertilized ovum in the uterus. Several of the commercially available gonadotropins can help in enhancing both male and female fertility as discussed below.

Specific Drugs

Menotropins (Menopur, Repronex). Menotropins are natural products obtained from the urine of postmenopausal women and then biologically standardized (international units) for FSH and LH activities in an approximate ratio of 1:1. Menotropins are used in males with primary (hypothalamic) or secondary (pituitary) hypogonadism to stimulate spermatogenesis. Patients must have been treated previously with human chorionic gonadotropin (hCG; a peptide hormone of placental origin that has activity very similar to LH, as discussed below) to effect masculinization through increased testosterone production. In females, menotropins and hCG are given sequentially for the purposes of inducing ovulation in women with either hypothalamic or pituitary hormonal dysfunction. The menotropins are given for 7-12 days, and after clinical evaluation (via ultrasound) indicates the presence of a mature follicle, a single dose of hCG is given to simulate the typical LH surge that normally triggers ovulation. Also, women use the combination of menotropins and hCG to promote the development of multiple follicles when they are participating in an IVF program requiring the recruitment of follicles.

Follitropins. Follitropins are hormonal products that consist entirely of FSH and are used to stimulate ovarian follicle growth in women who do not have primary ovarian failure. In the absence of an adequate endogenous LH surge, hCG must be given following the use of follitropins to stimulate ovulation.

Urofollitropins (Bravelle). Urofollitropin, a natural product like the menotropins, is obtained from the urine of postmenopausal women and then highly purified so as to contain only FSH, reportedly with only small amounts of LH. Urofollitropin is used for its ability to stimulate follicle development in women undergoing drug-induced pituitary suppression (GnRH antagonist or superagonist) for purposes of IVF (i.e., multiple follicle development or egg donation). When the target number and size of ovarian follicles is achieved, as determined by ultrasound, hCG is administered so as to effect ovulation, and the oocytes are retrieved for IVF.

This drug is also indicated for women who have infertility caused by polycystic ovary syndrome, which generally is observed clinically as enlarged, cystic ovaries containing relatively small follicles. These patients often develop hirsutism, as their androgen and LH levels appear elevated while their FSH levels are low. The early exposure to these improper hormone levels may be causing the follicular atresia.[20]

Lately, it has become desirable to have a nonnatural source of pure FSH. It is believed that exposure to increased amounts of LH early in follicular development, as would be the case with menotropins, is detrimental to fertility. Also, urofollitropin is derived from menopausal urine, and the supply of this natural product is limited and contains variable levels of urine-derived contaminant proteins.[21] These problems have given rise to recombinant forms of FSH.

Follitropin α and follitropin β are human FSH preparations produced by rDNA technology. The production of rhFSH in a Chinese hamster ovary (CHO) cell line has proved to be particularly challenging. Follitropin α was the first heterodimeric glycoprotein to be produced by rDNA technology. Before the product of rDNA origin was available for infertility treatment, FSH was isolated from urine at less than 5% purity.

Follitropin α (Gonal-F, Gonal-F RFF, Gonal-F RFF Pen). Follitropin α is a human FSH preparation of rDNA origin. Because FSH is a glycoprotein, alterations in the carbohydrate side chain attachments afford different isoforms, which leads to different pharmacokinetic and pharmacodynamic properties. Because it is of recombinant origin and not isolated from urine, it is free of any additional substances, such as urinary proteins and LH.

Like urofollitropin, follitropin α is marketed for promoting the development of multiple follicles that can then be induced to ovulate, via hCG administration, so that the oocytes can be collected for IVF. It is also used in women who wish to become pregnant and are anovulatory because of polycystic ovary syndrome, in whom it can enhance follicle maturation before hCG administration for final ovulation.

Men with infertility can also benefit from therapy with follitropin α if their infertility is related to hypothalamic or pituitary hormonal dysfunction and not primary testicular failure because it induces spermatogenesis. Just as with therapy using menotropins, pretreatment with hCG is performed for 3 months to achieve serum testosterone levels within the normal range before hCG and follitropin α therapy.

Follitropin β (Follistim AQ). Follitropin β is a human FSH preparation of rDNA origin that differs chemically from natural FSH and follitropin α only by slight changes in the composition of the carbohydrate side chains. In fact, the primary and tertiary structures of both follitropins α and β are indistinguishable from those of natural human FSH. Furthermore, bioassays and physiochemical studies indicate that follitropins α and β are indistinguishable from each other. Therefore, follitropin β is approved for the same indications as follitropin α.

Lutropin α (Luveris). Lutropin α is the first pure human LH preparation and is of rDNA origin. According to physicochemical and biologic assays, it is indistinguishable from human LH of natural origin. It is indicated for use in infertile women who are undergoing ART, specifically those with severe LH deficiency. It is meant to be coadministered with follitropin α so as to stimulate follicular growth in these women. When the follicles are of correct size, as determined by ultrasound examination, hCG is administered to stimulate ovulation.

Adrenocorticotropic Hormone (H.P. Acthar Gel). The anterior pituitary, under the influence of the hypothalamic hormone hCRF, releases ACTH, a single-chain peptide of 39 amino acids (also known as corticotropin). The sequence of 24 amino acid residues beginning from the amino terminus contains all the biologic activity of the parent. The remaining 15 C-terminal residues confer species specificity, as well as enhance the stability of ACTH toward proteolytic cleavage. Amino acids 1-24, which are critical for ACTH activity, are identical in humans, pigs, sheep, and cattle, whereas these species differ only slightly from each other in the final 15 amino acids. The main action of ACTH on the adrenal cortex involves the release of the glucocorticoid hormone hydrocortisone and the mineralocorticoid hormone aldosterone.

Commercial ACTH is obtained from natural sources and is available in 16% gelatin (repository gel) to prolong its release after SC or intramuscular injection. ACTH has both anti-inflammatory and immunosuppressant properties, which contributes to its use in the treatment of acute exacerbations of multiple sclerosis.

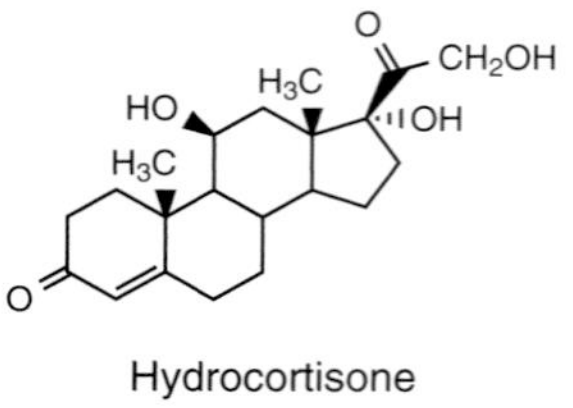
O
CH_2OH
H_3C
HO
OH
H_3C
O

Hydrocortisone

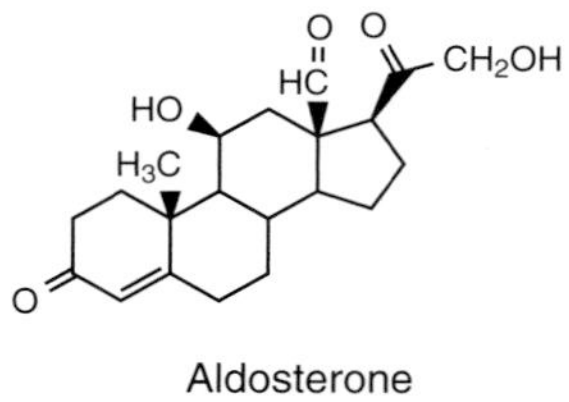
O
O
HC
CH_2OH
HO
H_3C
O

Aldosterone

Cosyntropin (Cortrosyn). Cosyntropin is a synthetic polypeptide consisting of amino acids 1 through 24 of human ACTH that are required for full biologic activity. Since it is of synthetic origin, it is less allergenic than ACTH of natural origin. Cosyntropin is used as a diagnostic agent in the screening of patients suspected of having adrenocortical insufficiency.

Thyrotropin (Thyrogen). Thyroid-stimulating hormone (thyrotropin) is a 28-30 kDa glycoprotein secreted by the anterior lobe of the pituitary gland that is necessary for the growth and function of the thyroid. A recombinant thyrotropin α useful for the detection and treatment of thyroid cancer was approved by the FDA in 1998.

Hormones Released From the Posterior Lobe of the Pituitary Gland

As previously discussed, the pituitary gland is responsible for the secretion of several peptide hormones, only two of which are released by the posterior lobe. In fact, these two hormones, oxytocin and vasopressin, are synthesized in neurons originating in the hypothalamus and are transported to the posterior pituitary for storage until release is required.

OXYTOCIN (PITOCIN). Oxytocin is a cyclic nonapeptide hormone and neurotransmitter containing a 20-membered tocin ring (from Cys1 to Cys6) and an acyclic tripeptide tail (from Pro7 to $GlyNH_29$). Like somatostatin, it contains a large ring that includes a disulfide bridge (Fig. 34.4). Oxytocin has uterotonic action, contracting the muscles of the uterus during gestation, and plays an important role in milk ejection. Exogenous oxytocin most commonly is

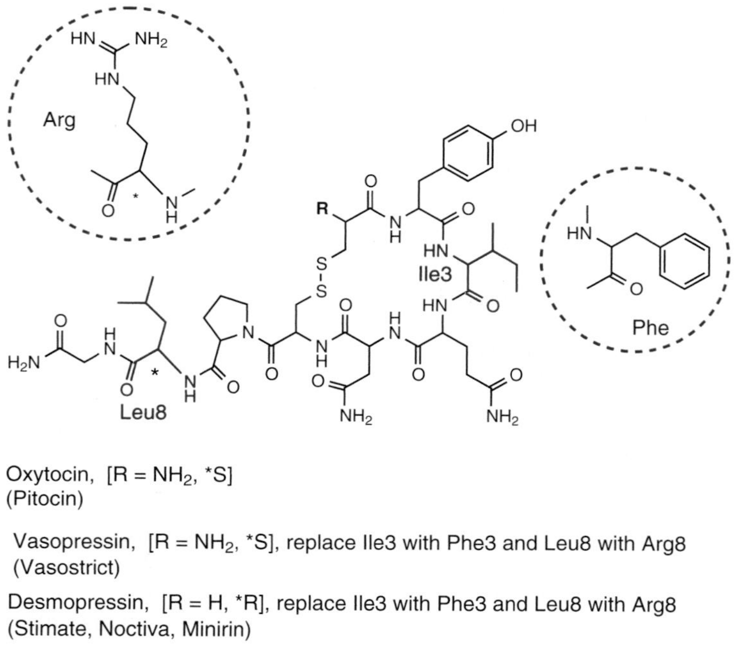
HN
NH_2
HN
Arg
OH
R
Ile3
Phe
H_2N
Leu8
NH_2
NH_2
Oxytocin, [R = NH_2, *S]
(Pitocin)
Vasopressin, [R = NH_2, *S], replace Ile3 with Phe3 and Leu8 with Arg8
(Vasostrict)
Desmopressin, [R = H, *R], replace Ile3 with Phe3 and Leu8 with Arg8
(Stimate, Noctiva, Minirin)

Figure 34.4 Structural relationship between oxytocin, vasopressin, and desmopressin.

used for induction of labor, wherein it improves uterine contractions to achieve early vaginal delivery for reasons of fetal or maternal well-being (e.g., preeclampsia, Rh factor problems, pregnancy that has exceeded 42 wk). It also finds use following delivery of the placenta because it promotes contraction and vasoconstriction and helps to control postpartum bleeding.

VASOPRESSIN (VASOSTRICT). Human vasopressin, or Arg-vasopressin, is chemically very similar to oxytocin and therefore sometimes is referred to as (Phe3, Arg8) oxytocin (Fig.34.4). The physiologic role of vasopressin is the regulation of water reabsorption in the renal tubules, and thus, it is often referred to as the antidiuretic hormone. In high doses, vasopressin promotes the contraction of arterioles and capillaries, resulting in an increase in blood pressure (thus the name vasopressin). An inadequate output of pituitary antidiuretic hormone can cause diabetes insipidus, which is characterized by the chronic excretion of large amounts of pale urine and results in dehydration and extreme thirst.

DESMOPRESSIN ACETATE (DDAVP). Desmopressin, as its acetate salt, is a synthetic analogue of vasopressin in which the N-terminal Cys is devoid of its α-amino function (1-desamino) and where Arg8 is present as its D-isomer (D-Arg8), thus the commercial acronym DDAVP (Fig. 34.4). The presence of D-Arg and the absence of the N-terminal amine in the desmopressin structure have contributed to its increased half-life, and it is available for oral, parenteral, or nasal use. It is used by all three of these routes to prevent or control polydipsia (excessive thirst), polyuria, and dehydration of patients with diabetes insipidus caused by a deficiency of vasopressin. It has also been approved for the treatment of nocturnal enuresis (bed-wetting), which is believed to be caused by an absence of the normal nighttime rise in vasopressin levels.

Desmopressin is known to cause an increase in both plasma factor VIII (antihemophilic factor) and plasminogen activator. Therefore, it is approved by the FDA for use, parenterally and nasally, in reducing spontaneous or trauma-induced bleeding episodes in patients with hemophilia A and type I von Willebrand disease, provided that their plasma factor VIII activity is greater than 5%. Stimate, the nasal spray used in treating bleeding disorders, is 15-fold the concentration of DDAVP nasal spray; the latter is used in treating diabetes insipidus.

Hormones of Placental Origin

If, after ovulation occurs in females, the liberated ovum is fertilized and then implants in the endometrium, the resulting placenta that forms between mother and fetus begins to release hCG, the function of which is to maintain and prolong the life of the ovarian corpus luteum. The corpus luteum is important for the continued production of progesterone. Progesterone is especially important because it prepares the uterus for pregnancy and helps in the maintenance of the placenta. hCG begins to appear in the maternal bloodstream and urine shortly after conception and implantation of the fertilized ovum. As a result of this early release of hCG, its detection in the urine forms the basis for the home pregnancy kits that have become so popular in the early detection of pregnancy.

HUMAN CHORIONIC GONADOTROPIN (HCG, PREGNYL). Placental hCG is a complex protein that consists of an α and β subunit. The α subunit consists of 92 amino acids that are identical in sequence with those found in both LH and FSH, whereas the β subunit contains 145 amino acids and is responsible for its biologic specificity. The biologic actions of hCG closely resemble those of LH, but the former has a longer half-life and minimal FSH activity.

Like LH, hCG stimulates the production of testosterone by the testes; therefore, it is used in treating male hypogonadism and to stimulate testicular descent in prepubertal cryptorchidism in young males 4-9 years of age. In treating infertility caused by pituitary dysfunction, hCG, in combination with menotropins (as previously discussed) or clomiphene, can induce ovulation and pregnancy in anovulatory females. This hCG, which is of natural origin, is purified from the urine of pregnant women.

Choriogonadotropin α (Ovidrel). Choriogonadotropin α is obtained by rDNA technology and is biologically and chemically identical to hCG of natural origin. Similar to hCG of natural origin, it is used for inducing ovulation in women with anovulatory infertility. Following proper pretreatment with a GnRH antagonist or superagonist to desensitize the pituitary, women participating in ART are treated with a follicle-stimulating agent (e.g., menotropins) to effect the final maturation of the follicles within the ovaries. Ultrasonograms are used to determine proper follicle maturation before the administration of choriogonadotropin α to induce ovulation. A distinct advantage of this product is that it can be self-administered by the patient via SC injection.

Hormone of Parathyroid Origin

The four parathyroid glands exist as two pairs, one pair of which is embedded on the back surface of each of the two lobes of the thyroid gland. These very small glands are responsible for the secretion of parathyroid hormone (PTH), the action of which is the regulation of both calcium and phosphate metabolism within bone and kidney. In humans, the Ca^{2+} concentration is carefully regulated, and when it falls below homeostatic levels, the parathyroid glands secrete PTH, an 84–amino acid, single-chain protein. Depending on whether exogenous PTH is administered intermittently or continuously, it can stimulate bone formation (osteoblastic activity) or breakdown (osteroclastic activity or resorption), respectively.

TERIPARATIDE (FORTEO). Teriparatide, a polypeptide prepared by rDNA techniques, consists of the first 34 amino acids from the N-terminal end of PTH. It has been shown to contain all the structural requirements for the full biologic activity of PTH. When teriparatide is administered daily by SC injection, it stimulates osteoblastic activity at the expense of osteoclastic activity, and this enhances bone formation. This is the basis for teriparatide's use in treating high-risk patients in danger of bone fracture resulting from osteoporosis, men with primary or hypogonadal osteoporosis, and women with postmenopausal osteoporosis.[22] It carries a Boxed Warning for increased risk of osteosarcoma.

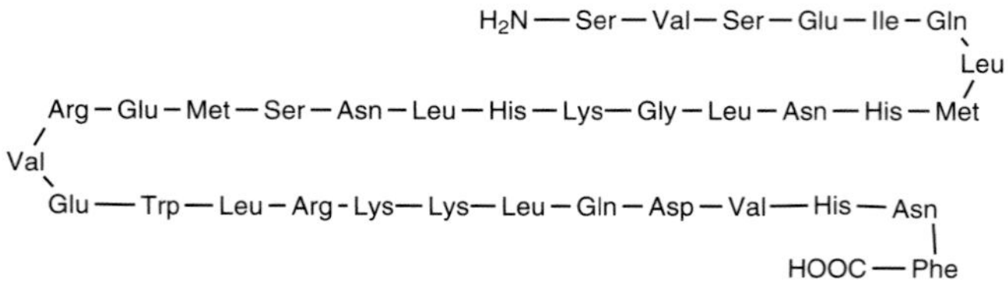

H_2N—Ser—Val—Ser—Glu—Ile—Gln—Leu—Met—His—Asn—Leu—Gly—Lys—His—Leu—Asn—Ser—Met—Glu—Arg—Val—Glu—Trp—Leu—Arg-Lys—Lys—Leu—Gln—Asp—Val—His—Asn—Phe—COOH

Teriparatide

Hormone Secreted by the Parafollicular C Cells of the Thyroid Gland

The majority of the thyroid gland contains follicular cells responsible for the production of the thyroid hormones. A second population of endocrine cells within the thyroid known as C (clear) cells, or parafollicular cells, produce the hormone calcitonin (CT), which has an opposing action to that of PTH in that it decreases the Ca^{2+} concentration in body fluids. It accomplishes this by inhibiting the activity of osteoclasts (i.e., decreasing Ca^{2+} release from bone by inhibiting bone resorption). The actual biosynthesis and release of CT is regulated by the concentration of Ca^{2+} in plasma; when it is high, CT secretion increases.

SALMON CALCITONIN (FORTICAL, MIACALCIN). Calcitonin is a single-chain polypeptide consisting of 32 amino acids (Fig. 34.5). Calcitonins obtained from different species are identical at seven of the first nine amino acids, contain Gly at position 28, and all terminate with Pro-NH_2. The C-terminal Pro amide (Pro-NH_2) is very important for the biologic function of CT, as is the disulfide bridge between Cys amino acids at positions 1 and 7. In contrast, the amino acids from 10 to 27 can be varied and seem to influence CT's potency, as well as its duration of action. Salmon CT differs from human CT at 16 amino acids.

Only salmon CT is commercially available for medical use because, on a weight basis, it is approximately 45-fold more potent than human CT. Salmon CT, in parenteral form, is approved for treating Paget disease of bone (generally seen in older persons; involves increased bone resorption and softening of bones), postmenopausal osteoporosis, and hypercalcemia of malignancy (multiple myeloma or advanced breast carcinoma). Salmon CT is also available in a nasal spray formulation, which is used exclusively in the treatment of postmenopausal osteoporosis (see Chapter 23).

Hormones of Endocrine Pancreatic Origin

The exocrine pancreas consists mostly (~99%) of gland cells known as pancreatic acini, which are responsible for secreting several digestive enzymes. The endocrine pancreas, or the remaining 1% of the gland, consists of a group of cells known as pancreatic islets or islets of Langerhans. Each of these islets consists of four distinct cell types, designated as α, β, γ, and δ cells. The α cells secrete glucagon, the β cells secrete insulin and amylin, the δ cells secrete a peptide that is identical to somatostatin of hypothalamic origin, and the γ cells secrete pancreatic polypeptide, of which little concerning its physiologic action is known. Insulin, glucagon, and somatostatin are essential in regulating carbohydrate, lipid, and amino acid metabolism. Insulin is responsible for promoting the storage of glucose as glycogen and effecting hypoglycemia, whereas glucagon mobilizes glucose from its glycogen stores and causes hyperglycemia. The primary action of somatostatin of hypothalamic origin is to inhibit the release of GH from the pituitary, but pancreatic somatostatin suppresses the production of both insulin and glucagon. Amylin, which is cosecreted with insulin from the β cells, has physiologic actions that include slowing of gastric emptying, suppression of postprandial glucagon secretion, reduction of food intake, and inhibition of the secretion of both stomach acid and pancreatic digestive enzymes.

SPECIFIC DRUGS

Insulin. Insulin has anabolic properties that include the stimulation of both skeletal muscle and liver cells to incorporate glucose and convert it to glycogen, to synthesize proteins from amino acids in the blood, and to

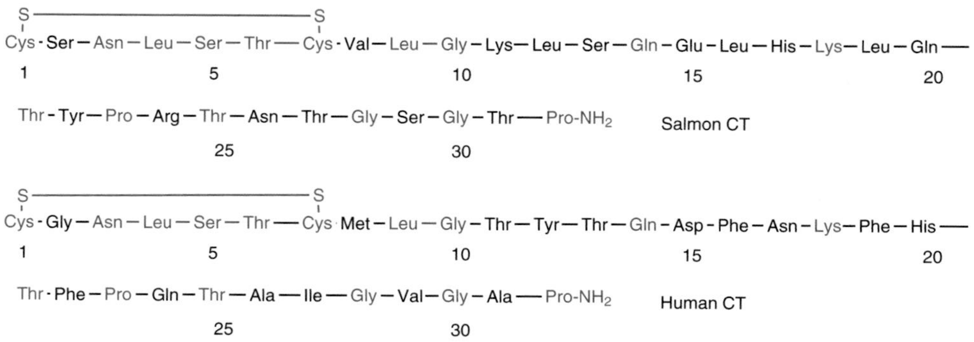

Salmon CT (S—S bridge between Cys 1 and Cys 7):

Cys-Ser—Asn—Leu—Ser—Thr—Cys-Val—Leu—Gly—Lys—Leu—Ser—Gln—Glu—Leu—His—Lys—Leu—Gln—Thr-Tyr—Pro—Arg—Thr—Asn—Thr—Gly—Ser—Gly—Thr—Pro-NH_2

Human CT (S—S bridge between Cys 1 and Cys 7):

Cys-Gly—Asn—Leu—Ser—Thr—Cys Met—Leu—Gly—Thr—Tyr—Thr—Gln—Asp—Phe—Asn—Lys—Phe—His—Thr-Phe—Pro—Gln—Thr—Ala—Ile—Gly—Val—Gly—Ala—Pro-NH_2

Figure 34.5 Primary structures of salmon and human calcitonin (CT). Similarities are highlighted in red.

act on fat cells to enhance their uptake of glucose and the synthesis of fat. In short, insulin encourages anabolism rather than catabolism because it promotes the synthesis of glycogen, proteins, and lipids. A deficiency of insulin, which characterizes the disease diabetes mellitus (DM), causes extreme changes in the entire metabolic pattern of individuals with the disease (see Chapter 20). Patients with DM often demonstrate elevated blood glucose levels, excess glucose in the urine, and failure to properly use carbohydrate and lipids. Untreated DM can be fatal. Even when treated, however, there can be numerous circulatory and renal complications, and some metabolic abnormalities may lead to blindness (diabetic retinopathy).

The human insulin molecule, consisting of 51 amino acids, has the structural characteristics of a large protein yet is only the size of a polypeptide. Two disulfide bonds (CysA7 to CysB7 and CysA20 to CysB19) link two polypeptide chains, with the A-chain consisting of 21 amino acids and the B-chain consisting of 30 amino acids. An additional disulfide loop is found in the A-chain between CysA6 and CysA11.

and Novolin products are produced using genetically modified strains of two different microorganisms. Humulin is prepared using recombinant *E. coli* bacteria. The pharmaceutical preparation is reported to contain less than 4 ppm of immunoreactive bacterial polypeptides that act as possible contaminants. Baker's yeast (*S. cerevisiae*) serves as the recombinant organism for the production of Novolin.

Studies in animals, healthy adults, and patients with type 1 DM have shown human insulin to have pharmacologic effects identical to those of purified porcine insulin. A comparable pharmacokinetic profile has also been shown. Human insulin, however, administered intramuscularly (IM) or IV, may have a slightly faster onset and slightly shorter duration of action when compared with purified porcine insulin in patients with diabetes. The usual precautions concerning toxic potentials observed with insulin of animal origin should be followed with rDNA human insulin. As would be expected, the recombinant product has been shown to be less immunogenic than nonhuman insulins.

Insulin remains the only treatment option for type 1 diabetes and is still widely used to treat patients with type 2 diabetes who do not respond adequately to other pharmacotherapies. Recombinant DNA technology has led to the development of insulin analogues that have greater utility in certain situations and may more closely resemble the normal diurnal pattern of insulin secretion. The newly engineered analogues have specific amino acid sequence modifications that improve absorption properties and biologic profiles. Insulin lispro (Humalog) has a more rapid onset and shorter duration of action than regular human insulin. Unlike regular insulin that must be injected 30-60 minutes before a meal, recombinant insulin lispro is effective when injected 15 minutes before a meal. The analogue differs from natural human insulin because the B-chain amino acids B28 Pro and B29 Lys are exchanged. Insulin aspart (Novolog), which is homologous with human insulin except for the single amino acid substitution of Asp for Pro at B28, is effective when injected 5-10 minutes before a meal.

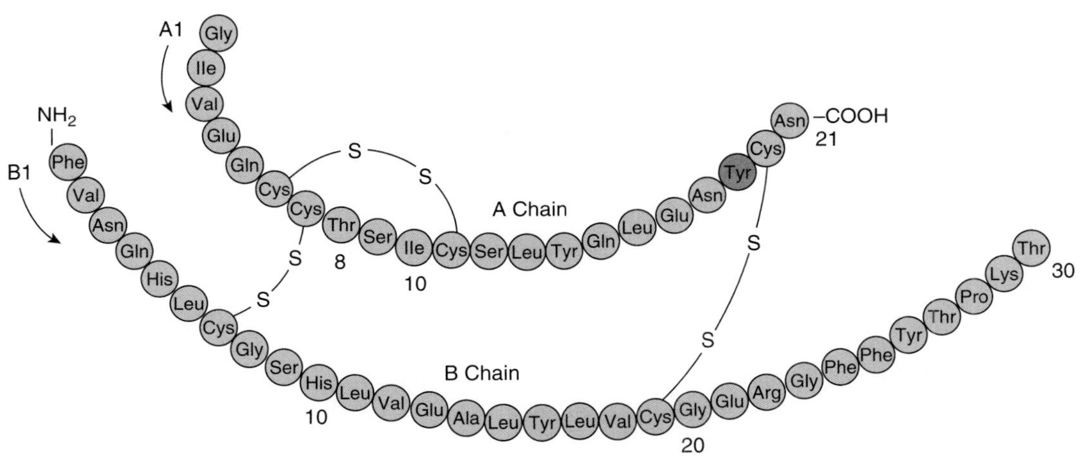

Primary structure of human insulin chains A and B

The primary sequences of insulin from several species are known, and porcine insulin is the closest to that of humans. Their A-chains are identical, and they differ only in their B-chains, with Ala30 (porcine) in place of Thr30 (human). Human and bovine insulin differ in each chain, with Ala8 and Val10 in the A-chain (bovine) and Ala30 in the B-chain (bovine). Recombinant insulin, approved in 1982 for the treatment of insulin-dependent diabetes, is the first FDA-approved rDNA drug. The biotechnology-derived insulin has several advantages over insulin derived from animal sources: (1) it has potentially fewer serious immune reactions, (2) it is pyrogen free, (3) it is not contaminated with other peptide hormones (e.g., glucagon, somatostatin, proinsulin) and (4) it can be produced in large amounts.

Human insulin of rDNA origin is available commercially as Humulin, Novolin, and several analogues, and they are classified based on their duration of action.[23] The Humulin

An ultra-long-acting agent, insulin glargine (Lantus, Toujeo) differs from human insulin in that the amino acid Asn at residue A21 is replaced by Gly, and two Arg residues are added to the C-terminus of the B chain. When administered SC, insulin glargine has a duration of action up to 24-48 hours. This change in action profile resulted from structural modifications that enhance the product's basicity, thus causing the product to precipitate at neutral pH post injection and increasing its duration of action.

Glucagon (GlucaGen). Glucagon, a 29–amino acid, straight-chain polypeptide of α-cell pancreatic origin, triggers liver glycogenolysis and gluconeogenesis, thereby elevating glucose levels. The principal action of glucagon is the liver-mediated release into the blood of abnormally high concentrations of glucose, which causes hyperglycemia. This means that glucagon has an effect on blood glucose levels that is the opposite of insulin.[24]

Glucagon of rDNA origin is now available. Replacing the bovine product with the rDNA-derived drug would eliminate the risk of acquiring bovine spongiform encephalopathy from glucagon therapy. Human glucagon of rDNA origin is marketed for the treatment of severe hypoglycemic reactions in patients with diabetes, as can occur when there is an overdose of insulin. In patients with type 1 diabetes, the increase in glucose resulting from glucagon administration may not be sufficient, and supplemental carbohydrates may need to be administered quickly, especially in children.

1 5 10 15
His-Ser-Gln-Gly-Thr-Phe-Thr-Ser-Asp-Tyr-Ser-Lys-Tyr-Leu-Asp-Ser
Thr-Asn-Met-Leu-Tyr-Gln-Val-Phe-Asp-Gln-Ala-Arg–Arg
25 20

Amino acid sequence of glucagon

AMYLIN. Amylin is a 37–amino acid peptide that is structurally similar to CT (Fig. 34.6). Amylin works together with insulin to regulate glucose concentrations after a meal. When in solution, amylin is viscous, is unstable, and tends to aggregate; therefore, it cannot be used parenterally and is not commercially available.

PRAMLINTIDE ACETATE (SYMLIN). Pramlintide acetate is a synthetic analogue of amylin with Pro substitutions at amino acids 25, 28, and 29 (Fig. 34.6). These substitutions change its physical properties such that it is can be formulated for SC injection. When pramlintide is used in combination with insulin, it slows gastric emptying, lowers blood glucose levels after meals, and affords a feeling of fullness that leads to decreased caloric intake and the potential for weight loss. Pramlintide has been approved for use in adults with type 1 or type 2 diabetes as an adjunct to insulin.[25]

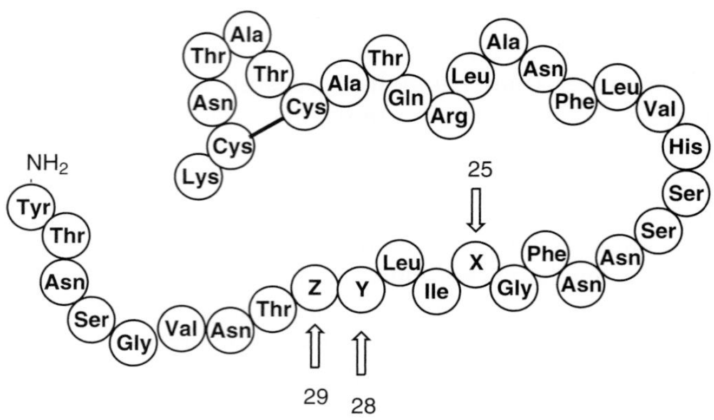

Amylin (human) X = Ala, Y = Z = Ser

Pramlintide (Symlin) X = Y = Z = Pro

Figure 34.6 Amino acid sequence of amylin and pramlintide.

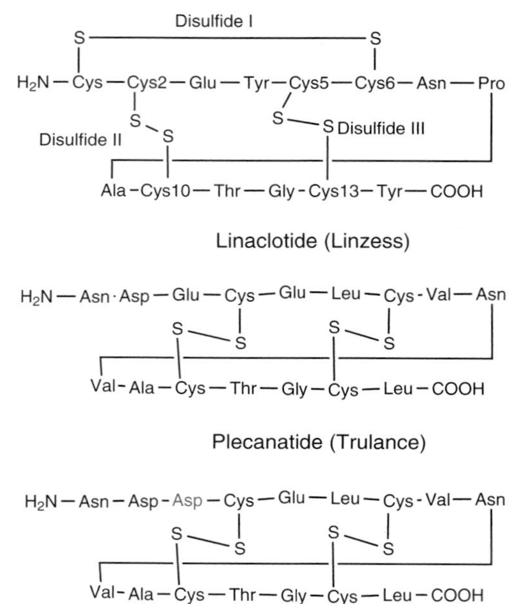

Uroguanylin

Figure 34.7 Amino acid sequences of guanylyl cyclase C agonists. Plecanatide contains Glu3 in place of Asp3 of uroguanylin.

Miscellaneous Peptidic Drugs

Specific Drugs

LINACLOTIDE (LINZESS). Linaclotide is a first-in-class, orally administered, locally acting, and minimally absorbed 14–amino acid peptide approved by the FDA in 2012 for the treatment of pain associated with irritable bowel syndrome accompanied by constipation (IBS-C) and for the treatment of chronic idiopathic constipation (CIC) (Fig. 34.7). Linaclotide achieves significant improvement in complete spontaneous bowel movements, abdominal pain, and other abdominal symptoms.

Linaclotide is a structural analogue of various naturally occurring guanylyl cyclase C (GC-C) agonists, including heat-stable bacterial enterotoxins produced by *Escherichia coli*, *Klebsiella* sp., and *Yersinia enterocloitica* which have the same 14–amino acids core, but in one case contains an additional pentapeptide sequence (Asn-Cys-Cys-Asn-Tyr-) attached to the N-terminal sequence of linaclotide. The heat-stable enterotoxins are responsible for the severe diarrhea produced by these organisms due to their agonist action at GC-C receptors. The intrachain disulfide bonds are required for activity, as well as for the reported stability toward acid and pepsin. Disulfide bonds II and III are essential for activity (Fig. 34.7). Linaclotide is relatively stable to gastric acid and is metabolized by carboxypeptidase A to a 13–amino acid peptide with removal of the C-terminal Tyr to an active metabolite, while remaining stable to further metabolism by pepsin. Linaclotide, and its active metabolite mimic the actions of the endogenous intestinal peptides guanylin (15 amino acids) and uroguanylin (16 amino acids) by activating GC-C on the intestinal epithelium. Activation of GC-C leads to increased intra- and extra-cellular levels of cGMP and activation of the cystic fibrosis transmembrane conductance regulator (CFTR) ion channel, resulting in increased levels of bicarbonate, chloride ions and water in the intestinal lumen and accelerated gastrointestinal transit.

The most common adverse reactions include diarrhea, abdominal pain, flatulence, and abdominal distension. It carries a Boxed Warning for pediatric use and is contraindicated in pediatric patients up to 6 years of age.[26-28]

PLECANATIDE (TRULANCE). Plecanatide is a newer GC-C agonist and the first uroguanylin analogue approved by the FDA in 2017 for the treatment of CIC (Fig. 34.7).[27] It has also been used for the treatment of irritable bowel syndrome with constipation (IBS-C). Although it is a peptidic drug, its site of action is in the upper gastrointestinal tract, and thus, it is orally active. It has minimal systemic exposure upon oral administration and can be administered with or without food.

UROGUANYLIN. Uroguanylin is a 16–amino acid peptide secreted by enterochromaffin cells in the duodenum and jejunum where, at pH 5-6, it binds the GC-C receptor and triggers the signaling cascade initiated by cGMP. This, in turn leads to fluid and electrolyte balance (Fig. 34.7). While linaclotide, a structural analogue of heat-stable bacterial enterotoxins, is a highly constrained structure with three disulfide bonds, plecanatide with its two disulfide bonds mimics uroguanylin in its flexibility and ability to activate GC-C receptor in a pH dependent manner. The two charged acid-sensing Asp/Glu amino acids at the N-terminus regulate the binding affinity to GC-C receptors in a pH-dependent manner (exhibit higher activity in the more acidic proximal small intestine and lower activity in the more basic distal small intestine and colon). Linaclotide on the other hand is pH independent due to lack of the requisite acidic amino acid residue at position 2.[29] Studies suggest that plecanatide assumes the most active conformation at pH 5, which is the pH of the proximal small intestine. One amino acid substitution in plecanatide (Asp3 vs. Glu3) results in stronger receptor binding.[30] Plecanatide is metabolized in the GI tract to an active metabolite by the hydrolysis of C-terminal Leu. The most common adverse effect is diarrhea which may be severe. Additional adverse effects consist of sinus and upper respiratory tract infections, bloating, gas, and increases in several liver biochemical tests.[28,29,31]

H_2N—His1-Asp—Gly—Ser—Phe—Ser—Asp—Glu—Met9

Asp20—Arg—Ala-Ala—Leu-Asn—Asp-Leu—Ile—Thr—Asn10

Phe·Ile-Asn-Trp-Leu·Ile-Glu-Val·Lys-Ile-Thr Asp32-COOH

Teduglutide (Gattex)

H_2N—Gly1—Gly—Val—Leu—Val—Gln—Pro—Gly8-COOH

Larazotide

Figure 34.8 Amino acid sequences of teduglutide and larazotide.

TEDUGLUTIDE (GATTEX). Teduglutide is a glucagon-like peptide-2 (GLP-2) agonist approved in 2012 for the treatment of adult patients with short bowel syndrome (SBS) who are dependent on parenteral nutrition (Fig. 34.8). SBS is a rare and potentially life-threatening condition in which nutrients are not properly absorbed because a large part of the small intestine is missing or has been surgically removed. GLP-2 is a 33–amino acid endogenous peptide hormone located at the carboxy terminus of proglucagon and secreted by intestinal enteroendocrine L-cells in the small and large intestines. GLP-2 helps compensate for a loss of absorptive and digestive capacity associated with SBS. Teduglutide was designed to be resistant to degradation by dipeptidyl peptidase IV (DPP-IV) by replacing Ala at position 2 of the N-terminus with Gly, and is manufactured using rDNA technology.[28]

LARAZOTIDE ACETATE. Larazotide is a locally acting, poorly absorbed, peptidic drug under late-stage clinical trials (NCT01396213) for the treatment of gastrointestinal disorders such as celiac disease (Fig. 34.8).[32] It is a first-in-class, orally active synthetic octapeptide, useful for the treatment of patients with celiac disease who are on a strict gluten-free diet. Its localized action in decreasing permeability of tight junctions occurs by blocking zonulin receptors and thereby preventing actin rearrangement in response to a range of different stimuli. Larazotide would be the first ever drug approved for celiac disease.

Enzymes

Tissue-Type Plasminogen Activator

The fibrinolytic system is activated in response to the presence of an intracellular thrombus or clot. The process of clot dissolution is initiated by the conversion of plasminogen to plasmin. Plasminogen activation is catalyzed by two endogenous and highly specific serine proteases, urokinase-type plasminogen activator, and tissue-type plasminogen activator (t-PA).

The mature human t-PA (alteplase) is a glycoprotein consisting of a single chain of 527 amino acids (Fig. 34.9). Its MW is approximately 70 kDa. Human t-PA contains 35 Cys residues assigned to 17 disulfide bonds. A serine protease domain of approximately 270 amino acids is located at the carboxy-terminal end of this protein. A fibronectin “finger” domain, two kringle domains, and an epidermal growth factor domain also are present. The t-PA

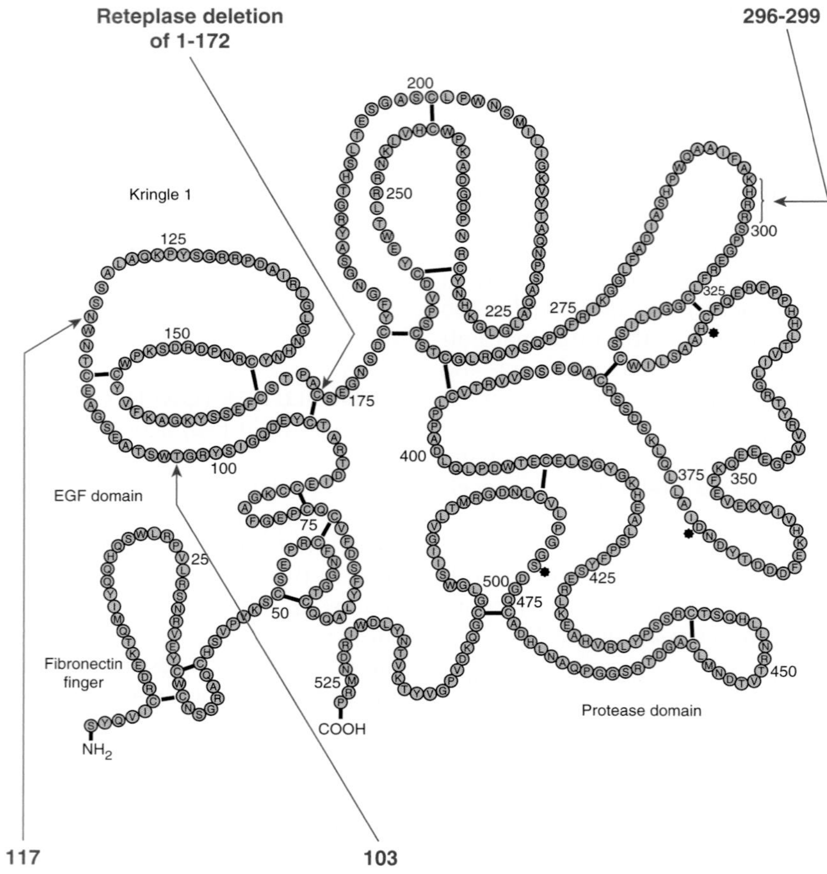

Figure 34.9 Schematic diagram of t-PA (alteplase), reteplase (removal of amino acids 1-172), and tenecteplase in which threonine-103 (T) is replaced with asparagine, asparagine-117 (N) is replaced with glutamine, and lysine-histidine-arginine-arginine (KHRR) at positions 296-299 are replaced with four alanines. Correctly folded and functional t-PA contains 17 intradomain disulfide bonds and consists of fibronectin finger (amino acids 4-50), EGF domain (amino acids 51-87), Kringle 1 (amino acids 88-175), Kringle 2 (amino acids 176-256), and Protease domain (amino acids 256-527). Adapted with permission from Nordt TK, Bode C. Thrombolysis:newer thrombolytic agents and their role in clinical medicineThrombolysis:newer thrombolytic agents and their role in clinical medicineThrombolysis:newer thrombolytic agents and their role in clinical medicine. *Heart.* 2003;89:1358-1362.

protease domain is approximately 35%-40% homologous with typical serine proteases, such as bovine trypsin and chymotrypsin.

Mammalian cells produce two t-PA variants of N-linked glycosylation, type 1 (at Asn117, 184, and 448) and type 2 (only at Asn117 and 448). The rate of fibrin-dependent plasminogen activation is twofold to threefold faster for type 2 compared with type 1. The cDNA obtained from a human melanoma cell line was expressed in CHO cells to achieve a glycosylated protein identical to the natural protein. Protein engineering studies have produced variant t-PA molecules with modified pharmacokinetics, affinity for fibrin, catalytic activity, and side effects.

Three rDNA thrombolytic agents are approved in the United States.[33] The first is alteplase, an enzyme equivalent to human t-PA (Fig. 34.9). It is indicated for the treatment of acute myocardial infarction (administered as a bolus), acute massive pulmonary embolism (administered by IV infusion), and ischemic stroke. It is the first fibrin-selective thrombolytic agent preferentially activating fibrinogen bound to fibrin. Thus, the thrombolytic effect is localized to a blood clot and avoids systemic activation of fibrinogen, preventing bleeding elsewhere in the body. Plasma t-PA concentrations are proportional to the rate of infusion. Alteplase is rapidly cleared from circulating plasma, with 50% cleared within 5 minutes after termination of infusion. The mechanisms for clearance of t-PA from the blood are poorly understood. Detectable levels of antibody against alteplase have been found in patients receiving the drug, although 12 days to 10 months later, antibody determinations have been negative.

The second agent, reteplase (Fig. 34.9), is a recombinant, nonglycosylated deletion mutation of human t-PA containing 355 of 527 amino acids of native t-PA. The drug is indicated for acute myocardial infarction and is given as a 10 U + 10 U double bolus.

The most recent addition to the marketed rDNA-derived t-PAs is tenecteplase (Fig. 34.9). This recombinant protein contains three modifications from natural human t-PA. In the kringle 1 domain of natural t-PA, Thr103 is replaced by Asn; the kringle 1 domain Asn117 is replaced by Gln; and in the protease domain, four amino acids (Lys, His, and two Arg residues) are replaced by four Ala residues. The drug is indicated for acute myocardial infarction.

Bleeding at the injection site is similar to that with alteplase, but there is a reduction in noncerebral bleeding complications. It is administered as a single, 5-second bolus.

DNase—Dornase α (Pulmozyme)

According to the Cystic Fibrosis Foundation, cystic fibrosis (CF) is the most common fatal genetic disorder, afflicting approximately 30,000 patients in the United States. Breakthrough treatments have increased the median survival age to close to 40 years. Cystic fibrosis patients develop thick mucus secretions and suffer from severe, frequent lung infections. Studies during the 1950s and 1960s determined that CF-related secretions in the lungs contained large amounts of DNA. Mucous-thickening DNA release resulted from an inflammatory response and ensuing white blood cell death. The enzyme DNase I specifically cleaves extracellular DNA, such as that found in the mucous secretion of CF patients, and has no effect on the DNA of intact cells. The FDA has approved a recombinant human DNase.

The enzyme DNase I is a glycoprotein containing 260 amino acids with an approximate MW of 37 kDa. The recombinant protein is expressed by genetically engineered CHO cells encoding for the native enzyme, although DNase I was not purified or sequenced from human sources at the time. A degenerate sequence, based on the sequence of bovine DNase (263 amino acids), was used to synthesize probes and screen a human pancreatic DNA library. The primary amino acid sequence of rhDNase is identical to native human DNase I.

The only FDA-approved DNase product, dornase α (inhalation solution), has been developed as a therapeutic agent for the management of CF. It is administered by nebulizer aerosol delivery systems.

Dornase α[34] is indicated for daily administration in conjunction with standard CF therapies to reduce the frequency of respiratory infections requiring parenteral antibiotics to improve pulmonary function. The breakdown of DNA in infected sputum results in improved airflow in the lung and reduced risk of bacterial infection. Although effective for the management of the respiratory symptoms of CF, dornase α is not a replacement for antibiotics, bronchodilators, and daily physical therapy. This product also finds application in treating chronic bronchitis.

Enzyme Replacement Therapy

Enzyme replacement therapy (ERT) is available for many of the lysosomal storage diseases, including Gaucher disease, Fabry disease, Pompe disease, mucopolysaccharidosis (MPS) type I (Hurler, Scheie, and Hurler/Scheie syndromes), MPS II (Hunter syndrome), and MPS VI (Maroteaux-Lamy syndrome).[35] The most frequent drug-related adverse events of ERT are infusion-related reactions. Antibodies formed against infused enzymes are usually of the immunoglobulin G (IgG) serotype. Signs and symptoms of infusion-related reactions (IRRs) can include cutaneous reactions, pyrexia, headache, and hypertension. The precise relationship between antibody formation and occurrence of IRRs is unclear. Not all IRRs are antibody mediated, and not all patients who develop antibodies develop IRRs.[35]

Imiglucerase (Cerezyme)

Type 1 Gaucher disease, the most common form, is an inherited disorder. Fewer than 1 in 40,000 people in the general population have Gaucher disease. Patients with the disease lack the normal form of the enzyme glucocerebrosidase. They cannot break down glucocerebroside, leading to its accumulation within the lysosomes. This leads to the poor functioning of macrophages and an accumulation of "Gaucher cells" in the spleen, liver, and bone marrow. Imiglucerase is an analogue of glucocerebrosidase produced by rDNA technology using mammalian cell culture system. The drug is a monomeric glycoprotein consisting of 497 amino acids (MW ~ 60 kDa), with four N-linked glycosylation sites, and differs from the human placental glucocerebrosidase by one amino acid (His495 replaces Arg). Imiglucerase carries out the normal function of the missing enzyme and has been shown to be safe in long-term safety studies.[36]

Alglucosidase α (Myozyme, Lumizyme)

Pompe disease, a rare genetic disorder affecting nearly 1 in every 40,000 births, is caused by the mutation in a gene that makes the α-glucosidase enzyme. It was the first disease to be identified as a lysosomal storage disorder. α-Glucosidase enzyme is responsible for the breakdown of glycogen to glucose. The lack of degradation results in the accumulation of glycogen in lysosomes in all tissues, most notably in skeletal and cardiac muscles. The disease is characterized as early-onset or late-onset Pompe disease based on age at the time of onset. Severe α-glucosidase deficiency manifests during infancy with rapidly progressing muscle weakness, hypotonia, and cardiomyopathy and eventually lethal muscle disorder. As with other lysosomal storage disorders, ERT is the patient's only hope.

Alglucosidase α was developed and launched in 2006 for the treatment of infants and children with Pompe disease.[37] Another alglucosidase α drug (Lumizyme) was approved by the FDA in 2010 for patients age 8 years and older with late-onset (noninfantile) Pompe disease. Alglucosidase α is a recombinant human enzyme produced by transfected CHO cells as a 110 kDa precursor that targets lysosomes via the mannose-6-phosphate receptor. Following endocytosis, the enzyme is transformed to its mature 76 kDa form that restores glycogen processing and reverses accumulation. Alglucosidase α therapy has been shown to improve cardiac and muscle function.

Idursulfase (Elaprase)

MPS II (Hunter syndrome), a disease with an incidence of approximately 1 in 162,000 births, is caused by the deficiency of the lysosomal enzyme iduronate-2-sulfatase. This enzyme is responsible for a crucial step in the degradation of two glycosaminoglycans (GAGs), dermatan sulfate and heparin sulfate, in the lysosomes of various cells. Iduronate-2-sulfatase deficiency causes an accumulation of GAGs in tissue, and the patient's only recourse is ERT. The clinical manifestations of this deficiency are short stature, joint stiffness, harsh facial features, hepatosplenomegaly, and progressive intellectual disability. Recombinant iduronate-2-sulfatase has been available in the United States since 2006. It is produced from HT-1080 cells for proper translational attachment of N-linked oligosaccharides and the crucial mannose-6-phosphate groups as the targeting phosphate into lysosomes.[38] In addition to being fully glycosylated with eight mannose-6-phosphate groups, the enzyme possesses sialylated moieties that improve its stability in circulation. For full activity, Cys59 must undergo modification to formylglycine. Idursulfase has been designated as an orphan product by the FDA.

Cytokines

Cytokines communicate in a dynamic cellular network during an immune/inflammatory response to an antigen. Lymphokine and monokine are the terms used for a cytokine derived from lymphocytes and macrophages, respectively. Chemokines are a group of at least 25 structurally homologous, low-molecular-weight cytokines that stimulate leukocyte movement and regulate the migration of leukocytes from the blood to tissues. Cytokines, usually released and targeted to produce a localized effect, regulate the growth, differentiation, and activation of the hematopoietic cells responsible for the maintenance of the immune response. A wide array of glycoproteins, including interferons, interleukins, hematopoietic growth factors, and tumor necrosis factors (TNFs), are cytokines. Cytokines can only act on target cells that express receptors for that cytokine. There are five families of cytokine receptor proteins: class I cytokine receptors, class II cytokine receptors, TNF receptors, chemokine receptors, and immunoglobulin superfamily receptors (Table 34.2).[39-43]

Interferons

The interferons are a family of cytokines discovered in the late 1950s with broad-spectrum antiviral and potential anticancer activity, making them biologic response modifiers. Biotherapy (the therapeutic use of any substance of biologic origin) of cancer is different than standard cytotoxic chemotherapy. That is, biotherapeutic agents belong to a group of compounds that enhance normal immune interactions (therefore, they also are immunomodulators) with cells in a specific or nonspecific fashion. Chemotherapeutics interact directly with the cancer cells themselves.

Table 34.2 The Five Families of Cytokine Receptors and Some Ligands

Receptor Families	Ligands
Class I cytokine receptors	IL-2, IL-7, IL-9, IL-11, IL-13, IL-15, GM-CSF, G-CSF
Class II cytokine receptors	INF-α, INF-β, INF-γ
Tumor necrosis factor receptors	TNF-α, TNF-β, CD30, CD40, FAS
Chemokine receptors	IL-8, RANTES, MIP-1, PF-4, MCAF
Immunoglobin superfamily receptors	IL-1, M-CSF

Three types of naturally occurring interferons have been found in small quantities: leukocyte interferon (IFN-α), produced by lymphocytes and macrophages; fibroblast interferon (IFN-β), produced by fibroblasts, epithelial cells, and macrophages; and immune interferon (IFN-γ), synthesized by $CD4^+$, $CD8^+$, and natural killer lymphocytes. Both IFN-α and IFN-β, also known as type I interferons, exhibit approximately 30% primary sequence homology but no structural similarity to IFN-γ, a type II interferon. All three are glycoproteins. Previously only available in low yields by chemical synthesis or isolation, several rDNA interferon pharmaceuticals now have been marketed in the United States including three IFN-α products, two IFN-β agents, and an IFN-γ drug.

INTERFERON-α. At least 24 different human genes producing 16 distinct mature IFN-α molecules with slight structural variations are known. Human IFN-α proteins generally are composed of either 165 or 166 amino acids. The two primary subtypes, IFN-α2a (Roferon-A) and IFN-α2b (Intron A), both contain 165 amino acids, differing only at position 23, with IFN-α2a containing a Lys residue and IFN-α2b an Arg residue at this position. They have MWs of approximately 19 kDa. Although cultures of genetically modified *E. coli* produce two recombinant FDA-approved IFN-α products, IFN-α2a and IFN-α2b, their method of purification differs. Purification of IFN-α2a includes affinity chromatography using a murine MAb, whereas that of IFN-α2b does not.

Interferon-α possesses complex antiviral, antineoplastic, and immunomodulating activities. Although the precise mechanism of action of IFN-α is not known, it is believed to interact with cell surface receptors to produce the biologic effects. The actions appear to result from a complex cascade of biologic modulation and pharmacologic effects that include the modulation of host immune responses, cellular antiproliferative effects, cell differentiation, transcription, and translation processes, and reduction of oncogene expression. Interferon-α is filtered through the glomeruli in the kidney and undergoes rapid proteolytic degradation during tubular reabsorption.

CONSENSUS INTERFERON (IFN ALFACON-1). Hepatitis C infection results in a chronic disease state in 50%-70% of cases and is now the most important known cause of chronic liver disease. Following the acute phase, as many as 80% of patients may progress to the chronic phase of the infectious disease. An estimated 20% of patients with a chronic form of the disease progress to cirrhosis. The only agents shown to be effective in the treatment of hepatitis C are the interferons. A unique recombinant molecule, a consensus IFN, known as IFN alfacon-1, has been approved for the treatment of chronic hepatitis C infection. It is a 19.5 kDa recombinant protein produced in *E. coli* and contains 166 amino acids in a relationship in which each amino acid position in the molecule contains the most commonly occurring amino acid among all the natural IFN-α subtypes. IFN alfacon-1 exhibits 5- to 10-fold higher biologic activity when compared to either IFN-α2a or IFN-α2b.

INTERFERON-β. Normally produced by fibroblasts, human IFN-β was first cloned and expressed in 1980; however, its instability made it unsuitable for clinical use. The more stable recombinant IFN-β1b (Betaseron), a 165–amino acid analogue of human IFN-β, differs from the native protein with a Ser residue substituted for Cys at position 17. The highly purified rDNA technology–derived product has an MW of 18.5 kDa. It is produced in a recombinant *E. coli.* Approved in 1993 by the FDA, IFN-β1b is indicated for the treatment of patients with exacerbating-remitting multiple sclerosis (MS). The National MS Society says that an estimated one million Americans have this disease, with nearly 85% of patients falling into the exacerbating-remitting category. A vial of recombinant IFN-β1b contains 0.3 mg of protein with dextrose and human albumin as stabilizers. The exact mechanism of action of IFN-β1b is not known. Its immunomodulating effects, however, may benefit patients with MS by decreasing the levels of endogenous IFN-γ. Levels of IFN-γ are believed to rise before and during acute attacks in patients with MS.

Whereas IFN-β1b of rDNA origin was the first to the market, IFN-β1a (Avonex) also is now available. IFN-β1a is produced in mammalian cells and has the same amino acid sequence and carbohydrate side chain as natural IFN-β. Recombinant IFN-β1a is administered to patients once weekly by intramuscular injection. This differs from the SC administration every other day of rDNA-produced IFN-β1b.

INTERFERON-γ. Human IFN-γ[44] is a single-chain glycoprotein with an MW of approximately 15.5 kDa. The cytokine mainly exists as a noncovalent dimer of differentially glycosylated chains in solution in vivo. Glycosylation does not appear to be necessary for biologic activity. The 140–amino acid IFN-γ1b (Actimmune) is produced by fermentation of a recombinant *E. coli*. IFN-γ1b and was approved in 1990 by the FDA.

IFN-γ1b possesses biologic activity identical to the natural human IFN-γ derived from lymphoid cells. Although all the IFNs share certain biologic effects, IFN-γ differs distinctly from IFN-α and IFN-β by its potent capacity to activate phagocytes involved in host defense. These activating effects include the ability to enhance the production of toxic oxygen metabolites within phagocytes, resulting in a more efficient killing of various microorganisms. This activity is the basis for the use of IFN-γ1b in the management of chronic granulomatous disease. Chronic granulomatous disease is a group of rare X-linked or autosomal genetic disorders of the phagocytic oxygen metabolite–generating system, leaving patients susceptible to severe infections. The drug extends the time that patients spend without being hospitalized for infectious episodes. Investigational applications of IFN-γ include the treatment of renal cell carcinoma, small-cell lung cancer, infectious disease, trauma, atopic dermatitis, asthma, allergies, rheumatoid arthritis, and venereal warts.

Interleukins

Interleukins are cytokines involved in immune cell communication. Synthesized by monocytes, macrophages, and lymphocytes, interleukins serve as soluble messengers between leukocytes. Currently, at least 18 interleukins have been observed. One of the most studied cytokines is interleukin (IL)-2, originally called T cell growth factor because of its ability to stimulate growth of T lymphocytes.

INTERLEUKIN-1. IL-1 is a major inflammatory mediator and exists in two forms: IL-1α and IL-1β. Each form is a product of two separate genes, but the two are related to each other structurally at a three-dimensional level. IL-1β is a systemic, hormone-like mediator intended to be released from cells, whereas IL-1α is primarily a regulator of intracellular events and mediator of local inflammation. The recombinant protein anakinra, which is an IL-1 receptor antagonist, and the fusion protein rilonacept, which blocks the excessive IL-1β signaling, are commercially available and described below.[45,46]

Anakinra (Kineret). Rheumatoid arthritis (RA) is a chronic, inflammatory disease affecting synovial joints. Patients with persistent, active disease are traditionally treated with disease-modifying antirheumatic drugs (DMARDs). IL-1 receptor antagonist is an endogenous cytokine that blocks the binding of proinflammatory cytokine IL-1 to its receptor, thereby balancing the cartilage destruction and bone resorption mediated by IL-1. Anakinra is the first recombinant human IL-1 receptor antagonist and differs from the native human protein in that it is not glycosylated and has an additional N-terminal Met residue (rmetHuIL-1 receptor antagonist). Anakinra, a 17.3 kDa recombinant protein expressed in *E. coli*, was approved in 2001 for treating the signs and symptoms and the joint-destructive components of RA.[45-47] However, the challenge for anakinra for occupying the large number of IL-1 receptors is formidable, as these receptors are expressed on all cells except red blood cells. Moreover, anakinra is rapidly excreted by the kidney, and blood levels are low after 24 hours. IL-1 receptors are also readily generated each day, necessitating a daily SC injection.

Rilonacept (Arcalyst). Cryopyrin-associated periodic syndromes are inherited disorders caused by mutations in the nucleotide-binding domain, leucine-rich family, pyrin domain containing-3 (*NLRP-3*) gene, which encodes the protein cryopyrin. Cryopyrin regulates the protease caspase-1 and controls activation of IL-1β. Mutations in the *NLRP-3* gene can cause an overactive inflammasome, resulting in excessive levels of activated IL-1β, which causes inflammation, joint pain, rash or skin lesions, fever and chills, eye redness or pain, and fatigue. Rilonacept is a 252 kDa recombinant fusion protein produced in CHO cells and approved by the FDA in 2008 for the long-term treatment of familial cold autoinflammatory syndrome and Muckle-Wells syndrome. These two cryopyrin-associated periodic syndromes are extremely rare, affecting approximately 300 people in the United States.

Rilonacept's mechanism of intervention involves blockade of excessive IL-1β signaling.[45,46,48] Rilonacept combines the extracellular binding domains of the human

IL-1 receptor component and IL-1 receptor accessory protein in a single chain, with two of these chains joined to the fragment crystallizable (Fc) portion of human IgG, creating a dimeric molecule. Rilonacept serves as an effective soluble IL-1β sink or trap, since the coupled receptor components bind IL-1β with higher affinity than either individual receptor. It exerts its effects through a multicomponent receptor system and is more effective than drugs that target only one of the components, such as the IL-1 receptor antagonist anakinra. With its weekly SC dosing regimen, rilonacept may have better patient compliance than anakinra.

Concomitant administration of other IL-1 blockers and anti–TNF-α agents has been associated with an increased risk of serious infection and neutropenia. Because IL-1 blockade may interfere with the immune response to infections, patients should not initiate rilonacept with an existing infection. Patients with chronic inflammation tend to have suppressed formation of CYP450 enzymes. Treatment with rilonacept is expected to normalize CYP450 distribution, so plasma levels of coadministered drugs that are CYP450 substrates with narrow therapeutic indexes should be carefully monitored for potential dose modification.

INTERLEUKIN-2. Human IL-2 is a 133–amino acid, 15.4 kDa protein that is O-glycosylated at a Thr in position 3. An intramolecular disulfide bond between Cys58 and Cys105 is essential for biologic activity. A recombinant version of IL-2 is marketed as aldesleukin as described below.[49,50]

Aldesleukin (Proleukin). Aldesleukin differs from the native protein by the absence of glycosylation, a lack of the N-terminal Ala residue at position 1 (132 amino acids), and the replacement of Cys with Ser at position 125 of the primary sequence. Sequence changes were accomplished by site-directed mutagenesis to the IL-2 gene before cloning and expression. Aldesleukin exists as noncovalent microaggregates with an average size of 27 recombinant IL-2 molecules. The recombinant drug possesses the biologic activity of the native protein.

Aldesleukin is used in cancer biotherapy as a biologic response modifier for the treatment of metastatic renal cell carcinoma and metastatic melanoma. Side effects are the major dose-limiting factor because aldesleukin is an extremely toxic drug. Aldesleukin should be restricted to patients with normal cardiac and pulmonary functions and administered in a hospital setting under the supervision of a qualified physician experienced in the use of anticancer agents.

INTERLEUKIN-2 FUSION PROTEIN. Using ligation chemistry approaches during the preparation of recombinant proteins, researchers have created biologically active molecules that combine the activities of two individual proteins into "fusion molecules." These fusion technologies hold promise for developing custom molecules expressing a wide variety of dual activities.

Denileukin Diftitox (Ontak). The FDA approved the fusion protein denileukin diftitox in 1999 for the treatment of patients with persistent or recurrent cutaneous T cell lymphoma (CTCL) whose malignant cells express the CD25 component of the IL-2 receptor.[51-53] CTCL is a general term for a group of low-grade, non-Hodgkin lymphomas (NHLs) affecting approximately 1,000 new patients per year. Malignant T cells manifest initially in the skin. Over time, there is systemic involvement. For many patients, CTCL is a persistent, disfiguring, and debilitating disease that requires multiple treatments. Malignant CTCL cells express one or more of the components of the IL-2 receptor. Thus, the IL-2 receptor may be a homing device to attract a "killer drug." Men are twice as likely as women to have the disease.

Denileukin diftitox is an rDNA-derived, cytotoxic IL-2 fusion protein that is composed of two different components: the first 389 amino acids of diphtheria toxin fused to amino acids 2-133 of human IL-2. Thus, the fusion protein binds to IL-2 receptors on neoplastic T cells and is internalized via receptor-mediated endocytosis, delivering diphtheria toxin directly to kill the CTCL target. Interestingly, although denileukin diftitox was originally thought to act primarily by binding to CD25, now that the components of IL-2 receptor are better delineated, it appears that clinical activity of denileukin diftitox is associated with the presence of CD122. It carries a Boxed Warning of severe infusion reactions and capillary leak syndrome.

INTERLEUKIN-11. IL-11 is a thrombopoietic growth factor that directly stimulates the proliferation of hematopoietic stem cells and megakaryocyte progenitor cells. This induces megakaryocyte maturation, resulting in increased platelet production. IL-11 is a 178–amino acid glycosylated cytokine produced by bone marrow stromal cells. Primary osteoblasts and mature osteoclasts express mRNAs for an IL-11 receptor (IL-11Rα). Thus, bone-forming cells and bone-resorbing cells are potential targets of IL-11. In 1997, the FDA approved oprelvekin, an rDNA-derived version of IL-11 produced in *E. coli*.

Oprelvekin (Neumega). Oprelvekin contains only 177 amino acids, lacking the amino terminal Pro of the native IL-11. Produced in *E. coli*, the cytokine analogue is nonglycosylated. Oprelvekin has potent thrombopoietic activity in animal models of compromised hematopoiesis. It is indicated for the prevention of thrombocytopenia following myelosuppressive chemotherapy. Pharmacists should monitor for possible fluid retention and electrolyte imbalance when it is used with chronic diuretic therapy.

Tumor Necrosis Factor

TNFs, a family of cytokines produced mainly by activated mononuclear phagocytes, have both beneficial and potentially harmful effects, mediating cytotoxic and inflammatory reactions. The TNFs are endogenous pyrogens capable of inducing chills, fever, and other flu-like symptoms. TNF-α, also called cachectin (and commonly referred to as TNF), and TNF-β, also called lymphotoxin, both bind to the same receptor and induce similar biologic activities. Biologic effects of TNF-α include selective toxicity against a range of tumor cells, mediation of septic shock, activation of elements of the immune system in response to gram-negative bacteria, and induction/regulation of inflammation. rDNA-derived TNF-α has been studied extensively, but it has not been developed into a useful drug.

ETANERCEPT (ENBREL). Etanercept is an rDNA-produced fusion protein that binds specifically to TNF and blocks its interaction with cell surface TNF receptors.[54,55] It is indicated for the treatment of moderate to severe active RA in adults and for juvenile RA in patients who have had an inadequate response to one or more DMARDs. It is a genetically engineered protein that includes two components. The extracellular, ligand-binding portion (p75) of the human TNF receptor is linked as a fusion protein to the Fc portion of the human IgG1 antibody. Each etanercept molecule binds specifically to two TNF molecules found in the synovial fluid of patients with RA, blocking the interaction of TNF with the TNF receptor. The drug inhibits both TNF-α and TNF-β. The Fc portion of the fusion protein helps to clear the etanercept-TNF complex from the body.

ABATACEPT (ORENCIA). With the recognition that T cells play a central role in the pathogenesis of RA, abatacept has been developed as a novel, rational approach to interfere with the upstream effector of the inflammation. This drug has the potential to meet the needs of patients who fail to respond adequately to existing therapy using traditional DMARDs such as methotrexate (MTX) or TNF-blocking agents. Abatacept is a soluble 92 kDa human fusion protein approved for the treatment of RA as a new class of DMARDs.[56] Structurally, abatacept consists of a fusion between the extracellular domain of human cytotoxic T-lymphocyte–associated antigen-4 (CTLA-4) linked to the modified Fc portion of human IgG1. Abatacept selectively modulates the CD80/CD86:CD28 costimulatory signal required for full T cell activation. By targeting the activation of T cells, an upstream event in the immune cascade that underlies RA, abatacept has the potential to impact multiple downstream aspects of RA immunogenesis, such as the production of cytokines, autoantibodies, and inflammatory proteins. The immunoglobulin portion of the abatacept serves as a handle to facilitate purification of the protein produced by rDNA technology in a mammalian cell expression system. It also enhances the solubility and serum half-life of the fusion protein. Serum half-life of 14.7 days is independent of dose, and rate of elimination remains constant, supporting the lack of antidrug antibody generation.

Abatacept was found to be well tolerated for up to 7 years of exposure in patients with RA who had an inadequate response to MTX or other traditional DMARDs or who failed to respond to treatment with anti-TNF agents.[57] The potential for increased risk of infection is an important safety concern in patients with RA receiving biologic therapies. During abatacept treatment, live vaccinations should be avoided because the drug may diminish the effectiveness of some immunizations, and anti-TNF agents should be avoided due to risk of infections.

Hematopoietic Growth Factors

Hematopoiesis is the complex series of events involved in the formation, proliferation, differentiation, and activation of red blood cells, white blood cells, and platelets. Hematopoietic growth factors are cytokines that regulate these events. Investigators have identified and cloned at least 20 factors, including IL-3 (or multi–colony-stimulating factor [CSF]), IL-4, IL-5, IL-6, IL-7, erythropoietin (EPO), granulocyte-macrophage colony-stimulating factor (GM-CSF), granulocyte colony-stimulating factor (G-CSF), macrophage colony-stimulating factor (M-CSF), and stem cell factor. Figure 34.10 summarizes the elaborate hematopoietic cascade. All blood cells originate within the bone marrow from a single class of pluripotent stem cells. In response to various external and internal stimuli, regulated by hematopoietic growth factors, stem cells give rise to additional new stem cells (self-renewal) and differentiate into mature, specialized blood cells.

ERYTHROPOIETIN—EPOETIN α (EPOGEN, PROCRIT). EPO,[58-60] a glycoprotein with an MW of 30-34 kDa produced by the kidney, stimulates the division and differentiation of erythroid progenitors in the bone marrow, increasing the production of red blood cells. Epoetin α (sometimes called rHuEPO-α), a recombinant EPO prepared from cultures of genetically engineered mammalian CHO cells, consists of the identical 165–amino acid sequence of endogenous EPO. The MW is approximately 30.4 kDa. The protein contains two disulfide bonds (linking Cys residues 7 with 161 and 29 with 33) and four sites of glycosylation (one O-site and three N-sites); the disulfide bonds and glycosylation are necessary for the hormone's biologic activity. Deglycosylated natural EPO and bacterial-derived EPO (without glycosylation) have greatly decreased in vivo activity, although in vitro activity is largely conserved. The sugars may play a role in thermal stability or the prevention of aggregation in vivo.

The marketed products are formulated as a sterile, colorless, preservative-free liquid for IV or SC administration. Epoetin α is indicated for the treatment of various anemias. Epoetin α also represents a major scientific advance in the treatment of patients with chronic renal failure, serving as replacement therapy for inadequate production of endogenous EPO by failing kidneys. Epoetin α may decrease the need for infusions in dialysis patients. By several mechanisms related to elevating the erythroid progenitor cell pool, epoetin α increases the production of red blood cells.

The manufacturer's full prescribing information should be consulted for dosing regimens, because the dose is titrated individually to maintain the patient's target hematocrit. The circulating half-life is 4-13 hours in patients with chronic renal failure. Peak serum levels are achieved within 5-24 hours following SC administration.

COLONY-STIMULATING FACTORS. The CSFs are glycoprotein cytokines that promote progenitor proliferation, differentiation, and some functional activation. The name "colony-stimulating factor" results from the fact that these proteins often are assayed by their ability to stimulate the formation of cell colonies in bone marrow cultures. The names added to "CSF" reflect the types of cell colonies that arise in these assays.

GRANULOCYTE COLONY-STIMULATING FACTOR—FILGRASTIM (NEUPOGEN). Recombinant DNA–derived G-CSF,[61-64] or filgrastim, was approved by the FDA in 1991

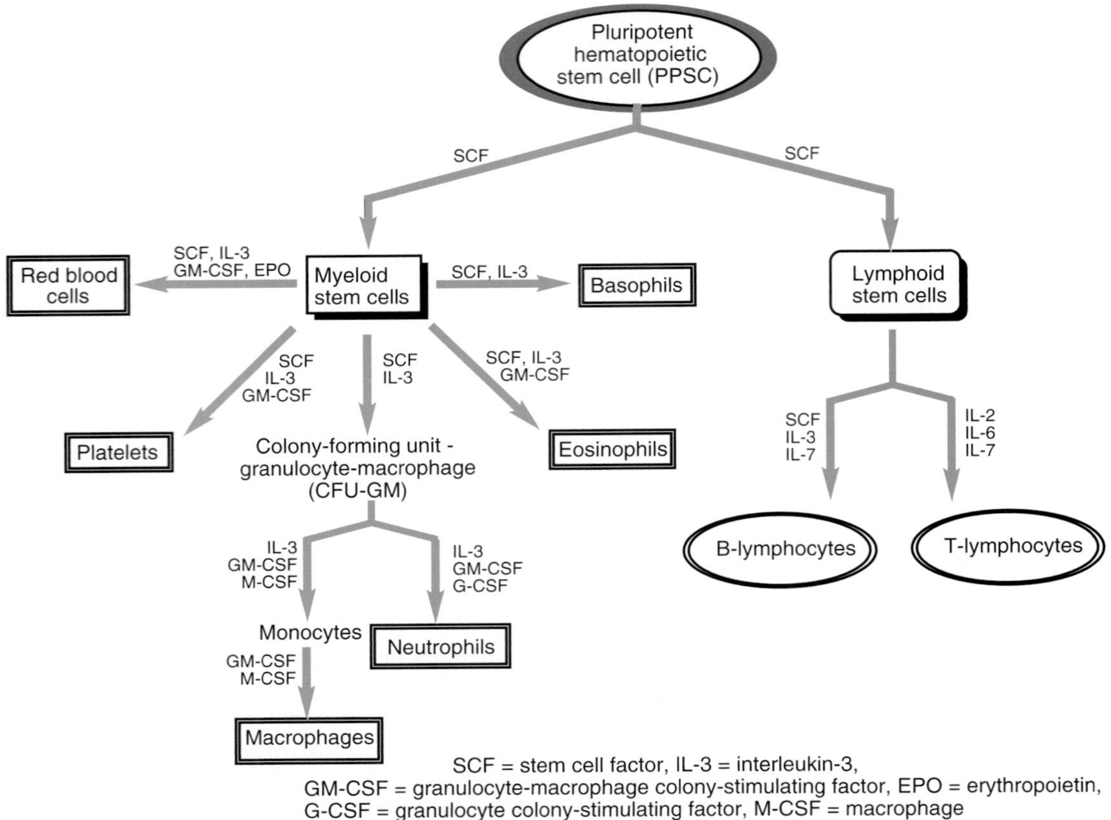

Figure 34.10 Schematic overview of hematopoiesis.

to decrease the incidence of infection in patients with non-myeloid malignancies who are receiving myelosuppressive anticancer drugs. Filgrastim is a 175–amino acid, single-chain protein with an MW of 18.8 kDa. Filgrastim, produced by a recombinant bacteria, differs from the endogenous human protein by the addition of a Met at the N-terminus (recombinant methionyl G-CSF is sometimes called r-metHuG-CSF) and the lack of glycosylation. Glycosylation, however, does not appear to be necessary for the biologic activity.

Filgastrim is administered by IV infusion or by SC injection or infusion. The drug is rapidly absorbed, with peak serum concentrations reached in 4-5 hours. The elimination half-life is approximately 3.5 hours.

Filgrastim is selective for the neutrophil lineage type of white blood cells, whereas GM-CSF is multilineage, stimulating progenitors of neutrophils, monocytes, basophils, and eosinophils. The drug reduces the period of neutropenia, the number of infections, and the number of days the patient is on antibiotics. Filgrastim generally is well tolerated, with medullary bone pain being the most frequently encountered side effect.

GRANULOCYTE-MACROPHAGE COLONY-STIMULATING FACTOR—SARGRAMOSTIM (LEUKINE). GM-CSF[61-64] has been produced by rDNA technology in the yeast *S. cerevisiae*. Sargramostim is a glycoprotein of 127 amino acids, differing from the endogenous human GM-CSF by substituting Leu at position 23. Also, the glycosylation pattern may differ from that of the native protein.

Cellular division, maturation, and activation are induced through the binding of GM-CSF to specific receptors expressed on the surface of target cells. On 2-hour IV infusion, the α half-life is 12-17 minutes, followed by a slower decrease (β half-life) of 2 hours.

Other Growth Factors

Growth factors are cytokines responsible for regulating cell proliferation, differentiation, and function. They act as intercellular signals. Each cell type's response is specific for each particular growth factor and differs from growth factor to growth factor. Platelet-derived growth factor (PDGF) is an endogenous growth-promoting protein that is released from cells involved in the healing process, and is evident at the cell proliferation stage of a healing open wound. A recombinant human (rH) PDGF B homodimer has been produced from genetically engineered *S. cerevisiae* cells. Becaplermin is the B-chain of the PDGF B protein. Thus, becaplermin is also referred to as rHPDGF-BB. The 25 kDa protein is formulated into a gel that mimics natural PDGF when applied to diabetic foot ulcers.

CLOTTING FACTOR VIII, FACTOR IX, AND ANTICOAGULANTS. Antihemophilic factor, or factor VIII, is required for the transformation of prothrombin (factor II) to thrombin by the intrinsic clotting pathway.[65] Hemophilia A, a lifelong bleeding disorder, results from a deficiency of factor VIII. Conventional biotherapy for the treatment of hemophilia A includes protein concentrates from human plasma collected by transfusion services or commercial organizations. Therefore, the concentrates may contain other native human proteins and microorganisms, such as viruses (e.g., HIV and hepatitis) derived from infected blood.

Four versions of recombinant factor VIII that are highly purified and microorganism-free proteins are now available. All four therapeutic proteins are produced by the insertion of cDNA encoding for the entire factor VIII protein into mammalian cells. The mature, heavily glycosylated protein is composed of 2,332 amino acids (293 kDa) and contains sulfate groups. Stability of the large protein is a concern because of degradation by proteases. The products have proved to be safe and effective for reducing bleeding time in patients. There is the possibility, however, of induction of inhibitors in previously untreated patients.

Hemophilia B results when a patient is deficient in specific clotting factor IX. It affects males primarily and makes up approximately 15% of all hemophilia cases. A recombinant human factor IX is now available.

Surgeons have used medicinal leeches (*Hirudo medicinalis*) for years to prevent thrombosis in fine vessels of reattached digits. Hirudin is the potent, specific thrombin inhibitor isolated from the leech. Lepirudin is an rDNA-derived (recombinant yeast) polypeptide that differs from the natural polypeptide, having a terminal Leu instead of Ile and missing the sulfate group at Tyr63.

Monoclonal Antibody Therapeutic Agents

Hybridoma technology and advanced antibody engineering has led to the design of an increasing number of site-directed therapeutic agents for the treatment and prevention of transplant rejection, therapy in rheumatoid arthritis, treatment of NHL, and other indications. These products are examples of murine (e.g., tositumomab), chimeric (e.g., cetuximab), human (e.g., panitumumab), and humanized (e.g., trastuzumab) MAbs, and they represent significant advances in pharmacotherapy. Murine MAbs are derived from mice. Chimeric MAbs contain 65%-90% human protein that is fused with the murine antibody variable region, which allows for functional complement activation and antibody-dependent cell-mediated cytotoxicity in humans. Variations of chimeric MAbs, such as partially humanized and de-immunized MAbs, are 95% human protein, and are composed of a few critical residues involved in the antigen binding site from the murine antibody or modified murine variable domains containing nonimmunogenic amino acid sequences, respectively. To prevent any human anti-mouse antibody (HAMA) response, fully humanized MAbs containing only human protein sequences have been developed from mice that have had human immunoglobulin genes placed in their genome.

Therapeutic MAbs (Table 34.3) can be divided into three main classes based on their mechanism of action: (1) MAbs as directed targeted therapy; these MAbs either block or stimulate a particular cell membrane molecule (e.g., growth factor signal receptor) or ligand (vascular endothelial growth factor [VEGF]) and thereby inhibit tumor growth or activate effector cells; (2) cytotoxicity by chaperoning cytotoxic molecules (immunoconjugates); these MAbs are conjugated to various cytotoxic molecules/atoms including chemotherapeutic drugs, radioisotopes such as yttrium-90, cellular toxins such as diphtheria toxin, or biologic agents such as IFN; and (3) modulating an immunologic mechanism; these MAbs exert their cytotoxic effects by antibody-dependent cell-mediated cytotoxicity or complement-dependent cytotoxicity.

Specific Drugs

CATUMAXOMAB (REMOVAB). Catumaxomab is a 180 kDa, chimeric murine IgG2a/rat IgG2b anti-EpCAM/anti-CD3, trifunctional MAb produced in the rat/mouse quadroma cell line.[66] The human epithelial cell adhesion molecule (EpCAM) protein is overexpressed on a variety of carcinomas, and its inhibition has emerged as a viable approach for the immunotherapy of cancer. In addition to targeting EpCAM, catumaxomab has anti-CD3 arm that targets the T cell antigen CD3; binding to the CD3 receptor activates T cells to release cytotoxic cytokines and to promote T cell–mediated lysis. The trifunctionality comes from an intact Fc region that selectively binds to FCg receptor–positive accessory cells, such as macrophages, dendritic cells, and natural killer cells that promote phagocytosis and antibody-dependent cell cytotoxicity. Catumaxomab was generated using a hybrid hybridoma or quadroma, where two hybridoma cells producing different MAbs are fused together to form a new hybrid cell that contains sets of genes encoding the two parent antibodies. Catumaxomab is used for the intraperitoneal treatment of malignant ascites in patients with EpCAM-positive carcinomas where standard therapy is not available or no longer feasible.

TRASTUZUMAB (HERCEPTIN). Advances in the understanding of tumor pathobiology and molecular biology have facilitated the development of targeted therapies, in particular in breast cancer. HER2 (or erbB2) is a transmembrane tyrosine kinase receptor that belongs to the epidermal growth factor receptor (EGFR) family. HER2 protein overexpression is observed in approximately 30% of primary breast cancers. Activated erbBs stimulate many intracellular signaling pathways, mainly the mitogen-activated protein kinase (MAPK) and the phosphatidylinositol 3-kinase (PI3K)-Akt pathways. In 1998, trastuzumab was approved by the FDA for clinical use largely based on a randomized clinical trial that compared cytotoxic chemotherapy alone with chemotherapy plus trastuzumab as a front-line treatment for patients with erbB2-overexpressing metastatic breast cancer.[67]

Trastuzumab is a recombinant humanized anti-erbB2 MAb that binds the extracellular domain of the erbB2 receptor and blocks intracellular signaling. Both cytostatic and cytotoxic mechanisms of action of trastuzumab were identified in preclinical studies. In vitro, downregulation of erbB2 disrupts receptor dimerization and signaling through the downstream PI3K cascade. It effectively prevents cell proliferation of the erbB2-overexpressing breast cancer SK-BR-3 cell line.

Table 34.3 U.S. FDA–Approved MAb Therapeutic Agents

Generic Name	Trade Name	MAb Type	Indication
Abciximab	ReoPro	Chimeric	Adjunct to percutaneous transluminal coronary angioplasty for prevention of acute cardiac complications
Adalimumab	Humira	Fully human	Rheumatoid arthritis
Adalimumab-Atto[a]	Amjevita	Fully human	Moderate to severe active rheumatoid arthritis, psoriatic arthritis, active ankylosing spondylitis
Alemtuzumab	Campath	Humanized	B cell chronic lymphocytic leukemia
Atezolizumab	Tecentriq	Humanized	Urothelial carcinoma (PD-1/PD-L1 inhibitor) (programmed death-ligand 1 inhibitor)
Avelumab	Bavencio	Fully human	PD-1/PD-L1 inhibitor approved for metastatic Merkel cell carcinoma
Basiliximab	Simulect	Chimeric	Prevention of transplant rejection
Belimumab	Benlysta	Fully human	Systemic lupus erythematosus plus standard therapy
Bevacizumab	Avastin	Humanized	Metastatic colorectal cancer
Bezlotoxumab	Zinplava	Fully human	Prevent *Clostridium difficile* reinfection (CDI)
Blinatumomab	Blincyto	Mouse	Acute lymphoblastic leukemia (ALL)
Brodalumab	Siliq	Fully human	Moderate-to-severe plaque psoriasis
Canakinumab	Ilaris	Fully human	Cryopyrin-associated periodic syndromes and Muckle-Wells syndrome
Catumaxomab	Removab	Chimeric	Malignant ascites
Certolizumab pegol	Cimzia	Humanized	Crohn's disease
Cetuximab	Erbitux	Chimeric	Colorectal cancer
Daratumumab	Darzalex	Fully human	Multiple myeloma (IgG1κ)
Denosumab	Prolia	Fully human	Postmenopausal osteoporosis
Dinutuximab	Unituxin	Chimeric	Neuroblastoma
Dupilumab	Dupixent	Humanized	Severe atopic dermatitis (eczema)
Durvalumab	Imfinzi	Humanized	Treat locally advanced or metastatic urothelial carcinoma
Eculizumab	Soliris	Fully human	Paroxysmal nocturnal hemoglobinuria
Efalizumab	Raptiva	Humanized	Psoriasis
Elotuzumab	Empliciti	Humanized	Multiple myeloma
Erenumab	Aimovig	Fully human	Migraine prevention
Etanercept	Enbrel	Fusion MAb	Rheumatoid and psoriatic arthritis and ankylosing spondylitis
Evolocumab	Repatha	Fully human	Hypercholesterolemia
Gemtuzumab	Mylotarg	Fusion MAb	Treatment of CD33-positive acute myeloid leukemia
Golimumab	Simponi	Fully human	Rheumatoid and psoriatic arthritis and ankylosing spondylitis
Ibritumomab tiuxetan	Zevalin	Murine	Non-Hodgkin lymphoma
Idarucizumab	Praxbind	Humanized	Reverses anticoagulant effects of dabigatran
Infliximab	Remicade	Chimeric	Crohn's disease

Table 34.3 U.S. FDA–Approved MAb Therapeutic Agents (Continued)

Generic Name	Trade Name	MAb Type	Indication
Infliximab-dyyb[a]	Inflectra	Chimeric	Crohn's disease, ulcerative colitis, rheumatoid arthritis, ankylosing spondylitis, psoriatic arthritis, plaque psoriasis.
Infliximab-abda[a]	Renflexis	Chimeric	Crohn's disease, ulcerative colitis, rheumatoid arthritis, ankylosing spondylitis, psoriatic arthritis, plaque psoriasis.
Ipilimumab	Yervoy	Fully human	Late-stage melanoma
Ixekizumab	Taltz	Humanized	Moderate to severe plaque psoriasis
Mepolizumab	Nucala	Humanized	Severe eosinophilic asthma
Natalizumab	Tysabri	Humanized	Multiple sclerosis
Necitumumab	Portrazza	Fully human	Metastatic squamous non–small-cell lung cancer (NSCLC)
Nivolumab	Opdivo	Fully human	Metastatic melanoma and advanced squamous non–small-cell lung cancer (NSCLC)
Obiltoxaximab	Anthim	Chimeric	Inhalational anthrax (in combination with appropriate anti-bacterial drugs)
Obinutuzumab	Gazyva	Humanized	Chronic lymphocytic leukemia (in combination with chlorambucil)
Ocrelizumab	Ocrevus	Humanized	Multiple sclerosis
Ofatumumab	Arzerra	Fully human	Chronic lymphocytic leukemia
Olaratumab	Lartruvo	Human IgG1 antibody	Soft tissue sarcoma (in combination with doxorubicin)
Palivizumab	Synagis	Humanized	Respiratory syncytial virus prophylaxis
Panitumumab	Vectibix	Fully human	First- or second-line treatment of metastatic colorectal cancer
Pembrolizumab	Keytruda	Humanized	Advanced or unresectable melanoma and treatment of non–small-cell lung cancer
Pertuzumab	Perjeta	Humanized	HER2-positive metastatic breast cancer
Ramucirumab	Cyramza	Fully human	Advanced or metastatic stomach or gastroesophageal junction cancer.
Ranibizumab	Lucentis	Fully human	Neovascular age-related macular degeneration
Reslizumab	Cinqair	Humanized	Maintenance treatment of severe asthma
Rituximab	Rituxan	Chimeric	B cell non-Hodgkin lymphoma
Sarilumab	Kevzara	Fully human	Rheumatoid arthritis
Secukinumab	Cosentyx	Fully human	Rheumatoid arthritis, ankylosing spondylitis, plaque psoriasis
Siltuximab	Sylvant	Chimeric	Multicentric Castleman disease (MCD) patients who are HIV negative
Tositumomab	Bexxar	Murine	Non-Hodgkin lymphoma
Trastuzumab	Herceptin	Humanized	Refractory breast cancer
Ustekinumab	Stelara	Fully human	Moderate to severe psoriasis
Vedolizumab	Entyvio	Humanized	Moderate to severe ulcerative colitis or Crohn's disease

[a]Biosimilar approvals.

Trastuzumab is administered as single-agent in women with erbB2-overexpressing metastatic breast cancer, including those who have progressed after chemotherapy.[67]

BEVACIZUMAB (AVASTIN). Angiogenesis, the process of developing new blood vessels from existing ones, is critical for tumor cell growth, survival, invasion, and metastasis. Numerous growth factors work in the tumor microenvironment to promote angiogenesis. Of these, VEGF may be among the most important, based on its specificity as an endothelial cell mitogen and the ability of many tumor types to produce it in physiologically relevant quantities. Oncogenic activation, loss of tumor suppressor factors, and tumor hypoxia lead to the upregulation of VEGF production. There are four isoforms of VEGF (A, B, C, and D) and three types of VEGF receptors (VEGFRs). Once produced, VEGF-A binds to two tyrosine kinase receptors, termed VEGFR-1 and VEGFR-2, which are predominantly located on the surface of vascular endothelial cells. VEGFR-2 appears to be the more important of the two receptors for mediating the angiogenic effects of VEGF, whereas VEGFR-1 may be a decoy receptor that modulates the amount of VEGF available for binding to VEGFR-2. VEGF and its receptors have emerged as anticancer targets based on their central and specific role in angiogenesis. In principle, VEGF-targeted therapy may inhibit tumor growth by blocking new vessel growth. Bevacizumab was approved in 2004 for the treatment of metastatic colorectal cancer in combination with fluorouracil-based chemotherapy.[68]

Bevacizumab, a 149 kDa recombinant humanized monoclonal IgG1 antibody (93% human, 7% murine sequences) directed against VEGF-A, is believed to globally prevent the binding of all VEGF isoforms to all VEGFRs. Bevacizumab is composed of two identical light chains (214 amino acids) and two heavy chains (453 amino acids) and is produced in a CHO cell expression system.[68] It carries a Boxed Warning for gastrointestinal perforation, surgery and wound healing complications, and hemorrhage.

PANITUMUMAB (VECTIBIX). EGFR, a transmembrane cell surface glycoprotein belonging to the subfamily of type I tyrosine kinase receptors, is overexpressed in certain human cancers including colon and rectum cancers. The binding of ligands such as EGF and transforming growth factor-α to EGFR triggers autophosphorylation and internalization of EGFR, thereby activating various signaling pathways involved in proliferation, angiogenesis, inhibition of apoptosis, and metastasis.

Panitumumab is a 147 kDa recombinant, fully human IgG2 anti-EGFR MAb produced in genetically engineered mammalian CHO cells. Panitumumab was discovered using Abgenix's XenoMouse technology and was approved by the FDA in 2006.[69] Proposed mechanisms explaining the antitumor activity of panitumumab include downregulation of EGFR expression resulting from receptor internalization, induction of apoptosis via inhibition of EGFR signaling pathways and induction of cell cycle arrest, induction of autophagy, and inhibition of angiogenesis.

Panitumumab is used in combination with chemotherapy for the treatment of metastatic colorectal cancer or as monotherapy for the treatment of chemotherapy-refractory metastatic colorectal cancer in patients with wild-type rather than mutant K-*ras* tumors. K-*ras* protein is a membrane bound G protein and is activated by receptor tyrosine kinases and is found to be mutated in 30%-40% of colorectal cancer patients.[70,71] Panitumumab has an acceptable tolerability profile when administered as monotherapy or in combination with chemotherapy. It is associated with dermatologic toxicity, which is a characteristic of EGFR inhibitors.

CETUXIMAB (ERBITUX). As discussed previously, EGFR overexpression is detected in many human cancers, including colorectal cancer. Cetuximab was approved in 2004 for the second-line treatment of colorectal cancer, either alone or in combination with chemotherapy. Cetuximab, a recombinant human/mouse chimeric MAb with an approximate MW of 152 kDa, is produced in mammalian murine myeloma cell culture. It binds specifically to the extracellular domain of the human EGFR on normal and tumor cells and competitively inhibits the binding of the EGF and other ligands, such as transforming growth factor-α. Binding of cetuximab to the EGFR blocks phosphorylation and activation of receptor-associated kinases, resulting in inhibition of cell growth, induction of apoptosis, decreased matrix metalloproteinase, and VEGF reduction. Cetuximab is eliminated by binding to EGFRs in various tissues, followed by internalization of the antibody-EGFR complex. It carries a Boxed Warning for serious infusion reactions and cardiopulmonary arrest.

OFATUMUMAB (ARZERRA). Chronic lymphocytic leukemia (CLL) is the most common adult leukemia and one of the most common malignant lymphoid diseases. Based on American Cancer Society's 2018 estimates, leukemia accounts for approximately 60,000 new cases and more than 24,000 deaths in the United States. CLL accounts for approximately 20,000 new cases with more than 4,500 deaths. CLL cells are malignant B cells that have low surface expression levels of CD20 molecules. B cells normally protect the body from invading pathogens by developing into plasma cells, which make antibodies. These antibodies directly inactivate pathogens or attach to pathogens to prepare them for destruction by other white blood cells. Ofatumumab received accelerated approval in 2009 for the treatment of patients with CLL refractory to fludarabine and alemtuzumab.

Ofatumumab is a fully human 149 kDa IgG1κ anti-CD20 MAb generated via transgenic mouse and hybridoma technology and is produced in a recombinant murine cell line (NS0) using standard mammalian cell culture and purification technologies.[72] Ofatumumab binds specifically to both the small and large extracellular loops of the CD20 molecule. Ofatumumab is highly potent in lysing B cells, which is presumably due to its binding to the membrane-proximal, small extracellular loop of the target CD20 protein and its slow release from the target molecule.[73] As with other human MAbs, ofatumumab induces both antibody-dependent cell-mediated cytotoxicity and complement-dependent cytotoxicity. It carries a Boxed Warning for severe allergic reactions and/or anaphylaxis and prolonged and severe cytopenia.

ALEMTUZUMAB (CAMPATH-1H). Alemtuzumab was introduced in 2001 for the treatment of patients with B-cell CLL who had been previously treated with alkylating agents and failed fludarabine therapy. Alemtuzumab is an rDNA-derived humanized IgG1κ MAb specific for the cell surface glycoprotein CD52 expressed on normal and malignant human peripheral-blood B and T lymphocytes, as well as natural killer cells, monocytes, macrophages, and tissues of the male reproductive system. It is produced in CHO cells and has an approximate MW of 150 kDa. The mechanism of action is not completely understood but involves a number of effects, including complement-mediated cell lysis, antibody-dependent cellular toxicity, and the induction of apoptosis.[74,75] It carries a Boxed Warning for hematologic toxicity, infusion reactions, and opportunistic infections.

IBRITUMOMAB TIUXETAN (ZEVALIN). Radioimmunotherapy is an innovative form of cancer therapy, combining an MAb against a specific target antigen with a source of radiation such as a radioisotope. Technical advances have made it possible to link radionuclides such as yttrium-90 (^{90}Y) to MAbs specifically to target radiation to lymphoma cells. Yttrium-90 is a β-emitting radionuclide that delivers 90% of its radiation (2.3 MeV) over a mean path length of 5 mm and has a half-life of 64 hours. These characteristics are particularly advantageous for treating bulky, poorly vascularized tumors and tumors with heterogeneous antigen expression. Ibritumomab tiuxetan therapeutic regimen became the first radioimmunotherapy approved by the FDA in 2002 for the treatment of NHL. Based on American Cancer Society's 2018 estimates, more than 70,000 new cases of NHL will be diagnosed in the United States and will account for nearly 20,000 deaths.

Ibritumomab tiuxetan, a 148 kDa radioimmunoconjugate, is a short-course therapy that uses immunobiologic and radiolytic mechanisms of action to destroy both dividing and nondividing tumor cells. Ibritumomab is a murine IgG1κ MAb produced in CHO cells. It is directed against the CD20 antigen found on the surface of malignant B lymphocytes in patients with B cell NHL, as well as on normal mature B lymphocytes. Tiuxetan, [N-[2-bis(carboxymethyl)amino]-3-(*para*-isothiocyanatophenyl) propyl]-[N-[bis(carboxy-methyl) amino-2-(methyl)-ethyl] glycine, forms a stable covalent thiourea-type linkage with the Lys and Arg residues of the antibody and can chelate a radionuclide via its carboxyl groups (Fig. 34.11). Ibritumomab tiuxetan can chelate indium-111 (^{111}In) for imaging or ^{90}Y for therapy. Thus, the antibody specifically targets radiation to CD20-positive cells while sparing normal nonlymphoid cells.

Ibritumomab tiuxetan is indicated for the treatment of patients with relapsed or refractory, low-grade, follicular, or transformed B cell NHL, including patients with rituximab-refractory follicular NHL. After ^{90}Y Zevalin enters the bloodstream, the MAb ibritumomab recognizes and attaches to the CD20 antigen, allowing β radiation emitted

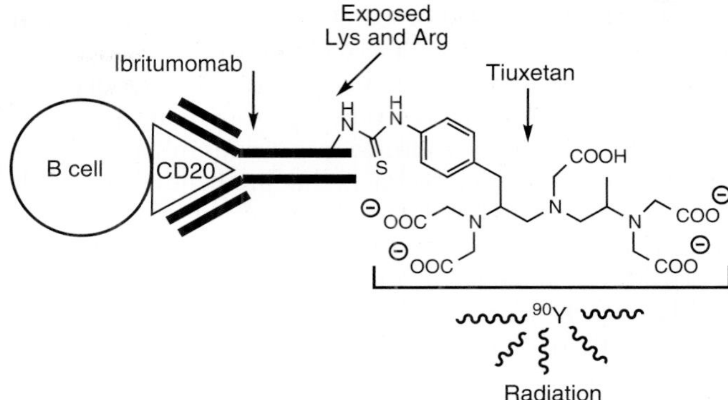

Figure 34.11 Structure of ibritumomab tiuxetan radioimmunoconjugate monoclonal antibody (MAb) and its binding to the target CD20 on the surface of the B cell.

by the ^{90}Y isotope to penetrate and damage the B cell, as well as neighboring cells.[76] It carries a Boxed Warning of acute infusion reactions, severe cutaneous and mucocutaneous reactions, and prolonged and severe cytopenia.

TOSITUMOMAB (BEXXAR). Tositumomab was introduced in 2003 as a novel radioimmunotherapeutic antibody for the treatment of B cell NHL. The therapeutic entity is composed of tositumomab and iodine-131 [(^{131}I)-tositumomab] which are covalently linked through Tyr residues. Tositumomab is a murine IgG2a λ monoclonal antibody directed against the CD20 antigen, which is found on the surface of normal and malignant B lymphocytes. Tositumomab is produced in an antibiotic-free culture of mammalian cells, and is composed of two murine λ2a heavy chains of 451 amino acids each and two λ light chains of 220 amino acids each. The approximate MW of tositumomab is 150 kDa.

Tositumomab's actions include induction of apoptosis, complement-dependent cytotoxicity, and antibody-dependent cellular cytotoxicity. Cell death is also associated with ionizing radiation from the radioisotope. ^{131}I has a half-life of 8 days and emits β particles and γ rays, the former being responsible for the antitumor activity. Thus the mechanisms of action of this radioimmunotherapeutic drug involve combining tumor-targeting ability of the cytotoxic MAb with patient-specific delivery of a radiation dose directly to the tumor cells. The radioimmunotherapeutic antibody is indicated for the treatment of CD20 antigen–expressing relapsed or refractory, low-grade, follicular, or transformed NHL, including patients with rituximab-refractory NHL.[76]

Storage of radioimmunotherapeutic drugs requires special considerations. The lead pot containing ^{131}I-tositumomab must be stored in a freezer at a temperature of −20°C or below until it is removed for thawing prior to administration to the patient. Thawed dosimetric and therapeutic doses of ^{131}I-tositumomab are stable for up to 8 hours at 2-8°C, or at room temperature. Any unused portion must be discarded according to federal and state laws. It carries a Boxed Warning for serious allergic reactions, prolonged and severe cytopenias, and radiation exposure.

CANAKINUMAB (ILARIS). Canakinumab was approved in 2009 for the treatment of cryopyrin-associated periodic syndromes, known as familial cold autoinflammatory syndrome and Muckle-Wells syndrome, in patients 4 years of age or older. The two syndromes are serious inherited autoimmune inflammatory disorders that are believed to result from cryopyrin-activated overproduction of IL-1β.

Canakinumab is a 150 kDa, fully human, IgG1 anti–IL-1β MAb produced in mouse hybridoma Sp2/0-Ag14 cell line by rDNA technology.[77] Compared to other drugs targeting IL-1β, such as anakinra and rilonacept, canakinumab possesses a less frequent dosing regimen and instigates fewer injection site reactions. Because IL-1β suppression can hinder the immune response, the labeling recommends that patients receive all recommended vaccinations before starting canakinumab therapy. No live vaccines should be administered during treatment with canakinumab, and patients should be tested for latent tuberculosis before receiving the drug. Similar to rilonacept, the labeling warns against the concomitant administration of canakinumab and TNF inhibitors, and therapeutic monitoring is recommended with concurrent administration of drugs that interact with the CYP450 system.

CERTOLIZUMAB PEGOL (CIMZIA). Crohn's disease is an immunologically mediated chronic relapsing inflammatory bowel disease that can potentially affect the entire gastrointestinal tract, but most commonly occurs in the terminal ileum and colon. Active Crohn's disease is associated with excessive levels of proinflammatory cytokines, including TNF-α. The incidence is on the rise in both developing and developed countries, with the rate in North America among the highest at 6-23 cases per 100,000 person-years.[78]

Certolizumab pegol is a TNF-α blocker approved for the treatment of moderate to severe Crohn's disease.[79,80] It is specifically indicated for reducing signs and symptoms and maintaining clinical response in adult patients who have had an inadequate response to conventional therapy. Certolizumab pegol is a 91 kDa humanized antibody fragment Fab' that is manufactured in *E. coli*, purified, and conjugated to PEG. The addition of the PEG moiety significantly enhances the plasma half-life of the antibody, allowing for less frequent dosing.

Certolizumab is the third anti–TNF-α biologic to be marketed for Crohn's disease behind infliximab and adalimumab, and it has a higher affinity than either of these drugs for TNF-α. Unlike the full-length antibodies infliximab and adalimumab, certolizumab pegol does not contain an Fc region and, therefore, does not induce complement activation, antibody-dependent cellular cytotoxicity, or apoptosis in vitro. As with other TNF-α inhibitors, the drug is associated with an increased risk of opportunistic infections and malignancy, and it carries a Boxed Warning for the risk of serious infections such as histoplasmosis.

GOLIMUMAB (SIMPONI). The proinflammatory cytokine TNF-α has been implicated as the primary mediator of articular inflammation in diseases such as RA, psoriatic arthritis, and ankylosing spondylitis. Targeting TNF-α has been a successful strategy in the intervention of a range of immunoinflammatory disorders. Golimumab is a 150 kDa, fully human, IgG1 anti-TNF MAb produced in murine Sp2/0 cell line. It was approved by the FDA in 2009.[81] Golimumab binds to both soluble and transmembrane forms of TNF-α, is the first once-monthly SC agent to enter the market, and is currently approved for the treatment of RA and psoriatic arthritis in combination with MTX and for treatment of ankylosing spondylitis. The drug is administered as an SC injection once a month. Live vaccines should not be administered while being treated with golimumab. The drug carries a Boxed Warning regarding the risk of serious infections including tuberculosis and invasive fungal infections, such as histoplasmosis. Furthermore, patients are also warned that lymphoma and other malignancies, some fatal, have been reported in children and adolescent patients treated with TNF blockers.

USTEKINUMAB (STELARA). Psoriasis is a chronic inflammatory disease that affects approximately 2%-3% of the world population. The most common form of the disease is plaque psoriasis. Conventional treatment options for psoriasis include topical corticosteroids, phototherapy, and systemic drugs, but all of these drugs have limitations. Ustekinumab is a fully human 149 kDa IgG1κ MAb developed in transgenic mouse and expressed in unspecified recombinant cell line. Ustekinumab inhibits IL-12 and IL-23 signaling by blocking p40 binding to IL-12/23 receptors. It was approved by the FDA in 2009 for the treatment of moderate to severe psoriasis in patients who cannot tolerate other treatment modalities with ease or in whom these modalities have failed.[82] As a human IgG1κ MAb, ustekinumab is expected to be degraded into small peptides and amino acids via catabolic pathways in the same manner as endogenous IgG. The mean half-life of ustekinumab ranges from 15 to 46 days across all psoriasis studies following IV and SC administration.

ECULIZUMAB (SOLIRIS). Paroxysmal nocturnal hemoglobinuria is a clonal hematopoietic stem cell disorder that is characterized by the production of abnormal red blood cells. Eculizumab, a fully humanized anti-CD5 MAb with an approximate MW of 148 kDa, is used for the treatment of patients with paroxysmal nocturnal hemoglobinuria to reduce hemolysis.[83,84] It is the first therapy to be introduced for this rare and life-threatening form of hemolytic anemia. Eculizumab is effective in controlling serum hemolytic activity and has been granted orphan drug status from both the FDA and European regulatory agencies. The drug carries a Boxed Warning for the potential increased risk of meningococcal infections, and requires patients to receive a meningococcal vaccine at least 2 weeks prior to receiving the first dose of eculizumab.

RANIBIZUMAB (LUCENTIS). Ranibizumab is a recombinant, fully humanized IgG1 MAb fragment produced by the *E. coli* expression system. It neutralizes all active forms of VEGF-A and is indicated for the treatment of neovascular age-related macular degeneration.[85,86] The full-length anti-VEGF-A MAb, bevacizumab, is approved for the treatment of colorectal cancer. The Fab domain of ranibizumab differs from the Fab domain of bevacizumab by six amino acids. The smaller size of ranibizumab (~48 kDa) is expected to facilitate retinal penetration and, hence, is more suitable for intraocular use. The binding of ranibizumab to VEGF-A prevents the interaction with its receptors (VEGFR-1 and VEGFR-2) on the surface of endothelial cells, thereby reducing endothelial cell proliferation, vascular leakage, and new blood vessel formation. Ranibizumab is administered once a month by intravitreal injection.

DENOSUMAB (PROLIA). Osteoporosis is a chronic, debilitating disease in which the bones become porous and break easily. Approximately 10 million people in the United States are estimated to have osteoporosis, and almost 43 million Americans are estimated to have low bone mass, placing them at increased risk for osteoporosis.[87] Receptor activator of nuclear factor-κB ligand (RANKL) is a protein expressed by osteoblasts and bone-lining cells that binds to receptor activator of nuclear factor-κB (RANK) receptors on osteoclast and osteoclast precursors. The RANKL/RANK complex stimulates osteoclast precursors to mature to osteoclasts and increases osteoclast activity on bone resorption. After menopause, as estrogen levels drop, RANKL levels increase. Denosumab, a 147 kDa fully human MAb produced in genetically engineered mammalian CHO cells, is specific for RANKL and was approved by the FDA in 2010 for the treatment of postmenopausal osteoporosis in women (see Chapter 23). By inhibiting RANKL, denosumab inhibits osteoclast-mediated bone resorption. Denosumab has been shown to increase bone mineral density and decrease fracture risk in postmenopausal women with osteoporosis.

BLINATUMOMAB (BLINCYTO). Blinatumomab is a constructed MAb approved in 2014 for the treatment of acute lymphoblastic leukemia (ALL) in patients with Philadelphia chromosome–negative B cell precursor ALL (Fig. 34.12). It is a bioengineered bispecific T cell engaging antibody (BiTE), which is expected to engage polyclonal T cells and CD19-expressing B cells common in most cases of ALL. It is responsible for bringing T cells close to malignant B cells to potentiate T cell-induced cytotoxicity toward the malignant cells. This is a result of its binding to the CD3 site on T cells and CD19 site of the B cells.

Blinatumomab is a nonglycosylated 55 kDa MAb, is administered as a single cycle continuous IV infusion for 4 weeks, and may be followed by multiple cycles at increased drug concentration. The drug has a mean half-life of 1.25 hours.

Adverse effects include life-threatening cytokine-release syndrome (fever, chills, hypotension, and shortness of breath) for which the preadministration of dexamethasone may prove valuable. Leukopenia and hypogammaglobulinemia has been reported in a high number of patients (~70%) leading to an increased risk of infection. CNS events including seizures and confusion have also been reported.[88] It carries a Boxed Warning for cytokine release syndrome and neurological toxicities.

OLARATUMAB (LARTRUVO). Olaratumab was approved in 2016 for the treatment of adults with soft tissue sarcoma (STS) in combination with doxorubicin. It is a platelet-derived growth factor receptor-α (PDGFRα)–blocking antibody. Mutations of this growth factor have been reported to increase in sarcomas and glioblastomas (non–small-cell lung cancers and gastrointestinal stromal tumors).

The binding of endogenous PDGF-AA, PDGF-BB, and PDGF-CC ligands to PDGFα receptors results in receptor dimerization, which in turn leads to intracellular transphosphorylation and signaling pathways resulting in cancer cell proliferation. Olaratumab is a human IgG1 MAb which binds with high infinity to human PDGFRα, inhibits the binding of these ligands, and also causes cellular internalization of the PDGFα receptor. It is administered via IV infusion over a 60 minutes period with a half-life of approximately 11 days. The most common adverse effects of the drug combination include nausea, fatigue, skeletal muscle pain, alopecia, vomiting, decreased appetite,

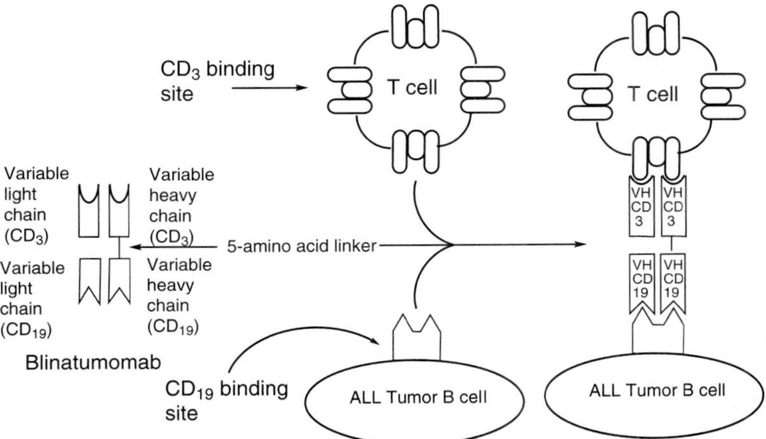

Figure 34.12 Representation of the mechanism of action of blinatumomab in which the drug binds to T cells and the ALL tumor B cell to initiate cytotoxic response.

abdominal pain, neuropathy, and headache. A number of blood abnormalities have also been reported (e.g., lymphopenia, neutropenia, thrombocytopenia, and elevated aPTT).[89] It carries a Boxed Warning for severe and life-threatening reactions.

BASILIXIMAB (SIMULECT). Basiliximab is a mouse-human chimeric MAb which is used in combination with other immunosuppressive drugs for the prevention of acute organ rejection in adult and pediatric renal transplant recipients. It targets the α chain of the IL-2 receptor (CD25), which is primarily expressed on the surface of activated T cells. It acts through a competitive mechanism by binding to the α chain of IL-2 receptor with high affinity, which leads to blockade of downstream cascade of events that would result in acute graft-versus-host disease (a-GVHD).[90,91] It carries a Boxed Warning related to the requirement of being prescribed only by physicians experienced in immunosuppression therapy and management of organ transplantation patients.

BELIMUMAB (BENLYSTA). Belimumab, approved by the FDA in 2011, is a fully human monoclonal IgG1λ antibody neutralizing soluble B cell–activating factor (BAFF). BAFF is a key factor for survival and maturation of B cells.[92] It is the first targeted therapy for systemic lupus erythematosus.

IPILIMUMAB (YERVOY). Ipilimumab received FDA approval in 2011 for the treatment of metastatic melanoma. It is an immunoglobulin G1 (IgG1)-κ produced in CHO cell culture using recombinant technology. It binds to cytotoxic T-lymphocyte-associated antigen 4 (CTLA-4) and blocks the interaction of CTLA-4 with CD80 and CD85 ligands. The CTLA-4 acts as an immune checkpoint that downregulates T cell activation pathways and thus prevents autoimmunity.[93] By inhibiting this function, ipilimumab potentiates the anticancer T cell response which results in unrestrained proliferation of T cells.[94,95] It is administered as a preservative-free solution via IV infusion. It carries a Boxed Warning for fatal immune-mediated adverse reactions.

Antibody Drug Conjugates

The field of antibody drug conjugates (ADCs) has exploded in the last two decades with the successful launching of a series of ADCs into the market and several more currently in clinical trials. The principles behind the design of new ADC therapeutics, including the linker technology and use of payloads to attach to an antibody directed toward an antigen expressed on a cell type of interest, are described in Chapter 5.

Specific Drugs

BRENTUXIMAB VEDOTIN (ADCETRIS). Brentuximab vedotin was approved by the FDA in 2011 for treatment of Hodgkin lymphoma in patients who have failed autologous stem cell transplant (ASCT) or ASCT ineligible patients who have failed on at least two prior chemotherapy regimens, and for second line treatment of systemic anaplastic large cell leukemia (ALCL). Brentuximab vedotin (MW = 153 kDa) is a CD-30–directed ADC. It contains three components: (1) the chimeric IgG1 antibody cAC10 that binds to CD30 protein expressed on the cancer cell surface, (2) the microtubule-disrupting cytotoxic component, monomethyl auristatin E (MMAE), and (3) a protease-cleavable linker that covalently attaches MMAE to cAC10 (Fig. 34.13).[96,97] MMAE is a synthetic analogue of dolastatin-10 that is covalently linked to the chimeric CD30 antibody cAC10 at Cys residues by a Val-citrulline dipeptide linker that contains a self-immolative *p*-aminobenzyl carbamate spacer. The Val-citrulline dipeptide undergoes cleavage by lysosomal enzymes such as cathepsin B, which leads to self-immolation of *p*-aminobenzyl carbamate and release of MMAE. Brentuximab vedotin has approximately four molecules of MMAE attached to each antibody molecule. The most common serious adverse effects include neutropenia, thrombocytopenia, and anemia and peripheral sensory and motor neuropathy. It is administered as an IV infusion. It carries a Boxed Warning of progressive multifocal leukoencephalopathy.

ADO-TRASTUZUMAB EMTANSINE (KADCYLA). Ado-trastuzumab emtansine was approved by the FDA in 2013 for the treatment of patients with HER2-positive metastatic breast cancer who previously received tratuzumab and a taxane, separately or in combination.[98] Ado-trastuzumab emtansine is an HER2-targeted ADC which contains the humanized anti-HER2 IgG1, trastuzumab, covalently linked at Lys residues with the maytansinoid DM1 via a noncleavable thioether linker MCC (4-[N-maleimidomethyl] cyclohexane-1-carboxylate). Emtansine refers to the MCC-DM1 complex.[97] Ado-trastuzumab emtansine contains an average of 3.5 DM1 molecules per antibody. The antibody component of the ADC binds to HER2-positive tumor cell surface and undergoes subsequent internalization via receptor-mediated endocytosis and releases the active cytotoxic DM1 moiety upon proteolytic degradation in the lysosome. DM1 disrupts the microtubule assembly/disassembly dynamics to produce cell cycle arrest and, ultimately, tumor cell death.[99] The most common side effects include fatigue, nausea, musculoskeletal pain, hemorrhage, thrombocytopenia, increased transaminases, headache, and constipation. It is administered as an IV infusion.

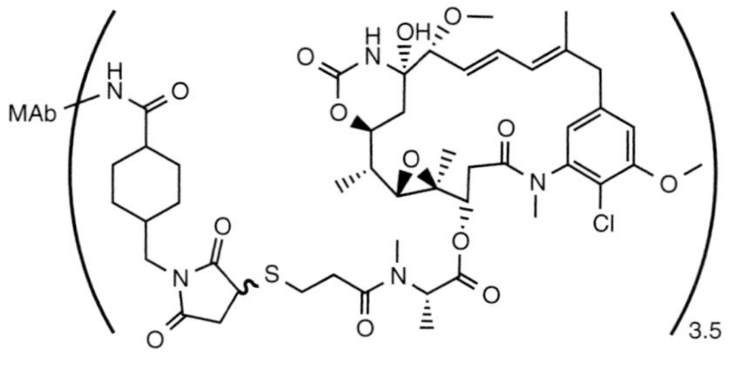

Ado-trastuzumab emtansine

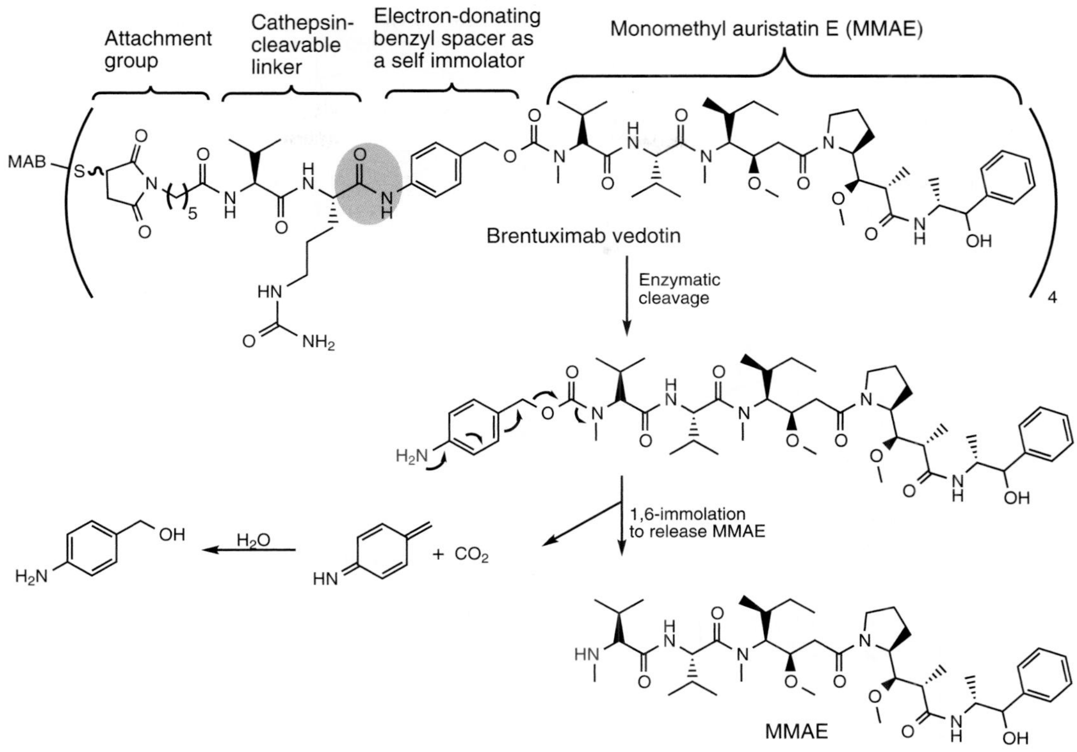

Figure 34.13 Structure of brentuximab vedotin and its self-immolative metabolism.

INOTUZUMAB OZOGAMICIN (BESPONSA). Inotuzumab ozogamicin (InO) was approved in 2017 for the treatment of adults with CD22-positive relapsed or refractory B cell precursor acute lymphoblastic leukemia (ALL). It is a CD22-directed antibody-drug conjugate consisting of three components: (1) the recombinant humanized immunoglobulin class G subtype 4 (IgG4) κ antibody inotuzumab, specific for human CD22, (2) N-acetyl-γ-calicheamicin that causes double-stranded DNA breaks, and (3) an acid-cleavable linker composed of the condensation product of 4-(4′-acetylphenoxy)-butanoic acid (AcBut) and 3-methyl-3-mercaptobutane hydrazide (known as dimethylhydrazide) that covalently attaches N-acetyl-γ-calicheamicin to inotuzumab.[97] Upon binding to CD22, InO internalizes into lysosomes where calicheamicin is released. Calicheamicin binds within the minor groove of DNA, which leads to double strand breaks and subsequent apoptosis as shown in Figure 34.14. InO has a molecular weight of 160 kDa with approximately six molecules of calicheamicin derivative molecules attached to each antibody molecule. The most common adverse reactions are thrombocytopenia, neutropenia, infection, anemia, leukopenia, fatigue, hemorrhage, pyrexia, nausea, headache, febrile neutropenia, increased transaminases, abdominal pain, increased γ-glutamyltransferase, and hyperbilirubinemia. It is administered as an IV infusion.

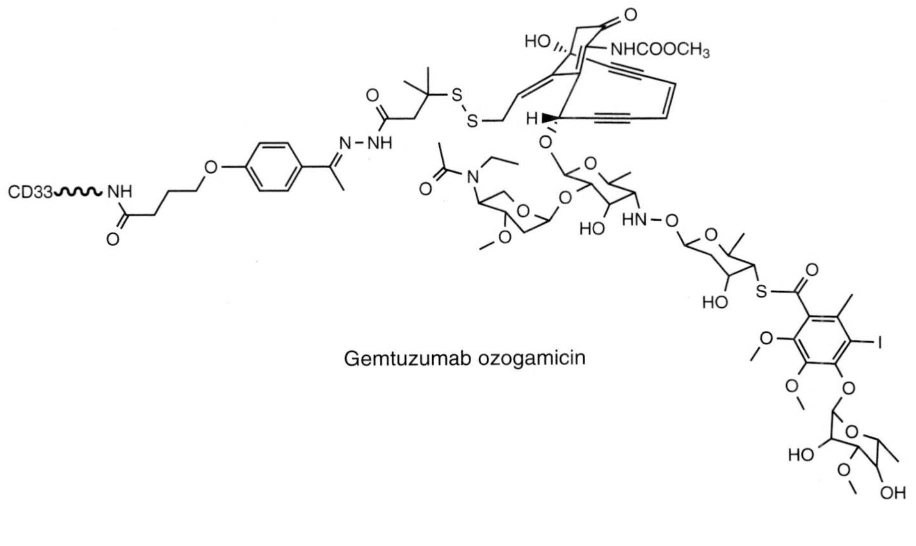

Gemtuzumab ozogamicin

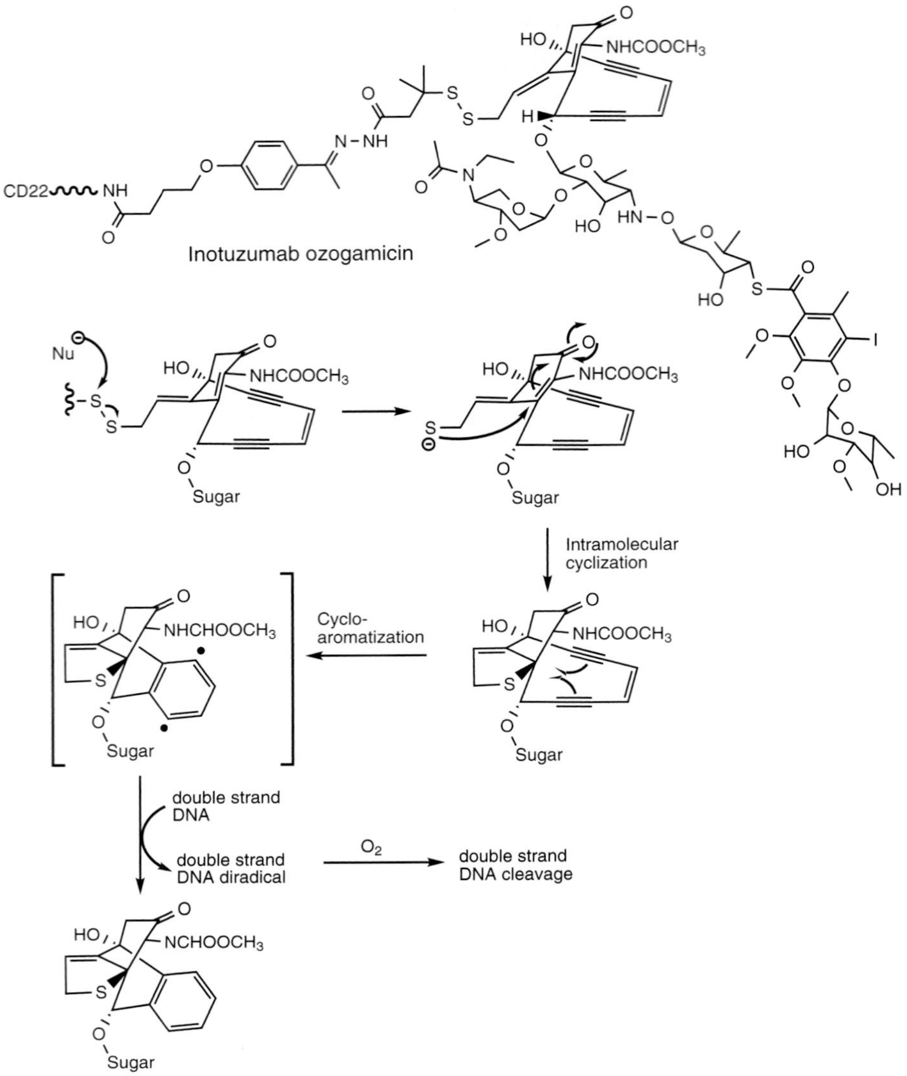

Figure 34.14 Structure of inotuzumab ozogamicin and molecular mechanism of DNA cleavage by calicheamicin.

Gemtuzumab Ozogamicin (Mylotarg). In 2017, the FDA approved gemtuzumab ozogamicin for the treatment of adults with newly diagnosed acute myeloid leukemia (AML) who carry CD33 antigen–overexpressing tumors and patients aged 2 years and older with CD33-positive AML who have experienced a relapse or who are refractory to first line therapy. It is an ADC comprised of a CD33-directed MAb that is covalently linked to the highly cytotoxic DNA-strand breaking N-acetyl-γ-calicheamicin. The molecular mechanism of activation of this ADC is similar to that of inotuzumab ozogamicin.[97] Gemtuzumab ozogamicin contains an average of 2-3 moles of calicheamicin derivatives per mole of gemtuzumab. Common side effects include fever, infection, nausea, vomiting, bleeding, constipation, rash, headache, fever, thrombocytopenia, swelling in the mouth, and neutropenia. It is administered as an IV infusion. It carries a Boxed Warning for hepatotoxicity, including severe hepatic veno-occlusive disease.

Antisense Oligonucleotides

Antisense oligonucleotides (ASO) are the oligonucleotides that bind to RNA through Watson-Crick base pairing and subsequently modulate the function of the targeted RNA. The modulating mechanisms of these oligonucleotides include (1) binding to RNA and interference with its function without facilitating RNA degradation and (2) promotion of RNA degradation through endogenous enzymes. The key aspects of ASO design include structural modifications to maintain the ability to recognize target RNA by Watson-Crick base pairing, enhanced resistance toward nucleolytic degradation, wide distribution to tissues, and preferential localization in the cellular compartments that contain target RNA of interest. Chemical approaches used to achieve the desired characteristics include modification of the phosphodiester backbone, heterocycle (base) and ribose sugar.

Fomivirsen was the first ASO to receive FDA approval. Fomivirsen, a 21-mer phosphorothioate oligodeoxynucleotide, was approved in 1998 for the treatment of cytomegalovirus (CMV) retinitis, a highly unmet therapeutic need. It was highly effective in ameliorating the symptoms of CMV retinitis. With the development of high-activity antiretroviral therapy (HAART), the number of CMV cases was dramatically reduced and drug production was stopped in 2006.

Mipomersen, an antisense 20-mer phosphorothioate 2′-methoxyethoxy gapmer targeted to coding region of the apoB mRNA, was approved by the FDA in 2013 for the treatment of homozygous familial hypercholesterolemia. The drug failed to generate enough sales, and its clinical fate is currently unclear.

Eteplirsen, a 30-mer phosphomorpholidate oligonucleotide, was approved for the treatment of Duchenne muscular dystrophy (DMD) in 2016, a controversial decision in which the FDA overruled its own scientists due to high unmet medical need. Eteplirsen (renamed Exondys 51) must produce positive outcomes data in more than 12 patients in order to retain its approval status for the treatment of this rare and devastating genetic disorder that affects approximately 1 in 3,600 male infants.

Nusinersen, an 18-mer phosphorothioate 2′-O-methoxyethoxy ASO with all cytidines methylated at position 5, was approved in 2016 and is the only ASO currently on the market. It is an orphan drug used for the treatment of spinal muscular atrophy, a rare genetic disease that affects approximately 1 in 10,000 infants each year.[100,101]

Specific Drugs

Nusinersen (Spinraza)

As noted above, nusinersen is approved for the treatment of pediatric and adult patients diagnosed with spinal muscular atrophy (SMA). SMA results from a genetic defect in the *SMN1* gene located in chromosome 5q, leading to a deficiency of survival motor neuron (SMN) protein. Low levels of SMN protein leads to loss of function of neuronal cells in the anterior horn of the spinal cord leading to muscular atrophy.

There are four classifications of the disease (SMA1-SMA4) related to the onset and severity of the condition. SMA1 (infantile—also known as Werdnig-Hoffmann disease) is nearly always fatal and is characterized by loss of motor neurons affecting many organs of the body. The respiratory system is especially affected leading to pneumonia and death. In patients with SMA, the *SMN1* gene is mutated such that it is not able to code correctly for the SMN protein. The reduced level of this critical protein ultimately leads to death of the motor neuron cells and a decrease in contractile activity. The *SMN2* gene is able to produce small amounts of SMN protein but, without exon 7 within the *SMN2* gene, the mRNA produces an SMN protein which is unstable and only displays partial functionality. Nusinersen directed to the *SMN2* gene promotes exon 7 retention via displacement of hnRNP proteins which normally works to silence exon 7. Thus, it is expected to promote additional functional SMN protein to offset the loss of *SMN1* gene–producing SMN protein.

Nusinersin is administered as a single intrathecal bolus and has a long half-life of 4-6 months. It is metabolized by exonuclease which hydrolyzes the 3′- to 5′ phosphodiester bonds. It is well-tolerated when administered intrathecally. The most common adverse effects consist of headache and backache.[102,103]

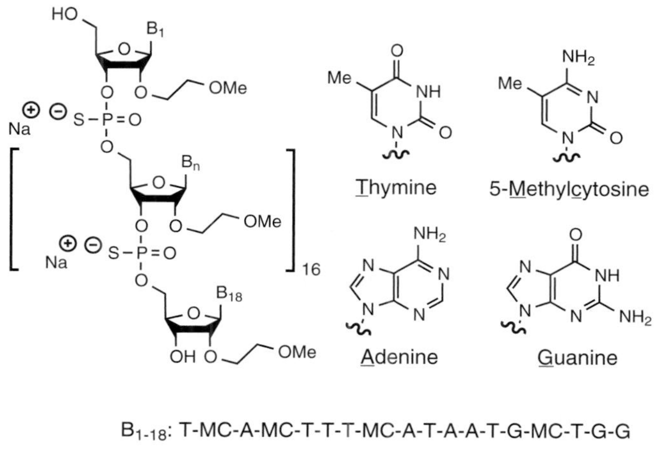

$B_{1\text{-}18}$: T-MC-A-MC-T-T-T-MC-A-T-A-A-T-G-MC-T-G-G

Nusinersen

PEPTIDE DRUG CONJUGATES (PDCs)

Peptides offer unique properties such as automated synthesis and high target affinity and specificity that make them attractive candidates for conjugation with drug molecules. Four major strategies for peptide conjugation include (1) conjugation of a pharmacologically active peptide with another active drug molecule, (2) conjugation of an active peptide with another entity designed to modify its pharmacokinetic properties, (3) conjugation of an active drug with a peptide designed to act as a targeting agent, and (4) conjugation of an active drug with a peptide designed to serve as a transmembrane delivery agent. A schematic representation of a peptide-drug conjugation strategy is provided in Figure 34.15.[3]

Peptide drug conjugates are comprised of three components: (1) the active drug molecule (which is sometimes a peptide), (2) the peptide navigating/targeting moiety, and (3) a linker that tethers these molecules. Since active drug is covalently linked to a peptide, PDCs are considered as prodrugs. PDCs have been receiving increased attention due to ease of synthesis of large quantities of peptides and their simple purification process. Furthermore, an array of tumor-targeting peptides have been recently disclosed for application in multiple types of cancers.[104] Two PDCs (D-Lys6-LHRH-doxorubicin[105] and angiopep-2-paclitaxel[106]) have been explored in phase III and II clinical trials, respectively.

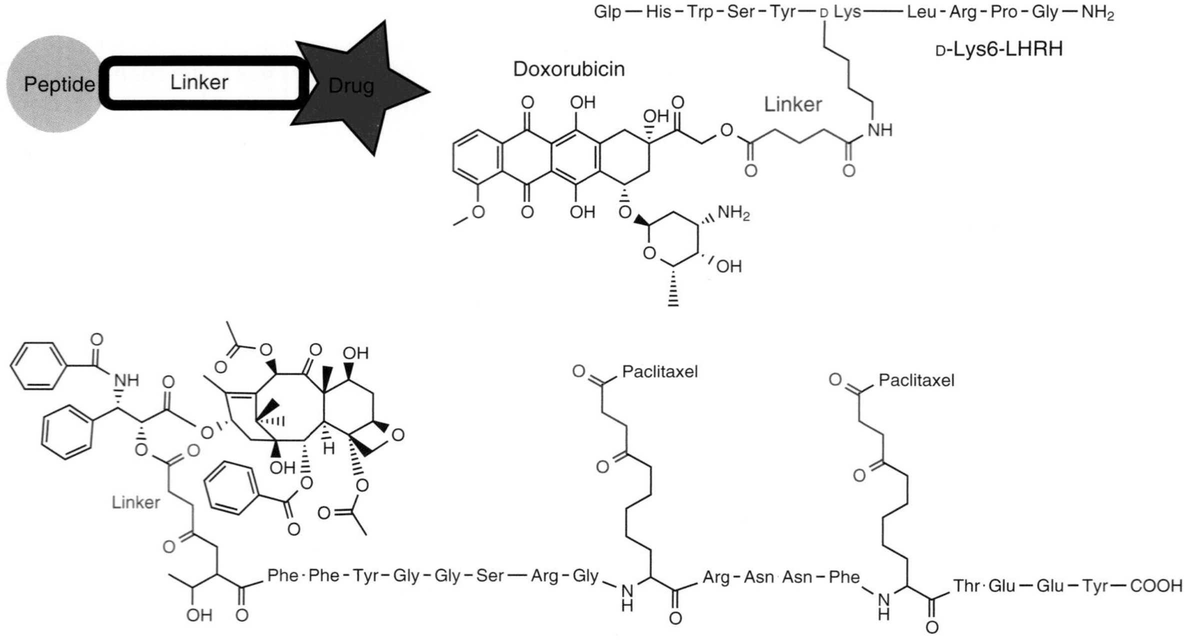

Figure 34.15 Schematic representation of peptide-drug conjugates and two (D-Lys6-LHRH-doxorubicin and angiopep-2-paclitaxel) clinically evaluated PDCs.

SUMMARY

The field of peptide and protein therapeutics has exploded in the last two decades with advances in a vast array of technologies that facilitate the discovery of novel peptides and proteins, as well as their conjugates with small molecules. The synthesis of moderately long peptides (30-50 amino acids long) through the use of modern solid-phase peptide synthesizer is now considered relatively routine. Improvement in automated purification systems is further increasing the throughput at this traditional bottleneck. Advances in predicting and preventing the potential for peptides and proteins to elicit immunogenic responses, along with innovations in their formulation and delivery, have further stimulated growth in peptide and protein therapeutics industry. The number of drugs in this category will continue to increase, providing patients with innovative new treatments across a wide range of therapeutic areas. An area of particular interest and opportunity for medicinal chemists is the development of technologies to produce novel antibody-drug conjugates (ADCs). ADCs combine the specificity of MAbs the with high cell-killing power of small cytotoxic molecules attached via a suitable linker. These revolutionary drug products hold the promise of targeting the disease while sparing the healthy tissue, bringing the concept of "magic bullet" closer to reality.

Structure Challenge

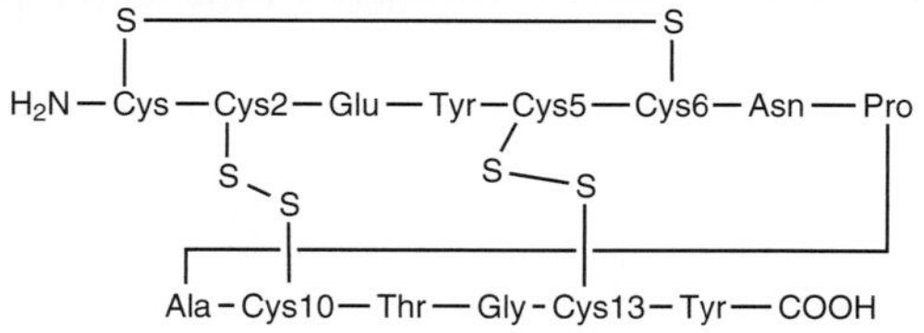

A

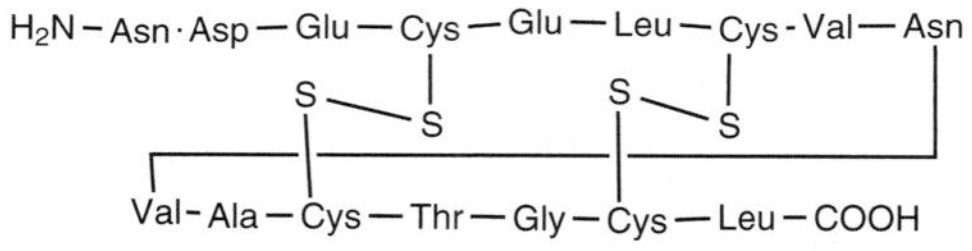

B

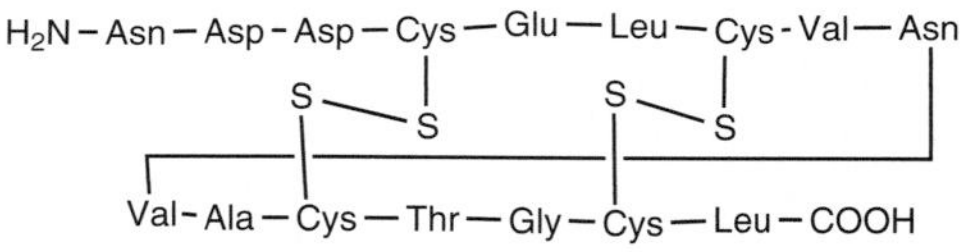

C

Structure Challenge—Continued

Conduct a structural analysis of the guanylyl cyclase receptor agonist peptides **a-c**.

1. Which of the three agonists is the most conformationally constrained? Explain why.
2. Which of the three agonists exhibit pH-dependent binding to the GC-C receptors? Explain based on their amino acid sequence.
3. Structure **b** has higher binding affinity for the GC-C receptor compared to structure **c**. What is the structural basis for this difference?

Structure Challenge Answers found immediately after References.

ACKNOWLEDGMENT

The authors wish to acknowledge the work of Drs. Ronald E. Reid and Robert D. Sindelar, who authored content used within this chapter in the 6th edition of this text.

REFERENCES

1. Banting FG, Best CH, Collip JB, Campbell WR, Fletcher AA. Pancreatic extracts in the treatment of diabetes mellitus. *Can Med Assoc J*. 1922;12:141-146.
2. Qvit N, Rubin SJS, Urban TJ, Mochly-Rosen D, Gross ER. Peptidomimetic therapeutics: scientific approaches and opportunities. *Drug Discov Today*. 2017;22:454-462.
3. Henninot A, Collins JC, Nuss JM. The current state of peptide drug discovery: back to the future? *J Med Chem*. 2018;61:1382-1414.
4. Usmani SS, Bedi G, Samuel JS, et al. THPdb: database of FDA-approved peptide and protein therapeutics. *PLoS One*. 2017;12:e0181748.
5. Chengalvala MV, Pelletier JC, Kopf GS. GnRH agonists and antagonists in cancer therapy. *Curr Med Chem Anticancer Agents*. 2003;3:399-410.
6. Conn PM, Crowley WF. Gonadotropin-releasing hormone and its analogues. *N Engl J Med*. 1991;324:93-103.
7. Padula AM. GnRH analogues–agonists and antagonists. *Anim Reprod Sci*. 2005;88:115-126.
8. Wilson AC, Meethal SV, Bowen RL, Atwood CS. Leuprolide acetate: a drug of diverse clinical applications. *Expert Opin Investig Drugs*. 2007;16:1851-1863.
9. Nestor JJ, Tahilramani R, Ho TL, McRae GI, Vickery BH. Potent, long-acting luteinizing hormone-releasing hormone antagonists containing new synthetic amino acids: N,N′-dialkyl-d-homoarginines. *J Med Chem*. 1988;31:65-72.
10. Reissmann T, Schally AV, Bouchard P, Riethmiiller H, Engel J. The LHRH antagonist cetrorelix: a review. *Hum Reprod Update*. 2000;6:322-331.
11. Klotz L. Degarelix acetate for the treatment of prostate cancer. *Drugs Today (Barc)*. 2009;45:725-730.
12. Brazeau P, Vale W, Burgus R, et al. Hypothalamic polypeptide that inhibits the secretion of immunoreactive pituitary growth hormone. *Science*. 1973;179:77-79.
13. Bauer W, Briner U, Doepfner W, et al. SMS 201-995: a very potent and selective octapeptide analogue of somatostatin with prolonged action. *Life Sci*. 1982;31:1133-1140.
14. Olsen JO, Pozderac RV, Hinkle G, et al. Somatostatin receptor imaging of neuroendocrine tumors with indium-111 pentetreotide (octreoscan). *Semin Nucl Med*. 1995;25:251-261.
15. Emeric-Sauval E. Corticotropin-releasing factor (CRF)–a review. *Psychoneuroendocrinology*. 1986;11:277-294.
16. Hintz RL. Untoward events in patients treated with growth hormone in the USA. *Horm Res*. 1992;38(suppl 1):44-49.
17. Cazares-Delgadillo J, Ganem-Rondero A, Kalia YN. Human growth hormone: new delivery systems, alternative routes of administration, and their pharmacological relevance. *Eur J Pharm Biopharm*. 2011;78:278-288.
18. Tritos NA, Biller BM. Pegvisomant: a growth hormone receptor antagonist used in the treatment of acromegaly. *Pituitary*. 2017;20:129-135.
19. Combarnous Y. Molecular basis of the specificity of binding of glycoprotein hormones to their receptors. *Endocr Rev*. 1992;13:670-691.
20. Homburg R, Giudice LC, Chang RJ. Polycystic ovary syndrome. *Hum Reprod*. 1996;11:465-466.
21. Lispi M, Bassett R, Crisci C, et al. Comparative assessment of the consistency and quality of a highly purified FSH extracted from human urine (urofollitropin) and a recombinant human FSH (follitropin alpha). *Reprod Biomed Online*. 2006;13:179-193.
22. Jiang Y, Zhao JJ, Mitlak BH, Wang O, Genant HK, Eriksen EF. Recombinant human parathyroid hormone (1-34) [teriparatide] improves both cortical and cancellous bone structure. *J Bone Miner Res*. 2003;18:1932-1941.
23. Jin X, Zhu DD, Chen BZ, Ashfaq M, Guo XD. Insulin delivery systems combined with microneedle technology. *Adv Drug Deliv Rev*. 2018;127:119-137.
24. Ceriello A, Genovese S, Mannucci E, Gronda E. Glucagon and heart in type 2 diabetes: new perspectives. *Cardiovasc Diabetol*. 2016;15:123.
25. Edelman S, Maier H, Wilhelm K. Pramlintide in the treatment of diabetes mellitus. *BioDrugs*. 2008;22:375-386.
26. McWilliams V, Whiteside G, McKeage K. Linaclotide: first global approval. *Drugs*. 2012;72:2167-2175.
27. Pitari GM. Pharmacology and clinical potential of guanylyl cyclase C agonists in the treatment of ulcerative colitis. *Drug Des Devel Ther*. 2013;7:351-360.
28. Fretzen A. Peptide therapeutics for the treatment of gastrointestinal disorders. *Bioorg Med Chem*. 2018;26:2863-2872.
29. Brancale A, Shailubhai K, Ferla S, Ricci A, Bassetto M, Jacob GS. Therapeutically targeting guanylate cyclase-C: computational modeling of plecanatide, a uroguanylin analog. *Pharmacol Res Perspect*. 2017;5:e00295.
30. Moroz E, Matoori S, Leroux JC. Oral delivery of macromolecular drugs: where we are after almost 100 years of attempts. *Adv Drug Deliv Rev*. 2016;101:108-121.
31. Thomas RH, Luthin DR. Current and emerging treatments for irritable bowel syndrome with constipation and chronic idiopathic constipation: focus on prosecretory agents. *Pharmacotherapy*. 2015;35:613-630.
32. Leffler DA, Kelly CP, Green PH, et al. Larazotide acetate for persistent symptoms of celiac disease despite a gluten-free diet: a randomized controlled trial. *Gastroenterology*. 2015;148:1311-1319. e1316.
33. Higgins DL, Bennett WF. Tissue plasminogen activator: the biochemistry and pharmacology of variants produced by mutagenesis. *Annu Rev Pharmacol Toxicol*. 1990;30:91-121.

34. Wagener JS, Kupfer O. Dornase alfa (pulmozyme). *Curr Opin Pulm Med*. 2012;18:609-614.
35. Burton BK, Whiteman DA. Incidence and timing of infusion-related reactions in patients with mucopolysaccharidosis type II (hunter syndrome) on idursulfase therapy in the real-world setting: a perspective from the hunter outcome survey (HOS). *Mol Genet Metab*. 2011;103:113-120.
36. Starzyk K, Richards S, Yee J, Smith SE, Kingma W. The long-term international safety experience of imiglucerase therapy for gaucher disease. *Mol Genet Metab*. 2007;90:157-163.
37. Hegde S, Schmidt M. Alglucosidase alfa. *Ann Rep Med Chem*. 2007;42:511-512.
38. Hegde S, Schmidt M. Idursulfase. *Ann Rep Med Chem*. 2007;42:520-522.
39. Arai KI, Lee F, Miyajima A, Miyatake S, Arai N, Yokota T. Cytokines: coordinators of immune and inflammatory responses. *Annu Rev Biochem*. 1990;59:783-836.
40. Pestka S, Krause CD, Walter MR. Interferons, interferon-like cytokines, and their receptors. *Immunol Rev*. 2004;202:8-32.
41. Rodriguez FH, Nelson S, Kolls JK. Cytokine therapeutics for infectious diseases. *Curr Pharm Des*. 2000;6:665-680.
42. Xing Z, Wang J. Consideration of cytokines as therapeutics agents or targets. *Curr Pharm Des*. 2000;6:599-611.
43. Urdal D. Cytokine receptors. *Ann Rep Med Chem*. 1991;26:221-228.
44. Todd AV, Fuery CJ, Impey HL, Applegate TL, Haughton MA. DzyNA-PCR: use of DNAzymes to detect and quantify nucleic acid sequences in a real-time fluorescent format. *Clin Chem*. 2000;46:625-630.
45. Molto A, Olive A. Anti-IL-1 molecules: new comers and new indications. *Joint Bone Spine*. 2010;77:102-107.
46. Hoffman HM. Therapy of autoinflammatory syndromes. *J Allergy Clin Immunol*. 2009;124:1129-1138; quiz 1139-1140.
47. Bernardelli P, Gaudilliere B, Vergne F. Anakinra. *Ann Rep Med Chem*. 2002;37:261.
48. Hegde S, Schmidt M. Rilonacept (genetic autoinflammatory syndromes). *Ann Rep Med Chem*. 2009;44:615-616.
49. Arenas-Ramirez N, Woytschak J, Boyman O. Interleukin-2: biology, design and application. *Trends Immunol*. 2015;36:763-777.
50. Conrad A. Interleukin-2–where are we going? *J Assoc Nurses AIDS Care*. 2003;14:83-88.
51. Hussar DA. New drugs of 1999. *J Am Pharm Assoc (Wash)*. 2000;40:181-221.
52. Piascik P. FDA approves fusion protein for treatment of lymphoma. *J Am Pharm Assoc (Wash)*. 1999;39:571-572.
53. Manoukian G, Hagemeister F. Denileukin diftitox: a novel immunotoxin. *Expert Opin Biol Ther*. 2009;9:1445-1451.
54. Hoy SM, Scott LJ. Etanercept: a review of its use in the management of ankylosing spondylitis and psoriatic arthritis. *Drugs*. 2007;67:2609-2633.
55. Newton RC, Decicco CP. Therapeutic potential and strategies for inhibiting tumor necrosis factor-alpha. *J Med Chem*. 1999;42:2295-2314.
56. Kaine JL. Abatacept for the treatment of rheumatoid arthritis: a review. *Curr Ther Res Clin Exp*. 2007;68:379-399.
57. Khraishi M, Russell A, Olszynski WP. Safety profile of abatacept in rheumatoid arthritis: a review. *Clin Ther*. 2010;32:1855-1870.
58. Faulds D, Sorkin EM. Epoetin (recombinant human erythropoietin). A review of its pharmacodynamic and pharmacokinetic properties and therapeutic potential in anaemia and the stimulation of erythropoiesis. *Drugs*. 1989;38:863-899.
59. Graber SE, Krantz SB. Erythropoietin: biology and clinical use. *Hematol Oncol Clin North Am*. 1989;3:369-400.
60. Mertelsmann R. Hematopoietins: biology, pathophysiology, and potential as therapeutic agents. *Ann Oncol*. 1991;2:251-263.
61. Blackwell S, Crawford J. Colony-stimulating factors: clinical applications. *Pharmacotherapy*. 1992;12:20s-31s.
62. Lieschke GJ, Burgess AW. Granulocyte colony-stimulating factor and granulocyte-macrophage colony-stimulating factor. *N Engl J Med*. 1992;327:28-35.
63. Petros WP. Pharmacokinetics and administration of colony-stimulating factors. *Pharmacotherapy*. 1992;12:32s-38s.
64. Smith SP, Yee GC. Hematopoiesis. *Pharmacotherapy*. 1992;12:11s-19s.
65. Piascik P. Use of Regranex gel for diabetic foot ulcers. *J Am Pharm Assoc (Wash)*. 1998;38:628-630.
66. Hegde S, Schmidt M. Catumaxomab. *Ann Rep Med Chem*. 2010;45:486-488.
67. Bernard-Marty C, Lebrun F, Awada A, Piccart MJ. Monoclonal antibody-based targeted therapy in breast cancer: current status and future directions. *Drugs*. 2006;66:1577-1591.
68. Press MF, Lenz HJ. EGFR, HER2 and VEGF pathways: validated targets for cancer treatment. *Drugs*. 2007;67:2045-2075.
69. Keating GM. Panitumumab: a review of its use in metastatic colorectal cancer. *Drugs*. 2010;70:1059-1078.
70. Gaedcke J, Grade M, Jung K, et al. KRAS and BRAF mutations in patients with rectal cancer treated with preoperative chemoradiotherapy. *Radiother Oncol*. 2010;94:76-81.
71. Castagnola P, Giaretti W. Mutant KRAS, chromosomal instability and prognosis in colorectal cancer. *Biochim Biophys Acta*. 2005;1756:115-125.
72. Cheson BD. Ofatumumab, a novel anti-CD20 monoclonal antibody for the treatment of B-cell malignancies. *J Clin Oncol*. 2010;28:3525-3530.
73. Sanford M, McCormack PL. Ofatumumab. *Drugs*. 2010;70:1013-1019.
74. Gawronski KM, Rainka MM, Patel MJ, Gengo FM. Treatment options for multiple sclerosis: current and emerging therapies. *Pharmacotherapy*. 2010;30:916-927.
75. Minagar A, Alexander JS, Sahraian MA, Zivadinov R. Alemtuzumab and multiple sclerosis: therapeutic application. *Expert Opin Biol Ther*. 2010;10:421-429.
76. Dillman RO. Radiolabeled anti-CD20 monoclonal antibodies for the treatment of B-cell lymphoma. *J Clin Oncol*. 2002;20:3545-3557.
77. Hegde S, Schmidt M. Canakinumab. *Ann Rep Med Chem*. 2010;45:484-485.
78. Ng SC, Shi HY, Hamidi N, et al. Worldwide incidence and prevalence of inflammatory bowel disease in the 21st century: a systematic review of population-based studies. *Lancet*. 2018;390:2769-2778.
79. Panes J, Gomollon F, Taxonera C, Hinojosa J, Clofent J, Nos P. Crohn's disease: a review of current treatment with a focus on biologics. *Drugs*. 2007;67:2511-2537.
80. Rivkin A. Certolizumab pegol for the management of Crohn's disease in adults. *Clin Ther*. 2009;31:1158-1176.
81. Hegde S, Schmidt M. Golimumab. *Ann Rep Med Chem*. 2010;45:503-505.
82. Chien AL, Elder JT, Ellis CN. Ustekinumab: a new option in psoriasis therapy. *Drugs*. 2009;69:1141-1152.
83. Charneski L, Patel PN. Eculizumab in paroxysmal nocturnal haemoglobinuria. *Drugs*. 2008;68:1341-1346.
84. Hegde S, Schmidt M. Eculizumab. *Ann Rep Med Chem*. 2008;43:468-469.
85. Blick SK, Keating GM, Wagstaff AJ. Ranibizumab. *Drugs*. 2007;67:1199-1206.
86. Chappelow AV, Kaiser PK. Neovascular age-related macular degeneration: potential therapies. *Drugs*. 2008;68:1029-1036.
87. Wright NC, Looker AC, Saag KG, et al. The recent prevalence of osteoporosis and low bone mass in the United States based on bone mineral density at the femoral neck or lumbar spine. *J Bone Miner Res*. 2014;29:2520-2526.
88. Portell CA, Wenzell CM, Advani AS. Clinical and pharmacologic aspects of blinatumomab in the treatment of B-cell acute lymphoblastic leukemia. *Clin Pharmacol*. 2013;5:5-11.

89. Chiorean EG, Sweeney C, Youssoufian H, et al. A phase I study of olaratumab, an anti-platelet-derived growth factor receptor alpha (PDGFRα) monoclonal antibody, in patients with advanced solid tumors. *Cancer Chemother Pharmacol.* 2014;73:595-604.
90. Onrust SV, Wiseman LR. Basiliximab. *Drugs.* 1999;57:207-213.
91. Massenkeil G, Rackwitz S, Genvresse I, Rosen O, Dorken B, Arnold R. Basiliximab is well tolerated and effective in the treatment of steroid-refractory acute graft-versus-host disease after allogeneic stem cell transplantation. *Bone Marrow Transplant.* 2002;30:899-903.
92. Schneider P, MacKay F, Steiner V, et al. Baff, a novel ligand of the tumor necrosis factor family, stimulates B cell growth. *J Exp Med.* 1999;189:1747-1756.
93. Fellner C. Ipilimumab (yervoy) prolongs survival in advanced melanoma: serious side effects and a hefty price tag may limit its use. *P T.* 2012;37:503-530.
94. O'Day SJ, Hamid O, Urba WJ. Targeting cytotoxic T-lymphocyte antigen-4 (CTLA-4): a novel strategy for the treatment of melanoma and other malignancies. *Cancer.* 2007;110:2614-2627.
95. Robert C, Ghiringhelli F. What is the role of cytotoxic T lymphocyte-associated antigen 4 blockade in patients with metastatic melanoma? *Oncologist.* 2009;14:848-861.
96. Okeley NM, Miyamoto JB, Zhang X, et al. Intracellular activation of SGN-35, a potent anti-CD30 antibody-drug conjugate. *Clin Cancer Res.* 2010;16:888-897.
97. Chari RV, Miller ML, Widdison WC. Antibody-drug conjugates: an emerging concept in cancer therapy. *Angew Chem Int Ed Engl.* 2014;53:3796-3827.
98. Verma S, Miles D, Gianni L, et al. Trastuzumab emtansine for HER2-positive advanced breast cancer. *N Engl J Med.* 2012;367:1783-1791.
99. Erickson HK, Lewis Phillips GD, Leipold DD, et al. The effect of different linkers on target cell catabolism and pharmacokinetics/pharmacodynamics of trastuzumab maytansinoid conjugates. *Mol Cancer Ther.* 2012;11:1133-1142.
100. Stein CA, Castanotto D. FDA-approved oligonucleotide therapies in 2017. *Mol Ther.* 2017;25:1069-1075.
101. Bolger CA, Murali Dhar TG, Pashine A, et al. *Medicinal Chemistry Reviews.* Vol. 52. 2016:531-599.
102. Zanetta C, Nizzardo M, Simone C, et al. Molecular therapeutic strategies for spinal muscular atrophies: current and future clinical trials. *Clin Ther.* 2014;36:128-140.
103. Chiriboga CA, Swoboda KJ, Darras BT, et al. Results from a phase 1 study of nusinersen (ISIS-SMN(Rx)) in children with spinal muscular atrophy. *Neurology.* 2016;86:890-897.
104. Kapoor P, Singh H, Gautam A, Chaudhary K, Kumar R, Raghava GP. Tumorhope: a database of tumor homing peptides. *PLoS One.* 2012;7:e35187.
105. Engel JB, Tinneberg HR, Rick FG, Berkes E, Schally AV. Targeting of peptide cytotoxins to LHRH receptors for treatment of cancer. *Curr Drug Targets.* 2016;17:488-494.
106. Li F, Tang S-C. Targeting metastatic breast cancer with ANG1005, a novel peptide-paclitaxel conjugate that crosses the blood-brain-barrier (BBB). *Genes Dis.* 2017;4:1-3.

Structure Challenge Answers

1. Peptide **a** has three disulfide bonds, while peptide analogues **b** and **c** have two disulfide bonds; therefore peptide **a** is more conformationally constrained than the other two peptides.
2. Peptides **b** and **c** demonstrate pH-dependent binding to GC-C receptors because of the presence of two charged acid-sensing amino acids at positions 2 and 3. Peptide **a**, on the other hand, is pH independent due to lack of the requisite acidic amino acid residue at position 2.
3. The presence of Glu3 in place of Asp3 in peptide **b** is responsible for its higher binding affinity for GC-C receptor compared to peptide **c**.

PART IV

DISEASE STATE MANAGEMENT

CHAPTER **35**

Coronary Artery Disease

Kimberly Beck and Marc W. Harrold

Drugs covered in this chapter:

- Abciximab
- Acebutolol
- Alirocumab
- Alteplase
- Amlodipine
- Argatroban
- Aspirin
- Atenolol
- Atorvastatin
- Betaxolol
- Bisoprolol
- Bivalirudin
- Bupropion
- Canagliflozin
- Canakinumab
- Cangrelor
- Carvedilol
- Cholestyramine
- Clopidogrel
- Diltiazem
- Empagliflozin
- Enalapril
- Enoxaparin
- Eplerenone
- Eptifibatide
- Everolimus
- Evolocumab
- Ezetimibe
- Fluvastatin
- Fondaparinux
- Hydrochlorothiazide
- Isosorbide dinitrate
- Isosorbide mononitrate
- Liraglutide
- Lomitapide
- Lovastatin
- Metoprolol
- Mipomersen
- Morphine
- Nicotine
- Nifedipine
- Nitroglycerin
- Pitavastatin
- Prasugrel
- Pravastatin
- Protamine
- Ranolazine
- Reteplase
- Rivaroxaban
- Rosuvastatin
- Simvastatin
- Tenecteplase
- Ticagrelor
- Tirofiban
- Unfractionated heparin
- Valsartan
- Varenicline
- Verapamil
- Vorapaxar

Abbreviations

AA arachidonic acid
ABI ankle-brachial index
ACC American College of Cardiology
ACCF American College of Cardiology Foundation
ACE angiotensin converting enzyme
ACEI angiotensin converting enzyme inhibitor
ACS acute coronary syndrome
ADP adenosine diphosphate
AHA American Heart Association
ALT alanine transaminase
AMI acute myocardial infarction
apoB apolipoprotein B
ARB angiotensin receptor blocker
ASA acetylsalicylic acid
ASCVD atherosclerotic cardiovascular disease
ASH American Society of Hypertension
ATP adenosine triphosphate
BMI body mass index
BMS bare metal stent
BP blood pressure
CABG coronary artery bypass graft
CAC coronary artery calcium
CAD coronary artery disease
cAMP cyclic adenosine monophosphate
CCB calcium channel blocker
CHD coronary heart disease
COX cyclooxygenase
cTNI cardiac troponin I
cTNT cardiac troponin T
CVD cardiovascular disease
DAPT dual antiplatelet therapy
DES drug-eluting stent
DOAC direct oral anticoagulant
ECG electrocardiogram
FDA U.S. Food and Drug Administration
GalNAc N-acetylgalactosamine
GERD gastroesophageal reflux disorder
GLP-1 glucagon-like peptide-1
GPIIb/IIIa glycoprotein IIb/IIIa
hCE human carboxylesterase
HDL high-density lipoprotein
HIT heparin-induced thrombocytopenia
HMG 3-hydroxy-3-methylglutaryl
HMGR HMG-CoA reductase
HMGRI HMG-CoA reductase inhibitor
HoFH homozygous familial hypercholesterolemia

Abbreviations—Continued

hsCRP high-sensitivity C-reactive protein
IHD ischemic heart disease
IL interleukin
ISA intrinsic sympathomimetic activity
IV intravenous
JNC8 Eighth Joint National Committee
LDL low-density lipoprotein
LMWH low molecular weight heparin
LVEF left ventricular ejection fraction
MACE major adverse cardiovascular events
M-CSF macrophage colony-stimulating factor
MI myocardial infarction
MIDAS metal ion-dependent adhesion site
MTTP microsomal triglyceride transport protein
nAChR nicotinic acetylcholine receptor
NHLBI National Heart, Lung, and Blood Institute
NO nitric oxide
NPC1L1 Niemann-Pick C1-Like 1
NRT nicotine replacement therapy
NSAID nonsteroidal antiinflammatory drug
NSTE-ACS non–ST-elevation acute coronary syndromes
NSTEMI non–ST-elevation myocardial infarction
PAR-1 protease-activated receptor-1
PCI percutaneous coronary intervention
PCSK9 proprotein convertase subtilisin/kexin type 9
PGH_2 prostaglandin H_2
PGI_2 prostaglandin I_2, prostacyclin
PPI proton pump inhibitor
RCA right coronary artery
RISC RNA-induced silencing complex
SC subcutaneous
siRNA small (or silencing) interfering RNA
SGLT2 sodium–glucose cotransporter 2
SNP single-nucleotide polymorphism
SPM specialized pro-resolving mediator
SR sustained-release
STEMI ST elevation myocardial infarction
Th T helper cells
TIMI Thrombolysis in Myocardial Infarction
tPA tissue plasminogen activator
Treg T cells
TXA_2 thromboxane A_2
UA unstable angina
UFH unfractionated heparin
VLDL very-low-density lipoprotein

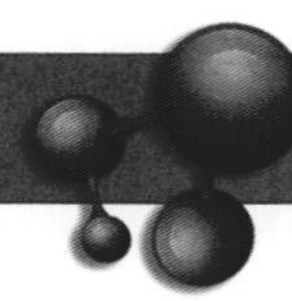

CLINICAL SIGNIFICANCE

DRUGS USED TO TREAT ACUTE CORONARY SYNDROMES (ACS)

Alexander J. Ansara, PharmD, BCPS—AQ Cardiology

Treatment guidelines from the American Heart Association outline the optimal interventional and pharmacological treatment approaches based on type of acute coronary syndrome (unstable angina, NSTEMI, and STEMI). While the underlying pathophysiology of plaque rupture is common to each ACS type, the extent of vessel occlusion and therefore myocardial tissue ischemia varies by ACS type. Patients with unstable angina do not have evidence of myocardial infarction but have myocardial ischemia that may lead to infarction if not urgently treated. Patients with NSTEMI have platelet-rich white clots that partially occlude coronary arteries, while STEMI patients have fibrin-rich red clots that result in complete culprit vessel occlusion. As such, emergent reperfusion therapy with fibrinolytics or PCI is essential for STEMI patients. Patients with UA and NSTEMI, however, can either be conservatively or invasively managed as dictated by risk-stratification.

The goals of acute management of ACS include the relief of symptoms and the reestablishment of coronary perfusion, thereby minimizing myocardial infarction size and preventing death and/or heart failure. As such, a variety of drug classes are utilized to optimize outcomes. Nonpharmacologic therapy with PCI, including balloon angioplasty and intracoronary stenting, is often combined with pharmacologic therapy to reestablish patency of occluded coronary arteries. In STEMI patients, either PCI or fibrinolytic therapy must be administered to improve survival by achieving TIMI-3 flow grade or normal coronary flow in which distal coronary beds fill completely.

Acutely, a variety of medications are necessary to treat ACS patients. Negative chronotropic medications that reduce heart rate, primarily β-adrenergic blockers, are necessary to lessen myocardial oxygen demand and blunt sympathetic outflow. Vasodilators such as nitrates lower systemic vascular resistance, dilate coronary arteries, and facilitate myocardial oxygen supply by directly relaxing smooth muscle cells of the vasculature. Antiplatelet agents including aspirin and $P2Y_{12}$ antagonists are necessary to minimize platelet activation by inhibiting the effects of TXA_2 and adenosine diphosphate, respectively, while parenteral anticoagulants inhibit thrombus propagation and platelet activation by inhibiting the effects of thrombin.

The treatment of ACS has evolved in recent years as advancements in intracoronary stenting and the development of more potent antiplatelet drugs have reduced the risk of recurrent cardiac events. More specifically, the invention and widespread utilization of drug-eluting stents has led to reductions in both the risk of restenosis and the need for revascularization procedures when compared to bare metal stents. Prasugrel and ticagrelor, $P2Y_{12}$ receptor antagonists that inhibit adenosine diphosphate-mediated platelet activation more extensively than clopidogrel, have been proven to significantly lower the risk of nonfatal myocardial infarction, death from cardiovascular causes, and stent thrombosis. Ticagrelor also demonstrated a reduction in all-cause mortality when compared to clopidogrel in the large prospective post-ACS PLATO trial.

When treating patients with ACS, clinicians should be mindful to optimize pharmacotherapeutic regimens at hospital discharge to reduce the risk of ACS recurrence, heart failure, and mortality. Medications proven to reduce the recurrence of major adverse cardiac events that should be prescribed at hospital discharge in post-ACS patients include β-adrenergic blockers, angiotensin-converting enzyme inhibitors (ACEIs) or angiotensin receptor blockers, high intensity HMG-CoA reductase inhibitor therapy, and dual antiplatelet therapy with the combination of aspirin and a $P2Y_{12}$ antagonist. In post-ACS patients whose ejection fraction is <40%, the use of aldosterone receptor antagonists are indicated to lessen the risk of mortality and hospitalization from heart failure.

Epidemiology and Economic Impact

Coronary artery disease (CAD), also called coronary heart disease (CHD) or ischemic heart disease (IHD), is the leading cause of death in the United States (US) and worldwide.[1,2] In 2015, CHD was the cause of 366,081 deaths in the United States.[3] The number of deaths due to CAD is increasing, despite a decrease in the age-specific death rate of IHD. The factors leading to the increased number of deaths caused by CAD are primarily an aging population and an increase in population growth.[1,2] The American Heart Association (AHA) projected that 16.8 million Americans had CAD in 2015, and an additional 7.2 million American are projected to have CAD in 2035 representing over 8% of the United States population.[4] Myocardial infarction (MI) is an outcome of CAD. In 2018, approximately 720,000 Americans will be hospitalized for the first time for a MI or death due to CAD, and an additional approximately 335,000 Americans will have a recurrent event due to CAD.[3]

It comes as no surprise that the prevalence of CAD increases with increasing age. In the United States, there are disparities in prevalence in CAD among gender, race, and ethnicity. Overall, male patients have a higher prevalence of CAD than female patients. Figure 35.1 shows the prevalence of CHD in US adults older than 20 years according to population group.[3] Socioeconomic status also affects the incidence of CHD. In patients younger than 65 years, regardless of education level, those with low income had a more than three times higher incidence of CHD than those with high income.[5]

CHD is an expensive disease. Direct medical costs in the United States associated with CAD were projected to be \$89 billion annually in 2015 and to rise to \$235 billion annually by 2035.[4] Indirect costs of CAD in the United States, which includes loss of productivity at work and home, were projected to be \$99 billion in 2015 and to increase to \$151 billion per year in 2035.[4] Spending per capita for IHD is significantly more for patients of age 65 years and older than for younger patients and IHD is the condition with the highest health care spending in this age-group.[6] Mean cost estimates for cardiovascular events and coronary revascularization procedures as a consequence of CAD, in 2013 values in the United States, are listed in Table 35.1.[7] The follow-up care required in the year after either unstable angina or myocardial infarction is significantly more expensive than the acute treatment of the event.

Pathogenesis of Coronary Artery Disease

CAD is used to describe a syndrome in which atherosclerotic plaque builds up within the walls of coronary arteries. As shown in Figure 35.2,[8] atherosclerotic plaque formation

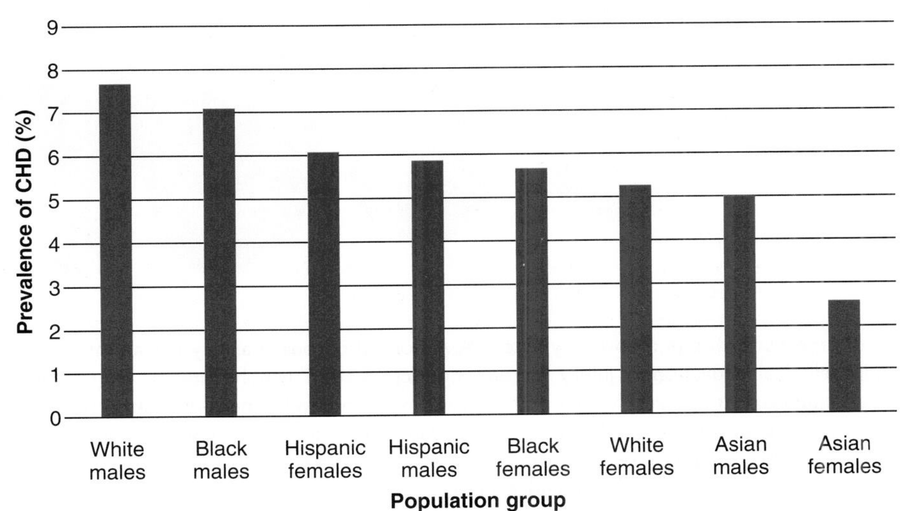

Figure 35.1 Prevalence of CHD, 2011–2014. Adapted from Benjamin EJ, Virani SS, Calloway CW, et al. Heart disease and stroke statistics-2018 update: a report from the American Heart Association. *Circulation*. 2018;137(12):e67-e492.

Table 35.1 Average Costs for Cardiovascular Events

Condition Treated or Procedure	Average Cost[a]
Acute Hospitalization for UA	$7,916
UA follow-up for 1 yr	$17,015
Acute Hospitalization for MI	$24,695
MI follow-up for 1 yr	$34,463
Acute CABG	$57,577
Acute PCI	$13,501

Adapted from Nicholson G, Gandra SR, Halbert RJ, et al. Patient-level costs of major cardiovascular conditions: a review of the international literature. *Clinicoecon Outcomes Res.* 2018;8:495-506.

[a]In US dollars

CABG, coronary artery bypass graph; MI, myocardial infarction; PCI, percutaneous coronary intervention; UA, unstable angina.

is a progressive chronic inflammatory disease. It begins with the diffusion of low-density lipoproteins (LDLs) into vessel walls in areas of intimal thickening where proteoglycan is found in the extracellular matrix.[9] LDLs are retained in these areas due to ionic bonding between negatively charged sugar groups in proteoglycan and a cluster of positively charged arginine and lysine residues on the apolipoprotein B (apoB) portion of lipoproteins.[9] Proteoglycan-bound LDLs in the intima are more prone to oxidation and oxidized LDLs trigger an inflammatory response.[9]

Inflammation of the endothelial lining of the cardiac vessel lumen causes increased permeability. Typically, the endothelial cells of an arterial vessel do not interact with leukocytes. The inflammatory response, however, activates endothelial cells to express leukocyte adhesion molecules, chemoattractant cytokines (chemokines), and macrophage colony–stimulating factor (M-CSF).[10–14] The chemokines secreted by the activated endothelial cells attract mostly monocytes and some T lymphocytes, which adhere to the adhesion molecules now expressed on the

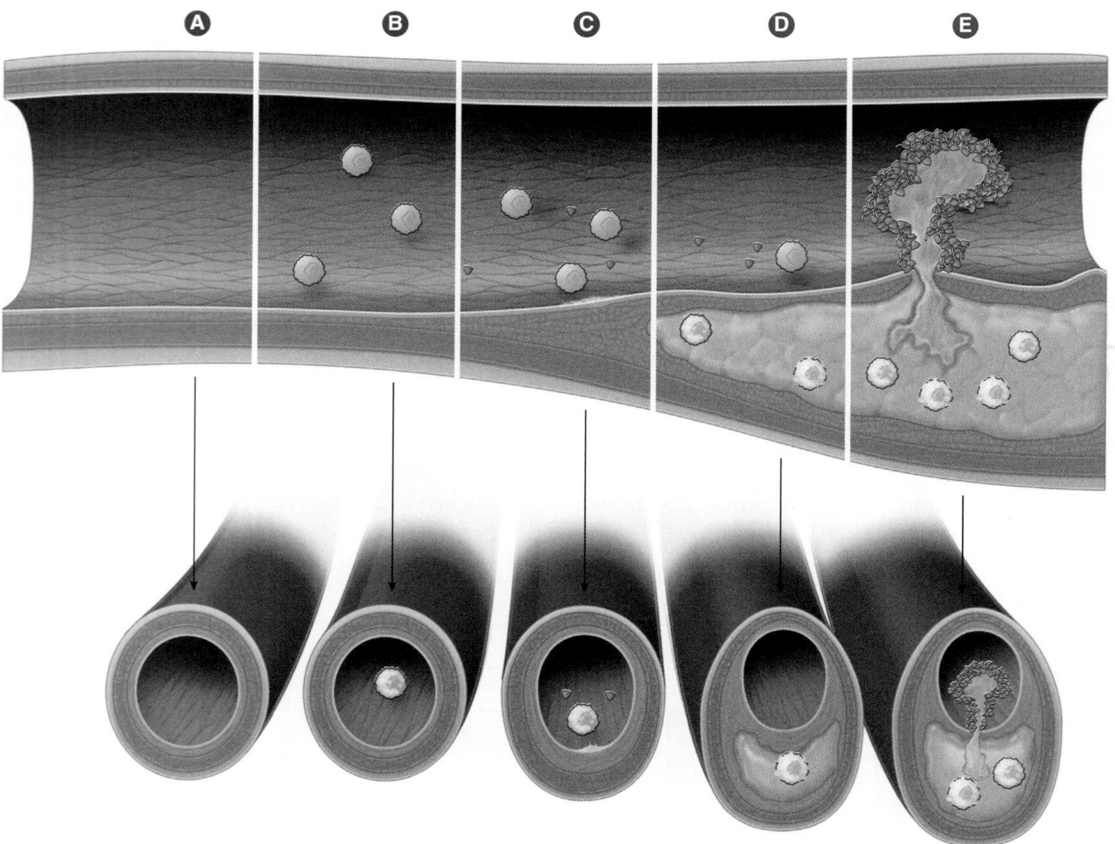

Figure 35.2 Pathogenesis of atherosclerosis in a coronary artery. A, A normal coronary artery has an intact endothelium surrounded by smooth muscle cells. B, Endothelial cell activation or injury recruits monocytes and T lymphocytes to the site of injury, leading to development of a fatty streak. C, Continued oxidative stress within a fatty streak leads to development of an atherosclerotic plaque. D, Macrophage apoptosis and continued cholesterol deposition cause further plaque organization and may induce the expression of additional inflammatory proteins and matrix metalloproteinases. At this stage, the cap of the fibroatheroma remains intact. E, Continued inflammation within an atherosclerotic plaque leads to thinning of the fibrous cap and, eventually, to plaque erosion or rupture. Exposure of plaque constituents to the bloodstream activates platelets and the coagulation cascade, with resulting coronary artery occlusion. From McCabe JM, Armstrong EJ. Integrative cardiovascular pharmacology: hypertension, ischemic heart disease, and heart failure. In: Golan DE, Armstrong EJ, Armstrong AW, eds. *Principles of Pharmacology: The Pathophysiologic Basis of Drug Therapy*. 4th ed. Philadelphia: Wolters-Kluwer Health; 2017:482, with permission.

endothelial luminal surface. This allows these leukocytes to migrate into the intimal layer of a coronary artery, triggering the immune response. Once in the intima, monocytes differentiate into macrophages and proliferate under the influence of M-CSF. Some of these macrophages exhibit a proinflammatory phenotype and secrete proinflammatory/proatherogenic cytokines, such as interleukin 1β (IL-1β) and IL-1β–induced IL-6.[11,12,15] Macrophages, within the intima, engulf lipids and change into foam cells. These lipid-filled foam cells cause fatty streaks within the lumen of a coronary artery, the first visible sign of atherosclerosis. Cholesterol continues to build up at the site of the atherosclerotic plaque forming a lipid core. A detailed discussion regarding the role of lipids in the formation of atherosclerotic plaques can be found in Chapter 19.

Cytokines and growth factors produced by foam cells, activated platelets, and endothelial cells within the atherosclerotic plaque stimulate vascular smooth muscle cells from the media of the vessel wall to infiltrate the atherosclerotic plaque and proliferate.[14] These smooth muscle cells produce collagen, elastin, and proteoglycans to form an extracellular matrix which gives structural integrity to the growing plaque and forms a collagen-rich fibrous cap over the surface that contains the atherosclerotic plaque.[11,14] Proinflammatory macrophages and foam cells secrete matrix metalloproteinases and other proteolytic enzymes that degrade collagen fibrils and other structures, which thins the fibrous cap, making it prone to rupture.

Like macrophages, T lymphocytes (or T cells) exhibit different functional phenotypes within the atherosclerotic lesion.[15] The phenotypes vary between proinflammatory/proatherogenic effector T cells, such as interferon-γ producing T helper (Th) cells, and antiinflammatory regulatory T cells (Treg). Within the atherosclerotic plaque, macrophage and T cells modulate the functional phenotype of each other.[15] For example, inflammation promoting Th cells shift the differentiation of intraplaque macrophages toward a proinflammatory phenotype that stimulates progression of the atherosclerotic plaque, whereas antiinflammatory Treg cells promote a resolution and repair macrophage phenotype that leads to regression of the atherosclerotic plaque and vice versa. Normally, the tissue inflammatory response is simultaneously linked to a resolution response which counterregulates the inflammatory response and repairs the damaged tissue.[15] The resolution response involves the action of its own set of antiinflammatory and repair inducing proteins, cytokines, and endogenous lipids called specialized pro-resolving mediators (SPMs).[15,16] SPMs include the omega-6 fatty acid derived lipoxins, and the omega-3 fatty acid derived resolvins, protectins, and maresins.[17] Overall, atherosclerosis is an imbalance of the inflammatory and resolving mechanisms where the balance tips toward the inflammatory mechanisms.[15]

The accumulating macrophages and foam cells within the lipid core undergo apoptosis (cell death), and typically the resultant debris is cleared by phagocytes in a process called efferocytosis. In an advancing atherosclerotic plaque, efferocytosis is impaired such that the lipid core evolves into a necrotic core due to the necrosis of the sequestered apoptotic foam cells and smooth muscle cells.[11,15] The necrotic core generates mediators that further contribute to inflammation, as well as mediators that are proteolytic, which makes the atherosclerotic plaque prone to rupture. When exposed to blood, thrombogenic mediators within the necrotic core, such as tissue factor, may trigger the formation of a vessel occluding thrombus.[16]

Angina

The progressive buildup of atherosclerotic plaque narrows the lumen (stenosis) of the affected coronary arteries leading to decreased myocardial tissue perfusion. When the lumen narrows to the extent that myocardial blood flow is no longer able to meet the oxygen demands of the heart, ischemia occurs leading to clinical symptoms. Ischemia is a critical loss of blood flow to tissue. Myocardial ischemia is due to an imbalance between myocardial oxygen demand and myocardial oxygen supply. The first clinical manifestation of chronic CAD is angina. Figure 35.3 illustrates the pathophysiology of angina.[8] Chronic stable angina is brief chest discomfort provoked by increased physical exertion or emotional stress. When the diameter of a coronary artery lumen is narrowed due to atherosclerotic stenosis by more than 70%, the vessel may be able to adequately supply the myocardial tissue with oxygen at rest.[18] With activity, however, as the demand for oxygen increases, the stenotic vessel is no longer able to meet the oxygen demands of the tissue and ischemia causing clinical symptoms ensues.

Endothelial dysfunction, as a result of atherosclerotic plaque formation, diminishes the ability of endothelial cells to increase vessel diameter in response to increased needs of the tissue.[18] Normal vascular endothelial cells secrete nitric oxide (NO) and prostacyclin (PGI_2). Action by both of these chemical mediators results in vasodilation by causing vascular smooth muscle relaxation. In contrast, sympathetic nervous system stimulation of vascular smooth muscle results in vasoconstriction. During increased physical activity or emotional stress, the sympathetic system is activated. Sympathetic stimulation results in increased heart rate, force of myocardial contraction, and vasoconstriction, which causes increased blood pressure (BP). In vessels with normally functioning endothelial cells, the increased sheering stress as a result of increased BP causes the secretion of NO and PGI_2 and vasodilation prevails. This enables increased coronary blood flow to meet the increase in oxygen demand. The dysfunctional endothelial cells of coronary vessels with atherosclerotic plaque have diminished ability to secrete NO and PGI_2. Consequently, these vessels exhibit vasoconstriction, in addition to reduced lumen diameter due to atherosclerotic plaque, which may contribute to the ischemic pain upon exertion exhibited in stable angina. The atherosclerotic plaque of chronic stable angina is characterized by a thick fibrous cap that is resistant to rupture.

Endothelial dysfunction also creates a prothrombotic environment on the surface of the atherosclerotic plaque. In addition to inducing vasodilation, NO and PGI_2 are inhibitors of platelet aggregation. Upon activation, platelets secrete serotonin, thromboxane A_2 (TXA_2), and adenosine diphosphate (ADP) which all stimulate platelet

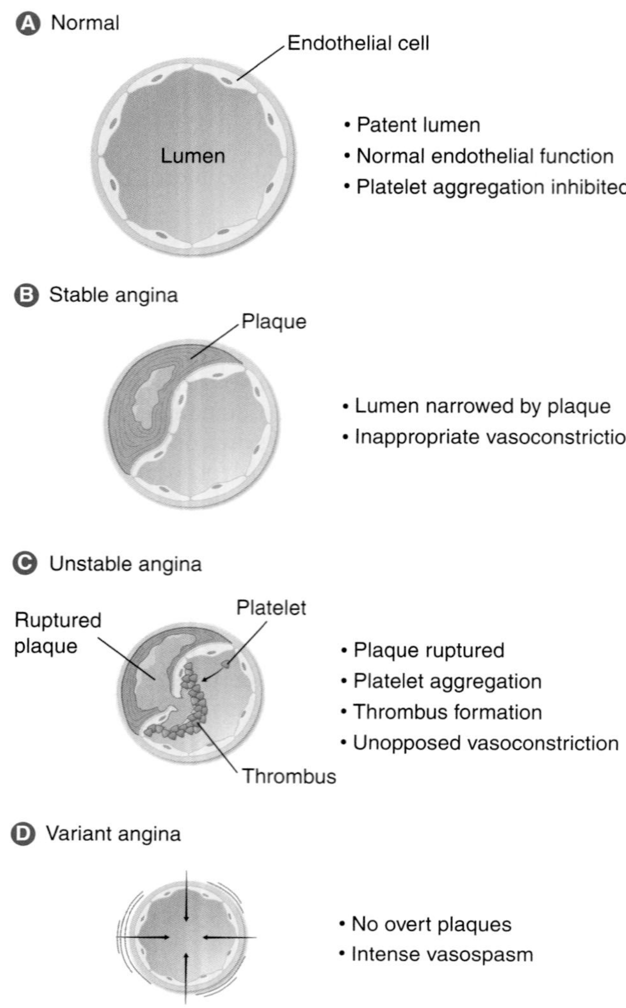

Figure 35.3 Pathophysiology of angina syndromes. A, Normal coronary arteries are widely patent, the endothelium functions normally, and platelet aggregation is inhibited. B, In stable angina, atherosclerotic plaque and inappropriate vasoconstriction (caused by endothelial damage) reduce the vessel lumen diameter and hence decrease coronary blood flow. C, In unstable angina, rupture of the plaque triggers platelet aggregation, thrombus formation, and vasoconstriction. Depending on the anatomic site of plaque rupture, this process can progress to non–Q wave (non-ST elevation) or Q wave (ST elevation) myocardial infarction. D, In variant angina, atherosclerotic plaques are absent, and ischemia is caused by intense vasospasm. From McCabe JM, Armstrong EJ. Integrative cardiovascular pharmacology: hypertension, ischemic heart disease, and heart failure. In: Golan DE, Armstrong EJ, Armstrong AW, eds. *Principles of Pharmacology: The Pathophysiologic Basis of Drug Therapy*. 4th ed. Philadelphia: Wolters-Kluwer Health; 2017:480, with permission.

aggregation. Serotonin and TXA_2 both cause smooth muscle contraction resulting in vasoconstriction. Serotonin and ADP released by aggregating platelets stimulate endothelial cells to release NO and PGI_2 in a finely balanced system such that in vessels with normally functioning endothelial cells, not only vasodilation, but also inhibition of platelet aggregation prevails. The diminished ability of dysfunctional endothelial cells to secrete NO and PGI_2 makes them unable to inhibit platelet aggregation. Furthermore, tissue factor expressed on damaged endothelial cells activates platelets and triggers the extrinsic coagulation pathway by forming an activated complex with factor VII (see Chapter 18 for a full discussion of the coagulation process). Normally, in order to keep the endothelial lining free of interactions with blood constituents and to maintain hemostasis, endothelial cells secrete a variety of anticoagulant factors. At the atherosclerotic plaque, the normal anticoagulant properties of endothelial cells are impaired allowing thrombosis to proceed unchecked.

When stenosis of a coronary artery vessel narrows the lumen more than 90%, even with maximum vasodilation, there may not be adequate blood flow to meet the oxygen needs of the myocardium at rest.[18] Intermittent chest pain at rest is a characteristic of unstable angina as a result of inadequate blood flow perfusing the myocardial tissue. The plaque is a dynamic entity and over time the fibrous surface may erode or rupture exposing subendothelial collagen and releasing thrombogenic mediators from the necrotic core that trigger platelet aggregation and the coagulation cascade. Vulnerable atherosclerotic plaques prone to rupture characteristically have a thin fibrous cap shielding a large lipid-rich necrotic core from the bloodstream. At the site of a ruptured atherosclerotic plaque, a thrombus may form which partially or completely occludes the coronary artery. The two mechanisms by which atherosclerotic plaque may partially or completely occlude a coronary vessel are accumulation of plaque to the extent that it obstructs blood flow to a critical point or formation of a thrombus at a site of ruptured or eroded plaque.[19] A summary of the mechanisms leading to thrombus formation in coronary arteries is shown in Figure 35.4.[20] Abrupt coronary artery occlusion causing myocardial ischemia results in several conditions categorized as acute coronary syndromes (ACS).

Acute Coronary Syndromes

This chapter will focus on ACS as the major consequences of CAD that can be treated. ACS are the result of a sudden reduction in coronary blood flow and include unstable angina (UA) and acute myocardial infarction (AMI). The majority of ACS result from disruption of an atherosclerotic plaque and formation of an intracoronary thrombus. Figure 35.5 summarizes the consequences of coronary thrombosis.[20]

If myocardial ischemia to a particular area of myocardial tissue persists for more than 20-30 minutes, necrosis (cell death) of the myocardial cells deprived of oxygen occurs. The area of cell death is called an infarct. The presence of the biomarkers cardiac-specific troponins I (cTnI) or T (cTnT) in the blood indicates myocardial necrosis with high sensitivity.[21] An ST-elevation MI (STEMI) is the result of a coronary artery that is totally occluded by a thrombus causing ischemia and tissue necrosis as indicated by the presence of serum cTnI or cTnT. As the name designates, STEMI is characterized by the presence of ST elevation on the electrocardiogram (ECG). Q waves may appear on the ECG in STEMI as time progresses.

Patients presenting with a clinical picture suggestive of ACS without an ST elevation on the ECG are likely to have either UA or non–ST-elevation MI (NSTEMI). UA and

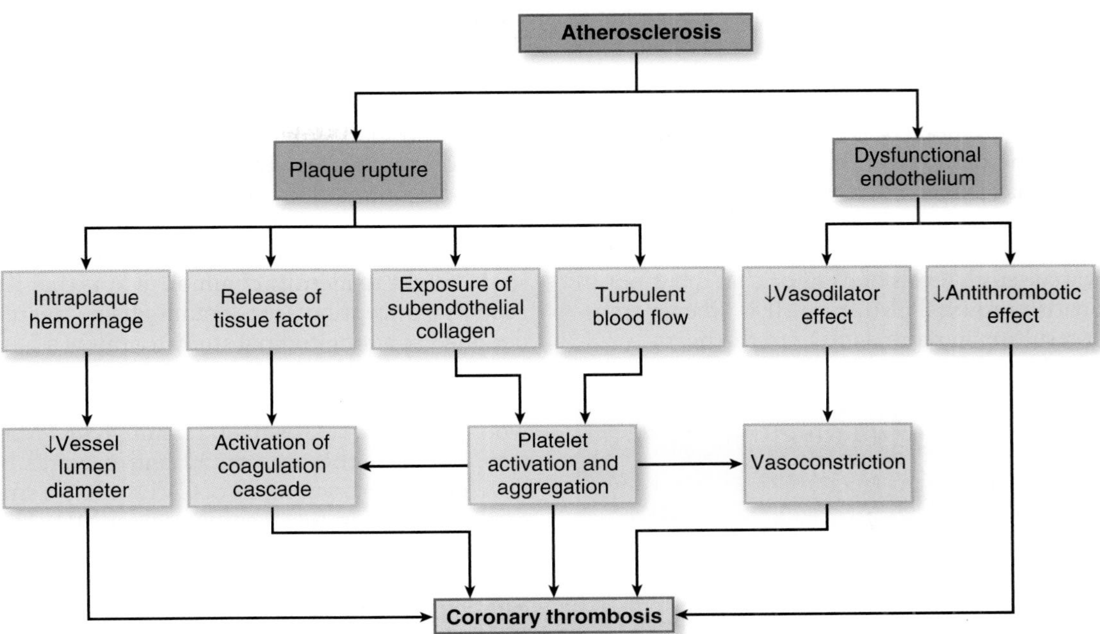

Figure 35.4 **Mechanisms of coronary thrombus formation. Factors that contribute to this process include plaque disruption (e.g., rupture) and inappropriate vasoconstriction and loss of normal antithrombotic defenses because of dysfunctional endothelium.** From Wilder J, Sabatine MS, Lilly LS. Acute coronary syndromes. In: Lilly LS, ed. *Pathophysiology of Heart Disease: A Collaborative Project of Medical Students and Faculty*. 6th ed. Philadelphia: Wolters-Kluwer; 2016:165, with permission.

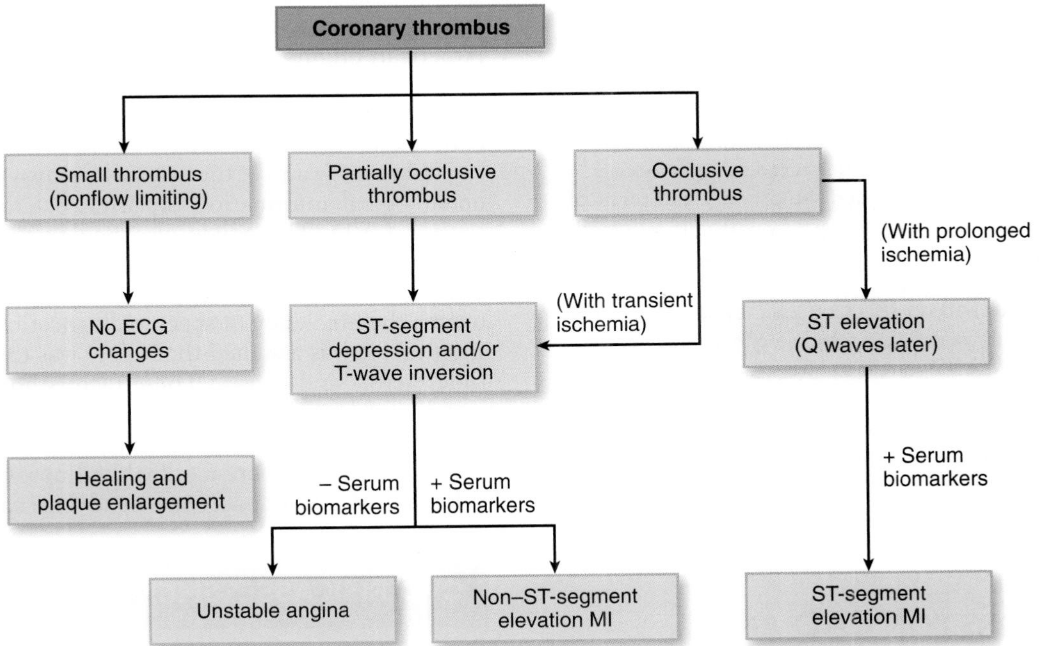

Figure 35.5 **Consequences of coronary thrombosis. A small thrombus formed on superficial plaque rupture may not result in symptoms or electrocardiogram (ECG) abnormalities, but healing and fibrous organization may incorporate the thrombus into the plaque, causing the atherosclerotic lesion to enlarge. A partially occlusive thrombus narrows the arterial lumen, restricts blood flow, and can cause unstable angina or a non–ST-elevation MI, either of which may result in ST-segment depression and/or T-wave inversion on the ECG. A totally occlusive thrombus with prolonged ischemia is the most common cause of ST-elevation MI, in which the ECG initially shows ST-segment elevation, followed by Q-wave development if early reperfusion is not achieved. An occlusive thrombus that recanalizes, or one that develops in a region served by adequate collateral blood flow, may result in less prolonged ischemia and a non–ST-elevation MI instead. Serum biomarkers of myocardial necrosis include cardiac-specific troponins I and T.** From Wilder J, Sabatine MS, Lilly LS. Acute coronary syndromes. In: Lilly LS, ed. *Pathophysiology of Heart Disease: A Collaborative Project of Medical Students and Faculty*. 6th ed. Philadelphia: Wolters-Kluwer; 2016:167, with permission.

NSTEMI are typically the result of a coronary artery that is partially occluded by thrombus formation or briefly totally occluded. UA and NSTEMI lack an ST elevation on the ECG by definition and are defined as non–ST-elevation acute coronary syndromes (NSTE-ACS). Specific ECG changes may not be observed in either UA or NSTEMI, although either may have ST-depression and/or T-wave inversion. The difference between UA and NSTEMI is that myocardial cell necrosis occurs in NSTEMI, as indicated by elevated serum levels of cTnI or cTnT, but not in UA. In comparison to NSTEMI, STEMI is a larger transmural infarct resulting in more damage to the heart.

TREATING ATHEROSCLEROSIS WITH ANTIINFLAMMATORY THERAPY

In the past several decades, the pathogenesis of atherosclerosis has evolved to include inflammation as a critical feature. The majority of the current drugs used to treat atherosclerosis focus on lowering lipid levels. Canakinumab is a recombinant human monoclonal antibody against the proinflammatory cytokine IL-1β. Canakinumab is FDA approved for the treatment of several autoimmune inflammatory disorders including systemic juvenile idiopathic arthritis. The recent Canakinumab Antiinflammatory Thrombosis Outcome Study (CANTOS) examined the effect of canakinumab in over 10,000 patients with previous myocardial infarction and a serum high-sensitivity C-reactive protein (hsCRP) level of 2 mg/L or higher.[22] hsCRP is a biomarker of inflammation that is associated with an increased risk of cardiovascular events, independent of serum lipid levels. The results of CANTOS showed that canakinumab, administered subcutaneously once every 3 months, decreased the primary end point of nonfatal MI, nonfatal stroke, or cardiovascular (CV) death. Canakinumab decreased levels of hsCRP and IL-6, an inflammatory cytokine also associated with increased risk of CV events, but had no effect on lipid levels.[22] While the cost ($64,000 per year[23]) and adverse effects likely preclude the use of canakinumab for the treatment of CAD, this study is important because it shows that treating inflammation is effective at reducing CV events associated with atherosclerosis. In the future, drugs that target the processes of inflammation involved in atherosclerosis to reduce CV events may come to fruition.

RISK FACTORS FOR CAD AND STRATEGIES TO REDUCE RISK

Framingham Study

In the 1940s and 1950s, the incidence of cardiovascular disease (CVD) became the leading cause of mortality in the United States, with one out of three men developing CVD before reaching 60 years of age. At that time, very little was known regarding the etiology of heart disease, stroke, and other related disorders; however, as the incidence and deaths continued to rise, it was clear that cohesive plans to prevent and treat CVD were sorely needed. Efforts began to focus on prevention and the identification of predisposing factors that could be modified. This backdrop led to the development of the Framingham Heart Study. Begun in 1948 under the direction of the National Heart Institute (currently known as the National Heart, Lung, and Blood Institute, NHLBI), this epidemiological study sought to identify common factors that lead to CVD. From its inception, the Framingham Heart Study was designed as a longitudinal study to follow a large cohort of patients over a long period of time.[24–26]

The original cohort consisted of 5,209 men and women who lived in the town of Framingham, Massachusetts, were between the ages or 30 and 62, and had not yet developed overt symptoms of CVD or had a stroke or myocardial infarction (*aka* heart attack or MI). These individuals participated in lifestyle interviews, extensive physical examinations, and laboratory tests every 2 years in order to gain appropriate data over an extended period of time. In 1971, the Framingham Study enrolled a second generation cohort consisting of the original cohort's adult children and their spouses, and in 2002 the Study enrolled a third generation cohort consisting of the grandchildren of the original cohort. Since Framingham was essentially a white middle class community in 1948, the first two cohorts did not provide a diverse community of participants. To rectify this situation, 507 men and women of African American, Hispanic, Asian, Indian, Pacific Islander, and Native American origins who were residents of Framingham and the surrounding towns were enrolled as the first Omni cohort of the Framingham Study in 1994. A second Omni cohort was enrolled in 2003.

The primary aim of the original Study was to gather epidemiological information on arteriosclerotic and hypertensive CVD. The Study also had two subsidiary aims: (1) to gather information on the prevalence of all forms of CVD in a standard, representative population and (2) to test the efficiency of specific diagnostic procedures. At the time, it was assumed that CVD was the result of multiple factors and causes. These factors and causes served as a list of hypotheses that were later verified as a result of this Study (Table 35.2). Many of the risk factors which contribute to CAD are modifiable. Improvement of these risk factors leads to a decrease in adverse cardiac events.

CVD RISK ASSESSMENT[27]

Tracy Sprunger, PharmD, BCPS

The American Heart Association (AHA) and the American College of Cardiology (ACC) recommend assessing cardiovascular risk factors beginning at the age of 20 years every 4-6 years. Patients with known atherosclerotic cardiovascular disease (ASCVD) are at significant risk of developing a future event, and it is important to recognize this history in your patient assessment. ASCVD includes ACS, history of MI, angina, coronary or other arterial revascularization, stroke, transient ischemic attack, or peripheral artery disease presumed to be of atherosclerotic origin. Patients without known ASCVD may still be at increased risk; therefore, modifiable ASCVD risk factors (smoking, dyslipidemia, hypertension, and diabetes mellitus) and nonmodifiable risks (age, race, and sex) should be assessed. Beginning at the age of 40 years, it is recommended to estimate a 10-year risk of developing a first hard ASCVD event (myocardial infarction, coronary heart disease, or stroke) every 4-6 years. The Pooled Cohort Equations are recommended by the ACC/AHA in non-Hispanic white and black patients and may be accessed via a web based link or downloadable calculator from the ACC website. http://tools.acc.org/ASCVD-Risk-Estimator-Plus/#!/calculate/estimate/. There are additional factors that influence a patient's risk and should be considered when evaluating a patients risk including; LDL–C > 160 mg/dL, family history of premature ASCVD, elevated lifetime ASCVD risk, abnormal coronary artery calcium (CAC) score or ankle-brachial index (ABI), or hs-CRP > 2 mg/L. Pharmacotherapy is often recommended in patients with a 10-year risk >7.5% to modify risk such as dyslipidemia or hypertension. By estimating risk, the pharmacist can establish an evidence-based treatment regimen designed to target modifiable risk factors as well as utilize the estimate to educate patients how risk may change as comorbid conditions and risk factors change. It is important to recognize that these calculations of risk are an estimate and should not replace clinical judgment.

Smoking Cessation

S-(−)-Nicotine

Table 35.2 Major Hypotheses of the Framingham Study[26]

CVD increases with age and occurs more frequently in males.
Patients with hypertension are more likely to develop CVD than those who do not.
Tobacco use increases the risk of developing CVD.
Alcohol use increases the risk of developing CVD.
Increased physical activity decreases the risk of developing CVD.
Increased body weight increases the risk of developing CVD.
Patients with diabetes mellitus have an increased risk of developing CVD.
Patients with gout have an increased risk of developing CVD.

While tobacco smoke causes most of the ill health effects associated with cigarette smoking, it is the nicotine that is addictive. *S*-(−)-Nicotine is the predominant isomer in tobacco smoke. The nicotine in cigarettes causes the dependence of smoking, in part, through its agonist activity on α4β2 neuronal nicotinic acetylcholine receptors (nAChRs) found in the highest concentration in the mesolimbic dopamine system in the brain. This is frequently referred to as the reward center in the brain. Stimulation of α4β2 nAChRs by nicotine in inhaled cigarette smoke depolarizes dopamine cell bodies in the ventral tegmental area which increases the release of dopamine in the nucleus accumbens reinforcing the addictive behavior of smoking.[28,29] Upon cessation of smoking, the resultant low levels of dopamine in the mesolimbic dopamine area, due to the lack of nicotine stimulation, is associated with craving and withdrawal symptoms. The first line treatments for smoking cessation include nicotine replacement therapy (NRT), varenicline oral tablets, and bupropion sustained-release (SR) tablets. While studies have shown that all three therapies are more effective than placebo in helping patients to quit smoking, a Cochrane meta-analysis concluded that more patients successfully quit smoking with varenicline therapy than with either NRT or bupropion.[30,31]

NRT

NRT is available in five different dosage forms including oral inhaler, chewing gum, oral lozenge, nasal spray, and extended release transdermal patch. The oral formulations and nasal spray provide rapid delivery of nicotine while the patch has a slower onset of nicotine delivery but a 24-hour duration. NRT delivers nicotine to the central nervous system in a lower concentration and at a much slower rate than tobacco smoke. NRT staves off the craving sensation for cigarettes and symptoms of nicotine withdrawal without introducing the toxic chemicals in cigarette smoke.

Nicotine undergoes extensive first-pass metabolism in the liver (Fig. 35.6) and, consequently, has poor oral bioavailability.[32,33] The major route of nicotine metabolism (70%-80%) is via CYP2A6 to form cotinine. Cotinine is further metabolized to *trans*-3′-hydroxycontinine which is the major metabolite found in urine. *Trans*-3′-hydroxycotinine and its O-glucuronide together represent 40%-60% of the nicotine metabolites found in urine. The NRT dosage forms all bypass first-pass metabolism via buccal absorption (chewing gum, oral lozenge, oral inhaler), absorption through the nasal mucosa (nasal spray), or transdermal absorption (patch).

Nicotine is dibasic containing a weak basic pyridine nitrogen with a pK_a of 3.1 and a pyrrolidine nitrogen with a pK_a of 8.0. Nicotine bound to an ion exchange resin, called nicotine polacrilex, is the active ingredient in chewing gum and oral lozenge NRT formulations. The gum and lozenge formulations also contain potassium or sodium bicarbonate and/or sodium carbonate to increase the salivary pH which facilitates buccal absorption of nicotine in the nonionized state.[34,35] Foods that decrease the pH of the saliva will decrease the buccal absorption of nicotine by

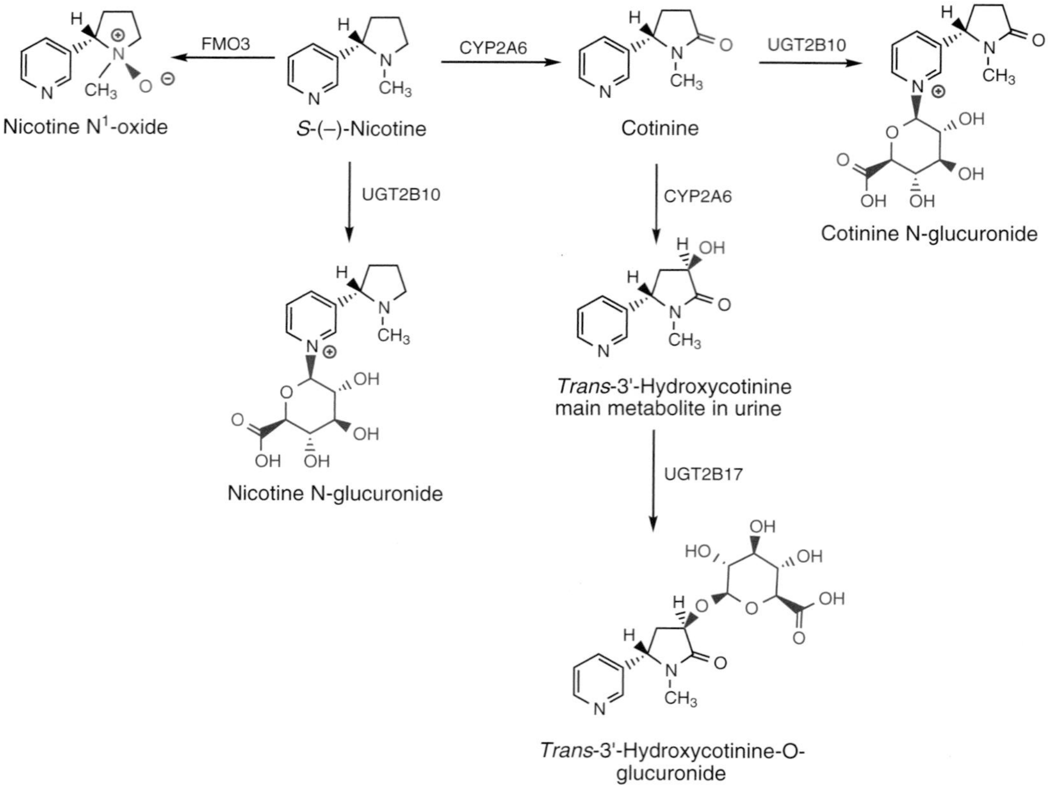

Nicotine N^1-oxide
FMO3
S-(−)-Nicotine
CYP2A6
Cotinine
UGT2B10
Cotinine N-glucuronide
UGT2B10
Nicotine N-glucuronide
CYP2A6
Trans-3'-Hydroxycotinine
main metabolite in urine
UGT2B17
Trans-3'-Hydroxycotinine-O-glucuronide

Figure 35.6 Major metabolic pathways of nicotine.

increasing the percentage of the ionized form. Therefore, patients should be counseled to drink only water 15 minutes prior to and during the use of oral NRT.[36] Coffee, fruit juices, and cola drinks, in particular, lower salivary pH and may decrease the buccal absorption of nicotine, decreasing the efficacy of oral NRT.

Most of the adverse effects associated with NRT are related to the dosage form including pruritus at the application site (patch), mouth and throat irritation (oral forms and nasal spray), and transient stinging of nasal mucosa, lacrimation, and sneezing (nasal spray).[37] The oral formulations and nasal spray may cause nausea and the patch may cause insomnia and vivid dreams.[37]

Varenicline

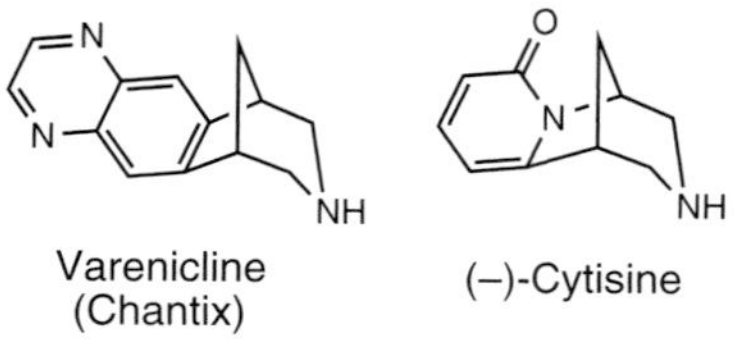

Varenicline
(Chantix)

(−)-Cytisine

Varenicline is an α4β2 nAChR partial agonist.[38] Based on the structure of the natural alkaloid (−)-cytisine and like other nicotinic compounds, varenicline possesses a nitrogen that will be charged at physiological pH and an electron deficient π-system. There are several key differences between nicotine and varenicline binding to the α4β2 nAChR (Fig. 35.7). The tertiary ammonium ion of nicotine forms a critical cation-π interaction with a key tryptophan residue designated "TrpB," and it is a hydrogen bond donor to the tryptophan backbone carbonyl oxygen.[39,43] The pyridine nitrogen of nicotine serves as a hydrogen bond acceptor. Alternately, the smaller secondary ammonium cation of varenicline allows it to form a cation-π interaction not only to TrpB in the α4β2 nAChR, but also to a tyrosine residue termed TyrC2.[40] Like nicotine, the secondary ammonium ion in varenicline is a hydrogen bond donor to the TrpB backbone carbonyl. Another difference is that the quinoxaline ring of varenicline does not serve as a hydrogen bond acceptor. Two factors contribute to this lack of hydrogen bond formation at the quinoxaline nitrogen of varenicline. First, the quinoxaline ring nitrogen is very weakly basic (pK_a 0.8) rendering it a poor hydrogen bond acceptor compared to the pyridine nitrogen (pK_a 3.1) in nicotine.[41] Additionally, the distance between the cationic center forming the cation-π interaction, and the aromatic nitrogen is longer in varenicline (5.75 Å) compared to the relationship in nicotine (4.36 Å).[41]

As an α4β2 nAChR partial agonist, varenicline stimulates a moderate and sustained release of dopamine in the mesolimbic region which is sufficient to stave off cigarette craving and nicotine withdrawal symptoms. Varenicline has a higher affinity for α4β2 nAChRs than nicotine. By competing with nicotine for binding to α4β2 nAChRs, varenicline antagonizes the full agonist effects of inhaled nicotine should the patient smoke during varenicline therapy, thereby inhibiting the dopamine "reward."

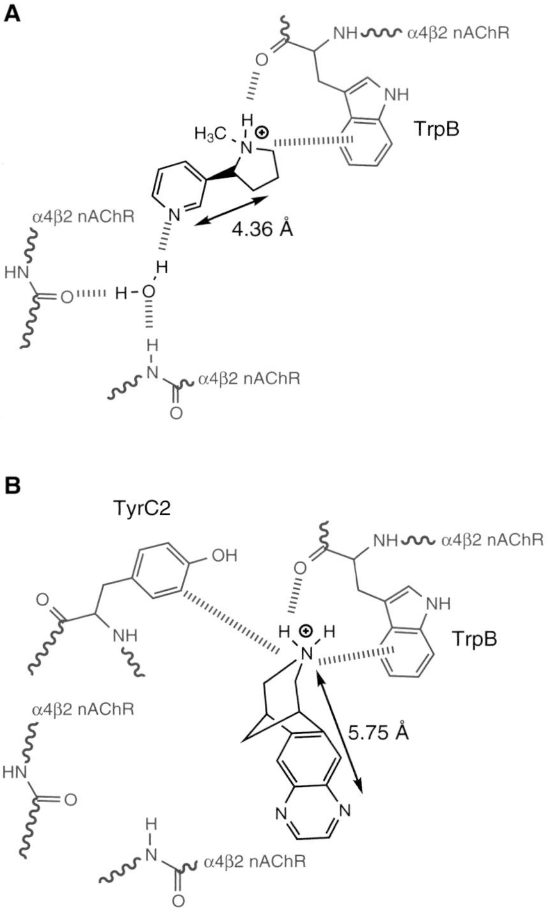

Figure 35.7 A model of nicotine (A) and varenicline (B) binding to the α4β2 nicotinic acetylcholine receptor (nAChR).[39–42] Binding sites within the α4β2 nAChR are noted in red.

Varenicline is not metabolized by CYP enzymes and is nearly exclusively excreted unchanged in the urine.[42] Varenicline neither inhibits nor induces CYP enzymes and has few drug-drug interactions. The most common adverse effect with varenicline is nausea.

Bupropion

Initially approved for the treatment of depression, bupropion, formulated as a 12-hour sustained-release tablet under the tradename Zyban, is another first-line agent for smoking cessation. The mechanism of action of bupropion in smoking cessation is unclear but likely involves several mechanisms including dopamine reuptake inhibition and norepinephrine reuptake inhibition in the central nervous system. Additionally, there is evidence that bupropion noncompetitively blocks the activation of neuronal nAChRs by nicotine potentially reducing its reinforcing properties.[44,45] More information about bupropion can be found in Chapter 11.

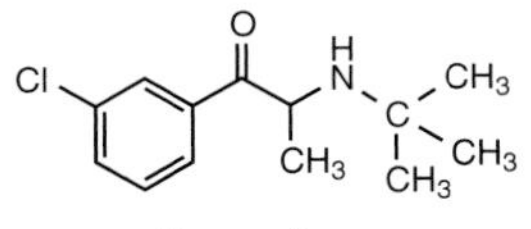

Bupropion
(Zyban)

Decrease Body Weight Mass

Obesity is defined as body mass index (BMI) ≥ 30, and overweight is defined as BMI of 25-29. The Global Burden of Disease 2015 Obesity Collaborators found that in 2015, 2.7 million (67.5%) of the 4 million deaths related to high BMI worldwide were due to CVD.[46] Of those deaths, just over 60% occurred among obese patients which means more than 1 million patients who died of high BMI-related deaths occurred in patients with a BMI less than 30. There is a statistically significant greater risk of IHD with every 5-unit increase in BMI across all 5-year age-groups from 25 to 80+ years, with the highest relative risk in the 25-30-year-old group (RR = 2.274; 95% CI 1.257 – 3.686).[46] In a pooled analysis of prospective observational studies, which included only patients who never smoked and had no identifiable chronic disease who survived 5 years after recruitment, patients with a BMI of 20-25 had the lowest overall risk of death.[46] A full discussion of drugs used to treat obesity is provided in Chapter 37.

Diabetes Mellitus

Diabetes mellitus is a well-established risk factor for CAD and it is an independent predictor of adverse outcomes (CAD death, MI, or urgent coronary revascularization for myocardial ischemia) after ACS.[47] Except for a 15% relative risk reduction for nonfatal MI, evidence to date suggests that intensive glucose control in patients with type 2 diabetes does not significantly decrease cardiovascular mortality or all-cause mortality.[48] The sodium-glucose cotransporter 2 (SGLT2) inhibitors empagliflozin and canagliflozin and glucagon-like peptide-1 (GLP-1) receptor agonist liraglutide have been shown to significantly decrease cardiovascular events in patients with type 2 diabetes who are at high risk for cardiovascular events.[49–51] Furthermore, empagliflozin and liraglutide have been shown to decrease mortality.[49,51] Including one of these agents to the treatment of patients with type 2 diabetes and established atherosclerotic vascular disease is part of the American Diabetes Association Standards of Medical Care.[52] A full discussion of each class of drugs to treat diabetes is provided in Chapter 20.

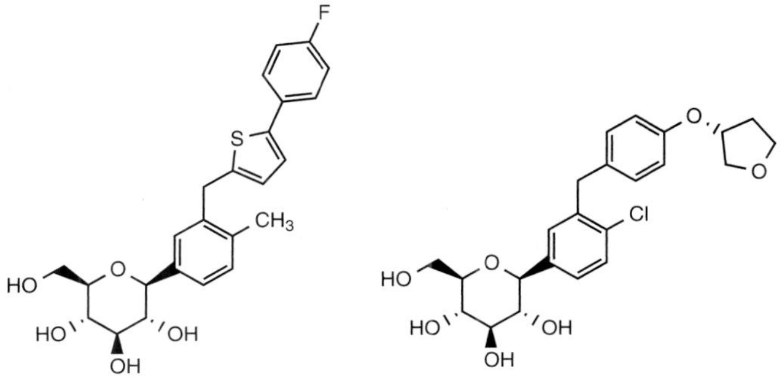

Canagliflozin
(Invokana)

Empagliflozin
(Jardiance)

Genetic and Lifestyle Factors

A link between CAD and familial patterns was first reported in 1938 and has since been confirmed by multiple large studies using data from parents, siblings, and other family members. A 2007 report identified genetic markers that significantly contribute to the risk of development of CAD.[53] Since that report, over 50 different single-nucleotide polymorphisms (SNPs) have been linked to an increased risk of CAD.[54]

A large amount of evidence supports the hypothesis that individuals who lead a healthy lifestyle are much less likely to develop CAD than those individuals who do not. Key factors in determining a healthy lifestyle include the absence of smoking, the prevention of obesity, adherence to regular physical activity, and a healthy diet.

A recent study examined the correlation between genetic risk factors and a healthy lifestyle. The study used data from over 50,000 patients who had been enrolled in three other longitudinal studies. A polygenic risk score was calculated using an analysis of up to 50 SNPs that were provided from the National Center for Biotechnology Information, and each individual was placed into one of three genetic risk groups: low genetic risk, intermediate genetic risk, or high genetic risk. A healthy lifestyle was based on the absence of smoking, a BMI less than 30, physical activity at least once weekly, and a healthy diet as outlined by the study parameters. The results of this study showed that genetic risk is independent of healthy lifestyle behaviors; however, within each genetic risk group, the adherence to a healthy lifestyle was associated with a decreased risk of CAD and related coronary events.[54]

Hypertension

Hypertension has been identified by the AHA, the American College of Cardiology (ACC), and the American Society of Hypertension (ASH) as a major independent risk factor of CAD in males and females of all races and ages.[55] The relationship between hypertension and the occurrences of MI, stroke, renal failure, and death have led to specific guidelines for the early detection and treatment of hypertension, with the overall goal of decreasing disease progression and increasing quality of life.[56] According to the 2014 report from the Eighth Joint National Committee (JNC8), adults >60 years of age should have a BP goal of less than 150/90 mm Hg. Due to insufficient evidence for a systolic goal in patients under 60 years of age and for a diastolic goal in patients under 30 years of age, a general recommendation for all patients under 60 years of age is a BP goal of 140/90 mm Hg.[56]

Studies have shown that elevations in BP differ as a function of age, with increases in diastolic BP predominating in younger patients and increases in systolic BP occurring more often in older patients. In patients <50 years of age, diastolic BP is more important in predicting CAD, whereas in patients >60 years of age, systolic BP is the more important predictor. Additionally, fatal CAD has been correlated to specific increases in BP. Over a BP range of 115/75-185/115 mm Hg, an increase in systolic BP of 20 mm Hg or an increase of diastolic BP of 10 mm Hg doubles the risk of a fatal event.[55]

The elevation of BP can be linked to a variety of genetic, physiological, metabolic, and environmental causes. From a genetic perspective, SNPs of angiotensin converting enzyme, the angiotensin II receptor, and angiotensinogen have been linked to increased BP. From a physiological perspective, increased activity of the sympathetic nervous system and/or the renin, angiotensin, aldosterone system have been shown to increase BP. Additionally, elevated BP can occur as a result of decreased activity or decreased release of vasodilators (e.g., nitric oxide), changes in natriuretic peptides, increased expression of inflammatory cytokines, and abnormalities in endothelial dysfunction. From metabolic and environmental perspectives, excessive dietary intake of sodium, inadequate dietary intake of potassium and calcium, increased exposure to psychosocial stress, insulin resistance, obesity, and diabetes mellitus all increase the risk of both elevated BP and CAD.[57,58]

Treatment of Hypertension

Guidelines for the management and treatment of high BP can be found in JNC8.[56] For patients who do not have either diabetes or chronic kidney disease, thiazide-type diuretics, angiotensin converting enzyme inhibitors (ACEI), angiotensin receptor blockers (ARB), and/or calcium channel blockers (CCB) are recommended as initial therapy either alone or in combination in nonblack patients. In black patients, initial therapy should include either thiazide-type diuretics or CCB either alone or in combination. These same guidelines hold true for all patients with diabetes without chronic kidney disease; however, in patients with diabetes and chronic kidney disease, the recommended initial therapy is an ACEI or an ARB either alone or in combination with a thiazide-type diuretic or CCB in all age-groups and races. The combination of an ACEI and an ARB should not be used due to a risk of increased adverse drug-related events.[59]

Patients who are not at their target BP goal after initial therapy and who have been adhering to medication and lifestyle changes should have their medications titrated and/or have additional drugs added. The current guidelines suggested that second and third line therapeutic alterations should maximize the combination use and dosages of the thiazide-type diuretics, ACEI, ARB, and CCB. If this fails to produce the desired BP goal, then additional pharmacological classes of drugs can be added. These include β-blockers, aldosterone antagonists, α_1-antagonists, and α_2-agonists.

While the above guidelines for the general treatment of hypertension recommend that β-blockers only be used after other drug classes have failed, their role in treating patients with CAD is much more prevalent. The ability of β-blockers to decrease the rate and contractility of the heart decreases oxygen demand and alleviates ischemia and angina in patients with ischemic heart disease. In comparing the available drugs, those that are selective for the β_1 receptor (e.g., atenolol, metoprolol) are preferred over those that are nonselective.[55]

A full discussion of each class of antihypertensive drugs is provided in Chapter 17. Examples of drugs from each major chemical/pharmacological class are provided in Figure 35.8. A summary of their mechanisms of actions and key adverse effects are provided in Table 35.3.[60–62]

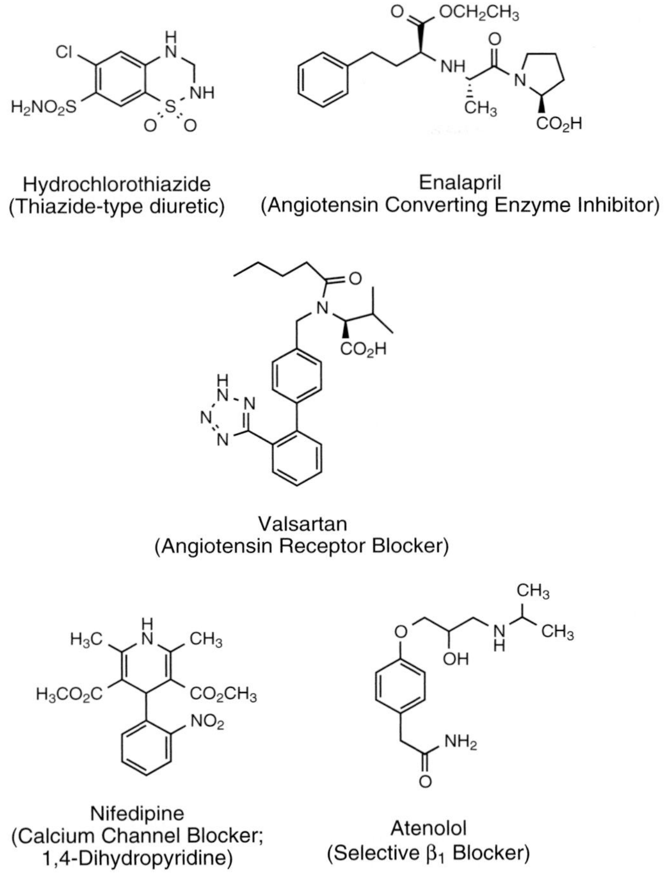

Hydrochlorothiazide (Thiazide-type diuretic)

Enalapril (Angiotensin Converting Enzyme Inhibitor)

Valsartan (Angiotensin Receptor Blocker)

Nifedipine (Calcium Channel Blocker; 1,4-Dihydropyridine)

Atenolol (Selective β_1 Blocker)

Figure 35.8 Examples of drug classes used to treat hypertension.

Atherosclerosis and Drug Therapy to Decrease the Risk of Coronary Artery Disease

As previously discussed in this chapter and in Chapter 19, dyslipidemia/hyperlipidemia has been strongly associated with atherosclerotic lesions and CAD. Current guidelines for lowering plasma LDL-cholesterol focus on the use of 3-hydroxy-3-methylglutaryl (HMG)-CoA reductase inhibitors, commonly known as statins, and other dietary and pharmacological/chemical classes of drugs, commonly known as nonstatin therapy.[63,64] These guidelines define four patient population groups that would benefit from the use of statins. The guidelines also identify other factors that need to be considered when recommending specific therapy. These include adherence, lifestyle, the control of other risk factors, the balance between risks and benefits of using a statin, the patient's preference for one medication over another, the total LDL reduction that is set as the patient's goal, and patient monitoring. For patients who develop statin intolerance or who fail to achieve their target LDL reduction, ezetimibe (an inhibitor of dietary cholesterol), bile acid sequestrants, proprotein convertase subtilisin/kexin type 9 (PCSK9) inhibitors, mipomersen (a microsomal triglyceride transfer protein inhibitor), and lomitapide (an apo B-100 protein translation inhibitor) can be used as optional interventions. Full discussions for all of these drugs and drug classes can be found in Chapter 19. An overview of the key structural features, pharmacological and therapeutic effects, and adverse effects/interactions/precautions are described below.

Table 35.3 Mechanisms of Action and Key Adverse Effects for Drugs Used to Treat Hypertension in Patients With CAD

Drug Class	Mechanism of Action	Key Adverse Effects
Thiazide-type diuretics	Blocks the chloride binding site of the Na^+/Cl^- symporter located in the distal convoluted tubule. This inhibits the reabsorption of sodium and chloride ions and enhances fluid excretion.	• Hypersensitivity reactions • Hypokalemia • Increase blood glucose levels
Angiotensin-converting enzyme inhibitors	Tripeptide substrate analogs that inhibit the conversion of angiotensin I (inactive decapeptide) to angiotensin II (active octapeptide).	• Hyperkalemia • Dry cough • Angioedema • Contraindicated during pregnancy
Angiotensin receptor blockers	Contain structural features that mimic the side chains of the amino acids present within the structure of angiotensin II. This allows the drugs to bind to the AT_1 receptor and act as receptor antagonists.	• Hyperkalemia • Contraindicated during pregnancy
Calcium channel blockers	Bind to specific receptor sites located within the central α_1 subunit of L-type, potential-dependent calcium channels and prevent the influx of calcium into the cell. This prevents excitation-contraction coupling resulting in vasodilation.	• Flushing • Hypotension • Nasal congestion • Palpitations (1,4-dihydropyridines) • Bradycardia (verapamil and diltiazem)
Selective β_1-Blockers	Bind to β_1-adrenergic receptors and block the binding of norepinephrine and epinephrine. This causes an inhibition of normal sympathetic effects and a reduction of blood pressure.	• Decreased exercise tolerance • Cold extremities • Impotence • Hypoglycemia (as well as masking the signs of hypoglycemia)

HMG-CoA Reductase Inhibitors

HMG-CoA reductase inhibitors (HMGRIs), commonly known as statins, prevent the biosynthesis of cholesterol by mimicking HMG-CoA (the substrate), mevinolin (the product), and/or the transition state that converts these two biomolecules (Fig. 35.9). All HMGRIs contain the highlighted 3,5-dihydroxy acid as part of their structure. While modifications and prodrugs are tolerated, this highlighted functional group is essential for activity and must be present within the liver and other extrahepatic cells that synthesize cholesterol.[65] Competitive inhibition of this enzyme causes an initial decrease in hepatic cholesterol. Compensatory mechanisms result in an enhanced expression of both HMG-CoA reductase and LDL receptors. The net result of all these effects is a slight to modest decrease in cholesterol synthesis, a significant increase in receptor-mediated LDL uptake, and an overall lowering of plasma LDL levels.[66]

Seven HMGRIs are currently available for the reduction of LDL levels. Based on the guidelines established in 2013, these drugs have been divided into three categories, "high-intensity," "moderate-intensity," and "lower-intensity" based upon doses given and the ability to decrease LDL cholesterol and the risk of atherosclerotic cardiovascular disease (ASCVD) (Table 35.4).[63] The basis for this differentiation came about through randomly controlled trials and two "critical questions" that focused on evidence for LDL cholesterol and non-HDL cholesterol goals for the primary and secondary prevention of ASCVD. There was a high level of evidence that atorvastatin 40-80 mg reduced ASCVD risk more than atorvastatin 10 mg, pravastatin 40 mg, or simvastatin 20-40 mg bid. The relative classifications were based on evidence in relative reductions in ASCVD risk as this related to the lowering of plasma LDL levels. No differentiations were made among the specific HMGRIs in each category. The percent reductions for LDL cholesterol shown in Table 35.4 came from a meta-analysis of data from 170,000 participants in multiple randomized trials.[67]

Common adverse effects of HMGRIs include abdominal pain, arthralgia, chest pain, constipation, diarrhea, dyspepsia, elevated hepatic enzymes, flatulence, headache, muscle cramps, myalgia, myopathy, nausea, rhabdomyolysis, rhinitis, sinusitis, and vomiting.[66,68] Of these, myalgia and myopathies are the most common, and potentially the most serious as they can lead to rhabdomyolysis, a rare condition involving massive muscle necrosis with secondary acute renal failure. While these muscle-related symptoms may occur, the development of true statin intolerance is uncommon. Patients who report muscle related symptoms need to be evaluated for scope as well as other potential causes. In general, statin-related myalgia or weakness tends to involve large proximal muscle groups as opposed to a single muscle. For patients who meet the above criteria, there are a number of ways to address this issue. First of all, the patient can be switched to a different statin, a lower dose, or a less intensive statin regimen. Second, statin therapy can be discontinued and then rechallenged to verify a causal effect. The term "statin intolerance" has not been universally defined; however, common criteria for this designation include unacceptable muscle-related discomfort, resolution with discontinuation, and reoccurrence with a rechallenge using at least two to three statins with different physicochemical properties at the lowest approved dose.[64]

Ezetimibe

Ezetimibe lowers plasma cholesterol levels by inhibiting the absorption of cholesterol at the brush border of the small intestine.[66,69] Specifically, it binds to the sterol transporter, Niemann-Pick C1-Like 1 (NPC1L1), located in the epithelial cells of small intestine. The 1,4-diaryl-β-lactam ring serves as a scaffold to orient the two aromatic rings and the aliphatic chain. The hydrophilic nature of the two hydroxyl groups is important for helping ezetimibe localize in the small intestine. Ezetimibe is selective in that it does not interfere with the absorption of triglycerides,

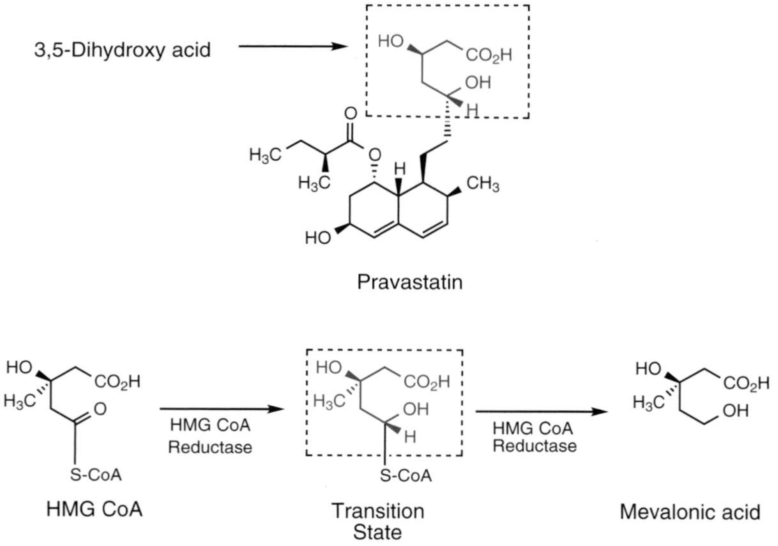

3,5-Dihydroxy acid

HO CO₂H OH H O H₃C O H₃C H CH₃ HO

Pravastatin

HO CO₂H H₃C O S-CoA — HMG CoA Reductase → HO CO₂H H₃C OH H S-CoA — HMG CoA Reductase → HO CO₂H H₃C OH

HMG CoA | Transition State | Mevalonic acid

Figure 35.9 Mechanism of action of the statin class of drugs as illustrated by pravastatin. The 3,5-dihydroxy acid portion of pravastatin is able to mimic the tetrahedral transition state produced by the enzyme HMG-CoA reductase.

Table 35.4 High-, Moderate-, and Low-Intensity Statin Therapy

High-Intensity Statin Therapy	Moderate-Intensity Statin Therapy	Low-Intensity Statin Therapy
Lowers LDL cholesterol by >50%	Lowers LDL cholesterol by 30% to <50%	Lowers LDL cholesterol by <30%
Atorvastatin 40-80 mg Rosuvastatin 20-40 mg	Atorvastatin 10-20 mg Fluvastatin 40 mg BID Fluvastatin XL 80 mg Lovastatin 40 mg Pitavastatin 2-4 mg Pravastatin 40-80 mg Rosuvastatin 5-10 mg Simvastatin 20-40 mg	Fluvastatin 20-40 mg Lovastatin 20 mg Pitavastatin 1 mg Pravastatin 10-20 mg Simvastatin 10 mg

Doses are once daily unless otherwise stated.

lipid-soluble vitamins, or other nutrients. The decreased absorption of cholesterol eventually leads to enhanced receptor-mediated LDL uptake similar to that seen with HMGRIs. When used as monotherapy, the decreased absorption of cholesterol causes a compensatory increase in cholesterol biosynthesis; however, it is insufficient to override the overall LDL-lowering effects of ezetimibe.

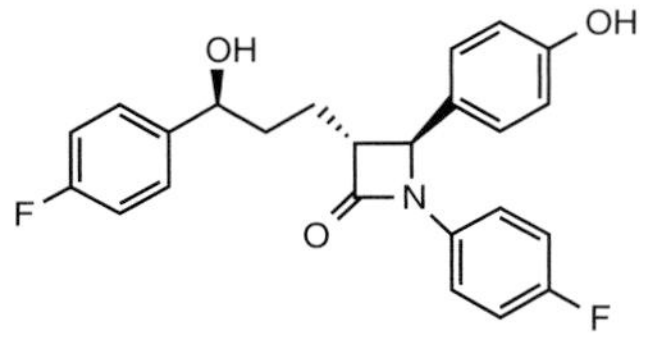

Ezetimibe
(Zetia)

The most common adverse effects seen with ezetimibe include abdominal pain, diarrhea, back pain, cough, pharyngitis, sinusitis, fatigue, and viral infection. Whenever ezetimibe is used in combination with an HMGRI, the incidence of myopathy does not increase above that seen with HMGRI monotherapy.[66,68] Ezetimibe generally does not interact with other drugs; however, aluminum and magnesium-containing antacids decrease the maximum plasma concentration of ezetimibe. Additionally, bile acid sequestrants will decrease the bioavailability of ezetimibe unless their administration is adequately spaced.

Bile Acid Sequestrants

Bile acid sequestrants, exemplified by cholestyramine, interfere with the normal enterohepatic circulation of bile acids and indirectly increase the clearance of LDL from the blood. The positively charged amines and quaternary nitrogen atoms present on the structures of bile acid sequestrants allows them to directly bind to negatively charged atoms or functional groups present on drug molecules or biomolecules.

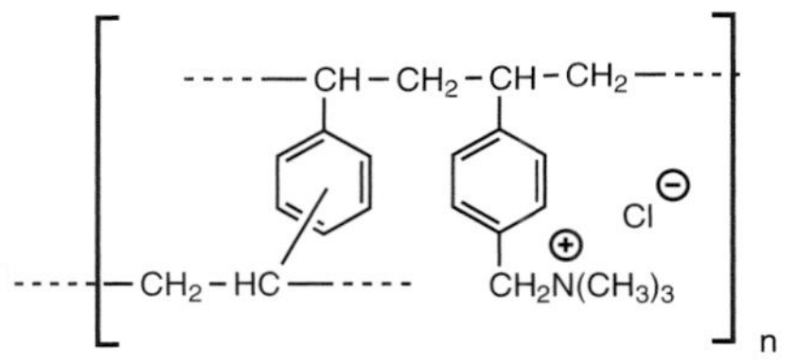

Cholestyramine
(Questran)

Bile acid sequestrants are not orally absorbed but act locally within the gastrointestinal tract to bind the two major bile acids, glycocholic acid and taurocholic acid, and greatly increase their fecal excretion. The decreased return of these acids to the liver causes an increase in the hepatic conversion of cholesterol to bile acids and a subsequent decrease in hepatic cholesterol. This in turn causes an increased expression of LDL receptors and an increased hepatic uptake of plasma LDL similar to that previously described for HMGRIs and ezetimibe. Compensatory responses also lead to the induction of HMG-CoA reductase and increased biosynthesis of cholesterol; however, similar to ezetimibe, these effects are insufficient to counteract the decrease in plasma LDL.[66,70,71]

Bile acid sequestrants are not orally absorbed; therefore, they produce minimal systemic side effects. The most frequently encountered adverse effect is constipation. This can be managed by increasing dietary fiber or using bulk-producing laxatives, such as psyllium. Other gastrointestinal symptoms include bloating, heartburn, nausea, eructation, and abdominal discomfort.[66,69] As a result of their mechanism of action, bile acid sequestrants can potentially bind with almost any other drug and decrease its oral absorption. Because bile acid sequestrants contain numerous positive charges, they are much more likely to bind to acidic compounds than to basic compounds or nonelectrolytes. To manage this potential drug interaction, it is recommended that all other oral medication should be administered at least 1 hour before or 4 hours after a bile acid sequestrant.[66,70]

Proprotein Convertase Subtilisin/Kexin Type 9 (PCSK9) Inhibitors

The hepatic enzyme, proprotein convertase subtilisin/kexin type 9 (PCSK9), is involved in cholesterol homeostasis and the maintenance of plasma LDL cholesterol levels. This is accomplished through the binding of PCSK9 to LDL receptors located on the surface of hepatocytes. The subsequent internalization of the PCSK9/LDL receptor complex leads to LDL receptor destruction and an increase in plasma LDL. This regulation is important for maintaining normal plasma LDL levels in healthy patients; however, it can contribute to hypercholesterolemia in other patients. Alirocumab (*Pradulent*) and evolocumab (*Repatha*) are human monoclonal IgG antibodies that bind to PCSK9 and inhibit its actions. Both drugs have been approved for treatment of hypercholesterolemia in individuals with severe forms of hereditary high cholesterol who cannot tolerate or who do not exhibit sufficient LDL lowering by HGMRIs.[69,72,73]

The clinical efficacy of PCSK9 inhibitors in lowering plasma cholesterol and decreasing the risk of cardiovascular events was shown in the FOURIER trial.[74] In this double-blind, placebo-controlled trial, patients who were already receiving statin therapy were randomly assigned to receive either evolocumab or placebo. Patients receiving evolocumab along with a statin for 48 weeks showed a 59% reduction in LDL cholesterol levels as compared to a statin and a placebo. The addition of evolocumab in patients receiving statin therapy also significantly reduced their risk of cardiovascular events by 15%-20% as compared with a placebo and a statin.

Both drugs are well tolerated but can cause injection-site reactions, muscle aches, rash, and itching. Flu-like symptoms, nasopharyngitis, allergic skin reactions, and cognitive effects (i.e., confusion, dementia, and memory impairment) may also occur. To date, there are no reported drug interactions with either alirocumab or evolocumab.[66]

Interestingly, the development of a related humanized monoclonal antibody, bocucizumab, was discontinued by the manufacturer due to the development of antidrug antibodies. Unlike alirocumab and evolocumab, which are fully human monoclonal IgG antibodies, bococizumab is humanized and contains a murine sequence that comprises approximately 3% of the monoclonal antibody. Numerous studies showed an appreciable reduction in LDL cholesterol after 12 weeks; however, this beneficial effect was significantly attenuated over time due to the development of anti–bococizumab antibodies. Additionally, bococizumab was associated with a substantially higher rate of injection site reactions than either evolocumab or alirocumab.[75]

PROSPECTIVE THERAPY: A MODIFIED siRNA TO BLOCK PCSK9 ACTIVITY. Small (or silencing) interfering RNA sequences (siRNAs) are naturally occurring biomolecules that function to regulate gene expression. The siRNAs, which are non-coding sequences, are formed through the processing and cleavage of longer double-stranded RNA sequences by an enzyme known as dicer. The cleavage produces RNA sequences that are 20-25 nucleotides in length and which have two non-paired nucleotides on each 3′ end. Once formed, the siRNA binds to an RNA-induced silencing complex (RISC). Each RNA strand of the siRNA serves a specific function. The guide-strand is complementary to the target mRNA, while the passenger-strand acts to stabilize the guide-strand and helps it to bind to the RISC. Once the siRNA is bound to the RISC, the passenger-strand is cleaved and removed, and the remaining guide-strand binds to the complementary target mRNA. Once this occurs, the target mRNA is destroyed, thus "silencing" its ability to produce the target protein or enzyme. Once the guide strand is bound (or loaded) to the RISC, it has a long half-life and can be used to destroy multiple versions of the target mRNA.[76–78]

Given the fact that a specific siRNA acts to degrade/destroy a specific mRNA thus inhibiting the formation of a specific enzyme or receptor, this class of biomolecules provides a potential alternative to attenuating the actions of proteins and enzymes. Unmodified siRNAs are unstable due to degradation by endo- and exonucleases. The major challenge in the development of siRNAs as drugs is to find chemical modifications that will enhance stability without compromising the selectivity and the ability to bind to the RISC. One example in which this challenge was met is the design, development, and synthesis of inclisiran. The general structure and the modifications within the double stranded RNA are shown below.

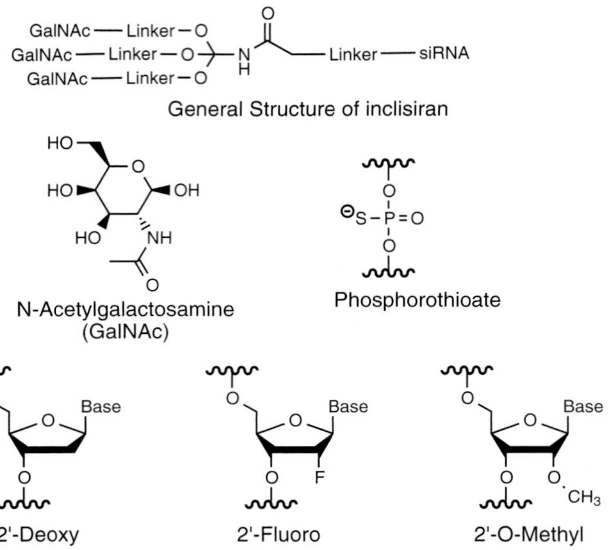

General Structure of inclisiran

N-Acetylgalactosamine (GalNAc)

Phosphorothioate

2'-Deoxy

2'-Fluoro

2'-O-Methyl

The left hand side of the structure contains three "arms," each of which is connected to an N-acetylgalactosamine (GalNAc). This section of the molecule has been referred to in the literature as a triantennary N-acetylgalactosamine. The major function of this portion of the molecule is to bind to the asialoglycoprotein receptor that is expressed on the surface of hepatocytes. Once the drug binds to this receptor, it is internalized and the linker portions of the drug are removed. The remaining siRNA binds to the RISC, targets the mRNA for PCSK9, and promotes its destruction. Similar to PCSK9 inhibitors, this action causes a decrease in plasma LDL levels. Several structural alterations provide chemical stability to the siRNA portion of inclisiran. The use of a phosphorothiolate group to link the nucleotides provides stability against endogenous peptidases, as compared to the natural phosphate linker. This structural variation is also seen in the structure of mipomersen, an antisense DNA drug discussed below. Variations of the ribose sugar also help to prevent degradation. While normal siRNAs are too unstable for therapeutic use, inclisiran has been shown to be active 6 months after a subcutaneous (SC) injection. Further tests to determine patient safety and tolerance need to be done; however, from a mechanistic standpoint, siRNAs appear to offer a promising new drug target.[78]

Drugs to Treat Homozygous Familial Hypercholesterolemia

Homozygous familial hypercholesterolemia (HoFH) results from genetic mutations of the LDL receptor in both parents. Patients with HoFH can develop severe hypercholesterolemia within the first two decades of life and can develop accelerated atherosclerosis and CAD.[79]

Mipomersen and lomitapide have been approved for the treatment of this rare genetic disorder. According to current therapeutic guidelines, these drugs are indicated for patients with HoFH who have a baseline LDL-C > 190 mg/dL and who have had an inadequate response to statins with or without ezetimibe and PCSK9 inhibitors.[64,69]

MIPOMERSEN. Mipomersen is a stable oligonucleotide that contains a modified DNA sequence that is complementary to the coding region of the mRNA for apo B-100. This complementary or antisense nature allows it to bind to the mRNA and create a 20 nucleotide hybrid DNA/mRNA sequence. This results in RNase-H mediated degradation of the mRNA and an inhibition of the production of the apo B-100 protein required for the synthesis of both LDL and very-low-density lipoprotein (VLDL).[66,80]

The chemical stability of mipomersen was achieved by two structural alterations. First, the phosphate oxygen atom was isosterically replaced with a sulfur atom. Second, 2′-O-(2-methoxyethyl) groups were added to the terminal five nucleotides at the 5′ and 3′ ends to inhibit nuclease action. The overall result of these modifications was an increase in the duration of the action that allows for once weekly SC administration.[80]

Injection site reactions, including erythema, pain, hematoma, pruritus, swelling, discoloration, and rash are the most common adverse effects seen with mipomersen. Other common adverse effects include elevations in serum ALT levels, flu-like symptoms, headache, and nausea. The most serious adverse effect is an increased risk of hepatotoxicity. To date, no clinically relevant drug interactions have been reported with mipomersen; however, caution should be exercised when using mipomersen in combination with other medications known to have potential for hepatotoxicity.[66,80]

LOMITAPIDE. Lomitapide inhibits the microsomal triglyceride transport protein (MTTP) located in the lumen of the endoplasmic reticulum. This prevents the assembly of apo-B–containing lipoproteins (i.e., VLDL and LDL) in both hepatocytes and enterocytes. The overall result of these actions is an initial decrease in the synthesis of chylomicrons and VLDL and an ultimate reduction in plasma LDL cholesterol. As compared to mipomersen, lomitapide can be administered orally; however, due to its high lipid solubility, lomitapide is extensively metabolized in the liver and has an overall low bioavailability (~7%). The major route of metabolism involves CYP3A4 oxidation; therefore interactions can occur with co-administered drugs that either inhibit or induce this isozyme.[66,81]

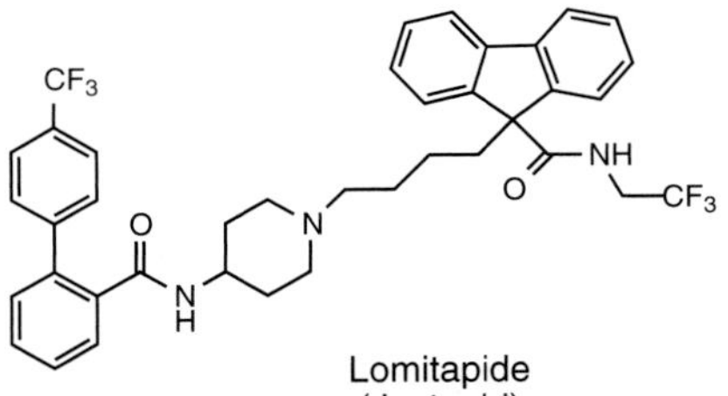

CF_3 O N H N O NH CF_3

Lomitapide
(Juxtapid)

The most commonly seen adverse effects of lomitapide involve the gastrointestinal tract and include abdominal discomfort, constipation, diarrhea, gastroesophageal reflux disorder (GERD), nausea, and vomiting. The most serious adverse effect is an increased risk of hepatotoxicity.[81]

THERAPEUTIC STRATEGIES FOR TREATING ACUTE CORONARY SYNDROMES

In 2014, a joint task force from the ACC and AHA published clinical practice guidelines for the management and treatment of patients with NSTE-ACS.[82] These guidelines discuss the initial evaluation and management of ACS, early hospital care, myocardial revascularization using percutaneous coronary intervention (PCI), post hospital care, and special patient groups. The following discussion summarizes the key aspects of drug medication use in patients with NSTE-ACS, as it pertains to their chemical and pharmacological actions.

Early Hospitalization Drug Therapy for NSTE-ACS

Following an initial clinical assessment and evaluation, patients who present with signs and symptoms of NSTE-ACS are normally admitted for inpatient hospital management. The treatment goals for these patients are immediate alleviation of ischemic symptoms and the prevention of an MI and death. Recommendations for treatment account for individual patient profiles and include oxygen therapy, antianginal drugs, analgesic therapy, high-intensity statins, ACEIs or ARBs, antiplatelet drugs, and anticoagulant drugs.

Antianginal Drugs

As previously discussed in this chapter, ischemia results from an imbalance between myocardial oxygen supply and demand. Thus the overall goal in treating ischemia can be met by either increasing oxygen supply or decreasing oxygen demand. Myocardial contractility, heart rate, and myocardial wall tension are the three major determinants of myocardial oxygen demand. Organic nitrates and calcium channel blockers can decrease myocardial wall tension through their ability to produce vasodilation, while β-adrenergic blockers and nondihydropyridine calcium channel blockers (i.e., verapamil and diltiazem) can decrease myocardial contractility and heart rate. All three chemical/pharmacological classes of drugs have been found to be therapeutically useful in treating angina.[62,83] An overview of their role in treating NSTE-ACS is provided below. Complete discussions of these classes of drugs can be found in Chapters 16 and 17.

ORGANIC NITRATES. Organic nitrates, exemplified below with nitroglycerin and isosorbide mononitrate, produce vasodilation in both coronary and peripheral vascular smooth muscles. The nitrates react with sulfhydryl groups in the vascular smooth muscle causing the ultimate production of nitric oxide. Nitric oxide then stimulates the production of cGMP leading to smooth muscle relaxation. This effect decreases cardiovascular preload and reduces ventricular wall tension. Nitrates can also dilate coronary arteries and redistribute coronary blood. Reflex responses may cause increases in heart rate and contractility; however, this can be managed through the combined use of a β-blocker.[62,83,84]

Nitroglycerin

Isosorbide mononitrate

Isosorbide mononitrate is available for oral use only, while nitroglycerin is available for oral, subcutaneous, topical, and IV use. The IV formulation is useful in patients with heart failure, hypertension, or symptoms not relieved with other formulations in combination with a β-blocker. The most common adverse effects seen with these drugs are vascular headaches, dizziness, weakness, and postural hypotension. It should be noted that all of these are simply natural extensions of their pharmacological effects. Nitrates are contraindicated in patients using a phosphodiesterase 5 inhibitor or riociguat.[62,66,83]

β-BLOCKERS

Selective β_1-adrenergic receptor antagonists (i.e., β_1-blockers) are recommended for patients who present with signs/symptoms of NSTE-ACS with the exception of patients who have signs of heart failure, evidence of a low-output state, are at an increased risk for cardiogenic shock, or have other contraindications. β_1-Blockers decrease myocardial contractility and heart rate, thus lowering the overall oxygen demand of the heart. Additionally, they have a hypotensive effect. Sustained-release metoprolol succinate, bisoprolol, and carvedilol (a mixed β- and α_1-blocker) are recommended in patients with NSTE-ACS, stabilized heart failure, and systolic dysfunction due to their proven clinical benefit in reducing mortality in this patient population.[82] The *para*-substitutions on metoprolol and bisoprolol allow for specific hydrogen bonding interactions with the β_1 receptor. All of these drugs lack the intrinsic sympathomimetic activity (ISA) seen with acebutolol and other nonselective β-blockers.[85] Two other selective β_1-blockers, atenolol and betaxolol, lack ISA and could potentially provide similar benefits.

Metoprolol Succinate

Bisoprolol

Carvedilol
(Used as racemate)

Common adverse reactions of β-blockers are decreased exercise tolerance, cold extremities, depression, sleep disturbance, hypoglycemia, and impotence. All of these adverse reactions are less severe in selective β_1-blockers. Selective β_1-blockers can be used in patients with chronic obstructive pulmonary disorder or asthma who are controlled by other medication and who do not have active bronchospasm. The use of β-blockers in patients with risk factors for shock can cause potential harm and thus should be avoided.[82,85]

CALCIUM CHANNEL BLOCKERS. From a chemical/pharmacological standpoint, calcium channel blockers can be classified as either 1,4-dihydropyridines or nondihydropyridines. As shown in Figure 35.10, amlodipine and nifedipine have a 1,4-dihydropyridine ring, while diltiazem and verapamil do not. All calcium channel blockers can produce peripheral vasodilation due to their ability to bind to specific receptor sites located within the central α_1 subunit of L type, potential-dependent channels and thus decrease calcium influx into the cell. The 1,4-dihydropyridines produce more vasodilation than the nondihydropyridines; however, the nondihydropyridines have significant cardiodepressive effects that are not seen with the 1,4-dihydropyridines. Both diltiazem and verapamil decrease AV nodal conduction and contractility.[62,83]

Diltiazem and verapamil are recommended in patients with NSTE-ACS who have recurring ischemia after the initial use of β-blockers and nitrates. Additionally, these two drugs are recommended as initial therapy in patients who have a contraindication to β-blockers, an absence of clinically significant left ventricular dysfunction, an increased risk of cardiogenic shock, an increased PR interval, or AV nodal block without a pacemaker. With the exception of immediate-release nifepidine, all calcium channel blockers are recommended to treat ischemic symptoms when β-blockers are contraindicated, fail to meet therapeutic goals, or cause unacceptable adverse reactions.

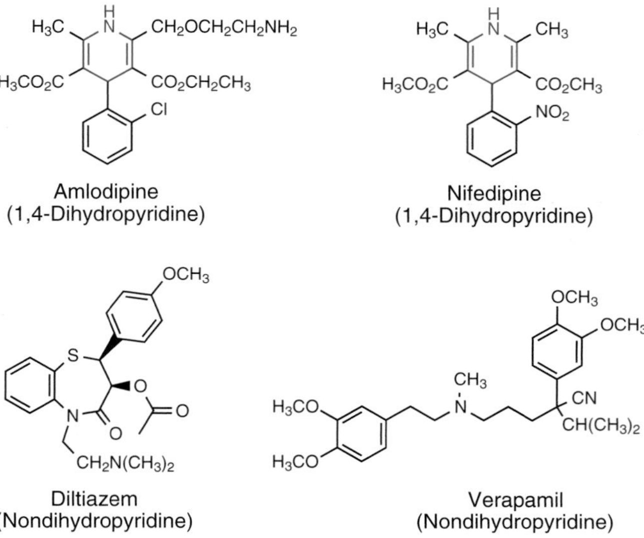

Figure 35.10 Examples of 1,4-dihydropyridines and the two nondihydropyridines, diltiazem and verapamil. The 1,4-dihydropyridine ring has been highlighted.

Immediate-release nifepidine is not recommended since it has been associated with a dose-related increase in mortality in patients with CAD.[82]

Common adverse effects seen with all calcium channel blockers are edema, flushing, hypotension, nasal congestion, headache, and dizziness. All of these are in part due to excessive vasodilation caused by these drugs. Additionally, reflex responses of the 1,4-dihydropyridines to vasodilation can result in palpitations, chest pain, and tachycardia. The use of a calcium channel blocker with a β-blocker can help minimize these compensatory responses.[62,66,83]

RANOLAZINE. Ranolazine is another antianginal drug that can be used in combination with drug classes discussed above. It is currently indicated for the treatment of chronic ischemia. It inhibits the late inward sodium current resulting in a reduction of intracellular sodium and calcium overload in ischemic cardiac myocytes. It has minimal effects on BP and heart rate, and it does not increase myocardial workload. The most common adverse effects seen with ranolazine are nausea, vomiting, dizziness, headache, and constipation. Ranolazine can cause a dose-related prolongation of the QTc interval.[66]

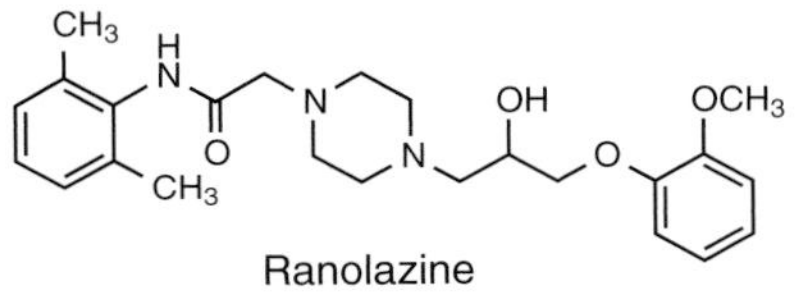

Ranolazine

Analgesic Therapy

In patients who continue to experience ischemic chest pain despite the optimal use of the drugs discussed above, IV morphine sulfate can be used to alleviate this discomfort. In addition to its analgesic and anxiolytic effects, morphine produces venodilation and a modest reduction in both heart rate and systolic BP. All of these hemodynamic effects are therapeutically beneficial to patients with NSTE-ACS. The use of morphine should be used judiciously in order to prevent known adverse effects (constipation, nausea, and vomiting) and serious complications (hypotension and respiratory depression).[82]

While the use of morphine does not appear to effect the actions of other classes of drugs used to treat ischemia, recent studies have shown that the coadministration of morphine with the oral antiplatelet $P2Y_{12}$ receptor antagonists, ticagrelor, clopidogrel, and prasugrel, causes a decreases their plasma concentration and their active metabolites. The exact mechanism of this drug interaction was not investigated in all studies; however, it is postulated that morphine interferes with the absorption of these drugs.[86–88] The overall effect of morphine on prasugrel appears to be much less than the other two $P2Y_{12}$ antagonists.[88] Given that $P2Y_{12}$ inhibitors are recommended in combination with aspirin as early treatment in patients with NSTE-ACS,[82] additional studies are needed in order to optimize the use of morphine with this class of drugs.

The use of nonsteroidal antiinflammatory drugs (NSAIDs) during early hospitalization is contraindicated due do their inhibition of the normal homeostasis of platelet function. Platelet aggregation is, in part, mediated through platelet-derived TXA_2. These effects are normally balanced through vascular endothelial prostacyclin production. Since platelets are anucleate, low-dose aspirin selectively decreases the production of TXA_2 without altering the production of prostacyclin and produces an antithrombotic effect. The use of an NSAID will nonselectively inhibit cyclooxygenase, decrease the concentrations of prostacyclin, and prevent the beneficial actions of aspirin.[82,89]

High-Intensity Statin Therapy

The use of statins for the prevention and risk reduction of atherosclerosis and CAD has been previously discussed. Once a patient has progressed and is diagnosed with NSTE-ACS, current recommendations state that the patient should either initiate or continue with high-intensity statins (Table 35.4) unless there is a contraindication. Clinical studies have shown that high-intensity statins reduce the rate of recurrent MI, the need for myocardial revascularization, the prevalence of stroke, and the overall mortality from coronary heart disease. The same level of reduction was not seen with mild- or low-intensity statin therapy.[63,82]

Inhibitors of the Renin-Angiotensin-Aldosterone Pathway

ACE inhibitors and ARBs have been shown to have beneficial cardiovascular effects beyond simply reducing BP and managing this risk factor. Specifically, they reduce mortality in patients with a recent MI and who have left ventricular (LV) dysfunction, i.e., less than 0.40 ejection fraction (EF). Additionally, they have been shown to reduce mortality and the incidence of heart failure in patients with normal LV function. Current guidelines recommend that ACE inhibitors should be started and continued indefinitely in all NSTE-ACS patients with a LVEF less than 0.40, as well as those with hypertension, diabetes mellitus, or stable chronic kidney disease unless there is a contraindication. ARBs may be used in place of ACEIs; however, these two classes of drugs should not be used in combination. Additionally, eplerenone, a selective aldosterone receptor blocker, has shown efficacy in decreasing long-term mortality when used as an adjunct in patients taking ACE inhibitors and β-blockers.[61,62,82]

Therapeutic Strategies for Treating Acute Coronary Syndromes

Antiplatelet Therapy in Patients With Definite or Likely NSTE-ACS

Platelet activation and aggregation are core components of coronary artery plaque formation and occlusion. Antiplatelet therapy is a cornerstone of the treatment of patients with ACS because it improves outcomes.

Currently, aspirin and $P2Y_{12}$ receptor antagonists are the most frequently used antiplatelet agents in patients with ACS. The role of the newest antiplatelet drug, vorapaxar, remains to be established. Although used for decades, use of glycoprotein IIb/IIIa inhibitors is on the decline due to the improved efficacy of newer drugs, but they still have their role in certain scenarios. All antiplatelet drugs are associated with a risk of bleeding which needs to be considered when prescribed for patients.

Aspirin

An immediate loading dose (162-325 mg) of non–enteric-coated chewable aspirin (acetylsalicylic acid, ASA) is first line therapy for patients with NSTE-ACS.[82] Subsequently, a maintenance dose of aspirin (81-162 mg/d) is recommended indefinitely because it decreases the incidence of recurrent MI and death in patients with NSTE-ACS.[90]

Aspirin
(Acetylsalicylic acid, ASA)

MECHANISM OF ANTIPLATELET ACTIVITY. Platelet aggregation plays a key role in the pathogenesis of atherosclerotic plaque and coronary artery thrombosis. Aspirin has antiplatelet activity by selectively and irreversibly inhibiting cyclooxygenase-1 (COX-1) at low doses (81-162 mg per day). The antiplatelet effect of aspirin occurs at doses that are more than 10- to 50-fold lower than doses required for analgesic, antipyretic, or anti-inflammatory activity.[91]

In platelets, COX-1 converts arachidonic acid (AA) to prostaglandin H_2 (PGH_2) which is further converted to TXA_2, a potent stimulator of platelet aggregation and inducer of vasoconstriction (Fig. 35.11). The mechanism by which TXA_2 causes platelet aggregation involves binding to discrete G-protein coupled TXA_2 receptors on the surface of platelets and is illustrated in Figure 35.12. Ultimately, the action of TXA_2 results in the activation of glycoprotein IIb/IIIa (GPIIb/IIIa) receptors on the surface of activated platelets. Each end of fibrinogen binds to GPIIb/IIIa receptors on neighboring platelets, linking platelets together causing platelet aggregation.

The active site of the COX enzymes is comprised of a long hydrophobic channel that accommodates AA for the ultimate conversion to prostaglandin H_2 (PGH_2).[92] The substrate binding site within the hydrophobic channel anchors AA in place via an ionic bond between the carboxylate of AA and the guanidinium side chain of Arg120. This ionic bond is reinforced with an electrostatic interaction between the same carboxylate and Tyr355. (The amino acid sequence numbering of COX enzymes typically refers to the ovine sequence.) Aspirin takes advantage of Arg120 and Tyr355 and binds in a similar manner as AA. This situates the acetyl group in close proximity to a serine residue

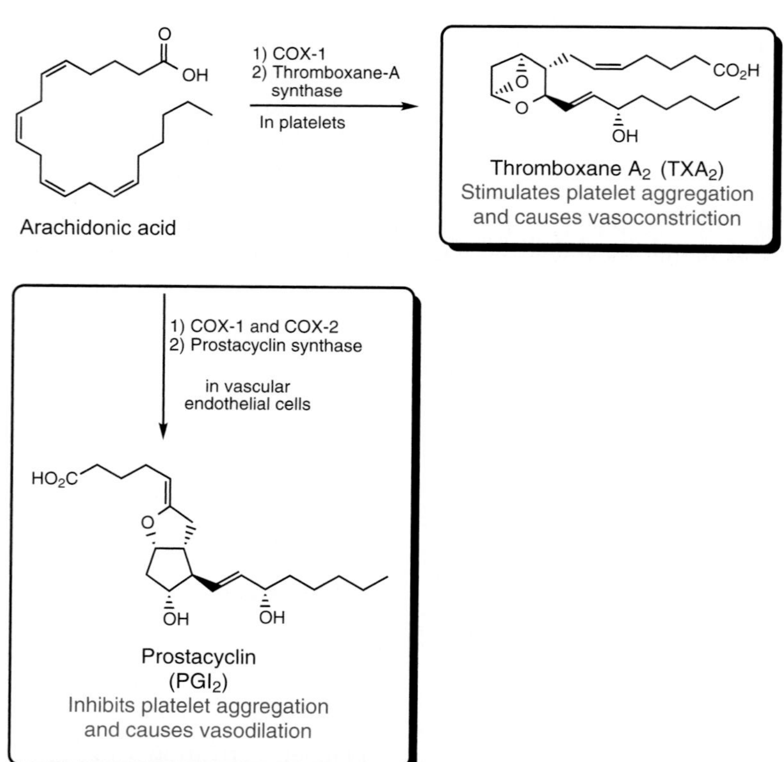

Figure 35.11 The biosynthesis of thromboxane A_2 and prostacyclin from arachidonic acid. Thromboxane A_2 and prostacyclin are synthesized predominantly in platelets and vascular endothelial cells, respectively.

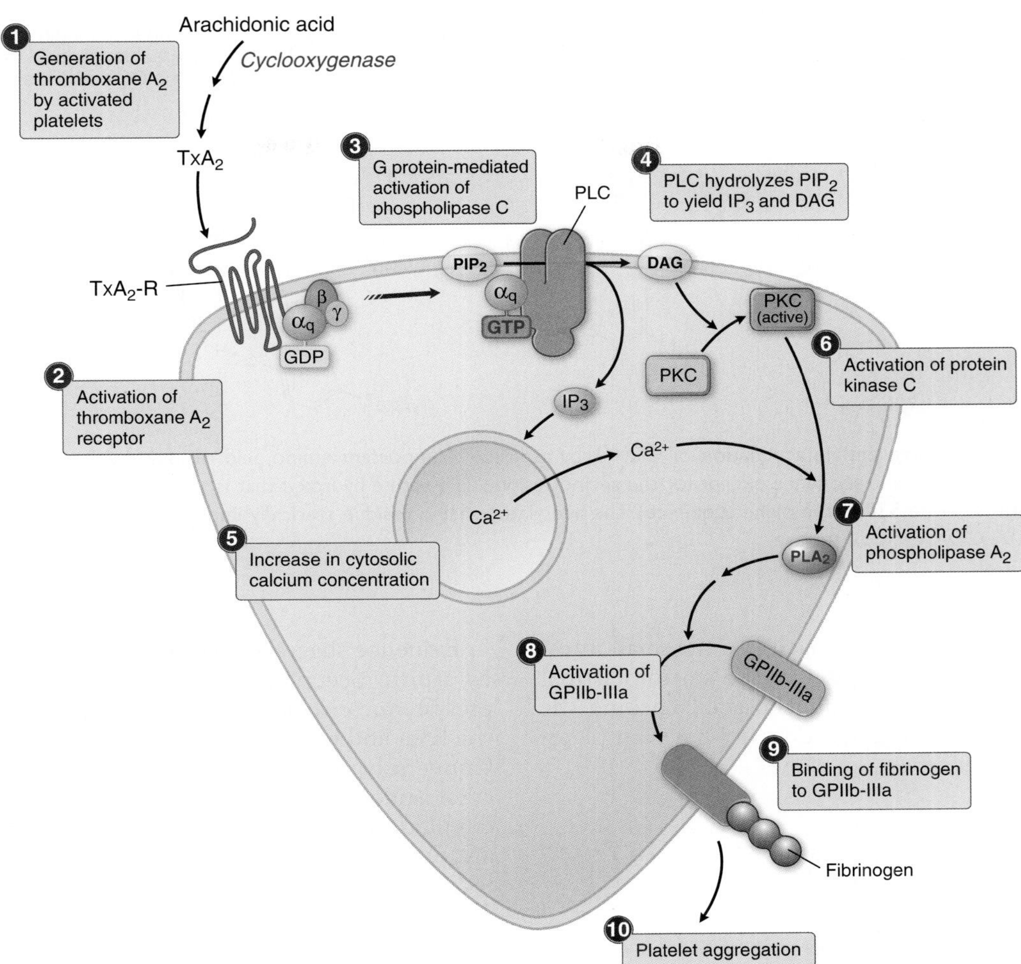

Figure 35.12 Platelet activation by thromboxane A_2. **1.** Thromboxane A_2 (TxA_2) is generated from arachidonic acid in activated platelets; cyclooxygenase catalyzes the committed step in this process. **2.** Secreted TxA_2 binds to the cell surface TxA_2 receptor (TxA_2-R), a G protein–coupled receptor. **3.** The Gα isoform of Gαq activates phospholipase C (PLC). **4.** PLC hydrolyzes phosphatidylinositol 4,5-biphosphate (PIP2) to yield inositol 1,4,-trisphosphate (IP_3) and diacylglycerol (DAG). **5.** IP_3 increases the cytosolic Ca2+ concentration by promoting vesicular release of Ca2+ into the cytosol. **6.** DAG activates protein kinase C (PKC). **7.** PKC activates phospholipase A2 (PLA2). **8.** Through an incompletely understood mechanism, activation of PLA2 leads to the activation of glycoprotein (GP) IIb-IIIa. **9.** Activated GPIIb-IIIa binds to fibrinogen. **10.** Fibrinogen cross-links platelets by binding to GPIIb-IIIa receptors on other platelets. This cross-linking leads to platelet aggregation and formation of a primary hemostatic plug. From Armstrong EJ, Golan DE. Pharmacology of hemostasis and thrombosis. In: Golan DE, Armstrong EJ, Armstrong AW, eds. *Principles of Pharmacology: The Pathophysiologic Basis of Drug Therapy*. 4th ed. Philadelphia: Wolters-Kluwer Health; 2017:407, with permission.

at position 529 in human COX-1 (Fig. 35.13).[92] Tyr385 forms a hydrogen bond to the carbonyl oxygen of the acetyl group on aspirin. It is suggested that Tyr385 stabilizes the resultant tetrahedral intermediate formed in the process of acetylating the serine hydroxyl at position 529.[93] By hydrogen bonding to the phenolic hydroxyl of Tyr385, Tyr348 increases the hydrogen bonding capacity of Tyr385 to the acetyl group on aspirin.[93] The formation of the acetylated serine hydroxyl at position 529 of human COX-1 (serine 516 in human COX-2) irreversibly inhibits the enzyme. This serine residue is not critical for the catalytic function of COX-1. Instead, the acetylated serine residue sterically impedes the entrance of AA to its binding site on the COX enzyme, thereby inhibiting the conversion of AA to PGH_2 and ultimately prostaglandins and TXA_2.[94]

Mature platelets contain only COX-1, and as platelets are fragments of megakaryocytes and lack a nucleus, they are unable to synthesize additional COX-1. Consequently, when platelet COX-1 is irreversibly inhibited by aspirin, TXA_2 synthesis is inhibited for the life of the platelet (8-10 d). In contrast, both COX-1 and COX-2 are present in vascular endothelial cells where PGI_2 is ultimately synthesized from AA predominantly by COX-2. Aspirin is 10-100 times more potent at inhibiting COX-1 than COX-2, and at low doses of aspirin, COX-2 remains functional.[92,95] Furthermore, vascular endothelial cells are capable of synthesizing COX-2. Therefore, with low-dose aspirin therapy, while TXA_2 activity is inhibited, PGI_2 activity remains such that the overall balance is an antiplatelet effect (Table 35.5).

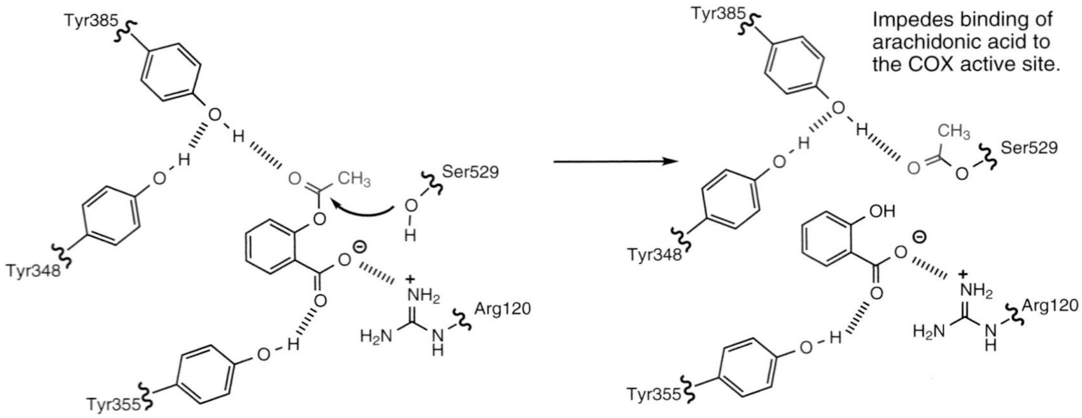

Figure 35.13 A model of irreversible acetylation of COX-1 by aspirin.[92–94] Important amino acid residues within COX-1 are noted and numbered according to the ovine sequence except for the serine residue. The serine hydroxyl that is acetylated by aspirin is at position 529 in human COX-1 (it is serine 530 in the ovine sequence). The acetylated serine residue sterically impedes binding of arachidonic acid to its binding site on COX. COX, cyclooxygenase

Aspirin is absorbed in the stomach and the small intestine. It is hydrolyzed via esterases in the gastrointestinal mucosa, liver, and plasma to salicylic acid. Lacking the critical acetyl group, salicylic acid does not have antiplatelet activity.

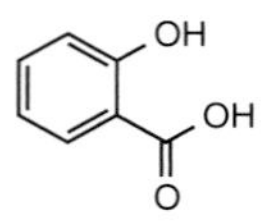

Salicylic acid

Table 35.5 Cyclooxygenase Activity and Thrombosis

Characteristic	Platelets	Vascular Endothelial Cells
COX isoform	COX-1	COX-1 and COX-2
Ability to synthesize COX	No	Yes
AA metabolite	TXA_2	PGI_2
Activity of AA metabolite	• Stimulates platelet aggregation • Induces vasoconstriction	• Inhibits platelet aggregation • Induces vasodilation
With low-dose aspirin therapy	TXA_2 synthesis is inhibited; antiplatelet activity results	PGI_2 synthesis and inhibition of platelet aggregation activity remains

Modified from Lipsky PE, Brooks P, Crofford CJ, et al. Unresolved issues in the role of cyclooxygenase-2 in normal physiologic processes and disease. *Arch Intern Med.* 2000;160:913-920.

AA, arachidonic acid; COX, cyclooxygenase; PGI_2, prostacyclin; TXA_2, thromboxane A_2.

Evidence suggests that most of the COX-1 inhibition by aspirin occurs in platelets in the portal system (the presystemic circulation) before aspirin is deacetylated in the liver and before it gets into the systemic circulation.[96] Conversely, inhibition of prostacyclin formation in vascular endothelial cells occurs by aspirin in the systemic circulation.[96] The oral bioavailability of regular immediate release aspirin tablets is 40%-50% and peak plasma levels are achieved 30-40 minutes after oral ingestion.[95] The oral bioavailability of enteric formulations of aspirin is reduced which may reduce the antiplatelet effect.[96–98] Furthermore, peak plasma levels of aspirin may not be achieved with enteric formulations until after 4 hours rendering this formulation inappropriate for the treatment of ACS.[97,98]

Greater than 95% of TXA_2 activity must be inhibited to achieve an antiplatelet effect. While doses of aspirin as low as 30 mg/d completely suppress platelet TXA_2 production within a week by cumulative acetylation of platelet COX-1, a general maintenance dose of 75 mg to 100 mg/d is recommended. In the United States, low-dose aspirin chewable tablets are available as 81 mg. In patients with ACS, who were not previously taking aspirin, a rapid and complete inhibition of TXA_2 stimulated platelet aggregation can be achieved with a loading dose of 162-325 mg.[95] With the normal turnover of platelets, platelet function fully returns by about 3 days after the last dose of aspirin; therefore, patient compliance with daily aspirin is required for antithrombotic effects. Even at low doses, inactivation of COX-1 by aspirin increases the risk of bleeding complications such as gastrointestinal bleeds and hemorrhagic strokes. These bleeding complications are the result of inhibition of TXA_2-induced platelet aggregation and decreased synthesis of COX-1 derived prostaglandin E_2 and PGI_2 which has cytoprotective effects on the gastric mucosa. The incidence of adverse effects of aspirin is dose related and increases at higher doses. Furthermore, at higher doses, aspirin loses COX-1 selectivity and also inhibits COX-2.

DRUG INTERACTIONS. Traditional NSAIDs, such as ibuprofen or naproxen, reversibly bind to COX 1 with higher affinity than aspirin; thereby preventing the irreversible inhibition of aspirin.[99,100] NSAIDs also inhibit COX-2. Therefore, when given concomitantly, NSAIDs circumvent the antiplatelet effects of aspirin at low doses.

$P2Y_{12}$ Receptor Antagonists

Independent of TXA_2, platelet aggregation can be induced by ADP. Platelets possess two types of ADP receptors (also called purinergic receptors), $P2Y_1$ and $P2Y_{12}$, but currently available therapeutic agents are only able to antagonize ADP at $P2Y_{12}$ receptors. Upon ADP binding to the Gi-protein coupled $P2Y_{12}$ receptors on the surface of platelets, adenylyl cyclase activity is inhibited resulting in a decrease in the concentration of cyclic adenosine monophosphate (cAMP) which leads to platelet shape change and expression of GPIIb/IIIa resulting in platelet aggregation (Fig. 35.14). ADP is released by activated platelets, thereby recruiting additional platelets to aggregate contributing to the thrombosis associated with CAD. Inhibiting the binding of ADP to $P2Y_{12}$ receptors and, consequently, inhibiting platelet aggregation, plays an important role in the treatment of ACS and as an adjunct to percutaneous coronary intervention (PCI).[82,101]

Treatment with the combination of low dose aspirin (81 mg) and an oral $P2Y_{12}$ antagonist, termed dual antiplatelet therapy (DAPT), is established as standard therapy for one year following an ACS or stent placement for the secondary prevention of ischemic events.[101] DAPT inhibits platelet aggregation stimulated by two different mediators, intervening in the TXA_2 and the ADP pathways. $P2Y_{12}$ receptor antagonists to date, used in the treatment of ACS, are represented by two general types, the thienopyridine prodrugs and the nucleoside/nucleotide

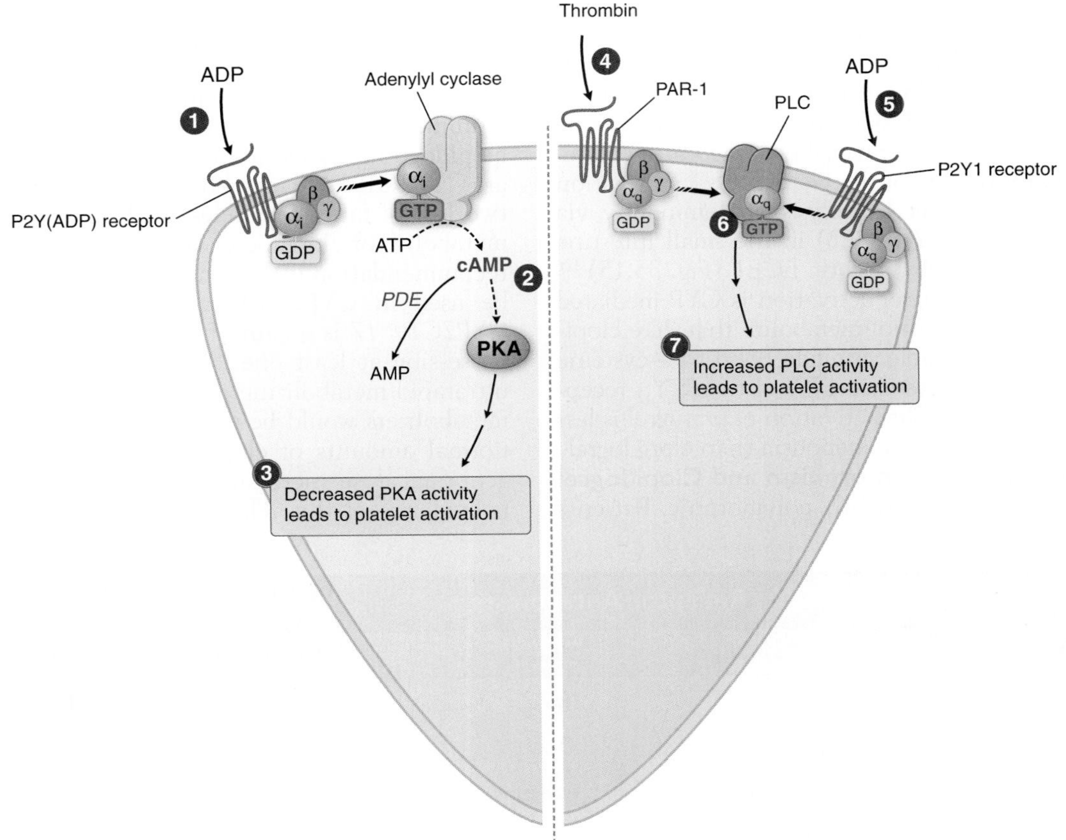

Figure 35.14 Platelet activation by ADP and thrombin. **Left panel: 1.** Binding of ADP to the P2Y(ADP) receptor (also called the $P2Y_{12}$ receptor) activates a Gi protein, which inhibits adenylyl cyclase. **2.** Inhibition of adenylyl cyclase decreases the synthesis of cAMP and hence decreases protein kinase A (PKA) activation (*dashed arrow*). cAMP is metabolized to AMP by phosphodiesterase (PDE). **3.** PKA inhibits platelet activation through a series of incompletely understood steps. Therefore, the decreased PKA activation that results from ADP binding to the P2Y(ADP) receptor causes platelet activation. **Right panel: 4.** Thrombin proteolytically cleaves the extracellular domain of protease-activated receptor 1 (PAR-1). This cleavage creates a new N-terminus, which binds to an activation site on PAR-1 to activate a Gq protein. **5.** ADP also activates Gq by binding to the P2Y1 receptor. **6.** Gq activation (by either thrombin or ADP) activates phospholipase C (PLC). **7.** PLC activation leads to platelet activation, as shown in Figure 35.12. Note that ADP can activate platelets by binding to either the P2Y(ADP) receptor (also called the $P2Y_{12}$ receptor) or the P2Y1 receptor, although evidence suggests that full platelet activation requires the participation of both receptors. From Armstrong EJ, Golan DE. Pharmacology of hemostasis and thrombosis. In: Golan DE, Armstrong EJ, Armstrong AW, eds. *Principles of Pharmacology: The Pathophysiologic Basis of Drug Therapy*. 4th ed. Philadelphia: Wolters-Kluwer Health; 2017:408, with permission.

analogs. Table 35.6 is a comparison of $P2Y_{12}$ receptor antagonists with regards to their mode of binding and key clinical attributes.

THIENOPYRIDINES. The thienopyridines, clopidogrel and prasugrel, are irreversible antagonists of the $P2Y_{12}$ receptor.

Clopidogrel (Plavix)

Prasugrel (Effient)

Mechanism of Irreversible $P2Y_{12}$ Receptor Antagonism. Clopidogrel and prasugrel are oral prodrugs and require activation in vivo (Fig. 35.15). The main route of metabolism (approximately 85%) of clopidogrel is hydrolysis of the methyl ester by human carboxylesterase 1 (hCE1) in the liver to the inactive carboxylic acid metabolite.[102] Activation of clopidogrel requires a two-step oxidation process involving multiple CYP enzymes in the liver.[103] The active thiol metabolite of clopidogrel forms a disulfide bond with a cysteine residue (cysteine 97 or cysteine 175) of the $P2Y_{12}$ receptor irreversibly antagonizing platelet aggregation for the life of the platelet.[104,105] Activation of prasugrel requires ester hydrolysis predominantly via human carboxylesterase 2 (hCE2) in the small intestine and to a limited degree by hepatic hCE1 (Fig. 35.15).[106] The second step of prasugrel activation is CYP mediated and generates the active thiol metabolite that, like clopidogrel, forms an irreversible disulfide bond to a cysteine residue (cysteine 97 or cysteine 175) of the $P2Y_{12}$ receptor.[105] Overall, the metabolic activation of prasugrel is less reliant on hepatic oxidative metabolism than clopidogrel.

CYP2C19 Genetic Polymorphism and Clopidogrel Activity. CYP2C19 is genetically polymorphic. Patients who possess one loss of function allele, most frequently *CYP2C19*2* and to a lesser extent *CYP2C19*3* among others, have a decreased metabolizing phenotype and are defined as intermediate metabolizers. Patients with two loss of function CYP2C19 alleles are considered poor metabolizers. Both steps necessary to produce the active metabolite of clopidogrel occur to a significant extent via CYP2C19. Studies have shown that patients with loss of function alleles exhibit decreased activation of clopidogrel resulting in decreased $P2Y_{12}$ antagonist activity thereby diminishing the platelet antiaggregatory effect.[107] Consequently, patients possessing at least one loss of function CYP2C19 allele would be expected to have an increase in major adverse cardiovascular events (MACE), defined as death from cardiovascular causes, MI, and stroke, when taking clopidogrel in the treatment or prevention of ACS. This has been observed in some studies, but has not been a universal finding, thus making the role of CYP2C19 testing unclear.[107–110] The current AHA/ACC guidelines do not include testing for CYP2C19 genotype for clopidogrel. However, the Clinical Pharmacogenetics Implementation Consortium (CPIC) does include guidelines for CYP2C19 testing and clopidogrel dosing.[111] Additionally, the Food and Drug Administration (FDA) has issued a boxed warning in the clopidogrel package insert indicating that patients who are CYP2C19 poor metabolizers (those patients who have two loss of function alleles) will form less of the active metabolite of clopidogrel at recommended doses.[112] The recommendation is that another $P2Y_{12}$ antagonist should be used in CYP2C19 poor metabolizers. Conversely, *CYP2C19*17* is a gain of function allele, and a patient possessing at least one *CYP2C19*17* allele exhibits an ultrarapid metabolizing phenotype. CYP2C19 ultrarapid metabolizers would be expected to produce higher than normal amounts of clopidogrel active metabolite with a normal dose increasing their risk of bleeding. There is evidence of this relationship,[113] but more studies are

Table 35.6 Comparison of $P2Y_{12}$ Receptor Antagonists

Characteristics	Clopidogrel	Prasugrel	Ticagrelor	Cangrelor
Prodrug	Yes	Yes	No	No
Route of administration	Oral	Oral	Oral	IV
Mode of binding to target	Irreversible	Irreversible	Reversible	Reversible
Dosing frequency	Once a day	Once a day	Twice a day	Bolus followed by continuous infusion
Onset of inhibition of platelet aggregation	2-6 hr	30 min to 4 hr	30 min to 2 hr	Within 2 min of infusion
Return of platelet function after discontinuing drug (time of withdrawal before CABG)	5 d	7 d	5 d	Within 1 hr

Modified from Bhatt DL, Golwala H. The timing of P2Y12 inhibitor initiation in the treatment of ACS? Does the evidence exist in this era? *J Am Coll Cardiol.* 2018;60:471-477.

CABG, coronary artery bypass graft surgery.

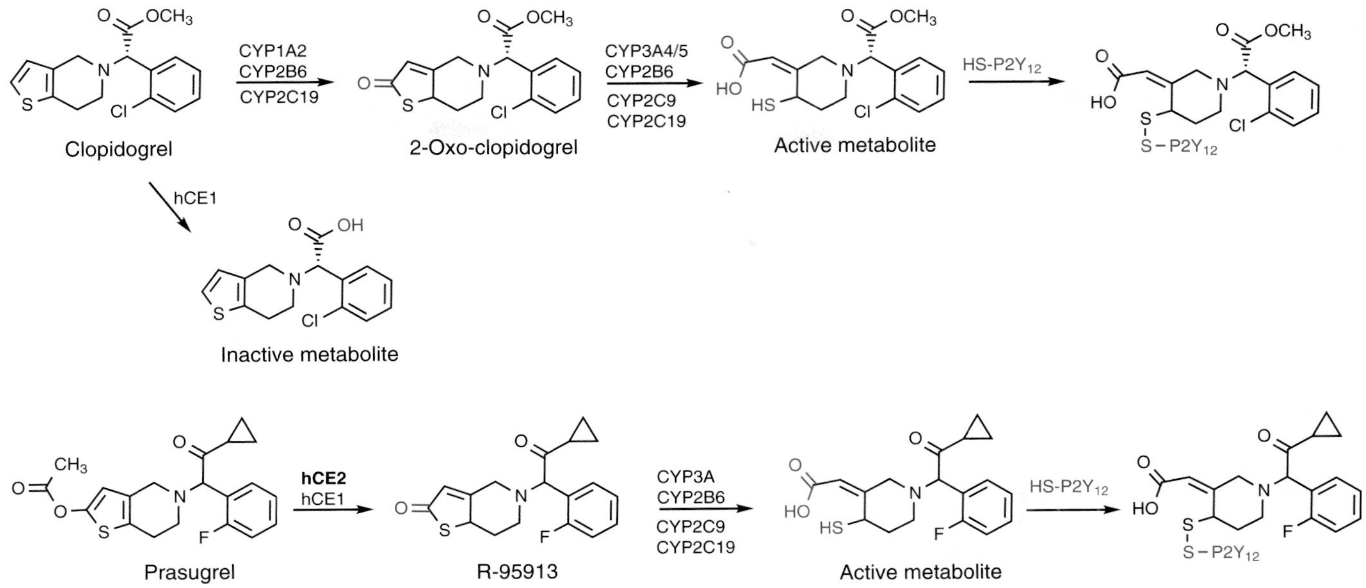

Figure 35.15 In vivo activation of clopidogrel and prasugrel. hCE1, human carboxyesterase 1; hCE2, human carboxyesterase 2; HS-$P2Y_{12}$, the thiol group of the cysteine residue at position 97 or 175 of the platelet surface $P2Y_{12}$ receptor.

needed in this area to establish the clinical significance. Prasugrel activation is not affected by CYP2C19 genetic polymorphism.

Drug Interactions. To reduce the risk of gastrointestinal bleeding, a proton pump inhibitor (PPI) is recommended for patients on DAPT with a history of gastrointestinal bleeding or at increased risk of gastrointestinal bleeding.[101] PPIs that strongly inhibit CYP2C19, most notably omeprazole and esomeprazole, inhibit the formation of the active thiol metabolite of clopidogrel and decrease its antiplatelet effect.[114,115] Whether or not this is clinically significant is unclear.[116] Several studies have shown no association between PPI use and risk of MACE with clopidogrel treatment.[116–118] Based on early studies, the FDA-approved product information states that concomitant use of omeprazole and esomeprazole should be avoided with clopidogrel and notes that dexlansoprazole, lansoprazole, and pantoprazole have less effect on the antiplatelet activity of clopidogrel.[112] Prasugrel is not associated with a clinically relevant interaction with PPIs.

Prasugrel Contraindications. Prasugrel has a more rapid onset of antiplatelet activity and is a more potent inhibitor of ADP induced platelet aggregation than clopidogrel.[119] Currently, the indication for prasugrel is for ACS patients undergoing PCI. In this patient population, the increased potency of prasugrel has been shown to decrease the rate of ischemic events, most notably myocardial infarction, to a greater extent than clopidogrel. Prasugrel is also associated with a higher incidence of major bleeding, including fatal bleeding, compared to clopidogrel.[120] Consequently, prasugrel has a boxed warning and is contraindicated in patients with a history of stroke or transient ischemic attack where the risk of harm outweighs any benefit.[121] Additionally, prasugrel should be avoided in patients at high risk of bleeding, such as patients of age 75 years or older and patients with body weight less than 60 kg.

NUCLEOSIDE/NUCLEOTIDE ANALOGS. Adenosine triphosphate (ATP) is a weak competitive antagonist of the $P2Y_{12}$ receptor, although it is not selective for $P2Y_{12}$ receptors. Ticagrelor and cangrelor were both designed based on the structure of ATP (Fig. 35.16) and they are both highly selective $P2Y_{12}$ antagonists that do not require bioactivation unlike the thienopyridines. They are direct, reversible, and competitive inhibitors of ADP binding to the $P2Y_{12}$ receptor resulting in platelet antiaggregatory activity.

Ticagrelor. Ticagrelor was designed to be an oral antiplatelet drug.[122] Before the design of ticagrelor, cangrelor had already been designed based on the structure of ATP as a short-acting water soluble solution for injection. For oral activity, the compound would need to be longer acting and more lipid soluble. Similar to the nucleoside portion of cangrelor, the design of ticagrelor started with a 5,7-substituted purine derivative. The triazolopyrimidine ring is a bioisosteric replacement for the purine ring. Replacing the ribose sugar with a dihydroxycyclopentane bioisostere maintained potency and eliminated the potentially labile glycosidic bond. From more than 6,000 analogs, the thiopropyl group at position 5 and the 1*R*,2*S*-*trans*-phenylcyclopropylamine at position 7 of the triazolopyrimidine ring were found to have optimal potency and metabolic stability. The affinity to the $P2Y_{12}$ receptor and metabolic stability were enhanced with the addition of 3,4 difluoro substituents on the phenyl ring of the substituent at position 7. The triphosphate chain in ATP and the modified phosphate chain in cangrelor would not be suitable for oral bioavailability because these side chains are highly ionized which precludes oral absorption, and they are metabolized rapidly via ectonucleotidases. The hydroxyethoxy group at the 2-position was found to be resistant to glucuronidation and had good oral bioavailability. *Ticagrelor (Clog P = 1.95)* is much more lipophilic

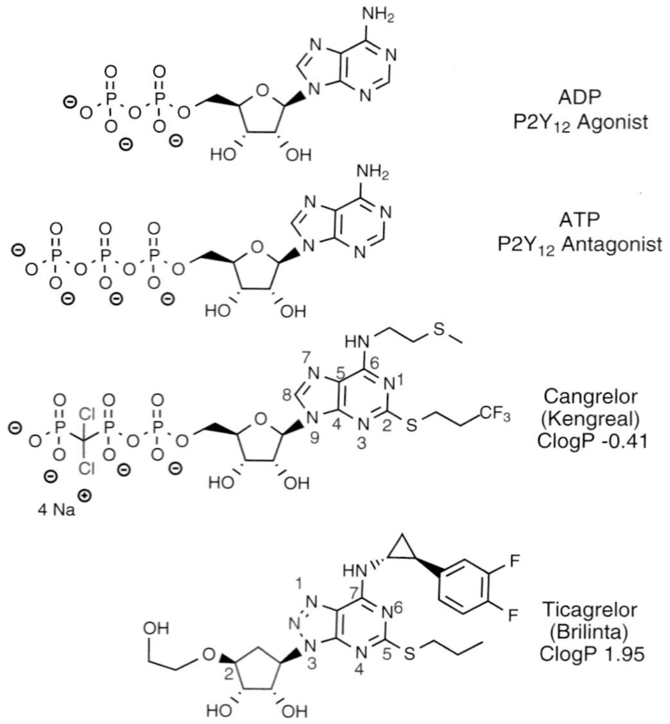

ADP
P2Y12 Agonist

ATP
P2Y12 Antagonist

Cangrelor
(Kengreal)
ClogP -0.41

Ticagrelor
(Brilinta)
ClogP 1.95

Figure 35.16 Nucleoside/nucleotide analogs as reversible $P2Y_{12}$ receptor antagonists. ADP, adenosine diphosphate; ATP, adenosine triphosphate. Modified from Dobesh PP, Oestreich JH. Ticagrelor: pharmacokinetics, pharmacodynamics, clinical efficacy, and safety. *Pharmacotherapy*. 2014;34:1077-1090.

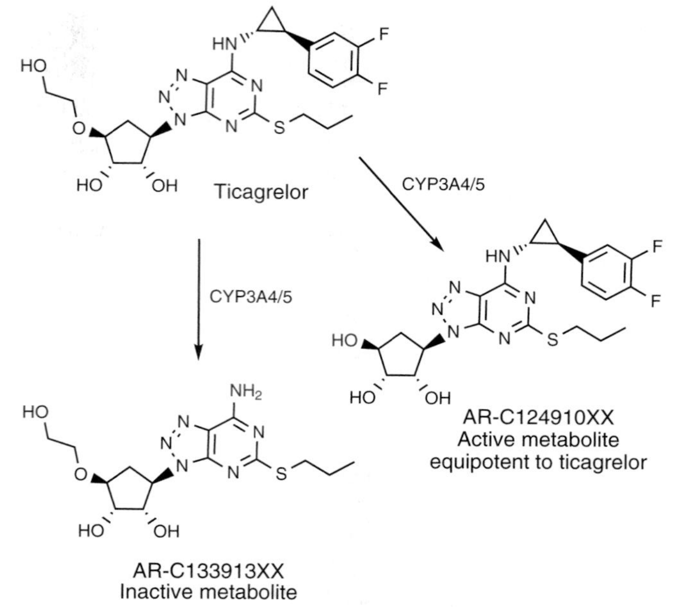

Ticagrelor

CYP3A4/5

CYP3A4/5

AR-C124910XX
Active metabolite
equipotent to ticagrelor

AR-C133913XX
Inactive metabolite

Figure 35.17 Metabolism of ticagrelor to active metabolite.

than cangrelor (Clog P = −0.41) which makes it amenable to oral absorption.[123] Lacking phosphate groups, ticagrelor is a nucleoside analog of ATP. Ticagrelor is also referred to as a cyclopentyltriazolopyrimidine. Ticagrelor has a fast onset similar to prasugrel and is dosed twice a day (Table 35.6).

Ticagrelor is a more potent inhibitor of platelet aggregation than clopidogrel.[124] As part of DAPT in patients with ACS, ticagrelor was shown to be more effective than clopidogrel in decreasing MACE in the international PLATO study, but was associated with a higher rate of non-coronary artery bypass graft major bleeding, including fatal intracranial bleeding.[125] Consequently, ticagrelor is contraindicated in patients with a history of intracranial bleeding.

A subgroup analysis of the data from the PLATO study showed that in the United States, ticagrelor showed a trend toward worse outcomes than clopidogrel.[126] One rationale for this regional difference is that more patients in the United States took a higher dose (≥300 mg/d) of aspirin than patients in the rest of the world. With ticagrelor, the lowest event rates were observed with low dose (<300 mg/d) aspirin. Therefore, ticagrelor was FDA approved with a boxed warning that maintenance doses of aspirin >100 mg/d decrease the effectiveness of ticagrelor.[127]

Oxidative metabolism, via CYP3A4 and CYP3A5, plays an important role in ticagrelor metabolism (Fig. 35.17).[128] The major plasma metabolite, AR-C124910XX, is the result of CYP3A4/5 mediated O-dealkylation of the hydroxyethoxy group of ticagrelor. AR-C124910XX is equipotent to ticagrelor and represents 30%-40% of the exposure to ticagrelor.[127,128] AR-C133913XX, the result of CYP3A4/5 mediated N-dealkylation of ticagrelor, and its glucuronide are the major urinary metabolites.[128] AR-C133913XX is inactive. Coadministration of strong inducers or inhibitors of CYP3A with ticagrelor may result in decreased efficacy or increased risk of bleeding, respectively, and should be avoided.[127]

Cangrelor. Cangrelor is a nucleotide analog of ATP that is administered intravenously (Fig. 35.16). The triphosphate chain of ATP is sequentially dephosphorylated via ectonucleotidases with the first dephosphorylation reaction liberating ADP, the potent inducer of platelet aggregation, via binding to the $P2Y_{12}$ receptor on the surface of platelets. The terminal phosphate anhydride oxygen of ATP was replaced with a dichloro-methylene group in cangrelor to prevent the hydrolysis to the proaggregatory diphosphate product.[129] Furthermore, the dichloro groups on the methylene bridge render the pK_a values within the triphosphate chain similar to those of ATP such that, like ATP, cangrelor exists as a tetraanion at physiological pH. The tetraanion is critical for high affinity to the $P2Y_{12}$ receptor and is important for conferring antagonist activity within the nucleotide template. The combination of the nonpolar trifluoromethyl thiopropyl group at position 2 of adenine and monoalkylation of the nitrogen at position 6 with a lipophilic methylthioethyl group led to cangrelor which has both high potency and a short half-life allowing rapid recovery of platelet aggregation capability.[129]

The most rapid acting of all the $P2Y_{12}$ antagonists (Table 35.6), cangrelor is administered as a bolus followed by infusion and inhibits platelet aggregation within 2 minutes. Cangrelor is rapidly dephosphorylated in vivo by ectonucleotidases to an inactive nucleoside metabolite and has a plasma half-life of

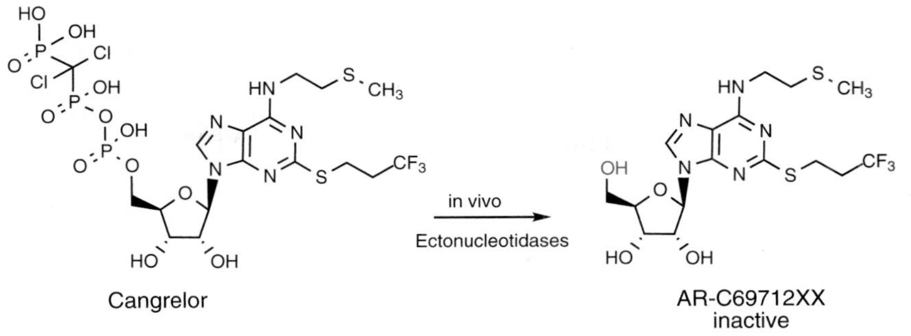

Cangrelor

in vivo

Ectonucleotidases

AR-C69712XX
inactive

Figure 35.18 Metabolism of cangrelor.

3-6 minutes (Fig. 35.18).[130] Upon discontinuing the infusion of cangrelor, platelet function returns to normal within an hour. The rapid onset/offset characteristics of cangrelor make it suitable for antiplatelet therapy just before and during PCI where it was found to decrease death, MI, ischemia-driven revascularization, and stent thrombosis at 48 hours more than clopidogrel without an increase in bleeding.[131]

Cangrelor has been found to block the irreversible binding of the thienopyridine active metabolites to the $P2Y_{12}$ receptor.[132] Therefore, when patients are transitioned from intravenous cangrelor to oral clopidogrel or prasugrel for continued antiplatelet therapy post-PCI, the thienopyridine must not be started until after the discontinuation of cangrelor infusion to insure effective antiplatelet activity.

Thrombin Protease-Activated Receptor-1 (PAR-1) Antagonist

In addition to being a key component of coagulation, thrombin is a potent inducer of platelet aggregation by binding predominantly to the PAR-1 receptor on the surface of platelets (Fig. 35.14). Thrombin is a serine protease that cleaves the N-terminus of the PAR-1 receptor when bound to it. The resultant new N-terminus bears a sequence that acts as a tethered ligand and activates the Gq protein coupled PAR-1 receptor.[133] Activation of the Gq protein stimulates phospholipase C which leads to platelet aggregation. Vorapaxar is an oral selective and competitive PAR-1 antagonist and the only marketed compound in this class to date. Vorapaxar blocks thrombin induced platelet aggregation. It was designed based on a lead structure discovered in a high-throughput screening program of analogs of the natural product (+)-himbacine (Fig. 35.19).[134,135] Vorapaxar has high affinity and a long dissociation half-life from the PAR-1 receptor of approximately 20 hours which is critical as it is competing with a tethered ligand.[135]

Vorapaxar is rapidly absorbed and has high oral bioavailability.[136] Vorapaxar completely inhibits (>80%) platelet aggregation stimulated by a thrombin receptor activating peptide within 1 week of initiating daily dosing. It has no effect on ADP induced platelet aggregation. With a terminal half-life of approximately of 173-269 hours, the antiplatelet effect of vorapaxar is essentially irreversible. Upon discontinuing daily dosing of vorapaxar, it takes 4-8 weeks to recover normal platelet function.[136] Vorapaxar specifically inhibits the platelet aggregatory effects of thrombin via PAR-1 antagonism and does not antagonize the effects of thrombin on the coagulation cascade. Therefore, vorapaxar has no effect on coagulation tests.[135,136]

In patients who have had an MI, when added to standard therapy of aspirin or DAPT, vorapaxar has been shown to decrease the rate of MACE, but there is an increase in bleeding, including intracranial bleeding.[137] Patients with a history of stroke had a significantly higher rate of intracranial bleeding with vorapaxar. As a result, vorapaxar was FDA approved with a box warning contraindicating its use in patients with a history of stroke.[138] More information about vorapaxar can be found in Chapter 18.

Intravenous GPIIb/IIIa Receptor Antagonists

GPIIb/IIIa is a platelet surface membrane protein of the integrin family which are cell adhesion molecules. Integrins are heterodimers comprised of two subunits,

(+)-Himbacine
Natural product
(PAR-1 inactive)

The active enantiomer
of a lead compound found
in high throughput screen
for the design of vorapaxar

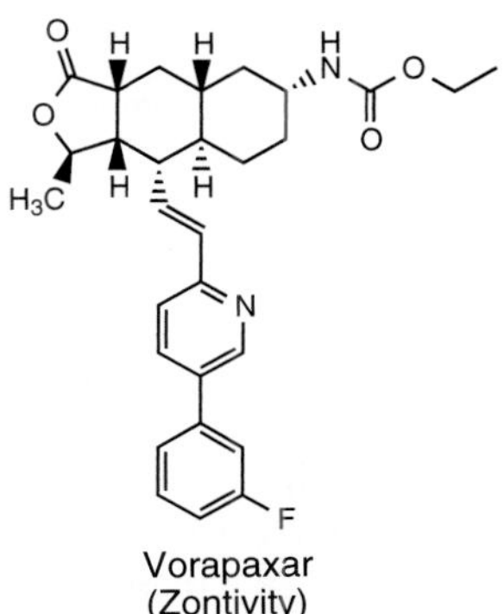

Figure 35.19 Structures of compounds leading to the design of the PAR-1 receptor antagonist vorapaxar.

an α subunit and a β subunit, noncovalently linked that traverse the cytoplasmic membrane with an extracellular domain and an intracellular cytoplasmic tail from each subunit. The α subunit of GPIIb/IIIa is IIb (or αIIb in integrin nomenclature), and the β subunit is IIIa (or β3 in integrin nomenclature).[139] GPIIb/IIIa receptors are platelet αIIbβ3 integrins. Platelet activation causes a change in the extracellular domain of the GPIIb/IIIa receptors from a resting low affinity conformation to a high affinity conformation that allows adhesive ligands to bind via arginine-glycine-aspartic acid (RGD) sequences. Fibrinogen possesses RGD sequences on each end. In this way, fibrinogen crosslinks activated platelets causing platelet aggregation. Fibrinogen also binds to GPIIb/IIIa via a Lys-Gln-Ala-Gly-Asp-Val sequence at the carboxy terminus of the gamma chains.[139,140] GPIIb/IIIa antagonists block the binding of fibrinogen thereby inhibiting platelet aggregation, independent of the mediator of platelet activation, resulting in an antithrombotic effect.

The three available GPIIb/IIIa antagonists were FDA approved in the 1990s. They vary widely in structure, and all are administered intravenously. They include the monoclonal antibody abciximab, a cyclic heptapeptide eptifibatide, and a nonpeptide small molecule tirofiban (Fig. 35.20). Abciximab binds to the GPIIb/IIIa receptor at an epitope located in the β3 subunit of the receptor. Although a monoclonal antibody, abciximab is not specific and also binds to two other integrins, αVβ3 and αMβ2. The two small molecule antagonists, eptifibatide and tirofiban, bind to GPIIb/IIIa in a drug-binding pocket located at the interface of the α and β subunits and they are both specific for GPIIb/IIIa (Fig. 35.21).[141]

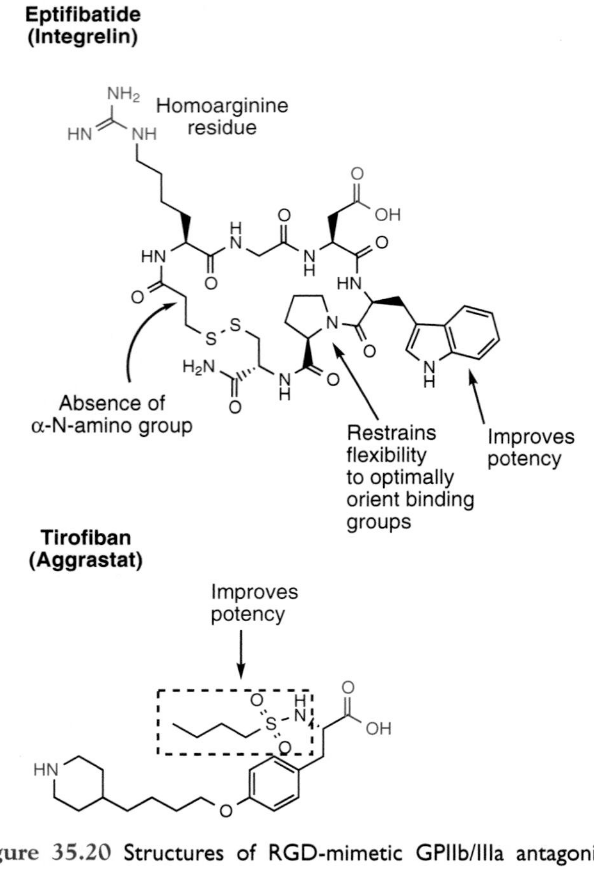

Figure 35.20 Structures of RGD-mimetic GPIIb/IIIa antagonists, eptifibatide and tirofiban.

The design of eptifibatide is based on a Lys-Gly-Asp (KGD) sequence found in the 73 amino acid snake venom peptide barbourin.[142] Barbourin inhibits the binding of adhesive proteins, such as fibrinogen, specifically to GPIIb/IIIa receptors. A KGD containing cyclic heptapeptide, with potent GPIIb/IIIa antagonist activity, was optimized to form eptifibatide. Modifying the ε-amino group of lysine to a guanidino group to form a homoarginine residue increased potency 5- to 10-fold and increased the specificity for GPIIb/IIIa over other integrins.[142] In this way, eptifibatide is mimicking the RGD sequence of the natural ligands of GPIIb/IIIa. The large hydrophobic tryptophan residue next to the aspartic acid residue further increased affinity. The proline residue of eptifibatide restrains conformational flexibility of the heptapeptide ring to optimally position the homoarginine, aspartic acid, and tryptophan residues within the drug binding pocket.[142] Removing the amino group of the N-terminus cysteine further improved potency.

Tirofiban, an L-tyrosine analog, was designed as a nonpeptide drug that maintains the distance between the basic moiety and the carboxylic acid similar to that in the RGD sequence.[143] It possesses a basic piperidine nitrogen that mimics the arginine in RGD or the lysine in the additional fibrinogen binding sequence. The basic homoarginine residue of eptifibatide and the basic piperidine nitrogen of tirofiban each form an ionic bond with Asp224 of the αIIb subunit.[141] The carboxylic acid group in both eptifibatide and tirofiban coordinates with an Mg^{2+} ion in the metal ion-dependent adhesion site (MIDAS) located in the β3 subunit.[141,144] The binding of the Mg^{2+} ion in the MIDAS involves the assistance of Glu220 in the β3 subunit and induces a conformational change to the GPIIb/IIIa receptor. The N-α-sulfonamide group of tirofiban is critical to its potent activity.

Table 35.7 is a comparison of the three GPIIb/IIIa antagonists.[139,145,146] While GPIIb/IIIa antagonists continue to be used during PCI, their use in the noninvasive treatment of NSTE-ACS has been supplanted by oral $P2Y_{12}$ antagonists.

ADVERSE EFFECTS. All three intravenous GPIIb/IIIa antagonists are associated with bleeding and thrombocytopenia. Thrombocytopenia associated with abciximab occurs in about 5% of patients and is thought to be due to antibodies to the murine portion of the Fab.[146,147] The incidence of thrombocytopenia associated with eptifibatide and tirofiban is lower than with abciximab and it occurs mainly via a different immune mechanism.[147,148] Binding of eptifibatide or tirofiban to GPIIb/IIIa causes a conformational change in the β3 subunit that exposes epitopes, called ligand-induced binding sites (LIBS).[148] Some patients have innate antibodies that recognize these LIBS causing platelet destruction leading to acute thrombocytopenia.[148] Due to the risk of thrombocytopenia, the platelet count needs to be monitored in patients on intravenous GPIIb/IIIa antagonists.

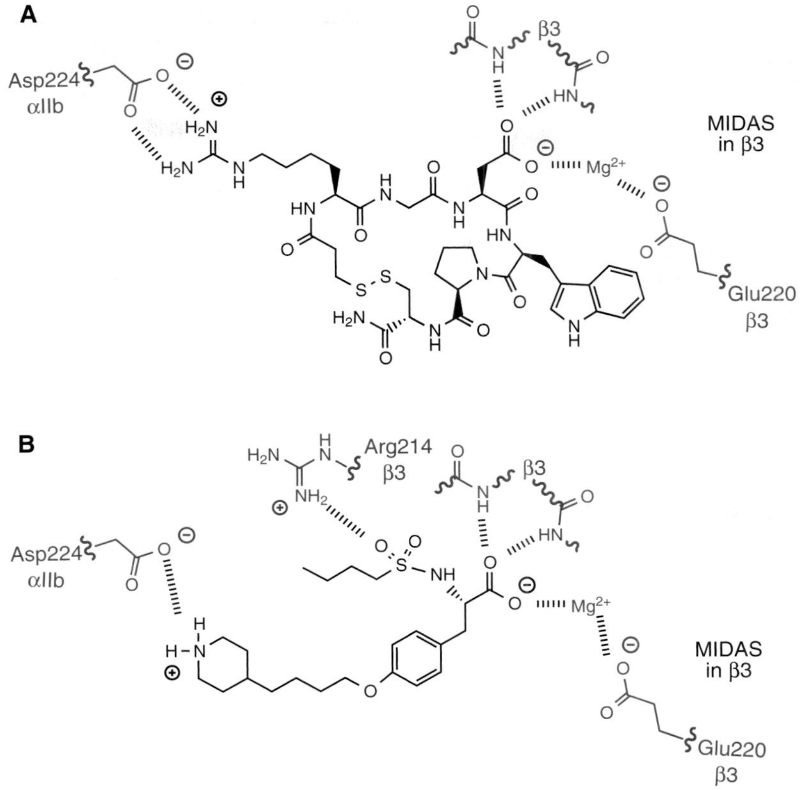

Figure 35.21 Important GPIIb/IIIa binding interactions with (A) eptifibatide and (B) tirofiban. MIDAS, metal ion–dependent adhesion site. Binding sites within the GPIIb/IIIa receptor are noted in red.

NON–RGD-MIMETIC ANTAGONIST OF GPIIB/IIIA ON THE HORIZON

Clinical studies of oral GPIIb/IIIa antagonists that contained an RGD mimic as part of their structure revealed that these compounds caused an increase in mortality and a risk of bleeding and thrombocytopenia.[139,148] One theory for the increase in mortality is that RGD-mimetic GPIIb/IIIa antagonists activate the GPIIb/IIIa receptor by inducing a high affinity conformation that facilitates fibrinogen binding.[148,149] Thus when plasma concentrations of the oral GPIIb/IIIa antagonists are subtherapeutic, patients are left in a prothrombotic state. This phenomenon is commonly referred to as "priming" the GPIIb/IIIa receptor for fibrinogen binding. The same conformational change is associated with causing thrombocytopenia. A key aspect of this conformational change is binding of Mg^{2+} in the MIDAS of GPIIb/IIIa by RGD-mimetic inhibitors.[144,150,151] RUC-4 is a non–RGD-mimetic antagonist of GPIIb/IIIa that does not bind to the Mg^{2+} in the MIDAS and, therefore, does not induce the above conformational change (Fig. 35.22).[150,151]

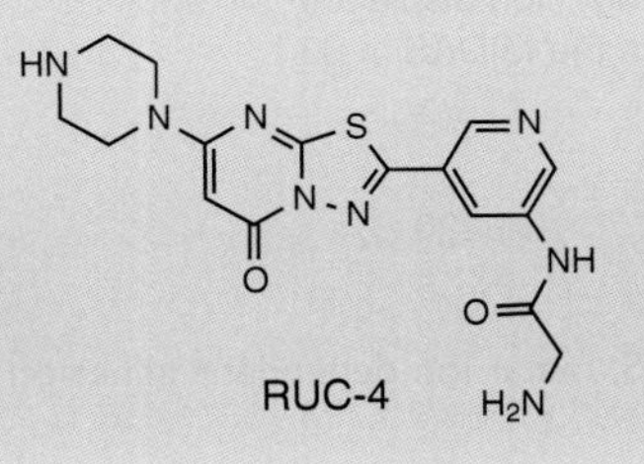

RUC-4 possesses a basic piperazine nitrogen and, like eptifibatide and tirofiban, forms an ionic bond with Asp224 of the αIIb subunit. The structure of RUC-4 lacks a carboxylic acid, but it possesses a primary amine that competes with Mg^{2+} and forms an ionic bond with Glu220 in the β3 subunit which is reinforced by a hydrogen bond between the charged nitrogen and a backbone carbonyl oxygen. In this way, RUC-4 displaces the Mg^{2+} ion from the MIDAS on the β3 subunit and holds the GPIIb/IIIa receptor in an inactive conformation that does not prime the receptor for fibrinogen binding and does not expose neoepitopes.[150,151] RUC-4 is under preclinical investigation as an intramuscular injection for pre–hospital administration in patients with STEMI.[151] Research in the area of non–RGD-mimetic antagonists of GPIIb/IIIa continues.[152,153]

Parenteral Anticoagulant Therapy in Patients With Definite NSTE-ACS

Atherosclerotic plaque rupture leading to coronary artery occlusion involves not only platelet aggregation, but also activation of the coagulation cascade. The coagulation cascade is triggered by the release of cells that express tissue factor from the necrotic core of the ruptured plaque and by tissue factor exposed on damaged endothelial cells. Tissue factor complexed with factor VIIa activates factor X. A complex of factors Xa, Va, and Ca^{2+} on anionic phospholipid membrane surfaces, converts

Table 35.7 Comparison of GPIIb/IIIa Receptor Antagonists

Characteristic	Abciximab	Eptifibatide	Tirofiban
Molecular description	Fab fragment of the chimeric human-murine monoclonal antibody c7E3 to GPIIb/IIIa	Cyclic heptapeptide	Nonpeptide small molecule
Molecular weight (Dalton)	47,615	832	495
Mechanism of action	Sterically blocks the binding of fibrinogen by binding to epitope in β3 subunit	Mimics RGD binding sequence of natural ligands	Mimics RGD-binding sequence of natural ligands
Affinity for αIIbβ3 (K_D)	5 nM	120 nM	15 nM
Mode of binding to target	Essentially irreversible	Reversible	Reversible
Selectivity for GPIIb/IIIa	No; also binds to αVβ3 and αMβ2—clinical relevance, if any, unclear	Yes	Yes
Plasma t1/2	10-30 min	~2.5 hr	~2.0 hr
Platelet-bound t1/2	Days	Seconds	Seconds
Excretion	Unknown, not renal	Renal	Renal and biliary
Return of platelet function after discontinuing drug	~48 hr	2-4 hr	2-4 hr

αMβ2, a leukocyte integrin; αVβ3, integrin receptor for vitronectin; K_D, dissociation constant; RGD, arginine-glycine-aspartic acid sequence.

prothrombin to thrombin (factor IIa). Among its many activities, thrombin converts soluble fibrinogen to insoluble fibrin and activates factor XIII which converts fibrin to crosslinked polymers forming the fibrin clot. Therefore, in addition to antiplatelet therapy, parenteral anticoagulation therapy is recommended for all patients with NSTE-ACS to inhibit thrombus propagation.[82] A full discussion of parenteral anticoagulant drugs is provided in Chapter 18. Structures of the anticoagulants used in the treatment of NSTE-ACS are provided in Figure 35.23. These include enoxaparin, unfractionated heparin (UFH), fondaparinux, bivalirudin, and argatroban. A comparison of their mechanisms of actions and key characteristics are provided in Table 35.8.[145,154–157] The 2014 AHA/ACC NSTE-ACS guidelines recommend UFH, enoxaparin, or fondaparinux for noninvasive medical therapy and UFH, enoxaparin, fondaparinux, or bivalirudin for PCI with stenting.[82]

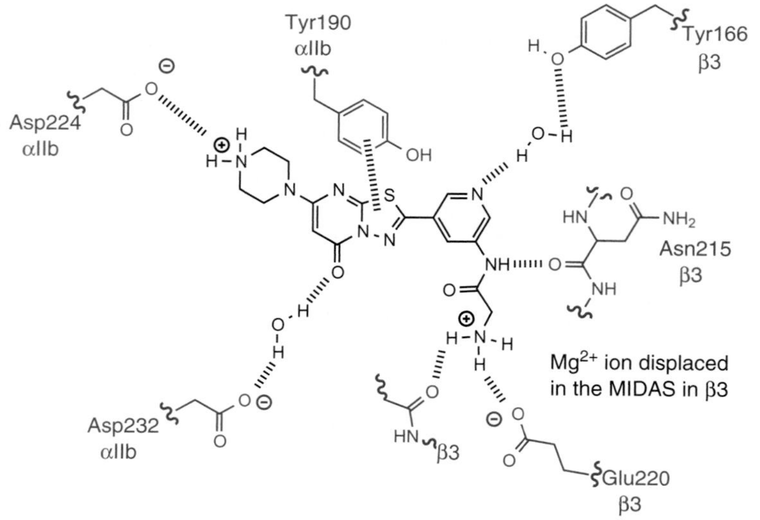

Figure 35.22 Binding interactions between the GPIIb/IIIa receptor and RUC-4. MIDAS, metal ion-dependent adhesion site. Binding sites within the GPIIb/IIIa receptor are noted in red.

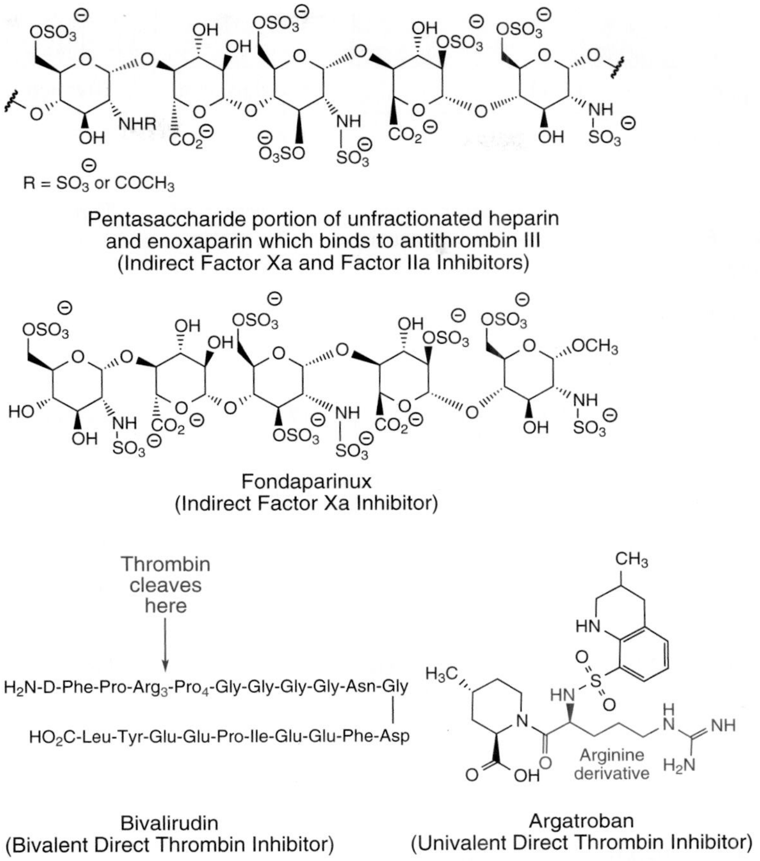

Figure 35.23 Parenteral anticoagulants used in the treatment of ACS.

UFH

Heparins are a mixture of acidic polymeric sugar fragments obtained from porcine intestinal mucosa. They indirectly elicit their anticoagulant activity by potentiating the catalytic activity of antithrombin III to inactivate factor Xa and factor IIa by about 1000 times. Via a specific pentasaccharide sequence (shown in Fig. 35.23), the negative charges on heparin form ionic bonds to positively charged lysine residues on antithrombin III. The heparin-antithrombin III complex produces a conformational change exposing the site on antithrombin III that interacts with factor Xa and factor IIa, resulting in their inactivation. The size of the heparin fragment dictates the action the fragment will exhibit. Anti-factor Xa activity requires fragments of at least the essential pentasaccharide unit to bind to antithrombin III. Heparin fragments of at least 18 saccharide units are required for anti-factor IIa activity. This includes the required pentasaccharide sequence to bind to antithrombin III along with an additional 13 saccharide unit required to bind to thrombin (factor IIa) for inactivation. UFH is a heterogeneous mixture of fragments from 3,000 to 30,000 Da. The average molecular weight of UFH fragments is 15,000 Da which is approximately 45 monosaccharide chains. Approximately one-third of the UFH fragments contain the required pentasaccharide sequence and virtually all of these fragments are capable of inactivating factor Xa or factor IIa resulting in a 1:1 ratio of anti-factor Xa to anti-factor IIa activity.

Enoxaparin

Enoxaparin is a low molecular weight heparin (LMWH) obtained from UFH by an alkaline depolymerization process of heparin benzyl ester producing a mixture composed of fragments with a mean molecular weight of 4,500, less than one-third the mean molecular weight of UFH.[67] Due to the smaller fragments, enoxaparin has fewer fragments that can elicit anti-factor IIa activity. Consequently, enoxaparin is more selective for anti-factor Xa activity exhibiting a 4:1 ratio of anti-factor Xa to anti-factor IIa activity. While enoxaparin is typically administered subcutaneously, in the treatment of ACS, a loading dose may be administered intravenously if a rapid anticoagulant response is needed. Enoxaparin is slightly more effective than UFH in the treatment of patients with NSTE-ACS.[19,82,158]

Fondaparinux

Fondaparinux is a synthetic analog modeled on the pentasaccharide sequence in heparin responsible for binding to antithrombin III. As such, it is too short to have anti-factor IIa activity. Therefore, fondaparinux elicits anti-factor Xa activity only.

Bivalirudin

Bivalirudin is a 20 amino acid peptide that acts as a bivalent direct thrombin inhibitor. After binding to the active site and to exosite 1 of thrombin, it is cleaved by thrombin between Arg3 and Pro4 regenerating

Table 35.8 Comparison of Parenteral Anticoagulants Used in the Treatment of NSTE-ACS

Characteristic	Enoxaparin	UFH	Fondaparinux	Bivalirudin	Argatroban
Molecular weight (Dalton)	Average 4,500	Average 15,000	1,508	2,180	508
Mechanism of action	4:1 Anti–factor Xa to Anti–factor IIa activity	1:1 Anti–factor Xa to anti–factor IIa activity	Indirect factor Xa inhibitor	Direct thrombin inhibitor	Direct thrombin inhibitor
Route of administration	SC (IV loading dose may be administered)	IV	SC	IV	IV
t1/2	3-6 hr	60-90 min (dose dependent)	17 hr	25 min	45 min
Excretion	Renal	Reticuloendothelial system	Renal	80% Enzymatic hydrolysis 20% Renal	Hepatic metabolism (CYP3A4/5)
Monitoring	NA	aPTT (ACT during PCI)	NA	aPTT (ACT during PCI)	aPTT (ACT during PCI)
Antidote	Partial reversal with protamine sulfate	Complete reversal with protamine sulfate	None	None	None
Incidence of HIT	<5%	<1%	No	No	No

ACT, activated clotting time; aPTT, activated partial thromboplastin time; HIT, heparin-induced thrombocytopenia; IV, intravenous; SC, subcutaneous.

thrombin. The half-life of bivalirudin is 25 minutes, which is the shortest plasma half-life of the parenteral anticoagulants.

Argatroban

Argatroban is an arginine derivative that is a univalent direct thrombin inhibitor. It is indicated for use in the prevention and treatment of thrombosis in patients with heparin-induced thrombocytopenia (HIT) and as an anticoagulant in patients with or at high risk of HIT undergoing PCI. Bivalirudin and fondaparinux may also be used in patients with a history of HIT.

DIRECT ORAL ANTICOAGULANTS (DOACS) IN THE SECONDARY PREVENTION OF ACS

The COMPASS trial found that rivaroxaban, an oral direct factor Xa inhibitor, in a dose of 2.5 mg twice a day, plus aspirin (100 mg daily) had a significantly lower incidence of MACE than aspirin (100 mg daily) alone in patients with a history of stable atherosclerotic vascular disease.[159] While there was a significant increase in major bleeding events in the rivaroxaban plus aspirin group, there was no significant difference in intracranial or fatal bleeding between the two groups. Overall, there was a net clinical benefit with the combination of rivaroxaban and aspirin. The rivaroxaban dose of 2.5 mg twice a day is a fourth of the dose indicated for stroke prophylaxis in atrial fibrillation.

Rivaroxaban (Xarelto)

During in-hospital treatment of ACS, patients are administered DAPT and parenteral anticoagulants. After acute treatment, despite continued DAPT, cardiovascular ischemic events after an ACS remain high. In an effort to decrease thrombosis in the months after an ACS, continuing to block the coagulation cascade, in addition to blocking platelet aggregation, is an area of research interest. Adding a DOAC to antiplatelet therapy for secondary prevention after an ACS has been studied with mixed results.[160,161] An increase in bleeding has been a problem with adding a DOAC to DAPT and in some cases a lack of efficacy in reducing ischemic events. Additional clinical studies to establish the role of DOACs in the secondary prevention of ACS in patients with a recent history of ACS are needed.[162]

Adverse Effects

Bleeding is an adverse effect of all parenteral anticoagulants. The acidic anionic nature of UFH allows rapid reversal of its anticoagulant effects with intravenous protamine sulfate. Protamine sulfate is a mixture of arginine rich cationic peptides, each approximately 30-32 amino acids in length, derived from the sperm of chum salmon harvested in Japanese fishing grounds.[163] Protamine forms a complex with UFH, via ionic bonds, completely neutralizing its anticoagulant effects. Protamine only partially reverses the anticoagulant effects of LMWH as protamine does not bind to the smaller heparin fragments within LMWH because they lack a sufficient number of anionic sulfate groups.[156] Consequently, protamine neutralizes the anti-factor IIa effects of LMWH, but does not completely reverse the anti-factor Xa activity of LMWH. Protamine has no effect on fondaparinux. There is no reversal agent for bivalirudin or argatroban.

After bleeding, HIT is the most important adverse effect associated with UFH. The longer fragments of UFH participate in nonspecific binding. In the case of HIT, polyanionic heparin fragments bind to the cationic platelet factor 4 (PF4) protein released from activated platelets.[156,157] The heparin-PF4 complex causes conformational changes exposing antigens that trigger IgG antibody formation. The immune response to the heparin-PF4 complex leads to thrombocytopenia with or without thrombosis. The incidence of HIT with LMWH is lower than with UFH. LMWH can complex with PF4, therefore, LMWH should be avoided in patients with HIT due to cross-reactivity with HIT antibodies.

The Role of Fibrinolytic Therapy in the Treatment of NSTE-ACS

The use of fibrinolytic agents offers no benefit in mortality and they increase the rate of intracranial hemorrhage, and fatal and nonfatal MI in patients with NSTE-ACS.[82] Consequently, fibrinolytics are contraindicated in the treatment of NSTE-ACS.

Invasive Strategies in the Treatment of NSTE-ACS

If a patient with UA is not adequately responding to medical therapy, they are evaluated as being at high risk for an adverse cardiac event, or if the patient is diagnosed with an NSTEMI, invasive coronary artery revascularization may be performed. This includes coronary angiography and revascularization with PCI and coronary artery bypass graft (CABG) surgery.

Drug Therapy Used in PCI

The predominant form of PCI is coronary stent placement. This involves the insertion of a catheter, with a deflated balloon surrounded by a collapsed metal mesh stent at the end, through a peripheral artery, such as the radial or femoral artery. The catheter is threaded into the site of the stenotic coronary vessel. The process of stent placement is summarized in Figure 35.24.

There are two types of stents, bare metal stents (BMS) and drug-eluting stents (DES). DES were designed to decrease restenosis that occurs with BMS.[164] DES are coated with a polymer of a drug, such as everolimus, that is released over time from approximately 30-120 days. Everolimus has immunosuppressant and antiproliferative activity preventing restenosis.

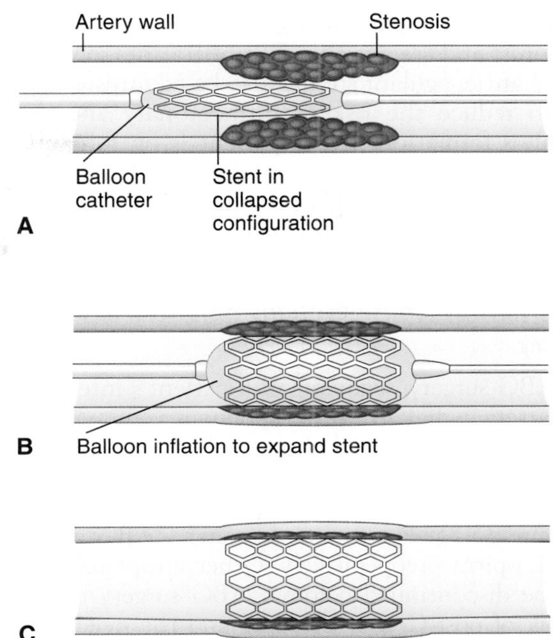

Figure 35.24 Placement of a coronary artery stent. A, A stent, in its original collapsed state, is advanced into the coronary stenosis on a balloon catheter. B, The balloon is inflated to expand the stent. C, The balloon is deflated, and the catheter is removed from the body, leaving the stent permanently in place. From Wilder J, Sabatine MS, Lilly LS. Ischemic heart disease. In: Lilly LS, ed. *Pathophysiology of Heart Disease: A Collaborative Project of Medical Students and Faculty.* 6th ed. Philadelphia: Wolters-Kluwer; 2016:158, with permission.

Everolimus

Dual antiplatelet therapy with aspirin and a loading dose of an oral $P2Y_{12}$ antagonist are standard therapy before PCI.[82] The AHA/ACC guidelines for NTSE-ACS, recommend GPIIb/IIIa antagonists for patients at high risk of ischemia, for example, patients who have an elevated troponin level, who are not adequately pretreated with clopidogrel or ticagrelor.[82] Cangrelor, which was FDA approved after the publication of the latest treatment guidelines for NSTE-ACS, is indicated as an adjunct to PCI in patients who are not already on a $P2Y_{12}$ antagonist and are not on a GPIIb/IIIa antagonist. A parenteral anticoagulant should also be administered before PCI to reduce the risk of intracoronary and catheter thrombus formation. If the patient is on fondaparinux, UFH must also be administered before PCI to prevent catheter thrombosis. UFH provides anti-factor IIa activity. After PCI, DAPT should be continued for at least 12 months in patients receiving a BMS or a DES.[82]

Drug Therapy Considerations Before CABG Surgery

In CABG surgery, segments of a patient's internal mammary artery, radial artery, or saphenous vein are grafted to divert blood flow around obstructed coronary arteries.[18,165] A bypass graft restores blood flow to the ischemic myocardial tissue in the area. Examples of CABGs are illustrated in Figure 35.25. Patients undergoing CABG are administered aspirin preoperatively. Other antiplatelet therapy must be discontinued before CABG surgery to decrease the risk of post-CABG bleeding and the need for blood transfusion. Clopidogrel and ticagrelor should be discontinued for at least 5 days, prasugrel for at least 7 days, eptifibatide and tirofiban for 2-4 hours, and abciximab at least 12 hours before elective CABG surgery (Tables 35.6 and 35.7).[82] When urgent CABG surgery is necessary, discontinuing clopidogrel and ticagrelor for at least 24 hours is recommended to decrease the risk of major bleeding.[82]

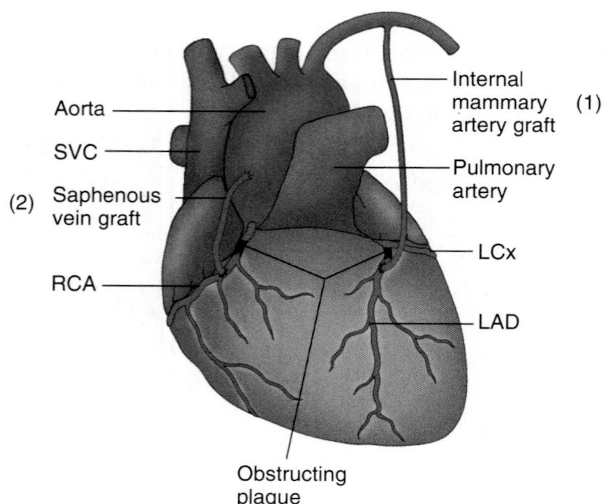

Figure 35.25 Coronary artery bypass graft (CABG) surgery. Two types of bypasses are illustrated: (1) the left internal mammary artery originates from the left subclavian artery, and in this schematic, it is anastomosed to the left anterior descending (LAD) coronary artery distal to obstructing plaque; (2) one end of a saphenous vein graft is sutured to the proximal aorta and the other end to the right coronary artery (RCA) distal to a stenotic segment. *LCx*, left circumflex artery; *SVC*, superior vena cava. From Wilder J, Sabatine MS, Lilly LS. Ischemic heart disease. In: Lilly LS, ed. *Pathophysiology of Heart Disease: A Collaborative Project of Medical Students and Faculty*. 6th ed. Philadelphia: Wolters-Kluwer; 2016:159, with permission.

Treatment of STEMI

STEMI is the result of complete occlusion of a coronary artery. Prompt reperfusion with either PCI or intravenous fibrinolytic therapy is indicated in patients with STEMI. The timing of reperfusion therapy is critical to limit myocardial tissue death. PCI is the treatment of choice when it can be performed within 90 minutes or less.[166] The drug therapy described above for PCI in patients with NSTE-ACS also applies to patients with STEMI.

Treatment with an oral β-blocker and ACEI in the first 24 hours, lipid management therapy, nitrates, calcium channel blockers, and morphine are all recommended for patients with STEMI as described above. Drug therapy for STEMI patients who require CABG surgery is as described above for CABG surgery in patients with NSTE-ACS.

Fibrinolytic Therapy in the Treatment of STEMI

In patients with STEMI and symptom onset within the previous 12 hours, the American College of Cardiology Foundation (ACCF)/AHA guidelines recommend fibrinolytic therapy, barring no contraindications, when PCI will be delayed by more than 120 minutes.[166] Fibrinolytic therapy should be administered intravenously within 30 minutes of hospital arrival. A full discussion of fibrinolytic agents is provided in Chapter 18. Alteplase, reteplase, and tenecteplase are the fibrinolytic agents approved for use in the treatment of STEMI.[145,157,166] Alteplase is recombinant human tissue plasminogen activator (tPA). Reteplase and tenecteplase are recombinant variants of human tPA with longer plasma half-lives than alteplase. Fibrinolytic agents convert plasminogen to plasmin which digests the fibrin clot of the occluded coronary artery. All three agents used in the treatment of STEMI are fibrin specific and activate fibrin-bound plasminogen more rapidly than plasminogen in the circulation.

Alteplase has a short half-life of 5 minutes, requiring it to be administered as a bolus injection followed by continuous infusion over 90 minutes.[145] The longer half-life of reteplase allows it to be administered as two bolus injections given 30 minutes apart. Tenecteplase is administered as a single bolus.

Adjunctive antithrombotic therapy is recommended with fibrinolytic therapy to improve coronary artery patency and to prevent reocclusion.[166] This includes antiplatelet therapy with aspirin and clopidogrel, and anticoagulant therapy with either UFH, enoxaparin, or fondaparinux.[166]

Adverse Effects

Bleeding is the most common adverse effect associated with fibrinolytic therapy. Intracranial hemorrhage is the most serious adverse effect of fibrinolytic therapy occurring in 0.5%-1% of patients.[164] Compared to tPA, tenecteplase causes less noncerebral bleeding.[157]

Clinical Scenario

Alexander J. Ansara, PharmD, BCPS – AQ Cardiology

SCENARIO

RM is a 59-year-old woman (70 kg) with a long-standing past history of smoking, hyperlipidemia, and hypertension who presented to the emergency department with severe substernal chest pain at rest that radiated to her jaw and left arm. Her pain "came and went" over the course of a few weeks prior to admission but had acutely worsened 2 hours prior to calling 9-1-1. She was given three sublingual nitroglycerin tablets in the ambulance, with no relief of angina symptoms, as well as four baby aspirin and a dose of morphine 3 mg IV. Her initial electrocardiogram demonstrated ST segment elevations of leads 2, 3, and aVF. Her first troponin was 0.07 ng/mL and she was given unfractionated heparin 5,000 units IV and ticagrelor 180 mg prior to being taken emergently to the cardiac catheterization lab for percutaneous coronary intervention (PCI). Angiography revealed 100% stenosis of her distal right coronary artery (RCA) and 50% stenosis of her mid left anterior descending coronary artery. She underwent successful RCA angioplasty and drug-eluting stent deployment with a post TIMI flow grade[a] of 3. Three hours later, RM is transferred to the cardiac intensive care unit where she is started on metoprolol 12.5 mg twice daily and atorvastatin 40 mg each evening. A ticagrelor regimen of 90 mg every 12 hours will be resumed as will aspirin 81 mg daily.

OUTCOME

The therapeutic goals of ACS are to emergently reestablish coronary blood flow, minimize infarct size, prevent death, and optimize treatment to reduce the future recurrence of ACS. In this case, PCI with intracoronary stenting was successful at re-establishing TIMI 3 flow grade in the fully occluded RCA vessel. Appropriate antiplatelet therapy was administered with an initial high dose of aspirin (325 mg) as well as a loading dose of the $P2Y_{12}$ antagonist, ticagrelor, which should be continued at 90 mg every 12 hours starting 12 hours after the loading dose. Aspirin 81 mg daily should be started the next day and DAPT with ticagrelor should be continued for a minimum of 12 months post stent deployment. Anticoagulation was provided with an unfractionated heparin bolus, but there is no need for long-term anticoagulation after the acute ACS treatment is completed. High-intensity statin therapy is warranted to further reduce mortality and recurrent ACS risk. High-intensity statin therapy includes atorvastatin at doses ≥40 mg or rosuvastatin at doses ≥20 mg daily. A β-blocker should be prescribed to reduce sympathetic outflow to prevent the detrimental effects of norepinephrine on neurohormonal cardiac remodeling, thereby lowering the risk of heart failure with reduce ejection fraction. Additionally, β-blockers lower heart rate to lessen myocardial oxygen demand and lower recurrent ACS risk. There is no preferred β-blocker for this patient, but cardioselective β-blockers are often preferred in patients at risk for obstructive pulmonary disease as this patient is given her history of smoking. Metoprolol and atenolol are appropriate cardioselective β-blockers and should be titrated to achieve a target heart rate of ≤60 beats per minute. Lastly, medications that block the detrimental effects of angiotensin II have been proven to reduce mortality in patients at high risk for coronary events. Chronic treatment with an ACEI is warranted and should be initiated when the patient is deemed to be hemodynamically stable.

Pharmacists play a pivotal role in ensuring that an optimal pharmacotherapeutic regimen is prescribed for post-ACS patients and that medications are dosed correctly without contraindications or potential for drug-drug interactions. Pharmacists also play an essential role in patient education. Post-ACS patients should be educated on the importance of compliance with DAPT, the role that each prescribed medication plays to reduce further cardiac risk, and potential adverse effects for which to monitor. Patients should be instructed only to utilize low-dose (81 mg) aspirin as higher doses increase bleeding risk and also potentially reduce the efficacy of ticagrelor. The appropriate use of rescue sublingual nitroglycerin tablets should be explained and patients should be instructed to carry it with them at all times. Signs and symptoms of recurrent ACS should also be reviewed. Lastly, cardiac rehabilitation should be recommended by the medical team and arranged prior to hospital discharge as it has proven to significantly reduce the risk of mortality from recurrent ACS.

Chemical Analysis found immediately after References.

[a]TIMI flow grades are a classification system for coronary artery blood flow established by the Thrombolysis in Myocardial Infarction (TIMI) Study Group. They range from TIMI flow grade 0 (complete occlusion) to TIMI flow grade 3 (normal flow).

REFERENCES

1. GBD 2016 Mortality and Causes of Death Collaborators. Global, regional, and national age-sex specific mortality for 264 causes of death, 1980–2016: a systematic analysis for the Global Burden of Disease Study 2016. *Lancet*. 2017;390:1151-1210.
2. Roth GA, Forouzanfar MH, Moran AE, et al. Demographic and epidemiologic drivers of global cardiovascular mortality. *N Engl J Med*. 2015;372:1333-1341.
3. Benjamin EJ, Virani SS, Calloway CW, et al. Heart disease and stroke statistics-2018 update: a report from the American Heart Association. *Circulation*. 2018;137:e67-e492.
4. American Heart Association, & American Stroke Association. *Cardiovascular Disease: A Costly Burden for America*. Projections through 2035; 2017. http://www.heart.org/idc/groups/heart-public/@wcm/@adv/documents/downloadable/ucm_491543.pdf. Accessed 21 January 2018.
5. Lewis MW, Khodneva Y, Redmond N, et al. The impact of the combination of income and education on the incidence of coronary heart disease in the prospective Reasons for Geographic and Racial Differences in Stroke (REGARDS) cohort study. *BMC Public Health*. 2015;15:1312-1322.
6. Dieleman JL, Baral R, Birger M, et al. US spending on personal health care and public health, 1996–2013. *JAMA*. 2016;316:2627-2646.

7. Nicholson G, Gandra SR, Halbert RJ, et al. Patient-level costs of major cardiovascular conditions: a review of the international literature. *Clinicoecon Outcomes Res*. 2018;8:495-506.
8. McCabe JM, Armstrong EJ. Integrative cardiovascular pharmacology: hypertension, ischemic heart disease, and heart failure. In: Golan DE, Armstrong EJ, Armstrong AW, eds. *Principles of Pharmacology: The Pathophysiologic Basis of Drug Therapy*. 4th ed. Philadelphia: Wolters-Kluwer Health; 2017:469-496.
9. Fogelstrand P, Borén J. *Nutr Metab Cardiovasc Dis*. 2012;22:1-7.
10. Libby P. *Am J Clin Nutr*. 2006;83(suppl):456S-460S.
11. Fog Bentson J, Otsuka F, Virmani R, Falk E. Mechanisms of plaque formation and rupture. *Circ Res*. 2014;114:1852-1866.
12. Head T, Daunet S, Goldschmidt-Clermont PJ. The aging risk and atherosclerosis: a fresh look at arterial homeostasis. *Front Genet*. 2017;8:216.
13. Sakakura K, Nakano M, Otsuka F, et al. Pathophysiology of atherosclerosis plaque progression. *Heart Lung Circ*. 2013;22:399-411.
14. Shahawy S, Libby P. Atherosclerosis. In: Lilly LS, ed. *Pathophysiology of Heart Disease: A Collaborative Project of Medical Students and Faculty*. 6th ed. Philadelphia, PA: Wolters-Kluwer; 2016:112-133.
15. Tabas I, Lichtman AH. Monocyte-macrophages and T cells in atherosclerosis. *Immunity*. 2017;47:621-634.
16. Libby P, Tabas I, Fredman G, Fisher EA. Inflammation and its resolution as determinants of acute coronary syndromes. *Circ Res*. 2014;114:1867-1879.
17. Dudzinski DM, Serhan CN. Pharmacology of eiscosanoids. In Golan DE, Armstrong EJ, Armstrong AW, eds. *Principles of Pharmacology: The Pathophysiologic Basis of Drug Therapy*. 4th ed. Philadelphia: Wolters-Kluwer Health; 2017:794-818.
18. Wilder J, Sabatine MS, Lilly LS. Ischemic heart disease. In: Lilly LS, ed. *Pathophysiology of Heart Disease: A Collaborative Project of Medical Students and Faculty*. 6th ed. Philadelphia: Wolters-Kluwer; 2016:134-161.
19. Anderson JL, Morrow DA. Acute myocardial infarction. *N Engl J Med*. 2017;376:2053-2064.
20. Wilder J, Sabatine MS, Lilly LS. Acute coronary syndromes. In: Lilly LS, ed. *Pathophysiology of Heart Disease: A Collaborative Project of Medical Students and Faculty*. 6th ed. Philadelphia: Wolters-Kluwer; 2016:162-191.
21. Alvin MD, Jaffe AS, Ziegelstein RC, et al. Eliminating creatine kinase – myocardial band testing in suspected acute coronary syndrome: a value-based quality improvement. *JAMA Intern Med*. 2017;177:1508-1512.
22. Ridker PM, Everett BM, Thuren JG, et al. Antiinflammatory therapy with canakinumab for atherosclerotic disease. *N Engl J Med*. 2017;377:1119-1131.
23. ILARIS. In: *Red Book Online (Electronic Version)*. Greenwood Village, Colorado: Truven Health Analytics; 2018. http://www.micromedexsolutions.com/. Accessed 27 March 2018.
24. Dawber TR. *The Framingham Study: The Epidemiology of Atherosclerotic Disease*. Cambridge, MA: Harvard University Press; 1980.
25. Dawber TR, Meadors GF, Moore FE. Epidemiological approaches to heart disease: the Framingham study. *Am J Pub Heal*. 1951;41:279-286.
26. Framingham Heart Study: A Project of the National Heart, Lung, and Blood Institute and Boston University. https://www.framinghamheartstudy.org/index.php. Accessed 14 March 2018.
27. 2013 ACC/AHA guideline on the assessment of cardiovascular risk: a report of the American College of Cardiology/American Heart Association task force on practice guidelines. *J Am Coll Cardiol*. 2014:63;2935-2959.
28. Picciotto MR, Kenny PJ. Molecular mechanisms underlying behaviors related to nicotine addiction. *Cold Spring Harb Perspect Med*. 2013;3:a012112.
29. Hays JT, Ebbert JO. Varenicline for tobacco dependence. *N Engl J Med*. 2008;359(19):2018-2024.
30. Cahill K, Stevens S, Perera R, et al. Pharmacological interventions for smoking cessation: an overview and network meta-analysis. *Cochrane Database Syst Rev*. 2013;(5):CD009329. doi:10.1002/14651858.CD009329.pub2.
31. Cahill K, Lindson-Hawley N, Thomas KH, et al. Nicotine receptor partial agonists for smoking cessation. *Cochrane Database Syst Rev*. 2016;(5):CD006103. doi:10.1002/14651858.CD006103.pub7.
32. Benowitz NL, Hugganen J, Jacob P. Nicotine chemistry, metabolism, kinetics, and biomarkers. *Handb Exp Pharmacol*. 2009;192:29-60.
33. Chen G, Giambrone NE, Lazarus P. Glucuronidation of trans-3′-hydroxycotinine by UGT2B17 and UGT2B10. *Pharmacogenet Genomics*. 2012;22:183-190.
34. Nicorette Nicotine Polacrilex Chewing Gum [OTC Drug Label]. Warren, NJ: GlaxoSmithKline; 2017. Available at https://www.accessdata.fda.gov/drugsatfda_docs/label/2017/018612s078,020066s059lbl.pdf. Accessed 26 May 2018.
35. Nicorette Nicotine Polacrilex Lozenge [OTC Drug Label]. Moon Park, PA: GlaxoSmithKline; 2015. Available at https://www.accessdata.fda.gov/drugsatfda_docs/label/2017/018612s078,020066s059lbl.pdf. Accessed 26 May 2018.
36. Barboza JL, Patel R, Patel R, et al. An update on the pharmacotherapeutic interventions for smoking cessation. *Expert Opin Pharmacother*. 2016;17:1483-1496.
37. Drugs for tobacco dependence. *Med Lett Drugs Ther*. 2016;58(1489):27-31.
38. Coe JW, Books PR, Vetelino MG, et al. Varenicline: an α4β2 nicotinic receptor partial agonist for smoking cessation. *J Med Chem*. 2005;48:3474-3477.
39. Blum AP, Lester HA, Dougherty DA. Nicotinic pharmacophore: the pyridine N or nicotine and carbonyl of acetylcholine hydrogen bond across a subunit interface to backbone NH. *Proc Natl Acad Sci USA*. 2010;107:13206-13211.
40. Post MR, Tender GS, Lester HA, Dougherty DA. Secondary ammonium agonists make dual cation-π interactions in α4β2 nicotinic receptors. *eNeuro*. 2017;4(2):ENEURO.0032-17.2017. doi:10.1523/ENEURO.0032-17.2017.
41. Tavares XDS, Blum AP, Nakamura DT, et al. Variations in binding among several agonists at two stoichiometries of the neuronal, α4β2 nicotinic receptor. *J Am Chem Soc*. 2012;134:11474-11480.
42. Faessel HM, Obach RS, Rollema H, et al. A review of the clinical pharmacokinetics and pharmacodynamics of varenicline for smoking cessation. *Clin Pharmacokinet*. 2010;49:799-816.
43. Xiu X, Puskar NK, Shanata JA, et al. Nicotine binding to brain receptors requires a strong cation-pi interaction. *Nature*. 2009;458:534-537.
44. Slemmer JE, Martin BR, Damaj MI. Bupropion is a nicotinic antagonist. *J Pharmacol Exp Ther*. 2000;295:312-327.
45. Warner C, Shoaib M. How does bupropion work as a smoking cessation aid? *Addict Biol*. 2005;10:219-231.
46. The GBD 2015 Obesity Collaborators. Health effects of overweight and obesity in 195 countries over 25 years. *N Engl J Med*. 2017;377:13-27.
47. Cavallari I, Cannon CP, Braunwald E, et al. Metabolic syndrome and the risk of adverse cardiovascular events after acute coronary syndrome. *Eur J Prev Cardiol*. 2018;25:830-838.
48. Rodriguez-Gutierrez R, Montori VM. Glycemic control for patients with type 2 diabetes mellitus our evolving faith in the face of evidence. *Circ Cardiovasc Qual Outcomes*. 2016:9:504-512. doi:10.1161/CIRCOUTCOMES.116.002901.
49. Zinman B, Wanner C, Lachin JM, et al. Empagliflozin, cardiovascular outcomes, and mortality in type 2 diabetes. *N Engl J Med*. 2015;373:2117-2128.
50. Neal B, Perkovic V, Mahaffey KW, et al. Canagliflozin and cardiovascular and renal event in type 2 diabetes. *N Engl J Med*. 2017;377:644-657.
51. Marso SP, Daniels GH, Brown-Frandsen K. Liraglutide and cardiovascular outcomes in type 2 diabetes. *N Engl J Med*. 2016;375:311-322.

52. American Diabetes Association. 9. Cardiovascular disease and risk management: standards of medical care in diabetes – 2018. *Diabetes Care*. 2018;41(suppl 1):S86-S104.
53. Samani NJ, Erdmann J, Hall AS, et al. Genomewide association analysis of coronary artery disease. *N Engl J Med*. 2007;357:443-453.
54. Khera AV, Emdin CA, Drake I, et al. Genetic risk, adherence to a healthy lifestyle, and coronary disease. *N Engl J Med*. 2016;375:2349-2358.
55. Rosendorff C, Lackland DT, Allison M, et al. Treatment of hypertension in patients with coronary artery disease. *Circulation*. 2015;131:e435-e470.
56. James PA, Oparil S, Carter BL, et al. 2014 evidence-based guideline for the management of high blood pressure in adults. *JAMA*. 2014;311(5):507-520.
57. Acelajado MC, Calhoun DA, Oparil S. Pathogenesis of hypertension. In: Black H, Elliott W, eds. *Hypertension: A Companion to Braunwald's Heart Disease*. 2nd ed. Philadelphia, PA: Elsevier Sanders; 2012:12-26.
58. Ding K, Kullo IJ. Genome-wide association studies for atherosclerotic vascular disease and its risk factors. *Circ Cardiovasc Genet*. 2009;2:63-72.
59. The ONTARGET Investigators. Telmisartan, ramipril, or both in patients at high risk for vascular events. *N Engl J Med*. 2008;358:1547-1559.
60. Reilly RF, Jackson EK. Regulation of renal function and vascular volume. In: Brunton LL, Chabner BA, Knollmann BC, eds. *Goodman and Gilman's the Pharmacological Basis of Therapeutics*. 12th ed. New York: McGraw-Hill; 2011:671-719.
61. Hilal-Dandan R. Renin and angiotensin. In: Brunton LL, Chabner BA, Knollman BC, eds. *Goodman & Gilman's the Pharmacological Basis of Therapeutics*. 12th ed. New York: McGraw-Hill; 2011:721-744.
62. Michel T, Hoffman BB. Treatment of myocardial ischemia and hypertension. In: Brunton LL, Chabner BA, Knollman BC, eds. *Goodman & Gilman's the Pharmacological Basis of Therapeutics*. 12th ed. New York: McGraw-Hill; 2011:745-788.
63. Stone NJ, Robinson JG, Lichtenstein AH, et al. 2013 ACC/AHA guideline on the treatment of blood cholesterol to reduce atherosclerotic cardiovascular risk in adults: a report of the American College of Cardiology/American Heart Association task force on practice guidelines. *Circulation*. 2014;129(suppl 2):S1-S45.
64. Lloyd-Jones DM, Morris PB, Ballantyne CM, et al. 2017 focused update of the 2016 ACC expert consensus decision pathway on the role of non-statin therapies for LDL-cholesterol lowering in the management of atherosclerotic cardiovascular disease risk. *J Am Coll Cardiol*. 2017;70(14):1785-1822.
65. Stokker GE, Hoffman WF, Alberts AW, et al. 3-Hydroxy-3-methylglutaryl–coenzyme A reductase inhibitors. 1. Structural modification of 5-substituted 3,5-dihydroxypentanoic acids and their lactone derivatives. *J Med Chem*. 1985;28:347-358.
66. *Clinical Pharmacology Online*. Gold Standard Elsevier; 2017. Available at http://clinicalpharmacology.com. Accessed May 2018.
67. Cholesterol Treatment Trialists Collaboration. Efficacy and safety of more intensive lowering of LDL cholesterol: a meta-analysis of data from 170,000 participants in 26 randomized trials. *Lancet*. 2010;376:1670-1681.
68. Facts & Comparisons eAnswers. St. Louis, MO: Wolters Kluwer Health. Available at http://www.wolterskluwercdi.com/facts-comparisons-online. Accessed May 2018.
69. Lipid-lowering drugs. *Med Lett*. 2016;58:133-140.
70. Bersot TP. Drug therapy for hypercholesterolemia and dyslipidemia. In: Brunton L, Chabner B, Knollman B, eds. *Goodman & Gilman's the Pharmacological Basis of Therapeutics*. 12th ed. New York: McGraw-Hill; 2011:877-908.
71. Cendella RJ. Cholesterol and hypocholesterolemic drugs. In: Craig CR, Stitzel RE, eds. *Modern Pharmacology with Clinical Applications*. 5th ed. Boston: Little, Brown and Company; 1997:279-289.
72. Praluent (Alirocumab) Prescribing Information. Regeneron Pharmaceuticals, Inc.; 2017. Available at http://products.sanofi.us/praluent/praluent.pdf.
73. Repatha (Evolocumab) Prescribing Information. Amgen Inc.; 2017. Available at https://pi.amgen.com/~/media/amgen/repositorysites/pi-amgen-com/repatha/repatha_pi_hcp_english.pdf.
74. Sabatine MS, Giugliano RP, Keech AC, et al. Evolocumab and clinical outcomes in patients with cardiovascular disease. *N Engl J Med*. 2017;376:1713-1722.
75. Ridker PM, Tardif JC, Amarenco P, et al. Lipid-reduction variability and antidrug-antibody formation with bococizumab. *N Engl J Med*. 2017;376:1517-1526.
76. Levin AA. Targeting therapeutic oligonucleotides. *N Engl J Med*. 2017;376:86-88.
77. Dana H, Mahmoodi GM, Mahmoodzadeh H, et al. Molecular mechanisms and biological functions of siRNA. *Int J Biomed Sci*. 2017;13:48-57.
78. Khvorova A. Oligonucleotide therapeutics—a new class of cholesterol-lowering drugs. *N Engl J Med*. 2017;376:4-7.
79. Raul FJ, Santos RD. Homozygous familial hypercholesterolemia: current perspectives on diagnosis and treatment. *Atherosclerosis*. 2012;223:262-268.
80. Kynamro (Mipomersen) Prescribing Information. Genzyme Corporation; 2016. Available at http://www.kynamro.com/media/pdfs/Kynamro_Prescribing_information.pdf.
81. Juxtapib (Lomitapide) Prescribing Information. Aegerion Pharmaceuticals; 2016. Available at http://www.juxtapidpro.com/prescribing-information.
82. Amsterdam EA, Wenger NK, Brindis RG, et al. 2014 AHA/ACC guideline for the management of patients with non-ST-elevation acute coronary syndromes: a report of the American College of Cardiology/American Heart Association task force on practice guidelines. *J Am Coll Cardiol*. 2014:64:e139-e228.
83. Talbert RL. Ischemic heart disease. Dipiro JT, Talbert RL, Yee GC, et al, eds. *Pharmacotherapy: A Pathophysiologic Approach*. 9th ed. New York: McGraw-Hill; 2014:141-173.
84. Ignarro LJ, Lippto H, Edwards JC, et al. Mechanism of vascular smooth muscle relaxation by organic nitrates, nitrites, nitroprusside and nitric oxide: evidence for the involvement of S-nitrosothiols as active intermediates. *J Pharmacol Exp Ther*. 1981;218:739-749.
85. Westfall TC, Westfall DP. Adrenergic agonists and antagonists. In: Brunton L, Chabner B, Knollman B, eds. *Goodman & Gilman's the Pharmacological Basis of Therapeutics*. 12th ed. New York: McGraw-Hill; 2011:277-333.
86. Kubica J, Adamski P, Ostrowska M, et al. Morphine delays and attenuates ticagrelor exposure and action in patients with myocardial infarction: the randomized, double-blind, placebo-controlled IMPRESSION trial. *Eur Heart J*. 2016;37:245-252.
87. Hobl E, Stimpfl T, Ebner J. Morphine decreases clopidogrel concentrations and effects: a randomized, double-blind, placebo-controlled trial. *J Am Coll Cardiol*. 2014;63:630-635.
88. Hobl E, Reiter B, Schoergenhofer C, et al. Morphine interaction with prasugrel: a double blind, cross-over trial in healthy volunteers. *Clin Res Cardiol*. 2016;105:340-355.
89. Grosser T, Smyth E, FitzGerald GA. Anti-inflammatory, antipyretic, and analgesic agents: pharmacotherapy of gout. In: Brunton L, Chabner B, Knollman B, eds. *Goodman & Gilman's the Pharmacological Basis of Therapeutics*. 12th ed. New York: McGraw-Hill; 2011:959-1004.
90. Baigent C, Blackwell L, Collins R, et al. Aspirin in the primary and secondary prevention of vascular disease: collaborative meta-analysis of individual participant data from randomized trials. *Lancet*. 2009;373:1849-1860.
91. Patrono C. Aspirin and human platelets: from clinical trials to acetylation of cyclooxygenase and back. *TIPS*. 1989;10:453-458.
92. Blobaum AL, Marnett LJ. Structural and functional basis of cyclooxygenase inhibition. *J Med Chem*. 2007;50:1425-1441.

93. Hochgesang GP, Rowlinson SW, Marnett LJ. Tyrosine-385 is critical for acetylation of cyclooxygenase-2 by aspirin. *J Am Chem Soc.* 2000;122:6514-6515.
94. Smith WL, DeWitt DL, Kraemer SA, et al. Structure-function relationships in sheep, mouse, and human prostaglandin endoperoxide G/H synthases. *Adv Prostaglandin Thromboxane Leukot Res.* 1990;20:14-21.
95. Patrono C, Garcia Rodriguez LA, Landolfi R, et el. Low-dose aspiring for the prevention of atherothrombosis. *N Engl J Med.* 2005;353:2373-2383.
96. Pedersen AK, FitzGerald GA. Dose-related kinetics of aspirin. *N Engl J Med.* 1984;311:1206-1211.
97. Grosser T, Fries S, Lawson JA, et al. Drug resistance and pseudoresistance: an unintended consequence of enteric coating aspirin. *Circulation.* 2013:127:377-385.
98. Haastrup PF, Gronlykke T, Jarbol DE. Enteric coating can lead to reduced antiplatelet effect of low-dose acetylsalicylic acid. *Basic Clin Pharmaol Toxicol.* 2015;116:212-215.
99. Li X, Fries S, Li R, et al. Differential impairment of aspirin-dependent platelet cyclooxygenase acetylation by nonsteroidal antiinflammatory drugs. *Proc Natl Acad Sci USA.* 2014;111:16830-16835.
100. Catella-Lawson F, Reilly MP, Kapoor SC, et al. Cyclooxygenase inhibitors and the antiplatelet effects of aspirin. *N Engl J Med.* 2001;345:1809-1817.
101. Levine GN, Bates ER, Bittl JA, et al. 2016 ACC/AHA guideline focused update on duration of dual antiplatelet therapy in patients with coronary artery disease: a report of the American College of Cardiology/American Heart Association task force on clinical practice guidelines. *J Am Coll Cardiol.* 2016;68:1082-1115.
102. Tang M, Mukundan M, Yang J, et al. Antiplatelet agents aspirin and clopidogrel are hydrolyzed by distinct carboxylesterases, and clopidogrel is transesterificated in the presence of ethyl alcohol. *J Pharmacol Exp Ther.* 2006;319:1467-1476.
103. Kazui M, Nishiya Y, Ishizuka T, et al. Identification of the human cytochrome P450 enzymes involved in the two oxidative steps in the bioactivation of clopidogrel to its pharmacologically active metabolite. *Drug Metab Dispos.* 2010;38:92-99.
104. Savi P, Zachayus JL, Delesque-Touchard N, et al. The active metabolite of clopidogrel disrupts P2Y12 receptor oligomers and partitions them out of lipid rafts. *Proc Natl Acad Sci USA.* 2006;103:11069-11074.
105. Algaier I, Jakubowski JA, Asai F, et al. Interaction of the active metabolite of prasugrel, R-138727, with cysteine 97 and cysteine 175 of the human $P2Y_{12}$ receptor. *J Thromb Haemost.* 2008;6:1908-1914.
106. Farid NA, Atsushi Kurihara A, Wrighton SA. Metabolism and disposition of the thienopyridine antiplatelet drugs ticlopidine, clopidogrel, and prasugrel in humans. *J Clin Pharmacol.* 2010;50:126-142.
107. Mega JL, Close SL, Wiviott SD, et al. Cytochrome P-450 polymorphisms and response to clopidogrel. *N Engl J Med.* 2009;360:354-362.
108. Brown SA, Pereira N. Pharmacogenomic impact of CYP2C19 variation on clopidogrel therapy in precision cardiovascular medicine. *J Pers Med.* 2018;8:E8. doi:10.3390/jpm8010008.
109. Pare G, Mehta SR, Yusuf S, et al. Effects of CYP2C19 genotype on outcomes of clopidogrel treatment. *N Engl J Med.* 2010;363:1704-1714.
110. Doll JA, Neely ML, Roe MT, et al. Impact of CYP2C19 metabolizer status on patients with ACS treated with prasugrel versus clopidogrel. *J Am Coll Cardiol.* 2016;67:936-947.
111. Scott SA, Sangkuhl K, Stein CM, et al. Clinical Pharmacogenetics Implementation Consortium guidelines for CYP2C19 genotype and clopidogrel therapy: 2013 update. *Clin Pharmacol Ther.* 2013;94:317-323.
112. Plavix (Clopidogrel Bisulfate) Tablets [Package Insert]. Bridgewater, NJ: Bristol-Myers Squibb/Sanofi Pharmaceuticals Partnership; 2017. Available at https://www.accessdata.fda.gov/drugsatfda_docs/label/2017/020839s068lbl.pdf. Accessed 26 May 2018.
113. Sibbing D, Koch W, Gebhard D, et al. Cytochrome 2C19*17 allelic variant, platelet aggregation, bleeding events, and stent thrombosis. *Circulation.* 2010;121:512-518.
114. Angiolillo DJ, Gibson CM, Cheng S, et al. Differential effects of omeprazole and pantoprazole on the pharmacodynamics and pharmacokinetics of clopidogrel in healthy subjects: randomized, placebo-controlled, crossover comparison studies. *Clin Pharmacol Ther.* 2011;89:65-74.
115. Frelinger AL, Lee RD, Mulford DJ, et al. A randomized, 2-period, crossover design study to assess the effects of dexlansoprazole, lansoprazole, esomeprazole, and omeprazole on the steady-state pharmacokinectics and pharmacodynamics of clopidogrel in healthy volunteers. *J Am Coll Cardiol.* 2012;59:1304-1311.
116. Melloni C, Washam JB, Jones WS, et al. Conflicting results between randomized trials and observational studies on the impact of proton pump inhibitors on cardiovascular events when coadministered with dual antiplatelet therapy: systematic review. *Circ Cardiovasc Qual Outcomes.* 2015;8:47-55.
117. O'Donague ML, Braunwald E, Antman EM, et al. Pharmacodynamic effect and clinical efficacy of clopidogrel and prasugrel with or without a proton-pump inhibitor: an analysis of two randomised trials. *Lancet.* 2009;374:989-997.
118. Gargiulo G, Costa F, Ariotti S, et al. Impact of proton pump inhibitors on clinical outcomes in patients treated with a 6- or 24-month dual-antiplatelet therapy duration: insights from the PROlonging Dual-antiplatelet treatment after Grading stent-induced Intimal hyperplasia studY trial. *Am Heart J.* 2016;174:95-102.
119. Jakubowski JA, Winters KJ, Naganuma H, et al. Prasugrel: a novel thienopyridine antiplatelet agent. A review of preclinical and clinical studies and the mechanistic basis for its distinct antiplatelet profile. *Cardiovasc Drug Rev.* 2007;25:357-374.
120. Wiviott SD, Braunwald E, McCabe CH, et al. Prasugrel versus clopidogrel in patients with acute coronary syndromes. *N Engl J Med.* 2007;357:2001-2015.
121. Effient (Prasugrel) Tablets [Package Insert]. Indianapolis, IN: Eli Lilly and Company; 2018. Available at https://www.accessdata.fda.gov/drugsatfda_docs/label/2018/022307s015lbl.pdf. Accessed 26 May 2018.
122. Springthorpe B, Bailey A, Barton P, et al. From ATP to AZD6140: the discovery of an orally active reversible P2Y12 receptor antagonist for the prevention of thrombosis. *Bioorg Med Chem Lett.* 2007;17:6013-6018.
123. Remko M, Remkova A, Broer R. A comparative study of molecular structure, pKa, Lipophilicity, solubility, absorption and polar surface area of some antiplatelet drugs. *Int J Mol Sci.* 2016;17:388. doi:10.3390/ijms17030388.
124. Storey RF, Husted S, Harrington RA, et al. Inhibition of platelet aggregation by AZD6140, a reversible oral P2Y12 receptor antagonist, compared with clopidogrel in patients with acute coronary syndromes. *J Am Coll Cardiol.* 2007;50:1852-1856.
125. Wallentin L, Becker RC, Budaj, et al. Ticagrelor versus clopidogrel in patients with acute coronary syndromes. *N Engl J Med.* 2009;361:1045-1057.
126. Mahaffey KW, Woidyla DM, Carroll K, et al. Ticagrelor compared with clopidogrel by geographic region in the Platelet Inhibition and Patient Outcomes (PLATO) trial. *Circulation.* 2011;124:544-554.
127. Brilinta (Ticagrelor) Tablets [Package Insert]. Wilmington, DE: AstraZeneca Pharmaceuticals LP. 2018. Available at https://www.accessdata.fda.gov/drugsatfda_docs/label/2018/022433s022lbl.pdf. Accessed 26 May 2018.
128. Zhou D, Andersson TB, Grimm SW. In vitro evaluation of potential drug-drug interactions with ticagrelor: cytochrome P450 reaction phenotyping, inhibition, induction, and differential kinetics. *Drug Metab Disp.* 2011;39:703-710.
129. Ingall AH, Dixon J, Bailey A, et al. Antagonists of the platelet P2T receptor: a novel approach to antithrombotic therapy. *J Med Chem.* 1999;42:213-220.

130. Walsh JA, Price MJ. Cangrelor for treatment of arterial thrombosis. *Expert Opin Pharmacother*. 2014;15:565-572.
131. Bhatt DL, Stone GW, Mahaffey KW. Effect of platelet inhibition with cangrelor during PCI in ischemic events. *N Engl J Med*. 2013;368:1303-1313.
132. Dovlatova NL, Jakubowski JA, Sugidachi A, et al. The reversible P2Y antagonist cangrelor influences the ability of the active metabolites of clopidogrel and prasugrel to produce irreversible inhibition of platelet function. *J Thromb Haemost*. 2008;6:1153-1159.
133. Armstrong EJ, Golan DE. Pharmacology of hemostasis and thrombosis. In: Golan DE, Armstrong EJ, Armstrong AW, eds. *Principles of Pharmacology: The Pathophysiologic Basis of Drug Therapy*. 4th ed. Philadelphia: Wolters-Kluwer Health; 2017:403-432.
134. Chackalamannil S, Xia Y, Greenlee WJ, et al. Discovery of potent orally active thrombin receptor (protease activated receptor 1) antagonists as novel antithrombotic agents. *J Med Chem*. 2005;48:5884-5887.
135. Chackalamannil S, Wang Y, Greenlee WJ, et al. Discovery of a novel, orally active himbacine-based thrombin receptor antagonist (SCH530348) with potent antiplatelet activity. *J Med Chem*. 2008;51:3061-3064.
136. Kosoglou T, Revderman L, Tiessen RG, et al. Pharmacodynamics and pharmacokinetics of the novel PAR-1 antagonist vorapaxar (formerly SCH 530348) in healthy subjects. *Eur J Clin Pharmacol*. 2012;68:249-258.
137. Morrow DA, Braunwald E, Bonaca MP, et al. Vorapaxar in the secondary prevention of atherothrombotic events. *N Engl J Med*. 2012;366:1404-1413.
138. Zontivity (Vorapaxar) Tablets [Package Insert]. Whitehouse Station, NJ: Merck Sharp & Dohme Corp; 2015. Available at https://www.accessdata.fda.gov/drugsatfda_docs/label/2015/204886s002lbl.pdf. Accessed 29 May 2018.
139. Bledza K, Smyth SS, Plow EF. Integrin αIIbβ3: from discovery to efficacious therapeutic target. *Circ Res*. 2013;112:1189-1200.
140. Scarborough RM, Gretler DD. Platelet glycoprotein IIb-IIIa antagonists as prototypical intergrin blockers: novel parenteral and potential oral antithrombotic agents. *J Med Chem*. 2000;43:3453-3473.
141. Xiao T, Takagi J, Coller BS, et al. Structural basis for allostery in integrins and binding to fibrinogen-mimetic therapeutics. *Nature*. 2004;432:59-67.
142. Scarborough RM, Naughton MA, Teng W, et al. Design of potent and specific integrin antagonists. Peptide antagonists with high specificity for glycoprotein IIb-IIIa. *J Biol Chem*. 1993;268:1066-1073.
143. Hartman GD, Egbertson MS, Halczenk W, et al. Non-peptide fibrinogen receptor antagonists. 1. Discovery and design of exosite inhibitors. *J Med Chem*. 1992;35:4640-4642.
144. Zhu J, Choi WS, McCoy JG, et al. Structure-guided design of a high-affinity platelet integrin αIIbβ3 receptor antagonist that disrupts Mg^{2+} binding to the MIDAS. *Sci Transl Med*. 2012;4:125ra32. doi:10.1126/scitranslmed.3003576.
145. Hogg K, Weitz JI. Blood coagulation and anticoagulant, fibrinolytic, and antiplatelet drugs. In: Brunton LL, Hilal-Dandan R, Knollmann BC, eds. *Goodman & Gilman's the Pharmacological Basics of Therapeutics*. 13th ed. New York: McGraw Hill; 2018:584-603.
146. King S, Short M, Harmon C. Glycoprotein IIb/IIIa inhibitors: the resurgence of tirofiban. *Vascul Pharmacol*. 2016;78:10-16.
147. Aster RH. Immune thrombocytopenia caused by glycoprotein IIb/IIIa inhibitors. *Chest*. 2005;127:53S-59S.
148. Bougie DW, Wilker PR, Wuitschick ED, et al. Acute thrombocytopenia after treatment with tirofiban or eptifibatide is associated with antibodies specific for ligand-occupied GPIIb/IIIa. *Blood*. 2002;100:2071-2076.
149. Chew DR, Bhatt DL, Topol EJ. Oral glycoprotein IIb/IIIa inhibitors: why don't they work? *Am J Cardiovasc Drugs*. 2001;1:421-428.
150. Bassler N, Loeffler C, Mangin P, et al. A mechanistic model for paradoxical platelet activation by ligand-mimetic alphaIIb beta3 (GPIIb/IIIa) antagonists. *Arterioscler Thromb Vasc Biol*. 2007;27:e9-e15.
151. Jiang J, McCoy JG, Shen M, et al. A novel class of ion displacement ligands as antagonists of the αIIbβ3 receptor that limit conformational reorganization of the receptor. *Bioorg Med Chem Lett*. 2014;24:1148-1153.
152. Li J, Vootukuri S, Shang Y, et al. RUC-4: a novel αIIbβ3 antagonist for pre-hospital therapy of myocardial infarction. *Arterioscler Thromb Vasc Biol*. 2014;34:2321-2329.
153. Miller LM, Pritchard JM, Macdonald SJF, et al. Emergence of small-molecule non-RGD-mimetic inhibitors for RGD integrins. *J Med Chem*. 2017;60:3241-3251.
154. Weitz JI. Low-molecular weight heparins. *N Engl J Med*. 1997;337:688-699.
155. Lovenox (Enoxaparin Sodium Injection) [Package Insert]. Bridgewater, NJ: Sanofi-Aventis U.S. LLC; 2017. Available at https://www.accessdata.fda.gov/drugsatfda_docs/label/2017/020164s110lbl.pdf. Accessed 12 June 2018.
156. Garcia DA, Baglin TP, Weitz JI, et al. Parenteral anticoagulants: antithrombotic therapy and prevention of thrombosis, 9th ed: American College of Chest Physicians evidence-based clinical practice guidelines. *Chest*. 2012;141:e24S-e43S.
157. Weitz JI. Hemostasis, thrombosis, fibrinolysis, and cardiovascular disease. In: Mann DL, Zipes DP, Libby P, Bonow RO, eds. *Braunwald's Heart Disease: A Textbook of Cardiovascular Medicine*. 10th ed. Vol. 2. Philadelphia: Elsevier; 2015:1809-1833.
158. Petersen JL, Mahaffey KW, Hasselblad V, et al. Efficacy and bleeding complications among patients randomized to enoxaparin or unfractionated heparin for antithrombin therapy in non-ST-segment elevation acute coronary syndromes: a systematic overview. *JAMA*. 2004;292:89-96.
159. Eikelboom JW, Connolly SJ, Bosch J, et al. Rivaroxaban with or without aspirin in stable cardiovascular disease. *N Engl J Med*. 2017;377:1319-1330.
160. Moon JY, Nagaraju D, Franchi F, et al. The role of oral anticoagulant therapy in patients with acute coronary syndrome. *Ther Adv Hematol*. 2017;8:353-366.
161. Chiarito M, Cao D, Cannata F, et al. Direct oral anticoagulants in addition to antiplatelet therapy for secondary prevention after acute coronary syndromes: a systematic review and meta-analysis. *JAMA Cardiol*. 2018;3:234-241.
162. Braunwald E. An important step for thrombocardiology. *N Engl J Med*. 2017;377:1387-1388.
163. Gucinski AC, Boyne MT, Keire DA. Modern analytics for naturally derived complex drug substances: NMR and MS tests for protamine sulfate from chum salmon. *Anal Bioanal Chem*. 2015;407:749-759.
164. Torrado J, Buckley L, Duran A, et al. Restenosis, stent thrombosis, and bleeding complications: navigating between Scylla and Charybdis. *J Am Coll Cardiol*. 2018;71:1676-1695.
165. Gaudino M, Benedetto U, Fremes S, et al. Radial-artery or saphenous-vein grafts in coronary-artery bypass surgery. *N Engl J Med*. 2018;378:2069-2077.
166. O'Gara PT, Kushner FG, Ascheim DD, et al. 2013 ACCF/AHA guideline for the management of ST-elevation myocardial infarction: a report of the American College of Cardiology Foundation/American heart association task force on practice guidelines. *Circulation*. 2013;127:e362-e425.

Clinical Scenario

CHEMICAL ANALYSIS

Kimberly Beck, Marc Harrold

DAPT inhibits two separate pathways that trigger platelet aggregation, TXA_2 and ADP. At low doses, aspirin selectively and irreversibly inhibits COX-1 by acetylating a serine residue in the COX-1 active site. This inhibits TXA_2 synthesis in platelets resulting in inhibition of platelet aggregation, but leaves the synthesis of PGI_2 by COX-2 in endothelial cells unaffected. PGI_2 is a potent inhibitor of platelet aggregation. Ticagrelor is a nucleoside analog of ATP and is a reversible antagonist of the ADP $P2Y_{12}$ receptor on the surface of platelets. The lipophilic nature of ticagrelor enables oral bioavailability.

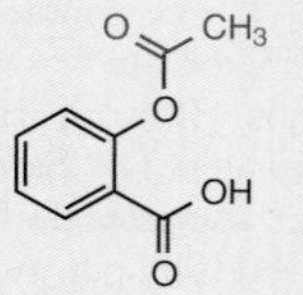

Aspirin

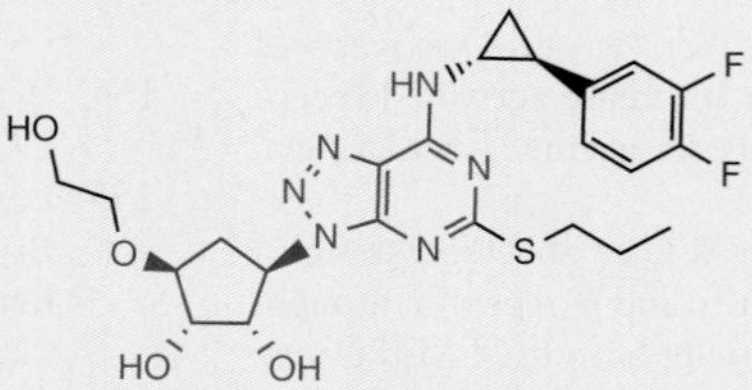

Ticagrelor

The patient was not previously on aspirin; therefore, she was initially started on one dose of 325 mg aspirin which immediately inhibits platelet TXA_2 synthesis. At this dose, aspirin loses COX-1 selectivity and also inhibits COX-2. Thus, the patient's maintenance dose will be low-dose aspirin to confer the full antithrombotic benefit of aspirin and to insure there is no interference with the efficacy of ticagrelor.

Atorvastatin and rosuvastatin contain the 3,5-dihydroxy acid required for competitive HMG-CoA reductase (HMGR) inhibition. The 3,5-dihydroxy acid group mimics the transition state between HMG-CoA and mevalonic acid. It binds to the HMGR active site with high affinity via an ionic bond with the carboxylic acid and a series of ion-dipole interactions between the enzyme and the two alcohol groups and the acid. The 4-fluorophenyl group is a key substituent for potency as it forms a cation-π interaction with the guanidinium group of Arg590. The isopropyl group participates in van der Waals attractions with the HMGR enzyme. Compared to other statins, there is an additional hydrogen bond between Ser565 and the amide carbonyl oxygen of atorvastatin and a sulfone oxygen of the sulfonamide in rosuvastatin, respectively. Rosuvastatin also forms an ion-dipole interaction between the guanidinium ion of Arg568 and the sulfone group. Due to enhanced interactions with the HMGR enzyme, atorvastatin and rosuvastatin are the most potent HMGRIs and are used in "high intensity" statin therapy to reduce LDL levels and for the secondary prevention of ASCVD.

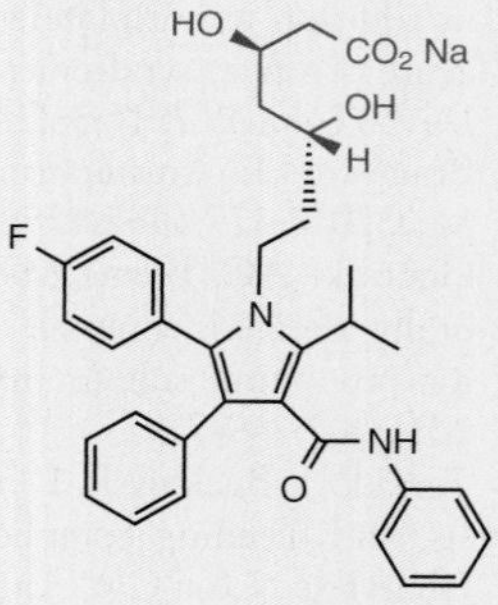

Atorvastatin

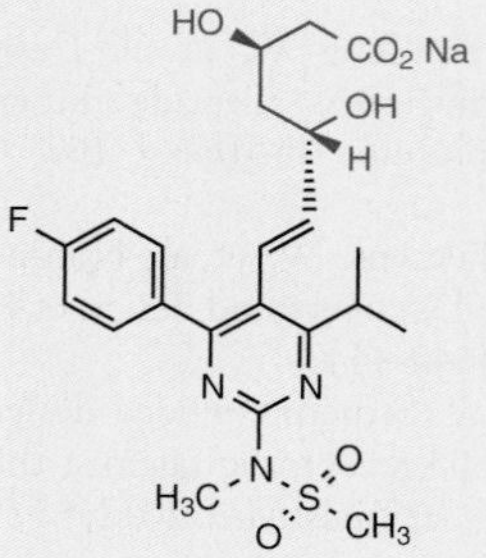

Rosuvastatin

The aryloxypropanolamine backbone of metoprolol and atenolol confers β-adrenergic antagonist activity. These compounds are devoid of α-adrenergic activity due to the N-isopropyl group which sterically impedes their binding to α-adrenergic receptors. Both of these drugs are β_1-selective due to the para-substituent and either would be appropriate for this patient. Metoprolol is relatively lipophilic and undergoes extensive hepatic metabolism, principally by CYP2D6. Therefore, a lower dose may be necessary in patients with hepatic impairment. Atenolol is hydrophilic and does not undergo hepatic metabolism. Approximately 50% of a dose of atenolol is orally absorbed and it is primarily excreted unchanged in the urine. Thus, patients with renal impairment may require a lower dose of atenolol.

Clinical Scenario—Continued

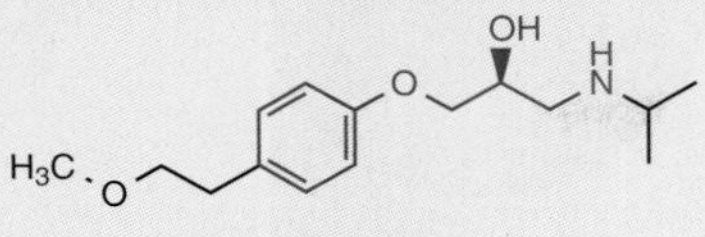

Metoprolol

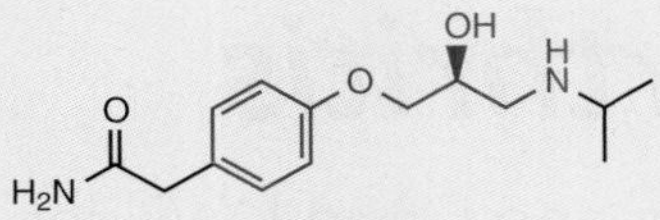

Atenolol

An example of an ACEI that would be appropriate for this patient is lisinopril. Lisinopril is an orally active ACEI with a long duration of action allowing once a day dosing. Unlike most ACEIs, lisinopril has sufficient oral absorption without being a prodrug. The di-zwitterion state of lisinopril in the duodenum gives it a net charge of zero which is an explanation for its satisfactory absorption through the GI mucosa despite its hydrophilic character. The tetrahedral carbon bound to a phenylethyl group, a carboxylic acid, and a secondary amine within the structure of lisinopril mimics the transition state of angiotensin I hydrolysis in the ACE active site. The phenylethyl group mimics the phenylalanine side chain in angiotensin I, the carboxylate anion binds to Zn^{2+}, and the secondary amine is in the same location as the labile amide nitrogen in angiotensin I. The ε-amino group of the lysine side chain of lisinopril forms an ionic bond with a glutamic acid residue within a side chain pocket on ACE. The carbonyl group participates in a hydrogen bond and the proline carboxylate anchors lisinopril to the ACE active site via an ionic bond with a lysine residue.

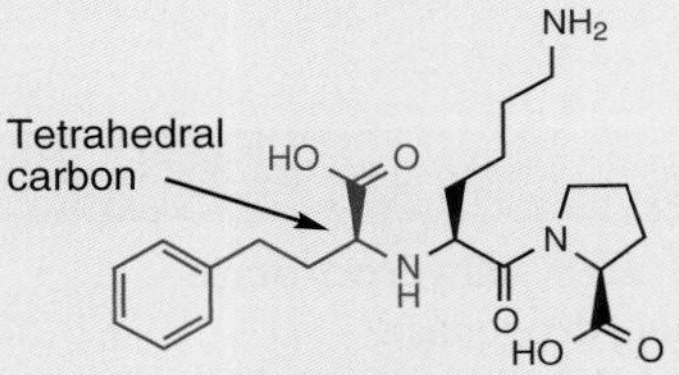

Lisinopril

Administration of sublingual nitroglycerin liberates NO in vivo. By binding to soluble guanylyl cyclase, NO stimulates the production of cGMP which results in smooth muscle relaxation and vasodilation of coronary and peripheral blood vessels. Nitroglycerin predominantly induces vasodilation of vessels in the venous system which reduces preload. To a lesser degree, nitroglycerin causes vasodilation of the vessels in the arterial system which reduces afterload. Both actions decrease myocardial oxygen demand. Dilation of coronary arteries by nitroglycerin increases myocardial oxygen supply. By decreasing myocardial oxygen demand and increasing myocardial oxygen supply, nitroglycerin can relieve myocardial ischemic pain.

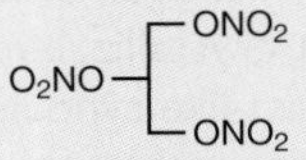

Nitroglycerin

CHAPTER 36

Rheumatoid Arthritis

Kristopher E. Boyle, Abby J. Weldon, and David J. Weldon

Drugs covered in this chapter:

TRADITIONAL OR SYNTHETIC DISEASE-MODIFYING ANTIRHEUMATIC DRUGS (SDMARDS)
- Baricitinib
- Chloroquine
- Hydroxychloroquine
- Leflunomide
- Methotrexate
- Sulfasalazine
- Tofacitinib

BIOLOGIC DMARDS (bDMARDS)

TUMOR NECROSIS FACTOR INHIBITORS (TNFI)
- Adalimumab
- Certolizumab pegol
- Etanercept
- Golimumab
- Infliximab

NON-TNFI BIOLOGIC DMARDS
- Abatacept
- Anakinra
- Rituximab
- Tocilizumab

Abbreviations

ACPA anti-citrullinated protein antibody
ACR American College of Rheumatology
ADCC antibody-dependent cellular cytotoxicity
AICAR aminoimidazole carboxamide ribonucleotide
APC antigen-presenting cell
5-ASA 5-aminosalicylic acid
ATIC AICAR transformylase/inosine monophosphate cyclohydrolase
bDMARD biologic disease-modifying antirheumatic drug
CBC complete blood count
CCP cyclic citrullinated peptides
CDAI clinical disease activity index
CDC complement-dependent cytotoxicity
CDR complementarity-determining regions
CoQ coenzyme Q
CQ chloroquine
CRP C-reactive protein
CTLA-4 cytotoxic T-lymphocyte antigen 4
DAS28 disease activity score 28
DC dendritic cell
DHFR dihydrofolate reductase
DHODH dihydroorotate dehydrogenase
DMARD disease-modifying antirheumatic drug
dTMP 2′-deoxythymidine monophosphate
dUMP 2′-deoxyuridine monophosphate
ESR erythrocyte sedimentation rate
EULAR European League Against Rheumatism
Fab fragment antigen binding
Fc fragment crystallizable
FLS fibroblast-like synoviocytes
GI gastrointestinal tract
GWAS genome-wide association studies
HCQ hydroxychloroquine
HLA human leukocyte antigen
hOAT human organic anion transporter
IFN interferon
IgG immunoglobulin G
IL interleukin
IL-1 interleukin 1
ILD interstitial lung disease
IL-1R interleukin 1 receptor
IL-1RA interleukin 1 receptor antagonist
IMP inosine monophosphate
IV intravenous
JAK Janus kinase
JIA juvenile idiopathic arthritis
LEF leflunomide
LT-β lymphotoxin beta
Mab monoclonal antibody
MCP-1 monocyte chemoattractant protein-1
MCP-4 monocyte chemoattractant protein-4
MHC major histocompatibility complex
MIP-1α macrophage inflammatory protein 1 alpha
MMP matrix metalloproteinases
MTX methotrexate
MTX-PG polyglutaminated methotrexate
NK natural killer cell
NSAID nonsteroidal anti-inflammatory drug
PAD peptidyl arginine deiminase
PAS or PASII patient activity scale
PTPN22 protein tyrosine phosphatase, nonreceptor type 22
RA rheumatoid arthritis
RANKL receptor activator of nuclear factor kappa-B ligand

Abbreviations—Continued

RAPID-3 routine assessment of patient index data-3
RF rheumatoid factor
rUMP ribonucleotide uridine monophosphate
SAM S-adenosylmethionine
SC subcutaneous
SDAI simple disease activity index
sDMARD synthetic disease-modifying anti-rheumatic drug
SSZ sulfasalazine
TB tuberculosis
THF tetrahydrofolate
TNF tumor necrosis factor
TNF-α tumor necrosis factor alpha
TNF-R2 tumor necrosis factor alpha receptor 2
TNFi tumor necrosis factor inhibitor
TTT treat-to-target
VLDLR very-low-density lipoprotein receptor

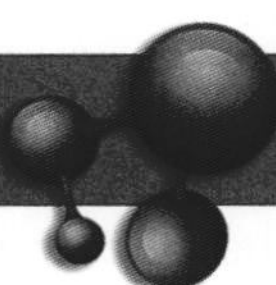

CLINICAL SIGNIFICANCE

Justin Kinney, PharmD

The synthetic disease-modifying antirheumatic drugs (sDMARD) are a unique class of small molecule agents that possess no structural properties in common from one agent to the next. Due to this, they do not possess a typical structure-activity relationship (SAR), and each individual drug operates by a different mechanism of action. The biologic DMARDs (bDMARDs), on the other hand, may possess common mechanisms of action (tumor necrosis factor inhibitors [TNFi], for instance) but biological macromolecules are not generally thought of as possessing an SAR either.

The sDMARDs interact with their cellular target's protein residues by a small number of relatively strong intermolecular interactions over a small surface area, such as hydrogen bonding interactions, ion-dipole interactions, or ion-ion interactions as well as weaker and less significant van der Waals and π-stacking interactions. These may be easily seen in some cases, such as methotrexate and its structural similarity to folic acid and the manner in which it binds to dihydrofolate reductase. The bDMARDs, with molecular weights often in excess of 100,000 g/mol, instead interact with their cellular targets by a large number of interactions over a very large molecular surface area. Each bDMARD is a protein, and its amino acid residues have attractive interactions with the amino acid residues of its cellular target. For instance, a cationic lysine residue on a bDMARD may bind to an anionic aspartic acid residue on the cellular target, or a phenylalanine on the bDMARD may be involved in a π-stacking interaction with a target tyrosine or tryptophan. It is important for clinicians to understand the scientific underpinnings of the mechanisms of action behind the drugs used to treat rheumatoid arthritis in addition to the important distinctions in use, efficacy, and side effects of the sDMARDs compared to the bDMARDs.

RHEUMATOID ARTHRITIS

Introduction

Rheumatoid arthritis (RA) is a chronic, systemic autoimmune inflammatory disease, which results in significant cartilage, bone, and joint damage.[1] Individuals with rheumatoid arthritis experience musculoskeletal loss of function, lowered quality and length of life, and a number of comorbidities. The most commonly involved joints are the wrists and hands, with larger joints less commonly affected. The condition results in inflamed, swollen, and painful joints that typically present symmetrically, with joints on both sides of the body involved. Disease onset is most frequent in middle age, and women are affected about 2.5 times more frequently than men. Rheumatoid arthritis has an incidence of 0.5%-1%, with a reduction in incidence from north to south and from urban to rural communities in the United States.[2,3]

Rheumatoid arthritis is a disease that can be traced to antiquity, with evidence of the disease dating back more than 4,000 years to skeletal remains of Native Americans of Tennessee, as well as to Egyptian mummies.[4] Certain Native American populations still have extraordinarily high incidence of the disease.[2] RA was exceptionally rare or absent in Europe before the 18th century, with the first reported case occurring in 1785.[5] It has been suggested that the importation of sugar to Europe from the West Indies during this time, and the attendant increase in periodontal disease and gingivitis (which has been correlated with increased rheumatoid arthritis risk), may have contributed to the introduction of RA to Europe in the 18th century.[6]

Risk factors for developing rheumatoid arthritis include a positive family history of the disease, and concordance rates in twins are increased. Rheumatoid arthritis is categorized as either seropositive, meaning that the patient's blood has tested positive for rheumatoid factor (RF) and/or anti-citrullinated protein antibodies (ACPAs), or seronegative. The heritability of rheumatoid arthritis is estimated as 40%-65% for seropositive disease, but only 20% for seronegative rheumatoid arthritis.[7,8] The most significant environmental risk factor is smoking, and it is associated with an increased risk of developing seropositive disease (RF or ACPA), as well as poor response to antirheumatic therapy.[9] Hormonal factors are also thought to be important, as there is an increased incidence of RA in women.[10] Use of birth control pills lowers the risk of developing RA by half. Men with RA have been found to have lower levels of testosterone than unaffected men. Lower socioeconomic and educational status is also correlated with

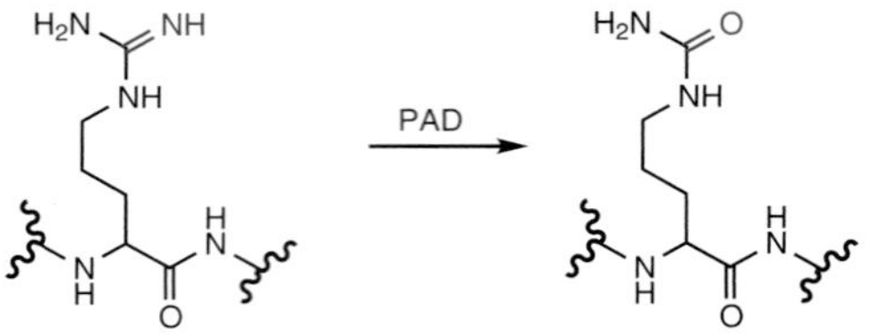

Figure 36.1 Protein citrullination with peptidyl arginine deiminase (PAD).

increased risk of developing RA.[11] As mentioned, gingivitis is present at about twice the rate in RA patients compared to the general population.[12] Notably, *Porphyromonas gingivalis*, the causative bacteria in gingivitis, is the only bacterium known to produce the enzyme peptidyl arginine deiminase (PAD), which is responsible for the citrullination of proteins, and may be correlated with the presence of ACPAs in RA patients. Protein citrullination by PAD is depicted in Figure 36.1.

Diagnosis and Disease Activity of RA

In patients who present with inflammatory arthritis, a physical examination and laboratory testing are performed to evaluate the clinical features of RA and to rule out other diseases that share overlapping features with RA. Systemic lupus erythematosus, psoriatic arthritis, scleroderma, polymyalgia rheumatica, Lyme arthritis, viral infection, gout, osteoarthritis, fibromyalgia, and inflammatory bowel disease can present with symptoms consistent with RA and must be excluded through differential diagnosis.

The diagnosis of RA may be made when more than one joint has inflammatory arthritis, serological testing is positive for RF and/or ACPA, elevated levels of the acute phase C-reactive protein (CRP) or the erythrocyte sedimentation rate (ESR) are observed, symptoms are present for more than 6 weeks, and conditions that cause inflammatory arthritis or other clinical features inconsistent with RA are excluded. The American College of Rheumatology and the European League Against Rheumatism (ACR/EULAR) developed the 2010 RA Classification Criteria by generating an algorithm that assigns a point value based on joint involvement, serology, acute phase reactants, and disease duration (Table 36.1). An RA classification is given when a total score of at least 6 out of 10 from the 4 categories listed above is reached. The goal of this classification system is to identify patients with symptoms of RA as early as possible in order to start therapy before erosive joint damage begins. If a patient does not meet these criteria, this does not mean that RA should be ruled out. Patients meeting the criteria but lacking both RF and ACPA can be classified as having seronegative RA. As symptoms persist, patients who were not initially classified with RA may meet the criteria upon repeated screening.

Table 36.1 2010 ACR/EULAR RA Classification Criteria for RA[a,13]

	Score
Joint Involvement	
1 large joint (shoulders, elbows, hips, knees or ankles)	0
2-10 large joints	1
1-3 small joints (with or without large joint involvement)	2
4-10 small joints (with or without large joint involvement)	3
>10 joints (at least 1 small joint involved)	5
Serology	
Negative RF and ACPA	0
Low-positive RF or CPA	2
High-positive RF or CPA	3
Acute-Phase Reactants	
Normal CRP and ESR	0
Abnormal CRP or ESR	1
Duration of Symptoms	
<6 wk	0
≥6 wk	1

[a]These criteria are recommended for newly presenting patients who have at least 1 joint with clinical synovitis that is not due to another condition. Patients with erosive joint disease typical of RA with a history compatible with prior fulfillment of the 2010 criteria should be classified as having RA. Patients should have a score of 6 or greater to meet the criteria for RA diagnosis.

The 2010 ACR/EULAR RA Classification Criteria was developed primarily for use in classifying RA patients for clinical trials and other research studies so that results from multiple studies could be compared.

Once a positive diagnosis of RA has been established, it is necessary to determine the level of disease activity for the patient. There are several scales of disease activity that are employed by clinicians that rank disease activity as in remission, low activity, moderate activity, or high activity. These scales include the Patient Activity Scale (PAS or PASII), the Routine Assessment of Patient Index Data 3 (RAPID-3), the Clinical Disease Activity Index (CDAI), the Simplified Disease Activity Index (SDAI), and the Disease Activity Score 28 (DAS28).[14] Treatment of RA is designed to bring the patient to either in remission or to low disease activity.

The Genetics of Rheumatoid Arthritis

Like many rheumatic diseases, RA is believed to arise from a combination of genetic and epigenetic susceptibility coupled with an environmental trigger that initiates disease progression. A clear and general cause of rheumatoid arthritis has remained elusive over several decades of study. Genetic risk factors are generally easier to study than environmental risk factors because genetic factors are present from conception and continue throughout life and are easily measured using current genetic technology. There has been an enormous increase in our knowledge of the genetic contributors underlying rheumatoid arthritis in the last 10 years.

It has been known for decades that rheumatoid arthritis has a genetic component. In one study conducted in Great Britain, 15% of sets of identical twins both had rheumatoid arthritis compared to 4% of fraternal twins in the same study, corresponding to 60% heritability for rheumatoid arthritis.[15] The sibling recurrence risk for a disease is the risk of recurrence in a sibling of a disease compared to the general population risk and has been found to be between 3% and 19% for rheumatoid arthritis.

Before the advent of modern genetic technology, researchers could assign only two genetic loci with confidence to RA—the *HLA-DRB1* and *PTPN22* genes. As with most autoimmune conditions, the HLA (human leukocyte antigen) region confers most of the genetic risk for the disease and accounts for about 60% of the genetic load in RA. Due to the strength of this correlation, the involvement of HLA was understood 30 years before the modern genetic era.[16] Both of these genes are correlated with immune function and are still considered the two largest genetic risk factors for rheumatoid arthritis. The *HLA-DRB1*0401* allele was the first HLA polymorphism associated with RA and is still the allele most strongly associated with RA in Caucasian populations.[16] Most of the risk alleles in the DRB1 region share a common sequence between positions 70 and 74, consisting of Gln or Lys-Arg-Arg-Ala-Ala. This consensus sequence is referred to as the shared epitope (SE), with the major variations at this allele that contribute to RA being **0401, *0101, *404, *0405, and *1001*.[17] Table 36.2 describes the relative risks for developing rheumatoid arthritis for several of these genotypes. Some combinations of *DRB1* alleles carry extremely high risk for RA, with the combination of *DRB1*0401* and **0404* carrying a relative risk of more than 30 in Caucasian populations. The **1001* allele has a one amino acid deviation from the shared epitope, with the substitution of an Arg at position 70, as does *DRB1*0901* which is commonly associated with RA in Asian populations.

Table 36.2 · Shared Epitope Relative Risks

DRB1 Genotype	Relative Risk
0101/DRX	2.3
0401/DRX	4.7
0404/DRX	5
0101/0401	6.4
0401/0404	31.3

The DRB1 protein belongs to the HLA class II beta chain paralogues and plays a central role in presenting peptides derived from extracellular proteins to T-helper cells. The five amino acid structural feature contained in the SE is located in the third hypervariable region on the α-helical region of the DRB1 protein and determines the shape of the groove responsible for binding foreign bodies. It is likely that a specific RA antigen, as yet unidentified but most probably an autoantigen, is presented to the immune system and elicits an improper immune response that triggers the progression of RA. Intense research efforts over many years have failed to unambiguously confirm the identity of the autoantigen target of the shared epitope. It is noteworthy, given the importance of ACPA's in RA, that citrullinated peptides appear to have a strong affinity for *DRB1*0401* alleles.[18] The shared epitope hypothesis is not a complete explanation of the HLA association with RA, as not all SE genotypes carry the same degree of genetic risk and the strength of the association varies in different populations. For instance, the SE does not appear to associate strongly with RA in African American populations.[19] Researchers have proposed a number of other hypotheses for the genetics of RA that may apply to certain individuals and populations, but these require additional experimental confirmation.

The *PTPN22* gene is also strongly associated with RA.[20,21] *PTPN22* (protein tyrosine phosphatase, nonreceptor type 22) is involved in immune response regulation, and mutations in *PTPN22* are associated with both increases and decreases in risk for autoimmune disease.[21] Allelic variants in *PTPN22* are also associated with type I diabetes, systemic lupus erythematosus, and autoimmune thyroid disease and are protective for Crohn's disease. A change in one of the binding sites in *PTPN22* (a change from arginine to tryptophan in codon 620) disrupts the association of *PTPN22* with Csk, an intracellular tyrosine kinase that plays an important role in the regulation of immune response.[20,22] Knockout of *PTPN22* in rodents leads to a dramatic increase in the activity of T cells.

More recently, genome-wide association studies (GWAS) looking at single nucleotide polymorphisms have found more than a hundred loci correlated with increased risk of rheumatoid arthritis, most of which are known to correlate with immune function.[23] The dominant influence derives from mutation of *HLA-DRB1* and *PTPN22*. New discoveries of genes involved in the pathogenesis of RA may provide novel targets for new therapies.

The Pathogenesis of Rheumatoid Arthritis

The Role of Immune Cells

Many immune cells are involved in joint inflammation resulting from RA, including B cells, T cells, monocytes and macrophages, dendritic cells (DC), plasma cells, and fibroblast-like synoviocytes (FLS) within the joint (Fig. 36.2). Synovial tissue samples from RA patients reveal an increased concentration of immune cells, with T cells having the highest incidence, followed by B cells, macrophages, and DCs having lower frequency, suggesting that these immune cells are involved in RA joint damage or that they are upstream mediators of the inflammatory cascade that leads to joint damage.[24] B cells play a pathogenic role in RA by producing autoantibodies such as RF (antibody against the Fc portion of immunoglobulin G [IgG]), anti-citrullinated protein antibodies, anti-carbamylated proteins, anti-acetylated proteins, and others.[25] B cells also contribute to RA by secreting cytokines that activate other immune cells in the joint and by acting as potent antigen-presenting cells that are able to stimulate T cells to differentiate into inflammatory T helper cells. Joint damage begins at the synovial membrane where immune cells infiltrate the synovium leading to hypertrophied synovial tissue that forms a pannus (an abnormal layer of fibrovascular tissue that erodes articular cartilage and bone).

The Role of Cytokines

Cytokines are a loosely defined category of small proteins important in cell signaling. The role of cytokines in the pathogenesis of RA is confirmed through the successful treatment of patients with targeted therapies against cytokines including tumor necrosis factor (TNF) and interleukins 1 and 6 (IL-1 and IL-6). During synovitis, immune cells infiltrate the synovium leading to the paracrine and autocrine secretion of inflammatory cytokines. TNF-α, IL-6, and IL-1 levels are elevated in RA patients. TNF-α is a proinflammatory cytokine that can induce multiple proinflammatory cytokines such as IL-1, IL-6, and IL-8. TNF-α also stimulates monocytes to produce matrix metalloproteinases (MMP). IL-1β, TNF-α, and IL-6 can activate endothelial cells, stromal cells, and chondrocytes; induce osteoclast activation and differentiation; and increase cellular infiltration of the joint. TNF-α acts in conjunction with IL-6 and IL-1β to increase production of pro-angiogenic factors leading to increased vascularization of the joint. IL-6 activates B cells, macrophages, and endothelial cells and induces a systemic response by promoting an acute phase response. IL-6 levels are elevated in the joints of RA patients and can result in endothelial activation, neutrophil activation, and chemotaxis, and activate osteoclasts and chondrocytes leading to a breakdown of the joint matrix and bone erosion. IL-1 activates immune cells, chondrocytes, and osteoclasts leading to inflammation and degradation of the joint. Multiple cytokines play an important role in the pathogenesis of RA through the activation, proliferation, and differentiation of immune cells.

The Role of Chemokines

Chemokines are a group of cytokines secreted by certain cells that induce chemotaxis in nearby responsive cells. Immune cells migrate to the synovium through the actions of chemokines and cellular adhesion molecules. Chemokines within the joint are produced by macrophages, fibroblast-like synoviocytes, and chondrocytes and can be induced by inflammatory cytokines such as TNF-α, IL-1, and IL-6. Elevated levels of the chemokines such as monocyte chemoattractant protein-4 (MCP-4), monocyte

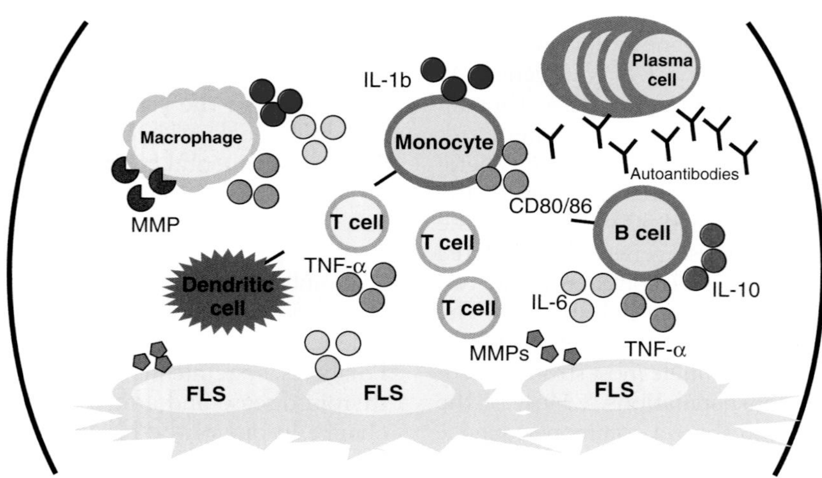

Figure 36.2 The role of immune cells in rheumatoid arthritis (RA). During inflammatory synovitis, immune cells infiltrate the joint and produce cytokines. These cytokines can activate many other immune cells involved in joint inflammation, including B cells, monocytes, dendritic cells, T cells, macrophages, and plasma cells. These cells produce further cytokines, chemokines and enzymes that ultimately result in joint damage and deformation.

chemoattractant protein 1 (MCP-1), macrophage inflammatory protein 1α (MIP-1α) and fractalkine are found in synovial fluid from RA patients. Increased levels of these chemokines in the synovial fluid suggest that they play an important role in the pathogenic recruitment of immune cells to the joint.[26] Chemokines can also stimulate fibroblast-like synoviocytes to secrete cytokines and matrix metalloproteinases, and collagenase, leading to the degradation of cartilage in the joint. In addition, chemokines can increase FLS cell proliferation leading to synovial hyperplasia.[27] In summary, chemokines play a role in the pathogenesis of RA through the recruitment of immune cells to the joint, by inducing the secretion of inflammatory cytokines and through increasing cell proliferation within the joint.

The deleterious effects of RA extend beyond the joint, and the inflammation resulting from many of the cytokines produced by RA patients affect vital organs and tissues. RA patients have a 2-fold higher risk of developing cardiovascular disease than the general population. RA is associated with systemic bone loss and increased risk of fracture. This increased risk of fracture is due to increased levels of inflammatory cytokines TNF, IL-6, and IL-1, leading to upregulation of receptor activator of nuclear factor kappa-B ligand (RANKL), which regulates the differentiation and activation of osteoclasts critical to bone resorption and remodeling. Lung disease, such as small airway disease and bronchial wall thickening, are more prominent in patients with longstanding RA. The risk of developing interstitial lung disease (ILD) is increased in RA patients compared to the general population and is associated with an older age at the time of RA onset and with greater RA severity. The cause of ILD in RA is unknown; however, the employment of RA therapies such as DMARDs (perhaps especially TNFi) and glucocorticoid use are associated with ILD development. Malignancies are also increased in RA patients. The risk of lymphoma is 2-fold higher in RA patients. Therapeutics, specifically TNFi, are also associated with lymphoma, melanoma, and nonmelanoma skin cancer risk.[28]

TREATMENT OF RHEUMATOID ARTHRITIS

There is no cure for RA, but recent advancements in the treatment of RA both improve symptoms and slow progression of the disease. The goals of treatment are to minimize pain and swelling, prevent cartilage and bone loss and deformity, and maintain healthy day-to-day function for the patient. The cornerstone of modern RA treatment is the use of disease-modifying antirheumatic drugs (DMARDs), which slow the progression of the disease. NSAIDs and steroids may be used to help manage pain.

Disease Modifying Antirheumatic Drugs

The DMARDs are a class of drugs employed to slow the progress of joint destruction in rheumatoid arthritis.[14] Many of these drugs have a similar impact in slowing rheumatoid arthritis disease progression, though they operate by a multitude of different mechanisms of action and are considered mostly unrelated except as they are employed to treat RA. Most DMARDs have both anti-inflammatory and immunomodulatory activity. They are generally divided into two main categories: traditional or synthetic DMARDs (sDMARD), which are synthetic small molecules, and biologic DMARDs (bDMARD) that are protein-based agents produced through genetic engineering. These agents are often used in combination, though the application of combination DMARD therapy for individual patients is not strictly defined. Combination therapy allows for a smaller dose of each drug than would be the case for a drug taken as a monotherapy and thus attenuates side effects that may result from larger drug doses. It is generally agreed that early introduction of DMARD therapy is advantageous in minimizing joint damage from RA.[29] While waiting for DMARDs to produce their full effects, which often takes weeks to months, NSAIDs are commonly employed to reduce inflammation and pain. NSAIDs do not slow the rate of disease progression but do reduce inflammation and pain. Steroids, which blunt immune response, may be used on a short-term basis until the beneficial effects of DMARD therapy take effect. Corticosteroid use effectively keeps inflammation at bay, but the deleterious effects of long-term steroid use make the goal of DMARD therapy to use DMARDs instead of—not in addition to—steroids.

Traditional or Synthetic DMARDs

METHOTREXATE. Methotrexate (MTX) is the most important and widely used DMARD, and it would be difficult to overstate its importance in the treatment of RA. Introduced in the 1950s as a treatment for cancer, its use as a treatment for RA has increased over the last 25 years and it is now considered the DMARD of choice. Methotrexate is also the cornerstone of combination DMARD therapy for RA.[14]

Methotrexate is a structural analogue of folic acid with substitutions on the pteridine group (–OH to $-NH_2$) and methylation of the aniline structure (Fig. 36.3). MTX is a substrate for many cellular efflux proteins. After transport into the cell, MTX is polyglutaminated (MTX-PG), which hinders drug efflux from the cell. Genetic polymorphisms can affect MTX influx, efflux, and polyglutamination and are believed to contribute to variable MTX response and toxicity.[30]

MTX and MTX-PG inhibit several important cellular enzymes, which result in the drug's anti-inflammatory and immunomodulatory effects (Fig. 36.4). MTX is best known as an inhibitor of dihydrofolate reductase (DHFR), and this is the primary mechanism of action responsible for MTX's anticancer activity when given at the much higher doses employed to treat cancer as opposed to RA.[31] Inhibition of DHFR results in decreased concentration of tetrahydrofolate (THF) and impaired cellular function and survival. DHFR is responsible for transmethylation reactions essential to many cellular functions and is responsible for the production of THF, which is converted to 5,10-methylene tetrahydrofolate

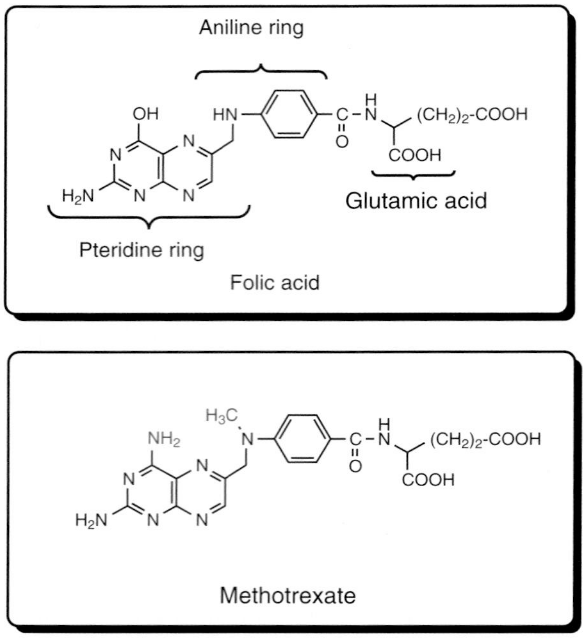

Aniline ring

Glutamic acid

Pteridine ring

Folic acid

Methotrexate

Figure 36.3 The structures of methotrexate and folic acid.

to become a methyl donor for the conversion of homocysteine to methionine. Methionine is then converted to S-adenosylmethionine (SAM), which is a methyl donor for epigenetic methylation reactions of DNA, as well as methylation of RNA, proteins, amino acids, and phospholipids. The most important of the methylation processes affected by the action of MTX is the production of the pyrimidine nucleobase 2′-deoxythymidine monophosphate (dTMP) from 2′-deoxyuridine monophosphate (dUMP) via the action of thymidylate synthetase (TYMS), an enzyme that is also inhibited by MTX, and its cofactor 5,10-methylene tetrahydrofolate. Inhibition of this process results in disrupted DNA synthesis and decreased cellular proliferation.

DHFR is also involved in the synthesis of the polyamines spermidine and spermine, which accumulate in the synovial fluid,[32] peripheral blood mononuclear cells,[33] and urine of RA patients.[34] Metabolism of polyamines produces toxic ammonia and hydrogen peroxide, which may impair lymphocyte function and contribute to the severity of RA.[35,36] Accumulation of polyamines in B cells increases production of RF in vitro.[31] Inhibition of DHFR by MTX is believed to result in a beneficial reduction in the amounts of polyamines present in RA patients.

MTX-PG inhibits aminoimidazole carboxamide ribonucleotide (AICAR) transformylase/IMP cyclohydrolase (ATIC), which mediates the conversion of AICAR to formyl-AICAR and then a further condensation to form inosine monophosphate (IMP). IMP is converted in a few steps to AMP.[37] Thus, MTX use results in increased intracellular and extracellular concentrations of adenosine, a potent inhibitor of inflammation.

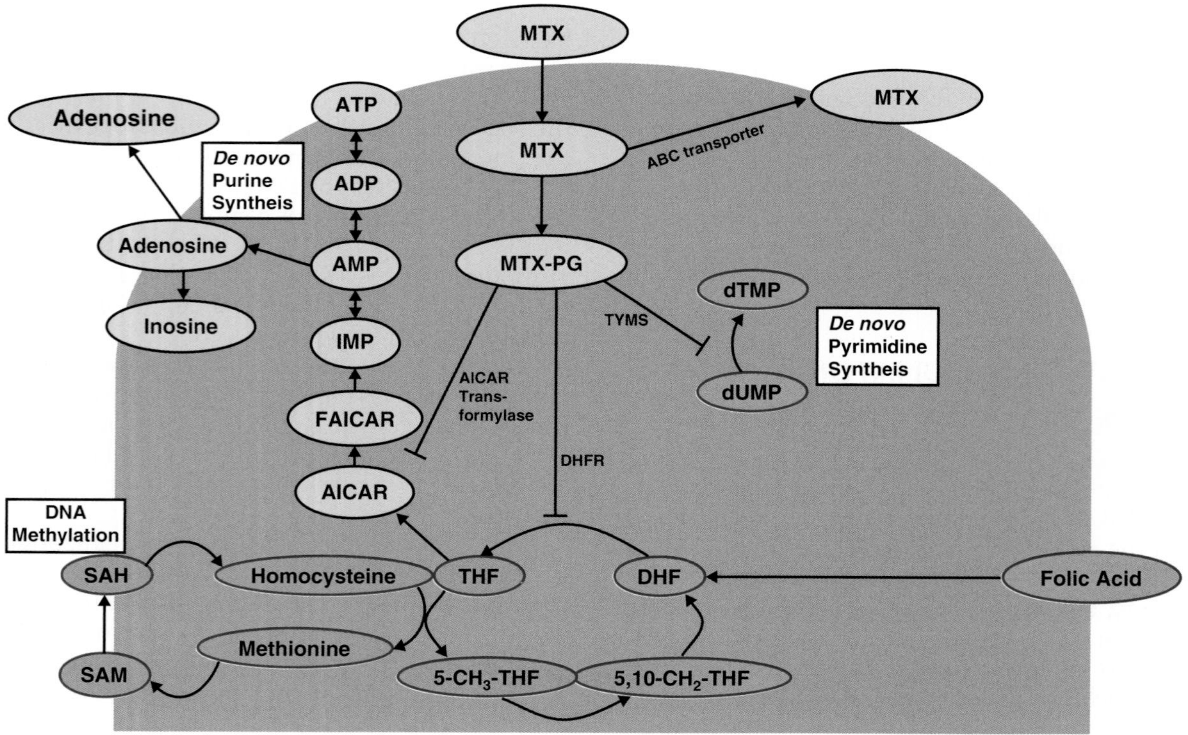

Figure 36.4 Several mechanisms of action contribute to the anti-inflammatory effects of methotrexate. Methotrexate inhibits de novo purine and pyrimidine synthesis, the methylation of DNA, and increases the level of adenosine leading to suppression of inflammation. ABC transporters, adenosine triphosphate–binding cassette transporters; ADP, adenosine diphosphate; AICAR, 5-aminoimidazole-4-carboxamide ribonucleotide; AMP, adenosine monophosphate; ATP, adenosine triphosphate; DHF, dihydrofolate; DHFR, dihydrofolate reductase; dTMP, deoxythymidine-5′-monophosphate; dUMP, deoxyuridine-5′-monophosphate; FAICAR, 10-formyl-AICAR; IMP, inosine monophosphate; MTX, methotrexate; MTX-PG, methotrexate polyglutamates; SAH, S-adenosylhomocysteine; SAM, S-adenosylmethionine; THF, tetrahydrofolate; TYMS, thymidylate synthase. Adapted from Cronstein BN. The mechanism of action of methotrexate. *Rheum Dis Clin North Am.* 1997;23(4):739-755.

MTX-PG inhibition of ATIC results in increased levels of adenosine via three other mechanisms. Increased amounts of AICAR resulting from ATIC inhibition in turn inhibit adenosine monophosphate deaminase, which leads to increased production of adenosine from AMP. Decreased conversion of adenosine to inosine due to inhibition of adenosine deaminase by AICAR results in accumulation of adenosine, and finally AICAR activation of ecto-5′-nucleotidase converts extracellular AMP to adenosine.[37]

Adenosine has tissue protective functions in response to harmful stimuli by inducing vasodilation and inhibiting inflammation.[38] Adenosine receptor ligation suppresses many inflammatory mediators, including IL-6, IL-8, IL-12, TNF, leukotriene B4, MIP-1α, and nitric oxide, and increases production of anti-inflammatory mediators IL-10 and IL-1 receptor antagonists.[31,39-41]

Methotrexate has been suggested to have a beneficial effect on cardiovascular health in RA patients, who have a higher incidence of cardiovascular disease compared to the general population and may protect against stroke, congestive heart failure, and acute myocardial infarction.[28] Adenosine's cardiovascular effects include negative inotropic and chronotropic effects, decreased adrenergic response, inhibition of vascular smooth muscle proliferation, and decreases in platelet aggregation. The beneficial effect of MTX on cardiovascular health likely arises from increases in adenosine production.

Pharmacology and Toxicity of Methotrexate. At the low doses typically employed in the treatment of RA (<15 mg/wk), MTX can be administered either orally or parenterally (SQ or IM). Absorption is rapid, peaking at 1-2 hours for oral administration, and at 0.1-1 hour for parenteral. The absorption of low-dose oral MTX is variable, and when the dose exceeds 15 mg/wk, absorption may diminish by as much as 30%.[42] Parenterally dosed MTX exhibits a linear increase in systemic levels with increasing dosage. Higher systemic levels of MTX in the treatment of rheumatoid arthritis have not been associated with increases in toxicity.[43,44] A recent study comparing parenteral versus oral administration of MTX at equivalent doses showed improved efficacy for parenteral administration.[45]

Orally administered MTX is not affected by food intake, though absorption may be affected by intestinal pathologies, such as malabsorptive conditions or inflammatory bowel disease.[46] Orally administered MTX is absorbed in the gastrointestinal tract (GI) and passes through the liver via the hepatic artery. For this reason, the parenteral route of administration is considered to have diminished likelihood of hepatotoxicity.

MTX is 50%-60% plasma protein bound and has a plasma half-life of 6 hours.[47] MTX can be displaced by highly protein-bound drugs, though this displacement has more clinical significance when MTX is employed in the treatment of cancer than with the lower doses employed for RA.

Intracellular polyglutamination of methotrexate produces MTX-PG, which is also biologically active. Methotrexate undergoes up to five glutaminations, with the mono- to pentaglutamate all biologically active. Once a stable dose of MTX has been achieved for a patient, the median time until 90% of the maximal steady-state concentration of MTX-PG was 27.5 weeks. Most MTX is excreted in urine within the first 12 hours, though MTX-PG is very slowly excreted from the cell and thus eliminated much more slowly. The estimated half-life for MTX-PG is 3.1 weeks, with MTX-PG3 the most common subtype (30% of total MTX-PG) and possessing an elimination half-life of 4.1 weeks.[48]

Numerous trials have compared the efficacy of methotrexate to other DMARDs in the treatment of rheumatoid arthritis.[49] MTX was found to be superior to placebo, auranofin and hydroxychloroquine and comparable to penicillamine, sulfasalazine, and IM gold. No trial has ever suggested than any other traditional DMARD is more efficacious than methotrexate.[50]

Despite the concerns resulting from toxicities associated with methotrexate therapy in the treatment of cancer, MTX is well tolerated when given once a week in the doses used in the treatment of RA. Most of the toxicities associated with MTX therapy are dose-dependent and related to folate deficiency, and respond well to folate replacement therapy. Other toxicities (e.g., pneumonitis) appear to be allergic or idiopathic, and usually require discontinuation of therapy.

Life-threatening drug interactions are known to occur between methotrexate and NSAIDs, probenecid, and penicillin G.[51] The NSAIDs (salicylate, ibuprofen, ketoprofen, piroxicam, and indomethacin), probenecid, and penicillin G dose dependently inhibit methotrexate elimination into urine by human organic anion transporters (hOAT1, hOAT3, and hOAT4). The inhibitory effects of these drugs on hOAT3 were comparable within therapeutically relevant plasma concentrations of unbound drugs. Thus, patients with rheumatoid arthritis should not take NSAIDs while taking methotrexate.

Methotrexate therapy requires monitoring of liver enzymes and is contraindicated in those with hepatic disease and in women considering pregnancy.

LEFLUNOMIDE. Leflunomide (Arava, LEF) is an isoxazole derivative that was discovered during an NSAID drug discovery program and that has potent immunomodulatory effects. It slows joint damage in adults who have moderately to severely active rheumatoid arthritis. It is chemically unrelated to any other immunosuppressant. Leflunomide is a prodrug and is rapidly and completely converted to its active α-cyanoenol metabolite teriflunomide in the GI tract and liver (Fig. 36.5).

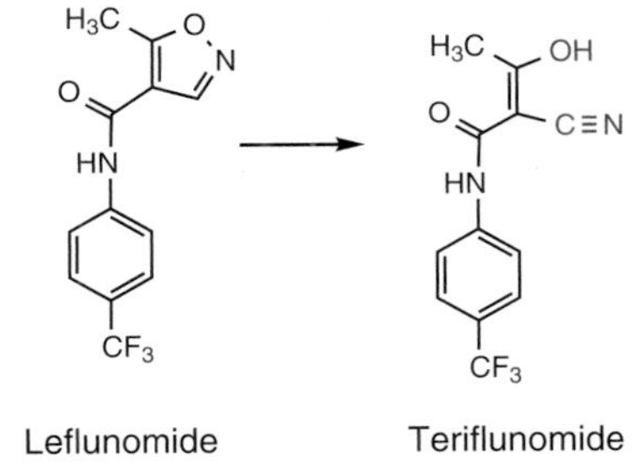

Figure 36.5 Leflunomide reductive activation to teriflunomide.

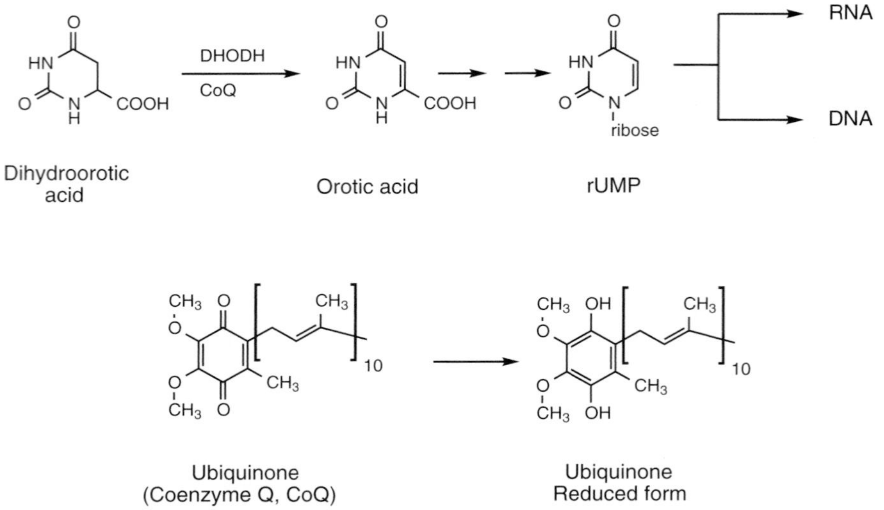

Figure 36.6 DHODH and ubiquinone reduction leading to formation of RNA and DNA.

As with methotrexate, the precise mechanism by which leflunomide operates in rheumatoid arthritis is not completely understood.[52] Leflunomide's action results in a net reduction of activated T cell and B cell lymphocytes, resulting in reduced antibody formation. At the concentration of teriflunomide achieved in patient use the primary effect appears to be inhibition of the enzyme dihydroorotate dehydrogenase (DHODH), which results in lowered pyrimidine synthesis. At higher concentrations, teriflunomide also inhibits phosphorylation by a number of tyrosine kinases involved in cell signal transduction.[53] It is unclear whether concentrations capable of eliciting this effect are achieved in vivo.

DHODH in combination with coenzyme Q (CoQ, ubiquinone) mediates the conversion of dihydroorotic acid to orotic acid in the mitochondria. Orotic acid then moves to the cytoplasm where it is phosphorylated to orotidine monophosphate, and then converted to ribonucleotide uridine monophosphate (rUMP) and ultimately to RNA and DNA. The reduction of dihydroorotic acid to orotic acid occurs concurrently with the reduction of its cofactor, coenzyme Q. Inhibition of DHODH lowers the quantity of rUMP produced and ultimately prevents the de novo synthesis of RNA and DNA (Fig. 36.6).[54,55]

Resting lymphocytes maintain their ribonucleotide requirements through salvage pathways and are largely unaffected by leflunomide.[56] When the T cell is activated, and the process of replication is initiated, the restricted pool of rUMP resulting from DHODH inhibition by teriflunomide triggers p53, which then translocates to the nucleus and initiates apoptosis and cell cycle arrest.

Leflunomide is administered as a once-daily dose, and its absorption is unaffected by food. Therapy can be initiated by a loading dose given over 3 days, and steady state is reached within 7 weeks after daily dosing. It undergoes primarily enterohepatic circulation, extending its duration of action. Cholestyramine can be used to enhance elimination in cases of toxicity.

SULFASALAZINE. Sulfasalazine (SSZ, occasionally SASP) was the first drug to be developed specifically for rheumatoid arthritis. Produced in 1938 in Sweden, SSZ was designed to possess both anti-inflammatory and antibacterial action because it was believed at the time that RA was caused by bacterial infection. SSZ is a conjugate of the anti-inflammatory 5-aminosalicylic acid (5-ASA) and the antibiotic sulfapyridine joined by an azo bond (Fig. 36.7). Sulfasalazine is converted to these two agents after reduction by colonic bacteria.

In spite of more than eight decades of use, the mechanism of action for sulfasalazine in the treatment of RA has not been fully elucidated, and it is likely that multiple different actions of the drug are in play. It was originally believed that alterations in gut flora resulting from the actions of sulfapyridine contributed to SSZ's therapeutic actions with RA. However, no correlation between gut flora and clinical response to SSZ has been discovered to date.[57] Additionally, a lack of evidence for an infectious cause of RA and the lack of efficacy of other sulfonamide antibiotics in the treatment of RA has caused this hypothesis to fall out of favor. Currently, SSZ is believed to operate via anti-inflammatory and immunomodulatory mechanisms.

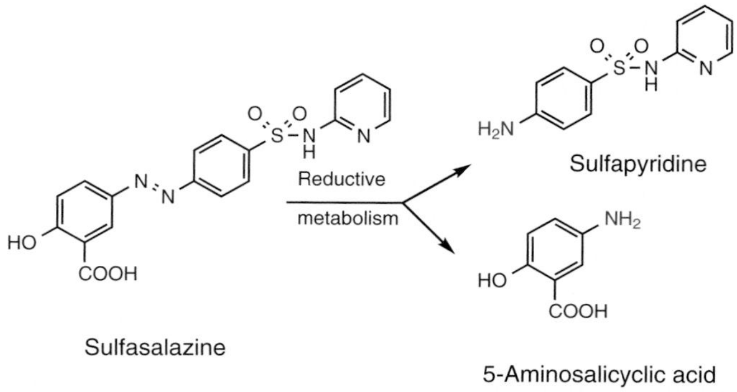

Figure 36.7 Sulfasalazine metabolism.

SSZ has several anti-inflammatory properties. In common with methotrexate, SSZ inhibits folate-dependent enzymes, including ATIC and DHFR, resulting in increased adenosine release.[58] This effect seems to be the effect of SSZ alone, as 5-ASA and sulfapyridine are inactive against these enzymes. Sulfasalazine also inhibits several enzymes involved in the arachidonic acid cascade, which further contributes to its anti-inflammatory properties.[59]

SSZ's immunomodulatory activities include inhibited T cell proliferation, natural killer (NK) cell activity, and B cell activation, with resultant reductions in immunoglobulin and RF production.[57] The intracellular quantities of many cytokines are also altered by SSZ, likely through the inhibition of NF-κB translocation to the nucleus.[60] NF-κB is an important transcription factor that promotes the production of many key cytokines and chemokines important to the immune response.

Following oral administration, sulfasalazine is poorly absorbed, with approximately 20% of the ingested sulfasalazine reaching the systemic circulation.[61] The remainder of the ingested dose is metabolized by colonic bacteria into its components, sulfapyridine and 5-ASA. Most of the sulfapyridine metabolized from sulfasalazine (60%-80%) is absorbed in the colon following oral administration, and approximately 25% of the 5-ASA metabolized from sulfasalazine is absorbed in the colon. The apparent volume of distribution of sulfasalazine in eight healthy volunteers was 64 L/kg, and that of sulfapyridine was 0.4-1.2 L/kg. Protein binding is approximately 99% for sulfasalazine, approximately 50% for sulfapyridine, and approximately 43% for 5-ASA. The absorbed sulfapyridine is acetylated and hydroxylated in the liver, followed by conjugation with glucuronic acid and, for 5-ASA, acetylation in the intestinal mucosal wall and the liver.[39] The elimination half-life is 5-10 hours for sulfasalazine and 6-14 hours for sulfapyridine, depending on acetylator status of the patient, and 0.6-1.4 hours for 5-ASA. Time to peak serum concentration is 1.5-6 hours for oral sulfasalazine and 9-24 hours for oral sulfapyridine; for enteric-coated tablets, time to peak serum concentration is 3-12 hours for sulfasalazine and 12-24 hours for sulfapyridine. Approximately 5% of sulfapyridine and 67% of 5-ASA are eliminated in feces, and 75%-91% of sulfasalazine and sulfapyridine metabolites are excreted in urine within 3 days, depending on the dosage form used. 5-ASA is excreted in urine mostly in acetylated form.

Sulfasalazine is used for the treatment of mild-to-moderate ulcerative colitis; as adjunct therapy in the treatment of severe ulcerative colitis; for the treatment of Crohn's disease; and for the treatment of rheumatoid arthritis or ankylosing spondylitis. Contraindications include hypersensitivity to sulfa drugs, salicylates, intestinal or urinary obstruction, and porphyria.

Antimalarials in the Treatment of RA: Chloroquine and Hydroxychloroquine. The aminoquinolines chloroquine (CQ) and hydroxychloroquine (HCQ) are antimalarial agents that have been employed in the treatment of rheumatoid arthritis since the early 1950s (Fig. 36.8). Quinine, the prototypical aminoquinoline antimalarial, was originally isolated from the Peruvian cinchona tree. The 4-aminoquinoline derivatives CQ and HCQ possess reduced toxicity relative to quinine and are the most commonly prescribed (though not the most effective) drugs for the treatment of malaria. CQ and HCQ are identical, except for the addition of a hydroxyl group on the terminal carbon of the aminoethyl functionality. Chloroquine is no longer employed in the treatment of RA due to corneal and renal toxicity, though most of the data available for the use of the aminoquinolines in the treatment of rheumatic disease relate to CQ. It is assumed that HCQ operates in a very similar fashion to CQ. Hydroxychloroquine is considered to be less effective as a DMARD compared to chloroquine. One to two months of treatment is necessary to observe beneficial effects for RA.

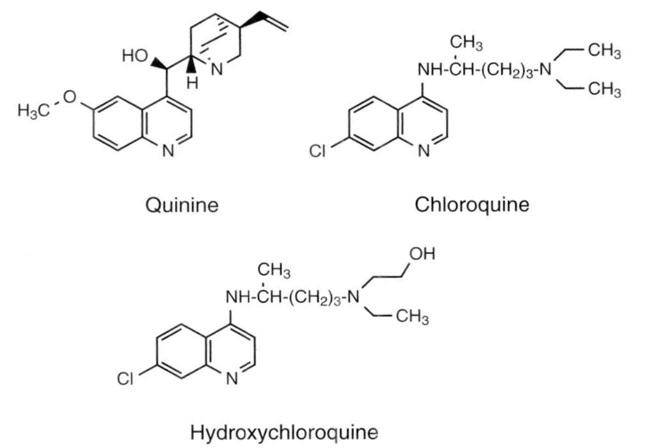

Quinine

Chloroquine

Hydroxychloroquine

Figure 36.8 Antimalarial medications used in the treatment of rheumatoid arthritis.

Though antimalarial agents have been employed as DMARDs in the treatment of RA for decades, their mechanism of action in the treatment of rheumatic disease remains unclear. CQ and HCQ have both immunomodulatory and anti-inflammatory properties, and both of these contribute to their beneficial effects. Both agents are weak bases and pass through cytoplasmic membranes to accumulate in cytoplasmic vesicles, where they increase the vesicle pH from 4.0 to 6.0 and interfere with acid-dependent cellular processes.[62,63] This change is postulated to have a number of immunomodulatory effects. Macrophages and monocytes require precise pH conditions for protein digestion and antigen recognition, and the raised pH caused by HCQ interferes with these processes.[64] The raised pH is also postulated to stabilize the lysosomal membrane and to slow antigen processing. Specifically, the increased pH in the endoplasmic reticulum affects class II major histocompatibility complex (MHC) molecules by stabilizing the invariant chains and preventing their displacement by low-affinity autoantigens. This leads to a decrease in antigen presentation. HCQ is also known to upregulate apoptosis of immune cells, specifically autoreactive lymphocyte clones that are involved in the pathological perpetuation of autoimmunity.[63]

Anti-inflammatory properties of the antimalarials involve inhibition of the arachadonic acid cascade by downregulation of phospholipases A2 and C. Additionally, HCQ blocks IL-1, IL-6, and interferon (IFN)-γ and may inhibit TNF.

TOFACITINIB. Tofacitinib (Xeljanz) is an orally active immunosuppressant used for treatment of moderate-to-severe rheumatoid arthritis in patients who have an inadequate response to, or are intolerant of, methotrexate. When added to methotrexate as a combination therapy, tofacitinib and adalimumab were noninferior in terms of efficacy and possessed similar tolerability.[65]

Tofacitinib is also being investigated for the treatment of inflammatory bowel disease, psoriasis, and for the prevention of transplant rejection, as well as other immunological diseases.

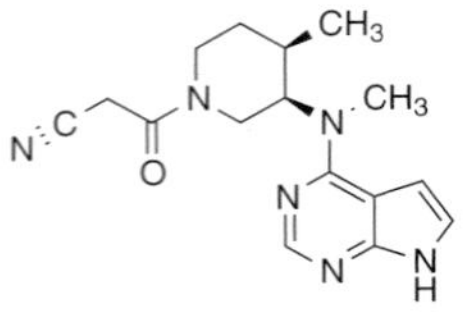

Tofacitinib (Xeljanz)

Tofacitinib specifically inhibits janus kinase (JAK) 1 and 3, interfering with the JAK-STAT pathway and blocking proinflammatory cytokine signaling, thus preventing the expression of both B and T cells.[66,67] Tofacitinib is approved in the United States, Japan, and Switzerland, but not in Europe because of concerns over safety and efficacy. Studies investigating the efficacy of tofacitinib suggest this new drug may be as effective as TNF-α inhibitors (TNFi). Dose-dependent decreases in white blood cell counts and increases in low-density lipoprotein cholesterol, high-density lipoprotein cholesterol, total cholesterol, and serum creatinine levels were observed in patients treated with tofacitinib. The most frequent treatment-related adverse events (<5%) were urinary tract infection, diarrhea, bronchitis, and headache. Some hepatic metabolism of tofacitinib by CYP3A4/5 and CYP2C19 in human liver microsomes and hepatocytes was observed. The low clearance of the drug in humans occurred via a combination of renal excretion of unchanged drug and low hepatic metabolic clearance. Volume of distribution in humans was 1.9 L/kg, with a terminal elimination half-life of 7 hours. Tofacitinib is given as a once- or twice-daily dose.

BARICITINIB. Baricitinib (Olumiant) is also an oral JAK inhibitor used in the treatment of RA. In this case, baricitinib specifically inhibits JAK1 and JAK2 with much less affinity for JAK3 relative to tofacitinib. The drug is currently approved in Europe and more recently received FDA approval in the United States for treatment of RA patients with moderately to severely active disease who have not responded to TNF antagonist therapies. Baricitinib is well absorbed and excreted largely unchanged, and inhibition of various CYP enzymes had no clinically relevant influence on baricitinib plasma concentrations. The most common side effects observed were increased cholesterol levels (in common with tofacitinib) and upper respiratory tract infections. An increase in herpes zoster was also observed in clinical trials of baricitinib.

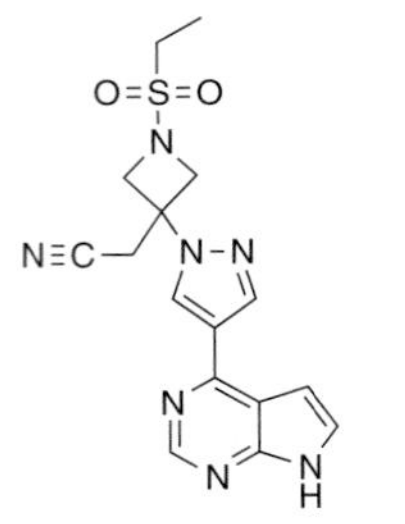

Baricitinib (Olumiant)

Biologic DMARDs

The treatment of RA has dramatically improved through the introduction of biologic DMARDs into the clinic. Several classes of biologic DMARDs have been developed to target multiple inflammatory mediators involved in the pathogenesis of RA, including inhibiting the cytokines TNF-α, IL-1, and IL-6. Other biologics carry out their immunomodulating effects by depleting B cells and blocking T cell activation. In contrast to most of the synthetic DMARDs, the biologic DMARDs are highly targeted therapies with specific and well-understood actions.

Substantial biotechnological efforts have gone into the development of high-affinity therapeutic antibodies that have target specificity while minimizing immunogenicity. These biotechnological processes are detailed in Chapter 5. Monoclonal antibodies (Mab) have important structural regions that can be manipulated to form highly specific therapeutics against a specific antigen (Fig. 36.9). The immunoglobulin G (IgG) class of antibodies are employed widely as therapeutics. IgG antibodies are glycoproteins that are composed of two different polypeptide chains—2 identical light (L) chains and 2 identical heavy (H) chains (Fig. 36.9). Disulfide bonds link together the two heavy chains and the light chain and heavy chain of each arm of the antibody. The amino-terminal end of each these chains is a highly variable (V) amino acid sequence, while the carboxy-terminal region is less variable and is referred to as constant (C). The variability of the V region provides for greater diversity in antigen-binding specificity of the Mab. Two functional fragments of immunoglobulins are responsible for antigen binding and interaction with effector molecules and cells. The Fc region (fragment crystallizable) is responsible for mediating the biological activity of the antibody through interactions with effector cells and consists of the CH_2 and CH_3 domains. The Fc portion of the Mab is not antigen specific and interacts with immune cells to determine whether the target is eliminated by complement-dependent cytotoxicity (CDC) or antibody dependent cell-mediated cytotoxicity (ADCC) clearance pathways. The fragment antigen-binding region (Fab fragment) consists of V_H, V_L, C_H1, and C_L and is the

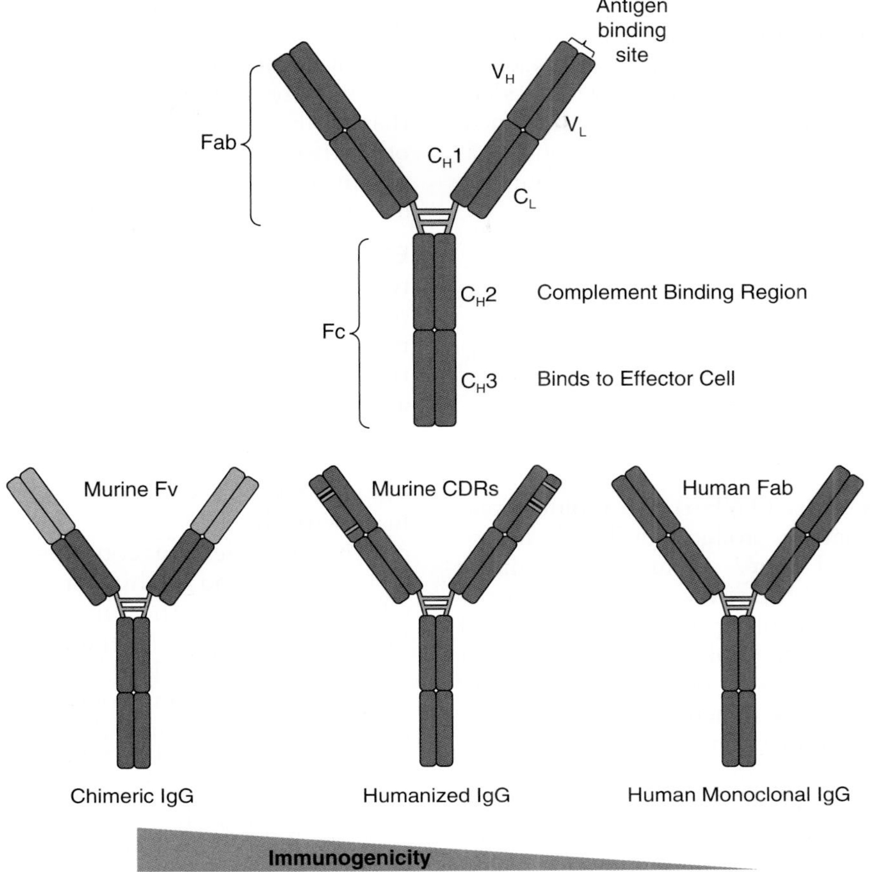

Figure 36.9 Monoclonal antibody structure and scale of immunogenicity.

region where antigen binds to the antibody. The variable region within the Fab fragment contains 6 hypervariable regions called the complementarity-determining regions (CDRs) that are responsible for antigen recognition. Each arm of the Fab binds a single antigen epitope. The immunogenicity of the Mab is largely determined by the murine component of the CDRs of the Fab, ranging from an entirely murine Fv (a chimeric antibody), to containing some murine CDRs (humanized) to fully human with no murine components. While Mab drugs demonstrate impressive specificity for their biological targets, the fact that the monoclonal antibody protein structure of many of these agents contains murine portions that can generate an immunogenic response impacts the efficacy of these therapeutics. The goal is to design a Mab with high target specificity while reducing immunogenicity by minimizing or eliminating the murine component of the Mab.

The nomenclature of monoclonal antibodies provides insight into the target for the drug as well as the source and potential immunogenicity of the Mab (Fig. 36.10). The prefix has no special meaning and is unique for each drug. Adalimumab and golimumab are both fully human Mabs that differ in chemical structure but have the same target; therefore a different prefix was used for each drug. The target substem refers to the tissue, pathogen, or protein target of the drug. For example, those drugs that target

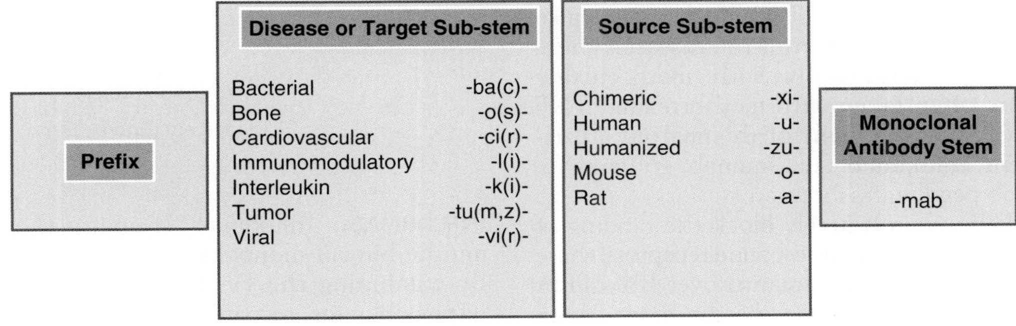

Figure 36.10 Monoclonal antibody nomenclature.

the immune system contain the substem -li-, such as ada**li**mumab. Drugs that target a specific interleukin have the substem -ki-, such as the interleukin-1 receptor antagonist, ana**ki**nra. The source sub-stem of the antibody name identifies the organism from which the antibody was obtained. Antibodies that are not fully human are recognized as foreign by the immune system and may illicit an immune response. The immune response can potentially cause the drugs to be ineffective and can result in adverse side effects including an allergic response. The more human a Mab is, the less likely it is to produce an immunogenic response. The source substem -xi- indicates the Mab is chimeric, -zu- is used to indicate a less immunogenic humanized Mab, and fully human Mab have the source substem -u- and are the least immunogenic source of antibodies.

Tumor Necrosis Factor Inhibitors

Tumor necrosis factor alpha (TNF-α) is a proinflammatory cytokine that is primarily produced by T cells, monocytes, and macrophages. TNF-α is an important mediator of local inflammation, and the release of TNF-α from T cells produces increased vascular permeability, release of nitric oxide with vasodilation, local activation of vascular endothelium, increased expression of adhesion molecules on endothelial blood vessels, and increased platelet activation and adhesion. TNF-α plays an important role in the pathogenesis of RA by stimulating the production of additional inflammatory cytokines such as IL-1 and IL-6 (both of which are targets of biologic DMARDs), by increasing the proliferation and the activation of immune effector cells, and by inducing chondrocytes and osteoclasts, ultimately leading to joint damage and deformity. Biologically active TNF exists in both soluble and membrane-bound forms, and all currently approved TNF inhibitors (TNFi) block both forms of TNF-α. Inhibiting TNF has been shown to reduce levels of inflammatory cytokines, chemokines, adhesion molecules, and matrix metalloproteinases within the joint.

Three different approaches have been developed to decrease TNF activity that have resulted in marketable drugs: administration of soluble TNF receptors (TNFRs; e.g., etanercept), use of PEGylated anti-TNF-α Fab fragments (e.g., certolizumab pegol), and treatment with anti-TNF-α antibodies (e.g., infliximab, adalimumab). These compounds are designed to target and neutralize the effects of TNF, and help to reduce pain and morning stiffness, and relieve tender or swollen joints, usually within 1 or 2 weeks after treatment begins. Evidence suggests that TNF blockers can also halt the radiographic progression of the disease. These medications work synergistically with methotrexate and therefore are often taken with methotrexate. TNF blockers approved for treatment of rheumatoid arthritis are etanercept, infliximab, adalimumab, golimumab, and certolizumab pegol.

Though all TNFi nonselectively block the binding of TNF to both soluble and membrane-bound receptors, these medications fail to be effective in treating over 30% of RA patients.[68] TNFi therapy failure may be the result of the immunogenicity of the TNFi or pharmacogenomic effects. Interestingly, the presence of antidrug antibodies against one TNFi does not preclude the use of another TNFi.[69] RA is a heterogeneous disease, and it is likely that in some patient populations additional proinflammatory cytokines and immune cells play a larger role in RA pathogenesis than TNF. Such patients may respond more favorably to other treatment regimens.[70] Other factors may also play a role in decreased patient response to TNFi treatment, such as a history of cigarette use and obesity.[69]

ETANERCEPT. Etanercept (Enbrel) is produced by recombinant DNA technology in a Chinese hamster ovary mammalian cell line and was the first biotechnology-derived drug to be introduced for the reduction of the signs and symptoms of moderate to severe active rheumatoid arthritis in patients who have not adequately responded to one or more of the synthetic DMARDs. It is a fusion protein comprising two recombinant 75-kDa TNF-receptor 2 (TNF-R2/p75) portions fused with the Fc domain of human IgG1. The Fc component of etanercept contains the CH2 domain, the CH3 domain, and the hinge region of IgG1, but not the CH1 domain from the Fab region of IgG1. Etanercept functions as a decoy receptor and can bind specifically to two molecules of TNF-α. It is able to bind both the soluble and membrane-bound forms of TNF-α and has been shown to induce ADCC-mediated cell death. Etanercept is the only TNFi that inhibits lymphotoxin-beta (LT-β), also known as TNF-β. Etanercept is administered as a clear and colorless subcutaneous injection at a dose of 25-50 mg once weekly or 25 mg twice weekly. Etanercept is available as a powder for injection in single-use vials containing 25 mg of the drug. It can be used as monotherapy or in combination with methotrexate. Etanercept has a half-life of 4.3 days and is FDA approved for both RA and JIA. In addition to risk of lymphomas, patients receiving etanercept have nervous system-based adverse events such as multiple sclerosis, myelitis, and optic neuritis.[71]

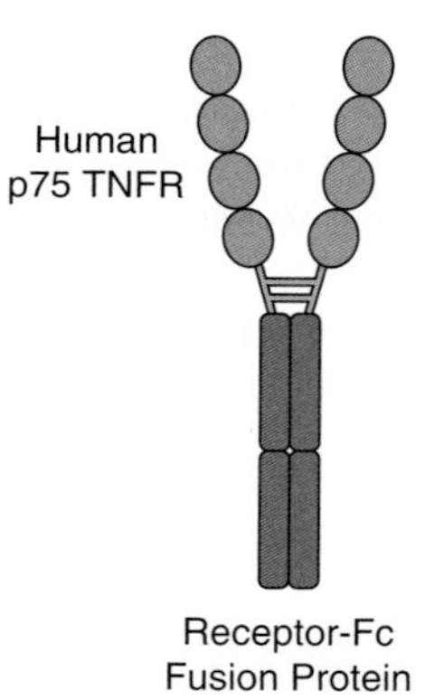

Etanercept (Enbrel, Erelzi)

INFLIXIMAB. Infliximab (Remicade) is a chimeric murine-human monoclonal antibody to human TNF-α. By combining the Fv domain of the mouse antibody responsible for recognizing TNF-α with parts of the human Fc domain of IgG1 (IgG1κ), the fused protein looks more like normal human IgG1, providing a better chance the fused protein will not be destroyed by the patient's own immune system. Infliximab binds specifically, with high affinity, to both the transmembrane and soluble forms of TNF-α in the blood, thus neutralizing its biologic activity and inducing both ADCC and CDC, resulting in the death of cells with bound infliximab antibodies. Infliximab is administered by IV infusion at a dose of 3 mg/kg every 8 weeks and has a half-life of 8-9.5 days. After treatment with infliximab, patients with rheumatoid arthritis exhibited reduced infiltration of inflammatory cells and TNF-α production in inflamed tissues and decreased levels of serum IL-6 and CRP compared to baseline. In psoriatic arthritis, treatment with infliximab resulted in a reduction in the number of T cells and blood vessels in the synovium and psoriatic skin as well as a reduction of macrophages in the synovium. Single IV infusions showed a linear relationship between the dose administered and the maximum serum concentration. The volume of distribution at steady-state was independent of dose and indicated that infliximab was distributed primarily within the vascular compartment. The terminal half-life of infliximab is 8.0-9.5 days. No systemic accumulation of infliximab occurred on continued repeated treatment at 4- or 8-week intervals.

Infliximab is supplied as a sterile, white, lyophilized powder formulated for IV infusion. Following reconstitution with sterile water for injection, the solution should be used immediately after reconstitution, because the vials do not contain antibacterial preservatives. The reconstituted solution should be colorless to light yellow and opalescent.

Infliximab is indicated for the treatment of rheumatoid arthritis in combination with methotrexate. Long-term use can be associated with the development of anti-infliximab antibodies (neutralizing antibodies), an effect that does not appear when it is used with methotrexate. Warnings associated with the use of infliximab include risks of autoimmunity, infections, and hypersensitivity reactions. Infliximab has also been associated with exacerbating congestive heart failure in already diagnosed patients. Patients may be pretreated with acetaminophen, antihistamines, and corticosteroids to reduce infusion reactions.

ADALIMUMAB. Adalimumab (Humira) is a recombinant human IgG1 monoclonal antibody targeted for soluble and membrane-bound forms of human TNF-α. Adalimumab is produced by recombinant DNA technology in a mammalian cell expression system using a protein-engineering strategy for creating a TNF-α antibody with human-derived, heavy- and light-chain variable regions (Fab) and human IgG1κ constant regions. Adalimumab works by targeting and binding TNF-α, thus neutralizing the effect of TNF-α, reducing the symptoms of rheumatoid arthritis, and slowing the progression of structural joint damage caused by the disease. Adalimumab is supplied in single-use, prefilled, glass syringes as a sterile, preservative-free, colorless solution for subcutaneous administration. The pharmacokinetic profile of adalimumab was linear over the dose range of 0.5-10.0 mg/kg following a single IV dose. The mean elimination half-life was approximately 2 weeks. Adalimumab is indicated for use in RA and JIA patients as a monotherapy or in combination with MTX.

GOLIMUMAB. Golimumab (Simponi and Simponi ARIA) is a recombinant human IgG1 monoclonal antibody that binds with high affinity and specificity to both soluble and membrane-bound forms of human TNF-α. Golimumab is produced by a murine hybridoma cell line with recombinant DNA technology. Golimumab (Simponi) is supplied as a single-use, preservative-free, sterile solution in a glass syringe for SC administration monthly. The IV version of golimumab (Simponi ARIA) is supplied as a colorless to light yellow sterile solution in preservative-free single use vials and is administered at a dose of 2 mg/kg every 8 weeks in combination with MTX. Golimumab exhibited approximately dose-proportional blood levels over the dose range of 0.1-10.0 mg/kg following a single IV dose. The mean terminal half-life of golimumab is approximately 2 weeks. The most notable advantage golimumab possesses over other TNFi is dosing (injected subcutaneously once a month, whereas adalimumab is injected subcutaneously every other week, etanercept is injected subcutaneously weekly, and infliximab is injected by IV infusion every 8 weeks).

CERTOLIZUMAB PEGOL. Certolizumab pegol (Cimzia) is a recombinant humanized Fab fragment conjugated to a 40-kDa polyethylene glycol that targets human TNF-α. The Fab fragment is manufactured utilizing *Escherichia coli*, purified and then conjugated to PEG2MAL40K (polyethylene glycol) to produce certolizumab pegol. The PEGylation does not elicit an immunogenic response and protects the Fab fragment from enzymatic digestion, as well as decreasing the production of neutralizing antibodies and increasing retention in the circulation. Certolizumab pegol has been shown to accumulate in inflamed tissues to a greater extent than other TNFi's, such as infliximab and adalimumab.[72-74] Certolizumab pegol lacks the Fc antibody region and therefore cannot fix complement, induce antibody-dependent cellular toxicity (ADCC), or cause apoptosis of activated immune cells. However, limited studies indicate that certolizumab induces non-apoptotic cell death mediated through transmembrane signaling.[75]

Certolizumab is supplied as 200 mg of lyophilized powder in a single-dose vial for reconstitution. The reconstituted solution is administered subcutaneously and has a terminal half-life of approximately 14 days. Metabolism of the Fab fragment is unknown, whereas the PEG moiety is excreted in urine. Certolizumab is indicated for the treatment of adults with moderate-to-severe rheumatoid arthritis as a monotherapy or in combination with MTX.

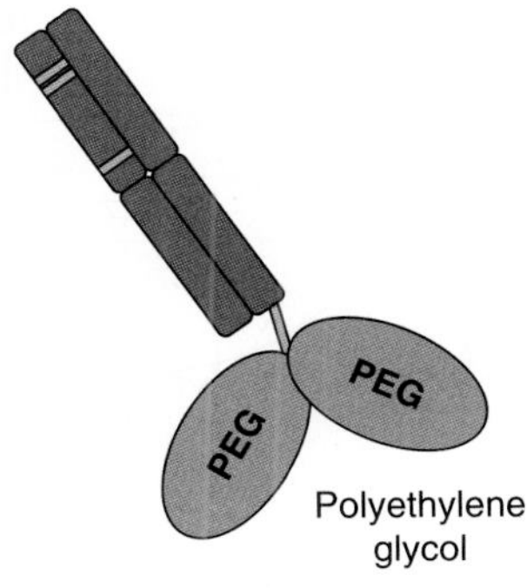

Certolizumab pegol (Cimzia)

Safety Profile for TNFi

Potential side effects of TNF antagonists include injection site irritation, blood disorders, lymphoma (primarily reported in adolescents), demyelinating diseases, increased risk of infection, and worsening of congestive heart failure (observed with infliximab). These drugs should not be taken if an active infection is present. A black-box warning was issued for all members of the TNFi class (etanercept, infliximab, adalimumab, golimumab, and certolizumab pegol) indicating an increased risk of developing serious infections that could lead to hospitalization or death. Most of the patients who developed serious infections were also being treated with an immunosuppressant, such as methotrexate or corticosteroids. TNFi treatment may reactivate latent tuberculosis, and patients should be screened for TB prior to initiating biologic therapy. Additional rescreening may be performed if the patient has TB risk factors.

Non-TNFi Biologic DMARDs

COSTIMULATION MODULATORS. Costimulatory molecules CD80 (also known as B7-1) and CD86 (B7-2) are expressed on antigen-presenting cells (APC), including B cells, monocytes, and dendritic cells. CD80 and CD86 are highly expressed on B cells from RA patients.[76] The increased expression of costimulatory molecules CD80 and CD86 is associated with an increase in the antigen-presenting capability of B cells and more efficient T cell activation. To become activated by an antigen, T cells require two signals that are delivered by APCs, referred to as costimulation. Regulation of costimulatory molecules is a mechanism whereby the immune system limits the extent of an immune response. If an unactivated APC (a cell that "presents" an antigen on its MHC that is recognized by the T-cell receptor (TCR)) presents an antigen to a T cell in the absence of an appropriate costimulatory signal, the T cell does not respond and becomes unreactive and nonresponsive to further antigenic stimuli (Fig. 36.11). The T-cell costimulatory activation pathway is initiated when an activated APC presents both an antigen and a costimulatory ligand, such as B7 (CD80 or CD86), that interacts with CD28 on the surface of the T cell to form B7-CD28 complex, initiating T-cell proliferation and differentiation in response to the antigenic stimulus. This stimulus causes the release of IL-2 that binds to the IL-2 receptor (IL-2R) on the T cell, further enhancing its activation. A counterbalance to CD28 is cytotoxic T-lymphocyte antigen-4 (CTLA-4), both of which are expressed on the surface of T cells. The CTLA-4, which is homologous with CD28, becomes expressed upon T-cell activation, where it then competes with CD28 for binding to B7 ligands on the surface of APCs. The B7 ligands bind with much greater affinity to CTLA-4 than to CD28, preventing delivery of the costimulatory signal. This built-in inhibition prevents T-cell activation from spiraling out of control. CTLA-4 is not expressed constitutively, and its expression is initiated upon T-cell activation. Eventually CD28 is downregulated and the T-cell activation cascade is halted. Since the formation of a B7-CD28 complex between the APC and the T cell results in T-cell proliferation and the release of inflammatory cytokines, whereas the B7–CTLA-4 interaction inhibits the T-cell responses, the design of a pharmacologic agent that prevents costimulation would preferentially inhibit only reactive T cells and be effective in the treatment of rheumatoid arthritis.

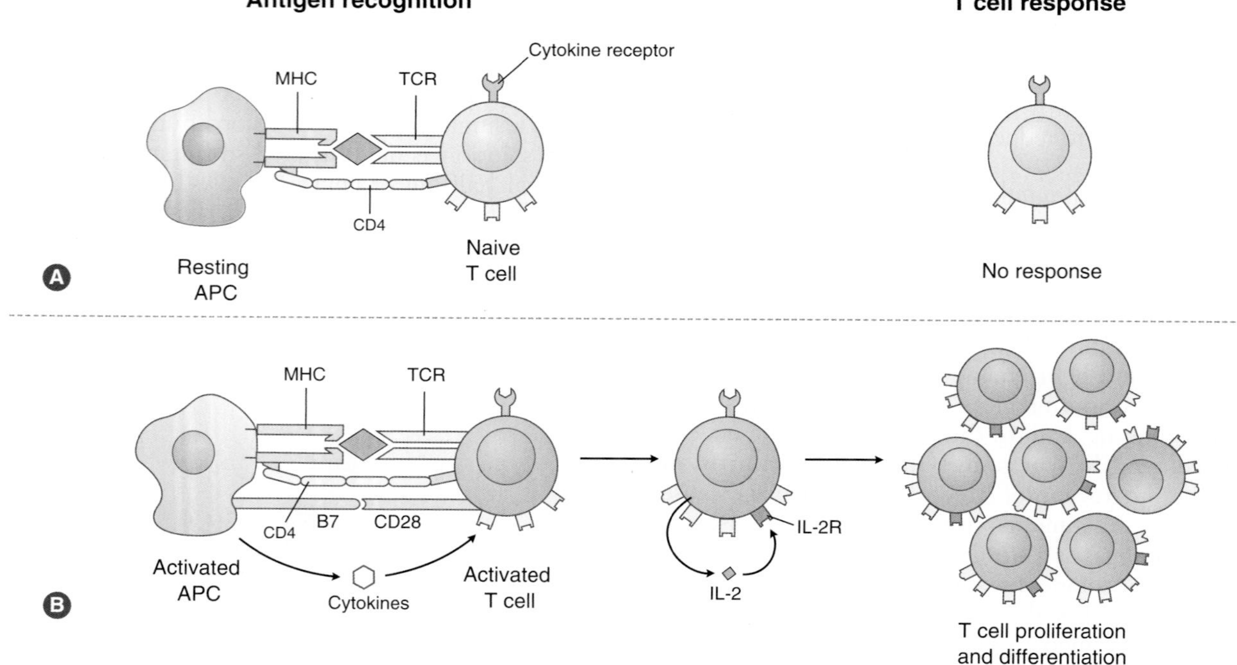

Figure 36.11 Costimulation in the T-cell activation pathway. A, No costimulation. B, With costimulation.

ABATACEPT. Abatacept (Orencia) is a novel chimeric CTLA-4–IgG1 fused protein created from the fusion of the extracellular domain of murine CTLA-4 with the modified heavy-chain constant region of human IgG1. Abatacept, therefore, acts like an antibody that binds with great affinity to CD80 and CD86, preventing these ligands from interacting with CD28 on activated T cells. In patients with rheumatoid arthritis, blocking this response by abatacept prevents the generation of positive costimulation signals and T-cell activation, thus suppressing the proliferation of reactive T cells and the release of tissue-destroying cytokines that produce the symptoms and signs of RA. The CTLA-4 portion of abatacept is responsible for the drug's affinity for B7 ligands. Abatacept has been shown to slow the damage to bones and cartilage of the joint and relieves the symptoms and signs of RA. Abatacept is administered as a subcutaneous injection or by IV infusion and has a half-life of 13-16 days. An induction phase is required for IV administration. Abatacept is approved for the treatment of RA and JIA as a monotherapy or in combination with MTX. The Corrona registry was used to compare the effectiveness of abatacept versus tocilizumab in patients with moderate-to-severe RA and that had prior exposure to TNFi. Patients who were treated with either abatacept or tocilizumab showed substantial improvement in disease activity with similar safety profiles.

IL-6 INHIBITION. Interleukin 6 (IL-6) is an inflammatory cytokine that is secreted by T cells and macrophages to stimulate immune response and is elevated both in the joint and systemically in RA patients. IL-6 induces the production of acute phase proteins such as CRP, promotes the differentiation of T cells into T effector cells and B cells into plasma cells, and stimulates RANKL in osteoblasts leading to osteoclast activation.

TOCILIZUMAB. Tocilizumab (Actemra) is a recombinant humanized anti-human IL-6 receptor (IL-6R) IgG1 monoclonal antibody that binds to both the soluble and membrane-bound forms of the IL-6R, preventing IL-6 signaling. Tocilizumab is administered by subcutaneous injection (half-life of 5-13 d) and by IV infusion (half-life 11-13 d). Patient response was similar for both forms of delivery.[77] In addition to its role in the inflammatory response, IL-6 also decreases blood lipid levels by increasing very-low-density lipoprotein receptor (VLDLR) expression.[78] Thus, treatment with tocilizumab is associated with increases in total cholesterol, triglycerides, and HDL levels, and a lipid monitoring plan is recommended for patients taking tocilizumab. Infections are the most common adverse reaction reported, and prescreening for TB is recommended. Gastrointestinal perforations have also been reported in patients with history of diverticulitis or on concomitant corticosteroid or NSAID treatment.[79]

IL-1 INHIBITION. IL-1α and IL-1β are inflammatory cytokines that are elevated in RA and have been shown to play a role in the pathogenesis of RA by activating monocytes, inducing fibroblast proliferation, and by activating both chondrocytes and osteoclasts leading to inflammation and cartilage and bone resorption and loss. The interleukin-1 receptor antagonist (IL-1RA) binds nonproductively to the IL-1R and prevents IL-1 from sending its signal to the cell.

ANAKINRA. Anakinra (Kineret), a recombinant human IL-1 receptor (IL-1R) antagonist, competitively blocks the cytokine IL-1 from binding and signaling through the IL-1R. Anakinra blocks the signaling of IL-1α and IL-1β through the IL-1R. Anakinra neutralizes the proinflammatory activity of IL-1 by competitively inhibiting the binding of IL-1 to IL-1RI, similar to the endogenous antagonist IL-1R antagonist. In vitro studies have shown that anakinra inhibits the induction of the inflammatory mediators nitric oxide, PGE2, and collagenase. Anakinra differs from native human IL-1RA in that it has the addition of a single methionine residue at its amino terminus. It is produced by recombinant DNA technology using an *E. coli* bacterial expression system. Anakinra is the first IL-1RA to be approved for use in adults with moderately to severely active rheumatoid arthritis who have not responded adequately to conventional DMARD therapy. It can be used either alone or in combination with methotrexate. Anakinra is supplied in single-use, prefilled, glass syringes as a sterile, clear, preservative-free solution that is administered daily as a subcutaneous injection. Potential side effects include injection site reactions, decreased white blood cell counts, headache, and an increase in upper respiratory infections. A slightly higher rate of respiratory infections in people who have asthma or chronic obstructive pulmonary disease has been observed. Persons with an active infection are advised not to use anakinra. Its elimination half-life after subcutaneous administration is 4-6 hours. The disadvantage of this bDMARD over others is the need for daily subcutaneous administration. Anakinra is not included in the 2015 ACR guidelines because of the lack of strong data of efficacy and infrequency of use.[14,80]

B Cell Depletion

B cells function to make antibodies, present antigens, secrete cytokines and chemokines, and generate memory B cells to enhance humoral immune response. Normal B cell function can become compromised when B cells become autoreactive and produce pathogenic autoantibodies, which leads to the downstream activation of additional immune mediators such as T cells. The presence of autoantibodies in RA patients indicates a breakdown in negative selection processes (the process of eliminating any B lymphocytes that are reactive to self antigens). The pathogenic role of B cells in RA was first identified with the discovery of RF (autoantibody against the Fc region of IgG antibodies) and the identification of anticyclic citrullinated peptides (anti-CCP) and more recently through the use of the B cell depletion as a therapy.[81,82]

RITUXIMAB. Rituximab (Rituxan) is a genetically engineered mouse-human chimeric anti-CD20 monoclonal IgG1 antibody that binds to CD20 antigen located exclusively on the surface of pre-B and mature B cells. Rituximab is produced by a mammalian cell (Chinese hamster ovary) culture system. The Fab portion of rituximab binds to CD20 on B cells, and the Fc portion induces mechanisms of B cell removal including ADCC, CDC, and apoptosis. In clinical trials, the majority of patients showed peripheral B-cell depletion for at least 6 months, followed by subsequent gradual recovery. A small proportion of patients (4%) had prolonged peripheral B-cell depletion lasting more than 3 years after a single course of treatment. Reduced total serum immunoglobulin levels (IgM, IgG, and IgA) have been observed 6 months post rituximab treatment. RA patients treated with rituximab showed decreased levels of inflammatory markers (IL-6 and CRP) and reductions in autoantibodies (anti-CCP, RF.) Of note, evidence of rituximab efficacy in RA is primarily from seropositive RA patients. Limited evidence is available for the efficacy of rituximab in seronegative RA patients. Rituximab has changed the treatment of rheumatoid arthritis by showing that targeted B-cell therapy in combination with methotrexate can reduce signs and symptoms of rheumatoid arthritis in adult patients with moderately to severely active rheumatoid arthritis who have had an inadequate response to one or more TNF antagonist therapies. Although B cells were once considered to be one of the main contributing factors in the pathogenesis of rheumatoid arthritis, recent evidence has shown that T cells, dendritic cells, and macrophages are also involved. Rituximab has rekindled interest in B cells, highlighting their importance in perpetuating the inflammatory process in seropositive patients and showing how they can interact with other cell types and contribute to joint inflammation.

Rituximab is a sterile, clear, colorless, preservative-free, liquid concentrate formulated for IV administration and has a median terminal half-life of approximately 18 days. For rheumatoid arthritis, rituximab is given as two 1,000-mg IV infusions separated by 2 weeks. Glucocorticoids are also recommended to reduce the incidence and severity of infusion reactions. Rituximab is given in combination with methotrexate. Its administration has been associated with hypersensitivity reactions (non–IgE-mediated reactions), which can respond to adjustments in the infusion rate and in medical management. People who have not found relief using TNF blockers might consider using rituximab. Side effects include flu-like symptoms such as fever, chills, and nausea. The response to killed vaccines may be reduced following rituximab therapy; therefore vaccines should be administered prior to therapy. Some people experience an "infusion-reaction complex," such as difficulty breathing and heart problems that can result in death.

Safety Concerns of Biologic DMARDs

The most significant safety concerns arising from the use of biologic DMARDs involve the impairment of defense mechanisms of the immune system. This increases the risk of developing serious infections in patients taking these medications. An increased risk of TB reactivation in patients treated with a TNFi has been shown.[83] ACR 2015 RA treatment guidelines recommend that all patients should be screened for TB prior to initiating biologic or tofacitinib therapy and additional rescreening be performed yearly if the patient has TB exposure risk factors. Live vaccines must be avoided while on biologic therapy. Additional infections have been reported resulting from the reactivation of herpes zoster, hepatitis B, and hepatitis C.

RA is a complex, systemic, and heterogeneous disease. Patients vary widely in disease severity and may present with severe destructive joint disease or a more slowly progressing form of the disease. Multiple immune cells, chemokines and cytokines play a role in the pathophysiology of RA, and variable responses to biologic DMARD therapies may reflect individual variations in the prominence of causative factors producing RA at the level of the individual patient. Variable clinical responses to biologic DMARDs targeting specific inflammatory mediators such as TNF-α, IL-1, and IL-6, as well as DMARDs depleting B cells and T cell costimulation inhibitors suggest that multiple mechanisms are likely responsible for the pathogenesis of RA.

Table 36.3 details the biologic DMARD name, cellular target, Mab structure, mechanism of action, method of administration, drug half-life, and approved usage of the drug.

Treatment Guidelines

The tool that clinicians currently use to guide pharmacologic treatment decisions is the 2015 ACR Guidelines for the Treatment of Rheumatoid Arthritis. The guideline authors considered the side effect profile, cost, and the perceived burden of taking DMARD therapies when developing these guidelines. The synthetic DMARDs included in the guidelines are methotrexate, leflunomide, hydroxychloroquine, and sulfasalazine, and the biologic DMARDS included are adalimumab, certolozumab pegol, etanercept, golimumab, infliximab, abatacept, rituximab, and tocilizumab. Other DMARDs were excluded due to infrequent use or lack of updated clinical studies.

A treat-to-target (TTT) strategy, where the patient is treated aggressively in order to reach and maintain the therapeutic goal of clinical remission or a reduction in disease activity, should be used to treat RA patients. The patient should be provided with the goals of the TTT approach and be able to evaluate the risks and benefits of this targeted and potentially aggressive approach. To determine if the desired target is reached, disease activity should be routinely monitored in patients using validated instruments and methodologies. The disease activity measures include several instruments to assess disease activity including the number of tender and swollen joints along with levels of inflammatory markers CRP and/or ESR. Ultimately, the goal of TTT is to provide patients with an optimized clinical treatment plan that will improve their symptoms and prevent joint damage, thereby maximizing long-term health and improving quality of life for the patient.[84]

For patients with early RA (disease duration ≤6 mo), a TTT strategy is highly recommended. DMARD monotherapy is recommended for patients with low, moderate, and high disease activity. If moderate or high disease activity persists after initiation of DMARD monotherapy, the use of combination synthetic DMARD (sDMARD) therapy (with or without glucocorticoids), TNFi (with or

Table 36.3 Biologic DMARD Summary Table

Drug	Target	Structure	Mechanism	Administration	Half-Life	Approved Usage
Etanercept	TNF-α, LTβ	Recombinant fusion protein TNF2R and IgG Fc	Decoy receptor binds to inhibits TNF-α/β	sc injection	4.3 d	Monotherapy or with MTX
Infliximab	TNF-α	Mouse-human chimeric IgG Mab	Mab binds to and inhibits TNF-α	iv infusion	8-9.5 d	With MTX
Adalimumab	TNF-α	Human Mab	Mab binds to and inhibits TNF-α	sc injection	14 d	Monotherapy or with MTX
Golimumab	TNF-α	Human Mab	Mab binds to and inhibits TNF-α	sc injection	14 d	With MTX
Certolizumab pegol	TNF-α	Pegylated humanized Fab fragment	Fab fragment binds to and inhibits TNF-α	sc injection	14 d	Monotherapy or with MTX
Abatacept	T cells	CTLA-4 fused to IgG Fc	Blocks costimulatory signal for T cell activation	sc injection iv infusion	14 d	Monotherapy or with MTX
Tocilizumab	IL-6	Humanized IL-6R Mab	Mab binds and inhibits IL-6R	sc injection iv infusion	5-13 d	Monotherapy or with MTX
Anakinra	IL-1	Recombinant human IL-R antagonist	Binds to IL-1R	sc injection	4-6 hr	Monotherapy or with MTX
Rituximab	B cells	Mouse-human chimeric Mab	Mab binds to CD20 positive B cells	iv infusion	18-32 d	With MTX

without MTX), or a non-TNFi biologic (with or without MTX) is recommended. If moderate to high disease activity persists, then the patient should be treated using the established RA algorithm.

For patients with established RA (disease duration ≥6 mo), a TTT strategy is also strongly recommended. MTX is the preferred DMARD for drug-naive established RA patients. Otherwise, the same strategy used for treating early RA patients with low, moderate, or high disease activity is recommended with the addition of tofacitinib (with or without MTX) as an alternative therapy if moderate or severe disease activity persisted following treatment with DMARD monotherapy.

If a patient fails to respond to a TNFi, then a non-TNF biologic or another TNFi is recommended. If the patient fails to respond to multiple TNFi's, then a non-TNF biologic or tofacitinib is conditionally recommended. Following a failure to respond to a non-TNF biologic, another non-TNF biologic should be used. If the patient continues to have no response or insufficient response to non-TNF biologics, then TNFi or tofacitinib should be used.

Recommendations for laboratory monitoring for RA patients on sDMARD therapy involve interval monitoring for complete blood count (CBC), liver transaminase levels, and serum creatinine levels in patients receiving MTX, LEF, SSZ, and HCQ. Initially, RA patients should be monitored monthly and as the treatment is established monitoring is recommended every 3 months. Patients receiving bDMARDs or tofacitinib should be screened for TB prior to beginning therapy and rescreened yearly if patients have risk factors for TB exposure.

The current RA treatment guidelines recommend that bDMARD therapy should be combined with MTX because this combination has greater efficacy than biologic monotherapy. If the patient experiences a disease flare or has a continuing high disease activity while on the DMARD treatment plan, short-term use of glucocorticoids at the lowest possible dose and duration is recommended.

In addition to these guidelines, other considerations are taken into account when deciding which therapeutic regimen to use. Less is known about long-term safety in newer DMARDs like tofacitinib compared to more established therapeutics such as MTX and TNFi's. Medication costs also play a role in which therapy is employed. More studies are needed to determine if the order or use of DMARD classes impacts therapeutic outcomes. For example, it is not known whether patients who fail to respond to one TNFi are more likely to benefit from switching to another TNFi or to a non-TNF biologic therapy. Recent studies indicate that switching to an alternative TNFi when a patient ceases to respond to an initial TNFi may improve disease activity, but that the response to a new TNFi will be less than the original TNFi. Emerging data suggest that patients with inadequate response to TNFi treatment have improved responses when treated with a non-TNFi biologic.[69]

Clinical Scenario

Justin Kinney, PharmD, Abby Weldon, PhD

SCENARIO

MM is 35-year-old woman with a history of established RA. She was prescribed adalimumab and methotrexate 3 months ago. She complains of morning stiffness that lasts more than an hour and swelling in her second and third metacarpophalangeal (MCP) joints and in her second and third proximal interphalangeal (PIP) joints in both hands. The patient indicates that the morning stiffness and joint swelling are interfering with her ability to carry out her duties as a nurse. Laboratory tests reveal an abnormal C-reactive protein. Serology testing reveals she is rheumatoid factor (RF) negative and anti-citrullinated protein antibody (ACPA) negative. Disease activity assessment using the SDAI reveals moderate disease activity. MM's past medical history includes hypertension, dyslipidemia, and RA. Since MM is not responding to her current DMARD therapy regimen, her physician has asked your advice regarding a change from adalimumab to a non-TNFi DMARD. The physician asks you for a recommendation between abatacept, tocilizumab, and rituximab.

OUTCOME AND ANALYSIS

Since the patient has moderate disease activity despite being treated with adalimumab and methotrexate for 3 months, the physician has decided to replace adalimumab with a non-TNFi DMARD. The physician has asked you for a recommendation between abatacept, tocilizumab, and rituximab.

Given the seronegative status of MM, rituximab would likely be a poor choice for her. Since autoantibodies are not present, this suggests that B cells are not playing a large role in disease pathology and there is not likely to be any large benefit for MM from the use of rituximab. Rituximab has not been shown to be beneficial for seronegative RA patients.

The choice between abatacept and tocilizumab is not as clear as was the case with rituximab since both would likely be helpful in alleviating the symptoms of MM's RA. Retrospective cohort studies have shown that both abatacept and tocilizumab were able to reduce disease activity in RA patients with similar safety profiles. Abatacept is a chimeric CTLA-4-IgG1 fused protein that directly inhibits T cell activation and subsequent inflammatory cytokine production. Abatacept is a chimeric biologic and therefore has the potential to be immunogenic. Immunogenicity is one of the main reasons for the loss of efficacy of biologics.

Tocilizumab is a humanized monoclonal antibody that blocks IL-6 signaling. Tocilizumab has been associated with increased blood cholesterol levels and abnormal liver function, as well as myelosuppression, and requires close monitoring. Due to MM's history of dyslipidemia, and the concomitant potential for liver issues with the methotrexate, tocilizumab should not be chosen for this patient. Furthermore, it should be avoided if MM confirms a history of diverticulitis or if she is on current NSAID therapy as there is an increased risk of bowel perforation with tocilizumab therapy.

Using the treat-to-target strategy, abatacept combined with methotrexate would be the best therapeutic option for this patient. Methotrexate will improve the efficacy of abatacept by reducing the potential of MM developing antidrug antibodies. Abatacept requires less monitoring and has a better side effect profile for MM. If abatacept is not providing adequate therapeutic effect by reducing disease activity in MM, then the side effect profile of tocilizumab would have to be weighed against the potential improvement in her RA.

REFERENCES

1. National Institutes of Health. Rheumatoid Arthritis. Available at https://www.niams.nih.gov/health--topics/rheumatoid--arthritis. Last Update Date 4/30/2017.
2. Alamanos Y, Voulgari PV, Drosos AA. Incidence and prevalence of rheumatoid arthritis, based on the 1987 American College of Rheumatology criteria: a systematic review. *Semin Arthritis Rheum.* 2006;36:182-188.
3. Silman AJ, Pearson JE. Epidemiology and genetics of rheumatoid arthritis. *Arthritis Res.* 2002;S265-S272.
4. Rothschild BM. *Tennessee Origins of Rheumatoid Arthritis.* Frank H. McClung Museum; 1991.
5. Arthritis Research Campaign. *Bones of Contention*; 1999. http://www.arc.org.uk/newsviews/arctdy/104/bones.htm.
6. Tang Q, Fu H, Qin B, et al. A possible link between rheumatoid arthritis and periodontitis: a systematic review and meta-analysis. *Int J Periodontics Restorative Dent.* 2017;37:79-86.
7. Firestein GS, McInnes IB. Immunopathogenesis of rheumatoid arthritis. *Immunity.* 2017;46:183-196.
8. Smolen JS, Aletaha D, McInnes IB. Rheumatoid arthritis. *Lancet.* 2016;388:2023-2038.

9. Liao KP, Alfredsson L, Karlson EW. Environmental influences on risk for rheumatoid arthritis. *Curr Opin Rheumatol*. 2009;21:279-283.
10. Pikwer M, Giwercman A, Bergström U, Nilsson JÅ, Jacobsson T, Turesson C. Association between testosterone levels and risk of future rheumatoid arthritis in men: a population-based case-control study. *Ann Rheum Dis*. 2014;73:573-579.
11. Parks CG, D'Aloisio AA, DeRoo LA, et al. Childhood socioeconomic factors and perinatal characteristics influence development of rheumatoid arthritis in adulthood. *Ann Rheum Dis*. 2013;72:350-356.
12. Mikuls TR, Payne JB, Yu F, et al. Periodontitis and Porphyromonas gingivalis in patients with rheumatoid arthritis. *Arthritis Rheumatol*. 2014;66:1090-1100.
13. Aletaha D, Neogi T, Silman AJ, et al. 2010 Rheumatoid arthritis classification criteria: an American College of Rheumatology/ European League against rheumatism collaborative initiative. *Arthritis Rheum*. 2010;62:2569-2581.
14. Singh JA, Saag KG, Bridges SL, et al. 2015 American College of Rheumatology guideline for the treatment of rheumatoid arthritis. *Arthritis Rheumatol*. 2016;68:1-26.
15. Silman AJ, MacGregor AJ, Thomson W, et al. Twin concordance rates for rheumatoid arthritis: results from a nationwide study. *Br J Rheumatol*. 1993;32:903-907.
16. Stastny P. Association of the B-cell alloantigen DRw4 with rheumatoid arthritis. *N Engl J Med*. 1978;298:869-871.
17. Gregersen PK, Silver J, Winchester RJ. The shared epitope hypothesis. An approach to understanding the molecular genetics of susceptibility to rheumatoid arthritis. *Arthritis Rheum*. 1987;30:1205-1213.
18. Hill JA, Southwood S, Sette A, Jevnikar AM, Bell DA, Cairns E. Cutting edge: the conversion of arginine to citrulline allows for a high-affinity peptide interaction with the rheumatoid arthritis-associated HLA-DRB1*0401 MHC class II molecule. *J Immunol*. 2003;171:538-541.
19. Hughes LB, Morrison D, Kelley JM, et al. The HLA-DRB1 shared epitope is associated with susceptibility to rheumatoid arthritis in African Americans through European genetic admixture. *Arthritis Rheum*. 2008;58:349-358.
20. Begovich AB, Carlton VE, Honigberg LA, et al. A missense single-nucleotide polymorphism in a gene encoding a protein tyrosine phosphatase (PTPN22) is associated with rheumatoid arthritis. *Am J Hum Genet*. 2004;75:330-337.
21. Gregersen PK, Lee HS, Batliwalla F, Begovich AB. PTPN22: setting thresholds for autoimmunity. *Semin Immunol*. 2006;18:214-223.
22. Bottini N, Musumeci L, Alonso A, et al. A functional variant of lymphoid tyrosine phosphatase is associated with type I diabetes. *Nat Genet*. 2004;36:337-338.
23. Okada Y, Wu D, Trynka G, et al. Genetics of rheumatoid arthritis contributes to biology and drug discovery. *Nature*. 2014;506:376-381.
24. Takakubo Y, Tamaki Y, Hirayama T, et al. Inflammatory immune cell responses and Toll-like receptor expression in synovial tissues in rheumatoid arthritis patients treated with biologics or DMARDs. *Clin Rheumatol*. 2013;32:853-861.
25. Derksen V, Huizinga TWJ, van der Woude D. The role of autoantibodies in the pathophysiology of rheumatoid arthritis. *Semin Immunopathol*. 2017;39:437-446.
26. Iwamoto T, Okamoto H, Toyama Y, Momohara S. Molecular aspects of rheumatoid arthritis: chemokines in the joints of patients. *FEBS J*. 2008;275:4448-4455.
27. Garcia-Vicuna R, Gómez-Gaviro MV, Domínguez-Luis MJ, et al. CC and CXC chemokine receptors mediate migration, proliferation, and matrix metalloproteinase production by fibroblast-like synoviocytes from rheumatoid arthritis patients. *Arthritis Rheum*. 2004;50:3866-3877.
28. Cutolo M, Kitas GD, van Riel PL. Burden of disease in treated rheumatoid arthritis patients: going beyond the joint. *Semin Arthritis Rheum*. 2014;43:479-488.
29. Aletaha D, Smolen JS. DMARD use in early rheumatoid arthritis. Lessons from observations in patients with established disease. *Clin Exp Rheumatol*. 2003;21:S169-S173.
30. Ranganathan P, McLeod HL. Methotrexate pharmacogenetics: the first step toward individualized therapy in rheumatoid arthritis. *Arthritis Rheum*. 2006;54:1366-1377.
31. Cronstein BN. The mechanism of action of methotrexate. *Rheum Dis Clin North Am*. 1997;23:739-755.
32. Yukioka K, Wakitani S, Yukioka M, et al. Polyamine levels in synovial tissues and synovial fluids of patients with rheumatoid arthritis. *J Rheumatol*. 1992;19:689-692.
33. Nesher G, Moore TL. The in vitro effects of methotrexate on peripheral blood mononuclear cells. Modulation by methyl donors and spermidine. *Arthritis Rheum*. 1990;33:954-959.
34. Furumitsu Y, Yukioka K, Kojima A, et al. Levels of urinary polyamines in patients with rheumatoid arthritis. *J Rheumatol*. 1993;20:1661-1665.
35. Flescher E, Bowlin TL, Ballester A, Houk R, Talal N. Increased polyamines may downregulate interleukin 2 production in rheumatoid arthritis. *J Clin Invest*. 1989;83:1356-1362.
36. Flescher E, Bowlin TL, Talal N. Regulation of IL-2 production by mononuclear cells from rheumatoid arthritis synovial fluids. *Clin Exp Immunol*. 1992;87:435-437.
37. Baggott JE, Vaughn WH, Hudson BB. Inhibition of 5-aminoimidazole-4- carboxamide ribotide transformylase, adenosine deaminase and 5′-adenylate deaminase by polyglutamates of methotrexate and oxidized folates and by 5-aminoimidazole-4-carboxamide riboside and ribotide. *Biochem J*. 1986;236:193-200.
38. Hasko G, Cronstein BN. Adenosine: an endogenous regulator of innate immunity. *Trends Immunol*. 2004;25:33-39.
39. Hasko G, Szabó C, Németh ZH, Kvetan V, Pastores SM, Vizi ES. Adenosine receptor agonists differentially regulate IL-10, TNF-alpha, and nitric oxide production in RAW 264.7 macrophages and in endotoxemic mice. *J Immunol*. 1996;157:4634-4640.
40. Krump E, Lemay G, Borgeat P. Adenosine A2 receptor-induced inhibition of leukotriene B4 synthesis in whole blood ex vivo. *Br J Pharmacol*. 1996;117:1639-1644.
41. Szabo C, Scott GS, Virág L, et al. Suppression of macrophage inflammatory protein (MIP)-1alpha production and collagen-induced arthritis by adenosine receptor agonists. *Br J Pharmacol*. 1998;125:379-387.
42. Hamilton RA, Kremer JM. Why intramuscular methotrexate may be more efficacious than oral dosing in patients with rheumatoid arthritis. *Br J Rheumatol*. 1997;36:86-90.
43. Pichlmeier U, Heuer KU. Subcutaneous administration of methotrexate with a prefilled autoinjector pen results in a higher relative bioavailability compared with oral administration of methotrexate. *Clin Exp Rheumatol*. 2014;32:563-571.
44. Schiff MH, Jaffe JS, Freundlich B. Head-to-head, randomised, crossover study of oral versus subcutaneous methotrexate in patients with rheumatoid arthritis: drug-exposure limitations of oral methotrexate at doses ≥15 mg may be overcome with subcutaneous administration. *Ann Rheum Dis*. 2014;73:1549-1551.
45. Braun J, Kästner P, Flaxenberg P, et al. Comparison of the clinical efficacy and safety of subcutaneous versus oral administration of methotrexate in patients with active rheumatoid arthritis: results of a six-month, multicenter, randomized, double-blind, controlled, phase IV trial. *Arthritis Rheum*. 2008;58:73-81.
46. Kremer JM, Hamilton RA. The effects of nonsteroidal antiinflammatory drugs on methotrexate (MTX) pharmacokinetics: impairment of renal clearance of MTX at weekly maintenance doses but not at 7.5 mg. *J Rheumatol*. 1995;22:2072-2077.
47. Herman RA, Veng-Pedersen P, Hoffman J, Koehnke R, Furst DE. Pharmacokinetics of low-dose methotrexate in rheumatoid arthritis patients. *J Pharm Sci*. 1989;78:165-171.
48. Dalrymple JM, Stamp LK, O'Donnell JL, Chapman PT, Zhang M, Barclay ML. Pharmacokinetics of oral methotrexate in patients with rheumatoid arthritis. *Arthritis Rheum*. 2008;58:3299-3308.
49. Tugwell P, Bennett K, Gent M. Methotrexate in rheumatoid arthritis. Indications, contraindications, efficacy, and safety. *Ann Intern Med*. 1987;107:358-366.

50. Felson DT, Anderson JJ, Meenan RF. Use of short-term efficacy/toxicity tradeoffs to select second-line drugs in rheumatoid arthritis. A metaanalysis of published clinical trials. *Arthritis Rheum.* 1992;35:1117-1125.
51. Chaner BL. *Dan, Cancer Chemotherapy and Biotherapy: Principles and Practices.* 4th ed. Philadelphia: Lippincott Williams and Wilkins; 2011.
52. Fox RI, Herrmann ML, Frangou CG, et al. Mechanism of action for leflunomide in rheumatoid arthritis. *Clin Immunol.* 1999;93:198-208.
53. Fox RI. Mechanism of action of leflunomide in rheumatoid arthritis. *J Rheumatol Suppl.* 1998;53:20-26.
54. Cao WW, Kao PN, Chao AC, Gardner P, Ng J, Morris RE. Mechanism of the antiproliferative action of leflunomide. A77 1726, the active metabolite of leflunomide, does not block T-cell receptor-mediated signal transduction but its antiproliferative effects are antagonized by pyrimidine nucleosides. *J Heart Lung Transplant.* 1995;14:1016-1030.
55. Silva HT, Cao W, Shorthouse R, Morris RE. Mechanism of action of leflunomide: in vivo uridine administration reverses its inhibition of lymphocyte proliferation. *Transplant Proc.* 1996;28:3082-3084.
56. Marijnen YM, de Korte D, Haverkort WA, den Breejen EJ, van Gennip AH, Roos D. Studies on the incorporation of precursors into purine and pyrimidine nucleotides via 'de novo' and 'salvage' pathways in normal lymphocytes and lymphoblastic cell-line cells. *Biochim Biophys Acta.* 1989;1012:148-155.
57. Smedegard G, Bjork J. Sulphasalazine: mechanism of action in rheumatoid arthritis. *Br J Rheumatol.* 1995;2:7-15.
58. Gadangi P, Longaker M, Naime D, et al. The anti-inflammatory mechanism of sulfasalazine is related to adenosine release at inflamed sites. *J Immunol.* 1996;156:1937-1941.
59. Tornhamre S, Edenius C, Smedegård G, Sjöquist B, Lindgren JA. Effects of sulfasalazine and a sulfasalazine analogue on the formation of lipoxygenase and cyclooxygenase products. *Eur J Pharmacol.* 1989;169:225-234.
60. Wahl C, Liptay S, Adler G, Schmid RM. Sulfasalazine: a potent and specific inhibitor of nuclear factor kappa B. *J Clin Invest.* 1998;101:1163-1174.
61. Molin L, Stendahl O. The effect of sulfasalazine and its active components on human polymorphonuclear leukocyte function in relation to ulcerative colitis. *Acta Med Scand.* 1979;206:451-457.
62. Cabral AR, Alarcon-Segovia D. Will some day PAPS fade into SLE? *Lupus.* 1996;5:4-5.
63. Wozniacka A, Carter A, McCauliffe DP. Antimalarials in cutaneous lupus erythematosus: mechanisms of therapeutic benefit. *Lupus.* 2002;11:71-81.
64. Espinoza LR, Jara LJ, Martinez-Osuna P, Silveira LH, Cuellar ML, Seleznick M. Refractory nephrotic syndrome in lupus nephritis: favorable response to indomethacin therapy. *Lupus.* 1993;2:9-14.
65. Fleischmann R, Mysler E, Hall S, et al. Efficacy and safety of tofacitinib monotherapy, tofacitinib with methotrexate, and adalimumab with methotrexate in patients with rheumatoid arthritis (ORAL Strategy): a phase 3b/4, double-blind, head-to-head, randomised controlled trial. *Lancet.* 2017;390:457-468.
66. Ghoreschi K, Jesson MI, Li X, et al. Modulation of innate and adaptive immune responses by tofacitinib (CP-690,550). *J Immunol.* 2011;186:4234-4243.
67. Flanagan ME, Blumenkopf TA, Brissette WH, et al. Discovery of CP-690,550: a potent and selective Janus kinase (JAK) inhibitor for the treatment of autoimmune diseases and organ transplant rejection. *J Med Chem.* 2010;53:8468-8484.
68. Moots RJ, Naisbett-Groet B. The efficacy of biologic agents in patients with rheumatoid arthritis and an inadequate response to tumour necrosis factor inhibitors: a systematic review. *Rheumatology (Oxford).* 2012;51:2252-2261.
69. Siebert S, Tsoukas A, Robertson J, McInnes I. Cytokines as therapeutic targets in rheumatoid arthritis and other inflammatory diseases. *Pharmacol Rev.* 2015;67:280-309.
70. Feldmann M, Maini RN. Anti-TNF therapy, from rationale to standard of care: what lessons has it taught us? *J Immunol.* 2010;185:791-794.
71. Kemanetzoglou E, Andreadou E. CNS demyelination with TNF-alpha blockers. *Curr Neurol Neurosci Rep.* 2017;17:36.
72. Acosta-Felquer ML, Rosa J, Soriano ER. An evidence-based review of certolizumab pegol in the treatment of active psoriatic arthritis: place in therapy. *Open Access Rheumatol.* 2016;8:37-44.
73. Goel N, Stephens S. Certolizumab pegol. *MAbs.* 2010;2:137-147.
74. Palframan R, Airey M, Moore A, Vugler A, Nesbitt A. Use of biofluorescence imaging to compare the distribution of certolizumab pegol, adalimumab, and infliximab in the inflamed paws of mice with collagen-induced arthritis. *J Immunol Methods.* 2009;348:36-41.
75. Nesbitt A, Fossati G, Bergin M, et al. Mechanism of action of certolizumab pegol (CDP870): in vitro comparison with other anti-tumor necrosis factor alpha agents. *Inflamm Bowel Dis.* 2007;13:1323-1332.
76. Amu S, Strömberg K, Bokarewa M, Tarkowski A, Brisslert M. CD25-expressing B-lymphocytes in rheumatic diseases. *Scand J Immunol.* 2007;65:182-191.
77. Burmester GR, Rubbert-Roth A, Cantagrel A, et al. A randomised, double-blind, parallel-group study of the safety and efficacy of subcutaneous tocilizumab versus intravenous tocilizumab in combination with traditional disease-modifying antirheumatic drugs in patients with moderate to severe rheumatoid arthritis (SUMMACTA study). *Ann Rheum Dis.* 2014;73:69-74.
78. Hashizume M, Yoshida H, Koike N, Suzuki M, Mihara M. Overproduced interleukin 6 decreases blood lipid levels via upregulation of very-low-density lipoprotein receptor. *Ann Rheum Dis.* 2010;69:741-746.
79. Curtis JR, Lanas A, John A, Johnson DA, Schulman KL. Factors associated with gastrointestinal perforation in a cohort of patients with rheumatoid arthritis. *Arthritis Care Res (Hoboken).* 2012;64:1819-1828.
80. Singh JA, Saag KG, Bridges SL, et al. 2015 American College of Rheumatology guideline for the treatment of rheumatoid arthritis. *Arthritis Care Res (Hoboken).* 2016;68:1-25.
81. Rantapaa-Dahlqvist S, de Jong BA, Berglin E, et al. Antibodies against cyclic citrullinated peptide and IgA rheumatoid factor predict the development of rheumatoid arthritis. *Arthritis Rheum.* 2003;48:2741-2749.
82. Silverman GJ, Carson DA. Roles of B cells in rheumatoid arthritis. *Arthritis Res Ther.* 2003;5:S1-S6.
83. Mariette X, Vencovsky J, Lortholary O, et al. The incidence of tuberculosis in patients treated with certolizumab pegol across indications: impact of baseline skin test results, more stringent screening criteria and geographic region. *RMD Open.* 2015;1:e000044.
84. Smolen JS, Aletaha D, Bijlsma JW, et al. Treating rheumatoid arthritis to target: recommendations of an international task force. *Ann Rheum Dis.* 2010;69:631-637.

CHAPTER 37

Nutrition and Obesity

David Wallace and Thomas L. Lemke

Drugs covered in this chapter[a]:

DRUGS
- Amphetamine
- Benzphetamine
- Diethylpropion
- Liraglutide
- Lisdexamfetamine
- Lorcaserin
- Naltrexone/bupropion
- Olestra
- Orlistat
- Phendimetrazine
- Phenmetrazine
- Phentermine
- Topiramate

MACRONUTRIENTS
- Acesulfame-K
- Aspartame
- *Cyclamate*
- Fatty acids
  - Saturated
  - Unsaturated (polyunsaturated)
- Fiber
- Glycogen
- Mogrosides
- Neotame
- Rebaudioside A
- Saccharin
- Starch
- Sucralose
- Xylitol

MICRONUTRIENTS
- Sodium chloride
- Vitamin A (retinal, retinol, carotenes)
- Biotin (B_7)
- Folic acid (B_9)
- Lutein
- Niacin (B_3)
- Pantothenic acid (B_5)
- Pyridoxine (B_6)
- Riboflavin (B_2)
- Thiamine (B_1)
- Vitamin B_{12} (cobalamin)
- Vitamin C (ascorbic acid)
- Vitamin D
- Vitamin E (tocopherols)
- Vitamin K

[a]Nutrients/drugs listed include those available inside and outside of the United States; the nutrient shown in italics is no longer available in the United States.

Abbreviations

ATP adenosine triphosphate
BMI body mass index
BMR basal metabolic rate
CHD coronary heart disease
CNS central nervous system
CoA coenzyme A
DIT diet-induced thermogenesis
DRI Dietary Reference Intake
DSHEA Dietary Supplement Health and Education Act
DV daily value
EEA energy of expenditure of activity
EPA eicosapentaenoic acid
FDA U.S. Food and Drug Administration
GI gastrointestinal
GRAS generally recognized as safe
HDL high-density lipoprotein
LDL low-density lipoprotein
NLEA Nutrition Labeling and Educational Act
OEI Obesity Education Initiative
PKU phenylketonuria
PUFA polyunsaturated fatty acid
RAE retinol activity equivalent
RDA Recommended Dietary Allowance
RDI Recommended Daily Intakes
ROS reactive oxygen species
RS resistant starch
SSRI selective serotonin reuptake inhibitor
TEE total energy expenditure
TFA *trans* fatty acid

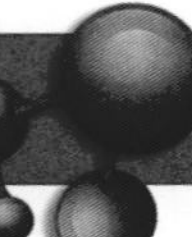

CLINICAL SIGNIFICANCE

David Wallace, PharmD

The application of medicinal chemistry knowledge presents in numerous decisions made by a pharmacist during his or her patient care activities, though it may not be obvious in the clinician's mind. The screening for and evaluation of drug interactions illustrates one situation where a pharmacist directly employs the understanding of medicinal chemistry in practice. An example is a drug interaction involving chelation, such as between a calcium carbonate supplement and levothyroxine, where the pharmacist must counsel the patient to separate the administration of the two medications by 4 hours so the latter is properly absorbed. More subtly a pharmacist will counsel a patient taking levodopa to spread out their dietary protein intake to diminish the competition for absorption from both the small intestine and across the blood-brain barrier.

Other applications of medicinal chemistry in patient care may be less directly apparent. For instance if a patient is a candidate for drug therapy treatment of obesity and has been diagnosed with diabetes mellitus type 2 and hypertension, liraglutide may be an appealing choice to the clinician because of its ability to augment weight loss, lower blood sugar, and not adversely affect blood pressure. Like any nutritional protein which is metabolized in the GI tract liraglutide is prone to both gastric pH and intestinal enzymes breakdown preventing its intact absorption. Thus, the patient with a severe fear of needles is not a candidate for liraglutide therapy. Another application may be screening patients for potential allergies to medication. While hypersensitivity reactions to amphetamine anorexiant derivatives seem to be very rare, it might be prudent to recommend avoiding phentermine use in a patient with a history of toxic epidermal necrolysis following exposure to amphetamine given the chemical structures similarities.

INTRODUCTION TO NUTRITION AND OBESITY

A startling statistic in the United States today is the high rate of Americans who are overweight or obese and the projection of where we will be in the near future. It has been projected by 2020 that an estimated 75% of Americans will meet the criteria for being overweight or obese. Childhood obesity is considered to be a national epidemic with nearly one in three children of age 2-19 years being classified as overweight or obese. The quality and length of life are directly related to body weight as is the potential for the development of a long list of disease states such as diabetes, coronary heart disease, hypertension, sleep apnea, osteoarthritis, various cancers, and psychological disorders. By the simplest definition, obesity occurs when energy intake exceeds energy expenditure, which in turn leads to abnormal amounts of triglycerides being stored in adipose tissue. The etiology of obesity brings together a number of contributing factors of which genetics has often been suggested. While a genetics predisposition does play a role in obesity (possibly as low as ~30%), the recent epidemic of obesity is probably not of genetic origin.[1] To a greater extent environment, socioeconomic status, reduced physical activity and a sedentary lifestyle, technology, and gender are all contributors to what are being seen in the Western world. Because energy intake and energy expenditure play such an important role in overweight and obesity, this chapter will begin with a brief discussion of nutrition, our source of energy intake, followed by methods of reducing caloric content of human nutrition, and finally pharmacotherapeutic treatment/prevention of overweight and obese conditions.

INTRODUCTION TO NUTRITION

Every living cell requires essential ingredients to survive. These essential ingredients are chemical substances, both organic and inorganic, that are not generally produced in the body or, if they are, they are not produced in sufficient quantities to meet cellular or body needs. These chemical substances are commonly referred to as nutrients, and the utilization of these substances for normal body development and growth is called nutrition. Poor nutrition can result from both insufficient quantities of nutrients and overconsumption of nutrients. Examples of diseases associated with low levels of nutrients are blindness (vitamin A deficiency), osteoporosis (vitamin D, calcium, and phosphate deficiencies), scurvy (vitamin C deficiency), and kwashiorkor (protein deficiency). Excessive intake of nutrients can lead to obesity and associated diseases. Nutritional balance will always be critical to overall body health and will be emphasized throughout this chapter. From our standpoint, nutrition is essential for body growth and maintenance and will be presented in this context.

NUTRIENT CLASSIFICATION

The nutrients essential to man and animals can be classified as macronutrients or micronutrients. Those chemicals that must be taken in large quantities are referred to as macronutrients, whereas those that are required in small quantities are referred to as micronutrients. The macronutrients consist of carbohydrates, fats, proteins, and water, whereas the micronutrients consist of vitamins and minerals. The quantities of macro- and micronutrients change with age. From conception until the mid-teens, the body undergoes considerable growth, and the quantities of nutrients required for good health will be high. From the teens throughout much of the remainder of life, nutrients are expected to maintain the structure of the body. In the elderly, the demand for some nutrients may actually decrease, although this may be more associated with reduced physical activity. During much of our adult life (20 yr of age and older), nutrition serves the role of maintaining the body by replacing essential chemicals lost due to normal turnover and supplying energy for running the body. The energy supplied to the body is primarily met through the macronutrients and, more specifically, by carbohydrates and fats. Body composition and weight will generally be relatively stable in an individual with good health, but depending on the eating habits and physical activity, serious medical issues may arise. The simplistic view of excessive body weight or the medical condition of obesity occurs when the intake of macronutrients exceeds the energy needs of the body and nutrients are put into storage. Carbohydrates are stored in the form of glycogen; amino acids, the absorbable form of protein, are stored in the form of protein; and fats are stored as triglycerides or lipids (Fig. 37.1).

The use of the terms lipids, fats, triglycerides, and fatty acids may be confusing and in some cases these terms are used interchangeably. In a true sense a lipid is a generic term referring to a substance that dissolves in an organic solvent. A lipid substance is a hydrophobic chemical, which includes fats and steroids as well as many other chemicals. A fat is a more specific term is also known as a triglyceride. The structure of a fat consists of glycerin to which three (tri) fatty acids are attached. Natural fatty acids are nonbranched hydrocarbons with an even number of carbons usually from 4 to 26 carbons.

Glycerin	Fatty acid	Triglyceride
H_2C-OH / $HC-OH$ / H_2C-OH	$R-C(=O)-OH$	$H_2C-O-C(=O)-R$ / $HC-O-C(=O)-R$ / $H_2C-O-C(=O)-R$

BODY ENERGY NEEDS

The energy needed to meet body demands is derived from ingested organic macronutrients. Specifically, carbohydrates, fats (hydrolysis products of a triglyceride), and proteins serve as potential energy sources, and the oxidative breaking of carbon-carbon and carbon-hydrogen bonds converts this potential energy into the body's energy carrier adenosine triphosphate (ATP) (Fig. 37.2). ATP in turn is used to carry out biochemical processes in the body such as muscle contraction for external work, vascular and heart contraction for blood flow, active transport of molecules and ions, biosynthesis of macromolecules, and a whole host of other cellular functions. The conversion of foods to energy (food energy) is not a very efficient process, and as a result, nearly half of the potential energy of the macronutrients is lost in the form of heat. The unit of measure of potential energy is that of the calorie (Cal or kcal) and is defined as the amount of energy required to heat 1 kg of water 1°C from 15 to 16°C. Note that the terminology *Cal* (spelled with an uppercase "C") replaces the older unit terminology *cal* (spelled with a lowercase "c"), which is 1/1,000 of a kcal. Nutritional labels report caloric content of foods in the form of calories (Cal). One may also see energy reported in joules or kilojoules (kJ) where 1 kcal equals 4.184 kJ, a standard set by the International System of Units. The hydrolysis of ATP, a phosphoric acid anhydride, releases approximately 12 kcal/mol and results from the exothermic hydrolysis of an anhydride bond and the resulting stabilization of the phosphate anion through resonance stabilization (Fig. 37.3).

The measure of potential energy present in any particular foodstuff can be determined experimentally by complete combustion of a particular foodstuff within an instrument called a calorimeter. The calorimeter consists of a combustion chamber submerged in a water bath. The foodstuff is combusted within the chamber, and the rise in water temperature is measured, which in turn indicates the energy released during combustion. On average, carbohydrates release 4.1 kcal/g, proteins release 4.2 kcal/g, and fats release 9.3 kcal/g of energy (Fig. 37.4). Several attributes can be noted by viewing the chemical structures of the macronutrients. Complete combustion of the carbon atoms in these molecules gives rise to carbon dioxide and water. Nitrogen within the structure of proteins is not oxidized and is not a source of energy. The carbons in carbohydrates are already in a partially oxidized form C—OH, as are several of the carbons in a protein C—NH, C═O, whereas a fatty acid, released from a triglyceride, has a large number of carbon-carbon and carbon-hydrogen bonds that are available for metabolism. Thus, by simple observation of the chemical structures of the macronutrients, one can see that fatty acids would be expected to have a significantly larger potential for generating energy.

Ideally, the amount of energy being generated from the macronutrients should equal the amount of energy needed to run and maintain the body. Actually, there are two sources of macronutrient calories; those arising from the external foods that are eaten are called exogenous

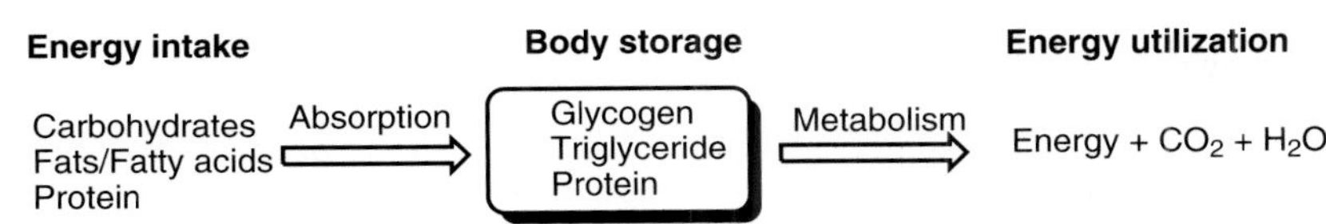

Figure 37.1 Diagrammatic representation of macronutrient absorption, storage, and utilization needed to run the body.

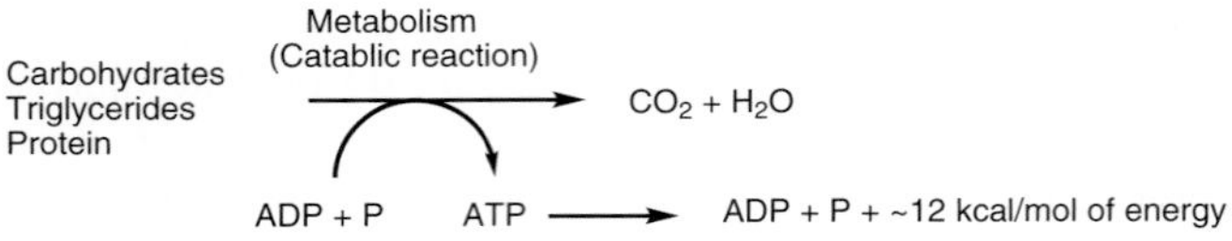

Figure 37.2 Conversion of foodstuff to adenosine triphosphate (ATP), the body's energy currency.

calories, and those calories that are found stored in the body are called endogenous calories (Fig. 37.5). In an attempt to quantify the number of calories expended on a daily basis, various calculations and formulas have been developed. In most cases, these calculations have either been too complicated to be of practical value or are only a rough approximation of actual caloric consumption. One simplistic approximate measure of calories needed to maintain the body at a resting state (i.e., energy needed for cellular metabolism plus energy for blood circulation and respiration) is the basal metabolic rate (BMR). Combining the BMR with the energy expenditure of activity (EEA), also known as the total energy expenditure (TEE), and the diet-induced thermogenesis (DIT) can give an estimate of daily energy needs, which if combined with an estimate of calories consumed will help the individual determine their balance between calorie intake and calorie expenditure. BMR calculations can be done with the formula shown in Equation 37.1. As indicated, the BMR is dependent on the gender of the individual and the individual's weight, height, and age.

Eq. 37.1

$$\text{BMR (in Cal/day for women)} = 655 + (9.6 \times W) + (1.8 \times H) - (4.7 \times A)$$

$$\text{BMR (in Cal/day for men)} = 66 + (13.7 \times W) + (5 \times H) - (6.8 \times A)$$

where, W, weight in kg of the individual (1 kg = 2.2 lbs); H, height in cm of the individual (1 in. = 2.54 cm); A, age of the individual.

A generalization can be made for lifestyle activities; for a sedentary lifestyle, the EEA is between 400 and 800 Cal/d; for a moderately active lifestyle, the EEA would be 1,200-1,800 Cal/d; and for an individual involved in heavy labor, the EEA would be 1,800-4,500 Cal/d. An energy expenditure calculator can be found at www.health-calc.com/diet/energy-expenditure-advanced. Table 37.1 lists a number of physical activities along with an approximation of the calorie expenditure. A third component of the calculation of daily caloric needs is DIT. The DIT is defined as the energy expenditure above basal fasting levels divided by the energy content of the food ingested over a 24-hour period and is expressed as a percentage.[2] The DIT is different for each nutrient, but normally, the DIT for a mixed diet is in the range of 10% of the total amount of energy ingested. The DIT is associated with the energy required for nutrient absorption, steps involved in metabolism, and storage of the absorbed nutrients. Ideally, the sum of the BMR, EEA, and DIT should equal the dietary daily intake so as to protect against weight gain or weight loss.

OVERWEIGHT AND OBESITY

Worldwide, overweight and obesity have become major health issues, and nowhere can this be seen more dramatically than in the United States. Various reports indicate that obesity continues to be a major health concern, Table 37.2.[3,4] Today, obesity is considered to be a chronic disease, which is directly or indirectly related to the other diseases, including coronary heart disease, hypertension, stroke, and type 2 diabetes, and various other conditions, including an increase in death rates. It has been reported that even among overweight individuals, the risk of death for middle-age men and women increases by 20%-40% compared with people who maintain a desirable weight.[5] By definition, obesity is defined as excessive body fat, whereas overweight is defined as excessive body weight composed of bone, muscle, fat, and water. It is generally agreed that men with more than 25% body fat and women with more than 30% body fat are obese. There are various methods for measuring body fat both directly and indirectly. Underwater weighing, also known as hydrodensitometry, and dual-energy X-ray absorptiometry can give direct

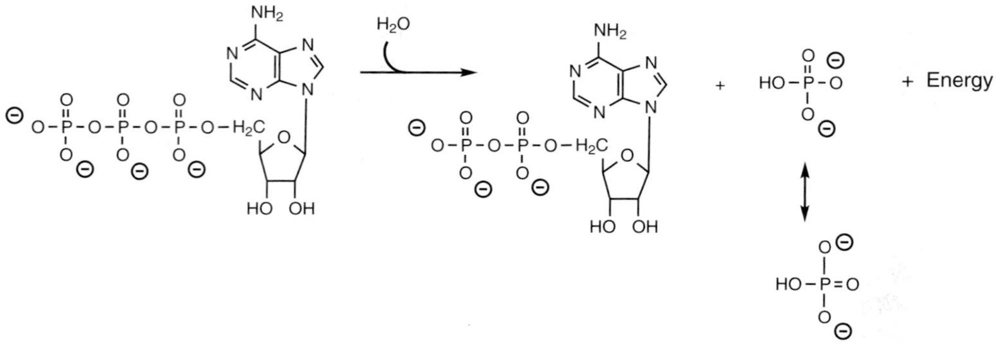

Figure 37.3 Energy release reaction involving adenosine triphosphate (ATP) hydrolysis to adenosine diphosphate (ADP) plus phosphate.

	Approximate energy released
Carbohydrate	4.1 kcal/g
Protein	4.2 kcal/g
Fatty acid	9.3 kcal/g

Figure 37.4 Potential energy derived from various foodstuffs.

measures of body fat content, but these methods tend to be expensive. More commonly used are the BMI calculation and waist circumference measurement, which give a good, but indirect, estimate of total body fat. The BMI is a simple calculation useful for adults and is shown in Equation 37.2.

Eq. 37.2

$$\text{BMI} = \text{Weight (kg)/Height (m)}^2$$

$$\text{BMI} = \text{Weight (lb)/Height (in)}^2 \times 703$$

In 1998, the NHLBI Obesity Education Initiative (OEI), citing a World Health Organization report from a year earlier, published the BMI breakpoints that are in use today.[6] Individuals with a BMI ≥18.5 but less than 25 are considered normal, individuals with a BMI of 25-29.9 are classified as overweight, and individuals with a BMI ≥30 are said to be obese. With a BMI ≥40, the person is considered to have extreme obesity or class 3 obesity. It should be noted that there are individuals who have a normal amount of body fat, but because of a high muscular content may have an "obese" BMI; this may be seen in athletes, especially football players. The elderly may actually have an underestimate of body fat based on BMI calculations because of the loss of muscle mass. However, in general, the BMI gives a good estimate of total body fat. Subsequent, guidelines for the treatment of obesity have maintained these cut points but have added additional BMI thresholds for initiating various therapeutic interventions based on presences of comorbid conditions. The relationship of BMI to potential health risks is shown in Table 37.3.

The presence of excessive abdominal fat can also be used as an indicator of health risk, and this is done through the measuring of waist circumference. The waist circumference gives a good measure of abdominal fat mass. The circumference is measured in the United States per the NHANES Anthropometry Procedures manual in a horizontal plane at the iliac crest (Fig. 37.6). Per the OEI, a high-risk waist circumference is >40 inches in a man and >35 inches in a woman. However, it should be noted these waist circumference cut points do not reflect ethnic differences. The International Diabetes Federation has set cut points of >94 cm (male) and >80 cm (female) for the Europid ethnic groups while Asian ethnic groups have lower cut point for males at >90 cm. These measurements also differ in that they follow the WHO measurement protocol, which determines waist circumference measured horizontally at the midpoint between the lower margin of the last palpable rib and the upper margin of the iliac crest at the midaxillary line.[7]

A commonly asked question is: To what extent are overweight and obesity related to genetics and environment? Current research appears to point to environment as a major contributor to overweight and obesity. A combination of increased calorie consumption and reduced physical activity over a long enough period of time leads to excessive body weight. As reported by Putnam et al,[8] between 1985 and 2000, the average consumption of calories increased by 12% or approximately 300 Cal/d. It was estimated that of this 300-calorie increase, fats and sugars accounted for 24% and

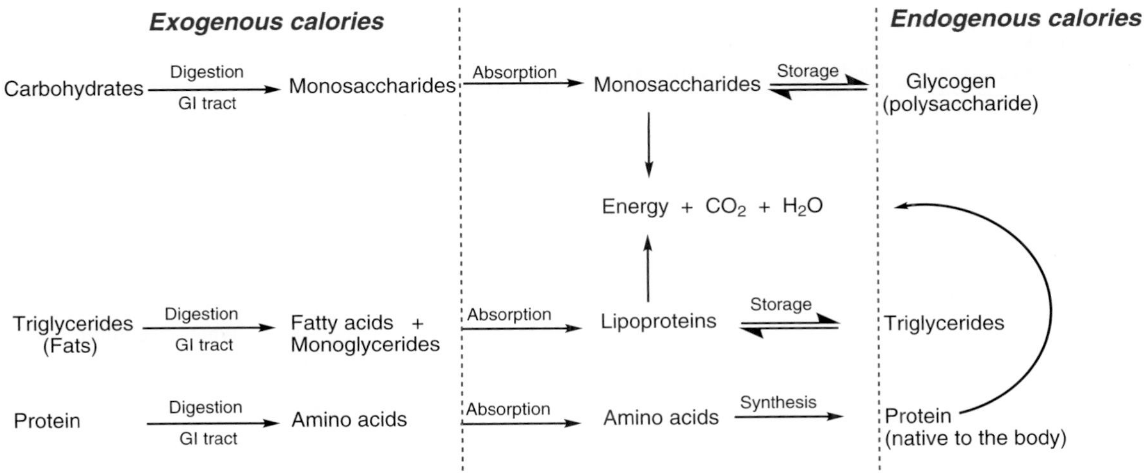

Figure 37.5 Digestion, absorption, and storage of macromolecules and conversion to energy. GI, gastrointestinal.

Table 37.1 Energy Expended During Typical Exercises[a]

Activity	Calories Used per Hour
Bicycling (6 mph)	240
Bicycling (12 mph)	410
Jogging (7 mph)	920
Running in place	650
Jumping rope	720
Swimming (50 yd/min)	500
Walking (2 mph)	240
Walking (3 mph)	320
Walking (4.5 mph)	440

[a]For a more detailed list of activities, see Appendix B in McArdle WD, Katch FI, Katch VL. *Sports and Exercise Nutrition*. 3rd ed. Baltimore: Lippincott Williams &Wilkins; 2009.

23%, respectively. An increase in 300 Cal/d without a compensatory increase in physical activity could lead to a weight gain of 22 lbs/yr. It was further reported in 2004 that an increase in fat intake occurred, while protein and carbohydrate intake remained unchanged. In another study, it was reported that between 1977 and 1996, food portions increased both inside and outside the home, resulting in increases in calories of salty snacks (93 kcal), soft drinks (49 kcal), hamburgers (97 kcal), French fries (68 kcal), and Mexican dishes (133 kcal).[9] An increase of 10 kcal/d could lead to an

Table 37.2 Estimates of Obesity in the United States.

	Obesity		
	Crude Prevalence	Age Adjusted	Class 3 Obesity
2013-2014			
Overall	37.9%		7.7%
Men	35.2%	35.0%	5.5%
Women	40.5%	40.4%	9.9%
2011-2014			
Preschool[a]		8.9%	
School[b]		17.5%	
Adolescents[c]		20.5%	

[a]Age 2-5 years.
[b]Age 6-11 years.
[c]Age 12-19 years.

Table 37.3 Relationship of Body Mass Index (BMI) to Health Risk

BMI Category	Health Risk	Risk Adjusted to Comorbidity
<25	Minimal	Low
25 to <27	Low	Moderate
27 to <30	Moderate	High
30 to <35	High	Very high
35 to <40	Very high	Extremely high

increase in body weight by 1 lb/yr. All of this suggests that an imbalance between calorie consumption and physical activity may contribute to the increase in body weight that now threatens the US population.

Food Labels

On May 27, 2016 the U.S. Food and Drug Administration (FDA) published a new set of rules governing Nutritional Facts labeling in the Federal Register.[10] Figure 37.7 illustrates an example of a typical food label in its present form and the proposed new label format.

Unfortunately, the exact date for conversion from the present label to the new label is uncertain. Compliance was listed as July 26, 2018, but that date has tentatively been changed to January 1, 2020. The goal of food labeling remains to help individuals manage their caloric and nutrient intake. Food labeling has remained unchanged for 20 years, while scientific information and new public health information have changed significantly. Changes listed in May 27, 2016, are shown in Table 37.4.

Other items which will continue to be listed include sodium and cholesterol in mgs and % daily value (DV) along with dietary fiber in grams and %DV. Protein will also continue to be listed in grams. Serving size must be based upon amount of foods and beverages that a person is actually eating. Package size must be included and for products that are larger than a single or multiple sittings, a "dual column" label with listed calories and nutrients

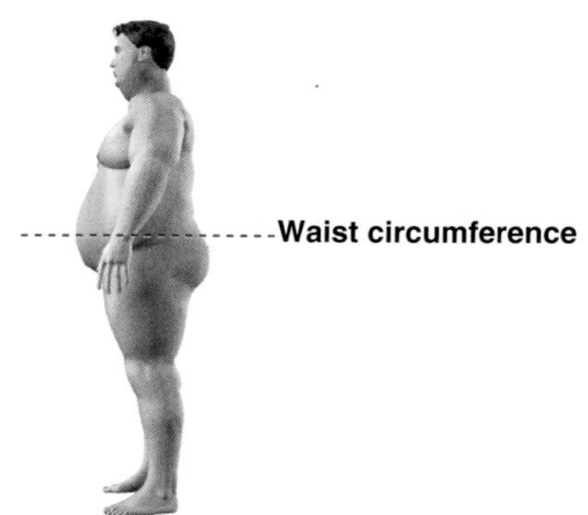

Figure 37.6 Measurement of waist circumference at iliac crest.

Nutrition Facts

Serving Size 2/3 cup (55g)
Servings Per Container About 8

Amount Per Serving	
Calories 230	Calories from Fat 72
	% Daily Value*
Total Fat 8g	**12**%
Saturated Fat 1g	**5**%
Trans Fat 0g	
Cholesterol 0mg	**0**%
Sodium 160mg	**7**%
Total Carbohydrate 37g	**12**%
Dietary Fiber 4g	**16**%
Sugars 1g	
Protein 3g	
Vitamin A	10%
Vitamin C	8%
Calcium	20%
Iron	45%

* Percent Daily Values are based on a 2,000 calorie diet. Your daily value may be higher or lower depending on your calorie needs.

	Calories:	2,000	2,500
Total Fat	Less than	65g	80g
Sat Fat	Less than	20g	25g
Cholesterol	Less than	300mg	300mg
Sodium	Less than	2,400mg	2,400mg
Total Carbohydrate		300g	375g
Dietary Fiber		25g	30g

Present label

Nutrition Facts

8 servings per container
Serving size 2/3 cup (55g)

Amount per serving	
Calories	**230**
	% Daily Value*
Total Fat 8g	**10%**
Saturated Fat 1g	**5%**
Trans Fat 0g	
Cholesterol 0mg	**0%**
Sodium 160mg	**7%**
Total Carbohydrate 37g	**13%**
Dietary Fiber 4g	**14%**
Total Sugars 12g	
Includes 10g Added Sugars	**20%**
Protein 3g	
Vitamin D 2mcg	10%
Calcium 260mg	20%
Iron 8mg	45%
Potassium 235mg	6%

* The % Daily Value (DV) tells you how much a nutrient in a serving of food contributes to a daily diet. 2,000 calories a day is used for general nutrition advice.

Proposed new label

Figure 37.7 Comparison of present food label with U.S. Food and Drug Administration (FDA)–proposed new label. From FDA website. https://www.fda.gov/Food/GuidanceRegulation/GuidanceDocumentsRegulatoryInformation/LabelingNutrition/ucm385663.htm. Accessed December 21, 2018.

in both "per serving" and "per package" basis must be included.

It should be noted that the U.S. Food and Drug Administration (FDA) has the authority to manage food labels and derives this authority from the Federal Food Drug and Cosmetic Act of 1938, the updated Nutrition Labeling and Educational Act of 1990 (NLEA), and the Dietary Supplement Health and Education Act of 1994 (DSHEA). The DVs are actually based on the highest Recommended Dietary Allowance (RDA) for the age or gender groups listed for RDAs and therefore would be a high-end recommendation. The RDAs are given in gram or milligram quantities, representing the average daily nutrient intake level required to meet the daily needs of an individual for good health, whereas the DV values are a percentage of the total daily requirements. These numbers are reviewed and updated by the Food and Nutrition Board of the Institute of Medicine, in partnership with Health Canada. RDAs, also referred to as the Recommended Daily Intakes (RDIs), have become part of broader dietary guidelines known as the Dietary Reference Intake (DRI), which is revised and updated continually and serves as the basis for determination of the %DV. Based on the most up-to-date scientific findings, the RDI may be greater than, lesser than, or equal to the older RDA numbers. Presently, the RDI is 300 g for total carbohydrates, 65 g for fats, and 50 g for protein

Table 37.4 Recommended Changes in Food Labels

Increased size of type for "calories"
List servings per container
Declare serving size
Bold print the number of calories per serving
Declare the amount and percent of daily value (DV) of vitamin D, calcium, iron, and potassium[a]
Add a footnote explaining the meaning of percent daily value (%DV)
Vitamin A and C will no longer be required to be listed
Sugar added in grams and %DV must be included[b]
The label will continue to require total fat, saturated fat, and *trans* fat[c]

[a]DV tells you how much a nutrient in a serving of food contributes to a daily diet. 2,000 Cal a day is used for general nutrition advice.

[b]Sugar added is defined as sugars either added during the processing of food or are packaged as such.

[c]*Trans* fats arising from partially hydrogenated oils has been reduced, but some *trans* fats are naturally occurring, and therefore this listing will continue. Industry can also petition the FDA for certain uses of partially hydrogenated oils which would then increase *trans* fats present.

(Table 37.5). The intent of these numbers and percentages is to help the consumer judge the nutritional value of a particular food by seeing the actual nutrient content in a serving of the food and the percentage of that nutrient toward reaching a 2,000-calorie daily intake for a cross section of American/Canadian consumers. It should be noted that carbohydrate and protein do not have a DV percent list, which is because there is no consensus on the quantitative intake of these two nutrients. However, because both carbohydrates and proteins are important and essential nutrients in the diet, their RDAs/RDIs are listed to help consumers manage their intake. Nutrients present in less than 500 mg/serving may be listed as 0.0 g and therefore may be present but need not be listed. Finally, it was not until 2003 that *trans* fatty acids were required to be reported. In 2015, the FDA formally determined that partially hydrogenated oils are not generally recognized as safe. And while the compliance date for manufactures to remove partially hydrogenated oils from their products has been extended, it is expected that the quantity of *trans* fatty acids will decrease since most *trans* fatty acids arise from partially hydrogenated oils once the compliance date has past.

MACRONUTRIENTS

To address the issue of overweight and obesity from the standpoint of overconsumption of calories, one must first identify the sources of calories within our foods. The macronutrients (carbohydrates, fats, and proteins) are the source of calories in our diet (Figs. 37.1 to 37.5). In fact, carbohydrates and fats are the usual organic nutrients from which the majority of our energy arise.

Carbohydrates

Carbohydrates are compounds composed of carbon, hydrogen, and oxygen and consist of simple monosaccharides such as glucose, galactose, and fructose; disaccharides such as sucrose (table sugar), maltose, and lactose (milk sugar); and polysaccharides such as starch, glycogen, and cellulose (Fig. 37.8). The absorbable form of a carbohydrate is the monosaccharide, or simple sugar; disaccharides and polysaccharides must first be hydrolyzed in the gastrointestinal (GI) tract before absorption.

Monosaccharide Absorption

Absorption of the very hydrophilic monosaccharides requires facilitated absorption/transport, both from the intestine and from body fluids into the cytoplasm of cells. Two families of membrane proteins involved in monosaccharide transport are the glucose transporter proteins (GLUT1 to GLUT5) and the Na^+-glucose cotransporters (SGLT1 to SGLT3). The GLUTs are 12 membrane–spanning proteins of approximately 500 amino acids found in red blood cells, the blood-brain barrier, liver cells, fat cells, and brush borders of the intestine. The role of these GLUT transporters is to

Table 37.5 Dietary Recommendations for Various Nutrients

			Micronutrients					
Macronutrients	**RDI[a]**	**RDI[b]**	**Vitamins**	**RDI[a]**	**RDI[b]**	**Minerals**	**RDI[a]**	**RDI[b]**
Carbohydrates	300 g	275 g	A	900 µg	900 µg	Sodium	2.4 g	2.3 g
Fiber	25 g	28 g	D	10 µg	20 µg	Potassium	3.5 g	4.7 g
Added sugar		50 g	E	30 IU	15 IU	Calcium	1.0 g	1.3 g
Total Fat	65 g	78 g	K	80 µg	120 µg	Iron	18 mg	18 mg
Saturated Fat	20 g	20 g	C	60 mg	90 mg	Phosphorus	1.0 g	1.25 g
Protein	50 g	50 g	Thiamin	1.5 mg	1.2 mg	Iodine	150 µg	150 µg
			Riboflavin	1.7 mg	1.3 mg	Magnesium	400 mg	400 mg
			Niacin	20 mg	16 mg	Zinc	15 mg	11 mg
			B6	2 mg	1.7 mg	Selenium	70 µg	55 µg
			Folate	400 µg	400 µg	Copper	2 mg	0.9 mg
			B12	6 µg	2.4 µg	Manganese	2 mg	2.3 mg
			Biotin	300 µg	30 µg	Chromium	120 µg	35 µg
			B5	10 mg	5 mg	Chloride	3.4 g	2.3 g

[a]Present RDI.
[b]Proposed new RDI.
RDI, Recommended Daily Intakes.

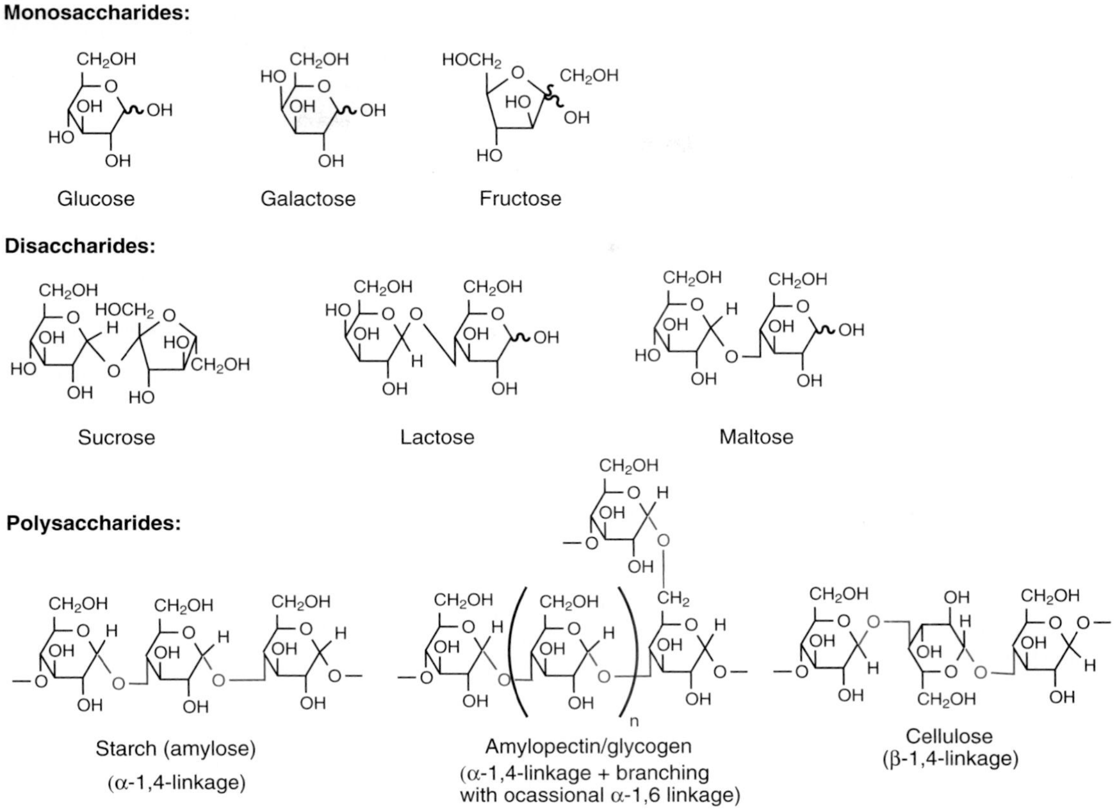

Monosaccharides:

Glucose Galactose Fructose

Disaccharides:

Sucrose Lactose Maltose

Polysaccharides:

Starch (amylose) (α-1,4-linkage)

Amylopectin/glycogen (α-1,4-linkage + branching with ocassional α-1,6 linkage)

Cellulose (β-1,4-linkage)

Figure 37.8 Structures of common carbohydrates.

facilitate the absorption of glucose and fructose. The SGLTs are 12 membrane–spanning proteins that are unrelated to the GLUTs, which exhibit high affinity for glucose following binding to sodium ion (Chapter 4). The SGLT1 is primarily expressed in the small intestine, whereas SGLT2 is expressed in the kidney, where they increase the absorption of glucose from the gut and reabsorb glucose from the kidney tubules, respectively. SGLTs also show affinity for galactose transport. Because monosaccharides account for the major source of energy to human cells, the role of GLUTs and SGLTs is quite important.

Disaccharide Metabolism

Disaccharides require hydrolysis to monosaccharides; for example, sucrose is hydrolyzed to glucose and fructose prior to absorption. Various enzymes present in the brush border of the intestine are involved in the hydrolytic process (i.e., sucrase-isomaltase, lactase-phlorizin hydrolase, maltase-glucoamylase, and trehalase).

Starch Metabolism

Starch is a polysaccharide of glucose that exists as a straight chain polymer called amylose with three or more glucose monomers linked via α-1,4-linkages and amylopectin, a highly branched polymer consisting of α-1,4-linkages together with α-1,6-linkages similar to what is seen in glycogen (Fig. 37.8). Amylose exists in a helix configuration. Starch is a major constituent of plants with various ratios of amylose to amylopectin (for example, potato is 20% amylose and 80% amylopectin; rice is 18.5% amylose and 81.5% amylopectin). The hydrolytic metabolism of starch begins in the oral cavity where α-amylase, which attacks the α-1,4-linkages, is secreted by the salivary glands and later by α-amylase secreted by the pancreas in the duodenum. Glucoamylase in the small intestine is also involved in starch hydrolysis. The result of amylase metabolism is that maltose and maltotriose (a three α-1,4 glucose unit molecule) are formed, at which point final hydrolysis occurs via the previously mentioned brush border disaccharidases, leading to formation of absorbable glucose.

Glycogen Synthesis and Metabolism

Glycogen is the human storage form for glucose, with storage occurring in the liver and muscle tissue. Once glucose is absorbed and phosphorylated to glucose-1-phosphate, it is then incorporated into glycogen through the action of glycogen synthase and glycogen branching enzyme. The structure of glycogen is similar to starch, with both α-1,4-links and α-1,6-links (Fig. 37.8). The process of glycogen formation differs from glycogen degradation. Glycogen hydrolysis occurs when the body requires energy, which involves a process of phosphorylation, transferase, and a debranching enzyme, leading to the release of glucose into the bloodstream.

Cellulose

Cellulose is a major polysaccharide found in plants (Fig. 37.8). It is a linear polymer of glucose but differs from starch by the fact that the linkage between the glucose monomeric units has the β-1,4-linkage, which increases the stability of the polymer through internal hydrogen bonding to produce a strong linear configuration. This configuration prevents hydrolytic metabolism by human enzymes that are specific for α-1,4-linkages. The β-1,4-linkage can be hydrolyzed by cellulase found in some bacteria, protozoa, fungi, and in bovine animals.

Fiber

Fiber or, more specifically, dietary fiber is made up of nondigestible oligosaccharides usually of plant origin, such as the polysaccharides cellulose and pectin (polysaccharide containing 1,4-α-D-galactosyluronic acid monomeric units), or complex material found in wood and cell walls of plants such as lignin (Table 37.6). There is no FDA definition of what a dietary fiber actually is. Fibers may be further classified as soluble fibers (water soluble) such as pectin or insoluble fibers such as cellulose, hemicellulose, and lignin.

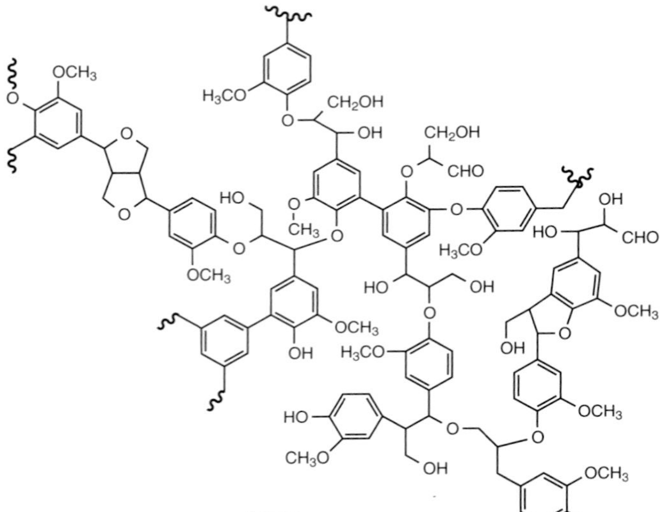

Lignin

As the name would imply, soluble fibers absorb and dissolve in water forming gels that are prone to fermentation by bacteria that are located in the colon, generating short-chain fatty acids, such as butyric acid, through the benefit of epithelial cells in the colon. Insoluble fibers create bulk, which is suggested to be beneficial via increased stomach transit time and a reduction of intestinal transit time. This is thought to decrease the urge to eat and cause a reduction in the ability for chemical absorption to occur from the intestine. Although evidence supporting the health benefits of dietary fibers is suggestive at best, there is general agreement that fiber in the diet can lower the incidence of obesity (creates a feeling of satiety),[11] reduce insulin resistance and the risk of type 2 diabetes, reduce the risk of heart disease (decrease cholesterol absorption from the intestine), and reduce the risk of colon cancer (decrease absorption of potential carcinogens from the gut). Insoluble fibers also act as bulk laxatives. The average American diet contains 12–15 g of fiber compared to 40–150 g of fiber in the diets of Africans and Indians. Recommendations for fiber content in the diet are presently 38 g/d for men under the age of 50 years, 30 g/d for men over the age of 50 years, 25 g/d for women under the age of 50 years, and 20 g/d for women over the age of 50 years. Recently, food manufacturers have been studying starches referred to as resistant starch (RS). Resistant starch is expected to resist digestion by amylase and amylopectinase in the small intestine but may be fermented in the colon. RS, therefore, would be expected to have the same health benefits claimed for the dietary fibers. Various classes of RS, some of which are natural while others are manufactured, are being investigated (informally classified as RS1 through RS5). Changes in crystalline structure of the RS, increases in branching and cross-linking within the starch, and starch-lipid complexes cause the starch to become more resistant to hydrolysis.[12,13] Unripe bananas contain approximate 50% RS.

Table 37.6 Classes of Dietary Fibers

Oligosaccharides	Source
Cellulose	Bran, legumes, peas, vegetables, cabbage, seeds, and apple skin
Hemicellulose	Bran and whole grains
Polyfructose	Oligofructans and insulin
Gums	Oatmeal, barley, and legumes
Pectin	Apples, strawberries, and citrus fruits
Resistant starches	Ripe bananas and potatoes
Nonsaccharide lignin	Root vegetables, wheat, fruits, strawberries

Although nondigestible fibers have little or no caloric value, the soluble fiber that is fermented in the colon can be a source of energy and is given a caloric value of 4 kcal/g.

Properties of Sugars

Sugar is defined as a sweet-tasting crystalline carbohydrate, and in most cases, when one refers to sugar, the person is referring to sucrose (table sugar), although glucose, galactose, lactose, and fructose are sugars having similar properties. Normally, carbohydrates make up 40%-70% of the human daily caloric intake, and the majority of the carbohydrates come in the form of starch, but sizable quantities of sucrose and lactose are also commonly found in the diet. It is estimated that the average American adult consumes 64 lb of sucrose/year, while children may consume as much as 140 lb/yr. Approximately one-third of sugar is ingested from the table sugar bowl, and two-thirds is found in commercially processed food, mostly as high-fructose corn syrup. The consumption of sugar has both a physiologic and a psychological basis. The perception of sweetness is detected by G protein–coupled receptors located in the taste buds on the tongue. Sweetness is one of the five basic tastes that the human body has evolved to detect, and humans crave sweet materials as a way of supplying the body with sufficient energy to meet the daily needs. However, children have been taught to crave sweet foods since sweets are commonly used to bribe children. As a result, we crave sweet foods, namely carbohydrates, in excess to what is actually needed for good health. Excessive intake of sucrose or high-fructose corn syrup is directly related to the development of tooth caries and indirectly related to the development of overweight and obesity, which in turn is related to the onset of type 2 diabetes. Although it might be assumed that a good approach to the health issues associated with excessive consumption of carbohydrates, sugars in particular, would be to reduce the intake of these macronutrients, it seems replacement is a more palatable strategy than restraint. Thus, because of the mounting concern regarding overweight and obesity and the need to reduce calorie intake and yet the desire to meet the craving for sweet substances, nonnutritive sweeteners have gained universal acceptance.

Table 37.7 Comparison of the Sweetness of Nutritive and Nonnutritive Sweeteners

	Sweetness	Calories per 100 g
Nutritive Sweetener		
Sucrose	100%	All mono- and disaccharides ~370
Glucose	60%-70%	
Fructose	110%-180%	
Maltose	33%-50%	
Galactose	15%-40%	
Xylitol	100%	~192
Nonnutritive Sweetener		
Saccharin	300X sucrose	0
Sodium cyclamate	30X sucrose	0
Aspartame	200X sucrose	~0.05
Neotame	7,000X sucrose	0
Acesulfame-K	200X sucrose	0
Sucralose	600X sucrose	0
Rebaudioside A	200X sucrose	0
Rebaudioside M	300X sucrose	0

Nonnutritive Sweeteners

Saccharin (Sweet'N Low)

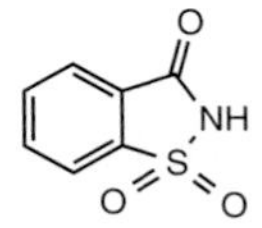

Saccharin

The history of saccharin began with its synthesis in 1878, and over the past 130 plus years, this food additive has been part of the human food scene. Saccharin's history has included a period when it was banned from the market as an adulterant only to be returned as a sugar substitute. It has had limited use directed toward diabetics, carried a warning as a possible carcinogen, and is now openly available for consumer use and a common ingredient in a host of food products. Saccharin's colorful history has recently been presented in a book titled *Empty Pleasures: The Story of Artificial Sweeteners from Saccharin to Splenda.*[14]

The properties of saccharin include a sweetness 300-fold that of sucrose with zero calories (Table 37.7). Saccharin does have a bitter aftertaste, a fact that makes saccharin less than the ideal nonnutritive sweetener, and instability to prolonged heating, thus limiting its use to nonbaked products. The bitter aftertaste has been masked by the addition of other sweeteners. The biggest health-related problem associated with saccharin was a scare resulting from the development of bladder cancer in male rats reported in 1977 and titled the "Canadian Rat Study." This study resulted in the banning of saccharin by the FDA, but the passage of the Saccharin Study and Labeling Act in 1977 by the US Congress allowed saccharin to remain on the market with the required label that saccharin-containing products were potentially carcinogenic. (*This product contains saccharin, which has been determined to cause cancer in laboratory animals.*) Saccharin-containing products retained this label until December 2000, when the warning label was removed following presentation of evidence that male rats are unique in that a combination of high bladder pH, high calcium phosphate concentrations, and a specific protein that favors crystal formation occurs in the presence of saccharin. The formation of microcrystals in the bladder of male rats causes damage to the bladder wall, which over an extended period of time led to tumor formation. These conditions do not exist in humans, and therefore, a threat of saccharin-induced tumors is not possible.[15]

Cyclamate (Sucaryl)

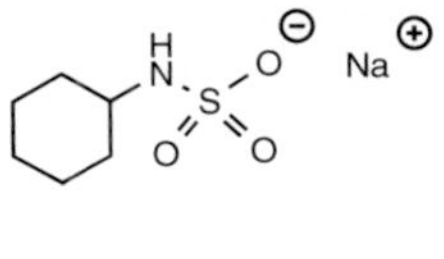

Cyclamate

Cyclamates were first synthesized in 1937 and reached the US market in the 1950s. This artificial sweetener has several advantages over saccharin in that it does not possess a bitter aftertaste and is stable to heat. The compound is 30-50 times sweeter than sucrose with zero caloric value (Table 37.9). During the 1960s, the cyclamates became very popular as nonnutritive sweeteners when directly added to foods, used in baked products, and added to soft drinks and canned fruits. In 1958, cyclamate was added to the generally recognized as safe (GRAS) list, but in 1969, the chemical was banned by the FDA for use in the United States due to what was reported to be the development of bladder cancer in rats possibly due to metabolism of cyclamate to cyclohexylamine. While studies to repeat these results were claimed by the manufacturer to be irreproducible, the chemical has never returned to the US market, although the chemical is still sold in many countries throughout the world.

Aspartame (Equal, NutraSweet) and Neotame

Aspartame   Neotame

In 1965, a chemist working at G.D. Searle & Company discovered that a compound composed of the methyl ester of the dipeptide of two natural amino acids, L-phenylalanine and L-aspartic acid, had an outstanding sweet taste. This dipeptide was later named aspartame. Coming at a time when both saccharin and cyclamate were facing intense scrutiny as synthetic, nonnutritive sweeteners, aspartame was seen as a potentially significant breakthrough in the nonnutritive sweetener market. The properties of aspartame included a sweetness 200-fold sucrose with no bitter aftertaste. A single serving of aspartame, equivalent to an equally sweet 180-calorie serving of sucrose, contains only 0.1 Cal (Table 37.9). While still not stable to prolonged heating, aspartame's other major attraction was the fact that it was composed of L-phenylalanine and L-aspartic acid, two naturally occurring amino acids. At a time when the consumer was (and still is) concerned about synthetic, unnatural chemicals, aspartame offered a marketing windfall. Present in the form of a dipeptide methyl ester, aspartame was first approved for marketing in 1974, but concerns about tumors, brain damage, and testing procedures delayed its introduction to the market until July 1981. By 1985, aspartame was consumed to the extent of 800 million pounds/yr, and 2 years later, it was estimated that aspartame appeared in more than 1,200 products.

Aspartame, being a dipeptide, is prone to hydrolytic metabolism, either in the intestine or mucus membrane of the intestinal lining, to produce phenylalanine, aspartic acid, and methanol (Fig. 37.9). This metabolism in turn raised the question of the safety of the products formed. Methanol, or wood alcohol, is a potential toxin when absorbed into the bloodstream, where it can be converted into formaldehyde and then to formic acid, which could potentially lead to systemic metabolic acidosis and blindness.[16] It was found that the quantity of formic acid detected in the urine (studies could not detect formic acid in the blood after aspartame administration) following large doses of aspartame generated less formic acid from the aspartame than that found after consuming some fruit juices.

The second concern for aspartame is the effect of phenylalanine on individuals who suffer from phenylketonuria (PKU). PKU is a genetic condition in which children are born with a deficiency of phenylalanine hydroxylase, an enzyme that converts phenylalanine into tyrosine. A lack of this enzyme leads to higher than normal levels of phenylalanine in the blood, which leads to formation of catabolic products such as phenylpyruvate and phenyllactate. These products can result in a reduced level of tyrosine and possibly the neurotransmitters formed from tyrosine (norepinephrine and dopamine). If not diagnosed within a few days of birth, PKU can lead to central nervous system (CNS) damage and mental retardation. The exact cause of the mental retardation is not known, but it is assumed that one or all of the abnormal conditions cited above may have a role in PKU. Although phenylalanine is still essential in PKU patients, a diet with low phenylalanine levels is important in the prevention of the serious outcomes of excessive phenylalanine in PKU patients. As a result, the consumption of aspartame by women during pregnancy who might give birth to a PKU infant and administering aspartame-containing foods to a child diagnosed with PKU

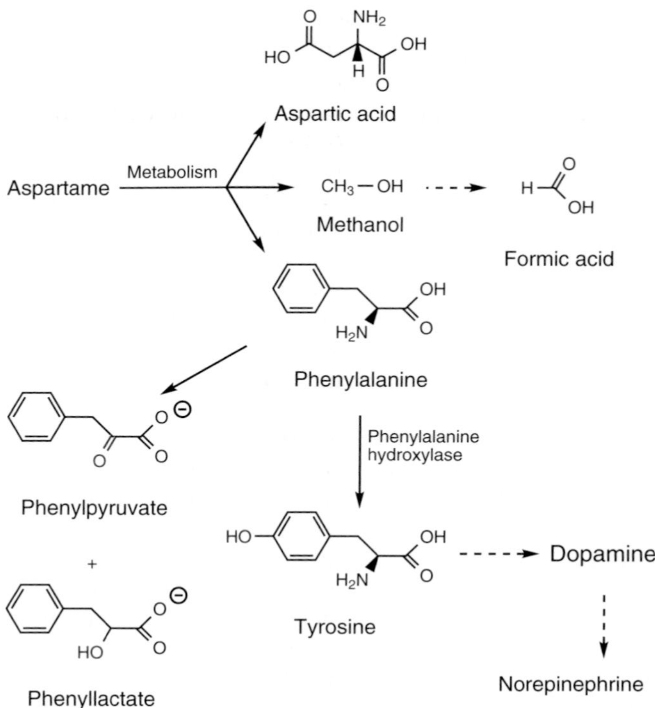

Figure 37.9 Metabolism of aspartame and its metabolites.

have raised concerns. Studies demonstrated that abusive doses of aspartame (200 mg/kg in an adult or 100 mg/kg in a child) or successive doses of aspartame (three 10 mg/kg doses in a child) did not lead to phenylalanine levels equal to or above those approved for adults or children with PKU.[16] These studies suggested that aspartame-containing foods and beverages are unlikely to have adverse effects on patients with PKU, although there is no reason for infants with or without PKU to be using nonnutritive sweeteners. Aspartame-containing foods contain a warning indicating its presence and its potential for harm in patients with PKU.

In 2002, an analogue of aspartame, neotame was approved for marketing in the United States. This compound differs from aspartame by the addition of a dimethylbutyl substituent on the nitrogen of aspartic acid. The result of this substitution is that sweetness is 30-fold greater than aspartame and from 7,000- to 13,000-fold greater than sucrose. Metabolism of neotame results in formation of methanol but significantly less phenylalanine and N-dimethylbutylaspartic acid. The nitrogen substitution also decreases the hydrolysis of the dipeptide, and only 20%-30% of the neotame is absorbed, presumably as the individual amino acids.[17] Since the sweetness of neotame is so much higher than aspartame, a much lower dose would be required to meet the desired sweetness of a neotame-containing food. As a result, it is estimated that the amount of methanol absorbed after an appropriate dose of neotame is approximately 1.3 mg/L, whereas the methanol content from some juices is calculated to be approximately 140 mg/L. The amount of phenylalanine produced from neotame is estimated to be 2.6 mg/d in an adult and 1.5 mg/d in a child, whereas the restricted diet content of phenylalanine for a child with PKU is set at 0.4-0.6 g/d, and the average adult consumes 2.5-10 g/d of phenylalanine. The amount of phenylalanine obtained from a dose of neotame would have a negligible effect on a patient with PKU. Presently, there do not appear to be any food products where neotame is declared as an ingredient. This may be due, however, to the fact that the amount of neotame used does not meet the FDA's threshold for declaration on food labeling.

Acesulfame-K (Sunett)

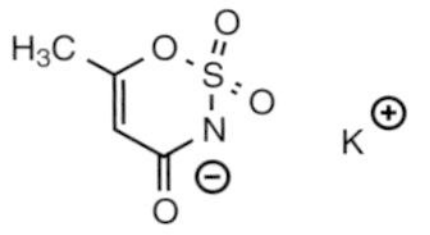

Acesulfame

Discovered in 1967, acesulfame-K is a nonnutritive sweetener that is approximately 200 times sweeter than sucrose and heat stable and therefore can be used in cooking and baking (Table 37.9). The compound is not metabolized and shows structural similarity to saccharin. Acesulfame-K is commonly used in combination with other sweeteners due to its bitter aftertaste, a property it has in common with saccharin (both chemicals affect the same bitter receptor).[18] The chemical was approved for use in the United States in 1988 in dry food, and by 2003, it was approved as a general purpose sweetener, allowing for its added use in carbonated and noncarbonated beverages.

Sucralose (Splenda)

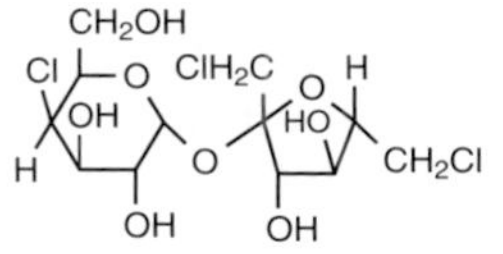

Sucralose

Sucralose is a synthetic derivative of sucrose in which three hydroxyl groups have been replaced with chlorine atoms. As a result, the compound is not metabolized by the body but retains the sweet taste of sucrose, and in fact, the sweetness is increased by approximate 600-fold. The chloride substitution, in addition to preventing the metabolism of sucralose, increases stability of the chemical to heat. Sucralose can be used in baking and cooking.[17] In 1999, sucralose was approved as a general purpose sweetener in the United States. Its general purpose use is indicative of its safety as judged by the FDA.

Rebaudioside A (Truvia, Rebiana, or Reb-A)

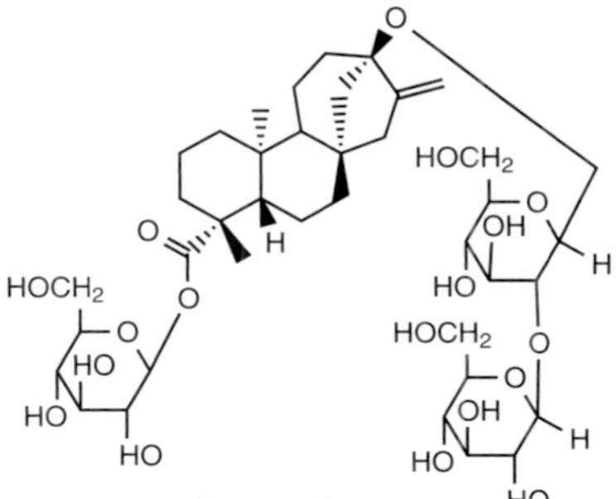

Stevioside

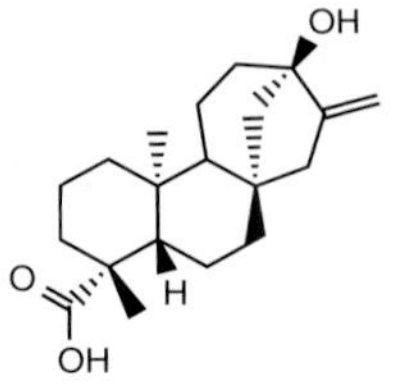

Steviol

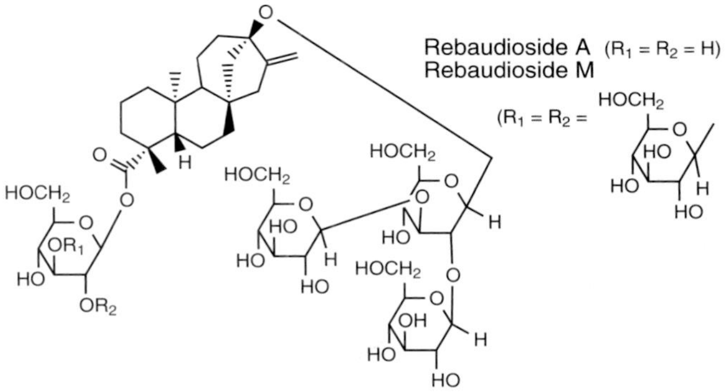

Rebaudioside A ($R_1 = R_2 = H$)
Rebaudioside M ($R_1 = R_2 =$ glucosyl)

For many centuries, the leaves of the stevia plant (*Stevia rebaudiana* Bertoni) have been used for their sweet taste,[17,19] but not until the last decade has commercial interest in this plant resulted in a marketed product derived from the stevia plant. Two major glycosides possess much of the sweet taste; these are stevioside and rebaudioside A, which has been developed and introduced onto the market as a nonnutritive sweetener. Rebaudioside A, known by the trade name Rebiana or Reb-A, is a diterpene glycoside that possesses a sweetness approximately 200-fold greater than sucrose (Table 37.9) and has zero calories. As a glycoside, it is prone to acid-catalyzed hydrolysis. At low pHs, stevioside can undergo hydrolysis by intestinal bacterial flora, leading to the formation of steviol, the aglycone component of the rebiosides. Human metabolic studies on stevioside have shown that only trace amounts of stevioside can be detected in blood and no steviol is detected. Because steviol has been shown to exhibit positive genetic toxicology as well as the ability to induce chromosome breakage in bacteria, stevioside, stevia extracts, and, to some extent, rebaudioside A have been studied in depth for their safety.[19,20] These studies have concluded that stevioside and rebaudioside A are not genotoxic or carcinogenic in vitro or in vivo and that the only cell-damaging effects of steviol occurred in in vitro studies at excessive concentrations.

In 2008, the FDA approved inclusion of rebaudioside A in the GRAS list as well as its use in foods and beverages as a nonnutritive sweetener. Prior to these approvals, rebaudioside A was available in the United States as a dietary supplement. In the single-component product Truvia, erythritol (a four-carbon polyhydroxy sugar alcohol) is added as a sweetener to mask the aftertaste of licorice, which appears to be associated with rebaudioside A. Erythritol itself has a caloric content of 0.2 kcal/g.

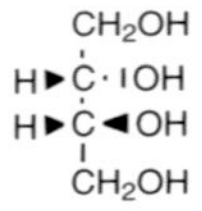

Erythritol

Rebaudioside M is presently under review for inclusion in the GRAS list. The chemical is derived from *Stevia rebaudiana* Bertoni and prepared by fermentation using a yeast from the saccharomycetaceae family. A significant property of Rebaudioside M is that it is pH stable at pH 3-8 and stable for 1 hour at temperature of 100°.

Xylitol

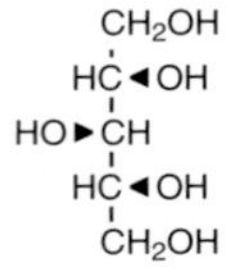

Xylitol

Xylitol is a polyol (a five-carbon polyhydroxy sugar alcohol) with structural similarity to glucose and erythritol. It has been used since the 1960s as a sugar substitute with a sweetness comparable to sucrose but with 40% fewer calories (Table 37.9). Xylitol is commonly found in chewing gums because it does not promote the development of dental caries or plaque formation and yet satisfies the need for sweetness. This property is due to the fact that the polyols are not metabolized to organic acids in the oral cavity. Xylitol can be added to the gum, and the gum can still be labeled as sugar "free."[17] Unfortunately, if consumed in large quantities, xylitol can have a laxative effect due to its poor absorption and water osmotic effect. Xylitol can be consumed by diabetics and will not affect blood sugar levels. Xylitol is found commonly in fruits such as raspberries and plums and can be prepared from the hydrogenation of xylose, which is found in corncobs and wood pulp.

Mogrosides (Nectresse)

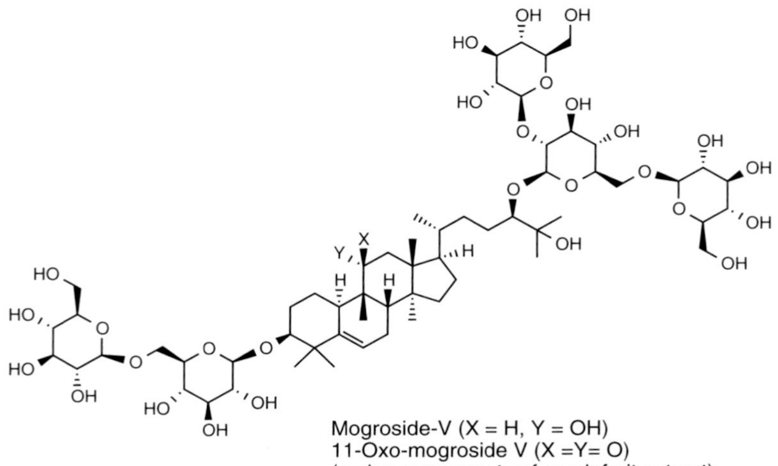

Mogroside-V (X = H, Y = OH)
11-Oxo-mogroside V (X = Y = O)
(major components of monk fruit extract)

The plant *Siraitia grosvenorii* found commonly in China and Thailand is an herbaceous perennial which produces a fruit known as luo han guo or the monk fruit (the fruit was used by Buddhist monks). The fruit is approximately 300 times sweeter than sugar and has been used for generations in cooling drinks and Chinese medicine (Table 37.9). The fruit is also known as a longevity fruit and comes from Chinese provinces, which are known for their inhabitance living beyond 100 years. The fruit extract has been approved by the FDA for inclusion on the GRAS list and there are no known toxicities associated with its use. The major components of the monk fruit are the mogrosides which are triterpene glycosides. Mogroside V and 11-oxo-mogroside V are the major mogrosides possessing the sweet taste found in the monk fruit. Both of these ingredients have been reported to exhibit antioxidant properties and act as scavengers of reactive oxygen species (ROS).[21,22] In vitro studies suggest that 11-oxo-mogroside V is a more potent scavenger of ROS than mogroside V. Monk fruit has been used to treat a variety of inflammatory conditions including acute and chronic bronchitis, gastritis, sore throats, and minor stomach and intestinal problems.

While monk fruit products are still available, the manufacturer of Nectresse has discontinued its sales due to disappointing sales.

Fats and Fatty Acids

Chemistry of Fats and Fatty Acids

By definition, a fat is a neutral molecule composed of three fatty acids attached to the alcohol glycerol, thus referred to as triglycerides, and represents a storage and transport form for fatty acids.

Glycerin

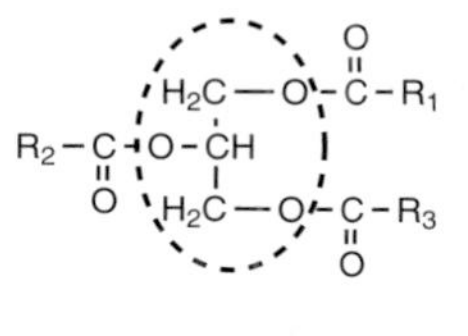

Triglyceride
(Fat)

Fatty acids themselves play multiple biologic roles, including the following: They are components of the cell wall, usually in the form of phospholipids, glycolipids, and fatty acid acetylated proteins; a high-energy source of calories; and hormone and intracellular messengers.

The fatty acids are classified based on the presence or absence of double bonds. The natural fatty acids with no double bonds are referred to as saturated fatty acids; they are totally saturated with hydrogen. The naturally occurring saturated fatty acids contain 12-24 carbon atoms (Fig. 37.10) and have an even number of carbon atoms, which results from the fact that they are biosynthesized from the two-carbon acetate unit. A second group of fatty acids is the monounsaturated fatty acids, consisting of palmitoleic acid (9Z-hexadecenoic acid) and oleic acid (9Z-octadecenoic acid). These acids have a single double bond, and it should be noted that the stereochemistry of these and other naturally occurring unsaturated fatty acids contain the *cis* or Z configuration. A third class of fatty acids are the polyunsaturated fatty acids (PUFAs) and consist of linoleic and linolenic acid (9Z,12Z-octadecadienoic acid and 9Z,12Z,15Z-octadecatrienoic acid, respectively). Additional fatty acids of nutritional significance are arachidonic acid (C20:4 *cis* double bonds), eicosapentaenoic acid (EPA) (C20:5 *cis* double bonds), and docosahexaenoic acid (C22 with 6 *cis* double

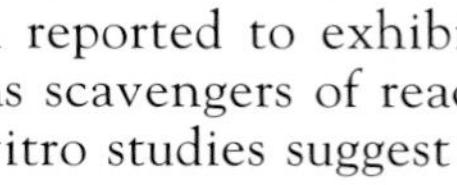

$H_3C-(CH_2)_x-C(=O)-OH$

x	Common name	Official name
10	Lauric acid	n-Dodecanoic acid
12	Myristic acid	n-Tetradecanoic acid
14	Palmitic acid	n-Hexadecanoic acid
16	Stearic acid	n-Octadecanoic acid
18	Arachidic acid	n-Eicosanoic acid
20	Behenic acid	n-Docosanoic acid
22	Lignoceric acid	n-Tetracosanoic acid

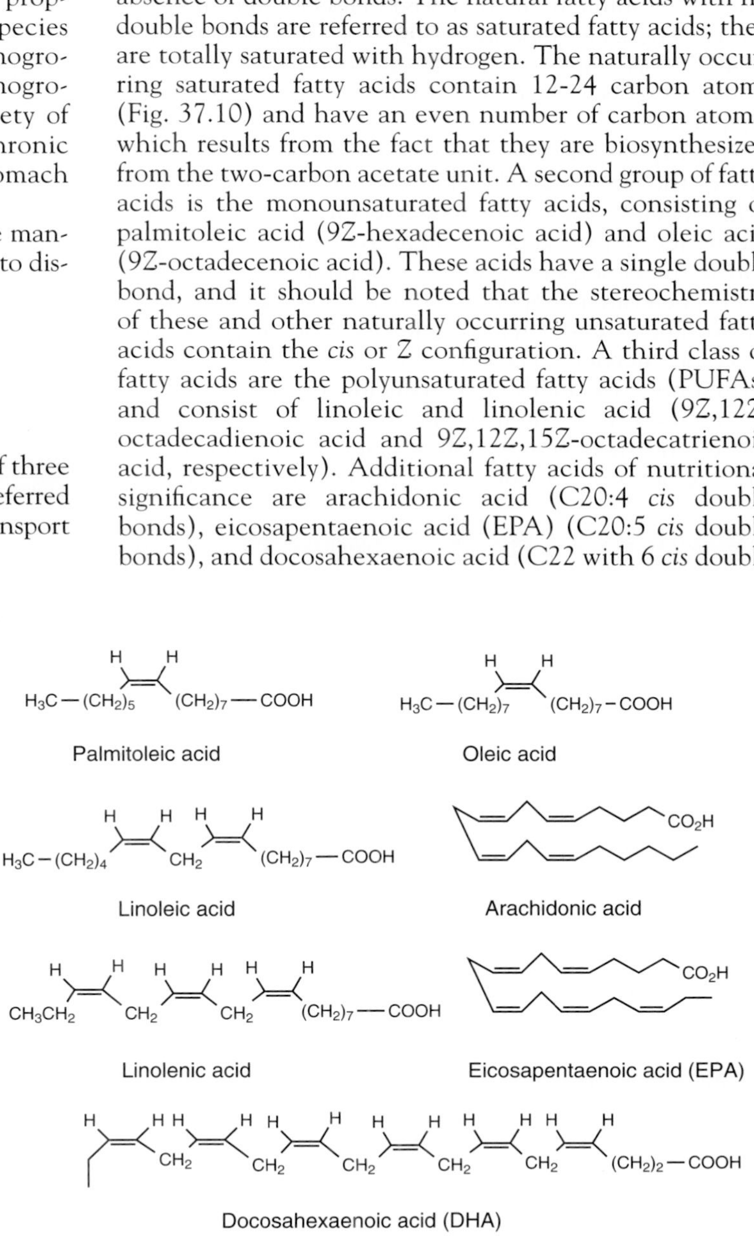

Palmitoleic acid

Oleic acid

Linoleic acid

Arachidonic acid

Linolenic acid

Eicosapentaenoic acid (EPA)

Docosahexaenoic acid (DHA)

Figure 37.10 Structures of unsaturated, monounsaturated, and polyunsaturated fatty acids (PUFAs).

bonds), which are shown in Figure 37.10. Fatty acids with a double bond three carbons from the end of the fatty acid chain are referred to as the ω-3 fatty acids in a commonly used nomenclature.

Physical-Chemical Properties

A distinguishing physical-chemical property of the various classes of fatty acids is that as the degree of unsaturation increases, the melting point decreases. The saturated fatty acids tend to be low-melting solids, whereas the unsaturated fatty acids and PUFAs are liquids (Table 37.8). The saturated fatty acids tend to be found in higher concentrations in animal fats, whereas the unsaturated and polyunsaturated fatty acids are found in high concentrations in vegetable oils (Table 37.9). It is interesting that as the consumer demand moves away from saturated fats and toward unsaturated fats that seed manufacturers are turning to genetically modified plant seeds to product plants that produce increased levels of monounsaturated fatty acids and reduced levels of saturated and polyunsaturated fatty acids.[23]

In part, this relates to a second physical-chemical property of the fatty acids. The fats containing saturated fatty acids generally have a more stable shelf-life and are stable at elevated temperatures to air oxidation. The PUFAs within the fat are susceptible to oxidation reactions, especially at elevated temperature (baking and frying temperatures). The oxidative reactions lead to rancidity, darkening in color, increased viscosity, and polymer formation. A commonly used method of reducing the concentration of the PUFA is through partial hydrogenation (leading to the hydrogenated oils). Catalytic hydrogenation involves a reversible addition of hydrogen and catalyst to the double bond followed by the irreversible addition of a second hydrogen to the initial double bond (Fig. 37.11). The reversibility of the initial step in the hydrogenation leads to loss of the hydrogen from the saturated carbon and formation of both the initial alkene and a new alkene with the more stable *trans* or *E* stereochemistry and, thus, formation of a *trans* fatty acid (TFA) impurity. The quantity of TFAs formed by catalytic hydrogenation can be reduced by changes in the conditions used for the hydrogenation process.[24] The 2006 report of a Canadian study, "Transforming the Food Supply: Report of the Trans Fat Task Force," submitted to the Minister of Health reports that of the fats present in food, the TFA levels may be as high as 24%-33% for bakery products, 20%-40% for margarines, and as high as 40% for snack foods, nachos, and nachos cheese sauces.[23] The concern is that TFA consumption increases the levels of low-density lipoprotein (LDL) cholesterol, reduces the level of high-density lipoprotein (HDL) cholesterol, and increases the ratio of total cholesterol to HDL cholesterol, which are measures that are associated with increased risk of coronary heart disease (CHD).[25] Other endogenous changes have been associated with TFA consumption including changes in triglyceride levels, promotion of inflammatory reactions, and endothelial dysfunction. Generally, *trans* fats composed of one or more TFAs attached to the glycerin backbone are not normally present in natural foods with the exception of small amounts in meats coming from cows,

Table 37.8 Melting Points of Saturated and Unsaturated Fatty Acids

$H_3C-(CH_2)_Z-\overset{O}{\overset{\|}{C}}-OH$ (I) $H_3C-(CH_2)_Y-(CH=CH-CH_2)_X-(CH_2)_W-COOH$ (II)

Common Name	z			mp (°C)
Saturated (I)				
Lauric acid	10			44
Myristic acid	12			58
Palmitic acid	14			63
Stearic acid	16			70
Unsaturated (II)	w	x	y	
Palmitoleic acid	6	1	5	−1
Oleic acid	6	1	7	4
Linoleic acid	6	2	4	−5
Linolenic acid	6	3	1	−12
Arachidonic acid	2	5	1	−49.5

Table 37.9 Approximate Percent of Fatty Acids in Various Food

Food	Saturated Fatty Acids %	Monounsaturated Fatty Acids %	Polyunsaturated Fatty Acids %
Butterfat	60	36	4
Pork fat	59	39	2
Beef	53	44	2
Chicken fat	39	44	21
Margarines[a]	20	40	40
Salmon oil	24	39	36
Corn oil	15	31	53
Soybean oil	14	24	53
Olive oil	14	75	11
Sunflower	10	22	66
Canola	7	61	22

Data from Nazir DJ, Moorecroft BJ, Mishkel MA. Fatty acid composition of margarines. *Am J Clin Nutrition*. 1976;29:331-339.

[a]Fatty acid content shows considerable variations between percentage of saturated fatty acids (palmitic acid and stearic acid), monounsaturated fatty acid (oleic acid), and polyunsaturated fatty acid(linoleic acid) as well as *cis/trans* ratio in various brand named mararines.

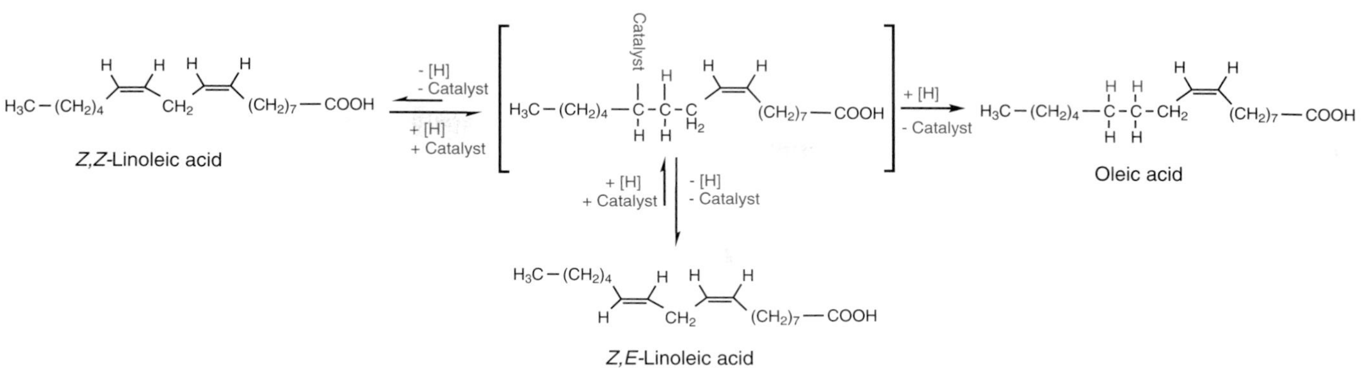

Figure 37.11 Catalytic hydrogenation of a polyunsaturated fatty acid to a monounsaturated fatty acid.

sheep, and other ruminants in which bacteria within the stomach of ruminants produce the TFAs. It is estimated that this accounts for approximately 0.5% of the total caloric intake. But commercially deep-fried foods, bakery products, packaged snack foods, margarines, and crackers prepared with *trans* fat–containing oils may increase the amount of *trans* fats in our diet, leading to 2%-3% of the total caloric intake being TFAs. Thus, considerable concern has been generated in the press, health professionals, and the public about the long-term effects of *trans* fats. This has led to changes in the manufacture of cooking oils and the use of oils containing *trans* fats including, in some cases, legislation outlawing the use of *trans* fat–containing oils. It has been suggested that a 2% increase in energy intake from TFAs could result in a 23% increase in the incidence of CHD.[26] Over the past several years, the presence of TFAs in food products has declined as indicated by the labeling of foods as having zero *trans* fats, although such a label does not guarantee zero grams per serving. The FDA allows a report of zero grams per serving if the food contains <500 mg/serving of *trans* fats. The FDA has ruled that food manufacturers had until June 18, 2018, to ensure that their products no longer contain partially hydrogenated oils for uses that have not been approved by the FDA.[27] As a result, the presence of *trans* fats in food are expected to be greatly reduced.

Fat and Fatty Acid Absorption

The major nutritional value of fats comes from the fatty acids, which upon metabolism are a high-density source of energy. In order for this to occur, the fat must be absorbed, transported via the bloodstream either to the cells in tissue where the energy is needed or to storage sites in adipose cells for future energy needs, and finally moved into a cell's mitochondria for metabolism, with the release of energy in the form of ATP units. This process is complicated by the fact that fats themselves cannot be transported across cell membranes due to their low hydrophilicity. Rather, a sequence of hydrolysis and ester formation occurs at various stages in the absorption-transport-storage-utilization process.

Consumed fats travel to the small intestine where they are emulsified with the aid of bile acids and are then hydrolyzed through the action of pancreatic lipase. The resulting fatty acids and glycerol can now be absorbed into the intestinal mucosa. At this point, the fat is reformed and, in the presence of apoproteins and cholesterol, is converted to chylomicrons (large lipoprotein particles consisting of 85%-92% triglycerides), which are capable of entering the bloodstream for transport to storage sites in adipocytes or muscle cells for utilization as an energy source. Once again, for transport into adipocytes or muscle cells, the fat must be hydrolyzed by lipases, absorbed across the cell membrane, and re-esterified to the triglycerol fat for storage in adipocytes or metabolized in the mitochondria of the muscle cell (myocytes).[28]

Mobilization of fats from adipocytes is a G protein–innervated process involving β-adrenergic receptors and various hormones including glucagon, epinephrine, and β-corticotropin. Release of fatty acids from the adipocytes into the bloodstream allows for the transport to myocytes with the aid of blood albumin and ultimately passive absorption into the myocytes. It should be noted that insulin can inhibit the release of fatty acids from adipocytes by inhibition of adenylyl cyclase. Once again, transport into the mitochondria from the cytoplasm requires esterification to a fatty acyl-coenzyme A (CoA), transport across the outer mitochondria membrane, transesterification to fatty acylcarnitine, transport across the inner mitochondria, and transesterification back to fatty acyl-CoA, which can now be metabolized in the Krebs cycle to carbon dioxide, water, and release of ATP.

Nutritional Properties

It is estimated that 35%-40% of the caloric intake in the United States comes in the form of fat, with greater than 90% of the fat being in the form of triglycerides (free fatty acids, cholesterol, and phospholipids represent the remaining amount of fat in the diet). This amounts to approximately 100-150 g/d of triglycerides. The RDI for fat is 65 g/d consisting of 20 g/d of saturated fats and 300 mg of cholesterol. This is based on a 2,000-calorie diet for an adult. Obviously the typical diet of 100-150 g/d of fat will lead to an excessive caloric intake of this macronutrient and an associated potential for overweight and obesity.

Fats have an essential role in the health of the body. In addition to being a major source of body energy (80%-90%), fatty acids are an endogenous source of cholesterol via acetyl-CoA units. Cholesterol is the precursor to hormones of the body (bile salts, vitamin D, sex hormones, and adrenocortical hormones). Phospholipids and unsaturated fatty acids are components of the cell membrane, and subcutaneous fats give the body thermal insulation. However, excessive quantities of fats are associated with significant human disease.

Health Issues

As already indicated, fats and fatty acids as a source of calories are associated with overweight and obesity, but this is true of any calorie source because a calorie is a calorie irrespective of whether it comes from fats, carbohydrates, or proteins. There are particular disease states in which evidence points to dietary fats as a major contributor to the condition. CHD, which includes ischemic heart disease, myocardial infarction, and angina pectoris, is a condition in which fats and cholesterol have a significant role (Chapter 19). Countries that have diets low in saturated fats and cholesterol have a low incidence of ischemic heart disease, whereas Western industrialized countries with high dietary fat intake show significant increases in heart disease. A strong link exists between high blood lipid levels (e.g., LDL) and atherosclerosis, which in turn is tied to CHD. A reversible relationship also exists between CHD and the lowering of blood lipid levels. Thus, a goal is to reduce total fat calories to less than 35% of caloric intake.

Epidemiologic studies suggest that colorectal cancer is correlated with high calorie intake, diets rich in meat protein, and elevated dietary fats and oils. Metabolic processes in the GI tract and low fiber in the diet have been suggested as possible mechanisms.

It is generally agreed that a relationship exists between fats and insulin resistance, leading to type 2 diabetes, and diets consisting of low fat content and high carbohydrate content are commonly recommended. Obesity is certainly considered a predisposing factor to type 2 diabetes, but other than fats being a significant source of calories, the relationship between diabetes and fats is tenuous. Animal studies support the relationship of saturated fats and decreased insulin sensitivity, but whether these studies can be carried over to humans is debatable. Because of the complexity of diets, human variability, and the lack of long-term studies, it is difficult to associate fats with type 2 diabetes, although evidence points to beneficial effects of low saturated fats, low *trans* fats, and high PUFA combined with high-fiber diets in reducing the risk of type 2 diabetes.[29]

Fats and Fatty Acid Substitution

As with carbohydrates, replacement of fats and fatty acids with nonfats or reduced-fat calories is desirable. Other than reducing the proportion of fats in the diet, the options for fat substitutes are far less than the choices available with sugar substitutes.

SKIMMED MILK. Skimmed milk is a dairy product in which nearly all of the butterfat is removed, whereas whole milk contains approximately 3.5 g of a mixture of fats in 100 g of fluid. The fatty acid content of whole milk consists of saturated fatty acids (palmitic acid [31%], myristic acid [12%], and stearic acid [11%]) and unsaturated fatty acids (oleic acid [24%], palmitoleic acid [4%], and linoleic acid [3%]). Various other milk products are available such as reduced-fat (2% fat) and low-fat milk (~1% fat). Because of the low fat content of skimmed milk, the caloric content of 100 g of skimmed milk is approximately 34 Cal compared with 64 Cal in 100 g of whole milk. Ice cream prepared from cow's milk contains from 10% to 19% fat, a varying content of cholesterol (~97 mg/100 g of ice cream), and a caloric content of approximately 274 Cal. In contrast, frozen yogurt made from skimmed milk has very little fat but may have significant calorie content due to added sucrose.

OLESTRA (OLEAN)

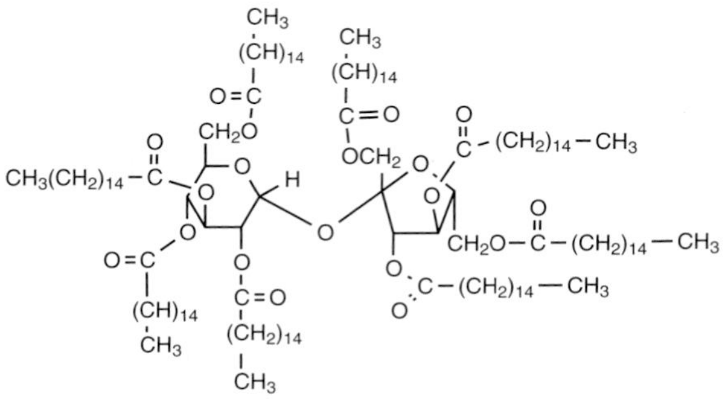

CH_3 $(CH)_{14}$ $O=C$ CH_2O CH_3 $(CH)_{14}$ $C=O$ OCH_2 $C-(CH_2)_{14}-CH_3$ $CH_3(CH_2)_{14}-C$ H $CH_2O-C-(CH_2)_{14}-CH_3$ $O=C$ $C=O$ $C-(CH_2)_{14}-CH_3$ $(CH)_{14}$ CH_3 $(CH_2)_{14}$ CH_3

Olestra

Olestra is composed of a sucrose nucleus with all of the alcohol groups substituted with stearic acid. As a result of the bulky substituents, the compound is not readily hydrolyzed to the fatty acids and sucrose; thus, olestra is advertised as a "fat-free" material. The properties of olestra include a high boiling point with stability to baking and cooking and a taste and feel similar to fat. As a result, olestra is used as a frying oil to prepare potato chips. Americans purchased more than 1.6 billion pounds of potato chips, pretzels, and microwave popcorn in 1999.[30] Olestra-prepared chips have 0 g of fat and 70 Cal, whereas an equivalent quantity of normally prepared chips has 10 g of fat and 160 Cal. The lower metabolism is associated with poor absorption of the olestra, and as a highly fatty material, it has the potential for dissolving and retaining the fat-soluble vitamins (vitamins A, D, E, and K), increasing the potential for hypovitaminosis of these vitamins. Most significantly, olestra causes cramping and loose stools, which have seriously affected the sales of olestra-containing products. To offset the potential for fat-soluble vitamin deficiencies, olestra-containing foods commonly are fortified with small amounts of the fat-soluble vitamins.

Various nondigestible fibers from oats have been developed that can be used in foods as fat replacements products, but these appear to have low commercial value at the present time.

Protein

The third major macronutrient is protein. As indicated earlier, proteins are essential to the body as a source of amino acids. Proteins, as a polymer of amino acids, are not absorbed as such but must be metabolized by peptidases in the GI tract to the monomeric amino acids and di- and tripeptides, which can then be absorbed from the GI tract via active transport. Protein makes up 12%-14% of our normal diet. The body's energy needs are met primarily by fat (~15 kg in the body), whereas carbohydrates in the form of glycogen give rise to immediate energy needs, but its presence in the body is quite small (~0.2 kg). Protein, in the form of muscle mass, accounts for approximately 6 kg of body weight and is a source of potential energy via metabolism to amino acids, which are converted into glucose through the biochemical process called gluconeogenesis. In general, proteins are used for body structure (muscle), hormones, and enzymes and as a source of nitrogen for the synthesis of key chemical components such as purine for RNA and DNA synthesis; only as a last resort will the body use protein as a source of energy.

Twenty amino acids are essential to the human body and are normally obtained from the proteins in the diet. Once absorbed, these essential amino acids can be used for protein synthesis through the action of DNA and RNA (see Chapter 5). The actual RDAs for individual amino acids are not known, and it is not possible to accurately determine the RDAs for proteins that have varying quantities of individual amino acids. It is generally accepted that males have an RDA of 45-63 g of protein/day, whereas females have an RDA of 44-50 g/d. These numbers are greatly affected by pregnancy and lactation in women (RDA may increase by as much as 50%), but can also be affected in both men and women by chronic stress, where the level of protein requirement will increase.

PHARMACOTHERAPY OF OVERWEIGHT AND OBESITY

Overweight and obesity are complex chronic conditions for which successful treatment is not easily attained. Although the cause of obesity and overweight can be easily defined as resulting from a chronic intake of calories in excess to what the body needs, the involvement of social, behavioral, cultural, physiologic, metabolic, and genetic factors makes treatment extremely difficult. Dieting and physical activity can normally produce a loss of weight, but the long-term maintenance of the desired body weight is extremely difficult. Health hazards are associated with both excessive body weight and weight cycling, which commonly occurs through the loss and regaining of weight. A comprehensive study of the issues and treatment of overweight and obesity was reported in 1997 by the National Heart, Lung, and Blood Institute Obesity Education Initiative titled "Clinical Guidelines on the Identification, Evaluation, and Treatment of Overweight and Obesity in Adults" in which drug therapy was addressed as being one of several methods that can be helpful to long-term treatment.[6] It would be over 15 years later until the "2013 AHA/ACC/TOS Guideline for the Management of Overweight and Obesity in Adults" was published. It maintained the cut points for therapeutic interventions established in the NHLBI guideline and recommend addressing targeted goals of other comorbid conditions as part of the weight loss goals.[31] Soon after, the 2015 publication of the "Pharmacological Management of Obesity: An Endocrine Society Clinical Practice Guideline" stressed the use of weight loss medication aid in the treatment of comorbid conditions while encouraging clinicians to consider the use of weight-losing or weight-neutral medications when treating other conditions in overweight or obese patients.[32] A year later, the "American Association of Clinical Endocrinologist and American College of Endocrinology Comprehensive Clinical Practice Guidelines for Medical Care of Patients with Obesity" sought to answer nine top level questions via a systematic evidenced base review of the literature. The AACE/ACE guidelines present clinicians with recommendations individualizing the selection of weight loss medications based on coexisting diseases and along with weight loss goals need for the tertiary prevention of obesity related illnesses in patients.[33]

The FDA-approved labeling for all medications indicated for weight loss states the medication should be used as an adjunct to or in conjunction with a reduced-calorie diet. The rapid increase in the publication of clinical practice guidelines for the treatment of obesity coincided with the growing evidence base as to the health impacts of obesity as well as the development of medications FDA approved for the long-term treatment of obesity. Orlistat was originally approved in 1999 by the FDA and, for many years, was the only agent for obesity that was not labeled for short-term use of "a few weeks."[34] Then in 2012, lorcaserin and phentermine/topiramate were approved followed in 2014 by liraglutide and naltrexone/bupropion bringing to five the number of agents indicated for long-term use in the pharmacologic treatment of obesity.[35-38]

Orlistat (Alli, Xenical)

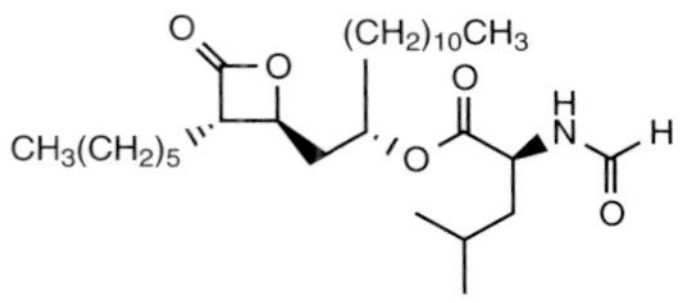

O (CH$_2$)$_{10}$CH$_3$ O H N H CH$_3$(CH$_2$)$_5$ O O

Orlistat

Orlistat, tetrahydrolipstatin, is a semisynthetic derivative of the natural product lipstatin produced by *Streptomyces toxytricini*. The compound acts as an irreversible inhibitor of pancreatic lipase and several other lipases and, as such, prevents the normal metabolic breakdown of fats, leading to reduced absorption of fatty acids from the GI tract.[39,40] Fecal fat loss increases by as much as 30% after treatment with orlistat, thus indicating that reduced activity of intestinal lipases increases the loss of undigested fats. Studies with porcine pancreatic lipase show that acylation of serine 152 is responsible for this inhibition of lipase activity (Fig. 37.12), [40] suggesting a similar mechanism for orlistat in human intestine. Orlistat itself is not absorbed to any appreciable extent and is lost from the body via the GI tract. In addition, drug interaction studies indicate that orlistat may interfere with the absorption of a wide spectrum of drugs, such as cyclosporin and some diabetes

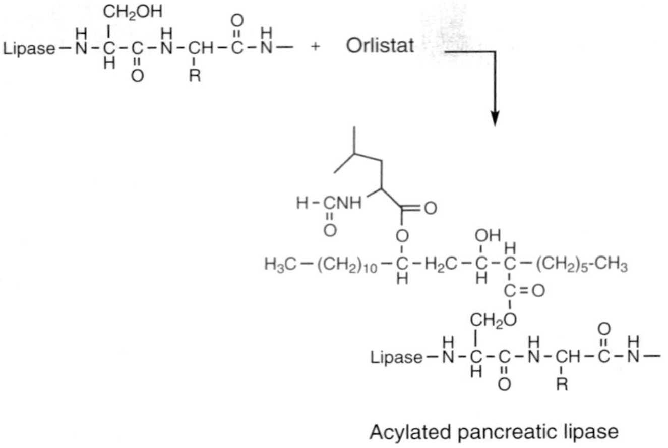

Figure 37.12 Irreversible acylation of a serine in pancreatic lipase by orlistat.

medications, levothyroxine and warfarin, and with the fat-soluble vitamins with the exception of vitamin E.[41]

As might be expected, the most common adverse events were associated with the lack of absorption of fats and consisted of oily stools, spotting bowel movements, stomach pain, and flatulence. A meta-analysis of 16 trials found that 80% of patients treated with orlistat reported at least one GI adverse event.[42] Additionally, it was noted that while on orlistat, obese patients showed a decrease in LDL and total cholesterol levels and that HbA_{1c} levels decreased in patients with type 2 diabetes.

Orlistat is available in a nonprescription product (Alli, 60 mg taken with each fat-containing meal up to 3 doses/d) and a prescription product (Xenical, 120 mg taken with each fat-containing meal up to 3 doses/d). Orlistat is used as an adjunct to diet and exercise and can be used for long-term therapy.

Anorexiants as Pharmacologic Agents in the Management of Obesity

The anorexiants, also known as anorectics or anorexigenics, antiobesity and appetite suppressants, constitute the starting place of pharmacologic therapy for obesity. These drugs are used as adjuncts in weight reduction programs under physician supervision for morbidly obese patients (BMI >40 kg/m^2) who are on a caloric reduction diet, exercise program, and behavioral therapy program, who may need to reduce weight over months or years. Appetite is clearly a very important instinct to promote survival.[43] Arguably any drug that would abolish appetite may carry a high mortality risk and may be unsuitable for clinical use. Because the human body uses various neurochemicals and hormones to protect its stores of fat (a reaction probably useful to our ancestors when food was scarce), a "silver bullet," or a way to completely circumvent this natural habit of protecting excess food stores, has not yet been found. As a result, anorexiants/antiobesity drugs are not a practical long-term solution for people who are overweight. Appetite suppressants should not be used in place of proper diet. For best results, these drugs must be used along with a medically approved diet and exercise program.

Sympathomimetic Amines

Introduction

The sympathomimetic anorexiants shown in Figure 37.13 are structurally and pharmacologically related to amphetamine and its closely related analogues. The sympathomimetic anorexiants are related to each other through the phenylpropylamine pharmacophore. Anorexiants are primarily intended to suppress the appetite, but most of the drugs in this class appear not to have a primary effect on appetite, but their appetite suppressant actions appear to be secondary to CNS stimulation and as CNS stimulants have a potential for abuse or addiction. As a result of the abuse potential amphetamine itself and many of its early analogues have very limited use as anorexiants.[44] Lisdexamfetamine, a recently approved drug, is a prodrug, which releases dextroamphetamine, but its use is limited to treatment of binge eating disorders. Because of the abuse potential the sympathomimetic agents are classified as schedule II, III, and IV, as determined by the Controlled Substances Act of 1971 (Fig. 37.13).

Mechanism of Action

The mechanism of action of the sympathomimetic amines when used to treat obesity remains unclear, but it is thought that these drugs act by releasing norepinephrine from storage vesicles in the adrenergic neuron and by blocking norepinephrine reuptake from the synapse. These drugs also act as reuptake inhibitors of dopamine, which is believed to be linked with their abuse and addiction potential. This class of compounds has no primary effect on the appetite brain center; rather, its appetite-suppressant action appears to be secondary to CNS stimulation. With the exception of phentermine, all of the sympathomimetics are chiral

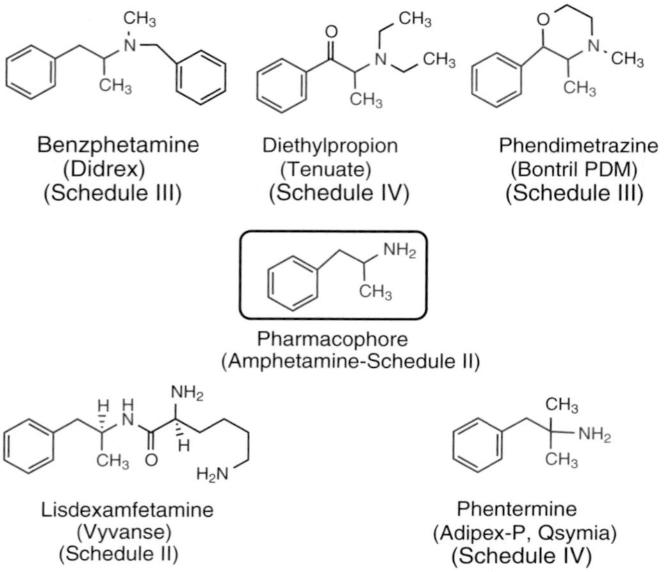

Figure 37.13 Sympathomimetic anorexiants.

compounds with the dextro isomer as in the case of dextroamphetamine exhibiting the psychostimulant and anorexiant activity.

Physicochemical and Pharmacokinetics Properties

All of the sympathomimetic anorexiants are available as water-soluble salts (i.e., hydrochlorides, tartrates, dimesylate). These compounds are readily absorbed and often extensively metabolized.

Metabolism

The symphathomimetics commonly undergo N-dealkylation as shown in Figure 37.14. The N-dealkylation products in general retain biological activity.[45,46]

Benzphetamine is primarily N-demethylated to N-benzylamphetamine and to the minor metabolites methamphetamine, amphetamine, and their hydroxylated metabolites. The appetite-suppressant effect of diethylpropion is due to its metabolic N-monodeethylation to ethocathinone.

Phenmetrazine, a previous approved and withdrawn anorexiant, has been replaced with phendimetrazine which in turn functions as a prodrug metabolically giving rise to low levels of phenmetrazine (~30%). Because of the slow conversion to phenmetrazine the abuse potential for this drug is reported to be reduced. Additionally, 30% of the administered drug is excreted unchanged.

As with phendimetrazine, lisdexamfetamine is a prodrug, which is metabolized to the active appetite-suppressant drug dextroamphetame to the extent of ~40%.

Clinical Applications

Sympathomimetic appetite suppressants are used in the short-term treatment of obesity (i.e., no more than 12 wk). Their appetite-reducing effect tends to decrease after a few weeks of treatment. These drugs should not be taken with other appetite suppressants due to the possibility of serious adverse effects. Lisdexamfetamine is specifically approved for treatment of binge eating disorders (BED) and for treatment of attention deficit hyperactivity disorder (ADHD) in children age 6 years or older. It should not be used to treat obesity in general.

EPHEDRINE, PSEUDOEPHEDRINE, AND PHENYLPROPANOLAMINE

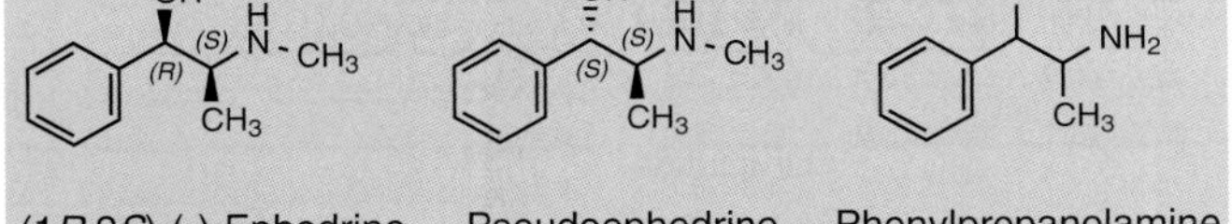

(1*R*,2*S*)-(-)-Ephedrine Pseudoephedrine Phenylpropanolamine

For a number of years over-the-counter dietary supplements and Internet products (Herbal Fen-Phen, PhenTrim, Phen-Cal, Xenadrine) contain ephedrine, which is derived from the ephedra herb, ma huang. Ephedra is one of a group of plants that are a source of ephedrine alkaloids, including ephedrine and pseudoephedrine. Ephedrine can cause a number of side effects, including rapid heartbeat, high blood pressure, psychosis, heart attacks, and seizures. Pseudoephedrine, a related stereoisomer of ephedrine, is commonly found in many antihistamines and cold medicines, has similar effects, and was sometimes used by dieters. Pseudoephedrine has also been used for its CNS stimulant properties. The structural similarity of pseudoephedrine to the amphetamines has made the drug a sought-after chemical precursor in the illicit manufacture of methamphetamine. As a result, in 2004, the FDA prohibited the sale of any dietary supplement containing ephedra/ephedrine in the United States due to an unreasonable risk to those who use it. In 2006, the FDA declared all dietary supplements containing ephedrine alkaloids to be adulterated and, therefore, illegal for marketing in the United States. For similar reasons in 2005, the FDA removed phenylpropanolamine from over-the-counter sale due to a proposed increased risk of stroke in younger women and because of its potential use in amphetamine manufacture; it is controlled by the Combat Methamphetamine Epidemic Act of 2005.

Serotonergic Agents

Early studies suggested that serotonin plays a significant role in promoting a feeling of fullness and loss of appetite and that a drug which increased the release of serotonin from vesicular storage sites and inhibited serotonin transporter reuptake from the synaptic cleft could be beneficial in treatment of obesity. This was evidenced by the early success of combining phentermine and fenfluramine or dexfenfluramine, popularly referred to Fen-Phen or Redux, in producing significant weight loss. However, both fenfluramine and dexfenfluramine were removed from the market due to safety fears regarding a potential link to heart valve damage and primary pulmonary hypertension. The damage was found to be a result of activity of fenfluramine and dexfenfluramine at the 5-HT_{2B} serotonin receptor in heart valves. More recently the drug lorcaserin, a selective serotonin agonist has been marketed as a treatment of chronic weight management in adults with an initial body mass index (BMI) >30 kg/m^2 or those with a BMI >27 kg/m^2 in the presence of one or more comorbid conditions. The drug should be used as an adjunct in combination with caloric diet reduction and exercise.

Lorcaserin Hydrochloride (Belviq)

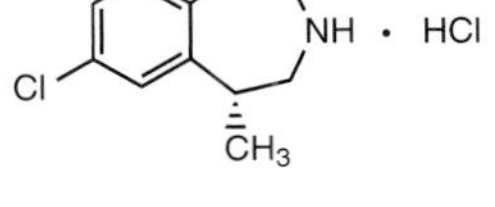

Lorcaserin

MECHANISM OF ACTION. Lorcaserin has a unique mechanism of action in that it acts as a specific agonist at $5HT_{2C}$ receptors, thus promoting satiety via decrease in food consumption. The site of action of lorcaserin is thought be

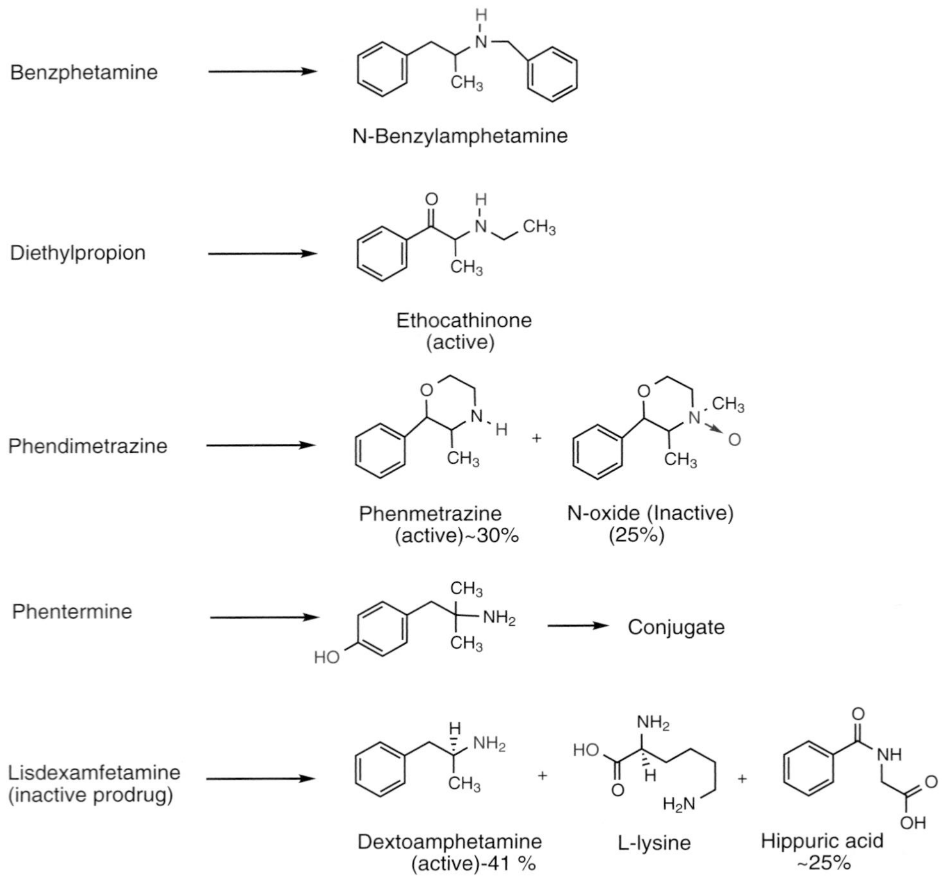

Figure 37.14 Metabolism of sympathomimetic anorexiants.

in the hypothalamus. Pharmacological studies have shown that lorcaserin does not produce significant agonist activity at $5HT_{2A}$ or $5HT_{2B}$ receptors at the dose indicated for weight reduction (10 mg bid). The significance of the latter is that $5HT_{2B}$ receptor stimulation has been associated with valvular heart disease as have previously used antiobesity drugs. Stimulation of $5HT_{2A}$ receptors has been associated with psychological disturbance leading to hallucinations. Once again the therapeutic dose of lorcaserin is considerably less than that necessary to produce significant $5HT_{2A}$ receptor stimulation.[47,48]

Pharmacokinetic Properties. Lorcaserin is readily absorbed via oral administration and is moderately bound to plasma protein (~70%). The drug reaches maximum steady state plasma concentrations within 2 hours and maximum CSF concentration within 6 hours. The drug is metabolized via oxidation and conjugation with various CYP isoforms being involved in the oxidation along with FMO. UDP-glucuronosyltransferase (UGT—various isoforms) and sulfotransferase (SULT) are involved in glucuronidation and sulfation, respectively (Fig. 37.15). The two major metabolites are M1 and M5 both of which are inactive.

Adverse Events. No major increases in mood-related adverse events were reported in the clinical studies. The most common adverse events reported include headache, dizziness, fatigue, nausea, dry mouth, and constipation.

Miscellaneous Classes of Anorexiants

Liraglutide (Saxenda)

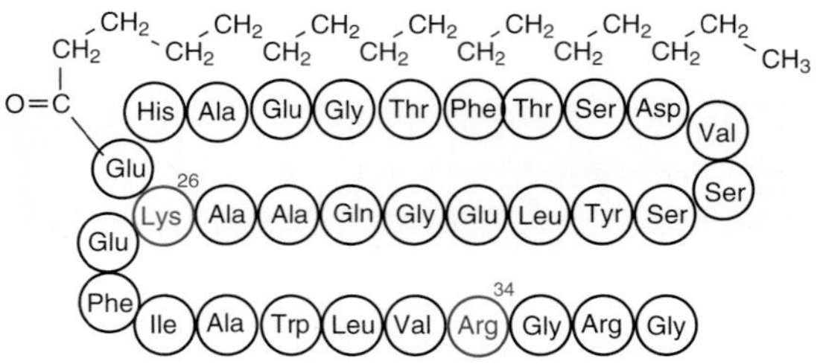

Liraglutide

Liraglutide has previously been approved under the trade name of Victoza for the treatment of diabetic patients who have not achieved glycemic control on metformin or a sulfonylurea. The clinical application for liraglutide has now been extended for use as an adjunct in treatment of

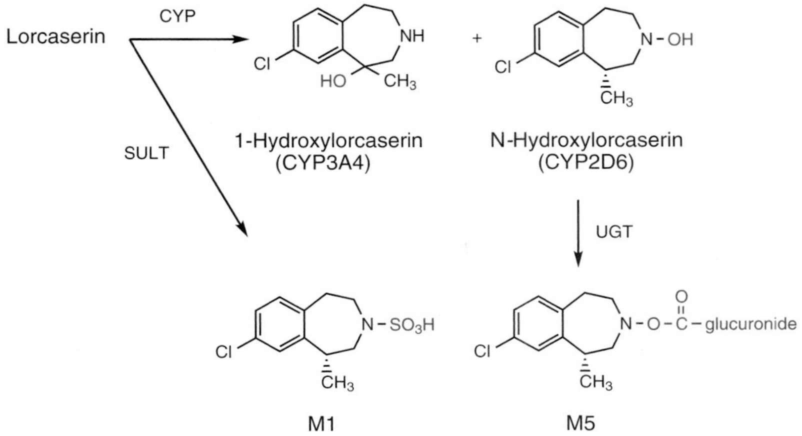

Figure 37.15 Metabolism of lorcaserin.

chronic weight management in adults with a BMI >30 kg/m[2] and those patients with a BMI 27 kg/m[2] or greater who have at least one weight-related comorbid condition marketed under the trade name Saxenda. It should be noted that the target dose for weight loss is 3 mg/d while the maximum daily dose for treating diabetes is 1.8 mg/d.

MECHANISM OF ACTION. In general, it is suggested that liraglutide act as an agonist at glucagon-like peptide 1 (GLP-1) receptors in specific regions within the hypothalamus leading to a reduction of food intake. Animal studies have shown direct stimulation on various neurons within the hypothalamus, but human studies have been unsuccessful in supporting these animal studies.[49]

PHARMACOKINETICS. The chemical modification of GLP-1 leading to liraglutide results in an improved half-life of 13 hours in comparison to that of GLP-1 (1.5-2 min). The drug demonstrates consider stability toward dipeptidyl peptidase 4 (DPP-4) and neutral endopeptidase (NEP) which normally metabolize GLP-1. As a peptide, liraglutide is administered subcutaneously. The drug exhibits an absolute bioavailability of ~55%. The presence of the palmitoyl glutamic acid substituent at position 26 increases plasma protein binding (>98%).

ADVERSE EFFECTS. Common adverse effects consist of nausea, vomiting, hypoglycemia, diarrhea, constipation, and decreased appetite. More severe adverse effects include thyroid C-cell tumors in patients with a personal or family history of medullary thyroid cancer, pancreatitis, and renal impairment. The drug is contraindicated during pregnancy.

Phentermine/Topiramate (Qsymia)

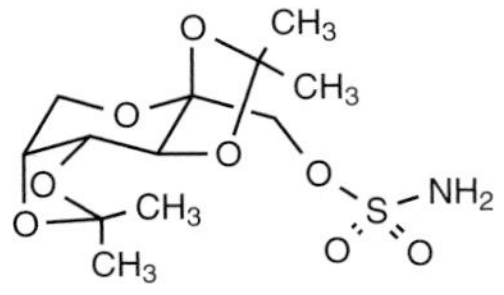

Topiramate

The fixed combination of the sympathomimetic phentermine (Fig. 37.13) with the extended release topiramate (a previously approved drug for treatment of epilepsy) has been approved by the FDA for the treatment of chronic weight management in adults with obesity. Significant weight loss had previously been observed in patients using topiramate for non–weight-associated conditions.

MECHANISM OF ACTION. The mechanism of action of topiramate in chronic weight management is unknown although both appetite suppression and satiety enhancement may be associated with one or more of the previously observed pharmacological actions of the drug. Among the actions of topiramate are those shown in Table 37.10.[50]

PHARMACOKINETICS. Topiramate is readily absorbed following oral administration. The drug is only moderately bound to plasma protein (14%-41%) and is primarily excreted unchanged in the urine (~70%). A number of metabolites have been identified but amount to less than 5% of the administered drug. The use of extended release topiramate improved the half-life of the drug.

Table 37.10 Pharmacological Actions of Topiramate

Receptor/ Substrate	Activity	Site
GABA-A receptors	Agonist	Central
Voltage-gated Na channel	Antagonist	Central/ peripheral
Carbonic anhydrase isoenzymes	Inhibitor	Systemic
Ca channels	Antagonist	Central/ peripheral
AMPA/kainate receptor	Antagonist	Central
CYP 2C19/CYP3A4	Inhibitor	Systemic

AMPA, α-amino-3-hydroxy-5-methyl-4-isoxazolepropionic acid; CYP, cytochrome P450; GABA, γ-aminobutyric acid.

ADVERSE EFFECTS. Common adverse effects include paraesthesia, dizziness, visual disturbances, insomnia, constipation, and dry mouth. Topiramate is contraindicated during pregnancy due to the reports of orofacial clefts in the fetus.

Naltrexone/Bupropion (Contrave)

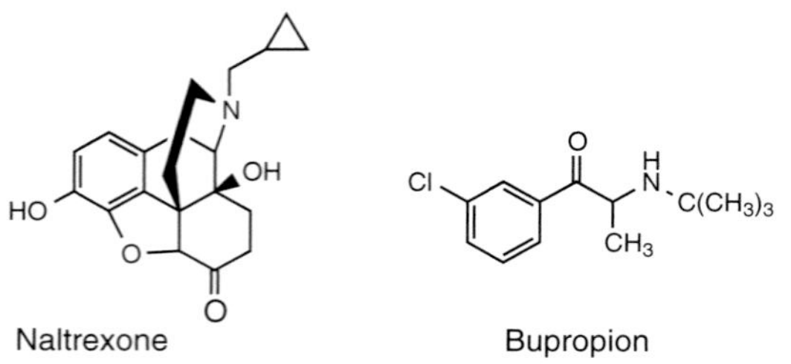

Naltrexone Bupropion

The combination of naltrexone, an opioid antagonist, with bupropion, a norepinephrine-dopamine reuptake inhibitor (NDRI), has proven effective for chronic weight management.

MECHANISM OF ACTION. While the mechanism of action is not known, it is thought that the combination modulates homeostatic hypothalamic melanocortin system with the nonhomeostatic mesolimbic dopamine (DA) reward system. This action may come about through increased firing frequency of the proopiomelanocortin (POMC) neurons in the hypothalamus by bupropion releasing α-melanocyte stimulating hormone (α-MSH) which binds to melanocortin-4 receptors (MC4Rs) located in the hypothalamus to decrease food intake and increase energy expenditure. POMC at the same time releases β-endorphin which inhibits its further release of α-MSH by its action on the μ-opioid receptor. Naltrexone's role is to blocks the μ-opioid receptor thus inhibiting the negative feedback process.[51]

The NDRI effect of bupropion may involve alterations in cortical reactivity to food cues, memory, and self-control. The combination exhibited synergistic action.

PHARMACOKINETIC. The pharmacokinetics and metabolism of bupropion and naltrexone are reported in Chapters 11 and 14 (Table 18.11 in Foye's 7th ed.).

ADVERSE EFFECTS. Common adverse effects include nausea, constipation, headache, vomiting, dizziness, insomnia, dry mouth, and diarrhea. A black box warning accompanies this combination warning of suicidal thoughts and behavior, a condition associated with bupropion.

Over-the-Counter Drugs and Herbal Remedies

People must be cautious when using any weight loss medications, including over-the-counter diet pills and herbal or so-called natural remedies. In the former, after the removal of phenylpropanolamine years ago, orlistat remains the only ingredient FDA approved for weight loss in nonprescription products. The latter, classified as dietary supplements, are statutorily not tightly controlled by the FDA, and thus it is up to the consumer to be aware of their effectiveness and safety. Examples of some products being sold over the Internet for weight loss are shown in Figure 37.16. Data published in Medline for chromium picolate, chitosan, glucomannan, and St. John's wort have failed to show evidence that these products are effective in weight loss.[52-54]

Adulteration of dietary supplements also occurs to an alarming degree. The FDA's Center for Drug Evaluation and Research maintains a list of "Tainted Products Marketed as Dietary Supplements" that it states represent just a small proportion of "potentially hazardous products with hidden ingredients marketed to consumers". A search spanning over a decade found that of 851 tainted products, 326 were categorized as weight loss. Of these, 207 contained undeclared sibutramine with desmethylsibutramine, phenolphthalein, orlistat, or fluoxetine found in a number of the adulterated products.[55]

MICRONUTRIENTS

Vitamins

Vitamins are organic chemicals found in microorganisms, plants, and animals, but not man, that are essential to man and higher animals for the maintenance of growth, physiologic function, metabolism, and reproduction. The role of vitamins in the body is to act as catalysts for the biochemical reactions of the body, and although they are not consumed in these reactions, vitamins do have a normal turnover and elimination and therefore must be continuously resupplied to the body. The reader is referred to a biochemistry textbook for a discussion of the molecular mechanisms involving vitamins, as well as earlier chapters in this text (see Chapter 18 for vitamin K and Chapter 23 for vitamin D). Also the reader is referred to the Suggested Reading: Vitamins at the end of this chapter. The RDIs for the vitamins are given in Table 37.5. It is not our intention to review all of the vitamins in depth, but rather to describe nutritional properties of a select few vitamins.

The vitamins are divided into fat-soluble and water-soluble vitamins based on their physical-chemical properties. The fat-soluble vitamins include vitamins A, D, E, and K, whereas all of the remaining vitamins are considered water soluble (the B complex vitamins: thiamine [vitamin B_1], riboflavin [vitamin B_2], niacin [vitamin B_3], pantothenic acid [vitamin B_5], pyridoxal/pyridoxine [vitamin B_6], cobalamin [vitamin B_{12}], folic acid, and biotin; and vitamin C). Diseases associated with the vitamins most commonly occur due to deficiencies of the vitamins (hypovitaminosis) (Table 37.11) but can also occur due to excessive quantities of a vitamin (hypervitaminosis). Because of the lack of water solubility, the fat-soluble vitamins can build up in the body and therefore are commonly associated with hypervitaminosis, but the water-soluble vitamins can also cause hypervitaminosis. Vitamin deficiencies can be classified as either primary hypovitaminosis or secondary hypovitaminosis. Primary hypovitaminosis is the result of inadequate diet because of a lack of foods containing the vitamins or an inadequate diet due to poor use of foods. The latter may occur if the individual is dieting and not consuming a balanced diet or possibly because of food faddism where a variety of foods are not being used. Secondary hypovitaminosis may be the result of poor

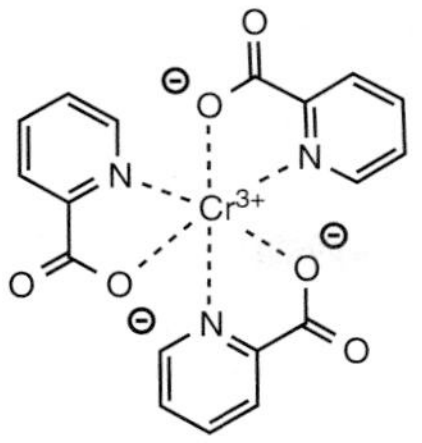

Chromium picolinate

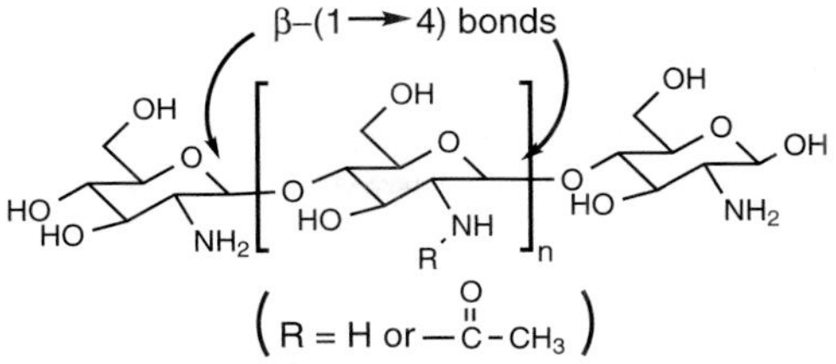

Chitosan (*D*-glucosamine polymers) with varying amounts N-acetyl-*D*-glucosamine

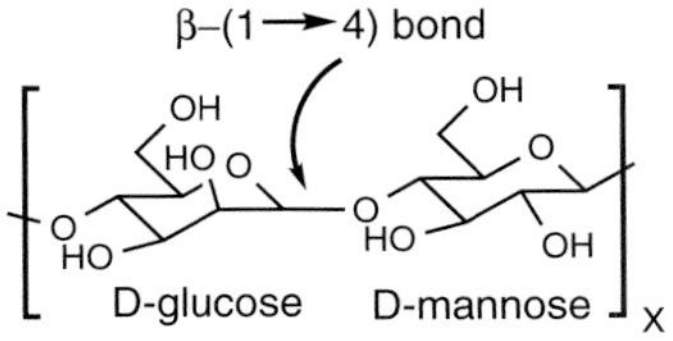

Glucomannan – mainly a straight chain polymer composed of D-mannose and D-glucose linked by β-(1→4) bonds

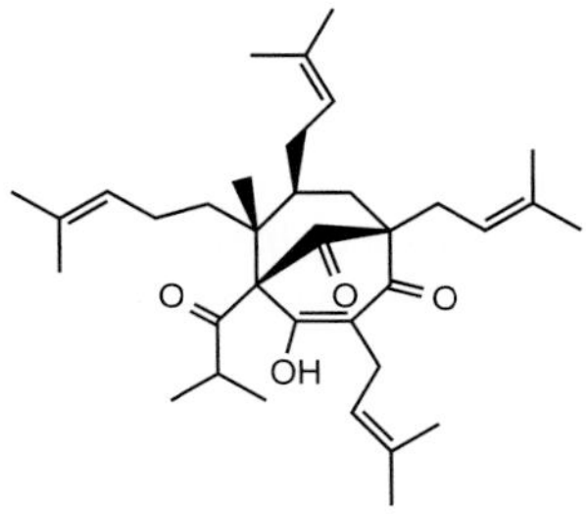

Hyperforin

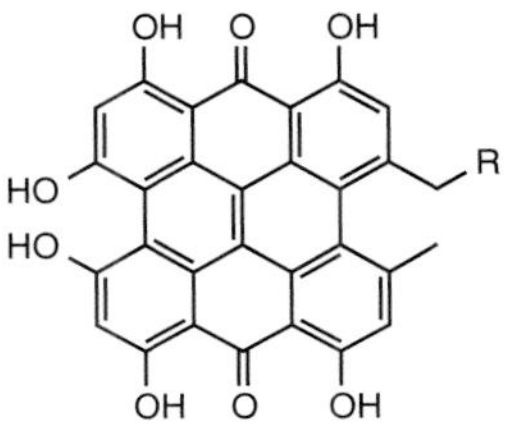

Hypericin (R = H)
Pseudohypericin (R = OH)

Major component of **St. John's wort**

Figure 37.16 Components of commonly available over-the-counter (OTC) dietary products.

health or chronic disease states. Examples might be hyperthyroidism, chronic diarrhea, liver disease, or diseases of the GI tract. There are times in the life of an individual when demands for vitamins increase, such as during pregnancy and lactation in the female when the RDIs for all nutrients increase. Unless an increase in vitamin consumption occurs, the female will suffer hypovitaminosis. The use of drugs can also result in hypovitaminosis. An alcoholic may experience both primary and secondary deficiencies. While consuming alcohol, an alcoholic may not be eating a balanced diet and thus is at risk for a primary deficiency. Alcohol also damages both the intestinal lining and the liver, and nutrients cannot be absorbed through the damaged mucosal membrane or properly used by a damaged liver.

Vitamin A (Retinol, Retinal, Carotenes)

Vitamin A and its precursors, the carotenes (classified as carotenoids—nonpolar carbon hydrogen molecules), are fat soluble and found in high concentrations in liver and fish oils, yellow and green leafy vegetables, eggs, and whole-milk products. β-carotene is also found in high levels in carrots and is highly lipophilic and readily absorbed. The carotenes, α- and β-carotene, are oxidatively converted into all-*trans*-retinal, which in turn can be converted into all-*trans*-retinol (Fig. 37.17), and thus the carotenes can be considered provitamin A's. *Trans*-retinol is generally considered the active form of vitamin A, whereas β-carotene has approximately half the activity of retinol, with α-carotene being a far less efficient source of vitamin A activity. Retinol is commonly found as a lipid-soluble ester with either palmitic acid or acetic acid. The carotinoids, a combination of all sources of vitamin A, have used various measures to define their biologic activity. Since 2001, the retinol activity equivalent (RAE) has been used, which defines 1 μg of RAE as equal to 1 mcg of all-*trans*-retinol and equal to 2 μg of β-carotene, which is equal to 12 μg of food-based β-carotene and 24 μg of other food-based all-*trans* provitamin A carotenoids. Presently, the recommendation is that men should receive a dose of 900 μg daily, whereas women should receive 700 μg/d. Of course, the female dose should be increased during pregnancy and lactation (770 and 1,300 μg, respectively).[56]

BIOLOGIC ACTION

Vision. One commonly thinks of vitamin A and its role in vision. A simplistic outline of the process of vision is shown in Figure 37.18. To initiate the process, *trans*-retinol is isomerized to 11-*cis*-retinol, which in turn is oxidized to 11-*cis*-retinal, the aldehyde that forms a Schiff base with the protein opsin to form rhodopsin, which is the functional form of vitamin A. The absorption of a photon of light by rhodopsin results in sodium conductance at a G protein–coupled receptor, leading to signaling in the visual center in the cortex via the optic nerve and release of opsin and *trans*-retinal, which is recycled through conversion back to *trans*-retinol. A deficiency of vitamin A (i.e., hypovitaminosis A) in the rods of the retina will initially lead to night blindness, nyctalopia, which is a reversible condition. Vitamin A deficiency in a child has much more severe consequences and is a leading cause of blindness (via xerophthalmia) in many Third World nations.

Other Effects of Vitamin A. Animal studies suggest additional roles for vitamin A in the development

Table 37.11 Vitamins, Outward Disease(s), and Common Sources and Roles

Vitamin	Specific Disease(s)	Source	Role
Fat Soluble			
Vitamin A	Xerophthalmia Nyctalopia	Yellow and green leafy vegetables, carrots, yellow fruits, fish oils, milk, fats, and egg yolk, apricots, peaches, and sweet potatoes	Necessary for normal eye function, integrity of the epithelium, synthesis of adrenocortical steroids
Vitamin D	Rickets Osteomalacia	Egg yolks, dairy products, fish, and UV light	Calcium absorption and bone formation
Vitamin E	Spinocerebellar ataxia Skeletal myopathy	Cereals, nuts, unsaturated oils, leafy green and yellow vegetables, milk, muscle meats, and butter	Health of sensory neurons leading to peripheral neuropathy if absent
Vitamin K	Pigmented retinopathy Hypoprothrombinemia	Synthesized in the intestinal tract by bacteria and found in leafy green vegetables	Involved in the blood-clotting process
Water Soluble			
Vitamin C (ascorbic acid)	Scurvy	Citrus fruits, cabbage, peppers, berries, melons, and salad greens	Prevents scurvy, necessary for proper bone and teeth formation
Vitamin B_1 (thiamine)	Beriberi Wernicke encephalopathy	Yeast, beans, brown rice, lean pork, whole-wheat bread, liver, and outer layers of seeds of plants or unrefined cereal grains	Prevents beriberi (leg edema, paralysis, muscle atrophy)
Vitamin B_2 (riboflavin)	Anemias	Liver, kidney, milk, yeast, heart, anaerobic fermenting bacteria, and many vegetables	Deficiency leads to lip lesions, seborrheic dermatitis
Vitamin B_3 (niacin)	Pellagra	Liver, kidney, lean meat, soybeans, wheat germ, broccoli, and avocados	Prevents pellagra (dermatitis, diarrhea, dementia)
Vitamin B_5 (pantothenic acid)	Rare, no specific disease	Muscle meats, outer layer of whole grains, broccoli, and avocados	Deficiencies are rare but may appear as numbness, paresthesia, and muscle cramps
Vitamin B_6 (pyridoxal)	Homocystinuria	Wheat germ, milk, yeast, liver	Prevents dermatitis sicca in adults and convulsions in infants, essential to biochemical reactions
Vitamin B_{12} (cobalamin)	Pernicious anemia	Liver, kidney, muscle meats	Prevents pernicious anemia
Folic acid	Megaloblastic anemia NTDs	Leafy vegetables, beans, peas, liver, kidney, baker's yeast, grains, various nuts, and sunflower seeds	Important for prevention of NTDs, necessary to DNA and RNA synthesis and other biochemical reactions
Biotin	Rare, no specific disease	Tomatoes, kidney, egg yolk, peanuts, chocolates, yeast, and liver	Deficiency causes myodermatitis, lassitude, gastrointestinal symptoms, and hyperesthesias, including muscle pain

NTD, neural tube defect; *UV*, ultraviolet.

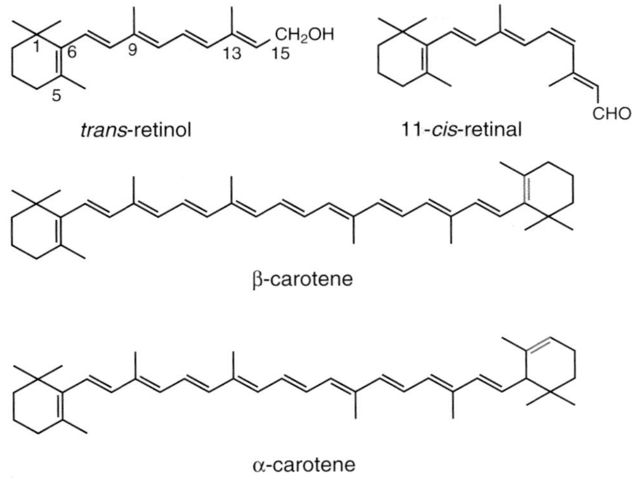

CH_2OH 1 6 9 13 15 5

trans-retinol

CHO

11-*cis*-retinal

β-carotene

α-carotene

Figure 37.17 Naturally occurring cartenoids.

of epithelial tissue, mucus-producing tissue, reproduction, and bone growth. Whether these activities relate to human conditions is not known, and the evidence appears to point to retinoic acid as being important for these actions. Carotenoids have also been suggested to function as antioxidants and therefore have been proposed as valuable agents in the prevention of heart disease and cancer. The data supporting this notion are weak at best. Specific carotenoid, lutein and its isomer zeaxanthin (classified as xanthophylls—polar carotenoids containing one or more oxygen atoms), as well as β-carotene in combination with vitamin E, vitamin C, and zinc have been claimed to show benefit in the treatment of age-related macular degeneration. Scientific evidence specifically supporting health claims for lutein and zeaxanthin continue to grow. A role, if it exists, centers on the antioxidant properties of these polyunsaturated chemicals and their potential for improvement in visual function and a reduced risk of age-related macular degeneration (AMD).[57,58] Both of these chemicals concentrate in the macula adding to their potential value in AMD. Studies

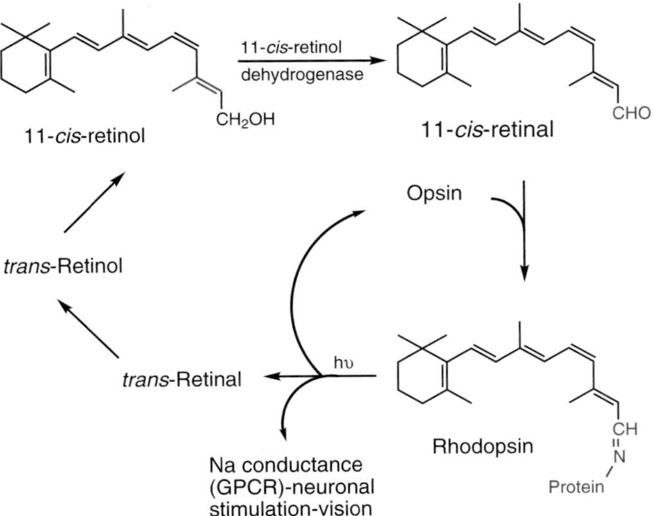

Figure 37.18 Role of vitamin A leading to visual signaling in the cortex.

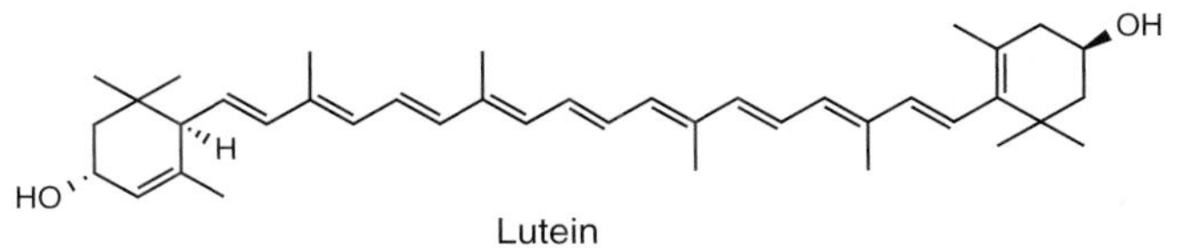

have shown that intake of lutein/zeaxanthin reduce the risk of early, intermediate, and advanced AMD. High quantities of lutein and zeaxanthin are found in green leafy vegetable (i.e., spinach, kale, and yellow carrots) and egg yolks. It should be noted that commercial forms of lutein can be found in the free form (as shown) or as esters, but only the free form is absorbable and esters require initial hydrolysis prior to absorption.

OH H HO

Lutein

OH HO

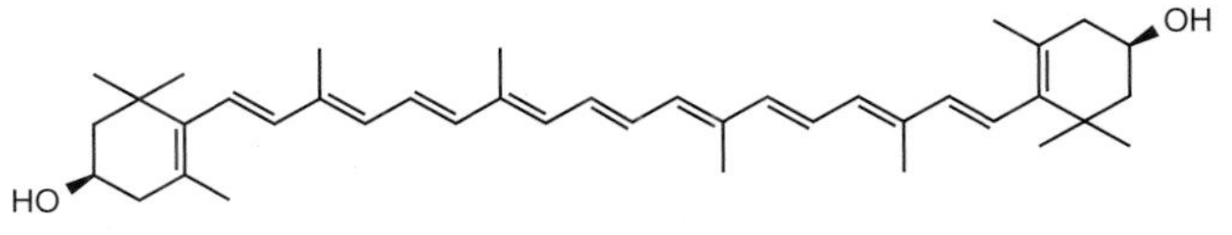

Zeaxanthin

ABSORPTION. The absorbable form of vitamin A is usually considered to be retinol. When vitamin A is administered as a retinol ester, hydrolysis is required in the intestine to release the free alcohol. If the source of vitamin A is β-carotene, oxidative cleavage is required to produce two molecules of retinal, which in turn are reduced to all-*trans*-retinol. Studies have shown that β-carotene can be absorbed as such, but quite inefficiently. Oxidative cleavage of β-carotene does not always occur symmetrically, in which case the yield of vitamin A is less than two molecules per molecule of β-carotene. Approximately 70%-90% of absorption of vitamin A occurs from the small intestine, with much of the vitamin A being transported to the liver for storage.

HYPERVITAMINOSIS A. Lay press publications claiming unsubstantiated benefits from vitamin A have resulted in consumers ingesting vitamin A in doses beyond normal daily requirements (doses as high as 25,000 IU or 7,500 μg). Because of the lipid nature of vitamin A, large quantities can be retained and stored in the body, leading to hypervitaminosis A. The signs and symptoms of hypervitaminosis A include headache, fatigue, insomnia, cracked bleeding lips, cirrhosis-like damage of the liver, birth defects, and yellow skin coloration. Adverse events associated with vitamin A will not normally be seen unless the vitamin is consumed in large quantities over an extended period of time, and these effects are reversible upon discontinuance of the vitamin. The upper safe limit for vitamin A consumption is considered to be 3,000 μg. The relationship between vitamin A and birth defects appears to be primarily associated with the intake of 13-*cis*-retinoic acid (Accutane), which is a known teratogen if consumed during the first trimester of pregnancy. There does not appear to be evidence that retinol, retinal, or β-carotene are sources of retinoic acid or 13-*cis*-retinoic acid, but cautious intake of vitamin A should be advised.

Vitamin D (Sunshine Vitamin, Calcitriol, Calciferols)

Vitamin D is an interesting fat-soluble vitamin because the vitamin can be synthesized in the body via a series of reactions including an ultraviolet-stimulated ring cleavage (ultraviolet B radiation) and hydroxylation reactions that occur in the liver and kidney (Fig. 37.19). Since the vitamin can be and is synthesized in the body, it should be considered a hormone rather than a vitamin. However, the absence of sufficient sunlight will lead to vitamin D–associated diseases, and therefore, additional quantities of vitamin D (actually its precursors) are required, and thus the vitamin nature of the calcitriol. Because the amount of sunlight that an individual receives can vary considerably, the actual daily needs for an individual can also vary considerably, and the recommended intake for vitamin D cannot be accurately defined. It is generally accepted that 5 μg (200 IU) is sufficient for those under the age of 50 years, with increased quantities for those between 51 and 70 years of age (400 IU) and those over 71 years (600 IU). However, clinicians are recommending up to 2,000 μg/d, especially for individuals living in the northern latitudes. A scan of the Internet shows that the consumer can purchase vitamin D_3 (cholecalciferol) in doses as high as 5,000 IU/dose.

BIOLOGIC ACTION. The major role of vitamin D is to regulate the serum levels of ionic calcium and phosphate, which in turn affects bone ossification and neuromuscular function. 7-Dehydrocholesterol is found in most tissues, but that which is in the epidermis can be cleaved (between the C9 and C10 position) by the energy of absorbed ultraviolet light (UV B—290-320 nm). Following isomerization, vitamin D_3 is formed and circulates in the blood (Fig. 37.19). In the liver, vitamin D_3 is hydroxylated to 25-hydroxycholecalciferol, the primary circulating form of vitamin D. Final activation of vitamin D occurs in the kidney where hydroxylation occurs at the 1-postion to give the active 1,25-dihydroxycholecalciferol (calcitriol). Calcitriol is transported through the serum into the target tissue of the intestine and bone where it governs the transcription of mRNA, leading to synthesis of proteins, which increase the absorption of calcium from the gut or resorption of calcium from the bones in conjunction with parathyroid hormone (see Chapter 23). The termination of the action of calcitriol occurs through further hydroxylation, leading to any of a number of tri- and tetrahydroxycholecalciferols (24-hydroxylation is shown in Fig. 37.19).

HYPOVITAMINOSIS D. Hypovitaminosis D, resulting from insufficient vitamin D serum levels, leads to poor absorption of calcium and phosphate from the intestine, which can result in mobilization of calcium from bones (resorption) in order to meet serum needs for the ion. In an infant, this can lead to rickets, whereas in an adult, osteomalacia will result. To prevent these conditions, it has become common practice to fortify milk and other food products with vitamin D as well as to recommend that women who breastfeed their infant

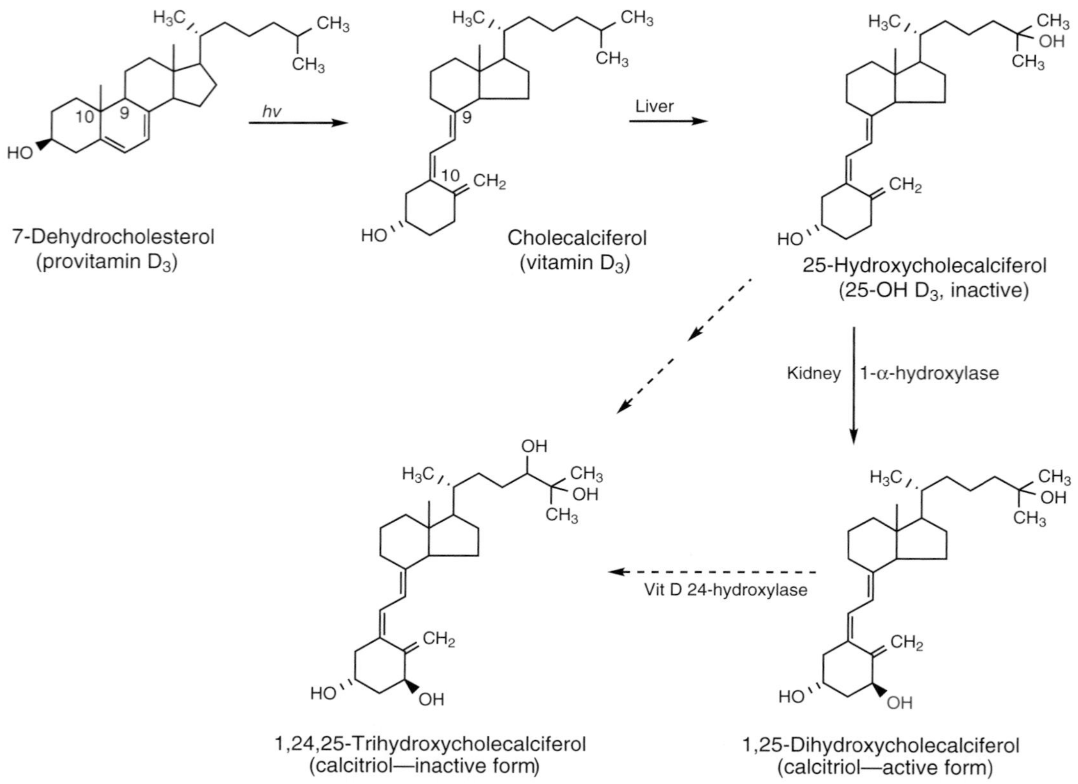

Figure 37.19 Bioactivation and inactivation of vitamin D.

should supplement their diet with vitamin D. There are indications that the vitamin D content of breast milk from many lactating women may be low in vitamin D. Hypovitaminosis D is common in the elderly due to the inability of the aged skin to form vitamin D_3 and because window glass filters out much of the beneficial ultraviolet light wavelengths (~90% of UV light below 300 nm). Hypovitaminosis D has also been found to be a factor in individuals with autoimmune diseases, such as diabetes, multiple sclerosis, irritable bowel syndrome, and rheumatoid arthritis, but the significance of the deficiency in these diseases has not been determined.

Hypervitaminosis D, resulting from consumption of high doses of vitamin D supplements, appears to be far less of a problem than earlier literature suggested, although doses of 10,000 IU/d or greater are considered problematic. High serum calcium levels increase the likelihood for precipitation of calcium salts in soft tissue such as the kidney and heart. This could lead to a decrease in renal function and kidney stones, although the more common symptoms of hypervitaminosis D include constipation, bone pains and stiffness, and confusion. Treatment of hypervitaminosis D consists of removal of the source of vitamin D and reduction in exposure to the sun along with hydration and diuresis.

Vitamin E (Tocopherols)

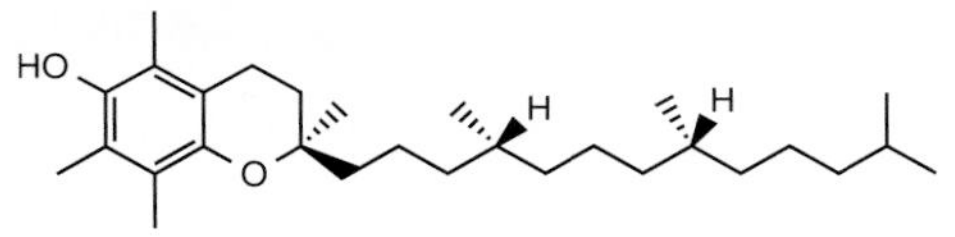

α-Tocopherol

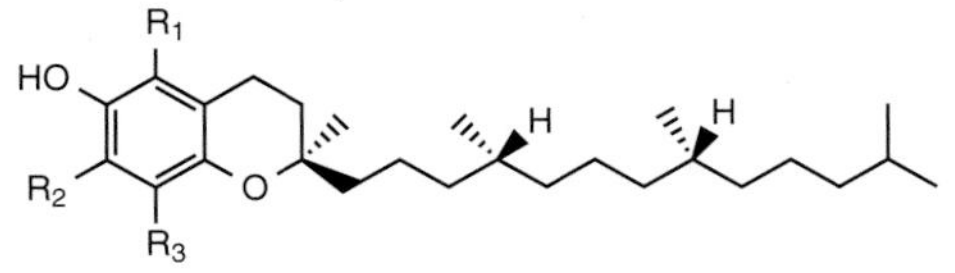

β-Tocopherol (R_2 = H, R_1 = R_3 = CH_3)
γ-Tocopherol (R_1 = H, R_2 = R_3 = CH_3)
δ-Tocopherol (R_1 = R_2 = H, R_3 = CH_3)

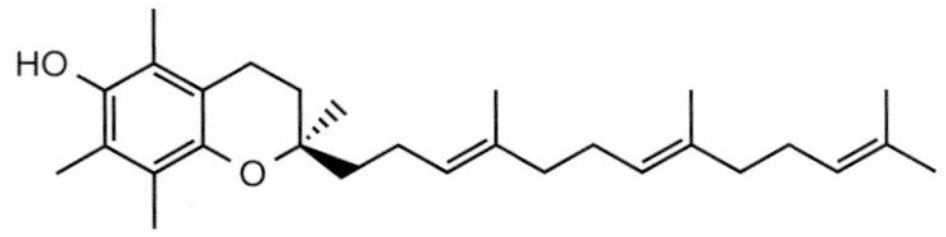

α-Tocotrienol

Vitamin E consists of a group of fat-soluble compounds composed of α-, β-, γ-, δ-tocopherol and α-, β-, γ-, δ-tocotrienol. α-Tocopherol and γ-tocopherol represent the two major tocopherols, whereas the tocotrienols are normally found in low concentrations in nature and are the unsaturated analogues of the respective tocopherols. Since the tocopherols have three chiral centers, a total of eight stereoisomers are possible for each of the tocopherols. The tocotrienols have only a single asymmetric center, resulting in two isomers for each of these products. Both the tocopherols and tocotrienols make up what is normally called vitamin E. The interest in vitamin E arose from studies of infertile male rats, which were shown to be deficient in a substance with vitamin E biologic activity. The substance was isolated and given the name of tocopherol, which is derived from the Greek words meaning "bring forth childbirth." Vitamin E is known as the antisterility vitamin, although there is no known correlation between low levels of vitamin E in male humans and infertility. The commercially available vitamin E may be a single isomer of one of the tocopherols or a mixture of tocopherols, although it is generally considered that α-tocopherol or *R,R,R*-α-tocopherol is the more active form of vitamin E. The tocotrienols may also be present in commercial vitamin E but far less is known about the effects of these materials. The tocopherols may come in the form of an ester of the primary alcohol with the acetate ester being a common form of the vitamin. The quantization of vitamin E is based on a direct analytical measure or an indirect biologic rat assay method.

BIOLOGIC ACTION. The search for a human function for vitamin E has not been an easy task. Vitamin E is ubiquitous in nature, and therefore, human deficiency in this vitamin is uncommon. The source of vitamin E include cereals, nuts, unsaturated oils, leafy green and yellow vegetables, milk, muscle meats, and butter (Table 37.11), although the distribution of the tocopherols and tocotrienols in nature is not uniform. Tocopherols are found in oils, seeds, leaves, and other green part of higher plants, whereas tocotrienols are limited to bran and germ fractions of certain seeds and cereals. In either case, nearly every diet will have a source of vitamin E. A reference to generic vitamin E would usually include products containing both tocopherols and tocotrienols. The difficulty of identifying a role for vitamin E has been that the lay press contains numerous articles claiming favorable actions for vitamin E, including improving wound healing without scaring, slowing down the aging process, protecting against various cancers, preventing heart disease, and improving the performance of athletes. Many of these claims are not substantiated by scientific studies, although a common thread linking these claims is that vitamin E has the chemical property of being a fat-soluble antioxidant. Located in cell membranes, vitamin E could act by virtue of its high reactivity toward reactive oxygen species (ROS), thus protecting cellular components from oxidation (antioxidant). A diagram representing the action of an antioxidant such as vitamin E is shown in Figure 37.20. The tocopherols are thought to protect PUFA from ROS-catalyzed reactions that result in lipid peroxide radicals, which through a series of chain reactions damage PUFA.

MECHANISM OF ANTIOXIDANT ACTIVITY. Vitamin E and especially α-tocopherol are substituted nicely to preferentially scavenge a lipid peroxyl radical. The mechanism and products of this reaction are shown in Figure 37.21. ROS can readily oxidize PUFA via abstraction of a hydrogen from the fatty acid, leaving behind a dienyl radical.[59] This dienyl radical combines

$$\text{Chemical A} \xrightarrow{\text{ROS}} \text{Oxidized Chemical A}$$

$$\text{Chemical A} + \text{Vitamin E} \xrightarrow{\text{ROS}} \text{Oxidized Vitamin E} + \text{Chemical A}$$

Figure 37.20 Vitamin E acting as an antioxidant to protect Chemical A. (ROS = reactive oxygen species.)

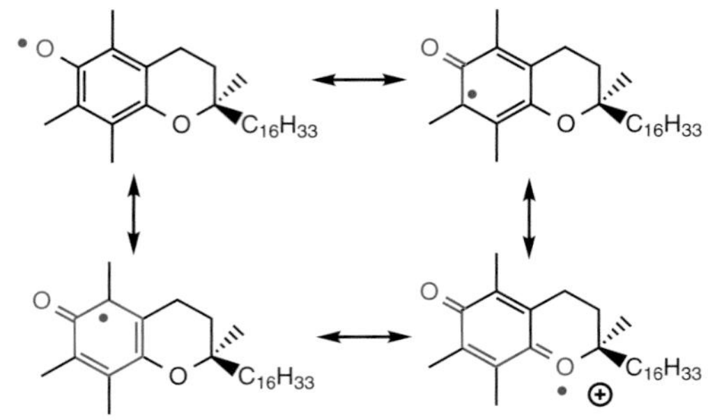

with oxygen to give a mixture of *cis/trans* lipid peroxyl radicals, which if left unchecked will lead to severe cellular damage through a series of hydrogen abstraction chain reactions with biomolecules (i.e., PUFA, DNA, RNA, etc.). In the presence of vitamin E, the lipid free radical abstracts a hydrogen from the phenolic group of α-tocopherol to produce a relatively stable tocopherol radical, thus effectively halting or chain-braking the auto-oxidation cascade of the PUFA. α-Tocopherol is very efficient in acting as an antioxidant by virtue of the stability of the α-tocopherol radical, which results from the chemical substituents attached to the chroman ring system. Stabilization of the α-tocopherol radical is increased by the electron-donating *ortho* methyl groups, with only α-tocopherol having methyls in both *ortho* positions. Additionally, resonance stabilization by the *para* oxygen in the chroman ring improved the stability of the α-tocopherol radical.[60,61]

Resonance stabilization of α-tocopherol radical

The quenching of the α-tocopherol radical leads to formation of α-tocopherolquinone and the epoxytoxopherones (Fig. 37.21).

ABSORPTION AND METABOLISM. The absorption of vitamin E, both the tocopherols and the tocotrienols, occurs readily provided that two conditions are met. First, if vitamin E is administered as an ester, the ester must initially be hydrolyzed. This is easily done by esterases present in the intestine. Second, absorption is dependent on the presence of bile acids in the GI tract. Bile acids favor micelle formation, which is essential for absorption of these fat-soluble materials.

REACTIVE OXYGEN SPECIES (ROS)

A variety of chemicals, found in the human body, possess the chemical property of being a reactive oxygen species. These include molecular oxygen, hydrogen peroxide, and the hydroxy radical.

Reactive oxygen species (ROS)

$$\cdot O{=}O\cdot + e^{\ominus} \longrightarrow {:}O{=}O\cdot^{\ominus} \quad \text{Superoxide radical anion}$$

Oxygen (an unpaired diradical)

$$O_2 + 2\,e^{\ominus} + 2\,H^{\oplus} \longrightarrow H_2O_2 \quad \text{Hydrogen peroxide}$$

$$HO{-}OH \longrightarrow 2\,HO\cdot \quad \text{Hydroxyl radical}$$

A characteristic of an ROS is that it is highly reactive due to the presence of or ability to produce a single unshared valance shell electron which is known as a free radical. Free radicals such as molecular oxygen, superoxide radical anion, or hydroxy radical are very reactive and can attack cellular components leading to oxidation by abstracting an electron from the cellular component. DNA, RNA, protein, and PUFA are all prone to oxidative reactions catalyzed by the ROS. Generally, the body has sufficient enzymes, such as catalase, superoxide dismutase, and ubiquinone (coenzyme Q_{10}) along with natural antioxidants such as vitamin E, vitamin C, vitamin A, carotenes, and lutein/zeaxanthin to protect the cell against damage from ROS. Under oxidative stress cellular damage may occur and some theories suggest that chronic damage to key components of the cell may account for various cancers, cardiovascular disease, and even the aging process.

A general characteristic of the fat-soluble vitamins is their high lipophilicity and the potential for hypervitaminosis to occur; however, in the case of vitamin E, hypervitaminosis is quite uncommon. This may be due to the fact that both the tocopherols and the tocotrienols are oxidized to more water-soluble chemicals that can be readily excreted from the body. The common metabolism consists of ω-oxidation of the lipophilic side chain of vitamin E followed by progressive shortening of the side chain through β-oxidation and the elimination of acetic and propionic

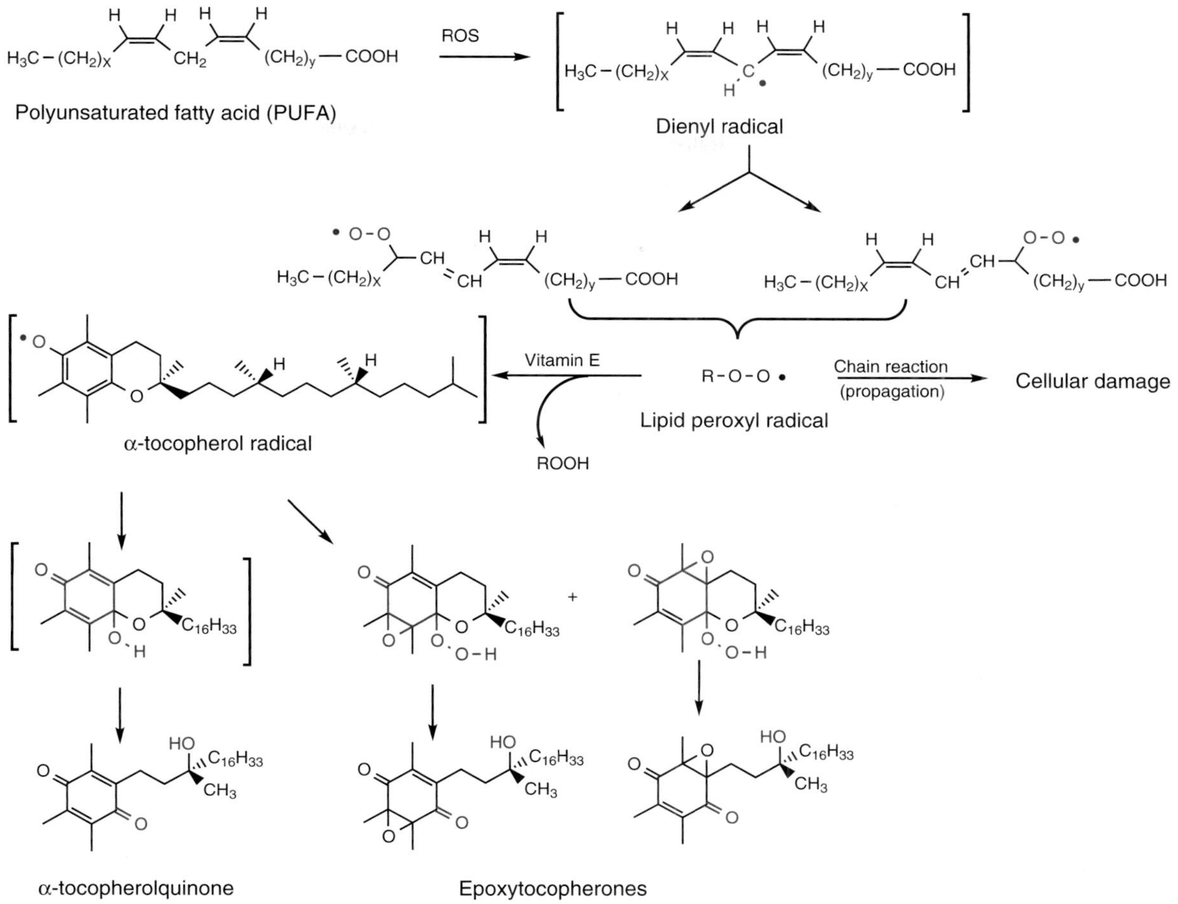

Polyunsaturated fatty acid (PUFA) — ROS → Dienyl radical

Lipid peroxyl radical R-O-O• — Chain reaction (propagation) → Cellular damage

Vitamin E → ROOH; α-tocopherol radical

α-tocopherolquinone   Epoxytocopherones

Figure 37.21 The action of vitamin E in decreasing cellular damage via reaction with polyunsaturated fatty acid (PUFA)–free radicals.

acids (Fig. 37.22). The final products of these oxidations are the hydroxychromans as shown in Figure 37.22.[62-64] The ω-oxidation and apparently the β-oxidations are catalyzed by CYP4F2, and these series of reactions also occur with the tocotrienols, although the rates of these reactions and the amount of each of the metabolites may differ. It should be noted that whether the side chain of the vitamin E is saturated or unsaturated similar metabolic products are formed (how or when the alkene is reduced is not presently known). Thus, the plasma level of the particular vitamin E derivative may differ depending on the tocopherols or tocotrienols that are administered, which in turn may affect the antioxidant benefit of vitamin E.

Vitamin K (Menadiones)

Vitamin K, the fourth of the fat-soluble vitamins, derives its name from the German word *koagulation* because of its role in blood coagulation and is similar to vitamin E in that there is no single chemical entity that possesses the biologic activity attributed to vitamin K (Fig. 37.23). The major activity associated with vitamin K is catalyzing a posttranslation carboxylation of several proteins that are involved in blood coagulation (Fig. 37.24 and see Chapter 18). The basic nucleus of all vitamin K compounds is the 2-methyl-1,4-naphthoquinone to which various chain lengths of the 5-carbon isoprenoid unit are attached at the 3-position.

Green plants produce phylloquinone or vitamin K_1, which represents a major dietary source of the vitamin. Bacteria, some of which live in the intestine, produce various chain length methaquinones, where *n* varies from 4 to 9, that are abbreviated MK-n, and these compounds are referred to as vitamin K_2. Animals, including man, but not bacteria, can synthesize MK-4 from phylloquinone as well as from menadione, which is a synthetic form of vitamin K.

The importance of vitamin K and its role in blood coagulation is that a major class of anticoagulants, the coumarins (Chapter 18), are active by virtue of their ability to block a key step in activation of prothrombin (Fig. 37.24).

SOURCES AND PROPERTIES OF VITAMIN K. As previously indicated, vitamin K is found in leafy green vegetables such as collards, spinach, and salad greens, which have the highest concentrations (300-400 μg/100 g), and from fats and oils such as soybean and canola oil (Table 37.11).[65,66] The RDA is rather low, being 1 μg/kg body weight/day, while the DRI varies considerably from approximately 2 μg/d for infants to 90-120 μg/d for females and males between the ages of 19 and 70 years. One might expect that vitamin K deficiencies would be uncommon since various foods and intestinal bacterial flora are sources of this vitamin, and although this is generally true, the bioavailability of phylloquinone is in the range of 15%-20%, and turnover of the

α-tocopherol
CYP4F2
CH_2OH
C_2H_5COOH
β-hydroxylation
CH_3COOH
Progressive β-oxidations and eliminations
α-carboxymethylhexylhydroxychroman (α-CMHHC)
α-carboxymethylbutylhydroxychroman (α-CMBHC)
α-carboxyethylhydroxychroman (α-CEHC)

Figure 37.22 Metabolism of α-tocopherol.

vitamin occurs rapidly. The absorption of dietary vitamin K occurs via the lymphatic system, whereas the metabolism of vitamin K is not well characterized.

Vitamin K toxicity has often been cited, and in fact, menadione is considered to be potentially toxic, a toxicity associated with interference with the functioning of glutathione. However, phylloquinone and the menaquinones have not been shown to produce toxic effects even at high doses.

Phylloquinone (Vitamin K_1)
Methaquinone-n (MK-n)
Isoprenoid unit
2-Methyl-1,4-naphthoquinone
Methaquinone-4 (MK-4)
Menadione

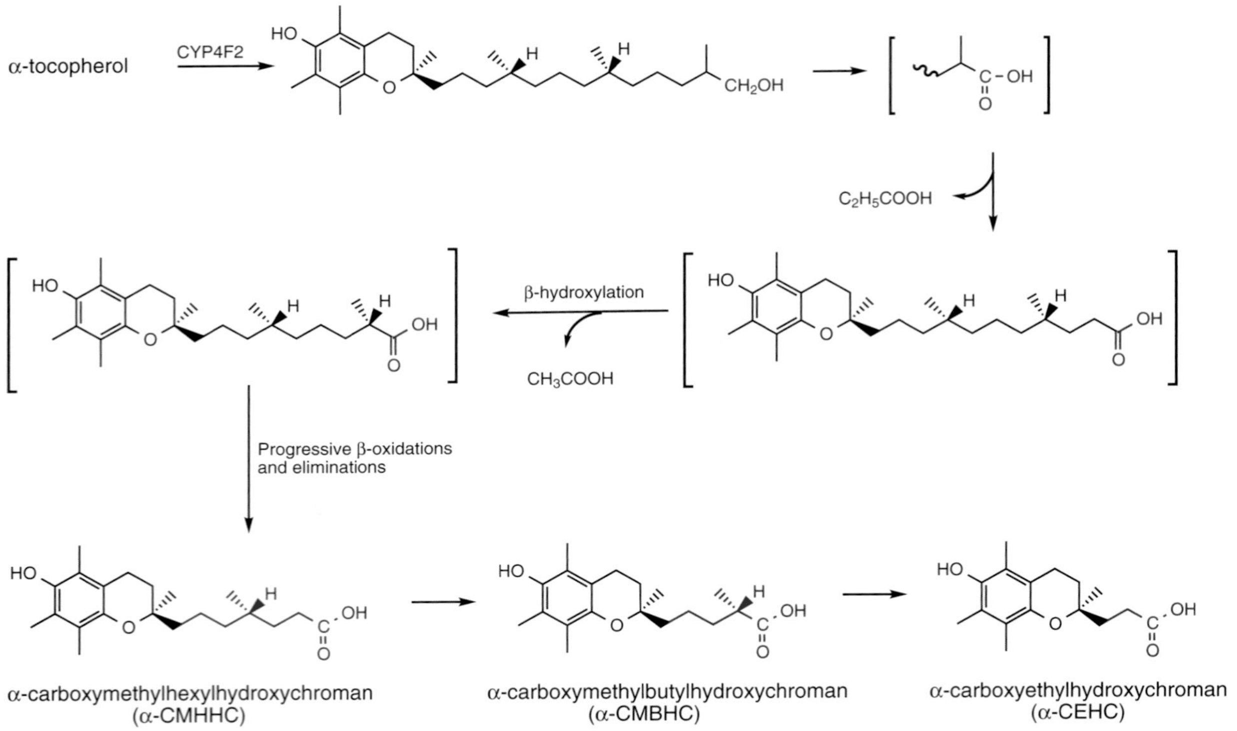

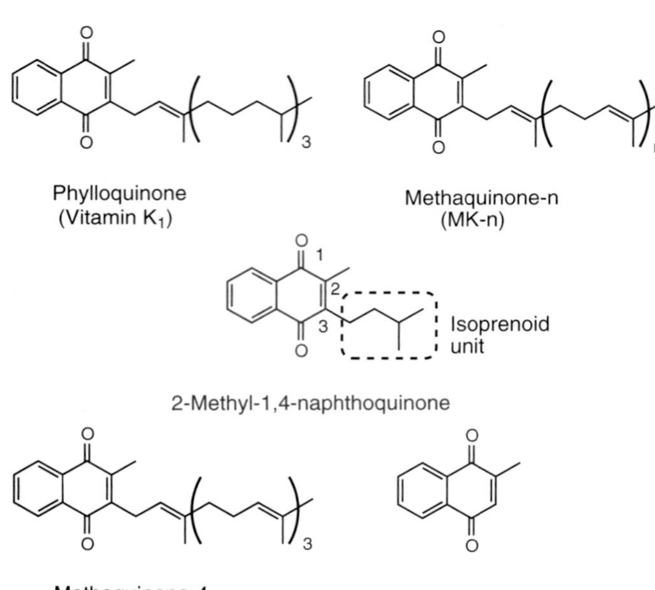

Figure 37.23 Structures of various vitamin K analogues.

Water-Soluble Vitamins

Vitamin C (Ascorbic Acid)

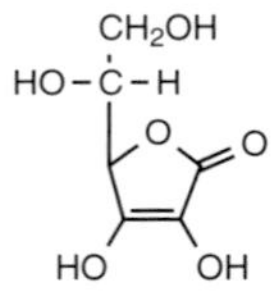

Ascorbic acid

Vitamin C, or ascorbic acid, is a water-soluble vitamin. The deficiency of vitamin C, known as scurvy, has a long history dating back to 3000 BC. Scurvy is a condition characterized by subcutaneous hemorrhage due to blood vessel rupture, commonly seen in the gingival, skin, and GI mucosa. With severe scurvy, loss of teeth, bone damage, internal bleeding, and infections occur, ultimately leading to death. Although the condition was described in the literature, it was not until the 1800s that its relationship to a chemical present in fruit juices became well known. It was another 100 years before Albert Szent-Gyorgyi identified and named the chemical in fruit juices that could prevent scurvy as ascorbic acid. Vitamin C is synthesized in plants from glucose and fructose, and most mammals can also synthesize this substance with the exception of humans, nonhuman primates, including guinea pigs, and several other animal species. Water-soluble vitamin C is often considered to be a vitamin that is not stored in the body and thus excessive levels will not build up in the body. Neither of these ideas is entirely correct. Vitamin

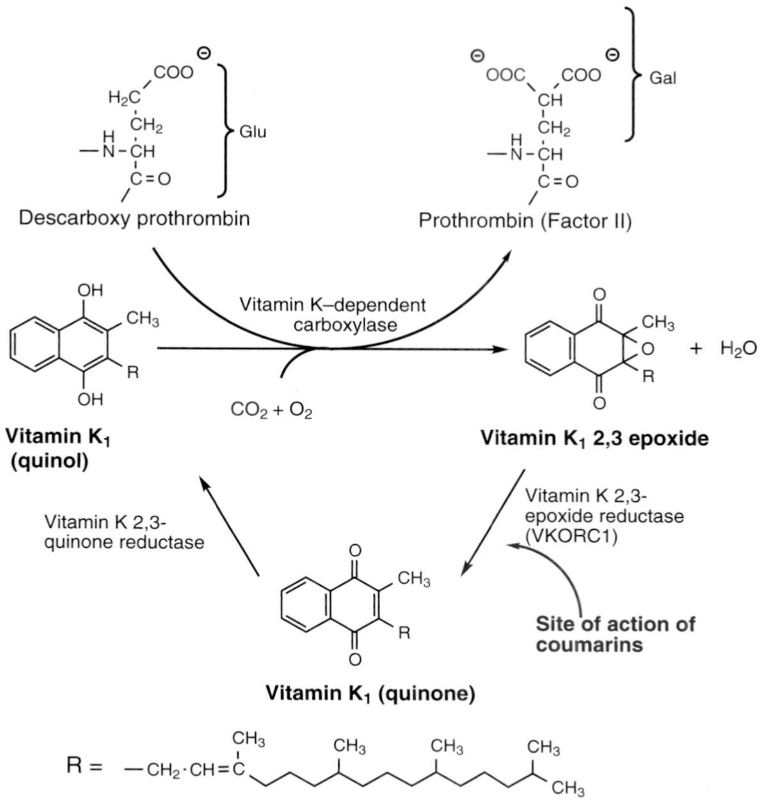

Figure 37.24 Posttranslational carboxylation reaction catalyzed by vitamin K_1.

C is stored in quantities sufficient to prevent scurvy for approximately 30-40 days, whereas large doses of vitamin C do have the potential for adverse effects (see below).

BIOLOGIC ACTION. Vitamin C is a water-soluble antioxidant by virtue of its ability to give up two electrons and in the process become oxidized (Fig. 37.25). The driving force for this activity resides in the fact that the ascorbyl free radical is stable and, with the loss of the second electron, ascorbic acid becomes dehydroascorbic acid, which following hydration is recycled back to ascorbic acid by reduction via glutathione. The relationship between the antioxidant property of vitamin C, and scurvy is not

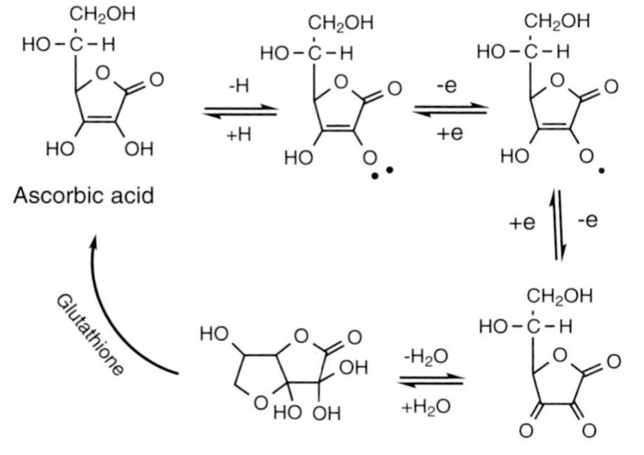

Figure 37.25 Antioxidant property of ascorbic acid.

known with certainty, but it is known that vitamin C is a cofactor in the hydroxylation of the amino acids proline and lysine, which are essential components of collagen. The hydroxylated amino acids have a role in stabilizing the helix structure of collagen, and therefore, deficiency of vitamin C may impair the proper function of collagen. Collagen is part of the structural make up of connective tissue; thus, vitamin C deficiency leads to gum deterioration and bleeding, adverse effects on bone integrity leading to teeth loss, and skin discoloration.

The antioxidant property of vitamin C has led to many suggestions as to additional biologic activity for vitamin C, which includes benefits in prevention of cardiovascular diseases. The atherosclerosis properties of LDL are thought to relate to the oxidation of LDL to a peroxy radical, which then plaques onto the walls of blood vessels. Vitamin C may inhibit the initial oxidation. Increased consumption of vitamin C has been reported to correspond to a reduction in ischemic heart disease and a reduction in hypertension. Increased plasma levels of vitamin C, associated with increased consumption of fruits and vegetables (common sources of vitamin C), have been linked with a decrease in various cancers including oral cavity, esophagus, stomach, colon, and lung cancers. Suppression of ROS or radical intermediates serves as the basis for these claims. Doses in the gram quantity are often recommended for these actions, but clinical data are normally absent or complicated by other factors such as the benefits derived from simply increasing the intake of fruits and vegetables in the diet. Linus Pauling championed the concept that vitamin C was beneficial in treating some terminally ill cancer patients and could prevent or promote the recovery from the common cold. Data did not support the use of doses of up to 10 g/d for terminally ill cancer patients. As to the benefit of vitamin C in treatment of the common cold, it is felt that vitamin C will not prevent the common cold but may hasten the recovery from the cold. There is some evidence showing that vitamin C may increase the body's production of interferons, which in turn possess antiviral activity, thus supporting the claim for benefit in the common cold and potentially the treatment of viral-associated cancers.

HYPERVITAMINOSIS C. The RDA for vitamin C is in the range of 60-75 mg/d, with higher amounts recommended for women during pregnancy and lactation and for smokers. Vitamin C–containing products are available with daily doses in the range of the RDAs all the way up to products that contain 1,000 mg per tablet or capsule. With such potent products available to the consumer, it is not uncommon for the patient to be consuming excessive quantities of vitamin C. High doses of vitamin C have been associated with increased oxalate excretion, with the potential for oxalate-based kidney stones, and will lower urine pH, affecting drug excretion. High doses, in the range of 3 g/d, may cause diarrhea and bloating, while even normal doses of vitamin C increase iron absorption, which in some individuals may cause health issues. Vitamin C prevents intestinal oxidation of ferrous ion to ferric ion, which is poorly absorbed from the GI tract. It should be noted that the ferrous (Fe^{2+}) state of iron is important for iron absorption.

Although vitamin C is an essential component in our diet, its role in good health and the biochemistry of the body is still not clear, and additional benefits may be elucidated in the future.

Thiamine

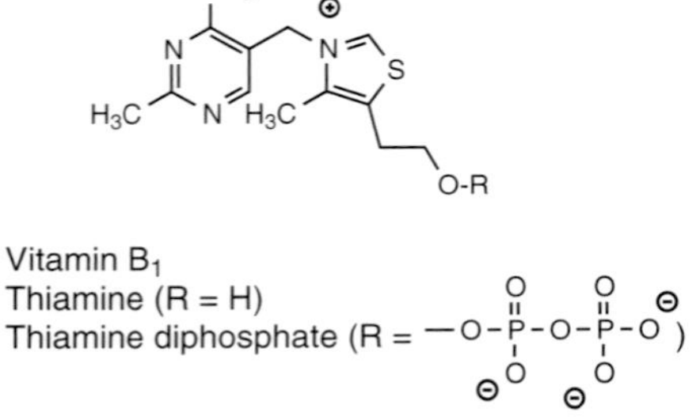

Vitamin B_1
Thiamine (R = H)
Thiamine diphosphate (R = $-O-P(=O)(O^-)-O-P(=O)(O^-)-O^-$)

Thiamine also known as thiamin or vitamin B_1 is a member of the vitamin B complex. Deficiency of this vitamin can lead to beriberi, Wernicke-Korsakoff syndrome and Korsakoff pyschosis. Death can occur as a result of severe and prolonged deficiencies of thiamine. The RDI and source and role are shown in Tables 37.5 and 37.11, respectively. Thiamine is essential as a coenzyme for a number of important enzyme systems in which a breaking of chemical bonds occur including carbon-carbon, carbon-sulfur, carbon-hydrogen, and carbon-nitrogen bonds. As a result, thiamine is important in the generation of energy. A more detailed discussion of the function and specific disease states resulting from thiamine deficiencies is presented by Butterworth.[67]

Riboflavin

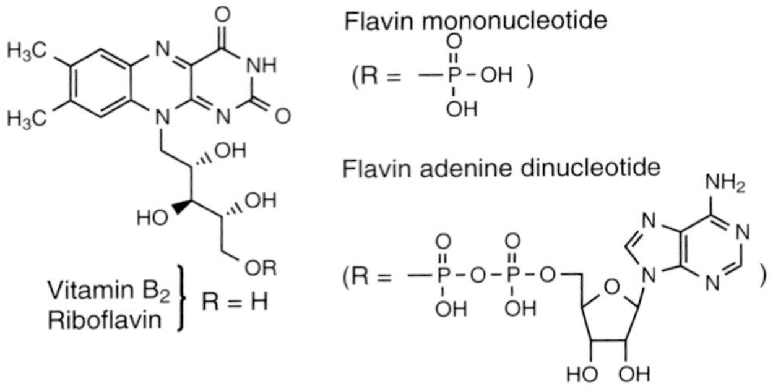

Vitamin B_2 / Riboflavin } R = H

Flavin mononucleotide (R = $-P(=O)(OH)-OH$)

Flavin adenine dinucleotide

Riboflavin (vitamin B_2), as with many of the other vitamins, is an important coenzyme with various proteins. Flavin mononucleotide (FMN) and flavin adenine dinucleotide (FAD) are important in electron transport complexes, oxidation reactions, as a cofactor with vitamin A, folic acid, niacin, and reduction reactions involving glutathione. The flavins have a yellow coloration and following light excitation has a phosphorescent characteristic representing a triplet state. As a result of this, the vitamin can be used during phototherapy of neonatal jaundice.[68]

DEFICIENCY (TABLE 37.11). Deficiency states are not common, but when they do occur these states are associated with deficiencies of other B complex vitamins, especially niacin, vitamin B_6, and thiamine. Symptoms include sore throat, hyperemia, pharyngeal edema, leg legions, and seborrheic dermatitis. In general, excessive intake of riboflavin will not result in disease since the vitamin in large doses is not readily absorbed from the GI tract and the vitamin is readily excreted via renal tubules.

Niacin

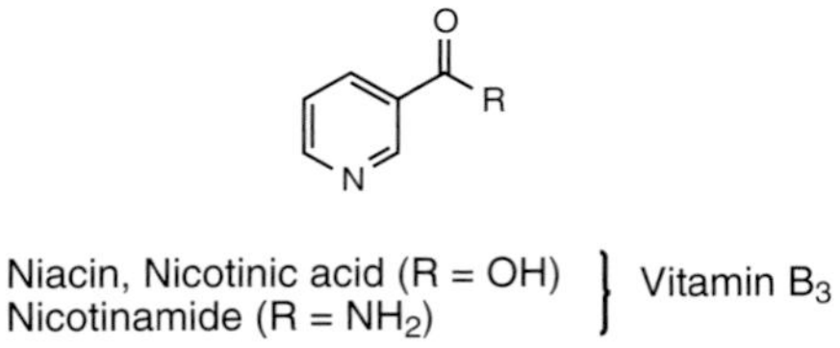

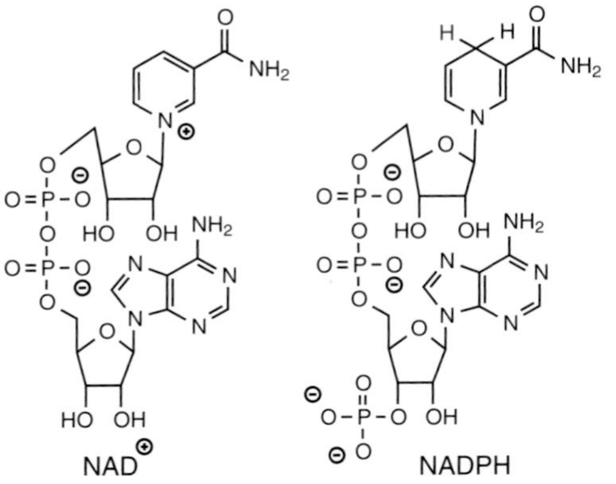

Niacin, Nicotinic acid (R = OH) } Vitamin B_3
Nicotinamide (R = NH_2)

NAD^+

NADPH

Niacin or nicotinamide (less commonly vitamin B_3) is useful in its own right as an over-the-counter (OTC) drug, while its biochemically active form acts as a coenzyme within nicotinamide adenine dinucleotide (NAD^+) and the reduced form of nicotinamide adenine dinucleotide phosphate (NADHP). The NAD^+ is the oxidizing form of this vitamin while the NADHP is the reducing form of the enzyme. The oxidation/reduction activity of this vitamin involves the hydrogen at the C4 position of niacin.

DEFICIENCY. The major disease state associated with deficiencies of niacin is pellagra, a condition associated with dermatitis, diarrhea, and dementia along with the hyperpigmentation of the skin, inflammation of the tongue and mouth, and disorders of the GI tract (Table 37.11). It is not just deficiencies of niacin that can bring about pellagra, but deficiencies of other vitamins (e.g., vitamin B_2 and B_6) can add to the problem. In fact treatment of tuberculosis with isoniazid can deplete vitamin B_6 and bring about niacin deficiency.

THERAPEUTIC USE OF NIACIN AND ITS MECHANISM OF ACTION. Along with the prevention of pellagra, niacin has been used in the recent past for the treatment of hyperlipidemia. Niacin's ability to lower plasma lipid levels through its action in the liver is based upon two actions: (1) modulation of triglyceride (TG) synthesis followed by the reduction of very-low-density lipoprotein (VLDL) and low-density lipoprotein (LDL) particles (Fig. 37.26); (2) niacin also decreased degradation of apo B degradation thus decreasing VLDL and LDL concentrations. This latter action appears to be associated with binding of niacin to the G protein–coupled receptor GRP109A.[69] It should be noted that the action of niacin involves nicotinic acid and not nicotinamide. However, niacin has failed to show a decrease in cardiovascular-related mortality and has failed to show a decrease in cardiovascular events.[70] This lack of reduction of clinical outcomes combined with several significant side effects have resulted in niacin being no longer recommended for routine primary or secondary prevention of atherosclerotic cardiovascular disease (ASCVD).

Finally, immediate released forms of niacin lead to severe flushing which is associated with the release of prostaglandin D_2 and E_2. The slow release dosage forms of niacin appear to reduce this adverse effect.

Pantothenic Acid

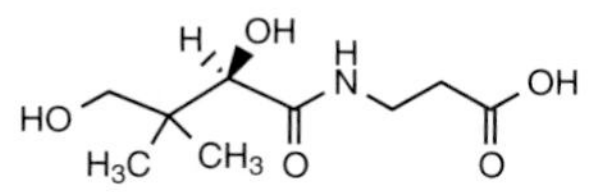

Vitmain B_5
Pantothenic acid

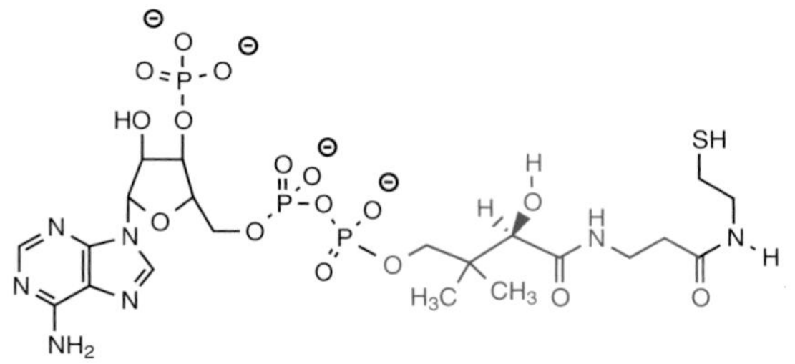

Coenzyme A

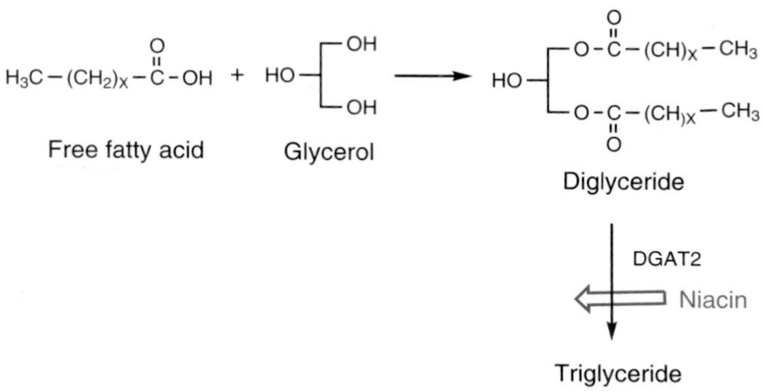

Free fatty acid + Glycerol → Diglyceride → (DGAT2, Niacin) → Triglyceride

Figure 37.26 The site of action of niacin on triglyceride synthesis.

Pantothenic acid is the centerpiece for coenzyme A (CoA) and as such is essential for the transfer of acetyl and acyl groups. CoA is important for β-oxidation of fatty acids and degradation of amino acids. Additionally, CoA is involved in the citric acid cycle through oxaloacetic acid and in cholesterol synthesis via hydroxyl-3-methylglutaryl-CoA. Most of the pantothenic acid is present in the body in the form of CoA.

The likelihood of a pantothenic acid deficiency is quite rare in part because of the ubiquitous nature of this vitamin (Table 37.11). Additionally, the vitamin is produced by intestinal microorganisms from which human absorption can occur.

Pyridoxine

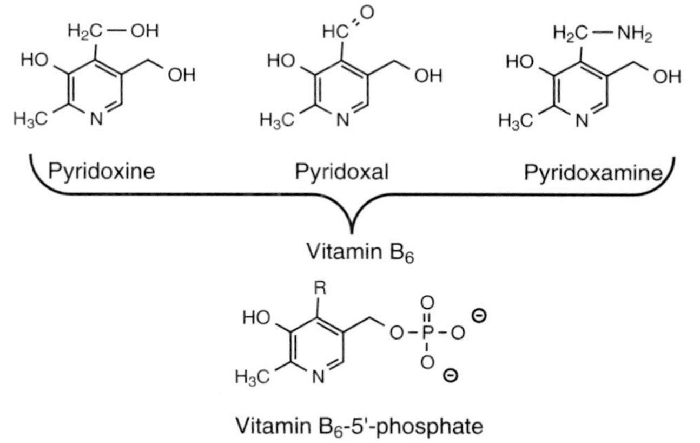

Pyridoxine — Pyridoxal — Pyridoxamine

Vitamin B_6

Vitamin B_6-5'-phosphate

The terminology of pyridoxine or vitamin B_6 actually refers to any of three interconverting compounds: pyridoxine, pyridoxal, or pyridoxamine. The phosphorylated derivatives are all considered active forms of vitamin B_6. Because all three compounds make up what are considered the active form of the vitamin, the preferred name for this vitamin is B_6. Information concerning the RDI and source and role are shown in Tables 37.5 and 37.11, respectively.

HYPOVITAMINOSIS B_6. Vitamin B_6 deficiencies are rare because of the broad number of sources of these vitamins, but low plasma levels may be seen in chronic alcoholics, with obese states, during pregnancy, and in patients with various bowl diseases. Occasionally deficiencies may be seen due to drug antagonism such as that reported for patients on isoniazid treatment for tuberculosis. Vitamin B_6 must be continuously ingested since as a water soluble vitamin it is lost from the body with a half-life of 15-20 days.

Over the years many unsubstantiated claims have appeared in the lay press encouraging patients to take in large doses of vitamin B_6. While unlikely, large doses of this vitamin consumed over extended periods of time can lead to sensory neuropathies, movement disorders, and GI symptoms such as nausea and heartburn. The symptoms are reversed upon removal of the vitamin.

BIOLOGIC ACTION. Pyridoxine is a coenzyme in more than 100 different enzyme systems. As examples of its role pyridoxal is involved in deamination reactions and decarboxylation reactions involving amino acids (Fig. 37.27). As indicated, vitamin B_6 is involved in the formation of the neurotransmitter dopamine.

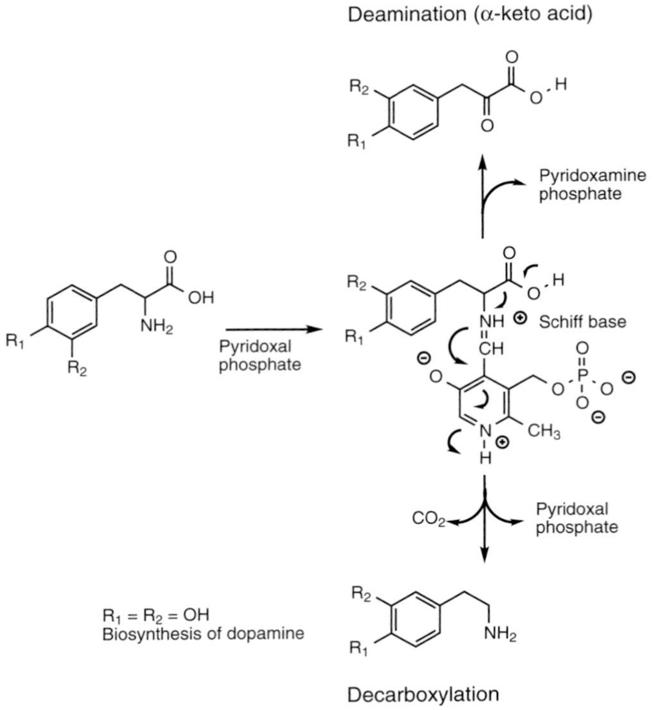

Vitamin B_{12} (Cobalamine)

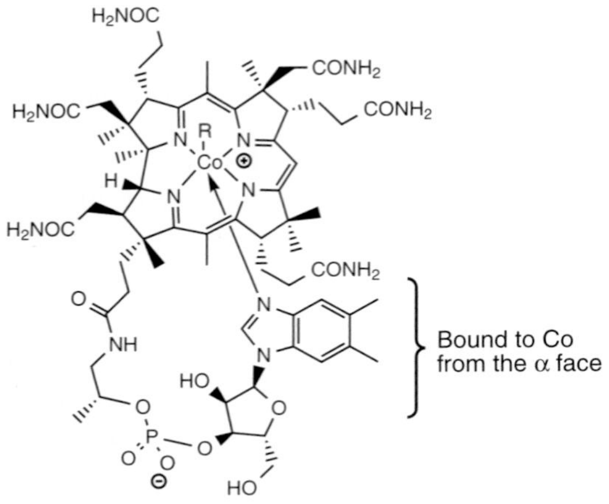

R = 5'-deoxyadenosyl	Adenosylcobalamin
CH_3	Methylcobalamin
OH	Hydroxocobalamin
CN	Cyanocobalamin

R group bound to Co from the β face

Figure 37.27 Vitamin B_6 involvement in deamination and decarboxylation reactions.

Vitamin B_{12} also referred to as cobalamine or cyanocobalamine has a long history of discovery, biology, and chemical nature. Its development resulted in the awarding of multiple Noble Prizes. Today it is recognized that vitamin B_{12} has a very specific role in the development and function of the brain, nervous system including myelinogenesis, formation of blood cells, and a variety of metabolic reactions.

The vitamin B_{12} utilized in vitamin supplements is produced via bacterial synthesis and contains the element cobalt positioned in the center of a corrin ring with its planar tetrapyrrole heterocycles. The cobalt exists in any of three oxidative states (e.g., +1, +2, +3).

HYPOVITAMINOSIS B_{12}. Deficiency states may result from a lack of the vitamin in the diet (primary deficiency) or poor absorption (secondary deficiency) associated with intestinal disorders. A common source of vitamin B_{12} is meat in which the vitamin is bound to protein, and thus the vitamin must first be released via digestion, which is facilitated by an acid media. Thus prolonged use of proton pump inhibitors could reduce the availability of vitamin B_{12} leading to lower plasma levels of the vitamin. Following digestive release the vitamin is transported via a number of intrinsic proteins as depicted in Figure 37.28.[71] Deficiency of any of these factors can lead to hypovitminosis.

Deficiencies of vitamin B_{12} are not easily discernable from deficiencies of folic acid since the two vitamins are involved in similar biochemical processes. Additionally clinical signs of a deficiency may take a considerable time to appear since body stores are slowly depleted. Deficiency of vitamin B_{12} and folic acid leads commonly to hematologic changes leading to pancytopenia resulting from abnormal DNA replication. Neurological damage resulting from vitamin B_{12} deficiencies can result in irreversible changes. The damage involves neuronal myelin ultimately leading to demyelination and neuronal cell death. Clinical symptoms include paresthesias of hands and feet, unsteadiness, decreased deep tendon reflexes, confusion, moodiness, and loss of memory. Delusions, hallucination, and psychosis may also be seen.

BIOLOGIC ACTION. Methylcobalamin is found primarily in the cytoplasm where it functions as a cofactor involved in the transfer of a methyl group from methyltetrahydrofolic acid to methionine, a reaction catalyzed by methionine synthase. Deoxyadenosylcobalamin in the mitochondria serves as a cofactor along with methylmalonyl-coenzyme A mutase to produce succinyl-CoA in propionate metabolism. It is through these two cobalamins that vitamin B_{12} carries out its essential actions.

Folic Acid (B_9)

pterodine

glutamate

p-aminobenzoic acid

Folic acid

Tetrahydrofolic acid

N^5,N^{10}-Methylene-tetrahydrofolic acid

N^5-Methyl-tetrahydrofolic acid

N^{10}-Formyl-tetrahydrofolic acid

Folic acid, occasionally referred to as vitamin B_9, and the activated forms of this vitamin tetrahydrofolic acid (THFA), N^5,N^{10}-methylenetetrahydrofolic acid, N^5-methyltetrahydrofolic acid, and N^{10}-formyltetrahydrofolic acid are involved in DNA and RNA synthesis, and metabolism of amino acids. The essential nature of this vitamin can be met by utilizing folic acid since the human body is capable of the reduction of folic acid via folate reductase leading initially to 5,6-dihydrofolic acid followed by a second reduction by the same enzyme to THFA. Bacteria are capable of the biosynthesis of folic acid from an activated pterodine, *p*-aminobenzoic acid, and glutamate. Recognizing the bacterial biosynthesis of folic acid and the human metabolism of folic acid to its active forms is essential in order to understand the mechanism of action of the antibacterial sulfonamides and trimethoprim (see Chapter 29) and the anticancer activity of methotrexate (see Chapter 33).

HYPOVITAMINOSIS. As indicated in the discussion of hypovitaminosis B_{12}, the close relationship of folic acid and vitamin B_{12} often makes it difficult to differentiate between disease states caused by one or the other of these vitamins. This is especially true with the condition of megaloblastic anemia or macrocytic anemia. On the other hand, folic acid deficiency normally does not lead to neurological diseases.

Folate deficiency has been associated with neural tube defects (e.g., spina bifida, encephaloceles, anencephaly), and it is now recommended that pregnant women or women expecting to become pregnant add a supplement of folic acid (400 μg).

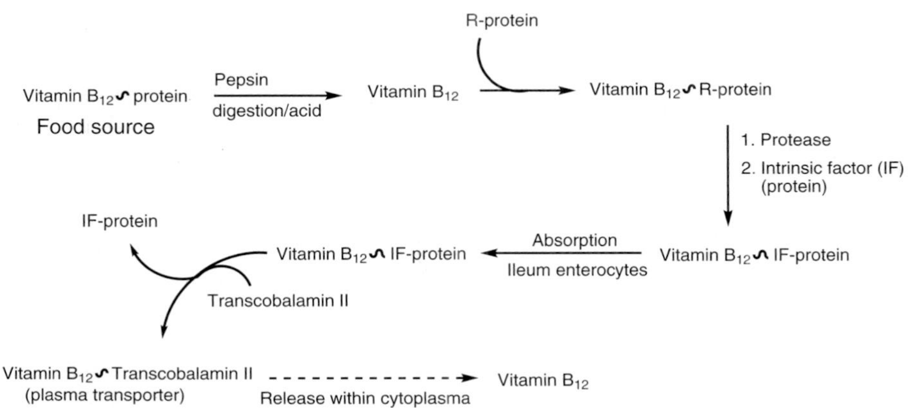

Figure 37.28 Transport and absorption of vitamin B_{12} into cellular cytoplasm.

BIOLOGIC ACTION. Folic acid is involved in the human body as a coenzyme or cosubstrate in which it supplies one-carbon units in the biosynthesis of purines through N^{10}-formyltetrahydrofolic acid and in the biosynthesis of thymine via N^5,N^{10}-methylenetetrahydrofolic acid. The synthesis of the essential amino acids serine/glycine interconversion through N^5,N^{10}-methylenetetrahydrofolic acid and methionine via N^5-methyltetrahydrofolic acid are folic acid dependent.

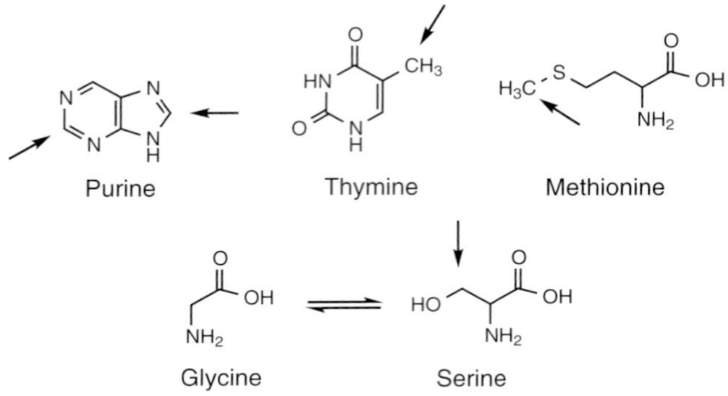

Purine Thymine Methionine

Glycine Serine

Arrow indicates methyl groups supplied by methylated THFA

Biotin

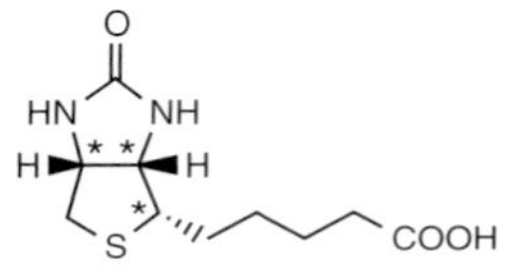

Biotin

Biotin, also known as vitamin B_7, has three asymmetric centers, but only the D-isomer as shown is active. Biotin is a cofactor in five carboxylase enzymes: α- and β-acetyl-coenzyme A (CoA) carboxylase, pyruvate carboxylase, propionyl-CoA carboxylase, and methylcrotonyl-CoA carboxylase. These enzymes catalyze reactions in which carboxybiotin is involved in carboxylation of various substrates as shown in Figure 37.29.

HYPOVITAMINOSIS BIOTIN. Biotin deficiencies are reported to be rare, and while biotin is reported to be essential for metabolism of fatty acids, glucose, and some amino acids, its association with particular disease states still remains unclear.[72] Conditions attributed to hypovitaminosis biotin are given in Table 37.11, the actual role of biotin in clinically defined diseases has still not been fully determined nor have toxicities associated with hypervitaminosis been shown.

Minerals

Sodium Chloride (Table Salt, NaCl)

The human body is composed of both organic and inorganic compounds. The inorganic nutrients generally are considered under the title of micronutrients and are too numerous to cover in this chapter. The essential minerals include calcium, chromium, copper, iodine, iron, magnesium, manganese, molybdenum, phosphorus, selenium, and zinc, along with the essential electrolytes of sodium, potassium, and chloride. This discussion will be limited to sodium and chloride ions.

DIETARY ROLE. Sodium ion, most commonly consumed in the form of sodium chloride, is essential for various roles in the body. What is not known is just how much sodium chloride represents the minimum amount needed for good health. It is estimated that Americans consume approximately 10-12 g/d, which qualifies it as the second most common food additive (~15 lb/yr). There is no RDA set for sodium chloride, although it is thought that an intake of less than 1,000 mg/d would meet the needs for a normal adult. The adequate intake and upper limit for sodium chloride are given as approximately 3.8 and 9.1 g/d, respectively, which would result in 1.5-3.6 g/d of sodium and 2.3-5.5 g/d of chloride (39.6% of sodium chloride is sodium and 60.4% of sodium chloride is chloride). The 2005 dietary guideline for sodium chloride consumption was established at 5.8 g/d (~1 teaspoon), or 2.3 g/d of sodium. The 2.3 g/d of sodium continues to be the desired goal as reported in the 2015-2020 Dietary Guidelines.[73]

The human appetite for sodium chloride has both a physiologic and an educated basis. Taste receptors in the oral cavity can detect a salty taste presumably as a means of encouraging and assuring the intake of sodium chloride. But the human also has an educated appetite for salt. Commercially processed food commonly has added sodium, usually in the form of sodium chloride, as a preservative but also to improve the taste. It is estimated that as much as 65%-85% of the daily consumed sodium chloride is present as "hidden salt" in processed food. In the case of baby food, sodium chloride may be added to meet the need to satisfy the parent who tastes the food rather than to meet a nutritional need of the child. As a result, the child grows up with a conditioned belief that a specific food must have a certain degree of saltiness, whether natural or "man enhanced." Many adults salt their food prior to tasting it because again they have a belief that the food must meet an expected level of saltiness.

The concern about sodium intake is not a new concern as indicated by the White House Conference on Food, Nutrition, and Health, which issued a report in 1969 in which the role of sodium in hypertension was emphasized. Since this report, additional reports and studies have appeared, all of which suggest that Americans need to reduce their intake of sodium in the form of sodium chloride and that high sodium intake is associated with elevated blood pressure, heart disease, stroke, congestive heart failure, and renal disease. In the 1980s, the FDA made an attempt to sensitize the public to this growing public health issue, which at best resulted in a public awareness of sodium intake from processed foods and resulted in some manufacturers producing low-salt products, but in general, attempts to actually reduce salt intake have failed. These efforts by the FDA were directed primarily at consumer education, and it

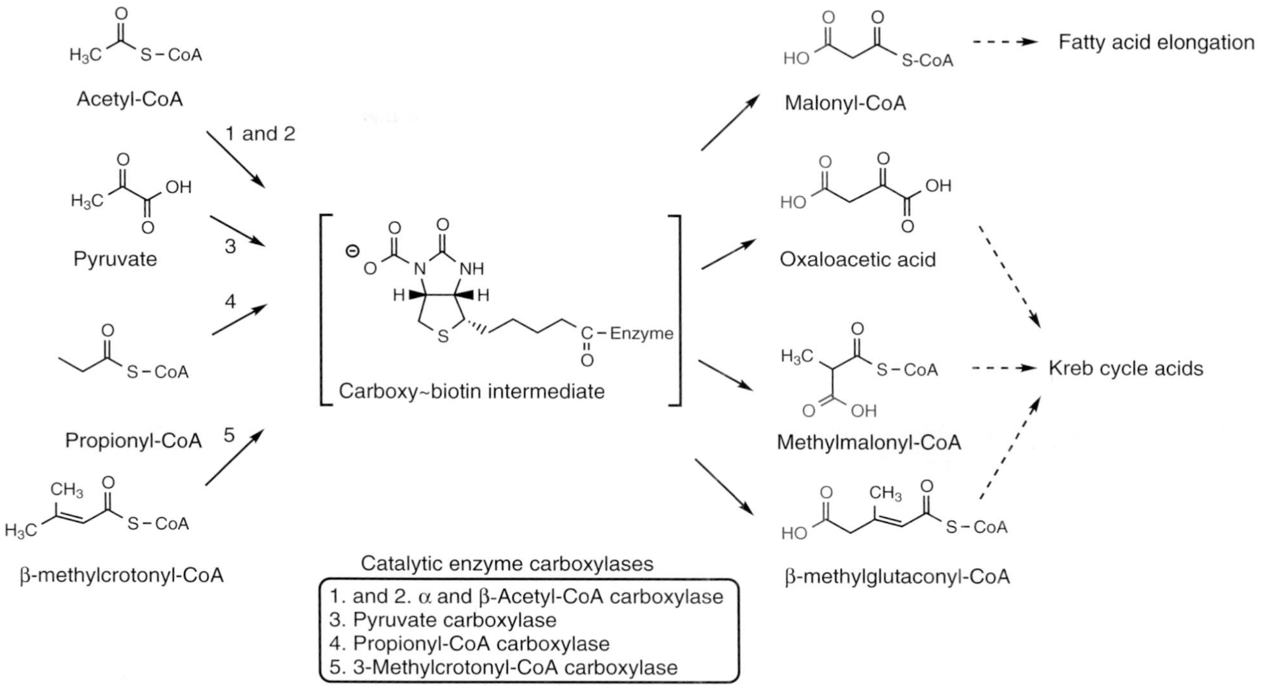

Acetyl-CoA

Pyruvate

Propionyl-CoA

β-methylcrotonyl-CoA

Carboxy~biotin intermediate

Malonyl-CoA → Fatty acid elongation

Oxaloacetic acid

Methylmalonyl-CoA → Kreb cycle acids

β-methylglutaconyl-CoA

Catalytic enzyme carboxylases

1. and 2. α and β-Acetyl-CoA carboxylase
3. Pyruvate carboxylase
4. Propionyl-CoA carboxylase
5. 3-Methylcrotonyl-CoA carboxylase

Figure 37.29 Reactions involving key mammalian biochemicals and carboxy bound biotin leading to fatty acids and carboxylic acids in the Krebs cycle.

was estimated that only about 30% of the consumers actually attempted to reduce sodium intake. In 2009, the Institute of Medicine Committee on Strategies to Reduce Sodium Intake convened and issued their report in 2010.[74] This comprehensive report and the more recent report[57] indicates that although dietary sources of sodium are plentiful, a major contributor to sodium intake is processed and restaurant foods, whereas sodium added to food from the salt shaker amounts to only 5% of the sodium consumed. The report reached the conclusion that standards for sodium intake need to be set by the FDA and that a progressive decrease in sodium content of processed food and restaurant food needs to occur but that this reduction needs to be done in a way acceptable to the consumer. It is also noted that sodium does appear in the GRAS list, giving the FDA authority to set standards, but that these standards need to be done within the confines of GRAS and that sodium should not be removed from GRAS. A total of five recommendations were made, and basically, the GRAS status of salt needs to be changed over time and in cooperation with the food industry. Throughout the changes in sodium content in foods, efforts need to be made to educate the public to the need for lowering sodium intake so as to lead to successful behavioral changes in the taste expectations of the public.

DIETARY SUPPLEMENTS

Two legislative acts that were passed by Congress in the 1990s have impacted nutrition in the United States. These are the NLEA of 1990 and the DSHEA of 1994. The NLEA allows companies, through petition to the FDA, to label their product with health claims linking food or food components to a reduced risk of a specific disease. The petitioning company is responsible for presenting evidence to support its claims. Among the claims that have appeared since this legislation went into effect are the following:

- Low sodium and a reduced risk of hypertension
- Calcium for the treatment of osteoporosis
- Fiber-containing grains and a reduction in the risk of cancer
- Fruits, vegetables, and grains and the prevention of coronary heart disease
- Folic acid and the prevention of neural tube defects
- Soy protein and the prevention of coronary heart disease
- Whole-grain foods and the prevention of specific cancers
- Dietary lipids as the cause of cancer
- Dietary sugar alcohols and protection of dental caries
- Soluble fibers and the prevention of heart disease

The second act, DSHEA, allows companies to introduce dietary supplements without FDA approval provided "there is a history of use or other evidence to establishing safety." This legislation allows "structure-function" claims but not health claims without supportive evidence. The manufacturer must show safety of ingredients. A dietary supplement is a product that contains dietary ingredients, is taken by mouth, and is intended to supplement one's diet. Such products include vitamins, minerals, herbs, enzymes, amino acids, and metabolites.

As a result of these acts, various classes of nutrients have appeared on the market including nutraceuticals, functional foods, and the official use of foods titled as "organic foods." Nutraceuticals are defined as dietary supplements, foods, or medical foods that possess health benefits and that are safe for human consumption in such quantities and such frequency as required to realize beneficial properties. A functional food is a product that is conveyed in a conventional food format and has health benefits. Through these acts, various natural products have appeared as dietary supplements including S-adenosylmethionine (SAM-e), plant stanols, soy protein in "milk" products, and a number of herbal products being sold as dietary supplements.

Structure Challenge

ANOREXIANTS USED IN THE MANAGEMENT OF OBESITY

The following chemicals have all found pharmacological benefit in treatment of obesity through various molecular mechanisms. Identify which agent(s) acts through the mechanism indicated.

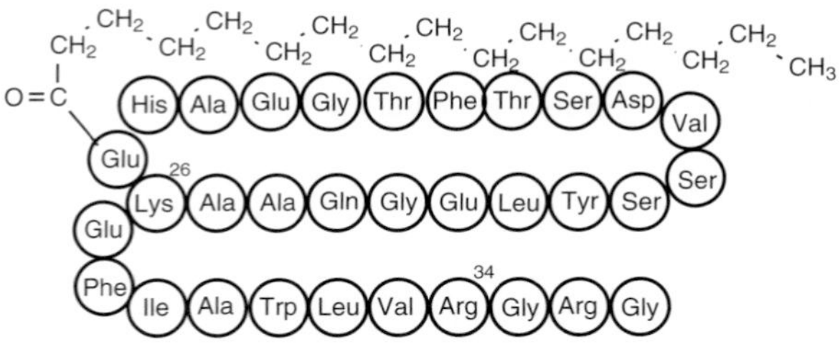

1 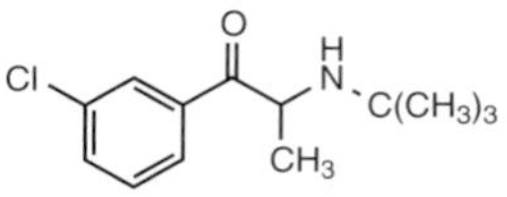 2 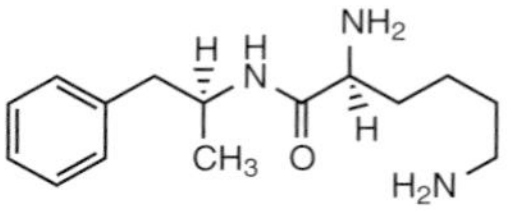 3 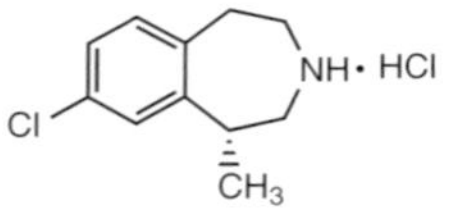 4 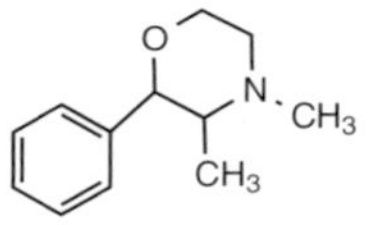 5 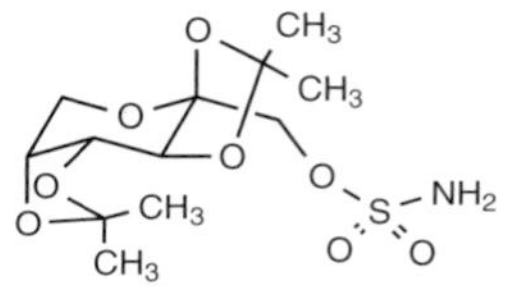 6

A. Acts as a sympathomimetic amine blocking norepinephrine reuptake. Highlight the pharmacophore.
B. Acts as a serotonin agonist.
C. Acts as a GLP-1 agonist.
D. Centrally active possibly as a GABA-A agonist

Structure challenge answers found immediately after References.

REFERENCES

1. Herrera BM, Keildson S, Lindgren CM. Genetics and epigenetics of obesity. *Maturitas*. 2011;69(1):41-49.
2. Westerterp KR. Diet induced thermogenesis. *Nutr Metab*. 2004;1:1-5.
3. Flegal KM, Kruszon-Moran D, Carroll MD, et al. Trends in obesity among adults in the United States, 2005 to 2014. *J Am Med Assoc*. 2016;315(21);2284-2291.
4. Ogden CL, Carroll MD, Fryar CD, et al. Prevalence of obesity amoung adults and youth: United States, 2011-2014. *NCHS Data Brief*. 2015;219. www.cdc.gov/nchs/data/databriefs/db219.pdf.
5. Adams KF, Schatzkin A, Harris TB, et al. Overweight, obesity, and mortality in a large prospective cohort of persons 50 to 71 years old. *N Engl J Med*. 2006;355:763-778.
6. National Heart, Lung, and Blood Institute Obesity Education Initiative. *Clinical Guidelines on the Identification, Evaluation, and Treatment of Overweight and Obesity in Adults*. Bethesda, MD: National Institutes of Health; 1998. NIH Publication No. 98-4083.
7. WHO. *Waist Circumference and Waist-Hip Ratio: Report of a WHO Expert Consultation*. Geneva: World Health Organization (WHO); 2011.
8. Putnam J, Allshouse J, Kantor LS. U.S. per capita food supply trends: more calories,refined carbohydrates, and fats. *Food Rev*. 2002;25:2-15.
9. Nielsen SJ, Popkin BM. Patterns and trends in food portion sizes, 1977–1998. *JAMA*. 2003;289:450-453.
10. https://www.fda.gov/food/guidanceregulation/guidance-documentsregulatory-information/labelingnutrition/ChangestotheNutritionFactsLabel. Accessed January 31, 2018.

11. Howarth NC, Saltzmen E, Roberts SB. Dietary fiber and weight regulation. *Nutr Rev*. 2001;59:129-139.
12. Kemsley J. New fibers for foods. *Chem Eng News*. 2010;88(49):38-40.
13. Ashwar BA, Gani A, Shah A, et al. Preparation, health benefits and applications of resistant starch – a review. *Starch*. 2016;68(3-4):278-301.
14. DeLaPena C. *Empty Pleasures: The Story of Artificial Sweeteners from Saccharin to Splenda*. Chapel Hill, NC: The University of North Carolina Press; 2010.
15. Whysmer J, Williams GM. Saccharin mechanistic data and risk assessment: urine composition, enhanced cell proliferation, and tumor promotion. *Pharmacol Ther*. 1996;71:225-252.
16. Stegink L. The aspartame story: a model for the clinical testing of a food additive. *Am J Clin Nutr*. 1987;46:204-215.
17. Kroger M, Meister K, Kava R. Low-calorie sweeteners and other sugar substitutes: a review of the safety issues. *Compr Rev Food Sci Food Safety* 2006;5:35-47.
18. Kuhn C, Bufe B, Winnig M, et al. Bitter taste receptors for saccharin and acesulfame-K. *J Neurosci*. 2004;24:10260-10265.
19. Brusick DJ. A critical review of the genetic toxicity of steviol and steviol glycosides. *Food Chem Toxicol*. 2008;46:S83-S91.
20. Pezzuto JM, Compadre CM, Swanson SM, et al. Metabolically-activated steviol, the aglycone of stevioside, is mutagenic. *Proc Natl Acad Sci USA*. 1985;82:2478-2482.
21. Shi H, Hiramatsu M, Komatsu, et al. Antioxidant property of fructus momordicae extract. *Biochem Mol Biol Int*. 1996;40(6):1111-1121.
22. Chen WJ, Wang J, Qi XY, et al. The antioxidant activities of natural sweeteners, mogrosides, from fruits of Siraitia grosvenori. *Int J Food Sci Nutr*. 2007;58(7):548-556.
23. Jacoby M. Sowing the seeds of oil customization. *Chem Eng News*. 2010;88(22):52-55.
24. Eller FJ, List GR, Teel JA, et al. Preparation of spread oils meeting U.S. Food and Drug Administration labeling requirements for trans fatty acids via pressure-controlled hydrogenation. *J Agric Food Chem*. 2005;53:5982-5984.
25. Health Canada. Transforming the Food Supply: Report of the Trans Fat Task Force submitted to the Minister of Health. Available at http://www.hc-sc.gc.ca/fn-an/nutrition/gras-trans-fats/tf-ge/tf-gt_rep-rap_e.html. Accessed February 2011.
26. Mozaffarian D, Katan MB, Ascherio A, et al. Trans fatty acids and cardiovascular disease. *N Engl J Med*. 2006;354:1601-1613.
27. https://www.fda.gov/food/ucm292278.htm. Accessed February 3, 2018.
28. Wiley. Tutorial on Fatty Acid Metabolism. Available at http://www.wiley.com/college/pratt/0471393878/student/animations/fatty_acid/index.html.
29. Hu FB, van Dam RM, Liu S. Diet and risk of type II diabetes: the role of types of fat and carbohydrates. *Diabetologia*. 2001;44:805-817.
30. Allshouse J, Frazao B, Turpening J. Are Americans turning away from lower fat salty snacks? *Food Rev*. 2002;25:37-43.
31. Jensen MD, Ryan DH, Apovian CM, et al. 2013 AHA/ACC/TOS guidelines for the management of overweight and obesity in adults. *J Am Coll Cardiol*. 2014;63:2985-3023.
32. Apovian CM, Aronne LJ, Bassesen DH, et al. Pharmacologic management of obesity: an endocrine society clinical practice guideline. *JCEM*. 2015;2:342-362.
33. Garvey WT, Mechanick JI, Brett EM, et al. American Association of Clinical Endocrinologists and American College of Endocrinology comprehensive clinical practice guidelines for medical care of patients with obesity. *Endocr Pract*. 2016;22(suppl 3):1-326.
34. https://www.accessdata.fda.gov/drugsatfda_docs/nda/99/020766a_xenical_appltr.pdf. Accessed June 14, 2018.
35. https://www.accessdata.fda.gov/drugsatfda_docs/nda/2012/022529Orig1s000Approv.pdf. Accessed June 14, 2018.
36. https://www.accessdata.fda.gov/drugsatfda_docs/nda/2012/022580Orig1s000Approv.pdf. Accessed June 14, 2018.
37. https://www.accessdata.fda.gov/drugsatfda_docs/nda/2014/206321Orig1s000Approv.pdf. Accessed June 14, 2018.
38. https://www.accessdata.fda.gov/drugsatfda_docs/nda/2014/200063orig1s000approv.pdf. Accessed June 14, 2018.
39. Hadvary P, Lengsfeld H, Wolfer H. Inhibition of pancreatic lipase in vitro by the covalent inhibitor tetrahydrolipstatin. *Biochem J*. 1988;256:357-361.
40. Hadvary P, Sidler W, Meister W, et al. The lipase inhibitor tetrahydrolipstatin binds covalently to the putative active site serine of pancreatic lipase. *J Biol Chem*. 1991;266:2021-2027.
41. McNeely W, Benfield P. Orlistat. *Drugs*. 1998;56:241-249.
42. Padwal RS, Li SK, Lau DC. Long-term pharmacotherapy for obesity and overweight. *Cochrane Database Syst Rev*. 2003;4:CD004094.
43. Centers for Disease Control and Prevention. *The Practical Guide: Identification, Evaluation and Treatment of Overweight and Obesity in Adults*. Druid Hills, GA: Centers for Disease Control and Prevention; 2000.
44. WebMD. Diet Pills and Prescription Weight Loss Drugs: How They Work. Available at http://www.webmd.com/diet/guide/weight-loss-prescription-weight-loss-medicine. Accessed June 8, 2011.
45. Inoue T, Suzuki S. The metabolism of 1-phenyl-2-(N-methyl-N-benzylamino)propane (benzphetamine) and 1-phenyl-2-(N-methyl-N-furfurylamino)propane (furfenorex) in man. *Xenobiotica*. 1986;16:691-698.
46. Rothman RB, Baumann MH. Therapeutic potential of monoamine transporter substrates. *Curr Top Med Chem*. 2006;6:1845-1859.
47. Halford JC, Boyland EJ, Lawton CL, et al. Serotonergic anti-obesity agents: past experience and future prospects. *Drugs*. 2011;71(17):2247-2255.
48. Colman E, Golden J, Roberts M, et al. The FDA's assessment of two drugs for chronic weight management. *N Engl J Med*. 2012;367:1577-1579.
49. Mancini MC, de Melo ME. The burden of obesity in the current world and the new treatments available: focus on liraglutide 3.0 mg. *Diabetol Metab Syndr*. 2017;9:44-58.
50. Cosentino G, Conrad AO, Uwaifo GI. Phentermine and topiramate for the management of obesity: a review. *Drug Des Devel Ther*. 2013;3(7):267-278.
51. Narayanaswami V, Dwoskin LP. Obesity: current and potential pharmacotherapeutics and targets. *Pharmacol Ther*. 2017;170:116-147.
52. Tian H, Guo X, Wang X, et al. Chromium picolinate supplementation for overweight or obese adults (review). *Cochrane Database Syst Rev*. 2013;11:CD010063.
53. Onakpoya I, Posadzki P, Ernst E. The efficacy of glucomannan supplementation in overweight and obesity: a systematic review and meta-analysis of randomized clinical trials. *J Am Coll Nutr*. 2014;33(1):70-78.
54. Egras AM, Hamilton WR, Lenz TL, Monaghan MS. An evidence-based review of fat modifying supplemental weight loss products. *J Obes*. 2011;2011:297315.
55. https://www.accessdata.fda.gov/scripts/sda/sdNavigation.cfm?sd=tainted_supplements_cder. Accessed June 25, 2018.
56. Ross AC. Vitamin A and carotenoids. In: Shils ME, Shike M, Ross AC, et al, eds. *Modern Nutrition in Health and Disease*. 10th ed. Philadelphia: Lippincott Williams & Wilkins; 2006.
57. Ranard KM, Jeon S, Mohn ES, et al. Dietary guidance for lutein: consideration for intake recommendations is scientifically supported. *Eur J Nutr*. 2017;56(3):S37-S42.
58. Gong X, Draper CS, Allison GS, et al. Effects of the macular carotenoid lutein in human retinal pigment epithelial cells. *Antioxidants (Basel)*. 2017;6(4):100. doi:10.3390/antiox6040100.
59. Porter NA, Caldwell SE, Mills KA. Mechanisms of free radical oxidation of unsaturated lipids. *Lipids*. 1995;30:277-290.
60. Kamal-Eldin A, Appelqvist L. The chemistry and antioxidant properties of tocopherols and tocotrienols. *Lipids*. 1996;31:671-701.
61. Liebler DC, Burr JA. Antioxidant stoichiometry and the oxidative fate of vitamin E in peroxyl radical. *Lipids*. 1995;30:789-793.
62. Sontag TJ, Parker RS. Cytochrome P450 omega-hydroxylase pathway of tocopherol catabolism novel mechanism of regulation of vitamin E status. *J Biol Chem*. 2002;277:25290-25296.
63. Birringer M, Pfluger P, Kluth D, et al. Identities and differences in the metabolism of tocotrienols and tocopherols in HepG2 cells. *J Nutr*. 2002;132:3113-3118.

64. Lodgea JK, Ridlingtonb J, Leonarda S, et al. Tocotrienols are metabolized to carboxyethyl hydroxychroman derivatives and excreted in human urine. *Lipids*. 2001;36:43-48.
65. Suttie JW. Vitamin K. In: Shils ME, Shike M, Ross AC, et al, eds. *Modern Nutrition in Health and Disease*. 10th ed. Philadelphia: Lippincott Williams & Wilkins; 2006.
66. Booth SL, Suttie JW. Dietary intake and adequacy of vitamin K. *J Nutr*. 1998;128:785-788.
67. Butterworth RF. Chapter 23 Thiamin. In: Shils ME, Shike M, Ross AC, et al, ed. *Modern Nutrition in Health and Disease*. 10th ed. Philadelphia: Lippincott Williams & Wilkins; 2006.
68. McCormick DB. Chapter 26 Riboflavin. In: Shils ME, Shike M, Ross AC, et al, ed. *Modern Nutrition in Health and Disease*. 10th ed. Philadelphia: Lippincott Williams & Wilkins; 2006.
69. Kamanna VS, Kashyap ML. Mechanism of action of niacin. *Am J Cardiol*. 2008;101(8):S20-S26.
70. Garg A, Sharma A, Krishnamoorthy P, et al. Role of niacin in current clinical practice: a systematic review. *Am J Med*. 2017;130:170-187.
71. Carmel R. Chapter 29 Cobalamin (vitamin B_{12}). In: Shils ME, Shike M, Ross AC, et al, eds. *Modern Nutrition in Health and Disease*. 10th ed. Philadelphia: Lippincott Williams & Wilkins; 2006.
72. Eng WK, Giraud D, Schlegel VL, et al. Identification and assessment of markers of biotin status in health adults. *Br J Nutr*. 2013;110(2):321-329.
73. U.S. Department of Health and Human Services and U.S. Department of Agriculture. *2015 –2020 Dietary Guidelines for Americans*. 8th ed.; 2015. Available at https://health.gov/dietaryguidelines/2015/guidelines/.
74. Henney JE, Taylor CL, Boon CS, eds. *Strategies to Reduce Sodium Intake in the United States*. *Institute of Medicine (US) Committee on Strategies to Reduce Sodium Intake*. Washington, DC: National Academies Press; 2010.

SUGGESTED READINGS: VITAMINS

Vitamin A through vitamin C in chapters 19-31. In: Shils ME, Shike M, Ross AC, et al, eds. *Modern Nutrition in Health and Disease*. 10th ed. Philadelphia: Lippincott Williams & Wilkins; 2006.

Deimling MJ, Khan MOF, Ortega GR. Chapter 28 Vitamins. In: Beale JM, Block JH, eds. *Wilson and Gisvold's Organic Medicinal and Pharmaceutical Chemistry*. 12th ed. Philadelphia: Wolters Kluwer/Lippincott Williams & Wilkins; 2011.

Brown MJ, Beier K. *Vitamin, B6 (Pyridoxine), Deficiency*. Source StatPearls [Internet]. Treasure Island (FL): StatPearls Publishing; 2017.

Structure Challenge Answers

A-3 and 5

3

5

B-4, C-1, D-6

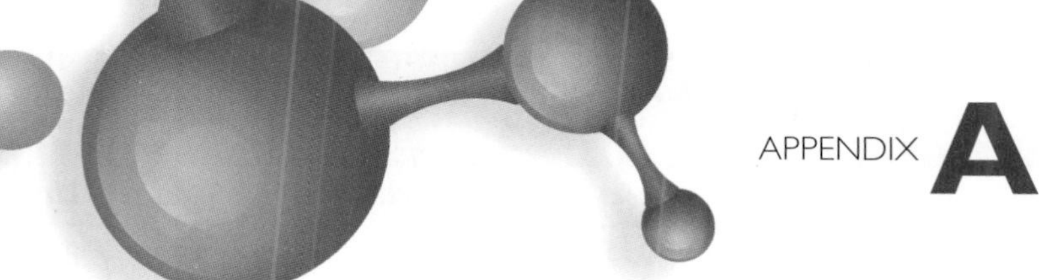

APPENDIX **A**

cLogP and cLogD$_{pH\ 7.4}$ Values of Selected Drugs[a]

David A. Williams

cLogP and cLogD$_{pH\ 7.4}$ for Selected Drugs[a]

Drug	cLogD$_{pH\ 7.4}$	cLogP
Abacavir	1.32	0.72
Abemaciclib	2.55	2.74
Acebutolol	−0.38	1.95
Acetaminophen	0.40	0.34
Acetazolamide	−0.81	−0.26
Acetylcysteine	−3.70	−0.15
Acetylsalicylic acid	−1.69	1.19
Acrivastine	0.99	4.55
Acyclovir	−1.47	−1.76
Albendazole	3.10	3.07
Albuterol	−1.52	0.01
Alectinib	4.89	5.59
Alendronic acid	−8.80	−3.52
Alfentanil	1.69	1.99
Alfuzosin	0.10	−1.00
Aliskiren	0.26	2.74
Allopurinol	−0.06	−0.46
Alprazolam	2.63	2.50
Alvimopan	0.55	3.38
Amantadine	−0.37	2.22
Ambrisentan	1.48	6.24
Amifostine	−4.35	−1.68
Amikacin	−9.81	−3.34

cLogP and cLogD$_{pH\ 7.4}$ for Selected Drugs[a] (Continued)

Drug	cLogD$_{pH\ 7.4}$	cLogP
Amiloride	−0.17	1.08
Aminocaproic acid	−3.45	−0.11
p-Aminosalicylic acid	−1.68	1.14
Amiodarone	5.41	8.89
Amitriptyline	2.96	4.92
Amlodipine	1.91	4.16
Amobarbital	−0.56	1.78
Amoxapine	1.70	2.35
Amoxicillin	−2.72	0.61
Amphetamine	−0.62	1.81
Amphotericin B	−2.24	1.16
Ampicillin	−2.38	1.35
Anakinra	−1.93	2.69
Anastrozole	2.68	0.97
Antipyrine	0.72	0.28
Apalutamide	1.38	1.30
Apixaban	0.87	0.48
Apomorphine	2.52	3.05
Apraclonidine	−0.04	0.29
Aprepitant	3.70	4.23
Argatroban	−0.47	2.56
Aripiprazole	4.99	5.59

(continued)

cLogP and cLogD$_{pH\ 7.4}$ for Selected Drugs[a] (Continued)

Drug	cLogD$_{pH\ 7.4}$	cLogP
Ascorbic acid	−4.99	−2.41
Atazanavir	4.61	5.20
Atenolol	−1.85	0.10
Atomoxetine	1.06	3.28
Atorvastatin	1.25	4.13
Atovaquone	2.49	6.18
Atropine	−0.61	1.53
Avibactam	−6.77	−3.20
Azacitidine	−2.30	−1.99
Azathioprine	−0.04	0.67
Azelastine	2.40	3.71
Aztreonam	−6.02	−0.66
Baclofen	−0.96	1.56
Balsalazide	−1.90	2.70
Beclomethasone	2.04	2.04
Benazepril	−0.71	3.86
Bendroflumethiazide	1.46	2.07
Benznidazole	1.09	0.91
Benzocaine		1.95
Benzphetamine	2.77	4.43
Benztropine	1.89	4.96
Bepotastine	0.85	3.67
Besifloxacin	−1.20	1.91
Betaxolol	0.76	2.69
Betrixaban	1.17	2.93
Bicalutamide	2.53	4.94
Bictegravir	−3.26	−1.26
Binimetinib	3.51	3.1
Bisoprolol	0.12	2.14
Bitolterol	3.23	5.25
Bortezomide	1.87	2.45
Brimonidine	0.70	0.96
Brinzolamide	−0.12	−0.65
Brivaracetam	0.61	0.88
Bosentan	1.53	1.15
Bromocriptine	3.45	5.15

cLogP and cLogD$_{pH\ 7.4}$ for Selected Drugs[a] (Continued)

Drug	cLogD$_{pH\ 7.4}$	cLogP
Brompheniramine	1.40	3.57
Bumetanide	0.03	2.78
Bupivacaine	2.68	3.64
Buprenorphine	3.48	3.43
Bupropion	2.88	3.47
Buspirone	2.60	3.43
Butabarbital	1.32	1.52
Butenafine	5.59	6.77
Butoconazole	6.44	6.88
Butorphanol	2.75	3.77
Caffeine	0.28	−0.13
Camptothecin	1.88	1.60
Canagliflozin	3.75	5.34
Candesartan	0.04	5.01
Captopril	−2.83	0.27
Carbachol	−4.02	−3.90
Carbamazepine	2.28	2.67
Carbidopa	−2.58	−0.19
Carbinoxamine	1.38	2.76
Cariprazine	4.56	4.98
Carisoprodol	1.93	2.15
Carteolol	−0.24	1.35
Carvedilol	3.04	4.11
Cefaclor	−3.63	0.10
Cefadroxil	−4.06	−0.09
Cefazolin	−4.02	1.13
Cefotaxime	−3.31	1.20
Celecoxib	3.23	4.21
Cephalexin	−3.63	0.65
Cetirizine	−0.55	2.16
Cevimeline	−0.44	1.23
Chlorambucil	0.56	3.10
Chloramphenicol	1.02	1.02
Chlorcyclizine	3.39	3.00
Chlordiazepoxide	2.36	2.16
Chlorhexidine	0.55	4.58

cLogP and cLogD$_{pH\ 7.4}$ for Selected Drugs[a] (Continued)

Drug	cLogD$_{pH\ 7.4}$	cLogP
Chloroprocaine	1.15	2.93
Chloroquine	1.74	4.69
Chlorothiazide	−0.21	−0.18
Chlorpheniramine	1.16	3.39
Chlorpromazine	3.42	5.20
Chlorpropamide	0.19	2.30
Chlorzoxazone	2.34	2.19/1.82 lactam
Ciclopirox	0.69	2.59
Cidofovir	−7.35	−3.37
Cilostazol	3.01	3.05
Cimetidine	0.40	0.07
Ciprofloxacin	−2.23	0.65
Citalopram	1.27	2.51
Cladribine	0.01	0.01
Clarithromycin	2.38	3.16
Clemastine	3.22	5.99
Clevidipine	5.11	5.46
Clindamycin	1.08	1.83
Clobazam	2.26	1.69
Clofarabine	−0.17	0.24
Clofibrate	3.53	3.32
Clomiphene	4.95	8.01
Clomipramine	3.31	5.39
Clonazepam	2.53	2.34
Clonidine	1.04	1.41
Clopidogrel	4.21	4.23
Clotrimazole	5.22	5.44
Clozapine	2.72	2.36
Cobimetinib	2.88	5.96
Cocaine	1.22	3.08
Codeine	0.28	1.20
Colchicine	1.10	0.92
Conivaptan	4.28	4.40
Cromolyn	−2.95	2.30
Cyclizine	2.47	2.41

cLogP and cLogD$_{pH\ 7.4}$ for Selected Drugs[a] (Continued)

Drug	cLogD$_{pH\ 7.4}$	cLogP
Cyclobenzaprine	2.89	5.00
Cyclopentolate	1.52	2.59
Cyclosporine	1.80	3.35
Cyproheptadine	3.51	6.41
Cytarabine	−2.17	−1.93
Dabigatran	−1.08	0.79
Dacarbazine	−1.50	−2.30
Daclatasvir	4.47	5.44
Danazol	4.33	4.70
Dantrolene	1.33	1.42
Dapagliflozin	2.48	4.42
Dapsone	1.08	0.94
Darifenacin	2.33	4.50
Darunavir	3.09	3.94
Daunorubicin	−0.29	2.92
Decitabine	−2.00	−1.93
Delafloxacin	−1.13	0.81
Delavirdine	0.78	−1.21
Desipramine	1.58	4.13
Desloratadine	2.14	6.77
Desvenlafaxine	0.89	2.26
Dexlansoprazole	2.40	2.76
Dexmedetomidine	2.80	3.10
Dexmethylphenidate	0.26	2.55
Dextroamphetamine	0.62	1.81
Dextromethorphan	1.86	4.11
Diacetylmorphine (heroin)	1.24	1.52
Diazepam	2.92	2.91
Diazoxide	1.23	1.08
Dibucaine	1.76	3.87
Diclofenac	1.37	4.06
Dicyclomine	3.42	6.05
Diethylpropion	1.66	2.95
Difenoxin	2.45	5.04
Diflunisal	1.16	4.44

(continued)

cLogP and cLogD$_{pH\ 7.4}$ for Selected Drugs[a] (Continued)

Drug	cLogD$_{pH\ 7.4}$	cLogP
Dihydroergotamine	2.57	3.53
Diltiazem	2.06	3.63
Diphenhydramine	2.34	3.66
Diphenoxylate	5.48	5.88
Dipyridamole	0.30	−1.22
Disopyramide	0.35	2.86
Dobutamine	−0.33	1.94
Dofetilide	0.83	1.56
Dolasetron	2.63	2.82
Donepezil	2.79	4.71
Dopamine	2.18	0.12
Doripenem	−4.53	−3.65
Dorzolamide	−0.36	−0.91
Doxazosin	1.46	0.65
Doxepin	2.50	3.86
Doxorubicin	−0.79	2.82
Doxycycline	−0.54	−3.29
Doxylamine	1.57	2.52
Dronedarone	3.98	7.58
Droperidol	3.34	3.51
Duloxetine	1.53	3.73
Dyclonine	2.68	4.67
Econazole	5.63	5.32
Edaravone	1.13	0.44
Edoxaban	1.24	1.12
Elagolix	3.29	7.20
Eluxadoline	0.58	4.35
Empagliflozin	2.46	3.38
Enalapril	1.57	2.43
Enalaprilat	−2.68	1.54
Encorafenib	1.48	2.7
Entacapone	−0.04	2.38
Ephedrine	−0.75	1.05
Epinephrine	−2.56	−0.63
Eravacycline	−2.39	1.55
Ergonovine	1.37	1.14

cLogP and cLogD$_{pH\ 7.4}$ for Selected Drugs[a] (Continued)

Drug	cLogD$_{pH\ 7.4}$	cLogP
Ergotamine	2.42	3.58
Ertugliflozin	3.95	6.49
Erythromycin	1.69	2.83
Esmolol	−0.08	1.91
Estrone	3.38	3.69
Ethacrynic acid	−0.31	3.36
Ethambutol	−2.13	−0.05
Ethosuximide	0.33	0.38
Etomidate	2.55	3.26
Eugenol	2.48	2.20
Fenfluramine	0.69	3.03
Fenoprofen	0.10	3.84
Fenoterol	0.45	3.89
Fentanyl	3.01	3.89
Fesoterodine	2.28	5.08
Fexofenadine	2.43	4.80
Finasteride	3.01	3.24
Flibanserin	3.44	4.07
Flurbiprofen	0.68	4.11
Fluoxetine	1.75	4.09
Fluphenazine	4.11	4.84
Flurazepam	1.20	3.99
Flutamide	3.14	3.72
Fluvoxamine	1.08	3.11
Formoterol	−0.05	1.57
Furosemide	−0.78	3.10
Gabapentin	−1.40	1.19
Galantamine	0.92	1.75
Gentamicin	−8.31	−2.23
Glecaprevir	0.34	1.71
Glibenclamide	1.85	3.75
Glimepiride	1.23	2.94
Glipizide	−0.12	2.01
Glutethimide	2.20	2.70
Grazoprevir	1.70	3.93
Guanabenz	10.11	2.57

cLogP and cLogD$_{pH\ 7.4}$ for Selected Drugs[a] (Continued)

Drug	cLogD$_{pH\ 7.4}$	cLogP
Guanfacine	1.56	1.12
Haloperidol	2.65	3.01
Homatropine	−0.76	1.57
Hydralazine	1.13	1.00
Hydrochlorothiazide	−0.02	−0.07
Hydrocodone	0.17	1.83
Hydrocortisone	1.66	1.43
Hydromorphone	0.24	1.06
Hydroxyzine	2.66	2.03
Hyoscyamine	−0.61	1.53
Ibuprofen	0.45	3.72
Ibutilide	1.55	4.17
Idarubicin	0.38	2.95
Ifosfamide	0.68	0.23
Iloperidone	2.72	3.81
Imipramine	2.68	4.80
Inamrinone	−0.35	−0.54
Indacaterol	2.13	3.88
Indapamide	2.15	2.10
Indinavir	3.03	2.88
Indomethacin	0.75	3.11
Iodoquinol	4.10	4.10
Irbesartan	1.25	4.50
Irinotecan	2.14	4.35
Isavuconazole	3.38	3.92
Isoniazid	−0.77	−0.77
Isoproterenol	−1.89	0.25
Isradipine	3.75	3.59
Itraconazole	4.96	4.35
Ivabradine	2.18	3.69
Ivacaftor	5.42	6.34
Ivermectin	6.21	6.61
Ivosidenib	1.21	3.4
Ixabepilone	2.44	1.77
Kanamycin	−7.93	−2.58

cLogP and cLogD$_{pH\ 7.4}$ for Selected Drugs[a] (Continued)

Drug	cLogD$_{pH\ 7.4}$	cLogP
Ketamine	2.07	2.18
Ketoconazole	3.49	3.55
Ketoprofen	0.06	2.81
Ketorolac	−0.44	2.08
Ketotifen	2.61	4.88
Labetalol	0.85	2.31
Lacosamide	0.82	0.90
Lamivudine	−0.98	−0.71
Lamotrigine	1.68	−0.19
Lansoprazole	2.40	2.76
Lapatinib	5.18	5.14
Leflunomide	2.20	1.95
Lenalidomide	−0.48	−1.39
Lenvatinib	2.98	3.39
Letrozole	2.22	1.91
Levobunolol	0.50	2.61
Levodopa	−2.70	−0.22
Levofloxacin	−2.08	0.84
Levomilnacipran	−1.09	1.23
Levorphanol	1.67	3.46
Levothyroxine	1.76	5.93
Lidocaine	1.80	2.36
Lifitegrast	−0.43	1.54
Lincomycin	−0.44	0.91
Linezolid	0.82	0.30
Liothyronine	1.54	5.08
Lisinopril	−1.80	1.19
Lofexidine	1.02	3.59
Loperamide	3.94	4.26
Lopinavir	5.24	6.26
Loratadine	5.32	5.94
Lorazepam	2.49	2.47
Losartan	1.29	3.56
Lovastatin	4.14	4.07
Loxapine	2.93	2.74

(continued)

cLogP and $cLogD_{pH\ 7.4}$ for Selected Drugs[a] (Continued)

Drug	$cLogD_{pH\ 7.4}$	cLogP
Macimorelin	1.11	2.64
Maprotiline	2.10	4.51
Maraviroc	1.49	3.60
Mecamylamine	−0.04	3.06
Meclizine	4.66	4.99
Meclofenamic acid	2.95	6.67
Mefenamic acid	2.04	5.33
Mefloquine	1.47	2.87
Meloxicam	−0.50	2.71
Melphalan	−1.03	1.79
Memantine	0.56	3.18
Meperidine	1.88	2.35
Mepivacaine	1.40	2.04
Meprobamate	0.82	0.70
Mercaptopurine	−2.70	−0.18
Meropenem	−4.09	−3.13
Mesalamine	−1.98	0.46
Metaproterenol	−1.78	0.13
Metaraminol	−2.07	0.07
Metaxalone	2.29	2.42
Metformin	−3.36	−2.31
Methadone	2.80	4.20
Methamphetamine	−0.57	1.94
Methazolamide	−0.02	0.13
Methenamine	0.99	2.17
Methohexital	2.06	2.36
Methotrexate	−5.22	−0.24
Methyclothiazide	1.19	1.76
Methyldopa	−2.39	−0.09
Methylergonovine	1.65	1.67
Methylphenidate	0.26	2.55
Methyl salicylate	2.43	2.23
Metoclopramide	0.55	2.22
Metolazone	2.42	1.57
Metoprolol	−0.25	1.79
Metronidazole	0.05	−0.01

cLogP and $cLogD_{pH\ 7.4}$ for Selected Drugs[a] (Continued)

Drug	$cLogD_{pH\ 7.4}$	cLogP
Metyrosine	−1.25	0.73
Mexiletine	1.23	2.16
Miconazole	6.13	5.93
Midazolam	3.35	3.93
Midostaurin	4.79	5.27
Miglustat	−0.84	0.46
Milnacipran	−1.09	1.23
Minocycline	−2.74	−0.65
Minoxidil	1.09	−0.41
Mirtazapine	2.40	2.75
Mitomycin	−0.36	0.49
Molindone	2.14	1.96
Montelukast	4.95	7.80
Morphine	−0.13	0.43
Moxidectin	7.29	8.43
Nabilone	7.25	7.05
Nadolol	−0.86	1.29
Nafcillin	−0.59	3.52
Nalbuphine	1.63	1.79
Naldemedine	0.45	5.24
Nalidixic acid	−0.32	1.19
Naloxone	1.42	1.45
Naltrexone	1.18	1.80
Naphazoline	1.35	3.88
Naproxen	0.45	3.00
Nebivolol	2.36	3.67
Nelfinavir	5.68	6.98
Netarsudil	2.78	3.53
Niacin/nicotinic acid	−2.60	0.15
Nicotinamide	−0.40	−0.11
Nicotine	−0.37	0.72
Niraparib	0.11	2.85
Nitrofurantoin	−0.26	−0.40
Nordefrin	−2.73	−0.53
Norepinephrine	−2.65	−0.88
Nortriptyline	2.28	5.62

cLogP and cLogD$_{pH\ 7.4}$ for Selected Drugs[a] (Continued)

Drug	cLogD$_{pH\ 7.4}$	cLogP
Nystatin	−1.95	1.81
Olanzapine	1.90	2.18
Olaparib	1.04	0.00
Olmesartan	−0.39	3.72
Olopatadine	1.54	3.14
Olsalazine	−0.12	3.94
Omeprazole	2.08	2.17
Ondansetron	2.43	2.07
Orphenadrine	2.72	4.12
Oseltamivir	0.63	1.50
Osimertinib	2.07	3.30
Oxacillin	−1.66	2.05
Oxaprozin	0.84	4.19
Oxazepam	2.06	2.31
Oxcarbazepine	1.87	1.44
Oxiconazole	6.07	5.83
Oxybutynin	3.72	5.19
Oxycodone	0.45	1.67
Oxymorphone	0.60	0.90
Ozenoxacin	1.75	3.41
Palbociclib	0.32	0.99
Paliperidone	0.88	1.52
Palonosetron	1.04	2.61
Panobinostat	10.5	3.62
Pantoprazole	1.45	1.69
Papaverine	3.16	3.74
Paroxetine	1.46	3.89
Penbutolol	1.80	4.17
Penciclovir	−1.50	−2.03
Penicillamine	−1.84	0.93
Penicillin G	−1.70	1.67
Penicillin V	−1.68	1.88
Pentamidine	−0.90	2.47
Pentazocine	2.26	4.53
Pentobarbital	1.91	2.05

cLogP and cLogD$_{pH\ 7.4}$ for Selected Drugs[a] (Continued)

Drug	cLogD$_{pH\ 7.4}$	cLogP
Pentostatin	−2.09	−2.40
Pentoxifylline	0.54	0.32
Perindopril	−0.46	03.36
Permethrin	6.47	7.15
Phendimetrazine	1.55	2.14
Phenelzine	0.51	1.2
Phenobarbital	1.19	1.67
Phenoxybenzamine	4.20	4.78
Phentermine	−0.17	2.15
Phentolamine	1.11	3.60
Phenylbutazone	0.59	3.16
Phenylephrine	−2.04	−0.03
Phenylpropanolamine	−1.15	0.81
Phenyl salicylate	0.81	3.70
Phenyltoloxamine	2.64	3.98
Phenytoin	2.38	2.52
Physostigmine	0.81	1.22
Pibrentasvir	7.72	8.71
Pilocarpine	0.24	−0.09
Pindolol	−0.32	1.97
Pioglitazone	1.53	2.94
Piperacillin	−2.72	1.88
Pirbuterol	−2.48	−0.83
Piroxicam	0.46	2.23
Pitavastatin	0.38	3.45
Pivampicillin	1.43	1.88
Posaconazole	3.70	2.25
Pralatrexate	−4.27	0.23
Pramipexole	−0.30	1.42
Pramoxine	2.93	3.48
Prasugrel	3.37	3.17
Pravastatin	−0.75	1.35
Praziquantel	2.71	2.44
Prazosin	1.11	0.04
Pregabalin	−1.75	1.12

(continued)

cLogP and $cLogD_{pH\ 7.4}$ for Selected Drugs[a] (Continued)

Drug	$cLogD_{pH\ 7.4}$	cLogP
Prilocaine	1.33	1.74
Primaquine	−0.56	2.67
Primidone	0.61	0.40
Probenecid	0.01	3.30
Procainamide	−0.65	1.10
Procaine	0.29	2.36
Procarbazine	0.26	0.77
Prochlorperazine	4.22	4.65
Promazine	2.69	4.69
Promethazine	3.10	4.78
Propafenone	1.45	3.93
Propantheline	−0.51	−1.77
Proparacaine	1.47	3.34
Propofol	3.88	4.16
Propoxycaine	1.34	3.26
Propranolol	1.15	3.10
Propylhexedrine	−0.19	3.04
Propylthiouracil	0.34	1.37
Protriptyline	1.85	5.06
Pseudoephedrine	−0.75	1.05
Pyrantel	0.40	1.51
Pyrazinamide	−0.17	−0.37
Pyridoxine	−0.69	−1.10
Pyrilamine	1.14	2.75
Pyrimethamine	2.36	2.75
Quazepam	4.35	4.06
Quinapril	4.32	−0.11
Quetiapine	2.29	1.57
Quinidine	1.17	3.44
Quinine	1.17	3.44
Rabeprazole	1.81	1.83
Raloxifene	4.40	6.88
Ramipril	−0.13	3.41
Ramelteon	3.07	2.57
Ranolazine	2.44	3.47
Ranitidine	−0.63	1.23

cLogP and $cLogD_{pH\ 7.4}$ for Selected Drugs[a] (Continued)

Drug	$cLogD_{pH\ 7.4}$	cLogP
Rasagiline	2.34	2.27
Remifentanil	1.81	2.05
Repaglinide	2.00	4.69
Reserpine	3.93	4.05
Ribavirin	−2.07	−2.26
Ribociclib	−0.15	−0.74
Rifampin	−0.28	1.09
Rifaximin	0.73	3.22
Riluzole	2.44	2.84
Rimantadine	−0.03	3.10
Risperidone	1.81	2.88
Ritonavir	5.09	5.28
Rivaroxaban	1.84	1.84
Rivastigmine	1.09	2.14
Rizatriptan	0.04	0.96
Ropinirole	1.21	3.19
Ropivacaine	4.21	4.39
Rosiglitazone	1.66	2.56
Rosuvastatin	−1.77	0.42
Rucaparib	0.38	2.85
Rufinamide	0.42	0.05
Saccharin	−1.29	0.90
Safinamide	2.09	2.37
Salicylamide	1.16	1.41
Salicylic acid	2.01	2.01
Salmeterol	1.98	3.07
Salsalate	0.44	3.05
Saquinavir	4.11	4.44
Sarecycline	−3.00	−1.04
Saxagliptin	−0.20	−0.14
Scopolamine	0.30	0.76
Secnidazole	0.23	0.33
Secobarbital	1.78	2.18
Selegiline	2.51	2.95
Serotonin	−1.71	0.21
Sertaconazole	6.76	7.49

cLogP and cLogD$_{pH\ 7.4}$ for Selected Drugs[a] (Continued)

Drug	cLogD$_{pH\ 7.4}$	cLogP
Sertraline	3.14	4.81
Sibutramine	2.90	5.43
Sildenafil	1.79	2.27
Silodosin	1.16	2.52
Simvastatin	4.60	4.41
Sitagliptin	1.09	1.30
Sofosbuvir	0.71	1.62
Solifenacin	2.16	3.70
Sorafenib	4.26	5.16
Sotalol	−1.63	0.32
Spironolactone	2.78	3.12
Stavudine	−0.67	−0.86
Stiripentol	2.80	3.39
Sufentanil	3.38	3.38
Sulconazole	5.97	5.66
Sulfadiazine	−0.79	−0.12
Sulfamethoxazole	−0.56	0.89
Sulfasalazine	0.22	3.18
Sulindac	0.33	3.59
Sumatriptan	−0.56	0.67
Tacrolimus	4.09	3.96
Tadalafil	1.88	1.43
Tafenoquine	1.84	4.89
Tamoxifen	5.51	7.88
Tamsulosin	0.77	2.24
Tapentadol	0.62	3.22
Telmisartan	4.01	7.73
Telotristat	1.07	4.79
Temazepam	2.11	2.19
Temozolomide	−0.99	−1.32
Terazosin	0.50	−0.96
Terbinafine	5.89	6.61
Terbutaline	−1.01	0.48
Tetrabenazine	3.12	3.48
Tetracaine	2.26	3.65

cLogP and cLogD$_{pH\ 7.4}$ for Selected Drugs[a] (Continued)

Drug	cLogD$_{pH\ 7.4}$	cLogP
Tetracycline	−3.55	−1.47
Tetrahydrocannabinol	7.25	7.68
Tetrahydrozoline	0.78	3.31
Thalidomide	0.48	0.54
Theobromine	−0.34	−0.72
Theophylline	0.11	−0.17
Thioguanine	−2.26	−0.12
Thiopental	2.48	2.99
Thioridazine	3.69	6.13
Thiothixene	3.34	3.94
Thiouracil	−0.98	−0.28
Tiagabine	2.45	5.69
Ticarcillin	−3.70	0.69
Ticlopidine	3.93	3.77
Timolol	−0.35	0.68
Tipiracil	−3.06	−1.37
Tipranavir	2.73	7.20
Tizanidine	0.94	0.65
Tobramycin	−9.45	−3.41
Tocainide	0.17	0.76
Tolazamide	0.43	1.71
Tolbutamide	1.22	4.07
Tolcapone	1.22	4.07
Tolmetin	−0.68	1.55
Tolnaftate	4.67	5.15
Tolterodine	2.57	5.77
Topiramate	2.16	2.97
Topotecan	0.68	1.08
Toremifene	5.56	7.82
Torsemide	1.44	3.53
Trabectedin	3.03	3.10
Tramadol	0.52	2.51
Trandolapril	0.17	3.97
Tranylcypromine	0.46	1.25
Trazodone	2.59	1.66

(continued)

cLogP and cLogD$_{pH\ 7.4}$ for Selected Drugs[a] (Continued)

Drug	cLogD$_{pH\ 7.4}$	cLogP
Triamterene	1.16	1.34
Triazolam	3.01	2.66
Trifluoperazine	4.34	5.11
Trihexyphenidyl	2.47	4.49
Trimethobenzamide	1.06	1.85
Trimethoprim	1.00	0.79
Trimipramine	3.04	5.15
Tripelennamine	0.91	2.84
Triprolidine	2.25	4.22
Tropicamide	1.54	1.15
Tubocurarine	−0.13	0.08
Valacyclovir	−1.49	−0.88
Valbenazine	3.59	4.31
Valganciclovir	−1.45	−1.28
Valproic acid	0.10	2.72
Valrubicin	3.64	6.31
Valsartan	−0.89	4.74
Vardenafil	1.83	2.65
Velpatasvir	6.18	6.78
Venetoclax	6.49	0.88
Venlafaxine	1.43	2.91

cLogP and cLogD$_{pH\ 7.4}$ for Selected Drugs[a] (Continued)

Drug	cLogD$_{pH\ 7.4}$	cLogP
Verapamil	2.38	3.90
Vigabatrin	−2.73	−0.10
Vilanterol	2.03	2.97
Vinblastine	3.68	4.18
Vincristine	2.60	2.82
Vinorelbine	4.69	4.69
Voriconazole	1.39	0.93
Vorinostat	1.20	0.86
Voxilaprevir	2.18	3.83
Warfarin	0.30	3.42
Xylometazoline	2.58	5.26
Zaleplon	1.45	0.87
Zanamivir	−6.03	−4.13
Zidovudine	−0.09	−0.53
Ziprasidone	3.40	4.00
Zolmitriptan	0.44	1.64
Zolpidem	3.07	3.07
Zonisamide	0.45	−0.16

[a]Calculated Log P values calculated on basis of unionized molecules and Log D$_{pH\ 7.4}$ distribution/partition coefficient calculated at pH 7.4, Advanced Chemical Development, Toronto, Canada, abstracted from ChemSpider Royal Society of Chemistry 2018.

REFERENCES FOR pK_a, cLogP AND cLogD

1. Albert A, Serjeant EP. *The Determination of Ionization Constants of Acids and Bases: A Laboratory Manual*. 3rd ed. New York: Chapman and Hall; 1984.
2. *cLogP and cLogD pH 7.4 Calculated From Advanced Chemical Development*. Toronto, Canada; 2018.
3. Florey K, ed. *Analytical Profiles of Drugs Substances*. New York: Academic Press; 1978.
4. Hansch C, Leo AJ. *Substituent Constants for Correlation Analysis in Chemistry and Biology*. New York: Wiley; 1979.
5. Hansch C, Sammes PG, Taylor JB, eds. *Comprehensive Medicinal Chemistry*. Vol 6. Oxford, UK: Pergamon Press; 1990.
6. O'Neil A, Heckelman PE, Koch CB, et al. *The Merck Index*. 14th ed. Rahway, NJ: Merck and Co; 2006.
7. Perrin DD, Dempsey B, Serjeant EP. *pKa Prediction for Organic Acids and Bases*. New York: Chapman and Hall; 1981.
8. Serjeant EP, Dempsey B. *Ionization Constants of Organic Acids in Aqueous Solution*. IUPAC Chemical Data Series. No. 23. Oxford, UK: Pergamon Press; 1979.
9. Sinko P. *Martin's Physical Pharmacy and Pharmaceutical Sciences*. 5th ed. Baltimore: Lippincott Williams & Wilkins; 2005.
10. Cheng T, Zhao Y, Li X, et.al. Computation of octanol–water partition coefficients by guiding an additive model with knowledge. *J Chem Inf Model*. 2007;47:2140-2148.

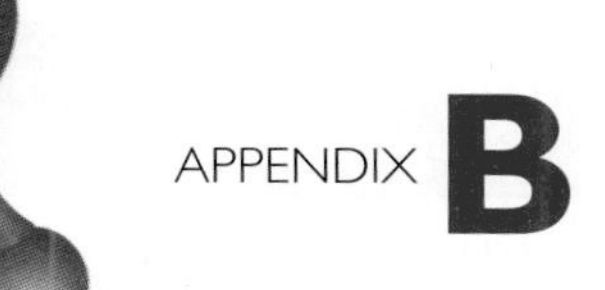

APPENDIX B

Predicted pK_a Values of Commonly Prescribed Drugs

S. William Zito and Victoria F. Roche

Predicted pK_a Values of Commonly Prescribed Drugs

Drugs	pK_a values	
	HA (unionized acid)	HB^+ (cationic acid)
Acetaminophen	9.46	
Acyclovir	7.99	2.63
Albuterol	9.4	10.1
Alendronic Acid	0.69	9.91
Allopurinol	7.83	2.57
Alprazolam		5.08
Amiodarone		8.47
Amitriptyline		9.76
Amlodipine		9.45
Amoxicillin	3.23	7.43
Anastrozole		2
Apixaban	13.12	
Aripiprazole	13.51	7.46
Atenolol		9.67
Atomoxetine		9.8
Atorvastatin	4.33	
Azithromycin	12.43	9.57
Baclofen	3.89	9.79

Predicted pK_a Values of Commonly Prescribed Drugs (Continued)

Drugs	pK_a values	
	HA (unionized acid)	HB^+ (cationic acid)
Benazepril	3.53	5.36
Benzonatate		3.47
Benztropine		9.54
Brimonidine		8.32
Bupropion		8.22
Buspirone		7.62
Carbidopa	2.35	5.66
Carvedilol		8.74
Cefdinir	1.74	7.45
Cefuroxime	3.15	
Celecoxib	10.7	
Cephalexin	3.45	7.44
Cetirizine	3.6	7.79
Chlorthalidone	8.76	
Ciprofloxacin	5.76	8.68
Citalopram		9.78
Clarithromycin	12.46	8.38
Clavulanic Acid	3.32	

(continued)

Predicted pK_a Values of Commonly Prescribed Drugs (Continued)

Drugs	pK_a values	
	HA (unionized acid)	HB$^+$ (cationic acid)
Clindamycin	12.41	7.55
Clobetasol	12.47	
Clonazepam	11.89	1.86
Clonidine		8.16
Clopidogrel		5.14
Cyclobenzaprine		9.76
Cyclosporine	11.83	
Dabigatran	3.18	12.52
Desvenlafaxine	10.11	8.87
Dexmethylphenidate		9.09
Diazepam		2.92
Diclofenac	4	
Digoxin	7.15	
Diltiazem	12.86	8.18
Donepezil		8.62
Doxazosin	12.67	7.24
Doxycycline	2.93	7.46
Duloxetine		9.7
Enalapril	3.67	5.2
Esomeprazole	9.68	4.77
Ethinylestradiol	10.33	
Estrone	10.33	
Ezetimibe	9.48	
Famotidine	9.29	8.38
Fluconazole	12.71	2.56
Fluoxetine		9.8
Fluticasone	12.19	
Furosemide	4.25	
Gabapentin	4.63	9.91
Gemfibrozil	4.42	
Glimepiride	2.23	
Glipizide	4.32	
Hydralazine		6.4
Hydrochlorothiazide	9.09	

Predicted pK_a Values of Commonly Prescribed Drugs (Continued)

Drugs	pK_a values	
	HA (unionized acid)	HB$^+$ (cationic acid)
Hydrocodone		8.61
Hydrocortisone	12.59	
Hydroxychloroquine		9.76
Hydroxyzine		7.82
Ibandronate	0.66	9.93
Ibuprofen	4.85	
Isosorbide	13.03	
Ketoconazole		6.75
Lamotrigine		5.87
Lansoprazole	9.35	4.16
Levalbuterol	10.12	9.4
Levocetirizine	3.59	7.42
Levodopa	1.65	9.06
Levofloxacin	5.45	6.2
Levothyroxine	0.27	9.43
Lisdexamfetamine		10.21
Lisinopril	3.17	10.21
Lithium carbonate	6.05	
Lorazepam	10.61	
Losartan	7.4	4.12
Meclizine		8.16
Meloxicam	4.47	0.47
Memantine		10.7
Metformin		12.33
Methocarbamol	13.6	
Methotrexate	3.41	2.81
Methylphenidate		9.09
Methylprednisolone	12.58	
Metoclopramide		9.04
Metoprolol		9.67
Minocycline		8.25
Mirtazapine		6.67
Modafinil	8.84	
Mometasone	12.49	

Predicted pK_a Values of Commonly Prescribed Drugs (Continued)

Drugs	pK_a values	
	HA (unionized acid)	HB$^+$ (cationic acid)
Montelukast	4.4	3.12
Morphine	10.26	9.12
Moxifloxacin	5.69	9.42
Naproxen	4.19	
Nebivolol	13.52	8.9
Nifedipine		5.33
Nystatin	3.62	9.11
Nortriptyline		10.47
Olmesartan	0.92	5.57
Pioglitazone	6.66	5.6
Pramipexole		10.31
Prasugrel		5.48
Pravastatin	4.21	
Prednisolone	12.59	
Prednisone	12.58	
Pregabalin	4.8	10.23
Promethazine		9.05
Propranolol		9.67
Quetiapine		7.06
Quinapril	3.7	5.2
Rabeprazole	9.35	4.24
Ramipril	3.75	5.2
Ranitidine		8.08
Risperidone		8.76
Rivaroxaban	13.6	
Ropinirole	13.24	10.17
Rosuvastatin	4.0	
Salmeterol	10.12	9.4
Sertraline		9.85
Sildenafil	7.27	5.97
Sitagliptin		8.78
Sulfamethoxazole	6.16	1.97
Sumatriptan	11.24	9.54
Tamsulosin	9.93	9.28

Predicted pK_a Values of Commonly Prescribed Drugs (Continued)

Drugs	pK_a values	
	HA (unionized acid)	HB$^+$ (cationic acid)
Temazepam	10.68	
Terazosin		7.24
Ticagrelor	12.94	2.93
Tiotropium	10.35	
Tizanidine		7.49
Tolterodine	10.28	11.01
Topiramate	11.09	
Tramadol	13.8	9.23
Trazodone		7.09
Triamterene		3.11
Trimethoprim		7.16
Valacyclovir	8.1	7.36
Valproic acid	5.14	
Valsartan	4.37	
Varenicline		9.73
Venlafaxine		8.91
Verapamil		9.68
Warfarin	6.33	
Zolpidem		5.65

From DrugBank: A Comprehensive Resource for In Silico Drug Discovery and Exploration. https://www.drugbank.ca/. Accessed May 14, 2019.

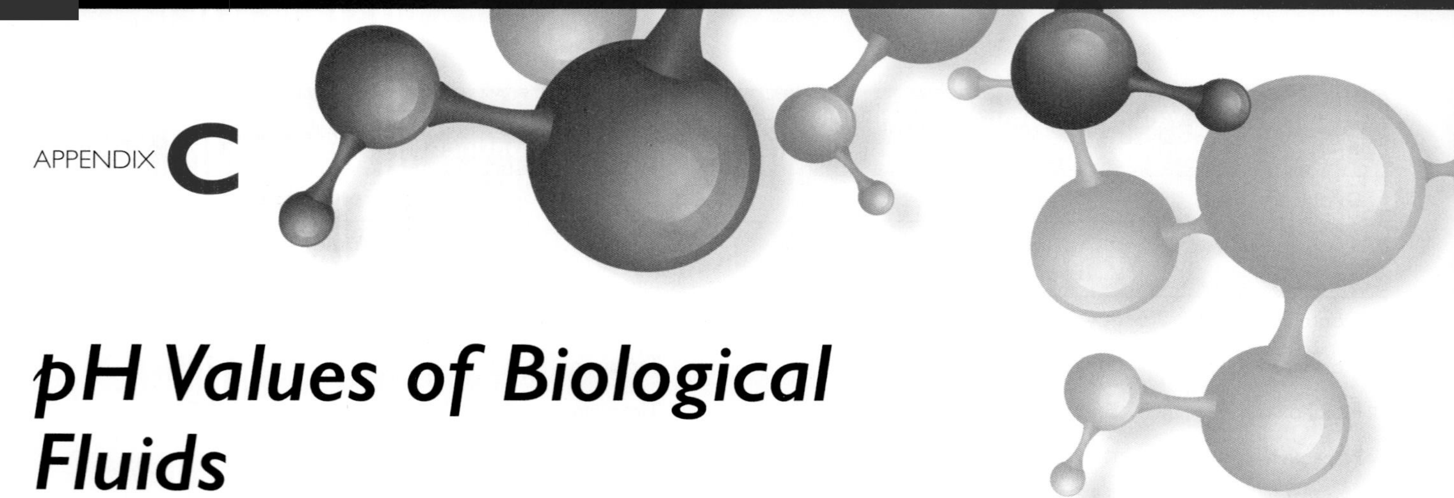

pH Values of Biological Fluids

David A. Williams

pH Values of Biological Fluids

Fluid	pH
Aqueous humor	7.2
Blood, arterial	7.4
Blood, venous	7.4
Blood, maternal umbilical	7.3
Cerebrospinal fluid	7.4
Colon[a]	
Fasting	5-8
Fed	5-8
Duodenum[a]	
Fasting	4.4-6.6
Fed	5.2-6.2
Feces[b]	7.1 (4.6-8.8)
Ileum[a]	
Fasting	6.8-8.6
Fed	6.8-8.0
Intestine, microsurface	5.3
Lacrimal fluid (tears)	7.4
Milk, breast	7.0
Muscle, skeletal[c]	6.0
Nasal secretions	6.0
Prostatic fluid	6.5
Saliva	6.4

pH Values of Biological Fluids (Continued)

Fluid	pH
Semen	7.2
Stomach[a]	
Fasting	1.4-2.1
Fed	3-7
Sweat	5.4
Urine	5.8 (5.5-7.0)
Vaginal secretions, premenopausal	4.5
Vaginal secretions, postmenopausal	7.0

[a]Reference: Dressman JB, Amidon GL, Reppas C, et al. Dissolution testing as a prognostic tool for oral drug absorption. *Pharm Res.* 1998;15:11-22.
[b]Value for normal, soft, formed stools. Hard stools tend to be more alkaline, whereas watery, unformed stools are acidic.
[c]Studies conducted intracellularly on the rat.

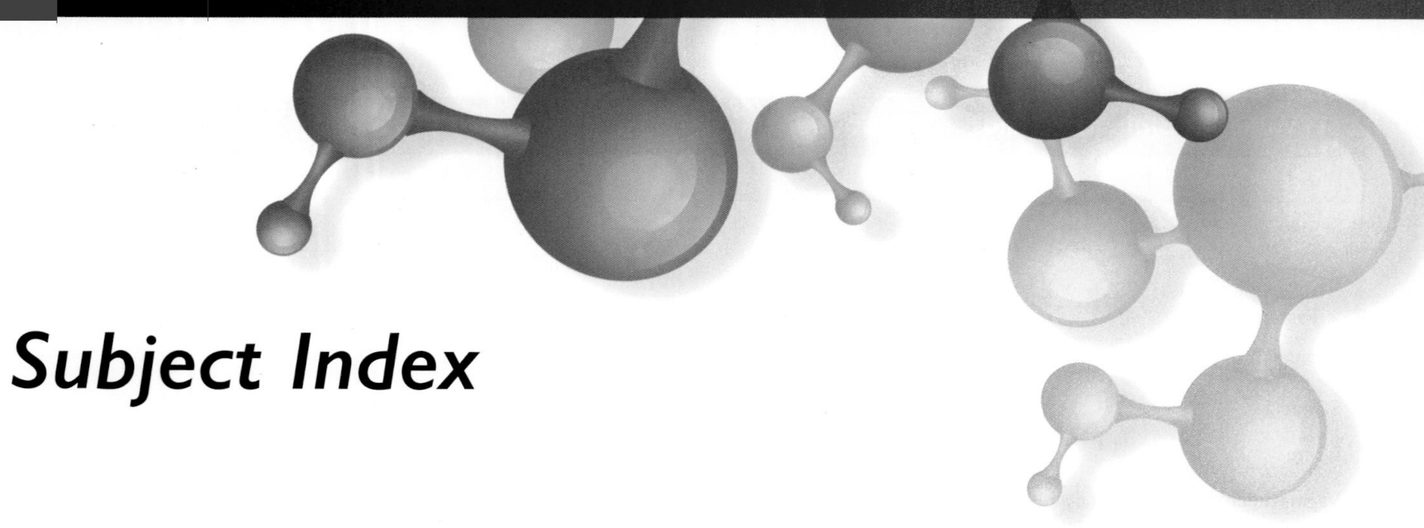

Subject Index

Note: Page numbers followed by "f" indicate figures, "t" indicate tables, and "b" indicate boxes.

A

B

C

D

E

F

G

H

I

O

P

Q

R

S

T

U

V

W

X

Y

Z

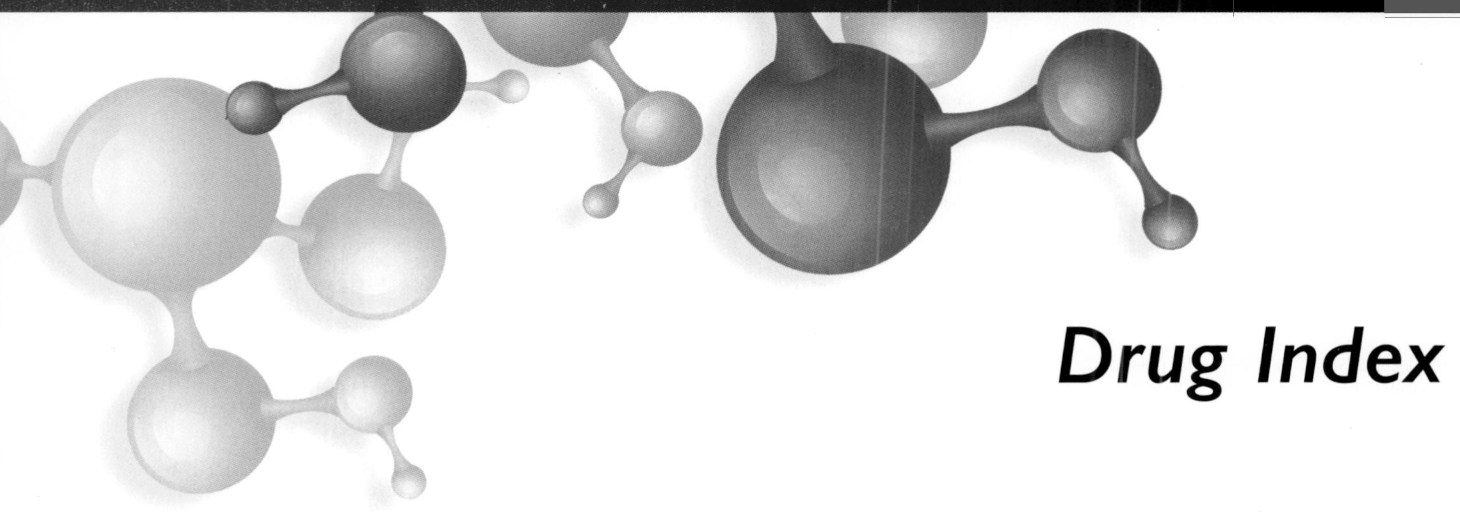

Drug Index

Note: Page numbers followed by "f" denotes figures, "t" denotes tables and "b" denotes boxes.

A

D

E

F

G

Q

R

S

T

U

V

W